Diseases of the

Breast

FOURTH EDITION

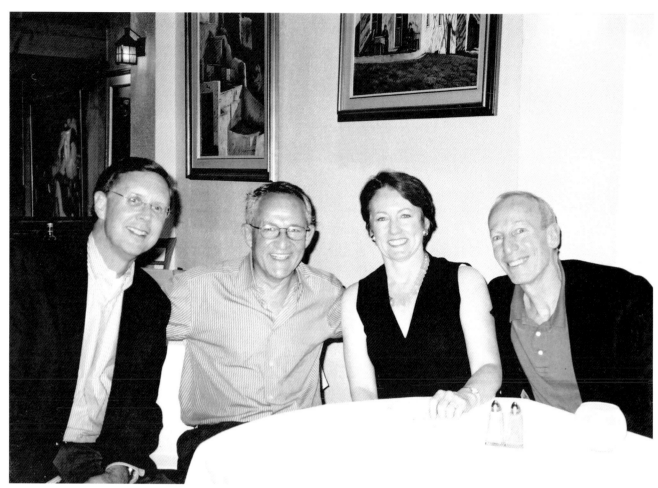

From left: Kent Osborne, Jay Harris, Monica Morrow, and Marc Lippman

Diseases of the

Breast

FOURTH EDITION

Edited by

Jay R. Harris, MD

Professor
Department of Radiation Oncology
Harvard Medical School
Chair
Department of Radiation Oncology
Dana-Farber Cancer Institute and
  Brigham Women's Hospital
Boston, Massachusetts

Marc E. Lippman, MD

Kathleen and Stanley Glaser Professor
Chairman, Department of Medicine
Leonard M. Miller School of Medicine
University of Miami
Miami, Florida

Monica Morrow, MD

Anne Burnett Windfohr Chair of Clinical
  Oncology
Chief, Breast Service
Memorial Sloan-Kettering Cancer Center
Professor of Surgery, Weill Medical
  College of Cornell University
New York, New York

C. Kent Osborne, MD

The Tina and Dudley Sharp Chair of
  Oncology
Professor of Medicine and Molecular and
  Cellular Biology
Director, Dan L. Duncan Cancer Center
Director, Lester and Sue Smith Breast
  Center
Baylor College of Medicine
Houston, Texas

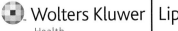

Wolters Kluwer | Lippincott Williams & Wilkins
Health

Philadelphia • Baltimore • New York • London
Buenos Aires • Hong Kong • Sydney • Tokyo

Executive Editor: Jonathan W. Pine, Jr.
Associate Director: Joyce Murphy
Project Manager: Alicia Jackson
Senior Manufacturing Manager: Benjamin Rivera
Senior Marketing Manager: Angela Panetta
Designer: Stephen Druding
Cover Designer: Bess Kiethas
Production Service: Aptara, Inc.

© 2010 by LIPPINCOTT WILLIAMS & WILKINS, a WOLTERS KLUWER business
530 Walnut Street
Philadelphia, PA 19106 USA
LWW.com

Third Edition © 2004 Lippincott Williams & Wilkins
Second Edition © 2000 Lippincott Williams & Wilkins
First Edition © 1996 Lippincott Raven

Printed in China

Library of Congress Cataloging-in-Publication Data

Diseases of the breast / edited by Jay R. Harris . . . [et al.]. — 4th ed.
      p. ; cm.
   Includes bibliographical references and index.
   ISBN 978-0-7817-9117-5
   1. Breast—Cancer. 2. Breast—Diseases. I. Harris, Jay R.
   [DNLM: 1. Breast Neoplasms—diagnosis. 2. Breast Neoplasms—therapy. 3. Breast Diseases. WP 870 D611 2009]
   RC280.B8D49 2009
   616.99'449—dc22

                                                                                 2009009897

Care has been taken to confirm the accuracy of the information presented and to describe generally accepted practices. However, the authors, editors, and publisher are not responsible for errors or omissions or for any consequences from application of the information in this book and make no warranty, expressed or implied, with respect to the currency, completeness, or accuracy of the contents of the publication. Application of the information in a particular situation remains the professional responsibility of the practitioner.

The authors, editors, and publisher have exerted every effort to ensure that drug selection and dosage set forth in this text are in accordance with current recommendations and practice at the time of publication. However, in view of ongoing research, changes in government regulations, and the constant flow of information relating to drug therapy and drug reactions, the reader is urged to check the package insert for each drug for any change in indications and dosage and for added warnings and precautions. This is particularly important when the recommended agent is a new or infrequently employed drug.

Some drugs and medical devices presented in the publication have Food and Drug Administration (FDA) clearance for limited use in restricted research settings. It is the responsibility of the health care provider to ascertain the FDA status of each drug or device planned for use in their clinical practice.

To purchase additional copies of this book, call our customer service department at (800) 638-3030 or fax orders to (301) 223-2320. International customers should call (301) 223-2300.

Visit Lippincott Williams & Wilkins on the Internet: at LWW.com. Lippincott Williams & Wilkins customer service representatives are available from 8:30 am to 6 pm, EST.

10 9 8 7 6 5 4 3 2 1

To the many thousands of women with breast cancer or at risk for the disease who participated in randomized clinical trials, without whom the improvements in care and a decrease in breast cancer mortality would not have been achieved.

Contents

Section I   Breast Anatomy and Development

Section II   Diagnosis and Management of Benign Breast Diseases

Section III   Breast Imaging and Image-Guided Biopsy Techniques

Section IV   Epidemiology and Assessing and Managing Risk

Section V   *In Situ* Carcinoma

Section VI   Pathology and Biological Markers of Invasive Breast Cancer

Section VII   Management of Primary Invasive Breast Cancer

Section VIII   Preoperative Systemic Therapy

Section IX   Special Therapeutic Problems

Section X   Evaluation after Primary Therapy and Management of Recurrent Breast Cancer

Section XI New Breast Cancer Therapeutic Approaches

Section XII Site-Specific Therapy of Metastatic Breast Cancer

Section XIII   Breast Cancer in Special Populations

Section XIV   Issues in Breast Cancer Survivorship

Section XV   Other Considerations

Preface

The previous three editions of *Diseases of the Breast* were intended as up-to-date, single-source multidisciplinary compilations of important knowledge on breast diseases, with a focus on breast cancer, presented in a form accessible to practicing clinicians. We have been gratified by the success of this effort, and for the fourth edition, we have similarly invited a diverse and distinguished group of experts to summarize the current knowledge about benign and malignant breast diseases, including their biology and epidemiology, clinical features, and management. The underlying premise for this book has been that multidisplinary care of the breast cancer patient is critical to achieve the best outcomes; furthermore, effective communication between pathologists, breast imagers, medical geneticists, nurses, psychologists, social services, and rehabilitation specialists as well as surgical, medical, and radiation oncologists is essential.

This fourth edition comes at a time when considerable progress has been made in the treatment of breast cancer. In the United States and in Western Europe, there has been a substantial decrease in the death rate from the disease, attributable to early detection with screening mammography and increasingly effective systemic treatment. It is now established that effective local treatment is also essential to decrease breast cancer mortality in addition to optimal local control. A key contributor to this decrease in breast cancer mortality has been the willingness of many thousands of women with breast cancer to participate in clinical trials and this edition is dedicated to them. Efforts have also been made to understand and improve the quality of life of breast cancer patients. The widespread use of sentinel node biopsy as an alternative to axillary lymph node dissection is a prominent example. Systemic therapy is increasingly targeted and less toxic, and advances in the molecular characterization of breast cancers have begun to explain the heterogeneity of the disease and allow for individualization of treatments. Radiation treatment has advanced by better incorporation of imaging modalities and more sophisticated irradiation techniques. While there has been progress in the treatment of breast cancer, many patients still die of the disease. Continued research into the biology, genetics, prevention, early diagnosis, and treatment of the disease is mandatory.

We hope that the Fourth Edition of *Diseases of the Breast* will be a useful resource for both clinicians and translational investigators. We highlight the rapid and substantial progress that has been made since the last edition that has reduced breast cancer mortality and provides optimism for additional advances in the near future.

Jay R. Harris, MD
Marc E. Lippman, MD
Monica Morrow, MD
C. Kent Osborne, MD

Preface to the First Edition

Interest in and knowledge about breast diseases, especially breast cancer, have increased greatly in recent years. A number of factors have contributed to this, the foremost of which are the high occurrence of breast cancer in westernized countries and the dramatic upswing in this incidence during the past few decades. Clinical investigators have also helped define various benign diseases of the breast and have described their management and relation to subsequent breast cancer development. Moreover, clinical trials performed throughout the world have contributed considerable information about the early detection and management of breast cancer using surgery, radiation therapy, and systemic therapies, including chemotherapy and hormonal interventions. Finally, rapid advances in the understanding of the molecular biology and genetics of both normal tissues and cancers have raised optimism that new, more specific methods can be developed to identify a woman's risk for breast cancer, to prevent or at least detect the disease at an earlier stage, and, failing this, to cure it with minimal toxicity. Ultimately a source of hope, these factors have nevertheless caused considerable anxiety in the population, as well as provided a proliferation of information important for clinicians dealing with diseases that strike the breast.

Diseases of the Breast is intended as a single-source compilation of the new knowledge on breast diseases presented in a form accessible to practicing clinicians. Although it is widely recognized that multidisciplinary interaction and information sharing are essential to effective clinical management of diseases of the breast, new developments are rapidly demonstrating that clinicians also need to be knowledgeable about advances in basic science. A prominent example of how advances in basic science can rapidly enter the clinical arena is the discovery of the first genetic mutations at specific loci shown to be associated with a high risk of breast cancer. Clinicians are now faced with patient questions about the nature and meaning of such testing as well as its risks and benefits. We believe that other advances in basic science will quickly be reflected in clinical practice.

For Diseases of the Breast, we invited a large, diverse, and distinguished group of experts to summarize the current knowledge about breast diseases, including clinical features, management, and underlying biologic and epidemiologic factors. In assembling these contributions, we have tried to make the book comprehensive and timely, as well as accessible to practicing clinicians. We believe that this book will also be an aid to basic and translational scientists concerned about a breast cancer problem by providing clinical information that can help focus their energies and talents. We hope that *Diseases of the Breast* will be a useful resource for both clinicians and scientists and will foster the understanding and communication necessary to provide optimal patient care and to rapidly achieve advances in managing diseases of the breast, especially breast cancer.

Jay R. Harris, MD
Marc E. Lippman, MD
Monica Morrow, MD
Samuel Hellman, MD

Contributors

Albert J. Aboulafia, MD, MBA
Assistant Clinical Professor
Department of Orthopaedic Surgery
University of Maryland
Co-Director Sarcoma Services
Department of Orthopaedic Surgery
Alvin and Lois Lapidus Cancer Center
Sinai Hospital of Baltimore
Baltimore, Maryland

David H. Abramson, MD
Associate Professor
Department of Surgery
New York Presbyterian Hospital
Weill-Cornell Medial College
Chief
Department of Surgery
Memorial Sloan-Kettering Cancer Center
New York, New York

D. Craig Allred, MD
Professor
Department of Pathology and
   Immunology
Washington University School of Medicine
Section Head
Department of Pathology
Washington University-Barnes Jewish
   Hospital
St. Louis, Missouri

Benjamin Olney Anderson, MD
Professor
Department of Surgery
University of Washington
Director
Department of Breast Health Clinic
Seattle Cancer Care Alliance
Seattle, Washington

Carlos L. Arteaga, MD
Professor of Medicine and Cancer
   Biology
Vanderbilt University
Director, Breast Cancer Program
Vanderbilt-Ingram Cancer Center
Nashville, Tennessee

Douglas W. Arthur, MD
Professor
Vice Chairman
Department of Radiation Oncology
Virginia Commonwealth University
Medical College of Virginia Hospitals
Richmond, Virginia

Alan Ashworth, PhD, FRS
Director
Breakthrough
Institute of Cancer Research
London, United Kingdom

Alvaro Moreno Aspitia, MD
Assistant Professor of Medicine
Department of Hematology/Oncology
Mayo Clinic
Jacksonville, Florida

Evandro de Azambuja, MD, PhD
Medical Director
Department of Breast Data Centre
Jules Bordet Institute
Brussels, Belgium

José Baselga, MD
Professor of Medicine
Vall d'Hebron University Hospital
Universitat Autonoma de Barcelona
Chariman
Vall d'Hebron Institute of Oncology
   (VHIO)
Vall d'Hebron University Hospital
Barcelona, Spain

Jennifer R. Bellon, MD
Assistant Professor
Department of Radiation Oncology
Harvard Medical School
Attending Physician
Department of Radiation Oncology
Dann-Farber Cancer Institute and
   Brigham and Women's Hospital
Boston, Massachusetts

Janet Sybil Biermann, MD
Associate Professor
Director of Musculoskeletal Oncology
Department of Orthopaedic Surgery
University of Michigan
Ann Arber, Michigan

Richard J. Bleicher, MD
Co-Director, Breast Fellowship
   Program
Associate Member
Department of Surgical Oncology
Fox Chase Cancer Center
Philadelphia, Pennsylvania

Susan K. Boolbol, MD
Assistant Professor of Surgery
Department of Surgery
Albert Einstein Medical College
Bronx, New York
Chief
Appel-Venet Comprehensive
   Breast Service
Beth Israel Medical Center
New York, New York

Glenn D. Braunstein, MD
Professor and Chairman
Department of Medicine
Cedar-Sinai Medical Center
Los Angeles, California

R. James Brenner, MD, JD
Professor
Department of Radiology
University of California-San Francisco
San Francisco, California
Director
Department of Breast Imaging
Bay Imaging Consultants-Alta Eden
   Division
Carol Ann Read Breast Health Center
Oakland, California

Thomas A. Buchholz, MD
Professor and Chair
Department of Radiation Oncology
The University of Texas M.D. Anderson
  Cancer Center
Houston, Texas

Nigel James Bundred, MD
Professor of Surgical Oncology
Department of Academic Surgery
University of Manchester
Consultant Surgeon
Nightingale Centre
Wythenshawe Hospital
Manchester, United Kingdom

Kristine Elizabeth Calhoun, MD
Assistant Professor
Department of Surgery
University of Washington
Assistant Professor
Department of Surgery
University of Washington Medical Center
Seattle, Washington

François Campana, MD
Chief of Service
Department of Radiotherapy
Institute Curie
Paris, France

Lisa A. Carey, MD
Associate Professor
Department of Medicine
University of North Carolina-Lineberger
  Comprehensive Cancer Center
Medical Director
University of North Carolina Breast
  Center
University of North Carolina Hospitals
Chapel Hill, North Carolina

Robert W. Carlson, MD
Professor of Medicine
Department of Medicine
Stanford University
Professor of Medicine
Department of Medicine
Stanford Hospital and Clinics
Stanford, California

Jenny C. Chang, MD
Professor
Breast Center
Baylor College of Medicine
Medical Director
Lester and Sue Smith Breast Center
Baylor Clinic
Houston, Texas

Nathan I. Cherney, MBBS
Associate Professor of Medicine
Department of Medicine
Ben Gurion University of the Negev
Norman Levan Chair of Humanistic
  Medicine
Director of Cancer Pain and Palliative
  Care
Department of Cancer Medicine
Shaare Zedek Medical Center
Jerusalem, Israel

Andrea L. Cheville, MD, MSLE
Associate Professor
Senior Associate Consultant
Department of Physical Medicine and
  Rehabilitation
Mayo Clinic
Rochester, Minnesota

Rowan T. Chlebowski, MD, PhD
Professor of Medicine
Davis Geffen School of Medicine
  at UCLA
Los Angeles, California
Chief
Division of Medical Oncology and
  Hematology
Harbor-UCLA Medical Center
Torrance, California

Hiram S. Cody III, MD
Professor
Department of Clinical Surgery
Weill Medical College of Cornell
  University
Attending Surgeon
Breast Service
Department of Surgery
Memorial Sloan-Kettering Cancer
  Center
New York, New York

Sara Cohen, OTR/L, CLT-LANA
Occupational Therapist Specialist
Department of Breast Service
Memorial Sloan-Kettering
  Cancer Center
New York, New York

Graham A. Colditz, MD, PhD
Niess-Gain Professor of Medicine
Associate Director
Department of Surgery
Washington University School of
  Medicine
Siteman Cancer Center
St. Louise, Missouri

Laura Christine Collins, MD
Assistant Professor
Department of Pathology
Harvard Medical School
Associate Director
Department of Pathology
Beth Israel Deaconess Medical
  Center
Boston, Massachusetts

Steven Come, MD
Associate Professor
Department of Medicine
Harvard Medical School
Associate Clinical Director,
  Hematology/Oncology
Department of Medicine
Beth Israel Deaconess Medical
  Center
Boston, Massachusetts

Carl D'Orsi, MD
Professor
Department of Radiology, Hematology/
  Oncology
Emory University School of Medicine
Director
Division of Breast Imaging Center
Emory University Hospital

Chau T. Dang, MD
Assistant Professor
Department of Medicine
New York Hospital-Cornell Medical
  Center
Assistant
Department of Medicine
Memorial Sloan-Kettering Cancer Center
New York, New York

Nancy E. Davidson, MD
Director
University of Pittsburgh Cancer Institute
Hillman Professor of Medicine
University of Pittsburgh
Director
University of Pittsburgh Medical Center
  Cancer Centers
University of Pittsburgh Medical Center
Pittsburgh, Pennsylvania

Lisa M. DeAngelis, MD
Professor
Department of Neurology
Weill Cornell Medical School
Chair
Department of Neurology
Memorial Sloan-Kettering Cancer Center
New York, New York

Angela DeMichele, MD, MSCE
Assistant Professor
Department of Medicine and
  Epidemiology
Co-Leader, Breast Cancer Program
Abramson Cancer Center
University of Pennsylvania
Philadelphia, Pennsylvania

Deborah A. Dillon, MD
Assistant Professor
Staff Pathologist
Department of Pathology
Harvard Medical School
Brigham and Women's Hospital
Boston, Massachusetts

**J. Michael Dixon, BSC(HOM), MBChB,
  MD, FRCS, FRCSGD, FRCPGD(HOM)**
Professor
Department of Surgery
Edinburgh Breast Unit
University of Edinburgh
Consultant Breast Surgeon
Edinburgh Breast Unit
Western General Hospital
Edinburgh, Scotland

Susan M. Domchek, MD
Associate Professor
Department of Medicine
University of Pennsylvania
Director
Cancer Risk Evaluation Program
Abramson Cancer Center
Philadelphia, Pennsylvania

Melinda Epstein, PhD
Department of Pathology
University of Southern California
Los Angeles, California

Francisco J. Esteva, MD, PhD
Associate Professor
Department of Medicine, Breast Medical
   Oncology
The University of Texas M.D. Anderson
   Cancer Center
Houston, Texas

Kathryn Evers, MD
Clinical Associate Professor
Department of Diagnostic Imaging
Temple University
Director of Breast Imaging
Department of Diagnostic Imaging
Fox Chase Cancer Center
Philadelphia, Pennsylvania

Rebecca Fisher, MD
Department of Neurology
Memorial Sloan-Kettering Cancer Center
New York, New York

David A. Flockhart, MD, PhD
Professor
Division of Clinical Pharmacology
Medical Genetics School of Medicine
Indiana University School of Medicine
Chief
School of Medicine
Division of Clinical Pharmacology School
   of Medicine
IU Simon Cancer Center
Indianapolis, Indiana

Alain Fourquet, MD
Chief
Department of Radiation Oncology
Institute Curie
Paris, France

Matthew T. Freedman, MD, MBA
Associate Professor
Department of Oncology
Lombardi Comprehensive Cancer
   Center
Georgetown University Medical
   Center
Washington, D.C.

Ronnie John Freilich, MD
Neurologist
Department of Neurology
Monash Medical Centre
Melbourne, Australia

Suzanne A. W. Fuqua, PhD
Professor
Department of Medicine and Molecular
   and Cellular Biology
Lester and Sue Smith Breast Center
Baylor College of Medicine
Houston, Texas

Susan M. Gapstur, MPH, PhD
Professor
Department of Preventive Medicine
Northwestern University
Chicago, Illinois

Richard D. Gelber, PhD
Professor
Department of Biostatistics
Harvard School of Public Health
Senior Biostatistician
Department of Biostatistics
Dana-Farber Cancer Institute
Boston, Massachusetts

Shari Gelber, MS, MSW
Biostatistician
Adult Oncology
Dana-Farber Cancer Institute
Boston, Massachusetts

Christophe Ginestier, PhD
Department of Internal Medicine
   Hematology/Oncology
University of Michigan Cancer Center
Ann Arbor, Michigan

Elizabeth S. Ginsburg, MD
Associate Professor
Department of Obstetrics, Gynecology
   and Reproductive Biology
Harvard Medical School
Medical Director, Assisted Reproductive
   Technologies Program
Department of Obstetrics and
   Gynecology
Brigham and Women's Hospital
Boston, Massachusetts

Armando E. Giuliano, MD
Clinical Professor of Surgery
University of California
Los Angeles, California
Director
John Wayne Cancer Institute
   (Breast Center)
Saint John's Health Center
Santa Monica, California

Aron Goldhirsch, MD
Professor of Medical Oncology
University of Bern
Bern, Switzerland
Director
Department of Medicine
European Institute of Oncology (EIO)
Milan, Italy

Mehra Golshan, MD
Assistant Professor
Department of Surgery
Harvard Medical School
Director of Breast Surgical Services
Department of Surgery
Brigham and Women's Hospital
Boston, Massachusetts

William J. Gradishar, MD
Professor
Department of Medicine
   Hematology/Oncology
Northwestern University
Director
Department of Breast Medical Oncology
Northwestern Memorial Hospital
Chicago, Illinois

Julie R. Gralow, MD
Associate Professor
Division of Medical Oncology
University of Washington
Director
Department of Breast Medical
   Oncology
Seattle Cancer Care Alliance
Seattle, Washington

Joe W. Gray, PhD
Associate Laboratory Director for Life
   and Environmental Sciences
Life Sciences Division Director
Life Sciences Division
Lawrence Berkeley National Laboratory
Berkeley, California
Adjunct Professor
Department of Laboratory Medicine
Helen Diller Family Comprehensive
   Cancer Center
University of California, San Francisco
San Francisco, California

Baiba J. Grube, MD
Associate
Department of Surgical Oncology/Breast
   Center
Yale Medical School
Breast Surgeon
Department of Surgical Oncology
Yale New Haven Hospital
New Haven, Connecticut

Anthony J. Guidi, MD
Chair
Department of Pathology
North Shore Medical Center
Salem, Massachusetts

Carolina Gutierrez, MD
Director of the Division of Breast
   Pathology
Director of the Division of Prognostic
   and Predictive Markers
Associate Professor of Pathology
Baylor College of Medicine
Houston, Texas

Bruce G. Haffty, MD
Professor and Chairman
Chairman/Chief
Department of Radiation Oncology
University of Medicine and Dentistry of
    New Jersey
Robert Wood Johnson Medical
    School/Cancer Institute of New Jersey
Robert Wood Johnson University
    Hospital
New Brunswick, New Jersey

Susan E. Hankinson, ScD
Associate Professor
Department of Medicine
Harvard Medical School
Principal Investigator of the NHS
Department of Chronic Diseases
Brigham & Women's Hospital
Boston, Massachusetts

Nora M. Hansen, MD
Associated Professor
Department of Surgery
Feinberg School of Medicine,
    Northwestern University
Director
Lynn Sage Comprehensive Breast Center
Department of Surgery
Prentice Women's Hospital of
    Northwestern Memorial Hospital
Chicago, Illinois

Douglas Hanto, MD, PhD
Lewis Thomas Professor of Surgery
Harvard Medical School
Chief
Division of Transplantation
Department of Surgery
Beth Israel Deaconess Medical Center
Boston, Massachusetts

Eleanor E. R. Harris, MD
Associate Professor
Department of Oncologic Sciences
University of South Florida
Associate Member and Clinical Director
Department of Radiation Oncology
H. Lee Moffit Cancer Center and
    Research Institute
Tampa, Florida

Jay R. Harris, MD
Professor
Department of Radiation Oncology
Harvard Medical School
Chair
Department of Radiation Oncology
Dana-Farber Cancer Institute and
    Brigham & Women's Hospital
Boston, Massachusetts

Daniel F. Hayes, MD
Professor
Department of Internal Medicine
Division of Hematology/Oncology
University of Michigan
Clinical Director
Breast Oncology Program
University of Michigan Comprehensive
    Cancer Center
Ann Arbor, Michigan

James A. Hayman, MD, MBA
Professor
Department of Radiation Oncology
University of Michigan
Associate Chair for Clinical Activities
Department of Radiation Oncology
University of Michigan Health System
Ann Arbor, Michigan

Laura Heiser, PhD
Staff Scientist
Division of Life Sciences
Lawrence Berkeley National Laboratory
Berkeley, California

Mark A. Helvie, MD
Professor
Director of Breast Imaging
Department of Radiology
University of Michigan Health System
Ann Arbor, Michigan

Dawn Hershman, MD, MS
Assistant Professor of Medicine and
    Epidemiology
Department of Medicine
Columbia University Medical Center
New York, New York

Bruce E. Hillner, MD
Professor of Medicine and Eminent
    University Scholar
Department of Internal Medicine
Virginia Commonwealth University
Member
Virginia Commonwealth Cancer Center
    and Medical Center
Richmond, Virginia

Susan G. Hilsenbeck, PhD
Professor
Department of Breast Cancer
Baylor College of Medicine
Houston, Texas

Gabriel N. Hortobagyi, MD
Professor and Chair
Department of Breast Medical Oncology
The University of Texas M.D. Anderson
    Cancer Center
Houston, Texas

Anthony Howell, MD
Muriel Edith Rickman Chair of Breast
    Cancer
Translation Research Facility 2
Paterson Institute for Cancer Research
Medical Oncologist
Medical Oncology
The Christie NHS Foundation Trust
Manchester, United Kingdom

Sacha J. Howell, MD, PhD
Breast Biology Group
Paterson Institute for Cancer
    Research
University of Manchester
Honorary Consultant
Department of Medical Oncology
The Christie NHS Foundation Trust
Manchester, United Kingdom

Clifford Hudis, MD
Attending Physician
Department of Medicine
Chief
Breast Cancer Medicine Services
Solid Tumor Division
Department of Medicine
Memorial Sloan-Kettering Cancer
    Center
New York, New York

Kevin S. Hughes, MD
Associate Professor
Harvard Medical School
Surgical Director, Breast Screening
Co-Director, Avon Comprehensive
    Breast Evaluation Center
Massachusetts General Hospital
Boston, Massachusetts

Kelly K. Hunt, MD
Professor
Department of Surgical Oncology
The University of Texas M.D. Anderson
    Cancer Center
Houston, Texas

David J. Hunter, MD, ScD
Vincent L. Gregory Professor of Cancer
    Prevention
Departments of Epidemiology and
    Nutrition
Harvard School of Public Health
Associate Epidemiologist
Department of Medicine
Brigham and Women's Hospital,
    Channing Laboratory
Boston, Massachusetts

Maria D. Iniesta, MD
Department of Internal Medicine
Division of Hematology/Oncology
Comprehensive Cancer Center
University of Michigan Health System
Ann Arbor, Michigan

Claudine Isaacs, MD
Associate Professor
Director, Clinical Breast Cancer Program
Departments of Medicine and Oncology
Georgetown University/Lombardi
    Comprehensive Cancer Center
Jess and Mildred Fisher Center for
    Familial Cancer Research
Washington, DC

Atif J. Khan, MD
Assistant Professor
Attending Physician
Department of Radiation Oncology
University of Medicine and Dentistry of
    New Jersey
Robert Wood Johnson Medical School/
    Cancer Institute of New Jersey
Robert Wood Johnson University
    Hospital
New Brunswick, New Jersey

Seema A. Khan, MD
Professor
Bluhm Family Professor of Cancer
  Research
Department of Surgery
Northwestern University/Feinberg
  School of Medicine
Co-Leader
Breast Program at Robert H. Lurie
  Comprehensive Cancer Center
Director
Bluhm Family Breast Cancer Early
  Detection and Prevention Center
Department of Surgery
Northwestern Memorial Hospital
Lynn Sage Comprehensive Breast
  Center
Chicago, Illinois

Nagi F. Khouri, MD
Associate Professor
Director
Division of Breast Imaging
Department of Radiology and Oncology
The Johns Hopkins University
Director
Division of Breast Imaging
Department of Radiology
The Johns Hopkins Hospital
Baltimore, Maryland

Kandice E. Kilbride, MD
Breast Surgeon
Breast Cancer Alliance of North Texas
Presbyterian Hospital of Dallas
Dallas, Texas

Janice Nam Kim, MD
Assistant Professor
Department of Radiation Oncology
University of Washington
Assistant Professor
Department of Radiation Oncology
Seattle Cancer Care Alliance
Seattle, Washington

Gretchen G. Kimmick, MD, MS
Associate Professor
Breast Oncology
Internal Medicine/Division of Medical
  Oncology
Department of Internal Medicine/
  Division of Medical Oncology
Duke University Medical Center
Durham, North Carolina

Tari A. King, MD
Assistant Professor
Department of Surgery
Weill Medical College of Cornell
  University
Assistant Attending Physician
Breast Service
Department of Surgery
Memorial Sloan-Kettering Cancer Center
New York, New York

Youlia M. Kirova, MD
Senior Radiation Oncologist
Department of Radiation Oncology
Institute Curie
Paris, France

Rita Kramer, MD
Associate Professor
Lester and Sue Smith Breast Center
Baylor College of Medicine
Houston, Texas

Sunil R. Lakhani, MD
Professor
Department of Molecular and Cellular
  Pathology School of Medicine
The University of Queensland Centre for
  Clinical Research
The University of Queensland
Professor
Department of Anatomical Pathology
Pathology Queensland Central
Royal Brisbane and Women's Hospital
Herston, Australia

Thomas J. Lawton, MD
Director
Seattle Breast Pathology Consultants
Seattle, Washington

Constance D. Lehman, MD, PhD
Professor and Vice Chair of Radiology,
  Section Head of Breast Imagining
Department of Radiology
University of Washington
Professor and Vice Chair of Radiology,
  Section Head of Breast Imaging
Department of Radiology
University of Washington Medical
  Center
Seattle, Washington

Constance D. Lehman, MD, PhD
Professor and Vice Chair of Radiology
Section Head of Breast Imaging
University of Washington
University of Washington Medical
  Center
Seattle, Washington

Michael T. Lewis, PhD
Assistant Professor
Department of Molecular and Cellular
  Biology
Baylor College of Medicine
Houston, Texas

Wenchi Liang, PhD
Assistant Professor
Department of Cancer Control Program
Georgetown University Medical Center
Washington, DC

Jennifer A. Ligibel, MD
Instructor
Department of Medicine
Harvard Medical School
Medical Oncologist
Department of Adult Oncology
Dana-Farber/Brigham and Women's
  Hospital
Boston, Massachusetts

Nancy U. Lin, MD
Instructor in Medicine
Harvard Medical School
Attending Physician
Department of Medical Oncology
Dana-Farber Cancer Institute
Boston, Massachusetts

Marc E. Lippman, MD
Kathleen and Stanley Glaser Professor
Chairman, Department of Medicine
Leonard M. Miller School of Medicine
University of Miami
Miami, Florida

Jennifer Keating Litton, MD
Assistant Professor
Department of Breast Medical Oncology
The University of Texas M.D. Anderson
  Cancer Center
Houston, Texas

Shelly S. Lo, MD
Assistant Professor of Medicine
Department of Medicine
Stritch School of Medicine
Assistant Professor
Department of Medicine
Loyola University Chicago
Maywood, Illinois

Charles L. Loprinzi, MD
Professor of Oncology
Director, NCCTG Cancer Control
  Program
Department of Oncology
Mayo Clinic
Rochester, Minnesota

Yanling Ma, MD
Assistant Professor
Department of Pathology
University of Southern California
Los Angeles, California

Eleftherios P. Mamounas, MD, MPH
Professor
Department of Surgery
Northeastern Ohio Universities College
  of Medicine
Rootstown, Ohio
Medical Director
Department of Cancer Center
Aultman Health Foundation
Canton, Ohio

Jeanne Mandelblatt, MD, MPH
Associate Director
Department of Oncology
Georgetown University Medical Center
Washington, DC

Robert E. Mansel, MB, MS
Chairman
Department of Surgery
Cardiff University
Chief
Department of Surgery
University Hospital of Wales
Cardiff, United Kingdom

Holly S. Mason, MD
Assistant Professor
Department of Surgery
Tufts University School of Medicine
Boston, Massachusetts
Director
Breast Surgical Services
Department of Surgery
Baystate Medical Center
Springfield, Massachusetts

Mary Jane Massie, MD
Professor
Department of Psychiatry
Weill Medical College of Cornell
    University
Attending Psychiatrist
Department of Psychiatry and
    Behavioral Sciences
Memorial Sloan-Kettering Cancer Center
New York, New York

Erica L. Mayer, MD, MPN
Instructor
Department of Medicine
Harvard Medical School
Staff Physician
Department of Medical Oncology
Dana-Farber Cancer Institue
Boston, Massachusetts

Craig D. McColl, MD
Staff Specialist in Neurology
Division of Medicine
Calvary Hospital
Bruce, Australia

Beryl A. McCormick, MD
Professor
Department of Medicine
Weill College/Cornell University
Clinical Director
Department of Radiation Oncology
Memorial Sloan-Kettering Cancer Center
New York, New York

Sarah A. McLaughlin, MD
Assistant Professor
Senior Assistant Consultant
Department of Surgery
Mayo Clinic Medical School
Jacksonville, Florida

Karen M. Meneses, PhD
Professor and Associate Dean for
    Research
School of Nursing, Center for Nursing
    Research
University of Alabama at Birmingham
Birmingham, Alabama

Steven J. Mentzer, MD
Professor
Department of Surgery
Harvard Medical School
Senior Thoracic Surgeon
Department of Surgery
Brigham and Women's Hospital
Boston, Massachusetts

Sofia D. Merajver, MD, PhD
Professor
Department of Internal Medicine
University of Michigan
Ann Arbor, Michigan

Rebecca Miksad, MD, MPH
Instructor
Department of Medicine
Harvard Medical School
Attending Physician
Division of Hematology/Oncology
Department of Medicine
Beth Israel Deaconess Medical Center
Boston, Massachusetts

Kathy D. Miller, MD
Associate Professor
Department of Hematology/Oncology
Indiana University
Indiana University Simon Cancer Center
Indianapolis, Indiana

Monica Morrow, MD
Anne Burnett Windfohr Chair of Clinical
    Oncology
Chief, Breast Service
Memorial Sloan-Kettering Cancer Center
Professor of Surgery, Weill Medical
    College of Cornell University
New York, New York

Hyman B. Muss, MD
Professor
Department of Medicine
University of North Carolina at Chapel
    Hill School of Medicine
Director
Geriatric Oncology
Division of Hematology/Oncology
Lineberger Comprehensive Cancer
    Center
Chapel Hill, North Carolina

Mary S. Newell, MD
Assistant Professor
Department of Radiology
Emory University
Assistant Director
Department of Breast Imaging
Emory University Hospital
Atlanta, Georgia

Lisa A. Newman, MD, MPH
Professor
Department of Surgery
University of Michigan
Director
Breast Care Center
University of Michigan Comprehensive
    Cancer Center
Ann Arbor, Michigan

Oded Olsha, MBBS
Breast Surgery Unit
Department of Surgery
Shaare Zedek Medical Center
Jerusalem, Israel

C. Kent Osborne, MD
The Tina and Dudley Sharp Chair of
    Oncology
Professor of Medicine and Molecular and
    Cellular Biology
Director, Dan L. Duncan Cancer Center
Director, Lester and Sue Smith Breast
    Center
Baylor College of Medicine
Houston, Texas

Michael P. Osborne, MD, MSurg
Director of Breast Program Continuum
    Cancer Centers of New York
Department of Surgery
Beth Israel Medical Center
New York, New York

Sumanta Kumar Pal, MD
Department of Medical Oncology and
    Experimental Therapeutics City of
    Hope Comprehensive Cancer Center
Duarte, California

Ann H. Partridge, MD, MPH
Assistant Professor
Department of Medicine
Harvard Medical School
Clinical Director, Breast Oncology Center
Department of Medical Oncology
Dana-Farber Cancer Institute
Boston, Massachusetts

Sameer A. Patel, MD
Associate Member, Plastic and
    Reconstructive Surgery
Department of Surgical Oncology
Fox Chase Cancer Center
Philadelphia, Pennsylvania

Mark D. Pegram, MD
Professor of Medicine
Department of Medicine, Hematology
    Oncology Division
Miller School of Medicine
Miami, Florida

Edith A. Perez, MD
Serene M. and Frances C. Durling
    Professor of Medicine
Department of Hematology/Oncology,
    Internal Medicine
Mayo Clinic
Jacksonville, Florida

Charles M. Perou, PhD
Associate Professor
Department of Genetics, and Pathology
    and Laboratory Medicine
University of North Carolina at Chapel
    Hill
Chapel Hill, North Carolina

Beth N. Peshkin, MS, CGC
Associate Professor
Senior Genetic Counselor
Department of Oncology
Georgetown University/Lombardi
    Comprehensive Cancer Center
Jess and Mildred Fisher Center for
    Familial Cancer Research
Washington, DC

Martine Piccart-Gebhart, MD, PhD
Professor
Department of Oncology
Universite Libre De
Head
Department of Medicine
Jules Bordet Institute
Brussels, Belgium

Michael F. Press, MD, PhD
Professor
Department of Pathology
University of Southern California
Los Angeles, California

Sofyan M. Radaideh, MD
Division of Hematology-Oncology
University of Texas Southwestern
    Medical Center
Dallas, Texas

James Michael Rae, PhD
Assistant Professor
Department of Internal Medicine
University of Michigan
Ann Arbor, Michigan

Naren R. Ramakrishna, MD, PhD
Instructor in Radiation Oncology
Radiation Oncology
Harvard Medical School
Chief, Division of CNS Radiation
    Oncology
Radiation Department
Brigham and Women's Hospital
Boston, Massachusetts

Priya Rastogi, MD
Assistant Professor
Department of Medicine
University of Pittsburgh
Medical Oncologist
Women's Cancer Center
University of Pittsburgh Cancer Institute
    at Magee-Women's Hospital
Pittsburgh, Pennsylvania

Jorge S. Reis-Filho, MD, PhD
Team Leader
Department of Molecular Pathology
The Breakthrough Breast Cancer
    Research Center
Institute of Cancer Research
London, United Kingdom

Mothaffar F. Rimawi, MD
Assistant Professor
Lester and Sue Smith Breast Center
Baylor College of Medicine
Houston, Texas

Jeffrey M. Rosen, PhD
C. C. Bell Professor
Department of Molecular and Cellular
    Biology
Baylor College of Medicine
Houston, Texas

Susan Orel Roth, MD
Professor
Department of Radiology
University of Pennsylvania School of
    Medicine
Hospital University of Pennsylvania
Philadelphia, Pennsylvania

Julia H. Rowland, PhD
Adjunct Associate Professor
Department of Psychiatry
Georgetown University School of
    Medicine
Washington, DC
Director, Office of Cancer Survivorship
Division of Cancer Control and
    Population Sciences
National Cancer Institute
Bethesda, Maryland

Michael S. Sabel, MD
Associate Professor
Department of Surgery
University of Michigan
Ann Arbor, Michigan

Rachel Schiff, MD
Associate Professor
Department of Medicine
Lester and Sue Smith Cancer Center
Baylor College of Medicine
Houston, Texas

Bryan P. Schneider, MD
Assistant Professor
Department of Hematology/Oncology
Indiana University
Indiana University Simon Cancer Center
Indianapolis, Indiana

Stuart J. Schnitt, MD
Professor
Department of Pathology
Harvard Medical School
Director
Division of Anatomic Pathology
Department of Pathology
Beth Israel Deaconess Medical Center
Boston, Massachusetts

Marc Schwartz, PhD
Associate Professor
Director, Cancer Control
Department of Oncology
Georgetown University/Lombardi
    Comprehensive Cancer Center
Jess and Mildred Fisher Center for
    Familial Cancer Research
Washington, DC

Brian J. Scott, MD
Clinical Assistant Professor
Department of Neurology
Tufts University
Boston, Massachusetts
Staff Physician
Department of Neurology
Laney Clinic Medical Center
Burlington, Massachusetts

Vanessa B. Sheppard, PhD, MA
Assistant Professor
Department of Oncology
Georgetown University Medical Center
Washington, DC

Lawrence N. Shulman, MD
Associate Professor
Department of Medicine
Harvard Medical School
Chief Medical Officer
Department of Medical Oncology
Dana-Farber Cancer Institute
Boston, Massachusetts

Peter T. Simpson, PhD
Department of Molecular and Cellular
    Pathology
The University of Queensland
Herston, Australia

Sonja Eva Singletary, MD
Professor
Department of Surgical Oncology
The University of Texas M.D. Anderson
    Cancer Center
Houston, Texas

George W. Sledge, Jr., MD
Professor of Medicine and Pathology
Department of Hematology/Oncology
Indiana University School of Medicine
Co-Director Breast Oncology Team
Department of Hematology/Oncology
Indiana University Simon Cancer Center
Indianapolis, Indiana

Jeffrey B. Smerage, MD, PhD
Assistant Professor
Department of Internal Medicine
University of Michigan Health System
Ann Arbor, Michigan

Ian E. Smith, MD, FRCP, FRCPE
Professor
Department of Medical Oncology,
    Breast Unit
The Royal Marsden NHS Foundation
    Trust
London, United Kingdom

Robert A. Smith, PhD
Director of Cancer Screening
Department of Cancer Control Sciences
American Cancer Society
Atlanta, Georgia

Lawrence J. Solin, MD
Chairman
Department of Radiation Oncology
Albert Einstein Medical Center
Philadelphia, Pennsylvania

Paul T. Spellman, PhD
Staff Scientist
Division of Life Sciences
Lawrence Berkeley National Laboratory
Berkeley, California

Vered Stearns, MD
Associate Professor
Department of Oncology
Johns Hopkins School of Medicine
Attending Physician
Sidney Kimmel Comprehensive Cancer
    Center
Johns Hopkins Hospital
Baltimore, Maryland

Nicole L. Stout, MPT, CLT-LANA
Lead Physical Therapist
Department of Breast Cancer
National Naval Medical Center
Bethesda, Maryland

Eric A. Strom, MD
Professor
Medical Director
Department of Radiation Oncology
Nellie B. Connall Breast Center
The University of Texas M.D. Anderson
    Cancer Center
Houston, Texas

Rulla May Tamimi, ScD
Assistant Professor
Department of Medicine
Harvard School of Medicine
Associate Epidemiologist
Channing Laboratory
Brigham and Women's Hospital
Boston, Massachusetts

Sing-Huang Tan, MD
Consultant
Department of Hematology/Oncology
National University Hospital
National University Health System
Singapore

Julia Tchou, MD, PhD
Assistant Professor
Department of Surgery
University of Pennsylvania
Philadelphia, Pennsylvania

Yee Lu Tham, MD
Assistant Professor
Department of Medicine
Baylor College of Medicine
Staff Oncologist
Department of Medicine
Michael E. DeBakey VA Medical Center
Houston, Texas

Richard Lee Theriault, DO
Professor
Department of Breast Medical Oncology
The University of Texas M.D. Anderson
    Cancer Center
Houston, Texas

Robert D. Timmerman, MD
Professor and Vice Chair
Department of Radiation Oncology
University of Texas Southwestern
Director of Stereotactic Radiotherapy
Moncrief Radiation Oncology Center
University of Texas Southwestern
    Medical Center
Dallas, Texas

Neal Stoddard Topham, MD
Chief Plastic and Reconstructive Surgery
Department of Surgical Oncology
Fox Chase Cancer Center
Philadelphia, Pennsylvania

Susan Urba, MD
Professor
Internal Medicine, Division of
    Hematology-Oncology
University of Michigan
Ann Arbor, Michigan

Kimberly J. Van Zee, MS, MD
Professor
Department of Surgery
Weill Medical College of Cornell
    University
Attending Surgeon
Department of Breast Service
Memorial Sloan-Kettering Cancer Center
New York, New York

Frank A. Vicini, MD
Clinical Professor
Department of Health Sciences
Oakland University
Rochester, Michigan
Chief of Oncology
Department of Oncology
William Beaumont Hospital
Royal Oak, Michigan

Victor G. Vogel, MD, MHS
Professor of Medicine and Epidemiology
Department of Medicine
University of Pittsburgh School of
    Medicine
Director of Breast Cancer Prevention
    Program
Women's Cancer Center
Magee Women's Hospital
Pittsburgh, Pennsylvania

Richard B. Wait, MD, PhD
Clinical Professor
Department of Surgery
Tufts University School of Medicine
Boston, Massachusetts
Chairman
Department of Surgery
Baystate Medical Center
Springfield, Massachusetts

Judy Wang, PhD
Assistant Professor
Department of Oncology
Georgetown University Medical Center
Washington, DC

Barbara L. Weber, MD
Vice President of Cancer Research
GlaxoSmith Kline Oncology
Collegeville, Pennsylvania

Susan P. Weinstein, MD
Assistant Professor
Department of Radiology
University of Pennsylvania Medical
    Center
Philadelphia, Pennsylvania

Patrick Y. Wen, MD
Associate Professor
Department of Neurology
Harvard Medical School
Clinical Director
Center for Neuro-Oncology
Dana-Farber Cancer Institute Brigham
    and Women's Cancer Center
Boston, Massachusetts

Julia R. White, MD
Professor
Radiation Oncology
Medical College of Wisconsin
Froedtert Memorial Lutheran Hospital
Milwaukee, Wisconsin

Max S. Wicha, MD
Distinguished Professor of Oncology
University of Michigan
Director
University of Michigan Comprehensive
    Cancer Center
Ann Arber, Michigan

Walter C. Willett, MD, DrPH
Professor and Chair
Department of Nutrition
Harvard School of Public Health
Boston, Massachusetts

Eric P. Winer, MD
Professor
Department of Medicine
Harvard Medical School
Chief
Division of Women's Cancer
Department of Medical Oncology
Dana-Farber Cancer Institute
Boston, Massachusetts

Kari B. Wisinski, MD
Assistant Professor
Department of Medicine
University of Wisconsin School of
    Medicine and Public Health
University of Wisconsin Hospitals and
    Clinics
Madison, Wisconsin

Antonio C. Wolff, MD
Associate Professor
Attending Physician
Department of Oncology
Johns Hopkins School of Medicine
Johns Hopkins Hospital
Baltimore, Maryland

Chapter 1
Breast Anatomy and Development

Michael P. Osborne and Susan K. Boolbol

Mammary glands are a distinguishing feature of mammals. Nursing of the young in the animal kingdom has many physiologic advantages for the mother, such as aiding postpartum uterine involution, and for the neonate, in terms of the transfer of immunity and bonding. It has become increasingly apparent that the advantages of nursing are substantial for both mother and child.

An understanding of the morphology and physiology of the breast, and the many endocrine interrelationships of both, is essential to the study of the pathophysiology of the breast and the management of benign, preneoplastic, and neoplastic disorders.

EMBRYOLOGY

During the fifth week of human fetal development, the ectodermal primitive milk streak, or "galactic band," develops from axilla to groin on the embryonic trunk (1). The ectoderm over the thorax invaginates into the surrounding mesenchyme, with subsequent epithelial budding and branching (2). In the region of the thorax, the band develops to form a mammary ridge, whereas the remaining galactic band regresses. Incomplete regression or dispersion of the primitive galactic band leads to accessory mammary tissues, found in 2% to 6% of women in the form of accessory nipples or axillary breast tissue.

At 7 to 8 weeks' gestation, a thickening occurs in the mammary anlage (milk hill stage), followed by invagination into the chest wall mesenchyme (disc stage) and tridimensional growth (globular stage). Further invasion of the chest wall mesenchyme results in a flattening of the ridge (cone stage) at 10 to 14 weeks' gestation. Between 12 and 16 weeks' gestation, mesenchymal cells differentiate into the smooth muscle of the nipple and areola. Epithelial buds develop (budding stage) and then branch to form 15 to 25 strips of epithelium (branching stage) at 16 weeks' gestation; these strips represent the future secretory alveoli (3). The secondary mammary anlage then develops, with differentiation of the hair follicle, sebaceous gland, and sweat gland elements, but only the sweat glands develop fully at this time. Phylogenetically, the breast parenchyma is believed to develop from sweat gland tissue. In addition, apocrine glands develop to form the Montgomery glands around the nipple. The developments described thus far are independent of hormonal influences.

During the third trimester of pregnancy, placental sex hormones enter the fetal circulation and induce canalization of the branched epithelial tissues (canalization stage) (4). This process continues from the 20th to the 32nd week of gestation. At term, 15 to 25 mammary ducts have been formed, with coalescence of approximately 10 major ducts and sebaceous glands near the epidermis (5). Parenchymal differentiation occurs at 32 to 40 weeks with the development of lobuloalveolar structures that contain colostrum (end-vesicle stage). A fourfold increase in mammary gland mass occurs at this time,

and the nipple–areolar complex develops and becomes pigmented. Externally the nipple is small and flattened, although rudimentary sebaceous glands and Montgomery tubercles are present. The circular smooth muscle fibers that lead to the erectile function of the nipple are developed by this stage.

In the neonate, the stimulated mammary tissue secretes colostral milk (sometimes called *witch's milk*), which can be expressed from the nipple for 4 to 7 days postpartum in most neonates of either sex. At birth, the withdrawal of maternal steroids results in the secretion of neonatal prolactin. It is this hormone that stimulates newborn breast secretion. In the newborn, colostral secretion declines over a 3- to 4-week period owing to involution of the breast after withdrawal of placental hormones. During early childhood, the end vesicles become further canalized and develop into ductal structures by additional growth and branching.

After birth, the male breast undergoes minimal additional development and remains rudimentary. In the female, the breasts undergo extensive further development, which is regulated by hormones that influence reproduction. The breast has reached its major development by 20 years of age and will usually begin to undergo atrophic changes in the fifth decade of life.

DEVELOPMENTAL ABNORMALITIES

The developmental abnormalities may be unilateral or bilateral and involve both the nipple and the breast or both. These abnormalities are usually isolated to the breast, but there are reports of being associated with a variety of other abnormalities. The most common association is with upper limb and urinary tract abnormalities.

Congenital Abnormalities

Polythelia and Polymastia

The most frequently observed abnormality seen in both sexes is an accessory nipple (polythelia). Ectopic nipple tissue may be mistaken for a pigmented nevus, and it may occur at any point along the milk streak from the axilla to the groin. The reported incidence of polythelia varies greatly in the literature. In a prospective study, Mimoumi et al. (6) found the incidence of polythelia to be 2.5%. Urbani and Betti (7) evaluated the association between polythelia and kidney and urinary tract malformations. These data indicate a significantly higher frequency of kidney and urinary tract malformations in patients with polythelia. This is a controversial issue, and many studies in the literature do not find any connection between polythelia and renal anomalies (8,9).

Rarely, accessory true mammary glands develop; these are most often located in the axilla (polymastia). During pregnancy and lactation, an accessory breast may enlarge; occasionally, if it has an associated nipple, the accessory breast may function.

Hypoplasia and Amastia

Hypoplasia is the underdevelopment of the breast; congenital absence of a breast is termed *amastia*. When breast tissue is lacking but a nipple is present, the condition is termed *amazia*. A wide range of breast abnormalities have been described and can be classified as follows (10,11):

> Unilateral hypoplasia, contralateral normal
> Bilateral hypoplasia with asymmetry
> Unilateral hyperplasia, contralateral normal
> Bilateral hyperplasia with asymmetry
> Unilateral hypoplasia, contralateral hyperplasia
> Unilateral hypoplasia of breast, thorax, and pectoral muscles (Poland's syndrome)

Most of these abnormalities are not severe. The most severe deformity, amastia or marked breast hypoplasia, is associated with hypoplasia of the pectoral muscle in 90% of cases (12), but the reverse does not apply. Of women with pectoral muscle abnormalities, 92% have a normal breast (13). Congenital abnormalities of the pectoral muscle are usually manifested by the lack of the lower third of the muscle and an associated deformity of the ipsilateral rib cage. The association among absence of the pectoral muscle, chest wall deformity, and breast abnormalities was first recognized by Poland in 1841. The original description, however, did not note the concomitant abnormalities of the hand (symbrachydactyly, with hypoplasia of the middle phalanges and central skin webbing) (14), and considerable controversy has evolved concerning the validity of the eponym for this congenital syndrome (15,16).

Athelia

The congenital absence of the nipple areolar complex is a rare entity and is usually associated with absence of the breast. This condition is typically associated with other anomalies.

Acquired Abnormalities

The most common—and avoidable—cause of amastia is iatrogenic. Injudicious biopsy of a precociously developing breast results in excision of most of the breast bud and subsequent marked deformity during puberty. The use of radiation therapy in prepubertal girls to treat either hemangioma of the breast or intrathoracic disease can also result in amastia. Traumatic injury of the developing breast, such as that caused by a severe cutaneous burn, with subsequent contracture, can also result in deformity.

NORMAL BREAST DEVELOPMENT DURING PUBERTY

Puberty in girls begins at the age of 10 to 12 years as a result of the influence of hypothalamic gonadotropin-releasing hormones secreted into the hypothalamic–pituitary portal venous system. The basophilic cells of the anterior pituitary release follicle-stimulating hormone and luteinizing hormone. Follicle-stimulating hormone causes the primordial ovarian follicles to mature into Graafian follicles, which secrete estrogens, primarily in the form of 17-estradiol. These hormones induce the growth and maturation of the breasts and genital organs (17). During the first 1 to 2 years after menarche, hypothalamic–adenohypophyseal function is unbalanced because the maturation of the primordial ovarian follicles does not result in ovulation or a luteal phase. Therefore, ovarian estrogen synthesis predominates over luteal progesterone synthesis. The physiologic effect of estrogens on the maturing breast is to stimulate

Table 1.1	PHASES OF BREAST DEVELOPMENT
Phase I Age: puberty	Preadolescent elevation of the nipple with no palpable glandular tissue or areolar pigmentation.
Phase II Age: 11.1 ± 1.1 yr	Presence of glandular tissue in the subareolar region. The nipple and breast project as a single mound from the chest wall.
Phase III Age: 12.2 ± 1.09 yr	Increase in the amount of readily palpable glandular tissue with enlargement of the breast and increased diameter and pigmentation of the areola. The contour of the breast and nipple remains in a single plane.
Phase IV Age: 13.1 ± 1.15 yr	Enlargement of the areola and increased areolar pigmentation. The nipple and areola form a secondary mound above the level of the breast.
Phase V Age: 15.3 ± 1.7 yr	Final adolescent development of a smooth contour with no projection of the areola and nipple.

From Tanner JM. *Wachstun und Reifung des Menschen.* Stuttgart: Georg Thieme erlag, 1962, with permission.

longitudinal growth of ductal epithelium. Terminal ductules also form buds that precede formation of breast lobules. Simultaneously, periductal connective tissues increase in volume and elasticity, with enhanced vascularity and fat deposition. These initial changes are induced by estrogens synthesized in immature ovarian follicles, which are anovulatory; subsequently, mature follicles ovulate, and the corpus luteum releases progesterone. The relative role of these hormones is not clear. In experimental studies, estrogens alone induce a pronounced ductular increase, whereas progesterone alone does not. The two hormones together produce full ductular–lobular–alveolar development of mammary tissues (17) The marked individual variation in development of the breast makes it impossible to categorize histologic changes on the basis of age (4). Breast development by age has been described by external morphologic changes. The evolution of the breast from childhood to maturity has been divided into five phases by Tanner (18), as shown in Table 1.1.

MORPHOLOGY

Adult Breast

The adult breast lies between the second and sixth ribs in the vertical axis and between the sternal edge and the midaxillary line in the horizontal axis (Fig. 1.1). The average breast measures 10 to 12 cm in diameter, and its average thickness centrally is 5 to 7 cm. Breast tissue also projects into the axilla as the axillary tail of Spence. The contour of the breast varies but is usually dome-like, with a conical configuration in the nulliparous woman and a pendulous contour in the parous woman. The breast is comprised of three major structures: skin, subcutaneous tissue, and breast tissue, with the last comprising both parenchyma and stroma. The parenchyma is divided into 15 to 20 segments that converge at the nipple in a radial arrangement. The collecting ducts that drain each segment are 2 mm in diameter, with subareolar lactiferous sinuses of 5 to 8 mm in diameter. Approximately 10 major collecting milk ducts open at the nipple (5).

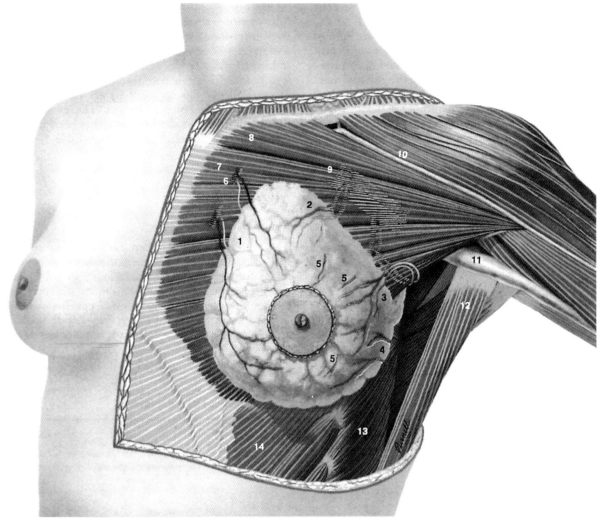

FIGURE. 1.1. Normal anatomy of the breast and pectoralis major muscle. 1. Perforating branches from internal mammary artery and vein; 2. Pectoral branches from thoracoacromial artery and vein; 3. External mammary branch from lateral thoracic artery and vein; 4. Branches from subscapular and thoracodorsal arteries and veins; 5. Lateral branches of third, fourth, and fifth intercostal arteries and veins; 6. Internal mammary artery and veins; 7. Sternocostal head of pectoralis major muscle; 8. Clavicular head of pectoralis major muscle; 9. Axillary artery and vein; 10. Cephalic vein; 11. Axillary sheath; 12. Latissimus dorsi muscle; 13. Serratus anterior muscle; 14. External abdominal oblique muscle.

The nomenclature of the duct system is varied. The branching system can be named in a logical fashion, starting with the collecting ducts in the nipple and extending to the ducts that drain each alveolus, as shown in Table 1.2. Each duct drains a lobe made up of 20 to 40 lobules. Each lobule consists of 10 to 100 alveoli or tubulosaccular secretory units (5,19). The stroma and subcutaneous tissues of the breast contain fat, connective tissue, blood vessels, nerves, and lymphatics.

The skin of the breast is thin and contains hair follicles, sebaceous glands, and eccrine sweat glands. The nipple, which is located over the fourth intercostal space in the nonpendulous breast, contains abundant sensory nerve endings, including Ruffini-like bodies and end bulbs of Krause. Moreover, sebaceous and apocrine sweat glands are present, but not hair follicles. The areola is circular and pigmented, measuring 15 to 60 mm in diameter. The Morgagni tubercles, located near the periphery of the areola, are elevations formed by openings of the ducts of the Montgomery glands. The Montgomery glands are large sebaceous glands capable of secreting milk; they represent an intermediate stage between sweat and mammary glands. Fascial tissues envelop the breast; the superficial pectoral fascia envelops the breast and is continuous with the superficial abdominal fascia of Camper. The undersurface of the breast lies on the deep pectoral fascia, covering the pectoralis major and anterior serratus muscles. Connecting these two fascial layers are fibrous bands (Cooper suspensory ligaments) that represent the "natural" means of support of the breast.

Vascular Anatomy of the Breast

The principal blood supply to the breast is derived from the internal mammary and lateral thoracic arteries. Approximately 60% of the breast, mainly the medial and central parts, is supplied by the anterior perforating branches of the internal mammary artery. Approximately 30% of the breast, mainly the upper, outer quadrant, is supplied by the lateral thoracic artery. The pectoral branch of the thoracoacromial artery; the lateral branches of the third, fourth, and fifth intercostal arteries; and the subscapular and thoracodorsal arteries all make minor contributions to the blood supply.

The principal veins involved in the venous drainage of the thoracic wall and the breast are the perforating branches of the internal thoracic vein, tributaries of the axillary vein, and perforating branches of posterior intercostal veins.

Table 1.2	NOMENCLATURE OF THE BREAST EPITHELIAL SYSTEM
Major ducts	Terminal ducts
Collecting ducts	Extralobular
Lactiferous sinuses	Intralobular
Segmental ducts	Lobules
Subsegmental ducts	Alveoli
Terminal duct–lobular unit	

Lymphatic Drainage of the Breast

Lymph Vessels

The lymphatic drainage of the breast is of great importance in the spread of malignant disease of the breast. The subepithelial or papillary plexus of the lymphatics of the breast is confluent with the subepithelial lymphatics over the surface of the body. These valveless lymphatic vessels communicate with subdermal lymphatic vessels and merge with the Sappey subareolar plexus. The subareolar plexus receives lymphatic vessels from the nipple and areola and communicates by way of vertical lymphatic vessels equivalent to those that connect the subepithelial and subdermal plexus elsewhere (20). Lymph flows unidirectionally from the superficial to deep plexus and from the subareolar plexus through the lymphatic vessels of the lactiferous ducts to the perilobular and deep subcutaneous plexus. The periductal lymphatic vessels lie just outside the myoepithelial layer of the duct wall (21). Flow from the deep subcutaneous and intramammary lymphatic vessels moves centrifugally toward the axillary and internal mammary lymph nodes. Injection studies with radiolabeled colloid (22) have demonstrated the physiology of lymph flow and have countered the old hypothesis of centripetal flow toward the Sappey subareolar plexus (23). Approximately 3% of the lymph from the breast is estimated to flow to the internal mammary chain, whereas 97% flows to the axillary nodes (24).

New insight into lymphatic anatomy and the physiology of lymph flow has been gained from sentinel lymph node studies. It has been observed that the dermal and parenchymal lymphatics drain to the same axillary lymph nodes that are the main basin for lymph draining from the breast (25–30). This might be expected considering the embryology of the breast described earlier in this chapter. Lymphoscintigraphic studies have also shown that deeper parenchymal or retromammary lymphatics preferentially drain to the internal mammary lymph nodes when compared to intradermal or subdermal injection (31–35). There has been controversy over the direction of parenchymal lymph flow in relation to the subareolar plexus. Isotope injection of technetium Tc 99m–labeled sulfur colloid into the subareolar region results in localization of isotope in the axillary sentinel lymph node (36–38). A detailed isotope study of subareolar injection and the lymphatic channels leading to the sentinel lymph node showed that in 90% of cases a single channel exited the areolar margin superiorly or laterally and terminated in an axillary sentinel lymph node (39). Secondary lymphatic channels exited the areola in 75% of cases. None entered the internal mammary lymph node chain.

Suami et al. (40) studied 24 breasts in 14 fresh human cadavers to examine the lymphatic drainage. Lymph collecting vessels were found evenly spaced at the periphery of the anterior upper torso draining radially into the axillary nodes. As identified in cross-section analysis, as these collecting vessels reached the breast some passed over and some through the breast parenchyma. Perforating lymph vessels that coursed beside the branches of the internal mammary vessels and drained into the ipsilateral internal mammary lymphatics were also found. Some of these findings are discordant with current knowledge and may explain some of the false-negative rates of sentinel lymph node biopsy.

Axillary Lymph Nodes

The topographic anatomy of the axillary lymph nodes has been studied as the major route of regional spread in primary mammary carcinoma. The anatomic arrangement of the axillary lymph nodes has been subject to many different classifications. The most detailed studies are those of Pickren (41), which show the pathologic anatomy of tumor spread. Axillary lymph nodes can be grouped as the apical or subclavicular nodes, lying medial to the pectoralis minor muscle, and the axillary vein lymph nodes, grouped along the axillary vein from the pectoralis minor muscle to the lateral limit of the axilla; the interpectoral (Rotter) nodes, lying between the pectoralis major and minor muscles along the lateral pectoral nerve (42,43); the scapular group, comprising the nodes lying along the subscapular vessels; and the central nodes, lying beneath the lateral border of the pectoralis major muscle and below the pectoralis minor muscle (Fig. 1.2). Other groups can be identified, such as the external mammary nodes lying over the axillary tail, intramammary lymph nodes, which are found in 28% of breasts (44), and the paramammary nodes located in the subcutaneous fat over the upper, outer quadrant of the breast.

An alternative method of delineating metastatic spread, for the purposes of determining pathologic anatomy and metastatic progression, is to divide the axillary lymph nodes into arbitrary levels (45). Level I lymph nodes lie lateral to the lateral border of the pectoralis minor muscle, level II nodes lie behind the pectoralis minor muscle, and level III nodes are located medial to the medial border of the pectoralis minor muscle (Fig. 1.3). These levels can be determined accurately only by marking them with tags at the time of surgery.

Internal Mammary Lymph Nodes

The internal mammary nodes lie in the intercostal spaces in the parasternal region. The nodes lie close to the internal mammary vessels in extrapleural fat and are distributed in the intercostal spaces, as shown in Figure 1.3. From the second intercostal space downward, the internal mammary nodes are separated from the pleura by a thin layer of fascia in the same plane as the transverse thoracic muscle. The number of lymph nodes described in the internal mammary chain varies. The nodes lie medial to the internal mammary vessels in the first and second intercostal spaces in 88% and 76% of cases, respectively, whereas they lie lateral to the vessels in the third intercostal space in 79% of cases. The prevalence of nodes in each intercostal space is as follows: first space, 97%; second space, 98%; third space, 82%; fourth space, 9%; fifth space, 12%; and sixth space, 62% (46). The pathologic anatomy of this route of lymphatic drainage in the spread of breast disease has been described by Handley and Thackray (47) and Urban and Marjani (48).

In the presence of nodal metastases, obstruction of the physiologic routes of lymphatic flow may occur, and alternative pathways may then become important. The alternative routes that have been described are deep, substernal, cross-drainage to the contralateral internal mammary chain (49,50); superficial presternal crossover, lateral intercostal, and mediastinal drainage (51); and spread through the rectus abdominis muscle sheath to

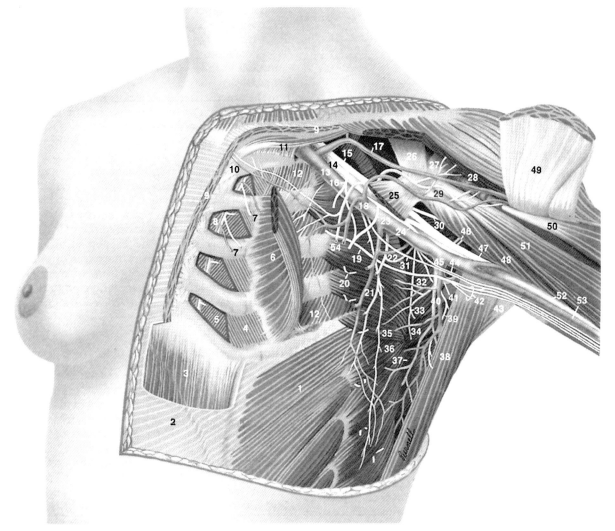

FIGURE 1.2. Chest wall muscles and vascular anatomy. 1. External abdominal oblique muscle; 2. Rectus sheath; 3. Rectus abdominis muscle; 4. Internal intercostal muscle; 5. Transverse thoracic muscle; 6. Pectoralis minor muscle; 7. Perforating branches from internal mammary artery and vein; 8. Internal mammary artery and vein; 9. Cut edge of pectoralis major muscle; 10. Sternoclavicular branch of thoracoacromial artery and vein; 11. Subclavius muscle and Halsted ligament; 12. External intercostal muscle; 13. Axillary vein; 14. Axillary artery; 15. Lateral cord of brachial plexus; 16. Lateral pectoral nerve (from the lateral cord); 17. Cephalic vein; 18. Thoracoacromial vein; 19. Intercostobrachial nerve; 20. Lateral cutaneous nerves; 21. Lateral thoracic artery and vein; 22. Scapular branches of lateral thoracic artery and vein; 23. Medial pectoral nerve (from medial cord); 24. Ulnar nerve; 25. Pectoralis minor muscle; 26. Coracoclavicular ligament; 27. Coracoacromial ligament; 28. Cut edge of deltoid muscle; 29. Acromial and humeral branches of thoracoacromial artery and vein; 30. Musculocutaneous nerve; 31. Medial cutaneous nerve of arm; 32. Subscapularis muscle; 33. Lower subscapular nerve; 34. Teres major muscle; 35. Long thoracic nerve; 36. Serratus anterior muscle; 37. Latissimus dorsi muscle; 38. Latissimus dorsi muscle; 39. Thoracodorsal nerve; 40. Thoracodorsal artery and vein; 41. Scapular circumflex artery and vein; 42. Branching of intercostobrachial nerve; 43. Teres major muscle; 44. Medial cutaneous nerve of forearm; 45. Subscapular artery and vein; 46. Posterior humeral circumflex artery and vein; 47. Median nerve; 48. Coracobrachialis muscle; 49. Pectoralis major muscle; 50. Biceps brachii muscle, long head; 51. Biceps brachii muscle, short head; 52. Brachial artery; 53. Basilic vein; 54. Pectoral branch of thoracoacromial artery and vein.

the subdiaphragmatic and subperitoneal plexus (the Gerota pathway). This last route allows the direct spread of tumor to the liver and retroperitoneal lymph nodes. Substernal crossover is demonstrable by isotope imaging of the lymph nodes and may be of significance in early breast cancer (52).

Muscular and Neural Anatomy

The important muscles in the region of the breast are the pectoralis major and minor, serratus anterior, and latissimus dorsi muscles, as well as the aponeurosis of the external oblique and rectus abdominis muscles (Fig. 1.2).

The pectoralis minor muscle arises from the outer aspect of the third, fourth, and fifth ribs and is inserted into the medial border of the upper surface of the coracoid process of the

scapula. The muscle is usually prefixed, rather than postfixed, and is innervated by the medial pectoral nerve, which arises mainly from the medial cord of the brachial plexus (cervical vertebra number, or C8, T1 segmental origin) and descends posteriorly to the muscle crossing the axillary vein anteriorly. The nerve enters the interpectoral space, passing through the muscle itself in 62% of cases and around the lateral border as a single branch in 38% of cases (53). Varying numbers of branches passing through the muscle provide motor supply to the lateral part of the pectoralis major muscle. The terms *medial* and *lateral* pectoral nerves are confusing: The standard terminology refers to their brachial plexus origin rather than their anatomic positions. Changes in terminology have been proposed but have not yet been generally accepted. The arrangement of these nerves is of particular importance in performing an axillary dissection.

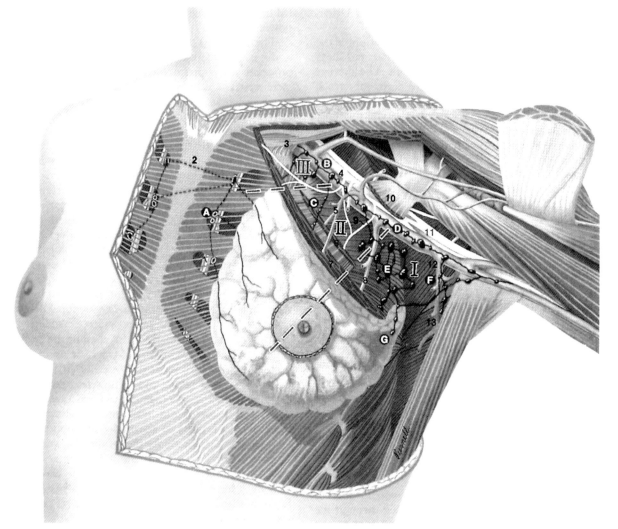

FIGURE 1.3. Lymphatic drainage of the breast showing lymph node groups and levels. 1. Internal mammary artery and vein; 2. Substernal cross-drainage to contralateral internal mammary lymphatic chain; 3. Subclavius muscle and Halsted ligament; 4. Lateral pectoral nerve (from the lateral cord); 5. Pectoral branch from thoracoacromial vein; 6. Pectoralis minor muscle; 7. Pectoralis major muscle; 8. Lateral thoracic vein; 9. Medial pectoral nerve (from the medial cord); 10. Pectoralis minor muscle; 11. Median nerve; 12. Subscapular vein; 13. Thoracodorsal vein; A. Internal mammary lymph nodes; B. Apical lymph nodes; C. Interpectoral (Rotter) lymph nodes; D. Axillary vein lymph nodes; E. Central lymph nodes; F. Scapular lymph nodes; G. External mammary lymph nodes; Level I lymph nodes: lateral to lateral border of pectoralis minor muscle; Level II lymph nodes: behind pectoralis minor muscle; Level III lymph nodes: medial to medial border of pectoralis minor muscle.

The serratus anterior muscle stabilizes the scapula on the chest wall. The muscle arises by a series of digitations from the upper eight ribs laterally; its origin from the first rib is in the posterior triangle of the neck. At its origin from the fifth, sixth, seventh, and eighth ribs, the serratus anterior muscle interdigitates with the origin of the external oblique muscle. The muscle inserts into the vertebral border of the scapula on its costal surface and is supplied by the long thoracic nerve of Bell (the nerve to the serratus anterior muscle). The origin of this important nerve is the posterior aspect of the C5, C6, and C7 roots of the brachial plexus. It passes posteriorly to the axillary vessels, emerging on the chest wall high in the medial part of the subscapular fossa. The nerve lies superficial to the deep fascia overlying the anterior serratus muscle and marks the posterior limit of dissection of the deep fascia. Preservation of the nerve to the serratus anterior muscle as it passes downward is essential to avoid "winging" of the scapula and loss of shoulder power.

The latissimus dorsi muscle, the largest muscle in the body, is characterized by a wide origin from the spinous processes and supraspinous ligaments of the seventh thoracic vertebra downward, including all the lumbar and sacral vertebrae. The muscle inserts, by a narrow tendon forming the posterior axillary fold, into a 2.5-cm insertion in the bicipital groove of the humerus. As the muscle spirals around the teres major muscle, the surfaces of the muscle become reversed to the point of insertion. The muscle is supplied by the thoracodorsal nerve (the nerve to the latissimus dorsi muscle), which arises from the posterior cord of the brachial plexus, with segmental origin from C6, C7, and C8. The nerve passes behind the axillary vessels, approaches the subscapular vessels from the medial side, and then crosses anterior to these vessels to enter the medial surface of the muscle. As the nerve passes through the axilla it is intimately involved in the scapular group of lymph nodes. Resection of the nerve does not result in any important cosmetic or functional defect; nevertheless, it should be preserved when possible.

An important landmark in the apex of the axilla is the origin of the subclavius muscle, which arises from the costochondral junction of the first rib. At the tendinous part of the lower border of this muscle, two layers of the clavipectoral fascia fuse together to form a well-developed band, the costocoracoid ligament, which stretches from the coracoid process to the first costochondral junction (the Halsted ligament). At this point, the axillary vessels (the vein being anterior and inferior to the artery) enter the thorax, passing over the first rib and beneath the clavicle. Many unnamed small branches enter the axillary vein at its lower border. Near the apex, a small artery, the highest thoracic artery, arises from the axillary artery and lies on the first and second ribs.

Muscular Abnormalities

Congenital absence of the sternocostal head of the pectoralis major muscle and its associated abnormalities (Poland's syndrome) has been described earlier in this chapter. In 5% of cadavers, a sternalis muscle can be found lying longitudinally between the sternal insertion of the sternocleidomastoid muscle and the rectus abdominis muscle. The pectoralis minor muscle is inserted into the head of the humerus as well as the coracoid process of the scapula in 15% of cases. Part of the tendon then passes between the two parts of the coracoacromial ligament to insert into the coracohumeral ligament. Rarely, the axillopectoral muscle arises as a separate part of the latissimus dorsi muscle and inferolaterally crosses the base of the axilla superficially, passing deep to the pectoralis major muscle to join its insertion or to continue to the coracoid process (the axillohumeral arch of Langer). This anatomic arrangement can cause compression of the axillary vessels (54) and difficulty in orientation during axillary dissection.

Microanatomy of Breast Development

The developing breast at puberty has been described in detail by Russo and Russo (55) as growing and dividing ducts that form club-shaped terminal end buds. Growing terminal end buds form new branches, twigs, and small ductules termed *alveolar buds* (Fig. 1.4). Alveolar buds subsequently differentiate into the terminal structure of the resting breast, named the *acines* by German pathologists or the *ductule* by Dawson (4). The term *alveolus* is best applied to the resting secretory unit, and *acines* to the fully developed secretory unit of pregnancy and lactation (55).

Lobules develop during the first few years after menarche. The alveolar buds cluster around a terminal duct and form type I (virginal) lobules, comprising approximately 11 alveolar buds lined by 2 layers of epithelium. Full differentiation of the mammary gland proceeds through puberty, takes many years, and may not be fully completed if interrupted by pregnancies.

Detailed microanatomic studies of the breast have shown the presence of three distinct types of lobules (55). Type I lobules, previously described, are the first generation of lobules that develop just after the menarche. The transition to type II and type III gradually results from continued sprouting of new

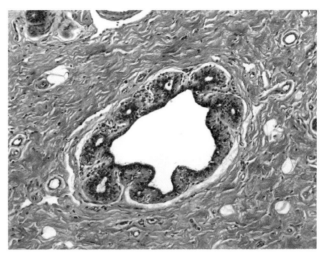

FIGURE 1.4. Normal duct in adolescent female breast. Rudimentary lobules are seen to be "budding" from the parent duct. Hematoxylin-eosin (H&E) stain. (Photomicrograph courtesy of Dr. Syed Hoda, M.D.)

alveolar buds. The characteristics of the four lobular types are described in Tables 1.3 and 1.4.

Russo et al. (56) recently determined that the breast tissue of women with invasive cancer and those with a familial pattern of breast cancer have an architectural pattern different from the control group of normal tissue. They also found that the *BRCA1* or related genes may have a functional role in the branching pattern of the breast during lobular development. This is seen mainly in the epithelial stroma interaction.

Microscopic Anatomy of the Adult Breast

In the immature breast, the ducts and alveoli are lined by a two-layer epithelium that consists of a basal cuboidal layer and a flattened surface layer. In the presence of estrogens at puberty and subsequently, this epithelium proliferates, becoming multilayered in the adult breast (Figs. 1.5 and 1.6). Three alveolar cell types have been observed: superficial (luminal) A cells, basal B cells (chief cells), and myoepithelial cells.

Superficial, or luminal, A cells are dark, basophilic-staining cells that are rich in ribosomes. Superficial cells undergo intercellular dehiscence, with swelling of the mitochondria, and become grouped, forming buds within the lumen. Basal B cells, or chief cells, are the major cell type in mammary epithelium. They are clear, with an ovoid nucleus without nucleoli. Where the basal cells are in contact with the lumen, microvilli occur on the cell membrane. Intracytoplasmic filaments are similar to those in myoepithelial cells, suggesting their differentiation toward that cell type. Myoepithelial cells are located around alveoli and small excretory milk ducts between the inner aspect of the basement membrane and the tunica propria. Myoepithelial

Table 1.3	CHARACTERISTICS OF HUMAN BREAST LOBULES					
Lobule Type	Lobule Area (mm^2)	Component Structures	Component Area ($\times 10^{-2}/mm^2$)	No. of Components/ Lobule	No. of Components/mm^2	No. of Cells/ Area Section
I	0.048 ± 0.0444	Alveolar bud	0.232 ± 0.090	11.20 ± 6.34	253.8 ± 50.17	32.43 ± 14.07
II	0.060 ± 0.026	Ductule	0.167 ± 0.035	47.0 ± 11.70	682.4 ± 169.0	13.14 ± 4.79
III	0.129 ± 0.049	Ductule	0.125 ± 0.029	81.0 ± 16.6	560.4 ± 25.0	11.0 ± 2.0
IV	0.250 ± 0.060	Acini	0.120 ± 0.050	180.0 ± 20.8	720.0 ± 150.0	10.0 ± 2.3

From Russo J, Russo IH. Development of human mammary gland. In: Neville MC, Daniel CW, eds. *The mammary gland.* New York: Plenum, 1987:67, with permission.

Table 1.4	PROLIFERATIVE ACTIVITY OF HUMAN BREAST TERMINAL DUCT–LOBULAR UNIT COMPONENTS AS MEASURED BY DNA-LABELING INDEX	
Structure		Index
Terminal end bud		15.8 ± 5.2
Type I lobule		5.5 ± 0.5
Type II lobule		0.9 ± 1.2
Type III lobule		0.25 ± 0.3
Terminal duct		1.2 ± 0.5

From Russo J, Russo IH. Development of human mammary gland. In: Neville MC, Daniel CW, eds. *The mammary gland.* New York: Plenum, 1987:67, with permission.

cells are arranged in a branching, star-like fashion. The sarcoplasm contains filaments that are 50 to 80 nm in diameter; these myofilaments are inserted by hemidesmosomes into the basal membrane. These cells are not innervated but are stimulated by the steroid hormones prolactin and oxytocin.

Anatomy of the Nipple and Breast Ducts

Recent advances exploring ductal lavage (57) and direct visualization of the ducts with breast endoscopy (58) have made the anatomy of the nipple clinically relevant. Utilizing six different approaches to examine the ductal anatomy, Love and Barsky (59) found that more than 90% of all nipple examined contained five to nine ductal orifices, generally arranged as a central group and a peripheral group. The central ducts did not extend in a radial fashion from the nipple as previously thought but traveled back from the nipple toward the chest wall. They also found that each nipple orifice communicated with a separate, nonanastomosing ductal system, which extended to the terminal duct lobular unit. Rusby et al. (60) prospectively examined nipples from mastectomy specimens. The median number of ducts was 23, but they found far fewer ductal orifices on the nipple surface. This study demonstrates that many ducts share a few common openings on the nipple surface and explains the discrepancy between the number of ductal openings on the nipple and the number of actual ducts.

There is evidence to suggest that both ductal and lobular carcinoma arises in the terminal duct lobular unit. Stolier and

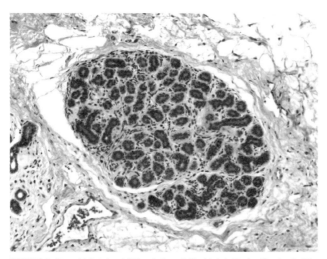

FIGURE 1.5. Normal lobule in adult female breast. The lobule is the functional unit of the breast. It is lined by two cell layers: inner epithelial layer and outer myoepithelial layer. The latter are inconspicuous on routine hematoxylin-eosin (H&E) stain such as this. (Photomicrograph courtesy of Dr. Syed Hoda, M.D.)

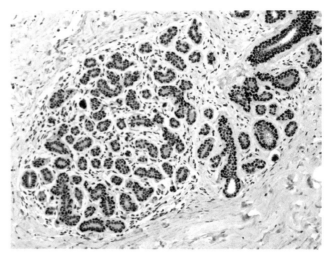

FIGURE 1.6. Normal lobule in adult female breast. p63 immunostain highlights the nuclei of the outer myoepithelial cell layer of the lobule. (Photomicrograph courtesy of Dr. Syed Hoda, M.D.)

Wang (61) examined 32 nipples of mastectomy specimens. In 29 of the specimens, there were no terminal duct lobular units identified. Three of the 32 specimens were found to have terminal duct lobular units. All terminal duct lobular units were found at the base of the nipple as opposed to near the tip. As interest in intraductal approaches and treatment increases so too will knowledge of ductal and nipple anatomy.

PHYSIOLOGY

Microscopy, Morphology, and the Menstrual Cycle

Histologic changes in the normal breast have been identified in relation to the endocrine variations of the menstrual cycle (62). Normal menstrual cycle–dependent histologic changes in both stroma and epithelium have been observed.

Cyclic changes in the sex steroid hormone levels during the menstrual cycle profoundly influence breast morphology. Under the influence of follicle-stimulating hormone and luteinizing hormone during the follicular phase of the menstrual cycle, increasing levels of estrogen secreted by the ovarian graafian follicles stimulate breast epithelial proliferation. During this proliferative phase, the epithelium exhibits sprouting, with increased cellular mitoses, RNA synthesis, increased nuclear density, enlargement of the nucleolus, and changes in other intercellular organelles. In particular, the Golgi apparatus, ribosomes, and mitochondria increase in size or number. During the follicular phase, at the time of maximal estrogen synthesis and secretion in midcycle, ovulation occurs. A second peak occurs in the midluteal phase, when luteal progesterone synthesis is maximal. Similarly, progestogens induce changes in the mammary epithelium during the luteal phase of the ovulatory cycles. Mammary ducts dilate, and the alveolar epithelial cells differentiate into secretory cells, with a partly monolayer arrangement. The combination of these sex steroid hormones and other hormones results in the formation of lipid droplets in the alveolar cells and some intraluminal secretion.

The changes in breast epithelium in response to hormones are mediated through either intracellular steroid receptors or membrane-bound peptide receptors. The presence of steroid receptors for estrogen and progestogens in the cytosol of normal mammary epithelium has been demonstrated (63). Through the binding of these hormones to specific receptors, the molecular changes, with their observed morphologic effects, are induced as physiologic changes. Similarly, membrane receptors are present to mediate the actions of prolactin. Increases in endogenous estrogen can also exert a histamine-like effect on the mammary microcirculation (64), resulting in an increased blood flow 3 to 4 days before menstruation, with an average increase in breast volume of 15 to 30 cm^3. Premenstrual breast fullness is attributable to increasing interlobular edema and enhanced ductular–acinar proliferation under the influence of estrogens and progestogens. With the onset of menstruation, after a rapid decline in the circulating levels of sex steroid hormones, secretory activity of the epithelium regresses.

Postmenstrually, tissue edema is reduced, and regression of the epithelium ceases as a new cycle begins, with concomitant rises in estrogen levels. Minimum breast volume is observed 5 to 7 days after menstruation. The cyclic changes in breast cellular growth rates are related to hormonal variations in the follicular and luteal phases of the menstrual cycle. Measurement of these changes can be made by observation and measurement of a variety of cellular and nuclear parameters:

- Histologic pattern
- Cellular morphology
- Nuclear morphology
- Mitoses
- Tritiated thymidine uptake
- Image cytometry
  - Nuclear area
  - Circumference
  - Boundary fluctuation
  - Chromatin granularity
  - Stain intensity
- Proliferation markers
  - Ki-67
  - Proliferating cell nuclear antigen
  - MIB1

Most observations have been made from surgical specimens, which are usually from women with breast abnormalities, or from autopsy specimens, which may have resulted in inconsistent and contradictory results.

Most studies have shown that breast epithelial cell proliferation increases in the second half (luteal phase) of the menstrual cycle (65–71).

A study of nuclear tritiated thymidine uptake in surgically excised breast tissue showed that peak uptake was during the luteal phase on days 22 to 24, coinciding with an increase in circulatory progesterone levels and a second peak of estrogen. The role of estrogen was considered unimportant because the preovulatory peak of estrogen was not associated with an increase in tritiated thymidine uptake (67). The possibility of a synergistic action between estrogen and progesterone would therefore be unlikely.

The role of estrogen and progesterone was subsequently studied in explants of human breast tissue implanted subcutaneously in nude mice (72). An increase in epithelial cell growth was observed 7 days after exposure to estrogen; progesterone had no effect, and a combination of estrogen and progesterone neither enhanced nor diminished the proliferative effect of estrogen. These observations may explain why proliferation increases during the luteal phase subsequent to the preovulatory estrogen peak.

Breast Changes during Pregnancy

During pregnancy, marked ductular, lobular, and alveolar growth occurs as a result of the influence of luteal and placental sex steroids, placental lactogen, prolactin, and chorionic gonadotropin (Fig. 1.4B). In experimental studies, these effects are observed when estrogen and progesterone cause a release

of prolactin by reducing the hypothalamic release of prolactin-inhibiting factor (PIF) (69). Prolactin in humans is also released progressively during pregnancy and probably stimulates epithelial growth and secretion (70,71). Prolactin increases slowly during the first half of pregnancy; during the second and third trimesters, blood levels of prolactin are three to five times higher than normal, and mammary epithelium initiates protein synthesis.

In the first 3 to 4 weeks of pregnancy, marked ductular sprouting occurs with some branching, and lobular formation occurs under estrogenic influence. At 5 to 8 weeks, breast enlargement is significant, with dilatation of the superficial veins, heaviness, and increasing pigmentation of the nipple–areolar complex. In the second trimester, lobular formation exceeds ductular sprouting under progestogenic influence. The alveoli contain colostrum but no fat, which is secreted under the influence of prolactin. From the second half of pregnancy onward, increasing breast size results not from mammary epithelial proliferation but from increasing dilatation of the alveoli with colostrum, as well as from hypertrophy of myoepithelial cells, connective tissue, and fat. If these processes are interrupted by early delivery, lactation may be adequate from 16 weeks of pregnancy onward.

At the beginning of the second trimester, the mammary alveoli, but not the milk ducts, lose the superficial layer of A cells. Before this, as in the nonpregnant woman, the two-layer structure is maintained. In the second and third trimesters, this monolayer differentiates into a colostrum–cell layer and accumulates eosinophilic cells, plasma cells, and leukocytes around the alveoli. As pregnancy continues, colostrum, composed of desquamated epithelial cells, accumulates. Aggregations of lymphocytes, round cells, and desquamated phagocytic alveolar cells (foam cells) may be found in colostrum; these are termed the *Donné corpuscles*.

Lactation

After parturition, an immediate withdrawal of placental lactogen and sex steroid hormones occurs. During pregnancy, these hormones antagonize the effect of prolactin on mammary epithelium. Concomitant to the abrupt removal of the placental hormones, luteal production of the sex steroid hormones also ceases. A nadir is reached on the fourth to fifth day postpartum; at this time, the secretion of PIF from the hypothalamus into the hypothalamoadenohypophyseal portal system decreases. This reduction in PIF secretion allows the transmembrane secretion of prolactin by pituitary lactotrophs. Sex steroid hormones are not necessary for successful lactation, and physiologic increases, such as may occur with postpartum ovulatory cycles, do not inhibit it.

Prolactin, in the presence of growth hormone, insulin, and cortisol, converts the mammary epithelial cells from a presecretory to a secretory state. During the first 4 or 5 days after giving birth, the breasts enlarge as a result of the accumulation of secretions in the alveoli and ducts (Fig. 1.7). The initial secretion is of colostrum, a thin, serous fluid that is, at first, sticky and yellow. Colostrum contains lactoglobulin, which is identical to blood immunoglobulins. The importance of these immunoglobulins is unknown; many maternal antibodies cross the placenta, transferring passive immunity to the fetus *in utero*. Fatty acids such as decadienoic acid, phospholipids, fat-soluble vitamins, and lactalbumin in colostrum have considerable nutritional value. After colostrum secretion, transitional milk and then mature milk are elaborated.

Mechanisms of Milk Synthesis and Secretion

The effects of prolactin are mediated through membrane receptors in the mammary epithelial cells. The release of prolactin is

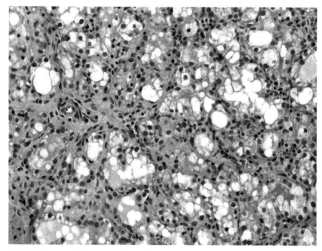

FIGURE 1.7. Lactating breast tissue. The glands within the lobules are enlarged and dilated. The stroma within the lobule is diminished. Secretory vacuoles are present within the individual lobular epithelial cells. Hematoxylin-eosin (H&E) stain. (Photomicrograph courtesy of Dr. Syed Hoda, M.D.)

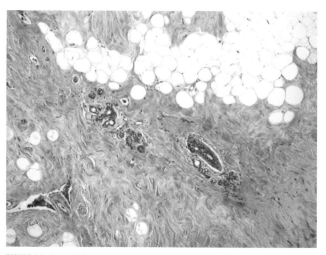

FIGURE 1.8. Atrophic breast tissue in a postmenopausal woman. Only a few atrophic ducts and lobules are present amid dense fibrous and fatty tissue. Hematoxylin-eosin (H&E) stain. (Photomicrograph courtesy of Dr. Syed Hoda, M.D.)

maintained and stimulated by suckling, as is the release of corticotrophin (adrenocorticotropic hormone). The mammary cells are cuboidal, depending on the degree of intracellular accumulation of secretions. The DNA and RNA of the nuclei increase, and abundant mitochondria, ribosomes, and rough endoplasmic reticulum, with a prominent Golgi apparatus, are apparent in the epithelial cells. Complex protein, mild fat, and lactose synthetic pathways are activated, as are water–ion transport mechanisms. These processes are initiated by the activation of hormone-specific membrane receptors. Changes in cyclic adenosine monophosphate stimulate milk synthesis through the induction of messenger and transfer RNA. Prolactin stimulates cyclic adenosine monophosphate–induced protein kinase activity, resulting in the phosphorylation of milk proteins. Polymerase activity and cellular transcription are enhanced (17).

Large fat vacuoles develop and move toward the apex of the cell. At the same time, the nucleus also moves toward the apex. As the water intake of the cell increases, longitudinal cellular striations may be observed. Ultimately, the vacuoles pass from the cell along with part of the cell membrane and cytoplasm; the apical cell membrane reconstitutes as secretion takes place.

Enhanced activity occurs during suckling. Fat is secreted chiefly through an apocrine mechanism, lactose is secreted through a merocrine mechanism, and the secretion of proteins occurs as a result of a combination of mechanisms. Ions enter the milk by diffusion and active transport. Relatively little holocrine secretion is thought to take place. The end result of secretion and subsequent intraductal dilution of extracellular fluid is milk, comprising a suspension of proteins—casein, β-lactalbumin, and β-lactoglobulin—and fat in a lactose–mineral solution. The white appearance of milk is due to emulsified lipids and calcium caseinate, whereas the yellow color of butterfat is due to the presence of carotenoids.

Mechanisms of Milk Ejection

The removal of milk by suckling is aided by active ejection. Sensory nerve endings in the nipple–areolar complex are activated by tactile stimuli. Impulses pass by way of sensory nerves through the dorsal roots to the spinal cord. In the spinal cord, impulses are relayed through the dorsal, lateral, and ventral spinothalamic tracts to the mesencephalon and lateral hypothalamus. Inhibition of PIF secretion permits the unimpeded secretion of prolactin from the anterior pituitary. Simultaneously,

through a different pathway in the paraventricular nucleus, the synthesis of oxytocin occurs. Oxytocin is released from the posterior pituitary neurovesicles by impulses traveling along the neurosecretory fibers of the hypothalamoneurohypophyseal tract. Oxytocin released into the systemic circulation acts on the myoepithelial cells, which contract and eject milk from the alveoli into the lactiferous ducts and sinuses. This phenomenon is specific to oxytocin, and changes in intramammary ductal pressures of 20 to 25 mm Hg may be observed in relation to peak blood levels. Oxytocin also acts on the uterus and cervix to promote involution. This effect may be stimulated by cervical dilatation and by vaginal stretching through the ascending afferent neural pathways (Ferguson reflex).

Complex neuroendocrine interactions determine normal lactation. An appreciation of these mechanisms is essential to the understanding of abnormalities and to the treatment of problems of lactation (17).

Menopause

Menopause is the result of the atresia of more than 400,000 follicles that are present in the ovaries of a female fetus at 5 months gestation. Declining ovarian function in late premenopause through the menopause leads to regression of epithelial structures and stroma. Menopausal involution of the breast results in reduction of both the number of ducts and lobules. Stromal changes dominate and fat deposition increases while the regression of connective tissue continues. The duct system remains, but the lobules shrink and collapse (Fig. 1.8). Lymphatic channels are also reduced in number in the postmenopausal breast (36). The last structures to appear with sexual maturity are the first ones to regress (17).

References

1. Hamilton NJ, Boyd JD, Mossman HW. *Human embryology.* Cambridge: Heffer, 1968:428.
2. Cardiff RD, Wellings SR. The comparative pathology of human and mouse mammary glands. *J Mammary Gland Biol Neoplasia* 1999;4:105.
3. Hughes ESR. Development of the mammary gland. *Ann R Coll Surg Engl* 1950;6:99.
4. Dawson EK. A histological study of the normal mamma in relation to tumour growth: I. Early development to maturity. *Edinb Med J* 1934;41:653.
5. Moffat DF, Going JJ. Three dimensional anatomy of complete duct systems in human breast: pathological and developmental implications. *J Clin Pathol* 1996;49:48.
6. Mimoumi R, Merlob P, Reisner SH. Occurrence of supernumerary nipples in newborns. *Am J Dis Children* 1983;137:952.

7. Urbani CE, Betti R. Accessory mammary tissue associated with congenital and hereditary nephrourinary malformations. *Int J Dermatol* 1996;35:349.
8. Grotto I, Browner-Elhanan K, Mimouni D, et al. Occurrence of supernumerary nipples in children with kidney and urinary tract malformations. *Pediatr Dermatol* 2001;40:637.
9. Jojart G, Seres E. Supernumerary nipple and renal anomalies. *Int Urol Nephrol* 1994;26:141.
10. Maliniac JW. *Breast deformities and their origin.* New York: Grune & Stratton, 1950:163.
11. Simon BE, Hoffman S, Kahn S. Treatment of asymmetry of the breasts. *Clin Plast Surg* 1975;2:375.
12. Trier WC. Complete breast absence. *Plast Reconstr Surg* 1965;36:430.
13. Pers M. Aplasias of the anterior thoracic wall, the pectoral muscle, and the breast. *Scand J Plast Reconstr Surg* 1968;2:125.
14. Beals RK, Crawford S. Congenital absence of the pectoral muscles. *Clin Orthop* 1976;119:166.
15. McDowell F. On the propagation, perpetuation and parroting of erroneous eponyms such as "Poland's syndrome." *Plast Reconstr Surg* 1977;59:561.
16. Ravitch MM. Poland's syndrome: a study of an eponym. *Plast Reconstr Surg* 1977;59:508.
17. Vorherr H. *The breast: morphology, physiology and lactation.* New York: Academic Press, 1974.
18. Tanner JM. *Wachstun und Reifung des Menschen.* Stuttgart: Georg Thieme Verlag, 1962.
19. Parks AG. The micro-anatomy of the breast. *Ann R Coll Surg Engl* 1959;25:235.
20. Spratt JS. Anatomy of the breast. *Major Probl Clin Surg* 1979;5:1.
21. Bonsor GM, Dossett JA, Jull JW. *Human and experimental breast cancer.* Springfield, IL: Charles C Thomas, 1961.
22. Turner-Warwick RT. The lymphatics of the breast. *Br J Surg* 1959;46:574.
23. Sappey MPC. *Injection preparation et conservation des vasseaux lymphatiques.* These pour le doctorat en medicine, no 241. Paris: Rignoux Imprimeur de la Faculte de Medecine, 1834.
24. Hultborn KA, Larsen LG, Raghnult I. The lymph drainage from the breast to the axillary and parasternal lymph nodes: studied with the aid of colloidal Au198. *Acta Radiol* 1955;43:52.
25. Lineham DC, Hill ADK, Akhurst T, et al. Intradermal radiocolloid and intraparenchymal blue dye injection optimize sentinel node identification in breast cancer patients. *Ann Surg Oncol* 1999;6:450.
26. Tanis PJ, Nieweg OE, Olmos RAV, et al. Anatomy and physiology of lymphatic drainage of the breast from the perspective of sentinel node biopsy. *J Am Coll Surg* 2001;192:399.
27. Nathanson SD, Nachna DL, Gilman D, et al. Pathways of lymphatic drainage from the breast. *Ann Surg Oncol* 2001;8:837.
28. Cody HS, Fey JV, Akhurst T, et al. Complementarity of blue dye and isotope in sentinel node localization for breast cancer: univariate and multivariate analysis of 966 procedures. *Ann Surg Oncol* 2001;8:13.
29. Boolbol SK, Key JV, Borgen PI, et al. Intradermal isotope injection: a highly accurate method of lymphatic mapping in breast carcinoma. *Ann Surg Oncol* 2001;8:20.
30. Vargas HI, Tolmos J, Agbunag RV, et al. A validation trial of subdermal injection compared with intraparenchymal injection for sentinel lymph node biopsy in breast cancer. *Am Surg* 2002;68:87.
31. Roumen RM, Geuskens LM, Valkenburg JG. In search of the true sentinel node by different injection techniques in breast cancer patients. *Eur J Surg Oncol* 1999;25:347.
32. Paganelli G, Galimberti V, Trifiro G, et al. Internal mammary node lymphoscintigraphy and biopsy in breast cancer. *Q J Nucl Med* 2002;46:138.
33. Shimazo K, Tamaki Y, Taguchi T, et al. Lymphoscintigraphic visualization of internal mammary node with subtumoral injection of radiocolloid in patients with breast cancer. *Ann Surg* 2003;237:390.
34. Feezor RJ, Kasraeian A, Copeland EM 3rd, et al. Sequential dermal-peritumoral radiocolloid injection for sentinel node biopsy for breast cancer: the University of Florida experience. *Am Surg* 2002;68:648; discussion 687.
35. Estourgie SH, Tanis PJ, Nieweg OE, et al. Should the hunt for internal mammary chain sentinel nodes begin? An evaluation of 150 breast cancer patients. *Ann Surg Oncol* 2003;10:935.
36. Kern KA. Sentinel lymph node mapping in breast cancer using subareolar injection of blue dye. *Eur J Surg Oncol* 1999;189:539.
37. Kern KA, Rosenberg R. Preoperative lymphoscintigraphy during lymphatic mapping for breast cancer: improved sentinel node imaging using subareolar injection of technetium 99m sulphur colloid. *J Am Coll Surg* 2000;191:479.
38. Klimberg V, Rubio I, Henry R, et al. Subareolar versus peritumoral injection for location of the sentinel lymph nodes. *Ann Surg* 2001;229:860.
39. Kern KA. Lymphoscintigraphic anatomy of sentinel lymphatic channels after subareolar injection of technetium 99m sulphur colloid. *J Am Coll Surg* 2001;193:601.
40. Suami H, Wei-Ren P, Mann GB, et al. The lymphatic anatomy of the breast and its implications for sentinel lymph node biopsy: a human cadaver study. *Ann Surg Oncol* 2008;15:863.
41. Pickren JW. Lymph node metastases in carcinoma of the female mammary gland. *Bull Roswell Park Mem Inst* 1956;1:79.
42. Grossman F. *Ueber die axillaren lymphdrusen.* Dissert. Berlin: 1896.
43. Rotter J. Zur topographic des mammacarcinoms. *Arch F Klin Chir* 1899;58:346.
44. Egan RL, McSweeney MB. Intramammary lymph nodes. *Cancer* 1983;51:1838.
45. Berg JW. The significance of axillary node levels in the study of breast carcinoma. *Cancer* 1955;8:776.
46. Stibbe EP. The internal mammary lymphatic glands. *J Anat* 1918;52:257.
47. Handley RS, Thackray AC. Invasion of internal mammary lymph nodes in carcinoma of the breast. *BMJ* 1954;1:161.
48. Urban JA, Marjani MA. Significance of internal mammary lymph node metastases in breast cancer. *AJR Am J Roentgenol* 1971;111:130.
49. Rouviere H. *Anatomie des lymphatiques de l'homme.* Paris: Masson, 1932.
50. Ege GN. Internal mammary lymphoscintigraphy. *Radiology* 1975;118:101.
51. Thomas JM, Redding WH, Sloane JP. The spread of breast cancer: importance of the intrathoracic lymphatic route and its relevance to treatment. *Br J Cancer* 1979;40:540.
52. Osborne MP, Jeyasingh K, Jewkes RF, et al. The preoperative detection of internal mammary lymph node metastases in breast cancer. *Br J Surg* 1979;66:813.
53. Moosman DA. Anatomy of the pectoral nerves and their preservation in modified mastectomy. *Am J Surg* 1980;139:883.
54. Boontje AH. Axillary vein entrapment. *Br J Surg* 1979;66:331.
55. Russo J, Russo IH. Development of human mammary gland. In: Neville MC, Daniel CW, eds. *The mammary gland.* New York: Plenum, 1987:67.
56. Russo J, Lynch H, Russo IH. Mammary gland architecture as a determining factor in the susceptibility of breast cancer. *Breast J* 2001;7:278.
57. Dooley WC, Ljung BM, Veronesi U, et al. Ductal lavage for the detection of cellular atypia in women at high risk for breast cancer. *J Natl Cancer Inst* 2001;93:1624.
58. Valdes EK, Boolbol SK, Cohen JM, et al. Clinical experience with mammary ductoscopy. *Ann Surg Onc* 2006; in press.
59. Love SM, Barsky SH. Anatomy of the nipple and breast ducts revisited. *Cancer* 2004;101:1947.
60. *Rusby JE, Brachtel EF, Michaelson JS, et al. Breast duct anatomy in the human nipple: three-dimensional patterns and clinical implications.* Breast Cancer Res Treat 2007;106:171.
61. Stolier AJ, Wang J. Terminal duct lobular units are scarce in the nipple: implications for prophylactic nipple-sparing mastectomy. *Ann Surg Oncol* 2008;15:438.
62. Vogel PM, Georgiade NG, Fetter BF, et al. The correlation of histologic changes in the human breast with the menstrual cycle. *Am J Pathol* 1981;104:23.
63. Wittliff JL, Lewko WM, Park DC, et al. Hormones, receptors and breast cancer. In: McGuire WL, ed. *Steroid binding proteins of mammary tissues and their clinical significance in breast cancer,* vol 10. New York: Raven, 1978:327.
64. Zeppa R. Vascular response of the breast to estrogen. *J Clin Endocrinol Metab* 1969;29:695.
65. Masters JRW, Drije JO, Scanisbrook JJ. Cyclic variation of DNA synthesis in human breast epithelium. *J Natl Cancer Inst* 1977;58:1263.
66. Meyer JS. Cell proliferation in normal breast ducts, fibroadenomas and other ductal hyperplasias measured by nuclear labeling with tritiated thymidine. *Hum Pathol* 1977;8:67.
67. Ferguson DJP, Anderson TJ. Morphological evaluation of cell turnover in relation to the menstrual cycle in the "resting" human breast. *Br J Cancer* 1981;44:177.
68. Longacre TA, Bartow SA. A correlative morphologic study of human breast and endometrium in the menstrual cycle. *Am J Surg Pathol* 1986;10:382.
69. Potter CS, Watson RJ, Williams GT, et al. The effect of age and menstrual cycle upon proliferative activity of the normal human breast. *Br J Cancer* 1988;58:163.
70. Going JJ, Anderson TJ, Battersby S, et al. Proliferative and secretory activity in human breast during natural and artificial menstrual cycles. *Am J Pathol* 1988;130:193.
71. Soderqvist G, Isaksson E, Schowltz BV, et al. Proliferation of breast epithelial cells in healthy women during the menstrual cycle. *Am J Obstet Gynecol* 1997;176:123.
72. Laidlaw IJ, Clarke RB, Howell A, et al. The proliferation of normal human breast tissue implanted into athymic nude mice is stimulated by estrogen but not progesterone. *Endocrinology* 1995;136:164.

Chapter 2
Molecular Mechanisms Regulating Breast Development

Jeffrey M. Rosen and Michael T. Lewis

In 1998 the National Cancer Institute Program Review Group Summary Report, titled "Charting the Course: Priorities for Breast Cancer Research," by Harold Moses and Nancy Davidson stated that "Our understanding of the biology and developmental genetics of the normal mammary gland is a barrier to progress . . . a more complete understanding of the normal mammary gland at each stage of development . . . will be a critical underpinning of continued advances in detecting, preventing and treating breast cancer" (1). A decade later, this statement has lost none of its poignancy.

Although there continues to be an explosion of new information related to mouse mammary gland development and function, recent progress in our understanding of human mammary gland development has been limited. Fortunately, evolutionary conservation of developmental and molecular mechanisms between rodents and humans appears to be the rule rather than the exception. Thus, it is likely that information gleaned from the mouse and rat can be translated directly to help elucidate the molecular mechanisms involved in the development of the human mammary gland.

Progress in understanding mouse mammary gland development has been driven primarily by the power of mouse genetics coupled with classical biological techniques, such as transplantation of mammary epithelium into the cleared mammary fat pad. Although these approaches are not directly applicable in humans, unique cell culture techniques and success with xenograft models of normal human breast epithelium transplanted into the humanized mammary fat pad of immunocompromised mice have provided new approaches to studying factors regulating development in the human breast (2). In particular, there has been considerable recent progress in identifying and isolating normal and malignant stem or progenitor cell populations in both the mouse and human mammary gland, as discussed in detail by Wicha et al. in this volume.

The ability to perform reconstitution experiments between isolated epithelium and stroma from the mammary glands of wild-type and genetically modified mice, and even chimeras between wild-type and null mammary epithelial cells (MECs), has helped elucidate paracrine signaling pathways important for mammary gland development. This chapter will focus on these recent advances in elucidating signaling pathways and cell lineages important in mammary gland development. Osborne and Boolbol (3) give a more general introduction to breast development in the human.

EMBRYONIC MOUSE MAMMARY GLAND DEVELOPMENT

Growth factor–mediated epithelial–mesenchymal interactions play a critical role in both embryonic and postnatal mammary gland development. The development of the embryonic mammary gland has similarities to other skin appendages, such as tooth buds, hair, and whisker follicles, in that the mammary rudiment develops as a consequence of sequential, reciprocal interactions between the epithelium and mesenchyme (4).

Establishment of the "Milk Line" or "Milk Streak"

The first morphological evidence of mammary gland development is the establishment of epidermal thickenings running anterior to posterior on either side of the trunk displaced off the ventral midline near the position of the hypaxial buds of the somites. These thickenings are referred to as the *milk streak* or *milk line* and are visible by embryonic day 10 or 11 (Fig. 2.1A). The milk line is defined molecularly by expression of *Wnt10b* mRNA.

Placode Induction

In the mouse, five pairs of ectodermal placodes or anlagen form (one pair in humans), and within a day these placodes form bulbs of epithelial cells that are morphologically and molecularly distinct from the surrounding epidermis. Dense mammary mesenchyme composed of two or three layers of tightly packed fibroblasts, envelop the developing mammary bud, appearing at embryonic day 13. The functions of this mesenchyme are to support growth of the epithelial bud and to regulate sexual dimorphism of the gland in response to testosterone. Posterior to the dense mammary mesenchyme lies the future fat pad, which is composed of preadipocytes. By embryonic day 14, the mammary mesenchyme expresses relatively high levels of androgen receptor (Fig. 2.1B). Androgens secreted by the testes in the male induce active regression of the mammary epithelial bud. In females the anlage continue to grow very slowly until embryonic day 16, when proliferation increases and the sprout of mammary epithelium begins to grow into the surrounding fat pad, opening to the nipple (Fig. 2.1C). At birth, only a rudimentary ductal tree consisting of a primary duct and 12 to 15 small branches of ductal epithelium is present (Fig. 2.1C), which persists in this rudimentary state until puberty (Fig. 2.1F).

One of the earliest genes known to be required for mammary gland development is the transcription factor TP63(p63), a member of the TP53(p53) gene family. p63 is required for mammalian epidermal development, and mice lacking the TP63 gene lose all stratified (5) squamous epithelia and their derivatives, including the mammary gland (6,7). The TP63 gene is transcribed from two different promoters, resulting in the expression of as many as six different protein isoforms with both activating and dominant negative functions. Different roles for specific p63 isoforms have been suggested not only in maintaining epithelial stem cell populations, but also in cellular differentiation and neoplasia (8). Using an antibody that recognizes all of these isoforms, p63 expression can be visualized in the embryonic day 16.5 mammary bud as well as the adjacent basal layer of the epidermis. The expression of keratin-14 (K14) is also readily detected in the mammary bud at this stage of embryonic development. One of the p63 isoforms, ΔNp63, has been shown to regulate the intranuclear expression of β-catenin (β-cat), and, therefore, influences the canonical Wnt signaling pathway (9). A different isoform, TAp63α, has been reported to increase the expression of the fibroblast growth-factor receptor 2 (FgfR2) (10), which is critical for mammary placode formation.

With respect to members of the fibroblast growth-factor (Fgf) family and their receptor tyrosine kinases, FgfR2IIIb, a specific isoform of FgfR2, is expressed in the mammary placode at embryonic day 11 or 12. Mice deficient for the FgfR2IIIb receptor, expressed in the epithelial cells, or its ligand, Fgf10, expressed in the surrounding mesenchyme lack induction of four out of five placodes (11). The mesenchyme that accumulates around the mammary buds also expresses Fgf7, another ligand for FgfR2IIIb, but mice deficient for Fgf7 do not appear to suffer any mammary defects (12).

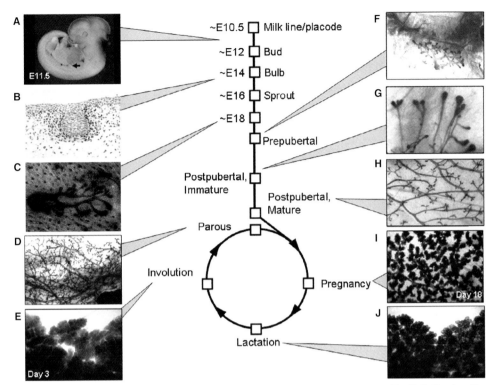

FIGURE 2.1. Overview of Mammary Gland Development. Selected phases of mammary gland development are identified in the schematic. Development can be divided into a linear phase (embryonic development through ductal maturity in the virgin) and a cyclical phase associated with pregnancy, lactation, and involution. **A:** Milk line and mammary placodes (*arrow*) in an embryonic (E) 11.5 day embryo identified by Wnt10b expression (*in situ* hybridization). Placodes 3 and 4 are visible. **B:** Bulb phase in an embryonic day 14 embryo. Note the condensed mammary mesenchyme around the bulb and prominent expression of androgen receptor (*brown stain*). **C:** Rudimentary mammary gland in an embryonic day 18 embryo showing modest branching. **D:** Parous gland after full involution. Morphology is similar to that found in mature virgin mammary glands. **E:** Early stage involuting mammary gland (day 3), while a significant cell death is occurring, there are only modest morphological differences between early involuting glands and lactating gland. **F:** Prepubescent mammary gland showing typical morphology observed from birth through puberty. **G:** Postpubertal, immature gland showing prominent terminal end buds and a simple branching pattern. **H:** Postpubertal, mature gland showing fully arborized ducts and blunt termini at the duct ends. **I:** Pregnancy. Gland is derived from an 18-day pregnant mouse. Alveoli are prominent, but not expanded. **J:** Lactation. Alveoli are large and expanded, nearly completely filling the available fat pad.

The importance of the Wnt signaling pathway in regulating embryonic mammary bud formation has been suggested by studies using a reporter mouse (TOPgal) in which β-catenin signaling can be visualized by the expression of a β-cat/TCF-driven β-galactosidase (β-gal) reporter gene, allowing the detection of β-gal positive cells as early as embryonic day 10 or 11 (13). Wnt10b and its downstream target Lef1, a member of the Lef/TCF family of transcription factors, are two early markers of the mammary placode. Deletion of *Lef1* results in the failure of mammary gland formation, as well as a number of other organs dependent on inductive mesenchymal–epithelial interactions, such as teeth, whiskers, and hair (14), similar to the TP63-null embryos. The functional importance of the Wnt pathway also has been demonstrated by the expression of an inhibitor of Wnt signaling, Dickkopf-1 from a K14 promoter in transgenic mice, which results in the absence of mammary buds. Thus, Wnt signaling through β-catenin appears to be essential for the formation of the mammary placode.

Recent studies also have revealed that loss of *Gli3* transcriptional repressor function leads to failure of mammary placode 3 and 5 formation during embryonic development (15,16). With respect to placode 3, elegant studies by Veltmaat et al. (16) have demonstrated that *Gli3* function is required in the hypaxial buds of thoracic somites as early as embryonic day 10.5 to induce somatic Fgf10 expression. As detailed above, this Fgf10 signal is received by the surface ectoderm via the FgfR2b receptor, where it then induces expression of Wnt10b in the mammary streak. Loss of *Gli3* leads to reduced Fgf10 expression, and failure to induce Wnt10b in the region corresponding to mammary

placode 3. Thus, at least for mammary gland 3, *Gli3* function is required in the somites to establish MEC identity, but *Gli3* function does not appear to be required in the epithelial cells themselves at these early phases of growth.

Elongation of the Mammary Sprout and Invasion of the Mammary Fat Pad Precursor

A reciprocal signaling pathway between the epithelium and the mesenchyme involves the parathyroid hormone–related peptide (PTHrP), which is expressed in the bud epithelium from embryonic day 11.5 to 18, and acts through its G-protein–coupled receptor PTHR1 in surrounding mesenchymal cells to induce the formation of the dense mammary mesenchyme. Mammary development of mice lacking either the ligand or receptor is arrested at approximately embryonic day 15, with a failure of sprout elongation (17). In the absence of PTHrP signaling, the MECs revert to an epidermal fate (18). These studies are selected examples of how reciprocal interactions between ligands and receptors expressed in both the mammary epithelium and mesenchyme regulate signaling pathways, which are essential for embryonic mammary gland development. For more comprehensive reviews, see Robinson (4) and Howard and Ashworth (19).

Finally, receptors for both estrogen and progesterone, which play an essential role for postnatal mammary gland development, are expressed in the embryonic mammary gland (20,21). However, no embryonic mammary phenotype has been reported for mice with ablation of either of the estrogen receptor (ER) or progesterone receptor (PR) isoforms (22–24).

DEFECTS IN HUMAN EMBRYONIC MAMMARY GLAND DEVELOPMENT

Ulnar-Mammary Syndrome

Spontaneous mutations in the T-box gene, *TBX3*, result in the human ulnar-mammary syndrome, a dominant developmental disorder characterized by abnormal forelimb and apocrine gland development. The phenotype of mutant mice lacking the mouse ortholog, *Tbx3*, also show a deficiency in mammary gland induction (25) as well as limb and other abnormalities. The *Tbx3* mutant mice also lack expression of *Wnt10b* and *Lef1*, suggesting that this transcription factor may be upstream of the Wnt signaling pathway.

Polythelia and Polymastia

Polythelia (supernumerary nipples) and polymastia (supernumerary mammary glands) in humans are surprisingly common birth defects, occurring in up to about 5% of the population (26). Most cases appear to be sporadic, but several hereditary forms are known. Curiously, many hereditary forms are associated with other developmental defects, particularly limb and digit defects (syndactyly or polydactyly), craniofacial defects (cleft lip, cleft palate), as well as with renal abnormalities. Some hereditary forms are associated with increased incidence of certain cancers (renal adenocarcinomas, Wilms' tumor) (5). The specific mutations responsible for sporadic or hereditary polythelia or polymastia are generally not known. Simpson-Golabi-Behmel syndrome is caused by an X-linked gene and has been associated with loss of *glypican-3 (GPC3)*, which is known to interact with *IGF2* (27).

A few mouse models of polythelia and polymastia have been identified. A spontaneous mutation in the *neuregulin-3 (Nrg3)* gene, which encodes a secreted ligand in the epithelial growth-factor (EGF) superfamily, leads to frequent loss of mammary placode 3, but also leads to supernumerary nipples (28). Nrg3 is expressed in the mesenchyme and signals to the surface ectoderm via binding to the ErbB4 receptor. Several other Nrg and ErbB receptors are also expressed in the embryonic mammary gland and associated mesenchyme in developmentally regulated and spatially restricted patterns, suggesting a complex interplay between epithelium and mesenchyme involving this signaling network (19).

POSTNATAL MAMMARY GLAND DEVELOPMENT: OVERVIEW

Postnatal development of the mammary gland is somewhat unusual in that it is under the influence of systemic steroid and peptide hormones, as well as local growth factors. This section will focus on the paracrine interactions between MECs and between the epithelium and stroma with emphasis on several new paradigms. Postnatal development (Fig. 2.1) consists of four tightly regulated stages: ductal morphogenesis from 3 to 9 weeks of age, lobuloalveolar proliferation and differentiation during pregnancy, synthesis and secretion of milk proteins and lipids at lactation, and involution of the secretory epithelium following weaning. Each stage depends on a critical balance between proliferation, differentiation, and apoptosis. With the advent of knock-out and transgenic mice models, the specific contributions of hormones, growth factors, and cell signaling

pathways are beginning to be mapped to these stages of mammary development (29,30).

Ductal Morphogenesis

In mice, the rudimentary ductal tree present at birth grows isometrically with the increase in size of the whole animal from to approximately 3 to 4 weeks of age (Fig. 2.1F). At this age, the ductal tree has not yet reached the lymph node in the inguinal (no. 4) gland that marks the first one third of the mammary fat pad. Removal of the endogenous epithelium at this age yields a "cleared fat pad," which provides a useful site for transplantation of mammary epithelium (31).

With the onset of puberty at approximately 3 to 4 weeks of age, rapid development of the rudimentary ductal epithelium is initiated in response to increasing levels of circulating hormones synthesized by the pituitary gland and the ovary, including estrogen, progesterone, and growth hormone (Fig. 2.1G). Ductal elongation is regulated by a balance between proliferation and apoptosis within multilayered club-shaped structures known as terminal end buds (TEB) located at the growing tips of elongating ducts (Figs. 2.1G and Fig. 2.2) (32).

The TEB is composed of two predominant epithelial cell types (Fig. 2.2A,B). The outermost layer of cells, known as *cap cells*, is in close contact to the basement membrane at the distal portion of the end bud. Cap cells are highly proliferative multipotent progenitor cells of the TEB and are thought to give rise to both preluminal cells and myoepithelial cells (Fig. 2.2C,D). Cap cells lack expression of ER, PR, and the prolactin receptor (PrlR), as well as intracellular junctions, and they are not polarized. The inner cell mass of the TEB is known as the *body cell layer*. Body cells differentiate into luminal epithelial cell types.

The body cell layer of the TEB can be divided into two zones: a proliferative zone and an apoptotic zone (Fig. 2.2A,C). It is thought that the programmed cell death within the innermost region of the body cell layer is the primary mechanism, resulting in the formation a hollow duct composed of a single layer of luminal epithelial cells (Fig. 2.2). Three genes, *Bim1*, *Bcl2*, and *Ptch1*, have been implicated in this process. Mutations in all three genes lead to inappropriate retention of cells near the neck of the TEB (33,34). As the ducts approach the edges of the fat pad, by approximately 8 to 9 weeks of age, the TEBs regress, typically leaving blunt-ended or rounded duct termini (although some terminal budding can be observed in some mouse strains) (Fig. 2.1H).

The virgin gland remains relatively growth quiescent until the onset of pregnancy or the administration of exogenous hormones such as estrogen and progesterone. Considerable progress has been made in modeling the process of lumen formation in three-dimensional cultures of nonmalignant and malignant MEC lines grown in a laminin-rich extracellular matrix preparation (Matrigel) and to study the role of oncogenes and integrin-mediated signaling on the regulation of apoptosis in these cultures (35–37). These three-dimensional culture models provide a valuable tool to study signaling pathways in a defined system, but whether the mechanisms involved in lumen formation are the same as those employed during ductal morphogenesis remain to be established.

Local Growth Factors and Ductal Morphogenesis

Local growth factors, such as EGF, insulin-like growth factor (IGF)-I, and transforming growth factor (TGF)-β, function downstream of systemic hormones and play critical roles in the regulation of ductal morphogenesis. In many cases these function were demonstrated by a series of classical experiments in which these growth factors were administered by slow-release pellets placed in the mammary fat pad adjacent to TEBs

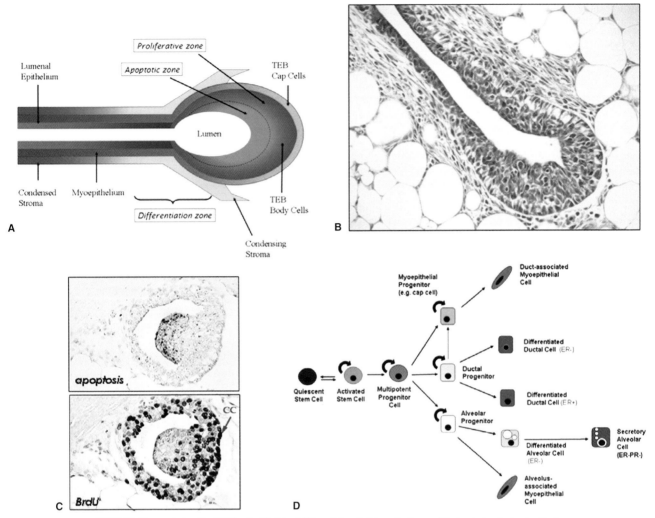

FIGURE 2.2. The terminal end bud (TEB) and epithelial cell differentiation. A: Schematic diagram of the terminal end bud and subtending duct. Characteristic cell layers are shown. The proliferative, apoptotic, and differentiation zones are identified. **B:** Histological preparation of a terminal end bud. **C:** Apoptotic (*top*) and proliferative (*bottom*) zones identified by terminal deoxynucleotidyl transferase-mediated dUTP biotin nick end labeling (TUNEL) staining and bromodeoxyuridine (BrdU) staining, respectively. (From Humphreys RC, Krajewska M, Krnacik S, et al. Apoptosis in the terminal endbud of the murine mammary gland: a mechanism of ductal morphogenesis. *Development* 1996;122:4013, with permission.) **D:** Hypothetical model for mammary epithelial cell differentiation. Differentiation events are shown by arrows. Self-renewal ability is shown by circular arrows.

(38–40). Further insight into the role of these local growth factors has been obtained by transplantation experiments in which knock-out and wild-type epithelium and stroma have been reconstituted (e.g., from wild-type and perinatal lethal EGF receptor knock-out mice). Using this latter approach, signaling through the stromal epidermal growth factor receptor has been shown to be necessary for ductal development (41).

Another example of stromal–epithelial crosstalk is illustrated by growth hormone regulation of IGF-I expression in the mammary stroma, which then acts on the IGF receptor (IGFR1) in the mammary epithelium. Deletion of IGFR results in embryonic lethality, but by transplantation of the mammary rudiment from embryonic day 17 to 18 lethal IGFR null mice into the cleared fat pad of wild-type recipients it has been possible to demonstrate that IGFR1 in the mammary epithelium is required for ductal outgrowth and proliferation in the TEBs (42).

A novel RhoGAP, p190-B, whose activity and localization is modulated by both integrin and IGF receptor signaling, has recently been shown to regulate the IGF signal transduction pathway and influence both embryonic epithelial or mesenchymal interactions as well as ductal outgrowth (43,44). The

importance of p190-B RhoGAP again was demonstrated by transplanting the mammary anlage from wild-type and *p190-B* heterozygous and null mice. This effect appears to be due at least in part to regulation of the levels of the insulin-receptor substrate molecules (IRS)-1 and IRS-2. Interestingly, IRS-2 is expressed in both the cap and body cells of the TEB, while IRS-1 expression appears to be confined to the body cells (45).

With respect to ER function, early studies using mammary tissues from immature wild-type and ERα–deficient mice (ERKO) mice transplanted into the kidney capsule originally indicated that stromal, but not epithelial ERα, was required for mammary gland ductal development. These results were surprising given that ERα, PR, and the PrlR are all expressed in the body cells of the TEB, thus it would appear likely that there should be some estrogenic effects directly on the epithelium. Accordingly, when MECs were isolated from adult ERKO mice or from wild-type counterparts and injected into epithelial-free mammary fat pads of 3-week-old female ERKO or wild-type mice, both stromal and epithelial ERα were shown to be required for complete mammary gland development. Subsequent studies showed that when the mice were treated with high doses of estrogen and progesterone, stromal ERα function was sufficient to allow regeneration of a full mammary gland (46) and that the original ERKO allele retained a certain level of ER function. More recently, Mallepell et al. (47) performed a series of elegant transplantation experiments using a new mouse line completely lacking ERα function to demonstrate that estrogen facilitates epithelial proliferation and morphogenesis by a paracrine mechanism and definitively demonstrated an absolute dependence on epithelial ERα for mammary ductal morphogenesis. Downstream, amphiregulin appears to be an essential paracrine mediator of ERα function (48,49). In addition, estrogens are known to enhance the stimulatory effects of IGF-I on proliferation in terminal end buds and ductal morphogenesis (39).

TGFβ is another local growth factor known to mediate epithelial–stromal interactions in ductal development. Expression of a dominant-negative TGFβ type II receptor in the mammary stroma results in increased branching in the mammary epithelium, suggesting an important role for TGFβ signaling as a negative regulator in branching morphogenesis. Additional studies have shown that TGFβ1 activity is regulated by ovarian hormones (50). Transplantation experiments comparing wild-type and TGFβ1 heterozygous mammary epithelium, which exhibit a greater than 90% reduction in TGFβ, in cleared fat pads suggests that this growth factor acts in an autocrine or juxtacrine manner to inhibit epithelial proliferation. More recent studies indicate that TGFβ is responsible for preventing proliferation of ER-expressing cells, which are normally not proliferative in adult mice and women (51). In addition, an interaction between the noncanonical Wnt family member, Wnt5a, and TGFβ to regulate ductal extension and lateral branching has been reported (52).

Several signaling pathways involved in neural development are now known to play important roles in mammary gland development. For example, the interaction between netrin-1 and neogenin, two molecules previously identified for their roles in axonal guidance in the nervous system, has also been shown to be involved in mammary gland morphogenesis (53). Netrin-1 is expressed in the preluminal body cells of the TEB, and its receptor, neogenin, is expressed in a complementary pattern in adjacent TEB cap cells. Loss of either gene resulted in disorganized TEBs. Thus, netrin-1 and its receptor, neogenin, may provide an adhesive rather than a guidance function during mammary morphogenesis. More recent studies also have established a novel role for SLIT2 as an adhesive cue, acting in parallel with netrin-1 to generate cell boundaries along ducts during bilayered tube formation (54).

The hedgehog (Hh) signal transduction pathway, important in the etiology of basal cell carcinoma, medulloblastoma, and other soft tissue cancers, has also been implicated in stromal–epithelial crosstalk and mammary gland development, regulation of mammary epithelial stem or progenitor cell, and in breast cancer (55,56). Heterozygous loss of *Patched-1* (*Ptch1*) and homozygous loss of *Gli2* in mouse models leads to ductal hyperplasias similar to those of the human breast. Both genes appear to function in the stroma (or in both epithelium and stroma) to regulate epithelial cell behavior. Transgenic overexpression of constitutively activated smoothened (Smo) lead to increased proliferation and an increased proportion of progenitor cell types (57). Transgenic overexpression of Gli1 in mammary epithelium leads to impaired alveolar differentiation (58).

Decreased *Ptch1* expression, and increased Smo expression have both been observed in a significant proportion of human breast cancers (57) and are consistent with increased Hh signaling. However, while *Ptch1* loss and transgenic *Smo* expression both lead to increased proliferation and ductal hyperplasia in mouse models, neither mutation leads to high frequency tumor formation.

The interaction between the mammary epithelium and the extracellular matrix (ECM) also plays a major role in branching morphogenesis (59). TEB bifurcation and sprouting of side branches from mature ducts both result in the formation of the branched mammary tree. ECM receptors, such as the discoidin domain receptor-1 (60), β1-integrin (61), as well as several metalloproteases capable of acting on the ECM (59), have all been shown to influence ductal morphogenesis. Inflammatory cells, such as macrophages and eosinophils, also appear to be important factors in this process. In mice lacking CSF1 and eotaxin, the populations of macrophages and eosinophils, respectively, in the mammary gland are depleted, resulting in impaired TEB formation, outgrowth into the surrounding fat pad, and decreased ductal branching (62).

Finally, the mammary gland is one of the few postnatal organs whose development is dependent on sprouting angiogenesis, with extensive new vasculature forming around the developing ductal tree, as well as during lobuloalveolar development (63,64). Thus, given the complexity of these interactions among local growth factors, ECM, inflammatory and endothelial cells, it is not surprising that it is difficult to adequately mimic these interactions even using optimized cell culture models containing ECM components. Functional microarray analysis applied to studying mammary gland organogenesis has identified specific gene expression profiles indicative of these diverse cell types present during mammary gland development (65,66).

Lobuloalveolar Development

Pregnancy induces proliferation of the secretory units of the mammary gland, alveoli, which originate from putative ductal progenitor cells (Fig. 2.2D) (67), and proliferate to eventually fill the entire stromal fat pad (Fig. 2.1I). DNA synthesis is initiated in the ductal epithelium early in pregnancy (day 3) before decreasing and being observed primarily in the developing alveoli, which are derived from these cells. Proliferation of the resulting alveoli per total number of MECs is maximal during the early pregnancy from days 6 to 10. By day 6 of pregnancy, fine secondary or tertiary branches with clusters of alveoli are apparent. By 10 days of pregnancy, the alveoli have begun to appear uniformly along the ductal network. By day 18 of pregnancy, the MEC population of the mammary gland accounts for approximately 90% of all cells; the entire fat pad has become filled with alveoli (Fig. 2.1I). Concurrent with proliferation, alveoli begin to functionally differentiate at midpregnancy, as assayed by the synthesis milk proteins, such as β-casein and whey acidic protein.

In addition to histological characterization and analysis of milk protein genes as markers of differentiation and as indicators of mammary gland function, three protein markers have been identified that distinguish different mammary keratin (K) K8/K18-positive luminal epithelial cells (68). The Na-K-Cl cotransporter 1 (NKCC1) and the water transporter aquaporin (AQP5) are both expressed in ductal cells in the mammary gland of virgin mice, but AQP5 was not detected in ductal cells during pregnancy. Interestingly, AQP5 is also detected in TEBs. NKCC1 is expressed basolaterally in the ductal cells in the virgin and pregnant glands, but its expression is decreased during pregnancy, and only low levels are detected in alveolar structures. In contrast, the Na-Pi type IIb transporter (Npt2b) is first observed in the apical membrane of the alveoli at day 15 of pregnancy and during lactation but is not detected in ductal cells. Thus, these three transporters provide useful markers to help distinguish changes in the luminal epithelium during mammary gland development, and antibodies against these transporters have provided extremely useful reagents in characterizing the mammary gland phenotype in several different knock-out mice (68).

The Importance of Hormone Receptor Patterning for Lobuloalveolar Development

Progesterone and prolactin (Prl) are the principal mediators of alveolar development in the mammary gland (69). Deletion of Prl, the PrlR, or PR completely inhibits alveolar development and ductal lateral branching, but does not compromise the process of ductal outgrowth and bifurcation significantly (24,70–72). Exogenous administration of P and Prl partially rescue lobuloalveolar development in ERKO mice (22). Two distinct progesterone receptor isoforms, PR-A and PR-B, transcribed from a single gene are expressed in the mammary gland. Analysis of mice null for either the PR-A or PR-B isoform (PRAKO and PRBKO mice, respectively) suggests that PR-B alone is sufficient to elicit normal proliferation and differentiation (73). Ductal side branching and lobuloalveolar development are markedly reduced in the PRBKO mice. Defects in both PrlR- and PR-mediated development have been localized to the mammary epithelium (70,71). As with ER, elegant PR +/+ and PRKO-*lacZ*-tagged (ROSA) MEC chimera reconstitution experiments have demonstrated that PR acts via a paracrine mechanism to induce alveolar proliferation (71). Alveolar development can be rescued if PRKO MEC mixed with PR +/+ MEC are reconstituted in close proximity within the cleared fat pads of syngeneic hosts, suggesting a paracrine mechanism of PR action (Fig. 2.3). Recombination of PR wild-type epithelium and PRKO stroma indicates that the stroma does not play a critical role in alveolar morphogenesis, further emphasizing the importance of epithelial–epithelial paracrine interactions, rather than epithelial–stromal interactions, in PR action. Interestingly, deletion of PR results in decreased cyclin D1 expression, providing one mechanism of impaired development in the PRKO mouse. Mice lacking cyclin D1 also display an epithelial cell-

autonomous defect in lobuloalveolar development (74,75). However, the effects of PR on cyclin D1 appear to occur in cells adjacent to those expressing the steroid receptor, again suggesting a paracrine mechanism (76). Disruption of steroid and PrlR patterning in certain knock-out mice results in an inhibition of lobuloalveolar development (77). The effect of PrlR on lobular development is mediated, in part, via a paracrine mechanism similar to that shown previously for ER and PR.

The spatial distribution of steroid receptors is critical to normal mammary gland development in humans and in rodents. For example, while the PR and ERα colocalize in over 96% of normal breast epithelial cells, proliferating cells in the adult are ERα and PR negative (Fig. 2.3) (78–80). Approximately, 25% to 30% of the ductal cells in the mature virgin are steroid receptor positive, and this distribution appears to be established during development as a consequence of the increase in progesterone levels (20). This nonuniform pattern of steroid receptors is also observed for PrlR (80), and it has been suggested, therefore, that ERα, PR, and PrlR are all colocalized in the same cells (81). The nonuniform pattern of PR expression along the mammary duct has been observed not only by immunostaining using specific anti-PR antibodies, but also by *in situ* hybridization to detect PR mRNA, and finally by using a unique lacZ reporter mouse to directly visualize PR promoter transcriptional activity. Confocal microscopy studies have revealed that the PR+ cells are not always directly adjacent to a proliferating cell, but are usually no more than two to three cells away from a PR+ cell, suggesting a paracrine mechanism controls MEC proliferation (Fig. 2.3). An analysis of PRKO and PrlR knock-out mice has suggested that there may be an autoregulatory pathway involved in the coexpression of ER, PR, and PrlR in ductal MEC (77).

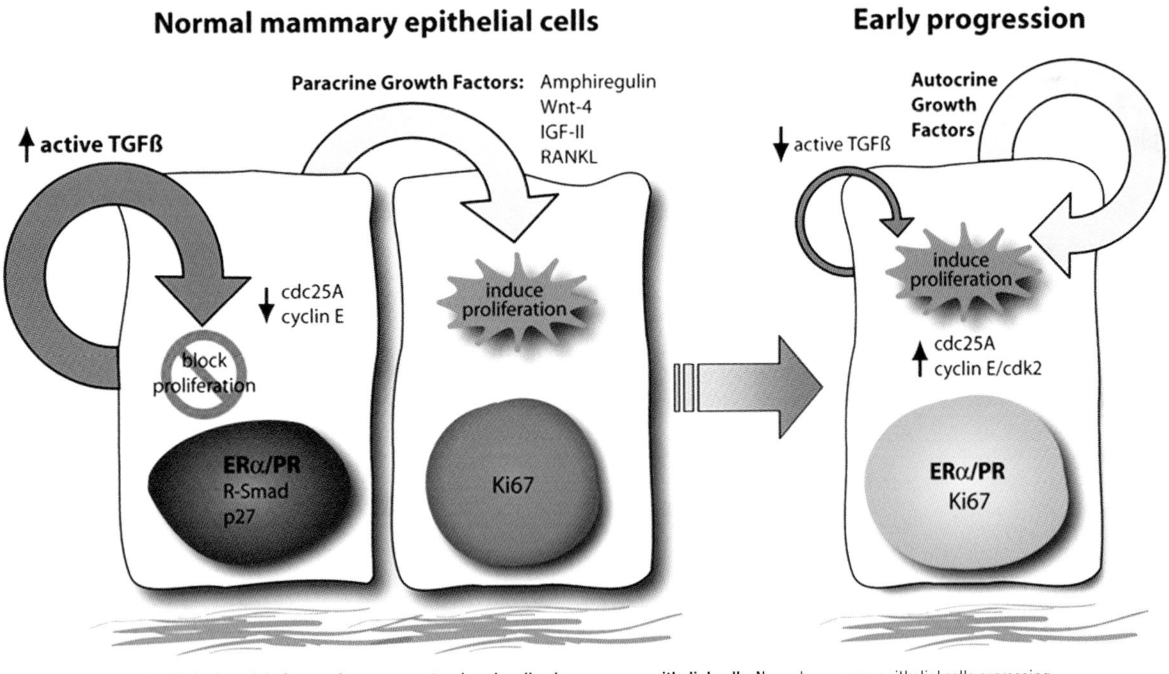

FIGURE 2.3. **A model of paracrine versus autocrine signaling in mammary epithelial cells.** Normal mammary epithelial cells expressing estrogen receptor (ER)α and progesterone receptor (PR) are restrained from proliferating, mediated by the growth-inhibitory actions of tumor growth factor (TGF)β signaling, active in this population. The steroid-receptor positive cells secrete local-acting growth factors to induce neighboring cells to divide in a paracrine fashion. In early breast cancer progression, this normal paracrine mechanism may switch to an autocrine loop, allowing steroid receptor positive cells to proliferate, possibly through the downregulation of active TGF-β signaling, leading to upregulation of cell cycle molecules such as cdc25A, cyclin E, and cdk2. (Figure and legend from Grimm SL, Rosen JM. Stop! In the name of transforming growth factor-beta: keeping estrogen receptor-alpha-positive mammary epithelial cells from proliferating. *Breast Cancer Res* 2006;8(4):106, with permission.)

Local Growth Factors as Paracrine Mediators of Lobuloalveolar Development

Establishment of the correct patterning of steroid and prolactin receptors in the mammary ducts is, therefore, required for local growth factors to stimulate the proliferation of nearby or adjacent steroid receptor negative MECs for normal lobuloalveolar development (Fig. 2.3). The phenotypic consequences of deletion of either PR or PrlR are quite similar (70,72), suggesting that their downstream signaling pathways likely converge at some point. In support of this hypothesis, gene arrays performed using these knock-out models have identified amphiregulin, IGF-II, Wnt-4, and receptor activator of nuclear factor κB (NF-κB) ligand (RANKL) as potential downstream targets of both pathways. Thus, as illustrated in Figure 2.3, members of the *IGF, EGF, Wnt* gene families, and RANKL may be the local growth factors that mediate the paracrine effects of progesterone and Prl. Support for this model has been obtained by the analysis of specific knock-out mice (48,76,82). The importance of the Wnt family of secreted glycoproteins was shown by ectopic expression of Wnt1, not normally expressed in the mammary gland, which rescued the lobuloalveolar defect in PRKO mice (82). Additional studies comparing mammary epithelium transplants from *Wnt4* null and wild-type donor mice into the cleared fat pad suggested that Wnt4 may act as a local mediator of progesterone action in early pregnancy. However, the defects in lobuloalveolar development observed in the Wnt4 null transplants were not seen in late pregnancy most likely due to compensation by other members of the Wnt gene family, such as Wnt5b.

The importance of EGF family members in regulating lobuloalveolar development has been obtained by the analysis of the triple knock-out of *TGF-α, EGF,* and *amphiregulin (AREG)* (83). In triple null glands, alveoli were poorly organized and undifferentiated, and milk protein gene expression was decreased. Again because of compensation by other family members, there are minimal effects of single deletions of these EGF family members. Estrogens have been shown to regulate directly amphiregulin expression (48).

Mice lacking RANKL or its receptor also fail to form lobuloalveolar structures during pregnancy (84). RANKL also appears to be an essential mediator of PR-dependent alveolar proliferation and survival (76) and was shown to be coexpressed in PR positive MECs, but not in the cyclin D1 proliferative cells. Studies using a mutant Ikkα (the Ikkα subunit of IκB kinase involved in the NF-κB signaling pathway) knock-in allele replacing serine residues with alanines in the activation loop have suggested that Ikkα is a critical intermediate in a pathway that controls mammary epithelial proliferation in response to RANKL signaling via cyclin D1 (85).

IGF-2 also has been suggested to be a mediator of prolactin-induced lobuloalveolar development (86,87). Ectopic IGF-2 expression restores alveologenesis in PrlR null epithelium, and lobuloalveolar development is retarded, but not prevented, in IGF-2-deficient MECs. IGF-1 and IGF-2 are also expressed in the mammary stroma (88) and may partially compensate for the loss of IGF-2 in the MECs. Alterations in the IGF signaling axis have been observed in the *CCAAT/enhancer binding protein (C/EBP) β* null mice, which also display an unusual pattern of steroid and prolactin gene expression as well as a defect in lobuloalveolar development (80).

A number of other transcription factors, specifically *GATA3* and *Elf5*, have also been shown recently to regulate luminal cell fate. For example, *GATA3* has been shown to be important for luminal cell differentiation (89,90), while the prolactin regulated *Elf5* transcription factor is required to establish the secretory alveolar lineage during pregnancy (91).

Thus, it appears that the precise patterning of steroid and prolactin receptors in the normal mammary gland is required

to elicit the appropriate paracrine response to local growth factors. A transition from a paracrine to an autocrine mechanism has been suggested to be an early step in preneoplastic progression (80). Supporting this hypothesis, ER-positive proliferating cells are rare in premenopausal lobules, but increase with age in the normal breast. However, the percentage of dual-expressing cells was significantly increased in all of the *in situ* proliferations examined, such as ductal carcinoma *in situ* (DCIS), and this correlated positively with the level of risk of developing breast cancer (92). Interestingly, in rodent models a similar increase in dual-expressing cells has been observed in aged rats, which could be prevented by an early exposure to estrogen and progesterone, which exerts protective effects similar to an early pregnancy (93).

In addition to the well-established roles of systemic steroid and peptide hormones and local growth factors on mammary gland development, recent studies have also established an important function for immune cell cytokines in mammary epithelial cell fate and function (94). Thus, the cytokines IL-4 and IL-13 using signal transducer and activator of transcription 6 (STAT6) as a downstream mediator appear to be critical for mammary gland differentiation and alveolar morphogenesis.

Lactation

The hormonal regulation of lactation has been reviewed by Neville et al. (95). Recently, gene expression profiling has been employed to decipher potential gene regulatory networks in lactation (96). Two general categories of hormones influencing lactation are defined: reproductive hormones, such as estrogen, progesterone, prolactin, placental lactogen, and oxytocin, and metabolic hormones, such as growth hormone, corticosteroids, thyroid hormone, and insulin all influence mammary gland development and lactation. For example, progesterone withdrawal at the end of pregnancy appears to trigger the closure of tight junctions and is required for the onset of lactation and secretion of milk proteins and lipids (97). Interestingly, PR expression is virtually absent from the mammary gland during lactation (20). The lactogenic hormones insulin, prolactin, and glucocorticoids regulate the expression of milk protein genes. At lactation oxytocin stimulates contraction of the myoepithelial cells in order to express milk through the nipple. Deletion of oxytocin impairs ejection of milk from alveoli, resulting in premature, milk stasis-induced apoptosis (98,99). Thyroid and growth hormone levels also influence lactation by both direct and indirect mechanisms, such as regulating nutrient uptake and increasing IGF-1 secretion from the stroma, respectively.

The importance of nutrient uptake in the mammary gland as a key regulator of lactation is nicely illustrated by studies in which the loss of *hypoxia inducible factor (HIF)-1α* impaired mammary differentiation and lipid secretion, culminating in lactation failure and striking changes in milk composition (100). These effects appear to be due in part for the requirement of HIF-1α to regulate the expression of the glucose transporter, GLUT1. During lactation, efficient glucose uptake is required for glycolysis, energy generation, and lactose synthesis. Unexpectedly, in these studies the deletion of *HIF-1α* did not appear to influence vascular density during pregnancy and lactation.

The control elements responsible for the hormonal, developmental, and cell-specific regulation of milk protein gene expression have been defined in both cell culture and transgenic mouse models (101). Clusters of transacting factor binding sites known as composite response elements (CoRE) are present in the proximal promoters and upstream enhancers of the casein and whey protein genes. The transcription factors that recognize and bind to these sites are not exclusively expressed in the mammary gland, and their DNA binding sites are often not the high affinity consensus binding sites identified for these factors. The CoRE contain multiple binding sites for several transcription factors, including C/EBPβ, NF1, STAT5, and the glucocorticoid receptor (GR). It appears that a combination of protein–DNA and protein–protein interactions is required to confer tissue and developmental-stage specific expression of the milk protein genes. Thus, to date there does not appear to be a "mammary-specific" transcription factor that regulates the identity of the mammary epithelial cells and milk protein gene expression.

Local Growth Factors and Cytokines also Regulate Mammary Gland Involution

Involution of the mammary gland following weaning is a multi-step process (102). Initially, milk stasis results in the induction of local factors that cause apoptosis in the alveolar epithelium. Next, after a prolonged absence of suckling, the consequent decline in circulating lactogenic hormone concentrations initiates remodeling of the mammary gland to resemble morphologically, but not genetically, the virgin-like state (66). Immediately following weaning, *TGFβ3* mRNA and protein are rapidly induced in the mammary epithelium, preceding the onset of apoptosis. Transplantation of neonatal mammary tissue derived from *TGFβ3* null mutant mice into syngenic hosts resulted in a significant inhibition of cell death compared to wild-type mice upon milk stasis (8). Transgenic mice overexpressing TGFβ3 under the control of the β-lactoglobulin promoter activated SMAD4 translocation to the nucleus and increased apoptosis. These results provide direct evidence that TGFβ3 is a local mammary factor induced by milk stasis that causes apoptosis in the mammary gland epithelium during involution.

Prolactin regulation of the Janus kinase (Jak)/STAT pathway, specifically the activation of STAT5, is critical both for mammary gland development and for the regulation of milk protein gene expression during lactation (103). However, at the onset of involution another STAT family member, STAT3, is specifically activated as evidenced by its tyrosine phosphorylation and nuclear translocation, while STAT5a is reciprocally inactivated (29). This switch appears to be triggered by milk stasis and is not dependent on changes in the level of circulating prolactin, thus suggesting it may be regulated by another local growth factor or cytokine. To address the function of *STAT3* in mammary epithelial apoptosis, a conditional knockout of *STAT3* using the Cre-lox recombination system has been generated, since germline deletion of *STAT3* results in early embryonic lethality (104). Following weaning, a decrease in apoptosis and a dramatic delay of involution occurred in STAT3 null mammary tissue. Mammary glands from *leukemia inhibitory factor (LIF)*-null mice, a cytokine known to activate STAT3, also exhibited delayed involution similar to the *STAT3* conditional knock-outs, suggesting that LIF may be the trigger for STAT3 activation (105).

A function for the NF-κB upstream regulator IκB kinase 2B (IKKB2) in apoptosis regulation in the normal regressing mammary gland recently has been reported (106). The IKKB2/NF-κB pathway was shown to be a regulator of TWEAK expression, which is a known ligand able to activate the death receptor, similar to the tumor necrosis factor (TNF).

Involution is normally associated with a significant increase in IGFBP-5 levels, which may be a direct or indirect transcriptional target of activated STAT3. IGFBP-5 has been suggested to induce apoptosis by sequestering IGF-1 to casein micelles, thereby inhibiting its survival function. Forced mammary gland involution also results in the decreased expression of IGF signaling molecules, such as insulin receptor substrates-1 and -2, critical docking molecules known to be required to transduce the signals from the IGF, and insulin receptors (107).

Decreased expression of IRS-1 and -2 are regulated by a post-transcriptional mechanism involving protein degradation, rather than by transcriptional control (45). Thus, several mechanisms are employed to inhibit the survival function of IGF-1 in order to facilitate involution. Likewise, overexpression of a constitutively activated Akt (protein kinase B), a known downstream target of the IGF signal transduction pathway, resulted in a marked delay in mammary gland involution and also provided a critical survival signal for mammary tumor progression (108,109). Thus, mutations that affect cell survival during mammary gland involution may play a significant role in the etiology of breast cancer.

CONCLUSION

Studies using genetically engineered mice coupled with the *in situ* analysis of specific signaling pathways have provided new insights into the molecular mechanisms regulating breast development. Thus, there is now a better understanding of the molecular mechanisms regulating the development of the embryonic mammary gland and by which systemic hormones and local growth factors regulate postnatal mammary gland development. Not surprisingly, many of these mechanisms appear to be conserved between the mouse mammary gland and human breast. Technologies such as RNA interference, multiphoton imaging of live cells, and high throughput microarray and proteomic analyses have been recently optimized and are powerful tools now being employed to help elucidate the mechanisms regulating mammary gland development and breast cancer progression. Thus, this is the beginning of an era where it should be possible to design targeted therapies based on the specific cell populations, giving rise to particular tumor types, and on signal transduction pathways either present or absent in the normal breast, which have been altered or inappropriately activated in breast cancer.

ACKNOWLEDGMENTS

Research in the authors' laboratories is supported by grants from the National Cancer Institute. The authors wish to thank Dr. Jacqueline Veltmaat for providing images of the embryonic mammary gland shown in Figure 2.1. Finally, the authors apologize to the many colleagues whose work was not cited because of space limitations.

References

1. Moses H, Davidson N. Charting the course: priorities for breast cancer research. *National Cancer Institute Program Review Group Summer Report*. Bethesda, MD: National Cancer Institute; 1998.
2. Kuperwasser C, Chavarria T, Wu M, et al. Reconstruction of functionally normal and malignant human breast tissues in mice. *Proc Natl Acad Sci U S A* 2004; 101(14):4966–4501.
3. Osborne M, Boolbol S. Breast anatomy and development. In: Harris JR, Lippman ME, Morrow M, Osborne CK, eds. *Diseases of the breast*, 4ed. Philadelphia: Lippincott Williams & Wilkins; 2009:1–11.
4. Robinson GW. Cooperation of signalling pathways in embryonic mammary gland development. *Nat Rev Genet* 2007;8(12):963–972.
5. Urbani CE, Betti R. Aberrant mammary tissue and nephrourinary malignancy. *Cancer Genet Cytogenet* 1996;87(1):88–89.
6. Mills AA, Zheng B, Wang XJ, et al. p63 is a p53 homologue required for limb and epidermal morphogenesis. *Nature* 1999;398(6729):708–713.
7. Yang A, Schweitzer R, Sun D, et al. p63 is essential for regenerative proliferation in limb, craniofacial and epithelial development. *Nature* 1999;398 (6729): 714–718.
8. Nguyen AV, Pollard JW. Transforming growth factor beta3 induces cell death during the first stage of mammary gland involution. *Development* 2000;127(14): 3107–3118.
9. Patturajan M, Nomoto S, Sommer M, et al. DeltaNp63 induces beta-catenin nuclear accumulation and signaling. *Cancer Cell* 2002;1(4):369–379.
10. Wu G, Nomoto S, Hoque MO, et al. DeltaNp63alpha and TAp63alpha regulate transcription of genes with distinct biological functions in cancer and development. *Cancer Res* 2003;63(10):2351–2357.

11. Mailleux AA, Spencer-Dene B, Dillon C, et al. Role of FGF10/FGFR2b signaling during mammary gland development in the mouse embryo. *Development* 2002; 129(1):53–60.
12. Cunha GR, Hom YK. Role of mesenchymal-epithelial interactions in mammary gland development. *J Mammary Gland Biol Neoplasia* 1996;1(1):21–35.
13. Chu EY, Hens J, Andl T, et al. Canonical Wnt signaling promotes mammary placode development and is essential for initiation of mammary gland morphogenesis. *Development* 2004;131(19):4819–4829.
14. van Genderen C, Okamura RM, Farinas I, et al. Development of several organs that require inductive epithelial-mesenchymal interactions is impaired in LEF-1-deficient mice. *Genes Dev* 1994;8(22):2691–2703.
15. Hatsell SJ, Cowin P. Gli3-mediated repression of hedgehog targets is required for normal mammary development. *Development* 2006;133(18):3661–3670.
16. Veltmaat JM, Relaix F, Le LT, et al. Gli3-mediated somitic Fgf10 expression gradients are required for the induction and patterning of mammary epithelium along the embryonic axes. *Development* 2006;133(12):2325–2335.
17. Wysolmerski JJ, Philbrick WM, Dunbar ME, et al. Rescue of the parathyroid hormone-related protein knockout mouse demonstrates that parathyroid hormone-related protein is essential for mammary gland development. *Development* 1998; 125(7):1285–1294.
18. Foley J, Dann P, Hong J, et al. Parathyroid hormone-related protein maintains mammary epithelial fate and triggers nipple skin differentiation during embryonic breast development. *Development* 2001;128(4):513–525.
19. Howard B, Ashworth A. Signalling pathways implicated in early mammary gland morphogenesis and breast cancer. *PLoS Genet* 2006;2(8):e112.
20. Ismail PM, Li J, DeMayo FJ, et al. A novel LacZ reporter mouse reveals complex regulation of the progesterone receptor promoter during mammary gland development. *Mol Endocrinol* 2002;16(11):2475–2489.
21. Lemmen JG, Broekhof JL, Kuiper GG, et al. Expression of estrogen receptor alpha and beta during mouse embryogenesis. *Mech Dev* 1999;81(1–2):163–167.
22. Bocchinfuso WP, Lindzey JK, Hewitt SC, et al. Induction of mammary gland development in estrogen receptor-alpha knockout mice. *Endocrinology* 2000;141(8): 2982–2994.
23. Dupont S, Krust A, Gansmuller A, et al. Effect of single and compound knockouts of estrogen receptors alpha (ERalpha) and beta (ERbeta) on mouse reproductive phenotypes. *Development* 2000;127(19):4277–4291.
24. Lydon JP, DeMayo FJ, Funk CR, et al. Mice lacking progesterone receptor exhibit pleiotropic reproductive abnormalities. *Genes Dev* 1995;9(18):2266–2278.
25. Davenport TG, Jerome-Majewska LA, Papaioannou VE. Mammary gland, limb and yolk sac defects in mice lacking Tbx3, the gene mutated in human ulnar mammary syndrome. *Development* 2003;130(10):2263–2273.
26. Schmidt H. Supernumerary nipples: prevalence, size, sex and side predilection—a prospective clinical study. *Eur J Pediatr* 1998;157(10):821–823.
27. Neri G, Gurrieri F, Zanni G, et al. Clinical and molecular aspects of the Simpson-Golabi-Behmel syndrome. *Am J Med Genet* 1998;79(4):279–283.
28. Howard B, Panchal H, McCarthy A, et al. Identification of the scaramanga gene implicates neuregulin3 in mammary gland specification. *Genes Dev* 2005;19(17): 2078–2090.
29. Hennighausen L, Robinson GW. Signaling pathways in mammary gland development. *Dev Cell* 2001;1(4):467–475.
30. Hennighausen L, Robinson GW. Information networks in the mammary gland. *Nat Rev Mol Cell Biol* 2005;6(9):715–725.
31. DeOme KB, Faulkin LJ, Bern HA, et al. Development of mammary tumors from hyperplastic alveolar nodules transplanted into gland-free mammary fat pads of female C3H mice. *Cancer Res* 1959;19:515–520.
32. Humphreys RC, Krajewska M, Krnacik S, et al. Apoptosis in the terminal endbud of the murine mammary gland: a mechanism of ductal morphogenesis. *Development* 1996;122(12):4013–4022.
33. Lewis MT, Ross S, Strickland PA, et al. Defects in mouse mammary gland development caused by conditional haploinsufficiency of patched-1. *Development* 1999;126(22):5181–5193.
34. Mailleux AA, Overholtzer M, Schmelzle T, et al. BIM regulates apoptosis during mammary ductal morphogenesis, and its absence reveals alternative cell death mechanisms. *Dev Cell* 2007;12(2):221–234.
35. Debnath J, Brugge JS. Modelling glandular epithelial cancers in three-dimensional cultures. *Nat Rev Cancer* 2005;5(9):675–688.
36. Debnath J, Mills KR, Collins NL, et al. The role of apoptosis in creating and maintaining luminal space within normal and oncogene-expressing mammary acini. *Cell* 2002;111(1):29–40.
37. Weaver VM, Lelievre S, Lakins JN, et al. β4 integrin-dependent formation of polarized three-dimensional architecture confers resistance to apoptosis in normal and malignant mammary epithelium. *Cancer Cell* 2002;2(3):205–216.
38. Coleman S, Daniel CW. Inhibition of mouse mammary ductal morphogenesis and down-regulation of the EGF receptor by epidermal growth factor. *Dev Biol* 1990;137(2):425–433.
39. Ruan W, Catanese V, Wieczorek R, et al. Estradiol enhances the stimulatory effect of insulin-like growth factor-I (IGF-I) on mammary development and growth hormone-induced IGF-I messenger ribonucleic acid. *Endocrinology* 1995;136(3):1296–1302.
40. Silberstein GB, Daniel CW. Reversible inhibition of mammary gland growth by transforming growth factor-beta. *Science* 1987;237(4812):291–293.
41. Sternlicht MD, Sunnarborg SW, Kouros-Mehr H, et al. Mammary ductal morphogenesis requires paracrine activation of stromal EGFR via ADAM17-dependent shedding of epithelial amphiregulin. *Development* 2005;132(17):3923–3933.
42. Bonnette SG, Hadsell DL. Targeted disruption of the IGF-I receptor gene decreases cellular proliferation in mammary terminal end buds. *Endocrinology* 2001;142(11):4937–4945.
43. Chakravarty G, Hadsell D, Buitrago W, et al. p190-B RhoGAP regulates mammary ductal morphogenesis. *Mol Endocrinol* 2003;17(6):1054–1065.
44. Heckman BM, Chakravarty G, Vargo-Gogola T, et al. Crosstalk between the p190-B RhoGAP and IGF signaling pathways is required for embryonic mammary bud development. *Dev Biol* 2007;309(1):137–149.
45. Lee AV, Zhang P, Ivanova M, et al. Developmental and hormonal signals dramatically alter the localization and abundance of insulin receptor substrate proteins in the mammary gland. *Endocrinology* 2003;144(6):2683–2694.
46. Mueller SO, Clark JA, Myers PH, et al. Mammary gland development in adult mice requires epithelial and stromal estrogen receptor alpha. *Endocrinology* 2002; 143(6):2357–2365.
47. Mallepell S, Krust A, Chambon P, et al. Paracrine signaling through the epithelial estrogen receptor alpha is required for proliferation and morphogenesis in the mammary gland. *Proc Natl Acad Sci U S A* 2006;103(7):2196–2201.
48. Ciarloni L, Mallepell S, Brisken C. Amphiregulin is an essential mediator of estrogen receptor alpha function in mammary gland development. *Proc Natl Acad Sci U S A* 2007;104(13):5455–5460.
49. LaMarca HL, Rosen JM. Estrogen regulation of mammary gland development and breast cancer: amphiregulin takes center stage. *Breast Cancer Res* 2007; 9(4):304.
50. Ewan KB, Shyamala G, Ravani SA, et al. Latent transforming growth factor-beta activation in mammary gland: regulation by ovarian hormones affects ductal and alveolar proliferation. *Am J Pathol* 2002;160(6):2081–2093.
51. Ewan KB, Oketch-Rabah HA, Ravani SA, et al. Proliferation of estrogen receptor-alpha-positive mammary epithelial cells is restrained by transforming growth factor-beta1 in adult mice. *Am J Pathol* 2005;167(2):409–417.
52. Roarty K, Serra R. Wnt5a is required for proper mammary gland development and TGF-beta-mediated inhibition of ductal growth. *Development* 2007; 134(21):3929–3939.
53. Srinivasan K, Strickland P, Valdes A, et al. Netrin-1/neogenin interaction stabilizes multipotent progenitor cap cells during mammary gland morphogenesis. *Dev Cell* 2003;4(3):371–382.
54. Strickland P, Shin GC, Plump A, et al. Slit2 and netrin 1 act synergistically as adhesive cues to generate tubular bi-layers during ductal morphogenesis. *Development* 2006;133(5):823–832.
55. Lewis MT. Hedgehog signaling in mouse mammary gland development and neoplasia. *J Mammary Gland Biol Neoplasia* 2001;6(1):53–66.
56. Lewis MT, Ross S, Strickland PA, et al. The Gli2 transcription factor is required for normal mouse mammary gland development. *Dev Biol* 2001;238(1):133–144.
57. Moraes RC, Zhang X, Harrington N, et al. Constitutive activation of smoothened (SMO) in mammary glands of transgenic mice leads to increased proliferation, altered differentiation and ductal dysplasia. *Development* 2007;134(6):1231–1242.
58. Fiaschi M, Rozell B, Bergstrom A, et al. Targeted expression of GLI1 in the mammary gland disrupts pregnancy-induced maturation and causes lactation failure. *J Biol Chem* 2007;282(49):36090–36101.
59. Wiseman BS, Werb Z. Stromal effects on mammary gland development and breast cancer. *Science* 2002;296(5570):1046–1049.
60. Vogel WF, Aszodi A, Alves F, et al. Discoidin domain receptor 1 tyrosine kinase has an essential role in mammary gland development. *Mol Cell Biol* 2001;21(8): 2906–2917.
61. Klinowska TC, Soriano JV, Edwards GM, et al. Laminin and beta1 integrins are crucial for normal mammary gland development in the mouse. *Dev Biol* 1999;215(1):13–32.
62. Gouon-Evans V, Rothenberg ME, Pollard JW. Postnatal mammary gland development requires macrophages and eosinophils. *Development* 2000;127(11): 2269–2282.
63. Djonov V, Andres AC, Ziemiecki A. Vascular remodelling during the normal and malignant life cycle of the mammary gland. *Microsc Res Tech* 2001;52(2): 182–189.
64. Welm BE, Freeman KW, Chen M, et al. Inducible dimerization of FGFR1: development of a mouse model to analyze progressive transformation of the mammary gland. *J Cell Biol* 2002;157(4):703–714.
65. Kouros-Mehr H, Werb Z. Candidate regulators of mammary branching morphogenesis identified by genome-wide transcript analysis. *Dev Dyn* 2006;235(12): 3404–3412.
66. Master SR, Hartman JL, D'Cruz CM, et al. Functional microarray analysis of mammary organogenesis reveals a developmental role in adaptive thermogenesis. *Mol Endocrinol* 2002;16(6):1185–1203.
67. Wagner KU, Boulanger CA, Henry MD, et al. An adjunct mammary epithelial cell population in parous females: its role in functional adaptation and tissue renewal. *Development* 2002;129(6):1377–1386.
68. Shillingford JM, Miyoshi K, Robinson GW, et al. Prototyping of mammary tissue from transgenic and gene knockout mice with immunohistochemical markers: a tool to define developmental lesions. *J Histochem Cytochem* 2003;51(5): 555–565.
69. Brisken C. Hormonal control of alveolar development and its implications for breast carcinogenesis. *J Mammary Gland Biol Neoplasia* 2002;7(1):39–48.
70. Brisken C, Kaur S, Chavarria TE, et al. Prolactin controls mammary gland development via direct and indirect mechanisms. *Dev Biol* 1999;210(1):96–106.
71. Brisken C, Park S, Vass T, et al. A paracrine role for the epithelial progesterone receptor in mammary gland development. *Proc Natl Acad Sci U S A* 1998;95(9): 5076–5081.
72. Horseman ND. Prolactin and mammary gland development. *J Mammary Gland Biol Neoplasia* 1999;4(1):79–88.
73. Mulac-Jericevic B, Mullinax RA, DeMayo FJ, et al. Subgroup of reproductive functions of progesterone mediated by progesterone receptor-B isoform. *Science* 2000;289(5485):1751–1754.
74. Fantl V, Edwards PA, Steel JH, et al. Impaired mammary gland development in Cyl-1(–/–) mice during pregnancy and lactation is epithelial cell autonomous. *Dev Biol* 1999;212(1):1–11.
75. Sicinski P, Donaher JL, Parker SB, et al. Cyclin D1 provides a link between development and oncogenesis in the retina and breast. *Cell* 1995;82(4):621–630.
76. Mulac-Jericevic B, Lydon JP, DeMayo FJ, et al. Defective mammary gland morphogenesis in mice lacking the progesterone receptor B isoform. *Proc Natl Acad Sci U S A* 2003;100(17):9744–9749.
77. Grimm SL, Seagroves TN, Kabotyanski EB, et al. Disruption of steroid and prolactin receptor patterning in the mammary gland correlates with a block in lobuloalveolar development. *Mol Endocrinol* 2002;16(12):2675–2691.
78. Clarke RB, Howell A, Potten CS, et al. Dissociation between steroid receptor expression and cell proliferation in the human breast. *Cancer Res* 1997;57(22): 4987–4991.
79. Russo J, Ao X, Grill C, et al. Pattern of distribution of cells positive for estrogen receptor alpha and progesterone receptor in relation to proliferating cells in the mammary gland. *Breast Cancer Res Treat* 1999;53(3):217–227.
80. Seagroves TN, Lydon JP, Hovey RC, et al. C/EBPbeta (CCAAT/enhancer binding protein) controls cell fate determination during mammary gland development. *Mol Endocrinol* 2000;14(3):359–368.

81. Hovey RC, Trott JF, Ginsburg E, et al. Transcriptional and spatiotemporal regulation of prolactin receptor mRNA and cooperativity with progesterone receptor function during ductal branch growth in the mammary gland. *Dev Dyn* 2001; 222(2):192–205.

82. Brisken C, Heineman A, Chavarria T, et al. Essential function of Wnt-4 in mammary gland development downstream of progesterone signaling. *Genes Dev* 2000;14(6):650–654.

83. Luetteke NC, Qiu TH, Fenton SE, et al. Targeted inactivation of the EGF and amphiregulin genes reveals distinct roles for EGF receptor ligands in mouse mammary gland development. *Development* 1999;126(12):2739–2750.

84. Fata JE, Kong YY, Li J, et al. The osteoclast differentiation factor osteoprotegerin-ligand is essential for mammary gland development. *Cell* 2000;103(1):41–50.

85. Cao Y, Bonizzi G, Seagroves TN, et al. IKKalpha provides an essential link between RANK signaling and cyclin D1 expression during mammary gland development. *Cell* 2001;107(6):763–775.

86. Brisken C, Ayyannan A, Nguyen C, et al. IGF-2 is a mediator of prolactin-induced morphogenesis in the breast. *Dev Cell* 2002;3(6):877–887.

87. Hovey RC, Harris J, Hadsell DL, et al. Local insulin-like growth factor-II mediates prolactin-induced mammary gland development. *Mol Endocrinol* 2003;17(3):460–471.

88. Wood TL, Richert MM, Stull MA, et al. The insulin-like growth factors (IGFs) and IGF binding proteins in postnatal development of murine mammary glands. *J Mammary Gland Biol Neoplasia* 2000;5(1):31–42.

89. Asselin-Labat ML, Sutherland KD, Barker H, et al. Gata-3 is an essential regulator of mammary-gland morphogenesis and luminal-cell differentiation. *Nat Cell Biol* 2007;9(2):201–209.

90. Kouros-Mehr H, Slorach EM, Sternlicht MD, et al. GATA-3 maintains the differentiation of the luminal cell fate in the mammary gland. *Cell* 2006;127(5):1041–1055.

91. Oakes SR, Naylor MJ, Asselin-Labat M-L, et al. The Ets transcription factor Elf5 specifies mammary alveolar cell fate. *Genes Dev* 2008;22:581.

92. Shoker BS, Jarvis C, Clarke RB, et al. Estrogen receptor-positive proliferating cells in the normal and precancerous breast. *Am J Pathol* 1999;155(6):1811–1815.

93. Sivaraman L, Hilsenbeck SG, Zhong L, et al. Early exposure of the rat mammary gland to estrogen and progesterone blocks co-localization of estrogen receptor expression and proliferation. *J Endocrinol* 2001;171(1):75–83.

94. Khaled WT, Read EK, Nicholson SE, et al. The IL-4/IL-13/Stat6 signalling pathway promotes luminal mammary epithelial cell development. *Development* 2007;134(15):2739–2750.

95. Neville MC, McFadden TB, Forsyth I. Hormonal regulation of mammary differentiation and milk secretion. *J Mammary Gland Biol Neoplasia* 2002;7(1):49–66.

96. Lemay DG, Neville MC, Rudolph MC, et al. Gene regulatory networks in lactation: identification of global principles using bioinformatics. *BMC Syst Biol* 2007; 1:56.

97. Nguyen DA, Parlow AF, Neville MC. Hormonal regulation of tight junction closure in the mouse mammary epithelium during the transition from pregnancy to lactation. *J Endocrinol* 2001;170(2):347–356.

98. Nishimori K, Young LJ, Guo Q, et al. Oxytocin is required for nursing but is not essential for parturition or reproductive behavior. *Proc Natl Acad Sci U S A* 1996;93(21):11699–11704.

99. Wagner KU, Young WS 3rd, Liu X, et al. Oxytocin and milk removal are required for post-partum mammary-gland development. *Genes Funct* 1997;1(4):233–244.

100. Seagroves TN, Hadsell D, McManaman J, et al. HIF1alpha is a critical regulator of secretory differentiation and activation, but not vascular expansion, in the mouse mammary gland. *Development* 2003;130(8):1713–1724.

101. Rosen JM, Wyszomierski SL, Hadsell D. Regulation of milk protein gene expression. *Annu Rev Nutr* 1999;19:407–436.

102. Stein T, Salomonis N, Gusterson BA. Mammary gland involution as a multi-step process. *J Mammary Gland Biol Neoplasia* 2007;12(1):25–35.

103. Miyoshi K, Shillingford JM, Smith GH, et al. Signal transducer and activator of transcription (Stat) 5 controls the proliferation and differentiation of mammary alveolar epithelium. *J Cell Biol* 2001;155(4):531–542.

104. Chapman RS, Lourenco PC, Tonner E, et al. Suppression of epithelial apoptosis and delayed mammary gland involution in mice with a conditional knockout of Stat3. *Genes Dev* 1999;13(19):2604–2616.

105. Kritikou EA, Sharkey A, Abell K, et al. A dual, non-redundant, role for LIF as a regulator of development and STAT3-mediated cell death in the mammary gland. *Development* 2003;130.3459–3468.

106. Baxter FO, Came PJ, Abell K, et al. IKKbeta/2 induces TWEAK and apoptosis in mammary epithelial cells. *Development* 2006;133(17):3485–3494.

107. Marshman E, Green KA, Flint DJ, et al. Insulin-like growth factor binding protein 5 and apoptosis in mammary epithelial cells. *J Cell Sci* 2003;116(Pt 4):675–682.

108. Hutchinson J, Jin J, Cardiff RD, et al. Activation of Akt (protein kinase B) in mammary epithelium provides a critical cell survival signal required for tumor progression. *Mol Cell Biol* 2001;21(6):2203–2212.

109. Schwertfeger KL, Richert MM, Anderson SM. Mammary gland involution is delayed by activated Akt in transgenic mice. *Mol Endocrinol* 2001;15:867–881.

110. Grimm SL, Rosen JM. Stop! In the name of transforming growth factor-beta: keeping estrogen receptor-alpha-positive mammary epithelial cells from proliferating. *Breast Cancer Res* 2006;8(4):106.

Chapter 3
Stem Cells in Breast Development and Carcinogenesis: Concepts and Clinical Perspectives

Christophe Ginestier and Max S. Wicha

Evidence is accumulating that many, if not all, malignancies possess a subcomponent of cancer cells that have stem cells properties that have been termed "cancer stem cells." Although the concept that cancers arise from the transformation of "germ cells" or "stem cells" was first proposed over 150 years ago (1), it is only recently that advances in stem cell biology have allowed for a more direct testing of the cancer stem cell hypothesis (2). To present and discuss this concept, it is crucial to define the term stem cell. *Stem cells* are cells that have the capacity to self-renew as well as to generate daughter cells that can differentiate into multiple cell lineages. Self-renewal may either be symmetric, in which a stem cell produces two daughter stem cells identical to itself, or asymmetric, in which the stem cell generates one stem cell and one progenitor cell. The new stem cell produced provides for maintenance of the stem cell compartment, whereas the progenitor cell goes through a series of cell divisions and differentiation steps to generate the terminally differentiated cell populations that form the bulk of an organ. Embryonic stem cells are pluripotent, able to differentiate into all derivatives of the three primary germ layers (ectoderm, endoderm, and mesoderm), whereas adult stem cells are multipotent, able to form all of the cell types that are found in the mature tissue of an organ. In the mammary gland, these differentiating cells generate three lineages: ductal epithelial cells, which line ducts; alveolar epithelial cells, which are the milk-producing cells; and myoepithelial cells, which are contractile cells lining ducts and alveoli.

Based on this definition, cancer stem cells retain key stem cell properties. These properties include self-renewal, which initiates and drives tumorigenesis. and differentiation, albeit aberrant, which contributes to cellular heterogeneity (3).

In breast cancer, the discovery of tumor cells that display stem cell properties provides a possible explanation as to why cancer may be so difficult to eradicate, as well as suggesting strategies for the targeting of this cell population. This chapter will examine the implications of the cancer stem cell hypothesis and enable an understanding of carcinogenesis, as well as its implications for developing new strategies for prevention and therapy of breast cancer.

IDENTIFICATION OF NORMAL BREAST STEM CELLS

The mammary gland is a unique organ that undergoes most of its development after birth and is regulated through multiple cycles of pregnancy. Normal breast stem cells provide the capacity for extensive cellular expansion associated with pregnancy as well as generating differentiated cells that support lactation.

The existence of stem cells in the normal breast was first demonstrated in rodent mammary glands (4). It was shown that epithelial fragments, which were marked by unique retroviral insertion sites, had the ability to repopulate mouse mammary glands upon serial transplantation. Recently, a functional mammary gland was generated from single adult breast stem cell (5,6). A single cell characterized as either cluster of differentiation (CD) $CD29^{high}/CD24^+$ or $CD49f^{high}/CD24^+$ was able to reconstitute a functional mammary gland, when this cell was transplanted into a cleared mouse mammary fat pad. The murine mammary stem cell does not express estrogen receptors (ER) or

progesterone receptors (PR) but is able to give rise to ER and PR expressing cells (7). This observation suggests that a complex hormonal paracrine signaling network regulates normal breast stem cells during mammary development (8).

Characterization of human breast stem cells has been facilitated by the development of *in vitro* culture systems that allow for propagation of these cells in an undifferentiated state. Previously, it had been found that primitive neuronal cells could be propagated as floating spherical colonies termed *neurospheres* (9). Based on this, Dontu et al. (10) hypothesized that adult breast stem cells might display anchorage-independent growth and utilized this property to develop a culture system for human mammary epithelial stem and progenitor cells. They demonstrated that such cells isolated from reduction mammoplasties when grown on nonadherent substrata in serum free conditions in the presence of growth factors generate spherical colonies that were termed *mammospheres*. Mammosphere-initiating cells have stem cell properties and are able to self-renew *in vitro* as well as differentiating into all three lineages found in the adult mammary gland. Furthermore, mammosphere-initiating cells are capable of generating human mammary structures when transplanted into the fat pads of immunosuppressed not otherwise specified/severe combined immunodeficiency (NOD/SCID) mice that had been "humanized" by introduction of human mammary fibroblasts (11).

Ginestier et al. (12) has recently described the expression of aldehyde dehydrogenase 1 (ALDH1) as a stem cell marker that can be utilized to isolate human mammary stem cells. ALDH1 is a detoxifying enzyme responsible for the oxidation of intracellular aldehydes. This enzyme may play a role in early differentiation of stem cells through its role in oxidizing retinol to retinoic acid (13,14). It is expressed in hematopoietic and neuronal stem and progenitor cells and can be detected utilizing an enzymatic assay (ALDEFLUOR; Aldagen, Durham, North Carolina) (15–19). Human mammary epithelial cells with a high enzymatic activity for ALDH (ALDEFLUOR positive), isolated from reduction mammoplasties, were able to reconstitute human mammary gland structures when implanted in the humanized fat pad of NOD/SCID mice. Using ALDH1 antibody to immunostain paraffin-embedded sections of human normal breast epithelium researchers identified a relatively rare population of ALDH1-positive cells located in the terminal ductal lobular units (TDLUs). ALDH1-positive cells appeared to form a bridge in the lumen that was located at the bifurcation point of side branches in the TDLUs (12). This is consistent with recently published data demonstrating that human stem/progenitor cells are localized in the ductal part of the TDLU structures (20).

The identification of mammary stem cell markers and the development of *in vitro* and murine models utilizing these cells should facilitate the study of adult breast stem cells elucidating their role in mammary development. Furthermore, defining the pathways that regulate mammary stem cell self-renewal and differentiation should shed light on events involved in breast carcinogenesis.

BREAST CARCINOGENESIS

Classical model of carcinogenesis can be described as *stochastic* or *random* in which any cell in an organ, such as the breast,

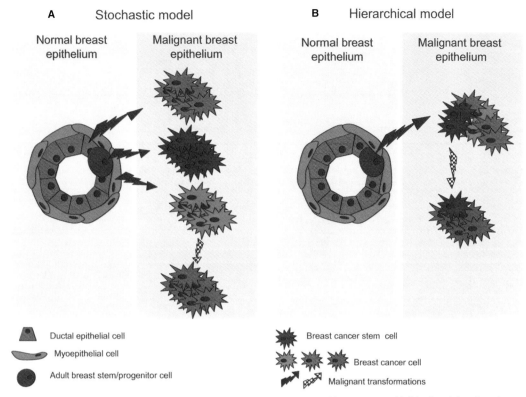

A   Stochastic model   **B**   Hierarchical model

Normal breast epithelium   Malignant breast epithelium   Normal breast epithelium   Malignant breast epithelium

Ductal epithelial cell

Myoepithelial cell

Adult breast stem/progenitor cell

Breast cancer stem cell

Breast cancer cell

Malignant transformations

FIGURE 3.1. Two Models of Breast Carcinogenesis. A: According to the stochastic model any mammary epithelial cell can be transformed by the right combination of mutations and resultant cancer cells of different phenotypes have extensive proliferation potential. **B:** According to the stem cell hierarchical model, cancers originate from the malignant transformation of a normal breast stem/progenitor cell. Most cancer cells have only limited proliferative potential, but cancer stem cells that have self-renewal capacity drive tumorigenesis.

can be transformed by the right combination of mutations (Fig. 3.1A). As a result, all or most of the cells in a fully developed cancer are equally malignant. Malignancies then progress through further mutation and clonal selection. The cancer stem cell hypothesis proposes a different model based on a hierarchical organization (2). According to this hypothesis, cancers originate from the malignant transformation of an adult stem cell through the deregulation of the normally tightly regulated self-renewal program. This leads to clonal stem cell expansion generating cells that then undergo further genetic or epigenetic alterations to become fully transformed (Fig. 3.1B). Consequently, tumors contain a cellular component of cancer stem cells that retains key stem cell properties that initiate and drive carcinogenesis. Recent studies in the hematopoietic system have demonstrated that cancer-causing mutations can also occur in more developmentally advanced, although still immature, progenitor cells. For example, overexpression of the *MLL-AF9* fusion gene in hematopoietic progenitors results in production of leukemia, which is driven by progenitor cells that acquire stem cell properties (21). Interestingly, these properties include the expression of self-renewal genes whose expression is normally restricted to hematopoietic stem cells.

Mouse models of breast carcinogenesis utilizing the mammary specific MMTV promoter have suggested that different oncogenes target mammary stem or progenitor cells. MMTV-Wnt1 transgenic mice developed tumors that expressed both epithelial and myoepithelial markers whereas MMTV/neu transgenic mice developed tumors that expressed only luminal differentiation marker (22,23). These data suggest that Wnt may affect primitive stem or progenitor cells, whereas Neu may target a committed luminal progenitor cell. These murine studies suggest that either mammary stem or progenitor cells may be targets for transformation. In the case of stem cells, this involves deregulation of self-renewal pathways, whereas for

progenitor cells, this involves the acquisition of the ability to self-renew a property normally limited to mammary stem cells (24). If similar events occur in human carcinogenesis, it could provide an explanation for aspects of molecular heterogeneity found in different human breast cancers.

Recent studies have suggested that breast stem cells may be targets for carcinogenesis. Liu et al. (24) demonstrated that *BRCA1*, involved in hereditary breast cancer, plays a role in the self-renewal and differentiation of breast stem cells. Knockdown of *BRCA1* in primary breast epithelial cells leads to an increase in cells displaying the stem or progenitor cell marker ALDH1 and a decrease in cells expressing luminal epithelial markers and estrogen receptor. In breast tissues from women with germline *BRCA1* mutations, entire lobules were detected that, although histologically normal, were positive for ALDH1 expression but negative for the expression of ER. Loss of heterozygosity for *BRCA1* was documented in these ALDH1-positive lobules but not in adjacent ALDH1-negative lobules. Because *BRCA1* also functions in DNA repair and in maintaining chromosome stability, the researchers proposed that loss of *BRCA1* function may produce genetically unstable stem or progenitor cells that serve as prime targets for further carcinogenic events. Similarly, Charles Holst et al. (25) have described hypermethylation and silencing of the p16^{INK4a} gene in morphologically normal breast epithelial cells. These cells acquired the ability to propagate *in vitro* without undergoing cellular senescence. Since p16^{INK4a} is known to be a downstream target of the polycomb gene *BMI1* that regulates stem cell self-renewal, it was proposed that breast carcinogenesis may be initiated by epigenetic changes such as silencing of p16^{INK4a}.

These studies lend support to the cancer stem cell hypothesis by suggesting that deregulation of stem cell self-renewal and differentiation may initiate hereditary as well as sporadic breast carcinomas. Furthermore, exploration of the mechanisms

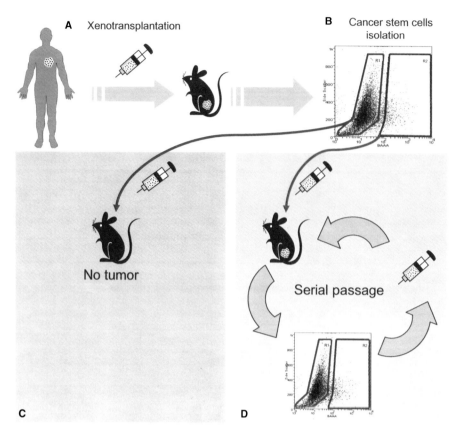

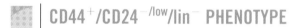

FIGURE 3.2. Isolation and characterization of breast cancer stem cells. A: The xenograft model involves introduction of tumor cells into the cleared fat pad of not otherwise specified/severe combined immunodeficiency (NOD/SCID) mice that have been humanized by the introduction of human mammary fibroblasts. **B:** When the xenograft is established, breast cancer stem cells can be separated from the rest of the tumor cells utilizing different techniques such as the ALDEFLUOR (Aldagen, Durham, North Carolina) assay. **C:** When transplanted, the cancer stem cell population initiates and maintains tumor growth upon serial passage, whereas the tumor cell population depleted of the cancer stem cell population fails to generate tumors (**D**).

that regulate stem cell self-renewal may lead to the development of new approaches for breast cancer prevention.

ISOLATION AND CHARACTERIZATION OF BREAST CANCER STEM CELLS

The isolation and characterization of cancer stem cells remains a challenge. In order to validate the method selected as an appropriate technique to isolate cancer stem cell, it is crucial to use assays that can assess the stem cell properties of self-renewal and differentiation. Presently, the most robust model for demonstrating these properties is the xenograft model based on the orthotopic injection of human cancer cells into the humanized cleared fat pad of immunodeficient mice. The cancer stem cell population initiates and maintains the tumor growth upon serial passage, whereas the tumor cell population depleted of cancer stem cells generates only limited growth that cannot sustain tumor growth upon serial transformation (Fig. 3.2). In addition to self-renewal, cancer stem cells retain the ability to differentiate, albeit abnormally, generating non–self-renewing cell populations that constitute the bulk of a tumor.

In vitro assays such as tumorosphere formation, have also been developed to enrich for cancer stem cells (26). This cell culture technique adapted for breast tumor tissue is based on the mammosphere technique (10). Tumorosphere-initiating cells have stem cell properties including the ability to survive and grow in suspension in serum-free conditions. In contrast, more differentiated tumor cells are anchorage-dependent and undergo anoikis in these conditions. The tumorosphere culture has also been used in different studies to screen for drugs capable of targeting the cancer stem cell populations (27,28).

In summary, a number of techniques have been utilized to enrich for and isolate breast cancer stem cells. Because of their simplicity, *in vitro* cancer stem cell assays provide an impor-

tant tool for mechanistic studies as well as for screening of agents. However, at this time, self-renewal can only be confirmed by serial passage in xenograft models. A potential limitation of these systems relates to the microenvironmental difference found in humans compared to NOD/SCID mice (29).

CD44$^+$/CD24$^{-/low}$/lin$^-$ PHENOTYPE

In order to identify human breast cancer stem cells, Al Hajj et al. (30) utilized techniques based on seminal studies identifying leukemic stem cells by Bonnet and Dick (31). Utilizing cell surface markers and flow cytometry, these authors identified a population of cells in human breast cancer that displayed cancer stem cell properties. This population was defined by the expression of cell surface markers (CD44$^+$/CD24$^{-/low}$/lin$^-$). As few as 200 of these cells were able to form tumors in NOD/SCID mice, whereas 20,000 cells that did not display this phenotype failed to generate tumors. The tumors formed in mice recapitulated the phenotypic heterogeneity of the initial tumor. The ability to serially transplant the tumors from an enriched stem cell population provides strong support for the existence of stem cells in breast cancers. CD44 appears to be also expressed in cancer stem cells in other tumor types including colon, pancreas, prostate, and head and neck (32–35).

SIDE POPULATION TECHNIQUE

There is evidence that immortalized breast cancer cell lines may also contain a cellular subcomponent with stem cell properties. Several techniques have been utilized to isolate this component including isolation of so-called side population (SP). This method is based on the overexpression of transmembrane transporters, such as the adenosine triphosphate (ATP)-binding cassettes molecule *ABCG2/BCRP1* in stem cells. These molecules actively exclude vital dyes such as Hoechst 33342 or Rhodamine 123, a property not found in differentiated cells that retain the dye (36). A side population was isolated from the MCF7 breast cancer cell line utilizing Hoechst dye exclusion. This population, representing 2% of the total cells, contained the tumorigenic fraction, as demonstrated by transplantation in NOD/SCID mice. Moreover, this fraction was able to generate tumors in mice that reconstituted the phenotypic heterogeneity present initially (37). A limitation of this technique is the cellular toxicity of Hoechst dye. Furthermore normal mouse mammary stem cells capable of reconstituting the mammary gland were not contained in the SP population.

 ## ALDEHYDE DEHYDROGENASE 1

As described previously, ALDH enzymatic activity has been recently used to isolate normal human breast stem and progenitors cells (12). Cancer cells that have high ALDH activity have been reported to display stem cell properties in leukaemia and multiple myeloma (15–19). Ginestier et al. (12) demonstrated that ALDEFLUOR-positive cells isolated from human breast cancer display properties of cancer stem cells. This was demonstrated by the ability of these cells, but not ALDEFLUOR-negative cells, to generate tumors in NOD/SCID mice. Serial passage of the ALDEFLUOR-positive cells generate tumors that recapitulate the phenotypic heterogeneity of the initial tumor. Interestingly, the ALDEFLUOR-positive cell population detected in breast tumors has a small overlap with the previously described cancer stem cell, CD44$^+$/CD24$^-$/lin$^-$ phenotype (30). In the tumors investigated, the overlap represented approximately 1% or less of the total cancer cell population. The ALDE-FLUOR-positive CD44$^+$/CD24$^-$/lin$^-$ cells appeared to be highly enriched in tumorigenic capability, being able to generate tumors from as few as 20 cells. ALDH1 immunostaining of paraffin-embedded specimens was utilize to identify breast cancer stem cells *in situ*. Analysis of ALDH1 expression in 577 human breast carcinomas showed that this stem or progenitor cell marker is a powerful predictor of poor clinical outcome and correlates with tumor histological grade, ER and PR negativity, proliferation index as assessed by Ki-67 expression, and *ERBB2* overexpression.

 ## THERAPEUTIC IMPLICATIONS OF BREAST CANCER STEM CELLS

Although advances have been made in the treatment of localized breast cancer, there has been less progress in the treatment of advanced metastatic disease. Some of this lack of progress may be due to the failure of current therapies to target cancer stem cells. Recent evidence suggests that breast cancer stem cells as well as cancer stem cells from other tumor types are relatively resistant to both radiation and chemotherapy. In MCF7 cells, the cancer stem cell-like subpopulation bearing the CD44$^+$CD24$^{-/low}$ phenotype has shown a relative radioresistance (38). The clinical relevance of these findings was demonstrated by recent neoadjuvant studies that documented an increase in CD44$^+$/CD24$^-$ breast cancer stem cells and tumorosphere-initiating cells following the administration of neoadjuvant chemotherapy (39).

There are several postulated mechanisms for the therapeutic resistance of cancer stem cells. These slow proliferating cells, making them resistant to cell cycle active chemotherapeutic agents. In addition, cancer stem cells express increased ATP-binding cassette proteins known to efflux chemotherapeutic drugs (40). Moreover, enzymes such as ALDH that are highly expressed in stem cells are able to metabolize chemotherapeu-

tic agents such as cyclophosphamide (41). Cancer stem cells may contribute to radioresistance through preferential activation of the DNA damage checkpoint response and an increase in DNA repair capacity. For example, it was demonstrated in glioma that the mechanism of resistance of brain cancer stem cells to radiation involves the cell-cycle-regulating proteins CHK1/CHK2 (42,43). Cancer stem cells may also express increased levels of antiapoptotic molecules such as survivin and BCL2 family proteins (44).

Tumor response is usually defined in the clinic as the shrinkage of a tumor by at least 50%. However, if cancer stem cells are inherently resistant to therapeutic agents and if these cells comprise only a minority of the tumor cell population, then shrinkage of tumors may reflect the effects of these agents on the differentiated cells in a tumor rather than the cancer stem cell population (3). This may explain why tumor regression in breast cancer does not correlate well with patient survival (45). The cancer stem cell concept suggests that significant improvements in clinical outcome will require effective targeting of the cancer stem cell population (Fig. 3.3).

There is increasing evidence that cancer stem cells may play an important role in mediating tumor metastasis. Balic et al. (46) demonstrated an increase in CD44$^+$/CD24$^-$ expressing cancer cells in metastatic bone marrow sites in patients with breast carcinoma. Studies are currently in progress to determine whether the expression of stem cell markers in micrometastasis to lymph nodes and bone marrow are predictive of development of distant disease. Charafe-Jauffret et al. (47) have recently reported the invasive and metastatic characteristics of cancer stem cells in inflammatory breast carcinomas (IBC). ALDEFLUOR-positive populations of an IBC cell line displayed increased invasive characteristics as well as increased ability to metastasize when injected systemically into NOD/SCID mice.

The presence of metastasis is the most important factor influencing the outcome of patients with invasive breast cancer. The development of therapies targeting the cancer stem cell population may provide new opportunities for the treatment of metastatic disease.

 ## OPPORTUNITIES FOR THE DEVELOPMENT OF THERAPIES TARGETING CANCER STEM CELLS

The need to design targeted therapeutics for breast cancers based on their molecular heterogeneity has long been recognized. For example, trastuzumab or more recently lapatinib has been used to target the intracellular signaling of *ERBB2*. These drugs have demonstrated clinical benefit in both the adjuvant and advanced breast cancer settings. The addition of trastuzumab to adjuvant chemotherapy reduces the recurrence rate by almost 50% (48). The efficiency of these therapies may be explained by the role of *ERBB2* in the regulation of the cancer stem cell population. Interestingly, in a series of 577 breast carcinomas Ginestier et al. (12) found a significant correlation between expression of the stem cell marker ALDH1 and *ERBB2*. Furthermore, Korkaya et al. (49) have recently found that *ERBB2* overexpression in normal human mammary epithelial cells as well as mammary carcinomas increases the proportion of stem cells as indicated by ALDH1 expression. The clinical relevance of this was demonstrated in a recent neoadjuvant breast cancer trial. Tumor regression induced by neoadjuvant chemotherapy was associated with an increase in CD44$^+$/CD24$^-$ cancer stem cells in residual tumors. In contrast, breast cancers with *ERBB2* amplification had an increased proportion of CD44$^+$/CD24$^-$ cells before treatment that was reduced by administration of the *ERBB2* inhibitor lapatinib

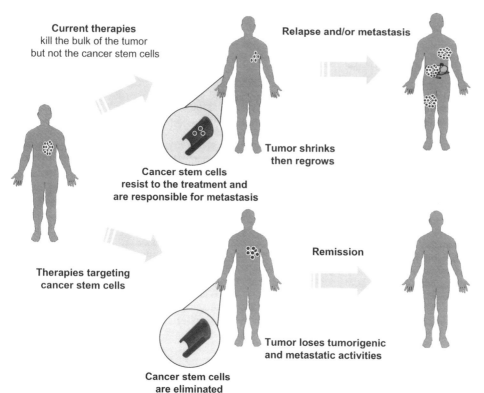

FIGURE 3.3. Therapeutics implications of breast cancer stem cells. Current therapies may shrink tumors by killing cells forming the tumor bulk. Because cancer stem cells are less sensitive to these therapies, they remain viable after therapy and re-establish the tumor. In contrast, therapies that target the cancer stem cell population limit tumor growth. Thus, even if cancer stem cell–directed therapies do not shrink tumors initially, they may eventually lead to cures. Furthermore, there is increasing evidence that cancer stem cells may play an important role in mediating tumor metastasis. The development of therapies targeting the cancer stem cell population may provide new opportunities to target metastatic disease.

(39). The clinical efficiency of *ERBB2* inhibitors provides evidence for the effectiveness of agents capable of targeting breast cancer stem cells. The elucidation of other pathways that regulate breast cancer stem cells, such as Notch and Hedgehog may provide new targets for therapeutic development.

Notch Pathway

The Notch pathway has been shown to play a role in mammary carcinogenesis in murine models, as well as in human mammary cancer. In mammals, there are four Notch receptors (Notch1 to Notch4), which interact with surface bound or secreted ligands (Delta-like 1, Delta-like 3, Delta-like 4, Jagged 1 and Jagged 2) (50). Upon ligand binding, Notch receptors are activated by serial cleavage events involving members of the ADAM protease family followed by intramembranous cleavage regulated by γ-secretase (presenilin). Following proteolitic cleavage, the intracellular domain of Notch translocates to the nucleus to act on downstream targets such as the Hes and Hey transcription factors (51). Evidence for the role of Notch signaling in mammary development has been provided by transgenic

models. In addition, Dontu et al. (27) demonstrated that Notch activation acts as a regulator of asymmetric cell fate decisions in human mammary cells by promoting mammary self-renewal. Approximately 40% of human breast cancers display reduced expression of the Notch inhibitor Numb (52). The accumulation of the intracellular domain of Notch1 (NICD1) and hence increased Notch signaling was detected in a significant proportion of human breast carcinomas. Notch pathway deregulation has been implicated in a preinvasive breast lesions including, ductal carcinoma *in situ* (DCIS), suggesting that aberrant activation of Notch signaling is probably an early event in breast cancer development. High expression of NICD1 in DCIS was also associated with an increased recurrence rate (53).

Since γ-secretase is necessary for Notch processing, γ-secretase inhibitors are able to inhibit Notch signaling (54). In medulloblastomas and T-cell leukemia, inhibitors of the γ-secretase deplete tumor stem cells and slow the growth of Notch-dependent tumors (55). Clinical trials utilizing γ-secretase inhibitors in combination with chemotherapy for women with advanced breast cancer are being initiated (Table 3.1). Such

Table 3.1	CLINICAL TRIALS TARGETING CANCER STEM CELLS		
Tumor Type	**Target**	**Drug**	**Investigator and Institution**
Acute myeloid leukemia	NF-κB	Parthenolide	C. Jordan, University of Rochester
Basal cell carcinoma and medulloblastoma	Hedgehog	Cyclopamine	F. J. de Sauvage, Genentech, Inc.
Breast	Notch	γ-secretase inhibitor (GSI)	A. Schott, University of Michigan, J. Chang, Baylor University
Glioblastoma	Chk1/Chk2	Debromohymenialdisine (DBH)	J. Rich, Duke University
Multiple myeloma	CD20-I^{125}	Bexxar	A. Jakuboviak, University of Michigan
Multiple myeloma	CD20	Rituximab	W. Matsui, Johns Hopkins University

trials will directly test the hypothesis that targeting breast cancer stem cells improves the therapeutic outcome in these women.

Hedgehog Pathway

The Hedgehog pathway is critical for many developmental processes. In the absence of Hedgehog, a cell-surface transmembrane protein Patched (PTCH) acts to prevent high expression and activity of a seven membrane spanning receptor Smoothened (SMO). When extracellular Hedgehog is present, it binds to and inhibits PTCH, allowing SMO to accumulate and inhibit the proteolytic cleavage of the Ci protein with subsequent activation of nuclear transcription factors including Gli1 and Gli2. In the mammary gland, the Hedgehog pathway is required for normal development. Alterations in Hedgehog signaling result in defects in both embryonic and postnatal mammary gland development. Activation of Hedgehog signaling either by mutation or misexpression of pathway members can lead to the development or progression of cancers in multiple organs (56). Utilizing *in vitro* culture systems and NOD/SCID mice, Liu et al. (11) demonstrated that hedgehog signaling mediated by the polycomb gene *BMI1* regulates the self-renewal of both normal and malignant human mammary stem cells. This process is blocked by specific inhibitors such as cyclopamine (11-deoxojervine). This compound has been shown to inhibited tumor growth in several mouse models. The development of cyclopamine analogs and other Hedgehog inhibitors is currently under way, and clinical trials utilizing these agents are in the planning stages (Table 3.1).

Other Pathways Regulating Breast Cancer Stem Cells

Other pathways that regulate the self-renewal and fate of cancer stem cells are being elucidated. In addition to pathways such as Wnt, Notch, and Hedgehog, known to regulate self-renewal of normal stem cells, tumor suppressor genes such as PTEN (phosphatase and tensin homolog on chromosome 10) and p53 have also been implicated in the regulation of normal and malignant breast stem cell self-renewal. It is believed that these pathways are deregulated in cancer stem cells, leading to uncontrolled self-renewal of these cells, which may generate tumors that are resistant to conventional therapies. Reduced PTEN expression is found in approximately 40% of human breast cancers (57). In addition, women with *BRCA1* germline mutations develop microdeletions of PTEN (58). PTEN has previously been shown to regulate self-renewal of hematopoietic and neuronal stem cells (59). There is preliminary evidence that deletion of PTEN has a similar effect on normal and malignant breast stem cells. PTEN is a lipid phosphatase that regulates PI-3 kinase/Akt signaling. This suggests that development of inhibitors of Akt or mammalian target of rapamycin (mTOR) signaling may be able to affect breast cancer stem cells. A number of mTOR inhibitors are in clinical development, and clinical trials using perifosine, an AKT inhibitor, are being initiated.

The tumor suppressor p53 has also been implicated in the regulation of stem cell self-renewal. The majority of human malignancies display either p53 mutation or dysregulation of the p53 pathway (60,61). In response to stress signal, such as ultraviolet irradiation and DNA damaging agents, p53 becomes activated to promote cell-cycle arrest or apoptosis. However, the p53 cascade also appears to play an important role in stem cell regulation. Cheng et al. (62) have recently reported that p53 suppresses self-renewal of adult neural stem cells. Cells from p53 null mice brain displayed increased neural stem cell proliferation *in vivo* and increased neurosphere formation compared to wild type mice. One of the p53 transcriptional target genes, p21, has been implicated in maintenance of hema-

topoietic stem cell (HSC) quiescence. In p21 null mice, baseline HSC self-renewal is increased. However, exposing animals to cell cycle specific myelotoxic injury resulted in premature death due to rapid depletion of HSCs. It is believed that p21 acts as a molecular switch regulating the cycling of stem cells. In its absence, increased cell cycling causes extensive cellular proliferation leading to exhaustion of HSCs. This suggests that development of drugs targeting p53 signaling may be able to affect cancer stem cells. MDM2 antagonists such as Nutlin could activate p53 and may offer a novel therapeutic approach to cancer (63). Interestingly the Notch inhibitor Numb has also recently been reported to regulate p53 through interactions with MDM2 (64). This suggests that the decreased Numb expression found in 40% of breast cancers may result in the simultaneous activation of Notch and down-regulation of p53 expression. Effective targeting of cancer stem cells in these tumors may require the combined use of agents designed to inhibit Notch and stimulate p53 signaling.

In summary, the cancer stem cell model suggests that it may be necessary to target and eliminate cancer stem cells in order to eradicate cancers. Drugs that interfere with stem cell self-renewal or survival may prove effective in targeting these cell populations. Since normal and tumoral stem cells share many common regulatory pathways, it will be critical to identify agents that have a therapeutic index between normal and cancer stem cells. A number of studies in mouse models suggest that this may be the case. For example, in a mouse model, PTEN deletion leads to the generation of mouse leukemias driven by leukemic stem cells. The mTOR inhibitor rapamycin specifically eliminated leukemic stem cells while stimulating self-renewal of normal hematopoietic stem cells (65). These and other studies support the feasibility of developing strategies to selectively target cancer stem cells. A number of agents targeting breast cancer stem cell self-renewal pathways are now entering early phase clinical trials (Table 3.1). These trials will provide a direct test of the cancer stem cell hypothesis.

References

1. Cohnheim J. (1839–1884) Experimental pathologist. *JAMA* 1968;206:1561–1562.
2. Wicha MS, Liu S, Dontu G. Cancer stem cells: an old idea—a paradigm shift. *Cancer Res* 2006;66:1883–1890.
3. Reya T, Morrison SJ, Clarke MF, et al. Stem cells, cancer, and cancer stem cells. *Nature* 2001;414:105–111.
4. Kordon EC, Smith GH. An entire functional mammary gland may comprise the progeny from a single cell. *Development* 1998;125:1921–1930.
5. Stingl J, Eirew P, Ricketson I, et al. Purification and unique properties of mammary epithelial stem cells. *Nature* 2006;439:993–997.
6. Shackleton M, Vaillant F, Simpson KJ, et al. Generation of a functional mammary gland from a single stem cell. *Nature* 2006;439:84–88.
7. Vaillant F, Asselin-Labat ML, Shackleton M, et al. The emerging picture of the mouse mammary stem cell. *Stem Cell Rev* 2007;3:114–123.
8. Ginestier C, Wicha MS. Mammary stem cell number as a determinate of breast cancer risk. *Breast Cancer Res* 2007;9:109.
9. Nicolis SK. Cancer stem cells and "stemness" genes in neuro-oncology. *Neurobiol Dis* 2007;25:217–229.
10. Dontu G, Abdallah WM, Foley JM, et al. *In vitro* propagation and transcriptional profiling of human mammary stem/progenitor cells. *Genes Dev* 2003;17:1253–1270.
11. Liu S, Dontu G, Mantle ID, et al. Hedgehog signaling and BMI-1 regulate self-renewal of normal and malignant human mammary stem cells. *Cancer Res* 2006; 66:6063–6071.
12. Ginestier C, Hur MH, Charafe-Jauffret E, et al. ALDH1 is a marker of normal and malignant human mammary stem cells and a predictor of poor clinical outcome. *Cell Stem Cell* 2007;1:555–567.
13. Sophos NA, Vasiliou V. Aldehyde dehydrogenase gene superfamily: the 2002 update. *Chem Biol Interact* 2003;143–144:5–22.
14. Yoshida A, Rzhetsky A, Hsu LC, et al. Human aldehyde dehydrogenase gene family. *Eur J Biochem* 1998;251:549–557.
15. Armstrong L, Stojkovic M, Dimmick I, et al. Phenotypic characterization of murine primitive hematopoietic progenitor cells isolated on basis of aldehyde dehydrogenase activity. *Stem Cells* 2004;22:1142–1151.
16. Corti S, Locatelli F, Papadimitriou D, et al. Identification of a primitive brain-derived neural stem cell population based on aldehyde dehydrogenase activity. *Stem Cells* 2006;24:975–985.
17. Hess DA, Meyerrose TE, Wirthlin L, et al. Functional characterization of highly purified human hematopoietic repopulating cells isolated according to aldehyde dehydrogenase activity. *Blood* 2004;104:1648–1655.
18. Hess DA, Wirthlin L, Craft TP, et al. Selection based on CD133 and high aldehyde dehydrogenase activity isolates long-term reconstituting human hematopoietic stem cells. *Blood* 2006;107:2162–2169.

19. Matsui W, Huff CA, Wang Q, et al. Characterization of clonogenic multiple myeloma cells. *Blood* 2004;103:2332–2336.
20. Villadsen R, Fridriksdottir AJ, Ronnov-Jessen L, et al. Evidence for a stem cell hierarchy in the adult human breast. *J Cell Biol* 2007;177:87–101.
21. Krivtsov AV, Twomey D, Feng Z, et al. Transformation from committed progenitor to leukaemia stem cell initiated by MLL-AF9. *Nature* 2006;442:818–822.
22. Li Y, Welm B, Podsypanina K, et al. Evidence that transgenes encoding components of the Wnt signaling pathway preferentially induce mammary cancers from progenitor cells. *Proc Natl Acad Sci U S A* 2003;100:15853–15858.
23. Smith GH. Stem cells and mammary cancer in mice. *Stem Cell Rev* 2005;1:215–223.
24. Liu S, Ginestier C, Charafe-Jauffret E, et al. *BRCA1* regulates human mammary stem/progenitor cell fate. *Proc Natl Acad Sci U S A* 2008;105:1680–1685.
25. Holst CR, Nuovo GJ, Esteller M, et al. Methylation of p16(INK4a) promoters occurs *in vivo* in histologically normal human mammary epithelia. *Cancer Res* 2003;63:1596–1601.
26. Ponti D, Costa A, Zaffaroni N, et al. Isolation and in vitro propagation of tumorigenic breast cancer cells with stem/progenitor cell properties. *Cancer Res* 2005;65:5506–5511.
27. Dontu G, Jackson KW, McNicholas E, et al. Role of Notch signaling in cell-fate determination of human mammary stem/progenitor cells. *Breast Cancer Res* 2004;6:R605–R615.
28. Yu F, Yao H, Zhu P, et al. Let-7 regulates self renewal and tumorigenicity of breast cancer cells. *Cell* 2007;131:1109–1123.
29. Polyak K. Breast cancer stem cells: a case of mistaken identity? *Stem Cell Rev* 2007;3:107–109.
30. Al-Hajj M, Wicha MS, Benito-Hernandez A, et al. Prospective identification of tumorigenic breast cancer cells. *Proc Natl Acad Sci U S A* 2003;100:3983–3988.
31. Bonnet D, Dick JE. Human acute myeloid leukemia is organized as a hierarchy that originates from a primitive hematopoietic cell. *Nat Med* 1997;3:730–737.
32. Collins AT, Berry PA, Hyde C, et al. Prospective identification of tumorigenic prostate cancer stem cells. *Cancer Res* 2005;65:10946–10951.
33. Dalerba P, Dylla SJ, Park IK, et al. Phenotypic characterization of human colorectal cancer stem cells. *Proc Natl Acad Sci U S A* 2007;104:10158–10163.
34. Li C, Heidt DG, Dalerba P, et al. Identification of pancreatic cancer stem cells. *Cancer Res* 2007;67:1030–1037.
35. Prince ME, Sivanandan R, Kaczorowski A, et al. Identification of a subpopulation of cells with cancer stem cell properties in head and neck squamous cell carcinoma. *Proc Natl Acad Sci U S A* 2007;104:973–978.
36. Kim M, Turnquist H, Jackson J, et al. The multidrug resistance transporter ABCG2 (breast cancer resistance protein 1) effluxes Hoechst 33342 and is overexpressed in hematopoietic stem cells. *Clin Cancer Res* 2002;8:22–28.
37. Patrawala L, Calhoun T, Schneider-Broussard R, et al. Side population is enriched in tumorigenic, stem-like cancer cells, whereas ABCG2+ and A. *Cancer Res* 2005;65:6207–6219.
38. Phillips TM, McBride WH, Pajonk F. The response of CD24(–/low)/CD44+ breast cancer-initiating cells to radiation. *J Natl Cancer Inst* 2006;98:1777–1785.
39. Li X, Lewis MT, Huang J, et al. Intrinsic resistance of tumorigenic breast cancer cells to chemotherapy. *J Natl Cancer Inst* 2008;100(9):672.
40. Dean M, Fojo T, Bates S. Tumour stem cells and drug resistance. *Nat Rev Cancer* 2005;5:275–284.
41. Bunting KD, Lindahl R, Townsend AJ. Oxazaphosphorine-specific resistance in human MCF-7 breast carcinoma cell lines expressing transfected rat class 3 aldehyde dehydrogenase. *J Biol Chem* 1994;269:23197–23203.
42. Bao S, Wu Q, McLendon RE, et al. Glioma stem cells promote radioresistance by preferential activation of the DNA damage response. *Nature* 2006;444:756–760.
43. Hambardzumyan D, Squatrito M, Holland EC. Radiation resistance and stem-like cells in brain tumors. *Cancer Cell* 2006;10:454–456.
44. Litingtung Y, Lawler AM, Sebald SM, et al. Growth retardation and neonatal lethality in mice with a homozygous deletion in the C-terminal domain of RNA polymerase II. *Mol Gen Genet* 1999;261:100–105.
45. Brekelmans CT, Tilanus-Linthorst MM, Seynaeve C, et al. Tumour characteristics, survival and prognostic factors of hereditary breast cancer from *BRCA2-*, *BRCA1-* and non-*BRCA1/2* families as compared to sporadic breast cancer cases. *Eur J Cancer* 2007;43:867–876.
46. Balic M, Lin H, Young L, et al. Most early disseminated cancer cells detected in bone marrow of breast cancer patients have a putative breast cancer stem cell phenotype. *Clin Cancer Res* 2006;12:5615–5621.
47. Charafe-Jauffret E, Ginestier C, Iovino F, et al. Tumor stem cells mediate the metastatic phenotype in inflammatory breast cancer. *J Exp Med* In press.
48. Slamon D, Pegram M. Rationale for trastuzumab (Herceptin) in adjuvant breast cancer trials. *Semin Oncol* 2001;28:13–19.
49. Korkaya H, Paulson A, Iovino F, et al. HER2 regulates the mammary stem/progenitor cell population driving tumorigenesis and invasion. *Oncogene* 2008;27:6120–6130.
50. Brennan K, Brown AM. Is there a role for Notch signalling in human breast cancer? *Breast Cancer Res* 2003;5:69–75.
51. Miele L, Golde T, Osborne B. Notch signaling in cancer. *Curr Mol Med* 2006;6:905–918.
52. Pece S, Serresi M, Santolini E, et al. Loss of negative regulation by Numb over Notch is relevant to human breast carcinogenesis. *J Cell Biol* 2004;167:215–221.
53. Farnie G, Clarke RB, Spence K, et al. Novel cell culture technique for primary ductal carcinoma *in situ*: role of Notch and epidermal growth factor receptor signaling pathways. *J Natl Cancer Inst* 2007;99:616–627.
54. Nickoloff BJ, Osborne BA, Miele L. Notch signaling as a therapeutic target in cancer: a new approach to the development of cell fate modifying agents. *Oncogene* 2003;22:6598–6608.
55. Chan SM, Weng AP, Tibshirani R, et al. Notch signals positively regulate activity of the mTOR pathway in T-cell acute lymphoblastic leukemia. *Blood* 2007;110:278–286.
56. Hatsell S, Frost AR. Hedgehog signaling in mammary gland development and breast cancer. *J Mammary Gland Biol Neoplasia* 2007;12:163–173.
57. Panigrahi AR, Pinder SE, Chan SY, et al. The role of PTEN and its signalling pathways, including AKT, in breast cancer; an assessment of relationships with other prognostic factors and with outcome. *J Pathol* 2004;204:93–100.
58. Saal LH, Gruvberger-Saal SK, Persson C, et al. Recurrent gross mutations of the PTEN tumor suppressor gene in breast cancers with deficient DSB repair. *Nat Genet* 2008;40:102–107.
59. Rossi DJ, Weissman IL. PTEN, tumorigenesis, and stem cell self-renewal. *Cell* 2006;125:229–231.
60. Hamroun D, Kato S, Ishioka C, et al. The UMD TP53 database and website: update and revisions. *Hum Mutat* 2006;27:14–20.
61. Soussi T. The p53 pathway and human cancer. *Br J Surg* 2005;92:1331–1332.
62. Cheng T, Rodrigues N, Shen H, et al. Hematopoietic stem cell quiescence maintained by p21cip1/waf1. *Science* 2000;287:1804–1808.
63. Wang W, El-Deiry WS. Restoration of p53 to limit tumor growth. *Curr Opin Oncol* 2008;20:90–96.
64. Colaluca IN, Tosoni D, Nuciforo P, et al. Numb controls p53 tumour suppressor activity. *Nature* 2008;451:76–80.
65. Yilmaz OH, Valdez R, Theisen BK, et al. PTEN dependence distinguishes haematopoietic stem cells from leukaemia-initiating cells. *Nature* 2006;441:475–482.

Chapter 4
Physical Examination of the Breast

Monica Morrow

Obtaining a careful history is the initial step in a breast examination. Regardless of the presenting complaint, baseline information regarding menstrual status and breast cancer risk factors should be obtained. The basic elements of a breast history are listed in Table 4.1. In premenopausal women, knowing the date of the last menstrual period and the regularity of the cycle is useful in evaluating breast nodularity, pain, and cysts. Postmenopausal women should be questioned about use of hormone replacement therapy, given that many benign breast problems are uncommon after menopause in the absence of exogenous hormones. Specific information about the patient's presenting complaint is then elicited. A breast lump is most often the clinical breast problem that causes women to seek treatment, and remains the most common presentation of breast carcinoma. Haagensen (1) observed that 65% of 2,198 breast cancer cases identified before the use of screening mammography presented as breast masses. Breast pain, a change in the size and shape of the breast, nipple discharge, and changes in the appearance of the skin are infrequent symptoms of carcinoma. The evaluation and management of these conditions are described in Chapters 5, 6, and 7. In general, the duration of symptoms, their persistence over time, and their fluctuation with the menstrual cycle should be assessed.

TECHNIQUE OF BREAST EXAMINATION

A woman must be disrobed from the waist up for a complete breast examination. Although attention to modesty is appropriate, and a gown or drape should be provided, inspection is an important part of the examination, and subtle abnormalities are best appreciated by comparing the appearance of both breasts. Breast examination should be done with the patient in both the sitting and supine positions, and care should be taken at all times to be gentle. The steps of a breast examination are illustrated in Figure 4.1.

The breasts should initially be inspected while the patient is in the sitting position with the arms relaxed (Fig. 4.1A). A comparison of breast size and shape should be made. If a size discrepancy is noted, its chronicity should be determined. Many women's breasts are not identical in size, and the finding of small size discrepancies is rarely a sign of malignancy. Differences in breast size that are of recent onset or progressive in nature, however, may be owing to both benign and malignant tumors, and require further evaluation (Fig. 4.2). Alterations in breast shape, in the absence of previous surgery, are of more concern. Superficially located tumors can cause bulges in the breast contour or retraction of the overlying skin. The skin retraction seen with superficial tumors may be caused by direct extension of tumor or fibrosis. Tumors deep within the substance of the breast that involve the fibrous septa (Cooper's ligaments) can also cause retraction. Retraction is not itself a prognostic factor except when caused by the direct extension of tumor into the skin and, for this reason, it is not a part of the

clinical staging of breast cancer (2). Although retraction is often a sign of malignancy, benign lesions of the breast, such as granular cell tumors (3) and fat necrosis (4), also cause retraction. Other benign causes of retraction include surgical biopsy and thrombophlebitis of the thoracoepigastric vein (Mondor's disease) (5) (Fig. 4.3).

The skin of the breasts and the nipples should also be carefully inspected. Edema of the skin of the breast (*peau d'orange*), when present, is usually extensive and readily apparent. Localized edema is frequently most prominent in the lower half of the breast and periareolar region, and is most noticeable when the patient's arms are raised. Although breast edema usually occurs as a result of obstruction of the dermal lymphatics with tumor cells, it can also be caused by extensive axillary lymph node involvement related to metastatic tumor, primary diseases of the axillary nodes, or axillary dissection. Some degree of breast edema is very common after irradiation of the breast and should not be considered abnormal in this circumstance. Erythema is another sign of a pathologic process that is evident on inspection (Fig. 4.4) . It may be caused by cellulitis or abscess in the breast, but a diagnosis of inflammatory carcinoma should always be considered. The erythema of inflammatory carcinoma usually involves the entire breast; it is distinguished from the inflammation caused by infection by the absence of breast tenderness and fever. A small percentage of large-breasted women have mild, dependent erythema of the most pendulous portion of the breast, a condition that resolves when they lie down, and that is of no concern.

Examination of the nipples should include inspection for symmetry, retraction, and changes in the character of the skin. The new onset of nipple retraction should be regarded with a high index of suspicion, except when it occurs immediately after cessation of breast-feeding. Ulceration and eczematous changes of the nipple may be the first signs of Paget's disease. The initial nipple abnormality may be limited in extent, but, if untreated, it progresses to involve the entire nipple.

After inspection with the arms relaxed, the patient should be asked to raise her arms to allow a more complete inspection of the lower half of the breasts (Fig. 4.5) . Inspection is completed with the patient contracting the pectoral muscles by pressing her hands against her hips. This maneuver often highlights subtle areas of retraction that are not readily apparent with the arms relaxed.

The next step in the examination is palpation of the regional nodes. Examination of the axillary and supraclavicular nodes is done optimally with the patient upright. The right axilla is examined with the physician's left hand while the patient's flexed right arm is supported (Fig. 4.1B). This position allows relaxation of the pectoral muscle and access to the axillary space, and is reversed to examine the left axilla. If lymph nodes are palpable, their size and character (soft, firm, tender) should be noted, as well as whether they are single, multiple, or matted together. An assessment of whether the nodes are mobile or fixed should also be made. Based on this

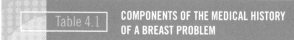

Table 4.1 **COMPONENTS OF THE MEDICAL HISTORY OF A BREAST PROBLEM**

All Women
- Age at menarche
- Number of pregnancies
- Number of live births
- Age at first birth
- Family history of breast cancer, including affected relative, age of onset, and presence of bilateral disease
- History of breast biopsies (and histologic diagnosis, if available)

Premenopausal Women
- Date of last menstrual period
- Length and regularity of cycles
- Use of oral contraceptives

Postmenopausal Women
- Date of menopause
- Use of hormone replacement therapy

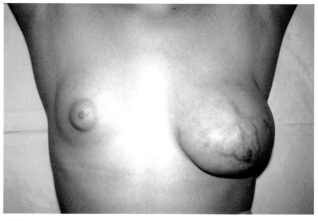

FIGURE 4.2. Marked breast asymmetry owing to a benign breast tumor.

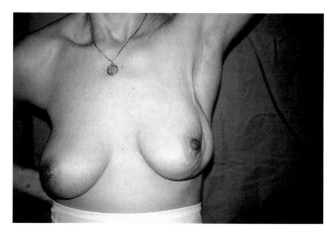

FIGURE 4.3. Breast retraction caused by thrombophlebitis of the thoracoepigastric vein (Mondor's disease). Seen is the characteristic pattern of lateral retraction superior to the nipple and crossing to the midline below the nipple.

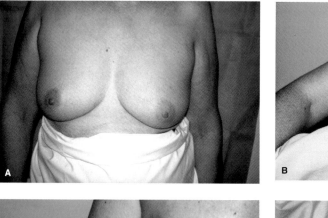

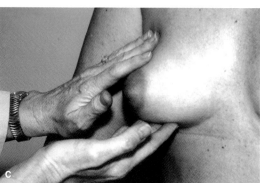

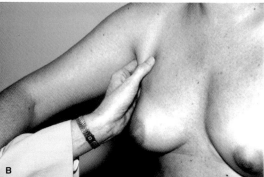

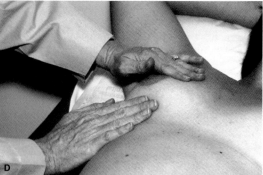

FIGURE 4.1. Inspection of the patient in the upright position with arms relaxed (A). Palpation of the axillary nodes (**B**). The patient's ipsilateral arm is supported to relax the pectoral muscle. Palpation of the breast in the upright position (**C**). Palpation of the breast in the supine position (**D**). The breast is stabilized with one hand.

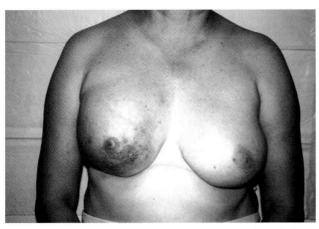

FIGURE 4.4. Signs of locally advanced breast cancer that are apparent on inspection: breast asymmetry, erythema and eczema owing to dermal involvement with tumor.

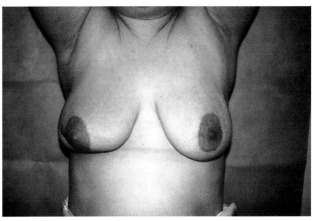

FIGURE 4.5. Retraction in the inferior right breast that is only apparent when the patient's arms are raised.

information, the physician can assess whether the nodes are clinically suspect. Many women have palpable axillary nodes secondary to hangnails, minor abrasions of the arm, or folliculitis of the axilla, and nodes that are small (<1 cm), soft, and mobile (especially if bilateral) should not be regarded with a high level of suspicion. In contrast, palpable supraclavicular adenopathy is uncommon and is an indication for further evaluation.

After the nodal evaluation is completed, palpation of the breasts should be done with the patient erect. Examination of the breast tissue in this position allows detection of lesions that might be obscured with the patient supine, such as those in the tail of the breast. The breast should be gently supported with one hand while examination is done with the flat portions of the fingers (Fig. 4.1C). Pinching breast tissue between two fingers always results in the perception of a mass and is a common error of inexperienced examiners and women attempting self-examination.

The breast examination is completed with the patient in the supine position and the ipsilateral arm raised above the head (Fig. 4.1D). In patients with extremely large breasts, it may be necessary to place a folded towel or a small pillow beneath the ipsilateral shoulder to elevate the breast, but this is not routinely necessary. The breast tissue is then systematically examined. Whether the examination is done using a radial search pattern or concentric circular pattern is unimportant, provided that the entire breast is examined. The examination should extend superiorly to the clavicle, inferiorly to the lower rib cage, medially to the sternal border, and laterally to the midaxillary line. Examination is done with one hand while the other hand stabilizes the breast. The degree of pressure needed to examine the breast tissue varies, but should not cause the patient discomfort.

One of the most difficult aspects of breast examination results from the nodular, irregular texture of normal breasts in premenopausal women. Normal breasts tend to be most nodular in the upper outer quadrants where the glandular tissue is concentrated, in the inframammary ridge area, and in the subareolar region. The characteristics that distinguish a dominant breast mass include the absence of other abnormalities of a similar character, density that differs from the surrounding breast tissue, and three dimensions. Generalized lumpiness is not a pathologic finding. Comparing the breasts is often helpful in determining whether a questionable area requires further evaluation. If the patient notices a mass that is not evident to the examiner, she should be asked to indicate the area of concern. The location of the perceived abnormality and the character of the breast tissue in the region should be described in the medical record. If uncertainty remains regarding the significance of an area of nodular breast tissue in a premenopausal woman, a repeat examination at a different time during the menstrual cycle may clarify the issue. If a dominant mass is identified, it should be measured, and its location, mobility, and character should be described in the medical record. The identification of a dominant mass is an indication for further evaluation. The steps in the evaluation of a palpable mass are described in Chapter 5.

References

1. Haagensen CD. *Diseases of the breast*. Philadelphia: WB Saunders; 1986:502.
2. American Joint Committee on Cancer. *Manual for staging of cancer.* 6th ed. New York: Springer; 2002:227.
3. Gold DA, Hermann G, Schwartz IS, et al. Granular cell tumor of the breast. *Breast Dis* 1989;2:211.
4. Adair F, Munzer J. Fat necrosis of the female breast. *Am J Surg* 1947;74:117.
5. Tabar L, Dean P. Mondor's disease: clinical, mammographic and pathologic features. *Breast* 1981;7:17.

Richard J. Bleicher

INTRODUCTION

The breast mass is the most common symptom of women presenting to breast centers, accounting for more than half of the complaints (1). Although most such lesions are benign, the presence of a mass can cause considerable anxiety because of the concern that cancer may be present. The most important task of the physician evaluating a breast mass is to exclude the presence of malignancy, and then provide an accurate diagnosis and explanation for the mass.

The presence of a mass should never be dismissed because of young age, male gender, or because of a lack of risk factors, such as a family history of cancer. Diagnostic delays of breast cancer are a common cause for litigation, and such claims are most commonly seen for non-Hispanic white women in their 40s who are premenopausal, married, have a history of fibrocystic change, and who are enrolled in a health maintenance organization (HMO) (2). Although delays in the diagnosis of a breast cancer may need to be 8 months or longer to be detrimental (3), no factor should override an expeditious and thorough evaluation, which must provide an explanation that is concordant with the patient's history, physical examination, imaging, and pathologic findings.

HISTORY

A thorough history is the first step in the proper evaluation of any breast mass. Historical elements must, at bare minimum, include a proper breast history, which includes current and prior symptoms, radiologic screening and diagnostic studies, and risk factors for cancer, including the patient's gynecologic and menstrual history. The cause of previous masses should be detailed, and specifics about any current and prior breast problems must include the character, frequency, severity, and duration of the issue.

Breast evaluation of benign and malignant disease nearly always includes diagnostic imaging. The complete history must therefore also include details about mammograms, ultrasounds, and magnetic resonance imaging (MRI), including the dates, findings, and follow-up for abnormalities on these studies. Although annual mammographic screening is currently recommended for average-risk women aged 40 years and older (4), many patients are either not aware of this recommendation or choose not to follow it. MRI is also recommended only as a screening modality in women whose lifetime risk is ≥20% to 25% (5), but MRI is still being used outside of this setting (5a).

Other symptoms, such as palpable lymph nodes, breast pain, skin changes, nipple inversion, and the character of any discharge (including color, bilaterality, number of ducts involved and spontaneity), should also be assessed, because these complete the history and may narrow the differential diagnosis of a dominant mass. Although a complete review of systems is often performed solely to satisfy reimbursement criteria, discussion of other organ systems may contribute substantially to understanding the current illness and to determine a patient's candidacy for certain treatments, especially if a mass is found to be malignant (Table 5.1).

Medical history may also shed light on current findings, either clarifying an ongoing process, or suggesting something that can recur over a woman's lifetime. Certain recurring entities may present as a mass; these include cancer and benign processes, such as pseudoangiomatous stromal hyperplasia, fibroadenomas, duct ectasia, mastitis, or abscess formation. A history of such lesions may assist in the differential diagnosis of a palpable mass because these can recur. Mass-forming lesions are listed in Table 5.2.

A discussion of the patient's surgical history, including breast surgeries and needle biopsies, often reminds patients to mention prior benign conditions, such as fibrocystic change, simple cysts, fibroadenomata, and fat necrosis. Knowledge of a patient's prior breast pathology and how these presented are important for overall assessment and to determine their risk of cancer. Often, patients are unfamiliar with specifics of their pathology and simply told that their prior biopsies are "benign," but the details are important because this lay description may encompass atypical hyperplasia (a lesion requiring further evaluation if recently diagnosed), lobular carcinoma *in situ* (LCIS, a high risk marker), or other entities that confer elevated risk. Pathology reports and slides may be of assistance to complete the evaluation if details are unclear.

In men, the history should include additional questions about hepatic dysfunction, sexual dysfunction, and current medications to rule out potential causes of gynecomastia, which can present as a central breast mass. Clearance of testosterone can be impaired by hepatic dysfunction, resulting in increased peripheral conversion of testosterone to estradiol and estrone, resulting in stimulation of the breast tissue and its hypertrophy. Sexual dysfunction may indicate abnormal testosterone levels. Medications (e.g., H_2 blockers and phenytoin) or drugs (e.g., marijuana) have also been associated with gynecomastia (6). Acute hypertrophy may also be painful, and associated symptoms should therefore be elicited.

PHYSICAL EXAMINATION

A presenting symptom that is designated as a new breast "mass" can span a variety of findings. This includes everything from a barely perceptible thickened region of the breast to a large fungating cancer or severe adenopathy. Physical examination is important before any diagnostic imaging so that (a) the study can be chosen and targeted appropriately and (b) the radiologist can best assist in evaluating what has been seen on examination.

Normal breast tissue demonstrates nodularity, which is often difficult to distinguish from an abnormal process, causing difficulty for patients as well as physicians. One study of 542 patients under 30 years of age referred for a breast mass found that among the 80% of masses detected by self-breast examination, only 53% were true masses, underscoring the difficulties seen in younger women (7). A second study by Morrow et al. (8) evaluating 605 patients under 40 years of age also found that masses were self-detected in 80% of the cases and, among those, only 27% had an identifiable cause other than fibrocystic change. Among masses felt to be true abnormalities on examination by the surgeon, 28% were false–positive findings.

In some cases, the physician will not detect any abnormality on the clinical breast examination even after focusing on the area of concern. In this situation, the patient should be reassured about the absence of worrisome findings and the physician should recheck to ensure that a screening mammogram

Table 5.1	EXAMPLES OF POTENTIAL CONTRIBUTIONS BY THE REVIEW OF SYSTEMS
System	**Contribution**
General	Fever suggests an inflammatory process.
Neurologic	Deficits suggest metastatic disease.
Pulmonary	Cough or compromise clarify operative candidacy.
Cardiac	Compromise may contraindicate operation or anthracycline chemotherapy.
	Inability to lie flat contraindicates whole breast radiotherapy.
Integument	Nipple changes suggest Paget's disease.
	Breast erythema and edema suggests mastitis, or breast cancer that is locally advanced or inflammatory.
	Symptoms of active collagen vascular disease contraindicate radiotherapy.
Musculoskeletal	Back or bone pain suggest metastatic disease.
	Inability to abduct the arm over the head may contraindicate whole breast radiotherapy.
Gynecologic	Active menses contraindicate aromatase inhibitor administration.
Hematologic	Frequent ecchymosis and bleeding suggest a need for preoperative evaluation.
	Deep venous thrombosis may contraindicate Tamoxifen therapy.

has been performed within the past year for the average-risk patient who is 40 years of age and older.

In other women, a subtle abnormality that remains ill defined is detected. Such a lesion, sometimes referred to as a breast "thickening," is one whose extent cannot be clearly defined in three dimensions. These poorly defined areas of prominence may represent a true abnormality within the breast parenchyma or, in many cases, may reflect the prominence of an underlying rib that elevates the normally nodular breast tissue superficial to it. With uncertainty about whether a finding represents a true mass, the clinician should compare it with the mirror-image location in the opposite breast and, if applicable, palpate that region of breast tissue again once it has been moved off the underlying bony prominence. If any level of concern remains, further imaging evaluation is required, and for those physicians whose experience evaluating breast masses is limited, a follow-up examination in 2 to 3 months after the initial visit is appropriate.

When the examination is complete, the patient can be characterized as having four possible findings:

1. No abnormality present
2. A thickening without the characteristics of a dominant mass
3. A dominant mass with benign characteristics on palpation
4. A dominant mass with malignant characteristics (Fig. 5.1).

Table 5.2	BREAST LESIONS THAT MAY PRESENT AS A PALPABLE ABNORMALITY
Fibrocystic change	Sarcomas, including phyllodes tumors
Simple and complex cysts	
Pseudoangiomatous stromal hyperplasia	Sarcoidosis
	Idiopathic granulomatous mastitis
Fat necrosis	
Lipomas	Hematomas
Abscesses	Seromas
Adenopathy	Mucoceles
Duct ectasia	Galactoceles
Fibroadenomata	Amyloidosis
Hamartomas	Focal fibrosis
Ductal carcinoma *in situ*	Lactating adenomas
Invasive carcinoma	Epidermal inclusion cysts
Gynecomastia	Lymphadenopathy

Documentation

Documentation of any findings present on physical examination should be done consistently and include a description of the superficial appearance of the breasts, including the skin, nipples, and areolae, as well as whether a mass or retractions can be detected by observation alone, or with movement. Exanthemas, nipple inversion, and the character of any discharge should be noted.

When documenting the characteristics of a mass, detail is of the utmost importance because it inherently conveys a level of concern and assists in the formulation of a differential diagnosis. Many women have diffusely nodular breasts and, therefore, the size of the mass and its location should be detailed. At minimum, the mass should be described by indicating the breast in question and the quadrant of the mass, although it is helpful to specify more detail whenever possible by utilizing tangents emanating from the nipple as numbers on the clock when facing the patient. The mass is also described by its distance from the nipple along that tangent, such as "a 2-cm left breast mass at the 4:00 position, 6 cm from the nipple." Other characteristics that should be specified include whether its borders are smooth or irregular, details about its consistency (e.g., being soft, firm, or scirrhous), and whether it is discrete or an indistinct thickening. Characteristics associated with malignancy should also be noted. These include fixation to the chest wall or skin, skin satellite nodules or edema of the skin (including *peau d'orange*), and ulceration. These characteristics are indicative of cancer and assist in its evaluation and staging.

The Axilla

The location of some masses may be difficult to distinguish as being present in the tail of the breast or the low axilla. Although normal lymph nodes are usually not palpable, small nonsuspicious lymph nodes may be detectable, often described as "shotty" nodes (the term originating from and referring to shot or pellets of lead and not "shoddy," as in poor quality). Lymph nodes can vary in size from several millimeters to several centimeters when abnormally enlarged, and tend to be discrete oblong nodules that have greater freedom of movement than breast parenchymal masses unless the nodes are fixed to one another or to the chest wall. These should also be described in detail, paying particular attention to the number of palpable nodes, fixation, laterality, and size.

The Male Breast

Men have considerably less breast tissue, except in those with gynecomastia. Most of the breast tissue is located behind the nipple–areola complex, and benign masses owing to abnormal breast enlargement are typically described as disclike or platelike. Eccentricity in relation to the central male breast should be noted because such lesions are more likely to be malignant. Despite less breast tissue and a predominance of centralized parenchyma, the examination and documentation for the male breast remains similar to the female examination.

RADIOLOGIC EXAMINATION

Mammography

Mammogram remains the standard for the evaluation of breast abnormalities, and is necessary even when a mass very clearly seems malignant. When a palpable abnormality is found, a diagnostic mammogram is performed, which consists of at least one view in addition to those taken in a screening study. A skin marker is placed over the palpable area of interest, and

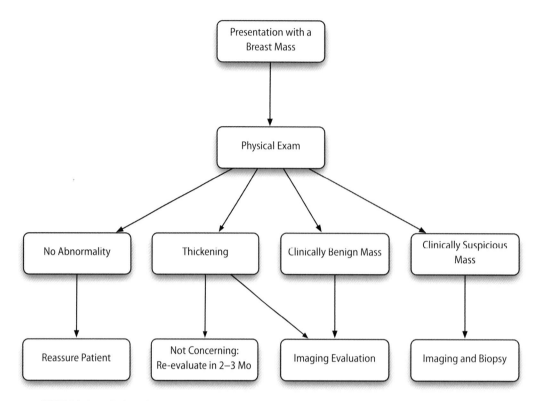

FIGURE 5.1.   General schema for initial evaluation of a mass on examination based upon its palpable characteristics. Upon presentation with the complaint of a mass, four findings can occur: (1) No abnormality noted, (2) a thickening which may be either not concerning or may be equivocal, (3) a clinically benign mass, or (4) a clinically suspicious mass. These characteristics determine the next appropriate step in evaluation. When the characteristics of a thickening are equivocal or uncertain, imaging is indicated.

additional views are taken if deemed appropriate by the radiologist. Mammographic imaging may be sufficient if a suspicious mass is found, corresponding to the area in question. If nothing is visualized on mammogram or if the mass appears to be benign, characterization by ultrasound is indicated, as mammograms typically miss approximately 10% to 25% of cancers detectable by physical examination regardless of tumor size (9,10), and they cannot differentiate solid from cystic abnormalities.

When possible, mammograms should be obtained before a biopsy of any mass because of the consequent mammographic changes that might occur. The two exceptions to this are in evaluating the pregnant and very young patient (covered below). Hann et al. (11) reviewed mammographic results immediately after stereotactic biopsy, and demonstrated, among 113 cases, that 76% of changes were due to the core biopsy, with 58 (51%) having a core-biopsy induced hematoma (11). In 31 (27%) lesions, the visualized lesion size changed, and in three cases (3%) hematoma obscured the ability to see calcifications at the site.

Prior mammograms from outside facilities should be obtained for comparison before any intervention. Review of all imaging by all treating physicians is critical for correlation to the palpable abnormality. If a breast cancer is diagnosed histologically without the use of bilateral imaging, the clinician should ensure that a bilateral mammogram has been obtained within the past 6 months to rule out evident multicentric or contralateral disease requiring simultaneous intervention, even if no other palpable findings are present on examination.

The inability to see a palpable mass on mammogram should prompt an ultrasound, but the inability to see the lesion on either set of imaging does not mean that the lesion should be disregarded. If the lesion is discrete, biopsy should be performed. MRI is sometimes performed as an additional step to evaluate a mass that is mammographically occult, although MRI adds little because it is a poor substitute for the required

pathologic diagnosis because of its lack of specificity (12). In addition, the sensitivity of MRI is insufficient to allow biopsy to be eliminated when a mass is detected clinically. A palpable mass not seen on mammogram or ultrasound should undergo needle biopsy as the next step.

Mammography in Men

Although mammography in men may confirm that a mass is of low clinical suspicion or assist in cases where body habitus makes a patient's physical examination more difficult, it generally adds little to the workup of the palpable breast mass. The physical examination in male patients is particularly important, largely because of the smaller amount of breast tissue that allows a prominence of male breast cancers on examination and the low prevalence of benign breast masses other than gynecomastia. In a Mayo Clinic study evaluating mammograms performed on men, 196 were performed for breast masses and other symptomatic complaints. Among these, one benign-appearing mammogram among 203 missed a cancer (0.5%), but all three cancers in this series presented with a discrete palpable mass, 2 associated with overlying retractions and 1 with interval enlargement and lymphadenopathy (13). In a series of 104 male patients with cancer, Borgen et al. (14) also reported that most patients presented with more than one symptom, including masses in 77, nipple retraction in 18, bloody discharge in 16, skin ulceration in 10, and others with Paget's disease, clinical inflammatory carcinoma, and fixed tumors. These series suggest that male cancers usually present with at least one suspicious physical examination findings, and although bilateral mammography may be considered in men once a cancer is suspected or diagnosed to rule out bilaterality, its role and benefit in the routine evaluation of the male breast mass has yet to be defined.

Ultrasound

Ultrasound enables directed characterization of an abnormality, but is not utilized as a screening study. Ultrasound is most commonly used to determine whether a breast mass is cystic or solid, and to characterize its appearance. Solid masses may appear benign or malignant, and cystic masses are characterized as simple or complex.

Cyst Evaluation

Cysts are most frequently seen in persons between the ages of 40 and 49 years (15), but account for only 10% of masses in women younger than 40, and 25% of masses in women overall (8,16). More than half of all women who have cysts develop more one than during their lifetime, which may present synchronously or metachronously (17). Detection of cysts on ultrasound requires their characterization either as simple cysts, containing a smooth thin wall that is well-circumscribed with few internal echoes, or as a complex cyst, which is defined as any cyst that does not meet these criteria (18). Ultrasound is 98% to 100% accurate for characterization of benign cysts when strict criteria are utilized (16,19). A cyst can be characterized as complex owing to the presence of a significant solid component, internal echoes or a fluid-debris level, scalloped or irregular borders, and the presence of septations. Complex cysts have an overall rate of malignancy as low as 0.3%, but complex cystic lesions containing a significant solid component have been reported to have an associated malignancy rate of up to 23% and so complex cysts are generally aspirated (20,21).

Cysts that appear simple on ultrasound have a negligible risk of cancer. Such cysts do not require aspiration unless the patient is symptomatic. In such cases, aspiration is performed to relieve the distension and discomfort and not for fluid evaluation. Complex cysts require aspiration to rule out bloody fluid, which is suggestive of malignancy. Benign cyst fluid is typically green, yellow, or brown, and should not be sent for cytology because dead epithelial cells present in that fluid may appear atypical despite the low likelihood of malignancy. One study evaluating 6,747 cysts in 4,105 women with nonbloody aspiration found no cancers in these women (15).

Ultrasound is often the only imaging study required for a clinically benign breast mass found in women younger than 35 years, because of the low risk of malignancy, and because breast density often precludes mammographic visualization in this age group. When breast cancer is diagnosed, bilateral mammograms remain standard and should be obtained to assess the presence of multicentric or bilateral disease. Digital mammography has demonstrated some benefit over analogue studies in younger women and in those with dense breasts (22), but in those who are the most difficult to assess, MRI may be of assistance because it is not affected by breast density (23).

In the young woman, masses that are benign to palpation may undergo an attempt at aspiration before ultrasonographic imaging. Those with nonbloody benign cyst aspirate in whom the aspiration resolves the palpable abnormality may undergo observation (17). When planning to perform an aspiration, one must be cognizant that a traumatic aspiration can cause a bloody aspirate or potentially a hematoma, leading to further unnecessary workup and making ultrasound assessment more difficult. It is therefore important only to attempt blind aspiration in cases where the lesion is easily accessible by minimal manipulation and few needle passes.

For those in whom the cyst recurs, repeat aspiration is acceptable, although with multiple recurrences, a mammogram (because of the small increase in risk of malignancy) and ultrasound (to further evaluate the cyst) should be considered, and excision is an option primarily reserved for a suspicious lesion or when repeat aspirations are no longer desired by the patient.

Solid Mass Evaluation

The physical examination is important in combination with imaging to assess solid lesions. One of the more common solid abnormalities seen in young women are fibroadenomas (24), but these have also been found in women in their 40s and 50s as in 9.5% of 42 women in one autopsy study (25) demonstrating that, although less common, they may be present in older women. These masses are typically round or multilobulated, firm or "rubbery" and nontender and freely mobile within the breast parenchyma. The physical examination for diagnosis of the fibroadenoma is helpful, but not definitive, as demonstrated by one study evaluating women less than 35 years of age in whom a clinical diagnosis of a fibroadenoma was made. After 14 masses among 110 were excluded for various reasons, including three patients found to have cancer by fine-needle aspiration (FNA), 92 women remained, among which 15 masses resolved spontaneously. Although imaging and histologic evaluation in this subset was not specified, in the remaining 77 women where the mass persisted, only 56 (72%) were confirmed histologically to be fibroadenomas by FNA (26).

Combining imaging and physical examination for evaluation of the palpable mass improves cancer detection over imaging alone. van Dam et al. (27) found, in their series of 201 patients, that ultrasound and mammogram each had respective sensitivities for cancer detection of 78% and 94% and specificities of 94% and 55%. When combining ultrasound, mammogram, and physical examination together, sensitivity increased to 97% for cancer detection, but with a decrease in specificity to only 49%. In the Sydney Breast Imaging Accuracy Study in which 240 women with, and 240 age-matched matched women without, cancer were evaluated, ultrasound had a 76% sensitivity for cancer and an 88% specificity, but most notable was the significant sensitivity advantage that ultrasound had over mammography in women aged 45 and younger (85% vs. 72%), suggesting that ultrasound is a critical addition to mammography in the evaluation of breast lesions in young women (28).

The common and benign fibroadenoma can, however, be difficult to distinguish from the uncommon and malignant phyllodes tumors by imaging. Bode et al. (29) reviewed ultrasonography and core biopsy with subsequent excision performed on 57 fibroadenomas and 12 phyllodes tumors, finding that 42% of the phyllodes tumors were initially felt to be benign on ultrasound, whereas 46% of the fibroadenomas were indeterminate or suspicious. This underscores the need for the triple test (see below), which is standard even when imaging suggests a benign solid mass (Fig. 5.2).

Magnetic Resonance Imaging

Few indications exist for MRI in the workup of breast masses. MRI is best suited for settings where standard imaging techniques are insufficient, or where a patient's elevated breast cancer risk outweighs the false–positive findings, costs, and disadvantages of the modality. The absence of a lesion noted on MRI does not negate the presence of a concerning mass on physical examination. MRI has an 85% negative predictive value for cancer in palpable masses containing calcifications, which drops to less than 80% when no calcifications are present (12). MRI is highly sensitive, but very nonspecific. One study of 1,909 women with a significant familial risk of cancer demonstrated a threefold increase in the number of unnecessary biopsies because of the MRI performed (30).

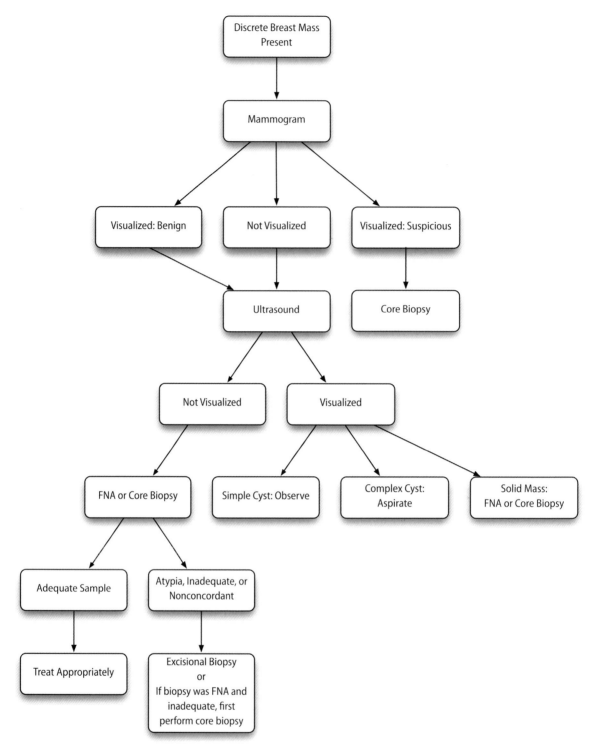

FIGURE 5.2. Specific schema for evaluation of a discrete mass on examination. Evaluation workflow, including imaging and tissue diagnosis, based upon the presence of a discrete mass on examination. If a mass is found to be clinically suspicious on examination, imaging should still be performed, but in such as case a tissue diagnosis is indicated, regardless of the imaging findings.

PATHOLOGIC EXAMINATION

Triple Test Evaluation

Masses found to be solid on imaging require triple-test evaluation, which refers to physical examination, radiologic examination, and needle biopsy, performed by core or FNA. The triple test requires concordance between the three aspects of evaluation and is not confirmatory if a mammogram does not visualize the lesion or if an FNA contains insufficient cells for diagnosis. The latter case mandates core needle biopsy for completion of the triple-test evaluation without surgery.

The triple test is performed even in cases where masses are considered benign on imaging because of the difficulties in distinguishing benign lesions, such as fibroadenomas from some malignant lesions, such as phyllodes tumors of low malignant potential (31), and because some carcinomas can have a benign appearance (32). In one series of 191 patients, Steinberg et al. (33) found the sensitivity and specificity of triple test to be 95.5% and 100%, respectively. In a smaller series of 46 lesions in 43 patients, concordance between the three modalities provided a positive predictive value and specificity of 100%, whereas nonconcordance dropped the positive predictive value to 64% (34). The triple test also saved an average of $1,412 per case in comparison with open biopsy, demonstrating that it provides accurate diagnostic results and is cost effective, despite the use of both imaging and pathologic evaluation. In one of the largest series evaluating the combination, benign triple tests in 2,184 patients demonstrated only 7 (0.32%) with carcinoma on follow-up.

Postbiopsy Follow-Up

Although the accuracy of the triple test is high, benign concordant results do not obviate further surveillance of a palpable mass. Serial examinations and imaging at 6-month intervals for 1 to 2 years are often recommended to ensure stability and growth should prompt surgical excision, especially in older women where benign masses are less frequently seen. Even fibroadenomas undergoing needle biopsy should be followed because those that are monoclonal have been reported on very rare occasions to transform into, or recur as, phyllodes tumors (35). No consensus exists regarding a threshold for excision when growth of a lesion occurs, although Gordon et al. (36) evaluated 179 masses in 173 patients under 50 years of age, and 15 masses in 14 patients who were 50 and older. The 95th percentile in women under 50 and the 90th percentile in those 50 and older for growth by ultrasound over 6 months were each 20% (36). They found that all masses excised with slower growth were benign, and recommended that a 6-month growth rate of 20% become the threshold above which excision should be performed. This threshold has not been universally adopted, however, and smaller growth rates may prompt excision because no data exist relating outcome to growth rates of masses initially diagnosed as benign.

The triple test has been found to be the most accurate combination of modalities, but anxiety over a palpable mass remains an indication for surgical excision once the relevant literature and data have been disclosed to the patient. Before performing a core biopsy to complete the triple test, there should be a discussion with the patient. The triple test implies observation if the biopsy is concordant and benign, and the consent process should clarify that the patient is comfortable with leaving the mass *in situ*.

Fine-Needle Aspiration

Fine-needle aspiration involves the use of a handheld syringe and needle to aspirate a tumor mass percutaneously to obtain cytology for evaluation. This was first described in detail by Martin and Ellis in 1930 (37), and is most commonly used for palpable breast lesions that do not require imaging to target the lesion. FNA has been established as a variably accurate method of diagnosis and clinicians should consequently perform validation of their own results. In a large meta-analysis of 29 studies comprised of 31,340 aspirations, the sensitivity of FNA varied from 65% to 98% and specificity ranged between 34% and 100% (38).

Fine-needle aspiration has the advantages of being easily performed with readily available equipment, requiring only a syringe and an appropriately sized needle. Its biggest limitations are that insufficient material may make proper diagnosis difficult, and FNA usually cannot rule out the presence of an invasive component for the uncommon mass that is pure ductal carcinoma *in situ* (DCIS). It also does not capture histologic architecture, making subtyping difficult, and it is inaccurate for some masses, such as hamartomas (39). FNA remains accurate

for the diagnosis of both palpable and nonpalpable suspicious lesions even after reduction mammoplasty where the clinical diagnosis may be more difficult (40).

Core Needle Biopsy

Core needle biopsy is associated with slightly greater discomfort and higher cost, but provides both more tissue than FNA and histologic architecture to better classify pathologic subtype. It is less morbid than excisional biopsy, and even in an early series of 104 lesions comparing core needle with excisional biopsy, the results were identical in 90% of lesions (41). Although overwhelming data have demonstrated that excisional biopsy should not be a contraindication to sentinel node biopsy (42–44), concern about excisional biopsy in lieu of core biopsy has existed because higher rates of sentinel node nonidentification were seen in some prospective sentinel node trials (45,46), further emphasizing the benefits of core over excisional biopsy.

In the case of malignancy, the presence of invasion can be more easily assessed with core biopsy than with FNA. Westenend et al. (46a) performed both FNA and core needle biopsy in 286 breast lesions of which 232 were palpable masses. FNA and core biopsy demonstrated no statistical differences in either sensitivity (92% and 88%, respectively), overall positive predictive value (100% and 99%, respectively), or the number of inadequate specimens (7% for both). The diagnostic differences were present in their specificity, which was higher at 90% for core biopsy (vs. 82% for FNA), and for the positive predictive value of suspicious lesions (100% vs. 78%), and atypia (80% vs. 18%). In a multi-institutional study by Parker et al. (47), among 1,363 lesions undergoing core and excisional biopsy under image guidance, only 15 (1.1%) false–negative core biopsies occurred, of which 12 were performed using stereotaxis, and 3 using ultrasound guidance. Although this study was performed for lesions detected by imaging, it underscores the value of utilizing imaging with core biopsy for those areas of thickening that are equivocal on examination. Core biopsy remains the current standard of care for evaluation of masses of the breast.

Incisional Biopsy

Incisional biopsy is performed only very rarely. This method of tissue sampling refers to the intentional surgical excision of only a portion of a mass. Palpable lesions requiring biopsy are typically removed by excising the entire lesion (see Excisional Biopsy, below). When a mass (e.g., a large adherent fungating cancer) is too large to excise *in toto*, a core biopsy or FNA is nearly always the preferred method of diagnosis, thereby avoiding the associated morbidity, including operative and anesthesia risks. Markers, such as estrogen and progesterone receptors, as well as HER2/neu overexpression can be obtained from core biopsy, also eliminating any need for incisional or excisional biopsy.

Excisional Biopsy

The surgical removal of a lesion in the breast with the intent to remove the entire lesion is referred to as an excisional biopsy. In 2008, excisional biopsy is no longer the standard of care for the initial diagnosis of palpable breast masses, except where needle biopsy is not feasible for technical reasons, is nonconcordant with imaging or examination, is nondiagnostic, or demonstrates a high-risk lesion, such as atypia.

Excisional biopsies, however, are all too often performed without specimen orientation for the pathologist. For those excisional biopsies that demonstrate a malignancy, lack of orientation may necessitate complete re-excision of the entire cavity for even a single positive margin. This results in needless resection of tissue (48), especially because orientation of excisional biopsy specimens is simple to perform. It is also inadvisable to perform intraoperative frozen section of an excisional biopsy because of the concerns about the accuracy of the analysis (49). Intraoperative assessment of an excised mass has few advantages other than to satisfy immediate physician and patient curiosity, and no change in definitive surgery (e.g., conversion from breast conservation to mastectomy) should ever be performed based on an initial result (50) and without an in-depth discussion about treatment options. The specific schema for imaging and treatment of a discrete mass is shown in Figure 5.2.

SPECIFIC CLINICAL SETTINGS

The Young Patient

Assessment of the young female patient with a breast mass poses a challenge because of (a) difficulties in imaging dense breast tissue, (b) the greater nodularity seen in those 30 and under whose breasts contain a lower proportion of fat, and (c) cosmetic and sexuality concerns about treatment tend to be greater in women of younger age (51). Malignancy is rare in women under 30, but complete evaluation of all masses is still required, including a tissue diagnosis in those masses found to be solid. In a large series of 542 women under 30 who presented with the complaint of a breast mass, 80% were detected by the patient, 53% were true masses, and 44% were confirmed by the surgeon on examination (7). Only 2% of cases were demonstrated to be malignant on biopsy, and among the benign lesions, the most common diagnosis was fibroadenoma, accounting for 72% of cases, with fibrocystic change next in frequency at 8%.

The evaluation and treatment of young women should proceed similarly to older women, although their increased breast density makes mammographic evaluation more difficult, and so ultrasound is the primary modality used to characterize a mass. If ultrasound demonstrates that the lesion in solid, core or fine needle biopsy is indicated and, if malignancy is found, bilateral mammographic evaluation should then be performed. Likewise, if a lesion that is discrete is not seen on ultrasound, mammographic evaluation may characterize the lesion, but needle biopsy (or excision, if not possible) should be performed as with any other age group. In the younger woman in whom a nonsuspicious lesion is less well defined, re-examination within 2 to 3 months at a different point during the menstrual cycle may demonstrate resolution of the lesion, implying fibrocystic change. If any question remains, needle biopsy should be performed, or if the lesion is too indistinct causing concern for sampling error, excision may be considered.

Care must be taken when excising lesions in younger adolescents. In addition to considering the cosmetic outcome of the scar that will be life-long for the patient, the central subareolar breast bud can be mistaken for a new breast mass. This subareolar breast tissue should be spared because this is the origin of the ducts and deposition of fat that becomes the mature breast in the adult. Surgical damage of the breast bud has been reported to cause breast hypoplasia and significant disfigurement (52).

Young male patients referred for breast masses are predominantly adolescents found to have gynecomastia. Welch et al. (53) reviewed all male breast patients at a large tertiary pediatric hospital who were referred for ultrasound. The patients were between 1 month and 18 years of age, and 72% of the 25 patients, between 7 and 18 years of age, were found to have gynecomastia, 13 of which were unilateral and 3 bilateral, but asymmetric. Two patients had galactoceles, and two

had hematomas postoperative from gynecomastia surgery, whereas duct ectasia, a periductal hemangioma, and a neurofibroma constituted the remaining masses. In most cases, adolescent male gynecomastia can be observed because it will resolve in adulthood.

The Pregnant Patient

The pregnant patient presenting with a breast mass poses a dilemma. During pregnancy, the proliferative effect of circulating hormones causes the breasts to become increasingly nodular and engorged, making the physical examination extremely difficult. A nodule found before pregnancy or early in its course should be evaluated promptly and not observed. This is because the increasing proliferation of glandular elements and consequent nodularity during pregnancy and lactation can potentially obscure an initial finding. Ultrasound is the imaging modality of choice, because this will determine whether a mass represents a simple cyst, a galactocele, an abscess, or a benign lymph node. Liberman et al. (54) evaluated 23 women with pregnancy-associated breast cancer and found that the sensitivity of mammography and ultrasound were 78% and 100%, respectively.

Even with shielding, mammography is thought by many to be contraindicated under any circumstance during pregnancy. This is incorrect, and most likely because of undue concern among physicians (55), despite its delivery of only 0.5 mGy to the fetus in comparison with the 1.0 mGy of normal background radiation that the fetus receives over the 9 months of pregnancy (54,55). Although MRI is safe, the gadolinium used as the contrast agent is contraindicated (56), leaving MRI without contrast as an option that is less optimal than ultrasound.

If the mass is solid, needle biopsy should be attempted before mammogram because mammography will not provide a definitive diagnosis of a solid mass. Core biopsy in the pregnant patient before mammography will also reduce unnecessary fetal irradiation, even though the consequent risk is low. If malignancy is diagnosed, bilateral mammography with fetal shielding is then appropriate.

Core biopsy is the best option for tissue sampling in the pregnant patient. FNA is more difficult to perform and is associated with a higher risk of false–positive findings during pregnancy owing to the proliferative changes that occur within the breast (57). Although core biopsy during pregnancy has the added risk of milk fistula (58), this should not deter or raise the threshold for its use in the evaluation of a palpable mass. In theory, core biopsy should have a lower risk of milk fistula than excisional biopsy, but this has not been proven. Excisional biopsy is not appropriate during pregnancy when core biopsy is an option because of its unnecessary morbidity and cost.

Ductal Carcinoma *IN SITU*

As with any malignancy, DCIS can be found in association with a mass, although it most commonly now presents as calcifications on mammogram without abnormal examination findings. Comedo DCIS is generally high grade and more likely to contain invasion, which is why it is the only subtype likely to present with a mass, and why it accounted for most DCIS cases detected before mammography was routinely used (59). One series of 452 palpable solid breast masses demonstrated five with pure DCIS on excision, representing 12% of the 41 cancers found (60).

Core needle biopsy is the current standard of care for the diagnosis of breast masses; however, 10% to 20% of lesions diagnosed as DCIS by core needle biopsy are found to be understaged on final excision, demonstrating invasion (61). Risk factors for the presence of invasion have been investigated in multiple series, some of which have correlated it to the presence of a mass on examination or on imaging (61–63). Meijnen et al. (64) evaluated 172 DCIS lesions diagnosed by core biopsy, and found that a mass on examination or a mass on imaging were the two most significant independent risk factors for the presence of invasion.

It remains unclear whether DCIS that presents as a mass in men also has a higher risk of invasion because the series have been too small and too few to make generalizations. In one small series of four men having DCIS, three had a mass as their presenting symptom (65), whereas Hittmair et al. (66) reviewed DCIS in men found with and without associated invasion. A palpable mass was present in 19 of 30 cases (63%) found to have invasion, but among the 84 cases of pure DCIS, 49 (58%) were also associated with a mass. This association may be one of several DCIS characteristics that cannot be generalized from women to men.

The Patient with a Personal History of Cancer

The patient who has a history of breast cancer has usually undergone either breast-conserving therapy (BCT) or mastectomy. In those women who have had BCT, surgical scarring and radiation-induced changes may make evaluation more difficult. Mammography after BCT is less sensitive overall and specifically in the quadrant of the prior surgery, which may explain why 45% of recurrences after BCT can only be detected by palpation (67). In the patient who has had a mastectomy without reconstruction, abnormal nodularity on examination is most commonly found in the scar or skin and should immediately undergo biopsy, as imaging is likely to add little to the evaluation. In those having had a mastectomy and reconstruction, ultrasound or MRI may assist in characterizing recurrences. Imaging may be of benefit in this setting so that adequate surgical planning can help to minimize any risk to the reconstruction.

OTHER MASS-FORMING LESIONS

Hematoma

Hematomas of the breast are most commonly reported as a result of iatrogenic intervention, either in evaluation of a breast lesion or subsequent to its treatment, although spontaneous hematomas have been reported (68). They have also been rarely reported to mimic carcinoma identically on presentation (69). Physicians most likely encounter breast hematomas on examination after core biopsy, where it may be difficult to determine whether a lesion is truly palpable or whether a thickening in that location is caused by a small amount of bleeding. Core needle biopsy can result in hematoma and, although significant bleeding is uncommon, a malignancy may be obscured in extreme examples (11,70). Some series note a postbiopsy hematoma rate of greater than 1% (47), although one study found hematomas in 51% of 113 lesions undergoing stereotactic core biopsy (11). When any question about a lesion's palpability exists, needle localization should be planned in case the thickened area is solely owing to hematoma and resolves by the date of surgery, leaving a nonpalpable mass.

The appropriate management of a hematoma varies with its presentation. A palpable mass may be present with or without ecchymosis, which can sometimes extend laterally to the chest wall, below the inframammary fold, and over to the opposite breast. In most cases, observation of the hematoma with supportive garments and analgesics other than nonsteroidal anti-inflammatory drug (NSAID) analgesics is sufficient, although hematomas in the postoperative period require a lower threshold for re-exploration. Expanding hematomas, in particular, should be explored and evacuated with the intent to achieve hemostasis.

Seroma

Seromas are localized regions of serous fluid that usually occur after iatrogenic intervention. In some cases, ultrasound may be required to differentiate a seroma from a solid nodule, depending on the degree of distension of the surrounding tissue. The breast contains an extensive lymphatic network, and excisional biopsy or lumpectomy cavities, total mastectomy sites, and axillary wounds may all develop seromas. Although these are advantageous at local breast excision sites by maintaining breast contour, large seromas may accumulate and create a palpable mass. When present after mastectomy, they can impede flap healing by interfering with their adherence to the chest wall. Finally, a postreconstruction seroma can create a palpable mass that is most easily evaluated with ultrasound (71).

Few data exist on what predisposes women undergoing BCT to develop significant breast seromas. Most investigations have focused on those that develop after axillary dissection, but factors that are known to contribute to seroma formation, generally, include the use of cautery (72), the extent of the dissection and amount of disease present, primary tumor size, patient weight, the use of chemotherapy, and the type of surgery performed (73). Seromas are usually of little consequence and confer few symptoms, but when they become bothersome to the patient they may be ameliorated with a small number of repeated aspirations (74).

Fat Necrosis

Fat necrosis is a phenomenon that is occasionally seen in the breast owing to its high fat content, and is significantly correlated with trauma or surgical intervention (75). Fat necrosis results from lipase-induced aseptic saponification of adipose tissue that can create mass lesions that are tough to distinguish from carcinoma. This difficulty was first documented in 1920 by Lee and Adair (76), who reported the case of a woman with a history of breast trauma who was later thought to have a breast carcinoma. This patient underwent a radical mastectomy, although the pathology only demonstrated fat necrosis and no evidence of malignancy.

An oil or lipid cyst, one manifestation of fat necrosis that can be seen on imaging, is composed of a confined pool of neutral lipid surrounded by a membrane. This pathognomonic finding is not present in all cases, but when evident, demonstrates a characteristic lucent center with a water-density rim which may calcify with time (77). Demonstration of such a lesion does not require further evaluation, especially with a history of trauma. Many cases of fat necrosis, however, do not present in this fashion and may contain calcifications or fibrosis which can appear as a spiculated mass, and may have a scirrhous feel on examination. Without a history of trauma or the presence of an oil cyst, and with any question remaining that makes the diagnosis uncertain, areas of potential fat necrosis should undergo core or excisional biopsy for confirmation (78). On diagnosis, no treatment is required.

Hamartomas

Hamartomas, previously known as fibroadenolipomas or lipofibroadenomas because of their components, are benign lesions which are often palpable as a mass and can grow to extremely large sizes (79,80), pushing the breast tissue outward as they grow rather than replacing it. Although they have been reported in men (81), they are most commonly seen in women, and traditionally appear mammographically as a fibrofatty mass, but can have a variable mammographic appearance (82). Ultrasound appearance is usually solid, but one series of 35 hamartomas demonstrated that these masses may have cystic regions, present in 24% of the cases (83). Although most hamartomas have a benign radiographic appearance, biopsy is recommended as with other solid masses to confirm the diagnosis.

Neither FNA nor core biopsy can accurately make the diagnosis of a hamartoma without correlation to imaging findings because of the variety of elements required to make a diagnosis. FNA, in particular, is insufficient, resulting at best in a diagnosis of a nonspecified, benign lesion (39) because the cytologic features overlap with other benign disease (84). Core biopsy also often yields an insufficient variety of tissue types for a diagnosis, and surgical excision may be required when imaging correlation is not performed to reach a definitive diagnosis. Hamartomas, on occasion, have been seen in association with atypia, as well as *in situ* and invasive malignancies (39,85), but correlation to these more concerning pathologic entities has not been found consistently enough to universally recommend surgical excision.

If the diagnosis of hamartoma is entertained on evaluation of a breast mass, mammograms should be obtained and core biopsy attempted, while providing the pathologist with the imaging and clinical findings. Surgical excision may be required for definitive diagnosis, and clear margins should be sought because of the possibility of recurrence (39). As with any large solid mass, discomfort or anxiety regarding the lesion is an indication for excision, as is enlargement on subsequent follow-up.

MANAGEMENT SUMMARY

- Palpable masses should never be dismissed because imaging is negative, because of young age, male gender, or because of a lack of risk factors, such as a family history of cancer, especially if the mass is discrete or suspicious.
- Mammography should be performed before biopsy of a solid mass. If further characterization is required, ultrasound characterizes whether it is cystic or solid, and suspicious or benign-appearing.
- MRI is of little benefit in the workup of a palpable breast mass.
- Core biopsy or FNA is the first-line modality of choice for sampling a breast mass. Excisional biopsy is no longer the standard of care when core or fine needle biopsy is feasible, and incisional biopsy is rarely beneficial.
- The triple test is the standard of care for evaluation of benign and malignant solid lesions, even when imaging appears benign.
- Cysts can be aspirated for confirmation of their benign nature or patient comfort, but cytology of benign, non-bloody cyst fluid is not sent, because it can confound the evaluation by appearing atypical when benign.
- Pregnant patients and those who are young pose a diagnostic challenge because of breast density. Ultrasound is the modality of choice for breast mass evaluation and a low threshold for prompt evaluation over observation should be maintained in gravid patients.

References

1. Hindle WH. Breast mass evaluation. *Clin Obstet Gynecol* 2002;45:750–757.
2. Zylstra S, D'Orsi CJ, Ricci BA, et al. Defense of breast cancer malpractice claims. *Breast J* 2001;7:76–90.
3. Barber MD, Jack W, Dixon JM. Diagnostic delay in breast cancer. *Br J Surg* 2004; 91:49–53.
4. Smith RA, Saslow D, Sawyer KA, et al. American Cancer Society guidelines for breast cancer screening: update 2003. *CA Cancer J Clin* 2003;53:141–169.
5. Saslow D, Boetes C, Burke W, et al. American Cancer Society guidelines for breast screening with MRI as an adjunct to mammography. *CA Cancer J Clin* 2007;57: 75–89.
5a. Bleicher RJ, Ciocca RM, Egleston BL, et al. The influence of routine pretreatment MRI on time to treatment, mastectomy rate, and positive margins. *In* Grunberg SM (ed): *Proc Am Soc Clin Oncol 2008 Breast Cancer Symposium*, Washington, DC: Cadmus Professional Publications 2008; 199.
6. Bland KI, Copeland EM. *The Breast. Comprehensive management of benign and malignant disorders.* St. Louis: Saunders, 2004.
7. Vargas HI, Vargas MP, Eldrageely K, et al. Outcomes of surgical and sonographic assessment of breast masses in women younger than 30. *Am Surg* 2005;71: 716–719.
8. Morrow M, Wong S, Venta L. The evaluation of breast masses in women younger than forty years of age. *Surgery* 1998;124:634–640; discussion 640–631.
9. Baker LH. Breast Cancer Detection Demonstration Project: five-year summary report. *CA Cancer J Clin* 1982;32:194–225.
10. Edeiken S. Mammography and palpable cancer of the breast. *Cancer* 1988;61: 263–265.
11. Hann LE, Liberman L, Dershaw DD, et al. Mammography immediately after stereotaxic breast biopsy: is it necessary? *AJR Am J Roentgenol* 1995;165:59–62.
12. Bluemke DA, Gatsonis CA, Chen MH, et al. Magnetic resonance imaging of the breast prior to biopsy. *JAMA* 2004;292:2735–2742.
13. Hines SL, Tan WW, Yasrebi M, et al. The role of mammography in male patients with breast symptoms. *Mayo Clin Proc* 2007;82:297–300.
14. Borgen PI, Wong GY, Vlamis V, et al. Current management of male breast cancer. A review of 104 cases. *Ann Surg* 1992;215:451–457; discussion 457–459.
15. Ciatto S, Cariaggi P, Bulgaresi P. The value of routine cytologic examination of breast cyst fluids. *Acta Cytol* 1987;31:301–304.
16. Hilton SV, Leopold GR, Olson LK, et al. Real-time breast sonography: application in 300 consecutive patients. *AJR Am J Roentgenol* 1986;147:479–486.
17. Hughes LE, Bundred NJ. Breast macrocysts. *World J Surg* 1989;13:711–714.
18. Stavros AT. *Breast ultrasound.* Philadelphia: Lippincott Williams & Wilkins, 2004.
19. Sickles EA, Filly RA, Callen PW. Benign breast lesions: ultrasound detection and diagnosis. *Radiology* 1984;151:467–470.
20. Berg WA, Campassi CI, Ioffe OB. Cystic lesions of the breast: sonographic-pathologic correlation. *Radiology* 2003;227:183–191.
21. Venta LA, Kim JP, Pelloski CE, et al. Management of complex breast cysts. *AJR Am J Roentgenol* 1999;173:1331–1336.
22. Pisano ED, Gatsonis C, Hendrick E, et al. Diagnostic performance of digital versus film mammography for breast-cancer screening. *N Engl J Med* 2005;353: 1773–1783.
23. Buchanan CL, Morris EA, Dorn PL, et al. Utility of breast magnetic resonance imaging in patients with occult primary breast cancer. *Ann Surg Oncol* 2005;12: 1045–1053.
24. Dupont WD, Page DL, Parl FF, et al. Long-term risk of breast cancer in women with fibroadenoma. *N Engl J Med* 1994;331:10–15.
25. Frantz VK, Pickren JW, Melcher GW, et al. Incidence of chronic cystic disease in so-called "normal breasts". A study based on 225 postmortem examinations. *Cancer* 1951;4:762–783.
26. Wilkinson S, Anderson TJ, Rifkind E, et al. Fibroadenoma of the breast: a follow-up of conservative management. *Br J Surg* 1989;76:390–391.
27. van Dam PA, Van Goethem ML, Kersschot E, et al. Palpable solid breast masses: retrospective single- and multimodality evaluation of 201 lesions. *Radiology* 1988;166:435–439.
28. Houssami N, Irwig L, Simpson JM, et al. Sydney Breast Imaging Accuracy Study: comparative sensitivity and specificity of mammography and sonography in young women with symptoms. *AJR Am J Roentgenol* 2003;180:935–940.
29. Bode MK, Rissanen T, Apaja-Sarkkinen M. Ultrasonography and core needle biopsy in the differential diagnosis of fibroadenoma and tumor phyllodes. *Acta Radiol* 2007;48:708–713.
30. Kriege M, Brekelmans CT, Boetes C, et al. Efficacy of MRI and mammography for breast-cancer screening in women with a familial or genetic predisposition. *N Engl J Med* 2004;351:427–437.
31. Foxcroft LM, Evans EB, Porter AJ. Difficulties in the pre-operative diagnosis of phyllodes tumours of the breast: a study of 84 cases. *Breast* 2007;16:27–37.
32. Meyer JE, Amin E, Lindfors KK, et al. Medullary carcinoma of the breast: mammographic and US appearance. *Radiology* 1989;170:79–82.
33. Steinberg JL, Trudeau ME, Ryder DE, et al. Combined fine-needle aspiration, physical examination and mammography in the diagnosis of palpable breast masses: their relation to outcome for women with primary breast cancer. *Can J Surg* 1996;39:302–311.
34. Vetto J, Pommier R, Schmidt W, et al. Use of the "triple test" for palpable breast lesions yields high diagnostic accuracy and cost savings. *Am J Surg* 1995;169: 519–522.
35. Valdes EK, Boolbol SK, Cohen JM, et al. Malignant transformation of a breast fibroadenoma to cystosarcoma phyllodes: case report and review of the literature. *Am Surg* 2005;71:348–353.
36. Gordon PB, Gagnon FA, Lanzkowsky L. Solid breast masses diagnosed as fibroadenoma at fine-needle aspiration biopsy: acceptable rates of growth at long-term follow-up. *Radiology* 2003;229:233–238.
37. Martin HE, Ellis EB. Biopsy by needle puncture and aspiration. *Ann Surg* 1930; 92:169–181.
38. Giard RW, Hermans J. The value of aspiration cytologic examination of the breast. A statistical review of the medical literature. *Cancer* 1992;69:2104–2110.
39. Tse GM, Law BK, Ma TK, et al. Hamartoma of the breast: a clinicopathological review. *J Clin Pathol* 2002;55:951–954.
40. Mitnick JS, Vazquez MF, Plesser KP, et al. Distinction between postsurgical changes and carcinoma by means of stereotaxic fine-needle aspiration biopsy after reduction mammaplasty. *Radiology* 1993;188:457–462.
41. Gisvold JJ, Goellner JR, Grant CS, et al. Breast biopsy: a comparative study of stereotaxically guided core and excisional techniques. *AJR Am J Roentgenol* 1994;162:815–820.
42. Haigh PI, Hansen NM, Qi K, et al. Biopsy method and excision volume do not affect success rate of subsequent sentinel lymph node dissection in breast cancer. *Ann Surg Oncol* 2000;7:21–27.
43. McMasters KM, Tuttle TM, Carlson DJ, et al. Sentinel lymph node biopsy for breast cancer: a suitable alternative to routine axillary dissection in multi-institutional practice when optimal technique is used. *J Clin Oncol* 2000;18:2560–2566.
44. Tafra L, Lannin DR, Swanson MS, et al. Multicenter trial of sentinel node biopsy for breast cancer using both technetium sulfur colloid and isosulfan blue dye. *Ann Surg* 2001;233:51–59.
45. Krag D, Weaver D, Ashikaga T, et al. The sentinel node in breast cancer—a multicenter validation study. *N Engl J Med* 1998;339:941–946.

46. Krag DN, Anderson SJ, Julian TB, et al. Technical outcomes of sentinel-lymph-node resection and conventional axillary-lymph-node dissection in patients with clinically node-negative breast cancer: results from the NSABP B-32 randomised phase III trial. *Lancet Oncol* 2007;8:881–888.

46a. Westenend PJ, Sever AR, Beekman-De Voider HJ, Liem SJ. A comparison of aspiration cytology and core needle biopsy in the evaluation of breast lesions. *Cancer*, Apr 25 2001;93(2):146–150.

47. Parker SH, Burbank F, Jackman RJ, et al. Percutaneous large-core breast biopsy: a multi-institutional study. *Radiology* 1994;193:359–364.

48. Gibson GR, Lesnikoski BA, Yoo J, et al. A comparison of ink-directed and traditional whole-cavity re-excision for breast lumpectomy specimens with positive margins. *Ann Surg Oncol* 2001;8:693–704.

49. Rosen PP. Pathological assessment of nonpalpable breast lesions. *Semin Surg Oncol* 1991;7:257–260.

50. Underwood JC, Parsons MA, Harris SC, et al. Frozen section appearances simulating invasive lobular carcinoma in breast tissue adjacent to inflammatory lesions and biopsy sites. *Histopathology* 1988;13:232–234.

51. Bleicher RJ, Abrahamse P, Hawley ST, et al. The influence of age on the breast surgery decision-making process. *Ann Surg Oncol* 2008;15:854–862.

52. Goyal A, Mansel RE. Iatrogenic injury to the breast bud causing breast hypoplasia. *Postgrad Med J* 2003;79:235–236.

53. Welch ST, Babcock DS, Ballard ET. Sonography of pediatric male breast masses: gynecomastia and beyond. *Pediatr Radiol* 2004;34:952–957.

54. Liberman L, Giess CS, Dershaw DD, et al. Imaging of pregnancy-associated breast cancer. *Radiology* 1994;191:245–248.

55. Ratnapalan S, Bona N, Chandra K, et al. Physicians' perceptions of teratogenic risk associated with radiography and CT during early pregnancy. *AJR Am J Roentgenol* 2004;182:1107–1109.

56. Coakley F, Gould R. Safety of imaging during pregnancy: guidelines for the use of CT and MRI during pregnancy and lactation. Available at http://www.radiology.ucsf.edu/instruction/abdominal/ab_handbook/05-CT_MRI_preg.html. Accessed December 25, 2007.

57. Mitre BK, Kanbour AI, Mauser N. Fine needle aspiration biopsy of breast carcinoma in pregnancy and lactation. *Acta Cytol* 1997;41:1121–1130.

58. Schackmuth EM, Harlow CL, Norton LW. Milk fistula: a complication after core breast biopsy. *AJR Am J Roentgenol* 1993;161:961–962.

59. Winchester DP, Jeske JM, Goldschmidt RA. The diagnosis and management of ductal carcinoma in-situ of the breast. *CA Cancer J Clin* 2000;50:184–200.

60. Osuch JR, Reeves MJ, Pathak DR, et al. BREASTAID: clinical results from early development of a clinical decision rule for palpable solid breast masses. *Ann Surg* 2003;238:728–737.

61. Jackman RJ, Burbank F, Parker SH, et al. Stereotactic breast biopsy of nonpalpable lesions. determinants of ductal carcinoma *in situ* underestimation rates. *Radiology* 2001;218:497–502.

62. Huo L, Sneige N, Hunt KK, et al. Predictors of invasion in patients with core-needle biopsy-diagnosed ductal carcinoma *in situ* and recommendations for a selective approach to sentinel lymph node biopsy in ductal carcinoma *in situ*. *Cancer* 2006;107:1760–1768.

63. King TA, Farr GH, Jr., Cederbom GJ, et al. A mass on breast imaging predicts coexisting invasive carcinoma in patients with a core biopsy diagnosis of ductal carcinoma in situ. *Am Surg* 2001;67:907–912.

64. Meijnen P, Oldenburg HS, Loo CE, et al. Risk of invasion and axillary lymph node metastasis in ductal carcinoma in situ diagnosed by core-needle biopsy. *Br J Surg* 2007;94:952–956.

65. Camus MG, Joshi MG, Mackarem G, et al. Ductal carcinoma *in situ* of the male breast. *Cancer* 1994;74:1289–1293.

66. Hittmair AP, Lininger RA, Tavassoli FA. Ductal carcinoma in situ (DCIS) in the male breast: a morphologic study of 84 cases of pure DCIS and 30 cases of DCIS associated with invasive carcinoma—a preliminary report. *Cancer* 1998;83: 2139–2149.

67. Orel SG, Troupin RH, Patterson EA, et al. Breast cancer recurrence after lumpectomy and irradiation: role of mammography in detection. *Radiology* 1992;183:201–206.

68. Kanegusuku MS, Rodrigues D, Urban LA, et al. Recurrent spontaneous breast hematoma: report of a case and review of the literature. *Rev Hosp Clin Fac Med Sao Paulo* 2001;56:179–182.

69. Huston TL, Tabatabai N, Eisen C, et al. Hematoma mimicking local recurrence of breast cancer. *Breast J* 2006;12:274–275.

70. Deutch BM, Schwartz MR, Fodera T, et al. Stereotactic core breast biopsy of a minimal carcinoma complicated by a large hematoma: a management dilemma. *Radiology* 1997;202:431–433.

71. Shestak KC, Ganott MA, Harris KM, et al. Breast masses in the augmentation mammaplasty patient: the role of ultrasound. *Plast Reconstr Surg* 1993;92: 209–216.

72. Porter KA, O'Connor S, Rimm E, et al. Electrocautery as a factor in seroma formation following mastectomy. *Am J Surg* 1998;176:8–11.

73. Gonzalez EA, Saltzstein EC, Riedner CS, et al. Seroma formation following breast cancer surgery. *Breast J* 2003;9:385–388.

74. Yamamoto D, Yamada M, Okugawa H, et al. A comparison between electrocautery and scalpel plus scissor in breast conserving surgery. *Oncol Rep* 2003;10: 1729–1732.

75. Bilgen IG, Ustun EE, Memis A. Fat necrosis of the breast: clinical, mammographic and sonographic features. *Eur J Radiol* 2001;39:92–99.

76. Lee BJ, Adair F. Traumatic fat necrosis of the female breast and its differentiation from carcinoma. *Ann Surg* 1920;72:188–195.

77. Evers K, Troupin RH. Lipid cyst: classic and atypical appearances. *AJR Am J Roentgenol* 1991;157:271–273.

78. Harrison RL, Britton P, Warren R, et al. Can we be sure about a radiological diagnosis of fat necrosis of the breast? *Clin Radiol* 2000;55:119–123.

79. Weinzweig N, Botts J, Marcus E. Giant hamartoma of the breast. *Plast Reconstr Surg* 2001;107:1216–1220.

80. Sanal HT, Ersoz N, Altinel O, et al. Giant hamartoma of the breast. *Breast J* 2006;12:84–85.

81. Ravakhah K, Javadi N, Simms R. Hamartoma of the breast in a man: first case report. *Breast J* 2001;7:266–268.

82. Helvie MA, Adler DD, Rebner M, et al. Breast hamartomas: variable mammographic appearance. *Radiology* 1989;170:417–421.

83. Wahner-Roedler DL, Sebo TJ, Gisvold JJ. Hamartomas of the breast: clinical, radiologic, and pathologic manifestations. *Breast J* 2001;7:101–105.

84. Herbert M, Schvimer M, Zehavi S, et al. Breast hamartoma: fine-needle aspiration cytologic finding. *Cancer* 2003;99:255–258.

85. Coyne J, Hobbs FM, Boggis C, et al. Lobular carcinoma in a mammary hamartoma. *J Clin Pathol* 1992;45:936–937.

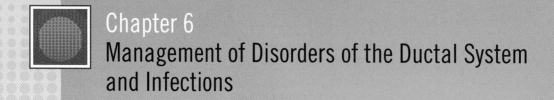

Chapter 6
Management of Disorders of the Ductal System and Infections

J. Michael Dixon and Nigel James Bundred

Disorders of the ductal system can present as nipple discharge, nipple inversion, breast mass, or periareolar infection.

 ## NIPPLE DISCHARGE

Nipple discharge accounts for approximately 5% of referrals to breast clinics (1). It is a frightening symptom because of the fear of breast cancer. Approximately 95% of women presenting to the hospital with nipple discharge have a benign cause for the discharge (2). Discharge associated with a significant underlying pathologic process is spontaneous, usually arises from a single duct, is persistent, troublesome, and is blood-stained or contains blood on testing. For this reason, the physician must establish whether the discharge is spontaneous or induced, whether it arises from a single or from multiple ducts, and whether it is from one or both breasts. The characteristics of the discharge also need to be defined: whether it is viscous or watery and whether it is serous, serosanguineous, bloody, clear, milky, green, or blue-black. The frequency of discharge and the amount of fluid also need to be assessed; this assessment is important for milky discharge, which should be considered to be galactorrhea only if it is copious and arises from multiple ducts of both breasts (3).

Investigations

Assessment includes performance of a complete physical examination (Chapter 4) to identify the presence or absence of a breast mass. During the examination, firm pressure should be applied around the areola to identify the site of any dilated duct (pressure over a dilated duct will produce the discharge); this is helpful in defining where an incision should be made for any subsequent surgery. The nipple is squeezed with firm digital pressure and, if fluid is expressed, the site and character of the discharge are recorded. Testing the discharge for hemoglobin determines whether blood is present. Less than 10% of patients who have a bloodstained discharge or who have a discharge containing moderate or large amounts of blood have an underlying malignancy. The absence of blood in nipple discharge is not an absolute indication that the discharge is not related to an underlying malignancy, as demonstrated in a recent series of 108 patients where the sensitivity of hemoccult testing was only 50% (4). Age is said to be an important predictor of malignancy; in one series, 3% of patients younger than 40 years of age, 10% of patients between ages 40 and 60 years, and 32% of patients older than 60 years who presented with nipple discharge as their only symptom were found to have cancers (5). Cytology of nipple discharge is of little value in determining whether duct excision should be performed. In two studies of 1,009 and 338 patients with nipple discharge, cytology sensitivity for malignancy was 34.6% (2) and 46.5% (6), respectively.

Two related techniques have emerged: ductal lavage, in which fluid-yielding nipple ducts are cannulated at their orifices and lavaged with saline while the breast is intermittently massaged (Chapter 21); and ductoscopy, in which discharging or fluid-yielding duct orifices are dilated and intubated with a microendoscope, and the lumen directly visualized. Both techniques have significant potential in terms of allowing repeated

sampling of ductal epithelium over time and diagnosing the cause of nipple discharge (7). Fiberoptic ductoscopy applied to 415 patients with nipple discharge was successful in identifying a lesion in 166 patients (40%) (8). Of these 166, 11 were subsequently shown to have ductal carcinoma *in situ* (DCIS); ductoscopy was suspect in 8, a sensitivity of 73%, with the specificity being 99% and the positive predictive value 80% (8). DCIS in this series tended to affect more peripheral ducts compared with papillomas. Numerous other small series have been published evaluating ductoscopy in nipple discharge (9–12). The sensitivity for malignancy in these other series varies from 81% (11) to 100% (9). Ductoscopy appears of particular value for directing duct excision (9,10) and for detecting deeper lesions that can be missed by blind central duct excision (11). Surgical resection of lesions visualized on ductoscopy is facilitated by simple transillumination of the skin overlying the lesion during ductoscopy. Lesions visualized by ductoscopy can be sampled; in one report, 38 of 46 women with biopsy-proved papillomas were observed for 2 years with no case of missed cancer becoming evident (11). Newer biopsy devices using vacuum assistance are now available for diagnostic assessment and can be ductoscope or sonographically guided (12).

Ductal lavage has been investigated as a method of increasing diagnostic accuracy in patients having ductoscopy. It increases cell yield approximately 100 times compared with analysis of discharge alone, averaging 5,000 cells per washed duct in one series (8). The sensitivity for cytology obtained by ductal lavage in this series was 64%, with a 100% positive predictive value. Another series reported a lower sensitivity of 50%, but a high specificity of 94.3% and a high overall accuracy rate (87.9%) (13). Both ductoscopy and ductal lavage remain investigative techniques, and the evidence that they have an important role in the detection of significant breast disease is limited to a few small series (7).

Imaging of the ductal tree by ductography or galactography can identify intraductal lesions. Although this investigation has only a 60% sensitivity for malignancy, a filling defect or duct cutoff has a high positive predictive value for the presence of either a papilloma or a carcinoma (2,14). In one report, ductography-directed excisions were significantly more likely than central duct excisions to identify a specific underlying lesion (15). The value of both ductography and ductoscopy is that they allow identification of the site of any lesion in younger women, allowing localization and excision of the causative lesion while retaining the ability to lactate.

Mammography has a high overall sensitivity for breast cancer, but not all malignant lesions that cause nipple discharge are visible mammographically and most patients with nipple discharge have negative mammograms (Chapter 12). In one recent series, the sensitivity of mammography for malignancy in patients with nipple discharge was only 57% (4). Nonetheless, mammography should be performed in women of appropriate age, because if a lesion is visualized it may help establish the cause of the discharge. Ultrasonography can sometimes identify papillomas and malignant lesions in the ducts close to the nipple, thus allowing Mammotome-directed excision by sonography (12,15,16) (Chapter 16). Patients with a visible lesion on ultrasonography were significantly more likely to have malignancy than those women with a negative scan in one series (15). Where a papilloma is visualized on imaging, vacuum-assisted

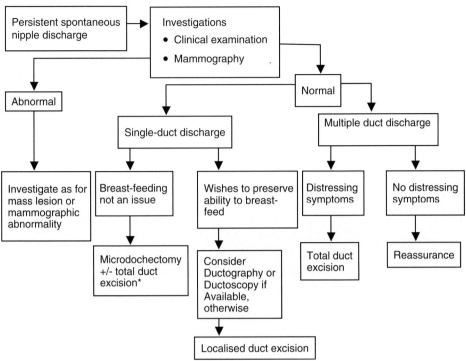

*See Indications section in Total Duct Excision

FIGURE 6.1. Investigation of nipple discharge.

core biopsy provides tissue for diagnosis and, in selected cases, can control symptoms by completely removing the lesion (12,16,17). In large papillomas, magnetic resonance imaging (MRI) may aid assessment of the presence of malignancy, which is more likely if an enhancing rim is seen, but histopathologic assessment remains essential. At the present time MRI has no role in the diagnosis of nipple discharge (Chapter 14).

If clinical examination demonstrates a mass lesion or mammography or ultrasonography raises suspicion of malignancy, then core biopsy of the lesion should be performed and the lesion managed appropriately (Section VII: Management of Primary Invasive Breast Cancer). Otherwise, when no abnormality is found on clinical or mammographic examination, patients are treated according to whether the discharge is from a single duct or multiple ducts (Fig. 6.1). Surgery is indicated in cases of spontaneous discharge from a single duct that is confirmed on clinical examination and has one of the following characteristics:

- Is bloodstained or contains moderate or large amounts of blood on testing
- Is persistent (occurs on at least two occasions per week)
- Is associated with a mass
- Is a new development in a woman older than 50 years of age, but is not thick or cheesy

Discharge from multiple ducts normally requires surgery only when it causes distressing symptoms, such as persistent staining of clothes (1). Some breast units adopt an age-related policy: Patients younger than age 30 years who have serous, serosanguineous, or watery discharge are observed, with microdochectomy reserved for cases in which discharge persists at review (18); patients older than 45 years of age are treated by a formal excision of the major duct system on the affected side; patients between 30 and 45 years of age are deemed suitable for either approach (18). The current evidence is that total duct excision is

more effective than microdochectomy at establishing a specific diagnosis and not missing any underlying malignancy in women more than 40 years of age (19). Nowadays, many units incorporate ductography and ductoscopy into their management protocols, particularly in younger women (Fig. 6.1). The problem is how to treat a patient with nipple discharge in whom imaging, including ductography or ductoscopy and ductal lavage, fails to identify any serious lesion. Because pathologic discharge is persistent and troublesome, a period of observation, particularly in younger women (≤35 years of age), is appropriate if the history of discharge is short. If spontaneous discharge persists (≥2 per week) at review 4 to 6 weeks later and discharge can be expressed from a single duct on examination, then surgical excision is indicated to treat and establish the cause of the discharge.

Causes of Nipple Discharge
Physiologic Causes

In two-thirds of nonlactating women, a small quantity of fluid can be expressed from the ducts of the nipple if the nipple is cleaned, the breast massaged, and gentle suction pressure applied (20,21). This fluid is physiologic secretion and varies in color from white to yellow to green to brown to blue-black (1); it is thought to represent apocrine secretion, the breast being a modified apocrine gland. These discharging ducts can be cannulated and lavaged with saline to obtain large numbers of epithelial cells (8). These cells can then be examined microscopically; ongoing studies are evaluating whether this may be a valuable technique to screen women at high risk (7). This physiologic secretion usually emanates from multiple ducts, and the discharge from each duct can vary in color. Women often first notice discharge after a warm bath or after nipple manipulation, and the discharge is not usually spontaneous or bloodstained. Once this condition is diagnosed, no specific treatment is required, and reassurance should be given.

Intraductal Papilloma

A true intraductal papilloma develops in one of the major sub-areolar ducts and is the most common lesion causing a serous or serosanguineous discharge. In approximately half of women with papillomas, the discharge is bloody; in the other half, it is serous (14). Papillomas should be differentiated from papillary hyperplasia, which affects the terminal duct lobular unit and can also cause nipple discharge. Central papillomas consist of epithelium covering arborescent fronds of fibrovascular stroma attached to the wall of the duct by a stalk. The covering epithelium has a two-cell population, with lining cuboidal or columnar cells covering an underlying layer of myoepithelial cells. A mass may be felt on examination in as many as one-third of cases (18). Occasionally, the papilloma is so close to the nipple that it can be seen in the orifice of the duct at the nipple. The treatment of choice is microdochectomy. A solitary papilloma is not thought to be a premalignant lesion (22) and is considered by some to be an aberration rather than a true disease process (1). Papillary lesions can be difficult to characterize on core biopsies. Any atypia is an indication for biopsy, but even benign papillary lesions on core are occasionally shown to be malignant following excision.

Multiple Intraductal Papillomas

In approximately 10% of cases of intraductal papilloma, multiple lesions are found; usually, two or three occur, often in the same duct. The term *multiple intraductal papilloma syndrome* is reserved for a rare and distinctive group of patients in whom one duct system is involved by large and often palpable papillomas with a peripheral distribution (20). Nipple discharge is less common in this group than in patients with a solitary intraductal papilloma. In one study, multiple papillomas were found to be associated with an increased risk of breast cancer (22), but any increased risk is almost certainly associated with areas of atypical epithelial hyperplasia rather than with the papillomas themselves (23). Repeated excision of papillomas in patients

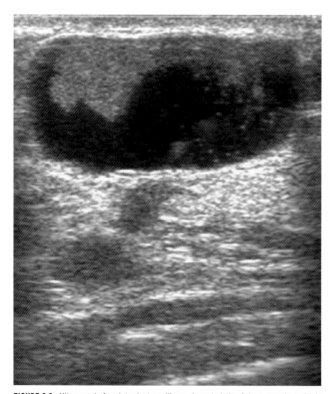

FIGURE 6.2. Ultrasound of an intraduct papilloma characteristic of those seen in multiple papilloma syndrome—such lesions can be excised by mammotomy.

with multiple intraductal papillomas involving a breast segment can result in significant breast asymmetry. One option in such patients is to excise such lesions using ultrasound guidance by a mammotome (Fig. 6.2). This provides sufficient material for the pathologist to assess whether all the lesions are benign.

Juvenile Papillomatosis

A rare condition, juvenile papillomatosis affects women between the ages of 10 and 44 years (24). The patient usually presents with a discrete mass lesion. In one series of 13 patients, 11 had peripheral and 2 central lesions (25). Three of the 13 presented with nipple discharge; 2 had a palpable peripheral mass lesion, and the third had nipple discharge alone. Treatment is by complete excision. Patients with this condition may be at some increased risk of subsequent breast cancer, and close clinical and radiological surveillance of any woman with this condition is indicated (26).

Carcinoma

An invasive or noninvasive cancer can cause nipple discharge. Only rarely does an invasive cancer cause nipple discharge in the absence of a clinical mass. In most series, DCIS is responsible for up to 10% of unilateral nipple discharges (2). Nipple discharge alone or in association with a mass or Paget's disease is the presenting feature in approximately one-third of symptomatic *in situ* cancers (27). With the advent of mammography, increasing numbers of noninvasive cancers are being detected and, overall, nipple discharge is the presenting symptom in 7% to 8% of cases of DCIS (Chapter 26). Scanty data exist on the frequency with which these *in situ* cancers are visible on mammography. A significant percentage are not visible on mammography and so mammography is unreliable in excluding malignancy (28–30). A diagnosis of invasive or noninvasive cancer is often established only by microdochectomy, but this operation is rarely, if ever, therapeutic. Traditionally, in patients with *in situ* and invasive cancer presenting with nipple discharge the nipple is excised as part of the surgical therapeutic procedure. This is based on the high rate of reported occult nipple–areolar complex involvement (31). A number of studies have demonstrated, however, that breast-conserving surgery can be performed in patients presenting with DCIS or invasive carcinoma and nipple discharge (32–36). Bauer et al. (33), in 1998, reported that 11 of 43 patients with breast cancer with nipple discharge were successfully treated by breast-conserving surgery. Obedian and Haffty (34) reported on 17 patients and Cabioglu et al. (31) reported on 24 patients. More recent publications have confirmed the success of such breast conserving surgery in such patients (35,36). In the study by Cabioglu et al. (31), nipple preserving surgery was successfully performed in one-half of all patients presenting with breast cancer and nipple discharge. There were no local recurrences in those patients who had radiotherapy postoperatively. Concerns about the safety of nipple preserving breast-conserving surgery in patients with nipple discharge were raised by the retrospective review of Obedian and Haffty (34). Local disease recurrence was noted in 6 of 17 patients with nipple discharge. Patients in this series who underwent central excisions incorporating the nipple had a lower recurrence rate than those patients who had conservation of the nipple–areolar complex. However, this difference did not reach significance. The problem with this series is that margins were not adequately documented in most patients. It cannot, therefore, be determined whether high local recurrence rates are attributable to residual tumour underneath the nipple. Although Cabioglu et al. (31) argue that long-term results obtained from larger series will be required before definitive conclusions can be drawn, they conclude that nipple preserving breast-conserving surgery can be performed safely if negative margins are achieved and appropriate radiotherapy or systemic therapies administered.

Bloody Nipple Discharge in Pregnancy

Nipple discharge with blood present, either visibly or cytologically, during pregnancy or lactation is common. In 20% of women who experience nipple discharge during pregnancy, blood is evident on testing (37). The likely cause is hypervascularity of developing breast tissue; it is benign, usually settles quickly and requires no specific treatment (38).

Galactorrhea

Galactorrhea should be diagnosed if there is copious bilateral milky discharge not associated with pregnancy or breast-feeding. A careful drug history should be taken because a number of drugs, particularly psychotropic agents, cause hyperprolactinemia. Blood should be taken to test for prolactin, and if prolactin levels are significantly elevated ($\geq$1,000 mU/L) in the absence of any drug cause, then a search for a pituitary tumor should be instituted (18). The diagnosis of hyperprolactinemia is suggested by a history of galactorrhea, amenorrhea, and relative infertility. Galactorrhea disappears after appropriate drug therapy or surgical removal of the adenoma. Appropriate drug therapy includes administration of cabergoline because bromocriptine produces significant side effects in up to one-third of patients. For patients with troublesome galactorrhea who are intolerant of medication, bilateral total duct ligation is effective but is rarely indicated.

Periductal Mastitis and Duct Ectasia

A variety of terms have been applied to the conditions now known as *periductal mastitis* and *duct ectasia.* Haagensen (39) first introduced the term *duct ectasia* and considered the condition to be an age-related phenomenon; he believed that breast ducts dilated with age and that stagnant secretions in these dilated ducts leaked into surrounding tissues to cause periductal mastitis. This description of events ignores the findings of all other authors that periductal inflammation predominates in young women, whereas duct dilatation increases in frequency with advancing age; the sequence of events described by Haagensen is therefore incorrect (40,41). If periductal mastitis and duct ectasia are related, then patients with duct ectasia would be expected to have a history of episodes of periductal mastitis. In a study of 186 patients with the clinical syndrome of duct ectasia, only 1 (0.5%) had a history of previous periductal mastitis; in contrast, 97 (70%) of 139 patients with the clinical syndrome of periductal mastitis reported a previous clinical episode of periductal mastitis (42).

Clinical Syndromes

Periductal mastitis is characterized clinically by episodes of periareolar inflammation with or without an associated mass, a periareolar abscess, and a mammary duct fistula. Nipple retraction can be seen early at the site of the affected duct and is often subtle (43). Nipple discharge can also occur and is often purulent.

The clinical features of duct ectasia include nipple retraction at the site of the shortened duct or ducts and cheesy, viscous, toothpaste like nipple discharge. Patients with green discharge from multiple ducts are often diagnosed as having duct ectasia, but most of these have leaking physiologic breast secretion. In one large series, periductal mastitis affected women between the ages of 18 and 48 years, whereas patients presented with duct ectasia between the ages of 42 and 85 years (42).

Etiology

Although parity and breast-feeding were thought at one time to be important factors in the etiology of duct dilatation (40), sub-sequent studies have not demonstrated any association between these factors and periductal mastitis or duct ectasia (44). Age is an important factor in the cause of duct ectasia; the frequency of the condition increases with age; in one postmortem study, 48% of women age 60 years or older had pathologic evidence of duct ectasia (45). Although early studies suggested that the lesions of both periductal mastitis and duct ectasia are sterile (39), when appropriate transport media are used, bacteria can be isolated from 83% of periareolar inflammatory masses and 100% of nonlactational abscesses and mammary duct fistulae (46). The organisms isolated are frequently anaerobic. In contrast, a study of duct ectasia lesions identified bacteria in only 1 of 11 patients, a finding indicating that these lesions are usually sterile (47).

An association between smoking and recurrent periareolar abscesses was first reported in 1988 (48). A subsequent study showed that heavy smokers are more likely to have abscess recurrence or subsequent mammary duct fistulae than light smokers or nonsmokers (49). Studies with carefully matched cases and controls have shown a significant excess of smokers among patients with clinically diagnosed periductal mastitis, but no excess of smokers among women with clinically diagnosed duct ectasia (42,50). Women with periductal mastitis are also more likely to be heavy smokers (50). How cigarette smoking causes periductal mastitis is unclear. Substances in cigarette smoke may either directly or indirectly damage the wall of subareolar ducts. Accumulation of toxic metabolites, such as lipid peroxidase, epoxides, nicotine, and cotinine in the breast ducts has been demonstrated to occur in smokers within 15 minutes of a woman starting to breast-feed (51,52). Smoking has also been shown to inhibit growth of gram-positive bacteria *in vivo* and *in vitro,* leading to an overgrowth of gram-negative bacteria (53). This may affect the normal bacterial flora and allow overgrowth of pathogenic aerobic and anaerobic gram-negative bacteria, and would explain the presence of these organisms in the lesions of periductal mastitis. Microvascular changes have also been recorded and may cause local ischemia (54). The combination of damage caused by toxins, microvascular damage by lipid peroxidases, and altered bacterial flora may be responsible for the clinical manifestations of periductal mastitis.

Etiologic data suggest that periductal mastitis and duct ectasia are separate conditions with different causes. Duct ectasia appears to be an involutionary phenomenon, whereas periductal mastitis is a disease in which smoking and bacteria are important causal factors.

Other Causes of "Nipple" Discharge

Other diseases of the nipple–areolar complex can present with "nipple" discharge, including nipple adenoma, eczema, Paget's disease, ulcerating carcinoma, and long-standing nipple inversion with maceration (18). Nipple adenoma is rare, but easy to diagnose. It usually presents with a bloodstained discharge or change in contour or color of the nipple. Occasionally, an ulcer develops. Clinically, there is a nondiscrete mass in the substance of the superficial layer of the nipple. Definitive treatment is complete excision (55). Eczema or dermatitis can sometimes involve the nipple and is usually caused by irritation from chemicals on clothes or in cosmetics. Eczema can be differentiated from Paget's disease in that eczema affects primarily the areola and only rarely spreads onto the nipple (56). In contrast, Paget's disease affects the nipple first and only secondarily affects the areola. Treatment for eczema is removal of any aggravating factor, such as perfumed soap or detergents, by the use of hypoallergenic washing materials for clothes and skin, and prescription of a short course of topical corticosteroids.

Long-standing nipple inversion with maceration is rare but is seen in elderly people (18). The injured skin produces a

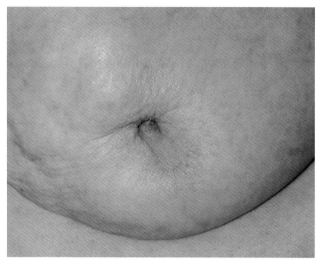

FIGURE 6.3. Nipple inversion from breast cancer.

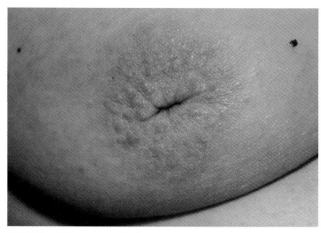

FIGURE 6.4. Slitlike nipple retraction from duct ectasia.

discharge, which can be purulent. Treatment is by careful cleaning of the affected area. Repeated nipple trauma caused by friction from rubbing of the clothes on the nipple from jogging and cycling is sometimes sufficiently severe to cause bleeding.

 ## NIPPLE INVERSION OR RETRACTION

The terms *inversion* and *retraction* are often used interchangeably, although some call the condition *inversion* only when the whole nipple is pulled in (Fig. 6.3), and use the term *retraction* when part of the nipple is drawn in at the site of a single duct to produce a slitlike appearance (1) (Fig. 6.4). These changes can be congenital or acquired. The acquired causes, in order of frequency, are duct ectasia, periductal mastitis, carcinoma, and tuberculosis.

All patients with acquired nipple inversion or retraction should have a full clinical examination and, if the patient is older than 35 years, a mammogram (57). Management depends on the presence or absence of a clinical or mammographic abnormality (Fig. 6.5). Central, symmetric, transverse slitlike

retraction is characteristic of benign disease; nipple inversion occurring in association with either breast cancer or inflammatory breast disease is more likely to involve the whole of the nipple and, in a breast cancer, to be associated with distortion of the areola when the breast is examined in different positions (Figs. 6.3 and 6.4). Benign nipple retraction requires no specific treatment, but can be corrected surgically if the patient requests it and the surgeon considers the operation appropriate. Usually, division or excision of the underlying breast ducts (total duct division or excision) is required; patients should be warned that they cannot breast-feed after this procedure.

 ## OPERATIONS FOR NIPPLE DISCHARGE OR RETRACTION
Microdochectomy

Microdochectomy is indicated for spontaneous, persistent single-duct discharge. Microdochectomy can be performed either through a radial incision across the areola or through a cir-

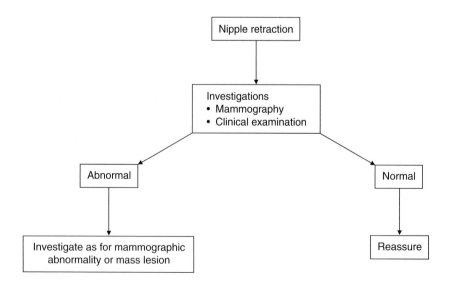

FIGURE 6.5. Management of nipple retraction.

cumareolar incision centered over the discharging duct. A circumareolar incision leaves a better cosmetic scar. The discharging duct is cannulated either with a probe or a blunt-ended needle following which methylene blue can be injected, thus allowing the involved duct to be identified under the surface of the nipple. The duct is dissected distally into the breast; a portion of the duct over a distance of at least 2 to 3 cm is removed because almost all significant disease affects the proximal 5 cm (14). If the remaining duct appears abnormal and dilated after the proximal portion of the duct is removed, the distal duct can be opened and any pathologic lesion in the remaining duct can be visualized and excised. This is an important maneuver because ductoscopy has taught that many significant lesions affect ducts some distance from the nipple. If performing a duct excision directed by ductoscopy, when an abnormality is visualized in the duct, the light is used to direct the surgical excision. Once the excision has been performed, the nipple should be squeezed gently to ensure that the discharging duct has been excised. Drains are not necessary after this procedure, and the skin is closed in layers with absorbable sutures.

Papillomas visible on ultrasonography can be removed by percutaneous vacuum-assisted core biopsy devices and this has been reported to be both diagnostic and therapeutic (12). Concerns, however, exist that such excisions might compromise full pathologic assessment, which is essential in papillary lesions. Current standard practice thus remains to biopsy lesions visualised on ultrasound and, if a papillary lesion is reported by the pathologist, to excise it surgically.

Total Duct Excision or Division

Total duct excision or division is indicated for multiple troublesome duct discharge or nipple eversion, and as treatment for periductal mastitis and its associated complications. Because the lesions of periductal mastitis usually contain organisms (Table 6.1), patients having operations for this condition should receive appropriate antibiotic treatment during the operation and for 5 days after surgery. Options for antibiotic therapy include amoxicillin–clavulanate or a combination of erythromycin and metronidazole hydrochloride. Some surgeons treat older women with single-duct discharge, but who no longer wish to breast-feed, with a total duct excision. The measure is taken so that if a condition, such as duct estasia, exists, which is likely to affect all the ducts underneath the nipple, a further episode of discharge from the treated breast will not develop. A circumareolar incision based at the 6-o'clock position is used unless a previous scar exists, in which case the same scar is reused. Dissection is performed under the areola down either side of the major ducts. Curved tissue forceps are passed around the ducts, and these are delivered into the wound. The

ducts are divided from the undersurface of the nipple and, if a total duct excision is being performed, a 2-cm portion of ducts is excised (57). For patients having cosmetic nipple eversion, the procedure can be performed through a small incision either at the areolar margin or at the base of the nipple and the ducts are divided sufficiently to ensure the nipple everts. If the operation is being performed for periductal mastitis, the back of the nipple must be cleared of all ducts up to the nipple skin because recurrence can occur when residual diseased ductal tissue is left (58). If the nipple was inverted before the operation, it is manually everted; only rarely are sutures required under the nipple to maintain nipple eversion. No drains are placed, and the wound is closed in layers with absorbable sutures. Patients should be warned before surgery that this operation results in significantly reduced nipple sensitivity in up to 40% of women (59).

◼ | BREAST INFECTION

Breast infection is much less common than it used to be. It is occasionally seen in neonates, but most commonly affects women between the ages of 18 and 50 years. In the adult, breast infection can be considered lactational or nonlactational. Infection can also affect the skin overlying the breast, and occurs either as a primary event or secondary to a lesion in the skin, such as a sebaceous cyst, or a more generalized condition, such as hidradenitis suppurativa. The organisms responsible for different types of breast infection and the most appropriate antibiotics with activity against these organisms are summarized in Table 6.1 (60). The guiding principle in treating breast infection is to give antibiotics as early as possible to stop abscess formation; if the infection or inflammation fails to resolve after one course of antibiotics, then abscess formation or an underlying cancer should be suspected (61).

Mastitis Neonatorum

Continued enlargement of the breast bud in the first week or two of life occurs in approximately 60% of newborns, and the gland may reach several centimeters in size before regressing. The enlarged breast bud can become infected, usually by *Staphylococcus aureus,* although *Escherichia coli* can sometimes cause this infection. In the early stage, antibiotics (flucloxacillin) can control infection; however, if a localized collection is evident on ultrasound, incision and drainage, placing a small stab incision as peripherally as possible so as not to damage the breast bud, is effective at producing resolution.

Table 6.1	ORGANISMS RESPONSIBLE FOR DIFFERENT TYPES OF BREAST INFECTION AND APPROPRIATE ANTIBIOTICS		
Type of Infection	Organism	No Penicillin Allergy	Penicillin Allergy
Neonatal	*Staphylococcus aureus* (rarely *Escherichia coli*)	Flucloxacillin (500mg four times daily)	Erythromycin (500mg twice daily)
Lactational	*S aureus* (rarely *S epidermidis* and streptococci)	Flucloxacillin (500mg four times daily)	Erythromycin (500mg twice daily)
Skin associated	*S aureus*	Flucloxacillin (500mg four times daily)	Erythromycin (500mg twice daily)
Non-Lactating	*S aureus*, enterococci, anaerobic streptococci, *Bacteroides* spp	Co-amoxiclav (375mg three times daily)	Combination of erythromycin (500mg twice daily) with metronidazole (200mg three times daily)

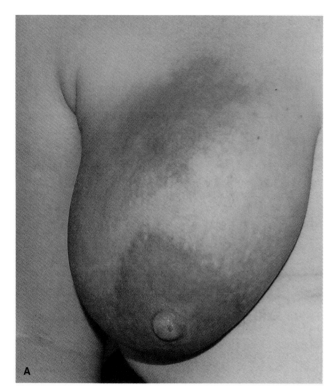
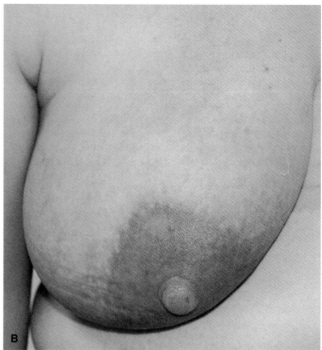

FIGURE 6.6. (**A**) Lactational breast infection: large abscess was present on ultrasound which was treated by aspiration with rapid resolution (**B**).

Lactational Infection

Lactational infection is less common today. The infection is usually caused by *S. aureus,* but it can also be caused by *Staphylococcus epidermidis* and *Streptococcus* species. Usually, the patient has a history of a cracked nipple or a skin abrasion, which results in a break in the body's defense mechanisms and an increase in the number of bacteria over the skin of the breast. These bacteria enter the breast through the nipple and infect poorly draining segments. Infection most commonly occurs following a first pregnancy in the first 6 weeks of breast-feeding or during weaning. Patients present with pain, erythema, swelling, tenderness, or systemic signs of infection. Clinically, the breast is swollen, tender, and erythematous; if an abscess is present, a fluctuant mass with overlying shiny, red skin may be seen (59) (Fig. 6.6). Axillary lymphadenopathy is not usually a feature. Patients can be toxic with pyrexia, tachycardia, and leukocytosis. Antibiotics given at an early stage usually control the infection and stop abscess formation. Because more than 80% of staphylococci are resistant to penicillin, flucloxacillin or amoxicillin–clavulanate are given, except in patients with a penicillin sensitivity, for whom erythromycin or clarithromycin is usually effective. Tetracycline, ciprofloxacin, and chloramphenicol should not be used to treat infection in breast-feeding women because they enter breast milk and may harm the child (59). Patients whose condition does not improve rapidly on antibiotic therapy require hospital referral and assessment with ultrasonography to determine whether pus is present and to exclude an underlying neoplasm. Inflammatory cancers can be difficult to differentiate from abscesses. If an abscess is evident on ultrasonography and the overlying skin is not thinned or necrotic, the abscess should be aspirated to dryness following injection of local anesthesia into the skin and the cavity irrigated with local anesthetic to minimize pain. The combination of repeated aspiration and oral antibiotics is usually effective at resolving local abscess formation and is the current treatment of choice for most breast abscesses (60–62). Aspiration should be repeated every 2 to 3 days until no further pus is obtained. Characteristically, the fluid aspirated changes from pus to serous fluid and then to milk. If the skin overlying the abscess is thinned and pus is visible on ultrasonography, then after application of local anesthetic cream and infiltration of local anesthetic into the overlying skin, a small incision (mini-incision) is made over the point of maximal fluctuation, and the pus is drained (60). The cavity can be irrigated with local anesthetic solution, which produces instant pain relief. Irrigation is continued daily until the incision site closes. If the skin overlying the abscess is necrotic, the necrotic skin is excised, which allows the pus to drain. Few lactational abscesses require drainage under general anesthesia, and neither the placement of drains nor wound packing after incision is necessary. Breast-feeding should be continued if possible because this promotes drainage of the engorged segment and helps resolve infection. The infant is not harmed by bacteria in the milk, nor by flucloxacillin, amoxicillin–clavulanate, or erythromycin. Patients who have incision and drainage of their breast abscesses performed under general anesthesia usually stop breast-feeding, whereas those who are treated by mini-incision or aspiration and antibiotic therapy can usually continue to breast-feed if they wish. Only rarely is it necessary to suppress lactation with cabergoline in patients with breast infection.

Nonlactational Infection

Nonlactational infections can be divided into those occurring centrally in the breast in the periareolar region and those affecting peripheral breast tissue.

Periareolar Infection

Periareolar infection is most commonly seen in young women; the mean age of occurrence is 32 years, and most are cigarette smokers. The underlying pathologic process is periductal mastitis (60,63). It can present as periareolar inflammation, with or without a mass, a periareolar abscess, or a mammary duct fistula. Associated nipple retraction, which can be quite subtle, may also be seen at the site of the diseased duct (54), and nipple discharge, which can be purulent, may be present. A patient presenting with periareolar inflammation without a mass should be treated with antibiotics that are active against both the aerobic and anaerobic bacteria seen in these lesions (64) (Table 6.1). If the infection does not resolve after one course of antibiotics, ultrasonography should be performed to determine whether a localized abscess is present. A patient who presents with or develops an abscess should be treated by recurrent aspiration and oral antibiotics or incision and drainage under local anesthesia. After resolution of the infective episode, patients older than age 35 years should have mammography performed, because very rarely infection can develop in association with comedo necrosis in an area of ductal carcinoma *in situ.* Up to half of patients with periareolar sepsis experience recurrent episodes of infection; the only effective long-term treatment for these women is removal of all the affected ducts (total duct excision). If this operation is performed carefully, it is usually curative (58). Rarely subareolar abscesses can be caused by actinomyces species, which can result in chronic subareolar abscess formation, which resolves following incision and drainage (65).

Mammary Duct Fistula

A mammary duct fistula is a communication between the skin, usually in the periareolar region, and a major subareolar breast duct (60) (Fig. 6.8). It is most commonly seen after incision and drainage of a nonlactational breast abscess, although it can occur after spontaneous discharge of a periareolar inflammatory mass or after biopsy of an area of periductal mastitis (66). Patients usually have preceding episodes of recurrent abscess formation and a puslike discharge through the fistula opening. Occasionally, more than one external opening is noted at the areolar margin, either from a single duct or from multiple affected ducts.

Treatment is surgical, consisting of either opening up the fistula tract and leaving it to granulate (66,67) or excising the fistula and affected duct or ducts (a total duct excision is usually required) and closing the wound primarily under appropriate antibiotic cover (68). The latter is the preferred treatment

method because it produces a much more satisfactory cosmetic outcome (68).

Peripheral Nonlactational Breast Abscess

Peripheral nonlactational breast abscesses are less common than periareolar abscesses and have been reported to be associated with a variety of underlying disease states, such as diabetes, rheumatoid arthritis, steroid treatment, and trauma (69). *S. aureus* is the organism usually responsible, but some abscesses contain anaerobic organisms. Peripheral nonlactational breast abscesses are three times more common in premenopausal women than in menopausal or postmenopausal women and in most no obvious underlying cause is evident; however, because infection associated with comedonecrosis has been reported following resolution of infection, mammography may be indicated in women older than 35 years. Systemic evidence of malaise and fever is usually absent. Management is the same as for other breast abscesses, with aspiration or incision and drainage (Fig. 6.7).

Skin-Associated Infection

Cellulitis of the breast, with or without abscess formation, is common, particularly in patients who are overweight, have large breasts, or have had previous surgery or radiation therapy (60). It is most common in the lower half of the breast, where sweat accumulates and intertrigo develops. *S. aureus* is the organism most commonly responsible for skin infection. Skin-associated infection can also occur in association with sebaceous cysts in the skin over the breast or can be seen in association with hidradenitis suppurativa (70). Hidradenitis is more common in smokers, and the same organisms are present in these lesions as in periductal sepsis (Table 6.1). Excision of the affected skin and grafting is effective in up to 50% of cases (61). For some women with large breasts and recurrent skin infection, reduction mammoplasty can be effective at preventing further episodes of infection.

Acute episodes of infection should be treated with appropriate antibiotics and, when an abscess is present, aspiration or incision and drainage should be performed. In patients with recurrent infections affecting the lower half of the skin of the breast, the area should be kept as clean and dry as possible; the area should be washed twice a day, creams and talcum

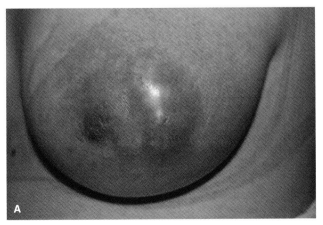
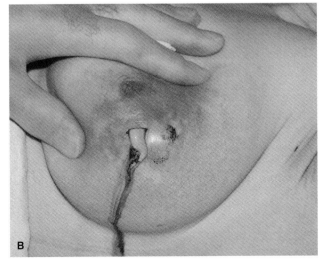

FIGURE 6.7. (**A**) Peripheral abscess: note the shiny thin skin. This abscess was treated by min-incision and drainage with resolution (**B**).

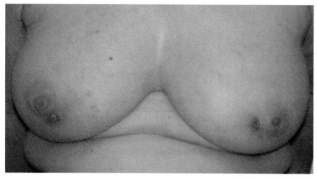

FIGURE 6.8. Mammary duct fistula. Bilateral mammary duct fistula. On each side the fistula is discharging in the periareolar region. The affected duct is pulled toward the fistula.

powders should be avoided, and cotton bras or a cotton T-shirt or vest worn inside the bra (60).

Other Rare Infections

Tuberculosis

Tuberculosis is rare in Western countries. The breast can be the primary site, but tuberculosis more commonly reaches the breast through lymphatic spread from axillary, mediastinal, or cervical nodes or directly from underlying structures, such as the ribs. Tuberculosis predominantly affects women in the latter part of their childbearing years. An axillary or breast sinus is present in up to 50% of patients. The most common presentation is that of an acute abscess resulting from infection of an area of tuberculosis by pyogenic organisms (60,61). Treatment is with local surgery and antitubercular drug therapy.

Primary actinomycosis (65), syphilis, mycotic, helminthic, and viral infections occasionally affect the breast, but are rare. *Molluscum contagiosum* can affect the areola and present as wartlike lesions.

Granulomatous Lobular Mastitis

Granulomatous lobular mastitis is characterized by non-caseating granulomata and microabscesses confined to the breast lobule (71,72). The condition presents as a firm mass, which is often indistinguishable from breast cancer, or as multiple or recurrent abscesses. Some patients with granulomatous lobular mastitis report that the mass is tender to touch and painful and the overlying skin is sometimes ulcerated (Fig. 6.9). Young women, often within 5 years of pregnancy, are most frequently affected (73). In contrast to periductal mastitis, it is common is Asian rather than white women and few are smokers. The role of organisms in the etiology of this condition is unclear, but one study isolated corynebacteria from 9 of 12 women with granulomatous lobular mastitis (74). The most common species isolated was the newly described *Corynebacterium kroppenstedtii*, followed by *Corynebacterium amycolatum* and *Corynebacterium tuberculostearicum*. These organisms are usually sensitive to penicillin and tetracycline; treatment should be based on sensitivities as reported by the local bacteriologic service. We have been unable to confirm these organisms in lesions of granulomatous lobular mastitis and antibiotics effective against these organisms do not produce resolution of this condition. For this reason, a search for the etiology of this condition continues. In patients presenting with a breast mass diagnosed on core biopsy as granulomatous lobular mastitis, excision of the mass should be avoided because it is often followed by persistent wound discharge and failure of the wound to heal. Current treatment involves establishing the diagnosis and observation because the condition usually resolves without specific treatment. Any abscesses that develop require aspiration or mini-incision and drainage. There is a strong tendency for this condition to recur, but eventually it does resolve spontaneously without treatment (60). Steroids have been tried without consistent success (72).

Factitial Disease

Cases of factitious abscess are occasionally seen. These patients usually have psychiatric problems, but some cases can appear quite plausible. Factitial disease should be suspected when peripheral abscesses persist or recur despite appropriate treatment (70). The condition can be difficult to treat because patients are often resistant to help and may be very manipulative.

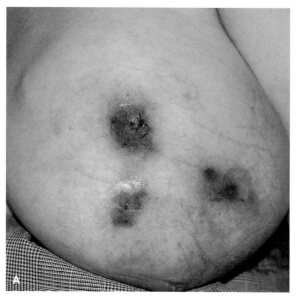
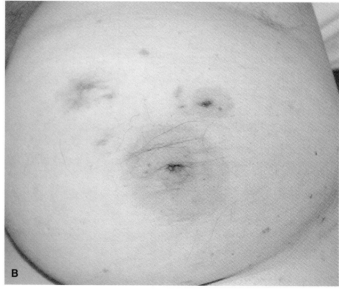

FIGURE 6.9. Granulomatous lobular mastitis at presentation (**A**) and following resolution (**B**).

References

1. Dixon JM, Mansel RE. Symptoms, assessment and guidelines for referral. ABC of breast diseases. *BMJ* 1994;309:722.
2. Ambrogetti D, Berni D, Catarzi S, et al. The role of ductal galactography in the differential diagnosis of breast carcinoma. *Radiol Med (Torino)* 1996;91:198.
3. Kleinberg D, Noel G, Frantz A. Galactorrhoea: a study of 235 cases including 48 with pituitary tumors. *N Engl J Med* 1977;296:589.
4. Simmons R, Adamovich T, Brennan M, et al. Nonsurgical evaluation of pathologic nipple discharge. *Ann Surg Oncol* 2003;10:113.
5. Selzer MH, Perloff LJ, Kelley RI, et al. Significance of age in patients with nipple discharge. *Surg Gynecol Obstet* 1970;131:519.
6. Groves AM, Carr M, Wadhera V, et al. An audit of cytology in the evaluation of nipple discharge: a retrospective study of 10 years' experience. *Breast* 1996;5:96.
7. Khan SA, Baird C, Staradub VL, et al. Ductal lavage and ductoscopy: the opportunities and the limitations. *Clin Breast Cancer* 2002;3:185.
8. Shen KW, Wu J, Lu JS, et al. Fiberoptic ductoscopy for breast cancer patients with nipple discharge. *Surg Endosc* 2001;15:1340.
9. Dooley WS. Routine operative breast endoscopy for bloody nipple discharge. *Ann Surg Oncol* 2002;9:920.
10. Dietz JR, Crowe JP, Grundfest S, et al. Directed duct excision by using mammary ductoscopy in patients with pathologic nipple discharge. *Surgery* 2002;132:582.
11. Matsunaga T, Ohta D, Misaka T, et al. Mammary ductoscopy for diagnosis and treatment of intraductal lesions of the breast. *Breast Cancer* 2001;8:213–221.
12. Govindarajulu S, Narreddy SR, Shere MH, et al. Sonographically guided mammotome excision of ducts in the diagnosis and management of single duct nipple discharge. *Eur J Surg Oncol* 2006;32:725–728.
13. Yamamoto D, Shoji T, Kawanishi H, et al. A utility of ductography and fiberoptic ductoscopy for patients with nipple discharge. *Breast Cancer Res Treat* 2001; 70:103.
14. Van Zee KJ, Ortega Perez G, Minnard E, et al. Preoperative galactography increases the diagnostic yield of major duct excision for nipple discharge. *Cancer* 1998;82:1874.
15. Cabioglu N, Hunt KK, Singletary SE, et al. Surgical decision making and factors determining a diagnosis of breast carcinoma in women presenting with nipple discharge. *J Am Coll Surg* 2003;196:354.
16. Guenin MA. Benign intraductal papilloma: diagnosis and removal at stereotactic vacuum-assisted directional biopsy guided by galactography. *Radiology* 2001;218: 576.
17. Dennis MA, Parker S, Kaske TI, et al. Incidental treatment of nipple discharge caused by benign intraductal papilloma through diagnostic mammotome biopsy. *AJR Am J Roentgenol* 2000;174:1263.
18. Hughes LE, Mansel RE, Webster DJT. Nipple discharge. In: Hughes LE, Mansel RE, Webster DJT, eds. *Benign disorders and diseases of the breast: concepts and clinical management,* 2nd ed. London: WB Saunders, 2000:171.
19. Sharma R, Dietz J, Wright H, et al. Comparative analysis of minimally invasive microductectomy versus major duct excision in patients with pathologic nipple discharge. *Surgery* 2005;138:591–596.
20. Sartorius OW, Smith HS, Morris P, et al. Cytologic evaluation of breast fluid in the detection of breast disease. *J Natl Cancer Inst* 1977;59:1073.
21. Wynder EL, Hill P, Laakso K, et al. Breast secretion in Finnish women. *Cancer* 1981;47:1444.
22. Haagensen CD, Bodian C, Haagensen DE. *Breast carcinoma risk and detection.* Philadelphia: WB Saunders, 1981:146.
23. Page DL, Anderson TJ. *Diagnostic histopathology of the breast.* Edinburgh, UK: Churchill Livingstone, 1987.
24. Rosen PP, Holmes G, Lesser ML, et al. Juvenile papillomatosis and breast carcinoma. *Cancer* 1985;55:1345.
25. Bazzocchi F, Santini D, Martinelli G, et al. Juvenile papillomatosis (epitheliosis) of the breast: a clinical and pathologic study of 13 cases. *Am J Clin Pathol* 1986; 86:745.
26. Rosen PP, Cantrell B, Mullen DL, et al. Juvenile papillomatosis (Swiss cheese disease) of the breast. *Am J Surg Pathol* 1980;4:3.
27. Bonser GM, Dossett JA, Jull JW. *Human and experimental breast cancer.* London: Pitman Medical, 1961.
28. Ito Y, Tamaki Y, Nakano Y, et al. Nonpalpable breast cancer with nipple discharge: how should it be treated? *Anticancer Res* 1997;17:791.
29. Fung A, Rayter Z, Fisher C, et al. Preoperative cytology and mammography in patients with single-duct nipple discharge treated by surgery. *Br J Surg* 1990;77: 1211.
30. Welsh M, Durrant D, Gonzales J, et al. Microdochectomy for discharge from single lactiferous duct. *Br J Surg* 1990;77:1213.
31. Cabioglu N, Krishnamurthy S, Kuerer HM, et al. Feasibility of breast-conserving surgery for patients with breast carcinoma associated with nipple discharge. *Cancer* 2004;101:508.
32. Ito Y, Tamaki Y, Nakano Y, et al. Nonpalpable breast cancer with nipple discharge: how should it be treated? *Anticancer Res* 1997;17:791.
33. Bauer RL, Eckhert KH Jr, Nemoto T. Ductal carcinoma in situ-associate nipple discharge: a clinical marker for locally extensive disease. *Ann Surg Oncol* 1998;5:452.
34. Obedian E, Haffty BG. Breast conserving therapy in breast cancer patients presenting with nipple discharge. *Int J Radiat Oncol Biol Phys* 2000;47:137.
35. Kato M, Oda K, Kubota T, et al. Non-palpable and non-invasive ductal carcinoma with bloody nipple discharge successfully resected after cancer spread was accurately diagnosed with three-dimensional computer tomography and galactography. *Breast Cancer* 2006;13:360.
36. Fitzal F, Mittlboeck M, Trischler H, et al. Breast-conserving therapy for centrally located breast cancer. *Ann Surg* 2008;247:470.
37. Kline TS, Lash SR. The bleeding nipple of pregnancy and postpartum: a cytologic and histologic study. *Am J Pathol* 1964;8:336.
38. Lafreniere R. Bloody nipple discharge during pregnancy: a rationale for conservative treatment. *J Surg Oncol* 1990;43:228.
39. Haagensen CD. Mammary-duct ectasia: a disease which may simulate carcinoma. *Cancer* 1951;4:749.
40. Bonser GM, Dossett JA, Jull JW. *Human and experimental breast cancer.* London: Pitman Medical, 1961:237.
41. Dixon JM. Periductal mastitis/duct ectasia. *World J Surg* 1989;13:715.
42. Dixon JM, Ravi Sekar O, Chetty U, et al. Periductal mastitis and duct ectasia: different conditions with different aetiologies. *Br J Surg* 1996;83:820.
43. Rees BI, Gravelle IH, Hughes LE. Nipple retraction in duct ectasia. *Br J Surg* 1977; 64:577.
44. Dixon JM, Anderson TJ, Lumsden AB, et al. Mammary duct ectasia. *Br J Surg* 1983;70:60.
45. Frantz VK, Pickren JW, Melcher GW, et al. Incidence of chronic cystic disease in so-called normal breast. *Cancer* 1950;4:762.
46. Bundred NJ, Dixon JM, Lumsden AB, et al. Are the lesions of duct ectasia sterile? *Br J Surg* 1985;72:844.
47. Aitken RJ, Hood J, Going JJ, et al. Bacteriology of mammary duct ectasia. *Br J Surg* 1988;75:1040.
48. Schafer P, Furrer G, Mermillod B. An association of cigarette smoking with recurrent subareolar breast abscesses. *Int J Epidemiol* 1988;17:810.
49. Bundred NJ, Dover MS, Coley S, et al. Breast abscesses and cigarette smoking. *Br J Surg* 1992;79:58.
50. Bundred NJ, Dover MS, Aluwihare N, et al. Smoking and periductal mastitis. *BMJ* 1993;307:772.
51. Wynder EL, Hill P. Nicotine and cotinine in breast fluid. *Cancer Lett* 1979;6:251.
52. Petrakis NL, Maack CA, Lee RE, et al. Mutagenic activity of nipple aspirates of breast fluid. *Cancer Res* 1980;40:188.
53. Ertel A, Eng R, Smith SM. The differential effect of cigarette smoke on the growth of bacteria found in humans. *Chest* 1991;100:628.
54. Bundred NJ. Surgical management of periductal mastitis. *Breast* 1988;7:79.
55. Hughes LE, Mansel RE, Webster DJT. The relationship between clinician and pathologist in benign breast disorders. In: *Benign disorders and diseases of the breast: concepts and clinical management,* 2nd ed. London: WB Saunders, 2000:49.
56. Dixon JM, Sainsbury JRC, Rodger A. Breast cancer: treatment of elderly patients and uncommon conditions—ABC of breast diseases. *BMJ* 1994;309:1292.
57. Kalbhen CL, Kezdi-Rogus PC, Dowling MP, et al. Mammography in the evaluation of nipple inversion. *AJR Am J Roentgenol* 1998;170:117.
58. Dixon JM, Kohlhardt SR, Dillon P. Total duct excision. *Breast* 1998;7:216.
59. Dixon JM. Breast surgery. In: Taylor EW, ed. *Infection in surgical practice.* Oxford: Oxford Medical Publications, 1992:187.
60. Dixon JM. Breast infection: ABC of breast diseases. *BMJ* 1994;309:946.
61. Hughes LE, Mansel RE, Webster DJT. Infections of the breast. In: Hughes LE, Mansel RE, Webster DJT, eds. *Benign disorders and diseases of the breast: concepts and clinical management,* 2nd ed. London: WB Saunders, 2000:187.
62. Dixon JM. Repeated aspiration of breast abscesses in lactating women. *BMJ* 1988;297:1517.
63. Dixon JM. Periductal mastitis and duct ectasia: an update. *Breast* 1998;7:128.
64. Dixon JM, Lee ECG, Greenall MJ. Treatment of periareolar inflammation associated with periductal mastitis using metronidazole and flucloxacillin: a preliminary report. *Br J Clin Pract* 1988;42:78.
65. Attar KH, Waghorn D, Lyons M, et al. Rare species of actinomyces as causative pathogens in breast abscess. *Breast* 2007;13:501–505.
66. Bundred NJ, Dixon JM, Chetty U, et al. Mammillary fistula. *Br J Surg* 1987;74:466.
67. Atkins HJB. Mammillary fistula. *BMJ* 1955;2:1473.
68. Dixon JM, Thompson AM. Effective surgical treatment for mammillary fistula. *Br J Surg* 1991;78:1185.
69. Rogers K. Breast abscess and problems with lactation. In: Smallwood JA, Taylor I, eds. *Benign breast disease.* London: Edward Arnold, 1990:96.
70. Hughes LE, Mansel RE, Webster DJT. Miscellaneous conditions. In: Hughes LE, Mansel RE, Webster DJT, eds. *Benign disorders and disease of the breast: concepts and clinical management,* 2nd ed. London: WB Saunders, 2000:231.
71. Going JJ, Anderson TJ, Wilkinson S, et al. Granulomatous lobular mastitis. *J Clin Pathol* 1987;40:535.
72. Howell JD, Barker P, Gazet J-C. Granulomatous lobular mastitis: report of a further two cases and a comprehensive literature review. *Breast* 1994;3:119.
73. Al-Khaffaf B, Knox F, Bundred NJ. Idiopathic granulomatous mastitis: a 25-year experience. *J Am Coll Surg* 2008;206:269–273.
74. Paviour S, Musaad S, Roberts S, et al. *Corynebacterium* species isolated from patients with mastitis. *Clin Infect Dis* 2002;35:1434.

Robert E. Mansel

Breast pain is one of the most common problems for which patients consult primary care physicians, gynecologists, and breast specialists. Patients mistakenly think the symptom is associated with early breast cancer, but once cancer has been ruled out, reassurance alone will resolve the problem in 86% of those with mild and 52% of those with severe mastalgia (1). A survey of screened women in the U. K. national program revealed that 69% had experienced severe breast pain, although only 3% had sought treatment (2). Ader et al. in 2001 (3) attempted to establish the prevalence in the community in the United States. In this study, 874 women between 18 and 44 years of age were recruited for interview by random number dialing in Virginia. Of these, 68% reported some cyclic mastalgia and, in 22% this was described as moderate or severe. Interestingly, patients on the oral contraceptive pill had less trouble, whereas there was a positive association with smoking, caffeine intake, and perceived stress. A study from the United States (4) showed the impact of breast pain among a population of 1,171 women attending a general obstetrics and gynecology clinic. Of these, 69% suffered regular discomfort and 36% had consulted a physician about their breast pain. Reading of the literature might suggest that the incidence of breast pain is different in many parts of the world, but these differences are mainly cultural in relation to the willingness of women to consult their physicians about breast pain.

The major clinical issue is to determine the impact on quality of life in patients complaining of breast pain, because this the primary reason for medication. Only rarely is intervention required, but, after appropriate patient selection, some may derive great benefit from treatment.

ETIOLOGY

Breast swelling is a frequent event in the late luteal phase of the menstrual cycle. Cyclic mastalgia is a more extreme form of this change, and researchers have sought endocrine abnormalities in those with severe breast pain, particularly measuring estradiol, progesterone, and prolactin (5). Sitruk-Ware et al. (6) suggested that inadequate corpus luteal function is an etiologic factor in women with benign breast disease, but this term has been used to include all nonmalignant breast conditions, blurring the distinction between a variety of benign breast conditions. In contrast, Walsh et al (7) found no evidence of progesterone deficiency during the luteal phase in those with mastalgia. The confusion in the literature between the symptom of breast pain, and the large number of variable pathologic descriptions of benign breast conditions has resulted in the belief that the condition is a "disease," rather than physiologic responses to menstrual cycles. In the aberrations of normal development and involution (ANDI) classification of benign conditions, mastalgia is regarded as a physiologic disorder arising from hormonal activity with little connection to cancer risk, or true pathologic conditions (8).

No consistent abnormality of estradiol has been reported in women with cyclic mastalgia; both normal levels (9) and elevated levels have been reported during the luteal phase (10). Baseline levels of prolactin are either normal or marginally elevated (9,10), but increased prolactin release was found after domperidone stimulation in severe cyclic mastalgia (11), possibly representing a stress response to prolonged pain.

Ecochard et al. (12) measured a range of personal and endocrine variables in 30 women with mastalgia and 70 control subjects. The women were more likely to report foot swelling or abdominal bloating (43% vs. 19%). Women with mastalgia had higher mean luteal levels of luteinizing hormone (LH) and follicle-stimulating hormone (FSH).

No histologic differences have been detected in biopsies from women with and without mastalgia (13). Immunohistochemical examination of biopsies from 29 women with mastalgia and 29 control subjects revealed no differences in expression of interleukin-6, interleukin-1β, and tumor necrosis factor (14).

CLASSIFICATION

Preece et al. (15) proposed a classification with six subgroups based on a prospective study of 232 patients with breast pain: cyclic mastalgia, duct ectasia, Tietze's syndrome, trauma, sclerosing adenosis, and cancer. This was subsequently simplified into two groups with noncyclic pain: true noncyclic breast pain and those with other causes of chest wall pain (16). Although an accurate diagnosis can be achieved on the basis of history and examination, patients with breast pain can be more simply assigned to one of three groups: cyclic breast pain (around 70%), noncyclic breast pain (20%), or extramammary pain (10%).

Khan and Apkarian (17) studied the differences between cyclic and noncyclic pain using standardized pain questionnaires, including the McGill Pain instrument in 271 women, and found that the level of pain described by the subjects was equivalent to chronic cancer pain, and just less than the pain of rheumatoid arthritis. They noted that women with cyclic pain tended to refer to heaviness and tenderness as found in the Preece study, whereas women with noncyclic pain related the severity to the area of breast involved (17).

EVALUATION

Important aspects of history-taking include the type of pain, relationship to menses, duration, location, and any other medical problems. The impact of the pain on the everyday activities of the patient, particularly sleep and work should be established, to assess the need for medication.

After inspection, the first aspect of the breast examination should be very gentle palpation of the breasts once the patient has indicated the site(s) of the pain. Having excluded discrete masses, a more probing evaluation should be performed, focusing on the site(s) of pain. After turning the patient half on her side, so that the breast tissue falls away from the chest wall, it may be possible to identify that the pain is arising from the underlying rib or costal cartilage. The pain can be reproduced by placing a fingertip on the affected rib and demonstrating to the patient its source.

Nodularity can be associated with mastalgia, but the extent is unrelated to pain severity; in younger women, the finding is so common that it should be considered within the spectrum of normality. If it is apparent that the pain, whether cyclic or noncyclic, is mammary in origin, the decision to treat is based on the subjective assessment of severity, together with the duration of symptoms. This assessment may be facilitated by a daily pain chart that assesses the timing and severity (semiquantitative scale) of the pain. Generally, there should be a history of pain of at least 4 months before hormonal therapy is indicated.

ROLE OF RADIOLOGY

The average age of women entered into trials of treatment for mastalgia is 32 years: In this age-group, mammography is not a standard adjunct to clinical evaluation. In the absence of a discrete lump, ultrasonography is also unlikely to give useful information, but any breast lump present requires triple assessment. No specific mammogram findings are associated with breast pain.

Recently, Peters et al. (18) reported results of ultrasonography in 212 asymptomatic women and 212 with mastalgia. Among the control subjects, the mean maximal duct dilatation was 1.8 mm compared with 2.34 mm in the 136 with cyclic pain and 3.89 mm in the 76 with noncyclic pain. Dilated ducts were found in all quadrants, but mostly in the retroareolar area, and dilatation did not alter during the menstrual cycle. A highly significant association was found between the extent of ductal dilatation and pain severity.

MONDOR'S DISEASE

Mondor's disease is a rare cause of breast pain, with diagnostic clinical features of local pain associated with a tender, palpable subcutaneous cord or linear skin dimpling (19). The cause is superficial thrombophlebitis of the lateral thoracic vein or a tributary. The condition resolves spontaneously. Mondor's disease can cause serious alarm because some patients assume that the skin tethering is secondary to an underlying carcinoma, so they are greatly relieved when informed of the benign nature of the condition.

In a series of 63 cases of Mondor's disease, no underlying pathologic process was found in 31 cases (20). Of the remaining 32, local trauma or surgical intervention was responsible in 15 (47%), an inflammatory process in 6 (19%), and carcinoma in 8 (25%). In view of this, mammography should be performed in women with Mondor's disease who are age 35 years or older to exclude an impalpable breast cancer.

PSYCHOSOCIAL ASPECTS

Several studies have confirmed that patients with severe mastalgia have psychological morbidity that may be the result rather than the cause of their breast pain. Preece et al. (21) used the Middlesex Hospital Questionnaire to compare patients with mastalgia, psychiatric patients, and minor surgical cases. No significant differences were found between the patients with breast pain and the surgical cases, and both scored significantly lower than psychiatric cases. Only the scores of patients who failed treatment approached those of psychiatric patients. In a small study of 25 women with severe mastalgia, using the Composite International Diagnostic Interview, 45 diagnoses were made in 21 patients (84%): anxiety (n = 17), panic disorder (n = 5), somatization disorder (n = 7), and major depression (n = 16) (22).

Downey et al. (23), using the Hospital Anxiety and Depression Scale (HADS), reported high levels of both anxiety and depression in 20 women with severe mastalgia. At Guy's Hospital, HADS was also used to evaluate 54 patients with mastalgia (24). The 33 women with severe pain manifested levels of anxiety and depression comparable with those in women with breast cancer before surgery. Those who responded to treatment had a significant improvement in psychosocial function, but the nonresponders continued to have high levels of distress.

Fox et al. (25) conducted a prospective trial in 45 women with mastalgia who kept pain diaries for 12 weeks, with half randomized to listen daily to a relaxation tape during weeks 5

to 8. Abnormal or borderline HADS scores were found at entry in 54%, and a complete or substantial reduction in pain score was measured in 25% of the control subjects and 61% of those randomized to relaxation therapy (p <.005).

MASTALGIA AND BREAST CANCER RISK

Because of the lack of precision in classification of benign breast conditions in older studies, it was difficult to determine whether breast pain led to an increased risk of subsequent breast cancer. Foote and Stewart (26) wrote in 1945, "Any point of view that one chooses to take concerning the relation of so-called cystic mastitis to mammary cancer can be abundantly supported from the literature."

Webber and Boyd (27) carried out a critical analysis of the 36 published papers that were available in English before 1984. They set 16 standards, including a description of the study population, a definition of benign disease, follow-up, and a description of the risk analysis. Of the 22 studies reporting an increase in risk, all met more of the standards than the 11 suggesting no increase in risk and the 3 drawing no conclusions.

Since then, a few studies have specifically examined the relation between cyclic mastalgia and breast cancer risk. Plu-Bureau et al. (28) conducted a case-control study among premenopausal women, 210 younger than 45 years of age with breast cancer, and 210 neighborhood control subjects, matched on year of birth, education level, and age at first full-term pregnancy. The unadjusted relative risk (RR) for cancer in those with cyclic mastalgia was 2.66, and after adjustment for family history, prior benign breast disease, and age at menarche, the RR was still significantly elevated at 2.12.

Goodwin et al. (29) recruited 192 women with premenopausal node-negative breast cancer and 192 age-matched premenopausal control subjects. Significant risk variables for breast cancer in the model were marital status, family history, number of years of smoking, prior breast biopsy (before cancer diagnosis), and mean cyclic change in breast tenderness. The odds ratio of cancer for cyclic mastalgia was 1.35, rising to 3.32 in those with severe pain.

Another indication of a possible link between mastalgia and cancer is the relationship between Wolfe grade of mammograms and breast pain (30). Deschamps et al. (31) determined the Wolfe grades of 1,394 women in the Canadian National Breast Screening Study. All completed a questionnaire, with mastalgia reported by 46%. The extent of dysplasia on mammograms was categorized as Dy2 (25% to 49%), Dy3 (50% to 74%), and Dy4 (≥75%). The odds ratio for a Dy3/4 rating was 1 for those who never had breast swelling and mastalgia, whereas it was 2.7 in those reporting both symptoms.

These epidemiologic studies have the problems of recall biases and unknown extent of histologic atypia in the patients who have not had biopsies. In most studies assessing risk using established algorithms, the presence of breast pain is not used as an independent variable in the calculations, unlike prior breast biopsy. That women attend a physician for breast pain, itself results in a higher rate of breast biopsy as noted in the study by Ader et al. (3).

TREATMENT TRIALS

Multiple treatments have been used in women with "benign breast disease," some of whom had nothing more than nodularity without tenderness. Patients with diffusely nodular breasts that are painless require nothing other than exclusion of significant pathology and can be discharged if no other indications for follow-up exist.

| Table 7.1 | PLACEBO-CONTROLLED, RANDOMIZED TRIALS OF TREATMENT FOR MASTALGIA WITH VISUAL ANALOG SCORING OF RESPONSE |

Agent	>20 Subjects/Arm	More Than 1 Trial	Side Effects[a]	Efficacy	References
Endocrine					
Goserelin	Yes	Yes	Yes	Yes	64
Danazol	Yes	Yes	Yes	Yes	42,43
Bromocriptine	Yes	Yes	Yes	Yes	46–49
Tamoxifen	Yes	Yes	No	Yes	56–59
Medroxyprogesterone acetate	No	No	No	No	54
Lynestrenol	No	No	No	No	32
Gestrinone	Yes	No	No	Yes	55
Lisuride	Yes	No	No	Yes	51
Isoflavone	No	No	No	Yes	65
Nonendocrine					
Fat reduction	No	No	No	Yes	35
Evening primrose oil	Yes	Yes	No	?	36–41
Mefenamic acid	No	No	No	No	33
Caffeine reduction	Yes	No	No	No	34
Vitamin E	Yes	No	No	No	31
Iodine	Yes	No	No	Yes	69–71
Agnus castus	Yes	No	No	Yes	68

[a]Side effects of sufficient severity that treatment was discontinued.

Treatment trials for breast pain should have well-documented breast pain classified into cyclic or not, measured with visual analog scales (VAS) or other rating scales, and ideally using each patient as her own control. Pain should have been present for a minimum of 6 months. The overall quality of most published studies has been poor with low numbers of patients recruited. Trials should be of double-blinded, placebo-controlled, randomized design and include a minimum of 20 patients in each arm. Some trials have met these criteria and defined effective drugs or interventions; results are summarized in Table 7.1.

The initial approach by most physicians is to advise reduction in alleged dietary factors associated with breast pain, such as caffeine or saturated fat intake, but the evidence for these interventions is poor. Diuretics are widely used by family physicians to oppose suggested water retention in the luteal phase of the cycle, but are ineffective.

Several agents have been found in controlled trials to be no better than placebo: vitamin E (32), lynestrenol (33), mefenamic acid (34), and caffeine reduction (35). This is perhaps not surprising because placebo-controlled trials report placebo response rates from 10% to 50%.

As an alternative, more complex approach, reduction in dietary fat can significantly reduce cyclic breast pain (36). Boyd et al. (36) entered 21 women with a minimum of 5 years of breast pain into a trial in which 11 were shown how to reduce their dietary fat content to 15% of total calories and 10 received general dietary advice. Those in the fat-reduction group had a significant reduction in breast pain. Although a nondrug intervention appeals to many patients, long-term dietary change is a difficult intervention to maintain.

A similar dietary approach of adding the long-chain unsaturated fatty acid gamma-linolenic acid, present in evening primrose oil and starflower oil, provides a nonendocrine approach, but with an efficacy that is questionable. Preece et al. (37) entered 103 women with mastalgia into a double-blinded, crossover study comparing evening primrose oil with placebo for 3 months, after which both groups received evening primrose oil capsules for a further 3 months. Cyclic pain was significantly diminished in those given evening primrose oil, but had no effect on noncyclic mastalgia.

In contrast, when Budeiri et al. (38) carried out a systematic literature search to determine the efficacy of evening primrose oil for premenstrual syndrome, they found no evidence of benefit. Both randomized, placebo-controlled trials reported no difference in response of the two groups (39,40). A more recent Dutch trial also failed to show an advantage for evening primrose oil (41).

In an attempt to resolve this question, one of the largest studies ever performed in both community and hospital patients involving a total of 555 patients was carried out, but with a different placebo arm to the previous trials. This trial failed to show any advantage of the active arms containing gamma linoleic acid, principally owing to the very large response of 40% reduction in symptoms in the placebo group (42). Despite this, many physicians advise their patients to try this product, which is widely available in nonprescription format, as an initial treatment of breast pain, because the incidence of side effects was very low in all the trials.

In cyclic mastalgia, most treatments have focused on reduction in estrogen or prolactin drive to the breast cells in the belief that hormonal overstimulation is the predominant factor in severe breast pain, although as noted above little evidence exists for this hypothesis.

Danazol, an impeded androgen, may relieve pain in up to 93% of patients (43,44), but with side effects that include nausea, depression, menstrual irregularity, and headaches in up to two-thirds of patients, sometimes leading to discontinuation of treatment. To reduce side effects, O'Brien and Abukhali (45) conducted a double-blinded, placebo-controlled trial of luteal-phase danazol in 100 women with premenstrual syndrome, including cyclic mastalgia. Danazol or placebo was given during the luteal phase for three cycles, with a significant pain reduction in those treated and similar side effects in both groups.

As an alternative to drugs, some physicians recommend a more supportive brassiere to relieve mastalgia. In a nonrandomized study of 200 Saudi women with mastalgia, 100 were given danazol 200 mg/day and 100 instructed to wear a sports brassiere (46). Pain was relieved in 85% of those who wore sports brassieres and in 58% of those given danazol, but of the latter group 42% had side effects and 15% stopped treatment.

Bromocriptine, a prolactin inhibitor, is also effective (47–49). In a multicenter European study of 272 women comparing bromocriptine, 2.5 mg twice daily, with placebo, significant symptom relief occurred in the treated group, but 29% dropped out because of side effects, mostly nausea and dizziness (50). Hinton et al. (51) conducted a double-blinded study in 47 women with severe breast pain given danazol, bromocriptine, or placebo (51). Those treated with bromocriptine and danazol had significantly better pain relief than the placebo group, but the best response was recorded in the danazol group.

Kaleli et al. (52) used the dopamine agonist lisuride maleate in a double-blinded, placebo-controlled trial, giving the randomized treatment for 2 months. There were 30 women in each treatment arm: Severity of mastalgia was monitored by VAS, but there was neither run-in period nor any pain severity threshold for trial entry. In patients with less pain, the response rate was 8 of 11 (73%) in the treated and 2 of 15 (13%) in the placebo arm. Among those with more severe pain, the respective response rates were 19 of 19 (100%) and 5 of 15 (33%). The main side effect was nausea, experienced by 17% of the treated and 10% of the control subjects. However the use of dopamine agents has been limited owing to problematic side effects.

The efficacy of progesterone vaginal cream has been investigated in two randomized trials (53,54). In a small study, McFadyen et al. (53) reported a minor, nonsignificant benefit for those women given placebo cream. In a larger trial with 80 participants, a greater than 50% reduction in pain was recorded in 22% of the placebo group and in 65% of those given progesterone-containing cream (54).

Maddox et al. (55) compared medroxyprogesterone acetate tablets, 20 mg/day in the luteal phase of the cycle, with placebo and found no difference in response rate or side effects in 26 women. In a multicenter, double-blinded, randomized trial, Peters (56) administered the synthetic 19-norsteroid gestrinone to 73 women and placebo to 72 control subjects. A significantly greater reduction in pain was seen in the gestrinone group, with side effects reported by 44% of the treated cases and 14% of the control subjects.

The agent tamoxifen, a partial estrogen antagonist and agonist, is effective in treating breast pain. In the first double-blinded, crossover, randomized trial, conducted at Guy's Hospital, pain relief occurred in 71% of those given tamoxifen and 38% of control subjects (57). After 3 months, nonresponders switched to the alternative treatment arm, and pain control was achieved in 75% of the tamoxifen group and 33% of the placebo group. The most common side effect of tamoxifen was hot flashes, occurring in 27%.

A similar placebo response was seen in the trial run by Messinis and Lolis (58), but among the group that received tamoxifen 10 mg, breast pain was controlled in 89%. In two trials that compared tamoxifen 10 mg, with 20 mg, similar response rates were seen, but side effects with the lower dose were substantially reduced (21% vs. 64%) (59). When tamoxifen was compared with danazol, similar response rates were seen, but Powles et al. (60) reported significantly more side effects in those given danazol (90% vs. 50%). Kontostolis et al. (61) reported hot flashes in 25% of those given tamoxifen 10 mg, and weight gain in 31% of the danazol-treated group. Sandrucci et al. (62) compared tamoxifen 10 mg with bromocriptine 7.5 mg daily: Pain relief was achieved in 18 of 20 (90%) of the tamoxifen group and in 17 of 20 (85%) of those given bromocriptine. Tamoxifen is now being used extensively in the management of breast pain, as an off-label drug because it is not currently licensed for use in benign breast conditions. The safety of this drug in patients without breast cancer is, however, well documented in the prevention trials involving large numbers of normal high risk women

(63). Furthermore, this review of the prevention trials confirms the reduction in benign breast conditions on the drug, which is consistent with the reduction in symptoms seen in the breast pain trials.

Alternative routes of delivery of tamoxifen or selective estrogen receptor modulators (SERMS) may be possible by the transcutaneous route, to reduce side effects by avoiding transhepatic passage. This approach has shown some promise using a gel containing 4-hydroxy tamoxifen applied to the breast morning and night (64). A placebo-controlled trial of this gel showed efficacy in cyclic mastalgia, particularly in the late luteal phase of the cycle, and showed a clear blunting of the luteal peak of cyclic breast pain (Fig. 7.1). It is clear that these series of studies of SERMS and the prevention studies confirm the active therapeutic role of these agents in benign conditions of the breast. These new agents are currently not licensed in the treatment of breast pain.

The relationship of the menstrual cycle in cyclic breast pain was further demonstrated by a randomized trial of the luteinizing hormone-releasing hormone (LHRH) agonist goserelin (Zoladex), which abolishes the menstrual cycle and thus removes the normal fluctuation in estradiol and progesterone. This large placebo-controlled trial of women with cyclic mastalgia treated with Zoladex for 6 months showed significant reduction in breast pain (65). The patients were then followed off treatment for 6 months and the breast pain gradually returned as did menstruation.

In a different approach, Ingram et al. (66) studied isoflavones derived from red clover to determine whether this phytoestrogen could relieve mastalgia. The 18 patients in the trial underwent a 2-month, single-blinded, placebo run-in phase, after which they received either placebo, isoflavone 40 mg, or isoflavone 80 mg. Pain scores for the final single-blinded month and the final double-blinded month were compared. In the placebo group, there was a 13% reduction, for the 40 mg/day group it was 44%, and for the 80 mg/day group it was 31%. No major side effects were reported, but the study needs repeating with larger numbers to determine the true efficacy of isoflavones.

ALTERNATIVE APPROACHES

Acupuncture has been used for the treatment of premenstrual syndrome (67) with some improvement of symptoms, but has not been used specifically for the treatment of mastalgia; double-blinded studies would be difficult to execute. At Guy's Hospital in an open pilot study, applied kinesiology was used in 88 women with self-rated moderate or severe mastalgia present for more than 6 months (68). This technique uses a type of pressure massage and is a hands-on technique based on improving lymphatic flow. Using self-rated pain scores, there was improvement in 60% and complete resolution in 18%, but this trial was not blinded, and not placebo controlled for obvious reasons.

A randomized trial of Vitus Agnus Castus extract (Castor Oil, Mastodynon), showed a modest fall in VAS scores on the plant extract (54% compared with 40% on placebo), with few side effects (Mastodynon) (69).

Ghent et al. (70) investigated the effect of iodine replacement in women with breast pain in three different studies, one of which was a randomized, double-blinded, placebo-controlled trial. The rationale was that iodine deficiency in Sprague-Dawley rats led to mammary epithelial hyperplasia and carcinoma (71). Participants were treated for 6 months with aqueous molecular iodine 0.07 to 0.09 mg/kg daily, or placebo composed of an aqueous mixture of brown vegetable dye and quinine. Pain improvement occurred in 11 of 33 (33%) of the placebo group and 15 of 23 (65%) of those given iodine. No side effects were reported. More recently Kessler (72) studied

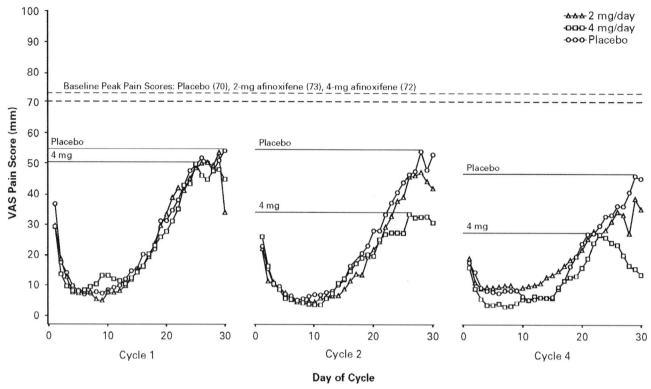

FIGURE. 7.1. Effect of topical 4-hydroxy tamoxifen gel on cyclical mastalgia. Randomized trial of 4-hydroxy tamoxifen gel (2 and 4 mg vs. placebo gel) applied to the breast for breast pain. Note the clear cyclical pattern of pain and the reduction of the peak luteal pain in cycle 4 by the 4-mg preparation. (From Mansel R, Goyal A, Nestour EL, et al. Afimoxifene [4-OHT] Breast Pain Research Group. A phase II trial of Afimoxifene [4-hydroxytamoxifen gel] for cyclical mastalgia in premenopausal women. *Breast Cancer Res Treat* 2007; 106[3]:389–397, with permission.)

supraphysiologic doses of iodine in cyclic mastalgia and reported that approximately 40% of patients obtained more than 50% reduction in breast pain on 3 to 6 mg iodine daily compared with 8% on placebo.

 ## EXTRA MAMMARY PAIN

Pain originating within the thorax or abdomen and referred to the breast area is managed by treatment of the underlying condition. Pain that originates from the thoracic wall (Tietze's syndrome or costochondritis), and localized specific tender areas in the breast, (trigger spots), can be managed by injection of steroid and local anesthetic (73). More recently, nonsteroidal analgesics have been used as topical gel applications and their use is supported by a large randomized trial of 108 women with both cyclic and noncyclic pain, which showed significant reduction in breast pain by diclofenac gel at 6 months compared with placebo gel (reduction in pain measured on visual analogue scale from 0 = no pain to 10 = intolerable pain; cyclic 5.87 with diclofenac versus 1.30 placebo; noncyclic 6.33 diclofenac versus 1.12 placebo, $p < .001$) (74).

 ## ROLE OF SURGERY

Severely distressed nonresponders to drug therapy may ask for mastectomy. This drastic step should not be undertaken before a full psychiatric assessment has been sought because without careful selection, surgical intervention will damage body image without achieving pain relief. Even after careful psychiatric assessment, excisional surgery should very rarely be undertaken because pain reduction is achieved in only a small num-

ber of patients (75). This is not surprising because the etiology of breast pain is poorly understood, and there are causes of pain that lie outside the breast tissue. In the author's experience the focus on pain will often move to body image after mastectomy and this leaves an unhappy patient who still complains of breast pain, which is clearly therapeutic failure.

 ## MANAGEMENT SUMMARY

- The essentials of treatment of women with breast pain are excluding serious underlying pathologic processes, making a diagnosis, and communicating this to the patient to reassure the majority. Only a small proportion (<10%) have problems of such severity and duration that specific treatment is necessary.

- If moderate or severe pain has been present for less than 6 months, a high probability exists of spontaneous remission after reassurance, and no specific treatment should be given.

- In women older than 35 years of age who have not had mammography within the past 12 months and are presenting with a new symptom, mammography should be carried out to exclude abnormalities that may be unrelated to the breast pain. The small group with severe, prolonged pain should be encouraged to keep a pain chart and return after 6 weeks. If the pain persists, treatment should be started with either tamoxifen or danazol. The former has fewer side effects and can be very effective. Although not licensed specifically for treatment of mastalgia, tamoxifen can be prescribed.

- Treatment should be given at a dosage of 10 mg/day for 3 months. If this achieves pain relief, the dose can be further reduced to 10 mg on alternate days for a further 3 months. For the few who do not respond, a higher dosage of 20 mg/day should be given.

- The very few who do not respond to this treatment should be switched to danazol or goserelin for 4 months.

References

1. Barros AC, Mottola J, Ruiz CA, et al. Reassurance in the treatment of mastalgia. *Breast J* 1999;5:162.
2. Leinster SJ, Whitehouse GH, Walsh PV. Cyclical mastalgia: clinical and mammographic observations in a screened population. *Br J Surg* 1987;74:220.
3. Ader DN, South-Paul J, Adera T, et al. Cyclical mastalgia: prevalence and associated health behavioural factors. *J Psychosom Obstet Gynaecol* 2001;22:71–76.
4. Ader DN, Browne MW. Prevalence and impact of cyclical mastalgia in a United States clinic-based sample. *Am J Obstet Gynecol* 1997;177:126–132.
5. Wang DY, Fentiman IS. Epidemiology and endocrinology of benign breast disease. *Breast Cancer Res Treat* 1985;6:5.
6. Sitruk-Ware LR, Sterkers N, Mowszowics I, et al. Inadequate corpus luteal function in women with benign breast disease. *J Clin Endocrinol Metab* 1977;44:771.
7. Walsh PV, Bulbrook RD, Stell PM, et al. Serum progesterone concentration during the luteal phase in women with benign breast disease. *Eur J Cancer Clin Oncol* 1984;20:1339.
8. Hughes LE, Mansel RE, Webster DJT. Aberrations of normal development and involution (ANDI): a new perspective on pathogenesis and nomenclature of benign breast disorders. *Lancet* 1987;2:1316.
9. Watt-Boolsen S, Andersen AN, Blichert-Toft M. Serum prolactin and oestradiol levels in women with cyclical mastalgia. *Horm Metab Res* 1981;13:700.
10. Walsh PV, McDicken IW, Bulbrook RD, et al. Serum oestradiol-17β and prolactin concentrations during the luteal phase in women with benign breast disease. *Eur J Cancer Clin Oncol* 1984;20:1345.
11. Kumar S, Mansel RE, Hughes LE, et al. Prolactin response to thyrotropin-releasing hormone stimulation and dopaminergic inhibition in benign breast disease. *Cancer* 1984;53:1311.
12. Ecochard R, Marret H, Rabilloud M, et al. Gonadotropin level abnormalities in women with cyclic mastalgia. *Eur J Obstet Gynecol* 2001;94:92.
13. Jorgensen J, Watt-Boolsen S. Cyclical mastalgia and breast pathology. *Acta Chir Scand* 1985;151:319.
14. Ramakrishnan R, Werbeck J, Khurana KK, et al. Expression of interleukin-6 and tumor necrosis factor alpha and histopathologic findings in painful and nonpainful breast tissue. *Breast J* 2003;9:91.
15. Preece PE, Hughes LE, Mansel RE, et al. Clinical syndromes of mastalgia. *Lancet* 1976;2:670.
16. Maddox PR, Harrison BJ, Mansel RE, et al. Non-cyclical mastalgia: an improved classification and treatment. *Br J Surg* 1989;76:901.
17. Khan SA, Apkarian AV. The characteristics of cyclical and non cyclical mastalgia: a prospective study using a modified McGill Pain Questionnaire. *Breast Cancer Res Treat* 2002;75:147–157.
18. Peters F, Diemer P, Mecks O, et al. Severity of mastalgia in relation to milk duct dilatation. *Am J Obstet Gynecol* 2003;101:54.
19. Mondor H. Tronculite sous-cutane subaigue de la paroi thoracique antro-latrale. *Memories Academies de Chirurgie* 1939;65:1271.
20. Catania S, Zurrida S, Veronesi P, et al. Mondor's disease and breast cancer. *Cancer* 1992;69:2267.
21. Preece PE, Mansel RE, Hughes LE. Mastalgia: psychoneurosis or organic disease? *BMJ* 1978;1:29.
22. Jenkins PL, Jamil N, Gateley C, et al. Psychiatric illness in patients with severe treatment-resistant mastalgia. *Gen Hosp Psychiatry* 1993;15:55.
23. Downey HM, Deadman JM, Davis C, et al. Psychological characteristics of women with cyclical mastalgin. *Breast Dis* 1993;6:99.
24. Ramirez AJ, Jarrett SR, Hamed H, et al. Psychological adjustment of women with mastalgia. *Breast* 1995;4:48.
25. Fox H, Walker LG, Heys SD, et al. Are patients with mastalgia anxious, and does relaxation help? *Breast* 1997;6:138.
26. Foote FW, Stewart FW. Comparative studies of cancerous versus non-cancerous breasts. *Ann Surg* 1945;121:6.
27. Webber W, Boyd N. A critique of the methodology of studies of benign breast disease and breast cancer risk. *J Natl Cancer Inst* 1986;77:397.
28. Plu-Bureau G, Thalabard JC, Sitruk-Ware R, et al. Cyclical mastalgia as a marker of breast cancer susceptibility: results of a case-control trial among French women. *Br J Cancer* 1992;65:945–949.
29. Goodwin PJ, DeBoer G, Clark RM, et al. Cyclical mastopathy and premenopausal breast cancer risk. *Breast Cancer Res Treat* 1994;33:63.
30. Wolfe JN. Risk for breast cancer development determined by mammographic parenchymal pattern. *Cancer* 1976;37:2486.
31. Deschamps M, Band PR, Coldman AJ, et al. Clinical determinants of mammographic dysplasia patterns. *Cancer Detect Prev* 1996;20:610.
32. Ernster VL, Goodson WH, Hunt TK, et al. Vitamin E and benign breast "disease": a double-blind randomized trial. *Surgery* 1984;97:490.
33. Colin C, Gaspard U, Lambotte R. Relationship of mastodynia with its endocrine environment and treatment in a double-blind trial with lynestrenol. *Archiv für Gynaekologie* 1978;225:7.
34. Gunston KD. Premenstrual syndrome in Capetown: II. A double-blind placebo-controlled study of the efficacy of mefenamic acid. *S Afr Med J* 1986;70:159.
35. Ernster VL, Mason L, Goodson WH, et al. Effects of caffeine-free diet on benign breast disease: a randomized trial. *Surgery* 1982;91:263.
36. Boyd NF, Shannon P, Kriukov V, et al. Effect of a low-fat high-carbohydrate diet on symptoms of cyclical mastopathy. *Lancet* 1988;2:128.
37. Preece PE, Hanslip JI, Gilbert L, et al. Evening primrose oil (Efamol) for mastalgia. In: Horrobin D, ed. *Clinical uses of essential fatty acids.* Montreal: Eden Press, 1982:147–154.
38. Budeiri D, Li Wan Po A, Dornan JC. Is evening primrose oil of value in the treatment of premenstrual syndrome? *Controlled Clinical Trials* 1996;17:60.
39. Collins A, Cerin, Coleman G, et al. Essential fatty acids in the treatment of premenstrual syndrome. *Obstet Gynecol* 1993;81:93.
40. Khoo SK, Munro C, Battistutta D. Evening primrose oil and treatment of premenstrual syndrome. *Med J Aust* 1990;153:189.
41. Blommers J, DeLange-deKlerk ESM, Kulk DJ, et al. Evening primrose oil and fish oil for severe chronic mastalgia: a randomized double-blind controlled trial. *Am J Obstet Gynecol* 2002;187:1389–1394.
42. Goyal A, Mansel RE. A randomized multicentre study of gamolenic acid (Efamast) with and without antioxidant vitamins and minerals in the management of mastalgia. *Breast J* 2005;11:41–47.
43. Mansel RE, Wisbey JR, Hughes LE. Controlled trial of the antigonadotrophin danazol in painful nodular benign breast disease. *Lancet* 1982;1:928.
44. Doberl A, Tobiassen T, Rasmussen T. Treatment of recurrent cyclical mastodynia in patients with fibrocystic breast disease. *Acta Obstet Gynecol Scand Suppl* 1984;123:177.
45. O'Brien PM, Abukhali IE. Randomized controlled trial of the management of premenstrual syndrome and premenstrual mastalgia using luteal phase-only danazol. *Am J Obstet Gynecol* 1999;180:18.
46. Abdel Hadi MSA. Sports brassiere: is it a solution for mastalgia? *Breast J* 2000;6:407.
47. Mansel RE, Preece PE, Hughes LE. A double-blind trial of the prolactin inhibitor bromocriptine in painful benign breast disease. *Br J Surg* 1978;65:724.
48. Blichert-Toft M, Nyobe Andersen AN, Hendriksen OB, et al. Treatment of mastalgia with bromocriptine: a double-blind cross-over study. *BMJ* 1979;1:237.
49. Durning P, Sellwood RA. Bromocriptine in severe cyclical breast pain. *Br J Surg* 1982;69:248.
50. Mansel RE, Dogliotti L. European multicentre trial of bromocriptine in cyclical mastalgia. *Lancet* 1990;335:190.
51. Hinton CP, Bishop HM, Holliday HW, et al. A double-blind controlled trial of danazol and bromocriptine in the management of severe cyclical breast pain. *Br J Clin Pract* 1986;40:326.
52. Kaleli S, Aydin Y, Erel CT, et al. Symptomatic treatment of premenstrual mastalgia in premenopausal women with lisuride maleate: a double-blind placebo-controlled randomized study. *Fertil Steril* 2001;75:718.
53. McFadyen IJ, Raab GM, Macintyre CCA, et al. Progesterone cream for cyclic breast pain. *BMJ* 1989;298:931.
54. Nappi C, Affinito P, Di Carlo C, et al. Double-blind controlled trial of progesterone vaginal cream treatment for cyclical mastodynia in women with benign breast disease. *J Endocrinol Invest* 1992;15:801.
55. Maddox PR, Harrison BJ, Horobin JM, et al. A randomized controlled trial of medroxyprogesterone acetate in mastalgia. *Ann R Coll Surg Engl* 1990;72:71.
56. Peters F. Multicentre study of gestrinone in cyclical breast pain. *Lancet* 1992;339:205.
57. Fentiman IS, Caleffi M, Brame K, et al. Double-blind controlled trial of tamoxifen therapy for mastalgia. *Lancet* 1986;1:287.
58. Messinis IE, Lolis D. Treatment of premenstrual mastalgia with tamoxifen. *Acta Obstet Gynecol Scand* 1988;67:307.
59. GEMB (Grupo de Estudio de Mastopatias Benignas). Tamoxifen therapy for cyclical mastalgia: dose randomized trial. *Breast* 1997;5:212.
60. Powles TJ, Ford HT, Gazet J-C. A randomized trial to compare tamoxifen with danazol for treatment of benign mammary dysplasia. *Breast Dis* 1987;2:1.
61. Kontostolis E, Stefanidis K, Navrozoglou I, et al. Comparison of tamoxifen with danazol for treatment of cyclical mastalgia. *Gynecol Endocrinol* 1997;11:393.
62. Sandrucci S, Mussa A, Festa V, et al. Comparison of tamoxifen and bromocriptine in management of fibrocystic breast disease: a randomized blind study. *Ann N Y Acad Sci* 1990;586:626.
63. Cuzick J, Powles T, Veronesi U, et al. Overview of the main outcomes in breast-cancer prevention trials. *Lancet* 2003;361:296–230.
64. Mansel RE, Goyal A, Le Nestour E, et al. (Afimoxifine (4-OHT) Breast Pain Research Group). A phase II trial of Afimoxifene (4-hydroxytamoxifen gel) for cyclical mastalgia in premenopausal women. *Breast Cancer Research and Treatment* 2007;106:389–397.
65. Mansel RE, Goyal A, Preece P, et al. European randomized, multicenter study of goserelin (Zoladex) in the management of mastalgia. *Am J Obstet Gynecol* 2004;191:1942–1949.
66. Ingram DI, Hickling C, West L, et al. A double-blind randomized controlled trial of isoflavones in the treatment of cyclical mastalgia. *Breast* 2002;11:170.
67. Habek D, Habek JC, Barbir A. Using acupuncture to treat premenstrual syndrome. *Arch Gynecol Obstet* 2007;267:23.
68. Gregory WM, Mills SP, Hamed HH, et al. Applied kinesiology for treatment of women with mastalgia. *Breast* 2001;10:15.
69. Halaska M, Gorkow C, Sieder C. Treatment of cyclical mastalgia with a solution containing a Vitex agnus castus extract: results of placebo controlled double-blind study. *Breast* 1999;8:175–181.
70. Ghent WR, Eskin BA, Low DA, et al. Iodine replacement in fibrocystic diseases of the breast. *Can J Surg* 1993;36:453.
71. Eskin BA. Iodine metabolism and breast cancer. *Trans N Y Acad Sci* 1970;32:911.
72. Kessler KH. The effect of supraphysiological levels of iodine on patients with cyclic mastalgia. *Breast J* 2004;10:328–336.
73. Crile G. Injection of steroids in painful breasts. *American Journal of Surgery* 1977;133:705.
74. Colak T, Ipek T, Kanik A, et al. Efficacy of topical nonsteroidal anti-inflammatory drugs in mastalgia treatment. *J Am Coll Surg* 2003;196:525–530.
75. Lloyd Davies E, Cochrane RA, Sweetland HM, et al. Is there a role for surgery in the treatment of mastalgia? *The Breast* 1999;8:285–288.

Richard B. Wait and Holly S. Mason

INTRODUCTION

Breast disease during pregnancy and lactation represents a clinical and diagnostic dilemma for the clinician. During this period, there is significant change to the breast parenchyma in the form of hormone-related hypertrophy and increased vascularity. These changes affect the clinical breast examination as well as alter the efficacy of current imaging modalities. Added to this is the need to balance concern for the mother with concern for the fetus. Breast cancer remains one of the most common types of cancer to be diagnosed during pregnancy or in the lactational period, with an incidence estimated to be 1 in 3,000 pregnancies (1–3) (see Chapter 68); however, benign breast disease is even more prevalent during pregnancy and lactation. It is critical for the physician to remain diligent in the evaluation of any breast abnormality in the pregnant or lactating patient. This chapter reviews the current state of the diagnosis and treatment of benign breast disease during pregnancy and lactation.

EVALUATION

Clinical Breast Examination

During the course of pregnancy, the pregnancy-related hormones (estrogen, progesterone, and prolactin) cause breast tissue to undergo significant changes that lead to increased volume and density (see Chapter 1). During the first trimester, the ratio of fatty tissue to glandular tissue decreases; as the volume of glandular tissue increases, so does the overall volume of the breast. As the pregnancy progresses, these changes intensify and make the evaluation of any breast abnormality more difficult. It is preferred, therefore, that the pregnant patient have a baseline clinical breast examination during the first trimester before these changes have occurred. As the number of women who become pregnant during their fourth decade increases, it is likely that more women will present already having had a baseline mammogram before becoming pregnant. A prior mammogram and any other imaging study obtained before pregnancy may help facilitate the evaluation of a new mass.

The pregnant patient who presents with a new mass or physical finding should be evaluated and followed very closely. If observation is chosen after completion of the appropriate workup (described later in this chapter), a short interval follow-up examination is indicated because delay in examination may allow pregnancy-related changes (volume or nodularity increase) to obscure the physical finding. Because the pregnant patient does not undergo the cyclic hormonal changes that the non-pregnant patient experiences, persistence of a mass after a short interval warrants further attention (Fig. 8.1). Ultimately, it is the responsibility of the clinician finding a breast mass to rule out a pregnancy-associated breast cancer.

Diagnostic Imaging Issues in Pregnancy and Lactation

When evaluating a pregnant patient, consideration must be give to minimizing exposure of ionizing radiation to the fetus. For this reason, ultrasonography is an ideal first option in the evaluation of a breast mass in this patient population. Ultrasound is a reliable means of differentiating a fluid-filled structure (cyst) versus a solid mass. It can assess the margins and shape of a solid mass, which may help differentiate a benign mass (e.g., lymph node or adenoma) from a malignancy. Ultrasound can easily guide aspiration of a cyst or percutaneous biopsy of a suspicious mass. An important benefit of ultrasound is that it is less affected by pregnancy-related changes than is mammography. Yang et al. (4) demonstrated that ultrasound had 100% sensitivity for identifying malignancy in a study of 20 women with breast cancer (Table 8.1). Similar results have been seen in other studies (5,6). For these reasons, ultrasound is the optimal first imaging study employed for a pregnancy-related breast mass.

The use of mammography in this patient population, on the other hand, remains controversial. Obvious concern exists about radiation exposure from mammography in pregnant patients. Estimates of ionizing radiation exposure to the mother remain at approximately 0.5 mGy per mammogram (5,7), but, with proper abdominal shielding, exposure to the fetus is considered negligible (8,9). Also affecting the utility of mammography, however, is the potential for lowered sensitivity owing to the increased density of the pregnant breast and the decrease in adipose tissue-to-breast parenchyma ratio (10). Several studies have contradicted this concept, demonstrating that an increase in mammographic density is not universally seen (11,12). Yang et al. (4) documented that a malignancy was visualized in 18 of 20 patients (90%) with breast cancer despite breast density issue. To improve the quality of the mammographic study in the lactating patient, the patient should empty her breast either by nursing or pumping just before having the study. Several studies have shown that ultrasound has consistently higher sensitivity rates as compared with mammography (see Table 8.1) (4–6,13,14). In general, mammography should not be the primary imaging tool if there is a suspicious physical examination finding in a pregnant patient; if a patient has a suspicious discrete mass on examination that is not visible on ultrasound, tissue diagnosis with percutaneous biopsy can be performed. Mammography is more useful in the lactating patient or in the newly-diagnosed pregnant patient to assess for calcifications or extent of disease.

Magnetic resonance imaging (MRI) of the breast has been used increasingly in the evaluation and treatment of breast cancer. At this time, however, it has not been well studied in the pregnant patient. Pregnancy-associated changes alter the ratio of parenchyma to adipose tissue, causing increased flow and permeability (15). In addition, gadolinium (the contrast agent used in breast MRI) crosses the placenta and, therefore, is a pregnancy category C drug. It is advised to wait until after first trimester if breast MRI is judged to be absolutely necessary (16,17). Gadolinium uptake in lactating breast tissue can mimic malignancy, however, and result in a false–positive study result (15). MRI is currently not indicated in the pregnant patient for these reasons.

Tissue Biopsy in the Pregnant and Lactating Patient

Percutaneous biopsy has become the standard of care for tissue diagnosis of any breast mass or imaging abnormality. Surgical incisional or excisional biopsy for diagnosis necessitates an

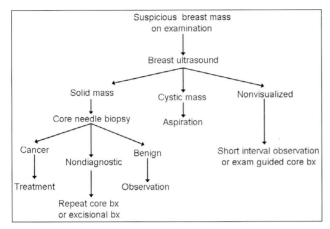

FIGURE 8.1. Flow diagram for management of clinically suspicious breast masses during pregnancy.

incision and potential need to return for more surgery if the biopsy reveals malignancy. The clinician must protect the fetus while ensuring appropriate treatment for the pregnant patient. In addition, minimal disruption of the ductal structures should be a goal to allow for lactation. An in-depth discussion of the risks and benefits of biopsy needs to be discussed with the patient to allow for informed consent.

For many years, fine needle aspiration biopsy (FNAB) was thought to be the best method of percutaneous tissue diagnosis. In the pregnant or lactating patient, the hormone-mediated hyperproliferation of ductal cells can, however, result in a false–positive diagnosis in the hands of an inexperienced cytopathologist (18,19). In addition, FNAB can miss the intended target, causing a false–negative result. Percutaneous core biopsy can be more accurate and will provide the cellular architecture needed for a more definitive diagnosis. Excisional biopsy should only be undertaken when there is a lack of concordance between clinical suspicion, imaging result, and percutaneous biopsy result (Fig. 8.1). If an excisional biopsy is intended in the pregnant patient, surgery should be carefully planned to minimize the risk to the fetus from anesthesia, including fetal monitoring if indicated. Local anesthesia alone is preferred method in these cases.

Care must be taken in this patient population to minimize operative complications. Gestational or lactational breast tissue is hypervascular, and meticulous hemostasis is mandatory with any intervention to prevent hematoma formation. Breast milk provides a good culture medium for bacteria and, therefore, efforts must be made to minimize the risk of infection (18). The lactating patient should either nurse or express milk regularly after a biopsy to prevent milk stasis. If infection should develop, antibiotics can be administered.

The development of a milk fistula, a tract between a lactiferous duct and the skin, is a potential complication of any percutaneous or surgical intervention. The risk of milk fistula, whether from FNA, core biopsy or excision, is not well documented, although case reports exist in the literature (20,21). Some clinicians suggest breast binding as a means of facilitating cessation of milk leakage, but this is not likely to succeed. Bromocriptine, a dopamine agonist that decreases prolactin levels, can be used to treat a milk fistula, but it is not routinely recommended (18,20). Cessation of lactation will allow the fistula tract to heal, and remains the only reliable method to control a milk fistula (20). If possible, the patient should stop lactation 1 week before the biopsy to minimize this risk.

CLINICAL PROBLEMS

Inflammatory and Infectious Problems in Pregnancy

Breast milk represents a lactose-rich culture medium and, thus, inflammatory or infectious problems remain the most common issues for the pregnant patient (22). Milk stasis, or poor emptying of milk from the breast, results from ineffective suckling, restriction of frequency of feeds, or blockage of milk ducts (23). Poor infant attachment to the breast can lead to cracking of the nipple epithelium, which is thought to allow bacteria to enter the breast in a retrograde direction via the terminal ducts, and it has been shown to be a risk factor for mastitis (24). Milk stasis, which provides a medium for bacterial growth and injury to the nipple, with subsequent bacterial translocation. Milk stasis can lead to a generalized infection (mastitis) with fever, redness, and tenderness, and it may also result in a breast abscess. *Staphylococcus aureus* is the most common organism (Table 8.2) and usually it can be treated with oral antibiotics (25). Other known risk factors for mastitis include age (<21 or >35 years) (26), primiparity (27), and a previous episode of mastitis (26). It is most important to continue the expression of breast milk to allow for complete emptying of the breast and symptom relief. Education concerning proper emptying, positioning of the infant, and nipple hygiene should be a key component to prevent future episodes of mastitis (23).

A breast abscess will not resolve with antibiotics alone, however, and further intervention is necessary. Ultrasound will help to differentiate mastitis from a breast abscess. Repeated aspiration can be successful and it can avoid a disfiguring incision and drainage (28). Aspirate cultures should be taken to ensure adequate antibiotic coverage. Skin and parenchymal biopsies should be considered to rule out inflammatory breast cancer (as seen in 3% of pregnant patients in a 1992 Memorial Sloan-Kettering series) (29) if no improvement is seen. Despite

		Imaging Study	Imaging Study
Table 8.1	**SENSITIVITY OF ULTRASONOGRAPHY AND MAMMOGRAPHY IN PREGNANT WOMEN[a]**		
Author	Number of Patients	Ultrasound	Mammography
Yang et al. 2006 (4)	23	100% (20 of 20)	90% (18 of 20)
Liberman et al. 1994 (5)	23	100% (6 of 6)	78% (18 of 23)
Ahn et al. 2006 (6)	22	100% (19 of 19)	86.7% (13 of 25)
Ishida et al. 1992 (13)	192	93% (39 of 42)	68% (34 of 50)
Samuels et al. 1998 (14)	19	100% (4 of 4)	63% (5 of 8[J8])

[a]Specificity data are not available. There is currently no data on the sensitivity of breast MRI in the pregnant patient.

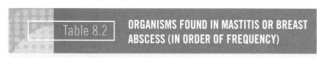

Table 8.2	ORGANISMS FOUND IN MASTITIS OR BREAST ABSCESS (IN ORDER OF FREQUENCY)

Staphylococcus aureus
Staphylococcus epidermidis
Streptococcus (alpha, beta and non-hemolytic)
Escherichia coli
Candida (rare)

(WHO, 19)

Table 8.3	FREQUENCY OF PATHOLOGY TYPES OF PREGNANCY-RELATED BREAST MASSES

Pathology	Collins et al. 1995 (31)	Son et al. 2006 (10)	Byrd et al. 1962 (41)	Slavin et al. 1993 (32)
All non-pregnancy benign neoplasms[a]	4/19	2/29	39/105	18/30
All pregnancy-related benign neoplasms	14/19	18/29	23/105	12/30
[b]Infection		9/29	7/105	
Benign or fibrocystic breast tissue	1/19		36/105	

[a]Tubular adenoma, fibroadenoma, hamartoma, adenofibroma, lipoma, papilloma, phyllodes tumor.
[b]Lactating adenoma, lobular hyperplasia, galactocele or other changes "coincident with pregnancy."

concerns of the risk to the infant from bacterial contamination in the breast milk (30), the World Health Organization currently does not recommend cessation of breast-feeding in the presence of a breast abscess (23).

Management of Solid Masses in Pregnancy and Lactation

Most solid masses in the pregnant or lactating patient are benign lesions, such as fibroadenomas and hamartomas, and often predate the pregnancy. Any cause for a breast mass in the nonpregnant or lactating woman can also exist in pregnancy or the postpartum period.

Lactating adenomas are the most common cause of breast masses in this patient population and arise owing to hormones associated with pregnancy and lactation (31). Lactating adenomas may be related to tubular adenomas, fibroadenomas, or hyperplasia (32). Biopsy can determine if a mass is a true lactating adenoma or is caused by lactational change in a pre-existing fibroadenoma (33). Ultrasound remains an effective tool in the evaluation of these benign masses (Fig. 8.1). Sumkin et al. (34) documented that the ultrasound features of lactating adenomas are benign (ovoid shape, well-defined margins, posterior acoustic enhancement), but nonspecific. Most of these lesions will involute once lactation has stopped, although excision may be required for those that do not. Hemorrhage or infarction will occur in 5% of lactating adenomas owing to vascular insufficiency seen occasionally in pregnancy-induced proliferative breast tissue (33). Lactating adenomas are not thought to be a risk factor for breast cancer (35), although there are case reports of breast cancer arising at the site of an excised lactating adenoma or occurring concurrent with a lactating adenoma (33,35,36).

Galactoceles are milk-filled cysts, which are thought to occur because of ductal obstruction during lactation (37). These usually present as tender masses; ultrasound can differentiate a galactocele from a solid mass. Asymptomatic patients can safely be observed. Local breast care, including ice packs and breast support, may help alleviate the discomfort, although aspiration provides the greatest likelihood of symptom relief (22). Rarely, galactoceles can become infected, but they can be effectively treated with repeated aspiration or drain placement in addition to appropriate antibiotics (28,38,39).

Localized breast infarction can occur in the pregnant or lactating breast and often results in a palpable mass that must be differentiated from breast cancer (40). Other benign breast lesions, such as fibroadenomas, lipomas, and papillomas, can occur in these patients and, overall, are just as likely to be the cause of a breast mass as pregnancy-related lesions (10,31,32,41) (Table 8.3).

Bloody Nipple Discharge

The presence of bloody nipple discharge creates significant patient anxiety because of its association with breast cancer. In the nonpregnant patient, the evaluation of bloody nipple discharge has been well-described (see Chapter 6). The workup in the pregnant or lactating patient remains controversial, however, because of the issues with imaging as previously discussed. As in the nonpregnant or lactating population, most bloody nipple discharge is of benign etiology.

Bloody nipple discharge can occur owing to the epithelial proliferation and new capillary formation that occurs during the second and third trimesters (22,42). A careful clinical breast examination should include obtaining a sample of discharge for cytology. The location of the draining duct should be carefully documented. If the examination does not reveal a palpable mass, retroareolar ultrasound can be undertaken. If cytology shows abnormal or atypical cells, further imaging with mammography and ductography should be performed to identify the lesion location, which then should be biopsied. Terminal duct excision remains an option but may predispose the patient to having difficulty with lactation with subsequent pregnancies.

Controversy arises in the evaluation of the patient with cytology that does not show any abnormality. Some authors suggest that observation is reasonable in patients without physical finding or abnormal cytology (43,44). Lafreniere (43) reported in her series of five patients that no malignancies were identified over a 2-year follow-up period. All patients had drainage from multiple ducts rather than a single orifice. On the other hand, King et al. (45) identified three women whose only presenting symptom was bloody nipple discharge and who were subsequently diagnosed with breast cancer. Because of this possibility, some authors support terminal duct excision in this patient population (42,45).

MANAGEMENT SUMMARY

- Although most problems related to the breast in the pregnant or lactating patient are of benign origin, a thorough clinical and imaging evaluation is mandatory to rule out malignancy.
- Ultrasound remains the imaging technique of choice for initial evaluation because of its safety and sensitivity.
- Percutaneous core biopsy is the preferred method to obtain a tissue diagnosis of a solid mass, although FNA remains an acceptable option. Although not the preferred method of diagnosis, surgical excision may be appropriate in certain circumstances. Surgical excision of a biopsy-proved benign mass should be deferred either

until pregnancy or lactation has been completed or until the risk to the fetus and mother can be minimized.

- The management of bloody nipple discharge remains controversial. It is considered mandatory to obtain a sample of the discharge for cytology. Abnormal discharge cytology should be treated appropriately; patients with normal cytology should be followed closely.
- Infectious or inflammatory problems remain a common cause of breast pathology during the pregnant or lactational period. Repeated aspiration with antibiotic therapy is an acceptable means of treating an abscess. If incision and drainage is undertaken, biopsy of the abscess wall is a reasonable undertaking for histologic evaluation and elimination of malignancy as a possible cause of the abscess.

References

1. Barnes DM, Newman LA. Pregnancy-associated breast cancer: a literature review. *Surg Clin North Am* 2007;87:417–430.
2. White TT. Prognosis of breast cancer for pregnant and nursing women. Analysis of 1,1413 cases. *Surg Gynecol Obstet* 1955;100:661–666.
3. Loibl S, von Minckwitz G, Gwyn K, et al. Breast carcinoma during pregnancy. International recommendations from an expert meeting. *Cancer* 2006;106: 237–246.
4. Yang WT, Dryden MJ, Gwyn K, et al. Imaging of breast cancer diagnosed and treated with chemotherapy during pregnancy. *Radiology* 2006;239:52–60.
5. Liberman L, Geiss CS, Dershaw DD, et al. Imaging of pregnancy-associated breast cancer. *Radiology* 1994;191:245–248.
6. Ahn B, Kim HH, Moon WK, et al. Pregnancy- and lactation-associated breast cancer: mammographic and sonographic findings. *J Ultrasound Med* 2003;22: 491–497.
7. Berlin L. Radiation exposure and the pregnant patient. *AJR Am J Roentgenol* 1996; 167:1377–1379.
8. Woo JC, Taechin Y, Hurd T. Breast cancer in pregnancy—a literature review. *Arch Surg* 2003;138:91–99.
9. Streffer C, Shore R, Kinermann G, et al. Biologic effects after prenatal irradiation (embryo and fetus). A report of the International Commission on Radiological Protection. *Ann ICRP* 2003;33:205–206.
10. Son EJ, Oh KK, Kim EK. Pregnancy-associated breast disease: radiologic features and diagnostic dilemmas. *Yonsei Med J* 2006;47:34–42.
11. Swinford AE, Adler DD, Garver KA. Mammographic appearance of the breasts during pregnancy and lactation: false assumptions. *Acad Radiol* 1998;5:467–472.
12. Hogge JP, de Paredes ES, Magnant CM, et al. Imaging and management of breast masses during pregnancy and lactation. *Breast J* 1999;5:272–283.
13. Ishida T, Yokoe T, Kasumi F, et al. Clinicopathological characteristics and prognosis of breast cancer patients associated with pregnancy and lactation: analysis of case control study in Japan. *Jpn J Cancer Res* 1992;83:1143–1149.
14. Samuels T, Liu F, Yaffe M, et al. Gestational breast cancer. *Can Assoc Radiol J* 1998;49:172–180.
15. Talele AC, Slantez PJ, Edminster WB, et al. The lactating breast: MRI findings and literature review. *Breast J* 2003;9:237–240.
16. Kanal E. Pregnancy and the safety of magnetic resonance imaging. *Magn Reson Imaging Clin N Am* 1994;2:309–317.
17. Oto A, Ernst R, Jesse MK, et al. Magnetic resonance imaging of the chest, abdomen, and pelvis in the evaluation of pregnant patients with neoplasms. *Am J Perinatol* 2007;24:243–250.
18. Petrek JA. Breast cancer during pregnancy. *Cancer* 1994;74:518–527.
19. Finley JL, Silverman JF, Lannin DR. Fine-needle aspiration cytology of breast masses in pregnant and lactating women. *Diagn Cytopathol* 1989;5:255–260.
20. Schackmuth EM, Harlow CL, Norton LW. Milk fistula: a complication after core biopsy. *AJR Am J Roentgenol* 1993;161:961–962.
21. Barker P. Milk fistula: an unusual complication of breast biopsy. *J R Coll Surg Edinb* 1988;33:106.
22. Scott-Conner CEH, Schorr SJ. The diagnosis and management of breast problems during pregnancy and lactation. *Am J Surg* 1995;170:401–405.
23. World Health Organization. Mastitis: causes and management. Geneva, WHO/FCH/CAH/00.13;2000.
24. Amir LH, Forster DA, Lumley J, et al. A descriptive study of mastitis in Australian breastfeeding women: incidence and determinants. *BMC Public Health* 2007; 7:62.
25. Niebyl J, Spence M, Parmely T. Sporadic (nonepidemic) puerperal mastitis. *J Reprod Med* 1978;20:97–100.
26. Jonsson S. Pulkkinen MO. Mastitis today: incidence, prevention and treatment. *Annales Chirugiae Et Gynaecologiae. Supplementum* 1994;208:84–87.
27. Kaufmann R, Foxman B. Mastitis among lactating women: occurrence and risk factors. *Soc Sci Med* 1991;33:701–705.
28. Dixon JM. Repeated aspirations of breast abscesses in lactating women. *BMJ* 1988;297:1517–1518.
29. Petrek JA, Dukoff R, Rogatko A. Prognosis of pregnancy-associated breast cancer. *Cancer* 1991;67:869–872.
30. Eschenbach DA. Acute postpartum infections. *Emerg Med Clin North Am* 1985;3: 87–115.
31. Collins JC, Liao S, Wile AG. Surgical management of breast masses in pregnant women. *J Reprod Med* 1995;40:785–788.
32. Slavin JC, Billson VR, Ostor AG. Nodular breast lesions during pregnancy and lactation. *Histopathology* 1993;22:481–485.
33. Baker TP, Lenert JT, Parker J et al. Lactating adenoma: a diagnosis of exclusion. *Breast J* 2001;7:354–357.
34. Sumkin JH, Perrone AM, Harris KM, et al. Lactating Adenoma: US Features and literature review. *Radiology* 1998;206:271–274.
35. Saglam A, Can B. Coexistence of lactating adenoma and invasive ductal adenocarcinoma of the breast in a pregnant woman. *J Clin Pathol* 2005;58:87–89.
36. Hertel BF, Zaloudek C, Kempson RL. Breast adenomas. *Cancer* 1976;37:2891–2905.
37. Winker JM. Galactocele of the breast. *Am J Surg* 1964;108:357–360.
38. Ghosh K, Morton MJ, Whaley DH, et al. Infected galactocele: a perplexing problem. *Breast J* 2004;10:159.
39. O'Hara RJ, Dexter SPL, Fox JN. Conservative management of infective mastitis and breast abscesses after ultrasonographic assessment. *Br J Surg* 1996;83:1413–1414.
40. Lucy JJ. Spontaneous infarction of the breast. *J Clin Pathol* 1975;28:937–943.
41. Byrd BF, Bayer DS, Robertson JC, et al. Treatment of breast tumors associated with pregnancy and lactation. *Ann Surg* 1962;155:940.
42. Psyrri A, Burtness B. Pregnancy-associated breast cancer. *Cancer J* 2005;11: 83–95.
43. Lafreniere R. Bloody nipple discharge during pregnancy: a rationale for conservative treatment. *J Surg Oncol* 1990;43:228–230.
44. Petrek JA. Abnormalities of the breast in pregnancy and lactation. In: Harris JR, ed. *Diseases of the breast*. 3rd ed. Philadelphia: Lippincott Williams & Wilkins, 2004:63–67.
45. King RM, Welch JS, Martin JK Jr, et al. Carcinoma of the breast associated with pregnancy. *Surg Gynecol Obstet* 1985;160:228–232.

Glenn D. Braunstein

Benign proliferation of the glandular tissue of the male breast constitutes the histologic hallmark of gynecomastia, which, if sufficiently great, appears clinically as palpable or visual enlargement of the breast. This condition, which is exceedingly common, may (a) be a sign of a serious underlying pathologic condition, (b) cause physical or emotional discomfort, or (c) be confused with other breast problems, most significantly carcinoma.

 ## PREVALENCE

Breast glandular proliferation commonly occurs in infancy, during puberty, and in older age. It has been estimated that between 60% and 90% of infants exhibit the transient development of palpable breast tissue owing to estrogenic stimulation from the maternal–placental–fetal unit. This stimulus for breast growth ceases as the estrogens are cleared from the neonatal circulation, and the breast tissue gradually regresses over a 2- to 3-week period. Although population studies have shown that the prevalence of pubertal gynecomastia varies widely, most have indicated that 30% to 60% of pubertal boys exhibit gynecomastia, which usually begins between 10 and 12 years of age, with the highest prevalence between 13 and 14 years of age (corresponding to Tanner stage III or IV of pubertal development), followed by involution that is usually complete by age 16 to 17 years (1–10). The percentage of men who exhibit gynecomastia increases with advancing age, with the highest prevalence found in the 50- to 80-year age range (Fig. 9.1). The prevalence of the condition in men ranges between 24% and 65%, with the differences between series being accounted for by the defining criteria and by the population studied (10–17).

PATHOGENESIS

No inherent differences appear to exist in the hormonal responsiveness of the male or female breast glandular tissue (9,18). The hormonal milieu, the duration and intensity of stimulation, and the individual's breast tissue sensitivity determine the type and degree of glandular proliferation. Under the influence of estrogens, the ducts elongate and branch, the ductal epithelium becomes hyperplastic, the periductal fibroblasts proliferate, and the vascularity increases. This histologic picture is found early in the course of gynecomastia and is often referred to as the *florid stage*. Acinar development is not seen in the male because it requires the presence of progesterone in concentrations found during the luteal phase of the menstrual cycle (18,19). Androgens exert an antiestrogen effect on rodent breast cancer models and the human MCF-7 breast cancer cell line; they are thought to antagonize at least some of the effects of estrogens in normal breast tissue (20,21). Accordingly, gynecomastia is usually considered to represent an imbalance between the breast-stimulatory effects of estrogen and the inhibitory effects of androgens. In fact, alterations in the estrogen-to-androgen ratio have been found in many of the conditions associated with gynecomastia. Such alterations can occur through a variety of mechanisms (Table 9.1; Fig. 9.2).

In men, the testes secrete 95% of the testosterone, 15% of the estradiol, and less than 5% of the estrone produced daily. Most of the circulating estrogens are derived from the extraglandular conversion of estrogen precursors by extragonadal tissues, including the liver, skin, fat, muscle, bone, and kidney (Fig. 9.2). These tissues contain the aromatase enzyme that converts testosterone to estradiol and androstenedione, an androgen primarily secreted by the adrenal glands, to estrone. Estradiol and estrone are interconverted in extragonadal tissues through the activity of the 17-ketosteroid reductase enzyme. This enzyme is also responsible for the interconversion of testosterone and androstenedione. When androgens and estrogens enter the circulation, either through direct secretion from gonadal tissues or from the sites of extragonadal metabolism, most are bound to sex hormone-binding globulin (SHBG), a protein derived primarily from the liver and one that has a greater affinity for androgens than for estrogens. The non-SHBG sex hormones circulate either in the free or unbound state or are weakly bound to albumin. These fractions are able to cross the plasma membrane of target cells and are bound to steroid receptors. Testosterone and dihydrotestosterone bind to the same hormone-responsive element. Each also binds to the hormone-responsive element of the appropriate genes, resulting in the initiation of transcription and hormone action. A similar sequence of events occurs after the binding of estradiol or estrone to the estrogen receptor (19).

From a pathophysiologic standpoint, an imbalance between estrogen and androgen concentrations or effects can occur as a result of abnormalities at several levels (Table 9.1; Fig. 9.2). Overproduction of estrogens from testicular or adrenal neoplasms or enhanced extraglandular conversion of estrogen precursors to estrogens can elevate the total estrogen concentration. Such extraglandular conversion can occur directly in the breast tissue. Indeed, increased aromatization of androgens to estrogens has been noted in pubic skin fibroblasts from some patients with idiopathic gynecomastia (22). Elevations of the absolute quantity of circulating free estrogens can occur if estrogen metabolism is slowed or if SHBG-bound estrogens are displaced from the protein. Conversely, decreased secretion of androgens from the testes—caused primary by defects in the testes or secondary to loss of tonic stimulation by pituitary gonadotropins, enhanced metabolic degradation of androgens, or increased binding of androgens to SHBG—results in decreases in free androgens that could antagonize the effect of estrogens on the breast glandular tissue. As noted previously, androgen and estrogen balance depends not only on the amount and availability of free androgens and estrogens but on their ability to act at the target tissue level. Thus, defects in the androgen receptor or displacement of androgens from their receptors by drugs with antiandrogenic effects (e.g., spironolactone) result in decreased androgen action and, hence, decreased estrogen antagonism at the breast glandular cell level. Finally, the inherent sensitivity of an individual's breast tissue to estrogen or androgen action may predispose some persons to development of gynecomastia even in the presence of apparently normal concentrations of estrogens and androgens.

 ## ASSOCIATED CONDITIONS

Tables 9.1 and 9.2 list the various conditions and drugs that have been associated with gynecomastia. Although the list is relatively long, almost two-thirds of the patients have either pubertal gynecomastia (approximately 25%), drug-induced gynecomastia (10% to 20%), or no underlying abnormality detected (idiopathic gynecomastia, approximately 25%). Most of the remainder have cirrhosis or malnutrition (8%), primary hypogonadism (8%), testicular tumors (3%), secondary

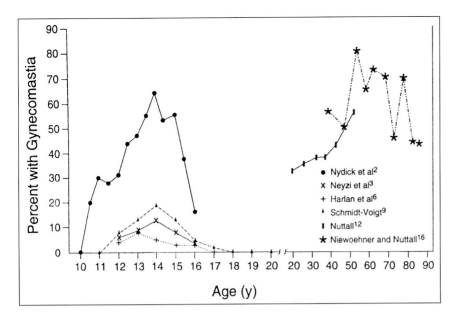

FIGURE 9.1. Prevalence of gynecomastia at various chronologic ages. Data were derived from multiple population studies (2,3,6,9,12,16). (Adapted from Braunstein GD. Pubertal gynecomastia. In: Lifshitz F, ed. *Pediatric endocrinology.* New York: Marcel Dekker, 1996:197–205, with permission.)

hypogonadism (2%), hyperthyroidism (1.5%), or renal disease (1%) (23). For most pathologic conditions, alterations in the balance between estrogen and androgen levels or action occur through several of the pathophysiologic mechanisms outlined in Table 9.1 and Figure 9.2. One of the best examples is the gynecomastia associated with spironolactone. This aldosterone antagonist inhibits the testicular biosynthesis of testosterone, enhances the conversion of testosterone to the less potent androgen androstenedione, increases the aromatization of testosterone to estradiol, displaces testosterone from SHBG (leading to an increase in its metabolic clearance rate), and binds to the androgen receptors in target tissues, thereby acting as an antiandrogen (24). For an in-depth discussion of

the pathophysiology of gynecomastia associated with each of the conditions listed in Tables 9.1 and 9.2, the reader is referred to primary sources and several reviews (14,18,19, 23,25–35).

 EVALUATION

Most patients with gynecomastia are asymptomatic, with the condition detected during a physical examination. Patients with recent onset of gynecomastia owing to drugs or one of the pathologic conditions noted in Tables 9.1 and 9.2, however, may present with breast or nipple pain and tenderness. Approximately

Table 9.1	CONDITIONS ASSOCIATED WITH GYNECOMASTIA AND THEIR PRIMARY PATHOPHYSIOLOGIC MECHANISMS

Physiologic
  Neonatal
  Pubertal
  Aging
Pathologic
  Idiopathic
  Drug induced (see Table 9.2)
  Increased serum estrogen
    Increased aromatization (peripheral and glandular)
      Sertoli cell (sex cord) tumors
      Testicular germ cell tumors
      Leydig cell tumors
      Adrenocortical carcinoma
      Hermaphroditism
      Obesity
      Hyperthyroidism
      Liver disease
      Testicular feminization
      Refeeding after starvation
      Primary aromatase excess
    Displacement of estrogen from sex hormone-binding globulin
      Spironolactone
      Ketoconazole
    Decreased estrogen metabolism
      Cirrhosis (?)
    Exogenous sources
      Topical estrogen creams and lotions

      Ingestion of estrogen
      Tree tea or lavender oils
    Eutopic hCG production
      Choriocarcinoma
    Ectopic hCG production
      Lung carcinoma
      Liver carcinoma
      Gastric carcinoma
      Kidney carcinoma
  Decreased testosterone synthesis
    Primary gonadal failure, congenital
      Anorchia
      Klinefelter's syndrome
      Hermaphroditism
      Hereditary defects in testosterone synthesis
    Primary gonadal failure, acquired
      Viral orchitis
      Castration
      Granulomatous diseases (including leprosy)
    Testicular failure owing to hypothalamic or pituitary disease
  Androgen resistance owing to androgen receptor defects
Other
  Chronic renal failure
  Chronic illness
  Spinal cord injury
  Human immunodeficiency virus
  Enhanced breast tissue sensitivity

hCG, human chorionic gonadotropin.
Adapted with permission from Mathur R, Braunstein GD. Gynecomastia: pathomechanisms and treatment strategies. *Horm Res* 1997;48:95–102.

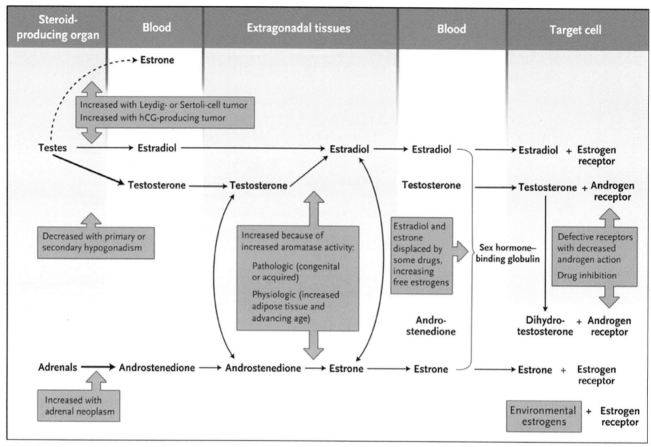

FIGURE 9.2. Pathways of estrogen and androgen production, action, and metabolism, and pathologic and physiologic changes that alter the pathways. (Adapted from Braunstein GD. Gynecomastia. *New Engl J Med* 2007;357:1229–1237, with permission.)

Table 9.2	DRUGS ASSOCIATED WITH GYNECOMASTIA

Hormones
Androgens and anabolic steroids[a]
Chorionic gonadotropin[a]
Estrogens and estrogen agonists[a]
Growth hormone

Antiandrogens or Inhibitors of Androgen Synthesis
Bicalutamide[a]
Cyproterone[az]
Flutamide[a]
Gonadotropin-releasing hormone agonists[a]
Nilutamide[a]

Antibiotics
Ethionamide
Isoniazid
Ketoconazole[a]
Metronidazole
Minocycline

Antiulcer Medications
Cimetidine[a]
Omeprazole
Ranitidine

Cancer Chemotherapeutic Agents
Alkylating agents[a]
Methotrexate
Vinca alkaloids
Combination chemotherapy

Cardiovascular Drugs
Amiodarone
Captopril
Digitoxin[a]

Digoxin
Diltiazem
Enalapril
Methyldopa
Nifedipine
Reserpine
Spironolactone[a]
Verapamil

Psychoactive Agents
Diazepam
Haloperidol
Phenothiazine
Tricyclic antidepressants

Drugs of Abuse
Alcohol
Amphetamines
Heroin
Marijuana
Methadone

Other
Auranofin
Diethylpropion
Domperidone
Etretinate
Highly active antiretroviral
   therapy (HAART)[a]
Metoclopramide
Penicillamine
Phenytoin
Sulindac
Theophylline

[a]A strong relation has been established. Other relations have been proposed on the basis of epidemiologic studies or challenge–rechallenge studies of individual patients or small groups of patients.

10% to 15% of patients recall a history of breast trauma just before or at the time of discovery of the breast enlargement (18,28). It is unclear whether breast trauma itself causes gynecomastia. It is likely that, in many patients with an antecedent history of trauma, the breast irritation from the trauma actually led to the discovery of preexisting gynecomastia. Although half of patients have clinically apparent bilateral gynecomastia, histologic studies have shown that virtually all patients have bilateral involvement (15). This discrepancy may be explained by asynchronous growth of the two breasts and differences in the amount of breast glandular and stromal proliferation.

Gynecomastia must be differentiated from other conditions that cause breast enlargement. Although neurofibromas, dermoid cysts, lipomas, hematomas, and lymphangiomas may enlarge portions of the breast, these abnormalities are usually easily distinguished from gynecomastia on historical or clinical grounds. The two conditions that are most important to differentiate are pseudogynecomastia and breast carcinoma. *Pseudogynecomastia* refers to enlargement of the breasts owing to fat deposition rather than to glandular proliferation. Patients with this condition often have generalized obesity and do not complain of breast pain or tenderness. In addition, the breast examination should allow the correct diagnosis (Fig. 9.3). The breasts are examined while the patient is lying on the back with hands behind the head. The examiner places a thumb on one side of the breast and the second finger on the other side. The fingers are then gradually brought together without more than superficial pressure being applied to the skin. Patients with gynecomastia have a rubbery or firm disc of tissue that extends concentrically out from the nipple and that either is easily palpated or offers some resistance to the apposition of the fingers, whereas those with pseudogynecomastia exhibit no such mound of tissue, and no resistance is felt as the fingers are brought together. Alternatively, flat palpation with the finger can be used to detect the glandular tissue.

Differentiation of gynecomastia from breast carcinoma usually can be accomplished through careful physical examination. Carcinoma of the breast in men is usually eccentric in location and unilateral (rather than subareolar and bilateral) and is hard or firm, whereas gynecomastia tends to be rubbery to firm in texture. Patients with carcinoma may also exhibit skin dimpling and nipple retraction; they are more likely to have a nipple discharge (10%) than are patients with gynecomastia and may present with axillary lymphadenopathy (28,36). If the two conditions cannot be differentiated on clinical grounds, then mammography, fine-needle aspiration (FNA) for cytologic examination, or open biopsy should be done. There is no increased risk of breast cancer in men with gynecomastia followed for 20 or more years (37). Data, however, indicate that the prevalence of Klinefelter's syndrome (XXY genotype) is increased up to 50-fold in men with breast cancer (38). In contrast, other studies have not found an increase in breast cancer risk in patients with Klinefelter's syndrome (39).

After a clinical diagnosis of gynecomastia has been made, several causes should be investigated through a thorough history and physical examination. A careful history of medication use is essential, specifically regarding ingestion of the drugs listed in Table 9.2. A history of liver or renal disease, especially if the patient has been receiving hemodialysis for the latter, may point to the underlying cause. A history of weight loss, tachycardia, tremulousness, diaphoresis, heat intolerance, and hyperdefecation, with or without the presence of a goiter, raises the possibility of hyperthyroidism. The patient should be evaluated for the signs and symptoms of hypogonadism, including loss of libido, impotence, decreased strength, and testicular atrophy. A careful examination for abdominal masses, which may be present in nearly one-half the patients with adrenocortical carcinoma, and a meticulous examination for testicular masses are essential parts of the evaluation.

The next step depends on the results of the clinical evaluation. If any of the drugs listed in Table 9.2 have been ingested, they should be discontinued and the patient reexamined in 1 month. If the drug was the inciting agent, then a decrease in breast pain and tenderness should occur during that time. If

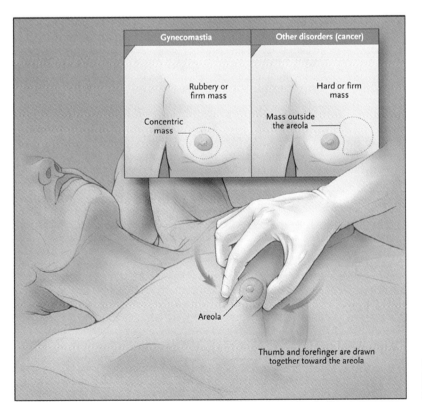

FIGURE 9.3. Differentiation of gynecomastia from pseudogynecomastia and other disorders by physical examination. (From Braunstein GD. Gynecomastia. *New Engl J Med* 2007;357:1229–1237, with permission.)

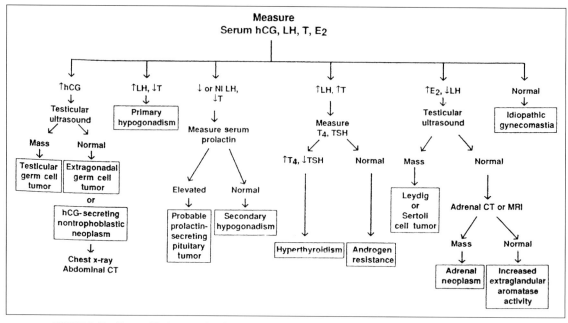

FIGURE 9.4. Algorithm providing interpretation of serum hormone levels and recommendations for further evaluation of patients with gynecomastia. CT, computed tomography; E_2, estradiol; hCG, human chorionic gonadotropin; LH, luteinizing hormone; MRI, magnetic resonance imaging; NI, normal; T, testosterone; T_4, thyroxine; TSH, thyroid-stimulating hormone. (From Braunstein GD. Gynecomastia. *N Engl J Med* 1993;328:490–495, with permission.)

the patient is of pubertal age and has an otherwise negative general physical and testicular examination, he probably has transient or persistent pubertal gynecomastia. Reexamination at 3-month intervals should determine whether the condition is transient or persistent. At this time, medical or surgical therapy should be considered. If, during routine clinical examination, an adult is found to have asymptomatic gynecomastia without the presence of underlying disease, biochemical assessments of liver, kidney, thyroid function and testosterone should be performed. In a patient with normal results, no further tests are necessary, but he should be reevaluated in 6 months. Conversely, if the gynecomastia is of recent onset or if the patient complains of pain or tenderness, additional studies—including measurements of serum concentrations of human chorionic gonadotropin (hCG), estradiol, testosterone, and luteinizing hormone—should be done, although the diagnostic yield is often low (40).

The algorithm outlined in Figure 9.4 can be used to discern the underlying abnormality, if any, that is responsible for the breast enlargement (22). An elevated level of hCG in the serum indicates the presence of a testicular or nongonadal germ cell tumor or, rarely, a nontrophoblastic neoplasm that secretes the hormone ectopically. Testicular ultrasonography should be done, and, if no testicular mass is found, a chest radiograph and abdominal computed tomographic scan or magnetic resonance imaging (MRI) study should be performed in an effort to localize an extragonadal hCG–producing tumor. Most nontrophoblastic tumors that secrete the hormone are bronchogenic, gastric, renal cell, or hepatic carcinomas. An elevated serum concentration of luteinizing hormone associated with a low testosterone level is indicative of primary hypogonadism, whereas a low testosterone level and a low or normal luteinizing hormone level suggest secondary hypogonadism owing to a hypothalamic or pituitary abnormality. Serum prolactin concentration should be determined in this situation to rule out a prolactin-secreting pituitary adenoma, which can cause hypogonadotropic hypogonadism. Elevated serum concentrations of luteinizing hormone and testosterone are found with hyperthyroidism and in patients with

various forms of androgen resistance caused by androgen receptor disorders. Thyroid function tests can distinguish between these conditions.

If an elevated serum estradiol level is found along with a normal or suppressed concentration of luteinizing hormone, testicular ultrasonography is indicated to rule out a Leydig cell, Sertoli cell, or sex cord testicular tumor. If the ultrasonogram is negative, a computed tomographic scan or MRI scan of the adrenal glands should be done to detect an estrogen-secreting adrenal neoplasm. If both the testes and adrenal glands appear normal, the increased estradiol level is probably caused by enhanced extraglandular aromatization of estrogen precursors to estrogens. In this situation, estrone levels are often relatively higher than estradiol concentrations. Finally, if all of these endocrine measurements are normal, the patient is considered to have idiopathic gynecomastia.

 PREVENTION

Two situations exist in which gynecomastia can be prevented. The first is in patients who require a medication. Avoidance of the drugs listed in Table 9.2 decreases the risk for drug-induced breast stimulation. Also, not all the therapeutic agents in the drug groups listed in the table cause gynecomastia to the same extent. For example, when considering the use of a calcium channel blocker in an older man, the clinician should remember that nifedipine has been associated with the highest frequency of gynecomastia, followed by verapamil, with diltiazem having the lowest association (25,41). Similarly, the incidence of gynecomastia in patients receiving histamine receptor or parietal cell proton pump blockers is highest with cimetidine, then ranitidine, and least with omeprazole (25,42). The second area of prevention occurs among patients with prostate cancer who are about to receive monotherapy with antiandrogens. Numerous studies have shown that prophylactic administration of the antiestrogen, tamoxifen, is superior to either the aromatase inhibitor, anastrozole, or low-dose breast irradiation (43–45).

TREATMENT

Discontinuation of the offending drug or correction of the underlying condition that altered the estrogen–androgen balance results in regression of gynecomastia in recent-onset breast growth. As was noted, histologic studies of the breast tissue from men with gynecomastia have shown a marked duct epithelial cell proliferation, inflammatory cell infiltration, increase in stromal fibroblasts, and enhanced vascularity early in the course of the disorder. It is during this proliferative, or florid, stage that patients may complain of breast pain and tenderness. This stage persists for a variable period, but usually lasts less than a year and is followed by spontaneous resolution or enters an inactive stage. There is a reduction in the epithelial proliferation, dilatation of the ducts, and hyalinization and fibrosis of the stroma (11,15,46). The inactive stage is usually asymptomatic. This histologic picture predominates in men whose gynecomastia is detected during a routine physical examination. When considering therapeutic approaches, it is important to appreciate that, after the inactive stage is reached, the gynecomastia is unlikely spontaneously to regress and is also unlikely to respond to medical therapies. Another important factor to consider is that most gynecomastia regresses spontaneously. Indeed, pubertal gynecomastia develops in a large proportion of boys, but very few exhibit persistent breast glandular enlargement. Similarly, in a group of patients with gynecomastia from various causes, 85% of untreated patients had spontaneous improvement (28). This finding emphasizes the difficulties in assessing the response to any medical intervention.

The indications for therapy are severe pain, tenderness, or embarrassment sufficient to interfere with the patient's normal daily activities. Surgical removal of the breast glandular and stromal tissue has been the mainstay of interventional therapy. Subcutaneous mastectomy through a periareolar incision with contouring of the breast by suction-assisted lipectomy and ultrasound-assisted liposuction to remove the subglandular adipose tissue are currently the surgical procedure that are usually performed (47,48). These techniques should be used as primary therapy in patients with long-standing gynecomastia and as definitive therapy in patients who fail to respond to a series of medical therapies.

Three types of medical therapy—androgens, antiestrogens, and aromatase inhibitors—have been tested in patients with gynecomastia. Because this condition has a high frequency of spontaneous regression, the decision of when to treat is often difficult. It is also difficult to assess the use of most medications that have been tried, given the small sample sizes and non-blinded, uncontrolled designs of most studies. Nevertheless, with the exception of early pubertal gynecomastia that has been present for less than 3 months, a trial of medical therapy for patients with moderate to severe symptoms is recommended (49).

Testosterone administration has not been shown to be more effective than placebo in patients with pubertal or idiopathic gynecomastia and it carries the risk of exacerbating the condition by being aromatized to estradiol (28). Micronized testosterone has, however, been shown in a double-blinded, placebo-controlled trial to reduce the prevalence of gynecomastia in men with liver cirrhosis after 6 months of therapy (50). Dihydrotestosterone, a nonaromatizable androgen, given either by injection or percutaneously, has been followed by a reduction in breast volume in 75% of patients, with complete resolution in approximately 15% (51). Responders had a decrease in breast tenderness within 1 to 2 weeks without side effects. The androgenic progestogen danazol has also been tried in uncontrolled trials and a single placebo-controlled study, with the latter showing a complete resolution in 23% of patients who received danazol and only a 12% response in those given placebo (52). Although the investigators believed that this drug was safe and well tolerated, other studies using danazol to treat other conditions have noted side effects, including edema, weight gain, acne, nausea, and muscle cramps.

The three antiestrogens that have been tested are clomiphene citrate, tamoxifen, and raloxifene. Response rates of 36% to 95% have been reported for clomiphene citrate, but two of the three systematic studies indicate that less than one-half of patients had a decrease in breast volume of 20% or more or were satisfied with the results (53–55). No side effects were noted by the investigators when the drug was used in dosages of 50 to 100 mg/day orally. In other settings, the drug has been associated with gastrointestinal distress and visual problems. Tamoxifen, given in dosages of 10 mg orally twice a day, has been studied in several uncontrolled as well as randomized, double-blinded studies (56–65). Partial response is found in approximately 80% of the patients studied and complete regression noted in up to 60% of the patients. None of the studies has reported major side effects that are clearly medication-related from tamoxifen given in these doses, and, in view of its safety, the author usually recommends a 3-month trial of the drug for patients with painful gynecomastia. Raloxifene was reported to be partially effective in treating 10 patients with pubertal gynecomastia, but additional studies are needed to assess the true effectiveness of this drug (64).

The aromatase inhibitor testolactone has been given to a small number of patients with pubertal gynecomastia for up to 6 months at a dose of 450 mg/day orally without side effects (66). The authors of this uncontrolled study report a decrease in breast size after 2 months of therapy, but insufficient data currently exist to recommend this drug as a first-line agent. Anecdotal reports of the use of more potent members of this class of medications, such as anastrozole or letrozole, showed some benefit in individual patients (49). A study that examined anastrozole in a large group of patients with pubertal gynecomastia in a randomized, double-blinded, placebo-controlled trial failed, however, to show a beneficial effect over placebo (67). In addition, anastrozole was found to be inferior to tamoxifen for preventing gynecomastia in patients with prostate cancer receiving antiandrogen monotherapy (47,48).

MANAGEMENT SUMMARY

- Gynecomastia, with its concentric enlargement of tissue radiating from beneath the nipple–areolar complex, needs to be differentiated from pseudogynecomastia (fatty breasts), cancer, and less common lesions.
- For a lesion that is unilateral, eccentric, or hard, breast cancer must excluded through mammography or FNA.
- Medications known to be associated with gynecomastia should be stopped or switched to another agent less likely to cause the problem. Breast pain and tenderness should remit within 1 month if the drug was the etiologic factor.
- If the patient is pubertal, a careful general physical and testicular examination should be performed and, if negative, the patient given reassurance, and seen again in 3 months.
- For breast enlargement that is of recent onset, is painful or tender, and hyperthyroidism or liver, adrenal, or testicular abnormalities are not present on physical examination, the clinician should measure serum concentrations of hCG, luteinizing hormone, estradiol, and free testosterone to differentiate among the pathologic causes of gynecomastia.
- If no reversible underlying cause is found and the patient has pain or tenderness or experiences embarrassment over the gynecomastia, a trial of medical therapy with tamoxifen or plastic surgical removal should be offered.

References

1. Jung FT, Shafton AL. Mastitis, mazoplasia, mastalgia, and gynecomastia in normal adolescent males. *Ill Med J* 1938;73:115–123.
2. Nydick M, Bustos J, Dale JH Jr, et al. Gynecomastia in adolescent boys. *JAMA* 1961;178:449–454.
3. Neyzi O, Alp H, Yalcindag A, et al. Sexual maturation in Turkish boys. *Ann Hum Biol* 1975;2:251–259.
4. Lee PA. The relationship of concentrations of serum hormones to pubertal gynecomastia. *J Pediatr* 1975;86:212–215.
5. Fara GM, DelCorvo G, Bernuzzi S, et al. Epidemic of breast enlargement in an Italian school. *Lancet* 1979;2:295–297.
6. Harlan WR, Grillo GP, Cornoni-Huntley J, et al. Secondary sex characteristics of boys 12 to 17 years of age: the U.S. Health Examination Survey. *J Pediatr* 1979;95: 293–297.
7. Moore DC, Schlaepfer LV, Paunier L, et al. Hormonal changes during puberty: V. Transient pubertal gynecomastia: abnormal androgen-estrogen ratios. *J Clin Endocrinol Metab* 1984;58:492–499.
8. Biro FM, Lucky AW, Huster GA, et al. Hormonal studies and physical maturation in adolescent gynecomastia. *J Pediatr* 1990;116:450–455.
9. Schmidt-Voigt J. Brustdruenschwellungen bei mannlichen Jugendlichen des Pubertatsalters (Pubertatsmakromastie). *Z Kinderheilkd* 1941;62:590–606.
10. Georgiadis E, Papandreou L, Evangelopoulou C, et al. Incidence of gynaecomastia in 954 young males and its relationship to somatometric parameters. *Ann Hum Biol* 1994;21:579–587.
11. Williams MJ. Gynecomastia: its incidence, recognition and host characterization in 447 autopsy cases. *Am J Med* 1963;34:103–112.
12. Nuttall FQ. Gynecomastia as a physical finding in normal men. *J Clin Endocrinol Metab* 1979;48:338–340.
13. Ley SB, Mozaffarian GA, Leonard JM, et al. Palpable breast tissue versus gynecomastia as a normal physical finding. *Clin Res* 1980;28:24A.
14. Carlson HE. Gynecomastia. *N Engl J Med* 1980;303:795–799.
15. Andersen JA, Gram JB. Male breast at autopsy. *APMIS* 1982;90:191–197.
16. Niewoehner CB, Nuttall FQ. Gynecomastia in a hospitalized male population. *Am J Med* 1984;77:633–638.
17. Murray NP, Daly MJ. Gynecomastia and heart failure: adverse drug reaction or disease process? *J Clin Pharm Ther* 1991;16:275–279.
18. Kanhai RCJ, Hage JJ, van Diest PJ, et al. Short-term and long-term histologic effects of castration and estrogen treatment on breast tissue of 14 male-to-female transsexuals in comparison with two chemically castrated men. *Am J Surg Pathol* 2000;24:74.
19. Wilson JD, Aiman J, MacDonald PC. The pathogenesis of gynecomastia. *Adv Intern Med* 1980;29:1–32.
20. Somboonporn W, Davis SR. Testosterone effects on the breast: implications for testosterone therapy for women. *Endocr Rev* 2004;25:374–388.
21. Dimitrakakis C, Zhou J, Wang J, et al. A physiologic role for testosterone in limiting estrogenic stimulation of the breast. *Menopause* 2003;10:292–298.
22. Bulard J, Mowszowicz I, Schaison G. Increased aromatase activity in pubic skin fibroblasts from patients with isolated gynecomastia. *J Clin Endocrinol Metab* 1987;64:618–623.
23. Braunstein GD. Gynecomastia. *N Engl J Med* 1993;328:490–495.
24. Rose LI, Underwood RH, Newmark SR, et al. Pathophysiology of spironolactone-induced gynecomastia. *Ann Intern Med* 1977;87:398–403.
25. Thompson DF, Carter JR. Drug-induced gynecomastia. *Pharmacotherapy* 1993;13: 37–45.
26. Reiter EO, Braunstein GD. Gynecomastia. In: Pescovitz OH, Eugster EA, eds. *Pediatric endocrinology: mechanisms, manifestations, and management.* Philadelphia: Lippincott Williams & Wilkins, 2004:349–359.
27. Mathur R, Braunstein GD. Gynecomastia: pathomechanisms and treatment strategies. *Horm Res* 1997;48:95–102.
28. Treves N. Gynecomastia. The origins of mammary swelling in the male: an analysis of 406 patients with breast hypertrophy, 525 with testicular tumors, and 13 with adrenal neoplasms. *Cancer* 1958;11:1083–1102.
29. Braunstein GD. Aromatase and gynecomastia. *Endocr Relat Cancer* 1999;6: 315–324.
30. Braunstein GD. Gynecomastia. *N Engl J Med* 2007;357:1229–1237.
31. Satoh T, Fujita KI, Munakata H, et al. Studies on the interactions between drugs and estrogen: analytical method for prediction system of gynecomastia induced by drugs on the inhibitory metabolism of estradiol using *Escherichia coli* coexpressing human CYP3A4 with human NADPH-cytochrome P450 reductase. *Anal Biochem* 2000;286:179–186.
32. Satoh T, Munakata H, Fujita K, et al. Studies on the interactions between drug and estrogen. II. On the inhibitory effect of 29 drugs reported to induce gynecomastia on the oxidation of estradiol at C-2 or C-17. *Biol Pharm Bull* 2003;26: 695–700.
33. Satoh T, Tomikawa Y, Takanashi K, et al. Studies on the interactions between drugs and estrogen. III. Inhibitory effects of 29 drugs reported to induce gynecomastia on the glucuronidation of estradiol. *Biol Pharm Bull* 2004;27:1844–1849.
34. Rahim S, Ortiz O, Maslow M, et al. A case-control study of gynecomastia in HIV-1-infected patients receiving HAART. *AIDS Read* 2004;14:23–24, 29–32, 35–40.
35. Henley DV, Lipson N, Korach KS, et al. Prepubertal gynecomastia linked to lavender and tea tree oils. *N Engl J Med* 2007;356:479–485.
36. Giordano SH, Buzdar AU, Hortobagyi GN. Breast cancer in men. *Ann Intern Med* 2002;137:678–687.
37. Olsson HL, Bladstrom A, Alm P. Gynecomastia and risk for malignant tumors—ca cohort investigation. *BMC Cancer* 2002;2:26.
38. Hultborn R, Hanson C, Knopf I, et al. Prevalence of Klinefelter's syndrome in male breast cancer patients. *Anticancer Res* 1997;17:4293–4297.
39. Hasle H, Mellemgaard A, Nielsen J, et al. Cancer incidence in men with Klinefelter syndrome. *Br J Cancer* 1995;71:416–420.
40. Bowers SP, Pearlman NW, McIntyre RC, Jr, et al. Cost-effective management of gynecomastia. *Am J Surg* 1998;176:638–641.
41. Tanner LA, Bosco LA. Gynecomastia associated with calcium channel blocker therapy. *Arch Intern Med* 1988;148:379–380.
42. Lindquist M, Edwards IR. Endocrine adverse effects of omeprazole. *BMJ* 1992; 305:451–452.
43. Boccardo F, Rubagotti A, Battaglia M, et al. Evaluation of tamoxifen and anastrozole in the prevention of gynecomastia and breast pain induced by bicalutamide monotherapy of prostate cancer. *J Clin Oncol* 2005;23:808–815.
44. Saltzstein D, Sieber P, Morris T, et al. Prevention and management of bicalutamide-induced gynecomastia and breast pain: randomized endocrinologic and clinical studies with tamoxifen and anastrozole. *Prostate Cancer Prostatic Dis* 2005;8: 75–83.
45. Perdona S, Autorino R, De Placido S, et al. Efficacy of tamoxifen and radiotherapy for prevention and treatment of gynaecomastia and breast pain caused by bicalutamide in prostate cancer: a randomised controlled trial. *Lancet Oncol* 2005;6: 295–300.
46. Nicolis GL, Modlinger RS, Gabrilove JL. A study of the histopathology of human gynecomastia. *J Clin Endocrinol Metab* 1971;32:173–178.
47. Rohrich RJ, Ha RY, Kenkel JM, et al. Classification and management of gynecomastia: defining the role of ultrasound-assisted liposuction. *Plast Reconstr Surg* 2003;111:909–923.
48. Tashkandi M, Al-Qattan MM, Hassanain JM, et al. the surgical management of high-grade gynecomastia. *Ann Plast Surg* 2004;53:17–20.
49. Gruntmanis U, Braunstein GD. Treatment of gynecomastia. *Curr Opin Invest Drug* 2001;2:643–649.
50. The Copenhagen Study Group for Liver Diseases. Testosterone treatment of men with alcoholic cirrhosis: a double-blind study. *Hepatology* 1986;6:807–813.
51. Kuhn JM, Roca R, Laudat MH, et al. Studies on the treatment of idiopathic gynaecomastia with percutaneous dihydrotestosterone. *Clin Endocrinol (Oxf)* 1983;19: 513–520.
52. Jones DJ, Davison DJ, Holt SD, et al. A comparison of danazol and placebo in the treatment of adult idiopathic gynecomastia: results of a prospective study in 55 patients. *Ann R Coll Surg Engl* 1990;72:296–298.
53. Stepanas AV, Burnet RB, Harding PE, et al. Clomiphene in the treatment of pubertal-adolescent gynecomastia: a preliminary report. *J Pediatr* 1977;90:651–653.
54. Plourde PV, Kulin HE, Santner SJ. Clomiphene in the treatment of adolescent gynecomastia: clinical and endocrine studies. *Am J Dis Child* 1983;137:1080–1082.
55. LeRoith D, Sobel R, Glick SM. The effect of clomiphene citrate on pubertal gynecomastia. *Acta Endocrinol (Copenh)* 1980;95:177–180.
56. Eversmann T, Moito J, von Werder K. Testosterone and estradiol levels in male gynecomastia: clinical and endocrine findings during treatment with tamoxifen. *Dtsch Med Wochenschr* 1984;109:1678–1682.
57. Parker LN, Gray DR, Lai MK, et al. Treatment of gynecomastia with tamoxifen: a double-blind crossover study. *Metabolism* 1986;35:705–708.
58. Alagaratnam TT. Idiopathic gynecomastia treated with tamoxifen: a preliminary report. *Clin Ther* 1987;9:483–487.
59. König R, Schönberger W, Neumann P, et al. Treatment of marked gynecomastia in puberty with tamoxifen. *Klin Padiatr* 1987;199:389–391.
60. McDermott MT, Hofeldt FD, Kidd GS. Tamoxifen therapy for painful idiopathic gynecomastia. *South Med J* 1990;83:1283–1285.
61. Staiman VR, Lowe FC. Tamoxifen for flutamide/finasteride-induced gynecomastia. *Urology* 1997;50:929–933.
62. Ting ACW, Chow LWC, Leung YF. Comparison of tamoxifen with danazol in the management of idiopathic gynecomastia. *Am Surg* 2000;66:38–40.
63. Kahn HN, Rampaul R, Blamey RW. Management of physiological gynaecomastia with tamoxifen. *Breast* 2004;13:61–65.
64. Lawrence SE, Faught KA, Vethamuthu J, et al. Beneficial effects of raloxifene and tamoxifen in the treatment of pubertal gynecomastia. *J Pediatr* 2004;145:71–76.
65. Hanavadi S, Banerjee D, Monypenny IJ, et al. The role of tamoxifen in the management of gynaecomastia. *Breast* 2006;15:276–280.
66. Zachmann M, Eiholzer U, Muritano M, et al. Treatment of pubertal gynaecomastia with testolactone. *Acta Endocrinol (Copenh)* 1986;279(Suppl):218–226.
67. Plourde PV, Reiter EO, Jou HC, et al. Safety and efficacy of anastrozole for the treatment of pubertal gynecomastia: a randomized, double-blind, placebo-controlled trial. *J Clin Endocrinol Metab* 2004;89:4428–4433.

Chapter 10

Pathology of Benign Breast Disorders

Stuart J. Schnitt and Laura Christine Collins

The term *benign breast disorders* encompasses a heterogeneous group of lesions that may present as a palpable mass, a nonpalpable abnormality detected on breast imaging studies, or an incidental microscopic finding. Some are discrete lesions, such as fibroadenoma and intraductal papilloma, but a large number of benign breast biopsies exhibit a mixture of histologic changes affecting the terminal duct lobular units. The two major goals in the pathologic evaluation of a benign breast biopsy are (a) to distinguish benign lesions from *in situ* and invasive breast cancer; and, (b) to assess the risk of subsequent breast cancer associated with the benign lesion(s) identified.

BENIGN BREAST DISEASE AND BREAST CANCER RISK: NONPROLIFERATIVE LESIONS, PROLIFERATIVE LESIONS WITHOUT ATYPIA, AND ATYPICAL HYPERPLASIAS

It has been known for many years that some benign breast lesions are more highly associated with breast cancer than others. Two types of studies have evaluated this relationship. In the first type, the prevalence of benign alterations in breasts with cancer was compared with their prevalence in breasts without cancer (1,2). While these studies demonstrated that some benign lesions are more common in cancer-containing breasts, the histologic co-existence of certain benign breast lesions with breast cancer is not sufficient to establish that those benign lesions impart an increased cancer risk.

More recent studies have evaluated the subsequent risk of developing breast cancer in patients who have had a benign breast biopsy and for whom long-term follow-up is available (3–20). In these studies, histologic sections of the benign biopsies were reviewed, and the type of benign lesions present were recorded and related to the risk of breast cancer. In some of these studies, it was also possible to study the interaction of the histologic findings with other factors, such as family history of breast cancer, time since biopsy, and menopausal status, in determining cancer risk. The results of these studies have provided important information regarding the risk of breast cancer associated with benign breast lesions and this information is useful in patient treatment, counseling and follow-up. These studies have further indicated that terms such as *fibrocystic disease, chronic cystic mastitis*, and *mammary dysplasia* are not clinically meaningful because they encompass a heterogeneous group of processes, some physiologic and some pathologic, with widely varying cancer risks (2,21,22).

The seminal study evaluating benign breast disease and cancer risk is the retrospective cohort study of Dupont et al (4,23). In their study, the slides of benign breast biopsies from more than 3,000 women in Nashville were reviewed, and the histologic lesions present were categorized using strictly defined criteria (4,23,24) into one of three categories: nonproliferative lesions, proliferative lesions without atypia, and atypical hyperplasias (Table 10.1). The risk of developing breast cancer was then determined for each of these groups. This system provides a pragmatic, clinically relevant approach to benign breast lesions and has been supported by a consensus conference of the College of American Pathologists (25). Studies from other groups have largely confirmed the initial observations of

the Nashville group and have extended these findings by providing important new information regarding benign breast disease and breast cancer risk (7,8,11,13,14,16–20) (Table 10.2).

Nonproliferative Lesions

Nonproliferative lesions, as defined by Dupont and Page (4), include cysts, papillary apocrine change, epithelial-related calcifications, and mild hyperplasia of the usual type.

Cysts are fluid-filled, round-to-ovoid structures that vary in size from microscopic to grossly evident (Fig. 10.1). *Gross cysts*, as defined by Haagensen (26), are those which are sufficiently large to produce palpable masses. Cysts are derived from the terminal duct lobular unit. The epithelium usually consists of two layers: an inner (luminal) epithelial layer and an outer myoepithelial layer. In some cysts, the epithelium is markedly attenuated or absent; in others, the lining epithelium shows apocrine metaplasia, characterized by granular eosinophilic cytoplasm and apical cytoplasmic protrusions ("snouts").

Papillary apocrine change is characterized by a proliferation of ductal epithelial cells in which all of the cells show apocrine features as described above. *Epithelial-related calcifications* are frequently observed in breast tissue and may be seen in normal ducts and lobules or in virtually any pathologic condition in the breast. It should also be noted that calcifications may also be seen in the breast stroma as well as in blood vessel walls. *Mild hyperplasia of the usual type* is defined as an increase in the number of epithelial cells within a duct that is less than four epithelial cells in depth. In this type of hyperplasia, the epithelial cells do not cross the lumen of the involved space.

In the original study of Dupont and Page (4), 70% of the biopsies showed nonproliferative lesions. The risk of subsequent breast cancer among these patients was not increased, compared with that of women who have had no breast biopsy (relative risk [RR], 0.89), even in patients with a family history of breast cancer (in a mother, sister, or daughter). The only group of patients in the nonproliferative category with an increased risk of developing breast cancer was that with gross cysts plus a family history of breast cancer. The relative risk with gross cysts alone was 1.5, but was 3.0 in patients with

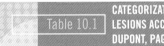

	CATEGORIZATION OF BENIGN BREAST LESIONS ACCORDING TO THE CRITERIA OF DUPONT, PAGE, AND ROGERS (4,17,18)
Table 10.1	

Nonproliferative
  Cysts
  Papillary apocrine change
  Epithelial-related calcifications
  Mild hyperplasia of the usual type
Proliferative lesions without atypia
  Moderate or florid ductal hyperplasia of the usual type
  Intraductal papilloma
  Sclerosing adenosis
  Fibroadenoma
Atypical hyperplasia
  Atypical ductal hyperplasia
  Atypical lobular hyperplasia

Table 10.2	RELATIVE RISK OF BREAST CANCER ACCORDING TO HISTOLOGIC CRITERIA OF BENIGN BREAST DISEASE IN FOUR STUDIES USING THE CRITERIA OF DUPONT, PAGE AND ROGERS (4,23,24)			
			Histologic Category	
Study	**Study Design**	**Nonproliferative**	**Proliferative Without Atypia**	**Atypical Hyperplasia**
Nashville (4)	Retrospective cohort	1	1.9 (1.9–2.3)	5.3 (3.1–8.8)
Nurses' Health Study (17)	Case-control	1	1.5 (1.2–2.0)	4.1 (2.9–5.8)
Breast Cancer Detection Demonstration Project (11)	Case-control	1	1.3 (0.8–2.2)	4.3 (1.7–11.0)
Mayo Clinic (16)	Retrospective cohort	1.3 (1.15–1.41)	1.9 (1.7–2.1)	4.2 (3.3–5.4)

Numbers in parentheses represent 95% confidence intervals.

gross cysts and a family history. It should be noted that, although Dupont and Page initially included fibroadenomas among the nonproliferative lesions, the results of a subsequent study by these investigators indicated a higher relative risk for breast cancer among patients with fibroadenoma than for patients with nonproliferative lesions (27). As a result, fibroadenomas are now included among the proliferative lesions without atypia (see section on Fibroadenomas).

Proliferative Lesions Without Atypia

Included within the group of proliferative lesions without atypia are *usual ductal hyperplasia* (28) (also known as *moderate or florid hyperplasias of the usual type*), *intraductal papillomas, sclerosing adenosis, and radial scars* (4,29). As noted above, *fibroadenomas* are now included in this category as well. Women who have had a benign breast biopsy showing proliferative lesions without atypia, as defined above, have a mildly elevated breast cancer risk, approximately 1.5 to 2.0 times that of the reference population (*intraductal papillomas, radial scars,* and *fibroadenomas* are discussed elsewhere in this chapter).

Usual ductal hyperplasias are intraductal epithelial proliferations more than four epithelial cells in depth. They are characterized by a tendency to bridge and often distend the involved space. The proliferation may have a solid, fenestrated or papillary architecture. If spaces remain within the duct lumen, they are irregular and variable in shape. These spaces are often slit-like and arranged around the periphery of the proliferation, with their long axes parallel to the basement membrane. The cells comprising this type of proliferation are cytologically benign and variable in size, shape, and orientation, and they often are arranged in a "swirling" pattern (Fig. 10.2). It is sometimes possible to discern multiple distinct cell populations, including epithelial cells, metaplastic apocrine cells, and myoepithelial cells.

Sclerosing adenosis is usually an incidental finding, but may present as a mammographic abnormality (microcalcifications, distorted architecture) or a mass lesion (also known as *nodular adenosis* or *adenosis tumor* [30]). This lesion is composed of distorted epithelial, myoepithelial, and sclerotic stromal elements arising in association with the terminal duct lobular unit. This lobulocentric pattern is key to the correct diagnosis of sclerosing adenosis and its variants, and is best appreciated at low power microscopic examination (Fig. 10.3). The epithelium in sclerosing adenosis may undergo apocrine metaplasia, and is then referred to as *apocrine adenosis* (31,32). The apocrine metaplastic cells may show cytologic atypia, raising the differential diagnosis of invasive carcinoma if the lesion is examined at high microscopic power without accounting for the lobulocentric architecture appreciated at low power (33). Sclerosing adenosis may also be involved by atypical lobular hyperplasia, lobular carcinoma *in situ*, atypical ductal hyperplasia (ADH), or ductal carcinoma *in situ* (DCIS) (34–37). Perineural "pseudoinvasion" may be present in approximately 2% of sclerosing adenosis cases and should not be confused with invasive carcinoma (38–40). Because of the distorted glandular pattern of sclerosing adenosis, this lesion may be confused with a low-grade invasive carcinoma, particularly tubular carcinoma. In contrast to the lobulocentric pattern of

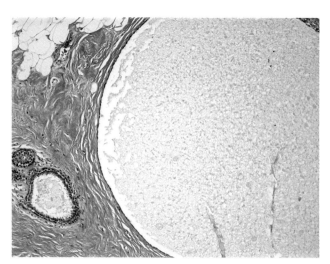

FIGURE 10.1. Cyst characterized by a large, dilated space filled with secretory material and lined by a flattened epithelial cell layer.

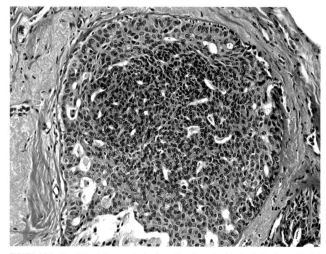

FIGURE 10.2. Usual ductal hyperplasia. A proliferation of cytologically benign epithelial cells fills and distends the duct. The nuclei vary in size, shape, and placement. The spaces within the duct are also variable in size and contour.

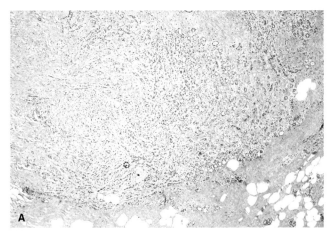
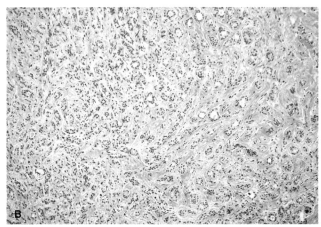

FIGURE 10.3. Sclerosing adenosis. A: Low power view demonstrates a lobulocentric proliferation of epithelial and stromal elements with scattered calcifications. **B:** Higher power view reveals glands and cords of epithelial cells entrapped in fibrotic stroma. The cells are cytologically benign, but the pattern simulates that of an invasive carcinoma.

sclerosing adenosis, tubular carcinoma is infiltrative in nature, however, and does not conform to the normal breast ductal and lobular microanatomy. Although sclerosing adenosis is composed of distorted, elongated or obliterated glands and tubules, tubular carcinoma is composed of angulated tubules with open lumens. The stroma of sclerosing adenosis is fibrotic or sclerotic compared with the desmoplastic stroma of invasive carcinoma. Importantly, as opposed to tubular carcinoma, sclerosing adenosis contains myoepithelial cells, which may be highlighted by immunohistochemistry.

Atypical Hyperplasias

Atypical hyperplasias have been defined as proliferative lesions of the breast which possess some, but not all, of the features of carcinoma *in situ* and are classified as either ductal or lobular type (4,23,24). *Atypical ductal hyperplasias* are lesions that have some of the architectural and cytologic features of low-grade DCIS, such as nuclear monomorphism, regular cell placement and round regular spaces, in at least part of the involved space. The cells may form tufts, micropapillations, arcades, bridges, solid, and cribriform patterns (28). A second cell population with features similar to those seen in usual ductal hyperplasia is also typically present (Fig. 10.4).

Atypical lobular hyperplasia (ALH) is composed of cells identical to those found in lobular carcinoma *in situ* (LCIS). These cells are monomorphic, evenly spaced, and dyshesive, with round or oval, usually eccentric nuclei and pale cytoplasm often with intracytoplasmic vacuoles (Fig. 10.5). Although criteria for the distinction between ALH and LCIS differ among experts, we utilize the criteria proposed by Page and Anderson (41) and diagnose ALH when the characteristic cells are present but less than one-half of the acini of a lobular unit are filled, distorted, or distended. In addition to involving lobular units, the cells of atypical lobular hyperplasia may also involve ducts (42).

It is important to note that with the increasing use of mammographic screening, atypical hyperplasias are being diagnosed more frequently than in the past. For example, when a biopsy is performed because of a palpable mass, atypical hyperplasia is seen in only about 2% to 4% of cases (4,43). In contrast, atypical hyperplasia was identified in 12% to 17% of biopsies performed because of the presence of mammographic microcalcifications (44,45).

Women who have had a benign breast biopsy that demonstrates atypical hyperplasia are at a substantially increased risk for developing breast cancer, approximately 3.5 to 5.0 times that of the reference population. Some studies have sug-

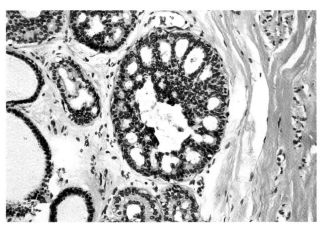

FIGURE 10.4. Atypical ductal hyperplasia. Near the center of this space is a proliferation of relatively uniform epithelial cells with monomorphic, round nuclei similar to those seen in low-grade ductal carcinoma *in situ*. However, these cells comprise only a portion of the proliferation within the space.

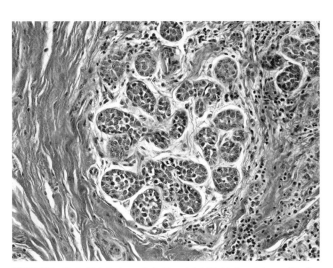

FIGURE 10.5. Atypical lobular hyperplasia. The acini of this lobule contain a proliferation of small uniform cells, which are dyshesive, and are identical to the cells that comprise lobular carcinoma *in situ*. However, the acini are not distended by this cellular proliferation.

Table 10.3	RELATIVE RISK OF BREAST CANCER ACCORDING TO TYPE OF ATYPICAL HYPERPLASIA		
Study/ Reference	All Atypical Hyperplasia[a]	Atypical Ductal Hyperplasia[a]	Atypical Lobular Hyperplasia[a]
Nashville (23)	5.3 (3.1–8.8)	4.7 (2.5–8.9)	5.8 (3.0–11.0)
Nashville (15)	—	—	3.1 (2.3–4.3)
Nurses' Health Study (17)	4.1 (2.9–5.8)	3.1 (2.0–4.8)	5.5 (3.3–9.2)
Mayo Clinic (19)	3.9 (3.0–4.9)	3.8 (2.5–5.6)	3.7 (2.5–5.3)

[a]Numbers in parentheses represent 95% confidence intervals.

gested that the risk associated with atypical lobular hyperplasia is greater than that associated with ADH (13,17,23), but others have not (15,19) (Table 10.3); at the present time this issue remains unresolved. Patients whose biopsies showed atypical lobular hyperplasia involving both lobules and ducts had a higher relative risk of developing cancer (RR, 6.8) than those with either atypical lobular hyperplasia alone (RR, 4.3) or those with only ductal involvement by atypical lobular hyperplasia (RR, 2.1) (42).

Columnar Cell Lesions and Flat Epithelial Atypia

Lesions of the breast characterized by enlarged terminal duct lobular units lined by columnar epithelial cells are being encountered increasingly in breast biopsies performed because of mammographic microcalcifications. Some of these lesions feature banal columnar cells in either a single layer (columnar cell change) or showing stratification and tufting, but without complex architectural patterns (columnar cell hyperplasia). In other columnar cell lesions, the lining cells exhibit cytologic atypia, most commonly of the low-grade, monomorphic type. Such lesions were included among lesions originally categorized by Azzopardi as "clinging carcinoma" (monomorphic type) (46), and were more recently included among lesions designated *flat epithelial atypia* (FEA) (Fig. 10.6) (28). The role of columnar cell lesions and, in particular, FEA in breast tumor progression is still emerging. FEA commonly coexists with well-developed examples of ADH, low-grade DCIS, and tubular carcinoma (47). These findings, in conjunction with the results

of recent genetic studies (47), suggest that FEA is a neoplastic lesion that may represent either a precursor to, or the earliest morphologic manifestation of, DCIS. The few available clinical outcome studies suggest, however, that the risk of progression of FEA to invasive cancer is extremely low, supporting the notion that categorizing such lesions as *clinging carcinoma* and managing them as if they were fully developed DCIS will result in overtreatment of many patients (47). Additional studies are needed to better understand the biological nature and the level of subsequent breast cancer risk associated with these lesions.

Factors Modifying Breast Cancer Risk in Women with Biopsy-Proven Benign Breast Disease

A number of factors appear to modify the breast cancer risk associated with biopsy-proved benign breast disease, including a family history of breast cancer, time since biopsy, menopausal status, and the appearance of the background breast tissue.

Family History

There is general agreement that the presence of a family history of breast cancer in a first-degree relative (mother, sister, or daughter) is associated with a slight increase in the breast cancer risk in women with proliferative lesions without atypia (4,11,16,18,23). The influence of family history on breast cancer risk in women with atypical hyperplasia is less clear, however. Dupont et al. (4,23) reported that the risk among patients with both atypical hyperplasia and a family history of breast cancer was twice that of women with atypical hyperplasia without a family history. Similarly, in a study conducted by the Breast Cancer Detection Demonstration Project (BCDDP), the presence of a positive family history substantially increased the breast cancer risk among women with atypical hyperplasia (11). In a recent update of the Nurses' Health Study (18) and in a recent study from the Mayo Clinic (16), the presence of a positive family history was not, however, associated with a further increase in breast cancer risk among women with atypical hyperplasia (Table 10.4). Additional studies are needed to clarify this important issue.

Time Since Biopsy

Information regarding the relationship between time since benign breast biopsy and breast cancer risk is available from several studies. In the Nashville study, women with proliferative lesions without atypia who remained free of breast cancer for 10 years after their benign breast biopsy were at no greater breast cancer risk than women of similar age without such a history. In addition, the breast cancer risk among women with atypical hyperplasia was greatest in the first 10 years after the benign breast biopsy (RR, 9.8) and fell to a relative risk of 3.6 after 10 years (48). In contrast, in an analysis of data from the Nurses' Health Study, the breast cancer risk among women with proliferative lesions without atypia was similarly elevated before *and* after 10 years following the benign breast biopsy (RR, 1.4 and 1.6, respectively). In addition, the risk associated with atypical hyperplasia was higher after 10 years (RR, 5.2) than in the first 10 years after the benign breast biopsy (RR, 3.3) (17). Similarly, in the Mayo Clinic study, an excess breast cancer risk was seen among women with biopsy-proved benign breast disease for at least 25 years after the benign breast biopsy (16). Among patients with atypical hyperplasia, the relative risk was persistently elevated beyond 15 years (19). More data are needed to clarify further the relationship between time since biopsy and breast cancer risk for women with benign breast disease, particularly for women with atypical hyperplasia.

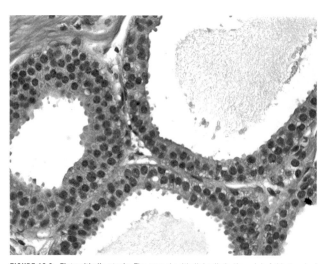

FIGURE 10.6. Flat epithelia atypia. The normal epithelial cells in the acini of this terminal duct are replaced by a population of columnar epithelial cells with round, monomorphic nuclei.

	Proliferative without Atypia		Atypical Hyperplasia	
Study	No Family history	Family History	No Family History	Family History
Nashville (4)	1.5 (1.2–1.9)	2.1 (1.2–3.7)	3.5 (2.3–5.5)	8.9 (4.8–17.0)
Nurses' Health Study (18)	1.5 (1.1–2.1)	2.5 (1.6–3.7)	4.3 (2.9–6.0)	5.4 (3.0–9.6)
Breast Cancer Detection Demonstration Project (11)	1.7 (0.9–3.2)	2.6 (1.0–6.4)	4.2 (1.4–12.0)	22.0 (2.3–203)
Mayo Clinic (16)	1.6 (~1.4–2.0)[a]	2.2 (~1.5–3.0)[a]	3.0 (~1.7–4.9)[a]	4.0 (~2.0–7.0)[a]

Table 10.4 EFFECT OF FAMILY HISTORY OF BREAST CANCER ON RELATIVE RISK OF BREAST CANCER

Numbers in parentheses represent 95% confidence intervals.
[a]95% confidence intervals estimated from Figure 2 in reference 16.

Menopausal Status

The risk of breast cancer among women with atypical hyperplasia appears to be influenced by the patient's menopausal status. In the BCDDP study, premenopausal women with a biopsy showing atypical hyperplasia were at a substantially higher breast cancer risk (RR, 12, 95% CI 1.0–68) than postmenopausal women with that diagnosis (RR, 3.3, 95% CI 1.1–10) (11). In the Nurses' Health Study, the breast cancer risk associated with atypical hyperplasia as a group was similar in premenopausal and postmenopausal women (RR, 3.9 and 3.8, respectively). Among premenopausal women, however, the risk associated with atypical lobular hyperplasia was greater than the risk associated with atypical ductal hyperplasia (RR, 7.3 and 2.7, respectively). In contrast, the risk associated with atypical lobular hyperplasia and atypical ductal hyperplasia were similar in postmenopausal women (RR, 3.4 and 4.0, respectively) (17). Of note, in both the BCDDP study and the Nurses' Health Study, the breast cancer risk among women with proliferative lesions without atypia did not vary according to menopausal status.

Another issue of clinical importance is the influence of postmenopausal hormone replacement therapy on the risk of breast cancer in women with biopsy-proved benign breast disease. Clinical follow-up studies have shown that women who take hormone replacement therapy are at increased risk for developing breast cancer (49). The use of hormone replacement does not, however, appear to further increase the risk in women with proliferative breast disease without atypia or in those with atypical hyperplasia (50). In an analysis from the Nurses' Health Study among women with proliferative lesions without atypia, the relative risks of breast cancer were similar for those women who never used postmenopausal hormones, who were past users, and who were current users (RR, 1.6, 2.1, and 1.9, respectively). Similarly, among women with atypical hyperplasia, the relative breast cancer risks were not significantly different for those who had not used hormone replacement, for past users, and for current users (RR, 3.4, 3.0, and 2.5, respectively) (51). Thus, the available data suggest that the use of hormone replacement therapy does not further increase the breast cancer risk among women with a history of biopsy-proved benign breast disease, even among those with atypical hyperplasia.

Background Breast Tissue

A study from the Mayo Clinic has suggested that the presence of lobular involution in the background breast tissue of a benign breast biopsy is associated with a significant decrease in the risk of breast cancer. Furthermore, in that study the presence of lobular involution modified the risk in women with proliferative lesions without atypia and in those with atypical hyperplasia. For example, the relative risk for the development of breast cancer was 7.8 (95% CI 3.6–14.8) for women with atypical hyperplasia without involution in the background breast tissue and 1.5 (95% CI 0.4–3.8) for those with both atypical hyperplasia and complete involution of the background breast tissue (20). Similar results have recently been reported for women enrolled in the Nurses' Health Study (52).

Laterality of Risk

Breast cancers that develop among women with atypical hyperplasia may occur in either breast. Overall, approximately 60% of cancers that develop in women with atypical hyperplasia occur in the ipsilateral breast; an excess of ipsilateral cancers is seen particularly in the first 10 years after the benign breast biopsy (16,17). Among women with atypical ductal hyperplasia, about 55% of cancers occur in the ipsilateral breast (16,17,23). Among those with atypical lobular hyperplasia, about 60% to 70% of the cancers occur in the ipsilateral breast (15,17). These observations suggest that the concept that atypical hyperplasias represent only risk indicators is overly simplistic and that, in at least some instances, these lesions may act as direct (albeit nonobligate) precursors to invasive breast cancer (53).

Consistency of Histologic Classification

The foregoing data provide compelling evidence that breast cancer risk varies with the histologic category of benign breast disease. They further indicate that the risk among women with biopsy-proven benign breast disease is influenced by other factors as well. To counsel individual patients properly, an understanding of the difference between relative risk and absolute risk is necessary (54). The *relative risk* for breast cancer represents the incidence of breast cancer among women within a certain subpopulation divided by the incidence of breast cancer in the reference population. The magnitude of the relative risk is highly dependent on the breast cancer incidence in both the study group and the reference population. In contrast, a woman's *absolute risk* of breast cancer is her probability of developing breast cancer during some specified time period. For example, although the relative risk for patients with atypical hyperplasia and a family history of breast cancer in the study of Dupont and Page was 8.9, only 20% of patients in this group had developed breast cancer 15 years after their benign biopsy. Eighty percent of patients with atypical hyperplasia but no family history, 4% of patients with proliferative lesions without atypia, and 2% of women with nonproliferative lesions developed breast cancer in 15 years (4).

Given the apparent clinical importance of distinguishing among the various types of benign breast disease, the ability of pathologists to categorize accurately and reproducibly such lesions and to distinguish them from carcinoma *in situ* is a matter of legitimate concern. This problem has been addressed in several studies (55–57). In one of these studies conducted by Rosai (55), five highly respected breast pathologists were asked to apply the criteria they used in their daily practice to categorize a series of proliferative breast lesions. Under these conditions, in not a single case did all five pathologists arrive at the same diagnosis and in only 18% of the cases did four of the five pathologists agree (55). The results of a subsequent study suggest that with standardization of histologic criteria among pathologists, interobserver variability in the diagnosis of proliferative breast lesions can be reduced. In that study, six experienced breast pathologists were instructed to use standardized diagnostic criteria (i.e., those of Page et al.) for categorizing a series of proliferative breast lesions. Complete agreement among all six pathologists was observed in 58% of the cases and all but one pathologist arrived at the same diagnosis in 71% (56). The results of these studies indicate that, although the use of standardized histologic criteria improves interobserver concordance in the diagnosis of proliferative breast lesions, even under these circumstances some lesions defy reproducible categorization, particularly the distinction between ADH and limited examples of low-grade DCIS.

Some authors have advocated that qualitative criteria should be supplemented by quantitative criteria to aid in the distinction between ADH and low-grade DCIS. For example, Page et al. (23) require that all of the features of low-grade DCIS be uniformly present throughout at least two separate spaces before DCIS is diagnosed. Lesions that have the qualitative features of low-grade DCIS that do not fulfill this quantitative criterion are categorized as ADH. Tavassoli and Norris (6) have suggested that the risk of breast cancer associated with very small foci of low-grade DCIS (i.e., <2 mm) is similar to that of ADH; therefore, they classify lesions that fulfill the qualitative criteria for low-grade DCIS but that are less than 2 mm in size as ADH (6).

Newer Methods to Assess Breast Cancer Risk

There is currently an active effort to determine if biological markers in benign breast biopsies might be useful in predicting breast cancer risk, either alone or in combination with histopathology (58–60). To date, a variety of biomarkers have been studied in this regard including estrogen receptor (ER), angiogenesis, p53 expression, *HER2/neu* expression, transforming growth factor (TGF)-β receptor II, and cyclooxygenase 2 (COX-2), among others.

In a study of ER expression in benign breast tissue, Khan et al. (61) found that the odds ratio for breast cancer in women with estrogen receptor positive benign epithelium was 3.2 in comparison with women with estrogen receptor negative benign breast tissue. In contrast, Gobbi et al. (62) found no significant differences in ER expression in usual-type hyperplasias of women who subsequently developed breast cancer compared with those who did not. Shabban et al. (63) have suggested that the ratio of ERα to ERβ in hyperplasias of the usual type is an important determinant of breast cancer risk. In that study, in women with hyperplasias of the usual type who developed invasive breast cancer the ERα-to-ERβ ratio was significantly higher that in those that did not develop breast cancer (63).

In a small pilot study, Guinebretiere et al. (64) found that increased angiogenesis in benign breast biopsies was associated with a significantly increased breast cancer risk, independent of the presence of atypical hyperplasia. Heffelfinger et al. (65) have also shown that some benign proliferative breast lesions are associated with angiogenesis in the surrounding stroma and that stromal vascularity associated with normal breast epithelium is greater in breasts with invasive cancer than in breasts without cancer. Finally, Viacava et al. (66) have demonstrated higher microvessel density counts in

association with usual and atypical ductal hyperplasias than in association with normal mammary glandular structures.

One study has suggested that p53 protein accumulation in benign breast tissue was associated with an increased breast cancer risk (RR, 2.6), even after adjustment for other breast cancer risk factors. In that study, no significant association was found between *HER2/neu* protein expression in benign breast tissue and increased breast cancer risk (67). In another study, however, *HER2/neu* gene amplification in benign breast tissue, as determined by the polymerase chain reaction, was associated with an increase in breast cancer risk, particularly among women with coexistent proliferative breast disease (68).

In another study, women with hyperplasia that showed loss of expression of TGF-β receptor II were found to have a greater risk of breast cancer than those whose hyperplasia showed prominent expression of this receptor protein (69). Most recently, Visscher et al. (70) reported that higher levels of COX-2 expression in atypical hyperplasias were associated with greater breast cancer risk.

A number of studies have also evaluated loss of heterozygosity, genomic copy number changes, and microsatellite instability in benign breast lesions. These studies have shown that at least some examples of usual ductal hyperplasia and atypical hyperplasia exhibit a variety of genomic alterations (58,71). The clinical significance of these observations is not yet clear, however. Finally, studies to identify patterns of gene expression or protein expression using expression profiling and proteomic technologies, respectively, are likely to provide important new insights into the molecular and genetic alterations involved in both neoplastic progression and breast cancer risk in women with benign breast lesions.

A number of follow-up studies evaluating benign breast disease and breast cancer risk have used diagnostic criteria other than those of the Nashville group for categorizing benign breast lesions (3,5,9,10,12). In some of these studies, information regarding the pathology findings in the benign breast biopsies was obtained from a review of the pathology reports only, without a slide review. In general, in these studies, proliferative lesions, particularly those categorized as atypical hyperplasia, have been associated with a higher breast cancer risk than other lesions, although the magnitude of this risk has varied among these studies. In a recent analysis of almost 12,000 women enrolled in the National Surgical Adjuvant Breast and Bowel Project breast cancer prevention (NSABP-P1) trial, women with a history of biopsy-proved "benign breast disease" had a fourfold greater risk of developing breast cancer than women without such a history. Information about the benign breast disease was obtained from review of pathology reports and no further details regarding the nature of the benign breast disease were reported (72).

In summary, the results of clinical follow-up studies indicate that most women who have a benign breast biopsy are not at increased risk for developing breast cancer. A substantially increased breast cancer risk is seen only in the small percentage of patients whose benign breast biopsies show atypical hyperplasia using strictly defined histologic and cytologic criteria. The role of biological and molecular markers to help assess breast cancer risk is not yet well defined but remains an area of active investigation.

SPECIFIC BENIGN LESIONS

Benign Neoplasms and Proliferative Lesions

Fibroadenomas

On gross examination, fibroadenomas are pseudoencapsulated and are sharply delimited from the surrounding breast tissue.

They are usually spherical or ovoid, but may be multilobulated. When cut, the tumor bulges above the level of the surrounding breast tissue. The cut surface is most typically gray-white, and small, punctate, yellow-to-pink soft areas and slitlike spaces are commonly observed. Occasionally, the tumor has a gelatinous, mucoid consistency.

Microscopically, fibroadenomas have both an epithelial and stromal component. The histologic pattern depends upon which of these components predominates. In general, the epithelial component consists of well-defined, glandlike and ductlike spaces lined by cuboidal or columnar cells with uniform nuclei. Varying degrees of epithelial hyperplasia are frequently observed. The stromal component consists of connective tissue that has a variable content of acid mucopolysaccharides and collagen (Fig. 10.7). In older lesions and in postmenopausal patients, the stroma may become hyalinized, calcified, or even ossified (ancient fibroadenoma). On rare occasions, mature adipose tissue or smooth muscle may comprise a portion of the stroma (46,73). The term *intracanalicular* has been used to describe tumors in which the stromal component compresses the glands into slitlike spaces, whereas *pericanalicular* tumors are those in which the rounded configuration of the glandular structures is maintained. In fact, these two patterns often coexist in the same lesion, and this distinction has no clinical significance.

Complex Fibroadenomas

Fibroadenomas that contain cysts larger than 3 mm in diameter, sclerosing adenosis, epithelial calcifications, or papillary apocrine change have been designated complex fibroadenomas. In a review of almost 2,500 fibroadenomas, such changes were seen in 23% of the cases. In one clinical follow-up study, complex fibroadenomas were reported to be associated with a greater subsequent breast cancer risk than fibroadenomas that lack such changes (27).

Juvenile Fibroadenomas

Most fibroadenomas in adolescents and younger women are of the usual type seen in older patients. A few present a different clinical and pathologic picture and are termed *juvenile fibroadenomas* (74–77). This term, however, has been used by different authors to describe different lesions. Some authors use the term to refer to fibroadenomatous lesions that grow rapidly and may show venous dilatation in the overlying skin. Such lesions may clinically resemble virginal hypertrophy, and only surgical exploration will reveal a circumscribed tumor (74–76). Microscopically, juvenile fibroadenomas are more

floridly glandular and have greater stromal cellularity than the more common adult-type fibroadenoma. Mies and Rosen (77) use the term *juvenile fibroadenomas* to refer to fibroadenomatous lesions that demonstrate severe epithelial hyperplasia which may border on carcinoma *in situ*. Nevertheless, these lesions behave in a clinically benign fashion.

Giant Fibroadenomas

Some tumors that are histologically typical fibroadenomas may attain great size. Several authors have used the terms *giant fibroadenoma* and *benign cystosarcoma phyllodes* synonymously, however, and have created considerable confusion regarding these entities. A lesion that has the microscopic appearance of a conventional fibroadenoma, but that is large, should still be classified as a fibroadenoma and may be treated adequately by enucleation. The major feature that distinguishes a cystosarcoma phyllodes (preferably called a phyllodes tumor) from a giant fibroadenoma is the cellularity of the stromal component in the former (46). It must be noted, however, that the distinction between these two entities may be extremely difficult in some cases. Because juvenile fibroadenomas may attain great sizes, some authors consider them to be variants of giant fibroadenomas (76).

Infarction

Fibroadenomas may undergo partial, subtotal, or total infarction. Pregnancy and lactation are the most common predisposing factors. It has been postulated that a relative vascular insufficiency in the face of increased metabolic activity in the breast underlies this phenomenon (46).

Involvement of Fibroadenomas by Atypical Hyperplasia

Atypical hyperplasia of both ductal and lobular types may occasionally be found within a fibroadenoma. In a study of almost 2,000 fibroadenomas, atypical hyperplasia was found in 0.81% of the cases (78). Of note, in that study, the presence of atypia in a fibroadenoma did not predict for the presence of atypical hyperplasia in the surrounding breast tissue, nor was it associated with a significant increase in the risk of subsequent breast cancer.

Involvement of Fibroadenomas by Carcinoma

This subject has been reviewed by Azzopardi (46) and by Pick and Iossifides (79). Infrequently, carcinoma occurs in association with a fibroadenoma. The most frequent type of carcinoma involving fibroadenomas is LCIS, but DCIS, invasive ductal, and invasive lobular carcinomas have also been observed. In almost half of the reported cases, the malignant tumor also involves the surrounding breast tissue. The prognosis of carcinoma limited to a fibroadenoma is excellent.

Adenomas

Adenomas of the breast are well-circumscribed tumors composed of benign epithelial elements with sparse, inconspicuous stroma (80). The last feature differentiates these lesions from fibroadenomas, in which the stroma is an integral part of the tumor. For practical purposes, adenomas can be divided into two major groups: tubular adenomas and lactating adenomas.

Tubular Adenomas

Tubular adenomas present in young women as well-defined, freely movable nodules that clinically resemble fibroadenomas (80). Gross examination reveals a well-circumscribed, tan-yellow, firm tumor. On microscopic examination, tubular adenomas are separated from the adjacent breast tissue by a pseudocapsule, and are composed of a proliferation of uniform, small tubular structures with a scant amount of intervening stroma. The tubules are composed of an inner epithelial layer

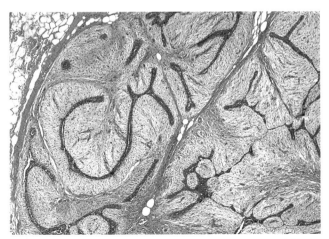

FIGURE 10.7. Fibroadenoma. The tumor is well circumscribed and is composed of benign glandular and stromal elements.

and an outer myoepithelial layer, and resemble normal breast acini, both at the light and ultrastructural level. The tubular lumens often contain eosinophilic material. In some cases, this pattern is admixed with that of a fibroadenoma, suggesting a relationship between the two tumors.

Lactating Adenomas (Nodular Lactational Hyperplasia)

Lactating adenomas present as one or more freely movable masses during pregnancy or the postpartum period (80). They are grossly well-circumscribed and lobulated, and on cut section appear tan and softer than tubular adenomas. On microscopic examination, these lesions have lobulated borders and are composed of glands lined by cuboidal cells with secretory activity, identical to the lactational changes normally observed in breast tissue during pregnancy and the puerperium. Although some authors believe that these lesions are the result of lactational changes superimposed on a preexisting tubular adenoma, others have suggested that they represent *de novo* lesions and are merely nodular foci of hyperplasia in the lactating breast.

O'Hara and Page (81) reviewed 42 breast adenomas that demonstrated lactational changes. They observed an overlapping spectrum of morphologic features in fibroadenomas with lactational changes and in lactating and tubular adenomas. These authors suggested that all these lesions may have a common pathogenesis.

Rarely, adenomatous tumors resembling dermal sweat-gland neoplasms are observed as primary lesions in the breast parenchyma (e.g., clear cell hidradenoma and eccrine spiradenoma) (79,82) or nipple (e.g., syringomatous adenoma) (83,84). Pleomorphic adenomas, histologically identical to those seen in the salivary glands and skin, have also been described in the breast (85–88). Although some of these lesions appear to arise from the breast tissue *de novo*, others appear to represent variants of intraductal papillomas (88).

Adenomas of the Nipple

Adenoma of the nipple has been described under a variety of names, including florid papillomatosis of the nipple ducts (89), subareolar duct papillomatosis (46), papillary adenoma of the nipple (90), and erosive adenomatosis of the nipple (91). It is not, strictly speaking, a true adenoma of the breast, as defined by Hertel et al. (80), because of its prominent stromal component.

On macroscopic examination, some adenomas of the nipple appear as solid, gray-tan, poorly demarcated tumors in the nipple and subareolar region; in other cases, no gross lesion is evident. Microscopically, the dominant feature is a proliferation of small glandlike structures. Solid and papillary proliferation of ductal epithelium is also usually evident; however, the papillary pattern may be inconspicuous or totally absent. In advanced lesions, glandular epithelium extends out onto the surface of the nipple. It is this phenomenon that results in the clinically apparent, reddish, granular appearance. Squamous epithelium frequently extends into the superficial regions of the involved ducts, sometimes with the formation of keratinaceous cysts. The lesions usually show considerable stromal fibrosis. This connective tissue may distort and entrap the epithelial elements, resulting in a pattern mimicking invasive carcinoma. The lesion is distinguishable from carcinoma by the preservation of a double layer of epithelium in the proliferating glands (an inner epithelial and outer myoepithelial cell layer), minimal nuclear atypia, absence of necrosis, and the overall low-power configuration. In problematic cases, immunohistochemical stains for myoepithelial cell markers may be of value in distinguishing a nipple adenoma (the glands of which are surrounded by myoepithelial cells) and invasive carcinoma (which lacks a myoepithelial cell component) (92).

A few cases of carcinoma associated with adenomas of the nipple have been reported (93–95). In most cases, however, adenomas of the nipple are entirely benign. Reports of recurrence most likely represent cases in which the initial resection failed to remove the lesion completely.

Syringomatous Adenoma of the Nipple

Syringomatous adenoma of the nipple is an uncommon benign breast lesion similar in histologic appearance to eccrine syringoma of the skin. The usual clinical presentation is as a mass lesion in the region of the nipple–areola complex. Microscopic examination reveals an infiltrative pattern of epithelial islands that are angulated or comma shaped, as well as tubular or solid in configuration. The glandular lumens are small or obliterated. Squamous metaplasia is usually present within a variable proportion of epithelial islands, which have an inconspicuous outer myoepithelial layer. The epithelial elements often "invade" into the smooth muscle of the nipple, mimicking invasive carcinoma (83,84,96,97).

It is important to distinguish syringomatous adenoma from the malignant lesions tubular carcinoma and low-grade adenosquamous carcinoma. The glandular structures of tubular carcinoma are mostly angulated with open lumens compared with the epithelial islands of syringomatous adenoma, which have smaller or absent lumens and often have characteristic "comma" or "tadpole" shapes. In addition, the glands of tubular carcinoma are composed of a single cell population as opposed to those of syringomatous adenoma, which have a variable amount of squamous metaplasia. Unlike syringomatous adenoma, tubular carcinoma often has associated DCIS. Low-grade adenosquamous carcinoma is virtually indistinguishable from syringomatous adenoma, but usually involves the deeper parenchyma of the breast. If low-grade adenosquamous carcinoma involves the nipple areola complex, the lesion may be impossible to distinguish from syringomatous adenoma.

Intraductal Papillomas

Intraductal papillomas can be divided into two major categories: solitary (central) papillomas and multiple (peripheral) papillomas.

Solitary intraductal papillomas are tumors of the major lactiferous ducts, most frequently observed in women 30 to 50 years of age. These lesions are generally less than 1 cm in diameter, usually measuring 3 to 4 mm. Occasionally, they may be as large as 4 or 5 cm. On gross examination, solitary intraductal papillomas are tan-pink, friable tumors within a dilated duct or cyst. A frankly papillary configuration may or may not be apparent. The tumor is usually attached to the wall of the involved duct by a delicate stalk, but it may be sessile. To identify the papilloma, the involved duct should be opened carefully, using a fine pair of scissors, until the tumor is exposed. Identification of the lesion may be facilitated by the placement of a suture at the end of the involved duct nearest the nipple. Randomly slicing through the excised tissue is not recommended, because a small lesion might be missed.

Microscopically, these tumors are composed of multiple, branching, and interanastomosing papillae, each with a central fibrovascular core and a covering layer of cuboidal to columnar epithelial cells. A myoepithelial cell layer is often discernible between the epithelial cells and the connective tissue stalk (Fig. 10.8). In some areas, the complex growth pattern of the papillae results in the formation of glandlike spaces. Variable amounts of fibrosis can result in the entrapment of epithelial elements, producing a pseudoinfiltrative pattern. The lesion designated *ductal adenoma*, appears to represent an extensively sclerotic variant of an intraductal papilloma (98,99). Florid epithelial proliferation is sometimes observed in intraductal papillomas. At times, the epithelial hyperplasia or fibrosis (or both) and the architectural distortion make it

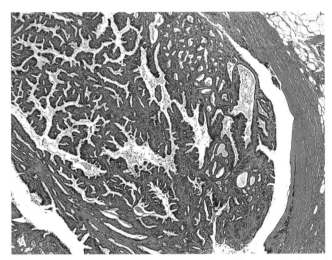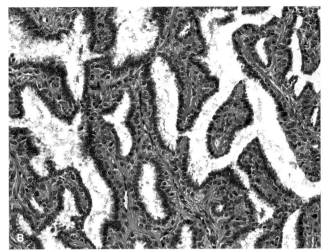

FIGURE 10.8. Intraductal papilloma. A: Low power view demonstrates the papillary lesion within a dilated duct. **B:** Higher power view demonstrates that the papillae are composed of fibrovascular cores covered by an epithelial cell layer (closer to the duct lumen) and a myoepithelial layer (closer to the cores).

extremely difficult to distinguish between benign papilloma and papillary DCIS. Features helpful in making this distinction have been elucidated by Kraus and Neubecker (100) and by Azzopardi (46).

Several additional features of solitary intraductal papillomas deserve emphasis. Papillomas can undergo partial or total infarction, often accompanied by distortion of the adjacent, viable epithelium and production of a pattern that may simulate invasive carcinoma. Squamous metaplasia has been observed in intraductal papillomas. In some cases, it accompanies infarction, but it has also been observed in the absence of infarction. This phenomenon may also result in a disturbing growth pattern that can be confused with carcinoma (101). Finally, some intraductal papillomas exhibit areas of atypia that range from foci resembling ADH to areas qualitatively similar to DCIS, most often low-grade. The classification of such lesions, particularly when the proliferation fulfills the qualitative criteria for the diagnosis of DCIS, varies among different authors. In general, the classification of such lesions has been based largely on the extent of the atypical proliferation within the papillary lesion. For example, Tavassoli (102) uses the designation *atypical papilloma* if the atypical changes involve less than one-third of the papilloma and *carcinoma arising in a papilloma* when the atypical population of cells involves at least a third but less than 90% of the lesion (102). Page et al. (103) have stated that the presence of "any area of uniform histology and cytology consistent with non-comedo DCIS" within a papilloma that is more than 3 mm in size should be considered DCIS within a papilloma, whereas foci with the same qualitative features which measure 3 mm or less in size are classified as a papilloma with atypia.

The clinical significance of atypia or DCIS in a papilloma is not well-defined. Some authors have reported a substantially increased risk (7.5-fold) for the subsequent development of breast cancer, predominantly in the ipsilateral breast (103), whereas others have found that the level of breast cancer risk associated with papillomas with atypia was similar to that of patients with ADH elsewhere in the breast (four- to fivefold) and that the risk was approximately equal in both breasts (104). Breast cancer risk is reported to be particularly high (sevenfold) among women with multiple papillomas with atypia (104).

The risk of subsequent breast cancer and local recurrence does not appear to be related to the extent of atypia or DCIS within the papilloma. In fact, the most important consideration is the presence of atypia or DCIS in the surrounding breast tissue because this appears to be more closely related to the risk

of recurrence than the qualitative features or extent of atypia within the papilloma itself (103,105).

Multiple (Peripheral) Intraductal Papillomas

Compared with solitary intraductal papillomas, multiple intraductal papillomas tend to occur in younger patients; they are less often associated with nipple discharge, are more frequently peripheral, and are more often bilateral. Most importantly, these lesions appear to be particularly susceptible to the development of carcinoma. In Haagensen's (26) series of 68 patients with multiple papillomas, simultaneous or subsequent carcinoma of the apocrine papillary and cribriform types was observed in 22 patients (32%). Another study in which surgically excised specimens from patients with intraductal papillomas were subjected to three-dimensional reconstruction confirms these observations (106). All 16 cases of multiple papillomas in the series were found to originate in the most peripheral portion of the duct system, the terminal duct lobular unit (TDLU). Furthermore, carcinoma was found to be associated with these multiple peripheral papillomas in six cases (37.5%). In contrast, no cases of carcinoma were found to be associated with solitary papillomas involving the large ducts. These findings suggest that peripheral papillomas, in contrast to solitary central papillomas, may be highly susceptible to malignant transformation.

Juvenile Papillomatosis (Swiss Cheese Disease)

Juvenile papillomatosis was first recognized as a clinicopathologic entity in 1980 by Rosen et al. (107). This lesion occurs most commonly in adolescents and young women (with a mean age of 23 years), but has been seen in women up to 48 years of age. Patients typically present with a painless mass which, on physical examination, is circumscribed, easily movable, and is most often considered to be a fibroadenoma.

On gross pathologic examination, the lesions range in size from 1 to 8 cm. Multiple cysts of up to 1 cm in diameter are generally apparent. The microscopic features of juvenile papillomatosis are not unique to this entity, and are all components previously described as part of *fibrocystic disease*. The constellation of histologic features, however, forms a characteristic complex. These lesions appear to be well-circumscribed, but not encapsulated, and are characterized by the following elements: duct papillomatosis, apocrine and nonapocrine cysts, papillary apocrine hyperplasia, sclerosing adenosis, and duct stasis. The epithelial proliferation in these lesions may be quite marked, and the cytologic and architectural features may approach those of DCIS.

Follow-up studies have suggested that juvenile papillomatosis is associated with an increased risk of breast cancer in the patient's female relatives, and that the patient herself may be at increased risk for developing carcinoma, particularly if the lesion is bilateral and the patient has a family history of breast cancer (108–111).

Microglandular Adenosis

Microglandular adenosis (MGA) is an uncommon lesion that may be found incidentally in breast tissue excised for other lesions, or it may present as a mass lesion (112–114). Most women in whom this lesion has been reported are older than 40 years of age, but patients as young as 28 years and as old as 82 years have been reported to have MGA (115). The importance of this lesion is that it may be mistaken for a well-differentiated (tubular) carcinoma on histological examination.

On gross examination, MGA has generally been described as an ill-defined area of firm, rubbery tissue. Microscopically, the lesion is characterized by a poorly circumscribed, haphazard proliferation of small, round glands in the breast stroma and adipose tissue. Unlike sclerosing adenosis, MGA does not have a lobulocentric, organoid configuration. As with tubular carcinoma, the glands are composed of a single cell layer and lack an outer myoepithelial layer. In contrast to tubular carcinoma, however, the glands are round (not angulated). The single layer of cuboidal epithelial cells has clear to slightly eosinophilic cytoplasm and small, regular nuclei, but the cells lack the apical secretory snouts that are characteristic of tubular carcinoma. The cells stain strongly for S100 protein, and the glands are surrounded by basement membrane material (116,117). Eosinophilic secretions are frequently present within the glandular lumina, and are periodic acid-Schiff (PAS) positive. When tubular carcinoma gland lumens contain material, it is usually calcified. As opposed to the desmoplastic stroma associated with tubular carcinoma, the stroma in MGA is typically composed of dense, relatively acellular collagen, which usually demarcates the lesion from the adjacent parenchyma. In some areas, the stroma is minimal and the proliferating glands lie exposed in adipose tissue (Fig. 10.9).

The relationship between MGA and cancer has been addressed in several studies (115,118–122). Simultaneous or subsequent carcinoma was reported in 4 of the 13 patients originally reported by Rosen et al. (113), 1 of the 11 patients described by Tavassoli and Norris (114), and none of

the 6 patients reported by Clement and Azzopardi (112). Rosenblum et al. (123) described seven cases of MGA associated with carcinoma. James et al. (118) noted carcinoma arising in, or in conjunction with, MGA in 14 of 60 cases (23%). A study by Koenig et al. (119) emphasized the potential importance of atypical MGA as a transitional form between typical MGA and carcinomas arising in this setting. At the present time, the recommended approach to the treatment of patients with MGA is complete, local excision of the lesion and careful follow-up.

Radial Scars

Radial scars were first recognized by Semb in 1928 (124). Linell et al. (125) proposed the name *radial scar* in 1980, which was a translation of Hamperl's *strahlige narben* introduced in 1975 (126). They have been described in the literature by a variety of other names, including sclerosing papillary proliferation, nonencapsulated sclerosing lesion, indurative mastopathy, and radial sclerosing lesion (88,127–130). The term "complex sclerosing lesion" is sometimes used for similar lesions larger than 1 cm in size or for those lesions with several fibroelastotic areas in close contiguity (41). The importance of these lesions is twofold. First, they may, on mammographic, gross, and microscopic examination, simulate breast carcinomas. Second, although the relationship between the presence of radial scars and subsequent breast cancer has long been a matter of controversy, recent evidence suggests that the presence of a radial scar is associated with an increased risk of subsequent breast cancer (131).

Radial scars are most often incidental microscopic findings in breast biopsies performed for other indications (128,131,132). Some are sufficiently large to be detected mammographically where they appear as spiculated masses that cannot be reliably distinguished from carcinomas (133). The reported incidence of radial scars varies from 4% to 28% (128,134,135). In a recent nested case-control study, radial scars were identified in 7% of benign breast biopsies reviewed (131). Several studies have found radial scars to be bilateral and multicentric (132,135,136), with these frequencies reported to be as high as 43% and 67%, respectively (135). They are often multiple, with as many as 31 lesions having been observed in a single breast (134).

On gross examination, radial scars are irregular, gray-white, and indurated with central retraction—an appearance identical to that of scirrhous carcinoma. On microscopic examination, radial scars are characterized by a central zone of fibroelastosis from which ducts and lobules radiate, exhibiting various benign alterations, such as microcysts, apocrine metaplasia, and proliferative changes, such as florid hyperplasia and papillomas. Within the central area of fibroelastotic stroma, smaller entrapped ducts are present, which are often distorted or angular in appearance (Fig. 10.10). These ducts are lined by one or more layers of epithelium and an outer myoepithelial cell layer. The presence of these myoepithelial cells may be confirmed immunohistochemically with markers such as smooth muscle myosin heavy chain, p63, and calponin (137–139). Radial scars may be involved by atypical hyperplasia (either ductal or lobular), and LCIS, DCIS, or invasive carcinoma may rarely be present.

The relationship between radial scars and breast cancer has interested investigators for many years. The observation that the entrapped epithelial elements within the central zone of fibroelastosis in radial scars may mimic tubular carcinoma (127–129,133,140–143) led several authors to postulate that radial scars represent an early phase in the development of some breast cancers (124,125,128,142,144). The presence of invasive, *in situ* carcinoma, or both in some radial scars has been cited as further support for the concept of their malignant potential (133,145,146). To define further the relationship

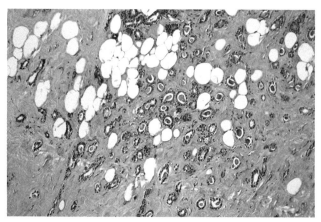

FIGURE 10.9. Microglandular adenosis, characterized by a haphazard proliferation of small glands composed of a single layer of epithelial cells. The glands are relatively rounded and many contain eosinophilic secretions in their lumens.

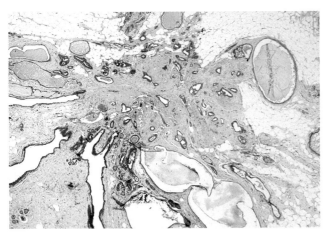

FIGURE 10.10. Radial scar. This lesion is characterized by a central fibroelastic core containing entrapped benign glands. Radiating from this core are ducts that show a variety of changes, including cysts and epithelial hyperplasia.

between radial scars and breast cancer, Sloane and Mayers (133) reviewed 126 radial scars and complex sclerosing lesions. They found that carcinoma and atypical hyperplasia were more common in radial scars larger than 6 to 7 mm than in smaller radial scars and in radial scars in women older than 50 years than in younger women. The similarity in appearance between radial scars and some cancers, and the coexistence of *in situ* or invasive carcinoma within some radial scars, although of interest, does not, however, provide conclusive evidence of a relationship. Studies of the frequency of radial scars in women with breast cancer compared with those without cancer have, however, yielded conflicting results regarding their potential premalignant nature (132,134–136).

Until recently, the malignant potential of radial scars postulated in these observational reports had not been validated by clinical follow-up studies. The few available follow-up studies that existed were characterized by small patient numbers and lack of suitable controls (127,130). The results of one case-control study suggest that women with a biopsy-proved radial scar are at increased risk for subsequent breast cancer. In that study, the presence of a radial scar was associated with a twofold increase in breast cancer risk, independent of the histologic category of benign breast disease (131). Moreover, the presence of a radial scar further increased the breast cancer risk in women with other types of proliferative breast disease, particularly those with proliferative lesions without atypia. In particular, among women with proliferative lesions without atypia, those with a radial scar had a relative risk of breast cancer of 3.0, whereas the relative risk of breast cancer in those without a radial scar was 1.5. No significant difference was noted between the number of women who developed cancer in the breast ipsilateral or contralateral to that of their original benign biopsy containing a radial scar (131). In a subsequent study, the increased breast cancer risk associated with radial scars was observed primarily in women over the age of 50 years and was largely attributable to the category of coexistent proliferative breast disease (147). Therefore, radial scars are probably best considered markers of generalized increased breast cancer risk. Given that *in situ* and invasive carcinomas appear to be more common in larger than smaller radial scars (133), the possibility that at least some radial scars represent direct cancer precursors must also be considered. In fact, these two possibilities are not mutually exclusive. Most authorities agree that the finding of radial scar on a core needle biopsy is an indication for excision (148–156).

The pathogenesis of radial scars is uncertain, as are the reasons for their association with an increased risk of breast cancer. It is attractive to postulate that a disturbance in the normal reciprocal stromal–epithelial interaction exists in radial scars. This may be a reflection of a more generalized perturbation of the interaction between stromal and epithelial cells in the breast, a phenomenon postulated to be important in breast cancer pathogenesis (157). Jacobs et al. (158) demonstrated by *in situ* hybridization that certain vascular stromal factors found in radial scars were similar to those in invasive carcinomas, raising the possibility that a similar disturbance in stromal–epithelial interactions is present in both lesions.

Granular Cell Tumor

Granular cell tumors are uncommonly found in the breast but, when present, simulate carcinoma on clinical, mammographic, and pathologic examination (159,160). These tumors occur more commonly in African American than white women, and typically appear between puberty and menopause, implicating some hormonal factor in their development. Granular cell tumors of the breast most commonly occur in the upper, inner quadrant in contrast to carcinomas, which occur most frequently in the upper, outer quadrant. Patients present with a palpable mass that may be associated with skin retraction or fixation to chest wall skeletal muscles. The similarity of granular cell tumors to carcinoma is also evident on mammographic examination, on which they resemble scirrhous carcinoma. Gross examination of the lesion reveals a gray-white to tan firm tumor that may be gritty when cut with a knife; these features further support the impression of carcinoma. Microscopically, these lesions are identical to granular cell tumors in other sites, consisting of a poorly circumscribed proliferation of cells in which the most characteristic feature is prominent granularity of the cytoplasm. On electron microscopic examination, these granules correspond to secondary lysosomes. The nuclei are small and uniform, and lack the features of malignant disease.

Granular cell tumors are almost invariably benign and are adequately treated by wide local excision. Rare cases of malignant granular cell tumors have been reported in both the breast and extramammary sites. Granular cell tumors were initially considered to be myogenic in origin (hence, their earlier designation as granular cell myoblastomas), but ultrastructural and immunohistochemical evidence supports a neurogenic origin for these tumors (160,161).

Fibromatosis

Fibromatosis of the breast, which is analogous to fibromatosis in other sites (e.g., desmoid tumors of the abdominal wall), is characterized by a locally invasive, nonencapsulated proliferation of well-differentiated spindle cells (162–169). These tumors have the capacity to recur locally if inadequately excised, but they do not metastasize. Although most cases are sporadic, mammary fibromatosis may be seen in association with familial adenomatous polyposis, Gardner's syndrome, or as part of a hereditary desmoid syndrome (166,167,169).

Patients typically present with a palpable mass which is sometimes associated with skin retraction or fixation to the underlying pectoral muscle. On mammography, these lesions are indistinguishable from carcinomas. Gross pathologic examination reveals an ill-defined, firm, gray-white lesion. Microscopically, fibromatoses consist of interlacing bundles of spindle-shaped cells surrounded by collagen. The cells show minimal to no cytologic atypia, and mitoses are only infrequently encountered. The proliferation tends to surround and entrap preexisting ducts and lobules without destroying them. Fibromatosis may exhibit keloid-like areas where collagen is increased, and the periphery of the lesion may be more cellular, with lymphocytic aggregates also present. The edges of the lesion infiltrate irregularly into the adjacent parenchyma. On electron microscopic and immunohistochemical examination, many of the tumor cells have the features of fibroblasts and myofibroblasts.

The proper treatment for fibromatosis consists of wide local excision. Although metastases have not been reported, lesions may recur locally. Zayid and Dehmis (170) described an exceptional case in which a patient was treated with mastectomy, subsequently developing multiple tumor recurrences in the chest wall, which ultimately resulted in her death.

MISCELLANEOUS BENIGN LESIONS

Lipomas

Lipomas consist of encapsulated nodules of mature adipose tissue. Although true lipomas occur in the breast, many lesions designated *lipoma* probably represent foci of fatty breast tissue without a true capsule. *Adenolipoma* is a term that has been applied to a benign fatty tumor of the breast containing entrapped lobular epithelial elements (46); however, such lesions are probably best considered hamartomas.

Vascular Lesions

Benign vascular lesions of the breast parenchyma are relatively uncommon and most often represent incidental microscopic findings. In a series of 550 mastectomy specimens from patients with breast carcinoma, the incidence of benign hemangiomas was 1.2% (171). Benign vascular lesions of the breast can be divided into four major categories: *perilobular hemangiomas, angiomatoses, venous hemangiomas, and hemangiomas involving the mammary subcutaneous tissue* (172–175). The major significance of these lesions is that they must be distinguished from angiosarcomas (176). Benign angiomatous lesions are almost always microscopic in size and lack interanastomosing channels, endothelial proliferation, and atypia. Complete excision is recommended for all vascular lesions of the breast. Atypical vascular lesions have been described in the skin of the breast and the mammary parenchyma in women who have been treated with conservative surgery and radiation therapy for breast cancer (177–179).

Pseudoangiomatous Stromal Hyperplasia

Pseudoangiomatous hyperplasia of the mammary stroma is a benign stromal proliferation that simulates a vascular lesion (180–182). The lesion is often seen as an incidental microscopic finding, but may present as a palpable mass. Microscopic examination reveals complex interanastomosing spaces, some of which have spindle-shaped stromal cells at their margins simulating endothelial cells. Ultrastructural examinations have demonstrated, however, that the spaces appear to be caused by separation and disruption of collagen fibers and that the associated spindle cells are myofibroblasts. The significance of this lesion is that it must be distinguished from a true vascular lesion, specifically, angiosarcoma.

Chondromatous Lesions

Chondromatous lesions of the breast are uncommon. Although chondromatous changes are most often seen in breast carcinomas and sarcomas, chondroid metaplasia may rarely be seen in fibroadenomas and intraductal papillomas. A few cases of *chondrolipoma* have also been reported (183,184), as has a single case of *choristoma* containing cartilage (185).

Leiomyoma

Leiomyomas of the breast are most often seen in the areolar region and rarely occur in the breast parenchyma (46). The histologic characteristics are the same as those of leiomyomas in other tissue.

Neural Lesions

Neurofibromas and neurilemmomas (schwannomas) are benign nerve sheath tumors. These lesions are most frequently seen in the breast in patients with neurofibromatosis and are most common in the areolar area (186).

Adenomyoepithelioma

Adenomyoepitheliomas are uncommon lesions considered variants of intraductal papilloma. They present as palpable masses that are grossly circumscribed. Microscopically, these lesions are usually multinodular and are composed of a combination of epithelial and myoepithelial elements. The myoepithelial cells may be polygonal or spindle shaped. These lesions are adequately treated by complete local excision (187–190). Lesions composed exclusively of myoepithelial cells *(myoepitheliomas)* have also been described (189,190).

Hamartoma

Hamartomas of the breast present as well-defined masses on physical examination and on mammography. Microscopically, these lesions are composed of an admixture of ducts, lobules, fibrous stroma and adipose tissue in varying proportions (191,192). Occasional lesions also contain smooth muscle *(myoid hamartomas)* (193). These lesions frequently go unrecognized by the pathologist, because histologically they resemble other benign or physiologic changes in the breast.

Myofibroblastoma

Myofibroblastomas are uncommon benign mesenchymal tumors. These lesions are typically well circumscribed and are most often composed of a proliferation of relatively uniform-appearing spindle cells in a densely collagenized stroma. The cells comprising the tumor show features of myofibroblasts on ultrastructural and immunohistochemical examination (169, 194,195).

Mucocele-like Lesion

Mucocele-like lesions are composed of mucin-containing cysts that often rupture, with resultant extravasation of mucin into surrounding stroma (196). The mucoid character of these lesions is usually evident on gross examination. The epithelium lining these cysts can range from benign (including flat or cuboidal epithelium and hyperplasia, including papillary) to atypical ductal hyperplasia to DCIS (197). The distinction between mucocele-like lesion and mucinous (colloid) carcinoma may be difficult, particularly if there are epithelial cells floating within the mucin. Therefore, these lesions must be completely excised and carefully examined histologically (with multiple sections if necessary) to rule out the possibility of an invasive mucinous carcinoma (196–200).

Collagenous Spherulosis

Collagenous spherulosis is most often an incidental microscopic finding in breast tissue removed for another abnormality. This lesion appears to be more frequent in breasts containing sclerosing lesions (e.g., radial scar or sclerosed papilloma).

Occasionally, collagenous spherulosis may calcify and present as mammographic microcalcifications. This lesion is characterized by aggregates of eosinophilic fibrillary, hyaline spherules, or both, which are surrounded by an inner myoepithelial layer and outer epithelial layers within the lobules. This arrangement gives rise to an appearance of a fenestrated or cribriform proliferation at low power microscopic examination. The spherules are composed of variable amounts of basement membrane-like material and type IV collagen and are positive for PAS and Alcian blue. This lesion is important to recognize because it must be distinguished from cribriform DCIS and adenoid cystic carcinoma (201).

REACTIVE/INFLAMMATORY LESIONS

Mammary Duct Ectasia (Periductal Mastitis)

Mammary duct ectasia occurs primarily in perimenopausal and postmenopausal women, and is characterized by dilatation of the subareolar ducts (26). Considerable controversy exists regarding the most appropriate name for this condition. This controversy has arisen because some authors consider ductal dilatation to be the primary event, whereas others consider the ectatic ducts to be the consequence of prior periductal inflammation.

Duct ectasia is a frequent pathologic finding in breast tissue obtained at autopsy and in surgically excised material. It has been observed on microscopic examination in 30% to 40% of women older than 50 years of age. Clinically evident disease, however, occurs much less frequently (202).

A wide spectrum of pathologic changes is observed in this condition. Cut section of the gross specimen often reveals dilated, thick-walled ducts that contain pasty, yellow-brown secretions. The intervening stroma may be fibrotic. On microscopic examination, some cases show prominent inspissation of lipid-rich material within ducts, accompanied by periductal inflammation. Rupture or leakage of these ducts results in release of this material into the adjacent stroma, with subsequent inflammation and fat necrosis. Plasma cells may be a prominent component of the periductal and stromal inflammatory infiltrate. It should be noted that many cases previously designated as plasma cell mastitis probably represent a stage in the evolution of duct ectasia. In other cases, the histologic picture is dominated by periductal fibrosis and ductal dilatation with minimal inflammation.

As alluded to earlier, the pathogenesis of this condition has not been fully established. Dixon et al. (202) suggested that the primary event is periductal inflammation and that duct ectasia is the ultimate outcome of this disorder. In support of this premise, they observed that inflammation around nondilated ducts predominates in younger patients with this condition, whereas duct dilatation and nipple retraction are more common in older patients (202). Thus, their postulated sequence of events in the evolution of this disease was that periductal inflammation leads to periductal fibrosis, which subsequently results in ductal dilatation. This group of investigators has also suggested that periductal mastitis and duct ectasia may represent two separate entities, based on differences between women with these two disorders with regard to age, clinical history, and smoking history (203).

Squamous Metaplasia of Lactiferous Ducts (Recurrent Subareolar Abscess, Zuska's Disease)

Keratinizing squamous epithelium normally extends into the orifices of the lactiferous ducts for 1 to 2 mm. If these keratinizing cells extend deeper into the ducts, keratin production

can result in ductal distention and eventual duct rupture, resulting in an intense inflammatory response and sterile abscess formation. Secondary bacterial colonization and infection may occur. A fistulous tract may also develop, typically opening at the edge of the areola. Appropriate treatment requires excision of the involved duct, which may also require excision of a portion of the nipple (204).

Fat Necrosis

The importance of fat necrosis is that it may closely simulate carcinoma, both clinically and on mammographic examination (26,205).

The macroscopic appearance of fat necrosis depends on its age. In early lesions, there is hemorrhage and indurated fat. With time, a rounded, firm tumor is formed. The cut surface of the lesion at this stage has a variegated, yellow-gray appearance with focal hemorrhage. Cavitation can subsequently occur, owing to liquefactive necrosis. The lesion may eventually be converted to a dense, fibrous scar or may remain a cystic cavity with calcification of its walls.

On microscopic examination, early lesions show cystic spaces surrounded by lipid-laden macrophages and foreign body-type giant cells with foamy cytoplasm (Fig. 10.11). A variable, acute inflammatory cell infiltrate may be present, and there may be focal hemorrhage. With time, there is fibroblastic proliferation with deposition of collagen. Scattered, chronic inflammatory cells are usually present, and focal hemosiderin deposition may be observed. Even in older lesions, scattered, foamy histiocytes and foreign body giant cells are usually discernible. A similar pathologic appearance may be seen after surgical trauma to the breast and after radiation therapy for carcinoma (see the section on pathologic changes associated with radiation therapy, below).

Reactions to Foreign Material

Foreign body-type granulomatous inflammation has been described following injection within the breast of a variety of substances, including paraffin and silicone. Clinically, these lesions generally appear as firm nodules that may be tender (205).

A variety of tissue reactions has been reported in association with mammary implants (206–210). One of these is the formation of a fibrous capsule in the surrounding tissue. In 10% to 40% of patients there is contracture of this capsule which results in breast tightness or firmness and deformation of the

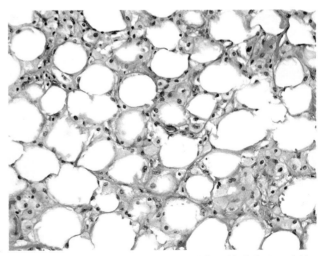

FIGURE 10.11. Fat necrosis. The fatty breast tissue is infiltrated by histiocytes containing foamy cytoplasm.

implant necessitating either capsulotomy or removal of the implant and the surrounding capsule. Histologic examination of the capsular tissue shows varying degrees of fibrosis, chronic inflammation, fat necrosis, granulation tissue, fibrin deposition, histiocytes, and foreign body giant cells, often with demonstrable silicone (and in some cases in which it has been used as part of the implant shell, polyurethane). In some cases, the capsule surrounding breast implants develops a cellular lining that histologically, immunohistochemically, and ultrastructurally resembles either normal synovium or synovium with papillary hyperplasia (proliferative synovitis) and has physiologic properties similar to synovium (211–214). This change has been variably described as *pseudoepithelialization*, *synovial metaplasia*, and *capsular synovial hyperplasia*. The factors associated with development of synovial-type metaplasia in this setting are not known. Some have suggested that this is a consequence of mechanical forces (e.g., micromotion and friction) between the implant and the surrounding tissue.

Mondor's Disease (Phlebitis of the Thoracoepigastric Vein)

Mondor's disease, or phlebitis of the thoracoepigastric vein, has been considered to be rare (215–217). On pathologic examination, there is phlebitis and periphlebitis. The obliterative endophlebitis is associated with varying degrees of thrombosis, and the adventitia and media may be completely destroyed in advanced cases.

Pathologic Changes Associated with Radiation Therapy for Carcinoma

Breast-conserving surgery, followed by radiation therapy, is now a common treatment for patients with early-stage breast cancer. The effects of therapeutic doses of ionizing radiation on the skin of the breast have been well-described, and are identical to the radiation-induced alterations occurring in skin from any irradiated site (218).

Fat necrosis can occur in the breast following local excision and radiation therapy for carcinoma. These lesions may be indistinguishable from carcinoma by clinical and radiographic examination, requiring complete histologic examination for accurate diagnosis (219). The most characteristic pathologic finding in breast tissue excised following primary radiation therapy for carcinoma is epithelial cell atypia in the TDLU, usually associated with varying degrees of lobular sclerosis and atrophy (Fig. 10.12) (220). These changes may be distinguished from carcinoma involving the TDLU by the preservation of polarity and cohesion, and by the absence of cellular proliferation and distention of the involved TDLU in areas of radiation-induced change. Similar epithelial changes have been described in patients treated with preoperative or neoadjuvant chemotherapy (221–223). Less frequently, epithelial atypia in large (extralobular) ducts, atypical fibroblasts in the stroma, and radiation-related vascular changes may be observed. Interestingly, stromal fibrosis, a characteristic feature of radiation effect in other organs, is so variable among both irradiated patients and nonirradiated control subjects that it is not, by itself, a reliable marker for radiation-induced injury in the breast.

Sarcoidosis

Involvement of the breast by sarcoidosis is rare, but when present, may clinically simulate a neoplasm (224–226). Histologically, the lesions consist of typical, noncaseating granulomas with varying numbers of giant cells present in the interlobular and intralobular connective tissue. A diagnosis of sarcoidosis should be made only after the exclusion of other causes of

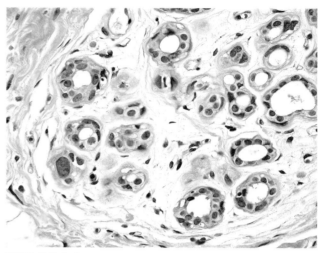

FIGURE 10.12. Radiation effects. This terminal duct lobular unit contains scattered enlarged epithelial cells with large, diffusely hyperchromatic nuclei. Cellular polarity is maintained and no evidence of cellular proliferation is present.

granulomatous inflammation, such as mycobacterial, fungal, and parasitic infections or reactions to foreign materials. Sarcoidosis should also be distinguished from *granulomatous mastitis*, a lesion in which the granulomas are associated with microabscesses and which may respond to corticosteroid therapy (227–230).

Lymphocytic Mastitis/Diabetic Mastopathy

Insulin-dependent diabetic patients occasionally develop breast masses that on histologic examination show a characteristic constellation of features (231–235). These include dense, keloid-like fibrosis, lymphocytic infiltrates in association with ducts and lobules (lymphocytic ductitis and lobulitis), lymphocytic vasculitis, and epithelioid fibroblasts in the stroma. Although the pathogenesis of this lesion is unknown, it may represent an autoimmune reaction. Similar histologic changes have been described in association with other autoimmune diseases, such as Hashimoto's thyroiditis and in patients with various types of autoantibodies in their serum (231).

References

1. Page DL, Dupont WD. Anatomic indicators (histologic and cytologic) of increased breast cancer risk. *Breast Cancer Res Treat* 1993;28(2):157–166.
2. Love SM, Gelman RS, Silen W. Sounding board. Fibrocystic "disease" of the breast—a nondisease? *N Engl J Med* 1982;307(16):1010–1014.
3. Kodlin D, Winger EE, Morgenstern NL, et al. Chronic mastopathy and breast cancer. A follow-up study. *Cancer* 1977;39(6):2603–2607.
4. Dupont WD, Page DL. Risk factors for breast cancer in women with proliferative breast disease. *N Engl J Med* 1985;312(3):146–151.
5. Carter CL, Corle DK, Micozzi MS, et al. A prospective study of the development of breast cancer in 16,692 women with benign breast disease. *Am J Epidemiol* 1988;128(3):467–477.
6. Tavassoli FA, Norris HJ. A comparison of the results of long-term follow-up for atypical intraductal hyperplasia and intraductal hyperplasia of the breast. *Cancer* 1990;65(3):518–529.
7. Palli D, Rosselli del Turco M, Simoncini R, et al. Benign breast disease and breast cancer: a case-control study in a cohort in Italy. *Int J Cancer* 1991;47(5):703–706.
8. London SJ, Connolly JL, Schnitt SJ, et al. A prospective study of benign breast disease and the risk of breast cancer. *JAMA* 1992;267(7):941–944.
9. Krieger N, Hiatt RA. Risk of breast cancer after benign breast diseases. Variation by histologic type, degree of atypia, age at biopsy, and length of follow-up. *Am J Epidemiol* 1992;135(6):619–631.
10. McDivitt RW, Stevens JA, Lee NC, et al. Histologic types of benign breast disease and the risk for breast cancer. The Cancer and Steroid Hormone Study Group. *Cancer* 1992;69(6):1408–1414.
11. Dupont WD, Parl FF, Hartmann WH, et al. Breast cancer risk associated with proliferative breast disease and atypical hyperplasia. *Cancer* 1993;71(4):1258–1265.

12. Bodian CA, Perzin KH, Lattes R, et al. Prognostic significance of benign proliferative breast disease. *Cancer* 1993;71(12):3896–3907.
13. Marshall LM, Hunter DJ, Connolly JL, et al. Risk of breast cancer associated with atypical hyperplasia of lobular and ductal types. *Cancer Epidemiol Biomarkers Prev* 1997;6(5):297–301.
14. Shaaban AM, Sloane JP, West CR, et al. Histopathologic types of benign breast lesions and the risk of breast cancer: case-control study. *Am J Surg Pathol* 2002; 26(4):421–430.
15. Page DL, Schuyler PA, Dupont WD, et al. Atypical lobular hyperplasia as a unilateral predictor of breast cancer risk: a retrospective cohort study. *Lancet* 2003; 361(9352):125–129.
16. Hartmann LC, Sellers TA, Frost MH, et al. Benign breast disease and the risk of breast cancer. *N Engl J Med* 2005;353(3):229–237.
17. Collins LC, Baer HJ, Tamimi RM, et al. Magnitude and laterality of breast cancer risk according to histologic type of atypical hyperplasia: results from the Nurses' Health Study. *Cancer* 2007;109(2):180–187.
18. Collins LC, Baer HJ, Tamimi RM, et al. The influence of family history on breast cancer risk in women with biopsy-confirmed benign breast disease: results from the Nurses' Health Study. *Cancer* 2006;107(6):1240–1247.
19. Degnim AC, Visscher DW, Berman HK, et al. Stratification of breast cancer risk in women with atypia: a Mayo cohort study. *J Clin Oncol* 2007;25(19):2671–2677.
20. Milanese TR, Hartmann LC, Sellers TA, et al. Age-related lobular involution and risk of breast cancer. *J Natl Cancer Inst* 2006;98(22):1600–1607.
21. Hutter RV. Goodbye to "fibrocystic disease" [editorial]. *N Engl J Med* 1985;312(3): 179–181.
22. Hughes LE, Mansel RE, Webster DJ. Aberrations of normal development and involution (ANDI): a new perspective on pathogenesis and nomenclature of benign breast disorders. *Lancet* 1987;2(8571):1316–1319.
23. Page DL, Dupont WD, Rogers LW, et al. Atypical hyperplastic lesions of the female breast. A long-term follow-up study. *Cancer* 1985;55(11):2698–2708.
24. Page DL, Rogers LW. Combined histologic and cytologic criteria for the diagnosis of mammary atypical ductal hyperplasia. *Hum Pathol* 1992;23(10):1095–1097.
25. Fitzgibbons PL, Henson DE, Hutter RV. Benign breast changes and the risk for subsequent breast cancer: an update of the 1985 consensus statement. Cancer Committee of the College of American Pathologists. *Arch Pathol Lab Med* 1998; 122(12):1053–1055.
26. Haagensen CD. *Diseases of the breast.* 3 ed. Philadelphia: WB Saunders, 1986.
27. Dupont WD, Page DL, Parl FF, et al. Long-term risk of breast cancer in women with fibroadenoma. *N Engl J Med* 1994;331(1):10–15.
28. Tavassoli FA, Hoefler H, Rosai J, et al. Intraductal Proliferative Lesions. In: Tavassoli FA, Devilee P, eds. *Pathology and genetics: tumours of the breast and female genital organs.* Lyon: IARC Press, 2003:63–73.
29. Jensen RA, Page DL, Dupont WD, et al. Invasive breast cancer risk in women with sclerosing adenosis. *Cancer* 1989;64(10):1977–1983.
30. Nielsen BB. Adenosis tumour of the breast—a clinicopathological investigation of 27 cases. *Histopathology* 1987;11(12):1259–1275.
31. Seidman JD, Ashton M, Lefkowitz M. Atypical apocrine adenosis of the breast: a clinicopathologic study of 37 patients with 8.7-year follow-up. *Cancer* 1996; 77(12):2529–2537.
32. Eusebi V, Damiani S, Losi L, et al. Apocrine differentiation in breast epithelium. *Adv Anat Pathol* 1997;4:139.
33. Carter DJ, Rosen PP. Atypical apocrine metaplasia in sclerosing lesions of the breast: a study of 51 patients. *Mod Pathol* 1991;4(1):1–5.
34. Fechner RE. Lobular carcinoma in situ in sclerosing adenosis. A potential source of confusion with invasive carcinoma. *Am J Surg Pathol* 1981;5(3):233–239.
35. Chan JK, Ng WF. Sclerosing adenosis cancerized by intraductal carcinoma. *Pathology* 1987;19(4):425–428.
36. Eusebi V, Collina G, Bussolati G. Carcinoma in situ in sclerosing adenosis of the breast: an immunocytochemical study. *Semin Diagn Pathol* 1989;6(2):146–152.
37. Fechner RE. Carcinoma in situ involving sclerosing adenosis. *Histopathology* 1996;28(6):570.
38. Taylor HB, Norris HJ. Epithelial invasion of nerves in benign diseases of the breast. *Cancer* 1967;20(12):2245–2249.
39. Davies JD. Neural invasion in benign mammary dysplasia. *J Pathol* 1973;109(3): 225–231.
40. Gould VE, Rogers DR, Sommers SC. Epithelial-nerve intermingling in benign breast lesions. *Arch Pathol* 1975;99(11):596–598.
41. Page DL, Anderson TJ. *Diagnostic histopathology of the breast.* Edinburgh, Scotland: Churchill Livingstone, 1987.
42. Page DL, Dupont WD, Rogers LW. Ductal involvement by cells of atypical lobular hyperplasia in the breast: a long-term follow-up study of cancer risk. *Hum Pathol* 1988;19(2):201–207.
43. Schnitt SJ, Wang HH. Histologic sampling of grossly benign breast biopsies. How much is enough? *Am J Surg Pathol* 1989;13(6):505–512.
44. Owings DV, Hann L, Schnitt SJ. How thoroughly should needle localization breast biopsies be sampled for microscopic examination? A prospective mammographic/pathologic correlative study. *Am J Surg Pathol* 1990;14(6):578–583.
45. Rubin E, Visscher DW, Alexander RW, et al. Proliferative disease and atypia in biopsies performed for nonpalpable lesions detected mammographically. *Cancer* 1988;61(10):2077–2082.
46. Azzopardi JG. *Problems in breast pathology.* Philadelphia: WB Saunders, 1979.
47. Schnitt SJ, Collins LC. Columnar cell lesions and flat epithelial atypia of the breast. *Seminars in Breast Disease* 2005;8:100–111.
48. Dupont WD, Page DL. Relative risk of breast cancer varies with time since diagnosis of atypical hyperplasia. *Hum Pathol* 1989;20(8):723–725.
49. Chen CL, Weiss NS, Newcomb P, et al. Hormone replacement therapy in relation to breast cancer. *JAMA* 2002;287(6):734–741.
50. Dupont WD, Page DL, Rogers LW, et al. Influence of exogenous estrogens, proliferative breast disease, and other variables on breast cancer risk. *Cancer* 1989; 63(5):948–957.
51. Byrne C, Connolly JL, Colditz GA, et al. Biopsy confirmed benign breast disease, postmenopausal use of exogenous female hormones, and breast carcinoma risk. *Cancer* 2000;89(10):2046–2052.
52. Baer H, Collins L, Connolly J, et al. Lobular involution and subsequent breast cancer risk: findings from the Nurses' Health Study. *Cancer* 2009, [epub ahead of print].
53. Reis-Filho JS, Lakhani SR. The diagnosis and management of pre-invasive breast disease: genetic alterations in pre-invasive lesions. *Breast Cancer Res* 2003;5(6): 313–319.
54. Dupont WD, Plummer WD, Jr. Understanding the relationship between relative and absolute risk. *Cancer* 1996;77(11):2193–2199.
55. Rosai J. Borderline epithelial lesions of the breast. *Am J Surg Pathol* 1991;15(3): 209–221.
56. Schnitt SJ, Connolly JL, Tavassoli FA, et al. Interobserver reproducibility in the diagnosis of ductal proliferative breast lesions using standardized criteria [see comments]. *Am J Surg Pathol* 1992;16(12):1133–1143.
57. Bodian CA, Perzin KH, Lattes R, et al. Reproducibility and validity of pathologic classifications of benign breast disease and implications for clinical applications [see comments]. *Cancer* 1993;71(12):3908–3913.
58. Krishnamurthy S, Sneige N. Molecular and biologic markers of premalignant lesions of human breast. *Adv Anat Pathol* 2002;9(3):185–197.
59. Shackney SE, Silverman JF. Molecular evolutionary patterns in breast cancer. *Adv Anat Pathol* 2003;10(5):278–290.
60. Arpino G, Laucirica R, Elledge RM. Premalignant and in situ breast disease: biology and clinical implications. *Ann Intern Med* 2005;143(6):446–457.
61. Khan SA, Rogers MA, Khurana KK, et al. Estrogen receptor expression in benign breast epithelium and breast cancer risk [see comments]. *J Natl Cancer Inst* 1998;90(1):37–42.
62. Gobbi H, Dupont WD, Parl FF, et al. Breast cancer risk associated with estrogen receptor expression in epithelial hyperplasia lacking atypia and adjacent lobular units. *Int J Cancer* 2005;113(5):857–859.
63. Shaaban AM, Jarvis C, Moore F, et al. Prognostic significance of estrogen receptor beta in epithelial hyperplasia of usual type with known outcome. *Am J Surg Pathol* 2005;29(12):1593–1599.
64. Guinebretiere JM, Le Monique G, Gavoille A, et al. Angiogenesis and risk of breast cancer in women with fibrocystic disease. *J Natl Cancer Inst* 1994;86(8): 635–636.
65. Heffelfinger SC, Yassin R, Miller MA, et al. Vascularity of proliferative breast disease and carcinoma in situ correlates with histological features. *Clin Cancer Res* 1996;2(11):1873–1878.
66. Viacava P, Naccarato AG, Bocci G, et al. Angiogenesis and VEGF expression in pre-invasive lesions of the human breast. *J Pathol* 2004;204(2):140–146.
67. Rohan TE, Hartwick W, Miller AB, et al. Immunohistochemical detection of c-erbB-2 and p53 in benign breast disease and breast cancer risk [see comments]. *J Natl Cancer Inst* 1998;90(17):1262–1269.
68. Stark A, Hulka BS, Joens S, et al. HER-2/neu amplification in benign breast disease and the risk of subsequent breast cancer. *J Clin Oncol* 2000;18(2):267–274.
69. Gobbi H, Arteaga CL, Jensen RA, et al. Loss of expression of transforming growth factor beta type II receptor correlates with high tumour grade in human breast *in situ* and invasive carcinomas. *Histopathology* 2000;36(2):168–177.
70. Visscher DW, Pankratz VS, Santisteban M, et al. Association between cyclooxygenase-2 expression in atypical hyperplasia and risk of breast cancer. *J Natl Cancer Inst* 2008;100(6):421–427.
71. Simpson PT, Reis-Filho JS, Gale T, et al. Molecular evolution of breast cancer. *J Pathol* 2005;205(2):248–254.
72. Wang J, Costantino JP, Tan-Chiu E, et al. Lower-category benign breast disease and the risk of invasive breast cancer. *J Natl Cancer Inst* 2004;96(8):616–620.
73. Goodman ZD, Taxy JB. Fibroadenomas of the breast with prominent smooth muscle. *Am J Surg Pathol* 1981;5(1):99–101.
74. Oberman HA. Breast lesions in the adolescent female. In: Sommers SC, Rosen PP, eds. *Pathology annual,* Part 1. Norwalk, CT: Appleton-Century-Crofts, 1979.
75. Nambiar R, Kutty MK. Giant fibro-adenoma (cystosarcoma phyllodes) in adolescent females—a clinicopathological study. *Br J Surg* 1974;61(2):113–117.
76. Ashikari R, Farrow JH, O'Hara J. Fibroadenomas in the breast of juveniles. *Surg Gynecol Obstet* 1971;132(2):259–262.
77. Mies C, Rosen PP. Juvenile fibroadenoma with atypical epithelial hyperplasia. *Am J Surg Pathol* 1987;11(3):184–190.
78. Carter BA, Page DL, Schuyler P, et al. No elevation in long-term breast carcinoma risk for women with fibroadenomas that contain atypical hyperplasia. *Cancer* 2001;92(1):30–36.
79. Pick PW, Iossifides IA. Occurrence of breast carcinoma within a fibroadenoma. A review. *Arch Pathol Lab Med* 1984;108(7):590–594.
80. Hertel BF, Zaloudek C, Kempson RL. Breast adenomas. *Cancer* 1976;37(6): 2891–905.
81. O'Hara MF, Page DL. Adenomas of the breast and ectopic breast under lactational influences. *Hum Pathol* 1985;16(7):707–712.
82. O'Connell P, Pekkel V, Fuqua SA, et al. Analysis of loss of heterozygosity in 399 premalignant breast lesions at 15 genetic loci. *J Natl Cancer Inst* 1998;90(9): 697–703.
83. Rosen PP. Syringomatous adenoma of the nipple. *Am J Surg Pathol* 1983;7(8): 739–745.
84. Jones MW, Norris HJ, Snyder RC. Infiltrating syringomatous adenoma of the nipple. A clinical and pathological study of 11 cases. *Am J Surg Pathol* 1989;13(3): 197–201.
85. Chen KT. Pleomorphic adenoma of the breast. *Am J Clin Pathol* 1990;93(6): 792–794.
86. Moran CA, Suster S, Carter D. Benign mixed tumors (pleomorphic adenomas) of the breast. *Am J Surg Pathol* 1990;14(10):913–921.
87. Ballance WA, Ro JY, el-Naggar AK, et al. Pleomorphic adenoma (benign mixed tumor) of the breast. An immunohistochemical, flow cytometric, and ultrastructural study and review of the literature. *Am J Clin Pathol* 1990;93(6):795–801.
88. Rosen PP, Oberman HA. *Tumors of the mammary gland.* Washington, DC: Armed Forces Institute of Pathology, 1993.
89. Jones DB. Florid papillomatosis of the nipple ducts. *Cancer* 1955;8:315.
90. Perzin KH, Lattes R. Papillary adenoma of the nipple (florid papillomatosis, adenoma, adenomatosis). A clinicopathologic study. *Cancer* 1972;29(4):996–1009.
91. Smith EJ, Kron SD, Gross PR. Erosive adenomatosis of the nipple. *Arch Dermatol* 1970;102(3):330–332.
92. Diaz NM, Palmer JO, Wick MR. Erosive adenomatosis of the nipple: histology, immunohistology, and differential diagnosis. *Mod Pathol* 1992;5(2):179–184.
93. Gudjonsdottir A, Hagerstrand I, Ostberg G. Adenoma of the nipple with carcinomatous development. *Acta Pathol Microbiol Scand [A]* 1971;79(6):676–680.
94. Bhagavan BS, Patchefsky A, Koss LG. Florid subareolar duct papillomatosis (nipple adenoma) and mammary carcinoma: report of three cases. *Hum Pathol* 1973; 4(2):289–295.
95. Rosen PP, Caicco JA. Florid papillomatosis of the nipple. A study of 51 patients, including nine with mammary carcinoma. *Am J Surg Pathol* 1986;10(2):87–101.

96. Ward BE, Cooper PH, Subramony C. Syringomatous tumor of the nipple. *Am J Clin Pathol* 1989;92(5):692–696.
97. Suster S, Moran CA, Hurt MA. Syringomatous squamous tumors of the breast. *Cancer* 1991;67(9):2350–2355.
98. Azzopardi JG, Salm R. Ductal adenoma of the breast: a lesion which can mimic carcinoma. *J Pathol* 1984;144(1):15–23.
99. Lammie GA, Millis RR. Ductal adenoma of the breast—a review of fifteen cases. *Hum Pathol* 1989;20(9):903–908.
100. Kraus FT, Neubecker RD. The differential diagnosis of papillary tumors of the breast. *Cancer* 1962;15:444–455.
101. Flint A, Oberman HA. Infarction and squamous metaplasia of intraductal papilloma: a benign breast lesion that may simulate carcinoma. *Hum Pathol* 1984; 15(8):764–767.
102. Tavassoli FA. *Pathology of the breast.* 2nd ed. Stamford, CT: Appleton and Lange, 1999.
103. Page DL, Salhany KE, Jensen RA, et al. Subsequent breast carcinoma risk after biopsy with atypia in a breast papilloma. *Cancer* 1996;78(2):258–266.
104. Lewis JT, Hartmann LC, Vierkant RA, et al. An analysis of breast cancer risk in women with single, multiple, and atypical papilloma. *Am J Surg Pathol* 2006; 30(6):665–672.
105. MacGrogan G, Tavassoli FA. Central atypical papillomas of the breast: a clinico-pathological study of 119 cases. *Virchows Arch* 2003;443(5):609–617.
106. Ohuchi N, Abe R, Kasai M. Possible cancerous change of intraductal papillomas of the breast. A 3-D reconstruction study of 25 cases. *Cancer* 1984;54(4): 605–611.
107. Rosen PP, Cantrell B, Mullen DL, et al. Juvenile papillomatosis (Swiss cheese disease) of the breast. *Am J Surg Pathol* 1980;4(1):3–12.
108. Rosen PP, Lyngholm B, Kinne DW, Beattie EJ, Jr. Juvenile papillomatosis of the breast and family history of breast carcinoma. *Cancer* 1982;49(12):2591–2595.
109. Rosen PP, Holmes G, Lesser ML, et al. Juvenile papillomatosis and breast carcinoma. *Cancer* 1985;55(6):1345–1352.
110. Bazzocchi F, Santini D, Martinelli G, et al. Juvenile papillomatosis (epitheliosis) of the breast. A clinical and pathologic study of 13 cases. *Am J Clin Pathol* 1986; 86(6):745–748.
111. Rosen PP, Kimmel M. Juvenile papillomatosis of the breast. A follow-up study of 41 patients having biopsies before 1979. *Am J Clin Pathol* 1990;93(5):599–603.
112. Clement PB, Azzopardi JG. Microglandular adenosis of the breast—a lesion simulating tubular carcinoma. *Histopathology* 1983;7(2):169–180.
113. Rosen PP. Microglandular adenosis. A benign lesion simulating invasive mammary carcinoma. *Am J Surg Pathol* 1983;7(2):137–144.
114. Tavassoli FA, Norris HJ. Microglandular adenosis of the breast. A clinicopathologic study of 11 cases with ultrastructural observations. *Am J Surg Pathol* 1983; 7(8):731–737.
115. Millis RR. Microglandular adenosis of the breast. *Adv Anat Pathol* 1995;2:10.
116. Diaz NM, McDivitt RW, Wick MR. Microglandular adenosis of the breast. An immunohistochemical comparison with tubular carcinoma. *Arch Pathol Lab Med* 1991;115(6):578–582.
117. Tavassoli FA, Bratthauer GL. Immunohistochemical profile and differential diagnosis of microglandular adenosis. *Mod Pathol* 1993;6(3):318–322.
118. James BA, Cranor ML, Rosen PP. Carcinoma of the breast arising in microglandular adenosis. *Am J Clin Pathol* 1993;100(5):507–513.
119. Koenig C, Dadmanesh F, Bratthauer GL, et al. Carcinoma arising in microglandular adenosis: an immunohistochemical analysis of 20 intraepithelial and invasive neoplasms. *Int J Surg Pathol* 2000;8(4):303–315.
120. Acs G, Simpson JF, Bleiweiss IJ, et al. Microglandular adenosis with transition into adenoid cystic carcinoma of the breast. *Am J Surg Pathol* 2003;27(8): 1052–1060.
121. Harmon M, Fuller B, Cooper K. Carcinoma arising in microglandular adenosis of the breast. *Int J Surg Pathol* 2001;9(4):344.
122. Salarieh A, Sneige N. Breast carcinoma arising in microglandular adenosis: a review of the literature. *Arch Pathol Lab Med* 2007;131(9):1397–1399.
123. Rosenblum MK, Purrazzella R, Rosen PP. Is microglandular adenosis a precancerous disease? A study of carcinoma arising in microglandular adenosis. *Lab Invest* 1985;52:57A.
124. Semb C. Pathologico-anatomical and clinical investigations of fibro-adenomatosis cystica mammae and its relation to other pathological conditions in the mamma, especially cancer. *Acta Chir Scand (Suppl)* 1928;64:1–484.
125. Linell F, Ljungberg O, Anderson I. Breast carcinoma. Aspects of early stages, progression and related problems. *Acta Pathol Microbiol Scand Suppl* 1980(272): 1–233.
126. Hamperl H. Strahlige narben und obliterierende mastopathie. Beitrage zur pathologischen histologie der mamma. XI. *Virchows Arch A Pathol Anat Histol* 1975;369(1):55–68.
127. Fenoglio C, Lattes R. Sclerosing papillary proliferations in the female breast. A benign lesion often mistaken for carcinoma. *Cancer* 1974;33(3):691–700.
128. Fisher ER, Palekar AS, Kotwal N, et al. A nonencapsulated sclerosing lesion of the breast. *Am J Clin Pathol* 1979;71(3):240–246.
129. Rickert RR, Kalisher L, Hutter RV. Indurative mastopathy: a benign sclerosing lesion of breast with elastosis which may simulate carcinoma. *Cancer* 1981; 47(3):561–571.
130. Andersen JA, Gram JB. Radial scar in the female breast. A long-term follow-up study of 32 cases. *Cancer* 1984;53(11):2557–2560.
131. Jacobs TW, Byrne C, Colditz G, et al. Radial scars in benign breast-biopsy specimens and the risk of breast cancer. *N Engl J Med* 1999;340(6):430–436.
132. Anderson TJ, Battersby S. Radial scars of benign and malignant breasts: comparative features and significance. *J Pathol* 1985;147(1):23–32.
133. Sloane JP, Mayers MM. Carcinoma and atypical hyperplasia in radial scars and complex sclerosing lesions: importance of lesion size and patient age. *Histopathology* 1993;23(3):225–231.
134. Wellings SR, Alpers CE. Subgross pathologic features and incidence of radial scars in the breast. *Hum Pathol* 1984;15(5):475–479.
135. Nielsen M, Jensen J, Andersen JA. An autopsy study of radial scar in the female breast. *Histopathology* 1985;9(3):287–295.
136. Nielsen M, Christensen L, Andersen J. Radial scars in women with breast cancer. *Cancer* 1987;59(5):1019–1025.
137. Bocker W, Bier B, Freytag G, et al. An immunohistochemical study of the breast using antibodies to basal and luminal keratins, alpha-smooth muscle actin, vimentin, collagen IV and laminin. Part I: Normal breast and benign proliferative lesions. *Virchows Arch A Pathol Anat Histopathol* 1992;421(4):315–322.
138. Bocker W, Bier B, Freytag G, et al. An immunohistochemical study of the breast using antibodies to basal and luminal keratins, alpha-smooth muscle actin, vimentin, collagen IV and laminin. Part II: Epitheliosis and ductal carcinoma in situ. *Virchows Arch A Pathol Anat Histopathol* 1992;421(4):323–330.
139. Damiani S, Ludvikova M, Tomasic G, et al. Myoepithelial cells and basal lamina in poorly differentiated *in situ* duct carcinoma of the breast. An immunocyto-chemical study. *Virchows Arch* 1999;434(3):227–234.
140. Bloodgood JC. Border-line breast tumors. Encapsulated and non-encapsulated cystic adenomata, observed from 1890–1931. *Am J Cancer* 1932;16:103–176.
141. Tremblay G, Buell RH, Seemayer TA. Elastosis in benign sclerosing ductal proliferation of the female breast. *Am J Surg Pathol* 1977;1(2):155–166.
142. Andersen JA, Carter D, Linell F. A symposium on sclerosing duct lesions of the breast. *Pathol Annu* 1986;21 Pt 2:145–179.
143. Weidner N. Benign breast lesions that mimic malignant tumors: analysis of five distinct lesions. *Semin Diagn Pathol* 1990;7(2):90–101.
144. Fisher ER, Palekar AS, Sass R, et al. Scar cancers: pathologic findings from the National Surgical Adjuvant Breast Project (protocol no. 4) - IX. *Breast Cancer Res Treat* 1983;3(1):39–59.
145. Frouge C, Tristant H, Guinebretiere JM, et al. Mammographic lesions suggestive of radial scars: microscopic findings in 40 cases. *Radiology* 1995;195(3): 623–625.
146. Douglas-Jones AG, Pace DP. Pathology of R4 spiculated lesions in the breast screening programme. *Histopathology* 1997;30(3):214–220.
147. Sanders ME, Page DL, Simpson JF, et al. Interdependence of radial scar and proliferative disease with respect to invasive breast carcinoma risk in patients with benign breast biopsies. *Cancer* 2006;106(7):1453–1461.
148. Jackman RJ, Nowels KW, Rodriguez-Soto J, et al. Stereotactic, automated, large-core needle biopsy of nonpalpable breast lesions: false-negative and histologic underestimation rates after long-term follow-up. *Radiology* 1999;210(3):799–805.
149. Dershaw DD, Morris EA, Liberman L, et al. Nondiagnostic stereotaxic core breast biopsy: results of rebiopsy. *Radiology* 1996;198(2):323–325.
150. Lee CH, Egglin TK, Philpotts L, et al. Cost-effectiveness of stereotactic core needle biopsy: analysis by means of mammographic findings. *Radiology* 1997;202(3): 849–854.
151. Lee CH, Philpotts LE, Horvath LJ, et al. Follow-up of breast lesions diagnosed as benign with stereotactic core-needle biopsy: frequency of mammographic change and false-negative rate. *Radiology* 1999;212(1):189–194.
152. Philpotts LE, Shaheen NA, Jain KS, et al. Uncommon high-risk lesions of the breast diagnosed at stereotactic core-needle biopsy: clinical importance. *Radiology* 2000;216(3):831–837.
153. Brenner RJ, Jackman RJ, Parker SH, et al. Percutaneous core needle biopsy of radial scars of the breast: when is excision necessary? *AJR Am J Roentgenol* 2002;179(5):1179–1184.
154. Cawson JN, Malara F, Kavanagh A, et al. Fourteen-gauge needle core biopsy of mammographically evident radial scars: is excision necessary? *Cancer* 2003; 97(2):345–351.
155. Douglas-Jones AG, Denson JL, Cox AC, et al. Radial scar lesions of the breast diagnosed by needle core biopsy: analysis of cases containing occult malignancy. *J Clin Pathol* 2007;60(3):295–298.
156. Doyle EM, Banville N, Quinn CM, et al. Radial scars/complex sclerosing lesions and malignancy in a screening programme: incidence and histological features revisited. *Histopathology* 2007;50(5):607–614.
157. Ronnov-Jessen L, Petersen OW, Bissell MJ. Cellular changes involved in conversion of normal to malignant breast: importance of the stromal reaction. *Physiol Rev* 1996;76(1):69–125.
158. Jacobs TW, Schnitt SJ, Tan X, Brown LF. Radial scars of the breast and breast carcinomas have similar alterations in expression of factors involved in vascular stroma formation. *Hum Pathol* 2002;33(1):29–38.
159. DeMay RM, Kay S. Granular cell tumors of the breast. In: Sommers SC, Rosen PP, eds. *Pathology annual,* Part 1. Norwalk, CT: Appleton-Century-Crofts, 1984.
160. Damiani S, Koerner FC, Dickersin GR, et al. Granular cell tumour of the breast. *Virchows Arch A Pathol Anat Histopathol* 1992;420(3):219–226.
161. Ingram DL, Mossler JA, Snowhite J, et al. Granular cell tumors of the breast. Steroid receptor analysis and localization of carcinoembryonic antigen, myoglobin, and S100 protein. *Arch Pathol Lab Med* 1984;108(11):897–901.
162. Gump FE, Sternschein MJ, Wolff M. Fibromatosis of the breast. *Surg Gynecol Obstet* 1981;153(1):57–60.
163. Ali M, Fayemi AO, Braun EV, Remy R. Fibromatosis of the breast. *Am J Surg Pathol* 1979;3(6):501–505.
164. Rosen Y, Papasozomenos SC, Gardner B. Fibromatosis of the breast. *Cancer* 1978;41(4):1409–1413.
165. Hanna WM, Jambrosic J, Fish E. Aggressive fibromatosis of the breast. *Arch Pathol Lab Med* 1985;109(3):260–262.
166. Wargotz ES, Norris HJ, Austin RM, et al. Fibromatosis of the breast. A clinical and pathological study of 28 cases. *Am J Surg Pathol* 1987;11(1):38–45.
167. Rosen PP, Ernsberger D. Mammary fibromatosis. A benign spindle-cell tumor with significant risk for local recurrence. *Cancer* 1989;63(7):1363–1369.
168. Devouassoux-Shisheboran M, Schammel MD, Man YG, et al. Fibromatosis of the breast: age-correlated morphofunctional features of 33 cases. *Arch Pathol Lab Med* 2000;124(2):276–280.
169. McMenamin ME, DeSchryver K, Fletcher CD. Fibrous lesions of the breast: a review. *Int J Surg Pathol* 2000;8(2):99–108.
170. Zayid I, Dihmis C. Familial multicentric fibromatosis—desmoids. A report of three cases in a Jordanian family. *Cancer* 1969;24(4):786–795.
171. Rosen PP, Ridolfi RL. The perilobular hemangioma. A benign microscopic vascular lesion of the breast. *Am J Clin Pathol* 1977;68(1):21–23.
172. Jozefczyk MA, Rosen PP. Vascular tumors of the breast. II. Perilobular hemangiomas and hemangiomas. *Am J Surg Pathol* 1985;9(7):491–503.
173. Rosen PP. Vascular tumors of the breast. III. Angiomatosis. *Am J Surg Pathol* 1985;9(9):652–658.
174. Rosen PP, Jozefczyk MA, Boram LH. Vascular tumors of the breast. IV. The venous hemangioma. *Am J Surg Pathol* 1985;9(9):659–665.
175. Rosen PP. Vascular tumors of the breast. V. Nonparenchymal hemangiomas of mammary subcutaneous tissues. *Am J Surg Pathol* 1985;9(10):723–729.
176. Donnell RM, Rosen PP, Lieberman PH, et al. Angiosarcoma and other vascular tumors of the breast. *Am J Surg Pathol* 1981;5(7):629–642.
177. Fineberg S, Rosen PP. Cutaneous angiosarcoma and atypical vascular lesions of the skin and breast after radiation therapy for breast carcinoma. *Am J Clin Pathol* 1994;102(6):757–763.

178. Requena L, Kutzner H, Mentzel T, et al. Benign vascular proliferations in irradiated skin. *Am J Surg Pathol* 2002;26(3):328–337.
179. Brenn T, Fletcher CD. Radiation-associated cutaneous atypical vascular lesions and angiosarcoma: clinicopathologic analysis of 42 cases. *Am J Surg Pathol* 2005;29(8):983–996.
180. Vuitch MF, Rosen PP, Erlandson RA. Pseudoangiomatous hyperplasia of mammary stroma. *Hum Pathol* 1986;17(2):185–191.
181. Ibrahim RE, Sciotto CG, Weidner N. Pseudoangiomatous hyperplasia of mammary stroma. Some observations regarding its clinicopathologic spectrum. *Cancer* 1989;63(6):1154–1160.
182. Powell CM, Cranor ML, Rosen PP. Pseudoangiomatous stromal hyperplasia (PASH). A mammary stromal tumor with myofibroblastic differentiation. *Am J Surg Pathol* 1995;19(3):270–277.
183. Kaplan L, Walts AE. Benign chondrolipomatous tumor of the human female breast. *Arch Pathol Lab Med* 1977;101(3):149–151.
184. Marsh WL Jr, Lucas JG, Olsen J. Chondrolipoma of the breast. *Arch Pathol Lab Med* 1989;113(4):369–371.
185. Metcalf JS, Ellis B. Choristoma of the breast. *Hum Pathol* 1985;16(7):739–740.
186. Cohen MB, Fisher PE. Schwann cell tumors of the breast and mammary region. *Surg Pathol* 1991;4:47–56.
187. Rosen PP. Adenomyoepithelioma of the breast. *Hum Pathol* 1987;18(12):1232–1237.
188. Young RH, Clement PB. Adenomyoepithelioma of the breast. A report of three cases and review of the literature. *Am J Clin Pathol* 1988;89(3):308–314.
189. Tavassoli FA. Myoepithelial lesions of the breast. Myoepitheliosis, adenomyoepithelioma, and myoepithelial carcinoma. *Am J Surg Pathol* 1991;15(6):554–568.
190. Erlandson RA, Rosen PP. Infiltrating myoepithelioma of the breast. *Am J Surg Pathol* 1982;6(8):785–793.
191. Oberman HA. Hamartomas and hamartoma variants of the breast. *Semin Diagn Pathol* 1989;6(2):135–145.
192. Daya D, Trus T, D'Souza TJ, et al. Hamartoma of the breast, an underrecognized breast lesion. A clinicopathologic and radiographic study of 25 cases. *Am J Clin Pathol* 1995;103(6):685–689.
193. Daroca PJ Jr., Reed RJ, Love GL, et al. Myoid hamartomas of the breast. *Hum Pathol* 1985;16(3):212–219.
194. Wargotz ES, Weiss SW, Norris HJ. Myofibroblastoma of the breast. Sixteen cases of a distinctive benign mesenchymal tumor. *Am J Surg Pathol* 1987;11(7):493–502.
195. Hamele-Bena D, Cranor ML, Sciotto C, et al. Uncommon presentation of mammary myofibroblastoma. *Mod Pathol* 1996;9(7):786–790.
196. Rosen PP. Mucocele-like tumors of the breast. *Am J Surg Pathol* 1986;10(7):464–469.
197. Ro JY, Sneige N, Sahin AA, et al. Mucocelelike tumor of the breast associated with atypical ductal hyperplasia or mucinous carcinoma. A clinicopathologic study of seven cases. *Arch Pathol Lab Med* 1991;115(2):137–140.
198. Weaver MG, Abdul-Karim FW. Mucinous lesions of the breast. A pathological continuum. *Pathol Res Pract* 1993;189(8):873–876.
199. Fisher ER, Palekar AS, Stoner F, Costantino J. Mucocele-like lesions and mucinous carcinoma of the breast. *Int J Surg Pathol* 1994;1:213.
200. Hamele-Bena D, Cranor ML, Rosen PP. Mammary mucocele-like lesions. Benign and malignant. *Am J Surg Pathol* 1996;20(9):1081–1085.
201. Clement PB, Young RH, Azzopardi JG. Collagenous spherulosis of the breast. *Am J Surg Pathol* 1987;11(6):411–417.
202. Dixon JM, Anderson TJ, Lumsden AB, et al. Mammary duct ectasia. *Br J Surg* 1983;70(10):601–603.
203. Dixon JM, Ravisekar O, Chetty U, et al. Periductal mastitis and duct ectasia: different conditions with different aetiologies. *Br J Surg* 1996;83(6):820–822.
204. Lester S. Subareolar abscess (Zuska's disease): a specific disease entity with specific treatment and prevention strategies. *Pathology Case Reviews* 1999;4(5):189–193.
205. Symmers W. The breasts. In: Symmers W, ed. *Systemic pathology*. Edinburgh: Churchill Livingstone, 1978.
206. Sanchez-Guerrero J, Schur PH, Sergent JS, et al. Silicone breast implants and rheumatic disease. Clinical, immunologic, and epidemiologic studies. *Arthritis Rheum* 1994;37(2):158–168.
207. Bridges AJ, Vasey FB. Silicone breast implants. History, safety, and potential complications. *Arch Intern Med* 1993;153(23):2638–2644.
208. Carter D. Tissue reaction to breast implants [Editorial; comment]. *Am J Clin Pathol* 1994;102(5):565–566.
209. Schnitt SJ. Tissue reactions to mammary implants: a capsule summary. *Adv Anat Pathol* 1995;2(1):24–27.
210. Noone RB. A review of the possible health implications of silicone breast implants. *Cancer* 1997;79(9):1747–1756.
211. Chase DR, Oberg KC, Chase RL, et al. Pseudoepithelialization of breast implant capsules. *Int J Surg Pathol* 1994;1:151–154.
212. Raso DS, Crymes LW, Metcalf JS. Histological assessment of fifty breast capsules from smooth and textured augmentation and reconstruction mammoplasty prostheses with emphasis on the role of synovial metaplasia. *Mod Pathol* 1994;7(3):310–316.
213. Emery JA, Spanier SS, Kasnic G Jr, et al. The synovial structure of breast-implant-associated bursae. *Mod Pathol* 1994;7(7):728–733.
214. Hameed MR, Erlandson R, Rosen PP. Capsular synovial-like hyperplasia around mammary implants similar to detritic synovitis. A morphologic and immunohistochemical study of 15 cases. *Am J Surg Pathol* 1995;19(4):433–438.
215. Honig C, Rado R. Mondor's disease–superficial phlebitis of the chest wall: a review of seven cases. *Ann Surg* 1961;153:589.
216. Fischl RA, Kahn S, Simon BE. Mondor's disease. An unusual complication of mammaplasty. *Plast Reconstr Surg* 1975;56(3):319–322.
217. Tabar L, Dean PB. Mondor's disease: clinical, mammographic, and pathologic features. *Breast J* 1981;7:18.
218. Fajardo LJ. *Pathology of radiation injury*. New York: Masson Publishing, 1982.
219. Clarke D, Curtis JL, Martinez A, et al. Fat necrosis of the breast simulating recurrent carcinoma after primary radiotherapy in the management of early stage breast carcinoma. *Cancer* 1983;52(3):442–445.
220. Schnitt SJ, Connolly JL, Harris JR, et al. Radiation-induced changes in the breast. *Hum Pathol* 1984;15(6):545–550.
221. Kennedy S, Merino MJ, Swain SM, et al. The effects of hormonal and chemotherapy on tumoral and nonneoplastic breast tissue. *Hum Pathol* 1990;21(2): 192–198.
222. Fisher ER, Wang J, Bryant J, et al. Pathobiology of preoperative chemotherapy: findings from the National Surgical Adjuvant Breast and Bowel (NSABP) protocol B-18. *Cancer* 2002;95(4):681–695.
223. Pinder SE, Provenzano E, Earl H, et al. Laboratory handling and histology reporting of breast specimens from patients who have received neoadjuvant chemotherapy. *Histopathology* 2007;50(4):409–417.
224. Gansler TS, Wheeler JE. Mammary sarcoidosis. Two cases and literature review. *Arch Pathol Lab Med* 1984;108(8):673–675.
225. Ross MJ, Merino MJ. Sarcoidosis of the breast. *Hum Pathol* 1985;16(2):185–187.
226. Fitzgibbons PL, Smiley DF, Kern WH. Sarcoidosis presenting initially as breast mass: report of two cases. *Hum Pathol* 1985;16(8):851–852.
227. Kessler E, Wolloch Y. Granulomatous mastitis: a lesion clinically simulating carcinoma. *Am J Clin Pathol* 1972;58(6):642–646.
228. DeHertogh DA, Rossof AH, Harris AA, et al. Prednisone management of granulomatous mastitis. *N Engl J Med* 1980;303(14):799–800.
229. Fletcher A, Magrath IM, Riddell RH, et al. Granulomatous mastitis: a report of seven cases. *J Clin Pathol* 1982;35(9):941–945.
230. Kessler EI, Katzav JA. Lobular granulomatous mastitis. *Surg Pathol* 1990;3:115–120.
231. Lammie GA, Bobrow LG, Staunton MD, et al. Sclerosing lymphocytic lobulitis of the breast—evidence for an autoimmune pathogenesis. *Histopathology* 1991;19(1):13–20.
232. Tomaszewski JE, Brooks JS, Hicks D, et al. Diabetic mastopathy: a distinctive clinicopathologic entity. *Hum Pathol* 1992;23(7):780–786.
233. Seidman JD, Schnaper LA, Phillips LE. Mastopathy in insulin-requiring diabetes mellitus. *Hum Pathol* 1994;25(8):819–824.
234. Morgan MC, Weaver MG, Crowe JP. Diabetic mastopathy: a clinicopathologic study in palpable and nonpalpable breast lesions. *Mod Pathol* 1995;8(4):349–354.
235. Ely KA, Tse G, Simpson JF, et al. Diabetic mastopathy. A clinicopathologic review. *Am J Clin Pathol* 2000;113(4):541–545.

Chapter 11
Screening for Breast Cancer

Robert A. Smith, Carl D'Orsi, and Mary S. Newell

In the mid-18th century Henri François LeDran proposed that breast cancer originated as a localized disease that subsequently spread via the lymphatics to the general circulation. According to Donegan (1), LeDran's recognition of the dominant course of breast cancer progression was pivotal and established the idea that surgery, if performed early, offered the potential to cure breast cancer. However, it was not until the early 20th century that experimental work with x-rays revealed occult breast disease, thereby establishing the potential for diagnosis before the earliest detection of a palpable mass (1,2). The evolution of the understanding of the natural history of breast cancer eventually led to population-based randomized trials of breast cancer screening (3), and ultimately the public health impetus to screen women for breast cancer with mammography (4,5).

Today there is widespread acceptance of the value of regular breast cancer screening as the single most important public health strategy to reduce mortality from breast cancer. In 1977 the first breast cancer screening guidelines were established during a Consensus Development Meeting on Breast Cancer Screening convened by the National Cancer Institute for the purpose of establishing evidence-based eligibility for participation in the Breast Cancer Detection Demonstration Project (BCDD) (6). Since then, all U.S. states have required insurance companies to address coverage for mammography, Medicare provides for annual mammography for all beneficiaries, and the National Committee on Quality Assurance (NCQA) has established breast cancer screening for women 40 years and older as one of the core national Health Plan Employer Data and Information Set (HEDIS) measures (7–9). In 2006 approximately 61% of women aged 40 or older reported having had a mammogram in the past year (10). Perhaps the most important measure of the success of the introduction of mammography as a routine part of women's preventive health care is that the death rate from breast cancer began to decline in 1989 and has declined each year since (11,12).

Before the availability of breast imaging, the control of breast cancer relied entirely on the success of treating symptomatic breast cancer. Today, breast cancer control is significantly influenced by the opportunity to diagnose breast cancer at a more favorable stage, due both to increased mammography utilization as well as increased awareness of the importance of reporting new symptoms promptly to a clinician (13,14). Although continued progress in the understanding of the epidemiology of breast cancer suggests the potential for risk reduction through lifestyle modification and chemoprevention, the latter specifically through several select estrogen-receptor modulators (SERMs) in higher-risk women (15,16), there still is no dependable preventive strategy, apart from prophylactic surgery in very high-risk women (17), which can measurably reduce the absolute risk of breast cancer or eliminate the need for regular screening. For the foreseeable future, early detection and appropriate treatment will remain the cornerstone of the disease-control strategy for breast cancer in average and high-risk women.

This chapter will discuss breast cancer screening in the context of basic screening principles, methodologic issues related to the evaluation of experimental studies of screening, as well as the evaluation of modern service screening, the current evidence of screening efficacy, and practical and clinical aspects of modern breast cancer screening and diagnosis in average and high-risk women.

 ## PRINCIPLES OF CANCER SCREENING

The primary goal of breast cancer screening on an individual or population basis is to distinguish among those who are likely and not likely to have the disease (18). The emphasis on *likelihood* underscores the limits of screening (i.e., screening examinations are *not* diagnostic examinations). It is inherent to the concept of screening that a person identified with an abnormality is then referred for further diagnostic testing to determine whether the disease truly is present. Further, the emphasis on likelihood also is important because screening tests have inherent and even practical limitations because the main purpose of screening is to test a large, defined asymptomatic population at an acceptable cost. In the case of breast cancer screening, the majority of screening interpretations are accurate, but it is inevitable that some women will be identified as possibly having breast cancer when they do not, and likewise, screening programs will fail to identify some women who do have the disease, including women who develop breast cancer before the age that routine screening should commence.

Before large numbers of asymptomatic individuals undergo routine testing for the presence of a chronic disease, certain conventional criteria should be met (19). First, the disease should be an important health problem. Second, there should be a period when the disease is detectable in an asymptomatic individual (i.e., a detectable preclinical phase, or *sojourn time*). Third, treatment at this early stage should offer better outcomes than if the disease were treated at a later stage. Fourth, the screening test must be effective and reasonably accurate. With respect to accuracy, ideally the test should achieve acceptable levels of sensitivity and specificity (i.e., the test should have good accuracy to detect breast cancer when it is present and also should correctly identify as normal the large majority of women without breast cancer). The importance of accuracy is self-evident, but the comparative consequence of a false-positive or false-negative test result may also be a consideration when determining thresholds of acceptable performance. Moreover, the complements of sensitivity and specificity (i.e., false negatives and false positives) can provide insights not only into what is being achieved in a screening program but what potentially could be achieved in the screening program with improvements in accuracy or program design. Finally, the test must be affordable and acceptable to targeted individuals and referring clinicians.

Screening for breast cancer meets each of these criteria well enough, although over the years mammography screening has been the subject of considerable debate, less over the fundamental question of the efficacy of screening, but rather operational issues related to screening, such as the age to begin and end screening (20–24), screening intervals (25,26), and financial and individual costs (27–29). In particular, as evidence accumulated supporting the value of screening for both younger and older women (26,30), debates have shifted from efficacy to effectiveness, with emphasis on monetary and psychosocial costs (31), including costs associated with false-positive results, particularly the anxiety experienced by women whose mammograms are interpreted as abnormal as well as those who undergo biopsy (32), and the chance that an abnormality identified on screening will result in a diagnosis of ductal carcinoma *in situ* (DCIS) (33), which some regard as largely overdiagnosis leading to overtreatment. The combination of these costs is regarded by some as too high, or at least as too high in some age groups of women, by others as acceptable or at least unavoidable, and by others as evidence of a need to strive for better performance (34,35). In order to summarize the current evidence for the efficacy and effectiveness of breast cancer screening, each of the previously mentioned criteria will be addressed, as well as key issues related to the status of breast cancer screening in clinical practice today.

DISEASE BURDEN

By a sizable margin, breast cancer is the most common malignancy diagnosed in women in the world and also the leading cause of cancer mortality among women (36). In the United States, breast cancer also is the most common malignancy diagnosed among women and the second leading cause of death from cancer (12). In fact, breast cancer alone accounts for approximately one in four (26%) new cancer cases in women each year (11). According to current incidence and mortality estimates, in a hypothetical cohort of U.S. women, approximately one in eight will be diagnosed with invasive breast cancer in her lifetime, approximately one in seven will be diagnosed with either invasive or *in situ* disease, and 1 in 35 will die from breast cancer (12). In the United States, breast cancer is the second most common cause of person-years of life lost to cancer among women, accounting for an estimated 795,000 years of premature mortality, and an average of 19.3 years of life lost per woman dying from this disease (12). This count does not include the years of diminished quality of life and lower productivity from the time of diagnosis, which are difficult to factor into disease burden measures but nonetheless are important to acknowledge.

Some additional aspects of the descriptive epidemiology of breast cancer are relevant to understanding current screening guidelines. The age-specific incidence of breast cancer increases with age. Breast cancer is rare before age 25 years and begins to increase steadily and more rapidly until menopause; after menopause age-specific rates continue to rise, but more gradually (Chapter 20, Fig. 2). This same pattern has been observed in other countries, although the rate of increase in age-specific rates after the age of menopause is greater in Western countries than in Asian countries (Chapter 20, Fig. 2) (37). The earliest age at which breast cancer screening with mammography is recommended for average risk women is age 40 (38,39), which is based in large part on the legacy of methodologic decisions related to choosing study populations for the randomized trials. Shapiro et al. (40) included women age 40 and older after they observed that more than one third of the premature mortality

from breast cancer occurred in women diagnosed between the ages of 40 and 49. With respect to disease burden, age-specific incidence rates and years of potential life lost due to a diagnosis of disease at and after a particular age are more relevant to programmatic decisions to offer screening than age-specific mortality rates.

SOJOURN TIME AND THE INFLUENCE OF EARLY INTERVENTION

The detectable preclinical phase, also known as the *sojourn time*, is the estimated duration of time that an occult tumor can be detected before the onset of symptoms (41). In a screening program, the *lead time* is the amount of time before the expected onset of symptoms actually gained by screening (Fig. 11.1). The breast cancer sojourn time will vary somewhat in individuals due to personal characteristics and tumor histology (42), but in the context of screening programs, the analysis of the randomized controlled trial (RCT) data has shown that the mean sojourn time (MST) and mean lead time primarily vary by age. Estimates of the MST vary in the literature and with method of calculation, but a consistent finding is that the breast cancer MST is not very long and lengthens with increasing age (43,44). Estimates of the MST range between 2.0 to 2.4 years in women aged 40 to 49, 2.5 to 3.7 years in women aged 50 to 59, and 3.5 to 4.2 years in women aged 60 to 69, and approximately 4.0 to 4.1 years in women 70 to 74 (44).

Knowledge of the MST is important for determining screening intervals in a breast cancer screening program. The sojourn time defines the upper limit of the lead time that might be gained and thus should provide most individuals undergoing *regular* screening with the opportunity to detect occult disease while still localized (41). When a screening interval exceeds the MST, there is increased potential for a higher rate of interval cancers (i.e., cancers that present with symptoms in the interscreening interval, thus with poorer prognosis in that subset of incident cases). Early evidence of the influence of MST on the interval cancer rate was seen in the Swedish Two-County study, which reported nearly twice the interval cancer rate in women aged 40 to 49 compared with women aged 50 and older when both groups were screened at intervals of 24 or more months (45).

The element of staging that is of particular importance in the context of screening is tumor size. Data on long-term survival are remarkably consistent between surveillance programs, trials, and demonstration projects, with each showing

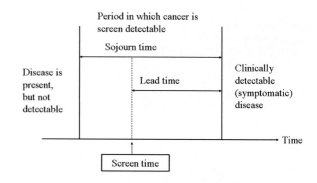

FIGURE 11.1. Schematic showing the detectable phase, sojourn time, and lead time for breast cancer.

an inverse association between tumor size and long-term survival (43,46). As tumor size increases, so too does the likelihood of metastases to the axillary lymph nodes and distant organs (5). Moreover, as Elkin et al. (47) have shown, trends in stage migration to smaller tumor sizes over a 20-year period (1975 to 1979 and 1995 to 1999) accounted for 61% and 28% of the improvement in relative survival for localized and regional disease, respectively (47).

EVALUATION OF BREAST CANCER SCREENING

Determining the efficacy of a screening test is best evaluated with a population-based RCT with a mortality end point. RCTs eliminate the potential biases in observational studies that may influence survival among screen-detected and non-screen-detected cases, most notably lead-time bias, length-bias sampling, and selection bias. Since screening will increase lead time and thus the length of survival compared with cases diagnosed after the onset of clinical symptoms, it is important to distinguish the actual improvements in survival from apparent improvements (18). As noted previously, the goal of screening is to gain lead time. If treatment before the onset of symptoms offers greater benefits, then improvements in survival should be associated with the lead time gained, and mortality should be lower in cases diagnosed by screening compared with cases diagnosed after the onset of symptoms. On the other hand, if lead time only advances the time of diagnosis and life is not extended because death occurs at the same point in the natural history of the disease among screen-detected and nonscreen-detected cases, then there is only the appearance of a greater survival duration. *Lead-time bias* occurs when increased survival is a function only of the time gained *before* the point at which diagnosis would have occurred in the absence of screening. It is important to not confuse lead time, which is the goal of screening, and lead-time bias, which is the false estimation of improved survival due simply to earlier diagnosis. *Length-bias sampling* refers to the tendency for screening to detect more slow-growing, less aggressive disease and to be less successful at detecting more aggressive, faster-growing disease. If screening selectively identifies cases at a lower risk of death, length-bias sampling can influence end results and exaggerate the benefit of screening. *Selection bias* refers to the tendency for individuals who are healthier, or more health conscious, and with a different probability of developing or dying from cancer, to participate in screening.

In a population-based RCT, these biases are eliminated, because randomization should result in equal distributions of these confounding factors in the groups invited and not invited to several rounds of screening. Lead-time bias is eliminated because disease-specific mortality in the group invited to screening is compared with mortality in the group not invited to screening at some future date after the starting point of the study, which is the same for both groups. Length-bias sampling and selection bias are eliminated because randomization into an invited and control group should ensure the same distribution of individuals with similar overall health status as well as underlying probabilities of developing cancer with faster- and slower-growing tumors. Because the analysis is based on mortality differences in the group invited to screening compared with the group receiving usual care rather than the subgroups that were and were not screened, most known and unknown biases can be eliminated or minimized. However, due to the degree of nonadherence with the randomization assignments, RCTs usually underestimate the true potential benefit of screening.

RANDOMIZED CONTROLLED TRIALS OF MAMMOGRAPHY SCREENING AND META-ANALYSES

Following are brief summaries of the major RCTs of breast cancer screening (Table 11.1). They represent study designs in which a large group of women was randomly assigned to a group that either would or would not receive an invitation to be screened for breast cancer. The first of these studies was initiated in the early 1960s, and for some RCTs follow-up still continues. Each RCT followed a somewhat different protocol, and the outcome in each has been influenced by a number of factors that have important implications for the interpretation of study results. These factors include the study methodology, the clinical protocol, participation rates in the study group (compliance), screening rates in the control group (contamination), and the number of screening rounds before an invitation to screening was extended to the control group. Other factors that likely influenced end results include the quality of the screening process, thresholds for diagnosis, follow-up mechanisms for women with an abnormality, and the quality of therapy. For these other factors, there are few insights into individual trials. It is also the case that, with the exception of the RCTs conducted in Canada (the National Breast Screening Study [NBSS-1] and [NBSS-2]) and the United Kingdom, none was specifically designed to evaluate the efficacy of breast cancer screening in age-specific subgroups (e.g., women aged 40 to 49).

Health Insurance Plan of New York

The Health Insurance Plan (HIP) study was initiated in December 1963 (3). It was the first RCT to evaluate the efficacy of breast cancer screening with clinical breast examination (CBE) and mammography. Approximately 62,000 women aged 40 to 64 were randomly assigned to two groups: The study group was offered annual CBE and two-view mammography (craniocaudal and mediolateral views) for 4 years, and the control group received usual care. Mammography was performed using general purpose x-ray machines, rather than the dedicated screen-film units that evolved in the 1970s and were used in subsequent RCTs. After 10 years from entry into the study, approximately 30% fewer breast cancer deaths were observed in the study group compared with the control group (48). At 18 years of follow-up, there were 23% fewer deaths (40). Given the primitive nature of the mammography technology used in the study, mammography and CBE contributed independently to breast cancer detection, with 33% of cases detected by mammography alone, 45% with CBE alone, and 22% with combined modalities.

Swedish Two-County Study

The largest RCT of breast cancer screening is the Swedish Two-County study, so-called because women were randomized within two counties in Sweden, study and control groups in Kopparberg (now Dalarna) and Ostergötland (49). The trial consisted of approximately 133,000 women aged 40 to 74 years, with approximately 77,000 women invited to the screening. The screening intervals differed by age, with women aged 40 to 49 invited every 24 months and women aged 50 and older invited every 33 months. The screening examination included only single-view mammography (mediolateral oblique view) using modern, dedicated mammography units. CBE was not included in the screening protocol. After 8, 11, 14, and 20 years of follow-up, approximately 30% to 32% fewer breast cancer deaths occurred in the study group invited to the screening compared with the control group (30,43,49,50).

Table 11.1	SUMMARY OF RANDOMIZED CONTROLLED TRIALS OF BREAST CANCER SCREENING							
Study (Duration)	Screening Protocol CBE (yes/no)[a]	Frequency No. Rounds	Study Population				Years of Follow-Up	RR (95% CI)
			Age	Subgroup	Invited	Control		
HIP study (1963–1969)	2 V MM CBE	Annually 4 rounds	40–64	40–49 50–64	14,432 16,568	14,701 16,299	18 18	0.77 (0.53–1.11) 0.80 (0.59–1.08)
Edinburgh (1979–1988)	1 or 2 V MM CBE (initial)	24 mos 4 rounds	45–64	45–49 50–64	11,755[b] 11,245	10,641[b] 12,359	14 10	0.83[b] (0.54–1.27) 0.85 (0.62–1.15)
Kopparberg (1977–1985)	1 V MM	24 mos 4 rounds	40–74	40–49 50–74	9,650 28,939	5,009 13,551	20 20	0.76 (0.42–1.40) 0.52 (0.39–0.70)
Ostergötland (1977–1985)	1 V MM	24 mos 4 rounds	40–74	40–49 50–74	10,240 28,229	10,411 26,830	20 20	1.06 0.65–1.76 0.81 (0.64–1.03)
Malmö (1976–1990)	1 or 2 V MM	18–24 mos 5 rounds	45–69	45–49 50–69	13,528[c] 17,134	12,242[c] 17,165	12.7 9	0.64[c] (0.45–0.89) 0.86 (0.64–1.16)
Stockholm (1981–1985)	1 V MM	28 mos 2 rounds	40–64	40–49 50–64	14,185 25,815	7,985 12,015	11.4 7	1.01 (0.51–2.02) 0.65 (0.4–1.08)
Gothenburg (1982–1988)	2 V MM	18 mos 5 rounds	39–59	39–49 50–59	11,724 9,276	14,217 16,394	12 13	0.56 (0.32–0.98) 0.91 (0.61–1.36)
CNBSS-1 (1980–1987)	2 V MM CBE	12 mos 4–5 rounds	40–49	40–49	25,214	25,216	11–16	1.07 (0.75–1.52)
CNBSS-2 (1980–1987)	2 V MM CBE	12 mos 4–5 rounds	50–59	50–59	19,711	19,694	13	1.02 (0.78–1.33)
UK Age Trial	1 V MM	12 mos	39–41 Until age 48		53,884	106,956	10	0.83 (0.66–1.04)

HIP, Health Insurance Plan of New York.
[a]1 V MM refers to one-view mammography of each breast; 2 V MM refers to two-view mammography of each breast; CBE refers to clinical breast examination.
[b]The Edinburgh trial included three separate groups of women 45–49 at entry: the first had 5,949 women in the invited group and 5,818 in the control group (with 14 years' follow-up); the next had 2,545 in the invited group and 2,482 in the control group (12 years' follow-up); and the third had 3,261 in the invited group and 2,341 in the control group (10 years' follow-up). Only the first group's results had been reported previously. New results are included for women 45–49.
[c]The Malmö trial included two groups of women aged 45–49 at entry: one group (MMST-I) received first-round screening in 1977–1978 and had 3,954 women in the invited group, 4,030 women in the control group; the second group (MMST-II) received first-round screening from 1978–1990 and had 9,574 women in the invited group, 8,212 women in the control group. Only the first group's results had been reported previously.

Malmö

In Malmö, Sweden, an RCT to evaluate the efficacy of breast cancer screening was initiated in 1976, designated the Malmö Mammographic Screening Trial I (51). Approximately 42,000 women aged 45 to 69 were randomized on the basis of birth cohort (women born between 1908 and 1932) into study and control groups. The study group was invited to receive screening at 18- to 24-month intervals for five rounds. Screening was carried out with either two-view mammography (craniocaudal and oblique views), or only the oblique view, alone depending on the breast density. CBE was not included in the screening protocol. No overall reduction in deaths was observed in the study group compared with the control group at 8 and 11 years of follow-up, although a nonsignificant 20% lower breast cancer mortality rate was observed for women aged 55 and older. Possible explanations include significant contamination in the control group, with approximately 25% of the control group

being screened with mammography during the study period, and a similar percentage of nonattenders in the study group, thus diluting the effect of an invitation to screening. Another factor that has been cited was the long period of enrollment and short period for follow-up (52). A second cohort of women born between 1933 and 1945, designated Malmö Mammographic Screening Trial II, were invited to be screened between 1978 and 1990. The most recent update reports only results of the combined cohorts for women younger than age 50 at the time of randomization. The investigators observed a statistically significant 36% reduction in breast cancer mortality among the group invited to screening (53).

Stockholm

The Stockholm RCT of breast cancer screening was initiated in 1981. Sixty thousand women aged 40 to 64 were randomized on the basis of birth date into a study group of approximately

40,000 women who would receive invitations to screening and a control group of 20,000 women who would receive usual care. The study consisted of only two rounds of screening with single-view mammography (oblique view) at a 28-month interval. CBE was not included in the screening protocol. At 7.4 years of follow-up there was a nonsignificant 29% fewer breast cancer deaths in the group invited to screening, and at 11.4 years of follow-up, the difference was 26%, also not statistically significant (54).

Gothenburg

The Gothenburg RCT of breast cancer screening was initiated in 1982 (55). Approximately 51,600 women aged 39 to 59 years were randomized into groups to be invited and not to be invited to five screening rounds. The screening interval was 18 months, and usually women were screened with two-view mammography (craniocaudal and mediolateral oblique views), unless prior screening examinations indicated such low breast density that single-view mammography was justified (approximately 30% of mammograms). CBE was not included in the screening protocol. The investigators observed a 44% statistically significant reduction in breast cancer mortality among women aged 39 to 49 after 11 years of follow-up. A nonsignificant 21% mortality difference was observed in the entire invited group (56), although statistically significant mortality reductions were observed for all ages groups with the exception of women ages 50 to 54.

Edinburgh

The Edinburgh RCT was initiated in 1979 and was an evaluation of the efficacy of CBE and mammography. The first examination utilized two-view mammography, and depending on initial findings, single-view mammography was often performed in subsequent screening rounds (57). CBE was done annually and mammography every 2 years. Eighty-seven general practices representing approximately 45,000 women were randomized into study and control groups, which later was determined to have led to unanticipated confounding by socioeconomic status. Women aged 45 to 64 in the study group received invitations to four rounds of screening with mammography. At 7 years of follow-up, a nonsignificant 17% fewer breast cancer deaths had occurred in the study group compared with the control group (58). At 14 years of follow-up, the Edinburgh investigators compared breast cancer mortality in the invited versus control group after applying a new adjustment for the socioeconomic differences between the general medical practices and observed a nonsignificant 21% mortality reduction (59). However, when breast cancer deaths after diagnosis occurring more than 3 years after the end of the study were censored, the mortality reduction increased to a statistically significant 29% fewer deaths in the group invited to screening compared with the control group. Censoring deaths occurring from cancers diagnosed more than 3 years after the end of the study was a reasonable methodologic adjustment because these breast cancers were outside of the range of the detectable preclinical phase and thus could not have been influenced by screening.

Canada: National Breast Screening Study 1

The Canadian RCT of the efficacy of breast cancer screening in women aged 40 to 49 was initiated in 1980 (60). It was designed specifically to test the efficacy of breast cancer screening in women in their 40s and consisted of four to five rounds of annual CBE and mammography, depending on time of entry into the study. After a physical examination that included CBE, women were invited to participate in the study, and volunteers were then randomized into a study group or control group.

Approximately 50,000 women participated in the study, with virtually equal numbers randomized to study and control groups. At 7 years of follow-up, approximately 36% more breast cancer deaths had occurred in the study group than in the control group. At 10.5 years of follow-up, the rate of excess mortality had declined to 14% (61), and at 11 to 16 years of follow-up, there still was 7% more breast cancer deaths in the group invited to screening compared with the group that received usual care (relative risk [RR] = 1.07, 95% confidence interval [CI] 0.75–1.52) (62).

This study and its conclusions have been controversial for a number of reasons, including study design (all study participants received a high-quality CBE before randomization), concerns about the randomization process and the quality of mammography, and the observation that there was a significant excess of patients with advanced tumors in the group invited to screening compared with the usual care group (60,63–66). More specifically, Tarone (65) has shown that the excess of patients in the NBSS-1 who had four or more positive nodes in the screening arm is statistically significant and inconsistent with the stage distribution of disease in all other trials, both in the first round and at the conclusion of the study. There is no plausible explanation for the excess of advanced tumors in the group invited to the screening, and an outside review of the randomization process reported that there was no persuasive evidence of irregularities (67). Others, however, cited numerous inconsistencies in the randomization process that had been overlooked by the reviewers (66). However, regardless of what is known and not known about the source of the imbalance of advanced cases in the group invited to screening compared with the control group, the excess of advanced cancers accounts for the higher breast cancer death rate in the screening arm, a difference that still is evident at the most recent follow-up.

Canada: National Breast Screening Study 2

The NBSS-2 was also initiated in 1980 and was a trial of the efficacy of breast cancer screening in women aged 50 to 59 (68). It was designed to test specifically the efficacy of breast cancer screening in this age group with mammography and CBE versus CBE alone and consisted of four rounds of annual examinations in the study and control groups. As with the NBSS-1, after a physical examination that included CBE, women were invited to participate in the study, and volunteers were then randomized into a study group or control group. Approximately 39,000 women participated in the study, with virtually equal numbers randomized to study and control groups. At 7 years of follow-up, there were only 3% fewer breast cancer deaths in the study group versus the control group. At 13 years of follow-up, women in the invited group had 2% more breast cancer deaths compared with women in the control group. The authors concluded that in women aged 50 to 59 years, the addition of annual mammography screening to physical examination has no impact on breast cancer mortality. The NBSS-2 has received less attention than the NBSS-1, but many of the same critiques have been cited.

United Kingdom Age Trial

In 1991, the UK Coordinating Committee on Cancer Research (UKCCCR) established a national multicenter RCT to evaluate the efficacy of screening women in their 40s (69). The trial was designed to overcome the potential bias associated with the age migration during the screening rounds when women in the upper age range of a group randomized in their 40s would reach their 50th birthday. If the benefit of mammography was truly age dependent, then it was important to confine the evaluation of the benefit to women in their 40s within that age range during the screening rounds. Thus, in the UK Age trial,

60,921 women aged 39 to 41 years were randomly assigned in the ratio 1:2 to an experimental group that would be invited to annual screening, and a control group that would receive usual care. The initial screening was with two-view mammography, with a single mediolateral oblique view in subsequent rounds (70). At a mean follow-up of 10.7 years there were 17% fewer breast cancer deaths in the group invited to screening compared with the control group (RR = 0.83, 95% CI, 0.66–1.04; p = .11). When the data were adjusted for noncompliance in the invited group, among women who actually underwent screening, a 24% mortality reduction was observed (RR = 0.76, 95% CI, 0.51–1.01) (70). The authors concluded that although neither comparison was statistically significant, the results were consistent with findings from other RCTs.

Mammography Trials, Meta-Analyses, and Age-Specific Benefits

Given the amount of experimental data from multiple RCTs, it would seem that defining screening policies and protocols would be relatively straightforward. This has not been the case. Over the years there has been considerable debate over the age to begin and end screening, the screening interval, and a small, but persistent presence of opinion that the detection of occult breast cancer is not beneficial (71).

Although the HIP study and the Swedish Two-County study provided clear and early evidence that mammography could reduce breast cancer mortality in women aged 50 and older, other trials did not provide the same level of convincing evidence. Furthermore, early evidence supporting the value of screening for women in their 40s was less clear. Although there was indirect evidence of a benefit both from the trials and observational studies, prior to 1997 no single trial had shown a statistically significant reduction in breast cancer deaths among women who were aged 40 to 49 at the time of randomization. Whereas the absence of definitive evidence of a benefit was persuasive to some that screening women under age 50 was ineffective (72), especially in light of early findings of an excess of breast cancer deaths in the NBSS-1, others were persuaded that the RCT results for women under age 50, especially the NBSS-1 findings, were anomalous (63). Supporters of screening women under age 50 argued that there was no obvious reason why breast cancer screening should be any less effective in younger versus older women, and the absence of a statistically significant benefit in the other RCTs likely was due to methodologic limitations in the design and protocols, particularly low statistical power in the trials for subgroup analysis (73).

To overcome the limits of small sample sizes for age-specific subgroups and to consider the totality of the evidence, investigators began to conduct meta-analyses of trial data, combining age-specific results from the various studies to overcome the limits of small sample sizes. There are five important observations about these meta-analyses to evaluate age-specific results. First, because of the long-standing controversy regarding screening in women aged 40 to 49, meta-analyses commonly were done separately for women in that age group and then for women aged 50 to 69. Second, as was the case with individual trials, benefits for women aged 50 and older appear early in the follow-up period, whereas they occur later for women aged 40 to 49. Third, with accumulating years of follow-up in the 40 to 49 group, the relative risk of breast cancer mortality steadily improves in the group invited to screening. Fourth, depending on inclusion and exclusion criteria and the duration of the follow-up period, meta-analysis results have shown considerable variation, but as would be expected, the magnitude of the benefit is less for all studies combined than for some individual studies. Fifth, the primary purpose of meta-analysis is to overcome the limitations of small sample sizes, and this was the initial purpose for combining the RCT data for women randomized in their 40s and to also compare age-specific outcomes for women younger and older than age 50. However, this early approach to reconcile the limitations of the trials for age-specific analyses has led to a tendency to presume that the true benefit of mammography is best estimated by combining the RCT results even when statistical power was adequate rather than carefully evaluating the RCTs on an individual basis. This pattern has led to mistaken summary conclusions, estimated from meta-analyses, that the true benefit of mammography is less than was estimated by some individual studies.

A detailed history of breast cancer meta-analyses and the still ongoing debate over age-specific benefits is not particularly informative except for those methodologic issues and conclusions that have endured over time and continue to influence the debates about breast cancer screening. In particular, these issues pertain to the longer period of follow-up before a statistically significant mortality reduction was observed in women aged 40 to 49 compared with women aged 50 or older, issues related to age at randomization versus age at breast cancer diagnosis, different inclusion and exclusion criteria for studies included in the meta-analyses, and variability in the duration of follow-up and the particular point estimates included in the analysis. Prior to 1997, meta-analyses of all RCT data showed a statistically significant reduction in breast cancer mortality of approximately 26% in women aged 50 years and older associated with an invitation to screening (74,75). These meta-analyses were carried out because some trials showed a statistically significant benefit from mammography, while others had not. The first age-specific analysis focused on women aged 40 to 49 at randomization was done by Kerlikowske et al. (75) in 1995, which showed a nonsignificant 17% mortality reduction with 10 to 12 years of follow-up. In that same year, a similar analysis by Smart et al. (76) showed a nonsignificant 16% mortality reduction in women aged 40 to 49 when all RCTs were included in the analysis, but a statistically significant 24% mortality reduction when the NBSS-1 was excluded from the analysis. The difference was due to the influence the NBSS-1 had on point estimate because of the size of the study and the unexplained excess breast cancer mortality in the group invited to screening. In 1997, with additional years of follow-up (10.5 to 18 years), and new data from the Malmö II and Gothenberg RCTs, Hendrick et al. demonstrated a statistically significant 18% mortality reduction in women aged 40 to 49 (RR = 0.82, 95% CI, 0.71–0.95) and a 24% mortality reduction in women aged 50 to 74 (RR = 0.76, 95% CI, 0.67–0.87) in an analysis that included all the RCTs (77). However, the meta-analysis for only the five Swedish trials, a more homogeneous group, showed 29% fewer breast cancer deaths in the 40 to 49 age group (RR = 0.71, 95% CI, 0.57–0.89) and a 26% mortality reduction for women aged 50 to 74 (RR = 0.74, 95% CI, 0.64–0.86). The most recent meta-analyses of the RCT data show a significant 15% reduction in breast cancer mortality with invitation to screening in women aged 40 to 49 (Fig. 11.2), a significant 22% reduction in breast cancer mortality with invitation to screening in women aged 50 to 74 (Fig. 11.3), and a significant 20% reduction in women aged 40 to 74 (not shown) (44).

Although the trial protocols shown in Table 11.1 do not provide much insight into the variability in trial results, Table 11.2 provides a clear indication of why some RCTs showed a significant mortality reduction and some did not. Table 11.2 shows the relative risks of node positive disease and of dying from breast cancer in each of the RCTs. The two measures are closely related and demonstrate that when screening reduces the incidence rate of advanced disease there will be a subsequent reduction in breast cancer deaths. Those RCTs that were not successful in reducing the incidence rate of advanced disease also did not demonstrate a reduction in breast cancer deaths. This same pattern of observing a strong association between the relative risk of being diagnosed with an advanced

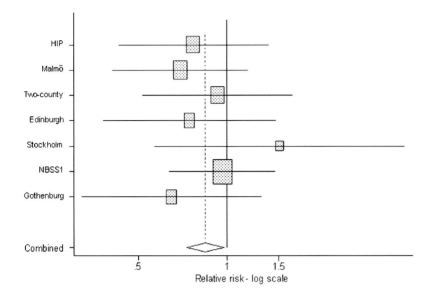

FIGURE 11.2. Breast cancer mortality results of the mammography randomized controlled trials in women aged 39 to 49 years. Overall relative risk (RR) is 0.85 (0.73, 0.98), with χ^2 for heterogeneity = 7.19 (p = .30). HIP, Health Insurance Plan of New York; NBSS, National Breast Screening Study.

breast cancer and the relative risk of dying from breast cancer in the RCTs is evident for both women aged 40 to 49 and women aged 50 or older at randomization.

One notable observation in the RCT data was that mortality differences in the 40 to 49 group appeared much later in the follow-up period compared with women aged 50 or older, and speculative reasons for these differences are a source of ongoing debate. Probably the most common argument discounting the observed benefit for women under age 50, which is a variant of the lower benefit argument, was the hypothesis that among women randomized in their 40s, it is only those women who were older than age 50 when their breast cancer was diagnosed that accounts for the appearance of lower mortality in the 40 to 49 age group (78). Because the analysis of age-specific mortality differences in trials is based on age at randomization (not age at diagnosis), at the conclusion of the invitations to screening, the group randomized in their 40s will include some women diagnosed with breast cancer *after* they have had a 50th birthday. According to this hypothesis, which has been referred to as "age migration" or "age creep," if a benefit from screening truly begins at age 50, then the observation of benefit for women in their 40s is more apparent than real, because it must be due to the benefit of diagnosing breast cancer after age 50 among women randomized in their 40s. Thus, according to this hypothesis, the observation that benefit is delayed is best explained by the time required to accumulate the age-migration cases and time required to observe a difference in mortality rates. For women randomized in their 50s, the benefit from screening was seen earlier in the follow-up period because they already were at an age when mammography is beneficial.

Whether or not there are differences in the age-specific benefit of mammography is an obviously important question, but one not easily answered with RCT data due to the fact that analyses based on age at diagnosis has a built-in bias. The purpose of screening is to diagnosis breast cancer earlier in its natural history, and thus, screening will advance the time of diagnosis to a younger age than when symptoms would be expected to appear. In an RCT, age at diagnosis will be influenced by the

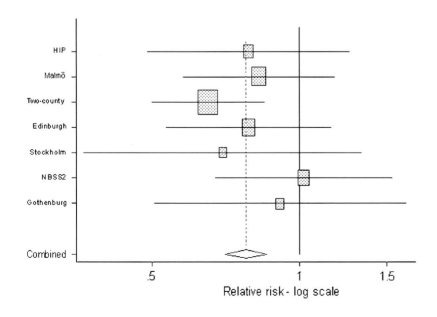

FIGURE 11.3. Breast cancer mortality results of the mammography randomized controlled trials in women aged 50 to 74 years. Overall relative risk (RR) is 0.78 (0.70, 0.85) with χ^2 for heterogeneity = 9.48 (p = .15). HIP, Health Insurance Plan of New York; NBSS, National Breast Screening Study.

Table 11.2	RELATIVE RISK OF BREAST CANCER MORTALITY AND OF INCIDENCE OF NODE POSITIVE DISEASE IN THE 8 MAMMOGRAPHY RANDOMIZED CONTROLLED TRIALS	
RCT	**RR Mortality**	**RR Node Positive**
HIP	0.78	0.85
Malmö	0.78	0.83
Two-county	0.68	0.73
Edinburgh	0.78	0.81
Stockholm	0.90	0.82
NBSS-1	0.97	1.20
NBSS-2	1.02	1.09
Gothenburg	0.79	0.80

RCT, randomized controlled trial; RR, relative risk; HIP, Health Insurance Plan of New York; NBSS, National Breast Screening Study.

study intervention (i.e., mammography) and thus is regarded as a pseudovariable (79). Analyzing RCT data by age at diagnosis introduces lead-time bias and complicates comparisons between the invited and not-invited group, especially if there is a particular age threshold that is the focus of the analysis. Although the question of age-specific benefits is important, to be properly addressed a trial would need to randomize a narrow age range of women (i.e., women aged 40 to 41) to an invited and not-invited group and follow them for the duration of interest (i.e., until age 50), thus avoiding age-creep. This is, in fact, the very design of the UK Age trial (70). Still, despite the methodologic problems introduced by examination of RCT data by age at diagnosis, the issue of age-migration or age-creep was pursued as an intuitive explanation for an observed benefit for women in their 40s.

In 1995 de Koning et al. (80) used published reports from the Swedish Two-County trial to develop a mathematical model to estimate the proportion of the observed mortality reduction in women randomized in their 40s that could be attributable to a diagnosis after age 50. They concluded that age migration in the group randomized in their 40s could account for 70% of the observed benefit and thus explain the late onset of benefit in this age group. In an accompanying editorial, Forrest and Alexander (78) acknowledged that this kind of analysis actually violates the underlying logic of RCT methodology (as described above), but if it were to be pursued, analysis of actual trial data rather than modeling would be preferable. Duffy et al. (81) subsequently evaluated actual Swedish Two-County data and compared cumulative mortality rates in the invited and control group by age at randomization and age at diagnosis. The analysis of actual trial data provided no support for the age migration hypothesis, and in fact, the relative mortality reduction among women randomized in their 40s was greater among those diagnosed before their 50th birthday than in women diagnosed after age 50. No support for this hypothesis was observed in a similar analysis of Gothenburg trial data (55). Despite lack of empirical support for the age-migration hypothesis and the fact that there are clear methodologic reasons why this sort of analysis of RCT data introduces bias, age-migration continues to be conjectured as a likely explanation of the observed benefit in younger women with increasing years of follow-up (70,82).

A clearer and more clinically intuitive explanation for the delay in benefit observed in the individual trials and meta-analyses can be seen in the effect trial screening protocols had on mortality trends when examined by tumor histology (30,83). As described above in the section Sojourn Time and the Influence of Early Intervention, the mean breast cancer sojourn time (i.e., potential lead time) is shorter in women younger than age 50 than in women older than age 50 (84). Because the majority of the trials screened women aged 40 to 49 at an interval of 24 months, faster tumor progression in women in this age group meant that they were less likely to benefit from mammography than would women aged 50 and older because the screening interval was too long.

The consequence of screening all women at the same 24-month interval becomes further evident when cumulative mortality trends in the Swedish Two-County trial are examined by age and tumor histology (30). When cumulative mortality trends are compared for ductal grade 3 tumors, a benefit begins to appear after 5 years among women aged 50 to 74 but is not evident in the follow-up period among women aged 40 to 49. These higher malignancy grade tumors are more aggressive, have a worse prognosis, and, compared with ductal grade 2, medullary and invasive lobular cancers, account for a higher proportion of breast cancer deaths that occur sooner after diagnosis. When comparing trends in the invited versus control group in the Swedish Two-County trial for ductal, grade 2, lobular, and medullary carcinoma, women aged 40 to 49 and 50 to 74 showed similar trends in cumulative mortality. Furthermore, for women both younger and older than age 50 who were diagnosed with these less aggressive cancers, the mortality benefit does not appear until after 7 to 8 years of follow-up, consistent with the observation that survival is better for these tumor types and the mortality that occurs will occur later. When examining the overall trend in cumulative mortality by age, these same trends are evident; in other words, for the groups invited to screening, a mortality benefit begins to emerge after approximately 5 years for women aged 50 to 74 and after 8 years for women aged 40 to 49. Results from Gothenburg, which screened women aged 39 to 49 at 18-month intervals, showed that the timing of the benefit in the younger age group, which appears at 6 to 8 years, is similar to that observed for women aged 50 and older (55). Additional insights into these observations come from earlier analysis of National Cancer Institute (NCI) Surveillance, Epidemiology, and End Results (SEER) data and Swedish Two-County data comparing long-term survival by tumor size, extent of disease, and histologic grade (46,85). When tumors are grouped by size, grade, and nodal involvement, there is little difference in observed survival by age.

Tabar et al. (42) have also observed that the incidence of grade 3 tumor at the time of diagnosis is higher in women younger than age 50 than in women aged 50 and older, indicating that one important difference between breast cancer in premenopausal women compared with postmenopausal women is less favorable histology. As shown in earlier and later analyses, the influence of tumor grade on survival becomes increasingly pronounced once tumors are greater than 10 mm in size (43). As a general rule, it is important to diagnose tumors at the earliest opportunity, but these data suggest that this goal is especially important in premenopausal women.

The fundamental conclusion that can be drawn from these data is that the common screening interval of 2 or more years in the trials contributed to sufficiently favorable lead times for most tumor types in women aged 50 and older and failed to provide that same benefit to the more aggressive tumors in women younger than age 50. The observation in the RCTs that some eventual benefit accrued to women aged 40 to 49 who were invited to the screening is a function of the heterogeneity of breast cancer.

These findings are further corroborated by the observed mortality reductions in premenopausal women in the Malmö and Gothenberg RCTs (53,55,56), as well as more recent observational studies (86,87) and the evaluation of service screening (88–90).

The evolution of our understanding of the interplay between the MST, the screening interval, and the ability to detect breast cancer at a favorable stage is one of the most fundamental lessons from the RCTs. Tabar et al. (45) reported that interval cancer rates were twice as high in the 40 to 49 age group compared with the 50 to 69 age group, an early indication that a 2-year screening interval was less effective in detecting occult breast cancer in women younger than age 50. If the screening interval is greater than the mean sojourn time, the potential for the program to reduce the rate of advanced disease is diminished because a higher proportion of cancers will progress undetected within the screening interval to the point at which they become clinically evident and appear as interval cancers. In Gothenburg, which screened women aged 40 to 49 every 18 months and showed a 44% reduction in breast cancer mortality, the proportional interval cancer incidence was only 18% in the first 12 months after a negative screen but increased to more than 50% in the period from 12 to 18 months (55). According to Sickles (91), in the University of California at San Francisco screening program, interval cancer rates for women aged 40 to 49 with annual screening are approximately equivalent to interval cancer rates in women aged 50 years and older who are screened every 2 years. Further evidence related to age-specific benefits will be discussed in the next section.

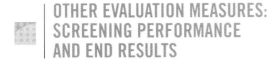

OTHER EVALUATION MEASURES: SCREENING PERFORMANCE AND END RESULTS

Sensitivity, Specificity, and Positive Predictive Value

The interpretation of a screening examination ultimately falls into one of two categories: normal or abnormal. These judgments, in turn, ultimately are divided among four categories based on either the determination or estimation of the underlying reality of having or not having breast cancer at the time of screening. At the time of screening, a normal interpretation may be a *true negative* or a *false negative*. A positive interpretation may be a *true positive* or a *false positive*. By convention, each of these initial findings is given a summary determination on the basis of the patient's status at 1 year after the screening examination and are defined as follows: true positive (TP)—cancer diagnosed within 1 year after biopsy recommendation based on an abnormal mammogram; true negative (TN)—no known cancer diagnosed within 1 year of a normal mammogram; false negative (FN)—cancer diagnosed within 1 year of a normal mammogram; false positive (FP)—no known cancer diagnosed within 1 year of an abnormal mammogram (92). There are three definitions of false positives: FP1 refers to a case recalled for additional imaging evaluation of an abnormal finding on a screening mammogram in which no cancer was found within 1 year or a recalled case was not shown to be malignant within 1 year. The additional imaging may take place at the same time as the screening examination or at a later date. FP2 refers to a case in which no known cancer was diagnosed within 1 year after an abnormal mammogram and recommendation for biopsy or surgical consultation. This definition is based on the recommendation for biopsy alone—a biopsy may or may not be done. FP3 refers to a case in which benign disease is found at biopsy within 1 year after an abnormal mammogram and biopsy. This last definition of false positive is similar to the definition proposed by the American College of Radiology (ACR) breast imaging reporting and data system, described later in the section on Quality Assurance (93).

These summary categories are the basic elements for measuring the performance of screening programs, and adherence to these definitions ensures that comparisons can be made across screening programs. Because the large majority of women who undergo mammography examinations do not have breast cancer, nearly all normal interpretations (true negatives) are accurate. True positives are obviously measured in the near term by biopsy results revealing invasive or *in situ* disease. False negatives or false positives are based on the assumption that cancer would have been detected, or was not present, on the basis of the presence or absence of histologic confirmation of disease within 1 or 2 years, depending on the screening interval. Variability in these definitions can have a significant influence on these summary measures. For example, a breast cancer detected due to the presence of symptoms within 1 year of the last normal mammogram would be regarded as an interval cancer, the previous mammogram would be redefined as a false negative, and each would be a measure of a failure of the screening program to detect a breast cancer. However, if an asymptomatic woman receives a follow-up screening mammogram close to, but before the end of, the 1- or 2-year duration since the last normal mammogram, to treat this finding as an interval cancer and to redefine the previous examination as a false negative is inconsistent with the quality assurance purpose of these measurements. Moreover, extending the duration of follow-up for several months beyond the interval also introduces measurement variability into these standard indicators and complicates comparisons across programs or imaging technologies.

Sensitivity

Sensitivity is a measure of the probability of detecting breast cancer when it is truly present. It is the proportion of patients found to have breast cancer within 1 year of screening who were identified as having an abnormality at the time of screening (sensitivity = TP/[TP + FN]). Another method of measuring sensitivity has been outlined by Day and Walter (94) and is based on the ratio of observed (invited group) to expected (control group) rates after omitting results from the first screening round as a basis for estimating the proportion of cases that would be expected to appear as clinical cancers. *Specificity* is the probability of correctly identifying a patient as normal when no cancer exists and is the proportion of all patients not found to have breast cancer within 1 year of screening who had a normal interpretation at the time of screening (specificity = TN/[TN + FP]). *Positive predictive value* (PPV) of a screening test is the proportion of all positive screening cases that result in a diagnosis of cancer and varies according to the criteria for a false-positive interpretation outlined above (PPV1–3 = TP/TP + FP1–3). According to the Agency for Health Care Research and Quality (AHRQ), approximate targets for PPV1 are 5% to 10%, whereas for PPV2 or PPV3 the target is 25% to 40% (92).

Sensitivity estimates derived from the trials and in other settings have shown that the sensitivity of mammography was higher in women aged 50 and older than in women aged 40 to 49 (84,95,96). For women in their 40s, sensitivity ranged from 53% to 81%, whereas for women who were 50 and older it ranged from 73% to 88% (72). These sensitivity estimates are based on a variety of screening protocols and screening intervals, of which the latter is likely to be the major factor in observed age group differences. When Swedish Two-County data are adjusted for the screening interval and the estimated age-specific mean sojourn time, the magnitude of these differences diminishes, with sensitivity estimated to be 86% for women aged 40 to 49 and approximately 93% for women aged 50 to 59 (97). Furthermore, service screening programs offer a glimpse into current estimates of sensitivity when screening intervals are actually tailored to the estimated sojourn time. In a screening program in Albuquerque, New Mexico, representing more than 100,000 women, sensitivity was 85.3% for women

Table 11.3	PERFORMANCE MEASURES FOR 3,603,832 SCREENING MAMMOGRAM EXAMINATIONS[a] FROM 1996 TO 2006			
	Performance Measures			
Age	Sensitivity (%)[b]	Specificity (%)[c]	PPV1 (%)	Recall Rate (%)[d]
40–44	70.8	89.8	1.5	10.3
45–49	74.3	89.8	2.3	10.3
50–54	78.4	90.9	3.3	9.2
55–59	81.6	91.5	4.6	8.8
60–64	80.0	91.9	5.4	8.4
65–69	82.5	92.4	6.3	8.0
70–74	82.9	93.1	7.9	7.3
75–89	84.5	93.6	9.8	6.9
Total	**80.2**	**91.4**	**4.3**	**8.9**

[a]Mammography examinations indicated by the radiologist to be for screening with bilateral views done and no other mammogram within the past 9 months among women without breast implants or a prior breast cancer diagnosis.
[b]The percentage of examinations with a positive interpretation (Breast Imaging Reporting and Data System [BI-RADS] category 0, 3 with recommendation for immediate follow-up, 4, or 5), with a tissue diagnosis of ductal carcinoma *in situ* (DCIS) or invasive cancer within 1 year and before the next screening mammography examination.
[c]The percentage of examinations with a negative interpretation (BI-RADS category 1, 2, or 3 with no recommendation for immediate follow-up), without a tissue diagnosis of cancer within one year or before the next screening examination, whichever occurs earlier.
[d]Recall rate equals the percentage of examinations with a positive interpretation (BI-RADS category 0, 3 with recommendation for immediate follow-up, 4, or 5).
From National Cancer Institute–funded Breast Cancer Surveillance Consortium co-operative agreement (U01CA63740 UC, U01CA86082, U01CA63736, U01CA70013, U01CA69976, U01CA63731, U01CA70040). Performance measures for 3,603,832 screening mammography examinations from 1996 to 2006 by age. Rockville, MD: National Cancer Institute, 2008.

aged 40 to 49 and 87.7% for women aged 50 and older (98). In the University of California at San Francisco screening program, the sensitivity was 86.7% for women aged 40 to 49 and 93.6% for women aged 50 to 59 (91). In each of these instances, a difference in the sensitivity of mammography in younger versus older women is still seen, but the data show that the sensitivity of the test in the two age groups is more similar than different when screening intervals reflect the underlying mean sojourn time, and that the effectiveness of screening gradually improves with increasing age (22). Performance data from the NCI's Breast Cancer Surveillance Consortium showing the performance measures for 3.6 million screening mammography examinations from 1996 to 2006 by age are shown in Table 11.3 (99).

A number of factors can influence sensitivity, including the screening interval, quality control factors, the interpretive skill of the reader, and host factors. The influence of age on sensitivity has already been discussed, both in terms of tumor growth rates and breast density. Breast density has a particularly strong influence on mammographic sensitivity.

There is a rich and growing literature on the influence of breast density on breast cancer risk and mammography performance. Boyd et al. (100) carried out three nested case-control studies of screened populations in Canada and observed both an increased risk of breast cancer associated with extensive breast density, but also a greater likelihood of breast cancer detection less than 12 months after the last normal mammogram. This association was particularly pronounced for women younger than the median study age of 56 years. In this age group, 26% of all breast cancers and half of cancers detected less than 12 months after the last normal mammogram were attributable to breast density of 50% or more.

Although breast density typically is greater in younger women than older women, hormone therapy is associated with increased density and reduced mammographic sensitivity in some older women (101,102). Mammographic density declines with increasing age, but at every age after the menopause, current postmenopausal hormone (PMH) users have greater mammographic breast density than former PHM users, which have greater mammographic breast density than never users

(Fig. 11.4) (102). Rosenberg et al. (103) examined data from the statewide tumor registry in New Mexico to determine the influence of hormone therapy on the sensitivity of mammography in women 65 years or older. Sensitivity was comparable in women without dense breasts regardless of whether the women used hormone therapy or not (83% vs. 86%). However, for women 65 or older with dense breasts, the sensitivity of mammography was lower among women taking hormone therapy compared with women not on hormone therapy (64% vs. 84%). Lower sensitivity in women taking hormone therapy also has been observed by others (104,105).

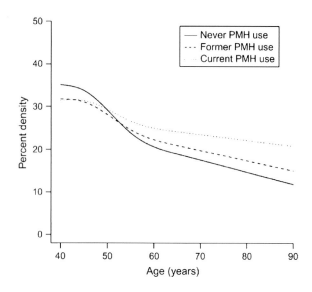

FIGURE 11.4. Longitudinal patterns of mammographic density by postmenopausal hormone (PMH) use and age among postmenopausal women, Minnesota Breast Cancer Family cohort, 1990 to 2003. (From Kelemen LE, Pankratz VS, Sellers TA, et al. Age-specific trends in mammographic density: the Minnesota Breast Cancer Family Study. *Am J Epidemiol* 2008;167: [9] 1027–1036, with permission.)

Although data indicate an influence of hormone therapy on breast density, not all women are affected. An analysis that included Dutch and United Kingdom hormone therapy users and never-users from the European Prospective Investigation into Cancer and Nutrition (EPIC) cohorts, mammograms before and during hormone therapy use and during a comparable period for never-users were assessed for changes in breast density. A mean decline in percentage of density was greater in never-users (7.3%) than in estrogen therapy only users (6.4%) and in combination hormone therapy users (3.5%), suggesting that hormone therapy use slows the normal process of change with increasing age from the dense pattern to the fatty pattern (106). The lack of sufficient evidence about the underlying mechanisms and influence on hormone therapy on breast density limits the ability to make specific recommendation regarding alternative screening strategies for older women who take hormone therapy or who have radiographically dense breasts. However, there are ongoing investigations attempting to improve screening performance with multimodal imaging in women with significant breast density.

Specificity

Specificity is also an important measure of the effectiveness of a screening program, and even small differences in program specificity can mean a large difference in program effectiveness and costs. Data from the NCI's Breast Cancer Surveillance Consortium, representing more than 3 million mammograms in hundreds of breast imaging facilities across the United States provide a good picture of comparative mammographic specificity by age (Table 11.3) (99). As is the case with sensitivity, the false-positive rate steadily improves with increasing age, which also is the case for the PPV. Because the prevalence of disease is lower in women in their 40s, the yield of cancers from mammography naturally is lower. Thus, although the rate of false-positive results based on additional mammographic views and referral for biopsy is very similar in younger and older women, the cost-effectiveness of screening improves with increasing age (26).

Although test specificity commonly receives less scrutiny than sensitivity, it is nonetheless an important measure because false-positive tests have both human and financial costs. A recent comparison of false-positive rates in the United Kingdom and the United States showed rates nearly twice as high in the United States compared with the United Kingdom (107). Although the authors were not able to directly measure factors associated with the difference, they speculate that the more organized elements of breast cancer screening in the United Kingdom (minimum volume requirements, structured feedback, double reading) and lack of malpractice concerns contribute to lower rates of false positives. An additional factor contributing to lower false-positive rates in the United Kingdom is likely to be regular attendance at the same facility. As Sickles (108) and Roelofs et al. (109) have shown, the recall rate of mammography is highly dependent on the ability to review films from previous examinations, which can reduce the callback rate by approximately 50%.

The extent of psychological and physical harms associated with false-positive mammography and, in particular, whether or not harms are lasting and have consequences for psychological well-being and subsequent screening have been the focus of a number of investigations (32). In general, the evidence suggests that some women experience anxiety related to screening and a greater percentage experience anxiety related to false-positive results. However, for most women psychological distress does not endure and does not have lasting consequences, either on stress or the likelihood of subsequent screening (110,111). A study by Schwartz et al. (31) revealed that women are aware of the likelihood of a false-positive result, accept false-positive results as a part of screening, and do not regard false positives as an important harm in the context of the underlying goal of early breast cancer detection (31).

As use of mammography has increased, concerns have been raised about detection, and overtreatment of DCIS (82,112). At this time, the majority of detected DCIS occur as a result of identification of small lesions on a mammogram that are perceived to be important, and it is not possible through image evaluation to either distinguish DCIS from invasive breast cancer or progressive DCIS from nonprogressive DCIS. The concern that some proportion of DCIS is nonprogressive has to be considered in the context of estimates that indicate that a substantial portion of DCIS is progressive. The actual fraction is unknown, and historical estimates from case series may not be generalizable to cases identified through mammographic screening (113). In one series, invasive breast cancer developed in over half of women with low-grade DCIS lesions identified on biopsy who were not treated (114). Furthermore, incomplete excision of DCIS or failure to excise DCIS associated with an invasive cancer is a predictor of local failure (115,116). In a recent evaluation of RCT and service screening data, Yen et al. (117) estimated the proportion of DCIS that was nonprogressive, and the proportion was higher on the first screening mammogram (37%) compared with subsequent screening mammograms (4%). These estimates indicated that overdiagnosis of DCIS does exist, but that it is a relatively small problem and confined mostly to the prevalent screen. According to Yen et al., a woman attending a prevalent screen is 19 times more likely to be diagnosed with a progressive DCIS lesion or invasive lesion compared with nonprogressive DCIS, and on subsequent screens she is 166 times more likely to be diagnosed with a progressive invasive or DCIS lesion than a nonprogressive lesion.

Breast Cancer Mortality versus All-Cause Mortality

Some investigators have asserted that studies of the efficacy of mammography should not focus on breast cancer mortality, but rather on all-cause mortality (118,119). There is concern that errors in the assignment of cause of death in an RCT are biased in favor of the group invited to screening. To avoid this bias, most RCTs guard against assignment error by having cause-of-death committees review deaths without knowledge of assignment to the intervention or control group. Further, although some diseases may pose challenges for determining underlying cause of death, breast cancer is not among them, so while the potential for error exists, it is not very large and certainly does not approach the level of a competing factor in the evaluation of the underlying cause of death (120). The second source of alleged bias with breast cancer mortality as an end point is the bias that would arise if there was a failure to identify deaths that occur from some other cause as a result of diagnosis and treatment of breast cancer (i.e., a cardiovascular death resulting from damage to the heart from radiation treatment for a nonlife threatening breast cancer detected by screening) (121). This bias would be more difficult to counteract because it depends on *a priori* knowledge of the presence or absence of collateral risk.

It is proper that the evaluation of a disease control intervention should consider not only whether deaths from the disease of interest are reduced, but also whether there were harms associated with the intervention that might themselves result in deaths. If a reduction in the disease-specific mortality rate is matched by an increase in the mortality rate from another cause due to diagnostic and therapeutic interventions, then there is an unfavorable balance of benefit to harm. However, critics of analyses of disease-specific mortality argue that the proper end point comparison is between the all-cause mortality rate in the entire experimental group and the control group, and this criticism has been applied to the evaluations of breast cancer screening studies. This comparison is illogical for several reasons. First, the ability to measure a statistically significant difference in all-cause mortality in an RCT would require trial sizes of more than a million women in each arm (122). Second, and more important, mammography cannot be expected to affect deaths in women who do not develop breast cancer. Although it is reasonable to compare the breast cancer mortality rate in the invited and control group, the proper comparison for differences in all-cause mortality is among the breast cancer cases in each group. Not only has it been demonstrated that there is a reduced risk of dying from breast cancer associated with an invitation to screening (RR = 0.69, 95% CI, 0.50–0.80), but also among women diagnosed with breast cancer, there is a reduced risk of dying from all causes associated with an invitation to screening (RR = 0.87, 95% CI, 0.78–0.99) (123). The fact that a statistically significant reduction in breast cancer mortality *and* a statistically significant reduction in all-cause mortality are evident is because mammography is an effective screening test, and because breast cancer is a leading cause of death in women aged 40 to 70. If the risk of dying from any of the leading causes of death in that age interval can be significantly reduced, then there should be a reduction in the risk of dying from "all causes," which indeed occurs as described above. Because breast cancer is a leading cause of premature mortality (12), a breast cancer death avoided through early detection, especially in younger women, results in a significant reduction in the risk of dying prematurely from all causes combined, since it is among the dominant causes of premature death.

The Number Needed to Screen to Prevent One Breast Cancer Death

The number needed to screen (NNS) is an epidemiological measure that is generally described as an indicator of the effectiveness of an intervention (124). It is similar to the number needed to treat (NNT), in that it is a measure of the number of individuals that need to be screened once or over a particular duration to prevent one adverse outcome, usually a death.

The NNS is a metric that increasingly is used as a comparative measure, as described above, but it also has been suggested as a key point of information for patient-shared decision making (26,125). Although estimating the NNS seems relatively straightforward, it has commonly been overestimated because several key measurement considerations have been overlooked. For example, Humphrey et al. (26) estimated the NNS to save one life based on meta-analysis data from an average of 14 years of follow-up in the breast cancer screening trials and arrived at an estimate of 1,224 women. However, since RCT data were used, their estimate actually is based on the "number needed to invite" rather than the NNS since mortality reductions in the RCTs are based on an intention to treat analysis (i.e., they are based on mortality differences between an invited and control group, not a screened and unscreened group). Another important consideration is that when expressing the NNS over a period of time, the time period should only include the period of active screening, not including the follow-up period. Tabar et al. (49,126) used Swedish Two-County data, with seven screening rounds and 20 years of follow-up, to estimate the NNS. Comparing the number of women screened during three screening rounds over 7 years and then the duration of follow-up, they estimated that for every 1,000 women screened, 2.15 breast cancer deaths were prevented, or put another way, the NNS over an average of three screening rounds to save one life was 465 (126). The suggestion from other estimates that 1,000 women would need to be screened annually for 10 years to prevent one death from breast cancer is inaccurate, since RCT point estimates typically derive from

studies of biennial screening for fewer than 10 rounds, leaving a woman to perhaps believe mistakenly that annual screening over a 10-year period will only provide her with a 1 in 1,000 chance of averting a premature death from breast cancer. The estimate from Tabar et al. (126) is closer to 1 in 350, which is more consistent with the underlying lifetime risk and the demonstrated value of screening.

 ## THE EVALUTION OF SERVICE SCREENING

The inherent limitations of the RCTs to estimate the benefits associated with screening with mammography and the desire to measure the contribution of modern mammography to reduce breast cancer mortality have resulted in new investigations focused on evaluating the impact of screening in the community setting, referred to as *service screening*. The evaluation of service screening can focus on both mortality reductions in the entire population, which somewhat simulates an intention to treat analysis, but also mortality reductions in women who actually attend community screening programs, which is a more relevant estimate of benefit to use to promote screening, and as noted above, to estimate the NNS. The evaluation of service screening also can be applied to estimate differences in mortality over time due to screening compared with improvements in therapy and increased awareness (88), although establishing the relative contribution of screening and non-screening factors is complex and can only be indirectly estimated.

There are a number of methodological issues that must be heeded in the evaluation of service screening, including:

1. Correct identification of when screening is initiated in a population;
2. Adjustment for the take-up period (i.e., the fact that it may take several years to invite an entire population to screening after the initiation of new policy);
3. Adjustment for the proportion of the population that may already be undergoing screening in an opportunistic setting;
4. The fact that a proportion of new breast cancer cases will be advanced at the time of the first mammogram; and
5. The need to distinguish screened and unscreened cohorts among the deaths from breast cancer after the onset of the program (88).

This last point is especially important, since failure to consider exposure to screening has led to erroneous conclusions about the lack of an influence of screening on breast cancer mortality after the introduction of screening (127). To illustrate, in a hypothetical 10-year period after the introduction of screening, a period when visible reductions in breast cancer mortality are anticipated, approximately half or more of the deaths from breast cancer will occur in women whose cancers will have been diagnosed before the beginning of that period (128).

There are several methodologies that can be applied to the evaluation of service screening programs. These include: (a) comparisons of the breast cancer mortality trends before and after screening has been introduced, (b) case control studies, and (c) contemporaneous comparisons of invited with not-yet-invited women during the early years of a screening program.

Gabe and Duffy (129) examined mammography service screening studies published between 1990 and 2004 that evaluated trends in breast cancer mortality associated with screening, or that compared trends in breast cancer mortality in screened and unscreened groups. Thirty-eight nonrandomized studies were identified, including 15 studies that attempted to measure time/trend descriptive epidemiologic results, eight cohort studies, seven case-control studies, four case series, and four non-RCT comparison studies. There was a range of estimated benefits observed in the service screening programs associated with (a) an invitation to screening, which simulates a trial, and (b) actual exposure to screening, and in some studies the benefits have significantly exceeded the results from the RCTs. Cohort study breast cancer mortality reductions associated with an invitation to screening ranged from 8% to 41%, while mortality reductions associated with actual exposure to screening ranged from 37% to 44%. Results from case-control studies observed mortality reductions associated with exposure to screening ranging from 25% to 58%. In the non-RCT comparative studies, breast cancer mortality reductions associated with an invitation to screening ranged from 6% to 27%, while mortality reductions associated with actual exposure to screening ranged from 33% to 43%. A wider range of breast cancer mortality reductions was observed in cohort studies and non-RCT comparative studies depending on whether the analysis was based on an invitation to screening or actual exposure to screening.

These data reveal a wide range of estimates of breast cancer mortality reductions associated with service screening, just as a wide range of mortality reductions was observed in the RCTs. These differences are expected and likely due to:

1. The greater logistical challenge of delivering screening to the population compared with a smaller study population;
2. Differences between a study population and the larger population in the underlying risk of disease and likelihood of adherence to screening protocols;
3. The wider range of experience and skills among a larger number of professionals delivering screening services;
4. Improvements in technology, technique, protocol, including the screening interval, and quality assurance over time; and
5. The duration that the screening program has been in place (129).

Indeed, long-term evaluation of the impact of breast cancer screening on population cause-specific mortality reveals that the duration of the program has a major influence on the magnitude of the benefit. In one analysis of service screening, those programs that had been in place the longest demonstrated the greatest reductions in the risk of dying from breast cancer compared with the prescreening period (130).

With respect to comparisons with a nonexposed group, or in comparisons between prescreening versus postscreening periods, advances in therapy and increased awareness and responsiveness to breast symptoms can also affect end results (88). Duffy et al. (128) compared breast cancer mortality in the prescreening and postscreening periods among women aged 40 to 69 in six counties and aged 50 to 69 in a seventh county. Adjusting for selection bias, they observed a 44% breast cancer mortality reduction in women who underwent screening, and a 39% breast cancer mortality reduction in the population associated with the policy of offering screening to the population. Because the authors were able to distinguish between screened and unscreened cohorts, they estimated that about two thirds of the observed mortality reductions were attributable to screening, with the remainder due to improvements in therapy and increased awareness. An analysis of service screening in the two counties where the Swedish Two-County trial took place (Dalarna and Ostergötland) compared the mortality rates from breast cancer in the 20 years following the introduction of screening with the corresponding rates in the 20 years preceding the introduction (i.e., prescreening and screening epochs) (89). Among women aged 40 to 69 exposed to screening, there was a statistically significant reduction (44%; RR = 0.56, 95% CI, 0.49–0.64) in mortality in the screening epoch compared to the prescreening epoch, and a 16% (RR = 0.84, 95% CI, 0.71–0.99) mortality reduction that was independent of screening (i.e., in women not exposed to screening). Among women aged 40 to 49 at the time of diag-

nosis, the investigators observed a statistically significant reduction (48%; RR = 0.52, 95% CI, 0.4–0.67) in breast cancer mortality among women exposed to screening, and a nonsignificant 19% reduction in women who were not screened. Several points are worth noting. First, these observations are based on mortality rates from incident tumors in the overall population, rather than case fatality rates. Second, the results are based on age at diagnosis and thus provide further evidence against the hypothesis that age-creep in the RCTs explains any apparent benefit from screening in premenopausal women. Third, in Sweden, women aged 40 to 54 are invited to screening every 18 months, and women aged 55 and older are invited every 24 months, based on the estimated MST. These data provide further confirmation that screening is not only beneficial in women aged 40 to 49, but is associated with the same mortality reduction observed in older women when the screening interval is tailored to the MST.

More extensive evaluations of service screening data have been conducted by the Swedish Organized Service Screening Evaluation Group (SOSSEG), which is a team of researchers representing local Swedish investigators and officials, but also researchers from the United States, United Kingdom, and Taiwan (130–132). Breast cancer mortality data from 13 areas in Sweden were evaluated in both the prescreening and screening epochs. The size of the total female population in the 13 areas was similar during the prescreening epoch (n~542,187) and in the screening epoch (n~566,423). Attendance rates ranged from 70% to 90%, and recall rates ranged from 2% to 5%. Including both the prescreening epoch and screening epoch, there were 6,231 breast cancer deaths available for analysis, including 4,778 deaths that were incidence-based deaths in the two epochs, 2,736 breast cancer deaths in the prescreening epoch from tumors diagnosed in that epoch, and 2,042 breast cancer deaths from tumors diagnosed in the screening epoch. For all 13 areas combined, and after adjustment for selection bias, there was a 43% reduction in incidence-based breast cancer mortality among women exposed to screening in the screening epoch compared with women in the prescreening epoch (Fig. 11.5). In the individual areas, the breast cancer mortality reductions ranged from 36% to 54%, and the number needed to screen to save one life varied from 188 (with 22 years of follow-up) to 862 (with 11 years of follow-up) (130). The

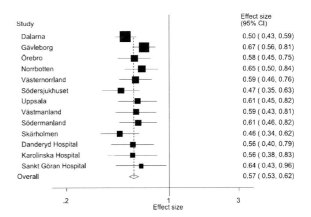

FIGURE 11.5. Relative risk of incidence-based breast cancer mortality for screened women in the screening epoch compared with the prescreening epoch, adjusted for self-selection bias. CI, confidence interval. (From Swedish Organized Service Screening Evaluation Group. Reduction in breast cancer mortality from organized service screening with mammography: 1. Further confirmation with extended data. *Cancer Epidemiol Biomarkers Prev* 2006;15[1]:45–51, with permission.)

SOSSEG has also evaluated the effect of service screening on the stage of presentation of breast cancers in Sweden (132). As noted earlier, a reduction in the incidence rate of advanced disease is a powerful surrogate for eventual breast cancer mortality reductions. Based on a total of 10,177,113 person-years of observation and 23,092 breast cancers, among women aged 40 to 49 exposed to screening, there was a significant 45% reduction in the risk of being diagnosed with a tumor greater than 2 cm in size compared with tumor sizes in the prescreening epoch (RR = 0.55, 95% CI, 0.46–0.66), and among women aged 50 to 69, a 33% reduction in being diagnosed with a tumor greater than 2 cm in size in the population exposed to screening compared with the population in the prescreening epoch (RR = 0.67, 95% CI, 0.62–0.72) (132). Figures 11.6 (A–C) and 11.7 (A–C) show the cumulative incidence of (A) lymph node positive disease, (B) tumors more than 2 cm, and (C) tumors stage II or worse by age group for the prescreening epoch, which varied by county from 1977 to 1993, and the population exposed and not exposed to screening in the screening epoch. As can been seen, for both women aged 40 to 49 and 50 to 69, exposure to screening is associated with a significantly lower rate of each tumor characteristic associated with advanced disease and worse prognosis (132).

The Screening Mammography Program of British Columbia (SMPBC) was established in 1988 and provides mammography to women aged 40 to 49 annually, and women aged 50 years and older every 2 years. Coldman et al. (90) evaluated outcomes in SMPBC participants (at least one mammogram) and compared them with expected incidence and survival rates among British Columbian women who had not participated in the program. During the period of evaluation (1988 to 2003), 598,690 women underwent 2,196,441 mammograms (average 3.7 screening examinations per woman). During the study period, 14,247 SMPBC participants were diagnosed with invasive breast cancer and 19,913 invasive breast cancers were diagnosed in nonparticipants. Expected incidence and survival rates were derived from nonparticipants. To address the issue of age-migration in women aged 40 to 49, both observed and expected rates also were recalculated among the group of women who had at least one mammogram in the program before age 50 to exclude any cases diagnosed after age 50. A breast cancer mortality ratio was calculated as the ratio of observed to expected mortality. The results for all ages showed a mortality ratio of 0.60 (95% CI, 0.55–0.65; *p* <.0001), and for women aged 40–49, the mortality ratio was 0.61 (95% CI, 0.52–0.71), and 0.63 (95% CI, 0.52–0.77) when cases diagnosed after age 50 were censored. There was no significant difference between the mortality ratios for women aged 40 to 49 versus 50 or older.

Insofar as additional RCTs of breast cancer screening are unlikely and would certainly strain ethical considerations if women were randomized to an unexposed group, the evaluation of service screening represents an important new development in measuring the impact of screening on breast cancer mortality. These data show that modern, high-quality, high-attendance, organized breast cancer screening can achieve breast cancer mortality reductions equal to or greater than those observed in the randomized trials. To the extent that these studies can address methodological challenges and reliably estimate the mortality reduction associated with exposure to screening, it is no longer appropriate to cite estimates of the benefit of mammography from analyses based on intention to treat comparisons. Although RCTs were necessary to evaluate the efficacy of mammography, they underestimate the benefit of mammography to women who attend screening, and especially underestimate the benefit in some age-specific groups.

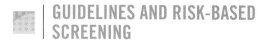

GUIDELINES AND RISK-BASED SCREENING

Mammography

By convention, in the United States most guidelines for breast cancer screening in average risk women recommend that women begin screening at age 40 (Table 11.4) (38,133). Guidelines that recommend screening beginning at age 50 are older have not recently been updated or are limited to the older trial evidence and the legacy of ideological debates over cost-effectiveness and the balance of benefits to harms (24). Beginning breast cancer screening exactly at age 40 is admittedly arbitrary. The American Cancer Society (134) and the U.S. Preventive Services Task Force (USPSTF) (38) both recommend that women begin regular screening mammography at age 40. The ACS recommends annual mammography beginning at age 40, whereas the USPSTF recommends mammography every 1 to 2 years. The difference in the recommendations primarily is due to the ACS's greater reliance on inferential evidence showing shorter MST's in women under age 50 compared with women age 50 and older, and the higher interval cancer rate in women under age 50 in the 12- to 24-month period. The USPSTF's recommendations are based on meta-analyses of RCT data that include trials that screened women at 12- and 24-month intervals. Since no trial has compared a 12- versus 24-month interval, no direct experimental evidence exists to measure the incremental benefit of a 12- versus 24-month screening interval for women under age 50.

Some have questioned the value of screening mammography in women older than age 70, based on both lack of evidence from RCTs (only one trial included women over the age of 70) and lower cost-effectiveness (134). The USPSTF found little evidence to question the effectiveness of breast cancer screening in women older than age 70, and apart from longer MSTs and slower rates of progression, there are few supporting data to indicate that breast cancer in older women is more likely to be indolent (26). Breast cancer is an important health problem in women over age 70, and although age-specific incidence declines after age 75 to 79, it never declines to a rate less than the rate in women aged 60 to 64 (359 per 10^5) (12). In the United States, breast cancer mortality rates continue to rise with increasing age, and the single largest age-specific increase occurs between the age group 80 to 84 versus 85 or older (137 vs. 185 per 10^5) (12). Badgwell et al. (134) utilized the linked SEER-Medicare database to evaluate the screening histories, stage at diagnosis, and survival of 12,358 women 80 years of age or less who had been diagnosed with breast cancer between 1996 and 2002. Patients were 37% less likely to present with late-stage cancer for each mammogram obtained during the 5-year period preceding diagnosis of breast cancer (odds ratio [OR] = 0.63, 95% CI, 0.63–0.67). Breast cancer–specific 5-year survival was 94% among regular users of mammography compared with 82% among nonusers. Less than half of the women in the study had three or more mammograms in the 5 years prior to diagnosis with breast cancer, and 22% had no screening history, although it is likely that some healthy screenee bias is occurring. Of greater concern is recent evidence that older women at higher risk of breast cancer due to a prior diagnosis of breast cancer are underutilizing surveillance mammography. Field et al. (136) examined the screening histories of 1,762 women aged 65 or older at the time of a diagnosis of earlier stage (I or II) breast cancer and found that annual mammography declined from year 1 (82%) to year 4 (65%), and the odds of routine surveillance were considerably higher for women who had routine visits to a surgeon or oncologist rather

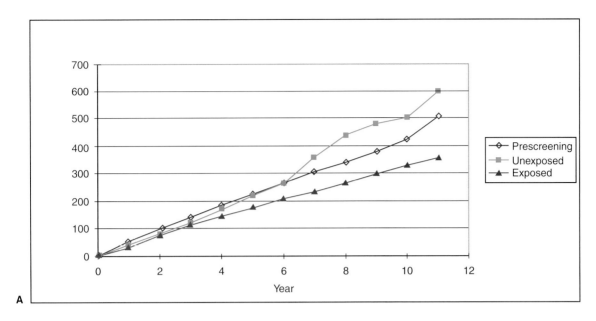

A

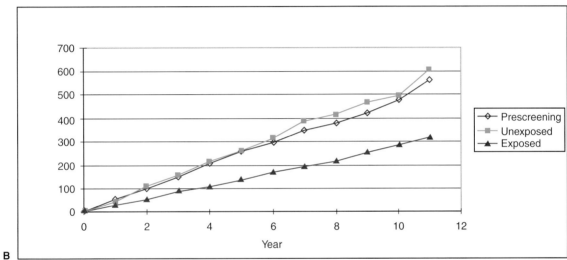

B

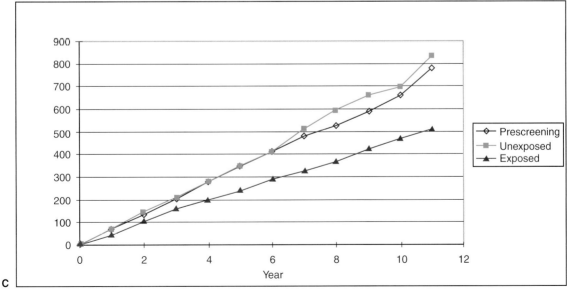

C

FIGURE 11.6. **A:** Cumulative incidence of lymph node positive disease, ages 40 to 49 years. **B:** Cumulative incidence of tumors of size greater than 2 cm, ages 40 to 49 years. **C:** Cumulative incidence of tumors stage II or worse, ages 40 to 49 years. Y-axis is cumulative incidence per 100,000. (From Swedish Organized Service Screening Evaluation Group. Effect of mammographic service screening on stage at presentation of breast cancers in Sweden. *Cancer* 2007;109[11]:2205–2212, with permission.)

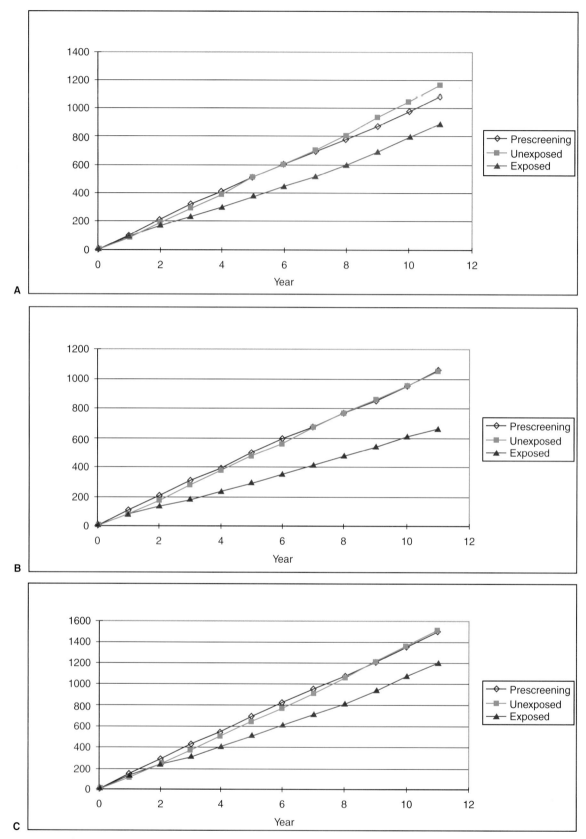

FIGURE 11.7. A: Cumulative incidence of lymph node positive disease, ages 50 to 69 years. **B:** Cumulative incidence of tumors of size greater than 2 cm, ages 50 to 69 years. **C:** Cumulative incidence of tumors stage II or worse, ages 50 to 69 years. Y-axis is cumulative incidence per 100,000. (From Swedish Organized Service Screening Evaluation Group. Effect of mammographic service screening on stage at presentation of breast cancers in Sweden. *Cancer* 2007;109[11]:2205–2212, with permission.)

| Table 11.4 | BREAST CANCER SCREENING GUIDELINES |

Age Group	ACS	ACR	NCI	USPSTF
Last update	2003–2007	2004	1997	2002
20–39	BSE optional; CBE every 3 yrs	No recommendation	No recommendation	No recommendation
40+	Begin annual mammography and yearly CBE at age 40	Begin annual mammography and yearly CBE at age 40	Mammography every 1–2 yrs for women in their 40s at average risk of breast cancer	Mammography every 1–2 yrs with or without annual CBE for women ages 40–69
Age to stop screening?	No upper age limit as long as a woman is in good health	No upper age limit as long as a woman is in good health	Upper age limit not addressed	Insufficient evidence to recommend for against screening after age 70
Women at greater than average risk	Women at higher risk should consult with their physician about beginning screening before age 40 Screening MRI is recommended for women with an approximately 20%–25% or greater lifetime risk of breast cancer, including women with a strong family history of breast or ovarian cancer and women who were treated for Hodgkin's lymphoma	Women at higher risk should consult with their physician about beginning screening before age 40, and to determine their mammography schedule in their 40s	Women at higher risk should consult with their physician about beginning screening before age 40, and to determine their mammography schedule in their 40s	Not addressed

ACS, American Cancer Society; ACR, American College of Radiology; NCI, National Cancer Institute; USPSTF, U.S. Preventive Services Task Force; BSE, breast self-examination; CBE, clinical breast examination; MRI, magnetic resonance imaging.

than a primary care provider, although mammography rates declined in all groups from year 1 to year 4.

The deciding issue about when to stop screening with mammography pertains to life expectancy and life-limiting comorbidity. Although average life expectancy for women in the United States born in 1950 is 71.1 years, at age 65 years, average longevity is an additional 20 years, at age 70, average life expectancy is 15.4 more years, and at age 75 years it is an additional 12.8 years (137). Although comorbidity increases with age, a significant percentage (75%) of the population older than age 65 rate their health as excellent, very good, or good (137). McPherson and Nissen (138) documented that only 13% of women over age 65 had multiple, severe comorbidities. Decisions about screening in older women should consider age, current health status, and a woman's preferences and values. According to the ACS, as long as a woman is in good health, she still is a candidate for breast cancer screening (133). This issue is also discussed in Chapter 91.

Physical Examinations: Clinical Breast Examination and Breast Self-Examination

Whereas some organizations recommend breast self-examination (BSE) and CBE in their screening guidelines, others do not, mostly because of the lack of clear evidence of their efficacy as a stand-alone examination or in combination with mammography. RCTs of screening have shown mortality reductions among women invited to screening that included either mammography or mammography in combination with CBE (3,49). In the HIP study and the Breast Cancer Demonstration Project (BCDDP), CBE was responsible for finding some cancers not detected by mammography (40,139). However, improvements in screening rates and the quality of mammography, as well as heightened awareness among women, have diminished the proportion of breast cancers diagnosed with CBE only or CBE and mammography. On all aspects of screening performance, CBE performs more poorly than mammography. Sensitivity of CBE in particu-

lar was estimated in a recent meta-analysis to be only 54% (140). While noting that two trials demonstrated breast cancer mortality reductions associated with the combination of mammography and CBE (3,59), the USPSTF concluded there was insufficient evidence to quantify the incremental benefits of adding CBE to mammography (38). This question of unique or added benefit is increasingly relevant since much of the RCT data related to the value of CBE combined with mammography derives from a period that predates modern breast imaging. The proportion of breast cancers not visible with modern, high-quality mammography appears to be considerably lower today than in the past (141–143). Oestreicher et al. (143) evaluated the sensitivity of CBE in 468 women diagnosed with breast cancer within a year of a screening CBE. Overall sensitivity was estimated to be 35%, but the majority of these cases (83.6%) also were detected by mammography. Among women with false-negative mammograms, 37% were detected by CBE, but overall, only 5.7% (n = 27) of breast cancers were diagnosed by CBE only. Sensitivity ranged from 17.2% for tumors 0.5 cm or less to 58.3% for tumors 2.1 cm or more and was lower in younger women and women with higher body weight. In a subsequent analysis of comparing the sensitivity of mammography and CBE, Oestreicher et al. (144) observed that the addition of CBE to mammography improved sensitivity by 4% overall (82% vs. 78%), and that the biggest increment was in women aged 50 to 59 with dense breasts (+6.8%). However, the addition of CBE to mammography screening also diminished specificity and PPV.

Despite the lack of unambiguous evidence for the contribution of CBE to reductions in breast cancer mortality, or its specific value in subsets of women for which mammography is less sensitive, there appears to be broad acceptance of the value of CBE as a complementary modality. Some breast cancers cannot be seen on a mammogram, or the mammographic examination may be enhanced if there is awareness of a palpable mass detected by CBE, although the presence of a palpable mass means that the patient should be undergoing a diagnostic rather than screening mammogram. For this reason, the ACS has recommended that

CBE should occur close to and before the occasion of a screening mammogram (133). Furthermore, recommendations from the former Agency for Health Care Policy and Research's (AHCPR, now AHRQ) "Quality Determinants of Mammography" strongly assert that a negative mammogram in the presence of a palpable mass does not rule out breast cancer (92). It should be stressed, however, that the value of CBE is determined by the quality of the examination, which is addressed in Chapter 4.

The goal of periodic BSE, as with CBE, is to detect palpable tumors The value of BSE historically has been viewed in a similar way to that of CBE, that is, it is a form of low-cost surveillance for breast changes that once noticed should be brought to the attention of a physician. An additional role of BSE is to increase awareness of normal breast composition and thus, heightened awareness of changes that may be detected during BSE or during normal activities.

The literature on the effectiveness of BSE as a detection modality has shown mixed results, but recent reviews have focused on the lack of direct evidence of benefit in two RCTs (145–149), and data indicating that the rate of benign biopsy, and thus harms, is higher in women who regularly perform BSE compared to women who do not regularly perform BSE (148). In the update of the USPSTF breast cancer screening guidelines, the task force concluded that the evidence is insufficient to recommend for or against teaching or performing routine BSE (38). The Canadian Task Force on Preventive Health Care went further and recommended against routine instruction in BSE in periodic health examinations based on fair evidence of no benefit, and good evidence of harm (i.e., false-positive results) (150). In an accompanying editorial to the Canadian report, Nekhlyudov and Fletcher (151) argued that the limitations in the RCT data and observational studies do not provide a sound basis for dismissing the value of BSE, and instead, advise that women should err on the side of prudence. The ACS guidelines recommend that women be informed about the benefits and limitations of BSE, and that they should be able to chose whether or not to practice BSE, but all women should be informed about the importance of prompt reporting of any new breast symptoms. Women who elect to practice BSE should have access to instruction, and should have their technique periodically reviewed (133).

Risk-Based Screening

For women at very high risk due to a significant family history of breast or ovarian cancer in first-degree relatives diagnosed premenopausally or confirmation of mutation carrier status on a breast cancer susceptibility gene in herself or a close family relative, more aggressive surveillance has been recommended based on evidence and expert opinion (Tables 11.4 and 11.5) (133,152,153). For women who carry a *BRCA* mutation, who are untested but have a first-degree relative who carries a *BRCA* mutation, or who have a lifetime risk of approximately 20% or greater based on pedigree analysis software that evaluates family history on both the maternal and paternal side, the ACS recommends annual mammography and magnetic resonance imaging (MRI) beginning at age 30 (153). This same recommendation also applies to women who have received mantle radiation to the chest between the ages 10 to 30 or who are known carriers of other high-risk genetic variants. Women with a prior diagnosis of breast cancer, DCIS, lobular neoplasia, or atypical hyperplasia might also reach a shared decision with their physicians to establish a program of more aggressive surveillance. Over time and with the accumulation of additional evidence, it is likely that screening recommendations can be further tailored to better meet the needs of higher risk subgroups.

For women who do not fall into these higher-risk categories, it has been proposed that informed decisions about screening should be made weighing comparative risks (e.g., cost, inconvenience, anxiety associated with false-positive results, harm

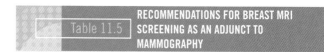

Table 11.5	RECOMMENDATIONS FOR BREAST MRI SCREENING AS AN ADJUNCT TO MAMMOGRAPHY

Recommend Annual MRI Screening (based on evidence)[a]
- *BRCA* mutation
- First degree relative of *BRCA* carrier but untested
- Lifetime risk ~ 20%–25% as defined by BRCAPRO, or other models that are largely dependent on family history

Recommend Annual MRI Screening (based on expert consensus opinion)[b]
- Radiation to chest between ages 10 and 30
- Li-Fraumeni syndrome and first-degree relatives
- Cowden and Bannayan-Riley-Ruvalcaba syndromes and first-degree relatives

Insufficient Evidence to Recommend for or Against MRI Screening[c]
- Lifetime risk 15%–25% as defined by BRCAPRO, or other models that are largely dependent on family history
- Lobular carcinoma *in situ* (LCIS) or atypical lobular hyperplasia (ALH)
- Atypical ductal hyperplasia (ADH)
- Heterogeneously or extremely dense breast on mammography
- Women with a personal history of breast cancer, including ductal carcinoma *in situ* (DCIS)

Recommend Against MRI Screening (based on expert consensus opinion)
- Women at less than 15% lifetime risk

MRI, magnetic resonance imaging.
[a]Evidence from nonrandomized screening trials and observational studies.
[b]Based on evidence of lifetime risk for breast cancer.
[c]Payment should not be a barrier. Screening decisions should be made on a case-by-case basis, as there may be particular factors to support MRI. More data on these groups are expected to be published soon.
From Saslow D, Boates C, Burke W, et al. American Cancer Society guidelines for breast screening with MRI as an adjunct to mammography. *CA Cancer J Clin* 2007;57(2):90–104.

associated with avoidable biopsy, etc.) and benefits (20, 38,133). The underlying message in this recommendation is that women should understand their risk of breast cancer, the benefit of screening, and what to expect when undergoing screening, including the comparative risk of harms associated with screening. Because the majority of women are not diagnosed with breast cancer in their lifetimes, they could choose to not be screened, be screened less often, or delay initiating screening in order to reduce their higher risk of a false-positive examination compared with a lower likelihood of being diagnosed with breast cancer (154). However, it should be understood that any of these choices increases the probability, however, low in the short term, of being diagnosed with an advanced breast cancer compared with the protective effect gained with routine screening. Further, individuals vary in the degree to which they wish to make individual decisions about screening and the degree to which they are able to comprehend esoteric information, and their doctors have variable ability to fully communicate these issues in a manner that ensures complete understanding (155,156).

Because breast cancer risk increases with increasing age, concerns about comparative risks and benefits associated with breast cancer screening in younger women have been raised. At an age when breast cancer risk is comparatively low, Gail and Rimer (154) have proposed that a woman's risk-factor profile could be used to make decisions about whether to begin screening before age 50. Their model, which is derived from BCDDP data, is based on the assumption that regular mammographic screening is justified for a 50-year-old woman with none of the important risk factors, whereas average individual risk is sufficiently low in the 40s to favor a greater degree of flexibility. Regular screening would be justified for women in their 40s if they have a prior history of breast cancer; atypical hyperplasia on a previous breast biopsy; two or more breast biopsies even with benign results; a known mutation on a breast cancer susceptibility gene; a mother, sister, or daughter previously diagnosed with breast cancer; or if they are age 45 to 49 with at least 75% breast density. For women in their 40s who do not fall into any of these categories, age at menarche, number of previous breast biopsies, and age at first live birth would be the bases for an informed decision about screening. For example, according to the authors, in a woman in her early 40s with no history of breast biopsies and age at first live birth younger than 30 years, delay would be an option. Based on their estimates, only approximately 10% of 40-year-old women would make a decision to be screened if this model were followed, compared with 68% by age 45 and 95% by age 49. Because breast cancer risk increases with increasing age, their model may prove useful for women who wish to make an informed, risk-based decision about when to begin screening. No data are included with this model to estimate the proportion of incident cases within specific ages that would be identified if all women followed this approach. However, in a retrospective evaluation of women in their forties diagnosed with breast cancer, McPherson and Nissen (138) applied both the estimation routines developed by Gail and Rimer (154) and observed that approximately 70% to 75% of women who developed breast cancer would have been recommended for screening based on the model results. Thus, although the model was effective in identifying a majority of the breast cancer cases, it is unknown whether it would be useful for making an informed decision at the individual level, especially since one in four women diagnosed with breast cancer would not have been recommended to undergo routine mammography.

Another tool available to help women understand their individual risk is an interactive computer program for breast cancer risk assessment that has come to be known as the *risk disk*. This risk assessment tool is available from NCI and was developed to determine eligibility for participation in the Breast Cancer Prevention Trial (157). These tools may have their greatest value in helping women understand individual risk against the backdrop of health education messages and articles in the media that emphasize risk as a basis for raising awareness about breast cancer prevention and early detection.

Are risk factors other than age useful for establishing screening intervals? Only one study has shown an association between a breast cancer risk factor and the length of the detectable preclinical phase. Duffy et al. (158) observed that postmenopausal women with a family history tended to have shorter sojourn times compared with women without a family history. These findings require further validation before they might be included in screening recommendations. However, any attempt to decide on the basis of risk factors whether to be screened more or less frequently than recommended guidelines would be a decision based on the underlying probability of disease, not the underlying probability of having a longer or shorter sojourn time.

On a population basis, risk-based screening for breast cancer has never been shown to have much potential to identify the majority of new cases by screening a subgroup of women at higher risk. In 1984 Solin et al. (159) reported on the screening experience of 17,543 women, for whom data on eight risk factors were collected (including any family history, prior breast biopsy, menstrual history, pregnancy history, lactation, and hormone use). They concluded that more than half of the 246 cases diagnosed would not have been detected if the program had screened only women with either prior breast biopsy or family history and that more than 40% would have been missed if the program had been limited to any one of the listed risk factors.

In 1987 Alexander et al. (160) reported similar findings from the analysis of Edinburgh trial data; by screening the 20% of the population at higher risk because of a prior biopsy or a family history in a mother or sister, only 30% of the first-round cancers would have been detected. When menopausal status and nulliparity or first birth after age 30 were included, the proportion of new cases that would have been detected in the first round increased to 29.6%. Again, concentrating on the more important risk factors would fail to identify the majority of prevalent cancers in an asymptomatic population.

Madigan et al. (161) recently reported population-attributable risk estimates for breast cancer using data from the National Health and Nutrition Examination Survey Epidemiologic Follow-Up Study. Using well-established risk factors, such as later age at first live birth, nulliparity, higher family income, and family history of breast cancer in first-degree relatives, these risk factors were associated with approximately 41% of breast cancer cases in the United States. In each of these instances, it is estimated that fewer than half of breast cancer cases would be identified by a risk-based screening strategy applying well-established risk factors.

QUALITY ASSURANCE

The usefulness of mammography is dependent on the proper use of dedicated mammography equipment, including positioning, breast compression, and appropriate technique settings (Fig. 11.8A–D), the diagnostic skills of the interpreter, prompt follow-up and appropriate action for examinations that are positive, and reducing barriers to the regular screening. These issues have been and are continually being addressed in an effort to promote safe and effective mass screening for early stage breast cancer.

As knowledge and use of mammography slowly increased after the beginning of early promotion efforts in the early 1980s, the nationwide evaluation of x-ray trends demonstrated a great variation in dose and image quality among mammography sites (162). Based on the reports findings and recommendations, the ACS approached the ACR to stimulate the development of quality standards for mammography facilities. With funding from the ACS, the voluntary ACR Mammography Accreditation Program (MAP) was established and began to accredit mammography facilities in August 1987 (163). The application process included a questionnaire to obtain information about personnel, volume, and type of examinations performed at the facility; assessment of the imaging system through evaluation of phantom images and dose delivery; and, most important, assessment of clinical images to evaluate positioning, contrast, compression, and image-label identifiers. Over time, greater understanding of the link between high-quality mammography and the goals of breast cancer screening led to new professional and regulatory initiatives.

Maryland was the first state to pass legislation pertaining to quality assurance in mammography. In 1986 Maryland required mammography examinations to be performed with machinery designed and built only for mammography. Use of these dedicated units was vastly superior to mammography performed on general purpose machines in terms of dosage and image quality. By 1993, 41 states and the District of Columbia had either passed legislation or established regulations addressing quality mammography (164).

Toward the end of 1990, the U.S. Congress added mammography to the benefit package for Medicare-eligible women and included quality standards for sites approved to provide services to Medicare beneficiaries (165). These standards were heavily influenced by the ACR MAP standards. Also in that year, Congress passed the Breast and Cervical Cancer Mortality Prevention Act of 1990 (PL 101-354), appropriating funds to the Centers for Disease Control and Prevention (CDC) for state programs to provide breast and cervical cancer screening to low-income women (166).

By the early 1990s, fewer than half of all mammography facilities had embraced voluntary accreditation, and the number of voluntary and regulatory standards for mammography

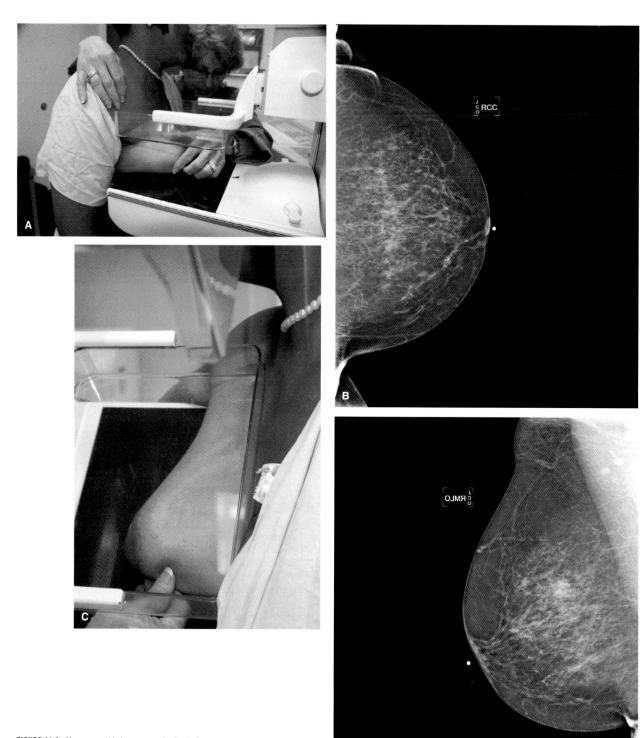

FIGURE 11.8. Mammographic images are obtained after the mammographic technologist carefully positions the breast on the image receptor and applies firm compression to the breast with a compression paddle in order to immobilize the breast and disperse overlapping tissue maximally. This is done in two nearly orthogonal projections: **A:** craniocaudal (cc) view, **B:** with resultant mammographic cc image; **C:** mediolateral oblique (MLO) view, **D:** with resultant mammographic MLO view.

was increasing. In order to ensure that women could depend on a uniform set of quality standards in all mammography facilities, Congress passed the Mammography Quality Standards Act (MQSA) in 1992. Under MQSA, all facilities offering mammography services would be required to be accredited by a private accrediting body, undergo an annual on-site inspection, and be certified by an agency designated by the Secretary of Health and Human Services. The following year, the U.S. Food and Drug Administration (FDA) was assigned the task of enforcing MQSA by establishing standards, regulations, inspection processes, compliant mechanisms, and penalties for failure to comply with the regulations.

At approximately the same time MQSA was enacted, the AHCPR convened a panel to produce clinical practice guidelines on the quality determinants of mammography for interpreting physicians, clinicians, and consumers (92). The panel considered the entire process involved in providing high-quality mammography to consumers, including (a) actions before the examination, which relate to scheduling, including triaging patients into screening or diagnostic examinations; (b) appropriate data to collect related to the patient's history and risk; (c) the roles of imaging team members, including qualifications; (d) machinery standards, dosage limitations, quality control procedures, and the importance of routine evaluation of clinical images and the imaging system; and (e) the communication of results to patients. The development of these clinical practice guidelines underscores the importance of factors beyond image quality that contribute to a high-quality examination.

In addition to determinants of a high-quality examination, the AHCPR panel addressed the critical issue of assessing outcome data from mammography facilities by use of medical audits. Data (both collected and derived) required for the basic medical audit include (a) the number and type of mammography examinations performed; (b) the recall rate; (c) the PPV of screening mammography, as well as the PPV of patients sent to biopsy for a mammographic abnormality; and (d) the stage of disease at diagnosis and the breast cancer detection rate per 1,000 women screened. A more advanced audit requires linkage to a breast cancer registry, which is not possible in most areas in the United States, and thus measuring sensitivity and specificity is not easily achieved in the average facility (167).

The final and arguably most critical step related to mammography quality is interpretation. One of the early major barriers to interpretation and communication of findings was the lack of a standardized language for mammographic features. Through the efforts of the ACR, with support from various clinical colleges, including the American College of Surgeons and the American College of Obstetrics and Gynecology, a multidisciplinary committee was established in the early 1990s to address the suboptimal and often confusing terminology and lack of cogent management recommendations found in mammography reports. The document produced by this committee is the Breast Imaging Reporting and Data System (BI-RADS) (168). BI-RADS is designed to standardize mammographic reporting, reduce confusion in breast imaging interpretations, and facilitate outcome monitoring. The system is divided into three sections:

1. *Breast imaging lexicon.* An illustrated review of all the findings seen on a mammogram with suggested terminology as well as guidance regarding whether the findings are worrisome for malignancy, are probably benign, or are definitely benign.
2. *Reporting system.* Provides an organized approach to image interpretation and reporting. Several sample reports are included to illustrate the suggested format for different mammographic scenarios.
3. *Follow-up outcome monitoring.* Describes minimum data to be collected and used to calculate important audit measures, allowing each radiologist to assess his or her overall performance in mammography interpretation.

There are seven categories in BI-RADS that cover all possible initial and summary interpretations. Category 0 is "assessment is incomplete." This category should be used on reports of screening mammograms that require further evaluation. After this evaluation is complete, or in the case of screening examinations that do not require assessment, there are five final categories. Category 1 is a "negative" examination. It does not require comment, and the patient is encouraged to return for routine screening in 1 year. Category 2 is a "benign finding." This is also a negative examination, but the interpreting physician may wish to describe a benign feature for subsequent reviewers. The patient is encouraged to return for routine screening in 1 year. Category 3 is for a "probably benign finding." This category is reserved for findings that have an extremely low probability of malignancy, as validated by clinical research (i.e., 2% or less) (169). It is not intended as an intermediate category between benign and malignant, but rather to denote a finding that has such a low probability of malignancy that a short-term follow-up, usually 6 months, is more appropriate than further diagnostic interventions. The interpreting physician, referring physician, and patient all have an interest in ensuring adherence with this recommendation, because neglecting the short-term follow-up results in adverse consequences in a small percentage of cases. The next two categories are those that warrant a biopsy. Category 4, "suspicious abnormality—biopsy should be considered," is for a lesion that has a definite possibility of being malignant. However, this category encompasses a broad spectrum of lesions (and resultant malignant probabilities), including those with a 2% likelihood (e.g., circumscribed mammographic mass containing low-level homogeneous echoes upon ultrasound) at one extreme to much more suspicious findings that approach the 95% malignant likelihood reserved for category 5 lesions. As a result, the fourth edition of BI-RADS describes a further division of category 4 into subcategories 4A ("low suspicion"), 4B ("intermediate suspicion"), and 4C ("moderate concern, but not classic"), for optional, internal use to help stratify this broad assessment category (168). Category 5, "highly suggestive of malignancy—appropriate action should be taken," is for a lesion that is virtually pathognomonic for malignancy. Category 6, "known malignancy," is reserved for mammograms with biopsy proven malignancy prior to definitive therapy. The fourth edition of BI-RADS released in 2003 was expanded to include lexicons for ultrasound and MRI.

OTHER SCREENING TESTS

The search for alternative methods of screening for breast cancer is stimulated by a desire to increase accuracy and to overcome some of the technical barriers associated with film screen mammography. Adjunctive modalities are not discussed here, but those with a possible use as a breast cancer screening tool are. Many screening methods have and are being suggested, including electrical impedance (170,171), light scanning (172), thermography (173), and infrared imaging (174). There has been no substantiation of a benefit accruing from these technologies for detection of early breast cancer in a screening situation. However, ultrasound, digital full-field mammography, and magnetic resonance (MR) mammography seem to hold promise in this regard.

Ultrasound Screening

The sensitivity of mammography is related to the radiographic density of the breast, with up to 98% sensitivity in women with predominantly fatty breasts to as low as 48% in women with extremely dense breasts (175–177). Ultrasonic imaging has been used for many years as an adjunct to mammography in women with a suspicious abnormality that is not easily or fully seen on the mammogram or to image an area of the breast that has such dense fibroglandular tissue that the ability of mammography to provide a clear image is limited. Ultrasound imaging is achieved by exposing the breast to high frequency sound waves, and then measuring the echo waves to produce a real-time image of the breast on a monitor. Although screening breast ultrasound is not a new concept, early results were not encouraging, with only 68% of clinically occult and mammographically demonstrated lesions seen on ultrasound (178).

With significant improvement of ultrasound technology, there was renewed interest in ultrasound screening for breast cancer detection. Four recent trials dating from 1995 to 2002 (177,179–181) collectively performed breast ultrasound on 37,085 women. These examinations were done with knowledge of the mammographic findings, were of a retrospective nature, or were done for areas of clinical concern. Overall, in these four studies the clinically or mammographically occult cancer detection rate was 3.4 per thousand and the positive predictive value (PPV2) for biopsy recommendation ranged from 3.1% to 10.5% (for comparison, the reported PPV2 for mammography in a large series was 31.5%) (182). The mean size of these mammographically and clinically occult malignancies was 9 mm, with almost all (94.5%) demonstrating invasion. The detection of ultrasound-only breast cancer was 27% in women with heterogeneously dense breasts but only 11% for women with a minimal amount of glandular tissue. In those women whose cancers were seen only sonographically, 93% had either heterogeneously dense or extremely dense parenchyma. Corsetti et al. (183) prospectively used whole-breast ultrasound to evaluate 9,157 asymptomatic women with dense breasts (BI-RADS density 3 or 4) and negative mammograms and showed general agreement with the above studies, with an incremental cancer detection rate (ultrasound-only detected) of 0.40%. In this subpopulation of women with dense breasts, ultrasound detected earlier-stage cancers than those detected by mammography and had greater sensitivity in women under age 50.

In an attempt to systematically evaluate screening ultrasound, a multicenter trial initiated by the ACR Imaging Network (ACRIN) began in the fall of 2003 (184). The trial enrolled women at higher than average risk for breast cancer who also had a predetermined level of breast density in order to select a population expected to harbor more malignancies than the average risk population. Although a mortality difference in women offered screening ultrasound and mammography versus mammography alone was not an end point due to both ethical and practical considerations, surrogate measures predictive of screening performance and breast cancer mortality (i.e., the cancer detection rate, tumor size and nodal status) were evaluated. In the study, 40 women were diagnosed with cancer: 20% of the cases (n = 8) were suspicious on both ultrasound and mammography; equal numbers (30%; n = 12) were suspicious on either mammography alone or ultrasound alone, and in 8 women (9 breasts), both ultrasound and mammography were normal. The diagnostic yield of breast cancer was 7.6 per 1,000 for mammography, and 11.8 for the combination of mammography and ultrasound, for an additional detection rate of 4.2 breast cancers per 1,000 women screened. Among 12 cancers detected by ultrasound alone, 11 (92%) were invasive with a median size of 10 mm, and 8 of the 9 lesions (89%) detected were node negative. While the addition of ultrasound improved the diagnostic yield in this high risk cohort, the cost in false positives and negative biopsies was considerable. The specificity for ultrasound alone was 91.8%, and for the combination of mammography and ultrasound, specificity was 89.4%. The PPV of a biopsy recommendation after a full diagnostic work-up was approximately 23% for mammography alone, 9% for ultrasound alone, and 11% for the combination of mammography and ultrasound.

There are many issues that must be evaluated prior to widespread utilization of screening ultrasound. At the most fundamental level, the main question related to the use of ultrasound for breast cancer screening centers on the degree to which the examination done alone or in combination with mammography results in reduced breast cancer mortality. This question is unlikely to ever be answered with a prospective RCT with a mortality end point. Berg et al. (184) observed a significant improvement in the diagnostic yield of small, node-negative cancers, many of which likely would have progressed to palpable, more advanced cancers if imaging had been done with mammography alone. Secondary questions are more opera-

tional and pertain to applications in select populations and whether the financial costs and the costs associated with higher rates of false positives generated by the addition of screening breast ultrasound to screening mammography are acceptable. The poor performance of mammography in the subgroup of higher risk women with dense breasts suggests that screening may require a combination of technologies that achieve a higher sensitivity, but at a cost of a higher false-positive rate (185). Although these costs are a basis for concern, additional research may identify strategies and protocols that will reduce the false-positive rate, and surveys of women have revealed that an excess biopsy rate is regarded as an acceptable cost of finding breast cancer early (31). An additional concern is the time required to perform ultrasound examinations. Although Kolb et al. (186) reported a mean time of 4 minutes for performing a complete bilateral screening ultrasound examination with a range of 1 minute 28 seconds to 9 minutes 46 seconds, the median time to perform a bilateral examination in the ACRIN study was 19 minutes, not including time for comparisons with previous examinations, discussing results with the patient, or creating a report (184). Careful determination of examination time is important since radiologist time is the most expensive component in the imaging chain.

Digital Mammography

All current routine screening of the breast is performed with dedicated equipment, due to the requirement of high spatial resolution and contrast for mammography. Digital techniques promise to fulfill these requirements. There are two general techniques of performing digital mammography. The first and less desirable method is digitizing a film screen mammogram. Although this allows for some of the desirable features of digital mammography, it also preserves some undesirable attributes of the film screen technique. The second method replaces the film screen cassette combination with a specialized detector capable of transforming the latent x-ray image into an electronic digital image. There are major benefits and significant barriers to digital mammography use for routine screening. Because there is no film processing involved, image acquisition is much faster, producing a mammogram in approximately 6 seconds as compared to the 90 to120 seconds required for film development. In a situation in which 40 or more screening examinations are done per day, this higher performance could increase throughput. Once a digital image is acquired, it can be manipulated to adjust contrast and brightness to the individual patient. Regions of interest may also be magnified. This can all be accomplished with the single x-ray exposure used to produce the original image and may be particularly useful in the dense breast, in which a masking effect for early cancer detection can exist (Fig. 11.9) (187).

The long-range expectation for full field digital mammography (FFDM) was that it would increase sensitivity for breast cancer detection over screen-film mammography (SFM) in women with dense breasts. In an early comparison of FFDM to SFM, Lewin et al. (188,189) reported on a prospective trial that directly compared the two technologies. Women 40 years of age and over who presented for screening were eligible and underwent both SFM and FFDM no more than 3 days apart performed by the same technologist. Each examination was interpreted independently by two radiologists reading equal numbers of SFMs and DDFMs. Most important, all findings, whether demonstrated on one or both techniques, were followed clinically and reasons for discrepant interpretations between the two techniques were tabulated. A total of 6,736 paired examinations were performed on 4,489 subjects. Forty-two cancers were detected, but no statistically significant difference between FFDM and SFM was observed (60% vs. 63%, respectively). However, the PPV3 for FFDM was significantly higher than for

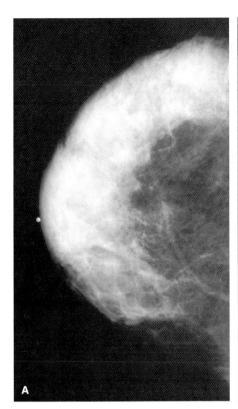 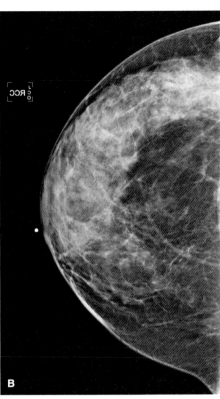

FIGURE 11.9. Using screen film technique (**A**), this patient's breast tissue appears dense and shows little intrinsic contrast, possibly allowing for obscuration of a cancer, which may be of similar attenuation to normal tissue. However, digital technique, used 1 year subsequent (**B**), provides improved dynamic range, resulting in greater tissue contrast.

SFM (30% vs. 19%). Thus, malignancy was more often found in woman who had been recalled and recommended for biopsy after diagnostic work-up based on initial digital technique compared with SFM technique. The reason for this finding is that the capacity of digital technology for image manipulation means that a significant proportion of suspicious findings can be resolved without requiring additional images. Thus, women recalled for diagnostic work-up following digital imaging typically will have a higher probability of malignancy.

The much-anticipated results of the Digital Mammographic Imaging Screening Trial (DMIST), a large multicenter trial prospectively comparing FFDM and SFM, became available in 2005 (190). Over 49,000 women were enrolled in the trial at 33 participating sites (data available for primary analysis in 42,760 patients), with the difference in sensitivity between FFDM and SFM being the primary end point of the study. Women underwent both FFDM and SFM and results were interpreted independently by two radiologists. Overall, the diagnostic accuracy of digital and film screen mammography was equivalent in both sensitivity and specificity. However, in women less than age 50, premenopausal or perimenopausal women, and women with heterogeneously or extremely dense tissue, FFDM displayed statistically significant greater sensitivity (70% vs. 51%; $p = .002$), with no difference in specificity compared to SFM. No variation in recall rates or biopsy rates between the two techniques was noted.

The observation that the overall performance of FFDM versus SFM was roughly equivalent, but that FFDM outperformed SFM in subgroups of women who were younger or who had dense breasts suggested that there also must be a subgroup of women for whom SFM had better performance than FFDM. In a follow-up analysis of the DMIST data, Pisano et al. (191) compared combinations of age, menopausal status, and breast density based on biopsy and other follow-up data. In the first report, the performance of FFDM was superior to SFM in three overlapping subgroups of women based on young age, menopausal status, and breast density (190). In the follow-up

report, the only subgroup in which FFDM outperformed SFM was the group of women who were under age 50, were pre- or perimenopausal, and who had dense breasts. As expected, SFM showed a nonsignificant advantage over FFDM for women aged 65 years or older with fatty breasts (191).

There are barriers to the use of digital mammography, of which perhaps the greatest is the method of display. The ability to manipulate the contrast and brightness of an image is essential in order to maximize the interpretive potential of this technology. This can be achieved only by interpreting digital mammograms on a high-resolution monitor. However, problems exist with this type of display. In order to detect subtle findings that may represent early malignancies, high contrast resolution is required. This, in turn, depends on the number of shades of gray demonstrated by the display. Film can depict 1,029 levels of gray. The digital receptor can generate 4,096 levels of gray. However, when this digital signal is fed into a monitor that can only demonstrate 256 levels of gray, the 4,096 gray levels generated by the digital receptor are compressed into 256 levels of gray on the monitor display. While the reader can view all the gray levels generated by the digital receptor by manipulating contrast at the monitor, it is still the case that the screen can display only 256 levels of gray at any one time. This limitation greatly affects efficiency for interpreting screening mammograms. Compounding this effect is the limited brightness of monitors versus the standard film viewer. With decreasing object size, as with findings related to early malignancy, the need for contrast increases if these findings are to be detected. In addition, contrast sensitivity will increase as the luminance or brightness of an object increases. Thus, if a monitor has limited ability to display many contrast levels at once and also has limited luminance, there is a potential disadvantage for detecting subtle signs of early cancers. An interesting study by Krupinski et al. (192) underscores the trade-offs that potentially exist with monitor interpretation. In their experiment, mixtures of subtle and negative cases were displayed with film on standard mammographic viewers and were also displayed digitally on a high-resolution monitor. Although the accuracy was no different for either viewing condition, the time required to determine that an examination was negative was twice as long on the monitor compared with the standard film viewer. Since the large majority of women undergoing screening do not have occult breast cancer and will have negative examinations, the monitor display could have a significant impact on screening efficiency. Although there are advantages of higher throughput, as mentioned above, the gains in patient flow may be nullified by the longer time to interpret the examination. As is the case with other new breast imaging modalities, targeting digital imaging to subgroups that are likely to benefit more from FFDM compared with SFM may be the most cost-effective use of digital imaging. Tosteson et al. (193) estimated that digital mammography targeted to women under age 50 and SFM to women aged 50 years and older was more cost-effective and resulted in more breast cancers detected and fewer breast cancer deaths than applying all SFM or all FFDM to the population, or specifically targeting FFDM on the basis of age and density.

Magnetic Resonance Imaging

The basis for contrast-enhanced MRI of the breast centers on the vascularity and vessel permeability difference of benign and malignant tumors. In general, benign lesions frequently are sparsely vascularized, whereas malignant breast tumors require additional blood supply, as they grow larger in size (194,195). The contrast agents used for MRI are paramagnetic agents and tend to concentrate in tissue with more abundant vasculature (196). Because these agents alter the MR signatures, the conspicuity of areas with greater blood supply than normal is enhanced. Neovascularity associated with malignant tumors as well as increased capillary permeability and local changes in osmolar pressure contribute to the enhancement characteristics of breast cancer (Fig. 11.10) (197).

MRI of the breast has reported sensitivity for breast cancer detection as high as 94% to 100% but with a much lower and wider range (37% to 97%) of specificity (198). Morris et al. (199) reported results of a screening trial of MRI in high-risk women (personal or family history of breast cancer, lobular carcinoma *in situ*, or atypical hyperplasia) with normal physical examination and mammographic findings. Among women who underwent biopsy based on MR findings, 24% had cancer, representing 4% of all women who were examined with MRI. The PPV for biopsy (PPV3) in this group of women was significantly higher in those with a family history of breast cancer compared to those without a family history, and higher also for those with both a personal and family history of breast cancer compared to women without this combination of risk factors.

Although screening MRI of the breast can detect occult malignancies, several factors must be taken into consideration. MRI is an expensive and invasive procedure requiring injection of a contrast agent (gadopentetate dimeglumine or similar agent). Additionally, the examination is contraindicated in women with pacemakers, aneurysm clips, or those who suffer with severe claustrophobia. Due to the lower specificity of

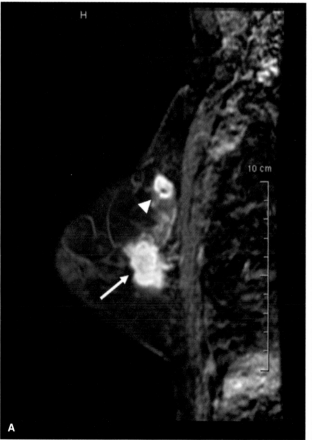
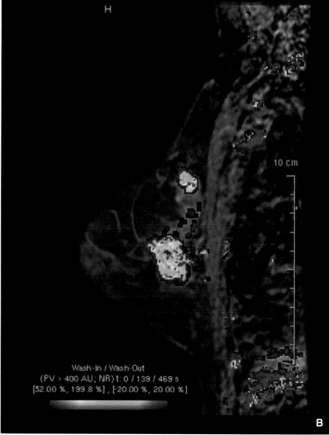

FIGURE 11.10. A: Sagittal magnetic resonance image of the breast shows a cancer (*arrow*) that is highly conspicuous due to its intense enhancement with contrast material. Note the second, smaller cancer (*arrowhead*), which was unsuspected and occult on mammogram. **B:** Same image with computer-assisted detection overlay. Any area of the breast that shows significant enhancement over baseline will be highlighted by color, the hue further outlining the specific pattern of enhancement, which can provide information about the benign versus malignant nature of the tissue in question.

breast MRI, the need to biopsy areas of MRI concern with no mammographic or ultrasound counterpart may be high and has the potential for increasing patient anxiety. The identification of abnormalities that require biopsy also requires a method to localize or sample these lesions percutaneously utilizing MR guidance. These biopsy systems are commercially available, but only recently are becoming widely available.

General screening for breast cancer with MRI deserves special mention. Screening implies the testing of a large population to identify the small subset that may have preclinical disease. As noted above in the section Principles of Cancer Screening, just as the decision to screen an asymptomatic population for disease must meet well-defined benchmarks, so too does the introduction of a new screening technology if it is to replace the existing standard bearer. When considering screening the large majority of average-risk women for breast cancer, MRI presently does not meet these conventional criteria as well as conventional mammography. MRI is much more costly at present than conventional mammography, is an invasive technique that requires injection of paramagnetic contrast agents, and there are not sufficient data regarding sensitivity and specificity. Thus, MRI should not be used in a pure screening setting for average-risk women until more data concerning test accuracy and reproducibility are available.

As noted above, in 2007, the American Cancer Society Breast Cancer Advisory Group published a set of recommendations to guide use of breast MRI as a screening adjunct to mammography in high-risk women (Table 11.5) (153). The guidelines summarize recommendations validated by evidence (e.g., *BRCA* mutation or first-degree relative of *BRCA* carrier; lifetime risk approximately 20% to 25% as defined by risk models that are capable of detailed pedigree analysis on both the maternal and paternal sides) or expert consensus opinion, but also outlined risk categories that, while elevated, had "insufficient evidence to recommend for or against MRI screening." Based on expert consensus, and as noted above, the guidelines recommend against MRI in average-risk women.

The use of mammography and MRI for women at very high risk due to known *BRCA* mutation status, and women at significantly elevated risk for other reasons, will benefit from additional research. One question that has been raised is whether the unique advantage of MRI in these women who are known mutation carriers principally is due to breast density, and if so, if breast density is reduced with increasing age, would mammography alone be sufficient for screening. A recent study of the comparative performance of mammography and MRI in a screening program for women at high risk for hereditary breast cancer, Bigenwald et al. (200) observed that sensitivity of mammography for invasive cancer was greater in women with fattier breasts compared with women with greater breast density, but still considerably lower than the sensitivity of MRI regardless of density. Further, density had no effect on the detection of DCIS, and a significant fraction of DCIS without calcifications was detected by MRI and not mammography. Bigenwald et al. conclude that women at high risk for hereditary breast cancer need to be screened with mammography and MRI regardless of breast density, which at this time suggests that there may not be an age at which these high-risk women can be screened with mammography alone. The observation that MRI detects synchronous breast cancer not found by mammography equally well in women with and without significant breast density provides additional support for continuing to screen with MRI in this high-risk subpopulation (201).

Double Reading and Computer-Aided Detection

Among the most persistent issues of concern associated with screening mammography are the variability of sensitivity and specificity of screening with mammography (202,203). Two methods that have been used in an attempt to increase accuracy are double reading and computer-aided detection (CAD). Interest in double-reading mammograms has been high since the early 1990s when several reports showed two readers significantly improved sensitivity compared with a single reader (193). The introduction and evolution of CAD held the promise of using computer algorithms to aid a single reader to not overlook areas of suspicion, in effect replacing the second reader with a computer. The evaluation of double reading and CAD generally compares the sensitivity and specificity of a single reader with the addition of a second reader or the CAD system (204). The evaluation of findings from investigations of double reading or CAD should always be based on changes in sensitivity and specificity, rather than area under the receiver operating curve (ROC). Although ROC analysis is informative, the ROC statistic represents the intersection between sensitivity and specificity. In other words, the ROC statistic may be the same for single reading and double reading or CAD based on sensitivity going up and specificity going down, or vice versa.

In general, research on double reading has shown improvements in sensitivity, with some accompanying degradation in specificity (205,206). Although there is wide variability in the manner in which double reading may be carried out, Taylor and Potts (204) concluded that double reading increased both the detection and recall rate, whereas double reading with arbitration increased the detection rate, but decreased the recall rate. The initial enthusiasm for the potential to improve sensitivity with double reading has been tempered by the growing appreciation that double reading in clinical practice may not live up to the potential identified in experimental settings, especially because double reading is more complicated than just two sequential interpretations and it adds costs. Without additional incentives, double reading is not likely to be commonly applied in the U.S. imaging practices.

The FDA approved CAD in 1998, and with the evolution of digital screening mammography, CAD is becoming commonly used in screening (207–209). Using detection algorithms for specific mammographic features associated with malignancy, CAD systems are able to identify these potential findings on the digitized x-ray image, or the digitized detector, and highlight those areas that the radiologist should scrutinize. This process in no way serves as a replacement for careful review of the images by the physician, but rather can serve as an adjunct to single-viewer reading. Taylor and Pott's (204) review of CAD studies concluded that it did not result in a significant improvement in the cancer detection rate, but that it did increase the recall rate. CAD systems vary in terms of overall accuracy, but they share in common greater sensitivity for calcifications and well-defined masses compared with small developing densities. In addition, the experience of the reader also has a significant influence on the influence of the CAD system, with inexperienced readers showing little improvement in sensitivity, but a marked decline in specificity (210). In one of the largest evaluations of CAD to date, Fenton et al. (211) examined the comparative performance of CAD systems over a 4-year period (1998 to 2002) with data from 222,135 women and approximately 430,000 mammograms in 43 facilities in three states, in which 7 of the 43 facilities had implemented CAD systems. The investigators observed a significant decline in specificity, a decline in the PPV, a nearly 20% increase in the biopsy rate, and a nonsignificant increase in sensitivity. Interestingly, a comparison of the facilities that had implemented CAD to those that had not revealed that those practices that implemented CAD tended to be characterized by interpreting physicians with less experience, suggesting that the marginal performance of CAD may have been influenced by less experienced interpreting physicians. In contrast, Gromet (212) reported the experience of a large, experienced practice that shifted from double reading to CAD. Over 230,000 mammographic examinations in a 4-year period were evaluated. Double reading improved sensitivity over single reading, with a small increase in the recall rate, while CAD slightly improved sensitivity over double reading, also with only a small increase in the recall rate. The accumulation of data to date indicates that CAD can be a useful tool when used by a reader who is experienced and competent at reading mammograms, but that it actually may decrease overall accuracy when used by an inexperienced reader (212).

CONCLUSION

Mammography is the cornerstone of the present state-of-the-art approach to the control of breast cancer. The decision to screen women for breast cancer is based on the importance of the disease as a risk to women's health, and the demonstrated ability of mammography to reduce morbidity and mortality from breast cancer by reducing the incidence rate of advanced disease. Although great progress has been made over the past two decades in establishing a screening and diagnostic infrastructure, the full potential of breast cancer screening as a disease control strategy remains unfulfilled. Although a majority of women aged 40 and older have had a mammogram, most women are not regularly screened at recommended intervals (213). In the United States, screening is commonly opportunistic rather than organized, and access is still a significant problem for medically underserved women. Further, low reimbursement and the risk of malpractice may be steadily eroding interest in specializing in mammography at a time when the size of the population needing breast imaging is increasing by more than a million women per year (214–217).

Evaluation of service screening data and RCT data, as well as long-term trends in survival by stage, clearly reveals that, at present, the greatest potential to save lives from breast cancer depends on initiating treatment while the disease is still localized. More fundamentally, for screening to be effective, the program must achieve a high degree of performance in reducing the incidence rate of advanced breast cancer. Once the decision to screen has been reached, screening programs should be carefully monitored, and attention should be devoted to using results to improve performance. In general, a breast cancer screening program must have high levels of participation and must achieve acceptable levels of performance in terms of sensitivity and specificity. In the coming years, there must be renewed efforts to monitor and increase access and to make the most of the current technology as newer screening modalities and emerging preventive strategies are anticipated.

References

1. Donegan WL. Introduction to the history of breast cancer. In: Donegan WL, Spratt JS, eds. *Cancer of the breast.* 4th ed. Philadelphia: WB Saunders, 1995:1–15.
2. Bassett LW, Gold RH, Kimme-Smith C. History of the technical development of mammography. In: Haus AG, Yaffe MJ, eds. *Syllabus: a categorical course in physics: technical aspects of breast imaging.* 2nd ed. Chicago: Radiological Society of North America, 1993:9–20.
3. Shapiro S, Strax P, Venet L. Periodic breast cancer screening in reducing mortality from breast cancer. *JAMA* 1971;215:1777–1785.
4. Shapiro S. Periodic screening for breast cancer: the HIP Randomized Controlled Trial. Health Insurance Plan. *J Natl Cancer Inst Monogr* 1997;22:27–30.
5. Tabar L, Duffy SW, Vitak B, et al. The natural history of breast carcinoma: what have we learned from screening? *Cancer* 1999;86(3):449–462.
6. Dodd GD. American Cancer Society guidelines from the past to the present. *Cancer* 1993;72[4 Suppl]:1429–1432.
7. Health Care Financing Administration. Medicare covers mammograms. Available at http://www.hcfa.gov/news/ncireq.htm. October 27, 1997.
8. National Committee for Quality Assurance. The Health Plan Employer Data and Information Set (HEDIS). Available at http://www.ncqa.org/programs/HEDIS/index.htm. January 19, 2004.
9. State Cancer Legislative Database Program. Breast cancer insurance reimbursement. Available at http://www.scld-nci.net/scld_products_data_breast.cfml. February 15, 2008.
10. Smith RA, Cokkinides V, Brawley OW. Cancer screening in the United States, 2008: a review of current American Cancer Society guidelines and cancer screening issues. *CA Cancer J Clin* 2008;58(3):161–179.
11. Jemal A, Siegel R, Ward E, et al. Cancer statistics, 2008. *CA Cancer J Clin* 2008;58(2):71–96.
12. Ries L, Melbert D, Krapcho M, et al. *SEER Cancer Statistics Review, 1975–2005.* Bethesda, MD: National Cancer Institute, 2008.
13. Chu KC, Tarone RE, Kessler LG, et al. Recent trends in U.S. breast cancer incidence, survival, and mortality rates [see comments]. *J Natl Cancer Inst* 1996;88(21):1571–1579.
14. Stockton D, Davies T, Day N, et al. Retrospective study of reasons for improved survival in patients with breast cancer in east Anglia: earlier diagnosis or better treatment [published erratum appears in *BMJ* 1997;314(7082):721] [see comments]. *BMJ* 1997;314(7079):472–475.
15. Willett LR, August DA, Carson JL. Breast cancer prevention. New options for patients and clinicians. *N J Med* 2002;99(9).27–34.
16. Hankinson SE, Colditz GA, Willett WC. Towards an integrated model for breast cancer etiology: the lifelong interplay of genes, lifestyle, and hormones. *Breast Cancer Res* 2004;6(5):213–218.
17. Fatouros M, Baltoyiannis G, Roukos DH. The predominant role of surgery in the prevention and new trends in the surgical treatment of women with *BRCA1/2* mutations. *Ann Surg Oncol* 2008;15(1):21–33.
18. Morrison A. *Screening in chronic disease.* New York: Oxford University Press, 1992.
19. Wilson JMG, Junger G. *Principles and practice of screening for disease.* Geneva: World Health Organization, 1968.
20. National Institutes of Health Consensus Development Panel. National Institutes of Health Consensus Development conference statement: breast cancer screening for women ages 40–49, January 21–23, 1997. National Institutes of Health Consensus Development Panel. *J Natl Cancer Inst* 1997;89(14):1015–1026.
21. Berry DA. Benefits and risks of screening mammography for women in their forties: a statistical appraisal. *J Natl Cancer Inst* 1998;90(19):1431–1439.
22. Smith RA. Breast cancer screening among women younger than age 50: a current assessment of the issues. *CA Cancer J Clin* 2000;50(5):312–336.
23. Walter LC, Covinsky KE. Cancer screening in elderly patients: a framework for individualized decision making. *JAMA* 2001;285(21):2750.
24. Qaseem A, Snow V, Sherif K, et al. Screening mammography for women 40 to 49 years of age: a clinical practice guideline from the American College of Physicians. *Ann Intern Med* 2007;146(7):511–515.
25. Michaelson JS, Kopans DB, Cady B. The breast carcinoma screening interval is important. *Cancer* 2000;88(6):1282–1284.
26. Humphrey LL, Helfand M, Chan BK, et al. Breast cancer screening: a summary of the evidence for the U.S. Preventive Services Task Force. *Ann Intern Med* 2002;137(5 Pt 1):347–360.
27. Salzmann P, Kerlikowske K, Phillips K. Cost-effectiveness of extending screening mammography guidelines to include women 40 to 49 years of age [published erratum appears in *Ann Intern Med* 1998;128(10):878] [see comments]. *Ann Intern Med* 1997;127(11):955–965.
28. Zappa M, Visioli CB, Ciatto S. Mammography screening in elderly women: efficacy and cost-effectiveness. *Crit Rev Oncol Hematol* 2003;46(3):235–239.
29. Stout NK, Rosenberg MA, Trentham-Dietz A, et al. Retrospective cost-effectiveness analysis of screening mammography. *J Natl Cancer Inst* 2006;98(1):774–782.
30. Tabar L, Chen HH, Fagerberg G, et al. Recent results from the Swedish Two-County trial: the effects of age, histologic type, and mode of detection on the efficacy of breast cancer screening. *J Natl Cancer Inst Monogr* 1997;22:43–47.
31. Schwartz LM, Woloshin S, Sox HC, et al. US women's attitudes to false positive mammography results and detection of ductal carcinoma *in situ*: cross sectional survey. *BMJ* 2000;320(7250):1635–1640.
32. Brewer NT, Salz T, Lillie SE. Systematic review: the long-term effects of false-positive mammograms. *Ann Intern Med* 2007;146(7):502–510.
33. Ernster VL, Ballard-Barbash R, Barlow WE, et al. Detection of ductal carcinoma *in situ* in women undergoing screening mammography. *J Natl Cancer Inst* 2002;94(20):1546–1554.
34. Fletcher SW, Elmore JG. Clinical practice. Mammographic screening for breast cancer. *N Engl J Med* 2003;348(17):1672–1680.
35. Scott HJ, Gale AG. Breast screening: PERFORMS identifies key mammographic training needs. *Br J Radiol* 2006;79(2):S127–S133.
36. Parkin DM, Bray F, Ferlay J, et al. Global cancer statistics, 2002. *CA Cancer J Clin* 2005;55(2):74–108.
37. Bray F, McCarron P, Parkin DM. The changing global patterns of female breast cancer incidence and mortality. *Breast Cancer Res* 2004;6(6):229–239.
38. U.S. Preventive Services Task Force. Screening for breast cancer: recommendations and rationale. *Ann Intern Med* 2002;137(5 Pt 1):344–346.
39. Smith RA, Saslow D, Sawyer KA, et al. American Cancer Society guidelines for breast cancer screening: update 2003. *CA Cancer J Clin* 2003;53(3):141–169.
40. Shapiro S, Venet W, Strax P, et al. *Periodic screening for breast cancer: the Health Insurance Plan project and its sequelae.* Baltimore: Johns Hopkins University Press, 1988.
41. Duffy SW, Chen HH, Tabar L, et al. Estimation of mean sojourn time in breast cancer screening using a Markov chain model of both entry to and exit from the preclinical detectable phase. *Stat Med* 1995;14(14):1531–1543.
42. Tabar L, Fagerberg G, Chen HH, et al. Tumour development, histology and grade of breast cancers: prognosis and progression. *Int J Cancer* 1996;66(4):413–419.
43. Tabar L, Vitak B, Chen HH, et al. The Swedish Two-County Trial twenty years later. Updated mortality results and new insights from long-term follow-up. *Radiol Clin North Am* 2000;38(4):625–651.
44. Smith RA, Duffy SW, Gabe R, et al. The randomized trials of breast cancer screening: what have we learned? *Radiol Clin North Am* 2004;42(5):793–806.
45. Tabar L, Faberberg G, Day NE, et al. What is the optimum interval between mammographic screening examinations? An analysis based on the latest results of the Swedish Two-County breast cancer screening trial. *Br J Cancer* 1987;55(5):547–551.
46. Ries L, Henson D, Harras A. Survival from breast cancer according to tumor size and nodal status. *Surg Oncol Clin North Am* 1994;3:35–50.
47. Elkin EB, Hudis C, Begg CB, et al. The effect of changes in tumor size on breast carcinoma survival in the U.S.: 1975–1999. *Cancer* 2005;104(6):1149–1157.
48. Shapiro S, Venet W, Strax P, et al. Ten- to fourteen-year effect of screening on breast cancer mortality. *J Natl Cancer Inst* 1982;69(2):349–355.
49. Tabar L, Fagerberg CJ, Gad A, et al. Reduction in mortality from breast cancer after mass screening with mammography. Randomised trial from the Breast Cancer Screening Working Group of the Swedish National Board of Health and Welfare. *Lancet* 1985;1(8433):829–832.

50. Tabar L, Fagerberg G, Duffy SW, et al. The Swedish Two-County trial of mammographic screening for breast cancer: recent results and calculation of benefit. *J Epidemiol Community Health* 1989;43(2):107–114.

51. Andersson I, Aspegren K, Janzon L, et al. Mammographic screening and mortality from breast cancer: the Malmö mammographic screening trial. *BMJ* 1988;297(6654):943–948.

52. Miettinen OS, Henschke CI, Pasmantier MW, et al. Mammographic screening: no reliable supporting evidence? *Lancet* 2002;359(9304):404–405.

53. Andersson I, Janzon L. Reduced breast cancer mortality in women under age 50: updated results from the Malmö Mammographic Screening Program. *J Natl Cancer Inst Monogr* 1997;22:63–67.

54. Frisell J, Lidbrink E, Hellstrom L, et al. Follow-up after 11 years—update of mortality results in the Stockholm mammographic screening trial. *Breast Cancer Res Treat* 1997;45(3):263–270.

55. Bjurstam N, Bjorneld L, Duffy SW, et al. The Gothenburg breast screening trial: first results on mortality, incidence, and mode of detection for women ages 39–49 years at randomization [comments]. *Cancer* 1997;80(11):2091–2099.

56. Bjurstam N, Bjorneld L, Warwick J, et al. The Gothenburg breast screening trial. *Cancer* 2003;97(10):2387–2396.

57. Roberts MM, Alexander FE, Anderson TJ, et al. The Edinburgh randomised trial of screening for breast cancer: description of method. *Br J Cancer* 1984;50(1):1–6.

58. Alexander FE, Anderson TJ, Brown HK, et al. The Edinburgh randomised trial of breast cancer screening: results after 10 years of follow-up. *Br J Cancer* 1994;70(3):542–548.

59. Alexander FE, Anderson TJ, Brown HK, et al. Fourteen years of follow-up from the Edinburgh randomised trial of breast cancer screening [comments]. *Lancet* 1999;353(9168):1903–1908.

60. Miller AB, Baines CJ, To T, et al. Canadian National Breast Screening Study: 1. Breast cancer detection and death rates among women aged 40 to 49 years [published erratum appears in *Can Med Assoc J* 1993;148(5):718] [comments]. *Can Med Assoc J* 1992;147(10):1459–1476.

61. Miller AB, To T, Baines CJ, et al. The Canadian National Breast Screening study: update on breast cancer mortality. *J Natl Cancer Inst Monogr* 1997; 22:37–41.

62. Miller AB, To T, Baines CJ, et al. The Canadian National Breast Screening Study-1: breast cancer mortality after 11 to 16 years of follow-up. A randomized screening trial of mammography in women age 40 to 49 years. *Ann Intern Med* 2002;137(5 Pt 1):305–312.

63. Burhenne LJ, Burhenne HJ. The Canadian National Breast Screening study: a Canadian critique. *AJR Am J Roentgenol* 1993;161(4):761–763.

64. Kopans DB, Feig SA. The Canadian National Breast Screening study: a critical review. *AJR Am J Roentgenol* 1993;161(4):755–760.

65. Tarone RE. The excess of patients with advanced breast cancer in young women screened with mammography in the Canadian National Breast Screening study. *Cancer* 1995;75(4):997–1003.

66. Boyd NF. The review of randomization in the Canadian National Breast Screening study. Is the debate over? *Can Med Assoc J* 1997;156(2):207.

67. Bailar JC, MacMahon B. Randomization in the Canadian National Breast Cancer Screening study. Report of a review team appointed by the National Cancer Institute of Canada. *Can Med Assoc J* 1997;156:213–215.

68. Miller AB, Baines CJ, To T, et al. Canadian National Breast Screening Study: 2. Breast cancer detection and death rates among women aged 50 to 59 years [published erratum appears in *Can Med Assoc J* 1993;148(5):718] [comments]. *Can Med Assoc J* 1992;147(10):1477–1488.

69. Moss S. A trial to study the effect on breast cancer mortality of annual mammographic screening in women starting at age 40. Trial Steering Group. *J Med Screen* 1999;6(3):144–148.

70. Moss SM, Cuckle H, Evans A, et al. Effect of mammographic screening from age 40 years on breast cancer mortality at 10 years' follow-up: a randomised controlled trial. *Lancet* 2006;368(9552):2053–2060.

71. Gotzsche PC, Olsen O. Is screening for breast cancer with mammography justifiable? *Lancet* 2000;355(9198):129–134.

72. Fletcher SW, Black W, Harris R, et al. Report of the International Workshop on Screening for Breast Cancer [comments]. *J Natl Cancer Inst* 1993;85(20):1644–1656.

73. Feig SA. Estimation of currently attainable benefit from mammographic screening of women aged 40–49 years. *Cancer* 1995;75(10):2412–2419.

74. Wald N, Chamberlain J, Hackshaw A. Report of the European Society of Mastology Breast Cancer Screening Evaluation Committee [published erratum appears in *Tumori* 1994;80(4):following 314]. *Tumori* 1993;79(6):371–379.

75. Kerlikowske K, Grady D, Rubin SM, et al. Efficacy of screening mammography. A meta-analysis [comments]. *JAMA* 1995;273(2):149–154.

76. Smart CR, Hendrick RE, Rutledge JH 3rd, et al. Benefit of mammography screening in women ages 40 to 49 years. Current evidence from randomized controlled trials [published erratum appears in *Cancer* 1995;75(11):2788. *Cancer* 1995;75(7):1619–1626.

77. Hendrick RE, Smith RA, Rutledge JH 3rd, et al. Benefits of screening mammography in women aged 40–49: a new meta-analysis of randomized control trials. *J Natl Cancer Inst Monogr* 1997;22:87–92.

78. Forrest AP, Alexander FE. A question that will not go away: at what age should mammographic screening begin? [editorial; comment]. *J Natl Cancer Inst* 1995;87(16):1195–1197.

79. Prorok PC, Hankey BF, Bundy BN. Concepts and problems in the evaluation of screening programs. *J Chron Dis* 1981;34:159–171.

80. de Koning HJ, Boer R, Warmerdam PG, et al. Quantitative interpretation of age-specific mortality reductions from the Swedish breast cancer-screening trials [comments]. *J Natl Cancer Inst* 1995;87(16):1217–1223.

81. Duffy SW, Day NE, Tabar L, et al. Markov models of breast tumor progression: some age-specific results. *J Natl Cancer Inst Monogr* 1997;22:93–97.

82. Sox H. Screening mammography for younger women: back to basics. *Ann Intern Med* 2002;137(5 Pt 1):361–362.

83. Organizing Committee and Collaborators. Breast cancer screening with mammography in women aged 40–49 Years. Report of the organizing committee and collaborators, Falun meeting, Falun, Sweden (21–22 March, 1996). *Int J Cancer* 1996;68:693–699.

84. Duffy SW, Chen HH, Tabar L, et al. Sojourn time, sensitivity and positive predictive value of mammography screening for breast cancer in women aged 40–49. *Int J Epidemiol* 1996;25(6):1139–1145.

85. Tabar L, Duffy SW, Burhenne LW. New Swedish breast cancer detection results for women aged 40–49. *Cancer* 1993;72[4 Suppl]:1437–1448.

86. Buist DS, Porter PL, Lehman C, et al. Factors contributing to mammography failure in women aged 40–49 years. *J Natl Cancer Inst* 2004;96(19):1432–1440.

87. Bucchi L, Ravaioli A, Foca F, et al. Incidence of interval breast cancers after 650,000 negative mammographies in 13 Italian health districts. *J Med Screen* 2008;15(1):30–35.

88. Tabar L, Vitak B, Tony HH, et al. Beyond randomized controlled trials: organized mammographic screening substantially reduces breast carcinoma mortality. *Cancer* 2001;91(9):1724–1731.

89. Tabar L, Yen MF, Vitak B, et al. Mammography service screening and mortality in breast cancer patients: 20-year follow-up before and after introduction of screening. *Lancet* 2003;361(9367):1405–1410.

90. Coldman A, Phillips N, Warren L, et al. Breast cancer mortality after screening mammography in British Columbia women. *Int J Cancer* 2007;120(5):1076–1080.

91. Sickles EA. Breast cancer screening outcomes in women ages 40–49: clinical experience with service screening using modern mammography. *J Natl Cancer Inst Monogr* 1997;22:99–104.

92. Bassett L, Hendrick R, Bassford T, et al. *Quality determinants of mammography. clinical practice guideline no. 13.* AHCPR Publication No. 95-0632. Rockville, MD: Agency for Health Care Policy and Research, Public Health Service, U.S. Department of Health and Human Services, 1994.

93. American College of Radiology BI-RADS Committee. *Illustrated breast imaging reporting and data system (BI-RADS).* 3rd ed. Reston, VA: American College of Radiology, 1998.

94. Day NE, Walter SD. Simplified models for screening: estimation procedures form mass screening programmes. *Biometrics* 1984;40:1–14.

95. Beam CA, Layde PM, Sullivan DC. Variability in the interpretation of screening mammograms by US radiologists. Findings from a national sample. *Arch Intern Med* 1996;156(2):209–213.

96. Beam CA, Conant EF, Sickles EA. Association of volume and volume-independent factors with accuracy in screening mammogram interpretation. *J Natl Cancer Inst* 2003;95(4):282–290.

97. Tabar L, Fagerberg G, Chen HH, et al. Efficacy of breast cancer screening by age. New results from the Swedish Two-County trial. *Cancer* 1995;75(10):2507–2517.

98. Linver MN, Paster SB. Mammography outcomes in a practice setting by age: prognostic factors, sensitivity, and positive biopsy rate. *J Natl Cancer Inst Monogr* 1997;22:113–117.

99. NCI-funded Breast Cancer Surveillance Consortium co-operative agreement (U01CA63740 UC, U01CA86082, U01CA63736, U01CA70013, U01CA69976, U01CA63731, U01CA70040). Performance measures for 3,603,832 screening mammography examinations from 1996 to 2006 by age. Rockville, MD: National Cancer Institute, 2008.

100. Boyd NF, Guo H, Martin LJ, et al. Mammographic density and the risk and detection of breast cancer. *N Engl J Med* 2007;356(3):227–236.

101. Carney PA, Miglioretti DL, Yankaskas BC, et al. Individual and combined effects of age, breast density, and hormone replacement therapy use on the accuracy of screening mammography. *Ann Intern Med* 2003;138(3):168–175.

102. Kelemen LE, Pankratz VS, Sellers TA, et al. Age-specific trends in mammographic density: the Minnesota Breast Cancer Family Study. *Am J Epidemiol* 2008; 167(9):1027–1036.

103. Rosenberg RD, Hunt WC, Williamson MR, et al. Effects of age, breast density, ethnicity, and estrogen replacement therapy on screening mammographic sensitivity and cancer stage at diagnosis: review of 183,134 screening mammograms in Albuquerque, New Mexico. *Radiology* 1998;209(2):511–518.

104. Laya MB, Larson EB, Taplin SH, et al. Effect of estrogen replacement therapy on the specificity and sensitivity of screening mammography [comments]. *J Natl Cancer Inst* 1996;88(10):643–649.

105. Mandelson MT, Oestreicher N, Porter PL, et al. Breast density as a predictor of mammographic detection: comparison of interval- and screen-detected cancers. *J Natl Cancer Inst* 2000;92(13):1081–1087.

106. van Duijnhoven FJ, Peeters PH, Warren RM, et al. Postmenopausal hormone therapy and changes in mammographic density. *J Clin Oncol* 2007;25(11):1323–1328.

107. Smith-Bindman R, Chu PW, Miglioretti DL, et al. Comparison of screening mammography in the United States and the United Kingdom. *JAMA* 2003;290(16):2129–2137.

108. Sickles EA. Successful methods to reduce false-positive mammography interpretations. *Radiol Clin North Am* 2000;38(4):693–700.

109. Roelofs AA, Karssemeijer N, Wedekind N, et al. Importance of comparison of current and prior mammograms in breast cancer screening. *Radiology* 2007;242(1):70–77.

110. Lampic C, Thurfjell E, Bergh J, et al. Short- and long-term anxiety and depression in women recalled after breast cancer screening. *Eur J Cancer* 2001;37(4):463–469.

111. Yasunaga H, Ide H, Imamura T, et al. Women's anxieties caused by false positives in mammography screening: a contingent valuation survey. *Breast Cancer Res Treat* 2007;101(1):59–64.

112. Ernster VL, Barclay J, Kerlikowske K, et al. Incidence of and treatment for ductal carcinoma *in situ* of the breast [comments]. *JAMA* 1996;275(12):913–918.

113. Morrow M, Harris JR. Ductal carcinoma in situ and microinvasive carcinoma. In: Harris JR, Lippman ME, Morrow M, et al., eds. *Diseases of the breast.* 2nd ed. Philadelphia: Lippincott Williams & Wilkins, 2000:383–402.

114. Page DL, Dupont WD, Rogers LW, et al. Continued local recurrence of carcinoma 15–25 years after a diagnosis of low grade ductal carcinoma *in situ* of the breast treated only by biopsy. *Cancer* 1995;76(7):1197–1200.

115. Connolly JL, Boyages J, Nixon AJ, et al. Predictors of breast recurrence after conservative surgery and radiation therapy for invasive breast cancer. *Mod Pathol* 1998;11(2):134–139.

116. Page DL, Simpson JF. Ductal carcinoma *in situ*—the focus for prevention, screening, and breast conservation in breast cancer. *N Engl J Med* 1999;340(19):1499–1500.

117. Yen MF, Tabar L, Vitak B, et al. Quantifying the potential problem of overdiagnosis of ductal carcinoma *in situ* in breast cancer screening. *Eur J Cancer* 2003;39(12):1746–1754.

118. Olsen O, Gotzsche PC. Cochrane review on screening for breast cancer with mammography. *Lancet* 2001;358(9290):1340–1342.

119. Black WC, Haggstrom DA, Welch HG. All-cause mortality in randomized trials of cancer screening. *J Natl Cancer Inst* 2002;94(3):167–173.

120. Health Council of The Netherlands. *The benefit of population screening for breast cancer with mammography.* The Hague: Health Council of The Netherlands. 2002.

121. Olsen O, Gotzsche P. Systematic review of screening for breast cancer with mammography. Available at http://image.thelancet.com/lancet/extra/fullreport.pdf. 2001.

122. Gail MH, Katki HA. Re: all-cause mortality in randomized trials of cancer screening. *J Natl Cancer Inst* 2002;94(11):862.

123. Tabar L, Duffy SW, Yen MF, et al. All-cause mortality among breast cancer patients in a screening trial: support for breast cancer mortality as an end point. *J Med Screen* 2002;9(4):159–162.

124. Rembold CM. Number needed to screen: development of a statistic for disease screening. *BMJ* 1998;317(7154):307–312.

125. Jorgensen KJ, Gotzsche PC. Presentation on websites of possible benefits and harms from screening for breast cancer: cross sectional study. *BMJ* 2004;328(7432):148.

126. Tabar L, Vitak B, Yen MF, et al. Number needed to screen: lives saved over 20 years of follow-up in mammographic screening. *J Med Screen* 2004;11(3):126–129.

127. Sjonell G, Stahle L. [Mammographic screening does not reduce breast cancer mortality]. *Lakartidningen* 1999;96(8):904–905.

128. Duffy SW, Tabar L, Chen HH, et al. The impact of organized mammography service screening on breast carcinoma mortality in seven Swedish counties. *Cancer* 2002;95(3):458–469.

129. Gabe R, Duffy SW. Evaluation of service screening mammography in practice: the impact on breast cancer mortality. *Ann Oncol* 2005;16[Suppl 2]:ii153–ii162.

130. Swedish Organized Service Screening Evaluation Group. Reduction in breast cancer mortality from organized service screening with mammography: 1. Further confirmation with extended data. *Cancer Epidemiol Biomarkers Prev* 2006;15(1):45–51.

131. Swedish Organized Service Screening Evaluation Group. Reduction in breast cancer mortality from the organised service screening with mammography: 2. Validation with alternative analytic methods. *Cancer Epidemiol Biomarkers Prev* 2006;15(1):52–56.

132. Swedish Organized Service Screening Evaluation Group. Effect of mammographic service screening on stage at presentation of breast cancers in Sweden. *Cancer* 2007;109(11):2205–2212.

133. Smith RA, Cokkinides V, Eyre HJ. American Cancer Society guidelines for the early detection of cancer, 2003. *CA Cancer J Clin* 2003;53(1):27–43.

134. Smith-Bindman R, Kerlikowske K, Gebretsadik T, et al. Is screening mammography effective in elderly women? *Am J Med* 2000;108(2):112–119.

135. Badgwell BD, Giordano SH, Duan ZZ, et al. Mammography before diagnosis among women age 80 years and older with breast cancer. *J Clin Oncol* 2008;26(15):2482–2488.

136. Field TS, Doubeni C, Fox MP, et al. Under utilization of surveillance mammography among older breast cancer survivors. *J Gen Intern Med* 2008;23(2):158–163.

137. National Center for Health Statistics. *Health, United States, 2007.* Hyattsville, MD: NCHS, 2007.

138. McPherson CP, Nissen MJ. Evaluating a risk-based model for mammographic screening of women in their forties. *Cancer* 2002;94(11):2830–2835.

139. Smart CR, Byrne C, Smith RA, et al. Twenty-year follow-up of the breast cancers diagnosed during the Breast Cancer Detection Demonstration project [comments]. *CA Cancer J Clin* 1997;47(3):134–149.

140. Barton MB, Harris R, Fletcher SW. The rational clinical examination. Does this patient have breast cancer? The screening clinical breast examination: should it be done? How? *JAMA* 1999;282(13):1270–1280.

141. Bobo J, Lee N. Factors associated with accurate cancer detection during a clinical breast examination. *Ann Epidemiol* 2000;10(7):463.

142. Newcomer LM, Newcomb PA, Trentham-Dietz A, et al. Detection method and breast carcinoma histology. *Cancer* 2002;95(3):470–477.

143. Oestreicher N, White E, Lehman CD, et al. Predictors of sensitivity of clinical breast examination (CBE). *Breast Cancer Res Treat* 2002;76(1):73–81.

144. Oestreicher N, Lehman CD, Seger DJ, et al. The incremental contribution of clinical breast examination to invasive cancer detection in a mammography screening program. *AJR Am J Roentgenol* 2005;184(2):428–432.

145. Foster RS Jr, Lang SP, Costanza MC, et al. Breast self-examination practices and breast-cancer stage. *N Engl J Med* 1978;299(6):265–270.

146. Greenwald P, Nasca PC, Lawrence CE, et al. Estimated effect of breast self-examination and routine physician examinations on breast-cancer mortality. *N Engl J Med* 1978;299(6):271–273.

147. Semiglazov VF, Moiseenko VM, Manikhas AG, et al. [Interim results of a prospective randomized study of self-examination for early detection of breast cancer (Russia/St. Petersburg/WHO)]. *Vopr Onkol* 1999;45(3):265–271.

148. Thomas DB, Gao DL, Ray RM, et al. Randomized trial of breast self-examination in Shanghai: final results. *J Natl Cancer Inst* 2002;94(19):1445–1457.

149. Kosters JP, Gotzsche P. Regular self-examination or physical examination for the early detection of breast cancer [review]. *Cochrane Library* 2008;(3):1–22.

150. Baxter N. Preventive health care, 2001 update: should women be routinely taught breast self-examination to screen for breast cancer? *Can Med Assoc J* 2001;164(13):1837–1846.

151. Nekhlyudov L, Fletcher SW. Is it time to stop teaching breast self-examination? *Can Med Assoc J* 2001;164(13):1851–1852.

152. Burke W, Daly M, Garber J, et al. Recommendations for follow-up care of individuals with an inherited predisposition to cancer. II. *BRCA1* and *BRCA2*. Cancer Genetics Studies Consortium. *JAMA* 1997;277(12):997–1003.

153. Saslow D, Boates C, Burke W, et al. American Cancer Society guidelines for breast screening with MRI as an adjunct to mammography. *CA Cancer J Clin* 2007;57(2):90–104.

154. Gail M, Rimer B. Risk-based recommendations for mammographic screening for women in their forties. *J Clin Oncol* 1998;16(9):3105–3114.

155. Lipkus IM, Samsa G, Rimer BK. General performance on a numeracy scale among highly educated samples. *Med Decis Mak* 2001;21(1):37–44.

156. Rimer BK, Halabi S, Sugg Skinner C, et al. The short-term impact of tailored mammography decision-making interventions. *Patient Educ Couns* 2001;43(3):269–285.

157. National Cancer Institute (NCI) and National Surgical Adjuvant Breast and Bowel Project (NSABP). Breast Cancer Risk Assessment Tool. Breast cancer risk assessment tool. Available at http://bcra.nci.nih.gov/brc/. January 10, 2003.

158. Duffy SW, Tabar L, Smith RA, et al. Risk of breast cancer and risks with breast cancer: the relationship between histologic type and conventional risk factors, disease progression, and survival. *Sem Breast Dis* 1999;2:292.

159. Solin L, Schwartz G, Feig S, et al. Risk factors as criteria for inclusion in breast cancer screening programs. In: Ames F, Blumenschein G, Montague E, eds. *Current controversies in breast cancer.* Austin: University of Texas Press, 1984:565–573.

160. Alexander F, Roberts M, Huggins A. Risk factors for breast cancer with applications to selection for the prevalence screen. *J Epid Comm Health* 1987;41:101–106.

161. Madigan MP, Ziegler RG, Benichou J, et al. Proportion of breast cancer cases in the United States explained by well-established risk factors. *J Natl Cancer Inst* 1995;87(22):1681–1685.

162. Conway BJ, Suleiman OH, Rueter FG, et al. National survey of mammographic facilities in 1985, 1988, and 1992 [comments]. *Radiology* 1994;191(2):323–330.

163. McLelland R, Hendrick RE, Zinninger MD, et al. The American College of Radiology Mammography Accreditation Program [comments]. *AJR Am J Roentgenol* 1991;157(3):473–479.

164. Fintor L, Alciati MH, Fischer R. Legislative and regulatory mandates for mammography quality assurance. *J Public Health Policy* 1995;16(1):81–107.

165. Hendrick RE, Smith RA, Wilcox PA, eds. *ACR accreditation and legislative issues in mammography.* Chicago: RSNA; 1993. In: Haus AG, Yaffee MJ, eds. Syllabus: A Categorical Course in Physics: Technical Aspects of Breast Imaging.

166. Centers for Disease Control. Update: National Breast and Cervical Cancer Early Detection Program—July 1991–September 1995. *MMWR Morb Mortal Wkly Rep* 1996;45(23):484–487.

167. Smith RA, Osuch JR, Linver MN. A national breast cancer database. *Radiol Clin North Am* 1995;33:1247–1257.

168. American College of Radiology. *BI-RADS Atlas:Breast Imaging and Reporting Data System.* 4th ed. Reston, VA: American College of Radiology, 2003.

169. Sickles EA. Management of probably benign lesions of the breast. *Radiology* 1996;193:582.

170. Cuzick J, Holland R, Barth V, et al. Electropotential measurements as a new diagnostic modality for breast cancer. *Lancet* 1998;352(9125):359–363.

171. Poplack SP, Tosteson TD, Wells WA, et al. Electromagnetic breast imaging: results of a pilot study in women with abnormal mammograms. *Radiology* 2007;243(2):350–359.

172. Monsees B, Destouet JM, Totty WG. Light scanning versus mammography in breast cancer detection. *Radiology* 1987;163(2):463–465.

173. Ng EY, Sudharsan NM. Computer simulation in conjunction with medical thermography as an adjunct tool for early detection of breast cancer. *BMC Cancer* 2004;4:17.

174. Cerussi AE, Berger AJ, Bevilacqua F, et al. Sources of absorption and scattering contrast for near-infrared optical mammography. *Acad Radiol* 2001;8(3):211–218.

175. Kerlikowske K, Grady D, Barclay J, et al. Effect of age, breast density, and family history on the sensitivity of first screening mammography [comments]. *JAMA* 1996;276(1):33–38.

176. Kerlikowske K, Carney PA, Geller B, et al. Performance of screening mammography among women with and without a first-degree relative with breast cancer. *Ann Intern Med* 2000;133(11):855–863.

177. Kolb TM, Lichy J, Newhouse JH. Comparison of the performance of screening mammography, physical examination, and breast US and evaluation of factors that influence them: an analysis of 27,825 patient evaluations. *Radiology* 2002;225(1):165–175.

178. Sickles EA, Filly RA, Callen PW. Breast cancer detection with sonography and mammography: comparison using state-of-the-art equipment. *AJR Am J Roentgenol* 1983;140(5):843–845.

179. Gordon PB, Goldenberg SL. Malignant breast masses detected only by ultrasound. A retrospective review. *Cancer* 1995;76(4):626–630.

180. Buchberger W, Niehoff A, Obrist P, et al. Clinically and mammographically occult breast lesions: detection and classification with high-resolution sonography. *Semin Ultrasound CT MR* 2000;21(4):325–336.

181. Kaplan SS. Clinical utility of bilateral whole-breast US in the evaluation of women with dense breast tissue. *Radiology* 2001;221(3):641–649.

182. Sickles EA, Miglioretti DL, Ballard-Barbash R, et al. Performance benchmarks for diagnostic mammography. *Radiology* 2005;235(3):775–790.

183. Corsetti V, Houssami N, Ferrari A, et al. Breast screening with ultrasound in women with mammography-negative dense breasts: evidence on incremental cancer detection and false positives, and associated cost. *Eur J Cancer* 2008;44(4):539–544.

184. Berg WA, Blume JD, Cormack JB, et al. Combined screening with ultrasound and mammography vs mammography alone in women at elevated risk of breast cancer. *JAMA* 2008;299(18):2151–2163.

185. Kuhl CK. The "coming of age" of nonmammographic screening for breast cancer. *JAMA* 2008;299(18):2203–2205.

186. Kolb TM, Lichy J, Newhouse JH. Occult cancer in women with dense breasts: detection with screening US—diagnostic yield and tumor characteristics. *Radiology* 1998;207(1):191–199.

187. Van Gils CH, Otten JD, Verbeek AL, et al. Mammographic breast density and risk of breast cancer: masking bias or causability? *Eur J Epidemiol* 1998;14:315–320.

188. Lewin JM, Hendrick RE, D'Orsi CJ, et al. Comparison of full-field digital mammography with screen-film mammography for cancer detection: results of 4,945 paired examinations. *Radiology* 2001;218(3):873–880.

189. Lewin JM, D'Orsi CJ, Hendrick RE, et al. Clinical comparison of full-field digital mammography and screen-film mammography for detection of breast cancer. *AJR Am J Roentgenol* 2002;179(3):671–677.

190. Pisano ED, Gatsonis C, Hendrick E, et al. Diagnostic performance of digital versus film mammography for breast-cancer screening. *N Engl J Med* 2005;353(17):1773–1783.

191. Pisano ED, Hendrick RE, Yaffe MJ, et al. Diagnostic accuracy of digital versus film mammography: exploratory analysis of selected population subgroups in DMIST. *Radiology* 2008;246(2):376–383.

192. Krupinski E, Roehrig H, Furukawa T. Influence of film and monitor display luminance on observer performance and visual search. *Acad Radiol* 1999;6(7):411–418.

193. Tosteson AN, Stout NK, Fryback DG, et al. Cost-effectiveness of digital mammography breast cancer screening. *Ann Intern Med* 2008;148(1):1–10.

194. Folkman J, Shing Y. Angiogenesis. *J Biol Chem* 1992;267(16):10931–10934.

195. Cosgrove DO, Kedar RP, Bamber JC, et al. Breast diseases: color Doppler US in differential diagnosis [comments]. *Radiology* 1993;189(1):99–104.

196. Strich G, Hagan PL, Gerber KH, et al. Tissue distribution and magnetic resonance spin lattice relaxation effects of gadolinium-DTPA. *Radiology* 1985;154(3): 723–726.

197. Brasch RC, Weinmann HJ, Wesbey GE. Contrast-enhanced NMR imaging: animal studies using gadolinium-DTPA complex. *AJR Am J Roentgenol* 1984;142(3): 625–630.

198. Orel SG, Schnall MD. MR imaging of the breast for the detection, diagnosis, and staging of breast cancer. *Radiology* 2001;220(1):13–30.

199. Morris EA, Liberman L, Ballon DJ, et al. MRI of occult breast carcinoma in a high-risk population. *AJR Am J Roentgenol* 2003;181(3):619–626.

200. Bigenwald RZ, Warner E, Gunasekara A, et al. Is mammography adequate for screening women with inherited BRCA mutations and low breast density? *Cancer Epidemiol Biomarkers Prev* 2008;17(3):706–711.

201. Lehman C, Gatsonis C, Kuhl CK, et al. MRI evaluation of the contralateral breast in women with a recently diagnosed breast cancer. *N Engl J Med* 2007;356(13): 1295–1303.

202. Elmore JG, Barton MB, Moceri VM, et al. Ten-year risk of false positive screening mammograms and clinical breast examinations [comments]. *N Engl J Med* 1998;338(16):1089–1096.

203. Elmore JG, Miglioretti DL, Reisch LM, et al. Screening mammograms by community radiologists: variability in false-positive rates. *J Natl Cancer Inst* 2002;94(18): 1373–1380.

204. Taylor P, Potts HW. Computer aids and human second reading as interventions in screening mammography: two systematic reviews to compare effects on cancer detection and recall rate. *Eur J Cancer* 2008;44(6):798–807.

205. Taplin SH, Rutter CM, Elmore JG, et al. Accuracy of screening mammography using single versus independent double interpretation. *AJR Am J Roentgenol* 2000;174(5):1257–1262.

206. Ciatto S, Del Turco MR, Risso G, et al. Comparison of standard reading and computer aided detection (CAD) on a national proficiency test of screening mammography. *Eur J Radiol* 2003;45(2):135–138.

207. Quinn M, Allen E. Changes in incidence of and mortality from breast cancer in England and Wales since introduction of screening. United Kingdom Association of Cancer Registries [comments]. *BMJ* 1995;311(7017): 1391– 1395.

208. Kalman BL, Reinus WR, Kwasny SC, et al. Prescreening entire mammograms for masses with artificial neural networks: preliminary results. *Acad Radiol* 1997; 4(6):405–414.

209. Freer TW, Ulissey MJ. Screening mammography with computer-aided detection: prospective study of 12,860 patients in a community breast center. *Radiology* 2001;220(3):781–786.

210. Ellis RL, Meade AA, Mathiason MA, et al. Evaluation of computer-aided detection systems in the detection of small invasive breast carcinoma. *Radiology* 2007; 245(1):88–94.

211. Fenton JJ, Taplin SH, Carney PA, et al. Influence of computer-aided detection on performance of screening mammography. *N Engl J Med* 2007;356(14): 1399–1409.

212. Gromet M. Comparison of computer-aided detection to double reading of screening mammograms: review of 231,221 mammograms. *AJR Am J Roentgenol* 2008;190(4):854–859.

213. Carney PA, Goodrich ME, Mackenzie T, et al. Utilization of screening mammography in New Hampshire. *Cancer* 2005;104(8):1726–1732.

214. Committee on Technologies for the Early Detection of Breast Cancer. *Mammography and beyond: developing technologies for the early detection of breast cancer*. Washington, DC: National Academy Press, 2001.

215. Bassett LW, Monsees BS, Smith RA, et al. Survey of radiology residents: breast imaging training and attitudes. *Radiology* 2003;227(3):862–869.

216. Committee on Improving Mammography Quality Standards. *Improving breast imaging quality standards*. Washington, DC: National Academy Press, 2005.

217. Farria DM, Schmidt ME, Monsees BS, et al. Professional and economic factors affecting access to mammography: a crisis today, or tomorrow? Results from a national survey. *Cancer* 2005;104(3):491–498.

Chapter 12
Imaging Analysis: Mammography

Mark A. Helvie

Mammography is widely practiced in the United States and internationally for screening and diagnostic indications. High-quality examinations and interpretations are necessary for successful practice. Mammography refers to the process of obtaining images of the breast utilizing low energy x-rays. Breast imaging is a more general term that encompasses mammography, breast sonography, breast magnetic resonance imaging (MRI), breast positron emission tomography (PET) scanning and other emerging technologies. Although it is convenient to discuss mammography independent of other breast imaging modalities, modern practice stresses an integrated approach of various imaging modalities, in particular, mammography, sonography, and more recently MRI.

This chapter will describe the basics of mammographic interpretation and usage in screening and common diagnostic situations. Efficacy of screening mammography, breast sonography, and MRI are covered in Chapters 11, 13, and 14, respectively.

Radiography of the breast has been performed for over 95 years. Although palpable breast cancer was often found to have characteristic mammographic findings, the application of mammography into practice was slow. The potential of mammography to detect clinically occult cancer led to international efforts to refine mammographic technique and eventually led to screening trials, primarily in northern European countries and North America. These showed mortality reduction in screened women, which formed the basis for the current National Cancer Institute and American Cancer Society recommendation for mammographic screening of women age 40 and older (1). The explosive increase in mammographic screening in the United States in the 1980s and 1990s was associated with extensive public scrutiny and regulation. Breast imaging is unique among imaging specialties to develop a standard lexicon and assessment categories to improve quality and communication between radiologist, referring physicians, and patients. Federal law (the Mammography Quality Standards Act [MQSA]) regulates mammographic equipment, quality operations, technologists, and interpreting physicians (2). Direct written reporting of mammographic results to patients is required. The U.S. Food and Drug Administration (FDA) performs annual on-site regulatory inspections. All sites, equipment, technologists, and reading physicians in the United States require FDA approval to perform and interpret mammograms.

TECHNIQUE

Basic understanding of radiologic physics is necessary for mammographic interpretation. A typical mammographic machine generates low energy (25 to 32 kVp) x-rays, utilizing a small (0.3 mm) focal spot source, typically molybdenum. The breast is compressed between an image receptor (film or digital detector) and a transparent plastic compression plate. Compression is used to minimize thickness and motion and is necessary to limit the radiation dose and improve image quality. X-rays are differentially absorbed by different types breast tissue. X-rays that are not absorbed pass through the breast and are detected by an image receptor. There are now two types of FDA-approved receptors: film screen and digital. In film-screen systems, the energy is eventually received by film, which is developed to produce a mammographic image similar to a photographic negative. In contrast, a digital detector receives the x-rays and electronically converts the energy into an electronic data set, which can be projected on a video monitor or printed as a film or stored and manipulated electronically similar to digital photography. The mammographic appearance of cancer such as calcifications or masses is not different, although each system may offer some theoretical advantages at displaying these findings (3,4). Dark areas on a mammogram represent areas with minimal absorption (fat), while white areas represent moderate absorption by fibroglandular tissue or extensive absorption by calcium. Resolution of modern film systems is 13 or greater line pairs per millimeter.

Image quality is affected by a host of factors including breast tissue density, compressed thickness, positioning, motion, focal spot size, detector performance, and radiation dose. Manufacturers attempt to maximize multiple factors to achieve optimum image quality at the lowest possible radiation dose. The FDA limits dose to 3 mGy (300 mrad) for an average thickness breast per exposure. Mammographic technical requirements are mandated by the MQSA. Passing a yearly facility on-site inspection by an FDA-approved agent is necessary to maintain operational accreditation. The mammographic technologists play a critical role in ensuring a quality screening program by optimizing mammographic positioning (5,6). The radiologist can only interpret the parts of the breast that have been included in the imaged field, so the skill of the technologist in maximizing positioning is essential for a quality mammogram. The American College of Radiology (ACR) reviews facility mammograms to assess positioning and technique prior to certification.

SCREENING VERSUS DIAGNOSTIC MAMMOGRAPHY

Screening mammography refers to obtaining routine mammographic images of asymptomatic women in order to detect cancer at a preclinical stage. This is the primary role of mammography. The goal of screening is high sensitivity for early cancer detection. *Diagnostic* mammography refers to mammography used to evaluate abnormal clinical findings, such as a breast mass, thickening, or nipple discharge. Diagnostic mammography also refers to obtaining incremental mammographic images (such as magnification views or spot views) for characterization of possible abnormalities detected by screening mammography at time of recall or call back (7). *Magnification* views employ smaller focal spots (0.1 mm) and larger subject to receptor distances and produce a 2× magnified image. *Spot* compression utilizes smaller compression paddles that focally decrease breast thickness in an area of concern. Unfortunately, the distinctions between screening and diagnostic mammography have been confused by definitions utilized for insurance billing purposes. An insurer may consider a woman with a prior biopsy of "fibrocystic disease" as "diagnostic" mammography for billing, even though that individual may have no current abnormal palpable findings. For the discussion here, screening mammography refers to the mammographic evaluation of an asymptomatic individual. In the United States, a screening study consists of two views craniocaudal (CC) and mediolateral oblique (MLO) of each breast. Usually, screening mammography is performed without the presence of the physician, with mammographic interpretation occurring later in a batch reading situation, which improves efficiency and allows for low-cost screening (8,9).

Screening Mammography Pyramid

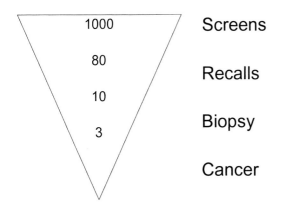

FIGURE 12.1. Simplified screening pyramid showing typical outcomes of 1,000 annually screened women of normal risk.

Not infrequently, findings are noted on screening mammography that require additional diagnostic imaging to resolve. This is analogous to a general practitioner referring a questionable skin lesion to a dermatologist for further evaluation. Only a small portion of women recalled for diagnostic imaging will have cancer. A simplified United States screening pyramid (Fig. 12.1) provides an overview of the screening process. Assuming a cancer incidence of 3 per 1,000 of annually screened women and a recall rate of 8%, the following outcome is expected for 1,000 normal risk women undergoing annual screening mammography: 920 of 1,000 (92%) will be normal and 80 of 1,000 (8%) will be recalled for diagnostic mammography or ultrasound. Of the 80 women who are recalled, 70 of 1,000 (7%) will be normal at diagnostic imaging and returned to mammographic screening and 10 of 1,000 (1%) will require tissue diagnosis for a mammographic abnormality. Of the 10 undergoing biopsy, 3 of 1,000 (0.3%) will be found to have cancer (10). These numbers are illustrative but will vary with incidence, screening frequency, recall rate, and biopsy rate.

MAMMOGRAPHIC INTERPRETATION

Mammographic interpretation is a difficult task that can be dichotomized into two basic processes: detection (perception) of a possible abnormality and characterization (classification, analysis) of a potential abnormality. The goal of image interpretation by screening is high-detection sensitivity, which requires the generation of false positives due to the nonspecific appearance of most small cancers. High sensitivity involves the ability to perceive potential abnormalities, only a fraction of which will prove to be cancer. Careful analysis of recalled patients by diagnostic imaging is necessary to evaluate a suspected lesion. With additional diagnostic mammography and ultrasound, a group of abnormalities of sufficient probability for malignancy will be recommended for biopsy. The commonly used U.S. threshold for biopsy is a probability of malignancy greater than or equal to 3% (11). Experienced readers can assign a reasonable probability of malignancy to a finding recommended for biopsy, but tissue diagnosis is necessary to confirm diagnosis even for lesions of very high probability. Mammographic appearances are seldom tissue specific.

Radiologists' Performance

Interpretation of mammographic images involves the art and science of medicine. The *New York Times* article has stated that "interpreting mammograms, even good ones, is considered the hardest task in radiology" (12). Although the recognition and characterization of classic large tumors is often straightforward, the detection of the small, subtle lesions can challenge the most expert reader. Interpretive variability exists for screening and diagnostic mammography. Key factors that influence overall performance include physician expertise, recall rates, observation time, biopsy rates, double reading, and computer-aided detection (CAD). The relationships between these parameters are complex.

Similar to other areas of human endeavor and medicine in particular, differences have been found among radiologists interpreting mammograms (13–23). Beam et al. (19), using an experimental model, found variation among practicing U.S. radiologists with overall sensitivity ranging from 59% to 100% and specificity 35% to 98%. Elmore et al. (20), in an enriched study population, noted 78% weighted agreement. Sickles et al. (15) reported higher cancer detection rates for specialists than generalists (6.0 per 1,000 vs. 3.4 per 1,000) within a single academic center in a retrospective clinical study. Specialists had higher volumes, more frequently participated in continuing medical education programs, and fellowship training, and more often participated in radiologic–pathologic correlation conferences than generalists. The influence of reading volume on performance has not been consistent. Beam et al. (19) tested 100 radiologists with an enriched study set of 148 mammograms with a 43% cancer incidence. He found reading volume not to be tightly associated with improved sensitivity. Rather complex multifactorial processes were found to be associated with expertise. Miglioretti et al. (23) reported better performance for readers of diagnostic mammography at academic centers, those concentrating their time in breast imaging, and those performing breast biopsies. Volume was not associated with performance. To date, no definite set of parameters completely predict reader expertise. Common associations with favorable interpretive skills and expertise include concentration in breast imaging, academic practice, continuing education, association with a multidisciplinary breast center, and practice audits (15,21,23). Reading a minimum of 480 mammographic cases per year is required by the U.S. Food and Drug Administration (FDA) to maintain certification.

Sensitivity and specificity are inversely related for any particular reader due to nonspecific appearance of early breast cancer. Sensitivity increases with recall rate over a range of recall rates. High sensitivity can only be achieved when a sufficient number of women are recalled from screening for additional diagnostic mammography and ultrasonography (14,22,24–27). The ideal balance between sensitivity and recall rate is controversial and reflects philosophy, cost, cultural issues, and medical–legal issues. Yankaskas et al. (25) demonstrated sensitivity increased from 65% at recall rates of 1.9% to 4.4% and to 80% sensitivity at recall rates of 8.9% to 13.4% in a study of practicing North Carolina radiologists. Karssemeijer et al. (14), in an enriched study population, found sensitivity for masses improved from approximately 35% at a 3% callback rate to 59% at a 20% callback rate. Gur et al. (27) noted improvements in sensitivity with increasing recall over a wide range (7.7% to 17.2%; $p < .05$) at a large clinical practice. On average, a 0.22 per 1,000 cancer detection rate improvement occurred for every 1% absolute increase in recall rate. Otten et al. (26), in an experimental situation, found 47% sensitivity improvement when false positive rate increased from 1% to 4%. Moskowitz (24) advocated callback rates of 10% to 12% for first screening mammograms and considered callback rates lower than 5% suboptimal. In the United States, callback rates of 5% to 15% are common. Rosenberg et al. (22) reported the middle 50%

recall rate for practicing U.S. radiologists to be 6.4% to 13.3% (mean 9.8%) for 2.5 million screening studies. European call-back rates are frequently lower. The Dutch breast cancer screening program has reported callback rates as low as 1.1% (14,26). Emphasis on specificity and low cost will limit recall rate. Emphasis on high sensitivity will increase callback rates.

Mammographic sensitivity increases with reader observation time. Nodine et al. (28) noted experienced mammographers made 71% of detections in the first 25 seconds but had continued true positive detections for approximately 80 seconds, albeit at a slower rate. Krupinski (29) observed the detection of subtle findings occurred later in observation cycle than obvious masses, which required longer visual dwell times. The threshold to initiate biopsy will influence cancer detection similar to recall rate thresholds. Higher thresholds for biopsy may be associated with higher false negative rates and lower sensitivity (27).

Double Reading

Double reading (DR) has been advocated as a method to detect abnormalities overlooked by a single reader. Most independent DR studies have demonstrated improvement in sensitivity at a cost of lowered specificity. A review of clinical independent DR studies shows detection rate improvements of 4% to 15% (30). However, recall rates (false positive) increased by 11% to 45%. One of the largest U.S. clinical DR studies showed a 6.7% increase in detection and a 11.5% increase in recall rate (31). These divergent trends for DR between sensitivity and specificity tend to balance accuracy. Taplin et al. (32), in an experimental study, showed independent DR improved sensitivity by 8.9% and decreased specificity by 13.6% similar to clinical trials. Accuracy, as determined by receiver operating characteristics (ROC) methods, did not change, suggesting that independent DR acted to shift the decision threshold toward sensitivity at the expense of specificity. DR with expert or consensus readers as the second reader appears to retain most improvements in sensitivity without large declines in specificity, but this outcome may reflect in part the expertise of the second reader.

Computer-Aided Detection

CAD systems use artificial computer intelligence in an attempt to act as a second reader. CAD mammographic systems are now commercially available. Like DR, most clinical CAD trials have shown improvement in sensitivity but declines in specificity. A CAD system functions as a second reader by placing "marks" on a mammographic site deemed suspicious. The radiologists then characterize these CAD detections. CAD can correctly identify approximately 60% to 80% of cancers with highest performance for microcalcifications. Unfortunately, CAD systems are very non-specific with two to four marks placed per every examination. It has been estimated that only 1 per 5,000 CAD marks will reflect a true positive finding, representing a unique cancer missed by the radiologist (30). The interactions between radiologist and CAD are complex but tend to mirror DR studies. Clinical studies with CAD show sensitivity improvements varying from 1.7% to 19.5% with declines in specificity as noted by increased recall rate of 0.1% to 26% (30). CAD's effect on accuracy has often been incompletely reported, so the determination whether CAD is increasing accuracy or shifting the threshold toward sensitivity has been questioned. Fenton et al. (33) showed accuracy as measured by ROC methods declined with incremental use of CAD in a retrospective clinical study of 429,345 mammograms. CAD improved sensitivity from 80.4% to 84% but resulted in loss of specificity from 90.2% to 87%. Sensitivity improvement for CAD was for ductal carcinoma *in situ* (DCIS). Invasive cancer detection decreased. The reason for this negative result is uncertain but based on other research may result from over reliance on CAD, change in radiologists reading patterns, spending less overall time in observation, and radiologists being overwhelmed with the large number of false-positive CAD marks. Although CAD remains controversial, it is in its infancy and its future is robust for detection and characterization tasks as a second reader. More effort will be required to improve the human interaction with CAD to reap its theoretical advantages. Advances in computer technology and artificial intelligence will continue at a rapid pace. Current CAD systems are best viewed as a second reader with moderate sensitivity and poor specificity. Overreliance on CAD should be avoided and may actually degrade overall reader performance if used incorrectly. CAD should never be used to discount a finding deemed by the radiologist to be suspicious.

 ## CHARACTERIZATION OF MAMMOGRAPHIC FINDINGS

Characterization is the process to determine if a suspected mammographic finding represents normal tissue, a benign finding, or potentially breast cancer. The goal of characterization is to establish a probability of malignancy and threshold the finding to determine if tissue sampling is required. This assessment is based on morphologic appearance of a finding and stability or change over time.

Mammography is not tissue specific. Some very low probability appearing abnormalities will prove to be malignant, and conversely, some high probability findings will be benign. Distinguishing between which lesions require biopsy and which can be followed involves thresholds. Most U.S. radiologists recommend biopsy for probability of cancer greater than or equal to 3% (11). Individual radiologists assess their thresholds by auditing their practices and by reviewing the frequency of malignancy for lesions recommended for biopsy (positive predictive value), their false-negative rate for lesions recommended for follow-up, tumor size, and stage (34). The U.S. Department of Health and Human Services has suggested the following as desirable goals for screening mammography, which have been attained by highly skilled experts: Positive predictive value for biopsy 25% to 40%, recall rate 5% to 10%, incident cancer detection 2 to 4 per 1,000, minimal cancer detection greater than 30%, stage 0, 1 greater than 50%, sensitivity greater than 85%, and specificity greater than 90% (10). Different patient populations will significantly impact the ability of a screening population to attain these goals.

FOOD AND DRUG ADMINISTRATION AND BREAST IMAGING REPORTING AND DATA SYSTEM FINAL ASSESSMENT CATEGORIES

In order to provide national uniformity for reporting and assessment of mammographic findings, the American College of Radiology developed a lexicon for final assessment classifications called the Breast Imaging Reporting and Data System (BI-RADS) (11). After analyzing a mammogram, radiologists classify their findings into one of five final assessment categories (2,11). MQSA requires the use of final assessment categories paralleling those of the American College of Radiology (2). This lexicon is now used internationally. The final assessment categories are presented in Table 12.1. The categories are as follows:

Category 1: negative,
Category 2: benign finding,
Category 3: probably benign finding,
Category 4: suspicious abnormality,
Category 5: highly suggestive of malignancy (risk ≥95%).

Category 4 can be subdivided by risk into 4A (low), 4B (intermediate), and 4C (moderate). Functionally, category 1 and 2 represent a normal mammogram without findings of malignancy.

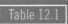

AMERICAN COLLEGE OF RADIOLOGY BREAST IMAGING REPORTING AND DATA SYSTEM (BI-RADS) ASSESSMENT CATEGORIES: MAMMOGRAPHY		

Complete Final Assessment Categories

Category 1	Negative	There is nothing to comment on. The breasts are symmetrical and no masses, architectural disturbances, or suspicious calcifications are present.
Category 2	Benign finding	Like Category 1, this is a "normal" assessment, but here, the interpreter chooses to describe a benign finding in the mammography report. Involuting, calcified fibroadenomas, multiple secretory calcifications, fat-containing lesions such as oil cysts, lipomas, galactoceles and mixed-density hamartomas all have characteristically benign appearances, and may be labeled with confidence. The interpreter may also choose to describe intramammary lymph nodes, vascular calcifications, implants or architectural distortion clearly related to a prior surgery while still concluding that there is no mammographic evidence of malignancy. Note that both Category 1 and Category 2 assessments indicate that there is no mammographic evidence of malignancy. Note that both Category 1 and Category 2 should be used when describing one or more specific benign mammographic findings in the report, whereas Category 1 should be used when no such findings are described.
Category 3	Probably benign finding; initial short interval follow-up suggested	A finding placed in this category should have less than a 2% risk of malignancy. It is not expected to change over the follow-up interval, but the radiologist would prefer to establish its stability. There are several prospective clinical studies demonstrating the safety and efficacy of initial short-term follow-up for specific mammographic findings. Three specific findings are described as being probably benign (the noncalcified circumscribed solid mass, the focal asymmetry and the cluster of round (punctate) calcifications; the latter is anecdotally considered by some radiologists to be an absolutely benign feature). All the published studies emphasize the need to conduct a complete diagnostic imaging evaluation before making a probably benign (Category 3) assessment; hence it is inadvisable to render such an assessment when interpreting a screening examination. Also, all the published studies exclude palpable lesions, so the use of a probably benign assessment for a palpable lesion is not supported by scientific data. Finally, evidence from all the published studies indicates the need for biopsy rather than continued follow-up when most probably benign findings increase in size or extent. While the vast majority of findings in this category will be managed with an initial short-term follow-up (6 months) examination followed by additional examinations until longer-term (2 years or longer) stability is demonstrated, there may be occasions where biopsy is done (patient wishes or clinical concerns).
Category 4	Suspicious abnormality; biopsy should be considered	This category is reserved for findings that do not have the classic appearance of malignancy but have a wide range of probability of malignancy that is greater than those in Category 3. Thus, most recommendations of breast interventional procedures will be placed within this category. By subdividing Category 4 into 4A, 4B, and 4C as suggested in the guidance chapter, it is encouraged that relevant probabilities for malignancy by indicated within this category so the patient and her physician can make an informed decision on the ultimate course of action.
Category 5	Highly suggestive of malignancy; appropriate action should be taken	These lesions have a high probability (7.95%) of being cancer. This category contains lesions for which one-stage surgical treatment could be considered without preliminary biopsy. However, current oncologic management may require percutaneous tissue sampling as, for example, when sentinel node imaging is included in surgical treatment or when neoadjuvant chemotherapy is administered at the outset.
Category 6	Known biopsy; proven malignancy; appropriate action should be taken	This category is reserved for lesions identified on the imaging study with biopsy proof of malignancy prior to definitive therapy.
Category 0 Incomplete	Need additional imaging evaluation and/or prior mammograms for comparison	Finding for which additional imaging evaluation is needed. This is almost always used in a screening situation. Under certain circumstances this category may be used after a full mammographic work-up. A recommendation for additional imaging evaluation may include, but is not limited to the use of spot compression, magnification, special mammographic views and ultrasound. Whenever possible, if the study is not negative and does not contain a typically benign finding, the current examination should be compared to previous studies. The radiologist should use judgment on how vigorously to attempt obtaining previous studies. Category 0 should only be used for old film comparison when such comparison is required to make a final assessment.

Routine screening mammography is recommended for follow-up Category 2 can include a normal finding, such as a calcified fibroadenoma, normal lymph node, or stable benign appearing calcifications. Category 3, probably benign, represents a finding of such low probability for malignancy that follow-up is recommended instead of biopsy. Multiple studies have established the risk of malignancy to be less than 2% (35–40). The risk of malignancy expresses itself generally over the first 2 years. Recommended management consists of a follow-up mammogram at 6 months following the initial examination with subsequent follow-up at 12 and 24 months unless biopsy is elected by the patient or physician. Diagnostic mammography should be performed prior to using the probably benign category. Most probably benign literature relates to nonpalpable mammographic findings. Categories 4 and 5 assessments are abnormalities that require tissue biopsy for diagnosis. These categories represent a broad range (3% to 100%) of risk for cancer, and experienced radiologists can render reasonable probability of malignancy estimates.

A category "incomplete" (BI-RADS 0) is used when a screening study requires additional imaging such as recall for diagnostic mammograms or comparison with older examinations prior to rendering a final assessment. An incomplete assessment is just that, incomplete. An incomplete examination should not be considered "abnormal" as most will be shown to be normal. Only after diagnostic imaging or comparison with older films can a category 1 to 5 final assessment be rendered. "Incomplete" has been used to categorize a normal mammogram in a setting of a palpable mass with assessment decision deferred to findings on ultrasonography. Although this is an acceptable use per FDA guidelines, it has lead to some confusion in the performance literature based upon BI-RADS codes alone. I prefer a definitive mammographic assessment as "negative" in this situation but recommend ultrasound examination of the palpable finding and report the sonographic finding independently. BI-RADS category 6, "known biopsy proven malignancy," can be used for cases with known malignant diagnosis.

Although BI-RADS reporting system has been favorably received, confusion can arise from patients and clinicians when a suspicious palpable or sonographic mass has a "negative" mammogram report. In these situations, tissue biopsy is recommended when the palpable or sonographic findings are suspicious even if the mammogram is negative. A negative mammogram in the presence of a suspicious clinical finding, suspicious ultrasonogram, or suspicious MRI, should never obviate a needed surgical biopsy. Mammography cannot rule out cancer.

MAMMOGRAPHIC APPEARANCE OF BREAST CANCER

There is a tendency to limit mammographic analysis to morphologic features. In practice, biologic change provides a separate axis of analysis from morphologic features. A group of four calcifications that have been present for 5 years and unchanged may be observed, while four new calcifications that were not present on a prior mammogram may be biopsied. Most mammographic cancers appear as masses, calcifications, distortion, or a combination of the three (41–44). Masses and calcification account for about 90% of all cancer appearances. Similar to the final assessment categories, a lexicon has been established by the ACR BI-RADS for describing and characterizing morphologic features (11). This lexicon use is not required by MQSA. The following discussion summarizes the lexicon. Mammographic interpretation remains a *visual* interpretation process and not a verbal descriptive process. The figures have been chosen to show a range of appearances of breast cancer, not just obvious cases.

Masses

Masses account for nearly half of all mammographic cancers. Masses refer to space occupying lesions that can be detected in two different projections. If a finding is only noted in a single CC view, it is referred to as a focal asymmetry. A focal asymmetry may or may not prove to be a "real" finding. Masses are characterized by their shape, margin, and density in order to determine a probability of malignancy.

Shape

Because of the infiltrative biologic nature of most breast cancers, irregular or lobular-shaped masses are more likely associated with malignancy than round or oval masses.

Margins

The margin between a mass and the surrounding breast tissue is the key feature for analysis of masses because it relates to the infiltrating pattern of cancer. Often, margins are obscured by breast tissue, rendering this evaluation impossible. Circumscribed, well-defined margins tend to represent a benign process (Figs. 12.2 and 12.3) such as cysts or fibroadenomas. Margins that are indistinct or microlobulated suggest infiltration into normal breast tissue and higher risk for malignancy. Smoothly marginated masses are usually subjected to ultrasound interrogation to assess if they represent a breast cyst for which no further intervention is required or a solid mass, which often requires biopsy. Masses with indistinct margins may also be interrogated with ultrasound to assess for size, character, and visibility for potential biopsy procedure. Masses with spiculated borders forming a stellate or star-type pattern of radiating lines are associated with the highest risk of malignancy. As shown in Figures 12.2 through 12.8, there is a continuum in appearance of malignant and benign masses.

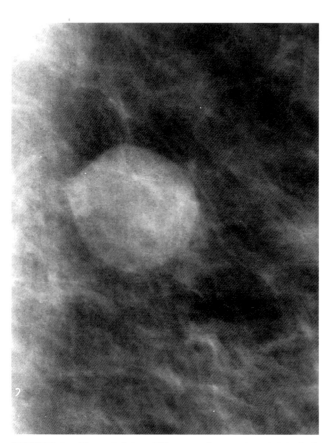

FIGURE 12.2. Smoothly marginated round 14-mm mass. Sonogram demonstrated a simple cyst.

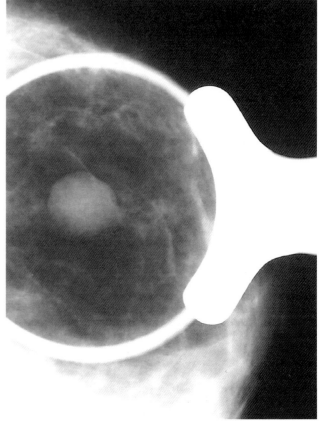

FIGURE 12.3. Spot compression view of a smoothly marginated mass proven to represent a fibroadenoma. Sonogram demonstrated a solid mass.

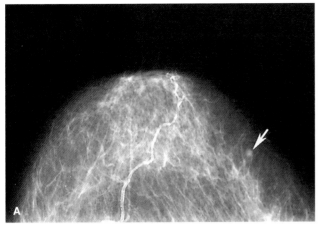

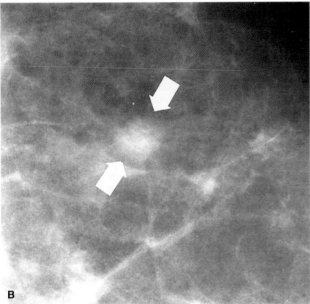

FIGURE 12.4. A: Craniocaudal screening view shows a new small focal asymmetry in the lateral aspect of the breast (*arrows*). **B:** Incidental note is made of artery calcification. Diagnostic spot compression magnification view confirms the presence of a 5-mm noncalcified mass (*arrows*). Invasive ductal carcinoma found at pathology.

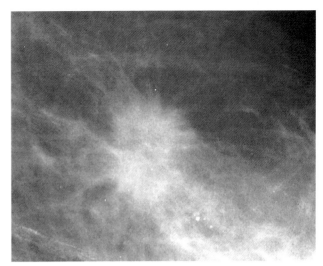

FIGURE 12.6. An 11-mm mass with spiculated borders and a few associated microcalcifications. Invasive ductal cancer and ductal carcinoma *in situ* found at pathology.

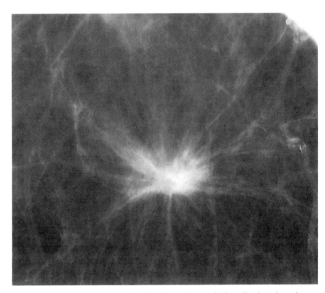

FIGURE 12.7. Mass with very spiculated borders shown to be invasive ductal carcinoma. Although the appearance is "classic" for carcinoma, most cancers found on mammography do not have a classic appearance.

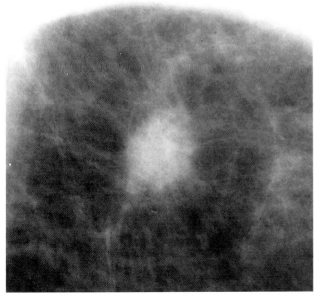

FIGURE 12.5. Spot compression view of a 10-mm mass with slightly irregular borders shown to represent invasive ductal carcinoma.

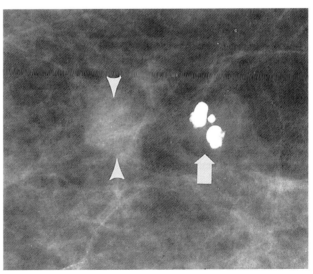

FIGURE 12.8. Unusual pairing of a classic fibroadenoma containing coarse calcifications (*arrow*) immediately adjacent to a 7-mm focal asymmetry (*arrow*) that was not present on prior screening mammogram. Although the asymmetry lacks characteristic morphology of cancer, it was not present in the previous examination and biopsy showed invasive cancer.

Mass Density

Lesions that are fat density (black on a mammogram) are benign and do not require tissue diagnosis. These typically represent lipomas or areas of traumatic fat necrosis with oil cyst formation. Certain circumscribed fat containing and fibroglandular density tissues may have appearance pathognomonic for a benign hamartoma and not require biopsy. Otherwise, density is of limited value in discriminating benign from malignant lesions, although high density is often a suspicious sign.

Calcifications

For reasons not entirely understood, calcifications are formed or are associated with breast carcinomas. Fortunately, calcifications are exquisitely detected by mammography, with particles as small as 50 μm being visible. Because calcium absorbs x-rays, they produce a bright white spot on a mammogram. This inherent contrast between calcification and background tissue is a significant reason why mammography is successful in detecting small tumors, especially those associated with DCIS. Mammography allows "elemental" imaging of calcifications. Calcifications can be seen reasonably well in dense breasts because calcium absorbs more x-ray energy than dense tissue. Unfortunately, many benign conditions such as fibrocystic change also produce breast calcifications, which at times mimic breast cancer calcifications. Some type of calcification is present on most mammograms. The radiologist is faced with a common problem regarding the nature and significance of calcifications. Magnification mammography is critical in characterizing calcifications. This allows better morphologic assessment of individual particles and clusters. Assessment of microcalcifications includes location, morphology, distribution, number, and biologic stability or progression. All of these factors are important in determining a risk of malignancy.

Location

Calcifications present within the skin may masquerade as parenchymal calcifications. These calcifications are typically small (<1 mm) with lucent centers. Radiologists can, with incremental imaging, prove with certainty that calcifications reside in the skin by tangential views. Dermal calcifications require no intervention. Other than dermal calcifications, location is of limited use in assessment.

Morphology

Artery calcifications appear as parallel lines associated with blood vessels and usually when established can be readily distinguished from linear calcifications of carcinoma. Large, coarse peripherally based "popcorn" calcifications are noted with fibroadenomas that are undergoing involution with age (Fig. 12.8). These also can be recognized as a specific benign entity and require no tissue diagnosis. Rod-like linear calcifications associated with benign ductal ectasia appear to fill ectatic ducts, are bilateral, and rather homogeneous (Fig. 12.9). In established cases, these calcifications provide no diagnostic dilemma. Early ductal ectatic calcifications may appear indistinguishable from DCIS. Calcifications containing lucent centers ("eggshell" or "rim" calcifications) are benign and associated with calcified fat necrosis and calcified cysts (Fig. 12.10). Dystrophic calcifications associated with fat necrosis often follow trauma such as surgery and irradiation. They are usually larger than 0.5 mm and have lucent centers. Calcifications that appear to layer with gravity are consistent with sedimenting calcifications within small cysts ("milk of calcium" or "microcystic adenosis"). They are ill defined on the CC view and are sharply defined on the lateral view with dependent linear calcifications within small cysts. Biopsy is not required.

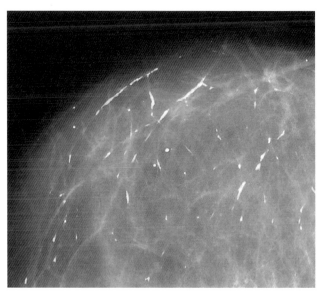

FIGURE 12.9. Benign calcifications associated with ductal ectasia. These needle-like calcifications are oriented toward the nipple in this postmenopausal woman.

Most calcifications associated with cancer are small (<0.5 mm) and often require magnification views for characterization. Malignant calcifications are notable for heterogeneity in size, shape, and geographic clustering. Malignant calcifications vary in appearance from subtle to obvious (Figs. 12.11 through 12.13) and may be associated with mass. Focal areas of amorphous indistinct calcifications are nonspecific in appearance and usually require tissue diagnosis. Positive predictive value for this type of calcification is about 20%.

High probability for cancer calcifications include pleomorphic or heterogeneous calcifications, which are fine linear or fine-linear branching calcifications conforming to a casting pattern of a duct. These calcifications are often associated with high-grade DCIS, with or without invasive cancer.

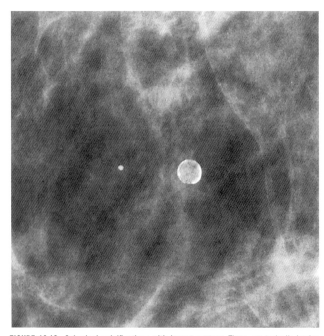

FIGURE 12.10. Spherical calcifications with lucent centers. These are typically benign calcifications associated with fat necrosis and calcified cysts.

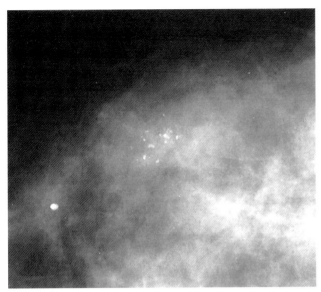

FIGURE 12.11. A 5-mm area of microcalcifications in a dense breast detected by screening mammography. Ductal carcinoma *in situ* found at pathology.

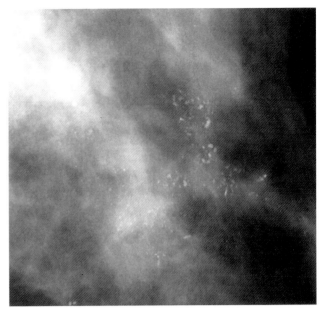

FIGURE 12.13. A 20-mm area of pleomorphic microcalcifcations in an extremely dense breast. Invasive ductal carcinoma found at pathology.

Number

Although no number absolutely distinguishes benign from malignant, attempts have been made to determine reasonable thresholds for clinical intervention based on number of calcifications in a cluster. Five or more clustered calcifications not typically benign have been a threshold advocated by some experienced readers for biopsy (45). Others have noted increased frequency of cancer with increasing number of calcification particles (46). Most radiologists incorporate number of calcifications in a cluster, their morphology, and change with time to form an assessment regarding the need to biopsy.

Distribution

Distribution of calcifications in addition to morphology, number, and biologic change helps establish a probability of malignancy.

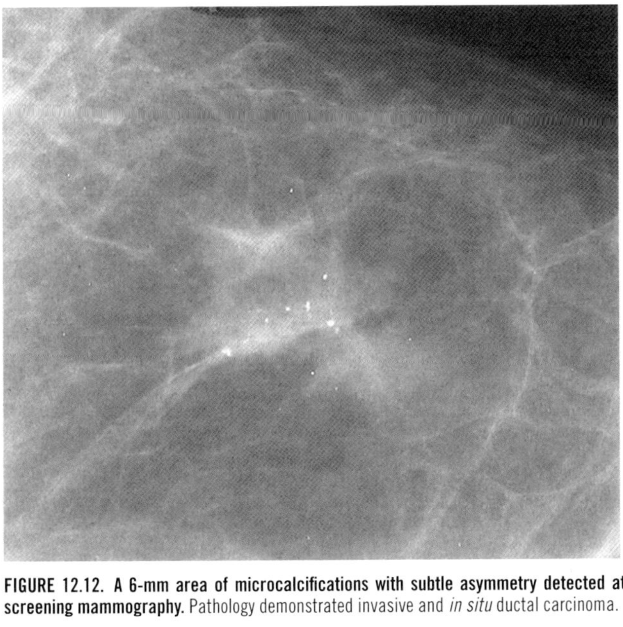

Grouped or clustered: Clustered calcifications refer to a group of calcifications in a less than 2 cm³ volume of tissue. Although "cluster" has historically been associated with malignancy, this term can be used as a neutral designator.

Linear: Calcifications that appear to be arranged within a line or duct imply a ductal origin. This is of moderate suspicion.

Segmental: Calcifications restricted to a segment or wedge-shaped portion of the breast may arise within a single ductal system and its branches. This is a distribution frequently associated with malignancy.

Diffuse/scattered: Calcifications that appear to be randomly distributed throughout the breast are referred to as diffuse or scattered. Compared to linear or segmental, scattered calcifications are associated with lower risk of malignancy. By chance, randomly distributed calcification will have areas of higher concentration of calcification particles and areas of fewer, not dissimilar to a shotgun pellet pattern. These more concentrated groups are viewed with less suspicion than a similar isolated group of calcification.

Architectural Distortion

Architectural distortion may be a very subjective appearance on a mammogram or a straightforward observation. Architectural distortion refers to an unusual pattern that includes spiculations and retraction (Fig. 12.14). Unless associated with an area of prior biopsy or area of prior infection, architectural distortion requires tissue diagnosis. A benign entity, radial sclerosing lesion, may have this appearance, but biopsy is necessary to establish histology. Skin retraction and nipple retraction carry significant risks of malignancy and require tissue biopsy.

Unusual Findings

Focal skin thickening may be associated with benign or malignant ideologies. Malignant causes would include inflammatory carcinoma (Fig. 12.15) and local skin thickening adjacent to a known carcinoma. Skin thickening may be present with benign conditions such as infection and venous obstruction. Clinical management assumes primary importance in these situations.

FIGURE 12.12. A 6-mm area of microcalcifications with subtle asymmetry detected at screening mammography. Pathology demonstrated invasive and *in situ* ductal carcinoma.

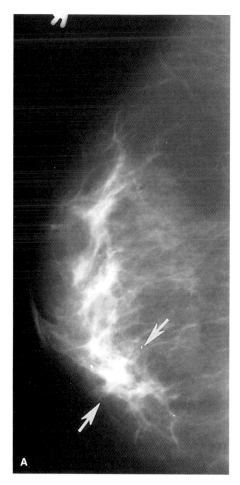

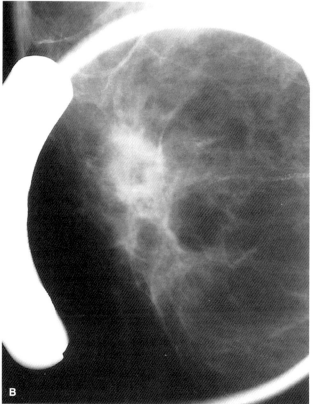

FIGURE 12.14. A: Subtle area of architectural distortion (*arrows*). **B:** Spot compression views demonstrate distortion with questionable mass to a better advantage. Invasive lobular carcinoma diagnosed at biopsy.

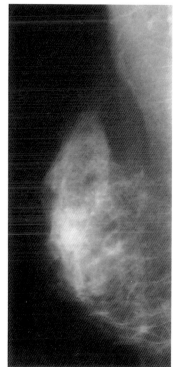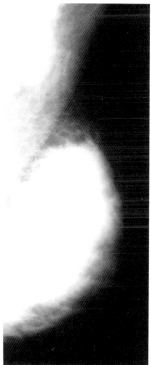

FIGURE 12.15. Bilateral mediolateral oblique mammographic views demonstrate increased density, pathologically dense axillary lymph nodes, and skin thickening on right. Inflammatory carcinoma diagnosed clinically.

Focal asymmetry describes an area that lacks the appearance of a true mass. Additional imaging and ultrasound may be required for characterization (Fig. 12.4), but this may be a very subtle manifestation of early breast cancer especially if it is a new finding.

ROLE OF THE MAMMOGRAPHY IN EVALUATION THE SYMPTOMATIC PATIENT

The evaluation of a symptomatic patient is common. Physical examination has poor specificity, with only 4% of symptomatic women found to have malignancy (23,47). The goal of mammography in this setting is to characterize the palpable finding and assess the balance of the breast. Breast ultrasound is used extensively in the setting of a symptomatic patient in addition to mammography. Use of standard practice guidelines is recommended for imaging and management of symptomatic women (48). A suspicious palpable finding should undergo surgical consultation even if imaging is negative.

Palpable Mass or Thickening

Individuals with a palpable breast abnormality such as a discrete mass or focal thickening should undergo diagnostic imaging prior to biopsy, since biopsy can alter mammographic and sonographic appearances. Women 30 years and older are recommended for mammography and sonography, women younger than 30 are initially evaluated with sonography, although mammography may be necessary in certain circumstances (48). Spot compression views of the palpable area increases sensitivity. Approximately 5% to 15% of patients with a palpable cancer will have a false-negative mammogram. This number is higher for women with extremely dense breasts and lower for women with extremely fatty breasts. An individual clinician may overestimate mammography performance due to the low incidence of cancer in the symptomatic population. Of a typical group of 250 diagnostic patients referred for mammography, there will be 10 cancers. Only 1 of the 250 will have cancer and a false-negative mammogram (assumes a 4 per 100 cancer incidence and a 10% false-negative rate), but this low number is due primarily to the low incidence of cancer rather than the superb performance of mammography. If the mammogram is negative, directed breast ultrasound is generally performed of the palpable area since most cancers with false-negative mammography will be identified as abnormal by sonography. A patient with a negative mammogram and negative ultrasound in the setting of a palpable finding is at very low risk of malignancy. The false-negative rate of combined ultrasound and mammograms at experienced breast centers is 0% to 3% (49–52). The management of patients with palpable findings with negative mammogram and ultrasound depends on the clinical assessment and patient issues. Suspicious palpatory findings should be biopsied even if imaging is negative. If biopsy is not elected for a very low clinical suspicion palpable findings with negative imaging, short-term clinical follow-up and imaging are recommended to assess for change (48).

Bloody or Serous Discharge

Mammographic sensitivity may be limited for intraductal cancer presenting as nipple discharge (53). Although sensitivity variability has been reported, a recent study showed sensitivity of 10% for mammography alone (53). If the mammogram is negative, retroareolar breast ultrasound can be performed to assess for intraductal masses or other findings. Some surgeons and radiologists recommend ductography prior to operative intervention. During ductography, a small needle is cannulated into the discharging duct and a iodinated contrast is injected. The resultant image will show delineation of the discharging duct (Fig. 12.16). Abnormalities on ductography include filling defects, obstructions, and cysts. Characterization of benign and

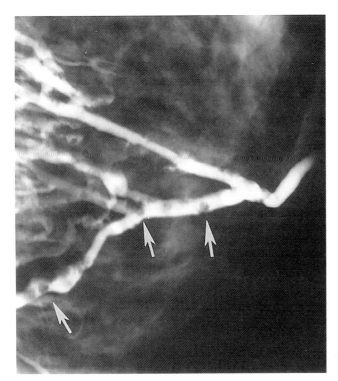

FIGURE 12.16. Ductogram performed for bloody nipple discharge. Multiple intraluminal irregular filling defects noted within the contrast filled (*white*) ductal system (*arrowheads*). Extensive ductal carcinoma *in situ* was found at surgical biopsy.

malignant filling defects by ductography is not sufficient to distinguish benign papilloma from DCIS. Filling defects or stenoses requires surgical excision to determine histologic cause. Rarely, a ductogram may demonstrate a distal intraductal mass, which may not be reached during routine retroareolar duct surgery. In this situation, the intraluminal mass can be localized for the surgeon to ensure proper excision. A negative ductogram, mammogram, or ultrasound in a setting of a clinically suspicious nipple discharge should not dissuade surgical excision (48).

Skin Changes or Inflammatory Breast Findings

Women presenting with inflammatory breast findings are referred for diagnostic mammography and often sonography. The distinction between inflammatory cancer and infection is frequently not possible by imaging alone as both may show skin changes, interstitial edema, and abnormal axillary lymph nodes (54). Unless a suspicious mass or calcification is found, which would direct biopsy, urgent clinical evaluation is recommended. Sonography may detect a fluid collection consistent with abscess, which can be confirmed with aspiration. For those women initially treated with antibiotics for suspected mastitis, very short-term clinical re-evaluation to ensure resolution is imperative. Early surgical consultation is recommended for nonresponders (48).

Axillary Lymph Node Presentation of Breast Cancer

Less than 1% of women with breast cancer will present with an axillary mass found to represent metastatic breast cancer in axillary lymph nodes with normal breast physical examination. Diagnostic mammography should be performed of both breasts to assess for occult breast cancer. If mammography is negative, breast MR has been advocated since up to 86% of such cases will demonstrate the breast primary by MR (55). Some radiologists perform whole breast sonographic screening at time of mammography to assess for an occult primary.

Symptomatic Pregnant and Lactating Women

Sonography is the initial imaging evaluation of pregnant and lactating women, many of whom have never been screened due to young age, although mammography may be also useful in some cases to assess for calcifications (56–58). Due to the extremely low fetal radiation dose, mammography is not contradicted when sonography or physical findings are suspicious for cancer. Mammographic sensitivity has been reported to be as high as 90%, albeit for large tumors (57). The radiation dose of a two-view mammogram to the uterus or fetus is less than 1 per 10,000 the breast dose (0.03 μGy or 0.003 mrad), which is further reduced by a factor of 2 to 7 with shielding (59). To put this dose in perspective, the natural background radiation exposure in the United States is about 1 mrem per day.

NEWLY DIAGNOSED BREAST CANCER

Diagnostic mammography has an important and critical role in evaluating the patient's eligibility for breast conservation therapy. Morrow (60) showed that diagnostic mammography, physical exam, and pathologic analysis could correctly determine 97% of patients' eligibility for breast conservation versus mastectomy. Extensive calcifications associated with DCIS by mammography are generally a contraindication to breast conservation therapy. Multicentric disease by mammography is also a contraindication to breast conservation therapy. Review of patients' mammograms after histologic diagnosis of breast cancer may change surgical management. Newman et al. (61) reported 10.7% patients had a change in management after mammographic review at a multidisciplinary academic center and 7% incremental detection of cancer. The impact on survival is unknown. Magnification mammography is routinely used in the setting of breast cancer manifested as microcalcifications to assess extent. Following lumpectomy with negative pathologic margins, mammography is recommended in cases with malignant calcifications to ensure excision. Suspicious residual calcifications should be subject to re-excision prior to radiation therapy. The use of MR is controversial and covered in Chapter 14.

BREAST-CONSERVATION–TREATED PATIENT SURVEILLANCE

Mammographic surveillance following breast conservation therapy (BCT) is typically performed at 6 months, 12 months, and then yearly, although variations exist and the optimal intervals have not been established. Because normal post-BCT changes can mimic cancer by mammography, the first mammogram can serve as a baseline for future evaluations. Typical findings such as mass, edema, and skin thickening are observed. Since these mammographic findings can be signs of malignancy, specificity of mammography is low, so aggressive mammographic interpretation at the first post-BCT examination in women with a margin negative cancer is not appropriate. The reported sensitivity of mammography for detection of in breast recurrence is variable (62). Voogd (63) showed only 25% of recurrences were detected solely by mammography between 1980 to 1992. More recently, Vapiwala et al. (64) reported 68% of local recurrences (including skin) were positive by mammography. The biopsy positive predictive value was higher for mammography than physical examination (65% vs. 40%) and was highest when both mammography and physical examination were abnormal (79%), showing the complementary role of imaging and physical examination. Mammographic surveillance following BCT for DCIS appears reasonable at detection of recurrences, although data are limited. Pinsky et al. (65) found 97% of recurrences after BCT for DCIS were apparent by mammography and 91% were minimal cancer (DCIS and invasive cancer <1 cm) at detection.

Symptomatic Males

Men presenting with palpable findings may undergo mammographic imaging, although some clinicians proceed directly to biopsy when the clinical findings are suspicious. The normal male breast is entirely fatty. Gynecomastia presents as retroareolar mammographic density without calcification that may be asymmetric. This often has a characteristic flame-like pattern of distribution and does not appear mass-like. Enlarged breast due to excessive adipose tissue (pseudogynecomastia) appears as fat on mammography and requires no further evaluation. The mammographic findings of male carcinoma are similar to female cancer, but microcalcifications are unusual (Fig. 12.17). Mammography is very sensitive for breast cancer detection due to the lack of breast tissue in most men, with negative predictive values of 99% to 100% reported (66,67). Because some unusual forms of gynecomastia may appear mass-like by mammography, biopsy is required in these cases to establish the diagnosis. Similar to women, a suspicious palpatory finding in the setting of a negative mammogram should not deter biopsy.

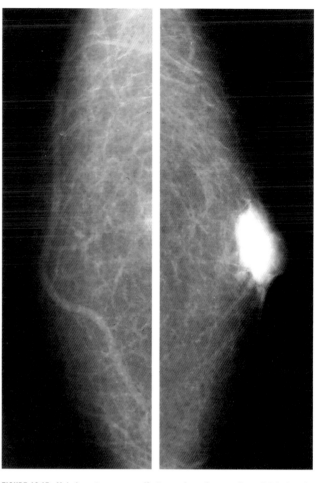

FIGURE 12.17. Male breast cancer manifest as an irregular mass immediately deep to the nipple on right. The patient's left mammogram is entirely fatty.

SCREENING: SPECIAL SITUATIONS

Screening mammography of high-risk women is performed in a manner similar to routine screening but at an earlier age. Early screening (prior to age 40) has been advocated for women treated with chest mantle radiation during youth, genetic carriers of breast cancer genes such as *BRCA1* and *BRCA2*, other genetic risks, and women with strong premenopausal family history with both annual mammography and MR (48,68). This screening may start as early as age 25. There are no randomized controlled trials to show survival benefit. Mammographic appearance of cancer in some high-risk groups may be similar to the population in general (69). However, because these are young women, mammography may be less sensitive due to higher frequency of dense breasts and possible aggressive tumor biology. The use of digital mammography in young women with dense breasts may improve sensitivity (4).

MAMMOGRAPHIC ASSESSMENT OF BREAST DENSITY AS A RISK FACTOR

Mammographic breast density is an independent risk factor for breast carcinoma (70–73). Fibroglandular tissue attenuates x-rays and produces a white (dense) area on a mammogram. Fatty areas of the breast do not attenuate x-rays as much and produce a dark (nondense) area on the mammogram.

Mammography cannot discriminate between density attributed to fibrotic tissue and that attributed to glandular tissue. Estimation of breast density can be made qualitatively using the four-category BI-RADS classification:

1. entirely fat,
2. scattered fibroglandular densities,
3. heterogeneously dense, and
4. extremely dense (11) (Fig. 12.18)

This density classification scheme was developed to address the issue of mammographic sensitivity rather than the estimation of risk. More quantitative measurements can be made with computer software programs (11,74). Thresholds between the white and nonwhite tissue are not absolute and will influence reproducibility and accuracy. Although these classifications have merit, there is variability among readers (75). Although breast density is correlated with risk, changes in breast density may or may not be associated with changing risk (76,77). Breast density has not been shown to be a causative factor for breast cancer.

 ## FACTORS AFFECTING MAMMOGRAPHIC SENSITIVITY

The ability of mammography to detect cancer varies greatly among patients. Factors affecting sensitivity and specificity include breast density, age, hormone replacement therapy, biologic subtypes of cancer, and breast thickness.

Breast Density

There is enormous variability in density among breasts, from those that are almost entirely fibroglandular in appearance to those that are almost entirely fatty in appearance (Fig. 12.18). About half of screened women have BI-RADS fatty or scattered density classification. Breast cancer attenuates x-rays and appears as a white density. A white density against a black (fatty) background is easy to detect (high signal to noise ratio). A white density cancer against a white background of fibroglandular tissue is difficult and in many situations, impossible to detect. The normal dense tissue camouflages the cancer. Extensive breast density has been associated with higher frequency of false-negative mammograms (78–82). Whether these differences relate entirely to imaging by the masking of cancers by dense tissue or to more aggressive tumor biology occurring in women with dense breasts is unknown. At the author's institution, mammographic sensitivity for fatty breasts is nearly 99% but may be as low as 69% for extremely dense breasts (82). The relative insensitivity of mammography in women with dense breasts is a significant limitation of the technique. Alternative methods of imaging these individuals with ultrasound, MRI, tomosynthesis, and digital mammography are ongoing investigations.

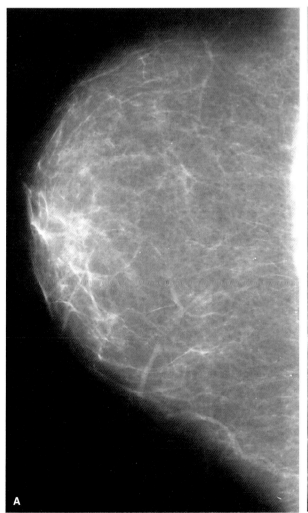
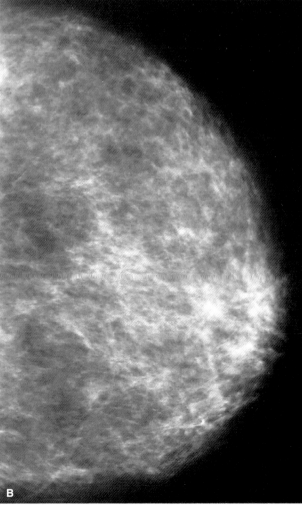

FIGURE 12.18. A: Spectrum of breast density showing fatty, scattered fibroglandular density **(B)**, heterogeneously dense, *(continued)*

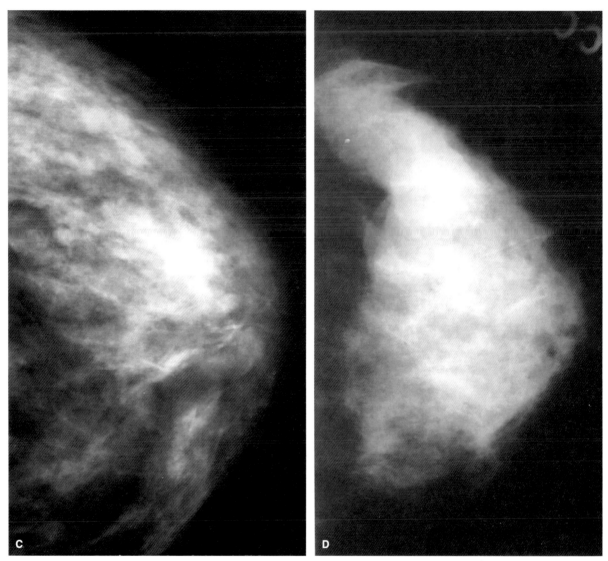

FIGURE 12.18. *(Continued).* **(C)**, and extremely dense **(D)**. Mammographic sensitivity is highest in fatty breasts and lowest in extremely dense breasts.

Age

Breast density generally declines with age. Variations exist to defy this trend, and postmenopausal hormone replacement therapy can reverse this trend so that age alone rarely is a useful factor in assessing mammographic density. Benign processes that mimic cancers such as fibrocystic changes are less common in the elderly. For these reasons the accuracy of mammography is highest in older women compared to younger women (23,81, 83,84).

Hormone Therapy

Hormone therapy is associated with increases in breast density (Fig. 12.19) in some women, especially those products containing estrogen and progestin (76). This may mask cancers and limit detection of developing asymmetries. Some drugs such as tamoxifen used for chemosuppression have been associated with a decrease in breast density. Theoretically, this should allow easier detection of malignancy.

Biologic Subtypes

Invasive lobular cancer (ILC) is difficult to detect by mammography prior to clinical presentation (85,86). The infiltrative pattern of ILC often does not produce a recognizable mass by mammography when small. Additionally, only 5% of ILC is associated with microcalcifications. ILC is detected at a larger size than invasive ductal carcinoma and represents a disproportionate number of false-negative mammograms. Invasive mucinous or medullary cancers and some anaplastic cancers may appear as a circumscribed mass mimicking benign conditions such as cysts or fibroadenomas and can produce mischaracterization. Detection is not affected. Sonographic evaluation demonstrates solid masses, and biopsy establishes the diagnosis.

Patient Factors

Achieving optimal mammographic position requires full patient cooperation. Portions of the breast may not be imaged, especially areas adjacent to the chest wall, which become a silent area for mammography (5,6). Mammographic image quality declines as breast thickness increases (6). The decline is due to loss of geometric sharpness, contrast, and increased motion. Breast thickness generally increases with body mass index (87). It is unknown if cancer detection is adversely effected. Breast implants, especially those placed anterior to the pectoral muscle, may limit mammographic sensitivity even when implant-displaced views are performed. The implant absorbs x-rays, which precludes mammographic display of portions of the breast.

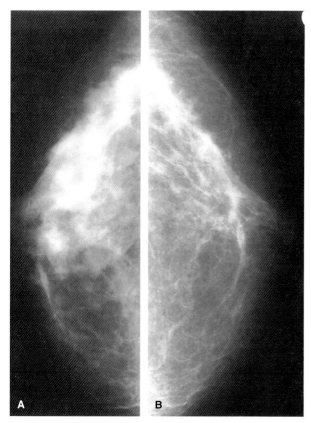

FIGURE 12.19. Effect of exogenous hormone therapy on breast density. Examinations are taken 1 year apart. **A:** Demonstrates increased density (category heterogeneously dense) while on hormone therapy. **B:** Demonstrates diminished breast density (category scattered fibroglandular density) off hormone therapy.

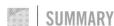 | SUMMARY

High-quality mammography has dramatically changed the evaluation of women for breast cancer in the past 20 years. Age appropriate routine screening mammography is recommended. Diagnostic breast imaging of symptomatic individuals can assist characterization of palpable findings. However, clinically suspicious abnormalities should be surgically evaluated even when breast-imaging examinations are normal.

References

1. National Cancer Institute. *NCI statement on mammography screening.* Bethesda, MD: NCI, 2002.
2. U.S. Department of Health and Human Services. Food and Drug Administration. Quality mammography standards. Final rule. *Fed Register* 1997;62:208.
3. Lewin JM, D'Orsi CJ, Hendrick RE, et al. Clinical comparison of full-field digital mammography and screen-film mammography for detection of breast cancer. *AJR Am J Roentgenol* 2002;179:671–677.
4. Pisano ED, Gatsonis C, Hendrick E, et al. Diagnostic performance of digital versus film mammography for breast-cancer screening. *N Engl J Med* 2005;353:1773–1783.
5. Bassett L, Hirbawi I, DeBruhl N, et al. Mammographic positioning: evaluation from the view box. *Radiology* 1993;188:803–806.
6. Helvie M, Chan H, Adler D, et al. Breast thickness in routine mammograms: effect on image quality and radiation dose. *AJR Am J Roentgenol* 1994;163:1371–1374.
7. Moskowitz M. Screening is not diagnosis. *Radiology* 1979;133:265–268.
8. Sickles E, Weber W, Galvin H, et al. Mammographic screening: how to operate successfully at low cost. *Radiology* 1986;160:95–97.
9. Bird R, McLelland R. How to initiate and operate a low-cost screening mammography center. *Radiology* 1986;161:43–47.
10. U.S. Department of Health and Human Services. *Quality determinants of mammography.* AHCPR Publication No. 95-0632. Clinical Practice Guideline 1994.
11. American College of Radiology. *Breast Imaging Reporting and Data System* (BI-RADS). Reston, VA: ACR, 2003.
12. Moss J, Steinhauer J. Mammogram clinic's flaws highlight gaps in U.S. rules. *New York Times* Oct. 22, 2002, p.A22.
13. Beam CA, Sullivan DC, Layde PM. Effect of human variability on independent double reading in screening mammography. *Acad Radiol* 1996;3:891–897.
14. Karssemeijer N, Otten J, Verbeek A, et al. Computer-aided detection versus independent double reading of masses on mammograms. *Radiology* 2003;227:192–200.
15. Sickles E, Wolverton D, Dee K. Performance parameters for screening and diagnostic mammography: specialist and general radiologists. *Radiology* 2002;224:861–869.
16. Thurfjell E, Lernevall K, Taube A. Benefit of independent double reading in a population-based mammography screening program. *Radiology* 1994;191:241–244.
17. Yankaskas B, Schell M, Bird R, et al. Reassessment of breast cancers missed during routine screening mammography: a community-based study. *AJR Am J Roentgenol* 2001;177:535–541.
18. Kopans D. The accuracy of mammographic interpretation. *N Engl J Med* 1994;331:1521–1522.
19. Beam C, Conant E, Sickles E. Association of volume and volume-independent factors with accuracy in screening mammogram interpretation. *J Natl Cancer Inst* 2003;95:282–290.
20. Elmore JG, Wells CK, Lee CH, et al. Variability in radiologists' interpretations of mammograms. *N Engl J Med* 1994;331:1493–1499.
21. Elmore JH, Miglioretti D, Carney P. Does practice make perfect when interpreting mammography? Part II. *J Natl Cancer Inst* 2003;95:250–252.
22. Rosenberg RD, Yankaskas BC, Abraham LA, et al. Performance benchmarks for screening mammography. *Radiology* 2006;241:55–66.
23. Miglioretti DL, Smith-Bindman R, Abraham L, et al. Radiologist characteristics associated with interpretive performance of diagnostic mammography. *J Natl Cancer Inst* 2007;99:1854–1863.
24. Moskowitz M. Retrospective reviews of breast cancer screening: what do we really learn from them? *Radiology* 1996;199:615–620.
25. Yankaskas BC, Cleveland RJ, Schell MJ, et al. Association of recall rates with sensitivity and positive predictive values of screening mammography. *AJR Am J Roentgenol* 2001;177:543–549.
26. Otten JDM, Karssemeijer N, Hendriks JHCL, et al. Effect of recall rate on earlier screen detection of breast cancers based on the Dutch performance indicators. *J Natl Cancer Inst* 2005;97:748–754.
27. Gur D, Sumkin J, Hardesty L, et al. Recall and detection rates in screening mammography. *Cancer* 2004;100:1590–1594.
28. Nodine CF, Mello-Thoms C, Kundel HL, et al. Time course of perception and decision making during mammographic interpretation. *AJR Am J Roentgenol* 2002;179:917–923.
29. Krupinski EA. Visual search of mammographic images: influence of lesion subtlety 1. *Acad Radiol* 2005;12:965–969.
30. Helvie MA. Improving mammographic interpretation: double reading and computer-aided diagnosis. *Radiol Clin North Am* 2007;45:801–811.
31. Harvey SC, Geller B, Oppenheimer RG, et al. Increase in cancer detection and recall rates with independent double interpretation of screening mammography. *AJR Am J Roentgenol* 2003;180:1461–1467.
32. Taplin SH, Rutter CM, Elmore JG, et al. Accuracy of screening mammography using single versus independent double interpretation. *AJR Am J Roentgenol* 2000;174:1257–1262.
33. Fenton JJ, Taplin SH, Carney PA, et al. Influence of computer-aided detection on performance of screening mammography. *N Engl J Med* 2007;356:1399–1409.
34. Sickles E, Ominsky S, Solitto R, et al. Medical audit of a rapid-throughput mammography screening practice: methodology and results of 27,114 examinations. *Radiology* 1990;175:323–327.
35. Helvie M, Pennes D, Rebner M, et al. Mammographic follow-up of low-suspicion lesions: compliance rate and diagnostic yield. *Radiology* 1991;178:155–158.
36. Sickles E. Nonpalpable, circumscribed, noncalcified solid breast masses: likelihood of malignancy based on lesion size and age of patient. *Radiology* 1994;192:439–442.
37. Sickles EA. Periodic mammographic follow-up of probably benign lesions: results in 3,184 consecutive cases. *Radiology* 1991;179:463–468.
38. Varas X, Leborgne J, Leborgne F, et al. Revisiting the mammographic follow-up of BI-RADS category 3 lesions. *AJR Am J Roentgenol* 2002;179:691–695.
39. Vizcaino I, Gadea L, Andreo L, et al. Short-term follow-up results in 795 nonpalpable probably benign lesions detected at screening mammography. *Radiology* 2001;219:475–483.
40. Rosen E, Baker J, Scott Soo M. Malignant lesions initially subjected to short-term mammographic follow-up. *Radiology* 2002;223:221–228.
41. Moskowitz M. The predictive value of certain mammographic signs in screening for breast cancer. *Cancer* 1983;51:1007–1011.
42. Ciatto S, Cataliotti L, Distante V. Nonpalpable lesions detected with mammography: review of 512 consecutive cases. *Radiology* 1987;165:99–102.
43. D'Orsi C, Kopans D. Mammographic feature analysis. *Semin Roentgenol* 1993;28:204–230.
44. Sickles E. Mammographic features of 300 consecutive nonpalpable breast cancers. *AJR Am J Roentgenol* 1986;176:661–663.
45. Egan R, McSweeney M, Sewell C. Intramammary calcifications without an associated mass in benign and malignant diseases. *Radiology* 1980;137:1–7.
46. de Lafontan B, Daures J, Salicru B, et al. Isolated clustered microcalcifications: diagnostic value of mammography—series of 400 cases with surgical verification. *Radiology* 1994;190:479–483.
47. Barton M, Elmore J, Fletcher S. Breast symptoms among women enrolled in a health maintenance organization: frequency, evaluation, and outcome. *Ann Intern Med* 1999;130:651–657.
48. National Comprehensive Cancer Network (NCCN). Breast cancer screening and diagnostic guidelines. 2007. Available at http://www.nccn.org/professionals/physician_gls/PDF/breast-screening.pdf. December 12, 2008.
49. Dennis M, Parker S, Klaus A, et al. Breast biopsy avoidance: the value of a normal mammogram and normal sonogram in the setting of a palpable lump. *Radiology* 2001;219:186–191.
50. Kaiser J, Helvie M, Blacklaw R, et al. Palpable breast thickening: role of mammography and US in cancer detection. *Radiology* 2002;223:839–844.
51. Moy L, Slanetz P, Moore R, et al. Specificity of mammography and US in the evaluation of a palpable abnormality: retrospective review. *Radiology* 2002;225:176–181.
52. Scott Soo M, Rosen E, Baker J, et al. Negative predictive value of sonography with mammography in patients with palpable breast lesions. *AJR Am J Roentgenol* 2001;177:1167–1170.

53. Adepoju LJ, Chun J, El-Tamer M, et al. The value of clinical characteristics and breast-imaging studies in predicting a histopathologic diagnosis of cancer or high-risk lesion in patients with spontaneous nipple discharge. *Am J Surg* 2005; 190:644–646.

54. Chow C. Imaging in inflammatory breast carcinoma. *Breast Dis* 2005,2006; 22:45–54.

55. Orel SG, Weinstein SP, Schnall MD, et al. Breast MR imaging in patients with axillary node metastases and unknown primary malignancy. *Radiology* 1999;212: 543–549.

56. Obenauer S, Dammert S. Palpable masses in breast during lactation. *Clin Imaq* 2007;31:1–5.

57. Ahn BY, Kim HH, Moon WK, et al. Pregnancy and lactation associated breast cancer: mammographic and sonographic findings. *J Ultrasound Med* 2003;22: 491–497.

58. Yang WT, Dryden MJ, Gwyn K, et al. Imaging of breast cancer diagnosed and treated with chemotherapy during pregnancy. *Radiology* 2006;239:52–60.

59. Sechopoulos I, Suryanarayanan S, Vedantham S, et al. Radiation dose to organs and tissues from mammography: Monte Carlo and phantom study. *Radiology* 2008;246(2):434–443.

60. Morrow M. Management of nonpalpable breast lesions. *Prin Pract Oncol* 1990; 4:1–11.

61. Newman E, Guest A, Helvie M, et al. Changes in surgical management resulting from case review at a breast cancer multidisciplinary tumor board. *Cancer* 2006; 107:2346–2351.

62. de Bock GH, Bonnema J, van Der Hage J, et al. Effectiveness of routine visits and routine tests in detecting isolated locoregional recurrences after treatment for early-stage invasive breast cancer: a meta-analysis and systematic review. *J Clin Oncol* 2004;22:4010–4018.

63. Voogd AC. Local recurrence after breast conservation therapy for early stage breast carcinoma. *Cancer* 1999;85:437–446.

64. Vapiwala N, Starzyk J, Harris EE, et al. biopsy findings after breast conservation therapy for early-stage invasive breast cancer. *Int J Radiat Oncol Biol Physics* 2007;69:490–497.

65. Pinsky RW, Rebner M, Pierce LJ, et al. Recurrent cancer after breast-conserving surgery with radiation therapy for ductal carcinoma in situ: mammographic features, method of detection, and stage of recurrence. *AJR Am J Roentgenol* 2007; 189:140–144.

66. Evans GFF, Anthony T, Appelbaum AH, et al. The diagnostic accuracy of mammography in the evaluation of male breast disease. *Am J Surg* 2001;181:96–100.

67. Patterson SK, Helvie MA, Aziz K, et al. Outcome of men presenting with clinical breast problems: the role of mammography and ultrasound. *Breast J* 2006;12: 418–423.

68. Saslow D, Boetes C, Burke W, et al. American Cancer Society guidelines for breast screening with MRI as an adjunct to mammography. *CA Cancer J Clin* 2007;57: 75–89.

69. Helvie M, Roubdioux M, Weber G, et al. Mammography of breast carcinoma in women who have the breast cancer gene *BRCA1*: initial experience. *AJR Am J Roentgenol* 1997;168:1599–1602.

70. Boyd NF, Dite GS, Stone J, et al. Heritability of mammographic density, a risk factor for breast cancer. *N Engl J Med* 2002;347:886–894.

71. Boyd N, Lockwood G, Byng J, et al. Mammographic densities and breast cancer risk. *Cancer Epidemiol Biomark Prevent* 1998;7:1133–1144.

72. Heine JJ, Malhotra P. Mammographic tissue, breast cancer risk, serial image analysis, and digital mammography, part 1. *Acad Radiol* 2002;9:298–316.

73. Vachon CM, Kuni CC, Anderson K, et al. Association of mammographically defined percent breast density with epidemiologic risk factors for breast cancer (United States). *Cancer Causes Control* 2000;11:653–662.

74. Zhou C, Chan H-P, Petrick N, et al. Computerized image analysis: estimation of breast density on mammograms. *Med Physics* 2001;28:1056–1069.

75. Martin KE, Helvie MA, Zhou C, et al. Mammographic density measured with quantitative computer-aided method: comparison with radiologists' estimates and BI-RADS categories. *Radiology* 2006;240:656–665.

76. Greendale GA, Reboussin BA, Slone S, et al. Postmenopausal hormone therapy and change in mammographic density. *J Natl Cancer Inst* 2003;95:30–37.

77. Chlebowski R, McTiernan A. Biological significance of interventions that change breast density. *J Natl Cancer Inst* 2003;95:4–5.

78. Barlow WE, Lehman CD, Zheng Y, et al. Performance of diagnostic mammography for women with signs or symptoms of breast cancer. *J Natl Cancer Inst* 2002; 94:1151–1159.

79. Kolb T, Lichy J, Newhouse J. Comparison of the performance of screening mammography, physical examination, and breast US and evaluation of factors that influence them: an analysis of 27,825 patient evaluations. *Radiology* 2002;225: 165–175.

80. Mandelson MT, Oestreicher N, Porter PL, et al. Breast density as a predictor of mammographic detection: comparison of interval- and screen-detected cancers. *J Natl Cancer Inst* 2000;92:1081–1087.

81. Rosenberg R, Hunt W, Williamson M. Effects of age, breast density, ethnicity, and estrogen replacement therapy on screening mammographic sensitivity and cancer stage at diagnosis: review of 183,134 screening mammograms in Albuquerque, New Mexico. *Radiology* 1998;92:1081–1087.

82. Roubidoux MA, Bailey JE, Wray LA, et al. Invasive cancers detected after breast cancer screening yielded a negative result: relationship of mammographic density to tumor prognostic factors. *Radiology* 2004;230:42–48.

83. Wilson T, Helvie M, August D. Breast cancer in the elderly patient: early detection with mammography. *Radiology* 1994;190:203–207.

84. Gabriel H, Wilson T, Helvie M. Breast cancer in women 65–74 years old: earlier detection by mammographic screening. *AJR Am J Roentgenol* 1997;168: 23–27.

85. Helvie M, Paramagul C, Oberman H, et al. Invasive lobular carcinoma: imaging features and clinical detection. *Invest Radiol* 1993;28:202–207.

86. Hilleren D, Andersson I, Lindholm K, et al. Invasive lobular carcinoma: mammographic findings in a 10-year experience. *Radiology* 1991;178:149–154.

87. Guest AR, Helvie MA, Chan H-P, et al. Adverse effects of increased body weight on quantitative measures of mammographic image quality. *AJR Am J Roentgenol* 2000;175:805–810.

Chapter 13
Breast Ultrasound

Nagi F. Khouri

The remarkable technological developments of ultrasound over the past 18 years have made it an indispensable tool in the evaluation of the breast (1). Ultrasound plays a role in almost every clinical or imaging problem of the breast. Ultrasound is highly accurate, readily available, and remains relatively financially accessible. This imaging technique contributes complementary information to other imaging modalities such as mammography and magnetic resonance imaging (MRI) and provides exclusive information not detected on a mammogram because of a clinical problem (lump, nipple discharge).

Indications for the use of breast ultrasound include:

- Characterization of palpable mass and distinction from lumpiness.
- Evaluation of mammographically detected mass, developing density, or focal asymmetry.
- Evaluation of a finding suspicious for cancer.
- Evaluation of extent of disease in a newly discovered breast cancer: multifocality, multicentricity, axillary adenopathy in the ipsilateral breast, and occult cancer in the contralateral breast.
- Evaluation of clinically significant nipple discharge.
- Evaluation of the inflamed breast: mastitis, abscess, or inflammatory carcinoma.
- Evaluation of the postoperative surgical bed.
- Evaluation of locally advanced breast cancer before, during, and after preoperative chemotherapy.
- Evaluation of MRI-detected, mammographically occult lesion (second-look ultrasound).
- Evaluation of possible problem with implants.
- Guidance for interventional procedures (discussed in Chapter 16).
- Screening for high-risk individuals with dense breasts (discussed in Chapters 11 and 14).

 ## EQUIPMENT

High-quality breast ultrasound requires the best equipment available. Optimal resolution must be achieved for both near field and far field. Spatial and contrast resolution must be optimal to better differentiate various types of tissues from each other and to enhance the conspicuity of discrete lesions.

A high-resolution, linear array, electronically focused high-frequency transducer of at least 10 MHz and a wide dynamic range are the minimum requirements, as recommended by the American College of Radiology (2). Transducers are available with frequencies ranging from 5 to 15 MHz. Technical advances in high-frequency transducer design allow high resolution of superficial structures and up to 4 cm of depth. Standoff pads are rarely needed to optimize near-field visualization. Occasionally, 5 MHz linear transducers are helpful in examining thick, noncompressible breasts, such as lactating or inflamed breasts, and in attempting better delineation of deep lesions. Conventional transducers measure 3.8 to 5 cm along the long axis. Extended or panoramic view, an option offered by some manufacturers, offers better visualization of large lesions or multiple adjacent lesions on one image (Fig. 13.1A).

Manufacturers continuously try to improve the resolution of ultrasound systems. Recent developments include automatic tissue optimization, spatial compounding, harmonics, elastography, and three-dimensional ultrasound.

Automatic tissue optimization is an algorithm that generates, at the press of a button, images that are optimized for the tissue components as they change from region to region.

Spatial compounding results from the transmission of ultrasound waves from different view angles on the transducer and subsequent reconstruction of the image. This results in a reduction of the speckle artifact, improved contrast, and a sharper image with better definition of lesion borders (Fig. 13.1B,C). Conversely, enhanced through transmission, seen with typical cysts, and shadowing, seen with cancer and dense solid masses, are reduced.

Harmonics improves signal-to-noise ratio by receiving only high-frequency echoes at double the transmitted frequency (3). Echoes not at high frequency are canceled, thereby reducing artifacts and resulting in improved resolution and a better image. Harmonics enhances the contrast between focal breast lesions and the surrounding tissues as well as the conspicuity, border definition, and content definition of lesions.

Color Doppler sonography allows an assessment of vascularization of a lesion in the breast and has been used to differentiate malignant from benign lesions (4–6). Although malignant tumors show vascularization more often than benign lesions, the presence or absence of vascularization is frequent enough in both types of lesions (Fig. 13.2A,B,C). This makes color Doppler an unreliable tool to differentiate benign from malignant lesions. Nevertheless, whenever blood flow is detected within a lesion in the breast, biopsy is almost always recommended, except in cases of a recognized lymph node.

Elastography's potential benefit in breast ultrasound is based on differences in compressibility between breast cancers and benign lesions (7,8). Although elastography is commercially available it remains an investigational tool. If found reliable, elastography may reduce the number of biopsies of benign lesions when the elasticity score indicates a high level of certainty for a benign mass. Ultrasound elasticity images are different from those of conventional ultrasound (Fig. 13.3A,B). For example, a benign lesion such as a fibroadenoma will appear smaller in the elasticity image than in conventional ultrasound; conversely, cancers appear larger in the elasticity image than in conventional ultrasound. Additional large-scale studies are needed to evaluate the contribution of elastography to patient care and management.

Three dimensional (3D) ultrasound, requiring a different transducer, offers visualization of any plane of a lesion once the 3D image is acquired. This helps solve the problem of nonstandardized documentation and subjective selection of images taken. In addition, the coronal plane, which is unique to 3D imaging, offers improved characterization of lesions by better demonstration of retraction and spiculation (Fig. 13.4A,B). In recent studies, 3D imaging was found to be superior to 2D imaging in terms of lesion contrast and characterization of the masses (9–11). Although the information obtained from 3D ultrasound is different from that of 2D ultrasound, diagnostic accuracy does not appear to be significantly different. Additional studies are still needed to evaluate this technology.

Unsuccessful in the 1980s, automated whole breast ultrasound is still a target for technological development in an attempt to overcome the drawbacks of current ultrasound technology manpower requirements. Exciting potential applications on the horizon include the fusion of modalities such as mammography with ultrasound.

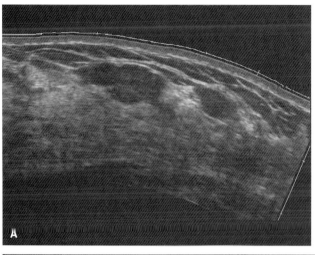

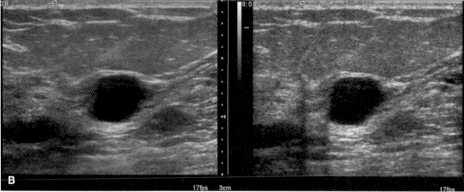

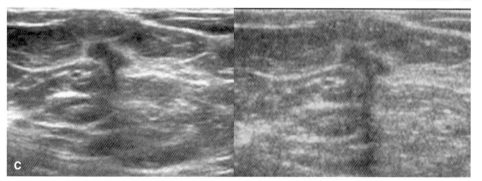

FIGURE 13.1. A: Panoramic Imaging. **B,C:** Comparison of spatial compound imaging (*left*) and standard high-resolution ultrasound shows reduced speckle and sharper image. **B:** Simple cyst. **C:** Cancer. (A and B reprinted with permission from Siemens Medical Solutions, Malvern, PA.)

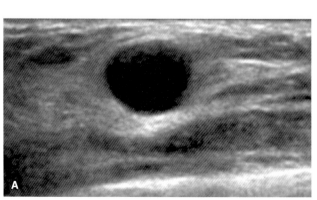

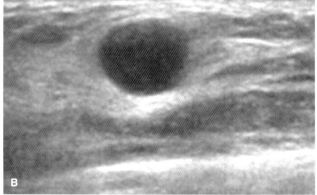

FIGURE 13.2. A 1-cm palpable well-defined cancer scanned with **(A)** high contrast appears anechoic, initially called a cyst, hypoechoic **(B)** with a higher dynamic range recognized to be solid, and *(continued)*

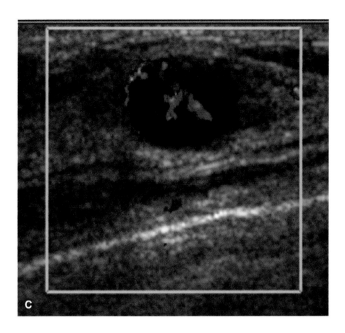

FIGURE 13.2. *Continued.* **(C)** vascular on Doppler.

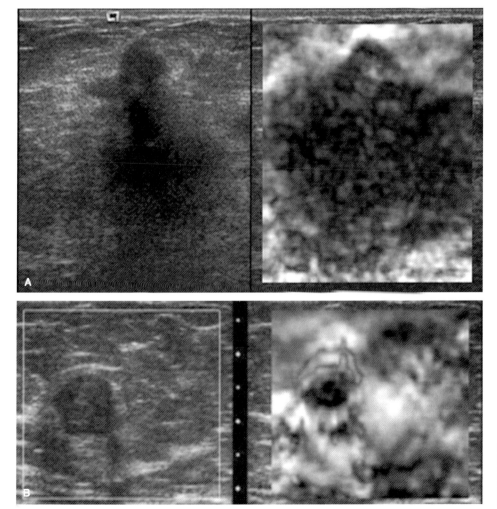

FIGURE 13.3. Elastography Images. A: A cancer that is larger on the elasticity image when compared with conventional ultrasound. **B:** Fibroadenoma smaller on the elasticity image. (Reprinted with permission from Siemens Medical Solutions, Malvern, PA.)

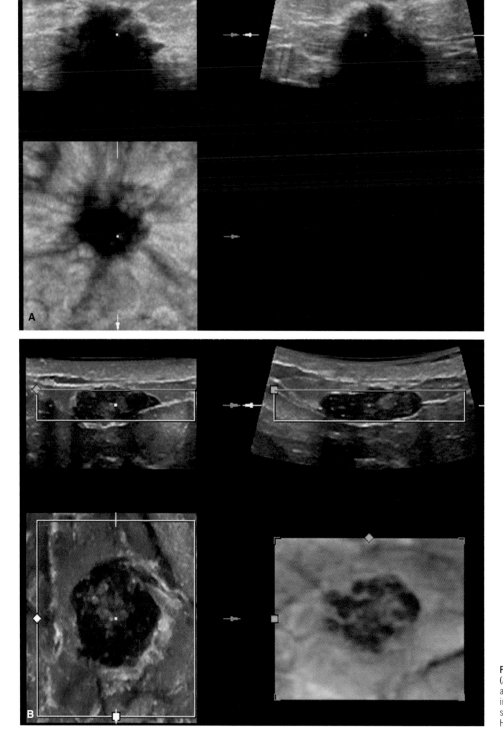

FIGURE 13.4. Three-dimensional imaging of (**A**) cancer and (**B**) fibroadenoma. Allows dynamic and multisectional imaging including coronal imaging (*bottom left*), which adds a new dimension. (Reprinted with permission from GE Healthcare, Wauwatosa, WI.)

An exciting development over the past 10 years has been the introduction of relatively high-quality compact ultrasound machines, which are relatively less expensive than the full-size units, allowing them to be more accessible. The wider availability of this technology may allow for earlier detection and diagnosis of breast cancer in countries with limited resources where screening mammography is unlikely to be introduced in the near future.

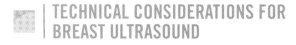

TECHNICAL CONSIDERATIONS FOR BREAST ULTRASOUND

Who Scans?

Who scans the patient: the physician or the technologist? There is no doubt that the physician responsible for correlating the imaging (mammographic and ultrasonic) and the physical findings should perform or at least participate in the ultrasound examination. In certain busy radiology practices, the technologist performs the ultrasound study. If the technologist is properly trained, he or she may do an adequate job in ultrasound screening or in evaluating a dominant finding on the mammogram, frequently accompanied by a limited evaluation by the breast imager. However, involving the breast imager may be critical to identifying small or subtle malignancies. Because of this, many practices have restricted breast ultrasound performance exclusively to the breast imager, despite the time commitment required.

Prior to Performing an Ultrasound Examination

Two steps must be performed before starting the ultrasound examination: measurement and physical examination.

Measurement

It is recommended that an accurate measurement be made of the location of a nonpalpable finding in relation to the nipple as seen on the mammogram (if one has been obtained). Measurement is particularly important in cases of a small or subtle finding. Because it is notoriously inaccurate to estimate the superior to inferior location based on the mediolateral oblique view, it is helpful to obtain a mediolateral or lateromedial view of the breast. This allows measurement of the distance of the lesion from the level of the nipple to the superior or inferior location on the lateral view, and to the medial or lateral location of the lesion on the craniocaudal view. Such measurement is usually quite accurate to within 1 cm, allowing detection of a subtle lesion, except in larger-breasted women, where the determination is less accurate and requires covering a larger area to find the lesion.

Physical Examination

A physical examination of the breast is recommended, either limited to the quadrant where a mammographic or palpable abnormality is noted or a more complete examination if there is a question of a palpable finding with a negative mammogram. Physical examination allows for a better feel of the overall texture of the breast and a comparison of both breasts. A description of the impression from the physical examination should be documented in the report. Breast imagers and all physicians who deal with the breasts would do well to develop their clinical breast examination skills, as would their patients.

Patient Positioning

The ideal position for ultrasound scanning is one that results in optimal thinning of the breast portion being examined. Varying the position of the patient can achieve this goal. Placing the wrist over the forehead is uniformly beneficial to all women because it spreads the breast tissue over the chest wall. The supine position is always optimal to examine the tissues medial to the 12 to 6 o'clock axis. Various degrees of changing obliquity, sometimes up to the decubitus position, are used to image the rest of the breast. For larger-breasted women, a semi-upright position or even a sitting position may be used to scan the upper part of the breast.

Examination Technique

The breast can be scanned in a number of ways (sagittal, transverse, radial, and antiradial). Consistency of method is advised. We have adopted antiradial screening as our survey technique, supplemented by sagittal and transverse scanning as warranted.

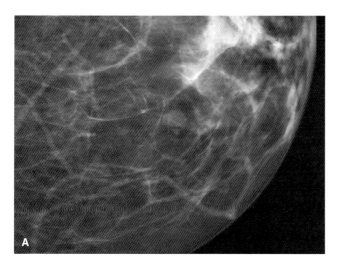

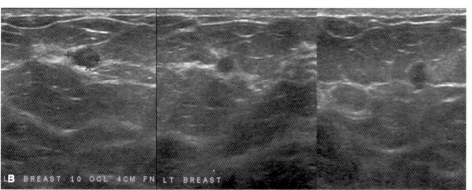

FIGURE 13.5. Value of rotating the transducer to analyze size and shape of mass. A: A 6-mm smooth, benign-appearing nodule in the medial left breast on mammogram. **B:** Three ultrasound images with different transducer orientations show images of increasing suspicion (*left to right*), making the mass highly suspicious, proven carcinoma.

Once a discrete lesion is suspected or detected (Fig. 13.5A,B), scan along different axes up to 360 degrees to differentiate a real lesion from a pseudolesion and to evaluate its morphology if a real lesion is confirmed. A fat lobule often mimics a discrete hypoechoic mass in one plane and merges with the adjacent fat in another. Baker et al. (12) illustrate in a pictorial essay a number of artifacts and pitfalls that every person who scans should be familiar with.

How many images should be obtained? For a typical cyst, a single image is sufficient, although one should look at it from various angles. For a solid mass, four to eight images may be required to document the size, shape, and characteristics of the lesion. Orthogonal planes are recommended and include radial and antiradial or longitudinal and transverse. In addition, maximal dimension sizes should be documented in two planes. Images with and without caliper should be obtained.

Extent of Scanning

The extent of the scanning depends on the clinical problem. It may be adequate to limit the scanning to the abnormal finding on the mammogram or to the palpable finding. However, in the presence of mammographic or ultrasonic findings strongly suspicious for cancer, it is important to scan the entire quadrant and possibly the entire breast to evaluate for multifocal or multicentric disease once the primary abnormality has been evaluated and documented (more discussion on this subject later). In this situation, the draining nodes, usually the axillary nodes and occasionally the subclavicular and internal mammary nodes, would be evaluated. This evaluation can be completed in one visit, but it may be preferable to conduct the primary evaluation and the appropriate core biopsy at one time and the breast staging evaluation at a different time.

Documentation

The report should include a description of the area scanned. The images should be labeled as to right or left breast. If no discrete finding is seen, the entire quadrant may need to be scanned and cited on the recorded images (e.g., RUO: right upper outer; RUI: right upper inner; RLI: right lower inner; RLO: right lower outer).

The documentation of a specific finding should include the o'clock position and a ruler measurement of the distance from the nipple. Documentation should indicate whether the finding is palpable or nonpalpable. Many small cancers are found to be palpable once their exact location has been established.

IMAGE ANALYSIS

Cystic Lesions: Simple Cysts versus Complicated Cysts

Breast cysts are common. A simple cyst is defined as a well-circumscribed, rounded or oval anechoic mass with a thin or imperceptible wall and posterior acoustic enhancement. Ultrasound is highly accurate in identifying a simple cyst. Unfortunately, many cysts and probably most cysts do not strictly meet all of the criteria to be called simple cysts either because the contents are not anechoic or because the wall is not uniformly imperceptible or thin or because of a lack of posterior enhancement (Fig. 13.6A–G). These are referred to as *complicated cysts* (the term *complex cyst* has also been used). Berg et al. (13) reviewed the sonographic features of 150 cystic lesions, correlating their sonographic appearance with pathologic findings. Other breast lesions contain fluid and must be distinguished from simple cysts because some of them may require intervention.

Internal echoes in what otherwise looks like a cyst preclude the diagnosis of a simple cyst. Internal echoes may be due to debris, protein, cholesterol, blood, inflammatory cells, or may be artifactual. It is relatively easy to recognize a complex cyst if the internal echoes are moving. There is a definite overlap in the appearance of cysts that contain nonmoving internal echoes because of thick fluid versus a solid mass that may be benign or malignant (depending on other characteristics). Solid masses that may be misinterpreted as cysts include fibroadenoma, papilloma, lymph nodes, and cancer. Turning color Doppler on allows one to confirm the solid nature of a mass if found to be vascular. One should not hesitate to insert a needle into a mass to determine whether it contains fluid or is solid. If it is solid, a biopsy can be scheduled or performed on the spot.

Thin septations are seen in multiloculated cysts or are mimicked by immediately adjacent cysts. Anterior reverberations are easily recognized as such, located beneath the anterior surface of the cyst.

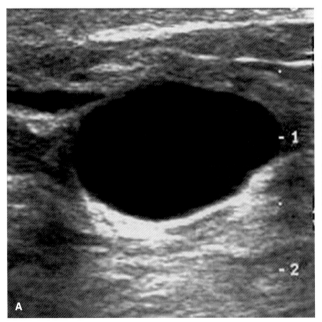

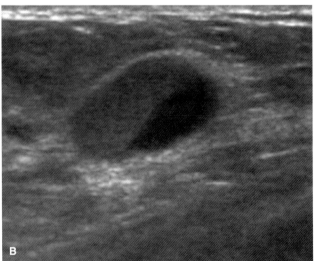

FIGURE 13.6. Cysts. A: Typical simple cyst. **B:** Acorn cyst, no action needed, may be followed, rarely aspirated. *(continued)*

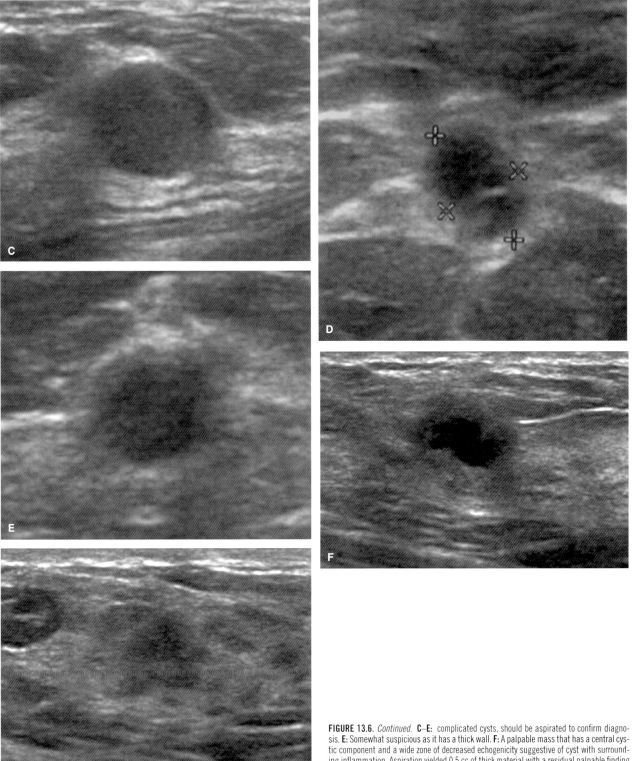

FIGURE 13.6. *Continued.* **C–E:** complicated cysts, should be aspirated to confirm diagnosis. **E:** Somewhat suspicious as it has a thick wall. **F:** A palpable mass that has a central cystic component and a wide zone of decreased echogenicity suggestive of cyst with surrounding inflammation. Aspiration yielded 0.5 cc of thick material with a residual palpable finding and persistent focal area of decreased echogenicity (**G**). Follow-up 6 weeks later showed disappearance of the mass and the ultrasonic finding.

There is not much controversy regarding how simple cysts should be managed. Indications for aspiration of simple cysts include palpable and tender cysts. Patients may also request aspiration of a cyst particularly if it is an only finding. Cytologic examination of the aspirated fluid is not necessary if the fluid is not bloody (14). If hemorrhagic fluid, either fresh or old, is obtained, it has been customary to send the fluid for cytologic examination, although the yield is very low. Some investigators have advocated injecting air into the cyst cavity after complete aspiration of the cyst to decrease the likelihood of recurrence (15). Otherwise simple cysts do not need to be aspirated nor have short-term follow-up. The patient should be advised to seek medical attention if anything palpable is felt and not to assume that it is a cyst.

Management of complicated cysts can vary greatly, depending on the ultrasound findings and criteria, the confidence and skills of the radiologist, and the patient's desires. With few exceptions, all palpable suspected complicated cysts should be aspirated for confirmation. Thick-walled cysts should all probably be aspirated. Nonpalpable suspected complicated cysts may be managed with short-term follow-up or aspiration, depending on whether single or multiple, the level of concern, the comfort of the patient and of the referring physician, and the reported level of uncertainty. Venta et al. (16) reviewed 308 complex cysts, half of which were followed and the other half aspirated or core biopsied. There was only one patient in whom a 3-mm focus of ductal carcinoma *in situ* was found on core biopsy. Their conclusion, based on their series, was that complex cysts can be managed with follow-up imaging rather than aspiration or biopsy.

Solid Masses: Benign versus Malignant

There are clearly criteria that would allow one to readily suspect that a solid mass is either benign or malignant. However, it is widely recognized that there is much overlap, so careful analysis is warranted to select those lesions that do not need to be biopsied when there is a very high probability (>98%) of benignity. If those lesions can be identified, they can be categorized under the American College of Radiology Breast Imaging Reporting and Data System (BI-RADS) 3 and be followed. Lesions that do not fit the 98% probability of benignity must be considered for biopsy.

It is critical to be familiar with all of the sonographic findings that malignant lesions can manifest. These reflect the morphologic characteristics of breast cancer tempered by the resolution of the ultrasound system. Many minimal and subtle manifestations of breast cancer are better appreciated during real-time scanning rather than in still images. Assessment can be based on both the review of the saved or printed images on the viewing monitors and the impression made during scanning.

Stavros et al. (17) prospectively classified 750 sonographically solid breast nodules as benign, indeterminate, or malignant, all proven by biopsy. Of those 750, 625 nodules (83%) were benign and 125 (17%) were malignant. Sixty-eight percent of malignant lesions were less than 1.5 cm in diameter and were not significantly different in size from the benign lesions. Benign criteria included absence of any malignant characteristics, intense homogeneous hyperechogenicity, a thin echogenic pseudocapsule with an elliptical shape, and the presence of up to two to three gentle lobulations (Table 13.1). The most com-

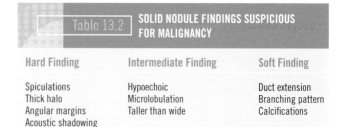

Table 13.2	SOLID NODULE FINDINGS SUSPICIOUS FOR MALIGNANCY		
Hard Finding		**Intermediate Finding**	**Soft Finding**
Spiculations		Hypoechoic	Duct extension
Thick halo		Microlobulation	Branching pattern
Angular margins		Taller than wide	Calcifications
Acoustic shadowing			

From Stavros AT, Rapp CL, Parker SH. *Breast ultrasound.* Baltimore: Lippincott Williams & Wilkins, 2003 p. 445–527, with permission.

mon benign diagnosis was that of a fibroadenoma in 54% of the benign lesions. Of the 750 nodules, 726 were also imaged mammographically, negative in 174 (24%), probably benign in 189 (26%), indeterminate in 313 (43%), and probably malignant or malignant in 50 (7%). Of the 125 proven malignant nodules (Table 13.2), the mammograms were classified as negative for 24 (19%) of the nodules, probably benign for 5 (4%), indeterminate for 59 (47%), and probably malignant and malignant in 37 (30%) (Fig. 13.7A–I).

Breast ultrasound sensitivity for malignancy was 98.4% and specificity was 67.8% (Table 13.3). Only 1.6% of malignant lesions were misclassified as benign by ultrasound criteria. The positive predictive value was 38%; the negative predictive value was 99.5%. Spiculation has the highest positive predictive value for cancer. Other sonographic characteristics of malignancy include nodules that are taller than they are wide, angular margins, marked hypoechogenicity, shadowing, calcification, duct

Table 13.1	SOLID NODULE FINDINGS INDICATIVE OF BENIGNITY

Pure and intensely hyperechoic texture
Elliptical shape (wider than tall)
Gently lobulated shape (three or fewer lobulations)
Complete thin capsule

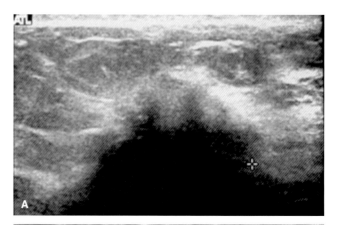

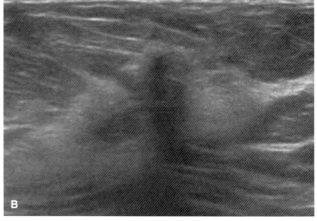

FIGURE 13.7. Typical Cancers. A,B: Irregular shape, indistinct margins, markedly hypoechoic with shadowing; both invasive ductal carcinoma. *(continued)*

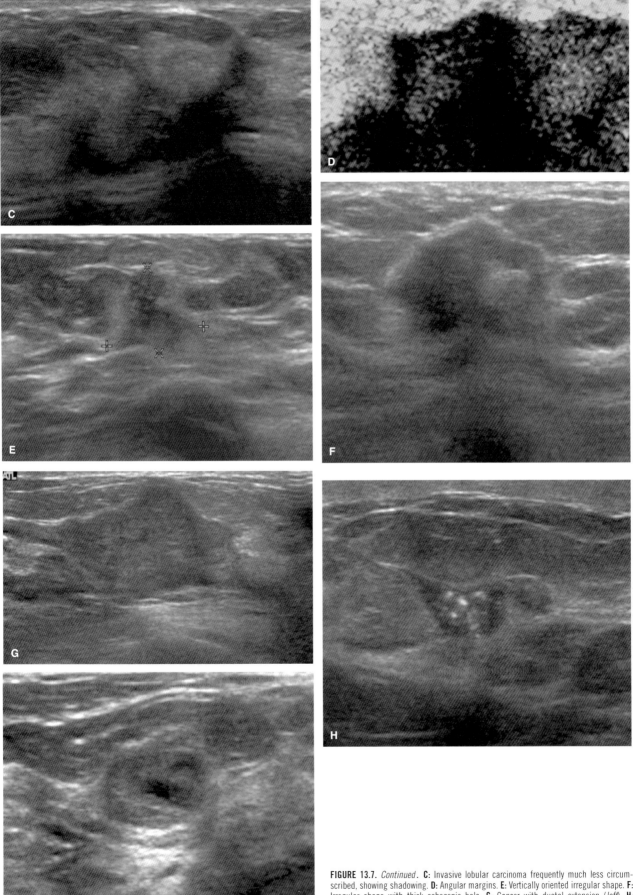

FIGURE 13.7. *Continued.* **C:** Invasive lobular carcinoma frequently much less circumscribed, showing shadowing. **D:** Angular margins. **E:** Vertically oriented irregular shape. **F:** Irregular shape with thick echogenic halo. **G:** Cancer with ductal extension (*left*). **H:** Multifocal invasive and *in situ* ductal carcinoma with ultrasound visualization of microcalcifications in mass. **I:** Well-circumscribed colloid carcinoma.

Table 13.3	DIAGNOSTIC SENSITIVITY, POSITIVE PREDICTIVE VALUE, AND ODDS RATIO FOR MALIGNANCY OF INDIVIDUAL FINDINGS[a]		
Sonographic Findings	Diagnostic Sensitivity (%)[b]	PPV[c] (%)	Odds Ratio (%)
Angular margins	90	59	1.8
Spiculations	36	87	2.7
Thick hyperechoic halo	35	74	1.9
Spiculations or thick halo	71	80	2.4
Acoustic shadowing	35	62	1.9
Marked hypoechoic appearance	49	64	1.9
Taller than wide	48	74	2.5
Microlobulations	92	50	1.5
Calcifications	40	53	1.6
Branch pattern	44	60	1.8
Duct extension	49	46	1.4

[a]Data from 1375 sonographic visually depicted solid nodules. Prevalence of cancer in nodule population was 32.8%.

[b]Diagnostic sensitivity should be distinguished from screening sensitivity, which will necessarily be lower than diagnostic sensitivity. Diagnostic sensitivity refers to percentage of sonographically depicted nodules correctly characterized as Breast Imaging Reporting and Data System (BI-RADS) 4 or 5. Screening sensitivity would be lower because some malignant lesions would not be sonographically depicted. The combined diagnostic sensitivity was 99.6%.

[c]PPV, positive predictive value.

extension, branch pattern, and microlobulation. Smaller cancers frequently are less obviously malignant looking or may have the same typical features as larger lesions (Fig. 13.8A–G). A lesion can be analyzed for benign characteristics only after determining that there is no malignant characteristic whatsoever. Rahbar et al. (18) reviewed 161 consecutive patients who underwent breast mass tissue sampling and reported on the application of benign and malignant ultrasound criteria by three experienced breast imagers. Interobserver variability was found among the readers, and 4 of 38 carcinomas were interpreted as benign, stressing the need for further exploration of the reproducibility of criteria analysis in various practices.

BREAST IMAGING REPORTING AND DATA SYSTEM

The BI-RADS classification was developed in 1993 to standardize the language of mammography reporting and to clarify communication among clinicians. To develop a similar classification for ultrasound, Mendelson et al. (19) published an initial draft of a breast ultrasound lexicon. A BI-RADS lexicon was adopted for breast ultrasound in 2003 for the same purpose (20). The sonographic BI-RADS lexicon includes sonographic descriptors of lesions for shape, orientation, margins, lesion

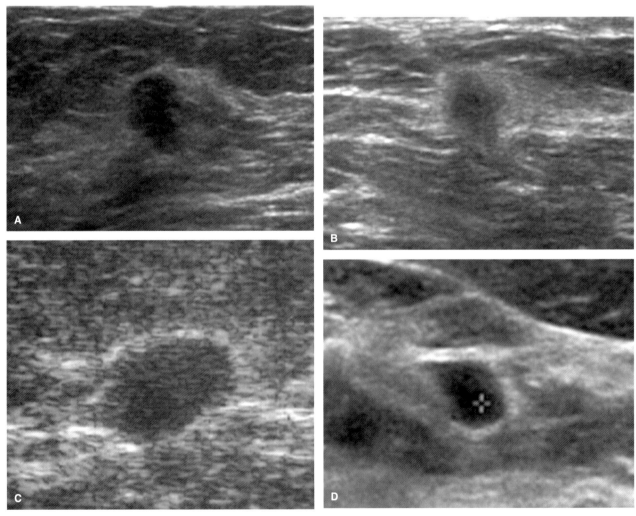

FIGURE 13.8. Small Cancers. A,B: Typical appearance of malignancies. Small lesions under 8 mm are frequently associated with fewer and more subtle signs of malignancy. **C:** Very subtle irregular contour. **D:** Well-defined with a tail, which makes it suspicious. (*continued*)

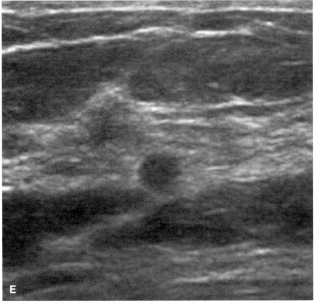

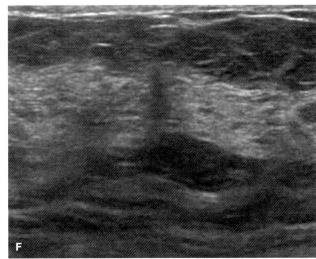

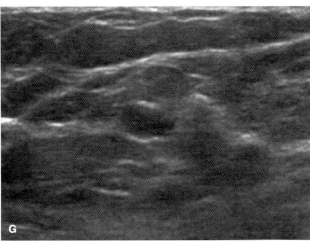

FIGURE 13.8. *Continued*. **E:** Very subtle irregular contour. **F:** Vertically oriented tiny zone of shadowing proven malignant on fine-needle aspiration biopsy, indicating a multicentric breast cancer in a patient with a known cancer in another quadrant. **G:** Cancer (6 × 4 mm) with very subtle irregular contours.

boundary, echo pattern, posterior acoustic features, and surrounding tissue alterations. On the basis of these descriptors, each lesion is assigned a final assessment category (Table 13.4). Hong et al. (21) reported on the positive and negative predictive values of the BI-RADS assessment of 403 solid breast lesions. The descriptors showing a high predictive value for malignancy include spiculated margins (86%), irregular shape (62%), and a nonparallel orientation (taller than wide) (69%). The descriptor that showed a high predictive value for a benign lesion include circumscribed margin (90%), parallel orientation (wider than tall) (78%), and oval shape (84%). Several other studies have validated the BI-RADS classification as helpful in distinguishing and classifying benign and malignant breast lesions (22,23).

SPECIFIC BREAST LESIONS

The most important task in analyzing the ultrasound features of discrete masses is to identify lesions that are typical of malignancy or possibly malignant, with no further attempt to correlate the histologic types of breast cancer. However, occasionally some ultrasonic features suggest a specific type. Invasive lobular carcinoma is frequently associated with focal areas of shadowing without a discrete mass (24). Medullary carcinomas and colloid carcinomas are frequently quite discrete and microlobulated. Medullary carcinomas and colloid carcinomas are usually markedly hypoechoic with good through transmission and associated increased vascularity. Colloid carcinoma is isoechoic and occasionally hyperechoic and also shows good through–transmission (1).

Ductal carcinoma *in situ* is most frequently manifested by clustered microcalcifications on the mammogram. Although there may not be much of a role for ultrasound in evaluating a tiny cluster of suspicious microcalcifications, ultrasound should be performed if there is a zone of increased density on the mammogram associated with the microcalcifications or if the microcalcifications are numerous or distributed over a long segment. Ductal carcinoma *in situ* is frequently associated with invasive carcinoma the larger the number of microcalcifications present, and, in its pure form, may also be associated with a soft tissue mass without invasion. Identification of ultrasonic findings of a mass or the associated microcalcifications allows the use of ultrasound-guided biopsy rather than stereotactic biopsy for the diagnosis (1,25).

Breast cancer in male patients accounts for less than 1% of all breast cancers. Frequently referred for the evaluation of a breast mass behind the nipple, most male patients will be diagnosed with unilateral or bilateral gynecomastia. The breast

Table 13.4	**FEATURE CATEGORIES AND DESCRIPTORS FOR MASSES, CALCIFICATIONS, AND OTHER BREAST LESIONS: BREAST IMAGING REPORTING AND DATA SYSTEM (BI-RADS)–ULTRASOUND (US)**

A. Background echotexture
   1. Homogeneous background echotexture: fat
   2. Homogeneous background echotexture: fibroglandular
   3. Heterogeneous background

B. Masses
   1. Shape: oval, round, irregular
   2. Orientation: parallel, not parallel
   3. Margin: circumscribed, not circumscribed (indistinct, angular, microlobulated, spiculated)
   4. Lesion boundary: abrupt interface, echogenic halo
   5. Echo pattern: anechoic, hyperechoic, complex, hypoechoic, isoechoic
   6. Posterior acoustic features: no posterior acoustic features, enhancement, shadowing, combined pattern
   7. Surrounding tissue: ducts, changes in Cooper ligaments, edema, architectural distortion, skin thickening, skin retraction/irregularity

C. Calcifications
   1. Macrocalcifications
   2. Microcalcifications out of mass
   3. Microcalcifications in mass

D. Special cases
   1. Clustered microcysts
   2. Complicated cysts
   3. Mass in or on skin
   4. Foreign body
   5. Lymph nodes: intramammary
   6. Lymph nodes: axillary

E. Vascularity
   1. Present or not present
   2. Present immediately adjacent to lesion
   3. Diffusely increased vascularity in surrounding tissue

BI-RADS Category 0: Incomplete. Need additional imaging evaluation.
BI-RADS Category 1: Negative. Routine follow-up.
BI-RADS Category 2: Benign finding. Routine follow-up.
BI-RADS Category 3: Probably benign finding. Short-term follow-up recommended.
BI-RADS Category 4: Suspicious abnormality. Biopsy should be considered.
BI-RADS Category 5: High probability of malignancy. Appropriate action should be taken.
BI-RADS Category 6: Proven malignancy. Appropriate action should be taken.

Reprinted with permission of the American College of Radiology. No other representation of this material is authorized without the expressed, written permission from the American College of Radiology.
American College of Radiology (ACR). ACR BI RADS-Mammography. 4th edition. ACR Breast Imaging Reporting and Data System, Breast Imaging Atlas; BI-RADS. Reston, VA. American College of Radiology; 2003.

mass in these cases is frequently firm. Gynecomastia on ultrasound is frequently associated with shadowing and requires careful attention to examination technique to distinguish gynecomastia from a cancer in the subareolar area (1). The location of a mass away from the nipple should raise suspicions. Mammographic and ultrasonic characteristics of men with breast cancer are similar to those of women with breast cancer. Cystic masses in men should raise suspicions for malignancy because simple cysts are rare in men (26,27).

Fibroadenoma

Fibroadenoma is the most common benign mass of the breast. Typically a fibroadenoma is hypoechoic and ellipsoid or oval and has homogeneous internal echoes and smooth margins, occasionally with slight lobulation and cystic components (28). Fibroadenomas are, however, frequently much less typical, being quite lobulated, with inhomogeneous internal echoes and associated with shadowing, overlapping with characteristics of malignant lesions. Fibroadenomas may also be entirely isoechoic and not recognizable on ultrasound (Fig. 13.9A–I).

Benign and Malignant Phyllodes Tumors

Phyllodes tumors (the term cystosarcoma phyllodes is a misnomer and should no longer be used) overlap frequently in appearance with fibroadenoma except that they are usually larger and may be fast growing. They may be rounded and may have an irregular contour. Tumors larger than 3 cm are more likely to be malignant and are frequently associated with cystic spaces (29).

Papillary Lesions

Benign papilloma, papilloma with atypia, and papillary carcinoma cannot be distinguished from one another by imaging criteria (30–32). They may present as an intraductal mass with or without nipple discharge, as a solid mass within the breast, as an intracystic mass, or as a cluster of microcalcifications. Papillary lesions are usually vascular. Management of papillary carcinoma and papilloma with atypia is surgical, but management of a benign papilloma on core biopsy remains a matter of debate because of varying reported associations with adjacent atypia or malignancy in resected benign papillomas (Fig. 13.10A–G).

SELECTED APPLICATIONS OF BREAST ULTRASOUND

Breast Lump with No Corresponding Mammographic Finding

It is rare to discover a cancer in a woman with entirely fatty breasts who has a lump and a negative mammogram, but it is not rare in women who have scattered fibroglandular tissue or dense breasts.

Whatever the breast density, ultrasound is indispensable in evaluating patients with a breast lump or question of a lump to explain the physical finding. Either the patient or the referring health care professional may feel the lump. It is extremely helpful if the clinician describes on the requisition the size of the lump, the o'clock location, and the distance from the nipple to

make sure that the problem in question is addressed. Although there is usually no disagreement about the presence of a discrete lump, women are commonly referred for evaluation of a breast lump for which there would be disagreement about whether the palpable finding constitutes lumpiness versus a discrete lump; hence the importance of clinical assessment by

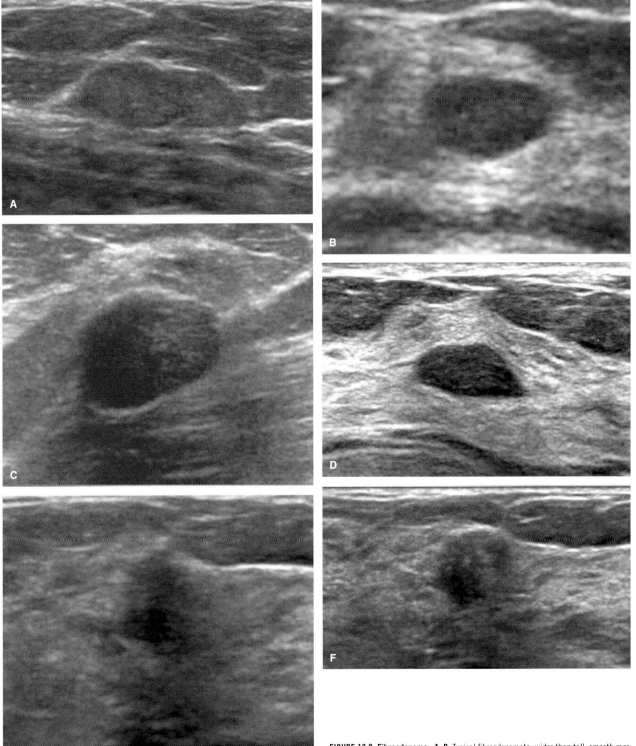

FIGURE 13.9. Fibroadenoma. A–D: Typical fibroadenomata: wider than tall, smooth margin, one or two lobulations, thin capsule. **E–H:** Proven fibroadenomata with several features of malignant lesions. **(E)** and **(G)** show irregular contours, shadowing, and what looks like duct extension. *(continued)*

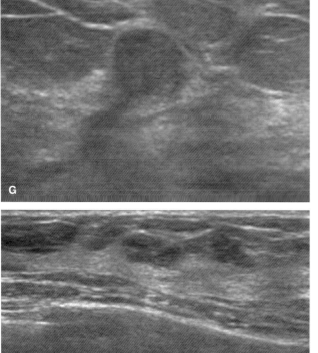

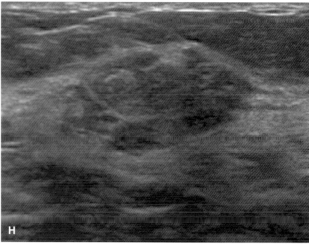

FIGURE 13.9. *Continued.* **I:** Isoechoic fibroadenoma easier to pick up during real-time scanning as discrete, corresponding to a small, well-defined mass on the mammogram.

the breast imager. If a discrete fluid-filled or solid mass is discovered, then a plan of action (aspiration, biopsy, or follow-up) can be recommended after complete analysis of the lesion. If no mass is seen on the ultrasound, every attempt must be made to explain the palpable finding, which may be due to a fat lobule, lipoma, or nodularity of the breast. This requires simultaneous scanning and palpation of the lump with the finger and often comparison with the contralateral breast. In addition, for premenopausal women, because many women have much greater breast lumpiness (more so in the upper outer quadrants, and occasionally asymmetric) in the premenstrual phase, it is important to indicate where the patient is in her menstrual cycle. Re-evaluation following menses may show dramatic regression of what may have been considered a discrete mass. Several studies (33,34) have shown that in the evaluation of a

palpable finding, the absence of a corresponding finding on the mammogram and ultrasound is associated with a very high negative predictive value (99.8%). Very rarely an MRI may need to be performed to provide additional reassurance if the clinical finding is too discrete. However, a biopsy should be considered if clinical suspicion is high or the mass is definitely a new finding.

Evaluation of Lumps in Very Young, or Pregnant or Lactating Women

Evaluation of a lump in women younger than age 30 or who are pregnant or lactating should start with ultrasound and most often should be limited to ultrasound only. Common

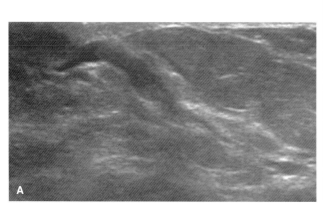

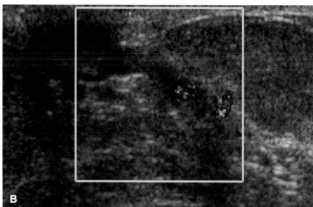

FIGURE 13.10. Papillary Lesions. A,B: Small intraductal vascular lesion in a patient with a spontaneous bloody nipple discharge; proven papilloma. *(continued)*

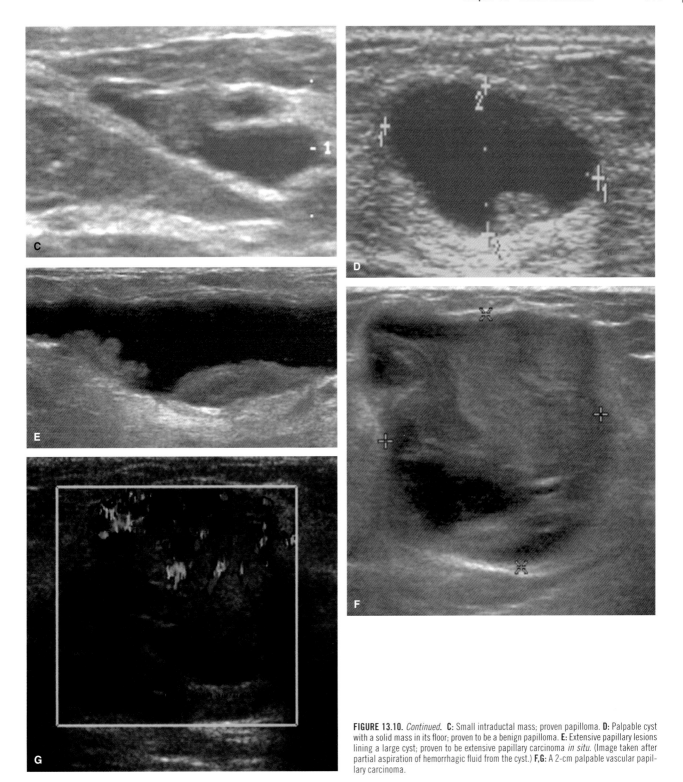

FIGURE 13.10. *Continued.* **C:** Small intraductal mass; proven papilloma. **D:** Palpable cyst with a solid mass in its floor; proven to be a benign papilloma. **E:** Extensive papillary lesions lining a large cyst; proven to be extensive papillary carcinoma *in situ.* (Image taken after partial aspiration of hemorrhagic fluid from the cyst.) **F,G:** A 2-cm palpable vascular papillary carcinoma.

lesions in these women are fibroadenoma, lactating adenoma, galactocele, cyst, and abscess. Malignancy is much less common. If the mass is considered benign by clinical examination and ultrasound criteria, then it can be aspirated, core biopsied, fine-needle aspirated (FNA), or followed. However, if the mass is considered highly suspicious for malignancy, then a mammogram can be obtained to evaluate the breast prior to a core

biopsy and particularly to look for microcalcifications. If the mass is considered indeterminate, it may be biopsied first because of the likelihood of a benign entity. The mammogram can always be performed several days after the biopsy.

Women between the ages of 30 and 40 should be managed in the same way as women older than 40; that is, starting with the diagnostic mammogram followed by ultrasound.

Morrow et al. (35) reported on their experience with 484 women younger than 40 referred with a breast lump. Dominant masses were confirmed by the surgeon in 36% of self-detected masses and in 29% of physician-detected masses. Carcinoma was found in 5%. These authors proposed an algorithm for the management of breast masses in young women that includes:

- If the physical examination reveals no evidence of a mass, the patient is reassured and no imaging is obtained.
- If there is clinical uncertainty as to lump versus lumpiness, ultrasound is obtained.
- If no mass is seen, the clinical examination is repeated in 2 to 4 months.
- In women 35 and older, a mammogram may be obtained based on the degree of suspicion, followed by appropriate imaging with ultrasound and biopsy as clinically warranted.

The authors stress the importance of clinical follow-up to identify the rare cases with false-negative indeterminate clinical examination with negative imaging studies. Confirmed masses are biopsied after appropriate imaging.

Regarding the imaging characteristics of breast cancer in younger women, Foxcroft et al. (36) reviewed the records of 239 women under the age of 40 diagnosed with breast cancer. A definite mass was present in 72% and ill-defined thickening in 15%. Seventy-two percent had mammographic abnormalities, and 92% of the cancers had a corresponding abnormality on ultrasound. In 14 cancers, the ultrasound appearance was indistinguishable from fibroadenoma and read as such, and 10 other cancers read as atypical fibroadenoma or were consistent with fibroadenoma.

Inflamed Breast

A common condition is the presentation of a woman with swelling, redness, and tenderness of one breast. Differential diagnosis includes mastitis, cellulitis, abscess, and inflammatory carcinoma. Ultrasound can be extremely helpful in discovering an underlying mass such as abscess or carcinoma, both of which require immediate intervention such as aspiration of an abscess, biopsy of a solid mass, or biopsy of the skin. Despite appropriate antibiotic therapy, abscesses may need to be aspirated on more than one occasion (Fig. 13.11A,B), which helps the abscess resolve progressively over the course of several weeks until it resolves completely. If no discrete mass is discovered and in the absence of any sign of malignancy such as adenopathy, it is appropriate to treat the patient with antibiotics and possibly cold compresses. With such treatment, mastitis or cellulitis shows significant improvement, usually within a couple of days. The patient should be followed clinically at close appropriate intervals and should return 4 to 6 weeks later for a complete breast evaluation. Lack of improvement after a short period (1 to 2 weeks) should raise questions about the greater probability of a malignancy rather than an inflammatory or infectious process.

Gunhan-Bilgen et al. (37) reviewed the records of 142 patients with inflammatory breast cancer. Ultrasound was found to be superior to mammography in documenting skin thickening and engorgement of the lymphatics and in identifying a mass or masses in the breast, with axillary adenopathy helping to narrow the differential diagnosis and proceeding to a biopsy when the clinical presentation is not clearly that of inflammatory carcinoma. MRI was not used in the study but is probably superior in depicting the findings of inflammatory carcinoma.

Clinically Significant Nipple Discharge

Nipple discharge is not an infrequent symptom. It may be spontaneous or elicited upon squeezing the nipple areolar complex. It may involve a single or multiple duct openings, and may be unilateral or bilateral. The discharge may be watery and clear, greenish, milky, serous, sticky, serosanguineous, or bloody. Nipple discharge due to fibrocystic change or duct ectasia is frequently greenish or milky, from multiple openings, and unilateral or bilateral. This type of discharge does not require investigation, except for spontaneous milky discharge, which is potentially associated with elevated serum prolactin levels in the right clinical setting. Clinically significant nipple discharge, on the other hand, is spontaneous or readily elicited, usually unilateral, clear, serous, serosanguineous, or bloody and from a

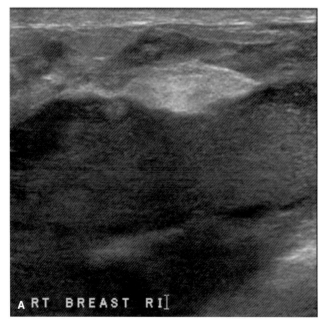

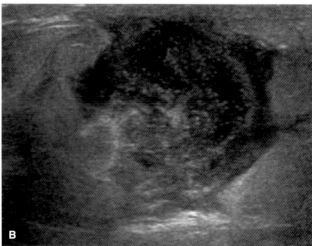

FIGURE 13.11. Abscess. A: *Staphylococcus* abscess yielded 80 cc of pus in a 23-year-old woman who had finished lactating. The abscess resolved entirely over 6 weeks and required two additional aspirations during that time, along with antibiotic therapy. **B:** *Staphylococcus* abscess yielded 5 cc of pus on aspiration; treated with antibiotic with no recurrence.

single duct opening. Such discharge is frequently associated with a papillary lesion, most commonly a benign papilloma rather than a papilloma with atypia or papillary carcinoma, and rarely ductal carcinoma. The discharge may sometimes be difficult to elicit when the patient presents with this complaint and there is a precise trigger point limited to a single o'clock position. Mammography is frequently not helpful except when such symptomatology is associated with ductal carcinoma either *in situ* or invasive. Galactography has been the traditional mode of investigation; contrast is injected to outline the discharging duct to identify and locate a potential growth within the duct. Increasingly ultrasound is used as the first modality after the mammogram to identify a small mass in the duct of concern (Fig. 13.11A–C). This type of ultrasound examination, focused on the periareolar area, requires meticulous technique to identify and follow segments of a duct all the way to the nipple (1). Papillary lesions are frequently associated with a vascular stalk distinct from sometimes confusing secretions in a duct.

Rissanen et al. (38) reported on 52 patients with clinically significant nipple discharge who eventually had surgical duct excision. Forty-seven patients (90%) had a benign lesion and 5 (10%) had cancer. Ultrasound visualized an intraductal mass in 36 (69%), dilated duct(s) without intraductal mass in 6 patients (12%), and no abnormality in 10 (19%). A full 80% of papillomatous lesions and only 10% of malignancies were visible on ultrasound. Whereas galactography can identify intraductal lesions of the cannulated duct only, breast ultrasound can identify multiple papillary lesions involving different duct systems and can delineate the extent of the lesion. Papillary lesions associated with a clinically significant nipple discharge, particularly lesions less than 5 mm, may be needle localized under ultrasound guidance for resection without necessarily a needle biopsy.

Second-Look Ultrasound after Breast MRI

There are many uses for breast MRI, including characterization of mammographically visible suspicious lesions, delineation of extent of breast cancer in the ipsilateral breast, evaluation of residual disease postlumpectomy or local recurrence, assessment of response to preoperative chemotherapy, detection of an occult primary carcinoma in patients with documented axillary carcinomatous adenopathy, contralateral breast evaluation in patients with a newly diagnosed breast cancer, and screening for high-risk individuals.

With the increasing use of breast MRI, mammographically occult enhancing lesions are being discovered on MRI with various levels of suspicion. These lesions are often recommended for biopsy. Second-look breast ultrasound is readily available and relatively inexpensive and should be used to find a correlate for the MRI-detected lesion.

There are technical challenges in attempting to correlate the MRI findings with ultrasound, particularly if they are small. Whereas the MRI examination is done in the prone position, the ultrasound examination is done in either the supine position or the oblique position or both. Careful extrapolation must be done regarding location, distance from lesion to nipple, and depth of the MRI finding. The size and shape of the MRI finding should also correspond to the finding seen on the ultrasound.

Frequently the corresponding lesions found on ultrasound are less conspicuous and not readily distinguishable from the surrounding tissues. Occasionally the ultrasound-detected lesion is so subtle that it precludes the feasibility of an ultrasound-guided core biopsy.

In a study published in *Radiology*, La Trenta et al. (39) reviewed 93 suspicious lesions detected on breast MRI, all mammographically occult, 19 of which eventually were proven malignant (20%). There was a sonographic correlate in 21 of the 93 (23%), 9 of which were found to be malignant (43%). Of those 93, 71 (56%) did not have a sonographic correlate and 10

(14%) were found to be malignant. Therefore, in the presence of an ultrasound correlate, a core biopsy should be performed in most cases unless the correlate has characteristics of a definitively benign lesion. If there is no ultrasound correlate, then the lesion should be biopsied under MRI guidance. Occasionally the MRI-detected lesion may be followed if the level of suspicion is low.

In pooling other similar studies, 16% to 42% of MRI-enhancing lesions turn out to be malignant, 23% to 65% are found to have an ultrasound correlate, 23% to 43% of those turn out to be malignant (40). In lesions without an ultrasound correlate, malignancy is discovered on MRI-guided biopsy in 8% to 56% of patients. Overall, 43% to 54% of MRI-detected, mammographically occult malignancies are discovered by second-look ultrasound. The rest are diagnosed by MRI-guided biopsy.

The wide range of percentages of malignant diagnoses in MRI-enhancing lesions probably reflects the current interreader variability of what constitutes a suspicious area of enhancement.

Implant-Related Findings

Palpable findings in women with silicone implants may be related to the implants or to the breast parenchyma. A bulge of the implants or a ridge that is felt can be easily confirmed with ultrasound. Clinical symptoms and physical findings, although nonspecific, frequently raise the question of damage to the integrity of the implants. Ultrasound has been shown to be very helpful in evaluating implant integrity (41): intact versus intracapsular or extracapsular rupture. When the implant is intact it has an anechoic interior and frequently anterior reverberations are also seen. Echogenic horizontal lines within the lumen of the implant are seen with intracapsular rupture, sometimes in a stepladder arrangement, representing the collapsed shell of the implant corresponding to the linguine sign described from MRI studies. Extracapsular rupture of an implant associated with free silicone leaking into the soft tissues of the breast is manifested by either an echogenic zone that is poorly defined posteriorly and has a well-defined anterior margin (best described as snowstorm, diagnostic of free silicone), or as a hypoechoic nodule, representing a silicone granuloma. These may sometimes be palpable and may present a diagnostic dilemma. Although MRI has been found to be more sensitive and specific in documenting implant status and the presence of leakage, with or without a mass, ultrasound is frequently utilized first to supplement mammographic findings and may solve the problem without MRI.

EVALUATION OF PATIENTS WITH BREAST CANCER

Breast Evaluation

The goal of the surgical treatment of breast cancer is to remove all cancerous tissue whether the patient is undergoing a lumpectomy or a mastectomy. Additional foci of cancer or a separate primary cancer can be discovered using ultrasound or MRI in the same quadrant as the primary cancer (multifocality) or in different quadrants of the affected breast (multicentricity). Holland et al. (42) in 1985 reported on the incidence of multifocality in 282 mastectomy specimens of 399 consecutive cases in patients who would have been candidates for breast conservation. In 56 patients (20%), additional foci were found within 2 cm and in 121 patients (43%), the tumor was found beyond 2 cm from the primary tumor. Several more recent studies have shown a 7% to 20% incidence of multifocality detected on MRI and a 7% to 10% incidence of multicentricity (43,44). The contribution of additional imaging on altering the management of the ipsilateral breast affected by cancer averages around 17%. The discovery of suspected multicentric breast cancer by imaging excludes the option of lumpectomy for treatment once tissue confirmation is established. Similarly, wide distribution of additional foci of carcinoma around the primary malignancy may influence the decision of surgical treatment toward mastectomy rather than lumpectomy. Berg et al. (45) in 2004 reported on a comparison of the diagnostic accuracy of mammography, clinical examination, ultrasound, and MRI in preoperative assessment of breast cancer in 177 malignant foci in 121 cancerous breasts. The sensitivity of mammography for invasive ductal carcinoma was 81%, and for invasive lobular carcinoma it was 34%. The sensitivity of ultrasound was higher: 94% and 86%, respectively. The sensitivity of MRI was highest: 95% and 96%, respectively. Similarly, recent data from the MRI literature have shown an incidence of mammographically occult contralateral breast cancer in 3.5% to 8% of patients with newly diagnosed breast cancer (46–48). Increasingly ultrasound evaluation is extended to the entire breast in patients with breast cancer and sometimes also includes the evaluation of the contralateral breast. These examination may be done on the first visit or on a return visit. Alternatively both breasts would be evaluated if an MRI is obtained.

Evaluation of Draining Lymph Nodes

The standard of care in evaluating newly diagnosed breast cancer patients includes assessment of the axilla with a sentinel lymph node biopsy. Patients who are candidates for primary surgical management with lumpectomy or mastectomy have the sentinel node biopsy performed at the time of the surgical resection of the cancer, either with frozen section immediately followed by lymph node dissection if the node is positive, or as a separate procedure several days later if permanent sections show cancer cells in the lymph node. Clinical examination of the axilla is notoriously unreliable. Ultrasound examination of the axilla is increasingly being used to identify patients with abnormal lymph nodes and to assess the contribution of FNA biopsy to patient management. If FNA biopsy shows a lymph node involved with metastatic disease, then the patient does not need sentinel lymph node biopsy and can proceed to lymph node dissection. This finding also opens the door to the option of preoperative therapy. On the other hand, if FNA biopsy is negative, the patient will still need a sentinel node biopsy (Fig. 13.12).

Morphologic criteria of metastatic lymph nodes include cortical changes such as thickening beyond 3 mm, rounded shape, and eccentric cortical bulge, as well as hilar changes such as displacement, compression, or complete disappearance of the hilum. Size is notoriously unreliable (Fig. 13.13A–F).

Several studies describe the accuracy and impact of ultrasound and FNA biopsy of axillary lymph nodes on the management of the patient with breast cancer (49–55). Ultrasound sensitivity varied from 35% to 87%, with a specificity of 48% to 97%. Sensitivity with T2 lesions is higher than with T1 lesions (67% vs. 35%). Sensitivity of axillary lymph node FNA biopsy varied from 43% to 95%, with a specificity of 97% to 100%. In a study by Jain et al. (53), published in 2008, 69 axillae were biopsied: 41 (60%) were positive, 4 (6%) were nondiagnostic, and 24 (34%) were negative on FNA biopsy. FNA had 89% sensitivity, 100% specificity, and 100% positive predictive value in patients with palpable or ultrasonographically suspicious nodes. The sensitivity dropped significantly for nonpalpable, ultrasonographically normal nodes (54%), whereas specificity and positive predictive value remained 100%. Twenty-three of

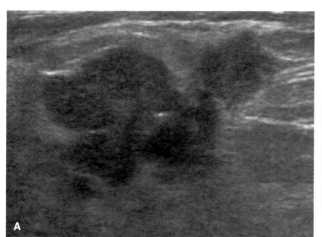

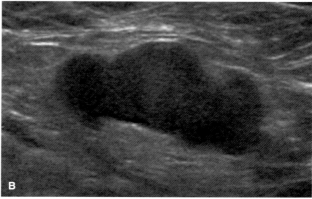

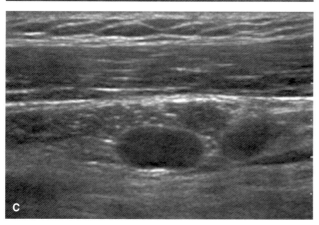

FIGURE 13.12. locally advanced breast cancer. Efficient work-up. This patient presented with palpable left breast mass **(A)** and palpable axillary nodes **(B)**. Ultrasound evaluation shows the cancer in the breast, enlarged lymph nodes in the axilla, and abnormal lymph nodes in the infraclavicular area **(C)**. Core biopsy of the mass in the breast was carried out, followed by fine-needle aspiration biopsy of the axillary lymph nodes. Computerized axial tomography of the chest, abdomen, and pelvis and a bone scan were ordered so that the patient could be scheduled to see the surgeon and a medical oncologist following those results, all within 10 days.

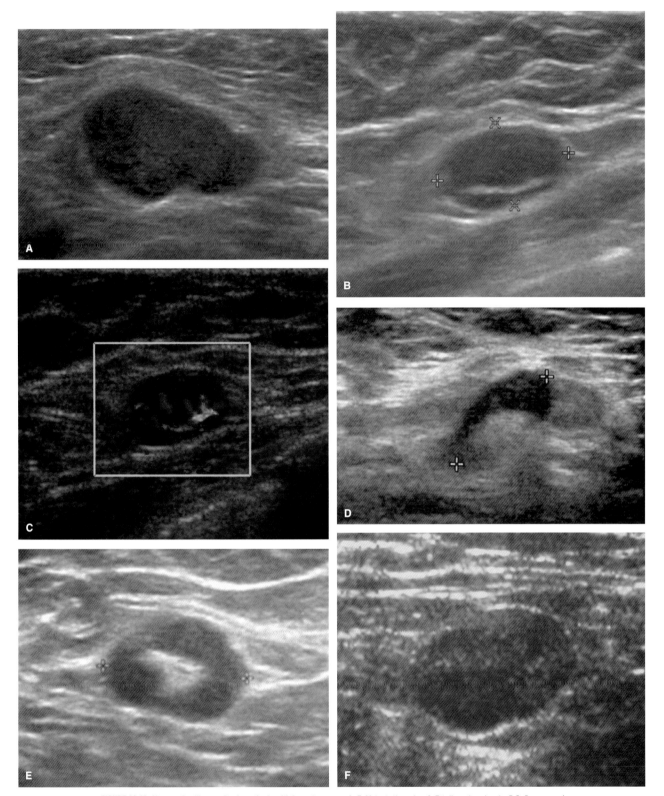

FIGURE 13.13. Abnormal axillary nodes in patients with breast cancer. A–F: Metastatic nodes. A: Totally replaced node. B,C: Compressed hilum, vascular node. D: Eccentric bulge of cortex. E: Diffusely prominent thick cortex. F: Appears to be an entirely replaced lymph node; fine-needle aspiration shows reactive node, proven surgically.

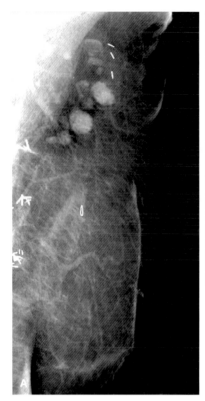
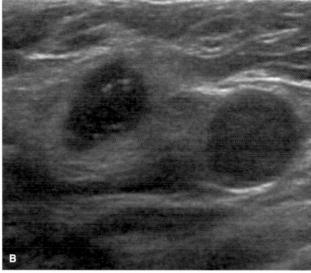

FIGURE 13.14. Skipped sentinel node? This patient had a left mastectomy for a 2.6-cm invasive ductal cancer (grade III/III), two negative sentinel nodes, and reconstruction of her breast. The patient presented 18 months later with a mass in her axilla that is proven to be two metastatic lymph nodes **(A,B)**. The nodes are located caudal to the clips left from her sentinel node. It is possible that the two metastatic lymph nodes were totally replaced at the time of her mastectomy and did not pick up the blue dye or the radiopharmaceutical agent at the time of the sentinel injection—a known cause for false-negative sentinel node. This case illustrates another reason to evaluate the axilla preoperatively in patients with breast cancer.

the 41 patients (56%) who had a positive FNA biopsy of axillary lymph node elected to proceed with preoperative chemotherapy before definitive surgery. The remaining 18 patients (44%) elected to proceed directly with surgery and axillary lymph node dissection. Twenty-five percent of the patients who had a negative FNA biopsy of the axilla turned out to have a positive sentinel lymph node.

Increasingly, in a number of institutions, ultrasound evaluation of the axilla has become part of the routine preoperative evaluation of patients with breast cancer (Fig. 13.14).

 ## SUMMARY

The continuous evolution of breast ultrasound technology has made it one of the most valuable and accurate tools in the evaluation of breast problems. Breast ultrasound can characterize the nature of a mammographic or palpable mass and can differentiate a solid mass from a cyst. Using multiple criteria, one can differentiate benign-looking masses from malignant ones and indeterminate ones. In the presence of breast cancer, ultrasound can provide additional valuable information regarding the local extent, the potential multicentricity, and the likelihood of axillary lymph node involvement. It plays a role in the evaluation of clinically significant nipple discharge and in patients who present with an inflamed breast. To take full advantage of the contributions of breast ultrasound technology, two conditions are important. First, the breast imager should pay particular attention to detail and be meticulous in technique. Second, because many ultrasound findings still lack 100% specificity, the imager should be skilled in performing the relevant aspiration and needle biopsy procedures to provide the best care to women, with minimal discomfort.

References

1. Stavros AT, Rapp CL, Parker SH. In: Stavros AT, ed. *Breast ultrasound.* Philadelphia: Lippincott Williams & Wilkins, 2003.
2. American College of Radiology. *Practice guideline for the performance of a breast ultrasound examination.* Reston, VA: American College of Radiology, 2007: 523–527.
3. Szopinski KT, Pajk AM, Wysocki M, et al. Tissue harmonic imaging: utility in breast sonography. *J Ultrasound Med* 2003;22:479–487.
4. Del Cura JL, Elizagaray E, Zabala R, et al. The use of unenhanced Doppler sonography in the evaluation of solid breast lesions. *AJR Am J Roentgenol* 2005;184: 1788–1794.
5. McNicholas MMJ, Mercer PM, Miller JC, et al. Color Doppler sonography in the evaluation of palpable breast masses. *AJR Am J Roentgenol* 1993;161:765–771.
6. Raza S, Baum JK. Solid breast lesions. evaluation with power Doppler US. *Radiology* 1997;203:164–168.
7. Itoh A, Ueno E, Tohno E, et al. Breast disease: clinical application of US elastography for diagnosis. *Radiology* 2006;239:341–350.
8. Burnside ES, Hall TJ, Sommer AM, et al. Differentiating benign from malignant solid breast masses with US stain imaging. *Radiology* 2007;245:401–410.
9. Watermann DO, Foldi M, Hanjalic-Beck A, et al. Three-dimensional ultrasound for the assessment of breast lesions. *Ultrasound Obstet Gynecol* 2005;25:592–598.
10. Cho KR, Seo BK, Lee JK, et al. A comparative study of 2D and 3D ultrasonography for evaluation of solid breast masses. *Eur J Radiol* 2005;54:365–370.
11. Cho N, Moon WK, Cha JH, et al. Differentiating benign from malignant solid breast masses: comparison of two-dimensional and three-dimensional US. *Radiology* 2006;240:26–32.
12. Baker JA, Soo MS, Rosen EL. Pictorial essay: artifacts and pitfalls in sonographic imaging of the breast. *AJR Am J Roentgenol* 2000; 176:1261–1266.
13. Berg WA, Campassi CI, Ioffe OB. Cystic lesions of the breast: sonographic-pathologic correlation. *Radiology* 2003;227:183–191.
14. Hindle WM, Arias RD, Florentine B, et al. Lack of utility in clinical practice of cytologic examination of nonbloody cyst fluid from palpable breast cysts. *Am J Obstet Gynecol* 2000;182:1300–1305.
15. Gizienski TA, Harvey JA, Sobel AH. Breast cyst recurrence after postaspiration injection of air. *Breast J* 2002;8(1):34–37.
16. Venta L, Kim J, Pelloski CE, et al. Management of complex breast cysts. *AJR Am J Roentgenol* 1999;173:1331–1336.
17. Stavros AT, Thickman D, Rapp CL, et al. Solid breast nodules: use of sonography to distinguish between benign and malignant lesions. *Radiology* 1995;196:123–134.
18. Rahbar G, Sie AC, Hansen GC, et al. Benign versus malignant solid masses: US differentiation. *Radiology* 1999;213:889–894.
19. Mendelson EB, Berg WA, Merritt CRB. Toward a standardized breast ultrasound lexicon, BI-RADS: Ultrasound. *Semin Roentgenol* 2001;36(3):217–225.
20. American College of Radiology (ACR). ACR BIRADS: ultrasound. In: *Breast imaging reporting and data system:breast imaging atlas.* 4th ed. Reston VA: American College of Radiology, 2003, p. 1–86.
21. Hong AS, Rosen EL, Soo MS, et al. BI-RADS for sonography: positive and negative predictive values of sonographic features. *AJR Am J Roentgenol* 2005;84: 1260–1265.
22. Lazarus E, Mainiero MB, Schepps B, et al. BI-RADS lexicon for US and mammography: interobserver variability and positive predictive value. *Radiology* 2006;239: 385–391.
23. Costantini M, Belli P, Lombardi R, et al. Characterization of solid breast masses: use of the sonographic breast imaging reporting and data system lexicon. *J Ultrasound Med* 2006;25:649–659.
24. Butler RS, Venta LA, Wiley EL, et al. Sonographic evaluation of infiltration lobular carcinoma. *AJR Am J Roentgenol* 1999;172:325–330.

25. Moon WK, Myung FS, Lee YF, et al. US of ductal carcinoma in situ. *Radiographics* 2002;22:269–281.
26. Yang WT, Whitman GJ, Yuen EHY, et al. Sonographic features of primary breast cancer in men. *AJR Am J Roentgenol* 2001;176:413–416.
27. Chen L, Chantra PK, Larsen LH, et al. Imaging characteristics of malignant lesions of the male breast. *Radiographics* 2006;26:993–1006.
28. Jackson VP, Rothschild PA, Kreipke DL, et al. The spectrum of sonographic findings of fibrodenoma of the breast. *Invest Radiol* 1986;21:34–40.
29. Liberman L, Bonaccio E, Hamele-Bena D, et al. Benign and malignant phyllodes tumors: mammographic and sonographic findings. *Radiology* 1996;198:121–124.
30. Soo MS, Williford ME, Walsh R, et al. Papillary carcinoma of the breast: imaging findings. *AJR Am J Roentgenol* 1995;164:321–326.
31. Liberman L, Feng TL, Susnik B. Case 35: intracystic papillary carcinoma with invasion. *Radiology* 2001;219:781–784.
32. Lam WWM, Chu WCW, Tang APY, et al. Role of radiologic features in the management of papillary lesions of the breast. *AJR Am J Roentgenol* 2006;186:1322–1327.
33. Dennis MA, Parker SH, Klaus AJ, et al. Breast biopsy avoidance: the value of normal mammograms and normal sonograms in the setting of a palpable lump. *Radiology* 2001;219:186–191.
34. Soo MS, Rosen EL, Baker JA, et al. Negative predictive value of sonography with mammography in patients with palpable breast lesions. *AJR Am J Roentgenol* 2001;177:1167–1170.
35. Morrow M, Wong S, Venta L. The evaluation of breast masses in women younger than forty years of age. *Surgery* 1998;124:634–641.
36. Foxcroft LM, Evans EB, Porter AJ. The diagnosis of breast cancer in women younger than 40. *Breast* 2004;13:297–306.
37. Gunhan-Bilgen I, Ustun EE, Memis A. Inflammatory breast carcinoma: mammographic, ultrasonographic, clinical, and pathologic findings in 142 cases. *Radiology* 2002;223:829–838.
38. Rissanen T, Reinikainen H, Apaja-Sarkkinen M. Breast sonography in localizing the cause of nipple discharge. *J Ultrasound Med* 2007;26:1031–1039.
39. LaTrenta LR, Menell JH, Morris EA, et al. Breast lesions detected with MR imaging: utility and histopathologic importance of identification with US. *Radiology* 2003;227:856–861.
40. Sim LSJ, Hendriks JHCL, Bult P, et al. US correlation for MRI-detected breast lesions in women with familial risk of breast cancer. *Clin Radiol* 2005;60:801–806.
41. Harris KM, Ganott MA, Shestak KC, et al. Silicone implant rupture: detection with US. *Radiology* 1993;187:761–768.

42. Holland R, Veling SHJ, Mravunac M, et al. Histologic multifocality of Tis, T1-2 breast carcinomas: implications for clinical trials of breast-conserving surgery. *Cancer* 1985;56:979–990.
43. Berg WA, Gilbreath PL. Multicentric and multifocal cancer: whole-breast US in preoperative evaluation. *Radiology* 2000;214:59–66.
44. Liberman L, Morris EA, Dershaw DD, et al. MR imaging of the ipsilateral breast in women with percutaneously proven breast cancer. *AJR Am J Roentgenol* 2003;180:901–910.
45. Berg WA, Gutierrez L, Ness-Aiver MS, et al. Diagnostic accuracy of mammography, clinical examination, US and MR imaging in preoperative assessment of breast cancer. *Radiology* 2004;233:830–849.
46. Liberman L, Morris EA, Kim CM, et al. MR imaging findings in the contralateral breast of women with recently diagnosed breast cancer. *AJR Am J Roentgenol* 2003;180:333–341.
47. Lee S, Orel S, Woo I, et al. MR imaging of the contralateral breast in patients newly diagnosed breast cancer: preliminary results. *Radiology* 2003;226:773–778.
48. Lehman CD, Gatsonis C, Kuhl CK et al. MRI Evaluation of the contralateral breast in women recently diagnosed with breast cancer. *N Engl J Med* 2007;356:1295–1303.
49. Mathijssen IMJ, Strijdhorst H, Kiestra SK, et al. Added value of ultrasound in screening the clinically negative axilla in breast cancer. *J Surg Oncol* 2006;94:364–367.
50. Khan A, Sabel MS, Nees A, et al. Comprehensive axillary evaluation in neoadjuvant chemotherapy patients with ultrasonography and sentinel lymph node biopsy. *Ann Surg Oncol* 2005;12(9):697–704.
51. Krishnamurthy S, Sneige N, Bedi DG, et al. Role of ultrasound-guided fine-needle aspiration of indeterminate and suspicious axillary lymph nodes in the initial staging of breast carcinoma. *Cancer* 2002;95:982–988.
52. Somasundar P, Gass J, Steinhoff M, et al. Role of ultrasound-guided axillary fine-needle aspiration in the management of invasive breast cancer. *Am J Surg* 2006;192:458–461.
53. Jain A, Haisfield-Wolfe M, Lange J, et al. The role of ultrasound-guided fine-needle aspiration of axillary nodes in the staging of breast cancer. *Ann Surg Oncol* 2008;15(2):462–471.
54. Ciatto S, Brancato B, Risso G, et al. Accuracy of fine needle aspiration cytology (FNAC) of axillary lymph nodes as a triage test in breast cancer staging. *Breast Cancer Res Treat* 2007;103(1):85–91.
55. Koelliker SL, Chung Maureen A, Mainiero Martha B, et al. Axillary lymph nodes: US-guided fine-needle aspiration for initial staging of breast cancer—correlation with primary tumor size. *Radiology* 2008;246:81–89.

Susan Orel Roth

Over the past two decades, tremendous advances have been made in magnetic resonance imaging (MRI) of the breast and MRI-guided breast interventional procedures. Technical requirements for optimal breast imaging, including the requirement for a breast MRI biopsy system, are now being defined as part of a voluntary American College of Radiology (ACR) breast MRI accreditation program. The ACR BI-RADS (Breast Imaging Reporting and Data System) lexicon for breast MRI has brought uniformity to the interpretation and reporting of breast MRI examinations. With advances in imaging technique, interpretation guidelines, and increasing availability of MRI breast biopsy systems, MRI of the breast is rapidly gaining popularity in clinical practice in both the diagnostic setting and, more recently, in the screening setting. The clinical indications for MRI of the breast, however, remain to be defined. There are clinical settings that have emerged where MRI, as an adjunct to mammography, appears to be the imaging study of choice. There are other clinical settings where MRI is being utilized with increasing frequency but where controversy persists.

TECHNICAL CONSIDERATIONS

In contrast to mammography, where the techniques for optimal imaging are well defined, now under the regulation of the Mammography Quality Standards Act (MQSA), overseen by the U.S. Food and Drug Administration (FDA) (1), the image quality of breast MRI studies has varied widely. There are many variables that can affect image quality, and there has been ongoing debate as to what is required for optimal MRI of the breast (2). In an effort to bring uniformity to the quality of breast MRI studies in the United States, the technical requirements for breast MRI examinations are currently being defined by the American College of Radiology voluntary MRI accreditation program. The requirements (as of January 2008) are detailed in the sections that follow.

High Field Magnet

Breast MRI studies should be performed on a high field (>1.0 T) magnet. There is a linear relationship between magnetic field strength and signal-to-noise ratio (SNR). With greater field strength, the SNR is higher, and higher spatial resolution images can be obtained with shorter acquisition times. Also, at high field, a homogeneous magnetic field can be achieved across both breasts, permitting homogeneous fat suppression (see below). Most clinical investigations of MRI of the breast have been performed on standard high field MRI systems (1 to 1.5 T), and, currently, clinical breast MRI studies are most commonly being performed on these high field systems. There is ongoing clinical investigation into imaging the breast at higher (3.0 T) magnetic field strength, with the potential for higher SNR and higher spatial and temporal resolution (3).

Dedicated Breast Coils

A dedicated breast surface coil must be used when performing breast MRI. Many different types of surface coils are available. At the Hospital of the University of Pennsylvania, a bilateral breast multicoil is utilized (4). This type of coil allows for parallel imaging techniques that can halve the image acquisition time through imaging both breasts simultaneously. The patient is examined in the prone position with the breast(s) gently compressed between two plates, which are placed along the medial and lateral sides of the breast. The compression minimizes patient motion and reduces the number of sagittal slices required to image the breasts and, thereby, reducing imaging time. This configuration also ensures that all of the breast tissue is close to one of the elements of the array, resulting in enhanced SNR. The compression should be applied gently, as firm compression can delay contrast uptake.

Intravenous Contrast

The cornerstone of breast MRI is imaging following the intravenous injection of a paramagnetic contrast agent (gadolinium chelate). Gadolinium is a T1 shortening agent. Following intravenous injection, accumulation of gadolinium in tissue reflects alterations in vascular density or vascular permeability. Most investigators report the use of a dose of 0.1 mmol/kg of body weight. The contrast is injected intravenously, usually as a bolus, followed by a saline flush. To ensure that the postcontrast images can be obtained immediately following the contrast injection, tuning and gain adjustments should be performed before the contrast is injected and should not be readjusted for the remainder of the postcontrast enhanced sequence.

Fat Suppression

In contrast to mammography, where lesion detectability is increased in a fatty background, on MRI, an enhancing lesion may not be detected as it becomes isointense to fat following the administration of intravenous contrast. Thus, the signal from fat needs to be eliminated. This can be accomplished with either active or passive fat suppression. the author and others prefer using "active" fat suppression where the signal from fat is removed prior to the injection of intravenous contrast. There are a variety of available fat suppression techniques (2,4,5). Alternatively, passive fat suppression can be accomplishing with postprocessing image subtraction (subtracting the precontrast from the postcontrast image) (6,7). This requires that there be no patient motion between the pre- and the postcontrast sequences. Both methods of fat suppression (chemical fat suppression and image postprocessing image subtraction) can be used together, and in the author's experience, this does aid in the detection of small enhancing lesions.

High Spatial and Temporal Resolution

Historically, investigators studying the differentiation of malignant from benign breast lesions were divided into two groups, the first being the "high temporal resolution" group where lesion characterization was based on contrast enhancement kinetics, which required high temporal resolution, and the "high spatial resolution" group, where lesion morphology was critical and required high spatial resolution (4–9). Unfortunately, high temporal and high spatial resolution are competing strategies, and choosing one was at the sacrifice of the other. Sensitivity for the detection of small enhancing foci improves with increasing

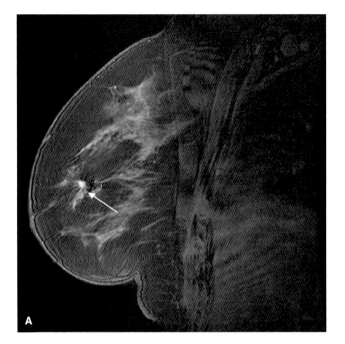

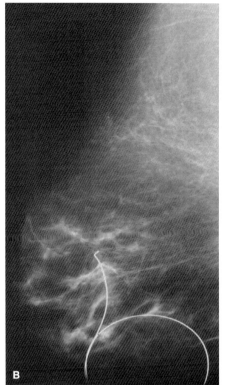

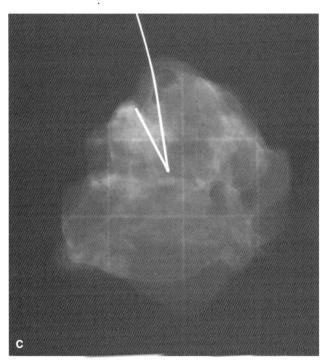

FIGURE 14.1. Magnetic resonance–guided wire localization for excisional biopsy. A: Sagittal magnetic resonance image (MRI) demonstrate the enhancing lesion (*arrow*) to be localized by the needle. **B:** Mediolateral oblique view mammograms show the tip of the hook wire to be in the central breast. There is no visible mammographic finding. **C:** Mammographic specimen radiograph reveals the hook wire but again, no mammographic finding is present. Pathology showed a 1-cm invasive ductal carcinoma.

spatial resolution, but this requires longer imaging times. On the other hand, the high temporal resolution needed for dynamic contrast enhancement is obtained at the cost of a loss of spatial resolution, signal to noise, or volume of the breast imaged. For optimal spatial resolution, a pixel size of less than 1.0 mm in each in-plane direction is necessary. For optimal temporal resolution, the first postcontrast images should be obtained in less than 2 minutes following contrast injection, with subsequent scans obtained over the following 5 to 7 minutes to evaluate the shape of the enhancement curve. The need to choose a high temporal resolution sequence versus a high spatial resolution sequence has been obviated by recent advances in MRI technology, specifically parallel imaging, which permits simultaneous imaging of both breasts with high temporal and spatial resolution.

Magnetic Resonance Imaging–Guided Localization and Biopsy Capability

The ability to perform MRI-guided interventional procedures will also be part of the ACR accreditation program. There will be malignant lesions detected on MRI that will be occult on mammography, sonography, and clinical examination. On the other hand, the majority of enhancing lesions recommended for biopsy will prove to be benign. With a technique that is highly sensitive but not highly specific, a needle localization or core needle biopsy system is needed to differentiate true positive enhancing malignant lesions from false-positive benign enhancing lesions. There are now several commercially available MRI compatible localization or biopsy systems.

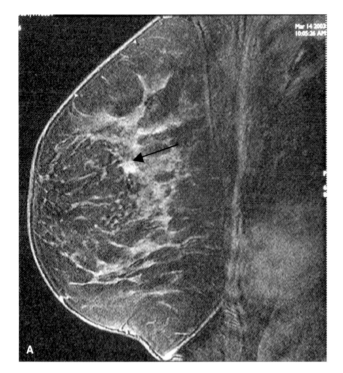

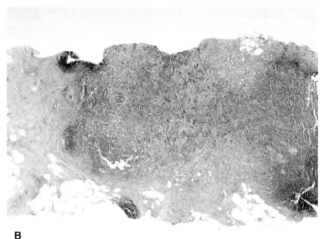

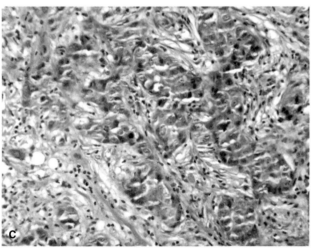

FIGURE 14.2. Magnetic resonance imaging (MRI)-guided core biopsy. A: Sagittal MRI of a 30-year-old *BRCA1* positive with a 6-mm peripherally enhancing lesion with irregular borders (*arrow*). **B,C:** Pathology reveals a high-grade invasive ductal carcinoma.

Historically, MRI-guided intervention was limited to needle localization followed by excisional biopsy. Several investigators have demonstrated the clinical utility of these systems (10–12) (Fig. 14.1). More recently, MRI-compatible core biopsy systems have become commercially available (Fig. 14.2). The advantages of MRI-guided core biopsy compared with needle localization and excisional biopsy are the same as for conventional core biopsy, the major advantages being a decrease in the number of benign excisional biopsies and a reduced number of surgical procedures for patients diagnosed with breast cancer. There have now been several studies demonstrating the feasibility and accuracy of MRI-guided core biopsy (13–16).

A major limitation of MRI-guided needle localization and core biopsy remains the inability to verify successful lesion removal or lesion sampling. In the case of needle localization, the lesion localized with MRI guidance is usually not visible with mammographic specimen radiography (Fig. 14.1). In the case of core biopsy, the ability to document successful sampling can be impossible due to the wash-out of contrast during the procedure (Fig. 14.3). Although a clip is placed following most MRI core biopsies, documentation of accurate clip placement can be difficult or impossible if the lesion is not visible at the end of the procedure.

It is possible for the lesion to have been displaced by the needle such that the lesion location and clip location are not the same. Careful radiologic and pathologic correlation is needed to determine if the pathology findings are concordant with the imaging findings. In any case where the MRI finding is highly suspicious but the pathology is benign, immediate repeat MRI is required. Whether short interval MRI follow-up should be performed in all cases with a nonspecific benign pathology result (i.e., fibrocystic changes or benign breast tissue) remains to be defined.

There has been clinical investigation into the use of directed "second-look" ultrasound following the MRI detection of a suspicious enhancing lesion. In those cases where the MRI-detected lesion is sonographically visible, an ultrasound-guided core biopsy could be performed in place of an MRI-guided biopsy. In a retrospective review, LaTrenta et al. (17) reported the results of directed ultrasound in 64 patients with 93 suspicious lesions identified on MRI. An ultrasound correlate was identified in 21 (23%) lesions, 19 of 76 (25%) focal masses and 2 of 17 (11%) nonmass lesions. Cancer was found in nine (43%) lesions. Among the lesions where ultrasound was negative, 10 (14%) yielded cancer (50% invasive and 50% ductal carcinoma *in situ* [DCIS]). Although ultrasound can be used to identify a subset of

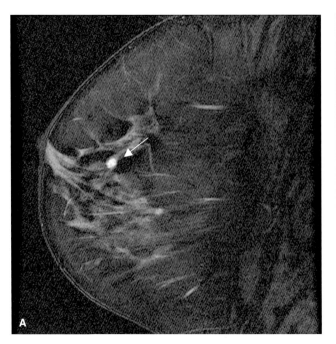

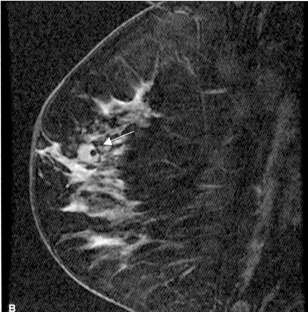

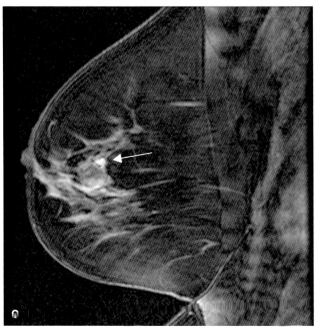

FIGURE 14.3. False-negative magnetic resonance–guided core biopsy. A: Sagittal magnetic resonance imaging (MRI) demonstrates a 7-mm enhancing mass (*arrow*). B: Postbiopsy MRI reveals a biopsy cavity (*arrow*) with no residual enhancing lesion identified. Pathology showed a 3 mm papilloma, which was not felt to be concordant with the imaging findings. C: Repeat MRI demonstrates the enhancing lesion (*arrow*) adjacent to the postbiopsy cavity. Invasive ductal carcinoma was found at MR-guided wire localization and excision.

MRI-detected suspicious lesions, there will be both invasive and noninvasive cancers that will be sonographically occult and thereby require MRI-guided biopsy for tissue diagnosis.

Image Interpretation

Following contrast administration, one or more areas of enhancement will often be identified in one or both breasts. These enhancing areas must then be further characterized: are any suspicious for breast cancer? Early investigation of contrast-enhanced MRI of the breast suggested that breast cancer consistently enhanced following the administration of intravenous contrast and that cancer could be differentiated from benign lesions with very high specificity based on differences in contrast kinetics (6–9). Further investigation, however, demonstrated that in addition to breast cancer, many benign lesions demonstrated contrast enhancement that overlapped with the enhancement of malignant lesions (5,18). Reported specificities of MRI have been

very variable, ranging from 37% to 97% (4). Contrast enhancement has been seen not only in cancer, but also in fibroadenoma, fibrocystic changes including sclerosing adenosis, fat necrosis, radial scar, mastitis, atypical ductal hyperplasia, and lobular neoplasia (Fig. 14.4). In addition, normal breast tissue may enhance following contrast enhancement. This enhancement has been shown to vary with different phases of the menstrual cycle, being greatest in weeks 1 and 4, lowest in week 2 (Fig. 14.5) (19). When using enhancement kinetics alone, it was shown in one study that up to three fourths of enhancing lesions with suspicious enhancement kinetics completely disappeared when the study was repeated at a different time in the menstrual cycle (19).

In attempting to differentiate enhancing lesions suspicious for breast cancer from those felt to be benign or likely benign, investigators have utilized differences in enhancement kinetics or morphologic features. Investigators who have studied the enhancement characteristics of benign and malignant lesions utilizing high temporal resolution techniques have described

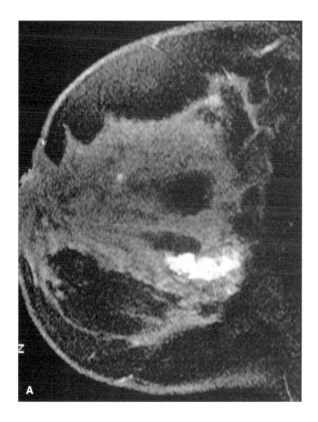
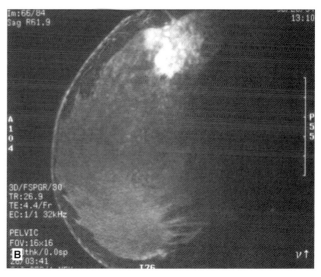
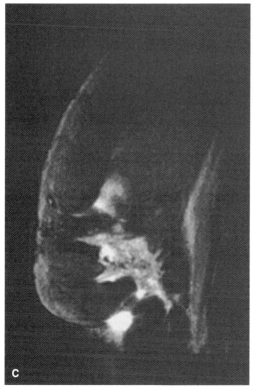
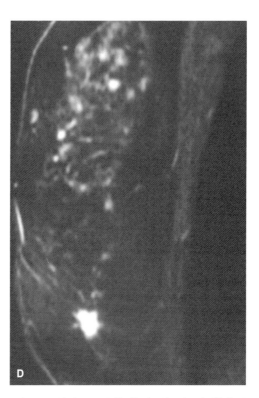

FIGURE 14.4. False-positive enhancing lesions. Contrast enhancement is demonstrated in (**A**) sclerosing adenosis, (**B**) chronic mastitis, (**C**) fat necrosis, and (**D**) radial scar.

both quantitative and qualitative methods for determining lesion enhancement (6–9,20–23). It has been suggested, based on the results of these studies, that enhancement kinetics can be used to differentiate malignant from benign lesions, where malignant lesions tend to demonstrate a rapid increase in signal intensity following contrast administration, often followed by a wash-out of contrast, while benign lesions tend to exhibit a slower, progressive rise in signal intensity over time (Fig. 14.6). Other investigators, however, have observed an overlap in the enhancement kinetics of benign and malignant lesions, which can be explained, at least in part, by histologic variability of both cancers and benign lesions (22).

A second approach for lesion characterization has utilized morphologic features identified on high spatial resolution

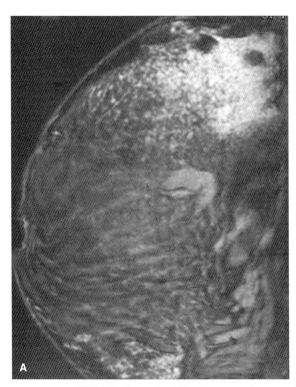
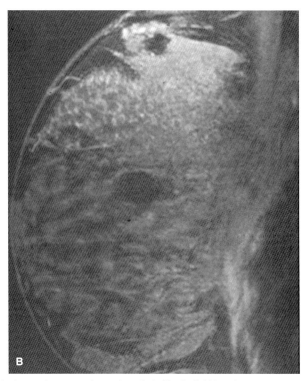

FIGURE 14.5. Hormonal variability of contrast enhancement. Sagittal magnetic resonance image of a patient with a family history of breast cancer reveals an area of regional enhancement in the superior breast, which was no longer present when the patient was imaged at a different time in her menstrual cycle.

images to differentiate lesions suspicious for malignancy from those that are benign or probably benign (4,5,18,24,25). Features that suggest the possibility of malignancy include a mass with irregular or spiculated borders, a mass with peripheral enhancement, an area of segmental or regional enhancement, and ductal enhancement (Fig. 14.7). Features suggesting benign disease include a mass with smooth or lobulated borders, a mass demonstrating minimal or no contrast enhancement, a mass with nonenhancing internal septations, and scattered foci (<5 mm in size) of enhancement (Fig. 14.8). An interpretation model encompassing multiple architectural features has been described, yielding a specificity of 80% (25).

It has become apparent that the integration of both kinetic and morphologic information may ultimately be needed in order to achieve optimal discrimination (26). As discussed above, with continued technical advances in breast coils and in imaging software, it is now possible to image with both high

Enhancement Kinetics

Fast

Medium

Slow

Persistent (C)

Plateau (B)

Washout (A)

FIGURE 14.6. Enhancement kinetics. Enhancement measured over time shows three enhancement curves: (**A**) wash-out of contrast commonly seen in cancer, (**B**) plateau enhancement seen in both malignant and benign lesions, and (**C**) persistent increasing enhancement common in benign lesions.

temporal and high spatial resolution so that both kinetics and lesion morphology can be used together for lesion evaluation.

In an effort to bring uniformity to breast MRI reports, an MRI breast imaging lexicon (BI-RADS) has been created through the efforts of the Susan Komen Foundation, the Public Health Service Office on Women's Health, and the ACR (27). The first version of the MRI breast lexicon was published by the ACR in 2003. The structure of the lexicon is similar to that used in mammography. Included in the MRI lexicon are lesion descriptors (using both morphology and enhancement kinetics), an overall impression, and final recommendation. A BI-RADS category 0 study is incomplete, where comparison with a previous MRI study or correlation with mammography or ultrasound is needed. A BI-RADS category 1 study is negative. A BI-RADS category 2 study demonstrates benign findings such as postsurgical or postradiation changes, cysts, or an enhancing lesion(s) with benign MRI characteristics. A BI-RADS category 3 study demonstrates an enhancing lesion(s) that is deemed to be probably benign and short-term interval follow-up, usually at 6 months, is recommended. Finally, a BI-RADS category 4 (suspicious) and 5 (highly suspicious) study demonstrate an enhancing lesion(s) for which a biopsy is recommended. The biopsy can be performed with MRI guidance if seen only on MRI, or with ultrasound guidance in those cases where the MRI finding can be identified on a directed ultrasound study.

Refinements to the first version of the BI-RADS lexicon for MRI are ongoing. Although lesion descriptors are well defined, additional clinical investigation is needed to gain a better understanding of how to interpret those studies where one or more enhancing lesions are detected that do not demonstrate morphologic features or a kinetic enhancement profile that is suspicious for malignancy. In these cases, it should be determined if the enhancement is normal, benign, or probably benign. In mammography, findings that should be placed into the probably benign category have been well studied. In clinical investigation, it has been demonstrated that the likelihood of a lesion classified as probably benign, BI-RADS category 3, but ultimately prove to be malignant should be less than 1% to 2% (28). For MRI, the type of enhancement that should be classified as probably benign as opposed to normal, benign, or suspicious remains unclear. In

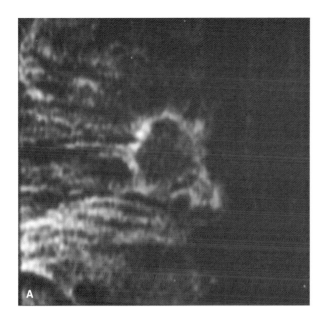

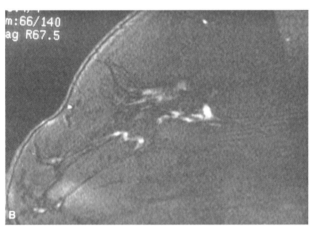

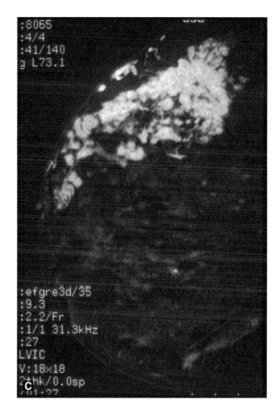

FIGURE 14.7. Morphologic features of malignant lesions. A: Peripheral enhancement and spiculated borders of invasive ductal carcinoma, (B) ductal enhancement, and (C) clumped segmental enhancement of ductal carcinoma *in situ*.

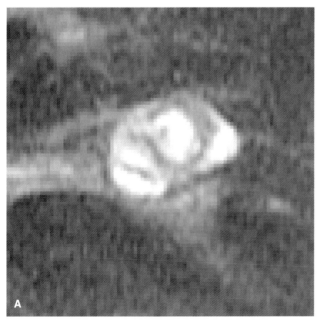

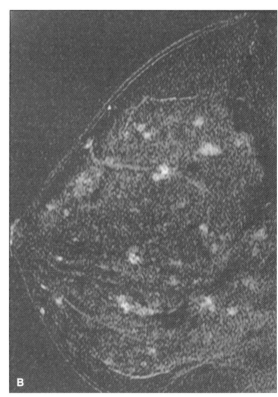

FIGURE 14.8. Morphologic features of benign lesions. A: Lobulated mass with nonenhancing septa and (B) scattered foci (<5 mm) of enhancement.

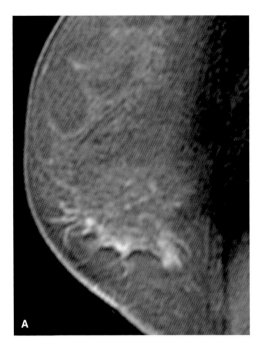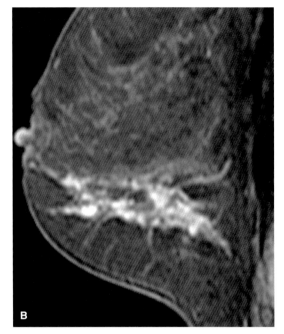

FIGURE 14.9. Breast cancer in lesion classified as Breast Imaging Reporting and Data System (BI-RADS) category 3. A: Sagittal magnetic resonance imaging (MRI) shows mild enhancement in the inferior breast. Six-month follow-up MRI was recommended. **B:** Progression of enhancement was identified at 6 months. Pathology revealed ductal carcinoma *in situ*. (Courtesy of Elizabeth Morris, MSKCC.)

contrast to mammography, there has been very little published on the outcome of lesions placed into the BI-RADS category 3. In a study of enhancing lesions classified as probably benign in high-risk women, Liberman et al. (29) reported that 89 of 367 (24%) women had one or more MRI findings classified as probably benign. Twenty women underwent biopsy and malignancy was found in 9 of 89 (10%) women. Five were DCIS and four were invasive cancers (Fig. 14.9). This percentage is much higher than would be accepted for a mammographic category 3 lesion. However, in a second study, Eby et al. (30) reported the outcome of probably benign findings in 809 consecutive MRI examinations. Twenty percent (160/809) were classified as probably benign. Only one (0.6%) cancer was found. The wide discrepancy in results between these two studies is likely, in large part, due to differences in patient populations, where the probability of malignancy of a probably benign lesion is higher in a population at high risk for the development of breast cancer.

CLINICAL INDICATIONS

Problem Solving: The Equivocal Mammogram, Ultrasound, or Physical Examination Finding

There are reports that MR imaging can be used as a problem-solving tool in the setting of equivocal imaging (mammography and/or ultrasound) findings (Fig. 14.10) or equivocal physical examination findings (Fig. 14.11) (31–33). MRI can be a very useful clinical tool when breast cancer is suspected, but the diagnosis cannot be established by means of conventional methods. MRI, however, should never be used in place of a full mammographic and sonographic evaluation.

Based on results of several studies demonstrating sensitivity of MRI for the detection of invasive cancer approaching 100%, it has been suggested that a negative MRI examination in the setting of equivocal imaging or physical examination findings virtually excludes the presence of invasive cancer (34). However, there have been multiple reports (24,31,36–40) documenting false-negative MRI cases, not only of noninvasive

cancer, but of invasive ductal cancer as well, including invasive lobular cancer. The reported false-negative rates of MRI range from 4% to 12% (37–39). As is true with a negative mammogram or a negative ultrasound study in a patient with a suspicious palpable abnormality, a negative MRI study should not preclude biopsy (Fig. 14.12).

Axillary Node Malignancy and Unknown Site of Primary Tumor

Occult primary breast cancer presenting as malignant axillary adenopathy represents less than 1% of breast cancers (40). The ability of mammography to identify a primary breast cancer in this clinical setting has been disappointing, with reported rates ranging from 0% to 56%. In contrast, MRI has demonstrated very high sensitivity for the detection of an ipsilateral breast cancer primary (41–43) in these patients. In a review of six studies, the overall sensitivity of MRI was 94% with a specificity of 94% to 100% and estimated positive predictive value was 90% (43). The results of these studies support the clinical use of MRI as the imaging study of choice in the setting of malignant axillary adenopathy and unknown site of primary tumor (Fig. 14.13). In this patient population, MRI offers the potential for breast cancer detection as well as staging, which can then be used to guide treatment planning. The identification of localized disease may offer some patients the option of breast-conservation therapy as an alternative to mastectomy. Follow-up of a small number of patients presenting with malignant axillary adenopathy and MRI-detected mammographically and clinically occult breast cancer who subsequently underwent lumpectomy and radiation therapy has demonstrated similar outcome to the expected outcome of patients who presented with breast cancer and positive axillary lymph nodes (44).

Monitoring Response to Chemotherapy

The clinical and mammographic detection of tumor response to chemotherapy can be impaired by chemotherapy-induced fibrosis (45). Given the high sensitivity of MRI for the detection of invasive cancer in the untreated breast, the potential use of MRI in the setting of preoperative chemotherapy has been

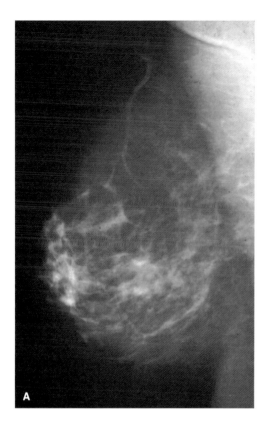

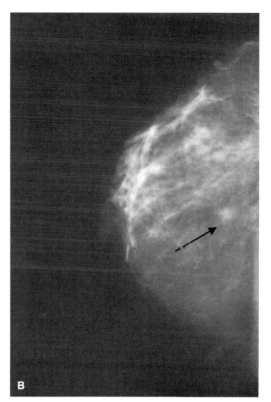

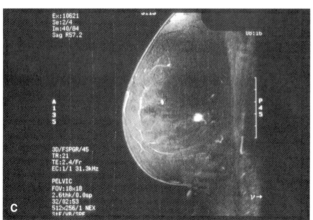

FIGURE 14.10. Magnetic resonance imaging (MRI) for problem solving. A: Mediolateral oblique (MLO) and (**B**) craniocaudad (CC) view mammogram demonstrates a density in the central breast on the CC view (*arrow*). This persisted on spot compression, but could not be identified on the ML or MLO views or on ultrasound examination. **C:** Sagittal MRI reveals an enhancing mass in the central breast. MRI-guided wire localization and excisional biopsy revealed invasive ductal carcinoma.

investigated in multiple clinical studies (46–54) (Fig. 14.14). It has been shown that MRI can provide evidence of response to therapy as early as 6 weeks following the initiation of chemotherapy, where contrast enhancement decreases before any change in tumor size can be detected (47). However, it has been demonstrated in multiple studies that the accuracy of MRI varies with the degree of response to chemotherapy (46–54). MRI appears to be highly accurate for the identification of cancers in nonresponders and in those with a partial response to chemotherapy, where residual tumor size predicted by MRI correlates closely with that found at surgery. In these patients, contrast enhancement tends to increase or decrease only slightly during chemotherapy. In responders, contrast enhancement decreases during chemotherapy. However, it has been shown that MRI may overestimate tumor response in those cases where the tumors responds well to chemotherapy. In some cases, MRI following treatment demonstrates no residual enhancing tumor, yet residual tumor nests, which may be extensive, are found at excision. The absence of enhancement even in the presence of residual invasive tumor is likely secondary to chemotherapy-induced decreased tumor vascular-

ization or decreased vascular permeability. It has also been demonstrated that the underestimation of residual tumor burden on MRI may vary with the chemotherapeutic agent. Tumors treated with a taxane-containing regimen are often underestimated (53). It is postulated that the underestimation of tumor volume by MRI is secondary to the numerous nests of tumor left following the taxane regimen compared with a more concentric tumor shrinkage with other chemotherapeutic agents. There have also been reports of overestimation of residual tumor burden on MRI that may be secondary to chemotherapy-induced reactive changes within the tumor (54).

Despite its limitations, MRI does appear, at the current time, to be the most accurate imaging method for evaluating response to chemotherapy (Fig. 14.3). However, the potential for MRI to overestimate tumor response must be considered when planning definitive surgical management following the end of treatment.

Breast Cancer Screening in Women at High Risk

In the mid- to late 1990s, six prospective, nonrandomized studies were initiated in The Netherlands, the United Kingdom,

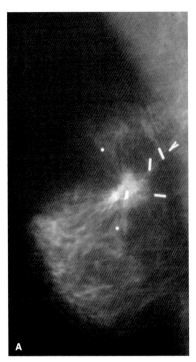
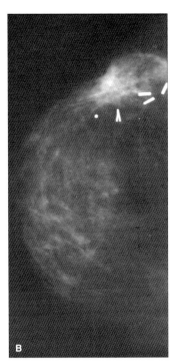
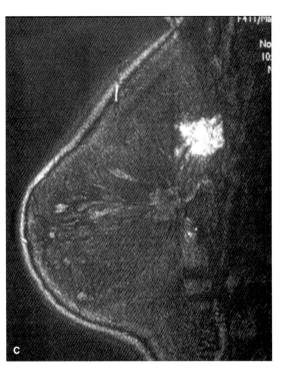

FIGURE 14.11. **Magnetic resonance imaging (MRI) for problem solving. A:** Mediolateral oblique (MLO) and (**B**) craniocaudad (CC) view mammograms is a patient 1-year status post–breast-conservation therapy with discomfort in the left axilla. Posttreatment changes are present but no suspicious finding is seen. Directed ultrasound of the left axillary tail and axilla revealed biopsy changes but no suspicious findings. **C:** Sagittal MRI reveals an enhancing mass posterior to the biopsy site. Pathology showed invasive ductal carcinoma.

Canada, Germany, the United States, and Italy to determine the benefit of adding annual MRI to film mammography for women genetically at high risk, defined as *BRCA1/BRCA2* mutation carriers or with at least a 20% probability of carrying a *BRCA1/BRCA2* mutation (55–60). The cancer detection rate in these studies ranged from 1.0% to 9.3% (average 5.7%).

Despite substantial differences in patient population (i.e., age, risk) and MRI technique, all reported significantly higher sensitivity for MRI compared with film mammography (or any of the other modalities) (Fig. 14.2). Overall, the studies reported a high sensitivity for MRI, ranging from 71% to 100% versus 16% to 40% for mammography in high-risk populations (61). Three studies

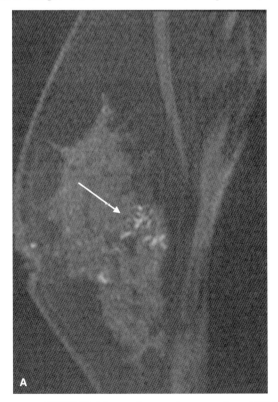
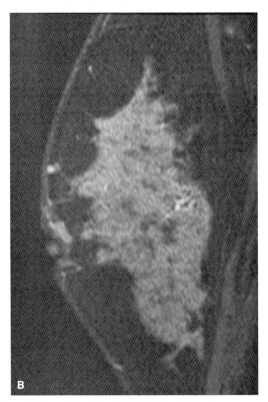

FIGURE 14.12. **False-negative magnetic resonance image (MRI).** MRI requested for evaluation of a patient with bloody nipple discharge and negative mammogram. **A:** Sagittal MRI reveals high signal fluid filled ducts (*arrow*) in the central breast. **B:** Sagittal MRI reveals diffuse glandular enhancement. In the absence of a focal area of enhancement, the study was interpreted as negative. Excisional biopsy revealed multifocal ductal carcinoma *in situ* in the central breast.

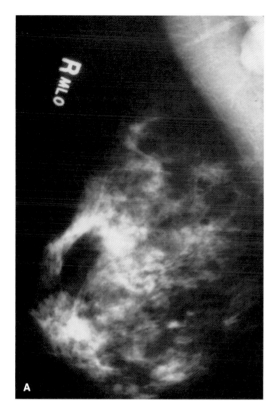

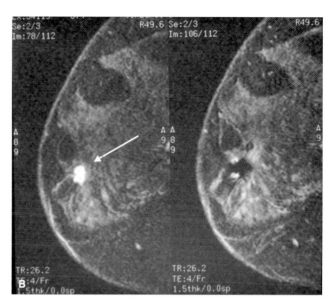

FIGURE 14.13. Axillary node malignancy. Magnetic resonance imaging (MRI) requested for evaluation of a patient presenting with malignant axillary adenopathy. **A:** mediolateral oblique view mammogram demonstrated heterogeneously dense breast tissue with no suspicious findings identified. **B:** Sagittal MRI reveals a 1-cm enhancing lesion (*arrow*) in the subareolar breast. MRI-guided wire localization and excisional biopsy revealed a 1-cm high-grade invasive ductal carcinoma with lymphatic invasion. The patient underwent breast-conservation therapy.

included ultrasound, which had sensitivity similar to mammography.

Although MRI has demonstrated high sensitivity for the detection of mammographic and clinically occult cancer in the clinical setting of high-risk screening, the limited specificity of MRI resulting in false-positive findings remains of concern. In the six screening studies, call-back rates for additional imaging ranged from 8% to 17%, and biopsy rates ranged from 3% to 15% (61). However, it has been reported that recall rates decreased in subsequent rounds of screening, where the prevalence screens had

the highest false-positive rates, which subsequently dropped to less than 10%. The call-back and biopsy rates of MRI were higher than for mammography in high-risk populations. Although the increased sensitivity of MRI lead to a higher call-back rate, it also lead to a higher number of cancers detected. The proportion of biopsies yielding a malignant diagnosis (positive predictive value) in these studies was 20% to 40% (61).

The potential for heightened patient anxiety following a false-positive MRI examination remains of concern. Results of relatively small studies have demonstrated variable degrees

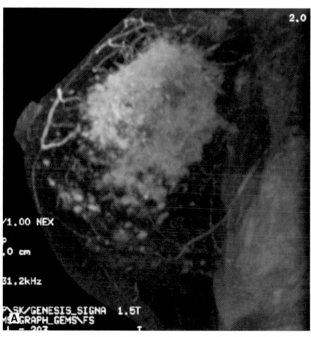

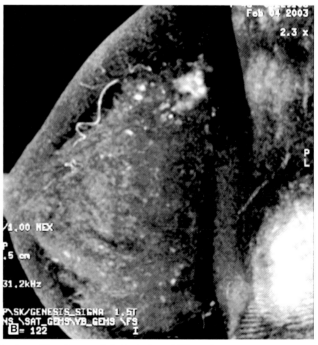

FIGURE 14.14. Magnetic resonance imaging (MRI) follow-up of locally advanced breast cancer. A: Contrast-enhanced MRI reveals a large enhancing mass. **B:** Sagittal MRI following chemotherapy demonstrates a marked reduction in tumor size.

of elevated anxiety in women following a false-positive MRI examination; however, most women continued to return for annual MRI screening (61). There has been anecdotal evidence that a false-positive MRI screening examination in a woman at high risk for the development of breast cancer may result in the request for prophylactic mastectomy. The actual frequency of prophylactic mastectomy secondary to a false-positive MRI study remains to be determined. Hoogerbrugge et al. (62) reported their experience in a study of 196 *BRCA* mutation carries who underwent screening with MRI. In this study, 41% (81/196) of women had at least one positive MRI or mammogram. The probability that a positive MRI result was a false positive was 83%. In patients with a prior preference for mastectomy, prophylactic mastectomy was performed in 89% in those with a false-positive MRI versus 66% with a negative MRI ($p = .06$). No significant difference was found in women with prior preference for surveillance.

Another concern surrounding screening MRI is the potential for high downstream costs when the MRI examinations yield false-positive results, leading to immediate recall MRI studies, short interval follow-up MRI studies, additional mammogram and ultrasound studies, and benign breast biopsies. There are limited data on the cost-effectiveness of MRI screening. In one study, the authors concluded that the cost per quality-adjusted life year (QALY) saved for annual MRI plus film mammography, compared with annual film mammography alone, varied by age and was more favorable in carriers of a mutation in *BRCA1* than *BRCA2* because *BRCA1* mutations confer higher cancer risk and higher risk of more aggressive cancers than *BRCA2* mutations. Estimated cost per QALY for women aged 35 to 54 years was $55,420 for women with a *BRCA1* mutation and $130,695 for women with a *BRCA2* mutation. The most important determinants of cost-effectiveness were breast cancer risk, sensitivity of mammography, cost of MRI, and quality of life gains from MRI (63). An evaluation of the cost-effectiveness in the United Kingdom showed that the incremental cost per cancer detected for women at approximately 50% risk of carrying a *BRCA* gene mutation was $50,911 for MRI combined with mammography over mammography alone. For known mutation carriers, the incremental cost per cancer detected decreased to $27,544 for MRI combined with mammography, compared with mammography alone (64).

Based on the results of the MRI screening trials, the American Cancer Society (ACS) is currently recommending annual screening breast MRI for women who have an approximately 20% to 25% or greater lifetime risk of breast cancer, including women with a strong family history of breast or ovarian cancer and women who were treated for Hodgkin's lymphoma (61). There are several risk subgroups for which the available data were felt to be insufficient to recommend for or against screening, including women with a personal history of breast cancer, biopsy demonstrated lobular carcinoma *in situ* (LCIS) or atypical hyperplasia, and extremely dense breasts on mammography. Clinical investigation into the potential role of MRI patients with a history of LCIS and atypia continues (65).

There is ongoing debate surrounding the use of MRI in the subgroup of patients with newly diagnosed breast cancer where MRI is being requested for screening of the contralateral breast. Historically, the reported incidence of synchronous bilateral breast cancer detected on physical examination or mammography is 3% to 6% (66). There are now multiple single institution and multicenter trial reports demonstrating the utility of MRI in the detection of mammographic and clinically occult synchronous contralateral cancers, with reported rates of approximately 3% to 19% of patients examined (67–70). Approximately half of the lesions detected on MRI have been invasive cancers and the other half have been DCIS (Figs. 14.15 and 14.16). In a recent report of 969 women with a recent diagnosis of unilateral breast cancer who underwent MRI as part of a multicenter trial, mammographic and clinically occult contralateral breast cancer was detected at MRI in 30 (3.1%)

women (69). The sensitivity of MRI was 91% and the specificity was 88%. The negative predictive value of MRI was 99%. A biopsy was performed in 12.5% of patients with a positive result in 24.8% of cases. Eighteen of 30 were invasive cancers.

Although MRI can be used to detect clinically and mammographically unsuspected synchronous bilateral breast cancer, questions remain. The clinical significance, specifically survival benefit, of the detection of these occult synchronous cancers, especially the noninvasive cancers, is not known (Fig. 14.16). Would the contralateral cancers detected on MRI be successfully treated in those patients who undergo systemic chemotherapy and, thus, never become clinically apparent? Furthermore, the detection of these contralateral cancers must be weighed against the added time, expense, and additional costs associated with MRI and MRI-guided biopsy in those cases where the MRI-detected lesions prove to be benign. Similar to the experience of false-positive MRI findings in the setting of high-risk screening, there has been anecdotal experience that some women will choose to undergo prophylactic mastectomy of the contralateral breast when a lesion is detected on MRI, even without tissue biopsy (Fig. 14.17) (64,65). The frequency of prophylactic mastectomy following a false-positive MRI examination remains to be determined.

Nipple Discharge

The incidence of malignancy in patients with clinically concerning nipple discharge ranges from 5% to 20% (71). The utility of cytology, mammography, ultrasound, and galactography have been limited. There have been a few reports, with relative small numbers of patients, demonstrating the potential of MRI to identify both malignant and benign lesions in this clinical setting (72–74). In a retrospective study performed at the Hospital of the University of Pennsylvania, evaluating MRI in 23 patients with nipple discharge, in 11 of 15 (73%) patients who underwent excisional biopsy, MRI findings correlated with histopathologic findings (72). MRI correctly identified four of six papillomas and one of two fibroadenomas as circumscribed masses (Fig. 14.18). MRI correctly identified six of seven malignancies as peripherally enhancing irregular masses or regional or ductal enhancement (Fig. 14.19). In a study of 55 patients with bloody nipple dischargethat compared MRI, galactography, and ultrasound, MRI demonstrated all malignancies (73). Four cases of DCIS were not seen at ultrasound and three malignant lesions were not seen at galactography. At MRI, segmental clumped enhancement had a positive predictive value of 100%, while a mass with smooth borders had a negative predictive value of 87.5%. The need for imaging in the setting of clinically concerning nipple discharge remains unclear. However, given the high sensitivity of MRI for the detection of breast cancer, if imaging is requested, mammography, to evaluate for calcifications, followed by MRI would be recommended at this time.

Breast Cancer Staging

There are multiple reports in the literature (5,41,74–87) documenting the ability of MRI to determine the extent of cancer within the breast more accurately than can be accomplished with conventional methods. Reported rates of MRI demonstrated that mammographically and clinically occult multifocal or multicentric cancer ranges from 16% to 37% (43). Clinical indications have included staging newly diagnosed breast cancer following core needle biopsy (Fig. 14.20) and identifying the extent of residual disease following excisional biopsy where tumor is identified at the margins of resection (Fig. 14.21). Given the potential of MRI to detect unsuspected multifocal or multicentric cancer, it has been suggested that the addition of MRI to the imaging work-up of patients with newly diagnosed breast cancer can aid in surgical planning and definitive treatment planning, with the potential to reduce the number of surgical procedures to obtain negative margins of resection or to

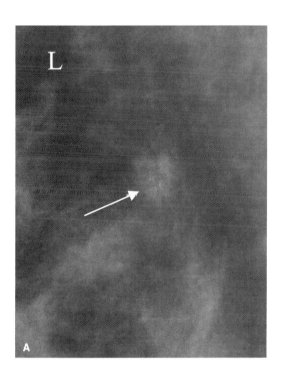

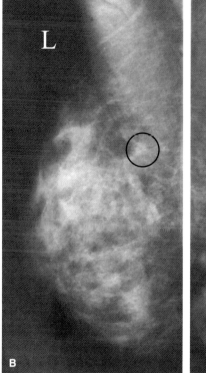

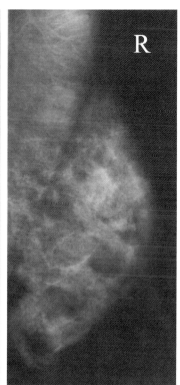

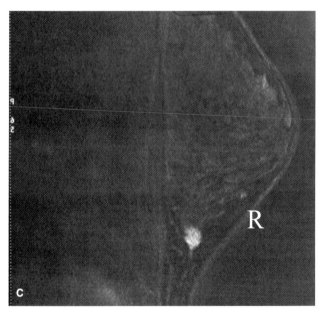

FIGURE 14.15. Magnetic resonance imaging (MRI)-detected synchronous, contralateral invasive breast cancer. A,B: Bilateral mammogram reveals a cluster of calcifications (*arrow and magnified in (B)*) that proved to be ductal carcinoma *in situ*. **C:** Sagittal MRI of the contralateral right reveals a 1-cm enhancing mass. The lesion was subsequently visualized with directed ultrasound examination, and ultrasound-guided core biopsy revealed invasive ductal carcinoma.

convert patients from planned breast-conservation therapy to mastectomy when multifocal or multicentric cancer is found.

Changes in therapy after MRI are reported in 8% to 20% of patients (43). In most cases, MRI allowed accurate assessment of extent of cancer, leading to better surgical planning (43). However, in cases where the enhancement proved to be benign, this resulted in unnecessary additional surgery. False-positive enhancement is the main downside of using MRI for breast cancer staging. One of the major limitations of MRI of the breast, as discussed earlier, is limited specificity (65% to 79%) due to the enhancement of many benign processes, including fibroadenomas, fat necrosis, fibrocystic changes, as well as presumably normal breast tissue (4). False-positive rates in the setting of breast cancer staging have varied among studies, with an average rate of approximately 20% (39). In a

study of 70 women with percutaneously diagnosed breast cancer who were being considered for breast-conserving therapy, MRI detected additional sites of cancer in the ipsilateral breast in 27% of patients (88). Biopsy was recommended for MRI detected additional lesions in the ipsilateral breast in 51% of women. The positive predictive value was 52%. Despite this relatively high positive predictive value, which is higher than the reported positive predictive value for mammography detected suspicious lesions (20% to −40%), overall, 24% of women were referred for biopsy of an MRI finding that proved to be benign (88). The positive predictive value was higher for lesions in the same quadrant as the index lesion as compared with lesions in different quadrants (64% vs. 31%). A similar finding was reported by Bedrosian et al. (89), where 75% of enhancing lesions in the same quadrant as the index cancer

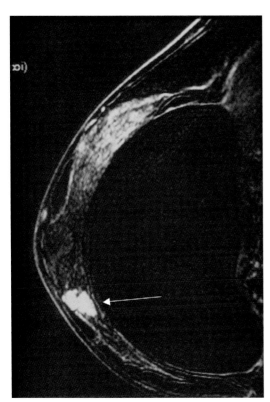

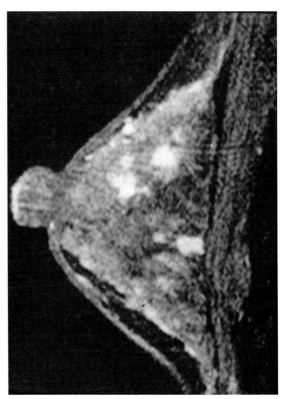

FIGURE 14.16. Magnetic resonance imaging (MRI)-detected synchronous, contralateral ductal carcinoma *in situ* (DCIS). A: Sagittal MRI in two patients with newly diagnosed breast cancer demonstrates contrast enhancement (*arrow*) in the contralateral breast. DCIS was found.

FIGURE 14.17. False-positive enhancement in the contralateral breast. Sagittal magnetic resonance imaging (MRI) of the contralateral breast in a patient with known breast cancer reveals multiple areas of enhancement. Based on the MRI findings alone, the patient was recommended to undergo bilateral mastectomy. At mastectomy, no tumor was found in the contralateral breast.

were malignant compared with 47% in a different quadrant. The identification of one or more additional enhancing lesions at a distance from the primary tumor may require an increase in the amount of tissue excised, a second excision elsewhere in the breast, or mastectomy (Fig. 14.22). This can be especially problematic when trying to determine which lesions, if any, require biopsy when multiple enhancing lesions distant from the primary tumor site are identified. The detection of additional enhancing lesions that prove to be benign may compromise the patient's cosmetic results for those who undergo breast conservation and may lead to an increased mastectomy rate. As is the case with false-positive MRI findings in the setting of high-risk screening, false-positive MRI findings in the

setting of breast cancer staging may result in high cost, increased patient anxiety and an increase in the mastectomy rate. The extent of these costs and the potential impact of patient management remain to be determined.

Magnetic Resonance Imaging Staging of the Ipsilateral Breast: What Question Remain to Be Answered?

Many questions surrounding the use of MRI for ipsilateral breast cancer staging remain unanswered. Because additional areas of cancer can be detected with MRI, will this prove to be

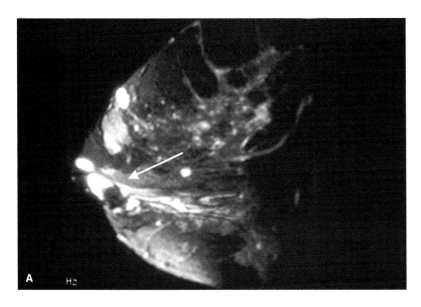

FIGURE 14.18. Nipple discharge. A: Sagittal fat suppressed T2 magnetic resonance image (MRI) demonstrated a low signal intensity mass (*arrow*) within a high signal intensity dilated duct. Sagittal (**B**) pre- and *(continued)*

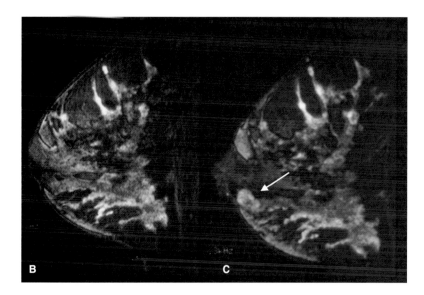

FIGURE 14.18. *Continued.* Sagittal (**B**) pre- and (**C**) postcontrast-enhanced, fat-suppressed MRI demonstrated mild enhancement of the intraductal mass (*arrow*). Excisional biopsy revealed a benign intraductal papilloma.

clinically important? Should treatment (i.e., breast-conserving therapy vs. mastectomy) be altered because MRI detects additional foci of cancer, especially in those cases where the foci prove to be tiny areas of DCIS (Fig. 14.23)? Would these foci of cancer identified on MRI be successfully treated with postoperative radiation therapy? In those cases where the additional foci of cancer detected on MRI are subsequently excised, might not these patients be ideally suited to breast-conserving therapy?

The data are clear that MRI permits detection of mammographically, sonographically, and clinically occult multifocal cancer in selected patients with presumed unifocal disease. But what is not known is whether this will translate into a decrease rate of local recurrence, improved relapse-free survival, and overall survival. To date, there have been no prospective randomized trials designed to answer these questions. The only information on the impact of staging MRI on outcome comes from single institution, retrospective studies. In a study of 346 patients, 65% of whom underwent breast-conserving therapy, Fischer et al. (90) reported a reduced rate of local failure for patients who underwent staging MRI compared with those who did not (1.2% vs. 6.5%; $p < .001$). This study, however, is limited

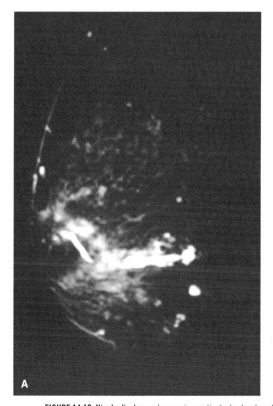

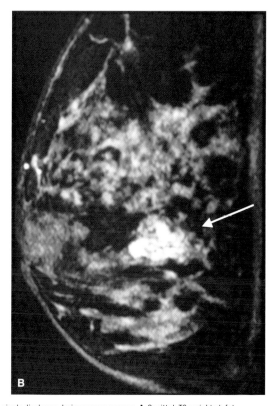

FIGURE 14.19. Nipple discharge. Images in a patient who developed nipple discharge during a mammogram. **A:** Sagittal, T2-weighted, fat suppressed magnetic resonance image (MRI) reveals fluid filled ducts in the central breast. **B:** Contrast-enhanced, fat-suppressed MRI reveals an area of regional enhancement (*arrow*) just posterior to the fluid filled ducts. MRI-guided wire localization and excisional biopsy revealed ductal carcinoma *in situ* with microinvasion.

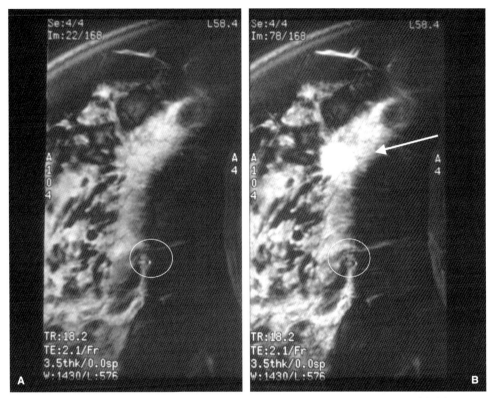

FIGURE 14.20. Magnetic resonance imaging (MRI) following stereotactic core biopsy of ductal carcinoma *in situ* **(DCIS).** Sagittal MRI demonstrates a 1.5-cm enhancing mass (**B,** *arrow*) several centimeters superior to the biopsy clip (**A, B** *circle*). The MRI-detected mass was subsequently identified on directed breast ultrasound examination. Excisional biopsy revealed a 1.5-cm invasive ductal carcinoma. Residual DCIS was found at the core biopsy site. No tumor was found between the core biopsy site and the invasive cancer.

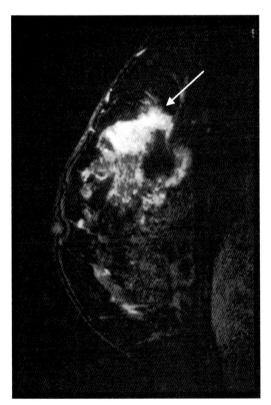

FIGURE 14.21. Magnetic resonance imaging (MRI) following excisional biopsy with positive margins of resection. Sagittal MRI demonstrates enhancement (*arrow*) along the superior margins of the seroma. Re-excision demonstrated residual tumor.

by failure to adjust for differences in tumor size, nodal status, and the use of systemic chemotherapy between groups. In a more recent study, Solin et al. (92), in a retrospective study of 756 women who underwent breast-conserving therapy (28% of whom had a staging MRI), reported no significant difference in 8-year rates of relapse-free survival (3% with MRI vs. 4% without MRI) and no significant difference in the 8-year rates of overall survival (94% with MRI vs. 95% without MRI). There are limitations to this study. It was a nonrandomized, retrospective study. There was a potential for bias as patients who underwent MRI tended to be young with dense breast tissue displayed on mammography. The value of MRI may have been underestimated as patients with extensive disease detected on MRI were excluded. Given the low rates of local failure, it may have been difficult to show an improvement in outcome in a single institution study.

Another unanswered question is whether there are subsets of patients most at risk for having multifocal or multicentric cancer who would benefit most from MRI. In a review of the literature, Van Goethem et al. (43) found that unsuspected multifocal or multicentric disease was most often observed in young or perimenopausal women or patients with larger (>5 cm) lesions, dense breast tissue on mammography, a first-degree family history, and invasive lobular cancer. Based on the current success of breast-conserving surgery, it is unlikely that MRI of the breast is warranted in all patients with newly diagnosed breast cancer. Furthermore, given the high cost and limited availability of breast MRI, it is unlikely that all patients with newly diagnosed breast cancer will have access to MRI. Even if the cost of MRI could be reduced and these imaging modalities do become widely available, which patients with breast cancer should undergo an MRI study

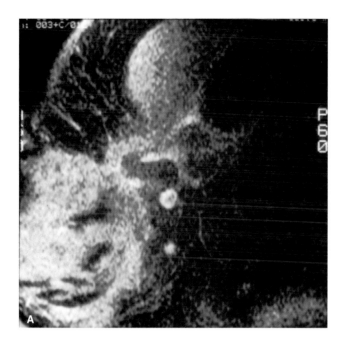

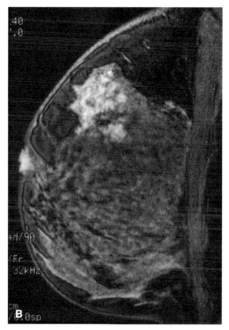

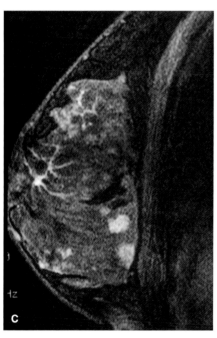

FIGURE 14.22. False-positive enhancement. Sagittal magnetic resonance images in three patients with newly diagnosed breast cancer shows enhancement in biopsy proven (**A**) fat necrosis, (**B**) fibrocystic changes, and (**C**) two fibroadenomas.

prior to surgery? And for those who do undergo this examination, what is the risk—benefit ratio? Additional clinical investigation is needed in attempt to find answers to these questions.

 CONCLUSION

Results from clinical investigations have demonstrated that MRI has very high sensitivity for the visualization of both invasive carcinoma and DCIS. Perhaps most important, MRI can enable the detection of breast cancer, both invasive and noninvasive disease, that is mammographically, sonographically, and clinically occult, offering the potential for improved cancer detection and cancer staging. Questions surrounding clinical indications for breast MRI remain. In the settings of an equivocal mammographic, sonographic, or physical examina-

tion findings, malignant axillary adenopathy with unknown site of primary tumor, and for monitoring the response of locally advanced cancer to chemotherapy, MRI appears to be indicated as an adjunct to mammography. The use of MRI for screening of women at high risk for the development of breast cancer is supported by the results of six clinical trials that demonstrate greater sensitivity of MRI compared with mammography for the detection of breast cancer. Based on the results of these studies, the American Cancer Society is currently recommending annual screening MRI in addition to annual screening mammography in women with a known *BRCA1* or *BRAC2* gene mutation, a greater than 20% lifetime risk of developing breast cancer, or a history of radiation therapy to the chest for Hodgkin's lymphoma. Despite this current recommendation, there is ongoing concern that false-positive studies may result in high downstream costs due to multiple short-interval follow-up MRI examinations, additional mam-

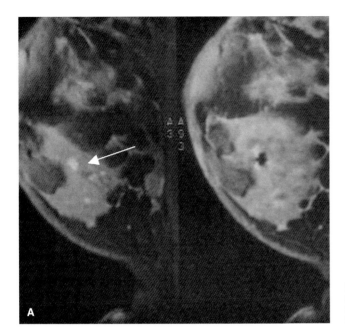

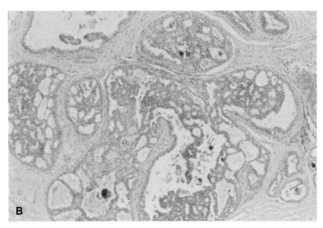

FIGURE 14.23. Magnetic resonance imaging (MRI) detected multifocal ductal carcinoma *in situ* (DCIS). A: Sagittal MRI demonstrates a 3-mm enhancing focus (*arrow*) in a patient with newly diagnosed DCIS in the ipsilateral breast. **B:** MRI-guided needle localization revealed a 3-mm focus of DCIS. The patient was advised to undergo mastectomy.

mogram and ultrasound studies, and a potentially high number of benign breast biopsies. It has also been demonstrated that false-positive MRI findings in this clinical setting may result in an increase of prophylactic mastectomies. Although the feasibility of using MRI for breast cancer screening in selected high-risk populations has been demonstrated, there are other patients at increased risk for the development of breast cancer, including those with a personal history of breast cancer and those with a history of atypia or LCIS who may ultimately benefit from the addition of screening MRI to screening mammography. But in these clinical settings, given the relatively limited published experience, screening MRI is not currently being recommended by the American Cancer Society. The use of MRI for breast cancer staging remains controversial. MRI is currently the most accurate imaging method for determining extent of disease in the ipsilateral breast. However, the detection of additional foci of breast cancer may not necessarily translate into better patient outcome. In some cases, the additional foci of breast cancer detected on MRI may have been successfully treated with breast irradiation, yet mastectomy is recommended. In those patients who do undergo breast-conserving therapy, it remains to be determined if preoperative staging with MRI will result in a decrease in local failure rate and improved overall survival. Given the low rate of local failure and the high rates of relapse-free and overall survival following breast-conservation therapy, it may be difficult to show a benefit with MRI. If MRI is to be used for staging, which patients with newly diagnosed breast cancer should undergo MRI and how the MRI findings should be incorporated in patient management remain to be defined. Furthermore, issues of technical quality, cost, and availability need to be addressed. Much has been learned about MRI of the breast as a method to detect, diagnose, and stage breast cancer. Clinical investigation has shown that MRI has tremendous potential for breast imaging, yet, there is more to be learned. This breast imaging modality continues to mature as clinical investigation continues.

References

1. Medical devices; performance standard for diagnostic x-ray systems; amendment. Department of Health and Human Services (HHS), Public Health Service (PHS), U.S. Food and Drug Administration (FDA). Final rule. *Fed Regist* 1999;64(127): 35924–35928.

2. Hylton NM, Kinkel K. Technical aspects of breast magnetic resonance imaging. *Top Magn Reson Imaging* 1998;9:3–16.

3. Kuhl CK. Breast MR imaging at 3T. *Magn Reson Imaging Clin North Am* 2007; 15(3):315–320.

4. Orel SG, Schnall MD. MR imaging of the breast: state of the art. *Radiology* 2001; 220:13–30.

5. Harms SE, Flamig DP, Hensley KL, et al. MR imaging of the breast with rotating delivery of excitation off resonance: clinical experience with pathologic correlation. *Radiology* 1993;187:493–501.

6. Kaiser WA, Zeitler E. MR imaging of the breast: fast imaging sequences with and without Gd-DTPA—preliminary observations. *Radiology* 1989;170:681–686.

7. Heywang SH, Wolf A, Pruss E, et al. MR imaging of the breast with Gd-DTPA: use and limitations. *Radiology* 1989;171:95–103.

8. Boetes C, Barentsz JO, Mus RD, et al. MR characterization of suspicious breast lesions with a gadolinium-enhanced turboFLASH subtraction technique. *Radiology* 1994;193:777–781.

9. Gilles R, Guinebretiere JM, Lucidarme O, et al. Nonpalpable breast tumors: diagnosis with contrast-enhanced subtraction dynamic MR imaging. *Radiology* 1994;191:625–631.

10. Orel SG, Schnall MD, Newman RW, et al. MR imaging–guided localization and biopsy of breast lesions: initial experience. *Radiology* 1994;193:97–102.

11. Kuhl CK, Elevelt A, Leutner CC, et al. Interventional breast MR imaging: clinical use of stereotactic localization and biopsy device. *Radiology* 1997;204: 667–675.

12. Morris EA, Liberman L, Dershaw DD, et al. Preoperative MR imaging-guided needle localization of breast lesions. *AJR Am J Roentgenol* 2002;179(6):1643.

13. Orel SG, Rosen M, Mies C, et al. MR imaging-guided 9-gauge vacuum-assisted core-needle breast biopsy: initial experience. *Radiology* 2006;238(1):54–61.

14. Liberman L, Bracero N, Morris E, et al. MRI-guided 9-gauge vacuum-assisted breast biopsy: initial clinical experience. *AJR Am J Roentgenol* 2005;185 (1):183–193.

15. Lehman CD, Deperi ER, Peacock S, et al. Clinical experience with MRI-guided vacuum-assisted breast biopsy. *AJR Am J Roentgenol* 2005;184(6):1782–1787.

16. Perlet C, Heywang-Kobrunner SH, Heinig A, et al. Magnetic resonance-guided, vacuum-assisted breast biopsy: results from a European multicenter study of 538 lesions. *Cancer* 2006;106(5):982–990.

17. LaTrenta LR, Menell JH, Morris EA, et al. Breast lesions detected with MR imaging: utility and histopathologic importance of identification with US. *Radiology* 2003; 227(3):856–861.

18. Orel SG, Schnall MD, LiVolsi VA, et al. Suspicious breast lesions: MR imaging with radiologic-pathologic correlation. *Radiology* 1994;190:485–493.

19. Kuhl CK, Bieling HB, Gieseke J, et al. Healthy premenopausal breast parenchyma in dynamic contrast-enhanced MR imaging of the breast: normal contrast medium enhancement and cyclical-phase dependency. *Radiology* 1997;203: 137–144.

20. Kuhl CK, Mielcareck P, Klaschik S, et al. Dynamic breast MR imaging: are signal intensity time course data useful for differential diagnosis of enhancing lesions? *Radiology* 1999;211:101–110.

21. Schimpfle MM, Ohmenhauser K, Sand J, et al. Dynamic 3D-MR mammography: is there a benefit of sophisticated evaluation of enhancement curves for clinical routine? *J Magn Reson Imaging* 1997;7:236–240.

22. Orel SG. Differentiating benign from malignant enhancing lesions identified at MR imaging of the breast: are time–signal intensity curves an accurate predictor? [editorial]. *Radiology* 1999;211:5–7.

23. Flickinger FW, Allison JD, Sherry RM, et al. Differentiation of benign from malignant breast masses by time-intensity evaluation of contrast-enhanced MRI. *Magn Reson Imaging* 1993;11:617–620.

24. Stomper PC, Herman S, Klippenstein DL, et al. Suspect breast lesions: findings at dynamic gadolinium-enhanced MR imaging correlated with mammographic and pathologic features. *Radiology* 1995;197:387–395.

25. Nunes LW, Schnall MD, Orel SG. Update of breast MR imaging architectural interpretation model. *Radiology* 2001;219(2):484–494.

26. Schnall MD, Blume J, Bluemke DA, et al. Diagnostic architectural and dynamic features at breast MR imaging: multicenter study. *Radiology* 2006;238(1):42–53.
27. Ikeda DM, Hylton NM, Kinkel K, et al. Development, standardization, and testing of a lexicon for reporting contrast-enhanced breast magnetic resonance imaging studies. *J Magn Reson Imaging* 2001;13(6):889–895.
28. Leung JW, Sickles EA. The probably benign assessment. *Radiol Clin North Am* 2007;45(5):773–789.
29. Liberman L, Morris EA, Benton CL, et al. Probably benign lesions at breast MRI: preliminary experience in high-risk women. *Cancer* 2003;15;98(2):377.
30. Eby PR, Demartini WB, Peacock S, et al. Cancer yield of probably benign breast MR examinations. *J Magn Reson Imaging* 2007;26(4):950–955.
31. Orel SG. High resolution MR imaging for the detection, diagnosis and staging of breast cancer. *Radiographics* 1998;18:903–912.
32. Dao TH, Rahmouni A, Campana F, et al. Tumor recurrence versus fibrosis in the irradiated breast: differentiation with dynamic gadolinium-enhanced MR imaging. *Radiology* 1993;187:752–755.
33. Lee CH, Smith RC, Levine JA, et al. Clinical usefulness of MR imaging of the breast in the evaluation of the problematic mammogram. *AJR Am J Roentgenol* 1999;173:1323–1329.
34. Kelcz F, Santyr G. Gadolinium-enhanced breast MRI. *Crit Rev Diagn Imaging* 1995;36:287–338.
35. Orel SG, Mendonca MH, Reynolds C, et al. MR imaging of ductal carcinoma in situ. *Radiology* 1997;202:413–420.
36. Gilles R, Zafrani B, Guinebretiere JM, et al. Ductal carcinoma in situ: MR imaging—histopathologic correlation. *Radiology* 1995;196:415–419.
37. Ghai S, Muradali D, Bukhanor K, et al. Nonenhancing breast malignancies on MRI: sonographic and pathologic correlation. *AJR Am J Roentgenol* 2005;185:481–487.
38. Boetes C, Strijk SP, Holland R, et al. False-negative MR imaging of malignant breast tumors. *Eur Radiol* 1997;7:1231–1234.
39. Teifke A, Hlawatsch A, Beier T, et al. Undetected malignancies of the breast: dynamic contrast-enhanced MR imaging at 1.0 T. *Radiology* 2002;224:881–888.
40. Solin LJ. Special considerations. In Fowble B, Goodman RL, Glick JH, et al., eds. *Breast cancer treatment: a comprehensive guide to management.* St. Louis, MO: Mosby-Yearbook, 1991:523–528.
41. Morris EA, Schwartz LH, Dershaw DD, et al. MR imaging of the breast in patients with occult primary breast carcinoma. *Radiology* 1997;205:437–440.
42. Orel SG, Weinstein SP, Schnall MD, et al. Breast MR imaging in patients with axillary node metastases and unknown primary malignancy. *Radiology* 1999;212:543–549.
43. Van Goethem M, Tjalma W, Schelfout I, et al. Magnetic resonance imaging in breast cancer. *Eur J Surg Oncol* 2006;32:901–910.
44. Chen C, Orel SG, Harris E, et al. Outcome after treatment of patients with mammographically occult, magnetic resonance imaging-detected breast cancer presenting with axillary lymphadenopathy. *Clin Breast Cancer* 2004;5:72–77.
45. Helvie MA, Joynt LK, Cody RL, et al. Locally advanced breast carcinoma: accuracy of mammography versus clinical examination in the prediction of residual disease after chemotherapy. *Radiology* 1996;198:327–332.
46. Partridge SC, Gibbs JE, Lu Y, et al. Accuracy of MR imaging for revealing residual breast cancer in patients who have undergone neoadjuvant chemotherapy. *AJR Am J Roentgenol* 2002;179:1193–1199.
47. Rieber A, Brambs HJ, Gabelmann A, et al. Breast MRI for monitoring response of primary breast cancer to neo-adjuvant chemotherapy. *Eur Radiol* 2002;12(7):1711–1719.
48. Cheung YC, Chen SC, Su MY, et al. Monitoring the size and response of locally advanced breast cancers to neoadjuvant chemotherapy (weekly paclitaxel and epirubicin) with serial enhanced MRI. *Breast Cancer Res Treat* 2003;78(1):51–58.
49. Belli P, Romani M, Costantini M, et al. Role of magnetic resonance imaging in the pre and postchemotherapy evaluation in locally advanced breast carcinoma. *Rays* 2002;27(4):279–290.
50. Bollet MA, Thibault F, Bouillon K, et al. Role of dynamic magnetic resonance imaging in the evaluation of tumor response to preoperative concurrent radiochemotherapy for large breast cancers: a prospective phase II study. *Int J Radiat Oncol Bio Phys* 2007;699(1):13–18.
51. Segra D, Krop IE, Garber JE, et al. Does MRI predict pathologic tumor response in women with breast cancer undergoing preoperative chemotherapy? *J Surg Oncol* 2007;96(6):474–480.
52. Wasser K, Sinn HP, Fink C, et al. Accuracy of tumor size measurement in breast cancer using MRI is influenced by histologic regression induced by neoadjuvant chemotherapy. *Eur Radiol* 2003;13:1213–1223.
53. Denis F, Desbiez-Bourcier AV, Chapiron C, et al. Contrast enhanced magnetic resonance imaging underestimates residual disease following neoadjuvant docetaxel based chemotherapy for breast cancer. *Eur J Surg Oncol* 2004;30: 1069–1076.
54. Kwong MS, Chung GG, Horvath LJ, et al. Postchemotherapy MRI overestimates residual disease compared with histopathology in responders to neoadjuvant therapy for locally advanced breast cancer. *Cancer J* 2006;12:212–221.
55. Kuhl CK, Schrading S, Leutner CC, et al. Mammography, breast ultrasound, and magnetic resonance imaging for surveillance of women at high familial risk for breast cancer. *J Clin Oncol* 2005;23:8469–8476.
56. Leach MO, Boggis CR, Dixon AK, et al. Screening with magnetic resonance imaging and mammography of a UK population at high familial risk of breast cancer: a prospective multicentre cohort study (MARIBS). *Lancet* 2005;365: 1769–1778.
57. Warner E, Plewes DB, Hill KA, et al. Surveillance of BRCA1 and BRCA2 mutation carriers with magnetic resonance imaging, ultrasound, mammography, and clinical breast examination. *JAMA* 2004;292:1317–1325.
58. Kriege M, Brekelmans CT, Boetes C, et al. Efficacy of MRI and mammography for breast-cancer screening in women with a familial or genetic predisposition. *N Engl J Med* 2004;351:427–437.
59. Lehman DC, Issacs C, Schnall MD, et al. Cancer yield of mammography, MR, and US in high-risk women: prospective multi-institution breast cancer screening study. *Radiology* 2007;244:381–388.
60. Sardinelli F, Podo F, A'Angolo G, et al. Multicenter comparative multimodality surveillance of women at genetic-familial high risk for breast cancer (HIBCRIT study): interim results. *Radiology* 2007;242:698–715.
61. Saslow D, Boetes C, Burke W, et al. American cancer society guidelines for breast cancer screening with MRI as an adjunct to mammography. *CA Cancer J Clin* 2007;57(2):75–89.
62. Hoogerbrugge N, Kamm YJ, Bult P, et al. The impact of a false-positive MRI on the choice for prophylactic mastectomy in BRCA mutation carriers is limited. *Ann Oncol* 2008;19(4):655–659.
63. Plevritis SK, Kurian AW, Sigal BM, et al. Cost-effectiveness of screening BRCA1/2 mutation carriers with breast magnetic resonance imaging. *JAMA* 2006;295:2374–2381.
64. Griebsch I, Brown J, Boggis C, et al. Cost-effectiveness of screening with contrast enhanced magnetic resonance imaging vs. X-ray mammography of women at a high familial risk of breast cancer. *Br J Cancer* 2006;95:801–810.
65. Port ER, Park A, Borgen PI, et al. MRI screening for breast cancer in high risk patients with LCIS and atypical hyperplasia. *Ann Surg Oncol* 2007;14: 151–157.
66. Bennion RS, Love SM. Treatment of breast disease in Bassett LW, Jackson VP, Jahan R, et al., eds. *Diagnosis of diseases of the breast.* Philadelphia: Saunders, 1997:521–545.
67. Lee CG, Orel SG, Woo H, et al. MR imaging screening of the contralateral breast in patients with newly diagnosed breast cancer: preliminary results. *Radiology* 2003; 226:773–778.
68. Liberman L, Morris EA, Kim CM, et al. MR imaging findings in the contralateral breast of women with recently diagnosed breast cancer. *AJR Am J Roentgenol* 2003;180:333–341.
69. Lehman CD, Gatsonis C, Kuhl CK, et al. MRI evaluation of the contralateral breast in women with recently diagnosed breast cancer. *N Engl J Med* 2007;356: 1295–1303.
70. Pediconi F, Catalano C, Roselli A, et al. Contrast-enhanced MR mammography for evaluation of the contralateral breast in patients with diagnosed unilateral breast cancer. *Radiology* 2007;243:670–680.
71. Tjalma W, Verslegers I. Nipple discharge and the value of MR imaging. *Eur J Obstet Gynecol Reprod Biol* 2004;115(2):234–236.
72. Orel SG, Dougherty CS, Reynolds C, et al. MR imaging in patients with nipple discharge: initial experience. *Radiology* 2000;216:248–254.
73. Nakahara H, Namba K, Wantanabe R, et al. A comparison of MR imaging, galactography, and ultrasonography in patients with nipple discharge. *Breast Cancer* 2003;10:320–329.
74. Yoshimoto M, Kasumi F, Iwase T, et al. Magnetic resonance galactography for a patient with nipple discharge. *Breast Cancer Res Treat* 1977;42:87–90.
75. Orel SG, Schnall MD, Powell CM, et al. Staging of suspected breast cancer: effect of MR imaging and MR-guided biopsy. *Radiology* 1995;196:115–122.
76. Boetes C, Mus RD, Holland R, et al. Breast tumors: comparative accuracy of MR imaging relative to mammography and US for demonstrating extent. *Radiology* 1995;197:43–47.
77. Essermann L, Hylton N, Yassa L, et al. Utility of magnetic resonance imaging in the management of breast cancer: evidence for improved preoperative staging. *J Clin Oncol* 1999;17:110–119.
78. Fischer U, Kopka L, Grabbe E. Breast carcinoma: effect of preoperative contrast-enhanced MR imaging on the therapeutic approach. *Radiology* 1999;213:881–888.
79. Weinstein SP, Orel SG, Heller R, et al. MR imaging of the breast in patients with invasive lobular carcinoma. *AJR Am J Roentgenol* 2001;176:399–406.
80. Rodenko GN, Harms SE, Pruneda JM, et al. MR imaging in the management before surgery of lobular carcinoma of the breast: correlation with pathology. *AJR Am J Roentgenol* 1996;167:1415–1419.
81. Orel SG, Reynolds C, Schnall MD. Breast carcinoma: MR imaging before reexcisional biopsy. *Radiology* 1997;205:429–436.
82. Fischer U, Baum F, Luftner-Nagel S. Preoperative MR imaging in patients with breast cancer: preoperative staging, effects on recurrence rates, and outcome analysis. *Magn Reson Imaging Clin North Am* 2006;14:351–362.
83. Liberman L. Breast MR imaging in assessing extent of disease. *Magn Reson Imaging Clin North Am* 2006;14:351–362.
84. Tillman G, Orel SG, Schnall MD, et al. Effect of breast magnetic resonance imaging on the clinical management of women with early-stage breast cancer. *J Clin Oncol* 2002;20:3413–3423.
85. Mann RM, Veltman J, Barentsz JO, et al. The value of MRI compared to mammography in the assessment of tumour extent in invasive lobular carcinoma. *Eur J Surg Oncol* 2008;34(2):135–142.
86. Beatty JD, Porter BA. Contrast-enhanced breast magnetic resonance imaging: the surgical perspective. *Am J Surg* 2007;193:600–605.
87. Bilmoria KY, Cambic A, Hansen NM, et al. Evaluating the impact of preoperative breast magnetic resonance imaging on the surgical management of newly diagnosed breast cancers. *Arch Surg* 2007;142:441–445.
88. Liberman L, Morris EA, Dershaw DD, et al. MR Imaging of the ipsilateral breast in women with percutaneously proven breast cancer. *AJR Am J Roentgenol* 2003, 180:901–910.
89. Bedrosian I, Schlencker J, Spitz FR, et al. Magnetic resonance imaging-guided biopsy of mammographically and clinically occult breast lesions. *Ann Surg Oncol* 2002;9(5):457–461.
90. Fischer U, Zachariae O, Baum F, et al. The influence of preoperative MRI of the breasts on recurrence rate in patients with breast cancer. *Eur Radiol* 2004;14: 1725–1731.
91. Solin LJ, Orel SG, Hwange W-T, et al. Relationship of breast magnetic resonance imaging to outcome after breast-conservation treatment with radiation for women with early-stage invasive breast carcinoma or ductal carcinoma in situ. *J Clin Oncol* 2008;26:468–473.

Chapter 15
Imaging: New Techniques

Matthew T. Freedman

The purpose of this chapter is to provide background information on the scientific basis of several proposed, but nonstandard, methods of breast imaging. Some of these are reasonable alternatives to current practice; others are novel methods under development. Novel methods of breast imaging are proposed with some frequency. Most are likely to be similar to those previously proposed by some other investigator. Understanding the scientific basis of several types of proposed methods should provide a basis for understanding new methods.

The chapter presents information on the physics and engineering that underlie breast imaging methods; bioinformatics, the display of complex information; supporting data from clinical studies; validating novel methods of breast imaging; and the potential applications of novel methods to clinical decisions.

Breast imaging can be used for six purposes: screening for cancer, diagnosis of a suspected finding, establishing the extent of disease, assessment of individual risk for development of breast cancer, monitoring the response to cancer therapy, and monitoring the response to preventive measures (dietary and pharmaceutical). A technique that is standard for one of these may be experimental for another.

The fundamental or conceptual goal in breast imaging is to separate the clinically relevant signal (usually the cancer) from the tissue that surrounds it. The clinically relevant signal may be the result of the water radiodensity in a mammogram compared with the surrounding fatty tissue, the difference in the speed of sound in different tissues in ultrasonography, the rate of proton spin relaxation in magnetic resonance imaging (MRI), hemoglobin in optical imaging, or some other signal. If the signal in a lesion is different from the background, detection is possible. For example, if cancer shows a different signal than benign processes, diagnosis of an indeterminate finding can be enhanced. If a method were able to separate clearly a small invasive breast cancer from a vascular fibroadenoma, biopsy of the fibroadenoma might be avoidable. Scientists, including physicists, biologists, and engineers, are working to develop imaging methods based on improved methods for detection or characterization of the signal, use of novel types of signals, and create new contrast agents.

Perhaps the greatest limit in devising better methods for breast imaging is the complexity of the background tissue that surrounds the clinically relevant signal. This background tissue is often similar in imaging characteristics to the cancer or other clinically relevant signal, masking disease. Normal breast tissues produce information with all imaging methods, and this information is shown in the images unless it has been filtered out. When the goal is to find a breast cancer, the method is useful if the breast cancer can be separated from the background of normal breast tissue.

techniques provide information on cellular function. Positron emission tomography (PET) imaging with ^{18}F-fluorodeoxyglucose (FDG) can be used to study glucose metabolism of breast tissues. ^{99m}Tc-Sestamibi (MIBI) can provide information about mitochondrial function and the P-glycoprotein adenosine triphosphate (ATP)-dependent transport mechanisms.

The newer approaches to breast imaging provide additional information on the molecular and metabolic processes and dynamic changes occurring in the breast tissues over time. Molecular imaging is intended to complement molecular medicine by providing images of the location where selected cellular events are occurring. As examples, magnetic resonance spectroscopy (MRS) can provide specific information about cell membranes and indirectly provide information about ischemia by identifying lactate and glucose utilization through measuring ATP and other phosphate compounds. Novel methods now under study in cell cultures and research animals can image cell surface receptors and demonstrate activity or lack of activity of a few intracellular pathways. Thermal, optical, and contrast-enhanced MRI methods can be used to show the physiologic changes in breast blood flow occurring over time, either spontaneous changes or in response to therapy. The breadth of these types of measurements will expand over the next few years.

U.S. Food and Drug Administration and New Techniques of Breast Imaging

In the United States of America, the U.S. Food and Drug Administration (FDA) controls the legal framework for the marketing of new medical devices and the use of pharmaceutical agents including those used as medical imaging contrast agents. Devices can receive premarket approval or can receive FDA clearance. To obtain FDA approval or clearance, companies submit documentation and request FDA approval or clearance. Devices and imaging contrast agents fall into several different categories with different requirements for review and approval.

FDA approval is based on statements made by the companies indicating claims about the device or imaging agents, indications for use, and data to support the claims. For the devices and methods described in this chapter, some have received FDA approval or clearance and others not. In some cases, part of a system is FDA approved or cleared, but not necessarily for a particular use in breast imaging. Before using a novel method for patient evaluation and care, one should ensure that it has received FDA approval or clearance for the purpose for which it will be used. Most of the methods mentioned in this chapter either are not FDA approved or the proposed uses go beyond the limits given in the FDA approval.

MOLECULAR, METABOLIC, AND FUNCTIONAL (PHYSIOLOGIC) IMAGING

Clinical imaging is evolving from an emphasis on structural information toward combined information on structure, metabolism, and function. Mammography provides images of breast structure. Ultrasonography is mainly used to image the structure of the breast, with physiologic information provided on vascular flow by Doppler recordings. Contrast-enhanced MRI combines structural information with dynamic measures of plasma flow and vascular permeability. Current nuclear tracer

PHYSICS AND ENGINEERING UNDERLYING BREAST IMAGING METHODS

Breast imaging is based on the detection of signal. Signal can be clinically relevant or not clinically relevant. The following sections discuss the types of signal, the methods for detecting signal, the components of a breast imaging signal, and then, in greater detail, each of the common types of signals used to image the breast.

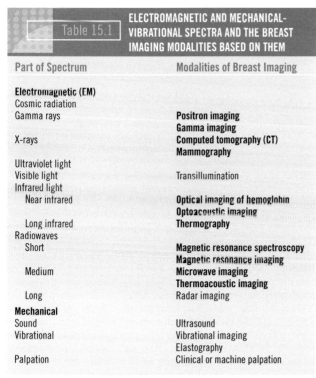

Table 15.1	ELECTROMAGNETIC AND MECHANICAL-VIBRATIONAL SPECTRA AND THE BREAST IMAGING MODALITIES BASED ON THEM
Part of Spectrum	Modalities of Breast Imaging
Electromagnetic (EM)	
Cosmic radiation	
Gamma rays	**Positron imaging**
	Gamma imaging
X-rays	**Computed tomography (CT)**
	Mammography
Ultraviolet light	
Visible light	Transillumination
Infrared light	
Near infrared	**Optical imaging of hemoglobin**
	Optoacoustic imaging
Long infrared	**Thermography**
Radiowaves	
Short	**Magnetic resonance spectroscopy**
	Magnetic resonance imaging
Medium	**Microwave imaging**
	Thermoacoustic imaging
Long	Radar imaging
Mechanical	
Sound	Ultrasound
Vibrational	Vibrational imaging
	Elastography
Palpation	Clinical or machine palpation

*Those toward the top have higher wave frequency and higher energy levels. The breast imaging modalities in bold type are discussed in this chapter.

Possible Types of Signal

Signals are caused by energy. The energy can be mechanical-vibrational or electromagnetic (EM). Almost all portions of the electromagnetic and vibrational spectra have been considered as potential methods for breast imaging. Table 15.1 lists many of the types of energies used and the imaging methods based on them. Table 15.2 lists the topics in this section.

Mechanical Signals

The mechanical signals used in breast imaging include low- and high-frequency sound (as seen with ultrasound imaging)

Table 15.2	TYPES OF SIGNALS

Types of signal
  Mechanical
  Electromagnetic (EM)
Source of energy
  Intrinsic
  Induced
Improving the detection of the signal
The components of a breast imaging system
Signals and potential signals used in breast imaging
  X-ray absorption and scattering
  High-frequency sound (ultrasound)
  Nuclear spin
  Vascular flow identification
    Contrast agents
    Electrical measurements
    Flow of hemoglobin
  Measures of cellular function
    Glucose metabolism
    Tissue oxygenation and hypoxia
    Mitochondrial activity: multidrug resistance

and continuous or intermittently applied pressure. Using pressure, one can record the pattern of deformation of a portion of the breast using ultrasound or MRI. The methods are called *sonoelastography* and *MR-elastography*. From these images, the elastic properties of tissues can be derived; these are related to measures of hardness and softness. There are also a few mechanical devices under development that use machine palpation of the breast to detect areas of hardness in the breast and use an image to record the location the machine measured.

Electromagnetic Signals

Types of electromagnetic signals used in breast imaging include gamma rays, x-rays, near infrared (NIR), visible light, microwaves, magnetic fields, and electrical fields. Measurements of this energy include intensity, spectral frequency, phase of the sinusoidal wave, and time of arrival. Each of these measurements can be changed by cancer and other clinically relevant structures in the breast.

Intrinsic and Induced Energy

The energy can be intrinsic to the tissue or induced from outside. Types of intrinsic energy include cellular electrical activity, autofluorescence, heat, and pulsations from blood flow. Induced energy can be mechanical or electromagnetic. Energy can be transmitted, absorbed, scattered, or changed in intensity, phase, or spectral frequency. A single imaging method can be used by itself or combined with other methods.

The signal can reflect changes in one frequency of energy, a group of specific frequencies, or a portion of a continuous spectrum of frequencies. The energy stream can be continuous, wavelike, or interrupted.

Improving the Detection of the Signal

Improved detection of the signal is not a simple task, and improvements usually are not achieved quickly. Mammography was first proposed in the 1920s, but it was not until the 1980s that proof of effectiveness was shown. Computer-aided detection of breast cancer on mammograms dates to the mid-1980s, but the first proof of its success in a screening setting was reported in 2001. Digital mammography development began in the early 1990s or earlier and was first commercially introduced in the United States in 2000. Strong proof for its effectiveness in a large clinical trial was published in 2005 (1).

One must guard against a rapid decision against new proposed technologies. If the ultrasonography of 1970 were proposed as a new method of breast imaging, it likely would have been rapidly rejected. In the 21st century, ultrasonography is one of the standard methods and is still showing rapid improvement in its technology. Although a few of the methods discussed in this chapter are of clear value and are commercially available, their place in the evaluation of patients remains incompletely defined. Other methods discussed in this chapter are considered not ready for standard use, but offer true potential to form part of the standard breast evaluation methods in the future.

Components of a Breast Imaging System

A breast imaging system contains several components, each of which can undergo modification and improvement. For successful imaging, energy must be able to both enter and leave the breast. This energy pattern must then be recorded. The recorded pattern often requires analog or digital processing to create information. This information then needs to be displayed and interpreted.

Not all systems incorporate all steps. In some cases, the image serves as little more that a graphic method to show the location from which the signal arises. In some cases, the image is dispensed with, leaving a measure of breast physiology or metabolism, with the location indicated in a verbal description or a handmade drawing, rather than an image recorded directly from the breast.

With standard methods of breast imaging, such as mammography and ultrasound, the image forms the basis of interpretation. With breast MRI, the image is combined with dynamic information on the wash-in and wash-out of contrast. With newer methods of breast imaging, the image conveys different information. Tissue structure can become less important; the image is used mainly to localize a physiological or metabolic process. With the novel methods, the image can be interpreted only if the method used to create it is known.

Signals and Potential Signals

The goal of breast imaging is to acquire information about the breast. The information can be about its structure or function. *Signal* is energy that carries information. *Noise* is energy that carries no information. Signal can be relevant or not relevant to the problem under investigation. Signal that is not relevant can be called background or normal tissue or clutter. A signal may be clinically relevant or not clinically relevant. Signal is clinically relevant when it provides information that is or may be of clinical use.

The electromagnetic and vibrational spectra of energies include most of the methods used or proposed to image the breast. These are listed in Table 15.1. Imaging with these portions of the energy spectrum requires that the energy can enter the breast, exit from the breast, and be able to be recorded. Not all of the EM and vibrational spectra meet those three requirements. Within the breast, the amount of energy can be reduced by absorption, scattering, and reflection. These changes in energy produce the data from which information can be derived.

Some of the signals that have been proposed as useful in breast imaging are discussed in the following sections.

X-Ray Absorption and Scattering

X-rays are absorbed and scattered as they pass through tissue. Different tissues may have different degrees of absorption and scattering. For example, fatty tissue in the breast absorbs and scatters x-rays less than fibroglandular tissue, and thus these two tissues can be distinguished on radiographs. Calcium absorbs and scatters more x-ray photons than fibroglandular tissue. Thus, fatty tissue, fibroglandular tissue, and calcifications can be separated on x-ray–produced images of the breast. Two types of x-ray images are made of the breasts: mammograms and computed tomograms (CTs). Breast cancer can sometimes contain calcifications that help in its identification. Breast cancer that does not contain calcifications has x-ray absorption and scattering characteristics very similar to normal fibroglandular tissue. Sometimes it can be identified by its shape, but in some cases it cannot be recognized. Because the signals from breast cancer and normal fibroglandular tissue are so similar on x-ray–produced images, other methods have been developed in which the signal from the breast cancer and normal fibroglandular tissue are different.

High-Frequency Sound (Ultrasound)

High-frequency sound (ultrasound) can be used to produce clinically relevant signals from the breast. Sound interacts with tissue in several different ways. Three different properties of the interaction of sound and tissue can be used to create images containing information:

1. Echoes occur at boundaries between tissues with differences in the speed of sound transmission. The reflective echoes can be formed into an image.
2. Tissues absorb ultrasound, and different tissues absorb ultrasound to different degrees. This differential absorption can be used to create an image.
3. Heterogeneity of tissue structures may produce many local echoes; homogeneity of tissue can result in a lack of local echoes. Homogeneity or heterogeneity of tissue echoes is used to help differentiate different types of tissue.

Breast cancers and normal fibroglandular tissues often differ in these three properties, allowing them to produce different patterns in ultrasonographic images. Thus, tissues that appear the same or similar on mammography, such as fibroglandular tissue and carcinoma, can be separated in many, but not all, cases. Fatty tissue in the breast and breast cancer can be quite similar on ultrasonographic images, and, therefore, not all breast cancers can be detected with ultrasonography.

Ultrasound can be produced at different frequencies. There are some frequency-dependent differences in the interactions of ultrasound with different tissues that might, in the future, allow some degree of clinically useful tissue characterization.

Doppler ultrasonographic imaging can be used to identify vascular flow. Ultrasound contrast media can help define the presence and amount of vascular flow to a breast mass.

Novel methods using ultrasound called optoacoustic and thermal acoustic imaging are described below. Sonoelastography is an additional novel method where changes in the echoes when a nodule is mechanically compressed can be used to characterize the hardness of the nodule.

Nuclear Spin

Spinning charged particles, such as hydrogen atoms and the protons in atomic nuclei, produce an electromagnetic signal. MRI uses this to produce images. Magnetic fields are used to align and then deflect the spinning protons. As the spinning protons return toward alignment, they release energy in the radio frequency range that can be recorded and used to produce an image. Different types of deflection of the alignment can be used, and the released energy can be recorded at different times, providing different images and information. This can accentuate the patterns of different tissues. Fatty tissue, fibroglandular tissue, and larger areas of benign calcification have different spin characteristics, allowing them to be distinguished. Breast cancer and fibroglandular tissue have spin characteristics that are quite similar on MRI obtained without contrast enhancement, but cancer often demonstrates greater vascularity and vascular permeability with contrast enhancement.

Vascular Flow

Invasive breast cancer usually has increased vascular flow. The presence of increased vascular flow can therefore be used as a marker indicating that a specific area of tissue is more likely to represent breast cancer. The finding of increased vascular flow is, however, also seen in some nonmalignant breast processes and benign tumors. Imaging of vascular flow can be separated into three separate components:

1. Increased plasma flow often demonstrated with the injection of contrast agents,
2. Increased flow of hemoglobin and red blood cells that can be detected using NIR optical imaging, and Doppler ultrasound, and
3. Detection of increased heat produced in the breast by inflow of blood (and increased metabolism) that can be detected with thermography.

Increased plasma flow can be demonstrated by the use of intravenous contrast agents. Agents approved by the FDA exist for MRI, CT, and ultrasonography. Experimental agents for these modalities and also for optical imaging are used in animal and human research. Increased vascular flow is often associated with increased vascular permeability, so the signals of increased vascular flow and vascular permeability are often combined when intravenous contrast agents are used. Patterns of plasma flow and vascular permeability can be analyzed mathematically for each volume element (voxel) of the image, creating a complex pattern of information.

There are contrast agents under development that are particulate, too large to pass out of the capillaries into the interstitial space, and one potentially could make agents that could pass through the spaces in tumor vessels while being too large to pass through normal capillaries. These experimental agents may provide improved ability to separate vascular flow from vascular permeability and, perhaps, separate the locations of normal capillaries from tumor vascular beds. These "intravascular only" agents have not yet been applied to breast imaging.

Electrical conductivity in the breast is increased in the presence of increased plasma flow and can be detected by electrical imaging. The increased flow of red blood cells can be shown by Doppler ultrasonographic techniques.

The flow of hemoglobin can be identified by optical imaging in which NIR light shows selective absorption by hemoglobin. Different NIR frequencies allow the partial separation of oxyhemoglobin and deoxyhemoglobin. Thermography measures the amount of heat radiated from the breast. Flowing blood is usually warmer than the breast tissue surrounding it. This difference in breast heat can be detected.

Electrical Activity

Two types of electrical activity in the breast can be detected: intrinsic and induced. Intrinsic electrical activity is the electrical activity at the cell membrane. Where there are more cells, this electrical activity is increased. There are limited data indicating that the electrical potential across the cell membrane in cancer is different than in benign tissue. The intrinsic electrical signals are quite weak, and, although they can be detected by electrodes implanted in the breast tissue, external measurement, at present, does not appear sufficiently sensitive.

Induced electrical activity is an area of active study. In these methods, electrical signals are applied to the body and are recorded from the skin surface of the breast. Areas of breast tissue that are more vascular and more cellular show increased activity. Two different components of the induced electrical activity can be measured: conductivity and capacitance. Each has several underlying factors. Conductivity appears to be mainly related to the vascularity of tissues; capacitance (also called permeativity) is mainly related to the number of cell membranes present and is therefore a sign of cellularity. Different frequencies of alternating current result in different patterns in different tissues, and analysis of conductivity and capacitance using different frequencies can, in experimental systems, enhance the differentiation of tissues.

Glucose Metabolism

There are at least three methods of measuring glucose metabolism. One can measure the uptake of a glucose-mimicking agent by cells, the ratio of ATP to adenosine diphosphate (ADP), and the heat produced in tissues by glucose metabolism.

FDG is a positron-emitting glucose analog that is transported into cells by the glucose transport pathway, but then fails to be metabolized, blocked after hexokinase phosphorylation from further metabolism. It provides a measure of glucose uptake by cells. Glucose uptake is increased in metabolically active cells.

Both normal glandular cells and cancer cells use glucose, but breast cancer cells are metabolically more active and have a higher uptake. Optical imaging agents reflecting glucose uptake in a way similar to that of FDG are under development.

MRS is a method of evaluating the chemical composition of both organic and inorganic compounds. Chemical compounds of several elements can be detected and measured. MRS of phosphorus-containing compounds can be used to detect and measure ATP and ADP. Thermography can measure the production of heat caused by glucose metabolism.

Tissue Oxygenation and Hypoxia

Optical imaging in the NIR region can, by measuring the absorption at several light frequencies, differentiate oxygenated hemoglobin and deoxygenated hemoglobin, providing a measure of oxygen extraction by tissue. In the presence of hypoxia, more lactate is produced, and this can be identified on MRS.

Mitochondrial Activity: Multidrug Resistance

MIBI is an agent that is concentrated in mitochondrial membranes based on P-glycoprotein ATP-dependent mechanisms. Its uptake is enhanced in regions of increased mitochondrial activity, and hence it can be used to aid in the identification of breast cancer. It is excreted by the multidrug resistance pathway, and this excretion is increased in cancers having the *MDR1* (*ABCB1*) and *MDR2* (*ABCB4*) genes.

Physical Principles Applied for Signal Detection

For a signal to be detected, it must "stand out" from the background in some way. The signal in the area of interest may be more intense or less intense than what surrounds it. The differences in signal between the areas of interest (often representing an abnormality) and the background tissue can be detected by intensity differences. These differences represent *contrast*. The stronger the signal differences, the easier it is to detect the area of interest. When contrast is high, smaller areas of interest can be detected, and areas of interest deeper in the tissues can be seen.

There are several physical processes that can result in differences between the area of interest and the background. Some of these are described in the following sections. Those discussed are listed in Table 15.3.

Absorption–Transmission of Energy

When energy is directed at an organ like the breast, some is reflected, some is absorbed, and some is transmitted. If the detection system is placed on the far side of the breast away from the source of energy, then the detection system is detecting the pattern of transmission. There is less transmission of energy where there is absorption. If the absorption is nonuniform, it

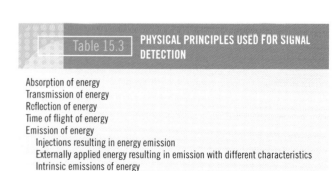

Table 15.3	PHYSICAL PRINCIPLES USED FOR SIGNAL DETECTION

Absorption of energy
Transmission of energy
Reflection of energy
Time of flight of energy
Emission of energy
    Injections resulting in energy emission
    Externally applied energy resulting in emission with different characteristics
    Intrinsic emissions of energy
Spectroscopy of energy

produces a pattern that may represent the pattern or distribution of the areas of interest. Thus, a mammogram represents a visible map of the transmission and absorption differences of x-rays. In optical imaging, different tissues and different molecules absorb light photons of specific frequencies to different degrees, creating a pattern. Using different light frequencies, the signals from oxyhemoglobin and deoxyhemoglobin can be partially separated, producing images of the distribution of these molecules in the breast.

Reflection of Energy

Tissues not only absorb energy, they can also reflect energy, and there are systems that can produce images of the breast by analyzing the patterns of reflection. The common forms of ultrasonography produce their images by reflection, although there are a few ultrasonographic systems that produce images by absorption–transmission. Optical imaging can be done with either reflection imaging or absorption–transmission imaging.

Time of Flight of Energy

The time it takes for packets of energy to pass through tissue can be recorded to make a series of timed images. This is called *time of flight* imaging. Energy has the properties of both discrete units called photons and continuous oscillating patterns called *waves*. When these photons and waves interact with tissue, some of them are scattered and some are transmitted without scattering. Some are scattered more and others are scattered less. It takes a certain amount of time for the photons and waves to pass through tissue. When there is no scattering, the transmission time is shorter than when the photons and waves are scattered. In addition, certain types of waves such as ultrasound waves are transmitted slower or faster depending on the frequency of the wave and the characteristics of the tissue. If one sends short bursts of energy into tissue and records the energy exiting the tissue, the time that it takes for the photons and waves to pass from the source of the energy to the detector can be measured and used to create timed images. In ultrasonographic reflective imaging (the common type of ultrasonographic imaging), this method is used to determine the depth of the surface causing the reflection. In optical imaging, it can be used to separate those photons that pass through the tissue with no scattering, minimal scattering, moderate scattering, and so forth. In optical imaging, scattering is one of the major causes of loss of resolution, so time-gated images could provide higher resolution and also show where there is less tissue of the type that scatters light photons of that frequency.

Emission of Energy

Emission of energy can occur by three general mechanisms. Materials that emit energy can be injected, externally applied energy fields can induce energy emissions of different types from those applied, and the energy from the intrinsic metabolic activity of tissues can be detected.

Injections Resulting in Energy Emission

Substances that directly emit energy can be injected (as with radioactive agents), or genes can be implanted in animals (and perhaps eventually in people) that can produce photons of light energy that can be recorded externally. The most common agents now used are radioactive compounds. In breast imaging, MIBI and FDG are two agents that are used in evaluation of breast lesions that may represent breast cancer. They are also used to follow women with breast cancer after therapy. In animals, there are several optical agents that can be used that emit light of specific frequencies. One method is to insert optical reporter genes into the animal genome that then stimulate the gene product to produce light. A luciferase gene can be inserted into implanted tumors and then stimulated to produce light by the injection of luciferin. An inserted gene can produce green fluorescent protein (GFP), a protein that appears green when stimulated with light of specific frequency. Other genes produce proteins of different colors, so it is possible to identify specific cells or tissues based on different colors of induced fluorescence. With gene therapy, one may eventually include therapeutic genes in a combined structure with genes inducing optically active proteins. By using this combination, one could identify the locations where the therapeutic genes have entered cells; the gene induced optical proteins would show that the therapeutic gene has likely been incorporated into the cellular genome.

Externally Applied Energy Fields Inducing Energy Emissions with Different Characteristics

In MR techniques, rapidly varying magnetic fields are used to produce the emission of electromagnetic energy that is recorded to produce an image. Because different tissues can emit different quantities and frequencies of energy, images of different tissues can be produced and spectroscopy can be used to analyze the different energy patterns. Microwave- and light-frequency applied energies can result in the production of ultrasound waves that can be used to produce an image. Light applied to tissues at one spectral frequency can interact with tissue and result in the emission of light at a different spectral frequency.

Intrinsic Emissions of Energy

Living tissues also have intrinsic emissions of energy. They produce and emit small amounts of light (called *autofluorescence*), electromagnetic energy (in part produced by the electrical activities of cells), and a moderate amount of thermal energy (from cellular metabolism). Each of these emissions can be measured.

Spectroscopy

Spectroscopy provides information on the quantity of energy at different energies and different frequencies. It can be used to separate different energy signals in imaging of radioactive materials, to record the different types of molecules in MR, and to record the transmission, absorption, and reflection patterns of light and ultrasound. Spectroscopic information can be derived from MR, optical methods, ultrasound signals, and electrical signals. It is likely that spectroscopy will be increasingly used in the future.

Enhancement of Signal

The clinically relevant signals and background tissue signals are often of low signal to background contrast. Several methods are used to enhance the extraction and contrast of clinically important signals. Most of these are based on computer processing of already recorded image data. These are called *postprocessing* methods. Table 15.4 lists the topics in this section.

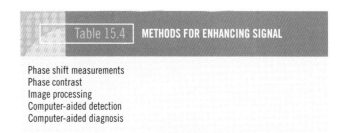

Table 15.4	METHODS FOR ENHANCING SIGNAL

Phase shift measurements
Phase contrast
Image processing
Computer-aided detection
Computer-aided diagnosis

Phase Shift and Phase Contrast

The energies used in breast imaging often include phase information. Phase results from the sinusoidal shaped wave of the energy. When the signal is delayed in only one part of an image, its phase is shifted compared to regions where the signal is not delayed. Light recorded after its transmission through, or reflection within, the breast can be analyzed according to phase. This can be used to separate light photons that have been delayed from those that are less delayed by their passage through tissues. When x-ray or ultrasound energy interacts with a tissue edge that is almost parallel to the direction of the energy, the direction of the energy slightly angled. Phase contrast is a physical property of boundaries in tissue that can be used to enhance the edges of tissue with both x-ray and ultrasonographic imaging (2,3).

Image Processing

Image processing is (usually) the use of computer processing algorithms to produce enhanced conspicuity of the differences between the areas of interest and the background. It can be applied to any image that is in computer-readable (digital) form. It can be used to decrease noise, increase contrast, increase the definition of edges between tissues, and increase conspicuity of objects. It is commonly used in digital mammography, ultrasonography, CT, MRI, and optical imaging.

Computer-Aided Detection

Computers can be programmed to mark areas that have features that to the computer algorithm resemble findings of disease. Thus, the computer programs can direct the radiologist's attention to breast microcalcifications, masses, and areas of architectural distortion, all findings that may indicate the presence of breast cancer (4–11). Computer aids have also been developed to assist in breast MRI interpretation and in ultrasound characterization of breast lesions.

Computer-Aided Diagnosis

Computer algorithms are under development that can help radiologists improve their classification of findings on mammograms and breast ultrasonographic examinations into benign and malignant (12–15). Similar methods of computer-aided diagnosis likely will be applied to aid in diagnosis from optical and other molecular imaging methods.

Contrast Media

Contrast media are agents that are administered to patients to increase the contrast between areas of interest and background tissues. There are various types that are used currently in clinical care, and others are under development in animals and tissue cultures. The types of contrast agents under development in animals will likely be used in patients in the future. Table 15.5 lists the types of contrast media discussed in this section.

X-Ray Contrast Media

X-ray contrast agents are commonly used in CT imaging. Most are compounds containing iodine. They are used to show vessels, regions of enhanced blood flow, and areas of increased tissue permeability to small molecules.

Ultrasonographic Contrast Media

Ultrasonographic contrast agents are used to increase the reflection of ultrasound during imaging. There are several types commercially available and others with additional fea-

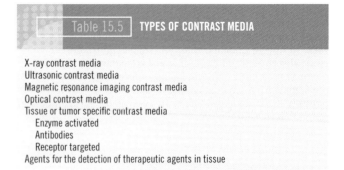

Table 15.5	TYPES OF CONTRAST MEDIA

X-ray contrast media
Ultrasonic contrast media
Magnetic resonance imaging contrast media
Optical contrast media
Tissue or tumor specific contrast media
   Enzyme activated
   Antibodies
   Receptor targeted
Agents for the detection of therapeutic agents in tissue

tures that are in clinical trials. The current agents, in general, are used to enhance images of blood flow in regions that may contain tumors. Experimentally, they can be used to measure the rate of blood flow into tumors as a method of monitoring the response to antiangiogenesis therapy.

Magnetic Resonance Imaging Contrast Media

Commercially available contrast agents relevant to breast cancer are intravenously injected and show areas of increased blood flow and tissue permeability to small molecules. Most are based on compounds of gadolinium.

Iron oxide nanoparticles have also been used as an experimental MRI contrast agent. They present a different picture than current vascular contrast agents because, once they have accumulated in tissues with increased capillary permeability, they remain there for hours to days, much longer than current contrast agents. This results in their progressive accumulation in tissues that have increased vascular permeability, resulting in increasing enhancement of tumors (16,17). Other iron oxide MR contrast agents accumulate in lymph nodes but are not yet reported in evaluating for axillary lymph node metastases in breast cancer (18–20).

Also under development are MR contrast agents that accumulate preferentially in malignant tumors based on antibodies to cell surface receptors. Other experimental contrast agents are small molecules that can bind to receptors on the cell surface or be transported intracellularly through molecular mechanisms. Work is under way to develop MR contrast agents that are actively accumulated in cells through cell wall mechanisms, such as the transferrin receptor (21,22). Artemov et al. (23) report on a contrast agent for imaging the *HER2/neu* receptor.

Optical Contrast Agents

There are several optical dyes used in research in optical imaging in animals and humans. In humans, indocyanine green and similar compounds are used to show regions of increased blood flow.

Tissue- or Tumor-Specific Contrast Agents

Enzyme Activated

Contrast agents that are activated by enzymes are under development for use in MRI, ultrasonographic imaging, and optical imaging. These agents place the contrast agent in a "cage" that is opened by enzymatic action.

Antibodies

Antibodies tagged with contrast agents are under development for use in MRI, ultrasonographic imaging, and optical imaging.

Receptor Targeted

Molecular imaging agents that target specific cell wall, mitochondrial membrane, and nuclear receptors are under development for MRI and optical imaging.

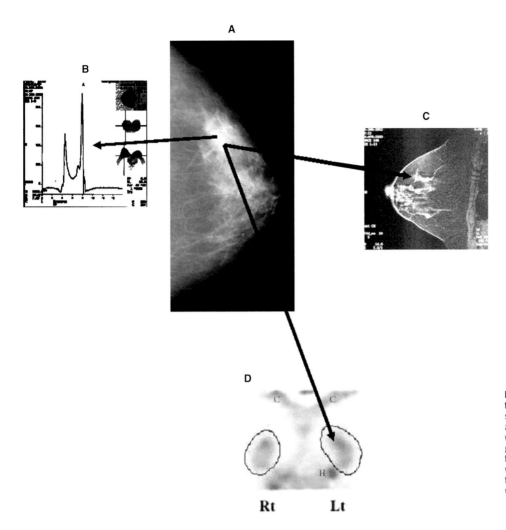

FIGURE 15.1. Invasive ductal carcinoma, multimodality imaging. (A), mammogram, **(B)**, MR spectroscopy, **(C)**, MR image, **(D)** FDG-PET. The arrows point to the same location in the breast where the index lesion is shown on the mammogram. Each image provides different information. Location coordinated information about voxels in the breast can be obtained sequentially, as in this case, or almost simultaneously, with, for example, multispectral optical imaging.

Detection of Therapeutic Agents in Tissue

Cancer therapy agents can be labeled in three general ways:

1. The delivery system can contain a mixture of the therapeutic compound and an imaging compound. Thus, the liposomes or antibodies used to transmit the therapeutic agent can be mixed with liposomes containing contrast or the same antibody linked to an imaging agent.
2. The therapeutic agent can be labeled with an isotope that provides the imaging substrate. A radioactive isotope of an element in the drug compound can be used for radiolabeling, or an MRS detectable agent such as ^{19}F can be used to label the compound for MRS detection.
3. An optical dye can be inserted into a gene used for gene therapy. Research in animals using these mechanisms is under way.

 ## BIOINFORMATICS: THE DISPLAY OF COMPLEX INFORMATION

This chapter has largely refrained from providing images of the breasts using the nonstandard methods discussed. This is because these nonstandard methods often involve a complexity of information beyond that seen in standard methods such as ultrasonography and mammography; the display methods are still evolving. A potentially useful approach is to think of the displayed image as a localizing image. It tells you where something is, but not what it is. No single image can provide all of the clinically relevant information about that location. Figure 15.1 is a composite image that demonstrates some of the multiple types of information that can be present at one location in the breast.

If one interprets the breast as a three-dimensional object composed of units of volume, then for each unit of volume in the breast, most of the nonstandard imaging methods provide multiple pieces of information about it. In computer language, the image is composed of volume elements (voxels). Each voxel represents a location. Each attribute of the image represents a dimension in multidimensional space. No single display can provide all of the information about that volume in the breast that is being studied. For example, optical imaging in the NIR region provides a spectrum of the absorption of light of different frequencies across the NIR region for each volume of tissue. From this absorption spectrum (Fig. 15.2), the amount of oxyhemoglobin, deoxyhemoglobin, water, and lipid can be derived and ratios calculated for each voxel. Each voxel therefore has multiple dimensions of information, and the information in each voxel can change over time. If one induces a cold stress or if one compresses and then releases compression, each voxel shows a time course of changes in the spectrum reflecting changes in the composition of each of these optically active substances. Spectral information on breast hemoglobin changes during the menstrual cycle. Therefore, depending on the process under study, the clinically useful image or images of the breast will change.

Bioinformatics is the science of the use of computers to analyze complex biologic information. Visualization of this information is a valuable adjunct to aid in the understanding of complex information. Tools for aiding in the visual interpretation of complex biomedical imaging data are under development, but are

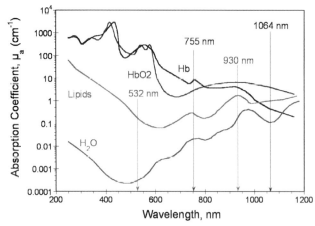

FIGURE 15.2. Near-infrared (NIR) absorption spectra of water, lipid, oxyhemoglobin, and deoxyhemoglobin. The y axis shows the absorption coefficient, the x axis shows the NIR wave length spectra. By choosing appropriate laser frequencies (in this chart 532 nm, 755 nm, 930 nm, and 1,064 nm), one can partially separate the component of each molecular type for each voxel in the breast, thus determining the amount of oxyhemoglobin, deoxyhemoglobin, water and lipid. (Courtesy of Alan Stein, M.D., and Seno Medical Instruments, Inc., San Antonio, Texas.)

still limited. Different groups approach the problem differently. In some instances, the "image" provides a numerical or color guide of the risk of malignancy; in other cases, the system provides several images, each displaying a specific characteristic of the breast composition. Dynamic curves can be provided to assist in breast MRI interpretation. Color-coded images can be used to reflect the rate of change of blood flow, temperature, or other defined attributes of the voxel. It is not yet known what type of information should be displayed to be of maximal benefit to the person interpreting the visualized information or how it should be displayed. An example of a colored image showing the areas with increased oxyhemoglobin is shown in Figure 15.3.

SUPPORTING DATA FROM CLINICAL STUDIES: EXAMPLES OF SPECIFIC METHODS OF NOVEL BREAST IMAGING

The following sections discuss specific types of novel breast imaging, including reports of clinical studies where they are available. The imaging methods discussed in the section are listed in Table 15.6.

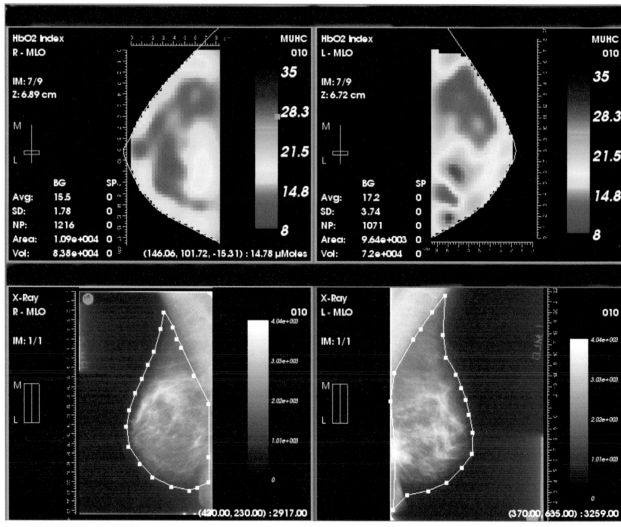

FIGURE 15.3. Color mapping of the amount of oxyhemoglobin in different parts of the breast. Corresponding mammogram views are provided. In the images to the right, one can see orange-red areas in the breast on the upper image corresponding to areas of increased oxyhemoglobin levels, a sign supportive of the diagnosis of breast cancer. (Courtesy of Mark A. Mallioux, ART Advanced Research Technologies, Inc., Montreal, Canada.)

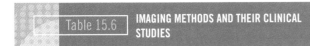

Table 15.6	IMAGING METHODS AND THEIR CLINICAL STUDIES

Optical imaging
Optoacoustic imaging
Thermoacoustic imaging
Microwave imaging
Electrical imaging and spectroscopy
Radioactive tracer imaging
   Sestamibi
   [8]F-fluorodeoxyglucose positron emission tomography
Computed tomography imaging
Thermography

Table 15.7	TOPICS ON OPTICAL IMAGING

Type of light
   Visible
   Near infrared (NIR)
Interactions with tissue
   Transmission
   Reflection
   Absorption
   Scattering
   Change in phase
Time for light transmission
   Time of flight
Modulation
   Continuous wave
   Superimposed low frequency
   Short pulses
Multispectral imaging
Optical dyes

Optical Imaging of the Breast

Overview

Optical imaging of the breast was first described in 1929 using transmission of visible light through the breast to create an image. Currently, after many years of research, optical imaging of the breast is now a rapidly expanding and promising area of inquiry. There are two main approaches: methods to image the breast—optical imaging—and methods to measure the absorption of one or several frequencies of light within the breast—optical spectroscopy. These may be combined or used separately. Current research shows that, in the future, optical imaging and spectroscopy methods may have important applications in four areas: (a) cancer risk assessment, (b) diagnosis of suspect lesions identified in the breast by other methods, (c) assessment of the response to preoperative chemotherapy, and (d) detection of local recurrence after local resection and radiation therapy. It has been suggested as a method for breast cancer screening, but information to evaluate this potential application is insufficient.

Most current optical methods utilize the NIR portion of the electromagnetic spectrum, a portion of the EM spectrum where the breast is relatively translucent, thus allowing the light to penetrate. Within the NIR spectrum, different tissues absorb at different light frequencies, as shown in Figure 15.2. This differential absorption permits multispectral imaging and enables oxyhemoglobin and deoxyhemoglobin, water, and lipid to be separately measured.

Fundamental Methods

There are several approaches to optical imaging of the breasts. Those described here are listed in Table 15.7. Optical imaging of the breast consists of two main approaches to illumination (transmission and reflection–scattering), two main types of light (visible and near infrared), and, for each type of light, three subtypes of modulation of the beams of light (continuous wave, superimposed lower wave frequency, and short pulses). Thus, there are 12 varieties of optical imaging. There are also three main methods of analysis of the light beam to create an image of the residual pattern of the light that remains after passing through the breast, so there are at least 36 possible combinations of factors in optical imaging.

Classes: Transmission and Reflection

The two main classes are transmission and reflection–scattering. Light can be transmitted through the breast and detected on the opposite side, or it can be beamed into the breast and the reflected and scattered light can then be detected on the same side of the breast as the input beam.

The main problem with transmission is that the light may not penetrate adequately through thick breasts, and scattering makes accurate localization more difficult. For transmission imaging, sensors for low light levels are needed.

For reflection–scattering, the main problem is in localizing the abnormality. The resolution of these systems appears to be less than for transmission systems. To aid in localization, optical methods are sometimes combined with ultrasound; when combined, the optical methods record physiology or pathophysiology and the ultrasound methods record location and size.

Types of Light: Visible Light and Near Infrared

There are two main types of light used: visible light and NIR. NIR at selected wavelengths can penetrate adequately into the breast. The main absorbing tissues of interest are oxyhemoglobin and deoxyhemoglobin, but at specific wavelengths information of lipid and water content can be estimated. By selecting the correct wavelengths, these molecules can be distinguished (Fig. 15.2 shows the NIR spectrum). There are also fluorescent dyes that absorb in the NIR range. If these dyes are injected, NIR light can cause these dyes to fluoresce, allowing localization and measurement. Rapid pulses of NIR light can, in interacting with tumors, create ultrasound signals based on the presence of oxyhemoglobin and deoxyhemoglobin. Visible-light breast imaging does not appear to be a current area of research interest, although visible light transmission imaging of the breast was the first method of optical breast imaging and was carefully studied in the past.

Changes in Light as It Passes through Tissue: Changes in Absorption, Scattering, Phase, and Time for Transmission

Three types of changes occur as light passes through tissue:

1. Some is absorbed and scattered, resulting in attenuation (decrease) in the amount or intensity of light.
2. The phase of the wave of light is changed so that if one compares the wave cycle of the initial light with that of the light as it exits tissue, the exiting light has its wave position (phase) offset compared with the original wave (24,25).
3. The time of transmission of light can be delayed because of scattering, providing information on the scattering characteristics of the tissues (26,27).

Types of Modulation: Continuous Wave, Superimposed Low Frequencies, and Short Pulses

Light consists of waves and particles. The light can be modulated in at least three ways: continuous wave, imposed lower frequency, and short pulses. *Continuous wave* is light oscillating at its inherent frequency with that resulting wavelength; because the wave is not interrupted, it is called continuous wave. Alternatively, the intensity of the light can be varied in a sinusoidal fashion thereby imposing a lower continuous wave frequency where shifts in phase may be more easily detected. *Short pulse light* results when the inherent continuous wave is rapidly turned on and off at a megahertz frequency. Short pulses are pulses or "packets" of light in which each induction and arrival time can be measured and filtered by the time it takes for the packet of light to arrive at its destination.

Combinations of Light: Multispectral Imaging

Light is electromagnetic radiation within a specific range of frequencies. Each of these frequencies has the potential to be absorbed or transmitted by tissues to a varying degree. Different molecules in the tissue absorb light at different frequencies, with different degrees of absorption. If more than one frequency is used in imaging, it is called *multispectral imaging*.

Since the absorption of oxygenated hemoglobin, deoxyhemoglobin, lipid, and water have different levels of absorption and scattering that vary according to the wavelength of NIR light, it is possible to create separate curves or pictures representing the quantity of each of these at specific points within the breast and then use these different patterns for analysis and diagnosis. Multispectral NIR imaging can be used to measure the blood volume, blood oxygen saturation, fat, and water content of the normal breast or portions of it (28,29), characteristics of tumors within the breast (29–31), and evidence of response to chemotherapy (29,32). Multispectral imaging offers the advantage that different molecules can be identified and measured separately.

Use of Optical Dyes

Optical dyes such as indocyanine green can be injected intravenously. The arrival time and pattern of persistence of these dyes can be observed optically and provide information similar to the measurements made with MRI when gadolinium compounds are injected. The phases that can be separated show vascular flow, tissue permeability, and wash-out. These patterns are similar to those seen with contrast-enhanced MRI and show some relationship to the benign or malignant nature of breast masses (33–37).

In the future, optical dyes with special properties may be developed that accumulate in specific tissues or that have more selective uptake based on their chemical structure. Such compounds could use antibodies to cause them to accumulate in specific types of tumors or contain dyes that are quenched (i.e., not visible) until acted on by specific cellular enzymes such as cathepsin and matrix metalloproteinase. Ebert et al. (38) report on the development of an NIR fluorescent dye that concentrates in breast cancer cell line xenographs in mice. Mahmood et al. (39) report on a NIR molecular probe used in mouse imaging that is quenched (not active) until acted on by tumor associated proteases for cathepsins B and H. Other similar agents are undergoing development and testing in animal models.

Measurements of Time of Flight

Grosenick et al. (40–42), as well as others, have developed methods to record the time delay of light photons transmitted through the breast. Delay is caused by scattering and should be greater where tumors are present. In a few cases, their findings suggest that edge artifacts are more common in the early arriving photons and that tumors are easier to detect in the image made from late-arriving photons. Up to three frequencies of NIR light are used for their analyses of absorption and scattering of the NIR light. Their method provides calculated results for hemoglobin concentration and scattering power, factors that showed differences between carcinomas and normal breast tissue.

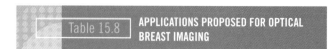

Table 15.8	APPLICATIONS PROPOSED FOR OPTICAL BREAST IMAGING

Measurement of breast density
Detection of the vascularity of tumors
Detection of breast tumors
Detection of axillary lymph node metastases

Potential Clinical Applications of Optical Breast Imaging

Optical imaging has been proposed for the following purposes: (a) measurements of breast density, (b) detection of the vascularity of tumors, (c) detection of breast tumors, and (d) detection of axillary lymph node metastases. These are listed in Table 15.8.

Measurements of Breast Density

Women with higher breast density are at greater risk for the development of breast cancer. Optical imaging can be used to determine water content, lipid content, and hemoglobin content. These may in turn show greater potential for risk assessment compared with current methods for the measurement of breast density on mammography. An important advantage of the use of optical measurements is that they involve no ionizing radiation. In addition, such methods, if proved to be effective, would likely have low costs and would be safe to use to assess breast cancer risk in women who, because of age, do not currently receive mammography.

As an example of such work, Cerussi et al. (43,44) used a seven-wavelength frequency-domain photon migration system to study 28 healthy, premenopausal and postmenopausal women, aged 18 to 64 years. Of these, six were on hormone replacement therapy (HRT). They found absorption and scattering differences that were age dependent. By measuring oxyhemoglobin, deoxyhemoglobin, lipid, and water content or ratios, they could determine breast involution. Both premenopausal women and postmenopausal women on HRT had similar profiles, and they were both different from women who were postmenopausal and not on HRT.

Intes (45) uses four NIR wavelengths to calculate water, lipid, oxyhemoglobin and deoxyhemoglobin levels. In a small number of subjects, measurements of the ratio of water to lipid correlated with mammographic breast density, suggesting that optical imaging could serve as a marker of risk similar to mammographic breast density.

Shah et al. (46) used multispectral functional optical spectroscopy to show changes with menstrual cycle, menopause, and hormone use. Their method uses multispectral imaging at 674, 803, 849, and 956 nm and can measure oxyhemoglobin, deoxyhemoglobin, total hemoglobin, tissue hemoglobin oxygen saturation, and total water content.

Simick and Lilge (47) and Blackmore et al. (48) report an ongoing project where breast optical spectroscopy is compared to mammographic density. Optical spectroscopy is measured by four transmission sites in each breast at multiple spectral frequencies. These are then analyzed for water, lipid, and hemoglobin content. These results are then compared to those of mammographic breast density measured on an ordinal scale by a single trained observer. Interest is in identifying women with breast density greater than 75%. In the more recent study, 292 women were evaluated and the two methods showed quite similar results with a resulting receiver operating characteristic (ROC) area under the curve of 0.922. Further work in this project is ongoing. This method of spectroscopy does not produce an image of the breast.

These studies indicate that optical spectroscopy is a promising method for identifying women with high breast parenchymal density and therefore at increased risk for breast cancer.

Detection of the Vascularity of Tumors

Optical imaging can detect the vascular flow to tumors and the degree of oxygen extraction by tumors. It thus provides information on the physiological state of tumors. As an example, Jiang et al. (49,50) computed absorption and scattering components of continuous wave NIR at 785 nm separately in nine subjects—six with benign or malignant tumors and three control subjects. Control subjects showed uniform patterns of both absorption and scattering. Malignant tumors showed increased absorption and increased scattering. The authors suggest that scattering may be due to cellular organelles in malignant tumors. Fibroadenomas showed increase absorption and a marked decrease in scattering, a pattern quite different from malignancy. This and other work suggests that chemotherapy-induced changes in tumor vascularity would be detectable using optical methods.

Heffer and Fantini (51) propose a method of measuring oxygen saturation in tissues and provide mathematical models and studies in phantoms to support the method.

A different method of studying vascular flow is to perform dynamic optical imaging (52). In one such approach, the breast is gently compressed and then optical imaging is used to measure the rate of return of blood to areas of the breast. The pattern of enhancement seen in normal breasts in the areas of glandular tissue is a sinusoidal pattern representing cardiac pulsation and respiratory effect. In areas of tumor, a blood concentration enhancement curve similar to that seen with contrast enhancement during MRI is seen. Only a small number of patients have been imaged, but the approach and its similarity to MRI enhancement curves is intriguing. The method, at least in its preliminary report, has low specificity.

Detection of Breast Tumors

Optical imaging can detect breast cancers. Franceschini et al. (25), for example, studied 15 patients with breast cancer. In 11, frequency-domain optical breast imaging showed the tumor location. These authors used 690- and 810-nm wavelengths and superimposed on them intensity changes at two frequencies close to, but slightly different from, 110 MHz. By analyzing the patterns from these two slightly different frequencies, they could extract lower frequencies that were used for their analyses. Reports to date do not provide sufficient information to determine the range of sizes of breast cancer that can be detected, and whether ductal carcinoma *in situ* (DCIS) can be detected reliably.

Eppstein et al. (33) suggest that enhancement of smaller tumors will occur after the intravenous injection of optical dyes such as indocyanine green. Fantini et al. (53) provided preliminary data on 131 patients of whom 60 had breast cancer. Although their optical imaging system used four NIR wavelengths, they reported preliminary data using one wavelength in their analysis. They calculated the sensitivity using two different methods. When analysis required that the lesion be identified on two views, sensitivity was 72% and specificity 52%. When the criteria for a true-positive result applied to one or two views, sensitivity was 88% and specificity 30%. The sizes of tumors were not reported.

Grosenick et al. (40–42) used time of flight NIR imaging to characterize breast cancers and compare their appearance to normal breast. They used pulses of light and recorded the data with time of arrival. No benign tumors or benign lesions were reported. In their two clinical site studies 154 patients suspected of having breast cancer were included. Optical images were obtained prospectively, but analyzed retrospectively, using x-ray mammograms or MR breast images for lesion localization. This method was able to visualize 92 of 102 carcinomas including 7 of 9 cases of DCIS, 68 of 72 cases of invasive ductal carcinoma, and 12 of 12 invasive lobular carcinomas. Their method, by using x-ray or MR breast images for localization, does not provide a measurement of optical imaging false positives. They do not provide information on specificity. They do not report the optical characteristics of benign breast tumors.

Intes (45) reported on a prototype system that uses four NIR frequencies to differentiate benign and malignant nodules. The system compares optical properties of the mammographically identified lesion with the area immediately surrounding the lesion. Water, hemoglobin, oxygen saturation, and lipid were measured. In a study of 23 cases, the deoxyhemoglobin content provided a statistically significant differentiation between benign and malignant lesions.

Tromberg et al. (29) and Chance et al. (31) have emphasized the use of NIR spectroscopy using small hand-held devices that measure the absorption spectra at several to multiple NIR frequencies. Tromberg et al. used a continuous NIR spectrum; Chance et al. used three wavelengths. Tromberg et al. measured the spectra in premenopausal women, both for normal breasts and breast tumors. Their study found significant differences in oxyhemoglobin, deoxyhemoglobin, water, and lipids when normal areas and tumors were compared. Their study also identified changes toward the normal pattern in the NIR spectra in one patient with a locally advanced tumor while that patient received chemotherapy.

Chance et al. (31) reported on a prospective two center study of 116 subjects where 44 had cancer verified by biopsy and histopathology. NIR recordings were made with an inexpensive probe using three NIR wavelengths. The aim of this study was to record total hemoglobin and the degree of oxygen desaturation reflecting the physiological parameters of tumor vascularity and hypermetabolism. The device does not produce an image of the tumor, only measures of its vascularity and the ratio of oxyhemoglobin and deoxyhemoglobin. Each subject served as her own control with comparisons made between normal areas of the involved breast and comparisons with the opposite breast and a model of normal breast vascularity. The molecular changes of tumors were detected in a tumor size range of 8 mm and larger. Most were less than 2 cm. The area under the ROC curve was 0.95; sensitivity was 96% with specificity of 93%. The authors propose that this device could provide an inexpensive portable method for the detection of breast cancer in underserved populations.

Optical Imaging for Tumors using Other Methods for Localization

One of the problems in optical imaging is that the size and depth of lesions that result in optical absorption is not known. This limits the accuracy of measurement of the physiologic and metabolic characteristics. For this reason, some investigators have combined optical imaging with other imaging methods to aid in analysis. Grosenick et al. (40–42) work in time of flight optical imaging and use information from mammography and breast MRI to improve the accuracy of the measurements.

Zhu et al. (54–56) have developed and are testing a combined optical imaging and ultrasound probe so that the optical imaging results can be correlated with the ultrasound image. This should allow more accurate measurements of the physiological and metabolic features of breast lesions. In a study of 65 women with 81 breast lesions, concurrent optical spectroscopy, ultrasound imaging, and image-guided core biopsy were performed. Biopsy documented eight invasive carcinomas 6 to 22 mm in size. Seven of the 8 carcinomas were 11 mm or less. Seventy-three benign lesions were present. Based on the optical analysis, the maximum and average hemoglobin concentrations were significantly higher in the malignant group than in the benign group. Assigning a threshold value for maximum hemoglobin concentration, optical spectroscopy had a sensitivity of 100%, specificity

96%, positive predictive value (PPV) 73%, negative predictive value (NPV) 100%. Work by this group is continuing.

Detection of Axillary Lymph Node Metastases

Optical dyes are currently in clinical use for sentinel lymph node identification for biopsy. MR contrast agents providing enhanced lymph node imaging have also been developed and are in clinical trials (18,20,57). In the future, these may be applied to axillary lymph node imaging.

Summary of Optical Imaging

Optical imaging is a developing technology for breast imaging that provides information not otherwise easily available. Measurements of oxyhemoglobin and deoxyhemoglobin can be obtained noninvasively from localized areas of the breast (e.g., breast tumors). In addition, in small series of patients, malignant tumors and fibroadenomas appear to have different light absorption characteristics. Injected optical dyes can be used to study blood flow, tissue permeability, and the rate of wash-out. These measurements are similar to those obtainable on MRI and, as with MRI, have shown a predictive association the benign and malignant nature of breast masses. The major limitation of optical imaging is related to the size of the cancers that can be detected. There does not yet appear to be sufficient information to determine the lower limit of size of malignant tumors that are detectable and the sensitivity of the method for tumors of various sizes. The area of light absorption is not directly related to the size of the tumor because the increase in blood flow often extends into the tissues surrounding the tumor and the light is scattered within the breast. Information on the rate of false-positive results and the nature of these false-positive detections does not seem to be available. Optical imaging may provide a method of breast cancer risk assessment similar to using measurements of mammographic breast density, but this needs further evaluation.

Optical imaging is a broad field with much exciting research and technical development ongoing. It may prove to be quite valuable in the field of breast imaging in the future, and has specific areas where it may be of great interest to breast cancer researchers today who are studying specific aspects of breast cancer metabolism and therapeutic response.

Optoacoustic and Thermoacoustic Tomography of the Breast

Optoacoustic and thermoacoustic tomography used rapidly pulsed energy transmitted into the breast to generate ultrasound signals where this energy interacts with breast tumors. Optoacoustic tomography uses NIR pulses to create ultrasound signals. Thermoacoustic tomography uses microwave pulses to generate ultrasound images.

Optoacoustic Tomography

Optoacoustic tomography of the breast is a developing technology for breast imaging that shows initial promising results (58–62). It is a hybrid method merging optical imaging and ultrasonography. As described in the previous section, NIR laser pulses have relatively low absorption in normal breast tissue, with absorption increased by the hemoglobin present in vessels in the breast, including that in breast tumors. Oxyhemoglobin and deoxyhemoglobin concentrations can be calculated. A major limitation of optical imaging is its relatively low spatial resolution. Optoacoustic tomography in preliminary work done in phantoms and a few human subjects appears to provide improved resolution compared with optical imaging while taking advantage of the optical absorptive properties of hemoglobin (60,63).

In optoacoustic tomography, high-frequency pulses of NIR light are transmitted into the breast. The NIR light is absorbed by hemoglobin, producing a small amount of heat that rapidly dissipates. By rapidly turning the laser on and off (measured in nanoseconds), the heat-generated expansion and contraction of the tissues can reach ultrasound frequencies, and this ultrasound is transmitted through the breast tissues to the skin surface where it can be recorded as ultrasound. This is then used to produce an image of the regions of the breast where hemoglobin is present. Early data have shown the difference between total oxyhemoglobin and deoxyhemoglobin (Fig. 15.4). In theory, it could provide images of injected optical dyes.

Studies have been performed in phantoms, a limited number of mastectomy specimens, and a few research subjects prebiopsy with suspect breast lesions. Only limited data on clinical utility are currently available.

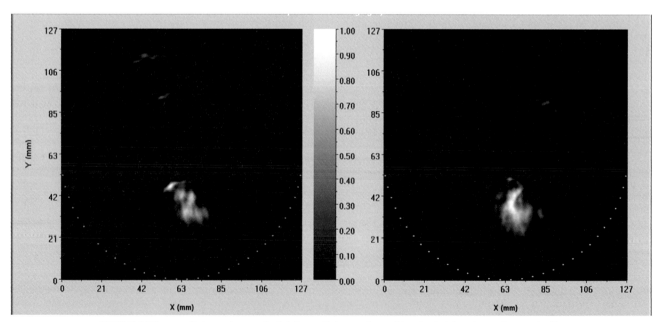

FIGURE 15.4. This composite image shows a pair of photoacoustic images of a small invasive ductal carcinoma. By measuring the absorption at different near-infrared (NIR) frequencies, two images can be calculated. The one on the left is of the oxyhemoglobin distribution, the one on the right is of the deoxyhemoglobin. From the images alone, it is not possible to tell which image is due to which form of hemoglobin; one needs information of the imaging parameters to understand how to interpret such images. (Courtesy of Alan Stein, M.D., and Seno Medical Instruments, Inc, San Antonio, Texas.)

Thermoacoustic Tomography

Thermoacoustic tomography is similar to optoacoustic tomography. In optoacoustic tomography, rapidly pulsed light is used to heat tissues. In thermoacoustic tomography, microwaves are used to create the rapid expansion and contraction of tissues, producing high-frequency sound that can then be used to produce an image. So far the mathematical principles have been explored and images have been produced in tissue samples and tissue-containing phantoms. *In vivo* images have not been reported (64–68).

Microwave Imaging of the Breast

Microwave imaging is under study as a potential method of breast imaging. It is based on the differences in dielectric properties between normal breast tissue and breast cancer. The dielectric constant varies for different microwave frequencies, with approximately a fivefold difference between normal breast tissue and breast cancer at the frequencies under study. Reconstruction methods have been tested in mathematical models and in tissue samples (69–71).

Initial clinical studies are under way. Initial work focused on defining the patterns seen in normal women's breasts (72,73). More recently, Poplack et al. (74) have reported initial results from a clinical study comparing electrical impedance breast spectroscopy, microwave spectroscopy, and NIR spectroscopy. Figure 15.5 shows images of invasive ductal carcinomas as localized by each of these methods. With both electrical impedance spectroscopy and microwave spectroscopy, measurements are made of conductivity and permittivity (capacitance); *permittivity* is the ability of the tissue to hold an electric charge. In this study, 150 participants were included. Different participants received different combinations of imaging methods. Subjects

with American College of Radiology Breast Imaging Reporting and Data System (BI-RADS) 1, 4, and 5 were included. Among the cancers, the mean size was 12 mm. As an interim summary of results, electrical impedance spectroscopy showed very good ability to separate normal from abnormal cases, but not in separating different types of abnormalities and separating them into likely benign and malignant categories. Microwave spectroscopy and NIR optical spectroscopy showed the potential to distinguish between normal and abnormal breasts and, in the presence of an abnormal (BI-RADS 4 or 5) mammogram, moderate ability to differentiate benign and malignant breast disease. The authors consider the work preliminary and it is continuing. Currently, their best results came from a combination of measurements from these three methods.

Imaging and Spectroscopy of the Electrical Activity of the Breast

Electrical impedance imaging of the breast has been under development for more than 20 years. Each tissue in the body has a specific range of electrical characteristics that can be used to define it. If two adjacent tissues have different characteristics, it is possible to identify that these two tissues are different and create an image resulting from the tissue differences. Differences in electrical properties between normal breast adipose tissue, glandular tissue, benign processes, and malignant tumors have been recorded. The topics discussed in this section are listed in Table 15.9.

Electrical Activity in the Breast: Physical Principles

Tissues differ in three main electrical features. First, there is a cell membrane potential that differs between the cells in normal,

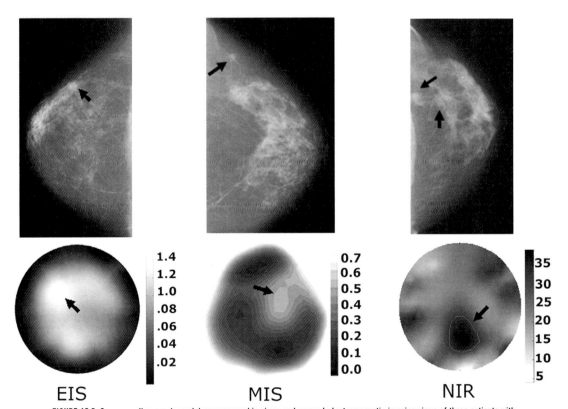

FIGURE 15.5. Corresponding craniocaudal mammographic views and coronal electromagnetic imaging views of three patients with invasive ductal carcinomas (*arrows*). As displayed in this image, electrical impedance spectroscopy (EIS) and microwave imaging spectroscopy (MIS) display the cancer location as a white area; the near infrared image (NIR) shows it as a dark area. The differences are due to the underlying interaction of the tissue with the electromagnetic radiation and on the choice of the researchers on the pattern of display. (From Poplack SP, Tosteson TD, Wells WA, et al. Electromagnetic breast imaging: results of a pilot study in women with abnormal mammograms. *Radiology* 2007;243[2]:350–359, with permission.)

Table 15.9	ELECTRICAL PROPERTIES OF THE BREAST

Electrical activity in the breast: physical principles
Clinical studies
    Detection and classification of breast tumors
    Assessment of breast cancer risk

fatty, and cancerous tissue. This can be detected by placing an electrode in the tissue and measuring the direct current that results. Second, there is the conduction of electrons through tissue. Tissues resist the flow of electrons, a property called *resistance*. Resistance is related to extracellular fluid, cellular density, and tissue vascularity. Third, tissues also act as capacitors. Capacitance (also called permittivity) is related to cell membrane density and intercellular tight boundaries. Alternating current flowing into and out of a capacitor results in a change in the phase of the signal, a property of reactance. If one applies an alternating current to the body, the combination of resistance and reactance can be measured. This combination of resistance and reactance is called *impedance*. In the breast, fatty tissue, glandular tissue, and breast cancer of various types (DCIS, invasive ductal carcinoma, and lobular carcinoma) differ in their impedance properties.

Although these electrical properties of tissue have been known for more than 30 years, converting laboratory data obtained from tissue samples into clinically useful systems for breast cancer detection has been quite slow but is now making important progress because of improvements in electronics and software design (72,74,75).

Electrical activity of the breast can be intrinsic or induced. Intrinsic electrical activity arises from cellular functions that maintain an electrical potential across the cell membrane. Extrinsically, an electrical current can be induced in the patient and measured over the breast. One can induce one electrical frequency or several. There are three components of this that can be measured: the amplitude of remaining electrical activity, differences of remaining activity according to electrical frequency, and phase as a measure of tissue capacitance. The transmission of electrical activity to the breast appears to depend mainly on vascularity; the phase shift (inductance resulting from capacitance) depends on the number of cell membranes in the local region of measurement.

Clinical Study Results

Electrical measurements have been proposed for the following uses: (a) detection of malignant tumors, (b) classification of tumors into those likely benign or likely malignant, (c) assessment of breast cancer risk.

Detection and Classification of Benign and Malignant Tumors

One system for electrical measurements of the breast using induced electrical activity has premarket approval from the FDA. It is approved for use to improve the classification of breast lesions that on mammograms classified to be BI-RADS 3 or low-suspicion BI-RADS 4. It is used for electrical impedance spectroscopy and measures both conductance and capacitance.

Recent clinical reports from a several groups provide data on its sensitivity and specificity. Melloul et al. (76) compared the value of MIBI and electrical impedance spectroscopy in 121 women. MIBI had an overall sensitivity of 89% and a specificity of 88%, with 100% sensitivity for breast tumors greater than 1 cm, but only 66% for tumors less than 1 cm. Electrical impedance spectroscopy had a sensitivity of 72% and a specificity of 67%.

Malich et al. (77) have provided three reports. First is a study of 52 women with sonographically or mammographically suspect findings. There were 29 malignant and 29 benign lesions in these women (some women had more than one lesion). All patients were also imaged with MRI. Two methods of electrical impedance imaging and spectroscopy were used: targeting the specific lesion and surveying the breast. When specific lesions were targeted this study showed a positive predictive value of 93% and a negative predictive value of 73%. The malignancies were midsized, averaging 17 mm, and none of the invasive cancers was less than 1 cm. In the surveys of the breasts there were 47 spots in 52 patients, which would suggest potential problems if this system were used for screening. Twenty-two of 29 malignancies were identified, but 25 of the spots were false-positive results. Artifacts such as signals from superficial skin lesions, poor skin contact, and air bubbles were reported as limitations.

A second report from the same group included 100 cases (with inclusion of the prior subjects) with ultrasonographic and MRI correlation (78). Fifty of 62 malignant lesions were identified by electrical impedance spectroscopy (sensitivity 81%). Twenty-four of 38 benign lesions were correctly identified as benign (specificity 63%). Ultrasonographic examination showed 52 lesions as suspect and 48 as not suspect (sensitivity 77%; specificity 89%). MRI could be performed on 90 of the 100 patients; its sensitivity was 98% and specificity 81%. The authors concluded that the use of the tested electrical impedance spectroscopy system supplemented the results of the ultrasonographic examination. A third report from the same group on 240 lesions consisting of 103 malignant lesions and 137 benign lesions showed a sensitivity of 87.8% and specificity of 66.4% (79).

The June 2002 issue of *IEEE Transactions on Medical Imaging* is a special issue on electrical impedance tomography. In this special issue there are four articles reporting on electrical studies of the breast. Glickman et al. (75) reported on a new algorithm for the analysis of the electrical impedance spectroscopy. This new system software (which has received FDA premarket approval) provides not only an image of the breast, but incorporates an automated analysis system that provides a color-coded guide to the likelihood of malignancy. Using this new algorithm, the system was trained with 83 carcinomas and 153 benign lesions. It was then verified on an independent test group including 87 carcinomas, 153 cases with benign lesions, and 356 asymptomatic volunteers. Using histology of the biopsied tissue as ground truth, the system had a sensitivity of 84% and a specificity of 52%. The advantage of this system is that it reduces some of the subjectivity involved in interpretation of the electrical impedance images.

A second article uses data obtained with the commercial electrical impedance spectroscopy system (80) and describes progress in methods for determining the three-dimensional localization of the source of the electrical impedance signal in breast phantoms. This system was then tested on existing data from patients. It shows a reasonable correlation of lesion depth as determined by ultrasonography, with the depth determined by the proposed algorithm. From the article, it is clear that additional work is still required. The authors suggest extending the range of recorded electrical frequencies, currently 100 Hz to 5 kHz, to the megahertz range to increase accuracy in determining tissue characteristics.

The third article reports results of studies of 26 subjects using a different system for measuring electrical impedance spectroscopy of the breast (81). In this experimental device, spectroscopic data ranging from 10 to 950 kHz is used to create cross-sectional images of the breast. Using visual inspection criteria, the system detected 83% of the BI-RADS 4 to 5 lesions. The authors' conclusion is that "multi-frequency electrical impedance imaging appears promising for detecting breast malignancies, but improvements must be made before the method reaches full potential." A more recent report on this system indicates that it may be more useful for breast cancer risk assessment and is discussed in the next section (74).

The fourth article describes yet another system for electrical imaging of the breast (82). In this case, only breast conductivity is used to create the images. The article reports the appearance of the breast during normal physiologic cycles. The authors report patterns reflecting different phases of the menstrual cycle, changes of pregnancy, lactation, and postmenopausal findings. The goal of this study was to determine the baseline appearances of the normal breast before proceeding to studies of the abnormal breast.

Studies of Potential Value as Measurements for Breast Cancer Risk

Several recent reports on electrical impedance spectroscopy have emphasized its potential value as a measure of risk for breast cancer. Poplack et al. (74) compared electrical impedance, microwave, and NIR spectroscopy and concluded that electrical impedance spectroscopy could separate those with normal breast tissue from those with abnormalities, but could not separate cancer from other types of breast abnormalities.

Three recent articles by Stojadinovic et al. (83–85) report on different (but overlapping) studies of electrical impedance spectroscopy with the analysis algorithm set to provide high specificity (rather than high sensitivity) in cancer detection. The proposed value in this would be in screening younger women, who are usually not screened with mammography, for breast cancer risk. In the largest study, they used separate populations to determine specificity and sensitivity. Among 390 women aged 30 to 45 referred for biopsy for suspected cancer, 87 had cancer; 52% of those were less than 20 mm in diameter and 23 were detected. Sensitivity was 26.4%. Of 1,751 asymptomatic women aged 30 to 39, 93 had positive studies. Specificity was 94.7%. The relative risk of a woman with a positive electrical impedance study compared to an age-appropriate risk of breast cancer in the normal population is 4.95. The authors consider this a sufficient elevation of risk to warrant additional breast evaluation in young women with positive studies. Although a specific electrical impedance spectroscopy system is FDA approved as a complement to mammography for BI-RADS 3 and low grade 4 lesions, its use for cancer risk assessment has not been approved by the FDA.

Summary of Electrical Measurements of the Breast

Electrical measurements of the breast have shown in reasonably sized clinical studies their value to help classify breast lesions into benign and malignant categories. One commercial system has received premarket approval from the FDA for this application. It is not yet determined how sensitive it will be to smaller cancers, although it can detect some unknown percentage of cancers less than 10 mm in size. For screening, current equipment highlights too many false-positive locations. Recent reports suggest that the method may be appropriate for assessing a woman's risk for breast cancer. Further development of the technology is expected to enhance its capabilities.

Radioactive Tracer Imaging of the Breast

Radioactive tracers are commonly used clinically. They are used for (a) the detection of malignant tumors in the breast, (b) determining the likely benign or malignant nature of breast tumors, (c) evaluating molecular and metabolic differences between malignant tumors, (d) evaluating the extent of malignancy in the breast, (e) identifying axillary nodal and other metastases. They have been proposed as methods to determine the potential or actual response of carcinomas to chemotherapy. These uses are listed in Table 15.10.

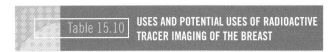

Table 15.10	USES AND POTENTIAL USES OF RADIOACTIVE TRACER IMAGING OF THE BREAST

Detection of malignant breast tumors
Determine likely benign or malignant nature
Evaluate molecular and metabolic differences
Evaluate extent of malignancy
Identify axillary nodal and other metastases
Determine reponse of carcinomas to chemotherapy

The two main agents are MIBI and FDG. Both tracers are used to study the total body with whole body large field of view imagers and localized small fields of views including the breast or the axillary lymph nodes. The small field of view imagers provide higher resolution in the breast and can detect smaller breast cancers and local lymph node metastases than the large field of view cameras. The large field of view cameras provide lower resolution images but can view the entire body for evidence of metastases. No data comparing imaging with MIBI and FDG in the same patients have been reported. Based on the physical characteristics of the two types of imaging, imaging with MIBI is likely to be less expensive. Imaging with FDG is likely to show smaller tumors and better define the extent of disease infiltrating the breast. In this section, MIBI and its clinical data are discussed first, followed by the discussion of FDG and its clinical data.

^{99m}Tc-Sestamibi

The uses of MIBI and FDG-PET are FDA approved for breast imaging. They are both used to assist in the evaluation of suspect lesions identified within the breast and the potential effectiveness and response of identified malignancies to chemotherapy. MIBI and FDG have, however, different pathways of interaction with carcinomas. Both depend on tumor vessels to transport them to the cell membrane, but, once there, they interact with cells differently. FDG is a glucose analog and is taken up by cells as though it were glucose. It then is blocked in the hexokinase pathway and accumulates in the cancer cells.

Cellular Mechanisms of ^{99m}Tc-Sestamibi Uptake and Excretion

MIBI shows a more complex pattern within the cellular pathways. It is used to both show that a breast finding is carcinoma and to evaluate a breast carcinoma for drug resistance (86). It is taken up as a lipophilic cation, probably by diffusion through the negative plasma membrane and mitochondrial membrane potentials into the cell and its mitochondria. Its uptake into mitochondria (in cells in culture) appears to be blocked by overexpression of the Bcl-2 antiapoptotic protein; Bcl-2 is associated with drug resistance. The excretion of MIBI from cells is enhanced by the overexpression of P-glycoprotein; and overexpression of P-glycoprotein is implicated in multidrug resistance. Thus, the failure of uptake of MIBI into carcinoma cells could indicate that there is decreased blood flow to the tumor or increased expression of Bcl-2. Once taken up, its more rapid excretion from cells could indicate P-glycoprotein overexpression indicative of multidrug resistance (86). For this reason, imaging using MIBI may be done at several time points to separately evaluate uptake and excretion (87). Imaging with MIBI, therefore, can be used both to identify carcinoma and its potential resistance to certain types of chemotherapies (86,88,89). MIBI imaging has been use as a predictor of response to neoadjuvant chemotherapy (90), but it is also reported to be ineffective for this purpose (91).

99mTc-Sestamibi for Clinical Detection of Carcinoma

The sensitivity of MIBI for the detection of breast cancer varies, in reported studies, from 72% to 91% and specificity from 63% to 88% (92–94). Greater sensitivity was shown for palpable lesions than for nonpalpable lesions (92), at least in part related to tumor size. Melloul et al. (76) conducted MIBI imaging in 121 women and reported an overall 89% sensitivity and 88% specificity, with 100% sensitivity for breast tumors greater than 1 cm, but only 66% for tumors less than 1 cm.

Brem et al. (95,96) reported on the use of a small field of view MIBI imager for invasive carcinoma and DCIS. They tested the system for use in high-risk screening and for the diagnosis of indeterminate mammographic and ultrasound abnormalities. In 22 cases of biopsy proven DCIS, 91% were detected, compared to 82% detected by mammography and 88% with contrast enhanced breast MRI (95). These differences were not statistically significant for this sample size. In a separate study (96), probably with some overlap of study populations, they reports on 23 women with 33 indeterminate breast lesions comparing contrast enhanced breast MRI with MIBI small field of view imaging. There were nine carcinomas confirmed by pathology. There were four areas of DCIS, three infiltrating ductal carcinomas, one invasive lobular carcinoma, and one invasive carcinoma with ductal and lobular features. One patient had two foci of carcinoma. Of these nine carcinomas, breast MRI detected nine and MIBI imaging eight (difference is not statistically significant). Important statistically significant differences were seen in specificity: breast MRI specificity was 25%, MIBI imaging was 71%. Brem et al. (97) also investigated the findings with a small field of view MIBI imager in 94 high-risk women with normal mammography (BI-RADS 1 or 2) and normal physical examination. Sixteen (17%) of these had abnormal scintimammograms. Of these 16, 2 had previously unidentified invasive cancers; both of these cancers were 9 mm in diameter at pathology examination. Nine had biopsies showing benign pathology. Of the remaining five, there were no focal ultrasound abnormalities and biopsy was not performed; follow-up of these five patients at 6 months with MIBI imaging showed no remaining abnormality. Although the size of these three studies is limited, the results suggest that MIBI with a small field of view imager could be of clinical use to investigate women with indeterminate findings on mammography that remain indeterminate after ultrasound. MIBI may not be suitable for screening women at high or low risk for breast cancer. A comparative screening study comparing MIBI with breast MRI in women at high risk would be of interest.

99mTc-Sestamibi and the Detection of Molecular Differences in Tumors

Studies have shown that there are molecular differences between tumors that take up MIBI and those that do not. Tumors with less response to chemotherapy have increased excretion of MIBI from mitochondria through the P-glycoprotein ATP-dependent transport mechanisms, and this is increased in cancers having the *MDR1* (*ABCB1*) and *MDR2* (*ABCB4*) genes (88,98–100). Tumors with these genes may not always be successfully imaged with MIBI. Nonimaged tumors also have a decreased apoptotic index and increased Bcl-2 levels (88).

Wilczek et al. (92) looked for early changes in MIBI uptake after chemotherapy as a possible predictor of chemotherapy response. Changes were seen only after the course of therapy had been completed, not earlier. Pusztai et al. (101) used MIBI imaging to determine those patients with P-glycoprotein positive tumors who might benefit from the use of tariquidar, a P-glycoprotein inhibitor. Limited tumor response treatment benefit was seen in two of five women who showed an increase in MIBI uptake after tariquidar.

18F-Fluorodeoxyglucose

The use of FDG to image the breasts is FDA cleared. FDG uptake is increased in both primary and metastatic breast cancer. FDG is currently used in evaluating undiagnosed lesions that could represent metastatic disease. It is also used for evaluating suspected in-breast recurrence of tumor after local excision. FDG imaging is under study as a diagnostic agent for indeterminate breast lesions suspected of being cancer (102,103), for staging cancer at the time of initial presentation, and for monitoring the response to therapy (104–106).

Clinical Studies of 18F-Fluorodeoxyglucose for Tumor Characterization

FDG is used both for tumor detection and detection of tumor margins. A recent multicenter trial using a small field of view dedicated breast imager showed overall sensitivity of 90% with a specificity of 86% (107). In this population of 77 women with 92 lesions, there were 48 cancers of which 11 were DCIS, 3 cases of atypical ductal hyperplasia, and 41 benign lesions. When patients with diabetes and lesions clearly benign on conventional imaging were removed, sensitivity was 91% with specificity 93%. Ten of 11 patients with DCIS showed positive FDG uptake. Figure 15.6 shows one of the images from this study. It shows increased tracer uptake in three lesions: an invasive ductal carcinoma with an axillary lymph node metastasis and contralateral DCIS. In addition, multiple small focal areas of uptake are seen in an area of diffuse multifocal invasive ductal carcinoma.

FDG-PET imaging has been proposed as a method for determining the boundaries of tumors at the time of surgical resection. In two reports, based on overlapping case samples, improved definition of the extent of tumor was found (107,108). In one of these, FDG-PET small field of view imaging correctly predicted those cases with positive margins in 6 of 8 cases (75%) and 11 of 11 cases with negative margins (100%) (108). FDG-PET has also been suggested as a method to guide biopsy in areas of diffuse calcification so that biopsy of those regions most metabolically active can be performed.

Experimental Radiotracer Imaging

Experimental work in animals indicates that radiotracers can potentially provide tumor-specific radioactive probes. Given the available variety of radioactive tracers, many compounds can be radiolabeled, and hence specific radioactive compounds can be used to localize tissues of interest. These radiotracers can be gamma emitters or positron emitters. They can be chemically bound to antibodies or structural ligands and can be made to target membrane and intracellular receptors or intracellular enzymes (109). Markers of amino acid metabolism such as 11C-methionine and 18F-labeled estradiol to image estrogen receptors are under study in animals (109).

Breast Computed Tomography

CT imaging of the breast can occur when the thorax is imaged for other purposes or with the direct intention to image the breasts. CT can be performed without or with contrast agents and can be done on standard CT machines or on research breast-specific CT devices. It can be used to determine the extent of a known tumor within the breast and to look for chest wall invasion. Research devices specifically made to image the breasts are under development as potential replacements for mammography.

CT to Define Tumor Extent

Contrast-enhanced CT (CECT) has been proposed as a potential method for determining the extent of breast cancer before breast-conserving therapy (110). Breast MRI has also been

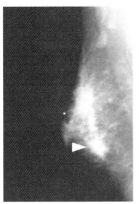 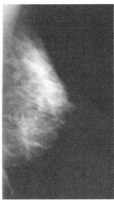 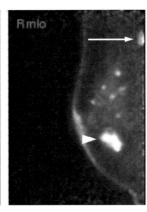 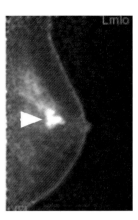

FIGURE 15.6. ^{18}F-fluorodeoxyglucose positron emission tomography (FDG-PET) small field of view images of both breasts in mediolateral oblique (MLO) projections. The MLO view of each breast is shown in the left pair of images. The FDG images are the pair to the right. In the left images, the right breast shows a focal irregular mass (*arrowhead*). Lymph nodes are present in the right axilla. In the pair of FDG images, the left image shows the right breast. The small arrowhead shows the area of FDG uptake in the index lesion that was invasive ductal carcinoma. The long arrow points to an area of uptake in a metastasis in an axillary lymph node. Lying between them, the small bright areas of whiteness represent foci of multicenter carcinoma. In the right FDG image, the large arrowhead points to an area of intermediate grade ductal carcinoma *in situ* (DCIS). (From Berg WA, Weinberg IN, Narayanan D, et al. High-resolution fluorodeoxyglucose positron emission tomography with compression ["positron emission mammography"] is highly accurate in depicting primary breast cancer. *Breast J* 2006;12[4]:309–323, with permission.)

proposed for this purpose. Uematsu et al. (110) report on 136 cases of invasive breast cancer evaluated by CECT. The results of the CTs were used to guide resection. Comparison of the CT slices with the pathology specimens was performed at 5-mm slice intervals through the specimens. The criterion used to judge correlations was whether the pathology-detected edge of the tumor extended 1 cm or more from the edge of the dominant mass. Using this criterion, CECT had a sensitivity of 70% and specificity of 89%. There were 10 false-positive tumors when the tumor extent was less than expected based on CECT. In seven, this was caused by benign pathologic lesions adjacent to the tumor. In three cases, the tumor was smaller than shown by CECT. There were 14 false-negative cases when the tumor extended beyond the limits of detection. In these cases, the tumor extending beyond the CT-detected margin was sparse.

Akashi-Tanaka et al. (111) reported on 122 women, of whom 44 demonstrated extensive intraductal tumor components histologically. The sensitivity for detection of intraductal spread by preoperative CECT was 88%, with a specificity of 79%.

Research on Computed Tomography Scanners Designed for Breast Imaging

Several groups are working to develop CT scanners designed to image the breast (112–114). A clinical study with one of these systems is under way and has been reported twice as the number of subjects increased (114,115). The radiation dose with this equipment is equivalent to two-view mammography. The series included 10 healthy women and 69 with BI-RADS 4 and 5 lesions (115). Overall, using subjective comparisons made by one breast imaging specialist, CT was reported as equivalent to mammography, performing significantly better for breast masses and significantly less well for microcalcifications. This system uses no breast compression; subjects found CT imaging significantly more comfortable. Most women in these series were imaged without intravenous contrast. Several were imaged with intravenous CT contrast with representative images presented in one study (114).

Potential Uses of Computed Tomography in Breast Imaging

Breast CT can be used as a diagnostic test to determine tumor extent competing with breast MRI. It is not sufficiently studied to determine its potential value compared to breast MRI. Dedicated breast CT, if confirmed to be at least equivalent to breast MRI, is likely to be less expensive and have higher acceptability to women because it does not require breast compression, is faster, and is less likely to induce feelings of claustrophobia.

As a screening test, dedicated breast CT shows promise, but further studies are needed. Because CT has more limited spatial resolution than mammography, microcalcifications are more difficult to identify.

Thermography: Imaging Breast Heat

Thermography has been proposed as a method for the detection of breast carcinoma, differentiating benign from malignant breast tumors, and to identify women at higher risk of developing breast carcinoma. The topics in this section are listed in Table 15.11.

The fundamental signal in thermography of the breast is heat. The wavelength of heat is in the mid- to far infrared region of the electromagnetic spectrum. Different devices can create temperature maps of the breast either by being placed in direct contact with the breast or by measuring the temperature of the breast surface at a distance as infrared light emissions. These are called contact and noncontact (or telethermography) systems. The temperature of the breast is related to the effect of blood flow into the breast, the intrinsic metabolic processes in the breast, and the dissipation of heat from the breast.

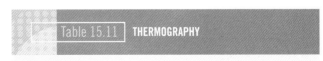

Table 15.11	THERMOGRAPHY

Basic prinicples
Types of thermography
   Contact
   Noncontact: telethermography
   Static thermography
   Dynamic thermography
Limitations of thermography
Recent clinical trial results
   Static thermography
   Dynamic thermography

Three different findings are used to evaluate the heat pattern on the surface of the breast: (a) the pattern and number of vessels compared between the two breasts, (b) the temperature of the vessels and skin surface, and (c) the dynamic pattern of heat over time. The temperature of the breast can be measured at one point in time, at multiple points in time, or can be monitored continuously (for example for 24 hours). Dynamic changes in breast temperature can be measured over a period of time without a specific intervention or after either (a) releasing breast compression or (b) cold-induced vasoconstriction from cooling the room air or by placing the hand in ice water. Abnormalities are recognized both by identifying patterns in a single breast that are abnormal and by recognizing differences in patterns between the two breasts.

Thermography of the breast has been under study for many years and was used clinically for screening and diagnosis at various sites into the 1970s. It has been proposed as a method for risk assessment (116). In the 1980s, its use decreased because of studies showing it to be insufficiently accurate and demonstrating the greater benefit of mammography as mammography improved. In the late 1990s, new developments in thermal imaging equipment resulted in systems that could detect smaller gradients in temperature at higher spatial and temporal resolution. The newer systems permit (a) smaller differences in temperature to be recorded, (b) smaller areas of temperature differences to be separated, and (c) the recording of dynamic changes in temperature as blood flows into or is pushed out of the breast by mechanical or thermal challenges.

The temperature at the breast surface can be affected by both intrinsic and extrinsic factors. To obtain a proper heat map of the breast, both the internal and the external factors should be controlled as closely as possible. To control the internal factors, the subject should be allowed to rest for approximately 15 minutes so that the internal heat production of the body is at or close to the basal metabolic rate. To control the external factors, the patient should be placed in a temperature-controlled room to equilibrate to the ambient temperature, clothing covering the breasts should be removed, with only a light, nonconstricting gown used for modesty (117,118). If dynamic thermography is used, then, after equilibration, a thermal stress may be applied.

Static and Dynamic Thermography

Thermography images can be obtained at one point in time (static thermography) or dynamically when a series of images is obtained after some intervention that could change the flow of blood to the breast.

Normal Patterns of Breast Heat Production

Xu and Wang (67) and Ng et al. (118) recorded the pattern of breast surface temperature variation in 50 normal menstruating women aged 21 to 45 over the course of one or more menstrual cycles. They showed that temperature varies over the cycle, increasing toward the onset of menstruation. To limit variability in temperature measurements, they recommend that breast thermograms should be obtained at the times when the temperature is most stable over several days. These times are at 5 to 12 days and around 21 days after the onset of menstruation. Various image analysis methods, including computer-based artificial neural network analysis, have been proposed as potential methods of enhancing the differences seen in the presence of cancer (119–122). Research with these computer methods suggests that the combination of a human observer and computer analysis will improve the accuracy of interpretation of breast thermography.

Dynamic Thermography

With dynamic thermography, the pattern of change in heat becomes an important factor in the analysis. Dynamic thermo-

grams can look at the spontaneous or physiologic variations in heat or at induced changes in breast perfusion that occur from thermal or mechanical stress. Anbar (123) describes the spontaneous changes that occur in breast temperature by looking at high-frequency variations in skin surface patterns. Such rapid changes are due to several factors, such as heart rate and vascular flow changes controlled by the autonomic nervous system and enzymatic production of nitric oxide. Both large- and small-area changes in heat production are seen with frequency variations from 0.01 to 10 Hz.

Parisky et al. (124) report on a dynamic thermography method in which the breast is cooled by blowing cool air on it, after which its thermal recovery is mapped. The method is used to determine the characteristics of abnormalities detected on mammography to aid in determining their likelihood of malignancy.

Giansanti (125) and Giansanti and Maccioni (126) have developed a wearable breast thermography unit placed in direct contact with the breast that will allow continuous monitoring for up to 24 hours. They propose that diurnal variations in the heat production of the breast may be a better indicator of breast disease. This work is still quite early and its clinical significance is not yet established.

Limitations of Breast Thermography

Breast thermograms record the temperature at the surface of the breast. This surface measurement reflects the pattern of heat within the breast, but the actual source in the depths of the breast is not visualized. Small cancers have increased blood flow and metabolic activity and can be imaged when they are close to the skin surface, but modeling suggests that the deeper a cancer is, the less likely it is to affect the thermogram for any given size (127). In patients with locally increased temperature, the area of increased temperature projected on the surface of the breast is often larger than the actual size of the cancer. In addition, there are conditions other than cancer that can have increased blood flow and metabolism, so that both malignant and benign processes can result in similar patterns.

Recent Clinical Trial Results

Static Thermography Clinical Trial Results

Ng et al. (121) and Ng and Kee (122) reported on an artificial neural network computer reanalysis of clinical thermograms of 90 subjects that were obtained using a static system for thermal imaging. In eight of the patients, there had been a prior mastectomy or severe deformity of one of the breasts. Of the 82 remaining, there were 30 patients with normal results on screening mammography, 48 with either complaints or mammographic abnormalities other than cancer, and 4 cases of invasive breast cancer. In measuring the difference between those with normal mammograms and those with breast complaints or abnormal mammograms (including the cancer cases) the neural network achieved an area under the ROC curve of 0.89 with point sensitivity of 81.2% and specificity of 88.2.

Koay et al. (119) reanalyzed 19 thermograms in women of whom 4 had cancer, 1 had fibrocystic disease, and 13 were clinically normal. In this limited population study, the artificial neural network correctly classified three of four cancers and all cancer-free cases.

Dynamic Thermography Clinical Trial Results

Anbar (123) reports on a mathematical model of breast heat in 104 subjects who were studied before surgery with dynamic thermography. There were 27 breast cancers and 77 benign lesions. Differences were found between the benign and malignant groups. In further study of 87 benign, 14 DCIS and 30 invasive cancer cases, clear separation was seen between the invasive cancers and benign lesions. Most of the DCIS cases were outside the 1.96 standard error bars of the benign lesions, but there was some overlap. Sensitivity and specificity are reported to be greater than 95%, but precise details were not included in this report.

Parisky et al. (124) reported on a recently completed clinical trial. The tested system uses dynamic thermal recording of the inflow of blood into the breast after breast cooling. In this clinical trial, 769 subjects with 875 sampled lesions, of which 187 were malignant, were evaluated with mammography and dynamic thermography. The study used an agreement and consensus method for image interpretation. Results are reported for those cases when the radiologists agreed on interpretation. For 110 masses, the sensitivity for correctly assigning the diagnosis of malignancy was 99% and the specificity 18%, with a 99% NPV. For all breast lesions, including microcalcifications, sensitivity was 97%, specificity 14%, NPV 95%, and PPV 27%.

Summary of Thermography of the Breast

The measurement of the temperature at the surface of the breast provides information on both the rate and volume of blood flow into local areas of the breast and the local production of heat by metabolic activity in the breast. It can provide both a static picture of heat and dynamic pictures of the change in temperature during mechanical or thermal stress. A number of clinical trials have been reported, as described above. In general, these trials point toward thermography having high sensitivity, but moderately low specificity. The studies fail to provide sufficient information on the size and other characteristics of the tumors. The appropriate role for thermography in clinical practice remains uncertain, but promising.

VALIDATING NOVEL METHODS OF BREAST IMAGING

This chapter has reviewed a series of novel methods for breast imaging. It represents only a sample of those methods under development by industry and academia. Given the large variety of methods under development, the question arises as to how to select among the proposed methods: Which should be funded for further research and which should receive priority for clinical trials?

A guiding principle of clinical medicine is to do no harm. Mammography is currently the best and best-proven method there is for finding small, curable breast cancers, but because of the problems with both its sensitivity and specificity and patient complaints about breast compression, a search is continuing for other methods. Currently, there are insufficient data to recommend replacing screening by mammography by any other technique. Contrast-enhanced MRI appears to be an excellent method for finding small invasive breast cancers, but the cost is high and in a screening setting, there are too many false-positive findings; contrast-enhanced MRI, however, may be of benefit when used as a supplement to or as a replacement for mammography for women carrying the *BRCA1* or *BRCA2* genes (128–130). The detection of DCIS with MRI is variable and often reported to be lower than for mammography.

The author suggests the following set of criteria for assessing and validating novel methods for imaging the breasts. First, there should be a clearly defined scientific basis, understandable by those knowledgeable in physics, engineering, and biology. There should be evidence that there is sufficient signal or potential signal so that a cancer could be detected against the background tissues. This evidence should be derived, in an ideal situation, from mathematical simulations and physical models as well as from clinical trials of human subjects. For

some systems that record dynamic or metabolic properties, physical models may not be a useful approach. For some methods, data from animal models could provide useful evidence.

Reports of simulations, physical models, and human subject data should include information on simulated and real breast cancers of different sizes, different depths in the breast, and in breast tissue backgrounds of fatty-replaced, moderately dense, and severely dense breasts. The method of reporting tumor size should be more accurate than palpable versus nonpalpable. Ideally, it should include the size estimated from the pathology specimen, and at a minimum by some other generally accepted imaging method such as MRI or ultrasonography. As appropriate, models and human data should consider the menstrual cycle. As appropriate, tumors of different malignant and benign types should be considered. At a minimum, fibroadenomas, vascular fibroadenomas, DCIS, invasive ductal carcinoma, lobular neoplasia, and invasive lobular carcinoma should be included in the studies and reported as separate groups as part of the validation studies.

Determining the appropriate sample size depends on the intended clinical use of the new imaging method. Devices proposed for screening for breast cancer have particular problems in validation if the intention is to show that the new device is better than mammography. This is because the frequency of breast cancer in a screening population is relatively low. Validation to show improved screening may require extrapolation from either very–high-risk populations or populations enriched with high-risk individuals. Showing equivalence to mammography may be easier than showing that the device is better. The recently reported comparison of digital and screen film mammography in screening used 49,528 subjects in a nonrandomized design (1). Validating a new method of screening on such sample sizes is likely to prove impractical in terms of cost and logistics.

For devices intended to show diagnostic improvement, sample sizes are more reasonable and statistical methods are well established.

Newer methods of targeted therapy will require improved and validated methods to determine, *in vivo*, the effectiveness of the therapy. Novel imaging methods have much to offer in this field, and optical methods, MRI, MRS, MIBI, and FDG-PET each have aspects that make them suitable for use in clinical trials. Molecular imaging agents that target the same pathway as the therapy may, as they are validated, become the best method for assessing targeted therapy. Imaging results can then be compared with pathology results and clinical follow-up.

SUMMARY

Potential Applications of Novel Methods to Clinical Decisions

Breast imaging can be used for six purposes: screening for cancer, diagnosis of a suspected finding, establishing the extent of disease, assessment of individual risk for development of breast cancer, monitoring the response to cancer therapy, and monitoring the response to preventive measures (dietary and pharmaceutical).

Screening for Breast Cancer

Mammography is the current best standard and there is evidence that contrast-enhanced MRI and perhaps ultrasonography, alone or in combination with mammography, will also become established for this purpose. New proposed methods for screening include optical imaging, radiotracer imaging, thermal imaging, and electrical recording. At present, there do not appear to have been clinical trials of sufficient size to justify current screening with any of the newer methods. There are sufficient data to support future research on the potential of these modalities for screening, but, for screening, these methods should remain in the research realm, not in the clinical.

Diagnosis of a Suspect Lesion in the Breast

The current standards are special mammographic views, ultrasonography, and contrast-enhanced MRI. There is sufficient evidence to support the use of FDG-PET for this purpose. MIBI combined with other methods is probably useful for this purpose. Optical imaging for this purpose is promising, but not as well established.

Establishing the Extent of Disease in the Breast

The current standard method is contrast-enhanced MRI. The publications on contrast enhanced CT, MIBI, and FDG suggest that these methods may also be quite effective.

Establishing the Extent of Disease Outside of the Breast

For axillary lymph nodes, the standard is probably sentinel node biopsy, supported either by optical dyes or radiotracers. There are some data suggesting that FDG-PET may be effective for this. In some cases, ultrasonography demonstrates tumor-containing axillary lymph nodes, but it does not detect all positive nodes. MRI contrast agents that accumulate in lymph nodes are still experimental, but the results in other lymph node areas are promising. Internal mammary nodes containing cancer metastases can be identified in some cases with contrast-enhanced MRI and FDG-PET. The sensitivity and specificity for these techniques are unknown. For distant metastases, the standard is changing from a three-test combination of contrast-enhanced MRI of the brain, CECT of the liver, and radiotracer imaging of the skeleton toward a single study with FDG-PET or PET-CT.

Assessment of Individual Risk

With respect to imaging, this is now evaluated by mammographic measurements of breast density. There are new methods for the measurement of breast density under development, including improved computer models based on mammography and x-ray dual-energy methods. Newer imaging modalities that may prove to be of use in the assessment of risk include several optical imaging methods. Older literature suggested that thermography may be useful for this, but only limited recent data are available.

Monitoring the Response to Cancer Therapy

Currently, MRI and ultrasonography are the standard methods used to look for changes in tumor size during chemotherapy. Molecularly targeted therapy may not result in a decrease in tumor size, so techniques that rely on measurements of tumor size without also measuring tumor physiology may not be sufficient. Methods under study that provide functional information and that have some supportive evidence include studies of contrast-enhanced MRI to look at changes in enhancement pattern, FDG-PET, MIBI, and optical methods. Targeted molecular imaging agents will likely prove useful for assessing tumor response, but this needs further validation.

Monitoring the Response to Preventive Measures (Dietary and Pharmaceutical)

There is research interest in identifying possible imaging biomarkers of response to chemopreventive and dietary preventive strategies for breast cancer. It has been shown that chemopreventive agents (raloxifene and tamoxifen) both result in decreased breast density (131). It has not been shown that this decrease in breast density correlates with chemopreventive effectiveness. Optical imaging and radiotracer imaging are other methods that may have some value for research on this problem.

References

1. Pisano ED, Gatsonis C, Hendrick E, et al. Diagnostic performance of digital versus film mammography for breast-cancer screening. *N Engl J Med* 2005;353 (17): 1773–1783.
2. Freedman MT, Lo SCB, Honda C, et al. Phase contrast digital mammography using molybdenum x-ray: clinical implications in detectability improvement. *Proc SPIE* 2003;5030:533–540.
3. Lo SCB, Hieh D, Lasser ME, et al. A C-scan transmission ultrasound based on a hybrid microelectronic sensor array and its physical performance. *Proc SPIE* 2001;4325:87–93.
4. Lo SCB, Lin JS, Freedman MT, et al. Application of artificial neural networks to medical image pattern recognition: detection of clustered microcalcifications on mammograms and lung cancer on chest radiographs. *J VLSI Sign Proc Sys* 1998; 18(241):250.
5. Lo SC, Li H, Wang Y, et al. A multiple circular path convolution neural network system for detection of mammographic masses. *IEEE Trans Med Imaging* 2002; 21(2):150–158.
6. Freedman MT, Lo SCB, Steller-Artz D, et al. Classification of false positives findings on computer aided detection of breast microcalcifications. *Proc SPIE Med Imaging* 1997;3034:853–859.
7. Malich A, Sauner D, Marx C, et al. Influence of breast lesion size and histologic findings on tumor detection rate of a computer-aided detection system. *Radiology* 2003;228(3):851–856.
8. Brem RF, Hoffmeister JW, Rapelyea JA, et al. Impact of breast density on computer-aided detection for breast cancer. *AJR Am J Roentgenol* 2005;184(2): 439–444.
9. Destounis SV, DiNitto P, Logan-Young W, et al. Can computer-aided detection with double reading of screening mammograms help decrease the false-negative rate? Initial experience. *Radiology* 2004;232(2):578–584.
10. Karssemeijer N, Otten JD, Verbeek AL, et al. Computer-aided detection versus independent double reading of masses on mammograms. *Radiology* 2003;227 (1):192–200.
11. Vyborny CJ, Doi T, O'Shaughnessy KF, et al. Breast cancer: importance of spiculation in computer-aided detection. *Radiology* 2000;215(3):703–707.
12. Kinnard LM, Lo SCB, Wang PC, et al. Separation of malignant and benign masses using image and segmentation features. *Proc SPIE Image Process* 2003;5032: 835–842.
13. Kinnard L, Lo SCB, Wang P, et al. Separation of malignant and benign masses using maximum-likelihood modeling and neural networks. *Proc SPIE Image Process* 2002;4684:733–741.
14. Drukker K, Giger ML, Vyborny CJ, et al. Computerized detection and classification of cancer on breast ultrasound. *Acad Radiol* 2004;11(5):526–535.
15. Drukker K, Horsch K, Giger ML. Multimodality computerized diagnosis of breast lesions using mammography and sonography. *Acad Radiol* 2005;12(8):970–979.
16. Basilion JP. Current and future technologies for breast cancer imaging. *Breast Cancer Res* 2001;3(1):14–16.
17. Hogemann-Savellano D, Bos E, Blondet C, et al. The transferrin receptor: a potential molecular imaging marker for human cancer. *Neoplasia* 2003;5(6):495–506.
18. Harisinghani MG, Barentsz J, Hahn PF, et al. Noninvasive detection of clinically occult lymph-node metastases in prostate cancer. *N Engl J Med* 2003;348(25): 2491–2499.
19. Harisinghani MG, Dixon WT, Saksena MA, et al. MR lymphangiography: imaging strategies to optimize the imaging of lymph nodes with ferumoxtran-10. *Radiographics* 2004;24(3):867–878.
20. Anzai Y, Piccoli CW, Outwater EK, et al. Evaluation of neck and body metastases to nodes with ferumoxtran 10-enhanced MR imaging: phase III safety and efficacy study. *Radiology* 2003;228(3):777–788.
21. Rydland J, BjOrnerud A, Haugen O, et al. New intravascular contrast agent applied to dynamic contrast enhanced MR imaging of human breast cancer. *Acta Radiol* 2003;44(3):275–283.
22. Pirollo KF, Dagata J, Wang P, et al. A tumor-targeted nanodelivery system to improve early MRI detection of cancer. *Mol Imaging* 2006;5(1):41–52.
23. Artemov D, Mori N, Ravi R, et al. Magnetic resonance molecular imaging of the HER-2/neu receptor. *Cancer Res* 2003;63(11):2723–2727.
24. Fantini S, Franceschini MA, Gaida G, et al. Frequency-domain optical mammography: edge effect corrections. *Med Phys* 1996;23(1):149–157.
25. Franceschini MA, Moesta KT, Fantini S, et al. Frequency-domain techniques enhance optical mammography: initial clinical results. *Proc Natl Acad Sci U S A* 1997;94(12):6468–6473.
26. Rinneberg H, Grosenick D, Wabnitz H. Detection and characterization of breast tumors by a laser pulse mammograph. In: *Proceedings of Inter-Institute Workshop on In Vivo Optical Imaging in the NIH.* Bethesda, MD: NIH, 2000:110.
27. Rinneberg H, Grosenick D, Moesta KT, et al. Scanning time-domain optical mammography: detection and characterization of breast tumors *in vivo*. *Technol Cancer Res Treat* 2005;4(5):483–496.
28. Durduran T, Choe R, Culver JP, et al. Bulk optical properties of healthy female breast tissue. *Phys Med Biol* 2002;47(16):2847–2861.
29. Tromberg BJ, Cerussi A, Shah N, et al. Imaging in breast cancer: diffuse optics in breast cancer: detecting tumors in pre-menopausal women and monitoring neoadjuvant chemotherapy. *Breast Cancer Res* 2005;7(6):279–285.
30. Durduran T, Choe R, Yu G, et al. Diffuse optical measurement of blood flow in breast tumors. *Opt Lett* 2005;30(21):2915–2917.
31. Chance B, Nioka S, Zhang J, et al. Breast cancer detection based on incremental biochemical and physiological properties of breast cancers: a six-year, two-site study. *Acad Radiol* 2005;12(8):925–933.

32. Cerussi A, Hsiang D, Shah N, et al. Predicting response to breast cancer neoadjuvant chemotherapy using diffuse optical spectroscopy. *Proc Natl Acad Sci U S A* 2007;104(10):4014-9.
33. Eppstein MJ, Dougherty DE, Hawrysz DJ, et al. Three-dimensional bayesian optical image reconstruction with domain decomposition. *IEEE Trans Med Imaging* 2001;20(3):147–163.
34. Ntziachristos V, Chance B. Probing physiology and molecular function using optical imaging: applications to breast cancer. *Breast Cancer Res* 2001;3(1):41–46.
35. Ntziachristos V, Hielscher AH, Yodh AG, et al. Diffuse optical tomography of highly heterogeneous media. *IEEE Trans Med Imaging* 2001;20(6):470–478.
36. Ntziachristos V, Yodh AG, Schnall M, et al. Concurrent MRI and diffuse optical tomography of breast after indocyanine green enhancement. *Proc Natl Acad Sci U S A* 2000;97(6):2767–2772.
37. Chance B. Near-infrared (NIR) optical spectroscopy characterizes breast tissue hormonal and age status. *Acad Radiol* 2001;8(3):209–210.
38. Ebert B, Sukowski U, Grosenick D, et al. Near-infrared fluorescent dyes for enhanced contrast in optical mammography: phantom experiments. *J Biomed Opt* 2001;6(2):134–140.
39. Mahmood U, Tung C, Bogdanov AJ, et al. Near-infrared optical imaging of protease activity for tumor detection. *Radiology* 1999;213:866–870.
40. Grosenick D, Wabnitz H, Moesta KT, et al. Concentration and oxygen saturation of haemoglobin of 50 breast tumours determined by time-domain optical mammography. *Phys Med Biol* 2004;49(7):1165–1181.
41. Grosenick D, Moesta KT, Moller M, et al. Time-domain scanning optical mammography: I. recording and assessment of mammograms of 154 patients. *Phys Med Biol* 2005;50(11):2429–2449.
42. Grosenick D, Wabnitz H, Moesta KT, et al. Time-domain scanning optical mammography: II. optical properties and tissue parameters of 87 carcinomas. *Phys Med Biol* 2005;50(11):2451–2468.
43. Cerussi AE, Berger AJ, Bevilacqua F, et al. Sources of absorption and scattering contrast for near-infrared optical mammography. *Acad Radiol* 2001;8(3):211–218.
44. Cerussi AE, Jakubowski D, Shah N, et al. Spectroscopy enhances the information content of optical mammography. *J Biomed Opt* 2002;7(1):60–71.
45. Intes X. Time-domain optical mammography SoftScan: initial results. *Acad Radiol* 2005;12(8):934–947.
46. Shah N, Cerussi AE, Eker C, et al. Noninvasive functional optical spectroscopy of human breast tissue. *Proc Natl Acad Sci U S A* 2001;98:4420–4425.
47. Simick MK, Lilge L. Optical transillumination spectroscopy to quantify parenchymal tissue density: an indicator for breast cancer risk. *Br J Radiol* 2005;78(935):1009–1017.
48. Blackmore KM, Knight JA, Jong R, et al. Assessing breast tissue density by transillumination breast spectroscopy (TIBS): an intermediate indicator of cancer risk. *Br J Radiol* 2007;80(955):545–556.
49. Jiang H, Xu Y, Iftimia N, et al. Three-dimensional optical tomographic imaging of breast in a human subject. *IEEE Trans Med Imaging* 2001;20(12):1334–1340.
50. Jiang H, Iftimia NV, Xu Y, et al. Near-infrared optical imaging of the breast with model-based reconstruction. *Acad Radiol* 2002;9(2):186–194.
51. Heffer EL, Fantini S. Quantitative oximetry of breast tumors: a near-infrared method that identifies two optimal wavelengths for each tumor. *Appl Opt* 2002;41(19):3827–3839.
52. Athanasiou A, Vanel D, Balleyguier C, et al. Dynamic optical breast imaging: a new technique to visualise breast vessels: comparison with breast MRI and preliminary results. *Eur J Radiol* 2005;54(1):72–79.
53. Fantini S, Heffer EL, Franceschini MA, et al. Optical mammography with intensity-modulated light. In: *Proceedings of Inter-Institute Workshop on In Vivo Optical Imaging at the NIH*. Bethesda, MD: NIH, 2000:111.
54. Zhu Q, Kurtzma SH, Hegde P, et al. Utilizing optical tomography with ultrasound localization to image heterogeneous hemoglobin distribution in large breast cancers. *Neoplasia* 2005;7(3):263–270.
55. Zhu Q, Cronin EB, Currier AA, et al. Benign versus malignant breast masses: optical differentiation with US-guided optical imaging reconstruction. *Radiology* 2005;237(1):57–66.
56. Zhu Q, Xu C, Guo P, et al. Optimal probing of optical contrast of breast lesions of different size located at different depths by US localization. *Technol Cancer Res Treat* 2006;5(4):365–380.
57. Harisinghani MG, Saksena MA, Hahn PF, et al. Ferumoxtran-10-enhanced MR lymphangiography: does contrast-enhanced imaging alone suffice for accurate lymph node characterization? *AJR Am J Roentgenol* 2006;186(1):144–148.
58. Andreev VG, Karabutov AA, Solomatin SV, et al. Opto-acoustic tomography of breast cancer with arc-array-transducer. *Proc SPIE Biomed Optoacoustics* 2000; 3916:36–47.
59. Andreev VG. Detection of ultrawide-band ultrasound pulses in optoacoustic tomography. *IEEE Trans Ultrason Ferroelectr Freq Control* 2003;50(10):1383–1390.
60. Oraevsky AA, Karabutov AA, Solomatin SV, et al. Laser optoacoustic imaging of breast cancer *in vivo*. *Proc SPIE Biomed Optoacoustics II* 2001;4256:6–15.
61. Oraevsky AA, Savateeva EV, Solomatin SV, et al. Optoacoustic imaging of blood for visualization and diagnostics of breast cancer. *Proc SPIE Biomed Optoacoustics* 2002;4618:81–93.
62. Oraevsky AA, Karabutov AA. *Biomedical photonics handbook*. Boca Raton, FL: CRC Press, 2003.
63. Niederhauser JJ, Jaeger M, Lemor R, et al. Combined ultrasound and optoacoustic system for real-time high-contrast vascular imaging in vivo. *IEEE Trans Med Imaging* 2005;24(4):436–440.
64. Wang LV, Zhao X, Sun H, et al. Microwave-induced acoustic imaging of biological tissues. *Rev Sci Instrum* 1999;70(9):3744–3748.
65. Xu M, Ku G, Wang LV. Microwave-induced thermoacoustic tomography using multi-sector scanning. *Med Phys* 2001;28(9):1958–1963.
66. Ku G, Wang LV. Scanning thermoacoustic tomography in biological tissues. *Med Phys* 2000;27(5):1195–1202.
67. Xu M, Wang LV. Time-domain reconstruction for thermoacoustic tomography in a spherical geometry. *IEEE Trans Med Imaging* 2002;21(7):814–822.
68. Xu Y, Xu M, Wang LV. Exact frequency-domain reconstruction for thermoacoustic tomography—II: Cylindrical geometry. *IEEE Trans Med Imaging* 2002;21(7):829–833.
69. Hagness SC, Taflove A, Bridges JE. Two-dimensional FDTD analysis of a pulsed microwave confocal system for breast cancer detection: fixed-focus and antenna-array sensors. *IEEE Trans Biomed Eng* 1998;45(12):1470–1479.
70. Fear EC, Li X, Hagness SC, et al. Confocal microwave imaging for breast cancer detection: localization of tumors in three dimensions. *IEEE Trans Biomed Eng* 2002;49(8):812–822.
71. Bulyshev AE, Semenov SY, Souvorov AE, et al. Computational modeling of three-dimensional microwave tomography of breast cancer. *IEEE Trans Biomed Eng* 2001;48(9):1053–1056.
72. Poplack SP, Paulsen KD, Hartov A, et al. Electromagnetic breast imaging: average tissue property values in women with negative clinical findings. *Radiology* 2004;231(2):571–580.
73. Meaney PM, Fanning MW, Raynolds T, et al. Initial clinical experience with microwave breast imaging in women with normal mammography. *Acad Radiol* 2007;14(2):207–218.
74. Poplack SP, Tosteson TD, Wells WA, et al. Electromagnetic breast imaging: results of a pilot study in women with abnormal mammograms. *Radiology* 2007; 243(2):350–359.
75. Glickman YA, Filo O, Nachaliel U, et al. Novel EIS postprocessing algorithm for breast cancer diagnosis. *IEEE Trans Med Imaging* 2002;21(6):710–712.
76. Melloul M, Paz A, Ohana G, et al. Double-phase ^{99m}Tc-sestamibi scintimammography and trans-scan in diagnosing breast cancer. *J Nucl Med* 1999;40(3):376–380.
77. Malich A, Fritsch T, Anderson R, et al. Electrical impedance scanning for classifying suspicious breast lesions: first results. *Eur Radiol* 2000;10(10): 1555–1561.
78. Malich A, Boehm T, Facius M, et al. Differentiation of mammographically suspicious lesions: evaluation of breast ultrasound, MRI mammography and electrical impedance scanning as adjunctive technologies in breast cancer detection. *Clin Radiol* 2001;56(4):278–283.
79. Malich A, Bohm T, Facius M, et al. Additional value of electrical impedance scanning: experience of 240 histologically-proven breast lesions. *Eur J Cancer* 2001; 37(18):2324–2330.
80. Scholz B. Towards virtual electrical breast biopsy: space-frequency MUSIC for trans-admittance data. *IEEE Trans Med Imaging* 2002;21(6):588–595.
81. Kerner TE, Paulsen KD, Hartov A, et al. Electrical impedance spectroscopy of the breast: clinical imaging results in 26 subjects. *IEEE Trans Med Imaging* 2002; 21(6):638–645.
82. Cherepenin VA, Karpov AY, Korjenevsky AV, et al. Three-dimensional EIT imaging of breast tissues: system design and clinical testing. *IEEE Trans Med Imaging* 2002;21(6):662–667.
83. Stojadinovic A, Nissan A, Gallimidi Z, et al. Electrical impedance scanning for the early detection of breast cancer in young women: preliminary results of a multicenter prospective clinical trial. *J Clin Oncol* 2005;23(12):2703–2715.
84. Stojadinovic A, Moskovitz O, Gallimidi Z, et al. Prospective study of electrical impedance scanning for identifying young women at risk for breast cancer. *Breast Cancer Res Treat* 2006;97(2):179–189.
85. Stojadinovic A, Nissan A, Shriver CD, et al. Electrical impedance scanning as a new breast cancer risk stratification tool for young women. *J Surg Oncol* 2008; 97(2):112–120.
86. Del Vecchio S, Zannetti A, Aloj L, et al. MIBI as prognostic factor in breast cancer. *Q J Nucl Med* 2003;47(1):46–50.
87. Kim IJ, Bae YT, Kim SJ, et al. Determination and prediction of P-glycoprotein and multidrug-resistance-related protein expression in breast cancer with double-phase technetium-99m sestamibi scintimammography visual and quantitative analyses. *Oncology* 2006;70(6):403–410.
88. Del Vecchio S, Zannetti A, Aloj L, et al. Inhibition of early ^{99m}Tc-MIBI uptake by Bcl-2 anti-apoptotic protein overexpression in untreated breast carcinoma. *Eur J Nucl Med Mol Imaging* 2003;30(6):879–887.
89. Del Vecchio S, Salvatore M. ^{99m}Tc-MIBI in the evaluation of breast cancer biology. *Eur J Nucl Med Mol Imaging* 2004;31[Suppl 1]:S88–S96.
90. Sciuto R, Pasqualoni R, Bergomi S, et al. Prognostic value of (99m)Tc-sestamibi washout in predicting response of locally advanced breast cancer to neoadjuvant chemotherapy. *J Nucl Med* 2002;43(6):745–751.
91. Travaini LL, Baio SM, Cremonesi M, et al. Neoadjuvant therapy in locally advanced breast cancer: ^{99m}Tc-MIBI mammoscintigraphy is not a reliable technique to predict therapy response. *Breast* 2007;16(3):262–270.
92. Wilczok B, Svensson L, Danielsson R, et al. ^{99m}Tc-exametazime as a breast tumor-seeking agent: comparison with ^{99m}Tc-sestamibi. *J Nucl Med* 2004;45(12): 2040–2044.
93. Bone B, Wiberg MK, Szabo BK, et al. Comparison of ^{99m}Tc-sestamibi scintimammography and dynamic MR imaging as adjuncts to mammography in the diagnosis of breast cancer. *Acta Radiol* 2003;44(1):28–34.
94. Khalkhali I, Baum JK, Villanueva-Meyer J, et al. (99m)Tc-sestamibi breast imaging for the examination of patients with dense and fatty breasts: multicenter study. *Radiology* 2002;222(1):149–155.
95. Brem RF, Fishman M, Rapelyea JA. Detection of ductal carcinoma *in situ* with mammography, breast specific gamma imaging, and magnetic resonance imaging: a comparative study. *Acad Radiol* 2007;14(8):945–950.
96. Brem RF, Petrovitch I, Rapelyea JA, et al. Breast-specific gamma imaging with ^{99m}Tc-sestamibi and magnetic resonance imaging in the diagnosis of breast cancer—a comparative study. *Breast J* 2007;13(5):465–469.
97. Brem RF, Rapelyea JA, Zisman G, et al. Occult breast cancer: Scintimammography with high-resolution breast-specific gamma camera in women at high risk for breast cancer. *Radiology* 2005;237(1):274–280.
98. Joseph B, Bhargava KK, Malhi H, et al. Sestamibi is a substrate for *MDR1* and *MDR2* P-glycoprotein genes. *Eur J Nucl Med Mol Imaging* 2003;30(7): 1024–1031.
99. Liu Z, Stevenson GD, Barrett HH, et al. Imaging recognition of multidrug resistance in human breast tumors using ^{99m}Tc-labeled monocationic agents and a high-resolution stationary SPECT system. *Nucl Med Biol* 2004;31(1): 53–65.
100. Liu Z, Stevenson GD, Barrett HH, et al. Imaging recognition of inhibition of multidrug resistance in human breast cancer xenografts using ^{99m}Tc-labeled sestamibi and tetrofosmin. *Nucl Med Biol* 2005;32(6):573–583.
101. Pusztai L, Wagner P, Ibrahim N, et al. Phase II study of tariquidar, a selective P-glycoprotein inhibitor, in patients with chemotherapy-resistant, advanced breast carcinoma. *Cancer* 2005;104(4):682–691.
102. Avril N, Rose CA, Schelling M, et al. Breast imaging with positron emission tomography and fluorine-18 fluorodeoxyglucose: use and limitations. *J Clin Oncol* 2000;18(20):3495–3502.

103. Avril N, Menzel M, Dose J, et al. Glucose metabolism of breast cancer assessed by ^{18}F-FDG PET: histologic and immunohistochemical tissue analysis. *J Nucl Med* 2001;42(1):9–16.
104. Krak NC, van der Hoeven JJ, Hoekstra OS, et al. Measuring [(18)F]FDG uptake in breast cancer during chemotherapy: comparison of analytical methods. *Eur J Nucl Med Mol Imaging* 2003;30(5):674–681.
105. Spaepen K, Stroobants S, Dupont P, et al. [(18)F]FDG PET monitoring of tumour response to chemotherapy: does [(18)F]FDG uptake correlate with the viable tumour cell fraction? *Eur J Nucl Med Mol Imaging* 2003;30(5):682–688.
106. Schelling M, Avril N, Nahrig J, et al. Positron emission tomography using [(18)F]fluorodeoxyglucose for monitoring primary chemotherapy in breast cancer. *J Clin Oncol* 2000;18(8):1689–1695.
107. Berg WA, Weinberg IN, Narayanan D, et al. High-resolution fluorodeoxyglucose positron emission tomography with compression ("positron emission mammography") is highly accurate in depicting primary breast cancer. *Breast J* 2006;12(4):309–323.
108. Tafra L, Cheng Z, Uddo J, et al. Pilot clinical trial of ^{18}F-fluorodeoxyglucose positron-emission mammography in the surgical management of breast cancer. *Am J Surg* 2005;190(4):628–632.
109. Berger F, Gambhir SS. Recent advances in imaging endogenous or transferred gene expression utilizing radionuclide technologies in living subjects: applications to breast cancer. *Breast Cancer Res* 2001;3(1):28–35.
110. Uematsu T, Sano M, Homma K, et al. Comparison between high-resolution helical CT and pathology in breast examination. *Acta Radiol* 2002;43(4):385–390.
111. Akashi-Tanaka S, Fukutomi T, Miyakawa K, et al. Contrast-enhanced computed tomography for diagnosing the intraductal component and small invasive foci of breast cancer. *Breast Cancer* 2001;8(1):10–15.
112. Glick SJ. Breast CT. *Annu Rev Biomed Eng* 2007;9:501–526.
113. Yang WT, Carkaci S, Chen L, et al. Dedicated cone-beam breast CT: feasibility study with surgical mastectomy specimens. *AJR Am J Roentgenol* 2007; 189(6):1312–1315.
114. Boone JM, Kwan AL, Yang K, et al. Computed tomography for imaging the breast. *J Mammary Gland Biol Neoplasia* 2006;11(2):103–111.
115. Lindfors KK, Boone JM, Nelson TR, et al. Dedicated breast CT: initial clinical experience. *Radiology* 2008;246:725–733.
116. Head JF, Elliott RL. Infrared imaging: making progress in fulfilling its medical promise. *IEEE Eng Med Biol Mag* 2002;21(6):80–85.
117. Sudharsan NM, Ng EY. Parametric optimization for tumour identification: bioheat equation using ANOVA and the Taguchi method. *Proc Inst Mech Eng [H]* 2000;214(5):505–512.
118. Ng EY, Ung LN, Ng FC, et al. Statistical analysis of healthy and malignant breast thermography. *J Med Eng Technol* 2001;25(6):253–263.
119. Koay J, Herry C, Frize M. Analysis of breast thermography with an artificial neural network. *Conf Proc IEEE Eng Med Biol Soc* 2004;2:1159–1162.
120. Tang X, Ding H. Asymmetry analysis of breast thermograms with morphological image segmentation. *Conf Proc IEEE Eng Med Biol Soc* 2005;2: 1680–1683.
121. Ng EY, Kee EC, Rajendra Acharya U. Advanced technique in breast thermography analysis. *Conf Proc IEEE Eng Med Biol Soc* 2005;1:710–713.
122. Ng EY, Kee EC. Advanced integrated technique in breast cancer thermography. *J Med Eng Technol* 2007;17:1–12.
123. Anbar M. Assessment of physiologic and pathologic radiative heat dissipation using dynamic infrared imaging. *Ann N Y Acad Sci* 2002;972.111–110.
124. Parisky YR, Sardi A, Hamm R, et al. Efficacy of computerized infrared imaging analysis to evaluate mammographically suspicious lesions. *AJR Am J Roentgenol* 2003;180(1):263–269.
125. Giansanti D. Improving spatial resolution in skin-contact thermography: comparison between a spline based and linear interpolation. *Med Eng Phys* 2008; 30(6):733–738.
126. Giansanti D, Maccioni G. Design and construction of a closed loop phantom for skin-contact thermography. *Med Eng Phys* 2008;30(1):41–47.
127. Ng EY, Sudharsan NM. An improved three-dimensional direct numerical modelling and thermal analysis of a female breast with tumour. *Proc Inst Mech Eng [H]* 2001;215(1):25–37.
128. Lehman CD, Blume JD, Weatherall P, et al. Screening women at high risk for breast cancer with mammography and magnetic resonance imaging. *Cancer* 2005;103(9):1898–1905.
129. Plevritis SK, Kurian AW, Sigal BM, et al. Cost-effectiveness of screening *BRCA1/2* mutation carriers with breast magnetic resonance imaging. *JAMA* 2006; 295(20):2374–2384.
130. Warner E, Plewes DB, Hill KA, et al. Surveillance of *BRCA1* and *BRCA2* mutation carriers with magnetic resonance imaging, ultrasound, mammography, and clinical breast examination. *JAMA* 2004;292(11):1317–1325.
131. Freedman M, San Martin J, O'Gorman J, et al. Digitized mammography: a clinical trial of postmenopausal women randomly assigned to receive raloxifene, estrogen, or placebo. *J Natl Cancer Inst* 2001;93(1):51–56.

Chapter 16
Image-Guided Biopsy of Nonpalpable Breast Lesions

Kathryn Evers

The increasing use of screening mammography has led to the detection of nonpalpable breast lesions (1), many of which require biopsy evaluation to determine if they represent breast cancer. Initially, complete evaluation of these lesions required localization under imaging guidance followed by surgical excision. This resulted in an exceedingly high cost in diagnosing carcinoma as many of these lesions were benign. It is estimated that there will be about 178,500 new cases of breast carcinoma diagnosed in the United States this year (2). If all eligible women followed the American Cancer Society's screening guidelines, it is estimated that there would be approximately 1 million biopsies recommended each year to diagnose mammographically detected abnormalities (3–5). Up to 80% of these biopsies will be benign (6). Given the high costs associated with surgical biopsy as well as the small risk of anesthesia with surgical excision, a more cost-effective method of diagnosing these imaging abnormalities was required (7).

Initial attempts to diagnose imaging-detected abnormalities utilized fine needle aspirates (FNA). Although these can be quite accurate, they have several disadvantages. The most important of these is a large number of inadequate or nondiagnostic specimens. In addition, trained cytopathologists are required to accurately interpret these samples, and invasive disease cannot be differentiated from *in situ* disease. FNA has been reported to be only 30% accurate in diagnosing lobular and tubular carcinomas (8). For these reasons, the use of FNA on a wide scale was impractical.

In the late 1980s and 1990s, large-core needle biopsy performed using either stereotactic or ultrasound guidance was proven to be a safe and accurate method to evaluate abnormalities found on imaging (9–11), with results comparable to those obtained at surgical excision (12). The use of core biopsy resulted in a more specific diagnosis than FNA and allowed assessment of invasion, grading of tumors, and immunohistochemistry to be performed (13). Initial results using 14-gauge automated biopsy needles were improved with the use of directional vacuum-assisted devices. These were later modified to allow lesions identified only on magnetic resonance imaging (MRI) examination to be sampled. The safety, accuracy, and decreased costs (14–17) associated with these procedures, performed under local anesthesia, allowed them to become the predominant method for diagnostic biopsy of nonpalpable breast lesions (18,19).

In order to ensure that minimum standards are met in the performance of stereotactic and ultrasound-guided core biopsies, accreditation programs have been developed by both the American College of Radiology (20) and the American College of Surgeons (21). It is likely that accreditation for stereotactic biopsy will be required as part of the Mammography Quality Services Act (MQSA). Although many sites have amiable working relationships regarding who will perform biopsies, competition exists at others (22,23).

This chapter will review the current indications for image-guided biopsy, with an emphasis on patient selection and the clinical significance of these procedures. The basic technical aspects of performance of these procedures will be discussed, as well as complications and controversies involving results of these biopsy procedures.

INDICATIONS

Prior to performing any image-guided biopsy for a nonpalpable finding, a complete imaging work-up should be performed (24).

Further imaging consisting of additional mammographic images or ultrasound should be completed. This will avoid attempting to biopsy pseudolesions caused by overlapping of densities or apparent clustering of calcifications that are actually widely scattered. Failure to recognize that an apparent abnormality is not a true lesion prior to biopsy may result in a biopsy with benign results that are felt to be discordant, leading to additional interventions. A review of stereotactic biopsies revealed that the biopsies were canceled due to the lack of a reproducible abnormality in 29% of 89 cases, reassessment of the lesion as probably benign in 19%, and the presence of simple cysts in 25% (21). A diagnostic work-up would have avoided the patient being scheduled for a biopsy and reduced patient anxiety. Another study looked at a group of 476 patients scheduled for stereotactic biopsy on a prone table (25). Sixty-four (13%) of these planned procedures were canceled. Extremely dense breast tissue, axillary location of the lesion, lesion located less than 15 mm from the chest wall, and extremely thin patient were all factors in the procedure being canceled. MRI should not be used to determine whether or not a lesion should be subjected to tissue sampling, as it is not sufficiently specific. The role of MRI in the evaluation of mammographic or ultrasound detected abnormalities is quite limited and should not be used routinely.

Mammography, ultrasound, and MRI examinations can be classified according to the level of suspicion for malignancy using the American College of Radiology (ACR) Breast Imaging Reporting and Data System (BI-RADS) (26). For mammograms, a final assessment category is required on all mammography reports by the MQSA. Although final assessment categories are not required for ultrasound or MRI interpretation, these categories are useful for evaluating the appropriateness of biopsy and to standardize patient treatment.

The final mammography assessment categories are:

> BI-RADS 1: Normal mammogram;
> BI-RADS 2: Benign finding;
> BI-RADS 3: Probably benign, short interval follow-up suggested;
> BI-RADS 4: Suspicious for malignancy;
> BI-RADS 5: Strongly suggestive of malignancy;
> BI-RADS 6: Imaging in a patient with a known malignancy; and
> BI-RADS 0: Additional imaging evaluation or comparison with previous films is suggested.

BI-RADS categories for ultrasound and breast MRI use the same system. Virtually all nonpalpable category 4 and 5 lesions will require biopsy as will category 3 lesions in anxious patients.

The role of core needle biopsy will logically depend on the degree of suspicion based on the imaging findings. Patients with probably benign (BI-RADS 3) lesions on any of the imaging modalities will have a less than 2% chance of malignancy based on the imaging characteristics and can be safely managed with a short interval, generally 6-month, follow-up. There have been suggestions that needle biopsy be used in the evaluation of these low-risk lesions in order to alleviate the anxiety of the women in this group. In addition to adding significantly to the cost of screening, a study evaluating patient stress reported that the overall stress experienced by women undergoing biopsy was significantly greater than that in the group who were followed with mammograms (27).

Percutaneous core biopsy is of great benefit to women with lesions that are of intermediate risk (BI-RADS 4). The majority of these lesions are benign and the costs associated with core biopsy are significantly less than the costs of a surgical excision. In addition, since these procedures are performed under local anesthesia, the risk of general anesthesia is eliminated.

Use of core biopsy for the diagnosis of nonpalpable abnormalities can decrease the number of trips to the operating room for many patients. Definitive surgery can be planned and axillary lymph node evaluation performed at the same surgery if this is required. Jackman et al. (28) reported that a single surgical procedure was required in 90% of patients when the cancer diagnosis was made via core biopsy versus 24% of patients when the diagnosis was made by surgical biopsy. Similar results have been shown in other studies (29).

The use of core biopsy is most beneficial in cases where the patient will require mastectomy or axillary sampling. Preoperative knowledge of the diagnosis allows all of the surgical options to be discussed and decisions made prior to surgery. This has generally replaced the use of frozen sections, with their inherent inaccuracies. In addition, receptor status and various biomarkers can be evaluated on the core biopsy samples (11,30), so if neoadjuvant chemotherapy is required, this can be tailored to the patient's tumor.

There is no good evidence that diagnosis using core biopsy results in an improvement in obtaining clear surgical margins. The literature is not definitive on this issue, with some reviews reporting no significant difference in the incidence of positive margins in cases diagnosed with core biopsy and those diagnosed with excisional biopsy following needle localization (31). Others report a decreased incidence of positive margins in patients diagnosed with image-guided core biopsy (32). In this review, this was directly related to a larger volume of tissue being removed at surgery in the group of patients diagnosed using core biopsy.

In patients with multiple suspicious lesions or lesions covering a large area of the breast, image-guided biopsy can be extremely useful. Multiple areas can be biopsied and decisions can be made preoperatively regarding whether breast conserving therapy is a reasonable option. In addition, it is much more efficient to sample multiple areas using core biopsy techniques than to perform multiple needle-localized excisional biopsies.

PATIENT SELECTION

There are certain limiting factors in selecting patients for image-guided biopsy. For those patients in whom stereotactic biopsy or MRI-guided core biopsy is contemplated, the patient must be able to remain motionless in the prone position for the period of time required to complete the procedure, usually a minimum of 15 to 20 minutes for a stereotactic biopsy and 30 minutes for an MRI-guided procedure. It is not possible to accurately target the area for biopsy in patients who cannot remain still, usually patients who are kyphotic, have respiratory problems, including chronic cough or who are extremely anxious. Patients with back pain or abdominal pain may also find it impossible to tolerate the required positioning. Weight and girth limits are most problematic for MRI-guided procedures. Usually obese patients are unable to have the diagnostic MRI examination performed. However, different tables have different weight limits and the bores of the machines are not of a uniform size. Patients who weigh over 350 pounds will not be able to have a biopsy performed on most prone stereotactic tables.

TECHNIQUE

Patient Preparation

Patients are generally asked to stop taking aspirin, nonsteroidal anti-inflammatory agents, and vitamin E for at least 1 week before the procedure. Patients who are anticoagulated with warfarin (Coumadin) are advised individually in consultation with their physicians regarding their medication. Core biopsies in patients who are anticoagulated can be safely performed when it has been impossible to stop the medication or when urgent biopsy is required (33). The data suggest that there is not an increased rate of hematoma formation in these patients, although the size of the hematoma may be slightly larger (33). Premedication with antibiotics in patients with mitral valve prolapse, prosthetic valves, or joint replacements is not generally necessary. Patients who are extremely anxious are advised to consult their physicians regarding premedication. The presence of an implant is not generally a contraindication to the procedure unless the lesion is immediately adjacent to the implant surface on imaging obtained with implant displacement (34).

Stereotactic Biopsy

Until the 1990s, stereotactic biopsy had essentially no role in the evaluation of nonpalpable mammographic findings. Although prone biopsy tables were available, these were used only to perform FNA and were not widely utilized in the United States. In 1990 Parker et al. (35) reported on using stereotactic technique and an automated biopsy gun. They reported that of 102 core biopsies performed, there was histologic agreement between the core samples and the surgically excised specimens in 97% of cases with no inadequate samples. The demonstration of decreased costs (1,15,36–38) and equivalent accuracy when compared with surgical excision allowed these procedures to become the standard of care for the diagnostic biopsy of nonpalpable breast lesions.

Both dedicated (prone) tables and units that add on to the diagnostic mammography unit can be successfully used for stereotactic biopsy (19,39–41), using either a 14-gauge biopsy needle or a directional vacuum-assisted device. The use of digital imaging is preferred, since it is important that the patient remain immobile, and this may be quite difficult if films need to be processed, as this prolongs the procedure. Prone tables permit the examination to be performed without the patient seeing the biopsy equipment because this is all underneath the table. Some patients also find it easier to remain immobile while in the prone position. In addition, as the patient is already recumbent, the risk of fainting as the result of a vasovagal reaction is reduced. However, prone biopsy tables are not only expensive but they also require a dedicated room, factors that may make them impractical for sites with a low volume of biopsies.

Add-on units initially required that patients be in the upright, usually sitting, position. With newer units, it is possible to perform biopsies with add on equipment and the patient in a decubitus position on a stretcher or reclinable mammography chair (42). With add-on units, there is a reported incidence of vasovagal reactions of about 2% (19). Add-on units have the advantages of being less expensive, requiring less space, and allowing the room to be used for routine mammography when biopsy is not being performed.

Regardless of the type of unit used, the performance of the biopsy is similar (Fig. 16.1). It must be possible to identify the abnormality on imaging in order to successfully perform a biopsy (39). Based on the location of the lesion and possible differences in the visibility of the lesion in different views, an approach for the biopsy is chosen. The breast must be maintained in compression throughout the examination.

The lesion is initially imaged in the center of a 5 × 5 cm cutout in a compression plate (Fig. 16.1A). Imaging at both +15 degrees and −15 degrees from the center line (stereotactic pair) is then obtained (Fig. 16.1B). The x- and y-axis of the abnormality are directly obtained from the images, while the depth of the lesion (z-axis) is calculated from the stereotactic pair using the principle of parallax. This calculation is performed by the computer within the apparatus. The housing of the machine is moved electronically to the x, y coordinates. After the area is appropriately cleansed and anesthetized with lidocaine, a nick is made in the skin to facilitate needle entry and the needle is placed to the predetermined depth. Needle position is confirmed with an additional stereo pair (prefire position). The needle is then rapidly advanced into the area of interest and an additional stereo pair is obtained (postfire images) (Fig. 16.1C). The position of the needle trough in relationship to the lesion is evaluated. Once needle placement has been confirmed, the biopsy samples are obtained. As the needle is placed parallel to the chest wall, there is no risk of possible incursion into the chest wall or pleural cavity. If there is uncertainty as to whether the lesion has been sampled, an additional stereo pair can be obtained after obtaining the samples and prior to removing the needle. Additional samples can

then be obtained if necessary. Most stereotactic breast biopsies are currently performed with directional vacuum-assisted biopsy devices. These are large core needles that are placed in the area of interest. The needle can be rotated through 360 degrees while within the breast, allowing the entire volume of tissue surrounding the needle to be sampled. Newer devices transport the tissue to a collection chamber, removing the need to manually remove tissue samples and permitting sampling to be accomplished within 1 to 2 minutes.

When stereotactic biopsy of calcifications is performed, specimen radiography should be performed to confirm that the calcifications have been removed (Fig. 16.1D). If there is concern that firing the needle will result in the excursion of the needle through the deep aspect of the breast and into the compression plate, it is possible to fire the gun before inserting it into the breast. However, this has been associated with an increased risk of a failed biopsy (43). In those cases where

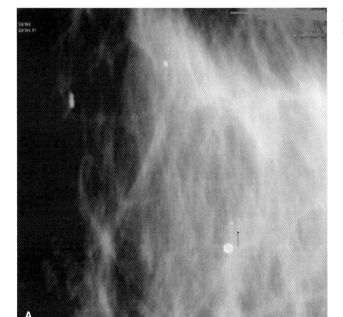

FIGURE 16.1. Stereotactic core needle biopsy of a cluster of indeterminate microcalcifications. A: Prebiopsy image of the calcifications to be sampled (*arrow*). **B:** Stereotactic pair obtained prior to the biopsy. The calcifications are marked with arrows. (*continued*)

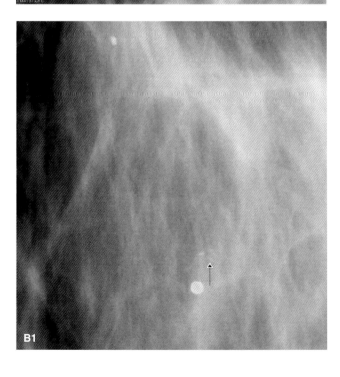

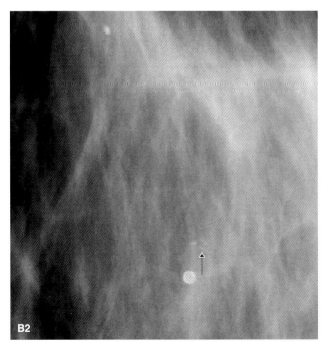

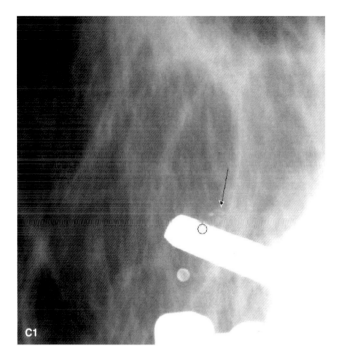

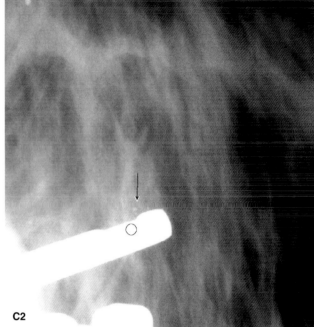

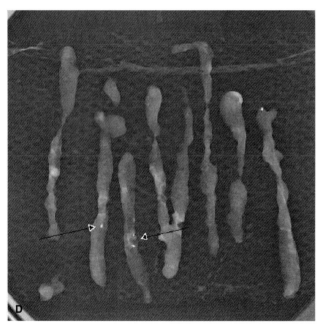

FIGURE 16.1. *Continued* **C:** Postfire stereo pair showing the calcifications (*arrows*) underlying the trough in the needle (*circle*). The needle is a 9-gauge vacuum-assisted probe. **D:** Specimen radiograph revealing the calcifications in the specimens (*arrows*). Histology revealed ductal carcinoma *in situ*.

suspicious calcifications involve a large portion of the breast, multiple areas can be sampled to determine if breast-conserving therapy can be attempted or if mastectomy will be required (44).

In women with small breasts, it may not be possible to perform a biopsy using the standard technique because there is insufficient tissue to allow the needle to be seated within the lesion. In general, the compressed breast needs to be more than 2-cm thick in order to perform a core biopsy. If the breast thickness is insufficient, most newer biopsy tables allow the biopsy to be done with a lateral arm. This allows the needle to be placed into the lesion in a direction parallel to, rather than through, the compression plate. No reports on the accuracy of biopsy using the lateral arm are available, but anecdotal reports suggest that this technique has an acceptable accuracy rate.

Ultrasound-Guided Core Biopsy

Core biopsy of lesions visible on ultrasound can be performed safely and easily using ultrasound guidance (Fig. 16.2). Although this chapter focuses on the evaluation of nonpalpable lesions, ultrasound guidance can also be used to improve the accuracy of core biopsy in the setting of a palpable mass (8,45). This technique is well accepted by patients because of the lack of compression, comfortable positioning, and lack of radiation. Once the technique has been mastered, it is faster and easier than stereotactic biopsy. As the needle and mass are both visualized in real time, adequate sampling is more consistently obtained. An accuracy rate of at least 96% has been reported using 14-gauge automated biopsy guns (46,47) and 98% to 100% using 11-gauge directional vacuum-assisted core devices

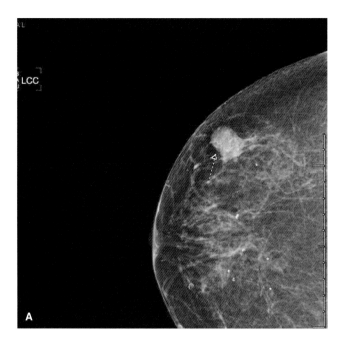

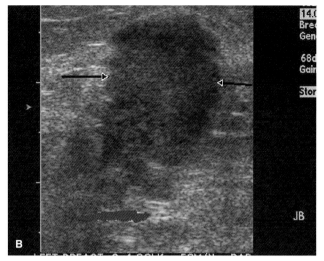

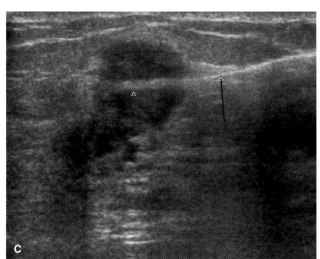

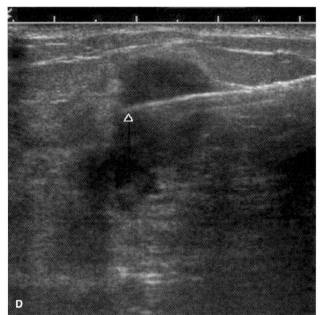

FIGURE 16.2. Ultrasound guided core biopsy. **A:** Single craniocaudad (CC) film from a mammogram showing the suspicious mass (*arrow*). **B:** Preliminary image revealing a hypoechoic mass (*arrow*) corresponding with the mammographic finding. **C:** Prefire image showing the needle tip (*arrow*) at the edge of the mass. Line within the mass (*arrowhead*) is air introduced during the administration of local anesthesia. **D:** Postfire image showing the needle with its tip (*arrow*) extending through the mass. Pathology revealed invasive ductal carcinoma.

(48,49). A recent large review found a long-term false-negative rate of 2.4% (31 of 1,312 core biopsies with benign results) using a 14-gauge biopsy system (47).

Ability to visualize the lesion is the major limitation to ultrasound-guided biopsy (50,51). It has been reported that more than 50% of lesions requiring biopsy cannot be visualized under ultrasound. These include small masses (<5 mm), calcifications and areas of architectural distortion. If a steep angle is used in attempting to biopsy a lesion, the needle may be difficult to visualize as the steep angle leads to less reflective echoes (46).

Masses that have been demonstrated to be noncystic are the most common lesions sampled, although calcifications may be seen and successfully biopsied using ultrasound guidance (52). If calcifications are the reason for biopsy, specimen radiography should be utilized to confirm that these have indeed been sampled.

The same equipment used for diagnostic ultrasound is used for ultrasound-guided interventional procedures. The transducers used should be of the highest frequency that permits adequate penetration of the tissue. A minimum of 7.5 MHz is required, although 10 or 12 MHz transducers are more commonly used. A linear array transducer is utilized to allow optimal visualization of the needle and the lesion during the procedure. As ultrasound imaging can be performed in an almost infinite number of projections, an approach to nearly any lesion can be utilized to safely and effectively perform the procedure. The approach should be as nearly parallel to the chest wall as possible to prevent inadvertent puncture of the chest wall and possible pneumothorax.

Prior to performing the procedure, the area in question should be imaged in two planes (46). If there is any question about whether the mass is a complex cyst, attempted aspiration can be performed. Once the area has been cleansed and anesthetized, it is possible to convert the attempted aspiration into a core biopsy if required. The patient should be placed in a position that is comfortable, with the ipsilateral arm placed over the head. This will keep the skin somewhat taut, simplifying needle entry. Placing the patient on her side or in an oblique position may move lesions away from the chest wall and shorten the distance from the skin to the mass. It is important that the operator as well as the patient be in a comfortable position.

A variety of needles can be used for ultrasound-guided biopsy. It is possible to perform FNA if desired. Most breast lesions are sampled as core biopsies. These can be performed either with an automated biopsy gun, usually a 14-gauge device, or with vacuum assistance using a 9- or 11-gauge needle. If multiple specimens are going to be obtained, consideration should be given to using a coaxial system, where the biopsy gun is placed through a large-core needle that is not removed after each sample.

Automated biopsy guns use a double-action needle that consists of an outer cutting cannula and an inner trocar with a sample notch. The needle is placed at the edge of the lesion to be sampled and is "fired" by pushing a button on the device. The biopsy gun rapidly advances the needle into the breast, obtaining a core of tissue in its excursion. As the gun is fired, a sample of tissue is cut by the outer cannula and stored in the sample notch. The needle is removed from the breast and the tissue sample is obtained from the needle. In order to ensure adequate sampling, at least four samples are usually obtained (53).

Hand-held directional, vacuum-assisted biopsy devices have been developed for ultrasound use. These have been found to be accurate (54) and are useful when either a larger volume of tissue is desired or when a lesion is to be completely removed. The only disadvantage to the use of these devices is increased cost. When these are utilized, the technique is quite similar to that used with the automated biopsy guns. Optimally the probe should be positioned at the posterior edge of the lesion so that shadowing from the probe does not obscure the mass. Placement of the needle varies slightly between devices, but in the postfire position the sample notch must be within the lesion. Some devices allow the needle to be "prefired" outside the breast and advanced until the sample notch is within the lesion. Some of these devices must be removed from the breast after each sample, while some allow multiple samples to be removed and stored in a collection chamber. The number of cores necessary to ensure adequate sampling when vacuum assistance is used has not been determined, however, it should be noted that each sample yields a greater volume of tissue than when the 14-gauge automated device is used. The major advantage of using the vacuum-assisted devices is that masses can be removed, such that no visible mass remains. This is not a substitute for a lumpectomy since margin status cannot be evaluated. However, this is an alternative method for removing fibroadenomas or other benign masses if this is deemed desirable. Markers can be placed after biopsy with either type of device with the marker placed either through a coaxial needle or with a separate needle puncture.

Correlation with the mammogram is essential if there is any question about the concordance between the findings on ultrasound and mammography. Placement of a marker at the time of ultrasound-guided biopsy followed by a postprocedure mammogram will allow any misidentifications to be promptly recognized. The reported rate of nonconcordance between ultrasound and mammography has been reported to be about 10% (55).

Magnetic Resonance Image–Guided Biopsy

Over the past decade, breast MRI has become widely incorporated into clinical practice. Contrast-enhanced MRI has been demonstrated to be extremely sensitive for the detection of breast carcinoma; however, it has a relatively low sensitivity (56–58). Although there is improving accuracy in diagnosis, there continues to be a huge range when comparing different centers and individual radiologists. The incorporation of computer-assisted detection (CAD) systems designed for breast MRI is improving the consistency of diagnosis for invasive carcinoma,

but there continue to be a large number of false-positive examinations. The reasons for this include a continued lack of guidelines for imaging protocols, variability in criteria for interpretation, patient selection, and the fact that benign lesions may enhance (59). Fibroadenomas, areas of hyperplasia, sclerosing adenosis, radial scars, and benign breast tissue may all enhance following the administration of contrast material (59–61). The criteria for diagnosing ductal carcinoma *in situ* (DCIS) remain a work in progress (62). In addition, malignant lesions occasionally do not enhance. MRI is generally not useful in determining if a mammographic abnormality requires biopsy because a negative MRI cannot ensure that a lesion is benign. MRI cannot be used as a replacement for mammography (57).

Breast MRI is best performed on a magnet with a field strength of at least 1.5 T. Improved signal-to-noise ratios and homogeneity of the field are seen when the examinations are performed on a 3-T magnet. A breast biopsy coil is required, as it is not possible to perform diagnostic quality work with a whole body coil. Imaging is performed in the prone position with the breast is light compression. Compression is necessary to immobilize the breast to reduce motion and to decrease the number of slices required to image the entire breast. The compression is much less than that used for mammography. Tight compression should not be used because this may inhibit blood flow into and out of the breast, potentially obscuring enhancing lesions. Most modern MRI units allow both breasts to be imaged at the same time. Although MRI has been found to be extremely sensitive for the detection of breast carcinoma (56,63), the specificity is lower, being reported as 50% to 70% in most series (59,63). A combination of the morphologic features of the lesion and the enhancement kinetics need to be used for accurate diagnosis (64–66). DCIS more commonly presents as nonmass enhancement and frequently does not demonstrate the same enhancement characteristics as invasive carcinoma (67,68).

Gadolinium intravenous contrast material is required to perform a diagnostic examination. Although the complication rates are low, gadolinium should not be used in patients with compromised renal function as nephrogenic sclerosing fibrosis (NSF), a potentially life-threatening complication, may occur. Imaging is performed both before and after the administration of the contrast material, with imaging performed at predetermined time intervals after injection.

MRI-guided procedures, while generally tolerated by the patient, are time-consuming, uncomfortable, and require the intravenous injection of contrast material. Abnormalities detected on MRI that are felt to require biopsy should first be evaluated with a second-look ultrasound to determine if the lesion can be visualized (69). In a review of 1,086 breast MRI cases, Teifke et al. (70) found that 30 of 54 lesions requiring biopsy could be identified on second-look ultrasound. LaTrenta et al. (71) found this to be the case in only 21 of 93 (23%) lesions identified on MRI. They further found that the likelihood of carcinoma was considerably higher in those lesions with an ultrasound correlate (43% vs. 14%) than without an ultrasound correlate. If there is an ultrasound correlate, biopsy should be performed under ultrasound guidance. There are a number of lesions that can only be detected on MRI (64), requiring that biopsy be performed under MRI guidance (72–77). Comparison of the results of MRI-guided core biopsy with the results of MRI-guided needle localization and excision (73,75,78,79) revealed the results to be comparable, making core biopsy an acceptable alternative. As normal breast tissue may enhance on MRI, some apparent lesions will have resolved prior to the date of proposed biopsy. The rate of canceled biopsy due to lesion resolution has been reported to be 4.7% to 6% (78,79).

The principles of MRI-guided biopsy are the same as those regarding stereotactic biopsy and ultrasound-guided core biopsy, with a few major differences. With both stereotactic and ultrasound-guided biopsy, the abnormality is evident both before and during the procedure. If the abnormality is sampled and not completely removed, it will be visualized on postprocedure imaging. With MRI, as contrast material washes out from the abnormal tissue, the lesion may be evident only on images obtained at beginning of the procedure. In addition, the presence of calcifications in stereotactic biopsy specimens can be confirmed on specimen radiography. There is no established method to confirm that the abnormality has been sampled when an MRI-guided biopsy is performed. There is one report of 12 cases of MRI-guided needle-localized excisional biopsies in which an abnormality could be seen on specimen radiography in five lesions (42%) (80). Sliced specimens were radiographed in 11 of these cases and the abnormality could be

identified in 9 of these (82%). It is not certain that this work will apply to core biopsies obtained using MRI guidance. As MRI biopsy is not performed if the lesion can be visualized on mammography or ultrasound, there is no simple test that can be used to reliably confirm that the proper area has been sampled.

Performance of an MRI-guided core biopsy will depend somewhat on the particular equipment available. Various grids are available that allow MRI safe biopsy devices to be placed in the area of interest. Newer CAD systems include a biopsy package that indicates the correct area to place the needle and the appropriate depth for the needle. When these systems are not available, the calculations can be made manually.

To perform the procedure (Fig. 16.3), MRI is performed with the patient in the prone position with the breast in light

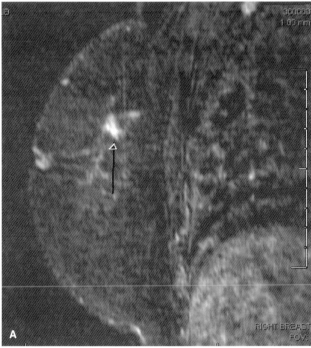

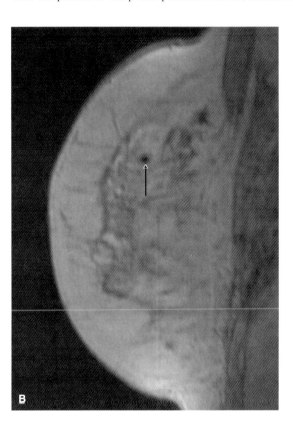

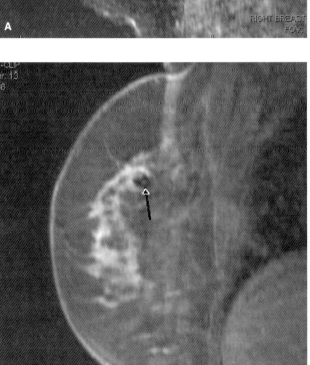

FIGURE 16.3. Magnetic resonance image (MRI)-guided core biopsy. **A:** Sagittal postcontrast subtraction MRI image showing a suspicious enhancing mass (*arrow*). **B:** Sagittal T1-weighted MRI showing the obturator in place (*arrow*). Mass can no longer be visualized. **C:** Postbiopsy sagittal imaging revealing cavity and a marker (*arrow*) at the biopsy site. Biopsy revealed invasive lobular carcinoma.

compression. Using most of the commercially available systems, the breast can be accessed from either the medial or lateral approach (78). The patient is removed from the magnet, the area of interest is identified, and the skin is cleansed and anesthetized. A nonmetallic sheath is placed over a large core (usually 9-gauge) needle and is inserted in this area to the appropriate depth. The needle is removed, a plastic trocar is inserted, and images are obtained to confirm that the parameters of needle placement and lesion location are concordant (Fig. 16.3B). The patient is then removed from the magnet and biopsy is performed using a vacuum-assisted device that is slightly modified so as to be MRI safe. These units have long tubing so that the actual unit can remain outside the MRI room. A nonmagnetic marker is placed at the biopsy site at the conclusion of the examination, and one additional scan is performed to confirm marker placement (Fig. 16.3C). Because the lesion cannot be visualized with the biopsy gun in place, it is advantageous to obtain multiple samples to maximize the chances of accurate sampling. This is impractical using an automated biopsy gun because it would require multiple needle insertions with repeat imaging after each insertion. Use of a vacuum-assisted system makes it possible to obtain a relatively large biopsy sample in a short period of time.

Mammographic imaging is performed following the biopsy to identify the position of the marker. Should excisional biopsy be required, needle localization can be performed under mammographic guidance using the marker as a guide rather than requiring an additional MRI examination.

As with all other imaging-guided procedures, correlation with pathology specimens is imperative. The appropriate rate of positive biopsies for a particular institution must be determined. The rate may vary depending on the indications for the examination, such that an acceptable biopsy rate for the very high-risk patients may be different from the biopsy rate for patients having MRI after the diagnosis of breast cancer. In most instances, the biopsy rate will not differ significantly from that used when evaluating biopsy rates using other modalities, with a 20% to 30% positive rate. In addition, MRI biopsy specimen reports must be correlated with the imaging findings to ensure that nonconcordant and probably concordant biopsy specimens are appropriately addressed. In a study by Lee et al. (81) of 342 MRI-guided, 9-gauge vacuum-assisted biopsies, there was imaging histologic discordance in 7% of the lesions. Surgical excision of these lesions revealed carcinoma in 30%.

COMPLICATIONS

Complications following needle-core biopsy procedures are unusual and are rarely serious. Bleeding, whether from difficulty obtaining hemostasis or hematoma formation, is the most common complication seen and has been reported in up to 3% of cases with an 11-guage vacuum-assisted system (33,82). Inadvertent nicking or biopsy of a blood vessel may occur. In almost all cases, hemostasis can be obtained by compressing the area for 10 to 15 minutes. Although some practices place a pressure dressing on the biopsy site, this is not generally necessary. In those cases where there is difficulty obtaining hemostasis, this may be helpful. Patients who have prolonged bleeding or who have a hematoma visible on the postprocedure mammogram should be advised that they may find a palpable abnormality following the procedure.

Infection is very unusual following biopsy, although it may occur if sterile technique is not maintained. The occurrence of infection may be more common in diabetics.

Occasionally stereotactic biopsies will be unsuccessful (83, 84). This may occur because the wrong area is targeted, the patient moves before the needle is placed, or needle placement is less than optimal. An analysis of the reasons for unsuccessful results when attempting to sample calcifications found that

failure to retrieve calcifications was more likely if the lesion was 5 mm in size or smaller, if the calcifications had an amorphous morphology, or if the biopsy gun was fired outside the breast (83). Others have identified significant bleeding as a factor in the failure to retrieve calcifications (82). Specimen radiography should be used routinely to identify calcifications within the sampled tissue (85,86). Failure to retrieve calcifications in the biopsy specimens is dependent not only on the number of specimens obtained, but on the type of biopsy system used. Failure to retrieve calcifications has been reported to occur approximately 16% of the time when 14-gauge automated biopsy guns are used, compared to 1% with 11-gauge vacuum-assisted systems (82).

It is imperative that the findings on the mammogram are correlated with the results of the biopsy to ensure that they are concordant. This is the responsibility of the person performing the biopsy. If these procedures are performed by a surgeon in conjunction with a breast imager, responsibility for correlating the findings should be assigned. It has been reported that discordant findings are more common when biopsy is performed for suspicious calcifications than for masses (87). If the biopsy attempt is not successful or the results are felt to be not concordant, either a repeat stereotactic biopsy or an excisional biopsy should be performed (87).

Follow-up mammograms are routinely performed in cases where the results of biopsy are benign. This is most commonly performed at 6 months following the procedure. In most cases, there is no distortion at the biopsy site (88). Lamm and Jackman (89) reported a mammographic density to be visible in 5 of 226 (2%) of cases after stereotactic biopsy with an 11-gauge vacuum-assisted device. If there has been a hematoma postoperatively, this may persist. Short-interval follow-up ultrasound or MRI is suggested when biopsy has been performed with ultrasound or MRI guidance.

False-negative diagnoses can occur. When ultrasound-guided biopsy has been performed, these are usually related to technical or sampling errors, unrecognized radiologic–histologic or ultrasound–mammography discordance, or lack of follow-up after a biopsy with benign results (46). If the results of biopsy are discordant or equivocal, including papillary lesions and lobular neoplasia, repeat biopsy should be undertaken (90). Sonographic follow-up at 6 months after biopsy and then annually for at least 2 years is recommended following an ultrasound-guided core needle biopsy with benign results to ensure stability of the findings (47).

CONCORDANCE AND ACCURACY

To avoid missing cancers, it is essential that the imaging findings be correlated with the pathology findings in all cases. False-negative results may occur with any biopsy. False-negative rates are low, reported as between 0.3% and 8%, although some of these series do not have complete follow-up (87,91–95). Reported false-negative rates are 0% to 8% for stereotactic biopsy performed with a 14-gauge needle (96,97), 3% for stereotactic biopsy performed with an 11-gauge vacuum-assisted system (98), and 0% to 8% for needle localization and excision (98,99). Orel et al. (75) reported a 2% false-negative rate in their initial experience in 85 cases of MRI-guided core biopsy. False-negative rates appear to decrease with increasing experience (98). These results compare favorably with reported rates of accuracy for needle-localized excisional biopsy, reported as a 0% to 18% overall miss rate with a mean of 2.6% (99).

If the findings on imaging are of low suspicion and the pathology is benign and concordant, the patient can be returned to imaging surveillance and surgical biopsy is not necessary. Some authors recommend annual imaging follow-up if the results are specific and concordant (such as fibroadenoma or lymph node) and a 6-month follow-up if the pathology is nonspecific (such as fibrocystic change) (100). Jackman et al. (91) recommend that follow-up be performed at 6 months for all cases of benign pathology. In most instances this should be followed by annual imaging for at least 2 years to ensure that the lesion does not progress (47). Patient compliance can be a problem in this regard, with only 54% of patients in one series adhering to the follow-up recommendations (101). If the imaging findings are highly suspicious, a benign pathology will be considered discordant and additional biopsy will be recommended. This can be performed either as a repeat attempt at image-guided biopsy or a surgical biopsy. Benign, nonspecific pathology findings, such as fibrocystic change, will be acceptable if the imaging findings are not highly suspicious and a 6-month imaging follow-up will be performed. On the other hand, if the imaging findings are highly suspicious, nonspecific pathology will not be acceptable.

Discordance between the imaging findings and the pathology report should result in a repeat biopsy, either as an image-guided core biopsy or as a surgical biopsy. It has been reported that up to 47% of these repeat biopsies will result in a cancer diagnosis (102). In other reported series, the incidence of cancers was considerably lower, on the order of 5% (103,104).

 ## MARKERS

Clips or markers should ideally be placed in or immediately adjacent to the biopsy cavity (105,106). This is generally easily accomplished when an ultrasound-guided biopsy is performed because the position of the marker can be verified in real time. When biopsies are performed with the breast in compression, as is the case with stereotactic or MRI-guided biopsies, markers may be displaced up to several centimeters from the biopsy site. This is because as the breast is released from compression, the marker may move along the needle track. This has been described as the *accordion effect* (107–109). This should be recognized on the postprocedure mammogram when a stereotactic biopsy has been performed, and if needle localization is necessary, appropriate corrections can be made (108). The final position should be evaluated on mammograms obtained after the procedure rather than on stereotactic images made while the breast is still in compression. Reports in the literature indicate that in approximately 10% of the cases the marker has been at least 2 cm from the biopsy site, with others reporting that 28% of clips were more than 1 cm from the biopsy site (108). In most cases, the markers remain in the location where they were placed. However, there have been occasional reports in the literature of delayed migration of markers (110–113). If needle localization and surgical excision is required, it is essential that the position of the marker in relationship to the biopsy site be confirmed and localization performed appropriately. This may require ignoring the marker that has migrated. Hematomas at the biopsy site may also contribute to displacement of the marker (113). Because most of the markers currently used are not clips and are therefore not fixed to tissue, displacement by a hematoma has the potential to permanently displace the marker from the biopsy site.

The placement of metallic clips within or immediately adjacent to a site of carcinoma prior to the institution of neoadjuvant chemotherapy has been demonstrated to be a useful technique to ensure that the area of tumor will be recognizable at the time of surgery. If the response to chemotherapy results in the tumor no longer being visualized on imaging, the marker may be the only way to localize the tumor bed (114,115). The marker can be placed at the time of core biopsy or may be placed at a later date independent of a biopsy procedure. Similarly, if a small lesion is sampled, especially if a vacuum-assisted device is used, there may be no recognizable abnormality on the postbiopsy images. If a small lesion is sampled, marker placement should be routinely employed.

 ## UNDERESTIMATION OF DISEASE

Underestimation of disease occurs when DCIS diagnosed on core biopsy is upgraded to invasive carcinoma on surgical excision or when atypical ductal hyperplasia (ADH) is upgraded to DCIS or invasive carcinoma at surgery. This may occur in up to 20% of cases (84,116). In one series, the risk for underestimation of DCIS was found to be greatest in lesions over 3 cm in size (117). However, there is improvement in the rate of ADH or DCIS underestimation when vacuum-assisted systems are used rather than automated core biopsy devices (118). When a 14-gauge automated core biopsy is used for diagnosis, the underestimation rate is 20% to 30% (11,119), compared with a 4% to 11% underestimation rate when the vacuum-assisted 11-gauge device is used (116,117,120). It is felt that the lower rate of underestimation with the larger needles is attributable to a larger volume of tissue acquired, resulting in decreased sampling error. It was hoped that the use of larger (8- or 9-gauge) core biopsy specimens would lead to a decrease in the rate of underestimation, however this has not proven to be the case (67,121). Lee et al. (67) reported on a series of 34 lesions of DCIS diagnosed at MRI-guided vacuum-assisted breast biopsy, 29 of which were DCIS and 5 were DCIS with possible microinvasion. In this series, 17% of the lesions diagnosed as DCIS and 80% of the lesions reported as DCIS with possible microinvasion were found to be invasive carcinoma at surgical excision. In this series, invasive carcinoma was more likely if the area of the lesion on MRI was 6 cm or greater. This study found no difference in the overall accuracy of directional vacuum-assisted biopsy with the use of 8-gauge versus 11-gauge systems. Similarly, there is upgrading to DCIS or invasive carcinoma in up to 20% of cases when ADH is diagnosed on core biopsy.

COMPLETE LESION REMOVAL

Lesion removal may inadvertently occur during core biopsy procedures of a small lesion. As long as a marker has been deployed at the biopsy site, this is not a problem even if the lesion is cancerous or a high-risk lesion that requires surgical removal. If a marker has not been placed, finding the site of biopsy can be difficult, since the immediate postbiopsy changes of air in the cavity or hematoma will resolve, leaving no residual indication of where the lesion was. When image-guided biopsies first became popular, there was no ability to place a marker when a 14-gauge needle was used. With the advent of 11-gauge vacuum-assisted biopsies, clips were designed that could be placed through the needle at the biopsy site. There are now various clips and markers that can be placed through any of the commercially available biopsy needles or can be placed independently. Although large cores of tissue can be obtained with 9-gauge vacuum-assisted devices, these cannot be used for the removal of malignant or premalignant lesions as there is no way to assess the margins of excision either for completeness of excision or orientation.

Although a lesion may be removed so that no imaging abnormality remains, this cannot be used as a therapeutic procedure for cancer. The margins cannot be assessed using this technique and needle-localized excisional biopsy will be required for definitive treatment.

Atypical Ductal Hyperplasia

ADH is a pathologic finding that is part of the spectrum between normal breast tissue and DCIS. There is not a sharp demarcation between ADH and DCIS, and the amount of tissue involved is one of the factors used in determining the final diagnosis. The implications of this diagnosis are described differently in the literature, depending on whether the diagnosis is made at surgical excision or core biopsy. Women who are diagnosed with ADH at surgery are believed to carry an increased risk of developing invasive breast carcinoma in either breast, but there is not thought to be an increased risk at the biopsy site (122,123). However, when ADH is diagnosed at core biopsy, surgical excision is routinely recommended as there have been reports of associated carcinoma being present in surgical excision specimens adjacent to the core biopsy site.

ADH is more commonly found when core biopsy is performed for calcifications than for masses. The rate of ADH on core biopsy specimens varies depending on the experience of the pathologist and the size of the needle used. The diagnosis of ADH can be expected in 3% to 7% of core biopsies performed for suspicious microcalcifications. Similar statistics are reported when the biopsy is performed for abnormal findings on MRI (67,73–75). Studies have demonstrated that when ADH is diagnosed on core biopsy, there is at least a 20% chance of this being upstaged on excisional biopsy of the area, with some authors reporting underestimation of disease in up to 58% of cases (67,84,91,124). This is reported to be considerably decreased when biopsy is performed with vacuum-assisted systems, reduced in one series from 24% when biopsy is performed with a 14-gauge biopsy needle to 19% when an 11-gauge vacuum-assisted system is used (118,125). Another series found carcinoma in 15% of biopsies with ADH diagnosed with 11-gauge vacuum-assisted biopsy (126). Lourenco et al. (121) found no significant difference in the rate of underestimation when 9-gauge or 11-gauge needles were used for vacuum-assisted stereotactic biopsy. The upstaging may be either to DCIS or to invasive carcinoma. ADH is therefore considered a high-risk lesion, so that when ADH is diagnosed on core biopsy, the general recommendation is for an excisional biopsy.

Atypical Lobular Hyperplasia and Lobular Carcinoma *In Situ*

The appropriate management of the core biopsy yielding a diagnosis of lobular neoplasia is controversial. This term includes a spectrum of proliferative changes ranging from atypical lobular hyperplasia (ALH) to lobular carcinoma *in situ* (LCIS). This is an uncommon diagnosis at core biopsy, with rates of 1.6% to 1.8% for lobular neoplasia (127,128), 0.2% to 1.2% for LCIS (18,129,130) and 0.05% to 3.3% for ALH (131,132). Lobular neoplasia has been regarded as a high-risk marker, conferring an increased risk of developing invasive carcinoma, usually invasive ductal carcinoma. This risk has been estimated at about 1% per year and is the same for both breasts. Recommendations for the appropriate management of LCIS have varied from bilateral mastectomy to routine surveillance (133). Additionally, pleomorphic forms of LCIS have been associated with invasive lobular carcinoma in proximity to the diagnosed LCIS. In part due to the uncertainties associated with the diagnosis of LCIS, some have suggested that excisional biopsy be performed when this is diagnosed at core biopsy.

Although lobular neoplasia has traditionally been felt to be an incidental finding in core biopsy done for other reasons, there have been studies suggesting that calcifications may be associated with this process (18,127,134). In one series of 15 cases of lobular neoplasia that were excised, one case of DCIS and three cases of ADH were found at surgical excision (127). All of these cases were associated with residual microcalcifications within the breast. Other suggested criteria for surgical excision include lesions with pathologic feature that overlap with those of DCIS, an associated high-risk lesion in the specimen and mammographic-pathologic discordance (127,129).

Mahoney et al. (18), in a review of 27 cases of lobular neoplasia diagnosed with 11-gauge vacuum-assisted biopsy, found that of the 20 patients who underwent subsequent surgical excision, there was a 19% upgrade to either DCIS or invasive cancer. Foster et al. (135), in a review of 35 patients, had similar findings with an upgrade rate of 17%. In a meta-analysis of the published data, Cohen (136) noted a 19% upgrade to DCIS or invasive carcinoma in 159 reported cases.

ALH has traditionally been considered a benign, nonspecific diagnosis on core biopsy and was considered part of the spectrum of fibrocystic change. As with LCIS, in cases with marked atypia, there may be an increased incidence of DCIS, invasive lobular, or invasive ductal carcinoma in the vicinity of the ALH. The reasons for this are uncertain. Given this reported increased incidence of malignancy, some authors have suggested that excisional biopsy follow the diagnosis of ALH on core biopsy (127,135). This suggestion remains controversial, as does the management of patients with core biopsies revealing LCIS (137).

 ## RADIAL SCAR

Radial scars, also known as complex sclerosing lesions, are hyperplastic lesions that present as areas of architectural distortion on mammography, radiographically indistinguishable from carcinoma. Pathologically, these lesions contain dense collagen centrally combined with peripheral ducts that are dilated and hyperplastic. It is not uncommon to find ductal hyperplasia, with or without atypia, papillomas, lobular neoplasia, and occasionally DCIS, within these lesions. There have been intermittent reports in the literature of an association between radial scar and tubular carcinoma (138–140).

Initially it was felt that potential radial scars should be subjected to excisional biopsy as the histologic evaluation of these lesions was difficult in small samples, with early reports of underestimation of disease in 40% of cases (91). With the ability to obtain larger core samples, the accuracy rate has improved, so that a review by Douglas-Jones et al. (141) showed a false-negative rate of 3.9%, making core biopsy an acceptable alternative to excision.

PAPILLARY LESIONS

Papillary lesions of the breast have a fibrovascular core that arborizes into branching frond-like papillae. These lesions protrude into the duct lumen. This category includes papilloma, atypical papilloma, intraductal papillary carcinoma, and invasive papillary carcinoma (142). These lesions may have similar morphologic features, making it difficult to differentiate benign from malignant papillary disease. These are relatively uncommon lesions, occurring in 3% to 5% of biopsy specimens (143).

Classification and further evaluation of papillary lesions remains controversial (75,143). Sydnor et al. (144) reviewed 63 cases diagnosed as papillary lesions at core biopsy. In this series, benign papilloma was associated with malignancy in only 3% of cases, while atypical papilloma was associated with malignancy in 67% of cases. This led them to recommend mammographic follow-up for lesions without atypia. Sohn et al. (145) agreed with this recommendation. In an earlier study, Mercado et al. (146) found underestimation of malignant papillary disease in 25% of patients with atypical papilloma and recommended excision only for lesions that are atypical or malignant on core biopsy. However, in a more recent series of 36 lesions diagnosed at core biopsy as papillary lesions without atypia and referred for surgical excision, Mercado et al. (147) reported 10 lesions upgraded to ADH and DCIS and recommended that papillary lesions be considered high-risk lesions requiring surgical excision.

SUMMARY

Image-guided biopsy has become the standard for diagnosing non-palpable abnormalities in the breast. It is less invasive and less expensive than surgical biopsy (148) with equivalent accuracy. As a large portion of the cost of any breast cancer screening program is associated with biopsies that are recommended for abnormalities found on imaging, use of core needle biopsy can significantly reduce these costs (15,149,150).

Widespread use of core needle biopsy techniques has changed recommended practice patterns. Since their incorporation into most practices in the 1990s, core biopsies have become the predominant tool for the diagnosis of both benign and malignant breast disease (38). A benign core biopsy with concordant imaging findings can allow surgical excision to be avoided, and in many cases can minimize the number of operations required for treatment of carcinoma. However, this is not always the case. In addition there are extremely anxious patients who prefer that surgical excision be performed, and for these patients this is the management option of choice. Some patients will be unable to tolerate stereotactic biopsy due to their inability to lie in the prone position.

As new technologies are developed for breast cancer diagnosis, it can be expected that core needle biopsy technique will be adapted to these examinations. Tumor ablation methods using imaging guidance and high-intensity–focused ultrasound (HIFU) and laser and cryoablation are being studied and may play a part in breast cancer therapy in the future.

MANAGEMENT SUMMARY FOR IMAGE-GUIDED BIOPSY OF NONPALPABLE BREAST LESIONS

- Most nonpalpable breast lesions can be successfully and accurately diagnosed using image-guided needle biopsy.
- Core needle biopsy is preferred over FNA because of fewer inadequate samples and the ability to obtain information about invasion and receptor status.
- If breast lesions are visible under ultrasound, this is the preferred imaging for biopsy guidance.
- Correlation of the imaging and pathology findings is imperative and nonconcordant cases must be appropriately addressed.
- Management of high-risk lesions remains controversial.

References

1. Groenewoud JH, Pijnappel RN, van den Akker-van Marle ME, et al. Cost-effectiveness of stereotactic large-core needle biopsy for nonpalpable breast lesions compared to open-breast biopsy. *Br J Cancer* 2004;90:383–392.
2. Jemal A, Siegel R, Ward E, et al. Cancer statistics, 2007. *CA Cancer J Clin* 2007;57:43–66.
3. Hall F. Screening mammography: potential problems on the horizon. *N Engl J Med* 1986;314:53–55.
4. Hall FM, Storella JM, Silverstone DZ, et al. Nonpalpable breast lesions: recommendations for biopsy based on suspicion of carcinoma at mammography. *Radiology* 1988;167:353–358.
5. Tersegno MM. Mammography: positive predictive value and true-positive biopsy rate. *AJR Am J Roentgenol* 1993;160:660–661.
6. Bernstein J. Role of stereotactic breast biopsy. *Sem Surg Oncol* 1996;12:290–299.
7. Yim JH, Barton P, Weber B, et al. Mammographically detected breast cancer: benefits of stereotactic core versus wire localization biopsy. *Ann Surg Oncol* 1996;63:1072–1078.
8. Yeow K-M, Lo Y-F, Wang C-S, et al. Ultrasound-guided core needle biopsy as an initial diagnostic test for palpable breast masses. *J Vasc Interv Radiol* 2001;12:1313–1317.
9. Brenner R, Bassett LW, Fajardo LL, et al. Stereotactic core-needle breast biopsy: a multi-institutional prospective trial. *Radiology* 2001;218:866–872.
10. Chen AM, Haffty BG, Lee CH. Local recurrence of breast cancer after breast conservation therapy in patients examined by means of stereotactic core-needle biopsy. *Radiology* 2002;225:707–712.
11. Rakha EA, Ellis IO. An overview of assessment of prognostic and predictive factors in breast cancer needle core biopsy specimens. *J Clin Pathol* 2007;60:1300–1306.
12. Riedl CC, Pfarl G, Memarsadeghi M, et al. Lesion miss rates and false-negative rates for 1,115 consecutive cases of stereotactically guided needle-localized open breast biopsy with long-term follow-up. *Radiology* 2005;237:847–853.
13. Shannon J, Douglas-Jones AG, Dallimore NS. Conversion to core biopsy in preoperative diagnosis of breast lesions: is it justified by the results? *J Clin Pathol* 2001;54:762–765.
14. Liberman L, Gougoutas CA, Zakowski MF, et al. Calcifications highly suggestive of malignancy: comparison of breast biopsy methods. *AJR Am J Roentgenol* 2001;177:165–172.
15. Liberman L, Sama MP. Cost-effectiveness of stereotactic 11-gauge directional vacuum-assisted breast biopsy. *AJR Am J Roentgenol* 2000;175:53–58.
16. Cipolla C, Fricano S, Vieni S, et al. Validity of needle core biopsy in the histological characterisation of mammary lesions. *Breast* 2006;15:76–80.
17. Alonso-Bartolome P, Vega-Bolivar A, Torres-Tabanera M, et al. Sonographically guided 11-G directional vacuum-assisted breast biopsy as an alternative to surgical excision: utility and cost study in probably benign lesions. *Acta Radiol* 2004;45:390–396.
18. Mahoney MC, Robinson-Smith TM, Shaughnessy EA. Lobular neoplasia at 11-gauge vacuum-assisted stereotactic biopsy: correlation with surgical excisional biopsy and mammographic follow-up. *AJR Am J Roentgenol* 2006;187:949–954.
19. Koskela AK, Sudah M, Berg MH, et al. Add-on device for stereotactic core-needle breast biopsy: how many biopsy specimens are needed for a reliable diagnosis? *Radiology* 2005;236:801–809.
20. Hendrick RD, Kimme-Smith C, Dershaw DD, et al. *Stereotactic breast biopsy quality control manual*. Reston, VA: American College of Radiology, 1999.
21. Dershaw D. Equipment, technique, quality assurance, and accreditation for imaging-guided breast biopsy procedures. *Radiol Clin North Am* 2000;38:773–789.
22. Winchester D. What's best for the patient. *Am J Surg* 2007;194:278.
23. Dowlatshahi K, Snider II, Lerner AG. Who should perform image-guided breast biopsy and treatment? *Am J Surg* 2007;194:275–277.
24. Philpotts LE, Lee CH, Horvath LJ, et al. Canceled stereotactic core-needle biopsy of the breast: analysis of 89 cases. *Radiology* 1997;205:423–428.
25. Verkooijen HM, Peeters PHM, Borel Rinkes IHM, et al. Risk factors for cancellation of stereotactic large core needle biopsy on a prone biopsy table. *Br J Radiol* 2001;74:1007–1012.
26. American College of Radiology. ACR Breast Imaging Reporting and Data System (BI-RADS): breast imaging atlas. Reston, VA: American College of Radiology, 2003.
27. Lindfors KK, O'Connor J, Acredolo CR, et al. Short-interval follow up mammography versus immediate core biopsy of benign breast lesions: assessment of patient stress. *AJR Am J Roentgenol* 1998;171:55–58.
28. Jackman RJ, Marzoni F, Finkelstein SL, et al. Benefits of diagnosing nonpalpable breast cancer with stereotactic large-core needle biopsy: lower costs and fewer operations. *Radiology* 1996;201:67–70.
29. Liberman L, Goodstine SL, Dershaw DD, et al. One operation after percutaneous diagnosis of nonpalpable breast cancer: frequency and associated factors. *AJR Am J Roentgenol* 2002;178:673–679.
30. Usami S, Moriya T, Kasajima A, et al. Pathological aspects of core needle biopsy for non-palpable breast lesions. *Breast Cancer* 2005;12:272–278.
31. Liberman L, LaTrenta LR, Dershaw DD, et al. Impact of core biopsy on the surgical management of impalpable breast cancer. *AJR Am J Roentgenol* 1997;169:1464–1465.
32. Whitten TM, Wallace T, Bird RE, et al. Image-guided core biopsy has advantages over needle localization biopsy for the diagnosis of nonpalpable breast cancer. *Am Surg* 1997;63:1072.
33. Melotti MK, Berg WA. Core needle breast biopsy in patients undergoing anticoagulation therapy: preliminary results. *AJR Am J Roentgenol* 2000;174:245–249.
34. Jackman RJ, Lamm RL. Stereotactic histologic biopsy in breasts with implants. *Radiology* 2002;222:157–164.
35. Parker SH, Lovin JD, Jobe WE, et al. Stereotactic breast biopsy with a biopsy gun. *Radiology* 1990;176:741–747.
36. Liberman L, Fahs MC, Dershaw DD, et al. Impact of stereotaxic core breast biopsy on cost of diagnosis. *Radiology* 1995;195:633–637.
37. Lee CH, Egglin TK, Philpotts L, et al. Cost-effectiveness of stereotactic core needle biopsy: analysis by means of mammographic findings. *Radiology* 1997;202:849–854.
38. Golub RM, Bennett Cl, Stinson T, et al. Cost minimization study of image-guided core biopsy versus surgical excisional biopsy for women with abnormal mammograms. *J Clin Oncol* 2004;22:2430–2437.
39. Jackman RJ, Marzoni FA Jr. Stereotactic histologic biopsy with patients prone: technical feasibility in 98% of mammographically detected lesions. *AJR Am J Roentgenol* 2003;180:785–794.
40. Wunderbaldinger P, Wolf G, Turetschek K, et al. Comparison of sitting versus prone position for stereotactic large-core breast biopsy in surgically proven lesions. *AJR Am J Roentgenol* 2002;178:1221–1225.
41. Georgian-Smith D, D'Orsi C, Morris E, et al. Stereotactic biopsy of the breast using an upright unit, a vacuum-suction needle, and a lateral arm-support system. *AJR Am J Roentgenol* 2002;178:1017–1024.
42. Welle GJ, Clark M, Loos S, et al. Stereotactic breast biopsy: recumbent biopsy using add-on upright equipment. *AJR Am J Roentgenol* 2000;175:59–63.
43. Liberman L, Smolkin JH, Dershaw DD, et al. Calcification retrieval at stereotactic, 11-gauge, directional, vacuum- assisted breast biopsy. *Radiology* 1998;208:251–260.
44. Morrow M, Strom EA, Bassett LW, et al. Standard for the management of ductal carcinoma in situ of the breast (DCIS). *CA Cancer J Clin* 2002;52:256–276.
45. Liberman L, Ernberg LA, Heerdt A, et al. Palpable breast masses: is there a role for percutaneous imaging-guided biopsy? *AJR Am J Roentgenol* 2000;175:779–787.
46. Youk JH, Kim E-K, Kim MJ, et al. Missed breast cancers at US-guided core needle biopsy: how to reduce them. *Radiographics* 2007;27:79–94.

47. Youk JH, Kim E-K, Kim MJ, et al. Sonographically guided 14-gauge core needle biopsy of breast masses: a review of 2,420 cases with long-term follow-up. *Am J Roentgenol* 2008;190:202–207.
48. Philpotts LE, Hooley RJ, Lee CH. Comparison of automated versus vacuum-assisted biopsy methods for sonographically guided core biopsy of the breast. *AJR Am J Roentgenol* 2003;180:347–351.
49. Cho N, Moon WK, Cha JH, et al. Sonographically guided core biopsy of the breast: comparison of 14-gauge automated gun and 11-gauge directional vacuum-assisted biopsy methods. *Korean J Radiol* 2005;6:102–109.
50. Fornage BD, Coan JD, David CL. Ultrasound-guided needle biopsy of the breast and other interventional procedures. *Radiol Clin North Am* 1992;30:167–185.
51. Georgian-Smith D, Shiels W. Freehand invasive sonography in breast: basic principles and clinical application. *Radiographics* 1996;16:149–161.
52. Soo MS, Baker JA, Rosen EL. Sonographic detection and sonographically guided biopsy of breast microcalcifications. *AJR Am J Roentgenol* 2003;180:941–948.
53. Crystal P, Koretz M, Shcharynsky S, et al. Accuracy of sonographically guided 14-gauge core-needle biopsy: results of 715 consecutive breast biopsies with at least 2-year follow-up of benign lesions. *J Clin Ultrasound* 2005;33:47–52.
54. Sebag P, Tourasse C, Rouyer N, et al. Value of vacuum assisted biopsies under sonography guidance: results from a multicentric study of 650 lesions. *J Radiol* 2006;87:29–34.
55. Conway WF, Hayes CW, Brewer WH. Occult breast masses: use of a mammographic localizing grid for US evaluation. *Radiology* 1991;181:143–146.
56. Bluemke DA, Gatsonis CA, Chen MH, et al. Magnetic resonance imaging of the breast prior to biopsy. *JAMA* 2004;292:2735–2742.
57. Berg WA, Gutierrez L, NessAiver MS, et al. Diagnostic accuracy of mammography, clinical examination, US, and MR imaging in preoperative assessment of breast cancer. *Radiology* 2004;233:830–849.
58. Fischer U, Kopka L, Grabbe E. Breast carcinoma: effect of preoperative contrast-enhanced MR imaging on the therapeutic approach. *Radiology* 1999;213:881–888.
59. Macura KJ, Ouwerkerk R, Jacobs MA, et al. Patterns of enhancement on breast MR images: interpretation and imaging pitfalls. *Radiographics* 2006;26:1719–1734.
60. Delille JP, Slanetz PJ, Yeh ED, et al. Physiologic changes in breast magnetic resonance imaging during the menstrual cycle: perfusion imaging, signal enhancement, and influence of the T1 relaxation time of breast tissue. *Breast J* 2005;11:236–241.
61. Kuhl CK, Bieling HB, Gieseke J, et al. Healthy premenopausal breast parenchyma in dynamic contrast-enhanced MR imaging of the breast: normal contrast medium enhancement and cyclical-phase dependency. *Radiology* 1997;203:137–144.
62. Jansen SA, Newstead GM, Abe H, et al. Pure ductal carcinoma *in situ*: kinetic and morphologic MR characteristics compared with mammographic appearance and nuclear grade. *Radiology* 2007;245:684–691.
63. Lee C. Problem solving MR imaging of the breast. *Radiol Clin North Am* 2004;42:919–934.
64. Bartella L, Liberman L, Morris EA, et al. Nonpalpable mammographically occult invasive breast cancers detected by MRI. *AJR Am J Roentgenol* 2006;186:865–870.
65. Schnall MD, Blume J, Bluemke DA, et al. Diagnostic architectural and dynamic features at breast MR imaging: multicenter study. *Radiology* 2006;238:42–53.
66. Kuhl CK, Mielcareck P, Klaschik S, et al. Dynamic breast MR imaging: are signal intensity time course data useful for differential diagnosis of enhancing lesions? *Radiology* 1999;211:101–110.
67. Lee J-M, Kaplan JB, Murray MP, et al. Underestimation of DCIS at MRI-guided vacuum-assisted breast biopsy. *AJR Am J Roentgenol* 2007;189:468–474.
68. Morris EA, Liberman L, Ballon DJ, et al. MRI of occult breast carcinoma in a high-risk population. *AJR Am J Roentgenol* 2003;181:619–626.
69. Kuhl CK. The current status of breast MR imaging. Part I. Choice of technique, image interpretation, diagnostic accuracy and transfer to clinical practice. *Radiology* 2007;244:356–378.
70. Teifke A, Lehr HA, Vomweg TW, et al. Outcome analysis and rational management of enhancing lesions incidentally detected on contrast-enhanced MRI of the breast. *AJR Am J Roentgenol* 2003;181:655–662.
71. LaTrenta LR, Menell JH, Morris EA, et al. Breast lesions detected with MR imaging: utility and histopathologic importance of identification with US. *Radiology* 2003;227:856–861.
72. Kuhl CK, Elevelt A, Leutner CC, et al. Interventional breast MR imaging: clinical use of a stereotactic localization and biopsy device. *Radiology* 1997;204:667–675.
73. Lehman CD, DePeri ER, Peacock S, et al. Clinical experience with MRI-guided vacuum-assisted breast biopsy. *AJR Am J Roentgenol* 2005;184:1782–1787.
74. Liberman L, Morris EA, Dershaw DD, et al. Fast MRI-guided vacuum-assisted breast biopsy: initial experience. *AJR Am J Roentgenol* 2003;181:1283–1293.
75. Orel SG, Rosen M, Mies C, et al. MR imaging-guided 9-gauge vacuum-assisted core-needle breast biopsy: initial experience. *Radiology* 2005;238:54–61.
76. Kuhl CK, Morakkabati N, Leutner CC, et al. MR imaging-guided large-core (14-gauge) needle biopsy of small lesions visible at breast MR imaging alone. *Radiology* 2001;220:31–39.
77. Lehman CD, Aikawa T. MR-guided vacuum-assisted breast biopsy: accuracy of targeting and success in sampling in a phantom model. *Radiology* 2004;232:911–914.
78. Causer PA, Piron CA, Jong RA, et al. MR imaging-guided breast localization system with medial or lateral access. *Radiology* 2006;240:369–379.
79. Morris EA, Liberman L, Dershaw DD, et al. Preoperative MR imaging—guided needle localization of breast lesions. *AJR Am J Roentgenol* 2002;178:1211–1220.
80. Erguvan-Dogan B, Whitman GJ, Nguyen VA, et al. Specimen radiography in confirmation of MRI-guided needle localization and surgical excision of breast lesions. *AJR Am J Roentgenol* 2006;187:339–344.
81. Lee J-M, Kaplan JB, Murray MP, et al. Imaging histologic discordance at MRI-guided 9-gauge vacuum-assisted breast biopsy. *AJR Am J Roentgenol* 2007;189:852–859.
82. Jackman RJ, Rodriguez-Soto J. Breast microcalcifications: retrieval failure at prone stereotactic core and vacuum breast biopsy—frequency, causes, and outcome. *Radiology* 2006;239:61–70.
83. Liberman L, Smolkin JH, Dershaw DD, et al. Calcification retrieval at stereotactic, 11-gauge, directional, vacuum-assisted breast biopsy. *Radiology* 1998;208:251–260.
84. Lomoschitz FM, Helbich TH, Rudas M, et al. Stereotactic 11-gauge vacuum-assisted breast biopsy: influence of number of specimens on diagnostic accuracy. *Radiology* 2004;232:897–903.
85. Margolin FR, Kaufman L, Jacobs RP, et al. Stereotactic core breast biopsy of malignant calcifications: diagnostic yield of cores with and cores without calcifications on specimen radiographs. *Radiology* 2004;233:251–254.
86. Pijnappel RM, van Dalen A, Borel Rinkes IHM, et al. The diagnostic accuracy of core biopsy in palpable and non-palpable breast lesions. *Eur J Radiol* 1997;24:120–123.
87. Liberman L, Dershaw DD, Glassman JR, et al. Analysis of cancers not diagnosed at stereotactic core breast biopsy. *Radiology* 1997;203:151–157.
88. Burbank F. Mammographic findings after 14-gauge automated needle and 14-gauge directional, vacuum-assisted stereotactic breast biopsies. *Radiology* 1997;204:153–156.
89. Lamm RL, Jackman RJ. Mammographic abnormalities caused by percutaneous stereotactic biopsy of histologically benign lesions evident on follow-up mammograms. *AJR Am J Roentgenol* 2000;174:753–756.
90. Berg WA. Image-guided breast biopsy and management of high-risk lesions. *Radiol Clin North Am* 2004;42:935–946.
91. Jackman RJ, Nowels KW, Rodriguez-Soto J, et al. Stereotactic, automated, large-core needle biopsy of nonpalpable breast lesions: false-negative and histologic underestimation rates after long-term follow-up. *Radiology* 1999;210:799–805.
92. Fajardo L. Cost-effectiveness of stereotaxic breast core needle biopsy. *Acad Radiol* 1996;3:S21–S23.
93. Dahlstrom JE, Jain S, Sutton T, et al. Diagnostic accuracy of stereotactic core biopsy in a mammographic breast cancer screening programme. *Histopathology* 1996;28:421–427.
94. Lee CH, Egglin TK, Philpotts L, et al. Cost-effectiveness of stereotactic core needle biopsy: analysis by means of mammographic findings. *Radiology* 1997;202:849–854.
95. Fuhrman GM, Cederbom G, Bolton JS, et al. Image-guided core-needle breast biopsy is an accurate technique to evaluate patients with nonpalpable imaging abnormalities. *Ann Surg* 1998;6:932–939.
96. Elvecrog EL, Lechner MC, Nelson MT. Nonpalpable breast lesions: correlation of stereotaxic large-core needle biopsy and surgical biopsy results. *Radiology* 1993;188:453–455.
97. Gisvold JJ, Goellner JR, Grant CS, et al. Breast biopsy: a comparative study of stereotaxically guided core and excisional techniques. *AJR Am J Roentgenol* 1994;162:815–820.
98. Pfarl G, Helbich TH, Riedl CC, et al. Stereotactic 11-gauge vacuum-assisted breast biopsy: a validation study. *AJR Am J Roentgenol* 2002;179:1503–1507.
99. Jackman RJ, Marzoni FJ Jr. Needle-localized breast biopsy: why do we fail? *Radiology* 1997;204:677–684.
100. Lee CH, Philpotts LE, Horvath LJ, et al. Follow-up of breast lesions diagnosed as benign with stereotactic core-needle biopsy: frequency of mammographic change and false-negative rate. *Radiology* 1999;212:189–194.
101. Goodman KA, Birdwell RL, Ikeda DM. Compliance with recommended follow-up after percutaneous breast core biopsy. *AJR Am J Roentgenol* 1998;170:89–92.
102. Dershaw DD, Morris EA, Liberman L, et al. Nondiagnostic stereotaxic core breast biopsy: results of re-biopsy. *Radiology* 1996;198:323–325.
103. Liberman L, Dershaw DD, Glassman JR, et al. Analysis of cancers not diagnosed at stereotactic core breast biopsy. *Radiology* 1997;203:151–157.
104. Jackman RJ, Nowels KW, Shepard MJ, et al. Stereotaxic large-core needle biopsy of 450 non-palpable breast lesions with surgical correlation in lesions with cancer or atypical hyperplasia. *Radiology* 1994;193:91–95.
105. Liberman L, Dershaw DD, Morris EA, et al. Clip placement after stereotactic vacuum-assisted breast biopsy. *Radiology* 1997;205:417–422.
106. Rosen EL, Baker JA, Soo MS. Accuracy of a collagen-plug biopsy site marking device deployed after stereotactic core needle breast biopsy. *AJR Am J Roentgenol* 2003;181:1295–1299.
107. Burbank F, Forcier N. Tissue marking clip for stereotactic breast biopsy: initial placement accuracy, long-term stability and usefulness as a guide for wire localization. *Radiology* 1997;205:407–415.
108. Rosen EL, Vo TT. Metallic clip deployment during stereotactic breast biopsy: retrospective analysis. *Radiology* 2001;218:510–516.
109. Liberman L, Dershaw DD, Morris EA, et al. Clip placement after stereotactic vacuum-assisted breast biopsy. *Radiology* 1997;205:417–422.
110. Burnside ES, Sohlich RE, Sickles EA. Movement of a biopsy-site marker clip after completion of stereotactic directional vacuum-assisted breast biopsy: case report. *Radiology* 2001;221:504–507.
111. Harris A. Clip migration within 8 days of 11-gauge vacuum-assisted stereotactic breast biopsy: case report. *Radiology* 2003;228:552 554.
112. Birdwell RL, Jackman RJ. Clip or marker migration 5–10 weeks after stereotactic 11-gauge vacuum-assisted breast biopsy: report of two cases. *Radiology* 2003;229:541–544.
113. Harris AT. Clip migration within 8 days of 11-gauge vacuum-assisted stereotactic breast biopsy: case report. *Radiology* 2003;228:552–554.
114. Dash N, Chafin SH, Johnson RR, et al. Usefulness of tissue marker clips in patients undergoing neoadjuvant chemotherapy for breast cancer. *AJR Am J Roentgenol* 1999;173:911–917.
115. Edeiken BS, Fornage BD, Bedi DG, et al. US-guided implantation of metallic markers for permanent localization of the tumor bed in patients with breast cancer who undergo preoperative chemotherapy. *Radiology* 1999;213:895–900.
116. Jackman RJ, Burbank F, Parker SH, et al. Stereotactic breast biopsy of nonpalpable lesions: determinants of ductal carcinoma in situ underestimation rates. *Radiology* 2001;218:497–502.
117. Brem RF, Schoonjans JM, Goodman SN, et al. Nonpalpable breast cancer: percutaneous diagnosis with 11- and 8-gauge stereotactic vacuum-assisted biopsy devices. *Radiology* 2001;219:793–796.
118. Burbank F. Stereotactic breast biopsy of atypical ductal hyperplasia and ductal carcinoma in situ lesions: improved accuracy with directional, vacuum-assisted biopsy. *Radiology* 1997;202:843–847.
119. Dillon MF, Quinn CM, McDermott EW, et al. Diagnostic accuracy of core biopsy for ductal carcinoma *in situ* and its implications for surgical practice. *J Clin Pathol* 2006;59:740–743.
120. Liberman L, Kaplan JB, Morris EA, et al. To excise or to sample the mammographic target: what is the goal of stereotactic 11-guage vacuum-assisted breast biopsy? *AJR Am J Roentgenol* 2002;179:679–683.

121. Lourenco AP, Mainiero MB, Lazarus E, et al. Stereotactic breast biopsy: comparison of histologic underestimation rates with 11- and 9-gauge vacuum-assisted breast biopsy. *AJR Am J Roentgenol* 2007;189:W275–W279.
122. Page DL, Dupont WD, Rogers LW, et al. Atypical hyperplastic lesions of the female breast: a long-term follow-up study. *Cancer* 1985;55:2698–2708.
123. Tavassoli F. Intraductal hyperplasia, ordinary and atypical. In: Tavassoli FA, ed. *Pathology of the breast*. Norwalk, CT: Appleton & Lange, 1992:155–191.
124. Winchester DJ, Bernstein JR, Jeske JM, et al. Upstaging of atypical ductal hyperplasia after vacuum-assisted 11-gauge stereotactic core needle biopsy. *Arch Surg* 2003;138:619–623.
125. Jackman RJ, Birdwell RL, Ikeda DM. Atypical ductal hyperplasia: can some lesions be defined as probably benign after stereotactic 11-gauge vacuum-assisted biopsy, eliminating the recommendation for surgical excision. *Radiology* 2002;224:548–544.
126. Adrales G, Turk P, Wallace T, et al. Is surgical excision necessary for atypical ductal hyperplasia of the breast diagnosed by mammotome? *Am J Surg* 2000;180: 313–315.
127. Berg WA, Mrose HE, Ioffe OB. Atypical lobular hyperplasia or lobular carcinoma in situ at core-needle breast biopsy. *Radiology* 2001;218:503–509.
128. Renshaw AA, Cartagena N, Derhagopian RP, et al. Lobular neoplasia in breast core needle biopsy specimens is not associated with an increased risk of ductal carcinoma *in situ* or invasive carcinoma. *Am J Clin Pathol* 2002;117:797–799.
129. Liberman L, Sama M, Susnik B, et al. Lobular carcinoma *in situ* at percutaneous breast biopsy: surgical biopsy findings. *AJR Am J Roentgenol* 1999;173:291–299.
130. Philpotts LE, Shaheen NA, Jain KS, et al. Uncommon high-risk lesions of the breast diagnosed at stereotactic core-needle biopsy: clinical importance. *Radiology* 2000;216:831–837.
131. Lechner MC, Jackman RJ, Brem RF, et al. Lobular carcinoma in situ and atypical lobular hyperplasia at percutaneous biopsy with surgical correlation: a multi-institutional study. *Radiology* 1999;213:106.
132. Irfan K, Brem RF. Surgical and mammographic follow-up of papillary lesions and atypical lobular hyperplasia diagnosed with stereotactic vacuum-assisted biopsy. *Breast J* 2002;8:230–233.
133. Newman L. Lobular carcinoma *in situ*: clinical management. In: Harris JR, ME Lippman, Morrow M, et al., eds. *Diseases of the breast*. 4th ed. Philadelphia: Lippincott Williams & Wilkins, 2009:ch. 25.
134. Georgian-Smith D, Lawton TJ. Calcifications of lobular carcinoma *in situ* in the breast: radiologic-pathologic correlation. *AJR Am J Roentgenol* 2001;176: 1255–1259.
135. Foster MC, Helvie MA, Gregory NE, et al. Lobular carcinoma *in situ* or atypical lobular hyperplasia at core-needle biopsy: is excisional biopsy necessary? *Radiology* 2004;231:813–819.
136. Cohen MA. Cancer upgrades at excisional biopsy after diagnosis of atypical lobular hyperplasia or lobular carcinoma *in situ* at core-needle biopsy: some reasons why. *Radiology* 2004;231:617–621.
137. Dershaw DD. Does LCIS or ALH without other high-risk lesions diagnosed on core biopsy require surgical excision? *Breast J* 2003;9:1–3.
138. de la Torre A, Lindholm K, Lingren A. Fine needle aspiration cytology of tubular breast carcinoma and radial scar. *Acta Cytol* 1994;38:884.
139. Jackman RJ, Finkelstein SL, Marzoni FA. Stereotaxic large-core needle biopsy of histologically benign nonpalpable breast lesions: false-negative results and failed follow-up. *Radiology* 1995;197:203–206.
140. Orel SG, Evers K, Yeh IT, et al. Radial scar with microcalcifications: radiologic-pathologic correlation. *Radiology* 1992;183:479–482.
141. Douglas-Jones AG, Denson JL, Cox AC, et al. Radial scar lesions of the breast diagnosed by needle core biopsy: analysis of cases containing occult malignancy. *J Clin Pathol* 2007;60:295–298.
142. Tavassoli F. Papillary lesions. In: Tavassoli FA, ed. *Pathology of the breast*. Norwalk, CT: Appleton & Lange, 1992:193–227.
143. Liberman L, Bracero N, Vuolo MA, et al. Percutaneous large-core biopsy of papillary breast lesions. *AJR Am J Roentgenol* 1999;172:331–337.
144. Sydnor MK, Wilson JD, Hijaz TA, et al. Underestimation of the presence of breast carcinoma in papillary lesions initially diagnosed at core-needle biopsy. *Radiology* 2006;242:58–62.
145. Sohn V, Keylock J, Arthurs Z, et al. Breast papillomas in the era of percutaneous needle biopsy. *Ann Surg Oncol* 2007;14:2979–2984.
146. Mercado CL, Hamele-Bena D, Singer C, et al. Papillary lesions of the breast: evaluation with stereotactic directional vacuum-assisted biopsy. *Radiology* 2001;221: 650–655.
147. Mercado CL, Hamele-Bena D, Oken SM, et al. Papillary lesions of the breast at percutaneous core-needle biopsy. *Radiology* 2006;238:801–808.
148. Liberman L, Feng TL, Dershaw DD, et al. US-guided core breast biopsy: use and cost-effectiveness. *Radiology* 1998;208:717–723.
149. Liberman L, Fahs MC, Dershaw DD, et al. Impact of stereotaxic core biopsy on cost of diagnosis. *Radiology* 1995;195:633–637.
150. Lindfors KK, Rosenquist CJ. Needle core biopsy guided with mammography: a study of cost effectiveness. *Radiology* 1994;190:217–222.

Monica Morrow

The evaluation of abnormal findings on a screening mammogram in an asymptomatic woman has been well characterized and usually begins with diagnostic mammography to confirm the presence of a persistent, abnormal finding and to characterize the degree of suspicion for carcinoma. As outlined in Chapter 12, the majority of abnormalities identified on a screening mammogram are resolved with a diagnostic work-up and only about 10% will require a tissue diagnosis. The interval of the lesion is an essential part of the evaluation as it reliably allows the identification of simple cysts that require no further intervention. Even in the case of calcifications, ultrasonography is useful to determine if there is an associated mass lesion. Visualization of the calcifications with ultrasound allows an ultrasound-guided biopsy to be performed, avoiding exposure to ionizing radiation and the need for breast compression during the biopsy procedure.

Although the characteristics of benign and malignant lesions differ on both mammography and ultrasonography, the currently accepted threshold for considering a biopsy in the United States is a probability of malignancy of 3% to 4% or more (1). It was initially hoped that magnetic resonance imaging (MRI) would reliably differentiate benign and malignant abnormalities, reducing the number of biopsies generated by screening programs. Studies have demonstrated that MRI lacks the sensitivity and specificity to substitute for a histologic diagnosis and should not be obtained for this purpose. In a multicenter trial of 821 women with clinical, mammographic, or ultrasound findings suspicious enough to warrant biopsy, Bluemke et al. (2) found that MRI had a sensitivity of 88.1% for the detection of cancer (95% confidence interval [CI], 84.6%–91.1%), a specificity of 67.4% (95% CI, 62.7%–71.9%), and a negative predictive value of 85.4% (95% CI, 81.1%–89.0%). The use of MRI as a screening tool is discussed in Chapter 11. At present, clear evidence of the benefit for MRI screening exists only for women at a very high risk of breast cancer development, such as those with known or suspected *BRCA1* and *BRCA2* mutations.

In contrast to the evaluation of an abnormality detected on a screening mammogram, where the characteristics of the lesion determine the appropriate work-up, in the patient with a diagnosis of carcinoma the imaging evaluation should be tailored to the clinical circumstances. The routine use of ultrasound and MRI in all women with breast cancer is unnecessary and has the potential to both increase the cost of care and delay treatment of the cancer. For example, in the woman with clinically or mammographically evident multicentric cancer, mastectomy is medically indicated (3) and additional imaging characterization of the size or extent of the lesions will not change management. The same is true of the patient with inflammatory breast cancer. In contrast, in the patient who presents with axillary adenopathy in whom a primary tumor is not evident clinically or mammographically, additional imaging to identify the primary tumor site has the potential to be a great benefit, as discussed in Chapters 14 and 69. The extent of the imaging evaluation that is needed to confirm that a woman is an appropriate candidate for breast-conserving therapy (BCT) is the subject of much debate. The potential roles of imaging in the patient with a diagnosis of cancer are listed in Table 17.1. With the exception of the synchronous diagnosis of contralateral cancer, it is apparent that there are no added benefits for additional imaging evaluation of the patient who desires or requires mastectomy. The outcomes of BCT in patients selected for the

procedure using diagnostic mammography, with or without ultrasound of the primary tumor, are well documented. Ten-year rates of ipsilateral breast tumor recurrence in patients treated with BCT in National Surgical Adjuvant Breast and Bowel Project (NSABP) trials between 1984 and 1994 ranged from 3.5% to 6.5% for node positive patients (4) and 4.8% to 10% for node negative patients (5). In spite of this, multiple studies examining the benefit of MRI in patient selection for BCT have documented that additional tumors are identified in 15% to 25% of patients (6–8). In these studies, the most common change in treatment as a result of the MRI findings was a mastectomy that would not otherwise have been done, in spite of the fact that the frequency with which additional tumors are identified on MRI far exceeds the 10-year local recurrence rates with BCT in similar patients not evaluated by MRI. Direct evidence that MRI decreases local failure rate after BCT is lacking. Solin et al. (9) retrospectively examined local failure rates after BCT in 215 women who had an MRI as part of their initial evaluation and 541 who did not. The 8-year rates of local failure were 3% and 4% for women with and without MRI, respectively.

Similar controversy exists regarding the benefits of whole breast ultrasound in the patient with cancer. Wilkinson et al. (10) studied 102 newly diagnosed cancer patients seen in a 6-month time period and identified additional tumor with ultrasonography in 19% of cases. Surgical therapy was changed in 8%, and the number of benign biopsies was not significantly increased compared to a control group treated 1 year previously who had targeted ultrasonography only. Berg et al. (7) identified additional carcinoma in 18% of 96 breasts with ultrasonography, although the extent was overestimated in 12%. In contrast, Golshan et al. (11) reported that in 426 patients with stage I or II breast cancer the findings of the whole breast ultrasound changed surgical management in only 2.8% of cases. The use of ultrasound in this population resulted in 63 benign biopsies, 351 studies that were normal, and the identification of 12 malignancies more than 1 cm distant from the known primary tumor. At present, there are no data for either whole breast ultrasound or MRI indicating that these examinations improve outcome by decreasing the incidence of local recurrence, decreasing the number of patients who require re-excision, or decreasing conversion from BCT to mastectomy.

Information on the proportion of women attempting BCT who ultimately require mastectomy due to failure to obtain negative margins is limited. In a population-based study of 1,338 women treated in 2005, BCT was attempted in 800 and was unsuccessful in 12% (12). However, two thirds of the patients who underwent mastectomy did so after a single lumpectomy attempt, making it unclear whether a re-excision would have allowed BCT. Whether additional imaging studies such as whole breast ultrasound or MRI will reduce the frequency of re-excisions to achieve negative margins is also unclear. In the population-based study of Morrow et al. (12), discussed above, 20% of patients undergoing successful BCT had re-excision. The rate of re-excision reported in the literature varies widely. However, it appears that much of the variation may be due to the lack of a standard, accepted definition of what constitutes a negative margin. In a population-based survey of 188 surgeons who were asked what margin width precludes the need for re-excision of a T2-infiltrating ductal tumor in a patient who will receive chemotherapy and radiation therapy, 13% accepted tumor not touching the ink, 35% required a margin greater than 2 mm,

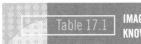

IMAGING EVALUATION IN THE PATIENT WITH KNOWN CANCER	
Imaging Role	**Clinical Correlate**
Accurately assess extent of disease	Decrease conversion from breast-conserving therapy to mastectomy
	Decrease number of re-excisions
Identify clinically occult multicentric disease	Decrease local recurrence
Identify residual disease postoperatively in cases of positive/unknown margins	Decrease negative re-excisions
Identify contralateral cancer	Synchronous treatment

36% greater than 5 mm, and 16% greater than 1 cm. A similar lack of consensus has been reported among radiation oncologists (13), with 46% of North American radiation oncologists accepting a negative margin as no tumor cells touching the inked surface, but only 28% of European radiation oncologists accepting this definition. This lack of agreement on what constitutes a negative margin and the uncertainty regarding the relationship between margin width and local control is unlikely to be resolved by the use of additional imaging techniques.

The other role of imaging in the woman with known cancer is to identify contralateral breast cancers. Lehman et al. (14) reported a 3.1% incidence of contralateral carcinoma identified by MRI within 12 months of initial cancer diagnosis, suggesting that MRI might allow synchronous rather than metachronous treatment of the opposite breast. This result is promising but does not take into account the 50% or greater reduction in contralateral breast cancer that occurs with adjuvant endocrine therapy or the 20% reduction seen with chemotherapy in the early breast cancer trialists collaborative group overview analysis (15). In the study of Solin et al. (9) a 6% incidence of contralateral breast cancer was seen at 8 years in both the MRI and non-MRI groups. Further data are needed to determine if the increased early detection of contralateral cancers with MRI reported by Lehman et al. translates into a longer term reduction in contralateral breast cancer incidence, or if these subclinical cancers are adequately treated with adjuvant systemic therapy. Although the routine use of MRI in the patient with breast cancer remains controversial, there are a number of clinical circumstances where it is clearly beneficial. These include women with known or suspected *BRCA1* and *BRCA2* mutations, identification of the primary tumor in patients presenting with axillary adenopathy, and in assessment of the response to preoperative or neoadjuvant chemotherapy. These are discussed in detail in Chapter 14.

Image-guided biopsy of nonpalpable breast lesions is a well-established technique that has been shown to be a reliable, cost-effective method of diagnosis. Histologic diagnoses on core biopsy associated with a significant risk of malignancy are well recognized, and these are detailed in Chapter 16. The use of surgical biopsy in these cases minimizes the risk of a missed cancer diagnosis. In a study of 318 patients undergoing 11-gauge vacuum-assisted biopsy between 1997 and 2001, the false-negative rate was 3.3%, which fell to 0.6% if the radiologist had done more than six biopsies. All of the missed cancers were identified at the time of biopsy due to discordance between the imaging findings and the histologic diagnosis or the failure to sample calcifications (16). The use of a needle biopsy for diagnosis allows the assessment of markers such as ER, PR, and *HER2*, avoids the placement of an incision on the breast prior to definitive local therapy and is the most cost-effective approach to diagnosis regardless of lesion type or degree of suspicion (17). In spite of this, a study of 5.5 million mammograms performed in two U.S.

government programs and the United Kingdom National Health Service between 1996 and 1999 found that 51% of the biopsies in the United States were surgical compared to 23% in the United Kingdom (18). There are a few indications for surgical biopsy as an initial diagnostic approach, with the most common being the inability to target the mammographic lesion. Although patients often express concerns that a surgical biopsy might be "safer," an explanation of the safeguards in place to avoid missing a cancer diagnosis when needle biopsy is done is usually sufficient to resolve these fears.

SUMMARY

- Screening mammography is the only imaging modality proven to reduce breast cancer mortality in asymptomatic women.
- MRI screening has been shown to be of benefit in the early diagnosis of cancer in *BRCA1* and *BRCA2* carriers.
- The evaluation of an abnormal screening mammogram includes additional diagnostic views, and in the case of masses or architectural distortions, an ultrasound to further characterize the lesion and determine the method of guidance for the biopsy.
- MRI lacks the sensitivity and specificity to substitute for a histologic diagnosis in patients with suspicious mammographic or ultrasound findings and should not be ordered for this purpose.
- Image-guided core biopsy is the diagnostic procedure of choice for the majority of nonpalpable abnormalities that require histologic sampling. Deployment of a clip at the time of biopsy allows reliable identification of the tumor site if the entire imaging target is removed with the biopsy and in the patient receiving neoadjuvant therapy.
- The imaging evaluation of the symptomatic patient is greatly enhanced by communication between clinicians and imagers. This allows placement of a marker on the area of clinical concern and a focused examination.
- Suspicious clinical findings warrant a histologic diagnosis unless imaging studies provide a definitive diagnosis (i.e., fat necrosis). The absence of imaging abnormalities does not obviate the need for a biopsy.
- The extent of the additional imaging work-up performed in a patient with known cancer should be tailored to the clinical scenario. When absolute indications for mastectomy are present (inflammatory carcinoma, multicentricity), attempts to further characterize the extent of the tumor are unwarranted.
- The ability of MRI or whole breast ultrasound to facilitate the selection of local therapy, aid in achieving negative margins, or reduce the rate of local recurrence in the conserved breast is unproven. At this time, these studies should not be considered a routine part of the presurgical evaluation.
- MRI and whole breast ultrasound may be useful in problem solving, for example when mammography cannot identify a primary tumor or its extent is unclear.

References

1. American College of Radiology. Bi-RADS Atlas breast imaging and reporting data system, 4th ed. Reston, VA, American College of Radiology, 2003.
2. Bluemke DA, Gatsonis CA, Chen MH, et al. Magnetic resonance imaging of the breast prior to biopsy. *JAMA* 2004;292:2735–2742.
3. Morrow M, Harris JR. Practice guideline for breast conservation therapy in the management of invasive breast carcinoma. *J Am Coll Surg* 2007;205:145–161.
4. Wapnir IL, Anderson SJ, Mamounas EP, et al. Prognosis after ipsilateral breast tumor recurrence and locoregional recurrences in five National Surgical Adjuvant Breast and Bowel Project node-positive adjuvant breast cancer trials. *J Clin Oncol* 2006;24:2028–2037.

5. Wapnir I, Anderson S, Mamounas E, et al. Survival after IBTR in NSABP node negative protocols B-13, B-14, B-19, B-20, and B-23. *J Clin Oncol* 2005;23:8s (abst517).

6. Bedrosian I, Mick R, Orel SG, et al. Changes in the surgical management of patients with breast carcinoma based on preoperative magnetic resonance imaging. *Cancer* 2003;98:468–473.

7. Berg WA, Gutierrez L, NessAiver MS, et al. Diagnostic accuracy of mammography, clinical examination, US, and MR imaging in preoperative assessment of breast cancer. *Radiology* 2004;233:830–849.

8. Deurloo EE, Peterse JL, Rutgers EJ, et al. Additional breast lesions in patients eligible for breast-conserving therapy by MRI: impact on preoperative management and potential benefit of computerised analysis. *Eur J Cancer* 2005;41: 1393–1401.

9. Solin LJ, Orel SG, Hwang WT, et al. Relationship of breast magnetic resonance imaging to outcome after breast-conservation treatment with radiation for women with early stage invasive breast carcinoma or ductal carcinoma *in situ*. *J Clin Oncol* 2008;26:386–391.

10. Wilkinson LS, Given-Wilson R, Hall T, et al. Increasing the diagnosis of multifocal primary breast cancer by the use of bilateral whole breast ultrasound. *Clin Radiol* 2005;60:573–578.

11. Golshan M, Fung BB, Wolfman J, et al. The effect of ipsilateral whole breast ultrasonography on the surgical management of breast carcinoma. *Am J Surg* 2003; 186:391–396.

12. Morrow M. Why do women get mastectomy? Results from a population-based study. *J Clin Oncol* 2007;25(185):285(abst605).

13. Taghian A, Mohiuddin M, Jagsi R, et al. Current perceptions regarding surgical margin status after breast-conserving therapy: results of a survey. *Ann Surg* 2005; 241:629–639.

14. Lehman CD, Gatsonis C, Kuhl CK, et al. MRI evaluation of the contralateral breast in women with recently diagnosed breast cancer. *N Engl J Med* 2007;356:1295–1303.

15. Early Breast Cancer Trialists' Collaborative Group (EBCTCG). Effects of chemotherapy and hormonal therapy for early breast cancer on recurrence and 15-year survival: an overview of the randomised trials. *Lancet* 2005;365:1687–1717.

16. Pfarl G, Helbich TH, Riedl CC, et al. Stereotactic 11-gauge vacuum-assisted breast biopsy: a validation study. *AJR Am J Roentgenol* 2002;179:1503–1507.

17. Golub RM, Bennett CL, Stinson T, et al. Cost minimization study of image-guided core biopsy versus surgical excisional biopsy for women with abnormal mammograms. *J Clin Oncol* 2004;22:2430–2437.

18. Smith-Bindman R, Chu PW, Miglioretti DL, et al. Comparison of screening mammography in the United States and the United Kingdom. *JAMA* 2003;290: 2129–2137.

Chapter 18
Inherited Genetic Factors and Breast Cancer

Alan Ashworth, Barbara L. Weber, and Susan M. Domchek

High-penetrance cancer susceptibility genes appear directly responsible for 5% to 10% of all breast cancers (1). Although much remains to be learned about the heritable factors involved, enormous strides have been made in understanding inherited susceptibility to this disease. These advances are based on the discovery and characterization of a number of genes responsible for the clustering of breast cancer in certain families. However, still, little is known about gene–gene and gene–environment interactions that likely modulate risk.

Given the strong influence of molecular genetics, there is a tendency to assume that familial clustering of disease invariably results from inherited predisposition. However, other explanations for familial clustering of breast cancer should be considered including (a) geographically limited environmental exposure to carcinogens, which might affect an extended family living in close proximity; (b) culturally motivated behavior that alters risk factor profile, such as age at first live birth; and (c) socioeconomic influences that, for example, might result in differing dietary exposures. In addition, multiple, complex inherited genetic factors likely influence the extent to which a risk factor for breast cancer plays a role in any one individual; such modifying effects are likely to be shared among genetically related members of an extended family. The epidemiology of breast cancer is discussed in greater detail in Chapter 20.

CLINICAL FEATURES OF HEREDITARY BREAST CANCER

Breast cancers caused by mutations in high-penetrance susceptibility genes have several distinctive clinical features: Age at diagnosis is considerably younger than in sporadic cases, the prevalence of bilateral breast cancer is higher, and associated tumors are noted in some families. Associated tumors may include ovarian, colon, prostate, pancreatic, and endometrial cancers, among others, as well as sarcomas (2) and breast cancer in male family members (3,4). Evidence reviewed later in this chapter also supports the notion that tumors arising in the setting of inherited mutations in susceptibility genes have different characteristics with regard to grade, estrogen receptor (ER) status, and molecular profile (5). Whether these cancers respond differently to treatment or are associated with a worse prognosis than sporadic tumors remains controversial.

EPIDEMIOLOGIC STUDIES OF FAMILIAL BREAST CANCER

The first attempts to determine the influence of family history on breast cancer risk were published in the first half of the 20th century (6,7). Although many of these studies have methodologic flaws, they consistently demonstrated a two- to threefold increase in breast cancer risk in mothers and sisters of patients

with breast cancer. The first large population-based study to estimate breast cancer risk associated with a family history was conducted in Sweden and involved 2,660 women (8). Within this study cohort, women with an affected relative had an increased breast cancer risk of 1.7 compared with those without. Relative risks (RR) of a similar magnitude were found in a Canadian population-based study (9) and in the U.S. Nurses' Health Study (10).

In the population-based Carolina Breast Cancer Study, 20% of individuals with breast cancer reported a first-degree relative with breast cancer, and 49% reported breast cancer in at least one relative of any type (11). The increased breast cancer incidence in this population, compared with that in the previously cited historical studies, as well as increases in both public awareness and the likelihood that women will discuss a diagnosis of breast cancer with family members, likely contributes to higher reporting of affected family members.

Anderson (12) was among the first to suggest that breast cancer was not a homogeneous disease and that the occurrence of breast cancer was not influenced by genetic factors in a uniform manner. He suggested that a small subset of families with a very high risk of developing breast cancer owing to a single genetic defect might be obscured in studies in which most breast cancer cases were multifactorial in origin. To emphasize the hereditary component, Anderson (12,13) assembled a database enriched for kindreds with a family history of breast cancer. The primary factors that increased risk within families were premenopausal status at time of diagnosis and bilateral disease.

By 1980, a significant body of evidence had accumulated supporting the presence of inherited factors responsible for familial clustering of breast cancer, and efforts shifted to determining the inheritance pattern of breast cancer within these families. In 1984, Williams and Anderson (14) examined 200 Danish pedigrees and provided the first evidence for an autosomal-dominant breast cancer susceptibility gene with age-related penetrance. This finding was supported 1988 by Newman et al. (15).

Although researchers are beginning to understand the influence of genetic factors on the incidence of breast cancer in largely white, Western populations of women, less is known about breast cancer risk attributable to inherited factors in other populations. The CARE study (Contraceptive and Reproductive Experience study), a population-based study, indicates that breast cancer risks for white and black women with a family history of the disease are similar through age 49. However, white women have a higher risk of breast cancer after this, and this risk increases as the number of affected first-degree relatives increases (16–18). Other studies in black women and the few studies that have examined breast cancer risk in Asian, Arab, and Hispanic women have concluded that a family history of breast cancer confers a similar magnitude of increased risk as is seen in white population-based studies (19–27).

How Much Breast Cancer Is Due to Inherited Susceptibility?

Two groups (26,28) have analyzed data from the Cancer and Steroid Hormone (CASH) study, a large case-control study initiated in 1981. In this study group, 11% of patients with breast cancer reported a first-degree relative with breast cancer, compared with 5% of control individuals (26). Using these data, Claus et al. (29) estimated that 36% of breast cancer cases in women aged 20 to 29 years are attributable to a single dominant susceptibility gene, with this fraction decreasing to less than 1% for women 80 years or older. Analysis of women diagnosed with breast cancer before age 40 years suggests that approximately 10% of such American women have a *BRCA1* mutation (30,31) whereas the prevalence of *BRCA2* mutations may be lower in this group (32). Results from several population-based studies of *BRCA1* and *BRCA2* mutations suggest that mutations in these genes account for 2.0% to 3.3% of breast cancer in a group of unselected women (11,18,33). In summary, current estimates place the percentage of breast cancer cases primarily attributable to inherited factors at 5% to 10%.

AUTOSOMAL DOMINANT INHERITANCE

To date, all studies of inherited susceptibility to breast cancer suggest that breast cancer susceptibility is transmitted in an autosomal-dominant mendelian fashion, and the identification of an increasing number of genes has borne out this modeling (1,34) (Table 18.1).

With a pattern of autosomal-dominant inheritance, an individual can have one of three possible genotypes: carrier of two nonmutant alleles (homozygous normal), or carrier of one (heterozygous) or two (homozygous) mutant alleles. The actual risk of developing breast cancer in a mutation carrier is based on the penetrance of the gene. Penetrance is the likelihood that the effect (phenotype) of a mutation (genotype) will

become clinically apparent. Individuals carrying two copies of an autosomal-dominant, disease–related gene are rare, partly because of the relative rarity of heterozygotes and partly because of the potential for a lethal defect in a homozygous affected fetus. Only one individual with two mutant *BRCA1* alleles (35) has been reported with none reported in the Ashkenazi Jewish and Icelandic populations where such occurrences are mathematically more likely (36). Given that a subsequent report demonstrating that an apparent homozygous *BRCA1* mutation was an artifact of polymerase chain reaction (PCR), the accuracy of this initial report is unclear (37). Biallelic (homozygous) deleterious mutations in *BRCA2* have been reported, however, in patients with Fanconi anemia type D1, a rare recessive disorder characterized by leukemia and birth defects (38). Finally, there are several reports of individuals who have both *BRCA1* and *BRCA2* mutations (39). Anecdotal observations suggest that these women develop more frequent and earlier cancers than single mutation carriers, but the number of such individuals identified is too small for definitive studies.

A 50% chance exists that an individual offspring will inherit a mutant copy of any given gene from a heterozygous parent. Therefore, on average, 50% of the related individuals in a family carry the mutant gene being transmitted. If the penetrance of the gene is high, the pedigree pattern for an autosomal-dominant disease is striking, with vertical inheritance and half the children of an affected parent also being affected, whereas none of the offspring of a homozygous normal parent are affected. This pedigree pattern also presupposes a low risk in the general population, which is not the case for breast cancer. As a result, breast cancer in women from families that have a known *BRCA1* mutation but who do not themselves carry the mutation is not uncommon. Such women are termed *phenocopies*, because they have the phenotype associated with the gene mutation but are noncarriers. This situation is illustrated in the pedigree shown in Figure 18.1, a typical pedigree of a family known to carry a mutation in *BRCA1*. As long as the gene being examined is not on the X or Y sex-determining

| Table 18.1 | GENETIC PREDISPOSITION TO BREAST CANCER |

Syndrome	Gene	Inheritance	Cancers	Other Features
Breast/Ovarian Cancer Syndrome	*BRCA1*	AD	Breast, Ovarian	
Breast/Ovarian Cancer Syndrome	*BRCA2*	AD	Breast, Ovarian Prostate, Pancreatic	Fanconi Anemia in Homozygotes
Breast, Ovarian, Li-Fraumeni Syndrome	*TP53*	AD	Breast, Brain, Soft Tissue Sarcomas, Osteosarcomas, Leukemia, Adrenocortical Carcinomas, Others	
Cowden Disease	*PTEN*	AD	Breast, Ovary, Follicular Thyroid Colon Cancer	Adenomas of Thyroid, Fibroids, Gastrointestinal Tract Polyps
Peutz-Jegher Syndrome	*STKII/LKB1*	AD	Gastrointestinal, Breast	Hamartomas of Bowel, Pigmentation of Buccal Mucosa, Digits
Ataxia-telangiectasia	*ATM*	AD	Breast	Homozygotes: Leukemia, Lymphoma Cerebellar Ataxia, Immune Deficiency, Telangiectasias
Site-specific Breast Cancer	*CHEK2*	AD	Breast Cancer	Low Penetrance
Muir-Torre Syndrome	*MSH2/MLH1*	AD	Colorectal, Breast	
Site-specific Breast Cancer	*PALB2*	AD (?)	Breast cancer	Low/Moderate Penetrance Fanconi Anemia in Homozygotes
Site-specific Breast Cancer	*BRIP1*	AD (?)	Breast Cancer	Low/Moderate Penetrance Fanconi anemia in homozygotes

Note: AD, autosomal dominant. Other low penetrance alleles have been detected using genome wide association studies. The affected gene in most cases is not known (34).

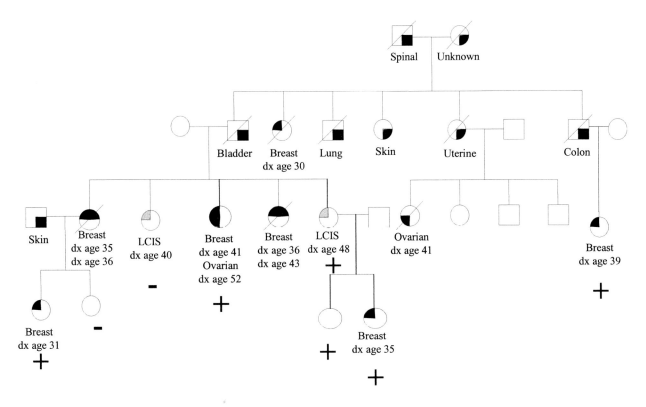

FIGURE 18.1. A kindred with a *BRCA1* mutation. □, Unaffected men; O, unaffected women; cancers are indicated with dark shading of symbols; , known *BRCA1* mutation carriers; , individuals who tested negative; all others are untested. Deceased individuals are indicated with a diagonal line through the symbol. One family member with lobular carcinoma *in situ* (LCIS) tested positive, and the other tested negative, consistent with previous reports suggesting LCIS is not a component of *BRCA1*-related cancer susceptibility.

chromosomes, the sex of the carrier is irrelevant. In the case of autosomal-dominant inheritance of breast cancer, significant sex-related differences in the penetrance of mutations exist. Therefore, although mutations occur equally in male and female populations, breast cancer is much more common in women with *BRCA1* or *BRCA2* mutations than in men, but male breast cancer is part of the spectrum of both *BRCA1* and *BRCA2*. However, the lifetime risk of breast cancer is clearly higher in male *BRCA2* carriers (lifetime risk estimate 5% to 10%) than male *BRCA1* carriers (1% to 5%) (40,41).

TUMOR SUPPRESSOR GENES

Two fundamental types of genetic alterations responsible for the development of the malignant phenotype are found in cancer cells: (a) activation of proto-oncogene producing a "gain of function" in the affected cell and (b) inactivation of tumor suppressor genes producing a "loss of function" in the cell. Some tumor suppressor genes are important in cell-cycle regulation, normally functioning as checks on cell growth; others are critical elements in the cellular response to DNA damage, preventing the propagation of mutations in other critical genes. Mutated tumor suppressor genes lose these regulatory functions, leading to malignant transformation. Because all individuals are born with two alleles of every gene, an explanation was needed, however, for the development of cancer in large numbers of individuals who had only a single inherited mutation in a tumor suppressor gene. In 1971, Knudson (42) put forth the "two-hit hypothesis," suggesting that cancer arises as a result of two genetic events occurring in the same cell, inactivating both copies of a given tumor suppressor gene. In the case of sporadic cancer (i.e., cancer occurring in women without a family history

of the disease), the likelihood that two events would occur in the same gene in the same cell is quite low. However, individuals from "cancer families" inherit an inactivating mutation in one allele of the implicated tumor suppressor gene in all cells (i.e., a germline mutation); therefore, only one somatic (noninherited) event is required to inactivate the single remaining copy, making the development of cancer a much more common event than in individuals born without the "first hit." Of particular relevance to breast cancer are the tumor suppressor genes *TP53*, *BRCA1*, and *BRCA2*.

HEREDITARY BREAST CANCER SYNDROMES

The study of clinical syndromes that include an increased incidence of breast cancer has provided insight into the mechanisms by which genetic mutations result in the development of cancer. The most frequently identified pedigrees contain site-specific breast cancer (i.e., breast cancer in these families is not found in association with inherited susceptibility to other cancers, such as ovarian) and are thought to represent the effect of a single genetic abnormality; *BRCA1* and *BRCA2* are the best studied examples. Breast cancer also has been noted to occur in association with other cancers. The occurrence of breast cancer in association with diverse childhood neoplasms in the Li-Fraumeni/SBLA (soft tissue and bony sarcomas, *b*rain tumors, *l*eukemias, and *a*drenocortical carcinomas) (43) syndrome and the association between breast and ovarian cancer represent some of the most intensively studied examples. An elevated frequency of breast cancer may occur in patients with hereditary syndromes that include nonmalignant manifestations as well, such as Cowden disease and Muir-Torre syndrome (44–46). An

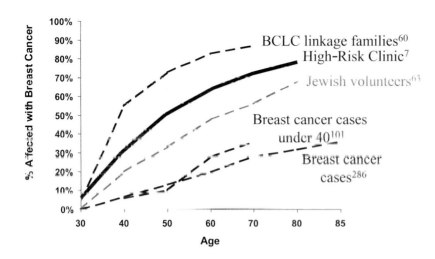

FIGURE 18.2. Breast cancer risk estimates associated with BRCA1 mutations vary depending on sample ascertainment. Breast cancer risks (penetrance) will be highest in families selected to have multiple affected family members for use in linkage studies (49) and lowest in population-based ascertainments (80,216). Sample sets collected in breast cancer risk evaluation clinics would be expected to be intermediate between these two ascertainments; recent data have confirmed that hypothesis (85). An ascertainment of Ashkenazi Jewish volunteers also falls between high- and low-risk penetrance estimates, again because this sample is likely a mix of population-based ascertainment and individuals who volunteer because they were aware of a strong family history (57).

increasing number of moderate risk genes—*ATM*, *CHEK2*, *PALB2*, and *BRIP1*—are being identified that lead to an increased risk of cancer of two- to fourfold (34). Finally, numerous common variants (population frequency 5% to 50%) in genes, which cause a very modest (1.25 to 1.65 fold) elevation in risk, are just starting to become part of the landscape of breast cancer susceptibility (34) (see also Chapter 20).

BRCA1 and BRCA2

In 1990, chromosome 17q21 was identified as the location of a susceptibility gene for early onset breast cancer, now termed *BRCA1* (47). Shortly thereafter, linkage between the genetic marker D17S74 on 17q21 and the appearance of ovarian cancer in several large kindreds was also demonstrated (48) (see Fig 18.1). Initial estimates suggested that *BRCA1* mutations were responsible for more than 90% of breast cancer cases in families with apparent autosomal-dominant transmission of breast cancer and at least one case of ovarian cancer, and 45% of cases in families with breast cancer only. However, the percentage of site-specific breast cancer cases attributed to *BRCA1* mutations rose to almost 70% if the median age at onset of breast cancer in the families was younger than 45 years (49), demonstrating the critical importance of the characteristics of a family to the likelihood that a *BRCA1* mutation will be detectable (see Fig 18.2). The *BRCA1* gene, identified in 1994 (50), encodes a novel protein now known to be important in the cellular response to DNA damage (51,52).

Initial progress toward the identification of a second breast cancer susceptibility gene came from a linkage analysis of 22 families with multiple cases of early-onset female breast cancer and at least one case of male breast cancer. Linkage between male breast cancer and polymorphic genetic markers on chromosome 13q12-13 identified the *BRCA2* locus (4). In 1995, the partial sequence of *BRCA2* and six germline mutations that truncated the putative *BRCA2* protein were identified (53). Shortly thereafter, the complete structure of the *BRCA2* gene was published (54).

BRCA1 is composed of 24 exons (coding regions) and is translated into a protein consisting of 1,863 amino acids (Fig. 18.3A). The coding region of *BRCA2* is 11.2 kb in length and is made up of 26 exons which produce a protein of 3,418 amino acids. The size of these genes is important from a clinical standpoint in the context of genetic testing, because this makes screening for mutations technically demanding and costly. Furthermore, the *BRCA1* gene contains a large number of repetitive elements that facilitate the generation of large dele-

tions and duplications. For example, disease-associated deletions account for 36% of *BRCA1* mutations in The Netherlands (55).

More than 500 coding region sequence variations have been detected in *BRCA1* and 250 in *BRCA2*. A listing and description of most known mutations is available on the Breast Cancer Information Core (BIC) website (*research.nhgri.nih.gov/bic/*) Several similarities between *BRCA1* and *BRCA2* are apparent. No mutation hot spots in either have been detected. Most unequivocally confirmed mutations reported to date are truncating mutations, adding little in the way of clues for defining functional regions. Finally, few mutations have been identified in either gene in sporadic breast cancers. It has been suggested, however, that the pathways in which the BRCA1 and BRCA2 proteins act may be disrupted in sporadic cancer, a phenotype that has been termed "BRCAness" (56).

Using direct mutation testing, several groups refined the estimates of mutation prevalence of *BRCA1* and *BRCA2* in less striking families (11,57,58). Estimates of *BRCA1* and *BRCA2* mutation prevalence in unselected patients with breast cancer are in the range of 2% to 3%. In a large population-based study of white and black cases (n = 1,628) and controls (n = 674) in North America ages 35 to 64, *BRCA1* mutations were detected in 2.4% of cases and 0.04% of controls, whereas *BRCA2* mutations were detected in 2.3% of cases and 0.4% of controls. *BRCA1* mutations were more common in white (2.9%) than black (1.4%) cases, whereas *BRCA2* mutations were slightly more frequent in black (2.6%), than white (2.1%) cases (11,18,33,58). In families identified through clinics treating high-risk breast cancer, *BRCA1* and *BRCA2* mutations are found in up to 55% of families with both breast and ovarian cancer (59) and up to 75% of families with both breast and ovarian cancer in the same individual, underscoring the importance of the family history in determining the likelihood that a *BRCA1* mutation is present (31,60–63).

Population Genetics of BRCA1 and BRCA2

The population genetics of *BRCA1* and *BRCA2* reflect several basic evolutionary principles. Each gene has undergone multiple independent mutations and these mutations have migrated with the populations in which they originally occurred. Certain *founder mutations* are known to exist in *BRCA1* and *BRCA2*, which have occurred in specific ethnic populations many generations in the past. They persist because the development of disease usually occurs after childbearing age, so individuals carrying these mutations are able to pass them on to subsequent

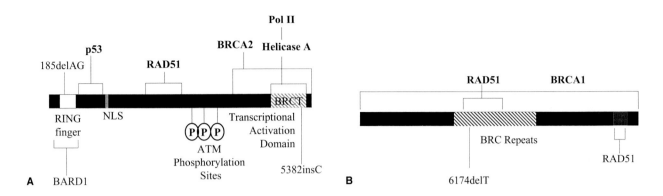

FIGURE 18.3. A: Functional domains of BRCA1. An idiogram of the 220-kd BRCA1 protein depicting known functional domains. Domains are shown as filled areas within the diagram. The two common mutations found in the Ashkenazi Jewish population (185delAG and 5382insC) are indicated. **B:** Functional domains of BRCA2. The carboxy terminal RAD51 binding site, and the central RAD51 binding BRC repeats are as depicted. The common mutation (6174delT) found in the Ashkenazi Jewish population is indicated (51,52).

generations with little impact of the mutated alleles on survival of the species.

Founder mutations have been identified in a number of populations. A comprehensive review by Szabo and King (36) reveals the similarities and differences in mutation rate, penetrance, and nature of the mutations among various population groups. The proportion of high-risk families with breast or ovarian cancer appears to vary widely by population group. Mutations in *BRCA1* are most common in Russia (79% of families with breast or ovarian cancer), as compared with Israel (47% of families) and Italy (29%). *BRCA2* mutations appear to be more common than *BRCA1* mutations only in Iceland, where a single mutation accounts for virtually all of the *BRCA2*-associated breast and ovarian cancer cases (64).

BRCA1 and *BRCA2* mutations among the Ashkenazi Jewish population are among the most intensively researched, because the presence of founder mutations facilitates these studies. The two Ashkenazi Jewish founder mutations in *BRCA1* are 185delAG and 5382insC, occurring in 1 in 8 and 1 in 12 individuals of Ashkenazi descent, respectively (65,66). One of these two mutations or 6174delT in *BRCA2* occurs in more than 2% of the Ashkenazi Jewish population (67,68). When compared with the estimated frequency of *BRCA1* mutations in an unselected white population of about 0.1% (58), this finding suggested the presence of a *founder effect* in the Ashkenazi Jewish population, documented with haplotype studies (69). Analysis of germline *BRCA1* mutations in several cohorts of Jewish women suggests that more than 20% of Jewish women developing breast cancer before age 40 years carry the 185delAG mutation (30,70). Even more strikingly, estimates suggest that 30% to 60% of all Ashkenazi Jewish women with ovarian cancer carry one of the *BRCA1* or *BRCA2* founder mutations (71–73). Up to 90% of mutations identified in women of Ashkenazi Jewish descent are one of the three founder mutations, although other *BRCA1* and *BRCA2* mutations have also been detected (39,74,75). Based on these data, individuals of Ashkenazi descent choosing to undergo genetic testing should first be tested for the three Ashkenazi Jewish founder mutations. Full sequencing can be reserved for those individuals at particularly high risk of having a *BRCA1* or *BRCA2* mutation.

Although still limited, data are now available on the prevalence of *BRCA1* and *BRCA2* mutations in some nonwhite populations. Interestingly, many *BRCA1* and *BRCA2* mutations in blacks appear unique to this ethnic or racial group (76). The probability of detecting a *BRCA1* or *BRCA2* mutation in a black woman with breast cancer is dependent on similar familial characteristics as those seen in the white population (age at breast cancer onset and the number of breast or ovarian cases in the family) (60,77). At present, genetic testing for *BRCA1* and *BRCA2* mutations in the black population is complicated by a high rate of variants of unknown significance (VUS), which are a problem in underrepresented minorities undergoing testing, but this issue has improved over time. Although in the past, 40% of blacks undergoing full sequencing at Myriad Genetics had a VUS (77), the number currently is approximately 20%, as an increasing number have been reclassified. Although this number remains quite high, progress has been made. Many of these variants of uncertain significance will undoubtedly be polymorphisms, but until this information is known, VUS will continue to complicate the interpretation of genetic testing results in the black population. More data are also becoming available from the Hispanic population, with similar features predicting pathogenic mutations. Interesting, there may be founder mutations in the Hispanic population, although further investigation of this is needed (78). Significant data from other ethnic groups or geographical areas are lacking.

Cancer Risks for BRCA1 and BRCA2 Mutation Carriers

Cancer risk estimates for *BRCA1* and *BRCA2* mutations carriers have been controversial (79). Estimates based on the highly penetrant families used to find these genes are high (as they were selected to be), likely owing to coexistent genetic and environmental modifiers that may increase the risk of disease. In studies of lower risk cohorts, such as population-based studies or cohorts of women with breast cancer unselected for family history, the lifetime risk of breast cancer was much lower (80,81). For this reason, the risk of breast cancer in *BRCA1* mutation carriers has been estimated to be as low as 36% (80) and as high 87% (49) (Fig. 18.2), with an estimate of pooled data of 65% (82,83). Estimates of contralateral breast cancer occurrence are as high as 60% (84). Cumulative risk of ovarian cancer in *BRCA1* carriers has been reported to be between 27% (58) and 45% (41,85,86), also with a significantly increased risk of fallopian tube cancer (85). In addition there have been reports of an increase in uterine and cervical cancer (2), stomach cancer (41), a two- to threefold increase in pancreatic cancer (2,85), a possible twofold increase in colon cancer (2), and a 17-fold risk of testicular cancer (41); however, these risks have not been consistently seen across studies. Prostate cancer risk does not appear increased, although the disease may occur at an earlier age. Male breast cancer is also seen in association with *BRCA1* mutations, with

Table 18.2	LIFETIME CANCER RISKS IN *BRCA1* AND *BRCA2* MUTATION CARRIERS					
Women	Women *BRCA1* (%)	Average *BRCA2* (%)	Men U.S. Women (%)	Men *BRCA1* (%)	Average *BRCA2* (%)	U.S. Men (%)
Breast	60–80	60–80	3	1–5	5–10	0.1
Ovarian	30–45	10–20	1–2	—	—	—
Colon	10–15	—	5–6	10–15	—	5–6
Pancreatic	2–3	3–5	1	2–3	3–5	1
Uterine	Increased	—	3	—	—	—
Cervical	Increased	—	1	—	—	—
Melanoma		3–5	1–2	—	3–5	1–2
Prostate	—	—	—	*	15–25*	16

*Although there is no convincing evidence of an overall increased risk of prostate cancer, men with *BRCA1* mutations may develop prostate cancer at a younger age than men in the general population. *BRCA2* mutations *are* associated with an increased risk of prostate cancer, which also can be of earlier onset.

an RR of more than 50 and a lifetime risk of approximately 1% to 5% (40,85). In the Myriad Genetics series, one-third of mutations found in families with male breast cancer were in *BRCA1*, and the remaining in *BRCA2* (39) (Table 18.2). Overall, *BRCA1* mutation carriers have a high cumulative lifetime risk of developing any cancer. A kin-cohort study performed in Ontario estimated that the lifetime risk of any cancer (to age 80) in a woman with a *BRCA1* mutation was 98% compared with 32% for a nonmutation carrier. For a male *BRCA1* mutation carrier, this risk was estimated at 59%, compared with a population risk of 40% (41).

BRCA2 has a cancer risk profile similar, but not identical, to *BRCA1*. Lifetime breast cancer risk for *BRCA2* mutation carriers is estimated to be 45% to 84%, with lifetime ovarian cancer risk in the range of 10% to 20% (41,82,83,87,88). *BRCA2* mutations are associated with a 6% lifetime risk of male breast cancer (1). Male *BRCA2* mutation carriers have an increased risk of prostate cancer, with an RR of 3 to 44 (3,64) and an RR of 7 in men younger than 65 years (3). Pancreatic cancer also is associated with *BRCA2* mutations (3,41), with an RR of 3.5. The incidence of *BRCA2* germline mutations in patients with familial pancreatic cancer (two first-degree relatives with pancreatic cancer) may be as high as 20% (89,90). *BRCA2* mutation carriers also appear to have an increased risk of stomach cancer (RR, 2.6), gallbladder and bile duct cancers (RR, 5.0), and

malignant melanoma (RR, 2.6) (3). Again, the lifetime risk of any cancer in *BRCA2* mutation carriers is high, estimated at 73% for women and 58% for men (41).

Genotype–Phenotype Correlations in BRCA1 and BRCA2

Several studies have attempted to establish correlations between specific *BRCA1* mutations and the types of cancer that subsequently develop. It was initially suggested that mutations in the 5' half of *BRCA1* predispose to both breast and ovarian cancer, whereas mutations closer to the 3' portion of the gene are predominantly associated with site-specific breast cancer (91,92). This was subsequently clarified by Thompson and Easton (88), who reported a lower risk of breast cancer with mutations in a central region of *BRCA1* relative to either end (Fig. 18.4A). For *BRCA2*, mutations in the *ovarian cancer cluster region* in the central portion of *BRCA2* are associated with a higher risk of ovarian cancer and a lower risk of breast cancer relative to mutations outside of this region (81,92–94) (Fig. 18.4B). Identification of specific genotype–phenotype correlations will ultimately aid clinicians in recommending appropriate screening, prevention, and treatment strategies in women with known mutations, but currently these data are too preliminary to be used in counseling such women.

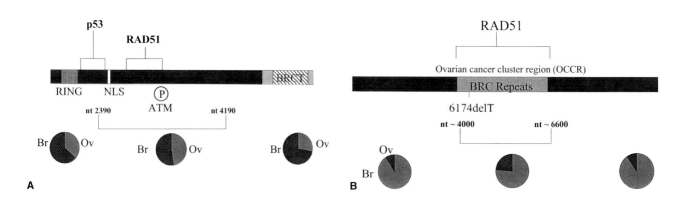

FIGURE 18.4. A: Genotype–phenotype correlations in *BRCA1*. The three regions of *BRCA1* for which there is evidence of differential risk of breast and ovarian cancer are as shown. The ratio of breast:ovarian cancer with mutations in the amino terminal region (nt 12389) is 64% breast:36% ovary. In the central region (nt 2390–4190), the relative risk of ovarian cancer increases significantly with a ratio of 52% breast:48% ovary, and carboxy mutations (4191–end) resemble those of the amino terminus at 72% breast:28% ovary (88). **B:** Genotype–phenotype correlations in *BRCA2*. As for *BRCA1*, the regions of differential risk of breast and ovarian cancer are as depicted. Mutations in *BRCA2* are associated with a lower overall risk for ovarian cancer, but the pattern seen in *BRCA1* is also seen in *BRCA2*, with the ratio of breast:ovarian cancer with mutations in the amino terminal region (nt 1–4000) being 89% breast:11% ovary, in the central region, corresponding to the previous described ovarian cancer cluster region (OCCR) (nt 4000–6000), the ratio is 77% breast:23% ovary, and in the carboxy terminal region (nt 6000–end), 90% breast:10% ovary (93).

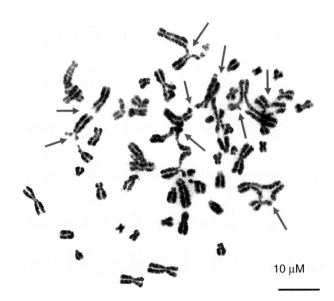

10 µM

FIGURE 18.5. BRCA2 deficient cells are highly sensitive to DNA cross-linking agents. Cells defective in BRCA2 function show a high degree of chromosome instability, including chromosome breaks and radial chromosomes (51,52,139). These aberrations accumulate spontaneously but are highly exacerbated by DNA damaging agents that induce DSBs, in particular DNA cross-linking agents. Shown here are the effects of treating CAPAN1 cells, which carry a loss of function c.6174delT BRCA2 allele and no wild-type allele, with the DNA cross-linking agent mitomycin C. Arrows indicate chromosomal aberrations.

Modifiers of BRCA1 and BRCA2 Mutations

Although germline mutations in *BRCA1* and *BRCA2* confer a high risk of breast cancer, variability in cancer risk has been observed among individuals both between and within families. The discovery of environmental or genetic factors that modify the penetrance of *BRCA1* and *BRCA2* mutations may clarify our understanding of their mechanism of action and provide additional information with which to counsel individuals with *BRCA1* and *BRCA2* mutations. Furthermore, factors that affect familial breast cancer risk in the general population could presumably affect breast cancer risk in *BRCA1* and *BRCA2* mutation carriers. By far, the most important modifiers identified for *BRCA1* and *BRCA2* mutation carriers are prophylactic oophorectomy and the use of tamoxifen for chemoprevention. Prophylactic oophorectomy decreases the risk of ovarian cancer by 95% but, importantly, also decreases the risk of breast cancer by 50% (95–99). The magnitude of the benefit of oophorectomy (and estrogen deprivation) on breast cancer risk is seen in both *BRCA1* and *BRCA2* mutation carriers, despite that 90% of *BRCA1*-related breast cancers are ER negative. A

recent prospective study has suggested that oophorectomy may have differential effects in *BRCA1* versus *BRCA2* mutation carriers, but more data are needed to quantify these differences (100). In retrospective studies, tamoxifen has been shown to decrease the risk of contralateral breast tumors by 50% in both *BRCA1* and *BRCA2* mutation carriers (101,102). To date, many reproductive factors have been examined as modifiers in *BRCA1* and *BRCA2* mutation carriers, including parity, age at first pregnancy, oral contraceptive use, and tubal ligation (96,103–109). Of all of these, perhaps the most clinically relevant are the protective effects of oral contraceptives on ovarian cancer risk, with the potential of a slight increase in breast cancer for *BRCA1* carriers (110–114).

Genetic factors are likely to modify the risk of cancer in *BRCA1* and *BRCA2* mutation carriers. Most studies examining this, however, have been limited in size and statistical power. Convincingly validated modifiers of *BRCA1* and *BRCA2* penetrance have yet to be identified. However, consortia of investigators are now being established to systematically investigate candidate genetic modifiers. One such group the Consortium of Investigators of Modifiers of *BRCA1* and *BRCA2* (CIMBA) contains about 30 affiliated groups who together have collected DNA and clinical data from approximately 10,000 *BRCA1* and 5,000 *BRCA2* mutation carriers (115). Initial results have provided support for the role of variants in the *RAD51* (116) and *AURKA* (117) genes in affecting penetrance in mutation carriers. The identification of proven genetic modifiers of breast cancer risk for *BRCA1* and *BRCA2* mutation carriers may prove useful to determine individualized risk of cancer among carriers.

Histopathology of BRCA1- and BRCA2-Associated Breast Tumors

In contrast to sporadic breast cancers, those arising in *BRCA1* mutation carriers are frequently, although not exclusively, negative for the estrogen receptor (ER) and the growth factor receptor, HER2, but mostly express basal cytokeratins (118–120). In support of this, gene expression profiling analysis indicates relative down-regulation of ER response genes and the up-regulation of proliferation-associated genes and basal cytokeratins. This phenotype leads to the clustering of these tumors with sporadic cancers of the basal-like subtype (5,121). A mechanism by which loss of *BRCA1* function likely mandates lack of ER and ER regulated gene expression has been suggested. Functional *BRCA1* appears necessary for the expression of ER by directly binding and transactivating the *ER* gene promoter. When *BRCA1* is lost in tumors, ER can no longer be expressed and, as a result, resistance to tamoxifen and other ER-directed therapies arises (122).

The association between *BRCA1* status and the so-called ER/PR/HER2-negative (triple negative) and basal-like phenotype

	All Histologies	Estrogen Receptor Positive			Estrogen Receptor Negative		
Age	(%)	Grade 1 (%)	Grade 2 (%)	Grade 3 (%)	Grade 1 (%)	Grade 2 (%)	Grade 3 (%)
<30	8	1.1	1.6	2.7	14.4	21.0	35.0
30–34	5	0.8	1.2	2.0	10.9	15.9	26.5
35–39	2	0.2	0.3	0.5	2.7	4.0	6.6
40–44	1.5	0.1	0.2	0.3	1.5	2.2	3.7
45–49	1	0.1	0.1	0.2	1.0	1.5	2.5
50–59	0.3	0.03	0.04	0.07	0.4	0.6	0.9

Table 18.3 | PREDICTED PROBABILITIES OF CARRYING A *BRCA1* MUTATION, BY AGE, ESTROGEN RECEPTOR STATUS, AND GRADE

From Lakhani SR, Van De Vijver MJ, Jacquamier J, et al. The pathology of familial breast cancer: predictive value of immunohistochemical markers estrogen receptor, progesterone receptor, HER-2, and p53 in patients with mutations in *BRCA1* and *BRCA2*. *J Clin Oncol* 2002;20:2310–2318, with permission.

means that a careful family history should be ascertained in young women with tumors of this type. A combined test using ER and basal keratin status has higher specificity and better predictive values than clinical algorithms alone; the results of the Breast Cancer Linkage Consortium study suggest that patients with ER negative or basal keratin-positive breast cancers have an odds ratio of approximately 148 of having a *BRCA1* mutation when compared with age-matched controls (119) (Table 18.3). Among women with triple negative breast cancer under 40 years of age, where family history is not known, more than 20% had a *BRCA1* mutation and this rises to nearly 30% when a woman under 50 years of age has a strong family history (123).

BRCA2 mutation-associated breast cancers typically differ from those arising in *BRCA1* mutation carriers and are generally much more similar to sporadic cases. Specific morphologic features, such as pushing margins and a greater degree of tubule formation, have been noted. The ER and HER2 status of tumors are not obviously different from the spectrum of sporadic invasive ductal cancers (124). A recent study has suggested, however, that *BRCA2*-associated tumors are of higher grade, are more frequently ER positive and are less likely to overexpress HER2 compared with control sporadic tumors matched for age and ethnicity. In summary *BRCA2* cancers tend to be a high grade proliferative form of luminal breast cancer. For further discussion of the pathology of breast cancer see Chapter 28.

Biological Function(s) of BRCA1 and BRCA2

BRCA1 and BRCA2 Proteins

BRCA1 is a nuclear protein with two important regions of sequence similarity to known functional motifs. These regions are the RING domain at the beginning of BRCA1 and the BRCT motif at the carboxyl terminus (Fig. 18.3A). The 42 amino acid RING domain (so-called because it was initially described in a *Really Interesting New Gene*) near the amino terminus of BRCA1 binds zinc (51,52). RING domains mediate interactions between proteins involved in polyubiquitination, a key cellular process regulating protein degradation that is essential in cell growth and differentiation (125). Two novel proteins, BAP1 (BRCA1 activator protein-1) and BARD1 (BRCA1-associated RING domain-1), have now been identified that bind the BRCA1 RING domain (126,127). The significance of the BRCA1–BAP1 interaction remains unclear, but the interaction of BRCA1 with BARD1 confers substantial ubiquitin ligase activity on the complex. The BRCA1–BARD1 heterodimer can therefore add polyubiquitin chains to specific lysine residues of other proteins, targeting those proteins for degradation (128,129). A number of proteins have been suggested to be ubiquitinated by the BRCA1–BARD1 heterodimer (130).

The BRCT (*br*east *c*ancer-1 *t*erminus) domain was first recognized as a cellular motif by its presence in BRCA1, but it is now known to be highly evolutionarily conserved and present in more than 40 other proteins involved in response to DNA damage, including scRAD9 in yeast and BARD1 (131,132). This domain functions as a phosphoprotein docking motif (52). The functional and clinical relevance of both the BRCT and RING domains is illustrated in that these two regions are the only portions of BRCA1 in which germline missense mutations have been shown unequivocally to confer a high risk of breast and ovarian cancer (133,134).

As with BRCA1, BRCA2 is a nuclear protein (135). However, the structure of BRCA2 initially provided fewer insights into its function (Fig. 18.3B). Subsequently, major structural motifs recognized in BRCA2 are the eight tandem BRC repeats in the central portion of the protein which mediate the critical interaction of BRCA2 and RAD51 (51–53). TR2, another binding site for RAD51, exists at the carboxyl terminus of BRCA2 (136,137).

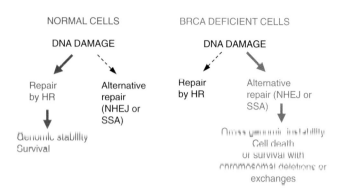

FIGURE 18.6. Loss of functional BRCA1 or BRCA2 affects the choice of DNA double-strand break repair pathway. DNA DSBs are repaired in normal cells, in part, by HR-based mechanisms. Functional BRCA1 and BRCA2 proteins are required for efficient repair by HR and genomic stability. In the absence of BRCA1 or BRCA2 alternative repair pathways, such as NHEJ and SSA, are utilized leading to cell death or survival with genomic damage (51,52,139).

The structure of a large portion of the C-terminus of BRCA2 has been determined, which revealed the presence of a single strand and double strand DNA binding domain (138).

Roles in the Response to DNA Damage

The *BRCA1* and *BRCA2* genes encode large proteins that likely function in multiple cellular pathways, including transcription, cell cycle regulation (51,52). However, it is the roles of BRCA1 and BRCA2 in the maintenance of genome stability DNA repair that has been best documented (52). Both proteins suppress illegitimate recombination and play important roles in the repair of double-stranded DNA breaks as a central part of this function. BRCA1 participates more broadly in this process than BRCA2 (e.g. Fig. 18.5), with a role both in sensing and signaling the presence of damaged DNA and in assisting in repair of the damage locally. When present in normal cells, BRCA1 enhances transcription of other important genes in the process, regulates the S, G_1, and G_{2M} checkpoints, ensuring that cells with damaged DNA do not replicate, alters chromatin structure and nucleosome organization at the local site of damage, facilitating access by repair complexes, and promotes use of the error-free repair pathway of homologous recombination (HR)-mediated repair rather than the error-prone process of nonhomologous end joining (NHEJ) (51,52,139).

BRCA2 has a more limited role in maintaining genome stability, functioning only at the local site of repair by regulating the activity of RAD51, an essential component of error-free HR-mediated repair of double-stranded breaks (52). In particular, BRCA2 affects the choice between the two HR subpathways—the conservative gene conversion (GC) mechanism and the error prone single-strand annealing (SSA). In BRCA2 mutant cells, GC is suppressed, leading to the preferential use of NHEJ and SSA. The physical interaction between BRCA2 and RAD51 is essential for error-free DSB repair. BRCA2 is required for the localization of RAD51 to sites of DNA damage, where RAD51 forms the nucleoprotein filament required for recombination. Foci of RAD51 protein are apparent in the nucleus after certain forms of DNA damage and these likely represent sites of repair by HR; BRCA2-deficient cells do not form RAD51 foci in response to DNA damage (140). Two different domains within BRCA2 interact with RAD51, the eight BRC repeats in the central part of the protein and a distinct domain, TR2, at the C-terminus. Recently, it has been proposed that BRC repeats hold RAD51 in an essentially inactive monomeric form and, when damage occurs, the BRCA2–RAD51 complex localizes to the site of DNA damage (136,137). Then, a critical serine in the C-terminus of BRCA2 becomes phosphorylated, activating TR2,

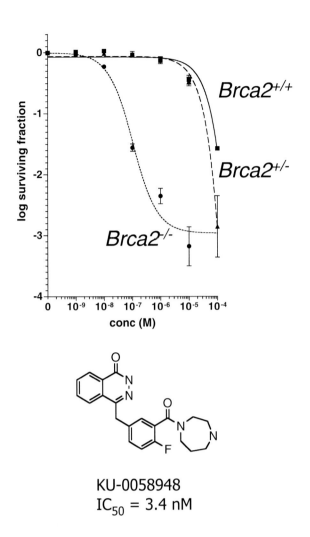

KU-0058948

$IC_{50} = 3.4$ nM

FIGURE 18.7. ***BRCA2*** **mutant cells are exquisitely sensitive to a potent PARP inhibitor (166,167).** Clonogenic survival curves of *BRCA2* wild-type, heterozygous and deficient mouse ES cells after exposure to a range of concentrations of the potent PARP inhibitor KU0058948. BRCA2 deficient cells are over 1,000-fold more sensitive than wild-type or heterozygous cells. KU0058948 is based around a phthalazin-1-one core and is a competitive inhibitor with respect to the PARP substrate NAD+ (166).

Other Functions of BRCA1

The role of BRCA1 as a transcriptional coactivator—a protein that facilitates transcription of genes in the presence of direct transcriptional activators—is a critical component of its ability to transduce signals, activating DNA damage response pathways. In unraveling this function, BRCA1 first was shown to interact with two key components of the cell transcription machinery of the cell, including the RNA polymerase holoenzyme (143). In addition, two groups characterized the carboxy-terminus BRCT repeats as transcriptional activation domains (144,145). Recently, BRCA1 has been shown to be an important factor in the transcriptional regulation of ER (122). In the absence of functional BRCA1, ER is no longer expressed and this is could be the explanation of the ER negative, basal, phenotype of tumors arising in *BRCA1* mutation carriers (5).

Influence of BRCA1 or BRCA2 Mutation Status on Breast Cancer Prognosis

The influence of *BRCA1* or *BRCA2* mutation status on breast cancer prognosis remains a controversial issue in part because of the diversity of the design of the studies that have been used. A review of most of these concluded that no convincing data, in women with breast cancer, suggest that *BRCA1* or *BRCA2* mutation status conferred adverse prognosis, other than for contralateral breast cancer occurrence (146). Since this review was published two other relevant studies have been reported. Moller et al. (147) studied patients who developed breast cancer while enrolled in prospective breast cancer surveillance programs because of strong family history of breast cancer and mutation status was confirmed by resequencing. *BRCA1* mutation was associated with worse prognosis even in classic low-risk node-negative patients. Rennert et al. (148) conducted a very large population study in Israel in which all new cases of invasive breast cancer in the country in 1987 and 1988 were sought. Case records and pathology samples were available on 1,545 women and tumor DNA was extracted and analyzed for the three Ashkenazi founder mutations in *BRCA1* and *BRCA2*. No difference in overall or breast cancer-specific survival was noted for *BRCA1* or *BRCA2* mutation carriers when compared with noncarriers. In contrast, *BRCA1*- and *BRCA2*-associated ovarian cancers have been consistently shown to have a better prognosis compared with sporadic cases (149–152).

The Influence of BRCA1 or BRCA2 Mutation Status on Response to Therapy

Rennert et al. (148) noted two important observations in subgroups of their large Israeli study. First, there was a statistically significant correlation between *BRCA1* mutation status and a more favorable prognosis in women receiving adjuvant chemotherapy when compared with noncarriers. Second, women presenting with tumors less than 2 cm had a worse prognosis if they were *BRCA1* carriers. This is intriguing, given the similar results of another retrospective study of similar design conducted in 505 Jewish women in New York and Montreal with small tumors suitable for breast-conserving surgery (153). Robson et al. (153) found the presence of an Ashkenazi founder mutation in *BRCA1* to be associated with adverse breast cancer survival when compared with noncarriers (62% at 10 years versus 86%; $p < .0001$). *BRCA1* status predicted breast cancer mortality only among women who did not receive chemotherapy (hazard ratio 4.8, 95% confidence interval 2.0–11.7; $p = .001$). Whether this phenomenon relates directly to *BRCA1* gene function or some other aspect of the basal-like breast cancer phenotype associated with *BRCA1* mutated breast cancer is not clear. A similar adverse prognosis normalized by an apparent increase in sensitivity to chemotherapy

which can then support RAD51 oligomerization and nucleoprotein filament formation. This filament can then invade and pair with a homologous DNA duplex, initiating strand exchange between the paired DNA molecules. The BRCA2 DBD domain also stimulates homologous pairing and the strand-exchange activities of RAD51, suggesting that BRCA2 might facilitate RAD51-mediated recombination by binding to the double-stranded DNA–single-stranded DNA (dsDNA–ssDNA) junction of the resected DSB (138, 140).

For both BRCA1 and BRCA2, it is the failure to faithfully repair DNA breaks that underlies the genomic instability in BRCA1 and BRCA2 mutant cells (Fig. 18.6). Cells defective in BRCA1 and BRCA2 function show a high degree of chromosome instability, including chromosome breaks and radial chromosomes (141,142). These aberrations accumulate spontaneously, but are exacerbated by DNA damaging agents that induce DSB, in particular DNA cross-linking agents. These observations eventually provided critical information for the identification of *FANCD2*, mutated in Fanconi anemia type D2, as *BRCA2* (38). This discovery was made in part owing to the observation that cells from patients from the Fanconi complementation group D2 have the same unusual chromosomal structures seen in BRCA2-deficient cells.

in sporadic basal-like breast cancer has also been reported in a small study (154) and sporadic basal-like breast cancers have been noted to have high response rates to anthracyclines-based chemotherapy, in common with the other major ER negative subtype, the HER2 positive cancers (155). Few data exist relating to *BRCA1* or *BRCA2* genotype-specific effects on normal tissue chemotherapy toxicity. Retrospective data suggest no evidence of increased complications (156). Taken together these data suggest that *BRCA1* mutation carriers who present with small and node-negative breast cancers may be at more significant risk of micrometastatic breast cancer than noncarriers. This may explain a worse prognosis if chemotherapy is avoided in what is regarded as a classically lower risk population. A greater sensitivity to adjuvant chemotherapy seems to correct for any adverse baseline prognosis. These data, while retrospective, may help inform discussions with regard to benefits of adjuvant chemotherapy in carriers with very small node-negative cancers, especially where evidence seems to indicate that the prognostic significance of pathologically normal lymph nodes seems to be lost in this type of tumour (157,158).

A potential concern, because of the role of *BRCA1* and *BRCA2* in the DNA damage response, is response to radiotherapy. A mature analysis of *BRCA1* and *BRCA2* carriers and matched controls treated with breast-conserving therapy and radiotherapy and followed for a median of 6 to 8 years has shown no increase in ipsilateral breast tumor recurrence in carriers who had had a prophylactic oophorectomy when compared with matched controls. An increase was noted in women who did not have prophylactic oophorectomy (159). As noted above, contralateral breast cancers were significantly more common in *BRCA1* and *BRCA2* mutation carriers than controls, whether or not prophylactic oophorectomy was performed. No evidence, however, indicates an increase in normal tissue radiation toxicity associated with carrier status (159,160).

What is the Most Effective Chemotherapy for BRCA1/BRCA2 Associated Breast Cancer?

A number of clinically used agents appear to be selective for killing cells defective in *BRCA1* or *BRCA2*. These include the DNA cross-linking agents (e.g., carboplatin, cisplatin, and mitomycin C) (142,161,162). This suggests an increased sensitivity to lesions that damage DNA in ways that interfere with DNA replication forks and which subsequently require DNA repair by homologous recombination for fork restart. This is consistent with the key role that *BRCA1* and *BRCA2* play in the Fanconi anemia network (38), the hallmark of which is extreme cellular sensitivity to DNA cross-linking agents.

It has been suggested that *BRCA1* may be required to mediate paclitaxel-induced cell death as loss of *BRCA1* function leads to microtubule stabilizing agent resistance (163). This contention is supported by uncontrolled, retrospective data from patients treated with taxane-based neoadjuvant therapy (164). The issue of taxane resistance remains controversial, however, because others have found increased sensitivity to taxanes in preclinical *BRCA1* deficient models (165). An international randomized phase II clinical study is now testing the efficacy of carboplatin and docetaxel in *BRCA1* and *BRCA2* carriers with advanced breast cancer (www.breakthrough.org.uk/researchcentre/clinical_trials/brca_trial/index.html) (139). For further discussion of the use of chemotherapy for the treatment of breast cancer see Chapter 49.

New Therapeutic Approaches to the Treatment of BRCA1-and BRCA2-Associated Cancers

New therapeutic strategies, based on synthetic lethality, have recently been put forward for the treatment of cancers arising in carriers of mutations in *BRCA1* or *BRCA2* (166,167). Synthetic lethality is defined as the situation when mutation in either of two genes individually has no effect, but combining the mutations leads to death (168). This effect can arise because of a number of different gene–gene interactions. Examples include two genes in separate semiredundant or cooperating pathways and two genes acting in the same pathway where loss of both critically affects flux through the pathway. The implication is that targeting one of these genes in a cancer where the other is defective should be selectively lethal to the tumor cells but not toxic to the normal cells. In principle, this should lead to a large therapeutic window (169).

The synthetic lethal pair in the approach that is being developed is the interaction between HR and the single strand break (SSB) DNA repair pathway (170). Endogenous base damage, including SSB, is the most common DNA aberration and it has been estimated that the average cell may repair 10,000 such lesions every day. Base excision repair (BER) is an important pathway for the repair of SSB and involves the sensing of the lesion followed by the recruitment of a number of other proteins. PARP-1 (Poly(ADP)Ribose Polymerase) is a critical component of the major *short-patch* BER pathway. PARP is an enzyme, discovered over 40 years ago (171), which produces large branched chains of poly(ADP) ribose (PAR) from NAD^+. In humans, there are 17 members of the PARP gene family, but most of these are poorly characterized (172,173). The abundant nuclear protein PARP-1 senses and binds to DNA nicks and breaks and these result in activation of catalytic activity causing poly(ADP)ribosylation of PARP-1 itself as well as other acceptor proteins, such as histones. This modification potentially signals the recruitment of other components of DNA repair pathways as well as modifying the activity of proteins (172,173). The highly negatively charged PAR that is produced around the site of damage may also serve as an antirecombinogenic factor.

PARP-1 inhibition causes failure of the repair of SSB lesions, but does not affect DSB repair (174). However, a persistent DNA SSB encountered by a DNA replication fork will cause stalling of the fork and may result in either fork collapse or the formation of a DSB (175). Therefore, loss of PARP-1 increases the formation of DNA lesions that might be repaired by GC. As loss of function of either *BRCA1* or *BRCA2* impairs GC (139), loss of PARP-1 function in a *BRCA1* or *BRCA2* defective background likely results in the generation of replication-associated DNA lesions normally repaired by sister chromatid exchange. This is likely to be the explanation of the observation that small molecules PARP inhibitors are highly selectively lethal to cells lacking functional *BRCA1* or *BRCA2* (Fig. 18.7).

These observations suggested a potential new mechanism-based approach for the treatment of patients with *BRCA1*- and *BRCA2*-associated cancers. In these patients, tumor cells lack wild-type *BRCA1* or *BRCA2*, but normal tissues retain a single wild-type copy of the relevant gene, potentially providing a large therapeutic window. This difference provides the rationale for inhibiting PARP to generate specific DNA lesions that require functional *BRCA1* and *BRCA2* for their repair. This approach is likely to be more specific and to have fewer side effects than standard cytotoxic chemotherapy, because PARP inhibitors are relatively nontoxic and do not directly damage DNA. A number of PARP inhibitors are in clinical development (176) and clinical trials are underway in *BRCA1* and *BRCA2* mutation carriers (177).

Mechanisms by which *BRCA2* mutated cells can acquire resistance to PARP inhibitors and platinum salts have recently been studied (178). These experiments have shown that mutagenic DNA pathways that are up-regulated in the absence of *BRCA2* function, may drive intragenic deletion events. These can rarely correct the effect of mutation on the open reading frame and restore expression of a functional *BRCA2* gene (178).

These rare events may then be selected for over time in a sensitive population. The potential clinical significance of these observations have been validated by demonstrating that DNA extracted from an ovarian cancer in a *BRCA2* mutation carrier that had become platinum refractory carried a revertant *BRCA2* allele (178). It is not yet clear which mutations in *BRCA1* or *BRCA2* may be susceptible to this process. It seems possible, however, that different mutations may revert at different rates, resulting in more or less sustained therapeutic benefit. These observations need further validation, but if this proves to be the case, it further suggests that platinum salts and PARP inhibitors may have their greatest benefits in low bulk early stage disease. Other new therapeutic approaches for breast cancer are discussed in Chapters 78–80.

OTHER BREAST CANCER SUSCEPTIBILITY GENES

TP53

Germline mutations in *TP53* result in Li Fraumeni Syndrome (LFS). First identified in 1969 in four kindreds with multiple childhood sarcomas and excessive cancer risks (43). Subsequent epidemiologic efforts have identified the major component neoplasms, including breast cancer, soft tissue sarcomas and osteosarcomas, brain tumors, leukemia, and adrenocortical carcinomas; several additional tumor types are likely to merit inclusion (179). Segregation analysis of families identified through a family member with sarcoma confirmed the autosomal dominant pattern of transmission of cancer susceptibility, with age-specific penetrance estimated to reach 90% by age 70 years (180). Nearly 30% of tumors in reported families occur before age 15 years (180). In 1990, germline *TP53* mutations were identified as the cause of LFS (181,182). Approximately 50% of carefully defined families have alterations identified in the *TP53* gene. The prevalence of germline *TP53* mutations in women with breast cancer diagnosed at younger than 40 years has been estimated at approximately 1% (182). Although an initial report suggested *CHEK2* mutations were responsible for some cases of LFS and LFS-like syndrome, this finding was not supported by much larger studies showing that *CHEK2* is a low-penetrance cancer susceptibility gene (183,184).

ATM

Ataxia-telangiectasia is an autosomal recessive disorder characterized by oculocutaneous telangiectasias, cerebellar ataxia, immune deficiency, and a predisposition to leukemia and lymphoma. Both copies of *ATM* (A-T, mutated) are mutated in patients with ataxia-telangiectasia (185). *ATM* is a member of a large family of protein kinases, and functions as a checkpoint in response to DNA damage, phosphorylating *TP53* and *BRCA1* in the presence of damaged DNA (186). Conflicting data have existed about whether female *ATM* heterozygotes have an increased risk for breast cancer. Initial studies examining family members of patients with ataxia-telangiectasia observed an increased number of breast cancer cases in obligate and predicted heterozygotes (187). However, the controls in the two largest studies had an unusually low incidence of breast cancer. Over the last decade, numerous studies have been performed in an attempt to assess the role of *ATM* mutation in breast cancer susceptibility (187). Most of these have been inconclusive owing to two factors: only small numbers of cases were included and, in general, the whole *ATM* gene was not screened because of its large size. In an attempt to overcome these limitations, Renwick et al. (188) screened the whole *ATM*

gene in 443 *BRCA1 and BRCA2* mutation negative familial breast cancer cases and 521 controls. Significantly more *bona fide* ataxia-telangiectasia causing mutations were found in the cases than the controls. These results convincingly establish *ATM* as a breast cancer susceptibility gene.

One controversy that has emerged as a result of the question of breast cancer risk in *ATM* heterozygotes is the use of mammography in women younger than 50 years. Concern over repeated mammography was raised based on data that *ATM* homozygotes (i.e., who have ataxia-telangiectasia) have increased DNA damage from ionizing radiation. This biological defect suggested that the use of mammography for cancer detection should be weighed against the possibility of inducing cancer as a result of radiation exposure. However, *ATM* mutations do not appear to contribute to breast cancers diagnosed following radiation therapy for Hodgkin disease (189,190) and do not seem to play a role in recurrence following radiation for breast cancer (191). Therefore, the magnitude of increased risk for breast cancer owing to mammography in *ATM* heterozygotes is unknown and presumably small, and the benefit of detecting a neoplasm in its early stages is large. Thus, almost uniform agreement is that screening mammography should be initiated when clinically appropriate regardless of concern over the presence of *ATM* mutations.

PTEN

Cowden disease is a rare inherited syndrome in which mutations in *PTEN* are transmitted in an autosomal-dominant pattern with variable penetrance. Malignant and benign lesions of the breast, along with hamartomas in the gastrointestinal tract; mucocutaneous lesions (including trichilemmomas, papillomatosis of the lips and oral mucosa, and acral keratoses); thyroid abnormalities, including goiters, adenomas, and follicular cancer; macrocephaly; uterine fibroids; and ovarian cysts and carcinomas characterize Cowden disease (44,192). Approximately 75% of affected women have either fibrocystic breasts or mammary fibroadenomas. A marked increase in breast cancer incidence as compared with the general population was first observed in a series of cases of families with Cowden disease (54) and, subsequently, it has been estimated that up to 25% to 50% of women with Cowden disease may develop invasive breast cancer (192). Male breast cancer also has been reported in families with Cowden disease, although infrequently (193). However, *PTEN* mutations are uncommon in families with a history of site-specific breast cancer (194).

STK11/LKB

Peutz-Jeghers syndrome, first described in the 1920s, is characterized by the occurrence of hamartomatous polyps in the small bowel and pigmented macules of the buccal mucosa, lips, fingers, and toes (195,196). It is an autosomal-dominant disorder that has been reported to occur in approximately 1 in 20,000 live births. More recently, it has been associated with an excess incidence of tumors involving the breast, gastrointestinal tract, ovary, testis, and uterine cervix (197,198). The gene mutated in Peutz-Jeghers syndrome has been identified on chromosome 19 (199) and is *STKII/LKB1*, a tumor suppressor gene that encodes a protein kinase. The association between mutations in *STKII/LKB1* and Peutz-Jeghers syndrome was subsequently confirmed in 20 additional families (200). Two studies have attempted to define the degree of cancer risk associated with the syndrome. Giardiello et al. (197) described a cohort of 31 patients followed from 1973 to 1985. Of patients 48% developed cancer during that interval: Four developed gastrointestinal tract cancer and ten developed non-gastrointestinal tract cancer, representing an RR 18 times that of the general population (197). Subsequently, another group of investigators reported an elevated risk of breast and gynecologic cancers in women with Peutz-Jeghers syndrome. In this cohort of 34 patients, the affected women had an RR of developing cancer of approximately 20, whereas male patients had a lower cancer risk, approximately sixfold that of the general population (198). These findings suggest that, despite its rare occurrence, Peutz-Jeghers syndrome is associated with an increased risk of breast cancer.

CHEK2

CHEK2 is located on chromosome 22, and encodes a cell-cycle checkpoint kinase that is implicated in DNA repair. An initial study suggested that families with LFS that lacked an identifiable *TP53* mutation had germline *CHEK2* mutations (183). Data, however, now provide strong evidence that *CHEK2* is not a high-penetrance cancer susceptibility gene in these families (184,201). The possibility that *CHEK2*, specifically the *CHEK2* 1100delC mutation, is associated with an increased risk of breast cancer was explored in a large multi-institutional study (184). In this study, 1,071 individuals from 718 families with breast cancer (defined as two or more cases, both diagnosed before age 60 years), 636 individuals with breast cancer unselected for family history (ascertained through the UK Case Control Study, the University of Pennsylvania Cancer Risk Evaluation Program, and the Erasmus Rotterdam Health and the Elderly Study), and 1,620 controls (from six studies in the United Kingdom, The Netherlands, and North America) were examined for the *CHEK2* mutation 1100delC. Those with familial breast cancer were known to be negative for *BRCA1* and *BRCA2* germline mutations. Of those with familial breast cancer, 5.1% carried a *CHEK2* 1100delC mutation, compared with 1.4% of sporadic breast cancers, and 1.1% of controls ($p < 10^{-7}$) providing evidence that germline *CHEK2* mutations confer a twofold risk of breast cancer (95% CI).

In addition, *CHEK2* 1100delC was found in 13.5% of individuals with breast cancer from families known to be negative for *BRCA1* or *BRCA2* mutations with at least one male breast cancer case (184). Thus, this mutation is associated with an RR of 10 for male breast cancer. Testing of 520 individuals from families with *BRCA1* or *BRCA2* mutations revealed no increase in *CHEK2* 1100delC frequency as compared with controls (1%), as might be expected, because they function in the same signaling pathway. Therefore, *CHEK2* 1100delC has been confirmed as a low-penetrance breast cancer susceptibility gene, with a high degree of statistical significance (184). At present, the clinical utility of testing for such a gene is unclear, particularly because further data demonstrate that *CHEK2* mutations are present in low frequency in North American cases and controls (202) and other *CHEK2* mutations do not seem to contribute to breast cancer risk (203). However, such low-penetrance genes may ultimately prove most useful as part of a risk assessment panel rather than an independent predictor of risk, such as *BRCA1* and *BRCA2*.

MLH1/MSH2

Muir-Torre syndrome, a variant of hereditary nonpolyposis colon cancer (HNPCC, also called *Lynch syndrome type II*) is the eponym given to the association between multiple skin tumors and multiple benign and malignant tumors of the upper and lower gastrointestinal and genitourinary tracts (46,204). Many of the manifestations of Muir-Torre syndrome are common lesions (basal cell carcinomas, keratoacanthomas, and colonic diverticula) in distributions similar to that in the general population, but with earlier age at onset in affected individuals. Women with the syndrome reportedly have an increased tendency to develop breast cancer, particularly after menopause, although lifetime risk has not been calculated (205). Multiple

genes responsible for HNPCC have been described, including *MLH1* and *MSH2* (206). Mutations in these genes are thought to lead to the development of HNPCC through accumulation of DNA replication errors and associated subsequent genome instability (206). Confirmation that Muir-Torre syndrome is a variant of HNPCC occurred with the identification of germline mutations in *MHS2* in individuals with the syndrome (207). A truncating mutation in *MLH1* also has been detected in a family with a history of Muir-Torre syndrome (208).

PALB2

PALB2 was originally identified as a protein which interacts with the N-terminal region of BRCA2 (209). This association is essential for BRCA2 function and PALB2 deficient cells are defective in double strand break repair HR. and sensitive to DNA cross-linking agents. These properties resemble genes involved in the Fanconi anemia network and in fact biallelic mutations in *PALB2* cause Fanconi anemia type N (210,211). A role for *PALB2* mutations in breast cancer susceptibility was established in two studies. Rahman et al. (212) identified five different monoallelic *PALB2* truncating mutations in 10 individuals with familial breast cancer; it was estimated that these mutations conferred a 2.3-fold elevated risk of breast cancer. In a separate study, a founder *PALB2* mutation in Finland was identified that appears to be associated with nearly a fourfold risk (213).

BRIP1

BRIP1 is a nuclear BRCA1 interacting protein originally referred to as BACH1 (214). This protein is a helicase and interacts with BRCA1 via the BRCT-motif and contributes to its DNA repair functions. As with PALB2, BRIP1 is implicated in Fanconi anemia; *BRIP1* is the *FANCJ* gene. Seal et al. (215) identified constitutional truncating mutations of the *BRIP1* gene in individuals with breast cancer from *BRCA1/BRCA2* mutation-negative families. These were significantly more common in this group than in a control population. It was estimated that *BRIP1* mutations confer a relative risk of breast cancer of about 2.

 ## FUTURE DIRECTIONS IN BREAST CANCER GENETICS

Following the identification of *BRCA1* and *BRCA2*, there is an improved understanding of cancer risks associated with these genes, and management strategies to reduce cancer risks based on clinical evidence have been developed. Further elucidation of the basic mechanisms involved in the pathogenesis of *BRCA1*- and *BRCA2*-related breast cancers may allow more targeted interventions to eliminate risks in individuals with germline mutations and may provide critical information regarding the development of sporadic tumors. The influence of modifying factors, both genetic and environmental, is being addressed because families with identical mutations can have marked variation in cancer phenotype. However, known breast cancer susceptibility genes account for less than 25% of the familial aggregation of breast cancer. Many other variants with moderate or low penetrance, some of them common, will be discovered. This will have considerable implications for risk assessment. The hope is that these advancements will improve the diagnosis and treatment of breast cancer in women affected with both inherited and sporadic forms of the disease.

References

1. Wooster R, Weber BL. Breast and ovarian cancer. *N Engl J Med* 2003;348: 2339–2347.

2. Thompson D, Easton D. Cancer incidence in BRCA1 mutation carriers. *J Natl Cancer Inst* 2002;94:1358–1365.

3. The Breast Cancer Linkage Consortium Cancer. Risks in BRCA2 mutation carriers. *J Natl Cancer Inst* 1999;91:1310–1316.

4. Wooster R, Neuhausen SL, Mangion J, et al. Localization of a breast cancer susceptibility gene, BRCA2, to chromosome 13q12-13. *Science* 1994;265:2088–2090.

5. Reis-Filho J, Turner N. Basal-like breast cancer and the BRCA1 phenotype. *Oncogene* 2006;25:5846–5853.

6. Lane-Clayton J. A further report on cancer of the breast, with special reference to its associated antecedent conditions. *Reports of the Ministry of Health, London: HM Stationary Office* 1926:32.

7. Wasink W. Cancer et heredite. *Genetika* 1935;17:103–144.

8. Adami HO, Hansen J, Jung B, et al. Characteristics of familial breast cancer in Sweden: absence of relation to age and unilateral versus bilateral disease. *Cancer* 1981;48:1688–1695.

9. Lubin JH, Burns PE, Blot WJ, et al. Risk factors for breast cancer in women in northern Alberta, Canada, as related to age at diagnosis. *J Natl Cancer Inst* 1982;68:211–217.

10. Bain C, Speizer FE, Rosner B, et al. Family history of breast cancer as a risk indicator for the disease. *Am J Epidemiol* 1980;111:301–308.

11. Newman B, Mu H, Butler LM, et al. Frequency of breast cancer attributable to BRCA1 in a population-based series of American women. *JAMA* 1998;279:915–921.

12. Anderson DE. Some characteristics of familial breast cancer. *Cancer* 1971;28:1500–1504.

13. Anderson DE. Breast cancer in families. *Cancer* 1977;40:1855–1860.

14. Williams WR, Anderson DE. Genetic epidemiology of breast cancer: segregation analysis of 200 Danish pedigrees. *Genet Epidemiol* 1984;1:7–20.

15. Newman B, Austin MA, Lee M, et al. Inheritance of human breast cancer: evidence for autosomal dominant transmission in high-risk families. *Proc Natl Acad Sci U S A* 1988;85:3044–3048.

16. Marchbanks PA, Mcdonald JA, Wilson HG, et al. The NICHD Women's Contraceptive and Reproductive Experiences Study: methods and operational results. *Ann Epidemiol* 2002;12:213–221.

17. Simon MS, Korczak JF, Yee CL et al. Breast cancer risk estimates for relatives of white and African American women with breast cancer in the Women's Contraceptive and Reproductive Experiences Study. *J Clin Oncol* 2006;24:2498–2504.

18. Malone KE, Daling JR, Doody DR, et al. Prevalence and predictors of BRCA1 and BRCA2 mutations in a population-based study of breast cancer in white and black American women ages 35 to 64 years. *Cancer Res* 2006;66:8297–8308.

19. Amos CI, Goldstein AM, Harris EL. Familiarity of breast cancer and socioeconomic status in blacks. *Cancer Res* 1991;51:1793–1797.

20. Schatzkin A, Palmer JR, Rosenberg L, et al. Risk factors for breast cancer in black women. *J Natl Cancer Inst* 1987;78:213–217.

21. Bondy M. Ethnic differences in familial breast cancer. *Proc Am Assoc Cancer Res* 1991;32(1316):221.

22. Kato I, Miura S, Kasumi F, et al. A case-control study of breast cancer among Japanese women: with special reference to family history and reproductive and dietary factors. *Breast Cancer Res Treat* 1992;24:51–59.

23. Weiss KM, Chakraborty R, Smouse PE, et al. Familial aggregation of cancer in Laredo, Texas: a generally low-risk Mexican-American population. *Genet Epidemiol* 1986;3:121–143.

24. Sattin RW, Rubin GL, Webster LA, et al. Family history and the risk of breast cancer. *JAMA* 1985;253:1908–1913.

25. Colditz GA, Willett WC, Hunter DJ, et al. Family history, age, and risk of breast cancer. Prospective data from the Nurses' Health Study *JAMA* 1993;270:338–343.

26. Zidan J, Diab M, Robinson E. Familial breast cancer [in Arabs]. *Harefuah* 1992;122:767–769, 819.

27. Ju W, Wang J, Li B, Li Z. An epidemiology and molecular genetic study on breast cancer susceptibility. *Chin Med Sci J* 2000;15:231–237.

28. Claus EB, Risch N, Thompson WD. Genetic analysis of breast cancer in the cancer and steroid hormone study. *Am J Hum Genet* 1991;48:232–242.

29. Claus EB, Schildkraut JM, Thompson WD, et al. The genetic attributable risk of breast and ovarian cancer. *Cancer* 1996;77:2318–2324.

30. FitzGerald MG, MacDonald DJ, Krainer M, et al. Germ-line BRCA1 mutations in Jewish and non-Jewish women with early-onset breast cancer. *N Engl J Med* 1996;334:143–149.

31. Couch FJ, DeShano ML, Blackwood MA, et al. BRCA1 mutations in women attending clinics that evaluate the risk of breast cancer. *N Engl J Med* 1997;336:1409–1415.

32. Krainer M, Silva-Arrieta S, FitzGerald MG, et al. Differential contributions of BRCA1 and BRCA2 to early-onset breast cancer. *N Engl J Med* 1997;336:1416–1421.

33. Anglian Breast Cancer Study Group. Prevalence and penetrance of BRCA1 and BRCA2 mutations in a population-based series of breast cancer cases. *Br J Cancer* 2000;83:1301–1308.

34. Stratton MR, Rahman N. The emerging landscape of breast cancer susceptibility. *Nat Genet* 2008;40:17–22.

35. Boyd M, Harris F, McFarlane R, et al. A human BRCA1 gene knockout [Letter]. *Nature* 1995;375:541–542.

36. Szabo CI, King MC. Population genetics of BRCA1 and BRCA2 [Editorial; comment]. *Am J Hum Genet* 1997;60:1013–1020.

37. Kuschel B, Gayther SA, Easton DF, et al. Apparent human BRCA1 knockout caused by mispriming during polymerase chain reaction: implications for genetic testing. *Genes Chromosomes Cancer* 2001;31:96–98.

38. Howlett NG, Taniguchi T, Olson S, et al. Biallelic inactivation of BRCA2 in Fanconi anemia. *Science* 2002;297:606–609.

39. Frank TS, Deffenbaugh AM, Reid JE, et al. Clinical characteristics of individuals with germline mutations in BRCA1 and BRCA2: analysis of 10,000 individuals. *J Clin Oncol* 2002;20:1480–1490.

40. Tai YC, Domchek S, Parmigiani G, et al. Breast cancer risk among male BRCA1 and BRCA2 mutation carriers. *J Natl Cancer Inst* 2007;99:1811–1814.

41. Risch HA, McLaughlin JR, Cole DE, et al. Population BRCA1 and BRCA2 mutation frequencies and cancer penetrances: a kin-cohort study in Ontario, Canada. *J Natl Cancer Inst* 2006;98:1694–706.

42. Knudson AG Jr. Mutation and cancer: statistical study of retinoblastoma. *Proc Natl Acad Sci U S A* 1971;68:820–823.

43. Li FP, Fraumeni JF. Soft-tissue sarcomas, breast cancer, and other neoplasms: familial syndrome? *Ann Intern Med* 1969;71:747.

44. Eng C. Will the real Cowden syndrome please stand up: revised diagnostic criteria. *J Med Genet* 2000;37:828–830.

45. Brownstein MH, Wolf M, Bikowski JB. Cowden's disease: a cutaneous marker of breast cancer. *Cancer* 1978;41:2393–2398.

46. Muir EG, Bell AJ, Barlow KA. Multiple primary carcinomata of the colon, duodenum, and larynx associated with kerato-acanthomata of the face. *Br J Surg* 1967;54:191–195.

47. Hall JM, Lee MK, Newman B, et al. Linkage of early-onset familial breast cancer to chromosome 17q21. *Science* 1990;250:1684–1689.

48. Narod SA, Feunteun J, Lynch HT, et al. Familial breast-ovarian cancer locus on chromosome 17q12-q23. *Lancet* 1991;338:82–83.

49. Easton DF, Bishop DT, Ford D, et al. Genetic linkage analysis in familial breast and ovarian cancer: results from 214 families. The Breast Cancer Linkage Consortium. *Am J Hum Genet* 1993;52:678–701.

50. Miki Y, Swensen J, Shattuck-Eidens D, et al. A strong candidate for the breast and ovarian cancer susceptibility gene BRCA1. *Science* 1994;266:66–71.

51. Venkitaraman AR. Cancer susceptibility and the functions of BRCA1 and BRCA2. *Cell* 2002;108:171–182.

52. Gudmundsdottir K, Ashworth A. The roles of BRCA1 and BRCA2 and associated proteins in the maintenance of genomic stability. *Oncogene* 2006;25:5864–5874.

53. Wooster R, Bignell G, Lancaster J, et al. Identification of the breast cancer susceptibility gene BRCA2. *Nature* 1995;378:789–792.

54. Tavtigian SV, Simard J, Rommens J, et al. The complete BRCA2 gene and mutations in chromosome 13q-linked kindreds. *Nat Genet* 1996;12:333–337.

55. Petrij-Bosch A, Peelen T, van Vliet M, et al. BRCA1 genomic deletions are major founder mutations in Dutch breast cancer patients. *Nat Genet* 1997;17:341–345.

56. Turner N, Tutt A, Ashworth A. Hallmarks of 'BRCAness' in sporadic cancers. *Nat Rev Cancer* 2004;4:814–819.

57. Struewing JP, Hartge P, Wacholder S, et al. The risk of cancer associated with specific mutations of BRCA1 and BRCA2 among Ashkenazi Jews. *N Engl J Med* 1997;336:1401–1408.

58. Whittemore AS, Gong G, Itnyre J. Prevalence and contribution of BRCA1 mutations in breast cancer and ovarian cancer: results from three U.S. population-based case-control studies of ovarian cancer. *Am J Hum Genet* 1997;60:496–504.

59. Martin AM, Blackwood MA, Antin-Ozerkis D, et al. Germline mutations in BRCA1 and BRCA2 in breast-ovarian families from a breast cancer risk evaluation clinic. *J Clin Oncol* 2001;19:2247–2253.

60. Stoppa-Lyonnet D, Laurent-Puig P, Essioux L, et al. BRCA1 sequence variations in 160 individuals referred to a breast/ovarian family cancer clinic. Institut Curie Breast Cancer Group. *Am J Hum Genet* 1997;60:1021–1030.

61. Shattuck-Eidens D, Oliphant A, McClure M, et al. BRCA1 sequence analysis in women at high risk for susceptibility mutations: risk factor analysis and implications for genetic testing. *JAMA* 1997;278:1242–1250.

62. Frank TS, Manley SA, Olopade OI, et al. Sequence analysis of BRCA1 and BRCA2: correlation of mutations with family history and ovarian cancer risk. *J Clin Oncol* 1998;16:2417–2425.

63. Shih HA, Couch FJ, Nathanson KL, et al. BRCA1 and BRCA2 mutation frequency in women evaluated in a breast cancer risk evaluation clinic. *J Clin Oncol* 2002;20:994–999.

64. Thorlacius S, Olafsdottir G, Tryggvadottir L, et al. A single BRCA2 mutation in male and female breast cancer families from Iceland with varied cancer phenotypes. *Nat Genet* 1996;13:117–119.

65. Tonin P, Serova O, Lenoir G, et al. BRCA1 mutations in Ashkenazi Jewish women. *Am J Hum Genet* 1995;57:189.

66. Struewing JP, Abeliovich D, Peretz T, et al. The carrier frequency of the BRCA1 185delAG mutation is approximately 1 percent in Ashkenazi Jewish individuals [published erratum in *Nat Genet* 1996;12(1):110]. *Nat Genet* 1995;11:198–200.

67. Oddoux C, Struewing JP, Clayton CM, et al. The carrier frequency of the BRCA2 6174delT mutation among Ashkenazi Jewish individuals is approximately 1%. *Nat Genet* 1996;14:188–190.

68. Roa BB, Boyd AA, Volcik K, et al. Ashkenazi Jewish population frequencies for common mutations in BRCA1 and BRCA2. *Nat Genet* 1996;14:185–187.

69. Neuhausen SL, Godwin AK, Gershoni-Baruch R, et al. Haplotype and phenotype analysis of nine recurrent BRCA2 mutations in 111 families: results of an international study. *Am J Hum Genet* 1998;62:1381–1388.

70. Offit K, Gilewski T, McGuire P, et al. Germline BRCA1 185delAG mutations in Jewish women with breast cancer. *Lancet* 1996;347:1643–1645.

71. Muto MG, Cramer DW, Tangir J, et al. Frequency of the BRCA1 185delAG mutation among Jewish women with ovarian cancer and matched population controls. *Cancer Res* 1996;56:1250–1252.

72. Abeliovich D, Kaduri L, Lerer I, et al. The founder mutations 185delAG and 5382insC in BRCA1 and 6174delT in BRCA2 appear in 60% of ovarian cancer and 30% of early-onset breast cancer patients among Ashkenazi women. *Am J Hum Genet* 1997;60:505–514.

73. Levy-Lahad E, Catane R, Eisenberg S, et al. Founder BRCA1 and BRCA2 mutations in Ashkenazi Jews in Israel: frequency and differential penetrance in ovarian cancer and in breast-ovarian cancer families. *Am J Hum Genet* 1997;60:1059–1067.

74. Kauff ND, Perez-Segura P, Robson ME, et al. Incidence of non-founder BRCA1 and BRCA2 mutations in high risk Ashkenazi breast and ovarian cancer families. *J Med Genet* 2002;39:611–614.

75. Phelan CM, Kwan E, Jack E, et al. A low frequency of non-founder BRCA1 mutations in Ashkenazi Jewish breast-ovarian cancer families. *Hum Mutat* 2002;20:352–357.

76. Olopade OI, Fackenthal JD, Dunston G, et al. Breast cancer genetics in African Americans. *Cancer* 2003;97:236–245.

77. Nanda R, Schumm LP, Cummings S et al. Genetic testing in an ethnically diverse cohort of high-risk women: a comparative analysis of BRCA1 and BRCA2 mutations in American families of European and African ancestry. *JAMA* 2005;294:1925–1933.

78. Weitzel JN, Lagos VI, Herzog JS et al. Evidence for common ancestral origin of a recurring BRCA1 genomic rearrangement identified in high-risk Hispanic families. *Cancer Epidemiol Biomarkers Prev* 2007;16:1615–1620.

79. Begg CB. On the use of familial aggregation in population-based case probands for calculating penetrance. *J Natl Cancer Inst* 2002;94:1221–1226.
80. Fodor FH, Weston A, Bleiweiss IJ, et al. Frequency and carrier risk associated with common BRCA1 and BRCA2 mutations in Ashkenazi Jewish breast cancer patients. *Am J Hum Genet* 1998;63:45–51.
81. Begg CB, Haile RW, Borg A, et al. Variation of breast cancer risk among BRCA1/2 carriers. *JAMA* 2008;299:194–201.
82. Antoniou A, Pharoah PD, Narod S, et al. Average risks of breast and ovarian cancer associated with BRCA1 or BRCA2 mutations detected in case series unselected for family history: a combined analysis of 22 studies. *Am J Hum Genet* 2003;72:1117–1130.
83. Antoniou AC, Pharoah PD, Narod S et al. Breast and ovarian cancer risks to carriers of the BRCA1 5382insC and 185delAG and BRCA2 6174delT mutations: a combined analysis of 22 population based studies. *J Med Genet* 2005;42: 602–603.
84. Ford D, Easton DF, Bishop DT, et al. Risks of cancer in BRCA1-mutation carriers. Breast Cancer Linkage Consortium. *Lancet* 1994;343:692–695.
85. Brose MS, Rebbeck TR, Calzone KA, et al. Cancer risk estimates for BRCA1 mutation carriers identified in a risk evaluation program. *J Natl Cancer Inst* 2002;94: 1365–1372.
86. Easton DF, Bishop DT, Ford D, et al. Breast and ovarian cancer incidence in BRCA1 mutation carriers. *Lancet* 1994;343:962.
87. Ford D, Easton DF, Stratton M, et al. Genetic heterogeneity and penetrance analysis of the BRCA1 and BRCA2 genes in breast cancer families. The Breast Cancer Linkage Consortium. *Am J Hum Genet* 1998;62:676–689.
88. Thompson D, Easton D. Variation in BRCA1 cancer risks by mutation position. *Cancer Epidemiol Biomarkers Prev* 2002;11:329–336.
89. Hahn SA, Greenhalf B, Ellis I, et al. BRCA2 germline mutations in familial pancreatic carcinoma. *J Natl Cancer Inst* 2003;95:214–221.
90. Murphy KM, Brune KA, Griffin C, et al. Evaluation of candidate genes MAP2K4, MADH4, ACVR1B, and BRCA2 in familial pancreatic cancer: deleterious BRCA2 mutations in 17%. *Cancer Res* 2002;62:3789–3793.
91. Gayther SA, Warren W, Mazoyer S, et al. Germline mutations of the BRCA1 gene in breast and ovarian cancer families provide evidence for a genotype-phenotype correlation. *Nat Genet* 1995;11:428–433.
92. Risch HA, McLaughlin JR, Cole DE, et al. Prevalence and penetrance of germline BRCA1 and BRCA2 mutations in a population series of 649 women with ovarian cancer. *Am J Hum Genet* 2001;68:700–710.
93. Thompson D, Easton D. Variation in cancer risks, by mutation position, in BRCA2 mutation carriers. *Am J Hum Genet* 2001;68:410–419.
94. Gayther SA, Mangion J, Russell P, et al. Variation of risks of breast and ovarian cancer associated with different germline mutations of the BRCA2 gene. *Nat Genet* 1997;15:103–105.
95. Rebbeck TR, Lynch HT, Neuhausen SL, et al. Prophylactic oophorectomy in carriers of BRCA1 or BRCA2 mutations. *N Engl J Med* 2002;346:1616–1622.
96. Rebbeck TR, Levin AM, Eisen A, et al. Breast cancer risk after bilateral prophylactic oophorectomy in BRCA1 mutation carriers. *J Natl Cancer Inst* 1999;91: 1475–1479.
97. Kauff ND, Satagopan JM, Robson ME, et al. Risk-reducing salpingo-oophorectomy in women with a BRCA1 or BRCA2 mutation. *N Engl J Med* 2002;346: 1609–1615.
98. Eisen A, Lubinski J, Klijn J et al. Breast cancer risk following bilateral oophorectomy in BRCA1 and BRCA2 mutation carriers: an international case-control study. *J Clin Oncol.* 2005;23:7491–7496.
99. Domchek SM, Friebel TM, Neuhausen SL et al. Mortality after bilateral salpingo-oophorectomy in BRCA1 and BRCA2 mutation carriers: a prospective cohort study. *Lancet Oncol* 2006;7:223–229.
100. Kauff ND, Domchek SM, Friebel TM et al. Risk-reducing salpingo-oophorectomy for the prevention of BRCA1- and BRCA2-associated breast and gynecologic cancer: a multicenter, prospective study. *J Clin Oncol* 2008 26:1331–1337.
101. Narod SA, Brunet JS, Ghadirian P, et al. Tamoxifen and risk of contralateral breast cancer in BRCA1 and BRCA2 mutation carriers: a case-control study. Hereditary Breast Cancer Clinical Study Group. *Lancet* 2000;356:1876–1881.
102. Gronwald J, Tung N, Foulkes WD, et al.Tamoxifen and contralateral breast cancer in BRCA1 and BRCA2 carriers: an update. *Int J Cancer* 2006;118:2281–2284.
103. Narod SA. Modifiers of risk of hereditary breast and ovarian cancer. *Nat Rev Cancer* 2002;2:113–123.
104. Narod SA, Goldgar D, Cannon-Albright L, et al. Risk modifiers in carriers of BRCA1 mutations. *Int J Cancer* 1995;64:394–398.
105. Jernstrom H, Lerman C, Ghadirian P, et al. Pregnancy and risk of early breast cancer in carriers of BRCA1 and BRCA2. *Lancet* 1999;354:1846–1850.
106. Rebbeck TR, Kantoff PW, Krithivas K, et al. Modification of BRCA1-associated breast cancer risk by the polymorphic androgen-receptor CAG repeat. *Am J Hum Genet* 1999;64:1371–1377.
107. Narod SA, Risch H, Moslehi R, et al. Oral contraceptives and the risk of hereditary ovarian cancer. Hereditary Ovarian Cancer Clinical Study Group. *N Engl J Med* 1998;339.424–428.
108. Narod SA, Sun P, Ghadirian P, et al. Tubal ligation and risk of ovarian cancer in carriers of BRCA1 or BRCA2 mutations: a case-control study. *Lancet* 2001;357: 1467–1470.
109. McLaughlin JR, Risch HA, Lubinski J et al. Reproductive risk factors for ovarian cancer in carriers of BRCA1 or BRCA2 mutations: a case-control study. *Lancet Oncol* 2007;8:26–34.
110. Ursin G, Henderson BE, Haile RW, et al. Does oral contraceptive use increase the risk of breast cancer in women with BRCA1/BRCA2 mutations more than in other women? *Cancer Res* 1997;57:3678–3681.
111. Narod SA, Dube MP, Klijn J, et al. Oral contraceptives and the risk of breast cancer in BRCA1 and BRCA2 mutation carriers. *J Natl Cancer Inst* 2002;94: 1773–1779.
112. Narod SA, Risch H, Moslehi R, et al. Oral contraceptives and the risk of hereditary ovarian cancer. Hereditary Ovarian Cancer Clinical Study Group. *N Engl J Med* 1998;339:424–428.
113. Brohet RM, Goldgar DE, Easton DF et al. Oral contraceptives and breast cancer risk in the international BRCA1/2 carrier cohort study: a report from EMBRACE, GENEPSO, GEO-HEBON, and the IBCCS Collaborating Group. *J Clin Oncol* 2007; 25:3831–3836.
114. Haile RW, Thomas DC, McGuire V et al. BRCA1 and BRCA2 mutation carriers, oral contraceptive use, and breast cancer before age 50. *Cancer Epidemiol Biomarkers Prev* 2006;15:1863–1870.
115. Chenevix-Trench G, Milne RL, Antoniou AL, et al. An international initiative to identify genetic modifiers of cancer risk in BRCA1 and BRCA2 mutation carriers: the Consortium of Investigators of Modifiers of BRCA1 and BRCA2 (CIMBA). *Breast Cancer Res* 2007;9:104.
116. Antoniou AC, Sinilnikova OM, Simard JE, et al. RAD51 135G→C modifies breast cancer risk among BRCA2 mutation carriers: results from a combined analysis of 19 studies. *Am J Hum Genet* 2007;81:1186–1200.
117. Couch FJ, Johnson MR, Rabe KG, et al. The prevalence of BRCA2 mutations in familial pancreatic cancer. *Cancer Epidemiol Biomarkers Prev* 2007;16: 342–346.
118. Lakhani SR, Van De Vijver MJ, Jacquemier J, et al. The pathology of familial breast cancer: predictive value of immunohistochemical markers estrogen receptor, progesterone receptor, HER-2, and p53 in patients with mutations in BRCA1 and BRCA2. *J Clin Oncol* 2002;20:2310–2318.
119. Lakhani SR, Reis Filho JS, Fulford L, et al. Prediction of BRCA1 status in patients with breast cancer using estrogen receptor and basal phenotype. *Clin Cancer Res* 2005;11:5175–5180.
120. Foulkes WD, Stefansson IM, Chappuis PO, et al. Germline BRCA1 mutations and a basal epithelial phenotype in breast cancer. *J Natl Cancer Inst* 2003;95: 1482–1485.
121. Sorlie T, Tibshirani R, Parker J, et al. Repeated observation of breast tumor subtypes in independent gene expression data sets. *Proc Natl Acad Sci U S A* 2003; 100:8418–8423.
122. Hosey AM, Gorski JJ, Murray MM, et al. Molecular basis for estrogen receptor alpha deficiency in BRCA1-linked breast cancer. *J Natl Cancer Inst* 2007;99: 1683–1694.
123. Kandel MJ, Stadler Z, Masciari S, et al. Prevalence of BRCA1 mutations in triple negative breast cancer (BC). *J Clin Oncol (Meeting Abstracts)* 2006;24:508.
124. Bane AL, Beck JC, Bleiweiss I, et al. BRCA2 mutation-associated breast cancers exhibit a distinguishing phenotype based on morphology and molecular profiles from tissue microarrays. *Am J Surg Pathol* 2007;31:121–128.
125. Kerr P, Ashworth A. New complexities for BRCA1 and BRCA2. *Curr Biol* 2001;11: R668–R676.
126. Jensen DE, Proctor M, Marquis ST, et al. BAP1: a novel ubiquitin hydrolase which binds to the BRCA1 RING finger and enhances BRCA1-mediated cell growth suppression. *Oncogene* 1998;16:1097–1112.
127. Wu LC, Wang ZW, Tsan JT, et al. Identification of a RING protein that can interact in vivo with the BRCA1 gene product. *Nat Genet* 1996;14:430–440.
128. Hashizume R, Fukuda M, Maeda I, et al. The RING heterodimer BRCA1–BARD1 is a ubiquitin ligase inactivated by a breast cancer-derived mutation. *J Biol Chem* 2001;276:14537–14540.
129. Ruffner H, Joazeiro CA, Hemmati D, et al. Cancer-predisposing mutations within the RING domain of BRCA1: loss of ubiquitin protein ligase activity and protection from radiation hypersensitivity. *Proc Natl Acad Sci U S A* 2001;98:5134–5139.
130. Starita LM, Parvin JD. Substrates of the BRCA1-dependent ubiquitin-ligase. *Cancer Biol Ther* 2006;5:137–141.
131. Soulier J, Lowndes NF. The BRCT domain of the S. cerevisiae checkpoint protein Rad9 mediates a Rad9-Rad9 interaction after DNA damage. *Curr Biol* 1999;9: 551–554.
132. Wu LC, Wang ZW, Tsan JT, et al. Identification of a RING protein that can interact in vivo with the BRCA1 gene product. *Nat Genet* 1996;14:430–440.
133. Monteiro AN, August A, Hanafusa H. Evidence for a transcriptional activation function of BRCA1 C-terminal region. *Proc Natl Acad Sci U S A* 1996;93: 13595–13599.
134. Vallon-Christersson J, Cayanan C, Haraldsson K, et al. Functional analysis of BRCA1 C-terminal missense mutations identified in breast and ovarian cancer families. *Hum Mol Genet* 2001;10:353–360.
135. Bertwistle D, Swift S, Marston NJ, et al. Nuclear location and cell cycle regulation of the BRCA2 protein. *Cancer Res* 1997;57:5485–5488.
136. Esashi F, Galkin VE, Yu X, et al. Stabilization of RAD51 nucleoprotein filaments by the C-terminal region of BRCA2. *Nat Struct Mol Biol* 2007;14:468–474.
137. Davies OR, Pellegrini L. Interaction with the BRCA2 C terminus protects RAD51-DNA filaments from disassembly by BRC repeats. *Nat Struct Mol Biol* 2007;14: 475–483.
138. Yang H, Jeffrey PD, Miller J, et al. BRCA2 function in DNA binding and recombination from a BRCA2-DSS1-ssDNA structure. *Science* 2002;297:1837–1848.
139. Tutt AN, Lord CJ, McCabe N, et al. Exploiting the DNA repair defect in BRCA mutant cells in the design of new therapeutic strategies for cancer. *Cold Spring Harb Symp Quant Biol* 2005;70:139–148.
140. Yuan SS, Lee SY, Chen G, et al. BRCA2 is required for ionizing radiation-induced assembly of Rad51 complex in vivo. *Cancer Res* 1999;59:3547–3551.
141. Patel KJ, Vu VP, Lee H, et al. Involvement of Brca2 in DNA repair. *Mol Cell* 1998; 1:347–357.
142. Tutt A, Bertwistle D, Valentine J, et al. Mutation in BRCA2 stimulates error-prone homology-directed repair of DNA double-strand breaks occurring between repeated sequences. *EMBO J* 2001;20:4704–4716.
143. Scully R, Anderson SF, Chao DM, et al. BRCA1 is a component of the RNA polymerase II holoenzyme. *Proc Natl Acad Sci U S A* 1997;94:5605–5610.
144. Chapman MS, Verma IM. Transcriptional activation by BRCA1. *Nature* 1996;382: 678–679.
145. Monteiro AN, August A, Hanafusa H. Evidence for a transcriptional activation function of BRCA1 C-terminal region. *Proc Natl Acad Sci U S A* 1996;93: 13595–13599.
146. Liebens FP, Carly B, Pastijn A, et al. Management of BRCA1/2 associated breast cancer: a systematic qualitative review of the state of knowledge in 2006. *Eur J Cancer* 2007;43:238–257.
147. Moller P, Evans DG, Reis MM, et al. Surveillance for familial breast cancer: differences in outcome according to BRCA mutation status. *Int J Cancer* 2007;121: 1017–1020.
148. Rennert G, Bisland-Naggan S, Barnett-Griness O, et al. Clinical outcomes of breast cancer in carriers of BRCA1 and BRCA2 mutations. *N Engl J Med* 2007; 357:115–123.
149. Rubin SC, Benjamin I, Behbakht K, et al. Clinical and pathological features of ovarian cancer in women with germ-line mutations of BRCA1. *N Engl J Med* 1996;335:1413–1416.
150. Boyd J, Sonoda Y, Federici MG, et al. Clinicopathologic features of BRCA-linked and sporadic ovarian cancer. *JAMA* 2000;283:2260–2265.
151. Cass I, Baldwin RL, Varkey T, et al. Improved survival in women with BRCA-associated ovarian carcinoma. *Cancer* 2003;97:2187–2195.

152. Chetrit A, Hirsh-Yechezkel G, Ben-David Y, et al. Effect of BRCA1/2 mutations on long-term survival of patients with invasive ovarian cancer: the national Israeli study of ovarian cancer. *J Clin Oncol* 2008;26:20–25.
153. Robson M, Levin D, Federici M, et al. Breast conservation therapy for invasive breast cancer in Ashkenazi women with BRCA gene founder mutations. *J Natl Cancer Inst* 1999;91:2112–2117.
154. Rodriguez-Pinilla SM, Sarrio D, Honrado E, et al. Prognostic significance of basal-like phenotype and fascin expression in node-negative invasive breast carcinomas. *Clin Cancer Res* 2006;12:1533–1539.
155. Rouzier R, Perou CM, Symmans WF, et al. Breast cancer molecular subtypes respond differently to preoperative chemotherapy. *Clin Cancer Res* 2005;11:5678–5685.
156. Shanley S, McReynolds K, Ardern-Jones A, et al. Acute chemotherapy-related toxicity is not increased in BRCA1 and BRCA2 mutation carriers treated for breast cancer in the United Kingdom. *Clin Cancer Res* 2006;12:7033–7038.
157. Rakha EA, El-Sayed ME, Green AR, et al. Prognostic markers in triple-negative breast cancer. *Cancer* 2007;109:25–32.
158. Foulkes WD, Metcalfe K, Hanna W, et al. Disruption of the expected positive correlation between breast tumor size and lymph node status in BRCA1-related breast carcinoma. *Cancer* 2003;98:1569–1577.
159. Pierce LJ, Levin AM, Rebbeck TR, et al. Ten-year multi-institutional results of breast-conserving surgery and radiotherapy in BRCA1/2-associated stage I/II breast cancer. *J Clin Oncol* 2006;24:2437–2443.
160. Shanley S, McReynolds K, Ardern Jones A, et al. Late toxicity is not increased in BRCA1/BRCA2 mutation carriers undergoing breast radiotherapy in the United Kingdom. *Clin Cancer Res* 2006;12:7025–7032.
161. Moynahan ME, Cui TY, Jasin M. Homology-directed dna repair, mitomycin-c resistance, and chromosome stability is restored with correction of a BRCA1 mutation. *Cancer Res* 2001;61:4842–4850.
162. Bhattacharyya A, Ear US, Koller BH, et al. The breast cancer susceptibility gene BRCA1 is required for subnuclear assembly of Rad51 and survival following treatment with the DNA cross-linking agent cisplatin. *J Biol Chem* 2000;275:23899–23903.
163. Kennedy RD, Quinn JE, Mullan PB, et al. The role of BRCA1 in the cellular response to chemotherapy. *J Natl Cancer Inst* 2004;96:1659–1668.
164. Byrski T, Gronwald J, Huzarski T, et al. Response to neo-adjuvant chemotherapy in women with BRCA1-positive breast cancers. *Breast Cancer Res Treat* 2008;108:289–296.
165. Zhou C, SmithJL, Liu J. Role of BRCA1 in cellular resistance to paclitaxel and ionizing radiation in an ovarian cancer cell line carrying a defective BRCA1. *Oncogene* 2003;22:2396–2404.
166. Farmer H, McCabe N, Lord CJ, et al. Targeting the DNA repair defect in BRCA mutant cells as a therapeutic strategy. *Nature* 2005;434:917–921.
167. Bryant HE, Schultz N, Thomas HD, et al: Specific killing of BRCA2-deficient tumours with inhibitors of poly(ADP-ribose) polymerase. *Nature* 2005;434:913–917.
168. Dobzhansky T. Genetics of natural populations. Xiii. Recombination and variability in populations of Drosophila pseudoobscura. *Genetics* 1946;31:269–290.
169. Kaelin WG Jr. The concept of synthetic lethality in the context of anticancer therapy. *Nat Rev Cancer* 2005;5:689–698.
170. Hoeijmakers JH. Genome maintenance mechanisms for preventing cancer. *Nature* 2001;411:366–374.
171. Chambon P, Weill JD, Mandel P. Nicotinamide mononucleotide activation of new DNA-dependent polyadenylic acid synthesizing nuclear enzyme. *Biochem Biophys Res Commun* 1963;11:39–43.
172. Ame JC, Spenlehauer C, de Murcia G. The PARP superfamily. *Bioessays* 2004;26:2525–2538.
173. Otto H, Reche PA, Bazan F, et al. In silico characterization of the family of PARP-like poly(ADP-ribosyl)transferases (pARTs). *BMC Genomics* 2005;6:139.
174. Noel G, Giocanti N, Fernet M, et al. Poly(ADP-ribose) polymerase (PARP-1) is not involved in DNA double-strand break recovery. *BMC Cell Biol* 2003;4:7.
175. Haber JE. DNA recombination: the replication connection. *Trends Biochem Sci* 1999;24:271–275.
176. Ratnam K, Low JA. Current development of clinical inhibitors of poly(ADP-ribose) polymerase in oncology. *Clin Cancer Res* 2007;13:1383–1388.
177. Yap TA, Boss DS, Fong PC, et al. First in human phase I pharmacokinetic (PK) and pharmacodynamic (PD) study of KU-0059436 (Ku), a small molecule inhibitor of poly ADP ribose polymerase (PARP) in cancer patients (p), including BRCA1/2 mutation carriers. *J Clin Oncol* 2007;25:3529.
178. Edwards S, Brough R, Lord CJ, et al. Resistance to therapy caused by intragenic deletion in BRCA2. *Nature* 2008;451:1111–1115.
179. Strong LC, Williams WR, Tainsky MA. The Li-Fraumeni syndrome: from clinical epidemiology to molecular genetics. *Am J Epidemiol* 1992;135:190–199.
180. Williams W, Strong L. Genetic epidemiology of soft tissue sarcomas in children. In: Muller H, Weber W, eds. *Familial cancer: first international research conference*. Basel: S Karger AG, 1985:151–153.
181. Malkin D, Li FP, Strong LC, et al. Germ line p53 mutations in a familial syndrome of breast cancer, sarcomas, and other neoplasms. *Science* 1990;250:1233–1238.
182. Martin AM, Kanetsky PA, Amirimani B, et al. Germline TP53 mutations in breast cancer families with multiple primary cancers: is TP53 a modifier of BRCA1? *J Med Genet* 2003;40:e34.
183. Bell DW, Varley JM, Szydlo TE, et al. Heterozygous germ line hCHK2 mutations in Li-Fraumeni syndrome. *Science* 1999;286:2528–2531.
184. Meijers-Heijboer H, van den Ouweland A, Klijn J, et al. Low-penetrance susceptibility to breast cancer due to CHEK2(*)1100delC in noncarriers of BRCA1 or BRCA2 mutations. *Nat Genet* 2002;31:55–59.
185. Savitsky K, Sfez S, Tagle DA, et al. The complete sequence of the coding region of the ATM gene reveals similarity to cell cycle regulators in different species. *Hum Mol Genet* 1995;4:2025–2032.
186. Shiloh Y. ATM and related protein kinases: safeguarding genome integrity. *Nat Rev Cancer* 2003;3:155–168.
187. Ahmed M, Rahman N. ATM and breast cancer susceptibility. *Oncogene* 2006;25:5906–5911.
188. Renwick A, Thompson D, Seal S, et al. ATM mutations that cause ataxia-telangiectasia are breast cancer susceptibility alleles. *Nat Genet* 2006;38:873–875.
189. Nichols KE, Levitz S, Shannon KE, et al. Heterozygous germline ATM mutations do not contribute to radiation-associated malignancies after Hodgkin's disease. *J Clin Oncol* 1999;17:1259.
190. Broeks A, Russell NS, Floore AN, et al. Increased risk of breast cancer following irradiation for Hodgkin's disease is not a result of ATM germline mutations. *Int J Radiat Biol* 2000;76:693–698.
191. Shafman TD, Levitz S, Nixon AJ, et al. Prevalence of germline truncating mutations in ATM in women with a second breast cancer after radiation therapy for a contralateral tumor. *Genes Chromosomes Cancer* 2000;27:124–129.
192. Eng C. Genetics of Cowden syndrome: through the looking glass of oncology. *Int J Oncol* 1998;12:701–710.
193. Fackenthal JD, Marsh DJ, Richardson AL, et al. Male breast cancer in Cowden syndrome patients with germline PTEN mutations. *J Med Genet* 2001;38:159–164.
194. Carroll BT, Couch FJ, Rebbeck TR, et al. Polymorphisms in PTEN in breast cancer families. *J Med Genet* 1999;36:94–96.
195. Jeghers H, McKusick V, Katz K. Generalized intestinal polyposis and melanin spots of the oral mucosa, lips and digits: a syndrome of diagnostic significance. *N Engl J Med* 1949;241:992–1005.
196. Peutz J. On a very remarkable case of familial polyposis of the mucous membrane of the intestinal tract and nasopharynx accompanied by peculiar pigmentation of the skin and mucous membrane. *Ned Tijdschr Geneeskd* 1921;10:134–146.
197. Giardiello FM, Welsh SB, Hamilton SR, et al. Increased risk of cancer in the Peutz-Jeghers syndrome. *N Engl J Med* 1987;316:1511–1514.
198. Boardman LA, Pittelkow MR, Couch FJ, et al. Association of Peutz-Jeghers-like mucocutaneous pigmentation with breast and gynecologic carcinomas in women. *Medicine (Baltimore)* 2000;79:293–298.
199. Hemminki A, Tomlinson I, Markie D. Localization of a susceptibility locus for PJS to 19p using comparative genomic hybridization and targeted linkage analysis. *Nat Genet* 1997;15:87–90.
200. Olschwang S, Markie D. Peutz-Jeghers disease: most, but not all, families are compatible with linkage to 19p13.3. *J Med Genet* 1998;35:42–44.
201. Sodha N, Houlston RS, Bullock S, et al. Increasing evidence that germline mutations in CHEK2 do not cause Li-Fraumeni syndrome. *Hum Mutat* 2002;20:460–462.
202. Offit K, Pierce H, Kirchhoff T, et al. Frequency of CHEK2*1100delC in New York breast cancer cases and controls. *BMC Med Genet* 2003;4:1.
203. Schutte M, Seal S, Barfoot R, et al. Variants in CHEK2 other than 1100delC do not make a major contribution to breast cancer susceptibility. *Am J Hum Genet* 2003;72:1023–1028.
204. Hall NR, Williams MA, Murday VA, et al. Muir-Torre syndrome: a variant of the cancer family syndrome. *J Med Genet* 1994;31:627–631.
205. Anderson DE. An inherited form of large bowel cancer: Muir's syndrome. *Cancer* 1980;45:1103–1107.
206. Rustgi AK. The genetics of hereditary colon cancer. *Genes Dev* 2007;21:2525–2538.
207. Kolodner RD, Hall NR, Lipford J, et al. Structure of the human MSH2 locus and analysis of two Muir-Torre kindreds for msh2 mutations. *Genomics* 1994;24:516–526.
208. Bapat B, Xia L, Madlensky L, et al. The genetic basis of Muir-Torre syndrome includes the hMLH1 locus [Letter]. *Am J Hum Genet* 1996;59:736–739.
209. Xia B, Sheng Q, Nakanishi T, et al. Control of BRCA2 cellular and clinical functions by a nuclear partner, PALB2. *Mol Cell* 2006;22:719–729.
210. Reid S, Schindler D, Hanenberg H, et al. Biallelic mutations in PALB2 cause Fanconi anemia subtype FA-N and predispose to childhood cancer. *Nat Genet* 2007;39:162–164.
211. Xia B, Dorsman JC, Ameziane N, et al. Fanconi anemia is associated with a defect in the BRCA2 partner PALB2. *Nat Genet* 2007;39:159–161.
212. Rahman N, Seal, S, Thompson D, et al. PALB2, which encodes a BRCA2-interacting protein is a breast cancer susceptibility gene. *Nat Genet* 2006;39:165–167.
213. Erkko H, Xia B, Nikkila J, et al. A recurrent mutation in PALB2 in Finnish cancer families *Nature* 2007;446:316–319.
214. Cantor SB, Bell DW, Ganesan S et al. BACH1, a novel helicase-like protein, interacts directly with BRCA1 and contributes to its DNA repair function. *Cell* 2001;105:149–160.
215. Seal S, Thompson D, Renwick A, et al. Truncating mutations in the Fanconi anaemia J gene BRIP1 are low-penetrance breast cancer susceptibility alleles. *Nat Genet* 2006;38:1239–1241.
216. Hopper JL, Southey MC, Dite GS, et al. Population-based estimate of the average age-specific cumulative risk of breast cancer for a defined set of protein-truncating mutations in BRCA1 and BRCA2. Australian Breast Cancer Family Study. *Cancer Epidemiol Biomarkers Prev* 1999;8:741–747.

Claudine Isaacs, Beth N. Peshkin, and Marc Schwartz

Genetic counseling and testing are increasingly being integrated into the management of women at increased risk for breast cancer. The group of women who have an elevated risk is very heterogeneous. Because breast cancer is such a common disease in North America and northern Europe, it is not uncommon to encounter families in which two or three women have had this disease. Thus, such clusters may be typical of *familial* breast cancer, particularly when the ages of onset are postmenopausal. *Genetic* or *hereditary* breast cancer, which is much less common, is usually characterized by two or more generations affected with breast and related cancers (e.g., ovarian cancer), often with a predisposition to early ages of onset. As discussed in this chapter, specific features of an individual's personal and family history can provide substantial clues about potential etiology. When family histories are suggestive of transmission of genetic risk, women at high risk and their family members may benefit from participation in genetic counseling and testing programs. Women at high risk can reduce their risk of cancer-related morbidity and mortality through increased surveillance and adoption of risk-reducing strategies. Noncarriers of risk-conferring mutations may be relieved of persistent worry. Despite these benefits, a number of psychological and social risks of testing exist that patients and providers must consider.

Although genetic counseling and testing for breast cancer have diffused into mainstream oncologic care, critical questions regarding cancer risks and the efficacy of some management options remain unanswered. These limitations in our knowledge create challenges for providers who must counsel patients about these issues and for the patients who face the decisions to undergo genetic testing. This chapter provides an overview of the medical and psychosocial issues that are relevant to this process. The focus of this chapter is on patients at high risk who have family histories consistent with inherited susceptibility to breast cancer and who have been deemed appropriate candidates for genetic testing by major medical organizations. In addition, we address the evaluation and management of women from families without an identifiable *BRCA1/2* mutation. We begin with a discussion of the characteristics of hereditary breast cancer followed by a discussion of the assessment of the likelihood that a family harbors a breast cancer-predisposing mutation. The genetic counseling process and testing issues are then reviewed. Finally, we discuss the medical and psychosocial management issues for high risk individuals and families.

 ## CLINICAL CHARACTERISTICS OF HEREDITARY BREAST CANCER

Most cases of hereditary breast cancer are attributable to mutations in *BRCA1* and *BRCA2* (*BRCA1/2*). Other hereditary breast cancer syndromes, caused by mutations in highly penetrant genes (noted in parentheses), account for less than 1% of all cases of breast cancer, and include Li-Fraumeni syndrome (*p53*), Cowden syndrome or *PTEN* hamartoma syndrome (*PTEN*), Peutz-Jeghers syndrome (*LKB1/STK11*), and hereditary diffuse gastric cancer syndrome (*CDH1/E-cadherin*). Mutations in other genes have also been identified, which may

act in concert with other gene mutations and environmental factors to confer a more modest risk of breast cancer. Examples of these lower penetrance genes include *ATM* and *CHEK2*.

A detailed discussion of the clinical manifestations associated with non-*BRCA1/2* mutations is covered elsewhere in this book. Because most women who present for genetic counseling are candidates for *BRCA1/2* testing, the following section focuses on cancer risks associated with mutations in these genes. Of note, most studies were conducted in primarily European white populations, so it is important to counsel individuals from other ethnic groups that the generalizability of penetrance estimates is not well established (1). In addition, we address cancer risks in families at high risk in which no mutation in *BRCA1/2* is identified.

BRCA1 AND *BRCA2* Cancer Risks

Breast and Ovarian Cancer Risks

The literature addressing cancer risks in *BRCA1* and *BRCA2* mutation carriers reveals a wide range of potential risks for breast and ovarian cancer which are considerably elevated over the U.S. general population risks of 7% and less than 1%, respectively, to age 70 (Table 19.1) (2). When reviewing these studies, it is important to consider various sources of ascertainment (e.g., through linkage testing versus direct genotyping, clinic-based versus unselected series, and selection through affected or unaffected cases or probands[1]) and the relative advantages and limitations of specific study designs. Most of these studies are retrospective in nature, therefore yielding less robust estimates of cancer risk from prospective cohorts—data which are expected to become available in the near future. In consideration of these factors, it is appropriate to inform patients about a range of reported risks in mutation carriers that is based on analysis of several studies. For example, the largest meta-analysis of studies published by Antoniou et al. (3) combined data from 22 international studies comprising more than 8,000 index cases affected with female (86%) or male (2%) breast cancer or epithelial ovarian cancer (12%). To be included, index cases were sampled independently of family history. The average cumulative breast cancer risk to age 70 years in *BRCA1* carriers was 65% (95% CI, 51%–75%), versus 45% (95% CI, 33%–54%) in *BRCA2* carriers (3). Interestingly, when families were ascertained through an index case diagnosed with breast cancer at an early age, especially before age 35 years, cumulative cancer risks were about 20% higher for *BRCA1* carriers (i.e., 87% risk of breast cancer (95% CI, 67%–95%) and 51% risk of ovarian cancer (95% CI, 9.1%–73%) versus 61% risk of breast cancer (41%–74%) and 32% for ovarian cancer (11%–49%) for families containing an older proband with breast cancer). When the index case was older, the *BRCA1*-associated breast cancer risks were similar to those identified through ovarian cancer probands. Similarly, in *BRCA2* families, the breast cancer risks were higher in families with breast cancer index cases versus ovarian cancer probands. Although breast cancer incidence was not impacted

---

[1]Proband refers to the first individual in the family to undergo genetic testing.

Table 19.1	ESTIMATED CANCER RISKS ASSOCIATED WITH *BRCA1* AND *BRCA2* MUTATIONS			
Cancer Type	Risk In *BRCA1/2* Carriers to Age 70 years (%)	General Population Risk to Age 70 years (%)	Comments	References
Breast	*BRCA1:* 50–75 *BRCA2:* 33–54	7	The incidence of breast cancer diagnosed <50 years is higher in *BRCA1* carriers compared with *BRCA2* carriers, but both groups have an increased risk of premenopausal breast cancer	(3–4)
Contralateral breast	40–65	0.5–1 per year of follow-up, leveling off at 20% at 20 years after follow-up	Over long follow-up periods, the risk of ipsilateral breast cancer is also elevated	(6–9,13–18)
Ovarian	*BRCA1:* 22–51 *BRCA2:* 4–21	<1	The incidence of ovarian cancer diagnosed <50 years is higher in *BRCA1* carriers, and overall rare in all carriers <40 years; risk of fallopian tube cancer is also substantially elevated	(3–4)
Colon	Unclear	2	If elevated, risk is small	(6,9,27,29–34)
Prostate	Probably elevated; absolute risk not well defined	8	Risk appears to be higher in *BRCA2* carriers and possibly in men <65 years	(9,27,35)
Male breast	<10	0.1	Risk appears to be higher in *BRCA2* carriers	(9,36,37)
Pancreatic	<5	0.5	Risk appears to be higher in *BRCA2* carriers	(6,9,25–28)

Note: Lifetime risks of cancer are approximate and are generally from birth to age 70 years. General population risks for most sites are derived from SEER data (2).

by the age of the index patient, *BRCA2*-associated ovarian cancer risks were higher when the proband had breast cancer before age 35. Another notable finding from these analyses was that the breast cancer incidence in *BRCA1* carriers increased with age, but starting at 50 years, the incidence remained somewhat constant. In *BRCA2* carriers, however, the incidence of breast cancer continued to rise. With respect to ovarian cancer, although these risks were higher for *BRCA2* carriers ascertained via an ovarian cancer index case (relative risk [RR] = 2.4, 95% CI, 0.74–8.1), this finding was not observed in *BRCA1* carriers (RR = 0.86, 95% CI, 0.42–1.8). These data also confirmed that ovarian cancer rates in women younger than 30 years are very low, but after that, risk rises more dramatically, especially for *BRCA1* carriers. Specifically, Antoniou et al. (3) reported the lifetime risk of ovarian cancer in *BRCA1* carriers to be 39% (95% CI, 22%–51%) and 11% (95% CI, 4.1%–18%) in *BRCA2* carriers (3).

Chen and Parmigiani (4) performed a meta-analysis of ten international mixed-ascertainment studies that included data from families at high risk as well as population-based series (4). The cumulative risks to age 70 for breast cancer were 57% (95% CI, 47%–66%) for *BRCA1* and 49% (95% CI, 40%–57%) for *BRCA2* and ovarian cancer risks of 40% (95% CI, 35%–46%) for *BRCA1* and 18% (95% CI, 13%–23%) for *BRCA2* mutation carriers. These data are roughly consistent with the findings of Antoniou et al. (3) and provide reasonable parameters for clinical use. In addition, Chen and Parmigiani (4) derived age-specific predicted mean breast and ovarian cancer risks for currently unaffected *BRCA1/2* mutation carriers based on their current age (20–60 years). These data, published in tabular form, may be useful in clinical counseling. For example, based on the table, it is estimated that a 30-year-old unaffected *BRCA1* carrier has a cumulative risk of breast cancer to age 40 of 10%; to age 50 it is 28%; to age 60 is 44%; and to age 70 it is 54%. In addition, her cumulative risk of ovarian cancer to age 40 is 2.2%; 8.7% to age 50; 22% to age 60; and 39% to age 70. Age-specific risks may be one important component to guide

decisions about the timing of risk management decision, such as prophylactic surgery.

These data underscore the complexity in providing an individualized risk assessment for *BRCA1/2* carriers. Emerging data suggest that family history may be used to guide risk assessment in that risks of breast cancer do appear to be higher in multicase families than in single-case families (5). It is important, however, to counsel individuals about features of the pedigree that may hamper risk assessment, such as small family size, few women in the family, limited or unverifiable cancer history data, and so forth. In addition, variation in risk is likely to be attributable in part to genetic and nongenetic risk factors (5), as addressed later in this chapter.

Second Malignancies after Breast Cancer

A hallmark of hereditary cancer is the predisposition toward multiple primary cancers. For example, *BRCA1* carriers who are affected with breast cancer have a 40% to 65% cumulative risk of contralateral breast cancer (6–8). The risks in *BRCA2* are comparable, at approximately 52% (95% CI, 42%–61%) (9). Most of this risk occurs in the first decade after diagnosis, estimated to be approximately 43% in *BRCA1* carriers and 35% in *BRCA2* carriers (10). The risk of contralateral breast cancer may be reduced substantially with the use tamoxifen, oophorectomy, or both (oophorectomy in premenopausal women) (10–12). This is discussed in greater detail in the section on management of mutation carriers with breast cancer. Of note, women with sporadic breast cancer have a 0.5% to 1.0% annual risk of contralateral breast cancer, leveling off at 20% at 20 years of follow-up (13). Although specific risks are difficult to quantify, it does appear that, over the long term, mutation carriers are at elevated risk of developing metachronous ipsilateral breast cancer (14–18).

A significant concern for *BRCA1/2* breast cancer survivors is the threat of developing ovarian cancer. Metcalfe et al. (19) reported that the 10-year actuarial risk of ovarian cancer in such patients was 12.7% and 6.8% for *BRCA1* and *BRCA2* carriers, respectively. Of note, the development of ovarian cancer was the cause of death in one-fourth of the patients with stage I breast cancer, underscoring the importance of considering the impact of mutation status in individuals who present with a malignancy.

Other Cancers

Importantly, primary fallopian tube cancer, although quite rare, is part of the tumor spectrum associated with *BRCA1* and *BRCA2* mutations (6,20). A related question that arises, particularly for surgical treatment, is whether carriers face an elevated risk of uterine cancer. Overall, it does not appear that *BRCA1/2* mutation carriers have an excess risk of this malignancy (9,21) unless they have used tamoxifen either as treatment or primary prevention (22). It has been suggested, however, that uterine serous papillary cancer (USPC) may be part of the tumor spectrum associated with *BRCA1/2* mutations (23,24). Controversy is ongoing about the association of uterine cancer with *BRCA1/2* mutations and the potential implications for surgical management.

Several studies have reported an association between pancreatic cancer and *BRCA2* mutations (9,25,26), whereas data are less clear about the risk associated with *BRCA1* mutations (6,27). In these studies, the overall number of carriers with pancreatic cancer is very low, so lifetime absolute risk calculations are difficult to make, but overall appear to be less than 5% (28).

With respect to colon cancer risk in mutation carriers, some studies have identified elevated risks (6,27,29) and others have not (9,30–34). Thus, it is likely that if an elevation in risk exists, it appears to be small. In addition, although increased relative risks for other cancer sites have been reported in carriers (e.g., melanoma and stomach) (6,9,27), additional studies need to verify these findings.

Cancers Affecting Males

Several, but not all, studies have demonstrated that prostate cancer risks are elevated in *BRCA1/2* carriers, with some data supporting higher risks in *BRCA2* carriers compared with *BRCA1* carriers (9,35) and in men younger than age 65 (9,27). The absolute risk in *BRCA2* carriers is difficult to pinpoint relative to general population risks, given the indolent nature of this disease. Male mutation carriers also have a substantially elevated risk of developing breast cancer. For example, a retrospective study utilizing data from 1,939 families, including 97 men with breast cancer, revealed that the cumulative risk of breast cancer at age 70 was 1.2% (95% CI, 0.22%–2.8%) and 6.8% (95% CI, 3.2%–12%) in *BRCA1* and *BRCA2* carriers, respectively (36). Although these risks are overall low, the relative risks, particularly up to age 50, are sizable. However, the median age at diagnosis has been reported to be 52 and 59 years, with the later onset occurring in *BRCA2* carriers (9,37).

Summary: BRCA1/2 Associated Cancer Risks

In summary, given the wide confidence intervals reported in most studies and the range of risks found in different populations, it is difficult to define the precise cancer risks for individual mutation carriers. In addition, whether genotype–phenotype correlations exist is not yet defined and, if so, how they translate into the provision of clinical risk assessments is also uncertain (see Risk Modifiers). Furthermore, although it is important to consider the limitations of pedigree analysis, a patient's family history may be useful to put risks in some context. Nonetheless, although the exact magnitude of cancer risks is not known, it remains clear that women with *BRCA1* and *BRCA2* mutations face a substantially elevated risk of early onset breast and ovarian cancer, with increased risks that persist throughout their lifetime.

Breast and Ovarian Cancer Risks in *BRCA1/2*-Negative Families

The ability to quantify cancer risks in *BRCA1/2*-negative (uninformative) families is hampered by limited research. A few key studies have, however, shed light on this important question. First, Kauff et al. prospectively followed 165 *BRCA1/2* negative families with site-specific breast cancer (i.e., three or more cases of breast cancer in the same lineage with one or more less than age 50) for a mean of 3.4 years (38). A threefold excess risk of breast cancer was noted, but no excess risk of ovarian cancer was noted. In a Finnish study, Eerola et al. (39) studied families with three or more cases of breast cancer: 23 *BRCA1/2*-positive families and 84 non-*BRCA1/2* families, with the latter including 14 families with ovarian cancer. The lifetime risk of breast cancer in unaffected women in *BRCA1/2* negative families was comparable to *BRCA1/2*-positive women, although slightly lower, and the risk of subsequent breast cancer was much lower in *BRCA1/2*-negative patients with breast cancer (8% vs. 25% in *BRCA1/2*-positive families). Importantly, the risk of ovarian cancer was not elevated in the uninformative families. In a Swedish population-based study of 181 *BRCA1/2*-negative families ascertained through a breast cancer case ≤40 years of age, the cumulative risk of breast cancer to age 70 for first-degree relatives was 12.8% (95% CI, 6.5%–15.7%), but when the family history contained at least one other close relative with breast cancer, the risk went up to 21.1% (95% CI, 11.1%–34.7%) (40). Another population-based study of young *BRCA1/2*-negative patients with breast cancer also revealed increased risks of breast cancer in relatives (41). None of the studies discussed above that assessed ovarian cancer risk found an elevation in *BRCA1/2*-negative families. However, Lee et al. (42) found that if a family is ascertained through a woman who has ovarian cancer, her close relatives may still face an elevated risk of ovarian cancer, although this risk is not well quantified. These results suggest that members of *BRCA*-negative families, especially those with site-specific breast cancer, have an increased incidence of breast cancer, but are likely not at a significant increased risk for ovarian cancer. For families with at least one documented case of ovarian cancer, the possibility must be considered that an undetected mutation in *BRCA1/2* exists, or that the proband tested may represent a phenocopy, as discussed later in this chapter.

CANCER RISK MODIFIERS

Genotype–Phenotype Correlations within *BRCA1* and *BRCA2*

Patients frequently ask whether mutation-specific data are available that may help individualize *BRCA1* or *BRCA2* risks. Although studies have suggested that genotype–phenotype correlations may exist, these data are not yet sufficiently substantiated to integrate into clinical counseling. With respect to *BRCA1*, studies have found that mutations occurring more distally within this gene may confer a significantly elevated risk of breast cancer (43) as well as lower ovarian cancer risks (44,45). These findings, however, have not been consistently replicated, particularly in studies of founder mutations in Ashkenazi Jews (46,47).

The data support a stronger genotype–phenotype association with *BRCA2* mutations. For example, a study of 164 families found that mutations occurring within the central region of the *BRCA2* gene, called the ovarian cancer cluster region

(OCCR), appeared to be associated with a lower risk of breast cancer (RR = 0.63, 95% CI, 0.46–0.84) and a higher risk of ovarian cancer (RR = 1.88, 95% CI, 1.08–3.33) (48). This OCCR region is thought to encompass *BRCA2* mutations affecting nucleotides 3059–4075 through 6503–6629, although the 5′ starting point may be with exon 3035 (48,49). Interestingly, in another study of unselected *BRCA2* carriers with ovarian cancer, first-degree relatives had ovarian, colon, stomach, pancreatic, or prostate cancer only when the proband's mutation was within the OCCR of exon 11, and an excess of breast cancers was observed when the mutation was outside of the OCCR (43). These findings suggest that mutations within the OCCR in *BRCA2* may confer a diminished risk of breast cancer (50) (i.e., not necessarily a higher risk of ovarian cancer) and that mutations within the region may be associated with a broader tumor spectrum altogether. In addition to mutation position, ethnicity may contribute to phenotypic variation. For example, Ashkenazi Jewish families with the 6174delT mutation were more likely to have a case of ovarian cancer and less likely to have a case of prostate cancer than non-Jewish families (49). Other hospital-based studies of unselected Jewish patients have shown that patients with ovarian cancer are about four times more likely to have this mutation compared with those with breast cancer (i.e., 14% vs. 3.6%) (46,51).

It is also important to note that some alterations in the *BRCA1* and *BRCA2* genes not classified as deleterious may be associated with more modest risks of breast and ovarian cancer. For example, a population-based case control study of Australian women showed that those with two copies of the N372H polymorphism in *BRCA2* had a 1.42-fold increased risk of breast cancer after adjustment for measured risk factors (52). Another study showed that two copies of this alteration also confer a similar increase in risk of ovarian cancer (53). It is possible that some *BRCA1/2* alterations presently classified as variants of unknown significance may confer modest risks of breast and ovarian cancer; however, particularly in high risk families, this finding may not be the sole cause for the observed cancers.

Further studies in *BRCA1* and *BRCA2* carriers are needed before these data can be used to refine risk estimates in the clinic. In addition, an understanding of putative molecular mechanisms for differential risks will further contribute to our understanding of genotype–phenotype correlations.

Modifier Genes

As discussed above, it is possible that specific mutations in the *BRCA1/2* genes are associated with variable cancer risks. It has also been observed, however, that polymorphisms within these genes may modulate risk for individuals with an identified deleterious mutation. For example, in *BRCA1* mutation carriers, the presence of a Gly1038 variant in the *BRCA1* wild-type allele modestly increased the risk of ovarian cancer (hazard ratio [HR], 1.50; 95% CI, 1.03–2.19) (54). An increasing body of research is focusing on how polymorphisms in other genes impact *BRCA1/2* cancer risks. To generate sample sizes with sufficient statistical power to detect effects of modifier genes, an international consortium of 30 groups has been formed, known as CIMBA (Consortium of Investigators of Modifiers of *BRCA1* and *BRCA2*) (55). By pooling data from approximately 15,000 mutation carriers, it is expected that this group will be able to confirm or refute studies of modifier genes in smaller populations. To date, the most well established genetic modifier of risk is a single nucleotide polymorphism (SNP) in the *RAD51* gene. This gene functions in repair of double-strand DNA breaks (56). Antoniou et al. (56) recently published a combined analysis of 19 studies on the effect of *RAD51* 135G→C, and concluded that there is an association with breast cancer risk in *BRCA2* carriers. Based on the estimated hazard ratio they obtained in CC homozygotes,

they postulated that the absolute risk of breast cancer to age 70 in the most recent birth cohort would be 90% in the CC homozygotes, and 51% in GG homozygotes. This risk differential, combined with other factors in a woman's history such as tamoxifen use and oophorectomy, could affect management options and decisions for *BRCA2* carriers.

Ongoing research in large sample sizes will be able to clarify inconsistent or unconfirmed data about the role of other risk modifiers, such as the CAG repeat length polymorphism in the androgen receptor gene; polymorphisms in the *p53* gene; and the PROGINS allele of the progesterone receptor gene (57).

In the future, it is very possible that individuals seeking information about their cancer risk may undergo a series of genetic tests that could help better tailor their risks. Thus, information about penetrance may be derived from data specific to an identified *BRCA1* or *BRCA2* mutation and any intragenic polymorphisms, as well as SNP or variants in other genes. In addition, other factors, such as a woman's reproductive history, hormone use, environmental risk factors, and utilization of risk-reducing measures, may be integrated into estimates of lifetime cancer risk.

Reproductive Factors

A central question has been whether reproductive factors that affect risk in the general population are applicable to *BRCA1/2* carriers. Although data are limited, several studies have suggested that early menarche may confer slightly elevated risks for breast cancer among *BRCA1/BRCA2* carriers (58–61). Data on parity and breast cancer risk are less consistent. For example, in two recent case-control studies, an association was found between increasing number of pregnancies and increased risk of breast cancer among *BRCA1* carriers (58) and *BRCA2* carriers (60,62). In contrast, Andrieu et al. (63) reported a protective effect of more pregnancies among *BRCA1* and *BRCA2* carriers over the age of 40 and Cullinane et al. (62) reported a modest protective effect for *BRCA1* carriers with a parity above 3. Several studies have demonstrated a protective effect of breast-feeding among *BRCA1* carriers (58,59,64). However, other studies have failed to detect such an effect (63).

The impact of parity on risk of ovarian cancer is inconsistent and controversial. Contrary to studies of the general population, several studies have suggested that increased parity might be a risk factor for ovarian cancer among *BRCA1/2* carriers. For example, in a recent matched case-control study with 794 cases and 2,424 controls, parity was associated with a 33% reduction in the odds of ovarian cancer among *BRCA1* carriers, but a nearly tripling of the odds of ovarian cancer among *BRCA2* carriers (65). These data are consistent with earlier studies which also reported increased risk associated with higher parity (66). However, consistent with literature in the general population, there have also been studies reporting a protective effect of increasing parity among mutation carriers (67).

Oral contraceptive use has been shown to be associated with an increased risk of breast cancer risk (68,69), and a decreased risk of ovarian cancer (65). An initial study indicated that tubal ligation reduced the risk of ovarian cancer in mutation carriers (70), whereas a subsequent study did not confirm this finding (65).

In summary, despite a growing literature on reproductive risk factors, the limited research to date and the inconsistent nature of the results, preclude definitive conclusions or concrete integration into risk assessments. Thus, clinical recommendations may not be affected by these factors.

Dietary and Lifestyle Interventions

A number of studies has focused on the impact of diet and other lifestyle interventions on breast cancer risk in mutation carriers. Total energy intake and weight gain during adulthood were shown to be related to an increased risk of breast cancer (71), and an inverse relationship between a healthful diet and breast cancer risk has been demonstrated (72). Smoking has also been examined and findings have been inconsistent, with one study showing a negative impact on breast cancer risk (73) and another showing no impact (74). Exercise has been addressed in two studies. Exercise during adolescence was shown to be associated with a lowered risk of breast cancer (75), whereas a second study showed no impact of vigorous or total activity in adult years (71). Additionally, one recent study found that alcohol did not impact breast cancer risk in carriers (76). As with reproductive history risk factors, most of these studies have been limited by small sample size and presently no definitive conclusions can be drawn regarding dietary factors or other lifestyle interventions on the cancer risks of mutation carriers. Nonetheless, it seems prudent to recommend a healthy diet, limited alcohol intake, exercise, and avoidance of smoking because these would also be anticipated to have benefits for overall health.

RISK ASSESSMENT/MUTATION PROBABILITY

Assessing *BRCA1/2* Carrier Probability

Cancer risk assessment encompasses several factors, including the likelihood that an individual or family harbors a gene mutation, the chance that an individual is a gene carrier based on mendelian analysis, and the cancer risks derived from estimates of gene penetrance. As discussed in the section Genetic Counseling Process, qualitative impressions of the pedigree are invaluable for identifying rare syndromes associated with hereditary breast cancer. However, for most women at moderate to high risk presenting for genetic counseling, consideration of *BRCA1/2* testing will be most appropriate. In this section, quantitative models for estimates of *BRCA1/2* carrier probability will be reviewed.

Approximately 5% to 10% of breast cancers arise as a result of an inherited susceptibility owing to alterations in a single highly penetrant gene. Among 237 families ascertained by the Breast Cancer Linkage Consortium, which contained at least four cases of female breast cancer (and no ovarian cancer), it was estimated that 28% were attributable to *BRCA1* mutations, 37% to *BRCA2* mutations, and 35% to unidentified gene mutations (77). In families with a history of breast or ovarian cancer, however, most (80%) were owing to *BRCA1* mutations, 15% to *BRCA2* mutations, and the remaining 5% to unidentified mutations (77). These data suggest that site-specific breast cancer is more genetically heterogeneous in origin than breast/ovarian cancer families, in which the presence of ovarian cancer is a significant predictor of whether a *BRCA1* or *BRCA2* mutation will be identified. These highly enriched families are not representative of those seen in clinical risk evaluation clinics, thus, the proportion of individuals testing positive in the latter settings will likely be lower (37,78,79). In fact, some models provide estimates for gene carrier probability based on data from clinical populations. The Couch model has been recently updated from the original one developed in 1997, in which calculations were based on only 169 familial breast cancer kindreds and assessed for *BRCA1* but not *BRCA2* carrier probability (80). The revised model, known as Penn II, is based on 966 tested families with at least two cases of breast or ovarian cancer from four high-risk breast cancer screening clinics in the United Kingdom and the United States (81). The model, which can be accessed online (82), uses logistic regression analysis to determine the likelihood of finding a *BRCA1* or *BRCA2* mutation in an individual and family. Strengths of the model include

the incorporation of third-degree relatives in the risk assessment (e.g., first cousins) as well as other *BRCA*-associated cancers (i.e., pancreatic, prostate, and male breast). If the proband is not affected, carrier probability can be determined by mendelian analysis. As expected, predictors of finding a mutation include the presence of breast cancer before age 50, male breast cancer, breast–ovarian double primaries, ovarian cancer, and Ashkenazi Jewish ancestry.

Data from the Frank or Myriad model are accessible as a user-friendly tool for determining carrier probability via tables derived from empirical rates of *BRCA1/2* mutation prevalence in over 20,000 consecutive gene analyses performed at a commercial laboratory (37). Data are presented according to age at diagnosis of breast or ovarian cancer, family history of these cancers, and the presence or absence of Ashkenazi Jewish ancestry. These data also underscore that the presence of ovarian cancer in the family increases the probability of testing positive and, in many cases, with comparable family history, Jewish individuals are more likely to harbor a *BRCA1/2* mutation than non-Jewish individuals. In families with multiple cases of breast and ovarian cancer, however, the impact of Jewish ancestry has a less significant effect on the likelihood of detecting a mutation. Of note, family history used for inclusion in these data was limited and often not verified. The tables are updated periodically and are downloadable from the internet to personal digital assistants (PDAs) and other portable devices (83).

A popular and well validated tool is a computer model called BRCAPRO, which uses Bayesian theory and family history information (e.g., affected status for breast or ovarian cancer, ages of affected and unaffected first- and second-degree relatives) to estimate *BRCA1/2* carrier probabilities as well as breast cancer risk (84–86). The model, which is frequently updated, also incorporates data about *BRCA1/2* mutation frequency and a range of *BRCA1/2* mutation penetrance figures based on published estimates. Strengths of the model include the ability to integrate multiple pieces of additional information into *BRCA1/2* carrier probability estimates, such as genetic testing results (for residual probability in the person tested or to account for the possibility of a phenocopy or uninformative result in an unaffected person), oophorectomy status, and breast tumor marker status, including estrogen and progesterone receptors and cytokines CK14 and CK5/6. Tumor markers indicating the triple negative or basaloid phenotype are predictors of *BRCA1* positivity (87). Of note, however, despite the establishment of ductal carcinoma *in situ* (DCIS) as part of the *BRCA1/2* tumor spectrum (88), at present, the program does not count DCIS as breast cancer (i.e., it factors in cases of invasive breast cancer only); therefore, carrier probability may be underestimated. Users may therefore wish to enter DCIS cases as invasive. Probabilities generated by this model vary based on which person is chosen for the analysis, so one could run the model on the person most likely to harbor a mutation (or who has the most affected relatives who will be captured within the model) and then calculate mendelian probabilities for other relatives. As with other models, a potential limitation of this model is that it tends to have better discrimination for carrier probability in high- versus low-risk families (89). Also, the model must be run on computer software, which requires entering a fair amount of information about the pedigree, which can be time consuming.

The Couch, Myriad, and BRCAPRO models, in addition to some older models, can be run concurrently through CancerGene software package, which is downloadable at no cost (90). However, other newly developed models are also available separately. The Manchester scoring system was developed based on empiric data from 921 non-Jewish British families (91,92). This model was developed to ascertain families with at least a 10% prior probability of having a *BRCA1* or *BRCA2* mutation for the purposes of clinical triage (91,92). The model assigns a score for *BRCA1* and *BRCA2* based on the presence of various cancers (i.e., female and male breast cancer, ovarian, prostate, and pancreatic) and, in most cases, the age of onset. Families with a score of at least 15 for one or the other genes meet the 10% threshold (92). Tables based on empiric data of actual genetic testing results may then be used to determine carrier probability for each gene (92). Limitations of the model include its lack of applicability to Ashkenazi Jewish individuals and that it may underestimate risk in small families or single affected breast cancer probands diagnosed at a young age.

The BOADICEA (Breast and Ovarian Analysis of Disease Incidence and Carrier Estimation Algorithm) model was developed using segregation analysis of breast and ovarian cancer in families identified through population-based series of breast cancer cases and multiple case families in the United Kingdom (93). The latest version is based on 2,785 families, including 537 with *BRCA1* or *BRCA2* mutations (93). A recent validation study of BOADICEA in 1,934 families seen in U.K. cancer genetics clinics showed that, when compared with four other commonly used models (Myriad, BRCAPRO, Manchester, and IBIS), it was the only one to accurately predict the overall observed number of *BRCA1/2* mutations (94). It also provided the best discrimination (i.e., between a carrier and noncarrier for an individual), although BRCAPRO performed similar to BOADICEA in this regard. As with the other models, it under predicted the presence of *BRCA1/2* mutations in the low-risk group. An internet version of the program is available, using the pedigree analysis software MENDEL, and is updated periodically by the University of Cambridge (BOADICEA Web application) (95). Strengths are that risk estimates computed by the model take into account the polygenic nature of hereditary breast cancer (i.e., implicating genes other than *BRCA1* and *BRCA2*), other cancers associated with *BRCA1/2* mutations, and risk modifiers that may affect *BRCA1/2* penetrance, and that the model allows for imputation of any family size (93). Of note, BOADICEA can be used to predict mutation carrier probabilities as well as cancer risks (93).

Another recently developed model is based on the International Breast Cancer Intervention Study and is referred to as IBIS or Tyrer-Cuzick (96). As with other tools, it is computer based; however, it is not yet widely available (97). Of importance, this model is applicable only to unaffected individuals with a family history of breast or ovarian cancer (first- and second-degree relatives are considered), and uses Bayesian calculations, *BRCA1/2* penetrance data from the Breast Cancer Linkage Consortium, and assumptions about the existence of a dominantly inherited low penetrance gene in calculating gene carrier probability. The model, however, also incorporates personal risk factors, such as age at menarche and menopause, age at first live childbirth, parity, height, and body mass index, as well as a history of breast conditions that may elevate risk (i.e., atypical hyperplasia and lobular carcinoma *in situ*, LCIS). These potential risk modifiers are incorporated into the genetic calculation, and are also used to estimate risk of breast cancer. Although the model has not undergone comprehensive validation, some studies have found that it outperforms other models in assessing breast cancer risk and accurately predicts breast cancer risk in *BRCA1/2*-positive families (98,99).

Application of Risk Models

Table 19.2 summarizes the *BRCA1/2* mutation probabilities for probands in three different pedigrees as determined by commonly used probability models. CancerGene software (90) was used to calculate the BRCAPRO probabilities and Myriad data. However, because CancerGene does not impute a full family structure (e.g., third-degree relatives such as cousins), Myriad data were also extracted from mutation prevalence tables (83).

Pedigree 1 (Fig. 19.1) is an example of a high-risk family, in that it contains four cases of breast cancer (one bilateral and two under the age of 50 years) in three generations and one case of ovarian cancer. Regardless of ancestry, BRCAPRO gives the highest carrier probability estimate (48% or 75%) although it does not consider the history of ovarian cancer in the proband's cousin (III-1; i.e., because she is a third-degree relative, her information is not entered in to the program). Similarly, the reason for the discrepancy in the Myriad probabilities is that the CancerGene value does not consider the cousin's history of ovarian cancer. Interestingly, the BRCAPRO calculations would be much lower if the paternal aunt was diagnosed with unilateral versus bilateral cancer, yielding probabilities for the proband (individual III-6) to be a *BRCA1/2* carrier of 56% if the family is Jewish and 14% if the family is not Jewish.

Pedigree 2 (Fig. 19.2) is also a highly suggestive family, with four cases of breast cancer, three under age 50 years, in three generations. Here again BRCAPRO does not factor in the affected cousin's diagnosis; nevertheless, this model yields the highest carrier probabilities. The difference between the two Myriad values arises because, on the prevalence tables, a distinction exists between having one relative diagnosed with breast cancer before age 50 versus more than one relative diagnosed with breast cancer before age 50. Because the cousin was not entered on CancerGene, the value derived from the Myriad table includes only the paternal aunt diagnosed younger than age 50 (II-2) and not the affected cousin (III-1).

| Table 19.2 | *BRCA1/2* MUTATION PROBABILITIES FOR SELECT PEDIGREES |

	Pedigree 1		Pedigree 2		Pedigree 3	
	Jewish (%)	Non-Jewish (%)	Jewish (%)	Non-Jewish (%)	Jewish (%)	Non-Jewish (%)
Penn II	54	26	41	19	27	13
Myriad[a]	24	16	24	16	12	7
Myriad[b]	51	39	38	30	12	7
BRCAPRO[a]	75	48	64	18	22	3

Combined probabilities of finding a *BRCA1* or *BRCA2* mutation for the proband indicated by an arrow in each pedigree. See text for model descriptions and references.
[a]Data from CancerGene, version 5, copyright University of Texas, 1998–2007 (90).
[b]Data from Myriad Genetic Laboratories, Mutation Prevalence Tables, Updated Spring 2006 (83).

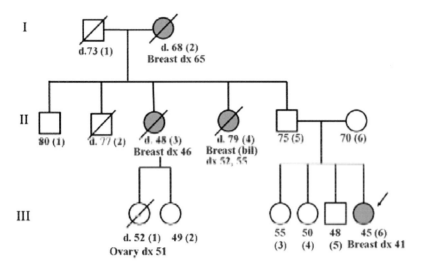

FIGURE 19.1 Pedigree 1, high risk breast/ovarian cancer family.

Finally, Pedigree 3 (Fig. 19.3) is an example of a moderately suggestive family history of the type commonly encountered in clinical practice. If the family is non-Jewish, all models yield a relatively low probability that the proband (III-1) will test positive, whereas, as expected, the probabilities are higher if the family is Jewish. Interestingly, if breast cancer tumor markers indicative of the basaloid phenotype are entered for the proband (e.g., estrogen and progesterone receptor negative, CK14 and CK5/6 positive), the probability of testing positive is substantially increased based on the BRCAPRO model (i.e., 40% if non-Jewish; 88% if Jewish). This finding underscores the emerging importance of considering breast cancer pathology in addition to family history, especially because this is a small family with few females in it.

These examples demonstrate several important concepts. First, quantitative probability estimates of *BRCA1/2* status may be highly variable, so it is important to understand the features of each model that could account for some of these differences, as well as the strengths and limitations of each model. Thus, carrier probability estimates must be interpreted in addition to a qualitative impression of the pedigree. In some cases, it might make more sense to calculate carrier probabil-

ity for someone in the family other than the proband. Such an approach might be useful if the proband is unaffected with breast or ovarian cancer (i.e., by calculating carrier probability for an affected individual, mendelian analysis can then be used to derive risks), or if there is a "higher risk" proband in the family (e.g., a woman with ovarian cancer, or who was diagnosed with breast cancer at a younger age). Finally, Jewish ancestry significantly impacts carrier probability, so it is critical to ascertain ethnic background when taking the pedigree. As pedigrees 1 and 2 underscore, paternal family history is also critical to ascertain. More detailed reviews of the applications and limitations of these models have are available (100–102).

Criteria for Genetic Counseling Referral

In general, it is recommended that individuals with a personal or family history of breast cancer be referred for genetic counseling, which includes a detailed risk assessment and discussion about the potential likelihood that genetic testing will provide informative results for medical management or for clarifying relatives' cancer risks. Although a threshold for

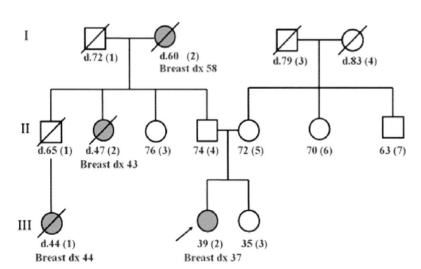

FIGURE 19.2. Pedigree 2, high risk site-specific breast cancer family.

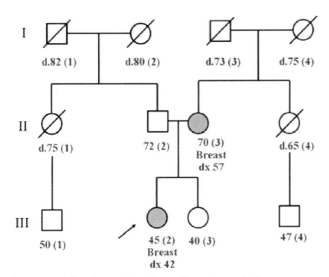

FIGURE 19.3. Pedigree 3, moderate risk site-specific breast cancer family.

potentially hereditary or familial cancers. We provide sample criteria for referral for consideration of *BRCA1/2* testing in Table 19.3.

THE GENETIC COUNSELING PROCESS

Genetic counseling is a critical part of the risk assessment and genetic testing process. In the latter, pre- and posttest counseling is important because of complexities in test result interpretation and discussion of medical management options, as well as the potential implications for family members. The process of genetic counseling, which encompasses everything from initial history taking to a review of the potential benefits, limitations, and risks of testing, is comprehensive in nature and is designed to facilitate informed decision-making (115).

Initial or pretest genetic counseling sessions involve a detailed review of the patient's family and medical history (111,116). The family history may be conveniently recorded in the form of a pedigree and should be updated periodically. Pedigrees should include information about maternal and paternal relatives encompassing at least three generations, if possible. With respect to cancer history, it is important to record all cancer or precancerous diagnoses, ages at diagnosis, laterality, treatment, and history of prophylactic or other related surgery. Review of pathology reports is important not only to verify diagnoses, but also to confirm whether certain histologies are present. For example, nonepithelial ovarian cancers, such as germ cell cancers, are not part of the tumor spectrum observed in *BRCA1/2* mutation carriers (117). Relevant environmental and exposure history is also important to note, as well as ethnic ancestry. In addition, current ages or ages at and causes of death, as well as other chronic medical conditions in unaffected and affected individuals, should also be indicated on the pedigree. For example, women who undergo oophorectomy at an early age who also have a positive family history of heart disease or osteoporosis may consider a more in-depth assessment of their own personal risk factors for these conditions so that they can discuss appropriate management options.

Analysis of the pedigree for hallmark features of hereditary cancer provides the basis for an accurate risk assessment. The two approaches to pedigree analysis are (a) a qualitative impression and (b) a quantitative estimate of carrier probability. A qualitative analysis is helpful to determine if a family history contains features suggestive of hereditary breast cancer, especially syndromes not attributable to *BRCA1/2* mutations.

BRCA1/2 carrier probability of 10% had been suggested several years ago (103), until the discrimination of models is improved, quantitative estimates combined with clinical judgment form the optimal basis for referral and risk assessment in clinical practice (104,105). Indeed, many organizations have published statements about the importance of genetic counseling for individuals at elevated cancer risk, and some contain specific criteria for genetic counseling referral. These groups include the American Society of Clinical Oncology (ASCO), the National Society of Genetic Counselors (NSGC), the National Comprehensive Cancer Network (NCCN), the United States Preventive Services Task Force (USPSTF), the National Institute for Health and Clinical Excellence (NICE), and others (103,106–112). In the United States, some third-party payers have established their own criteria for genetic counseling and testing (100). Also of note is that in countries with government-funded testing programs (e.g., Australia, France, Germany, The Netherlands, and the United Kingdom), genetic testing may be available at no cost to individuals who meet specific eligibility criteria (113). In addition, Hampel et al. (114) provide detailed criteria for identifying individuals at moderate to high risk of developing breast cancer and other

| Table 19.3 | CRITERIA FOR REFERRAL FOR GENETIC COUNSELING OF INDIVIDUALS AT INCREASED RISK FOR *BRCA1/2*-ASSOCIATED HEREDITARY BREAST CANCER[a,b] |

- Personal history of breast cancer diagnosed ≤ 40
- Personal history of breast cancer diagnosed ≤ 50 and Ashkenazi Jewish ancestry
- Personal history of breast cancer diagnosed ≤ 50 and at least one first- or second-degree relative with breast cancer ≤ 50 and/or epithelial ovarian cancer
- Personal history of breast cancer and two or more relatives on the same side of the family with breast cancer and/or epithelial ovarian cancer
- Personal history of epithelial ovarian cancer, diagnosed at any age, particularly if Ashkenazi Jewish
- Personal history of male breast cancer particularly if at least one first- or second-degree relative with breast cancer and/or epithelial ovarian cancer
- Relatives of individuals with a deleterious *BRCA1/2* mutation

[a]Close relatives of individuals with the history mentioned in the table are appropriate candidates for genetic counseling. It is optimal to initiate testing in an individual with breast or ovarian cancer prior to testing at-risk relatives.
[b]Criteria modified from NCCN (109).

For example, early onset breast cancer in the presence of a sarcoma, adrenocortical cancer, or childhood cancer is suggestive of Li-Fraumeni syndrome (118). In addition, the genetic counselor can also determine if factors in the family history may make it difficult to discern a pattern of hereditary cancer, thus limiting the utility of some quantitative models of risk assessment. Small family size, few women in the family, premature deaths, and lack of knowledge regarding medical history, are all potential limitations of pedigree analysis. For example, Weitzel et al. (119) found that in families containing a proband with breast cancer before age 50 and a limited family structure, three commonly used risk assessment models did not accurately predict BRCA1/2 carrier probability.

As discussed previously, various models exist to predict the likelihood that an individual harbors a BRCA1 or BRCA2 mutation. Again, these data need to be interpreted in the context of a specific pedigree. The mode of inheritance of the syndrome in question (usually autosomal dominance) and attendant risks are also important to review.

Another critical aspect of pretest counseling is a psychosocial assessment, along with a discussion about the review of the possible benefits, risks, and limitations of genetic testing (116). Although no individual can imagine fully how he or she might react on learning a test result, having this discussion beforehand can at least begin to prepare individuals for different responses and enable them to mobilize coping, support, and informational resources ahead of time. It is also helpful to clarify expectations about what the patient hopes to learn from genetic testing, and how he or she may handle uncertainties associated with test result interpretation. Discussing risk perception, attitudes toward cancer screening and prevention, past health behaviors, impact of relatives' diagnosis, and current and past psychiatric history can help frame discussions about goals, coping strategies, and decision-making (116).

Potential benefits of testing include the reduction of uncertainty because of increased knowledge. In addition, results may help facilitate more informed decision-making about medical options, including prophylactic surgery. Although such surgery may be undertaken by women who have never had a diagnosis of cancer, data about the risk of ipsilateral and contralateral breast cancers in BRCA1/2 carriers could potentially impact the surgical decision-making of high-risk, newly diagnosed patients with breast cancer who choose to learn their genetic status preoperatively (120).

Frequently, the choice to be tested may also be motivated by a desire to obtain information for other family members. For patients with cancer who are very ill or actively in treatment, this reason may be their only motivation to pursue genetic testing, because the medical implications to them may be inconsequential. Among individuals of childbearing age, concern about transmitting their mutation to future children may also exist (121). It is important to address reproductive concerns in the context of genetic counseling, especially as options such as prenatal testing and preimplantation genetic diagnosis become more widely available (122). Decision-making around these issues can be very complex and fraught with ethical dilemmas; thus, genetic counseling can be instrumental in helping patients clarify their own values and preferences (123).

A limitation of testing is the possibility that results may not be informative. Although no significant physical risks are associated with genetic testing, psychosocial risks must be taken into consideration. A common reason that individuals decline genetic testing in the United States is fear of genetic discrimination in the areas of health and life insurance and employment (124,125). However, in practice, few cases of genetic discrimination have been documented. In addition, it is important that individuals considering genetic testing are informed about current national and state or local laws that provide some protection against genetic discrimination (126,127). In May 2008,

the Genetic Information Nondiscrimination Act (GINA) [H.R. 493] was signed into law in the United States, which provides protection against discrimination based on genetic information for those with individual and group health insurance plans, and in employment settings (126). It is also encouraging that BRCA1/2 testing, which can cost up to approximately $3,000, is often a covered expense by many insurance companies in the United States.

Although studies have not demonstrated significant adverse emotional effects of testing, as described in the section on psychosocial issues, it is not uncommon for mutation carriers to experience some feelings of distress, anxiety, or sadness, which is usually manageable without clinical intervention and which dissipates over time (128). Although many individuals pursue testing for the sake of obtaining information for family members, the decision to disseminate one's test results and the ensuing ramifications can cause strain among relatives. It is not uncommon for those with true negative results to feel a combination of relief and survivor guilt for being spared a burden that other relatives may experience. In addition, the role of information gatekeeper may be overwhelming for some individuals as they try to attend also to their own needs for support. Through the process of genetic counseling, at-risk individuals can be identified from the pedigree, and the process of family communication may be facilitated with the provision of educational material and, for example, sample letters that can be modified and sent to relatives, for those wishing to use that means of notification.

Thus, in considering the complexities involved in genetic counseling and testing, and the potential for testing to have a significant impact on an individual and his or her family, an integral part of the informed consent process involves discussion of these issues before genetic testing. Post-test genetic counseling provides an opportunity to review pertinent information and may serve to help individuals begin to assimilate their results. Specially trained genetic counselors and nurses can provide these services to interested patients, often in combination with a multidisciplinary team of professionals, such as oncologists, surgeons, geneticists, and psychologists.

Issues in Test Result Interpretation

Regardless of which hereditary breast cancer syndrome is suspected within a family, the degree to which testing will be informative is always maximized by first testing an individual in the family who is most likely to carry a mutation (e.g., a woman diagnosed with breast cancer before age 50 or ovarian cancer). The sensitivity and specificity of testing are important considerations when selecting a laboratory. BRCA1/2 testing is the most frequently ordered test for hereditary breast or ovarian cancer susceptibility, with more than 200,000 individuals tested (129). Myriad Genetic Laboratories, which holds the patents on these genes, offers forward and reverse sequencing of coding exons and adjacent base pairs in noncoding intronic regions (130). This type of testing can detect frameshift and nonsense (i.e., protein truncating) mutations, which are known to be deleterious, as well as other types of mutations that are associated with increased cancer risks (130). In addition, sequence variants may also be identified. Such variants that are known to be inconsequential (e.g., nonprotein truncating changes that occur in approximately 1% of a control population without data suggesting clinical significance) are not reported (130). If identified, however, the following classifications are reported for variants: *suspected deleterious*, which are likely but not definitively proven to be risk conferring; *favor polymorphism*, which are likely but not definitively proven to be of no clinical consequence; and those of *uncertain significance* where insufficient data exist for classification (130). Although unclassified variants are relatively uncommon (i.e., approximately

8% of samples submitted to Myriad for comprehensive testing), they may occur with increased frequency in specific ethnic groups (e.g., 14% in black or Caribbean probands) (131). It is critical that providers counsel patients appropriately about these results and retain the ability to recontact them if the variant becomes reclassified. Of note, a useful database for finding out how many times a gene alteration has been reported and how it is classified is maintained by the Breast Cancer Information Core (BIC) (132).

In addition to full sequencing, all samples submitted for comprehensive *BRCA1* and *BRCA2* analysis through Myriad are now also analyzed for the presence of 5 *BRCA1* genomic rearrangements. Although the addition of this rearrangement panel is thought to bring the analytical sensitivity and specificity of comprehensive testing to a value approaching 100%, clinically significant mutations (e.g., other genomic rearrangements and mutations that affect RNA transcript processing) may still occur in an estimated 3% to 4% of patients (130). Also through Myriad, patients at very high risk automatically undergo testing for large rearrangements in *BRCA1* and *BRCA2*, known as BART testing, which further increases the sensitivity of testing; however, these mutations occur very rarely (in approximately 3% of very high risk families) (133). Patients may also opt to pay for this additional testing.

When a deleterious mutation is not identified in the proband after full testing, such results are considered to be indeterminate or uninformative. If an affected individual at high risk is the first to be tested in the family, a negative result could arise owing to a number of possibilities, such as

1. A mutation could be present in the gene/s analyzed, but was not detectable by the method/s used.
2. A rare mutation in another gene or genes could be implicated, for which testing may or may not be available.
3. The individual tested developed sporadic cancer.

With respect to the latter possibility, it is important to bear in mind that phenocopies can occur within families. That is, a proband with breast cancer who tests negative for *BRCA1/2* mutations may represent a sporadic occurrence within a hereditary breast cancer family. Smith et al. (134) studied 277 families with deleterious *BRCA1/2* mutations and identified 28 women with breast cancer in these families who did not harbor the familial mutation. If, in fact, an excess breast cancer risk exists among mutation negative women in a *BRCA1*- or *BRCA2*-positive family, a topic which has been debated, it could be attributable to mutations in modifier genes or correlated environmental factors, such as parity and oral contraceptive use (134–136). Of note, ovarian cancer is less likely to be a phenocopy given that it occurs much less frequently than breast cancer and is a significant predictor of finding a deleterious mutation within a family (37).

Founder Mutations in Ashkenazi Jews and Other Ethnic Groups

Targeted testing for specific mutations may also be appropriate based on a patient's ethnicity. The occurrence of recurrent or "founder" mutations is pronounced in individuals of Ashkenazi (central or eastern European) Jewish descent. In this population, three mutations occur with increased frequency: 187delAG and 5385insC in *BRCA1* and 6174delT in *BRCA2*. Whereas the general population frequency of *BRCA1/2* mutations in the United States is 1/1,250, in Ashkenazi Jews, the incidence of these founder mutations is 1/77 (137). Not surprisingly, the incidence of these founder mutations is substantially higher when selected Jewish populations are studied, such as young patients with breast or ovarian cancer (46,47,138). For this reason, individuals with a relative who

carries one of these mutations should still be tested for all three mutations if they have Ashkenazi Jewish ancestry on both sides of their family (139). It is important to note that these mutations do not occur exclusively in Ashkenazi Jews. In addition, nonfounder mutations have been reported in this ethnic group. In the largest series of Jewish individuals to undergo full *BRCA1/2* testing, Frank et al. (37) reported that 74 (10%) of 737 tested individuals had deleterious mutations, including 16 nonfounder mutations. Most of these individuals had a personal or family history of breast or ovarian cancer. Excluding the 5 individuals who also had non-Jewish ancestry, only 11 (2%) of 737 had a nonfounder mutation. Kauff et al. (140) studied 70 Jewish women with a personal history of breast or ovarian cancer who may have also had a family history of these cancers. Here, three (4%) tested positive for a deleterious nonfounder mutation. Thus, most Ashkenazi Jewish individuals who test positive will have one of the three founder mutations. At this time, it is not possible to predict which features of the family history will make it more likely that a nonfounder mutation will be identified. However, individuals who have a high prior probability of testing positive based on models such as BRCAPRO (e.g., if calculated as though the family was non-Jewish), or who have qualitative features within the family history that are highly suggestive of a mutation (e.g., more than one case of ovarian cancer, male breast cancer, or pancreatic cancer) should consider pursuing comprehensive testing if they three founder mutations are ruled out (141).

Founder mutations have also been described in other European and non-European populations, such as those with Icelandic, Norwegian, Dutch, or French Canadian ancestry (142). It is important for clinicians to determine whether targeted testing is appropriate. For most non-Ashkenazi Jewish individuals in the United States, targeted testing is not indicated. Importantly, when an Ashkenazi Jewish proband tests negative for founder mutations, although this does not definitively rule out an inherited susceptibility, in some instances, such a result can be very reassuring. For example, an Ashkenazi Jewish woman diagnosed with breast cancer at age 45 and no family history of breast or ovarian cancer or other features suggestive of hereditary cancer (based on an expansive and informative pedigree) can be reassured that her breast cancer probably developed sporadically. However, if that same woman had a family history containing multiple cases of early onset breast or ovarian cancer, the possibility of another *BRCA1* or *BRCA2* mutation or a mutation in a different gene would also have to be considered, and her result would be less "informative."

Testing for a Familial Mutation

Finally, once a mutation in a cancer susceptibility gene is identified, relatives may be offered testing for only the single mutation. One exception to this is for Ashkenazi Jewish individuals, who should generally be tested for all three founder mutations regardless of which one is segregating in the family. Indeed, families with more than one mutation and cases of double heterozygotes have been reported (141,143). Therefore, it may be important to determine if testing for additional founder mutations is appropriate. In general, testing for a familial mutation yields definitive information: A deleterious (positive) test result is obtained, with the attendant cancer risks, or the result is classified as a true negative, in which the patient can be reassured that cancer risks are thought to be equivalent to those observed in the general population. It is critical, however, to assess other potential risk factors, such as environmental factors and history on the side of family in which the mutation is not segregating (i.e., the family history of the other parent). If cases of cancer are present, and especially if these are suggestive of an inherited predisposition, the patient may still have an elevated risk of cancer and his or her medical management plan may need to take this into account.

To illustrate concepts in result interpretation, consider Pedigree 2 (Fig. 19.2). If the proband (III.2) underwent full *BRCA1/2* testing, including testing for large rearrangements, and no mutation was identified, this finding is considered to be uninformative given that this family history is strongly consistent with hereditary breast cancer. Although the likelihood is low that the proband's cancer is a phenocopy (given her young age at diagnosis), this possibility could be further discounted if her affected cousin had also tested negative for *BRCA1/2* mutations. In high risk Ashkenazi Jewish families, in which testing for the three founder mutations is relatively inexpensive, it may be prudent to offer testing to more than one affected individual especially if the proband was diagnosed with breast cancer postmenopausally.

The family history is not suggestive of any other hereditary breast cancer syndrome, although it is possible that families such as this may harbor rarely occurring mutations in genes, such as *CHEK2* or *PALB2*, or multiple low penetrance gene mutations may be present (144–146). One challenging clinical issue in families such as this is how they should be counseled about the risk of ovarian cancer, especially because there is no family history of this cancer. Relatives of the proband should be made aware of the fact that neither gene testing nor the family history indicates a basis for an elevated ovarian cancer risk. Although an unidentified mutation could be present that may be associated with a heightened risk for ovarian cancer, studies have suggested that women in *BRCA1/2*-negative, site-specific breast families do not have an excess risk of ovarian cancer (38,39,42).

If the affected proband (III.2) in Figure 19.2 was found to carry a variant of uncertain significance, and it was subsequently not identified in her father, this finding suggests that the mutation is not likely to be associated with heightened cancer risks as it is not segregating on the side of the family with multiple cases of breast cancer. If this observation can be replicated in numerous families, the accumulation of such data in conjunction with statistical approaches, such as Bayesian analyses, would add further credence to this assumption (147). Except to assist in the determination of a variant's significance, at-risk relatives should not be offered testing for a variant because it provides no further information about their risk of developing cancer.

If individual III.2 is found to harbor a *BRCA2* mutation, and her sister (III.3) subsequently tests negative for this mutation (true negative), the sister's chance of developing breast or ovarian cancer is reduced to that observed in the general population. This example underscores the importance of offering genetic testing to an affected individual first. If, however, the proband's sister (III.3) was the first person in the family to undergo *BRCA1/2* testing and tested negative, at that point, it would not be clear whether this result would be attributable to the fact that she did not inherit a mutation segregating in her family or whether a *BRCA1* or *BRCA2* mutation does not exist in this family. In this scenario, rather than a test result providing reassurance, the patient would have to be counseled that she is still considered to be at high risk for breast cancer.

In summary, there are several possible outcomes of genetic testing. There are two types of definitive test results: (a) a *positive* result refers to the identification of a deleterious mutation associated with increased cancer risks; and (b) a *true negative* result means that a mutation previously identified in a blood relative has been ruled out. Even among highly selected probands, the most commonly obtained result is one that is *indeterminate* or *uninformative*. These classifications mean that a deleterious mutation has not been identified in the family, and the prospect of an inherited susceptibility cannot be definitively ruled out. Given the complexities in test result inter-

pretation, it is important that it be done in the context of an individual's medical and family history, especially given that critical medical management may hinge on an accurate risk assessment.

Psychosocial Outcomes of *BRCA1/2* Genetic Testing

The advent of *BRCA1/2* testing was accompanied by considerable concern about the potential for adverse psychosocial outcomes in this already distressed population (148). In the 12 years since *BRCA1/2* testing became available, more than 200,000 individuals have been tested (129). A growing literature has begun to evaluate the psychosocial impact of learning one's *BRCA1/2* mutation status.

Studies evaluating the short-term impact of genetic testing demonstrate substantial decreases in distress and anxiety among women who learn that they do not carry a *BRCA1/2* mutation (149–151). The short-term impact on women who receive positive test results is less consistent. Although many studies suggest increased distress and anxiety immediately following receipt of a positive *BRCA1/2* test result (150–154), others demonstrate stable levels of distress and anxiety (149,155). This combination of decreased distress among those receiving negative test results and stable or increased distress among those who receive positive results yields significant short-term differences in distress between these groups.

Despite these short-term differences, little evidence suggests increased distress, anxiety, or depression among *BRCA1/2* carriers over the longer term. Studies have typically reported no change or a decrease in distress within the first 6-months to 2 years following genetic testing. For example, a recent study examining the trajectory of distress in the 18-months following testing reported no changes in distress overall among carriers and a decrease in distress among carriers who had been previously affected with breast cancer (156). Other studies with follow-up periods of 6 months to 5 years have also found stable distress in those found positive (128,157–162). In contrast, the receipt of a definitive negative test result has been associated with either no change (156) or significant long-term reductions in distress (128).

Although these studies are reassuring, need for caution exists in interpreting these results owing to the wide variability in emotional responses to testing and the select nature of research samples to date. For example, a number of studies have shown that individuals who report high levels of distress or poor quality of life before testing are substantially more likely to report ongoing distress following a positive test result (156,161,163,164). Further, more research is needed to determine whether the largely positive outcomes associated with genetic testing in controlled research programs can be replicated in community settings in which extensive genetic counseling may not always be provided (165). Finally, the participants in most of these studies have been overwhelmingly white, well-educated, and of high socioeconomic status. However, a recent report that focused on the impact of *BRCA1/2* among black patients suggests comparable outcomes to previous studies (160).

ETHICAL ISSUES IN GENETIC COUNSELING AND TESTING FOR HEREDITARY BREAST CANCER

Genetic counseling and testing for hereditary cancer risk often raises many complex issues because of the uncertain but often predictive nature of information obtained; potential risks and limitations of testing; and that genetic test results, especially positive results, have implications not just for the persons tested, but for their family members as well. In this section, the following major themes will be highlighted: (a) the importance of informed consent; (b) predictive testing in children; (c) duty to warn; and (d) duty to recontact.

First, to maximize the likelihood that patients make fully autonomous decisions about genetic testing, including a full appreciation of the potential benefits, limitations, risks, and implications of testing, it is imperative that informed consent is obtained before testing. The process of genetic counseling can be conceptualized as a means through which patients are consented. It is comprehensive in nature, not only encompassing information, potential implications, and options, but it also includes a discussion of the psychosocial and familial aspects of testing (106,111,115,166). It is advisable that patients sign a written consent form outlining pertinent information before undergoing genetic testing, regardless of whether they are obtaining it through a clinical program or research (167).

An issue that has garnered a significant amount of attention recently is the issue of testing children for susceptibility to adult onset cancers. Most professional societies agree that genetic testing for minors should occur when medical benefits accrue in childhood (106,168–170). With respect to hereditary breast cancer syndromes, childhood cancers are a feature of Li-Fraumeni syndrome and, although no approach for screening of the associated cancers has proven efficacy, a case for *p53* testing could be made to relieve parental worry and unnecessary medical procedures in the at-risk child (171). With respect to *BRCA1/2* testing, however, other factors may play into testing decisions, such as the child's readiness and interest in genetic testing, particularly for "mature minors"; the impact on the family unit and relationships with parents and siblings; the desire to obtain relief from true negative test results (which of course must be balanced against the possibility of testing positive for a familial mutation); and the impact on autonomous decision-making for the child once he or she reaches adulthood (168,170,172,173). *BRCA1/2* testing in minors remains controversial and, to date, a rare event. However, it is important for clinicians to explore the issue of family communication about genetic testing and to be sensitive to concerns that parents and adolescents may have about future cancer risk and the associated implications.

Another matter related to family communication concerns the delineation of moral responsibilities of individuals to inform their relatives about genetic risk and the ethical obligations of clinicians to ensure that relatives of the tested patient are informed about this risk (i.e., the so called "duty to warn"). Studies have shown that the rate of *BRCA1/2* test result disclosure to adult relatives, especially first-degree relatives, is generally high (174,175). However, the clinician's role in informing at-risk relatives when the tested individual does not is unclear. On one hand, patient autonomy and respect for privacy are important, but there are circumstances when it might be argued that providing benefit (e.g., the potential to reduce worry and distress and to provide information for medical management) and avoiding harm (e.g., avoidance of unnecessary screening or risk-reducing surgery) may be compelling ethical arguments for overriding patient autonomy. From a legal standpoint, the well-known Tarasoff case set the precedent for a breach of confidentiality between health care provider and patient when imminent harm can be prevented (176). In this case from 1976, a patient discussed with his psychotherapist his intention to kill a woman, which he ultimately did. The therapist in this case did not warn the woman of impending danger, but this ruling allows for patient confidentiality to be overridden to avoid harm. However, subsequent case law in the United States has not been consistent with respect to whether a clinician's obligation is fulfilled by informing patients about potential risks to relatives or whether relatives need to be informed directly (177,178). Indeed, the logistics of identifying and directly contacting relatives often prove to be prohibitive. In the United

States another legal consideration is raised by the HIPAA Privacy rule, which prohibits disclosure of "individually identifiable health information," which would include genetic testing results (179). It is not clear how this regulation impacts public health mandates to override confidentiality in the setting of a serious health threat (180). Many organizations have developed position statements that outline circumstances in which it may be permissible to override patient confidentiality based on the seriousness of the condition in question and immediacy of risk to relatives, the ability to identify at-risk relatives, and the potential benefit versus harm of disclosing to relatives (181–183). Despite the lack of clear guidance about this issue, it is important that clinicians explain familial implications of genetic testing during pre- and post-test genetic counseling, and consider inserting language into consent forms about the role that the provider and patient will play in identifying and notifying at-risk relatives, including circumstances, if any, under which patient confidentiality may be breached. Although clinicians may not be involved in direct notification of relatives, facilitating this process by giving patients resources (e.g., educational material, sample letters, or text for e-mails) can be very helpful. If it becomes necessary to override a patient's wishes about disclosure, consultation with an ethics committee or legal counsel may be in order (167).

Finally, given the many developments in cancer genetics, the issue of whether or when to recontact patients has been raised (184). For example, just since the third edition of this book was published, several important developments have occurred that are of clinical relevance to patients, including data about the efficacy of magnetic resonance imaging (MRI) screening in *BRCA1/2* mutation carriers and the availability of large rearrangement testing in the genes for those with prior uninformative test results. Thus, it is important that clinicians encourage patients to maintain up-to-date contact information. In addition, it could be specified that patients check in with the clinic at defined time intervals or for them to check reliable resources for important updates (167,184).

In summary, genetic counseling and testing for hereditary cancer risk may yield many potential benefits to individuals and their families. In some instances, however, patient values and preferences and the possibility of adverse outcomes need to be balanced carefully when considering ethically challenging issues.

MANAGEMENT OF HEREDITARY BREAST CANCER

Over the past few years, much data has emerged regarding the benefit of various screening and prevention options in those with an inherited susceptibility to cancer and other women at high risk. This section summarizes current knowledge regarding the benefits and limitations of these interventions. The management options for unaffected *BRCA1/2* mutation carriers will be discussed first, followed by a review of the impact of *BRCA1/2* status on treatment of patients with breast cancer, and finally we will summarize management options for *BRCA1/2*-negative families and those with other hereditary breast cancer syndromes. It is important to note that most of the recommendations for screening or risk reduction in this group of women at high risk are based on nonrandomized data or expert opinion (109,185).

Management of Unaffected *BRCA1/2* Carriers

In general, management options for women at increased risk for hereditary breast cancer include screening, prevention interventions, or both. The recommendations for an individual woman may change over time, particularly with regard to her desire for future childbearing. With respect to breast cancer, given the generally good prognosis associated with this disease

Table 19.4	RESULTS FROM PROSPECTIVE STUDIES OF MAMMOGRAPHY AND BREAST MRI FOR HIGH RISK WOMEN					
			Breast MRI		Mammography	
Study (year)	No. Subjects (% BRCA1/2 carrier)	No. of Cancers	Sensitivity (%)	Specificity (%)	Sensitivity (%)	Specificity (%)
Tilanus-Linthorst, 2000 (191)	109 (11)	3	100	94	NR	NR
Kriege, 2004 (187)	1909 (18.3)	51	71	90	40	45
Warner, 2004 (192)	236 (100)	22	77	95	36	99.8
Leach, 2005 (189)	649 (18)	35	77	81	40	93
Kuhl, 2005 (188)	529 (8.1)	43	91	97	33	97
Sardanelli, 2007 (190)	278 (60)	18	94	NR	59	NR

MRI, magnetic resonance imaging; NR, not reported.

and the known benefit of cancer screening options, the choice between screening and prevention is often a personal one, made by each woman (109).

Breast Cancer

Screening Options

The current breast cancer screening guidelines for women with a known inherited susceptibility to cancer include monthly breast self-examinations beginning at age 18, semiannual clinician performed breast examinations beginning at age 25, and annual mammograms and MRI beginning at age 25 or individualized based on earliest age of onset in the family (109,110,186).

Until recently, the breast cancer screening guidelines for mutation carries did not include breast MRI. Over the last decade, however, a number of prospective studies have emerged demonstrating that breast MRI had a higher sensitivity than mammography for the detection of invasive breast cancer in this group of women at high risk. This finding prompted the incorporation of this screening modality in the management recommendations of *BRCA1/2* carriers and other women at high risk. Studies from a number of different countries in Europe and North America demonstrated that MRI had a sensitivity of 71% to 100% and specificity of 81% to 97%, whereas mammography had sensitivity of 33% to 59% and specificity of 93% to 99.8% (Table 19.4). Several of these studies, however, noted that false–positive MRI results were quite frequent, with MRI having a positive predictive value that ranged from 7% to 63%. It is important to note that a number of technical and other factors limit the widespread use of MRI. Optimal breast MRI requires a dedicated breast coil, a well-established imaging technique, radiologic expertise in the interpretation of these studies, and the ability to perform MRI-guided biopsies. Additionally, to further minimize the likelihood of false–positive findings in studies, breast MRI in premenopausal women should be performed on days 7 to 14 of the menstrual cycle.

A number of outstanding issues remain. First, although studies have demonstrated that breast cancers detected by MRI tend to be small and frequently node negative (187–192), no data exist on the impact of this screening modality on breast cancer mortality. The role of MRI for the detection of DCIS is also somewhat controversial. Studies in women at high risk suggest that MRI is not as sensitive for the detection of DCIS as is mammog-

raphy (187–189,192). However, a recent single institution study of more than 7,000 women not selected for family history referred for breast MRI found that MRI detected 92% of the cases of pure DCIS, whereas mammography diagnosed only 53% (p <.0001) (193). The role of ultrasound has also been examined, but, in most studies, it has been shown to have inferior sensitivity to either mammography or MRI (190,194). Finally, although a concern has been raised that radiation exposure either in the form of prior chest x-ray or mammograms may increase the risk of breast cancer in mutation carriers (195), most data do not support this association (196,197). Thus, in summary it is not currently recommended that annual screening mammography be omitted in mutation carriers.

Risk Reduction Options

Many women at increased risk for hereditary breast cancer choose prevention interventions as an alternative to screening or, in some cases, in addition to screening. Options for unaffected women include risk-reducing or prophylactic surgery and chemoprevention. The two surgical options for risk reduction are bilateral mastectomy and bilateral salpingo-oophorectomy.

Risk-Reducing Mastectomy

Studies have examined the role of risk-reducing mastectomy (RRM) in mutation carriers and demonstrated that this is a very effective means of breast cancer prevention. Rebbeck et al. (198) conducted a multi-institution, case-control study of 483 mutation carriers from the Prevention and Observation of Surgical End Points Study Group (PROSE) study group. With a median follow-up of 6.4 years, 2 of 105 carriers (1.9%) who underwent risk-reducing mastectomy developed breast cancer as compared with 184 of 378 age-matched controls (48.7%) (adjusted hazard ratio [HR] 0.05 [95% CI, 0.01–0.22]) (198). When the analysis was restricted to carriers with intact ovaries, risk-reducing mastectomy was associated with a 90% reduction in risk (95% CI, 0.02–0.38). The group at the Rotterdam Family Cancer Clinic recently updated their experience with risk-reducing bilateral or contralateral mastectomy in 358 women with either known *BRCA1/2* mutations (N = 236) or at risk for hereditary breast cancer (N = 122) (199). The women in this study underwent skin-sparing mastectomy often accompanied by immediate reconstruction. With a median follow-up of 4.5 years, 1 case of metastatic breast cancer developed in a previously unaffected woman who had undergone risk-reducing mastectomy. The mastectomy specimens were carefully examined for the presence of occult malignancy, which was identified in 10 of the 358 women (2.8%). Invasive cancer was detected in three, whereas DCIS was seen in five, and LCIS in two. These cases were equally distributed among women with known *BRCA1/2* mutations and those at increased risk with no known heritable condition, and in women previously affected and unaffected with breast cancer.

Given the risk of occult malignancy, it has been suggested that mutation carriers planning RRM undergo MRI, sentinel node procedure, or both. Studies examining the rate of occult invasive malignancy in prophylactic mastectomy specimens (200) and modeling studies (201), suggest that routine MRI and sentinel node procedure in this setting are neither cost-effective nor would they would minimize the risk of complications. Thus, at present, routine sentinel node procedure and MRI are not recommended before RRM.

A number of surgical techniques are available, including total or simple mastectomy which involves removal of both breasts and the overlying skin; skin-sparing mastectomy in which both breasts are removed but the overlying skin is preserved; subcutaneous mastectomy entailing removal of both breasts with preservation of overlying skin and nipple and areolar complexes; and modified radical mastectomy, which is a total mastectomy with axillary node dissection. At present, outside of the setting of a clinical trial, total mastectomy or skin-sparing mastectomy are considered the procedures of choice because it is felt subcutaneous mastectomy results in significant residual breast tissue with sparing of the nipple–areolar complex.

Risk Reducing Bilateral Salpingo-Oophorectomy

A number of studies have evaluated the impact of risk-reducing salpingo-oophorectomy on subsequent risk of breast cancer and demonstrated that *BRCA1/2* carriers who underwent this procedure at age less than 50 had a significant reduction in their breast cancer risk (12,202–204). A prospective study from Memorial Sloan-Kettering Cancer Center of 170 *BRCA12* carriers followed for a median of 2 years, found that 3 of the 98 carriers who underwent salpingo-oophorectomy developed breast cancer as compared with 8 of the 72 women who chose surveillance (*p* − .07) (203). Similarly, a multi-institution study of 241 *BRCA12* carriers from the PROSE followed for about 8 years observed that breast cancer developed in 21% of those who had undergone bilateral salpingo-oophorectomy as compared with 42% of those who had not undergone this procedure BEGIN(HR = 0.47, 95%, CI, 0.29–0.77) (12). Recent data suggest that there may be a differential protective effect of this procedure on breast cancer risk in *BRCA1* versus *BRCA2* carriers. A prospective study of 368 *BRCA1* and 229 *BRCA2* carriers found that risk-reducing bilateral salpingo-oophorectomy (RRSO) resulted in a 72% reduction in risk of breast cancer in *BRCA2* carriers (HR = 0.28, 95% CI, 0.08–0.92, p = .036) as compared with a nonsignificant 39% reduction in *BRCA1* carriers (HR = 0.61, 95% CI, 0.30–1.12, p = .16) (11). However, a retrospective international case-control study of 1,439 *BRCA1/2* carriers with breast cancer and 1,866 *BRCA1/2* unaffected *BRCA1/2* carriers, found that prior history of oophorectomy conferred greater protection against breast cancer for *BRCA1* carriers than *BRCA2* carriers (56% reduction in *BRCA1* carriers [OR = 0.44, 95% CI, 0.29–0.66] vs. 46% reduction in *BRCA2* carriers [OR = 0.57, 95% CI, 0.28–1.15]) (202). Thus, at present, the data are somewhat conflicting. However, if future studies confirm a differential effect in *BRCA* carriers, recommendations will need to be based on the gene that is mutated.

BRCA1/2 carriers who choose to undergo prophylactic oophorectomy at a young age frequently consider taking hormone replacement therapy (HRT) to deal with the consequences of premature menopause. Data from the PROSE study group suggest that short-term use of HRT did not alter the protective effect of RRSO on breast cancer risk. Of the 155 carriers who underwent RRSO, 60% reported use of HRT, most of whom were under age 50, and these women had a 63% reduction in their risk of breast cancer as compared with a 62% reduction for the group as a whole (204). There were insufficient data to determine conclusively if there was a differential effect of estrogen alone versus estrogen and progesterone. Thus, mutation carriers who undergo RRSO before the age of natural menopause can consider short term HRT, but such therapy should not extend beyond age 50, the age after which it has been shown to increase breast cancer risk in the general population (205). Additionally, nonhormonal interventions to reduce menopausal symptoms and the management of other medical issues, such as bone health, should be considered.

Chemoprevention

Data from the NSABP P1 Breast Cancer Prevention Trial, the International Breast Cancer Intervention Study (IBIS-I), and the Study of Tamoxifen and Raloxifene (STAR) demonstrate that 5 years of the selective estrogen receptor modulators (SERM) tamoxifen and raloxifene reduce the risk of breast cancer by 30% to 50% in healthy women at increased risk for this disease based on a family history, age, and certain high-risk conditions, such as LCIS or atypical hyperplasia (206–210). However, limited information exists regarding the role of such agents in reducing the risk of breast cancer in mutation carriers. Given that SERM have only been demonstrated to decrease the risk of hormone receptor positive breast cancer in these studies, it has been postulated that these agents may be more effective in *BRCA2* carriers who tend to develop hormone receptor positive breast cancer as opposed to *BRCA1* carriers who more frequently have hormone receptor negative disease (211,212). This hypothesis was supported by a study in which genetic analysis was performed on 288 of the NSABP P1 participants who developed breast cancer cases (209). Only 19 (6.6%) were found to carry disease-conferring mutations. Tamoxifen was associated with a decrease in risk of breast cancer among *BRCA2* carriers (RR = 0.32, 95% CI, 0.06–1.56), but no reduction in risk among *BRCA1* carriers (RR = 1.67, 95% CI, 0.32–10.7). Of note, the study included only small numbers of carriers (8 *BRCA1* and 11 *BRCA2* carriers) and, thus, was not powered to address adequately the impact of tamoxifen in *BRCA1/2* carriers.

In contradistinction, other studies support the notion that endocrine interventions that reduce estrogen levels result in a lower risk of breast cancer in both *BRCA1* and *BRCA2* carriers. As previously described, bilateral salpingo-oophorectomy, if performed before age 50, reduces the risk of breast cancer in carriers by about 50% (11,12,203). Additionally, a number of studies have found that tamoxifen significantly reduced the risk of contralateral and ipsilateral breast cancer in *BRCA1* and *BRCA2* carriers. A study of 491 *BRCA1/2* carriers with breast cancer found that carriers who reported receiving tamoxifen were 41% less likely to develop contralateral breast cancer as compared with those who did not take the medication (HR = 0.59, 95% CI, 0.35–1.01). Of note, the risk reduction associated with tamoxifen was similar for *BRCA1* and *BRCA2* carriers. A case-control study by Gronwald et al. (213) matched 285 *BRCA1/2* carriers with bilateral breast cancer with 751 carriers affected with unilateral breast cancer, and demonstrated that the use of tamoxifen was associated with a 55% reduction in the odds of contralateral breast cancer (OR = 0.45, 95% CI, 0.29–0.70). This protective effect of tamoxifen was noted both for *BRCA1* carriers (OR = 0.48, 95% CI, 0.29–0.79) and *BRCA2* carriers (OR = 0.39, 95% CI, 0.16–0.94). Additionally, a retrospective cohort study of mutation carriers undergoing breast-conserving therapy performed by Pierce et al. (15) also noted that tamoxifen use resulted in a significant reduction in the rate of contralateral breast cancer (HR = 0.31, *p* = .05).

Studies have also examined the possibility of an additive effect of RRSO and tamoxifen in mutation carriers with invasive breast cancer. Metcalfe et al. (10) found that *BRCA1/2* mutation carriers less than age 50 who took tamoxifen and underwent RRSO reduced their contralateral breast cancer risk by 91% compared with a 41% risk reduction associated with tamoxifen alone and a 59% reduction associated with PBSO alone (HR = 0.09, 95% CI, 0.01–0.68). Gronwald et al (213) however, did not observe an additive protective effect of tamoxifen in women who had previously undergone bilateral oophorectomy, although the number of women in this subset was small (n = 26). Further investigations should clarify whether tamoxifen and oophorectomy work synergistically to reduce breast cancer risk. In summary, when counseling mutation carriers about the use of tamoxifen as a risk-reducing agent, it is important that they be informed that insufficient data currently exist to define clearly the benefit of such therapy. Ongoing trials are addressing the role of aromatase inhibitors as well as other agents. At present, no data exist regarding the potential benefit of raloxifene or aromatase inhibitors in mutation carriers.

Ovarian Cancer

Screening Options

It is recommended that mutation carriers who have not had prophylactic oophorectomy undergo concurrent semiannual transvaginal ultrasound (TVUS) and CA-125 beginning at age 35 or 5 to 10 years younger than the earliest age of onset of ovarian cancer in the family. For premenopausal women, it is recommended these studies be performed between days 1 and 10 of the menstrual cycle (109). It is important to note, however, that the benefit of such interventions is currently unclear. A number of ongoing trials are addressing the utility of screening with CA-125 and TVUS, both in the general population and in women at high risk. CA-125 has typically been considered abnormal if over 35 U/mL. However, it has also been suggested that the change over time of CA-125 compared with the patient's baseline (the risk of ovarian cancer algorithm or ROCA) may be a more accurate indicator of risk (214). The U.K. Collaborative Trial of Ovarian Cancer Screening accrued more than 200,000 normal-risk postmenopausal women and randomized them to no screening, annual CA-125 via ROCA followed by TVUS, if indicated, or TVUS as the first-line test. It is anticipated that results will be available in 2012. In the United States, the Prostate, Lung, Colorectal, and Ovarian (PLCO) screening trial has enrolled more than 75,000 postmenopausal women and randomized them to either no ovarian cancer screening or CA-125 performed at baseline and then annually for 5 years and TVUS performed at baseline and annually for 3 years. This study completed accrual in 2000 and all subjects have now completed their screening. Given the elevated risk of ovarian cancer in women with *BRCA1* and *BRCA2* mutations, studies in these high-risk women are typically single-arm trials. The Cancer Genetics Network, in collaboration with the Gynecologic Oncology Group (GOG), the Early Detection Research Network (EDRN) and the NCI Ovarian Specialized Program on Research Excellence groups (SPORE) is conducting a single arm study of CA-125 analyzed ROCA collected every 3 to 6 months with referral for TVUS if indicated. More than 2,300 women have been accrued to this study. Additionally, the U.K. Familial Ovarian Cancer Screening Study is performing

CA-125 with ROCA analyses every 4 months, with referral to TVUS for abnormal findings.

Further data from these large prospective trials are needed to shed light on the utility of CA-125 screening in this high-risk group of women. In the absence of these data, however, it is still recommended that mutation carriers who have not undergone salpingo-oophorectomy perform the screening outlined above. Additionally, studies are evaluating the utility of additional serum markers (215,216) and the current Cancer Genetics Network-led trial has prospectively collected serum for analysis of novel markers.

Risk Reduction Options

Risk-Reducing Bilateral Salpingo Oophorectomy

Risk-reducing bilateral salpingo-oophorectomy is strongly recommended for mutation carriers who have completed childbearing and are more than 35 years of age. Two pivotal studies published in 2002 demonstrated the strong protective effect of this intervention. Among 551 *BRCA1* and *BRCA2* carriers followed for more than 8 years, fallopian tube, ovarian cancer, or primary peritoneal carcinomatosis developed in 8 of the 259 (3.1%) subjects who had undergone RRSO as compared with 58 of the 292 (19.9%) who had not undergone this procedure (HR = 0.04, 95% CI, 0.01–0.16) (12). Similarly, in a prospective study of 170 *BRCA1* and *BRCA2* carriers over the age of 35 followed for 2 years, cancer of the fallopian tubes or ovaries or primary peritoneal carcinomatosis was diagnosed in 5 of the 83 women choosing surveillance as opposed to 1 of the 98 women who underwent salpingo-oophorectomy (*p* = .04) (203). In a recently published study updating data from the above two studies, 498 *BRCA1* carriers and 294 *BRCA2* carriers were prospectively followed for a median of 38 months. An 88% reduction in risk of *BRCA*-associated gynecologic malignancies was noted in those electing RRSO (3 of 509) as compared with surveillance (12 of 283) (HR = 0.12, 95% CI, 0.03–0.41). The benefit appeared to be more marked in *BRCA1* carriers (HR = 0.15, 95% CI, 0.04–0.56) than in *BRCA2* carriers (HR = 0, 95% CI not estimable) (11). Additionally, an international study of 1,828 *BRCA1/2* carriers demonstrated that, with a median follow-up of 3.5 years, RRSO was associated with an 80% reduction in risk of *BRCA*-associated gynecologic malignancies (HR = 0.20, 95% CI, 0.07–0.58; *p* = .003) (217). Of note, this study estimated a 4.3% cumulative incidence of peritoneal carcinomatosis at 20 years in those undergoing RRSO. In addition to the residual risk of peritoneal carcinomatosis after RRSO, studies have demonstrated that occult malignancies, including cancer of the fallopian tubes, occur in 2% to 10% of women at the time of risk-reducing surgery (12,203,218,219). This finding underscores the importance of removal of the fallopian tubes at the time of risk-reducing surgery as well as the significance of careful examination of the specimen for occult malignancy. Data from a prospective study also suggest that RRSO is associated not only with a reduction in breast and ovarian cancer incidence but also a reduction in disease related mortality (220). Further studies are needed to confirm this critically important finding.

A number of arguments have been made in support of the notion that hysterectomy is indicated in mutation carriers at the time of RRSO. Given the risk of fallopian tube cancer, concern has been raised that a small portion of the proximal fallopian tube remains if hysterectomy is not performed, thus resulting in a residual increased risk of fallopian tube cancer. However, two studies examining fallopian tube cancers indicate that more than 90% occur in the distal or mid-portion of the tube (218,221), suggesting that the occurrence of a proximal fallopian tube cancer would be a very unlikely event. Some reports have suggested an increased incidence of uterine carcinoma in mutation carriers (24,27), whereas others have not confirmed an elevated risk of serous uterine cancer (21,222). Additionally, a recent case-control study indicated an increased incidence of uterine cancer among mutation carriers taking tamoxifen (22). Given conflicting findings regarding the risk of uterine cancer in mutation carriers and lack of data on the impact of tamoxifen-related endometrial cancer on mortality, it remains unclear if the risk-to-benefit ratio favors hysterectomy. A final issue to be considered, centers on the type of HRT after RRSO. In carriers undergoing hysterectomy, estrogen alone could be used; however it is unclear if the findings from the Women's Health Initiative indicating greater safety of estrogen alone as compared with estrogen and progesterone apply to mutation carriers undergoing premature menopause for whom brief duration of HRT is being considered. Thus, carriers should consider this information at the time they are undergoing RRSO, but at present, hysterectomy is not routinely recommended.

Chemoprevention

Oral contraceptives are known to decrease the risk of ovarian cancer in the general population (223). As discussed previously, in the section on cancer risk modifiers, a recently published large case-control study demonstrated that oral contraceptive use reduced the risk ovarian cancer in *BRCA1* and *BRCA2* carriers (65). However, data from The International *BRCA1/2* Carrier Cohort Study, a retrospective study of 1,593 mutation carriers, indicate that both current and past use of oral contraceptives was associated with an increased risk of breast cancer (HR = 1.47, 95% CI, 1.16–1.87) (68). Thus, based on current data, it remains difficult to make recommendations for or against the use of oral contraceptives.

Male Breast Cancer

It is recommended that male *BRCA1/2* carriers perform monthly breast self-examination, undergo semiannual clinical breast examination, and consider undergoing baseline mammogram followed by annual mammogram if gynecomastia is present or baseline study reveals parenchymal or glandular breast density (109).

Prostate Cancer

It is recommended that male mutation carriers follow the general screening guidelines for prostate cancer (109).

Other Cancers

No specific guidelines exist for the management of pancreatic cancer risk. On an individualized basis, carriers can consider participating in studies of pancreatic cancer screening, especially if they have a family history of pancreatic cancer. Such studies may include imaging studies (e.g., endoscopic ultrasound or endoscopic retrograde cholangiopancreatography) with or without biomarker assessment (e.g., CA-19-9), although the role of the latter appears to be very limited in asymptomatic individuals (224). Novel strategies are also being evaluated. Additionally, it is generally recommended that carriers undergo annual skin examination with a dermatologist.

Management of Breast Cancer Patients with *BRCA1* or *BRCA2* Mutations

Breast Cancer

Phenotype

Histopathologically, *BRCA1*-associated breast cancers have been consistently noted to be both more frequently high grade

(225,226) and more frequently estrogen and progesterone receptor negative (211,227,228). In addition, these tumors exhibit more lymphocytic infiltration and continuous pushing margins than is typically seen in sporadic breast cancer (229) and more frequently have medullary or atypical medullary features (225,227). Although it had been thought that DCIS occurred infrequently in *BRCA1* carriers, more recent studies indicate that DCIS should be considered part of the tumor spectrum in both *BRCA1* and *BRCA2* carriers. For example, in a study examining the rate of DCIS (with or without associated invasive breast cancer) among women presenting for genetic counseling and testing, DCIS was seen 37% of *BRCA1/2* carriers as compared with 34% of noncarriers (88). On molecular analyses, *BRCA1*-associated breast cancers showed an increased incidence of *p53* mutations (211,230), but a decreased incidence of overexpression of *erb*B-2 (211,231,232).

Studies examining *BRCA2*-associated breast cancers have demonstrated that these appear to be similar to sporadic breast cancer with respect to hormone receptor status (228,233,234). In addition, two studies observed excess numbers of tubulolobular or pleomorphic lobular carcinomas in *BRCA2* carriers (235,236), but a third study did not confirm this finding (237). In addition, in contrast to *BRCA1*, *BRCA2*-associated breast cancers did not exhibit any differences in expression of p53 or *erb*B-2 (211).

Breast Cancer Prognosis

Investigations have focused on whether the observed phenotypic differences between sporadic and *BRCA1/2*-associated breast cancers have prognostic implications. There has been variability in the findings of these studies, as well as the methodologies employed. More recent studies have sought to overcome survival biases that could hinder the interpretability of the findings by genotyping tumor blocks from all Jewish women diagnosed over a specified timeframe and correlating the findings with clinical outcome. Rennert et al. (228) obtained data on all incident cases of invasive breast cancer diagnosed between January 1987 and December 1988 in the Israeli National Cancer Registry. DNA was extracted from available blocks and tested for the three founder mutations in those of Ashkenazi Jewish descent. A total of 1,545 subjects had tumor specimens available for analysis as well as clinical and pathologic records. *BRCA1* or *BRCA2* mutations were identified in 10% of the subjects. The 10-year survival rate was 49% for *BRCA1* carriers, 48% for *BRCA2* carriers, and 51% for noncarriers. The hazard ratio for death from breast cancer adjusted for age, tumor size, nodal status, and metastasis did not differ between *BRCA1* carriers (HR = 0.76, 95% CI, 0.45–1.30, *p* = 31), or *BRCA2* carriers (HR = 1.31, 95% CI, 0.8–2.15, *p* = .28) compared with noncarriers. Interestingly, among those receiving chemotherapy, a nonstatistically significant trend was seen for improved survival in *BRCA1* carriers (10-year survival of 71% in carriers vs. 46% in noncarriers; HR = 0.48, 95% CI, 0.19–1.21, *p* = 0.12) and the interaction term between *BRCA1* status and chemotherapy was significant for overall survival (*p* = .02). Additionally, a survival disadvantage was seen for *BRCA1* carriers with tumors less than 2 cm in size (*p* = .04). In a study by Robson et al. (234), tumor blocks of 496 Jewish women diagnosed between 1980 and 1995 who underwent breast-conserving surgery were analyzed. Founder mutations were identified in 11% of the women and 10-year breast cancer specific survival was significantly worse in *BRCA1* carriers than noncarriers (62% vs. 86%, *p* <.001), but not in those with *BRCA2* mutations (84% vs. 86%, *p* = .76). However, *BRCA1* status predicted for a worse outcome only in those not receiving chemotherapy. In a study by El-Tamer et al. (233), in which 487 tumor blocks were tested for the founder mutations, the 5- and

10-year overall and breast cancer specific survival was not found to differ between *BRCA1* carriers, *BRCA2* carriers, and noncarriers. The interpretation of the above studies is hampered by the lack of data on other well-recognized prognostic factors, such as estrogen receptor/progesterone receptor (ER/PR) status of the tumors. In a study from the high-risk clinic at Rotterdam, the prognosis of 223 patients with *BRCA1*-associated breast cancer was compared with that of 446 controls with sporadic breast cancer matched for age and year at diagnosis (227). On multivariate analysis, no difference in breast cancer specific survival was seen (HR = 1.29, 95% CI, 0.85–1.97). When the analysis was restricted to women who underwent testing within 2 years of diagnosis to minimize longevity bias, no differences in breast cancer specific survival were seen in *BRCA1* carriers versus noncarriers. Based on these data, mutation status should currently not be viewed as an independent predictor of clinical outcome. Thus, mutation status should not be used to influence systemic therapy decisions.

Local Treatment

Although the increased risk of contralateral breast cancer in *BRCA1/2* mutation carriers with breast cancer is well-established, it is less clear whether *BRCA1/2* carriers incur greater risks for ipsilateral cancer if treated with breast-conserving therapy. Additionally, concerns regarding increased radiation sensitivity and potential impact on cosmesis in mutation carriers have been raised. A recent review article noted that among 17 studies examining the risk of in-breast tumor recurrence in genetic cohorts as opposed to those with sporadic disease, 5 noted an increased risk, whereas 12 did not (238). Many of these studies however, did not factor in the impact of either tamoxifen or oophorectomy on subsequent risk of breast cancer. In a study by Pierce et al. (15), which compared 160 *BRCA1/2* carriers with breast cancer who underwent breast-conserving therapy with 445 matched controls with sporadic breast cancer, no overall difference in rate of ipsilateral recurrence at 10 years was noted. However, when women who had undergone prophylactic oophorectomy were excluded from the analysis, mutation carriers had significantly higher rates of ipsilateral recurrence (*p* = .03). The metachronous ipsilateral breast cancers in carriers were more commonly located in a quadrant other than that of the primary lesion and tended to be associated with longer time to recurrence, suggesting that these represented second primary cancer rather than an in-breast tumor recurrence. Additionally, in this study, no negative impact on cosmesis was observed.

Two additional studies prospectively examined the risk of ipsilateral breast cancer in *BRCA1/2* carriers (10,16). A study of 188 mutation carriers who underwent breast-conserving therapy identified an 11.5% 10-year risk of metachronous ipsilateral breast cancer (10). Another recent prospective study of 87 women with *BRCA1/2* mutations observed an 11.2%, 13.6%, and 23.4% risk of ipsilateral breast cancer at 5, 10, and 15 years, respectively (16). Thus, breast-conserving therapy is an appropriate local treatment option for mutation carriers with newly diagnosed breast cancer. Nonetheless, it is important that these women understand that they face increased risks for both contralateral and likely ipsilateral new breast cancers. Thus, some mutation carriers with a new diagnosed breast cancer may wish to consider bilateral mastectomy to minimize their risk of developing a new primary.

Systemic Treatment

As discussed, current data regarding the impact of *BRCA1/2* status on breast cancer related prognosis are inconclusive and, thus, mutation status should not factor into the decision-making process regarding systemic treatment options. It is possible that in the future, choice of systemic therapy may be influenced by genetic information because preclinical data suggest that *BRCA*-associated breast cancers may have enhanced sensitivity to certain chemotherapeutic agents such as platinum (239). The increased efficacy of platinum agents is thought to be a possible explanation for the improved survival seen in *BRCA*-associated ovarian cancers as compared with sporadic disease (240). In addition, hope is that a novel class of drugs Poly(ADP-ribose) polymerase-1 (PARP-1) inhibitors, may be particularly effective in *BRCA* mutation-associated breast cancer. PARP-1 is an enzyme involved in the repair of single-strand DNA (ssDNA) breaks through base excision repair. In PARP-1 deficient states, ssDNA breaks may go on to become double strand DNA (dsDNA) breaks. The repair of dsDNA breaks is dependent on *BRCA1*- and *BRCA2*-mediated processes. Thus in *BRCA*-deficient cells, it is hypothesized that PARP-1 inhibition will result in accumulation of dsDNA breaks, ultimately leading to apoptosis (241,242). Clinical trials tailoring systemic therapy to *BRCA* mutation status are currently ongoing.

Screening and Risk Reduction Options for Second Malignancies

Mutation carriers with a breast cancer diagnosis are at increased risk of developing a second breast cancer and ovarian cancer (see section on Clinical Characteristics). As previously noted, up to 25% of mutation carriers with stage I breast cancer will subsequently succumb to ovarian cancer (19). Thus, it is recommended that the screening and prevention guidelines for breast and ovarian cancer as described in the prior section on management of unaffected mutation carrier, be utilized. It is important to note that these must be individualized and balanced, incorporating information on the underlying prognosis related to the breast cancer.

Management of *BRCA1/2*-Negative Hereditary Breast Cancer Families

For members of *BRCA1/2*-negative hereditary breast cancer families, an individualized approach to cancer screening and prevention based on personal and family history is recommended. It is helpful to separate these families into those with site-specific breast cancer and those that include both breast and ovarian cancer. As discussed, families with site-specific breast cancer appear to have an increased incidence of breast cancer, but are likely not at a significant increased risk for ovarian cancer (38–40). Thus, for families meeting these criteria, it is recommended that they follow the same breast cancer screening and prevention guidelines as for *BRCA1/2* carriers. However, in these families, the benefit of management directed specifically at ovarian cancer risk reduction and screening is unclear, because the findings from the above studies suggest that they are not at significantly increased risk for ovarian cancer. It is important to remember that bilateral oophorectomy before age 50 is associated with a reduction in risk of breast cancer, in mutation carriers (11,12) as well as in those without a defined mutation (243). Nonetheless, further studies are required to address more fully the risk-to-benefit ratio of ovarian risk reduction strategies in *BRCA1/2*-negative site-specific breast cancer. For *BRCA1/2*-negative families with family histories of multiple cases of breast cancer (i.e., three to four or more cases breast cancer before age 60) and other *BRCA*-associated cancers, such as ovarian cancer, male breast cancer, or multiple cases of pancreatic cancer or melanoma, it is recommended they follow the same management guidelines as outlined above for *BRCA1* and *BRCA2* carriers.

UTILIZATION AND PSYCHOSOCIAL IMPACT OF MEDICAL MANAGEMENT OPTIONS

Risk-Reducing Surgery

For *BRCA1/2* testing to lead to the anticipated reductions in breast and ovarian cancer mortality, receipt of a positive test result must be followed by the adoption of appropriate behavioral management strategies. One such strategy is risk reducing mastectomy. Evidence suggests wide cultural variation in utilization of RRM and wide variability depending on the carrier's personal breast cancer history. Studies of unaffected women conducted in the United States have found rates of RRM ranging from 0% to 15% in the first 12 to 24 months following the receipt of a positive *BRCA1/2* test result (244–247). In contrast, studies conducted outside of the United States have reported much higher rates of RRM, ranging from 9% to 54% (158,248–250). Explanations for the discrepancies between U.S. women and women from other countries are not clear, but likely are related to cultural differences, differing physician attitudes toward prophylactic surgery, and differences across health care systems (250,251).

Although the use of RRM is relatively rare among unaffected mutation carriers in the United States, the rate of contralateral RRM among mutation carriers previously affected with breast cancer is substantially higher. For example, we found that among breast cancer survivors who sought genetic testing at varying times following their diagnosis, 18% of *BRCA1/2* mutation carriers opted for contralateral RRM in the year following testing (252). In an earlier study, we reported that 48% of patients newly diagnosed with breast cancer who learned that they carried a *BRCA1* or *BRCA2* mutation at the time of their diagnosis opted for an immediate RRM (120). In European studies, rates of contralateral RRM among women affected with breast cancer have ranged from 35% to 65% (248,253,254).

In addition to reducing the risk of ovarian cancer, RRSO also reduces the risk of breast cancer when performed premenopausally (11,12). In our own research, 27% of mutation carriers obtained RRSO within 12 months of result disclosure (255). More recent studies have, however, reported higher rates ranging from 21% to 65% in U.S. studies (256,257) and from 31% (162) to more than 70% (158,258) in European studies.

There have been few studies examining the factors associated with the use of RRM and RRSO or the outcomes of such surgery. Studies suggest that being age 50 or less (248,254), being a parent (254), receipt of a positive test result at diagnosis or *before* diagnosis (120,259–261), physician recommendation to consider contralateral prophylactic mastectomy (CPM) (120) have all been associated with the receipt of RRM. Older age (244,250,254), carrying a *BRCA1* (as opposed to *BRCA2*) mutation (255), having a family history of ovarian cancer (255), lower education (258), and having elevated perceived risk for ovarian cancer (255,262) have all been found to predict receipt of prophylactic oophorectomy.

The limited research on psychosocial outcomes of risk-reducing surgery has found high levels of satisfaction and little distress following prophylactic mastectomy (263–265). For example, at 1 year postdiagnosis, we found no differences in distress or quality of life among affected women who did and did not opt for prophylactic mastectomy at the time of their initial diagnosis (266). Similarly, Madalinska et al. (267) found no quality of life differences among women who did and did not opt for RRSO. Despite these generally positive outcomes, some women do report an adverse impact of risk-reducing surgery. For example, among breast cancer patients who opted for RRM, one-third reported a negative impact on body appearance, 26% reported a diminished sense of femininity, 23% reported negative effects on sexual relationships, and 17% reported diminished self-esteem. Patients who reported such outcomes also reported greater dissatisfaction with their decision to have RRM (263,268).

Surveillance

Carriers who do not opt for risk-reducing surgery are advised to participate in breast and ovarian cancer screening beginning at age 25 to 35 (109). Initial studies suggested that adherence to breast cancer screening was suboptimal. Lerman et al (245) reported that 6 months following testing only 60% of carriers who were due for a mammogram reported receiving one. This is comparable to our own research in which only 59% of carriers received a mammogram within 12 months of testing (246). More recent studies, however, have reported substantially higher rates of mammography for carriers, ranging from 82% to 95% (158,247). Studies directly comparing mammography adherence among carriers and noncarriers have found increased adherence among carriers (158,244,247). There are few data on the utilization of MRI screening among carriers. However, as more centers begin to recommend annual MRI to mutation carriers, the use of MRI within this population will need to be evaluated.

Results for ovarian cancer screening reflect lower rates of adherence. The low rates of ovarian cancer screening reported among carriers reflect the lack of acceptance of ovarian cancer screening among most health professionals. In our own research, 43% of carriers reported an annual CA-125 and 40% an annual TVUS (255). Lower rates have been reported in previous studies (245).

Chemoprevention

Another important decision for mutation carriers concerns whether to utilize chemopreventive agents. As yet, however, few data exist regarding the utilization of chemopreventive agents or participation in chemoprevention trials among carriers. However, two recent studies have reported rates of clinical use of chemopreventive agents (i.e., tamoxifen and raloxifene) ranging from 1% (250) to 12% (249) of Australian and Canadian *BRCA1/2* carriers, respectively. Additional research is needed to determine the clinical utilization of these and other chemopreventive agents among *BRCA1/2* carriers.

Summary: Psychological, Behavioral, and Medical Outcomes of BRCA1/2 Testing

The findings reviewed in this section suggest that, despite a modest increase in distress in the short term, serious long-term adverse psychosocial outcomes among carriers are rare. However, a number of factors have been demonstrated to predict distress following the receipt of *BRCA1/2* test results. Thus, it may be possible to identify individuals who are at risk for adverse outcomes and to target these individuals for enhanced psychosocial support during and following the genetic counseling process. Further, given the complex medical decisions that must be made following a positive *BRCA1/2* test result, additional decision-making support may be beneficial for some *BRCA1/2* mutation carriers. A number of such decision aids have been developed for women at high risk and *BRCA1/2* mutation carriers. We found that a decision aid delivered following the receipt of positive test results has helped participants to make more informed decisions about how to manage their breast cancer risk (269).

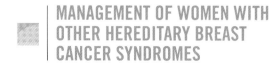

MANAGEMENT OF WOMEN WITH OTHER HEREDITARY BREAST CANCER SYNDROMES

Li-Fraumeni Syndrome

Li-Fraumeni syndrome (LFS) is a rare, highly penetrant auto-somal-dominant condition characterized primarily by soft tissue sarcomas, osteosarcomas, leukemias, brain tumors, adrenocortical malignancies, and early onset breast cancer (118,270). Mutations in the tumor suppressor gene *p53* have been documented in up to 70% of families with LFS (271). It has been estimated that 50% of carriers will develop some form of cancer by age 30 years and 90% by age 70 years (272). In particular, the occurrence of breast cancer in these families is remarkable. In a report of 24 families with a history of LFS, including 200 individuals, 45 women developed breast cancer, of whom 73% were diagnosed before age 45 years (273). Multiple breast cancers were diagnosed in about 25% of these women, and more than 25% had other additional primary tumors. Many of these cancers have occurred in the field of radiation treatment (273,274). Therefore, such risks may affect treatment options for *p53* carriers diagnosed with breast cancer (118). In women, surveillance for breast cancer with monthly breast self-examination beginning at age 18, semiannual clinical breast examinations beginning at age 20 to 25 or 5 to 10 years before the first breast cancer in the family, and annual mammogram or breast MRI starting at age 20 to 25 is recommended. Additionally, risk-reducing mastectomy should also be discussed on an individual basis. Participation in clinical trials with novel imaging is encouraged (109).

Additionally, beginning at age 20 to 25 years, an annual comprehensive physical examination is recommended with particular focus on rare cancers (3). Otherwise, surveillance can be tailored based on the family history, and prompt follow up of suggestive symptoms is urged (120). Proven strategies for screening for most of the component cancers of this syndrome, however, are not available, especially for the childhood cancers. Moreover, ethical issues surrounding the testing of minors should be carefully explored before testing children is undertaken.

Cowden Syndrome

Cowden syndrome is a rare, although potentially under-recognized, autosomal-dominant condition characterized by multiple hamartomatous lesions and an increased risk of early onset breast cancer and thyroid cancer (275). Mutations in the *PTEN* gene have been identified in at least 80% of patients who meet diagnostic criteria for Cowen syndrome (276). The lifetime risk of breast cancer is between 25% and 50%, with most cases diagnosed before age 50 (277–279). In addition, up to 75% of women with Cowden syndrome have been observed to have a variety of benign breast conditions, including ductal hyperplasia, intraductal papillomatosis, adenosis, lobular atrophy, fibroadenomas, and fibrocystic changes (278,280). An increased incidence of bilateral disease has been observed for benign and malignant conditions (278). Management of breast cancer risk includes monthly breast self-examination beginning at age 18, semiannual clinical breast examination beginning at age 20 to 25 or 5 to 10 years before the first breast cancer in the family, and annual mammogram and breast MRI starting at age 30 to 35 is recommended or 5 to 10 years younger than the earliest known breast cancer in the family. Risk-reducing mastectomy should also be discussed on an individual basis. The management recommendations for other malignancies include blind endometrial aspirations annually at age 35 to 40 or 5 years earlier than the earliest case of endometrial cancer in the family, annual comprehensive physical examination beginning at age 18 with particular focus on breast and thyroid examinations, annual urinalysis and consideration for annual urine cytology, baseline thyroid ultrasound at age 18 with consideration for annual examination, and finally consideration of annual dermatologic examination (109).

Peutz-Jeghers Syndrome

Peutz-Jeghers syndrome (PJS), arising from mutations in *STK11* and as yet other unidentified gene(s), is an autosomal-dominant condition characterized by hamartomatous polyps in the gastrointestinal tract and by mucocutaneous melanin deposits in the buccal mucosa, lips, fingers, and toes (201,202). With respect to extraintestinal cancers, the most significant risk is for breast cancer, with a lifetime risk estimated to be about 55%, which approaches that observed in *BRCA1* and *BRCA2* carriers (283). Although overall few cases have been reported, onset before age 50 years and bilateral disease is not uncommon (283–285). The risk of ovarian cancer, estimated at about 20%, is significant, but many of these are nonepithelial sex cord tumors (283). Women also face elevated risks for uterine cancer (283). Thus, in addition to the special surveillance for colon and other associated findings, women should consider heightened surveillance for breast, uterine, and ovarian cancers (282,283,286).

Hereditary Diffuse Gastric Cancer

Hereditary diffuse gastric cancer, an autosomal-dominant cancer predisposition syndrome, attributable to mutations in *CDH1* (*E-cadherin*), is associated with diffuse gastric cancer and female lobular breast cancer (287,288). Based on multicase families, it has been estimated that the cumulative risk to age 80 of gastric cancer is 67% and 83% in males and females, respectively (289). The cumulative risk of breast cancer in women to age 80 is 39%; however, this estimate assumes that they do not develop gastric cancer or that they survive it long term (289). No specific recommendations for breast cancer screening exist; however, it is advisable that these women follow the same screening recommendations as women with hereditary breast cancer owing to *BRCA1* or *BRCA2* mutations. It is important to note that lobular breast cancers are typically more difficult to detect on mammography. Studies suggest that MRI may be more accurate in this setting (290). Given that lobular carcinomas are frequently hormone receptor positive, chemoprevention with tamoxifen or raloxifene is a very reasonable option. Additionally, risk-reducing mastectomy can be considered.

CHEK2

CHEK2 (cell cycle checkpoint kinase 2) plays a role in cell-cycle arrest and DNA repair (291). One of the most commonly identified variants in the *CHEK2* gene is a small deletion (1100delC), which is found predominantly in individuals of northern and eastern European descent (146). A recent meta-analysis of breast cancer risk associated with this specific mutation reported that, among pedigrees with "familial breast cancer" (i.e., one case of female breast cancer with one or more relatives with breast cancer, including male breast cancer, or ovarian cancer), the cumulative risk of breast cancer to age 70 was 37% (95% CI, 26%–56%) (146). Although this risk roughly compares with those reported in *BRCA1* and *BRCA2* carriers, it is important to bear in mind that the studies used in the analysis used a variety of ascertainment methods, which may have biased estimates of penetrance (146,292). In addition, the full spectrum of cancers associated with this and other specific variants in *CHEK2* is not fully defined (146,292). For these reasons, routine clinical testing for *CHEK2* mutations has not been recommended (292). Moreover, it is unclear whether other low penetrance genes could contribute to familial breast cancer risks in *BRCA1/2*-negative families in addition to potential *CHEK2* mutations and what management strategies are optimal (292). Given that most *CHEK2*-related breast cancers are hormone receptor positive, chemoprevention with tamoxifen or raloxifene should be considered (293).

SUMMARY

Most individuals with a family history of breast cancer have a familial rather than hereditary basis to their disease. For women with hereditary breast cancer, *BRCA1* and *BRCA2* mutations account for most cases. Mutations in these genes are associated with a significantly elevated risk of early onset breast and ovarian cancer. In addition, other cancers may be seen with an increased frequency in mutation carriers. Models based on cancer history, family history, and ethnic background are available to guide clinicians in estimating the likelihood that an individual harbors a risk-conferring mutation. Over the last decade, data from prospective studies have emerged demonstrating a strong protective effect of bilateral salpingo-oopherectony and bilateral mastectomy on cancer incidence. Additionally, it is now recommended that women with a hereditary predisposition to breast cancer alternate annual breast MRI with mammogram. Because of the complexities involved in decision-making about genetic testing and medical management, genetic counseling is critical before and after undergoing testing. Further studies on genetic and environmental cancer risk modifiers, genotype–phenotype correlations, and the impact of cancer screening and prevention options are underway and will continue to provide greater insight into the features and management of individuals at high risk.

MANAGEMENT SUMMARY

- *BRCA1/2* carriers face significantly elevated risks of early onset breast and ovarian cancer as well as increased risk of pancreatic, prostate, and male breast cancer.
- Decisions regarding more intensive screening versus prevention are often personal, based on a careful balancing of the relative risks and benefits of the various options.
- Breast cancer screening recommendations include annual mammogram alternating with annual breast MRI. MRI should be performed at a center with expertise in this technique.
- Breast cancer prevention options can be combined with more intensive screening and include RRSO (if performed before age 50), risk reducing mastectomy, and tamoxifen for *BRCA2* carriers. The data on the benefit of tamoxifen in *BRCA1* carriers are less clear.
- For management of ovarian cancer risk, bilateral salpingo-oophorectomy after age 35 and once childbearing is complete is strongly recommended. Short-term HRT before age 50 can be considered.
- For women who have not undergone salpingo-oophorectomy, semiannual CA-125 and TVUS are recommended, beginning at age 35 or 5 years younger than the earliest age of onset of ovarian cancer in the family. However, no data currently exist to support a benefit of screening for ovarian cancer.
- Male mutation carriers should perform monthly breast self-examination, have semiannual clinical breast examination and consider annual mammography. It is recommended that they also follow the general population guidelines for prostate cancer screening.

- Mutation carriers should consider annual skin examination, which could be on an individualized basis, and consider participating in studies on pancreatic cancer screening.
- Mutation status does not impact breast cancer management in *BRCA1/2* carriers, but mutation carriers need to consider their risks of second malignancy and should follow similar guidelines to those outlined above for unaffected carriers.
- Recommendations for management of members of hereditary breast cancer families who have undergone genetic testing and tested negative for *BRCA1/2* mutations need to be individualized based on their personal and family history.
- The management options for breast cancer for women with other hereditary breast cancer syndromes are generally similar to those for *BRCA1/2* carriers.

References

1. Olopade OI. Genetics in clinical cancer care: a promise unfulfilled among minority populations. *Cancer Epidemiol Biomarkers Prev* 2004;13:1683–1686.
2. National Institutes of Health, National Cancer Institute. Surveillance Epidemiology and End Results (SEER). http://seer.cancer.gov/faststats/. 2008 [online]. Accessed Dec. 15, 2008.
3. Antoniou A, Pharoah PD, Narod S, et al. Average risks of breast and ovarian cancer associated with BRCA1 or BRCA2 mutations detected in case Series unselected for family history: a combined analysis of 22 studies. *Am J Hum Genet* 2003;72:1117–1130.
4. Chen S, Parmigiani G. Meta-analysis of BRCA1 and BRCA2 penetrance. *J Clin Oncol* 2007;25:1329–1333.
5. Begg CB, Haile RW, Borg A, et al. Variation of breast cancer risk among *BRCA1/2* carriers. *JAMA* 2008;299:194–201.
6. Brose MS, Rebbeck TR, Calzone KA, et al. Cancer risk estimates for BRCA1 mutation carriers identified in a risk evaluation program. *J Natl Cancer Inst* 2002;94:1365–1372.
7. Easton DF, Ford D, Bishop DT. Breast and ovarian cancer incidence in BRCA1-mutation carriers. Breast Cancer Linkage Consortium. *Am J Hum Genet* 1995;56:265–271.
8. Marcus JN, Watson P, Page DL, et al. Hereditary breast cancer: pathobiology, prognosis, and BRCA1 and BRCA2 gene linkage. *Cancer* 1996;77:697–709.
9. Breast Cancer Linkage Consortium. Cancer risks in BRCA2 mutation carriers. The Breast Cancer Linkage Consortium. *J Natl Cancer Inst* 1999;91:1310–1316.
10. Metcalfe K, Lynch HT, Ghadirian P, et al. Contralateral breast cancer in BRCA1 and BRCA2 mutation carriers. *J Clin Oncol* 2004;22:2328–2335.
11. Kauff ND, Domchek SM, Friebel TM, et al. Risk-reducing salpingo-oophorectomy for the prevention of BRCA1- and BRCA2-associated breast and gynecologic cancer: a multicenter, prospective study. *J Clin Oncol* 2008;26:1331–1337.
12. Rebbeck TR, Lynch HT, Neuhausen SL, et al. Prophylactic oophorectomy in carriers of BRCA1 or BRCA2 mutations. *N Engl J Med* 2002;346:1616–1622.
13. Dawson LA, Chow E, Goss PE. Evolving perspectives in contralateral breast cancer. *Eur J Cancer* 1998;34:2000–2009.
14. Haffty BG, Harrold E, Khan AJ, et al. Outcome of conservatively managed early-onset breast cancer by BRCA1/2 status. *Lancet* 2002;359:1471–1477.
15. Pierce LJ, Levin AM, Rebbeck TR, et al. Ten-year multi-institutional results of breast-conserving surgery and radiotherapy in BRCA1/2-associated stage I/II breast cancer. *J Clin Oncol* 2006;24:2437–2443.
16. Robson M, Svahn T, McCormick B, et al. Appropriateness of breast-conserving treatment of breast carcinoma in women with germline mutations in BRCA1 or BRCA2: a clinic-based series. *Cancer* 2005;103:44–51.
17. Seynaeve C, Verhoog LC, van de Bosch LM, et al. Ipsilateral breast tumour recurrence in hereditary breast cancer following breast-conserving therapy. *Eur J Cancer* 2004;40:1150–1158.
18. Turner BC, Harrold E, Matloff E, et al. BRCA1/BRCA2 germline mutations in locally recurrent breast cancer patients after lumpectomy and radiation therapy: implications for breast-conserving management in patients with BRCA1/BRCA2 mutations. *J Clin Oncol* 1999;17:3017–3024.
19. Metcalfe KA, Lynch HT, Ghadirian P, et al. The risk of ovarian cancer after breast cancer in BRCA1 and BRCA2 carriers. *Gynecol Oncol* 2005;96:222–226.
20. Aziz S, Kuperstein G, Rosen B, et al. A genetic epidemiological study of carcinoma of the fallopian tube. *Gynecol Oncol* 2001;80:341–345.
21. Levine DA, Lin O, Barakat RR, et al. Risk of endometrial carcinoma associated with BRCA mutation. *Gynecol Oncol* 2001;80:395–398.
22. Beiner ME, Finch A, Rosen B, et al. The risk of endometrial cancer in women with BRCA1 and BRCA2 mutations. A prospective study. *Gynecol Oncol* 2007;104:7–10.
23. Biron-Shental T, Drucker L, Altaras M, et al. High incidence of BRCA1-2 germline mutations, previous breast cancer and familial cancer history in Jewish patients with uterine serous papillary carcinoma. *Eur J Surg Oncol* 2006;32:1097–1100.
24. Lavie O, Hornreich G, Ben Arie A, et al. BRCA germline mutations in Jewish women with uterine serous papillary carcinoma. *Gynecol Oncol* 2004;92:521–524.
25. Hahn SA, Greenhalf B, Ellis I, et al. BRCA2 germline mutations in familial pancreatic cancer. *J Natl Cancer Inst* 2003;95:214–221.
26. Murphy KM, Brune KA, Griffin C, et al. Evaluation of candidate genes MAP2K4, MADH4, ACVR1B, and BRCA2 in familial pancreatic cancer: deleterious BRCA2 mutations in 17%. *Cancer Res* 2002;62:3789–3793.
27. Thompson D, Easton DF. Cancer Incidence in BRCA1 mutation carriers. *J Natl Cancer Inst* 2002;94:1358–1365.

28. Liede A, Karlan BY, Narod SA. Cancer risks for male carriers of germline mutations in BRCA1 or BRCA2: a review of the literature. *J Clin Oncol* 2004;22:735–742.

29. Ford D, Easton DF, Bishop DT, et al. Risks of cancer in BRCA1-mutation carriers. Breast Cancer Linkage Consortium. *Lancet* 1994,343.692–695.

30. Johannsson O, Loman N, Moller T, et al. Incidence of malignant tumours in relatives of BRCA1 and BRCA2 germline mutation carriers. *Eur J Cancer* 1999;35:1248–1257.

31. Lin KM, Ternent CA, Adams DR, et al. Colorectal cancer in hereditary breast cancer kindreds. *Dis Colon Rectum* 1999;42:1041–1045.

32. Niell BL, Rennert G, Bonner JD, et al. BRCA1 and BRCA2 founder mutations and the risk of colorectal cancer. *J Natl Cancer Inst* 2004;96:15–21.

33. Peelen T, de Leeuw W, van Lent K, et al. Genetic analysis of a breast-ovarian cancer family, with 7 cases of colorectal cancer linked to BRCA1, fails to support a role for BRCA1 in colorectal tumorigenesis. *Int J Cancer* 2000;88:778–782.

34. Struewing JP, Hartge P, Wacholder S, et al. The risk of cancer associated with specific mutations of BRCA1 and BRCA2 among Ashkenazi Jews. *N Engl J Med* 1997;336:1401–1408.

35. Kirchhoff T, Kauff ND, Mitra N, et al. BRCA mutations and risk of prostate cancer in Ashkenazi Jews. *Clin Cancer Res* 2004;10:2918–2921.

36. Tai YC, Domchek S, Parmigiani G, et al. Breast cancer risk among male BRCA1 and BRCA2 mutation carriers. *J Natl Cancer Inst* 2007;99:1811–1814.

37. Frank TS, Deffenbaugh AM, Reid JE, et al. Clinical characteristics of individuals with germline mutations in BRCA1 and BRCA2: analysis of 10,000 individuals. *J Clin Oncol* 2002;20:1480–1490.

38. Kauff ND, Mitra N, Robson ME, et al. Risk of ovarian cancer in BRCA1 and BRCA2 mutation-negative hereditary breast cancer families. *J Natl Cancer Inst* 2005;97:1382–1384.

39. Eerola H, Pukkala E, Pyrhonen S, et al. Risk of cancer in BRCA1 and BRCA2 mutation-positive and -negative breast cancer families (Finland). *Cancer Causes Control* 2001;12:739–746.

40. Loman N, Bladstrom A, Johannsson O, et al. Cancer incidence in relatives of a population-based set of cases of early-onset breast cancer with a known BRCA1 and BRCA2 mutation status. *Breast Cancer Res* 2003;5:R175–R186.

41. Dite GS, Jenkins MA, Southey MC, et al. Familial risks, early-onset breast cancer, and BRCA1 and BRCA2 germline mutations. *J Natl Cancer Inst* 2003;95:448–457.

42. Lee JS, John EM, McGuire V, et al. Breast and ovarian cancer in relatives of cancer patients, with and without BRCA mutations. *Cancer Epidemiol Biomarkers Prev* 2006;15:359–363.

43. Risch HA, McLaughlin JR, Cole DE, et al. Prevalence and penetrance of germline BRCA1 and BRCA2 mutations in a population series of 649 women with ovarian cancer. *Am J Hum Genet* 2001;68:700–710.

44. Gayther SA, Warren W, Mazoyer S, et al. Germline mutations of the BRCA1 gene in breast and ovarian cancer families provide evidence for a genotype-phenotype correlation. *Nat Genet* 1995;11:428–433.

45. Thompson D, Easton D. Variation in BRCA1 cancer risks by mutation position. *Cancer Epidemiol Biomarkers Prev* 2002;11:329–336.

46. Moslehi R, Chu W, Karlan B, et al. BRCA1 and BRCA2 mutation analysis of 208 Ashkenazi Jewish women with ovarian cancer. *Am J Hum Genet* 2000;66:1259–1272.

47. Satagopan JM, Offit K, Foulkes W, et al. The lifetime risks of breast cancer in Ashkenazi Jewish carriers of BRCA1 and BRCA2 mutations. *Cancer Epidemiol Biomarkers Prev* 2001;10:467–473.

48. Thompson D, Easton D. Variation in cancer risks, by mutation position, in BRCA2 mutation carriers. *Am J Hum Genet* 2001;68:410–419.

49. Lubinski J, Phelan CM, Ghadirian P, et al. Cancer variation associated with the position of the mutation in the BRCA2 gene. *Fam Cancer* 2004;3:1–10.

50. Al Saffar M, Foulkes WD. Hereditary ovarian cancer resulting from a non-ovarian cancer cluster region (OCCR) BRCA2 mutation: is the OCCR useful clinically? *J Med Genet* 2002;39:e68.

51. Warner E, Foulkes W, Goodwin P, et al. Prevalence and penetrance of BRCA1 and BRCA2 gene mutations in unselected Ashkenazi Jewish women with breast cancer. *J Natl Cancer Inst* 1999;91:1241–1247.

52. Spurdle AB, Hopper JL, Chen X, et al. The BRCA2 372 HH genotype is associated with risk of breast cancer in Australian women under age 60 years. *Cancer Epidemiol Biomarkers Prev* 2002;11:413–416.

53. Auranen A, Spurdle AB, Chen X, et al. BRCA2 Arg372 Hispolymorphism and epithelial ovarian cancer risk. *Int J Cancer* 2003;103:427–430.

54. Ginolhac SM, Gad S, Corbex M, et al. BRCA1 wild-type allele modifies risk of ovarian cancer in carriers of BRCA1 germ-line mutations. *Cancer Epidemiol Biomarkers Prev* 2003;12:90–95.

55. Chenevix-Trench G, Milne RL, Antoniou AC, et al. An international initiative to identify genetic modifiers of cancer risk in BRCA1 and BRCA2 mutation carriers: the Consortium of Investigators of Modifiers of BRCA1 and BRCA2 (CIMBA). *Breast Cancer Res* 2007;9:104.

56. Antoniou AC, Sinilnikova OM, Simard J, et al. RAD51 135G—>C modifies breast cancer risk among BRCA2 mutation carriers: results from a combined analysis of 19 studies. *Am J Hum Genet* 2007;81:1186–1200.

57. Milne R, Chenevix-Trench G. Breast cancer risk modifiers. In: Isaacs C, Rebbeck TR, eds. *Hereditary breast cancer*. New York, NY: Informa Healthcare, 2008:207–231.

58. Gronwald J, Byrski T, Huzarski T, et al. Influence of selected lifestyle factors on breast and ovarian cancer risk in BRCA1 mutation carriers from Poland. *Breast Cancer Res Treat* 2006;95:105–109.

59. Jernstrom H, Lubinski J, Lynch HT, et al. Breast-feeding and the risk of breast cancer in BRCA1 and BRCA2 mutation carriers. *J Natl Cancer Inst* 2004;96:1094–1098.

60. Kotsopoulos J, Lubinski J, Lynch HT, et al. Age at first birth and the risk of breast cancer in BRCA1 and BRCA2 mutation carriers. *Breast Cancer Res Treat* 2007;105:221–228.

61. Tryggvadottir L, Olafsdottir EJ, Gudlaugsdottir S, et al. BRCA2 mutation carriers, reproductive factors and breast cancer risk. *Breast Cancer Res* 2003;5:R121–R128.

62. Cullinane CA, Lubinski J, Neuhausen SL, et al. Effect of pregnancy as a risk factor for breast cancer in BRCA1/BRCA2 mutation carriers. *Int J Cancer* 2005;117:988–991.

63. Andrieu N, Goldgar DE, Easton DF, et al. Pregnancies, breast-feeding, and breast cancer risk in the International BRCA1/2 Carrier Cohort Study (IBCCS). *J Natl Cancer Inst* 2006;98:535–544.

64. Kotsopoulos J, Lubinski J, Lynch HT, et al. Age at menarche and the risk of breast cancer in BRCA1 and BRCA2 mutation carriers. *Cancer Causes Control* 2005;16:667–674.

65. McLaughlin JR, Risch HA, Lubinski J, et al. Reproductive risk factors for ovarian cancer in carriers of BRCA1 or BRCA2 mutations: a case-control study. *Lancet Oncol* 2007;8:26–34.

66. Narod SA, Goldgar D, Cannon-Albright L, et al. Risk modifiers in carriers of BRCA1 mutations. *Int J Cancer* 1995;64:394–398.

67. Modan B, Hartge P, Hirsh-Yechezkel G, et al. Parity, oral contraceptives, and the risk of ovarian cancer among carriers and noncarriers of a BRCA1 or BRCA2 mutation. *N Engl J Med* 2001;345:235–240.

68. Brohet RM, Goldgar DE, Easton DF, et al. Oral contraceptives and breast cancer risk in the international BRCA1/2 carrier cohort study: a report from EMBRACE, GENEPSO, GEO HEBON, and the IBCCS Collaborating Group. *J Clin Oncol* 2007;25:3831–3836.

69. Jernstrom H, Loman N, Johannsson OT, et al. Impact of teenage oral contraceptive use in a population-based series of early-onset breast cancer cases who have undergone BRCA mutation testing. *Eur J Cancer* 2005;41:2312–2320.

70. Narod SA, Sun P, Ghadirian P, et al. Tubal ligation and risk of ovarian cancer in carriers of BRCA1 or BRCA2 mutations: a case-control study. *Lancet* 2001;357:1467–1470.

71. Nkondjock A, Robidoux A, Paredes Y, et al. Diet, lifestyle and BRCA-related breast cancer risk among French-Canadians. *Breast Cancer Res Treat* 2006;98:285–294.

72. Nkondjock A, Ghadirian P. Diet quality and BRCA-associated breast cancer risk. *Breast Cancer Res Treat* 2007;103:361–369.

73. Breast Cancer Family Registry, Kathleen Cuningham Consortium for Research into Familial Breast Cancer (Australasia), Ontario Cancer Genetics Network (Canada). Smoking and risk of breast cancer in carriers of mutations in BRCA1 or BRCA2 aged less than 50 years. *Breast Cancer Res Treat* 2007.

74. Ghadirian P, Lubinski J, Lynch H, et al. Smoking and the risk of breast cancer among carriers of BRCA mutations. *Int J Cancer* 2004;110:413–416.

75. King MC, Marks JH, Mandell JB. Breast and ovarian cancer risks due to inherited mutations in BRCA1 and BRCA2. *Science* 2003;302:643–646.

76. McGuire V, John EM, Felberg A, et al. No increased risk of breast cancer associated with alcohol consumption among carriers of BRCA1 and BRCA2 mutations ages <50 years. *Cancer Epidemiol Biomarkers Prev* 2006;15:1565–1567.

77. Ford D, Easton DF, Stratton M, et al. Genetic heterogeneity and penetrance analysis of the BRCA1 and BRCA2 genes in breast cancer families. The Breast Cancer Linkage Consortium. *Am J Hum Genet* 1998;62:676–689.

78. Martin AM, Blackwood MA, Antin-Ozerkis D, et al. Germline mutations in BRCA1 and BRCA2 in breast-ovarian families from a breast cancer risk evaluation clinic. *J Clin Oncol* 2001;19:2247–2253.

79. Shih HA, Couch FJ, Nathanson KL, et al. BRCA1 and BRCA2 mutation frequency in women evaluated in a breast cancer risk evaluation clinic. *J Clin Oncol* 2002;20:994–999.

80. Couch FJ, DeShano ML, Blackwood MA, et al. BRCA1 mutations in women attending clinics that evaluate the risk of breast cancer. *N Engl J Med* 1997;336:1409–1415.

81. Domchek SM, Blackwood MA, Tweed AJ, et al. University of Pennsylvania BRCA1/BRCA2 prediction model. Poster presented at the NCI sponsored "Cancer Risk Prediction Models: A Workshop on Development, Evaluation, and Application," May 20–21, 2004, Washington, DC.

82. University of Pennsylvania. The Penn II BRCA1 and BRCA2 Mutation Risk Evaluation Model. https://www.afcri.upenn.edu:8022/itacc/penn2/. 2008. Accessed Dec. 15, 2008. [online].

83. Myriad Genetic Laboratories. BRCA risk calculator and mutation prevalence tables. www.myriadtests.com/provider/mutprev.htm. 2006 [online]. Accessed Dec. 15, 2008.

84. Berry DA, Parmigiani G, Sanchez J, Schildkraut J, Winer E. Probability of carrying a mutation of breast-ovarian cancer gene BRCA1 based on family history. *J Natl Cancer Inst* 1997;89:227–238.

85. Berry DA, Iversen ES, Jr., Gudbjartsson DF, et al. BRCAPRO validation, sensitivity of genetic testing of BRCA1/BRCA2, and prevalence of other breast cancer susceptibility genes. *J Clin Oncol* 2002;20:2701–2712.

86. Parmigiani G, Berry D, Aguilar O. Determining carrier probabilities for breast cancer-susceptibility genes BRCA1 and BRCA2. *Am J Hum Genet* 1998;62:145–158.

87. Lakhani SR, Reis-Filho JS, Fulford L, et al. Prediction of BRCA1 status in patients with breast cancer using estrogen receptor and basal phenotype. *Clin Cancer Res* 2005;11:5175–5180.

88. Hwang ES, McLennan JL, Moore DH, et al. Ductal carcinoma *in situ* in BRCA mutation carriers. *J Clin Oncol* 2007;25:642–647.

89. Parmigiani G, Chen S, Iversen ES, Jr., et al. Validity of models for predicting BRCA1 and BRCA2 mutations. *Ann Intern Med* 2007;147:441–450.

90. UT Southwestern Medical Center. CancerGene. http://www8.utsouthwestern.edu/utsw/cda/dept47829/files/65844.html. 2008 [online]. Accessed Dec. 15, 2008.

91. Evans DG, Eccles DM, Rahman N, et al. A new scoring system for the chances of identifying a BRCA1/2 mutation outperforms existing models including BRCAPRO. *J Med Genet* 2004;41:474–480.

92. Evans DG, Lalloo F, Wallace A, Rahman N. Update on the Manchester Scoring System for BRCA1 and BRCA2 testing. *J Med Genet* 2005;42:e39.

93. Antoniou AC, Cunningham AP, Peto J, et al. The BOADICEA model of genetic susceptibility to breast and ovarian cancer: updates and extensions. *Br J Cancer* 2008;98:1457–1466.

94. Antoniou A, Hardy R, Walker L, et al. Predicting the likelihood of carrying a BRCA1 or BRCA2 mutation: validation of BOADICEA, BRCAPRO, IBIS, Myriad and the Manchester scoring system using data from UK genetics clinics. *J Med Genet* 2008; 45:425–431.

95. University of Cambridge, Genetic Epidemiology Unit. BOADICEA Web application (BWA). http://www.srl.cam.ac.uk/genepi/boadicea/boadicea_home.html. 2008 [online]. Accessed Dec. 15, 2008.

96. Tyrer J, Duffy SW, Cuzick J. A breast cancer prediction model incorporating familial and personal risk factors. *Stat Med* 2004;23:1111–1130.

97. IBIS. Tyrer-Cuzick (IBIS Breast Cancer Risk Evaluation Tool, RiskFileCalc version 1.0, copyright 2004). Available by contacting IBIS: ibis@cancer.org.uk. 2004 [online].

98. Amir E, Evans DG, Shenton A, et al. Evaluation of breast cancer risk assessment packages in the family history evaluation and screening programme. *J Med Genet* 2003;40:807–814.

99. Mann GJ, Thorne H, Balleine RL, et al. Analysis of cancer risk and BRCA1 and BRCA2 mutation prevalence in the kConFab familial breast cancer resource. *Breast Cancer Res* 2006;8:R12.
100. Culver J, Lowstuter K, Bowling L. Assessing breast cancer risk and BRCA1/2 carrier probability. *Breast Dis* 2006;27:5–20.
101. Domchek SM, Eisen A, Calzone K, et al. Application of breast cancer risk prediction models in clinical practice. *J Clin Oncol* 2003;21:593–601.
102. Walker L, Eeles R. Risk prediction in breast cancer. In: Isaacs C, Rebbeck TR, eds. *Hereditary breast cancer.* New York, NY: Informa Healthcare, 2008;19–33.
103. American Society of Clinical Oncology. Statement of the American Society of Clinical Oncology: genetic testing for cancer susceptibility, Adopted on February 20, 1996. *J Clin Oncol* 1996;14:1730–1736.
104. Domchek SM, Antoniou A. Cancer risk models: translating family history into clinical management. *Ann Intern Med* 2007;147:515–517.
105. Kauff ND, Offit K. Modeling genetic risk of breast cancer. *JAMA* 2007;297: 2637–2639.
106. American Society of Clinical Oncology. American Society of Clinical Oncology policy statement update: genetic testing for cancer susceptibility. *J Clin Oncol* 2003; 21:2397–2406.
107. Klimberg VS, Galandiuk S, Singletary ES, et al. Society of Surgical Oncology: statement on genetic testing for cancer susceptibility. Committee on Issues and Governmental Affairs of the Society of Surgical Oncology. *Ann Surg Oncol* 1999;6:507–509.
108. Lancaster JM, Powell CB, Kauff ND, et al. Society of Gynecologic Oncologists Education Committee statement on risk assessment for inherited gynecologic cancer predispositions. *Gynecol Oncol* 2007;107:159–162.
109. National Comprehensive Cancer Network. NCCN Clinical Practice Guidelines in Oncology. Genetic/familial high-risk assessment: breast and ovarian—v.1.2008. http://www.nccn.org/professionals/physician_gls/PDF/genetics_screening.pdf. 2008 [online]. Accessed Dec. 15, 2008.
110. National Institutes of Health and Clinical Excellence (NICE). NICE Clinical Guideline 41: Familial breast cancer: the classification and care of women at risk of familial breast cancer in primary, secondary, and tertiary care. October 2006. http://www.nice.org.uk/nicemedia/pdf/CG41NICEguidance.pdf. 2006 [online]. Accessed Dec. 15, 2008.
111. Trepanier A, Ahrens M, McKinnon W, et al. Genetic cancer risk assessment and counseling: recommendations of the national society of genetic counselors. *J Genet Couns* 2004;13:83–114.
112. United States Preventive Services Task Force. Genetic risk assessment and BRCA mutation testing for breast and ovarian cancer susceptibility: recommendation statement. *Ann Intern Med* 2005;143:355–361.
113. Meiser B, Gaff C, Julian-Reynier C, et al. International perspectives on genetic counseling and testing for breast cancer risk. *Breast Dis* 2006;27:109–125.
114. Hampel H, Sweet K, Westman JA, et al. Referral for cancer genetics consultation: a review and compilation of risk assessment criteria. *J Med Genet* 2004;41: 81–91.
115. McKinnon WC, Baty BJ, Bennett RL, et al. Predisposition genetic testing for late-onset disorders in adults. A position paper of the National Society of Genetic Counselors. *JAMA* 1997;278:1217–1220.
116. Brown KL, Moglia DM, Grumet S. Genetic counseling for breast cancer risk: general concepts, challenging themes and future directions. *Breast Dis* 2006;27: 69–96.
117. Boyd J, Sonoda Y, Federici MG, et al. Clinicopathologic features of BRCA-inked and sporadic ovarian cancer. *JAMA* 2000;283:2260–2265.
118. Birch JM, Hartley AL, Tricker KJ, et al. Prevalence and diversity of constitutional mutations in the p53 gene among 21 Li-Fraumeni families. *Cancer Res* 1994;54: 1298–1304.
119. Weitzel JN, Lagos VI, Cullinane CA, et al. Limited family structure and BRCA gene mutation status in single cases of breast cancer. *JAMA* 2007;297:2587–2595.
120. Schwartz MD, Lerman C, Brogan B, et al. Impact of BRCA1/BRCA2 counseling and testing on newly diagnosed breast cancer patients. *J Clin Oncol* 2004;22: 1823–1829.
121. Staton AD, Kurian AW, Cobb K, et al. Cancer risk reduction and reproductive concerns in female BRCA1/2 mutation carriers. *Fam Cancer* 2007.
122. Offit K, Kohut K, Clagett B, et al. Cancer genetic testing and assisted reproduction. *J Clin Oncol* 2006;24:4775–4782.
123. Peshkin BN, Nusbaum RH, DeMarco TA. Genetic counseling about reproductive options for hereditary cancer: what is the standard of care? *J Clin Oncol* 2007;25: 911–912.
124. Armstrong K, Calzone K, Stopfer J, et al. Factors associated with decisions about clinical BRCA1/2 testing. *Cancer Epidemiol Biomarkers Prev* 2000;9:1251–1254.
125. Peterson EA, Milliron KJ, Lewis KE, et al. Health insurance and discrimination concerns and BRCA1/2 testing in a clinic population. *Cancer Epidemiol Biomarkers Prev* 2002;11:79–87.
126. National Human Genome Research Institute. NHGRI policy and legislation database. http://www.genome.gov/10002007 2008 [online]. Accessed Dec. 15, 2008.
127. United States statutes at large. Health Insurance Portability and Accountability Act of 1996. Public Law 104-191. http://aspe.hhs.gov/admnsimp/pl104191.htm [online]. *US Stat Large* 1996;110:1936–2103. Accessed Dec. 15, 2008.
128. Schwartz MD, Peshkin BN, Hughes C, et al. Impact of BRCA1/BRCA2 mutation testing on psychologic distress in a clinic-based sample. *J Clin Oncol* 2002;20: 514–520.
129. Myriad Genetic Laboratories. Myriad Genetics Annual Report 2007. http://www.myriad.com/downloads/Myriad-Annual-Report-2007.pdf. 2007 [online] Accessed Dec. 15, 2008.
130. Myriad Genetic Laboratories. BRACAnalysis Technical Specifications, updated August 4, 2006. http://www.myriadtests.com/provider/doc/BRACAnalysis-Technical-Specifications.pdf. 2006 [online]. Accessed Dec. 15, 2008.
131. Easton DF, Deffenbaugh AM, Pruss D, et al. A systematic genetic assessment of 1,433 sequence variants of unknown clinical significance in the BRCA1 and BRCA2 breast cancer-predisposition genes. *Am J Hum Genet* 2007;81: 873–883.
132. National Human Genome Research Institute. An open access on-line breast cancer mutation data base. http://research.nhgri.nih.gov/bic/. 2008 [online]. Accessed Dec. 15, 2008.
133. Wenstrup R, Judkins T, Eliason K, et al. Molecular genetic testing for large genomic deletion and duplication mutations in the BRCA1 and BRCA2 genes for hereditary breast and ovarian cancer [Abstract 10513]. 2007 ASCO Annual Meeting Proceedings (post-meeting edition). *J Clin Oncol* 2007;25 (18 Suppl).
134. Smith A, Moran A, Boyd MC, et al. Phenocopies in BRCA1 and BRCA2 families: evidence for modifier genes and implications for screening. *J Med Genet* 2007; 44:10–15.
135. Goldgar D, Venne V, Conner T, et al. BRCA phenocopies or ascertainment bias? *J Med Genet* 2007;44:e86.
136. Gronwald J, Cybulski C, Lubinski J, et al. Phenocopies in breast cancer 1 (BRCA1) families: implications for genetic counselling. *J Med Genet* 2007;44:e76.
137. Chen S, Iversen ES, Friebel T, et al. Characterization of BRCA1 and BRCA2 mutations in a large United States sample. *J Clin Oncol* 2006;24:863–871.
138. Satagopan JM, Boyd J, Kauff ND, et al. Ovarian cancer risk in Ashkenazi Jewish carriers of BRCA1 and BRCA2 mutations. *Clin Cancer Res* 2002;8:3776–3781.
139. Friedman E, Bar-Sade BR, Kruglikova A, et al. Double heterozygotes for the Ashkenazi founder mutations in BRCA1 and BRCA2 genes. *Am J Hum Genet* 1998;63:1224–1227.
140. Kauff ND, Perez-Segura P, Robson ME, et al. Incidence of non-founder BRCA1 and BRCA2 mutations in high risk Ashkenazi breast and ovarian cancer families. *J Med Genet* 2002;39:611–614.
141. Rubinstein WS. Roles and responsibilities of a medical geneticist. *Fam Cancer* 2007.
142. Ferla R, Calo V, Cascio S, et al. Founder mutations in BRCA1 and BRCA2 genes. *Ann Oncol* 2007;18(Suppl 6):vi93–vi98.
143. Leegte B, van der Hout AH, Deffenbaugh AM, et al. Phenotypic expression of double heterozygosity for BRCA1 and BRCA2 germline mutations. *J Med Genet* 2005;42:e20.
144. Nusbaum R, Vogel KJ, Ready K. Susceptibility to breast cancer: hereditary syndromes and low penetrance genes. *Breast Dis* 2006;27:21–50.
145. Tischkowitz M, Xia B, Sabbaghian N, et al. Analysis of PALB2/FANCN-associated breast cancer families. *Proc Natl Acad Sci U S A* 2007;104:6788–6793.
146. Weischer M, Bojesen SE, Ellervik C, et al. CHEK2*1100delC genotyping for clinical assessment of breast cancer risk: meta-analyses of 26,000 patient cases and 27,000 controls. *J Clin Oncol* 2008;26:542–548.
147. Petersen GM, Parmigiani G, Thomas D. Missense mutations in disease genes: a Bayesian approach to evaluate causality. *Am J Hum Genet* 1998;62:1516–1524.
148. Biesecker BB, Boehnke M, Calzone K, et al. Genetic counseling for families with inherited susceptibility to breast and ovarian cancer. *JAMA* 1993;269:1970–1974.
149. Lerman C, Narod S, Schulman K, et al. BRCA1 testing in families with hereditary breast-ovarian cancer. A prospective study of patient decision making and outcomes. *JAMA* 1996;275:1885–1892.
150. Lodder L, Frets PG, Trijsburg RW, et al. Psychological impact of receiving a BRCA1/BRCA2 test result. *Am J Med Genet* 2001;98:15–24.
151. Meiser B, Butow P, Friedlander M, et al. Psychological impact of genetic testing in women from high-risk breast cancer families. *Eur J Cancer* 2002;38:2025–2031.
152. Cella D, Hughes C, Peterman A, et al. A brief assessment of concerns associated with genetic testing for cancer: the Multidimensional Impact of Cancer Risk Assessment (MICRA) questionnaire. *Health Psychol* 2002;21:564–572.
153. Tercyak KP, Lerman C, Peshkin BN, et al. Effects of coping style and BRCA1 and BRCA2 test results on anxiety among women participating in genetic counseling and testing for breast and ovarian cancer risk. *Health Psychol* 2001;20:217–222.
154. van Roosmalen MS, Stalmeier PF, Verhoef LC, et al. Impact of BRCA1/2 testing and disclosure of a positive test result on women affected and unaffected with breast or ovarian cancer. *Am J Med Genet A* 2004;124:346–355.
155. van Dijk S, Timmermans DR, Meijers-Heijboer H, et al. Clinical characteristics affect the impact of an uninformative DNA test result: the course of worry and distress experienced by women who apply for genetic testing for breast cancer. *J Clin Oncol* 2006;24:3672–3677.
156. Reichelt JG, Moller P, Heimdal K, et al AA. Psychological and cancer-specific distress at 18 months post-testing in women with demonstrated BRCA1 mutations for hereditary breast/ovarian cancer. *Fam Cancer* 2008.
157. Arver B, Haegermark A, Platten U, et al. Evaluation of psychosocial effects of pre-symptomatic testing for breast/ovarian and colon cancer pre-disposing genes: a 12-month follow-up. *Fam Cancer* 2004;3:109–116.
158. Claes E, Evers-Kiebooms G, Decruyenaere M, et al. Surveillance behavior and prophylactic surgery after predictive testing for hereditary breast/ovarian cancer. *Behav Med* 2005;31:93–105.
159. Foster C, Watson M, Eeles R, et al. Predictive testing for BRCA1/2 in a UK clinical cohort: three year follow-up. *Br J Cancer* 2007;96:718–724.
160. Kinney AY, Bloor LE, Mandal D, et al. The impact of receiving genetic test results on general and cancer-specific psychologic distress among members of an African-American kindred with a BRCA1 mutation. *Cancer* 2005;104: 2508–2516.
161. Smith AW, Dougall AL, Posluszny DM, et al. Psychological distress and quality of life associated with genetic testing for breast cancer risk. *Psychooncology* 2008;17: 767–773.
162. Watson M, Foster C, Eeles R, et al. Psychosocial impact of breast/ovarian (BRCA1/2) cancer-predictive genetic testing in a UK multi-centre clinical cohort. *Br J Cancer* 2004;91:1787–1794.
163. Schlich-Bakker KJ, Ausems MG, Schipper M, et al. BRCA1/2 mutation testing in breast cancer patients: a prospective study of the long-term psychological impact of approach during adjuvant radiotherapy. *Breast Cancer Res Treat* 2007.
164. van Oostrom I, Meijers-Heijboer H, Duivenvoorden HJ, et al. Prognostic factors for hereditary cancer distress six months after BRCA1/2 or HNPCC genetic susceptibility testing. *Eur J Cancer* 2007;43:71–77.
165. Chen WY, Garber JE, Higham S, et al. BRCA1/2 genetic testing in the community setting. *J Clin Oncol* 2002;20:4485–4492.
166. Offit K, Thom P. Ethical and legal aspects of cancer genetic testing. *Semin Oncol* 2007;34:435–443.
167. Peshkin BN, Burke W. Bioethics of genetic testing for hereditary breast cancer. In: Isaacs C, Rebbeck TR, eds. *Hereditary breast cancer.* New York, NY: Informa Healthcare, 2008:35–51.
168. Points to consider: ethical, legal, and psychosocial implications of genetic testing in children and adolescents. American Society of Human Genetics Board of Directors, American College of Medical Genetics Board of Directors. *Am J Hum Genet* 1995;57:1233–1241.
169. Borry P, Stultiens L, Nys H, et al. Presymptomatic and predictive genetic testing in minors: a systematic review of guidelines and position papers. *Clin Genet* 2006;70:374–381.
170. Nelson RM, Botkjin JR, Kodish ED, et al. Ethical issues with genetic testing in pediatrics. *Pediatrics* 2001;107:1451–1455.

171. Strahm B, Malkin D. Hereditary cancer predisposition in children: genetic basis and clinical implications. *Int J Cancer* 2006;119:2001–2006.
172. Duncan RE, Delatycki MB. Predictive genetic testing in young people for adult-onset conditions: where is the empirical evidence? *Clin Genet* 2006;69:8–16.
173. Elger BS, Harding TW. Testing adolescents for a hereditary breast cancer gene (BRCA1): respecting their autonomy is in their best interest. *Arch Pediatr Adolesc Med.*
174. Hughes C, Lerman C, Schwartz M, et al. All in the family: evaluation of the process and content of sisters' communication about BRCA1 and BRCA2 genetic test results. *Am J Med Genet* 2002;107:143–150.
175. Julian-Reynier C, Eisinger F, Chabal F, et al. Disclosure to the family of breast/ovarian cancer genetic test results: patient's willingness and associated factors. *Am J Med Genet* 2000;94:13–18.
176. Tarasoff v. Regents of the University of California. 1 Jul 1976. *West's California Reporter* 1976;131:14–42.
177. Pate v. Threlkel. *West's Southern Reporter* 1995;661:278–282.
178. Safer v. Estate of Pack. *Atlantic Reporter* [illegible]
179. Hustead JL, Goldman J. Genetics and privacy. *Am J Law Med* 2002;28:285–307.
180. Offit K, Groeger E, Turner S, et al. The "duty to warn" a patient's family members about hereditary disease risks. *JAMA* 2004;292:1469–1473.
181. American Society of Human Genetics. ASHG statement. Professional disclosure of familial genetic information. The American Society of Human Genetics Social Issues Subcommittee on Familial Disclosure. *Am J Hum Genet* 1998;62:474–483.
182. American Medical Association. Code of medical ethics: opinion E 2.131: disclosure of familial risk in genetic testing. http://www.ama-assn.org/ama/pub/category/print/11963.html. 2003 [online]. Accessed March 2008.
183. Godard B, Hurlimann T, Letendre M, et al. Guidelines for disclosing genetic information to family members: from development to use. *Fam Cancer* 2006;5:103–116.
184. Hunter AG, Sharpe N, Mullen M, et al. Ethical, legal, and practical concerns about recontacting patients to inform them of new information: the case in medical genetics. *Am J Med Genet* 2001;103:265–276.
185. Burke W, Daly M, Garber J, et al. Recommendations for follow-up care of individuals with an inherited predisposition to cancer. II. BRCA1 and BRCA2. Cancer Genetics Studies Consortium. *JAMA* 1997;277:997–1003.
186. Kuschel B, Hauenstein E, Kiechle M, et al. Hereditary breast and ovarian cancer - current clinical guidelines in Germany. *Breast Care* 2006;1:8–14.
187. Kriege M, Brekelmans CT, Boetes C, et al. Efficacy of MRI and mammography for breast-cancer screening in women with a familial or genetic predisposition. *N Engl J Med* 2004;351:427–437.
188. Kuhl CK, Schrading S, Leutner CC, et al. Mammography, breast ultrasound, and magnetic resonance imaging for surveillance of women at high familial risk for breast cancer. *J Clin Oncol* 2005;23:8469–8476.
189. Leach MO, Boggis CR, Dixon AK, et al. Screening with magnetic resonance imaging and mammography of a UK population at high familial risk of breast cancer: a prospective multicentre cohort study (MARIBS). *Lancet* 2005;365:1769–1778.
190. Sardanelli F, Podo F, D'Agnolo G, et al. Multicenter comparative multimodality surveillance of women at genetic-familial high risk for breast cancer (HIBCRIT study): interim results. *Radiology* 2007;242:698–715.
191. Tilanus-Linthorst MM, Obdeijn IM, Bartels KC, et al. First experiences in screening women at high risk for breast cancer with MR imaging. *Breast Cancer Res Treat* 2000;63:53–60.
192. Warner E, Plewes DB, Hill KA, et al. Surveillance of BRCA1 and BRCA2 mutation carriers with magnetic resonance imaging, ultrasound, mammography, and clinical breast examination. *JAMA* 2004;292:1317–1325.
193. Kuhl CK, Schrading S, Bieling HB, et al. MRI for diagnosis of pure ductal carcinoma in situ: a prospective observational study. *Lancet* 2007;370:485–492.
194. Lehman CD, Isaacs C, Schnall MD, et al. Cancer yield of mammography, MR, and US in high-risk women: prospective multi-institution breast cancer screening study. *Radiology* 2007;244:381–388.
195. Andrieu N, Easton DF, Chang-Claude J, et al. Effect of chest X-rays on the risk of breast cancer among BRCA1/2 mutation carriers in the international BRCA1/2 carrier cohort study: a report from the EMBRACE, GENEPSO, GEO-HEBON, and IBCCS Collaborators' Group. *J Clin Oncol* 2006;24:3361–3366.
196. Goldfrank D, Chuai S, Bernstein JL, et al. Effect of mammography on breast cancer risk in women with mutations in BRCA1 or BRCA2. *Cancer Epidemiol Biomarkers Prev* 2006;15:2311–2313.
197. Narod SA, Lubinski J, Ghadirian P, et al. Screening mammography and risk of breast cancer in BRCA1 and BRCA2 mutation carriers: a case-control study. *Lancet Oncol* 2006;7:402–406.
198. Rebbeck TR, Friebel T, Lynch HT, et al. Bilateral prophylactic mastectomy reduces breast cancer risk in BRCA1 and BRCA2 mutation carriers: the PROSE Study Group. *J Clin Oncol* 2004;22:1055–1062.
199. Heemskerk-Gerritsen BA, Brekelmans CT, Menke-Pluymers MB, et al. Prophylactic mastectomy in BRCA1/2 mutation carriers and women at risk of hereditary breast cancer: long-term experiences at the Rotterdam Family Cancer Clinic. *Ann Surg Oncol* 2007;14:3335–3344.
200. Black D, Specht M, Lee JM, et al. Detecting occult malignancy in prophylactic mastectomy: preoperative MRI versus sentinel lymph node biopsy. *Ann Surg Oncol* 2007;14:2477–2484.
201. Boughey JC, Cormier JN, Xing Y, et al. Decision analysis to assess the efficacy of routine sentinel lymphadenectomy in patients undergoing prophylactic mastectomy. *Cancer* 2007;110:2542–2550.
202. Eisen A, Lubinski J, Klijn J, et al. Breast cancer risk following bilateral oophorectomy in BRCA1 and BRCA2 mutation carriers: an international case-control study. *J Clin Oncol* 2005;23:7491–7496.
203. Kauff ND, Satagopan JM, Robson ME, et al. Risk-reducing salpingo-oophorectomy in women with a BRCA1 or BRCA2 mutation. *N Engl J Med* 2002;346:1609–1615.
204. Rebbeck TR, Friebel T, Wagner T, et al. Effect of short-term hormone replacement therapy on breast cancer risk reduction after bilateral prophylactic oophorectomy in BRCA1 and BRCA2 mutation carriers: the PROSE Study Group. *J Clin Oncol* 2005;23:7804–7810.
205. Chlebowski RT, Hendrix SL, Langer RD, et al. Influence of estrogen plus progestin on breast cancer and mammography in healthy postmenopausal women: the Women's Health Initiative Randomized Trial. *JAMA* 2003;289:3243–3253.
206. Cuzick J, Forbes J, Edwards R, et al. First results from the International Breast Cancer Intervention Study (IBIS-I): a randomised prevention trial. *Lancet* 2002;360:817–824.
207. Cuzick J, Forbes JF, Sestak I, et al. Long-term results of tamoxifen prophylaxis for breast cancer—96-month follow-up of the randomized IBIS-I trial. *J Natl Cancer Inst* 2007;99:272–282.
208. Fisher B, Costantino JP, Wickerham DL, et al. Tamoxifen for prevention of breast cancer: report of the National Surgical Adjuvant Breast and Bowel Project P-1 Study. *J Natl Cancer Inst* 1998;90:1371–1388.
209. King MC, Wieand S, Hale K, et al. Tamoxifen and breast cancer incidence among women with inherited mutations in BRCA1 and BRCA2: National Surgical Adjuvant Breast and Bowel Project (NSABP-P1) Breast Cancer Prevention Trial. *JAMA* 2001;286:2251–2256.
210. National Cancer Institute. Study of Tamoxifen and Raloxifene (STAR) Trial. http://www.cancer.gov/star. 2006 [online].
211. Lakhani SR, Van De Vijver MJ, Jacquemier J, et al. The pathology of familial breast cancer: predictive value of immunohistochemical markers estrogen receptor, progesterone receptor, HER-2, and p53 in patients with mutations in BRCA1 and BRCA2. *J Clin Oncol* 2002;20:2310–2318.
212. Verhoog LC, Brekelmans CT, Seynaeve C, et al. Survival and tumour characteristics of breast-cancer patients with germline mutations of BRCA1. *Lancet* 1998;351:316–321.
213. Gronwald J, Tung N, Foulkes WD, et al. Tamoxifen and contralateral breast cancer in BRCA1 and BRCA2 carriers: an update. *Int J Cancer* 2006;118:2281–2284.
214. Menon U, Skates SJ, Lewis S, et al. Prospective study using the risk of ovarian cancer algorithm to screen for ovarian cancer. *J Clin Oncol* 2005;23:7919–7926.
215. Moore RG, Brown AK, Miller MC, et al. The use of multiple novel tumor biomarkers for the detection of ovarian carcinoma in patients with a pelvic mass. *Gynecol Oncol* 2008;108:402–408.
216. Zhang Z, Yu Y, Xu F, et al. Combining multiple serum tumor markers improves detection of stage I epithelial ovarian cancer. *Gynecol Oncol* 2007;107:526–531.
217. Finch A, Beiner M, Lubinski J, et al. Salpingo-oophorectomy and the risk of ovarian, fallopian tube, and peritoneal cancers in women with a BRCA1 or BRCA2 mutation. *JAMA* 2006;296:185–192.
218. Callahan MJ, Crum CP, Medeiros F, et al. Primary fallopian tube malignancies in BRCA-positive women undergoing surgery for ovarian cancer risk reduction. *J Clin Oncol* 2007;25:3985–3990.
219. Powell CB, Kenley E, Chen LM, et al. Risk-reducing salpingo-oophorectomy in BRCA mutation carriers: role of serial sectioning in the detection of occult malignancy. *J Clin Oncol* 2005;23:127–132.
220. Domchek SM, Friebel TM, Neuhausen SL, et al. Mortality after bilateral salpingo-oophorectomy in BRCA1 and BRCA2 mutation carriers: a prospective cohort study. *Lancet Oncol* 2006;7:223–229.
221. Alvarado-Cabrero I, Young RH, et al. Carcinoma of the fallopian tube: a clinicopathological study of 105 cases with observations on staging and prognostic factors. *Gynecol Oncol* 1999;72:367–379.
222. Goshen R, Chu W, Elit L, et al. Is uterine papillary serous adenocarcinoma a manifestation of the hereditary breast-ovarian cancer syndrome? *Gynecol Oncol* 2000;79:477–481.
223. Rosenberg L, Palmer JR, Zauber AG, et al. A case-control study of oral contraceptive use and invasive epithelial ovarian cancer. *Am J Epidemiol* 1994;139:654–661.
224. Brand RE, Lerch MM, Rubinstein WS, et al. Advances in counselling and surveillance of patients at risk for pancreatic cancer. *Gut* 2007;56:1460–1469.
225. Breast Cancer Linkage Consortium. Pathology of familial breast cancer: differences between breast cancers in carriers of BRCA1 or BRCA2 mutations and sporadic cases. Breast Cancer Linkage Consortium. *Lancet* 1997;349:1505–1510.
226. Brekelmans CT, Seynaeve C, Bartels CC, et al. Effectiveness of breast cancer surveillance in BRCA1/2 gene mutation carriers and women with high familial risk. *J Clin Oncol* 2001;19:924–930.
227. Brekelmans CT, Seynaeve C, Menke-Pluymers M, et al. Survival and prognostic factors in BRCA1-associated breast cancer. *Ann Oncol* 2006;17:391–400.
228. Rennert G, Bisland-Naggan S, Barnett-Griness O, et al. Clinical outcomes of breast cancer in carriers of BRCA1 and BRCA2 mutations. *N Engl J Med* 2007;357:115–123.
229. Lakhani SR, Jacquemier J, Sloane JP, et al. Multifactorial analysis of differences between sporadic breast cancers and cancers involving BRCA1 and BRCA2 mutations. *J Natl Cancer Inst* 1998;90:1138–1145.
230. Phillips KA, Nichol K, Ozcelik H, et al. Frequency of p53 mutations in breast carcinomas from Ashkenazi Jewish carriers of BRCA1 mutations. *J Natl Cancer Inst* 1999;91:469–473.
231. Phillips KA, Andrulis IL, Goodwin PJ. Breast carcinomas arising in carriers of mutations in BRCA1 or BRCA2: are they prognostically different? *J Clin Oncol* 1999;17:3653–3663.
232. Quenneville LA, Phillips KA, Ozcelik H, et al. HER-2/neu status and tumor morphology of invasive breast carcinomas in Ashkenazi women with known BRCA1 mutation status in the Ontario Familial Breast Cancer Registry. *Cancer* 2002;95:2068–2075.
233. El Tamer M, Russo D, Troxel A, et al. Survival and recurrence after breast cancer in BRCA1/2 mutation carriers. *Ann Surg Oncol* 2004;11:157–164.
234. Robson ME, Chappuis PO, Satagopan J, et al. A combined analysis of outcome following breast cancer: differences in survival based on BRCA1/BRCA2 mutation status and administration of adjuvant treatment. *Breast Cancer Res* 2004;6:R8–R17.
235. Armes JE, Egan AJ, Southey MC, et al. The histologic phenotypes of breast carcinoma occurring before age 40 years in women with and without BRCA1 or BRCA2 germline mutations: a population-based study. *Cancer* 1998;83:2335–2345.
236. Marcus JN, Watson P, Page DL, et al. BRCA2 hereditary breast cancer pathophenotype. *Breast Cancer Res Treat* 1997;44:275–277.
237. Agnarsson BA, Jonasson JG, Bjornsdottir IB, et al. Inherited BRCA2 mutation associated with high grade breast cancer. *Breast Cancer Res Treat* 1998;47:121–127.
238. Liebens FP, Carly B, Pastijn A, et al. Management of BRCA1/2 associated breast cancer: a systematic qualitative review of the state of knowledge in 2006. *Eur J Cancer* 2007;43:238–257.
239. Kennedy RD, Quinn JE, Mullan PB, et al. The role of BRCA1 in the cellular response to chemotherapy. *J Natl Cancer Inst* 2004;96:1659–1668.
240. Chetrit A, Hirsh-Yechezkel G, Ben David Y, et al. Effect of BRCA1/2 mutations on long-term survival of patients with invasive ovarian cancer: the national Israeli study of ovarian cancer. *J Clin Oncol* 2008;26:20–25.

241. Bryant HE, Schultz N, Thomas HD, et al. Specific killing of BRCA2-deficient tumours with inhibitors of poly(ADP-ribose) polymerase. *Nature* 2005;434: 913–917.

242. Farmer H, McCabe N, Lord CJ, et al. Targeting the DNA repair defect in BRCA mutant cells as a therapeutic strategy. *Nature* 2005;434:917–921.

243. Olson JE, Sellers TA, Iturria SJ, et al. Bilateral oophorectomy and breast cancer risk reduction among women with a family history. *Cancer Detect Prev* 2004;28: 357–360.

244. Botkin JR, Smith KR, Croyle RT, et al. Genetic testing for a BRCA1 mutation: prophylactic surgery and screening behavior in women 2 years post testing. *Am J Med Genet A* 2003;118:201–209.

245. Lerman C, Hughes C, Croyle RT, et al. Prophylactic surgery decisions and surveillance practices one year following BRCA1/2 testing. *Prev Med* 2000;31: 75–80.

246. Peshkin BN, Schwartz MD, Isaacs C, et al. Utilization of breast cancer screening in a clinically based sample of women after BRCA1/2 testing. *Cancer Epidemiol Biomarkers Prev* 2002;11:1115–1118.

247. Scheuer L, Kauff N, Robson M, et al. Outcome of preventive surgery and screening for breast and ovarian cancer in BRCA mutation carriers. *J Clin Oncol* 2002;20:1260–1268.

248. Lodder LN, Frets PG, Trijsburg RW, et al. One year follow-up of women opting for presymptomatic testing for BRCA1 and BRCA2: emotional impact of the test outcome and decisions on risk management (surveillance or prophylactic surgery). *Breast Cancer Res Treat* 2002;73:97–112.

249. Metcalfe KA, Snyder C, Seidel J, et al. The use of preventive measures among healthy women who carry a BRCA1 or BRCA2 mutation. *Fam Cancer* 2005;4: 97–103.

250. Phillips KA, Jenkins MA, Lindeman GJ, et al. Risk-reducing surgery, screening and chemoprevention practices of BRCA1 and BRCA2 mutation carriers: a prospective cohort study. *Clin Genet* 2006;70:198–206.

251. Julian-Reynier CM, Bouchard LJ, Evans DG, et al. Women's attitudes toward preventive strategies for hereditary breast or ovarian carcinoma differ from one country to another: differences among English, French, and Canadian women. *Cancer* 2001;92:959–968.

252. Graves KD, Peshkin BN, Halbert CH, et al. Predictors and outcomes of contralateral prophylactic mastectomy among breast cancer survivors. *Breast Cancer Res Treat* 2007;104:321–329.

253. Evans DG, Lalloo F, Hopwood P, et al. Surgical decisions made by 158 women with hereditary breast cancer aged <50 years. *Eur J Surg Oncol* 2005;31: 1112–1118.

254. Meijers-Heijboer EJ, Verhoog LC, Brekelmans CT, et al. Presymptomatic DNA testing and prophylactic surgery in families with a BRCA1 or BRCA2 mutation. *Lancet* 2000;355:2015–2020.

255. Schwartz MD, Kaufman E, Peshkin BN, et al. Bilateral prophylactic oophorectomy and ovarian cancer screening following BRCA1/BRCA2 mutation testing. *J Clin Oncol* 2003;21:4034–4041.

256. Lynch HT, Snyder C, Lynch JF, et al. Patient responses to the disclosure of BRCA mutation tests in hereditary breast-ovarian cancer families. *Cancer Genet Cytogenet* 2006;165:91–97.

257. Ray JA, Loescher LJ, Brewer M. Risk-reduction surgery decisions in high-risk women seen for genetic counseling. *J Genet Couns* 2005;14:473–484.

258. Madalinska JB, van Beurden M, Bleiker EM, et al. Predictors of prophylactic bilateral salpingo-oophorectomy compared with gynecologic screening use in BRCA1/2 mutation carriers. *J Clin Oncol* 2007;25:301–307.

259. Meijers-Heijboer H, Brekelmans CT, Menke-Pluymers M, et al. Use of genetic testing and prophylactic mastectomy and oophorectomy in women with breast or ovarian cancer from families with a BRCA1 or BRCA2 mutation. *J Clin Oncol* 2003;21:1675–1681.

260. Stolier AJ, Fuhrman GM, Mauterer L, et al. Initial experience with surgical treatment planning in the newly diagnosed breast cancer patient at high risk for BRCA-1 or BRCA-2 mutation. *Breast J* 2004;10:475–480.

261. Weitzel JN, McCaffrey SM, Nedelcu R, et al. Effect of genetic cancer risk assessment on surgical decisions at breast cancer diagnosis. *Arch Surg* 2003;138: 1323–1328.

262. Antill YC, Reynolds J, Young MA, et al. Screening behavior in women at increased familial risk for breast cancer. *Fam Cancer* 2006;5:359–368.

263. Frost MH, Schaid DJ, Sellers TA, et al. Long-term satisfaction and psychological and social function following bilateral prophylactic mastectomy. *JAMA* 2000;284: 319–324.

264. Hatcher MB, Fallowfield L, A'Hern R. The psychosocial impact of bilateral prophylactic mastectomy: prospective study using questionnaires and semistructured interviews. *BMJ* 2001;322:76.

265. Stefanek ME, Helzlsouer KJ, Wilcox PM, et al. Predictors of and satisfaction with bilateral prophylactic mastectomy. *Prev Med* 1995;24:412–419.

266. Tercyak KP, Peshkin BN, Brogan BM, et al. Quality of life after contralateral prophylactic mastectomy in newly diagnosed high-risk breast cancer patients who underwent BRCA1/2 gene testing. *J Clin Oncol* 2007;25:285–291.

267. Madalinska JB, Hollenstein J, Bleiker E, et al. Quality-of-life effects of prophylactic salpingo-oophorectomy versus gynecologic screening among women at increased risk of hereditary ovarian cancer. *J Clin Oncol* 2005;23:6890–6898.

268. Frost MH, Slezak JM, Tran NV, et al. Satisfaction after contralateral prophylactic mastectomy: the significance of mastectomy type, reconstructive complications, and body appearance. *J Clin Oncol* 2005;23:7849–7856.

269. Schwartz MD, Valdimarsdottir HB, DeMarco TA, et al. Randomized trial of a decision aid for BRCA1/BRCA2 mutation carriers: impact on measures of decision making and satisfaction. *Health Psychol.* In press.

270. Li FP, Fraumeni JF, Jr., Mulvihill JJ, et al. A cancer family syndrome in twenty-four kindreds. *Cancer Res* 1988;48:5358–5362.

271. Varley JM, McGown G, Thorncroft M, et al. Germ-line mutations of TP53 in Li-Fraumeni families: an extended study of 39 families. *Cancer Res* 1997;57: 3245–3252.

272. Malkin D. The Li-Fraumeni syndrome. *Cancer: principles and practice of oncology updates* 1993;7:1–14.

273. Hisada M, Garber JE, Fung CY, et al. Multiple primary cancers in families with Li-Fraumeni syndrome. *J Natl Cancer Inst* 1998;90:606–611.

274. Limacher JM, Frebourg T, Natarajan-Ame S, et al. Two metachronous tumors in the radiotherapy fields of a patient with Li-Fraumeni syndrome. *Int J Cancer* 2001;96:238–242.

275. Eng C. Will the real Cowden syndrome please stand up: revised diagnostic criteria. *J Med Genet* 2000;37:828–830.

276. Marsh DJ, Coulon V, Lunetta KL, et al. Mutation spectrum and genotype-phenotype analyses in Cowden disease and Bannayan-Zonana syndrome, two hamartoma syndromes with germline PTEN mutation. *Hum Mol Genet* 1998;7:507–515.

277. Brownstein MH, Wolf M, Bikowski JB. Cowden's disease: a cutaneous marker of breast cancer. *Cancer* 1978;41:2393–2398.

278. Schrager CA, Schneider D, Gruener AC, et al. Clinical and pathological features of breast disease in Cowden's syndrome: an underrecognized syndrome with an increased risk of breast cancer. *Hum Pathol* 1998;29:47–53.

279. Starink TM, van der Veen JP, Arwert F, et al. The Cowden syndrome: a clinical and genetic study in 21 patients. *Clin Genet* 1986;29:222–233.

280. Eng C. Genetics of Cowden syndrome: through the looking glass of oncology. *Int J Oncol* 1998;12:701–710.

281. Jenne DE, Reimann H, Nezu J, et al. Peutz-Jeghers syndrome is caused by mutations in a novel serine threonine kinase. *Nat Genet* 1998;18:38–43.

282. Tomlinson IP, Houlston RS. Peutz-Jeghers syndrome. *J Med Genet* 1997;34: 1007–1011.

283. Giardiello FM, Brensinger JD, Tersmette AC, et al. Very high risk of cancer in familial Peutz-Jeghers syndrome. *Gastroenterology* 2000;119:1447–1453.

284. Boardman LA, Thibodeau SN, Schaid DJ, et al. Increased risk for cancer in patients with the Peutz-Jeghers syndrome. *Ann Intern Med* 1998;128: 896–899.

285. Trau H, Schewach-Millet M, Fisher BK, et al. Peutz-Jeghers syndrome and bilateral breast carcinoma. *Cancer* 1982;50:788–792.

286. McGrath DR, Spigelman AD. Preventive measures in Peutz-Jeghers syndrome. *Fam Cancer* 2001;1:121–125.

287. Brooks-Wilson AR, Kaurah P, Suriano G, et al. Germline E-cadherin mutations in hereditary diffuse gastric cancer: assessment of 42 new families and review of genetic screening criteria. *J Med Genet* 2004;41:508–517.

288. Caldas C, Carneiro F, Lynch HT, et al. Familial gastric cancer: overview and guidelines for management. *J Med Genet* 1999;36:873–880.

289. Pharoah PD, Guilford P, Caldas C. Incidence of gastric cancer and breast cancer in CDH1 (E-cadherin) mutation carriers from hereditary diffuse gastric cancer families. *Gastroenterology* 2001;121:1348–1353.

290. Boetes C, Veltman J, van Die L, et al. The role of MRI in invasive lobular carcinoma. *Breast Cancer Res Treat* 2004;86:31–37.

291. Bartek J, Lukas J. Chk1 and Chk2 kinases in checkpoint control and cancer. *Cancer Cell* 2003;3.421–429.

292. Offit K, Garber JE. Time to check CHEK2 in families with breast cancer? *J Clin Oncol* 2008;26:519–520.

293. Schmidt MK, Tollenaar RA, de Kemp SR, et al. Breast cancer survival and tumor characteristics in premenopausal women carrying the CHEK2*1100delC germline mutation. *J Clin Oncol* 2007;25:64–69.

Chapter 20
Nongenetic Factors in the Causation of Breast Cancer

Walter C. Willett, Rulla May Tamimi, Susan E. Hankinson, David J. Hunter, and Graham A. Colditz

Breast cancer has an enormous impact on the health of women. Approximately 178,480 women are diagnosed with invasive breast cancer annually in the United States, accounting for approximately 32% of all incident cancers among women (1,2). Each year, 40,000 women die of breast cancer, making it the second leading cause of cancer deaths among U.S. women, after lung cancer, and the leading cause of death among women aged 40 to 55 years. Breast cancer is rare among men, with only 2,030 incident cases and 450 deaths estimated for the United States in 2007 (1). The lifetime risk of being diagnosed with breast cancer through age 85 years for an American woman is approximately 1 in 8, or 12.5%, whereas the lifetime risk of dying from breast cancer is approximately 3.4% (3).

This chapter begins with a description of the marked variations in breast cancer rates among populations and over time. Decades of research have led to a substantial understanding of the factors involved in the development of breast cancer; known and suspected risk factors are reviewed and considered in relation to etiologic mechanisms leading to breast cancer. The contribution that known risk factors make to the existing variations in rates is considered; this contribution is central to the question of whether unidentified pollutants or dietary factors explain the current high rates in the United States. Because of the major investments in breast cancer research, the means for preventing a substantial fraction of breast cancer now exists; strategies that can be adopted by individual women, their health care providers, and societies and governments as a whole are examined.

DESCRIPTIVE EPIDEMIOLOGY OF BREAST CANCER

High- and Low-Risk Populations

The incidence of female breast cancer varies markedly between countries, being highest in the United States, western and northern Europe, intermediate in southern and eastern Europe and South America, and lowest in Asia and Africa (4,5). From 2000 to 2005, the age-adjusted incidence rate of breast cancer varied by about a factor of five among countries (Fig. 20.1) (6). However, incidence rates have been rising in traditionally low-incidence Asian countries, particularly in Japan, Singapore, and urban areas of China, as these regions are making the transition toward a Western style of economy and pattern of reproductive behavior (7,8). As a result of unfavorable trends in these countries, the international gap in breast cancer incidence has narrowed since 1970 (9).

Age–Incidence Curve of Breast Cancer Risk

Breast cancer is extremely rare among women younger than 20 years and is uncommon among women younger than 30 years. Incidence rates increase sharply with advancing age, however, and become substantial before age 50 years. From 2000 to 2004, the incidence of breast cancer among American women aged 30 to 34 years was 25 per 100,000 and increased to 190 per 100,000 among women aged 45 to 49 years (10). The rate of increase in breast cancer incidence continues throughout life but slows somewhat around ages 45 to 50 years, strongly suggesting the involvement of reproductive hormones in breast

cancer etiology because non–hormone-dependent cancers do not exhibit this change in slope of the incidence rate curve around the time of menopause (11). By age 70 to 74 years, the incidence of breast cancer among American women rises to 455 per 100,000 (2). The shape of the age–incidence curve in low- and intermediate-risk populations is similar to that of the United States, although the absolute rates are lower at each age (12) (Fig. 20.2).

Racial and Ethnic Groups within the United States and Studies of Migrants

According to recent data from the Surveillance, Epidemiology, and End Results (SEER) registries (10), the lifetime risk of breast cancer for white women in the United States is 12.8%, approximately 1 in 8, whereas that for black women is 10.1%, slightly less than 1 in 10. Between 2000 and 2004, the overall age-adjusted incidence rate of breast cancer among white women in the United States averaged 137 per 100,000 women, whereas the corresponding rate among black women averaged 118 per 100,000 women (10). However, these age-adjusted figures conceal a crossover pattern in which the risk of breast cancer at a young age is modestly higher among black women than white women. At older ages, incidence rates for white women are substantially higher than those among black women (Fig. 20.2).

Unlike that of most other illnesses, the lifetime risk of breast cancer is positively associated with higher socioeconomic status. This association is largely explained by the known reproductive risk factors (13); women in lower socioeconomic strata are more likely to have more children and to have them at younger ages than women in higher socioeconomic strata. It is likely that much, if not all, of the black and white differences in breast cancer rates among older women reflect racial differences in social class distribution (14) and, thus, in the distribution of established reproductive risk factors. The modestly higher incidence rates of breast cancer among young black women relative to young white women are consistent with the hypothesis of a short-term increase in breast cancer risk immediately following pregnancy, although the overall lower lifetime risk of breast cancer among black women is consistent with the hypothesis of a long-term benefit of early and repeated pregnancy (15). The effect of these reproductive factors on breast cancer risk is described in greater detail in the following section on modeling. Although black women have a lower probability of developing breast cancer over their lifetime, their risk of dying from breast cancer is the same or perhaps even slightly higher than white women (3.12% vs. 3.39% for black and white women, respectively). Black women have poorer 5-year survival rates from breast cancer at all ages of diagnosis compared with white women (3). This poorer survival can be attributed, in part, to the tendency of black women to be diagnosed at later stages of disease (3). In addition, evidence indicates that molecularly defined subtypes of breast cancer associated with poor prognosis, specifically basal-like tumors, are more likely to occur among black women (16).

Breast cancer incidence rates among Asian, Hispanic, and Native American women in the United States are considerably lower than those of (non-Hispanic) white women (3). The magnitude of the difference in incidence rates among various ethnic groups often depends on migrant status. For instance, breast

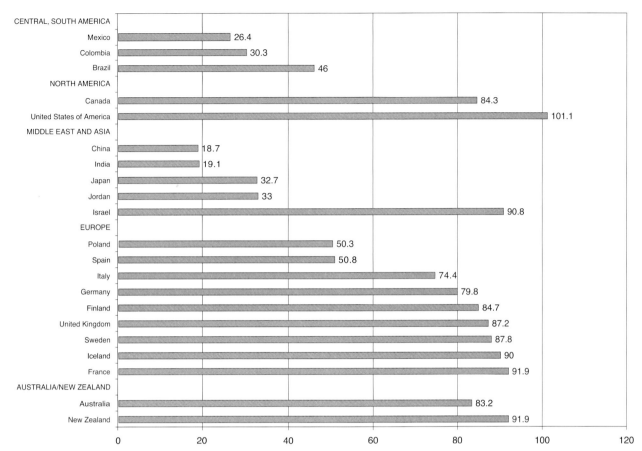

FIGURE 20.1. International variation in breast cancer incidence among women, from 2000 to 2005, per 100,000 women-years, age adjusted to the world standard. (Data from GLOBOCAN 2002; Ferlay J, Bray P, Pisani P, Parkin DM. *Cancer incidence, mortality and prevalence worldwide.* Lyon, France: IARCPress, 2004.)

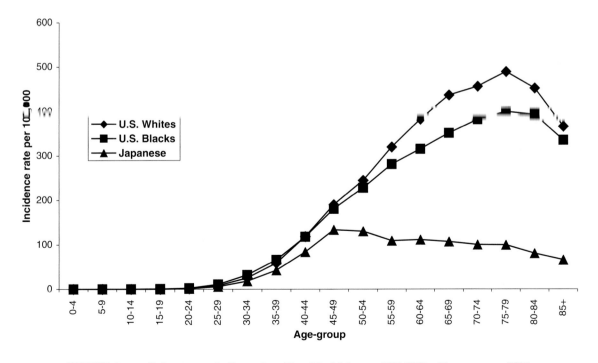

FIGURE 20.2. Age-specific breast cancer incidence rates, white and black U.S women (2000–2004) and Japanese women (2006). (Data for U.S. women from Surveillance, Epidemiology, and End Results (SEER) Program (www.seer.cancer.gov), National Cancer Institute, DCCPS, Surveillance Research Program, Cancer Statistics Branch; data for Japanese women from Cancer Statistics in Japan (http://www.ncc.go.jp/).)

cancer incidence for Chinese–American and Japanese–American women from 1973 to 1986 was about 50% lower for those born in Asia and about 25% lower for those born in the United States compared with U.S.-born white women (17). Among Filipino residents of the United States, the incidence rate of breast cancer was nearly identical between foreign-born and U.S.-born women, and both were less than half that of U.S.-born white women. Compared with Chinese women living in the mainland, Singapore, and Hong Kong, Asian-born Chinese women living in the United States had an almost twofold higher annual rate of breast cancer, and U.S.-born Chinese women had a higher rate still (5,17). The pattern for Japanese women was similar (17).

These findings are consistent with a large body of literature showing increases in breast cancer incidence following migration from a low-risk country to the United States (18–23). Ziegler et al. (23) noted a sixfold gradient in risk of breast cancer among Asian women, depending on recency of migration. Asian–American women with three or four grandparents born in the West were at highest risk, whereas women who were born in rural areas of Asia and whose length of residence in the United States was a decade or less were at lowest risk. Although the studies of breast cancer risk among migrants have focused almost exclusively on migrants from low-risk to high-risk countries and have shown convergence of rates, data also suggest that a convergence of rates similarly occurs when migrants move from high-risk to low-risk countries. For instance, Kliewer and Smith (24), reporting on immigrants to Australia and Canada, note that immigrant groups coming from countries where breast cancer mortality rates were higher than those of native-born women often showed a decrease in mortality. Such findings strongly suggest that factors associated with the lifestyle or environment of the destination country influence breast cancer risk and are consistent with a positive relationship between length of time in the destination country and adoption of that country's lifestyle. For example, among immigrants, the fertility rate and the average number of children born tend to converge to the rates of the destination country (25,26).

Geographic Variation in the United States

Breast cancer incidence and mortality rates vary within the United States, although to a much smaller degree than among other countries. During the 1980s, the incidence of breast cancer in the San Francisco Bay Area was somewhat higher than that for the rest of the United States, and international comparisons based on data from this decade led to an often-quoted statement that white women in the San Francisco Bay Area had the highest incidence of breast cancer in the world (6,27). Based on the most recent SEER data (10), the age-adjusted annual incidence rate among white women in the San Francisco area (147 per 100,000) is now surpassed by that of white women in Seattle (Puget Sound), where the age-adjusted incidence rate is 152 per 100,000. The incidence of breast cancer is also above the national average among white women in the northeastern United States (age-adjusted incidence rate for Connecticut is 140 per 100,000) (10). Recent reports have concluded that the high incidence of breast cancer in the San Francisco area and in the Northeast can likely be accounted for by regional differences in the prevalence of known risk factors, including parity, age at first full-term pregnancy, age at menarche, and age at menopause (27–31).

Among the 17 SEER registry sites, the lowest age-adjusted incidence rates among white women are found in rural Georgia (116 per 100,000), Utah (117 per 100,000), and New Mexico (118 per 100,000) (12). Again, regional differences in reproductive risk factors largely explain these lower rates. The variation in age-adjusted incidence rates for black women across the geographic sites ranges from 68.5 per 100,000 in New Mexico to 130 per 100,000 in Kentucky.

Geographic differences in breast cancer mortality parallel those in incidence, with mortality highest in the urban Northeast and West and lowest in the South and Midwest (12). Figure 20.3 illustrates these regional differences from 1990 to 1994. Notably, these differences have remained remarkably constant over the past 50 years. Geographic differences in the prevalence of established risk factors explain much of the geographic differences in

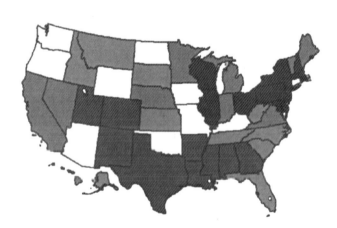

Mortality rate / 100,000 age-adjusted
1970 US population

- 26.58 to 30.48 (11)
- 25.72 to 26.58 (10)
- 24.84 to 25.72 (11)
- 24.13 to 24.84 (10)
- 21.98 to 24.13 (9)
- Sparse Data (0)

FIGURE 20.3. Age-adjusted breast cancer mortality rates for women (white) by state from 1990 to 1994. (Data from Devesa SS, Grauman DJ, Blot WJ, et al. *Atlas of cancer mortality in the United States*, 1950–1994. Washington, DC: U.S. Government Printing Office, 1999. National Institutes of Health publication no. 99-4564.)

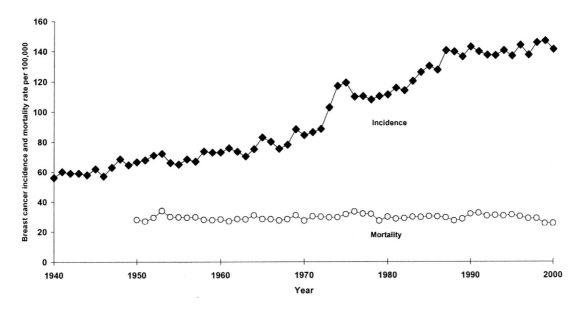

FIGURE 20.4. Age-standardized incidence of breast cancer and mortality rates in Connecticut from 1940 to 2000. (Data from Surveillance Epidemiology, and End Results Program, Cancer Incidence, and Mortality Rates.)

mortality. In 1987, age-adjusted mortality ratios among women 50 years and older were 1.15, 1.18, and 1.30 in the West, Midwest, and Northeast, respectively, compared with the South. After adjustment for established breast cancer risk factors, these mortality ratios fell to 1.13, 1.08, and 1.13, respectively (31).

Trends in Incidence and Mortality

Incidence rates of breast cancer have steadily increased in the United States since the 1930s (Fig. 20.4), when formal record-keeping began in Connecticut, until very recently. Between 1950 and 2000, the age-adjusted incidence rate rose by an average of 1.4% per year in this state (32), which has the oldest cancer registry in continuous operation. This represents a cumulative increase of about 70% over the 50 years. During the 1980s, incidence rates rose more sharply. Data from the SEER program, which began collecting data from different registries across the country in 1973, confirm the trends in incidence portrayed in the Connecticut registry since that time. Increases have occurred in all age groups since 1935, although the mag-nitude of increase has been greater for older women. In recent decades, incidence rates have increased more sharply among younger black women than white women; according to recent SEER data (2), between 1975 and 2000, incidence rates among black women younger than 50 years increased by 22% com-pared with a cumulative increase of 10% for white women younger than 50 years. Among women 50 years and older, the cumulative increase was 40% for both black and white women. Between 2001 and 2004, incidence rates of breast cancer decreased by approximately 3.5% per year.

Several studies have examined whether the increase in breast cancer incidence in the United States has resulted from the increasing use of screening mammography (33 38). Because screening causes at most a transient increase in inci-dence, and because its use was limited before the 1980s, it can explain little of the long-term increase between the 1930s and the 1980s. During the 1980s, however, the increased inci-dence was almost entirely because of an increase in localized disease and in tumors measuring less than 2 cm in diameter; the incidence of tumors 2 cm or larger remained stable. These findings, as well as the recently observed decrease in mortal-

ity for white women (discussed later in this chapter), suggest that the increase in use of screening mammography accounts for part of the recent increase in breast cancer incidence (36,39). The continued increase in breast cancer rates during the 1990s may be owing in part to increased use of hormone replacement therapy, obesity, and mammography screening. The decline in rates observed between 2000 and 2004 may reflect decreases in both mammographic screening and post-menopausal hormone use after publication of results from the Women's Health Initiative (WHI) randomized trial in 2002 (40,41).

Trends in breast cancer mortality are of major public health interest, but their interpretation is complex because they reflect the combined effects of trends in underlying risk of breast can-cer, changes in screening practices, and effectiveness of treat-ment. Further, mortality rates lag behind changes in breast can-cer incidence, screening, and treatment by at least 5 to 10 years (42). Age-adjusted mortality rates in the United States were rel-atively stable between the 1950s and the mid-1980s, when an overall decline was first noted (39). Mortality rates in the late 1980s began to decline slightly (about 1% per year). Rates through the 1990s declined somewhat more (3% decline per year) (2,43), perhaps because of enhanced treatment and screening. These overall trends obscure important variation by age and race, however. Since the 1970s, mortality rates have fallen for younger white women, and this decline has acceler-ated since the late 1980s. From 1973 to 1995, the cumulative decline in mortality rates for white women younger than 60 years has been more than 20%, with much of this decline occur-ring since 1988. In contrast to these trends among younger white women, mortality rates for white women 60 years and older increased slowly during the 1970s and 1980s, although since the late 1980s, mortality has also begun to decline in this age group (39,42). The trends in breast cancer mortality among black women have been unfavorable; between the 1970s and 1990, mortality rates increased for black women in all age-groups (42), and only recently is there evidence of a decline, but to a lesser extent than what is observed in white women (Fig. 20.5). From 1995 to 2004, breast cancer death rates have declined by 2.4% per year in white compared with 1.6% in black women (44).

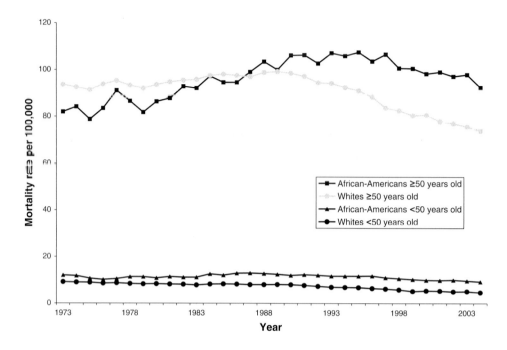

FIGURE 20.5. Trends in breast cancer mortality for white and black women in the United States by age-group. (Data from Surveillance, Epidemiology and End Results (SEER) Program (www.seer.cancer.gov) Limited-Use Data (1973–2005), National Cancer Institute, DCCPS, Surveillance Research Program, Cancer Statistics Branch, released April 2008, based on the November 2007 submission.)

Trends in Incidence and Mortality around the World

Since the 1950s, breast cancer incidence has been increasing in many of the lower risk countries and in high-risk Western countries. Some of the recent increases in incidence in high-risk populations may be owing to greater use of mammography, as in the United States. This appears to be the case in Sweden (45) and in England and Wales (46). Breast cancer incidence rates have nearly doubled in recent decades in traditionally low-risk countries such as Japan (7,12) and Singapore (8) and in the urban areas of China (47). Dramatic changes in lifestyle in such regions brought about by growing economies, increasing affluence, and increases in the proportion of women in the industrial workforce have had an impact on the population distribution of established breast cancer risk factors, including age at menarche and fertility, as well as nutritional status (48). These changes have resulted in a convergence toward the risk factor profile of Western countries (48).

Trends in breast cancer mortality around the world have largely paralleled the trends in incidence. Over recent decades, mortality has been increasing in both high-risk and lower risk populations, although since the 1990s mortality has recently declined slightly in the United Kingdom, The Netherlands, and Sweden, similar to the recent decline observed in the United States (4,49). As in the United States, some of the downturn in mortality in these countries may result from more widespread use of screening mammography and adjuvant chemotherapy during the 1980s (49,50). Countries with a recent downturn in mortality are generally those with the highest incidence and mortality rates, whereas those countries with mortality rates that are still increasing tend to be those with the lowest mortality (49). For instance, among European countries, Poland and Spain have had the lowest mortality rates, and these rates are continuing to rise. Thus, a convergence of breast cancer mortality rates may be occurring internationally, in part reflecting an international convergence of reproductive factors (49).

 REPRODUCTIVE FACTORS

This section addresses reproductive factors during the course of a woman's life in relation to the risk of breast cancer. An underlying concept is that ovarian hormones initiate breast development and that subsequent monthly menstrual cycles induce regular breast cell proliferation. Puberty is a critical period during breast development. The onset of puberty is marked by a surge of hormones that induces regular breast cell proliferation. This pattern of cell division terminates with menopause, as indicated by cessation of ovulation and menstrual periods.

Menarche

Menarche represents the development of the mature hormonal environment for a young woman and the onset of monthly cycling of hormones that induce ovulation, menstruation, and cell proliferation within the breast and endometrium. Earlier age at menarche has been consistently associated with increased risk of breast cancer (51). Most studies suggest that age at menarche is related to both premenopausal and postmenopausal breast cancer, although the magnitude of effect appears to be greater for premenopausal than postmenopausal women (52). In a pooled analysis of 7,764 premenopausal women and 16,467 postmenopausal women, each additional year in delay of menarche was associated with a 9% decrease in premenopausal breast cancer and a 4% decrease in postmenopausal breast cancer (53). In addition, age at menarche is inversely associated with both ER+/PR+ and ER-/PR- breast tumors, although the protective effect of late age at menarche is greater for hormone receptor positive tumors (54).

Although menarche is most clearly related to the onset of ovulation, some studies suggest that hormone levels may be higher through the reproductive years among women who have early menarche (55). In addition, early menarche may be associated with earlier onset of regular ovulatory menstrual cycles and hence greater lifetime exposure to endogenous hormones (56). Whether the levels of ovarian hormones or their cyclic characteristics are the underlying influence on breast cancer risk is unsettled (11); both likely play a role.

Menstrual Cycle Characteristics

Shorter cycle length has been quite consistently related to greater risk of breast cancer (51), although not all studies support this relation (57). Shorter cycle length during ages 20 to 39 years may be associated with higher risk of breast cancer, perhaps because the shorter cycle length is associated with a greater number of cycles and more time spent in the luteal phase when both estrogen and progesterone levels are high. Long and irregular cycles may also be related to reduced risk of breast cancer (57).

Ovulatory infertility, an indicator of infertility owing to hormonal causes, has not been consistently related to risk of breast cancer, although one cohort study suggested a substantially lower risk among women with this condition (relative risk [RR] = 0.4 compared with women with no infertility history) (57). The significant inverse association seen in this study may be related to the young age of the cohort and thoroughness of investigation of the cause of infertility in this group of health professionals.

Pregnancy and Age at First Full-term Pregnancy

Nulliparous women are at increased risk of breast cancer compared with parous women. This risk is evident after age 40 to 45 years, but not for breast cancer diagnosed at younger ages. In most epidemiologic studies, a younger age at first full-term pregnancy predicts a lower lifetime risk of breast cancer (51). The reduction in risk following pregnancy compared with nulliparous women is not immediate, but takes approximately 10 to 15 years to manifest (58). In fact, risk of breast cancer is increased for the first decade following first pregnancy (15,59,60). The proliferation of breast cells during the first pregnancy results in differentiation into mature breast cells prepared for lactation; this may also lead to growth of mutated cells and excess risk over the next decade. Epidemiologic evidence for the transient excess risk after the first pregnancy is consistent. Less clear is the presence of a transient increase in risk after subsequent pregnancies; some studies suggest an adverse effect (61) but others do not (60).

The first pregnancy is associated with permanent changes in the glandular epithelium and with changes in the biologic properties of the mammary cells. After the differentiation of pregnancy, epithelial cells have a longer cell cycle and spend more time in the G_1 phase, the phase that allows for DNA repair (62). The longer the interval from menarche to first pregnancy, the greater the adverse effect of the first pregnancy (15). The later the age at first full-term pregnancy, the more likely that DNA mistakes have occurred that will be propagated with the proliferation of mammary cells during pregnancy. The susceptibility of mammary tissue to carcinogens decreases after the first pregnancy, reflecting the differentiation of the mammary gland. This is also seen in the age-dependent susceptibility of the breast to radiation, reviewed later in this chapter.

Number and Spacing of Births

A higher number of births is consistently related to lower risk of breast cancer; each additional birth beyond the first reduces long-term risk of breast cancer. Although in some analyses, this has not been independent of earlier age at first birth, the overall evidence indicates an independent effect of greater parity (63). In addition to a protective effect of higher parity, several studies now indicate that more closely spaced births are associated with

lower lifetime risk of breast cancer (60,64). This may be owing to the breast having less time to accumulate DNA damage before it attains maximal differentiation by repeated pregnancies.

Lactation

As early as 1926, it was proposed that a breast never used for lactation is more liable to become cancerous (65). Two major biologic mechanisms are proposed to induce the protective effect; breast-feeding may result in further terminal differentiation of the breast epithelium and lactation delays the resuming of ovulatory menstrual cycles after pregnancy. Ecological studies demonstrate a consistency with the patterns of international variation in breast cancer incidence: Rates are lower in populations where breast-feeding is both common and of long duration. The overall evidence from case-control and cohort studies supports a reduction in risk with longer duration of breast-feeding, but the findings have varied substantially in the level of risk reduction. Some of the differences may relate to the pattern of breast-feeding; for example, whether feeding was exclusively from the breast or supplemented with other food, which needs to be evaluated further. A pooled analysis from almost 50 studies in 30 countries, reported an overall 4% reduction in risk per 12 months of breast-feeding for all parous women (66). The authors estimate that if women in developed countries had the number of births and lifetime duration of breast-feeding of women in developing countries, cumulative incidence of breast cancer by age 70 years would be reduced by as much as 60%. About two-thirds of this reduction would be related to breast-feeding (66).

Social norms regarding parity and breast-feeding in the American culture have limited our ability even to study this potential preventive behavior; the population who breast-feeds at all is small, and the group who breast-feeds over an extended period is even smaller. For example, despite the strong recommendation of the American Academy of Pediatrics that infants be breast-fed through the first 6 months of life because of the unequivocal benefit to the infant (67), by 2000 more than 60% of infants were ever breast-fed, but only 27% were receiving breast milk at 6 months of age (68). Among non-Hispanic blacks and Mexican–Americans, reported rates of breast-feeding were lower than those among non-Hispanic whites (69).

Spontaneous and Induced Abortion

Close to one-fourth of all clinically identified pregnancies in the United States end as induced abortions (70), and for women whose pregnancies continue for 0 to 20 weeks, the probability of spontaneous abortion ranges from 8% to 12% (68). It has been suggested that breast cells are the most vulnerable to mutation when breast tissue consists of rapidly growing and undifferentiated cells, such as during adolescence and pregnancy. In early pregnancy, the number of undifferentiated cells increases as rapid growth of the breast epithelium is taking place. If the pregnancy continues to term, these cells differentiate by the third trimester, and thus, the number of cells susceptible to malignancy decreases. The interruption of the differentiation of breast cells that takes place as the result of spontaneous and induced abortions has been hypothesized to increase a woman's risk of developing breast cancer (69). This hypothesis appears to be supported by a meta-analysis that included data from 28 published reports on induced abortion and breast cancer incidence (71). This analysis, based largely on case-control studies, contains the underlying serious potential for bias in retrospective studies of the relation between abortion and breast cancer. Induced abortion can be an extremely sensitive topic, and reporting on abortion history by women with a life-threatening condition such as breast cancer may be more complete than reporting by women without breast cancer.

By far the largest study on the association between breast cancer and abortion was a population-based cohort study made up of 1.5 million Danish women born April 1, 1935, through March 31, 1978 (72). Of these women, 280,965 (18.4%) had had one or more induced abortions. After adjusting for potential confounders of age, parity, age at delivery of first child, and calendar period, the risk of breast cancer for women with a history of induced abortion was not different from that of women who had not had an induced abortion (RR = 1.0, 95% confidence interval [CI], 0.94 1.06). In addition, no trend in risk was noted with increasing number of induced abortions in a woman's history. Similarly, no association between induced abortion and breast cancer incidence was observed in four prospective cohort studies, including the Iowa Women's Study (73), the Shanghai Textile Workers Study (74), the European Prospective Investigation into Cancer and Nutrition (75) and the Nurses' Health Study II (NHSII) (76). Taken as a whole and accounting for the limitations of the case-control study design, the available evidence does not support any important relation between induced abortion and risk of breast cancer. In 2003, the Early Reproductive Events and Breast Cancer Workshop, convened by the National Cancer Institute to assess the state of evidence between reproductive factors and breast cancer, recognized that spontaneous and induced abortions are not associated with breast cancer risk (77).

Age at Menopause

Early studies of age at menopause and risk of breast cancer focused on women who had undergone bilateral oophorectomy at a young age; these women have a greatly reduced risk of breast cancer (78,79). Women with bilateral oophorectomy before age 45 years have approximately half the risk of breast cancer compared with those with a natural menopause at 55 years or older. On average, the risk of breast cancer increases by some 3% per year of delay in age at menopause. Although some studies suggest the effect of age at menopause decreases with advancing age at breast cancer diagnosis (80), this may reflect greater error in recall of age at menopause as women are further removed from the event (81). Adjustment for error in recall removes this apparent decrease in the effect of menopause with advancing age.

The reduction in risk of breast cancer with early menopause is likely owing to the reduction of breast cell division with the termination of menstrual cycles and the decline in endogenous hormone levels, which become substantially lower than during the premenopausal years.

Models of Reproductive Factors and Breast Cancer Incidence

Biomathematical models are derived by translating a series of hypotheses about biologic process involved in carcinogenesis into mathematical terms. The classic models of carcinogenesis proposed by Armitage and Doll (82) and by Moolgavkar and Knudson (83) are the best known. Armitage and Doll noted that the gradient of 6 to 1 (i.e., 6 units increase in the logarithm of death rate per unit increase in logarithm of age) was more or less consistent across 17 cancer sites, but also noted a deficit in mortality from breast cancer among older women. They attributed this to a reduction during middle life in the rate of production of one of the later changes in the process of carcinogenesis (82). Pike et al. (59) reviewed the epidemiologic evidence in the early 1980s and proposed a model of tissue aging that accounted for the relation between reproductive risk factors and breast cancer incidence. Ultimately, models will ideally be developed that take into account all known risk factors.

The mathematical model proposed by Pike et al. (59) was based on the observed age-incidence curve, and on the known relations of ages at menarche, first birth, and menopause to the risk of breast cancer. The model proposed by Pike et al. (59) is built on earlier work by Moolgavkar and Knudson (83), who fitted mathematical parameters to breast cancer incidence data from several countries. The Pike et al. model related breast cancer rates to the growth of the breast. The model allowed a short-term increase in risk with first pregnancy followed by a subsequent decrease in risk. Finally, at menopause the breast begins an involutional process that is thought to reflect a decrease in cell turnover and eventual disappearance of epithelium. The original Pike et al. model, however, did not include terms for the second or subsequent births or for the spacing of pregnancies, nor did it easily accommodate pregnancies after age 40 years. Although there has been controversy about whether the bearing of additional children beyond the first reduces the risk of breast cancer, substantial evidence reviewed earlier indicates that both the number of births and their spacing are associated with risk: The greater the number of births and the closer they are spaced, the lower a woman's risk of breast cancer.

An extension of the Pike et al. model of breast cancer incidence utilized prospective data from the Nurses' Health Study (15,60,84), and added a term to summarize the spacing of births. Nonlinear models produced parameters that were difficult to interpret (60), but a subsequent modification allowed ready estimation of RR (15), thus making the results more accessible to epidemiologists and clinicians familiar with the RR as measure of the relation between an exposure and disease. Before menopause, the incidence of breast cancer increased 1.7% for a 1-year increase in age at first birth. Closer spacing of births was related to significantly reduced risk of breast cancer. For each additional year of delay between the first and second births, for example, the risk of breast cancer increased by 0.4%. The increase in risk with first pregnancy originally observed with this modified Pike model has since been documented in a prospective study from Sweden (61) and in an analysis from an international case-control study (85). The effect of age at first and subsequent births on breast cancer incidence was still greater after menopause (Fig. 20.6).

According to the extended Pike et al. (59) model, a parous woman with a single birth at age 35 years has a 34% increase in breast cancer incidence at the time of the birth relative to a

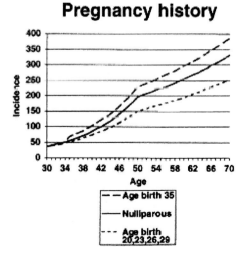

FIGURE 20.6. Age-specific incidence of breast cancer for three hypothetical women. (Data from Colditz G, Rosner B. Cumulative risk of breast cancer to age 70 years according to risk factor status: data from the Nurses' Health Study. *Am J Epidemiol* 2000;152:950–964, with permission.)

nulliparous woman (84). The excess risk goes down very slowly over time. Even at age 70 years such a woman has excess risk versus a nulliparous woman. In sum, the cumulative risk to age 70 is 16% greater than that of a nulliparous woman. Conversely, a parous woman with an early age at first birth (20 years) and multiple births conceived at a young age has a slight excess risk immediately after the first birth relative to the nulliparous woman (RR = 1.10), which slowly diminishes over time, reaching equality at age 32 years and continuing to decline until menopause (age 50 years), at which time the RR is 0.82. Because the relationship between breast cancer incidence and reproductive history changes with age, cumulative incidence, rather than age-specific incidence, is a useful summary (Fig. 20.6). Compared with a nulliparous woman, a woman with one birth at age 35 years has a 16% excess risk over the age period 30 to 70 years, whereas the woman with births at ages 20, 23, and 26 years has a 27% decrease in risk over the similar age period (84).

In the original Pike et al. model (59), factors associated with reduced risk of breast cancer were each considered to slow the rate of "breast tissue aging," which correlates with the accumulation of molecular damage in the pathway to breast cancer. In the Rosner and Colditz (15,84) extension of the Pike et al. model, the rate of tissue aging was highest between menarche and first birth, consistent with the hypothesis that this is the period when the breast is most vulnerable to mutagenesis. The transient increase in the risk of breast cancer associated with the first pregnancy is followed by a 20% decrease in the rate of breast tissue aging (15). This observation helps explain the *cross-over* effect in certain subgroups of women; around menopause, rates of one subgroup that were initially higher drop below rates of a second subgroup. For instance, using data from New York State, Janerich and Hoff (86) showed a cross-over in breast cancer incidence between single and married women at age 42, such that married women had a higher incidence before this age and lower mortality thereafter (86). A similar cross-over of incidence has been reported for black and white women in the United States (14,87), consistent with the distribution of age at first birth by race. Over many decades, pregnancy rates have been higher and age at first birth has been younger for black women than for white women (88).

The age–incidence curve from biomathematical models of reproductive events and breast cancer incidence also mirrors the observed patterns of breast cancer incidence across many countries. In China and many developing countries, the estimated number of births in the early 1960s was 6.5 births per woman (89), which is not associated with a late age at first birth. Also, the average age at menarche in China was about 17 years, even through the 1960s (90). Fitting the Rosner and Colditz model with menarche at age 16 years, first birth at age 19 years, 6 births spaced a year apart, and age at menopause 50 years, we estimate an annual rate of breast cancer incidence for 65-year-old Chinese women is 93.6 per 100,000. For the cohort of U.S. women born between 1921 and 1925, the average age at menarche was approximately 13.5 years, the median age at first birth was 23 years, the mean number of children was 3, and the mean interval between births was 3 years (91). Considering these characteristics, and holding age at menopause constant at 50 years, the annual rate of breast cancer incidence predicted for a 65-year-old U.S. woman is 279 per 100,000—close to the observed SEER rate of 300 per 100,000 for women of this age, and approximately three times the rate for Chinese women. Applying this model to typical reproductive patterns for women from low-incidence countries suggests that reproductive factors alone account for more than half of the international variation in the risk of breast cancer (92).

The extension of the Rosner and Colditz model to include history of benign breast disease, height, weight, alcohol intake, and type of postmenopausal hormone used, in addition to reproduc-

tive factors and family history, gives a model that compares favorably to the Gail model for risk prediction (93). Furthermore, this extended model has been applied to the evaluation of risk factors for estrogen-receptor (ER)-positive and ER-negative breast cancer. Incidence of ER-positive/progesterone receptor (PR)-positive tumors increases at 11.0% per year during premenopausal years and at 4.6% per year after natural menopause. In contrast, the incidence of ER-negative/PR-negative tumors increases at 5.0% per year during premenopausal years and 1.3% after natural menopause. The one-time adverse effect of first pregnancy is present for ER-negative/PR-negative breast cancer, but not ER-positive/PR-positive tumors. Parity shows a strong inverse association with ER-positive/PR-positive tumors (RR = 0.6 for four births at 20, 23, 26, and 29 vs. nulliparous), but not ER-negative/PR-negative tumors (RR = 1.1 for four births vs. nulliparous). Other risk factors, including benign breast disease, family history of breast cancer, alcohol use, and height, show consistent relations with both ER-positive/PR-positive and ER-negative/PR-negative breast cancer, whereas body mass index after menopause is related to incidence of PR-positive but not PR-negative tumors. The concordance statistic (indicating predictive ability of the model) adjusted for age was 0.64 (95% CI = 0.63–0.66) for ER-positive/PR-positive tumors, and for ER-negative/PR-negative the concordance statistic was 0.61 (95% CI = 0.58–0.64) (94).

Risk Prediction

Breast cancer incidence models have been applied to predict the risk of breast cancer over a defined time period, for instance, 5 or 10 years. The larger the number of risk factors considered, the higher the likelihood the prediction model will separate those at risk of disease from those who are not as likely to develop disease. As Wald notes (95), however, to be useful as a screening test or an individual marker of risk or to identify those who will develop disease and those who will not, the magnitude of association for a predictor must be on the order of 10 or higher comparing extreme quintiles for a detection rate of 20%. No prediction models for breast cancer have achieved this level of discrimination to date.

Ottman et al. (96) published a simple model in 1983 that calculates a probability of breast cancer diagnosis for mothers and sisters of breast cancer patients. They used life-table analysis to estimate the cumulative risks to various ages based on two groups of patients from the Los Angeles County Cancer Surveillance Program, then derived a probability within each decade between ages 20 and 70 for mothers and sisters of the patients, according to the age of diagnosis of the patient and whether the disease was bilateral or unilateral.

Because risk factors can change over the life course, (e.g., weight gain, change in alcohol intake, menopausal status, use of postmenopausal hormones for some years), it becomes more helpful to consider the impact of all these risk factors on breast cancer cumulative risk up to a given age (e.g., 70 or 75). This approach has been developed for breast cancer risk according to family history (97), and the prediction of *BRCA1* carrier status (98,99), but more general applications joining carrier status and lifestyle factors remain limited (100).

The complex nature of breast cancer incidence, with many possibly time-dependent risk factors, requires prediction models that account for this variation over time. These are now shown to outperform traditional approaches that fit indicator variables with fixed effects across time (93). In addition, the log-incidence model of Rosner and Colditz (15) performs significantly better than the commonly used Gail model (605) for total breast cancer incidence that includes only five variables (age, age at menarche, age at first birth, number of benign breast biopsies, and family history). Growing emphasis is placed on mammographic breast density as a contributor to risk prediction (101,102) and, although models have incorporated this measure, none yet includes the details of reproductive risk factors, specific type of postmenopausal hormone therapy used, and breast cancer incidence.

The efficacy of chemoprevention for breast cancer is clearly shown for ER-positive disease reducing risk by 50% (103). Given the need to balance risks and benefits when implementing a tamoxifen-based chemoprevention strategy (104), a model that successfully identifies women at increased risk of ER-positive breast cancer will, therefore, improve the risk-to-benefit ratio. Rosner and Colditz have applied their log incidence model to breast cancers classified according to receptor status and reported that the area under the receiver operating characteristic (ROC) curve adjusted for age was 0.630 (95% CI, 0.616–0.644) for ER-positive/PR-positive tumors and was 0.601 (95% CI, 0.575–0.626) for ER-/PR- tumors, indicating adequate discriminatory accuracy. On the other hand, when we fit the Gail model to the same data set it had performance characteristics that were somewhat lower than the Rosner and Colditz model with values of 0.578 for total cancer and 0.57 for ER-positive/PR-positive tumors. The difference between the area under the ROC for the Rosner and Colditz model versus the Gail model for total breast cancer was statistically significant ($p < .0001$), indicating that the more complete modeling of risk factors across the life course could be more useful for discriminating among those women at high and low risk of breast cancer.

ENDOGENOUS SEX HORMONES AND RISK OF BREAST CANCER

Several lines of evidence have long suggested that sex hormones play a central role in the etiology of breast cancer. As noted earlier, rates of breast cancer increase rapidly in the premenopausal years, but the rate of increase slows sharply at the time of menopause, when estrogen levels decline rapidly. In addition, several reproductive variables that alter hormone status affect risk of breast cancer; for example, early age at menarche and late age at menopause are associated with increased risk of breast cancer, whereas parity is inversely associated with risk. After menopause, adipose tissue is the major source of estrogen and obese postmenopausal women have both higher levels of endogenous estrogen and a higher risk of breast cancer (105). In animals, estrogens, progesterone, and prolactin all promote mammary tumors. Also, hormonal manipulations, such as antiestrogens (e.g., tamoxifen) are useful in the treatment of breast cancer and reduce breast cancer incidence in women at high risk (106–108).

Methodologic Issues in Studies of Endogenous Hormones and Breast Cancer Risk

In contrast to clinical needs where discerning grossly abnormal from normal hormone levels is the focus, epidemiologic studies are usually aimed at detecting modest differences within the normal range of levels. Considerable laboratory error has been reported in studies of assay reproducibility, with several hormones being measured poorly by some laboratories (109,110). Low reproducibility could result in true (and important) exposure or disease associations being missed. Varying sensitivities and specificities of different laboratory assays also have made comparison of results between studies difficult (111,112). For example, in studies of plasma estradiol, mean levels in control subjects have ranged from 9 (113) to 28 (114) pg/mL. Although these differences may result in part from differences in characteristics of study subjects (i.e., differences in adiposity), a substantial component is likely owing to the use of varying laboratory methods.

Several hormones, particularly estrogens, fluctuate markedly over the menstrual cycle. In some early studies, hormone levels were measured in samples collected without regard to the menstrual cycle phase, thus adding considerable *noise* to the comparison of hormone levels between breast cancer cases and controls. This noise could mask true associations or, because of chance differences in the distribution of cycle phase between cases and controls, could result in associations that do not truly exist. More recent studies have tended to collect all samples at approximately the same time in the cycle, have matched on cycle day, or have carefully controlled for cycle day in the analysis—an appropriate strategies.

For both logistic and financial reasons, in most epidemiologic studies only a single blood sample can be collected per study subject. Whether a single sample can reflect long-term hormone levels (generally the exposure of greatest etiologic interest) is therefore an important issue. In several studies, repeated blood samples were collected over a 1- to 3-year period in postmenopausal women and the correlation between the samples calculated. Overall, steroid hormones were reasonably stable, with intraclass correlations ranging from 0.5 to 0.9 (115–118). This level of reproducibility is similar to that found for other biologic variables, such as blood pressure and serum cholesterol measurements, all parameters that are considered reasonably measured and that are consistent predictors of disease in epidemiologic studies. Data on premenopausal women are more limited, although follicular or luteal estrogens were reasonably reproducible over a 3-year period (119), and androgens have been reasonably correlated over a several year period (116,117,119). Data on circulating levels of insulin-like growth factors also indicates substantial stability over a several year period (119,120).

Over the last decade, a number of well-conducted prospective studies have assessed the role of circulating hormone levels and breast cancer risk; their findings are summarized below.

Estrogens

Estradiol, considered the most biologically active endogenous estrogen, circulates in blood either unbound ("free") or bound to sex hormone-binding globulin or albumin. Free or bioavailable (free plus albumin-bound) estradiol is thought to be readily available to breast tissue and, thus, may be more strongly related to risk than total estradiol. Postmenopausally, estrone is the source of most circulating estradiol, and estrone sulfate is the most abundant circulating estrogen (121). Both normal and malignant breast cells have sulfatase and 17-β-dehydrogenase activity (122). Thus, estrone and estrone sulfate could serve as ready sources of intracellular estradiol.

In 2002, a pooled analysis was published consisting of all prospective studies of endogenous estrogens and androgens in postmenopausal women that had been available at that time (123). Data were from nine prospective studies with a total of 663 breast cancer cases and 1,765 healthy controls; none of the women were using exogenous hormones at blood collection. The risk of breast cancer increased with increasing estrogen levels. For example, the relative risks (95% CI) for increasing quintiles of estradiol level, all relative to the lowest quintile, were 1.4 (1.0–2.0), 1.2 (0.9–1.7), 1.8 (1.3–2.4), and 2.0 (1.5–2.7). Estrone, estrone sulfate, and free estradiol were similarly related to risk. No significant heterogeneity in results was noted between the studies. Subsequent to the pooled analysis, several additional prospective studies have been published and all have supported these findings (124–126). Further, urinary hormone levels have been assessed in relation to breast cancer in two prospective studies (127,128) and, in each, positive associations were observed.

The association between circulating estrogens and breast cancer risk appears to be stronger for estrogen and progesterone receptor-positive tumors, with little association for hormone receptor-negative tumors (126). In the one detailed study of this issue, for estradiol, the top versus bottom category RR (95% CI) was 3.3 (2.0–5.4) for ER-positive/PR-positive tumors (p-trend <0.001), and 1.0 (0.4–2.4; p-trend = 0.46) for ER-negative/PR-negative tumors. These data are in line with findings from the tamoxifen and raloxifene trials, where risk of only ER-positive tumors was reduced (107,129) and also from epidemiologic studies of obesity and breast cancer where stronger associations have been noted for ER-positive tumors.

Whether the association between plasma estrogens and postmenopausal breast cancer is similar in women at varying levels of breast cancer risk has been addressed in two recent studies. The first was conducted in the high-risk population of the National Surgical Adjuvant Breast and Bowel Project Cancer Prevention Trial (P-1) with 89 cases and 141 noncases enrolled in the placebo arm of the trial (130). In P-1, high risk was defined as having at least a 1.66% 5-year risk of breast cancer as estimated from the Gail model (131). No association was observed between estradiol levels and breast cancer risk: The relative risk for the top (vs. bottom) quartile of levels was 0.96 (95% CI, 0.47–1.95). In contrast, in the Nurses' Health Study cohort (with >400 cases and 800 controls) (132), women were classified as high or low risk in several ways: according to family history of breast cancer, by their 5-year modified Gail risk score, and by their 5-year Rosner and Colditz risk score (84). Overall, the associations of plasma estrogens with breast cancer were robust across risk categories regardless of which metric was used to define risk. Thus, the data from this larger cohort suggest that circulating estrogens are predictive of risk in women at low and at high risk of breast cancer; however, confirmation in other studies is needed.

Only one prospective study has addressed whether circulating estradiol levels are associated with breast cancer risk even in women using postmenopausal hormones (estrogen only or estrogen plus a progestin) (133). Modest positive associations with estradiol and free estradiol were observed (top vs. bottom quartile RR for estradiol = 1.3, 0.9–2.0, 95% CI, p-trend = 0.20, and for free estradiol = 1.7, 1.1–2.7, p-trend = 0.06). Interestingly, these associations were stronger among women who were older (e.g., estradiol RR = 2.8, 95% CI, 1.5–5.0), who were leaner (estradiol RR = 1.8, 95% CI, 1.1–3.0) and who had the longest duration of nonuse of hormones since menopause (estradiol RR = 2.8, 95% CI, 1.4–5.6). Thus, although women using postmenopausal hormones have a different hormonal profile than nonusers, plasma estradiol concentrations appear to be associated, albeit more modestly, with breast cancer in this group of women.

Data on premenopausal estrogen levels and breast cancer risk are more limited, in large part because of the complexities related to sampling during the menstrual cycle. Seven prospective studies have been published to date, although 5 of the 7 had fewer than 80 cases (range 14–79 cases) and, not surprisingly, no significant associations with plasma estrogens were observed in the 5 small studies (134–138). Two much larger studies have recently been published. In the first, conducted in the the European Prospective Investigation into Cancer and Nutrition (EPIC) cohort, with 285 breast cancer cases and 555 controls, one blood sample was collected per woman and the day in the menstrual cycle was recorded (139). Controls were matched to cases on age and phase of the menstrual cycle at blood collection (defined in five categories). Comparisons between case and control hormone levels were based on residuals from Spline Regression Models; the residuals indicated how much an individual's hormone level deviated from the predicted hormone levels on that day. Overall, no association was observed for either estradiol or estrone (e.g., top to bottom quartile comparison RR = 1.0, 95% CI, 0.7–1.5 for estradiol). In the second large prospective study, conducted within the

NHSII, both early follicular and mid-luteal samples were collected from each woman (140). The analysis included 197 cases with 394 controls also matched on age and luteal day. Follicular, but not luteal, total and free estradiol were significantly associated with breast cancer risk (top to bottom quartile comparison RR = 2.1, 95% CI, 1.1–4.1 for follicular total estradiol). No association was observed with either estrone or estrone sulfate (in either phase of the cycle). Clearly, additional data, with careful matching of cases and controls and detailed evaluation by timing in the menstrual cycle, are needed.

Estrogen Metabolites

A woman's pattern of estrogen metabolism also has been hypothesized to influence her breast cancer risk. Estradiol and estrone can be metabolized through several pathways, including the 16-α and 2- (and 4-) hydroxy pathways (141). Products of these pathways have markedly different biologic properties, and opposing hypotheses have been proposed concerning their influence on risk (141). Few epidemiologic studies have examined estrogen metabolites and postmenopausal breast cancer risk, and they have assessed only 2-OH estrone, 16α-OH estrone, and the 2:16α-OH estrone ratio. In the two prospective assessments among premenopausal women, nonsignificant inverse associations with the 2-:16α-OH estrone ratio were observed in each. Five prospective studies of either urinary (142–144) or serum (145) metabolite levels among postmenopausal women who were not using postmenopausal hormones (N = 42) (142) to N = 272) (145), also observed no significant associations for 2-OH estrone, 16α-OH estrone or their ratio and breast cancer risk. Cumulatively, the data to not support an important relationship with these metabolites and risk, however, more comprehensive assessments, including other biologically active metabolites (e.g., 4-OH estrogens) are needed.

Androgens and Breast Cancer Risk

Androgens have been hypothesized to increase breast cancer risk, either directly, by increasing the growth and proliferation of breast cancer cells, or indirectly, by their conversion to estrogen (56). In animal and *in vitro* experiments, androgens either increase or decrease cell proliferation, depending on the model system (146). Dehydroepiandrosterone (DHEA) administered to rodents can decrease tumor formation. In humans, DHEA may act like an antiestrogen premenopausally, but an estrogen postmenopausally in stimulating cell growth (147); this, in part, because of the estrogenic effect of its metabolite, 5-androstene-3b,17b-diol, also can bind to the estrogen receptor (148).

In postmenopausal women, the best summary of evidence on circulating androgens and breast cancer risk is from the pooled analysis of nine prospective studies described above (123) along with the recently published report from the EPIC study (124). In the pooled analysis, testosterone was positively associated with breast cancer risk: The relative risks (95% CI) for increasing quintile category (all relative to the lowest quintile of levels) were 1.3 (1.0–1.9), 1.6 (1.2–2.2), 1.6 (1.1–2.2), and 2.2 (1.6–3.1). Findings were generally similar for several other androgens measured. In EPIC, similar positive associations were observed for each of the androgens assessed. In each of these analyses, when estradiol was added to the statistical models, relative risks for the androgens were only modestly attenuated, suggesting some independent effect of circulating androgens on breast cancer risk. Interpretation of these data is complicated, however, because of possible differences between estradiol and the androgens in terms of assay precision, hormone stability within woman over time, and intracellular conversion of androgens to estrogens which cannot be accounted for in epidemiologic analyses.

The association of plasma testosterone levels and subsequent breast cancer risk also was positive and of the same general magnitude in women using postmenopausal hormones (133). In the two studies previously described, the association between circulating testosterone and breast cancer across categories of predicted breast cancer risk has been addressed. No association was observed between testosterone levels and breast cancer risk in the P-1 trial with 89 cases and 141 noncases (RR for top versus bottom quartile = 0.5, 95% CI, 0.2–1.1) (130), although the association was noted to be quite robust in the larger NHS cohort (132).

Among premenopausal women, although data are much more limited, prospective nested case-control studies are consistent in showing a positive association, of similar magnitude to that reported among postmenopausal women, between circulating androgen levels and risk of breast cancer (137,139, 140,149).

Progesterone

Progesterone exerts powerful influences on breast physiology and can influence tumor development in rodents (150). Based largely on indirect evidence, progesterone has been hypothesized both to decrease breast cancer risk by opposing estrogenic stimulation of the breast (150) and to increase risk because breast mitotic rates are highest in the luteal (high progesterone) phase of the menstrual cycle (56). In three large prospective studies, results have not been consistent with inverse (139,149) and no association (140) reported. However, progesterone levels vary substantially throughout the menstrual cycle and are difficult to measure in the context of large epidemiologic studies, hence further assessments with better measures are warranted. In postmenopausal women, only a single prospective study has been conducted and no association found (126).

Prolactin

Prolactin receptors have been found on more than 50% of breast tumors (151), and prolactin can increase the growth of both normal and malignant breast cells *in vitro* (152). Cumulatively, substantial laboratory evidence suggests that prolactin could play a role in mammary carcinogenesis (153) by promoting cell proliferation and survival (154–157), increasing cell motility (158), and supporting tumor vascularization (153,159). Because prolactin is influenced by both physical and emotional stress (160,161), levels in women with breast cancer may not reflect their predisease levels. Thus, evaluation of this association in prospective studies is particularly important.

Prolactin levels and risk of breast cancer has been evaluated in several studies to date (125,134,135,162–166). Most, although not all (125), studies have observed a significant positive association, with case numbers ranging from 26 (135) to 1,539 (164). In by far the largest study to date, an updated analysis within the NHS and NHSII cohorts with 1,539 cases (premenopausal and postmenopausal women combined), a modest but significant association was observed across quartiles of prolactin level, with a top (vs. bottom) quartile RR = 1.4, 95% CI, 1.0–1.9, p-trend = 0.05 (164). In this analysis, the association of prolactin with breast cancer did not differ by menopausal status (p = .95). The association was stronger for invasive cases (top vs. bottom quartile RR = 1.4, 95% CI, 1.1–1.7, p-trend = 0.001) than *in situ* cases (comparable RR = 1.2, 95% CI, 0.8–1.6, p-trend = 0.43). In addition, the association was significantly different by ER or PR status of the tumor (p-heterogeneity = 0.03) with RR for top versus bottom quartiles of 1.6, 95% CI, 1.3–2.0, p-trend <0.001 for ER-positive/PR-positive, 1.7, 95% CI, 1.0–2.7, p-trend = 0.06 for ER-positive/PR-negative, and 0.9, 95% CI, 0.6–1.3, p-trend = 0.70 for ER-negative/PR-negative. There

were too few ER-negative/PR-positive cases to evaluate separately. Cumulatively, epidemiologic data support a role for prolactin in the etiology of breast cancer.

Insulin-like Growth Factor

Insulin-like growth factor I (IGF-I) is a protein hormone with structural homology to insulin. The growth hormone–IGF-I axis can stimulate proliferation of both breast cancer and normal breast epithelial cells (167). Rhesus monkeys treated with growth hormone or IGF-I show histologic evidence of mammary gland hyperplasia. In addition, positive associations have been observed between breast cancer and birth weight as well as height, which are both positively correlated with IGF-I levels (168). In several meta-analyses of prospective epidemiologic studies published up to that time, a positive relationship was reported between circulating IGF-I and premenopausal breast cancer (comparing the 75th with the 25th percentile OR = 1.65, 95% CI, 1.26–2.08 (169), but not with postmenopausal breast cancer (169,170). In this same meta-analysis, high levels of IGF binding protein-3 (IGFBP-3) were also associated with increased premenopausal breast cancer (comparing the 75th with the 25th percentile OR = 1.51, 95% CI, 1.01–2.27) (169).

Subsequent to these meta-analyses, several large prospective studies have reported results that do not support the earlier findings (171). Rinaldi et al. (172) reported no association between IGF-I and breast cancer in women under the age of 50, but a positive modest association among older women in EPIC. In the NHSII, Schernhammer et al. (173) also reported no association between IGF-I, and IGFBP-3 with premenopausal breast cancer. An updated analysis of the NHS found that circulating IGF-I levels were only modestly associated with breast cancer risk among premenopausal women, but not among postmenopausal women (174). An updated analysis of the New York University Women's Health Study reported a significant twofold positive association with circulating IGF in premenopausal women, consistent with their initial findings (175). The most recent prospective data, from an Australian cohort, showed no association of IGF-I with In another interesting study, mothers with high pregnancy IGF levels were observed to be at higher risk of breast cancer compared with women with lower IGF levels during pregnancy; the positive association appeared strongest among uniparous women (177). Reasons for inconsistencies between studies are not known, but they may involve differences in study populations assessed (e.g., by age or time period of follow-up) and variability in the IGF assay methodology.

Insulin

Insulin is a known mitogen and circulating levels have been evaluated in relation to subsequent breast cancer risk. Some studies evaluated insulin levels in fasting or nonfasting subjects, others assessed c-peptide levels, which is a marker of insulin secretion. Among premenopausal women, overall no consistent associations have been observed between insulin levels and breast cancer risk (120,178–180). Similarly postmenopausal women, where at least 6 studies with over 1,200 postmenopausal cases have been published, no consistent associations have been reported (120,179–183).

Melatonin

Laboratory evidence in conjunction with recent epidemiologic data suggests a possible relation between melatonin and breast cancer risk. *In vitro* studies, although not entirely consistent (184), find that both pharmacologic and physiologic doses of melatonin reduce the growth of malignant cells of the breast

(185–189). In rodent models pinealectomy boosts tumor growth (190), whereas exogenous melatonin administration exerts anti-initiating (191) and oncostatic activity (192–195) in various chemically induced cancers. The hormone could influence risk through antimitotic or antioxidant activity (196), by modulating cell-cycle length through control of the p53-p21 pathway (189), or by reducing estrogen levels (197,198). Only two prospective studies have assessed the association between urinary 6-sulfatoxymelatonin levels (a metabolite of melatonin) and breast cancer risk. In the first, where a 24-hour urine sample was collected, no association between levels and breast cancer was observed (199). In the second, where a first morning sample was used to assess exposure, a significant inverse association was noted (200). Which melatonin exposure measure is superior is unknown, although the first morning urine sample may be better at detecting potential differences between subjects in the nocturnal duration or peak of melatonin levels. Additional studies are clearly needed. There is relatively consistent indirect evidence from observational studies for an association between night work and breast cancer risk (201). Night work is associated with substantially reduced melatonin levels (202,203). Two retrospective studies of flight attendants with occupational exposure to light at night linked employment time to an increased breast cancer risk (204,205). Two nationwide record linkage studies (206,207) and a retrospective case-control study (197) associated night work with an approximately 50% higher breast cancer risk. In the only two prospective studies, working 20 to 30 or more years of rotating night work as a nurse was associated with an increased risk of breast cancer (208,209).

ORAL CONTRACEPTIVES

Since oral contraceptives were first introduced in the 1960s, they have been used by millions of women (210). Most combined oral contraceptives contain ethinyl estradiol (or mestranol, which is metabolized to ethinyl estradiol) and a progestin. The estrogen dose in oral contraceptives has ranged from at least 100 mg in 1960 to 20 to 30 mg, the doses most commonly used today; during this same time period, at least nine different progestins have been used (211,212). Patterns of use also have changed considerably over time, with both increasing durations of use and a trend toward earlier age at first use. More than 50 epidemiologic studies have evaluated the relationship between oral contraceptive use and breast cancer risk.

Most studies have observed no significant increase in breast cancer risk even with long durations of use. Individual data from 54 epidemiologic studies were collected and analyzed centrally (80). In this large pooled analysis, in which data from 53,297 women with and 100,239 women without breast cancer were evaluated, no overall relationship was observed between duration of use and risk of breast cancer. Similar findings were generally observed when long-term use was evaluated among either postmenopausal women or women over the age of 45 years. However, before the pooled analysis, findings for long-term use among young women were not as consistent or reassuring. In two meta-analyses, summary relative risks for long duration of use in young women were 1.5 (213) and 1.4 (214). The greatest increase tended to be observed in the youngest women, generally those less than 35 years of age; this observation also was noted in several more case-control studies.

In the pooled analysis (80), current and recent users of oral contraceptives had an increased risk of breast cancer (for current vs. never-users, RR = 1.24). This increased risk disappeared within 10 years of stopping oral contraceptive use (RR by years since stopping use vs. never use: 1–4 years, 1.16; 5–9 years, 1.07; 10–14 years, 0.98; more than 15 years, 1.03) (Fig. 20.7). When the investigators evaluated both time since last

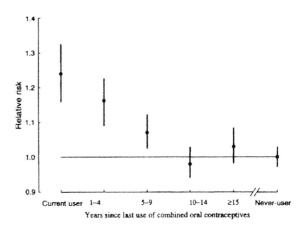

FIGURE 20.7. Relative risk (RR) of breast cancer by time since last use of combined oral contraceptives. (Reproduced from Collaborative Group on Hormonal Factors in Breast Cancer. Breast cancer and hormonal contraceptives: collaborative reanalysis of individual data on 53,297 women with breast cancer and 100,239 women without breast cancer from 54 epidemiological studies. *Lancet* 1996;347:1713–1727, with permission.)

use and duration of use, they observed a modestly increased risk only among current and recent users, and no independent effect of long duration of use on the risk of breast cancer even among very young women. Thus, the increased risk of breast cancer observed among young, long-term users of oral contraceptives in past individual studies (and meta-analyses) appears primarily owing to recency of use rather than to duration. These data suggest that oral contraceptives may act as late-stage promoters. Importantly, current and recent users, the women who appear to have a modest increase in risk, are generally young (<45 years of age) and, thus, have a low absolute risk of breast cancer. Hence, a modest increase in their risk will result in few additional cases of breast cancer. Nevertheless, this apparently increased risk among current and recent users should be considered in deciding whether to use oral contraceptives. On the basis of these data in conjunction with supporting laboratory evidence, the International Agency for Research on Cancer (IARC) classified oral contraceptives as carcinogenic to humans (i.e., group 1 carcinogens) in 2005 (215).

Because any influence of oral contraceptives on the breast has been hypothesized to be greatest before the cellular differentiation that occurs with a full-term pregnancy (216), a number of investigators have evaluated the effect of oral contraceptive use before a first full-term pregnancy. In both meta-analyses, the summary relative risk indicated a modest increase in risk with long-term use (213,214). In the pooled analysis (80), a significant trend of increasing risk with first use before age 20 years was observed. Among women ages 30 to 34 years, the relative risk associated with recent oral contraceptive use was 1.54 if use began before age 20 years and 1.13 if use began at age 20 years or older. Overall, no consistent evidence was found of a differential effect according to type or dose of either estrogen or progestin, but few studies had examined this issue (56).

Possible interactions with other breast cancer risk factors were evaluated in detail for the first time in the collaborative pooling project (80). In this study, the investigators defined oral contraceptive use in terms of recency and age at first use, rather than "ever use," as done in most previous individual studies. Overall, the relationship between oral contraceptive use and breast cancer did not vary appreciably by family history of breast cancer, weight, alcohol intake, or other breast cancer risk factors. In women with *BRCA1* and *BRCA2* mutations, a modest positive association between oral contraceptive use and breast cancer also has been observed (217–219). In contrast to data from the worldwide pooled analysis (80), however, the increase was not seen primarily among current and recent users; study findings were sufficiently variable that the particular aspect of exposure associated with risk in this group of women is as yet uncertain.

Until the time of the pooled analysis published in 1996, limited data existed regarding the influence of the newer oral contraceptive formulations on breast cancer risk (80). The Women's CARE Study, a large population-based, case-control study with 4,575 breast cancer cases and 4,682 controls enrolled in the mid-1990s, also examined the risk of breast cancer associated with oral contraceptives among different subgroups of women (220). In this study, no increased risk of breast cancer was seen among current users or former users regardless of estrogen dose. This study found no increased risk among women with a family history or those who initiated use at an early age. In addition, the risk of breast cancer did not appear to vary by duration, dose, or type of progestin (220).

Progestin only contraceptives include progestin-only pills ("mini-pill"), depot-medroxyprogesterone (DMPA, an injectable contraceptive), and implantable levonorgestrel (Norplant); few epidemiologic studies have evaluated their association with breast cancer risk. To date, longer-term users of the progestin-only pill have been observed to have either a similar or lower risk of breast cancer than never users (221). In the most comprehensive study of DMPA (222,223), no significant increase in risk was observed with increasing duration of use (for more than 3 years of use vs. never use, RR = 0.9). No data are available on the long-term use of Norplant, a long-acting contraceptive that is implanted subdermally, because it was introduced in the United States only in 1990. Further epidemiologic research is needed for each of these drugs.

POSTMENOPAUSAL HORMONE USE

Postmenopausal estrogens have been used for more than half a century. By the mid-1970s, almost 30 million prescriptions were being filled annually in the United States (224). A challenge in studying the relationship between postmenopausal hormones and breast cancer is the substantial variation in formulations and patterns of use that has occurred over time. By the time sufficient use of one type of hormone has occurred to allow a detailed epidemiologic evaluation, new formulations were already being introduced.

The possible relation between postmenopausal estrogen use and risk of breast cancer has been investigated in more than three dozen epidemiologic studies over the past 30 years. Most of these studies have been summarized in six meta-analyses (225–230) and a large pooled analysis (231). Subsequently, data from randomized, controlled trials have confirmed the epidemiologic relations of hormone therapy to increased risk of breast cancer and IARC has now classified estrogen plus progestin therapy as a human carcinogen (232). A summary of these findings, plus a more detailed discussion of several of the most important and most recent studies, is provided below. Particular attention is focused on use of estrogen alone versus estrogen plus progestin therapy.

Any Use

All meta-analyses have concluded that overall, ever users of postmenopausal estrogens have little or no increase in risk of breast cancer compared with women who have never used this therapy. Depending on the inclusion criteria for the meta-analyses, the RR estimates across studies range from 1.01 to 1.07. The RR observed in the pooled analysis was 1.14 (231). However, as for oral contraceptives, ever use is a poor measure of exposure because it fails to distinguish between short and long duration and recent and past users, nor does it distinguish type of hormone therapy used.

Duration of Use

In the meta-analyses, significant increases in risk of approximately 30% to 45% with more than 5 years of use have been observed. In updated results from the NHS (233), with 1,935 breast cancer cases, an excess risk of breast cancer was limited to women with current or very recent use of postmenopausal hormones. Within this group, the risk increased with longer duration of use and was statistically significant among current users who have used for 5 or more years (e.g., compared with never users of postmenopausal hormones, for ≥10 years of use RR = 1.47, 95% CI, 1.22–1.76) (233). Risk is greater for users of estrogen plus progestin compared with users of estrogen alone (234–236). These epidemiologic results were corroborated by the Women's Health Initiative, a randomized, controlled trial of estrogen plus progestin use that showed a significant increase in risk of breast cancer with duration of use of this hormone combination (40). Given the high dropout and noncompliance with therapy during the trial, analysis of compliers showed a substantially greater increase in risk with duration of therapy (237), closer to that observed in epidemiologic studies which by their nature evaluate risk among compliers or users of hormone therapy.

Recency of Use

Data on recency of use have been sparse because many studies do not distinguish current from past users. One meta-analysis calculated an RR for current use of 1.63 for women with natural menopause and 1.48 for women with surgical menopause. In a second, the summary RR was 1.40 (95% CI, 1.20–1.63) comparing current with never users. In the report from the NHS cohort (233), an excess risk of breast cancer was limited to women with current or very recent use of postmenopausal hormones. In the Breast Cancer Detection Demonstration Project (BCDDP) cohort, a positive association with invasive breast cancer was noted among current users with 5 to 15 or more years of use (238).

These relationships were evaluated in considerable detail in the pooled analysis that combined results of 51 epidemiologic studies (231). Importantly, in these analyses, women with an uncertain age at menopause were excluded (e.g., women with simple hysterectomies) because inadequate accounting for age at menopause in the analysis can lead to substantial attenuation of the observed relationships between postmenopausal hormone use and breast cancer risk (239). The investigators observed a statistically significant association between current or recent use of postmenopausal hormones and risk of breast cancer; the positive association was strongest among those with the longest duration of use (Fig. 20.8). For example, among women who used postmenopausal hormones within the previous 5 years (compared with never users of postmenopausal hormones), the RR for duration of use were 1.08 for 1 to 4 years of use, 1.31 for 5 to 9 years, 1.24 for 10 to 14 years, and 1.56 for 15 years or more of use. No significant increase in breast cancer risk was noted for women who had quit using postmenopausal hormones 5 or more years in the past, regardless of their duration of use.

Type, Dose, and Mode of Delivery of Estrogen

Limited data are available regarding the effects of dose or type of estrogen on breast cancer risk. Again, the best data come from the pooled analysis (231). No significant differences in the RR were observed according to either the type of estrogen used (conjugated estrogen vs. other) or the estrogen dose (<0.625

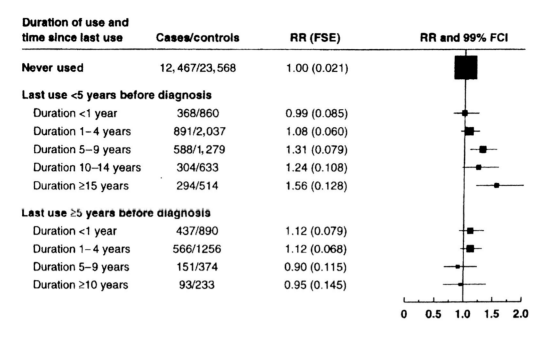

Duration of use and time since last use	Cases/controls	RR (FSE)	RR and 99% FCI
Never used	12,467/23,568	1.00 (0.021)	
Last use <5 years before diagnosis			
Duration <1 year	368/860	0.99 (0.085)	
Duration 1–4 years	891/2,037	1.08 (0.060)	
Duration 5–9 years	588/1,279	1.31 (0.079)	
Duration 10–14 years	304/633	1.24 (0.108)	
Duration ≥15 years	294/514	1.56 (0.128)	
Last use ≥5 years before diagnosis			
Duration <1 year	437/890	1.12 (0.079)	
Duration 1–4 years	566/1256	1.12 (0.068)	
Duration 5–9 years	151/374	0.90 (0.115)	
Duration ≥10 years	93/233	0.95 (0.145)	

FIGURE 20.8. Relative risk (RR) of breast cancer for different durations of use of hormone replacement therapy. Relative risk is shown in comparison with that of those who never used hormone replacement therapy, stratified by study, age at diagnosis, time since menopause, body mass index, parity, and the age of the woman at the time her first child was born. "Last use ≥5 years before diagnosis" includes current users. Floated standard error (FSE) and floated CI (FCI) were calculated from floated variation for each exposure category. Any comparison between groups must take variation into account. Each analysis is based on aggregate data from all studies. Black squares indicate relative risk, area of which is proportional to amount of information contributed (i.e., to inverse of variance of logarithm of relative risk). Lines indicate 99% FCI (lines are white when 99% FCI are so narrow as to be entirely within width of square). (Reproduced from Collaborative Group on Hormonal Factors in Breast Cancer. Breast cancer and hormone replacement therapy: collaborative reanalysis of data from 51 epidemiologic studies of 52,705 women with breast cancer and 108,411 women without breast cancer. *Lancet* 1997;350: 1047–1059, with permission.)

vs. ≥1.25 mg), although some modest differences in estimates suggested that further evaluation is warranted.

Although the effect of estrogen use on breast cancer risk could be reasonably hypothesized to vary by mode of estrogen delivery (e.g., patch estrogen, by avoiding the first pass effect in the liver, does not increase sex hormone binding globulin (SHBG) to the extent that oral preparations do), no important differences are observed in the largest study to date; The Million Women Study included more than 40,000 users of transdermal estrogen and observed no significant difference in relative risk of breast cancer (1.24) compared with that among the 60,000 users of oral therapy (1.32) (236).

Risk According to Breast Cancer Risk Factor Profile

The risk associated with postmenopausal hormone use was assessed in a number of specific subgroups in the pooled analysis (231). Risk did not appear to vary according to reproductive history, alcohol intake, smoking history, or family history of breast cancer. However, the RR associated with 5 or more years of postmenopausal hormone use were highest among the leanest women (p for heterogeneity = 0.001); this interaction has been consistently observed (236,240,241). Risk of unopposed estrogen therapy is also more clearly observed to increase with duration of use among women with bilateral oophorectomy than those without (240), again consistent with precise statistical control for underlying risk of breast cancer as age at menopause is more accurately assessed in women undergoing bilateral oophorectomy than in those who have hysterectomy without oophorectomy (242). This consistent finding that risk of unopposed estrogen is attenuated among overweight and

obese women may account for the apparent lower risk of breast cancer among women in the WHI trial of unopposed estrogen, given the overweight and obese population included in the trial (243).

Use of Estrogen Plus Progestin

The addition of a progestin to estrogen regimens has become increasingly common because it minimizes or eliminates the increased risk of endometrial hyperplasia and cancer associated with using unopposed estrogens. In the United States, by the mid-1980s, almost 30% of postmenopausal hormone prescriptions included a prescription for progestin (244). The impact of an added progestin to the risk of breast cancer has been evaluated only in the last 20 years.

Two of the first studies to assess this relationship suggested that the addition of a progestin could decrease breast cancer risk (245,246). These studies were small, however, and potentially important confounders (e.g., age and parity) were not accounted for in the analyses. Since this time, several additional studies have assessed this relationship and together indicate that a protective effect of typical doses used in postmenopausal hormone therapy can be ruled out (231). Prospective studies reporting on this relationship had similar findings. Bergkvist et al. (247) observed an RR of 4.4 (95% CI, 0.9–22.4) among women who used estrogen plus progestin (E&P) for 6 or more years compared with never users. Women using hormones for a shorter duration did not appear to be at increased risk, but confidence intervals again were wide and did not exclude either a modest increase or a decrease in risk. In findings from the NHS (233), in which among women using progestins, about two-thirds used 10 mg of medroxyprogesterone for 14 or fewer days per month, the RR associated with current E&P use versus never use was 1.4 (95% CI, 1.2–1.7). The Breast Cancer Demonstration Project found that the risk of breast cancer went up by about 1% for every year that women took estrogen alone and about 8% for every year that they took estrogen plus progestin (248). Although these yearly increases in risk seem minimal, their accumulation over time is of concern. For example, if women take estrogen with progestin for 10 years, their risk of breast cancer will be 80% higher than if they had never used hormones (249). For both types of therapy, however, this increase in risk begins to drop after hormone use stops (231). In the pooled analysis (231), data on the postmenopausal hormone formulation were available from only 39% of women, and only 12% of these reported using E&P. The RR associated with 5 or more years of recent use, relative to never use, was 1.53. More recent case-control studies also support this increase in risk with combination E&P (250,251).

In addition to their effect on breast cancer, postmenopausal hormones also have a major impact on other aspects of women's health. Results from the Women's Health Initiative (a large randomized clinical trial) definitively show that after 5 years of use, E&P does more overall harm to women than good (40), although the WHI studied only one type and dose of E&P (Prempro); because widespread use of E&P is relatively recent, few data are available to evaluate the effect of different formulations, doses, or schedules of use of progestin on risk of breast cancer (252,253). The British Million Women Study with more than 9,000 cases of breast cancer during follow-up again confirms the excess risk of breast cancer among women currently using combination E&P and notes this is a significantly greater relative risk than among women using estrogen alone. Risk increased with duration of use, but did not vary significantly according to the progestagen content or whether use was sequential or continuous (236). The possibility remains that the dose of progestagen is important, but variation in studies to date has not allowed rigorous and valid comparisons.

Receptor Status and Histologic Subtypes of Breast Cancer

Consistent evidence from larger epidemiologic studies shows combination estrogen plus progestin and unopposed estrogen therapy are associated with increased risk of ER-positive breast cancer (254). Although the WHI did not observe any significant difference in the distribution of invasive cancer by receptor status, the trial had limited power to detect an association with fewer than 500 cases of breast cancer. Some have suggested that risk is limited to lobular subtypes of breast cancer (255), but most evidence does not support this claim and, given the higher proportion of receptor-positive tumors in lobular rather than ductal cancers, a stronger relative risk observed for lobular cancer (254) would be expected for this subset of breast cancers.

Decline in Breast Cancer Incidence

Numerous studies in the United States and internationally have reported on the decline in breast cancer incidence after 2002. Based on data from the San Francisco mammography registry, prescribing of E&P peaked in 1999. Before publication of the Heart and Estrogen/Progestin Replacement Study (HERS) the use of hormone therapy was increasing at 1% per quarter, but declined by 1% per quarter after the publication (256). This decline in prescribing continued until the publication of the WHI in 2002, at which point a more substantial decline of 18% per quarter was observed. The peak and decline through 1999 to 2002 is concordant with the HERS report (257) in 1998 showing a significant increase in coronary heart disease (CHD) in the first year of therapy among women with prevalent coronary disease, and in addition, no long-term benefit in reducing

CHD (258). The growing epidemiologic evidence published since 2000 on the adverse effects of combination therapy on breast cancer added further evidence against the use of this therapy. Based on a prevalence of use of E&P in California, Clarke et al. (259) estimate a population attributable risk (PAR or the proportion of cases caused by E&P) of up to 11% based on a prevalence of use of 30% and a relative risk of 1.4. Given that substantially higher relative risks of 2 or more have been reported (236), this estimate of the PAR is conservative. Assuming a prevalence of use of 17.5%, the average reported for California in 2001 (259), a relative risk of 1.49 gives a PAR of 7.9% and a relative risk of 2.0 gives a PAR of 14.9%.

Evidence for breast cancer incidence rates now clearly shows a parallel drop in breast cancer consistent with the pattern of decreased prescribing. The rigorous, state-of-the-art analysis by Jemal et al. (260) using joint point analysis and drawing on SEER incidence data from 1975 through 2003 shows a significant decrease in incidence of invasive breast cancer from 1999 to 2003 in all 5-year age groups from 45 years and above, and a sharp decrease largely limited to ER-positive tumors in age groups 50 to 69 between 2002 and 2003. Furthermore, although others have suggested that a 1% to 3% drop in screening mammography may account for this drop in incidence, Jemal et al. show strong evidence against this. If screening was to account for a drop in incidence, rates of *in situ* disease would also need to drop because they are almost only detected by mammography. Before screening becoming widespread, Jemal et al. show *in situ* rates were low and rose with the uptake of screening to plateau from 1999 through 2003. The lack of a drop in *in situ* cancer offers compelling evidence that a reduction in screening does not account for the drop in incidence of invasive breast cancer.

Others have analyzed SEER data over a shorter period (41) or draw on the unique resources of the California tumor registry and the health maintenance organization (HMO) data sets (261) to show similar relations between change in hormone therapy and a decrease in breast cancer incidence. Most recently, Robbins and Clarke (262) have evaluated the change in prescribing as estimated from the California Health Interview Survey (CHIS) for almost 3 million non-Hispanic white women aged 45 to 74, against the change in breast cancer incidence across 58 counties in California. This thoughtful analysis shows that from 2001 to 2004, incidence declined by 8.8% in the counties with the smallest E&P reductions, by 13.9% in those with intermediate reductions, and by 22.6% in counties with the largest reductions in combination postmenopausal hormone therapy (262). Between 2001 and 2003, CHIS data did not show any significant change in the proportion of women who reported having a mammogram in the previous 2 years, adding further evidence against this as a plausible major explanatory factor in the observed declines in incidence. Analysis of women undergoing routine mammography in San Francisco rules out a drop in screening as a cause of the decrease in incidence and confirms other reports of the changes in incidence of invasive breast cancer (263). Even more evidence in support of this relation between decrease in E&P and breast cancer comes from declines in incidence that parallel those in the United States as reported in New Zealand (264), and Germany (265). Based on these data and the IARC classification of E&P as a carcinogen, we can conclude that removal of E&P acting as a promoter accounts for this rapid drop in incidence (266).

Summary of Postmenopausal Hormone Use and Breast Cancer Risk

Although some aspects of the relationship between postmenopausal hormones and breast cancer risk remain unresolved, several areas of clear agreement have emerged. The finding of no increase in risk comparing ever users with never users is consistent and reassuring. However, much of that observation reflects the experience among short-term users and hormone use in the past, predominantly unopposed estrogen.

Overall, the findings also indicate an increased risk in two important subgroups of users: users of long duration and current users. In general, users of long duration are more likely to be current users, so in many studies these two groups overlap substantially. From a biological perspective, these are the groups one would most expect to demonstrate a relation with breast cancer risk because exogenous estrogens appear to act as a promoter at a late stage.

The increase in breast cancer risk associated with E&P use appears considerably greater than that for use of estrogen alone. The impact on risk of differing progestins and patterns of use of progestins remains to be resolved.

GENETIC SUSCEPTIBILITY TO BREAST CANCER

Hereditary Syndromes

Family history of breast cancer is an accepted risk factor for breast cancer; however, the proportion of breast cancer estimated to be caused by rare highly penetrant genes, such as BRCA1 and BRCA2 is less than 10% (267), perhaps as low as 3% (268). A few highly penetrant genes and hereditary syndromes for breast cancer are described below; however, a more extensive discussion of this topic is covered in Chapter 18. Among 2,389 incident cases of breast cancer occurring in the Nurses' Health Study between 1976 and 1988, the age-adjusted RR associated with having a maternal history of breast cancer was 1.8 (95% CI 1.5–2.0) (269). This risk rose to 2.1 if the mother's breast cancer was diagnosed before age 40. Having a sister with breast cancer was associated with an RR of 2.3, and this rose to 2.5 for having both and mother and a sister with breast cancer. Risk of developing breast cancer by age 70 for a woman 30 years of age with both a mother and sister history of breast cancer was estimated to be 17.5%. Segregation analyses of breast-cancer susceptible families showed that inheritance in these families is consistent with an autosomal-dominant mode of inheritance (270). These families represent a heterogeneous group of syndromes, such as the Li-Fraumeni syndrome (a disorder that includes predisposition to sarcomas, lung cancer, brain cancer, leukemia, lymphoma, and adrenal-cortical carcinoma), Cowden disease (a syndrome involving mucocutaneous and gastrointestinal lesions and breast cancer), and a syndrome called by some "early onset breast cancer" (270) in which breast cancer often occurs in the 20s and 30s. The molecular basis for certain of these syndromes has been established. The Li-Fraumeni syndrome is caused by germline mutations in the p53 gene (271). Cowden syndrome is caused by germline mutations of the PTEN gene (272). Rare deletion mutations in CHEK2 increase breast cancer risk (273). The breast cancer susceptibility gene on chromosome 17q was called BRCA1 and was cloned in 1994 (274). A second breast cancer susceptibility locus, BRCA2, was localized on chromosome 13q and cloned in 1995 (275). Estimates of the cumulative lifetime risk of breast cancer in BRCA1 and BRCA2 carriers range from about 85% (estimated from the families selected for linkage analysis) to 50% or even less (estimated from population-based studies) (267). The higher estimates from the linkage analysis studies could be owing to higher penetrance mutations in these families, or to ascertainment bias resulting in failure to select families in which BRCA1 and BRCA2 mutations are present but do not give rise to a sufficiently striking breast cancer predisposition to qualify for enrollment into the linkage studies. In case series from "high risk" clinics to which women with a notable family history of breast cancer are referred, BRCA1 mutations may be responsible for 20% to 30% of early-onset breast cancer (276). However, estimates in unselected breast cancer cases are much lower, in the range of 2% to 3% (276,277). Estimates for BRCA2 tend to be lower (276). In unpublished data from the NHS only 2 of 192 consecutive cases had truncation mutations in BRCA1, and 1 of 192 had a truncation mutation in BRCA2. Genetic testing and management of patients with highly penetrant mutations is discussed in Chapter 19.

"Sporadic" and Later-onset Breast Cancers

As the high-penetrance genes responsible for single gene disorders have been found, the field of genetic epidemiology has seen a shift to studies using unrelated controls, often described as association studies. This has been largely motivated by the lack of power in family-based studies if allele penetrance is low, because few members of even large families will be affected. Additional parameters can be calculated in association studies; for instance, to assess the population attributable risk for alleles associated with familial risk or specific allelic variants, it is necessary to screen population-based case series.

Low Penetrance Alleles and Breast Cancer Risk

Until recently, the main method used in the search for these low penetrance alleles has been the candidate gene approach in which polymorphic variants in genes that plausibly influence breast cancer risk are assessed in conventional epidemiologic studies (i.e., case-control or cohort studies). The principal candidates studied have been genes involved in steroid hormone metabolism, carcinogen metabolism genes, and genes that may influence cell proliferation. Despite a large number of positive reports of association in a single study, few of these reports have been replicated (278). The failure to replicate initially positive findings has been ascribed to a variety of factors, including publication bias, the "winner's curse" phenomenon (the first report of an association is often more positive than subsequent studies), underpowered studies, multiple comparisons, and genetic heterogeneity (278). The major problem with candidate gene studies may be the low prior probability associated with any specific candidate gene chosen from among the approximately 20,500 human genes. Despite this, when all published studies are combined, approximately 20% to 30% of association studies yield statistically significant pooled estimates, usually of modest effects (278,279). Until recently, none of these replicated positives have applied to breast cancer. Recent results from the Breast Cancer Association Consortium suggest a nonsynonymous polymorphism in CASP8 may be associated with lower risk of breast cancer (280).

Whole Genome Single Nucleotide Polymorphism Scans and Cancer Susceptibility

In contrast to the candidate gene approach, genome-wide association studies (GWAS) offer the potential to conduct a comprehensive and unbiased search for modest associations (281). The generation of a draft sequence of the human genome led to subsequent efforts to define the spectrum of variability in the sequence. The largest such effort, the International HapMap, released the genotypes of its second stage late in 2005, and it provides a database of common single nucleotide polymorphisms (SNP) (defined as SNP with minor allele frequency, minor allele frequency (MAF), >5%) at an average spacing of every 1,250 bases across the 3 billion base pairs of genomic sequence (282). Analysis of this dataset indicates that more than 90% of the nearly 10 million common SNP estimated to exist are highly correlated with at least one other SNP (a phenomenon known as *linkage disequilibrium*). This observation suggests that much of the information on genetic variation can be extracted with the genotyping of a carefully chosen subset of SNP called *tagSNP*, which can serve as surrogates for untested SNP. The informativeness of a set of tagSNP can be increased by selecting SNP that maximize the r^2 to untyped SNP in a region, and further increased by ranking SNP according to the number of proxies they have (283). The extent of diversity in population genetics history is evident in the substantial differences in patterns of linkage disequilibrium between the three continental populations studied in the International HapMap Project, namely, European, East Asian and West African. For example, in the East Asian and European populations 500,000 to 600,000 tagSNP are required to capture approximately 90% or more of common SNP variation. For the African population, this subset may be twice as large because the inter-SNP correlations are on average lower. Thus, in populations of European ancestry, assessment of 500,000 to 600,000 tagSNP in an adequate number of cases and controls should permit genome-wide studies of susceptibility to specific cancers and cancer-related quantitative traits.

Replication in Whole Genome SNP Studies

Testing 500,000 or more independent SNP at conventional levels of statistical significance will generate a very large number of *statistically significant* results. Consideration of other factors, such as whether an SNP is in a known candidate gene pathway, or a candidate genomic region (identified for instance, by previous linkage analyses or cytogenetic abnormalities in tumors) might be useful in advancing SNP of interest, but because so little is known about most of the genes in the genome, this exercise will only apply to a small portion of genic regions. Thus, although there is considerable novelty for the first whole genome scan conducted for a specific disease, the reality is that it does not do much more than identify a list of SNP for further testing in follow-up replication studies.

Simulations, however, have shown that carefully designed multistage studies in which the best candidate SNP identified in the first stage are advanced in subsequent studies of comparable cases and controls, maintain high statistical power and enable a substantial decrease in genotyping cost (284,285).

Results from Three Genome-wide Scans of Breast Cancer

Results from three GWAS (286–288) for breast cancer were published in 2007. The three studies identified six loci as strongly associated with breast cancer risk, four of which contained genes (*FGFR2*, *TNRC9*, *MAP3K1* and *LSP1*) plausibly related to breast cancer. Larger scale replication of the Cancer Genetic Markers of Susceptibility-Nurses' Health Study (CGEMS-NHS) scan is underway with more than 28,000 variants being tested in more than 4,000 cases in a large-scale, second stage of a multistage design; these data should be available in 2008. The variants identified so far have all had modest effect sizes (RR = 1.2–1.6 per allele), emphasizing the need for large-scale replication. Studies have also been mainly conducted in postmenopausal breast cancer cases. In the CGEMS-NHS (287), the RR for SNP in *FGFR2* for premenopausal women in the NHSII were similar to those in postmenopausal and older-onset breast cancer case series, demonstrating the generalizability of the findings for this gene to premenopausal cases. The strongest association observed in a fourth GWAS, conducted among women of Ashkenazi Jewish ancestry, was with *FGFR2*; this analysis also suggested a new locus at chromosome 6q22 (289).

These findings, and additional loci that will almost certainly be discovered in further follow-up of these and further GWAS,

have established new loci that collectively are likely to robustly identify a much larger fraction of women at modest genetic risk of breast cancer, than the very small fraction at very high risk identifiable through analysis of the high penetrance genes such as *BRCA1* and *BRCA2*. Deriving the appropriate risk prediction models, and then understanding how they can be applied clinically, will be a substantial challenge over the next several years.

 ## DIETARY FACTORS

Nutritional factors have been prominent among the hypothesized environmental determinants of breast cancer that account for the large variation in breast cancer incidence around the world and the large increases in rates among the offspring of migrants from countries with low incidence to countries with high incidence. The dominant hypothesis has been that high-fat intake increases risk. In this section, evidence for this relationship is reviewed and alternative hypotheses are suggested.

Dietary Fat and Breast Cancer

Animal Studies

High-fat diets have long been known to increase the occurrence of mammary tumors in rodents. However, the interpretation of these and other animal data is controversial. Fat is the most energy-dense macronutrient (9 kcal/g compared with 4 kcal/g for protein and carbohydrate); thus, high-fat diets tend to be higher in energy intake unless care is taken to keep energy intake constant. Many animal experiments have not done this, resulting in confounding of fat consumption by energy intake. In a meta-analysis of diet and mammary cancer experiments in mice, Albanes (290) observed a weak inverse association with fat composition (adjusted for energy), whereas total energy intake was positively associated with mammary tumor incidence. Freedman et al. (291) conducted a similar meta-analysis of experiments in both rats and mice and reported that both higher fat intake and higher caloric intake independently increase mammary tumor incidence. In studies specifically designed to determine the independent effects of fat and energy intake, the effect of fat was either weak in relation to that of energy intake (292) or nonexistent (293). Furthermore, the relevance to human experience of rodent models in which animals are given high doses of specific carcinogens, to which humans are rarely exposed, is questionable. Notably, in a very large study of rats and mice fed substantially different amounts of corn oil without administration of a carcinogen, no effect of fat intake was found on spontaneous mammary cancer incidence (294). In a case-control study in dogs, fat intake, which ranged from 10% to 70% of energy, was not associated with risk of breast cancer (295). The clearest message from the animal data is the importance of total energy intake and the need to consider energy balance in epidemiologic studies.

International Correlation (Ecologic) Studies

The dietary fat hypothesis is largely based on the observation that national per capita fat consumption is highly correlated with breast cancer mortality rates (296). A serious problem with ecologic comparisons of diet and breast cancer is the potential for confounding by known and suspected breast cancer risk factors. National fat consumption per capita is highly correlated with level of economic development; thus, any factor that characterizes affluent Western countries would also be correlated with national rates of breast cancer. Prentice et al. (297) found that the ecologic relation between fat consumption and breast cancer incidence rates was still statistically significant after adjustment for Gross National Product (GNP) per capita and average age at menarche. However, other breast cancer risk factors such as low parity, late age at first birth, greater body fat, and lower levels of physical activity are more prevalent in Western countries and would be expected to confound the association with dietary fat. Thus, there is good reason to question whether the international correlation between fat intake and breast cancer represents a causal relationship.

Secular Trends

Estimates of per capita fat consumption based on *food disappearance* data (the food available rather than the amount actually eaten) and breast cancer incidence rates have both increased substantially in the United States during the 20th century. Surveys based on measures of actual individual intake, rather than food disappearance, indicate, however, that consumption of fat as a percentage of energy has declined in the last several decades, a time during which breast cancer incidence has increased. Higher dietary fat consumption has been implicated in the increase in breast cancer incidence in Japan since 1950. However, this increase could also be owing to the increasing prevalence of reproductive and other lifestyle risk factors that characterize Western populations.

The famine that occurred in Norway during World War II provided a natural experiment on the effects of nutritional deprivation on breast cancer risk (298). Women who were adolescents during the famine have subsequently experienced a reduction in breast cancer risk (about 13% lower) at all ages. These data on time trends indicate the sensitivity of breast cancer rates to nutritional and lifestyle factors, but do not specifically support a role of dietary fat.

Data from special populations with distinct dietary patterns are valuable, because adherence to a particular diet over many years may represent a more stable long-term exposure than that applicable to most free-living adults whose diet may change substantially over time. Because these populations often have unusual distributions of nondietary potential risk factors, such as alcohol consumption, smoking, and reproductive behavior, care must be taken in attributing differences in cancer rates to diet alone. Seventh-Day Adventists, who consume relatively small amounts of meat and other animal products, have substantially lower rates of colon cancer, but only slightly lower breast cancer rates than other U.S. white women of similar socioeconomic status (299). Breast cancer rates among British nuns who ate no meat, or very little meat, were similar to rates among single women from the general population (300), also suggesting no substantial association exists between animal fat and risk of breast cancer.

Case-control Studies

In a typical case-control study of diet and breast cancer, the diet before diagnosis reported by women with breast cancer (cases) is compared with the diet reported by women who have not been diagnosed with breast cancer. An early large study was that of Graham et al. (301), who used a food frequency questionnaire to compare the fat intake of 2,024 women with breast cancer with that reported by 1,463 female controls seen at the hospital with benign conditions. Animal fat and total fat intake were almost identical in the two groups. In a meta analysis, Howe et al. (302) summarized the results from 12 smaller case-control studies, including 4,312 cases and 5,978 controls. The overall pooled RR for a 100-g increase in daily total fat intake was 1.35; the risk was somewhat stronger for postmenopausal women (RR = 1.48). Because the average total fat consumption is about 70 g/day for U.S. women, a reduction in fat intake as large as 100 g would be impossible for almost all women. The results of this pooled analysis suggest that even if the reported

positive association were correct, the RR for readily achievable changes in total fat intake would be relatively small; for example, the reduction in risk for a 20-g/day decrease among postmenopausal women (corresponding to a decrease from 40% to 29% of calories for a typical middle-aged women) would be only about 0.9. Furthermore, RR of this magnitude in case-control studies may easily be owing to selection bias (the controls are drawn from a population with a different distribution of fat intake than the distribution in the population that gave rise to the cases) or recall bias (the cases, knowing their diagnosis, differentially misreport their prediagnosis diet) (303).

Cohort Studies

In a cohort (prospective) study, the diets of a large group of women are measured and the subsequent rates of breast cancer among those with different levels of dietary factors are compared. Selection bias should not be a problem because the population that gave rise to the cases is known (the starting members of the cohort), and recall bias should not occur because dietary information is collected before knowledge of disease. The results for postmenopausal breast cancer (for which fat intake has been hypothesized to be strongest because the international differences are greatest for this group) from prospective studies with at least 200 incident cases of breast cancer are shown in Table 20.1 (304–315). The number of breast cancer cases in these studies is similar to the number in the pooled analysis of case-control studies referred to earlier, and the size of the comparison series (i.e., noncases) is much larger. In not a single study was a significant association with total fat intake observed (comparing the highest with the lowest category of total fat intake). A collaborative pooled analysis has been conducted that included most of the prospective studies shown in Table 20.1 that included 4,980 cases of breast cancer among 337,819 women (316). In addition to providing great statistical precision, the pooled analysis allowed standard analytic approaches to be applied to all studies, an examination of a wider range of fat intake, and a detailed evaluation of interactions with other breast cancer risk factors. Overall, no association was observed between intake of total, saturated, monounsaturated, or polyunsaturated fat and risk of breast cancer. As noted in Figure 20.9, no reduction in risk was seen even for fat intakes as low as 20% of energy. When the relatively few women with fat intake lower than 15% of energy were examined, their risk of breast cancer was actually increased twofold; this could not be accounted for by other dietary or nondietary factors.

Substudies were available for each cohort in the pooled analysis in which the measurement errors of the dietary questionnaires were quantified and these were used to adjust the overall RR and CI to take into account errors in measuring diet. Without correction, the RR for a 25-g/day increment in fat intake was 1.02 (95% CI, 0.94–1.11). After accounting for measurement error, the RR was 1.07 (95% CI, 0.86–1.34). The upper bound of the adjusted 95% CI excludes the RR of 1.4 to 1.5 predicted by the international correlations. In calculations based on a series of theoretic assumptions, Prentice (316a) has claimed that the pooled analysis of breast cancer failed to find a positive association because the measurement error correction did not account for underreporting of fat by more obese women. However, actual studies do not support this assumption, and the other predictions based on this theoretic model are also not supported by the data (317). In analyses with extended follow-up of these cohorts (7,329 cases of breast cancer), the lack of association with total fat intake was confirmed (RR for an increment of 5% of energy from fat per day = 1.00) (95% CI, 0.98–1.03) (318). In the NHS, additional analyses have been conducted with 20 years of follow-up (3,537 postmenopausal cases) (319); up to six assessments of fat intake

Table 20.1	RESULTS FROM LARGE PROSPECTIVE STUDIES OF TOTAL AND SATURATED FAT INTAKE AND RISK OF BREAST CANCER				
				Relative Risk (95% CI) (High vs. Low Category)	
Study (Reference)	Total No. in Cohort	Years of Follow-Up	No. of Cases	Total Fat	Saturated Fat
Nurses' Health Study (314)	89,494	8	1,439	0.86 (0.67–1.08)	0.86 (0.73–1.02)
Nurses' Health Study (305)	88,795	14	2,956	0.97 (0.94–1.00)[a]	0.94 (0.88–1.01)[a]
Canadian Study (307)	56,837	5	519	1.30 (0.90–1.88)	1.08 (0.73–1.60)
New York State Cohort (304)	17,401	7	344	1.00 (0.59–1.70)	1.12 (0.78–1.61)[b]
Iowa Women's Study (308)	32,080	4	408	1.13 (0.84–1.51)	1.10 (0.83–1.46)
Dutch Health Study (312)	62,573	3	471	1.08 (0.73–1.59)	1.39 (0.94–2.06)
Adventists Health Study (310)	20,341	6	193		1.21 (0.81–1.81)
Swedish Mammography Screening Cohort (315)	61,471	6	674	1.00 (0.76–1.32)	1.09 (0.83–1.42)
Breast Cancer Detection Demo Project (313)	40,022	5	996	1.07 (0.86–1.32)	1.12 (0.87–1.45)
California Teachers Study (306)	115,526	2	711	0.8 (0.6–1.2)	0.8 (0.6–1.2)
NIH–AARP study (311)	188,736	4	3,501	1.11 (1.0–1.24)	1.18 (1.06–1.31)
Malmö Diet Cohort (309)	11,726	10	342	1.36 (0.96–1.94)	—

[a]Animal fat.
[b]Continuous.

were available, which substantially improves the measurement of long-term dietary intake. The RR for a 5% increase in percentage of energy from total fat was 0.98 (95% CI, 0.95–1.00), and no suggestion of any reduction in risk was seen for fat intakes even lower than 20% of energy (305). Thus, the prospective studies provide strong evidence that no major relation exists between total dietary fat intake over a wide range during midlife and breast cancer incidence. It remains possible that total fat intake during childhood or early adult life may affect breast cancer risk decades later. Notably, in the NHSII, which was established to evaluate the influence of dietary and other potential risk factors earlier in life, intake of animal fat (but not vegetable fat) before menopause was positively associated with risk of breast cancer (320). This finding, which needs to be replicated, was mainly caused by consumption of red meat and high-fat dairy products.

Intervention Studies

Some have suggested that the relation between dietary fat and breast cancer can be established only by randomized trials of fat reduction. In the WHI, 48,835 women were randomly assigned either to reduce their total fat intake to 20% of calories from fat or to their regular diet (321). After 8 years of follow-up, the RR for the low fat compared with the control group was 0.91; 95% CI, 0.83-1.0, p = .09), indicating so significant benefit of the intervention. However, as has been the experience in other large dietary intervention trials (322), maintaining compliance with a diet very different from prevailing food consumption habits proved to be difficult, and the reported difference in fat intake between groups was only 8% of energy at year 6 rather than the 14% of energy anticipated. Moreover, self-reported compliance in dietary intervention studies tends to be over reported, and no differences were seen between groups in blood levels of high-density lipoprotein (HDL) cholesterol or triglycerides (323). Because reduction in dietary fat would be expected to reduce HDL cholesterol and increase triglycerides (324), this lack of effect on blood lipids suggests that the WHI did not really address the dietary fat and breast cancer hypothesis, despite being the most expensive study ever conducted. Prentice et al. (321) suggested that, even though not significant, the slightly lower (9%) risk of breast cancer in the low fat group may represent a real effect of fat reduction that may become significant with longer follow-up. Even if a significant effect were to be seen, it would not be possible, however, to conclude that this was owing to reduction in dietary fat because there was an approximately 1.5 kg weight loss in the low fat group, which is typically seen with intensive dietary interventions independent of percentage of energy from dietary fat

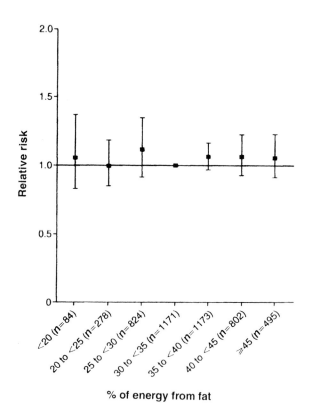

FIGURE 20.9. Pooled relative breast cancer risk and 95% confidence intervals (CI) associated with percentage of energy derived from fat intake. (Reproduced from Hunter DJ, Spiegelman D, Adami HO, et al. Cohort studies of fat intake and the risk of breast cancer: a pooled analysis. *N Engl J Med* 1996;334:356–361, with permission.)

(325). This degree of weight loss, although modest, could account for most of a 9% difference in breast cancer risk (326). Furthermore, as pointed out by the WHI investigators, women in the dietary intervention group were counseled to adopt a dietary pattern that is high in fruits, vegetables, and grain products and low in total fat and saturated fat (327). Thus, the trial is unable to distinguish between a decrease in risk owing to increased intake of fruit, vegetable, and grains or a decrease because of lower fat intake. Also, this trial could not address whether dietary fat reduction at an earlier age may reduce breast cancer risk. The lack of association with fat intake in the 20-year follow-up of the NHS (319) suggests that insufficient follow-up time is not a likely explanation for the nonsignificant results of the WHI trial. Another trial of fat reduction among women at high risk of breast cancer is ongoing in Canada (328).

Type of Fat

In addition to overall fat intake, specific types of fat could differentially affect risk of breast cancer. In most animal studies, diets high in polyunsaturated fat (linoleic acid), but typically at levels beyond human exposure, have clearly increased the occurrence of mammary tumors. As noted earlier, however, a positive association has not been found in prospective epidemiologic studies (318).

Some animal studies have suggested that monounsaturated fat, in the form of olive oil, may be protective relative to other sources of energy (329); the abundant antioxidants in this oil could contribute to this effect. In a Spanish study specifically undertaken because of the high consumption of olive oil and low breast cancer rates in this population, no association was observed with total fat intake (330). Higher intake of olive oil was, however, associated with reduced risk of breast cancer. Similar inverse associations with olive oil or monounsaturated fat were seen in case-control studies in Greece, Italy, and Spain (331). In the pooled analysis of cohort studies (318), saturated fat (compared with carbohydrate) was weakly associated with higher risk of breast cancer (RR for 5% of energy = 1.09, 95% CI, 1.00–1.19), and compared with monounsaturated fat, the RR was 1.18 (95% CI, 0.99–1.42).

High intake of N3-fatty acids from marine oils has inhibited the occurrence of mammary tumors in animals. However, case-control and cohort studies generally have not found intake of N3-fatty acids or fish (the major source of long-chain N3-fatty acids) to be associated with lower risk of breast cancer (305,331).

Height, Weight, and the Risk of Breast Cancer

As noted earlier, energy restriction powerfully reduces mammary tumor incidence in rodents (290,291). This relationship is difficult to evaluate directly in humans because estimates by adults of their energy intake, especially during childhood, are unlikely to be sufficiently precise and any analysis would also need to account for physical activity with high accuracy. However, because children who experience energy deprivation during growth do not attain their full potential height, attained height may be used as a proxy for childhood energy intake, although this is not a specific indicator because protein restriction and genetic factors also affect stature. In Japan, for instance, a substantial increase in average height has occurred during the 20th century, presumably because of improved nutrition. Among countries, height is positively correlated with breast cancer rates (332), supporting the hypothesis that childhood and adolescent energy intake may influence breast cancer rates decades later.

Most of the case-control and cohort studies of attained height and risk of breast cancer suggest a modest positive association (333). In a follow-up of the National Health and Nutrition Examination Survey-I (NHANES-I) population in which women at risk for malnutrition had been oversampled, a nearly twofold increase in risk was observed across the range for weights (334). Height was positively associated with later age at menarche (protective against breast cancer) and late age at first birth, low parity, higher socioeconomic status, and alcohol use (risk factors for breast cancer), suggesting that height may be confounded by other cancer risk factors (334). However, controlling for these variables in multivariate analyses had little influence on the association between height and breast cancer. In a pooled analysis of large cohort studies (4,385 cases among 337,819 women), the RR for an increment of 5 cm of height were 1.02 (95% CI, 0.96–1.10) for premenopausal women and 1.07 (95% CI, 1.03–1.12) for postmenopausal women (335) (Fig. 20.10) and, in a recent meta-analysis of 15 published cohort studies, the RR for a 5-cm increment was 1.11 (95% CI 1.09–1.13) among postmenopausal women and 1.09 (1.05–1.14) among premenopausal women (336). In the studies of Vatten and Kvinnsland (337,338), the positive trend between height and risk of breast cancer was most nearly linear in the birth cohort of women who lived through their peripubertal period during World War II (1929–1932), a time in which food was scarce and average attained greater height reduced. Collectively, these data provide convincing evidence that attained greater height is associated with a modest increased risk of breast cancer.

Age at menarche, an established risk factor for breast cancer, provides a second indirect indicator of energy balance during childhood. Nutritional factors, in particular energy balance, appear to be the major determinants of age at menarche. In prospective studies among young girls, the major predictors of age at menarche were weight, height, and body fatness (339–342). A marginally significant inverse association between dietary fat and age at menarche was seen in one study (341), but no relation was observed in others. The potential for energy balance to influence breast cancer risk through age at menarche is greater than might be appreciated by examining the distribution of this variable in modern Western countries. Although the average age at menarche in these countries is now 12 to 13 years, in rural China the typical age has been approximately 17 to 18 years (343), similar to that of Western countries 200 years ago. An effect of growth rate on breast cancer risk may begin even before birth, because an inverse relation between birth weight and breast cancer risk has been observed, mainly in premenopausal women (344,345).

The relation between preadolescent body fatness and risk of breast cancer appears to be complex; although greater adiposity reduces the age at menarche, adiposity at this age has been associated with lower rather than greater risk of breast cancer (344,346). Notably, in the NHSII cohort, women who were the most overweight at ages 5 and 10 had only half the risk of breast cancer before menopause compared with those who were the leanest at these ages (346), and adjustment for age at menarche had little effect on this association. This finding has been hypothesized to be owing to earlier differentiation of breast tissue and reduced susceptibility to carcinogens (344), but further examination of these relationships is needed.

The mechanisms by which age at menarche and attained height are related to risk of breast cancer are probably multiple. Early onset of menstrual cycles exposes the breast to ovarian hormones at a younger age and for a longer duration over a lifetime. Also, in several studies, an early age at menarche has been associated with higher estrogen levels at later ages (347). Height has been suggested to be a surrogate for mammary gland mass (348), which may be related to higher risk, or it may be a surrogate for exposure to high levels of IGF-I or other anabolic hormones during childhood. IGF-I is directly involved in regulation of growth during childhood and is hypothesized to increase risk of breast cancer, although the relation of blood levels during adulthood to cancer risk is complex and remains

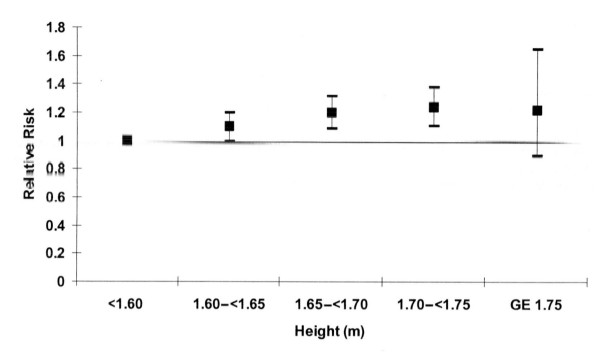

FIGURE 20.10. Results of prospective studies of the association between height and breast cancer. (Reproduced from van den Brandt PA, Spiegelman D, Yaun SS, et al. Pooled analysis of prospective cohort studies on height, weight, and breast cancer risk. *Am J Epidemiol* 2000;152:514–527, with permission.)

unsettled (173). IGF-I levels are determined, in part, by genetic factors, but energy restriction reduces IGF-I levels, and infusion of IGF-I appears to negate the effects of energy restriction tumorigenesis in animals (349). Also, high consumption of dairy products increases blood levels of IGF-1 (350–356) and, in addition, it appears to accelerate growth in height (355,357). However, data on milk consumption during childhood and risk of breast cancer are limited.

Weight and Weight Change during Adulthood

Attained weight and weight change in adults provide sensitive measures of the balance between long-term energy intake and expenditure. Although the relation between these variables and breast cancer risk has been complex and confusing, recent findings provide a coherent picture and indicate a major contribution of weight gain during adulthood to risk of postmenopausal breast cancer risk. Two reproducible findings have been particularly enigmatic: (a) In affluent Western populations with high rates of breast cancer, measures of body fatness have been *inversely* related to risk of premenopausal breast cancer, and (b) body fatness has been only weakly related to postmenopausal breast cancer risk despite strong associations between body fat and endogenous estrogen levels.

The inverse relation between body weight (typically used as body mass index [BMI], calculated as weight in kilograms divided by height in squared meters, to account for variation in height) and incidence of premenopausal breast cancer has been consistently seen in recent prospective studies (241,335) and in a meta-analysis of 14 cohort studies (336). In the most recent meta-analysis, the RR for a 2-unit increment in BMI was 0.94 (95% CI, 0.92–0.95) (336). Little relation of BMI to breast cancer mortality has been observed in premenopausal women, probably because delayed detection and diagnosis in heavier women counterbalances the lower incidence among heavier women. Heavier premenopausal women, even at the upper limits of what are considered to be healthy weights, have more

irregular menstrual cycles and increased rates of anovulatory infertility (358), suggesting that their lower risk may be owing to fewer ovulatory cycles and less exposure to ovarian hormones. Increased rates of menstrual irregularity and anovulatory infertility are also seen among very lean women, but such women are uncommon in Western populations. Although irregular menstrual cycles have been associated with reduced risk of breast cancer (57), adjustment for details of menstrual characteristics accounted for little of the inverse relation between BMI and risk of premenopausal breast cancer (359). This suggests that other factors, yet to be determined, account for most of the lower risk of breast cancer among overweight premenopausal women.

In both case-control and prospective studies conducted in affluent Western countries, the association between BMI and risk of breast cancer among postmenopausal breast cancer has often been only weakly positive or nonexistent (302,333, 335). The lack of a stronger association has been surprising because obese postmenopausal women have plasma levels of endogenous estrogens nearly twice as high as those of lean women, because of conversion of androstenedione to estrogens in adipose tissue, as well as lower levels of SHBG (360). The lack of a stronger positive association appears to be owing to two factors. First, as with the protective effect of early pregnancy, the reduction in breast cancer risk associated with being overweight in early adult life appears to persist through later life (241,361). Thus, an elevated BMI in a postmenopausal woman represents two opposing risks: a protective effect owing to the correlation between early weight and postmenopausal weight and an adverse effect owing to elevated estrogens after menopause. For this reason, weight *gain* from early adult life to after menopause should be more strongly related to postmenopausal breast cancer risk than would attained weight. Indeed, the relation between weight gain and risk of postmenopausal breast cancer has been consistently supported by both case-control (362–364) and prospective studies (241,336,361,365,366). A second reason for

Weight Change, Hormone Use and Postmenopausal Breast Cancer

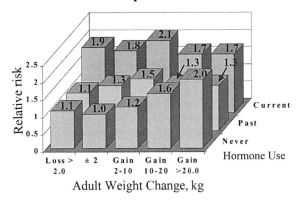

FIGURE 20.11. Relative risk (RR) of breast cancer by adult weight change and hormone use among postmenopausal women. (Reproduced from Huang Z, Hankinson SE, Colditz GA, et al. Dual effects of weight and height gain on breast cancer risk. *JAMA* 1997;278: 1407–1411, with permission.)

failing to appreciate a greater adverse effect of excessive weight or weight gain on risk of postmenopausal breast cancer is that the use of postmenopausal hormones obscures the variation in endogenous estrogens because of adiposity and elevates breast cancer risk regardless of body weight (241,366). To appreciate fully the impact of weight or weight gain, an analysis should be limited to women who never used postmenopausal hormones. Thus, among women who never used postmenopausal hormones in the NHS, those who gained 25 kg or more after age 18 years had double the risk of breast cancer compared with women who maintained their weight within 2 kg (241) (Fig. 20.11). In this population, the combination of either using postmenopausal hormones or gaining weight after age 18 years accounted for one-third of postmenopausal breast cancer cases. Greater BMI has generally been more strongly associated with breast cancer mortality than with incidence (241,367). This may relate to greater difficulty in detecting small tumors in fatter breasts, which could influence prognosis, as well as the greater endogenous estrogen levels.

The relation between body weight and breast cancer risk among lower risk mainly non-Western countries is somewhat different in higher risk countries (368). In general, the inverse relation between weight and premenopausal breast cancer risk has not been observed, and the association between weight and postmenopausal risk has been stronger. This difference is likely to be owing to the lower prevalence of overweight among premenopausal women in these low-risk countries; few women are likely to be sufficiently overweight to cause anovulation and a reduction in premenopausal breast cancer risk. As a result, BMI after menopause would only reflect the adverse effects of high endogenous estrogens, unopposed by a residual protective effect owing to correlation with overweight in early adult life.

In summary, as in animal studies, energy balance appears to play an important but complex role in the causation of human breast cancer. During childhood, rapid growth rates accelerate the occurrence of menarche, an established risk factor, and result in greater attained stature, which has been consistently associated with increased risk. During early adult life, overweight is associated with a lower incidence of breast cancer before menopause, but no reduction in breast cancer mortality. Weight gain after age 18 years is associated with a graded

and substantial increase in postmenopausal breast cancer that is seen most clearly in the absence of hormone replacement therapy.

Dietary Fiber

Diets high in fiber have been hypothesized to protect against breast cancer, perhaps because of inhibition of the intestinal reabsorption of estrogens excreted via the biliary system. A high-fiber diet was associated with reduced incidence of mammary cancer in animals (329). Dietary fiber includes crude fiber that is excreted unchanged, and various soluble fiber fractions that may have different biologic effects. In a meta-analysis of 10 case-control studies with estimates of dietary fiber intake, a statistically significant RR of 0.85 for a 20-g/day increase in dietary fiber was observed (302). Prospective studies have been less supportive (314,369–373). In the NHS, for example, the association between total dietary fiber intake and subsequent breast cancer incidence (1,439 cases) was very close to null (314), suggesting that any protective effect of dietary fiber is unlikely to be large. The possibility remains, however, that certain subfractions of fiber intake may be relevant to breast cancer causation.

Micronutrients

Vitamin A

Vitamin A consists of preformed vitamin A (retinol, retinyl esters, and related compounds) from animal sources and certain carotenoids found primarily in fruits and vegetables that are partially converted to retinol in the intestinal epithelium (carotenoid vitamin A). Many carotenoids are potent antioxidants and, thus, may provide a cellular defense against reactive oxygen species, which damage DNA. Vitamin A is also a regulator of cell differentiation and may prevent the emergence of cells with a malignant phenotype. Retinol inhibits the growth of human breast carcinoma cells *in vitro* (374), and retinyl acetate reduces breast cancer incidence in some rodent models (375).

Human studies of vitamin A intake and breast cancer have mostly been case-control studies; thus, their interpretation is limited by uncertainty about the extent to which selection and recall bias may have altered the observed associations. In the earliest large case-control study of total vitamin A intake (retinol plus carotenoids vitamin A) (301), an RR of 0.8 between the highest quartile of vitamin A consumption and the lowest was seen, with a significant inverse trend in risk with increased vitamin A consumption. In a meta-analysis of nine other case-control studies with data on vitamin A intake (302), a significant protective association between total vitamin A and breast cancer was reported. When preformed vitamin A and carotenoids were examined separately, however, the data from these case-control studies are more strongly supportive of a protective association for carotenoid vitamin A than for preformed vitamin A. More recently, specific carotenoids have been examined in case-control studies (376). Inverse associations were observed between dietary intakes of β-carotene and lutein/zeaxanthin and risk of breast cancer in premenopausal women.

The limited available prospective data suggest a possible modest inverse relation between vitamin A and breast cancer. In a cohort of Canadian women (519 cases) (371), a marginally significant protective association between total vitamin A intake and breast cancer was seen, with both preformed vitamin A and β-carotene contributing to the inverse association. With 14 years of follow-up in the NHS (2,697 cases), an inverse association with total vitamin A was seen only among premenopausal women (377). This inverse association was primarily accounted for by carotenoid sources of vitamin A; when specific carotenoids were examined, intakes of β-carotene and lutein/zeaxanthin were associated with reduced risk, but intake of lycopene was not. The inverse associations with specific carotenoids were strongest among women with a family history of breast cancer. In an extended follow-up of the Canadian cohort (1,452 cases), and in a Swedish cohort (1,271 cases), little overall association was seen between intake of carotenoids and breast cancer (378,379).

An alternative to the dietary assessment of vitamin A intake is the measurement of vitamin A compounds in blood. Most studies have assessed blood retinol, however, and are minimally informative about vitamin A intake in well-nourished populations because the liver maintains relatively constant blood retinol concentrations. Blood levels of β-carotene do reflect β carotene intake, however. Little consistency exists among these studies (333,380), however, probably related in part to their small size. In three of the largest studies based on bloods collected before diagnosis, low levels of β-carotene and other carotenoids were associated with an approximately twofold increase in risk of breast cancer (381–383).

Thus, available data are suggestive, but not conclusive, of a modest protective effect of vitamin A intake on breast cancer, although the evidence is stronger for benefits of carotenoid sources of vitamin A. Also, evidence of benefit is stronger for premenopausal women. It is possible that other anticarcinogens in vegetables and fruits, including carotenoids such as lutein, are responsible for the apparent benefits. Ideally, the effect of vitamin A supplements, in the form of either preformed vitamin A or carotenoids, should be evaluated in randomized trials. In a randomized trial of fenretinide, a powerful synthetic retinoid, in the prevention of contralateral breast cancer among women already diagnosed with a first breast cancer, no overall effect was seen (384), although a significant benefit was seen in premenopausal women. The Women's Health Study of 40,000 female health professionals is a randomized trial designed to test whether β-carotene or vitamin E supplements reduce breast cancer risk. However, the β-carotene arm was terminated in 1996 after reports from trials in Finland and the United States that β-carotene supplements appeared to increase risk of lung cancer among smoking men. Thus, data from randomized trials on specific carotenoids and breast cancer risk, particularly among premenopausal women, may never be available. In lieu of such data, further prospective studies of blood levels of carotenoids and breast cancer are desirable.

Vitamin E

Vitamin E is also an antioxidant and has inhibited mammary tumors in rodents in some, but not all, experiments (385). Although relatively few studies have assessed the association between dietary vitamin E intake and breast cancer, none of the published prospective studies has reported a significant inverse association (371,377,378,386). In the largest of these (377), no evidence was seen of a protective effect with use of vitamin E supplements, even at high doses for a long duration. In a 10-year randomized trial using 600 IU of vitamin E on alternate days, there was no effect on breast cancer incidence (387).

Vitamin C

Vitamin C (ascorbic acid) is also an antioxidant and can block the formation of carcinogenic nitrosamines. Few animal studies have assessed the effect of vitamin C on mammary cancer;

in a study in rats, no effect of ascorbic acid was seen on the growth of either transplanted or dimethyl benzanthracene-induced mammary tumors (388).

In a meta-analysis of nine case-control studies with data on vitamin C (302), a significant inverse association (RR = 0.7 for each 300-mg/day increase in vitamin C) was observed. In prospective studies, however, no significant overall association between intake of vitamin C and breast cancer was observed (369,371,377,378,386,389). In the 14-year follow-up of the NHS, no evidence of any reduction in risk was seen with long-term use of vitamin C supplements (377). Thus, the available prospective data do not support benefits of high vitamin C intake for reducing breast cancer risk.

Vitamin D

Vitamin D and its metabolites can reduce cell proliferation, enhance apoptosis, and inhibit tumor progression in animal models (390). Epidemiologic studies provide some support for a reduced risk of breast cancer with higher intake, particularly in premenopausal women (391–393). However, vitamin D is unique among nutrients in that the dominant source is obtained by the action of sunlight on a precursor molecule in the skin, rather than by diet. Plasma levels of 25-OH vitamin D (25(OH)D) provide an integrated biomarker of vitamin D from all sources that can be used in epidemiologic studies. Although many studies have shown an inverse relation between plasma 25-OH vitamin D levels and risk of colon cancer (394), the epidemiologic evidence is much more limited for breast cancer. In the largest prospective study to date, women in the highest quintile of 25(OH)D had a RR of 0.73 (95% CI = 0.49–1.07; P-trend = 0.06) compared with those in the lowest quintile (395). Because 25-OH vitamin D levels can be readily increased by supplements, resolution of the relationship between vitamin D and risk of breast cancer should be a high priority.

Selenium

Selenium, an important component of the antioxidant enzyme glutathione peroxidase, inhibits cell proliferation and, in animal studies, protects against a variety of cancers, although usually at high levels of intake (396). Ecologic studies have shown strong inverse associations between county-specific (in the United States) and national measures of selenium exposure and breast cancer rates (397). Selenium intake cannot be measured accurately by means of dietary assessment in geographically dispersed populations because of the high variability in the selenium content of individual foods, depending on the geographic area in which the foods were grown. However, selenium levels in tissues such as blood and toenails do reflect selenium intake (398) and thus provide an informative measure of diet.

Several studies using these biomarkers of selenium intake have been performed. In most prospective studies (399–401), no association between toenail selenium and risk of breast cancer has been observed. Of the prospective studies, only that of Knekt et al. (402) from Finland showed any evidence of an increased risk among women in the lowest category of selenium. Because Finland at that time had extremely low selenium intakes, this observation is consistent with the possibility that a threshold exists below which low selenium intake does increase breast cancer risk. In a small randomized trial, breast cancer was the only malignancy that occurred more often among those receiving selenium supplements (403). Taken together, these data suggest that increases in selenium intake are unlikely to reduce risk of breast cancer

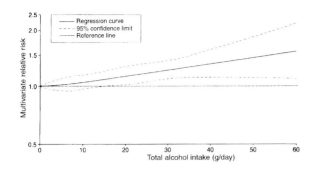

FIGURE 20.12. Nonparametric regression for the relationship between total alcohol intake and breast cancer. One drink of beer, wine, or liquor equals 12 to 15 g of alcohol. (From Smith-Warner SA, Spiegelman D, Yaun S-S, et al. Alcohol and breast cancer in women: a pooled analysis of cohort studies. *JAMA* 1998;279:535–540, with permission.)

in countries with existing moderate or high levels of selenium intake.

Other Dietary Constituents

Alcohol

Substantial evidence now supports the existence of a positive association between alcohol consumption and breast cancer risk (336).

In a pooled analysis of the six largest cohort studies with data on alcohol and dietary factors (404), the risk of breast cancer increased monotonically with increasing intake of alcohol (Fig. 20.12) with no statistical evidence of heterogeneity among studies. For a 10-g/day increase in alcohol, breast cancer risk increased by 9% (95% CI, 4%–13%), and a small but statistically significant excess is seen at even one drink per day (404–406). In this and other analyses, adjustment for known breast cancer risk factors and dietary variables hypothesized to be related to breast cancer had little impact on the association with alcohol. In the collective literature, beer, wine, and liquor all contribute to the positive association (380,404,407), strongly suggesting that alcohol *per se* is responsible for the increased risk.

Whether reducing alcohol consumption in middle life will decrease risk of breast cancer is an important practical issue. In one early report (408), women who drank before age 30 years and later stopped experienced a similar elevation in risk compared with those who continued to drink. However, in a large study designed to address this issue (409), recent consumption of three or more drinks per day was associated with an RR of 2.2, whereas the RR was 0.9 for consumption of three or more drinks per day from ages 16 to 29 years. This suggests that recent adult drinking may be more important than drinking patterns earlier in life and that a reduction in consumption in midlife should reduce risks of breast cancer.

In intervention studies, consumption of approximately two alcoholic drinks per day increased total and bioavailable estrogen levels in premenopausal women (410), and single doses of alcohol acutely increased plasma estradiol levels in postmenopausal women (411), suggesting a mechanism by which alcohol may increase breast cancer risk. In a cross-sectional study, alcohol intake was associated with elevated plasma levels of estrone sulfate, a long-term indicator of estrogen status (360), which in turn has been associated with future risk of breast cancer (113). In several large, prospective studies, high intake of folic acid appeared to mitigate the excess risk of breast cancer caused by alcohol, although a formal test of interaction was not statistically significant in the EPIC study (407,412–414). This relationship was confirmed using plasma folic acid levels (415). Because alcohol inactivates folic acid metabolites and low folate levels are associated with increased misincorporation of uracil into DNA, this finding suggests another possible mechanism for the adverse effects of alcohol.

Of all the associations between dietary factors and breast cancer risk, the relation with alcohol is by far the most consistent. This association has been observed in many diverse populations, and rigorous attempts to account for this relation by other variables have been unsuccessful. Moreover, the effect of alcohol on endogenous estrogen levels provides a plausible mechanism. Together, this body of data provides strong evidence for a causal relationship between alcohol consumption and breast cancer risk. However, the public health implications of this knowledge are complicated by the fact that consumption of one to two alcoholic beverages per day is almost certainly protective against cardiovascular disease. Because cardiovascular disease is the leading cause of death among women, moderate drinking is associated overall with a modest reduction in total mortality (416). Although still complex, reduction of daily alcohol consumption appears to be one of relatively few methods for actively reducing breast cancer risk, whereas many methods exist to reduce risk of cardiovascular disease. For women choosing to consume alcohol regularly, use of a multivitamin to assume adequate folic acid intake appears prudent.

Caffeine

Considerable speculation that caffeine may be a risk factor for breast cancer followed a report that women with benign breast disease experienced relief from symptoms after eliminating caffeine from their diet. Most case-control studies, however, have not observed evidence of a positive association with breast cancer. In prospective studies, no increase in breast cancer risk has been seen (369,417–419) and, in one (420), a weak, but significant, inverse association between caffeine consumption and breast cancer risk was observed. Similarly, no evidence for an association between tea consumption and risk of breast cancer has been seen in epidemiologic studies (380). Thus, the epidemiologic evidence is not compatible with any substantial increase in breast cancer risk associated with drinking coffee or tea.

Phytoestrogens

Phytoestrogens in soy products have attracted scientific and popular attention, in part because they are highly consumed in Asian countries, such as Japan and China, which have low rates of cancer (421). These compounds, which include daidzen and genistein, can bind ER but are much less potent than estradiol. In principle, these substances may, thus, act like tamoxifen by blocking the action of endogenous estrogens to reduce breast cancer risk. Dietary supplementation with a large amount of soy protein slightly lengthened menstrual cycle (422), which would be predicted to decrease breast cancer risk only minimally. Also, soy protein consumption is not the primary explanation for low rates breast cancer in Japan and China because rates are similarly low in other parts of China, elsewhere in Asia, and in many developing countries where soy and related foods are not regularly used. In case-control studies in Singapore (423) and China (424), and in Asian Americans (425), intake of soy products, particularly during adolescence, was associated with lower risk of breast cancer. However, in two other case-control studies in China (426,427) and in a prospective study from Japan (428), little relation was seen. Conceivably, phytoestrogens in high doses could even increase overall estrogenic activity among postmenopausal women with low levels of endogenous estrogens. In case-control and cohort studies that have been conducted so far, no clear association between consumption of soy products and risk of breast cancer has been seen, although there is some suggestion of benefit with consumption at young ages (429,430).

Another group of compounds formed from glucosinolates found in cruciferous vegetables (e.g., broccoli, cauliflower, cabbage) are hypothesized to alter the balance of estrogen metabolism toward less potent forms, but data on humans have not been supportive (431). The possibility that phytochemicals that block estrogen function or modulate estrogen metabolism may provide a nontoxic means of altering breast cancer risk deserves further study, but the available evidence is inconclusive at present.

Specific Foods

Foods contain an extremely complex mix of essential nutrients and other compounds that could individually or collectively influence breast cancer risk in ways that may not be detected by the study of individual nutrients. Thus, an examination of foods and food groups in relation to risk of breast cancer could be informative. However, because the foods examined in most studies are too numerous to be reported individually, published results are likely to reflect a bias toward reporting findings that are statistically significant or that fit preexisting hypotheses.

Inverse associations between intakes of fruits and vegetables and breast cancer risk have been reported in a notably large number of case-control studies (380). These associations have been more consistent for vegetables than for fruits and for green vegetables in particular. However, in the pooled analysis of eight large prospective studies (7,377 cases among 351,825 women), only weak and nonsignificant associations were seen with increasing consumption of fruit and vegetables (431). Comparing highest with lowest quartiles, RR were 0.93 (95% CI, 0.86–1.00) for total fruits, 0.96 (95% CI, 0.89–1.04) for total vegetables, and 0.93 (95% CI, 0.86–1.00) for total fruits plus vegetables. A thorough search among specific fruits and vegetables and botanical groups did not reveal any significant associations. A similar lack of association was seen in a large multicentered cohort study in Europe (432).

Associations between red meat consumption and risk of breast cancer have been reported sporadically (433). However, in the pooled analysis of large cohort studies (7,379 cases) (406), no association was seen with consumption of red meat, white meat, or dairy products. In an analysis that retrospectively assessed degree of cooking (434), consumption of well-done red meat was associated with breast cancer incidence. This will require evaluation in prospective analyses. In a prospective study among premenopausal women, intake of red meat was associated with a twofold increase in risk of breast cancers that were positive for estrogen and progesterone receptors (320). Fat *per se* was not associated with breast cancer risk, suggesting that other constituents of red meat consumed early in adult life may increase breast cancer risk. Although a protective effect of fish consumption has been suggested in a few studies, the overall evidence from case-control and cohort studies suggests little relationship (406). Intake of nuts and legumes has received limited attention in reports on diet and breast cancer, but in general, no relation has been seen (380).

Diet and Breast Cancer Survival

Whether diet is related to the occurrence of breast cancer, if postdiagnosis diet were related to risk of recurrence or survival, then dietary modifications might assist in breast cancer treatment. Several studies (435) have examined dietary fat intake before breast cancer diagnosis in relation to survival by following up the cases from breast cancer case-control studies; results have been inconsistent. Because the original interest was the relation of diet to breast cancer incidence, the investigators were at pains to assess diet before diagnosis. This approach is unsatisfactory, however, if the question is whether diet after diagnosis has an influence on survival, because women may make major changes in their diet after receiving the diagnosis. In one study of diet after diagnosis (albeit in the 1 to 5 months immediately after the diagnosis), no association was seen between dietary fat intake and survival (436). Among premenopausal women, higher consumption of butter, margarine, and lard after diagnosis was associated with greater likelihood of reoccurrence (437). In a larger study, diet was assessed before and after breast cancer diagnosis (438). Greater fat intake after diagnosis was associated with a nonsignificantly worse survival outcome. Higher protein consumption, mainly from poultry, fish, and dairy sources, was, however, related to a better prognosis, even after controlling for protein consumption before diagnosis. In the same study, neither alcohol consumption nor vitamin A intake was associated with survival. Although overall dietary patterns after diagnosis were not associated with breast cancer mortality in this cohort, a prudent dietary pattern was associated with lower mortality, and Western pattern with higher mortality, from causes other than breast cancer (439). This is important because with early diagnosis and good treatment, most women will survive their breast cancer, but they remain at risk for diseases of women in general.

Several randomized trials have been conducted among women with early stage breast cancer to determine the effects of dietary change on recurrence or mortality. In one trial, 2,437 women with breast cancer were randomized to a low-fat diet or their usual diet and followed for an average of 5 years (440). Dietary fat intake was reduced to 33 g/day in the intervention group compared with 51 g/day in the control group, and weight was also 6 pounds lower in the intervention group. In a preliminary report, 9.8% of women in the intervention group experienced a relapse compared with 12.4% of women in the control group (RR = 0.76, 95% CI, 0.60 to 0.98, p = .077 for stratified log rank test and p = .034 for adjusted Cox model analysis). These results were suggestive of a possible benefit of the intervention, but not conclusive, but it is not possible to know whether any benefit is owing to weight loss (potentially owing to the intense intervention because the overall evidence does not support a specific benefit of fat reduction on body weight) or to fat reduction *per se*. Further follow-up of the study population is planned. Dietary fat intake was lower in the intervention than in the control group (fat grams/day at 12 months, 33.3 [95% CI, 32.2–34.5] vs. 51.3 [95% CI, 50.0–52.7], respectively; *p* <.001), corresponding to a statistically significant (*p* = .005), 6-pound lower mean body weight in the intervention group. A total of 277 relapse events (local, regional, distant, or ipsilateral breast cancer recurrence or new contralateral breast cancer) have been reported in 96 of 975 (9.8%) women in the dietary group and 181 of 1,462 (12.4%) women in the control group. The hazard ratio of relapse events in the intervention group compared with the control group was 0.76 (95% CI, 0.60–0.98, *p* = .077 for stratified log rank and *p* = .034 for adjusted Cox model analysis).

In another trial among 3,088 women, one group was assigned to a diet high in fruits, vegetables, and fiber and low in fat (441). During an average of 7.3 years of follow-up, 256 women in the intervention group (16.7%) versus 262 in the comparison group (16.9%) developed an invasive breast cancer event (RR = 0.96; 95% CI, 0.80–1.14; p = .63), and 155 women in the intervention group (10.1%) versus 160 women in the control group (10.3%) died (RR = 0.91; 95% CI, 0.72–1.15; p = .43). The increase in fruit and vegetable consumption was large, and documented by a 50% increase in blood carotenoid level, but the reported difference in fat intake was small (−15%), so this study primarily tested the benefit of increasing fruit and vegetable intake. At this point, both observational data (442), and the results of a low-fat dietary intervention trial (440) suggest that avoidance of weight gain after diagnosis of breast cancer will improve prognosis.

Summary of Diet and Breast Cancer

The role of specific dietary factors in breast cancer causation is not completely resolved. Enthusiasm for the hypothesis that dietary fat intake was responsible for the high rates of breast cancer in Western countries was based largely on the weakest form of epidemiologic evidence—ecologic correlation studies. Results from prospective studies and the WHI trial do not support the concept that fat intake in middle or later life has a major relation to breast cancer risk. High-energy intake in relation to physical activity, which accelerates growth and the onset of menstruation during childhood, leads to weight gain in middle life and, thus, can contribute substantially to breast cancer risk. These effects of energy balance clearly account for an important part of international differences in breast cancer rates. Some evidence suggests that carotenoids or other compounds in carotenoid-rich foods may reduce breast cancer risk modestly, but these findings are not conclusive and deserve further consideration. Alcohol intake is the best established specific dietary risk factor for breast cancer, and studies demonstrating that even moderate alcohol intake increases endogenous estrogen levels provide a potential mechanism, thus supporting a causal interpretation. Hypotheses relating childhood and adolescent diet to breast cancer risk decades later will be more difficult to test. Nevertheless, evidence can be considered conclusive that breast cancer risk can be reduced by avoiding weight gain during adult years and by limiting alcohol consumption. Some evidence suggests that limiting intake of red meat during early adult life and replacing saturated fat with monounsaturated fat may reduce the risk of breast cancer, and this will reduce risk of coronary heart disease.

PHYSICAL ACTIVITY

Regular physical activity has been hypothesized to prevent breast cancer and, in 2002, the International Agency on Cancer Research concluded that there was "convincing" evidence that physical activity reduces the risk of breast cancer (443). A number of potential mechanisms have been proposed, including changes in menstrual cycle characteristics, lowering sex hormones and insulin-like growth factors, and improving immune function (444,445). The mechanisms by which physical activity reduces exposure to hormones vary by period of life. Young girls participating in strenuous athletic training, such as running and ballet dancing, have delayed menarche (446–448), which is known to reduce the risk of breast cancer, and even moderate-intensity physical activity may delay menstruation (341). This effect of activity at young ages may be reflected in lower body weight and body fat, both of which are determinants of delayed menstruation (342,446). A later menarche is associated with a later onset of regular ovulatory cycles and lower serum estrogen concentrations during adolescence (449). Once menstruation has been established, anovulatory and irregular menstrual cycles may be more common among moderately and strenu-

ously active women than among inactive women (339,448,450), although there is disagreement regarding the degree to which the intensity of physical activity influences menstrual abnormalities (451). Further, a substantial degree of ovarian dysfunction may occur even among physically active women who appear to have normal menstrual cycles (452). Among older women, levels of past and current physical activity influence fat stores (446,447,452–455), which after the menopause are primary sites of conversion of androstenedione to estrogen (456,457).

A number of epidemiologic studies have reported an inverse association between physical activity and postmenopausal breast cancer, although the evidence is less consistent for premenopausal breast cancer (444,445,458–461). A number of aspects regarding this association remain unclear, however. Methodologic differences in physical activity assessment are likely to have contributed to inconsistencies in study results. Studies have differed in the ages at which physical activity was assessed; methods for measuring intensity, frequency, and duration of physical activity; definition and categorization of physical activity levels (including consideration of only recreational, or recreational and occupational, activity); and age at breast cancer diagnosis. Results have varied, however, even among studies that have tried to assess physical activity at similar times in life using similar tools.

One of the strongest reductions in breast cancer risk associated with increased physical activity was reported in a population-based, case-control study of women younger than 40 years (462). The RR was 0.42 (95% CI, 0.27–0.64) comparing women with a lifetime average of 3.8 hours or more of physical activity per week with those with an average of 0 hours per week. This was the first study explicitly devoted to the relationship between physical activity and breast cancer, and it was also the first to use a detailed physical activity assessment instrument to quantify the average number of hours per week of recreational physical activity over the reproductive life span, beginning at menarche. Activities such as housework, gardening, and easy walking not for the explicit purpose of physical exercise were not counted in the measure of physical activity. These researchers concluded from their various analyses that lifelong physical activity is the critical exposure of interest with regard to breast cancer risk.

Since publication of this study, at least nine other studies (461,463–470) have assessed the relationship between lifetime physical activity and breast cancer risk. In one of these studies (471), in contrast to the study reported on earlier, no association between lifetime physical activity and breast cancer risk was found for premenopausal women. Among postmenopausal women, recreational physical activity was not associated with breast cancer risk, whereas household and occupational physical activity was inversely associated with risk (OR = 0.57, 95% CI, 0.41–0.79; and OR = 0.59, 95% CI, 0.44–0.81), comparing highest to lowest quartiles of household and occupational activity, respectively. The findings of inverse associations with household and occupational physical activity, but not with recreational activity, suggest that residual confounding by sociodemographic and reproductive factors are at least partly responsible for the observed inverse relationships.

A case-control study conducted among premenopausal and postmenopausal women in urban Shanghai (468) found significant inverse dose-response relationships between years of (recreational) exercise participation and breast cancer risk, as well as between lifetime occupational activity and breast cancer risk. In contrast, a case-control study nested within the Women's Health Study (467), which also assessed lifetime physical activity (recreational only), found no association between physical activity (lifetime or at any specific time in life) and breast cancer risk.

It has been hypothesized that high levels of physical activity during adolescence are particularly important with respect to influencing breast cancer risk. A retrospective cohort study of college alumnae (472) found that women who had been former college athletes had a 40% lower risk of breast cancer later in life than their nonathletic peers (OR = 0.61, 95% CI, 0.44–0.84). However, other studies that have examined the association between physical activity during adolescence and breast cancer risk have found little evidence for a protective effect.

In contrast to the detailed measurement of lifetime physical activity employed by some of the studies mentioned earlier, a relatively simple measure of physical activity was used in a prospective cohort study of Norwegian women aged 30 to 54 years at baseline (173). Over a period of 3 to 5 years, women were administered two surveys about their current patterns of physical activity during leisure hours; they were asked to rank themselves on a 4-point scale with respect to activity level. The RR was 0.63 (95% CI, 0.42–0.95) for consistently active women compared with consistently sedentary women. This result, besides being one of the strongest RR reported in the literature, is the strongest reported in any cohort study.

There would be obvious public health significance to an association between a modifiable lifestyle risk factor such as physical activity and breast cancer. Already at least 30 observational epidemiologic studies of this issue have been conducted, a number of them published since 2000 (465,467–469,471,472,474–482). Despite the wealth of data on the subject, it is difficult to come to a clear conclusion on the topic given numerous methodologic issues. These issues include the resolution of whether a critical lifetime period exists during which increased physical activity exerts its strongest effect on breast cancer risk, or whether lifetime physical activity is the critical exposure of interest for most women. It is also unclear if the effects of physical activity on breast cancer differ in particular subgroups of women. For example, studies have suggested the association is modified by family history of breast cancer (463,464,469), menopausal status (459), or BMI (469,483). A second important issue relates to the quantification of physical activity, and how information on frequency, intensity, duration, and time span of activity can and should be combined into a single measure or a small number of measures that can be readily modeled. A third issue pertains to the validity of women's reports of past physical activity. In case-control studies, random error in recall of past activity levels that is not dependent on disease status would be expected, on average, to dilute any inverse association that might truly exist. If errors are differential by disease status, however, findings may be biased in either direction away from their true point estimates. A fourth issue concerns the need to consider recreational, occupational, and household physical activity together. In studies of physical activity, the potential exists for confounding by reproductive characteristics for several reasons. Women in physically active jobs are more likely to be of lower socioeconomic status and, thus, may be more likely to have a lower risk reproductive profile. Women with higher levels of household activity may be more likely to be homemakers with children, and thus, again, to have a lower risk reproductive profile. Women with higher levels of recreational physical activity may be more likely to have lower levels of occupational and household activity; they may be more likely to be of higher socioeconomic status than women with lower levels of recreational activity and, thus, to have a higher risk reproductive profile. It is difficult in observational studies to control thoroughly for such potential confounding. Finally, although a hormonal mechanism linking physical activity and breast cancer risk has been postulated, few data exist relating physical activity over sustained periods to lower endogenous ovarian hormone levels. Available studies have been very short term, based on small numbers of women, and often limited to comparisons between young women who engage in high levels of activity and inactive young women.

Although numerous studies have examined the association between physical activity and risk of breast cancer, a number of issues remain unsettled. Most case-control studies have reported decreased risks, whereas cohort studies have been less consistent in their finding. The weight of the collective evidence, however, suggests that regular physical activity modestly protects against breast cancer (443), and this is most evident for postmenopausal breast cancer. Evidence relating higher physical activity to risk of postmenopausal breast cancer is strong because of the important role of activity in controlling weight gain, an important cause of postmenopausal breast cancer. This, in addition to many other benefits of staying lean and fit, provides sufficient justification for including regular physical activity in daily life.

IONIZING RADIATION

More is probably known about radiation-induced breast cancer than about any other radiation-induced malignancy, with the possible exception of radiation-induced leukemia. The knowledge that ionizing radiation to the chest in cumulative moderate to high doses (e.g., 1–3 Gy) at young ages substantially increases breast cancer risk comes from several lines of evidence, including atomic bomb survivor studies, studies of diagnostic or therapeutic uses of radiation, and occupational studies.

Among survivors of the atomic bombing of Hiroshima and Nagasaki (484), breast cancer risk was strongly associated with an estimated breast tissue dose of radiation. Further, the RR of breast cancer associated with each radiation dose depended heavily on the age at the time of the bombing, being highest for women exposed before age 10 years. For women exposed after age 40 years, there was no significant elevation in subsequent breast cancer risk.

Studies of diagnostic radiation have revealed a similar pattern of excess risk of breast cancer associated both with higher doses and with younger ages at exposure. In a study of women who received substantial radiation to the chest as a result of repeated fluoroscopic examinations for tuberculosis (485), the maximal excess risk was among women with first exposure between the ages of 10 and 14 years, whereas women first exposed at age 35 years or later had virtually no excess risk. Girls examined frequently for scoliosis with full spinal x-ray study also faced an increased risk of breast cancer later in life (486).

Studies of therapeutic radiation for nonmalignant and malignant disease have revealed the same pattern. In a study of women exposed to radiation therapy to the chest as treatment for Hodgkin disease (487), the excess risk of breast cancer again was dependent on dose and age at irradiation. In a study of radiation treatment of breast cancer and development of second breast cancers (488), risk of second cases was significantly elevated (above its already high level) among women who underwent radiation at younger than 45 years. Women who are heterozygous for the *ATM* gene are hypothesized to be at increased risk of both breast cancer and radiation-induced breast cancer (489). One report (490), however, found no *ATM* mutations in women with contralateral breast cancer and failed to support the hypothesis that *ATM* carriers account for a significant fraction of breast cancer cases that arose in women after radiation therapy. Studies of women who have developed subsequent breast cancer after radiation therapy for Hodgkin disease also reported no association with *ATM* heterozygosity (491).

Studies of radionuclide therapy have shown that women treated with such regimens have an increased risk of breast cancer later in life. A German study of young persons injected with radium-224 for bone diseases in 1945 to 1955 showed subsequent high rates of bone cancer, and an increased risk of breast cancer was observed in both women and men in the cohort (492).

Occupational studies provide a final set of evidence about radiation-induced breast cancer. Increased breast cancer incidence was observed among some groups of women who in the early part of the 20th century painted watch dials and gauges with radium-226 (493); such increased risk has also been observed among women in China who pioneered in the fields of radiology and medical x-ray work (494). Some of this excess may have been owing to higher breast cancer risk profiles of the women in such occupations, that is, a higher proportion of them tended to be nulliparous in comparison to the general population of women. The slightly increased risk of breast cancer observed among women who worked during World War II as x-ray technologists might have been owing to nulliparity; a disproportionate number of Catholic nuns were in these cohorts (495). Studies of women employed in subsequent times as x-ray technologists have not found this increased risk of breast cancer (496,497).

The risk associated with infrequent low-dose radiation exposure to the chest has been difficult to quantify, because the expected excess of breast cancers is small relative to the background risk (485). Thus, the risk of breast cancer associated with low-dose radiation, such as mammography, has been estimated by extrapolating the dose–response relationship from studies of women exposed to higher doses of radiation (498). In this way, less than 1% of all cases of breast cancer have been estimated to result from diagnostic radiography (498).

Genetic variation in DNA repair genes may modify the risk of breast cancer associated with low to moderate exposures of ionizing radiation (499). Initial studies among women with *BRCA1* and *BRCA2* mutations genes involved in the repair of double strand breaks, have reported inconsistent finding on the effect of exposure to mammography and chest x-ray study on breast cancer risk among mutation carriers (500–502).

Additional studies of genetic variation and low-dose exposure to radiation may yield useful information about which women face an identifiably higher risk of radiation-induced breast cancer from mammographic surveillance.

ENVIRONMENTAL POLLUTION

Evidence of geographic variation in incidence and mortality rates of breast cancer within the United States, the steady increase in incidence over time, and the identification of suspected breast cancer clusters have stimulated interest in the possibility that industrial chemicals or electromagnetic fields may be environmental risk factors for breast cancer. The experimental and epidemiologic evidence for the associations of certain specific synthetic chemicals with breast cancer are considered in the following sections and have been comprehensively reviewed with detailed citations elsewhere (503–505).

Organochlorines

Epidemiologic studies of breast cancer and environmental exposures to synthetic chemicals have concentrated on biologically persistent organochlorines. This class of compounds includes pesticides, such as 2,2-bis(*p*-chlorophenyl)-1,1,1-trichloromethane (DDT), chlordane, hexachlorocyclohexane (HCH, lindane), hexachlorobenzene (HCB), kepone, and mirex; industrial chemicals, such as polychlorinated biphenyls (PCB) and polybrominated biphenyls (PBB); and dioxins (polychlorinated dibenzofurans [PCDF] and polychlorinated dibenzodioxin [PCDD]), produced as combustion byproducts of PCB or contaminants of pesticides. Many of these chemicals are weak estrogens and are, therefore, hypothesized to increase breast cancer risk by mimicking endogenous estradiol. Furthermore, they are excreted in breast milk, suggesting that ductal and other cells in the breast are directly exposed. Other compounds, specifically the dioxins and some PCB congeners, exhibit antiestrogenic activity; therefore, despite the established carcinogenicity of dioxin at other anatomic sites in animal tests, they might be protective against breast cancer.

The organochlorines are highly lipophilic and resistant to metabolism. Thus, many of these compounds bioaccumulate in the food chain and persist in the body. These chemicals can be measured in breast milk, adipose tissue, and blood. Most of the epidemiologic literature on organochlorines focuses on DDT, DDE (1,1-dichloro-2,2,-bis(*p*-dichlorophenyl)ethylene, the main metabolite of DDT), and PCB because they are among the most persistent in humans. The general population was thought to be exposed to these compounds predominantly through ingestion of fish, dairy products, and meat. Almost everyone in the United States has had some measurable exposure; however, the average body burden of some of these chemicals (e.g., DDT) has been decreasing with time since the cessation of their production in this country (1972 for DDT and 1977 for PCB).

Although a positive correlation of age-specific breast cancer mortality rates in Israel with trends in DDT and other pesticide contamination in milk has been reported (506), estimates were based on only 2 years of data. With more extensive mortality and incidence data, no association was observed (507). In a study of PCB-contaminated fatty fish from the Baltic Sea, breast cancer rates among fishermen's wives from the contaminated east coast were higher than rates among fishermen's wives from the noncontaminated west coast (RR = 1.35, 95% CI, 0.98–1.86) (508). However, there was no control for other known breast cancer risk factors. In a recent study of consumption of sports fish in the United States Great Lakes region, (sports fish in this region have been shown to be a source of exposure to PCB and organochorine residues), no association was observed across all women studied (N = 1,481 cases); however, a positive association was observed among premenopausal women (n = 386, RR = 1.70; 95% CI, 1.16–2.50) (509). An accidental explosion in 1976 in a chemical plant near Seveso, Italy, provided the opportunity to evaluate exposure to high levels of dioxin. Breast cancer incidence during the decade after the accident in the areas closest to the accident was slightly but not significantly lower than expected (510).

Studies of occupational exposure to organochlorines have not supported an association with increased breast cancer risk. Fewer cases were observed than expected in studies of women occupationally exposed to phenoxy herbicides and PCB. A twofold increase of breast cancer mortality was found in facilities with herbicide and dioxin exposures (511), but only 7% of the patients worked in high-exposure areas. These studies are limited by difficulties of exposure assessment and the small numbers of women employed in the occupations with greatest exposure.

The results of small case-control studies of organochlorine levels and breast cancer risk have been mixed. In a large European case-control study (265 cases), a significantly inverse trend between levels of adipose DDE and risk of breast cancer was observed after controlling for known breast cancer risk factors; the authors did not evaluate PCB (512). In a case-control study in Buffalo, New York, lipid-adjusted serum levels of DDE, HCB, mirex, and total PCB were evaluated among 154 incident breast cancer cases and 192 community controls. No evidence was found of a positive association between any of these compounds and breast cancer risk with the possible exception of less chlorinated PCB (513). Lopez-Carrillo et al. (514) analyzed serum DDE levels in a case-control study in Mexico, where the pesticide is still in use. Serum DDE levels were not associated with risk of breast cancer. However, in one small study, contrary to expectation, the levels of octachlorinated dibenzo-*p*-dioxin (OCDD) were slightly elevated in the cases (515), although no differences were observed for six other polychlorinated dibenzo-*p*-dioxin isomers. In a large case-control study conducted on Long Island, New York, no association with breast cancer risk was seen for blood levels of DDE, chlordane, dieldrin, or common PCB congeners (516). Black women have been shown in some studies to have higher levels of exposure to these chemicals; however, in a case-control study of 355 breast cancer cases, no elevation in risk was seen for those with the highest serum levels of a PCB or organochlorine pesticide residues (517).

Several prospective studies have used stored blood samples collected before diagnosis to evaluate the relationship between DDE and total PCB with breast cancer (518–520). In a cohort in New York City of 14,290 women, a strong association between serum DDE levels and risk of breast cancer was initially reported (520), but no relation was seen with longer follow-up (521). No association with PCB levels was observed in this cohort. In a prospective study of 57,040 San Francisco Bay area women who had provided blood in the late 1960s, when DDT and PCB were still in production (519), 50 white, 50 black, and 50 Asian breast cancer cases occurring after blood draw and before 1991 were selected and compared with 150 age- and ethnicity-matched control women. Risk of breast cancer was not associated with either DDE or PCB level when all ethnic groups were combined, although nonsignificant elevated risks were observed for DDE for blacks and whites. Among 236 breast cancer cases and their matched controls in the NHS, there no evidence was seen of a positive association of breast cancer with either DDE or PCB (518). The multivariate RR for women in the highest quintile compared with women in the lowest were 0.72 (95% CI, 0.4–1.4) for DDE and 0.66 (95% CI, 0.32–1.37) for PCB. For women in the highest quintiles of both DDE and PCB, the RR was 0.43 (95% CI, 0.13–1.44) for joint exposure. In further follow-up in this cohort, adding an additional 143 postmenopausal cases, results were similar (522). A pooled study reanalyzing data from the five large studies in the northeast has also found no association between PCB and DDE levels and breast cancer risk when comparing the highest and lowest quintiles (504). In a large nested case-control study from Denmark, concentrations of 14 pesticides and 18 PCB measured in adipose tissue samples collected at baseline, no association was seen for any of these chemicals with breast cancer risk among 409 postmenopausal cases; a lower risk of ER-negative cancer was seen in the highest category of exposure for several of the PCBs and organochlorines (523). In a recent nested case-control study of 129 cases diagnosed an average of 17 years after they had blood drawn shortly after childbirth at an average age of 26 years, a positive associations were observed for serum DDT levels and early life breast cancer risk (524).

In summary, recent large studies have not found evidence of increased breast cancer risk among postmenopausal women associated with blood levels of DDE or total PCB; however, a small effect will always be difficult to exclude, as will hypotheses relating to specific subgroups, such as premenopausal women. All available studies address exposure to organochlorines in the decade or two before enrollment; it will be very difficult to obtain data to address the hypothesis that childhood or even *in utero* exposure is associated with breast cancer risk 50 or more years afterward. Nonetheless, organochlorines appear unlikely to be an important breast cancer risk factors or an explanation for secular changes in breast cancer rates.

Electromagnetic Fields

Electromagnetic fields (EMF) have been proposed to alter breast cancer risk, perhaps by altering melatonin secretion by the pineal gland. Although animal evidence is suggestive, few data address the relation of melatonin levels to human breast cancer risk. Exposure to light at night suppresses melatonin secretion and, in some studies, breast cancer risk has been lower among blind women (525,526). Gathering high-quality

epidemiologic data on EMF and nocturnal light exposure is challenging and these hypotheses are unlikely to be resolved definitively anytime soon. Evidence of an elevated risk of male breast cancer associated with presumed occupational EMF exposure based on job title has been observed in some studies, but these results are based on small numbers of cases. No evidence of an increased risk of breast cancer was observed in the studies that also included female employees. In case-control studies designed specifically to study occupational exposure to EMF and breast cancer in women, small increases in risk have been inconsistently observed. However, in those studies misclassification of exposure is a major concern. Because classifications are based on subjects' *usual* occupation, often obtained from death certificates, duration of exposure and personal work tasks could not be accounted for in most of the studies and adjustment for known breast cancer risk factors was limited or entirely absent.

The general population is exposed to EMF primarily from power lines, transformer substations, and electrical appliance use. In an initial 1987 study of mortality from all cancer subtypes and residential wiring configurations, a statistically significant elevation in female breast cancer incidence was associated with magnitude of exposure at the current residence (527). Other studies in Britain, The Netherlands, and Taiwan did not observe an association between female breast cancer deaths and residence in the vicinity of electricity transmission facilities. Again, these studies are limited by the indirect methods used to assess EMF exposure.

Use of electric blankets (produced before 1990) throughout the night approximately doubles an individual's average exposure to EMF, because the blanket is placed close to the body. In one case-control study, the use of electric blankets continuously throughout the night was associated with marginally significant increases for postmenopausal breast cancer (OR = 1.46, 95% CI, 0.96–2.20) (528) and for premenopausal breast cancer (OR = 1.43, 95% CI, 0.94–2.17) (529). However, in a recent large case-control study of breast cancer in women younger than 55 years, no association was seen (530), and no association was seen in retrospective or prospective analyses within the large NHS cohort (531), or in the large Long Island case-control study based on 1,354 cases (532).

In 2001, IARC conducted a formal review of the available evidence and concluded that the evidence at that time was inadequate to assess the effects of magnetic fields and breast cancer. Since that report, five additional studies of occupational exposure and four of residential exposure have been conducted (533). At present, the biological plausibility and most recent epidemiologic studies do not support an important relation between EMF exposure and breast cancer risk (533).

Active and Passive Smoking

The relation between active cigarette smoking and risk of breast cancer has been extensively evaluated in both case-control and cohort studies; collectively, the data provide strong evidence against any major overall relationship. It has been hypothesized that initiation of smoking early in adolescence, when breast tissue may be maximally sensitive to carcinogenic influences, may be a factor, although study results have been inconsistent (505,534,535). Among large, prospective cohort studies, evidence suggests a positive association with long-term smoking before the first birth (536–538). In the Norwegian-Swedish Women's Lifestyle and Health Cohort Study of more than 100,000 participants, women who initiated smoking during their teenage years and continued to smoke for 20 or more years were at an increased risk of breast cancer (comparing women who initiated smoking before age 15 to never smokers RR = 1.48, 95% CI, 1.03–2.13) (537). This increased risk of breast cancer was not observed among women who smoked for 20 or more years, but started smoking after their first birth. These results are consistent with the hypothesis that breast tissue is particularly susceptible to carcinogens between early puberty and the first full-term pregnancy (62).

Passive smoking has been suggested to be an important risk for breast cancer in part because sidestream smoke contains more carcinogenic activity per milligram than mainstream smoke. In a cohort study of cancer mortality among Japanese women exposed to passive smoke at home, a slight and insignificant risk elevation was seen (crude RR = 1.3, 95% CI, 0.8–2.0) (539,540). In several case-control studies, increases in risk of breast cancer have been seen, but usually without evidence of a dose response. Despite these positive associations, it is difficult to reconcile the absence of an effect of heavy smoking for decades with an effect of exposure to much lower amounts of environmental smoke. A likely explanation for the positive association seen in case-control studies is methodologic bias related to the selection of controls or the retrospective recall of exposure to passive smoke. In a large prospective study, neither active nor passive smoking was associated with any appreciable risk of breast cancer (541).

Silicone Breast Implants

Most studies examining the relation of silicone breast implants with breast cancer risk have actually reported lower rates of breast cancer among women with implants (542–547); thus, a direct association between silicone breast implants and the occurrence of breast cancer is unlikely.

Early anecdotal reports (548–551) of breast cancer among women whose breasts had been augmented with silicone raised concerns about a causal link with the disease. Since then, a number of observational studies, both case control and cohort, have been conducted. Most of these studies have found *reduced* breast cancer risk among women with implants compared with either the general population or women without implants. Reported reductions in risk in some of these studies have been large (on the order of 50% or 60%). A large retrospective cohort study (552), 10,778 women who had breast implants before 1989 and 3,214 comparison women who had had plastic surgery not involving silicone during the same time responded to a medical questionnaire. In analyses based on external and internal comparisons, the women who had had breast implants were not at elevated risk of breast cancer. The overall standardized incidence ratio (SIR) comparing breast cancer incidence among the breast implant cohort with the Atlanta SEER incidence rates was 0.89 (95% CI, 0.8–1.1) (552). The RR of breast cancer comparing the implant cohort with the comparison group of other patients who had undergone plastic surgery was 0.79 (95% CI, 0.6–1.1). There was no statistically significant heterogeneity in risk according to age or calendar year in which implants were received (in part, this calendar-year variable was a surrogate for the type of implant), and there was no variation in risk of breast cancer by preimplantation chest or cup size. There was indication of a slight decrease in risk of breast cancer in both the external and the internal comparisons during the initial 10-year period following breast implantation. This likely reflects a preimplantation screening or selection bias. The authors note that characteristics of patients who had breast implants could predispose to the discovery of a lower risk of breast cancer among such women; these characteristics include small breasts and thinness. In a follow-up of 2,763 women who underwent cosmetic breast implant surgery in Denmark on average about 15 years previously, breast cancer incidence was nonsignificantly reduced compared with a comparison series of 1,736 who had other forms of plastic surgery (547). In a large series of 24,588 women who underwent bilateral augmentation mammoplasty in Quebec or Ontario, breast cancer rates were actually significantly lower after a median of about 15 years,

than among women who had other forms of plastic surgery (544). In both these studies, results were similar when restricted to women who received silicone implants.

In summary, strong epidemiologic evidence indicates that breast implants do not lead to increased risk of breast cancer. Further, findings of significantly decreased risks in some studies probably reflect a combination of short duration of follow-up after implantation (i.e., bias owing to preimplantation screening and selection for women who do not have breast abnormalities) and favorable breast cancer risk profiles of women who tend to seek breast augmentation.

Summary of Evidence on Environmental Pollution and Breast Cancer Risk

In general, current evidence does not support any substantial relationship between exposure to human made chemicals or electrical fields in the environment and breast cancer risk. The best recent evidence in prospective analyses does not support an association between exposure to organochlorines and breast cancer risk. Although occupational studies of EMF exposure have been inconclusive, residential studies imply that no risk is associated with overhead power lines. Overall increases in breast cancer incidence caused by active or passive smoking are not supported by prospective data, but modest increases owing to smoking at early ages cannot be excluded.

Although other environmental exposures that have not been identified may warrant evaluation, with the exception of ionizing radiation, no environmental exposure can be confidently labeled as a cause of breast cancer based on current evidence.

OCCUPATION

A review of 115 studies published between 1971 and 1994 (553) found little support for an association between specific occupations and breast cancer risk. Limited evidence suggested that cosmetologists, beauticians, and pharmaceutical manufacturing workers had a modestly elevated risk of breast cancer, but conclusions were not possible because of lack of adequate exposure data. Although ionizing radiation is a recognized risk factor for breast cancer and studies conducted in the early part of the century confirmed this, none of the more recent studies of radiation workers, including x-ray technicians, workers at uranium fuel plants, and atomic energy plants found an elevation of breast cancer risk among women in these occupations. The few studies carried out on specific occupational agents have not provided any evidence of association. In particular, although organic solvents may increase risk of various cancers in animals, women who worked in dry cleaning or shoe manufacturing, or who were exposed to trichloroethylene did not have an elevated risk of breast cancer (553).

Despite much literature on occupation as a risk factor, most studies have simply examined associations between occupational title and breast cancer risk; specific information on exposure to potential carcinogens was collected in only a few studies. Although some studies collected detailed information on lifetime occupational history, often broad occupational groupings representing only the most recent occupation were used in analyses. Further, most studies have not controlled adequately for known breast cancer risk factors, in particular, reproductive factors, that are likely confounders of any observed association with occupation (554). Employment outside the home, and in a specific occupation, is likely to be highly correlated with educational attainment and socioeconomic status, and thus with reproductive characteristics. In the few studies that have controlled for sociodemographic and reproductive risk, breast cancer risk did not vary across occupational groups. In contrast, a consistent finding across studies that were unable to control for important confounders has been an increased breast cancer risk among more highly educated women, rather than a consistently observed association for any specific occupation. Thus, further analyses of occupational titles without consideration of known breast cancer risk factors or actual workplace exposures are unlikely to be informative.

MEDICAL HISTORY

A variety of diseases and medications are known or suspected to cause or to be associated with modifications of hormones and growth factors and, thus, may influence breast cancer risk (555). Type 2 diabetes has been suggested to increase the risk of breast cancer. Hyperinsulinemia, as occurs in adult-onset diabetes, may promote breast cancer because insulin may be a growth factor for human breast cancer cells (556). Further, insulin levels are inversely related to levels of SHBG, and, thus, are positively related to available estrogens and androgens (555). Many studies have lacked information about the type and severity of diabetes, making the interpretation of the various findings difficult (555). In the prospective NHS, women with type 2 diabetes had a modestly elevated incidence of breast cancer (hazard ratio [HR]= 1.17, 95% CI, 1.01–1.35) (557). This association was limited to postmenopausal women and was more predominant for risk of ER-positive disease (HR = 1.21, 95% CI, 1.01–1.47). In a case-control investigation of subclinical diabetes, hyperinsulinemia with insulin resistance was a significant risk factor for breast cancer, independent of weight or body fat distribution (558). Dietary factors are important in the insulin resistance syndrome; studies have found that both dietary glycemic index and glycemic load are positively associated with breast cancer risk. A more recent case-control study found that a history of diabetes mellitus was associated with a 50% increase in postmenopausal breast cancer, again independent of weight (555). Further studies of the relationship between breast cancer and insulin resistance are warranted because insulin resistance is increasing sharply in many populations and is modifiable through increases in physical activity, dietary changes, and maintenance of a lean body weight.

Women with a diagnosis of thyroid cancer were reported more likely to develop breast cancer than women without such a diagnosis; this association was first noted in 1966 (559). A study published in 2001 (560) sought to overcome the problem of small sample size that plagued many of the previous studies by using SEER registry data from 1973 to 1994. In this analysis, premenopausal white women who had thyroid carcinoma were more likely to develop breast cancer 5 to 20 years later than women without a diagnosis of thyroid carcinoma (RR = 1.41, 95% CI, 1.18 1.68). No evidence was found of such increased risk among postmenopausal white women. Point estimates of RR were elevated in both premenopausal and postmenopausal black women (RR = 1.54, 95% CI, 0.66–3.03 and RR = 1.29, 95% CI, 0.52–2.67, respectively), but statistical power was poor because of low numbers. No increased risk was seen of subsequent thyroid cancer following an initial diagnosis of breast cancer, suggesting that a woman's susceptibility to breast cancer after thyroid cancer may be related to treatment of the thyroid cancer rather than to genetic or environmental susceptibility to these two cancers simultaneously.

Strong evidence suggests that nonsteroidal anti-inflammatory drugs (NSAID), including aspirin, inhibit colon carcinogenesis in humans (561,562), thereby providing a rationale to investigate an inhibitory role of NSAID in breast carcinogenesis. However, the association between NSAID use and breast cancer is unclear. In a large case-control study (563), women who had used an NSAID three or more times per week for at least 1 year were at decreased risk of breast cancer compared with nonusers (OR = 0.66). Similarly, the observational study of the WHI, found that regular NSAID users (2+ tablets/week) had a 21% decreased risk of breast cancer (RR = 0.79; 95% CI, 0.60–1.04) (564). In contrast, a large prospective study (565), found no relationship with regular or heavy use of aspirin compared with nonusers. The California Teachers Study also observed no overall association between regular NSAID use and incidence of breast cancer (566). Unanswered questions remain regarding the effect of regular NSAID use for long durations, the effect of different doses, and the effects of different nonaspirin NSAID (567).

A growing body of literature suggests that statins have antitumor activity by interrupting cell-cycle progression and inducing apoptosis. Statins are a class of lipid-lowering drugs prescribed for the prevention of cardiovascular disease. A meta-analysis of randomized trials (568) and two large prospective studies (569,570) suggests that statins as a group are not associated with breast cancer incidence. However, one study reported that the hydrophobic class of statins (e.g., simvastatin and lovastatin) were associated with an 18% (HR = 0.82, 95% CI, 0.70–0.97) reduction in breast cancer incidence (569). Further evaluation of specific classes of statins and long-term use are necessary.

A history of eclampsia, preeclampsia, or pregnancy-induced hypertension has been associated with a reduced risk of breast cancer in parous women in at least two case-control studies (571,572) and one cohort study (573). Further, women born to mothers who had preeclamptic pregnancies also appear to have reduced risk of breast cancer (574). Explanations for these findings have focused on hormone-related factors: Women who develop preeclampsia have been found to have relatively low estrogen levels during pregnancy, and the lower exposure to estrogens *in utero* may confer a benefit to the female fetus in terms of lifetime breast cancer risk reduction (574). High levels of α-fetoprotein, a glycoprotein with antiestrogenic properties, are associated with preeclampsia and, thus, may mediate the association between preeclampsia and reduced breast cancer risk in female offspring (574). Nonspecific cellular immune responses may be involved as well (575,576).

Epstein-Barr virus (EBV) is the most ubiquitous viral (herpes) infection among humans, with more than 90% of the adult population worldwide affected by it. In most individuals, the persistent infection remains asymptomatic, but a few individuals develop EBV-associated tumors, including Burkitt lymphoma and Hodgkin lymphoma. Based on several lines of evidence, it has been hypothesized (577–579) that breast carcinoma is also an EBV-associated tumor. However, the limited data on the relationship between EBV and breast cancer are conflicting (580–586). For instance, Bonnet et al. (580) detected the EBV genome by polymerase chain reaction (PCR) in 51% of 100 primary invasive breast carcinomas, whereas the virus was detected in only 10% of a sample of healthy tissues adjacent to the tumors. Further, the virus was more frequently associated with the most aggressive tumors. Other studies have found no molecular or immunohistochemical evidence for an association between EBV and the development of breast carcinoma (581,583,584,587,588). Results of at least one study (589) suggest that EBV DNA detected in breast carcinoma tissues is likely related to the presence of EBV-infected lymphocytes in the tumor stroma; it does not indicate infection of the tumor cells with the virus and, thus, breast carcinoma is not an EBV-associated tumor.

At least two studies reported that selective serotonin reuptake inhibitors (SSRI) and tricyclic antidepressants promote mammary tumors in rodents (590,591). Epidemiologic studies in humans have produced inconsistent results. One study conducted before SSRI were widely available found an increased breast cancer risk among tricyclic antidepressant users (592). A more recent study also found such an increased risk (593). One study found a decreased risk of breast cancer among tricyclic antidepressant users (594), although some studies have found no association (595,596). Research findings are similarly inconsistent for SSRI. Two studies that employed prescription databases to assess exposure found no association between SSRI use and breast cancer risk (595,597), although a study that relied on self-report of medication usage found an elevated risk of breast cancer among recent SSRI users (596). Future epidemiologic studies of this topic must control adequately for possibly strong confounders, such as alcohol use and obesity, which may be associated with use of antidepressants, and should rely on an objective assessment of medication usage, because patients with cancer may be more likely to recall medication use those without cancer. Further, the indication for antidepressant use may itself be associated with increased cancer risk, and depression may be an early symptom of occult cancer.

Cytotoxic drugs, used in the treatment of cancer, may exert their own carcinogenic effects. One category of cytotoxic drugs, alkylating agents, may lead to an increased risk of solid tumors, including breast cancer, although evidence for this hypothesis is weak (598).

ETIOLOGIC SUMMARY

Much is known about the behavioral factors that influence breast cancer risk, and more recently the links between these factors and the pathophysiology of the disease have become clearer. Known and suspected risk factors are described in Table 20.2, grouped by reproductive, hormonal, nutritional, and other variables. Approximate strengths of association are also given for specific comparisons. These comparisons are somewhat arbitrary because many of these risk factors are continuous variables and the RR will depend on the levels chosen for comparison. For example, we have compared ages at menarche of 15 years with 11 years, but the RR would be stronger if age 17 years were contrasted with age 11 years. Although most of these risk factors are established with a high degree of certainty, some such as high prolactin levels, low physical activity, and low consumption of monounsaturated fat will require further research for confirmation.

Mechanisms linking known and suspected risk factors to the development of breast cancer are known with varying levels of certainty. Early events involve mutations of breast stem cells. These mutations can be inherited (e.g., mutations in *BRCA1, BRCA2*, or *p53*) or acquired, such as by exposure to ionizing radiation. At present little evidence indicates that classic chemical car-

cinogens play an important role in human breast cancer by causing early mutations; oxidative damage from endogenous metabolism is hypothesized to contribute to DNA damage (599), but the importance of this mechanism is difficult to quantify. To the extent that oxidative damage is important, dietary antioxidants might reduce the risk and higher intake of monounsaturated fat will result in cell structures that are less easily oxidized. Low availability of folic acid, which is exacerbated by high alcohol intake, leads to the incorporation of uracil rather than thymine into DNA and can be a cause of DNA damage. Pregnancy appears to render the breast substantially less susceptible to somatic mutations, although the exact mechanisms are unclear; thus, earlier first pregnancies will minimize the period of susceptibility. Vitamin A also plays a role in maintaining cell differentiation, but it may be that only very low intakes are related to increased risk.

A high endogenous estrogen level is well established as an important cause of breast cancer, and many known risk factors operate through this pathway. The additional contribution of cyclic estrogen exposure (as opposed to continuously high levels) is less clear, and much available evidence indicates that progestins add to breast cancer risk. Factors that increase lifetime exposure to estrogens and progestins include early age at menarche, regular ovulation, and late menopause. Lactation and overweight during young adult life result in anovulation and this probably accounts for most of their protective effects. Extreme underweight also causes anovulation and would be expected to reduce risk, but direct evidence is lacking. Alcohol consumption increases endogenous estrogen levels and may, at least in part, account for the observed increase in risk among regular drinkers. The increase in risk of breast cancer among current or recent users of oral contraceptives is also presumably owing to their estrogenic (and probable progestational) effects. After menopause, the major determinants of estrogen exposure are the amount of body fat and use of postmenopausal hormones; these are both important risk factors for breast cancer. Increases in physical activity can delay the onset of menarche and can reduce risk of breast cancer by helping to control weight gain.

Estrogens, by their mitotic effect on breast cells, appear to accelerate the development of breast cancer at many points along the progression from early mutation to metastasis and death. By increasing cell multiplication, estrogens may also increase the probability that DNA lesions become mutations. Although earlier exposure to high estrogen levels during adolescence increases risk decades later, a reduction in levels late in life abruptly reduces risk, whether this be by castration, cessation of postmenopausal hormones, or the administration of

Table 20.2	**RISK FACTORS FOR BREAST CANCER AND APPROXIMATE STRENGTH OF ASSOCIATION**		
Reproductive Factors	**Hormonal Factors**	**Nutritional/Lifestyle Factors**	**Others Factors**
Early age at first period+	OC use (current vs. none)+	Obesity (>30 BMI vs. <25) Premenopausal− Postmenopausal+	Family history (mother and sister)[a]+++
Age at first birth (>35 vs.<20)++ No. of births (0 vs. one child)+	Estrogen replacement (10+ years vs. none)+ Estrogen plus progesterone replacement (>5 years vs. none)++	Adult weight gain (postmenopausal)++ Alcohol (one or more drink/day vs. none)+	Family history (first-degree relative)[b]++ Jewish heritage (yes vs. no)+
Age at menopause (5-year increment)+	High blood estrogens or androgens (postmenopause)+++	Height (>5 feet 7 inches)+	Ionizing radiation (yes vs. no)+
Breast-feeding (>1 year vs. none)−	High blood prolactin++	Physical activity (>3 hours/week)− Monounsaturated fat[c]− (vs. saturated fat)	Benign breast disease (MD diagnosed)[d] ++

Note: BMI, body mass index; OC, oral contraceptives; +, relative risk (RR) = 1.1–1.4; ++, RR = 1.5–2.9; +++, RR = 3.0–6.9; −, RR = 0.7–0.8.
[a]Two first-degree relatives who have a history of breast cancer before age 65 years versus no relative.
[b]First-degree relative who has a history of breast cancer before age 65 years versus no relative.
[c]Upper quartile (top 25%) versus lower quartile (lowest 25%).
[d]Clinically recognized chronic cystic, fibrocystic, or other benign breast disease versus none.

antiestrogens. Other growth factors in addition to estrogens, particularly IGF-I and prolactin, also appear to contribute to risk of breast cancer, but these relationships are less firmly established.

Although this broad outline of breast carcinogenesis is unlikely to change substantially with further research, many details are incomplete and other contributing factors will probably be documented. For example, genetic polymorphisms yet to be identified are likely to contribute to variation in endogenous levels of, or responsiveness to, estrogens, IGF-I, and prolactin. Dietary and other behavioral determinants of these factors are incompletely defined. Also, other molecular mechanisms, such as DNA repair and apoptosis, are thought to be important in carcinogenesis in general, but the extent to which exogenous factors influence these processes in the context of human breast cancer is not known.

ATTRIBUTABLE RISK: THE QUANTITATIVE CONTRIBUTION OF KNOWN RISK FACTORS

As noted early in this chapter, the search for specific breast cancer risk factors has been stimulated by the large differences in rates of breast cancer among countries and by changes in rates among migrating populations and within countries over time. The extent to which known risk factors account for these differences in rates is, therefore, of considerable interest. An often-quoted estimate is that only 30% of breast cancer cases are explained by known risk factors (600,601). This has been widely used to suggest that other major risk factors remain to be discovered, in part fueling the search for environmental pollutants that may be responsible. A study of population attributable risks in a nationwide survey estimated, however, that at least 45% to 55% of breast cancer cases in the United States may be explained by later age at first birth, nulliparity, family history of breast cancer, higher socioeconomic status, earlier age at menarche, and prior benign breast disease (602). In another analysis, parity and age at menarche, first birth, and menopause appeared to explain more than half of the difference between breast cancer rates in China and in the United States (92). Among postmenopausal women, just the combination of weight gain after age 18 years and use of postmenopausal hormones accounted for approximately one-third of breast cancer incidence (241). Among women who do not use postmenopausal hormones, weight gain from age 18 accounts for 24.2% of postmenopausal breast cancer (603). Combined with the reproductive variables, this would clearly account for most of the international differences.

A precise determination of the degree to which changes in the prevalence of known breast cancer risk factors account for the increases in breast cancer rates over time is difficult. Changes in age at first birth do not appear to account for appreciable increases in overall U.S. breast cancer rates through 1990, although more delayed childbearing by women born after 1950 should ultimately contribute to an approximately 9% increase in rates (604). Since the 1940s, adiposity, use of postmenopausal hormones, and alcohol consumption by women have, however, increased dramatically. Although further work is needed to quantify these contributions to the secular trends, novel risk factors are not required to account for substantial increases in breast cancer rates.

COMMUNICATING RISK TO PATIENTS

Women and their health care providers are increasingly exposed to information on epidemiologic risk factors for breast cancer,

benefits of prevention strategies, and treatment options. The Gail et al. model of breast cancer risk prediction (605) is increasingly used by clinicians to assess breast cancer risk for women with differing risk factor profiles. This model has been validated, but appears to identify as high risk only a few women who will go on to develop breast cancer (606). Evidence suggests, however, that the understanding of personal risk by women is poor. For example, in a sample of women with a family history of breast cancer, more than two-thirds of women overestimated their lifetime risk of breast cancer, even after participating in a counseling session (607). The overestimation of risk was substantial and perhaps could lead to inappropriate behaviors, such as overscreening, excessive breast self-examination, or inappropriate decisions regarding prophylactic mastectomy or other strategies.

Factors that appear to influence perception of risk include numeracy (608). Women with higher numeracy scores had significantly higher accuracy in gauging the benefits of mammography. Importantly, when discussing risk and risk reduction, research indicates that both absolute risk and RR must be included in the message to maximize the accuracy of risk perception. A presentation must present probabilities about a variety of possible outcomes in a comprehensible manner. It must also attempt to counter *side effect aversion*, a phenomenon we have investigated in detail (609,610). Furthermore, any tool that aids the presentation of risks and benefits must address potential misperceptions about the magnitudes of breast cancer risks, and it must not overwhelm people with the complexity of reducing risk with, for example a SERM (607,611,612). Although more effective formats for presentation of risk and benefits are required, the evidence supports discussion of "risk in 1,000 women exactly like you," as well as the magnitude of risk reduction, perhaps as a percentage.

PREVENTION OF BREAST CANCER

Approaches for the primary prevention of breast cancer according to period of life are discussed here briefly and are considered in more detail elsewhere (613). Although the major reasons for the high rates of breast cancer in affluent Western populations are largely known, this knowledge does not necessarily translate easily into strategies for breast cancer prevention. Some risk factors (e.g., age at menarche) are well established, but difficult to modify; some (e.g., postmenopausal hormone use) are well established and carry risks and benefits; and others (e.g., replacing saturated fat with monounsaturated fat) are unproven, although suggested by some data, but have other strong benefits that justify the strategy, with reduction in breast cancer being a possible additional benefit. Also, known risk factors for breast cancer are modest in magnitude; RR are usually in the range of 1.3 to 1.8 for attainable changes. Although these RR are far less dramatic than that between smoking and lung cancer, they should still be considered important. To provide perspective, the RR of death from breast cancer for women who do not have mammography compared with those who receive regular mammograms is about 1.3. As we give great importance and resources to the provision of mammography, the avoidance of a risk factor with a similar magnitude of effect should have even higher priority because this prevents both the occurrence and the need for treatment of breast cancer as well as death. When considering primary prevention, it is important to remember that even small changes at the individual level can produce substantial changes in the population rates of disease (614).

Some strategies for prevention can be implemented by individuals themselves, but the health system and governments and society as a whole can take actions that will influence importantly rates of breast cancer. In Table 20.3 possible prevention

Table 20.3	**POSSIBLE STRATEGIES AND LEVELS OF ACTION FOR PRIMARY PREVENTION OF BREAST CANCER**		
Strategy	Individual	Health System	Society/Government
Delay menarche	Provide parental support for recreational activity and limit television watching	Encourage regular activity	Provide daily physical activity in schools and safe play environment
Breast-feed	Breast-feed at least 6 months/pregnancy	Encourage lactation	Provide infant child care at work and/or long maternal leaves
Limit alcohol	Limit intake to several drinks/week	Provide education	Develop social norms for low alcohol intake by women
Avoid long-term estrogen therapy, especially if combined with progestagens	Limit use to treatment of symptoms	Educate patients on risks and benefits	
Avoid adult weight gain	Engage in regular physical activity, moderately restrain total calorie intake	Counsel patients on the importance of avoiding weight gain	Provide safe environment for pedestrians and bicycle riding; provide work-site and community recreational facilities
Eat five servings of fruit and vegetables per day; replace saturated fat with olive, canola, and other oils high in monounsaturated fat	Make healthy dietary choices	Encourage healthy diets	Provide healthy choices in work site and schools, and provide best current information on diet and health

strategies are listed, along with actions that can be taken at these different levels to reduce rates of breast cancer.

Early onset of menarche in the United States and other affluent countries is largely the result of rapid growth and weight gain of children related to an abundant food supply, excellent sanitation, and low levels of physical activity (including sitting in school). Much of this is desirable for many reasons, and there is no reasonable expectation that we could or would want to increase the average age at menarche to 17 years, as has been typical in rural China. Yet, generally desirable increases in physical activity, such as greater recreational activities, have been associated with modest delays in age at menarche (341,615) and, thus, should contribute to reductions in breast cancer. The amount of time spent watching television is a major determinant of excessive weight gain by children (616,617) and, thus, an appropriate focus for reducing risk of breast cancer and future cardiovascular disease and diabetes. Society, through the provision of daily physical activity in schools and safe environments for recreational activity, must play a major role in these efforts.

Early age at first birth will substantially reduce breast cancer, but the societal trends are in the opposite direction because of delay of childbirth until after educational programs are completed and careers are established. Further, unplanned early pregnancies and more than an average of two completed pregnancies per woman have undesirable social and ecologic consequences. Nevertheless, a social norm that encouraged carefully planned first pregnancies at the beginning of advanced education and career development would reduce breast cancer rates. This would require major behavioral changes and social supports, such as for childcare, to be practical on a widespread basis. Because of the complex social changes needed for this to be a practical strategy for breast cancer prevention, and potential undesirable consequences, we have not included it in Table 20.3.

At least 6 months of lactation is recommended for optimal infant health (67) and evidence suggests this will modestly reduce the risk of breast cancer, particularly among premenopausal women. Improved physician counseling (618) can encourage this practice, but changes at workplaces to allow breast-feeding and longer maternity leaves will also be needed for many women to adopt this practice.

Alcohol consumption has a complex mix of desirable and adverse health effects, one being an increase in breast cancer. Individuals should make decisions considering all the risks and

benefits, but for a middle-aged woman who drinks alcohol on a daily basis, reducing intake is one of relatively few behavioral changes that is likely to reduce risk of breast cancer. Taking a multiple vitamin containing folic acid greatly reduces risks of neural tube defects and may prevent coronary artery disease (619) and colon cancer (620), and growing evidence suggests this may mitigate the excess risk of breast cancer owing to alcohol use (415). Thus, taking a multiple vitamin appears sensible for women who do elect to drink regularly.

Postmenopausal hormone use, as with alcohol consumption, involves a complex trade-off of benefits and risks. From the standpoint of breast cancer risk, the optimal strategy would be to use estrogens not at all or at most for a few years to relieve menopausal symptoms. Most importantly, combined use of estrogen plus progestin for more than 1 year should be avoided. The range of options, however, is rapidly increasing with the demonstration that tamoxifen and valoxifene, two selective estrogen receptor modulators, can be effective in the primary prevention of breast cancer. Physicians will need to play a key role in advising women in this rapidly evolving field.

Avoiding weight gain during adult life can importantly reduce risk of postmenopausal breast cancer, as well as cardiovascular disease and many other conditions. Individual women can reduce weight gain by exercising regularly and moderately restraining caloric intake. Health care providers play an important role in counseling patients throughout adult life about the importance of weight control. However, the incorporation of greater physical activity into daily life will be difficult for many persons unless governments provide a safer and more accessible environment for pedestrians and bicycle riders. The provision of work-site and community exercise facilities can also contribute importantly.

Specific aspects of diet that influence risk of breast cancer are not yet well established, but available evidence generally suggests that replacing saturated and transfat with monounsaturated fat may reduce risk. Increasing fruit and vegetable intake may reduce breast cancer risk, although the impact appears to be modest at best. These are reasonable strategies to pursue, however, because they will reduce the risk of cardiovascular and other diseases, and a slightly reduced risk of breast cancer may be an added benefit. Physicians can assess dietary habits and provide guidance, and governmental policies influence diets in many ways. Providing the best current information on diet and health is one such role.

With demonstration that tamoxifen and probably other selective ER modulators can be effective in the primary prevention of breast cancer (106,108), chemoprevention has become an option for women at elevated risk. Many other pharmacologic agents are being evaluated and are likely to increase the alternatives. The availability of effective chemopreventive agents raises many questions about the optimal criteria for use of these drugs. Evaluation of an individual woman's risk of breast cancer has become much more important because this risk can now be modified. Until recently, risk has been based primarily on an evaluation of family and reproductive history and history of benign breast disease. New information on risk based on genotype, detailed histologic characteristics of benign breast disease (621), and serum hormone levels (113) now allows a much more powerful prediction of risk for an individual woman. Screening for elevated estrogen levels in postmenopausal women to help identify those who would most benefit from an estrogen antagonist, as is done for serum cholesterol, may become part of medical practice. Physicians will play a key role in keeping current on this rapidly developing area and counseling patients appropriately.

In summary, available evidence provides a basis for a number of strategies that can reduce risk of breast cancer, although some of these represent complex decision making. Attainable objectives can make an important impact on individual risk of breast cancer. However, the collective implementation of all lifestyle strategies will not reduce population rates of breast cancer to the very low levels of traditional agrarian societies because the magnitude of the necessary changes is unrealistic or undesirable. Thus, a role will exist for hormonal and other chemopreventive interventions that may be appropriate for women at particularly high risk and, potentially, for wide segments of the population because few women can be considered to have very low risk. Together, the modification of nutritional and lifestyle risk factors and the judicious use of chemopreventive agents can have a major impact on incidence of this important disease.

References

1. Jemal A, Siegel R, Ward E, et al. Cancer statistics, 2007. *CA Cancer J Clin* 2007;57:43–66.
2. Weir HK, Thun MJ, Hankey BK, et al. Annual report to the nation on the status of cancer, 1975–2000, featuring the uses of surveillance data for cancer prevention and control. *J Natl Cancer Inst* 2003;95:1276–1299.
3. National Cancer Institute. SEER cancer statistics review, 1973–1995: National Center for Health Statistics, 1998.
4. Garcia M, Jemal A, Ward, EM, et al. *Journal of global cancer facts & figures 2007*. Atlanta, GA: American Cancer Society, 2007.
5. Parkin DM, Muir CS. Cancer incidence in five continents. Comparability and quality of data. *International Agency for Research on Cancer (IARC)* Lyon, France *Sci Publ* 1992;45–173.
6. Ferlay J, Pisani FBP, Parkin, DN. GLOBOCAN 2002. Cancer incidence, mortality and prevalence worldwide. IARC CancerBase No. 5, version 2.0: IARCPress, Lyon, 2004.
7. Nagata C, Kawakami N, Shimizu H. Trends in the incidence rate and risk factors for breast cancer in Japan. *Breast Cancer Res Treat* 1997;44:75–82.
8. Seow A, Duffy SW, McGee MA, et al. Breast cancer in Singapore: trends in incidence 1968–1992. *Int J Epidemiol* 1996;25:40–45.
9. Hoover R. Geographic, migrant, and time trend patterns. In: Fortner J, ed. *Accomplishments in cancer research*. New York: Lippincott-Raven, 1996.
10. Surveillance, Epidemiology, and End Results (SEER) Program (www.seer.cancer.gov) Limited-use data (1973–2005), National Cancer Institute, DCCPS, Surveillance Research Program, Cancer Statistics Branch, released April 2008, based on the November 2007 submission.
11. Pike MC, Spicer DV, Dahmoush L, et al. Estrogens, progestogens, normal breast cell proliferation, and breast cancer risk. *Epidemiol Rev* 1993;15:17–35.
12. Tominaga S, Aoki, K, Fujimoto I, et al. *Cancer mortality and morbidity statistics: Japan and the world—1994*. Tokyo: Japan Scientific Societies Press, 1994.
13. Heck KE, Pamuk ER. Explaining the relation between education and postmenopausal breast cancer. *Am J Epidemiol* 1997;145:366–372.
14. Krieger N. Social class and the black/white crossover in the age-specific incidence of breast cancer: a study linking census-derived data to population-based registry records. *Am J Epidemiol* 1990;131:804–814.
15. Rosner B, Colditz G A. Nurses' health study: log-incidence mathematical model of breast cancer incidence. *J Natl Cancer Inst* 1996;88:359–364.
16. Carey LA, Perou CM, Livasy CA, et al. Race, breast cancer subtypes, and survival in the Carolina Breast Cancer Study. *JAMA* 2006;295:2492–502.
17. Stanford JL, Herrinton LJ, Schwartz SM, et al. Breast cancer incidence in Asian migrants to the United States and their descendants. *Epidemiology* 1995;6:181–183.
18. Dunn J E. Cancer epidemiology in populations of the United States—with emphasis on Hawaii and California—and Japan. *Cancer Res* 1975;35:3240–3245.
19. Kolonel LN. Cancer patterns of four ethnic groups in Hawaii. *J Natl Cancer Inst* 1980;65:1127–1139.
20. Shimizu H, Ross RK, Bernstein L, et al. Cancers of the prostate and breast among Japanese and white immigrants in Los Angeles County. *Br J Cancer* 1991;63:963–966.
21. Tominaga S. Cancer incidence in Japanese in Japan, Hawaii, and western United States. *Natl Cancer Inst Monogr* 1985;69:83–92.
22. Yu H, Harris RE, Gao YT, et al. Comparative epidemiology of cancers of the colon, rectum, prostate and breast in Shanghai, China versus the United States. *Int J Epidemiol* 1991;20:76–81.
23. Ziegler RG, Hoover RN, Pike MC, et al. Migration patterns and breast cancer risk in Asian-American women. *J Natl Cancer Inst* 1993;85:1819–1827.
24. Tiirner EM, Smith KR. Breast cancer mortality among immigrants in Australia and Canada. *J Natl Cancer Inst* 1995;87:1154–1161.
25. Bouchardy C. *Cancer in Italian migrant populations*. France. International Agency for Research on Cancer (IARC) *Sci Publ* 1993;149–159.
26. Young C. Changes in demographic behaviour of migrants in Australia and the transition between generations. *Pop Studies* 1991;45:67–89.
27. Robbins AS, Brescianini S, Kelsey JL. Regional differences in known risk factors and the higher incidence of breast cancer in San Francisco. *J Natl Cancer Inst* 1997;89:960–965.
28. Centers for Disease Control and Prevention. Breast cancer on Long Island, New York. Washington, DC: U.S. Department of Health and Human Services; 1992.
29. Gammon MD, Neugut AI, Santella RM, et al. The Long Island Breast Cancer Study Project: description of a multi-institutional collaboration to identify environmental risk factors for breast cancer. *Breast Cancer Res Treat* 2002;74:235–254.
30. Radiology American College of Radiology Breast imaging reporting and data systems (BI-RADS). Reston, VA: American College of Radiology, 1998.
31. Sturgeon SR, Schairer C, Gail M, et al. Geographic variation in mortality from breast cancer among white women in the United States. *J Natl Cancer Inst* 1995;87:1846–1853.
32. Connecticut Tumor Registry. *Cancer incidence in Connecticut*. Vol. 2003. Connecticut: Department of Public Health, 2002.
33. Feuer EJ, Wun LM. How much of the recent rise in breast cancer incidence can be explained by increases in mammography utilization? A dynamic population model approach. *Am J Epidemiol* 1992;136:1423–1436.
34. Lantz PM, Remington PL, Newcomb PA. Mammography screening and increased incidence of breast cancer in Wisconsin. *J Natl Cancer Inst* 1991;83:1540–1546.
35. Liff JM, Sung JF, Chow WH, et al. Does increased detection account for the rising incidence of breast cancer? *Am J Public Health* 1991;81:462–465.
36. Miller BA, Feuer EJ, Hankey BF. The increasing incidence of breast cancer since 1982: relevance of early detection. *Cancer Causes Control* 1991;2:67–74.
36a. Prentice RL. Measurement error and results from analytic epidemiology: dietary fat and breast cancer *J Nati Cancer Inst* 1996;88(23)1738–1747.
37. Miller BA, Feuer EJ, Hankey BF. Recent incidence trends for breast cancer in women and the relevance of early detection: an update. *CA Cancer J Clin* 1993;43:27–41.
38. White E, Lee CY, Kristal AR. Evaluation of the increase in breast cancer incidence in relation to mammography use. *J Natl Cancer Inst* 1990;82:1546–1552.
39. Chu KC, Tarone RE, Kessler LG, et al. Recent trends in U.S. breast cancer incidence, survival, and mortality rates. *J Natl Cancer Inst* 1996;88:1571–1579.
40. Rossouw JE, Anderson GL, Prentice RL, et al. Risks and benefits of estrogen plus progestin in healthy postmenopausal women: principal results From the Women's Health Initiative randomized controlled trial. *JAMA* 2002;288:321–333.
41. Ravdin PM, Cronin KA, Howlader N, et al. The decrease in breast-cancer incidence in 2003 in the United States. *N Engl J Med* 2007;356:1670–1674.
42. Chevarley F, White E. Recent trends in breast cancer mortality among white and black US women. *Am J Public Health* 1997;87:775–781.
43. Wingo PA, Cardinez CJ, Landis SH, et al. Long-term trends in cancer mortality in the United States, 1930–1998. *Cancer* 2003;97:3133–3275.
44. American Cancer Society. *Breast cancer facts & figures 2007–2008*. Atlanta: American Cancer Society, 2007.
45. Persson I, Bergstrom R, Barlow L, et al. Recent trends in breast cancer incidence in Sweden. *Br J Cancer* 1998;77:167–169.
46. Quinn M, Allen E. Changes in incidence of and mortality from breast cancer in England and Wales since introduction of screening. United Kingdom Association of Cancer Registries. *BMJ* 1995;311:1391–1395.
47. Jin F, Shu XO, Devesa SS, et al. Incidence trends for cancers of the breast, ovary, and corpus uteri in urban Shanghai, 1972–1989. *Cancer Causes Control* 1993;4:355–360.
48. Althuis MD, Dozier JM, Anderson WF, et al. Global trends in breast cancer incidence and mortality 1973–1997. *Int J Epidemiol* 2005;34:405–412.
49. Hermon C, Beral V. Breast cancer mortality rates are levelling off or beginning to decline in many western countries: analysis of time trends, age-cohort and age-period models of breast cancer mortality in 20 countries. *Br J Cancer* 1996;73:955–960.
50. Beral V, Hermon C, Reeves G, et al. Sudden fall in breast cancer death rates in England and Wales. *Lancet* 1995;345:1642–1643.
51. Kelsey JL, Gammon MD John EM. Reproductive factors and breast cancer. *Epidemiol Rev* 1993;15:36–47.
52. Clavel-Chapelon F. Differential effects of reproductive factors on the risk of pre- and postmenopausal breast cancer. Results from a large cohort of French women. *Br J Cancer* 2002;86:723–727.
53. Clavel-Chapelon F, Gerber M. Reproductive factors and breast cancer risk. Do they differ according to age at diagnosis? *Breast Cancer Res Treat* 2002;72:107–115.
54. Ma H, Bernstein L, Pike MC, et al. Reproductive factors and breast cancer risk according to joint estrogen and progesterone receptor status: a meta-analysis of epidemiological studies. Breast *Cancer Res* 2006;8:R43.
55. MacMahon B, Trichopoulos D, Brown J, et al. Age at menarche, urine estrogens and breast cancer risk. *Int J Cancer* 1982;30:427–431.
56. Bernstein L, Ross RK. Endogenous hormones and breast cancer risk. *Epidemiol Rev* 1993;15:48–65.
57. Garland CF, Hunter DJ, Colditz GA, et al. Menstrual cycle characteristics and history of ovulatory infertility in relation to breast cancer risk in a large cohort of U.S. women. *Am J Epidemiol* 1998;147:636–643.
58. Bruzzi P, Negri E, La Vecchia C, et al. Short term increase in risk of breast cancer after full term pregnancy. *BMJ* 1998;297:1096–1098.

59. Pike MC, Krailo MD, Henderson BE, et al. 'Hormonal' risk factors, 'breast tissue age' and the age-incidence of breast cancer. *Nature* 1983;303:767–770.
60. Rosner B, Colditz GA, Willett WC. Reproductive risk factors in a prospective study of breast cancer: the Nurses' Health Study. *Am J Epidemiol* 1994;139:819–835.
61. Lambe M, Hsieh C, Trichopoulos D, et al. Transient increase in the risk of breast cancer after giving birth. *N Engl J Med* 1994;331:5–9.
62. Russo J, Tay LK, Russo IH. Differentiation of the mammary gland and susceptibility to carcinogenesis. *Breast Cancer Res Treat* 1982;2:5–73.
63. La Vecchia C, Negri E, Boyle P. Reproductive factors and breast cancer: an overview. *Soz Praventivmed* 1989;34:101–107.
64. Trichopoulos D, Hsieh CC, MacMahon B, et al. Age at any birth and breast cancer risk. *Int J Cancer* 1983;31:701–704.
65. Lane-Claypon JE. *A further report on cancer of the breast, with special reference to its associated antecedent conditions.* London: Ministry of Health, 1926.
66. Ventura S, Taffel S. Collaborative Group on Hormonal Factors in Breast Cancer Breast Cancer and breastfeeding: collaborative reanalysis of individual data from 47 epidemiological studies in 30 countries, including 50302 women with breast cancer and 96,973 women without the disease. *Lancet* 2002;360:187–195.
67. Committee on Nutrition, American Academy of Pediatrics. *Pediatric nutrition handbook*. Elk Grove Village, IL, 1993.
68. Kline J, Stein Z, Susser M. *Conception to birth, epidemiology of prenatal development*. New York, NY: Oxford University Press, 1989.
69. Krieger N. Exposure, susceptibility, and breast cancer risk: a hypothesis regarding exogenous carcinogens, breast tissue development, and social gradients, including black/white differences, in breast cancer incidence. *Breast Cancer Res Treat* 1989;13:205–223.
70. Ventura S, Taffel S, Mosher W, et al. *Trends in pregnancies and pregnancy rates: estimates for the United States, 1980–1992*. Hyattsville, MD: National Center for Health Statistics, 1995.
71. Brind J, Chinchilli VM, Severs WB, et al. Induced abortion as an independent risk factor for breast cancer: a comprehensive review and meta-analysis. *J Epidemiol Community Health* 1996;50:481–496.
72. Melbye M, Wohlfahrt J, Olsen JH, et al. Induced abortion and the risk of breast cancer. *N Engl J Med* 1997;336:81–85.
73. Lazovich D, Thompson JA, Mink PJ, et al. Induced abortion and breast cancer risk. *Epidemiology* 2000;11:76–80.
74. Ye Z, Gao DL, Qin Q, et al. Breast cancer in relation to induced abortions in a cohort of Chinese women. *Br J Cancer* 2002;87:977–981.
75. Reeves GK, Kan SW, Key T, et al. Breast cancer risk in relation to abortion: results from the EPIC study. *Int J Cancer* 2006;119:1741–1745.
76. Michels KB, Xue F, Colditz GA, et al. Induced and spontaneous abortion and incidence of breast cancer among young women: a prospective cohort study. *Arch Intern Med* 2007;167:814–820.
77. Early Reproductive Events and Breast Cancer Workshop. Summary Report: Early Reproductive Events and Breast Cancer Workshop; Bethesda, MD 2003.
78. Lilienfeld AM. The relationship of cancer of the female breast to artificial menopause and martial status. *Cancer* 1956;9:927–934.
79. Trichopoulos D, MacMahon B, Cole P. Menopause and breast cancer risk. *J Natl Cancer Inst* 1972;48:605–613.
80. Breast cancer and hormonal contraceptives: collaborative reanalysis of individual data on 53,297 women with breast cancer and 100,239 women without breast cancer from 54 epidemiological studies. Collaborative Group on Hormonal Factors in Breast Cancer. *Lancet* 1996;347:1713–1727.
81. Colditz GA, Stampfer MJ, Willett WC, et al. Reproducibility and validity of self-reported menopausal status in a prospective cohort study. *Am J Epidemiol* 1987;126:319–325.
82. Armitage P, Doll R. The age distribution of cancer and a multi-stage theory of carcinogenesis. *Br J Cancer* 1954;8:1–12.
83. Moolgavkar SH, Knudson AG Jr. Mutation and cancer: a model for human carcinogenesis. *J Natl Cancer Inst* 1981;66:1037–1052.
84. Colditz GA, Rosner B. Cumulative risk of breast cancer to age 70 years according to risk factor status: data from the Nurses' Health Study. *Am J Epidemiol* 2000; 152:950–964.
85. Hsieh C, Pavia M, Lambe M, et al. Dual effect of parity on breast cancer risk. *Eur J Cancer* 1994;30A:969–973.
86. Janerich DT, Hoff MB. Evidence for a crossover in breast cancer risk factors. *Am J Epidemiol* 1982;116:737–742.
87. Gray GE, Henderson BE, Pike MC. Changing ratio of breast cancer incidence rates with age of black females compared with white females in the United States. *J Natl Cancer Inst* 1980;64:461–463.
88. Census, U.S. Census Bureau *Fertility of American women: June 1983*. Washington, DC: U.S. Department of Commerce, Bureau of the Census, 1983.
89. Bank W. *Social indicators of development 1993*. Baltimore: Johns Hopkins University Press, 1993.
90. Chen J, Campbell T, Junyao L, et al. Diet, life-style, and mortality in China: a study of the characteristics of 65 Chinese counties. Oxford, England: Oxford University Press, 1990.
91. Rogers CC. Fertility of American women: June 1983. *Curr Popul Rep Popul Charact* 1983:1–63.
92. Colditz G. A biomathematical model of breast cancer incidence: the contrubution of reproductive factors to variation in breast cancer incidence. In: Fortner J, Sharp P, eds. *Accomplishments in cancer research 1996*. Philadelphia: Lippincott-Raven, 1996:116–121.
93. Rockhill B, Byrne C, Rosner B, et al. Breast cancer risk prediction with a log-incidence model: evaluation of accuracy. *J Clin Epidemiol* 2003;56:856–861.
94. Colditz G, Rosner B, Chen WY, et al. Risk factors for breast cancer: according to estrogen and progesterone receptor status. *J Natl Cancer Inst* 2004:96: 218–228.
95. Wald N, Hackshaw A, Frost C. When can a risk factor be used as a worthwhile screening test? *BMJ* 1999;319:1562–1565.
96. Ottman R, Pike MC, King MC, et al. Practical guide for estimating risk for familial breast cancer. *Lancet* 1983;2:556–558.
97. Claus EB, Risch N, Thompson WD. The calculation of breast cancer risk for women with a first degree family history of ovarian cancer. *Breast Cancer Res Treat* 1993;28:115–120.
98. Berry DA, Iversen ES Jr, Gudbjartsson DF, et al. BRCAPRO validation, sensitivity of genetic testing of BRCA1/BRCA2, and prevalence of other breast cancer susceptibility genes. *J Clin Oncol* 2002;20:2701–2712.
99. Parmigiani G, Berry D, Aguilar O. Determining carrier probabilities for breast cancer-susceptibility genes BRCA1 and BRCA2. *Am J Hum Genet* 1998;62: 145–158.
100. Tyrer J, Duffy SW, Cuzick J. A breast cancer prediction model incorporating familial and personal risk factors. *Stat Med* 2004;23:1111–1130.
101. Barlow WE, White E, Ballard-Barbash R, et al. Prospective breast cancer risk prediction model for women undergoing screening mammography. *J Natl Cancer Inst* 2006;98:1204–1214.
102. Chen J, Pee D, Ayyagari R, et al. Projecting absolute invasive breast cancer risk in white women with a model that includes mammographic density. *J Natl Cancer Inst* 2006;98:1215–1226.
103. Fisher B, Costantino J, Wickerham D, et al.; National Surgical Adjuvant Breast and Bowel Project Investigators. Tamoxifen for prevention of breast cancer: report of the National Surgical Adjuvant Breast and Bowel Project P-1 study. *J Natl Cancer Inst* 1998;90:1371–1388.
104. Gail MH, Costantino JP, Bryant J, et al. Weighing the risks and benefits of tamoxifen treatment for preventing breast cancer. *J Natl Cancer Inst* 1999;91: 1829–1846.
105. Key TJ, Appleby PN, Reeves GK, et al. Body mass index, serum sex hormones, and breast cancer risk in postmenopausal women. *J Natl Cancer Inst* 2003;95: 1218–1226.
106. Cummings SR, Eckert S, Krueger KA, et al. The effect of raloxifene on risk of breast cancer in postmenopausal women: results from the MORE randomized trial. Multiple Outcomes of Raloxifene Evaluation. *JAMA* 1999;281:2189–2197.
107. Cuzick J, Powles T, Veronesi U, et al. Overview of the main outcomes in breast-cancer prevention trials. *Lancet* 2003;361:296–300.
108. Fisher B, Costantino JP, Wickerham DL, et al. Tamoxifen for prevention of breast cancer: report of the National Surgical Adjuvant Breast and Bowel Project P-1 Study. *J Natl Cancer Inst* 1998;90:1371–1388.
109. Hankinson SE, Manson JE, London SJ, et al. Laboratory reproducibility of endogenous hormone levels in postmenopausal women. *Cancer Epidemiol Biomarkers Prev* 1994;3:51–56.
110. Potischman N, Falk RT, Laiming VA, et al. Reproducibility of laboratory assays for steroid hormones and sex hormone-binding globulin. *Cancer Res* 1994;54: 5363–5367.
111. Dowsett M, Folkerd E. Deficits in plasma oestradiol measurement in studies and management of breast cancer. *Breast Cancer Res* 2005;7:1–4.
112. Stanczyk FZ, Lee JS, Santen RJ. Standardization of steroid hormone assays: why, how, and when? *Cancer Epidemiol Biomarkers Prev* 2007;16:1713–1719.
113. Hankinson SE, Willett WC, Manson JE, et al. Plasma sex steroid hormone levels and risk of breast cancer in postmenopausal women. *J Natl Cancer Inst* 1998; 90:1292–1299.
114. Toniolo PG, Levitz M, Zeleniuch-Jacquotte A, et al. A prospective study of endogenous estrogens and breast cancer in postmenopausal women. *J Natl Cancer Inst* 1995;87:190–197.
115. Hankinson SE, Manson JE, Spiegelman D, et al. E. Reproducibility of plasma hormone levels in postmenopausal women over a 2–3-year period. *Cancer Epidemiol Biomarkers Prev* 1995;4:649–654.
116. Micheli A, Muti P, Pisani P, et al. Repeated serum and urinary androgen measurements in premenopausal and postmenopausal women. *J Clin Epidemiol* 1991;44:1055–1061.
117. Muti P, Trevisan M, Micheli A, et al. Reliability of serum hormones in premenopausal and postmenopausal women over a one-year period. *Cancer Epidemiol Biomarkers Prev* 1996;5:917–922.
118. Toniolo P, Koenig KL, Pasternack BS, et al. Reliability of measurements of total, protein-bound, and unbound estradiol in serum. *Cancer Epidemiol Biomarkers Prev* 1994;3:47–50.
119. Missmer SA, Spiegelman D, Bertone-Johnson ER, et al. Reproducibility of plasma steroid hormones, prolactin, and insulin-like growth factor levels among premenopausal women over a 2- to 3-year period. *Cancer Epidemiol Biomarkers Prev* 2006;15:972–978.
120. Muti P, Quattrin T, Grant BJ, et al. Fasting glucose is a risk factor for breast cancer: a prospective study. *Cancer Epidemiol Biomarkers Prev* 2002;11:1361–1368.
121. Roberts KD, Rochefort JG, Bleau G, et al. Plasma estrone sulfate levels in postmenopausal women. *Steroids* 1980;35:179–187.
122. Pasqualini JR, Chetrite G, Blacker C, et al. Concentrations of estrone, estradiol, and estrone sulfate and evaluation of sulfatase and aromatase activities in pre- and postmenopausal breast cancer patients. *J Clin Endocrinol Metab* 1996;81: 1460–1464.
123. Key T, Appleby P, Barnes I, et al. Endogenous sex hormones and breast cancer in postmenopausal women: reanalysis of nine prospective studies. *J Natl Cancer Inst* 2002;94:606–616.
124. Kaaks R, Rinaldi S, Key TJ, et al. Postmenopausal serum androgens, oestrogens and breast cancer risk: the European prospective investigation into cancer and nutrition. *Endocr Relat Cancer* 2005;12:1071–1082.
125. Manjer J, Johansson R, Berglund G, et al. Postmenopausal breast cancer risk in relation to sex steroid hormones, prolactin and SHBG (Sweden). *Cancer Causes Control* 12003;4:599–607.
126. Missmer SA, Eliassen AH, Barbieri RL, et al. Endogenous estrogen, androgen, and progesterone concentrations and breast cancer risk among postmenopausal women. *J Natl Cancer Inst* 2004;96:1856–1865.
127. Key TJ, Wang DY, Brown JB, et al. A prospective study of urinary oestrogen excretion and breast cancer risk. *Br J Cancer* 1996;73:1615–1619.
128. Onland-Moret NC, Kaaks R, van Noord PA, et al. Urinary endogenous sex hormone levels and the risk of postmenopausal breast cancer. *Br J Cancer* 2003;88:1394–1399.
129. Martino S, Cauley JA, Barrett-Connor E, Powles, et al. Continuing outcomes relevant to Evista: breast cancer incidence in postmenopausal osteoporotic women in a randomized trial of raloxifene. *J Natl Cancer Inst* 2004;96:1751–1761.
130. Beattie MS, Costantino JP, Cummings SR, et al. Endogenous sex hormones, breast cancer risk, and tamoxifen response: an ancillary study in the NSABP Breast Cancer Prevention Trial (P-1). *J Natl Cancer Inst* 2006;98:110–115.
131. Costantino JP, Gail MH, Pee D, et al. Validation studies for models projecting the risk of invasive and total breast cancer incidence. *J Natl Cancer Inst* 1999;91: 1541–1548.
132. Eliassen AH, Missmer SA, Tworoger SS, et al. Endogenous steroid hormone concentrations and risk of breast cancer: does the association vary by a woman's predicted breast cancer risk? *J Clin Oncol* 2006;24:1823–1830.

133. Tworoger SS, Missmer SA, Barbieri RL, et al. Plasma sex hormone concentrations and subsequent risk of breast cancer among women using postmenopausal hormones. *J Natl Cancer Inst* 2005;97:595–602.
134. Helzlsouer KJ, Alberg AJ, Bush TL, et al. A prospective study of endogenous hormones and breast cancer. *Cancer Detect Prev* 1994;18:79–85.
135. Kabuto M, Akiba S, Stevens RG, et al. A prospective study of estradiol and breast cancer in Japanese women. *Cancer Epidemiol Biomarkers Prev* 2000;9:575–579.
136. Rosenberg CR, Pasternack BS, Shore RE, et al. Premenopausal estradiol levels and the risk of breast cancer: a new method of controlling for day of the menstrual cycle. *Am J Epidemiol* 1994;140:518–525.
137. Thomas HV, Key TJ, Allen DS, et al. A prospective study of endogenous serum hormone concentrations and breast cancer risk in premenopausal women on the island of Guernsey. *Br J Cancer* 1997;75:1075–1079.
138. Wysowski DK, Comstock GW, Helsing KJ, et al. Sex hormone levels in serum in relation to the development of breast cancer. *Am J Epidemiol* 1987;125:791–799.
139. Kaaks R, Berrino F, Key T, et al. Serum sex steroids in premenopausal women and breast cancer risk within the European Prospective Investigation into Cancer and Nutrition (EPIC). *J Natl Cancer Inst* 2005;97:755–765.
140. Eliassen AH, Missmer SA, Tworoger SS, et al. Endogenous steroid hormone concentrations and risk of breast cancer among premenopausal women. *J Natl Cancer Inst* 2006;98:1406–1415.
141. Yager JD, Liehr JG. Molecular mechanisms of estrogen carcinogenesis. *Annu Rev Pharmacol Toxicol* 1996;36:203–232.
142. Meilahn EN, De Stavola B, Allen DS, et al. Do urinary oestrogen metabolites predict breast cancer? Guernsey III cohort follow-up. *Br J Cancer* 1998;78:1250–1255.
143. Muti P, Bradlow HL, Micheli A, et al. Estrogen metabolism and risk of breast cancer: a prospective study of the 2:16alpha-hydroxyestrone ratio in premenopausal and postmenopausal women. *Epidemiology* 2000;11:635–640.
144. Wellejus A, Olsen A, Tjonneland A, et al. Urinary hydroxyestrogens and breast cancer risk among postmenopausal women: a prospective study. *Cancer Epidemiol Biomarkers Prev* 2005;14:2137–2142.
145. Cauley JA, Zmuda JM, Danielson ME, et al. Estrogen metabolites and the risk of breast cancer in older women. *Epidemiology* 2003;14:740–744.
146. Liao DJ, Dickson RB. Roles of androgens in the development, growth, and carcinogenesis of the mammary gland. *J Steroid Biochem Mol Biol* 2002;80:175–189.
147. Ebeling P, Koivisto VA. Physiological importance of dehydroepiandrosterone. *Lancet* 1994;343:1479–1481.
148. Seymour-Munn K, Adams J. Estrogenic effects of 5-androstene-3 beta, 17 beta-diol at physiological concentrations and its possible implication in the etiology of breast cancer. Endocrinology 1983;112:486–491.
149. Micheli A, Muti P, Secreto G, et al. Endogenous sex hormones and subsequent breast cancer in premenopausal women. *Int J Cancer* 2004;112:312–318.
150. Kelsey JL. A review of the epidemiology of human breast cancer. *Epidemiol Rev* 1979;1:74–109.
151. Partridge RK, Hahnel R. Prolactin receptors in human breast carcinoma. *Cancer* 1979;43:643–646.
152. Malarkey WB, Kennedy M, Allred LE, et al. Physiological concentrations of prolactin can promote the growth of human breast tumor cells in culture. *J Clin Endocrinol Metab* 1983;56:673–677.
153. Clevenger CV, Furth PA, Hankinson SE, et al. The role of prolactin in mammary carcinoma. *Endocr Rev* 2003;24:1–27.
154. Gutzman JH, Miller KK, Schuler LA. Endogenous human prolactin and not exogenous human prolactin induces estrogen receptor alpha and prolactin receptor expression and increases estrogen responsiveness in breast cancer cells. *J Steroid Biochem Mol Biol* 2004;88:69–77.
155. Liby K, Neltner B, Mohamet L, et al. Prolactin overexpression by MDA-MB-435 human breast cancer cells accelerates tumor growth. *Breast Cancer Res Treat* 2003;79:241–252.
156. Perks CM, Keith AJ, Goodhew KL, et al. Prolactin acts as a potent survival factor for human breast cancer cell lines. *Br J Cancer* 2004;91:305–311.
157. Schroeder MD, Symowicz J, Schuler LA. PRL modulates cell cycle regulators in mammary tumor epithelial cells. *Mol Endocrinol* 2002;16:45–57.
158. Maus MV, Reilly SC, Clevenger CV. Prolactin as a chemoattractant for human breast carcinoma. *Endocrinology* 1999;140:5447–5450.
159. Struman I, Bentzien F, Lee H, et al. Opposing actions of intact and N-terminal fragments of the human prolactin/growth hormone family members on angiogenesis: an efficient mechanism for the regulation of angiogenesis. *Proc Natl Acad Sci U S A* 1999;96:1246–1251.
160. Herman V, Kalk WJ, de Moor NG, et al. Serum prolactin after chest wall surgery: elevated levels after mastectomy. *J Clin Endocrinol Metab* 1981;52:148–151.
161. Yen SSC, Jaffe RB. *Reproductive endocrinology*. Philadelphia: WB Saunders, 1991.
162. Hankinson SE, Willett WC, Michaud DS, et al. Plasma prolactin levels and subsequent risk of breast cancer in postmenopausal women. *J Natl Cancer Inst* 1999;91:629–634.
163. Tworoger SS, Eliassen AH, Rosner B, et al. Plasma prolactin concentrations and risk of postmenopausal breast cancer. *Cancer Res* 2004;64:6814–6819.
164. Tworoger SS, Eliassen AH, Sluss P, et al. A prospective study of plasma prolactin concentrations and risk of premenopausal and postmenopausal breast cancer. *J Clin Oncol* 2007;25:1482–1488.
165. Tworoger SS, Sluss P, Hankinson SE. Association between plasma prolactin concentrations and risk of breast cancer among predominately premenopausal women. *Cancer Res* 2006;66:2476–2482.
166. Wang DY, De Stavola BL, Bulbrook RD, et al. Relationship of blood prolactin levels and the risk of subsequent breast cancer. *Int J Epidemiol* 1992;21:214–221.
167. Pollak MN, Schernhammer ES, Hankinson SE. Insulin-like growth factors and neoplasia. *Nat Rev Cancer* 2004;4:505–518.
168. Pollak M, Beamer W, Zhang JC. Insulin-like growth factors and prostate cancer. *Cancer Metastasis Rev* 1998;17:383–390.
169. Renehan AG, Zwahlen M, Minder C, et al. Insulin-like growth factor (IGF)-I, IGF binding protein-3, and cancer risk: systematic review and meta-regression analysis. *Lancet* 2004;363:1346–1353.
170. Fletcher O, Gibson L, Johnson N, et al. Polymorphisms and circulating levels in the insulin-like growth factor system and risk of breast cancer: a systematic review. *Cancer Epidemiol Biomarkers Prev* 2005;14:2–19.
171. Renehan AG, Harvie M, Howell A. Insulin-like growth factor (IGF)-I, IGF binding protein-3, and breast cancer risk: eight years on. *Endocr Relat Cancer* 2006;13:273–278.
172. Rinaldi S, Peeters PH, Berrino F, et al. IGF-I, IGFBP-3 and breast cancer risk in women: The European Prospective Investigation into Cancer and Nutrition (EPIC). *Endocr Relat Cancer* 2006;13:593–605.
173. Schernhammer ES, Holly JM, Hunter DJ, et al. Insulin-like growth factor-I, its binding proteins (IGFBP-1 and IGFBP-3), and growth hormone and breast cancer risk in The Nurses' Health Study II. *Endocr Relat Cancer* 2006;13:583–592.
174. Schernhammer ES, Holly JM, Pollak MN, et al. Circulating levels of insulin like growth factors, their binding proteins, and breast cancer risk. *Cancer Epidemiol Biomarkers Prev* 2005;14:699–704.
175. Rinaldi S, Toniolo P, Muti P, et al. IGF-I, IGFBP-3 and breast cancer in young women: a pooled re-analysis of three prospective studies. *Eur J Cancer Prev* 2005;14:493–496.
176. Baglietto L, English DR, Hopper JL, et al. Circulating insulin-like growth factor-I and binding protein-3 and the risk of breast cancer. *Cancer Epidemiol Biomarkers Prev* 2007;16:763–768.
177. Lukanova A, Toniolo P, Zeleniuch-Jacquotte A, et al. Insulin-like growth factor I in pregnancy and maternal risk of breast cancer. *Cancer Epidemiol Biomarkers Prev* 2006;15:2489–2493.
178. Eliassen AH, Tworoger SS, Mantzoros CS, et al. Circulating insulin and c-peptide levels and risk of breast cancer among predominately premenopausal women. *Cancer Epidemiol Biomarkers Prev* 2007;16:161–164.
179. Toniolo P, Bruning PF, Akhmedkhanov A, et al. Serum insulin-like growth factor-I and breast cancer. *Int J Cancer* 2000;88:828–832.
180. Verheus M, Peeters PH, Rinaldi S, et al. Serum C-peptide levels and breast cancer risk: results from the European Prospective Investigation into Cancer and Nutrition (EPIC). *Int J Cancer* 2006;119:659–667.
181. Kaaks R, Lundin E, Rinaldi S, et al. Prospective study of IGF-I, IGF-binding proteins, and breast cancer risk, in northern and southern Sweden. *Cancer Causes Control* 2002;13:307–316.
182. Keinan-Boker L, Bueno De Mesquita HB, Kaaks R, et al. Circulating levels of insulin-like growth factor I, its binding proteins -1, -2, -3, C-peptide and risk of postmenopausal breast cancer. *Int J Cancer* 2003;106:90–95.
183. Mink PJ, Shahar E, Rosamond WD, et al. Serum insulin and glucose levels and breast cancer incidence: the atherosclerosis risk in communities study. *Am J Epidemiol* 2002;156:349–352.
184. Panzer A, Lottering ML, Bianchi P, et al. Melatonin has no effect on the growth, morphology or cell cycle of human breast cancer (MCF-7), cervical cancer (HeLa), osteosarcoma (MG-63) or lymphoblastoid (TK6) cells. *Cancer Lett* 1998;122:17–23.
185. Cos S, Fernandez F, Sanchez-Barcelo EJ. Melatonin inhibits DNA synthesis in MCF-7 human breast cancer cells *in vitro*. *Life Sci* 1996;58:2447–2453.
186. Cos S, Fernandez R, Guezmes A, et al. Influence of melatonin on invasive and metastatic properties of MCF-7 human breast cancer cells. *Cancer Res* 1998;58:4383–4390.
187. Cos S, Mediavilla MD, Fernandez R, et al. Does melatonin induce apoptosis in MCF-7 human breast cancer cells *in vitro*? *J Pineal Res* 2002;32:90–96.
188. Hill SM, Blask DE. Effects of the pineal hormone melatonin on the proliferation and morphological characteristics of human breast cancer cells (MCF-7) in culture. *Cancer Res* 1988;48:6121–6126.
189. Mediavilla MD, Cos S, Sanchez-Barcelo EJ. Melatonin increases p53 and p21WAF1 expression in MCF-7 human breast cancer cells in vitro. *Life Sci* 1999;5:415–420.
190. Tamarkin L, Cohen M, Roselle D, et al. Melatonin inhibition and pinealectomy enhancement of 7,12-dimethylbenz(a)anthracene-induced mammary tumors in the rat. BEGIN*Cancer Res* 1981;41:4432–4436.
191. Musatov SA, Anisimov VN, Andre V, et al. Effects of melatonin on N-nitroso-N-methylurea-induced carcinogenesis in rats and mutagenesis in vitro (Ames test and COMET assay). *Cancer Lett* 1999;138:37–44.
192. Anisimov VN, Kvetnoy IM, Chumakova NK, et al. Intestinal melatonin-containing cells and serum melatonin level in rats with 1,2-dimethylhydrazine-induced colon tumors. *Exp Toxicol Pathol* 1999;51:47–52.
193. Anisimov VN, Popovich IG, Zabezhinski MA. Melatonin and colon carcinogenesis: I. Inhibitory effect of melatonin on development of intestinal tumors induced by 1,2-dimethylhydrazine in rats. *Carcinogenesis* 1997;18:1549–53.
194. Cini G, Coronnello M, Mini E, et al. Melatonin's growth-inhibitory effect on hepatoma AH 130 in the rat. *Cancer Lett* 1998;125:51–9.
195. Mocchegiani E, Perissin L, Santarelli L, et al. Melatonin administration in tumor-bearing mice (intact and pinealectomized) in relation to stress, zinc, thymulin and IL-2. *Int J Immunopharmacol* 1999;21:27–46.
196. Brzezinski A. Melatonin in humans. *N Engl J Med* 1997;336:186–195.
197. Davis S, Mirick DK, Stevens RG. Night shift work, light at night, and risk of breast cancer. *J Natl Cancer Inst* 2001;93:1557–1562.
198. Stevens RG, Davis S. The melatonin hypothesis: electric power and breast cancer. *Environ Health Perspect* 1996;104;Suppl 1:135–140.
199. Travis RC, Allen DS, Fentiman IS, et al. Melatonin and breast cancer: a prospective study. *J Natl Cancer Inst* 2004;96:475–482.
200. Schernhammer ES, Hankinson SE. Urinary melatonin levels and breast cancer risk. *J Natl Cancer Inst* 2005;97:1084–1087.
201. Megdal SP, Kroenke CH, Laden F, et al. Night work and breast cancer risk: a systematic review and meta-analysis. *Eur J Cancer* 2005;41:2023–2032.
202. Graham C, Cook MR, Gerkovich MM, et al. Examination of the melatonin hypothesis in women exposed at night to EMF or bright light. *Environ Health Perspect* 2001;109:501–507.
203. Zeitzer JM, Dijk DJ, Kronauer R, et al. Sensitivity of the human circadian pacemaker to nocturnal light: melatonin phase resetting and suppression. *J Physiol* 2000;526;Pt 3:695–702.
204. Pukkala E, Auvinen A, Wahlberg G. Incidence of cancer among Finnish airline cabin attendants, 1967–1992. *BMJ* 1995;311:649–652.
205. Rafnsson V, Tulinius H, Jonasson JG, et al. Risk of breast cancer in female flight attendants: a population-based study (Iceland). *Cancer Causes Control* 2001;12:95–101.
206. Hansen J. Increased breast cancer risk among women who work predominantly at night. *Epidemiology* 2001;12:74–77.
207. Tynes T, Hannevik M, Andersen A, et al. Incidence of breast cancer in Norwegian female radio and telegraph operators. *Cancer Causes Control* 1996;7:197–204.
208. Schernhammer ES, Kroenke CH, Laden F, et al. Night work and risk of breast cancer. *Epidemiology* 2006;17:108–111.

209. Schernhammer ES, Laden F, Speizer FE, et al. Rotating night shifts and risk of breast cancer in women participating in the nurses' health study. *J Natl Cancer Inst* 2001;93:1563–1568.
210. Committe on the Relationship Between Oral Contraceptives and Breast Cancer. *Oral contraceptives and breast cancer*. Washington, DC: Institute of Medicine, 1991.
211. Annegers JF. Patterns of oral contraceptive use in the United States. *Br J Rheumatol* 1989;28;Suppl 1:48–50.
212. Burkman RT. Oral contraceptives: current status. *Clin Obstet Gynecol* 2001;44: 62–72.
213. Romieu I, Berlin JA, Colditz G. Oral contraceptives and breast cancer. Review and meta-analysis. *Cancer* 1990;66:2253–2263.
214. Thomas DB. Oral contraceptives and breast cancer: review of the epidemiologic literature. *Contraception* 1991;43:597–642.
215. Cogliano V, Grosse Y, Baan R, et al. Carcinogenicity of combined oestrogen-progestagen contraceptives and menopausal treatment. *Lancet Oncol* 2005;6:552–553.
216. Russo J, Gusterson BA, Rogers AE, et al. Comparative study of human and rat mammary tumorigenesis. *Lab Invest* 1990;62:244–278.
217. Brohet RM, Goldgar DE, Easton DF, et al. Oral contraceptives and breast cancer risk in the international BRCA1/2 carrier cohort study: a report from EMBRACE, GENEPSO, GEO-HEBON, and the IBCCS Collaborating Group. *J Clin Oncol* 2007;25:3831–3836.
218. Haile RW, Thomas DC, McGuire V, et al. BRCA1 and BRCA2 mutation carriers, oral contraceptive use, and breast cancer before age 50. *Cancer Epidemiol Biomarkers Prev* 2006;15:1863–1870.
219. Narod SA, Dube MP, Klijn J, et al. Oral contraceptives and the risk of breast cancer in BRCA1 and BRCA2 mutation carriers. *J Natl Cancer Inst* 2002;94:1773–1779.
220. Marchbanks PA, McDonald JA, Wilson HG, et al. The NICHD Women's Contraceptive and Reproductive Experiences Study: methods and operational results. *Ann Epidemiol* 2002;12:213–221.
221. Stanford JL, Thomas DB. Exogenous progestins and breast cancer. *Epidemiol Rev* 1993;15:98–107.
222. Breast cancer and depot-medroxyprogesterone acetate: a multinational study. WHO Collaborative Study of Neoplasia and Steroid Contraceptives. *Lancet* 1991;338:833–838.
223. Waaler HT, Lund E. Association between body height and death from breast cancer. *Br J Cancer* 1983;48:149–150.
224. Kennedy DL, Baum C, Forbes MB. Noncontraceptive estrogens and progestins: use patterns over time. *Obstet Gynecol* 1985;65:441–446.
225. Colditz GA, Egan KM, Stampfer MJ. Hormone replacement therapy and risk of breast cancer: results from epidemiologic studies. *Am J Obstet Gynecol* 1993; 168:1473–1480.
226. Dupont WD, Page DL. Menopausal estrogen replacement therapy and breast cancer. *Arch Intern Med* 1991;151:67–72.
227. Grady D, Rubin SM, Petitti DB, et al. Hormone therapy to prevent disease and prolong life in postmenopausal women. *Ann Intern Med* 1992;117:1016–1037.
228. Sillero-Arenas M, Delgado-Rodriguez M, Rodigues-Canteras R, et al. Menopausal hormone replacement therapy and breast cancer: a meta-analysis. *Obstet Gynecol* 1992;79:286–294.
229. Steinberg KK, Smith SJ, Thacker SB, et al. Breast cancer risk and duration of estrogen use: the role of study design in meta-analysis. *Epidemiology* 1994;5:415–421.
230. Steinberg KK, Thacker SB, Smith SJ, et al. A meta-analysis of the effect of estrogen replacement therapy on the risk of breast cancer. *JAMA* 1991;265:1985–1990.
231. Collaborative Group on Hormonal Factors in Breast Cancer. Breast cancer and hormone replacement therapy: collaborative reanalysis of data from 51 epidemiological studies of 52,705 women with breast cancer and 108,411 women without breast cancer. *Lancet* 1997;350:1047–1059.
232. International Agency for Research on Cancer. Combined estrogen-progestogen postmenopausal therapy. Combined Estrogen-progestogen Contraceptives and Combined Estrogen-progestogen Menopausal Therapy 91. Lyon, France: International Agency for Research on Cancer, 2007.
233. Colditz GA, Hankinson SE, Hunter DJ, et al. The use of estrogens and progestins and the risk of breast cancer in postmenopausal women. *N Engl J Med* 1995; 332:1589–1593.
234. Schairer C, Lubin J, Troisi R, et al. Menopausal estrogen and estrogen-progestin replacement therapy and breast cancer risk. *JAMA* 2000;283:485–491.
235. Ross RK, Paganini-Hill A, Wan P, et al. Effect of hormone replacement therapy on breast cancer: estrogen versus estrogen plus progestin. *JNCI* 2000;92:328–332.
236. Beral V. Breast cancer and hormone-replacement therapy in the Million Women Study. *Lancet* 2003;362:419–427.
237. Anderson GL, Chlebowski RT, Rossouw JE, et al. Prior hormone therapy and breast cancer risk in the Women's Health Initiative randomized trial of estrogen plus progestin. *Maturitas* 2006;55:103–115.
238. Schairer C, Byrne C, Keyl PM, et al. Menopausal estrogen and estrogen-progestin replacement therapy and risk of breast cancer (United States). *Cancer Causes Control* 1994;5:491–500.
239. Rockhill B, Colditz GA, Rosner B. Bias in breast cancer analyses due to error in age at menopause. *Am J Epidemiol* 2000;151:404–408.
240. Chen WY, Manson JE, Hankinson SE, et al. Unopposed estrogen therapy and the risk of invasive breast cancer. *Arch Intern Med* 2006;166:1027–1032.
241. Huang Z, Hankinson SE, Colditz GA, et al. Dual effects of weight and weight gain on breast cancer risk. *JAMA* 1997;278:1407–1411.
242. Colditz GA, Stampfer MJ, Willett WC, et al. Reproducibility and validity of self-reported menopausal status in a prospective cohort study. *Am J Epidemiol* 1987; 126:319–325.
243. Anderson GL, Limacher M, Assaf AR, et al. Effects of conjugated equine estrogen in postmenopausal women with hysterectomy: the Women's Health Initiative randomized controlled trial. *JAMA* 2004;291:1701–1712.
244. Hemminki E, Kennedy DL, Baum C, et al. Prescribing of noncontraceptive estrogens and progestins in the United States, 1974–1986. *Am J Public Health* 1988; 78:1479–1481.
245. Gambrell RD Jr., Maier RC, Sanders BI. Decreased incidence of breast cancer in postmenopausal estrogen-progestogen users. *Obstet Gynecol* 1983;62:435–443.
246. Nachtigall LE, Nachtigall RH, Nachtigall RD, et al. Estrogen replacement therapy II: a prospective study in the relationship to carcinoma and cardiovascular and metabolic problems. *Obstet Gynecol* 1979;54:74–79.
247. Bergkvist L, Adami HO, Persson I, et al. The risk of breast cancer after estrogen and estrogen-progestin replacement. *N Engl J Med* 1989;321:293–297.
248. Schairer C, Lubin J, Troisi R, et al. Menopausal estrogen and estrogen-progestin replacement therapy and breast cancer risk. *JAMA* 2000;283:485–491.
249. Willett WC, Colditz G, Stampfer M. Postmenopausal estrogens—opposed, unopposed, or none of the above. *JAMA* 2000;283:534–535.
250. Newcomb PA, Titus-Ernstoff L, Egan KM, et al. Postmenopausal estrogen and progestin use in relation to breast cancer risk. *Cancer Epidemiol Biomarkers Prev* 2002;11:593–600.
251. Ross RK, Paganini-Hill A, Wan PC, et al. Effect of hormone replacement therapy on breast cancer risk: estrogen versus estrogen plus progestin. *J Natl Cancer Inst* 2000;92:328–332.
252. Colditz GA. Relationship between estrogen levels, use of hormone replacement therapy, and breast cancer. *J Natl Cancer Inst* 1998;90:814–823.
253. Fletcher SW, Colditz GA. Failure of estrogen plus progestin therapy for prevention. *JAMA* 2002;288:366–368.
254. Colditz GA. Estrogen, estrogen plus progestin therapy, and risk of breast cancer. *Clin Cancer Res* 2005;11:909s–917s.
255. Li CI, Anderson BO, Daling JR, et al. Trends in incidence rates of invasive lobular and ductal breast carcinoma. *JAMA* 2003;289:1421–1424.
256. Haas JS, Kaplan CP, Gerstenberger EP, et al. Changes in the use of postmenopausal hormone therapy after the publication of clinical trial results. *Ann Intern Med* 2004;140:184–188.
257. Hulley S, Grady D, Bush T, et al. Randomized trial of estrogen plus progestin for secondary prevention of coronary heart disease in postmenopausal women. Heart and Estrogen/progestin Replacement Study (HERS) Research Group. *JAMA* 1998;280:605–613.
258. Grady D, Herrington D, Bittner V, et al. Cardiovascular disease outcomes during 6.8 years of hormone therapy: Heart and Estrogen/progestin Replacement Study follow-up (HERS II). *JAMA* 2002;288:49–57.
259. Clarke CA, Purdie DM, Glaser SL. Population attributable risk of breast cancer in white women associated with immediately modifiable risk factors. *BMC Cancer* 2006;6:170.
260. Jemal A, Ward E, Thun MJ. Recent trends in breast cancer incidence rates by age and tumor characteristics among U.S. women. *Breast Cancer Res* 2007;9:R28.
261. Clarke CA, Glaser SL, Uratsu CS, et al. Recent declines in hormone therapy utilization and breast cancer incidence: clinical and population-based evidence. *J Clin Oncol* 2006;24:e49–50.
262. Robbins A, Clarke C. Regional changes in hormone therapy use and breast cancer incidence, California, 2001–2004. *J Clin Oncol* 2007;25:3437–3438.
263. Kerlikowske K, Miglioretti DL, Buist DS, et al. Declines in invasive breast cancer and use of postmenopausal hormone therapy in a screening mammography population. *J Natl Cancer Inst* 2007;99:1335–1339.
264. Johnston M. *Breast cancer drop linked to fall in use of HRT*. New Zealand: Herald, 2006.
265. Katalinic A, Rawal R. Decline in breast cancer incidence after decrease in utilisation of hormone replacement therapy. *Breast Cancer Res Treat* 2008;107:427–430.
266. Colditz GA. Decline in breast cancer incidence due to removal of promoter: combination estrogen plus progestin. *Breast Cancer Res* 2007;9:108.
267. Whittemore AS. The Eighth AACR American Cancer Society Award lecture on cancer epidemiology and prevention. Genetically tailored preventive strategies: an effective plan for the twenty-first century? American Association for Cancer Research. *Cancer Epidemiol Biomarkers Prev* 1999;8:649–658.
268. Lux MP, Fasching PA, Beckmann MW. Hereditary breast and ovarian cancer: review and future perspectives. *J Mol Med* 2006;84:16–28.
269. Colditz GA, Willett WC, Hunter DJ, et al. Family history, age, and risk of breast cancer. Prospective data from the Nurses' Health Study. *JAMA* 1993;270:338–343.
270. Lynch H. Hereditary breast cancer: surveillance and management implications. *Breast diseases: a year book quarterly*. 1993:12–15.
271. Malkin D, Li FP, Strong LC, et al. Germ line p53 mutations in a familial syndrome of breast cancer, sarcomas, and other neoplasms. *Science* 1990;250:1233–1238.
272. Liaw D, Marsh DJ, Li J, et al. Germline mutations of the PTEN gene in Cowden disease, an inherited breast and thyroid cancer syndrome. *Nat Genet* 1997;16: 64–67.
273. Walsh T, Casadei S, Coats KH, et al. Spectrum of mutations in BRCA1, BRCA2, CHEK2, and TP53 in families at high risk of breast cancer. *JAMA* 2006;295: 1379–1388.
274. Miki Y, Swensen J, Shattuck-Eidens D, et al. A strong candidate for the breast and ovarian cancer susceptibility gene BRCA1. *Science* 1994;266:66–71.
275. Wooster R, Bignell G, Lancaster J, et al. Identification of the breast cancer susceptibility gene BRCA2. *Nature* 1995;378:789–792.
276. DeMichele A, Weber B. Chapter 16, Inherited genetic factors. In: Harris JR, editor. *Diseases of the Breast*, second edition. Philadelphia: Lippincott Williams & Wilkins; 2000;221–236.
277. Newman B, Mu H, Butler LM, et al. Frequency of breast cancer attributable to BRCA1 in a population-based series of American women. *JAMA* 1998;279: 915–921.
278. Lohmueller KE, Pearce CL, Pike M, et al. Meta-analysis of genetic association studies supports a contribution of common variants to susceptibility to common disease. *Nat Genet* 2003;33:177–182.
279. Ioannidis JP, Ntzani EE, Trikalinos TA, et al. Replication validity of genetic association studies. *Nat Genet* 2001;29:306–309.
280. Cox A, Dunning AM, Garcia-Closas M, et al. A common coding variant in CASP8 is associated with breast cancer risk. *Nat Genet* 2007;39:352–358.
281. Hirschhorn JN, Daly MJ. Genome-wide association studies for common diseases and complex traits. *Nat Rev Genet* 2005;6:95–108.
282. International HapMap Consortium. A haplotype map of the human genome. *Nature* 2005;437:1299–1320.
283. de Bakker PI, Yelensky R, Pe'er I, et al. Efficiency and power in genetic association studies. *Nat Genet* 2005;37:1217–1223.
284. Lin DY. Evaluating statistical significance in two-stage genomewide association studies. *Am J Hum Genet* 2006;78:505–509.
285. Skol AD, Scott LJ, Abecasis GR, et al. Joint analysis is more efficient than replication-based analysis for two-stage genome-wide association studies. *Nat Genet* 2006;38:209–213.
286. Easton DF, Pooley KA, Dunning AM, et al. Genome-wide association study identifies novel breast cancer susceptibility loci. *Nature* 2007;447:1087–1093.
287. Hunter DJ, Kraft P, Jacobs KB, et al. A genome-wide association study identifies alleles in FGFR2 associated with risk of sporadic postmenopausal breast cancer. *Nat Genet* 2007;39:870–874.

288. Stacey SN, Manolescu A, Sulem P, et al. Common variants on chromosomes 2q35 and 16q12 confer susceptibility to estrogen receptor-positive breast cancer. *Nat Genet* 2007;39:865–869.
289. Gold B, Kirchhoff T, Stefanov S, et al. Genome-wide association study provides evidence for a breast cancer risk locus at 6q22.33. *Proc Natl Acad Sci U S A* 2008;105:4340–4345.
290. Albanes D. Total calories, body weight, and tumor incidence in mice. *Cancer Res* 1987;47:1987–1992.
291. Freedman LS, Clifford C, Messina M. Analysis of dietary fat, calories, body weight, and the development of mammary tumors in rats and mice: a review. *Cancer Res* 1990;50:5710–5719.
292. Ip C. Quantitative assessment of fat and caloric as risk factors in mammary carcinogenesis in an experimental model. In: Mettlin C. J., Aoki K., eds. *Recent progress in research on nutrition and cancer: proceedings of a workshop sponsored by the International Union Against Cancer*, Nagoya, Japan. Wiley-Liss, Inc. 1989:107–117.
293. Beth M, Berger MR, Aksoy M, et al. Comparison between the effects of dietary fat level and of calorie intake on methylnitrosourea-induced mammary carcinogenesis in female SD rats. *Int J Cancer* 1987;39:737–744.
294. Appleton BS, Landers RE. Oil gavage effects on tumor incidence in the National Toxicology Program's 2-year carcinogenesis bioassay. *Adv Exp Med Biol* 1986;206:99–104.
295. Sonnenschein EG, Glickman LT, Goldschmidt MH, et al. Body conformation, diet, and risk of breast cancer in pet dogs: a case-control study. *Am J Epidemiol* 1991;133:694–703.
296. Armstrong B, Doll R. Environmental factors and cancer incidence and mortality in different countries, with special reference to dietary practices. *Int J Cancer* 1975;15:617–631.
297. Prentice RL, Kakar F, Hursting S, et al. Aspects of the rationale for the Women's Health Trial. *J Natl Cancer Inst* 1988;80:802–814.
298. Tretli S, Gaard M. Lifestyle changes during adolescence and risk of breast cancer: an ecologic study of the effect of World War II in Norway. *Cancer Causes Control* 1996;7:507–512.
299. Phillips RL, Garfinkel L, Kuzma JW, et al. Mortality among California Seventh-Day Adventists for selected cancer sites. *J Natl Cancer Inst* 1980;65:1097–1107.
300. Kinlen LJ. Meat and fat consumption and cancer mortality: A study of strict religious orders in Britain. *Lancet* 1982;1:946–949.
301. Graham S, Marshall J, Mettlin C, et al. Diet in the epidemiology of breast cancer. *Am J Epidemiol* 1982;116:68–75.
302. Howe GR, Hirohata T, Hislop TG, et al. Dietary factors and risk of breast cancer: combined analysis of 12 case-control studies. *J Natl Cancer Inst* 1990;82:561–569.
303. Giovannucci E, Stampfer MJ, Colditz GA, et al. A comparison of prospective and retrospective assessments of diet in the study of breast cancer. *Am J Epidemiol* 1993;137:502–511.
304. Graham S, Hellmann R, Marshall J, et al. Nutritional epidemiology of postmenopausal breast cancer in western New York. *Am J Epidemiol* 1991;134:552–566.
305. Holmes MD, Hunter DJ, Colditz GA, et al. Association of dietary intake of fat and fatty acids with risk of breast cancer. *JAMA* 1999;281:914–920.
306. Horn-Ross PL, Hoggatt KJ, West DW, et al. Recent diet and breast cancer risk: the California Teachers Study (USA). *Cancer Causes Control* 2002;13:407–415.
307. Howe GR, Friedenreich CM, Jain M, et al. A cohort study of fat intake and risk of breast cancer. *J Natl Cancer Inst* 1991;83:336–340.
308. Kushi LH, Sellers TA, Potter JD, et al. Dietary fat and postmenopausal breast cancer. *J Natl Cancer Inst* 1992;84:1092–1099.
309. Mattisson I, Wirfalt E, Wallstrom P, et al. High fat and alcohol intakes are risk factors of postmenopausal breast cancer: a prospective study from the Malmo diet and cancer cohort. *Int J Cancer* 2004;110:589–597.
310. Mills PK, Beeson WL, Phillips RL, et al. Dietary habits and breast cancer incidence among Seventh-day Adventists. *Cancer* 1989;64:582–590.
311. Thiebaut AC, Kipnis V, Chang SC, et al. Dietary fat and postmenopausal invasive breast cancer in the National Institutes of Health-AARP Diet and Health Study cohort. *J Natl Cancer Inst* 2007;99:451–462.
312. van den Brandt PA, van't Veer P, Goldbohm RA, et al. A prospective cohort study on dietary fat and the risk of postmenopausal breast cancer. *Cancer Res* 1993;53:75–82.
313. Velie E, Kulldorff M, Schairer C, et al. Dietary fat, fat subtypes, and breast cancer in postmenopausal women: a prospective cohort study. *J Natl Cancer Inst* 2000;92:833–839.
314. Willett WC, Hunter DJ, Stampfer MJ, et al. Dietary fat and fiber in relation to risk of breast cancer. An 8-year follow-up. *JAMA* 1992;268:2037–2044.
315. Wolk A, Bergstrom R, Hunter D, et al. A prospective study of association of monounsaturated fat and other types of fat with risk of breast cancer. *Arch Intern Med* 1998;158:41–45.
316. Hunter DJ, Spiegelman D, Adami HO, et al. Cohort studies of fat intake and the risk of breast cancer—a pooled analysis. *N Engl J Med* 1996,334:356–361.
316a. Prentice RL. Measurement error and results from analytic epidemiology: dietery fat and breast cancer. *J Natl Cancer Inst* 1996;88:1738–1747.
317. Hunter DJ, Spiegelman D, Willett W. Dietary fat and breast cancer. *J Natl Cancer Inst* 1998;90:1303–1306.
318. Smith-Warner SA, Spiegelman D, Adami HO, et al. Types of dietary fat and breast cancer: a pooled analysis of cohort studies. *Int J Cancer* 2001;92:767–774.
319. Kim EH, Willett WC, Colditz GA, et al. Dietary fat and risk of postmenopausal breast cancer in a 20-year follow-up. *Am J Epidemiol* 2006;164:990–997.
320. Cho E, Chen WY, Hunter DJ, et al. Red meat intake and risk of breast cancer among premenopausal women. *Arch Intern Med* 2006;166:2253–2239.
321. Prentice RL, Caan B, Chlebowski RT, et al. Low-fat dietary pattern and risk of invasive breast cancer: the Women's Health Initiative Randomized Controlled Dietary Modification Trial. *JAMA* 2006;295:629–642.
322. Willet WC. *Nutritional Epidemiology*. New York: Oxford University Press, 1998.
323. Howard BV, Van Horn L, Hsia J, et al. Low-fat dietary pattern and risk of cardiovascular disease: the Women's Health Initiative Randomized Controlled Dietary Modification Trial. *JAMA* 2006;295:655–666.
324. Willett W, Stampfer M, Chu NF, et al. Assessment of questionnaire validity for measuring total fat intake using plasma lipid levels as criteria. *Am J Epidemiol* 2001;154:1107–1112.
325. Michels KB, Willett WC. The Women's Health Initiative Randomized Controlled Dietary Modification Trial: a post-mortem. *Breast Cancer Res Treat* 2008;10:S11.
326. Eliassen AH, Colditz GA, Rosner B, et al. Adult weight change and risk of postmenopausal breast cancer. *JAMA* 2006;296:193–201.
327. Freedman L, Prentice R, Clifford C, et al. Dietary fat and breast cancer: where we are. *J Natl Cancer Inst* 1993;85:764–765.
328. Sutherland HJ, Carlin K, Harper W, et al. A study of diet and breast cancer prevention in Canada: why healthy women participate in controlled trials. *Cancer Causes Control* 1993;4:521–528.
329. Cohen LA, Kendall ME, Zang E, et al. Modulation of N-nitrosomethylurea-induced mammary tumor promotion by dietary fiber and fat. *J Natl Cancer Inst* 1991,83.496–501.
330. Martin Moreno JM, Willett WC, Gorgojo L, et al. Dietary fat, olive oil intake and breast cancer risk. *Int J Cancer* 1994;58:774–780.
331. Willett WC. Specific fatty acids and risks of breast and prostate cancer: dietary intake. *Am J Clin Nutr* 1997;66:1557S–1563S.
332. Micozzi MS. Nutrition, body size, and breast cancer. *Yearbook Phys Anthropol* 1985;28:175–206.
333. Hunter DJ, Willett WC. Diet, body size, and breast cancer. *Epidemiol Rev* 1993;15:110–132.
334. Swanson CA, Jones DY, Schatzkin A, et al. Breast cancer risk assessed by anthropometry in the NHANES I epidemiological follow-up study. *Cancer Res* 1988;48:5363–5367.
335. van den Brandt PA, Spiegelman D, Yaun SS, et al. Pooled analysis of prospective cohort studies on height, weight, and breast cancer risk. *Am J Epidemiol* 2000;152:514–527.
336. World Cancer Research Fund, American Institute for Cancer Research. Food, Nutrition, Physical activity, and the prevention of cancer: a global perspective. Washington, D.C: American Institute for Cancer Research, 2007.
337. Vatten LJ, Kvinnsland S. Body height and risk of breast cancer. A prospective study of 23,831 Norwegian women. *Br J Cancer* 1990;61:881–885.
338. Vatten LJ, Kvinnsland S. Prospective study of height, body mass index and risk of breast cancer. *Acta Oncol* 1992;31:195–200.
339. Bernstein L, Ross RK, Lobo RA, et al. The effects of moderate physical activity on menstrual cycle patterns in adolescence: implications for breast cancer prevention. *Br J Cancer* 1987;55:681–685.
340. Maclure M, Travis LB, Willett W, et al. A prospective cohort study of nutrient intake and age at menarche. *Am J Clin Nutr* 1991;54:649–656.
341. Merzenich H, Boeing H, Wahrendorf J. Dietary fat and sports activity as determinants for age at menarche. *Am J Epidemiol* 1993;138:217–224.
342. Meyer F, Moisan J, Marcoux D, et al. Dietary and physical determinants of menarche. *Epidemiology* 1990;1:377–381.
343. Chen J, Campbell TC, Junyao L, et al. *Diet, life-style, and mortality in China: a study of the characteristics of 65 Chinese counties*. Oxford, England: Oxford University Press, 1990.
344. Hilakivi-Clarke L, Forsen T, Eriksson JG, et al. Tallness and overweight during childhood have opposing effects on breast cancer risk. *Br J Cancer* 2001;85:1680–1684.
345. Michels KB, Trichopoulos D, Robins JM, et al. Birthweight as a risk factor for breast cancer. *Lancet* 1996;348:1542–1546.
346. Baer HJ, Colditz GA, Rosner B, et al. Body fatness during childhood and adolescence and incidence of breast cancer in premenopausal women: a prospective cohort study. *Breast Cancer Res* 2005;7:R314–R325.
347. Kelsey JL, H.-R. P. Breast cancer: magnitude of the problem and descriptive epidemiology. *Epidemiol Rev* 1993;15:7–16.
348. Trichopoulos D, Lipman RD. Mammary gland mass and breast cancer risk. *Epidemiology* 1992;3:523–526.
349. Dunn SE, Kari FW, French J, et al. Dietary restriction reduces insulin-like growth factor I levels, which modulates apoptosis, cell proliferation, and tumor progression in p53-deficient mice. *Cancer Res* 1997;57:4667–4672.
350. Barr SI, McCarron DA, Heaney RP, et al. Effects of increased consumption of fluid milk on energy and nutrient intake, body weight, and cardiovascular risk factors in healthy older adults. *J Am Diet Assoc* 2000;100:810–817.
351. Giovannucci E, Pollak M, Liu Y, et al. Nutritional predictors of insulin-like growth factor I and their relationships to cancer in men. *Cancer Epidemiol Biomarkers Prev* 2003;12:84–89.
352. Heaney RP, McCarron DA, Dawson-Hughes B, et al. Dietary changes favorably affect bone remodeling in older adults. *J Am Diet Assoc* 1999;99:1228–1233.
353. Holmes MD, Pollak MN, Willett WC, et al. Dietary correlates of plasma insulin-like growth factor I and insulin-like growth factor binding protein 3 concentrations. *Cancer Epidemiol Biomarkers Prev* 2002;11:852–861.
354. Hoppe C, Molgaard C, Juul A, et al. High intakes of skimmed milk, but not meat, increase serum IGF-I and IGFBP-3 in eight-year-old boys. *Eur J Clin Nutr* 2004;58.1211 1216.
355. Hoppe C, Udam TR, Lauritzen L, et al. Animal protein intake, serum insulin-like growth factor I, and growth in healthy 2.5-year-old Danish children. *Am J Clin Nutr* 2004;80:447–452.
356. Norat T, Dossus L, Rinaldi S, et al. Diet, serum insulin-like growth factor-I and IGF-binding protein-3 in European women. *Eur J Clin Nutr* 2007;61:91–98.
357. Wiley AS. Does milk make children grow? Relationships between milk consumption and height in NHANES 1999–2002. *Am J Hum Biol* 2005;17:425–441.
358. Rich-Edwards JW, Goldman MB, Willett WC, et al. Adolescent body mass index and infertility caused by ovulatory disorder. *Am J Obstet Gynecol* 1994;171:171–177.
359. Michels KB, Terry KL, Willett WC. Longitudinal study on the role of body size in premenopausal breast cancer. *Arch Intern Med* 2006;166:2395–2402.
360. Hankinson SE, Willett WC, Manson JE, et al. Alcohol, height, and adiposity in relation to estrogen and prolactin levels in postmenopausal women. *J Natl Cancer Inst* 1995;87:1297–1302.
361. Barnes-Josiah D, Potter JD, Sellers TA, et al. Early body size and subsequent weight gain as predictors of breast cancer incidence (Iowa, United States). *Cancer Causes Control* 1995;6:112–118.
362. Trentham-Dietz A, Newcomb PA, Egan KM, et al. Weight change and risk of postmenopausal breast cancer (United States). *Cancer Causes Control* 2000;11:533–542.
363. Wenten M, Gilliland FD, Baumgartner K, et al. Associations of weight, weight change, and body mass with breast cancer risk in Hispanic and non-Hispanic white women. *Ann Epidemiol* 2002;12:435–444.

364. Ziegler RG, Hoover RN, Nomura AM, et al. Relative weight, weight change, height, and breast cancer risk in Asian-American women. *J Natl Cancer Inst* 1996;88:650–660.
365. Le Marchand L, Kolonel LN, Earle ME, et al. Body size at different periods of life and breast cancer risk. *Am J Epidemiol* 1988;128:137–152.
366. Morimoto LM, White E, Chen Z, et al. Obesity, body size, and risk of postmenopausal breast cancer: the Women's Health Initiative (United States). *Cancer Causes Control* 2002;13:741–751.
367. Petrelli JM, Calle EE, Rodriguez C, et al. Body mass index, height, and postmenopausal breast cancer mortality in a prospective cohort of U.S. women. *Cancer Causes Control* 2002;13:325–332.
368. Pathak DR, Whittemore AS. Combined effects of body size, parity, and menstrual events on breast cancer incidence in seven countries. *Am J Epidemiol* 1992; 135:153–168.
369. Graham S, Zielezny M, Marshall J, et al. Diet in the epidemiology of postmenopausal breast cancer in the New York State Cohort. *Am J Epidemiol* 1992; 136:1327–1337.
370. Nicodemus KK, Jacobs DR Jr., Folsom AR. Whole and refined grain intake and risk of incident postmenopausal breast cancer (United States). *Cancer Causes Control* 2001;12:917–925.
371. Rohan TE, Howe GR, Friedenreich CM, et al. Dietary fiber, vitamins A, C, and E, and risk of breast cancer: a cohort study. *Cancer Causes Control* 1993;4:29–37.
372. Terry P, Jain M, Miller AB, et al. No association among total dietary fiber, fiber fractions, and risk of breast cancer. *Cancer Epidemiol Biomarkers Prev* 2002;11: 1507–1508
373. Giles GG, Simpson JA, English DR, et al. Dietary carbohydrate, fibre, glycaemic index, glycaemic load and the risk of postmenopausal breast cancer. *Int J Cancer* 2006;118:1843–1847.
374. Fraker LD, Halter SA, Forbes JT. Growth inhibition by retinol of a human breast carcinoma cell line *in vitro* and in athymic mice. *Cancer Res* 1984;44:5757–5763.
375. Moon RC, McCormick DL, Mehta RG. Inhibition of carcinogenesis by retinoids. *Cancer Res* 1983;43:2469s–2475s.
376. Freudenheim JL, Marshall JR, Vena JE, et al. Premenopausal breast cancer risk and intake of vegetables, fruits, and related nutrients. *J Natl Cancer Inst* 1996; 88:340–348.
377. Zhang S, Hunter DJ, Forman MR, et al. Dietary carotenoids and vitamins A, C, and E and risk of breast cancer. *J Natl Cancer Inst* 1999;91:547–556.
378. Michels KB, Holmberg L, Bergkvist L, et al. Dietary antioxidant vitamins, retinol, and breast cancer incidence in a cohort of Swedish women. *Int J Cancer* 2001; 91:563–567.
379. Terry P, Jain M, Miller AB, et al. Dietary carotenoids and risk of breast cancer. *Am J Clin Nutr* 2002;76:883–888.
380. World Cancer Research Fund AI. f. C. R. Food, nutrition and the prevention of cancer: a global perspective. Washington, D.C.: American Institute for Cancer Research, 1997.
381. Sato R, Helzlsouer KJ, Alberg AJ, et al. Prospective study of carotenoids, tocopherols, and retinoid concentrations and the risk of breast cancer. *Cancer Epidemiol Biomarkers Prev* 2002;11:451–457.
382. Toniolo P, Van Kappel AL, Akhmedkhanov A, et al. Serum carotenoids and breast cancer. *Am J Epidemiol* 2001;153:1142–1147.
383. Tamimi RM, Hankinson SE, Campos H, et al. Plasma Carotenoids, Retinol, and Tocopherols and Risk of Breast Cancer. *Am J Epidemiol* in press 2004.
384. Veronesi U, De Palo G, Marubini E, et al. Randomized trial of fenretinide to prevent second breast malignancy in women with early breast cancer. *J Natl Cancer Inst*, 1999;91:1847–1856.
385. King MM, McCay PB. Modulation of tumor incidence and possible mechanisms of inhibition of mammary carcinogenesis by dietary antioxidants. *Cancer Res* 1983;43:2485s–2490s.
386. Verhoeven DT, Assen N, Goldbohm RA, et al. Vitamins C and E, retinol, betacarotene and dietary fibre in relation to breast cancer risk: a prospective cohort study. *Br J Cancer* 1997;75:149–155.
387. Cook NR, Lee IM, Gaziano JM, et al. Low-dose aspirin in the primary prevention of cancer: the Women's Health Study: a randomized controlled trial. *JAMA* 2005;294:47–55.
388. Abul-Hajj YJ, Kelliher M. Failure of ascorbic acid to inhibit growth of transplantable and dimethylbenzanthracene induced rat mammary tumors. *Cancer Lett* 1982;17:67–73.
389. Kushi LH, Fee RM, Sellers TA, et al. Intake of vitamins A, C, and E and postmenopausal breast cancer. The Iowa Women's Health Study. *Am J Epidemiol* 1996;144:165–174.
390. Colston KW, Berger U, Coombes RC. Possible role for vitamin D in controlling breast cancer cell proliferation. *Lancet* 1989;1:188–191.
391. Bertone-Johnson ER. Prospective studies of dietary vitamin D and breast cancer: more questions raised than answered. *Nutr Rev* 2007;65:459–466.
392. Rohan T. Epidemiological studies of vitamin D and breast cancer. *Nutr Rev* 2007;65:S80–S83.
393. Lin J, Manson JE, Lee IM, et al. Intakes of calcium and vitamin D and breast cancer risk in women. *Arch Intern Med* 2007;167:1050–1059.
394. Wu K, Feskanich D, Fuchs CS, et al. A nested case control study of plasma 25-hydroxyvitamin D concentrations and risk of colorectal cancer. *J Natl Cancer Inst* 2007;99:1120–1129.
395. Bertone-Johnson ER, Hankinson SE, Bendich A, et al. Calcium and vitamin D intake and risk of incident premenstrual syndrome. *Arch Intern Med* 2005;165: 1246–1252.
396. Ip C. The chemopreventive role of selenium in carcinogenesis. *Adv Exp Med Biol* 1986;206:431–447.
397. Clark LC. The epidemiology of selenium and cancer. *Fed Proc* 1985;44:2584–2589.
398. Hunter DJ. Biochemical indicators of dietary intake. In: Willett WC., ed. *Nutritional Epidemiology*, New York: Oxford University Press, 1990:143–216.
399. Hunter DJ, Morris JS, Stampfer MJ, et al. A prospective study of selenium status and breast cancer risk. *JAMA* 1990;264:1128–1131.
400. Mannisto S, Alfthan G, Virtanen M, et al. Toenail selenium and breast cancer-a case-control study in Finland. *Eur J Clin Nutr* 2000;54:98–103.
401. van den Brandt PA, Goldbohm RA, van't Veer P, et al. Toenail selenium levels and the risk of breast cancer. *Am J Epidemiol* 1994;140:20–26.
402. Knekt P, Aromaa A, Maatela J, et al. Serum vitamin A and subsequent risk of cancer: cancer incidence follow-up of the Finnish Mobile Clinic Health Examination Survey. *Am J Epidemiol* 1990;132:857–870.
403. Clark LC, Combs GF Jr., Turnbull BW, et al. Effects of selenium supplementation for cancer prevention in patients with carcinoma of the skin. A randomized controlled trial. Nutritional Prevention of Cancer Study Group. *JAMA* 1996;276: 1957–1963.
404. Smith-Warner SA, Spiegelman D, Yaun SS, et al. Alcohol and breast cancer in women: a pooled analysis of cohort studies. *JAMA* 1998;279:535–540.
405. International Agency on Cancer Research. Alcoholic beverage consumption. Lyon, France: IARC, 2007.
406. Missmer SA, Smith-Warner SA, Spiegelman D, et al. Meat and dairy food consumption and breast cancer: a pooled analysis of cohort studies. *Int J Epidemiol* 2002;31:78–85.
407. Tjonneland A, Christensen J, Olsen A, et al. Alcohol intake and breast cancer risk: the European Prospective Investigation into Cancer and Nutrition (EPIC). *Cancer Causes Control* 2007;18:361–373.
408. Harvey EB, Schairer C, Brinton LA, et al. Alcohol consumption and breast cancer. *J Natl Cancer Inst* 1987;78:657–661.
409. Longnecker MP, Newcomb PA, Mittendorf R, et al. Risk of breast cancer in relation to lifetime alcohol consumption. *J Natl Cancer Inst* 1995;87:923–929.
410. Reichman ME, Judd JT, Longcope C, et al. Effects of alcohol consumption on plasma and urinary hormone concentrations in premenopausal women. *J Natl Cancer Inst* 1993;85:722–727.
411. Ginsburg ES, Walsh BW, Gao X, et al. The effect of acute ethanol ingestion on estrogen levels in postmenopausal women using transdermal estradiol. *J Soc Gynecol Investig* 1995;2:26–29.
412. Rohan TE, Jain MG, Howe GR, et al. Dietary folate consumption and breast cancer risk. *J Natl Cancer Inst* 2000;92:266–269.
413. Sellers TA, Kushi LH, Cerhan JR, et al. Dietary folate intake, alcohol, and risk of breast cancer in a prospective study of postmenopausal women. *Epidemiology* 2001;12:420–428.
414. Zhang S, Hunter DJ, Hankinson SE, et al. A prospective study of folate intake and the risk of breast cancer. *JAMA* 1999;281:1632–1637.
415. Zhang SM, Willett WC, Selhub J, et al. Plasma folate, vitamin B_6, vitamin B_{12}, homocysteine, and risk of breast cancer. *J Natl Cancer Inst* 2003;95:373–380.
416. Fuchs CS, Stampfer MJ, Colditz GA, et al. Alcohol consumption and mortality among women. *N Engl J Med* 1995;332:1245–1250.
417. Folsom AR, McKenzie DR, Bisgard KM, et al. No association between caffeine intake and postmenopausal breast cancer incidence in the Iowa Women's Health Study. *Am J Epidemiol* 1993;138:380–383.
418. Snowdon DA, Phillips RL. Coffee consumption and risk of fatal cancers. *Am J Public Health* 1984;74:820–823.
419. Vatten LJ, Solvoll K, Loken EB. Coffee consumption and the risk of breast cancer. A prospective study of 14,593 Norwegian women. *Br J Cancer* 1990;62: 267–270.
420. Ganmaa D, Willett WC, Li TY, et al. Coffee, tea, caffeine and risk of breast cancer: A 22-year follow-up. *Int J Cancer* 2008;122:2071–2076.
421. Steinmetz KA, Potter JD. Vegetables, fruit, and cancer. II. Mechanisms. *Cancer Causes Control* 1991;2:427–442.
422. Cassidy A, Bingham S, Setchell K. Biological effects of plant estrogens in premenopausal women. *FASEB J* 1993;7:A866(abst.).
423. Lee HP, Gourley L, Duffy SW, et al. Dietary effects on breast-cancer risk in Singapore. *Lancet* 1991;337:1197–1200.
424. Shu XO, Jin F, Dai Q, et al. Soyfood intake during adolescence and subsequent risk of breast cancer among Chinese women. *Cancer Epidemiol Biomarkers Prev* 2001;10:483–488.
425. Wu AH, Wan P, Hankin J, et al. Adolescent and adult soy intake and risk of breast cancer in Asian-Americans. *Carcinogenesis* 2002;23:1491–1496.
426. Yuan JM, Wang QS, Ross RK, et al. Diet and breast cancer in Shanghai and Tianjin, China. *Br J Cancer* 1995;71:1353–1358.
427. Yuan JM, Yu MC, Ross RK, et al. Risk factors for breast cancer in Chinese women in Shanghai. *Cancer Res* 1988;48:1949–1953.
428. Key TJ, Sharp GB, Appleby PN, et al. Soya foods and breast cancer risk: a prospective study in Hiroshima and Nagasaki, Japan. *Br J Cancer* 1999;81:1248–1256.
429. Duffy C, Cyr M. Phytoestrogens: potential benefits and implications for breast cancer survivors. *J Womens Health (Larchmt)* 2003;12:617–631.
430. Trock BJ, Hilakivi-Clarke L, Clarke R. Meta-analysis of soy intake and breast cancer risk. *J Natl Cancer Inst* 2006;98:459–471.
431. Smith-Warner SA, Spiegelman D, Yaun SS, et al. Intake of fruits and vegetables and risk of breast cancer: a pooled analysis of cohort studies. *JAMA* 2001;285: 769–776.
432. van Gils CH, Peeters PH, Bueno-de-Mesquita HB, et al. Consumption of vegetables and fruits and risk of breast cancer. *JAMA* 2005;293:183–193.
433. Toniolo P, Riboli E, Shore RE, et al. Consumption of meat, animal products, protein, and fat and risk of breast cancer: a prospective cohort study in New York. *Epidemiology* 1994;5:391–397.
434. Zheng W, Gustafson DR, Sinha R, et al. Well-done meat intake and the risk of breast cancer. *J Natl Cancer Inst* 1998;90:1724–1729.
435. Holmes M, Hunter D, Willett W. Reducing breast cancer risk in women, In: B. Stoll ed., *Dietary guidelines: Dordrecht*, vol. 75. Boston: Kluwer Academic Publishers, 1995:248.
436. Newman SC, Miller AB, Howe GR. A study of the effect of weight and dietary fat on breast cancer survival time. *Am J Epidemiol* 1986;123:767–774.
437. Hebert JR, Hurley TG, Ma Y. The effect of dietary exposures on recurrence and mortality in early stage breast cancer. *Breast Cancer Res Treat* 1998;51:17–28.
438. Holmes MD, Stampfer MJ, Colditz GA, et al. Dietary factors and the survival of women with breast carcinoma. *Cancer* 1999;86:826–835.
439. Kroenke CH, Fung TT, Hu FB, et al. Dietary patterns and survival after breast cancer diagnosis. *J Clin Oncol* 2005;23:9295-9303.
440. Chlebowski RT, Blackburn GL, Thomson CA, et al. Dietary fat reduction and breast cancer outcome: interim efficacy results from the Women's Intervention Nutrition Study. *J Natl Cancer Inst* 2006;98:1767–1776.
441. Pierce JP, Natarajan L, Caan BJ, et al. Influence of a diet very high in vegetables, fruit, and fiber and low in fat on prognosis following treatment for breast cancer: the Women's Healthy Eating and Living (WHEL) randomized trial. *JAMA* 2007;298:289–298.
442. Kroenke CH, Chen WY, Rosner B, et al. Weight, weight gain, and survival after breast cancer diagnosis. *J Clin Oncol* 2005;23:1370–1378.
443. International Agency for Research on Cancer. *Weight control and physical activity*. Lyon: IARC Press, 2002.

444. Friedenreich CM, Orenstein MR. Physical activity and cancer prevention: etiologic evidence and biological mechanisms. *J Nutr* 2002;132:3456S 3464S.

445. Vainio H, Kaaks R, Bianchini F. Weight control and physical activity in cancer prevention: international evaluation of the evidence. *Eur J Cancer Prev* 2002;11 Suppl 2: S94–S100.

446. Frisch RE, Gotz-Welbergen AV, McArthur JW, et al. Delayed menarche and amenorrhea of college athletes in relation to age of onset of training. *JAMA* 1981; 246:1559–1563.

447. Frisch RE, Wyshak G, Vincent L. Delayed menarche and amenorrhea in ballet dancers. *N Engl J Med* 1980;303:17–19.

448. Malina RM, Spirduso WW, Tate C, et al. Age at menarche and selected menstrual characteristics in athletes at different competitive levels and in different sports. *Med Sci Sports* 1978;10:218–222.

449. Apter D, Vihko R. Early menarche, a risk factor for breast cancer, indicates early onset of ovulatory cycles. *J Clin Endocrinol Metab* 1983;57:82–86.

450. Harlow SD, Matanoski GM. The association between weight, physical activity, and stress and variation in the length of the menstrual cycle. *Am J Epidemiol* 1991;133:38–49.

451. Cumming DC, Wheeler GD, Harber VJ. Physical activity, nutrition, and reproduction. *Ann N Y Acad Sci* 1994;709:55–76.

452. Broocks A, Pirke KM, Schweiger U, et al. Cyclic ovarian function in recreational athletes. *J Appl Physiol* 1990;68:2083–2086.

453. Bullen BA, Skrinar GS, Beitins IZ, et al. Induction of menstrual disorders by strenuous exercise in untrained women. *N Engl J Med* 1985;312:1349–1353.

454. Feicht CB, Johnson TS, Martin BJ, et al. Secondary amenorrhoea in athletes. *Lancet* 1978;2:1145–1146.

455. Russell JB, Mitchell D, Musey PI, et al. The relationship of exercise to anovulatory cycles in female athletes: hormonal and physical characteristics. *Obstet Gynecol* 1984;63:452–456.

456. Cauley JA, Gutai JP, Kuller LH, et al. The epidemiology of serum sex hormones in postmenopausal women. *Am J Epidemiol* 1989;129:1120–1131.

457. Siiteri PK. Adipose tissue as a source of hormones. *Am J Clin Nutr* 1987;45:277–282.

458. Monninkhof EM, Elias SG, Vlems FA, et al. Physical activity and breast cancer: a systematic review. *Epidemiology* 2007;18:137–157.

459. Friedenreich CM. Physical activity and breast cancer risk: the effect of menopausal status. *Exerc Sport Sci Rev* 2004;32:180–184.

460. McTiernan A, Ulrich C, Slate S, et al. Physical activity and cancer etiology: associations and mechanisms. *Cancer Causes Control* 1998;9:487–509.

461. Gammon MD, Schoenberg JB, Britton JA, et al. Recreational physical activity and breast cancer risk among women under age 45 years. *Am J Epidemiol* 1998;147:273–280.

462. Bernstein L, Henderson BE, Hanisch R, et al. Physical exercise and reduced risk of breast cancer in young women. *J Natl Cancer Inst* 1994;86:1403–1408.

463. Bernstein L, Patel AV, Ursin G, et al. Lifetime recreational exercise activity and breast cancer risk among black women and white women. *J Natl Cancer Inst* 2005;97:1671–1679.

464. Carpenter CL, Ross RK, Paganini-Hill A, et al. Effect of family history, obesity and exercise on breast cancer risk among postmenopausal women. *Int J Cancer* 2003;106:96–102.

465. Friedenreich CM, Bryant HE, Courneya KS. Case-control study of lifetime physical activity and breast cancer risk. *Am J Epidemiol* 2001;154:336–347.

466. John EM, Horn-Ross PL, Koo J. Lifetime physical activity and breast cancer risk in a multiethnic population: the San Francisco Bay area breast cancer study. *Cancer Epidemiol Biomarkers Prev* 2003;12:1143–1152.

467. Lee IM, Cook NR, Rexrode KM, et al. Lifetime physical activity and risk of breast cancer. *Br J Cancer* 2001;85:962–965.

468. Matthews CE, Shu XO, Jin F, et al. Lifetime physical activity and breast cancer risk in the Shanghai Breast Cancer Study. *Br J Cancer* 2001;84:994–1001.

469. Verloop J, Rookus MA, van der Kooy K, et al. Physical activity and breast cancer risk in women aged 20–54 years. *J Natl Cancer Inst* 2000;92:128–135.

470. Yang D, Bernstein L, Wu AH. Physical activity and breast cancer risk among Asian-American women in Los Angeles: a case-control study. *Cancer* 2003;97:2565–2575.

471. Friedenreich CM, Courneya KS, Bryant HE. Relation between intensity of physical activity and breast cancer risk reduction. *Med Sci Sports Exerc* 2001;33:1538–1545.

472. Wyshak G, Frisch RE. Breast cancer among former college athletes compared to non-athletes: a 15-year follow-up. *Br J Cancer* 2000;82:726–730.

473. Thune I, Brenn T, Lund E, et al. Physical activity and the risk of breast cancer. *N Engl J Med* 1997;336:1269–1275.

474. Dirx MJ, Voorrips LE, Goldbohm RA, et al. Baseline recreational physical activity, history of sports participation, and postmenopausal breast carcinoma risk in the Netherlands Cohort Study. *Cancer* 2001;92:1638–1649.

475. Friedenreich CM, Courneya KS, Bryant HE. Influence of physical activity in different age and life periods on the risk of breast cancer. *Epidemiology* 2001;12:604–612.

476. Gilliland FD, Li YF, Baumgartner K, et al. Physical activity and breast cancer risk in hispanic and non-hispanic white women. *Am J Epidemiol* 2001;154:442–450.

477. Lee IM, Rexrode KM, Cook NR, et al. Physical activity and breast cancer risk: the Women's Health Study (United States). *Cancer Causes Control* 2001;12:137–145.

478. Luoto R, Latikka P, Pukkala E, et al. The effect of physical activity on breast cancer risk: a cohort study of 30,548 women. *Eur J Cancer Prev* 2000;16:973–980.

479. Moore DB, Folsom AR, Mink PJ, et al. Physical activity and incidence of postmenopausal breast cancer. *Epidemiology* 2000;11:292–296.

480. Moradi T, Nyren O, Zack M, et al. Breast cancer risk and lifetime leisure-time and occupational physical activity (Sweden). *Cancer Causes Control* 2000;11:523–531.

481. Shoff SM, Newcomb PA, Trentham-Dietz A, et al. Early-life physical activity and postmenopausal breast cancer: effect of body size and weight change. *Cancer Epidemiol Biomarkers Prev* 2000;9:591–595.

482. Steindorf K, Schmidt M, Kropp S, et al. Case-control study of physical activity and breast cancer risk among premenopausal women in Germany. *Am J Epidemiol* 2003;157:121–130.

483. Breslow RA, Ballard-Barbash R, Munoz K, et al. Long-term recreational physical activity and breast cancer in the National Health and Nutrition Examination Survey I epidemiologic follow-up study. *Cancer Epidemiol Biomarkers Prev* 2001;10:805–808.

484. Tokunaga M, Land CE, Tokuoka S, et al. Incidence of female breast cancer among atomic bomb survivors, 1950–1985. *Radiat Res* 1994;138:209–223.

485. Miller AB, Howe GR, Sherman GJ, et al. Mortality from breast cancer after irradiation during fluoroscopic examinations in patients being treated for tuberculosis. *N Engl J Med* 1989;321:1285–1289.

486. Morin Doody M, Lonstein JE, Stovall M, et al. Breast cancer mortality after diagnostic radiography: findings from the U.S. Scoliosis Cohort Study. *Spine* 2000;25:2052–2063.

487. Hancock SL, Tucker MA, Hoppe RT. Breast cancer after treatment of Hodgkin's disease. *J Natl Cancer Inst* 1993;85:25–31.

488. Boice JD Jr, Harvey EB, Blettner M, et al. Cancer in the contralateral breast after radiotherapy for breast cancer. *N Engl J Med* 1992;326:781–785.

489. Lavin M. Role of the ataxia-telangiectasia gene (ATM) in breast cancer. A-T heterozygotes seem to have an increased risk but its size is unknown. *BMJ* 1998;317:486–487.

490. Shafman TD, Levitz S, Nixon AJ, et al. Prevalence of germline truncating mutations in ATM in women with a second breast cancer after radiation therapy for a contralateral tumor. *Genes Chromosomes Cancer* 2000;27:124–129.

491. Nichols KE, Levitz S, Shannon KE, et al. Heterozygous germline ATM mutations do not contribute to radiation-associated malignancies after Hodgkin's disease. *J Clin Oncol* 1999;17:1259.

492. Nekolla EA, Kellerer AM, Kuse-Isingschulte M, et al. Malignancies in patients treated with high doses of radium-224. *Radiat Res* 1999;152: S3–S7.

493. Stebbings JH, Lucas HF, Stehney AF. Mortality from cancers of major sites in female radium dial workers. *Am J Ind Med* 1984;5:435–459.

494. Wang JX, Inskip PD, Boice JD Jr., et al. Cancer incidence among medical diagnostic x-ray workers in China, 1950–1985. *Int J Cancer* 1990;45:889–895.

495. Morin Doody M, Mandel JS, Linet MS, et al. Mortality among Catholic nuns certified as radiologic technologists. *Am J Ind Med* 2000;37:339–348.

496. Boice JD Jr., Mandel JS, Doody MM. Breast cancer among radiologic technologists. *JAMA* 1995;274:394–401.

497. Doody MM, Mandel JS, Lubin JH, et al. Mortality among United States radiologic technologists, 1926–1990. *Cancer Causes Control* 1998;9:67–75.

498. Evans JS, Wennberg JE, McNeil BJ. The influence of diagnostic radiography on the incidence of breast cancer and leukemia. *N Engl J Med* 1986;315:810–815.

499. Bhatti P, Struewing JP, Alexander BH, et al. Polymorphisms in DNA repair genes, ionizing radiation exposure and risk of breast cancer in U.S. Radiologic technologists. *Int J Cancer* 2008;122:177–182.

500. Andrieu N, Easton DF, Chang-Claude J, et al. Effect of chest X-rays on the risk of breast cancer among BRCA1/2 mutation carriers in the international BRCA1/2 carrier cohort study: a report from the EMBRACE, GENEPSO, GEO-HEBON, and IBCCS Collaborators' Group. *J Clin Oncol* 2006;24:3361–3366.

501. Narod SA, Lubinski J, Ghadirian P, et al. Screening mammography and risk of breast cancer in BRCA1 and BRCA2 mutation carriers: a case-control study. *Lancet Oncol* 2006;7:402–406.

502. Goldfrank D, Chuai S, Bernstein JL, et al. Effect of mammography on breast cancer risk in women with mutations in BRCA1 or BRCA2. *Cancer Epidemiol Biomarkers Prev* 2006;15:2311–2313.

503. Adami HO, Lipworth L, Titus-Ernstoff L, et al. Organochlorine compounds and estrogen-related cancers in women. *Cancer Causes Control* 1995;6:551–566.

504. Laden F, Collman G, Iwamoto K, et al. 1,1-Dichloro-2,2-bis(p-chlorophenyl)ethylene and polychlorinated biphenyls and breast cancer: combined analysis of five U.S. studies. *J Natl Cancer Inst* 2001;93:768–776.

505. Laden F, Hunter DJ. Environmental risk factors for female breast cancer. *Annu Rev Public Health* 1998;19:101–123.

506. Westin JB, Richter E. The Israeli breast-cancer anomaly. *Ann N Y Acad Sci* 1990;609:269–279.

507. Shames LS, Munekata MT, Pike MC. Re: Blood levels of organochlorine residues and risk of breast cancer. *J Natl Cancer Inst* 1994;86:1642–1643.

508. Rylander L, Hagmar L. Mortality and cancer incidence among women with a high consumption of fatty fish contaminated with persistent organochlorine compounds. *Scand J Work Environ Health* 1995;21:419–426.

509. McElroy JA, Kanarek MS, Trentham-Dietz A, et al. Potential exposure to PCBs, DDT, and PBDEs from sport-caught fish consumption in relation to breast cancer risk in Wisconsin. *Environ Health Perspect* 2004;112:156–162.

510. Bertazzi A, Pesatori AC, Consonni D, et al. Cancer incidence in a population accidentally exposed to 2,3,7,8-tetrachlorodibenzo-para-dioxin. *Epidemiology* 1993;4:398–406.

511. Manz A, Berger J, Dwyer JH, et al. Cancer mortality among workers in chemical plant contaminated with dioxin. *Lancet* 1991;338:959–964.

512. van't Veer P, Lobbezoo IE, Martin Moreno JM, et al. DDT (dicophane) and postmenopausal breast cancer in Europe: case-control study. *BMJ* 1997;315:81–85.

513. Moysich KB, Ambrosone CB, Vena JE, et al. Environmental organochlorine exposure and postmenopausal breast cancer risk. *Cancer Epidemiol Biomarkers Prev* 1998;7:181–188.

514. Lopez-Carrillo L, Blair A, Lopez Cervantes M, et al. Dichlorodiphenyltrichloroethane serum levels and breast cancer risk: a case-control study from Mexico. *Cancer Res* 1997;57:3728–3732.

515. Hardell L, Lindstrom G, Liljegren G, et al. Increased concentrations of octachlorodibenzo-p-dioxin in cases with breast cancer—results from a case-control study. *Eur J Cancer Prev* 1996;5:351–357.

516. Gammon MD, Santella RM, Neugut AI, et al. Environmental toxins and breast cancer on Long Island. I. Polycyclic aromatic hydrocarbon DNA adducts. *Cancer Epidemiol Biomarkers Prev* 2002;11:677–685.

517. Gatto NM, Longnecker MP, Press MF, et al. Serum organochlorines and breast cancer: a case-control study among African-American women. *Cancer Causes Control* 2007;18:29–39.

518. Hunter DJ, Hankinson SE, Laden F, et al. Plasma organochlorine levels and the risk of breast cancer. *N Engl J Med* 1997;337:1253–1258.

519. Krieger N, Wolff MS, Hiatt RA, et al. Breast cancer and serum organochlorines: a prospective study among white, black, and Asian women. *J Natl Cancer Inst* 1994;86:589–599.

520. Wolff MS, Toniolo PG, Lee EW, et al. Blood levels of organochlorine residues and risk of breast cancer. *J Natl Cancer Inst* 1993;85:648–652.

521. Wolff MS, Zeleniuch-Jacquotte A, Dubin N, et al. Risk of breast cancer and organochlorine exposure. *Cancer Epidemiol Biomarkers Prev* 2000;9:271–277.

522. Laden F, Hankinson SE, Wolff MS, et al. Plasma organochlorine levels and the risk of breast cancer: an extended follow-up in the Nurses' Health Study. *Int J Cancer* 2001;91:568–574.
523. Bowers JL, Lanir A, Metz KR, et al. 23Na- and 31P-NMR studies of perfused mouse liver during nitrogen hypoxia. *Am J Physiol* 1992;262: G636–G644.
524. Cohn BA, Wolff MS, Cirillo PM, et al. DDT and breast cancer in young women: new data on the significance of age at exposure. *Environ Health Perspect* 2007; 115:1406–1414.
525. Feychting M, Osterlund B, Ahlbom A. Reduced cancer incidence among the blind. *Epidemiology* 1998;9:490–494.
526. Hahn RA. Profound bilateral blindness and the incidence of breast cancer. *Epidemiology* 1991;2:208–210.
527. Wertheimer N, Leeper E. Magnetic field exposure related to cancer subtypes. *Ann N Y Acad Sci* 1987;502:43–54.
528. Vena JE, Graham S, Hellmann R, et al. Use of electric blankets and risk of postmenopausal breast cancer. *Am J Epidemiol* 1991;134:180–185.
529. Vena JE, Freudenheim JL, Marshall JR, et al. Risk of premenopausal breast cancer and use of electric blankets. *Am J Epidemiol* 1994;140:974–979.
530. Gammon MD, Schoenberg JB, Britton JA, et al. Electric blanket use and breast cancer risk among younger women. *Am J Epidemiol* 1998;148:556–563.
531. Laden F, Neas LM, Tolbert PE, et al. Electric blanket use and breast cancer in the Nurses' Health Study. *Am J Epidemiol* 2000;152:41–49.
532. Kabat GC, O'Leary ES, Schoenfeld ER, et al. Electric blanket use and breast cancer on Long Island. *Epidemiology* 2003;14:514–520.
533. Feychting M, Forssen U. Electromagnetic fields and female breast cancer. *Cancer Causes Control* 2006;17:553–558.
534. Walker MP, Jahnke GD, Snedeker SM, et al. 32P-postlabeling analysis of the formation and persistence of DNA adducts in mammary glands of parous and nulliparous mice treated with benzo[a]pyrene. *Carcinogenesis* 1992;13: 2009–2015.
535. Welp EA, Weiderpass E, Boffetta P, et al. Environmental risk factors of breast cancer. *Scand J Work Environ Health* 1998;24:3–7.
536. Al-Delaimy WK, Cho E, Chen WY, et al. A prospective study of smoking and risk of breast cancer in young adult women. *Cancer Epidemiol Biomarkers Prev* 2004;13:398–404.
537. Gram IT, Braaten T, Terry PD, et al. Breast cancer risk among women who start smoking as teenagers. *Cancer Epidemiol Biomarkers Prev* 2005;14:61–66.
538. Reynolds P, Hurley S, Goldberg DE, et al. Active smoking, household passive smoking, and breast cancer: evidence from the California Teachers Study. *J Natl Cancer Inst* 2004;96:29–37.
539. Hirayama T. Cancer mortality in nonsmoking women with smoking husbands based on a large-scale cohort study in Japan. *Prev Med* 1984;13:680–690.
540. Wells AJ. Breast cancer, cigarette smoking, and passive smoking. *Am J Epidemiol* 1991;133:208–210.
541. Egan KM, Stampfer MJ, Hunter D, et al. Active and passive smoking in breast cancer: prospective results from the Nurses' Health Study. *Epidemiology* 2002; 13:138–145.
542. Brinton LA, Brown SL. Breast implants and cancer. *J Natl Cancer Inst* 1997;89: 1341–1349.
543. Brinton LA, Malone KE, Coates RJ, et al. Breast enlargement and reduction: results from a breast cancer case-control study. *Plast Reconstr Surg* 1996;97: 269–275.
544. Brisson J, Holowaty EJ, Villeneuve PJ, et al. Cancer incidence in a cohort of Ontario and Quebec women having bilateral breast augmentation. *Int J Cancer* 2006;118:2854–2862.
545. Bryant H, Brasher P. Breast implants and breast cancer—reanalysis of a linkage study. *N Engl J Med* 1995;332:1535–1539.
546. Deapen DM, Bernstein L, Brody GS. Are breast implants anticarcinogenic? A 14-year follow-up of the Los Angeles Study. *Plast Reconstr Surg* 1997;99: 1346–1353.
547. Friis S, Holmich LR, McLaughlin JK, et al. Cancer risk among Danish women with cosmetic breast implants. *Int J Cancer* 2006;118:998–1003.
548. Lewis CM. Inflammatory carcinoma of the breast following silicone injections. *Plast Reconstr Surg* 1980;66:134–136.
549. Maddox A, Schoenfeld A, Sinnett HD, et al. Breast carcinoma occurring in association with silicone augmentation. *Histopathology* 1993;23:379–382.
550. Morgenstern L, Gleischman SH, Michel SL, et al. Relation of free silicone to human breast carcinoma. *Arch Surg* 1985;120:573–577.
551. Okubo M, Hyakusoku H, Kanno K, et al. Complications after injection mammaplasty. *Aesthetic Plast Surg* 1992;16:181–187.
552. Brinton LA, Lubin JH, Burich MC, et al. Breast cancer following augmentation mammoplasty (United States). *Cancer Causes Control* 2000;11:819–827.
553. Goldberg MS, Labreche F. Occupational risk factors for female breast cancer. a review. *Occup Environ Med* 1996;53:145–156.
554. Calle EE, Murphy TK, Rodriguez C, et al. Occupation and breast cancer mortality in a prospective cohort of U.S. women. *Am J Epidemiol* 1998;148:191–197.
555. Talamini R, Franceschi S, Favero A, et al. Selected medical conditions and risk of breast cancer. *Br J Cancer* 1997;75:1699–1703.
556. Freiss G, Prebois C, Rochefort H, et al. Anti-steroidal and anti-growth factor activities of anti-estrogens. *J Steroid Biochem Mol Biol* 1990;37:777–781.
557. Michels KB, Solomon CG, Hu FB, et al. Type 2 diabetes and subsequent incidence of breast cancer in the Nurses' Health Study. *Diabetes Care* 2003;26:1752–1758.
558. Bruning PF, Bonfrer JM, van Noord PA, et al. Insulin resistance and breast-cancer risk. *Int J Cancer* 1992;52:511–516.
559. Chalstrey LJ, Benjamin B. High incidence of breast cancer in thyroid cancer patients. *Br J Cancer* 1966;20:670–675.
560. Chen AY, Levy L, Goepfert H, et al. The development of breast carcinoma in women with thyroid carcinoma. *Cancer* 2001;92:225–231.
561. Giovannucci E, Egan KM, Hunter DJ, et al. Aspirin and the risk of colorectal cancer in women. *N Engl J Med* 1995;333:609–614.
562. Rosenberg L, Palmer JR, Zauber AG, et al. A hypothesis: nonsteroidal anti-inflammatory drugs reduce the incidence of large-bowel cancer. *J Natl Cancer Inst* 1991;83:355–358.
563. Harris RE, Namboodiri KK, Farrar WB. Nonsteroidal antiinflammatory drugs and breast cancer. *Epidemiology* 1996;7:203–205.
564. Harris RE, Chlebowski RT, Jackson RD, et al. Breast cancer and nonsteroidal anti-inflammatory drugs: prospective results from the Women's Health Initiative. *Cancer Res* 2003;63:6096–6101.
565. Egan KM, Stampfer MJ, Giovannucci E, et al. Prospective study of regular aspirin use and the risk of breast cancer. *J Natl Cancer Inst* 1996;88:988–993.
566. Marshall SF, Bernstein L, Anton-Culver H, et al. Nonsteroidal anti-inflammatory drug use and breast cancer risk by stage and hormone receptor status. *J Natl Cancer Inst* 2005;97:805–812.
567. Rosenberg L. Aspirin and breast cancer: no surprises yet. *J Natl Cancer Inst* 1996;88:941–942.
568. Bonovas S, Filioussi K, Tsavaris N, et al. Use of statins and breast cancer: a meta-analysis of seven randomized clinical trials and nine observational studies. *J Clin Oncol* 2005;23:8606–8612.
569. Cauley JA, McTiernan A, Rodabough RJ, et al. Statin use and breast cancer: prospective results from the Women's Health Initiative. *J Natl Cancer Inst* 2006; 98:700–707.
570. Eliassen AH, Colditz GA, Rosner B, et al. Serum lipids, lipid-lowering drugs, and the risk of breast cancer. *Arch Intern Med* 2005;165:2264–2271.
571. Polednak AP, Janerich DT. Characteristics of first pregnancy in relation to early breast cancer. A case-control study. *J Reprod Med* 1983;28:314–318.
572. Thompson WD, Jacobson HI, Negrini B, et al. Hypertension, pregnancy, and risk of breast cancer. *J Natl Cancer Inst* 1989;81:1571–1574.
573. Vatten LJ, Romundstad PR, Trichopoulos D, et al. Pre-eclampsia in pregnancy and subsequent risk for breast cancer. *Br J Cancer* 2002;87:971–973.
574. Vatten LJ, Romundstad PR, Odegard RA, et al. Alpha-foetoprotein in umbilical cord in relation to severe pre-eclampsia, birth weight and future breast cancer risk. *Br J Cancer* 2002;86:728–731.
575. Pacheco-Sanchez M, Grunewald KK. Body fat deposition: effects of dietary fat and two exercise protocols. *J Am Coll Nutr* 1994;13:601–607.
576. Polednak AP. Pre-eclampsia, autoimmune diseases and breast cancer etiology. *Med Hypotheses* 1995;44:414–418.
577. Labrecque LG, Barnes DM, Fentiman IS, et al. Epstein-Barr virus in epithelial cell tumors: a breast cancer study. *Cancer Res* 1995;55:39–45.
578. Sugawara Y, Mizugaki Y, Uchida T, et al. Detection of Epstein-Barr virus (EBV) in hepatocellular carcinoma tissue: a novel EBV latency characterized by the absence of EBV-encoded small RNA expression. *Virology* 1999;256:196–202.
579. Yasui Y, Potter JD, Stanford JL, et al. Breast cancer risk and "delayed" primary Epstein-Barr virus infection. *Cancer Epidemiol Biomarkers Prev* 2001;10:9–16.
580. Bonnet M, Guinebretiere JM, Kremmer E, et al. Detection of Epstein-Barr virus in invasive breast cancers. *J Natl Cancer Inst* 1999;91:1376–1381.
581. Chu JS, Chen CC, Chang KJ. In situ detection of Epstein-Barr virus in breast cancer. *Cancer Lett* 1998;124:53–57.
582. Fina F, Romain S, Ouafik L, et al. Frequency and genome load of Epstein-Barr virus in 509 breast cancers from different geographical areas. *Br J Cancer* 2001;84:783–790.
583. Glaser SL. Correspondence re: Yasui et al, Breast cancer risk and "delayed" primary Epstein-Barr virus infection. 2001;10:9–16. *Cancer Epidemiol Biomarkers Prev* 2003;12:73–74.
584. Glaser SL, Ambinder RF, DiGiuseppe JA, et al. Absence of Epstein-Barr virus EBER-1 transcripts in an epidemiologically diverse group of breast cancers. *Int J Cancer* 1998;75:555–558.
585. Grinstein S, Preciado MV, Gattuso P, et al. Demonstration of Epstein-Barr virus in carcinomas of various sites. *Cancer Res* 2002;62:4876–4878.
586. McCall SA, Lichy JH, Bijwaard KE, et al. Epstein-Barr virus detection in ductal carcinoma of the breast. *J Natl Cancer Inst* 2001;93:148–150.
587. Brink AA, van Den Brule AJ, van Diest P, et al. Re: detection of Epstein-Barr virus in invasive breast cancers. *J Natl Cancer Inst* 2000;92:655–656.
588. Hemminki K, Dong C. Re: detection of Epstein-Barr virus in invasive breast cancers. *J Natl Cancer Inst* 1999;91:2126–2127.
589. Herrmann K, Niedobitek G. Epstein-Barr virus-associated carcinomas: facts and fiction. *J Pathol* 2003;199:140–145.
590. Brandes LJ, Arron RJ, Bogdanovic RP, et al. Stimulation of malignant growth in rodents by antidepressant drugs at clinically relevant doses. *Cancer Res* 1992;52:3796–3800.
591. Hilakivi-Clarke L, Wright A, Lippman M. Neonatal antidepressant treatment promotes DMBA-induced mammary tumor growth. *Proc Am Assoc Cancer Res* 1993; 34:84.
592. Wallace RB, Sherman BM, Bean JA. A case-control study of breast cancer and psychotropic drug use. *Oncology* 1982;39:279–283.
593. Sharpe CR, Collet JP, Belzile E, et al. The effects of tricyclic antidepressants on breast cancer risk. *Br J Cancer* 2002;86:92–97.
594. Danielson DA, Jick H, Hunter JR, et al. Nonestrogenic drugs and breast cancer. *Am J Epidemiol* 1982;116:329–332.
595. Dalton SO, Johansen C, Mellemkjaer L, et al. Antidepressant medications and risk for cancer. *Epidemiology* 2000;11:171–176.
596. Kelly JP, Rosenberg L, Palmer JR, et al. Risk of breast cancer according to use of antidepressants, phenothiazines, and antihistamines. *Am J Epidemiol* 1999;150: 861–868.
597. Wang PS, Walker AM, Tsuang MT, et al. Antidepressant use and the risk of breast cancer: a non-association. *J Clin Epidemiol* 2001;54:728–734.
598. Schottenfeld D, Fraumeni J Jr. *Cancer epidemiology and prevention.*, New York: Oxford University Press, 1996:1521.
599. Ames BN, Gold LS, Willett WC. The causes and prevention of cancer. *Proc Natl Acad Sci U S A* 1995;92:5258–5265.
600. Davis DL, Bradlow HL. Can environmental estrogens cause breast cancer? *Sci Am* 1995;273:167–172.
601. FitzGerald MG BJ, Hegde SR, Unsal H, et al. Heterozygous ATM mutations do not contribute to early onset of breast cancer. *Nat Genet* 1997;15:307–310.
602. Madigan MP, Ziegler RG, Benichou J, et al. Proportion of breast cancer cases in the United States explained by well-established risk factors. *J Natl Cancer Inst* 1995;87:1681–1685.
603. Eliassen AH, Colditz G, Rosner B, et al. Adult weight change and risk of postmenopausal breast cancer. *JAMA* 2006;296:193–201.
604. White E. Projected changes in breast cancer incidence due to the trend toward delayed childbearing. *Am J Public Health* 1987;77:495–497.
605. Gail MH, Brinton LA, Byar DP, et al. Projecting individualized probabilities of developing breast cancer for white females who are being examined annually. *J Natl Cancer Inst* 1989;81:1879–1886.
606. Rockhill B, Spiegelman D, Byrne C, et al. Validation of the Gail et al. model of breast cancer risk prediction and implications for chemoprevention. *J Natl Cancer Inst* 2001;93:358–366.

607. Lerman C, Lustbader E, Rimer B, et al. Effects of individualized breast cancer risk counseling: a randomized trial. *J Natl Cancer Inst* 1995;87:286–292.

608. Schwartz LM, Woloshin S, Black WC, et al. The role of numeracy in understanding the benefit of screening mammography. *Ann Intern Med* 1997;127:966–972.

609. Waters EA, Weinstein ND, Colditz GA, et al. Aversion to side effects in preventive medical treatment decisions. *Br J Health Psychol* 2007;12:383–401.

610. Waters EA, Weinstein ND, Colditz GA, et al. Reducing aversion to side effects in preventive medical treatment decisions. *J Exp Psychol Appl* 2007;13:11–21.

611. Smith BL, Gadd MA, Lawler C, et al. Perception of breast cancer risk among women in breast center and primary care settings: correlation with age and family history of breast cancer. *Surgery* 1996;120:297–303.

612. Davis S, Stewart S, Bloom J. Increasing the accuracy of perceived breast cancer risk: results from a randomized trial with Cancer Information Service callers. *Prev Med* 2004;39:64–73.

613. Colditz GA, Frazier AL. Models of breast cancer show that risk is set by events of early life: prevention efforts must shift focus. *Cancer Epidemiol Biomarkers Prev* 1995;4:567–571.

614. Rose G. Strategy of prevention: lessons from cardiovascular disease. *Br Med J (Clin Res Ed)* 1981;282:1847–1851.

615. Mosian J, Meyer F, Gingras S. Leisure, physical activity and age at menarche. *Medicine Sci Sports Exerc* 1991;23:1170–1175.

616. Berkey CS, Rockett HR, Gillman MW, et al. One-year changes in activity and in inactivity among 10- to 15-year-old boys and girls: relationship to change in body mass index. *Pediatrics* 2003;111:836–843.

617. Gortmaker SL, Dietz WH Jr, Cheung LW. Inactivity, diet, and the fattening of America. *J Am Diet Assoc* 1990;90:1247–1252, 1255.

618. Freed GL, Clark SJ, Sorenson J, et al. National assessment of physicians' breast feeding knowledge, attitudes, training, and experience. *JAMA* 1995;273:472–476.

619. Rimm E, Willett W, Manson J, et al. Folate and vitamin B6 intake and risk of myocardial infarction among U.S. women (Abstract). *Am J Epidemiol* 1996;143(Suppl):S36.

620. Giovannucci E, Stampfer MJ, Colditz GA, et al. Multivitamin use, folate, and colon cancer in women in the Nurses' Health Study. *Ann Intern Med* 1998;129:517–524.

621. Jacobs TW, Byrne C, Colditz G, et al. Radial scars in benign breast biopsy specimens and the risk of breast cancer. *N Engl J Med* 1999;340:430–436.

Chapter 21
Management of Other High Risk Patients

Seema A. Khan and Susan M. Gapstur

Breast cancer risk can be attributed to three broad categories of risk factors: increasing age, lifetime estrogen exposure (endogenous and exogenous), and genetic susceptibility. These major factors play a critical role in breast epithelial transformation and appear to converge in the phenotypic expression of proliferative precursor lesions of the breast epithelium, as observed in the unaffected breasts of women who are genetically susceptible (e.g., *BRCA* mutation carriers), as well as women at risk for the so-called *sporadic* breast cancer. This chapter focuses on the identification and management of women at higher than average risk for sporadic breast cancer; management of women who are genetically susceptible, and those with lobular carcinoma *in situ* is covered in Chapters 19 and 25. The discussions of breast cancer risk below will apply to women who do not carry mutations of known breast cancer susceptibility genes. Additionally, a full discussion of the epidemiology of sporadic breast cancer can be found in Chapter 20, and these risk factors are reviewed here only from the perspective of identification and management of individuals (rather than populations) at risk for breast cancer.

The management of women at increased risk for breast cancer includes (a) identification of women at high risk (or risk estimation); (b) recommendations for life-style modifications that may reduce risk; (c) a plan for breast surveillance; (d) discussion of pharmacologic prevention; and (e) discussion of prophylactic mastectomy (if appropriate and sought by the patient).

IDENTIFICATION OF HIGH RISK WOMEN

Age

The relation of age to breast cancer risk is discussed fully in Chapter 20, but it is worthwhile noting here that breast cancer risk estimation for individuals is heavily influenced by age. Incidence rates rise sharply with age, starting in the mid-to-late 30s; all currently used statistical risk estimation models relate the known relative risk (RR) for a particular risk factor to the age-specific breast cancer frequency in that population. This is important to recognize in terms of breast cancer risk management, because a 5-year risk estimate of 1.7% using the Gail model-2 (National Cancer Institute [NCI] Breast Cancer Risk Assessment Tool) has been widely used as a benchmark measure of breast cancer risk. The 5-year breast cancer Gail model probability for an average woman 45 years of age is 1%, whereas the similar estimate for an average woman 65 years of ages 2%. Thus, a 45-year-old woman who has a 5-year breast cancer probability of 1.7% is at higher life-time risk than her 65-year-old counterpart. As the same 45-year-old woman ages, however, if she does not acquire any new risk factors and does not develop breast cancer, her estimated risk declines and approaches the average risk for her age group. Thus longer-term risk estimates (e.g., 10- or 20-year estimates) may be a more useful framework for risk counseling.

Estrogen-related Risk Factors

A wide array of established risk factors for breast cancer relates to endogenous lifetime estrogen exposure. These include young age at menarche, late age at first full-term pregnancy, no exposure to lactation, and late age at menopause.

Other well-established risk factors also appear to operate through the endocrine axis: postmenopausal obesity is associated with increased aromatization of androgenic precursors in adipose tissue, lower sex hormone-binding globulin, and higher free estradiol (1). Physical activity in adolescence delays menarche and the onset of ovulatory cycles; later in life, it protects against obesity and may operate through other mechanisms as well (2). Moderate to heavy alcohol consumption is associated with higher circulating sex steroid levels and may retard the hepatic metabolism of hormones (3).

In general, the contribution of these individual risk factors to overall risk is modest, and relative risk estimates for each of these factors from most studies are in the range of 1.5 to 2.0. It is therefore difficult to apply this information to individual risk estimation unless it is incorporated into multifactorial statistical models, the prototype of which is the Gail model (4), validated in the Breast Cancer Prevention Trial (5). More recently developed models (Tyrer-Cusick) do include additional endocrine risk factors (age at menarche, use of postmenopausal hormone therapy, height, weight) and family history (6). Breast cancer risk estimation is discussed more fully below.

Mammographic Density

The radiographic appearance of the breast varies according to differences in the relative distributions of fat and fibroglandular tissues, where fat appears dark and radiographically dense areas appear light (Fig. 21.1). A substantial body of evidence now shows that extensive mammographic breast density is strongly associated with an increased risk factor of breast cancer. The RR for the highest category of breast density (>75% of breast area is dense) has been reproducible across several large studies. In a recent meta-analysis, the RR for the highest density category ranges from 3.25 to 6.49 in eight incidence studies published since 1995 (7). Additionally, Boyd et al. (8), reported results of a study in which they combined data from three nested case-control studies including 1,112 women who participated in breast cancer screening programs. In that study, women with density in 75% or more of the mammogram had a 4.7-fold (95% CI, 3.0–7.4) higher risk of breast cancer compared with women with density in less than 10% of the mammogram. A particularly high risk was, however, associated with density for women whose cancer was detected within 12 months of the screening mammogram (RR = 17), suggesting that density might mask the cancer. Based on these results, it is important to identify women who have extensive mammographic density among whom alternative imaging techniques might be useful for earlier detection.

The importance of mammographic density as a strong and independent risk factor for breast cancer is amplified by its high prevalence, with about one-third of the general population of women displaying dense areas of 50% or greater on mammography (7). Because of this prevalence, the fraction of breast cancer cases attributable to high mammographic density is in the range of 16% to 32% (9), and higher in premenopausal women (8). Thus, the impact of breast density on cancer risk is far stronger than any of the known endocrine-related risk factors, and in the same range as the risk associated with atypical proliferative lesions of the breast.

Breast density may also be a potentially useful surrogate intermediate marker for studies of breast cancer prevention because it reflects (at least partially) the cumulative hormonal

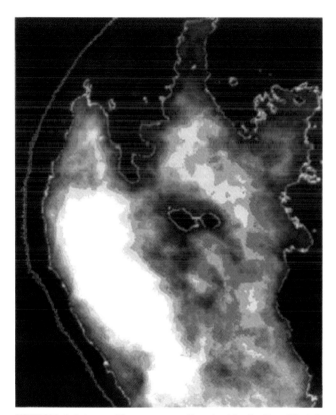

FIGURE 21.1. Technique used to measure area of breast and density. The *red line* indicates edge of breast image as viewed on monitor after digitization, and the *green line* delineates the area of density. (From Boyd NF, Byng JW, Jong RA, et al. Quantitative classification of mammographic densities and breast cancer risk: results from the Canadian National Breast Screening Study. *J Natl Cancer Inst* 1995;87(9):670–675, with permission.)

exposure of a woman. This is most evident in that the use of combination postmenopausal hormone therapy (PMHT) increases the percent breast density (10,11), and tamoxifen therapy reduces it (12), as does ovarian suppression with a gonadotrophin-releasing hormone agonist in premenopausal women (13). However, studies examining the correlation between serum sex steroid levels and mammographic density have not shown any consistent associations, with one large recent study showing no relationship between circulating sex steroid levels and mammographic density (14). It would be of interest to determine if local breast estradiol levels (e.g., those in nipple aspiration fluid) are related more closely to breast density than circulating levels; these studies are ongoing. On the other hand, mammographic density and serum sex steroids (estradiol and testosterone) may have independent and additive effects on breast cancer risk as suggested by a recently reported case-control study nested within the Nurses' Health Study (NHS) (15). Other hints that mammographic density is modulated by the endocrine environment come from the significant correlation between mammographic density and serum insulin-like growth factor-1 (IGF-1) that has been observed in some, but not all, studies of premenopausal women (16,17). Prolactin is another potentially important hormone in breast carcinogenesis; higher levels in the serum are associated with increased breast cancer risk in both pre- and postmenopausal women (18), and several studies now suggest an association between serum prolactin levels and mammographic density (16,19).

Studies relating breast density to histologic findings have shown that high mammographic density is associated with an increased risk for atypical hyperplasia (20). However, in breast epithelial samples obtained from high risk women using random fine needle aspiration (FNA), no correlation was seen between

cytologic atypia or cell proliferation (measured by Ki-67 labeling) and mammographic density (21). Quantitative microscopy of the autopsied breast shows relationships between mammographic density and total nuclear area, epithelial and nonepithelial nuclear area, glandular structures, and amount of collagen (22). Similarly, in reduction mammoplasty samples, the epithelial cell volume was concentrated in areas of high density connective tissue, and was significantly related to the mammographic density. No clear biological explanation exists, however, for the association of breast density with cancer risk, and much remains to be done to incorporate the measurement and modulation of mammographic density into algorithms for breast cancer risk assessment and prevention.

Breast Epithelial Hyperplasia

The present paradigm for the development of breast cancer suggests that, in the breast, as in other epithelial organs, the etiologic pathways of malignancy converge in the occurrence of breast epithelial hyperplasia or intraepithelial neoplasia (IEN) (23). This concept is supported by data going back several decades, relating benign breast disease (specifically, epithelial proliferation) to an increased risk of subsequent breast cancer; several studies have shown that the breast cancer risk for women with hyperplasia without atypia is approximately twofold greater than for women without; and the risk associated with atypical hyperplasia is increased approximately fourfold (24–27). The specific lesions included in the category of hyperplasia without atypia consist of moderate or florid duct hyperplasia, intraductal papilloma, sclerosing adenosis, and radial scar. The lesions usually included in the category of atypical proliferation include atypical duct hyperplasia (ADH), atypical lobular hyperplasia (ALH), atypical papilloma, and columnar cell change with atypia (see Chapter 23 for more detail). In a large retrospective cohort from Nashville, Tennessee, a strong interaction between atypical hyperplasia and a positive family history for breast cancer was observed, so that the risk associated with a history of a first-degree relative with breast cancer and atypical hyperplasia was increased almost 10-fold (24). Two recent studies do not substantiate these findings, however, and no significant interaction between a finding of atypical hyperplasia and positive family history was observed (27,28). Although a more marked risk increase with ALH than ADH was suggested in the Nashville and Nurses' cohorts, recent results from the Mayo Clinic cohort do not show a difference in risk between ADH and ALH. However, an increasing number of atypical foci, the presence of calcifications in the histologic material, and the combination of ADH and ALH, all raise risk significantly over that observed in the absence of these findings (29) (Fig. 21.2).

Despite the consistently increased risk seen with typical and atypical epithelial proliferation in the breast, most women with these findings do not develop breast cancer (e.g., 80% of the 330 women with atypical hyperplasia in the Mayo cohort remained free of breast cancer over a mean follow-up period of almost 14 years). A number of authors have attempted to identify molecular factors that might improve the specificity of risk assessment, so that preventive interventions can be targeted to a more purified high-risk group. Despite a number of potential risk biomarkers, little progress has been made in prospective validation of these. Most immunohistochemical markers that have been examined so far suggest a RR of 2 to 3, and include proteins, such as estrogen receptor (30), p53 (31), ERBB2 (HER2/nue) (32). Markers that have been recently discovered through gene array approaches appear more promising, and include carcinoembryonic antigen cell adhesion molecule 6 (CEACAM-6) (33), which (in a small study) was found to be expressed at a far higher frequency in ADH lesions from women who subsequently developed breast cancer, compared

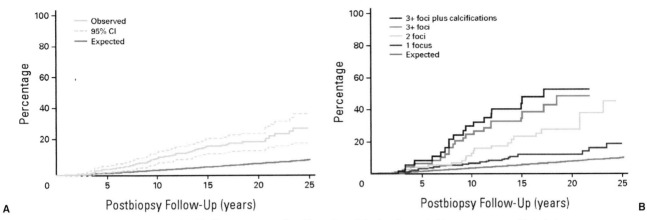

FIGURE 21.2. A: Cumulative risk of breast cancer over time. Observed cumulative breast cancer incidence among women with atypical hyperplasia, with 95% represented by *stippled lines*. Expected breast cancer events were calculated by applying age- and calendar period-stratified person-years of observation to corresponding Iows Surveillance, Epidemiology, and End Results breast cancer incidence rates. Observed and expected events cumulated after accounting for death as a computing risk. **B**: Observed and expected cumulative breast cancer incidence among women with atypical hyperplasia, stratified by number of foci of atypia and histologic presence of calcifications. (From Degnim AC, Visscher DW, Berman HK, et al. Stratification of breast cancer risk in women with atypia: a Mayo cohort. *J Clin Oncol* 2007;25(19):2671–2677. Epub 2007 June 11, with permission.)

with ADH lesions from women who remained cancer-free. Presently, no validated risk biomarkers exist in breast epithelial lesions, and the morphologic diagnosis of atypical hyperplasia and lobular carcinoma *in situ* remains the strongest tissue-based marker of breast cancer risk.

BREAST EPITHELIAL SAMPLING IN ASYMPTOMATIC, HIGH RISK WOMEN

Until recently, atypical hyperplasia has been identified only in women who developed breast lumps or mammographic findings that required biopsy. In such populations, the prevalence of atypical hyperplasia in an older series of open surgical biopsies was 3.5% (34), but ranges from 4.3% (35) to 9% (36) in a series of core needle biopsies for mammographic findings. Autopsy studies suggest that the prevalence of occult atypical IEN is 12.5% (37), and could be as high 26% (38), depending on the detail of the sampling. Good evidence, therefore, indicates that the prevalence of occult breast IEN is significantly higher than that suggested by surgical biopsy data.

The recent interest in techniques for the sampling of epithelium from clinically normal breasts is motivated by the expectation that an improved ability to identify occult IEN would lead to improvements in our ability to assess individual risk. Valid methods of breast epithelial sampling have another important application—the potential for the development of surrogate endpoints for the occurrence of malignancy, which are notably lacking in the field of breast cancer prevention at the moment. Although significant progress has occurred in this area over the last decade or so, breast epithelial sampling of asymptomatic women remains a research tool, with no specific application in the clinical management of women at high risk. The state of the field is briefly summarized below.

Methods of Noninvasive, Minimal Sampling of the Healthy High-risk Breast

The noninvasive, minimal sampling techniques available include two which obtain fluid and cells from ductal lumina (nipple aspiration fluid and ductal lavage) and two which obtain epithelial and stromal cells via random fine or core needle biopsy.

Nipple aspiration fluid (NAF): Nipple fluid contains cells that are exfoliated into the ductal lumen and can be collected at the

duct orifice by suction-aspiration. It is well tolerated, inexpensive, and produces samples that are paucicellular (or acellular) but rich in proteins and hormones. It was first evaluated by Papanicoloau in the 1950s (39), with the goal of breast cancer detection; and was subsequently furthered by Sartorius (40), who developed a breast pump device designed to improve nipple fluid yield from asymptomatic women. The method in use today involves breast massage, dekeratinization of the nipple, and suction-aspiration with a commercially available device (e.g., Cytyc Hologic Corporation, Bedford, MA). Nipple aspiration fluid ranging from 1µl to hundreds of µl can typically be obtained from 40% to 80% of women, with higher success rates in premenopausal women. It is typically collected at the nipple in a graduated capillary tube (41).

Ductal lavage (DL) is an extension of NAF, designed to overcome the problems of scant cellularity in NAF samples, and to sample the entire length of the ductal tree (42). The procedure involves application of a topical anesthetic or periareolar infiltration with lidocaine; the elicitation of nipple fluid, as described above, cannulation of each fluid-yielding duct (non-fluid-yielding ducts can also be cannulated) with a single lumen catheter (Cytyc Health Corporation, Boxborough, MA) and lavage with normal saline. The lavage effluent is fixed, centrifuged to recover a cell pellet, and cytologic smears prepared.

Random FNA (rFNA), is performed in the clinically and radiologically normal breast in healthy women at high risk. It is an approach that assumes a field change in the high-risk breast and does not rely on site-specific sampling. First tested in Utah (43,44), major work in this area has subsequently been reported from University of Kansas by Fabian et al. (45), who have modified the original technique of Ward et al. (43,44). After local anesthesia with buffered lidocaine with epinephrine, eight to ten passes are made per breast with a 21-gauge needle introduced at two locations (periareolar, upper outer and upper inner quadrants). Samples from both breasts are pooled. With the prophylactic use of vitamin K, use of buffered lidocaine, postprocedure cold packs, and tight-fitting sports bras, hematomas are rare, and the procedure is generally well tolerated.

Random core needle biopsy (rCNB), with the availability of spring-loaded core needle biopsy devices, has become a possible approach to breast epithelial sampling. Some data exist in terms of the utility of this approach for tissue acquisition for biomarker studies (46,47), but there is no published information on its use in risk assessment. In one biomarker study, up to seven cores were obtained from each subject, through the same skin incision. On average, three of the six to seven cores per subject contained epithelium, the rest being fatty. The investigators were able to count 3,000 cells per case after Ki-67 labeling, by combining a mean of 11 core-cut sections per subject. They did not find any significant difference in pre- and post-treatment Ki-67 labeling indices (47).

OCCULT INTRAEPITHELIAL NEOPLASIA AND BREAST CANCER RISK

The concept of epithelial sampling by nipple aspiration in relation to breast cancer risk was pioneered by Wrensch et al (48,49), who published a series of reports through the 1970s to the present, characterizing nipple fluid yield and cytologic findings in healthy women. In two cohorts studied by this group, NAF yield varied considerably (85% for the first cohort and 40% for the second) (48,49). In the first cohort, women who produced NAF and had cytologic evidence of hyperplasia developed breast cancer at 2.5-fold higher rate (95% CI, 1.1–5.5), which increased to 4.9-fold (95% CI, 1.7–13.9) when cytologic atypia was present (Fig. 21.3). Women who did not produce NAF were the reference group. In the second cohort, accrued between 1981 and 1991, the RR was 2.0 (95% CI, 1.3–3.3) for the hyperplasia and atypical hyperplasia groups combined, because no cancers occurred in the 22 women with atypical hyperplasia.

Ductal lavage was introduced with the expectation that it would perform better than NAF in the identification of occult IEN. When compared with NAF, DL samples consistently provide a higher cell yield, but at significantly greater cost in supplies, time, and patient discomfort (50) The utility of ductal lavage for breast cancer risk assessment is currently being investigated in a multicenter study where 500 women identified to be at high risk for breast cancer undergo DL at 6 month intervals for a 3-year period.

The notion that occult IEN exists in women at high risk and can be identified through random needle sampling techniques was substantiated by findings from a study of rFNA performed by Fabian et al. in 486 women at high risk women (median 5-year Gail model estimate of 4%). These women were followed for a median of 45 months after rFNA, and evidence showed that hyperplasia with atypia on random FNA equates with an increased short-term risk of breast cancer (Fig. 21.3). Hyperplasia with atypia was present in the initial FNA in 21% of women, and was predictive of the probability of developing breast cancer independent of a 10-year Gail risk. The proportion of women with atypical proliferation in this study was similar to that reported in rFNA samples from the normal breasts of a group of women with contralateral breast cancer, where the atypia rate was 16% (51). Good separation of cumulative 3-year breast cancer incidence rates was achieved by using a combination of Gail risk and rFNA atypia: Women with both an above-median Gail risk and hyperplasia with atypia on rFNA had an incidence rate of 15%, those with only an above-median Gail risk had a 3-year incidence of 4%, and those with a below-median Gail risk had no cancers detected in the first 3 years of follow-up.

Practical Utility of Identifying Occult Intraepithelial Neoplasia

The identification of occult IEN remains, for the moment, in the realm of clinical research, because both of the long-term studies demonstrating the value of occult IEN for breast cancer risk prediction (NAF and rFNA) came from single institutions and have not been replicated. Further, these institutions have the benefit of highly developed cytologic expertise, an important issue because the reproducibility of cytologic assessment of these minimal samples is questionable. For women whose risk estimate would be changed by a finding of occult atypia, data regarding the decision-making value of this information are beginning to appear. Although Port et al. (52) reported that only 5% of women seen in a high-risk clinic accepted tamoxifen therapy, an analysis of accrual patterns to the Breast Cancer Prevention Trial and the STAR trial (Study of Tamoxifen and Raloxifene) show that 36% of women with a history of atypical IEN were willing to participate, compared with 21% of those without a history of breast IEN (53). Data from our institution show a similar trend for acceptance of prophylactic tamoxifen, in that the acceptance rate in 68 women at high risk who were offered tamoxifen because of a history of atypical IEN was 53%, compared with 29% of 65 women who were high risk for other reasons (*p* = .008) (54).

BIOMARKER EVALUATION IN BREAST EPITHELIAL SAMPLES

Biomarker assessment in breast epithelial samples can potentially add precision to risk estimation, as discussed above; however, the validation of potential risk biomarkers has proved challenging. Molecular markers of risk were evaluated in rFNA studies, and a final three-test set (Epidermal growth factor receptor (EGFR), Estrogen Receptor (ER), p53), was an independently significant predictor of epithelial atypia (*p* <.001) (45). With cancer occurrence as the outcome, however, only atypia and Gail risk remain significant. More recent studies have focused on novel biomarkers, such as DNA hypermethylation of gene promoters, measured both in rFNA and

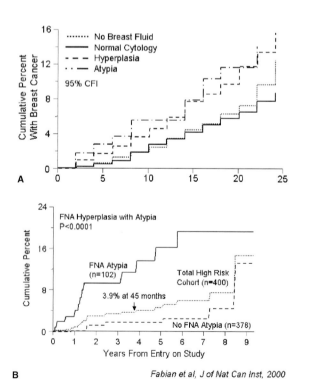

Fabian et al, J of Nat Can Inst, 2000

FIGURE 21.3. Breast cancer incidence rates in healthy women showing epithelial atypia. **A:** Combined results from two cohorts undergoing nipple aspiration fluid collection at the University of California, San Francisco. 1973–99 and 1981–99. (Wrensch et al., *J Natl Cancer Inst* 2002, reproduced with permission.) **B:** Breast Cancer Incidence rates in high-risk women with and without evidence of atypical hyperplasia in randomfine needle aspiration samples at the Kansas University Medical Center. (Fabian et al., *J Natl Cancer Inst* 2000, reproduced with permission). NAF: Nipple Aspiration Fluid. FNA: Fine Needle Aspiration.

DL samples. Early results are encouraging. These show that DNA methylation profiles perform better than cytologic evaluation in the detection of cancer cells in DL samples (55), and are associated with cytologic atypia and Gail risk in rFNA samples (56,57).

The reversibility of biomarkers in short-term phase II or III studies of chemopreventive intervention has not been demonstrated so far, although attempts have been made, using surrogate endpoints related to cell morphology and biomarker expression in rFNA samples (45,58). In a more recent single-arm study with letrozole as the intervention in postmenopausal women, Ki-67 labeling did decrease significantly in the post-treatment samples, but the lack of an untreated control arm renders interpretation difficult (59) . Nevertheless, Ki-67 labeling is a promising intermediate endpoint based on its validation in neoadjuvant breast cancer therapy trials, where post-treatment Ki-67 is a strong independent predictor of clinical outcomes (60).

ESTIMATION OF RISK FOR SPORADIC BREAST CANCER

Breast cancer risk estimation has acquired a practical importance with the availability of proven methods of risk reduction, which are logically targeted to women at high risk. As discussed above, epidemiologic investigations over the past half-century defined a number of breast cancer risk factors, and numerical estimation of group or individual breast cancer risk has become possible through the development of statistical models that incorporate these risk factors to compute the probability of breast cancer development. The first of these was developed by Gail and colleagues, who used data collected during the Breast Cancer Detection and Demonstration Project (61), and combined several known risk factors: age at menarche, age at first full-term pregnancy, number of first-degree relatives with breast cancer, number of surgical breast biopsies, and whether the biopsy showed atypical hyperplasia. Specific probability estimates were then calculated using age and race-specific frequencies of breast cancer in the population, recognizing that uncertainty was greater in non-European women because baseline data were not as robust. This model has been validated prospectively (62,63), and risk assessment using statistical models has been adopted as a standard clinical tool in many institutions. It is available at http://www.cancer.gov/bcrisktool/.

Although use of the Gail model has led to very precise prediction of rates of breast cancer occurrence in groups of women (5) (i.e., it is well calibrated for populations), the ability to identify individual women who will develop breast cancer (in other words, its discriminatory ability) remains poor. The discriminatory ability of a model is measured by the concordance statistic, which is equivalent to the area under the curve (AUC) in a receiver-operator curve (ROC) analysis, and examines the sensitivity and specificity of a given test at different thresholds. Thus, the concordance statistic or AUC measures the overall accuracy of the model, and for a perfect model should approach 1.0, whereas for a useful model should be 0.8 or greater. A concordance statistic of 0.5 would imply a model that predicts as well as chance (e.g., flipping a coin). The concordance statistic for the Gail model in the Nurses Health Study was 0.58 (95% CI, 0.56–0.60). Only 3.3% of women who developed breast cancer in the Nurses' cohort had a risk above the threshold recommended for preventive intervention with tamoxifen (64). In addition, the model overestimates risk in young, unscreened women and underestimates risk in women over 59 years of age (65). More recently recognized sources of risk, such as mammographic density, and use of hormone replacement therapy (HRT) are not included. Finally, it is a model that is well-calibrated for

sporadic breast cancer risk, but does not address many of the attributes of family history associated with inherited susceptibility syndromes, (age at onset, bilaterality of cancer, affected second-degree relatives, and history of ovarian cancer).

Since the validation of the Gail model, several other models have been developed that attempt to incorporate features of breast cancer risk applicable to both the genetic and the environmental–endocrine components. The Tyrer-Cuzick model (6) incorporates a number of endocrine risk factors, including age at menopause and use of hormones for postmenopausal women, height, weight, and a family history that includes information on extended family, age at onset, and ovarian cancer information (available at http://www.ems-trials.org/riskevaluator/). The model calculates personal risk over 10 years and life-time (presented in comparison to population risk); and computes the probability of *BRCA1* and *BRCA2* mutations. In the International Breast Cancer Intervention Study (IBIS-I) trial, the number of observed cancers did not differ significantly from the number predicted (66); in a separate high-risk cohort in Manchester, the model had a discriminatory accuracy of 0.762, compared with 0.735 for the Gail model (67). Prospective validation is expected from the IBIS-II trial, where postmenopausal women at high risk are being randomized to anastrozole or placebo.

Adding Mammographic Density

Given the strong impact of mammographic density on breast cancer risk, efforts are under way to incorporate this important risk factor into predictive models. Gail et al. have incorporated mammographic density data on 7,500 women from the BCDDP into the Gail-2 model, and have found that their new model remains well-calibrated in a set of 1,744 white women, with a modest increase in discriminatory power. The average age-specific concordance was 0.643 for the new model, in comparison with 0.596, for Gail-2 model (68). A second model, including mammographic density, has been developed by Barlow et al. (69), using data from the Breast Cancer Surveillance Consortium. For premenopausal women, significant risk factors included age, breast density, a positive family history of breast cancer, and a prior breast procedure. The fitted model had a concordance statistic of 0.631 (95% CI, 0.618—0.644), compared with 0.607 (95% CI, 0.592—0.621) when breast density was excluded. For postmenopausal women, the concordance statistic for the overall model was 0.624 (95% CI, 0.619—0.630). When breast density was excluded, the concordance statistic decreased to 0.605 (95% CI, 0.600–0.611). The addition of mammographic density, therefore, seems to improve the risk estimation modestly, but these models still require prospective validation.

Risk Estimation for Black Women

The Gail model/NCI risk assessment tool underestimates risk in women of African ancestry (70). A modification of the Gail model has been developed by Gail et al. using 1,600 African American case-control pairs from the Women's Contraceptive and Reproductive Experiences (CARE) study (71). Five-year breast cancer risk estimates from the CARE model and the NCI Breast Cancer Risk Assessment Tool show good agreement in younger women, but estimates for older women (>45 years) are higher with the CARE model. The calibration of the CARE model was tested in the 14,059 black women who entered the WHI without a prior history of breast cancer, 350 of whom developed invasive breast cancer over a mean 7-year follow-up period. The number of women predicted to develop breast cancer with the CARE model (323) was not significantly different from the number observed, with an observed-to-expected (O/E) ratio of = 1.08 (95% CI, 0.97–1.20). This held up for most categories, with the exception of women with a prior history of benign breast biopsy, where the O/E was significantly lower than observed, indicating underestimation of the breast cancer risk. For women who had one benign breast biopsy and for those who had two or more biopsy examinations were 1.51 (95% CI, 1.20–1.92) and 1.65 (95% CI, 1.16–2.35), respectively. Among those screened for the STAR trial, the models agreed for 83% of the AA women screened, but 14.5% of women were risk eligible for the trial when screened with the NCI Breast Cancer Risk Assessment Tool compared with 30.3% with the CARE model.

Estimation of Risk by Hormone Receptor Status

For the implementation of targeted risk reduction with selective estrogen receptor modulators (SERM), such as tamoxifen, which are effective only in the prevention of estrogen receptor (ER)-positive breast cancer, the identification of women specifically at risk for ER-positive disease is highly desirable. For women with a prior history of breast cancer, the hormone receptor status of the first primary tumor may predict that of a future second primary, as evidenced in a pooled analysis of contralateral breast cancers observed in National Surgical Adjuvant Breast and Bowel Project (NSABP) treatment trials (72). Among women who had not received tamoxifen, there was strong concordance between the ER status of the first and second primary cancers: 89% of those with an ER-positive primary cancer had an ER-positive contralateral breast cancer and 70% with an ER-negative primary breast cancer had an ER-negative contralateral breast cancer (for the association between primary and contralateral ER status, OR = 14.8, 95% CI, 3.8–74.3). In a subsequent study from Baylor College of Medicine, the ER concordance between first and second primaries was 88% when the first primary was ER-positive; but when the first primary was ER-negative, only 25% of women developed an ER-negative second primary (73). Among patients who received tamoxifen, both studies showed that the ER status of the second primary was not predicted by that of the first primary. Thus, in almost 90% of women who develop a second primary cancer, this will be ER-positive if the first tumor was ER-positive and they do not receive tamoxifen.

Among unaffected women, modest associations were seen between the risk for ER-positive disease and European ancestry, postmenopausal obesity, and post menopausal hormone therapy (74–76). High serum hormone levels have also been associated with the risk of ER-positive breast cancer (77–79). In the WHI cohort, the discriminatory accuracy of the Gail model was 0.58 overall (95% CI, 0.56–0.60), but was slightly better for women who developed ER-positive breast cancer (0.60, 95% CI, 0.58–0.62). For the prediction of ER-negative breast cancer, the model performed no better than chance (80). The AUC for the Gail model in the WHI is seen in Figure 21.4. Thus, with the possible exception of an ER-positive first primary tumor, no indicator of risk exists for ER-positive breast cancer that is sufficiently specific to select women for endocrine prevention strategies on this basis.

MANAGEMENT OF WOMEN AT HIGHER THAN AVERAGE RISK

Once a woman has been determined to be at high risk, but is not a mutation carrier, the management issues to be considered include counseling regarding life-style factors that may modify risk, surveillance for early detection of breast cancer, and pharmacologic interventions to reduce risk. The discussion of prophylactic mastectomy in the nonmutation carrier should be undertaken with women to wish to explore this option, but this is best initiated by the patient rather than the physician.

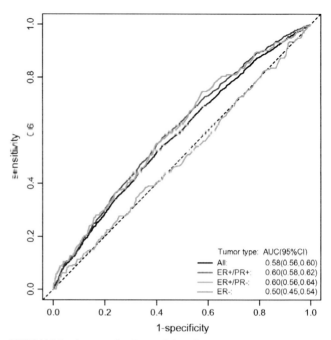

FIGURE 21.4. Receiver operating characteristic analysis and corresponding area under the curve (AUC) statistics for Gail model of prediction of invasive breast cancer risk by receptor status evaluated on the Women's Health Initiative clinical trial cohort. ER, estrogen receptor; PR, progesterone receptor; CI, confidence interval.

Surveillance

Physical examination is the most basic form of breast cancer surveillance and remains an important part of the surveillance plan. It is generally recommended twice or thrice a year in women at high risk, and can be shared between her various physicians (e.g., gynecologist, breast surgeon, internist) or may be performed by the same practitioner. In many offices, experienced physician extenders can provide this service with a high level of competence. Self-examination should be encouraged, although it is of uncertain utility in the early detection of breast cancer. Women, however, should be encouraged to learn the topography of their own breasts so that a change is easily noted.

Annual mammography remains the mainstay of breast surveillance, although its relatively poor performance in young women at high risk has led to the evaluation of other imaging modalities: whole breast ultrasound (WBUS) and magnetic resonance imaging (MRI). The evidence for WBUS utility in breast surveillance remains unproven; in one study of WBUS with a yield of 13 per 1,000 in the high-risk group, compared with 4.6 per 1,000 in standard risk women. The operator dependence of US, the time required for WBUS, and the cost are likely, however, to remain barriers to the wide-scale implementation of this technique. On the other hand, targeted US is routinely used for problem solving as an adjunct to mammography.

The addition of breast MRI to mammography and US in the surveillance of women at high risk has been evaluated in several studies and good consensus is that it adds to the effectiveness of breast surveillance for women with *BRCA* mutations, and those with a high probability of being mutation carriers (see Chapters 14 and 19). However, the addition of MRI to the surveillance regimen of women at risk for sporadic breast cancer is still controversial. In 2007, the American Cancer Society published guidelines for the incorporation of breast MRI in the surveillance regimen of women at increased risk of breast cancer (82). It should be noted that MRI is recommended for women who have a life-time breast cancer risk of 20% to 25% as estimated with BRCAPRO or other models that largely utilize family history. However, the BRCAPRO model estimates carrier probability rather than life-time risk of breast cancer occurrence, and other models that utilize family history are not prospectively validated outside of their original populations. These guidelines *do not* include women who have a 20% to 25% lifetime risk using the Gail model. The poor discriminatory power of available models has been discussed above, and poses an obvious problem in selecting women for MRI screening based on these. The huge expense of MRI and the burden of multiple repeat imaging examinations and biopsies generated needs to be considered along with the lack of evidence that MRI utilization in these populations improves survival or other cancer-related outcomes.

The American Cancer Society and the Nation Cancer Comprehensive Network (NCCN) guidelines are in agreement that there is not sufficient evidence to recommend use of MRI in women with high-risk epithelial lesions.

RISK-REDUCING INTERVENTIONS

Modifiable Breast Cancer Risk Factors

Despite the vast amount of information available on features that may increase the risk of developing breast cancer, few of these are modifiable, and therefore most cannot be exploited for breast cancer risk reduction. Of those that are modifiable, high lifetime physical activity is associated with a lower risk of breast cancer; during adolescence, physical activity is associated with delayed menarche and delay in the establishment of regular ovulatory cycles. Later in life, a beneficial effect of physical activity has been observed in several recent studies (83). Postmenopausal obesity too should be modifiable, and high-risk women who are obese should be directed toward weight control, because the combination of increased physical activity and caloric restriction are likely to have salutary effects on both breast cancer risk and overall health. Among the reproductive risk factors, lactation appears to be protective against breast cancer (84). Women who accumulate a life-time exposure to lactation of at least 15 months have a lower risk for breast cancer after adjusting for other risk factors. Every 12-month period of lactation decreases risk by 4.3%, as estimated in a meta-analysis of more than 50,000 breast cancer cases and 100,000 controls from 30 countries. The relative benefit of lactation was homogenous across countries. Women who are in child-bearing age should therefore be encouraged to nurse their children for as long a period as feasible.

Alcohol use is clearly modifiable, although there does not appear to be any difference in risk according to timing of alcohol consumption during young, middle, or late adulthood, and no clear evidence indicates that a decrease in alcohol use later in life will reduce breast cancer risk. Nevertheless, as in recommendations for diet, weight control, and physical activity, advice regarding moderation of alcohol use is generally well placed. Evidence indicates an interaction between menopausal hormone use and alcohol use, so that women who consume two or more drinks daily and also use hormones are at higher risk than those exposed to either factor alone (85). Thus, women on postmenopausal hormones should be particularly cautioned against regular alcohol use.

It is not clear whether mammographic density is modifiable through lifestyle changes. Clearly, a large genetic component exists to the determinants of mammographic density (86,87). In a study of a low-fat dietary intervention, no change in breast density was observed (88), and no specific dietary patterns were associated with high density (89). No specific associations were seen with physical activity in a large epidemiologic study (90) or in a study of Dutch women (91). Physical activity may be difficult to measure reliably, however, and measures of sedentary time may be more reliable. A trend of increased breast density was seen with extreme inactivity in Hispanic women in Chicago (92), with those describing more than 3.5 sedentary hours daily displaying greater dense area on mammogram. When breast density does change, breast cancer risk appears to change with it (93).

Current users of combination postmenopausal hormone therapy clearly experience an increased risk of breast cancer (94). The risk elevation appears to dissipate once hormone use is discontinued and, therefore, women at high risk should be advised to abstain from use of combination hormone therapy except for the control of menopausal symptoms, and then to use these in the lowest effective dose for the shortest possible time. In addition, it is reasonable to target hormone replacement to specific symptoms (e.g., for vaginal dryness, low-dose vaginal estrogen replacement results in a far lower systemic exposure than oral therapy).

Pharmacologic Intervention

The clinical trials of breast cancer prevention are discussed fully in Chapter 22. Briefly, the first generation of randomized prevention trials in the United States and Europe tested tamoxifen against placebo. The largest of these, the Breast Cancer Prevention Trial (BCPT) of the NSABP, enrolled healthy high-risk pre- and postmenopausal women, and showed a 49% reduction in the frequency of invasive breast cancer among those assigned to the tamoxifen arm, compared with the placebo arm. This landmark study led to the establishment of tamoxifen, the prototypic selective estrogen receptor modulator (SERM), as a method to reduce risk of breast cancer in women who had a 5-year breast cancer risk of 1.7% or greater as estimated by the Gail model. This successful outcome, confirmed by the IBIS-I trial, led to the successor STAR (P-2) trial of the NSABP which tested tamoxifen against the second generation SERM raloxifene (in postmenopausal women only). The third generation of breast cancer prevention trials are now ongoing, also in postmenopausal women, testing aromatase inhibitors against placebo (exemestane in the MAP.3 trial and anastrozole in the IBIS-II trial). The risks and benefits of these agents are discussed below, along with guidelines for the selection of prophylactic therapy in specific sets of high-risk women.

Tamoxifen

Tamoxifen remains the standard of care for premenopausal women who are risk eligible for pharmacologic prevention and willing to accept it. It should also be considered in hysterectomized postmenopausal women because of the lesser ductal carcinoma *in situ* (DCIS) protection seen with raloxifene in the STAR, Multiple Outcomes of Raloxifene Evaluation (MORE), and Continuing Outcomes Relevant to Evista (CORE) trials, and discussed in more detail below. The 7-year updated results of the BCPT show that the cumulative rate of invasive breast cancer was reduced from 42.5 per 1,000 women in the placebo group to 24.8 per 1,000 women in the tamoxifen group (RR = 0.57 95% CI, 0.46–0.70) (95). The IBIS-1 trial, which had a similar design to the BCPT but somewhat different entry criteria (the Gail model risk estimate was not used to determine eligibility, and a larger fraction of women had a family history for breast cancer), demonstrated a generally similar, although smaller benefit. With a mean follow-up of 8 years, the incidence rate in the tamoxifen group was 27% lower than in the placebo group with (RR = 0.73, 95% CI, 0.58–0.91, $p = .004$) (96). The benefits of tamoxifen therefore include a one-half to one-third reduction in the risk of invasive breast cancer; a similar reduction in the risk of noninvasive breast cancer; a one-third reduction in the risk of new benign breast biopsies (97); a reduction in mammographic density (98); and a reduction in osteoporotic fractures (seen in the

BCPT only with a significant 32% reduction in osteoporotic fractures (95). Women who are at high risk because of a history of atypical hyperplasia appear to derive a greater benefit from tamoxifen therapy, with a risk reduction of 46% (95). These women also seem to be more willing to accept recommendations for tamoxifen chemoprophylaxis (54) and, therefore, are good candidates for treatment. A particular concern for women contemplating tamoxifen therapy is the duration of tamoxifen benefit. This appears to be long-lived, judging from the overview data reported by the Early Breast Cancer Trialists' Group, where incidence rates remain lower in women who used 5 years of tamoxifen therapy going out to 15 years, and confirmed by the long-term results of the IBIS-I trial, where the reduction in breast cancer incidence in the tamoxifen arm is maintained to the same degree or better in the second 5-year period following cessation of tamoxifen therapy (96).

The possibility that the standard 20 mg dose of tamoxifen is not required for therapeutic efficacy has been considered by Decensi et al. (99) in phase II, biomarker-based trials to examine the effect of dose reductions of tamoxifen. In a presurgical study of women with ER-positive invasive breast cancer, a daily dose of 20 mg was compared with doses of 5 mg and 1 mg. There was equivalent reduction in tumor cell proliferation in all three groups, and serum biomarkers, such as sex hormone-binding globulin, fibrinogen, antithrombin III, and decreases in insulin-like growth factor showed a significant dose-response relationship, suggesting potentially lower for toxicity at lower doses. Additional data regarding the efficacy of lower dose tamoxifen are needed, however, before this can be used clinically.

Raloxifene

The uterine toxicity of tamoxifen seen in the BCPT led to the P-2 trial of the NSABP, designed to test the second generation SERM raloxifene against tamoxifen, with the expectation that it would be equally efficacious, but would have little or no uterine toxicity. Because of a lack of safety data on raloxifene in premenopausal women, the trial was restricted to postmenopausal women, with entry criteria otherwise being generally similar to the BCPT (see Chapter 22 for details). This trial established raloxifene as the preventive agent of choice for postmenopausal women with an intact uterus, because it was as effective as tamoxifen in preventing invasive breast cancer, but was generally better tolerated. The RR for noninvasive cancer in the raloxifene arm of the STAR trial was 1.40; (95% CI, 0.98–2.00). Intuitively, the mechanism for a reduction in invasive and noninvasive cancer risk should be similar, so this is a somewhat anomalous finding. However, the MORE, CORE, and Raloxifene Use for the Heart (RUTH) trials also did not show a reduction in the risk of noninvasive breast cancer, although the number of noninvasive events in those studies was very small. The efficacy of raloxifene for DCIS risk reduction therefore remains unproven at the moment. For the hysterectomized postmenopausal woman, the decision between tamoxifen and raloxifene would be a trade-off between the generally better tolerability of raloxifene and the better performance of tamoxifen against DCIS.

Newer Selective Estrogen Receptor Modulators

Third (arzoxifene) and fourth (acolbifene) generation SERMS are under investigation for bone mass preservation, and early phase breast cancer prevention trials suggest efficacy based on biomarker endpoints (100).

Options for Women at High Risk for ER-Positive Breast Cancer

Because SERMS reduce risk of ER-positive breast cancer specifically, with no impact on the risk of ER-negative breast cancer, the risk-to-benefit ratio of SERM use could be improved by the selection of women specifically at risk for ER-positive breast cancer. This concept was explored in an Italian trial testing tamoxifen against placebo in hysterectomized women which did not show an overall benefit for tamoxifen. A *post hoc* analysis looking at breast cancer risk reduction among women at specifically high risk for ER-positive breast cancer did show a benefit for this group (101). Women at risk for ER-positive cancer were identified through the presence of endocrine risk factors (height, age at menarche, age at first term pregnancy, oophorectomy). Supporting data come from a subset analysis of the MORE trial, where women with the highest quartile of serum estradiol levels were both at highest risk and derived the greatest benefit from raloxifene therapy (79). But a similar subset analysis by NSABP investigators showed no difference in breast cancer risk of BCPT participants by estradiol levels, and no differential benefit of tamoxifen therapy (102). Attempts to identify women specifically at risk for ER-positive cancer are discussed above; at this time, there is no basis for denying a woman tamoxifen therapy because of a predicted risk of ER-negative disease.

Toxicity

The uptake of tamoxifen therapy among women at high risk has been highly variable (52,54). A major reason for this is the toxicity profile of tamoxifen, with documented increases in the risk of uterine malignancy (mainly endometrial carcinoma, but also a suggestion of increases in uterine sarcoma) (103). The risk of tamoxifen-induced uterine neoplasia increases with age, with body mass index (BMI), with increasing duration of tamoxifen use (particularly over 5 years) and with prior use of postmenopausal hormone therapy. The increased risk of uterine carcinoma in the tamoxifen arm of the BCPT was seen primarily in older women; women aged 49 years or younger did not experience a significant excess of this problem (RR = 1.42, 95% CI, 0.55–3.81). In women aged 50 years or older, there was a substantially higher frequency of uterine malignancy (RR = 5.33, 95% CI, 2.47–13.17). Annual uterine surveillance with Papanicolaou smears and pelvis examination is therefore mandatory for women with intact uteri who are using tamoxifen, with additional testing (transvaginal ultrasound, uterine biopsies) reserved for those with symptoms, such as uterine bleeding, or abnormalities on clinical surveillance.

The uterine toxicity of tamoxifen is seen largely in older women, with little if any increase in women under age 50 (95). This problem has therefore been largely resolved by raloxifene, and should be less of a barrier to SERM chemoprevention. In the STAR trial, women taking raloxifene developed fewer uterine carcinomas (RR = 0.62; 95% CI, 0.35–1.08), and the frequency of other uterine events (hyperplasia, hysterectomy) was markedly and significantly lower (104). In hysterectomized women, however, it is not clear that raloxifene is superior to tamoxifen overall, because the risk of DCIS occurrence, which is clearly reduced by tamoxifen, does not seem to be affected by raloxifene.

The risk of thromboembolic disease (TED) associated with tamoxifen is increased approximately twofold, (IBIS-I, NSABP P-1). With raloxifene, the risk of deep vein thrombosis and pulmonary embolism may be lower than with tamoxifen but the risk of stroke and transient ischemic attacks is similar (104). Several attempts have been made to identify specific subgroups with higher risk of TED who should not be offered SERM therapy. Obese women and those with recent surgery, fracture, or immobilization are at increased risk of thrombotic events. However, women with factor V leidin or prothrombin G20210→A (PT20210) mutations do not have an added risk with SERM therapy (105,106). Notably, most thromboembolic events occur early in the course of treatment (within 36 months of initiation) (105). Thus, increased risk of TED needs to be factored into the SERM therapy decision by women who have risk factors for it (e.g., overweight, smokers, wheelchair confined), and it seems reasonable to advise women on tamoxifen therapy to discontinue use approximately 2 weeks before major surgery, but screening women who are SERM candidates for factor V leidin or thrombin mutations is not warranted.

The quality of life side effects, such as hot flashes and vaginal symptoms, as well as the perceived association of tamoxifen use with weight gain and depressive symptoms, has resulted in low rates of tamoxifen acceptance by both pre- and postmenopausal women who are risk-eligible for tamoxifen. The concomitant use of postmenopausal hormone therapy does not appear to alleviate hot flashes (107), and data from the Italian and Marsden trials where hormone therapy was allowed, suggest that this interferes with the benefit of tamoxifen therapy. In the Italian trial, the use of HRT increased the risk of breast cancer, as expected in view of previous epidemiologic findings, and the use of tamoxifen in women using HRT seemed to reduce the risk of breast cancer to that of nonusers of HRT (108). Additionally (although, there are no specific data to this effect), concern is that the uterine and thromboembolic toxicity of SERM use would increase if SERMS were combined with estrogen with or without progesterone. The use of low-dose vaginal estradiol supplements (either estradiol-coated rings, or low-dose estradiol tablets) for vaginal symptoms has not been formally evaluated in relation to breast cancer risk, but is reasonable in women with vaginal symptoms, because the systemic estrogen exposure with these preparations is extremely low and, unlike estrogen-containing vaginal creams, serum estradiol levels are not affected. The alleviation of hot flashes with selective serotonin uptake inhibitors (SSRI) is helpful for many women on tamoxifen therapy (109). Recent data regarding the deleterious effects of these compounds on CYP2D6 activity and, therefore, the formation of the active tamoxifen metabolites endoxifen and 4-hydoxytamoxifen suggest that SSRI therapy should be used with caution. Gabapentin is an alternative agent in women with severe hot flashes (110).

Aromatase Inhibitors

Aromatase inhibitors (AI) are promising breast cancer prevention agents since the recent Arimidex, Tamoxifen Alone or in Combination (ATAC) trial (see Chapter 48) showed a greater reduction in the frequency of new contralateral breast primary tumors in the anastrozole versus the tamoxifen arm of this larger randomized trial in which women with stage I and II breast cancer were randomized to anastrozole, tamoxifen, or the combination. The incidence of contralateral new primaries was reduced by a further 40% compared with tamoxifen (HR = 0.60; 0.42–0.85, p = .004). It is probable, therefore, that aromatase inhibitors will provide better protection against postmenopausal ER-positive breast cancer than SERMS. Two AI are currently being tested against placebo in phase III randomized trials: exemestane in the MAP.3 and anastrozole in the IBIS-II trials. Details of these and other prevention trials can be obtained at http://www.cancer.gov/search/ResultsClinicalTrials.aspx?protocolsearchid=4488377. Additional data regarding the impact of anastrozole on contralateral breast events in women with DCIS are anticipated from the NSABP B-35 and IBIS II trials. Ongoing trials will provide good data regarding the risk-to-benefit balance of these agents in healthy women (particularly, the frequency of arthralgias, bone loss, fractures, loss of libido, vaginal dryness, and cardiovascular safety). Until then, the use of AI for primary prevention should be restricted to those women who are at significant risk (e.g., a history of lobular carcinoma *in situ* [LCIS]) and a have contraindication to SERM therapy (e.g., a history of deep vein thrombosis). AI may also be considered for primary prevention in women who have been

on a SERM for breast cancer prophylaxis, but continue to develop new atypical lesions of the breast.

Risk-reducing Mastectomy

For selected women at high risk for breast cancer who are either not good candidates for pharmacologic risk reduction, or are highly motivated to reduce risk to the lowest level possible, prophylactic mastectomy may be a reasonable consideration. This is discussed in full in Chapter 19. Indications for risk-reducing mastectomy have been outlined by the Society of Surgical Oncology (111), and indications include

1. Mutations in *BRCA1* and *BRCA2* or other genetic susceptibility genes
2. Strong family history with no demonstrable mutation
3. Histological risk factors
4. Difficult surveillance

In the setting of a strong family history, genetic evaluation should be strongly encouraged, because if the source of the increased breast cancer incidence in a family can be attributed to a known mutation, individuals who then test negative can be reassured that they are in a population at risk and may be dissuaded from bilateral prophylactic mastectomy. If a mutation cannot be identified following testing of the appropriate affected individuals in the family, mutations in as yet unidentified genes may be responsible and, after appropriate counseling, prophylactic mastectomy can be undertaken. The family history pattern in this setting would be similar to *BRCA* mutation families (e.g., early age of onset, at least two generations involved). Women with histologic risk factors (atypical hyperplasia, LCIS) should first be given a full explanation of the risks and benefits of SERM therapy for chemoprevention, because this subset derives a particularly large benefit from it. Prophylactic mastectomy in this setting should be reserved for women who have contraindications to SERM therapy or are unwilling to take it, and yet seek a substantial reduction in breast cancer risk. The last indication (difficult surveillance) should be an unusual indication, which has been tempered further in recent years by the availability of MRI, which can be factored into the surveillance plan of women with a *BRCA* carrier probability of 30% or greater.

The option of risk-reducing mastectomy with nipple preservation has received attention recently, with several reported series showing that the procedure is feasible, with survival of the nipple–areolar complex in a high proportion of women (112). The long-term safety of this procedure is not established, however, and with the known possibility of new primary breast cancer following subcutaneous mastectomy (63), meticulous attention needs to be paid to complete resection of breast tissue (including the axillary tail) if this procedure is undertaken for risk reduction.

MANAGEMENT SUMMARY

- Women at risk for sporadic breast cancer are a heterogenous population and include those with endocrine and life-style risk factors, proliferative breast disease, and lesser degrees of family history.
- Breast cancer risk can be quantitated using a variety of statistical models, which generally perform well for groups of women, but lack discriminatory power for individuals.
- Improved precision may result from the addition of mammographic density measurement, and the use of minimally invasive techniques to sample breast epithelium, but these remain investigational at present.
- Women at increased risk should be counseled about modifiable risk factors: long-term lactation by women in childbearing age, regular physical activity, the avoidance of

more than light alcohol use, and the limitation of post-menopausal hormone use to the alleviation of symptoms with lowest possible dose for the shortest possible time.

- Surveillance for this group of patients includes annual mammography, directed ultrasound, and magnetic resonance imaging for those with dense breast tissue (after a full discussion of risks and benefits, including the likely need for additional imaging and biopsies).
- Pharmacologic intervention to reduce breast cancer risk consists of tamoxifen for premenopausal women, and raloxifene for postmenopausal women. Hysterectomized postmenopausal women should be given the option of tamoxifen or raloxifene, with a discussion of the difference in DCIS risk reduction with the two drugs.
- Prophylactic mastectomy should be reserved for those at markedly increased lifetime risk (e.g., ≥30%) who are unable or unwilling to take risk-reducing medication, and seek prophylactic mastectomy as a way to manage their risk.

References

1. Vona-Davis L, Howard-McNatt M, Rose DP. Adiposity, type 2 diabetes and the metabolic syndrome in breast cancer. *Obes Rev* 2007;8:395–408.
2. Friedenreich CM, Orenstein MR. Physical activity and cancer prevention: etiologic evidence and biological mechanisms. *J Nutr* 2002;132:3456S–64S.
3. Kendall A, Folkerd EJ, Dowsett M. Influences on circulating oestrogens in postmenopausal women: relationship with breast cancer. *J Steroid Biochem Mol Biol* 2007;103:99–109.
4. Gail MH, Brinton LA, Byar DP, et al. Projecting individualized probabilities of developing breast cancer for white females who are being examined annually [see comments]. *J Natl Cancer Inst* 1989;81:1879–1886.
5. Fisher B, Constantino JP, Wickerham DL, et al. Tamoxifen for prevention of breast cancer: report of the National Surgical Adjuvant Breast and Bowel Project P-1 Study. *J Natl Cancer Inst* 1998;90:1371–1388.
6. Tyrer J, Duffy SW, Cuzick J. A breast cancer prediction model incorporating familial and personal risk factors. *Stat Med* 2004;23:1111–1130.
7. McCormack VA, dos SS, I. Breast density and parenchymal patterns as markers of breast cancer risk: a meta-analysis. *Cancer Epidemiol Biomarkers Prev* 2006; 15:1159–1169.
8. Boyd NF, Guo H, Martin LJ, et al. Mammographic density and the risk and detection of breast cancer. *N Engl J Med* 2007;356:227–236.
9. Byrne C, Schairer C, Wolfe J, et al. Mammographic features and breast cancer risk: effects with time, age, and menopause status. *J Natl Cancer Inst* 1995;87: 1622–1629.
10. Greendale GA, Reboussin BA, Sie A, et al. Effects of estrogen and estrogen-progestin on mammographic parenchymal density. Postmenopausal Estrogen/Progestin Interventions (PEPI) Investigators. *Ann Intern Med* 1999;130:262–269.
11. Rutter CM, Mandelson MT, Laya MB, et al. Changes in breast density associated with initiation, discontinuation, and continuing use of hormone replacement therapy. *JAMA* 2001;285:171–176.
12. Cuzick J, Warwick J, Pinney E, et al. Tamoxifen and breast density in women at increased risk of breast cancer. *J Natl Cancer Inst* 2004;96:621–628.
13. Spicer DV, Ursin G, Parisky YR, et al. Changes in mammographic densities induced by a hormonal contraceptive designed to reduce breast cancer risk. *J Natl Cancer Inst* 1994;86:431–436.
14. Verheus M, Peeters PH, van Noord PA, et al. No relationship between circulating levels of sex steroids and mammographic breast density: the Prospect-EPIC cohort. *Breast Cancer Res* 2007;9:R53.
15. Tamimi RM, Byrne C, Colditz GA, et al. Endogenous hormone levels, mammographic density, and subsequent risk of breast cancer in postmenopausal women. *J Natl Cancer Inst* 2007;99:1178–1187.
16. Boyd NF, Stone J, Martin LJ, et al. The association of breast mitogens with mammographic densities. *Br J Cancer* 2002;87:876–882.
17. Bremnes Y, Ursin G, Bjurstam N, et al. Endogenous sex hormones, prolactin and mammographic density in postmenopausal Norwegian women. *Int J Cancer* 2007;121:2506–2511.
18. Tworoger SS, Eliassen AH, Sluss P, et al. A prospective study of plasma prolactin concentrations and risk of premenopausal and postmenopausal breast cancer. *J Clin Oncol* 2007;25:1482–1488.
19. Greendale GA, Huang MH, Ursin G, et al. Serum prolactin levels are positively associated with mammographic density in postmenopausal women. *Breast Cancer Treat* 2007;105:337–346.
20. Boyd NF, Jensen HM, Cooke G, et al. Relationship between mammographic and histological risk factors for breast cancer. *J Natl Cancer Inst* 1992;84:1170–1179.
21. Khan QJ, Kimler BF, O'Dea AP, et al. Mammographic density does not correlate with Ki-67 expression or cytomorphology in benign breast cells obtained by random periareolar fine needle aspiration from women at high risk for breast cancer. *Breast Cancer Res* 2007;9:R35.
22. Li T, Sun L, Miller N, et al. The association of measured breast tissue characteristics with mammographic density and other risk factors for breast cancer. *Cancer Epidemiol Biomarkers Prev* 2005;14:343–349.
23. Shaughnessy JA, Kelloff GJ, Gordon GB, et al. Treatment and prevention of intraepithelial neoplasia: an important target for accelerated new agent development: recommendations of the American Association for Cancer Research Task Force on the Treatment and Prevention of Intraepithelial Neoplasia. *Clin Cancer Res* 2002;8:314–446.
24. Dupont WD, Page DL. Risk factors for breast cancer in women with proliferative breast disease. *N Engl J Med* 1985;312:146–151.
25. Carter CL, Corle DK, Micozzi MS, et al. A prospective study of the development of breast cancer in 16,692 women with benign breast disease. *Am J Epidemiol* 1988;123,3:467–477.
26. London SJ, Connolly JL, Schnitt SJ, et al. A prospective study of benign breast disease and the risk of breast cancer. *JAMA* 1992;267:941–944.
27. Hartmann LC, Sellers TA, Frost MH, et al. Benign breast disease and the risk of breast cancer. *N Engl J Med* 2005;353:229–237.
28. Collins LC, Baer HJ, Tamimi RM, et al. The influence of family history on breast cancer risk in women with biopsy-confirmed benign breast disease: results from the Nurses' Health Study. *Cancer* 2006;107:1240–1247.
29. Degnim AC, Visscher DW, Berman HK, et al. Stratification of breast cancer risk in women with atypia: a Mayo cohort study. *J Clin Oncol* 2007;25:2671–2677.
30. Khan SA, Rogers MA, Khurana KK, et al. Estrogen receptor expression in benign breast epithelium and breast cancer risk [see comments]. *J Natl Cancer Inst* 1998;90:37–42.
31. Rohan TE, Hartwick W, Miller AB, et al. Immunohistochemical detection of c erbB-2 and p53 in benign breast disease and breast cancer risk [see comments]. *J Natl Cancer Inst* 1998;90:1262–1269.
32. Stark A, Hulka BS, Joens S, et al. HER-2/neu amplification in benign breast disease and the risk of subsequent breast cancer. *J Clin Oncol* 2000;18:267–274.
33. Poola I, Shokrani B, Bhatnagar R, et al. Expression of carcinoembryonic antigen cell adhesion molecule 6 oncoprotein in atypical ductal hyperplastic tissues is associated with the development of invasive breast cancer. *Clin Cancer Res* 2006;12:4773–4783.
34. Dupont WD, Page DL. Risk factors for breast cancer in women with proliferative breast disease. *N Engl J Med* 1985;312:146–151.
35. Brown TA, Wall JW, Christensen ED, et al. Atypical hyperplasia in the era of stereotactic core needle biopsy. *J Sur Oncol* 1998;67:168–173.
36. Liberman L, Cohen MA, Dershaw DD, et al. Atypical ductal hyperplasia diagnosed at stereotaxic core biopsy of breast lesions: an indication for surgical biopsy. *AJR Am J Roentgenol* 1995;164(5):1111–1113.
37. Bhathal PS, Brown RW, Lesueur GC, et al. Frequency of benign and malignant breast lesions in 207 consecutive autopsies in Australian women. *Br J Cancer* 1985;51:271–278.
38. Nielsen M, Thomsen JL, Primdahl S, et al. Breast cancer and atypia among young and middle-aged women: a study of 110 medicolegal autopsies. *Br J Cancer* 1987;56:814–819.
39. Papanicolaou GN, Holmquist DG, Bader GM, et al. Exfoliative cytology of the human mammary gland and its value in the diagnosis of cancer and other diseases of the breast. *Cancer* 1958;11:2:377–409.
40. Sartorius OW, Smith HS, Morris P, et al. Cytologic evaluation of breast fluid in the detection of breast disease. *J Natl Cancer Inst* 1977;59:1073–1080.
41. Sauter ER, Ross E, Daly M, et al. Nipple aspirate fluid: a promising non-invasive method to identify cellular markers of breast cancer risk. *Br J Cancer* 1997;76: 494–501.
42. Dooley WC, Ljung B-M, Veronesi U, et al. Ductal lavage for detection of cellular atypia in women at high risk for breast cancer. *J Natl Cancer Inst* 2001;93:1624–1632.
43. Skolnick MH, Cannon-Albright LA, Goldgar DE, et al. Inheritance of proliferative breast disease in breast cancer kindreds. *Science* 1990;250:1715–1720.
44. Marshall CJ, Schumann GB, Ward JH, et al. Cytologic identification of clinically occult proliferative breast disease in women with a family history of breast cancer. *Am J Clin Pathol* 1991;95:157–165.
45. Fabian CJ, Kimler BF, Zalles CM, et al. Short-term breast cancer prediction by random periareolar fine-needle aspiration cytology and the Gail Risk Model. *J Natl Cancer Inst* 2000;92:1217–1227.
46. Mansoor N, Ip C, Stomper PC. Yield of terminal duct lobule units in normal breast stereotactic core biopsy specimens: implications for biomarker studies. *Breast J* 2000;6:220–224.
47. Harper-Wynne C, Ross G, Sacks N, et al. Effects of the aromatase inhibitor letrozole on normal breast epithelial cell proliferation and metabolic indices in postmenopausal women: a pilot study for breast cancer prevention. *Cancer Epidemiol Biomarkers Prev* 2002;11:614–621.
48. Wrensch MR, Petrakis NL, King EB, et al. Breast cancer incidence in women with abnormal cytology in nipple aspirates of breast fluid. *Am J Epidemiol* 1992;135: 130–141.
49. Wrensch MR, Petrakis NL, Miike R, et al. Breast cancer risk in women with abnormal cytology in nipple aspirates of breast fluid. *J Natl Cancer Inst* 2001;93: 1791–1798.
50. Khan SA, Lankes HA, Patil DB, et al. Serial ductal lavage for biomarker assessment in a Phase 2 prevention study with tamoxifen. (ASCO Annual Meeting Proceedings Part I.) *J Clin Oncol* ASCO Meeting Abstracts 2007;25.1509. [Abstract] (18S):6-20-0207.
51. Khan SA, Masood S, Miller L, et al. Random fine needle aspiration of the breast of women at increased breast cancer risk, and standard risk controls. *Breast J* 1989;4(6):409–419.
52. Port ER, Montgomery LL, Heerdt AS, et al. Patient reluctance toward tamoxifen use for breast cancer primary prevention. *Ann Surg Oncol* 2001;8:580–585.
53. Vogel VG, Costantino JP, Wickerham DL, et al. Re: tamoxifen for prevention of breast cancer: report of the National Surgical Adjuvant Breast and Bowel Project P-1 Study. *J Natl Cancer Inst* 2002;94:1504.
54. Tchou J, Hou N, Rademaker A, et al. Acceptance of tamoxifen chemoprevention by physicians and women at risk. *Cancer* 2004;100:1800–1806.
55. Fackler MJ, Malone K, Zhang Z, et al. Quantitative multiplex methylation-specific PCR analysis doubles detection of tumor cells in breast ductal fluid. *Clin Cancer Res* 2006;12:3306–3310.
56. Bean GR, Scott V, Yee L, et al. Retinoic acid receptor-beta2 promoter methylation in random periareolar fine needle aspiration. *Cancer Epidemiol Biomarkers Prev* 2005;14:790–798.
57. Lewis CM, Cler LR, Bu DW, et al. Promoter hypermethylation in benign breast epithelium in relation to predicted breast cancer risk. *Clin Cancer Res* 2005;11:166–172.
58. Fabian CJ, Kimler BF, Brady DA, et al. A phase II breast cancer chemoprevention trial of oral alpha-difluoromethylornithine: breast tissue, imaging, and serum and urine biomarkers. *Clin Cancer Res* 2002;8:3105–3117.
59. Fabian CJ, Kimler BF, Zalles CM, et al. Reduction in proliferation with six months of letrozole in women on hormone replacement therapy. *Breast Cancer Res Treat* 2007;106(1):75–84.

60. Dowsett M, Smith IE, Ebbs SR, et al. Prognostic value of Ki67 expression after short-term presurgical endocrine therapy for primary breast cancer. *J Natl Cancer Inst* 2007;99:167–170.
61. Baker LH. Breast Cancer Detection Demonstration Project: five-year summary report. *CA Cancer J Clin* 1982;32:194–225.
62. Costantino JP, Gail MH, Pee D, et al. Validation studies for models projecting the risk of invasive and total breast cancer incidence. *J Natl Cancer Inst* 1999;91:1541–1548.
63. Hartmann LC, Schaid DJ, Woods JE, et al. Efficacy of bilateral prophylactic mastectomy in women with a family history of breast cancer [see comments]. *N Engl J Med* 1999;340:77–84.
64. Rockhill B, Spiegelman D, Byrne C, et al. Validation of the Gail et al. model of breast cancer risk prediction and implications for chemoprevention. *J Natl Cancer Inst* 2001;93:358–366.
65. Bondy ML, Lustbader ED, Halabi S, et al. Validation of a breast cancer risk assessment model in women with a positive family history. *J Natl Cancer Inst* 1994;86:620–625.
66. Cuzick J, Forbes J, Edwards R, et al. First results from the International Breast Cancer Intervention Study (IBIS-I): a randomised prevention trial. *Lancet* 2002;360:817–824.
67. Amir E, Evans DG, Shenton A, et al. Evaluation of breast cancer risk assessment packages in the family history evaluation and screening programme. *J Med Genet* 2003;40:807–814.
68. Chen J, Pee D, Ayyagari R, et al. Projecting absolute invasive breast cancer risk in white women with a model that includes mammographic density. *J Natl Cancer Inst* 2006;98:1215–1226.
69. Barlow WE, White E, Ballard-Barbash R, et al. Prospective breast cancer risk prediction model for women undergoing screening mammography. *J Natl Cancer Inst* 2006;98:1204–1214.
70. Bondy ML, Newman LA. Breast cancer risk assessment models: applicability to African-American women. *Cancer* 2003;97:230–235.
71. Gail MH, Costantino JP, Pee D, et al. Projecting individualized absolute invasive breast cancer risk in African American women. *J Natl Cancer Inst* 2007;99:1782–1792.
72. Swain SM, Wilson JW, Mamounas EP, et al. Estrogen receptor status of primary breast cancer is predictive of estrogen receptor status of contralateral breast cancer. *J Natl Cancer Inst* 2004;96:516–523.
73. Arpino G, Weiss HL, Clark GM, et al. Hormone receptor status of a contralateral breast cancer is independent of the receptor status of the first primary in patients not receiving adjuvant tamoxifen. *J Clin Oncol* 2005;23:4687–4694.
74. Gorla SR, Hou N, Acharya S, et al. Can we identify women at high risk for receptor (ER) positive breast cancer. *Ann Surg Oncol* 2004;11(2):S99.
75. Colditz GA, Rosner BA, Chen WY, et al. Risk factors for breast cancer according to estrogen and progesterone receptor status. *J Natl Cancer Inst* 2004;96:218–228.
76. Rosenberg LU, Einarsdottir K, Friman EI, et al. Risk factors for hormone receptor-defined breast cancer in postmenopausal women. *Cancer Epidemiol Biomarkers Prev* 2006;15:2482–2488.
77. Missmer SA, Eliassen AH, Barbieri RL, et al. Endogenous estrogen, androgen, and progesterone concentrations and breast cancer risk among postmenopausal women. *J Natl Cancer Inst* 2004;96:1856–1865.
78. Miyoshi Y, Tanji Y, Taguchi T, et al. Association of serum estrone levels with estrogen receptor-positive breast cancer risk in postmenopausal Japanese women. *Clin Cancer Res* 2003;9:2229–2233.
79. Cummings SR, Duong T, Kenyon E, et al. Serum estradiol level and risk of breast cancer during treatment with raloxifene. *JAMA* 2002;287:216–220.
80. Chlebowski RT, Anderson GL, Lane DS, et al. Predicting risk of breast cancer in postmenopausal women by hormone receptor status. *J Natl Cancer Inst* 2007;99:1695–1705.
81. Crystal P, Strano SD, Shcharynski S, et al. Using sonography to screen women with mammographically dense breasts. *AJR Am J Roentgenol* 2003;181:177–182.
82. Saslow D, Boetes C, Burke W, et al. American Cancer Society guidelines for breast screening with MRI as an adjunct to mammography. *CA Cancer J Clin* 2007;57:75–89.
83. Bernstein L, Patel AV, Ursin G, et al. Lifetime recreational exercise activity and breast cancer risk among black women and white women. *J Natl Cancer Inst* 2005;97:1671–1679.
84. Breast cancer and breastfeeding: collaborative reanalysis of individual data from 47 epidemiological studies in 30 countries, including 50302 women with breast cancer and 96,973 women without the disease. *Lancet* 2002;360:187–195.
85. Nielsen NR, Gronbaek M. Interactions between intakes of alcohol and postmenopausal hormones on risk of breast cancer. *Int J Cancer* 2008;122:1109–1113.
86. Boyd NF, Dite GS, Stone J, et al. Heritability of mammographic density, a risk factor for breast cancer. *N Engl J Med* 2002;347:886–894.
87. Vachon CM, Sellers TA, Carlson EE, et al. Strong evidence of a genetic determinant for mammographic density, a major risk factor for breast cancer. *Cancer Res* 2007;67:8412–8418.
88. Martin LJ, Greenberg CV, Kriukov V, et al. Effect of a low-fat, high-carbohydrate dietary intervention on change in mammographic density over menopause. *Breast Cancer Res Treat* 2008: epub ahead of print.
89. Vachon CM, Kushi LH, Cerhan JR, et al. Association of diet and mammographic breast density in the Minnesota breast cancer family cohort. *Cancer Epidemiol Biomarkers Prev* 2000;9:151–160.
90. Peters TM, Ekelund U, Leitzmann M, et al. Physical activity and mammographic breast density in the EPIC-Norfolk cohort study. *Am J Epidemiol* 2008;167(5):579–585.
91. Suijkerbuijk KP, Van Duijnhoven FJ, van Gils CH, et al. Physical activity in relation to mammographic density in the Dutch prospect-European prospective investigation into cancer and nutrition cohort. *Cancer Epidemiol Biomarkers Prev* 2006;15:456–460.
92. Gapstur SM, Lopez P, Colangelo LA, et al. Associations of breast cancer risk factors with breast density in Hispanic women. *Cancer Epidemiol Biomarkers Prev* 2003;12:1074–1080.
93. Kerlikowske K, Ichikawa L, Miglioretti DL, et al. Longitudinal measurement of clinical mammographic breast density to improve estimation of breast cancer risk. *J Natl Cancer Inst* 2007;99:386–395.
94. Chlebowski RT, Hendrix SL, Langer RD, et al. Influence of estrogen plus progestin on breast cancer and mammography in healthy postmenopausal women: the Women's Health Initiative Randomized Trial. *JAMA* 2003;289:3243–3253.
95. Fisher B, Costantino JP, Wickerham DL, et al. Tamoxifen for the prevention of breast cancer. current status of the National Surgical Adjuvant Breast and Bowel Project P-1 study. *J Natl Cancer Inst* 2005;97:1652–1662.
96. Cuzick J, Forbes JF, Sestak I, et al. Long-term results of tamoxifen prophylaxis for breast cancer—96-month follow-up of the randomized IBIS-I trial. *J Natl Cancer Inst* 2007;99:272–282.
97. Tan-Chiu E, Wang J, Costantino JP, et al. Effects of tamoxifen on benign breast disease in women at high risk for breast cancer. *J Natl Cancer Inst* 2003;95:302–307.
98. Cuzick J, Warwick J, Pinney E, et al. Tamoxifen and breast density in women at increased risk of breast cancer. *J Natl Cancer Inst* 2004;96:621–628.
99. Decensi A, Robertson C, Viale G, et al. A randomized trial of low-dose tamoxifen on breast cancer proliferation and blood estrogenic biomarkers. *J Natl Cancer Inst* 2003;95:779–790.
100. Fabian CJ, Kimler BF, Anderson J, et al. Breast cancer chemoprevention phase I evaluation of biomarker modulation by arzoxifene, a third generation selective estrogen receptor modulator. *Clin Cancer Res* 2004;10:5403–5417.
101. Veronesi U, Maisonneuve P, Rotmensz N, et al. Tamoxifen for the prevention of breast cancer: late results of the Italian Randomized Tamoxifen Prevention Trial among women with hysterectomy. *J Natl Cancer Inst* 2007;99:727–737.
102. Beattie MS, Costantino JP, Cummings SR, et al. Endogenous sex hormones, breast cancer risk, and tamoxifen response: an ancillary study in the NSABP Breast Cancer Prevention Trial (P-1). *J Natl Cancer Inst* 2006;98:110–115.
103. Cohen I. Endometrial pathologies associated with postmenopausal tamoxifen treatment. *Gynecol Oncol* 2004;94:256–266.
104. Vogel VG, Costantino JP, Wickerham DL, et al. Effects of tamoxifen vs raloxifene on the risk of developing invasive breast cancer and other disease outcomes: the NSABP Study of Tamoxifen and Raloxifene (STAR) P-2 trial. *JAMA* 2006;295:2727–2741.
105. Abramson N, Costantino JP, Garber JE, et al. Effect of Factor V Leiden and prothrombin G20210→A mutations on thromboembolic risk in the national surgical adjuvant breast and bowel project breast cancer prevention trial. *J Natl Cancer Inst* 2006;98:904–910.
106. Duggan C, Marriott K, Edwards R, et al. Inherited and acquired risk factors for venous thromboembolic disease among women taking tamoxifen to prevent breast cancer. *J Clin Oncol* 2003;21:3588–3593.
107. Sestak I, Kealy R, Edwards R, et al. Influence of hormone replacement therapy on tamoxifen-induced vasomotor symptoms. *J Clin Oncol* 2006;24:3991–3996.
108. Veronesi U, Maisonneuve P, Sacchini V, et al. Tamoxifen for breast cancer among hysterectomised women. *Lancet* 2002;359:1122–1124.
109. Loprinzi CL, Sloan JA, Perez EA, et al. Phase III evaluation of fluoxetine for treatment of hot flashes. *J Clin Oncol* 2002;20:1578–1583.
110. Loprinzi CL, Kugler JW, Barton DL, et al. Phase III trial of gabapentin alone or in conjunction with an antidepressant in the management of hot flashes in women who have inadequate control with an antidepressant alone: NCCTG N03C5. *J Clin Oncol* 2007;25:308–312.
111. Giuliano AE, Boolbol S, Degnim A, et al. Society of Surgical Oncology: position statement on prophylactic mastectomy. Approved by the Society of Surgical Oncology Executive Council, March 2007. *Ann Surg Oncol* 2007;14:2425–2427.
112. Sacchini V, Pinotti JA, Barros AC, et al. Nipple-sparing mastectomy for breast cancer and risk reduction: oncologic or technical problem? *J Am Coll Surg* 2006;203:704–714.

Priya Rastogi, Shelly S. Lo, and Victor G. Vogel

Chemoprevention can be defined as the use of specific natural or synthetic chemical agents to reverse, suppress, or prevent the progression of premalignant lesions to invasive carcinoma (1,2). Tamoxifen is classified as a first-generation selective estrogen receptor modulator (SERM). It is a proven treatment for breast cancer, which has encouraged its testing as a chemopreventive agent in healthy women. Four randomized, prospective clinical trials listed in Table 22.1 have used tamoxifen as a chemopreventive agent for breast cancer. Two of the trials, the National Surgical Adjuvant Breast and Bowel Project (NSABP) Breast Cancer Prevention Trial (BCPT) (3) and the International Breast Cancer Intervention Study I (IBIS-I) (4), showed a reduction in breast cancer risk with tamoxifen. Early results from the Royal Marsden Hospital (RMH) Tamoxifen Chemoprevention Trial (5,6), a pilot study for the IBIS-I trial, and the initial analysis of the Italian Tamoxifen Prevention Study (7–9) revealed no decrease in the incidence of breast cancer in women using tamoxifen. Longer follow-up or reanalysis of subgroups of women at risk revealed a breast cancer risk-reduction benefit in these trials as well.

Raloxifene is a second-generation SERM that prevents loss of bone mineral density and has been shown in several randomized trials to reduce the risk of invasive breast cancer in postmenopausal women, both at usual risk and at increased risk for breast cancer (10).

In this chapter, we review data from each of the four tamoxifen studies, as well as the studies of raloxifene, and we examine the differences among the trials and their impact on the primary prevention of breast cancer. We also review additional strategies under investigation for reducing the incidence of breast cancer in women at increased risk and make recommendations for their management.

THE BREAST CANCER PREVENTION TRIAL

In 1992, The National Cancer Institute (NCI) in collaboration with the NSABP launched the BCPT P-1 (3). The primary aim of this trial was to determine whether tamoxifen prevented invasive breast cancer in women at increase risk. Women eligible for the trial were 60 years or older, were 35 to 59 years of age with a 5-year predicted risk of breast cancer of at least 1.66%, or had a history of lobular carcinoma *in situ* (LCIS). Risk was estimated using the model developed by Gail et al. (11). During 5 years of recruitment, 13,388 women entered the trial and were randomly assigned to receive tamoxifen (20 mg daily) or placebo therapy.

The trial was stopped when statistical significance was achieved in a number of study end points after a median follow-up time was 54.6 months. Among the 13,175 women with evaluable end points, 368 invasive and noninvasive breast cancers occurred. As shown in Table 22.2, there was a 49% reduction in overall risk of invasive breast cancer. There were 175 cases of invasive breast cancer in the placebo group, compared with 89 in the tamoxifen group (risk ratio [RR] = 0.51; 95% confidence interval [CI], 0.39–0.66; $p < .00001$). The annual event rate for invasive breast among women taking tamoxifen was 3.4 per 1,000 women compared with 6.8 per 1,000 women taking placebo. For noninvasive breast cancer, the reduction in risk was 50% (Fig. 22.1). There

were 69 cases in women receiving placebo and 35 in those receiving tamoxifen ($p < .002$).

After 7 years of follow-up in BCPT (12), the cumulative rate of invasive breast cancer was reduced from 42.5 per 1,000 women in the placebo group to 24.8 per 1,000 women in the tamoxifen group, and the cumulative rate of noninvasive breast cancer was reduced from 15.8 per 1,000 women in the placebo group to 10.2 per 1,000 women in the tamoxifen group (63%). Risks of pulmonary embolism were approximately 11% lower than in the original report, and risks of endometrial cancer were about 29% higher, but these differences were not statistically significant (Fig. 22.2). The net benefit achieved with tamoxifen varied according to age, race, and level of breast cancer risk.

The BCPT revealed that substantial net benefit accrues for women with a diagnosis of either LCIS or atypical hyperplasia who take tamoxifen. Among women with a history of LCIS, the reduction in risk was 56%, and among women with a history of atypical hyperplasia, the reduction in risk was 86%. In the 7-year follow-up period, tamoxifen reduced the occurrence of estrogen receptor (ER)-positive tumors by 69%, but no difference in the occurrence of ER-negative tumors was seen.

ROYAL MARSDEN HOSPITAL CHEMOPREVENTION TRIAL

The RMH Chemoprevention Trial was initiated in 1986 as a preliminary pilot trial for the IBIS-I trial (5,6). The aim of this randomized placebo-controlled trial was to assess whether tamoxifen would prevent breast cancer in healthy women at increased risk of breast cancer based on family history. Each of 2,471 participants between the ages of 30 and 70 years had at least one first-degree relative younger than 50 years with breast cancer, one first-degree relative with bilateral breast cancer, or one affected first-degree relative of any age and another affected first- or second-degree relative. Women were allowed to use hormone replacement therapy (HRT) during the study. Between October 1986 and April 1996, 2,494 women were randomized to receive tamoxifen (20 mg/day) or placebo for up to 8 years. The primary end point was the occurrence of breast cancer. The median follow-up was 70 months.

In initial reports, a total of 70 invasive and noninvasive breast cancers occurred among the women in this trial. The frequency of breast cancer was the same for women receiving tamoxifen or placebo (tamoxifen, 34; placebo, 36; RR = 1.06, 95% CI, 0.7–1.7) (5,6). After 20 years of blinded follow-up (median follow-up 13 years), the trial reported a statistically significant decrease in ER-positive tumors (13) to a magnitude similar to the other reported prevention studies (14).

INTERNATIONAL BREAST INTERVENTION STUDY I

In the IBIS-I trial, eligible women had risk factors for breast cancer indicating at least a twofold RR for ages 45 to 70 years, a fourfold RR for ages 40 to 44 years, and approximately a tenfold RR for ages 35 to 39 years (4). Risk factors used included a combination of family history, LCIS, atypical hyperplasia, nulliparity, and benign breast biopsies; risk was

Table 22.1   TAMOXIFEN CHEMOPREVENTION TRIALS

Trial	Subject Characteristics	Population	No. Randomized	Intended Duration of Treatment (years)	Total Breast Cancers (Invasive and Noninvasive)	Breast Cancer Risk Reduction
Breast Cancer Prevention Trial (BCPT, NSABP P-1)	High breast cancer risk (age ≥60 years or a combination of risk factors using the Gail model); 39% <50 years	≥1.66% 5-years risk	13,388	5	Tamoxifen: 124 Placebo: 244	Overall: 49% Ductal carcinoma *in situ*: 50% With prior lobular carcinoma *in situ*: 55% With prior atypical hyperplasia: 86%
Royal Marsden Hospital Chemoprevention Trial	Family history of breast cancer <50 yr or two or more affected first-degree relatives	Family history of breast cancer	2,494	5–8	Tamoxifen: 62 Placebo: 75	Overall: no reduction
International Breast Intervention Study I	Women aged 35 to 70 yrs who were at increased risk for breast cancer	>twofold relative risk	7,152	5	Tamoxifen: 69 Placebo: 101	Overall: 32%
Italian Tamoxifen Prevention Study	Women with hysterectomy (48% bilateral oophorectomy); Median age: 51 yrs	Normal risk, hysterectomy	5,408	5	Tamoxifen: 34 Placebo: 45	Overall: no reduction; In the high-risk subseta[a]: 82%
All tamoxifen prevention trials			28,442		Tamoxifen: 289 Placebo: 465	Overall: 38% Estrogen receptor-positive invasive: 48%

[a]The high-risk subset included women taller than 160 cm, with at least one functioning ovary, menarche at age 13 years, and no pregnancy before age 24 years.
Adapted from Cuzick J, Powles T, Veronesi U, et al. Overview of the main outcomes in breast-cancer prevention trials. *Lancet* 2003;361:296–300, with permission.

Table 22.2   AVERAGE ANNUAL EVENT RATES FOR INVASIVE BREAST CANCER AND ENDOMETRIAL CANCER BY RISK CATEGORY

	No. of Events		Rate per 1,000 Women			
Patient Characteristic	Placebo	Tamoxifen	Placebo	Tamoxifen	Risk Ratio	95% Confidence Interval
All women Age (years)	175	89	6.76	3.43	0.51	0.39–0.66
≤49	68	38	6.7	3.77	0.56	0.37–0.85
50–59	50	25	6.28	3.10	0.49	0.29–0.81
≥60	57	26	7.33	3.33	0.45	0.27–0.74
History of lobular carcinoma *in situ*						
No	157	81	6.41	3.30	0.51	0.39–0.68
Yes	18	8	12.99	5.69	0.44	0.16–1.06
History of atypical hyperplasia						
No	152	86	6.44	3.61	0.56	0.42–0.73
Yes	23	3	10.11	1.43	0.14	0.03–0.47
5-year predicted breast cancer risk (%)						
2.00	35	13	5.54	2.06	0.37	0.18–0.72
2.01–3.00	42	29	5.18	3.51	0.68	0.41–1.11
3.01–5.00	43	27	5.88	3.88	0.66	0.39–1.09
≥5.01	55	20	13.28	4.52	0.34	0.19–0.58
First-degree relatives with breast cancer (n)						
0	38	17	6.45	2.97	0.46	0.24–0.84
1	90	46	6.00	3.03	0.51	0.35–0.73
2	37	20	8.68	4.75	0.55	0.30–0.97
≥3	10	6	13.72	7.02	0.51	0.15–1.55
Invasive endometrial cancer						
<49 yrs	8	9	1.09	1.32	1.21	0.41–3.60
≥50 yrs	7	27	0.76	3.05	4.01	1.70–10.90

From Fisher B, Costantino JP, Wickerham DL, et al. Tamoxifen for prevention of breast cancer: report of the National Surgical Adjuvant Breast and Bowel Project P-1 study. *J Natl Cancer Inst* 1998;90:1371–1388, with permission.

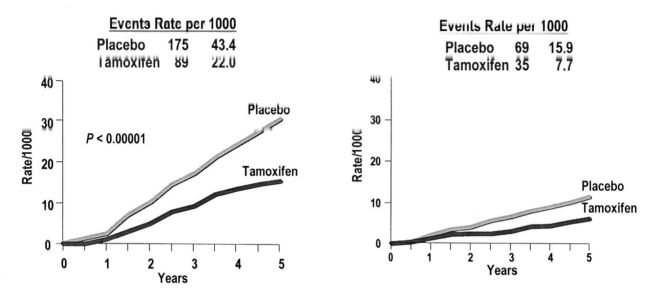

FIGURE 22.1. Rates of invasive and noninvasive breast cancer in the National Surgical Adjuvant Breast and Bowel Project Breast Cancer Prevention trial. (From Fisher B, Costantino JP, Wickerham DL, et al. Tamoxifen for prevention of breast cancer: report of the National Surgical Adjuvant Breast and Bowel Project P-1 Study. *J Natl Cancer Inst* 1998;90:1371–1388, with permission.)

quantified using a unique risk model (15). Approximately 60% had two or more first-degree relatives with breast cancer, and 60% of the study cohort had a 10-year risk of developing breast cancer of between 5% and 10%. One-third of women had hysterectomies previously; HRT use was permitted during the trial and approximately 40% of women used HRT at some point during this trial. The primary end point was the incidence of breast cancer, including ductal carcinoma *in situ* (DCIS).

A total of 7,139 women were included in the analysis; their baseline characteristics are shown in Table 22.3. After a median follow-up of 50 months, 170 breast cancers were diagnosed (including DCIS). The rate was 32% lower in the tamoxifen group than in the placebo group ($p = .01$). Women in the BCPT with 5-year risks between 2% and 5% experienced a reduction of breast cancer risk of 32% to 34%, a result

identical to the reduction reported in IBIS-I. The reduction in risk of ER-positive invasive tumors in IBIS-I was 31%, and there was no reduction in the risk of ER-negative tumors, a result similar to that observed in the BCPT. A summary of the long-term follow-up results by treatment subgroups is shown in Figure 22.3.

After a median follow-up of 96 months after randomization in IBIS-I (16), there was a 27% reduction in the risk of breast cancer. These rates are depicted in Figure 22.4. The risk-reducing effect of tamoxifen was fairly constant for the entire follow-up period, no lessening of benefit was observed for up to 10 years after randomization, and side effects of tamoxifen did not continue after the 5-year treatment period. A nonstatistically significant interaction was seen between HRT use among women in IBIS-I and treatment, and the data are shown in Table 22.4. Among women who never used HRT

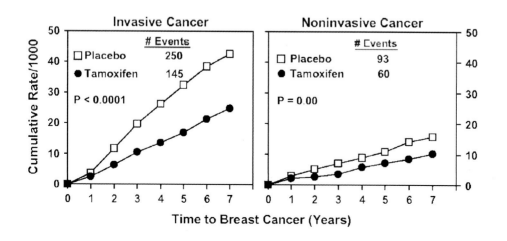

FIGURE 22.2. Cumulative rates per 1,000 women of invasive and noninvasive breast cancers in National Surgical Adjuvant Breast and Bowel Project P-1 (NSABP P-1) participants by treatment group. (From Fisher B, Costantino JP, Wickerham DL, et al. Tamoxifen for the prevention of breast cancer: current status of the National Surgical Adjuvant Breast and Bowel Project P-1 Study. *J Natl Cancer Inst* 2005;97: 1652–1662, with permission.)

Table 22.3	BASELINE CHARACTERISTICS AND HORMONE REPLACEMENT THERAPY USE IN THE INTERNATIONAL BREAST INTERVENTION STUDY-I TRIAL	
Demography	Placebo (n = 3,566)	Tamoxifen (n = 3,573)
Mean (SD) age (yrs)	50.8 (6.7)	50.7 (7.0)
Postmenopausal	1,740 (48.8%)	1,761 (49.3%)
Hormone replacement therapy use		
Before entry	1,443 (40.5%)	1,469 (41.1%)
During trial	1,399 (39.2%)	1,445 (40.4%)
Ever	1,783 (50.0%)	1,849 (51.7%)
Anthropometry		
Mean (SD) height (cm)	162.9 (6.4)	162.8 (6.6)
Mean (SD) weight (kg)	71.4 (14.0)	71.7 (14.5)
Mean (SD) body mass index (kg/m²)	26.9 (5.1)	27.0 (5.3)
Hysterectomy		
All	1,283 (36.0%)	1,232 (34.5%)
With both ovaries retained	737 (20.7%)	711 (19.9%)
One ovary removed	207 (5.8%)	229 (6.4%)
Both ovaries removed	327 (9.2%)	281 (7.9%)

SD, standard deviation.
Data are number of women and percent in each group unless otherwise stated.
From Cuzick J, Forbes J, Edwards R, et al. First results from the International Breast Cancer Intervention Study (IBIS-I): a randomised prevention trial. *Lancet* 2002;360:817–823, with permission.

or who used it only before the trial, there was a statistically significant reduction in ER-positive breast cancers in the tamoxifen group compared with the placebo group. For women who ever used HRT during the trial, no clear benefit of tamoxifen was seen in reducing the risk of breast cancer, either overall or for ER-positive tumors. The risk reduction observed may be smaller in this study as compared with the NSABP P-1 study because patients enrolled onto IBIS-I were allowed to take HRT during the trial and because few women in IBIS-I had atypical hyperplasia where a large reduction in incidence of invasive breast cancer was seen in the P-1 trial.

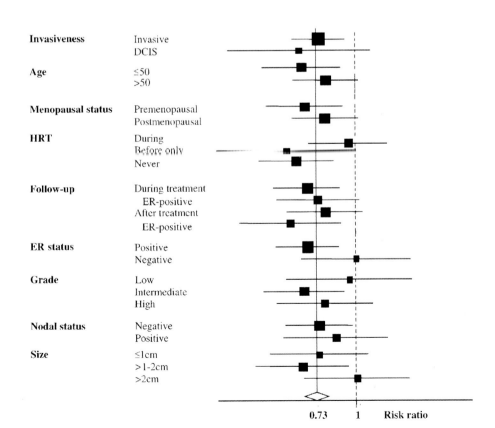

FIGURE 22.3. Risk ratios for breast cancer according to different subgroups of tumors and women. *Solid vertical line* shows overall effect, and *diamond* shows overall 95% confidence interval. *Horizontal lines* show 95% confidence interval for the specific group. The areas of the *boxes* are inversely proportional to variance of estimate. (From Cuzick J, Forbes JF, Sestak I, et al. Long-term results of tamoxifen prophylaxis for breast cancer—96-month follow-up of the randomized IBIS-I trial. *J Natl Cancer Inst* 2007;99:272–282, with permission.)

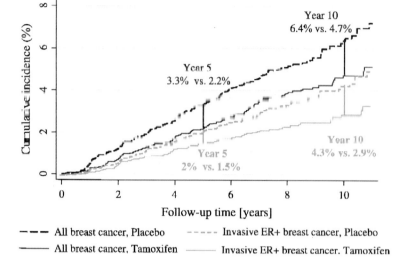

FIGURE 22.4. Cumulative incidence rates for all breast cancers and invasive estrogen receptor (ER)–positive breast cancers according to treatment arm. (From Cuzick J, Forbes JF, Sestak I, et al. Long-term results of tamoxifen prophylaxis for breast cancer—96-month follow-up of the randomized IBIS-I trial. *J Natl Cancer Inst* 2007;99:272–282, with permission.)

THE ITALIAN TAMOXIFEN PREVENTION STUDY

The Italian Tamoxifen Prevention Study evaluated tamoxifen in healthy women between the ages of 35 and 70 years (7–9). Because of the potential side effect of endometrial cancer, the study was restricted to women who had undergone a hysterectomy. The data-monitoring committee decided to end recruitment early primarily because 26% of women dropped out of this study; 5,408 women were randomized to receive tamoxifen (20 mg/day) or placebo for 5 years. Among the 5,378 women with complete data, 48.3% had a bilateral oophorectomy, and 18.2% had at least one first-degree relative or an aunt with breast cancer. As in IBIS-I, women were allowed to take HRT during the study. The primary end points were reduction in the frequency of, and the mortality rate from, breast cancer. At a median follow-up of 46 months, a nonsignificant difference was noted in the incidence of breast cancer when comparing the treatment groups.

An update of the Italian Tamoxifen Trial was reported in 2002 with an extended median follow-up of 81.2 months (8). A nonsignificant 24% reduction in breast cancer incidence was seen. In women who took HRT at some time during the trial, the cumulative frequency of breast cancer was 0.92% among women in the tamoxifen group and 2.58% among women in the placebo group. The updated data support the original conclusion that tamoxifen provides some benefit in the prevention of breast cancer, but the difference was not significant among women at normal or slightly reduced risk of the disease.

In an additional subgroup analysis (9), Italian investigators identified a group of women at increased risk for ER-positive breast cancer. This group included women taller than 160 cm (the median height of the group), with at least one functioning ovary, who had menarche no older than 13 years, and who had no full-term pregnancy before 24 years of age. In this high-risk group, the risk of breast cancer was increased threefold over that of the low-risk group, and tamoxifen reduced the incidence of breast cancer in the high-risk group

Table 22.4	RISK OF BREAST CANCER BY TREATMENT ARM ACCORDING TO HORMONE REPLACEMENT THERAPY (HRT) USE AND ESTROGEN RECEPTOR (ER) STATUS[a]

		Rate per 1,000 Woman-Years		
HRT Use	Placebo (n = 3,575)	Placebo	Tamoxifen	RR (95% CI)
During Trial				
All (including DCIS)	69	6.00	5.52	0.92 (0.65–1.31)
ER-positive	43	3.73	3.34	0.89 (0.57–1.41)
ER-negative	9	0.78	0.92	1.18 (0.44–3.21)
Only Before or Never				
All (including DCIS)	126	7.38	4.58	0.62 (0.46–0.83)
ER-positive	77	4.51	2.23	0.49 (0.32–0.74)
ER-negative	25	1.46	1.27	0.86 (0.46–1.61)

CI: confidence interval; DCIS: ductal carcinoma *in situ*; RR, risk ratio.
[a]ER status was evaluated only for invasive tumors.
From Cuzick J, Forbes JF, Sestak I, et al. Long-term results of tamoxifen prophylaxis for breast cancer—96-month follow-up of the randomized IBIS-I trial. *J Natl Cancer Inst* 2007;99:272–282, with permission.

by 77%, but had no effect in the low-risk group (17). This trial demonstrated that appropriate selection of women at high risk for developing hormone receptor-positive breast cancer led to benefit from tamoxifen intervention. The update after 11 years of follow-up confirmed the group's finding that tamoxifen, in addition to estrogen replacement therapy, is protective against breast cancer development, although this approach is not used in North America and is called into question by the IBIS-I results.

ADVERSE EVENTS ASSOCIATED WITH SELECTIVE ESTROGEN RECEPTOR MODULATORS

Major adverse events reported in the BCPT and the IBIS-I trial are summarized in Table 22.5 and Figure 22.5.

Uterine Malignancies

In the BCPT, women who received tamoxifen had a 2.5-fold greater risk of developing invasive endometrial cancer than women who received placebo (3) (Table 22.2). The average annual rate per 1,000 women was 2.30 in the group taking tamoxifen and 0.91 in the group receiving placebo. The increased risk was seen predominantly in women who were older than 50 years. All the invasive endometrial cancers that occurred among women receiving tamoxifen were classified as stages 0 or I according to the International Federation of Gynecology and Obstetrics (FIGO). The 7-year update quoted an approximate threefold risk, again seen predominantly among women aged 50 years and older. Most cases remained FIGO stage I (12). All the women affected with endometrial cancer in the IBIS-I trial were postmenopausal at diagnosis; most cases were in women older than 50 years at the time of randomization (16). Subsequent reports from women using tamoxifen in the adjuvant treatment setting have shown an increase in uterine sarcomas as well, but the prognosis of women with uterine sarcomas or adenocarcinomas who had taken tamoxifen is no worse than that for women not exposed to tamoxifen (18).

Thromboembolic Events

In the BCPT, there was an increase in the number of thromboembolic events among women taking tamoxifen, particularly

| Table 22.5 | SERIOUS TOXICITIES REPORTED IN THE BREAST CANCER PREVENTION TRIAL AND THE INTERNATIONAL BREAST INTERVENTION STUDY-I TRIAL (NOT ALL TOXICITIES WERE REPORTED BY AGE OR AT ALL FOR IBIS-I) | | | | | |

Age-Group and Symptom	Breast Cancer Prevention Trial			International Breast Intervention Trial-I		
	Placebo Arm Proportion (%)	Tamoxifen Arm Proportion (%)	Relative Risk (Tamoxifen/Placebo)	Placebo Arm Proportion (%)	Tamoxifen Arm Proportion (%)	p-Value
35–49 yrs						
Cold sweats	15.90	22.90	1.44			
Vaginal discharge	46.29	62.55	1.35	14.6	28.6	<.0001
Vaginal dryness				18.0	20.9	.10
Pain in intercourse	23.88	31.57	1.32			
Night sweats	59.58	74.16	1.24			
Hot flashes	65.54	81.28	1.24	54.1	68.0	<.0001
50–59 yrs						
Cold sweats	16.11	27.00	1.68			
Vaginal discharge	32.51	53.47	1.64			
Vaginal dryness				22.6	22.9	.10
Genital itching	36.93	45.24	1.23			
Night sweats	62.77	75.88	1.21			
Bladder control (laugh)	47.67	56.94	1.19			
Hot flashes				48.8	69.0	<.0001
≥60 yrs						
Vaginal bleeding	4.64	10.92	2.35			
Vaginal discharge	19.82	45.81	2.31			
Genital itching	32.05	40.96	1.28			
Hot flashes	51.51	63.59	1.23			
Bladder control (laugh)	49.88	56.49	1.13			
Overall						
Vaginal discharge	34.13	54.77	1.60			
Cold sweats	14.77	21.40	1.45			
Genital itching	38.29	47.13	1.23			
Night sweats	54.92	66.80	1.22			
Hot flashes	65.04	77.66	1.19	67.7	81.8	<.0001
Pain in intercourse	24.13	28.19	1.17			
Bladder control (laugh)	46.65	52.51	1.13			
Bladder control (other)	47.79	52.83	1.11			
Weight loss	41.97	44.94	1.07			
Vaginal bleeding	21.26	21.96	1.03			

Adapted from Day R, Ganz PA, Costantino JP, et al. Health-related quality of life and tamoxifen in breast cancer prevention: a report from the National Surgical Adjuvant Breast and Bowel Project P-1 Study. *J Clin Oncol* 1999;17:2659–2669; and Cuzick J, Forbes J, Edwards R, et al. First results from the International Breast Cancer Intervention Study (IBIS-I): a randomised prevention trial. *Lancet* 2002;360:817–823, with permission.

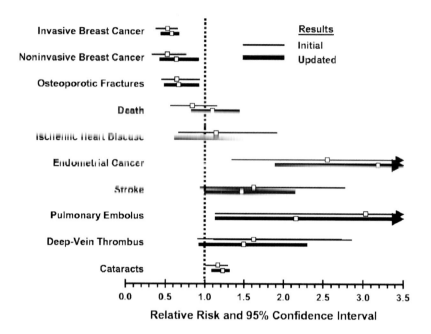

FIGURE 22.5. Comparison of relative risks (with 95% confidence intervals) of benefits and undesirable effects of tamoxifen from the initial and updated results of the National Surgical Adjuvant Breast and Bowel Project P-1. (From Fisher B, Costantino JP, Wickerham DL, et al. Tamoxifen for the prevention of breast cancer: current status of the National Surgical Adjuvant Breast and Bowel Project P-1 Study. *J Natl Cancer Inst* 2005;97:1652–1662, with permission.)

among women 50 years or older (3). The events reported through 7 years of follow-up are summarized in Table 22.6. During active treatment in IBIS-I, the rate of venous thromboembolic events was higher in the tamoxifen group than in the placebo group. Of these events, 25% occurred within 3 months of major surgery or after a long duration of immobility; 20 were in the tamoxifen group (*p* = .004). There was no indication of any synergy between tamoxifen and HRT and some evidence for a negative interaction (16). No differences were found in the numbers of cerebrovascular accidents, myocardial infarctions, or other vascular events.

Side effects in the tamoxifen group in IBIS-I occurred much less frequently after completion of the active treatment period than during active treatment. As in BCPT, deep-vein thrombosis and pulmonary embolism were more than twice as likely in the tamoxifen arm than in the placebo arm during active treat-

ment but not after tamoxifen was stopped. The preventive effect of tamoxifen appears to persist for at least 10 years.

The increase in thromboembolic events associated with tamoxifen appears to be mediated by a decrease in the circulating endogenous anticoagulants antithrombin-III (AT-III) and protein C. It is estimated that tamoxifen use decreases AT-III levels by 9% and protein C levels by 1.12 µg/mL (19). The reductions in AT-III and protein C were greater in postmenopausal women. In NSABP P-1, venous thromboembolic events occurred in 28 women (deep vein thrombosis in 22 and pulmonary emboli in 6) who were taking placebo and in 53 women (deep vein thrombosis in 35 and pulmonary emboli in 18) who were taking tamoxifen (RR = 1.90). Excessive risk for venous thromboembolic events was observed only in the first 36 months of therapy. Age, smoking, and race did not affect the risk of thromboembolic events, but women with clotting had a

Table 22.6	EVENTS AND INCIDENCE RATES OF VASCULAR-RELATED EVENTS IN THE PLACEBO AND TAMOXIFEN GROUPS OF THE BREAST CANCER PREVENTION TRIAL AFTER 7 YEARS BY AGE AT STUDY ENTRY

Type of Event by Age at Study Entry (y)	Events (n)		Rate per 1,000 Women		Difference[a]	RR[b]	95% CI
	Placebo	Tamoxifen	Placebo	Tamoxifen			
Stroke	50	71	1.23	1.75	−0.52	1.42	0.97–2.08
≤49	8	9	0.50	0.57	−0.07	1.13	0.39–3.36
≥50	42	62	1.70	2.50	−0.80	1.47	0.97–2.22
Transient ischemic attack	34	31	0.84	0.76	0.08	0.91	0.54–1.52
≤49	7	4	0.44	0.25	0.19	0.57	0.12–2.25
≥50	27	27	1.10	1.09	0.01	0.99	0.56–1.76
Pulmonary embolism	13	28	0.32	0.69	−0.37	2.15	1.08–4.51
≤49	2	4	0.13	0.25	−0.12	2.01	0.29–22.19
≥50	11	24	0.44	0.96	−0.52	2.16	1.02–4.89
DVT[b]	34	49	0.84	1.21	−0.37	1.44	0.91–2.30
≤49	12	16	0.76	1.01	−0.25	1.34	0.59–3.10
≥50	22	33	0.89	1.33	−0.44	1.49	0.84–2.68

DVT, deep-vein thrombosis.
[a]Rate in the placebo group minus rate in the tamoxifen group.
[b]Risk ratio for women in the tamoxifen group relative to women in the placebo group. RR: risk ratio; CI: confidence interval.
From Fisher B, Costantino JP, Wickerham DL, et al. Tamoxifen for the prevention of breast cancer: current status of the National Surgical Adjuvant Breast and Bowel Project P-1 Study. *J Natl Cancer Inst* 2005;97:1652–1662, with permission.

higher body mass index (BMI) than women without (BMI = 30 kg/m² vs. 27 kg/m² *p* <.001). Neither AT-III nor protein C levels was examined in NSABP P-1, but factor V Leiden, prothrombin PT20210 mutations, or both were found in 9 women (4 on tamoxifen and 5 on placebo) with venous thromboembolic events and in 20 control subjects (9 on tamoxifen and 11 on placebo). No associations were found, however, between risk of venous thromboembolic events and mutation status in either treatment group (20). Venous thromboembolic disease among women at increased risk for breast cancer who are tak-

ing tamoxifen is thus associated with increased BMI, but not with factor V leiden or prothrombin PT20210 mutations. Screening women at risk for breast cancer for factor V leiden and prothrombin PT20210 mutations appears to offer no benefit, therefore, in determining the risk of tamoxifen-associated thromboembolic events. Gail et al. (21) calculated an excess of 15 deep venous thromboses (DVT) and 15 pulmonary emboli (PE) per 10,000 women treated with tamoxifen for 5 years.

The benefits and risks of tamoxifen therapy stratified by risk of breast cancer and race are shown in Figure 22.6.

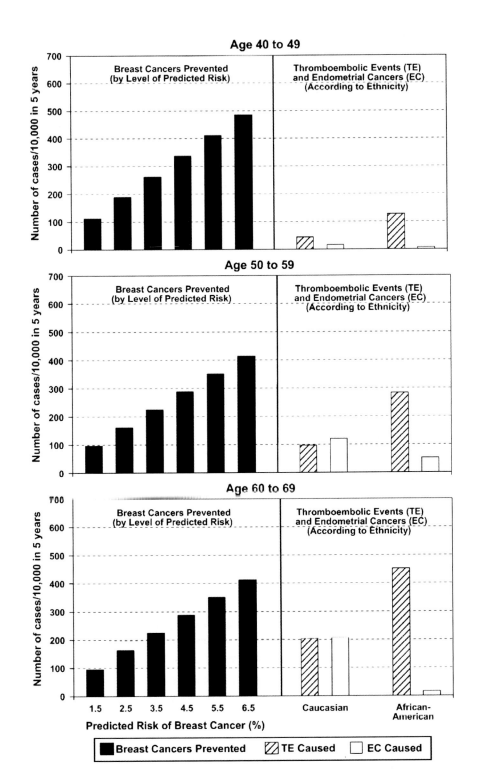

FIGURE 22.6. Benefits and risks associated with tamoxifen use for breast cancer risk reduction. Numbers of breast cancers prevented by tamoxifen in cases per 10,000 women over 5 years by 10-year age group and by level of predicted risk (**left**). Numbers of thromboembolic events and endometrial cancers caused by tamoxifen in cases per 10,000 women over 5 years, by ethnicity (**right**) (From Fisher B, Costantino JP, Wickerham DL, et al. Tamoxifen for the prevention of breast cancer: current status of the National Surgical Adjuvant Breast and Bowel Project P-1 Study. *J Natl Cancer Inst* 2005;97:1652–1662, with permission.)

Quality of Life and Other Events

The NSABP investigators evaluated quality-of-life data among 11,064 women recruited over the first 24 months of the BCPT (22). They analyzed depression using the Center for Epidemiological Studies Depression (CES-D) scale (23), and they used the Medical Outcomes Study 36-Item Short Form Health Status Survey (MOS SF-36) and sexual functioning scale (24), as well as a symptom checklist (25,26) to assess outcomes. They found no differences when comparing placebo and tamoxifen groups for the proportion of participants scoring above a clinically significant level on the CES-D scale. Likewise, they found no differences between groups for the MOS SF-36 summary physical and mental scores. As shown in Table 22.5, the proportion of women reporting symptoms was consistently higher in the tamoxifen group, however, and was associated with vasomotor and gynecologic symptoms. Significant increases were found in the proportion of women taking tamoxifen who reported problems with sexual functioning at a definite or serious level, although overall rates of sexual activity remained similar between the two groups. Weight gain and depression, two clinical problems anecdotally associated with tamoxifen treatment, were not increased in frequency in the BCPT.

A statistically marginal increase of approximately 14% in the rate of cataract development was seen among women taking tamoxifen who were free of cataracts at the time of entry into the BCPT (3). The only symptomatic differences between the placebo and the tamoxifen group were bothersome hot flashes and vaginal discharge.

Among the women in the IBIS-I trial, the only major symptomatic side effect grouping that showed differences was vasomotor and gynecologic symptoms, which were about 21% higher in the tamoxifen than the placebo group, and breast complaints, which were 22% lower (4). There were higher proportions of hot flashes, vaginal discharge, and abnormal vaginal bleeding in the tamoxifen group. Rates of pelvic ultrasonography, dilatation and curettage, and hysteroscopy were also significantly higher, and there were more women with endometrial polyps. The hysterectomy rate was 2.7% in the placebo group and 4.2% in the tamoxifen group ($p = .002$). In premenopausal women, ovarian cysts and amenorrhea were more than twice as common in those taking tamoxifen. At the 1-year follow-up, the mean weight gain was similar for the two groups. Reports of vaginal thrush were substantially increased in the tamoxifen group in both premenopausal and postmenopausal women. No difference was found in the frequency of cataracts or other eye complaints.

The IBIS-I investigators initially reported that the death rate from all causes was significantly higher in the tamoxifen group than in the placebo group (4), but this was not a primary outcome for the trial, and no single cause of death was predominant among the women treated with tamoxifen. In the 7-year follow-up analysis, this excess mortality was no longer seen (16).

EFFECT OF TAMOXIFEN ON THE INCIDENCE OF BENIGN BREAST DISEASE

The NSABP investigators examined the effect of tamoxifen treatment on the incidence of benign breast disease and on the number of breast biopsies among the women in the BCPT (27). They included women who had undergone a breast biopsy and had histologic diagnoses of adenosis, cyst, duct ectasia, fibrocystic disease, fibroadenoma, fibrosis, hyperpla-

sia, or metaplasia. Overall, tamoxifen treatment reduced the risk of benign breast disease by 28%. Compared with placebo, tamoxifen resulted in 29% fewer biopsies, and this risk reduction occurred predominantly in women younger than 50 years.

In IBIS-I, the rate of benign breast disease was 31% lower in the tamoxifen group than in the placebo group, similar to the findings in BCPT. The effect was mostly seen in premenopausal women. Reports of breast pain were also reduced by 32% in the tamoxifen group (4).

EFFECT OF TAMOXIFEN ON CARRIERS OF PREDISPOSING GENETIC MUTATIONS

Women with a mutation in *BRCA1* or *BRCA2* have a high risk of developing breast cancer and of contralateral cancer after the initial diagnosis of breast cancer. Tamoxifen protects against contralateral breast cancer in the general population, but whether it protects against contralateral breast cancer in *BRCA1* or *BRCA2* mutation carriers is not known. Prophylactic oophorectomy reduces the risk of invasive breast cancer among women with either *BRCA1* or *BRCA2* mutations by nearly 50% (28).

To investigate the effect of tamoxifen among women with predisposing genetic mutations, Narod et al. (29) compared 209 women with bilateral breast cancer and *BRCA1* or *BRCA2* mutations (bilateral disease cases) who had received or not received tamoxifen with 384 women with unilateral disease and *BRCA1* or *BRCA2* mutations (controls) in a matched case-control study. Age and age at diagnosis of breast cancer (range, 24 to 74 years) were much the same in bilateral disease cases and controls, and both groups had been followed for the same time for a second primary breast cancer. *BRCA2*-associated tumors are more likely to be ER positive (29), although stage-adjusted recurrence and death rates are reported to be nonsignificantly better for *BRCA2* cases. The reduction in contralateral breast cancer associated with tamoxifen use was 50%. Tamoxifen protected against contralateral breast cancer for carriers of *BRCA1* mutations (62% reduction) and for those with *BRCA2* mutations (37% reduction). In women who used tamoxifen for 2 to 4 years, the risk of contralateral breast cancer was reduced by 75%. ER status was available for only a few patients. In such patients with bilateral disease, 16 (29%) of 56 who had first primary cancers and 22 (30%) of 74 who had contralateral breast cancers were ER positive. Of the women who did not receive tamoxifen, 27% of contralateral tumors were ER positive and, of those who received tamoxifen, 50% of contralateral tumors were ER positive. Therefore, tamoxifen use reduced the risk of contralateral breast cancer in women with pathogenic mutations in either the *BRCA1* or the *BRCA2* gene.

In the BCPT, the investigators examined the incidence of breast cancer among women with *BRCA1* or *BRCA2* mutations, comparing those who received tamoxifen with the incidence of breast cancer among those receiving placebo (30). Of the 288 breast cancer cases with evaluable DNA, 19 (6.6%) inherited either *BRCA1* or *BRCA2* mutations as determined by complete gene sequencing. Of eight patients with *BRCA1* mutations, five received tamoxifen and three received placebo (no significant difference). Of 11 patients with *BRCA2* mutations, however, 3 received tamoxifen and 8 received placebo (62% reduction in risk).

In cost-to-benefit analyses, prophylactic oophorectomy or mastectomy, as well as tamoxifen therapy, all confer therapeutic advantage in reducing the risk of breast cancer. Among women with a diagnosis of invasive breast cancer and a *BRCA* mutation, 30-year-old, early-stage breast cancer patients gain

0.4 to 1.3 years of life expectancy from tamoxifen therapy compared with 0.2 to 1.8 years from prophylactic oophorectomy and 0.6 to 2.1 years from prophylactic contralateral mastectomy (31). Decreased gene penetrance, older age, and poorer prognosis from the primary breast cancer attenuate the gains in life expectancy. A 30-year-old woman without breast cancer could prolong her survival beyond that associated with surveillance alone by use of preventive measures. Using data from the tamoxifen risk-reduction trials and the genetics literature, Grann et al. (32) and Hershman et al. (33) estimated that a mutation carrier would gain 1.8 years of life by using tamoxifen, 2.6 years with prophylactic oophorectomy, 4.6 years with both tamoxifen and prophylactic oophorectomy, 3.5 years with prophylactic mastectomy, and 4.9 years with both surgeries. She could prolong her quality-adjusted survival by 2.8 years with tamoxifen, 4.4 years with prophylactic oophorectomy, 6.3 years with tamoxifen and oophorectomy, and 2.6 years with mastectomy, or with both surgeries. The benefits of all of these strategies would decrease if they were initiated in a woman more than 30 years of age. Women who test positive for *BRCA1/2* mutations may therefore derive greater survival and quality adjusted survival benefits from chemoprevention, prophylactic surgery, or a combination of the two. Using such estimates of gains in life expectancy may help both women and their physicians consider the uncertainties, risks, and advantages of these interventions and lead to more informed choices about cancer prevention strategies.

SUMMARY OF THE EFFECT OF TAMOXIFEN ON THE INCIDENCE OF BREAST CANCER

As summarized in Table 22.1, the combined results from the four tamoxifen prevention trials show a 38% (95% CI, 28–46; p <.0001) reduction in breast cancer incidence (14). ER-positive breast cancers are decreased by 48% (95% CI, 36–58; p <.0001), but there is no reduction in the incidence of ER-negative breast cancers. Age has no effect on the degree of breast cancer reduction. Rates of endometrial cancer are increased in all the tamoxifen prevention trials, and the excess risk is seen in women older than 50 years. Venous thromboembolic events are increased in all of the tamoxifen prevention studies. Overall, there has been no effect on all-cause mortality in the

tamoxifen prevention trials, but the trials were neither designed nor statistically powered to assess mortality as an outcome.

Clinical Monitoring of Patients Taking Tamoxifen for Risk Reduction

Women need to be informed of the increased frequency of vasomotor and gynecologic symptoms and problems of sexual functioning that are associated with tamoxifen use. When tamoxifen therapy is recommended, women should be counseled to seek prompt medical attention if they experience any gynecologic symptoms, such as menstrual irregularities, vaginal bleeding, change in vaginal discharge, or pelvic pain or pressure (34). There is insufficient evidence, however, for or against the use of transvaginal ultrasound or endometrial sampling for the early detection of endometrial cancer, and the American College of Obstetrics and Gynecology recommends that women on tamoxifen should have annual gynecologic examinations with Papanicolaou tests and pelvic examinations. Any abnormal bleeding should be evaluated with appropriate diagnostic testing. Routine screening with complete blood cell count or chemical blood tests is not indicated because no hematologic or hepatic toxic effects attributable to tamoxifen were demonstrated in the BCPT or in clinical trials using tamoxifen as adjuvant therapy. Because of the modest increase in the risk of cataracts and cataract surgery among women on tamoxifen compared with women taking placebo, women taking tamoxifen should be questioned about symptoms of cataracts during follow-up and should discuss with their health care provider the value of periodic eye examinations.

REDUCTION OF BREAST CANCER INCIDENCE WITH RALOXIFENE

A number of clinical trials have been conducted to assess the benefit of raloxifene on osteoporosis and fracture. These are listed in Table 22.7. After the publication of the results of the BCPT, these osteoporosis trials also reported data related to the incidence of invasive breast cancer among women taking raloxifene compared with those taking placebo.

The Multiple Outcomes for Raloxifene Evaluation (MORE) trial randomized 7,705 postmenopausal women younger than 81 years (mean age = 66.5 years) with osteoporosis to raloxifene

Table 22.7	BREAST CANCER RISK REDUCTION IN STUDIES OF RALOXIFENE			
Study	MORE	CORE	RUTH	STAR
Number of women taking raloxifene	5,129	3,570	5,044	9,745
Number of women in the comparison group	2,576	1,703	5,057	9,726
Comparison drug	Placebo	Placebo	Placebo	Tamoxifen
Mean age at study entry	66.5	66.2	67.5	58.5
Average follow-up time	40 mos	48 mos	5.6 yrs	47 mos
Number of breast cancers in the raloxifene group	13	40	553	168
Event rate in the raloxifene group (per 1,000 woman-years)	0.9	1.4	1.5	4.4
Number of breast cancers in the comparison group	27	58	533	163
Event rate in the comparison group (per 1,000 woman-years)	3.6	4.2	2.7	4.3
Risk reduction (hazard rate or risk ratio) and 95% confidence interval	0.24 (0.13-0.44)	0.34 (0.22-0.50)	0.56 (0.38-0.83)	Not reported

CORE, Continuing Outcomes Relevant to Evista; MORE, Multiple Outcomes for Raloxifene Evaluation; RUTH, Raloxifene Use for The Heart; STAR, Study of Tamoxifen and Raloxifene.
From Vogel VG. Raloxifene: a second-generation selective estrogen receptor modulator for reducing the risk of invasive breast cancer in postmenopausal women. *Women's Health* 2007;3: 139-153, with permission.

or placebo (35,36). The primary aim of the MORE study was to test whether 3 years of raloxifene reduced the risk of fracture in postmenopausal women with osteoporosis, and the occurrence of breast cancer was a secondary end point. Women were excluded if they took estrogens within 6 months of randomization and were not permitted to take concomitant estrogen replacement therapy with the study drug. With a median follow-up of 40 months, raloxifene reduced the risk of invasive breast cancer by 76% in postmenopausal women with osteoporosis, largely accounted for by a 90% reduction in ER-positive breast cancer. Raloxifene did not reduce the risk of ER-negative breast cancer. There was no apparent decrease in ER-negative cancers. In addition, raloxifene decreased the risk of vertebral fractures and decreased low-density lipoprotein cholesterol levels. Raloxifene did not increase the risk of endometrial cancer, but it was associated with a threefold increase in thromboembolic events. More women in the raloxifene group reported increased rates of hot flashes, leg cramps, and peripheral edema.

The Continuing Outcomes Relevant to Evista (CORE) trial was designed to evaluate the efficacy of an additional 4 years of raloxifene therapy in preventing invasive breast cancer in women who participated in the MORE trial (37). CORE was a multicenter, double-blind, placebo-controlled clinical trial. The CORE trial was conducted in the subset of the MORE women who agreed to participate in what was an extension of the MORE trial, with a change in the primary end point from vertebral fracture incidence to invasive breast cancer. A secondary objective of the CORE trial was to examine the effect of raloxifene (60 mg/day) on the incidence of invasive ER-positive breast cancer. Women who had been randomly assigned to receive raloxifene (either, 60 or 120 mg/day) in MORE were assigned to receive raloxifene (60 mg/day) in CORE (n = 3,510), and women who had been assigned to receive placebo in MORE continued on placebo in CORE (n = 1,703). Women in the raloxifene group had a 59% reduction in the incidence of all invasive breast cancer compared with women in the placebo group and a 66% reduction in the incidence of invasive ER-positive breast cancers compared with women in the placebo group. By contrast, the incidence of invasive ER-negative breast cancer in women who received raloxifene was not statistically significantly different from that in women who received placebo. The overall incidence of breast cancer, regardless of invasiveness, was reduced by 50% in the raloxifene group compared with the placebo group.

For the 7,705 women in the MORE trial, the total number of reported breast cancers from randomization in MORE to the end of their participation in either MORE or CORE was 121 (56 cancers in the raloxifene group and 65 cancers in the placebo group). During these 8 years, 40 invasive breast cancers were reported in the raloxifene group and 58 invasive breast cancers were reported in the placebo group. Thus, the raloxifene group had a 66% reduction in the incidence of invasive breast cancer compared with the placebo group. During these 8 years, the raloxifene group had a 76% reduction in the incidence of invasive ER-positive breast cancer compared with the placebo group. There was no difference in the incidence rates of invasive ER-negative breast cancer between the raloxifene group and the placebo group. During the 8 years of the MORE and CORE trials, the overall incidence of breast cancer, both *in situ* and invasive, was reduced by 58% in the raloxifene group compared with the placebo group (37,38) The CORE trial provides additional results that indicate that raloxifene reduces breast cancer incidence in postmenopausal women with osteoporosis.

THE RUTH TRIAL

The Raloxifene Use for The Heart (RUTH) trial was a randomized, double-blind, placebo-controlled trial whose primary objectives

were to determine the effect of raloxifene compared with placebo on the incidence of both coronary events and invasive breast cancer (39). A total of 10,101 postmenopausal women with coronary heart disease or at increased risk for coronary heart disease were randomized to raloxifene (60 mg/day) or placebo and followed for a median of 5.6 years. There was a 44% decreased incidence of invasive breast cancer in the raloxifene group. There was a 55% decreased incidence in ER-positive invasive breast cancers in the raloxifene group. No significant difference, however, was found between treatment groups in the incidence of ER-negative invasive breast cancers.

THE STAR TRIAL

Data from the osteoporosis trials, along with substantial laboratory evidence, indicated that raloxifene could reduce the incidence of primary breast cancer (10). To compare the relative effects and safety of raloxifene and tamoxifen on the risk of developing invasive breast cancer and other disease outcomes, the NSABP conducted the Study of Tamoxifen and Raloxifene (STAR) trial, a prospective, double-blind, randomized clinical trial that began July 1, 1999 in nearly 200 clinical centers throughout North America (40). Patients were 19,747 postmenopausal women (mean age 58.5 years) with increased 5-year breast cancer risk (mean risk, 4%) as estimated by the Gail model. Participants were randomly assigned to receive either tamoxifen (20 mg/day) or raloxifene (60 mg/day) over 5 years. Outcomes of interest were incidence of invasive breast cancer, uterine cancer, noninvasive breast cancer, bone fractures, and thromboembolic events. The trial was designed to assess statistical equivalence of the two therapies and was powered to report data when 327 cases of invasive breast cancer occurred.

After a median of 3.2 years of therapy in the trial, there were 163 cases of invasive breast cancer in women assigned to tamoxifen and 168 in those assigned to raloxifene (incidence, 4.30/1,000 vs. 4.41/1,000; RR = 1.02; 95% CI, 0.82–1.28). The cumulative incidence through 72 months for the two treatment groups was 25.1 and 24.8 per 1,000 for the tamoxifen and raloxifene groups, respectively (p = .83). These data are shown in Figure 22.7. When the treatment groups were compared by baseline categories of age, history of LCIS, history of atypical hyperplasia, Gail model 5-year predicted risk of breast cancer (11,41), and the number of relatives with a history of breast cancer, the pattern of no differential effect by treatment assignment remained consistent. There were no differences between the treatment groups in regard to distributions by tumor size, nodal status, or estrogen receptor level.

Fewer cases of noninvasive breast cancer were seen in the tamoxifen group (57 cases) than in the raloxifene group (80 cases). Cumulative incidence through 6 years was 8.1 per 1,000 in the tamoxifen group and 11.6 in the raloxifene group. About 36% of the cases were LCIS and 54% were DCIS, with the balance being mixed types. The pattern of fewer cases among the tamoxifen group was evident for both LCIS and DCIS.

Quality of Life in the STAR Trial

In the STAR trial, patient-reported symptoms were collected from all participants using a 36-item symptom checklist such as that used in the NSABP Breast Cancer Prevention Trial (22). Quality of life was measured with the Medical Outcomes Study Short-Form Health Survey (SF-36), the CES-D, and the Medical Outcomes Study Sexual Activity Questionnaire as in the BCPT in a substudy of 1,983 participants with a median follow-up of about 5 years. Questionnaires were administered before treatment, every 6 months for 60 months, and at 72 months. Primary quality of life end points were the SF-36 physical (PCS) and mental (MCS) component summaries (42).

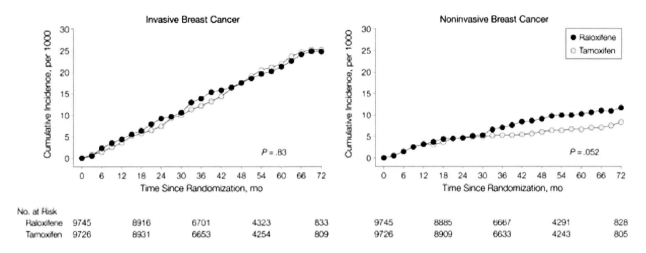

FIGURE 22.7. Cumulative incidence of invasive and noninvasive breast cancer in the National Surgical Adjuvant Breast and Bowel Project Study of Tamoxifen and Raloxifene (NSABP STAR) trial. (From Vogel VG, Costantino JP, Wickerham DL, et al. Effects of tamoxifen vs. raloxifene on the risk of developing invasive breast cancer and other disease outcomes: The NSABP Study of Tamoxifen and Raloxifene (STAR) P-2 Trial.)

Among women in the quality-of-life analysis in STAR, mean PCS, MCS, and CES-D scores worsened modestly throughout the study, with no significant difference between the tamoxifen and raloxifene groups. Sexual function was slightly better for participants assigned to tamoxifen. Of the women in the symptom assessment analyses, those in the raloxifene group reported greater mean symptom severity over 60 months of assessments than the women in the tamoxifen group for musculoskeletal problems, dyspareunia, and weight gain. Women in the tamoxifen group reported greater mean symptom severity for gynecologic problems, vasomotor symptoms, leg cramps, and bladder control symptoms. No significant differences existed, however, between the tamoxifen and raloxifene groups in patient-reported outcomes for physical health, mental health, and depression, although the tamoxifen group reported better sexual function. Although mean symptom severity was low among these postmenopausal women, those in the tamoxifen group reported more gynecologic problems, vasomotor symptoms, leg cramps, and difficulty with bladder control, whereas women in the raloxifene group reported more musculoskeletal problems, dyspareunia, and weight gain.

Adverse Events in the STAR Trial

In the STAR trial, there were 36 cases of uterine cancer with tamoxifen and 23 with raloxifene, a difference that approached statistical significance. No differences were found for other invasive cancer sites, for ischemic heart disease events, or for stroke (40). Thromboembolic events (i.e., PE and DVT) occurred 30% less often in the raloxifene group. The absolute rate of venous thromboembolism was significantly lower among women assigned to raloxifene (2.6/1,000 women annually) than among those assigned to tamoxifen (3.7/1,000 women annually). The cumulative incidence of serious clotting events at 6 years was 21.0 per 1,000 for the tamoxifen group and 16.0 per 1,000 for raloxifene group (Fig. 22.8). PE and DVT occurred in 54 versus

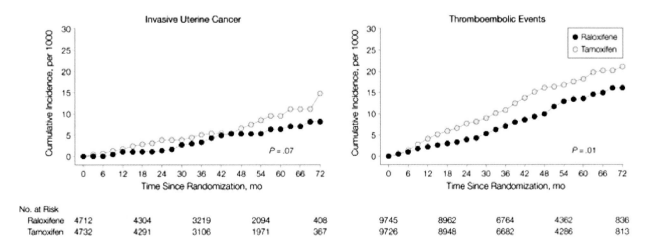

FIGURE 22.8. Cumulative incidence of invasive uterine cancer and thromboembolic events in the NSABP STAR trial. From Vogel VG, Costantino JP, Wickerham DL, et al. Effects of tamoxifen vs. raloxifene on the risk of developing invasive breast cancer and other disease outcomes: The NSABP Study of Tamoxifen and Raloxifene [STAR] P-2 Trial. *JAMA* 2006;295:2727–2741, with permission.

35 women (36% fewer with raloxifene) and in 87 versus 65 women (26% fewer with raloxifene) assigned to tamoxifen and raloxifene, respectively. Although no significant difference was found in the rates of death from any cause or total stroke according to group assignment, raloxifene was associated with a 50% increased risk of fatal stroke.

The number of osteoporotic fractures was similar with tamoxifen and raloxifene. There were 21% fewer cataracts and 18% fewer cataract surgeries in the women taking raloxifene. No difference was seen in the total number of deaths or in causes of death

SERUM HORMONE LEVELS AS INDICATORS OF RISK

In a study of elderly women with osteoporosis, the investigators reported that higher serum levels of estradiol increased the risk of developing breast cancer, and treatment with raloxifene reduced the breast cancer risk more in women with higher estradiol levels than in women with very low levels (43,44). Women assigned to the placebo group had a breast cancer risk of 0.6% if their estradiol level was undetectable compared with 3% in women with estradiol levels of more than 10 pmol/L ($p =$ .005). Women with estradiol levels of more than 10 pmol/L had a 6.8 times higher risk of developing breast cancer than women with undetectable estradiol levels. In women treated with raloxifene, those with the highest serum estradiol concentrations had the greatest absolute risk reduction in breast cancer compared with women with similar levels in the placebo group. In women with estradiol levels of more than 10 pmol/L randomized to raloxifene, there was a 76% risk reduction of breast cancer compared with women randomized to placebo, but no significant effect was seen in those with undetectable estradiol levels. It must be noted that a portion of women without breast cancer had their serum estradiol levels measured and reported in this study, but the data suggest that serum estradiol levels may, nevertheless, identify women who will benefit from therapy with SERM to reduce their risk of breast cancer.

Within the Nurses' Health Study, a large, prospective evaluation of more than 176,000 registered nurses in the United States, 418 women with breast cancer were identified and compared with control women without breast cancer (45). Multivariate relative risks for breast cancer were calculated by unconditional logistic regression, adjusting for matching and breast cancer risk factors. Estrone sulfate was statistically significantly associated with breast cancer risk among women with low (<1.66%) and high (≥2.52%) Gail model predicted risk. Testosterone results were similar across groupings of predicted risk, with two times the risk in the fourth versus the first quartile. Estradiol appeared more strongly associated with breast cancer in women with higher predicted risk compared with women with lower risk, indicating that higher levels of endogenous estrogens and testosterone may be associated with increased breast cancer risk, regardless of predicted risk or family history of breast cancer.

Contrary to these results, NSABP investigators carried out a case-cohort study among 275 postmenopausal women without breast cancer who were enrolled in the BCPT and treated with tamoxifen or placebo for 69 months (46). Estradiol, testosterone, and sex hormone-binding globulin were measured using radioimmunoassay in baseline plasma samples. Relative risks and 95% confidence intervals for invasive breast cancer were estimated for each quartile of sex hormone level using Cox proportional hazards models. In contrast to the results from the Nurses' Heath Study, median plasma levels of estradiol, testosterone, and sex hormone-binding globulin were similar between the cases of breast cancer and the unaffected control groups. Furthermore, the risk of developing breast cancer for women in the placebo group was not associated with sex hormone levels. The reduced risk of invasive breast cancer in tamoxifen-treated women compared with placebo-treated women was also not associated with sex hormone levels, and these data do not support the use of endogenous sex hormone levels to identify women who are at particularly high risk of breast cancer and who are most likely to benefit from chemoprevention with tamoxifen.

Although the data from BCPT do not suggest that hormone levels can further stratify risk, the data from the Nurses' Health Study indicate a continuum of serum hormone levels that are directly correlated with the risk of developing invasive breast cancer. It is possible that there is a plateau in circulating hormone concentrations in BCPT, given that the mean quantitative risk scores among the participants was high. The nurses' data suggest a continuum of hormone levels that peaks among those women who are at highest risk, but these observations do not yet prove that endogenous hormones will better serve to select women at moderate risk of breast cancer who are better candidates for chemoprevention interventions than quantitative risk assessment (e.g., with the Gail model) alone (11). Their use is not yet routine in clinical risk assessment.

AROMATASE INHIBITORS

In postmenopausal women, the main source of estrogen is derived from the peripheral conversion of androstenedione, produced by the adrenal glands, to estrone and estradiol in breast, muscle, and fat tissue. This conversion requires the aromatase enzyme (47). In postmenopausal women, estrogen is synthesized in these peripheral tissues and circulates at a relatively low and constant level. The selective aromatase inhibitors (AI) markedly suppress the concentration of estrogen in plasma via inhibition or inactivation of aromatase. The use of AI is restricted to postmenopausal women, however, because in premenopausal women, high levels of androstenedione compete with AI at the enzyme complex such that estrogen synthesis is not completely blocked. Moreover, the initial decrease in estrogen levels causes a reflex increase in gonadotrophin levels, provoking ovarian hyperstimulation, thereby increasing aromatase in the ovary and consequently overcoming the initial blockade. Unlike tamoxifen, AI lack partial estrogen agonist activity and, therefore, are not associated with an increased risk for the development of endometrial cancer.

Anastrozole and letrozole are reversible, nonsteroidal inhibitors of the aromatase enzyme, whereas exemestane is an irreversible steroidal inhibitor. AI have significant antitumor activity in postmenopausal breast cancer patients, and a number of randomized trials have evaluated the adjuvant use of aromatase inhibitors in postmenopausal women. The largest and most mature AI adjuvant therapy trial was the Arimidex, Tamoxifen Alone, or in Combination (ATAC) trial that compared 5 years of anastrozole with 5 years of tamoxifen as initial adjuvant therapy (48,49). The trial included 9,366 postmenopausal women with localized breast cancer. The ATAC trial enrolled 9,366 postmenopausal women with early breast cancer. The first interim analysis at a median follow-up of 33 months showed an improved disease-free survival. Side effects, such as vaginal bleeding, vaginal discharge, cerebrovascular events, venous thromboembolic events, hot flashes, and incidence of endometrial cancer, were significantly decreased in the anastrozole arm. Anastrozole was associated with more musculoskeletal events and fractures compared with the tamoxifen arm. Importantly, in regard to the potential use of AI for reduction of breast cancer risk, the incidence of contralateral breast cancer was reduced by 58% with anastrozole when compared with tamoxifen. The updated data at 47 and 100 months continued to show that anastrozole was superior to tamoxifen in reducing the incidence of new ER-positive breast cancer, but the results were not as dramatic as the initial report, with only a 40% reduction in the risk of contralateral breast cancer (50).

Similar results were reported in the reduction of the risk of contralateral, second breast primary tumors by letrozole when it was used following 5 years of tamoxifen in the extended adjuvant therapy of early, postmenopausal breast cancer. The National Cancer Institute of Canada (NCIC) Clinical Trials Group MA-17 Trial compared letrozole with placebo after 5 years of tamoxifen and demonstrated a 46% relative reduction of new primary contralateral breast cancers among women treated with letrozole (51).

Aromatase inhibitors are yet to be approved by the U.S. Food and Drug Administration (FDA) for the chemoprevention of breast cancer, but data from the adjuvant setting have provided the rationale for study of their potential use as chemopreventive agents (52). Ongoing randomized, placebo-controlled trials investigating the use of third-generation aromatase inhibitors in the chemoprevention of breast cancer in postmenopausal women include the NCIC Clinical Trials Group MAP3 trial Exemestane in Preventing Cancer in Postmenopausal Women at Increased Risk of Developing Breast Cancer (ExCel), and the International Breast Cancer Intervention Study-II (IBIS-II) trial (53). The North American MAP3 study randomizes patients to exemestane or placebo in patients who refuse treatment with a SERM, and the international IBIS-II trial compares anastrozole for 5 years versus placebo for chemoprevention in patients at increased risk. The only study of an aromatase inhibitor versus a SERM, the proposed NSABP P-4 study, Study to Evaluate Letrozole versus Raloxifene (STELLAR) was not funded by the NCI. Long-term safety and quality of life will be important end points in these studies. Until they are completed, it is not appropriate to use AI to reduce the risk of breast cancer in postmenopausal women. For the reasons we have shown, AI have no role in treating or preventing breast cancer in premenopausal women.

RETINOIDS

Retinoids have been studied as chemopreventive agents in clinical trials because of their established role in regulating cell growth, differentiation, and apoptosis in preclinical models (54). Experimental evidence suggests that retinoids affect gene expression both directly, by activating or repressing specific genes, and indirectly, by interfering with different signal transduction pathways. Induction of apoptosis is a unique feature of fenretinide, the most widely studied retinoid in clinical trials of breast cancer chemoprevention because of its selective accumulation in breast tissue and its favorable toxicologic profile.

The Istituto Nazionale dei Tumouri in Milan began a multicenter, phase III, randomized risk-reduction trial using fenretinide in 1987 (55). Eligible patients were women with stage I breast cancer, aged 33 to 70 years, who had been operated on for breast cancer within the previous 10 years and who had received no systemic adjuvant therapy. Women were randomly assigned to receive either no treatment or fenretinide given orally at a daily dose of 200 mg for 5 years. A placebo control arm was not included in the study. A 3-day drug interval at the end of each month was recommended to allow retinol recovery and to minimize impairment of dark adaptation.

The main outcome measure was the occurrence of contralateral breast cancer as the first malignant event. The secondary end point was the incidence of ipsilateral breast cancer local recurrence in the same quadrant or the occurrence of a second breast malignancy in a different quadrant from the primary tumor. Accrual closed in July 1993, below the expected

sample size of 3,500, because a US NCI alert recommended the administration of adjuvant systemic treatment for patients with node-negative breast cancer.

The Italian investigators reported a median follow-up of 14 years of 1,739 women aged 30 to 70 years (872 in the fenretinide arm and 867 in the observation arm) (56). These data represented 60% of the initial cohort of 2,867 women, and the main efficacy end point was second primary breast cancer (contralateral or ipsilateral). The number of second breast cancers was 168 in the fenretinide arm and 190 in the control arm (hazard ratio [HR] = 0.83, 95% CI, 0.67–1.03). There were 83 events in the fenretinide arm and 126 in the observation arm in premenopausal women (HR = 0.62, 95% CI, 0.46–0.83), and 85 and 64 events in postmenopausal women (HR = 1.23, 95% CI, 0.63–2.40). Risk reduction associated with fenretinide was greater among younger women, being 50% in women aged 40 years or younger and was not seen among women older than 55 years. No differences were reported for cancers in other organs, distant metastases, or survival. It appears that fenretinide induces a significant risk reduction of second breast cancer in premenopausal women.

The most frequently reported adverse events associated with fenretinide were diminished dark adaptation that occurred in about 15% of women and skin or mucosal dryness in 4% to 5%, along with uncommon pruritus, urticaria, and dermatitis. Gastrointestinal symptoms occurred in 11% of subjects and were mainly owing to dyspeptic syndrome or nausea. Eye symptoms included ocular dryness, disorders of lacrimation, and conjunctivitis. In total, about 4% of women had to stop fenretinide because of severe adverse events. Despite the encouraging preliminary results regarding reduction of breast cancer risk, however, fenretinide is not approved for the reduction of breast cancer risk in the United States.

Retinoids are vitamin A analogues that bind nuclear receptors retinoic acid receptors and retinoid X receptors. Retinoid X receptor-selective retinoids (also referred to as rexinoids) represent more effective and tolerable agents for the prevention of ER-negative breast cancers (57). A more selective rexinoid, LG100268, interacts with the SERM arzoxifene to prevent the development of ER-positive breast cancer in rats and may be an efficacious chemopreventive agent that is potentially more tolerable than other rexanoids for the prevention of ER-negative breast cancer.

STATINS

The statins are a class of cholesterol-lowering drugs commonly used by persons aged 50 years and older, and atorvastatin is among the 10 most commonly prescribed drugs in the United States. A growing body of laboratory data suggests that the statins may have chemopreventive potential against cancer at various sites, including colon, lung, breast, and prostate (58). Individual, mostly retrospective, studies have found sometimes large reductions in the risk of breast cancer associated with the use of statin therapy but dose, duration, and type of statin used were often not factored into the analyses. Nevertheless, statin users were half as likely to develop breast cancer as were women who were not statin users in some reports. It is possible, however, that the lower breast cancer incidence in statin users may have been caused by a deficit of breast cancers in the placebo groups rather than an excess in the treatment groups. Some published studies, however, have actually shown an increased risk of breast cancer with statin use. Thus, not all data support a protective effect of statins against breast cancer. Detection bias is a possible explanation for the higher risk observed for carcinoma *in situ* or early-stage cancer compared with invasive breast cancer.

A meta-analysis of seven large randomized trials and nine observational studies revealed no evidence that statin use affected breast cancer risk (59). This conclusion was limited by the relatively short follow-up times of the studies analyzed. In the randomized trials, nearly 60% of patients were taking pravastatin, a hydrophilic statin optimized for liver uptake (60) with decreased systemic distribution compared with lipophilic statins, such as simvastatin; grouping all statins together in a meta-analysis may, therefore, mask true effects. Prospective analysis of the Women's Health Initiative data confirmed that lower breast cancer incidence depends on differences in statin type, with lipophilic statins being associated with decreased risk of breast cancer development, whereas other agents are not (61). Only three of the nine observational studies were specifically designed to study breast cancer. In addition, the use of replacement estrogen may have modulated the effects of statins in several of the studies, as did lack of assessment of duration of statin use and failure to consider clinically important breast cancer subtypes, such as estrogen and progesterone receptor status (62).

Additionally, data from three large retrospective studies and one large prospective study were not included in the meta-analyses, as they had not yet been published. For example, analysis of retrospective data from the Nurses' Health Study (63) as well as a large retrospective population-based study (64) found no difference in breast cancer risk with statin use. One retrospective study found a protective benefit of statins (RR = 0.49) that increased with increasing duration of statin use (65).

Statins are safe, nontoxic, and effective drugs for most patients who use them to lower their cholesterol, and laboratory evidence indicates that statins have anticancer effects. However, until a randomized placebo-controlled trial is designed to evaluate their effect in preventing breast cancer, it is not appropriate to use statins for the reduction of breast cancer risk.

 PREVENTING ESTROGEN RECEPTOR-NEGATIVE BREAST CANCER

Estrogen receptor-negative breast cancer accounts for 20% to 30% of breast cancer and has a poor prognosis. With the success of SERM therapy in preventing ER-positive breast cancer, selecting novel chemopreventive agents for ER-negative breast cancer has now attracted more attention (66). A new generation of chemopreventive agents is being developed that modulate the nonendocrine biochemical pathways that are involved in regulating the growth of normal and malignant cells independent of ER status. Agents that target these pathways may thus inhibit the development of ER-negative breast cancer. Such agents include retinoids, tyrosine kinase inhibitors, selective cyclooxygenase (COX)-2 inhibitors, and others.

For example, the main target of nonsteroidal anti-inflammatory drugs (NSAID) is COX that consists of two isoforms, COX-1 and COX-2. COX enzymes catalyze the conversion of arachidonic acid to prostaglandin G2 (PGG2), which is further catalyzed by the peroxidase activity of COX to PGH2, a common precursor for all other prostanoids (66). Aberrant expression of COX-2 and prostaglandins has been observed in many cancers, including colon and breast cancers, and 40% of human breast cancers show overexpression of COX-2. COX-2 expression, in turn, is correlated with HER-2 protein levels, suggesting that overexpression of COX-2 is involved in breast cancer development.

Numerous studies have tested the cancer preventive effect of various NSAID and selective COX-2 inhibitors, and some selective COX-2 inhibitors significantly reduce the incidence and multiplicity of rat mammary tumors. COX-2 inhibitors carry a potential risk, however, for increased occurrence of thrombotic cardiovascular events, including a slight increase in the risk of heart attacks. These rare but serious side effects likely will limit the widespread use of COX-2 inhibitors as cancer prevention agents.

Carcinogenesis is a multistep process, and animal studies demonstrate that a combination of different agents has synergistic effect in reducing the mammary tumor growth and development. Effective prevention of breast cancer may, therefore, require the use of multiple agents that act through different mechanisms against cancer. Clinical evidence suggests that overexpression of growth factor receptors in breast cancer, especially those of the EGFR/HER-2 family, is associated with resistance to endocrine therapy and, in particular, to tamoxifen. Inhibition of EGFR signaling can overcome resistance to tamoxifen and fulvestrant and delay the emergence of therapeutic resistance. Activation of certain downstream kinase signaling molecules (e.g., MAPK and AKT) may also be associated with endocrine resistance, so that targeting these signaling elements or their downstream effectors with agents such as monoclonal antibodies, tyrosine kinase inhibitors, Raf kinase inhibitors, farnesyl transferase inhibitors, and mTOR inhibitors may modulate endocrine response and delay resistance (67). Ongoing clinical studies are examining whether combining endocrine therapy with a variety of novel targeted therapies may help overcome endocrine resistance and improve treatment outcomes. A more complete blockade of growth factor receptor pathways may be needed to more effectively overcome endocrine resistance. Thus, either multiple signaling inhibitors or agents with multiple kinase targeting capabilities may need to be tested together with endocrine therapy.

SUMMARY OF CLINICAL RECOMMENDATIONS USING SELECTIVE ESTROGEN RECEPTOR MODULATORS FOR REDUCTION OF BREAST CANCER RISK

An analysis conducted in 2003 combined the results of the BCPT, IBIS-I, RMH, and Italian trials investigating chemopreventive therapy for breast cancer (16). Overall, the trials demonstrated that tamoxifen decreased breast cancer incidence by 38% ($p < .0001$), and estrogen receptor-positive tumors by 48% ($p < .0001$). In postmenopausal women, age had no apparent effect on the degree of breast cancer reduction. Rates of endometrial cancer were increased with tamoxifen in all prevention trials, although most of the excess risk occurred in women more than 50 years of age and no excess deaths resulted from either endometrial or other cancers. As reviewed above, there was no observed decrease in estrogen-receptor-negative tumors. Venous thromboembolism was increased in all the tamoxifen prevention trials, and no excess deaths occurred from cardiac or vascular events, except for pulmonary embolism. The risk of the thrombotic side effects of tamoxifen may be reduced by the concomitant use of low-dose aspirin (although this has not been confirmed in prospective studies).

Based on results from the BCPT, the FDA approved the use of tamoxifen for breast cancer risk reduction in women who are 35 years or older and have a 5-year risk of 1.66% or more as determined by the Gail et al. model (11,21). The Gail model has been modified recently to improve the predictive value in black patients (68) and can be obtained at www.cancer.gov/bcrisktool to quantify risk among potentially eligible subjects.

The risks and benefits of tamoxifen depend on age and on a woman's specific risk factors for breast cancer. The absolute risks from tamoxifen for endometrial cancer, stroke, pulmonary embolism, and deep vein thrombosis increase with

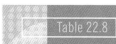

Table 22.8	SELECTING PATIENTS TO USE SELECTIVE ESTROGEN RECEPTOR MODULATORS (SERM) FOR REDUCTION OF BREAST CANCER RISK

Women in Whom SERM Can Be Considered for Risk Reduction

History of lobular carcinoma *in situ*

History of atypical ductal or lobular hyperplasia

Premenopausal women with mutations in either the *BRCA1* or the *BRCA2* gene

Premenopausal women ≥35 yrs of age with 5-yr probability of breast cancer ≥1.66%

Postmenopausal women with Gail model 5-yr probability of breast cancer ≥1.66% and significant benefit-to-risk profile

Women at increased risk without a uterus

Women in Whom Caution Should Be Used When Considering the Use of SERM

History of stroke, transient ischemic attack, deep venous thrombosis, pulmonary embolus

History of cataracts or cataract surgery

Current use of hormone replacement therapy

Adapted from Chlebowski RT, Col N, Winer EP, et al. American Society of Clinical Oncology technology assessment of pharmacologic interventions for breast cancer risk reduction including tamoxifen, raloxifene, and aromatase inhibition. *J Clin Oncol* 2002;20:1–17, with permission.

age, as does the protective effect of tamoxifen on fractures (21). Tamoxifen also has its greatest clinical benefit with less severe side effects in women who do not have a uterus and in women at higher risk of breast cancer. Tables and decision aids are available to describe the risks and benefits of tamoxifen and to identify classes of women for whom the benefits outweigh the risks (21). Tamoxifen is most beneficial for younger women with an elevated risk of breast cancer. Published quantitative analyses can assist health care providers and women in weighing the risks and benefits of tamoxifen for reducing breast cancer risk. These considerations are summarized in Table 22.8.

In 2002, the American Society of Clinical Oncology Technology Assessment Working Group published a comprehensive formal literature review of available data on breast cancer risk-reduction strategies with tamoxifen and raloxifene (69). They concluded that women with a defined 5-year projected risk of breast cancer of 1.66% or greater (i.e., the risk of the average, 60 year-old white, North American female) may be offered 20 mg of tamoxifen daily for up to 5 years for risk reduction. Thus, most women aged 60 years or older would fall within the group that may be offered tamoxifen for chemoprevention. However, the Working Group asserted that the greatest clinical benefit was observed when tamoxifen was given to younger, premenopausal women, women without a uterus, and in women with a higher risk for breast cancer. They recommended that, in all circumstances, tamoxifen use should be discussed as part of an informed decision-making process with careful consideration of individually calculated risks and benefits. Because of a lack of sufficient data, aromatase inhibitors were not recommended for chemoprevention outside clinical trials.

The U.S. Preventive Services Task Force (USPSTF) published its recommendations for the chemoprevention of breast cancer in 2002 (70). The task force found fair evidence that treatment with tamoxifen can significantly reduce the risk of invasive, ER-positive breast cancer in women at high risk, and that the likelihood of benefit increased with a higher risk of breast cancer. As with the ASCO Working Group, they did not recommend the routine use of tamoxifen or raloxifene for women at low or average risk, because the potential harms may outweigh the benefits. The USPSTF advised discussing chemoprevention with women at high risk of breast cancer and low risk for adverse events, and informing such patients of the potential benefits and harms of chemoprevention.

As reviewed in this chapter, tamoxifen can be used in carriers of *BRCA1* and *BRCA2* mutations who do not desire prophylactic mastectomy. The drug may be more effective in carriers of *BRCA2* mutations who are more likely to develop ER-positive cancers, but no prospective, randomized data are available to address the question. Beginning tamoxifen at younger ages (<45 years) is preferable than older ages because of the risk-to-benefit considerations already described, earlier initiation of benefit, and a lower likelihood of inducing menopausal symptoms. When tamoxifen is used, it should be given for 5 years. Combinations of tamoxifen with other agents have not been evaluated for either safety or efficacy. Women who elect prophylactic mastectomy to reduce their risk should not take tamoxifen to further decrease their risk because few data exist to suggest an additional benefit.

Raloxifene is a unique SERM with distinct activity and toxicity profiles. Extensive experience from prospective investigations has established its safety and efficacy in the management of postmenopausal osteoporosis, and it has neither apparent beneficial nor adverse effects on coronary heart disease (39). Four prospective, clinical trials have established its benefit in reducing the risk of invasive breast cancer (35–37,39,40), and it offers safety advantages when compared with tamoxifen in postmenopausal women who are at increased risk for breast cancer. Symptomatic side effects are acceptable as reported in the large, prospectively blinded clinical populations. The risk of other cancers, fractures, ischemic heart disease, and stroke are similar for both raloxifene and tamoxifen. Raloxifene at a dose of 60 mg orally daily for 5 years thus offers an alternative to tamoxifen for the reduction of breast cancer risk in high-risk postmenopausal women.

POPULATION BENEFITS OF CHEMOPREVENTION

Of the more than 65 million women aged 35 to 79 years without reported breast cancer in the United States in 2000, more than 10 million women would be eligible for tamoxifen chemoprevention using widely accepted definitions of eligibility (71). The percentage of eligible women varies by race, with 19% of white women, 6% of black women, and 3% of Hispanic women being eligible. Of the more than 50 million white women in the United States aged 35 to 79 years, nearly 2.5 million would have a positive benefit–risk index for tamoxifen chemoprevention. No similar calculations have been published for raloxifene, but its more favorable toxicity profile in regard to both thrombosis and uterine effects suggest that it will have a larger net benefit than tamoxifen in postmenopausal women.

Conservative cost modeling predicts that tamoxifen prolongs the average survival of women initiating use at ages 35, 50, and 60 years by 70, 42, and 27 days, respectively (33). It prolongs survival even more for those in the highest risk groups, especially those with atypical hyperplasia (202, 89, and 45 days, respectively). Tamoxifen use extends quality-adjusted survival by 158, 80, and 50 days by age category, respectively, in women with atypical hyperplasia.

The benefits are greater if tamoxifen is initiated before age 50 years rather than after, and if the breast cancer risk reduction conferred by tamoxifen lasts longer than 5 years. Chemoprevention with tamoxifen costs $46,619 per life-year saved for women who started at age 35; for women over age 50, it costs more than $50,000 per life-year saved (72). Although tamoxifen use appears to improve long-term survival and quality-adjusted survival among women who are at increased risk of breast cancer, this benefit diminishes with age. The data indicate that tamoxifen is cost-effective in comparison with other cancer treatment strategies for younger women only. No cost analyses have been published that evaluate the utility of raloxifene in the risk-reduction setting.

 MANAGEMENT SUMMARY

- Premenopausal women more than 35 years of age with Gail model risks of breast cancer greater than 1.67% in 5 years or lobular carcinoma *in situ* should be offered tamoxifen for the reduction of breast cancer risk.
- When used for reducing the risk of breast cancer, tamoxifen should be given in a dose of 20 mg once daily, the dose that was used in the large randomized breast cancer risk-reduction trials reported to date. Alternative doses and schedules have not been evaluated for either safety or efficacy.
- No study has evaluated the optimal age at which to begin tamoxifen to reduce breast cancer risk; premenopausal women at increased risk derive the greatest net benefit because of the absence of increased risks for either thromboembolic events or uterine cancer in this group.
- In Europe, tamoxifen is not recommended as a preventive agent, except possibly in very high-risk women wishing to avoid or delay prophylactic mastectomy.
- Because the risk of clotting increases with age, and because both stroke and pulmonary embolism are potentially life-threatening consequences of tamoxifen therapy, careful consideration must be given to risks versus benefits in older postmenopausal women who are considering tamoxifen for risk reduction.
- Early ambulation following surgery, discontinuation of tamoxifen in the perioperative setting, and the use of concomitant low-dose aspirin may be helpful (but as yet unproved) methods of thromboembolism prevention.
- Chemoprevention with a SERM may be particularly beneficial to women with atypical hyperplasia, a 5-year Gail model risk of more than 5%, lobular carcinoma *in situ*, or two or more first-degree relatives with breast cancer based on the published data reviewed in this chapter.
- No primary prevention studies have evaluated the optimal duration of tamoxifen therapy for reducing the risk of breast cancer. Ongoing clinical trials in the adjuvant therapy setting will determine whether using tamoxifen for more than 5 years would be beneficial. No trials are being conducted or are planned to examine the ideal duration of therapy in the risk-reduction setting.
- IBIS-I study data suggest that the benefit from tamoxifen chemoprevention extends beyond treatment into the post-treatment period.
- Absolute contraindications to tamoxifen use for risk reduction include a history of deep venous thrombosis or pulmonary embolism, a history of stroke or transient ischemic attack, and a history of uncontrolled diabetes, hypertension, or atrial fibrillation.
- Women currently taking estrogen, progesterone, androgens, or birth control pills should discontinue these medications before initiating tamoxifen therapy based on the data from the IBIS-I trial.
- Pregnant women or women who may become pregnant should also avoid tamoxifen.
- Raloxifene 60 mg orally daily for 5 years offers an acceptable alternative to tamoxifen for the reduction of breast cancer risk in high-risk postmenopausal women and is associated with lower associated risks of both benign and malignant uterine events as well as significantly less thromboembolic toxicity.
- Raloxifene should not be used in premenopausal women because there are neither efficacy nor toxicity data for women using raloxifene before menopause.

References

1. Sporn MB, Suh N. Chemoprevention of cancer. *Carcinogenesis* 2000;21:525–530.
2. Sporn MB, Suh N. Chemoprevention: an essential approach to controlling cancer. *Nat Rev Cancer* 2002;2:537–543.
3. Fisher B, Costantino JP, Wickerham DL, et al. Tamoxifen for prevention of breast cancer: Report of the National Surgical Adjuvant Breast and Bowel Project P-1 Study. *J Natl Cancer Inst* 1998;90:1371–1388.
4. Cuzick J, Forbes J, Edwards R, et al. First results from the International Breast Cancer Intervention Study (IBIS-I): a randomised prevention trial. *Lancet* 2002;360:817–823.
5. Powles T, Eeles R, Ashley S, et al. Interim analysis of the incidence of breast cancer in the Royal Marsden Hospital tamoxifen randomized chemoprevention trial. *Lancet* 1998;352:98–101.
6. Powles TJ. The Royal Marsden Hospital (RMH) trial: key points and remaining questions. *Ann N Y Acad Sci* 2001;949:109–112.
7. Veronesi U, Maisonneuve P, Costa A, et al. Prevention of breast cancer with tamoxifen: preliminary findings from the Italian randomised trial among hysterectomised women. *Lancet* 1998;352:93–97.
8. Veronesi U, Maisonneuve P, Sacchini V, et al. Tamoxifen for breast cancer among hysterectomized women. *Lancet* 2002;359:1122–1124.
9. Veronesi U, Maisonneuve P, Rotmensz N, et al. Italian randomized trial among women with hysterectomy: tamoxifen and hormone-dependent breast cancer in high-risk women. *J Natl Cancer Inst* 2003;95:160–165.
10. Vogel VG. Raloxifene: a second-generation selective estrogen receptor modulator for reducing the risk of invasive breast cancer in postmenopausal women. *Women's Health* 2007;3:139–153.
11. Gail MH, Brinton LA, Byar DP, et al. Projecting individualized probabilities of developing breast cancer for white females who are being examined annually. *J Natl Cancer Inst* 1989;81:1879–1886.
12. Fisher B, Costantino JP, Wickerham DL, et al. Tamoxifen for the prevention of breast cancer: current status of the National Surgical Adjuvant Breast and Bowel Project P-1 Study. *J Natl Cancer Inst* 2005;97:1652–1662.
13. Powles TJ. Twenty-Year Follow-up of the Royal Marsden Randomized, Double-Blinded Tamoxifen Breast Cancer Prevention Trial. *J Natl Cancer Inst* 2007;99:283–290.
14. Cuzick J, Powles T, Veronesi U, et al. Overview of the main outcomes in breast-cancer prevention trials. *Lancet* 2003;361:296–300.
15. Tyrer J, Duffy SW, Cuzick J. A breast cancer prediction model incorporating familial and personal risk factors. *Stat Med* 2004;23:1111–1130.
16. Cuzick J, Forbes JF, Sestak I, et al. Long-term results of tamoxifen prophylaxis for breast cancer—96-month follow-up of the randomized IBIS-I trial. *J Natl Cancer Inst* 2007;99:272–282.
17. Veronesi U, Maissonneuv P, Rotmensz N, et al. Tamoxifen for the prevention of breast cancer: late results of the Italian randomized tamoxifen prevention trial among women with hysterectomy. *J Natl Cancer Inst* 2007;99:727–737.
18. Wickerham DL, Fisher B, Wolmark N, et al. Association of tamoxifen and uterine sarcoma. *J Clin Oncol* 2002;20:2758–2760.
19. Cushman M, Constantino JP, Bovill EG, et al. Effect of tamoxifen on venous thrombosis risk factors in women without cancer: the Breast Cancer Prevention Trial. *Br J Haematol* 2003;120:109–116.
20. Abramson N, Constantino JP, Garber JE, et al. Effect of Factor V Leiden and prothrombin G20210 → A mutations on thromboembolic risk in the national surgical adjuvant breast and bowel project breast cancer prevention trial. *J Natl Cancer Inst* 2006;98:904–910.
21. Gail MH, Costantino JP, Bryant J, et al. Weighing the risks and benefits of tamoxifen treatment for preventing breast cancer. *J Natl Cancer Inst* 1999;91:1829–1846.
22. Day R, Ganz PA, Costantino JP, et al. Health-related quality of life and tamoxifen in breast cancer prevention. A report from the National Surgical Adjuvant Breast and Bowel Project P-1 Study. *J Clin Oncol* 1999;17:2659–2669.
23. Radloff LS. The CES-D Scale: a self-report depression scale for research in the general population. *Applied Psychological Measures* 1977;1:385–401.
24. Sherbourne CD. Social functioning: sexual problems measures. In: Stewart AL, Ware JE, eds. *Measuring functioning and well-being: The Medical Outcomes Study approach*. Durham, NC: Duke University Press, 1992:194–204.
25. McHorney CA, Ware JE Jr, Lu JF, Sherbourne CD. The MOS 36-item Short-Form Health Survey (SF-36), III: tests of data quality, scaling assumptions, and reliability across diverse patient groups. *Med Care* 1994;32:40–66.
26. McHorney CA, Ware JE Jr, Rogers W, et al. The validity and relative precision of MOS short- and long-form health status scales and Dartmouth COOP charts: results from the Medical Outcomes Study. *Med Care* 1992;30(5 Suppl):MS253–MS265.
27. Tan-Chiu E, Wang J, Constantino JP, et al. Effects of tamoxifen on benign breast disease in women at high risk for breast cancer. *J Natl Cancer Inst* 2003;95:302–307.
28. Rebbeck TR, Lynch HT, Neuhausen SL, et al. Prophylactic oophorectomy in carriers of BRCA1 or BRCA2 mutations. *N Engl J Med* 2002;346:1616–1622.
29. Narod SA, Brunet JS, Ghadirian P, et al. Tamoxifen and risk of contralateral breast cancer in BRCA1 and BRCA2 mutation carriers: a case-control study. Hereditary Breast Cancer Clinical Study Group. *Lancet* 2000;356:1876–1881.
30. King MC, Wieand S, Hale K, et al. Tamoxifen and breast cancer incidence among women with inherited mutations in BRCA1 and BRCA2: National Surgical Adjuvant Breast and Bowel Project (NSABP-P1) Breast Cancer Prevention Trial. *JAMA* 2001;286:2251–2256.
31. Schrag D, Kuntz KM, Garber JE, et al. Life expectancy gains from cancer prevention strategies for women with breast cancer and BRCA1 or BRCA2 mutations. *JAMA* 2000;283:617–624.
32. Grann VR, Jacobson JS, Thomason D, et al. Effect of prevention strategies on survival and quality-adjusted survival of women with BRCA1/2 mutations: an updated decision analysis. *J Clin Oncol* 2002;20:2520–2529.
33. Hershman D, Sundararajan V, Jacobson JS, et al. Outcomes of tamoxifen chemoprevention for breast cancer in very high-risk women: a cost-effectiveness analysis. *J Clin Oncol* 2002;20:9–16.
34. Chlebowski RT, Col N, Winer EP, et al. American Society of Clinical Oncology technology assessment of pharmacologic interventions for breast cancer risk reduction including tamoxifen, raloxifene, and aromatase inhibition. *J Clin Oncol* 2002;20:1–17.
35. Cummings SR, Eckert S, Krueger KA, et al. The effect of raloxifene on risk of breast cancer in postmenopausal women: results from the MORE randomized trial. *JAMA* 1999;281:2189–2197.

36. Cauley JA, Norton L, Lippman ME, et al. Continued breast cancer risk reduction in postmenopausal women treated with raloxifene: 4-year results from the MORE trial. *Breast Cancer Res Treat (Netherlands)* 2001;65:125–134.

37. Martino S, Cauley JA, Barrett-Connor E, et al. Continuing outcomes relevant to Evista: breast cancer incidence in postmenopausal osteoporotic women in a randomized trial of raloxifene. *J Natl Cancer Inst* 2004;96:1751–1761.

38. Mershon J, Yeo A, Qu Y, et al. Cumulative effects of raloxifene on the incidence of breast cancer over 8 years in postmenopausal women with osteoporosis. San Antonio Breast Cancer Symposium 2007. *Breast Cancer Res Treat* 2007;106, (Suppl 1):S180. Abstract #4042.

39. Barrett-Connor E, Mosca L, Collins P, et al. Raloxifene Use for The Heart (RUTH) Trial Investigators. Effects of raloxifene on cardiovascular events and breast cancer in postmenopausal women. *N Engl J Med* 2006;355:125–137.

40. Vogel VG, Costantino JP, Wickerham DL, et al. Effects of tamoxifen vs. raloxifene on the risk of developing invasive breast cancer and other disease outcomes: The NSABP Study of Tamoxifen and Raloxifene (STAR) P-2 Trial. *JAMA* 2006;295: 2727–2741.

41. Gail MH, Costantino JP. Validating and improving models for projecting the absolute risk of breast cancer. *J Natl Cancer Inst* 2001;93:334–335.

42. Land SR, Wickerham DL, Costantino JP, et al. Patient-reported symptoms and quality of life during treatment with tamoxifen or raloxifene for breast cancer prevention: The NSABP Study of Tamoxifen and Raloxifene (STAR) P-2 Trial. *JAMA* 2006;295:2742–2751.

43. Lippman ME, Krueger KA, Eckert S, et al. Indicators of lifetime estrogen exposure: effect on breast cancer incidence and interaction with raloxifene therapy in the Multiple Outcomes of Raloxifene Evaluation study participants. *J Clin Oncol* 2001;19:3111–3116.

44. Cummings SR, Tu D, Kenyon E, et al. Serum estradiol level and risk of breast cancer during treatment with raloxifene. *JAMA* 2002;287:216–220.

45. Eliassen AH, Missmer SA, Tworoger SS, et al. Endogenous steroid hormone concentrations and risk of breast cancer: does the association vary by a woman's predicted breast cancer risk? *J Clin Oncol* 2006;24:1823–1830.

46. Beattie MS, Costantino JP, Cummings SR, et al. Endogenous sex hormones, risk of breast cancer, and response to tamoxifen: an ancillary study in the NSABP Breast Cancer Prevention Trial (P-1). *J Natl Cancer Inst* 2006;98:110–115.

47. Simpson ER, et al. Aromatase cytochrome P450, the enzyme responsible for estrogen biosynthesis. *Endocr Rev* 1994;15:342–355.

48. Baum M, Buzdar A, Cuzik M, et al. Anastrozole alone or in combination with tamoxifen versus alone for adjuvant treatment of postmenopausal women with early stage breast cancer: results of the ATAC (arimidex, tamoxifen alone or in combination) trial efficacy and safety update analyses. *Cancer* 2003;98:1802–1810.

49. Howell A, et al., Results of the ATAC (arimidex, tamoxifen, alone or in combination) trial after completion of 5 years' adjuvant treatment for breast cancer *Lancet* 2005;365:60–62.

50. The Arimidex, Tamoxifen, Alone or in Combination (ATAC) Trialists' Group. Effect of anastrozole and tamoxifen as adjuvant treatment for early-stage breast cancer: 100-month analysis of the ATAC trial. *Lancet Oncol* 2008;9:45–53.

51. Goss PE, Ingle JN, Martino S, et al., A randomized trial of letrozole in postmenopausal women after five years of tamoxifen therapy for early-stage breast cancer. *N Engl J Med* 2003;349:1793–1802.

52. Ingle JN. Endocrine therapy trials of aromatase inhibitors for breast cancer in the adjuvant and prevention settings. *Clin Cancer Res* 2005;11:900s–905s.

53. Goss PE, Strasser-Weippl K. Aromatase inhibitors for chemoprevention. *Best Practice Res Clin Endocrinol Metabol* 2004;18:113–130.

54. Zanardi S, Serrano D, Argusti A, et al. Clinical trials with retinoids for breast cancer chemoprevention. *Endocr Rel Cancer* 2006;13:51–68.

55. Veronesi U, De Palo G, Marubini E, et al. Randomized trial of fenretinide to prevent second breast malignancy in women with early breast cancer. *J Natl Cancer Inst* 1999;91:1847–1856.

56. Veronesi U, Mariani L, Decensi A, et al. Fifteen-year results of a randomized phase III trial of fenretinide to prevent second breast cancer. *Ann Oncol* 2006;17:1065–1071.

57. Li Y, Zhang Y, Hill J, et al. The rexinoid LG100268 prevents the development of preinvasive and invasive estrogen receptor–negative tumors in MMTV-erbB2 mice. *Clin Cancer Res* 2007;13:6224–6231.

58. Vogel VG. Can statin therapy reduce the risk of breast cancer? *J Clin Oncol* 2005;23:8553–8555.

59. Bonovas S, Filioussi K, Tsavaris N, et al. Use of statins and breast cancer: a meta-analysis of seven randomized clinical trials and nine observational studies. *J Clin Oncol* 2005;23:8606–8612.

60. Sprague JR, Wood ME. Statins and breast cancer prevention: time for randomized controlled trials. *J Clin Oncol* 2006;24:2129–2130.

61. Cauley JA, McTiernan A, Rodabough RJ, et al. Statin use and breast cancer: prospective results from the Women's Health Initiative. *J Natl Cancer Inst* 2006;98:700–707.

62. Kumar AS, Benz CC, Shim VV, et al. Estrogen receptor-negative breast cancer is less likely to arise among lipophilic statin users. *Cancer Epidemiol Biomarkers Prev* 2008;17:1028–1033.

63. Eliassen AH, Colditz GA, Rosner B, et al. Serum lipids, lipid-lowering drugs, and the risk of breast cancer. *Arch Intern Med* 2005;165:2264–2271

64. Boudreau DM, Yu O, Miglioretti DL, et al. Statin use and breast cancer risk in a large population-based setting. *Cancer Epidemiol Biomarkers Prev* 2007;16:416–421.

65. Kochhar R, Khurana V, Bejjanki H. Statins to reduce breast cancer risk: a case control study in U.S. female veterans. ASCO Annual Meeting Proceedings 2005. *J Clin Oncol* 2005;23:514 [Abstract].

66. Li Y, Brown PH. Translational approaches for the prevention of estrogen receptor-negative breast cancer. *Eur J Cancer Prev* 2007;16:203–215.

67. Massarweh S, Schiff R. Unraveling the mechanisms of endocrine resistance in breast cancer: new therapeutic opportunities. *Clin Cancer Res* 2007;13:1950–1954.

68. Gail MH, Costantino JP, Pee D, et al. Projecting individualized absolute invasive breast cancer risk in African American women. *J Natl Cancer Inst* 2007;99:1782–1792.

69. Chlebowski RT, et al., American Society of Clinical Oncology technology assessment of pharmacologic interventions for breast cancer risk reduction including tamoxifen, raloxifene, and aromatase inhibition, *J Clin Oncol* 2002;20:3328–3343.

70. Kinsinger LS, Harris R, Woolf SH, et al. Chemoprevention of breast cancer: a summary of the evidence for the U.S. Preventive Services Task Force. *Ann Intern Med* 2002;137:E59–E69.

71. Freedman AN, Graubard BI, Rao SR, et al. Estimates of the number of U.S. women who could benefit from tamoxifen for breast cancer chemoprevention. *J Natl Cancer Inst* 2003;95:526–532.

72. Grann VR, Sundararajan V, Jacobson JS, et al. Decision analysis of tamoxifen for the prevention of invasive breast cancer. *Cancer J* 2000;6:169–178.

Chapter 23
Pathology and Biological Features of Premalignant Breast Disease

D. Craig Allred

The human breast is capable of producing a very large number histologically defined abnormalities of growth. However, only a handful appear to have any significance as risk factors or precursors of breast cancer. One of the first attempts to incorporate these premalignant lesions into a comprehensive model of breast cancer evolution was published by Wellings and Jensen (1–3) over 30 years ago. The model was based primarily on the evidence of gradual histological continuity and proposed that the cellular origin of breast cancers occurs in the normal terminal duct lobular unit (TDLU) and that the putative precursors represent a nonobligatory series of increasingly abnormal stages that progress to cancer over long periods of time, probably decades in most cases (Fig. 23.1).

The key stages in the model are generically referred to as hyperplasias, atypical hyperplasias, *in situ* carcinomas, and invasive carcinomas, but there are multiple lineages and subtypes. In the largest so-called ductal lineage (representing about 80% of all breast cancers), the terminology of hyperplasias is diverse and still evolving (discussed below), while the other stages are referred to as atypical ductal hyperplasia (ADH), ductal carcinoma *in situ* (DCIS), and invasive ductal carcinoma (IDC). IDCs are also referred to as no-special-type or not-otherwise-specified invasive breast cancers (IBCs) to distinguish them from the major so-called special histological subtypes, which include invasive tubular, mucinous, medullary, and lobular carcinomas. However, all of the special subtypes except lobular carcinomas can be considered as subtypes of IDC in the sense that they appear to evolve from the same precursors. The progression of the lobular lineage (representing the remaining 20% of carcinomas) is histologically relatively distinct, and the key precursors in this setting are referred to as atypical lobular hyperplasia (ALH) and lobular carcinoma *in situ* (LCIS). However, the practice of referring to breast cancers as ductal or lobular implies that they originate and reside in ducts and lobules, respectively, which is a historical misconception in the sense that both lineages are thought to arise from progenitor cells in normal TDLUs and both can occupy ducts and lobules (4). Furthermore, many IBCs show complex combinations of ductal (including special subtypes) and lobular features, emphasizing that these histology-based classifications, while very useful, oversimplify enormous diversity.

The Wellings-Jensen model has withstood the test of time in the sense of remaining generally consistent with information gained by other investigators. For example, other pathological studies have shown that the putative precursors are much more common in cancerous than noncancerous breasts, consistent with a precursor role (5–7). Epidemiological studies have shown that women with a history of these lesions in a previous biopsy are at increased relative risk for developing breast cancer, ranging from about 1.5-fold for hyperplasias, to 5-fold for ADH and ALH, to 10-fold or higher for DCIS and LCIS, and precursors must also be risk factors, although the opposite is not always true (7–17). Some studies suggest that the elevated risks associated with ADH, ALH, and LCIS are equal in both breasts, implying that they are only risk factors (9,11). However, these lesions (especially ALH and LCIS) are often multifocal and bilateral (2,3,6), so it is possible for them to be both risk factors and precursors, and their wide distribution suggests that they may be initiated during early breast development. Recent comprehensive studies of ALH and LCIS place the majority of the risk in the ipsilateral breast, supporting a precursor role (18–23), although the apparently equal bilateral risk associated with ADH remains an enigma. DCIS is usually a localized disease with a predominately ipsilateral risk for developing IBC, consistent with the notion that DCIS is a relatively advanced and committed precursor (14,24,25). Some of the most compelling evidence comes from recent laboratory studies showing that the putative precursors share identical genetic abnormalities with breast cancers, especially when they occur in the same breasts (26–31), as well as histological and biological similarities with genetically engineered mouse models (32–37).

There are important general characteristics that distinguish one stage from the next in the Wellings-Jensen model that accumulate and increase with progression. The transition from TDLUs to hyperplasias is characterized by increased growth due to epithelial hyperplasia. Alterations of cell adhesion and polarity distinguish ADH from hyperplasias as the epithelium begins to pile up and distend acini. DCIS is characterized by further growth and the appearance of enormously increased histological and biological diversity compared to earlier precursors. Invasion into surrounding stroma defines the transition of DCIS to IBC. The remainder of this chapter reviews some of the histological and biological features associated with these stages and transitions.

NORMAL BREAST EPITHELIUM

A large majority of normal epithelium in the adult female human breast resides within TDLUs, which, as the name implies, are composed of the smallest terminal branch of the ductal system ending in a grape-like cluster of acini whose primary function is to produce milk (Fig. 23.1). Carcinomas and their precursors are composed of transformed epithelial cells. Whether all epithelium has the potential to transform or only epithelial stem cells or progenitor cells is currently unknown and a major topic of research and debate. Regardless of their identity, the cells clearly undergo many adaptive, epigenetic, and genetic alterations leading to increased growth and progression.

The hormone estrogen plays a central role in regulating the growth and differentiation of normal breast epithelium (38–40). Its effects are mediated by estrogen receptor alpha (ERα) functioning primarily as a nuclear transcription factor.

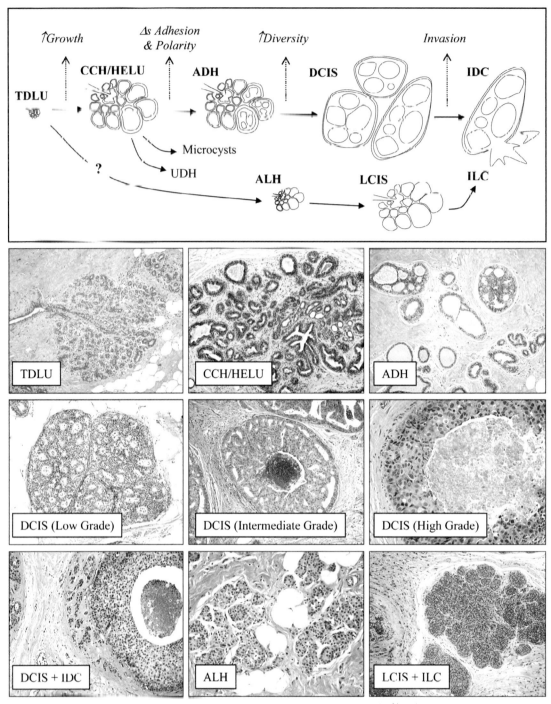

FIGURE 23.1. The Wellings-Jensen model of breast cancer evolution proposes that the cellular origin of breast cancers occurs in the normal terminal duct lobular unit (TDLU) and that the putative precursors represent a nonobligatory series of increasingly abnormal stages that progress to cancer over long periods of time, probably decades in most cases (see text for a detailed description). Briefly, the key stages in the so-called ductal lineage (representing about 80% of all breast cancers) are referred to as columnar cell hyperplasia (CCH) or hyperplastic enlarged lobular units (HELUs), atypical ductal hyperplasia (ADH), ductal carcinoma *in situ* (DCIS), and invasive ductal carcinoma (IDC). The stages in the so-called lobular lineage (representing the remaining 20% of carcinomas) are referred to as atypical lobular hyperplasia (ALH), lobular carcinoma *in situ* (LCIS), and invasive lobular carcinoma (ILC).

Estrogen-activated ERα stimulates cell proliferation and regulates the expression of many other genes, including the progesterone receptor (PR). PR mediates the effects of the hormone progesterone, which also participates in regulating growth and differentiation in normal cells (38). Many additional factors referred to as coactivators and corepressors modulate the functions of these hormone receptors (41). See Chapter 29 of this book for a more detailed discussion of the biology of ERα.

Many studies have shown that, for women of all ages combined, an average of about 30% of normal breast epithelial cells express ERα (Fig. 23.2) (42–46). In premenopausal women, the rate is somewhat lower (10% to 20% ERα-positive cells) and varies with the menstrual cycle, being twice as high in the follicular as the luteal phase (43,45). The average rate in postmenopausal women is higher (50% to 60% ERα-positive cells) and relatively stable in the absence of hormone replacement therapy (43).

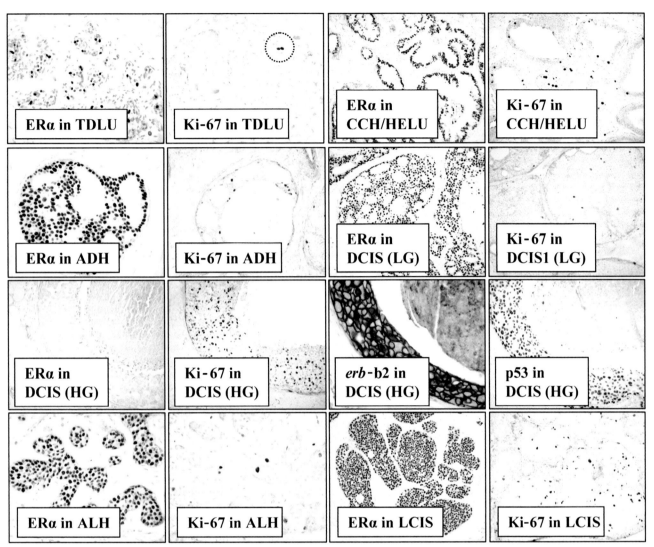

FIGURE 23.2. Standard prognostic biomarkers in premalignant breast lesions. Photomicrographs showing examples of standard prognostic biomarkers assessed by immunohistochemistry in premalignant breast lesions, including estrogen receptor alpha (ERα), proliferation (Ki-67 proliferation-associated marker), erb-b2 oncoprotein, and p53 tumor suppressor gene product (see text for detailed a description). TDLU, terminal duct lobular unit; CCH/HELU, columnar cell hyperplasia/hyperplastic enlarged lobular unit; DCIS, ductal carcinoma *in situ;* LG, low grade; HG, high grade; ALH, atypical lobular hyperplasia; LCIS, lobular carcinoma *in situ.*

Proliferation averages about 2% in normal cells (Fig. 23.2) (43,46–54). It also fluctuates with the menstrual cycle and is about twofold higher in the luteal than follicular phase, which is opposite to ERα, suggesting that the mitogenic effect of estrogen is indirect and partially mediated by downstream interactions such as that between progesterone and PR (38,55). Proliferation also varies with menopausal status and is significantly higher in premenopausal than postmenopausal breasts (averaging about 2.5% and 1.5%, respectively) (43). Proliferating normal epithelial cells are almost always (>95%) ERα negative and, conversely, ERα-positive normal cells are rarely (<5%) proliferating (38,56), and there is evidence that proliferation in these cells is being actively suppressed by transforming growth factor α1 (TGF-α1) activity (57). In a general way, homeostasis of growth in normal cells is a highly regulated balance between cell proliferation and cell death or apoptosis. Apoptosis is also partially regulated by estrogen-activated ERα, and average rates are higher in premenopausal (0.8%) than postmenopausal (0.4%) breast epithelial cells (43).

Recent studies have shown that histologically normal-appearing breast epithelial cells are not always normal at the molecular level, and some of these morphologically silent biological abnormalities may predispose the cells to premalignant or malignant transformation. For example, clonal allelic imbalances (chromosomal gains and losses) have been observed in normal breast epithelium (58–60). Although the overall frequency of imbalances is quite low, it is significantly higher in normal cells adjacent to cancer cells than normal cells at a distance (58). Some of these genetic defects may be shared with the adjacent cancer (58), although the majority are not and appear to be random (59). Other studies have shown that breast tissue, especially in women at high risk for breast cancer, may contain patches of histologically normal appearing cells in which activity of the p16 tumor suppressor gene is suppressed (61–63). Compared to adjacent cells with normal p16 function, these cells show increased proliferation and elevated expression of cyclooxygenase 2 (COX-2), and the latter appears to be associated with the development of many types of cancers. There are likely to be many other acquired and inherited molecular abnormalities in otherwise normal appearing cells to explain the dramatically different risks of developing breast cancer between women.

HYPERPLASIAS

The enlargement of normal TDLUs by hyperplastic epithelial cells is one of the most common abnormalities of growth in the adult female human breast (43,64–66). These hyperplastic enlarged lobular units (HELUs) are often multifocal, bilateral, and up to 100-fold larger (volume and numbers of cells) than the TDLUs they evolve from, representing a major alteration of growth (Fig. 23.1) (43). The majority of HELUs are lined by one or two layers of crowded columnar epithelial cells, but many exhibit more diverse histological features, contributing to the complex terminology that has evolved to describe them (43,64–66). Currently, they are most commonly referred to as columnar cell lesions (CCLs), which encompass several putative subtypes including columnar cell change (CCC; characterized by a generally single layer of hyperplastic columnar epithelium), columnar cell hyperplasia (CCH; characterized by stratified hyperplastic columnar epithelium), and CCLs with cytological atypia, sometimes referred to as flat epithelial atypia (FEA), among others (64–66). As mentioned, however, they often show variable combinations of these histological features and more that can be difficult to subclassify in a reproducible manner (67), so CCH or HELUs (or both) seem like reasonable general terms in the sense that they convey the salient features common to most of them (i.e., enlargement of TDLUs and proximal ducts by hyperplastic predominately columnar epithelial cells).

The idea that CCH/HELUs might be precursors of breast cancer was proposed as far back as the early 1900s, if not earlier (65,68,69), and it is supported by pathological studies showing that they are much more common in cancerous than noncancerous breasts (2,3), epidemiological studies showing that they are weak (about 1.5-fold) risk factors for developing breast cancer (7,12,70), and more recent laboratory studies showing that they may share identical genetic abnormalities (e.g., allelic imbalances) with cancer in the same breast, although the overall frequency of these abnormalities appears to be quite low (28). It is currently unknown whether the cytological atypia occasionally observed in CCH/HELUs is associated with significantly higher risk for developing breast cancer than the majority without atypia, although in some preliminary studies up to 20% with atypia identified on core biopsies were associated with cancer in follow-up excisions (64, 71–75), which is worrisome, leading some authors to advocate follow-up excisions in this setting (64). However, not all studies find a significant relationship between CCH/HELUs with atypia and cancer (7,76,77), so the jury is still out on this issue (66,78). It seems likely that some CCH/HELUs may indeed represent relatively high-risk lesions, but it is possible that histological features alone may not always be sufficient to identify them.

Wellings and Jensen proposed that CCH/HELUs (which they referred to as atypical lobules type A) are precursors of ADH primarily because of the striking gradual histological continuity between them. Similar continuity is also observed between CCH/HELUs and other alterations of growth in the breast, including microcysts (often with apocrine change) and usual ductal hyperplasia (UDH) (3,7,43,65). However, most CCH/HELUs probably remain stable or become cystic based on the higher incidence of these lesions compared to UDH and (especially) ADH. UDH has also been identified as a weak (approximately 1.5-fold) risk factor for developing breast cancer (9), but the absence of convincing histological continuity with cancer and recent immunohistochemical (IHC) studies suggesting that the progenitor cells in UDH may be different from CCH/HELUs and ADH suggest that UDH may be a side branch of the family tree of ductal cancers

(79,80), and their risk may be due to shared ancestry with CCH/HELUs.

The underlying causes of the hyperplasia leading to CCH/HELUs are unknown. Some evidence suggests that estrogen may be involved, including the observations that CCH/HELUs are more common in premenopausal compared to postmenopausal breasts (3) and in cancerous compared to noncancerous breasts (3,7) where increased estrogen exposure is such a strong risk factor for developing cancer (81). Several recent studies have shown highly elevated expression of ERα in the epithelial cells lining CCH/HELUs (Fig. 23.2) (28,43,64). Essentially all CCH/HELUs express ERα in some cells, and 80% to 90% show very high levels in nearly all cells, which is about threefold above normal (43). They also show a corresponding threefold increase and decrease in average proliferation (about 5%) (Fig. 23.2) and apoptosis (about 0.2%), respectively, although the ranges of these phenomena are quite large (43). Since estrogen, mediated by ERα, stimulates proliferation (38) and suppresses apoptosis (82) in normal cells, elevated ERα in CCH/HELUs may be a fundamental alteration leading to increased growth, although the cause of the elevation is unknown. A recent study in mice overexpressing ERα in normal murine breast epithelium noted the rapid development of hyperplasias, which occasionally progressed to cancer (83), supporting the idea that elevated ERα may be partially responsible for the development and progression of CCH/HELUs. Similar to ERα, recent studies have shown that PR is also highly elevated in CCH/HELUs (28,43), which may also contribute to their growth.

Recent studies have also shown a fivefold increase in the average percentage of ERα-positive proliferating cells in CCH/HELUs (43), suggesting that the regulation of proliferation in these cells is altered or that other pathways have been activated that stimulate proliferation independent of receptor expression. A similar increase in ERα-positive proliferating cells is observed in more advanced precursors (e.g., ADH and DCIS) and IBCs (38,56,84), consistent with the notion that CCH/HELUs are an earlier stage of the same continuum.

Recent microarray studies have identified some of the other pathways and genes that may be involved in the development of CCH/HELUs including, especially, the *erb-b* tyrosine kinases (TKs) (85). For example, compared to normal epithelium, the cells lining CCH/HELUs show a prominent uniform decrease in the expression of epidermal growth factor (EGF) and increase in amphiregulin (AREG), which are important in differentiation of adult breast and embryonic breast development, respectively (85–87). Interestingly, EGF and AREG are both ligands for the *erb-b1* TK receptor (also referred to as the epidermal growth factor receptor). However, the levels of *erb-b1* do not appear to change significantly, nor do the levels of the other *erb-b* TK receptors, including *erb-b2* (also referred to as *HER2* or *ERBB2*), which is amplified and overexpressed in about 20% of DCIS and IBCs. Certain other alterations common in DCIS and IBCs, such as mutation of the p53 tumor suppressor gene, are also rarely if ever observed in CCH/HELUs (28).

Because CCH/HELUs are so common in the population and share important biological characteristics such as highly elevated ERα, their beginnings seem more likely to reflect alterations of development or differentiation than genetic defects *per se*. This idea is supported by the microarray evidence of suppressed differentiation and reactivated embryonic developmental pathways and by the generally low frequency of genetic alterations identified so far. Regardless, the end result is increased growth, creating fertile soil for accumulating random genetic defects, leading to diversity and progression to other types of lesions, including more committed breast cancer precursors such as ADH.

ATYICAL HYPERPLASIAS

ADH and ALH are the two major types of histologically defined atypical hyperplastic lesions with premalignant potential currently recognized in the breast, although, as mentioned, additional research may demonstrate that CCH/HELUs with cytological atypia represent another. They are both rare and their incidence is roughly equal (each is found in 2% to 3% of benign biopsies performed for mammographic abnormalities and even less in random breasts) (3,51,88).

Histologically, ADH are characterized by small, uniform, mildly atypical hyperplastic epithelial cells that pile up on themselves, frequently in cribriform arrangements, mildly distending the ducts and acini they occupy, which are often found within or around CCH/HELUs (Fig. 23.1). Well-differentiated (low-grade) DCIS are characterized by a greater extent of essentially the same features, and the histological distinction between them is based primarily on extent of disease and is entirely artificial (89). By definition, ADH are very small (e.g., <2 mm).

Relatively little is known about the biological features of ADH, primarily because they are so rare, small, and there are few if any representative animal models. However, a few things have been learned, primarily from IHC studies of formalin-fixed paraffin-embedded tissue (FFPET) samples from human patients. For example, IHC studies have shown that essentially 100% of ADH express high levels of ER((Fig. 23.2) and PR in nearly all cells, which is three- to fourfold higher than the average in normal cells (46,90). Average proliferation (about 5%) is also increased two- to threefold above that observed in normal cells (Fig. 23.2) (91,92), and the majority of ER(/PR-positive cells are proliferating (56,84), which is unlike normal and similar to cancer cells. Preliminary studies also suggest that average apoptosis in ADH is decreased two- to threefold relative to normal (93,94), so growth appears to be accomplished through increased proliferation and decreased cell death. These characteristics are all very similar to CCH/HELUs, which is not surprising in the sense that they are thought to be precursors of ADH. The reciprocal changes in the expression of EGF and AREG observed in microarray studies of CCH/HELUs are also present in ADH (85).

The ability of the epithelial cells in ADH to detach from the basement membrane and grow on top of themselves within ducts and acini probably represents a seminal event in the progression from a primarily polyclonal (i.e., CCH/HELUs) to a monoclonal (i.e., ADH) neoplasm, although the fundamental causes are unknown. This idea is reinforced by the relatively high incidence (>50%) of clonal allelic imbalances observed in ADH compared to CCH/HELUs, many of which are shared with DCIS and IBCs, especially when they occur in the same breast, which makes sense if ADH is indeed a precursor of these lesions (1,27,31,95–100). Many chromosomal locations are involved in these imbalances (at least 30 genetic loci on 10 chromosomes) and, although there are a few hot spots with relatively high frequency (e.g., losses on 16q and 17p and gains on 6q), the overall pattern is heterogeneous and the average frequency per lesion is generally low, substantially below that observed DCIS and IBC (27,31). Consistent with this, recent microarray studies also show many similarities in gene expression profiles between ADH, DCIS, and IBC from the same breasts, and only a few stage-specific alterations have been identified (101).

Among the alterations that do appear to distinguish ADH from more advanced lesions are the absence of amplification of the *erb*-b2 oncogene (102–106) and mutation of the p53 tumor suppressor gene (107–109), which are both found in substantial subsets of DCIS and IBC, but even these may have caveats. For example, one study found low-level amplification of *HER2* in the absence of protein overexpression in 50% of ADH from cancer-

ous breasts (106). Another found elevated expression of the signal transduction molecule 14-3-3 zeta in a subset of ADH, which is known to down-regulate p53 expression and perhaps mimic the tumor-promoting effect of mutations (110). Yet another recent study found elevated expression of the COX-2 enzyme in a subset of ADH, and the levels were directly correlated with the risk of developing breast cancer (111). COX-2 is tumorigenic in several preclinical models of various types of cancers (112) and it is elevated in a third or more of clinical breast cancers (113).

ALH, the other major type of atypical hyperplasia, is also characterized histologically by a population of small, uniform, generally well-differentiated epithelial cells, but, unlike ADH, they tend to grow in TDLUS as small solid clusters of loosely cohesive cells, mildly distending the acini (Fig. 23.1) (114). They also occasionally extend into proximal ducts, undermining the normal epithelium (so-called Pagetoid spread). There is no obvious hyperplastic precursor analogous to CCH/HELUs for ALH, and the extent of disease varies from minimal to extensive. Similar to ADH and low-grade DCIS, the diagnostic distinction between ALH and LCIS is artificial and based on extent of disease. By definition, ALH are very small (e.g., involving less than half the acini in a TDLU) (114) and are confined to proximal ducts (115), although some authors consider the latter as LCIS (24). The quantitative continuum of ALH and LCIS is sometimes referred to as lobular neoplasia (116).

Knowledge about the biological characteristics of ALH is very limited for the same reasons as with ADH (rare, small, and no animal models). At least one IHC study of FFPET clinical samples showed that the majority (>90%) express high levels of ERα in nearly all cells (Fig. 23.2) (117). However, several studies have evaluated standard prognostic biomarkers in LCIS (described below), finding highly elevated expression of ERα and PR, low proliferation rates, and normal *erb*-b2 and p53, and the results are probably very similar in ALH. A few studies have assessed allelic imbalances in ALH, finding clonal alterations on several chromosomes (1,98,99,118–120). One loss stands out on chromosome 16q (>50% incidence), which encompasses the E-cadherin gene. This gene encodes a cell adhesion molecule and loss of protein expression, which is nearly universal in ALH and may be fundamental in its development (118,119). Surprisingly, ADH and ALH are both identified in up to 15% of breast biopsies with atypical hyperplasia (88,121), and preliminary studies showing shared chromosomal imbalances suggest that they may be genetically related in unsuspected ways (121).

IN SITU CARCINOMAS

DCIS and LCIS are the two major types of *in situ* carcinomas currently recognized in the breast, although, as mentioned, some CCH/HELUs with cytological atypia may represent another (66,78). DCIS are common, accounting for 20% to 25% of all newly diagnosed breast cancers (122,123). Most DCIS are detected by screening mammography, and they were rare (<5%) prior to such screening (102,122–125). LCIS are rare, accounting for only about 2% to 3% of all newly diagnosed breast cancers, and they are usually encountered incidentally in biopsies or excisions performed for other reasons (126–128).

DCIS show a broad continuum of histological diversity ranging from very well to very poorly differentiated (19,129–132), although, in clinical practice, they are often simply divided into two (e.g., noncomedo vs. comedo) or sometimes three (e.g., low vs. intermediate vs. high grade) categories, which fails to convey this diversity (Fig. 23.1) (132,133). Earlier precursors (i.e., CCH/HELUs and ADH), as they are currently defined, are generally well differentiated, so substantial diversity appears to emerge at the stage of DCIS during breast cancer evolution, although there are still inconsistencies and unknowns. For

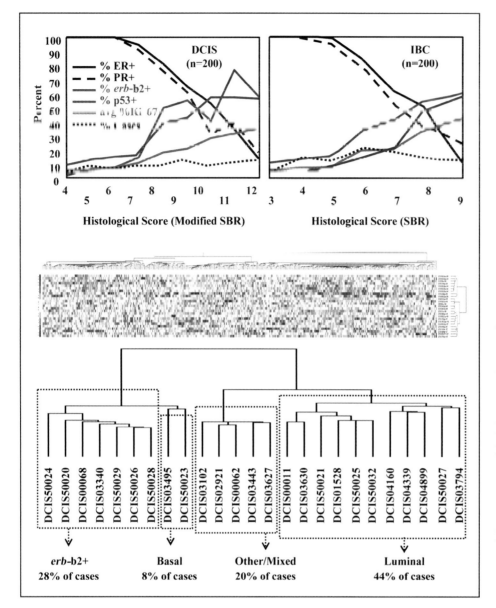

FIGURE 23.3. Standard prognostic biomarkers and intrinsic subtypes in ductal carcinoma *in situ* (**DCIS**). Pure DCIS (upper left histogram) shows a broad distribution of histological differentiation ranging from 4 (the best differentiated) to 12 (the most poorly differentiated), based on a recent study of 200 consecutive cases. SBR, Scarff-Bloom-Richardson. (From Allred DC, Wu Y, Mao S, et al. Ductal carcinoma *in situ* and the emergence of diversity during breast cancer evolution. *Clin Cancer Res* 2008;14:370–378.) Virtually all well-differentiated cases are strongly positive for estrogen receptor alpha (ERα) and progesterone receptor (PR). Receptor-positive cases gradually decline to about 20% in the most poorly differentiated. In contrast, *erb*-b2 and p53 positive cases (amplified/overexpressed and mutated/overexpressed, respectively) are observed in less than 10% of well-differentiated DCIS but gradually increase to about 60% in the most poorly differentiated. Average proliferation rate (% Ki-67 positive cells) also gradually increase from less than 5% to over 30%. Invasive breast cancers (IBCs) show nearly identical phenotypes (upper right histogram), as well as the DCIS component of the IBCs, which is present in nearly all cases (not shown). DCIS also show a similar distribution of luminal, basal, and *erb*-b2+ intrinsic subtypes as observed in previous microarray studies of IBCs (heat map and dendrogram in lower portion of figure).

example, ADH is widely regarded as the nonobligate precursor of low-grade/noncomedo DCIS because they show similar well-differentiated features, but not of high-grade/comedo DCIS, because of their dissimilar poorly differentiated features, leading to speculation that the latter pursue a different course of evolution from occult precursors, and the evolution of intermediate-grade lesions is essentially ignored.

There are strong correlations between histological differentiation in DCIS and standard prognostic biomarkers (Fig. 23.3). Nearly all well-differentiated or low-grade DCIS express high levels of ER and PR in nearly all cells (19,90,129,130,134–143). The proportion of cases expressing these receptors gradually declines to about 20% in the most poorly differentiated lesions, and there is also a decrease in the average proportion of positive cells (129). Alterations of erb-b2 (amplifications or overexpression) (102,105, 107,125,129,134,138,143–153) and p53 (mutations or overexpression) (108,129,134,135,140,142,143,146,153–160) are rare (5% to 10%) in well-differentiated DCIS, but gradually increase to about 60% in the most poorly differentiated lesions (Fig. 23.2). Average proliferation also gradually increases from about 5% to 35% from lowest to highest grade (Fig. 23.2) (129,134,143,146, 149,161,162). Apoptosis varies in the same direction from less

than 1% to over 5% (93,163,164). Apoptosis is quite low (average <1%) in normal cells and earlier precursors, and the substantially elevated levels observed in higher grade DCIS, which obviously have a large positive growth imbalance, points out that the equilibrium between cell proliferation and death may not always be accurately portrayed by the static methods used to measure these dynamic processes.

The correlations between histological differentiation and standard biomarkers in DCIS are nearly identical in IBCs (Fig. 23.3), as well as in the DCIS component of IBCs, which is present in nearly all cases (129). Thus, diversity for these features appears to evolve first in DCIS and is later propagated to IBC, which was proposed at least a decade ago (165). Although these features do not appear to influence the ultimate ability of DCIS to progress to invasive disease, they are associated with the rate of progression, as demonstrated by studies showing a much higher rate of short-term local recurrence in higher-grade DCIS compared to lower-grade lesions treated by lumpectomy, although the rates converge with longer follow-up (166). DCIS and IBCs have also been shown to be very similar at the high resolution of global gene expression evaluated by microarrays and other high throughput technologies, including

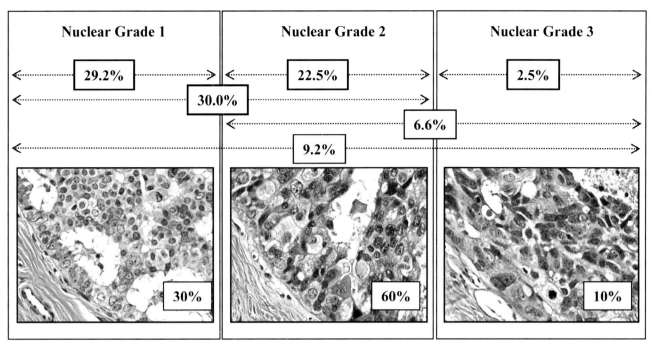

FIGURE 23.4. Histological diversity within ductal carcinoma *in situ* (DCIS). Diversity of histological nuclear grades *within* individual cases of DCIS, based on a recent study of 120 consecutive cases. (From Allred DC, Wu Y, Mao S, et al. Ductal carcinoma *in situ* and the emergence of diversity during breast cancer evolution. *Clin Cancer Res* 2008;14:370–378.) Nearly 50% of cases showed two or more areas with different nuclear grades, which is probably an underestimate since such a small volume of tumor (<1%) was evaluated.

similar distributions of the so-called luminal, basal, and *erb*-b2 intrinsic subtypes (Fig. 23.3) (101,129,167,168).

Understanding the source, magnitude, and characteristics of the diversity in DCIS is important clinically because it may influence the rate of progression to IBC, the sensitivity to specific therapies, and point to new strategies for breast cancer prevention. One compelling hypothesis is that higher-grade DCIS gradually evolve from lower-grade DCIS and, thus, indirectly from ADH, by accumulating random genetic abnormalities over time. This is essentially the hypothesis of *clonal evolution*, which is sometimes regarded as being contrary to the "cancer stem cell" hypothesis (169–171). However, both ideas are based on persuasive evidence and, hopefully, future studies will reconcile some of the apparent inconsistencies (169,170).

Epidemiological evidence supporting this hypothesis comes from studies showing that ADH is a risk factor for developing all histological grades and subtypes of IDCs and, thus, the biological characteristics associated with these histological features (172). If DCIS is the precursor of IDCs, which seems likely, then ADH is probably also a risk factor for the development of DCIS independent of its histological and biological characteristics, although this has not been directly demonstrated because there are no appropriate clinical databases to support such studies.

The enormous range of histological and biological diversity between cases of DCIS also argues against the notion that ADH is a precursor of low-grade but not high-grade lesions in the sense that it fails to explain the cellular origin of the majority of DCIS and because low-grade and high-grade DCIS do not really exist as distinct categories (129). Gradual change from well to poorly differentiated seems more likely for the majority of cases. This argument is based on studies using conventional methodologies that only provide information about the worst differentiated areas or averages of histological and biological features, and they are unable to convey internal diversity. However, if higher-grade do evolve from lower-grade DCIS, then there must be diversity within individual tumors at some point in time and, indeed, recent studies using more refined

methods have shown that at least 50% contain areas showing different histological growth patterns and nuclear grades (Fig. 23.4) (129,173). Furthermore, at least a third of these cases also show diversity for important biological features, including intrinsic subtypes, (luminal, basal, *erb*-b2) when comparing areas with different histological features within individual tumors (Fig. 23.5) (129). The presence and magnitude of internal diversity is highly correlated with mutation of p53, which leads to genetic instability (174,175), suggesting that randomly acquired defects with this outcome (and there are many possibilities) may enable or accelerate the development of diversity in DCIS. The presence of this diversity also suggests that there is considerable plasticity during tumor progression, and presumably regions with different characteristics would compete for dominance and eventually the most aggressive or poorly differentiated area would prevail. Well-differentiated DCIS may progress to more poorly differentiated DCIS by this general mechanism, and it seems likely that similar mechanisms are at work in IBCs as well. In addition, this mechanism may be responsible for the development of a substantial proportion of ERα-negative breast cancers from ERα-positive precursors (i.e., DCIS and IBCs). If true, it suggests that hormonal chemoprevention (e.g., tamoxifen) in high-risk women may eventually decrease both ERα-positive and ERα-negative breast cancers.

Other evidence supporting the idea that higher-grade evolve from lower-grade DCIS comes from studies showing that diversity increases with time. For example, a diagnosis of DCIS was rare (5%) before but common (20% to 25%) after the introduction of screening mammography (122,123). On average, DCIS was much larger and more poorly differentiated in the premammography era than it is today (102,123–125), which is also true for IBCs (123,124,176). These changes are consistent with the idea that early detection by screening mammography identifies lower-grade lesions before they progress to a higher grade.

Studies of allelic imbalance by loss of heterozygosity and comparative genomic hybridization have shown that nearly all DCIS contain multiple clonal genetic abnormalities. The

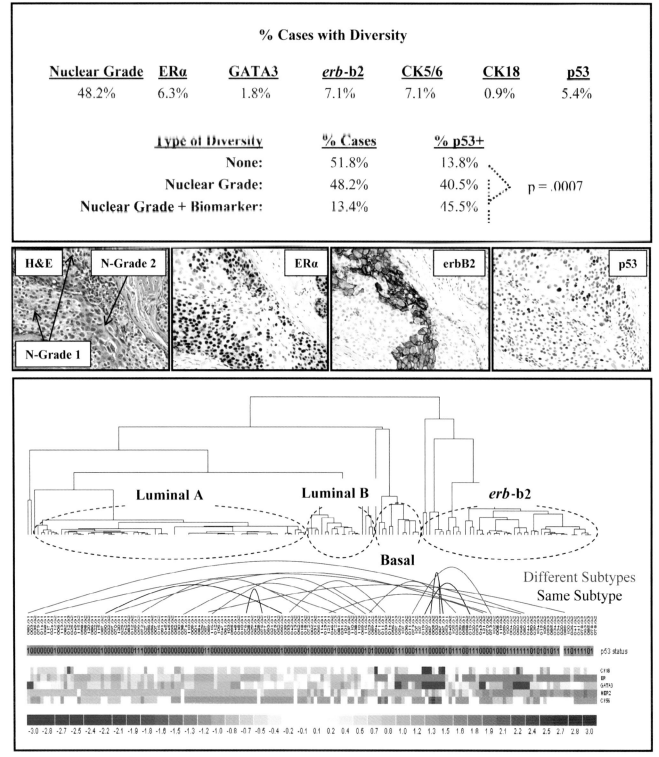

FIGURE 23.5. Histological and molecular diversity within ductal carcinoma *in situ* (DCIS). Diversity of histological nuclear grades, biomarkers, and intrinsic subtypes within individual cases of DCIS, based on a recent study of 120 consecutive cases. (From Allred DC, Wu Y, Mao S, et al. Ductal carcinoma *in situ* and the emergence of diversity during breast cancer evolution. *Clin Cancer Res* 2008;14:370–378.) Nearly 50% of cases showed two or more areas with different nuclear grades. Furthermore, nearly a third of these cases also showed internal diversity (positive to negative or the opposite) for one or more biomarkers when comparing areas with different nuclear grades. For example, the photomicrographs show a DCIS with cells of different nuclear grades (grades 1 and 2) in the same duct. The different cells show reciprocal expression of estrogen receptor alpha (ERα) and *erb*-b2, while both are positive (i.e., mutated) for p53. Mutation of p53, which results in genetic instability, was highly correlated with the presence and magnitude of any type of diversity. The majority of cases with internal diversity of nuclear grade and biomarkers also showed two or more intrinsic subtypes (luminal, basal, *erb*-b2). All of this diversity shows that that there is considerable plasticity during tumor progression and presumably different areas would compete for dominance and eventually the most aggressive would prevail. Higher grade DCIS may gradually evolve from lower grade DCIS by this general mechanism, and it is likely that similar evolution is present in invasive breast cancers. H&E, hematoxylin-eosin stained; N-grade, nuclear grade; GATA3; GATA binding protein 3; CK5/6, cytokeratin 5/6; CK18, cytokeratin 18.

complexity of the imbalances is very large, involving at least 100 genetic loci on 17 chromosomes (27,30,36,37,79,177–184), which rivals that observed in IBCs. Although this complexity suggests that there is a prominent randomness to the damage, there are hot spots on chromosomes 16q, 17p, and 17q where the overall incidence exceeds 40% (27,36). Interestingly, the identity of the majority of defects appears to be independent of histological differentiation, although the absolute number of defects is higher in more poorly differentiated lesions (27,36,129). One of the hot spots (17p loss) spans the p53 locus, and DCIS with this defect shows at least twice the frequency of imbalances as those without (129), again suggesting that genetic instability and the passage of time are plausible mechanisms for the progression of lower-grade to higher-grade DCIS.

LCIS is the other major type of *in situ* carcinoma. As mentioned, its histological features are qualitatively similar to ALH, but quantitatively greater in extent, and the distinction is artificial (Fig. 23.1) (114,185). Far less is known about the biological alterations in LCIS than DCIS, although several studies have characterized standard prognostic biomarkers. Nearly all (90% to 100%) LCIS express high levels of ERα in nearly all cells (Fig. 23.2) (18,43,137,141,164,186–189), and a large majority (80% to 90%) also express PR in a majority of cells (186). Alterations of *erb*-b2 (104,105,150,152,186,190–192) and p53 are both rare (about 5%) (186,193,194). Proliferation is very low, averaging about 2%, similar to normal epithelium (Fig. 23.2) (186–188,190). Several studies have also evaluated allelic imbalance in LCIS (29,118–120,186,195,196). The majority (>75%) of cases show chromosomal losses or gains that collectively involve at least 13 chromosomes and, interestingly, several overlap with those observed in DCIS. The most frequent (>60% incidence) imbalance involves loss of 16q (29,119,121). As mentioned in the discussion of ALH, this loss encompasses the E-cadherin gene, which is an important cell adhesion molecule, and it may be fundamental to lobular neoplasia, although it is also observed at somewhat lower frequency in ADH and DCIS (27,186). However, a large majority (about 90%) of ALH and LCIS also show a complete loss of protein expression for E-cadherin, while a similar majority of ADH and DCIS express it at high levels. The loss at 16q is often associated with mutation of the other allele in LCIS, although the latter appears to be much less frequent in ALH (119,197).

See Chapters 24 to 26 of this book for more discussion of DCIS and LCIS.

PROGRESSION TO INVASION

The progression of *in situ* to invasive carcinomas is one of the most important steps in breast cancer evolution because it transforms an essentially harmless growth into a potentially lethal disease. The cellular and molecular alterations responsible for tumor invasion are a fascinating and evolving story (198,199), which is far beyond the scope of this chapter, although a few general comments are relevant. For one, the vast majority of molecular alterations identified in the epithelium of *in situ* and invasive breast cancers are identical (27,101,168), which is surprising in the sense that invasion is such an enormous difference. This is true at any level of technological resolution ranging from individual mutations to global gene expression profiles. Obviously, however, there must be differences responsible for invasion, but they have been surprisingly difficult to identify so far. One of the most important advances in this field is the relatively recent understanding that surrounding stromal cells are playing an active critical role in tumor invasion (200). There are many types of stromal cells in

the breast, including fibroblasts, smooth muscle, endothelium, neurons, and macrophages, among others. Collectively, they perform many functions, including the secretion of extracellular matrix, which consists of many structural and regulatory proteins. In response to traumatic tissue injury, many of these cells and proteins are activated to enable wound healing (201). Interestingly, there are many similarities between the stroma of invasive carcinomas and healing wounds (202,203). For example, carcinoma-associated fibroblasts (CAFs) from several types of tumors, including breast cancer, show elevated expression of many growth factors involved in wound healing, as well as other similarities (204,205). CAFs can even promote benign epithelial cells to form invasive carcinomas in certain xenografts models (206), which is an unequivocal demonstration of the importance of stromal cells to tumor progression. Clonal genetic alterations (e.g., mutations, allelic imbalances, etc.) are essentially always found in the epithelium of invasive carcinomas (170,207), but rarely if ever in the stromal cells (207–209). These epithelial alterations are central to the development and progression of carcinomas, including progression to invasion, although the specific alterations that activate the stroma are largely unknown and the focus of considerable research today.

SUMMARY

Most breast cancers appear to evolve in a nonobligatory manner from normal cells through a series of increasingly abnormal stages or precursor lesions over long periods of time, probably decades in most cases. The key stages in this progression are generically referred to as hyperplasias, atypical hyperplasias, *in situ* carcinomas, and invasive carcinomas. There are important general characteristics that distinguish one stage from the next that accumulate and increase with progression. The transition from normal cells to hyperplasias is characterized by increased growth due to epithelial hyperplasia. Hyperplasias are very common and may be due to delayed differentiation rather than genetic damage *per se*, creating fertile soil for the accumulation of random genetic mutations, leading to diversity and progression to more advanced clonal precursors. Alterations of cell adhesion and polarity distinguish atypical hyperplasias from hyperplasias as the epithelium begins to pile up and distend acini. *In situ* carcinomas are characterized by further growth and the appearance of enormously increased histological and biological diversity compared to earlier precursors, which may be accelerated by acquiring mutations resulting in genetic instability. Invasion into surrounding stroma defines the transition from *in situ* to invasive carcinomas and genetic alterations in tumor epithelium appear to induce the participation of stromal cells in this process. Identifying the biological alterations associated with early precursors before the development of substantial diversity may reveal effective strategies for preventing the majority of breast cancers, and some progress has already been made. For example, ERα is highly elevated in nearly all early precursors, and drugs targeting this receptor (e.g., tamoxifen) reduce breast cancer by 50% in recent chemoprevention trials of high risk women (210,211). Unfortunately, most defects responsible for the development and progression of premalignant breast disease remain unknown and, hopefully, future studies will shed light on these important issues.

ACKNOWLEDGMENTS

This work was supported by the Breast Cancer Research Foundation.

References

1. Allred DC, Hilsenbeck SG, Mohsin SK. Biologic features of human premalignant breast disease. In: Harris JR, Lippman ME, Morrow M, et al. eds. *Diseases of the breast*. 3rd ed. Philadelphia: Lippincott Williams & Wilkins, 2004:512–513.
2. Wellings RR, Jensen HM. On the origin and progression of ductal carcinoma in the human breast. *J Natl Cancer Inst* 1973;50:1111–1118.
3. Wellings SR, Jensen HM, Marcum RG. An atlas of subgross pathology of the human breast with special reference to possible precancerous lesions. *J Natl Cancer Inst* 1975;55:231–273.
4. Rudland PS. Epithelial stem cells and their possible role in the development of the normal and diseased breast. *Histol Histopath* 1993;8:385–404.
5. Alpers CE, Wellings SR. The prevalence of carcinoma *in situ* in normal and cancer-associated breasts. *Hum Pathol* 1985;16:796–807.
6. Foote FW, Stewart FW. Comparative studies of cancerous versus noncancerous breasts. *Ann Surg* 1945;121:6–53, 197–222.
7. Shaaban AM, Sloane JP, West CR, et al. Breast cancer risk in usual ductal hyperplasia is defined by estrogen receptor-alpha and Ki-67 expression. *Am J Pathol* 2002;160:597–604.
8. Dupont WD, Page DL. Risk factors for breast cancer in women with proliferative breast disease. *N Engl J Med* 1985;312:146–151.
9. Dupont WD, Parl FF, Hartmann WH, et al. Breast cancer risk associated with proliferative breast disease and atypical hyperplasia. *Cancer* 1993;71:1258–1265.
10. London SJ, Connolly JL, Schnitt SJ, et al. A prospective study of benign breast disease and the risk of breast cancer. *JAMA* 1992;267:941–944.
11. Page DL, Dupont WD. Anatomic indicators (histologic and cytologic) of increased breast cancer risk. *Breast Cancer Res Treat* 1993;28:157–166.
12. Page DL, Dupont WD, Rogers LW. Breast cancer risk of lobular-based hyperplasia after biopsy: "ductal" pattern lesions. *Cancer Detect Prev* 1986;9:441–448.
13. Page DL, Dupont WD, Rogers LW, et al. Atypical hyperplastic lesions of the female breast. A long-term follow-up study. *Cancer* 1985;55:2698–2708.
14. Page DL, Dupont WD, Rogers LW, et al. Intraductal carcinoma of the breast: follow-up after biopsy only. *Cancer* 1982;49:751–758.
15. Page DL, Zwaag RV, Rogers LW, et al. Relation between component parts of fibrocystic disease complex and breast cancer. *J Natl Cancer Inst* 1978;61: 1055–1063.
16. Palli D, del Turco MR, Simonciini R, et al. Benign breast disease and breast cancer: a case-control study in a cohort in Italy. *Int J Cancer* 1991;47:703–706.
17. Degnim AC, Visscher DW, Berman HK, et al. Stratification of breast cancer risk in women with atypia: a Mayo cohort study. *J Clin Oncol* 2007;25:2671–2677.
18. Middleton LP, Grant S, Stephens T, et al. Lobular carcinoma *in situ* diagnosed by core needle biopsy: when should it be excised? *Mod Pathol* 2003;16:120–129.
19. Ottensen GL, Christensen IJ, Larsen JK, et al. Carcinoma *in situ* of the breast: correlation of histopathology to immunohistochemical markers and DNA ploidy. *Breast Cancer Res Treat* 2000;60:219–226.
20. Page DL, Schuyler PA, Dupont WD, et al. Atypical lobular hyperplasia as a unilateral predictor of breast cancer risk: a retrospective cohort study. *Lancet* 2003;361:125–129.
21. Selim AA, El-Ayat G, Wells CA. Immunohistochemical localization of gross cystic disease fluid protein-15, -24 and -44 in ductal carcinoma *in situ* of the breast: relationship to the degree of differentiation. *Histopathology* 2001;39:198–202.
22. Shin SJ, Rosen PP. Excisional biopsy should be performed if lobular carcinoma *in situ* is seen on needle core biopsy. *Arch Pathol Lab Med* 2002;126:697–701.
23. Li CI, Malone KE, Saltzman BS, et al. Risk of invasive breast carcinoma among women diagnosed with ductal carcinoma *in situ* and lobular carcinoma *in situ*, 1988–2001. *Cancer* 2006;106:2104–2112.
24. Bestill WL Jr, Rosen PP, Lieberman PH, et al. Intraductal carcinoma: long-term follow-up after treatment by biopsy alone. *JAMA* 1978;239:1863–1867.
25. Rosen PP, Braun DW Jr, Kinne DE. The clinical significance of preinvasive breast carcinomas. *Cancer* 1980;46[Suppl 4]:919–925.
26. Moinfar F, Man YG, Arnould L, et al. Concurrent and independent genetic alterations in the stromal and epithelial cells of mammary carcinoma: implications for tumorigenesis. *Cancer Res* 2000;60:2562–2566.
27. O'Connell P, Pekkel V, Fuqua SAW, et al. Analysis of loss of heterozygosity in 399 premalignant breast lesions at 15 genetic loci. *J Natl Cancer Inst* 1998;90: 697–703.
28. Simpson PT, Gale T, Reis-Filho JS, et al. Columnar cell lesions of the breast: the missing link in breast cancer progression? A morphological and molecular analysis. *Am J Surg Pathol* 2005;29:734–746.
29. Hwang SE, Nyante SJ, Yi Chen Y, et al. Clonality of lobular carcinoma *in situ* and synchronous invasive lobular carcinoma. *Cancer* 2004;100:2562–2572.
30. Waldman FM, DeVries S, Chew KL, et al. Chromosomal alterations in ductal carcinomas *in situ* and their *in situ* recurrences. *J Natl Cancer Inst* 2000;92: 313–320.
31. Larson PS, de las Morenas A, Cerda SR, et al. Quantitative analysis of allele imbalance supports atypical ductal hyperplasia lesions as direct breast cancer precursors. *J Pathol* 2006;209:307–316.
32. Cardiff RD. Genetically engineered mouse models of mammary intraepithelial neoplasia. *J Mammary Gland Biol Neoplasia* 2000;5:421–437.
33. Medina D. The preneoplasitc phenotype in murine mammary tumorigenesis. *J Mammary Gland Biol Neoplasia* 2000;5:393–407.
34. Miller FR. Xenograft models of premalignant breast disease. *J Mammary Gland Biol Neoplasia* 2000;5:379–391.
35. Amari M, Moriya T, Ishida T, et al. Loss of heterozygosity analyses of asynchronous lesions of ductal carcinoma *in situ* and invasive ductal carcinoma of the human breast. *Jpn J Clin Oncol* 2003;33:556–562.
36. Hwang ES, DeVries S, Chew KL, et al. Patterns of chromosomal alterations in breast ductal carcinoma *in situ*. *Clin Cancer Res* 2004;10:5160–5167.
37. Smeds J, Warnberg F, Norberg T, et al. Ductal carcinoma *in situ* of the breast with different histopathological grades and corresponding new breast tumour events: analysis of loss of heterozygosity. *Acta Oncol* 2005;44:41–49.
38. Anderson E, Clarke RB. Steroid receptors and cell cycle in normal mammary epithelium. *J Mammary Gland Biol Neoplasia* 2004;9:3–13.
39. Henderson BE, Ross R, Bernstein L. Estrogens as a cause of human cancer: the Richard and Hindau Rosenthal Foundation Award Lecture. *Cancer Res* 1988;48: 246–253.
40. Pike MC, Spicer DV, Dahmoush L, et al. Estrogens, progestins, normal breast cell proliferation, and breast cancer risk. *Epidemiol Rev* 1993;15:17–35.
41. Hall JM, McDonnell DP. Coregulators in nuclear estrogen receptor action: from concept to therapeutic targeting. *Mol Interv* 2005;5:343–357.
42. Allegra JC, Lippman ME, Green L, et al. Estrogen receptor values in patients with benign breast disease. *Cancer* 1979;44:228–231.
43. Lee S, Mohsin SK, Mao S, et al. Hormones, receptors, and growth in hyperplastic enlarged lobular units: early potential precursors of breast cancer. *Breast Cancer Res* 2006;8(1):R6.
44. Peterson OW, Hoyer PE, van Deurs B. Frequency and distribution of estrogen receptor-positive cells in normal, nonlactating human breast tissue. *J Natl Cancer Inst* 1986;77:343–349.
45. Ricketts D, Turnbull L, Tyall G, et al. Estrogen and progesterone receptors in the normal female breast. *Cancer Res* 1991;51:1817–1822.
46. Schmitt FC. Multistep progression from an oestrogen-dependent growth towards an autonomous growth in breast carcinogenesis. *Eur J Cancer* 1995;31A: 2049–2052.
47. Ferguson DJP, Anderson TJ. Morphological evaluation of cell turnover in relation to the menstrual cycle in the "resting" human breast. *Br J Cancer* 1981;44: 177–181.
48. Going JJ, Anderson TJ, Battersby S, et al. Proliferative and secretory activity in human breast during natural and artificial cycles. *Am J Pathol* 1988;130: 193–201.
49. Joshi K, Smith JA, Perusinghe N, et al. Cell proliferation in the human mammary epithelium: differential contribution by epithelial and myoepithelial cells. *Am J Pathol* 1986;124:199–206.
50. Kamel OW, Franklin WA, Ringus JC, et al. Thymidine labeling index and Ki-67 growth fraction in lesions of the breast. *Am J Pathol* 1989;134:107–113.
51. Longacre TA, Bartow SA. A correlative morphologic study of human breast and endometrium in the menstrual cycle. *Am J Surg Pathol* 1986;10:382–393.
52. Meyer JS. Cell proliferation in normal human breast ducts, fibroadenomas, and other ductal hyperplasias measured by nuclear labeling with tritiated thymidine. *Hum Pathol* 1977;8:67–81.
53. Potten CS, Watson RJ, Williams GT, et al. The effect of age and menstrual cycle upon proliferative activity of the normal human breast. *Br J Cancer* 1988;58: 163–170.
54. Russo J, Calaf GRL, Russo IH. Influence of age and gland topography on cell kinetics of normal breast tissue. *J Natl Cancer Inst* 1987;78:413–418.
55. Anderson E. The role of oestrogen and progesterone receptors in human mammary development and tumorigenesis. *Breast Cancer Res* 2002;4:197–201.
56. Clarke RB, Howell A, Potten CS, et al. Dissociation between steroid receptor expression and cell proliferation in the human breast. *Cancer Res* 1997;57: 4987–4991.
57. Ewan KBR, Oketch-Rabah HA, Ravani SA, et al. TGF-β1 restrains proliferation of estrogen receptor-α–positive mammary epithelial cells. *Am J Pathol* 2005;167: 409–417.
58. Deng G, Lu Y, Zlotnikov G, et al. Loss of heterozygosity in normal tissue adjacent to breast carcinomas. *Science* 1996;274:2057–2059.
59. Larson PS, de las Morenas A, Bennett SR, et al. Loss of heterozygosity or allele imbalance in histologically normal breast epithelium is distinct from loss of heterozygosity or allele imbalance in co-existing carcinomas. *Am J Pathol* 2002;161: 283–290.
60. Larson PS, Schlechter BL, de las Morenas A, et al. Allele imbalance, or loss of heterozygosity, in normal breast epithelium of sporadic breast cancer cases and *BRCA1* gene mutation carriers is increased compared with reduction mammoplasty tissues. *J Clin Oncol* 2005;23:8613–8619.
61. Bean GR, Bryson AD, Pilie PG, et al. Morphologically normal-appearing mammary epithelial cells obtained from high-risk women exhibit methylation silencing of INK4a/ARF. *Clin Cancer Res* 2007;13:6834–6841.
62. Crawford YG, Gauthier ML, Joubel A, et al. Histologically normal human mammary epithelia with silenced p16(INK4a) overexpress COX-2, promoting a premalignant program. *Cancer Cell* 2004;5:263–273.
63. Holst CR, Nuovo GJ, Esteller M, et al. Methylation of p16(INK4a) promoters occurs *in vivo* in histologically normal human mammary epithelia. *Cancer Res* 2003;63:1596–1601.
64. Feeley L, Quinn CM. Columnar cell lesions of the breast. *Histopathology* 2008;52: 11–19.
65. Nasser SM. Columnar cell lesions: current classification and controversies. *Semin Diagn Pathol* 2004;21:18–24.
66. Schnitt SJ. Flat epithelial atypia—classification, pathologic features and clinical significance. *Breast Cancer Res* 2003;5:263–268.
67. Tan PH, Ho BC, Selvarajan S, et al. Pathological diagnosis of columnar cell lesions of the breast: are there issues of reproducibility? *J Clin Pathol* 2005;58:705–709.
68. Bloodgood JC. Senile parenchymatous hypertrophy of female breast. Its relation to cyst formation and carcinoma. *Surg Gynecol Obstet* 1906;3:721–730.
69. Cheatle GL. Cysts, and primary cancer in cysts, of the breast. *Br J Surg* 1920;8: 149–166.
70. McLaren BK, Gobbi H, Schuyler PA, et al. Immunohistochemical expression of estrogen receptor in enlarged lobular units with columnar alteration in benign breast biopsies: a nested case-control study. *Am J Surg Pathol* 2005;29:105–108.
71. Bandyopadhyay S, Chivukula M, Dabbs DJ. Significance of atypical columnar cell change in core needle biopsies of breast. *Mod Pathol* 2007;20:23A.
72. Eradat J, Shamonki JM, Bassett LW, et al. Columnar cell lesions in breast core needle biopsy and the predictive value for unsampled ductal carcinoma. *Mod Pathol* 2007;20:30A.
73. Guerra-Wallace MM, Christensen WN, White RI. A retrospective study of columnar alteration with prominent apical snouts and secretions and the association with cancer. *Am J Surg* 2004;188:395–398.
74. Kunju LP, Kleer CG. Significance of flat epithelial atypia on mammatome core needle biopsy: should it be excised? *Hum Pathol* 2007;38:35–41.
75. Purdy KE, Nasser A, Logani S. Columnar cell lesions (CCL) with and without atypia in needle core biopsy of the breast: when is excision appropriate? *Mod Pathol* 2007;20:46A.
76. Eusebi V, Feudale E, Foschini MP, et al. Long-term follow-up of *in situ* carcinoma of the breast. *Semin Diagn Pathol* 1994;11:223–235.
77. BijKer N, Peterse JL, Duchateau L, et al. Risk factors for recurrence and metastasis after breast-conserving therapy for ductal carcinoma *in situ*: analysis of European Organization for Research and Treatment of Cancer Trial 10853. *J Clin Oncol* 2001;19:2263–2271.
78. Schnitt SJ. Columnar cell lesions of the breast: pathological features and clinical significance. *Curr Diagn Pathol* 2004;10:193–203.

79. Boecker W, Buerger H, Schmitz K, et al. Ductal epithelial proliferations of the breast: a biological continuum? Comparative genomic hybridization and high-molecular-weight cytokeratin expression patterns. *J Pathol* 2001;195:415–421.
80. Boecker W, Moll R, Dervan P, et al. Usual ductal hyperplasia of the breast is a committed stem (progenitor) cell lesion distinct from atypical ductal hyperplasia and ductal carcinoma *in situ*. *J Pathol* 2002;198:458–467.
81. Martin AM, Weber BL. Genetic and hormonal risk factors in breast cancer. *J Natl Cancer Inst* 2000;92:1126–1135.
82. Gompel A, Somai S, Chaouat M, et al. Hormonal regulation of apoptosis in breast cells and tissues. *Steroids* 2000;65:593–598.
83. Frech MS, Halama ED, Tilli MT, et al. Deregulated estrogen receptor alpha expression in mammary epithelial cells of transgenetic mice results in the development of ductal carcinoma *in situ*. *Cancer Res* 2005;65:681–685.
84. Shocker BS, Jarvis C, Clarke RB, et al. Estrogen receptor-positive proliferating cells in the normal and precancerous breast. *Am J Pathol* 1999;155:1811–1815.
85. Lee S, Medina D, Tsimelzon A, et al. Alterations of gene expression in the development of early hyperplastic precursors of breast cancer. *Am J Pathol* 2007;171:252–262.
86. Luetteke NC, Qiu TH, Fenton SE, et al. Targeted inactivation of the EGF and amphiregulin genes reveals distinct roles for EGF receptor ligands in mouse mammary gland development. *Development* 1999;126:2739–2750.
87. Troyer KL, Lee DC. Regulation of mouse mammary gland development and tumorigenesis by the ERBB signaling network. *J Mammary Gland Biol Neoplasia* 2001;6:7–21.
88. Arpino G, Allred DC, Mohsin SK, et al. Lobular neoplasia on core-needle biopsy—clinical significance. *Cancer* 2004;101:242–250.
89. Rogers LW. Epithelial hyperplasia: atypical ductal hyperplasia. In: Page DL, Anderson TJ, eds. *Diagnostic histopathology of the breast*. Edinburgh: Churchill Livingstone, 1987:137–145.
90. Barnes R, Masood S. Potential value of hormone receptor assay in carcinoma *in situ* of breast. *Am J Clin Pathol* 1990;94:533–537.
91. De Potter CR, Praet MM, Slavin RE, et al. Feulgen DNA content and mitotic activity in proliferative breast disease: a comparison with ductal carcinoma *in situ*. *Histopathology* 1987;7:1307–1319.
92. Hoshi K, Tokunaga M, Mochizuki M, et al. Pathological characterization of atypical ductal hyperplasia of the breast. *Jpn J Cancer Chemother* 1995;22[Suppl 1]:36–41.
93. Bai M, Agnantis NJ, Sevasti K, et al. *In vivo* cell kinetics in breast carcinogenesis. *Breast Cancer Res* 2001;3:276–283.
94. Prosser J, Hilsenbeck SG, Fuqua SAW, et al. Cell turnover (proliferation and apoptosis) in normal epithelium and premalignant lesions in the same breast. *Lab Invest* 1997;76:119(abst124A).
95. Amari M, Suzuki A, Moriya T, et al. LOH analyses of premalignant and malignant lesions of human breast: frequent LOH in 8p, 16q, and 17q in atypical ductal hyperplasia. *Oncol Rep* 1999;6:1277–1280.
96. Chauqui RF, Zhuang Z, Emmert-Buck MR, et al. Analysis of loss of heterozygosity on chromosome 11q13 in atypical ductal hyperplasia and *in situ* carcinoma of the breast. *Am J Pathol* 1997;150:297–303.
97. Lakhani SR, Collins N, Stratton MR, et al. Atypical ductal hyperplasia of the breast: clonal proliferation with loss of heterozygosity on chromosomes 16q and 17p. *J Clin Pathol* 1995;48:611–615.
98. Rosenberg CL, de las Morenas A, Huang K, et al. Detection of monoclonal microsatellite alterations in atypical breast hyperplasia. *J Clin Invest* 1996;98:1095–1100.
99. Rosenberg CL, Larson PS, Romo JD, et al. Microsatellite alterations indicating monoclonality in atypical hyperplasias associated with breast cancer. *Hum Pathol* 1997;28:214–219.
100. Tsuda H, Takarabe T, Akashi-Tanaka S, et al. Pattern of chromosome 16q loss differs between an atypical proliferative lesion and an intraductal or invasive ductal carcinoma occurring subsequently in the same area of the breast. *Mod Pathol* 2001;14:382–388.
101. Ma XJ, Salunga R, Tuggle JT, et al. Gene expression profiles of human breast cancer progression. *Proc Natl Acad Sci U S A* 2003;100:5974–5979.
102. Allred DC, Clark GM, Molina R, et al. Overexpression of *HER-2/neu* and its relationship with other prognostic factors change during the progression of *in situ* to invasive breast cancer. *Hum Pathol* 1992;23:974–979.
103. De Potter CR, van Daele S, van de Vijer MJ, et al. The expression of the *neu* oncogene product in breast lesions and in normal fetal and adult human tissues. *Histopathology* 1989;15:351–362.
104. Gusterson BA, Machin LG, Gullick WJ, et al. c-*erb*B-2 expression in benign and malignant breast disease. *Br J Cancer* 1988;58:453–457.
105. Lodato RF, Maguire Jr HC, Greene MI, et al. Immunohistochemical evaluation of c-*erb*B-2 oncogene expression in ductal carcinoma *in situ* and atypical ductal hyperplasia of the breast. *Mod Pathol* 1990;3:449–454.
106. Xu R, Perle MA, Inghirami G, et al. Amplification of *HER-2/neu* gene in *HER-2/neu*-overexpressing and -nonexpressing breast carcinomas and their synchronous benign, premalignant, and metastatic lesions detected by FISH in archival material. *Mod Pathol* 2002;15:116–124.
107. Barnes DM, Hanby AM, Gillett CE, et al. Abnormal expression of wild type p53 protein in normal cells of a cancer family patient. *Lancet* 1992;340:259–263.
108. Chitemere M, Andersen TI, Hom R, et al. TP53 alterations atypical ductal hyperplasia and ductal carcinoma *in situ* of the breast. *Breast Cancer Res Treat* 1996;41:103–109.
109. Umekita Y, Takasaki T, Yoshida H. Expression of p53 protein in benign epithelial hyperplasia, atypical ductal hyperplasia, non-invasive and invasive mammary carcinoma: an immunohistochemical study. *Virchows Arch* 1994;424:491–494.
110. Danes CG, Wyszomierski SL, Lu J, et al. 14-3-3 zeta down-regulates p53 in mammary epithelial cells and confers luminal filling. *Cancer Res* 2008;68:1760–1767.
111. Visscher DW, Pankratz VS, Santisteban M, et al. Association between cyclooxygenase-2 expression in atypical hyperplasia and risk of breast cancer. *J Natl Cancer Inst* 2008;100:421–427.
112. Howe LR. Cyclooxygenase/prostaglandin signaling and breast cancer. *Breast Cancer Res* 2007;9:210–219.
113. Ristimaki A, Sivula A, Lundin J, et al. Prognostic significance of elevated cyclooxygenase-2 expression in breast cancer. *Cancer Res* 2002;62:632–635.
114. Rogers LW. Epithelial hyperplasia: atypical lobular hyperplasia. In: Page DL, Anderson TJ, eds. *Diagnostic histopathology of the breast*. Edinburgh: Churchill Livingstone, 1987:145–156.
115. Page DL, Kidd TE, Jr., Dupont WD, et al. Lobular neoplasia of the breast: higher risk for subsequent invasive cancer predicted by more extensive disease. *Hum Pathol* 1991;22:1232–1239.
116. Haagensen CD, Lane N, Lattes R, et al. Lobular neoplasia (so-called lobular carcinoma *in situ*) of the breast. *Cancer* 1978;42:737–769.
117. Nonni A, Zagouri F, Sergentanis TN, et al. Immunohistochemical expression of estrogen receptors alpha and beta in lobular neoplasia. *Virchows Arch* 2007;451:893–897.
118. Mastracci TL, Shadeo A, Colby SM, et al. Genomic alterations in lobular neoplasia: a microarray comparative genomic hybridization signature for early neoplastic proliferation in the breast. *Genes Chromosomes Cancer* 2006;45:1007–1017.
119. Mastracci TL, Tjan S, Bane AL, et al. E-cadherin alterations in atypical lobular hyperplasia and lobular carcinoma *in situ* of the breast. *Mod Pathol* 2005;18:741–751.
120. Nayar R, Zhuang Z, Merino MJ, et al. Loss of heterozygosity on chromosome 11q13 in lobular lesions of the breast using tissue microdissection and polymerase chain reaction. *Hum Pathol* 1997;28:277–282.
121. Mohsin SK, Arbab R, Allred DC. Are synchronous atypical ductal hyperplasia and atypical lobular hyperplasia (which are common) genetically related? *Mod Pathol* 2005;18:44A(abst189).
122. Ernster VL, Barclay J. Increases in ductal carcinoma *in situ* (DCIS) of the breast in relation to mammography: a dilemma. *Natl Cancer Inst Monogr* 1997;22:151–156.
123. Ries LAG, Eisner MP, Kosary CL. *SEER cancer statistics review 1975–2000*. Bethesda, MD: National Cancer Institute, 2003.
124. Society AC. *Breast cancer facts and figures 2005–2006*. Atlanta: American Cancer Society, 2005.
125. van de Vijver MJ, Peterse JL, Mooi WJ, et al. Neu-protein overexpression in breast cancer. Association with comedo-type ductal carcinoma *in situ* and limited prognostic value in stage II breast cancer. *N Engl J Med* 1988;319:1239–1245.
126. Anderson BO, Rinn K, Georgian-Smith D, et al. Lobular carcinoma *in situ*. In: Silverstein MJ, Recht A, Lagios MD, eds. *Ductal carcinoma of the breast*. Philadelphia: Lippincott, 2002:615–634.
127. Schnitt SJ, Morrow M. Lobular carcinoma *in situ*: current concepts and controversies. *Semin Diagn Pathol* 1999;16:209–223.
128. Wood WC. Management of lobular carcinoma *in situ* and ductal carcinoma *in situ* of the breast. *Sem Oncol* 1996;23:446–452.
129. Allred DC, Wu Y, Mao S, et al. Ductal carcinoma *in situ* and the emergence of diversity during breast cancer evolution. *Clin Cancer Res* 2008;14:370–378.
130. Leong AS, Sormunen RT, Vinyuvat S, et al. Biologic markers in ductal carcinoma *in situ* and concurrent infiltrating carcinoma. A comparison of eight contemporary grading systems. *Am J Clin Pathol* 2001;115:709–718.
131. Mack L, Kerkvliet N, Doig G, et al. Relationship of a new histological categorization of ductal carcinoma *in situ* of the breast with size and the immunohistochemical expression of p53, c-*erb* B2, bcl-2, and Ki-67. *Hum Pathol* 1997;28:974–979.
132. Moreno A, Lloveras B, Figueras A, et al. Ductal carcinoma *in situ* of the breast: correlation between histologic classifications and biologic markers. *Mod Pathol* 1997;10:1088–1092.
133. Silverstein MJ, Cohlan BF, Gierson ED, et al. Duct carcinoma *in situ*: 227 cases without microinvasion. *Eur J Cancer* 1992;28:630–634.
134. Albonico G, Querzoli P, Feretti S, et al. Biophenotypes of breast carcinoma *in situ* defined by image analysis of biological parameters. *Path Res Pract* 1996;192:117–123.
135. Bose S, Lesser ML, Norton L, et al. Immunophenotype of intraductal carcinoma. *Arch Pathol Lab Med* 1996;120:81–85.
136. Chaudhuri B, Crist KA, Mucci S, et al. Distribution of estrogen receptor in ductal carcinoma *in situ* of the breast. *Surgery* 1993;113:134–137.
137. Giri DD, Dunda SAC, Nottingham JF, et al. Oestrogen receptors in benign epithelial lesions and intraduct carcinomas of the breast: an immunohistological study. *Histopathology* 1989;15:575–584.
138. Helin HJ, Helle MJ, Kallioneimi OP, et al. Immunohistochemical determination of estrogen and progesterone receptors in human breast carcinoma: correlation with histopathology and DNA flow cytometry. *Cancer* 1989;63:1761–1767.
139. Karayiannakis AJ, Bastounis EA, Chatzigianni EB, et al. Immunohistochemical detection of oestrogen receptors in ductal carcinoma *in situ* of the breast. *Eur J Surg Oncol* 1996;22:578–582.
140. Leal CB, Schmitt FC, Bento MJ, et al. Ductal carcinoma *in situ* of the breast. Histologic categorization and its relationship to ploidy and immunohistochemical expression of hormone receptors, p53, and c-erbB-2 protein. *Cancer* 1995;75:2123–2131.
141. Pallis L, Wilking N, Cedermark B, et al. Receptors for estrogen and progesterone in breast carcinoma *in situ*. *Anticancer Res* 1992;12:2113–2115.
142. Poller DN, Roberts EC, Bell JA, et al. p53 protein expression in mammary ductal carcinoma *in situ*: relationship to immunohistochemical expression of estrogen receptor and c-erbB-2 protein. *Hum Pathol* 1993;24:463–468.
143. Zafrani B, Leroyer A, Fourquet A, et al. Mammographically detected ductal *in situ* carcinoma of the breast analyzed with a new classification. A study of 127 cases: correlation with estrogen and progesterone receptors, p53, and c-erbB-2 proteins, and proliferative activity. *Semin Diagn Pathol* 1994;11:208–214.
144. Barnes DM, Meyer JS, Gonzalez JG, et al. Relationship between c-erbB-2 immunoreactivity and thymidine labeling index in breast carcinoma *in situ*. *Breast Cancer Res Treat* 1991;18:11–17.
145. Bartkova J, Barnes DM, Millis RR, et al. Immunohistochemical demonstration of c-erbB-2 protein in mammary ductal carcinoma *in situ*. *Hum Pathol* 1990;21:1164–1167.
146. Bobrow LG, Happerfield LC, Gregory WM, et al. The classification of ductal carcinoma *in situ* and its association with biological markers. *Semin Diagn Pathol* 1994;11:199–207.
147. De Potter CR, Foschini MP, Schelfhout AM, et al. Immunohistochemical study of neu protein overexpression in clinging *in situ* duct carcinoma of the breast. *Virchows Arch A Pathol Anat* 1993;422:375–380.
148. De Potter CR, Schelfhout A-M, Verbeeck P, et al. neu-Overexpression correlates with extent of disease in large cell ductal carcinoma *in situ* of the breast. *Hum Pathol* 1995;26:601–606.
149. Poller DN, Silverstein MJ, Galea M, et al. Ductal carcinoma *in situ* of the breast: a proposal for a new simplified histological classification association between cellular proliferation and c-erbB-2 protein expression. *Mod Pathol* 1994;7:257–262.
150. Ramachandra S, Machin L, Ashley S, et al. Immunohistochemical distribution of c-erbB-2 in *in situ* breast carcinoma: a detailed morphological analysis. *J Pathol* 1990;161:7–14.

151. Schimmelpenning H, Eriksson ET, Pallis L, et al. Immunohistochemical c-erbB-2 proto-oncogene expression and nuclear DNA content in human mammary carcinoma *in situ*. *Am J Clin Pathol* 1992;97[Suppl]:S48–S52.

152. Somerville JE, Clarke LA, Biggart JD. c-erbB-2 overexpression and histological type of *in situ* and invasive breast carcinomas. *J Clin Pathol* 1992;45:16–20.

153. Tsuda H, Iwaya K, Fukutomi T, et al. p53 mutations and c-erbB-2 amplification in intraductal and invasive breast carcinomas of high histologic grade. *Jpn J Cancer Res* 1993;84:394–401.

154. Eriksson ET, Schmmelpenning H, Aspenblad U, et al. Immunohistochemical expression of the mutant p53 protein and nuclear DNA content during the transition from benign to malignant breast disease. *Hum Pathol* 1994;25:1228–1233.

155. O'Malley FP, Vnencak-Jones CL, Dupont WD, et al. p53 mutations are confined to the comedo type ductal carcinoma *in situ* of the breast. Immunohistochemical and sequencing data. *Lab Invest* 1994;71:67–72.

156. Balan PR, Scott DJ, Perry RH, et al. p53 protein expression in ductal carcinoma *in situ* (DCIS) of the breast. *Breast Cancer Res Treat* 1997;42:283–290.

157. Schmitt FC, Leal D, Lopes C. p53 protein expression and nuclear DNA content in breast intraductal proliferations. *J Pathol* 1995;176:233–241.

158. Siziopikou KP, Prioleau JE, Harris JR, et al. Bcl-2 expression in the spectrum of preinvasive breast lesions. *Cancer* 1996;77:499–506.

159. Siziopikou KP, Schnitt SJ. MIB-1 proliferation index in ductal carcinoma *in situ* of the breast: relationship to the expression of the apoptosis-regulating proteins bcl-2 and p53. *Breast J* 2000;6:100–106.

160. Walker RA, Dearing SJ, Lane DP, et al. Expression of p53 protein in infiltrating and *in situ* breast carcinomas. *J Pathol* 1991;165:203–211.

161. Locker AP, Horrocks C, Gilmour AS, et al. Flow cytometric and histological analysis of ductal carcinoma *in situ* of the breast. *Br J Surg* 1990;77:564–567.

162. Meyer JS. Cell kinetics of histologic variants of *in situ* breast carcinoma. *Breast Cancer Res Treat* 1986;7:171–180.

163. Bodis S, Siziopikou KP, Schnitt SJ, et al. Extensive apoptosis in ductal carcinoma *in situ* of the breast. *Cancer* 1996;77:1831–1835.

164. Harn HJ, Shen KL, Yueh KC, et al. Apoptosis occurs more frequently in intraductal carcinoma than in infiltrating duct carcinoma of human breast cancer and correlates with altered p53 expression: detected by terminal-deoxynucleotidyl-transferase-mediated dUTP-FITC nick end labelling (TUNEL). *Histopathology* 1997;31:534–539.

165. Gupta SK, Douglas-Jones AG, Morgan JM, et al. The clinical behavior of breast carcinoma is probably determined at the preinvasive stage (ductal carcinoma *in situ*). *Cancer* 1997;80:1740–1745.

166. Solin LJ, Kurtz J, Forquet A, et al. Fifteen-year results of breast-conserving surgery and definitive breast irradiation for the treatment of ductal carcinoma *in situ* of the breast. *J Clin Oncol* 1996;14:754–763.

167. Hannemann J, Velds A, Halfwerk JB, et al. Classification of ductal carcinoma *in situ* by gene expression profiling. *Breast Cancer Res* 2006;8:R61.

168. Porter D, Lahti-Domenici J, Keshaviah A, et al. Molecular markers in ductal carcinoma *in situ* of the breast. *Mol Cancer Res* 2003;1:362–375.

169. Polyak K. Is breast tumor progression really linear? *Clin Cancer Res* 2008;14:339–341.

170. Polyak K. Breast cancer: origins and evolution. *J Clin Invest* 2007;117:3155–3163.

171. Campbell LL, Polyak K. Breast tumor heterogeneity: cancer stem cells or clonal evolution? *Cell Cycle* 2007;6:2332–2338.

172. Jacobs TW, Byrne C, Colditz G, et al. Pathologic features of breast cancers in women with previous benign breast disease. *Am J Clin Pathol* 2001;115:362–369.

173. Lennington WJ, Jensen RA, Dalton LW, et al. Ductal carcinoma *in situ* of the breast. Heterogeneity of individual lesions. *Cancer* 1994;73:118–124.

174. Levine AJ. p53, the cellular gatekeeper for growth and division. *Cell* 1997;88:323–331.

175. Perez-Losada J, Mao JH, Balmain A. Control of genomic instability and epithelial tumor development by the p53-Fbxw7/Cdc4 pathway. *Cancer Res* 2005;65:6488–6492.

176. Magne N, Roillon RA, Castadot P, et al. Different clinical impact of estradiol receptor determination according to the analytic method: a study on 1940 breast cancer patients over a period of 16 consecutive years. *Breast Cancer Res Treat* 2006;95:179–184.

177. Aldaz CM, Chen T, Sahin A, et al. Comparative allelotype of *in situ* and invasive human breast cancer: high frequency of microsatellite instability in lobular breast carcinomas. *Cancer Res* 1995;55:3976–3981.

178. Chappell SA, Walsh T, Walker RA, et al. Loss of heterozygosity at chromosome 6q in preinvasive and early invasive breast carcinomas. *Br J Cancer* 1997;75:1324–1329.

179. Fujii H, Marsh C, Cairns P, et al. Genetic divergence in the clonal evolution of breast cancer. *Cancer Res* 1996;56:1493–1497.

180. Fujii H, Szumel R, Marsh C, et al. Genetic progression, histologic grade, and allelic loss in ductal carcinoma *in situ* of the breast. *Cancer Res* 1996;56:5260–5265.

181. Man S, Ellis IO, Sibbering M, et al. High levels of allele loss at the FHIT and ATM genes in non-comedo ductal carcinoma *in situ* and grade I tubular invasive breast cancers. *Cancer Res* 1996;56:5484–5489.

182. Munn KE, Walker RA, Varley JM. Frequent alterations of chromosome 1 in ductal carcinoma *in situ* of the breast. *Oncogene* 1995;10:1653–1657.

183. Radford DM, Fair KL, Phillips NJ, et al. Allelotyping of ductal carcinoma *in situ* of the breast: deletion of loci on 8p, 13q, 16q, 17p and 17q. *Cancer Res* 1995;55:3399–3405.

184. Stratton MR, Collins N, Lakhani SR, et al. Loss of heterozygosity in ductal carcinoma *in situ* of the breast. *J Pathol* 1995;175:195–201.

185. Rogers LW. Carcinoma *in situ* (CIS): lobular carcinoma *in situ*. In: Page DL, Anderson TJ, eds. *Diagnostic histopathology of the breast.* Edinburgh: Churchill Livingstone, 1987:174–184.

186. Mohsin SK, O'Connell P, Allred DC, et al. Biomarker profile and genetic abnormalities in lobular carcinoma *in situ*. *Breast Cancer Res Treat* 2005;90:249–256.

187. Querzoli P, Albonico G, Ferretti S, et al. Modulation of biomarkers in minimal breast carcinoma: a model for human breast carcinoma progression. *Cancer* 1998;83:89–97.

188. Rudas M, Neumayer R, Gnant M, et al. p53 protein expression, cell proliferation and steroid hormone receptors in ductal and lobular *in situ* carcinomas of the breast. *Eur J Cancer* 1997;33:39–44.

189. Pertschuk LP, Kim DS, Nayer K, et al. Immunocytochemical estrogen and progestin receptor assays in breast cancer with monoclonal antibodies. Histopathologic, demographic, and biochemical correlations and relationship to endocrine response and survival. *Cancer* 1990;66:1663–1670.

190. Fisher ER, Costantino J, Fisher B, et al. Pathologic findings from the National Surgical Adjuvant Breast Project (NSABP) protocol B-17. *Cancer* 1996;78:1403–1416.

191. Midulla C, Giovagnoli MR, Valli C, et al. Correlation between ploidy status, erb-B2 and p53 immunohistochemical expression in primary breast carcinoma. *Analyt Quant Cytol Histol* 1995;17:157–162.

192. Porter PL, Garcia R, Moe R, et al. c-erbB-2 oncogene protein in *in situ* and invasive lobular breast neoplasia. *Cancer* 1991;68:331–334.

193. Domagala W, Striker G, Szadowska A, et al. p53 protein and vimentin in invasive ductal NOS breast carcinoma: relationship with survival and sites of metastases. *Eur J Cancer* 1994;30A:1527–1534.

194. Younes M, Lebovitz RM, Bommer KE, et al. p53 accumulation in benign breast biopsy specimens. *Hum Pathol* 1995;26:155–158.

195. Lakhani SR, Collins N, Sloane JP, et al. Loss of heterozygosity in lobular carcinoma *in situ* of the breast. *Mol Pathol* 1995;48:M74–M78.

196. Lu Y-L, Osin P, Lakhani SR, et al. Comparative genomic hybridization analysis of lobular carcinoma *in situ* and atypical lobular hyperplasia and potential roles for gains and losses of genetic material in breast neoplasia. *Cancer Res* 1998;58:4721–4727.

197. De Leeuw WJ, Berx G, Vos CB, et al. Simultaneous loss of E-cadherin and catenins in invasive lobular breast cancer and lobular carcinoma *in situ*. *J Pathol* 1997;183:404–411.

198. Wittekind C, Neid M. Cancer invasion and metastasis. *Oncology* 2005;69[Suppl 1]:14–16.

199. Duffy MJ, McGowan PM, Gallagher WM. Cancer invasion and metastasis: changing views. *J Pathol* 2008;214:283–293.

200. Bissell MJ, Radisky D. Putting tumours in context. *Nat Rev Cancer* 2001;1:46–54.

201. Tuxhorn JA, Ayala GE, Rowley DR. Reactive stroma in prostate cancer progression. *J Urol* 2001;166:2472–2483.

202. Park CC, Bissell MJ, Barcellos-Hoff MH. The influence of the microenvironment on the malignant phenotype. *Mol Med Today* 2000;6:324–329.

203. Barcellos-Hoff MH, Ravani SA. Irradiated mammary gland stroma promotes the expression of tumorigenic phenotype by unirradiated epithelial cells. *Cancer Res* 2000;60:1254–1260.

204. Frazier KS, Grotendorst GR. Expression of connective tissue growth factor mRNA in the fibrous stroma of mammary tumors. *Int J Biochem Cell Biol* 1997;29:153–161.

205. Kalluri R, Zeisberg M. Fibroblasts in cancer. *Nat Rev Cancer* 2006;6:392–401.

206. Olumi AF, Grossfeld GD, Hayward SW, et al. Carcinoma-associated fibroblasts direct tumor progression of initiated human prostatic epithelium. *Cancer Res* 1999;59:5002–5011.

207. Allinen M, Beroukhim R, Cai L, et al. Molecular characterization of the tumor microenvironment in breast cancer. *Cancer Cell* 2004;6:17–32.

208. Hu M, Yao J, Cai L, et al. Distinct epigenetic changes in the stromal cells of breast cancers. *Nat Genet* 2005;37:899–905.

209. Qiu W, Hu M, Sridhar A, et al. No evidence of clonal somatic genetic alterations in cancer-associated fibroblasts from human breast and ovarian carcinomas. *Nat Genet* 2008;40:650–655.

210. Fisher B, Costantino JP, Wickerham DL, et al. Tamoxifen for prevention of breast cancer: report of the National Surgical Adjuvant Breast and Bowel Project P-1 study. *J Natl Cancer Inst* 1998;90:1371–1388.

211. Vogel VG, Costantino JP, Wickerham DL, et al. Effects of tamoxifen vs raloxifene on the risk of developing invasive breast cancer and other disease outcomes: the NSABP Study of Tamoxifen and Raloxifene (STAR) P-2 trial. *JAMA* 2006;295:2727–2741.

Chapter 24
Lobular Carcinoma *In Situ:* Biology and Pathology

Peter T. Simpson, Jorge S. Reis-Filho, and Sunil R. Lakhani

Atypical lobular hyperplasia (ALH) and lobular carcinoma *in situ* (LCIS) are relatively uncommon lesions of the breast. They were first described over 60 years ago and have been subject to extensive characterization in the literature ever since. However, despite this long time span, there remain problems and confusion surrounding the most appropriate terminology and classification for these lesions, their biological significance (risk indicator vs. precursor for invasive cancer), and the best course of long-term management following diagnosis. This chapter discusses the historical perspective alongside recent clinicopathological and molecular developments that have enhanced our understanding of this fascinating entity.

LCIS was first described as an "atypical proliferation of acinar cells" by Ewing in 1919 (1). Foote and Stewart (2) subsequently described this distinctive entity and coined the term lobular carcinoma *in situ* in 1941 (2), choosing the name to emphasize the morphologic similarities between the cells of LCIS and those of frankly invasive lobular carcinoma (ILC). They recognized parallels with ductal carcinoma *in situ* (DCIS): foci of neoplastic cells that were still contained within a basement membrane. In some cases they observed LCIS occurring in conjunction with an ILC and hypothesized that the LCIS, in a manner akin to DCIS, would represent an established step along the pathway to development of invasive cancer. They therefore recommended mastectomy as the standard form of treatment, a management plan that was adopted for many years. Subsequently, the term ALH was introduced to describe morphologically similar but less well-developed lesions. The term lobular neoplasia (LN) was introduced by Haagensen et al. (3) in 1978 to cover the full range of proliferation within the spectrum, including both ALH and LCIS.

LN is now a well-established group of histopathologic entities in the classification of breast neoplasia, and, as predicted by Foote and Stewart, follow-up over many years does show a clear increased risk of breast carcinoma (4). However, many studies have established that the risk conferred by a diagnosis of LCIS is not as high as that of high-grade DCIS and that only a small proportion of LCIS progress to invasive breast cancer (5–8). A diagnosis of ALH or LCIS today is often perceived as a risk indicator for subsequent carcinoma, rather than a true precursor. As a result, radical surgical treatment has fallen out of favor, but there is a lack of consensus on what the most appropriate management of patients diagnosed with ALH or LCIS should be. Recommendations for treatment vary from follow-up with regular mammography to follow-up alone or simply no action (3,9–11). This view has been changing in the past few years, with several lines of evidence suggesting that LCIS is indeed a nonobligate precursor lesion (as well as a risk indicator) for carcinoma (12–17), a finding that has significant implications for the management of patients diagnosed with this disease. In fact there are several studies now advocating surgical excision following the diagnosis of LCIS in core needle biopsy (CNB) (18,19).

EPIDEMIOLOGY AND NATURAL HISTORY

Diagnosis of LCIS most frequently occurs in women aged 40 to 50 years (<10% of patients with LCIS are postmenopausal) (3,4), which is a decade earlier than the age of those diagnosed with DCIS. Calculating the true incidence of LCIS has proven to be challenging. There are no specific clinical abnormalities, in particular no palpable lump, and, because most LCIS is not associated with microcalcifications, it is usually undetectable by mammography (20,21). When examining a pathologic specimen, there are no macroscopic features characteristic of LCIS to guide tissue sampling. The diagnosis of LCIS is therefore often made as an incidental, microscopic finding in breast biopsy performed for other indications. For these reasons, the true incidence of LCIS in the general population is unknown, and many asymptomatic women presumably go undiagnosed. The incidence of LCIS in otherwise benign breast biopsy is documented as between 0.5% to 3.8% (3,4).

Characteristically, LCIS is both multifocal and bilateral in a large percentage of cases. Over 50% of patients diagnosed with LCIS show multiple foci in the ipsilateral breast, and roughly 30% of patients have further LCIS in the contralateral breast (22–24). Such multifocality in a clinically nondetectable lesion is one of the reasons why planning subsequent management has proven problematic and contentious. This clinical presentation (multifocal and bilateral), together with evidence from epidemiological studies (25–30), suggests that there is an underlying genetic predisposition for the development of LCIS. The gene(s) involved and the pattern of inheritance remain unclear (see below).

LCIS can also be considered a risk indicator, conferring an increased rate of development of invasive carcinoma of about 1% to 2% per year, with a lifetime risk of 30% to 40% (3,31,32). Page et al. (4,33) documented that the relative risk for development of subsequent breast cancer was different in women diagnosed with ALH compared with LCIS. Patients diagnosed with ALH have a four- to fivefold higher risk than the general population (i.e., women, of comparable age who have had a breast biopsy performed with no atypical proliferative disease diagnosed) (33,34). This relative risk appears doubled to 8 to 10 times for LCIS (4). Thus, although LN is a helpful term for collectively describing this group of lesions, specific classification into ALH and LCIS, may still be justified or preferable in terms of risk stratification and management decisions. Although ALH and LCIS have been shown to confer different relative risks of invasive breast cancer development, distinguishing the two lesions is, at least partly, subjective. For some experts the differences between these two categories of LN are expressed more easily in words than in actual practice (35).

In a meta-analysis of nine separate studies evaluating the outcome of a new diagnosis of LCIS, 228 patients were identified. Of these, a proportion underwent either unilateral or bilateral mastectomy. On follow-up, 15% of 172 patients (who did not undergo unilateral mastectomy as primary treatment) had invasive carcinoma in the ipsilateral breast and 9.3% of 204 patients had invasive carcinoma in the contralateral breast (31). The development of contralateral breast cancer is more likely in patients diagnosed with LCIS than in those without LCIS (30,36–38). The risk for development of breast cancer was therefore considered to be bilateral (22), and there are data to suggest that this risk is similar for both breasts (10,31,39). However, other studies demonstrate that carcinoma is more likely to develop in the ipsilateral compared with the contralateral breast (14,33,40–44), supporting the view that ALH and LCIS act both as risk indicators and as precursor lesions.

The time to the development of invasive cancer in an individual patient after a diagnosis of LCIS is difficult to predict. Page et al. (4) documented that in two thirds of women in whom invasive cancer developed, it did so within 15 years of biopsy. In a separate study, in over 50% of patients in whom cancer developed, it did so between 15 and 30 years after biopsy, with an average interval of 20.4 years (41). This extended time span may have significant implications for planning patient follow-up.

Both invasive ductal carcinoma (IDC) and ILC occur with LCIS, a fact that some have used to suggest that LCIS is not a true precursor lesion. However, the incidence of ILC occurring with LCIS is significantly greater than without (10,45). The coexistence of DCIS and LCIS may explain the IDC component observed, whereby DCIS and not LCIS is the likely precursor lesion (46,47). The role of LCIS as a nonobligate precursor to ILC has been demonstrated in many studies (4,12,14,33,34,48), being supported by the epidemiologic data outlined above, the morphologic similarity between cells of ALH or LCIS and lobular carcinoma, and the development of tumors in regions localized to ALH or LCIS. Molecular data also provide strong circumstantial evidence in support of the hypothesis that LCIS is a precursor lesion (see below), in particular concordant chromosomal abnormalities (15,17,49,50) and identical mutations in matched LCIS and ILC from the same patients (16).

HISTOLOGICAL FEATURES AND CLASSIFICATION

LCIS is composed of acini filled with a monomorphic population of small, round, polygonal, or cuboidal cells, with a thin rim of clear cytoplasm and a high nuclear-to-cytoplasmic ratio (2,51) (Figs. 24.1–24.4) The nuclei are uniform and the chromatin fine and evenly dispersed. Nucleoli when present are inconspicuous. A characteristic cytological feature is the presence of cells containing clear vacuoles, known as intracytoplasmic lumina or magenta bodies (Figs. 24.1 and 24.4). When they are identified in a fine-needle aspirate (FNA) from the breast, such cells strongly suggest the presence of a lobular lesion (including ALH, LCIS, and ILC) (52,53); however, the

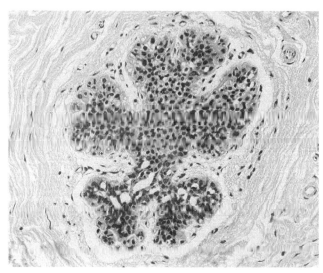

FIGURE 24.2. Typical appearance of a lobular unit distended by lobular carcinoma *in situ*.

presence of intracytoplasmic vacuoles in a breast FNA does not warrant a diagnosis of lobular carcinoma. The cells are loosely cohesive, regularly spaced, and fill and distend the acini; however, overall lobular architecture is maintained (2,51). Glandular lumina are usually not seen in fully developed cases, and mitoses and necrosis are uncommon. Pagetoid spread, where the neoplastic cells extend along adjacent ducts between intact overlying epithelium and underlying basement membrane, is also frequently seen (51,54) (Figs. 24.3 and 24.4).

For a diagnosis of LCIS, Page et al. (55) stated that more than half the acini in an involved lobular unit must be filled and distended by the characteristic cells, leaving no central lumina. For practical purposes, distention translates as eight or more cells present in the cross-sectional diameter of an acinus. A lesion is regarded as ALH when it is less well developed and less extensive than these criteria, for instance, when the characteristic cells only partly fill the acini, with only minimal or no distention of the lobule (Fig. 24.4). Lumina may still be identified, and the number of acini involved is less than half. Myoepithelial cells

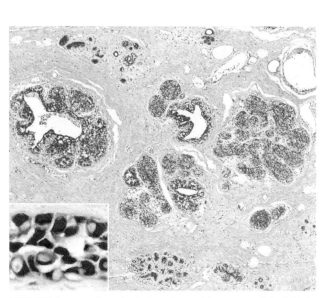

FIGURE 24.1. Low-power (scanning electron microscopic) appearance of classic lobular carcinoma *in situ*, showing filling and distension of lobules. Normal lobules are seen at the top and bottom center of the picture for comparison. Inset shows typical cytologic detail of the cells with prominent intracytoplasmic lumina and a magenta body.

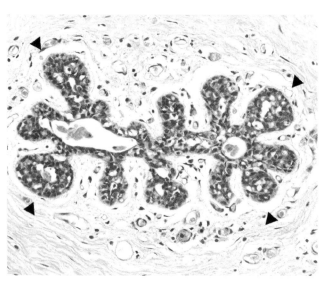

FIGURE 24.3. Pagetoid spread. Lobular carcinoma *in situ* cells (*arrowheads*) are seen growing beneath, and displacing inward, the luminal epithelium of a duct.

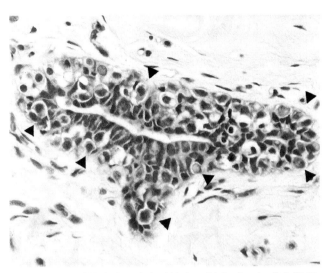

FIGURE 24.4. Atypical lobular hyperplasia. A lobular unit is focally and partially filled by characteristic cells with intracytoplasmic lumina (*arrowheads*).

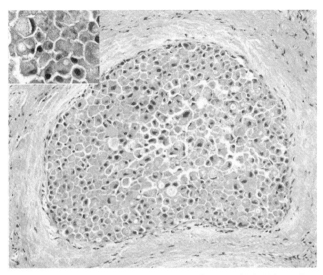

FIGURE 24.5. Pleomorphic lobular carcinoma *in situ.* The duct is filled with large, discohesive cells showing apocrine features, intracytoplasmic lumina, and occasional signet ring cells (detailed in insert).

may be seen admixed with the neoplastic population. Clearly, the differentiation between ALH and LCIS on these criteria is rather arbitrary and prone to interobserver and intraobserver variability. Therefore, the use of the term LN to encompass the whole range of changes, and remove this variability, may be preferable for diagnostic purposes. However, to date, the term has not gained widespread use among pathologists. As discussed above, one justification for continuing to use the ALH and LCIS terminology is that ALH has been shown to be associated with a lower risk of subsequent invasive carcinoma compared with LCIS (4,33,34). The cells contained in classic ALH or LCIS, as described previously, can also be referred to as type A cells. A well-recognized subtype of LCIS is an architecturally similar lesion containing cells with mild to moderately large nuclei, some increase in pleomorphism, and more abundant cytoplasm. These cells are known as type B cells.

A more recently described entity is that of pleomorphic LCIS (PLCIS) (56). These lesions are characterized by large cells displaying marked pleomorphism, with eccentrically-placed nuclei with nucleoli and eosinophilic cytoplasm. Occasionally, PLCIS may be composed of signet ring cells. In contrast to what has been reported for the classic variant, apocrine differentiation at the morphologic and immunohistochemical levels is very frequent in PLCIS (56) (Fig. 24.5). In fact, some advocate that partial or overt apocrine differentiation is one of the most common features of *bona fide* PLCIS. The cells are often more discohesive than in classic LCIS, and central necrosis and calcification in lobules are not uncommonly found. PLCIS is often encountered in conjunction with cytologically similar invasive pleomorphic lobular carcinoma and, occasionally, areas of transition between the two can be observed. Sneige et al. (56) have described type B cells as containing nuclei that are up to twice the size of a lymphocyte (type A cells are 1 to 1.5 times larger), whereas PLCIS nuclei are typically four times larger and harbor more prominent nucleoli. Recognition of the pleomorphic subtype is important because the combination of cellular features, necrosis, and calcification can lead to difficulty in differentiation from DCIS.

A further system for classification of these lesions has been proposed using the terminology lobular intraepithelial neoplasia (LIN), with subdivision, based on morphologic criteria and clinical outcome, into three grades—LIN 1, LIN 2, LIN 3—with LIN 3 representing the PLCIS end of the spectrum (48). The proposal is that risk of subsequent invasive carcinoma will be related to increasing grade of LIN. There is, as yet, no consensus of opinion on this grading system, despite it being described in the latest World Health Organization classification (57). In view of the rapid evolution in technology, especially in molecular pathology and high-throughput analysis methods, the classification systems are likely to undergo change as further data are incorporated. Hence, at present, it would not seem prudent to introduce yet another interim classification.

DIFFERENTIAL DIAGNOSIS

A few well-known pitfalls can occasionally cause diagnostic difficulty in the diagnosis of LCIS. Poor tissue preservation may lead to an artefactual appearance of discohesive cells in a lobular unit, resulting in overdiagnosis of LCIS. Similarly, foci of lactational change containing intracytoplasmic lipid droplets, or clear cell metaplasia, may superficially resemble ALH or LCIS if not recognized. Another difficulty arises when LCIS is growing in some types of benign breast lesions (i.e., sclerosing adenosis and radial scar), which clinically and radiologically can present as a mass. The histologic appearance of LCIS in association with these lesions may be misleading, with distortion of lobular units and a rather sclerotic stroma. The combination of abnormal architecture and proliferative lobular cells can easily be diagnosed as an invasive carcinoma by the unwary. In this situation, immunohistochemistry to demonstrate the myoepithelial cell layer, in particular with a combination of nuclear (e.g., p63) and cytoplasmic (e.g., smooth muscle myosin heavy chain or calponin) myoepithelial markers, or basement membrane is useful in making the distinction.

Perhaps the most important, and also the most difficult, differential diagnosis of both classic LCIS and PLCIS is with DCIS, especially DCIS of the solid, low nuclear-grade type (46,58,59). A diagnosis of DCIS carries wholly different management implications for a patient because it usually mandates surgical excision or radiation therapy as definitive treatment, whereas LCIS may arguably warrant no further action. Correct identification, therefore, is essential. However, distinction of LCIS from low-grade solid DCIS is challenging because morphologically they may be remarkably similar especially when DCIS involves the acini (termed cancerization of lobules) with minimal or no lobular distortion. Morphologic indicators include nuclear size and pleomorphism, which may be greater in DCIS (although this is less useful when dealing with PLCIS), the presence of secondary lumen formation, and cellular cohesion, which also points to a ductal lesion rather than LCIS (46,58). Immunohistochemical analysis of the lesion can prove useful in making the distinction. E-cadherin, β-catenin, and p120 catenin (see below) are typically absent or aberrant in ALH or LCIS but present on the membrane of neoplastic cells in DCIS (46,58,60–62). Occasionally, lesions show an overlapping range of morphologic features along with variable expression of immunohistochemical markers. This suggests that LCIS and low-grade solid DCIS may truly coexist within the same duct lobular unit. In these circumstances, differentiation between the two is often not possible and both diagnoses should be given. How patients should be managed in these unresolved cases remains a challenge, but pragmatically, they will receive treatment as for DCIS.

MOLECULAR PATHOLOGY

Molecular studies have been instrumental in highlighting the role of E-cadherin inactivation in the development of lobular lesions and in supporting the notion that ALH and LCIS are in fact nonobligate precursors for the development of invasive cancer rather than being simply risk indicators for invasive disease. Further molecular analyses focused on the peculiar biological and clinical features of LCIS, for example, the multifocal and bilateral presentation and the extended time (~15 years) to progress to invasive cancer, will be important to refine the long-term management of patients diagnosed with LCIS.

Immunophenotype

The immunohistochemical profile of ALH, LCIS, and PLCIS is compared to that of low- and high-grade DCIS in Table 24.1. All subtypes of LCIS are associated with strong expression of estrogen receptor alpha (ERα), ER-beta (ERβ), and progesterone receptor (PR) in the majority of neoplastic cells (60% to 90% of cases positive) (63–65). Most LCIS do not express biomarkers typically associated with an aggressive phenotype, being negative for *HER2* overexpression and gene amplification, p53 (as defined by >10% of neoplastic cells) and exhibiting a low proliferative (Ki-67) index. This profile is consistent whether LCIS is associated with invasive carcinoma or not (pure LCIS) (63) and also with ILC. Despite their high grade, PLCIS are often ER or PR positive but also harbor more frequent *HER2* gene amplification and overexpression, p53 immunohistochemical positivity (as a surrogate for p53 mutation), and a higher proliferative index. Given

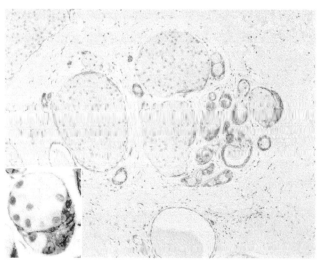

FIGURE 24.6. E-cadherin immunohistochemical staining in lobular carcinoma *in situ*. The outer rim of myoepithelial cells show strong membrane staining, whereas the lobular carcinoma *in situ* cells filling the lumen, are uniformly negative.

the characteristic apocrine features of PLCIS, it is not surprising that these lesions are often positive for GCDFP-15 (gross cystic disease fluid protein-15) (56,66).

E-Cadherin Immunohistochemistry in Lobular Neoplasia

Lobular proliferations (*in situ*, invasive and pleomorphic types) characteristically show loss or marked down-regulation of the transmembrane protein E-cadherin in more than 95% of cases (Fig. 24.6); whereas luminal epithelial cells and most ductal proliferations (atypical ductal hyperplasia [ADH], DCIS, and IDC) exhibit positive staining by immunohistochemistry (16,48,56,58, 67–74). E-cadherin mediates calcium-dependent cell–cell adhesion, hence its loss of function is strongly implicated in the characteristic discohesive nature of lobular neoplastic cells. The mechanisms involved in E-cadherin down-regulation are discussed below. Some authors have advocated the use of E-cadherin as an adjunct antibody to differentiate LCIS and DCIS, particularly in challenging situations such as solid *in situ* proliferations with indeterminate features (56,58,59,67,75,76). The authors

	ALH	LCIS	Low Grade DCIS	PLCIS	High Grade DCIS
Table 24.1			**SUMMARY OF IMMUNOHISTOCHEMICAL MARKER STATUS**		
ER	+	+	+	+/–	–/+
PR	+	+	+	+/–	–/+
HER2	–	–	–	–/+	+/–
E-cadherin	–	–	+ (membranous)	–	+ (membranous)
β-catenin	–	–	+ (membranous)	–	+ (membranous)
p120	– (cytoplasmic)	– (cytoplasmic)	+ (membranous)	– (cytoplasmic)	+ (membranous)
GCDFP-15	–/+	–/+	–/+	+/–	–/+
p53	–/+	–/+	–/+	+/–	+/–
Ki-67	Low	Low	Low	Moderate-high	High

(From Vogel VG. Raloxifene: a second-generation selective estrogen receptor modulator for reducing the risk of invasive breast cancer in postmenopausal women. *Women's Health* 2007;3:139-153, with permission.)
ALH, atypical lobular hyperplasia; LCIS, lobular carcinoma *in situ*; DCIS, ductal carcinoma *in situ*; PLCIS, pleomorphic LCIS; ER, estrogen receptor; PgR, progesterone receptor; GCDFP-15, gross cystic disease fluid protein-15; −/+, often negative though sometimes positive; +/−, often positive though sometimes negative.

suggested that (a) cases with positive E-cadherin staining should be considered as DCIS, (b) cases negative for E-cadherin should be classified as LCIS, and (c) in circumstances where a mixed pattern of positively and negatively stained cells are observed, the lesion should be classified as a mixed lesion (58). As the management of patients differs with regard to DCIS or LCIS, especially when found at the surgical margins, then correct classification is important. Some validation for using E-cadherin in classification comes from clinical-pathological studies of patients having pure LCIS in CNB, where E-cadherin positive LCIS was associated with a higher risk for development of invasive carcinoma compared to E-cadherin negative LCIS (11,77).

There are some issues with this practice if it is applied in the wrong context due to a lack of both an understanding of the biology behind E-cadherin but also a detailed inspection of staining. Some lobular carcinomas are positive for E-cadherin, so misinterpretation of "aberrant" positive staining may lead some pathologists to exclude a diagnosis of lobular carcinoma in favor of a ductal carcinoma, despite the morphology suggesting otherwise, and hence leading to misclassification of the tumor. To highlight this issue, Da Silva et al. (78) studied the molecular basis for E-cadheirn positivity in ILC and demonstrated that admixed with positive cells were also aberrantly (incomplete membrane, cytoplasmic, or Golgi staining) stained cells and aberrant β-catenin staining, suggesting the E-cadherin was probably nonfunctional, which was supported by a mutation found by gene sequencing. In addition, triple negative (ER, PR, and *HER2* negative) and basal-like breast cancers often lack or display aberrant E-cadherin expression (79).

Down-regulation of E-cadherin coincides with the loss or aberrant expression of β-catenin, α-catenin, and p120(ctn), molecules that complex with the cytoplasmic domain of E-cadherin, and these staining patterns can also be used to differentiate lobular from ductal lesions. β-catenin, α-catenin, and p120(ctn) show membranous localization by immunohistochemistry in normal luminal epithelial cells and most ductal proliferations, whereas in lobular neoplasia β-catenin and α-catenin typically show complete loss of expression, although aberrant staining in the cytoplasm or Golgi has been noted and p120 shows cytoplasmic localization. These staining patterns are observed in all stages of lobular neoplasia, from ALH to associated metastases, including in PLCIS and PLC, and were shown to be directly mediated by inactivation of E-cadherin from the cell membrane (60–62,72,74,78,80,81). E-cadherin, β-catenin, and p120 are therefore useful discriminators between lobular and ductal proliferations, although it must be said that most but not all lesions in each category conform to this.

Molecular Aspects of E-Cadherin Inactivation

Lobular and low-grade ductal proliferations have remarkably similar immunohistochemical and molecular genetic features, suggesting they evolve along closely related pathways of development that are distinct from high-grade carcinomas (82). A common finding between lobular and low-grade ductal lesions is the loss of chromosome arm 16q, which occurs in a high proportion of cases as an early event in neoplastic development. The candidate tumor suppressor gene(s) of this deletion is yet to be identified in low-grade ductal lesions, whereas in lobular lesions it has been shown to be the *CDH1* gene (16q22.1), which encodes for E-cadherin. E-cadherin inactivation or down-regulation occurs via a combination of genetic, epigenetic, or transcriptional mechanisms. Loss of chromosome 16q is usually accompanied by truncating mutations or gene promoter methylation, leading to biallelic inactivation of the gene and loss of protein expression (16,68,69,72,83,84). Gene mutations have been identified in ALH, LCIS, ILC, and PLC but are rare in bona fide IDC (68,74,84–87). Identical *CDH1* truncating mutations have been found in LCIS and associated ILC, supporting the role

of LCIS as a precursor for invasive carcinoma (16). In a small study, the frequency of *CDH1* mutations in pure ALH was reported to be lower than that detected in pure LCIS (74). This was unexpected because E-cadherin expression is already down-regulated at the stage of ALH. There are considerable data on the transcriptional regulation of E-cadherin via a number of different transcription factors, and this has recently been specifically described in lobular tumors via activation of transforming growth factor β (TGF-β) pathway and Snail and Slug up-regulation (78) and by zinc finger E-box binding homeobox1 (*ZEB1*) (88), as well as in some IDC (87).

Evidence for E-cadherin inactivation being directly related to the lobular phenotype has been demonstrated in a mouse tumor model with conditional mutation of E-cadherin and epithelial-specific knock-out of p53. Mammary tumors and metastases that developed had a strong morphological resemblance to human lobular carcinoma (89), however, this model had some significant differences, in particular lack of ER and PR expression, presence of *Trp53* gene mutations, and positivity for basal keratins, which are features not typically associated with LN and ILC.

CDH1 gene mutations have been linked to the pathogenesis of diffuse gastric carcinoma, which have similar growth features to lobular carcinomas. In fact, approximately one third of patients with diffuse gastric cancer associated with a familial predisposition harbor a germline mutation in *CDH1* (90,91). The clinical presentation of LCIS (multifocal and bilateral) and data from epidemiological studies suggest that lobular neoplasia is associated with a familial predisposition (25–29), yet the gene(s) involved in this predisposition remains unclear. Despite the clear pathogenetic role of E-cadherin in lobular proliferations, germline mutations of *CDH1* play a limited role in familial LCIS and ILC (92–96). Evidence suggests that *BRCA1*, *BRCA2*, *MLH1*, and *MSH2* (27,97,98) germline mutations are also not significantly involved in the pathogenesis of familial lobular neoplasms, yet there is an association between *CHEK2* U157T mutation and familial predisposition to lobular carcinomas (99).

Whole Genome Molecular Genetics of Lobular Neoplasia

Molecular genetic alterations occurring in lobular proliferations have been characterized by comparative genomic hybridization (CGH) and loss of heterozygosity (LOH) studies (50,100,101). These analyses have helped confirm the clonal nature of LCIS and its role as a precursor in the development of ILC (15,17,102,103). Chromosomal CGH analysis demonstrated that LCIS and ALH (49) are genetically similar, with both lesions harboring recurrent loss of material from 16p, 16q, 17p, and 22q and gain of material from 6q, alterations that are also identified in ILCs (49,104,105). Microarray-based CGH provides a higher resolution analysis of copy number changes across the whole genome (106). Array CGH analysis demonstrated that ILC harbor highly recurrent gain (>80% of cases) of 1q and 16p and loss of 16q (17,107,108). Other alterations occur less frequently, and this heterogeneity may account for the variable biological and clinical nature of lobular proliferations. For example, loss of 11q was found in approximately 50% of ILC (17,102,107), and genomic amplifications at 8p12-p11.2 and 11q13 were found in approximately 30% ILC. These alterations were already present in LCIS (17), suggesting they are early genetic events in development of these tumors. The target genes affected can vary from case to case since, for example, the amplifications are complex and variable (109,110), however, fibroblast growth factor receptor 1 (FGFR1; 8p12-p11.2) and cyclin D1 (11q13) overexpression are frequently associated with these amplifications (107,111). In one study, pure ALH harbored a surprisingly high level of genetic instability compared to pure LCIS (112) and lobular lesions from other studies (17,49,105,113). This was interpreted as a mechanism by which most pure ALH develop high-level genetic change and die off rather than acquire select genetic changes allowing progression to LCIS and ILC (112). PLCIS and PLC are genetically related entities, highlighting the precursor role of PLCIS in the development PLC (81) akin to the relationship between LCIS and ILC. They have similar genomic profiles to LCIS and ILC (81,104) including gain of 1q and 16p and loss of 11q and 16q. However, they also harbor amplification of genomic loci involving oncogenes associated with an aggressive phenotype, such as *MYC* (8q24) and *HER2* (17q12) (56,81,114).

Clearly loss of 16q plays a crucial and very early role in the pathogenesis of lobular and low-grade ductal neoplasia (17,49,50,60,63,74,82,101,103,115–117), contributing to the loss of E-cadherin in lobular neoplasia, as described above. It is unclear whether loss of other tumor suppressor genes mapping to this region play a role in the biology of lobular carcinomas, and the genes from this region that are important in the development of low-grade ductal carcinomas remain elusive (118–120). Two candidate tumor suppressor genes located closely to E-cadherin (*CDH1*) on 16q, Dipeptidase 1 (*DPEP1*) and CCCTC-binding factor (*CTCF*), were recently shown to be down-regulated in LCIS relative to normal luminal epithelial cells (121), suggesting they may play a role in LCIS development.

CLINICAL IMPLICATIONS

With the advent of national breast cancer screening programs around the world, there has been a vast increase in the number of investigations, including CNB, performed for screen-detected abnormalities. In a proportion of cases this will inevitably lead to detection of LN in an otherwise healthy, asymptomatic individual. Interestingly, the studies addressing the presence of ALH and LCIS on CNBs or screen-detected lesions have also changed the perception regarding the radiologic appearance of these lesions in mammograms (21,122–124). From a historical point of view, ALH and LCIS were considered lesions without associated mammographic changes (124); however, several studies have demonstrated that calcifications may be found in up to 40% of ALH and LCIS and that the pleomorphic variant is more frequently associated with mammographically detected microcalcifications (21,122–124).

LN is infrequently seen as the sole diagnostic finding in CNBs, accounting for 0.5% to 2.9% of biopsies taken for histological assessment of mammography detected lesions (18,19,122,124–132). Peer reviewed data and prospective analyses of LN in CNB are limited and, therefore, most of the management recommendations have been based more on pragmatism than scientific evidence. Until recently (13,122, 133,134), most authors agreed that excision should be performed in cases of LN diagnosed on a CNB when:

1. There is another lesion present, which would itself be an indication for surgical excision, on the core biopsy (e.g., ADH or a radial scar);
2. There is discordance between clinical, radiological, and pathological findings;
3. There is an associated mass lesion or an area of architectural distortion;
4. The LN showed mixed histological features with difficulty in distinguishing the lesion from DCIS, or show a mixed E-cadherin staining pattern;
5. The morphology was consistent with that of the pleomorphic variant of lobular neoplasia.

However, it should be noted that the above approach has not been universally applied. For instance, some units have been recommending and undertaking surgical diagnostic surgical excision of all LN for many years (18), while other groups were

excising only those cases defined as above, and in particular those with radiological, surgical, or pathological discordance. In the past 2 years, North American authors have suggested that LN should be perceived as "high–risk" and recommended excision of all cases due to the underestimation of cancer in up to 33% of LN diagnosed on CNB (19,131). Interestingly, in a recent study, Esserman et al. (135) analysed a series of 26 cases of LN diagnosed on CNB that were followed by excision biopsy and observed that invasive carcinoma was only found in cases where the initial diagnosis was of diffuse LN, suggesting that the extent of LN in the core biopsy may also be associated with the presence of invasive carcinoma.

Although it is important to avoid unnecessary diagnostic surgery for patients when LN is the sole finding in a CNB, the risk of associated malignancy in the adjacent breast at the time of diagnosis should be noted. Some have advocated that a multidisciplinary approach for such cases is essential (136), and that each case must be assessed individually. It should be noted that the paucity of large prospective studies to define accurately the risk of further aggressive lesions is problematic in clinical management. Despite the rather limited data on PLCIS, there is circumstantial evidence to suggest that these lesions are more frequently associated as higher risk lesions and may have a more aggressive clinical behavior than classic LN; therefore, many would recommend that such cases should subjected to further excision.

ACKNOWLEDGMENTS

The authors are grateful to Leonard Da Silva for critical review of this chapter.

References

1. Ewing, J. *Neoplastic diseases.* 1st edition. Philadelphia: WB Saunders, 1919.
2. Foote FW, Stewart SF. Lobular carcinoma *in situ*. *Am J Pathol* 1941;491–495.
3. Haagensen CD, Lane N, Lattes R, et al. Lobular neoplasia (so-called lobular carcinoma *in situ*) of the breast. *Cancer* 1978;42:737–769.
4. Page DL, Kidd TE Jr, Dupont WD, et al. Lobular neoplasia of the breast: higher risk for subsequent invasive cancer predicted by more extensive disease. *Hum Pathol* 1991;22:1232–1239.
5. Goldstein NS, Vicini FA, Kestin LL, et al. Differences in the pathologic features of ductal carcinoma *in situ* of the breast based on patient age. *Cancer* 2000; 88:2553–2560.
6. Ringberg A, Idvall I, Ferno M, et al. Ipsilateral local recurrence in relation to therapy and morphological characteristics in patients with ductal carcinoma *in situ* of the breast. *Eur J Surg Oncol* 2000;26:444–451.
7. Silverstein MJ, Poller DN, Waisman JR, et al. Prognostic classification of breast ductal carcinoma-*in-situ*. *Lancet* 1995;345:1154–1157.
8. Skinner KA, Silverstein MJ. The management of ductal carcinoma *in situ* of the breast. *Endocr Relat Cancer* 2001;8:33–45.
9. Wheeler JE, Enterline HT. Lobular carcinoma of the breast *in situ* and infiltrating. *Pathol Annu* 1976;11:161–188.
10. Wheeler JE, Enterline HT, Roseman JM, et al. Lobular carcinoma *in situ* of the breast. Long-term follow-up. *Cancer* 1974;34:554–563.
11. Goldstein NS, Kestin LL, Vicini FA. Clinicopathologic implications of E-cadherin reactivity in patients with lobular carcinoma *in situ* of the breast. *Cancer* 2001;92:738–747.
12. Lakhani, SR. *In situ* lobular neoplasia: time for an awakening. *Lancet* 2003; 361:96.
13. Simpson PT, Gale T, Fulford LG, et al. The diagnosis and management of pre-invasive breast disease: pathology of atypical lobular hyperplasia and lobular carcinoma *in situ*. *Breast Cancer Res* 2003;5:258–262.
14. Page DL, Schuyler PA, Dupont WD, et al. Atypical lobular hyperplasia as a unilateral predictor of breast cancer risk: a retrospective cohort study. *Lancet* 2003;361:125–129.
15. Etzell JE, Devries S, Chew K, et al. Loss of chromosome 16q in lobular carcinoma *in situ*. *Hum Pathol* 2001;32:292–296.
16. Vos CB, Cleton-Jansen AM, Berx G, et al. E-cadherin inactivation in lobular carcinoma *in situ* of the breast: an early event in tumorigenesis. *Br J Cancer* 1997; 76:1131–1133.
17. Shelley Hwang E, Nyante SJ, Yi Chen Y, et al. Clonality of lobular carcinoma *in situ* and synchronous invasive lobular carcinoma. *Cancer* 2004;100:2562–2572.
18. O'Driscoll D, Britton P, Bobrow L, et al. Lobular carcinoma *in situ* on core biopsy—what is the clinical significance? *Clin Radiol* 2001;56:216–220.
19. Elsheikh TM, Silverman JF. Follow-up surgical excision is indicated when breast core needle biopsies show atypical lobular hyperplasia or lobular carcinoma *in situ*: a correlative study of 33 patients with review of the literature. *Am J Surg Pathol* 2005;29:534–543.
20. Sapino A, Frigerio A, Peterse JL, et al. Mammographically detected *in situ* lobular carcinomas of the breast. *Virchows Arch* 2000;436:421–430.

21. Georgian-Smith D, Lawton TJ. Calcifications of lobular carcinoma *in situ* of the breast: radiologic-pathologic correlation. *AJR Am J Roentgenol* 2001;176:1255–1259.
22. Urban JA. Bilaterality of cancer of the breast. Biopsy of the opposite breast. *Cancer* 1967;20:1867–1870.
23. Rosen PP, Senie R, Schottenfeld D, et al. Noninvasive breast carcinoma: frequency of unsuspected invasion and implications for treatment. *Ann Surg* 1979;189:377–382.
24. Rosen PP, Braun DW Jr, Lyngholm B, et al. Lobular carcinoma *in situ* of the breast: preliminary results of treatment by ipsilateral mastectomy and contralateral breast biopsy. *Cancer* 1981;47:813–819.
25. Arpino G, Bardou VJ, Clark GM, et al. Infiltrating lobular carcinoma of the breast: tumor characteristics and clinical outcome. *Breast Cancer Res* 2004;6:R149–R156.
26. Allen-Brady K, Camp NJ, Ward JH, et al. Lobular breast cancer: excess familiality observed in the Utah Population Database. *Int J Cancer* 2005;117:655–661.
27. Lakhani SR, Gusterson BA, Jacquemier J, et al. The pathology of familial breast cancer: histological features of cancers in families not attributable to mutations in *BRCA1* or *BRCA2*. *Clin Cancer Res* 2000;6:782–789.
28. Claus EB, Risch N, Thompson WD, et al. Relationship between breast histopathology and family history of breast cancer. *Cancer* 1993;71:147–153.
29. Claus EB, Stowe M, Carter D. Family history of breast and ovarian cancer and the risk of breast carcinoma *in situ*. *Breast Cancer Res Treat* 2003;78:7–15.
30. Claus EB, Stowe M, Carter D, et al. The risk of a contralateral breast cancer among women diagnosed with ductal and lobular breast carcinoma *in situ*: data from the Connecticut Tumor Registry. *Breast* 2003;12:451–456.
31. Andersen JA. Lobular carcinoma *in situ* of the breast. An approach to rational treatment. *Cancer* 1977;39:2597–2602.
32. Bauer TL, Pandelidis SM, Rhoads JE Jr. Five-year survival of 100 women with carcinoma of the breast diagnosed by screening mammography and needle-localization biopsy. *J Am Coll Surg* 1994;178:427–430.
33. Page DL, Dupont WD, Rogers LW, et al. Atypical hyperplastic lesions of the female breast. A long-term follow-up study. *Cancer* 1985;55:2698–2708.
34. Dupont WD, Page DL. Risk factors for breast cancer in women with proliferative breast disease. *N Engl J Med* 1985;312:146–151.
35. Fisher ER, Land SR, Fisher B, et al. Pathologic findings from the National Surgical Adjuvant Breast and Bowel Project: twelve-year observations concerning lobular carcinoma *in situ*. *Cancer* 2004;100:238–244.
36. Webber BL, Heise H, Neifeld JP, et al. Risk of subsequent contralateral breast carcinoma in a population of patients with *in-situ* breast carcinoma. *Cancer* 1981;47:2928–2932.
37. Habel LA, Moe RE, Daling JR, et al. Risk of contralateral breast cancer among women with carcinoma *in situ* of the breast. *Ann Surg* 1997;225:69–75.
38. Haagensen CD, Lane N, Bodian C. Coexisting lobular neoplasia and carcinoma of the breast. *Cancer* 1983;51:1468–1482.
39. Chuba PJ, Hamre MR, Yap J, et al. Bilateral risk for subsequent breast cancer after lobular carcinoma-*in-situ*: analysis of surveillance, epidemiology, and end results data. *J Clin Oncol* 2005;23:5534–5541.
40. Li CI, Malone KE, Saltzman BS, et al. Risk of invasive breast carcinoma among women diagnosed with ductal carcinoma *in situ* and lobular carcinoma *in situ*, 1988–2001. *Cancer* 2006;106:2104–2112.
41. Rosen PP, Kosloff C, Lieberman PH, et al. Lobular carcinoma *in situ* of the breast. Detailed analysis of 99 patients with average follow-up of 24 years. *Am J Surg Pathol* 1978;2:225–251.
42. Ottesen GL, Graversen HP, Blichert-Toft M, et al. Carcinoma *in situ* of the female breast. 10 year follow-up results of a prospective nationwide study. *Breast Cancer Res Treat* 2000;62:197–210.
43. Ottesen GL, Graversen HP, Blichert-Toft M, et al. Lobular carcinoma *in situ* of the female breast. Short-term results of a prospective nationwide study. The Danish Breast Cancer Cooperative Group. *Am J Surg Pathol* 1993;17:14–21.
44. Marshall LM, Hunter DJ, Connolly JL, et al. Risk of breast cancer associated with atypical hyperplasia of lobular and ductal types. *Cancer Epidemiol Biomarkers Prev* 1997;6:297–301.
45. Abdel-Fatah TM, Powe DG, Hodi Z, et al. High frequency of coexistence of columnar cell lesions, lobular neoplasia, and low grade ductal carcinoma *in situ* with invasive tubular carcinoma and invasive lobular carcinoma. *Am J Surg Pathol* 2007;31:417–426.
46. Maluf H, Koerner F. Lobular carcinoma *in situ* and infiltrating ductal carcinoma: frequent presence of DCIS as a precursor lesion. *Int J Surg Pathol* 2001;9:127–131.
47. Rosen PP. Coexistent lobular carcinoma *in situ* and intraductal carcinoma in a single lobular-duct unit. *Am J Surg Pathol* 1980;4:241–246.
48. Tavassoli FA. *Pathology of the breast*. 2nd edition. Norwalk, CT: Appleton and Lange, 1999.
49. Lu YJ, Osin P, Lakhani SR, et al. Comparative genomic hybridization analysis of lobular carcinoma *in situ* and atypical lobular hyperplasia and potential roles for gains and losses of genetic material in breast neoplasia. *Cancer Res* 1998;58:4721–4727.
50. Reis-Filho JS, Lakhani SR. The diagnosis and management of pre-invasive breast disease: genetic alterations in pre-invasive lesions. *Breast Cancer Res* 2003;5:313–319.
51. Schnitt SJ, Morrow M. Lobular carcinoma *in situ*: current concepts and controversies. *Semin Diagn Pathol* 1999;16:209–223.
52. Leach C, Howell LP. Cytodiagnosis of classic lobular carcinoma and its variants. *Acta Cytol* 1992;36:199–202.
53. Ustun M, Berner A, Davidson B, et al. Fine-needle aspiration cytology of lobular carcinoma *in situ*. *Diagn Cytopathol* 2002;27:22–26.
54. Page DL, Dupont WD, Rogers LW. Ductal involvement by cells of atypical lobular hyperplasia in the breast: a long-term follow-up study of cancer risk. *Hum Pathol* 1988;19:201–207.
55. Page DL, Anderson TJ, Rogers LW. Carcinoma *in situ* (CIS). In: Page DL, Anderson TJ, eds. *Diagnostic histopathology of the breast*. New York: Churchill Livingston, 1987:157–192.
56. Sneige N, Wang J, Baker BA, et al. Clinical, histopathologic, and biologic features of pleomorphic lobular (ductal-lobular) carcinoma *in situ* of the breast: a report of 24 cases. *Mod Pathol* 2002;15:1044–1050.
57. Tavassoli FA, Millis RR, Boecker W, et al. Lobular neoplasia. In: Tavassoli FA, Devilee P, eds. World Health Organization Classification of Tumours. Pathology and genetics of tumours of the breast and female genital organs. Lyon: IARC Press, 2003:60–62.
58. Jacobs TW, Pliss N, Kouria G, et al. Carcinomas *in situ* of the breast with indeterminate features: role of E-cadherin staining in categorization. *Am J Surg Pathol* 2001;25:229–236.
59. Maluf HM. Differential diagnosis of solid carcinoma *in situ*. *Semin Diagn Pathol* 2004;21:25–31.
60. Sarrio D, Perez-Mies B, Hardisson D, et al. Cytoplasmic localization of p120ctn and E-cadherin loss characterize lobular breast carcinoma from preinvasive to metastatic lesions. *Oncogene* 2004;23:3272–3283.
61. Dabbs DJ, Bhargava R, Chivukula M. Lobular versus ductal breast neoplasms: the diagnostic utility of p120 catenin. *Am J Surg Pathol* 2007;31:427–437.
62. Dabbs DJ, Kaplai M, Chivukula M, et al. The spectrum of morphomolecular abnormalities of the E-cadherin/catenin complex in pleomorphic lobular carcinoma of the breast. *Appl Immunohistochem Mol Morphol* 2007;15:260–266.
63. Mohsin SK, O'Connell P, Allred DC, et al. Biomarker profile and genetic abnormalities in lobular carcinoma *in situ*. *Breast Cancer Res Treat* 2005;90:249–256.
64. Rudas M, Neumayer R, Gnant MF, et al. p53 protein expression, cell proliferation and steroid hormone receptors in ductal and lobular *in situ* carcinomas of the breast. *Eur J Cancer* 1997;33:39–44.
65. Middleton LP, Perkins GH, Tucker SL, et al. Expression of ERalpha and ERbeta in lobular carcinoma *in situ*. *Histopathology* 2007;50:875–880.
66. Eusebi V, Magalhaes F, Azzopardi JG. Pleomorphic lobular carcinoma of the breast: an aggressive tumor showing apocrine differentiation. *Hum Pathol* 1992;23:655–662.
67. Bratthauer GL, Moinfar F, Stamatakos MD, et al. Combined E-cadherin and high molecular weight cytokeratin immunoprofile differentiates lobular, ductal, and hybrid mammary intraepithelial neoplasias. *Hum Pathol* 2002;33:620–627.
68. Roylance R, Droufakou S, Gorman P, et al. The role of E-cadherin in low-grade ductal breast tumourigenesis. *J Pathol* 2003;200:53–58.
69. Droufakou S, Deshmane V, Roylance R, et al. Multiple ways of silencing E-cadherin gene expression in lobular carcinoma of the breast. *Int J Cancer* 2001;92:404–408.
70. Gamallo C, Palacios J, Suarez A, et al. Correlation of E-cadherin expression with differentiation grade and histological type in breast carcinoma. *Am J Pathol* 1993;142:987–993.
71. Rasbridge SA, Gillett CE, Sampson SA, et al. Epithelial (E-) and placental (P-) cadherin cell adhesion molecule expression in breast carcinoma. *J Pathol* 1993;169:245–250.
72. De Leeuw WJ, Berx G, Vos CB, et al. Simultaneous loss of E-cadherin and catenins in invasive lobular breast cancer and lobular carcinoma *in situ*. *J Pathol* 1997;183:404–411.
73. Sarrio D, Moreno-Bueno G, Hardisson D, et al. Epigenetic and genetic alterations of *APC* and *CDH1* genes in lobular breast cancer: relationships with abnormal E-cadherin and catenin expression and microsatellite instability. *Int J Cancer* 2003;106:208–215.
74. Mastracci TL, Tjan S, Bane AL, et al. E-cadherin alterations in atypical lobular hyperplasia and lobular carcinoma *in situ* of the breast. *Mod Pathol* 2005;18:741–751.
75. Maluf HM, Swanson PE, Koerner FC. Solid low-grade *in situ* carcinoma of the breast: role of associated lesions and E-cadherin in differential diagnosis. *Am J Surg Pathol* 2001;25:237–244.
76. Goldstein NS, Bassi D, Watts JC, et al. E-cadherin reactivity of 95 noninvasive ductal and lobular lesions of the breast. Implications for the interpretation of problematic lesions. *Am J Clin Pathol* 2001;115:534–542.
77. Reis-Filho JS, Cancela Paredes J, Milanezi F, et al. Clinicopathologic implications of E-cadherin reactivity in patients with lobular carcinoma *in situ* of the breast. *Cancer* 2002;94:2114–2115(author reply 2115–2116).
78. Da Silva L, Parry S, Reid L, et al. Aberrant expression of E-cadherin in lobular carcinomas of the breast. *Am J Surg Pathol* 2008;32(5):773–783.
79. Mahler-Araujo B, Savage K, Parry S, et al. Reduction of E-cadherin expression is associated with non-lobular breast carcinomas of basal-like and triple negative phenotype. *J Clin Pathol* 2008;61:615–620.
80. Rieger-Christ KM, Pezza JA, Dugan JM, et al. Disparate E-cadherin mutations in LCIS and associated invasive breast carcinomas. *Mol Pathol* 2001;54:91–97.
81. Reis-Filho JS, Simpson PT, Jones C, et al. Pleomorphic lobular carcinoma of the breast: role of comprehensive molecular pathology in characterization of an entity. *J Pathol* 2005;207:1–13.
82. Simpson PT, Reis-Filho JS, Gale T, et al. Molecular evolution of breast cancer. *J Pathol* 2005;205:248–254.
83. Berx G, Cleton-Jansen AM, Nollet F, et al. E-cadherin is a tumour/invasion suppressor gene mutated in human lobular breast cancers. *Embo J* 1995;14:6107–6115.
84. Berx G, Cleton-Jansen AM, Strumane K, et al. E-cadherin is inactivated in a majority of invasive human lobular breast cancers by truncation mutations throughout its extracellular domain. *Oncogene* 1996;13:1919–1925.
85. Palacios J, Sarrio D, Garcia-Macias MC, et al. Frequent E-cadherin gene inactivation by loss of heterozygosity in pleomorphic lobular carcinoma of the breast. *Mod Pathol* 2003;16:674–678.
86. Lei H, Sjoberg-Margolin S, Salahshor S, et al. *CDH1* mutations are present in both ductal and lobular breast cancer, but promoter allelic variants show no detectable breast cancer risk. *Int J Cancer* 2002;98:199–204.
87. Cheng CW, Wu PE, Yu JC, et al. Mechanisms of inactivation of E-cadherin in breast carcinoma: modification of the two-hit hypothesis of tumor suppressor gene. *Oncogene* 2001;20:3814–3823.
88. Aigner K, Dampier B, Descovich L, et al. The transcription factor ZEB1 (deltaEF1) promotes tumour cell dedifferentiation by repressing master regulators of epithelial polarity. *Oncogene* 2007;26:6979–6988.
89. Derksen PW, Liu X, Saridin F, et al. Somatic inactivation of E-cadherin and p53 in mice leads to metastatic lobular mammary carcinoma through induction of anoikis resistance and angiogenesis. *Cancer Cell* 2006;10:437–449.
90. Guilford P, Hopkins J, Harraway J, et al. E-cadherin germline mutations in familial gastric cancer. *Nature* 1998;392:402–405.
91. Kaurah P, MacMillan A, Boyd N, et al. Founder and recurrent *CDH1* mutations in families with hereditary diffuse gastric cancer. *JAMA* 2007;297:2360–2372.
92. Keller G, Vogelsang H, Becker I, et al. Diffuse type gastric and lobular breast carcinoma in a familial gastric cancer patient with an E-cadherin germline mutation. *Am J Pathol* 1999;155:337–342.
93. Rahman N, Stone JG, Coleman G, et al. Lobular carcinoma *in situ* of the breast is not caused by constitutional mutations in the E-cadherin gene. *Br J Cancer* 2000;82:568–570.
94. Masciari S, Larsson N, Senz J, et al. Germline E-cadherin mutations in familial lobular breast cancer. *J Med Genet* 2007;44:726–731.
95. Salahshor S, Haixin L, Huo H, et al. Low frequency of E-cadherin alterations in familial breast cancer. *Breast Cancer Res* 2001;3:199–207.

96. Schrader KA, Masciari S, Boyd N, et al. Hereditary diffuse gastric cancer: association with lobular breast cancer. *Fam Cancer* 2008;7(1):73–82.
97. Stone JG, Coleman G, Gusterson B, et al. Contribution of germline *MLH1* and *MSH2* mutations to lobular carcinoma *in situ* of the breast. *Cancer Lett* 2001;167:171–174.
98. Pathology of familial breast cancer: differences between breast cancers in carriers of *BRCA1* or *BRCA2* mutations and sporadic cases. Breast Cancer Linkage Consortium. *Lancet* 1997;349:1505–1510.
99. Huzarski T, Cybulski C, Domagala W, et al. Pathology of breast cancer in women with constitutional *CHEK2* mutations. *Breast Cancer Res Treat* 2005;90:187–189.
100. Kallioniemi A, Kallioniemi OP, Sudar D, et al. Comparative genomic hybridization for molecular cytogenetic analysis of solid tumors. *Science* 1992;258:818–821.
101. Reis-Filho JS, Simpson PT, Gale T, et al. The molecular genetics of breast cancer: the contribution of comparative genomic hybridization. *Pathol Res Pract* 2005;201:713–725.
102. Nayar R, Zhuang Z, Merino MJ, et al. Loss of heterozygosity on chromosome 11q13 in lobular lesions of the breast using tissue microdissection and polymerase chain reaction. *Hum Pathol* 1997;28:277–282.
103. Lakhani SR, Collins N, Sloane JP, et al. Loss of heterozygosity in lobular carcinoma *in situ* of the breast. *Clin Mol Pathol* 1995;48:M74–M78.
104. Nishizaki T, Chew K, Chu L, et al. Genetic alterations in lobular breast cancer by comparative genomic hybridization. *Int J Cancer* 1997;74:513–517.
105. Gunther K, Merkelbach-Bruse S, Amo-Takyi BK, et al. Differences in genetic alterations between primary lobular and ductal breast cancers detected by comparative genomic hybridization. *J Pathol* 2001;193:40–47.
106. Albertson DG, Pinkel D. Genomic microarrays in human genetic disease and cancer. *Hum Mol Genet* 2003;12[Spec no 2]:R145–R152.
107. Reis-Filho JS, Simpson PT, Turner NC, et al. FGFR1 emerges as a potential therapeutic target for lobular breast carcinomas. *Clin Cancer Res* 2006;12:6652–6662.
108. Loo LW, Grove DI, Williams EM, et al. Array comparative genomic hybridization analysis of genomic alterations in breast cancer subtypes. *Cancer Res* 2004;64:8541–8549.
109. Gelsi-Boyer V, Orsetti B, Cervera N, et al. Comprehensive profiling of 8p11-12 amplification in breast cancer. *Mol Cancer Res* 2005;3:655–667.
110. Ormandy CJ, Musgrove EA, Hui R, et al. Cyclin D1, EMS1 and 11q13 amplification in breast cancer. *Breast Cancer Res Treat* 2003;78:323–335.
111. Reis-Filho JS, Savage K, Lambros MB, et al. Cyclin D1 protein overexpression and CCND1 amplification in breast carcinomas: an immunohistochemical and chromogenic *in situ* hybridisation analysis. *Mod Pathol* 2006;19:999–1009.
112. Mastracci TL, Shadeo A, Colby SM, et al. Genomic alterations in lobular neoplasia: a microarray comparative genomic hybridization signature for early neoplastic proliferation in the breast. *Genes Chromosomes Cancer* 2006;45:1007–1017.
113. Weber-Mangal S, Sinn HP, Popp S, et al. Breast cancer in young women (< or = 35 years): Genomic aberrations detected by comparative genomic hybridization. *Int J Cancer* 2003;107:583–592.
114. Middleton LP, Palacios DM, Bryant BR, et al. Pleomorphic lobular carcinoma: morphology, immunohistochemistry, and molecular analysis. *Am J Surg Pathol* 2000;24:1650–1656.
115. Buerger H, Otterbach F, Simon R, et al. Different genetic pathways in the evolution of invasive breast cancer are associated with distinct morphological subtypes. *J Pathol* 1999;189:521–526.
116. Roylance R, Gorman P, Hanby A, et al. Allelic imbalance analysis of chromosome 16q shows that grade I and grade III invasive ductal breast cancers follow different genetic pathways. *J Pathol* 2002;196:32–36.
117. Roylance R, Gorman P, Harris W, et al. Comparative genomic hybridization of breast tumors stratified by histological grade reveals new insights into the biological progression of breast cancer. *Cancer Res* 1999;59:1433–1436.
118. Powell JA, Gardner AE, Bais AJ, et al. Sequencing, transcript identification, and quantitative gene expression profiling in the breast cancer loss of heterozygosity region 16q24.3 reveal three potential tumor-suppressor genes. *Genomics* 2002;80:303–310.
119. Rakha EA, Green AR, Powe DG, et al. Chromosome 16 tumor-suppressor genes in breast cancer. *Genes Chromosomes Cancer* 2006;45:527–535.
120. van Wezel T, Lombaerts M, van Roon EH, et al. Expression analysis of candidate breast tumour suppressor genes on chromosome 16q. *Breast Cancer Res* 2005;7:R998–R1004.
121. Green AR, Krivinskas S, Young P, et al. Loss of expression of chromosome 16q genes DPEP1 and CTCF in lobular carcinoma *in situ* of the breast. *Breast Cancer Res Treat* 2008. In press.
122. Jacobs TW, Connolly JL, Schnitt SJ. Nonmalignant lesions in breast core needle biopsies: to excise or not to excise? *Am J Surg Pathol* 2002;26:1095–1110.
123. Middleton LP, Grant S, Stephens T, et al. Lobular carcinoma *in situ* diagnosed by core needle biopsy: when should it be excised? *Mod Pathol* 2003;16:120–129.
124. Crisi GM, Mandavilli S, Cronin E, et al. Invasive mammary carcinoma after immediate and short-term follow-up for lobular neoplasia on core biopsy. *Am J Surg Pathol* 2003;27:325–333.
125. Shin SJ, Rosen PP. Excisional biopsy should be performed if lobular carcinoma *in situ* is seen on needle core biopsy. *Arch Pathol Lab Med* 2002;126:697–701.
126. Renshaw AA, Cartagena N, Derhagopian RP, et al. Lobular neoplasia in breast core needle biopsy specimens is not associated with an increased risk of ductal carcinoma *in situ* or invasive carcinoma. *Am J Clin Pathol* 2002;117:797–799.
127. Renshaw AA, Cartagena N, Schenkman RH, et al. Atypical ductal hyperplasia in breast core needle biopsies. Correlation of size of the lesion, complete removal of the lesion, and the incidence of carcinoma in follow-up biopsies. *Am J Clin Pathol* 2001;116:92–96.
128. Renshaw AA, Derhagopian RP, Martinez P, et al. Lobular neoplasia in breast core needle biopsy specimens is associated with a low risk of ductal carcinoma *in situ* or invasive carcinoma on subsequent excision. *Am J Clin Pathol* 2006;126:310–313.
129. Bauer VP, Ditkoff BA, Schnabel F, et al. The management of lobular neoplasia identified on percutaneous core breast biopsy. *Breast J* 2003;9:4–9.
130. Dmytrasz K, Tartter PI, Mizrachy H, et al. The significance of atypical lobular hyperplasia at percutaneous breast biopsy. *Breast J* 2003;9:10–12.
131. Mahoney MC, Robinson-Smith TM, Shaughnessy EA. Lobular neoplasia at 11-gauge vacuum-assisted stereotactic biopsy: correlation with surgical excisional biopsy and mammographic follow-up. *AJR Am J Roentgenol* 2006;187:949–954.
132. Liberman L, Sama M, Susnik B, et al. Lobular carcinoma *in situ* at percutaneous breast biopsy: surgical biopsy findings. *AJR Am J Roentgenol* 1999;173:291–299.
133. Lakhani SR, Audretsch W, Cleton-Jensen AM, et al. The management of lobular carcinoma *in situ* (LCIS). Is LCIS the same as ductal carcinoma *in situ* (DCIS)? *Eur J Cancer* 2006;42:2205–2211.
134. Reis-Filho JS, Pinder SE. Non-operative breast pathology: lobular neoplasia. *J Clin Pathol* 2007;60:1321–1327.
135. Esserman LE, Lamea L, Tanev S, et al. Should the extent of lobular neoplasia on core biopsy influence the decision for excision? *Breast J* 2007;13:55–61.
136. Lee AH, Denley HE, Pinder, SE, et al. Excision biopsy findings of patients with breast needle core biopsies reported as suspicious of malignancy (B4) or lesion of uncertain malignant potential (B3). *Histopathology* 2003;42:331–336.

Chapter 25
Lobular Carcinoma *In Situ:* Clinical Management

Kandice E. Kilbride and Lisa A. Newman

HISTORICAL BACKGROUND AND PATHOLOGY

The contemporary perception of lobular carcinoma *in situ* (LCIS) as a risk factor for breast cancer, as opposed to being a direct precursor lesion, has evolved gradually over the past several decades. In 1941 Foote and Stewart (1) published their landmark study of LCIS, describing a relatively rare entity within the broad spectrum of breast pathologic processes characterized by an "alteration of lobular cytology." The now well-established histologic features of LCIS were based on findings present in 14 of 300 cancerous mastectomy specimens (4.67%) from Memorial Hospital in New York City; in 2 cases (0.67%) this was described as "typical LCIS" fulfilling "strict" criteria; in another 2 the LCIS was scanty in amount; and in the remaining 10 cases, it was intermediate in extent. Foote and Stewart described this aberration of normal breast architecture as being notable for "the presence of a lobule or group of lobules in which . . . [t]he nuclei tend to be rather clear; they show no hyperchromatism. The cytoplasm is apt to be opaque, somewhat acidophilic, and occasionally vacuolated. The compact, orderly arrangement of the epithelium of the normal lobule gives place to a decided looseness, a loss of cohesion." These pathologists also documented the tendency for this disturbance of the terminal duct–lobular units to be diffuse, and they furthermore ascertained its occult nature, reporting that "it is always a disease of multiple foci" and that "there is no way by which it can be recognized grossly" (1).

Numerous subsequent studies have reiterated the pathologic hallmarks of LCIS: a proliferation of pale and slightly eosinophilic cells that are occasionally vacuolated and contain small, uniform nuclei. These cells pack the acinar units, resulting in varying degrees of terminal duct–lobular distention. Although Foote and Stewart appreciated the noninfiltrative nature of LCIS, the coexisting cancers in the study specimens coupled with the multicentric pattern were influential factors in leading the investigators to conclude that mastectomy is the indicated management. Twenty-six years later, however, McDivitt et al. (2) updated the Memorial Hospital experience and reported the long-term outcome of 50 patients with LCIS, 8 of whom were managed by unilateral mastectomy and 42 by local excision only. This study revealed evidence of LCIS as a risk factor for future breast cancer on either side: At 10 years, the cumulative breast cancer risk was 15% on the breast sampled for biopsy and 10% on the contralateral side; at 15 years, the corresponding risks were 27% and 15%; and at 20 years, the risks were 35% and 25%, respectively.

Emerging data throughout the 1970s yielded disparate recommendations for optimal management of LCIS. Haagensen et al. (3) reviewed and reclassified 5,560 benign breast biopsy specimens from the Columbia-Presbyterian Medical Center in New York, and identified 210 that contained foci of LCIS. After a mean follow-up of 14 years (range, 1 to 42 years), breast cancer developed in 16.7%, and the risk to either breast was equivalent. These findings stressed the cumulative long-term and bilateral risk of subsequent breast cancer, prompting the investigators to become proponents of an observation-only strategy for patients with LCIS. They also advocated replacement of the term LCIS with "lobular neoplasia" to minimize the association with frankly malignant breast tumors. Wheeler et al. (4) drew similar conclusions based on data from the University of Pennsylvania. Conversely, Rosen et al. (5) evaluated 84 cases of LCIS from Memorial Hospital treated by biopsy only; with an average 24-year follow-up, breast cancer developed in 29 (34.5%) of these patients, and the subsequent cancers were equally distributed in laterality relative to the sampled breast. These data led to a recommendation that LCIS be treated by ipsilateral mastectomy with low axillary dissection and contralateral breast biopsy (a strategy that is rarely, if ever, used today). The current treatment strategies include observation and risk reduction with bilateral mastectomy or chemoprevention (see below).

The detection of atypical lobular hyperplasia (ALH), a lesion quite comparable pathologically with LCIS, has further complicated efforts to develop a unified approach to the management of LCIS. ALH involves a microscopic pattern similar to that of LCIS, but is generally less extensive in the terminal ducts and lobules. As defined by Page et al. (6), a diagnosis of LCIS mandates that at least half of the spaces in a given lobule be distended by the characteristic cells. Because the distinction between LCIS and ALH can be fairly subjective, it has been suggested that they both be discussed within the context of the more general pathologic category of "lobular neoplasia" or "lobular intraepithelial neoplasia" (6–8). In contrast, some investigators have combined ALH with atypical ductal hyperplasia (ADH) (9,10) in the collective category of "atypical hyperplasia." Occasionally, discrepancies arise in the histopathologic interpretation of lesions representing ductal versus lobular patterns of atypia, and atypia versus *in situ* carcinomas, leading some investigators to recommend that these borderline lesions be evaluated collectively as "mammary intraepithelial neoplasia" (11). In response to these inconsistent approaches, several pathologists have advocated use of a standardized set of descriptive criteria to classify these lesions in the hope of minimizing interobserver variability (12,13). This chapter presents epidemiologic and management data on both LCIS and ALH, with distinctions made between the two lesions whenever possible.

Tissue involved with the process of lobular neoplasia is typically positive for estrogen receptor staining and negative for *HER2/neu* overexpression (14–17). Advances in molecular technology have revealed provocative findings regarding the pathogenesis of LCIS. Several investigators have reported the consistent loss of E-cadherin expression in both LCIS and invasive lobular cancer; this transmembrane protein is involved with cell-to-cell adhesion, and its genetic code is located on chromosome 16q. Absence of this cell adhesion function is probably related to the diffuse nature of lobular breast disease, and E-cadherin negativity serves as a fairly reliable means of distinguishing ductal from lobular patterns of disease at both the *in situ* and invasive stages. Other studies of lobular neoplasia have demonstrated loss of chromosomal material from 16p, 17p, and 22q, as well as gain of material on 1q and 6q (18–26). Recent evaluation using genetic fingerprinting has implicated *CDH1* and *CTCF* as tumor suppressor genes in the development of LCIS (24). It has also been suggested that sequential alterations in genetic content may account for the direct progression of some LCIS lesions into invasive lobular cancers (25), and can be used to distinguish classic LCIS from ductal carcinoma *in situ* (DCIS) and pleomorphic LCIS lesions (26).

Table 25.1	DETECTION OF LOBULAR NEOPLASIA: INCIDENCE AND PREVALENCE RATES

Study (Reference), Year	Study Population	Number Lobular Neoplasia/Total	Prevalence	Features
Wheeler (4), 1974	4,898 consecutive breast biopsies, retrospectively reviewed	57/138 8/4,898 30/3,570	4.3% 1.8% 0.8%	LCIS LCIS + cancer LCIS only
Anderson et al. (27), 1977	3,299 benign breast biopsies, retrospectively reviewed	52/3,299 47/3,294	1.5% 1.4%	All cases No prior history of cancer
Rosen et al. (28), 1978	8,609 consecutive benign breast biopsies, retrospectively reviewed	117/8,069 99/8,609	1.4% 3.8%	LCIS + other pathology LCIS only
Haagensen et al. (3), 1978	5,560 benign breast biopsies, retrospectively reviewed	211/5,560	3.8%	LCIS/LN
Page et al. (29), 1985[a]	10,542 benign breast biopsies, retrospectively reviewed	169/10,542	1.6%	ALH
Page et al. (6), 1991	10,542 benign breast biopsies, retrospectively reviewed	48/10,542	0.5%	LCIS
Li et al. (30), 2002	SEER Program	NA	0.9/100,000 person-yrs 2.8/100,000 person-yrs 3.2/100,000 person-yrs	1987–80, LCIS 1987–89, LCIS 1996–98, LCIS
Hoogerbrugge et al. (33), 2003	67 prophylactic mastectomy cases (66% *BRCA* mutation carriers)	17/67 25/67	25% 37%	LCIS ALH
Kauff et al. (34), 2003	24 prophylactic mastectomy cases (all *BRCA* mutation carriers)	1/24 3/24	4% 13%	LCIS ALH
Khurana et al. (36), 2000	35 prophylactic mastectomy cases	4/35	11.4%	ALH
Page et al. (38), 2003	17,170 benign breast biopsies	457/17,170	2.7%	ALH
Adem et al. (39), 2003	440 unilateral prophylactic mastectomy specimens[b] 64 prophylactic mastectomy cases (all *BRCA* mutation carriers)	22/440 1/64	5% 1.2%	LN LN
Dotto et al. (37), 2008	516 bilateral reduction mammoplasty specimens	17/516	3.3%	LN

LCIS, lobular carcinoma *in situ*; ALH, atypical lobular hyperplasia; LN, lobular neoplasia; SEER, Surveillance, Epidemiology, and End Results.
[a]Number of ALH cases estimated, based on 1.6% prevalence.
[b]Patients with a unilateral breast cancer undergoing bilateral mastectomy.

PREVALENCE AND NATURAL HISTORY

In general, lesions of lobular neoplasia are incidental findings detected when a biopsy is being performed to evaluate some other pattern of fibrocystic or malignant breast disease. The absence of any gross clinical or mammographic features specifically associated with these entities creates difficulty in accurately quantifying incidence. Table 25.1 demonstrates the relatively low prevalence (0.5% to 4.3%) of LCIS based on retrospective reviews of benign breast biopsies (3,4,6,26–31,33–38). Prevalence rates are higher when cancerous biopsies are included. Incidental detection rates of LCIS are also higher (4% to 25%) in two studies reporting the pathologic findings in prophylactic mastectomy specimens from high-risk women (34,35). Autopsy setudies have a potential age bias in favor of older cases in series of natural cause deaths, or favoring younger age in forensic series (34,35). Kauff et al. (34) described findings in a forensic autopsy series of 490 nonpregnant women, 76% of whom were younger than 55 years of age, and found only 2 cases (0.4%) each of LCIS and ALH. A review by Frykberg (35) of 19 published series (1989 to 1999) involving biopsy results for 10,499 nonpalpable, mammographically detected breast abnormalities revealed LCIS identified in 1.1% of all cases and in 5.7% of those cases where a malignancy was diagnosed.

Li et al. (30) estimated the incidence of LCIS to be 0.9/100,000, based on Surveillance, Epidemiology, and End Results

data in 1978 to 1980. They later reported a 2.6-fold increase from 1980 to 2001; the bulk of this increased LCIS burden was seen among women aged 50 to 69. Proposed explanations include an increase in number of screen-motivated biopsies, calcifications on mammogram associated with LCIS, and use of postmenopausal hormone replacement therapy (HRT) during that time (39). Many physicians question whether the incidence of LCIS will continue to increase, as the use of HRT in postmenopausal women has declined since the publication of the Women's Health Initiative Randomized Controlled Trial in 2002 (32). This has been associated with a parallel decrease in incidence of invasive breast cancer over the same period (40), but no findings have been reported to date regarding LCIS.

Prevalence of ALH appears to be slightly higher than that of LCIS, ranging from 1.6% to 2.7% in retrospective reviews of benign breast biopsies (29,37), 3.3% in reduction mammoplasty specimens (36), and 11% to 37% (33–36) in prophylactic mastectomy cases.

As shown in Table 25.2, studies providing long-term follow-up data reveal several consistent patterns that strengthen the perception of lobular neoplasia as a marker of increased bilateral breast cancer risk (2–4,6,27–29,37,39,42–52). The median age of women found to harbor lobular neoplasia falls in the fifth decade of life, approaching 10 years younger than the most common age range for diagnosis of invasive breast cancer. These same studies demonstrate the rising cumulative

Table 25.2	BREAST CANCER RISK FOLLOWING A DIAGNOSIS OF LOBULAR NEOPLASIA

	Study (Reference)	N	Comparison Population	Age at Diagnosis (yrs)	Follow-Up (yrs)	Number Develop CA (%)	Relative Risk	Ipsilateral Cancer (%)	Contralateral Cancer (%)	Invasive Lobular Histology
LCIS	McDivitt et al.[a] (2), 1967	50	NA	44.3	1–23	16 (32)	NR	50	NR	NR
LCIS	Wheeler et al.[b] (4), 1974	32	NA	43.9	17.5	4 (12.5)	NR	25	75	NR
LCIS	Andersen[c] (27), 1977	44	Copenhagen general population	46	15.9	13 (27.7)	11.9	69	31	NR
LCIS	Rosen et al.[d] (28), 1978	84	Connecticut general population	45	24	29 (34.5)	9	66	55	45%
LCIS	Haagensen et al.[e] (3), 1978	210	Connecticut general population	45–49	14	35 (16.7)	7.2	54	54	54%
LCIS	Salvadori et al. (42), 1991	78	Lombardy, Italy general population	49	4.8	5 (6.4)	10.3	100	0	0%
LCIS	Page et al. (6), 1991	39	Atlanta general population	45	19	9 (11)	6.9	60	40	7/10 (70%)
LCIS	Ottensen et al.[f] (43), 1993	69	Danish general population	47	5.8	15 (21.7)	11	100	0	3/8 (38%)
LCIS	Singletary[g] (44), 1994	45	NA	49	10	3 (6.7)	NR	66	33	0%
LCIS	Carson et al.[h] (45), 1994	51	NA	48	6.9	4 (7.8)	NR	75	NR	NR
LCIS	Chuba et al. (46), 2005	4,853	SEER database	45–49	10	350 (7.2)	2.4	46	54	81/350 (23.1%)
LCIS	Li et al. 39), 2006	4,490	Women with DCIS	54.3	NA	282 (6.2)	5.3	72	41	119/242 (49%)
LCIS	Chun et al. (47), 2006	307	NY general population	47	5	24 (30)	1.71	NR	NR	NR
ALH	Marshall et al. (52), 1997	49	Women with hx of BBD	43	10	11 (25.6)	5.3	64	NR	NR
ALH	Page et al.[i] (29), 1985	126	Atlanta general population	46	17.5	16 (12.7)	4.2	69	31	3/16 (19%)
ALH	Page et al. (48), 1988	146	Atlanta general population	44	17	16 (11)	2.7	NR	NR	NR
ALH	Shaaban et al.[j] (49), 2002	17	Controls with benign breast bx	49.4	5.8	NA	4.55	NR	NR	NR
ALH	Page et al.[k] (38), 2003	252	Nashville women with hx of BBD	46–55	NR	50 (19.8)	3.1	75	29	NR
ALH	Collins et al. (50), 2007	56	Nurses with hx of BBD	43.5	9.1	NR	5.49	61	NR	NR
ALH	Degnim et al. (51), 2007	175	Women with hx of BBD	58	13.7	34 (19.4)	3.67	Similar	Similar	NR

LCIS, lobular carcinoma *in situ*; SEER, Surveillance, Epidemiology, and End Results; DCIS, ductal carcinoma *in situ*; BBD, Benign Breast Disease; hx, history of; bx, biopsy;
ALH, atypical lobular hyperplasia; NA, not applicable; NR, not reported.
[a]Eight patients treated with immediate ipsilateral mastectomy; two patients lost to follow-up.
[b]Seven patients underwent mastectomy at time of LCIS diagnosis.
[c]Forty-four cases of LCIS initially treated with biopsy only; 2 patients developed subsequent bilateral cancer.
[d]Eighty-four of 99 LCIS cases with follow-up information; 7 patients developed subsequent bilateral cancer; 1 patient with unknown laterality of subsequent cancer.
[e]One patient with breast cancer prior to LCIS diagnosis; patients ages reported in 5-yr intervals.
[f]Eight patients with invasive recurrences.
[g]Two cases subsequent cancer occurred in residual breast tissue following prophylactic mastectomy.
[h]Three of four subsequent cancers with invasive histology; laterality not reported for DCIS.
[i]One of 16 subsequent cancers bilateral.
[j]Case control study; 674 benign breast biopsies (120 with subsequent breast cancer and age-matched controls).
[k]Age reported in 10-year intervals; 2 of 50 subsequent breast cancers cases with unknown laterality; 2 of 50 bilateral.

incidence rates of invasive carcinoma among women with a history of LCIS, averaging approximately 1% per year; the risk is expressed nearly equally for either breast. On average, the subsequent invasive cancer is characterized by an invasive lobular histology in only one quarter to one half of cases. The relative risk of breast cancer for women with LCIS compared with the general population of women without atypical proliferative breast disease ranges from 6.9 to 12. As shown by Haagensen et al. (3), this risk may increase substantially (from 5.0 to 10.0) in the presence of a family history of breast cancer occurring in a first degree relative. Interestingly, studies by Page et al. (6) showed no effect of family history on the risk conferred by LCIS, although the relative risk associated with ALH doubled (4.2 to 8.4) when compounded by breast cancer occurring within the immediate family (29). Page et al. (48) also demonstrated that extension of ALH foci to involve the ductal units also increased the subsequent risk of breast cancer. Data from the Nurses' Health Study indicate that ALH may confer a relatively higher risk for premenopausal compared with postmenopausal breast cancer (52). Finally, Page et al. (38) characterized ALH as having risk-associated features intermediate between those of ADH and LCIS; they noted that the age of presentation ranged from 31 to 55 years, relative risk for subsequent breast cancer was 3.1, and 75% of cancers occurred in the breast ipsilateral to where the ALH was detected. Lakhani (53) aptly summarized these findings as demonstrating that lobular neoplastic lesions are "precursors (albeit non-obligate) as well as risk indicators."

MANAGEMENT OPTIONS

Lobular neoplasia is a marker of abnormal proliferative activity in the breasts bilaterally. This is particularly relevant for LCIS, where the risk to either side approaches equivalence. Any rational management strategy must address this bilateral risk and would therefore include the following steps.

Observation

Close observation using clinical examination and mammography is the strategy selected by most patients. This is a reasonable and safe approach, as most women with LCIS will avoid a breast cancer diagnosis despite the increase in relative risk. As shown by Carson et al. (45), 4 of 51 women with LCIS choosing observation developed breast cancer, and all were detected at an early stage by mammographic screening. Port et al. (54) recently reported a study evaluating the use of breast magnetic resonance imaging (MRI) as a screening tool in high-risk patients, specifically those with a history of LCIS or atypical hyperplasia. Their data suggested that there was no added benefit in use of screening MRI in patients with atypical hyperplasia, and only a small benefit (4%) was seen in patients with LCIS.

Bilateral Prophylactic Mastectomy

The efficacy of bilateral prophylactic mastectomy (BPM) in reducing breast cancer risk and breast cancer mortality by approximately 90% was defined by Hartmann et al. (55), in their careful scrutiny of outcome among high-risk women (defined by family history) treated at the Mayo Clinic. However, a meta-analysis conducted more than 10 years ago revealed that although breast cancers developed in 16.4% of patients with LCIS managed with observation, the disease-related mortality rate was 2.8%, which was only slightly higher than the breast cancer mortality rate of 0.9% reported for the patients treated with BPM (56). A recent retrospective case-cohort study evaluating the efficacy of BPM in a community practice setting (57) showed a 95% reduction in the occurrence of breast cancer

in high-risk women; however, the absolute underlying risks of breast cancer and mortality were low.

Chemoprevention

Two large trials have been conducted by the National Surgical Adjuvant Breast and Bowel Project (NSABP) to address the use of chemoprevention for risk reduction in women with increased risk of developing breast cancer. The NSABP P-01 study was a prospective clinical trial which randomized 13,388 high-risk women older than 35 years of age to tamoxifen or placebo. In 1998, with a median follow-up of 54.6 months, the study was unblinded early because of the magnitude of the difference in breast cancer incidence between the two arms; tamoxifen reduced the incidence of breast cancer by 49% ($p < .001$) (58). Recent analysis with median follow-up of 74 months reported similar results; tamoxifen reduced the incidence of invasive cancer by 43% compared to placebo ($p < .001$). Subset analysis revealed that 413 of the participants randomized to placebo and 416 of those randomized to tamoxifen had a history of LCIS; breast cancers were detected in 38 and 9 women in each of these groups, respectively, consistent with a 46% reduction in breast cancer risk afforded by tamoxifen. In the 1,200 study participants with a history of atypical hyperplasia, tamoxifen reduced the incidence of breast cancer by a statistically significant 86% in the initial report (relative risk [RR] = 0.14, 95% confidence interval [CI], 0.03–0.47). The results persisted with the follow-up analysis; the reduction in breast cancer events in this group was 75% (RR = 0.25, 95% CI, 0.10–0.52). The study results did not specify the proportions of ductal versus lobular patterns of atypical hyperplasia among study participants (59).

The NSABP Study of Tamoxifen and Raloxifene (STAR) P-2 trial (60,61) compared the efficacy of these two drugs in the chemoprevention of breast cancer in 19,747 high-risk postmenopausal women. At a median follow-up of 3.9 years, similar rates of invasive cancer were reported in both groups (163 cases of invasive cancer in the tamoxifen group and 168 in the raloxifene group) (RR = 1.02, 95% CI, 0.82–1.28). Subset analysis of women with LCIS and atypical hyperplasia yielded similar results. In the 1,998 participants with a history of LCIS, 33 cases of invasive cancer were noted in each treatment group (RR = 0.98, 95% CI, 0.58–1.63). Those patients with LCIS had the highest risk of developing cancer than any other subgroup, with 9.61 to 9.83 cases per 1,000 participants. In the 2,186 patients with a history of atypical hyperplasia (no distinction was made between ductal and lobular histology), 41 breast cancer events were seen in the tamoxifen group and 47 in the raloxifene group (RR = 1.12, 95% CI, 0.72–1.74). The authors concluded that raloxifene is as effective as tamoxifen in decreasing risk of invasive breast cancer in all subgroups (61).

 ## SPECIAL TOPICS IN THE TREATMENT OF LOBULAR CARCINOMA *IN SITU*

Pleomorphic Lobular Carcinoma *In Situ*

Pleomorphic LCIS (PLCIS) is a relatively uncommon variant of LCIS characterized by medium to large pleomorphic cells containing eccentric nuclei, prominent nucleoli, and abundant eosinophilic cytoplasm. Adjacent ducts may be involved with PLCIS cells in pagetoid spread. As with classic LCIS, it is usually estrogen-receptor positive but negative for E-cadherin and *HER2/neu* staining; immunohistochemical testing for gross cystic disease fluid protein 15 (GCDFP-15) is also positive in this lesion (62,63). There is a higher proliferation rate and higher percentage of p53 protein positivity than seen in classic LCIS, which are indicative of aggressive behavior (62). PLCIS can be associated with central necrosis, and this may result in microcalcifications on mammogram (63,64). It may be difficult to distinguish PLCIS from DCIS; lack of E-cadherin staining may be helpful. PLCIS may have a relatively high incidence of coexisting invasive lobular cancer, and it has also been described in association with the fairly aggressive pattern of pleomorphic invasive lobular carcinoma (65). When PLCIS is detected, it is therefore prudent to conduct a meticulous histopathologic scrutiny for invasion. There is no consensus regarding therapy for PLCIS; however, most recommend treatment similar to patients with DCIS, with excision to negative margins with or without radiotherapy (62).

Breast-Conserving Therapy in the Presence of Lobular Carcinoma *In Situ*

Because LCIS is a marker of diffuse and bilateral proliferative activity in the breast, the presence of LCIS coexisting with invasive cancer provokes questions regarding the oncologic safety of breast-conservation therapy. As Table 25.3 demonstrates, studies designed to address the impact of LCIS on locoregional disease control have had mixed results (66–71); equivalent rates of in-breast tumor recurrence and overall survival have been reported regardless of whether LCIS was associated with the primary invasive cancer. However, Sasson et al. (68) and Jolly et al. (70) reported an increase in rates of ipsilateral breast tumor recurrence at 10 years in patients with LCIS who had chosen breast-conserving therapy. This difference was not evident at 5-year follow-up, suggesting that the LCIS was actually a marker for an increased risk for development of second primaries. It has been suggested that the presence of LCIS at the margin is associated with increased locoregional failure (72), but data regarding this are limited. Lumpectomy margins should be free of invasive carcinoma and DCIS, but re-excision

for LCIS at the margins does not appear to be warranted at this time. As shown by a review of 460 breast conservation cases by Fowble et al. (73), the presence of ALH coexisting with invasive cancer had no effect on risk of local recurrence, distant relapse, or contralateral new primary cancer.

Lobular Carcinoma *In Situ* Diagnosed on Core Needle Biopsy

It has become standard practice to recommend open excisional biopsy after detection of atypical hyperplasia on a core needle biopsy so that sampling error and risk of missing coexisting DCIS or invasive cancer will be minimized. When "pure" LCIS is found in a needle biopsy specimen, the primary concern should focus on whether some additional pathologic process is present in the biopsy specimen that would explain the clinical or imaging feature that prompted the biopsy, because LCIS would not account for any physical findings or radiographic abnormalities. The need for further surgical tissue sampling has been challenged in the setting of LCIS or ALH detected in a core needle biopsy specimen because some investigators have found very low rates of significant disease when the follow-up excisional biopsy was performed.

The recent use of large-bore, vacuum-assisted biopsy devices has also led clinicians to question the need for follow-up excisional biopsy in this setting. No series has directly compared the incidence of invasive cancers at follow-up excision for lobular neoplasia on core needle biopsy based on gauge; however, Margenthaler et al. (74) did find a significant difference in the rate of upgrade to cancer at excisional biopsy with the use of smaller-caliber biopsy devices. In contrast, in the study reported by Mahoney et al. (75), 27 core needle biopsies were done exclusively with 11-gauge, vacuum-assisted devices and were still upgraded to a diagnosis of cancer in 19%.

		Moran and Haffty[a] (66), 1998	Abner et al.[a] (67), 2000	Sasson et al.[a] (68), 2001	Carolin et al. (72), 2002	Ben-David et al.[a,b] (69), 2005	Jolly et al.[a] (70), 2006	Ciocca et al.[a] (71), 2008
Feature								
Number of subjects	LCIS present	51	137	65	105	64	56	290
	LCIS absent	1,045	1,044	1,209	(31 BCT) 115 (38 BCT)	121	551	2607
Primary histology invasive lobular or mixed ductal-lobular	LCIS present	53%	69%	51%	39%	58%	66%	47%
	LCIS absent	5%	5%	2%	9%	34%	6%	4%
Synchronous bilateral cancer	LCIS present	17%	NR	NR	2%	NR	NR	NR
	LCIS absent	8%	NR	NR	3%	NR	NR	NR
Follow-up (yrs)	LCIS present	10.6	8	6.3 for all	6.0	3.6	8.7 for all	5.2 for all
	LCIS absent	11.4	5.8		6.3	3.9		
Local recurrences	LCIS present	23%	12%[c]	5% at 5 yrs 29% at 10 yrs 3% at 5 yrs 6% at 10 yrs	16.7%	1.6%	14% at 10 yrs	4.8%
	LCIS absent	16%	13%[c]		18.9%	1.7%	7% at 10 yrs	3.8%
Overall survival	LCIS present	67%	84%	NR	80.2%	NR	NR	NR
	LCIS absent	72%	74%	NR	77.1%	NR	NR	NR
Subsequent contralateral new primary breast cancer	LCIS present	NR	6%	4%	22.2%	3.1%	NR	NR
	LCIS absent	NR	3%	3%	21.6%	0.8%	NR	NR

Table 25.3 STUDIES EVALUATING LCIS COEXISTING WITH INVASIVE CARCINOMA

NR, not reported; LCIS, lobular carcinoma *in situ*; BCT, (breast-conservation therapy).
[a]All BCT cases.
[b]Study was a matched pair analysis.
[c]Study compared local recurrences for 1,111 lumpectomy cases with "absent/scanty" LCIS component versus 70 lumpectomy cases with "moderate/marked" LCIS component.

Table 25.4	RISK OF CANCER DETECTED ON OPEN EXCISIONAL BIOPSY FOLLOWING PERCUTANEOUS CORE NEEDLE BIOPSY REVEALING LOBULAR NEOPLASIA AS THE PRIMARY PATHOLOGY

Study (Reference)	Number Cases Lobular Neoplasia/ Total Core Biopsy Cases (%)	Pathology on Core Biopsy (No. Cases)	Subsequent Excisional Biopsies	Number Upgraded to Cancer (invasive and *in situ*) on Excisional Biopsy (%)
Liberman et al. (78), 1999	16/1,315 (1.2)	LCIS (4)	0	0 (0)
		LCIS + other benign pathology (12)	12	2 (17)
Philpotts et al. (79), 2000	5/1,230 (0.4)	LCIS (1)	1	1 (100)
		LCIS + ALH (4)	4	0 (0)
Burak et al. (80), 2000	6/851 (0.7)	ALH (6)	6	1 (17)
Georgian-Smith and Lawton (64), 2001	7/NR	LCIS (7)	7	2 (28)
Berg et al. (81), 2001	25/1,400 (1.8)	ALH (15)	7	1 (14)
		LCIS (10)	8	0 (0)
Renshaw et al. (77), 2002	71/4,297 (1.7)	ALH (35)	6	0 (0)
		LCIS (36)	9	0 (0)
Shin and Rosen (82), 2002	20/NR	LCIS (8)	8	2 (25)
		ALH (5)	5	0 (0)
Irfan and Bren (83), 2002	7/212 (3.3)	ALH (7)	7	1 (14)
Verkooijen[a] (84), 2002	26/871 (3.0)	ALH, LCIS, ADH (26)	26	6 (23)
Dmytrasz et al. (85), 2003	13/766 (1.7)	ALH (13)	6	3 (50)
Bauer et al. (86), 2003	43/1,460 (2.9)	ALH (13)	7	1 (14)
Yeh et al. (87), 2003	15/1,836 (0.8)	ALH (12)	12	1 (8)
		LCIS (3)	3	0 (0)
Middleton et al. (76), 2003	35/2,337 (1.5)	ALH (17)	6	4 (67)
		LN (4)	2	0 (0)
		LCIS (14)	9	2 (22)
Crisi et al. (88), 2003	35/NR	ALH (3)	3	0 (0)
		ALH + LCIS (4)	4	0 (0)
		LCIS (9)	9	2 (22)
Foster et al. (89), 2004	35/6,081 (0.6)	ALH (20)	14	2 (14)
		LCIS (15)	12	4 (33)
Arpino et al. (90), 2004	106/2,053 (5.2)	ALH or LCIS (45)	21	4 (33)
Elsheikh and Silverman (91), 2005	33/NR	ALH (20)	20	5 (25)
		LCIS (13)	13	4 (31)
Mahoney et al. (75), 2006	27/1,819 (1.5)	ALH (15)	10	1 (10)
		LCIS (9)	8	3 (38)
		ALH+LCIS (3)	2	1 (50)
Margenthaler et al. (74), 2006	111/3,486 (0.32)	ALH (21)	19	3 (16)
		LCIS (20)	16	4 (25)
Karabakhtsian et al. (92), 2007	92/NR	ALH (63)	63	5 (8)
		LCIS (19)	19	4 (21)
		ALH+LCIS (10)	10	1 (10)
Lavoue et al. (93), 2007	70/4,062 (1.7)	Classic LN[b] (42)	42	7 (17)
		Pleomorphic LN (10)	10	3 (30)
Bowman et al.[c] (94), 2007	504/NR	ALH (197)	124	18 (15)
		LCIS (134)	94	20 (21)

LCIS, lobular carcinoma *in situ*; ALH, atypical lobular hyperplasia; NR, not reported; LN, lobular neoplasia.
[a]Core biopsy findings described as "high risk," without any further stratification into specific categories.
[b]Classic LN = ALH or LCIS.
[c]Meta-analysis of studies looking at ALH/LCIS on core biopsy with subsequent excisional biopsy.

As shown in Table 25.4, the preponderance of the data reveals that the completely benign cases cannot be reliably predicted (64,76–94), and therefore follow-up excisional biopsy is the definitive management. One recent study revealed a 38% rate of upstaging to DCIS or invasive cancer based on open excisional biopsy of nine cases where LCIS was the highest level of pathology on preoperative needle biopsy (75). A more selective approach has been advocated based on coexisting findings within the needle biopsy specimen and concordance of the pathology findings with the clinical impression of biopsied lesion. With LCIS, most reported cases of malignant breast findings on subsequent biopsy occurred in the setting of either suspicious mass lesions or calcifications that prompted the biopsy initially (74,76,78); however, others reported there are no consistent breast-imaging features that distinguished the lesions that were upgraded to cancer (75,89–91). Pleomorphic variants of LCIS would also warrant a routine follow-up excisional biopsy for further tissue evaluation (64).

MANAGEMENT SUMMARY

- LCIS is an uncommon pathologic finding in the general female population (0.5% to 4.3% of benign breast biopsies), and it is a marker of increased breast cancer risk. Subsequent cancer risk approaches 1% per year and is bilateral.
- ALH is pathologically similar to LCIS, it but is a risk factor for subsequent breast cancer that is expressed more strongly on the breast ipsilateral to the site of ALH detection.
- Management strategies of patients with lobular neoplasia must address the increased risk to both breasts. Observation with close surveillance is chosen by most patients; those who develop breast cancer do so at an early stage. Chemoprevention with tamoxifen or raloxifene decreases the risk of invasive cancer significantly in patients with lobular neoplasia. Bilateral prophylactic mastectomy reduces risk by approximately 90%, but should be reserved for those patients at highest risk due to family history and other factors.
- The presence of LCIS coexistent with an invasive cancer is not a contraindication to breast-conserving therapy, and at this time, it is not necessary to attempt wide local excision for margin control when LCIS is detected at the margins.
- LCIS is not associated with any mammographic or clinically apparent breast abnormalities; therefore, LCIS detected in a percutaneous core needle biopsy specimen should motivate a search for some other pathologic finding to explain the original biopsy target. This will generally involve open surgical excision to rule out the presence of a coexisting malignancy.

References

1. Foote F, Stewart F. Lobular carcinoma in situ: a rare form of mammary cancer. *Am J Pathol* 1941;17:491–499.
2. McDivitt RW, Hutter RV, Foote FW Jr, et al. In situ lobular carcinoma: a prospective follow-up study indicating cumulative patient risks. *JAMA* 1967;201:82–86.
3. Haagensen CD, Lane N, Lattes R, et al. Lobular neoplasia (so-called lobular carcinoma *in situ*) of the breast. *Cancer* 1978;42:737–769.
4. Wheeler JE, Enterline HT, Roseman JM, et al. Lobular carcinoma *in situ* of the breast: long-term followup. *Cancer* 1974;34:554–563.
5. Rosen PP, Groshen S, Kinne DW, et al. Contralateral breast carcinoma: an assessment of risk and prognosis in stage I (T1N0M0) and stage II (T1N1M0) patients with 20-year follow-up. *Surgery* 1989;106:904–910.
6. Page DL, Kidd TE Jr, Dupont WD, et al. Lobular neoplasia of the breast: higher risk for subsequent invasive cancer predicted by more extensive disease. *Hum Pathol* 1991;22:1232–1239.
7. Bratthauer GL, Tavassoli FA. Lobular intraepithelial neoplasia: previously unexplored aspects assessed in 775 cases and their clinical implications. *Virchows Arch* 2002;440:134–138.
8. Helvie MA, Hessler C, Frank TS, et al. Atypical hyperplasia of the breast: mammographic appearance and histologic correlation. *Radiology* 1991;179:759–764.
9. Dupont WD, Page DL. Risk factors for breast cancer in women with proliferative breast disease. *N Engl J Med* 1985;312:146–151.
10. Dupont WD, Parl FF, Hartmann WH, et al. Breast cancer risk associated with proliferative breast disease and atypical hyperplasia. *Cancer* 1993;71:1258–1265.
11. Rosai J. Borderline epithelial lesions of the breast. *Am J Surg Pathol* 1991;15:209–221.
12. Schnitt SJ, Connolly JL, Tavassoli FA, et al. Interobserver reproducibility in the diagnosis of ductal proliferative breast lesions using standardized criteria. *Am J Surg Pathol* 1992;16:1133–1143.
13. Jensen RA, Dupont WD, Page DL. Diagnostic criteria and cancer risk of proliferative breast lesions. *J Cell Biochem Suppl* 1993;17G:59–64.
14. Bur ME, Zimarowski MJ, Schnitt SJ, et al. Estrogen receptor immunohistochemistry in carcinoma in situ of the breast. *Cancer* 1992;69:1174–1181.
15. Ramachandra S, Machin L, Ashley S, et al. Immunohistochemical distribution of c-erbB-2 in *in situ* breast carcinoma: a detailed morphological analysis. *J Pathol* 1990;161:7–14.
16. Porter PL, Garcia R, Moe R, et al. C-erbB-2 oncogene protein in *in situ* and invasive lobular breast neoplasia. *Cancer* 1991;68:331–334.
17. Shoker BS, Jarvis C, Sibson DR, et al. Oestrogen receptor expression in the normal and pre-cancerous breast. *J Pathol* 1999;188:237–244.
18. Lu YJ, Osin P, Lakhani SR, et al. Comparative genomic hybridization analysis of lobular carcinoma in situ and atypical lobular hyperplasia and potential roles for gains and losses of genetic material in breast neoplasia. *Cancer Res* 1998;58:4721–4727.
19. Nayar R, Zhuang Z, Merino MJ, et al. Loss of heterozygosity on chromosome 11q13 in lobular lesions of the breast using tissue microdissection and polymerase chain reaction. *Hum Pathol* 1997;28:277–282.
20. Etzell JE, Devries S, Chew K, et al. Loss of chromosome 16q in lobular carcinoma in situ. *Hum Pathol* 2001;32:292–296.
21. Newsham IF. The long and short of chromosome 11 in breast cancer. *Am J Pathol* 1998;153:5–9.
22. Buerger H, Simon R, Schafer KL, et al. Genetic relation of lobular carcinoma in situ, ductal carcinoma in situ, and associated invasive carcinoma of the breast. *Mol Pathol* 2000;53:118–121.
23. Lakhani SR, Collins N, Stratton MR, et al. Atypical ductal hyperplasia of the breast: clonal proliferation with loss of heterozygosity on chromosomes 16q and 17p. *J Clin Pathol* 1995;48:611–615.
24. Green AR, Krivinskas S, Young P, et al. Loss of expression of chromosome 16q genes *DPEP1* and *CTCF* in lobular carcinoma *in situ* of the breast. *Breast Cancer Res Treat* 2008. In press.
25. De Leeuw WJ, Berx G, Vos CB, et al. Simultaneous loss of E-cadherin and catenins in invasive lobular breast cancer and lobular carcinoma in situ. *J Pathol* 1997;183:404–411.
26. Raju U, Lu M, Sethi S, et al. Molecular classification of breast carcinoma *in situ*. *Curr Genomics* 2006;7(8):523–532.
27. Andersen JA. Lobular carcinoma in situ of the breast: an approach to rational treatment. *Cancer* 1977;39:2597–2602.
28. Rosen PP, Kosloff C, Lieberman PH, et al. Lobular carcinoma *in situ* of the breast: detailed analysis of 99 patients with average follow-up of 24 years. *Am J Surg Pathol* 1978;2:225–251.
29. Page DL, Dupont WD, Rogers LW, et al. Atypical hyperplastic lesions of the female breast: a long-term follow-up study. *Cancer* 1985;55:2698–2708.
30. Li CI, Anderson BO, Daling JR, et al. Changing incidence of lobular carcinoma *in situ* of the breast. *Breast Cancer Res Treat* 2002;75:259–268.
31. Li CI, Daling JR, Malone KE. Age-specific incidence rates of in situ breast carcinomas by histologic type, 1980 to 2001. *Cancer Epid Biomark Prev* 2005;14(4):1008–1011.
32. Writing Group for the Women's Health Initiative Investigators. Risks and benefits of estrogen plus progestin in healthy postmenopausal women. *JAMA* 2002;288(3):321–333.
33. Hoogerbrugge N, Bult P, de Widt-Levert LM, et al. High prevalence of premalignant lesions in prophylactically removed breasts from women at hereditary risk for breast cancer. *J Clin Oncol* 2003;21:41–45.
34. Kauff ND, Brogi E, Scheuer L, et al. Epithelial lesions in prophylactic mastectomy specimens from women with *BRCA* mutations. *Cancer* 2003;97:1601–1608.
35. Frykberg ER. Lobular carcinoma in situ of the breast. *Breast J* 1999;5:296–303.
36. Khurana KK, Loosmann A, Numann PJ, et al. Prophylactic mastectomy: pathologic findings in high-risk patients. *Arch Pathol Lab Med* 2000;124:378–381.
37. Dotto J, Kluk M, Geramizadeh B, et al. Frequency of clinically occult intraepithelial and invasive neoplasia in reduction mammoplasty specimens: a study of 516 cases. *Int J Surg Path* 2008;16(1):25–30.
38. Page DL, Schuyler PA, Dupont WD, et al. Atypical lobular hyperplasia as a unilateral predictor of breast cancer risk: a retrospective cohort study. *Lancet* 2003;361:125–129.
39. Li CI, Malone KE, Saltzman BS, et al. Risk of invasive breast carcinoma among women diagnosed with ductal carcinoma in situ and lobular carcinoma *in situ*, 1988–2001. *Cancer* 2006;106(10):2104–2112.
39. Adem C, Reynolds C, Soderberg CL, et al. Pathologic characteristics of breast parenchyma in patients with hereditary breast carcinoma, including *BRCA1* and *BRCA2* mutation carriers. *Cancer* 2003;97:1–11.
40. Katalinic A, Rawal R. Decline in breast cancer incidence after decrease in utilisation of hormone replacement therapy. *Breast Cancer Res Treat* 2008;107(3):427–430.
41. Bartow SA, Pathak DR, Black WC, et al. Prevalence of benign, atypical, and malignant breast lesions in populations at different risk for breast cancer: a forensic autopsy study. *Cancer* 1987;60:2751–2760.
42. Salvadori B, Bartoli C, Zurrida S, et al. Risk of invasive cancer in women with lobular carcinoma *in situ* of the breast. *Eur J Cancer* 1991;27:35–37.
43. Ottesen GL, Graversen HP, Blichert-Toft M, et al. Lobular carcinoma in situ of the female breast: short-term results of a prospective nationwide study. The Danish Breast Cancer Cooperative Group. *Am J Surg Pathol* 1993;17:14–21.
44. Singletary SE. Lobular carcinoma in situ of the breast: a 31-year experience at the University of Texas M. D. Anderson Cancer Center. *Breast Dis* 1994;7:157–163.
45. Carson W, Sanchez-Forgach E, Stomper P, et al. Lobular carcinoma *in situ*: observation without surgery as an appropriate therapy. *Ann Surg Oncol* 1994;1:141–146.
46. Chuba PJ, Hamre MR, Yap J, et al. Bilateral risk for subsequent breast cancer after lobular carcinoma in situ: Analysis of Surveillance, Epidemiology, and End Results Data. *J Clin Oncol* 2005;23:5534–5541.
47. Chun J, El-Tamer M, Joseph KA, et al. Predictors of breast cancer development in a high-risk population. *Am J Surg* 2006;192:474–477.
48. Page DL, Dupont WD, Rogers LW. Ductal involvement by cells of atypical lobular hyperplasia in the breast: a long-term follow-up study of cancer risk. *Hum Pathol* 1988;19:201–207.
49. Shaaban AM, Sloane JP, West CR, et al. Histopathologic types of benign breast lesions and the risk of breast cancer: case-control study. *Am J Surg Pathol* 2002;26:421–430.
50. Collins LC, Baer HJ, Tamimi RM, et al. Magnitude and laterality of breast cancer risk according to histologic type of atypical hyperplasia: results from the Nurses Health Study. *Cancer* 2007;109(2):180–187.
51. Degnim AC, Visscher DW, Berman HK, et al. Stratification of breast cancer risk in women with atypical: a Mayo cohort study. *J Clin Oncol* 2007;25(19):2671–2677.

52. Marshall LM, Hunter DJ, Connolly JL, et al. Risk of breast cancer associated with atypical hyperplasia of lobular and ductal types. *Cancer Epidemiol Biomark Prev* 1997;6:297–301.
53. Lakhani SR. *In-situ* lobular neoplasia: time for an awakening. *Lancet* 2003;361:96.
54. Port E, Park A, Borgen PI, et al. Results of MRI screening for breast cancer in high risk patients with LCIS and atypical hyperplasia. *Ann Surg Oncol* 2007;14(3): 1051–1057.
55. Hartmann LC, Schaid DJ, Woods JE, et al. Efficacy of bilateral prophylactic mastectomy in women with a family history of breast cancer. *N Engl J Med* 1999; 340:77–84.
56. Bradley SJ, Weaver DW, Bouwman DL. Alternatives in the surgical management of *in situ* breast cancer: a meta-analysis of outcome. *Am Surg* 1990;56:428–432.
57. Geiger AM, Yu O, Herrinton LJ, et al. A population-based study of bilateral prophylactic mastectomy efficacy in women at elevated risk for breast cancer in community practices. *Arch Intern Med* 2005;165:516–520.
58. Fisher B, Costantino JP, Wickerham DL, et al. Tamoxifen for prevention of breast cancer: report of the National Surgical Adjuvant Breast and Bowel Project P-1 Study. *J Natl Cancer Inst* 1998;90:1371–1388.
59. Fisher B, Costantino JP, Wickerham DL, et al. Tamoxifen for the prevention of breast cancer: current status of the National Surgical Adjuvant Breast and Bowel Project P-1 Study. *J Natl Cancer Inst* 2005;97(22):1652–1662.
60. Vogel VG, Costantino JP, Wickerham DL, et al. Re: tamoxifen for prevention of breast cancer: report of the National Surgical Adjuvant Breast and Bowel Project P-1 Study. *J Natl Cancer Inst* 2002;94:1504.
61. Vogel VG, Costantino JP, Wickerham DL, et al. Effects of tamoxifen vs. raloxifene on the risk of developing invasive breast cancer and other disease outcomes: the NSABP study of tamoxifen and raloxifene (STAR) P-2 trial. *JAMA* 2006;295(23). 2727–2739.
62. Sneige N, Wang J, Baker BA, et al. Clinical, histopathologic, and biologic features of pleomorphic lobular (ductal-lobular) carcinoma *in situ* of the breast: a report of 24 cases. *Mod Pathol* 2002;15:1044–1050.
63. Sapino A, Frigerio A, Peterse JL, et al. Mammographically detected in situ lobular carcinomas of the breast. *Virchows Arch* 2000;436:421–430.
64. Georgian-Smith D, Lawton TJ. Calcifications of lobular carcinoma in situ of the breast: radiologic-pathologic correlation. *AJR Am J Roentgenol* 2001;176: 1255–1259.
65. Bentz JS, Yassa N, Clayton F. Pleomorphic lobular carcinoma of the breast: clinicopathologic features of 12 cases. *Mod Pathol* 1998;11:814–822.
66. Moran M, Haffty BG. Lobular carcinoma in situ as a component of breast cancer: the long-term outcome in patients treated with breast-conservation therapy. *Int J Radiat Oncol Biol Phys* 1998;40:353–358.
67. Abner AL, Connolly JL, Recht A, et al. The relation between the presence and extent of lobular carcinoma *in situ* and the risk of local recurrence for patients with infiltrating carcinoma of the breast treated with conservative surgery and radiation therapy. *Cancer* 2000;88:1072–1077.
68. Sasson AR, Fowble B, Hanlon AL, et al. Lobular carcinoma in situ increases the risk of local recurrence in selected patients with stages I and II breast carcinoma treated with conservative surgery and radiation. *Cancer* 2001;91:1862–1869.
69. Ben-David MA, Kleer CG, Paramagul C, et al. Is lobular carcinoma *in situ* as a component of breast carcinoma a risk factor for local failure after breast conserving therapy? *Cancer* 2005;106(1):28–34.
70. Jolly S, Kestin LL, Goldstein NS, et al. The impact of lobular carcinoma *in situ* in association with invasive breast cancer on the rate of local recurrence in patients with early stage breast cancer treated with breast conserving therapy. *Int J Rad Oncol Biol Phys* 2006;66(2):365–371.
71. Ciocca R, Li T, Freedman G, et al. The presence of lobular carcinoma *in situ* does not increase local recurrence in patients treated with breast-conserving therapy. Meeting of the Society of Surgical Oncology. *Ann Surg Oncol* 2008;15(8): 2263–2271.
72. Carolin KA, Tekyi-Mensah S, Pass HA. Lobular carcinoma *in situ* and invasive cancer: the contralateral breast controversy. *Breast J* 2002;8:263–268.
73. Fowble B, Hanlon AL, Patchefsky A, et al. The presence of proliferative breast disease with atypia does not significantly influence outcome in early-stage invasive breast cancer treated with conservative surgery and radiation. *Int J Radiat Oncol Biol Phys* 1998;42:105–115.
74. Margenthaler JA, Duke D, Monsees BS, et al. Correlation between core biopsy and excisional biopsy in breast high-risk lesions. *Am J Surg* 2006;192:534–537.
75. Mahoney MC, Robinson-Smith TM, Shaughnessy EA. Lobular neoplasia at 11-gauge vacuum-assisted stereotactic biopsy: correlation with surgical excisional biopsy and mammographic follow-up. *AJR Am J Roentgenol* 2006;187:949–954.
76. Middleton LP, Grant S, Stephens T, et al. Lobular carcinoma in situ diagnosed by core needle biopsy: when should it be excised? *Mod Pathol* 2003;16:120–129.
77. Renshaw AA, Cartagena N, Derhagopian RP, et al. Lobular neoplasia in breast core biopsy specimens is not associated with an increased risk of ductal carcinoma *in situ* or invasive carcinoma. *Am J Clin Pathol* 2002;117:797–799.
78. Liberman L, Sama M, Susnik B, et al. Lobular carcinoma in situ at percutaneous breast biopsy: surgical biopsy findings. *AJR Am J Roentgenol* 1999;173:291–299.
79. Philpotts LE, Shaheen NA, Jain KS, et al. Uncommon high risk lesions of the breast diagnosed at stereotactic core-needle biopsy: clinical importance. *Radiology* 2000;216:831–837.
80. Burak WE Jr, Owens KE, Tighe MB, et al. Vacuum-assisted stereotactic breast biopsy: histologic underestimation of malignant lesions. *Arch Surg* 2000;135:700–703.
81. Berg WA, Mrose HE, Ioffe OB. Atypical lobular hyperplasia or lobular carcinoma *in situ* at core-needle breast biopsy. *Radiology* 2001;218:503–509.
82. Shin SJ, Rosen PP. Excisional biopsy should be performed if lobular carcinoma *in situ* is seen on needle core biopsy. *Arch Pathol Lab Med* 2002;126:697–701.
83. Irfan K, Brem RF. Surgical and mammographic follow-up of papillary lesions and atypical lobular hyperplasia diagnosed with stereotactic vacuum-assisted biopsy. *Breast J* 2002;8:230–233.
84. Verkooijen HM. Diagnostic accuracy of stereotactic large-core needle biopsy for nonpalpable breast disease: results of a multicenter prospective study with 95% surgical confirmation. *Int J Cancer* 2002;99:853–859.
85. Dmytrasz K, Tartter PI, Mizrachy H, et al. The significance of atypical lobular hyperplasia at percutaneous breast biopsy. *Breast J* 2003;9:10–12.
86. Bauer VP, Ditkoff BA, Schnabel F, et al. The management of lobular neoplasia identified on percutaneous core breast biopsy. *Breast J* 2003;9:4–9.
87. Yeh IT, Dimitrov D, Otto P, et al. Pathologic review of atypical hyperplasia identified by image-guided breast needle core biopsy: correlation with excision specimen. *Arch Pathol Lab Med* 2003;127:49–54.
88. Crisi GM, Mandavilli S, Cronin E, et al. Invasive mammary carcinoma after immediate and short-term follow-up for lobular neoplasia on core biopsy. *Am J Surg Pathol* 2003;27:325–333.
89. Foster M, Helvie MA, Gregory N, et al. Is excisional biopsy necessary if percutaneous core needle biopsy shows lobular carcinoma *in situ* or atypical lobular hyperplasia? *Radiology* 2004;231:813–819.
90. Arpino G, Allred DC, Mohsin SK, et al. Lobular neoplasia on core needle biopsy—clinical significance. *Cancer* 2004;101(2):242–250.
91. Elsheikh TM, Silverman JF. Follow-up surgical excision is indicated when breast core needle biopsies show atypical lobular hyperplasia or lobular carcinoma *in situ*: a correlative study of 33 patients with review of the literature. *Am J Surg Path* 2005;29(4):534–543.
92. Karabakhtsian RG, Johnson R, Sumkin J, et al. The clinical significance of lobular neoplasia on breast core biopsy. *Am J Surg Path* 2007;31(5):717–723.
93. Lavoue V, Graesslin O, Classe JM, et al. Management of lobular neoplasia diagnosed by core needle biopsy: study of 52 biopsies with follow-up surgical excision. *Breast* 2007;16:533–539.
94. Bowman K, Munoz A, Mahvi D, et al. Lobular neoplasia diagnosed at core biopsy does not mandate surgical excision. *J Surg Res* 2007;142:275–280.

Monica Morrow and Jay R. Harris

Ductal carcinoma *in situ* (DCIS), also known as intraductal carcinoma, is an entity distinct in both its clinical presentation and its biologic potential from lobular carcinoma *in situ* (LCIS), the other lesion classified as noninvasive carcinoma. Previously, DCIS was an uncommon lesion that was routinely cured by mastectomy, and little attention was given to defining its natural history or exploring alternative local treatments. The widespread use of screening mammography has resulted in a significant increase in the rate of detection of DCIS, and the acceptance of breast-conserving therapy for the treatment of invasive carcinoma has raised questions about the routine need for mastectomy for a lesion that may be only precancerous. The proportion of women with mammographically detected DCIS in whom invasive carcinoma will develop within their lifetimes is uncertain. This uncertainty has led to debate as to whether all DCIS should be regarded as early stage carcinoma and treated with either mastectomy or lumpectomy and irradiation, or whether excision alone can be used to treat some DCIS.

PRESENTATION

DCIS has various clinical presentations. In the past, most DCIS was gross or palpable. Today, an abnormal mammographic result is by far the most common presentation of DCIS. DCIS usually appears as clustered microcalcifications. DCIS also presents as pathologic nipple discharge, with or without a mass, and may be identified as an incidental finding in a breast biopsy performed to treat or diagnose another abnormality. DCIS may also present as Paget's disease, an entity that is discussed in detail in Chapter 66. Today, an abnormal mammographic result is the most common presentation of DCIS. DCIS usually appears as clustered microcalcifications. In a retrospective review of 190 consecutive women with DCIS, 62% had calcifications, 22% had soft tissue changes, and in 16% no mammographic findings were present (1). In many reports of mammographically directed biopsies, DCIS accounts for one half or more of the malignancies identified (2–4). Pandya et al. (5) compared the features of DCIS lesions treated from 1969 to 1985 with those treated from 1986 to 1990. During this time, clinical presentations of DCIS fell from 81% of cases to 20% of cases, and grade 3 lesions increased from 24% to 33% of cases. In a similar study from The Netherlands Cancer Institute, histologic grade was equally distributed between screen-detected and symptomatic DCIS (6).

The use of screening mammography has resulted in a remarkable increase in the incidence (or detection rate) of DCIS (7). Between 1975 and 2004, age-adjusted DCIS incidence rates rose from 5.8 to 32.5 per 100,000 women, a 560% increase. In comparison, the incidence of invasive breast cancer increased by only 18% in the same time period (7). Incidence rates, however, were relatively stable between 1998 and 2004. This increase in the incidence of DCIS was observed for women both younger and older than 50 years, although the increase was greater for older women. This increase was observed for both white and African American women. In 2004, *in situ* carcinoma accounted for 20.6% of breast cancers diagnosed in white women, and 20.2% of those diagnosed in black women in the Surveillance, Epidemiology, and End Results (SEER) registries (7). The percentage of screen-detected cancers that are DCIS appears to be higher in younger women than in their older counterparts. Ernster et al. (8), analyzing data on 653,833 mammograms performed as part of the National Cancer Institute's Breast Cancer Surveillance Consortium in 1996 and 1997, found that DCIS accounted for 28.2% (95% confidence interval [CI], 23.9%–32.5%) of screen-detected cancers in women aged 40 to 49 years, compared with 16% (95% CI, 13.3%–18.7%) in women aged 70 to 84 years.

The dramatic increase in the number of DCIS cases seen in the past 30 years has led some authors to suggest that screening results in the detection of biologically indolent DCIS that is unlikely to become clinically significant during a woman's lifetime. The data discussed earlier, indicating a stable or higher frequency of grade 3 lesions in the screen-detected patients, argues against this interpretation. However, in the period between 1997 and 2001, rates of comedo DCIS were stable or decreasing, while rates of noncomedo DCIS increased across all age groups (7). A number of studies have also examined risk factors for DCIS and invasive carcinoma to see if these are similar. Gapstur et al. (9) examined prospectively collected risk factor data from the 37,105 women in the Iowa Women's Health Study. After a follow-up of 11 years, 1,520 carcinomas had developed in this cohort, including 175 cases of DCIS. No differences in risk factors for DCIS and infiltrating carcinoma were observed. Similar findings have been reported in case-control studies that have addressed this issue (10,11).

DISTRIBUTION OF TUMOR IN THE BREAST

The distribution of tumor in the breast is a critical consideration in selecting appropriate local therapy for patients with DCIS. The reported incidence of multicentricity in mastectomy specimens from patients with DCIS varies considerably and has ranged from 0% to 47% (12,13). These studies of multicentricity were conducted before the widespread use of screening mammography, and these data probably cannot be extrapolated to the small (often <1 cm), mammographically detected lesions commonly seen today, particularly since in these studies, the frequency of multicentricity appeared to be related to the size of the index lesion (12). Multicentricity has also been noted to be more frequent in micropapillary DCIS than in other histologic subtypes (14,15).

More recent studies suggest that, in most cases, true multicentricity in DCIS is rare. Holland and Hendriks (16) studied 119 mastectomy specimens containing DCIS by a subgross pathologic-mammographic technique. In all but one case, the tumor was confined to a single "segment" of the breast. Clear-cut multicentric distribution (defined in this study as foci of DCIS separated by 4 cm or more of uninvolved breast tissue) was seen in only one patient. Faverly et al. (17), using stereomicroscopic three-dimensional analysis to define the growth pattern of DCIS in the mammary duct system, studied 60 mastectomy specimens containing DCIS. They found that in the segment of breast involved by DCIS, growth was continuous in some cases and discontinuous in others. Overall, 50% of cases showed a continuous growth pattern and 50% showed a discontinuous pattern, characterized by uninvolved breast tissue between foci of DCIS ("gaps"). In most instances, these gaps were small (<5 mm in 82% of cases), and the likelihood of finding such gaps was related to the degree of differentiation of the lesion. Whereas 90% of the cases of poorly differentiated DCIS grew in a continuous manner without gaps, only 30% of well-differentiated lesions and 45% of intermediately differentiated lesions were continuous. This information has important implications when considering what constitutes an adequate margin of excision in DCIS. The findings in these two studies indicate that, in most cases, DCIS involves the breast in a segmental distribution, and truly multicentric disease is uncommon. In some cases, however, the segment involved by DCIS may be quite large. For example, in the study of Holland and Hendriks, although 86% of the DCIS lesions were nonpalpable and were detected mammographically, 46% were larger than 3 cm. One study of clonality in DCIS supports the contention that most DCIS is clonal, at least with regard to comedo lesions (18). In that study, clonality was assessed in widely separated sites of comedo-type DCIS in the same breast. Each of these widely separated sites was found to show inactivation of the same X chromosome–linked phosphoglycerokinase allele, suggesting an origin from the same clone. The incidence of nipple involvement in patients with DCIS has been evaluated in a few studies and appears to be related to the method of detection of the lesion. For example, Contesso et al. (19) found nipple involvement in 49% of 117 mastectomy specimens from patients in whom DCIS presented primarily with a palpable mass, nipple discharge, or Paget's disease. In contrast, Lagios et al. (12) found involvement of the nipple in 8 of 40 mastectomy specimens (20%) from patients with DCIS, most of whom presented with mammographic calcifications or had DCIS as an incidental finding. Of these eight cases, five were Paget's disease and three had lactiferous duct involvement.

The incidence of nipple involvement in DCIS has become more clinically relevant due to recent interest in nipple-sparing mastectomy.

The incidence of occult invasion, either near the primary tumor or in other parts of the breast, has also been examined in mastectomy series. The reported incidence of occult invasion ranges from 0% to 26% (20). Differences in the completeness of the initial biopsy and the extent of pathologic sampling of the biopsy specimen are responsible for some of this variation. In the current era of diagnosis of DCIS with image-guided biopsy, failure to identify invasive carcinoma prior to complete excision of the lesion remains a problem. Even when large-gauge, vacuum-assisted biopsy devices are used to establish the diagnosis of DCIS, invasive carcinoma is found in approximately 20% of cases. DCIS presenting with a clinical or mammographic mass, larger lesion size, and high histologic grade are associated with a greater likelihood of invasion in many studies (21–23).

NATURAL HISTORY

The major issue in the management of DCIS is the risk of progression to invasive carcinoma. Few clinically relevant data are available to address this question, primarily because DCIS has traditionally been treated with mastectomy. In addition, most DCIS cases for which long-term follow-up is available were either very low-grade lesions, initially thought to be benign, or gross DCIS, a form that may not be equivalent to the mammographically detected DCIS more commonly seen today.

Indirect support for the hypothesis that DCIS is a precursor lesion for invasive cancer is obtained from the investigation of tumors that have both an invasive and an *in situ* component. In one such study of 21 tumors, all of the cases with loss of heterozygosity of chromosome 11q13 in the DCIS component had the same loss in the corresponding invasive component (24). In another similar study of 305 tumors with both components, the

expression of tumor markers was almost identical in the two components (25).

A study of gene expression profiles demonstrated that low-grade DCIS had very similar profiles to low-grade invasive cancer, which were different from the profiles for high-grade DCIS and high-grade invasive cancer (25). These data suggest that many of the genetic alterations seen in invasive cancer are already present in DCIS. Also, these data suggest that low-grade DCIS is more likely to progress to low-grade invasive cancer than to high-grade DCIS (26).

More direct support is available from long-term follow-up data from several small series of women found to have DCIS on review of biopsy specimens that were originally classified as benign. No attempt was made to assess margin status in these studies, lesion size was unknown, and the completeness of excision is uncertain. Page et al. (27) identified 25 such cases in a review of 11,760 breast biopsies. Invasive carcinoma developed in 7 of these 25 women (28%) at intervals of 3 to 10 years (mean, 6.1 years) after biopsy. This incidence of carcinoma represents a relative risk of 11 compared with that of age-matched control subjects from the Third National Cancer Survey for white women in Atlanta. With follow-up to 24 years, the relative risk of carcinoma remained constant (28). In a similar study, Rosen et al. (29) described 30 women with untreated DCIS; complete follow-up was available only for 15. Seven invasive cancers occurred at a mean of 9.7 years after the diagnosis of DCIS. This corresponded to an incidence of 27% if all cases are included, or 53% if only patients with complete follow-up are considered. In both the Page et al. and Rosen et al. reports, all subsequent carcinomas were in the index breast and usually in the vicinity of the biopsy site. In a similar report, Eusebi et al. (30) described 28 cases of DCIS with an 11% incidence of invasive carcinoma at a median follow-up of 16.7 years. Eusebi et al. (31) later reported on 80 cases of DCIS followed for a mean of 17.5 years, only two of which were high grade. Eleven patients had invasive carcinoma and five had recurrent DCIS, for a total recurrence rate of 20%. The risk of invasive carcinoma was twice that of the general population. In all these studies, most cases included were low-grade, non-comedo lesions representing one extreme of the histologic spectrum of DCIS.

Further information on the natural history of DCIS can be obtained from autopsy studies. Alpers and Wellings (32) assessed a series of 185 randomly selected breasts from 101 women examined by a subgross sampling technique. One or more foci of DCIS were found in only 11 cases (6%). This finding was unrelated to age: DCIS was identified in 3 of 56 women (5%) age 49 years or younger; in 7 of 70 women (10%) between the ages of 50 and 69; and in 1 of 59 women (2%) older than 70 years. In a study with similar methodology, Bartow et al. (33) performed breast examinations on 519 women aged 14 years or older. Only one case of DCIS was identified; five occult invasive carcinomas were found. These findings suggest that DCIS is not commonly seen in asymptomatic women in the way that prostate cancer is commonly seen in elderly asymptomatic men. In contrast, information is also available from prophylactic mastectomies in women at hereditary risk of breast cancer (most of whom are *BRCA1* or *BRCA2* positive). In one series, among 67 women at hereditary risk of breast cancer, DCIS was noted in 15% of patients undergoing prophylactic mastectomy. The incidence of DCIS was considerably higher in patients older than 40 years compared with younger patients. Among a smaller series of 24 patients, all of whom had mutations in *BRCA1* or *BRCA2*, DCIS was noted in 13% of patients undergoing prophylactic mastectomy. In both series, a wide range of other premalignant lesions was noted. Taken together, these findings suggest that DCIS is a *bona fide* precursor to invasive cancer but not necessarily an obligate precursor (26,34).

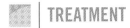
TREATMENT

The uncertainty regarding the natural history of DCIS has resulted in a wide range of local treatment practices, ranging from excision alone to mastectomy. In the past, making comparisons among the retrospective reports was difficult because of differences in patient populations, lack of standardization of surgical and radiotherapeutic techniques, and changes in treatment practices over time. There is now a significant body of data from prospective, randomized trials in well-characterized populations of women with DCIS that provides information about the risks of local recurrence and death after treatment with lumpectomy alone, and lumpectomy and radiation therapy (RT). Clinical trials have also evaluated the benefit of hormonal therapy in patients with DCIS.

Mastectomy

Mastectomy is a curative treatment in approximately 98% to 99% of patients with either gross or mammographically detected DCIS. Patients whose initial biopsies showed DCIS, but for whom invasive carcinoma was later identified in the mastectomy specimens, were excluded from these reports. Recurrences after mastectomy are almost all invasive carcinomas and may present as either local recurrence or distant metastases without evidence of local recurrence. In a study of 430 women undergoing mastectomy for DCIS between 1992 and 2005, the 12-year probability of an invasive local recurrence was 0.5% and the probability of breast cancer–specific mortality was 0.8% (35). A meta-analysis of 1,574 mastectomies reported a recurrence rate of 1.4% (95% CI, 0.7–2.1) (36), of which 76% were invasive cancers. Even when skin-sparing mastectomy is used, local recurrence is uncommon. Local recurrence was observed in 3.3% of 223 patients undergoing skin-sparing mastectomy for DCIS reported by Carlson et al. (37). Treatment failure after mastectomy for DCIS may be due to unsampled or unrecognized invasive carcinoma that results in local recurrence or distant metastases, or it may be due to incomplete removal of breast tissue. Residual breast tissue has the potential for development of a new carcinoma that would be manifested as a "local recurrence." The fact that most local recurrences after mastectomy occur in the first 5 years after mastectomy, however, suggests that most recurrences are due to undiagnosed invasive carcinoma rather than the malignant transformation of residual breast tissue.

Mastectomy is a highly effective treatment for DCIS, but it is a radical approach to a lesion that may not progress to invasive carcinoma during the patient's lifetime. It seems somewhat paradoxical that a woman with a palpable invasive carcinoma should be able to preserve her breast, whereas the "reward" for screening and early detection of DCIS is a mastectomy. The acceptance of breast-conserving therapy for the treatment of invasive carcinoma led to its use as a treatment for DCIS. However, no randomized trial has ever compared the treatment of DCIS by mastectomy with treatment by breast-conserving approaches, and no such trial is likely to occur. In some cases, the assumption has been made that because these two treatments result in equivalent survival for patients with invasive carcinoma, the same is true for patients with DCIS. This assumption is flawed because of the fundamental difference in the risk of metastatic disease for patients with invasive carcinoma and those with DCIS. In DCIS, unlike invasive cancer, the risk of metastases at diagnosis is negligible, and an invasive local recurrence carries with it the potential risk of breast cancer mortality. Therefore, the incidence of invasive recurrence and the results of salvage therapy should determine the suitability of breast-conserving approaches as a treatment for DCIS.

Excision and Radiation Therapy

Four randomized clinical trials have assessed the benefit of RT after excision in patients with DCIS (38–41) (Table 26.1). The first of these, National Surgical Adjuvant Breast and Bowel Project (NSABP) B-17, included 818 patients with localized DCIS who were randomized to excision or excision and breast RT (40). RT consisted of 5,000 cGy of irradiation over 5 weeks to the breast. Patients were required to have histologically negative surgical margins, defined as no tumor-filled ducts at an inked surface. Eighty percent of the women in the study had their DCIS detected by mammographic screening. The second trial, performed by the European Organisation for Research and Treatment of Cancer (EORTC), enrolled 1,002 patients with similar characteristics and treatment. Seventy-one percent of the women in the study had their DCIS detected by mammographic screening (38). The first results of the third trial by the United Kingdom Coordinating Committee on Cancer Research included a total of 1,701 patients who were entered into a 2 × 2 factorial-designed trial testing both RT and tamoxifen (41). Individual institutions were given the opportunity to participate in the 2 × 2 design or either of the two-way randomizations (RT vs. no RT; tamoxifen vs. no tamoxifen). This design may allow for potential imbalances between the arms in the two-way comparisons. The results of the RT part of the trial are shown in Table 26.1, and the results relating to tamoxifen alone are given later. The final study, from the Swedish Breast Cancer group, included 1,067 patients, 79% of whom had screen-detected DCIS. In contrast to the other three studies discussed, 20% of patients in this study had positive or unknown margins (42).

The results of the four trials testing RT after excision are reasonably similar. In aggregate, they demonstrate that:

1. RT reduces ipsilateral breast tumor recurrence (IBTR) by approximately 50% to 60%.
2. Approximately 50% of recurrences after excision alone are invasive and 50% are DCIS.
3. RT reduces both invasive and DCIS recurrences by approximately 50% to 60%.

Table 26.1 | **RESULTS OF RANDOMIZED CLINICAL TRIALS TESTING RADIATION THERAPY AFTER EXCISION**

Study (Reference)	No. of Patients	Median Follow-Up (mos)	IBTR E (%)	IBTR RT (%)
NSABP B-17 12-yr results (40)	813	128	32	16
EORTC 10853 10-yr results (38)	1,010	126	26	15
U.K. Trial 4.4-yr results (41)	1,030	53	14	6
SweDCIS (42)	1,046	96 (mean)	27	12

RT, radiation therapy; E, excision; NSABP, National Surgical Adjuvant Breast and Bowel Project; EORTC, European Organisation for Research and Treatment of Cancer; IBTR, ipsilateral breast tumor recurrence; DCIS, ductal carcinoma *in situ.*

4. The 50% to 60% reduction with RT is persistent through 12 years of follow-up, as seen in the NSABP trial B-17.
5. With RT, the annual rate of an invasive recurrence is 0.5% to 1% per year.
6. No survival benefit was seen for RT.
7. Subgroups of patients not benefiting from RT could not be identified.

The 50% to 60% reduction in IBTR seen in these trials is lower than the 70% to 75% reduction seen in the trials of similar RT after excision of invasive cancer. The reasons for this are not clear. It is not surprising that no survival benefit was seen in these studies, given the very favorable outcome for patients with localized DCIS, the available follow-up, and limited sample sizes. These trials were not designed to detect a small improvement in survival. Any possible survival benefit for RT would be mediated through its reduction in invasive recurrences. At 12 years in the NSABP trial, the absolute reduction in invasive recurrence is approximately 11% (40). Because these events are often delayed, additional follow-up in these trials and a meta-analysis of their results will be necessary to assess whether a survival benefit with RT is present. This information will be particularly important in view of the findings of the meta-analysis of trials of breast-conserving surgery with or without radiation in invasive carcinoma that demonstrated a reduction in breast cancer–specific mortality in the irradiated group after 15 years of follow-up (43). This issue is discussed in detail in the chapter on invasive breast carcinoma.

There are two randomized clinical trials that assess the benefit of tamoxifen in DCIS: one in patients treated with breast RT and one in patients treated with excision alone. The NSABP B-24 trial randomized 1,804 patients with DCIS treated by lumpectomy and RT to tamoxifen 20 mg daily for 5 years or placebo (44). Entry into the trial did not require either negative margins of resection or testing of the DCIS for hormone receptors. The latest published results of this trial are shown in Table 26.2 (40). With a median follow-up of 82 months, the addition of tamoxifen reduced the rate of an IBTR by 31% ($p = .02$), of an ipsilateral invasive breast tumor recurrence by 47% ($p = .01$), of an ipsilateral DCIS breast tumor recurrence by only 15% ($p = $ not significant [NS]), of a contralateral invasive cancer or DCIS by 47% ($p = .01$), and of any breast tumor event by 37% ($p = .01$). Age at diagnosis was significantly associated with a higher risk of IBTR and a greater absolute benefit from tamoxifen, although the proportional risk reductions (32.7% for women aged 50 years or younger, 30.1% for those over 50) were similar. Given the 50% reduction in invasive IBTR with RT and the further 50% reduction by adding tamoxifen, the overall reduction with RT combined with tamoxifen is approximately 75%, with a 7-year absolute rate of an invasive IBTR of 2.6%.

However, the reduction in IBTR seen with the addition of tamoxifen to RT in DCIS is considerably less than the reduction seen in IBTR in invasive cancer (see discussion in Chapter 40). The inclusion of patients with both estrogen receptor (ER)-positive and ER-negative DCIS into NSABP B-24 may partially account for this.

The NSABP has presented follow-up data on the results of B-24 based on the subset of patients for whom ER could be assessed (Table 26.3) (47). ER results were available in 676 of the 1,804 patients in the trial. Overall, 77% of the 676 patients had ER-positive DCIS. The benefit of adding tamoxifen to RT in patients with DCIS deemed to be ER positive (n = 480) in reducing all breast events (ipsilateral or contralateral DCIS or invasive cancer) was 59%, compared with a reduction of 37% in the overall patient population. The number of patients deemed to have ER-negative DCIS was small (n = 146), but no or little benefit for adding tamoxifen was seen in this group (Fig. 26.1).

The first results of the trial by the United Kingdom Coordinating Committee on Cancer Research provided information on the utility of tamoxifen added to excision alone. The results of the RT part of the trial were discussed previously, and the results relating to tamoxifen are shown in Table 26.4 (41). In this trial, the addition of tamoxifen after excision alone had no significant benefit in reducing IBTR; if anything, the rate of invasive IBTR was higher (relative risk = 1.3; $p = $ NS) with the addition of tamoxifen. The 2×2 factorial design of the trial, however, may have resulted in imbalances in the treatment arms, and only 33% of patients in the tamoxifen group received RT. Studies in invasive carcinoma support a synergistic effect between tamoxifen and RT (46).

These two trials taken together suggest that tamoxifen added to RT is effective in reducing IBTR, particularly invasive IBTR, although this effect appears to be limited to ER-positive patients, and that tamoxifen added to excision alone is not very effective in reducing IBTR. These results are similar to the effects of tamoxifen in patients with invasive cancer. Further information on the effect of tamoxifen on IBTR in patients treated by excision alone will be available from the Intergroup CE5194 trial (discussed in the section Breast-Conserving Surgery Alone, below). The benefits of tamoxifen compared to an aromatase inhibitor in patients with DCIS treated with excision and RT will be addressed in NSABP B-35, which has completed accrual of 3,000 patients with ER-positive or progesterone receptor (PR)–positive DCIS and negative margins receiving breast irradiation and randomized to treatment with tamoxifen or the aromatase inhibitor anastrozole. The International Breast Cancer Intervention Study (IBIS-II) trial is also comparing tamoxifen and anastrozole in 4,000 patients recruited from multiple European sites.

Table 26.2	**SEVEN-YEAR RESULTS OF NSABP PROTOCOL B-24 TESTING THE ADDITION OF TAMOXIFEN TO LUMPECTOMY AND RADIATION THERAPY (MEDIAN FOLLOW-UP TIME 82 MOS)**				
	IBTR	Invasive IBTR	DCIS IBTR	Contralateral Events	All Events
Excision + RT (n = 899)	18.4%	9.0%	9.4%	8.3%	28.2%
Excision + RT + tamoxifen (n = 899)	12.8%	4.8%	8.0%	4.4%	17.7%
RR	0.69	0.53	0.85	0.53	0.63
p-value	0.02	0.01	NS	0.01	0.0003

NSABP, National Surgical Adjuvant Breast and Bowel Project; RT, radiation therapy; RR, hazard rate in the group treated with tamoxifen divided by the rate in the placebo group; IBTR, ipsilateral breast tumor recurrence; DCIS, ductal carcinoma *in situ*.
From Fisher B, Land S, Mamounas E, et al. Prevention of invasive breast cancer in women with ductal carcinoma *in situ*: an update of the national surgical adjuvant breast and bowel project experience. *Semin Oncol* 2001;28:400–418.

NSABP B-24 Trial Based on ER Status

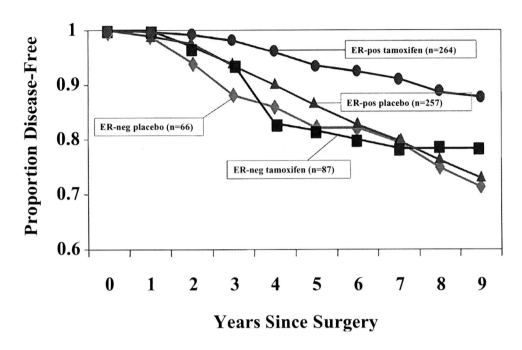

FIGURE 26.1. **Time to First Breast Event.** NSABP, National Surgical Adjuvant Breast and Bowel Project; ER, estrogen receptor.

Table 26.3	SITES AND FREQUENCY OF FIRST BREAST CANCER EVENTS BY ESTROGEN RECEPTOR AND TREATMENT			
	ER-Negative		**ER-Positive**	
	Placebo (n = 84)	Tamoxifen (n = 62)	Placebo (n = 243)	Tamoxifen (n = 237)
All events	22 (26%)	14 (23%)	56 (23%)	24 (10%)
Ipsilateral	15 (18%)	11 (17%)	32 (13%)	16 (7%)
Contralateral	5 (6%)	3 (5%)	20 (8%)	8 (3%)
Other	2 (2%)	0 (0%)	4 (2%)	0 (0%)

Median follow-up is 8.7 years (NSABP B-24). Reduction in all breast events is 59% for ER positive (0.0002) and 20% for ER negative (0.51).
NSABP, National Surgical Adjuvant Breast and Bowel Project; ER, estrogen receptor.
From Allred DC, Bryant J, Land S. Estrogen receptor expression as a predictive marker of effectiveness of tamoxifen in the treatment of DCIS: findings from NSABP Protocol B-24. *Br Cancer Res Treat* 2002;76-S36(abst)

Table 26.4	CRUDE RESULTS OF THE UNITED KINGDOM CLINICAL TRIAL TESTING TAMOXIFEN AFTER EXCISION ALONE (MEDIAN FOLLOW-UP IS 53 MOS.)			
	IBTR	Invasive IBTR	DCIS IBTR	All Events
Excision alone	13%	4%	9%	15%
Excision + tamoxifen	11%	5%	6%	12%
RR	1.32	0.73	0.80	—
p-value	0.26	0.10	0.11	—

RR, hazard rate in the group treated with tamoxifen divided by the rate in the placebo group; IBTR, ipsilateral breast tumor recurrence; DCIS, ductal carcinoma *in situ*; All events, including DCIS or invasive cancer in the contralateral breast.
From Houghton J, George WD, Cuzick J, et al. Radiotherapy and tamoxifen in women with completely excised ductal carcinoma *in situ* of the breast in the UK, Australia, and New Zealand: randomised controlled trial. *Lancet* 2003;362:95–102.)

Table 26.5	RESULTS OF CONSERVATIVE SURGERY AND RADIATION FOR MAMMOGRAPHICALLY DETECTED DUCTAL CARCINOMA *IN SITU*							
		Actuarial Breast Recurrence (%)			Cause-Specific Survival (%)			
Study (Reference)	No. of Patients	5-yr	8-yr	10-yr	5-yr	8-yr	10-yr	Median Follow-Up (yrs)
NSABP B-17 (40,47)	411	10.0	12.1	16.7	98.0	98.0	7.5 (mean)
Kuske et al. (51)	44	7.0	—	—	—	—	—	4.0
Fowble et al. (48)	110	1.0	—	15.0	100	—	100	5.3
Kestin et al. (50)	146	8.0	—	9.2	100	—	99.2	7.2
Hiramatsu et al. (49)	54	2.0	—	23.0	—	—	96.0	6.2
Sniege et al. (53)	31	0.0	—	8.0	—	—	—	7.2
Silverstein et al. (52)	133[a]	7.0	—	19.0	—	—	97.0	7.8
Collaborative Group (56)	110	7.0	—	14.0	100	—	96.0	9.3

NSABP, National Surgical Adjuvant Breast and Bowel Project.
[a]Eighty-nine of these patients had mammographically detected cancers.

A number of nonrandomized studies of breast-conserving therapy have been helpful in defining (a) long-term results of treatment, (b) prognostic factors for recurrence, and (c) outcome of salvage treatment for local recurrence (Table 26.5) (44,47–55). An international collaboration of radiation oncology programs provided the long-term results on excision and RT in 422 patients with mammographically detected DCIS (56). With a median follow-up of 9.4 years, they observed an actuarial rate of local recurrence of 6% at 5 years, 11% at 10 years, and 16% at 15 years, or approximately 1% per year through 15 years. This annual rate is lower than the annual rate seen with excision and RT in the NSABP trials of approximately 1.8% per year. Also, this result represents a similar annual rate of local recurrence, but a more protracted risk period for subsequent invasive cancer than that after conservative surgery and RT for invasive cancer, where the annual rate of local recurrence declines after approximately 8 years. In the international collaborative study (56), approximately half of the recurrences were invasive and half were DCIS, with a similar median time to the event. Of note, the cause-specific survival at 15 years for patients with DCIS treated with excision and RT was 96%, while overall survival was 87%.

A collaboration of radiation oncology programs in France also provided long-term results on excision and RT in 515 patients with DCIS and excision alone in 190 patients (57). With a median follow-up of 7 years, they observed an actuarial rate of local recurrence of 12.6% at 7 years, and 18.2% at

10 years with RT, and of 32.4% at 7 years, and 43.8% at 10 years for excision alone. These results are similar to the outcomes seen in NSABP B-17.

A number of studies have addressed prognostic factors for local recurrence in patients treated for DCIS by either excision alone or excision and RT. In reviewing these various prognostic factors, a comparison is made with the results of breast-conserving therapy for invasive cancer. Detailed pathologic reviews have been provided for the NSABP B-17 and EORTC 10853 trials (58,59). Margin status is seen in almost all studies to be associated with local recurrence, although the magnitude of the association is variable (Table 26.6). In a report on the experience at Yale in 230 patients treated with excision and RT, there was no association between margins and local recurrence (60). On the other hand, in the experience of Silverstein in southern California, there was a strong association between margin status and local recurrence in a retrospective review of 260 patients treated with excision and RT. With a median follow-up of 105 months, the crude incidence of local recurrence was 30% when margins were less than 1 mm, 17% when they were 1 to 9 mm, and only 2% when they were greater than 10 mm (52,61). One reason for the inconsistent association between margin status and local recurrence may be the variability and sampling error in determining margin status between different institutions. It has also been suggested that the generally weak association may be due to the failure to consider the amount of DCIS near the margin (62). A meta-analysis of the

Table 26.6	ANNUAL LOCAL RECURRENCE RATE[a] IN RELATION TO MARGINS AND TREATMENT							
	Excision Alone				Excision and Radiation Therapy			
Study (Reference)	Negative (%)	Close (%)	Close/Positive (%)	Positive (%)	Negative (%)	Close (%)	Close/Positive (%)	Positive (%)
NSABP at 8 yrs (59)	4.7	—	—	7.2	1.9	—	—	2.5
EORTC at 5.4 yrs (58)	2.9	—	5.9	—	2.0	—	3.0	—
Solin et al. at 9.4 yrs (56)	—	—	—	—	0.9	0.7	—	2.4
Cutuli et al. at 7 yrs (57)	—	—	—	—	1.4	—	—	3.6

[a]If annual hazard is not provided, the estimate is the actuarial rate at X years divided by X.

Table 26.7	ANNUAL LOCAL RECURRENCE RATE*a* IN RELATION TO AGE FOLLOWING EXCISION AND RADIATION THERAPY							
	Age (%)							
Study (Reference)	<35	<40	40–49	<50	>40	40–60	50–59	>60
NSABP at 5 yrs (59)	4	—	—	3.0	—	—	2.2	1.8
EORTC at 5.4 yrs (58)	—	4.1	—	—	2.0	—	—	—
Solin et al. at 9.4 yrs (56)	—	3.1	1.3	—	—	—	0.8	0.6
Cutuli et al. at 7 yrs (57)	—	4.1	—	—	—	1.9	—	1.1

*a*If annual hazard is not provided, the estimate is the actuarial rate at X years divided by X.

impact of margin width on local failure in DCIS included 5,500 patients, 3,606 from randomized trials and the remainder from nonrandomized reports. In all trials, the relative risk of IBTR for those with negative margins was 0.36 (95% CI, 0.27–0.47; $p < 0.0001$) compared to those with positive margins. In combined data from randomized and nonrandomized studies, the relative risk of IBTR for a 2-mm or greater margin was 0.53 (95% CI, 0.26–0.96; $p < .05$) compared to a lesser margin, but no significant difference in IBTR for 2-mm margins and those greater than 5 mm was noted (63). Taken together, these studies demonstrate that margin status is useful. The rate of local recurrence is lower with negative margins compared with positive or uncertain margins. However, the precise margin in millimeters required is uncertain. These results are similar to those seen with breast-conserving therapy for invasive cancer (see the discussion in Chapter 40).

Age has been more consistently associated with local recurrence (Table 26.7). Young patients consistently have a higher rate of local recurrence than older patients (64,65). In particular, patients younger than 40 years of age appear to have a higher rate of local recurrence than older patients. A similar trend is seen after breast-conserving therapy for invasive cancer. The reasons for this association are not clear. One study found that younger patients had smaller excision volumes and a greater proportion of high–nuclear-grade tumor and central necrosis than older patients (66). Another study did not find a difference in pathologic features, but found that young patients were more likely to have *HER2/neu*–positive lesions than older patients (67), while an analysis from the Swedish trial (42) suggested a smaller reduction in the risk of local recurrence from RT in younger women.

Histologic characteristics of DCIS have been evaluated by many as prognostic factors for local recurrence, and the results are variable. This is due in part to variations in the definition of grade and the presence of necrosis. In the EORTC trial, the local recurrence rate at 5.4 years was 8% for low-grade lesions, 14% for moderate-grade lesions, and 18% for high-grade lesions (58). In the NSABP B-17 trial at 8 years, the local recurrence rate was 11% for low-grade lesions without necrosis, 15% for low-grade lesions with necrosis, and 15% for high-grade lesions with necrosis (59). The presence of necrosis was also seen as a significant factor in the Yale experience. The 10-year rate of local recurrence was 22% in patients with necrosis and only 7% in those without necrosis (60).

Size of the DCIS has also been evaluated by many as a prognostic factor, and consistent results have not been seen. In part this is because the measurement of lesion size is considerably more difficult for DCIS than for invasive cancer. With DCIS, there is typically no gross lesion, unlike the situation with invasive cancer. Also, the size of DCIS is underestimated by its mammographic extent. Full assessment of size requires serial embedding and sampling of the entire specimen, a procedure

that is not routinely performed. In the EORTC trial, there was no relationship between size and local recurrence, whereas in the NSABP B-17 trial, the local recurrence rate was only 5% for lesions less than 5 mm and 11% for lesions measuring 5 to 10 mm when size was measured mammographically. It is likely that size and margins are confounded and have an inverse relationship, in that, small lesions are more likely to have clearly negative margins. Size is not a significant factor for local recurrence after breast-conserving therapy for invasive cancer.

Data are beginning to emerge on whether markers predict for local recurrence. In one case-control study of patients treated with breast-conserving surgery with or without radiation therapy, local recurrence was greater with *HER2/neu*–positive lesions than *HER2/neu*–negative lesions, and with ER-negative lesions than with ER lesions. p21 positivity also predicted for local recurrence (68). Among a group of patients treated with breast-conserving surgery alone, abrogated response to cellular stress was found to be common in DCIS with recurrence and is a defining characteristic of basal-like invasive tumors. Of the nine DCIS patients with high expression of p16 and low Ki-67, all developed recurrence (69).

Because half of the local failures seen after breast-conserving therapy for DCIS are invasive carcinoma, the outcome of salvage treatment of these recurrences is important. Solin et al. (70) described 41 cases of local recurrence in 422 cases of mammographically detected DCIS treated with excision plus irradiation. The median time to local failure was 4.8 years, and the median follow-up after salvage treatment was 4.5 years. In 18 patients, the recurrence was DCIS, in 22 the recurrence was invasive ductal carcinoma, and in 1 patient, the recurrence was invasive lobular carcinoma. In 86% the local recurrence was detected by mammography with or without findings on physical examination. All but five patients underwent salvage mastectomy. Twelve patients were known to have received systemic therapy at the time of local recurrence. Overall, 4 years after local recurrence, 11% of patients had distant metastases and 7% had died of breast cancer. Among patients with an invasive local recurrence, 19% of patients had distant metastases and 13% had died of breast cancer by 4 years. In contrast, none of the patients with a DCIS local recurrence had distant metastases or died of breast cancer. Similar findings were reported by Lee et al. (35). Their study population consisted of 31 patients with an invasive local recurrence after excision and RT, 29 patients after excision alone, and 3 patients after mastectomy. With a median follow-up of 77 months after an invasive local recurrence, the 12-year actuarial rate for distant metastases was 15% and the 12-year rate for breast cancer mortality was 12%. These studies point out the potential for distant metastases for patients in whom an invasive local recurrence develops after breast-conserving therapy and the need to minimize this event when managing a patient with DCIS.

| Table 26.8 | RESULTS OF TREATMENT OF DUCTAL CARCINOMA *IN SITU* WITH EXCISION ALONE |

Study (Reference)	No. of Patients	Follow-Up (mos)	No. of Recurrences (%)	Invasive Recurrences (%)
Arnesson and Olsen (71)	169	80[a]	16/22 (5/10-yr actuarial)	36
Carpenter et al. (72)	28	38[b]	10	20
Eusebi et al. (30)	80	210[b]	20	69
Lagios (73)	79	135[b]	22 (15-yr actuarial)	58
Schwartz (74)	256	66.5[a]	28/50 (5/10-yr actuarial)	37
Lee et al. (35)	496	54[a]	31 (12-yr actuarial)	34

[a]Median.
[b]Mean.

Breast-Conserving Surgery Alone

In spite of the four prospective, randomized trials that have demonstrated that the addition of RT to excision significantly decreases IBTR, interest persists in treatment of some subsets of women with DCIS by excision alone. A number of concerns about the randomized trials have been cited to support this interest including: (a) detailed tissue processing and the method of pathologic evaluation was not specified in the study protocols, (b) postexcision mammography was not mandated to document complete removal of calcifications, and (c) the impact of margin width on the benefit of RT was not assessed. A number of retrospective studies, usually including a highly select group of patients with small mammographically detected tumors of low histologic grade, have suggested that DCIS can be treated with excision alone with a high rate of local control.

A number of these studies are shown in Table 26.8 (30,71–74). Lagios (75) reported on 79 patients with mammographically detected tumors treated by excision alone, with a mean tumor size of 7.8 mm. After a mean follow-up of 135 months, the local recurrence rate was 22%. Recurrence occurred in 39% of patients with grade 3 lesions compared with 6% of those with grade 1 lesions. Recurrence was also less common in patients with margins greater than 1 cm in size. Silverstein et al. (76) developed the Van Nuys Prognostic Index (VNPI), a retrospectively derived risk classification that assigns a value of 1 to 3 to tumor size, margin width, and histologic classification to define three risk groups with scores of 3 or 4 (low risk), 5 to 7 (intermediate), and 8 or 9 (high risk). In retrospective analyses, no benefit for radiation was seen in the low-risk subgroup, where the local failure rate was only 2% regardless of treatment. The index was developed using retrospective data on 254 patients and was validated using retrospective data on a small series of 79 patients from another institution. The use of the classification system depends on the reproducibility of the individual components. Because the histologic classification scheme and method of tumor measurement are not in universal, or even routine, use, this is a significant issue. Equally important is the fact that the patients used to develop this index were treated over a long time span, from 1972 to 1995. However, treatment with excision alone was used in more recent years, whereas treatment with excision and irradiation was more common in the past. This suggests that the low rate of local recurrence seen after excision alone may be due to improvements in mammographic and pathologic evaluation. Hiramatsu et al. (49) reported that incidence of local recurrence 6.5 years after excision and irradiation decreased from 12% to 2% when patients treated between 1976 and 1985 were compared with those treated between 1985 and 1995, although radiation technique did not change.

Attempts by others to validate the VNPI have not confirmed the reports of Silverstein et al. The VNPI was applied to a retrospective series of 367 patients by de Mascarel et al. (77). Of the 134 patients in the low-scoring VNPI group who did not receive RT, 9% had recurrence after a median follow-up of 79 months, compared with 2% in the report of Silverstein et al. (76). The VNPI has subsequently been modified to include patient age, with age cutoffs of less than 40 years (score 3), 40 to 60 years (score 2), and greater than 60 years (score 1). In a retrospective analysis of 538 patients treated with breast-conserving therapy, those with the lowest VNPI score (4, 5, or 6) were not found to benefit from breast irradiation (78). Like the original VNPI, this classification system has not been prospectively validated by another group.

More recently, Silverstein et al. (79) suggested that any DCIS lesion, regardless of size or grade, that could be excised with a margin of 1 cm in all directions did not require RT or tamoxifen. This approach eliminates the problems of consistent size measurement and histologic grade that are inherent in the VNPI. In a retrospective review of 469 patients, Silverstein et al. (79) found no statistically significant decrease in local failure with the use of RT in patients whose tumors were excised to a margin width of 10 mm or greater. However, RT did have an effect on this group. The relative risk of recurrence was decreased by 50%, but this did not reach statistical significance owing to the small sample size. In addition, in this retrospective study, patients treated by excision alone were followed for a shorter time than those receiving RT, and their tumors were significantly larger. MacAusland et al. (80) retrospectively analyzed 222 patients treated with excision alone using the original VNPI classification (76), the age modified VNPI (78), and margin width of 1 cm or greater (79). With a median follow-up of 4.6 years, the crude rate of IBTR was 8.6%. At 5 years, IBTR rates were not statistically different for the low, intermediate, or high-risk groups using any of the three Van Nuys models.

Updated results of widely excised DCIS (>1 cm margins) are available from the Macdonald et al. (81). Among 212 patients treated with excision alone, the 12-year probability of any breast recurrence was 14%, and the 12-year probability of an invasive recurrence was 3.4%. Among the 60 patients treated with excision and radiation therapy, there was only one recurrence and it was an invasive recurrence.

The Dana-Farber/Harvard Cancer Center conducted a single-arm, prospective trial of wide excision alone beginning in 1994. Entry criteria included DCIS of predominant grade 1 or 2 with a mammographic extent of no greater than 2.5 cm and final margins of at least 1 cm. Tamoxifen was not permitted. The accrual goal was 200 patients; in July 2002 the study closed to further accrual at 157 patients because the number of local recurrences met the stopping rules (82). The median patient age was 51 years, and the median follow-up was 40 months (range, 0 to 82 months). Thirteen patients had local recurrence as the first site of failure between 7 and 63 months. Another patient had ipsilateral local recurrence (DCIS) after a contralateral DCIS. The rate of ipsilateral local recurrence as first site of failure was 2.4% per patient-year (95% CI, 1.3%–4.1%), corresponding to a 5-year rate of 12.5%. Nine patients recurred with DCIS and four with invasive disease. Twelve local recurrences were detected mammographically, and one was palpable. Ten were in the same quadrant as the initial DCIS and three were elsewhere in the ipsilateral breast. No patients had positive axillary nodes at local recurrence and none have developed metastatic disease. The local recurrence rate per patient-year was 5.2% for patients 60 years and older, and no greater than 2.1% for all other age groups.

The first results of a prospective, single arm, multi-institutional study (Intergroup CE5194) examining the role of excision alone in the treatment of DCIS have been reported. Eligibility criteria for this study included DCIS greater than or equal to 3 mm in size, excised with a margin width of 3 mm or more as determined by sequential sectioning and complete embedding (83). The study was open to patients with low- or intermediate-grade DCIS 2.5 cm or less in size, and high-grade DCIS (defined as nuclear grade 3 with necrosis) up to 1 cm in size. A postexcision mammogram was required for all participants. The characteristics of the study patients are summarized in Table 26.9. At a median follow-up of 5 years, the IBTR rate was 13.7% (95% CI, 6.2%–21.1%) for patients with high-grade DCIS, while IBTR occurred in 6.8% (95% CI, 4.4%–9.1%) of those with low or intermediate grade DCIS. In both groups, 50% of the recurrences were invasive cancers. The incidence of contralateral breast cancer in the low- and high-grade groups was 3.5% and 4.2%, respectively. Caution should be exercised in interpreting these results to mean that treatment with wide excision alone is appropriate for patients who do not have high-grade lesions. Studies of patients treated with excision and RT have shown that while early IBTR is more common in high-grade DCIS, after 10 years of follow-up, IBTR rates do not differ on the basis of grade (54). The prospective data from both of the studies discussed suggest that even in highly selected patients, there is a substantial local recurrence rate when treatment is with wide excision alone despite margins of 1 cm or more. These results are not in concordance with those of Silverstein et al. (79,81) and suggest that further work is needed to reliably identify favorable subgroups for wide excision alone.

Management of the Axilla

Incidence rates reported for axillary nodal involvement in patients given the diagnosis of DCIS range from 0% to 7% (54,84–86), with the higher rates noted in studies performed in the premammography era, when most patients with DCIS presented with a palpable mass. In such cases, invasion is undoubtedly present but is either not recognized by the pathologist or is undetected because of sampling error. Axillary lymph node involvement in patients with DCIS detected by mammography is a rare event. In one series of 189 patients with DCIS, most of whose tumors were detected by mammography alone, none showed metastases on axillary dissection (84).

In a National Cancer Database review of 10,946 patients with DCIS who had an axillary dissection between 1985 and 1991, only 406 (3.6%) were found to have axillary metastases (86). Based on these findings, axillary dissection in DCIS was largely abandoned. The widespread use of sentinel node biopsy for invasive carcinoma and the observation that immunohistochemistry allows the detection of tumor cells in lymph nodes determined to be negative by hematoxylin and eosin (H&E) staining (87) have reopened the debate on the value of nodal sampling in patients with DCIS. Pendas et al. (88) reported on

Table 26.9	**PATIENT CHARACTERISTICS IN E5194, A PROSPECTIVE TRIAL OF WIDE EXCISION IN DUCTAL CARCINOMA *IN SITU***	
	Low/Intermediate Grade	High Grade
No. of patients	579	101
Median tumor size	6 mm	7 mm
Margin >1 cm	46%	48%
Margin >5 cm	67%	75%
Tamoxifen planned	31%	31%

From Hughes L, Wang M, Page D. Five-year results of intergroup study E5194: local excision alone (without radiation treatment) for selected patients with ductal carcinoma *in situ* (DCIS). *Breast Cancer Res Treat* 2006:100[Suppl 1]:S15.

87 patients with DCIS undergoing sentinel node biopsy. Metastases were found by H&E staining in two and by immunohistochemistry in an additional three. No additional tumor-bearing nodes were identified by axillary dissection. Klauber-DeMore et al. (89) observed that 2 patients in their series of 76 women with DCIS had H&E-detected nodal metastases and 7 had metastases detected only by immunohistochemistry. Two of these patients had foci of invasion retrospectively identified in the DCIS lesions, and one-third had contralateral invasive breast cancer. Only one patient with an H&E-detected metastasis without an invasive carcinoma was identified. In a retrospective study by Lara et al. (90) in which the axillary nodes of patients with DCIS were examined with immunohistochemistry, 13% of patients were found to have nodal involvement. However, nodal involvement by immunohistochemistry was not predictive of the risk of local, regional, or distant recurrence at 10 years.

More recent data from the NSABP B-17 and B-24 studies document that the risk of axillary recurrence in patients treated with breast-conservation therapy with or without RT and with or without tamoxifen is extremely low (91). In the NSABP B-17 trial the axillary recurrence rate was 0.83 per 1,000 patient-years, and in the NSABP B-24 trial the axillary recurrence rate was 0.36 per 1,000 patient-years. These low rates of clinical recurrence do not justify the routine use of sentinel node biopsy in DCIS, particularly in view of data from the American College of Surgeons Z10 trial indicating that at 6 months of follow-up in 5,327 patients undergoing sentinel node biopsy, 9% reported paresthesias and 7% had lymphedema (92).

Most would agree that sentinel node biopsy should be performed in patients undergoing mastectomy for DCIS since the opportunity for sentinel node biopsy is lost if it is not performed at the time of the mastectomy. In addition, many of these patients have large areas of DCIS where the risk of sampling error and failure to diagnose invasive carcinoma is high. Gross or clinically evident DCIS and DCIS that is "suspicious" for microinvasion are also circumstances in which invasive carcinoma is frequently found and where sentinel node biopsy should be considered. The use of immunohistochemistry is not recommended for evaluation of the sentinel node in DCIS since the prognostic significance of these cells is uncertain (93,94).

TREATMENT SELECTION IN DUCTAL CARCINOMA *IN SITU*

The available information on DCIS suggests that, although all patients can be treated with mastectomy, many are candidates for treatment with excision and irradiation, and a smaller group may be appropriately treated with excision alone. The initial step in treatment selection is to determine, on the basis of the history and physical examination, imaging, and pathologic findings, whether the patient is a candidate for a breast-conserving approach. If so, the risks and benefits and what is entailed in breast-conserving surgery with or without radiation, as well as mastectomy (including reconstruction), should be described in detail. The risk of local recurrence, particularly an invasive recurrence, is a major focus of this discussion because regardless of the type of local therapy selected, the risk of breast cancer–specific mortality is extremely low. Guidelines for the selection of local therapy in DCIS have been developed by a joint committee of the American College of Surgeons, American College of Radiology, and the College of American Pathologists.

Absolute indications for mastectomy include multicentric DCIS or diffuse, malignant-appearing microcalcifications covering an area too large to encompass with a cosmetic resection (95). The persistence of tumor at resection margins after a reasonable number of surgical attempts is also an indication for mastectomy. Although DCIS lesions are not clinically detectable, they may be quite large. Morrow et al. (96) found that contraindications to breast-conserving surgery were present in 33% of patients with DCIS compared with only 10% of patients with stage I invasive carcinoma. Extensive disease that could not be encompassed with a cosmetic resection was the major contraindication to breast-conserving therapy in those with DCIS.

Most patients who require mastectomy can be identified before surgery with a careful imaging evaluation to determine the extent of the lesion. Holland et al. (97) have reported that the extent of poorly differentiated DCIS assessed by microscopy correlated well with the extent of the lesion evaluated radiologically, but the mammographic appearance of well-differentiated DCIS substantially underestimated the microscopic extent. However, the routine use of magnification views as part of the mammographic evaluation allowed the detection of additional calcifications that reduced the discrepancy between the pathologically and mammographically determined extent of well-differentiated DCIS. The role of magnetic resonance imaging (MRI) in the patient with DCIS is controversial. In the International Breast MRI Consortium study, the sensitivity of MRI for the detection of DCIS was 73%, significantly lower than the 90.9% observed for invasive cancer (98). In contrast, Kuhl et al. (99) reported that of 167 women diagnosed with DCIS who had undergone both MRI and mammography, 92% were diagnosed by MRI compared with 56% diagnosed by mammography ($p <.0001$). Of the 89 cases of high grade DCIS, 48% were diagnosed by MRI but missed by mammography. However, small studies suggest that MRI often overestimates the size of DCIS lesions (100,101), potentially resulting in unnecessary mastectomies. Most importantly, there is no evidence of improved clinical outcomes in patients selected for breast-conserving therapy with MRI. In a retrospective study from the University of Pennsylvania, the incidence of local recurrence and contralateral cancer was compared in 756 patients with DCIS or invasive carcinoma, 251 who had an MRI and 541 who had not undergone MRI prior to treatment selection. The 8-year incidence of local recurrence was 3% and 4% in patients with and without an MRI examination, respectively, while the incidence of contralateral cancer was 6% in both groups (102). At present, MRI cannot be considered part of the routine preoperative evaluation of the woman with DCIS. In patients who appear to have localized DCIS suitable for treatment with a breast-conserving approach, mammographically occult DCIS extensive enough to require mastectomy is uncommon. Some studies have suggested that micropapillary DCIS (14,15) and DCIS presenting as pathologic nipple discharge (103) are more likely to be extensive in the breast than other histologic subtypes or presentations. Although these findings do not represent a contraindication to breast conservation in patients who are otherwise suitable candidates, they should be considered when discussing the possibility of additional surgery if lumpectomy is attempted.

Needle localization should be used to guide the surgical excision; if the calcifications are extensive, bracketing wires are useful to aid in complete excision. Specimen mammography is essential to confirm the excision of calcifications. In cases in which calcifications are extensive or there is any doubt about residual microcalcifications in the breast based on a comparison of the specimen mammogram and the diagnostic mammogram or DCIS approaches the edge of the surgical specimen, postexcision mammograms are useful to document the removal of all suspect calcifications. Gluck et al. (104) performed postexcision mammograms, including spot compression views, on 43 women who required re-excision because of positive or unknown margins after a diagnosis of breast carcinoma. Twenty-eight patients had DCIS; the positive predictive value of residual calcifications as an indicator of residual tumor was 0.67 and increased to 0.9 when more than five calcifications were present. Even when the margins are negative, postexcision mammography can demonstrate residual calcifications indicative of the need for further resection (105). In most patients, a postexcision mammogram can be obtained within 2 to 4 weeks after surgery

For the woman who appears to have mammographically localized DCIS and is a candidate for breast conservation, a decision regarding the magnitude of benefit that will be obtained from RT cannot be made until the lesion has been excised and a pathology report is available. To facilitate decision making, a detailed pathologic evaluation is necessary. The evaluation should include inking of the specimen and measurement of both specimen and tumor size (if there is a gross lesion) before sectioning. Because accurate measurement of microscopic DCIS is often difficult, reporting the number of blocks in which DCIS is present and the number of blocks examined, as well as its largest single extent in any one slide, is often useful. The correlation of microcalcifications with DCIS (i.e., whether calcifications are present in the DCIS or in adjacent breast tissue), as well as the margin status, should be noted. If margins are involved, the extent of involvement should be stated; when margins are negative, proximity of the lesion to the margin should be noted.

As discussed previously, four prospective, randomized trials have demonstrated that in women with DCIS, the use of postoperative RT reduces the risk of recurrence compared with treatment by excision alone, by 50% to 60%. These trials have identified young patient age (<40 years) and, to a lesser extent, clinical presentations of DCIS, and the presence of comedo necrosis as factors predictive of higher rates of recurrence that are useful for identifying patient groups likely to achieve the greatest absolute benefit from RT (38–41).

Evidence from the NSABP B-24 trial indicates that tamoxifen is beneficial in women with ER-positive DCIS. This is consistent with a large body of data on the effect of tamoxifen in invasive cancer. The authors routinely use ER and PR status determined by immunohistochemistry for decision making regarding the use of tamoxifen in DCIS. The most favorable risk–benefit ratio for tamoxifen use is in premenopausal women with two breasts at risk. The combination of tamoxifen and RT maximally reduces the risk of ipsilateral breast recurrence. Tamoxifen is an option, but not a necessity, for the treatment of DCIS, which should be discussed with women with ER-positive disease who do not have contraindications to the drug. For patients with ER-positive DCIS, the combined effects of tamoxifen and breast RT reduced the risk of an invasive recurrence by approximately 85%. In NSABP B-17, the 12-year rate of an invasive recurrence was 18%, which would be reduced to only approximately 2% to 3% with combined tamoxifen and breast RT. In spite of this, an examination of tamoxifen usage among 1,622 patients treated for unilateral DCIS at eight National Comprehensive Cancer Network Centers between 1997 and 2003 demonstrated that only 41% received tamoxifen. Factors significantly associated with receipt of tamoxifen included diagnosis after July 1999, breast-conserving therapy in patients under age 70 years, receipt of RT, prior hysterectomy, and no history of vascular disease. However, the use of tamoxifen in patients undergoing breast-conserving therapy varied from 34% to 74% between centers (106).

The NSABP has completed a clinical trial in postmenopausal women with DCIS treated with lumpectomy and RT and then randomized to tamoxifen or anastrozole (NSABP B-35), but results are not available at this time. A similar trial outside the United States (IBIS-II–DCIS) is accruing patients, with a planned end of accrual in December 31, 2010.

In light of these findings, the authors approach patients before surgery with the assumption that breast irradiation will be a part of their treatment if they choose breast-conserving therapy. Contraindications to RT, as for invasive cancer, include prior therapeutic irradiation to the ipsilateral breast, diagnosis early in pregnancy, and active scleroderma or systemic lupus erythematosus. Large areas of DCIS that cannot be excised to clearly negative margins with an acceptable cosmetic outcome should prompt a discussion of mastectomy. An adequate excision is of particular concern in patients younger than 40 years of age with high-grade, ER-negative DCIS because of their higher baseline risk of recurrence and lack of benefit from tamoxifen. In patients who are candidates for breast irradiation, the final decision about the risks and benefits of RT and tamoxifen in an individual case is made when the final pathology report is available. Although it is clear that there are some patients who receive a small absolute benefit from either irradiation or tamoxifen, the final decision regarding the use of RT and tamoxifen is heavily influenced by the patient's perception of what level of benefit is meaningful to her. The ability to treat local recurrence with further breast preservation using re-excision and RT is one of the potential benefits of initial treatment with excision alone. However, local recurrence is psychologically traumatic, and only 44% of patients who had recurrence after initial treatment by excision alone in the NSABP B-17 trial chose breast-conserving surgery again (47). Furthermore, approximately 50% of recurrences are invasive and carry a risk of distant metastasis.

What constitutes an adequate negative margin for breast-conserving surgery has been the source of much debate. As previously discussed, convincing data to support a reduction in the rate of local recurrence when negative margins of more than 1 to 2 mm are obtained is lacking. In light of this, the authors do not believe that a single margin width is appropriate for all patients. Factors to consider when making a decision regarding the need for re-excision include the following:

1. The amount of DCIS close to the margin. Extensive DCIS is clearly of more concern than a single duct that is separate from the main area of DCIS.
2. Which margin is close or involved. "Close" margins on the anterior and posterior specimen surfaces are of no concern if there is no residual breast tissue in these areas. Those within the parenchyma (i.e., medial, lateral, superior, inferior) have the potential for more disease to be present.
3. Findings on postoperative mammography. Residual calcifications and close margins mandate re-excision.
4. Other factors, such as patient age, that affect the risk of recurrence.

In general, margins 1 mm or less warrant re-excision, although if this would necessitate mastectomy or sacrifice of the nipple areolar complex, the decision is made on a case-by-case basis. There is uncertainty regarding the number of re-excisions that should be performed in an effort to obtain negative margins for breast-conserving therapy. In a study of 2,770 patients, 13% with DCIS, treated between 1981 and 2006, the risk of local recurrence based on the number of surgical excisions required to obtain negative margins was examined. At a median follow-up of 73 months, the actuarial rates of local

recurrence at 5 and 10 years were 2.5% and 5.0%, respectively, in patients undergoing a single excision, and 4.9% and 5.6% for those having two or more re-excisions ($p = .02$). In multivariate analysis, the number of re-excisions was not a significant predictor of local recurrence (107). However, a histologic diagnosis of DCIS was a predictor of the need for re-excision when compared to a diagnosis of infiltrating ductal carcinoma.

The available data suggest that patient knowledge of the risks and benefits of local therapy options is low, and patient participation in the decision-making process is limited. Katz et al. (108) performed a population-based survey of 1,884 women diagnosed with DCIS or invasive carcinoma in 2002. The mastectomy rate was 30% and did not vary between women diagnosed with invasive carcinoma or DCIS. Greater patient involvement in the decision-making process was significantly correlated with receipt of mastectomy; only 5% of white women who stated that their surgeon made the surgical decision received mastectomy, compared with 17% of women who shared the decision with their surgeon, and 27% of women who stated that they made the treatment decision ($p < .001$). In a study limited to the 659 women with DCIS (109), those with high-grade lesions greater than 2 cm in size were most likely to undergo mastectomy (53%), although mastectomy was recommended in only 28% of this group. Patient concerns about the receipt of radiation and about recurrence were strongly correlated with mastectomy.

The use of sentinel node biopsy is reserved for patients undergoing mastectomy. If a presurgical diagnosis of DCIS is made by percutaneous core needle biopsy, invasive carcinoma is found in approximately 20% of cases at the time of surgical excision (79,110–112). As discussed previously, invasion is more frequent in large areas of DCIS, and the performance of a mastectomy precludes subsequent sentinel node biopsy. In patients undergoing breast conservation, sentinel node biopsy can be selectively applied to the subset of women found to have invasive carcinoma after surgical excision.

In summary, the term DCIS encompasses a heterogeneous group of lesions of varying malignant potential. In the future, advances in research may allow researchers to reliably identify those lesions that have the propensity to recur locally as invasive cancer and those that will display the metastatic phenotype. Until this goal is reached, therapy must be directed toward minimizing the risk of local recurrence while maintaining quality of life. The appropriate therapeutic strategy will vary based on both patient and disease characteristics, as well as patient preferences.

MICROINVASIVE CARCINOMA

One of the most important goals in the histologic examination of DCIS lesions is the identification of foci of stromal invasion because, in general, the therapeutic algorithm for patients with pure DCIS differs from that for patients with DCIS and associated invasive breast cancer. A frequently encountered problem in the examination of such specimens is the identification of the smallest foci of invasive carcinoma, or *microinvasion*. Although this diagnosis often appears in surgical pathology reports, this term has not been applied in a consistent, standardized manner, and the histologic diagnosis of microinvasion is not straightforward and is often problematic for the pathologist.

In the 2002 edition of the American Joint Committee on Cancer (AJCC) *Cancer Staging Manual* (113), microinvasion is defined as "the extension of cancer cells beyond the basement membrane into the adjacent tissues with no focus more than 0.1 cm in greatest dimension." Lesions that fulfill this definition are staged as T1mic, a subset of T1 breast cancer. The staging manual further states, "When there are multiple foci of microinvasion, the size of only the largest focus is used to classify the microinvasion," and that the size of the individual foci should not be added together. This is only the second edition of the AJCC staging manual that recognizes a specific T substage for microinvasion. Unfortunately, widely varying definitions of microinvasion have been used in the past, and some of these definitions differ substantially from that offered in the AJCC staging manual. For example, microinvasion has been variously defined as (a) DCIS with "evidence of stromal invasion" (111), (b) "DCIS with limited microscopic stromal invasion below the basement membrane, but not invading more than 10% of the surface of the histologic sections examined" (115); and (c) "breast cancer cells confined to the duct system of the breast with only a microscopic focus of malignant cells invading beyond the basement membrane of the duct as determined by light microscopy" (116). This lack of a uniform definition for microinvasion has clearly contributed to the confusion regarding this entity.

The identification of microinvasion in a lesion that is primarily DCIS can be difficult for the pathologist because a variety of patterns in DCIS may be misconstrued as stromal invasion. Lesions that are commonly mistaken for microinvasion include: (a) DCIS involving lobules ("cancerization of lobules"); (b) branching of ducts; (c) distortion or entrapment of involved ducts or acini by fibrosis; (d) inflammation present in association with and obscuring involved ducts or acini; (e) crush artifact; (f) cautery effect; (g) artifactual displacement of DCIS cells into the surrounding stroma or adipose tissue due to tissue manipulation or a prior needling procedure; and (h) DCIS involving benign sclerosing processes, such as radial scars, complete sclerosing lesions, and sclerosing adenosis (30,117–121). Although the presence of stromal desmoplasia and inflammation should heighten the suspicion of invasion, these phenomena are present so often in association with high-grade DCIS without demonstrable invasion that their presence cannot be depended on to make this distinction.

Another potential problem with the pathologic diagnosis of microinvasion relates to tissue sampling. Previous published studies of microinvasion have generally failed to indicate how much of a given specimen was submitted for microscopic evaluation. Thus, some lesions categorized as microinvasive based on limited tissue sampling could actually represent frankly invasive carcinomas in which the largest area of invasion was not submitted for histologic evaluation or was not represented on the slides because the cancer was deeper in the blocks. Given the problems with the definition and pathologic diagnosis of microinvasion, the controversy surrounding the clinical significance of this lesion should not be surprising. The incidence of microinvasive cancer is reported to range from 0.68% to 2.4% of cases (122), and as with DCIS, microinvasion is being diagnosed more frequently because of the increased use of screening mammography. To treat patients properly with microinvasive carcinoma, one must know whether this lesion behaves like DCIS, invasive carcinoma, or something in between. The behavior of microinvasive carcinoma is difficult to determine because of the variety of definitions used in the past.

As illustrated in Table 26.10, sentinel lymph node metastases are infrequent in microinvasive carcinoma, occurring in 6% to 10% of patients when the current AJCC definition of microinvasion is used (89,123–126), and approximately half of the metastases detected were micrometastases. The limited available long-term follow-up data on patients with microinvasive carcinoma suggest that the prognosis after surgical treatment is excellent. Rosner et al. (115) reported on 36 cases of DCIS with microinvasion treated between 1976 and 1987. Thirty-three patients underwent mastectomy. At a mean follow-up of 57 months, all patients remained free of disease. Wong et al. (116) also observed no treatment failures at a median follow-up of 47 months, and Kinne et al. (127) reported a 94% disease-free survival rate at a median follow-up of 11.5

Table 26.10	INCIDENCE OF SENTINEL LYMPH NODE INVOLVEMENT IN PATIENTS WITH MICROINVASION	
Author, Year (Reference)	No. of Patients	No. Node-Positive (%)
Klauber-DeMore et al. 2000 (89)	31	3 (10)
Intra et al. 2003 (124)	41	4 (10)
Katz et al. 2006 (125)	21	2 (9)
Zavagno et al. 2007 (126)	43	4 (9)
Gray et al. 2007 (123)	77	5 (6)

years. Most patients in these reports were treated with mastectomy. Solin et al. (128) reported on the outcome of 39 patients treated with breast-conserving surgery and RT. With a median follow-up of 55 months, the overall survival rate was 97%. However, nine patients (23%) had a recurrence in the breast. Outcome was compared for patients with microinvasive carcinoma, patients with DCIS, and patients with node-negative invasive carcinoma treated during the same period. Patients with microinvasive carcinoma were found to have a higher local recurrence rate than those with pure DCIS or those with invasive carcinoma, and a survival rate intermediate between the two groups. In a retrospective study, Silverstein and Lagios (129) compared 24 patients with microinvasion to 909 patients with pure DCIS and observed no difference in local recurrence, disease-free survival, or overall survival.

From the limited information available on microinvasive carcinoma, several tentative conclusions may be drawn. First, because of variability in the definition of microinvasion, results from the literature are applicable to an individual patient only if microinvasion is defined in the same way. The incidence of axillary node metastases is low but sufficient to warrant sentinel node biopsy. This is particularly true when the diagnosis of microinvasion is made by core needle biopsy and the amount of invasive carcinoma remaining in the breast is unknown, and in cases where multiple foci of microinvasion are present. Survival of patients with microinvasive carcinoma seems to be intermediate between that of patients with pure DCIS and that of patients with small invasive carcinomas. The use of breast-conserving treatment in these patients should follow the same guidelines for careful mammographic and pathologic evaluation, and the requirement for negative margins of resection as for patients with an extensive intraductal component–positive invasive carcinoma.

MANAGEMENT SUMMARY

- DCIS represents a heterogeneous group of lesions of varying malignant potential.
- Pathologic or molecular factors that predict which DCIS will progress to invasive cancer have not been identified.
- Appropriate treatment options for DCIS are primarily determined by the extent of disease in the breast.
- A detailed mammographic evaluation of the extent of DCIS is essential for treatment planning. The role of MRI is uncertain.
- Total mastectomy is curative for 98% to 99% of patients with DCIS.
- Patients with localized DCIS are candidates for treatment with excision and RT. Negative margins (no DCIS on ink) reduce the risk of local recurrence.
- A margin width that maximizes local control has not been identified. Margins of 2 to 3 mm are commonly used due to the discontinuous growth of some DCIS lesions.

- Subsets of DCIS patients who do not benefit from RT have not been reproducibly identified.
- Tamoxifen appears to be of benefit primarily in ER-positive DCIS. The combination of tamoxifen and RT maximizes local control, with the most favorable risk–benefit ratio seen in premenopausal women with two breasts at risk.
- Sentinel lymph node biopsy is not routinely indicated in DCIS. In women undergoing mastectomy for extensive DCIS, a sentinel lymph node biopsy obviates the need for axillary dissection if invasion is found and is recommended.
- Nodal metastases are present in 6% to 10% of patients with microinvasive carcinoma, and sentinel lymph node biopsy is indicated when the results will influence subsequent treatment.
- A detailed discussion of the pros and cons of the various treatment options is needed to allow each woman with DCIS to make an informed treatment choice.

References

1. Ikeda DM, Andersson I. Ductal carcinoma in situ: atypical mammographic appearances. *Radiology* 1989;172:661–666.
2. Alexander HR, Candela FC, Dershaw DD, et al. Needle-localized mammographic lesions. Results and evolving treatment strategy. *Arch Surg* 1990;125:1441–1444.
3. Morrow M, Schmidt R, Cregger B, et al. Preoperative evaluation of abnormal mammographic findings to avoid unnecessary breast biopsies. *Arch Surg* 1994; 129:1091–1096.
4. Silverstein MJ, Gamagami P, Colburn WJ, et al. Nonpalpable breast lesions: diagnosis with slightly overpenetrated screen-film mammography and hook wire-directed biopsy in 1,014 cases. *Radiology* 1989;171:633–638.
5. Pandya S, Mackarem G, Lee A, al e. Ductal carcinoma *in situ*: the impact of screening on clinical presentation and pathologic features. *Breast J* 1998;4:146.
6. Meijnen P, Peterse JL, Oldenburg HS, et al. Changing patterns in diagnosis and treatment of ductal carcinoma *in situ* of the breast. *Eur J Surg Oncol* 2005;31: 833–1839.
7. Ries LAG, Melbert D, Krapcho M, et al., eds. *SEER cancer statistics review, 1975–2004*. Bethesda, MD: National Cancer Institute, 2007.
8. Ernster VL, Barclay J, Kerlikowske K, et al. Incidence of and treatment for ductal carcinoma in situ of the breast. *JAMA* 1996;275:913–918.
9. Gapstur SM, Morrow M, Sellers TA. Hormone replacement therapy and risk of breast cancer with a favorable histology: results of the Iowa Women's Health Study. *JAMA* 1999;281:2091–2097.
10. Claus EB, Stowe M, Carter D. Breast carcinoma in situ: risk factors and screening patterns. *J Natl Cancer Inst* 2001;93:1811–1817.
11. Kerlikowske K, Barclay J, Grady D, et al. Comparison of risk factors for ductal carcinoma *in situ* and invasive breast cancer. *J Natl Cancer Inst* 1997;89:76–82.
12. Lagios MD, Westdahl PR, Margolin FR, et al. Duct carcinoma *in situ*. Relationship of extent of noninvasive disease to the frequency of occult invasion, multicentricity, lymph node metastases, and short-term treatment failures. *Cancer* 1982;50: 1309–1314.
13. Schwartz GF, Patchefsky AS, Finklestein SD, et al. Nonpalpable *in situ* ductal carcinoma of the breast. Predictors of multicentricity and microinvasion and implications for treatment. *Arch Surg* 1989;124:29–32.
14. Bellamy CO, McDonald C, Salter DM, et al. Noninvasive ductal carcinoma of the breast: the relevance of histologic categorization. *Hum Pathol* 1993;24:16–23.
15. Patchefsky AS, Schwartz GF, Finkelstein SD, et al. Heterogeneity of intraductal carcinoma of the breast. *Cancer* 1989;63:731–741.
16. Holland R, Hendricks J. Microcalcifications associated with ductal carcinoma *in situ*: mammographic-pathologic correlation. *Semin Diagn Pathol* 1994;11:181.
17. Faverly DR, Burgers L, Bult P, et al. Three dimensional imaging of mammary ductal carcinoma *in situ*: clinical implications. *Semin Diagn Pathol* 1994;11:193–198.
18. Noguchi S, Motomura K, Inaji H, et al. Clonal analysis of predominantly intraductal carcinoma and precancerous lesions of the breast by means of polymerase chain reaction. *Cancer Res* 1994;54:1849–1853.
19. Contesso G, Mouriesse H, Petit JY. Non-palpable breast cancer: the point of view of the pathologist. *J Belge Radiol* 1990;73:329–333.
20. van Dongen JA, Fentiman IS, Harris JR, et al. In-situ breast cancer: the EORTC consensus meeting. *Lancet* 1989;2:25–27.
21. Houssami N, Ciatto S, Ellis I, et al. Underestimation of malignancy of breast core-needle biopsy: concepts and precise overall and category-specific estimates. *Cancer* 2007;109:487–495.
22. Jackman RJ, Burbank F, Parker SH, et al. Stereotactic breast biopsy of nonpalpable lesions: determinants of ductal carcinoma in situ underestimation rates. *Radiology* 2001;218:497–502.
23. Kettritz U, Rotter K, Schreer I, et al. Stereotactic vacuum-assisted breast biopsy in 2,874 patients: a multicenter study. *Cancer* 2004;100:245–251.
24. O'Connell P, Pekkel V, Fuqua SA, et al. Analysis of loss of heterozygosity in 399 premalignant breast lesions at 15 genetic loci. *J Natl Cancer Inst* 1998;90:697–703.
25. Warnberg F, Nordgren H, Bergkvist L, et al. Tumour markers in breast carcinoma correlate with grade rather than with invasiveness. *Br J Cancer* 2001;85:869–874.
26. Hoogerbrugge N, Bult P, de Widt-Levert LM, et al. High prevalence of premalignant lesions in prophylactically removed breasts from women at hereditary risk for breast cancer. *J Clin Oncol* 2003;21:41–45.
27. Page DL, Dupont WD, Rogers LW, et al. Intraductal carcinoma of the breast: follow-up after biopsy only. *Cancer* 1982;49:751–758.
28. Page DL, Dupont WD, Rogers LW, et al. Continued local recurrence of carcinoma 15–25 years after a diagnosis of low grade ductal carcinoma *in situ* of the breast treated only by biopsy. *Cancer* 1995;76:1197–1200.
29. Rosen PP, Braun DW Jr, Kinne DE. The clinical significance of pre-invasive breast carcinoma. *Cancer* 1980;46:919–925.
30. Eusebi V, Foschini MP, Cook MG, et al. Long-term follow-up of *in situ* carcinoma of the breast with special emphasis on clinging carcinoma. *Semin Diagn Pathol* 1989;6:165–173.
31. Eusebi V, Feudale E, Foschini MP, et al. Long-term follow-up of *in situ* carcinoma of the breast. *Semin Diagn Pathol* 1994;11:223–235.
32. Alpers CE, Wellings SR. The prevalence of carcinoma *in situ* in normal and cancer-associated breasts. *Hum Pathol* 1985;16:796–807.
33. Bartow SA, Pathak DR, Black WC, et al. Prevalence of benign, atypical, and malignant breast lesions in populations at different risk for breast cancer. A forensic autopsy study. *Cancer* 1987;60:2751–2760.
34. Kauff ND, Brogi E, Scheuer L, et al. Epithelial lesions in prophylactic mastectomy specimens from women with *BRCA* mutations. *Cancer* 2003;97:1601–1608.
35. Lee LA, Silverstein MJ, Chung CT, et al. Breast cancer-specific mortality after invasive local recurrence in patients with ductal carcinoma-*in-situ* of the breast. *Am J Surg* 2006;192:416–419.
36. Boyages J, Delaney G, Taylor R. Predictors of local recurrence after treatment of ductal carcinoma in situ: a meta-analysis. *Cancer* 1999;85:616–628.
37. Carlson GW, Page A, Johnson E, Nicholson K, Styblo TM, Wood WC. Local recurrence of ductal carcinoma *in situ* after skin-sparing mastectomy. *J Am Coll Surg* 2007;204:1074–1078.
38. Bijker N, Meijnen P, Peterse JL, et al. Breast-conserving treatment with or without radiotherapy in ductal carcinoma-*in-situ*: ten-year results of European Organisation for Research and Treatment of Cancer randomized phase III trial 10853—a study by the EORTC Breast Cancer Cooperative Group and EORTC Radiotherapy Group. *J Clin Oncol* 2006;24:3381–3387.
39. Emdin SO, Granstrand B, Ringberg A, et al. SweDCIS: Radiotherapy after sector resection for ductal carcinoma *in situ* of the breast. Results of a randomised trial in a population offered mammography screening. *Acta Oncol* 2006;45:536–543.
40. Fisher B, Land S, Mamounas E, et al. Prevention of invasive breast cancer in women with ductal carcinoma *in situ*: an update of the national surgical adjuvant breast and bowel project experience. *Semin Oncol* 2001;28:400–418.
41. Houghton J, George WD, Cuzick J, et al. Radiotherapy and tamoxifen in women with completely excised ductal carcinoma *in situ* of the breast in the UK, Australia, and New Zealand: randomised controlled trial. *Lancet* 2003;362:95–102.
42. Holmberg L, Garmo H, Granstrand B, et al. Absolute risk reductions for local recurrence after postoperative radiotherapy after sector resection for ductal carcinoma *in situ* of the breast. *J Clin Oncol* 2008;26:1247–1252.
43. Clarke M, Collins R, Darby S, et al. Effects of radiotherapy and of differences in the extent of surgery for early breast cancer on local recurrence and 15-year survival: an overview of the randomised trials. *Lancet* 2005;366:2087–2106.
44. Fisher B, Dignam J, Wolmark N, et al. Tamoxifen in treatment of intraductal breast cancer: National Surgical Adjuvant Breast and Bowel Project B-24 randomised controlled trial. *Lancet* 1999;353:1993–2000.
45. Allred DC, Bryant J, Land S. Estrogen receptor expression as a predictive marker of effectiveness of tamoxifen in the treatment of DCIS: findings from NSABP Protocol B-24. *Br Cancer Res Treat* 2002;76:S36(abst).
46. Fisher B, Bryant J, Dignam JJ, et al. Tamoxifen, radiation therapy, or both for prevention of ipsilateral breast tumor recurrence after lumpectomy in women with invasive breast cancers of one centimeter or less. *J Clin Oncol* 2002;20:4141–4149.
47. Fisher B, Dignam J, Wolmark N, et al. Lumpectomy and radiation therapy for the treatment of intraductal breast cancer: findings from National Surgical Adjuvant Breast and Bowel Project B-17. *J Clin Oncol* 1998;16:441–452.
48. Fowble B, Hanlon AL, Fein DA, et al. Results of conservative surgery and radiation for mammographically detected ductal carcinoma in situ (DCIS). *Int J Radiat Oncol Biol Phys* 1997;38:949–957.
49. Hiramatsu H, Bornstein BA, Recht A, et al. Local recurrence after conservative surgery and radiation therapy for ductal carcinoma *in situ*: possible importance of family history. *Cancer J Sci Am* 1995;1:55–61.
50. Kestin LL, Goldstein NS, Martinez AA, et al. Mammographically detected ductal carcinoma in situ treated with conservative surgery with or without radiation therapy: patterns of failure and 10-year results. *Ann Surg* 2000;231:235–245.
51. Kuske RR, Bean JM, Garcia DM, et al. Breast conservation therapy for intraductal carcinoma of the breast. *Int J Radiat Oncol Biol Phys* 1993;26:391–396.
52. Silverstein MJ, Barth A, Poller DN, et al. Ten-year results comparing mastectomy to excision and radiation therapy for ductal carcinoma *in situ* of the breast. *Eur J Cancer* 1995;31A:1425–1427.
53. Sneige N, McNeese MD, Atkinson EN, et al. Ductal carcinoma *in situ* treated with lumpectomy and irradiation: histopathological analysis of 49 specimens with emphasis on risk factors and long term results. *Hum Pathol* 1995;26:642–649.
54. Solin LJ, Kurtz J, Fourquet A, et al. Fifteen-year results of breast-conserving surgery and definitive breast irradiation for the treatment of ductal carcinoma *in situ* of the breast. *J Clin Oncol* 1996;14:754–763.
55. Solin LJ, Recht A, Fourquet A, et al. Ten-year results of breast-conserving surgery and definitive irradiation for intraductal carcinoma (ductal carcinoma *in situ*) of the breast. *Cancer* 1991;68:2337–2344.
56. Solin LJ, Fourquet A, Vicini FA, et al. Mammographically detected ductal carcinoma *in situ* of the breast treated with breast-conserving surgery and definitive breast irradiation: long-term outcome and prognostic significance of patient age and margin status. *Int J Radiat Oncol Biol Phys* 2001;50:991–1002.
57. Cutuli B, Cohen-Solal-le Nir C, de Lafontan B, et al. Breast-conserving therapy for ductal carcinoma *in situ* of the breast: the French Cancer Centers' experience. *Int J Radiat Oncol Biol Phys* 2002;53:868–879.
58. Bijker N, Peterse JL, Duchateau L, et al. Risk factors for recurrence and metastasis after breast-conserving therapy for ductal carcinoma-*in-situ*: analysis of European Organization for Research and Treatment of Cancer Trial 10853. *J Clin Oncol* 2001;19:2263–2271.
59. Fisher ER, Dignam J, Tan-Chiu E, et al. Pathologic findings from the National Surgical Adjuvant Breast Project (NSABP) eight-year update of Protocol B-17: intraductal carcinoma. *Cancer* 1999;86:429–438.
60. Rodrigues N, Carter D, Dillon D, et al. Correlation of clinical and pathologic features with outcome in patients with ductal carcinoma *in situ* of the breast treated with breast-conserving surgery and radiotherapy. *Int J Radiat Oncol Biol Phys* 2002;54:1331–1335.
61. Nakamura S, Woo C, Silberman H, et al. Breast-conserving therapy for ductal carcinoma *in situ*: a 20-year experience with excision plus radiation therapy. *Am J Surg* 2002;184:403–409.

62. Vicini FA, Kestin LL, Goldstein NS, et al. Relationship between excision volume, margin status, and tumor size with the development of local recurrence in patients with ductal carcinoma-*in-situ* treated with breast-conserving therapy. *J Surg Oncol* 2001;76:245–254.
63. Dunne C, Burke JP, Morrow M, Kell MR. The effect of margin status on local recurrence following breast conservation and radiation therapy for DCIS. *J Clin Oncol*, in press.
64. Jhingran A, Kim JS, Buchholz TA, et al. Age as a predictor of outcome for women with DCIS treated with breast-conserving surgery and radiation: the University of Texas M. D. Anderson Cancer Center experience. *Int J Radiat Oncol Biol Phys* 2002;54:804–809.
65. Vicini FA, Recht A. Age at diagnosis and outcome for women with ductal carcinoma-*in-situ* of the breast: a critical review of the literature. *J Clin Oncol* 2002;20:2736–2744.
66. Goldstein NS, Vicini FA, Kestin LL, et al. Differences in the pathologic features of ductal carcinoma *in situ* of the breast based on patient age. *Cancer* 2000;88:2553–2560.
67. Rodrigues NA, Dillon D, Carter D, et al. Differences in the pathologic and molecular features of intraductal breast carcinoma between younger and older women. *Cancer* 2003;97:1393–1403.
68. Provenzano E, Hopper JL, Giles GG, et al. Biological markers that predict clinical recurrence in ductal carcinoma *in situ* of the breast. *Eur J Cancer* 2003;39:622–630.
69. Gauthier ML, Berman HK, Miller C, et al. Abrogated response to cellular stress identifies DCIS associated with subsequent tumor events and defines basal-like breast tumors. *Cancer Cell* 2007;12:479–491.
70. Solin LJ, Fourquet A, Vicini FA, et al. Salvage treatment for local recurrence after breast-conserving surgery and radiation as initial treatment for mammographically detected ductal carcinoma *in situ* of the breast. *Cancer* 2001;91:1090–1097.
71. Arnesson LG, Olsen K. Linkoping experience. In: Silverstein MJ, ed. *Ductal carcinoma in situ of the breast*. Baltimore: Williams & Wilkins, 1997:363–378.
72. Carpenter R, Boulter PS, Cooke T, et al. Management of screen detected ductal carcinoma in situ of the female breast. *Br J Surg* 1989;76:564–567.
73. Lagios MD. The Lagios experience. In: Silverstein MJ, ed. *Ductal carcinoma in situ of the breast*. Philadelphia: Lippincott Williams & Wilkins, 2002:303–207.
74. Schwartz GF. Treatment of subclinical DCIS by local excision and surveillance: an updated personal experience. In: Silverstein MJ, ed. *Ductal carcinoma in situ of the breast*. Philadelphia: Lippincott Williams & Wilkins, 2002:308–321.
75. Lagios MD. Lagios experience. In: Silverstein MJ, ed. *Ductal carcinoma in situ of the breast*. Baltimore: Williams & Wilkins, 1997:363–364.
76. Silverstein MJ, Lagios MD, Craig PH, et al. A prognostic index for ductal carcinoma *in situ* of the breast. *Cancer* 1996;77:2267–2274.
77. de Mascarel I, Bonichon F, MacGrogan G, et al. Application of the Van Nuys prognostic index in a retrospective series of 367 ductal carcinomas in situ of the breast examined by serial macroscopic sectioning: practical considerations. *Breast Cancer Res Treat* 2000;61:151–159.
78. Silverstein MJ. The University of Southern California Van Nuys Prognostic Index. In: Silverstein MJ, ed. *Ductal carcinoma in situ of the breast*. 2nd edition. Philadelphia: Lippincott Williams & Wilkins, 2002:459–473.
79. Silverstein MJ, Lagios MD, Groshen S, et al. The influence of margin width on local control of ductal carcinoma in situ of the breast. *N Engl J Med* 1999;340:1455–1461.
80. MacAusland SG, Hepel JT, Chong FK, et al. An attempt to independently verify the utility of the Van Nuys Prognostic Index for ductal carcinoma *in situ*. *Cancer* 2007;110:2648–2653.
81. Macdonald HR, Silverstein MJ, Lee LA, et al. Margin width as the sole determinant of local recurrence after breast conservation in patients with ductal carcinoma *in situ* of the breast. *Am J Surg* 2006;192:420–422.
82. Wong JS, Gadd MA, Gelman R, et al. Wide excision alone for ductal carcinoma in situ (DCIS) of the breast. *Proc Am Soc Clin Oncol* 2003;22(abst44).
83. Hughes L, Wang M, Page D. Five-year results of intergroup study E5194: local excision alone (without radiation treatment) for selected patients with ductal carcinoma *in situ* (DCIS). *Breast Cancer Res Treat* 2006;100[Suppl 1]:515.
84. Silverstein MJ, Gierson ED, Waisman JR, et al. Axillary lymph node dissection for T1a breast carcinoma. Is it indicated? *Cancer* 1994;73:664–667.
85. von Rueden DG, Wilson RE. Intraductal carcinoma of the breast. *Surg Gynecol Obstet* 1984;158:105–111.
86. Winchester DP, Menck HR, Osteen RT, et al. Treatment trends for ductal carcinoma *in situ* of the breast. *Ann Surg Oncol* 1995;2:207–213.
87. Giuliano AE, Dale PS, Turner RR, et al. Improved axillary staging of breast cancer with sentinel lymphadenectomy. *Ann Surg* 1995;222:394–399.
88. Pendas S, Dauway E, Giuliano R, et al. Sentinel node biopsy in ductal carcinoma *in situ* patients. *Ann Surg Oncol* 2000;7:15–20.
89. Klauber-DeMore N, Tan LK, Liberman L, et al. Sentinel lymph node biopsy: is it indicated in patients with high-risk ductal carcinoma-in-situ and ductal carcinoma-*in-situ* with microinvasion? *Ann Surg Oncol* 2000;7:636–642.
90. Lara JF, Young SM, Velilla RE, et al. The relevance of occult axillary micrometastasis in ductal carcinoma *in situ*: a clinicopathologic study with long-term follow-up. *Cancer* 2003;98:2105–2113.
91. Julian TB, Land SR, Fourchotte V, et al. Is sentinel node biopsy necessary in conservatively treated DCIS? *Ann Surg Oncol* 2007;14:2202–2208.
92. Wilke LG, McCall LM, Posther KE, et al. Surgical complications associated with sentinel lymph node biopsy: results from a prospective international cooperative group trial. *Ann Surg Oncol* 2006;13:491–500.
93. Fitzgibbons PL, Page DL, Weaver D, et al. Prognostic factors in breast cancer. College of American Pathologists Consensus Statement 1999. *Arch Pathol Lab Med* 2000;124:966–978.
94. Lyman GH, Giuliano AE, Somerfield MR, et al. American Society of Clinical Oncology guideline recommendations for sentinel lymph node biopsy in early-stage breast cancer. *J Clin Oncol* 2005;23:7703–7720.
95. Morrow M, Harris JR. Practice guideline for the management of ductal carcinoma *in-situ* of the breast. *J Am Coll Surg* 2007;205:145–161.
96. Morrow M, Bucci C, Rademaker A. Medical contraindications are not a major factor in the underutilization of breast conserving therapy. *J Am Coll Surg* 1998;186:269–274.
97. Holland R, Hendriks JH, Vebeek AL, et al. Extent, distribution, and mammographic/histological correlations of breast ductal carcinoma *in situ*. *Lancet* 1990;335:519–522.
98. Bluemke DA, Gatsonis CA, Chen MH, et al. Magnetic resonance imaging of the breast prior to biopsy. *JAMA* 2004;292:2735–2742.
99. Kuhl CK, Schrading S, Bieling HB, et al. MRI for diagnosis of pure ductal carcinoma in situ: a prospective observational study. *Lancet* 2007;370:485–492.
100. Arjan P, van der Velden G, Boetes C, et al. The value of magnetic resonance imaging in diagnosis and size assessment of *in situ* and small invasive breast carcinoma. *Am J Surg* 2006;192:172–178.
101. Esserman LJ, Kumar AS, Herrera AF, et al. Magnetic resonance imaging captures the biology of ductal carcinoma *in situ*. *J Clin Oncol* 2006;24:4603–4610.
102. Solin LJ, Orel SG, Hwang WT, et al. Relationship of breast magnetic resonance imaging to outcome after breast-conservation treatment with radiation for women with early-stage invasive breast carcinoma or ductal carcinoma *in situ*. *J Clin Oncol* 2008;26:386–391.
103. Bauer RL, Eckhert KH, Jr., Nemoto T. Ductal carcinoma *in situ*-associated nipple discharge: a clinical marker for locally extensive disease. *Ann Surg Oncol* 1998;5:452–455.
104. Gluck BS, Dershaw DD, Liberman L, et al. Microcalcifications on postoperative mammograms as an indicator of adequacy of tumor excision. *Radiology* 1993;188:469–472.
105. Aref A, Youssef E, Washington T, et al. The value of postlumpectomy mammogram in the management of breast cancer patients presenting with suspicious microcalcifications. *Cancer J Sci Am* 2000;6:25–27.
106. Yen TW, Kuerer HM, Ottesen RA, et al. Impact of randomized clinical trial results in the national comprehensive cancer network on the use of tamoxifen after breast surgery for ductal carcinoma *in situ*. *J Clin Oncol* 2007;25:3251–3258.
107. O'Sullivan MJ, Li T, Freedman G, et al. The effect of multiple reexcisions on the risk of local recurrence after breast conserving surgery. *Ann Surg Oncol* 2007;14:3133–3140.
108. Katz SJ, Lantz PM, Zemencuk JK. Correlates of surgical treatment type for women with noninvasive and invasive breast cancer. *J Women Health Gend Based Med* 2001;10:659–670.
109. Katz SJ, Lantz PM, Janz NK, et al. Patterns and correlates of local therapy for women with ductal carcinoma-*in-situ*. *J Clin Oncol* 2005;23:3001–3007.
110. Burbank F. Stereotactic breast biopsy of atypical ductal hyperplasia and ductal carcinoma *in situ* lesions: improved accuracy with directional, vacuum-assisted biopsy. *Radiology* 1997;202:843–847.
111. Jackman RJ, Nowels KW, Shepard MJ, et al. Stereotaxic large-core needle biopsy of 450 nonpalpable breast lesions with surgical correlation in lesions with cancer or atypical hyperplasia. *Radiology* 1994;193:91–95.
112. Morrow M, Venta L, Stinson T, et al. Prospective comparison of stereotactic core biopsy and surgical excision as diagnostic procedures for breast cancer patients. *Ann Surg* 2001;233:537–541.
113. American Joint Committee on Cancer. *AJCC cancer staging manual*. 6th ed. New York: Springer, 2002.
114. Schuh ME, Nemoto T, Penetrante RB, et al. Intraductal carcinoma. Analysis of presentation, pathologic findings, and outcome of disease. *Arch Surg* 1986;121:1303–1307.
115. Rosner D, Lane WW, Penetrante R. Ductal carcinoma in situ with microinvasion. A curable entity using surgery alone without need for adjuvant therapy. *Cancer* 1991;67:1498–1503.
116. Wong JH, Kopald KH, Morton DL. The impact of microinvasion on axillary node metastases and survival in patients with intraductal breast cancer. *Arch Surg* 1990;125:1298–1302.
117. Fisher ER. Pathobiological considerations relating to the treatment of intraductal carcinoma (ductal carcinoma *in situ*) of the breast. *CA Cancer J Clin* 1997;47:52–64.
118. Kerner H, Lichtig C. Lobular cancerization: incidence and differential diagnosis with lobular carcinoma *in situ* of breast. *Histopathology* 1986;10:621–629.
119. Oberman HA, Markey BA. Noninvasive carcinoma of the breast presenting in adenosis. *Mod Pathol* 1991;4:31–35.
120. Youngson BJ, Cranor M, Rosen PP. Epithelial displacement in surgical breast specimens following needling procedures. *Am J Surg Pathol* 1994;18:896–903.
121. Youngson BJ, Liberman L, Rosen PP. Displacement of carcinomatous epithelium in surgical breast specimens following stereotaxic core biopsy. *Am J Clin Pathol* 1995;103:598–602.
122. Hoda SA, Chiu A, Prasad ML, et al. Are microinvasion and micrometastasis in breast cancer mountains or molehills? *Am J Surg* 2000;180:305–308.
123. Gray RJ, Mulheron B, Pockaj BA, et al. The optimal management of the axillae of patients with microinvasive breast cancer in the sentinel lymph node era. *Am J Surg* 2007;194:845–849.
124. Intra M, Zurrida S, Maffini F, et al. Sentinel lymph node metastasis in microinvasive breast cancer. *Ann Surg Oncol* 2003;10:1160–1165.
125. Katz A, Gage I, Evans S, et al. Sentinel lymph node positivity of patients with ductal carcinoma *in situ* or microinvasive breast cancer. *Am J Surg* 2006;191:761–766.
126. Zavagno G, Belardinelli V, Marconato R, et al. Sentinel lymph node metastasis from mammary ductal carcinoma *in situ* with microinvasion. *Breast* 2007;16:146–151.
127. Kinne DW, Petrek JA, Osborne MP, et al. Breast carcinoma *in situ*. *Arch Surg* 1989;124:33–36.
128. Solin LJ, Fowble BL, Yeh IT, et al. Microinvasive ductal carcinoma of the breast treated with breast-conserving surgery and definitive irradiation. *Int J Radiat Oncol Biol Phys* 1992;23:961–968.
129. Silverstein MJ, Lagios MD. Ductal carcinoma in situ with microinvasion. In: Silverstein MJ, ed. *Ductal carcinoma in situ of the breast*. Philadelphia: Lippincott Williams & Wilkins, 2002:523–529.

Pathology and Biological Markers
of Invasive Breast Cancer

Chapter 27
Breast Cancer Genomics

Paul T. Spellman, Laura Heiser, and Joe W. Gray

Breast cancer is predominantly a disease of the genome with cancers arising and progressing through accumulation of aberrations that alter the genome—by changing DNA sequence, copy number, and structure in ways that that contribute to diverse aspects of cancer pathophysiology. Classic examples of genomic events that contribute to breast cancer pathophysiology include inherited mutations in *BRCA1*, *BRCA2*, *TP53*, and *CHK2* that contribute to the initiation of breast cancer, amplification of *ERBB2* (formerly HER2) and mutations of elements of the PI3-kinase pathway that activate aspects of epidermal growth factor receptor (*EGFR*) signaling and deletion of CDKN2A/B that contributes to cell cycle deregulation and genome instability. It is now apparent that accumulation of these aberrations is a time-dependent process that accelerates with age (1). Although American women living to an age of 85 have a 1 in 8 chance of developing breast cancer, the incidence of cancer in women younger than 30 years is uncommon. This is consistent with a multistep cancer progression model whereby mutation and selection drive the tumor's development, analogous to traditional Darwinian evolution (2,3). In the case of cancer, the driving events are changes in sequence, copy number, and structure of DNA and alterations in chromatin structure or other epigenetic marks.

Our understanding of the genetic, genomic, and epigenomic events that influence the development and progression of breast cancer is increasing at a remarkable rate through application of powerful analysis tools that enable genome-wide analysis of DNA sequence and structure, copy number, allelic loss, and epigenomic modification. Application of these techniques to elucidation of the nature and timing of these events is enriching our understanding of mechanisms that increase breast cancer susceptibility, enable tumor initiation and progression to metastatic disease, and determine therapeutic response or resistance. These studies also reveal the molecular differences between cancer and normal that may be exploited to therapeutic benefit or that provide targets for molecular assays that may enable early cancer detection, and predict individual disease progression or response to treatment. This chapter reviews current and future directions in genome analysis and summarizes studies that provide insights into breast cancer pathophysiology or that suggest strategies to improve breast cancer management.

CANCER GENOME SEQUENCE

Mutations and Polymorphisms

The discovery of germ-line and somatic mutations has long been a critical component of cancer research. Driven by increasingly powerful normal and tumor DNA sequencing capabilities, a substantial number of germ-line and somatic mutations and polymorphisms have been associated with an increased risk of breast cancer and with aspects of breast cancer pathogenesis.

To date, DNA sequence-based studies have established associations between germ-line mutations in *TP53*, *BRCA1*, *BRCA2*, and *PTEN* with high breast cancer risk and mutations in *CHEK2*, *ATM*, *NBS1*, *RAD50*, *BRIP1*, and *PALB2* with approximately twofold increased breast cancer risk (4). In addition, genome-wide analyses of single nucleotide polymorphisms have established associations between polymorphisms in *FGFR2*, *TNRC9*, *MAP3K1*, and *LSP1* with significant but modestly increased breast cancer risk (5).

Early DNA sequence analyses of primary tumors and cell lines revealed somatic mutations that contribute strongly to breast cancer pathophysiology. These include mutations such as *TP53*, *CDH1*, and *PIK3CA* that are commonly mutated in breast cancer (from COSMIC http://www.sanger.ac.uk/genetics/CGP/cosmic/). The human genome project proved the viability of sequencing entire genomes and since that time, it has been an obvious goal to search systematically for the mutations that drive cancer. Recent work from groups at the Sanger Center (6), Johns Hopkins University (7), and The Cancer Genome Atlas (8) highlight just how achievable this goal is, and what we can expect to learn when it is completed.

New Discovery Approaches

The critical issue is to determine which genes, when mutated, are responsible for cancer pathophysiology. Two approaches have been proposed to identify statistically significant recurrent mutations. One approach is to target specific classes of genes in a large survey of samples (100s), which provides the ability to detect rare but still recurrent mutational events. The other approach is to sequence all genes in a limited number of samples (~10) to identify the common mutational events that drive tumorigenesis. The result of these studies has been to show that (a) a relatively large number of mutated genes (>20) are likely to be driving each individual cancer and (b) hundreds of genes can act as drivers of breast cancer in total. Examining the functions of genes that can drive cancer when mutated has shown that they may not always be in genes predicted to harbor oncogenic or tumor suppressor functions.

Sequencing tumor DNA to identify somatic mutations is technically and logistically complicated (Fig. 27.1). Work published to date has used industry standard dideoxy chain termination-based sequencing (9). The standard approach is to use polymerase chain reaction (PCR) to amplify each exon of the gene to be sequenced and then sequence each exon individually. For example, sequencing 1,000 typical genes with 10 exons each, in 100 samples entails 1,000,000 DNA sequencing reactions covering approximately 150 million basepairs (bp) of total DNA sequence, which is a substantial amount of work. These sequences are compared with the reference human genome and if they do not match are flagged as possible mutations. It is

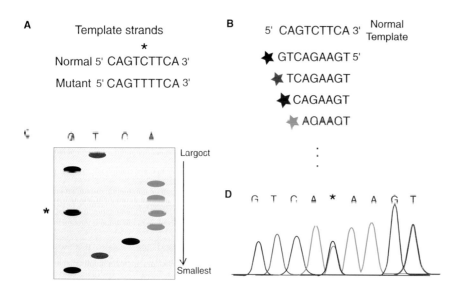

FIGURE 27.1. Sanger DNA sequencing using florescent chain terminators. A: Template DNA from tumor or normal cells is used to synthesize complementary molecules (**B**) that are terminated with differentially fluorescently labeled deoxyribose nucleotide triphosphates (dNTPs). Chain terminating nucleotides are present at a much lower concentration than normal nucleotides. If a chain terminator is incorporated no additional bases can be added and a DNA chain of a fixed length is created, tagging the molecule with a particular fluorescent dye that indicates a certain nucleotide. **C:** Chain terminated molecules are put in a gel-filled capillary, which allows smaller molecules to move through it more easily than larger molecules. In the presence of an electric field, DNA, which is negatively charged, migrates toward the positive electrode which is placed on the opposite end of the capillary from the side that is loaded. Before reaching the end of the capillary the molecules pass in front of a detector, which records the color of the fluorescence. **D:** Fluorescent spectra are analyzed so the DNA sequence can be interpreted; in the trace shown, the fifth base from the left is a mixture of G (*black*) and A (*green*) rather than a single peak of one color.

critical to note that there will be thousands of sequences in the tumor different than the reference genome caused by sequencing errors and normal sequence polymorphisms. Each potential mutation must be resequenced to ensure it is not an error and then the tumor and normal sequence must be compared to ensure that the variation from the reference genome is not a polymorphism.

Technically, Sanger sequencing is challenging because each reaction produces a single electropherogram that is the average sequence of all DNA molecules that are PCR amplified at that region. This is critical because DNA from tumors is not uniform, being contaminated by normal tissue and by heterogeneity within the tumor itself. In some rare cases a tumor may be homozygous for a mutation (caused by loss of heterozygosity see below), but in most cases tumors are heterozygous for a mutation, meaning that the electrophoretic trace will have two peaks at a given base pair. As the ratio of mutated to normal sequence decreases, the ability to detect a mutation correspondingly decreases. Typically, Sanger sequencing cannot reliably detect mutant alleles that are less than 30% of the total (8).

The Sanger Center (10) performed a screen to identify mutations in kinases predicated on two assumptions (a) kinases are key regulators of cell signaling and (b) targeted inhibition of kinases is a well-understood process, which is amenable to therapeutic intervention making genes that are mutated in the survey useful drug targets. In a survey of all 518 kinase genes across 210 diverse human cancers (including 16 breast cancers), they observed more than 900 nonsynonomous somatic mutations that altered the amino acid sequence of a kinase. Not all of the mutations are actually responsible for cancer, however, and the identification of those mutations that drive cancer (versus those that are random passengers) is a critical question. Through the use of selection pressure analysis (based on comparing the rate of synonymous mutations that did not change amino acid sequence with nonsynonymous, those that change the amino acid sequence), the Sanger Center group estimated that most (~80%) of the observed mutations were passenger mutations that did not influence the development of the cancer. This meant that in the 210 cancers they sequenced they identified approximately 150 mutations in protein kinase genes that were likely to drive oncogenesis. The overall power of the effort was not sufficient to estimate which genes are oncogenic drivers (most genes showed only single mutations), but it was possible to rank the genes as shown in Table 27.1. Many of the genes with the highest selection pressures (and overall ranking) are either known to be involved in cancer

through genetics or previous mutation studies (e.g., *ATM*, *FGFR2*, and *STK11*) (11–13), or have homologs that are known to be involved in oncogenesis (e.g., *MAP2K4*).

The Johns Hopkins group took the complementary approach. They sequenced every gene in 11 breast cancer cell lines samples as a discovery phase (7,14) followed by a validation phase of 24 breast tumor samples in which they sequenced only those genes that showed mutations in the discovery phase. Part of the rationale for the limited number of samples was to be genomically complete but another part was a resource limitation; the Johns Hopkins group used cell lines of which only a few matched the normal DNA is available. Sequencing cell lines for the discovery phase makes the sequencing traces more easily interpreted because there is neither normal DNA contamination nor tumor heterogeneity. The results of these studies were revolutionary, suggesting that hundreds, and possibly thousands, of genes have the potential to promote cancer when mutated. Further, individual breast tumors are likely to harbor 20 or more somatic mutations that are responsible for that specific cancer. These observations caused considerable controversy, but have now been generally accepted and new evidence from sequencing other tumor types has strengthened this argument (15,16).

Recent Results

Nearly 10% of all human genes in these discovery efforts harbored mutations in the discovery screen. This seems extraordinarily high but the background mutation rate of the tumors is roughly one mutation per megabase of genomic DNA (which corresponds to about 3,000 random mutations in the genome) that it is not wholly unexpected. The validation phase, however proved truly remarkable; 167 genes harbored mutations in both the discovery and validation phases, which is approximately 1% of all human genes. Beyond the large numbers of genes observed to be mutated, two key observations emerge from this analysis: first, many recurrent mutations occur in genes that are not obviously related to cancer (i.e., the glycosylase GALNT5 and the transglutaminase TGM3); second and more importantly, many of the mutations appear to be clustered in pathways. For example, at least seven biological pathways, including *ATM* signaling and apoptosis induction, show significant levels of mutation (17) (Table 27.2). The observation that particular pathways are significantly mutated provides a framework in which to understand their functional significance, and further suggests that a few key pathways may be especially critical for the development of oncogenesis.

Table 27.1	MUTATION PREVALENCE IN THE KINASE SCREEN. EACH GENE IS RANKED BY ITS MUTATION FREQUENCY AND SELECTIVE PRESSURE. THE TOP 20 GENES ARE SHOWN		
Gene	Ranking	Selection Pressure	Number of Nonsynonymous Mutations
TTN	1	2.0	63
BRAF	2	8.4	8
ATM	3	2.9	10
TAF1L	4	3.6	8
ERN1	5	4.5	6
MAP2K4	6	8.7	4
CHUK	7	5.4	5
FGFR2	8	5.1	5
NTRK3	9	4.8	5
MGC42105	10	7.1	4
TGFBR2	11	5.9	4
EPHA6	12	3.9	5
FLJ23074	13	5.4	4
ITK	14	4.9	4
DCAMKL3	15	4.7	4
STK11	16	7.2	3
PAK7	17	4.2	4
STK6	18	6.0	3
BRD2	19	3.8	4
RPS6KA2	20	3.7	4

Adapted from Greenman C, Stephens P, Smith R, et al. Patterns of somatic mutation in human cancer genomes. *Nature* 2007;446:153–158, with permission.

The next step, which is still in its infancy, is to relate the patterns of mutation to clinical outcome and treatment. For genes previously known to drive breast cancer when mutated, such as *TP53*, *PIK3CA*, and *PTEN*, the relationship between mutation and outcome for breast cancer has been examined and shown to be significant (18–20). In fact, conditional analysis of the activating mutation of *PIK3CA* (the catalytic subunit of PI3-kinase) or inactivating events of its negative regulator *PTEN*, provided better discrimination of outcome than mutation of either gene alone (Fig. 27.2).

STRUCTURAL ANALYSIS OF THE CANCER GENOME

Metaphase Chromosome Analysis

One of the most methodologically challenging questions in breast carcinomas is to understand the structural organization

of a tumor genome. This is a critical area of research, which can easily be evidenced by the large number of chromosomal fusion events that drive malignancies in the leukemias and lymphomas. Recurrent mutations have become even more interesting since the recent identification of recurrent gene fusion events including *TMPRSS-ERG* in prostate cancer (21).

Analyses of metaphase chromosome spreads from cultures of human tumors using classic banding techniques provided the first views of the extent of structural rearrangements that exist in human breast cancers. The catalogue by Mitelman et al. (22) provides a comprehensive assessment of breast cancer chromosome changes discovered using this approach. The general structural and numerical chaos is clear from these studies, but the approach is difficult because of the difficulty of preparing metaphase spreads of sufficiently high-quality metaphase chromosome preparations to allow identification of rearrangements with confidence.

The introduction of fluorescence *in situ* hybridization (FISH) with whole chromosome probes (23,24) and the subsequent development of combinatorial multicolor labeling and analysis (25–27) substantially simplified the identification interpretation of these complex karyotypic rearrangements. Molecular cytogenetic analyses using whole chromosome analysis techniques are, however, limited in resolution to a few million base pairs by the complex organization of DNA along chromosomes. FISH, with multiple, region-specific probes, enables high resolution mapping of the structures of numerical and structural chromosome abnormalities. However, this approach is not well suited to discovery or high-resolution analysis of complex structural aberrations.

The development of end sequence profiling (ESP) and paired end deep sequencing more generally have revolutionized analysis of structural aberrations in human breast cancers. Genome sequencing methodologies have used the paired end read technology since its proof of principle in sequencing *de novo* genomes (28,29). Pair end reads, where DNA sequence from both ends of a longer piece of DNA (with known sequence length) allow the information of the sequences to be organized in useful ways, primarily to provide larger *clone coverage* of

Table 27.2	PATHWAYS WITH SIGNIFICANT MUTATIONS IN BREAST CANCER		
Pathway	Observed Mutations (N)	Expected Mutations (N)	Significance Score
dsRNA induced gene expression	20	0.3	23.87
Interferon signaling	22	0.5	22.70
ATM signaling	25	0.8	22.37
BRCA1/2	24	1.4	15.68
Apoptosis signaling	20	0.8	16.13
Apoptosis induction	8	1.1	1.76
Fas and TNF	11	1.9	2.13

RNA, double-stranded RNA; TNF, tumor necrosis factor.
Adapted from Lin J, Gan CM, Zhang X, et al. A multidimensional analysis of genes mutated in breast and colorectal cancers. *Genome Res* 2007;17:1304–1318, with permission.

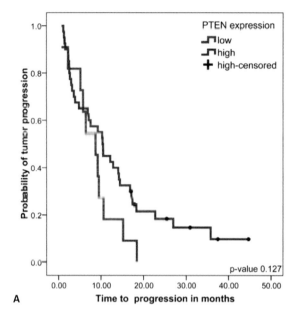

A

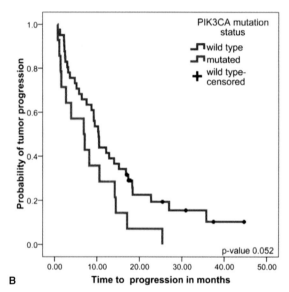

B

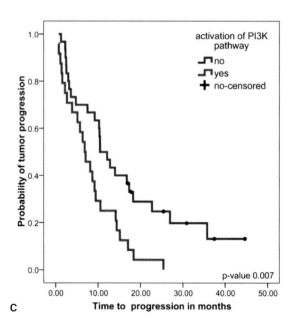

C

the genome or to span intermediary sequences that are common repeat elements (nearly one-half of the human genome). A diagram of paired end read methods is provided in Figure 27.3. Paired end reads have historically been performed on highly size-restricted pieces of DNA (either DNA clones of 1–10 kb), fosmids (of 50 kb), or bacterial artificial chromosome (BAC) of (~150 kb). The longer the insert, the greater the clone coverage. A total of 2,000 BAC each 150 kb in length would provide average one-fold (1X) clone coverage of the entire genome (~3 gigabases) whereas it would require 3 million, 1-kb clones to perform the same. If the goal is to understand which large regions of the genome are hooked together, larger inserts are more effective. As a note, insert lengths above 3 kb are sufficient to bridge most common repetitive sequences.

Initial work in the area of cancer genome structure discovery published in 2003 (30) involved reconstruction of the genomes of cancers by aligning paired end BAC reads against the human genome and searching for cases in which the ends do not map to consistent locations. Those clones that violate genome assembly indicate the presence of a rearrangement in the cancer genome (or an artifact in the BAC DNA library construction). These possibilities can be separated if multiple BACs with different end sequences support the same rearrangement (Fig. 27.3).

New work is ongoing both to identify rearrangement breakpoints and to reconstruct the likely genome of the cancer (31,111). These reconstructions may aid in understanding tumor evolution and disease progression, and may identify new therapeutic targets or interventions. New DNA sequences created in the tumor genome might even be targets for patient-directed personalized therapy if gene fusions create novel proteins or chimeric transcripts that can be targeted with emerging small interfering RNA (siRNA)-based therapeutics (32).

New sequencing technologies have obviated the BAC-based approaches developed in the previous decade. The new methods still perform paired end reads but, compared with conventional Sanger-based sequencing, the costs have dropped more than 1,000 fold, meaning that it is cheaper to sequence 1,000,000 3-kb DNA paired-end fragments than 2,000 BACs. As prices drop further, to the estimated $1,000 genome, evaluating the structures of genomes will become even easier. The first example of this exciting new work from the Sanger Center group in lung cancer (33) has shown what these observations are likely to allow (Fig. 27.4). In just two cell lines, 103 somatic rearrangements were observed, including chromosomal fusions, tandem duplications, and inverted duplications. The deep sequencing approach provides both structural data and very high resolution copy number data, because the number of sequencable reads is proportional to the DNA copy number.

GENOME COPY NUMBER

Comparative genomic hybridization (CGH) is a hybridization-based analysis strategy that maps changes in genome copy number onto a normal representation of the genome. In CGH, DNA from a test tumor is labeled and hybridized to a normal genome representation and the amount of bound, labeled tumor DNA relative to that for a normal genome is measured along the genome representation as an indication of relative

FIGURE 27.2. Mutations affecting breast cancer outcome. Mutations in either of two components of the PI3K pathway are more predictive than outcomes of individual analysis of mutations as assayed by Kaplan-Meier plots. **A:** Disruptions in *PTEN* activity or (**B**) mutations in *PIK3CA* are significantly less strongly associated with poor outcome than (**C**) the unified status of both *PIK3CA* and *PTEN*. (Adapted from Berns K, Horlings HM, Hennessy BT, et al. A functional genetic approach identifies the PI3K pathway as a major determinant of trastuzumab resistance in breast cancer. *Cancer Cell* 2007;12:395–402, with permission.)

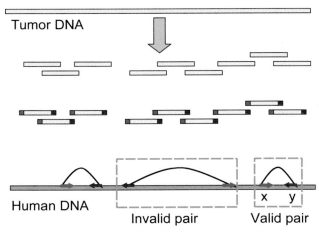

FIGURE 27.3. End sequence profiling (ESP). The principle of ESP is that given a piece of genomic DNA from within a known size distribution, the sequence of the two ends should map to the reference human genome in a particular orientation and within a certain distance. An invalid pair of sequences indicates the potential for a rearrangement. Practically, if more than one pair of sequences indicates the same aberration it has a high probability of being true. (Adapted from Raphael BJ, Volik S, Yu P, et al. A sequence-based survey of the complex structural organization of tumor genomes. *Genome Biol* 2008;9:R59, with permission.)

genome copy number. CGH is particularly informative because it provides a direct link between a genome copy number abnormality and its gene content.

The first CGH analyses mapped changes of recurrent aberrations onto normal metaphase chromosomes (34). This approach, however, was quickly supplanted by array CGH in which the genome representation was replaced by arrays of nucleic acid probes (35,36). Initially these arrays were composed of cloned probes, such as yeast artificial chromosome (YAC), BAC (35), and complementary DNA (cDNA) (37). Eventually, however, it was demonstrated that CGH could be accomplished by hybridization to arrays of synthetic oligonucleotides (38). This enabled use of commercial arrays so that today, commercially available oligonucleotide arrays that carry millions of probes are in common use. Current platforms provide kilobase pair resolution (39). In addition, some platforms have been developed to allow allele-specific discrimination so that the analysis yields allele-specific copy number information. Prominent commercial platforms are listed in Table 27.3.

Individual Tumor Genome Landscapes

One of the remarkable features of breast cancer genomes is the extent of abnormality within individual tumors. Figure 27.5 shows a typical breast cancer CGH profile with copy number abnormalities caused by gains or losses of single copies of portions of the genome, homozygous deletions, and high-level

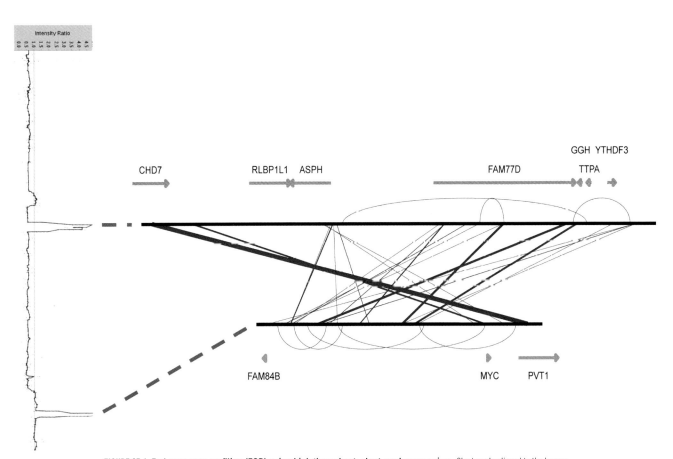

FIGURE 27.4. End sequence profiling (ESP) using high throughput, short read sequencing. Short reads aligned to the human genome estimate copy number and illustrate structural aberrations at the inter- and intra-chromosomal level. A plot of copy number reads that align to chromosome 8 from two regions of chromosome 8 NCI-H2171 are shown is graphed on the left. Intensity ratio corresponds to copy number estimates with two regions that appear at approximately 20 copies. These regions of the genome are shown in linear chromosomal order (x-axis) with the position of known genes drawn and with blue lines showing observed intra-chromosomal fusion events. Numerous events are observed to join various portions of these amplified regions. (Adapted from Campbell PJ, Stephens PJ, Pleasance ED, et al. Identification of somatically acquired rearrangements in cancer using genome-wide massively parallel paired-end sequencing. *Nat Genet* 2008;40:722–729, with permission.)

Table 27.3	COMMONLY USED COMMERCIAL ARRAY CGH PLATFORMS		
Manufacturer		Array Element Size	Allele Specific?
Affymetrix http://www.affymetrix.com		24 mer	Yes
Illumina http://www.illumina.com		50 mer	Yes
Agilent http://www.chem.agilent.com		60 mer	No
Roche Nimblegen http://www.nimblegen.com		Flexible	Possible

CGH, comparative genomic hybridization.

amplification. It is not unusual to find as much as 30% of a breast cancer genome present at abnormal copy number. The extent of the abnormalities may encompass entire chromosomes or as little as a few hundred base pairs. In general, the low-level copy number abnormalities tend to extend over significant parts of the genome, whereas homozygous losses and high-level amplifications involve relatively narrow parts of the genome. These differences in genomic extent of abnormality may reflect the mechanisms by which the abnormalities arise. Low-level copy number gains and losses involving whole chromosomes or chromosome arms may be caused by errors in chromosomal segregation—for example, owing to centrosome dysfunction (40). On the other hand, homozygous deletions and high-level amplifications are evidence of strong and active selection for or against regions of the genome that are particularly important in the pathophysiology of the disease—for example, by bridge-breakage-fusion (41) or through production and amplification of extrachromosomal elements (42).

Another remarkable feature of breast cancer genomes is the extent of variation between tumors. Figure 27.6, for example, shows CGH profiles for two breast tumors with similar clinical characteristics. One genome shows almost no aberrations whereas the other is *shattered* and displays numerous regions of high-level amplification and homozygous deletion. Some of these aberrations—both structural (43) and numerical (39)—are extremely complex. Complex aberrations (39) of closely spaced aberrations have been referred to as "firestorms." In most tumors, the aberrations accumulate during a relatively restricted portion of tumorigenesis and change slowly thereafter. In fact, the CGH profiles of metastatic tumors typically are similar to the profiles of the primary tumors from which they arise—even though the time between primary tumor and metastatic tumor development may be decades (44,45).

Recurrent Aberrations

The ability to map genome copy number abnormalities onto a normal representation of the genome facilitates identification of recurrent aberrations because many tumor profiles can be integrated onto the same representations. Figure 27.7, for example, shows the frequencies of recurrent copy number gains, losses, and amplifications in 145 primary breast tumors measured using BAC array CGH (46) as well as the locations of 9 regions of recurrent high-level amplification involving regions of chromosomes 8, 11, 12, 17, and 20. Numerous CGH studies in the last 5 years support the general locations of recurrent copy number increases involving chromosomes depicted in Figure 27.7 as well as the observation that relatively few parts of the genome are not abnormal in at least 15% of breast tumors (37,39,46–56). Recent studies using high-resolution oligonucleotide array CGH have defined the extents of these regions of recurrent abnormality with subgene resolution and demonstrate the existence of an increasing number of aberrations that involve very small regions of the genome that were missed with lower resolution technologies (39,57,58).

Integrative analyses of gene expression and genome copy number data indicate that expression levels of greater than 10% of the entire genome are deregulated by these recurrent abnormalities in breast cancers (46,53). Interestingly, a recent meta-analysis of 5,918 malignant epithelial tumors showed that the copy number gains involving 1q, 3q, 5p, 7q, 8q, 17q, and 20q, and losses at, 4q, 13q, 17p, and 18q found in breast cancer were also common in many other epithelial neoplasias (59). This suggests that these abnormalities may be generally important in carcinogenesis and it is consistent with the observation that the ensemble of genes deregulated by low-level genome copy number abnormalities preferentially affects genes that may contribute to increased metabolic fitness (46).

Several studies have compared recurrent genome copy number changes between clinicopathologic subtypes. These studies showed significant differences between estrogen receptor-positive (ER+) and ER-negative (ER−) tumors (60), between subtypes defined by transcriptional profiling (e.g., basal, ERBB2, luminal A and luminal B) (46,56) and tumors defined according to histologic features (e.g., ductal vs. lobular) (61). For example, higher numbers of gains or losses are associated with the basal-like, ER− tumor subtype, whereas high-level DNA amplification is more frequent in luminal-B subtype tumors (46,56). Interestingly, aging does not seem to influence the recurrent abnormality content (62).

A growing number of publications in breast cancer and other tumor types suggest that the pattern of recurrent abnormalities is also influenced by the presence of germ-line mutations, polymor-

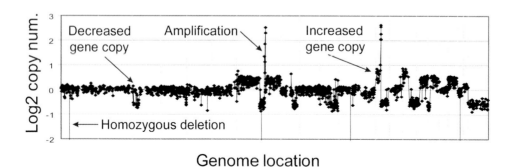

FIGURE 27.5. Genome copy number abnormalities measured using comparative genomic hybridization (CGH). Log 2 relative copy number is displayed along the genome with chromosome 1 to the left and chromosomes 22 and X to the right. *Vertical lines* show the chromosome boundaries. Relative copy number gains show as significant excursions above zero and losses show as significant excursions below zero.

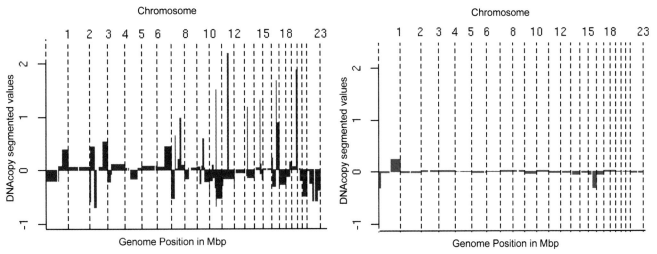

FIGURE 27.6. Comparative genomic hybridization (CGH) profiles measured for two clinically similar breast tumors after analysis using circular binary segmentation (113). Data are displayed as described in Figure 27.5. Relative copy number values for one tumor are displayed in *red* and the other in *blue*.

phisms, or both that influence aspects of the DNA repair machinery. For example, breast tumors in which p53 (52) or *BRCA1* (63,64) are aberrant tend to accumulate more abnormalities than do tumors with normal p53 and *BRCA1* function. Moreover, the pattern of recurrent aberrations is different in tumors that arise in individuals with *BRCA1* mutations than in sporadic tumors (63,64). Studies in mouse models also support the concept that the underlying individual genotype influences the spectrum of aberrations that arise. For example, CGH studies of five mouse models of breast cancer induced by wild-type and mutated forms of oncogenic *ERBB2* or the polyomavirus middle T antigen (PyMT) showed that the pattern of genome copy number abnormalities was strongly influenced by the driving oncogene (65).

 GENOME INSTABILITY AND EVOLUTION

Genome instability in solid tumors is thought to enable accumulation of the spectrum of genomic abnormalities needed for tumor progression (67–68). Tools, such as CGH, demonstrate the result of instability and show that the number of aberrations increases during tumor progression. The cartoon in Figure 27.8, for example, suggests that aberrations measured using CGH in breast cancer tend to increase dramatically during progression to ductal carcinoma *in situ* (DCIS) (69). CGH analyses do not, however, provide a direct measure of instability because they only show aberrations that are present in *most* of the cells in the tumor.

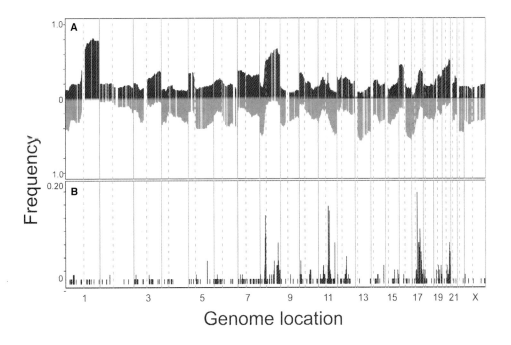

FIGURE 27.7. Recurrent genome copy number aberrations in breast cancer. Panel **A.** Frequencies of recurrent genome copy number changes in 145 breast cancers. Frequencies of copy number gains are plotted as positive values and frequencies of copy number losses are plotted as negative values. Panel **B.** Frequencies of amplification. Data from the same 145 tumors is plotted showing only the positions and frequencies of amplification events in the tumors (note the frequent amplifications at 8, 11, and 17). Data in both panels are plotted as a function of genome location as described in Figure 27.5. (Adapted from 46).

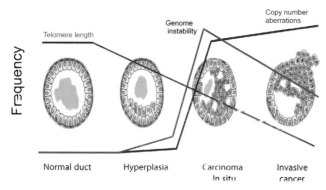

FIGURE 27.8. Schematic diagram of changes in number of genome copy number abnormalities measured using comparative genomic hybridization (CGH) (*blue*), genome instability measured using fluorescence *in situ* hybridization (FISH) (*black*) and relative telomere length (*red*). (Adapted from Chin K, de Solorzano CO, Knowles D, et al. In situ analyses of genome instability in breast cancer. *Nat Genet* 2004;36:984–988, with permission.)

Studies of the rate of instability in breast cancers assessed in thick tissue sections using FISH with chromosome-specific probes (69) showed that variability was low in normal ductal epithelium and usual ductal hyperplasia (UDH) but remarkably high in DCIS. Variability remained high in invasive cancer (IC). DCIS and IC also showed regions of increased overall ploidy. The variations in genome copy number in DCIS and IC were dramatic between adjacent cells, suggesting that the copy number changes were not the result of clonal evolution but rather were the result of continuing high instability. The instability observed in DCIS was similar to that observed in cultures of breast epithelial cells (70) and in epithelial cells in mice lacking protective telomere function (71–73). Quantitative FISH analyses of relative telomere length during breast cancer progression show decreasing telomere length during the period leading up to the time of increased instability, as detected using FISH and the rapid accumulation of chromosome aberrations as measured by CGH (69).

MECHANISMS OF ABERRATION FORMATION

The remarkable genomic complexity and diversity in the genome sequence, structure, and copy number observed in breast cancers raises the question of how these aberrations form. It is likely that several mechanisms are involved.

Telomere Crisis

One important issue to understand is the remarkable increase in genome instability and number of numerical and structural aberrations that occur during transition to DCIS. A likely explanation is that breast cancers begin with hyperplastic growth—likely initiated by epigenomic events (40,74,75)—in cells lacking functional telomerase. This causes progressive telomere loss and culminates in loss of protective telomere function and dramatically increased genome instability. In most cases, this is the end of the story because the dysfunctional cells die. Rarely, however, the genome instability may produce a genomic composition that reactivates telomerase and confers a proliferative advantage; DCIS or IC is the result. The extremely low probability of progressing through telomere crisis and reactivating telomerase would explain why hyperplasia, although it has many of the proliferative hallmarks of cancer, is associated with only modest cancer risk (76). The stochastic nature of passage through telomere crisis may explain, in large part, the remarkable variation in genome composition between individuals.

The modest changes in the spectrum of genome copy number abnormalities observed as breast cancers progress from DCIS to metastatic cancer (77,78) is in seeming contradiction to the continued high rate of instability observed in DCIS and IC. One possible explanation is that most of the genome copy number abnormalities observed in this study leave the cells at a proliferative disadvantage relative to a genomically unstable *tumor initiating* population that maintains the overall genotype during progression. This possibility is supported by analyses of breast cancer cell lines grown *in vitro* and as xenografts in which the average genome copy number profiles for such cultures or tumors measured using CGH evolve very slowly although FISH analyses demonstrate dramatic genome instability (69).

Although the telomere crisis model explains the large variation in genome composition between individual tumors, it does not explain recurrent aberrations. It seems likely that recurrent aberrations are the result of positive and negative selection during the progression process. This is clearly established for strong oncogenes and tumor suppressor genes that are associated with high level amplification (e.g., *ERBB2*, *MYC*, *CCND1*) and homozygous deletions (e.g., *CDKN2A* and *PTEN*). However, it is likely also the case for low level aberrations. Evidence of this is the observation that these aberrations preferentially deregulate genes associated with increased metabolic activity (69).

Of course the selection process also is influenced by the environment and the genotype of the individual in which the cancer arises. For example, breast tumors in which p53 or *BRCA1/2* are mutationally inactivated accumulate more abnormalities than do tumors with wild-type p53 and *BRCA1*. Studies in other tumor types implicate other DNA repair genes as modulators of genome copy number abnormality accumulation. Studies in mouse models also support the concept that the underlying individual genotype influences the spectrum of aberrations that arise. For example, CGH studies of five mouse models of breast cancer induced by wild-type and mutated forms of oncogenic ERBB2 or the PyMT showed distinctive, oncogene-associated patterns of genome copy number abnormality. Likewise, CGH analyses of oncogene-induced mouse pancreatic islet cell carcinomas showed that the individual genetic background strongly influenced genome copy number formation (79).

Microenvironment-related factors, such as expression of matrix metalloproteinases (MMP) in the stromal compartment (80,81), also strongly influence tumorigenesis and the onset of genome instability.

GENOME TARGETED THERAPIES AND MARKERS

Clinical Markers

Several recurrent genome aberrations have been associated with poor outcome. Examples of prognostic markers reported to date for breast cancer include (a) association of the total number of genome copy number aberrations with reduced survival duration (82); (b) gain of 3q as a stronger predictor of recurrence in lymph node-negative invasive cancer (83); (c) simultaneous chromosome 1q gain and 16q loss as a predictor of slow proliferation (84); (d) gain of chromosome 3q, 9p, 11p, and 11q and loss of 17p associated with short-term survival (85); (e) gain of 11q13, 12q24, 17, and 18p associated with metastasis-free survival (82); (f) gain at 8q24 associated with mutational status of p53 and reduced survival duration (52); (g) increased DNA copy number of *RAB25* associated with markedly decreased disease-free survival or overall survival (86); and (h) amplification and overexpression of 66 genes in regions of amplification at 8p11, 8q24, 11q13, 17q21, and 20q13 with reduced survival duration (56) and the presence of aberration hotspots or *fire storms* (39).

Therapeutic Targets

Several recurrently aberrant genes associated with reduced survival duration and other aspects of breast cancer pathophysiology have been suggested as therapeutic targets in breast cancer. Amplified genes implicated as therapeutic targets include *ERBB2* (87), *TOP2A*, (88), *CCND1* and *EMS1* (89), *MYC* (90), *ZNF217* (91), *RAB25* (86), *MDM2* (92), *TBX2* (93), *RPS6KB1*, and the microRNA mir-21 (94). More recently, correlative analyses of gene expression and high-level amplification have identified 66 genes in regions of amplification that are associated with reduced survival duration that are candidate therapeutic targets, 9 of which (*FGFR1, IKBKB, ERBB2, PROCC, ADAM9, FNTA, ACACA, PNMT*, and *NR1D1*) were predicted to be drugable (46). Recurrent mutations or deletions in breast cancers include TP53 (95), *PIK3CA* (96), *PTEN* (97), *BRCA1* (98), and *BRCA2* (99).

Recurrent genomic aberrations in breast cancer are attractive targets because they are events for which strong evidence indicates positive selection so the tumors may be *addicted* to the aberration. In addition, aberrations are not present in normal tissues so that therapies against them are likely to be relatively nontoxic. *ERBB2* is the prototypic genome-based therapeutic target (100,101). This receptor tyrosine kinase is highly amplified in about 30% of human breast cancers and the antibody, trastuzumab (102), and the small molecule inhibitor, lapatinib (103), have proved to be clinically effective against tumors in which *ERBB2* is amplified. One of the advantages of aberration-targeted therapies is that markers can be readily developed to identify tumors carrying the aberration that are most likely to respond to therapy. In the case of *ERBB2*-targeted therapies, FISH with probes to *ERBB2* readily identify tumor to be treated (104). Following this lead, therapies directed against tumors with aberrations involving *TP53* (105), *MDM2* (106), *TOP2A* (107), PI3-kinase mutations (*PTEN* and *PIK3CA*) (108), and *BRCA1* (109) are now being developed or tested. Clearly, the development of aberration-targeted therapy is only beginning.

FUTURE: WHAT DO WE NEED TO KNOW?

Application genome-wide analysis tolls, such as CGH and high throughput sequencing, are revealing the recurrent aberrations that contribute to breast cancer genesis and progression. They also are demonstrating the existence of hundreds of low-frequency aberrations. We also are beginning to understand how these aberrations influence the expression of coding and noncoding transcripts to influence cancer pathophysiology. We do not know, however, how these aberrations cooperate with each other (or substitute for each other) and with epigenomic aberrations to result in the overall cancer phenotype. We do not know how the aberrations arise during progression. And we do not know how the aberrations contribute to the development of drug resistance—especially in metastatic disease.

Progression Map

Recent genome-wide, high resolution breast cancer analyses so far have focused mostly on assessment of aberrations in invasive breast cancers and breast cancer cell lines. This provides a working aberration *parts list* and identifies aberrations that may be useful as prognostic or predictive markers or as therapeutic targets. They have not, however, provided substantial information about how these aberrations arise and evolve during progression. This information will come from longitudinal integrated "omic" analyses of genome aberration appearance during tumor progression. Studies in mouse models can provide some information, but studies of changes during the evolution of individual human tumors will be invaluable. This will require a long-term, sustained effort from the breast cancer research community to collect the necessary samples and continued refinement of large-scale omic analysis technologies so they are capable of analyzing the small amounts of neoplastic tissue that may be available at early stages of evolution.

Drug Resistance

Less than 30% of women with metastatic breast cancer will survive 5 years. This is in contrast to treatment of early disease where outcomes have improved greatly over the last decade. Dozens of next generation therapies are being designed to target these aberrations. The best developed of these in breast cancer are trastuzumab and lapatinib, which target ERBB2-positive tumors. The responses to these agents, even when combined with conventional chemotherapeutic agents, are not, however, durable in patients with metastatic disease and long-term survival is rare. It seems likely that current treatment strategies fail because these strategies do not take into account the genomic and epigenomic aberrations that contribute to resistance in metastatic breast cancer, resistance-related homeostatic, or feedback loops induced by pathway-targeted therapies and factors unique to the metastatic microenvironments in the bone marrow, lung, liver, and brain that contribute to therapeutic resistance. Development of a detailed "omic" understanding of drug-resistant, metastatic cancer will greatly facilitate treatment of this important aspect of the disease. This will require development of clinical trials in which samples of metastatic breast tissue suitable for large-scale omic analysis are acquired before and after development of drug resistance as well as the development of experimental model systems that mirror the aberrations that contribute to resistance.

Model Systems

Development of well-characterized human and murine model systems in which these aberrations function singly and together will be essential to sort out aberration function. Manipulations of gene function in the compendium of mouse breast cancer models being developed by the National Cancer Institute (NCI) Mouse Models of Human Cancer Consortium (http://emice.nci.nih.gov/) and the collections of well-characterized human breast cancer cell lines mirroring the aberrations found in human tumors (110) will facilitate these efforts.

ACKNOWLEDGMENTS

This work was supported by the National Institutes of Health (NIH) (CA58207, CA112970, CA126477), by the Director, Office of Science, Office of Biological and Environmental Research, of the U.S. Department of Energy under Contract No. DE–AC02–05CH11231, and the Avon foundation. The content of this publication does not necessarily reflect the views or policies of the Department of Health and Human Services, nor does the mention of trade names, commercial products, or organization imply endorsement by the U.S. Government.

References

1. Wun LM, Merrill RM, Feuer EJ. Estimating lifetime and age-conditional probabilities of developing cancer. *Lifetime Data Anal* 1998;4:169–186.
2. Foulds L. The experimental study of tumor progression: a review. *Cancer Res* 1954;14:327–339.
3. Nowell PC. The clonal evolution of tumor cell populations. *Science* 1976;194: 23–28.
4. Walsh T, King MC. Ten genes for inherited breast cancer. *Cancer Cell* 2007;11: 103–105.

5. Easton DF, Pooley KA, Dunning AM, et al. Genome-wide association study identifies novel breast cancer susceptibility loci. *Nature* 2007;447:1087–1093.
6. Stephens P, Edkins S, Davies H, et al. A screen of the complete protein kinase gene family identifies diverse patterns of somatic mutations in human breast cancer. *Nat Genet* 2005;37:590–592.
7. Wood LD, Parsons DW, Jones S, et al. The genomic landscapes of human breast and colorectal cancers. *Science* 2007;318:1108–1113.
8. Cancer Genome Atlas Network. Comprehensive genomic characterization defines human glioblastoma genes and core pathways. *Nature* 2008;455:1061–1068.
9. Sanger F, Coulson AR. A rapid method for determining sequences in DNA by primed synthesis with DNA polymerase. *J Mol Biol* 1975;94:441–448.
10. Greenman C, Stephens P, Smith R, et al. Patterns of somatic mutation in human cancer genomes. *Nature* 2007;446:153–158.
11. Katoh M. Cancer genomics and genetics of FGFR2 [Review]. *Int J Oncol* 2008;33:233–237.
12. Ahmed M, Rahman N. ATM and breast cancer susceptibility. *Oncogene* 2006;25:5906–5911.
13. Campeau PM, Foulkes WD, Tischkowitz MD. Hereditary breast cancer: new genetic developments, new therapeutic avenues. *Hum Genet* 2008;124:31–42.
14. Wood LD, Calhoun ES, Silliman N, et al. Somatic mutations of GUCY2F, EPHA3, and NTRK3 in human cancers. *Hum Mutat* 2006;27:1060–1061.
15. Jones AM, Mitter R, Springall R, et al. A comprehensive genetic profile of phyllodes tumours of the breast detects important mutations, intra-tumoral genetic heterogeneity and new genetic changes on recurrence. *J Pathol* 2008;214:533–544.
16. Parsons DW, Jones S, Zhang X, et al. An integrated genomic analysis of human glioblastoma multiforme. *Science* 2008;321:1807–1812.
17. Lin J, Gan CM, Zhang X, et al. A multidimensional analysis of genes mutated in breast and colorectal cancers. *Genome Res* 2007;17:1304–1318.
18. Langerod A, Zhao H, Borgan O, et al. TP53 mutation status and gene expression profiles are powerful prognostic markers of breast cancer. *Breast Cancer Res* 2007;9:R30.
19. Berns K, Horlings HM, Hennessy BT, et al. A functional genetic approach identifies the PI3K pathway as a major determinant of trastuzumab resistance in breast cancer. *Cancer Cell* 2007;12:395–402.
20. Bertheau P, Turpin E, Rickman DS, et al. Exquisite sensitivity of TP53 mutant and basal breast cancers to a dose-dense epirubicin-cyclophosphamide regimen. *PLoS Med* 2007;4:e90.
21. Mehra R, Tomlins SA, Shen R, et al. Comprehensive assessment of TMPRSS2 and ETS family gene aberrations in clinically localized prostate cancer. *Mod Pathol* 2007;20:538–544.
22. Mitelman F, Johansson B, Mertens F. *Mitelman database of chromosome aberrations in cancer.* 2002. http://CGAP.NCI.NIH.GOV/Chromosomes/Mitelman.
23. Pinkel D, Landegent J, Collins C, et al. Fluorescence in situ hybridization with human chromosome-specific libraries: detection of trisomy 21 and translocations of chromosome 4. *Proc Natl Acad Sci U S A* 1988;85:9138–9142.
24. Lichter P, Cremer T, Tang CJ, et al. Rapid detection of human chromosome 21 aberrations by *in situ* hybridization. *Proc Natl Acad Sci U S A* 1988;85:9664–9668.
25. Speicher MR, Gwyn Ballard S, Ward DC. Karyotyping human chromosomes by combinatorial multi-fluor FISH. *Nat Genet* 1996;12:368–375.
26. Liyanage M, Coleman A, du Manoir S, et al. Multicolour spectral karyotyping of mouse chromosomes. *Nat Genet* 1996;14(3):312–315.
27. Schrock E, du Manoir S, Veldman T, et al. Multicolor spectral karyotyping of human chromosomes. *Science* 1996;273:494–497.
28. Fleischmann RD, Adams MD, White O, et al. Whole-genome random sequencing and assembly of Haemophilus influenzae Rd. *Science* 1995;269:496–512.
29. Myers EW, Sutton GG, Delcher AL, et al. A whole-genome assembly of Drosophila. *Science* 2000;287:2196–2204.
30. Volik S, Zhao S, Chin K, et al. End-sequence profiling: sequence-based analysis of aberrant genomes. *Proc Natl Acad Sci U S A* 2003;100:7696–7701.
31. Bashir A, Volik S, Collins C, et al. Evaluation of paired-end sequencing strategies for detection of genome rearrangements in cancer. *PLoS Comput Biol* 2008;4:e1000051.
32. Shen Y. Advances in the development of siRNA-based therapeutics for cancer. *IDrugs* 2008;11:572–578.
33. Campbell PJ, Stephens PJ, Pleasance ED, et al. Identification of somatically acquired rearrangements in cancer using genome-wide massively parallel paired-end sequencing. *Nat Genet* 2008;40:722–729.
34. Kallioniemi A, Kallioniemi OP, Sudar D, et al. Comparative genomic hybridization for molecular cytogenetic analysis of solid tumors. *Science* 1992;258:818–821.
35. Pinkel D, Seagraves R, Sudar D, et al. High resolution analysis of DNA copy number variation using comparative genomic hybridization to microarrays. *Nat Genet* 1998;20:207–211.
36. Solinas-Toldo S, Lampel S, Stilgenbauer S, et al. Matrix-based comparative genomic hybridization: biochips to screen for genomic imbalances. *Genes Chromosomes Cancer* 1997;20:399–407.
37. Pollack JR, Perou CM, Alizadeh AA, et al. Genome-wide analysis of DNA copy-number changes using cDNA microarrays. *Nat Genet* 1999;23:41–46.
38. Lucito R, Healy J, Alexander J, et al. Representational oligonucleotide microarray analysis: a high-resolution method to detect genome copy number variation. *Genome Res* 2003;13:2291–2305.
39. Hicks J, Krasnitz A, Lakshmi B, et al. Novel patterns of genome rearrangement and their association with survival in breast cancer. *Genome Res* 2006;16:1465–1479.
40. Berman H, Zhang J, Crawford YG, et al. Genetic and epigenetic changes in mammary epithelial cells identify a subpopulation of cells involved in early carcinogenesis. *Cold Spring Harb Symp Quant Biol* 2005;70:317–327.
41. McClintock B. The production of homozygous deficient tissues with mutant characteristics by means of the aberrant mitotic behavior of ring-shaped chromosomes. *Genetics* 1938;23:315–376.
42. Kanda T and Wahl G. The dynamics of acentric chromosomes in cancer cells revealed by GFP-based chromosome labeling strategies. *J Cell Biochem Suppl* 2000;35:107–114.
43. Volik S, Raphael BJ, Huang G, et al. Decoding the fine-scale structure of a breast cancer genome and transcriptome. *Genome Res* 2006;16:394–404.
44. Kuukasjarvi T, Karhu R, Tanner M, et al. Genetic heterogeneity and clonal evolution underlying development of asynchronous metastasis in human breast cancer. *Cancer Res* 1997;57:1597–1604.
45. Nishizaki T, DeVries S, Chew K, et al. Genetic alterations in primary breast cancers and their metastases: direct comparison using modified comparative genomic hybridization. *Genes Chromosomes Cancer* 1997;19:267–272.
46. Chin K, DeVries S, Fridlyand J, et al. Genomic and transcriptional aberrations linked to breast cancer pathophysiologies. *Cancer Cell* 2006;10:529–541.
47. Adelaide J, Finetti P, Bekhouche I, et al. Integrated profiling of basal and luminal breast cancers. *Cancer Res* 2007;67:11565–11575.
48. Hermsen MA, Baak JP, Meijer GA, et al. Genetic analysis of 53 lymph node-negative breast carcinomas by CGH and relation to clinical, pathological, morphometric, and DNA cytometric prognostic factors. *J Pathol* 1998;186:356–362.
49. Tirkkonen M, Tanner M, Karhu R, et al. Molecular cytogenetics of primary breast cancer by CGH. *Genes Chromosomes Cancer* 1998;21:177–184.
50. Moore E, Magee H, Coyne J, et al. Widespread chromosomal abnormalities in high-grade ductal carcinoma *in situ* of the breast. Comparative genomic hybridization study of pure high-grade DCIS. *J Pathol* 1999;187:403–409.
51. Richard F, Pacyna-Gengelbach M, Schluns K, et al. Patterns of chromosomal imbalances in invasive breast cancer. *Int J Cancer* 2000;89:305–310.
52. Jain AN, Chin K, Borresen-Dale AL, et al. Quantitative analysis of chromosomal CGH in human breast tumors associates copy number abnormalities with p53 status and patient survival. *Proc Natl Acad Sci U S A* 2001;98:7952–7957.
53. Pollack JR, Sorlie T, Perou CM, et al. Microarray analysis reveals a major direct role of DNA copy number alteration in the transcriptional program of human breast tumors. *Proc Natl Acad Sci U S A* 2002;99:12963–12968.
54. Naylor TL, Greshock J, Wang Y, et al. High resolution genomic analysis of sporadic breast cancer using array-based comparative genomic hybridization. *Breast Cancer Res* 2005;7:R1186–R1198.
55. Fridlyand J, Snijders AM, Ylstra B, et al. Breast tumor copy number aberration phenotypes and genomic instability. *BMC Cancer* 2006;in press.
56. Bergamaschi A, Kim YH, Wang P, et al. Distinct patterns of DNA copy number alteration are associated with different clinicopathological features and gene-expression subtypes of breast cancer. *Genes Chromosomes Cancer* 2006;45:1033–1040.
57. Staaf J, Lindgren D, Vallon-Christersson J, et al. Segmentation-based detection of allelic imbalance and loss-of-heterozygosity in cancer cells using whole genome SNP arrays. *Genome Biol* 2008;9:R136.
58. Komatsu A, Nagasaki K, Fujimori M, et al. Identification of novel deletion polymorphisms in breast cancer. *Int J Oncol* 2008;33:261–270.
59. Baudis M. Genomic imbalances in 5,918 malignant epithelial tumors: an explorative meta-analysis of chromosomal CGH data. *BMC Cancer* 2007;7:226.
60. Loo LW, Grove DI, Williams EM, et al. Array comparative genomic hybridization analysis of genomic alterations in breast cancer subtypes. *Cancer Res* 2004;64:8541–8549.
61. Nishizaki T, Chew K, Chu L, et al. Genetic alterations in lobular breast cancer by comparative genomic hybridization. *Int J Cancer* 1997;74:513–517.
62. Yau C, Fedele V, Roydasgupta R, et al. Aging impacts transcriptomes but not genomes of hormone-dependent breast cancers. *Breast Cancer Res* 2007;9:R59.
63. Wessels LF, van Welsem T, Hart AA, et al. Molecular classification of breast carcinomas by comparative genomic hybridization: a specific somatic genetic profile for BRCA1 tumors. *Cancer Res* 2002;62:7110–7117.
64. van Beers EH, van Welsem T, Wessels LF, et al. Comparative genomic hybridization profiles in human *BRCA1* and *BRCA2* breast tumors highlight differential sets of genomic aberrations. *Cancer Res* 2005;65:822–827.
65. Hodgson JG, Malek T, Bornstein S, et al. Copy number aberrations in mouse breast tumors reveal loci and genes important in tumorigenic receptor tyrosine kinase signaling. *Cancer Res* 2005;65:9695–9704.
66. Lengauer C, Kinzler KW, Vogelstein B. Genetic instabilities in human cancers. *Nature* 1998;396:643–649.
67. Loeb KR, Loeb LA. Significance of multiple mutations in cancer. *Carcinogenesis* 2000;21:379–385.
68. Myung K, Chen C, Kolodner RD. Multiple pathways cooperate in the suppression of genome instability in Saccharomyces cerevisiae. *Nature* 2001;411:1073–1076.
69. Chin K, de Solorzano CO, Knowles D, et al. *In situ* analyses of genome instability in breast cancer. *Nat Genet* 2004;36:984–988.
70. Romanov S, Kozakliewicz B, Holst C, et al. Normal human mammary epithelial cells spontaneously escape senescence and acquire genomic changes. *Nature* 2001;409:633–637.
71. Artandi SE, Chang S, Lee SL, et al. Telomere dysfunction promotes non-reciprocal translocations and epithelial cancers in mice. *Nature* 2000;406:641–645.
72. Artandi SE, DePinho RA. A critical role for telomeres in suppressing and facilitating carcinogenesis. *Curr Opin Genet Dev* 2000;10:39–46.
73. Chang S, Khoo C, DePinho RA. Modeling chromosomal instability and epithelial carcinogenesis in the telomerase-deficient mouse. *Semin Cancer Biol* 2001;11:227–239.
74. Bean GR, Bryson AD, Pilie PG, et al. Morphologically normal-appearing mammary epithelial cells obtained from high-risk women exhibit methylation silencing of INK4a/ARF. *Clin Cancer Res* 2007;13:6834–6841.
75. Crawford YG, Gauthier ML, Joubel A, et al. Histologically normal human mammary epithelia with silenced p16(INK4a) overexpress COX-2, promoting a premalignant program. *Cancer Cell* 2004;5:263–273.
76. Dupont WD, Page DL. Risk factors for breast cancer in women with proliferative breast disease. *N Engl J Med* 1985;312:146–151.
77. Kuukasjarvi T, Tanner M, Pennanen S, et al. Genetic changes in intraductal breast cancer detected by comparative genomic hybridization. *Am J Pathol* 1997;150:1465–1471.
78. Waldman FM, DeVries S, Chew KL, et al. Chromosomal alterations in ductal carcinomas *in situ* and their in situ recurrences. *J Natl Cancer Inst* 2000;92:313–320.
79. Hager JH, Hodgson JG, Fridlyand J, et al. Oncogene expression and genetic background influence the frequency of DNA copy number abnormalities in mouse pancreatic islet cell carcinomas. *Cancer Res* 2004;64:2406–2410.
80. Sternlicht MD, Lochter A, Sympson CJ, et al. The stromal proteinase MMP3/stromelysin-1 promotes mammary carcinogenesis. *Cell* 1999;98:137–146.
81. Rizki A, Weaver VM, Lee SY, et al. A human breast cell model of preinvasive to invasive transition. *Cancer Res* 2008;68:1378–1387.
82. Aubele M, Auer G, Braselmann H, et al. Chromosomal imbalances are associated with metastasis-free survival in breast cancer patients. *Anal Cell Pathol* 2002;24:77–87.

83. Janssen EA, Baak JP, Guervos MA, et al. In lymph node-negative invasive breast carcinomas, specific chromosomal aberrations are strongly associated with high mitotic activity and predict outcome more accurately than grade, tumour diameter, and oestrogen receptor. *J Pathol* 2003;201:555–561.

84. Farabegoli F, Hermsen MA, Ceccarelli C, et al. Simultaneous chromosome 1q gain and 16q loss is associated with steroid receptor presence and low proliferation in breast carcinoma. *Mod Pathol* 2004;17:449–455.

85. Blegen H, Will JS, Ghadimi BM, et al. DNA amplifications and aneuploidy, high proliferative activity and impaired cell cycle control characterize breast carcinomas with poor prognosis. *Anal Cell Pathol* 2003;25:103–114.

86. Cheng KW, Lahad JP, Kuo WL, et al. The RAB25 small GTPase determines aggressiveness of ovarian and breast cancers. *Nat Med* 2004;10:1251–1256.

87. Slamon D, Clark G, Wong S, et al. Human breast cancer: Correlation of relapse and survival with amplification of the *HER-2/neu* oncogene. *Science* 1987;235: 177–182.

88. Al-Kuraya K, Novotny H, Bavi P, et al. HER2, TOP2A, CCND1, EGFR and C-MYC oncogene amplification in colorectal cancer. *J Clin Pathol* 2007;60:768–772.

89. Fantl V, Smith R, Brookes S, et al. Chromosome 11q13 abnormalities in human breast cancer. *Cancer Surv* 1993;18:77–94.

90. Escot C, Theillet C, Lidereau R, et al. Genetic alteration of the c-myc protooncogene (MYC) in human primary breast carcinomas. *Proc Natl Acad Sci U S A* 1986;83:4834–4838.

91. Collins C, Rommens JM, Kowbel D, et al. Positional cloning of ZNF217 and NABC1: genes amplified at 20q13.2 and overexpressed in breast carcinoma. *Proc Natl Acad Sci U S A* 1998;95:8703–8708.

92. Courjal F, Cuny M, Rodriguez C, et al. DNA amplifications at 20q13 and MDM2 define distinct subsets of evolved breast and ovarian tumours. *Br J Cancer* 1996; 74:1984–1989.

93. Sinclair CS, Adem C, Naderi A, et al. TBX2 is preferentially amplified in *BRCA1*- and *BRCA2*-related breast tumors. *Cancer Res* 2002;62:3587–3591.

94. Haverty PM, Fridlyand J, Li L, et al. High-resolution genomic and expression analyses of copy number alterations in breast tumors. *Genes Chromosomes Cancer* 2008;47:530–542.

95. Tennis M, Krishnan S, Bonner M, et al. p53 Mutation analysis in breast tumors by a DNA microarray method. *Cancer Epidemiol Biomarkers Prev* 2006;15:80–85.

96. Samuels Y, Wang Z, Bardelli A, et al. High frequency of mutations of the *PIK3CA* gene in human cancers. *Science* 2004;304:554.

97. Li J, Yen C, Liaw D, et al. PTEN, a putative protein tyrosine phosphatase gene mutated in human brain, breast, and prostate cancer. *Science* 1997;275: 1943–1947.

98. Futreal PA, Liu Q, Shattuck-Eidens D, et al. *BRCA1* mutations in primary breast and ovarian carcinomas. *Science* 1994;266:120–122.

99. Wooster R, Bignell G, Lancaster J, et al. Identification of the breast cancer susceptibility gene *BRCA2. Nature* 1995;378:789–792.

100. Ross JS, Fletcher JA. The *HER-2/neu* oncogene in breast cancer: prognostic fFactor, predictive factor, and target for therapy. *Oncologist* 1998;3:237–252.

101. Slamon D, Pegram M. Rationale for trastuzumab (Herceptin) in adjuvant breast cancer trials. *Semin Oncol* 2001;28:13–19.

102. Vogel CL, Cobleigh MA, Tripathy D, et al. First-line Herceptin monotherapy in metastatic breast cancer. *Oncology* 2001;61:37–42.

103. Moy B, Goss PE. Lapatinib: current status and future directions in breast cancer. *Oncologist* 2006;11:1047–1057.

104. Kallioniemi OP, Kallioniemi A, Kurisu W, et al. *ERBB2* amplification in breast cancer analyzed by fluorescence *in situ* hybridization. *Proc Natl Acad Sci U S A* 1992;89:5321–5325.

105. Heise C, Sampson-Johannes A, Williams A, et al. ONYX-015, an E1B gene-attenuated adenovirus, causes tumor-specific cytolysis and antitumoral efficacy that can be augmented by standard chemotherapeutic agents. *Nat Med* 1997;3: 639–645.

106. Wang H, Nan L, Yu D, et al. Antisense anti-MDM2 oligonucleotides as a novel therapeutic approach to human breast cancer: in vitro and in vivo activities and mechanisms. *Clin Cancer Res* 2001;7:3613–3624.

107. Burgess DJ, Doles J, Zender L, et al. Topoisomerase levels determine chemotherapy response *in vitro* and *in vivo. Proc Natl Acad Sci U S A* 2008;105:9053–9058.

108. Hennessy BT, Smith DL, Ram PT, et al. Exploiting the PI3K/AKT pathway for cancer drug discovery. *Nat Rev Drug Discov* 2005;4:988–1004.

109. Rottenberg S, Jaspers JE, Kersbergen A, et al. High sensitivity of BRCA1-deficient mammary tumors to the PARP inhibitor AZD2281 alone and in combination with platinum drugs. *Proc Natl Acad Sci U S A* 2008;105:17079–17084.

110. Neve RM, Chin K, Fridlyand J, et al. A collection of breast cancer cell lines for the study of functionally distinct cancer subtypes. *Cancer Cell* 2006;10:515–527.

111. Raphael BJ, Volik S, Yu P, et al. A sequence-based survey of the complex structural organization of tumor genomes. *Genome Biol* 2008;9:R59.

Chapter 28
Pathology of Invasive Breast Cancer

Deborah A. Dillon, Anthony J. Guidi, and Stuart J. Schnitt

Invasive breast cancers constitute a heterogeneous group of lesions that differ with regard to their clinical presentation, radiographic characteristics, pathologic features, and biological potential. The most widely used classification of invasive breast cancers, and that used in this chapter (with minor modifications), is that of the World Health Organization (1). This classification scheme is based on the growth pattern and cytologic features of the invasive tumor cells and does not imply histogenesis or site of origin within the mammary duct system. For example, although the classification system recognizes invasive carcinomas designated *ductal* and *lobular*, this is not meant to indicate that the former originates in extralobular ducts and the latter in lobules. In fact, subgross whole organ sectioning has demonstrated that most invasive breast cancers arise in the terminal duct lobular unit, regardless of histologic type (2).

The most common histologic type of invasive breast cancer by far is invasive (infiltrating) ductal carcinoma (3–5). In fact, the diagnosis of invasive ductal carcinoma is a diagnosis by default, because this tumor type is defined as a type of cancer not classified into any of the other categories of invasive mammary carcinoma (1). To further emphasize this point, and to distinguish these tumors from invasive breast cancers with specific or special histologic features (e.g., invasive lobular, tubular, mucinous, medullary, and other rare types), some authorities prefer the term *infiltrating ductal carcinoma*, not otherwise specified (NOS) (3), infiltrating carcinoma of no special type (NST) (5), or invasive ductal carcinomas, NOS (1) . In this chapter, the terms invasive ductal carcinoma, infiltrating ductal carcinoma, and infiltrating or invasive carcinoma of no special type are used interchangeably.

The distribution of histologic types of invasive breast cancer has varied among published series (Table 28.1). These differences may be related to a number of factors, including the nature of the patient population and variability in the confines of definition for the different histologic types. In general, special type cancers comprise approximately 20% to 30% of invasive carcinomas, and at least 90% of a tumor should demonstrate the defining histologic characteristics of a special type cancer to be designated as that histologic type (5,6).

The widespread use of screening mammography has had a dramatic impact on the nature of invasive breast cancers encountered in clinical practice (7–11). The value of mammography in detecting more cases of ductal carcinoma *in situ* (DCIS), smaller invasive breast cancers, and fewer cancers with axillary lymph node involvement is well recognized. Mammography, however, has also resulted in a change in the distribution of the histologic features of the invasive breast cancers detected. In particular, special type cancers (particularly tubular carcinomas) (12–16) and cancers of lower histologic grade (17–20) have been more frequently observed in mammographically screened populations than in patients who present with a palpable mass, particularly in the prevalent round of screening (21,22).

Most invasive breast cancers have an associated component of *in situ* carcinoma, although the extent of the *in situ* component varies considerably (23). The prevailing view has long been that the invasive carcinomas derive from the *in situ* component. This is based not only on the frequent coexistence of the two lesions, but on the histologic similarities between the invasive and *in situ* components within the same lesion. For example, a number of studies have clearly documented that low-grade invasive cancers are most often associated with low-grade DCIS, and high-grade invasive cancers with high-grade

in situ lesions (24–26). In addition, studies evaluating profiles of biological markers and genetic abnormalities have shown that coexisting invasive and *in situ* carcinomas often share the same immunophenotype and genetic alterations (27–31). Recent gene expression profiling studies have confirmed this observation (32,33).

The routine pathologic examination of invasive breast cancers has now extended beyond simply determining and reporting the histologic type of the tumor. Although histologic typing provides important prognostic information in and of itself (34), other morphologic features that are evaluable on routine histologic sections are also of prognostic value. In this chapter, the various histologic types of invasive breast cancer will be discussed as will pathologic features important in the assessment of prognosis (prognostic factors) and response to therapy (predictive factors).

INVASIVE (INFILTRATING) DUCTAL CARCINOMA

As noted above, invasive ductal carcinomas represent the single largest group of invasive breast cancers. Although these tumors are most commonly encountered in pure form, a substantial minority exhibit admixed foci of other histologic types. In one series of 1,000 invasive breast cancers, such combinations of invasive ductal carcinoma and other types were seen in 28% of cases (3). The classification of tumors composed primarily of invasive ductal carcinoma with a minor component consisting of one or more other histological types is problematic. Some authorities categorize such lesions as invasive ductal carcinomas (or invasive carcinomas of no special type) and simply note the presence of the other types (5), whereas others classify them as "mixed" (6).

Clinical Presentation

Invasive ductal carcinomas most often present as a palpable mass, mammographic abnormality, or both. No clinical or mammographic characteristics distinguish invasive ductal carcinomas from other histologic types of invasive cancer. Rarely, these lesions present with Paget disease of the nipple.

Gross Pathology

The classic macroscopic appearance of invasive ductal carcinoma is that of a scirrhous carcinoma, characterized by a firm, sometimes rock-hard mass which on cut section has a gray-white gritty surface (Fig. 28.1). This consistency and appearance is owing to the desmoplastic tumor stroma and not the neoplastic cells themselves. Some invasive ductal carcinomas are composed primarily of tumor cells with little desmoplastic stromal reaction, and such lesions are grossly tan and soft. Although most invasive ductal cancers have a stellate or spiculated contour with irregular peripheral margins, some lesions have rounded, pushing margins, and still others are grossly well-circumscribed.

Histopathology

The microscopic appearance of invasive ductal carcinomas is highly heterogeneous with regard to growth pattern, cytologic

Table 28.1	HISTOLOGIC TYPES OF INVASIVE BREAST CANCER IN FOUR LARGE SERIES BEFORE THE WIDESPREAD USE OF MAMMOGRAPHIC SCREENING								
		Histologic Type (%)							
Study	No. of Cancers	Ductal[a]	Lobular	Medullary	Mucinous	Tubular	Tubular Mixed	Mixed	Other
Fisher et al.[3]	1,000	53	5	6	2	1	—	32	—
Rosen[4]	857	75	10	9	2	2	—	—	—
Ellis et al.[6]	1,547	49	16	3	1	2	14	14	2
Edinburgh[5]	Not stated	70	10	5	2	3	—	2	8

[a]In some series, designated "not otherwise specified" (NOS) or "no special type" (NST).

features, mitotic activity, stromal desmoplasia, extent of the associated DCIS component, and contour. Variability in histologic features may even be seen within a single case. The tumor cells can be arranged as glandular structures, as nests, cords, or trabeculae of various sizes, or as solid sheets. Foci of necrosis are evident in some cases and may be extensive. Cytologically, the tumor cells range from those that show little deviation from normal breast epithelial cells to those exhibiting marked cellular pleomorphism and nuclear atypia. Mitotic activity can range from imperceptible to marked. Stromal desmoplasia is inapparent to minimal in some cases. At the other end of the spectrum, some tumors show such prominent stromal desmoplasia that the tumor cells constitute only a minor component of the lesion. Similarly, some invasive ductal carcinomas have no identifiable component of DCIS, whereas in others, the *in situ* carcinoma is the predominant component of the tumor. Finally, the microscopic margins of these cancers can be infiltrating, pushing, circumscribed, or mixed.

Recognizing that invasive ductal carcinomas are a histologically diverse group of lesions, many investigators have attempted to stratify them based on certain microscopic features. The most common method to subclassify invasive ductal carcinomas is grading, which may be based solely on nuclear features (nuclear grading) or on a combination of architectural and nuclear characteristics (histologic grading). In nuclear grading, the appearance of the tumor cell nuclei is compared with those of normal breast epithelial cells. The nuclear grading system most commonly employed is that of Black et al. (35,36). In this system, nuclei are classified as well differentiated, intermediately differentiated, and poorly differentiated. It is unfortunate that the numerical designation used for these

three grades is the opposite of that used for histologic grading (i.e., well-differentiated nuclei are considered grade 3 and poorly differentiated nuclei grade 1). In current practice, however, histologic grading is the method of grading most often used. In histologic grading, breast carcinomas are categorized based on the evaluation of three features: tubule formation, nuclear pleomorphism, and mitotic activity. The histologic grading system currently in most widespread use is that of Elston and Ellis (37). This system is a modification of the grading system proposed by Bloom and Richardson in 1957, but provides strictly defined criteria that are lacking in the original description. Tubule formation, nuclear pleomorphism, and mitotic activity are each scored on a 1-3 scale. The sum of the scores for these three parameters provides the overall histologic grade, such that tumors in which the sum of the scores is 3 to 5 are designated grade 1 (well-differentiated), those with score sums of 6 and 7 are designated grade 2 (moderately differentiated), and those with score sums of 8 and 9 are designated grade 3 (poorly differentiated) (Fig. 28.2; Table 28.2). The prognostic significance of histologic grading is discussed below (see section on Prognostic Factors).

The expression of biologic markers, such as estrogen and progesterone receptors, growth factors, oncogene and tumor suppressor gene products, and other markers is highly variable in invasive ductal carcinomas, which might be anticipated from their histologic heterogeneity.

Clinical Course and Prognosis

Although invasive ductal carcinomas have the poorest prognosis of all invasive breast cancers, even within this group prognostically favorable subsets can be identified, as discussed below.

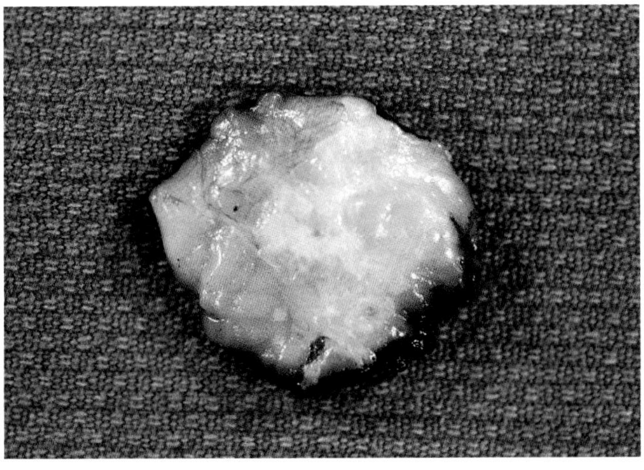

INVASIVE (INFILTRATING) LOBULAR CARCINOMA

Invasive lobular carcinomas constitute the second most frequent type of invasive breast cancer. In most series, these tumors account for approximately 5% to 10% of invasive breast carcinomas (3–5,38,39). The reported incidence of this tumor type has ranged, however, from under 1% to as high as 20% (34). Some of this difference may be related to differences in patient populations. Much of this variability appears, however, to be related to differences in diagnostic criteria. In particular, since the "classic" form of invasive lobular carcinoma was first described by Foote and Foote (40), a variety of authors have described invasive breast cancers that they consider variants of invasive lobular carcinoma (39,41–51), thereby expanding the spectrum of this histologic type and accounting for a higher incidence of invasive lobular carcinoma in more recent series than in the past. In addition, recent studies have suggested that

FIGURE 28.1. Cut surface of an excision specimen containing an invasive ductal carcinoma. The tumor appears as an irregular area of whitish tissue.

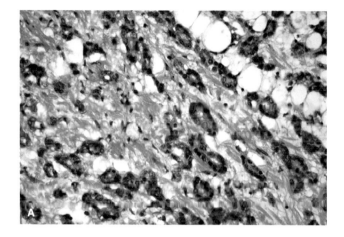
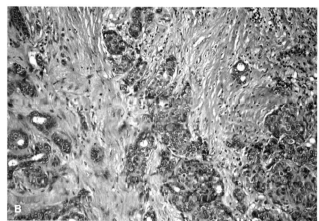
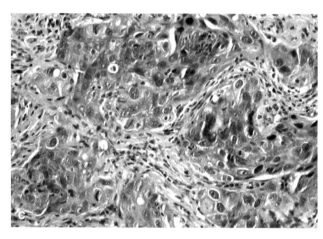

FIGURE 28.2. Invasive ductal carcinoma. A: Histologic grade 1. **B:** Histologic grade 2. **C:** Histologic grade 3.

the increase in the frequency of invasive lobular carcinoma may be partly related to the use of postmenopausal hormone replacement therapy (52–55).

Invasive lobular carcinomas are characterized by multifocality in the ipsilateral breast and appear to be more often bilateral than other types of invasive breast cancer, although the reported range of bilaterality has been broad (6% to 47%) (3,38,56–61). In two clinical follow-up studies of patients with

invasive lobular carcinoma, however, the incidence of subsequent contralateral breast cancer among patients with invasive lobular carcinoma was similar to that of patients with invasive ductal carcinoma (62,63).

Lobular carcinoma *in situ* (LCIS) co-exists with invasive lobular carcinoma in most cases (38,39,44,46,64–66). Overall, approximately 70% to 80% of cases of invasive lobular carcinoma contain foci of LCIS (67).

Table 28.2	HISTOLOGIC GRADING SYSTEM FOR INVASIVE BREAST CANCERS (ELSTON AND ELLIS MODIFICATION OF BLOOM AND RICHARDSON GRADING SYSTEM)

Components of Grade	Score
Tubules	
>75% of tumor composed of tubules	1 point
10–75% of tumor composed of tubules	2 points
<10% of tumor composed of tubules	3 points
Nuclear grade	
Nuclei small and uniform	1 point
Moderate variation in nuclear size and shape	2 points
Marked nuclear pleomorphism	3 points
Mitotic rate	
Dependent on microscope field area	1–3 points
Histologic Grade	**Total points**
1 (well differentiated)	3–5
2 (moderately differentiated)	6–7
3 (poorly differentiated)	8–9

Adapted from Black MM, Speer FD. Nuclear structure in cancer tissues. *Surg Gynecol Obstet* 1957;105:97.

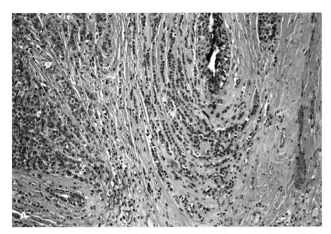
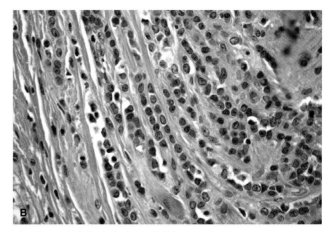

FIGURE 28.3. Invasive lobular carcinoma, classic type. **A:** Linear strands of tumor cells infiltrate the stroma. **B:** Higher power view to demonstrate cytologic detail. The tumor cells have small, relatively uniform nuclei.

Clinical Presentation

Invasive lobular carcinoma may present as a palpable mass or a mammographic abnormality with characteristics similar to those of invasive ductal carcinomas (i.e., discrete, firm mass on palpation; spiculated mass on mammogram). However, both the findings on physical examination and the mammographic appearance of invasive lobular carcinomas may be quite subtle. On physical examination, only a vague area of thickening or induration may be noted, without definable margins. Mammographic findings may be equally subtle, with many invasive lobular carcinomas appearing as poorly defined areas of asymmetric density with architectural distortion, and others revealing no mammographic abnormalities, even in the presence of a palpable mass (68–73). In fact, the extent of the tumor may be substantially underestimated by both physical examination and mammography.

Gross Pathology

Some invasive lobular carcinomas appear as firm, gritty, gray-white masses, indistinguishable from invasive ductal carcinomas. In other cases, however, no mass is grossly evident and the breast tissue may have only a rubbery consistency. In still other cases, no abnormality is evident on visual inspection or on palpation of the involved breast tissue and the presence of carcinoma is revealed only on microscopic examination.

Histopathology

Invasive lobular carcinomas as a group show distinctive cytologic features and patterns of tumor cell infiltration of the stroma. The *classic form* is characterized by small, relatively uniform neoplastic cells that invade the stroma singly and in a single-file pattern that results in the formation of linear strands (Fig. 28.3) (38–40,46,47,74). These cells frequently encircle mammary ducts in a targetoid manner. Furthermore, the tumor cells may infiltrate the breast stroma and adipose tissue in an insidious fashion, invoking little or no desmoplastic stromal reaction. This feature accounts for the difficulty in detecting some invasive lobular carcinomas on physical examination, mammography, and gross pathologic examination. The nuclei of the neoplastic cells are usually small, show little variation in size, and are often eccentric. Mitotic figures are infrequent. The cells may contain intracytoplasmic lumina which, in some, may be sufficiently large to

impart a signet ring cell appearance. In the classic form of invasive lobular carcinoma, cells with a signet ring configuration comprise only a small proportion of the tumor cell population. Many examples of invasive lobular carcinoma (as well as LCIS) are characterized histologically by tumor cells that are loosely cohesive. This phenotype is likely related to the fact that *in situ* and invasive lobular carcinomas typically show loss of expression of the adhesion molecule E-cadherin (75–78), owing in many cases to mutations in the gene encoding this protein (78,79) or to loss of heterozygosity on chromosome 16q22.1, the region of the E-cadherin gene (80). This feature distinguishes lobular carcinomas from ductal-type carcinomas which characteristically exhibit E-cadherin protein expression, albeit to a variable degree (75–77).

Variant forms of invasive lobular carcinoma differ from the classic form with regard to architectural or cytologic features. In the solid and alveolar variants, the cells comprising the lesion have features characteristic of the classic form of invasive lobular carcinoma, but differ from it with regard to the growth pattern of the tumor cells (39,41,43,44,47,81). In the *solid form*, the neoplastic cells grow in large confluent sheets with little intervening stroma (Fig. 28.4) (39,41,46,47,66). The *alveolar form* is characterized by tumor cells that grow in groups of 20 or more cells. These cellular aggregates are separated from one another by a delicate fibrovascular stroma

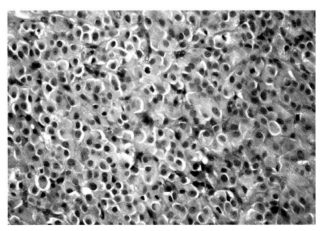

FIGURE 28.4. Invasive lobular carcinoma, solid type. The tumor cells grow in a confluent sheet with little intervening stroma.

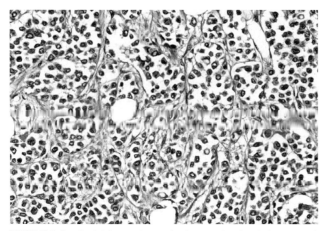

FIGURE 28.5. Invasive lobular carcinoma, alveolar type. Loosely cohesive tumor cell aggregates are separated by delicate fibrous septa.

(Fig. 28.5) (39,41,46,47,66). Although a *trabecular variant* has also been described (39), considerable overlap exists between this pattern and that seen in the classic form of invasive lobular carcinoma. A *tubulolobular variant* has been described, in which some of the tumor cells invade in the linear strands characteristic of the classic form of invasive lobular carcinoma, whereas others form small tubules that tend to have rounded to ovoid contours (43,81). These tubules are smaller and less angulated than those seen in tubular carcinoma (see below). Although originally considered to be a variant of invasive lobular carcinoma, more recent data show that most of these cases display membrane immunoreactivity for E-cadherin, supporting a ductal phenotype (82,83). In other variants, the invasive pattern is similar to that seen in the classic form of invasive lobular carcinoma, but the cytologic features differ. In the *pleomorphic variant*, the neoplastic cells are larger and exhibit more nuclear variation than that seen in the classic form of invasive lobular carcinoma (Fig. 28.6) (48–51). Although signet ring cell forms can be seen in the classic type of invasive lobular carcinoma as well as in some examples of invasive ductal carcinoma (45,84), tumors that are composed of a prominent component of signet ring cells that otherwise have the characteristic features of invasive lobular carcinoma are considered to represent the *signet ring cell variant* of invasive lobular carcinoma (42,45,85–87). *Histiocytoid carcinoma*

is an apocrine variant of invasive lobular carcinoma where the tumor cells have a histiocyte-like appearance with abundant foamy pale eosinophilic cytoplasm and mild nuclear atypia. The cells are periodic acid-Schiff (PAS) and diastase positive and stain for gross cystic disease fluid protein 15 (GCDFP-15) by immunohistochemistry (88–91). Several authors have recognized a *mixed* category of invasive lobular carcinomas. This term is generally used to designate lesions in which no single pattern comprises more than 80% to 85% of the lesion (5,66,92). However, Dixon et al. (60) also included in their *mixed* group the pleomorphic variant (60).

The relative frequency of these various lobular subtypes is difficult to discern because not all subtypes have been recognized in all series (Table 28.3). In addition, patient selection criteria varied among these studies. In the series of Dixon et al., among 103 invasive lobular carcinomas, 30% were of the classic type, 22% were solid, 19% were alveolar, and 29% were mixed lesions (60). In the experience of Ellis et al. (6), 40% of invasive lobular carcinomas were of the classic type, 10% were solid type, 4% were alveolar, 6% were tubulolobular, and 40% were mixed. In contrast, in a study from Memorial Sloan-Kettering Cancer Center, 176 of 230 invasive lobular carcinomas (77%) were of the classic type and the remainder were variants: 10 (4%) solid, 14 (6%) alveolar, and 30 (13%) mixed (66). The pleomorphic variant is particularly uncommon with only 9 cases identified among 843 invasive carcinomas in one series (50).

Classic invasive lobular carcinomas typically show expression of estrogen and progesterone receptors (ER and PR) and rarely show HER2 protein overexpression or gene amplification (93) or accumulation of the p53 gene product (94). Gross cystic disease fluid protein 15 expression is seen in about one-third of all invasive lobular carcinomas, but is present in most lesions that show prominent signet ring cell features (95). Although pleomorphic lobular carcinomas are also frequently ER- and PR- positive, they also frequently show abnormalities in HER2, myc, and p53, consistent with their aggressive clinical behavior (51,96,97).

Clinical Course and Prognosis

Several aspects of the clinical course of invasive lobular carcinomas merit consideration. First, a number of studies have noted differences in the pattern of metastatic spread between invasive lobular and invasive ductal carcinomas. In particular, metastases to the lungs, liver, and brain parenchyma appear to be less common in patients with lobular than ductal cancers (98–101). In contrast, lobular carcinomas have a greater propensity to metastasize to the leptomeninges, peritoneal surfaces, retroperitoneum, gastrointestinal tract, reproductive organs, and bone (98). In fact, most cases of carcinomatous meningitis in patients with metastatic breast cancer occur in patients with lobular cancers (98,99,101–103). Peritoneal metastases can appear as numerous small nodules studding the peritoneal surfaces in a manner similar to that seen in ovarian carcinoma (45,98,99,101). Metastases to the stomach can produce an appearance that simulates an infiltrative (linitis plastica) type of primary gastric carcinoma (104,105). Involvement of the uterus can result in vaginal bleeding (106), whereas metastatic tumor in the ovary can produce ovarian enlargement and the appearance of a Krukenberg tumor.

Whether or not invasive lobular carcinomas differ in overall prognosis from invasive ductal carcinomas is difficult to determine owing partially to variations in the application of histologic criteria for the diagnosis of invasive lobular carcinoma. The prognosis for patients with invasive lobular carcinoma as a group has, however, not consistently been shown to differ from that of patients with invasive ductal carcinoma (107). Several studies have suggested that the prognosis for the classic form of invasive lobular carcinoma is better than the solid

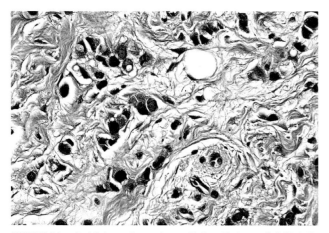

FIGURE 28.6. Invasive lobular carcinoma, pleomorphic type. The tumor cells infiltrate the stroma in linear strands, similar to those seen in the classic type of invasive lobular carcinoma. However, the cells in this lobular variant show considerable nuclear pleomorphism, in contrast to the small, monomorphic nuclei characteristic of the classic type of invasive lobular carcinoma (compare with Fig. 28.3B).

		Subtypes				
Study	No. Invasive Lobular Carcinomas	Classic	Solid	Alveolar	Tubulolobular	Mixed
Dixon et al. (44)	103	30	22	19	Not included	29
Ellis et al. (6)	243	40	10	4	6	40
DiCostanzo et al. (60)	230	77	4	6	Not included	13

Table 28.3 FREQUENCY OF INVASIVE LOBULAR CARCINOMA SUBTYPES IN SERIES WITH MORE THAN 100 PATIENTS

variant (6,60,66) and that the tubulolobular variant has a particularly favorable prognosis (6). Attempts to assess prognostic differences between classic and variant forms of invasive lobular carcinoma have been limited, however, by the small numbers of patients in the variant subgroups in virtually all of the published series as well as failure in some series to stratify patients by stage, and the results across studies have been inconsistent. Some studies have suggested that the classic form of invasive lobular carcinoma is associated with a more favorable prognosis than invasive ductal carcinoma (6,66,108). However, in the study of DiCostanzo et al. (66), a prognostic advantage for invasive lobular carcinomas over invasive ductal cancers was seen only among patients with stage I disease (66). Available evidence suggests that the pleomorphic variant (48–50) and the signet ring cell variant (when defined as lesions in which greater than 10% of the neoplastic cells are of the signet ring cell type) (87) appear to be associated with a particularly poor clinical outcome.

Numerous clinical follow-up studies have indicated that patients with invasive lobular carcinoma can be adequately treated with conservative surgery and radiation therapy following a complete gross excision of the tumor, with local recurrence rates comparable to those seen in patients with invasive ductal carcinoma (109).

 INVASIVE CARCINOMAS WITH DUCTAL AND LOBULAR FEATURES

A small proportion of invasive breast cancers are not readily classifiable as either ductal or lobular. This was acknowledged by Azzopardi (67), who noted that "infiltrating ductal and infiltrating lobular carcinoma cannot be separated quite as easily as is implied by much of the literature." In his experience, such tumors accounted for about 4% of invasive breast cancers (67). Tumors with such indeterminate histologic features were noted in 2.2% of 11,036 cancers studied by Sastre-Garau et al. (62), 2.6% of the 879 cancers in a study by Weiss et al. (110), and 4.4% of 1337 invasive cancers reviewed by Peiro et al. (63). Ellis et al. (6) noted that 4.7% of 1,536 invasive cancers had mixed ductal and lobular features.

In our experience, invasive cancers may be difficult to categorize definitively as either ductal or lobular for a variety of reasons. First, some cancers show distinct areas of invasive ductal carcinoma and invasive lobular carcinoma, but also exhibit foci that appear to represent a transition between the two patterns. Although such lesions may be categorized as *mixed*, this designation ignores the transitional component. Second, some lesions are composed of cells that have cytologic features of invasive lobular carcinoma, but infiltrate the stroma in a manner that more closely resembles that of invasive ductal carcinoma than of any of the described lobular variants. Third, some lesions have cytologic features that are more typical of invasive ductal carcinomas, but invade the

stroma in a single-file pattern. Although some such lesions represent the pleomorphic variant of invasive lobular carcinoma (48–50), others do not show the degree of nuclear variability required for that diagnosis. Finally, some invasive cancers have both cytologic and architectural features that are intermediate between those of invasive ductal and invasive lobular carcinomas. Immunohistochemical staining for E-cadherin and cytokeratin 8 has been proposed as a useful adjunct in making the distinction between ductal and lobular carcinomas in histologically problematic or indeterminate cases (111). That it may be difficult for the pathologist to categorize a given lesion as ductal or lobular in some cases should not be surprising in view of reports suggesting that some invasive ductal carcinomas exhibit cytogenetic alterations that are similar to those seen in invasive lobular carcinomas (80,112,113).

Given the heterogeneous nature of the lesions included in this group, data on clinical features and outcome of patients with invasive carcinomas with ductal and lobular features are difficult to interpret. In three series, however, lesions designated as having both ductal and lobular features were not distinctive in their rate of local recurrence or distant failure when compared with those in patients with invasive ductal or invasive lobular carcinomas (62,67,110).

 TUBULAR CARCINOMA

Tubular carcinoma is a special type cancer that is typically associated with limited metastatic potential and an excellent prognosis. The reported incidence of tubular carcinoma varies, depending on the histologic definition and the method of cancer detection used in the study population. In most studies performed before the widespread use of screening mammography, tubular carcinomas accounted for less than 1% to 4% of all breast cancers (3,114–118). These tumors, however, account for a much higher proportion of cancers detected in mammographically screened populations, with incidence rates ranging from 7.7% to 27% (12–16,119–122).

Clinical Presentation

The mean age at presentation for patients with tubular carcinoma is in the early sixth decade (range 23–89 years) (114–118,123–138). Historically, most tubular carcinomas were detected as palpable lesions (131). Most (60% to 70%), however, now present as nonpalpable mammographic abnormalities (118,134,135). Not infrequently, tubular carcinomas are discovered incidentally in biopsies performed for unrelated reasons. Lagios et al. (127) reported that 40% of patients with tubular carcinoma had a positive family history of breast cancer in a first-degree relative, a significantly higher rate than that observed in patients with other types of breast cancer (127). However, this strong association with family history has not been observed by others (139). Rare examples of tubular carcinoma have been reported in men (123,140).

Mammographic abnormalities have been reported in most (80%) patients with tubular carcinomas, most often in the absence of palpable abnormalities. However, mammographically occult tubular carcinomas are not infrequent (134). When a mammographic abnormality is present, it is usually a mass lesion, and is only occasionally associated with microcalcifications. The mass may be irregular, round, oval, or lobulated. The mammographic characteristics of most tubular carcinomas were described as "highly suggestive of malignant tumor" in one study; however, 10% were interpreted as "low to moderate probability" of being a malignant tumor (134). Most tubular carcinomas have spiculated margins, and cannot be distinguished radiologically from infiltrating ductal carcinomas.

Gross Pathology

Pure tubular carcinomas are typically small, with an average diameter less than 1.0 cm in most series (119,125,126,130, 136–138). Tubular carcinomas detected by screening mammography are typically smaller than palpable lesions (118,127,135), and pure tumors are smaller, on average, than tumors composed of mixtures of tubular carcinoma and other histologic types (131). Grossly, tubular carcinomas are firm, spiculated lesions that are indistinguishable from infiltrating ductal carcinomas.

Histopathology

Tubular carcinomas are characterized by a proliferation of well-formed glands or tubules produced by a single layer of epithelial cells without a myoepithelial cell component. These tubules tend to be ovoid in shape and have sharply angular contours with tapering ends, and open lumens. The cells comprising these tubules are characterized by low-grade nuclear features and are usually polarized toward the lumen, often exhibiting apical cytoplasmic "snouting" (Fig. 28.7). Tubular carcinomas should not be confused with invasive ductal carcinomas with gland-like structures in which the cells are typically less well-differentiated (74). The stroma of tubular carcinomas usually has desmoplastic features, and prominent elastosis may be present in some cases (141). General agreement now is that more than 90% of the tumor should exhibit this characteristic morphology to be categorized as a *pure* tubular carcinoma (5,6), and tumors with less than 90% tubular elements are generally referred to as *mixed* tubular carcinomas. The proportion required for this diagnosis in published studies has varied, however, from 75% to 100%.

Most tubular carcinomas have an associated component of ductal carcinoma *in situ* (118,124,125,130,131,135). The DCIS

seen in association with tubular carcinoma is usually of low nuclear grade, with cribriform, micropapillary, papillary, or solid patterns, and does not typically comprise a large proportion of the tumor mass. In addition, flat epithelial atypia is often found in the vicinity of tubular carcinomas (142). Lobular carcinoma in situ is also observed in association with tubular carcinoma, but only in a minority of cases (115,117,125,127,131,135). The frequency of multifocality and multicentricity in tubular carcinoma is difficult to determine owing to varying definitions and methods of specimen sampling employed by different investigators. In one report in which 17 mastectomy specimens with tubular carcinomas were examined using the Egan serial subgross method (143), Lagios et al. (127) found a 56% incidence of multicentricity, defined in that study as carcinoma of any type present 5 cm from the index lesion. This incidence was significantly greater than a control group composed of mastectomy specimens containing breast cancers of other types (127). The incidence of contralateral breast cancers in patients with tubular carcinomas ranges from 4.5% to 38% (116,118,124,125,127,128,131,136,144). The 38% incidence of contralateral breast cancers reported in one study was significantly greater than that seen in patients with other types of breast cancer (127).

The expression of various biologic markers in tubular carcinomas generally reflects the well-differentiated nature and good prognosis associated with these lesions. Estrogen receptor positivity has been reported in 70% to 100% of tubular carcinomas, and progesterone receptor positivity in 60% to 83% (118,136,137,145–148). In addition, these lesions are almost always diploid, have a low proliferative rate, and rarely show HER2 overexpression or p53 protein accumulation (148–151). In one study of six tubular carcinomas, all but one was associated with uncomplicated cytogenetic abnormalities, compared with the complex abnormalities exhibited by most breast cancers of no special type (152). In addition, when compared with invasive carcinomas of no special type, tubular carcinomas exhibit fewer overall chromosomal changes; more often they show losses of 16q and less often losses of 17p (153).

Because these lesions are extremely well-differentiated, several benign entities (e.g., sclerosing adenosis, radial scars, complex sclerosing lesions, and microglandular adenosis) may enter into the differential diagnosis. In such cases, the use of adjunctive immunohistochemical stains may be necessary to arrive at the correct diagnosis (154–157).

Clinical Course and Prognosis

The reported incidence of axillary lymph node metastases in patients with tubular carcinomas ranges from 0 to 30%

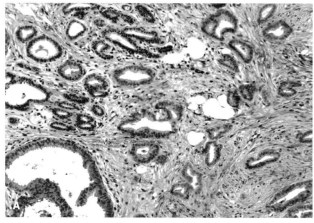
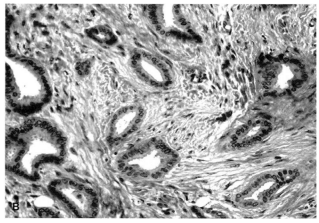

FIGURE 28.7. Tubular carcinoma. A: This tumor is composed of well-formed glandular structures in a desmoplastic stroma. **B:** The glands, or tubules, are elongated, and some have tapering ends. Numerous cytoplasmic "snouts" are evident at the luminal aspect of the tumor cells.

(114–119,124–138,144,158), and the reason for this wide range is multifactorial. Perhaps most important is variation in the histologic definition used in different studies. Many studies have shown an inverse relationship between the degree of tubular differentiation and the incidence of lymph node metastases (115,117,124,127,128,131,133,137). Nevertheless, even patients with *pure* tubular carcinomas have nodal metastases in up to 15% of cases (136). As with other types of breast cancer, however, the size of the tumor strongly influences the likelihood of axillary metastases. Winchester et al. (136) reported that 67% of tubular carcinomas associated with nodal metastases were greater than the median size of 1.0 cm. The relative infrequency of nodal disease in patients with small tubular carcinomas has led some investigators to advocate abandoning axillary lymph node dissection in these patients (118,137).

With regard to survival, all studies suggest that patients with tubular carcinoma have a good prognosis, albeit to a variable degree (6,114–119,124–138,144,158–161). In the randomized, prospective National Surgical Adjuvant Breast and Bowel Project-B06 (NSABP-B06) trial, 1,090 node-negative and 651 node-positive patients were classified with regard to histologic type, and the "favorable" category included 120 patients with tubular carcinoma (161). Both node-negative and node-positive patients in the favorable category experienced significantly greater overall survival at 10 years compared with other patients in a univariate analysis, and favorable histology proved to be an independent predictor of survival in node-negative patients by multivariate analysis (161). Similar improved survival rates in patients with tubular carcinoma were reported in a series of 1,621 patients, although these patients were not stratifed by node status (6). In this latter study, even patients with *tubular mixed* tumors (which were defined as stellate cancers composed of cells typical of invasive ductal carcinoma but with central tubules identical to tubular carcinoma) experienced significantly better overall survival compared with patients with invasive ductal carcinoma (6). In addition, two series, one examining patients with node-negative early-stage breast cancer treated with mastectomy, and the other examining early-stage patients treated with breast-conserving therapy, both reported that patients with tubular carcinoma had significantly lower rates of distant recurrences compared with patients with invasive ductal carcinoma (159,160).

Other investigators have suggested that even patients with node-positive tubular carcinoma have a relatively good prognosis. When tubular carcinoma does metastasize to axillary lymph nodes, usually one and seldom more than three level I nodes are involved (117,118,127,130,135,136). Furthermore, several investigators have concluded that the presence of nodal disease in patients with tubular carcinoma does not affect disease-free or overall survival in these patients (115,136,162).

Two reports examined the use of conservative surgery and radiation therapy in a total of 46 patients with tubular carcinoma. In these studies, no significant differences were seen in local recurrence rates when patients with tubular carcinomas were compared with patients with invasive ductal carcinoma (110,160,163). Although it is tempting to speculate that at least some patients with tubular carcinoma may be adequately treated with local excision alone (i.e., without radiation therapy), currently insufficient data exist to consider this a standard treatment option.

MUCINOUS CARCINOMA

Mucinous carcinoma (also known as colloid carcinoma) is another special type of cancer that is associated with a relatively favorable prognosis. The reported incidence of mucinous carcinoma varies, depending on the histologic criteria. Most studies have indicated that less than 5% of invasive breast carcinomas have a mucinous component and of these, less than half represent pure mucinous carcinomas (164–166).

Clinical Presentation

The mean age at presentation for patients with mucinous carcinoma is in the seventh or early eighth decade in most studies (range 21–94 years), and is greater than that for patients with breast cancers of no special type (164,165,167–175). Most patients with mucinous carcinoma included in published reports presented with palpable tumors. More recent reports suggest, however, that a substantial proportion of patients with mucinous carcinoma (30% to 70%) present with nonpalpable mammographic abnormalities (176,177).

Mammographically, mucinous carcinomas are most often poorly defined or lobulated mass lesions that are rarely associated with calcification (176–179). Wilson et al. (176) reported that pure mucinous carcinomas were more often associated with a circumscribed, lobulated contour than the irregular borders characteristic of tumors with a mixture of mucinous and nonmucinous components (176). In addition, mammographically occult mucinous carcinomas are not infrequent, accounting for 4 of 23 (17%) of cases in one study (178). On ultrasound examination, mucinous carcinomas are typically hypoechoic mass lesions (179).

Gross Pathology

Mucinous carcinomas average approximately 3 cm in size, with a wide range reported in the literature (180). In some studies, tumors composed exclusively of mucinous features are smaller, on average, than mixed tumors (172,176). Mucinous carcinomas have a distinctive gross appearance. These lesions are typically circumscribed and have a variably soft, gelatinous consistency, and a glistening cut surface. Lesions with a greater amount of fibrous stroma may have a firmer consistency.

Histopathology

The hallmark of mucinous carcinomas is extracellular mucin production. The extent of extracellular mucin varies from tumor to tumor, however. Typically, tumor cells in small clusters, sheets, or papillary configurations are dispersed within pools of extracelluar mucin (Fig. 28.8). This characteristic histology should comprise at least 90% of the tumor (or 100% according to some) (6) to qualify for the diagnosis of mucinous carcinoma. Mucinous neoplasms intermixed with other nonmucinous histologic features are classified as *mixed* mucinous tumors. The cellularity of mucinous carcinomas is variable, and some tumors are relatively paucicellular; in these cases, the differential diagnosis includes mucocele-type tumors, which are benign lesions characterized by cystically dilated ducts associated with rupture and extravasation of mucin into the stroma (181,182). The cells comprising mucinous carcinomas are usually of low or intermediate nuclear grade. Many studies have documented the presence of cytoplasmic argyrophilic granules in a significant subset of lesions, although this finding does not appear to be clinically meaningful (166). Mucinous carcinomas are often accompanied by a DCIS component that may have a papillary, micropapillary, cribriform, or even a comedo pattern. In some cases, the DCIS may also exhibit prominent extracellular mucin production (180).

The expression of various biological markers in mucinous carcinomas generally reflects the good prognosis associated with these lesions. Estrogen receptor positivity has been reported in 86% to 92% of tumors (145,147,173), and progesterone receptor positivity in 63% to 68% (146–148). In addition, mucinous carcinomas usually do not overexpress the HER2 oncoprotein (0 to 4% of cases) or show p53 protein accumulation (18% of cases)

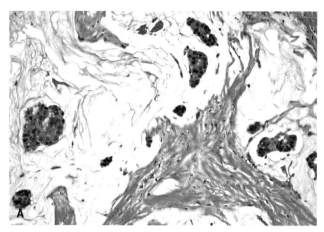
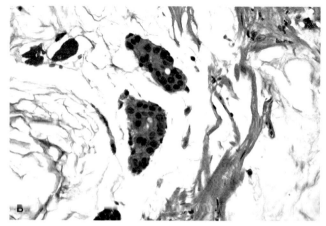

FIGURE 28.8. Mucinous carcinoma. A: The tumor is composed of clusters of neoplastic cells dispersed in mucous pools. **B:** In this specimen, the neoplastic cells have intermediate-grade nuclei.

(148–151). DNA studies of 26 pure mucinous carcinomas revealed that 25 (96%) were diploid compared with only 8 of 19 mixed tumors (42%). The rate of diploidy among the mixed tumors was comparable to that seen in breast cancers of no special type (183). In a review examining the karyotypic analysis of 20 mucinous carcinomas, 17 exhibited simple chromosomal abberrations in comparison to the complex aberrations typically associated with breast cancers of no special type (152). A more recent study has also confirmed that mucinous carcinomas show substantially fewer chromosomal abnormalities than invasive carcinomas of no special type (184).

Clinical Course and Prognosis

The incidence of axillary lymph node metastases in pure mucinous carcinomas, although variable (range 4% to 39%, average 15%), is significantly less than the incidence of node positivity seen in mixed mucinous tumors (38% to 59%) or breast cancers of no special type (43% to 63%) (164,165,167–173). Some investigators have questioned the necessity of performing lymph node dissections in patients with mucinous carcinoma, particularly if 100% of the tumor shows typical mucinous histology (171,172).

With regard to survival, 38 patients with mucinous carcinoma were enrolled in the NSABP-B06 trial, and they experienced the same significantly increased survival as patients with tubular carcinoma, particularly in the node-negative group (161). Similar results were reported by Ellis et al. (6) in their retrospective series; however, these patients were not stratified by nodal status. Survival data reported in most other retrospective reports suggest that, to a variable degree, patients with mucinous carcinoma experience decreased recurrence rates and increased short- and long-term survival compared with patients with mixed mucinous carcinomas and breast cancers of no special type (164–173,185). Several studies have noted that a significant number of late recurrences are seen in patients with mucinous carcinoma (170,186), with one report documenting a recurrence 30 years after initial treatment (186). A report utilizing the Surveillance, Epidemiology and End Results (SEER) database compared 20-year survival data from 11,422 patients with mucinous carcinoma and patients with invasive ductal carcinoma diagnosed between 1973 and 2002 (174,175). Similar to the studies cited above, this report indicated that the patients with mucinous carcinoma present most often with localized disease (86%), with only 12% having regional lymph node involvement and 2% with distant metastases at the time of diagnosis. Although no significant differences were seen in overall survival, survival at 10, 15, and 20 years for mucinous carcinoma was 89%, 85%, and 81%, respectively, compared with 72%,

66%, and 62% for invasive ductal carcinoma. The most significant prognostic factors in multivariate analyses were nodal status, then age, tumor size, PR status, and nuclear grade (175). In addition, two series, one examining patients with node-negative early-stage breast cancer treated with mastectomy (with 20-year follow-up), and the other examining those with early-stage treated with breast-conserving therapy (with 10-year follow-up), both reported that patients with mucinous carcinoma had significantly lower rates of distant recurrences compared with patients with invasive ductal carcinoma (159,160).

Three studies have examined the use of conservative surgery and radiation therapy in a total of 38 patients with mucinous carcinoma, and report no significant differences in local recurrence rates compared with patients with invasive ductal carcinoma (110,160,187). Given the relatively good prognosis for patients with mucinous carcinoma, some authors have raised the question of whether radiation therapy can be safely omitted after breast-conserving surgery in patients with this tumor type (172). Presently, however, insufficient data exist on which to base such a recommendation.

Mucinous carcinomas have rarely been associated with unusual metastatic manifestations, including mucin embolism resulting in fatal cerebral infarcts (188,189), and pseudomyxoma peritonei (190).

MEDULLARY CARCINOMA

Medullary carcinomas have been reported to account for less than 5% to 7% of all invasive breast cancers but in our experience are much less frequent than this (180). Some studies have indicated that this type of breast cancer has a favorable prognosis, despite its aggressive histologic appearance (191–198). Considerable controversy exists regarding the appropriate histologic definition of medullary carcinoma, as well as the reproducibility of this diagnosis among pathologists. As a result, the prognostic implications of this diagnosis are uncertain (191–205).

Clinical Presentation

Patients with medullary carcinoma usually present at a relatively younger age than patients with other breast cancers: The mean age at presentation is in the late fifth and early sixth decade, with a wide age range reported (191–198). Most patients with medullary carcinoma present with a palpable mass, usually in the upper outer quadrant (198). Of interest, some patients with this tumor type exhibit axillary lymphadenopathy at the time of presentation suggesting the presence of metastatic disease.

However histologic examination of the lymph nodes in such cases typically reveals benign reactive changes (206,207). Rare examples of medullary carcinoma have been reported in male patients (194). A number of studies have found an association between mutations in the *BRCA1* breast cancer susceptibility gene and the occurrence of medullary carcinomas and invasive ductal carcinomas with medullary features (208–211).

To some degree, the mammographic features of medullary carcinoma reflect the pathologic features, although they are not specific. Most lesions are associated with a moderately well-defined mass unassociated with calcifications (207,212). A significant proportion of cases of medullary carcinoma are, however, associated with an ill-defined margin. Moreover, most mammographically well-circumscribed cancers are infiltrating ductal carcinomas rather than medullary carcinomas (213). On ultrasound examination, medullary carcinomas are generally well-circumscribed, frequently lobulated, and hypoechoic (212,213).

Gross Pathology

The mean size of medullary carcinomas is similar to that of breast cancers of no special type (180). Grossly, these lesions are well-circumscribed, soft, tan-brown to gray tumors that bulge above the cut surface of the specimen. A multinodular appearance may be appreciated in some cases. Areas of hemorrhage, necrosis, or cystic degeneration may be present in tumors of any size, but prominent necrosis is usually seen in larger tumors.

Histopathology

Three similar but distinct classification systems for the histologic diagnosis of medullary carcinomas have been proposed by Ridolfi et al. (193), Wargotz et al. (196), and Pedersen et al. (197). All three classification schemes recognize the following attributes of medullary carcinomas, but the relative importance and the mandatory nature of each are stressed to a different degree: (a) syncytial growth pattern of the tumor cells in more than 75% of the tumor, (b) admixed lymphoplasmacytic infiltrate, (c) microscopic circumscription, (d) grade 2 or 3 nuclei, and (e) absence of glandular differentiation (Fig. 28.9). Tumors that lack a variable number of these characteristics (depending on the system used) are either classified as "atypical medullary carcinoma," or invasive ductal carcinoma. The Ridolfi system (193) has the most stringent and the Pedersen system (197) the least stringent criteria. Most recently the World Health Organization (WHO) proposed the following criteria for the diagnosis of medullary carcinoma: syncytial growth pattern (>75%), absence of glandular structures, diffuse moderate to marked lymphoplasmacytic infiltrate, moderate to marked

nuclear pleomorphism and complete histological circumscription (1). Regardless of the classification system used, however, medullary carcinoma is frequently overdiagnosed (203,214). Studies assessing the reproducibility and prognostic implications of the various classification systems have yielded conflicting results, and are summarized below.

In addition to the histologic features listed above, medullary carcinomas may be associated with a DCIS component (usually composed of cells that are morphologically similar to the invasive component), hemorrhage, tumor necrosis, cystic degeneration, and various types of metaplasia of the tumor cells, most often squamous metaplasia (180). There does not appear to be an increased incidence of multicentricity or contralateral cancers in patients with medullary carcinoma (195).

The expression of various biological markers in medullary carcinomas is more reflective of the aggressive histologic features of these tumors than of the favorable prognosis reported by some investigators (191–198). Estrogen receptor positivity has been reported in only 0 to 33% of medullary carcinomas (145–147,198,201), and progesterone receptor positivity in 0 to 36% (145–147,198). DNA studies performed in conjunction with various NSABP protocols, demonstrated that 85% of medullary carcinomas are aneuploid (201). A recent review of the karyotypic analysis of 14 examples of medullary carcinoma revealed complex chromosomal alterations in 9 (64%), which was a significantly greater proportion than that seen in tubular and mucinous carcinomas (152). In addition, medullary carcinomas are associated with p53 protein accumulation in most cases (151) and HER2 overexpression has been reported in 0 to 14% of lesions (149,150).

Recent tissue microarray studies of breast cancers diagnosed as medullary or with medullary features have shown that a basal-like phenotype is much more commonly associated with these tumors than with other grade 3 invasive ductal carcinomas (215,216). Gene expression profiling studies have compared patterns of gene expression in 22 cancers diagnosed as medullary carcinoma with 44 high-grade invasive ductal carcinomas. Results of these studies showed that 95% of medullary carcinomas displayed a basal-like profile, similar to that seen in the basal group of invasive ductal carcinomas. Compared with the basal group of invasive ductal carcinomas, however, medullary carcinomas showed less expression of genes involved in smooth muscle differentiation and greater expression of genes on 12p13 and 6p21, regions known to contain genes involved in pluripotency. Together, these findings suggest that medullary carcinomas and carcinomas with medullary features represent a subset of basal-like breast cancers (217). Studies using array comparative genomic hybridization (CGH) have begun to clarify further the similarities

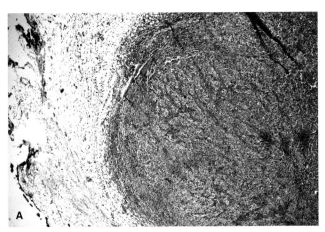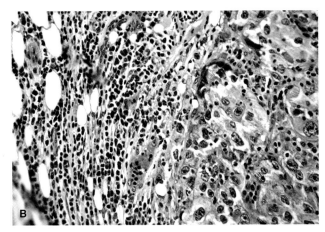

FIGURE 28.9. Medullary carcinoma. A: Low-power photomicrograph demonstrating the well-circumscribed border of the tumor. **B:** The tumor cells show high-grade nuclear features, and a prominent admixture of lymphocytes and plasma cells is seen.

and differences between cancers diagnosed as medullary and other basal-like carcinomas. In one study, medullary carcinomas and other basal-like carcinomas were both characterized by 1q and 8q gains and X losses, with medullary carcinomas typically showing greater chromosomal instability and a wider spectrum of chromosomal gains and losses (218).

Clinical Course and Prognosis

Although studies have differed in the histologic criteria used, most studies indicate that the incidence of axillary lymph node metastases is lower in patients with medullary carcinomas (19% to 46%) than in those with atypical medullary carcinomas (30% to 52%) or invasive ductal carcinomas (29% to 65%) (193–196,198).

Data regarding survival rates in patients with medullary carcinoma must be interpreted with an understanding of the histologic criteria used for diagnosis. Most pathologists currently use the histologic criteria set forth by Ridolfi et al. (193), who reported a significantly better 10-year survival rate for 57 patients with medullary carcinoma (84%) compared with 79 patients with atypical medullary carcinomas (74%), and 56 patients with nonmedullary carcinomas (63%). A later study by Wargotz et al., using slightly modified criteria, reported 5-year survival rates of 95% for 24 patients with medullary carcinoma, 80% for 16 patients with atypical medullary carcinoma, and 70% for 10 patients with breast cancers of no special type (196). A subsequent study using the Ridolfi criteria confirmed these findings, and reported 10-year survival rates of 92% for 26 patients with medullary carcinoma, 53% for 23 patients with atypical medullary carcinoma, and 51% for 46 patients with breast cancers other than medullary carcinoma (195). Several other reports have called these earlier findings into question, however. Pedersen et al. (200) examined the prognostic implications of each of the criteria put forth by Ridolfi, and found many to be poorly reproducible or to lack prognostic significance. Furthermore, the authors could not demonstrate a survival advantage in patients with medullary carcinoma as defined using these criteria (200). These authors proposed their own classification and suggested it yielded superior prognostic information (197,198). Similarly, using Ridolfi's criteria, Ellis et al. could not demonstrate a significant difference in the 10-year survival rates for patients with medullary carcinoma (51%) compared with patients with atypical medullary carcinoma (55%) and patients with carcinoma of no special type (47%), although patients with medullary carcinoma did demonstrate a more favorable survival rate when compared with patients with grade 3 tumors of no special type (6). Moreover, in a review of the NSABP experience, Fisher et al. (201) analyzed survival data for 198 patients with medullary carcinomas and 149 patients with atypical medullary carcinomas enrolled in multiple trials, and reported that node-negative patients with medullary carcinoma and node-positive patients with medullary carcinoma treated with chemotherapy experienced modestly improved survival rates compared with control patients with breast cancers of no special type. This improved survival was not observed, however, in untreated node-positive patients, although the sample sizes in this group were small (201). The authors concluded that "the prognosis of typical medullary cancer is not as 'good' as previously perceived" (201).

In addition to the clinical follow-up studies which question a favorable prognosis for medullary carcinoma, several recent studies have also questioned the practical applicability of the diagnostic criteria. Specifically, several studies have been published in which a number of pathologists (including those with expertise in breast pathology) failed to attain acceptable consensus in diagnosing medullary carcinomas using the Ridolfi criteria (199,202,203). In one of these studies (203), a direct comparison was made between the criteria advocated by Ridolfi (193), Wargotz (196), and Pedersen (197). In that study,

the criteria of Pedersen were the most reproducible. However, none of the three classification systems were related to axillary lymph node status or overall survival (203). In contrast, a clinical follow-up study examining a relatively small number of patients with medullary carcinoma suggested that the Ridolfi classification is superior to the Pedersen classification system in predicting improved survival (205).

In summary, although there may be patients with medullary carcinoma who have improved survival compared with patients with breast cancers of no special type, the ability of pathologists to identify reliably and reproducibly this subset of patients is suboptimal. It is essential that clinicians be aware of these limitations when confronted with a pathology report suggesting the diagnosis of medullary carcinoma. Given the difficulty in diagnosing these lesions, it could be argued that treatment decisions, particularly those related to the use of adjuvant chemotherapy, should not rest solely on assumptions regarding the prognostic implications of medullary carcinoma.

The results of the use of breast-conserving therapy in patients with medullary carcinoma have been reported in three studies with a total of 72 patients (110,160,187). The local recurrence rates in the two studies with a median follow-up of approximately 5 years were 4% (187) and 7% (110). However, in one study with a 10-year median follow-up, local recurrences were observed in 5 of 17 patients (29%) (160). In all three studies, no significant differences were found in local recurrence rates among patients with medullary carcinoma compared with patients with invasive ductal carcinoma. Recent data comparing 46 cases with medullary histology and 1,444 invasive ductal carcinomas have also demonstrated similar rates of local control in the two groups (219). Thus, the available limited data suggest that conservative surgery and radiation therapy is appropriate local treatment for patients with medullary carcinoma.

 # INVASIVE CRIBRIFORM CARCINOMA

Invasive cribriform carcinoma is a well-differentiated cancer that shares some morphologic features with tubular carcinoma, and is also associated with a favorable prognosis. Approximately 5% to 6% of invasive breast cancers show at least a partial invasive cribriform component (220,221).

Clinical Presentation

Most patients with invasive cribriform carcinoma present in the sixth decade (range 19 to 86 years) (220,221). A case of invasive cribriform carcinoma has been reported in the male breast (222). A significant proportion of invasive cribriform carcinomas were mammographically occult in a recent study (223). The remaining lesions showed nonspecific mammographic findings, usually spiculated masses with or without calcification (223).

Gross Pathology

No distinctive gross features of invasive cribriform carcinoma have been described.

Histopathology

Invasive cribriform carcinomas are characterized by tumor cells that invade the stroma in a cribriform, or fenestrated growth pattern similar to that seen in the cribriform pattern of DCIS (Fig. 28.10). These tumors often show admixtures of other histologic patterns of invasive breast cancer, particularly tubular carcinoma, which is seen in 17% to 23% of cases. The classic variant of invasive cribriform carcinoma, described by Page et al. (220), is defined as a tumor composed of an exclusively invasive cribriform pattern, or a tumor with more than 50%

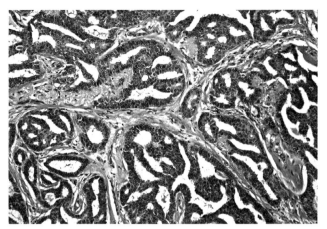

FIGURE 28.10. Invasive cribriform carcinoma. The tumor cells invade the stroma in nests that have a fenestrated growth pattern, similar to that seen in the cribriform pattern of ductal carcinoma *in situ*.

invasive cribriform features in which the remainder of the tumor exhibits features of tubular carcinoma. Tumors with any component of nontubular carcinoma were described as "mixed" in that study. Venable (221) subdivided cases into pure invasive cribriform carcinoma (12 of 62), lesions with 50% to 99% cribriform features (20 of 62), and lesions with less than 50% cribriform features (30 of 62) (221). The cribriform component of these lesions was associated with low or intermediate grade nuclear features. Significant nuclear pleomorphism, when present, was only seen in the non-cribriform component. In both studies, most invasive cribriform carcinomas were associated with DCIS, usually of the cribriform type. The average size of these tumors was relatively large, and varied from 3.1 cm (range 1 to 14 cm) for the classical variant of cribriform carcinoma, to 4.2 cm (range 2 to 9 cm) for tumors of mixed histology (220).

Venable et al. (221) reported that all 16 tumors in which the cribriform component constituted more than 50% of the tumor were positive for ER, whereas 11 of 16 (69%) were also positive for PR (221). In the six examples of invasive cribriform carcinoma examined in a recent study, none were associated with the overexpression of the HER2 oncoprotein (149). Little is known regarding the expression of other biological markers in invasive cribriform carcinoma.

The main lesion to distinguish from invasive cribriform carcinoma is the cribriform pattern of DCIS. It is clearly important not to confuse a purely *in situ* carcinoma with one that is invasive. The proportion of invasive and *in situ* cribriform components within a tumor is also important, however, with regard to sizing accurately the invasive component and also determining whether the invasive tumor has an extensive intraductal component (224). Invasive cribriform carcinoma ignores normal breast architecture and infiltrates between ducts and lobules, in contrast to DCIS which maintains the normal ductal and lobular architecture. In contrast to cribriform DCIS where the involved spaces have smooth, rounded contours, the infiltrating glands of invasive cribriform carcinoma have irregular, sharp and angulated borders. The stroma in invasive cribriform carcinoma tends to be desmoplastic compared with that associated with cribriform DCIS. Lastly, the main distinguishing feature is the lack of myoepithelial cells surrounding the glandular islands of invasive cribriform carcinoma, in contrast to their presence in cribriform DCIS.

Clinical Course and Prognosis

In the series of Page et al. (220), none of the 35 lesions categorized as the classic variant of invasive cribriform carcinoma

exhibited lymphatic or vascular space invasion, compared with 3 of 16 (19%) tumors with mixed histology. In that study, axillary lymph node metastases were seen in 14% of patients with classic cribriform carcinoma and 16% of patients with tumors of mixed histology (220). In the Venable et al. series (221), 37% of patients with pure invasive cribriform carcinoma had axillary lymph node metastases, compared with 48% to 50% of patients with tumors of mixed histology. With a median follow-up interval of 14.5 years, Page et al. (220) reported no deaths related to invasive cribriform carcinoma in patients with the classic variant (although one patient had a recurrence in axillary and supraclavicular lymph nodes), but 38% (6 of 16) of patients with tumors of mixed histology died of their disease. Similarly, Venable et al. (221) reported that with 5 years of follow-up, no patient with tumors composed of 50% or greater cribriform features died of disease, compared with a 7% death rate (2 of 30) for patients with tumors with less than 50% cribriform features. The authors of both studies stated that even though patients with pure, or classic lesions did better than patients with mixed tumors, even the latter group experienced significantly better overall survival compared with control groups that included patients with tumors without a cribriform component.

The relatively good prognosis in invasive cribriform carcinoma was confirmed by Ellis et al. (6), who reported a 10-year survival of 91% in 13 patients, compared with a 47% 10-year survival for patients with invasive carcinoma of no special type.

 ## INVASIVE PAPILLARY CARCINOMA

Invasive papillary carcinomas are rare, and most of the published literature concerning papillary carcinomas of the breast include both invasive and *in situ* papillary lesions (225–231). Although published series suggest that these tumors comprise from less than 1% to 2% of invasive breast cancers (232,233), in our experience invasive papillary carcinomas are more infrequent that this.

Clinical Presentation

Invasive papillary carcinomas are diagnosed predominantly in postmenopausal patients. Fisher et al. (232) noted a disproportionate number of cases in non-white women. Similar to medullary carcinomas, they noted that a significant proportion of patients with invasive papillary carcinoma exhibit axillary lymphadenopathy suggestive of metastatic disease, but which on pathologic examination is caused by benign reactive changes (232).

Mammographically, invasive papillary carcinoma is usually characterized by nodular densities which may be multiple, and are frequently lobulated (233–235). These lesions are often hypoechoic on ultrasound (235). One study noted the difficulty in distinguishing between intracystic papillary carcinoma, intracystic papillary carcinoma with invasion, and invasive papillary carcinoma (235).

Gross Pathology

Fisher et al. reported that invasive papillary carcinoma is grossly circumscribed in two-thirds of cases (232). Other invasive papillary carcinomas are grossly indistinguishable from invasive breast cancers of no special type.

Histopathology

Of the 1,603 breast cancers reviewed in the NSABP-B04 study, 38 had papillary features, and all but 3 of these were *pure*, without an admixture of other invasive histologic types.

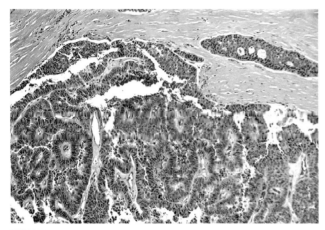

FIGURE 28.11. Invasive papillary carcinoma. The tumor cells are organized around fibrovascular cores.

Microscopically, invasive papillary carcinomas are characteristically circumscribed, show delicate or blunt papillae, as well as focal solid areas of tumor growth (Fig. 28.11). The cells typically show amphophilic cytoplasm, but may have apocrine features, and also may exhibit apical snouting of cytoplasm similar to tubular carcinoma. The nuclei of tumor cells are typically intermediate grade, and most tumors are histologic grade 2 (232). Tumor stroma is not abundant in most cases, and occasional cases show prominent extracellular mucin production. Calcifications, although not usually mammographically evident, are commonly seen histologically, but usually are present in associated DCIS. DCIS is present in more than 75% of cases, and usually, but not exclusively, has a papillary pattern. In some lesions in which both the invasive and *in situ* components have papillary features, it may be difficult to determine the relative proportion of each. Lymphatic vessel invasion has been noted in one-third of cases. Microscopic involvement of skin or nipple was present in 8 of 35 cases (23%), but Paget disease of the nipple was not observed (232).

Estrogen receptor positivity was observed in all five cases of invasive papillary carcinoma examined in one study, and progesterone receptor positivity in four of five (80%) (145). In a review of cytogenetic findings in five examples of invasive papillary carcinoma, three (60%) exhibited relatively simple cytogenetic abnormalities (152). In addition, none of the four examples of papillary carcinomas examined in two reports were associated with p53 protein accumulation or HER2 oncoprotein overexpression (149,151).

Clinical Course and Prognosis

Only limited data are available on the prognostic significance of invasive papillary carcinoma (161,232,236). Among 35 patients with this tumor in the NSABP-B04 trial, after 5-year median follow-up, only 3 treatment failures occurred, including 1 patient who died from metastatic papillary carcinoma. These survival data were similar to those reported in patients with pure tubular and mucinous carcinomas in this study (232). A later publication updating the NSABP-B04 results at 15 years revealed that patients with favorable histology tumors (including invasive papillary carcinomas) still had significantly better survival in univariate analysis, but tumor histology was not an independent predictor of survival in multivariate analysis (236). However, patients with node-negative disease with invasive papillary carcinomas enrolled in the NSABP-B06 trial experienced improved survival after 10 years follow-up compared with patients with carcinomas of no special type, and tumor histology was an independent predictor of survival in multivariate analysis (161).

INVASIVE MICROPAPILLARY CARCINOMA

Invasive micropapillary carcinoma is a relatively recently described entity that, unlike invasive papillary carcinoma, appears to be associated with a relatively poor prognosis (237–242). Tumors with pure micropapillary carcinoma comprised 1.7% of cases in one study (240) and 2.7% in another (238).

Clinical Presentation

The mean age at presentation for patients with invasive micropapillary carcinoma is 54 to 62 years (range 36 to 92 years) (237,238,241,242). In one study, 7 of 9 patients (78%) presented with a palpable mass, and 2 of 9 (22%) were mammographically detected (237). As with carcinomas of no special type, these lesions most frequently arise in the upper outer quadrant of the breast (237).

The mammographic features of this tumor type have not been well defined. Of two mammographically detected lesions in one study, one was described as a "suspicious soft tissue lesion," and the other was decribed as "suspicious microcalcifications" (237).

Gross Pathology

In a report describing nine examples of invasive micropapillary carcinoma, seven were solitary, one was multifocal, and two were not grossly apparent (237). No distinguishing gross features have been described. The median size was reported as 1.5 cm in one study (range 0.8 to 3 cm), and 4.9 cm in a second study (237,238). A more recent study of 80 cases reported a mean size of 2 cm (range 0.1 to 10 cm) (241). These sizes are significantly larger than invasive carcinomas of no special type (238).

Histopathology

In most reported cases, invasive micropapillary carcinomas have been admixed to a variable degree with invasive carcinomas of no special type or, in a few cases, with mucinous carcinoma. Unlike other special type carcinomas, however, the prognostic implications appear to be the same whether the micropapillary component is present focally or diffusely within the tumor (238,242). The lesions are characterized by clusters of cells in a micropapillary or tubular-alveolar arrangement that appear to be suspended in a clear space, or, in some cases, a mucinous or aqueous-type fluid. These micropapillary clusters, unlike *true* papillary lesions, lack fibrovascular cores (Fig. 28.12). The cell clusters appear to have an "inside-out" arrangement, with the apical surface polarized to the outside. The overall appearance of invasive micropapillary carcinoma may mimic serous papillary carcinomas of the ovary, or may simulate lymphatic or vascular space invasion (237). True lymphatic or vascular space invasion has been reported in 33% to 67% of cases, and may be extensive (237,238,241). Cytologically, the cells comprising the invasive micropapillary carcinoma usually have low to intermediate grade nuclei. Most tumors (67% to 70%) are associated with a DCIS component with micropapillary and cribriform patterns (237,238). A few cases (33%) have shown calcifications histologically (237).

In a recent large analysis, an invasive micropapillary component was found in 6% of all breast carcinomas (242). However, this component usually made up a small proportion of the overall tumor, involving less than 20% of the tumor mass in 53% of these cases (242).

Some immunohistochemical studies of invasive micropapillary carcinoma have reported that 72% to 75% were positive for ER, and 45% were positive for PR. HER2 overexpression was observed in 36% of cases, and p53 protein accumulation was

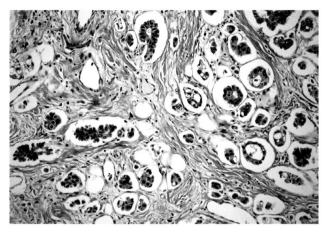

FIGURE 28.12. Invasive micropapillary carcinoma. Clusters of neoplastic cells, some forming glands, are present in clear spaces separated by fibrovascular tissue.

seen in 12% of cases, with 66% bcl-2 positive (243,244). A recent study of 62 cases of invasive micropapillary carcinoma of the breast demonstrated 18 tumors to be estrogen receptor-positive (32%), 11 to be progesterone receptor-positive (20%), with HER2 overexpression in 53 (95%) and p53 oncoprotein expression in 39 (70%) (245). Immunohistochemical positivity with Wilm tumor antigen 1 (WT-1) is rarely seen in breast cancer and can be useful in distinguishing metastatic micropapillary carcinoma of breast from papillary serous adenocarcinoma of the gynecologic tract in difficult cases (246).

Clinical Course and Prognosis

In a study of 27 patients with pure invasive micropapillary carcinoma, axillary lymph node metastases were seen in all 27 patients, compared with 66% of patients with invasive carcinoma of no special type (238). Furthermore, four or more lymph nodes were involved in 82% of cases and, on average, nine lymph nodes were positive for metastatic carcinoma. Follow-up information was available for 12 patients, and of these, 6 died an average of 22 months after their initial treatment (238). In a more recent study of 80 cases of invasive micropapillary carcinoma, 47 (72%) of 65 cases with axillary lymph node dissections had positive lymph nodes (241). Another recent study which analyzed both pure invasive micropapillary carcinoma and those present mixed with other histologic patterns, found axillary lymph node metastases present in 77% of cases. The metastases were typically multiple, with 51% of cases having three or more positive nodes (242). Importantly, these authors found no significant difference in lymph node status, ER status, tumor size, tumor grade or lymphatic vascular invasion between tumors with predominant versus focal invasive micropapillary components. Interestingly, the clinical outcome of tumors with invasive micropapillary histology did not differ from infiltrating ductal carcinomas of similar stage (i.e., nodal status) (242). These findings suggest that, although carcinomas with an invasive micropapillary component typically present with higher stage disease than that in patients with invasive carcinoma of no special type, when adjusted for stage, the prognosis of these two groups is similar.

 ## METAPLASTIC CARCINOMA

Metaplastic carcinomas represent a morphologically heterogeneous group of invasive breast cancers in which a variable portion of the glandular epithelial cells comprising the tumor have undergone transformation into an alternate cell type—either a nonglandular epithelial cell type (e.g., squamous cell) or a mesenchymal cell type (e.g., spindle cell, chondroid, osseous,

myoid). Numerous published reports describe various aspects of metaplastic carcinomas, and numerous appellations have been applied to the various tumors comprising this group (247–276). However, no uniformly agreed on classification scheme for these tumors exists. The WHO recently proposed classifying metaplastic carcinomas as either purely epithelial or mixed epithelial and mesenchymal. Metaplastic carcinomas are uncommon lesions, representing less than 5% of all breast cancers. The prognostic implications of metaplastic carcinomas are difficult to define, and may relate, to some degree, to the type of metaplasia present, as discussed below.

Clinical Presentation

Patients with metaplastic carcinoma are similar to patients with invasive carcinoma of no special type with regard to their age at presentation, the manner in which their tumors are detected, and the location within the breast in which these tumors arise (261,262). Most patients present with a single palpable lesion that not infrequently is associated with rapid growth of short duration (262). In one study, skin fixation was noted in 9 of 26 patients (35%), and fixation to deep tissues was noted in 6 of 26 patients (23%) (261).

The mammographic appearance of metaplastic carcinoma is not specific. Most are fairly circumscribed, noncalcified lesions, which in some cases appear benign (270). Some show both a circumscribed portion and a spiculated portion, which in one study correlated with the metaplastic and invasive epithelial components, respectively (270,271). Foci of osseous metaplasia may be detected mammographically in a subset of cases.

 ## GROSS PATHOLOGY

The gross appearance of metaplastic carcinomas is not distinctive, and these tumors can either be well-circumscribed or show an indistinct or irregular border. Cystic degenerative changes are not infrequent, particularly in lesions with squamous differentiation. In general, metaplastic carcinomas tend to be relatively large tumors, compared with invasive carcinomas of no special type, with a mean size of 3.9 cm (range 1.2 to 10 cm) reported in one recent study (268).

Histopathology

Microscopically, metaplastic carcinomas are highly distinctive, but vary in the types and extent of metaplastic changes. Most reports divide metaplastic carcinomas into two broad categories: those that show squamous differentiation (247–254) and those that feature heterologous elements, such as cartilage, bone, muscle, adipose tissue, vascular elements, and even melanocytes, among others (Figs. 28.13–28.15) (260–270,276). Investigators at the Armed Forces Institute of Pathology categorize metaplastic carcinomas into five categories: squamous cell carcinomas (254), spindle cell carcinomas (258), carcinosarcomas (264), matrix-producing carcinomas (263), and carcinomas with osteoclast-like giant cells (267), although others consider this last group a separate entity.

Squamous differentiation can range from well to poorly differentiated. In some tumors composed primarily of squamous cells, there is prominent cystic degeneration. In such cases, parts of the tumor may be composed of squamous epithelial-lined cysts resembling benign epidermal inclusion cysts. Spindle-cell differentiation is common in metaplastic carcinomas, and is frequently seen in association with squamous differentiation. The term "spindle cell carcinoma" has been used by some investigators to describe metaplastic carcinomas in which most of the tumor shows this growth pattern (255–258). Recently, a low-grade metaplastic breast tumor composed of

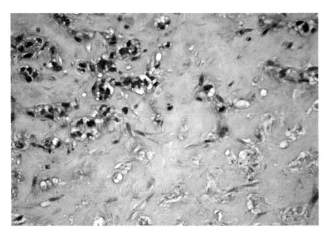

FIGURE 28.13. Metaplastic carcinoma with chondroid metaplasia. A small area of conventional invasive ductal carcinoma is present at the left side of this photomicrograph. The major portion of this tumor, however, is composed of neoplastic cells in a chondroid matrix.

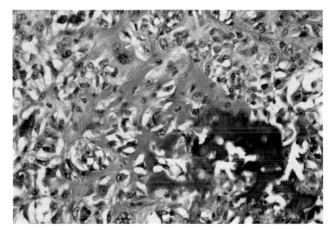

FIGURE 28.14. Metaplastic carcinoma with osseous metaplasia. Although some of this neoplasm shows features of invasive ductal carcinoma (**Left**), foci of osteoid formation are evident.

spindle cells that resemble those seen in fibromatosis has been described (277–279). One report of this rare tumor has noted an association with a high rate of local recurrence, but no distant or regional metastasis (253). Others, however, have noted cases in which the tumor has metastasized (254,279). The most common heterologous types of metaplastic carcinoma show chondroid or osseous differentiation. In these tumors, the cartilage and bone may appear histologically benign or frankly malignant, resembling chondrosarcoma and osteosarcoma, respectively. If the heterologous metaplastic component of a particular tumor predominates, the differential diagnosis must include a sarcoma, either primary or metastatic. The correct diagnosis in such cases may require extensive tissue sampling to demonstrate epithelial elements. In some cases, immunohistochemical staining for epithelial markers, such as cytokeratin, may be required for proper diagnosis. Although this is often helpful in tumors with spindle cell differentiation, not all metaplastic carcinomas show expression of epithelial markers, particularly those with heterologous differentiation. The results of immunohistochemical staining for other markers have been even more variable and this subject has recently been reviewed in detail (107). Finally, ultrastructural analysis may be of value to demonstrate epithelial features that may not be evident on routine light microscopic examination (107).

Low grade adenosquamous carcinoma, an unusual subtype of metaplastic carcinoma, appears to represent a distinct clinico-pathologic entity (273–275). These tumors are typically smaller

than other metaplastic carcinomas, with a median size between 2 and 2.8 cm (range 0.5 to 8.6 cm) (273,274). They exhibit a firm, yellow cut surface with irregular borders. Histologically, these tumors are well-differentiated and show epidermoid differentiation and a peculiar collagenized, lamellated stroma. Areas of squamous differentiation are present in most tumors, and are admixed with areas of glandular differentiation (Fig. 28.16). The glands often show elongated, compressed lumens, which may suggest syringomatous differentiation. Microcysts filled with keratinaceous material may be present. DCIS is usually not seen.

The differential diagnosis of low-grade adenosquamous carcinoma includes syringomatous adenoma of the nipple (see Chapter 10), reactive squamous metaplasia and tubular carcinoma. As discussed below, these lesions may be locally aggressive, but have a relatively good prognosis when compared with other metaplastic carcinomas (273–275).

The frequency of DCIS seen in association with metaplastic carcinoma varies among published reports. In lesions characterized by a prominent mesenchymal component in which a true sarcoma is in the differential diagnosis, the presence of DCIS argues in favor of metaplastic carcinoma.

Estrogen and progesterone receptor studies in metaplastic carcinomas are typically negative, regardless of the histologic subtype examined. A review of the literature shows that only 13 of 115 metaplastic carcinomas (11%) were positive for ER, and only 5 of 77 (6%) were positive for PR (254,256–258, 262–265,268,269,275). Using flow cytometry, Pitts et al. (265)

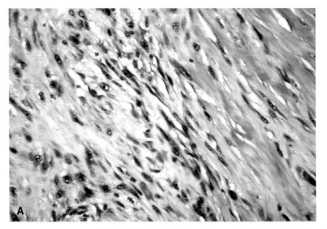

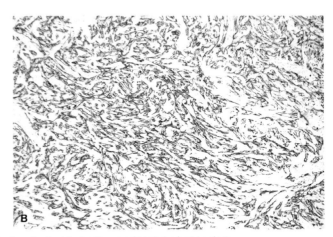

FIGURE 28.15. Metaplastic carcinoma, spindle cell type. A: Hematoxylin and eosin-stained sections reveal interlacing fascicles of spindle cells without evidence of epithelial differentiation. **B:** Immunoperoxidase stain for keratin reveals that most of the tumor cells show immunoreactivity for this protein, characteristic of cells with an epithelial phenotype.

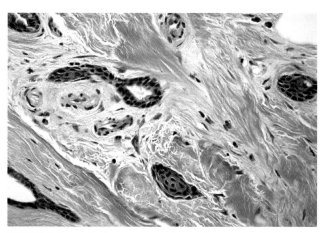

FIGURE 28.16. Low-grade adenosquamous carcinoma. The tumor shows foci of glandular and squamous differentiation. The neoplastic cells have low-grade nuclear features.

reported that 6 of 8 (75%) metaplastic carcinomas were aneuploid or tetraploid. Similarly, using Feulgen-stained sections from 12 examples of metaplastic carcinoma, Flint et al. (271) reported that the epithelial component demonstrated aneuploidy in all cases, whereas the mesenchymal elements were aneuploid in 11 of 12 (92%) (271). In addition, in one study 61% of metaplastic carcinomas with heterologous elements demonstrated p53 protein accumulation, and 11% demonstrated HER2 overexpression (268). In contrast, Drudis et al. (275) reported that 46% of low-grade adenosquamous carcinomas overexpressed HER2, and 13% showed p53 protein accumulation (275).

Clonality in metaplastic carcinomas has been assessed using microdissection techniques and evaluation of loss of heterozygosity at multiple chromosomal loci (272). In one study, all six cases of metaplastic carcinoma demonstrated identical clonality of the epithelial and mesenchymal components, and the same clone was also identified in nearby DCIS in one case. The authors concluded that the mesenchymal component of these lesions arose from mutation of the epithelial component (272).

Clinical Course and Prognosis

The reported frequency of axillary lymph node metastases in patients with squamous or spindle cell carcinomas ranges from 6% to 54% of cases (254,258,259,262). In patients with metaplastic carcinoma with heterologous elements, lymph node metastases have been noted in 6% to 31% of cases (259, 261–263,265,268).

In most cases, the routes of metastatic dissemination in metaplastic carcinomas are similar to those seen in breast cancers of no special type, including lymphatic spread to axillary lymph nodes rather than the hematogenous spread characteristic of mammary sarcoma. Metastatic lesions may demonstrate either an epithelial phenotype, the metaplastic phenotype, or both.

Survival data reported in various studies are difficult to compare owing to the relatively small numbers of patients included in the studies; differences in tumor types, in treatment and follow-up intervals, and in the use of appropriate control groups; and the paucity of studies that stratify patients by stage. Nevertheless, in patients with squamous or spindle cell carcinomas, reported overall survival rates have ranged from 43% to 86% (254,258,259,262). In patients with metaplastic carcinomas with heterologous elements, the reported overall survival rates range from 38% to 69% (259,261,263,265,268). One of these studies stratified patients by stage, and reported that the overall survival rate at 5 years was 56% for stage I patients, 26% for stage II patients, and 18% for stage III patients (261). In addition, Chhieng et al. (268) evaluated 32 patients with meta-

plastic carcinoma with heterologous elements, and follow-up information was available in 29 of these patients. The authors reported that metastases developed in six patients (21%) after an average follow-up of 6.25 years. The 5-year survival rate was 60%. The authors compared these patients with a control group of 112 patients with invasive ductal carcinoma matched for age at diagnosis, tumor size, and nodal status. Although patients with metaplastic carcinoma experienced a longer time to recurrence and a relatively better 5-year survival, the difference was not statistically significant (268).

In summary, the available data suggest that the prognosis for patients with metaplastic carcinoma is not appreciably different from that of invasive carcinomas of no special type when tumor size and stage are taken into consideration. The one exception among the variants of metaplastic carcinoma that does appear to have prognostic implications is low-grade adenosquamous carcinoma. Among 16 patients with low-grade adenosquamous carcinoma who had lymph node dissections performed, only one (6%) had evidence of metastatic disease (in a single lymph node) (273,274). Only 1 of 43 patients included in both studies experienced distant metastases. In one study, four of eight patients treated with excision alone developed a local recurrence (273). In a second study, local recurrence after excision alone was seen in 5 of 19 (26%) patients (274). Details regarding the margin status in these reports are not provided, however. Although it is possible that these lesions may be adequately treated with wide excision alone, it seems most prudent to use conventional local therapy for these patients until further data become available. The use of conservative surgery and radiation therapy for patients with other types of metaplastic carcinoma should also follow the same guidelines used for patients with conventional types of invasive breast cancer.

INVASIVE CARCINOMA WITH ENDOCRINE DIFFERENTIATION

Some invasive breast cancers show evidence of endocrine differentiation at the morphologic level, histochemical level, immunohistochemical level, or some combination of these. In addition, in rare instances, breast carcinomas can secrete hormonal products which cause clinical symptoms.

Clinical Presentation

With the exception of the very rare functioning endocrine tumor that results in clinical manifestations caused by hormone production and secretion (280–284), carcinomas with endocrine differentiation do not demonstrate unique clinical manifestations (285–298). Most of these tumors have been diagnosed in female patients, but endocrine tumors have also been reported in male patients (288,289,291,299), and some types may be proportionally more common in male patients than in female patients (291,292). In most studies, the median age of patients and the locations in which these tumors arise in the breast are similar to those seen in invasive cancers of no special type, with the exception of one study in which the most common location was subareolar (295).

Distinctive mammographic or ultrasound characteristics of invasive carcinomas with endocrine differentiation have not been reported.

Gross Pathology

Invasive carcinomas with endocrine differentiation are not associated with distinctive gross characteristics, and the reported mean size in most studies is similar to invasive cancers of no special type.

Histopathology

Carcinomas with endocrine differentiation represent a heterogeneous group of neoplasms. This is related to the fact that *endocrine differentiation* is defined differently in various studies. Most reports refer to *argyrophilic* carcinomas, which are defined as lesions that demonstrate distinctive granular material in the cytoplasm of tumor cells (argyrophilic granules) when stained with histochemical stains such as the Grimelius stain. Argyrophilic granules, however, reflect endocrine differentiation in some, but not all, cases (285–292). Argyrophilic carcinomas have been reported to account for 3.3% to as much as 52% of all breast carcinomas. This wide range is likely related to methodologic differences in histochemical staining and interpretation and, possibly, differences in patient selection (285–288,294). Argyrophilic carcinomas can be associated with a variety of histologic appearances, including tumors with no overt morphologic evidence of endocrine differentiation (usually invasive ductal carcinoma or mucinous carcinoma), tumors with histologic features suggestive, but not diagnostic, of endocrine differentiation, and tumors that show the organoid growth pattern with uniform epithelioid or spindle cells arranged in trabeculae and ribbon-like configurations diagnostic of carcinoid tumors (282–297). It must be noted, however, that tumors with typical endocrine morphology may fail to demonstrate histochemical evidence of argyrophilia (293). Furthermore, although most tumors with morphologic evidence of neuroendocrine differentiation also demonstrate immunoreactivity for one or more specific endocrine markers, such as chromogranin or synaptophysin, many *argyrophilic* tumors are negative for these markers by immunohistochemistry (289,292,296). Therefore, argyrophilic carcinomas clearly represent a heterogeneous group of tumors, only some of which should be considered as showing true endocrine differentiation.

A recent study evaluated endocrine differentiation in a series of breast carcinomas using modern immunohistochemical techniques for neuron-specific enolase, chromogranin A, and synaptophysin (298). These authors found immunopositivity for more than one endocrine marker in 11% of cases. None of the tumors, however, showed more than 50% tumor cells positive for the neuroendocrine markers. In fact, immunostaining for neuron-specific enolase, chromogranin, and synaptophysin was found in less than 5% of tumor cells in 82%, 90%, and 87% of cases, respectively. No significant association was noted between endocrine differentiation and tumor size, grade, or stage. In addition, overall or disease-free survival did not differ among patients with tumors with or without endocrine differentiation (298). This has led some authorities to propose separating breast carcinomas with endocrine differentiation into cases with focal endocrine differentiation (e.g., in the aforementioned study) from those with overwhelming endocrine differentiation (300). The latter tumors usually have distinct clinicopathologic features, and are usually found in older patients, and show differentiation typical of endocrine tumors at other sites.

With regard to tumors that show histologic evidence of endocrine differentiation by routine light microscopy, several distinct morphologic subtypes have been recognized. Although there is debate regarding the histogenesis of such lesions, primary tumors that are morphologically indistinguishable from carcinoid tumors occurring elsewhere in the body can arise in the breast, and these tumors comprise less than 1% of all breast cancers (Fig. 28.17) (293). These tumors must be distinguished from metastatic carcinoids, which occasionally involve the breast (301–306), and may even initially present as breast masses (305). In some cases, the presence of DCIS in the region of the tumor can assist with this differential diagnosis. In equivocal cases, a clinical evaluation to rule out an alternate primary site may be required.

At the other end of the endocrine spectrum are primary breast carcinomas that are indistinguishable from small-cell

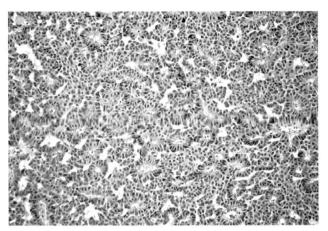

FIGURE 28.17. Carcinoid tumor. This tumor is composed of nests of cells that focally form acinar structures. The nuclei are small and uniform, and the cytoplasm is eosinophilic and granular. This histologic appearance is identical to that seen in carcinoid tumors in other sites.

neuroendocrine (oat cell) carcinomas in other sites (287, 307–313). Again, these tumors must be distinguished from metastatic small-cell neuroendocrine carcinoma involving the breast, and a clinical evaluation to rule out an alternate primary site, such as the lung, may be required (314,315).

Only limited information is available regarding the expression of biological markers in invasive carcinomas with endocrine differentiation. Of 20 tumors from four studies in which estrogen and progesterone receptor data were provided, 19 (95%) were positive for ER, and 15 (75%) were positive for PR (286,290,297,316). Jablon et al. (297) performed flow cytometric DNA studies on two carcinoid tumors, and reported diploidy in one and aneuploidy in the other. Wilander et al. (317) performed DNA studies on four examples of argyrophilic carcinoma unassociated with morphologic evidence of neuroendocrine differentiation, and reported that all four cases were diploid. In a study of nine mammary small-cell carcinomas, five were positive for estrogen and progesterone receptors, all were positive for bcl2, and all were negative for HER2 (313). In a follow-up study, these same authors found 2 of 10 small-cell carcinomas positive for thyroid transcription factor-1 and 11 of 11 positive for E-cadherin (318). A recent molecular analysis of two cases of mammary small-cell carcinoma found genetic changes in these cases that resembled those seen in both invasive ductal breast carcinoma and in pulmonary small-cell carcinoma (319).

Clinical Course and Prognosis

No significant difference appears to exist in the incidence of axillary lymph node metastases in patients with invasive carcinoma with endocrine differentiation compared with patients with invasive carcinoma of no special type. With regard to survival data, some of the retrospective reports provide limited follow-up data, but it is difficult to reach firm conclusions regarding the prognostic implications of endocrine differentiation in invasive breast cancer because of the relatively small numbers of patients included in the studies, differences in the definition of *endocrine differentiation*, differences in treatment and follow-up intervals, the lack of appropriately matched control groups, and the lack of studies that stratify patients by stage. Nevertheless, with regard to patients with argyrophilic tumors and carcinoid tumors, the available data do not point to any difference in prognosis from that of patients with invasive cancers of no special type. On the other hand, as may be expected based on the behavior of small-cell carcinoma arising from other sites, most (287,303,305), but not all (306,313), reports indicate an aggressive clinical course in patients with primary small-cell carcinoma of the breast.

One study has examined the use of breast-conserving treatment for patients with endocrine carcinomas. In that study, three patients with node-negative carcinoid tumors were treated by excision alone and followed for 15 months to 7 years (297), and no recurrences were observed. In a recent study of nine patients with small-cell carcinoma, three underwent mastectomy and six had breast-conserving therapy (lumpectomy) (313). Two of nine patients developed metastases; all patients were alive at 3 to 35 months of follow-up. Firm conclusions cannot however be drawn from these anecdotal data and patients with invasive breast cancers with endocrine differentiation should be treated in a manner appropriate for the size and stage of the lesion.

 ## ADENOID CYSTIC CARCINOMA

Adenoid cystic carcinoma is a rare and morphologically distinct form of invasive carcinoma which has been the subject of numerous published reports (320–347). These tumors comprise 0.1% of all breast cancers (325,330), and are associated with an excellent prognosis.

Clinical Presentation

The median age of patients with adenoid cystic carcinoma varies among studies, but is usually in the sixth or early seventh decade, with a wide age range reported. In most reports, these tumors present as a palpable mass with most lesions discovered in the subareolar or central region of the breast (323,325,340,345). Skin involvement has been reported in rare cases (329). These lesions are rarely multicentric, and the incidence of contralateral breast cancers does not appear increased. Rarely, this tumor has been reported in male patients (327,333,336,345).

Mammographically, these tumors can appear as well-defined lobulated masses, ill-defined masses, or spiculated lesions (213). Some adenoid cystic carcinomas present with mammographic microcalcifications, whereas others are mammographically occult (343).

Gross Pathology

The reported size range of adenoid cystic carcinomas is broad. In one recent study, the mean size was 1.8 cm (345). Grossly, these tumors are usually circumscribed and nodular; however, the microscopic extent of the lesion may be appreciably greater than the grossly evident lesion in 50% to 65% of cases (332–334, 341,343–345).

Histopathology

Histologically, these tumors are similar to adenoid cystic carcinomas that arise in the salivary glands, and are composed of epithelial cells with variable degrees of glandular, squamous, and sebaceous differentiation, myoepithelial cells, and characteristic collections of acellular basement membrane material (Fig. 28.18) (342,343). The epithelial component can assume variable architectural patterns, including solid, cribriform, tubular, and trabecular configurations. Recently, a solid variant of adenoid cystic carcinoma in which the cells display prominent basaloid features has been described (348). Some of these patterns may raise the differential diagnosis of *in situ* or invasive cribriform carcinoma, or benign conditions, such as collagenous spherulosis (330,349,350). Immunohistochemical studies have documented the presence of true lumens in the glandular com-

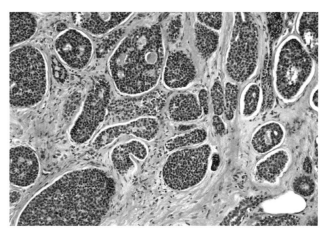

FIGURE 28.18. Adenoid cystic carcinoma. In this specimen, the invasive tumor cells grow in a cribriform pattern. Intraluminal aggregates of basement membrane material are present.

ponent, lined by cytokeratin-positive cells with intact polarity, as well as pseudolumens surrounded by cells immunohistochemically consistent with myoepithelial cells (344). Associated DCIS is seen in a few cases. Perineural invasion is also seen in some cases and may be prominent. Lymphatic vessel invasion is only rarely identified (343).

Scattered reports indicate that these tumors are usually ER- and PR-negative (145,331,332,334,338,343,346). However, ER positivity rates of 26% (345) and 46% (347) were reported in two other series. In addition, 92% to 100% of cases studied have been diploid (334,347) and these lesions have a low proliferative rate (347). Only one of four tumors demonstrated p53 mutations using the polymerase chain reaction (334). Several recent reports indicate that the cells of almost all adenoid cystic carcinomas express c-kit (351–353).

Clinical Course and Prognosis

Patients with adenoid cystic carcinoma usually have an excellent prognosis. Only rare instances of axillary lymph node metastases have been reported (334–336,340). Distant metastases are also infrequent (320,337–341,347,348), and death caused by adenoid cystic carcinoma is exceedingly rare (340). Nevertheless, Ro et al. (340) proposed using the histologic grading system employed for adenoid cystic carcinomas of salivary glands, and reported that the grading system provided prognostically useful information. The prognostic utility of this grading system, however, has been disputed (334,345).

Only sporadic reports are seen of breast-conserving treatment for patients with adenoid cystic carcinoma. Although local recurrences following excision alone have been described (322,326,328,337,340,345), details regarding microscopic margin status are rarely provided. At the present time, treatment of patients with adenoid cystic carcinoma should follow the same guidelines as those of other invasive breast cancers.

 ## INVASIVE APOCRINE CARCINOMA

Although many invasive breast cancers of various types show some evidence of apocrine differentiation, less than 1% of invasive breast carcinomas demonstrate pure apocrine features (i.e., exhibit cytologic characteristics that resemble apocrine sweat glands) (354). Although the morphologic features of these tumors are distinctive, available evidence suggests that patients with these tumors have the same prognosis as patients with invasive breast cancers of no special type.

Clinical Presentation

Patients with apocrine carcinomas are similar in age and mode of presentation to patients with invasive carcinoma of no special type, with the exception of one report in which 7 of 34 patients (21%) demonstrated skin involvement by tumor (355). Only rare examples of apocrine carcinoma have been reported in male patients (356). There is a low reported incidence of multifocal lesions or contralateral tumors (356,357).

The mammographic characteristics of apocrine carcinomas are not distinctive (213). Most tumors present as masses with ill-defined margins, and microcalcifications are infrequent (358). In addition, the ultrasound findings associated with these tumors are nonspecific (213).

Gross Pathology

No distinctive gross findings are associated with apocrine carcinoma, and the size distribution is similar to invasive carcinomas of no special type (356,357).

Histopathology

In contrast, the histologic features of apocrine carcinoma are highly distinctive (91,354–363). The invasive patterns are usually those seen in invasive ductal carcinoma, but in some cases, lesions with apocrine cytology can exhibit a pattern of invasion more characteristic of invasive lobular carcinomas (363). One variant with a distinctive discohesive and diffusely infiltrative pattern has been designated as having "myoblastoid" or "histiocytoid" features (91) and, in some cases, this lesion may mimic a granular cell tumor. Cytologically, the tumor cells have cytoplasm that is abundant and eosinophilic, with obvious granularity in some cases. The nuclei vary in grade, but typically show prominent nucleoli (Fig. 28.19). Associated DCIS, which may have apocrine features, is frequently seen. Extensive lymphatic vessel invasion, including dermal lymphatic involvement, was identified in 4 of 34 cases (12%) in one study (355).

Apocrine carcinomas characteristically show immunostaining for gross cystic disease fluid protein 15 (95). Five of 18 (28%) apocrine carcinomas described in three studies were positive for ER (146,354,357). In addition, some apocrine carcinomas show expression of androgen receptors (364). DNA studies using Feulgen-stained tissue sections demonstrated that 14 of 17 apocrine carcinomas were aneuploid, and the remainder were diploid (363). These data may be skewed, however, because all but two of the tumors analyzed were high grade. In addition, only 1 of 5 (20%) apocrine carcinomas exhibited p53 protein accumulation by immunohistochemistry (151).

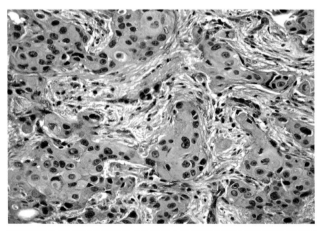

FIGURE 28.19. Apocrine carcinoma. The tumor cells show abundant eosinophilic granular cytoplasm.

Clinical Course and Prognosis

Patients with apocrine carcinoma do not appear to have a significantly different incidence of axillary lymph node involvement at presentation compared with patients with invasive carcinoma of no special type. Furthermore, a number of studies have compared patients with apocrine carcinoma with control patients with invasive carcinomas of no special type, matched for stage, and no appreciable differences in disease-free or overall survival were observed (355,357,359,365). These observations have led some to conclude that apocrine carcinomas are more a morphologic curiosity than a distinct clinicopathologic entity.

SECRETORY CARCINOMA

Secretory carcinoma is an exceedingly rare form of invasive breast carcinoma that accounts for less than .01% of all breast cancers (366). Although secretory carcinomas occur over a wide age range, they account for a substantial number of primary breast cancers diagnosed in childhood, and thus have also been referred to as "juvenile" carcinomas. In most cases, secretory carcinomas are associated with an indolent clinical course.

Clinical Presentation

Secretory carcinomas present over a wide age range (3 to 73 years) with a median age in the third decade (366–386). Most cases reported have been in female patients, but rare cases have occurred in male patients (366,378,379,384,385), including several examples in association with gynecomastia (378,385). Most lesions are detected as palpable masses, and these can arise anywhere in the breast, with no obvious site predilection. No association has been documented with underlying medical conditions or hormonal abnormalities. In addition, no increased incidence of a positive family history of breast cancer has been reported in patients with secretory carcinoma. Only rare cases have been reported to be multicentric (380), and there does not appear to be an increased incidence of contralateral breast cancer in these patients.

Mammographic abnormalities associated with secretory carcinoma in adults have not been described in detail. On ultrasound examination, these lesions sometimes appear as hypoechoic lesions with heterogeneous internal echo texture and posterior acoustic enhancement, similar to a fibroadenoma (213).

Gross Pathology

Secretory carcinomas are typically grossly circumscribed. A broad size range has been reported, with a median size of 3 cm noted in one relatively large series (371).

Histopathology

Histologically, these lesions are characterized by a proliferation of relatively low-grade tumor cells that form glandular structures and microcystic spaces filled with a vacuolated, lightly eosinophilic secretion (Fig. 28.20). The tumor cells have abundant eosinophilic or clear cytoplasm. DCIS is frequently present in association with the invasive component, and can be of the solid, cribriform, or papillary patterns, most often with low-grade nuclear features.

Sporadic reports regarding hormone receptor status in secretory carcinoma indicate that approximately one-third of cases are ER-positive, and three-quarters are PR-positive (366,376,377,381,383). In addition, DNA studies indicate that

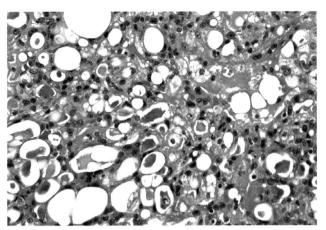

FIGURE 28.20. Secretory carcinoma. The tumor cells form glandular spaces, many of which contain eosinophilic secretions.

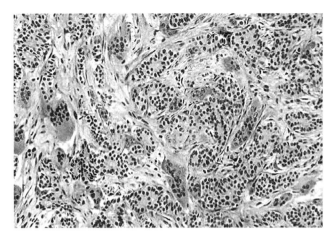

FIGURE 28.21. Invasive carcinoma with osteoclast-like giant cells. The epithelial component of this tumor forms solid nests and glands and has low-grade nuclear features. Numerous multinucleated giant cells resembling osteoclasts are admixed with the neoplastic epithelial cells.

virtually all secretory carcinomas are diploid or near diploid (366,383,384).

Clinical Course and Prognosis

Most patients with secretory carcinoma have stage I disease and an indolent clinical course. Nevertheless, approximately one-quarter to one-third of the reported cases of secretory carcinomas have been associated with axillary lymph node metastases, and this ratio holds true in both younger and older age groups (366,369,371,373,374,379,385). Most axillary metastases involve three or fewer lymph nodes.

Most of the reported cases do not provide adequate follow-up data, and so it is difficult to estimate the recurrence rates of patients with secretory carcinoma. Local recurrence in the breast (367,368,370,371,373,379) and chest wall (383) have been reported, and the interval between initial treatment and recurrence can be quite prolonged. Some of these recurrences were seen in patients treated with excision alone.

Distant metastases are rare, but do occur in patients with secretory carcinoma and have resulted in patient deaths in rare instances (371,379). Neither the efficacy of conservative surgery and radiation therapy nor the role of adjuvant chemotherapy in patients with secretory carcinoma has been defined.

MISCELLANEOUS RARE INVASIVE BREAST CANCERS

Invasive Carcinoma with Osteoclast-like Giant Cells

Invasive carcinoma with osteoclast-like giant cells is characterized by an invasive epithelial component with admixed giant cells that morphologically resemble osteoclasts and have the phenotypic features of histiocytes on immunohistochemical and ultrastructural analysis (387–398). The clinical features of patients with these tumors, and their location within the breast are similar to patients with invasive carcinomas of no special type. Invasive carcinoma with osteoclast-like giant cells is associated with a benign appearance, both mammographically (390,397) and grossly, owing to the presence of circumscribed borders. On macroscopic examination, these lesions are typically circumscribed, fleshy, and brown in color caused by recent and remote hemorrhage and benign vascular proliferation. The epithelial component of the tumor is usually moderately to poorly differentiated invasive ductal carcinoma (Fig. 28.21), but osteoclast-like giant cells have been reported in invasive lobular carcinomas and

most other special type cancers (389,391,393,394,398,399). The giant cell component can be, but is not invariably, present in metastatic lesions (394). Although the prognostic significance of this unusual lesion is not known with certainty, available evidence suggests that these tumors do not appear to be any more or less aggressive than breast cancers of no special type.

Invasive Carcinoma with Choriocarcinomatous Features

Invasive carcinoma with choriocarcinomatous features is an exceedingly rare form of breast cancer. Only two reports have described the presence of choriocarcinomatous elements (i.e., trophoblastic differentiation) admixed with conventional breast carcinomas (400,401). The choriocarcinomatous component was associated with invasive ductal carcinoma in one case (400), and metastatic mucinous carcinoma in the second (401). The choriocarcinomatous elements in these tumors produce human chorionic gonadotropin (400). If choriocarcinomatous features are encountered in a breast tumor, the differential diagnosis should include choriocarcinoma metastatic to the breast, because several such cases have been reported (402).

So-called Lipid-rich and Glycogen-rich Carcinomas

Variable amounts of lipid, glycogen, or both are commonly present in the cytoplasm of breast cancer cells. A small proportion of breast carcinomas are, however, characterized by tumor cells that contain abundant lipid or abundant glycogen within their cytoplasm. These lesions have been termed lipid-rich carcinomas (403–407) and glycogen-rich carcinomas (407–415), respectively. On routine light microscopy, the tumor cells comprising these lesions show vacuolated, clear cell cytoplasmic features, because the lipid and glycogen is dissolved during tissue processing. Neither lipid-rich nor glycogen-rich carcinomas, however, appear to be distinct clinicopathologic entities and the importance of recognizing these lesions lies in that they may mimic other forms of malignancy, particularly metastatic renal cell carcinoma.

Mucinous Cystadenocarcinoma

Mucinous cystadenocarcinoma is a recently described variant of invasive breast carcinoma that is morphologically indistinguishable from mucinous cystadenocarcinoma of the ovary or pancreas (416). Although these tumors may be associated with the extravasation of mucin, they are otherwise morphologically distinct from conventional mucinous carcinoma of the breast and, therefore, are considered separately. The importance of recognizing these tumors is that they must be distinguished from metastatic lesions in the breast, particularly those of ovarian origin (417). The prognostic significance of primary mucinous cystadenocarcinoma of the breast is currently unknown.

Carcinoma of the Male Breast

Rare in those under 30 years of age, carcinoma of the breast in men arises at a later age than in women and is approximately 100 times less frequent than carcinoma of the female breast. It is more frequent in certain parts of the world, such as Egypt, where it is related to chronic liver disease secondary to schistosomiasis. Hormonal factors play a probable causal role in fewer cases than in women, and radiation exposure and genetic factors may therefore be more important (418–420). An association has also been noted with Klinefelter syndrome (421), gynecomastia (422), and prostate cancer. The last of these associations is difficult to evaluate because of both the use of estrogens to treat prostate cancer (423) and the likelihood of prostate cancer to metastasize to the breast, where it may be confused with primary breast cancer (424,425). All the histologic types of carcinoma encountered in the female breast may be seen in the male breast, but they often exhibit poorer differentiation. Familial cases have been reported (426).

Grossly, the tumor infiltrates the small mammary gland, as well as the skin and the pectoral fascia. Ulceration of the overlying skin is common. Infiltrating ductal carcinoma is the most common histologic type, but all types of carcinoma have been reported. Although the prognosis of male breast cancer has been reported to be poorer than that of breast cancer in female patients, this may be largely related to more advanced disease stage at presentation (427). Male breast cancers are almost always ER- and PR-positive, most are positive for androgen receptors and bcl2, and about 20% to 50% are positive for HER2, p53, or both (428–430). In one study HER2 and p53 positivity were found to be independent adverse prognostic indicators (429). Treatment in most reported series has been radical mastectomy with adjuvant radiotherapy and chemotherapy, as necessary.

▨ EXTRAMAMMARY MALIGNANCIES METASTATIC TO THE BREAST

Numerous reports exist of metastatic tumors involving the breast. Secondary tumor deposits in the breast may emanate from the contralateral breast (431), or from virtually any nonmammary site. In one series, metastases to the breast from nonmammary malignancies comprised 1.2% of all malignancies diagnosed in the breast (315). Because many nonmammary malignancies can mimic the features of usual or unusual types of primary breast tumors, it can be very difficult to distinguish between the two in a subset of cases, particularly with no history of a prior nonmammary malignancy. Nevertheless, this distinction is critical for appropriate patient management.

Metastatic lesions involving the breast almost never occur in the absence of metastases to other sites, even when the breast metastasis is the first clinically detected site. When metastases are detected in the breast, a solitary unilateral lesion is present in 85% of cases; multiple lesions are present in 10% of cases, and diffuse involvement of the breast occurs in 5% of cases (432). The presence of tumor in ipsilateral axillary lymph nodes does not necessarily imply that the malignancy is a primary breast

tumor, because metastatic deposits simultaneously involving the breast and axillary lymph nodes are not infrequent (432).

Although metastatic lesions in the breast can mimic the mammographic appearance of primary breast cancers, they are more likely to be multiple, bilateral, and exhibit well-defined margins without evidence of spiculation (213,417,432). Mammographic microcalcifications associated with metastatic lesions are rare, but have been reported in association with metastatic ovarian tumors (417,433–436). On ultrasound examination, metastatic tumors involving the breast are usually round or ovoid masses with some degree of lobulation, and variable internal echoes (213).

Metastatic tumors to the breast have a variable gross appearance, depending on the type of metastasis. In general, however, these lesions may be single or multiple, and are generally well-demarcated from the surrounding breast parenchyma. The histologic and cytologic appearance of these neoplasms is related to the site of origin of the primary tumor. Metastatic lesions most frequently described in the breast include malignant melanoma (315,431,432,437–440), lung carcinoma (314,315,432,441–443), prostate carcinoma (425,444–449), and carcinoid tumors from a variety of primary sites (301–306,450–455). Less frequent metastases to the breast include ovarian carcinoma (417,433–436), gastric carcinoma (431,456), renal cell carcinoma (431,456–458), thyroid carcinoma (459), various malignant tumors from the head and neck (432,460), various types of sarcoma (417,431,432,439,461,462), colorectal carcinoma (463), medulloblastoma (464), neuroblastoma (438), malignant mesothelioma (442), carcinoma of the urinary bladder (431), endometrial carcinoma (438), cervical carcinoma (465), chloroma (431), and choriocarcinoma (402,466).

To a variable degree, the histologic features of many of the aforementioned tumors may mimic a primary breast carcinoma. Therefore it is important that the pathologist consider the possibility of metastasis in cases with unusual clinical, mammographic, or pathologic features. It is also imperative that any relevant information (e.g., a history of prior malignancy or simultaneous unexplained masses occurring elsewhere) is conveyed to the pathologist. If a tumor displays unusual histologic findings that raise the possibility of a metastasis, the pathologist may opt to additionally sample the tumor to look for areas more typical of primary breast carcinoma and for foci of associated DCIS. In addition, immunohistochemical stains for a variety of markers may be helpful in defining a tumor as being of mammary or nonmammary origin.

▨ MOLECULAR TUMOR CLASSIFICATION

Gene expression profiling studies have identified at least four major breast cancer subtypes: luminal A, luminal B, HER2, and basal-like (467,468). These subtypes differ with regard to their patterns of gene expression, clinical features, response to treatment, and outcome. Luminal A and luminal B cancers generally have a good prognosis and show high expression of hormone receptors and associated genes. Together, these two subtypes account for approximately 70% of all breast cancers. The luminal B cancers tend to be higher grade than the luminal A cancers and some may overexpress HER2. Both luminal A and luminal B cancers tend to respond to endocrine therapy, with luminal A cancers showing the greatest response. Response of the luminal cancers to chemotherapy is variable, with the luminal B cancers generally showing better response.

The HER2 cancers show high expression of HER2 and low expression of ER and associated genes. They account for approximately 15% of all breast cancers and are generally ER- or PR-negative. HER2 cancers are more likely to be high grade and lymph node positive. These cancers show the best response to trastuzumab and to anthracycline-based chemotherapy, but overall have a poor prognosis.

One of the most interesting findings of these studies is the elucidation of basal-like breast cancers, which are associated with a particularly poor prognosis. The basal-like breast cancers show high expression of basal epithelial genes and basal cytokeratins, low expression of ER and ER-associated genes as well as low expression of HER2. They constitute approximately 15% of all breast cancers and are often referred to as *triple negative* cancers, because they are invariably ER-, PR-, and HER2-negative. The basal-like tumor phenotype is especially common in African-American women and is also the most common phenotype of *BRCA1*-associated breast cancers. Basal-like cancers have a poor prognosis and are not amenable to treatment with either endocrine therapy or trastuzumab because they are hormone receptor-negative and do not show HER2 overexpression or amplification.

Although the classification of breast cancers using gene expression profiling is of interest, for practical purposes, three immunohistochemical markers (i.e. ER, PR and ERBB2) can be used as surrogates to approximate these various molecular subtypes. In general, luminal cancers are ER- or PR-positive and HER2-negative, HER2 cancers are ER- or PR-negative and HER2 positive, and basal-like cancers are ER- or PR-negative and HER2-negative (so called *triple negative*). It should be noted, however, that although most basal-like cancers are triple negative, not all triple negative cancers are basal-like. The use of additional immunostains (particularly cytokeratin 5/6 and epidermal growth factor receptor) can be used to further refine the categorization of basal-like cancers (469).

In addition to its important role in the classification of breast cancers, expression profiling has been used to grade invasive breast cancers. In one recent study, histologic grade 3 invasive breast cancers and histologic grade 1 invasive breast cancers were found to have distinct gene expression patterns. In contrast, no distinct expression signature was found for histologic grade 2 tumors. Of interest, gene expression profiling was able to stratify patients with histologic grade 2 tumors into good and poor prognosis groups (470).

PATHOLOGIC FEATURES OF BREAST CANCER IN PATIENTS WITH *BRCA1* and *BRCA2* Mutations

Considerable recent interest has focused on the pathology of the breast cancers that develop in women with a genetic predisposition to this disease as a result of mutations in the breast cancer susceptibility genes *BRCA1* and *BRCA2*. Recognition of histologic features that may indicate a genetic predisposition might be useful for providing insight into the function of these genes and as an aid in identifying patients in whom screening for these genetic abnormalities might provide a high yield. General agreement is that most *BRCA1*-related cancers are basal-like carcinomas. With regard to individual histologic features, cancers associated with *BRCA1* mutations have a significantly higher mitotic rate, a larger proportion of the tumor with a continuous pushing margin, and more lymphocytic infiltration than sporadic breast cancers. In addition, *BRCA1*-related cancers are less often ER- and PR-positive and less often HER2-positive; they are more often aneuploid, more often have a high S-phase fraction, and more often show accumulation of the p53 protein than sporadic breast cancers (209,471–475). High expression of cytokeratin 5/6, P-cadherin and cell-cycle proteins cyclins A, B1, and E, and SKP2 is also characteristic of the *BRCA1* phenotype (209,473,476). It should be noted, however, that none of these features, singly or in combination, uniquely identifies a cancer as being related to a

BRCA1 mutation (477). Despite this constellation of adverse features, most studies suggest that the clinical outcome of patients with *BRCA1*-related cancers appears to be similar to that of patients with sporadic breast cancer (478).

The histologic features reported in *BRCA2*-related breast cancers have been less consistent (479). Some studies note a significantly higher proportion of tubular-lobular group cancers (including tubular, lobular, tubulolobular, and invasive cribriform carcinomas) than in other patients (480,481). Another group, however, has found tubular carcinomas to be less common in *BRCA2* mutation carriers (482). In another small study, the pleomorphic variant of invasive lobular carcinoma was related to *BRCA2* mutation (211). Some investigators have reported that *BRCA2*-related cancers tend to be of high histologic grade (482,483), whereas others have not noted a significant difference in histologic grade when *BRCA2*-related cancers are compared with controls (484). In the largest study to date, Bane et al. (485) looked at 64 *BRCA2*-associated breast cancers and 185 *BRCA* mutation-negative age and ethnicity matched controls (485). In this series, most *BRCA2* associated cancers were invasive ductal carcinomas, with lobular carcinomas showing similar frequency in the two groups. *BRCA2* tumors were less likely to be grade I/III (6% vs. 19% in controls) and more likely to be grade III/III (60% vs. 39% in controls) and, in general, showed pushing rather than infiltrative margins. Controlling for tumor grade, *BRCA2*-associated cancers were more often positive for ER and less likely to express basal cytokeratin or overexpress HER2. *BRCA2*-associated tumors and controls overall showed no difference in expression of p53, bcl2, MIB1, or cyclin D1 (485). Other investigators have also found the basal phenotype to be rare in *BRCA2*-associated cancers, but have associated expression of cyclin D1 with *BRCA2* tumors (209). Available data on clinical outcome for patients with *BRCA2*-associated cancers also suggest no difference exists relative to patients with sporadic breast cancer (478).

HISTOPATHOLOGIC PROGNOSTIC FACTORS

Currently, considerable interest is in identifying biological, molecular, and genetic markers that may be useful to help assess the prognosis of patients with invasive breast cancer. This is discussed in other chapters. However, a considerable amount of useful prognostic information can be obtained from routine pathologic examination of specimens containing breast cancer, without the need for special diagnostic procedures, equipment, or reagents. Clinical follow-up studies have repeatedly demonstrated that features such as axillary lymph node status, tumor size, histologic type, histologic grade, and lymphatic vessel invasion represent powerful and independent prognostic indicators. Other factors have also been shown to provide important prognostic information in many studies (486–488). In fact, these traditional prognostic factors should be considered the standard against which any new prognostic factors are measured.

Axillary Lymph Node Status

Uniform agreement is that the status of the axillary lymph nodes is the single most important prognostic factor for patients with breast cancer and that disease-free and overall survival decrease as the number of positive lymph nodes increases. Nevertheless, there remain a number of important open issues regarding axillary lymph node evaluation. First, methods for the pathologic examination of these lymph nodes are not standardized. For example, although some pathologists entirely submit grossly uninvolved lymph nodes for histologic examination, others subject only a single section from such lymph nodes to microscopic scrutiny (489). This, in turn, could result in the misclassification of some node-positive cases as node-negative. In addition, although sentinel lymph node biopsy is now widely used to evaluate the status of the axilla (490), methods for examination of sentinel nodes is also highly variable (491). Another as yet unanswered clinical question concerns the significance of axillary lymph node micrometastases, particularly those identified exclusively by the use of immunohistochemistry (490,492). Approximately 10% to 20% of patients considered to be node-negative by conventional examination of the axillary lymph nodes have identifiable tumor cells in these nodes as determined by serial sectioning, immunohistochemical staining, or both methods. Studies that have sought to evaluate the significance of axillary micrometastases have differed with regard to patient population, treatment, methods to detect tumor cells, and length of follow-up. Virtually all studies with more than 100 patients have shown that the presence of micrometastases detected by serial sectioning, immunohistochemistry, or both methods is associated with a small, but significant decrease in disease-free or overall survival (493–495). Most of these studies have been retrospective, however, and were not initially designed to address this question. Furthermore, in some of these studies, it is not clear if the prognostic significance of micrometastases is independent of other factors, such as tumor size or lymphatic vessel invasion. The clinical significance of axillary lymph node micrometastases and isolated tumor cells detected by immunohistochemistry is currently being evaluated in a number of randomized clinical trials and it is likely that these trials will provide important information about this issue. Until then, most experts agree that it is premature to recommend the routine use of immunohistochemistry to evaluate either sentinel or nonsentinel lymph nodes (490,496).

Tumor Size

Numerous studies have demonstrated that the size of an invasive breast cancer is one of the most powerful prognostic factors for both axillary lymph node involvement and clinical outcome. In a study of almost 25,000 breast cancer cases, Carter et al. (497) demonstrated a linear relationship between tumor size and axillary nodal involvement as well as between tumor size and survival. The prognostic significance of tumor size is independent of axillary lymph node status and is a particularly valuable prognostic indicator in women with node-negative disease (497–499) (Tables 28.4 and 28.5). A number of studies have suggested that even among patients with breast cancers 2 cm and smaller (T1), assessment of tumor size permits further stratification of patients with regard to the likelihood of axillary lymph node involvement and outcome. In a study of 644 patients with T1 breast cancer from Memorial Sloan-Kettering Cancer Center, the likelihood of axillary nodal involvement was 11% for tumors 0.1 to 0.5 cm, 15% for lesions 0.6 to 1.0 cm, 25% for tumors 1.1 to 1.3 cm, 34% for tumors 1.4 to 1.6 cm, and 43% for cancers that were 1.7 to 2.0 cm (500). Furthermore, among node-negative patients treated by mastectomy without

Table 28.4	FIVE-YEAR SURVIVAL RATES (IN PERCENT) ACCORDING TO TUMOR SIZE AND AXILLARY LYMPH NODE STATUS		
	Lymph Node Status		
Tumor Size (cm)	Negative	1–3 Positive	≥ 4 Positive
<2	96.3	87.4	66.0
2–5	89.4	79.9	58.7
>5	82.2	73.0	45.5

Adapted from Fowler CA, Nicholson S, Lott M, et al. Choriocarcinoma presenting as a breast lump. *Eur J Surg Oncol* 1995;21(5):576–578.

Table 28.5	FIVE-YEAR SURVIVAL RATES ACCORDING TO TUMOR SIZE IN PATIENTS WITH AXILLARY NODE–NEGATIVE BREAST CANCER	
Tumor Size (cm)	No. Patients	5-year Survival (%)
<0.5	269	99.2
0.5–0.9	701	98.3
1.0–1.9	1,668	95.3
2.0–2.9	4,010	90.6
3.0–3.9	2,072	86.2
4.0–4.9	845	84.6
>5.0	809	82.2

Adapted from Fowler CA, Nicholson S, Lott M, et al. Choriocarcinoma presenting as a breast lump. *Eur J Surg Oncol* 1995;21(5):576–578.

adjuvant systemic therapy, those with cancers 1 cm or smaller had a 20-year recurrence-free survival rate of 88%, significantly higher than the 72% recurrence-free survival rate observed for patients with tumors 1.1 to 2.0 cm in size (159). Substantial variation is seen, however, in the reported rates of axillary node involvement and clinical outcome for patients with small tumors, particularly tumors that are 1cm and smaller (501,502) and not all investigators have observed that patients with tumors 1 cm and smaller have significantly lower rates of axillary node involvement and disease recurrence than those with tumors between 1 and 2 cm (503,504). Nonetheless, most studies have reported a very favorable clinical outcome for node-negative patients with tumors 1 cm and smaller, with 5- to 10-year disease-free survival survival rates of 90% or greater (16).

Several studies have suggested that the prognostic significance of size may be related to the method of cancer detection. For example, Silverstein et al. (505,506) reported that for every substage among the T1 tumors and among T2 tumors, nonpalpable lesions were less likely to have axillary node involvement than palpable lesions. In that study, positive axillary lymph nodes were seen in 2 of 51 (4%) nonpalpable T1a lesions (≤0.5 cm) and in 3 of 50 (6%) palpable T1a tumors. Among T1b lesions (0.51 to 1.0 cm), the frequency of positive nodes was 7% among the 92 nonpalpable lesions compared with 23% among the 143 palpable cancers. In patients with T1c lesions (1.1 to 2.0 cm) the frequency of positive lymph nodes was 16% for nonpalpable lesions compared with 31% for palpable tumors. Among patients with T2 tumors (2.1 to 5.0 cm), axillary nodes were involved in 23% of patients with nonpalpable lesions and in 48% of those with palpable tumors. Arnesson et al. (507) also reported that detection mode had an impact on axillary lymph node involvement in breast cancers 1 cm or smaller. In that series, lymph nodes were involved in 9% of the 221 T1a and T1b tumors detected by mammographic screening compared with 20% of the 89 clinically detected lesions ($p <.03$). Halverson et al. (508) examined 168 patients with T1a and T1b breast cancer and assessed the relationship between tumor palpability and nodal status. In contrast to the studies cited above, these investigators reported a similar frequency of axillary lymph node metastases in both palpable and nonpalpable clinically occult cancers and concluded that palpability of the tumor is not a significant prognostic factor in predicting axillary node positivity. Given the current widespread use of screening mammography, this subject is of great interest and merits further study. Whether the detection mode of the cancer is related to outcome, particularly in smaller lesions, has not been studied extensively. In one study that addressed the relationship between mode of detection and survival in node-negative T1a and T1b lesions, palpable tumors had a worse prognosis than mammographically detected lesions (509). In another study of T1a and T1b cancers, although a trend was noted for poorer outcome in the group that had been diagnosed clinically compared with the group of patients who had mammographically detected lesions, the difference was not statistically significant (507).

Accurate measurement of breast cancer size is essential to provide the most clinically meaningful information. However, studies of the significance of tumor size in breast cancer have used various methods to determine size, including clinical measurement, mammographic assessment, gross measurement, microscopic measurement of the entire lesion, and microscopic measurement of only the invasive component. In some studies, the method used to measure the tumor is not stated. This may at least partially explain differences in rates of axillary node involvement and clinical outcome in various studies. Now general agreement is that the most clinically significant measure of tumor size is the size of the invasive component of the lesion as determined from microscopic evaluation. In fact, the most recent edition of the *AJCC Cancer Staging Manual* states that "the pathologic tumor size for the T classification is a measurement of only the invasive component" (510). This approach appears to be justified because several studies have indicated that, in many cases, there are substantial differences in the size of the lesion as determined from gross pathologic examination and the size determined from microscopic measurement of the invasive component, particularly for small lesions. For example, in one series of 118 patients in whom the gross tumor size was measured as 2 cm or smaller, the gross tumor size was smaller than the microscopic size in 31%, larger in 46%, and the same in only 22% of cases (501). In 35% of these cases, the gross and microscopic tumor sizes differed by more than 3 mm. Similar discrepancies between gross and microscopic size were seen when the analysis was limited to those lesions in which the gross tumor size was measured as smaller than 1 cm. Of greatest importance, however, is the observation that the microscopic size of the invasive component of the tumor is the one that is most closely correlated with prognosis (501,511).

One important, but unresolved issue for both pathologists and clinicians is how to assess and report the tumor size in lesions that have more than one focus of invasive cancer, because it is not known if the prognosis is related to the largest single focus or to the cumulative volume of invasive cancer. Some evidence suggests that invasive carcinomas with multiple foci of invasion have higher rates of axillary lymph node involvement than those lesions characterized by a single focus of invasion (81,512,513). Additional studies are needed to determine with certainty if the number of lymph node metastases might be predicted best by the aggregate size of the invasive foci. At the present time, it seems most prudent for the pathologist to measure microscopically the size of each focus of invasive cancer and report the individual sizes, rather than adding them together.

Histologic Type

Some histologic types of breast cancer are associated with a particularly favorable clinical outcome (6,159). Special type tumors that have consistently been shown to have an excellent prognosis include tubular, invasive cribriform, mucinous, and adenoid cystic carcinomas. Some authors also place tubulolobular carcinomas and papillary carcinomas in this group. Moreover, Rosen et al. (159) have shown that the 20-year recurrence-free survival of special type tumors 1.1 to 3.0 cm in size is similar to that of invasive ductal carcinomas 1 cm and smaller (87% and 86%, respectively). Strict diagnostic criteria must be used, however, in order to observe the favorable outcome reported for these lesions.

Histologic Grade

The importance of tumor grading as a prognostic factor in patients with breast cancer has been clearly demonstrated in numerous clinical outcome studies. These studies have repeatedly shown higher rates of distant metastasis and poorer survival in patients with higher grade (poorly differentiated) tumors, independent of lymph node status and tumor size (17,161,486–489,514–523).

In fact, tumor grading has been shown to be of prognostic value even in patients with breast cancers 1 cm and smaller (502). Although a variety of methods of nuclear and histologic grading have been used in these studies, the grading method in most widespread clinical use at the present time is the histologic grading system of Elston and Ellis (520). These authors advocate the use of histologic grading for all types of invasive breast cancer, acknowledging, however, that histologic grade partially defines some of these histologic types (e.g., tubular carcinomas are by definition grade 1 and medullary carcinomas are grade 3 lesions). These authors have also pointed out, however, that the combination of histologic type and grade provides a more accurate assessment of prognosis than does histologic type alone (524).

The results of a study of 1,081 invasive breast cancers from patients treated with conservative surgery and radiation therapy at the Joint Center for Radiation Therapy in Boston illustrate the value of this histologic grading system and also illustrate some important caveats in the interpretation of grading data. In that study, time to distant recurrence was greatest for grade 1 cancers and least for grade 3 tumors (Fig. 28.22). Furthermore, in a polychotomous logistic regression analysis, increasing tumor grade was associated with a significantly

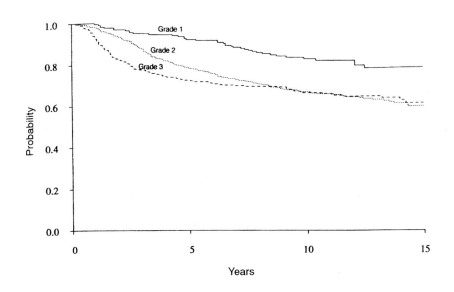

FIGURE 28.22. Kaplan-Meier curves indicating time to distant failure for 1,081 patients with invasive breast cancer according to histologic grade.

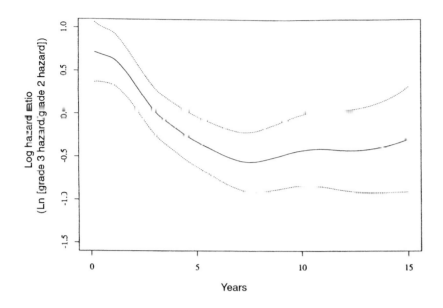

FIGURE 28.23. Hazard ratio for distant recurrence for patients with histologic grade 3 tumors compared with those with grade 2 tumors. Distant recurrence is greater for patients with grade 3 tumors than for those with grade 2 tumors when the curve is above zero, and less for those with grade 3 than for those with grade 2 when the curve is below zero (*dotted lines* represent 95% confidence limits).

increased risk of distant metastasis at 10 years (522). However, the hazard ratios for distant failure among the three grades were not constant over time. In particular, the risk of distant metastasis was highest for grade 3 tumors only within the first 3 years of follow-up. Beyond that time, the risk of metastasis associated with grade 2 tumors was actually greater than the risk associated with grade 3 cancers (Fig. 28.23). These observations emphasize that in interpreting data relating histologic grade to clinical outcome, the length of follow-up must be taken into consideration. They further suggest that grade may be best viewed as an indicator of time to recurrence rather than absolute rate of recurrence.

Some studies have suggested that histologic grade may provide useful information with regard to response to chemotherapy and may, therefore, be of value as a predictive factor as well as a prognostic indicator. The results of several studies have suggested that the presence of high histologic grade is associated with a better response to certain chemotherapy regimens than low histologic grade (525,526). Although basal-like carcinomas ("triple negative") are associated with shorter relapse-free and overall survival, they are associated with high response rates to neoadjuvant chemotherapy (527,528).

A frequent criticism of the use of histologic grading is that this assessment is subjective and, as a consequence, prone to considerable interobserver variability (529–531). Most of the studies that have suggested this have used grading systems that lack precisely defined criteria and/or did not attempt to educate the participating pathologists in the use of the system evaluated. Recent studies have indicated that the use of strict criteria and guidelines for histologic grading can result in acceptable levels of interobserver agreement and also identify areas that might benefit from refinement. In one of these studies, six pathologists each graded 75 invasive ductal carcinomas using the Elston and Ellis grading system (532). Moderate to substantial agreement was found for the overall histologic grade. Substantial agreement was also found with regard to tubule formation, moderate agreement for mitotic count, and near moderate agreement for nuclear pleomorphism as determined by generalized kappa statistics. These authors concluded that this grading system is suitable for use in clinical practice and suggested that efforts to improve agreement on nuclear grading would be of value in further fostering agreement in histologic grading. In another study, a substantial level of agreement (kappa statistic 0.70) was found among 25

pathologists who used the Elston and Ellis grading system, albeit in a small number of cases (533).

Lymphatic Vessel Invasion

Lymphatic vessel invasion has been shown in numerous studies to be an important and independent prognostic factor (Fig. 28.24). Its major clinical value at this time is in identifying node-negative patients at increased risk for axillary lymph node involvement (16,534–540) and adverse outcome (519,536,537,541,542). The identification of lymphatic vessel invasion may be of particular importance in patients with T1, node-negative breast cancers, because this finding may permit the identification of a subset of patients at increased risk for axillary lymph node involvement and distant metastasis in this group with otherwise favorable prognosis. For example, in one recent study, lymphatic vessel invasion was the only clinical or pathologic factor associated with lymph node metastasis in patients with tumors 1 cm and smaller (T1a,b). In that study, lymph node involvement was present in 4 of 7 patients whose tumors showed lymphatic vessel invasion (57%) compared

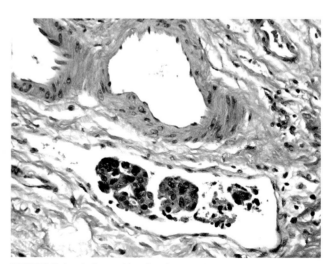

FIGURE 28.24. Lymphatic vessel invasion. A tumor embolus is present in a thin-walled, endothelial-lined space.

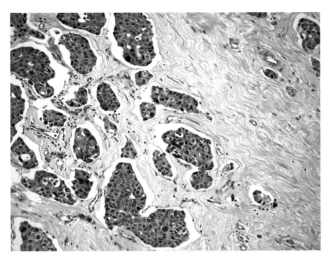

FIGURE 28.25. Retraction artifact. Tumor cells are present in artifactual tissue spaces, created by retraction of the surrounding stroma. These spaces lack an endothelial lining.

with only 1 of 100 patients without lymphatic vessel invasion (502). In another study of 461 patients with T1, node-negative breast cancer, patients with tumors lacking lymphatic vessel invasion had a 20-year survival rate of 81% compared with 64% for those whose tumors exhibited lymphatic vessel invasion (159). Similar findings have been reported by others (509,543,544), even when the analysis is restricted to the subset of T1 breast cancers that are 1 cm and smaller (509,542).

As with histologic grade, the ability of pathologists to reproducibly identify lymphatic vessel invasion has been challenged. For example, in one study, three pathologists concurred on the presence or absence of lymphatic vessel invasion in only 12 of 35 cases (545). A higher level of interobserver agreement has been noted, however, in other studies (534–537,544). In one of these studies in which stringent criteria were used, an 85% level of overall agreement between two pathologists was found for the presence or absence of lymphatic vessel invasion (534). The use of strict criteria for the identification of lymphatic vessel invasion is, therefore, imperative. In particular, retraction of the stroma is not uncommonly seen around nests of invasive cancer cells, and care should be taken not to interpret this as lymphatic vessel invasion erroneously (Fig. 28.25).

A number of investigators have evaluated the use of immunohistochemical stains for endothelial cells (including stains for factor VIII-related antigen, CD34, Ulex europaeus agglutinin I, and blood group isoantigens) and basement membrane components as an aid in the identification of lymphatic vessel invasion (546–553). These stains have been of limited value in this context, however. In particular, immunostains for blood group isoantigens and Ulex are not specific for endothelial cells and show reactivity with normal and malignant mammary epithelial cells in some cases. False–negative staining is not infrequently seen with the vascular endothelial markers, particularly factor VIII-related antigen (546,553). CD34 is not specific for endothelial cells because anti-CD34 antibodies can stain stromal cells around tumor cell nests and blood vessels (553). Immunostains for the basement membrane components laminin and type IV collagen are unable to distinguish between vascular structures and mammary ducts and lobules (546). Recently, a monoclonal antibody that recognizes lymphatic endothelium (D2-40) has been described and appears to facilitate the detection of lymphatic vessel invasion in routinely processed tissue sections (554–556). The clinical value of this antibody, however, remains to be determined. Thus, at the present time, lymphatic vessel invasion is best assessed on routine hematoxylin and eosin-stained sections using strict diagnostic criteria.

Other Factors

A number of other histologic factors have been reported to have prognostic value in patients with invasive breast cancer. The presence of *blood vessel invasion* (i.e., invasion of veins and arteries) has been reported to have an adverse effect on clinical outcome. In the long-term follow-up study from Memorial Sloan-Kettering Cancer Center, blood vessel invasion was identified in 14% of patients with T1N0 cancers and in 22% with T1N1 lesions using elastic tissue stains (519). A significantly worse outcome was seen for patients with, than those without, blood vessel invasion in both groups in that study. A broad range in the reported incidence of blood vessel invasion exists, however, ranging from under 5% to almost 50% (3,538,543,544,557–561). This is owing to a variety of factors, including the nature of the patient population, the criteria and methodology used to determine the presence of blood vessel invasion, and the occasional difficulty in distinguishing blood vessels from mammary ducts. Some studies use the term *blood vessel invasion* to denote those vascular structures that possess a muscular or elastic tissue component in their wall, whereas others include in addition thin-walled vessels of capillary caliber, many of which probably represent lymphatic spaces. Furthermore, some studies have based the evaluation for blood vessel invasion on examination of hematoxylin and eosin stained sections, whereas others have used elastic tissue stains. In our experience, invasion of arterial and venous caliber vascular structures is uncommon.

The prognostic significance of *tumor necrosis* has also been investigated in a number of studies (544,562–565). In most studies, the presence of necrosis has been associated with an adverse effect on clinical outcome (562–565), although in one of these studies, necrosis was associated with a worse prognosis only within the first 2 years after diagnosis (564). A number of issues must be addressed before tumor necrosis is accepted as an important prognostic factor. First, the extent of necrosis that must be present to be considered clinically significant requires more precise definition. Second, the presence of necrosis is highly correlated with other features associated with a poor prognosis, such as larger tumor size and high histologic grade (522,562), and it is not clear if the adverse prognostic influence of necrosis is independent of these other factors. Additional studies using multivariate analysis will be needed to address this question.

The relationship between clinical outcome and the extent of *mononuclear inflammatory cell infiltrate* in association with invasive breast cancers has also been investigated. The presence of a prominent mononuclear cell infiltrate has been correlated in some studies with high histologic grade (522). The prognostic significance of this finding is controversial, however, with some studies noting an adverse effect of a prominent mononuclear cell infiltrate on clinical outcome (36,566–569) and others observing either no significant effect or a beneficial effect (518,543,566,570).

The presence of *perineural invasion* is sometimes observed in invasive breast cancers. This phenomenon is often seen in association with lymphatic vessel invasion, but it has not been shown to be an independent prognostic factor (107).

The *extent of ductal carcinoma in situ* associated with invasive cancers has also been studied as a potential prognostic factor. Numerous investigators have shown that the presence of an extensive intraductal component is a prognostic factor for local recurrence in the breast in patients treated with conservative surgery and radiation therapy when the status of the excision margins is unknown. More recent studies have indicated, however, that this factor is not an independent predictor of local recurrence following conservative surgery and radiation therapy when the microscopic margin status is taken into consideration (109). Silverberg and Chitale (23) reported an inverse relationship between the amount of DCIS and both the risk of axillary lymph node metastasis and the 5-year survival rate in a series of patients with invasive ductal carcinoma treated by mastectomy (23). In another series of 573 patients with invasive ductal carcinoma treated by mastectomy, no significant relationship was noted between the extent of intraductal involvement and either recurrence or survival (571). Similarly, among 533 patients with invasive carcinoma treated with conservative surgery and radiation therapy, the presence of an extensive intraductal component was not associated with the risk of distant metastasis in a multiple logistic regression analysis (572). Therefore, although the extent of associated DCIS is a consideration in the local management of patients treated with breast-conserving therapy, it does not appear to be a significant prognostic factor with regard to distant metastasis or survival.

Combining Prognostic Factors

Although a variety of prognostic factors have been reported for patients with invasive breast cancer, how best to integrate these factors to assess patient outcome and formulate therapeutic decisions is an unresolved issue (573). Several authors have developed prognostic indices for this purpose, which take into account various combinations of factors. One of these, the Nottingham Prognostic Index, takes into consideration tumor size, lymph node status, and histologic grade. This index has been used to stratify patients with breast cancer into good, moderate, and poor prognostic groups with annual mortality rates of 3%, 7%, and 30%, respectively (574). Another group of investigators has proposed a prognostic index that combines tumor size, lymph node status, and mitotic index (morphometric prognostic index) (575). This index has been shown to be a useful prognostic discriminator for premenopausal patients with both node-negative and node-positive disease. Although prognostic indices such as these have not yet been widely accepted into clinical practice, they represent important attempts to refine prognostication in patients with invasive breast cancer.

 # CONTENTS OF THE FINAL SURGICAL PATHOLOGY REPORT

The final surgical pathology report for specimens containing invasive breast cancer should include, in addition to the diagnosis, information needed for staging and therapeutic decision-making (576,577). The information used by clinicians in determining treatment options varies among different institutions. At a minimum, however, every surgical pathology report for specimens containing an invasive breast cancer should include the type of specimen submitted, laterality, specimen size, tumor size, histologic type, histologic grade, presence or absence of lymphatic vessel invasion, presence or absence of an extensive intraductal component (EIC), the status of the microscopic margins, and lymph node status (if applicable). In addition, for specimens removed because of the presence of mammographically detected microcalcifications, it is important to note the location of the calcifications (i.e., in association with invasive cancer, carcinoma *in situ*, benign breast ducts and lobules, stroma or blood vessels). If ancillary studies are in progress (e.g., hormone receptor assays, HER2, other prognostic markers), this should also be documented in the final report. The use of standardized, synoptic-type reports, either in addition to or in place of a narrative report, is encouraged (576,577).

References

1. Ellis IO, Schnitt SJ, Sastre-Garau X, Bussolati G,. Invasive breast carcinoma. In: Tavassoli FA, Devilee P, ed. *Tumours of the breast and female genital organs.* Lyon: IARC Press, 2003:13–59.
2. Wellings SR, Jensen HM, Marcum RG. An atlas of subgross pathology of the human breast with special reference to possible precancerous lesions. *J Natl Cancer Inst* 1975;55(2):231–273.
3. Fisher ER, Gregorio RM, Fisher B, et al. The pathology of invasive breast cancer. A syllabus derived from findings of the National Surgical Adjuvant Breast Project (protocol no. 4). *Cancer* 1975;36(1):1–85.
4. Rosen PP. The pathological classification of human mammary carcinoma: past, present, and future. *Ann Clin Lab Sci* 1979;9(2):144–156.
5. Page DL, Anderson TJ. *Diagnostic histopathology of the breast.* Edinburgh, Scotland: Churchill Livingstone, 1987.
6. Ellis IO, Galea M, Broughton N, et al. Pathological prognostic factors in breast cancer. II. Histological type. Relationship with survival in a large study with long term follow-up. *Histopathology* 1992;20(6):479–489.
7. Cady B, Stone MD, Schuler JG, et al. The new era in breast cancer. Invasion, size, and nodal involvement dramatically decreasing as a result of mammographic screening. *Arch Surg* 1996;131(3):301–308.
8. Tabar L, Duffy SW, Vitak B, et al. The natural history of breast carcinoma: what have we learned from screening? *Cancer* 1999;86(3):449–462.
9. Gilliland FD, Joste N, Stauber PM, et al. Biologic characteristics of interval and screen-detected breast cancers. *J Natl Cancer Inst* 2000;92(9):743–749.
10. Porter PL, El-Bastawissi AY, Mandelson MT, et al. Breast tumor characteristics as predictors of mammographic detection: comparison of interval- and screen-detected cancers. *J Natl Cancer Inst* 1999;91(23):2020–2028.
11. Ernst MF, Roukema JA, Coebergh JW, et al. Breast cancers found by screening: earlier detection, lower malignant potential or both? *Breast Cancer Res Treat* 2002;76(1):19–25.
12. Stierer M, Rosen HR, Weber R, et al. Long term analysis of factors influencing the outcome in carcinoma of the breast smaller than one centimeter. *Surg Gynecol Obstet* 1992;175(2):151–160.
13. Cowan WK, Kelly P, Sawan A, et al. The pathological and biological nature of screen-detected breast carcinomas: a morphological and immunohistochemical study. *J Pathol* 1997;182(1):29–35.
14. Mustafa IA, Cole B, Wanebo HJ, et al. The impact of histopathology on nodal metastases in minimal breast cancer. *Arch Surg* 1997;132(4):384–390; discussion 390–391.
15. Tan P, Cady B, Wanner M, et al. The cell cycle inhibitor p27 is an independent prognostic marker in small (T1a, b) invasive breast carcinomas. *Cancer Res* 1997;57(7):1259–1263.
16. Chen YY, Connolly JL, Harris J, et al. Predictors of axillary lymph node metastases (ALNM) in patients with breast cancers 1 cm or smaller (T1a, b): Implications for axillary dissection (Meeting Abstract). *Mod Pathol* 1998;78:17A.
17. Henson DE, Ries L, Freedman LS, Carriaga M. Relationship among outcome, stage of disease, and histologic grade for 22,616 cases of breast cancer. The basis for a prognostic index. *Cancer* 1991;68(10):2142–2149.
18. Rosner D, Lane WW. Should all patients with node-negative breast cancer receive adjuvant therapy? Identifying additional subsets of low-risk patients who are highly curable by surgery alone. *Cancer* 1991;68(7):1482–1494.
19. Tabar L, Fagerberg G, Duffy SW, et al. Update of the Swedish two-county program of mammographic screening for breast cancer. *Radiol Clin North Am* 1992;30(1):187–210.
20. Newcomer LM, Newcomb PA, Trentham-Dietz A, et al. Detection method and breast carcinoma histology. *Cancer* 2002;95(3):470–477.
21. Anderson TJ, Lamb J, Donnan P, et al. Comparative pathology of breast cancer in a randomised trial of screening. *Br J Cancer* 1991;64(1):108–113.
22. Ellis IO, Galea MH, Locker A. Early experience in breast cancer screening: emphasis on development of protocols for triple assessment. *Breast* 1993;2:148–153.
23. Silverberg SG, Chitale AR. Assessment of significance of proportions of intraductal and infiltrating tumor growth in ductal carcinoma of the breast. *Cancer* 1973;32(4):830–837.
24. Lampejo OT, Barnes DM, Smith P, et al. Evaluation of infiltrating ductal carcinomas with a DCIS component: correlation of the histologic type of the *in situ* component with grade of the infiltrating component. *Semin Diagn Pathol* 1994;11(3):215–222.
25. Moriya T, Silverberg SG. Intraductal carcinoma (ductal carcinoma *in situ*) of the breast. A comparison of pure noninvasive tumors with those including different proportions of infiltrating carcinoma. *Cancer* 1994;74(11):2972–2978.
26. Gupta SK, Douglas-Jones AG, Fenn N, et al. The clinical behavior of breast carcinoma is probably determined at the preinvasive stage (ductal carcinoma *in situ*). *Cancer* 1997;80(9):1740–1745.
27. Ravdin PM. Biomarkers. In: Silverstein MJ, ed. *Ductal carcinoma in situ of the breast.* Baltimore: Williams & Wilkins, 1997:51–57.
28. Lakhani SR, Stratton MR, Poller DN. Cytogenetics and molecular biology. In: Silverstein MJ, ed. *Ductal carcinoma in situ of the breast.* Baltimore: Williams & Wilkins, 1997:77–91.
29. O'Connell P, Pekkel V, Fuqua SA, et al. Analysis of loss of heterozygosity in 399 premalignant breast lesions at 15 genetic loci. *J Natl Cancer Inst* 1998;90(9):697–703.
30. Lakhani SR. The transition from hyperplasia to invasive carcinoma of the breast. *J Pathol* 1999;187(3):272–278.
31. Buerger H, Otterbach F, Simon R, et al. Different genetic pathways in the evolution of invasive breast cancer are associated with distinct morphological subtypes. *J Pathol* 1999;189(4):521–526.
32. Porter DA, Krop IE, Nasser S, et al. A SAGE (serial analysis of gene expression) view of breast tumor progression. *Cancer Res* 2001;61(15):5697–5702.
33. Ma XJ, Salunga R, Tuggle JT, et al. Gene expression profiles of human breast cancer progression. *Proc Natl Acad Sci U S A* 2003;100(10):5974–5979.
34. Simpson JF. Predictive utility of the histopathologic analysis of carcinoma of the breast. *Adv Pathol Lab Med* 1994;7:107.
35. Black MM, Speer FD. Nuclear structure in cancer tissues. *Surg Gynecol Obstet* 1957;105:97.
36. Cutler SJ, Black MM, Mork T, et al. Further observations on prognostic factors in cancer of the female breast. *Cancer* 1969;24(4):653–667.
37. Elston CW, Ellis IO. Assessment of histologic grade. In: Elston CW, Ellis IO, eds. *The breast.* Edinburgh: Churchill Livingstone, 1998:365–384.
38. Wheeler JE, Enterline HT. Lobular carcinoma of the breast in situ and infiltrating. *Pathol Annu* 1976;11:161–188.
39. Martinez V, Azzopardi JG. Invasive lobular carcinoma of the breast: incidence and variants. *Histopathology* 1979;3(6):467–488.
40. Foote FW, Jr, Foote FW. A histologic classification of carcinoma of the breast. Surgery 1946;19:74.

41. Fechner RE. Histologic variants of infiltrating lobular carcinoma of the breast. *Hum Pathol* 1975;6(3):373–378.
42. Steinbrecher JS, Silverberg SG. Signet-ring cell carcinoma of the breast. The mucinous variant of infiltrating lobular carcinoma? *Cancer* 1976;37(2):828–840.
43. Fisher ER, Gregorio RM, Redmond C, et al. Tubulolobular invasive breast cancer: a variant of lobular invasive cancer. *Hum Pathol* 1977;8(6):679–683.
44. Van Bogaert LJ, Maldague P. Infiltrating lobular carcinoma of the female breast. Deviations from the usual histopathologic appearance. *Cancer* 1980;45(5):979–984.
45. Merino MJ, Livolsi VA. Signet ring carcinoma of the female breast: a clinicopathologic analysis of 24 cases. *Cancer* 1981;48(8):1830–1837.
46. Dixon JM, Anderson TJ, Page DL, et al. Infiltrating lobular carcinoma of the breast. *Histopathology* 1982;6(2):149–161.
47. du Toit RS, Locker AP, Ellis IO, et al. Invasive lobular carcinomas of the breast—the prognosis of histopathological subtypes. *Br J Cancer* 1989;60(4):605–609.
48. Eusebi V, Magalhaes F, Azzopardi JG. Pleomorphic lobular carcinoma of the breast: an aggressive tumor showing apocrine differentiation. *Hum Pathol* 1992; 23(6):655–662.
49. Weidner N, Semple JP. Pleomorphic variant of invasive lobular carcinoma of the breast. *Hum Pathol* 1992;23(10):1167–1171.
50. Bentz JS, Yassa N, Clayton F. Pleomorphic lobular carcinoma of the breast: clinicopathologic features of 12 cases. *Mod Pathol* 1998;11(9):814–822.
51. Middleton LP, Palacios DM, Bryant BR, et al. Pleomorphic lobular carcinoma: morphology, immunohistochemistry, and molecular analysis. *Am J Surg Pathol* 2000;24(12):1650–1656.
52. Chen CL, Weiss NS, Newcomb P, et al. Hormone replacement therapy in relation to breast cancer. *JAMA* 2002;287(6):734–741.
53. Li CI, Malone KE, Porter PL, et al. Relationship between long durations and different regimens of hormone therapy and risk of breast cancer. *JAMA* 2003;289 (24):3254–3263.
54. Li CI, Anderson BO, Daling JR, et al. Trends in incidence rates of invasive lobular and ductal breast carcinoma. *JAMA* 2003;289(11):1421–1424.
55. Daling JR, Malone KE, Doody DR, et al. Relation of regimens of combined hormone replacement therapy to lobular, ductal, and other histologic types of breast carcinoma. *Cancer* 2002;95(12):2455–2464.
56. Ashikari R, Huvos AG, Urban JA, et al. Infiltrating lobular carcinoma of the breast. *Cancer* 1973;31(1):110–116.
57. Lesser ML, Rosen PP, Kinne DW. Multicentricity and bilaterality in invasive breast carcinoma. *Surgery* 1982;91(2):234–240.
58. Tinnemans JG, Wobbes T, van der Sluis RF, et al. Multicentricity in nonpalpable breast carcinoma and its implications for treatment. *Am J Surg* 1986;151(3): 334–338.
59. Gump FE, Shikora S, Habif DV, et al. The extent and distribution of cancer in breasts with palpable primary tumors. *Ann Surg* 1986;204(4):384–390.
60. Dixon JM, Anderson TJ, Page DL, et al. Infiltrating lobular carcinoma of the breast: an evaluation of the incidence and consequence of bilateral disease. *Br J Surg* 1983;70(9):513–516.
61. Arpino G, Bardou VJ, Clark GM, et al. Infiltrating lobular carcinoma of the breast: tumor characteristics and clinical outcome. Breast *Cancer Res* 2004;6(3): R149–R156.
62. Sastre-Garau X, Jouve M, Asselain B, et al. Infiltrating lobular carcinoma of the breast. Clinicopathologic analysis of 975 cases with reference to data on conservative therapy and metastatic patterns. *Cancer* 1996;77(1):113–120.
63. Peiro G, Bornstein BA, Connolly JL, et al. The influence of infiltrating lobular carcinoma on the outcome of patients treated with breast-conserving surgery and radiation therapy. *Breast Cancer Res Treat* 2000;59(1):49–54.
64. Newman W. Lobular carcinoma of the female breast. Report of 73 cases. *Ann Surg* 1966;164(2):305–314.
65. Davis RP, Nora PF, Kooy RG, et al. Experience with lobular carcinoma of the breast. Emphasis on recent aspects of management. *Arch Surg* 1979;114(4): 485–488.
66. DiCostanzo D, Rosen PP, Gareen I, et al. Prognosis in infiltrating lobular carcinoma. An analysis of "classical" and variant tumors. *Am J Surg Pathol* 1990; 14(1):12–23.
67. Azzopardi JG. *Problems in breast pathology*. Philadelphia: WB Saunders, 1979.
68. Mendelson EB, Harris KM, Doshi N, et al. Infiltrating lobular carcinoma: mammographic patterns with pathologic correlation. *AJR Am J Roentgenol* 1989;153 (2):265–271.
69. Hilleren DJ, Andersson IT, Lindholm K, et al. Invasive lobular carcinoma: mammographic findings in a 10-year experience. *Radiology* 1991;178(1):149–154.
70. Le Gal M, Ollivier L, Asselain B, et al. Mammographic features of 455 invasive lobular carcinomas. *Radiology* 1992;185(3):705–708.
71. Helvie MA, Paramagul C, Oberman HA, et al. Invasive lobular carcinoma. Imaging features and clinical detection. *Invest Radiol* 1993;28(3):202–207.
72. Krecke KN, Gisvold JJ. Invasive lobular carcinoma of the breast: mammographic findings and extent of disease at diagnosis in 184 patients. *AJR Am J Roentgenol* 1993;161(5):957–960.
73. White JR, Gustafson GS, Wimbish K, et al. Conservative surgery and radiation therapy for infiltrating lobular carcinoma of the breast. The role of preoperative mammograms in guiding treatment. *Cancer* 1994;74(2):640–647.
74. The world Health Organization Histological Typing of Breast Tumors—Second edition. The World Organization. *Am J Clin Pathol* 1982;78(6):806–816.
75. Moll R, Mitze M, Frixen UH, et al. Differential loss of E-cadherin expression in infiltrating ductal and lobular breast carcinomas. *Am J Pathol* 1993;143(6): 1731–1742.
76. Rasbridge SA, Gillett CE, Sampson SA, et al. Epithelial (E-) and placental (P-) cadherin cell adhesion molecule expression in breast carcinoma. *J Pathol* 1993;169(2):245–250.
77. Palacios J, Benito N, Pizarro A, et al. Anomalous expression of P-cadherin in breast carcinoma. Correlation with E-cadherin expression and pathological features. *Am J Pathol* 1995;146(3):605–612.
78. De Leeuw WJ, Berx G, Vos CB, et al. Simultaneous loss of E-cadherin and catenins in invasive lobular breast cancer and lobular carcinoma in situ. *J Pathol* 1997;183(4):404–411.
79. Berx G, Cleton-Jansen AM, Strumane K, et al. E-cadherin is inactivated in a majority of invasive human lobular breast cancers by truncation mutations throughout its extracellular domain. *Oncogene* 1996;13(9):1919–1925.
80. Nishizaki T, Chew K, Chu L, et al. Genetic alterations in lobular breast cancer by comparative genomic hybridization. *Int J Cancer* 1997;74(5):513–517.
81. Green I, McCormick B, Cranor M, et al. A comparative study of pure tubular and tubulolobular carcinoma of the breast. *Am J Surg Pathol* 1997;21(6):653–657.
82. Kuroda H, Tamaru J, Takeuchi I, et al. Expression of E-cadherin, alpha-catenin, and beta-catenin in tubulolobular carcinoma of the breast. *Virchows Arch* 2006;448(4):500–505.
83. Esposito NN, Chivukula M, Dabbs DJ. The ductal phenotypic expression of the E-cadherin/catenin complex in tubulolobular carcinoma of the breast: an immunohistochemical and clinicopathologic study. *Mod Pathol* 2007;20(1):130–138.
84. Hull MT, Seo IS, Battersby JS, Csicsko JF. Signet-ring cell carcinoma of the breast: a clinicopathologic study of 24 cases. *Am J Clin Pathol* 1980;73(1):31–35.
85. Raju U, Ma CK, Shaw A. Signet ring variant of lobular carcinoma of the breast: a clinicopathologic and immunohistochemical study. *Mod Pathol* 1993;6(5): 516–520.
86. Eltorky M, Hall JC, Osborne PT, et al. Signet-ring cell variant of invasive lobular carcinoma of the breast. A clinicopathologic study of 11 cases. *Arch Pathol Lab Med* 1994;118(3):245–248.
87. Frost AR, Terahata S, Yeh IT, et al. The significance of signet ring cells in infiltrating lobular carcinoma of the breast. *Arch Pathol Lab Med* 1995;119(1):64–68.
88. Eusebi V, Betts C, Haagensen DE Jr, et al. Apocrine differentiation in lobular carcinoma of the breast: a morphologic, immunologic, and ultrastructural study. *Hum Pathol* 1984;15(2):134–140.
89. Allenby PA, Chowdhury LN. Histiocytic appearance of metastatic lobular breast carcinoma. *Arch Pathol Lab Med* 1986;110(8):759–760.
90. Walford N, ten Velden J. Histiocytoid breast carcinoma: an apocrine variant of lobular carcinoma. *Histopathology* 1989;14(5):515–522.
91. Eusebi V, Foschini MP, Bussolati G, et al. Myoblastomatoid (histiocytoid) carcinoma of the breast. A type of apocrine carcinoma. *Am J Surg Pathol* 1995;19(5):553–562.
92. Pinder SE, Elston CW, Ellis IO. Invasive carcinoma—usual histological types. In: Elston CW, Ellis IO, eds. *The reast*. Edinburgh: Churchill Livingstone, 1998: 283–337.
93. Porter PL, Garcia R, Moe R, et al. C-erbB-2 oncogene protein in in situ and invasive lobular breast neoplasia. *Cancer* 1991;68(2):331–334.
94. Domagala W, Markiewski M, Kubiak R, et al. Immunohistochemical profile of invasive lobular carcinoma of the breast: predominantly vimentin and p53 protein negative, cathepsin D and oestrogen receptor positive. *Virchows Arch A Pathol Anat Histopathol* 1993;423(6):497–502.
95. Mazoujian G, Bodian C, Haagensen DE Jr, et al. Expression of GCDFP-15 in breast carcinomas. Relationship to pathologic and clinical factors. *Cancer* 1989;63(11):2156–2161.
96. Radhi JM. Immunohistochemical analysis of pleomorphic lobular carcinoma: higher expression of p53 and chromogranin and lower expression of ER and PgR. *Histopathology* 2000;36(2):156–160.
97. Reis-Filho JS, Simpson PT, Jones C, et al. Pleomorphic lobular carcinoma of the breast: role of comprehensive molecular pathology in characterization of an entity. *J Pathol* 2005;207(1):1–13.
98. Harris M, Howell A, Chrissohou M, et al. A comparison of the metastatic pattern of infiltrating lobular carcinoma and infiltrating duct carcinoma of the breast. *Br J Cancer* 1984;50(1):23–30.
99. Lamovec J, Bracko M. Metastatic pattern of infiltrating lobular carcinoma of the breast: an autopsy study. *J Surg Oncol* 1991;48(1):28–33.
100. Borst MJ, Ingold JA. Metastatic patterns of invasive lobular versus invasive ductal carcinoma of the breast. *Surgery* 1993;114(4):637–641; discussion 41–42.
101. Dixon AR, Ellis IO, Elston CW, et al. A comparison of the clinical metastatic patterns of invasive lobular and ductal carcinomas of the breast. *Br J Cancer* 1991;63(4):634–635.
102. Smith DB, Howell A, Harris M, et al. Carcinomatous meningitis associated with infiltrating lobular carcinoma of the breast. *Eur J Surg Oncol* 1985;11(1):33–36.
103. Lamovec J, Zidar A. Association of leptomeningeal carcinomatosis in carcinoma of the breast with infiltrating lobular carcinoma. An autopsy study. *Arch Pathol Lab Med* 1991;115(5):507–510.
104. Cormier WJ, Gaffey TA, Welch TA, et al. Linitis plastica caused by metastatic lobular carcinoma of the breast. *Mayo Clinic Proc* 1980;55:747.
105. Battifora H. Metastatic breast carcinoma to the stomach simulating linitis plastica. *Appl Immunohistochem* 1994;2:225.
106. Kumar NB, Hart WR. Metastases to the uterine corpus from extragenital cancers. A clinicopathologic study of 63 cases. *Cancer* 1982;50(10):2163–2169.
107. Rosen PP. *Rosen's breast pathology*. 2nd ed. Philadelphia, PA: Lippincott-Raven, 2001.
108. Silverstein MJ, Lewinsky BS, Waisman JR, et al. Infiltrating lobular carcinoma. Is it different from infiltrating duct carcinoma? *Cancer* 1994;73(6):1673–1677.
109. Schnitt S. Morphologic risk factors for local recurrence in patients with invasive breast cancer treated with conservative surgery and radiation therapy. *Breast J* 1997;3:261.
110. Weiss MC, Fowble BL, Solin LJ, et al. Outcome of conservative therapy for invasive breast cancer by histologic subtype. *Int J Radiat Oncol Biol Phys* 1992; 23(5):941–947.
111. Lehr HA, Folpe A, Yaziji H, et al. Cytokeratin 8 immunostaining pattern and E-cadherin expression distinguish lobular from ductal breast carcinoma. *Am J Clin Pathol* 2000;114(2):190–196.
112. Roylance R, Gorman P, Harris W, et al. Comparative genomic hybridization of breast tumors stratified by histological grade reveals new insights into the biological progression of breast cancer. *Cancer Res* 1999;59(7):1433–1436.
113. Roylance R, Gorman P, Papior T, et al. A comprehensive study of chromosome 16q in invasive ductal and lobular breast carcinoma using array CGH. *Oncogene* 2006;25(49):6544–6553.
114. Tobon H, Salazar H. Tubular carcinoma of the breast. Clinical, histological, and ultrastructural observations. *Arch Pathol Lab Med* 1977;101(6):310–316.
115. Cooper HS, Patchefsky AS, Krall RA. Tubular carcinoma of the breast. *Cancer* 1978;42(5):2334–2342.
116. Carstens PH. Tubular carcinoma of the breast. A study of frequency. *Am J Clin Pathol* 1978;70(2):204–210.
117. Parl FF, Richardson LD. The histologic and biologic spectrum of tubular carcinoma of the breast. *Hum Pathol* 1983;14(8):694–698.
118. McBoyle MF, Razek HA, Carter JL, et al. Tubular carcinoma of the breast: an institutional review. *Am Surg* 1997;63(7):639–44; discussion 44–45.
119. Patchefsky AS, Shaber GS, Schwartz GF, et al. The pathology of breast cancer detected by mass population screening. *Cancer* 1977;40(4):1659–1670.

120. Report of the Working Group to Review the National Cancer Institute-American Cancer Society Breast Cancer Detection Demonstration Projects. *J Natl Cancer Inst* 1979;62(3):639–709.
121. Rajakariar R, Walker RA. Pathological and biological features of mammographically detected invasive breast carcinomas. *Br J Cancer* 1995;71(1):150–154.
122. Feig SA, Shaber GS, Patchefsky A, et al. Analysis of clinically occult and mammographically occult breast tumors. *AJR Am J Roentgenol* 1977;128(3):403–408.
123. Taxy JB. Tubular carcinoma of the male breast: report of a case. *Cancer* 1975;36(2):462–465.
124. Carstens PH, Huvos AG, Foote FW Jr, et al. Tubular carcinoma of the breast: a clinicopathologic study of 35 cases. *Am J Clin Pathol* 1972;58(3):231–238.
125. Oberman HA, Fidler WJ, Jr. Tubular carcinoma of the breast. *Am J Surg Pathol* 1979;3(5):387–395.
126. Eusebi V, Betts CM, Bussolati G. Tubular carcinoma: a variant of secretory breast carcinoma. *Histopathology* 1979;3(5):407–419.
127. Lagios MD, Rose MR, Margolin FR. Tubular carcinoma of the breast: association with multicentricity, bilaterality, and family history of mammary carcinoma. *Am J Clin Pathol* 1980;73(1):25–30.
128. Peters GN, Wolff M, Haagensen CD. Tubular carcinoma of the breast. Clinical pathologic correlations based on 100 cases. *Ann Surg* 1981;193(2):138–149.
129. van Bogaert LJ. Clinicopathologic hallmarks of mammary tubular carcinoma. *Hum Pathol* 1982;13(6):558–562.
130. McDivitt RW, Boyce W, Gersell D. Tubular carcinoma of the breast. Clinical and pathological observations concerning 135 cases. *Am J Surg Pathol* 1982;6(5):401–411.
131. Deos PH, Norris HJ. Well-differentiated (tubular) carcinoma of the breast. A clinicopathologic study of 115 pure and mixed cases. *Am J Clin Pathol* 1982;78(1):1–7
132. Carstens PH, Greenberg RA, Francis D, et al. Tubular carcinoma of the breast. A long term follow-up. *Histopathology* 1985;9(3):271–280.
133. Gadaleanu V, Galatar N, Tzortzi E. Tubular carcinoma of the breast. *Morphologie et embryologie* 1985;31(3):197–204.
134. Elson BC, Helvie MA, Frank TS, et al. Tubular carcinoma of the breast: mode of presentation, mammographic appearance, and frequency of nodal metastases. *AJR Am J Roentgenol* 1993;161(6):1173–1176.
135. Leibman AJ, Lewis M, Kruse B. Tubular carcinoma of the breast: mammographic appearance. *AJR Am J Roentgenol* 1993;160(2):263–265.
136. Winchester DJ, Sahin AA, Tucker SL, et al. Tubular carcinoma of the breast. Predicting axillary nodal metastases and recurrence. *Ann Surg* 1996;223(3):342–347.
137. Berger AC, Miller SM, Harris MN, et al. Axillary dissection for tubular carcinoma of teh breast. *Breast J* 1996;2:204.
138. Feig SA, Shaver GS, Patchefsky AS. Tubular carcinoma of the breast: mode of presentation, mammographic appearance and pathologic correlation. *Diagn Radiol* 1993;129:311.
139. Claus EB, Risch N, Thompson WD, et al. Relationship between breast histopathology and family history of breast cancer. *Cancer* 1993;71(1):147–153.
140. Visfeldt J, Scheike O. Male breast cancer. I. Histologic typing and grading of 187 Danish cases. *Cancer* 1973;32(4):985–990.
141. Tremblay G. Elastosis in tubular carcinoma of the breast. *Arch Pathol* 1974;98(5):302–307.
142. Schnitt SJ, Collins LC. Columnar cell lesions and flat epithelial atypia of the breast. *Semin Breat Dis* 2005;8:100–111.
143. Egan RL, Ellis JT, Powell RW. Team approach tthe study of diseases of the breast. *Cancer* 1969;23(4):847–854.
144. Taylor HB, Norris HJ. Well-differentiated carcinoma of the breast. *Cancer* 1970;25(3):687–692.
145. Reiner A, Reiner G, Spona J, et al. Histopathologic characterization of human breast cancer in correlation with estrogen receptor status. A comparison of immunocytochemical and biochemical analysis. *Cancer* 1988;61(6):1149–1154.
146. Helin HJ, Helle MJ, Kallioniemi OP, et al. Immunohistochemical determination of estrogen and progesterone receptors in human breast carcinoma. Correlation with histopathology and DNA flow cytometry. *Cancer* 1989;63(9):1761–1767.
147. Stierer M, Rosen H, Weber R, et al. Immunohistochemical and biochemical measurement of estrogen and progesterone receptors in primary breast cancer. Correlation of histopathology and prognostic factors. *Ann Surg* 1993;218(1):13–21.
148. Diab SG, Clark GM, Osborne CK, et al. Tumor characteristics and clinical outcome of tubular and mucinous breast carcinomas. *J Clin Oncol* 1999;17(5):1442–1448.
149. Soomro S, Shousha S, Taylor P, et al. c-erbB-2 expression in different histological types of invasive breast carcinoma. *J Clin Pathol* 1991;44(3):211–214.
150. Somerville JE, Clarke LA, Biggart JD. c-erbB-2 overexpression and histological type of *in situ* and invasive breast carcinoma. *J Clin Pathol* 1992;45(1):16–20.
151. Rosen PP, Lesser ML, Arroyo CD, et al. p53 in node-negative breast carcinoma: an immunohistochemical study of epidemiologic risk factors, histologic features, and prognosis. *J Clin Oncol* 1995;13(4):821–830.
152. Adeyinka A, Mertens F, Idvall I, et al. Cytogenetic findings in invasive breast carcinomas with prognostically favourable histology: a less complex karyotypic pattern? *Int J Cancer* 1998;79(4):361–4.
153. Waldman FM, Hwang ES, Etzell J, et al. Genomic alterations in tubular breast carcinomas. *Hum Pathol* 2001;32(2):222–226.
154. Flotte TJ, Bell DA, Greco MA. Tubular carcinoma and sclerosing adenosis: the use of basal lamina as a differential feature. *Am J Surg Pathol* 1980;4(1):75–77.
155. Ekblom P, Miettinen M, Forsman L, et al. Basement membrane and apocrine epithelial antigens in differential diagnosis between tubular carcinoma and sclerosing adenosis of the breast. *J Clin Pathol* 1984;37(4):357–363.
156. O'Leary TJ, Mikel UV, Becker RL. Computer-assisted image interpretation: use of a neural network to differentiate tubular carcinoma from sclerosing adenosis. *Mod Pathol* 1992;5(4):402–405.
157. Eusebi V, Foschini MP, Betts CM, et al. Microglandular adenosis, apocrine adenosis, and tubular carcinoma of the breast. An immunohistochemical comparison. *Am J Surg Pathol* 1993;17(2):99–109.
158. Kouchoukos NT, Ackerman LV, Butcher HR, Jr. Prediction of axillary nodal metastases from the morphology of primary mammary carcinomas. Guide to operative therapy. *Cancer* 1967;20(6):948–960.
159. Rosen PP, Groshen S, Kinne DW, et al. Factors influencing prognosis in node-negative breast carcinoma: analysis of 767 T1N0M0/T2N0M0 patients with long-term follow-up. *J Clin Oncol* 1993;11(11):2090–2100.
160. Haffty BG, Perrotta PL, Ward BE, et al. Conservatively treated breast cancer: outcome by histologic subtype. *Breast J* 1997;3:7.
161. Fisher ER, Anderson S, Redmond C, et al. Pathologic findings from the National Surgical Adjuvant Breast Project protocol B-06. 10-year pathologic and clinical prognostic discriminants. *Cancer* 1993;71(8):2507–2514.
162. Cabral AH, Recine M, Paramo JC, et al. Tubular carcinoma of the breast: an institutional experience and review of the literature. *Breast J* 2003;9(4):298–301.
163. Thurman SA, Schnitt SJ, Connolly JL, et al. Outcome after breast-conserving therapy for patients with stage I or II mucinous, medullary, or tubular breast carcinoma. *Int J Radiat Oncol Biol Phys* 2004;59(1):152–159.
164. Norris HJ, Taylor HB. Prognosis of mucinous (gelatinous) carcinoma of the breast. *Cancer* 1965;18:879.
165. Silverberg SG, Kay S, Chitale AR, et al. Colloid carcinoma of the breast. *Am J Clin Pathol* 1971;55(3):355–363.
166. Rasmussen BB. Human mucinous breast carcinomas and their lymph node metastases. A histological review of 247 cases. *Pathol Res Pract* 1985;180(4):377–382.
167. Clayton F. Pure mucinous carcinomas of breast: morphologic features and prognostic correlates. *Hum Pathol* 1986;17(1):34–38.
168. Rasmussen BB, Rose C, Christensen IB. Prognostic factors in primary mucinous breast carcinoma. *Am J Clin Pathol* 1987;87(2):155–160.
169. Komaki K, Sakamoto G, Sugano H, et al. Mucinous carcinoma of the breast in Japan. A prognostic analysis based on morphologic features. *Cancer* 1988;61(5):989–996.
170. Toikkanen S, Kujari H. Pure and mixed mucinous carcinomas of the breast: a clinicopathologic analysis of 61 cases with long-term follow-up. *Hum Pathol* 1989;20(8):758–764.
171. Andre S, Cunha F, Bernardo M, et al. Mucinous carcinoma of the breast: a pathologic study of 82 cases. *J Surg Oncol* 1995;58(3):162–167.
172. Fentiman IS, Millis RR, Smith P, et al. Mucoid breast carcinomas: histology and prognosis. *Br J Cancer* 1997;75(7):1061–1065.
173. Avisar E, Khan MA, Axelrod D, et al. Pure mucinous carcinoma of the breast: a clinicopathologic correlation study. *Ann Surg Oncol* 1998;5(5):447–451.
174. Northridge ME, Rhoads GG, Wartenberg D, et al. The importance of histologic type on breast cancer survival. *J Clin Epidemiol* 1997;50(3):283–290.
175. Di Saverio S, Gutierrez J, Avisar E. A retrospective review with long term follow-up of 11,400 cases of pure mucinous breast carcinoma. *Breast Cancer Res Treat* 2008;111(3):541–547.
176. Wilson TE, Helvie MA, Oberman HA, et al. Pure and mixed mucinous carcinoma of the breast: pathologic basis for differences in mammographic appearance. *AJR Am J Roentgenol* 1995;165(2):285–289.
177. Cardenosa G, Doudna C, Eklund GW. Mucinous (colloid) breast cancer: clinical and mammographic findings in 10 patients. *AJR Am J Roentgenol* 1994;162(5):1077–1079.
178. Goodman DN, Boutross-Tadross O, Jong RA. Mammographic features of pure mucinous carcinoma of the breast with pathological correlation. *Can Assoc Radiol J* 1995;46(4):296–301.
179. Chopra S, Evans AJ, Pinder SE, et al. Pure mucinous breast cancer-mammographic and ultrasound findings. *Clin Radiol* 1996;51(6):421–424.
180. Rosen PP, Oberman HA. *Tumors of the mammary gland*. Washington, DC: Armed Forces Institute of Pathology, 1993.
181. Rosen PP. Mucocele-like tumors of the breast. *Am J Surg Pathol* 1986;10(7):464–469.
182. Ro JY, Sneige N, Sahin AA, et al. Mucocelelike tumor of the breast associated with atypical ductal hyperplasia or mucinous carcinoma. A clinicopathologic study of seven cases. *Arch Pathol Lab Med* 1991;115(2):137–140.
183. Toikkanen S, Eerola E, Ekfors TO. Pure and mixed mucinous breast carcinomas: DNA stemline and prognosis. *J Clin Pathol* 1988;41(3):300–303.
184. Fujii H, Anbazhagan R, Bornman DM, et al. Mucinous cancers have fewer genomic alterations than more common classes of breast cancer. *Breast Cancer Res Treat* 2002;76(3):255–260.
185. Scopsi L, Andreola S, Pilotti S, et al. Mucinous carcinoma of the breast. A clinicopathologic, histochemical, and immunocytochemical study with special reference to neuroendocrine differentiation. *Am J Surg Pathol* 1994;18(7):702–711.
186. Sharnhorst D, Huntrakoon M. Mucinous carcinoma of the breast: recurrence 30 years after mastectomy. *South Med J* 1988;81:656.
187. Kurtz JM, Jacquemier J, Torhorst J, et al. Conservation therapy for breast cancers other than infiltrating ductal carcinoma. *Cancer* 1989;63(8):1630–1635.
188. Deck JH, Lee MA. Mucin embolism to cerebral arteries: a fatal complication of carcinoma of the breast. *Can J Neurol Sci* 1978;5(3):327–330.
189. Towfighi J, Simmonds MA, Davidson EA. Mucin and fat emboli in mucinous carcinomas. Cause of hemorrhagic cerebral infarcts. *Arch Pathol Lab Med* 1983;107(12):646–649.
190. Hawes D, Robinson R, Wira R. Pseudomyxoma peritonei from metastatic colloid carcinoma of the breast. *Gastrointest Radiol* 1991;16(1):80–82.
191. Richardson WW. Medullary carcinoma of the breast. A distinctive tumor type with a relatively good prognosis following radical mastectomy. *Br J Cancer* 1956;10:415.
192. Bloom HJ, Richardson WW, Field JR. Host resistance and survival in carcinoma of breast: a study of 104 cases of medullary carcinoma in a series of 1,411 cases of breast cancer followed for 20 years. *BMJ* 1970;3(716):181–188.
193. Ridolfi RL, Rosen PP, Port A, et al. Medullary carcinoma of the breast: a clinicopathologic study with 10 year follow-up. *Cancer* 1977;40(4):1365–1385.
194. Maier WP, Rosemond GP, Goldman LI, et al. A ten year study of medullary carcinoma of the breast. *Surg Gynecol Obstet* 1977;144(5):695–698.
195. Rapin V, Contesso G, Mouriesse H, et al. Medullary breast carcinoma. A reevaluation of 95 cases of breast cancer with inflammatory stroma. *Cancer* 1988;61(12):2503–2510.
196. Wargotz ES, Silverberg SG. Medullary carcinoma of the breast: a clinicopathologic study with appraisal of current diagnostic criteria. *Hum Pathol* 1988;19(11):1340–1346.
197. Pedersen L, Holck S, Schiodt T, et al. Medullary carcinoma of the breast, prognostic importance of characteristic histopathological features evaluated in a multivariate Cox analysis. *Eur J Cancer* 1994;30A(12):1792–1707.
198. Pedersen L, Zedeler K, Holck S, et al. Medullary carcinoma of the breast. Prevalence and prognostic importance of classical risk factors in breast cancer. *Eur J Cancer* 1995;31A(13–14):2289–2295.
199. Pedersen L, Holck S, Schiodt T, et al. Inter- and intraobserver variability in the histopathological diagnosis of medullary carcinoma of the breast, and its prognostic implications. *Breast Cancer Res Treat* 1989;14(1):91–99.

200. Pedersen L, Zedeler K, Holck S, et al. Medullary carcinoma of the breast, proposal for a new simplified histopathological definition. Based on prognostic observations and observations on inter- and intraobserver variability of 11 histopathological characteristics in 131 breast carcinomas with medullary features. *Br J Cancer* 1991;63(4):591–595.
201. Fisher ER, Kenny JP, Sass R, et al. Medullary cancer of the breast revisited. *Breast Cancer Res Treat* 1990;16(3):215–229.
202. Rigaud C, Theobald S, Noel P, et al. Medullary carcinoma of the breast. A multicenter study of its diagnostic consistency. *Arch Pathol Lab Med* 1993;117(10): 1005–1008.
203. Gaffey MJ, Mills SE, Frierson HF Jr, et al. Medullary carcinoma of the breast: interobserver variability in histopathologic diagnosis. *Mod Pathol* 1995;8(1):31–38.
204. Crotty TB. Medullary carcinoma: is it a reproducible and prognostically significant type of mammary carcinoma? *Adv Anat Pathol* 1996;3:179.
205. Jensen ML, Kiaer H, Andersen J, et al. Prognostic comparison of three classifications for medullary carcinomas of the breast. *Histopathology* 1997;30(6):523–532.
206. Schwartz GF. Solid circumscribed carcinoma of the breast. *Ann Surg* 1969; 169(2):165–173.
207. Neuman ML, Homer MJ. Association of medullary carcinoma with reactive axillary adenopathy. *AJR Am J Roentgenol* 1996;167(1):185–186.
208. Shousha S. Medullary carcinoma of the breast and *BRCA1* mutation. *Histopathology* 2000;37(2):182–185.
209. Honrado E, Benitez J, Palacios J. The molecular pathology of hereditary breast cancer: genetic testing and therapeutic implications. *Mod Pathol* 2005;18(10): 1305–1320.
210. Lakhani SR, Jacquemier J, Sloane JP, et al. Multifactorial analysis of differences between sporadic breast cancers and cancers involving *BRCA1* and *BRCA2* mutations. *J Natl Cancer Inst* 1998;90(15):1138–1145.
211. Armes JE, Egan AJ, Southey MC, et al. The histologic phenotypes of breast carcinoma occurring before age 40 years in women with and without *BRCA1* or *BRCA2* germline mutations: a population-based study. *Cancer* 1998;83(11): 2335–2345.
212. Meyer JE, Amin E, Lindfors KK, et al. Medullary carcinoma of the breast: mammographic and US appearance. *Radiology* 1989;170(1 Pt 1):79–82.
213. Kopans DB. *Breast imaging*. 2nd ed. Philadelphia: Lippincott-Raven Publishers, 1997.
214. Rubens JR, Lewandrowski KB, Kopans DB, et al. Medullary carcinoma of the breast. Overdiagnosis of a prognostically favorable neoplasm. *Arch Surg* 1990; 125(5):601–604.
215. Rodriguez-Pinilla SM, Rodriguez-Gil Y, Moreno-Bueno G, et al. Sporadic invasive breast carcinomas with medullary features display a basal-like phenotype: an immunohistochemical and gene amplification study. *Am J Surg Pathol* 2007; 31(4):501–508.
216. Jacquemier J, Padovani L, Rabayrol L, et al. Typical medullary breast carcinomas have a basal/myoepithelial phenotype. *J Pathol* 2005;207(3):260–268.
217. Bertucci F, Finetti P, Cervera N, et al. Gene expression profiling shows medullary breast cancer is a subgroup of basal breast cancers. *Cancer Res* 2006;66(9): 4636–4644.
218. Vincent-Salomon A, Gruel N, Lucchesi C, et al. Identification of typical medullary breast carcinoma as a genomic sub-group of basal-like carcinomas, a heterogeneous new molecular entity. *Breast Cancer Res Treat* 2007;9:R24.
219. Vu-Nishino H, Tavassoli FA, Ahrens WA, et al. Clinicopathologic features and long-term outcome of patients with medullary breast carcinoma managed with breast-conserving therapy (BCT). *Int J Radiat Oncol Biol Phys* 2005;62(4): 1040–1047.
220. Page DL, Dixon JM, Anderson TJ, et al. Invasive cribriform carcinoma of the breast. *Histopathology* 1983;7(4):525–536.
221. Venable JG, Schwartz AM, Silverberg SG. Infiltrating cribriform carcinoma of the breast: a distinctive clinicopathologic entity. *Hum Pathol* 1990;21(3):333–338.
222. Nishimura R, Ohsumi S, Teramoto N, et al. Invasive cribriform carcinoma with extensive microcalcifications in the male breast. *Breast Cancer* 2005;12(2): 145–148.
223. Stutz JA, Evans AJ, Pinder S, et al. The radiological appearances of invasive cribriform carcinoma of the breast. Nottingham Breast Team. *Clin Radiol* 1994; 49(10):693–695.
224. Boyages J, Recht A, Connolly JL, et al. Early breast cancer: predictors of breast recurrence for patients treated with conservative surgery and radiation therapy. *Radiother Oncol* 1990;19(1):29–41.
225. Gatchell FG, Dockerty MB, Clagett OT. Intracystic carcinoma of the breast. *Surg Gynecol Obstet* 1958;106:347.
226. Czernobilsky B. Intracystic carcinoma of the female breast. *Surg Gynecol Obstet* 1967;124(1):93–98.
227. McKittrick JE, Doane WA, Failing RM. Intracystic papillary carcinoma of the breast. *Am Surg* 1969;35(3):195–202.
228. Hunter CE, Jr., Sawyers JL. Intracystic papillary carcinoma of the breast. *South Med J* 1980;73(11):1484–1486.
229. Carter D, Orr SL, Merino MJ. Intracystic papillary carcinoma of the breast. After mastectomy, radiotherapy or excisional biopsy alone. *Cancer* 1983;52(1): 14–19.
230. Lefkowitz M, Lefkowitz W, Wargotz ES. Intraductal (intracystic) papillary carcinoma of the breast and its variants: a clinicopathological study of 77 cases. *Hum Pathol* 1994;25(8):802–809.
231. Leal C, Costa I, Fonseca D, et al. Intracystic (encysted) papillary carcinoma of the breast: a clinical, pathological, and immunohistochemical study. *Hum Pathol* 1998;29(10):1097–1104.
232. Fisher ER, Palekar AS, Redmond C, Barton B, Fisher B. Pathologic findings from the National Surgical Adjuvant Breast Project (protocol no. 4). VI. Invasive papillary cancer. *Am J Clin Pathol* 1980;73(3):313–322.
233. Schneider JA. Invasive papillary breast carcinoma: mammographic and sonographic appearance. *Radiology* 1989;171(2):377–379.
234. Mitnick JS, Vazquez MF, Harris MN, et al. Invasive papillary carcinoma of the breast: mammographic appearance. *Radiology* 1990;177(3):803–806.
235. McCulloch GL, Evans AJ, Yeoman L, et al. Radiological features of papillary carcinoma of the breast. *Clin Radiol* 1997;52(11):865–868.
236. Fisher ER, Costantino J, Fisher B, et al. Pathologic findings from the National Surgical Adjuvant Breast Project (Protocol 4). Discriminants for 15-year survival. National Surgical Adjuvant Breast and Bowel Project Investigators. *Cancer* 1993;71(6 Suppl):2141–2150.
237. Siriaunkgul S, Tavassoli FA. Invasive micropapillary carcinoma of the breast. *Mod Pathol* 1993;6(6):660–662.
238. Luna-More S, Gonzalez B, Acedo C, et al. Invasive micropapillary carcinoma of the breast. A new special type of invasive mammary carcinoma. *Pathol Res Pract* 1994;190(7):668–674.
239. Middleton LP, Tressera F, Sobel ME, et al. Infiltrating micropapillary carcinoma of the breast. *Mod Pathol* 1999;12(5):499–504.
240. Paterakos M, Watkin WG, Edgerton SM, et al. Invasive micropapillary carcinoma of the breast: a prognostic study. *Hum Pathol* 1999;30(12):1459–1463.
241. Walsh MM, Bleiweiss IJ. Invasive micropapillary carcinoma of the breast: eighty cases of an underrecognized entity. *Hum Pathol* 2001;32(6):583–589.
242. Nassar H, Wallis T, Andea A, et al. Clinicopathologic analysis of invasive micropapillary differentiation in breast carcinoma. *Mod Pathol* 2001;14(9): 836–841.
243. Luna-More S, de los Santos F, Breton JJ, et al. Estrogen and progesterone receptors, c-erbB-2, p53, and Bcl-2 in thirty-three invasive micropapillary breast carcinomas. *Pathol Res Pract* 1996;192(1):27–32.
244. Luna-More S, Casquero S, Perez-Mellado A, et al. Importance of estrogen receptors for the behavior of invasive micropapillary carcinoma of the breast. Review of 68 cases with follow-up of 54. *Pathol Res Pract* 2000;196(1):35–39.
245. Pettinato G, Manivel CJ, Panico L, et al. Invasive micropapillary carcinoma of the breast: clinicopathologic study of 62 cases of a poorly recognized variant with highly aggressive behavior. *Am J Clin Pathol* 2004;121(6):857–866.
246. Lee AH, Paish EC, Marchio C, et al. The expression of Wilms' tumour-1 and Ca125 in invasive micropapillary carcinoma of the breast. *Histopathology* 2007;51(6):824–828.
247. Cornog JL, Mobini J, Steiger E, Enterline HT. Squamous carcinoma of the breast. *Am J Clin Pathol* 1971;55(4):410–417.
248. Hasleton PS, Misch KA, Vasudev KS, et al. Squamous carcinoma of the breast. *J Clin Pathol* 1978;31(2):116–124.
249. Toikkanen S. Primary squamous cell carcinoma of the breast. *Cancer* 1981; 48(7):1629–1632.
250. Bogomoletz WV. Pure squamous cell carcinoma of the breast. *Arch Pathol Lab Med* 1982;106(2):57–59.
251. Eggers JW, Chesney TM. Squamous cell carcinoma of the breast: a clinicopathologic analysis of eight cases and review of the literature. *Hum Pathol* 1984; 15(6):526–531.
252. Shousha S, James AH, Fernandez MD, et al. Squamous cell carcinoma of the breast. *Arch Pathol Lab Med* 1984;108(11):893–896.
253. Eusebi V, Lamovec J, Cattani MG, et al. Acantholytic variant of squamous-cell carcinoma of the breast. *Am J Surg Pathol* 1986;10(12):855–861.
254. Wargotz ES, Norris HJ. Metaplastic carcinomas of the breast. IV. Squamous cell carcinoma of ductal origin. *Cancer* 1990;65(2):272–276.
255. Gersell DJ, Katzenstein AL. Spindle cell carcinoma of the breast. A clinocopathologic and ultrastructural study. *Hum Pathol* 1981;12(6):550–561.
256. Merino MJ, LiVolsi VA, Kennedy S, et al. Spindle-cell carcinoma of the breast: a clinicopathologic, ultrastructural and immunohistochemical study of eight cases. *Surg Pathol* 1988;1:193.
257. Bauer TW, Rostock RA, Eggleston JC, et al. Spindle cell carcinoma of the breast: four cases and review of the literature. *Hum Pathol* 1984;15(2):147–152.
258. Wargotz ES, Deos PH, Norris HJ. Metaplastic carcinomas of the breast. II. Spindle cell carcinoma. *Hum Pathol* 1989;20(8):732–740.
259. Huvos AG, Lucas JC Jr, Foote FW Jr. Metaplastic breast carcinoma. Rare form of mammary cancer. *N Y State J Med* 1973;73(9):1078–1082.
260. Kahn LB, Uys CJ, Dale J, et al. Carcinoma of the breast with metaplasia to chondrosarcoma: a light and electron microscopic study. *Histopathology* 1978;2(2): 93–106.
261. Kaufman MW, Marti JR, Gallager HS, et al. Carcinoma of the breast with pseudosarcomatous metaplasia. *Cancer* 1984;53(9):1908–1917.
262. Oberman HA. Metaplastic carcinoma of the breast. A clinicopathologic study of 29 patients. *Am J Surg Pathol* 1987;11(12):918–929.
263. Wargotz ES, Norris HJ. Metaplastic carcinomas of the breast. I. Matrix-producing carcinoma. *Hum Pathol* 1989;20(7):628–635.
264. Wargotz ES, Norris HJ. Metaplastic carcinomas of the breast. III. Carcinosarcoma. *Cancer* 1989;64(7):1490–1499.
265. Pitts WC, Rojas VA, Gaffey MJ, et al. Carcinomas with metaplasia and sarcomas of the breast. *Am J Clin Pathol* 1991;95(5):623–632.
266. Foschini MP, Dina RE, Eusebi V. Sarcomatoid neoplasms of the breast: proposed definitions for biphasic and monophasic sarcomatoid mammary carcinomas. *Semin Diagn Pathol* 1993;10(2):128–136.
267. Wargotz ES, Norris HJ. Metaplastic carcinomas of the breast: V. Metaplastic carcinoma with osteoclastic giant cells. *Hum Pathol* 1990;21(11):1142–1150.
268. Chhieng C, Cranor M, Lesser ME, et al. Metaplastic carcinoma of the breast with osteocartilaginous heterologous elements. *Am J Surg Pathol* 1998;22(2):188–194.
269. Brenner RJ, Turner RR, Schiller V, et al. Metaplastic carcinoma of the breast: report of three cases. *Cancer* 1998;82(6):1082–1087.
270. Patterson SK, Tworek JA, Roubidoux MA, et al. Metaplastic carcinoma of the breast: mammographic appearance with pathologic correlation. *AJR Am J Roentgenol* 1997;169(3):709–712.
271. Flint A, Oberman HA, Davenport RD. Cytophotometric measurements of metaplastic carcinoma of the breast: correlation with pathologic features and clinical behavior. *Mod Pathol* 1988;1(3):193–197.
272. Zhuang Z, Lininger RA, Man YG, et al. Identical clonality of both components of mammary carcinosarcoma with differential loss of heterozygosity. *Mod Pathol* 1997;10(4):354–362.
273. Rosen PP, Ernsberger D. Low-grade adenosquamous carcinoma. A variant of metaplastic mammary carcinoma. *Am J Surg Pathol* 1987;11(5):351–358.
274. Van Hoeven KH, Drudis T, Cranor ML, et al. Low-grade adenosquamous carcinoma of the breast. A clinocopathologic study of 32 cases with ultrastructural analysis. *Am J Surg Pathol* 1993;17(3):248–258.
275. Drudis T, Arroyo C, Van Hoeven KH, et al. The pathology of low grade adenosquamous carcinoma of the breast. An immunohistochemical study. *Pathology Annual* 1994;29(Pt2):181–197.
276. Ruffolo EF, Koerner FC, Maluf HM. Metaplastic carcinoma of the breast with melanocytic differentiation. *Mod Pathol* 1997;10(6):592–596.
277. Gobbi H, Simpson JF, Borowsky A, et al. Metaplastic breast tumors with a dominant fibromatosis-like phenotype have a high risk of local recurrence. *Cancer* 1999;85(10):2170–2182.

278. Sneige N, Yazyji H, Mandavilli SR, et al. Low-grade (fibromatosis-like) spindle cell carcinoma of the breast. *Am J Surg Pathol* 2001;25(8):1009–1016.
279. Carter MR, Hornick JL, Lester S, et al. Spindle cell (sarcomatoid) carcinoma of the breast: a clinicopathologic and immunohistochemical analysis of 29 cases. *Am J Surg Pathol* 2006;30(3):300–309.
280. Mavligit GM, Cohen JL, Sherwood LM. Ectopic production of parathyroid hormone by carcinoma of the breast. *N Engl J Med* 1971;285(3):154–156.
281. Coombes RC, Easty GC, Detre SI, et al. Secretion of immunoreactive calcitonin by human breast carcinomas. *BMJ* 1975;4(5990):197–199.
282. Kaneko H, Hojo H, Ishikawa S, et al. Norepinephrine-producing tumors of bilateral breasts: a case report. *Cancer* 1978;41(5):2002–2007.
283. Cohle SD, Tschen JA, Smith FE, et al. ACTH-secreting carcinoma of the breast. *Cancer* 1979;43(6):2370–2376.
284. Woodard BH, Eisenbarth G, Wallace NR, et al. Adrenocorticotropin production by a mammary carcinoma. *Cancer* 1981;47(7):1823–1827.
285. Partanen S, Syrjanen K. Argyrophilic cells in carcinoma of the female breast. *Virchows Arch A Pathol Anat Histol* 1981;391(1):45–51.
286. Clayton F, Sibley RK, Ordonez NG, et al. Argyrophilic breast carcinomas: evidence of lactational differentiation. *Am J Surg Pathol* 1982;6(4):323–333.
287. Toyoshima S. Mammary carcinoma with argyrophil cells. *Cancer* 1983;52(11): 2129–2138.
288. Fetissof F, Dubois MP, Arbeille-Brassart B, et al. Argyrophilic cells in mammary carcinoma. *Hum Pathol* 1983;14(2):127–134.
289. Bussolati G, Papotti M, Sapino A, et al. Endocrine markers in argyrophilic carcinomas of the breast. *Am J Surg Pathol* 1987;11(4):248–256.
290. Maluf HM, Zukerberg LR, Dickersin GR, et al. Spindle-cell argyrophilic mucin-producing carcinoma of the breast. Histological, ultrastructural, and immunohistochemical studies of two cases. *Am J Surg Pathol* 1991;15(7):677–686.
291. Scopsi L, Andreola S, Saccozzi R, et al. Argyrophilic carcinoma of the male breast. A neuroendocrine tumor containing predominantly chromogranin B (secretogranin I). *Am J Surg Pathol* 1991;15(11):1063–1071.
292. Scopsi L, Andreola S, Pilotti S, et al. Argyrophilia and granin (chromogranin/secretogranin) expression in female breast carcinomas. Their relationship to survival and other disease parameters. *Am J Surg Pathol* 1992;16(6):561–576.
293. Fisher ER, Palekar AS. Solid and mucinous varieties of so-called mammary carcinoid tumors. *Am J Clin Pathol* 1979;72(6):909–916.
294. Taxy JB, Tischler AS, Insalaco SJ, et al. "Carcinoid" tumor of the breast. A variant of conventional breast cancer? *Hum Pathol* 1981;12(2):170–179.
295. Azzopardi JG, Muretto P, Goddeeris P, et al. 'Carcinoid' tumours of the breast: the morphological spectrum of argyrophil carcinomas. *Histopathology* 1982;6(5): 549–569.
296. Bussolati G, Gugliotta P, Sapino A, et al. Chromogranin-reactive endocrine cells in argyrophilic carcinomas ("carcinoids") and normal tissue of the breast. *Am J Pathol* 1985;120(2):186–192.
297. Jablon LK, Somers RG, Kim PY. Carcinoid tumor of the breast: treatment with breast conservation in three patients. *Ann Surg Oncol* 1998;5(3):261–264.
298. Miremadi A, Pinder SE, Lee AH, et al. Neuroendocrine differentiation and prognosis in breast adenocarcinoma. *Histopathology* 2002;40(3):215–222.
299. Feczko JD, Rosales RN, Cramer HM, et al. Fine needle aspiration cytology of a male breast carcinoma exhibiting neuroendocrine differentiation. Report of a case with immunohistochemical, flow cytometric and ultrastructural analysis. *Acta Cytol* 1995;39(4):803–808.
300. Sapino A, Bussolati G. Is detection of endocrine cells in breast adenocarcinoma of diagnostic and clinical significance? *Histopathology* 2002;40(3):211–214.
301. Kashlan RB, Powell RW, Nolting SF. Carcinoid and other tumors metastatic to the breast. *J Surg Oncol* 1982;20(1):25–30.
302. Ordonez NG, Manning JT Jr, Raymond AK. Argentaffin endocrine carcinoma (carcinoid) of the pancreas with concomitant breast metastasis: an immunohistochemical and electron microscopic study. *Hum Pathol* 1985;16(7):746–751.
303. Fishman A, Kim HS, Girtanner RE, et al. Solitary breast metastasis as first manifestation of ovarian carcinoid tumor. *Gynecol Oncol* 1994;54(2):222–226.
304. Moreno A, Gonzalo MA, Sarasa JL, et al. Bilateral breast metastases as the first manifestation of an occult ileocecal carcinoid. *Medicina Clinica* 1995;104(13): 515–516.
305. Wozniak TC, Naunheim KS. Bronchial carcinoid tumor metastatic to the breast. *Ann Thorac Surg* 1998;65(4):1148–1149.
306. Rubio IT, Korourian S, Brown H, et al. Carcinoid tumor metastatic to the breast. *Arch Surg* 1998;133(10):1117–1119.
307. Yogore MG 3rd, Sahgal S. Small cell carcinoma of the male breast: report of a case. *Cancer* 1977;39(4):1748–1751.
308. Wade PM Jr, Mills SE, Read M, et al. Small cell neuroendocrine (oat cell) carcinoma of the breast. *Cancer* 1983;52(1):121–125.
309. Jundt G, Schulz A, Heitz PU, et al. Small cell neuroendocrine (oat cell) carcinoma of the male breast. Immunocytochemical and ultrastructural investigations. *Virchows Arch A Pathol Anat Histopathol* 1984;404(2):213–221.
310. Papotti M, Gherardi G, Eusebi V, et al. Primary oat cell (neuroendocrine) carcinoma of the breast. Report of four cases. *Virchows Arch A Pathol Anat Histopathol* 1992;420(1):103–108.
311. Francois A, Chatikhine VA, Chevallier B, et al. Neuroendocrine primary small cell carcinoma of the breast. Report of a case and review of the literature. *Am J Clin Oncol* 1995;18(2):133–138.
312. Carlson HJ, Trujillo YP, Taxy JB. Prolonged survival in a case of small cell carcinoma of the breast. *Breast J* 1996;2:160–163.
313. Shin SJ, DeLellis RA, Ying L, et al. Small cell carcinoma of the breast: a clinicopathologic and immunohistochemical study of nine patients. *Am J Surg Pathol* 2000;24(9):1231–1238.
314. Deeley TJ. Secondary deposits in the breast. *Br J Cancer* 1965;19(4):738–743.
315. Hajdu SI, Urban JA. Cancers metastatic to the breast. *Cancer* 1972;29(6): 1691–1696.
316. Birsak CA, Janssen PJ, van Vroonhoven CC, et al. Sex steroid receptor expression in 'carcinoid' tumors of the breast. *Breast Cancer Res Treat* 1996;40(3):243–249.
317. Wilander E, Lindgren A, Nister M, et al. Nuclear DNA and endocrine activity in carcinomas of the breast. *Cancer* 1984;54(6):1016–1018.
318. Shin SJ, DeLellis RA, Rosen PP. Small cell carcinoma of the breast—additional immunohistochemical studies. *Am J Surg Pathol* 2001;25(6):831–832.
319. Hoang MP, Sahin AA, Ordonez NG, et al. *HER-2/neu* gene amplification compared with HER-2/neu protein overexpression and interobserver reproducibility in invasive breast carcinoma. *Am J Clin Pathol* 2000;113(6):852–859.
320. Nayer HR. Cylindroma of the breast with pulmonary metastases. *Dis Chest* 1957;31:324.
321. Wilson WB, Spell JP. Adenoid cystic carcinoma of breast: a case with recurrence and regional metastasis. *Ann Surg* 1967;166(5):861–864.
322. Cavanzo FJ, Taylor HB. Adenoid cystic carcinoma of the breast. An analysis of 21 cases. *Cancer* 1969;24(4):740–745.
323. Friedman BA, Oberman HA. Adenoid cystic carcinoma of the breast. *Am J Clin Pathol* 1970;54(1):1–14.
324. Eisner B. Adenoid cystic carcinoma of the breast. *Pathologia Europaea* 1970;3:357.
325. Anthony PP, James PD. Adenoid cystic carcinoma of the breast: prevalence, diagnostic criteria, and histogenesis. *J Clin Pathol* 1975;28(8):647–655.
326. Qizilbash AH, Patterson MC, Oliveira KF. Adenoid cystic carcinoma of the breast. Light and electron microscopy and a brief review of the literature. *Arch Pathol Lab Med* 1977;101(6):302–306.
327. Hjorth S, Magnusson PH, Blomquist P. Adenoid cystic carcinoma of the breast. Report of a case in a male and review of the literature. *Acta Chir Scand* 1977;143(3):155–158.
328. Peters GN, Wolff M. Adenoid cystic carcinoma of the breast. Report of 11 new cases: review of the literature and discussion of biological behavior. *Cancer* 1983;52(4):680–686.
329. Wells CA, Nicoll S, Ferguson DJ. Adenoid cystic carcinoma of the breast: a case with axillary lymph node metastasis. *Histopathology* 1986;10(4):415–424.
330. Sumpio BE, Jennings TA, Merino MJ, et al. Adenoid cystic carcinoma of the breast. Data from the Connecticut Tumor Registry and a review of the literature. *Ann Surg* 1987;205(3):295–301.
331. Lamovec J, Us-Krasovec M, Zidar A, et al. Adenoid cystic carcinoma of the breast: a histologic, cytologic, and immunohistochemical study. *Semin Diagn Pathol* 1989;6(2):153–164.
332. Due W, Herbst WD, Loy V, et al. Characterisation of adenoid cystic carcinoma of the breast by immunohistology. *J Clin Pathol* 1989;42(5):470–476.
333. Miliauskas JR, Leong AS. Adenoid cystic carcinoma in a juvenile male breast. *Pathology* 1991;23(4):298–301.
334. Pastolero G, Hanna W, Zbieranowski I, et al. Proliferative activity and p53 expression in adenoid cystic carcinoma of the breast. *Mod Pathol* 1996;9(3):215–219.
335. Lusted D. Structural and growth patterns of adenoid cystic carcinoma of breast. *Am J Clin Pathol* 1970;54(3):419–425.
336. Verani RR, Van der Bel-Kahn J. Mammary adenoid cystic carcinoma with unusual features. *Am J Clin Pathol* 1973;59(5):653–658.
337. Lim SK, Kovi J, Warner OG. Adenoid cystic carcinoma of breast with metastasis: a case report and review of the literature. *J Natl Med Assoc* 1979;71(4):329–330.
338. Zaloudek C, Oertel YC, Orenstein JM. Adenoid cystic carcinoma of the breast. *Am J Clin Pathol* 1984;81(3):297–307.
339. Koller M, Ram Z, Findler G, et al. Brain metastasis: a rare manifestation of adenoid cystic carcinoma of the breast. *Surg Neurol* 1986;26(5):470–472.
340. Ro JY, Silva EG, Gallager HS. Adenoid cystic carcinoma of the breast. *Hum Pathol* 1987;18(12):1276–1281.
341. Herzberg AJ, Bossen EH, Walther PJ. Adenoid cystic carcinoma of the breast metastatic to the kidney. A clinically symptomatic lesion requiring surgical management. *Cancer* 1991;68(5):1015–1020.
342. Tavassoli FA, Norris HJ. Mammary adenoid cystic carcinoma with sebaceous differentiation. A morphologic study of the cell types. *Arch Pathol Lab Med* 1986; 110(11):1045–1053.
343. Rosen PP. Adenoid cystic carcinoma of the breast. A morphologically heterogeneous neoplasm. *Pathology Annual* 1989;24(Pt 2):237–254.
344. Kasami M, Olson SJ, Simpson JF, et al. Maintenance of polarity and a dual cell population in adenoid cystic carcinoma of the breast: an immunohistochemical study. *Histopathology* 1998;32(3):232–238.
345. Kleer CG, Oberman HA. Adenoid cystic carcinoma of the breast: value of histologic grading and proliferative activity. *Am J Surg Pathol* 1998;22(5):569–575.
346. Trendell-Smith NJ, Peston D, et al. Adenoid cystic carcinoma of the breast: a tumour commonly devoid of oestrogen receptors and related proteins. *Histopathology* 1999;35(3):241–248.
347. Arpino G, Clark GM, Mohsin S, et al. Adenoid cystic carcinoma of the breast: molecular markers, treatment, and clinical outcome. *Cancer* 2002;94(8):2119–2127.
348. Shin SJ, Rosen PP. Solid variant of mammary adenoid cystic carcinoma with basaloid features: a study of nine cases. *Am J Surg Pathol* 2002;26(4): 413–420.
349. Clement PB, Young RH, Azzopardi JG. Collagenous spherulosis of the breast. *Am J Surg Pathol* 1987;11(6):411–417.
350. Harris M. Pseudoadenoid cystic carcinoma of the breast. *Arch Pathol Lab Med* 1977;101(6):307–309.
351. Azoulay S, Lae M, Freneaux P, et al. KIT is highly expressed in adenoid cystic carcinoma of the breast, a basal-like carcinoma associated with a favorable outcome. *Mod Pathol* 2005;18(12):1623–1631.
352. Mastropasqua MG, Maiorano E, Pruneri G, et al. Immunoreactivity for c-kit and p63 as an adjunct in the diagnosis of adenoid cystic carcinoma of the breast. *Mod Pathol* 2005;18(10):1277–1282.
353. Crisi GM, Marconi SA, Makari-Judson G, et al. Expression of c-kit in adenoid cystic carcinoma of the breast. *Am J Clin Pathol* 2005;124(5):733–739.
354. Mossler JA, Barton TK, Brinkhous AD, et al. Apocrine differentiation in human mammary carcinoma. *Cancer* 1980;46(11):2463–2471.
355. d'Amore ES, Terrier-Lacombe MJ, Travagli JP, et al. Invasive apocrine carcinoma of the breast: a long term follow-up study of 34 cases. *Breast Cancer Res Treat* 1988;12(1):37–44.
356. Bryant J. Male breast cancer: a case of apocrine carcinoma with psammoma bodies. *Hum Pathol* 1981;12(8):751–753.
357. Abati AD, Kimmel M, Rosen PP. Apocrine mammary carcinoma. A clinicopathologic study of 72 cases. *Am J Clin Pathol* 1990;94(4):371–377.
358. Gilles R, Lesnik A, Guinebretiere JM, et al. Apocrine carcinoma: clinical and mammographic features. *Radiology* 1994;190(2):495–497.
359. Frable WJ, Kay S. Carcinoma of the breast. Histologic and clinical features of apocrine tumors. *Cancer* 1968;21(4):756–763.
360. Yates AJ, Ahmed A. Apocrine carcinoma and apocrine metaplasia. *Histopathology* 1988;13(2):228–231.
361. Lee BJ, Pack GT, Scharnagel I. Sweat gland cancer of the breast. *Surg Gynecol Obstet* 1933;54:975–996.
362. Eusebi V, Millis RR, Cattani MG, et al. Apocrine carcinoma of the breast. A morphologic and immunocytochemical study. *Am J Pathol* 1986;123(3):532–541.

363. Raju U, Zarbo RJ, Kubus J, et al. The histologic spectrum of apocrine breast pro-liferations: a comparative study of morphology and DNA content by image analy-sis. *Hum Pathol* 1993;24(2):173–181.

364. Gatalica Z. Immunohistochemical analysis of apocrine breast lesions. Consistent over-expression of androgen receptor accompanied by the loss of estrogen and progesterone receptors in apocrine metaplasia and apocrine carcinoma *in situ*. *Pathol Res Pract* 1997;193(11–12):753–758.

365. Tanaka K, Imoto S, Wada N, et al. Invasive apocrine carcinoma of the breast: clin-icopathologic features of 57 patients. *Breast J* 2008;14(2):164–168.

366. Lamovec J, Bracko M. Secretory carcinoma of the breast: light microscopical, immunohistochemical and flow cytometric study. *Mod Pathol* 1994;7(4):475–479.

367. McDivitt RW, Stewart FW. Breast carcinoma in children. *JAMA* 1966;195(5):388–390.

368. Oberman HA, Stephens PJ. Carcinoma of the breast in childhood. *Cancer* 1972;30(2):470–474.

369. Byrne MP, Fahey MM, Gooselaw JG. Breast cancer with axillary metastasis in an eight and one-half-year-old girl. *Cancer* 1973;31(3):726–728.

370. Sullivan JJ, Magee HR, Donald KJ. Secretory (juvenile) carcinoma of the breast. *Pathology* 1977;9(4):341–346.

371. Tavassoli FA, Norris HJ. Secretory carcinoma of the breast. *Cancer* 1980;45(9):2404–2413.

372. Masse SR, Rioux A, Beauchesne C. Juvenile carcinoma of the breast. *Hum Pathol* 1981;12(11):1044–1046.

373. Botta G, Fessia L, Ghiringhello B. Juvenile milk protein secreting carcinoma. *Virchows Arch A Pathol Anat Histol* 1982;395(2):145–152.

374. Karl SR, Ballantine TV, Zaino R. Juvenile secretory carcinoma of the breast. *J Pediatr Surg* 1985;20(4):368–371.

375. d'Amore ES, Maisto L, Gatteschi MB, et al. Secretory carcinoma of the breast. Report of a case with fine needle aspiration biopsy. *Acta Cytol* 1986;30(3):309–312.

376. Abe R, Masuda T. Secretory carcinoma of the breast in a Japanese woman. *Jpn J Surg* 1986;16(1):52–55.

377. Ferguson TB Jr, McCarty KS Jr, Filston HC. Juvenile secretory carcinoma and juvenile papillomatosis: diagnosis and treatment. *J Pediatr Surg* 1987;22(7):637–639.

378. Roth JA, Discafani C, O'Malley M. Secretory breast carcinoma in a man. *Am J Surg Pathol* 1988;12(2):150–154.

379. Krausz T, Jenkins D, Grontoft O, et al. Secretory carcinoma of the breast in adults: emphasis on late recurrence and metastasis. *Histopathology* 1989;14(1):25–36.

380. Richard G, Hawk JC 3rd, Baker AS Jr, et al. Multicentric adult secretory breast carcinoma: DNA flow cytometric findings, prognostic features, and review of the world literature. *J Surg Oncol* 1990;44(4):238–244.

381. Dominguez F, Riera JR, Junco P, et al. Secretory carcinoma of the breast. Report of a case with diagnosis by fine needle aspiration. *Acta Cytol* 1992;36(4):507–510.

382. Serour F, Gilad A, Kopolovic J, et al. Secretory breast cancer in childhood and adolescence: report of a case and review of the literature. *Med Pediatr Oncol* 1992;20(4):341–344.

383. Mies C. Recurrent secretory carcinoma in residual mammary tissue after mas-tectomy. *Am J Surg Pathol* 1993;17(7):715–721.

384. Pohar-Marinsek Z, Golouh R. Secretory breast carcinoma in a man diagnosed by fine needle aspiration biopsy. A case report. *Acta Cytol* 1994;38(3):446–450.

385. Kuwabara H, Yamane M, Okada S. Secretory breast carcinoma in a 66 year old man. *J Clin Pathol* 1998;51(7):545–547.

386. Furugaki K, Nagai E, Shinohara M, et al. Secretory carcinoma of the breast in an elderly woman: report of a case. *Surg Today* 1998;28(2):219–222.

387. Factor SM, Biempica L, Ratner I, et al. Carcinoma of the breast with multinucle-ated reactive stromal giant cells. A light and electron microscopic study of two cases. *Virchows Arch A Pathol Anat Histol* 1977;374(1):1–12.

388. Sugano I, Nagao K, Kondo Y, et al. Cytologic and ultrastructural studies of a rare breast carcinoma with osteoclast-like giant cells. *Cancer* 1983;52(1):74–78.

389. Fisher ER, Palekar AS, Gregorio RM, et al. Mucoepidermoid and squamous cell carcinomas of breast with reference to squamous metaplasia and giant cell tumors. *Am J Surg Pathol* 1983;7(1):15–27.

390. Holland R, van Haelst UJ. Mammary carcinoma with osteoclast-like giant cells. Additional observations on six cases. *Cancer* 1984;53(9):1963–1973.

391. Nielsen BB, Kiaer HW. Carcinoma of the breast with stromal multinucleated giant cells. *Histopathology* 1985;9(2):183–193.

392. McMahon RF, Ahmed A, Connolly CE. Breast carcinoma with stromal multinucle-ated giant cells—a light microscopic, histochemical and ultrastructural study. *J Pathol* 1986;150(3):175–179.

393. Ichijima K, Kobashi Y, Ueda Y, et al. Breast cancer with reactive multinucleated giant cells: report of three cases. *Acta Pathol Jpn* 1986;36(3):449–457.

394. Tavassoli FA, Norris HJ. Breast carcinoma with osteoclastlike giant cells. *Arch Pathol Lab Med* 1986;110(7):636–639.

395. Athanasou NA, Wells CA, Quinn J, et al. The origin and nature of stromal osteo-clast-like multinucleated giant cells in breast carcinoma: implications for tumour osteolysis and macrophage biology. *Br J Cancer* 1989;59(4):491–498.

396. Phillipson J, Ostrzega N. Fine needle aspiration of invasive cribriform carcinoma with benign osteoclast-like giant cells of histiocytic origin. A case report. *Acta Cytol* 1994;38(3):479–482.

397. Viacava P, Naccarato AG, Nardini V, et al. Breast carcinoma with osteoclast-like giant cells: immunohistochemical and ultrastructural study of a case and review of the literature. *Tumori* 1995;81(2):135–141.

398. Takahashi T, Moriki T, Hiroi M, et al. Invasive lobular carcinoma of the breast with osteoclastlike giant cells. A case report. *Acta Cytol* 1998;42(3):734–741.

399. Agnantis NT, Rosen PP. Mammary carcinoma with osteoclast-like giant cells. A study of eight cases with follow-up data. *Am J Clin Pathol* 1979;72(3):383–389.

400. Saigo PE, Rosen PP. Mammary carcinoma with "choriocarcinomatous" features. *Am J Surg Pathol* 1981;5(8):773–778.

401. Green DM. Mucoid carcinoma of the breast with choriocarcinoma in its metas-tases. *Histopathology* 1990;16(5):504–506.

402. Alvarez RD, Gleason BP, Gore H, et al. Coexisting intraductal breast carcinoma and metastatic choriocarcinoma presenting as a breast mass. *Gynecol Oncol* 1991;43(3):295–299.

403. Aboumrad MH, Horn RC, Fine G. Lipid-secreting mammary carcinoma: report of a case associated with Paget's disease of the nipple. *Cancer* 1963;16:521.

404. Ramos CV, Taylor HB. Lipid-rich carcinoma of the breast. A clinicopathologic analysis of 13 examples. *Cancer* 1974;33(3):812–819.

405. van Bogaert LJ, Maldague P. Histologic variants of lipid-secreting carcinoma of the breast. *Virchows Arch A Pathol Anat Histol* 1977;375(4):345–353.

406. Lapey JD. Lipid-rich mammary carcinoma—diagnosis by cytology. Case report. *Acta Cytol* 1977;21(1):120–122.

407. Dina R, Eusebi V. Clear cell tumors of the breast. *Semin Diagn Pathol* 1997;14(3):175–182.

408. Hull MT, Priest JB, Broadie TA, et al. Glycogen-rich clear cell carcinoma of the breast: a light and electron microscopic study. *Cancer* 1981;48(9):2003–2009.

409. Benisch B, Peison B, Newman R, et al. Solid glycogen-rich clear cell carcinoma of the breast (a light and ultrastructural study). *Am J Clin Pathol* 1983;79(2):243–245.

410. Fisher ER, Tavares J, Bulatao IS, et al. Glycogen-rich, clear cell breast cancer: with comments concerning other clear cell variants. *Hum Pathol* 1985;16(11):1085–1090.

411. Hull MT, Warfel KA. Glycogen-rich clear cell carcinomas of the breast. A clinico-pathologic and ultrastructural study. *Am J Surg Pathol* 1986;10(8):553–559.

412. Sorensen FB, Paulsen SM. Glycogen-rich clear cell carcinoma of the breast: a solid variant with mucus. A light microscopic, immunohistochemical and ultra-structural study of a case. *Histopathology* 1987;11(8):857–869.

413. Toikkanen S, Joensuu H. Glycogen-rich clear-cell carcinoma of the breast: a clin-icopathologic and flow cytometric study. *Hum Pathol* 1991;22(1):81–83.

414. Hayes MM, Seidman JD, Ashton MA. Glycogen-rich clear cell carcinoma of the breast. A clinicopathologic study of 21 cases. *Am J Surg Pathol* 1995;19(8):904–911.

415. Kuroda H, Sakamoto G, Ohnisi K, et al. Clinical and pathological features of glyco-gen-rich clear cell carcinoma of the breast. *Breast Cancer* 2005;12(3):189–195.

416. Koenig C, Tavassoli FA. Mucinous cystadenocarcinoma of the breast. *Am J Surg Pathol* 1998;22(6):698–703.

417. Bohman LG, Bassett LW, Gold RH, et al. Breast metastases from extramammary malignancies. *Radiology* 1982;144(2):309–312.

418. Mabuchi K, Bross DS, Kessler, II. Risk factors for male breast cancer. *J Natl Cancer Inst* 1985;74(2):371–375.

419. Casagrande JT, Hanisch R, Pike MC, et al. A case-control study of male breast cancer. *Cancer Res* 1988;48(5):1326–1330.

420. Wolman SR, Sanford J, Ratner S, et al. Breast cancer in males: DNA content and sex chromosome constitution. *Mod Pathol* 1995;8(3):239–243.

421. Evans DB, Crichlow RW. Carcinoma of the male breast and Klinefelter's syn-drome: is there an association? *CA Cancer J Clin* 1987;37(4):246–251.

422. Heller KS, Rosen PP, Schottenfeld D, et al. Male breast cancer: a clinicopathologic study of 97 cases. *Ann Surg* 1978;188(1):60–65.

423. Schlappack OK, Braun O, Maier U. Report of two cases of male breast cancer after prolonged estrogen treatment for prostatic carcinoma. *Cancer Detect Prev* 1986;9(3–4):319–322.

424. Sobin LH, Sherif M. Relation between male breast cancer and prostate cancer. *Br J Cancer* 1980;42(5):787–790.

425. Yan Z, Hummel P, Waisman J, et al. Prostatic adenocarcinoma metastatic to the breasts: report of a case with diagnosis by fine needle aspiration biopsy. *Urology* 2000;55(4):590.

426. Kozak FK, Hall JG, Baird PA. Familial breast cancer in males. A case report and review of the literature. *Cancer* 1986;58(12):2736–2739.

427. Donegan WL, Redlich PN, Lang PJ, et al. Carcinoma of the breast in males: a mul-tiinstitutional survey. *Cancer* 1998;83(3):498–509.

428. Rayson D, Erlichman C, Suman VJ, et al. Molecular markers in male breast car-cinoma. *Cancer* 1998;83(9):1947–1955.

429. Pich A, Margaria E, Chiusa L. Oncogenes and male breast carcinoma: c-erbB-2 and p53 coexpression predicts a poor survival. *J Clin Oncol* 2000;18(16):2948–2956.

430. Wang-Rodriguez J, Cross K, Gallagher S, et al. Male breast carcinoma: correla-tion of ER, PR, Ki-67, Her2-Neu, and p53 with treatment and survival, a study of 65 cases. *Mod Pathol* 2002;15(8):853–861.

431. Sandison AT. Metastatic tumors in the breast. *Br J Surg* 1959;47:54–58.

432. Toombs BD, Kalisher L. Metastatic disease to the breast: clinical, pathologic, and radiographic features. *AJR Am J Roentgenol* 1977;129(4):673–676.

433. Moncada R, Cooper RA, Garces M, et al. Calcified metastases from malignant ovarian neoplasm. Review of the literature. *Radiology* 1974;113(1):31–35.

434. Laifer S, Buscema J, Parmley TH, et al. Ovarian cancer metastatic to the breast. *Gynecol Oncol* 1986;24(1):97–102.

435. Duda RB, August CZ, Schink JC. Ovarian carcinoma metastatic to the breast and axillary node. *Surgery* 1991;110(3):552–556.

436. Yamasaki H, Saw D, Zdanowitz J, et al. Ovarian carcinoma metastasis to the breast case report and review of the literature. *Am J Surg Pathol* 1993;17(2):193–197.

437. Pressman PI. Malignant melanoma and the breast. *Cancer* 1973;31(4):784–792.

438. Silverman JF, Feldman PS, Covell JL, et al. Fine needle aspiration cytology of neo-plasms metastatic to the breast. *Acta Cytol* 1987;31(3):291–300.

439. Sneige N, Zachariah S, Fanning TV, et al. Fine-needle aspiration cytology of metastatic neoplasms in the breast. *Am J Clin Pathol* 1989;92(1):27–35.

440. Cangiarella J, Symmans WF, Cohen JM, et al. Malignant melanoma metastatic to the breast: a report of seven cases diagnosed by fine-needle aspiration cytology. *Cancer* 1998;84(3):160–162.

441. Kelly C, Henderson D, Corris P. Breast lumps: rare presentation of oat cell carci-noma of lung. *J Clin Pathol* 1988;41(2):171–172.

442. McCrea ES, Johnston C, Haney PJ. Metastases to the breast. *AJR Am J Roentgenol* 1983;141(4):685–690.

443. Nielsen M, Andersen JA, Henriksen FW, et al. Metastases to the breast from extra-mammary carcinomas. *Acta Pathol Microbiol Scand [A]* 1981;89(4):251–256.

444. Salyer WR, Salyer DC. Metastases of prostatic carcinoma to the breast. *J Urol* 1973;109(4):671–675.

445. Hartley LC, Little JH. Bilateral mammary metastases from carcinoma of the prostate during oestrogen therapy. *Med J Aust* 1971;1(8):434–436.

446. Scott J, Robb-Smith AH, Burns I. Bilateral breast metastases from carcinoma of the prostate. *Br J Urol* 1974;46(2):209–214.

447. Benson WR. Carcinoma of the prostate with metastases to the breast and testes. *Cancer* 1957;10:1235.

448. Malek GH, Madsen PO. Carcinoma of the prostate with unusual metastases. *Cancer* 1969;24(1):194–197.

449. Wilson SE, Hutchinson WB. Breast masses in males with carcinoma of the prostate. *J Surg Oncol* 1976;8(2):105–112.
450. Harrist TJ, Kalisher L. Breast metastasis: an unusual manifestation of a malignant carcinoid tumor. *Cancer* 1977;40(6):3102–3106.
451. Turner M, Gallager HS. Occult appendiceal carcinoid. Report of a case with fatal metastases. *Arch Pathol* 1969;88(2):188–190.
452. Schurch W, Lamoureux E, Lefebvre R, et al. Solitary breast metastasis: first manifestation of an occult carcinoid of the ileum. *Virchows Arch A Pathol Anat Histol* 1980;386(1):117–124.
453. Hawley PR. A case of secondary carcinoid tumours in both breasts following excision of primary carcinoid tumour of the duodenum. *Br J Surg* 1966;53(9):818–820.
454. Landon G, Sneige N, Ordonez NG, et al. Carcinoid metastatic to breast diagnosed by fine-needle aspiration biopsy. *Diagn Cytopathol* 1987;3(3):230–233.
455. Lozowski MS, Faegenburg D, Mishriki Y, et al. Carcinoid tumor metastatic to breast diagnosed by fine needle aspiration. Case report and literature review. *Acta Cytol* 1989;33(2):191–194.
456. Silverman EM, Oberman HA. Metastatic neoplasms in the breast. *Surg Gynecol Obstet* 1974;138(1):26–28.
457. Chica GA, Johnson DE, Ayala AG. Renal cell carcinoma presenting as breast carcinoma. *Urology* 1980;15(4):389–390.
458. Kannan V. Fine-needle aspiration of metastatic renal-cell carcinoma masquerading as primary breast carcinoma. *Diagn Cytopathol* 1998;18(5):343–345.
459. Cristallini EG, Ascani S, Nati S, et al. Breast metastasis of thyroid follicular carcinoma. *Acta Oncol* 1994;33(1):71–73.
460. Nunez DA, Sutherland CG, Sood RK. Breast metastasis from a pharyngeal carcinoma. *J Laryngol Otol* 1989;103(2):227–228.
461. Breitbart AS, Harris MN, Vazquez M, et al. Metastatic hemangiopericytoma of the breast. *New York State Journal of Medicine* 1992;92(4):158–160.
462. Howarth CB, Caces JN, Pratt CB. Breast metastases in children with rhabdomyosarcoma. *Cancer* 1980;46(11):2520–2524.
463. Alexander HR, Turnbull AD, Rosen PP. Isolated breast metastases from gastrointestinal carcinomas: report of two cases. *J Surg Oncol* 1989;42(4):264–266.
464. Baliga M, Holmquist ND, Espinoza CG. Medulloblastoma metastatic to breast, diagnosed by fine-needle aspiration biopsy. *Diagn Cytopathol* 1994;10(1):33–36.
465. Speert H, Greeley AV. Cervical cancer with metastasis to the breast. *Am J Obstet Gynecol* 1948;55:894.
466. Fowler CA, Nicholson S, Lott M, et al. Choriocarcinoma presenting as a breast lump. *Eur J Surg Oncol* 1995;21(5):576–578.
467. Sorlie T, Perou CM, Tibshirani R, et al. Gene expression patterns of breast carcinomas distinguish tumor subclasses with clinical implications. *Proc Natl Acad Sci U S A* 2001;98(19):10869–10874.
468. Brenton JD, Carey LA, Ahmed AA, et al. Molecular classification and molecular forecasting of breast cancer: ready for clinical application? *J Clin Oncol* 2005;23(29):7350–7360.
469. Nielsen TO, Hsu FD, Jensen K, et al. Immunohistochemical and clinical characterization of the basal-like subtype of invasive breast carcinoma. *Clin Cancer Res* 2004;10(16):5367–5374.
470. Sotiriou C, Wirapati P, Loi S, et al. Gene expression profiling in breast cancer: understanding the molecular basis of histologic grade to improve prognosis. *J Natl Cancer Inst* 2006;98(4):262–272.
471. Turner NC, Reis-Filho JS. Basal-like breast cancer and the *BRCA1* phenotype. *Oncogene* 2006;25(43):5846–5853.
472. Lakhani SR, Reis-Filho JS, Fulford L, et al. Prediction of *BRCA1* status in patients with breast cancer using estrogen receptor and basal phenotype. *Clin Cancer Res* 2005;11(14):5175–5180.
473. Arnes JB, Brunet JS, Stefansson I, et al. Placental cadherin and the basal epithelial phenotype of *BRCA1*-related breast cancer. *Clin Cancer Res* 2005;11(11):4003–4011.
474. Pinilla SM, Honrado E, Hardisson D, et al. Caveolin-1 expression is associated with a basal-like phenotype in sporadic and hereditary breast cancer. *Breast Cancer Res Treat* 2006;99(1):85–90.
475. Foulkes WD, Metcalfe K, Sun P, et al. Estrogen receptor status in *BRCA1*- and *BRCA2*-related breast cancer: the influence of age, grade, and histological type. *Clin Cancer Res* 2004;10(6):2029–2034.
476. Foulkes WD, Brunet JS, Stefansson IM, et al. The prognostic implication of the basal-like (cyclin E high/p27 low/p53+/glomeruloid-microvascular-proliferation+) phenotype of *BRCA1*-related breast cancer. *Cancer Res* 2004;64(3):830–835.
477. Henderson IC, Patek AJ. Are breast cancers in young women qualitatively distinct? *Lancet* 1997;349(9064):1488–1489.
478. Rennert G, Bisland-Naggan S, Barnett-Griness O, et al. Clinical outcomes of breast cancer in carriers of *BRCA1* and *BRCA2* mutations. *N Engl J Med* 2007;357(2):115–123.
479. Lakhani SR, Van De Vijver MJ, Jacquemier J, et al. The pathology of familial breast cancer: predictive value of immunohistochemical markers estrogen receptor, progesterone receptor, HER-2, and p53 in patients with mutations in *BRCA1* and *BRCA2*. *J Clin Oncol* 2002;20(9):2310–2318.
480. Marcus JN, Watson P, Page DL, et al. Hereditary breast cancer: pathobiology, prognosis, and *BRCA1* and *BRCA2* gene linkage. *Cancer* 1996;77(4):697–709.
481. Marcus JN, Page DL, Watson P, et al. *BRCA1* and *BRCA2* hereditary breast carcinoma phenotypes. *Cancer* 1997;80(3):543–556.
482. Pathology of familial breast cancer: differences between breast cancers in carriers of *BRCA1* or *BRCA2* mutations and sporadic cases. Breast Cancer Linkage Consortium. *Lancet* 1997;349(9064):1505–1510.
483. Agnarsson BA, Jonasson JG, Bjornsdottir IB, et al. Inherited *BRCA2* mutation associated with high grade breast cancer. *Breast Cancer Res Treat* 1998;47(2):121–127.
484. Marcus JN, Watson P, Page DL, et al. *BRCA2* hereditary breast cancer pathophenotype. *Breast Cancer Res Treat* 1997;44(3):275–277.
485. Bane AL, Beck JC, Bleiweiss I, et al. *BRCA2* mutation-associated breast cancers exhibit a distinguishing phenotype based on morphology and molecular profiles from tissue microarrays. *Am J Surg Pathol* 2007;31(1):121–128.
486. Mansour EG, Ravdin PM, Dressler L. Prognostic factors in early breast carcinoma. *Cancer* 1994;74(1 Suppl):381–400.
487. Weidner N, Cady B, Goodson WH, 3rd. Pathologic prognostic factors for patients with breast carcinoma. Which factors are important. *Surg Oncol Clin N Am* 1997;6(3):415–462.
488. Donegan WL. Tumor-related prognostic factors for breast cancer. *CA Cancer J Clin* 1997;47(1):28–51.
489. Fitzgibbons PL, Page DL, Weaver D, et al. Prognostic factors in breast cancer. College of American Pathologists Consensus Statement 1999. *Arch Pathol Lab Med* 2000;124(7):966–978.
490. Schwartz GF, Giuliano AE, Veronesi U. Proceedings of the consensus conference on the role of sentinel lymph node biopsy in carcinoma of the breast, April 19–22, 2001, Philadelphia, Pennsylvania. *Cancer* 2002;94(10):2542–2551.
491. Turner R. Histopathologic processing of the sentinel lymph node. *Semin Breats Dis* 2002;5:35–40.
492. Carter BA, Simpson JF, Jensen RA, et al. Significance of and redefinition of types of micrometastases in the sentinel node. *Semin Breast Dis* 2002;5:41–46.
493. Dowlatshahi K, Fan M, Snider HC, et al. [illegible] breast carcinoma: reviewing the dilemma. *Cancer* 1997;80(7):1188–1197.
494. Liberman L. Pathologic analysis of sentinel lymph nodes in breast carcinoma. *Cancer* 2000;88(5):971–977.
495. Colleoni M, Rotmensz N, Peruzzotti G, et al. Size of breast cancer metastases in axillary lymph nodes: clinical relevance of minimal lymph node involvement. *J Clin Oncol* 2005;23(7):1379–1389.
496. Allred DC, Elledge RM. Caution concerning micrometastatic breast carcinoma in sentinel lymph nodes. *Cancer* 1999;86(6):905–907.
497. Carter CL, Allen C, Henson DE. Relation of tumor size, lymph node status, and survival in 24,740 breast cancer cases. *Cancer* 1989;63(1):181–187.
498. McGuire WL, Tandon AK, Allred DC, et al. How to use prognostic factors in axillary node-negative breast cancer patients. *J Natl Cancer Inst* 1990;82(12):1006–1015.
499. Koscielny S, Tubiana M, Le MG, et al. Breast cancer: relationship between the size of the primary tumour and the probability of metastatic dissemination. *Br J Cancer* 1984;49(6):709–715.
500. Rosen PP, Groshen S. Factors influencing survival and prognosis in early breast carcinoma (T1N0M0-T1N1M0). Assessment of 644 patients with median follow-up of 18 years. *Surg Clin North Am* 1990;70(4):937–962.
501. Abner AL, Collins L, Peiro G, et al. Correlation of tumor size and axillary lymph node involvement with prognosis in patients with T1 breast carcinoma. *Cancer* 1998;83(12):2502–2508.
502. Chen YY, Schnitt SJ. Prognostic factors for patients with breast cancers 1 cm and smaller. *Breast Cancer Res Treat* 1998;51(3):209–225.
503. Quiet CA, Ferguson DJ, Weichselbaum RR, et al. Natural history of node-negative breast cancer: a study of 826 patients with long-term follow-up. *J Clin Oncol* 1995;13(5):1144–1151.
504. Fisher B, Redmond C. Systemic therapy in node-negative patients: updated findings from NSABP clinical trials. National Surgical Adjuvant Breast and Bowel Project. *J Natl Cancer Inst Monogr* 1992(11):105–116.
505. Silverstein MJ, Gierson ED, Waisman JR, et al. Predicting axillary node positivity in patients with invasive carcinoma of the breast by using a combination of T category and palpability. *J Am Coll Surg* 1995;180(6):700–704.
506. Barth A, Craig PH, Silverstein MJ. Predictors of axillary lymph node metastases in patients with T1 breast carcinoma. *Cancer* 1997;79(10):1918–1922.
507. Arnesson LG, Smeds S, Fagerberg G. Recurrence-free survival in patients with small breast cancer. An analysis of cancers 10 mm or less detected clinically and by screening. *Eur J Surg* 1994;160(5):271–276.
508. Halverson KJ, Taylor ME, Perez CA, et al. Management of the axilla in patients with breast cancers one centimeter or smaller. *Am J Clin Oncol* 1994;17(6):461–466.
509. Lee AK, Loda M, Mackarem G, et al. Lymph node negative invasive breast carcinoma 1 centimeter or less in size (T1a,bNOMO): clinicopathologic features and outcome. *Cancer* 1997;79(4):761–71.
510. *AJCC cancer staging manual*. 6th ed. New York: Springer, 2002.
511. Seidman JD, Schnaper LA, Aisner SC. Relationship of the size of the invasive component of the primary breast carcinoma to axillary lymph node metastasis. *Cancer* 1995;75(1):65–71.
512. Andea AA, Bouwman D, Wallis T, et al. Correlation of tumor volume and surface area with lymph node status in patients with multifocal/multicentric breast carcinoma. *Cancer* 2004;100(1):20–27.
513. Coombs NJ, Boyages J. Multifocal and multicentric breast cancer: does each focus matter? *J Clin Oncol* 2005;23(30):7497–7502.
514. NIH Consensus Conference. Treatment of early-stage breast cancer. *JAMA* 1990;265:391–395.
515. Goldhirsch A, Glick JH, Gelber RD, et al. Meeting highlights: International Consensus Panel on the Treatment of Primary Breast Cancer. *J Natl Cancer Inst* 1998;90(21):1601–1608.
516. Davis BW, Gelber RD, Goldhirsch A, et al. Prognostic significance of tumor grade in clinical trials of adjuvant therapy for breast cancer with axillary lymph node metastasis. *Cancer* 1986;58(12):2662–2670.
517. Contesso G, Mouriesse H, Friedman S, et al. The importance of histologic grade in long-term prognosis of breast cancer: a study of 1,010 patients, uniformly treated at the Institut Gustave-Roussy. *J Clin Oncol* 1987;5(9):1378–1386.
518. Le Doussal V, Tubiana-Hulin M, Friedman S, et al. Prognostic value of histologic grade nuclear components of Scarff-Bloom-Richardson (SBR). An improved score modification based on a multivariate analysis of 1,262 invasive ductal breast carcinomas. *Cancer* 1989;64(9):1914–1921.
519. Rosen PP, Groshen S, Saigo PE, et al. Pathological prognostic factors in stage I (T1N0M0) and stage II (T1N1M0) breast carcinoma: a study of 644 patients with median follow-up of 18 years. *J Clin Oncol* 1989;7(9):1239–1251.
520. Elston CW, Ellis IO. Pathological prognostic factors in breast cancer. I. The value of histological grade in breast cancer: experience from a large study with long-term follow-up. *Histopathology* 1991;19(5):403–410.
521. Page DL. Prognosis and breast cancer. Recognition of lethal and favorable prognostic types. *Am J Surg Pathol* 1991;15(4):334–349.
522. Nixon AJ, Schnitt SJ, Gelman R, et al. Relationship of tumor grade to other pathologic features and to treatment outcome of patients with early stage breast carcinoma treated with breast-conserving therapy. *Cancer* 1996;78(7):1426–1431.
523. Roberti NE. The role of histologic grading in the prognosis of patients with carcinoma of the breast: is this a neglected opportunity? *Cancer* 1997;80(9):1708–1716.
524. Pereira H, Pinder SE, Sibbering DM, et al. Pathological prognostic factors in breast cancer. IV: Should you be a typer or a grader? A comparative study of two histological prognostic features in operable breast carcinoma. *Histopathology* 1995;27(3):219–226.
525. Pinder SE, Murray S, Ellis IO, et al. The importance of the histologic grade of invasive breast carcinoma and response to chemotherapy. *Cancer* 1998;83(8):1529–1539.

526. Fisher ER, Redmond C, Fisher B. Pathologic findings from the National Surgical Adjuvant Breast Project. VIII. Relationship of chemotherapeutic responsiveness to tumor differentiation. *Cancer* 1983;51(2):181–191.

527. Keam B, Im SA, Kim HJ, et al. Prognostic impact of clinicopathologic parameters in stage II/III breast cancer treated with neoadjuvant docetaxel and doxorubicin chemotherapy: paradoxical features of the triple negative breast cancer. *BMC Cancer* 2007;7:203.

528. Colleoni M, Viale G, Zahrieh D, et al. Chemotherapy is more effective in patients with breast cancer not expressing steroid hormone receptors: a study of preoperative treatment. *Clin Cancer Res* 2004;10(19):6622–6628.

529. Stenkvist B, Westman-Naeser S, Vegelius J, et al. Analysis of reproducibility of subjective grading systems for breast carcinoma. *J Clin Pathol* 1979;32(10):979–985.

530. Delides GS, Garas G, Georgouli G, et al. Intralaboratory variations in the grading of breast carcinoma. *Arch Pathol Lab Med* 1982;106(3):126–128.

531. Harvey JM, de Klerk NH, Sterrett GF. Histological grading in breast cancer: interobserver agreement, and relation to other prognostic factors including ploidy. *Pathology* 1992;24(2):63–68.

532. Frierson HF, Jr., Wolber RA, Berean KW, et al. Interobserver reproducibility of the Nottingham modification of the Bloom and Richardson histologic grading scheme for infiltrating ductal carcinoma. *Am J Clin Pathol* 1995;103(2):195–198.

533. Dalton LW, Page DL, Dupont WD. Histologic grading of breast carcinoma. A reproducibility study. *Cancer* 1994;73(11):2765–2770.

534. Pinder SE, Ellis IO, Galea M, et al. Pathological prognostic factors in breast cancer. III. Vascular invasion: relationship with recurrence and survival in a large study with long-term follow-up. *Histopathology* 1994;24(1):41–47.

535. Orbo A, Stalsberg H, Kunde D. Topographic criteria in the diagnosis of tumor emboli in intramammary lymphatics. *Cancer* 1990;66(5):972–977.

536. Rosen PP. Tumor emboli in intramammary lymphatics in breast carcinoma: pathologic criteria for diagnosis and clinical significance. *Pathology Annual* 1983;18 Pt 2:215–232.

537. Davis BW, Gelber R, Goldhirsch A, et al. Prognostic significance of peritumoral vessel invasion in clinical trials of adjuvant therapy for breast cancer with axillary lymph node metastasis. *Hum Pathol* 1985;16(12):1212–1218.

538. Lauria R, Perrone F, Carlomagno C, et al. The prognostic value of lymphatic and blood vessel invasion in operable breast cancer. *Cancer* 1995;76(10):1772–1778.

539. Fein DA, Fowble BL, Hanlon AL, et al. Identification of women with T1-T2 breast cancer at low risk of positive axillary nodes. *J Surg Oncol* 1997;65(1):34–39.

540. Chadha M, Chabon AB, Friedmann P, et al. Predictors of axillary lymph node metastases in patients with T1 breast cancer. A multivariate analysis. *Cancer* 1994;73(2):350–353.

541. Nealon TF Jr, Nkongho A, Grossi C, et al. Pathologic identification of poor prognosis stage I (T1N0M0) cancer of the breast. *Ann Surg* 1979;190(2):129–132.

542. Leitner SP, Swern AS, Weinberger D, et al. Predictors of recurrence for patients with small (one centimeter or less) localized breast cancer (T1a,b N0 M0). *Cancer* 1995;76(11):2266–2274.

543. Rosen PP, Saigo PE, Braun DW Jr, et al. Predictors of recurrence in stage I (T1N0M0) breast carcinoma. *Ann Surg* 1981;193(1):15–25.

544. Roses DF, Bell DA, Flotte TJ, et al. Pathologic predictors of recurrence in stage 1 (TlN0M0) breast cancer. *Am J Clin Pathol* 1982;78(6):817–820.

545. Gilchrist KW, Gould VE, Hirschl S, et al. Interobserver variation in the identification of breast carcinoma in intramammary lymphatics. *Hum Pathol* 1982;13(2):170–172.

546. Lee AK, DeLellis RA, Silverman ML, et al. Lymphatic and blood vessel invasion in breast carcinoma: a useful prognostic indicator? *Hum Pathol* 1986;17(10):984–987.

547. Bettelheim R, Mitchell D, Gusterson BA. Immunocytochemistry in the identification of vascular invasion in breast cancer. *J Clin Pathol* 1984;37(4):364–366.

548. Lee AK, DeLellis RA, Rosen PP, et al. ABH blood group isoantigen expression in breast carcinomas—an immunohistochemical evaluation using monoclonal antibodies. *Am J Clin Pathol* 1985;83(3):308–319.

549. Lee AK, DeLellis RA, Wolfe HJ. Intramammary lymphatic invasion in breast carcinomas. Evaluation using ABH isoantigens as endothelial markers. *Am J Surg Pathol* 1986;10(9):589–594.

550. Martin SA, Perez-Reyes N, Mendelsohn G. Angioinvasion in breast carcinoma. An immunohistochemical study of factor VIII-related antigen. *Cancer* 1987;59(11):1918–1922.

551. Saigo PE, Rosen PP. The application of immunohistochemical stains to identify endothelial-lined channels in mammary carcinoma. *Cancer* 1987;59(1):51–54.

552. Ordonez NG, Brooks T, Thompson S, et al. Use of Ulex europaeus agglutinin I in the identification of lymphatic and blood vessel invasion in previously stained microscopic slides. *Am J Surg Pathol* 1987;11(7):543–550.

553. Hanau CA, Machera H, Meittinen M. Immunohistochemical evaluation of vascular invasion in carcinomas with five different markers. *Appl Immunohistochem* 1993;1:46.

554. Kahn HJ, Bailey D, Marks A. Monoclonal antibody D2-40, a new marker of lymphatic endothelium, reacts with Kaposi's sarcoma and a subset of angiosarcomas. *Mod Pathol* 2002;15(4):434–440.

555. Arnaout-Alkarain A, Kahn HJ, Narod SA, et al. Significance of lymph vessel invasion identified by the endothelial lymphatic marker D2-40 in node negative breast cancer. *Mod Pathol* 2007;20(2):183–191.

556. Mohammed RA, Martin SG, Gill MS, et al. Improved methods of detection of lymphovascular invasion demonstrate that it is the predominant method of vascular invasion in breast cancer and has important clinical consequences. *Am J Surg Pathol* 2007;31(12):1825–1833.

557. Rosen PP, Saigo PE, Braun DW, et al. Prognosis in stage II (T1N1M0) breast cancer. *Ann Surg* 1981;194(5):576–584.

558. Bell JR, Friedell GH, Goldenberg IS. Prognostic significance of pathologic findings in human breast carcinoma. *Surg Gynecol Obstet* 1969;129(2):258–262.

559. Kister SJ, Sommers SC, Haagensen CD, et al. Re-evaluation of blood-vessel invasion as a prognostic factor in carcinoma of the breast. *Cancer* 1966;19(9):1213–1216.

560. Sampat MB, Sirsat MV, Gangadharan P. Prognostic significance of blood vessel invasion in carcinoma of the breast in women. *J Surg Oncol* 1977;9(6):623–632.

561. Weigand RA, Isenberg WM, Russo J, et al. Blood vessel invasion and axillary lymph node involvement as prognostic indicators for human breast cancer. *Cancer* 1982;50(5):962–969.

562. Fisher ER, Palekar AS, Gregorio RM, et al. Pathological findings from the national surgical adjuvant breast project (Protocol No. 4). IV. Significance of tumor necrosis. *Hum Pathol* 1978;9(5):523–530.

563. Carter D, Pipkin RD, Shepard RH, et al. Relationship of necrosis and tumor border to lymph node metastases and 10-year survival in carcinoma of the breast. *Am J Surg Pathol* 1978;2(1):39–46.

564. Gilchrist KW, Gray R, Fowble B, et al. Tumor necrosis is a prognostic predictor for early recurrence and death in lymph node-positive breast cancer: a 10-year follow-up study of 728 Eastern Cooperative Oncology Group patients. *J Clin Oncol* 1993;11(10):1929–1935.

565. Parham DM, Hagen N, Brown RA. Simplified method of grading primary carcinomas of the breast. *J Clin Pathol* 1992;45(6):517–520.

566. Stenkvist B, Bengtsson E, Dahlqvist B, et al. Predicting breast cancer recurrence. *Cancer* 1982;50(12):2884–2893.

567. Black MM, Barclay TH, Hankey BF. Prognosis in breast cancer utilizing histologic characteristics of the primary tumor. *Cancer* 1975;36(6):2048–2055.

568. Alderson MR, Hamlin I, Staunton MD. The relative significance of prognostic factors in breast carcinoma. *Br J Cancer* 1971;25(4):646–656.

569. Berg JW. Morphological evidence for immune response to breast cancer. An historical review. *Cancer* 1971;28(6):1453–1456.

570. Dawson PJ, Ferguson DJ, Karrison T. The pathological findings of breast cancer in patients surviving 25 years after radical mastectomy. *Cancer* 1982;50(10):2131–2138.

571. Rosen PP, Kinne DW, Lesser M, et al. Are prognostic factors for local control of breast cancer treated by primary radiotherapy significant for patients treated by mastectomy? *Cancer* 1986;57(7):1415–1420.

572. Park C, Misumori M, Recht A, et al. The relationship between pathologic margin status and outcome after breast conserving therapy. *Int J Radiat Oncol Biol Phys* 1998;42 (Suppl):125.

573. McGuire WL, Clark GM. Prognostic factors and treatment decisions in axillary-node-negative breast cancer. *N Engl J Med* 1992;326(26):1756–1761.

574. Galea MH, Blamey RW, Elston CE, et al. The Nottingham Prognostic Index in primary breast cancer. *Breast Cancer Res Treat* 1992;22(3):207–219.

575. van Diest PJ, Baak JP. The morphometric prognostic index is the strongest prognosticator in premenopausal lymph node-negative and lymph node-positive breast cancer patients. *Hum Pathol* 1991;22(4):326–330.

576. Recommendations for the reporting of breast carcinoma. Association of Directors of Anatomic and Surgical Pathology. *Am J Clin Pathol* 1995;104(6):614–619.

577. Henson DE, Oberman HA, Hutter RV. Practice protocol for the examination of specimens removed from patients with cancer of the breast: a publication of the Cancer Committee, College of American Pathologists. Members of the Cancer Committee, College of American Pathologists, and the Task Force for Protocols on the Examination of Specimens from Patients with Breast Cancer. *Arch Pathol Lab Med* 1997;121(1):27–33.

Chapter 29
Clinical Aspects of Estrogen and Progesterone Receptors

Rachel Schiff, C. Kent Osborne, and Suzanne A. W. Fuqua

HISTORICAL PERSPECTIVE

In the early 1960s, radiolabeled estrogens were first observed to be preferentially concentrated in estrogen target organs—observations that gave rise to the concept of an "estrogen receptor" (1). Since then, it has become clear that many human breast cancers are dependent on estrogen, progesterone, or both for their growth. This stimulatory effect is mediated through the estrogen receptors (*ER α and β*, collectively called *ER*) and progesterone receptors (*PR A and B*), and probably not coincidentally, both are found relatively overexpressed in most malignant breast tissue. The concept of targeted therapy directed toward molecular components preferentially overexpressed by breast cancer cells has become a popular one. The ER, even before its discovery, was, however, the therapeutic target for the first breast cancer systemic therapy using surgical oophorectomy more than 100 years ago (2). Following the cloning of the receptors for estrogen and progesterone, there has been a massive effort to understand the mechanisms of hormone action for these receptors. Our goal is not to review the molecular intricacies of these nuclear receptor transcriptional networks, which are reviewed elsewhere (3), but instead to focus on their clinical usefulness. Thus, this chapter briefly assesses receptor action, and then reviews the utility of ER and PR for the clinical management of breast cancer, discussing methodologies used to measure these receptors, especially as they relate to assessing clinical outcome and selecting appropriate therapy.

BIOLOGY OF ESTROGEN RECEPTORS AND PROGESTERONE RECEPTORS

Structure–Function Relationship

The ER belong to a family of nuclear hormone receptors that function as transcription factors when they are bound to their respective ligands. Cloning of human ERα (4,5), ERβ (6), and PR (7), showed that each of these receptors share a common structural and functional organization; their functional domains are designated A through F (Fig. 29.1). Classic ER (now called *ERα*) contains 595 amino acids (*aa*) with a central DNA binding domain (DBD), along with a carboxyl-terminal hormone binding domain (HBD). Binding of hormone to ERα facilitates activation of the receptor and its binding to estrogen response elements present in the promoter of estrogen-responsive genes. The two ERs and PR are also complexed with a number of coregulatory proteins that coordinately act to influence the transcription of estrogen-responsive genes. Through DNA binding, the ERs influence the expression of estrogen-responsive genes, such as the two PR isoforms, and other key components important for mitogenic signaling and cell survival.

Regulation

Mechanisms regulating ERα and β function include differential usage of upstream untranslated exons, the splicing of their messenger RNA (mRNA), and post-translational modifications. At least seven different promoters have been described for

ERα, as reviewed by Kos et al. (8). The human ERβ promoter is less well characterized in the breast (9). It has been proposed that the multiple alternative promoters account for tissue-specific expression of ERα and ERβ levels in tumors, but further studies are required. Fuqua et al. (10,11) were the first to demonstrate that alternative RNA splicing generated truncated forms of ERα with significant functional consequences, and that alternative splicing was common in breast tumors; there have been reports of alternatively spliced forms of ERβ with altered function as well (12). Although some of these spliced forms have been reported to correlate with various clinical parameters in breast cancer (13), none are recommended for use as prognostic or predictive tumor markers.

Post-translational Modifications

Post-translational modifications of ER and PR play key roles in regulating their function. Several laboratories have evaluated receptor phosphorylation. Among the multiple kinases that can phosphorylate ERα are p38 mitogen-activated protein kinase (*MAPK*), cyclin A-CDK2, CDK7, c-Src, and pp90[rsk1] (14–18). ERα can also be differentially phosphorylated by a number of important signaling molecules, such as Akt (also known as protein kinase B), and extracellular regulated kinase (*Erk*) 1/2 MAPK, resulting in diverse responses to ligands (19). For example, direct phosphorylation of ERα serine (*S*) 167 by Akt and S118 by Erk1/2 can result in acquired resistance to the antiestrogen tamoxifen, and ligand-independent activation of ERα (20–22). The effects of ERα phosphorylation at S118 are complex; although phosphorylated (*p*) S118 immunostaining predicted a better likelihood of response to endocrine treatment in invasive breast cancers (23), pS118 levels were elevated in patients who had relapsed following tamoxifen treatment compared with pretreatment biopsies (24), suggesting that pS118 could play some role in the emergence of endocrine resistance. A recent report also suggested that endocrine therapy decreases S118 phosphorylation on ERα, and therefore that pS118 levels could be used as a surrogate marker to monitor treatment efficacy (25).

Protein kinase A (*PKA*) signaling mediates phosphorylation of ERα S236, which enhances DNA binding (26,27). Phosphorylation of S305 is mediated by both PKA and p21-activated kinase 1 (*PAK-1*) signaling, which impacts estrogen hypersensitivity and tamoxifen responsiveness (28–30); whether these two kinases directly phosphorylate ERα at S305 is not clear, however. It is likely that these phosphorylation events are complex and interdependent. For instance, phosphorylation at ERα S305 can regulate the subsequent phosphorylation of S118 (31). Because a number of different signaling pathways are probably active in tumors, and a variety of ER activities, such as receptor turnover, cellular localization, and transcriptional activity can all be influenced by receptor phosphorylation, then single phosphorylation site measurements may not afford a complete understanding of the deregulated ER activities that may be dominant in a particular tumor. The clinical utility of measuring simultaneous ERα phosphorylation has not yet been demonstrated.

It has been reported that both of the PR-A and B isoforms can be phosphorylated at multiple serine residues (n >14), with distinct groups of these sites coordinately regulated by ligands or kinases (32). Only a few proteins have been documented as authentic kinases for PR. Specifically, cyclin A-CDK2 and casein kinase II have been shown to phosphorylate PR-B at

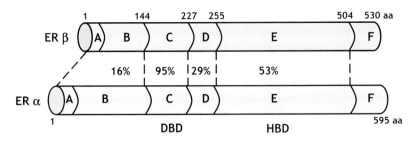

FIGURE 29.1. A schematic diagram showing estrogen receptor (ER)α functional domains and a comparison of ERα and ERβ structures. ERα contains 595 amino acids (aa) with the functional domains labeled A through F and a central DNA binding domain (DBD) and hormone binding domain (HBD). ERβ contains 530 aa, and the degree of homology between ERβ and ERα is shown as percentages. Region A–B is important for hormone-independent ER transcription, region C is the DBD, region D is the hinge domain, region E is the HBD responsible for hormone-dependent transcription, and region F is important for modulation of ER activity.

several sites in a cell cycle-dependent manner (33–35). But how PR serine phosphorylation regulates its function is not well developed. We do know that PR can be phosphorylated in breast cancer cells at S400 by CDK2, which regulates both PR activity and its localization in the absence of ligand (36), and it has recently been shown that similar to ERα, phosphorylation of PR can regulate ligand hypersensitivity (37). Thus, for both PR and ERα, a potential clinical utility exists for dissecting the roles of phosphorylation on receptor function.

Ubiquitination is the reversible covalent bonding of highly conserved ubiquitin molecules to lysine residues on client proteins. It is known that the ubiquitin-proteasome pathway can regulate ERα protein levels and response to ligand (38). On ligand binding to ERα, ubiquitin binds the receptor on lysine residues within the ligand-binding domain (LBD), inducing ubiquitin-mediated proteasomal degradation (38). ERα ubiquitination is important for transcriptional activity (39). It also appears that the lysines (K) 302 and 303 residues in the ERα hinge domain are important residues that regulate basal degradation by the proteasome (40).

ERα can be differentially affected by post-translational modifications either singly or in combination—phosphorylation and acetylation are examples. ERα can be acetylated on lysines, with the conserved ERα residues K266, K268, K299, K302, and K303 being the most important (41). Acetylation of K266 and K268 may have opposing effects compared with the acetylation of K302 and K303; K266 and K268 acetylations induced DNA-binding and ligand-dependent activation (42), but acetylation of K302 and K303 inhibited ERα ligand-dependent activation (41). It has also been reported that the K302/303 sites may not be acetylated in the full-length protein; therefore, there is some controversy as to which lysines are most important *in vivo*. Convincing data, however, indicate that the phosphorylation status of ERα S305 coordinately regulates the acetylation of the K302/303 residues, which suggests a physiologic relevance of these specific post-translational events (28).

The small ubiquitin-like modifier protein 1 (SUMO-1) covalently and reversibly binds to target proteins with the assistance of conjugating enzymes. Ligand-dependent sumoylation can occur on lysine residues as well, again within the ERα hinge domain (43). Thus, the hinge domain is a target of extensive post-translational modifications. Sumoylation also regulates the transcriptional activity of ER and PR (43,44). The same ERα lysine residues that are acetylated can also be sumolyated, including K266, K268, K302, and K303, suggesting a tight regulatory pathway governing the occupation of these residues adjacent to phosphorylation events at S305, with the processes of ubiquitination, acetylation and sumoylation. Finally, a recent report has shown that the K303 ERα residue can alter methylation at K302 (45). It is possible that acetylation of K303 attenuates ER-driven transcription, not just from antagonism via acetylation, but also by inhibition of K302 methylation and subsequent destabilization of ERα. In summary, indeed numerous and possibly coordinate post-translational modifications occur in ER and PR, and it can be predicted that as antibodies become available to these modifications, then they should be evaluated for clinical utility.

Estrogen Receptor Gene Alterations

Relatively few mutations have been reported in the ERα gene, surprising because many clinical therapeutic resistance mechanisms involve mutation of the target. A mutation that causes a single amino acid change in the ERα hinge domain (lysine 303 to arginine, called *K303R ERα*), has been reported in about a third of premalignant breast hyperplasias (46). The mutation represents a somatic, gain-of-function mutation arising in the breast resulting in a receptor that is hypersensitive to the growth effects of estrogen. More recently, utilizing a sensitive primer-extension sequencing technique, it has been demonstrated that the K303R ERα mutation was present in half of invasive breast tumors, and it was associated with older age, larger tumor size, lymph-node positive disease, and poor outcomes in univariate analyses (47). These patients were all untreated with adjuvant therapy; the role of this mutation in treatment resistance is currently under study. Preliminary results suggest, however, that the mutation may confer resistance to the aromatase inhibitor (AI) anastrozole via upregulation of the phosphatidylinositol-3-OH kinase (PI3K)/Akt pathways (48), and block tamoxifen antagonist action when engaged in crosstalk with growth factor receptor signaling pathways (49). Confirmatory studies are needed in this exciting new area of research.

Four other studies reported that the mutation was not present in invasive cancers (50–53); however, it has been convincingly demonstrated that the detection method used, standard dye-terminator sequencing, was not sensitive for detection of this specific mutation in ERα (47). In comparison, Conway et al. (54) have identified this mutation in only 6% of breast cancers using a different gel electrophoresis detection method. In a recent report, the K303R mutation was also found to be significantly associated with a first-degree family history of breast cancer, suggesting that the mutation might be involved in driving the proliferation of some breast tumors (46,55). Therefore, although the absolute frequency of this mutation remains to be established, it is present in a significant number of breast cancer samples.

Molecular analysis of the K303R ERα mutation has shown that the mutated arginine (R) at the 303 position allows ERα to be more highly phosphorylated by PKA signaling (e.g., the mutation creates a more efficient substrate sequence for PKA) (28). The K303R mutation is also a more efficient substrate for K302 methylation by enhancing its stability (45). These data, along with the extensive post-translational modifications that occur surrounding the mutation site described in the previous section, indicate that the K303/S305 residues play important roles in ERα action in the breast. The role of ER or PR mutations in breast cancer may be underappreciated to date because few metastatic lesions have been sequenced for mutations (56,57). The collection of accessible metastatic lesions from tumors unresponsive to treatment, combined with the use of alternative sequencing strategies to replace standard dye-terminator approaches, is recommended for an accurate assessment of whether specific ERα mutations could be involved in treatment resistance.

Whether the estrogen receptor gene locus (*ESR1*) is a target for increased gene copy number (amplification) has been controversial. Amplification is known to be a common mechanism for cancer cells to increase the expression of genes critical for cell growth or survival. Large deletions, rearrangements, or gene amplification in ERα are reportedly infrequent in breast cancer (58). Recent improvements in the detection of small amplifications using fluorescent *in situ* hybridization (FISH) have allowed, however, for a revisit of the question of genetic alterations in ESR1. One group has reported that more than 30% of breast tumors have ESR1 alterations (59). Amplifications between primary and metastatic tumors appear to be concordant, and tumors with ESR1 gene amplification also express higher levels of ERα by immunohistochemistry (60). Interestingly, preliminary results suggest that ESR1 amplification may predict resistance to adjuvant tamoxifen in postmenopausal women with ERα-positive breast cancer (61), a result which awaits confirmation by other groups.

Genomic Activity

It is well known that ER and PR function as tissue-specific and ligand-dependent transcription factors, which indicates that receptors do not act alone in their diversified activities, and require additional factors for their action. This concept led to the first discovery of ER coregulatory proteins by Dr. Bert O'Malley's laboratory over 10 years ago (62). The Nuclear Receptor Signaling Atlas (NURSA) website (www.nursa.org) now lists over 170 known nuclear receptor coregulatory proteins (63). Briefly, we know that in the absence of hormone, histone deacetylase (HDAC) and the receptor corepressors N-CoR and SMRT are bound to the receptor. Histone deacetylation silences or inhibits transcription by causing DNA to wrap more tightly around the core histone proteins. When hormone then binds to the receptor, the activated receptor complex displaces the repressor proteins and acetyltransferases, such as CBP/p300 (calcium binding protein) and PCAF (p300/CBP associated factor), are recruited to the complex along with coactivator proteins such as the p160 coactivator (steroid receptor coactivator [SRC1], transcriptional inhibitory factor [TIF2], amplified in breast 1 [AIB1]) complex. The acetyltransferases add acetyl groups to histones, loosening their interaction with DNA, which exposes important residues to the basal transcriptional machinery. The coactivators appear to cycle on and off the promoter during hormone treatment (64). Therefore, there is a dynamic and complex array of proteins present on estrogen-regulated promoters, many of which are involved in chromatin remodeling that coordinately contribute to the hormonal regulation of gene expression. Phosphorylation of ER coregulators is important in communicating growth factor and other signaling effects to the ER pathway (65).

Phosphorylation of coactivators can augment their activity on ER-dependent transcription, even in the absence of ligand or in the presence of antiestrogens, by increasing their subcellular nuclear localization, their interaction with the ER, and their ability to recruit other transcriptional coregulators, such as the CBP/p300 coactivator, to the receptor–promoter complex. Several key signaling kinases phosphorylate members of the p160 SRC family of coactivators, and especially AIB1, which is often gene-amplified or overexpressed in breast tumor cells (66). The clinical significance of AIB overexpression in tamoxifen resistance has been shown in a retrospective study demonstrating a poor disease-free survival for patients receiving adjuvant tamoxifen whose tumors express high levels of both the ERBB2 (formerly, HER2) oncogene, and the ER coactivator AIB1 (67,68). Agonist activity may manifest itself in tissues where corepressor expression is low, or perhaps mixed antiestrogens such as tamoxifen enable the receptor to interact with both corepressors and coactivators simultaneously. Thus, it may be the relative balance of bound coregulators that ultimately determines response to therapy. Of note is that many of the coregulatory proteins themselves have enzymatic activities, and are targets during tumorigenesis (69); however, a discussion of the molecular details of this area is beyond the scope of this chapter. Receptor coregulatory proteins are reviewed elsewhere (70).

Nongenomic Activities

In addition to the recognized ER genomic activity to alter gene expression in the nucleus, referred to as *nuclear initiated steroid signaling* (NISS), rapid effects of estrogens (71) and plasma membrane estrogen binding sites (72) were first described decades ago. Numerous later studies have revealed that in response to their ligands, ER, as well as PR and other nuclear receptors, can mediate signaling cascades originating from the membrane or the cytoplasm through direct interaction with, and activation of, signal transduction mediators (73,74). This nongenomic ER action (also called rapid, non-nuclear, nonclassic, or *membrane-initiated steroid signaling* [MISS]) occurs within seconds to a few minutes, and is independent of gene transcription. Such rapid responses to ER have been found in both classic and nonclassic target cells, including bone, neural, uterine, fat, and endothelial cells (73,75). It is now evident that in some of these tissues, such as bone and vasculature endothelium, nongenomic activity is the predominant type of estrogen signaling (76,77). Increasing evidence, however, also suggests the importance of the biological consequences of this estrogen-induced rapid signaling for the growth and survival of breast cancer cells (78–84).

The identity of the receptors mediating the nongenomic actions of steroids, their subcellular localization, and the precise mechanism by which they operate are all topics of active research that still raise some controversy. As recently reported and reviewed (85,86) for progesterone and glucocorticoid-induced rapid effects, much evidence now supports the existence of distinct nonclassic receptors as well as classic receptor forms which may also be present in the membrane or the cytoplasm. In contrast, many studies using immunohistochemical, biochemical, and genetic approaches clearly implicate a small subpopulation of the classic ERα and β subtypes located outside the nucleus or closely related nonclassic short forms of ERα (77,87–89) as the transducers of rapid estrogen signaling (83,90). Membrane receptors distinct from the classic ER, especially the G protein-coupled receptor 30 (GPR30), may also play a role in the rapid effects of estrogen (91–94). Membrane and cytoplasmic ER transmit their signals through kinase cascades, including growth factor receptors and cellular tyrosine kinases and their downstream kinase pathways (95), and also through calcium, cyclic adenosine monophosphate (cAMP), and other second messengers (73,83,96–98), ultimately to regulate transcription in the nucleus (99–102). Furthermore, membrane-initiated ER activity via growth factor signaling cascades can, in turn, modulate the activity of nuclear ER and its sensitivity to endocrine therapy (103,104) as we will further discuss below.

Estrogen receptor is now considered a central component of the membrane signal (73,83). Membrane ER may exist as a cytoplasmic entity tethered to the inner face of the plasma membrane bilayer through binding to proteins of lipid rafts, scaffold or adaptor proteins (83,105–108), or possibly through associating with other membrane receptors, such as insulin-like growth factor receptor (IGF-1R) (95,109), epidermal growth factor receptor (EGFR) (110), or ERBB2 (106,111). Studies using antibodies (112–114) or membrane-impermeant estrogen conjugates (115,116) suggest, however, that ER may also exist as transmembrane proteins. ERα in endothelial cells has been shown to reside in the caveolae, membrane signaling organelles that contain growth factor receptors and numerous other signaling molecules. Recent work has shown that palmitoylation within a highly conserved sequence in the ligand binding (E) domain of ER (Fig. 29.1) is crucial for its association with the key protein caveolin-1 for membrane translocation and for activation of rapid signaling (117). A role for additional domains in the amino terminus of the receptor has, however, also been reported to mediate its membrane localization and nongenomic signaling (109,118). Recent evidence also points to a role of ERs in the mitochondria, where they mediate cell survival signaling. (83,119,120).

Laboratory studies using breast cancer culture models have shown that endogenous membrane ER can directly or indirectly activate various growth factor receptors, including EGFR, ERBB2, and IGF-1R (83,95,121–123). This pathway involves sequential activation of G-proteins, the cellular tyrosine kinase c-Src, and matrix metalloproteinases (MMP), followed by the release of heparin-binding EGF-like growth factor (HB-EGF). HB-EGF, in turn binds to and activates adjacent EGFR and its downstream kinase cascades (e.g., Ras/Mek/MAPK and PI3K/Akt) (81,95,124). These downstream kinases sequentially phosphorylate and thereby activate components of the transcriptional machinery, including ER itself and its coregulators, resulting in potentiation of nuclear ER transcriptional activity (21,65,103,104,122,125). Therefore, ER genomic and nongenomic functions complement each other to promote proliferative and survival signaling in breast cancer (Fig. 29.2).

Both nongenomic and genomic activities of ER are dependent on estrogen for their activation. Although selective estrogen receptor modulators (SERMs), such as tamoxifen, usually inhibit estrogen's effects on genomic ER activity (antagonist activity), they have estrogen-like effects (agonist activity) on nongenomic ER functions (104). This activation of rapid ER effects by tamoxifen may contribute to endocrine therapy resistance (Fig. 29.2). In addition, similar to the genomic activity of ER, its nongenomic activity is also influenced by other cellular ER coregulatory proteins and by other pathways functioning in a given tumor. Increased expression of tyrosine kinase receptors (TKRs), such as in tumors amplified for ERBB2, can significantly augment ER nongenomic activity in response to both estrogen and tamoxifen (104,126–128). In preclinical models it has been shown that long-term treatment with tamoxifen facilitates translocation of the ER out of the nucleus and enhances its interaction with EGFR, ERBB2, or both (123,129). Activation of the ERBB pathway by tamoxifen in tumors that also express ER could explain the reduced benefit of tamoxifen in these patients.

Growth Factor and Estrogen Receptor Crosstalk—Implications for Hormone Resistance

The molecular crosstalk between growth factors, other signaling pathways, and the ER pathway is indeed bidirectional. Although this multilevel crosstalk seems to be important for the natural activity of these pathways under physiological conditions, recent studies also demonstrate the importance of this crosstalk in breast cancer etiology and progression (130), especially in modulating ER activity and tumor response to endocrine therapies (131–133). An important example is the bidirectional interaction between ER and the TKR pathway EGFR/ERBB2. Nuclear/genomic ER can activate growth factor pathways by increasing the expression of ligands (i.e., transforming growth factor [TGF] α, amphiregulin), receptors (i.e., IGF-1),

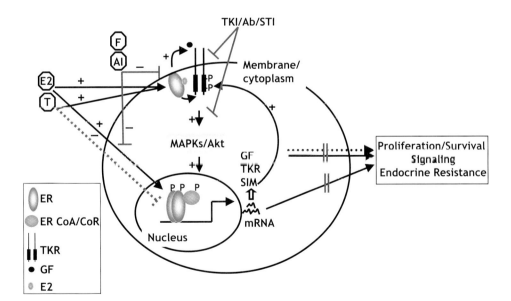

FIGURE 29.2. Bidirectional cross-talk between estrogen receptor (ER) and growth factor (GF) signaling pathways. The ER pathway, through both nongenomic actions (membrane and cytoplasmic, **top**) and genomic actions (nuclear, **bottom**) can activate, transmit, and amplify growth factor (GF) and cellular signaling, which are important for breast tumor cell proliferation and survival (see text for details). Estrogen (*E2*) can stimulate both ER activities; potent antiestrogens, such as fulvestrant (*F*), and estrogen deprivation strategies, such as aromatase inhibitors (*AI*), mostly block them; and mixed antiestrogens such as the selective estrogen receptor modulator (SERM) tamoxifen (*T*) inhibit the genomic action, but at the same time may induce ER nongenomic activity. Growth factor signaling pathways, in turn, phosphorylate (*P*) different components of the ER pathway (ER itself and its coregulatory proteins [*CoA*, coactivators, and *CoR*, corepressors]) and activate ER-dependent gene transcription (genomic activity). Overexpression or activation of tyrosine kinase receptors (*TKR*) (e.g., ERBB2, see text) can further augment both nongenomic and genomic functions of ER, thus leading to a stimulatory cycle and endocrine resistance, especially resistance to agents such as tamoxifen. Blockade of these growth factor pathways either by antibodies (*Ab*), by tyrosine kinase inhibitor (*TKI*) small molecules, or by other signal transduction inhibitors (*STI*) can restore tamoxifen's inhibitory properties and can delay or prevent resistance to other forms of endocrine therapy in model systems. This approach is currently being tested in the clinic. SIM, signaling intermediate molecules.

or other signaling intermediate molecules (SIM) (i.e., insulin receptor substrate-1 [IRS-1]) which are estrogen regulated and important for growth factor activity (134) (Fig. 29.2). Nongenomic ER activity is augmented in tumors that have high levels of the TKR ERBB2 (104,135,136). Membrane ER bound by estrogen or SERM can rapidly activate the ERBB pathway. In turn, signaling through the ERBB pathway can activate the transcriptional function of ER in the nucleus by phosphorylating coactivators and corepressors, as well as ER itself (104) (Fig. 29.2).

This increased crosstalk may further negate the efficacy of various hormonal therapies and especially of SERMs, such as tamoxifen, where tumor resistance involves an altered balance of the agonist versus the antagonist actions of the agents. Indeed, compelling clinical and experimental evidence suggests that breast tumors with increased expression of growth factor signaling components, particularly of the EGFR/ERBB2 pathway, are associated with a poor response to tamoxifen (68,137–143)—in preclinical systems tamoxifen can actually stimulate the growth of ERBB2-overexpressing tumors (104,138,144), whereas estrogen deprivation or the potent antiestrogen fulvestrant, which more effectively inhibit both activities of the ER, can still effectively suppress growth of these tumors (145). Interestingly, three published neoadjuvant endocrine therapy trials similarly demonstrate relatively high short-term response rates to aromatase inhibitors in ERBB2-overexpressing tumors, whereas responses to tamoxifen are few (146–148). Recent data from the adjuvant setting with disease-free survival (DFS) as the end point failed, however, to confirm this differential benefit of AI over tamoxifen in ERBB2-positive tumors (149,150). Increased estrogen-independent proliferation reported in ERBB2-positive primary breast cancers after neoadjuvant AI (151), may explain this discrepancy. Estrogen deprivation, by inhibiting both the genomic and nongenomic effects of ER, may cause a short term reduction in tumor growth, but over time increasing ERBB2 activity may result in more rapid tumor progression. These data suggest that successful treatment of ER-positive/ERBB2-positive tumors will require a blockade of both pathways (104,145,152,153).

Despite that ER and ERBB receptors can amplify each other's signals, these pathways can also provide inhibitory functions. ER activation downregulates the expression of the ERBB receptor family, including EGFR1 and ERBB2 (154,155), whereas ERBB signaling can downregulate the expression of ER and PR (153,156–161). It has been shown that blocking ER can then upregulate the expression of EGFR and ERBB2, perhaps contributing to resistance to ER-targeted therapy. Similarly, blocking the ERBB pathways can upregulate the expression of ER, providing an alternative survival pathway for the cell and causing resistance to ERBB-targeted therapy. Acquired resistance to tamoxifen in tumors that initially express low levels of EGFR and ERBB2 is indeed associated with increased EGFR/ERBB2, including ERBB2 gene amplification (139,142,162–164). Likewise, resistance to ERBB2 therapy, again both experimentally and in the clinical setting, is occasionally associated with increased ER expression (153,165,166).

Collectively, this substantial bidirectional crosstalk suggests the possibility that in some breast cancers a simultaneous blockade of both ER and ERBB signaling pathways, or of other pertinent deregulated cellular signaling networks, may be required to bypass resistance mechanisms and achieve optimal treatment benefit. Results from multiple studies in various preclinical models indeed imply that targeting the EGFR/ERBB2 pathway using specific monoclonal antibodies or tyrosine kinase inhibitors in combination with endocrine therapy can restore tamoxifen's antagonistic effects and antitumor activity, overcoming *de novo* resistance and significantly delaying or preventing the emergence of acquired resistance to various

endocrine therapies (104,138,139,142,167–169). Two recently reported randomized phase II trials comparing tamoxifen with or without gefitinib and anastrozole with or without gefitinib support this idea (170,171).

THE IMPORTANCE OF RECEPTORS IN CLINICAL BREAST CANCER

Approximately 30% to 40% of patients with ER-positive metastatic disease will respond to first-line hormonal therapies, and another 20% will experience disease stabilization (172–174). We also know that adjuvant hormonal therapy can halve the recurrence rate of patients with ER-positive breast cancer (175). Hormonal therapy is relatively nontoxic and responses can last for many years in some patients with metastatic disease. Thus, hormonal therapies offer many significant advantages to particular subsets of breast cancer patients. All endocrine therapies target the ER signaling pathway. The ER pathway can be targeted either by strategies that act on the receptor itself (i.e., selective ER modulators, such as tamoxifen, or potent pure antagonists that can degrade the receptor, such as fulvestrant), and by approaches that deprive the receptor of estrogen (i.e., AI and ovarian ablation). It is well accepted that the measurement of ER and PR levels in patients can select those tumors most likely to benefit from hormonal agents.

METHODS FOR MEASURING ESTROGEN AND PROGESTERONE RECEPTORS

Assessment of ER and PR status is an essential factor in the evaluation of breast cancers. Although ER and PR status provides prognostic information, currently the major clinical value of determining them is to assess the likelihood that a patient will respond to hormonal therapies (176). Early studies used radiolabeled ligand-binding assays, such as the dextran-coated charcoal (DCC) method, which was rigorously validated and standardized in the United States. These methods were replaced in the 1990s with immunohistochemical (IHC) assays, which have not been standardized or rigorously validated. This lack of standardization and validation may contribute to the relatively high error rate in some studies when ER is measured by IHC.

Dextran-coated Charcoal Ligand Binding Assay

The first prototypical assays used routinely in the clinical setting were performed on tumor cytosols derived by extraction methods. Tumor cytosols were incubated with radiolabeled steroid (estrogen or progestin), and the results reported as femtomoles (fmol) of receptor protein per milligram (mg) of total cytosol protein from Scatchard plots (177). Several disadvantages of the DCC assay exist, however, including tumor cellularity and heterogeneity, and the requirement for fresh or snap-frozen tissue. After standardization of these methods was accomplished by a National Cancer Institute (NCI)-funded quality control program in the 1980s, most laboratories defined positives as 10 fmol/mg or greater protein, borderline positive as more than 3 to 9, and negative as less than 3. These assays provide an overall score for the entire fragment of the tumor including neoplastic and non-neoplastic cells, and may give false results depending on the relative proportion of cancer versus other cell types within the tumor. Breast cancers display a broad dynamic range in ER and PR expression using these assays, and the magnitude of benefit from hormonal therapy is significantly related to the quantity of protein in the tumor (178). Mammographic screening has dramatically reduced the average size of breast cancer below that required for the assay, so today it has become impossible to prospectively collect enough tissue to sustain routine ER and PR measurements using DCC assays.

Immunohistochemical Assays

With the development of specific, reliable, and commercially available ER and PR antibodies (179,180), and the development of robust IHC technologies, IHC assays have replaced DCC to measure receptor levels. IHC allows for the precise determination of receptor status at the individual cell level, accommodating the problem of tissue heterogeneity within the tumor. IHC assays are less labor intensive and less expensive than extraction assays. They are also amenable to small tumors, and allow for the morphologic correlation of receptor status with histologic evaluation. Importantly, they can be performed on retrospectively collected, formalin-fixed, paraffin-embedded tissue, including archival tissues and fine-needle biopsies, and on frozen tissue as well. Additionally, IHC is not affected by bound ligand (a problem with the DCC assay in pre-or perimenopausal patients). IHC is performed by first treating thin sections of tissue using a variety of antigen retrieval methods, followed by incubation of the tissue with a primary antibody directed against ER or PR. Then a number of secondary detection systems, such as the use of secondary antibodies that have been conjugated to an enzyme (e.g., horseradish peroxidase), can be used to amplify the chromogenic signal. The sections can finally be counterstained and viewed microscopically. For both ER and PR, the staining produces a predominant nuclear stain, and considerable heterogeneity in staining can exist within the malignant epithelium.

Comparison of Assay Methods and Standardization

When hormone receptor status of tumors determined by IHC assay has been compared with that determined by extraction assays, discordances between 10% and 30% have been reported for both ER and PR status (181–183). This low level of discordance is remarkable given the variability in antibodies, techniques, and scoring systems applied in clinical IHC assays. Hormone receptor status determined by IHC assay has

consistently been found to have similar prognostic and predictive value as that determined using extraction assay (184,185) and, in some cases, superior ability to predict hormone response in patients (186,187). Using well-defined, randomized clinical trial cohorts and a central pathology laboratory to investigate concordance between the two assays, Regan et al. (188) recently reported that, for ER status, concordance was higher among postmenopausal women (88%), than among premenopausal patients (81%). In contrast, concordance for PR status was lower in postmenopausal patients (76% vs. 80% premenopausal). In this study, IHC assay appeared to increase the fraction of ER- or PR-positive tumors, most likely because of the overall higher sensitivity of this assay.

Immunohistochemical staining, however, can be highly affected by a variety of preanalytic factors, particularly the efficiency of antigen retrieval and the time of tissue fixation (189–191). Hormone receptors degrade in unfixed tissue, and tissue sitting at room temperature for 4 to 5 hours loses a significant amount of ER. A consensus development panel of the National Institutes of Health (NIH) convened in 2000 recommended that any ER staining in breast cancers should be sufficient to consider a tumor as ER-positive, and that patient is therefore a suitable candidate for endocrine therapy (192). The number of factors and assay details that affect ER IHC results highlight, however, the need for standardization of clinical IHC assays for determining hormone receptor status.

The most recent American Society of Clinical Oncology (ASCO) guidelines on the use of tumor markers were published in 2007 (193). This panel of experts acknowledged that deficits remain in the standardization of ER and PR IHC assays, and that further efforts were required for defining reproducibility and accuracy. They agreed with previous recommendations that ERα and PR should continue to be measured on every primary invasive breast cancer, and may be measured on metastatic lesions if the results could influence therapy decision-making. The ultimate utility of receptor status resides in its ability to predict clinical outcome, and several clinically validated IHC assays have been developed. One of the most highly developed manual scoring systems for hormone receptor IHC assays is called the *Allred Score* (AS) (187,194–196). This semiquantitative scoring system (Fig. 29.3) consists of a proportion score (*PS*) which represents the estimated proportion of positive-staining tumor cells (scores ranging from 0 to 5), and an intensity score (*IS*) which represents the average intensity of positive

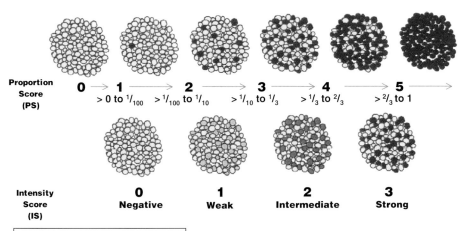

FIGURE 29.3. Schematic depicting the Allred scoring system. Proportion score (PS) range 0 to 5, intensity score (IS) range 0 to 3, Total score (TS = PS + IS) range 0, 2 to 8. (From Phillips T, Murray G, Wakamiya K, et al. Development of standard estrogen and progesterone receptor immunohistochemical assays for selection of patients for antihormonal therapy. *Appl Immunohistochem Mol Morphol* 2007;15:325–331, with permission.)

Total Score (TS) = PS + IS
(TS range = 0, 2-8)

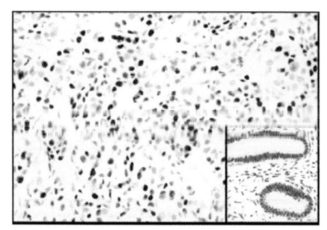

FIGURE 29.4. Photomicrograph of a representative invasive breast cancer tissue sample immunostained for estrogen receptor (ER) (magnification, ×200). ER-positive cells show a dark brown or black nuclear signal. Using this field, this tumor would get a total immunohistochemistry (IHC) score of 6 (proportion score [= 4] + intensity score [= 2]). The *inset* shows human endocervix tissue, which was used as a positive control because of its easy availability and relatively stable reactivity. (From Harvey JM, Clark GM, Osborne CK, et al. Estrogen receptor status by immunohistochemistry is superior to the ligand-binding assay for predicting response to adjuvant endocrine therapy in breast cancer. *J Clin Oncol* 1999;17:1474–1481. Reprinted with permission from the American Society of Clinical Oncology.)

tumor cells (scores ranging from 0 to 3). The proportion and intensity scores are added to obtain a total score (*TS ranging from 0 to 8*). A photomicrograph of a representative invasive breast cancer sample immunostained for ERα with a total AS of 6 is shown in Figure 29.4. It has been proposed that the AS facilitates discrimination between positive and negative results at low receptor expression levels. A total score between 3 and 8 is considered ERα-positive, which represents either 10% weakly staining nuclei or 1% intermediately staining nuclei. Using the AS, approximately 71% of samples were determined to be ERα-positive in a cohort of more than 1,900 primary breast cancers (187). A comparison of ER status results as determined by AS and DCC in this study is shown in Table 29.1. It has also been estimated that 62% of tumors coexpress ERα and β, about 14% to 15% stain for either receptor, and approximately 9% are completely negative for ERα using the AS method (Fig. 29.5) (197). The AS system may only be applicable when using IHC methodology similar to that in which the scoring system was developed. Although IHC assays for ERβ have been developed (197,198), no consensus exists on the

use of ERβ in routine clinical practice. Studies suggest that tumors expressing abundant ERβ respond better to tamoxifen (199,200).

Using both the AS and a manual estimate of the percentage of ER-positive tumor cells in a series of 800 breast cancers, it has been reported that ER staining using different methodology has a bimodal frequency distribution (Fig. 29.6) (201). Most breast cancers were either entirely ERα-negative or unambiguously ERα-positive; weak ERα-positivity was rare. These results are similar to what has been reported by others using percentage positivity scoring in a series of more than 5,900 breast cancers (202). In this series, most tumors were diffusely positive or completely negative for ER. Of all these breast cancers, 75% were positive for ERα and 55% were positive for PR. The frequency of hormone receptor positivity is summarized in Table 29.2, and a summary of the relationship of ER and PR to histologic subtypes is shown in Table 29.3. These results raise the question of whether quantitative measurement of receptors is necessary because the threshold was binary (completely negative or unequivocally positive) in these large studies. Others, however, have disagreed with this conclusion, and propose that these IHC assays may be too sensitive, having lost the semiquantitation that correlated well with clinical outcome when the DCC assay and earlier well-validated IHC assays were used (Fig. 29.7) (172,187,203). Thus, a more quantitative measurement of hormone receptor status might be of interest. To this aim, automated systems have been developed for quantifying ERα, and there appears to be good concordance between these imaging systems (203,204). Of note, the frequency distribution from these automated systems is continuous, similar to that obtained with DCC assay. Many pathologists agree that one priority should be to improve the quality of widespread IHC testing, possibly through guidelines from the College of American Pathology and the American Society of Clinical Oncology, such as those established for ERBB2 clinical testing (205). Recently, just such a committee has been established and recommendations are eagerly anticipated.

RNA-Based Assays

Because IHC scores of receptor status using highly sensitive methodology can be dichotomous, accurate quantization may be better suited for RNA-based assays, such as quantitative reverse transcription-polymerase chain reaction (qRT-PCR). The development of the robust 21 gene Onco*type* DX qRT/PCR predictive assay using fixed tissue material is evidence that it is possible to measure ERα and PR RNA levels reliably from archived tissues (206). Badve et al. (207) have compared

| Table 29.1 | **COMPARISON OF ER STATUS RESULTS, AS DETERMINED BY AS AND DCC IN 1,982 PRIMARY BREAST CANCER CASES** |

	Patients				Ligand Binding Results (fmol/mg protein)		
IHC Score	**No.**	**%**	**Mean**	**SD**	**Median**	**Minimum**	**Maximum**
0	517	26	10	49	1	0	758
2	67	3	50	100	8	0	548
3	117	6	59	95	23	0	623
4	190	10	67	73	39	0	428
5	320	16	104	139	56	0	1549
6	370	19	141	158	89	0	1181
7	318	16	193	215	142	0	1798
8	83	4	282	312	185	0	1439

ER, estrogen receptor; AS, Allred Score; DCC, Dextran-coated charcoal; SD standard deviation.
Adapted from Harvey JM, Clark GM, Osborne CK, et al. Estrogen receptor status by immunohistochemistry is superior to the ligand-binding assay for predicting response to adjuvant endocrine therapy in breast cancer. *J Clin Oncol* 1999;17:1474–1481, with permission.

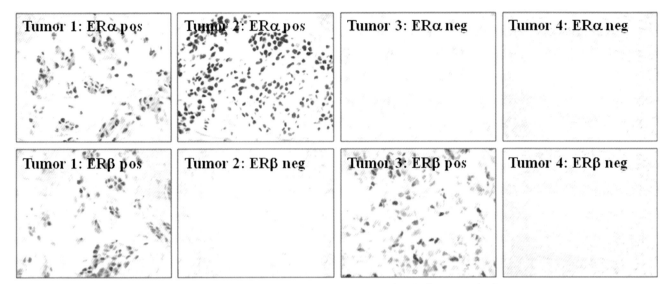

FIGURE 29.5. Immunohistochemistry (IHC) of four representative breast tumors from the tissue array using the estrogen receptor (ER)α 6F11 antibody or the ERβ-specific 14C8 antibody. Tumors representative of the different subgroups are included: tumor 1—ERα-positive/ERβ-positive; tumor 2—ERα-positive/ERβ-negative; tumor 3—ERα-negative/ERβ-positive; and tumor 4—ERα-negative/ERβ-negative. (From Fuqua SA, Schiff R, Parra I, et al. Estrogen receptor beta protein in human breast cancer: correlation with clinical tumor parameters. *Cancer Res* 2003;63:2434–2439, with permission.)

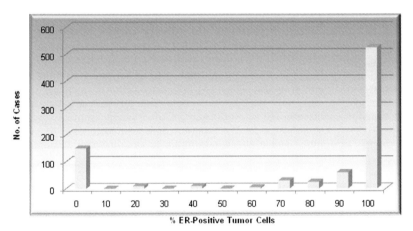

FIGURE 29.6. A frequency distribution of the percentage of cells showing nuclear staining for estrogen receptor among 825 primary breast cancers. (From Collins LC, Botero ML, Schnitt SJ. Bimodal frequency distribution of estrogen receptor immunohistochemical staining results in breast cancer: an analysis of 825 cases. *Am J Clin Pathol* 2005;123:16–20, with permission. 2005 American Society of Clinical Pathology.)

Table 29.2 STATUS OF ER AND PR IN 5,497 CASES OF INFILTRATING MAMMARY CARCINOMA IN HISTOLOGIC SPECIMENS

Receptor	No. (%)
ER+	4,100 (75)
PR+	3,016 (55)
ER+/PR+	3,016 (55)
ER+/PR−	1,084 (20)
ER−/PR−	1,397 (25)
ER−/PR+	0 (0)

ER, estrogen receptor; PR, progesterone receptor; +, positive; −, negative.
Adapted from Nadji M, Gomez-Fernandez C, Ganjei-Azar P, et al. Immunohistochemistry of estrogen and progesterone receptors reconsidered: experience with 5,993 breast cancers. *Am J Clin Pathol* 2005;123:21–27, with permission.

Table 29.3 RELATIONSHIP OF ER AND PR TO HISTOLOGIC SUBTYPES OF MAMMARY CARCINOMA

Type of Carcinoma	ER Positive		PR Positive	
Infiltrating ductal, not otherwise specified (n = 4,396)	3,255	74%	2,330	53%
Tubular (n = 237)	237	100%	225	95%
Colloid (n = 184)	184	100%	133	72%
Papillary (n = 44)	44	100%	35	80%
Apocrine (n = 40)	0	0%	0	0%
Medullary (n = 96)	0	0%	0	0%
Metaplastic (n = 120)	0	0%	0	0%
Infiltrating lobular (n = 380)	380	100%	293	77%

ER, estrogen receptor; PR, progesterone receptor; data are given as number (percentage).
Adapted from Nadji M, Gomez-Fernandez C, Ganjei-Azar P, et al. Immunohistochemistry of estrogen and progesterone receptors reconsidered: experience with 5,993 breast cancers. *Am J Clin Pathol* 2005;123:21–27, with permission.

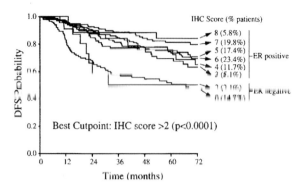

Patients receiving any endocrine therapy (n = 777)

IHC Score (% patients)

8 (5.8%)
7 (19.8%)
5 (17.4%)
6 (23.4%) — ER positive
4 (11.7%)
3 (5.1%)

2 (2.1%)
0 (14.7%) — ER negative

Best Cutpoint: IHC score >2 (p<0.0001)

FIGURE 29.7. Univariate disease-free survival (DFS) curves for all possible total immuno-histochemical (IHC) scores in patients receiving any adjuvant endocrine therapy (almost always tamoxifen). An IHC score >2 was the optimal cut point for predicting cut point for predicting significantly improved outcome ($p < .0001$), and this value was used to define estrogen receptor (ER) positivity throughout the study. (From Harvey JM, Clark GM, Osborne CK, et al. Estrogen receptor status by immunohistochemistry is superior to the ligand-binding assay for predicting response to adjuvant endocrine therapy in breast cancer. *J Clin Oncol* 1999;17:1474–1481, with permission.)

central laboratory IHC (using AS) and qRT-PCR for measuring ERα and PR levels in samples from Eastern Cooperative Oncology Group (ECOG) 2197 (207). There was a high degree of concordance between central IHC and qRT-PCR for both ER and PR status (Fig. 29.8). This agrees with a number of other studies that have shown a high degree of concordance between the two assays, particularly for ERα (208–210). In ECOG 2197 samples, measuring ERα by qRT-PCR was statistically superior to IHC in predicting relapse in tamoxifen-treated, ERα-positive patients (207). For PR, IHC outperformed RNA-based assays. In

this same series of patients, they found that the Oncotype DX RT-PCR assay exhibited a continuous distribution of expression over a 3,000-fold and 1,000-fold range, respectively, for ER and PR (207). In conclusion, qRT-PCR is an alternative method for determining hormone receptor status, which remains to be fully validated but which may circumvent the limitations of nonstandardized IHC assays. These techniques are discussed in detail in Chapter 32.

Another strategy under investigation is to augment the predictive value of hormone receptor mRNA levels with estrogen-regulated gene signatures determined by RNA microarray analysis (211,212). Profiling with expression arrays allows for the simultaneous assessment of thousands of mRNA species, rather than a single gene, such as ER, in tumor samples and may make individualized diagnosis and treatment possible in the future. Using microarray analysis of 142 breast tumor samples, Gong et al. (213) found a significant correlation between ER mRNA expression levels and ER IHC levels determined by the AS (Fig. 29.9). Several groups have developed gene expression-based predictors of ER and PR positivity, which can significantly predict outcomes (214–216). Additional studies are needed to address whether multigene signatures will indeed outperform individual biomarkers for prediction of patient outcome and tumor response.

ESTROGEN AND PROGESTERONE RECEPTORS IN THE CLINICAL MANAGEMENT OF PATIENTS WITH BREAST CANCER

Estrogen receptors and PR can be utilized as both predictive and prognostic factors. A prognostic factor is any measurable parameter available at the time of surgery that correlates with disease-free or overall survival after local therapy. As such, it is indicative of the inherent biological aggressiveness of a tumor and is correlated with the natural history of the disease.

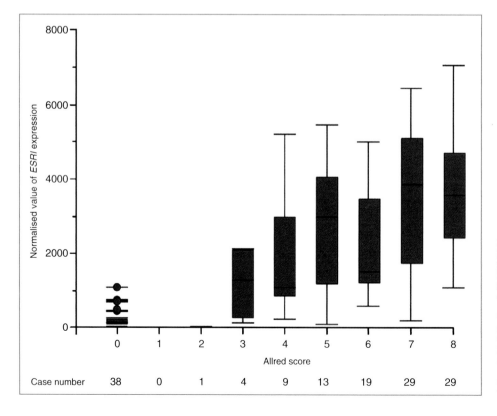

| Case number | 38 | 0 | 1 | 4 | 9 | 13 | 19 | 29 | 29 |

FIGURE 29.8. Box plots showing correlation between estrogen receptor gene locus (ESR1) messenger RNA (mRNA) expression and immunohistochemical (IHC) Allred scores in 142 samples. *Rectangles* = IQR (25th and 75th percentiles). *Horizontal line within rectangle* = median. *Outer boundary brackets* = 2.5th and 97.5th percentiles. *Circles* = individual samples outside range. IQR, interquartile range (From Yun Gong, Kai Yan, Feng Lin, et al. *Lancet Oncol* 2007;8:203–211. Determination of oestrogen-receptor status and ERBB2 status of breast carcinoma: a gene-expression profiling study. By Yun Gong, Kai Yan, Feng Lin, et al. with permission from Elsevier.)

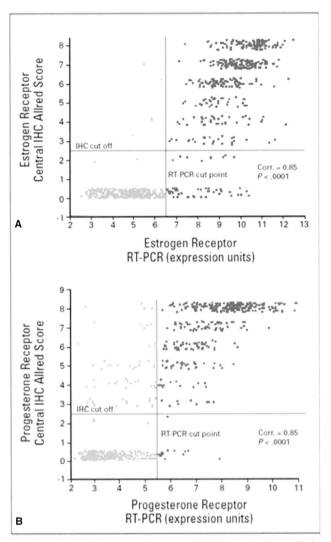

FIGURE 29.9. The distribution of expression by central IHC (Allred score) and expression by central RT-PCR using Onco*type* DX. A: Estrogen receptor expression. **B:** Progesterone receptor expression. Corr, Spearmen rank correlation; IHC, immunohistochemistry; RT-PCR, reverse-transcriptase polymerase chain reaction. (From Badve SS, Baehner FL, Gray RP, et al. Estrogen- and progesterone-receptor status in ECOG 2197: comparison of immunohistochemistry by local and central laboratories and quantitative reverse transcription polymerase chain reaction by central laboratory. *J Clin Oncol* 2008;26:2473–2481, with permission.)

In contrast, a predictive factor indicates the likelihood of a response to a given therapy—in the case of ER and PR, endocrine therapy. It should be noted that prognostic and predictive traits are not mutually exclusive, and some factors, such as ER and PR, as well as others such as ERBB2, are both prognostic and predictive. Given that up to two-thirds of invasive breast cancers of women aged younger than 50 years are ER- or PR-positive, and approximately 80% of tumors in women more than 50 years of age are ER-positive (217,218), understanding of the predictive and prognostic role of ER and PR has significant clinical implications.

The predictive value of ER and PR was established first in the advanced-disease setting, mainly by the DCC method, which detects ERα and PR-A and B, as discussed above. In current breast cancer practice, however, the status of ER and PR is mostly valuable in assessing the benefit and determining the use of endocrine therapy in the adjuvant setting. These two biomarkers are measured at present by the IHC method, which can selectively recognize, at least in the case of ER, the different subtypes of the receptor. The prognostic and predictive role

of ERβ is much less characterized than ERα and, for clinical purposes, only ERα is presently measured. Any reference to ER in this chapter hereafter in the context of studies using IHC refers to the α subtype alone, unless otherwise specified. As mentioned above, IHC assays for PR are perhaps even more challenging than those for ER. PR has two isoforms (A and B) that appear to function differently, and the more aggressive, tamoxifen-resistant tumors are those with a high A to B isoform ratio (219). The various antibodies currently used in IHC assays recognize different epitopes, with some identifying only one of the isoforms and some identifying both (220). This complexity might account for some of the recently observed discrepancies regarding PR's predictive and prognostic value among various adjuvant trials (see below).

Estrogen and Progesterone Receptors as Predictive Factors for Hormonal Therapy in Advanced Disease

Many trials testing multiple regimens have been conducted in advanced or metastatic breast cancer (MBC) to identify treatments that may improve response rates and survival. Despite some advances and the recent incorporation of new agents into the clinical practice, median survival of patients with MBC is still only 2 to 3 years (221,222) with very few patients—2%—surviving 20 years after the diagnosis of metastases (223). Pioneering studies carried out in the early 1970s were the first to suggest that ER status might be a predictor of response to endocrine therapy in advanced breast cancer (224). These early studies clearly indicated that ER-positive disease has a much higher response rate to a variety of hormonal therapies with only very rare responses in ER-negative tumors (224). Successive larger and better controlled studies performed over the next 30 years validated these original observations (172,173,225–227). This work has largely demonstrated that approximately 50% to 60% of all ER-positive patients respond to first-line hormonal therapy, with tumors either regressing or stabilizing. In contrast, only 5% to 10% of ER-negative patients respond (228,229), and these responses may represent false–negative receptor assay results. All metastatic patients receiving endocrine treatment eventually progress, but they often benefit from a new second-line endocrine therapy that lacks cross resistance with the primary agent (230). ER status is also important in predicting benefit from second-line and subsequent hormonal therapeutics. Although clinical benefits gradually decline, they remain in the 20% to 30% range (231–233), and treatment provides palliation, improved quality of life, and prolonged survival. Very few ER-negative patients respond to second-line therapy.

In the past decade, third-generation aromatase inhibitors (AIs) were approved as a first-line treatment for postmenopausal patients with MBC and, more recently, as treatment for early breast cancer as well (234,235). Several large randomized trials have demonstrated that AIs are at least as effective as tamoxifen in MBC patients (225,229,236–238). Meta-analysis of randomized controlled trials that compared several generations of AIs with standard hormonal treatments has further demonstrated that inhibition of aromatase—especially with third-generation AIs—is associated with statistically significantly improved survival in patients with MBC (239). To address the relationship between hormone receptor status and treatment outcome in MBC patients, Buzdar et al. (240) have reviewed the data on the AIs anastrozole and letrozole from some of these phase III trials (Table 29.4). With some limitations, the overall data conclude that positive hormone receptor status (ER, PR, or both) is of great importance in determining an improvement in time to progression (TTP) with the use of first-line treatment with these AIs (240) (Table 29.4).

Table 29.4	OBJECTIVE RESPONSE AND CLINICAL BENEFIT IN OVERALL PATIENT POPULATIONS AND HORMONE RECEPTOR-POSITIVE SUBGROUPS OF AROMATASE INHIBITOR TRIALS IN THE ADVANCED DISEASE

	Objective Response (%)[a]			Clinical Benefit (%)[b]			Median TTP (Months)			Median Survival (Months)		
Anastrozole Trials	AN	TAM	p	AN	TAM	p	AN	TAM	P	AN	TAM	p
TARGET (n = 668)	33	33	NS	50	50	NS	8.2	8.0	0.011	30.6	40.0	NA
North American (n = 353)	21	17	NS	59	46	0.0098	11.1	5.6	0.0006	10.1	38.6	NA
Combined Analysis (overall population n = 1,021)	29	27	NS	57	52	0.1129	8.5	7.0	0.103	39.2	40.1	NA
Combined Analysis (Patients with ER- and/or PR positive tumors) (n = 611/1021;60%)	28	24	NA	59	50	0.016	10.7	6.4	0.022	40.8	41.3	NS
Letrozole trial	LET	TAM	p	LET	TAM	p	LET	TAM	P	LET	TAM	P
Overall population (n = 907)	32	21	.0002	50	38	.0004	9.4	6.0	<.0001	34.0	30.0	NS

AN, anastrozole; ER, estrogen receptor; LET, letrozole; NA, data not available; NS, not significant; PR, progesterone receptor; TAM, tamoxifen; TTP, time to progression.
[a]Objective response includes complete or partial responders.
[b]Clinical benefit includes a complete or partial response or stabilization of ≥24 weeks.
Adapted from Buzdar AU, Vergote I, Sainsbury R. The impact of hormone receptor status on the clinical efficacy of the new-generation aromatase inhibitors: a review of data from first-line metastatic disease trials in postmenopausal women. *Breast J* 2004;10:211–217, with permission from Blackwell Publishing.

Although still somewhat controversial in current breast cancer pathology, many studies have confirmed that within the group of ER-positive tumors, the *quantity* of ER present in the tumor is an important factor. As mentioned above and later, for practical or technical reasons in both research and clinical settings, it is simpler to label tumors as either ER negative or positive. In actuality, however, ER concentration is a continuous variable. Response rates to endocrine therapies are, as expected, also continuous and are directly related to the level of the protein. Furthermore, low ER levels can also reflect active growth factor receptor signaling in the cell (156,159–161) that may jeopardize ER activity or provide alternative survival signals. When measured carefully, increasing ER by IHC (for ERα), as by DCC, is significantly associated with improved response and longer survival in MBC (Table 29.5) (172,221,240–242).

To improve the ability to predict the responsiveness of tumors to endocrine therapy, other tumor biomarkers, in addition to the quantity of ER, can also be utilized. Because a response to endocrine therapy requires a functioning ER pathway, it was hypothesized that measuring additional markers that reflect the integrity of the pathway, such as PR, an ER-regulated gene, will assist in predicting response to endocrine therapy more accurately than simply evaluating the presence

Table 29.5	RELATIONSHIP OF ESTROGEN RECEPTOR AND PROGESTERONE RECEPTOR LEVEL TO CLINICAL BENEFIT FROM ENDOCRINE THERAPY IN ADVANCED DISEASE

Estrogen Receptor Level, Ligand-Binding Assay (fmol/mg)[a]	N (Total = 415)	Response Rate	
<3.0	22	5%	
3.0–10.0	76	18%	
10.1–30.0	219	37%	
30.1–300.0	63	78%	
>300.0	35	77%	

Estrogen Receptor Level, Immunohistochemistry[b]	N (Total = 205)	Response Rate	Time to Treatment Failure
Negative	20	25%	5 months
Intermediate	54	46%	4 months
High	131	66%	10 months

Progesterone Receptor Level, Immunohistochemistry[b]	N (Total = 204)	Response Rate	Time to Treatment Failure
Negative	69	46%	5 months
Intermediate	78	55%	7 months
High	57	70%	10 months

[a]Estrogen receptor data in top panel adapted from Bezwoda W, Esser J, Dansey R, et al. The value of estrogen and progesterone receptor determinations in advanced breast cancer. *Cancer* 1991;68:867–872.
[b]Estrogen receptor data in middle panel and progesterone receptor data in bottom panel adapted from Elledge R, Green S, Pugh R, et al. Estrogen receptor (ER) and progesterone receptor (PR) by ligand-binding assay compared with ER, PR, pS2 by immunohistochemistry in predicting response to tamoxifen in metastatic breast cancer: a Southwest Oncology Group Study. *Int J Cancer* 2000;89:111–117.

or absence of only the ER protein (243). Indeed, in the metastatic setting, multiple clinical trials, including large prospective studies, have confirmed this notion and shown that, as with ER, increasing PR levels are also associated with better response, longer time to treatment failure, and longer survival (172,226,244) (Table 29.5). One of the first prospectively designed studies to validate a biomarker in breast cancer confirmed that quantitative measurement of PR by either the DCC method or by IHC was an independent predictive marker for response to tamoxifen (226,241). It should be mentioned, however, that more recent clinical research, including in both the adjuvant (see below) and neoadjuvant settings, suggests a more complex relationship between PR levels and response to endocrine therapy. For example, a neoadjuvant trial has documented a response rate that increases through an intermediate range of PR levels, but then decreases at the highest levels (146). It should be further emphasized that, although ER and PR are correlated, in the metastatic setting PR does provide valuable information independent of ER (226), with response rate higher by one-third in patients with ER-positive, PR-positive tumors in comparison with patients with ER-positive, PR-negative tumors. With an advanced understanding of the biology of ER and PR, it has become clear that PR status and its loss may provide important information regarding both the biology and responsiveness of tumors to endocrine and other therapies, as will be discussed later.

It has long been recognized that the hormone receptor status of metastases does not always correlate with that of the primary tumor, with approximately 20% to 30% conversion rate from ER-positive to ER-negative and much less frequently from ER-negative to ER-positive at relapse (242,245–247). Indeed, the receptor status of the metastasis may be more predictive of response. One small study showed that, although 74% of patients with ER-positive primary tumors whose recurrent tumors retained ER expression responded to endocrine therapy, only 12% of patients with ER-positive primaries and ER-negative metastases likewise responded (247). Similar discordances between hormone receptor content of primary breast cancer versus MBC have also been recently documented in several other studies (228,248,249), and loss of ER was associated with a significantly shorter median survival in one of these studies (228). The metastatic tumor ER status was shown to be a better predicator of survival than the primary tumor ER status. In biopsies from patients who developed resistance to tamoxifen, changes in hormone receptor status, as well as in other signaling pathway molecules, such as ERBB2, have also recently been documented (162). Similarly to ER, and perhaps even at a higher rate, a significant proportion of PR-positive tumors also lose PR expression in their metastasis (250), and loss of PR in sequential biopsies, particularly with intervening endocrine therapy, is associated with poorer survival as compared with patients retaining PR (251). Different explanations have been suggested for this discordance, including (a) intratumor heterogeneity of breast cancer, which can lead to clonal selection of different clones with distinct hormone receptor properties that can change over time; (b) changes within single cells themselves as an adaptive mechanism for treatment; (c) tumor dedifferentiation with the development of metastasis; or (d) technical laboratory difficulties in hormone receptor assessment of small biopsy specimens. Regardless of the cause, the high level of this discordance between both ER and PR for primary and metastatic disease emphasizes the necessity for the integration, at progression, of a sequential biopsy and biomarker analysis (improved decision-making in the management of advanced breast cancer).

Using the DCC for receptor analysis in MBC, a small subset of these tumors—approximately 5%—is classified as ER-negative, PR-positive. The existence of this group is still debatable (see below) and its detection could be attributed to false–negative ER results, or could indicate an actual unique biology and pathway activation in these tumors resulting in repression of ER and activation of PR independent of ER. Nevertheless, trials in metastatic disease suggest that these tumors still benefit from endocrine therapy (252), although some data suggest that they may have a somewhat worse clinical outcome than ER-positive tumors (253).

Estrogen and Progesterone Receptors in Predicting the Benefit of Adjuvant Therapy

Endocrine Therapy

Clearly, both ER and PR are predictive markers for response to endocrine therapy in patients with metastatic disease. It is critical to understand whether and how hormone receptor status of the primary tumors in women with early-stage breast cancer can be utilized to estimate the benefit of adjuvant hormonal therapy.

The Oxford overview of trials of women with early breast cancer who were randomized to adjuvant tamoxifen versus no tamoxifen provides important data for determining the relationship of ER and PR status and clinical benefit from endocrine therapy (175,254). The latest Oxford meta-analysis cycle (2000–2005) includes data from more than 48,000 women in 56 randomized clinical trials of tamoxifen with follow-up of at least 15 to 20 years, and additional data from nearly 32,000 more women who were randomized to different durations of tamoxifen (175). The findings from this latest overview, as from the previous one, clearly and unquestionably indicate that ER status is a significant predictive factor of benefit to 5 years of adjuvant tamoxifen. A significant reduction in the annual odds of recurrence and death (Fig. 29.10) was shown in women with definitive ER-positive tumors, but not those with ER-poor (ER-negative) tumors. Most ER data in the meta-analysis were based on DCC that had been standardized and validated, at least in the United States. Similar fundamental differences of responses by ER status were also observed in more recent large prospective trials and other pooled analyses of several cooperative group trials (175,255–257), again showing that tamoxifen is efficient in reducing the risk of distant relapse, death, and even contralateral breast cancer (Table 29.6) (Chapter 48), but only in patients whose original tumors were ER-positive (175,254,258–260). How ER status of the original tumor can predict the contralateral tumor's benefit from tamoxifen is somewhat puzzling, because it is well accepted that contralateral breast cancer is a second event independent of the first tumor (261). Some studies, however, still support a plausible association between primary and synchronous or metachronous contralateral tumors (262,263), and this intriguing quandary deserves further investigation.

Just as is seen in advanced disease, the degree of the benefit from tamoxifen in early-stage disease is also directly correlated with the amount of the tumor's ER. This phenomenon is, as mentioned before, not surprising, and it has been shown by measuring ER by either DCC or by IHC (187,241,254) (Table 29.7). Women with tumors having greater than 100 fmol/mg of protein experience greater reductions in recurrence from 5 years of tamoxifen therapy in comparison with patients with lower ER. Furthermore, recent studies that measured ER by qRT-PCR retrospectively in central archive samples of adjuvant trials have also confirmed the significance of ER quantitation (207,264). As such, findings from the National Surgical Adjuvant Breast and Bowel Project (NSABP) B-14 biomarker study have shown that, although quantitative ER expression by qRT-PCR in

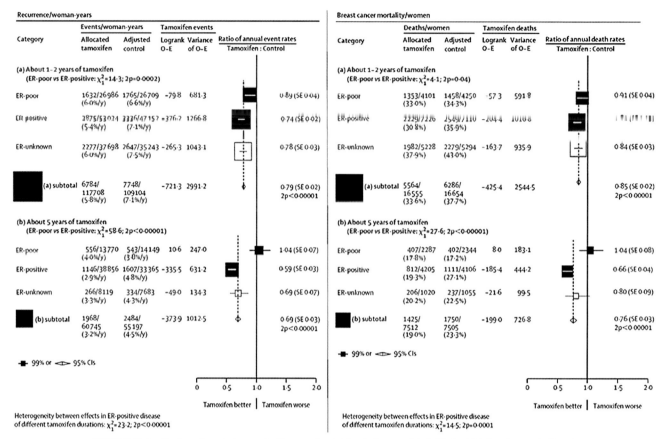

FIGURE 29.10. Results of a meta-analysis assessing the proportional risk reduction associated with about 1 to 2 or 5 years of adjuvant tamoxifen therapy, according to estrogen receptor (ER) status. The size of the *squares* reflects the relative size of the sample, and the *horizontal lines extending from each square* reflect the 99% confidence interval for the offset. The *vertical dashed line in the diamond* is the point estimate of the meta-analysis, and the *ends of the diamond* represent the 95% confidence intervals. Patients were randomized to receive adjuvant tamoxifen or no adjuvant tamoxifen. Women with ER-positive tumors received substantial benefit from 5 years of tamoxifen treatment. E, expected; O, observed; SE, standard error. (From Early Breast Cancer Trialists' Collaborative Group. Effects of chemotherapy and hormonal therapy for early breast cancer on recurrence and 15-year survival: an overview of the randomized trials. *Lancet* 2005;365:1702. Reprinted with permission from Elseveir.)

ER-positive, placebo-treated patients was not strongly prognostic, quantitative ER was the best single predictor of tamoxifen benefit (264). A similar positive relationship between ER levels and response to tamoxifen, as measured by Ki67 suppression, was also shown in the neoadjuvant setting (265).

Although ER positivity is clearly a good predictor of response both in the adjuvant setting and for metastatic disease, in an early meta-analysis ER-negative women treated with adjuvant tamoxifen also appeared to experience a small yet significant benefit (266). The most recent meta-analyses with longer follow-up and a larger patient population, however, did not confirm this observation. In the 2005 meta-analysis, among women with ER-negative disease, some benefit did appear in the trials of 1 to 2 years of tamoxifen, but not in the trials of 5 years of treatment. Although one may speculate that endocrine therapy may exert an effect not mediated through the tumor ER or PR and thus genuinely affect hormone receptor-negative tumors, a more probable explanation is that the benefits in ER-negative tumors are largely a result of false–negative ER measurements in some of the early trials of 1 to 2 years of tamoxifen (175).

The proven efficacy of AIs in advanced breast cancer has led to the development of multiple clinical trials evaluating their role in the adjuvant setting (see Chapter 48). Results are available for eight of these studies, which include more than 25,000 women, which were recently reviewed (267) (see also Chapter 48). Compared with a reference arm of 5 years of tamoxifen, these studies have focused on (a) an up-front AI (the Arimidex, Tamoxifen, Alone or in Combination [ATAC]) (268,269) and the Breast International Group (BIG) 1-98 (270,271) trials; (b) a sequential approach of switching to AI after 2 to 3 years of tamoxifen (Intergroup Exemestane Study [IES]) (272,273), Austrian Breast and Colorectal Cancer Study Group (ABCSG) trial 8 (274), Arimidex-Nolvadex (ARNO 95) trial (274, 275), and the Italian tamoxifen anastrozole (ITA)

Table 29.6	CONTRALATERAL BREAST CANCER INCIDENCE WITH TAMOXIFEN ACCORDING TO ESTROGEN RECEPTOR STATUS	
Study	No Tamoxifen	Tamoxifen
Intergroup study 0102[258,259]		
ER−	22/583	26/577
ER+	40/762	19/768
National Surgical Adjuvant Breast and Bowel Project B-23[260]		
ER−	19/992	18/990
Early Breast Cancer Trialists' Collaborative Group 1998[254]		
ER+/unk	260/5092	172/5137
ER−	57/1690	56/1645

ER, estrogen receptor; unk, unknown.

Table 29.7	RELATIVE REDUCTION IN RECURRENCE AND MORTALITY BY 5 YEARS OF ADJUVANT TAMOXIFEN ACCORDING TO LEVEL OF ESTROGEN RECEPTOR—OVERVIEW 1998	
	Reduction in Recurrence	Reduction in Mortality
ER+ (10–100 fmol/mg)	43% (±5)	23% (±6)
ER++ (>100 fmol/mg)	60% (±6)	36% (±7)

Values in parentheses are 95% confidence intervals.
Adapted from Early Breast Cancer Trialists' Collaborative Group. Tamoxifen for early breast cancer: an overview of the randomised trials. Early Breast Cancer Trialists' Collaborative Group. *Lancet* 1998;351:1451–1467.

study (276,277)]; and (c) extended AI hormonal therapy beyond 5 years of tamoxifen (the MA.17) (278,279) and NSABP B-33 (280) studies, and ABCSG trial 6a (281).

Findings from these studies have challenged the earlier standard of a 5-year duration of tamoxifen alone, and AIs are now becoming a standard component in the treatment of many postmenopausal women (267) (see Chapter 48). With these new treatment options, however, many questions remain about how to integrate these treatments to provide optimal therapy to individual patients. Identification of tumor and patient variables that might help tailor endocrine therapy, such as differentiating the relative benefits from an AI versus tamoxifen and determining the best sequential regimen, is an area of active research. A recent study of a subset of samples from the monotherapy arms of the ATAC trial (anastrozole versus tamoxifen) that were retrospectively collected and centrally tested (TransATAC) has recently been reported (150). This large study was international and only about one third of the blocks were obtained, most coming from patients entered from the United Kingdom. Analysis of quantitative ER by IHC revealed only a marginally significant relationship between ER level and time to recurrence (TTR) (150), with the effect less strong for tamoxifen ($p = .078$) than for anastrozole-treated patients ($p = .0009$). No significant interaction was noted between ER level and the relative benefit from anastrozole over tamoxifen treatments (150). The reason why this study, in contrast to the overview (254) and to analyses based on quantified ER mRNA (264), failed to detect a relationship between ER levels and tamoxifen outcome within the ER-positive population is still not clear, but may be related to technical aspects of the IHC assay.

Prognostic and predictive values of ER were also recently reported for the monotherapy arms (letrozole versus tamoxifen) of the BIG 1-98 trial, (282). Disease-free survival was statistically significantly different according to ER expression among more than 3,500 patients whose tumors were assessed centrally. Similar to the ATAC's results, no statistical

evidence of differential treatment effect according to ER status was detected between letrozole and tamoxifen ($p = .12$) (282).

Progesterone receptor status in advanced disease, as discussed above, has consistently been predictive of response to endocrine treatment (172,226,244). In contrast, in both the 1998 and the 2005 meta-analyses of early breast cancer, among women with ER-positive tumors, (175,254), knowing PR status did not offer additional information in predicting the benefit from adjuvant tamoxifen therapy, with the possible exception of the small subgroup of patients whose tumors are ER-negative/PR-positive (Table 29.8). Patients in this group did experience risk reduction from treatment, whereas those in the ER-negative/PR-negative group did not. Because of the small number of patients in this group, the results, however, must be viewed somewhat cautiously. Furthermore, although several studies have suggested that tumors in this small subset are biologically different from ER-positive/PR-positive tumors and represent a group of tumors with worse clinicopathologic features and clinical outcome (143,253,283–285), it is still debatable whether this group truly exists, or whether it represents tumors that are indeed ER-positive, but have been misclassified owing to technical challenges (285).

Relatively few studies included measurements of PR in the meta-analyses. Furthermore, assessing PR accurately can be even more challenging than ER. It may well be that owing to lack of standardization and quality control in the hundreds of contributing institutions, the data regarding PR in the meta-analyses included misclassification of tumors similar to the problem with ER in the early meta-analyses. PR measurement errors could explain the failure of PR to predict tamoxifen response in the overview. To better address the question of whether PR status, along with ER status, is useful in predicting the relative benefit from adjuvant tamoxifen, and to minimize the potential effect of measurement errors, a large retrospective study investigated the effect of PR status using a robust database. Of the 12,000 patients in this data set, most (98%) received tamoxifen, and ER

Table 29.8	RELATIVE CHANGE IN ANNUAL ODDS OF RECURRENCE AND MORTALITY ASSOCIATED WITH 5 YEARS OF ADJUVANT TAMOXIFEN THERAPY BY BOTH ESTROGEN RECEPTOR AND PROGESTERONE RECEPTOR STATUS—OVERVIEW 2005 [175]		
	N	Change in Recurrence (%)	Change in Mortality (%)
ER+/PR+	5700	−40 (±4)	−26 (±5)
ER+/PR−	2000	−41 (±6)	−26 (±7)
ER−/PR+	787	− 8 (±15)	−13 (±17)
ER−/PR−	3300	+13 (±8)	+12 (±9)

ER, estrogen receptor; PR, progesterone receptor.
Values in parentheses are 95% confidence intervals.
Adapted from Early Breast Cancer Trialists' Collaborative Group. Effects of chemotherapy and hormonal therapy for early breast cancer on recurrence and 15-year survival: an overview of the randomized trials. *Lancet* 2005;365:1687–1717.

Table 29.9	RELATIVE RISK OF RECURRENCE AND MORTALITY FROM ADJUVANT ENDOCRINE THERAPY BY BOTH ESTROGEN RECEPTOR AND PROGESTERONE RECEPTOR STATUS		
	Database 1[a] (N = 1,688)		Database 2[b] (N = 10,444)
	Relative Risk of Recurrence	Relative Risk of Death	Relative Risk of Death
ER−/PR−	1	1	1
ER+/PR−	0.75 (0.47–1.18)	0.62 (0.43–0.91)	0.68 (0.57–0.82)
ER+/PR+	0.47 (0.30–0.78)	0.42 (0.29–0.60)	0.53 (0.44–0.63)

ER, estrogen receptor; PR, progesterone receptor.
[a]Database 1: Medical Oncology Program Project Database.
[b]Database 2: Specialized Program of Research Excellence Database.
Values in parentheses are 95% confidence intervals.
Adapted from Bardou V, Arpino G, Elledge R, et. al. Progesterone receptor status significantly improves outcome prediction over estrogen receptor alone for adjuvant endocrine therapy. *J Clin Oncol* 2003;21:1973–1979.

and PR levels were measured by DCC at two central laboratories using identical methods and quality control measures (286). In a multivariate analysis including nodal status, tumor size, age, and ER and PR status, patients who received tamoxifen and had ER-positive/PR-positive tumors experienced a 15% to 30% lower risk of recurrence and death than patients who had ER-positive/PR-negative tumors (Table 29.9). This PR effect was both highly significant and independent of ER level, whether considered as a dichotomous or continuous variable. Other large studies of adjuvant tamoxifen have confirmed that PR, along with ER, is an important predictor of the benefits of endocrine therapy (140,283,287–289).

Likewise, a recent subset analysis from the MA.17 trial, which randomized postmenopausal women after 5 years of tamoxifen to the AI letrozole versus placebo, has also found that the benefit of letrozole over placebo was confined to ER-positive/PR-positive tumors and was not seen in the ER-positive/PR-negative tumors (290) (Table 29.10). It should be recognized, however, that a growing body of evidence now suggests that PR, as measured by both IHC and RT-PCR, is primarily prognostic (143,264) and, therefore, it is also possible that the poorer outcome of PR-negative patients on tamoxifen (or other endocrine therapies) is largely a result of their poorer prognosis, and that both PR-positive and PR-negative patients

may still gain significant benefits from tamoxifen. This possibility is inconsistent with the results in metastatic disease where PR has been confirmed as a predictive factor for tamoxifen objective response.

Laboratory and clinical studies have suggested that PR loss is multifactorial (157), but one significant cause is downregulation of its expression as a result of hyperactive growth factor signaling. Indeed, a report following the study mentioned above (286), in which the clinical and biological features of ER-positive/PR-negative tumors were compared with ER-positive/PR-positive tumors (291), showed that three times as many ER-positive/PR-negative tumors as ER-positive/PR-positive tumors expressed EGFR, and 50% more overexpressed ERBB2. Furthermore, among all patients treated with tamoxifen in this analysis, EGFR and ERBB2 predicted inferior outcomes, but results varied by PR status. Among tamoxifen-treated patients with ER-positive/PR-positive tumors, EGFR or ERBB2 status was not correlated with worse DFS. In contrast, among women with ER-positive/PR-negative tumors, both EGFR expression and ERBB2 overexpression were associated with a higher probability of recurrence on adjuvant tamoxifen. These data strongly support the idea that PR negativity may, in fact, reflect increased growth factor signaling (see below), which by itself is known to reduce the efficacy of endocrine therapy.

Table 29.10	RELATIVE RISK OF RECURRENCE FROM ADJUVANT TRIALS WITH AROMATASE INHIBITORS ACCORDING TO PROGESTERONE RECEPTOR STATUS	
	Relative Risk of Recurrence by PR Status in ER+	
Clinical Trials/Analysis	ER+/PR+	ER+/PR−
Upfront AI		
ATAC (Local laboratories) (Ans vs. Tam)[292]	0.84 (0.69–1.02)	0.43 (0.31–0.61)
TransATAC (Central analysis) (Ans vs. Tam)[150]	0.72 (0.52–1.01)	0.68 (0.40–1.17)
BIG 1-98 (Central) (Let vs. Tam)[282]	0.70 (0.57–0.85)	0.84 (0.54–1.31)
Sequential (Switching) AI Trials		
IES (Exem vs. Tam)[273]	0.77 (0.63–0.94)	0.73 (0.53–1.00)
ABC SG-8/ARNO95 (Ans vs. Tam)[274]	0.66 (0.46–0.93)	0.42 (0.19–0.92)
Extended Endocrine Therapy with AI		
MA.17 (Let vs. Placebo)[290]	0.49 (0.36–0.67)	1.21 (0.63–2.34)

AI, aromatase inhibitor; AN, anastrozole; ER, estrogen receptor; Exem, exemestane HR, hazard ratio; Let, letrozole; PR, progesterone receptor; Tam, tamoxifen.
Values in parentheses are 95% confidence intervals.

An initial report from the ATAC trial suggested that the relatively greater benefit of anastrozole over tamoxifen was in the subset of PR-negative tumors (292) (Table 29.10). This intriguing observation was consistent with the proposed biology of ER-positive/PR-negative tumors. These data, however, were not confirmed in the later TransATAC study that analyzed a subset of patients (about one-third of the total patient population) largely from the United Kingdom (150). Similarly, results from BIG 1-98 (282), IES (273), and the ARNO/ABCSG (274) trials have also found no effect of PR expression on the relative efficacy of AI over tamoxifen (Table 29.10), although patients in the latter two trials did not receive an AI until after several years on tamoxifen when PR status may well have changed owing to the drug. As mentioned, IHC assays for PR are more problematic than those for ER. PR has two isoforms (A and B) that appear to function differently, and tumors with a high A-to-B isoform ratio are more aggressive. DCC assays recognize both isoforms. The multiple different primary antibodies currently used in IHC assays recognize different epitopes, with some identifying only one of the isoforms and some identifying both (220). Clearly, the debate on PR status's prediction of endocrine therapy benefits, and in particular of response to specific endocrine treatments, requires further study. In the meantime, PR status should not be used today to select endocrine therapy.

As discussed above, diverse cellular signaling networks in patients' tumors, in addition to ER itself, are probably key elements in response to different types of endocrine therapies. These other molecular pathways, either via interacting with and modulating the ER pathway or by providing an alternative mitogenic and survival stimulus for the cells, can cause resistance to endocrine therapy. Thus, the simple presence of ER may not necessarily assure ER functional activity or response to endocrine therapy. In the past decade, a few multigene predictive scores have been developed to improve the prediction value of ER and help determine patients' expected benefit from endocrine therapy (see Chapter 32) (293,294). Examples of these assays are the 21-gene qRT-PCR-based assay Oncotype DX (295), which in addition to ER mRNA, also measures several downstream ER-regulated genes, ERBB2, and several proliferation genes; the 81-gene tamoxifen-resistance profile (296); the 200-gene ER reporter endocrine sensitivity index (SET [sensitivity index]) developed from genes whose expression is highly associated with ER (297); the two-gene signature (294); the estrogen-regulated gene signature (215); and others (298). Currently, no predictive profile has been validated and approved as a predictive assay for endocrine therapy, although many of these assays are under active development and clinical validation (see Chapter 32). Importantly however, as ample data from these studies together suggest that mRNA-based ER measurements provide more readily quantifiable results than ER IHC (213) (264), these multigene assays also hold the promise of providing valuable prognostic and predictive information regarding ER as an individual component. In fact, clinical reports from Oncotype DX now also include separate reports for ER, PR, and ERBB2 based on quantified mRNA levels.

Estrogen Receptor and Response to Chemotherapy

Growing evidence suggests that patients with endocrine-responsive breast cancers benefit less from adjuvant chemotherapy, including modern day taxane-based chemotherapies, than those with endocrine unresponsive disease (299). Laboratory evidence further suggests that ER- or PR-positive breast cancer cells are more resistant to taxanes (300,301). Data also suggest that patients with tumors that are most endocrine-responsive (ER and PR-positive/ERBB2-negative) may receive little or no chemotherapy benefit even if they have a higher risk of recurrence because of positive lymph nodes. This effect of ER was first

observed 30 years ago (302), and, although not all studies since then agree, most evidence does suggest that ER-positive tumors are less sensitive to a variety of chemotherapy regimens. Some of the studies that fail to show an effect of ER included premenopausal patients and are, therefore, confounded by the endocrine effects of chemotherapy-induced ovarian ablation in this subset (303–306). As an example, a large trial of taxotene, doxorubicin (adriamycin) and cyclophosphamide (TAC) versus 5-FU (fluorouracil), adriamycin and cyclophosphamide (FAC) was interpreted as showing an advantage for TAC regardless of ER status (306). More than half of the patients on this study were premenopausal, however, and TAC was associated with a greater incidence of chemotherapy-induced amenorrhea. Thus, the advantage for TAC in the ER-positive subset could be owing to its endocrine therapy effects. Neoadjuvant chemotherapy trials show a major difference by ER status in pathologic complete response (path CR) to chemotherapy (307). Path CR in the ER-negative subset often exceeds 20% to 30%, whereas that in ER-positive patients is typically less than 5%.

The meta-analysis of all adjuvant chemotherapy trials does support the hypothesis that ER-negative tumors are impacted much more by chemotherapy than are ER-positive tumors (175). In postmenopausal patients, where the ovarian ablative effects of chemotherapy are not relevant, the proportional benefits of chemotherapy in reducing recurrence and mortality of ER-negative patients are twice that for ER-positive patients. Although the meta-analysis does show a statistically significant modest benefit for adjuvant chemotherapy in postmenopausal women with ER-positive tumors, it has not reported an analysis of ER combined with other factors used to define endocrine responsiveness, such as ER level, PR status, or ERBB2 amplification. Based on the meta-analysis and other individual trials, one can conclude that patients with tumors classified simply as ER-positive do receive some benefit from adjuvant chemotherapy.

A recent summary of several Cancer and Leukemia Group B (CALGB) and Breast Cancer Inter-group modern chemotherapy trials evaluated the effects of ER status on patient outcome (255). Compared with the least effective chemotherapy regimen in this sequential series of trials, only ER-negative patients had a statistically significant reduction in relative risk of recurrence and mortality, either by increasing the dose of doxorubicin, by adding taxanes to the standard adriamycin and cyclophosphamide (AC) regimen, or by using dose-dense adjuvant chemotherapy. There was a trend for benefit from these increasingly aggressive adjuvant chemotherapy regimens in ER-positive patients, although this benefit did not reach statistical significance. A follow-up study from the same group that considered both ER and ERBB2 status showed that paclitaxel did not benefit patients with ERBB2-negative, ER-positive breast cancers, but did benefit those whose tumors were ERBB2-positive, regardless of ER status (308).

The International Breast Cancer Study Group (IBCSG) recently defined three categories of endocrine responsiveness: highly endocrine-responsive tumors defined as those with high levels of both ER and PR; incompletely endocrine-responsive tumors defined by low expression of ER and PR or by loss of one but not both receptors; and an endocrine nonresponsive group defined as tumors having no detectable expression of steroid hormone receptors (309). Based on their analyses, the St. Gallen Expert Consensus Panel recommended that chemotherapy be considered along with trastuzumab for patients with ERBB2-positive disease and that chemotherapy be considered also for patients with incompletely endocrine responsive or endocrine nonresponsive tumors. Patients with highly endocrine responsive tumors, particularly if they have a lower risk of relapse and lack ERBB2 amplification, might be considered for endocrine adjuvant therapy alone.

Although tumors with high levels of ER and PR and with absent ERBB2 (highly endocrine responsive) seem to receive little benefit from adjuvant chemotherapy, multigene profiles, such as the Oncotype 21-gene profile, may identify a larger group

Table 29.11	SITE AND FREQUENCY OF BREAST CANCER EVENTS IN DUCTAL CARCINOMA *IN SITU* BY ESTROGEN RECEPTOR STATUS AND TAMOXIFEN TREATMENT			
	ER Negative		ER Positive	
	Placebo (n = 84)	Tamoxifen (n = 62)	Placebo (n = 242)	Tamoxifen (n = 227)
All events	26%	22%	21%	10%
Ipsilateral breast	18%	18%	13%	7%
Contralateral breast	6%	5%	8%	3%

ER, estrogen receptor.
From Allred D, Land B, Paik S, et al. Estrogen receptor expression as a predictive marker of the effectiveness of tamoxifen in the treatment of DCIS: findings from NSABP Protocol B-24 [Abstract]. *Breast Cancer Res Treat* 2002;76[Suppl 1]:S36.

of patients for whom chemotherapy is ineffective. Patients with ER-positive tumors who also had a low risk 21-gene recurrence score received no benefit from CMF (cyclophosphamide, methotrexate and 5-fluorouracil)-based chemotherapy (206,310). A more recent preliminary report from the Southwest Oncology Group evaluating patients from a large intergroup study of node-positive, postmenopausal women with ER-positive tumors showed no benefit from the addition of cyclophosphamide, doxorubicin (adriamycin), and fluorouracil (5-Fu) (CAF) adjuvant chemotherapy to tamoxifen in patients who were strongly ER-positive and ERBB2-negative (311). When these same patients were analyzed using the 21-gene assay, a low risk score identified an even larger group of these node-positive patients who failed to benefit from adjuvant CAF, despite having a relatively high risk of recurrence. Although none of these reports were from prospective trials that would provide level 1 evidence, the cumulative data at least indicate that the benefit of chemotherapy in highly endocrine-responsive patients must be small, perhaps nil, and these data should be discussed with patients when making decisions about adjuvant chemotherapy.

Collectively, these data indicate that quantitative measurement of both ER and PR is beneficial in the management of women with early-stage breast cancer and should represent a minimal standard of care (193). It is clear, however, that more standardization and quality assurance programs for measuring ER and PR should be broadly adopted in clinical practice. Furthermore, it is also evident that many questions remain as to how better to refine and tailor adjuvant endocrine therapy in the individual patient. Better understanding of the predictive and prognostic roles of ER and PR, quantitatively and qualitatively, is imperative to enhance patients' benefit from the growing selection of treatment options and strategies now available in the adjuvant setting. Multigene assays will be increasingly used to augment or replace hormone receptor assays to improve personalized diagnosis and treatment.

Estrogen Receptor in Noninvasive Breast Cancer

Similar to invasive breast cancer, the presence of hormone receptors is important in determining the benefit of tamoxifen, and presumably other endocrine therapies, in the treatment of ductal carcinoma *in situ* (DCIS). The recognition that adjuvant tamoxifen reduces local, regional, and distant disease in patients diagnosed with invasive breast cancer led to the NSABP B-24 study, which randomized 1,804 patients with DCIS undergoing excision and radiation for 5 years of adjuvant tamoxifen versus placebo (312). Overall in the tamoxifen treatment group there was a 37% reduction in all breast cancer events. Tumor blocks on 676 patients were analyzed or reviewed by a central laboratory for ER by IHC (313). Of

patients, 77% were ER-positive and 23% were ER-negative. After 8.7 years of follow-up, the benefits of tamoxifen—up to 50% reduction in risk seen in a number of categories—were confined to those patients whose original DCIS expressed ER, with little if any reduction in the group with ER-negative DCIS (313) (Table 29.11). Although the overall number of patients was small and results should be confirmed by additional clinical trials, in light of the clear data from the B-24 study and the overwhelming data showing the relationship between ER expression and benefit from endocrine therapy in invasive breast cancer, measuring ER and PR in patients with DCIS to facilitate the decision-making process seems reasonable. Updates from the latest ASCO Breast Tumor Markers Guideline conclude, however, that in DCIS patients who are candidates for endocrine therapy, data are yet insufficient to recommend routine measurement of ER and PR for therapy recommendation (193), a conclusion owing in part, perhaps, to the fact that the studies of B-27 have not been published.

Estrogen and Progesterone Receptors as Prognostic Factors

Although in clinical practice ER is most valuable as a predictive factor, it can also be used as a prognostic factor. Rates of recurrence within the first 5 years in women with ER-positive tumors who did not receive systemic therapy after surgery are lower by 5% to 10% in comparison with ER-negative patients (314–316). Studies with longer follow-up suggest, however, that ER may be a time-dependent variable, such that as more time elapses, the difference in the rate of relapse and death significantly diminishes and eventually disappears (317–321). Because ER is not associated with nodal metastases and its prognostic significance reduces over time, it is possible that ER status predicts a more indolent and slower growing tumor with longer time to disease recurrence rather than the ultimate metastatic potential of the tumor.

In addition to being a prognostic factor itself, ER is also associated with a number of other established prognostic factors. ER-positive tumors are more frequently found in older patients (217,322); they are well-differentiated histologically (323), have a lower fraction of dividing cells (324), are more often diploid (324), and are less likely to exhibit a mutation, loss, high expression, or amplification of breast cancer-related genes such as TP53 (325,326), *ERBB2* (143,327,328), or EGFR (143,159,329, 330,331). ER positivity is also associated with the luminal subtype of breast cancers, based on molecular gene expression profiling (see Chapter 32). It is clear, however, that the luminal subtype, like the ER-positive group itself, is heterogeneous, with a continuum ranging from the more indolent luminal Aa tumors, through the intermediate Ab subgroup, to the more aggressive luminal B subtype (332,333). Interestingly, mRNA levels for ER (and PR) are inversely correlated with this continuum (333), although quantitative ER levels by qRT-PCR, based on the NSABP B-14 Oncotype DX study, are not prognostic (264).

The frequency of ER expression in malignant diseases varies across racial and ethnic groups. Although the biology behind this phenomenon is unclear, the receptor expression is consistently higher in U.S. whites and Asian-Americans than in blacks or Hispanics (334–336). Additionally, the rate of ER positivity is also greater among men with breast cancer than in women (336,337), and in screen-detected versus clinically detected cancers (338).

The incidence of ER-positive breast cancer had been rising (339,340), possibly because of the use of postmenopausal hormone therapy, screening mammography, more sensitive assays, and other unknown reasons. Following the substantial drop in the use of postmenopausal hormone therapy in the past several years, a significant decrease in breast cancer occurrence has been observed (175,341). It is too early to know whether the proportion of ER-negative new primary breast cancers will increase. ER status is also prognostic for the site of metastasis. Typically, ER-positive tumors tend to have metastases in bone, soft tissue, or the reproductive and genital tracts more frequently, whereas metastases in patients with ER-negative status are more often visceral or in the brain (321,342). That ER is associated with such a host of other good biological features offers a rationale for its association with a better short-term prognosis.

The utility of PR as a prognostic factor is less established, although it is an area of continued interest, and both old and recent studies strongly support this notion (143,286,315, 343–345), although other data do not (346). Recent results using quantitative PR levels measured by qRT-PCR do indicate that PR status is strongly prognostic. Unlike ER, PR levels are more likely to be higher or positive in young or premenopausal women, probably at least in part as a result of greater estrogen stimulation. It is also lower in blacks and Hispanics as compared with white women (336). Among ER-positive tumors, PR-positive tumors are likely to be smaller in size, to have a lower S-phase fraction, and to be less aneuploid (291). ER-positive/PR-negative tumors, in comparison to ER-positive/PR-positive tumors, have twice as many DNA copy number changes, including specific regions of gain or loss (347). PR loss correlates with the aggressive luminal B breast cancer subtype (347), with EGFR and ERBB2 expression (143,291,331), and with a gene expression signature of the PI3K/Akt/mTOR oncogenic pathway (347). These features also correlate with resistance to endocrine therapy. Overall, even considering the difficulties in measuring PR, which can explain some of the variability in study results, it is becoming clear that PR negativity may be a marker of a more aggressive distinct tumor subtype.

 CONCLUSIONS

Estrogen receptors and PR play a critical role in the development and the progression of breast cancer. Continuing progress in understanding the biology of these receptors emphasizes the complexity of their signaling networks which interact with multiple other survival and proliferation pathways in the cell.

Estrogen receptors and PR have proven usefulness in the clinical management of breast cancer. They should be measured in all breast tumor specimens, including the primary lesion in the breast and metastatic lesions when they occur. Assays have become simpler and cheaper, and thus more readily available for all patients. Currently used IHC assays are deficient, however, and a critical need exists for standardization of these assays, establishment of quality control procedures, and identification of a validated scoring system. The emerging

availability of more quantitative ER and PR assays in the clinic, using either new imaging tools or strategies that measure mRNA levels, has potential advantages compared with present IHC methods and these may become the assays of choice in the future. Ultimately, however, given the complexity of ER and PR biology, one should reasonably expect that even perfect assays for ER and PR alone would not be predictive of response to endocrine therapy in all patients. Multigene and proteomic signatures are likely to replace single-gene assays in the future.

TABLE OF RELEVANT WEBSITES

Estrogen Receptor (ER) Background	http://en.wikipedia.org/wiki/Estrogen_receptor
Progesterone Receptor (PR) Background	http://en.wikipedia.org/wiki/Progesterone_receptor
Receptor Coregulatory Proteins	http://www.nursa.org/
Arimidex, Tamoxifen Alone or in Combination (ATAC) Trial	http://www.cancer.gov/clinicaltrials/results/ATAC1204
ER Immuno-histochemical (IHC) Assays	http://www.cap.org/apps/cap.portal?_nfpb=true&cntvwrPtlt_actionOverride=%2Fportlets%2FcontentViewer%2Fshow&_windowLabel=cntvwrPtlt&cntvwrPtlt%7BactionForm.contentReference%7D=cap_today%2Ffeature_stories%2F0108_estrogen.html&_state=maximized&_pageLabel=cntvwr
ER IHC Methods	http://www.breastcenter.tmc.edu/research/cores/path/services/er.htm
PR IHC Methods	http://www.breastcenter.tmc.edu/research/cores/path/services/pr.htm

References

1. Jensen EV, Desombre ER, Kawashima T, et al. Estrogen-binding substances of target tissues. *Science* 1967;158:529–530.
2. Beatson C. On the treatment of inoperable cases of carcinoma of the mamma: suggestions for a new method of treatment, with illustrative cases. *Lancet* 1896;2:104–107.
3. O'Malley BW. A life long search for the molecular pathways of steroid hormone action. *Mol Endocrinol* 2005;19:1402–1411.
4. Green S, Walter P, Greene G, et al. Cloning of the human oestrogen receptor cDNA. *J Steroid Biochem* 1986;24:77–83.
5. Walter P, Green S, Greene G, et al. Cloning of the human estrogen receptor cDNA. *Proc Natl Acad Sci U S A* 1985;82:7889–7893.
6. Mosselman S, Polman J, Dijkema R. ER beta: identification and characterization of a novel human estrogen receptor. *FEBS Lett* 1996;392:49–53.
7. Misrahi M, Atger M, d'Auriol L, et al. Complete amino acid sequence of the human progesterone receptor deduced from cloned cDNA. *Biochem Biophys Res Commun* 1987;143:740–748.
8. Kos M, Reid G, Denger S, et al. Minireview: genomic organization of the human ERalpha gene promoter region. *Mol Endocrinol* 2001;15:2057–2063.
9. Hirata S, Shoda T, Kato J, Hoshi K. The multiple untranslated first exons system of the human estrogen receptor beta (ER beta) gene. *J Steroid Biochem Mol Biol* 2001;78:33–40.
10. Fuqua SA, Fitzgerald SD, Allred DC, et al. Inhibition of estrogen receptor action by a naturally occurring variant in human breast tumors. *Cancer Res* 1992;52:483–486.
11. Fuqua SA, Fitzgerald SD, Chamness GC, et al. Variant human breast tumor estrogen receptor with constitutive transcriptional activity. *Cancer Res* 1991;51:105–109.
12. Treeck O, Juhasz-Boess I, Lattrich C, et al. Effects of exon-deleted estrogen receptor beta transcript variants on growth, apoptosis and gene expression of human breast cancer cell lines. *Breast Cancer Res Treat* 2008;110:507–520.
13. Herynk MH, Fuqua SA. Estrogen receptor mutations in human disease. *Endocr Rev* 2004;25:869–898.
14. Joel PB, Smith J, Sturgill TW, et al. pp90rsk1 regulates estrogen receptor-mediated transcription through phosphorylation of Ser-167. *Mol Cell Biol* 1998;18:1978–1984.
15. Lee H, Bai W. Regulation of estrogen receptor nuclear export by ligand-induced and p38-mediated receptor phosphorylation. *Mol Cell Biol* 2002;22:5835–5845.

16. Rogatsky I, Trowbridge JM, Garabedian MJ. Potentiation of human estrogen receptor alpha transcriptional activation through phosphorylation of serines 104 and 106 by the cyclin A-CDK2 complex. *J Biol Chem* 1999;274:22296–22302.
17. Chen D, Washbrook E, Sarwar N, et al. Phosphorylation of human estrogen receptor alpha at serine 118 by two distinct signal transduction pathways revealed by phosphorylation-specific antisera. *Oncogene* 2002;21:4921–4931.
18. Arnold SF, Obourn JD, Jaffe H, et al. Phosphorylation of the human estrogen receptor by mitogen-activated protein kinase and casein kinase II: consequence on DNA binding. *J Steroid Biochem Mol Biol* 1995;55:163–172.
19. Likhite VS, Stossi F, Kim K, et al. Kinase-specific phosphorylation of the estrogen receptor changes receptor interactions with ligand, deoxyribonucleic acid, and coregulators associated with alterations in estrogen and tamoxifen activity. *Mol Endocrinol* 2006;20:3120–3132.
20. Campbell RA, Bhat-Nakshatri P, Patel NM, et al. Phosphatidylinositol 3-kinase/Akt mediated activation of estrogen receptor alpha: a new model for anti-estrogen resistance. *J Biol Chem* 2001;276:9817–9824.
21. Kato S, Endoh H, Masuhiro Y, et al. Activation of the estrogen receptor through phosphorylation by mitogen-activated protein kinase. *Science* 1995;270:1491–1494.
22. Lee H, Jiang F, Wang Q, et al. MEKKI activation of human estrogen receptor alpha and stimulation of the agonistic activity of 4-hydroxytamoxifen in endometrial and ovarian cancer cells. *Mol Endocrinol* 2000;14:1882–1896.
23. Murphy LC, Niu Y, Snell L, et al. Phospho-serine-118 estrogen receptor-alpha expression is associated with better disease outcome in women treated with tamoxifen. *Clin Cancer Res* 2004;10:5902–5906.
24. Sarwar N, Kim JS, Jiang J, et al. Phosphorylation of ERalpha at serine 118 in primary breast cancer and in tamoxifen-resistant tumours is indicative of a complex role for ERalpha phosphorylation in breast cancer progression. *Endocr Relat Cancer* 2006;13:851–861.
25. Zoubir M, Mathieu MC, Mazouni C, et al. Modulation of ER phosphorylation on serine 118 by endocrine therapy: a new surrogate marker for efficacy. *Ann Oncol* 2008;19:1402–1406.
26. Chen D, Pace PE, Coombes RC, et al. Phosphorylation of human estrogen receptor alpha by protein kinase A regulates dimerization. *Mol Cell Biol* 1999;19:1002–1015.
27. Zwart W, Griekspoor A, Rondaij M, et al. Classification of anti-estrogens according to intramolecular FRET effects on phospho-mutants of estrogen receptor alpha. *Mol Cancer Ther* 2007;6:1526–1533.
28. Cui Y, Zhang M, Pestell R, et al. Phosphorylation of estrogen receptor alpha blocks its acetylation and regulates estrogen sensitivity. *Cancer Res* 2004;64:9199–9208.
29. Wang RA, Mazumdar A, Vadlamudi RK, et al. P21-activated kinase-1 phosphorylates and transactivates estrogen receptor-alpha and promotes hyperplasia in mammary epithelium. *EMBO J* 2002;21:5437–5447.
30. Michalides R, Griekspoor A, Balkenende A, et al. Tamoxifen resistance by a conformational arrest of the estrogen receptor alpha after PKA activation in breast cancer. *Cancer Cell* 2004;5:597–605.
31. Rayala SK, Talukder AH, Balasenthil S, et al. P21-activated kinase 1 regulation of estrogen receptor-alpha activation involves serine 305 activation linked with serine 118 phosphorylation. *Cancer Res* 2006;66:1694–1701.
32. Clemm DL, Sherman L, Boonyaratanakornkit V, et al. Differential hormone-dependent phosphorylation of progesterone receptor A and B forms revealed by a phosphoserine site-specific monoclonal antibody. *Mol Endocrinol* 2000;14:52–65.
33. Zhang Y, Beck CA, Poletti A, et al. Identification of phosphorylation sites unique to the B form of human progesterone receptor. In vitro phosphorylation by casein kinase II. *J Biol Chem* 1994;269:31034–31040.
34. Zhang Y, Beck CA, Poletti A, et al. Phosphorylation of human progesterone receptor by cyclin-dependent kinase 2 on three sites that are authentic basal phosphorylation sites in vivo. *Mol Endocrinol* 1997;11:823–832.
35. Knotts TA, Orkiszewski RS, Cook RG, et al. Identification of a phosphorylation site in the hinge region of the human progesterone receptor and additional amino-terminal phosphorylation sites. *J Biol Chem* 2001;276:8475–8483.
36. Pierson-Mullany LK, Lange CA. Phosphorylation of progesterone receptor serine 400 mediates ligand-independent transcriptional activity in response to activation of cyclin-dependent protein kinase 2. *Mol Cell Biol* 2004;24:10542–10557.
37. Daniel AR, Qiu M, Faivre EJ, et al. Linkage of progestin and epidermal growth factor signaling: phosphorylation of progesterone receptors mediates transcriptional hypersensitivity and increased ligand-independent breast cancer cell growth. *Steroids* 2007;72:188–201.
38. Nawaz Z, Lonard DM, Dennis AP, et al. Proteasome-dependent degradation of the human estrogen receptor. *Biochemistry* 1999;96:1858–1862.
39. Tateishi Y, Kawabe Y, Chiba T, et al. Ligand-dependent switching of ubiquitin-proteasome pathways for estrogen receptor. *EMBO J* 2004;23:4813–4823.
40. Berry NB, Fan M, Nephew KP. Estrogen receptor alpha hinge-region lysines 302 and 303 regulate receptor degradation by the proteasome. *Mol Endocrinol* 2008;22:1535–1551.
41. Wang C, Fu M, Angeletti RH, et al. Direct acetylation of the estrogen receptor alpha hinge region by p300 regulates transactivation and hormone sensitivity. *J Biol Chem* 2001;276:18375–18383.
42. Kim MY, Woo EM, Chong YT, et al. Acetylation of estrogen receptor alpha by p300 at lysines 266 and 268 enhances the deoxyribonucleic acid binding and transactivation activities of the receptor. *Mol Endocrinol* 2006;20:1479–1493.
43. Sentis S, Le Romancer M, Bianchin C, et al. Sumoylation of the estrogen receptor alpha hinge region regulates its transcriptional activity. *Mol Endocrinol* 2005;19:2671–2684.
44. Daniel AR, Faivre EJ, Lange CA. Phosphorylation-dependent antagonism of sumoylation derepresses progesterone receptor action in breast cancer cells. *Mol Endocrinol* 2007;21:2890–2906.
45. Subramanian K, Jia D, Kapoor-Vazirani P, et al. Regulation of estrogen receptor alpha by the SET7 lysine methyltransferase. *Mol Cell* 2008;30:336–347.
46. Fuqua SA, Wiltschke C, Zhang QX, et al. A hypersensitive estrogen receptor-alpha mutation in premalignant breast lesions. *Cancer Res* 2000;60:4026–4029.
47. Herynk MH, Parra I, Cui Y, et al. Association between the estrogen receptor alpha A908G mutation and outcomes in invasive breast cancer. *Clin Cancer Res* 2007;13:3235–3243.
48. Barone I, Cui Y, Herynk M, Ando S, et al. The K303R ERa mutation confers resistance to an aromatase inhibitor. *Endocrine Society* 2008.
49. Giordano C, Ando S, Cui Y, et al. Growth factor activation decreases responsiveness to tamoxifen in cells expressing the K303R ERa mutation. *Endocrine Society* 2008.
50. Zhang Z, Yamashita H, Toyama T, et al. Estrogen receptor alpha mutation (A-to-G transition at nucleotide 908) is not found in different types of breast lesions from Japanese women. *Breast Cancer* 2003;10:70–73.
51. Tebbit CL, Bentley RC, Olson JA Jr, et al. Estrogen receptor alpha (ESR1) mutant A908G is not a common feature in benign and malignant proliferations of the breast. *Genes Chromosomes Cancer* 2004;40:51–54.
52. Tokunaga E, Kimura Y, Maehara Y. No hypersensitive estrogen receptor-alpha mutation (K303R) in Japanese breast carcinomas. *Breast Cancer Res Treat* 2004;84:289–292.
53. Davies MP, O'Neill PA, Innes H, et al. Hypersensitive K303R oestrogen receptor-alpha variant not found in invasive carcinomas. *Breast Cancer Res* 2005;7:R113–R118.
54. Conway K, Parrish E, Edmiston SN, et al. The estrogen receptor-alpha A908G (K303R) mutation occurs at a low frequency in invasive breast tumors: results from a population-based study. *Breast Cancer Res* 2005;7:R871–R880.
55. Conway K, Parrish E, Edmiston SN, et al. Risk factors for breast cancer characterized by the estrogen receptor alpha A908G (K303R) mutation. *Breast Cancer Res* 2007;9:R36.
56. Zhang QX, Borg A, Wolf DM, et al. An estrogen receptor mutant with strong hormone-independent activity from a metastatic breast cancer. *Cancer Res* 1997;57:1244–1249.
57. Fuqua SA. The role of estrogen receptors in breast cancer metastasis. *J Mammary Gland Biol Neoplasia* 2001;6:407–417.
58. Watts CKW, Handel ML, King RJD, et al. Oestrogen receptor gene structure and function in breast cancer. *J Steroid Biochem Mol Biol* 1992;41:529–536.
59. Holst F, Stahl PR, Ruiz C, et al. Estrogen receptor alpha (ESR1) gene amplification is frequent in breast cancer. *Nat Genet* 2007;39:655–660.
60. Holst F, Haas H, Nottbohm A, et al. Patterns of estrogen receptor alpha (ER) protein expression and ESR1 gene amplification in primary and metastatic breast cancer. *Breast Cancer Res Treat* 2007;106:S34.
61. Ejlertsen B, Nielsen K, Rasmussen B, et al. Amplification of ESR1 may predict resistance to adjuvant tamoxifen in postmenopausal patients with hormone receptor positive breast cancer. *Breast Cancer Res Treat* 2007;106:S34.
62. Onate SA, Tsai SY, Tsai MJ, et al. Sequence and characterization of a coactivator for the steroid hormone receptor superfamily. *Science* 1995;270.
63. Lanz RB, Jericevic Z, Zuercher WJ, et al. Nuclear Receptor Signaling Atlas (www.nursa.org): hyperlinking the nuclear receptor signaling community. *Nucleic Acids Res* 2006;34:D221–D226.
64. Shang Y, Hu X, DiRenzo J, et al. Cofactor dynamics and sufficiency in estrogen receptor-regulated transcription. *Cell* 2000;103:843–852.
65. Font de Mora J, Brown M. AIB1 is a conduit for kinase-mediated growth factor signaling to the estrogen receptor. *Mol Cell Biol* 2000;20:5041–5047.
66. Anzick SL, Kononen J, Walker RL, et al. AIB1, a steroid coactivator amplified in breast and ovarian cancer. *Science* 1997;277:965–968.
67. Kirkegaard T, McGlynn LM, Campbell FM, et al. Amplified in breast cancer 1 in human epidermal growth factor receptor - positive tumors of tamoxifen-treated breast cancer patients. *Clin Cancer Res* 2007;13:1405–1411.
68. Osborne CK, Bardou V, Hopp TA, et al. Role of the estrogen receptor coactivator AIB1 (SRC-3) and HER-2/neu in tamoxifen resistance in breast cancer. *J Natl Cancer Inst* 2003;95:353–361.
69. Hermanson O, Glass CK, Rosenfeld MG. Nuclear receptor coregulators: multiple modes of modification. *Trends Endocrinol Metab* 2002;13:55–60.
70. McKenna NJ, O'Malley BW. Minireview: nuclear receptor coactivators—an update. *Endocrinology* 2002;143:2461–2465.
71. Selye H. Correlations between the chemical structure and the pharmacological actions of the steroids. *Endocrinology* 1942;30:437–453.
72. Pietras RJ, Szego CM. Specific binding sites for oestrogen at the outer surfaces of isolated endometrial cells. *Nature* 1977;265:69–72.
73. Moriarty K, Kim KH, Bender JR. Minireview: estrogen receptor-mediated rapid signaling. *Endocrinology* 2006;147:5557–5563.
74. Wehling M, Losel R. Non-genomic steroid hormone effects: membrane or intracellular receptors? *J Steroid Biochem Mol Biol* 2006;102:180–183.
75. Ho KJ, Liao JK. Nonnuclear actions of estrogen. *Arterioscler Thromb Vasc Biol* 2002;22:1952–1961.
76. Kousteni S, Chen JR, Bellido T, et al. Reversal of bone loss in mice by nongenotropic signaling of sex steroids. *Science* 2002;298:843–846.
77. Li L, Haynes MP, Bender JR. Plasma membrane localization and function of the estrogen receptor alpha variant (ER46) in human endothelial cells. *Proc Natl Acad Sci U S A* 2003;100:4807–4812.
78. Migliaccio A, Castoria G, Di Domenico M, et al. Sex steroid hormones act as growth factors. *J Steroid Biochem Mol Biol* 2002;83:31–35.
79. Migliaccio A, Piccolo D, Castoria G, et al. Activation of the Src/p21ras/Erk pathway by progesterone receptor via cross-talk with estrogen receptor. *EMBO J* 1998;17:2008–2018.
80. Razandi M, Pedram A, Levin ER. Plasma membrane estrogen receptors signal to antiapoptosis in breast cancer. *Mol Endocrinol* 2000;14:1434–1447.
81. Razandi M, Pedram A, Park ST, et al. Proximal events in signaling by plasma membrane estrogen receptors. *J Biol Chem* 2003;278:2701–2712.
82. Pietras RJ, Marquez-Garban DC. Membrane-associated estrogen receptor signaling pathways in human cancers. *Clin Cancer Res* 2007;13:4672–4676.
83. Levin ER, Pietras RJ. Estrogen receptors outside the nucleus in breast cancer. *Breast Cancer Res Treat* 2008;108:351–361.
84. Razandi M, Alton G, Pedram A, et al. Identification of a structural determinant necessary for the localization and function of estrogen receptor alpha at the plasma membrane. *Mol Cell Biol* 2003;23:1633–1646.
85. Zhu Y, Bond J, Thomas P. Identification, classification, and partial characterization of genes in humans and other vertebrates homologous to a fish membrane progestin receptor. *Proc Natl Acad Sci U S A* 2003;100:2237–2242.
86. Boonyaratanakornkit V, McGowan E, Sherman L, et al. The role of extranuclear signaling actions of progesterone receptor in mediating progesterone regulation of gene expression and the cell cycle. *Mol Endocrinol* 2007;21:359–375.
87. Figtree GA, McDonald D, Watkins H, et al. Truncated estrogen receptor alpha 46-kDa isoform in human endothelial cells: relationship to acute activation of nitric oxide synthase. *Circulation* 2003;107:120–126.
88. Wang Z, Zhang X, Shen P, et al. Identification, cloning, and expression of human estrogen receptor-alpha36, a novel variant of human estrogen receptor-alpha66. *Biochem Biophys Res Commun* 2005;336:1023–1027.
89. Wang Z, Zhang X, Shen P, et al. A variant of estrogen receptor-α, hER-α 36: transduction of estrogen- and antiestrogen-dependent membrane-initiated mitogenic signaling. *Proc Natl Acad Sci U S A* 2006;103:9063–9068.

90. Levin ER. Cellular functions of plasma membrane estrogen receptors. *Steroids* 2002;67:471–475.

91. Filardo EJ. Epidermal growth factor receptor (EGFR) transactivation by estrogen via the G-protein-coupled receptor, GPR30: a novel signaling pathway with potential significance for breast cancer. *J Steroid Biochem Mol Biol* 2002;80:231–238.

92. Albanito L, Sisci D, Aquila S, et al. Epidermal growth factor induces G protein-coupled receptor 30 expression in estrogen receptor-negative breast cancer cells. *Endocrinology* 2008;149:3799–3808.

93. Filardo EJ, Quinn JA, Sabo E. Association of the membrane estrogen receptor, GPR30, with breast tumor metastasis and transactivation of the epidermal growth factor receptor. *Steroids* 2008;73:870–873.

94. Kleuser B, Malek D, Gust R, et al. 17-β-Estradiol inhibits transforming growth factor-β signaling and function in breast cancer cells via activation of extracellular signal-regulated kinase through the G protein coupled receptor 30. *Mol Pharmacol* 2008;74(6):1533–1543.

95. Song RX, Zhang Z, Chen Y, et al. Estrogen signaling via a linear pathway involving insulin-like growth factor I receptor, matrix metalloproteinases, and epidermal growth factor receptor to activate mitogen-activated protein kinase in MCF-7 breast cancer cells. *Endocrinology* 2007;148:4091–4101.

96. Cato AC, Nestl A, Mink S. Rapid actions of steroid receptors in cellular signaling pathways. *Sci STKE* 2002;2002:RE9.

97. Song RX, McPherson RA, Adam L, et al. Linkage of rapid estrogen action to MAPK activation by ERalpha-Shc association and Shc pathway activation. *Mol Endocrinol* 2002;16:116–127.

98. Szego CM, Davis JS. Adenosine 3',5'-monophosphate in rat uterus: acute elevation by estrogen. *Proc Natl Acad Sci U S A* 1967;58:1711–1718.

99. Duan R, Xie W, Li X, et al. Estrogen regulation of c-fos gene expression through phosphatidylinositol-3-kinase-dependent activation of serum response factor in MCF-7 breast cancer cells. *Biochem Biophys Res Commun* 2002;294:384–394.

100. Pratt MA, Satkunaratnam A, Novosad DM. Estrogen activates raf-1 kinase and induces expression of Egr-1 in MCF-7 breast cancer cells. *Mol Cell Biochem* 1998;189:119–125.

101. Watters JJ, Campbell JS, Cunningham MJ, et al. Rapid membrane effects of steroids in neuroblastoma cells: effects of estrogen on mitogen activated protein kinase signaling cascade and c-fos immediate early gene transcription. *Endocrinology* 1997;138:4030–4033.

102. Watters JJ, Chun TY, Kim YN, et al. Estrogen modulation of prolactin gene expression requires an intact mitogen-activated protein kinase signal transduction pathway in cultured rat pituitary cells. *Mol Endocrinol* 2000;14:1872–1881.

103. Stoica GE, Franke TF, Moroni M, et al. Effect of estradiol on estrogen receptor-alpha gene expression and activity can be modulated by the ErbB2/PI 3-K/Akt pathway. *Oncogene* 2003;22:7998–8011.

104. Shou J, Massarweh S, Osborne CK, et al. Mechanisms of tamoxifen resistance: increased estrogen receptor-HER2/neu cross-talk in ER/HER2-positive breast cancer. *J Natl Cancer Inst* 2004;96:926–935.

105. Lu Q, Pallas DC, Surks HK, et al. Striatin assembles a membrane signaling complex necessary for rapid, nongenomic activation of endothelial NO synthase by estrogen receptor alpha. *Proc Natl Acad Sci U S A* 2004;101:17126–17131.

106. Marquez DC, Chen HW, Curran EM, et al. Estrogen receptors in membrane lipid rafts and signal transduction in breast cancer. *Mol Cell Endocrinol* 2006;246:91–100.

107. Wong CW, McNally C, Nickbarg E, et al. Estrogen receptor-interacting protein that modulates its nongenomic activity crosstalk with Src/Erk phosphorylation cascade. *Proc Natl Acad Sci U S A* 2002;99:14783–14788.

108. Wyckoff MH, Chambliss KL, Mineo C, et al. Plasma membrane estrogen receptors are coupled to endothelial nitric-oxide synthase through Galpha(i). *J Biol Chem* 2001;276:27071–27076.

109. Song RX, Barnes CJ, Zhang Z, et al. The role of Shc and insulin-like growth factor 1 receptor in mediating the translocation of estrogen receptor alpha to the plasma membrane. *Proc Natl Acad Sci U S A* 2004;101:2076–2081.

110. Marquez DC, Lee J, Lin T, et al. Epidermal growth factor receptor and tyrosine phosphorylation of estrogen receptor. *Endocrine* 2001;16:73–81.

111. Pietras RJ, Arboleda J, Reese DM, et al. HER-2 tyrosine kinase pathway targets estrogen receptor and promotes hormone-independent growth in human breast cancer cells. *Oncogene* 1995;10:2435–2446.

112. Watson S. Real life—and a bit more. *Nurs Stand* 1999;13:13.

113. Pappas TC, Gametchu B, Watson CS. Membrane estrogen receptors identified by multiple antibody labeling and impeded-ligand binding. *FASEB J* 1995;9:404–410.

114. Zivadinovic D, Watson CS. Membrane estrogen receptor-alpha levels predict estrogen-induced ERK1/2 activation in MCF-7 cells. *Breast Cancer Res* 2005;7:R130–R144.

115. Stevis PE, Deecher DC, Suhadolnik L, et al. Differential effects of estradiol and estradiol-BSA conjugates. *Endocrinology* 1999;140:5455–5458.

116. Harrington WR, Kim SH, Funk CC, et al. Estrogen dendrimer conjugates that preferentially activate extranuclear, nongenomic versus genomic pathways of estrogen action. *Mol Endocrinol* 2006;20:491–502.

117. Pedram A, Razandi M, Sainson RC, et al. A conserved mechanism for steroid receptor translocation to the plasma membrane. *J Biol Chem* 2007;282:22278–88.

118. Barletta F, Wong CW, McNally C, et al. Characterization of the interactions of estrogen receptor and MNAR in the activation of cSrc. *Mol Endocrinol* 2004;18:1096–1108.

119. Chen JQ, Yager JD, Russo J. Regulation of mitochondrial respiratory chain structure and function by estrogens/estrogen receptors and potential physiological/pathophysiological implications. *Biochim Biophys Acta* 2005;1746:1–17.

120. Pedram A, Razandi M, Wallace DC, Levin ER. Functional estrogen receptors in the mitochondria of breast cancer cells. *Mol Biol Cell* 2006;17:2125–2137.

121. Lee AV, Guler BL, Sun X, et al. Oestrogen receptor is a critical component required for insulin-like growth factor (IGF)-mediated signalling and growth in MCF-7 cells. *Eur J Cancer* 2000;36(Suppl 4):109–110.

122. Schiff R, Massarweh SA, Shou J, et al. Cross-talk between estrogen receptor and growth factor pathways as a molecular target for overcoming endocrine resistance. *Clin Cancer Res* 2004;10:331S–336S.

123. Pancholi S, Lykkesfeldt A, Hilmi C, et al. ERBB2 influences the subcellular localization of the estrogen receptor in tamoxifen-resistant MCF-7 cells leading to the activation of Akt and p90RSK. *Endocr Relat Cancer* 2008;15(4):985–1002.

124. Razandi M, Alton G, Pedram A, et al. Identification of a structural determinant necessary for the localization and function of estrogen receptor alpha at the plasma membrane. *Mol Cell Biol* 2003;23:1633–1646.

125. Martin MB, Franke TF, Stoica GE, et al. A role for Akt in mediating the estrogenic functions of epidermal growth factor and insulin-like growth factor I. *Endocrinology* 2000;141:4503–4511.

126. Figtree GA, Webb CM, Collins P. Tamoxifen acutely relaxes coronary arteries by an endothelium-, nitric oxide-, and estrogen receptor-dependent mechanism. *J Pharmacol Exp Ther* 2000;295:519–523.

127. Kumar R, Wang RA, Mazumdar A, et al. A naturally occurring MTA1 variant sequesters oestrogen receptor-alpha in the cytoplasm. *Nature* 2002;418:654–657.

128. Kumar R, Wang RA, Bagheri-Yarmand R. Emerging roles of MTA family members in human cancers. *Semin Oncol* 2003;30:30–37.

129. Fan P, Wang J, Santen RJ, et al. Long-term treatment with tamoxifen facilitates translocation of estrogen receptor alpha out of the nucleus and enhances its interaction with EGFR in MCF-7 breast cancer cells. *Cancer Res* 2007;67:1352–1360.

130. Ali S, Coombes RC. Endocrine-responsive breast cancer and strategies for combating resistance. *Nat Rev Cancer* 2002;2:101–112.

131. Nicholson RI, McClelland RA, Robertson JF, et al. Involvement of steroid hormone and growth factor cross-talk in endocrine response in breast cancer. *Endocr Relat Cancer* 1999;6:373–387.

132. Schiff R, Massarweh S, Shou J, et al. Breast cancer endocrine resistance: how growth factor signaling and estrogen receptor coregulators modulate response. *Clin Cancer Res* 2003;9:447S–4454S.

133. Schiff R, Massarweh SA, Shou J, et al. Advanced concepts in estrogen receptor biology and breast cancer endocrine resistance: implicated role of growth factor signaling and estrogen receptor coregulators. *Cancer Chemother Pharmacol* 2005;56(Suppl 1):10–20.

134. Weinstein-Oppenheimer CR, Burrows C, Steelman LS, et al. The effects of beta-estradiol on Raf activity, cell cycle progression and growth factor synthesis in the MCF-7 breast cancer cell line. *Cancer Biol Ther* 2002;1:256–262.

135. Yang Z, Barnes CJ, Kumar R. Human epidermal growth factor receptor 2 status modulates subcellular localization of and interaction with estrogen receptor alpha in breast cancer cells. *Clin Cancer Res* 2004;10:3621–3628.

136. Chung YL, Sheu ML, Yang SC, et al. Resistance to tamoxifen-induced apoptosis is associated with direct interaction between Her2/neu and cell membrane estrogen receptor in breast cancer. *Int J Cancer* 2002;97:306–312.

137. Benz CC, Scott GK, Sarup JC, et al. Estrogen-dependent, tamoxifen-resistant tumorigenic growth of MCF-7 cells transfected with HER2/neu. *Breast Cancer Res Treat* 1992;24:85–95.

138. Kurokawa H, Lenferink AE, Simpson JF, et al. Inhibition of HER2/neu (erbB-2) and mitogen-activated protein kinases enhances tamoxifen action against HER2-overexpressing, tamoxifen-resistant breast cancer cells. *Cancer Res* 2000;60:5887–5894.

139. Nicholson RI, Hutcheson IR, Harper ME, et al. Modulation of epidermal growth factor receptor in endocrine-resistant, estrogen-receptor-positive breast cancer. *Ann N Y Acad Sci* 2002;963:104–115.

140. Tovey S, Dunne B, Witton CJ, et al. Can molecular markers predict when to implement treatment with aromatase inhibitors in invasive breast cancer? *Clin Cancer Res* 2005;11:4835–4842.

141. Arpino G, Green SJ, Allred DC, et al. HER-2 amplification, HER-1 expression, and tamoxifen response in estrogen receptor-positive metastatic breast cancer: a Southwest Oncology Group study. *Clin Cancer Res* 2004;10:5670–5676.

142. Massarweh S, Osborne CK, Creighton CJ, et al. Tamoxifen resistance in breast tumors is driven by growth factor receptor signaling with repression of classic estrogen receptor genomic function. *Cancer Res* 2008;68:826–833.

143. Dowsett M, Houghton J, Iden C, et al. Benefit from adjuvant tamoxifen therapy in primary breast cancer patients according to oestrogen receptor, progesterone receptor, EGF receptor and HER2 status. *Ann Oncol* 2006;17:818–826.

144. Dowsett M. Overexpression of HER-2 as a resistance mechanism to hormonal therapy for breast cancer. *Endocr Relat Cancer* 2001;8:191–195.

145. Massarweh S, Osborne CK, Jiang S, et al. Mechanisms of tumor regression and resistance to estrogen deprivation and fulvestrant in a model of estrogen receptor-positive, HER-2/neu-positive breast cancer. *Cancer Res* 2006;66:8266–8273.

146. Ellis MJ, Coop A, Singh B, et al. Letrozole is more effective neoadjuvant endocrine therapy than tamoxifen for ErbB-1- and/or ErbB-2-positive, estrogen receptor-positive primary breast cancer: evidence from a phase III randomized trial. *J Clin Oncol* 2001;19:3808–3816.

147. Zhu L, Chow LW, Loo WT, et al. Her2/neu expression predicts the response to antiaromatase neoadjuvant therapy in primary breast cancer: subgroup analysis from celecoxib antiaromatase neoadjuvant trial. *Clin Cancer Res* 2004;10:4639–4644.

148. Smith IE, Dowsett M, Ebbs SR, et al. Neoadjuvant treatment of postmenopausal breast cancer with anastrozole, tamoxifen, or both in combination: the Immediate Preoperative Anastrozole, Tamoxifen, or Combined with Tamoxifen (IMPACT) multicenter double-blind randomized trial. *J Clin Oncol* 2005;23:5108–5116.

149. Rasmussen BB, Regan MM, Lykkesfeldt AE, et al. Adjuvant letrozole versus tamoxifen according to centrally-assessed ERBB2 status for postmenopausal women with endocrine-responsive early breast cancer: supplementary results from the BIG 1-98 randomised trial. *Lancet Oncol* 2008;9:23–28.

150. Dowsett M, Allred C, Knox J, et al. Relationship between quantitative estrogen and progesterone receptor expression and human epidermal growth factor receptor 2 (HER-2) status with recurrence in the Arimidex, Tamoxifen, Alone or in Combination trial. *J Clin Oncol* 2008;26:1059–1065.

151. Ellis MJ, Tao Y, Young O, et al. Estrogen-independent proliferation is present in estrogen-receptor HER2-positive primary breast cancer after neoadjuvant letrozole. *J Clin Oncol* 2006;24:3019–3025.

152. Arpino G, Gutierrez C, Weiss H, et al. Treatment of human epidermal growth factor receptor 2-overexpressing breast cancer xenografts with multiagent HER-targeted therapy. *J Natl Cancer Inst* 2007;99:694–705.

153. Xia W, Bacus S, Hegde P, et al. A model of acquired autoresistance to a potent ErbB2 tyrosine kinase inhibitor and a therapeutic strategy to prevent its onset in breast cancer. *Proc Natl Acad Sci U S A* 2006;103:7795–7800.

154. Newman SP, Bates NP, Vernimmen D, et al. Cofactor competition between the ligand-bound oestrogen receptor and an intron 1 enhancer leads to oestrogen repression of ERBB2 expression in breast cancer. *Oncogene* 2000;19:490–497.

155. Yarden RI, Wilson MA, Chrysogelos SA. Estrogen suppression of EGFR expression in breast cancer cells: a possible mechanism to modulate growth. *J Cell Biochem Suppl* 2001;(Suppl 36):232–246.

156. Bayliss J HA, Vishnu P, Kathleen D, et al. Reversal of the estrogen receptor negative phenotype in breast cancer and restoration of anti-estrogen response. *Clin Cancer Res* 2007;13:7029–7036.

157. Cui X, Schiff R, Arpino G, Osborne CK, Lee AV. Biology of progesterone receptor loss in breast cancer and its implications for endocrine therapy. *J Clin Oncol* 2005;23:7721–7735.
158. Cui X, Zhang P, Deng W, et al. Insulin-like growth factor-I inhibits progesterone receptor expression in breast cancer cells via the phosphatidylinositol 3-kinase/Akt/mammalian target of rapamycin pathway: progesterone receptor as a potential indicator of growth factor activity in breast cancer. *Mol Endocrinol* 2003;17:575–588.
159. Konecny G, Pauletti G, Pegram M, et al. Quantitative association between HER-2/neu and steroid hormone receptors in hormone receptor-positive primary breast cancer. *J Natl Cancer Inst* 2003,95.142–153.
160. Lopez-Tarruella S, Schiff R. The dynamics of estrogen receptor status in breast cancer: re-shaping the paradigm. *Clin Cancer Res* 2007;13:6921–6925.
161. Oh AS, Lorant LA, Holloway JN, et al. Hyperactivation of MAPK induces loss of ERalpha expression in breast cancer cells. *Mol Endocrinol* 2001;15:1344–1359.
162. Gutierrez MC, Detre S, Johnston S, et al. Molecular changes in tamoxifen-resistant breast cancer: relationship between estrogen receptor, HER-2, and p38 mitogen-activated protein kinase. *J Clin Oncol* 2005;23:2469–2476.
163. Meng S, Tripathy D, Shete S, et al. HER-2 gene amplification can be acquired as breast cancer progresses. *Proc Natl Acad Sci U S A* 2004;101:9393–9398. Epub 2004 Jun 11.
164. Lipton A, Leitzel K, Ali SM, et al. Serum HER-2/neu conversion to positive at the time of disease progression in patients with breast carcinoma on hormone therapy. *Cancer* 2005;104:257–263.
165. Munzone E, Curigliano G, Rocca A, et al. Reverting estrogen-receptor-negative phenotype in HER-2-overexpressing advanced breast cancer patients exposed to trastuzumab plus chemotherapy. *Breast Cancer Res* 2006;8:R1.
166. Rimawi MF, Mohsin SK, Gutierrez MC, Arpino G, et al. Inhibiting the growth factor receptor (GFR) pathway preserves and enhances the expression of the estrogen receptor (ER) in HER-2/neu (HER2) over-expressing human breast tumors and xenografts [Abstract]. San Antonio Breast Cancer Symposium; 2005; San Antonio, Texas. *Breast Cancer Res Treat*;2005;94:S8.
167. Chu I, Blackwell K, Chen S, et al. The dual ErbB1/ErbB2 inhibitor, lapatinib (GW572016), cooperates with tamoxifen to inhibit both cell proliferation- and estrogen-dependent gene expression in antiestrogen-resistant breast cancer. *Cancer Res* 2005;65:18–25.
168. Witters L, Engle L, Lipton A. Restoration of estrogen responsiveness by blocking the HER-2/neu pathway. *Oncol Rep* 2002;9:1163–1166.
169. Dowsett M, Nicholson RI, Pietras RJ. Biological characteristics of the pure antiestrogen fulvestrant: overcoming endocrine resistance. *Breast Cancer Res Treat* 2005;93(Suppl 1):S11–S18.
170. Osborne K, Neven P, Dirix L, et al. Randomized phase II study of gefitinib (IRESSA) or placebo in combination with tamoxifen in patients with hormone receptor positive metastatic breast cancer [Abstract 2067]. San Antonio Breast Cancer Symposium; 2007; San Antonio, TX: *Breast Cancer Res Treat* 2007;106S:107.
171. Cristofanilli M, Valero V, Mangalik A, et al. A phase II multicenter, double-blind, randomized trial to compare anastrozole plus gefitinib with anastrozole plus placebo in postmenopausal women with hormone receptor-positive (HR+) metastatic breast cancer (MBC) [Abstract 1012]. 2008 American Society of Clinical Oncology Annual Meeting. 05/30/08–06/03/08, Chicago, IL. *J Clin Oncol* 2008;26(Suppl. May 20).
172. Bezwoda WR, Esser JD, Dansey R, et al. The value of estrogen and progesterone receptor determinations in advanced breast cancer. Estrogen receptor level but not progesterone receptor level correlates with response to tamoxifen. *Cancer* 1991;68:867–872.
173. Manni A, Arafah B, Pearson OH. Estrogen and progesterone receptors in the prediction of response of breast cancer to endocrine therapy. *Cancer* 1980;46:2838.
174. McClelland RA, Berger U, Miller LS, et al. Immunocytochemical assay for estrogen receptor: relationship to outcome of therapy in patients with advanced breast cancer. *Cancer Res* 1986;46:4241s.
175. Early Breast Cancer Trialists' Collaborative Group (EBCTCG) Effects of chemotherapy and hormonal therapy for early breast cancer on recurrence and 15-year survival: an overview of the randomised trials. *Lancet* 2005;365:1687–1717.
176. McGuire WL. Hormone receptors: their role in predicting prognosis and response to endocrine therapy. *Semin Oncol* 1978;5:428–433.
177. McGuire WL, De La Garza M, Chamness GC. Evaluation of estrogen receptor assays in human breast cancer tissue. *Cancer Res* 1977;37:637–639.
178. Bezwoda WR, Esser JD, Dansey R, et al. The value of estrogen and progesterone receptor determinations in advanced breast cancer. *Cancer* 1991;68:867–872.
179. King WJ, Greene GL. Monoclonal antibodies localize oestrogen receptors in the nuclei of target cells. *Nature* 1984;307:745–747.
180. Logeat F, Hai MT, Milgrom E. Antibodies to rabbit progesterone receptor: cross-reaction with human receptor. *Proc Natl Acad Sci U S A* 1981;78:1426–1430.
181. Pertschuk LP, Kim DS, Nayer K, et al. Immunocytochemical estrogen and progestin receptor assays in breast cancer with monoclonal antibodies. Histopathologic, demographic, and biochemical correlations and relationship to endocrine response and survival. *Cancer* 1990;66:1663–1670.
182. Beck T, Weikel W, Brumm C, et al. Immunohistochemical detection of hormone receptors in breast carcinomas (ER-ICA, PgR-ICA): prognostic usefulness and comparison with the biochemical radioactive-ligand-binding assay (DCC). *Gynecol Oncol* 1994;53:220–227.
183. Stierer M, Rosen H, Weber R, et al. Comparison of immunohistochemical and biochemical measurement of steroid receptors in primary breast cancer: evaluation of discordant findings. *Breast Cancer Res Treat* 1998;50:125–134.
184. Fisher ER, Anderson S, Dean S, et al. Solving the dilemma of the immunohistochemical and other methods used for scoring estrogen receptor and progesterone receptor in patients with invasive breast carcinoma. *Cancer* 2005;103:164–173.
185. Molino A, Micciolo R, Turazza M, et al. Prognostic significance of estrogen receptors in 405 primary breast cancers: a comparison of immunohistochemical and biochemical methods. *Breast Cancer Res Treat* 1997;45:241–249.
186. Barnes DM, Harris WH, Smith P, et al. Immunohistochemical determination of oestrogen receptor: comparison of different methods of assessment of staining and correlation with clinical outcome of breast cancer patients. *Br J Cancer* 1996;74:1445–1451.
187. Harvey JM, Clark GM, Osborne CK, et al. Estrogen receptor status by immunohistochemistry is superior to the ligand-binding assay for predicting response to adjuvant endocrine therapy in breast cancer. *J Clin Oncol* 1999;17:1474–1481.
188. Regan MM, Viale G, Mastropasqua MG, et al. Re-evaluating adjuvant breast cancer trials: assessing hormone receptor status by immunohistochemical versus extraction assays. *J Natl Cancer Inst* 2006;98(21):1571–1581.
189. Rhodes A, Jasani B, Balaton AJ, et al. Study of interlaboratory reliability and reproducibility of estrogen and progesterone receptor assays in Europe. Documentation of poor reliability and identification of insufficient microwave antigen retrieval time as a major contributory element of unreliable assays. *Am J Clin Pathol* 2001;115:44–58.
190. Goldstein NS, Ferkowicz M, Odish E, et al. Minimum formalin fixation time for consistent estrogen receptor immunohistochemical staining of invasive breast carcinoma. *Am J Clin Pathol* 2003;120:86–92.
191. Vassallo J, Pinto GA, Alvarenga JM, et al. Comparison of immunoexpression of 2 antibodies for estrogen receptors (1D5 and 6F11) in breast carcinomas using different antigen retrieval and detection methods. *Appl Immunohistochem Mol Morphol* 2004;12:177–182.
192. Eifel P, Axelson JA, Costa J, et al. National Institutes of Health Consensus Development Conference Statement: adjuvant therapy for breast cancer, November 1–3, 2000. *J Natl Cancer Inst* 2001;93:979–989.
193. Harris L, Fritsche H, Mennel R, et al. American Society of Clinical Oncology 2007 update of recommendations for the use of tumor markers in breast cancer. *J Clin Oncol* 2007;25:5287–5312.
194. Allred DC, Clark GM, Elledge R, et al. Association of p53 protein expression with tumor cell proliferation rate and clinical outcome in node-negative breast cancer. *J Natl Cancer Inst* 1993;85:200–206.
195. Phillips T, Murray G, Wakamiya K, et al. Development of standard estrogen and progesterone receptor immunohistochemical assays for selection of patients for antihormonal therapy. *Appl Immunohistochem Mol Morphol* 2007;15:325–331.
196. Mohsin SK, Weiss H, Havighurst T, et al. Progesterone receptor by immunohistochemistry and clinical outcome in breast cancer: a validation study. *Mod Pathol* 2004;17:1545–1554.
197. Fuqua SA, Schiff R, Parra I, et al. Estrogen receptor beta protein in human breast cancer: correlation with clinical tumor parameters. *Cancer Res* 2003;63:2434–2439.
198. Carder PJ, Murphy CE, Dervan P, et al. A multi-centre investigation towards reaching a consensus on the immunohistochemical detection of ERbeta in archival formalin-fixed paraffin embedded human breast tissue. *Breast Cancer Res Treat* 2005;92:287–293.
199. Hopp TA, Weiss HL, Parra IS, et al. Low levels of estrogen receptor beta protein predict resistance to tamoxifen therapy in breast cancer. *Clin Cancer Res* 2004;10:7490–7499.
200. Honma N, Horii R, Iwase T, et al. Clinical importance of estrogen receptor-beta evaluation in breast cancer patients treated with adjuvant tamoxifen therapy. *J Clin Oncol* 2008;26:3727–3734.
201. Collins LC, Botero ML, Schnitt SJ. Bimodal frequency distribution of estrogen receptor immunohistochemical staining results in breast cancer: an analysis of 825 cases. *Am J Clin Pathol* 2005;123:16–20.
202. Nadji M, Gomez-Fernandez C, Ganjei-Azar P, et al. Immunohistochemistry of estrogen and progesterone receptors reconsidered: experience with 5,993 breast cancers. *Am J Clin Pathol* 2005;123:21–27.
203. Rimm DL, Giltnane JM, Moeder C, et al. Bimodal population or pathologist artifact? *J Clin Oncol* 2007;25:2487–2488.
204. Gokhale S, Rosen D, Sneige N, et al. Assessment of two automated imaging systems in evaluating estrogen receptor status in breast carcinoma. *Appl Immunohistochem Mol Morphol* 2007;15:451–455.
205. Wolff AC, Hammond ME, Schwartz JN, et al. American Society of Clinical Oncology/College of American Pathologists guideline recommendations for human epidermal growth factor receptor 2 testing in breast cancer. *J Clin Oncol* 2007;25:118–145.
206. Paik S, Shak S, Tang G, et al. A multigene assay to predict recurrence of tamoxifen-treated, node-negative breast cancer. *N Engl J Med* 2004;351:2817–2826.
207. Badve SS, Baehner FL, Gray RP, et al. Estrogen- and progesterone-receptor status in ECOG 2197: comparison of immunohistochemistry by local and central laboratories and quantitative reverse transcription polymerase chain reaction by central laboratory. *J Clin Oncol* 2008;26:2473–2481.
208. Cronin M, Pho M, Dutta D, et al. Measurement of gene expression in archival paraffin-embedded tissues: development and performance of a 92-gene reverse transcriptase-polymerase chain reaction assay. *Am J Pathol* 2004;164:35–42.
209. Esteva FJ, Sahin AA, Cristofanilli M, et al. Prognostic role of a multigene reverse transcriptase-PCR assay in patients with node-negative breast cancer not receiving adjuvant systemic therapy. *Clin Cancer Res* 2005;11:3315–3319.
210. Ma XJ, Hilsenbeck SG, Wang W, et al. The HOXB13:IL17BR expression index is a prognostic factor in early-stage breast cancer. *J Clin Oncol* 2006;24:4611–4619.
211. Perou CM, Sorlie T, Eisen MB, et al. Molecular portraits of human breast tumours. *Nature* 2000;406:747–752.
212. van't Veer LJ, Dai H, van de Vijver MJ, et al. Gene expression profiling predicts clinical outcome of breast cancer. *Nature* 2002;415:530–536.
213. Gong Y, Yan K, Lin F, et al. Determination of oestrogen-receptor status and ERBB2 status of breast carcinoma: a gene-expression profiling study. *Lancet Oncol* 2007;8:203–211.
214. Dressman MA, Walz TM, Lavedan C, et al. Genes that co-cluster with estrogen receptor alpha in microarray analysis of breast biopsies. *Pharmacogenomics J* 2001;1:135–141.
215. Oh DS, Troester MA, Usary J, et al. Estrogen-regulated genes predict survival in hormone receptor-positive breast cancers. *J Clin Oncol* 2006;24:1656–1664.
216. Abba MC, Hu Y, Sun H, et al. Gene expression signature of estrogen receptor alpha status in breast cancer. *BMC Genomics* 2005;6:37.
217. Anderson WF, Chatterjee N, Ershler WB, et al. Estrogen receptor breast cancer phenotypes in the Surveillance, Epidemiology, and End Results database. *Breast Cancer Res Treat* 2002;76:27–36.
218. Clark GM, Osborne CK, McGuire WL. Correlations between estrogen receptor, progesterone receptor, and patient characteristics in human breast cancer. *J Clin Oncol* 1984;2:1102–1109.
219. Hopp TA, Weiss HL, Hilsenbeck SG, et al. Breast cancer patients with progesterone receptor PR-A-rich tumors have poorer disease-free survival rates. *Clin Cancer Res* 2004;10:2751–2760.
220. Mote PA, Johnston JF, Manninen T, et al. Detection of progesterone receptor forms A and B by immunohistochemical analysis. *J Clin Pathol* 2001;54: 624–630.
221. Nicolini A, Giardino R, Carpi A, et al. Metastatic breast cancer: an updating. *Biomed Pharmacother* 2006;60:548–556.
222. Smith TJ, Davidson NE, Schapira DV, et al. American Society of Clinical Oncology 1998 update of recommended breast cancer surveillance guidelines. *J Clin Oncol* 1999;17:1080–1082.

223. Greenberg PA, Hortobagyi GN, Smith TL, et al. Long-term follow-up of patients with complete remission following combination chemotherapy for metastatic breast cancer. *J Clin Oncol* 1996;14:2197–2205.
224. McGuire W, Carbone P, Sears M, et al. Estrogen receptors in human breast cancer: an overview. In: McGuire W, Vollmer E, Carbone P, eds. *Estrogen receptor in human breast cancer*. New York: Raven Press, 1975.
225. Nabholtz JM, Buzdar A, Pollak M, et al. Anastrozole is superior to tamoxifen as first-line therapy for advanced breast cancer in postmenopausal women: results of a North American multicenter randomized trial. Arimidex Study Group. *J Clin Oncol* 2000;18:3758–3767.
226. Ravdin PM, Green S, Dorr TM, et al. Prognostic significance of progesterone receptor levels in estrogen receptor-positive patients with metastatic breast cancer treated with tamoxifen: results of a prospective Southwest Oncology Group study. *J Clin Oncol* 1992;10:1284–1291.
227. Robertson JF, Bates K, Pearson D, et al. Comparison of two oestrogen receptor assays in the prediction of the clinical course of patients with advanced breast cancer. *Br J Cancer* 1992;65:727–730.
228. Lower EE, Glass EL, Bradley DA, et al. Impact of metastatic estrogen receptor and progesterone receptor status on survival. *Breast Cancer Res Treat* 2005;90:65–70.
229. Mouridsen H, Gershanovich M, Sun Y, et al. Phase III study of letrozole versus tamoxifen as first-line therapy of advanced breast cancer in postmenopausal women: analysis of survival and update of efficacy from the International Letrozole Breast Cancer Group. *J Clin Oncol* 2003;21:2101–2109.
230. Dodwell D, Wardley A, Johnston S. Postmenopausal advanced breast cancer: options for therapy after tamoxifen and aromatase inhibitors. *Breast* 2006;15:584–594.
231. Dombernowsky P, Smith I, Falkson G, et al. Letrozole, a new oral aromatase inhibitor for advanced breast cancer: double-blind randomized trial showing a dose effect and improved efficacy and tolerability compared with megestrol acetate. *J Clin Oncol* 1998;16:453–461.
232. Lonning PE, Taylor PD, Anker G, et al. High-dose estrogen treatment in postmenopausal breast cancer patients heavily exposed to endocrine therapy. *Breast Cancer Res Treat* 2001;67:111–116.
233. Buzdar A, Jonat W, Howell A, et al. Anastrozole, a potent and selective aromatase inhibitor, versus megestrol acetate in postmenopausal women with advanced breast cancer: results of overview analysis of two phase III trials. Arimidex Study Group. *J Clin Oncol* 1996;14:2000–2011.
234. Goss P, von Eichel L. Summary of aromatase inhibitor trials: the past and future. *J Steroid Biochem Mol Biol* 2007;106:40–48.
235. Briest S, Davidson NE. Aromatase inhibitors for breast cancer. *Rev Endocr Metab Disord* 2007;8:215–228.
236. Bonneterre J, Thurlimann B, Robertson JF, et al. Anastrozole versus tamoxifen as first-line therapy for advanced breast cancer in 668 postmenopausal women: results of the Tamoxifen or Arimidex Randomized Group Efficacy and Tolerability study. *J Clin Oncol* 2000;18:3748–3757.
237. Mouridsen H, Gershanovich M, Sun Y, et al. Superior efficacy of letrozole versus tamoxifen as first-line therapy for postmenopausal women with advanced breast cancer: results of a phase III study of the International Letrozole Breast Cancer Group. *J Clin Oncol* 2001;19:2596–2606.
238. Nabholtz JM, Bonneterre J, Buzdar A, et al. Anastrozole (Arimidex) versus tamoxifen as first-line therapy for advanced breast cancer in postmenopausal women: survival analysis and updated safety results. *Eur J Cancer* 2003;39:1684–1689.
239. Mauri D, Pavlidis N, Polyzos NP, et al. Survival with aromatase inhibitors and inactivators versus standard hormonal therapy in advanced breast cancer: meta-analysis. *J Natl Cancer Inst* 2006;98:1285–1291.
240. Buzdar AU, Vergote I, Sainsbury R. The impact of hormone receptor status on the clinical efficacy of the new-generation aromatase inhibitors: a review of data from first-line metastatic disease trials in postmenopausal women. *Breast J* 2004;10:211–217.
241. Elledge RM, Green S, Pugh R, et al. Estrogen receptor (ER) and progesterone receptor (PgR), by ligand-binding assay compared with ER, PgR and pS2, by immuno-histochemistry in predicting response to tamoxifen in metastatic breast cancer: a Southwest Oncology Group Study. *Int J Cancer* 2000;89:111–117.
242. Robertson JF. Oestrogen receptor: a stable phenotype in breast cancer. *Br J Cancer* 1996;73:5–12.
243. Horwitz KB, McGuire WL. Predicting response to endocrine therapy in human breast cancer: a hypothesis. *Science* 1975;189:726–727.
244. Pertschuk LP, Feldman JG, Eisenberg KB, et al. Immunocytochemical detection of progesterone receptor in breast cancer with monoclonal antibody. Relation to biochemical assay, disease-free survival, and clinical endocrine response. *Cancer* 1988;62:342–349.
245. Hull DF, Clark GM, Osborne CK, et al. Multiple estrogen receptor assays in human breast cancer. *Cancer Res* 1983;43:413–416.
246. Spataro V, Price K, Goldhirsch A, et al. Sequential estrogen receptor determinations from primary breast cancer and at relapse: prognostic and therapeutic relevance. The International Breast Cancer Study Group (formerly Ludwig Group). *Ann Oncol* 1992;3:733–740.
247. Kuukasjarvi T, Kononen J, Helin H, et al. Loss of estrogen receptor in recurrent breast cancer is associated with poor response to endocrine therapy. *J Clin Oncol* 1996;14:2584–2589.
248. Broglio K, Moulder SL, Hsu L, et al. Prognostic impact of discordance/concordance of triple-receptor expression between primary tumor and metastasis in patients with metastatic breast cancer [Abstract 1001]. 2008 American Society of Clinical Oncology Annual Meeting. 05/30/08–06/03/08, Chicago IL, *J Clin Oncol*, 2008;26(Suppl. May 20).
249. MacFarlane R, Speers C, Masoudi H, et al. Molecular changes in the primary breast cancer versus the relapsed/metastatic lesion from a large population-based database and tissue microarray series [Abstract 1000]. 2008 American Society of Clinical Oncology Annual Meeting. 05/30/08–06/03/08, Chicago, IL *J Clin Oncol* 2008;26(Suppl May 20).
250. Brankovic-Magic M, Jankovic R, Neskovic-Konstantinovic Z, et al. Progesterone receptor status of breast cancer metastases. *J Cancer Res Clin Oncol* 2002;128: 55–60.
251. Gross GE, Clark GM, Chamness GC, et al. Multiple progesterone receptor assays in human breast cancer. *Cancer Res* 1984;44:836–840.
252. Osborne CK, Yochmowitz MG, Knight WA, 3rd, et al. The value of estrogen and progesterone receptors in the treatment of breast cancer. *Cancer* 1980;46:2884–2888.
253. Keshgegian AA, Cnaan A. Estrogen receptor-negative, progesterone receptor-positive breast carcinoma: poor clinical outcome. *Arch Pathol Lab Med* 1996; 120:970–973.
254. Tamoxifen for early breast cancer: an overview of the randomised trials. Early Breast Cancer Trialists' Collaborative Group. *Lancet* 1998;351:1451–1467.
255. Berry DA, Cirrincione C, Henderson IC, et al. Estrogen-receptor status and outcomes of modern chemotherapy for patients with node-positive breast cancer. *JAMA* 2006;295:1658–1667.
256. Saphner T, Tormey DC, Gray R. Annual hazard rates of recurrence for breast cancer after primary therapy. *J Clin Oncol* 1996;14:2738–2746.
257. Dignam JJ, Dukic VM, Anderson SJ, et al. Time-dependent patterns of recurrence after early stage breast cancer: preliminary observations and methodological issues [Abstract 536]. 2007 American Society of Clinical Oncology Annual Meeting 2007. Jun 1–5; Chicago, IL Proceedings Part I. *J Clin Oncol*;2007;vol. 25,18S:536.
258. Hutchins LF, Green S, Ravdin P, et al. CMF versus CAF with and without tamoxifen in high-risk node-negative breast cancer patients and a natural history follow-up study in low-risk node-negative patients: first results of intergroup trial INT 0102 [Abstract]. American Society of Clinical Oncology,1998. *Proceeding of the American Society of Clinical Oncology* 1998;17:2.
259. Hutchins LF, Green SJ, Ravdin PM, et al. Randomized, controlled trial of cyclophosphamide, methotrexate, and fluorouracil versus cyclophosphamide, doxorubicin, and fluorouracil with and without tamoxifen for high-risk, node-negative breast cancer: treatment results of Intergroup Protocol INT-0102. *J Clin Oncol* 2005;23:8313–8321.
260. Fisher B, Anderson S, Tan-Chiu E, et al. Tamoxifen and chemotherapy for axillary node-negative, estrogen receptor-negative breast cancer: findings from National Surgical Adjuvant Breast and Bowel Project B-23. *J Clin Oncol* 2001;19:931–942.
261. Arpino G, Weiss HL, Clark GM, et al. Hormone receptor status of a contralateral breast cancer is independent of the receptor status of the first primary in patients not receiving adjuvant tamoxifen. *J Clin Oncol* 2005;23:4687–4694.
262. Swain SM, Wilson JW, Mamounas EP, et al. Estrogen receptor status of primary breast cancer is predictive of estrogen receptor status of contralateral breast cancer. *J Natl Cancer Inst* 2004;96:516–523.
263. Wedam SB, Swain SM. Contralateral breast cancer: where does it all begin? *J Clin Oncol* 2005;23:4585–4587.
264. Baehner FL, Habel LA, Quesenberry CP, et al. Quantitative RT-PCR analysis of ER and PR by Oncotype DX™ indicates distinct and different associations with prognosis and prediction of tamoxifen benefit [Abstract 45]. San Antonio Breast Cancer Symposium;2006. *Breast Can Res Treat*;2006;100:S21.
265. Dowsett M, Ebbs SR, Dixon JM, et al. Biomarker changes during neoadjuvant anastrozole, tamoxifen, or the combination: influence of hormonal status and HER-2 in breast cancer—a study from the IMPACT trialists. *J Clin Oncol* 2005;23:2477–2492.
266. Early Breast Cancer Trialists' Collaborative Group. Systemic treatment of early breast cancer by hormonal, cytotoxic, or immune therapy. 133 randomised trials involving 31,000 recurrences and 24,000 deaths among 75,000 women. *Lancet* 1992;339:1–15.
267. Lin NU, Winer EP. Advances in adjuvant endocrine therapy for postmenopausal women. *J Clin Oncol* 2008;26:798–805.
268. Baum M, Budzar AU, Cuzick J, et al. Anastrozole alone or in combination with tamoxifen versus tamoxifen alone for adjuvant treatment of postmenopausal women with early breast cancer: first results of the ATAC randomised trial. *Lancet* 2002;359:2131–2139.
269. Howell A, Cuzick J, Baum M, et al. Results of the ATAC (Arimidex, Tamoxifen, Alone or in Combination) trial after completion of 5 years' adjuvant treatment for breast cancer. *Lancet* 2005;365:60–62.
270. Coates AS, Keshaviah A, Thurlimann B, et al. Five years of letrozole compared with tamoxifen as initial adjuvant therapy for postmenopausal women with endocrine-responsive early breast cancer: update of study BIG 1-98. *J Clin Oncol* 2007;25:486–492.
271. Thurlimann B, Keshaviah A, Coates AS, et al. A comparison of letrozole and tamoxifen in postmenopausal women with early breast cancer. *N Engl J Med* 2005;353:2747–2757.
272. Coombes RC, Hall E, Gibson LJ, et al. A randomized trial of exemestane after two to three years of tamoxifen therapy in postmenopausal women with primary breast cancer. *N Engl J Med* 2004;350:1081–1092.
273. Coombes RC, Kilburn LS, Snowdon CF, et al. Survival and safety of exemestane versus tamoxifen after 2–3 years' tamoxifen treatment (Intergroup Exemestane Study): a randomised controlled trial. *Lancet* 2007;369:559–570.
274. Jakesz R, Jonat W, Gnant M, et al. Switching of postmenopausal women with endocrine-responsive early breast cancer to anastrozole after 2 years' adjuvant tamoxifen: combined results of ABCSG trial 8 and ARNO 95 trial. *Lancet* 2005;366:455–462.
275. Kaufmann M, Jonat W, Hilfrich J, et al. Improved overall survival in postmenopausal women with early breast cancer after anastrozole initiated after treatment with tamoxifen compared with continued tamoxifen: the ARNO 95 Study. *J Clin Oncol* 2007;25:2664–2670.
276. Boccardo F, Rubagotti A, Guglielmini P, et al. Switching to anastrozole versus continued tamoxifen treatment of early breast cancer. Updated results of the Italian tamoxifen anastrozole (ITA) trial. *Ann Oncol* 2006;17(Suppl 7):vii10–vii14.
277. Boccardo F, Rubagotti A, Puntoni M, et al. Switching to anastrozole versus continued tamoxifen treatment of early breast cancer: preliminary results of the Italian Tamoxifen Anastrozole Trial. *J Clin Oncol* 2005;23:5138–5147.
278. Goss PE, Ingle JN, Martino S, et al. Randomized trial of letrozole following tamoxifen as extended adjuvant therapy in receptor-positive breast cancer: updated findings from NCIC CTG MA.17. *J Natl Cancer Inst* 2005;97:1262–1271.
279. Goss PE. Preventing relapse beyond 5 years: the MA.17 extended adjuvant trial. *Semin Oncol* 2006;33:S8–S12.
280. Mamounas E, Jeong J-H, Wickerham L, et al. Benefit from exemestane (EXE) as extended adjuvant therapy after 5 years of tamoxifen (TAM): intent-to-treat analysis of NSABP B-33 [Abstract 49]. San Antonio Breast Cancer Symposium, 2006. San Antonio, Texas. *Breast Can Res Treat*,2006,100(Suppl 1)S22.
281. Jakesz R, Samonigg H, Greil R, et al. Extended adjuvant treatment with anastrozole: results from the Austrian Breast and Colorectal Cancer Study Group Trial 6a (ABCSG-6a) [Abstract 527]. 2005 American Society of Clinical Oncology Annual Meeting, 2005; May 13–17, Orlando, Florida. *J Clin Oncol* 2005;23:10S.
282. Viale G, Regan MM, Maiorano E, et al. Prognostic and predictive value of centrally reviewed expression of estrogen and progesterone receptors in a randomized trial comparing letrozole and tamoxifen adjuvant therapy for postmenopausal early breast cancer: BIG 1-98. *J Clin Oncol* 2007;25:3846–3852.
283. Rakha EA, El-Sayed ME, Green AR, et al. Biologic and clinical characteristics of breast cancer with single hormone receptor positive phenotype. *J Clin Oncol* 2007;25:4772–4778.

284. Dunnwald LK, Rossing MA, Li CI. Hormone receptor status, tumor characteristics, and prognosis: a prospective cohort of breast cancer patients. *Breast Cancer Res* 2007;9:R6.

285. De Maeyer L, Van Limbergen E, De Nys K, et al. Does estrogen receptor negative/progesterone receptor positive breast carcinoma exist? *J Clin Oncol* 2008;26:335–336; author reply 6–8.

286. Bardou VJ, Arpino G, Elledge RM, et al. Progesterone receptor status significantly improves outcome prediction over estrogen receptor status alone for adjuvant endocrine therapy in two large breast cancer databases. *J Clin Oncol* 2003;21. 1973–1979.

287. Ferno M, Stal O, Baldetorp B, et al. Results of two or five years of adjuvant tamoxifen correlated to steroid receptor and S-phase levels. South Sweden Breast Cancer Group, and South East Sweden Breast Cancer Group. *Breast Cancer Res Treat* 2000;58:00570.

288. Jakesz R, Samonigg H, Hausmaninger H. Progesterone receptor quality and level have a significant prognostic and predictive impact in pre- and postmenopausal patients with hormone-responsive breast cancer: six-year results of ABCSG trials 5 and 6 [Abstract].;*Breast Cancer Res Treat* 2002;76(Suppl 1):S45.

289. Lamy PJ, Pujol P, Thezenas S, et al. Progesterone receptor quantification as a strong prognostic determinant in postmenopausal breast cancer women under tamoxifen therapy. *Breast Cancer Res Treat* 2002;76.65–71.

290. Goss PE, Ingle JN, Martino S, et al. Efficacy of letrozole extended adjuvant therapy according to estrogen receptor and progesterone receptor status of the primary tumor: National Cancer Institute of Canada Clinical Trials Group MA.17. *J Clin Oncol* 2007;25:2006–20011.

291. Arpino G, Weiss H, Lee AV, et al. Estrogen receptor-positive, progesterone receptor-negative breast cancer: association with growth factor receptor expression and tamoxifen resistance. *J Natl Cancer Inst* 2005;97:1254–1261.

292. Dowsett M, Cuzick J, Wale C, et al. Retrospective analysis of time to recurrence in the ATAC trial according to hormone receptor status: an hypothesis-generating study. *J Clin Oncol* 2005;23:7512–7517.

293. Pusztai L, Mazouni C, Anderson K, et al. Molecular classification of breast cancer: limitations and potential. *Oncologist* 2006;11:868–877.

294. Kok M, Linn SC, Van Laar RK, et al. Comparison of gene expression profiles predicting progression in breast cancer patients treated with tamoxifen. *Breast Cancer Res Treat* 2009;113:275–283.

295. Sparano JA, Paik S. Development of the 21-gene assay and its application in clinical practice and clinical trials. *J Clin Oncol* 2008;26:721–728.

296. Jansen MP, Foekens JA, van Staveren IL, et al. Molecular classification of tamoxifen-resistant breast carcinomas by gene expression profiling. *J Clin Oncol* 2005; 23:732–740.

297. Symmans WF, Sotiriou C, Anderson SK, et al. Measurements of estrogen receptor and reporter genes from microarrays determine receptor status and time to recurrence following adjuvant tamoxifen therapy [Abstract 308]. San Antonio Breast Cancer Symposium, 2005. San Antonio, Texas. *Breast Cancer Res Treat*; 2005;94(Suppl 1):S32.

298. Loi S, Haibe-Kains B, Desmedt C, et al. Predicting prognosis using molecular profiling in estrogen receptor-positive breast cancer treated with tamoxifen. *BMC Genomics* 2008;9:239.

299. Henry NL, Hayes DF. Can biology trump anatomy? Do all node-positive patients with breast cancer need chemotherapy? *J Clin Oncol* 2007;25:2501–2503.

300. Schmidt M, Bremer E, Hasenclever D, et al. Role of the progesterone receptor for paclitaxel resistance in primary breast cancer. *Br J Cancer* 2007;96:241–247.

301. Sui M, Huang Y, Park BH, et al. Estrogen receptor alpha mediates breast cancer cell resistance to paclitaxel through inhibition of apoptotic cell death. *Cancer Res* 2007;67:5337–5344.

302. Lippman ME, Allegra JC, Thompson EB, et al. The relation between estrogen receptors and response rate to cytotoxic chemotherapy in metastatic breast cancer. *N Engl J Med* 1978;298:1223–1228.

303. Andre F, Broglio K, Roche H, et al. Estrogen receptor expression and efficacy of docetaxel-containing adjuvant chemotherapy in patients with node-positive breast cancer: results from a pooled analysis. *J Clin Oncol* 2008;26:2636–2643.

304. De Laurentiis M, Cancello G, D'Agostino D, et al. Taxane-based combinations as adjuvant chemotherapy of early breast cancer: a meta-analysis of randomized trials. *J Clin Oncol* 2008;26:44–53.

305. Mamounas EP, Bryant J, Lembersky BC, et al. Paclitaxel after doxorubicin plus cyclophosphamide as adjuvant chemotherapy for node-positive breast cancer: results from NSABP B-28. *J Clin Oncol* 2008;23:3686–3696.

306. Martin M, Pienkowski T, Mackey J, et al. Adjuvant docetaxel for node-positive breast cancer. *N Engl J Med* 2005;352:2302–2313.

307. Mazouni C, Kau SW, Frye D, et al. Inclusion of taxanes, particularly weekly paclitaxel, in preoperative chemotherapy improves pathologic complete response rate in estrogen receptor-positive breast cancers. *Ann Oncol* 2007;18:874–880.

308. Hayes DF, Thor AD, Dressler LG, et al. HER2 and response to paclitaxel in node-positive breast cancer. *N Engl J Med* 2007;357:1496–1506.

309. Goldhirsch A, Wood WC, Gelber RD, Coates AS, et al. Progress and promise: highlights of the international expert consensus on the primary therapy of early breast cancer 2007. *Annals of Oncology* 2007;18:1133–1144.

310. Paik S, Tang G, Shak S, et al. Gene expression and benefit of chemotherapy in women with node-negative, estrogen receptor-positive breast cancer. *J Clin Oncol* 2006;24:3726–3734.

311. Albain K, Barlow W, Shak S, et al. Prognostic and predictive value of the 21-gene recurrence score assay in postmenopausal, node-positive, ER-positive breast cancer (S8814, INT0100). Presented at the 30th Annual San Antonio Breast Cancer Symposium; December 13–16, 2007; San Antonio, TX. Abstract 10.

312. Fisher B, Dignam J, Wolmark N, et al. Tamoxifen in treatment of intraductal breast cancer: National Surgical Adjuvant Breast and Bowel Project B-24 randomised controlled trial. *Lancet* 1999;353:1993–2000.

313. Allred DC, Bryant J, Land S, et al. Estrogen receptor expression as a predictive marker of the effectiveness of tamoxifen in the treatment of DCIS: findings from NSABP Protocol B-24 [Abstract]. San Antonio Breast Cancer Symposium, December 2002. San Antonio, Texas. *Breast Cancer Res Treat* 2002; 76(Suppl 1):S36.

314. Crowe JP, Hubay CA, Pearson OH, et al. Estrogen receptor status as a prognostic indicator for stage I breast cancer patients. *Breast Cancer Res Treat* 1982;2: 171–176.

315. Fisher B, Redmond C, Fisher ER, et al. Relative worth of estrogen or progesterone receptor and pathologic characteristics of differentiation as indicators of prognosis in node negative breast cancer patients: findings from National Surgical Adjuvant Breast and Bowel Project Protocol B-06. *J Clin Oncol* 1988;6:1076–1087.

316. McGuire WL, Tandon AK, Allred DC, et al. How to use prognostic factors in axillary node-negative breast cancer patients. *J Natl Cancer Inst* 1990;82:1006–1015.

317. Adami H-O, Graffman S, Lindgren A, et al. Prognostic implication of estrogen receptor content in breast cancer. *Breast Cancer Res Treat* 1985;5:293–300.

318. Costa SD, Lange S, Klinga K, et al. Factors influencing the prognostic role of estrogen and progesterone receptor levels in breast cancer—results of the analysis of 670 patients with 11 years of follow up. *Eur J Cancer* 2002;38:1329–1334.

319. Hilsenbeck SG, Ravdin PM, de Moor CA, et al. Time-dependence of hazard ratios for prognostic factors in primary breast cancer. *Breast Cancer Res Treat* 1998;52:227–237.

320. Schmitt M, Thomssen C, Ulm K, et al. Time-varying prognostic impact of tumour biological factors urokinase (uPA), PAI-1 and steroid hormone receptor status in primary breast cancer. *Br J Cancer* 1997,76.306 311.

321. Hess KR, Pusztai L, Buzdar AU, et al. Estrogen receptors and distinct patterns of breast cancer relapse. *Breast Cancer Res Treat* 2003;78:105–118.

322. Diab SG, Elledge RM, Clark GM. Tumor characteristics and clinical outcome of elderly women with breast cancer. *J Natl Cancer Inst* 2000;92:550–556.

323. Fisher ER, Osborne CK, McGuire WL, et al. Correlation of primary breast cancer histopathology and estrogen receptor content. *Breast Cancer Res Treat* 1981.1. 37–41.

324. Wenger CR, Beardslee S, Owens MA, et al. DNA ploidy, S-phase, and steroid receptors in more than 127,000 breast cancer patients. *Breast Cancer Res Treat* 1993;28:9–20.

325. Elledge RM, Fuqua SA, Clark GM, et al. Prognostic significance of p53 gene alterations in node-negative breast cancer. *Breast Cancer Res Treat* 1993;26:225–235.

326. Falette N, Paperin MP, Treilleux I, et al. Prognostic value of P53 gene mutations in a large series of node-negative breast cancer patients. *Cancer Res* 1998;58: 1451–1455.

327. Andrulis IL, Bull SB, Blackstein ME, et al. neu/erbB-2 amplification identifies a poor-prognosis group of women with node-negative breast cancer. Toronto Breast Cancer Study Group. *J Clin Oncol* 1998;16:1340–1349.

328. Tandon AK, Clark GM, Chamness GC, et al. HER-2/neu oncogene protein and prognosis in breast cancer. *J Clin Oncol* 1989;7:1120–1128.

329. Bolla M, Chedin M, Souvignet C, et al. Estimation of epidermal growth factor receptor in 177 breast cancers: correlation with prognostic factors. *Breast Cancer Res Treat* 1990;16:97–102.

330. Ferrero JM, Ramaioli A, Largillier R, et al. Epidermal growth factor receptor expression in 780 breast cancer patients: a reappraisal of the prognostic value based on an eight-year median follow-up. *Ann Oncol* 2001;12:841–846.

331. Lal P, Tan LK, Chen B. Correlation of HER-2 status with estrogen and progesterone receptors and histologic features in 3,655 invasive breast carcinomas. *Am J Clin Pathol* 2005;123:541–546.

332. Sorlie T, Perou CM, Tibshirani R, et al. Gene expression patterns of breast carcinomas distinguish tumor subclasses with clinical implications. *Proc Natl Acad Sci U S A* 2001;98:10869–10874.

333. Finetti P, Cervera N, Charafe-Jauffret E, et al. Sixteen-kinase gene expression identifies luminal breast cancers with poor prognosis. *Cancer Res* 2008;68: 767–776.

334. Chu KC, Anderson WF. Rates for breast cancer characteristics by estrogen and progesterone receptor status in the major racial/ethnic groups. *Breast Cancer Res* Treat 2002;74:199–211.

335. Elledge RM, Clark GM, Chamness GC, et al. Tumor biologic factors and breast cancer prognosis among white, Hispanic, and black women in the United States. *J Natl Cancer Inst* 1994;86:705–712.

336. Joslyn SA. Hormone receptors in breast cancer: racial differences in distribution and survival. *Breast Cancer Res Treat* 2002;73:45–59.

337. Muir D, Kanthan R, Kanthan SC. Male versus female breast cancers. A population-based comparative immunohistochemical analysis. *Arch Pathol Lab Med* 2003;127:36–41.

338. Ernst MF, Roukema JA, Coebergh JW, et al. Breast cancers found by screening: earlier detection, lower malignant potential or both? *Breast Cancer Res Treat* 2002;76:19–25.

339. Li CI, Daling JR, Malone KE. Incidence of invasive breast cancer by hormone receptor status from 1992 to 1998. *J Clin Oncol* 2003;21:28–34.

340. Pujol P, Hilsenbeck SG, Chamness GC, et al. Rising levels of estrogen receptor in breast cancer over 2 decades. *Cancer* 1994;74:1601–1606.

341. Ravdin PM, Cronin KA, Howlader N, et al. The decrease in breast-cancer incidence in 2003 in the United States. *N Engl J Med* 2007;356:1670–1674.

342. Koenders PG, Beex LV, Langens R, et al. Steroid hormone receptor activity of primary human breast cancer and pattern of first metastasis. The Breast Cancer Study Group. *Breast Cancer Res Treat* 1991;18:27–32.

343. Clark GM, McGuire WL, Hubay CA, et al. Progesterone receptors as a prognostic factor in Stage II breast cancer. *N Engl J Med* 1983;309:1343–1347.

344. Huseby RA, Ownby HE, Brooks S, et al. Evaluation of the predictive power of progesterone receptor levels in primary breast cancer: a comparison with other criteria in 559 cases with a mean follow-up of 74.8 months. The Breast Cancer Prognostic Study Associates. *Henry Ford Hospital Medical Journal* 1990;38:79–84.

345. Loi S, Haibe-Kains B, Desmedt C, et al. Definition of clinically distinct molecular subtypes in estrogen receptor-positive breast carcinomas through genomic grade. *J Clin Oncol* 2007;25:1239–1246.

346. Stierer M, Rosen H, Weber R, et al. A prospective analysis of immunohistochemically determined hormone receptors and nuclear features as predictors of early recurrence in primary breast cancer. *Breast Cancer Res Treat* 1995;36:11–21.

347. Creighton CJ, Osborne CK, van de Vijver MJ, et al. Molecular profiles of progesterone receptor loss in human breast tumors. *Breast Cancer Res Treat* 2008; 68:7493–5501.

Chapter 30

ERBB2 Testing: Assessment of Status for Targeted Therapies

Melinda Epstein, Yanling Ma, and Michael F. Press

In 2007 an estimated 178,480 women were diagnosed with breast carcinoma and approximately 40,460 women died from the disease (1). Breast cancer is the most frequently diagnosed cancer in women and ranks second among causes for cancer-related death in women. Although the ability to identify and diagnose breast cancer in women has improved markedly, the subsequent treatment and outcome for these patients has been variable. Until recently, treatment decisions for breast cancer patients have been based predominantly on the anatomic extent of the disease, with relatively little consideration of the underlying biological mechanisms responsible for the malignant behavior of breast cancer. As a result, patients with a similar extent of disease have been treated in a similar fashion with surgery, radiation therapy, and chemotherapy.

During the last two decades, however, breast and other cancers have been shown to result from molecular genetic alterations, either inherited or acquired. Many of these molecular genetic alterations have been identified and characterized and many are known to play important roles in the pathways associated with one or more of the following characteristics of cancer: self-sufficiency in growth signals, insensitivity to antigrowth signals, sustained angiogenesis, limitless replicative potential and tissue invasion and metastasis. All of these cellular characteristics are considered to be hallmarks of cancer cells (2). Cancer cells depend on these genetic alterations, thus providing a powerful potential for therapeutic intervention. Amplification of the human epidermal growth factor receptor type 2 (ERBB2, formerly HER2) gene in human breast cancers is one example of an acquired molecular alteration on which human breast cancer cells depend for maintenance of a fully malignant phenotype.

ERBB2 (also known as *neu* oncogene) amplification with resultant ERBB2 protein overexpression has been shown to play a role in sustaining multiple cancer pathways, including self-sufficiency in growth signals, sustained angiogenesis, increased cell division, and enhanced invasion (3–9). Inhibition of ERBB2 membrane signaling in these cancer cells through administration of humanized anti-ERBB2 antibodies (trastuzumab [Herceptin]) or administration of small molecule inhibitors of ERBB2 tyrosine kinase activity (lapatinib [Tykerb]) is associated with improved patient outcomes for women with both primary and metastatic disease (10–17). Because these improvements in outcome are only documented in women whose breast cancers have alterations in the ERBB2 gene or protein product, accurate clinical testing for ERBB2 amplification or overexpression has become an important clinical consideration. The importance of this issue is reflected by the fact that the American Society of Clinical Oncology (ASCO) recommends routine testing of only three predictive markers, estrogen receptor (ER), progesterone receptor (PR), and ERBB2 in women diagnosed with primary, invasive breast carcinomas.

ASSOCIATION OF ERBB2 AMPLIFICATION WITH ERBB2 OVEREXPRESSION

The ERBB2 gene encodes a 185 kDa monomeric protein also known as phosphoprotein 185 (p185^{ERBB2}). The ERBB2 protein is a receptor tyrosine kinase that is classified as a member of the epidermal growth factor receptor (EGFR) family of tyrosine kinases based on significant homology to EGFR (18–20). ERBB2 is a membrane protein expressed at low levels in all epithelial cells in normal fetal and adult tissues (21).

The ERBB2 gene is amplified, or increased in copy number, in approximately 25% of human breast cancers (22,23) as well as a variable percentage of ovarian (23), bladder, endometrial (24), salivary gland (25), and gastric cancers (26). ERBB2 gene amplification has been associated with pathologically increased levels of expression of ERBB2 messenger RNA (mRNA) and p185^{ERBB2} protein product (23). Although ERBB2 gene copy and expression level were originally found to be closely associated in 90% of frozen breast cancer specimens (23), subsequent work by the same investigators has demonstrated a near complete concordance between the ERBB2 amplification status and expression status in frozen tissue samples (27). The 10% of breast cancers that were originally discordant cases were predominantly stromal-rich breast cancers that were classified as nonamplified, overexpression breast cancers. ERBB2 gene amplification status had been originally determined by Southern hybridization in these stromal-rich breast cancers and dilution of tumor DNA by more abundant normal DNA resulted in Southern blots that failed to show ERBB2 gene amplification owing to the dilution of tumor DNA by the more abundant normal DNA. Reanalysis of these same cases by fluorescence *in situ* hybridization (FISH) permitted a nucleus-by-nucleus evaluation of the ERBB2 gene copy number and demonstrated ERBB2 gene amplification in the tumor cell nuclei of these cases that were previously considered not to be amplified (by Southern blot), but had overexpression by Northern hybridization, Western Immunoblot, and frozen section immunohistochemical assay (23). Therefore, one can conclude, when working with frozen tissue specimens, there is a close association between ERBB2 gene amplification status and overexpression status. That is, when the ERBB2 gene is not amplified, then the products of the gene are not increased and overexpression is not observed. Similarly, when ERBB2 gene is amplified, overexpression is consistently observed. Although this close association can be demonstrated in frozen tissue samples, tissue fixation and paraffin-embedding of these same specimens leads to difficulties in analysis of protein expression, especially by immunohistochemistry (23,28–30). This problem will be addressed subsequently in this chapter when we discuss clinical assay methods for assessment of ERBB2 status.

CLINICAL IMPORTANCE OF ERBB2 GENE AMPLIFICATION AND OVEREXPRESSION STATUS

ERBB2 gene amplification or overexpression is a prognostic marker of poor outcome in the absence of adjuvant treatment and an important predictive marker of responsiveness to certain treatments. The ERBB2 alteration has been associated with an increased rate of metastasis, decreased time to recurrence, and decreased overall survival (22,23,31). ERBB2 gene amplification was significantly associated with shorter disease-free survival and shorter overall survival in primary, invasive, node-negative breast cancer patients treated with surgery alone, without chemotherapy, without hormone therapy, and without radiation therapy in the adjuvant setting (32). ERBB2 is a prognostic marker independent of nodal status, tumor size, grade, and hormone receptor status (32).

As a predictive marker, ERBB2 amplification or overexpression has been correlated with responsiveness to anthracycline-based chemotherapy (33), paclitaxel-containing chemotherapy (34), and, most importantly, trastuzumab (Herceptin) and lapatinib (Tykerb) anti-ERBB2 targeted therapies. Currently, patients with ERBB2-positive tumors are treated with therapy directed against the ERBB2 protein. Both trastuzumab, a humanized antibody directed against the extracellular domain of the ERBB2 membrane protein, and lapatinib ditosylate, a dual tyrosine kinase inhibitor of EGFR and ERBB2, are currently approved by the U.S. Food and Drug Administration (FDA) for use in the treatment of ERBB2-positive breast cancers. Trastuzumab is approved for use in treatment of both metastatic and primary, invasive ERBB2-positive breast cancer. Lapatinib is approved for the treatment of ERBB2-positive metastatic breast cancer that is unresponsive to trastuzumab. Recently concluded clinical trials have shown lapatinib to be efficacious in the treatment of trastuzumab-naïve, ERBB2-positive, metastatic breast cancers (12). Clinical trials are in progress to evaluate its utility in primary breast cancer. Several other biological agents directed at ERBB2 or the ERBB2 pathway are currently in development.

Substantial preclinical and clinical evidence indicates that only breast cancers with ERBB2 amplification or overexpression respond to ERBB2-directed therapies, such as trastuzumab and lapatinib. This is especially true of trastuzumab. Monoclonal antibodies directed to the extracellular domain of ERBB2 inhibit the growth of ERBB2 overexpression, but not low ERBB2 expression, tumor cells (15,35–40). Anti-ERBB2 antibodies inhibit the growth of tumor xenografts and transformed cells that overexpress the ERBB2 receptor (35–37,41–43). However, these antibodies only inhibit the proliferation of human breast cancer cell lines that overexpress ERBB2 receptor (44,45). Similarly, clinical benefit from trastuzumab, the first humanized monoclonal antibody directed against ERBB2, is restricted to patients with ERBB2-positive breast cancer (14,46). Clinical trials have shown significantly improved clinical outcomes for women with ERBB2 amplified or overexpression breast cancers, but not for women with breast cancers lacking this alteration (11,14,17,30,47). Although lapatinib is a dual tyrosine kinase inhibitor, blocking both ERBB2 and epidermal growth factor receptor (EGFR or ERBB1) tyrosine kinase activity in model systems and cell lines, early findings show it is efficacious only in women with ERBB2 amplification or overexpression, not EGFR expressing, breast cancers (16). Inaccurate assessment of ERBB2 status can lead to the inappropriate treatment of breast cancer patients in both the adjuvant and metastatic settings and subject patients to unnecessary risk. Errors in testing can also lead to the erroneous conclusion that women with ERBB2-*negative* tumors respond to ERBB2-targeted therapy, whereas reanalysis of these same cancers confirms that errors in testing of approximately 10% of the breast cancers led to this mistaken conclusion (16). Cardiac toxicity is a serious concern in patients with early-stage disease who are treated with both trastuzumab and anthracycline-containing chemotherapy. For these reasons, accurate determination of ERBB2 alterations in breast carcinomas, if present, are of crucial importance. Because trastuzumab is only effective in patients with ERBB2-positive disease and that inaccurate assessment of ERBB2 status can lead to the inappropriate treatment of breast cancer patients, it is critical for clinical laboratory tests to distinguish accurately the women with ERBB2-positive breast cancers and women with breast cancers that do not express the therapeutic target.

DETECTION OF ERBB2 ALTERATIONS

In 1998, the humanized mouse 4D5 monoclonal antibody trastuzumab, directed against the human epidermal growth factor receptor type-2 (ERBB2) (38), was approved for the treatment of ERBB2-positive metastatic breast cancer. These patients had been selected for entry to the registrational clinical trials of trastuzumab with an immunohistochemical assay method, known as the *Clinical Trials Assay* (CTA) (11,17). The CTA used two different antibodies, 4D5 (the mouse monoclonal antibody used to produce humanized trastuzumab) and CB11 (a mouse monoclonal antibody). Antigen retrieval techniques were used for both antibodies in the CTA. However, because the CTA was not considered appropriate for commercialization, a second immunohistochemistry (IHC) assay method, the Dako HercepTest, was developed for commercial testing of ERBB2 status to select women for treatment with trastuzumab. This companion IHC assay method to assess ERBB2 membrane staining was approved by the FDA based on a 79% concordance rate (95% confidence interval [CI], 76%, 82%) between the immunostaining results of the CTA and the immunostaining results of the HercepTest for 548 breast cancer specimens from the National Cancer Institute Cooperative Breast Cancer Tissue Resource, a group of tumors that lacked clinical outcome information. Subsequently, a fluorescence *in situ* hybridization assay method was also approved by the FDA to identify women whose breast cancers had ERBB2 gene amplification for selection to trastuzumab therapy. This approval was based on a blinded, retrospective analysis of archival tissue sections from the breast cancers of women entered in the H0648 and H0650 registrational trials (11,14,17). Currently, two IHC assay methods (Dako's HercepTest, Ventana's Pathway) and three FISH assays (Abbott's PathVysion, Ventana's Inform, and Dako's PHarmDx) are approved by the FDA to select women for trastuzumab therapy. In addition, a silver enhanced *in situ* hybridization (SISH) assay has been approved in Europe.

Because ERBB2 gene amplification is directly correlated with ERBB2 expression levels at the mRNA and protein levels, determination of ERBB2 status could potentially be made at any of these levels and should correspond to the ERBB2 status determined with any of the other measures. Although this is approximated when frozen tissues are used, the use of formalin-fixed, paraffin-embedded tissues for these determinations introduces practical problems that result in some errors in ERBB2 characterization, especially when IHC is used to assess ERBB2 status. We will briefly review the various methods used to assess ERBB2 in breast cancer specimens, and then compare and contrast the results obtained with different methods of analysis, especially between IHC and FISH. A summary of these techniques is provided in Table 30.1.

CLINICAL ASSAYS FOR ASSESSMENT OF ERBB2 STATUS

Although ERBB2 status has been determined by using frozen tissue to assess the gene with extracted DNA, the transcript with extracted RNA, and the protein in tissue or cell lysates with determined ERBB2 status highly concordant among these assays in frozen tissues, the current clinical use of paraffin-embedded tissue restricts the type of ERBB2 analyses that can be performed to relatively few choices. These choices for formalin-fixed, paraffin-embedded tissues include FISH, CISH, and SISH to determine gene amplification status; quantitative real-time reverse transcriptase-polymerase chain reaction (RQ-PCR) analysis and microarray-based RNA expression profiles (RNA-EP) to determine ERBB2 mRNA expression status (48,49); and IHC to determine ERBB2 protein overexpression status. The most popular of these methods is IHC with approximately 85% to 90% of primary ERBB2 assessments being performed with it. The second most popular method for assessment is FISH with use of 10% to 15% of assays for ERBB2 status performed with this assay method, approximately equally divided between primary ERBB2 FISH testing and

| Table 30.1 | SUMMARY OF ASSAYS USED TO DETERMINE ERBB2 STATUS IN TISSUE SPECIMENS |

Parameter	ERBB2 Protein					ERBB2 Gene		
	Immunohistochemistry			FISH			CISH	SISH
Assay	CTA	HercepTest	Pathway	PathVysion	INFORM	PharmDx	SPoT-Light	EnzMet GenePro
Manufacturer	Home-brew Assay	Dako	Ventana	Abbott	Ventana	Dako	Invitrogen/Zymed	Ventana
Methodology	CB11 and 4D5 Monoclonal Antibodies	A085 Polyclonal Antibody	CB11 Monoclonal Antibody	Fluorescent ERBB2 and chromosome 17 centromere probes	Biotin labeled ERBB2 probe and fluorescently labeled avidin	Direct fluorescence probes for ERBB2 and chromosome 17 centromere copy number	Digoxigenin labeled ERBB2 DNA probe and detection via anti-digoxigenin antibody followed by antimouse peroxidase	Dinitro-Phenol ERBB2 Probe with detection by enzyme metallo-graphy
Status	Research Assay used in trastuzumab clinical trials	FDA-approved	FDA-approved	FDA-approved	FDA-approved	FDA-approved	Kit available in United States as Research Use Only	Kit available in United States as Research Use Only

CISH, chromogen *in situ* hybridization; CTA, clinical trial assay; FISH, fluorescence *in situ* hybridization; SISH, silver enhanced *in situ* hybridization.
Table modified from Wolff AC, Hammond ME, Schwartz JN, et al. American Society of Clinical Oncology/College of American Pathologists guideline recommendations for human epidermal growth factor receptor 2 testing in breast cancer. *Journal of Clinical Oncology.* 25(1):118–145, 2007, with permission.

"reflex" FISH testing after primary IHC testing yields an immuno-staining score of IHC 2+. Messenger RNA assays for ERBB2 status in the clinical setting are used almost exclusively by Genomic Health in their Oncotype DX assay. Because these analyses are performed only by Genomic Health, they will not be addressed further.

IMMUNOHISTOCHEMISTRY

Immunohistochemistry uses antibodies that recognize antigenic determinants of the full-length ERBB2 protein to assess indirectly and qualitatively the overall level of ERBB2 protein expression in paraffin-embedded tumor samples (Figs. 30.1 and 30.2). Overexpression of the ERBB2 protein by IHC is associated with a poor patient prognosis because of increased metastatic potential, and it is an independent predictor of disease-free and overall survival in patients with breast cancer containing this alteration (22,23,50–54).

The CTA (55) was the first clinical assay developed to select women for entry into the clinical trials investigating trastuzumab therapy in metastatic breast cancer patients (11,17) (Fig. 30.1). The HercepTest (Dako, Carpenteria, California) and the CB11 IHC assays (Pathway, Ventana Medical Systems, Tucson, Arizona), the two current IHC assays approved by the FDA for determination of ERBB2 status, were modeled on the CTA and were approved by the FDA through concordance studies. The HercepTest was approved by the FDA based on a direct comparison of the agreement rate, or concordance, with the CTA. As summarized above, the agreement rate between these assay methods was 79%. The Ventana Pathway assay uses one of the two antibodies used in the original CTA, the CB11 anti-ERBB2 antibody, as the detection antibody in this assay method. The Pathway IHC method was approved by the FDA based on a 92.4% concordance (95% CI 89.6%, 94.7%) with the HercepTest.

The HercepTest utilizes a rabbit anti-human ERBB2 polyclonal antibody to detect the ERBB2 protein, whereas the CB11 assay uses a murine antihuman monoclonal antibody. The scoring of immunostaining intensity for both of these assay methods is modeled after scoring in the original CTA. The microscopic appearance of the immunostained tumor cell membranes is subjectively graded by a pathologist on a scale of 0 to 3+ with 0 and 1+ considered low expression, 2+ considered indeterminate, and 3+ considered overexpression. To reduce the subjective variation in scoring by different pathologists, a series of cell line controls are used in parallel to provide a comparison with a negative control (0) (MDA-MB-231 cells), a slightly positive control (1+) (MDA-MB-175 cells), and a strongly positive control (3+) sample (SKBR3 cells) for Dako reagents. Alternately, a different set of cell lines is available for Ventana reagents, including a negative control (0) (MCF7 cells), a slightly positive control (1+) (T47D cells), a moderately positive control (2+) (MDA-MB-453), and a strongly positive control (3+) (BT474 cells). Previously, IHC2+ immunostaining was also considered to be overexpression, but these cases were found to have a highly variable proportion with ERBB2 gene amplification and it was decided by the College of American Pathologists (CAP) and, more recently, by a joint guideline from the ASCO and the CAP that these cases should be considered *indeterminate* and *reflexed* to FISH for evaluation of ERBB2 gene amplification to determine the status of the case (56,57). The original CTA and HercepTest scoring system required a minimum of 10% of tumor cells to be immunostained with a particular intensity for scoring at a particular level; however, the newer ASCO-CAP guidelines require the use of 30% as the proportion of tumor cells stained to achieve a particular staining level (56,57). No objective published data demonstrate the need for 10% as a suitable scoring minimum nor were objective data offered for a change from 10% to 30% as the minimum needed for assessment of a particular score such as IHC 3+. In fact, in frozen tissues nearly all of the tumor cells in a given breast cancer show the same level of immunostaining, either 1+, 2+, or 3+ (23,58). ERBB2 immunostain heterogeneity is observed almost exclusively in fixed, paraffin-embedded tissue

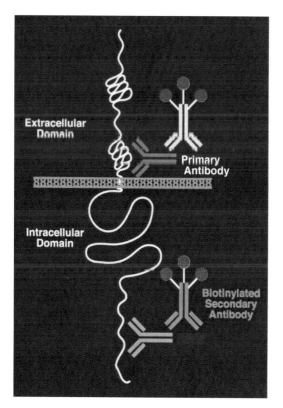

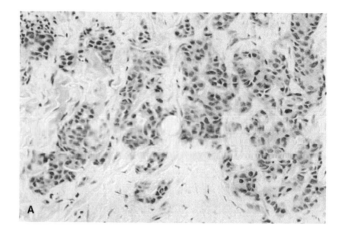

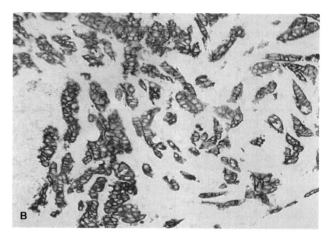

FIGURE 30.1. Schematic illustration of the Clinical Trials Assay (CTA) to assess ERBB2 expression by immunohistochemistry. In the CTA two different primary anti-ERBB2 monoclonal antibodies are used on sequential sections, not on the same section as illustrated in this schematic drawing. One of the primary anti-ERBB2 antibodies, 4D5, is the mouse monoclonal antibody that was humanized to synthesize trastuzumab. This antibody (*blue*) recognizes an extracellular domain of the ERBB2 protein. The other antibody, CB11 (*green*), recognizes an intracellular domain of the ERBB2 protein. These antibodies are each identified by biotinylated secondary antimouse IgG antibodies (*yellow and purple*) decorated with horseradish peroxidase (*red*). The site of ERBB2 is recognized by light microscopic identification of a diaminobenzidine reaction product deposited by the action of horseradish peroxidase. (Courtesy of Allison Bruce and Genentech)

samples (23,58). Nevertheless, both the HercepTest and Pathway assays have been shown to be approximately 90% accurate at assigning the known, molecularly determined status of breast cancer specimens (29).

The use of IHC to determine ERBB2 status is appealing for several reasons (Table 30.2). ERBB2 IHC tests are simple, rapid, relatively inexpensive and are easily accommodated by existing surgical pathology laboratory practices. In addition, pathologists have an established familiarity with the IHC technique and reagents. However, application of IHC to assess ERBB2 status is problematic for a number of reasons (Table 30.2). The clinical assays are performed on fixed, paraffin-embedded (FPE) tissues and ERBB2 IHC analyses of this type of material is associated with several problems (23,28, 29,58,59). Tissue handling, fixation, and processing can greatly affect immunoreactivity of tissue antigens (28,60,61). It has been proposed that loss of the ERBB2 antigen may occur in up to 20% of ERBB2-positive samples owing to formalin fixation or storage of unstained sections before use for IHC (61). ERBB2 positivity by IHC in FFPE tissues is dependant on the ERBB2 antibody used for the protocol (28). Some antibodies have been found to correctly detect only 25% or fewer of the known highly (more than fivefold) ERBB2 amplified or overexpressed breast cancers, whereas two are able to detect more than 95% of the known highly amplified or overexpressed breast cancers as overexpressed in paraffin-embedded tissue samples (29). In another study, 95% of the tumors examined were ERBB2-positive using the CB11 test but only 84% of these same tumor samples were ERBB2-positive using the HercepTest (62).

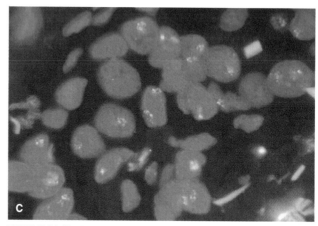

FIGURE 30.2. Infiltrating ductal carcinoma breast cancer with ERBB2 gene amplification and overexpression. A formalin-fixed, paraffin-embedded breast cancer is characterized (**A**) for histopathology by hematoxylin-and-eosin staining, (**B**) for ERBB2 protein overexpression by immunohistochemistry (IHC 3+), and (**C**) for ERBB2 gene amplification by FISH.

Interpretation of IHC is inherently subjective and qualitative. This leads to observer variability and affects the accuracy of results using the IHC technique (63). Considerable evidence now indicates that IHC performance is poorly controlled "in the real world" (56,57,59, 64–66). The ASCO-CAP guidelines draw attention to this with the alarming claim that "20% of ERBB2 assays performed in the field were incorrect" (56,57). The United Kingdom National External Quality Assurance Scheme (UK-NEQAS, see http://www.ukneqasicc.ucl.ac.uk/neqasicc.shtml) documents performance of diagnostic laboratories within the United Kingdom and across Europe and Asia and includes participants from the United States. Data from this scheme shows a

Table 30.2	ADVANTAGES AND DISADVANTAGES OF ERBB2 TESTING METHODS				
	ERBB2 Testing Methods				
	Immunohistochemistry (IHC)	Fluorescence *In Situ* Hybridization (FISH)	Chromogenic *In Situ* Hybridization (CISH)	Silver Enhanced *In Situ* Hybridization (SISH)	Enzyme Linked Immunosorbent Assay (ELISA)
Advantages	• Simple and rapid protocol • Relatively inexpensive • Easily accommodated by existing surgical pathology laboratories • Established familiarity with technique and reagents	• DNA relatively insensitive to tissue handling or variation in fixative type or fixation time • Quantitative scoring • Gene copy number can be individually assessed • Increased accuracy in determination of ERBB2 status relative to IHC	• Subtractive probes reduce nonspecific hybridization caused by repetitive DNA sequences • Staining is permanent and does not decay, allowing tissue to be archived • Signal assessed with light microscope • Permits concurrent analysis of tissue morphology	• Highly sensitive • No amplification stage so fewer reagents required relative to FISH and CISH • Staining is permanent and does not decay, allowing tissue to be archived • Quantitative scoring • Signal assessed with light microscope	• Only technique FDA approved to measure soluble ERBB2 extracellular domain (ECD) in patient serum or plasma • Real-time determination of ERBB2 status • Quantitative
Disadvantages	• Only 90% accurate • Restricted to FFPE tissue • Results influenced by immunoreactivity, which is altered by tissue handling, fixation, and processing • Accuracy dependent on ERBB2 antibody utilized • Interpretation is subjective and qualitative • Pathologic expertise required	• Two-day protocol • Signal fades with storage • Specialized equipment (i.e., fluorescence microscope, dark room) • Increased reagent expense relative to IHC • Pathologic expertise to distinguish benign and malignant nuclei	• Increased time and reagent expense relative to IHC • Pathologic expertise required • Gene copy number cannot be individually assessed, therefore qualitative assessment	• Increased time and reagent expense relative to IHC • Pathologic expertise required	• Source of ERBB2 ECD remains unknown • Lack of direct correlation between tumor burden and ERBB2 ECD level

FFPE, formalin-fixed, paraffin-embedded.

marked difference between the levels of acceptable performance for IHC-based assays. Remarkably, only between 57% and 65% of participants using the Dako HercepTest demonstrated acceptable performance (J. Bartlett personal communication). Although computerized image analysis could reduce the subjective nature of the pathologist scoring, it cannot address the preanalytic variability owing to tissue fixation and processing. Despite these issues, IHC remains the favored technique to determine the ERBB2 status of patients in the majority of laboratories.

 ## *IN SITU* HYBRIDIZATION

A variety of *in situ* hybridization (ISH) techniques, such as FISH, CISH, and SISH have been used to determine ERBB2 gene amplification status in paraffin-embedded tissue sections (32,67–69) (Figs. 30.2–30.4).

ERBB2 Gene Amplification by Fluorescence *In Situ* Hybridization

Fluorescence *in situ* hybridization is the second most frequently used technique for determination of the ERBB2 status. As described above, a strong correlation exists between ERBB2 protein overexpression and ERBB2 gene amplification. Similar to ERBB2 overexpression, amplification of the ERBB2 gene is associated with unfavorable tumor characteristics, such as high nuclear grade and decreased expression of the estrogen and progesterone receptors, and decreased overall and disease-free survival (22,23,70,71).

Currently three FISH tests have been approved by the FDA for selecting patients for treatment with the humanized monoclonal antibody trastuzumab: the PathVysion test (Abbott-Vysis Inc.,

Downers Grove, Illinois) (29,59), the PharmDx FISH test (Dako) (72,73), and the INFORM test (Ventana Medical Systems) (29). The PathVysion and PharmDx tests are dual-probe assays, utilizing both a fluorescent tag-labeled DNA probe specific for the ERBB2 gene and a fluorescent tag-labeled chromosome 17 centromere-specific enumeration probe (CEP) (29,59,72). These probes are hybridized to tissue sections under high stringency conditions (Fig. 30.3) and ERBB2 gene amplification status is assessed by enumeration of ERBB2 gene copy signals and chomosome 17 centromere signals. When the ratio of ERBB2 gene copies to chromosome 17 centromere copies is greater than or equal to 2.0, ERBB2 is considered amplified, whereas those with ratios less than 2 are considered nonamplified (16,32, 56–58). Although a FISH ratio of 2.0 was recommended by the manufacturers and the FDA as the cutoff value for ERBB2 amplification, the recent ASCO-CAP guidelines recommend and CAP now requires accredited laboratories to use 2.2 as the cutoff for amplification and consider FISH ratios between 1.8 and 2.2 to be *indeterminate*. Although the original FISH ratio of 2.0 correlates well with overexpression and has been supported by a number of studies of ERBB2 gene amplification as a prognostic marker (23,32,74) and a predictive marker of responsiveness to trastuzumab (14,46,47) and lapatinib (10,12,16), the ASCO-CAP guidelines committee offered no objective data for this change in cutoff ratio (56,57). Fortunately, only approximately 2% of unselected breast cancers have FISH ratios in this indeterminate region (58,59). Alternatively, the INFORM test utilizes an automated system and a single fluorescent tag-labeled DNA probe specific for the ERBB2 gene (72,73). As defined by the manufacturer and recommended by the FDA, a tumor sample with more than 4 signals per nucleus is considered ERBB2 amplified and the use of this average ERBB2 signal number is supported by published studies (32). In contrast, the ASCO-CAP guidelines recommend and CAP requires accredited laboratories to use 6.0 ERBB2

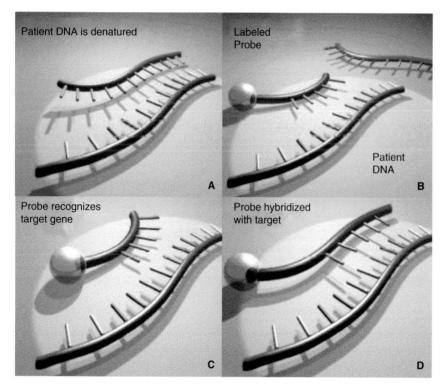

FIGURE 30.3. Schematic illustration of the fluorescence *in situ* hybridization (FISH) technique. Characterization of ERBB2 gene copy number involves a series of steps. Initially, the DNA-associated proteins are removed before probe hybridization with proteinase digestion of all proteins. Subsequently, the double-stranded DNA of the breast cancer is denatured by heating to separate the DNA strands (**A**). A DNA probe encoding the ERBB2 sequence and directly labeled with a fluorescent tag is incubated with the tissue section (**B**) under high-stringency conditions so the ERBB2 probe binds specifically to the genomic ERBB2 sequence (**C**) and remains bound to this site following high stringency washes to permit enumeration of the number of ERBB2 gene copies in each nucleus. (From Hicks D, Tubbs R. Assessment of the ERBB2 status in breast cancer by fluorescence *in situ* hybridization: a technical review with interpretive guidelines *Hum Pathol* 2005;36:250–261, with permission.).

copies per tumor cell nucleus as the minimum required for gene amplification with average ERBB2 copy numbers of 4.0 to 6.0 per tumor cell nucleus to be considered indeterminate (56,57), again without data to support a need for this change.

Both disadvantages and advantages exist with FISH (Table 30.2). The method requires 2 days to perform rather than 1 day as required by IHC. FISH requires a fluorescence microscope, is interpreted in a dark-room by a pathologist, and fluorescent signals fade on storage over a period of weeks to months. Because of the increased time as well as the use of more expensive reagents, FISH is more expensive than IHC. A disadvantage is that some high-volume laboratories use med-

ical technicians, not pathologists, to interpret the signals in tumor cells leading to some errors in scoring (16), probably related to the technician's inability to distinguish tumor cell nuclei from nuclei of benign reactive cells in some biopsies. An advantage of FISH is that DNA is more stable than protein and, therefore, is relatively insensitive to tissue handling or variations in fixative type or fixation time (75). Indeed, most hybridization failures encountered while performing FISH because of tissue fixation can be remedied by altering the amount of time that samples are exposed to protease digestion solution during the prehybridization phase of the analysis. This relative stability of DNA in FFPE tissues is probably responsi-

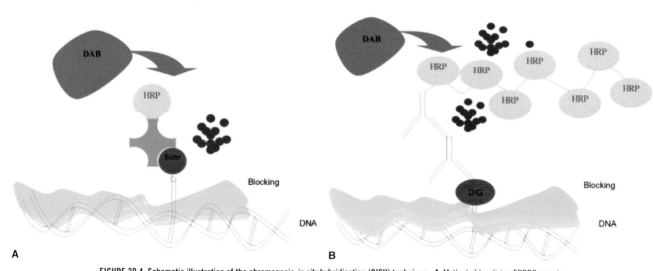

FIGURE 30.4. Schematic illustration of the chromogenic *in situ* hybridization (CISH) technique. A: Method of localizing ERBB2 gene in tissue sections involves the use of a biotin-labeled ERBB2 DNA probe to hybridize specifically with denatured genomic ERBB2 genetic sequence. The biotin of the hybridized probe is secondarily recognized by horseradish peroxidase (HRP)-labeled avidin. Finally, polymerization of diaminobenzidine (DAB) is catalyzed by HRP to produce a brown precipitate that is microscopically visualized. **B:** Alternatively, a digoxigen-labeled ERBB2 DNA probe is hybridized with genomic ERBB2 sequence. The digoxigen label is bound by an anti-dig mouse monoclonal antibody which is, subsequently, recognized by a secondary antimouse IgG rabbit or goat antibody labeled with HRP. The site of this secondary antibody is identified by reaction with DAB to produce a brown precipitate that is identified microscopically. (From Lambros MB, Natrajan R, Reis-Filho JS. Chromogenic and fluorescent in situ hybridization in breast cancer. *Hum Pathol* 2007;38:1105–1122, with permission.)

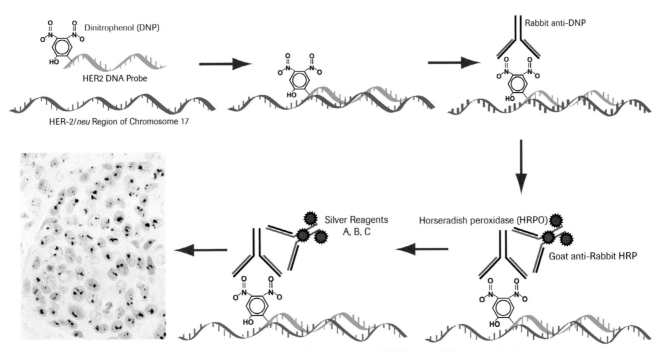

FFIGURE 30.5. Schematic illustration of the silver enhanced *in situ* hybridization (SISH) technique. SISH is accomplished through horse-radish peroxidase catalysis of silver ions to metallic silver leading to the deposition of metal nanoparticles at the site of a target gene hybridized to a DNA probe. SISH detection works as follows: A dinitrophenol (DNP)-labeled probe (**upper left**), either ERBB2-specific or chromosome 17 centromere-specific, binds to the genomic DNA target (**upper center**). A monoclonal rabbit anti-DNP linker antibody binds to the DNP hapten (**upper right**). The site of this primary antibody is recognized by a second antibody, a goat antirabbit antibody that is labeled with a horseradish peroxidase-labeled (HRP) multimer (**lower right**). Silver reagents are added to the tissue section, resulting in the deposition of metal nanoparticles at the site of the HRP (**lower center**), which allow visualization of the *in situ* hybridization signal (**lower left**). (Reproduced with permission from Ventana Medical Systems, Tucson, Arizona.)

ble for the increased accuracy of the FISH method relative to IHC (58,59,76). A second advantage of FISH is that results are quantitative and, therefore, interpretation is less subjective. Variability rates between independent observers using FISH is significantly better than IHC (77–80).

ERBB2 Gene Amplification by Chromogenic *In Situ* Hybridization

A modified *in situ* hybridation technique, chromogenic *in situ* hybridization was developed in 2000 by Tanner et al. and confirmed in multiple laboratories (67,81–85). CISH uses a digoxigenin (DIG)-labeled DNA probe corresponding to the ERBB2 sequence to localize the ERBB2 gene in the nuclei of cells (Fig. 30.4). The DIG CISH probe is hybridized to a tissue section and detected using a fluorescein (FITC)-conjugated anti-DIG antibody followed by a horseradish peroxidase (HRP)-conjugated anti-FITC antibody. The tissue is then treated with diaminobenzidine (DAB), an HRP substrate, staining the region where the probe is bound (85,86). The brown DAB reaction product labels the site of ERBB2 gene copies that can then be assessed using a standard light microscope. In a second indirect method, the CISH probe is labeled with biotin and hybridized with the tissue section (Fig. 30.4). The tissue is then treated with HRP conjugated avidin and detected with DAB as in the first method described (86). Regardless of which indirect method is utilized, traditional CISH is a single color assay and an additional slide must be used to determine centromere copy number using a chromosome 17 centromeric probe (86). In addition, CISH does not, in general, permit assessment of the number of ERBB2 gene copies present in amplified breast cancers because a single large aggregate of reaction product is deposited in the tumor cell nuclei when substantial increased copy number is present.

Numerous studies have indicated a good concordance between CISH and FISH with regard to *amplified* versus *not amplified* results in paraffin-embedded breast carcinomas.

Hanna and Kwok (87) examined ERBB2 amplification levels by both FISH and CISH and correlated these results with IHC scores. In IHC-negative patients, the concordance rate between FISH and CISH was 97%. In IHC-positive patients (3+) the concordance rate was 98%. For patients with 2+ IHC score the concordance rate between FISH and CISH remained high at 93% (87). Similar concordance rates have been reported by other laboratories (81–83,85,88–91).

There are several advantages to the CISH technique compared with FISH (Table 30.2). First, CISH probes are generated using subtractive probe technology (85). Using this technology, repetitive DNA sequences that can cause nonspecific hybridization are removed. Therefore, the final probes are very specific and do not require any blocking of nonspecific hybridization with Cot-1 DNA as in traditional FISH assays (85). Second, because the CISH method uses chromogens instead of fluorochromes to label probes, tissue staining is permanent, signals are nonbleaching, and they do not decay over time (86). This allows samples to be archived indefinitely. Third, with the CISH technique gene-copy signals can be assessed using a standard light microscope, removing the need for a fluorescence microscope, in turn decreasing the cost of the assay (86). Finally, because a light microscope is used to analyze CISH results, CISH permits concurrent analysis of tissue morphology. However, CISH has the disadvantage, described above, that the number of ERBB2 gene copies cannot be individually enumerated in breast cancers with ERBB2 gene amplification because the DAB reaction product results in a large, brown aggregate of reaction product deposited in tumor cell nuclei rather than individual discrete signals that can be counted.

ERBB2 Gene Amplification by Silver Enhanced *In Situ* Hybridization

Silver enhanced *in situ* hybridization (SISH) is an additional modified *in situ* hybridization technique used to detect gene amplification (Fig 30.5). Instead of being based directly on the traditional FISH technique, SISH is based on an autometallographic procedure called gold facilitated autometallographic *in situ* hybridization (GOLDFISH) first described by Tubbs et al. (6) in 2002 and Hainfeld et al. in 2000 (92). Briefly, in GOLDFISH a biotin-labeled probe is hybridized to a tissue section. A catalyzed reporter deposition/tyramide signal amplification (CARD/TSA) reaction is then used to amplify the probe signal (93). The sensitivity of the CARD/TSA technique was first demonstrated by Zehbe et al. (93) who utilized the method to detect single copies of the human papillomavirus (HPV) in cell lines. The tissue is finally treated with nanogold particles covalently linked to streptavidin and incubated with GoldEnhance particles that are deposited onto the nanogold particles, making the signal visible by light microscopy (92,94).

Silver enhanced *in situ* hybridization also relies on the action of the peroxidase enzyme linked to a metal to deposit metallic particles at the site of a probe. SISH differs from GOLDFISH in several ways. First, SISH utilizes silver particles instead of gold. Second, the silver particles in SISH are not placed around a metallic core, such as Nanogold, but are deposited as a result of direct action of peroxidase on a substrate linked to the metal. Third, SISH does not contain an amplification step in the procedure, such as the CARD/TSA reaction.

Several advantages exist to the SISH technique (Table 30.2). SISH is a sensitive method for detecting gene amplification (68). SISH does not require CARD/TSA amplification. Thus, fewer reagents are required for SISH than for FISH or CISH. Finally, similar to CISH, because no flurochromes are used to label SISH probes, resulting signals are permanent, not light sensitive, do not decay over time, and may be read using a standard light microscope.

Enzyme-linked Immunosorbent Assay for Assessment of ERBB2 Extracellular Domain in Serum or Plasma

In contrast to IHC, FISH, and alternative FISH techniques, this next technique to determine a patient's ERBB2 status is not performed directly on the tumor tissue but on the patient's serum or plasma. Since 1991, both manual and automated enzyme linked immunosorbent assays (ELISA) have been used to measure the amount of soluble ERBB2 protein extracellular domain (ECD) that is cleaved from cells and shed into patient serum (95) or plasma (96). Because a strong correlation exists between manual and automated results (97–100), both types of assays have been approved by the FDA to manage and monitor women diagnosed with metastatic breast cancer (100).

ERBB2 ECD can be detected in the plasma of healthy women and ECD levels increase in women diagnosed with both primary and metastatic breast cancer (95,96,101). High concentrations of shed ERBB2 ECD in serum correlate with ERBB2 overexpression (102), increased tumor size (103), higher relapse rates, and poor clinical response to hormone therapy and chemotherapy in patients with metastatic breast cancer (104–106). High ERBB2 ECD levels are also associated with sensitivity to therapy with trastuzumab (107).

The ERBB2 ECD test has been suggested as an alternative method to determine a patient's ERBB2 status. This testing method is the only protocol that allows for real-time determination of ERBB2 status and is currently the only way to monitor changes in ERBB2 levels after surgery (100). However, ERBB2 ECD tests are not established as useful in the diagnosis of ERBB2-positive breast cancer or in predicting responsiveness to therapies and disease outcome. The results of this test are quantitative and, because the FDA established a cutoff of 15 µg/L, not open to subjective interpretation (100). Unlike IHC and FISH, it is impossible to determine the source of the ERBB2 protein fragment when utilizing this method. Thus,

high baseline levels of ERBB2 ECD may not be caused by the direct shedding of the ERBB2 ECD by tumor, but may be attributed to individual variations in receptor density, tumor burden, the rate of ECD cleavage and release into circulation, and the subsequent degradation of the protein fragment (62,104). In addition, only moderate concordance (87.1%) is found between serum ERBB2 ECD levels and tissue ERBB2 levels as measured by IHC and FISH (107,108). Fornier et al. (62) not only observed elevated ERBB2 ECD levels in breast cancer patients with ERBB2-positive disease but also among patients with tumors that did not show ERBB2 overexpression or gene amplification. The ERBB2 ECD ELISA assay is useful for monitoring recurrent disease among women with established ERBB2-positive breast cancers.

COMPARISON OF TESTS FOR ASSESSMENT OF ERBB2 STATUS

Accurate determination of ERBB2 status is critical in the selection of adjuvant and neoadjuvant therapy for women diagnosed with invasive breast carcinoma as well as women with metastatic disease. Only patients with tumors that overexpress ERBB2 or exhibit gene amplification are candidates for treatment with targeted therapies directed against the ERBB2 protein. In patients diagnosed with metastatic breast cancer, clinical benefit from trastuzumab is restricted to ERBB2-positive tumors as demonstrated by FISH (14). Patients whose breast cancers have gene amplification by FISH but lack overexpression by IHC (IHC ≤2+), the IHC false–negative cases, show a clinical benefit from the addition of ERBB2-targeted therapies to chemotherapy (14,16). In contrast, those patients with breast cancers lacking ERBB2 gene amplification by FISH but having IHC 3+ immunostaining, the IHC false–positive cases, show no significant incremental benefit of ERBB2-targeted therapies beyond that of chemotherapy alone (16). Therefore, differences in the laboratory methods used to assess ERBB2 status are potentially important. These differences and similarities in ERBB2 status by FISH and IHC, the concordance rate, for determination of ERBB2 status are discussed in this section.

As stated previously, assessment of frozen tissue samples shows a direct relationship between ERBB2 gene amplification and ERBB2 protein overexpression. When the ERBB2 gene is amplified, there is consistent concordant overexpression of the receptor. In contrast, when the ERBB2 gene is not amplified, no increase in receptor expression is observed in frozen tissue samples or in breast cancer cell lines. The association between ERBB2 gene amplification and protein overexpression has been clearly demonstrated in frozen tissue samples using both IHC and FISH assays. In fixed paraffin-embedded tissue samples, however, equivalent results have only been consistently observed when utilizing FISH. Indeed, the fixation and embedding processes often lead to difficulties and inconsistencies in determining ERBB2 status, especially when utilizing IHC (23,28–30). This preanalytical variability owing to tissue fixation and processing in addition to the observer variability and subjective interpretation of IHC often leads to discordance between IHC and FISH (56,57,63). Because most tissue used to determine ERBB2 status has been fixed and embedded, this discordance impacts the selection of patients for targeted therapy.

Trastuzumab is a humanized monoclonal antibody that binds with high affinity to the ECD of the ERBB2 receptor. This biologic agent is designed to target cells dependent on ERBB2 signaling. Trastuzumab is effective only in breast cancers that overexpress ERBB2 and depend on activation of this pathway for their growth (17,47). Likewise, lapatinib, a small molecule, dual kinase inhibitor of both the epidermal growth factor receptor (ERBB1) and ERBB2, is only effective in patients diagnosed

Table 30.3 FREQUENCY OF ERBB2 GENE AMPLIFICATION (%) IN EACH IHC IMMUNOSTAINING CATEGORY (0, 1+, 2+ AND 3+) BY STUDY[a]

ERBB2 Gene Amplification Rate According to IHC Score[b]

0	1+	2+	3+	Number In Study[c]	IHC Method	Study Citation
0%	0%	17%	89%	100	Dako HercepTest	Hoang et al., *Am J Clin Pathol* 2000;113(6):852.
1.8%[e]		35.9%	100%	750	Dako Ab Unspecified	Ridolfi et al., *Mod Pathol* 2000;13(8):866.
3.5%	66.2%	97.1%	99%	2857	Dako HercepTest	Simon et al., *J Natl Cancer Inst* 2001;93(15):1141.
0%	2.2%	38.2%	91.4%	189	Dako A0485 Ab	Wang et al., *Am J Clin Pathol* 2001;116(4):495.
0%	5.7%	18.2%	100%	170	Homebrew Ab	Kobayashi et al., *Hum Pathol* 2002;33(1):21.
3.8%	8.5%	42.2%	100%	198	Dako HercepTest	McCormick et al., *Am J Clin Pathol* 2002;117(6):935.
3%	7%	24%	89%	1,575	Clinical Trials Assay	Perez et al., *Mayo Clin Proc* 2002;77(2):148.
0%	0%	0%	89.8%	119	Dako HercepTest	Roche et al., *J Natl Cancer Inst* 2002;94(11):855.
0.7%[e]		48.1%	94.1%	426	Dako HercepTest	Dowsett et al., *J Pathol* 2003;199(4):418.
4.2%[e]		6.1%	49%	102	Dako HercepTest	Hammock et al., *Hum Pathol* 2003;34(10):1043.
1.1%	3.1%	26.5%	89.7%	2,279	Dako HercepTest	Lal et al., *Am J Clin Pathol* 2004;121(5):631.
0%[e]		20%	90%	360	Dako HercepTest	Mrozkowiak et al., *Pol J Pathol* 2004;55(4):165.
0%[e]		15%	79%	600	Dako HercepTest	Varshney et al., *Am J Clin Pathol* 2004;121(1):70.
2.8%[e]		17%	91.6%	2,913	Dako A0485 Ab	Yaziji et al., *JAMA* 2004;291(16):1972.
3%	7%	24%	89%	529	Clinical Trials Assay	Dybdal et al., *Breast Cancer Res Treat* 1005;93:3–11.
6.9%[e]		31.8%	90%	114	Dako HercepTest	Ellis et al., *J Clin Pathol* 2005;58(7):710.
2.4%[e]		72%	100%	215	Dako HercepTest	Lottner et al., *J Pathol* 2005;205(5):577.
3.6%	6.1%	16.7%	78.1%	2249	Dako HercepTest and Ventana Pathway Assay	Press et al., *Clin Cancer Res* 2005;11(18):6598.
12.5%	6.7%	7%	52.4%	108	Dako HercepTest	Ciampa et al., *Appl Immunohistochem Mol Morphol* 2006;14(2):132.
0%	0%	12.2%	91.6%	289	Dako HercepTest	Hofmann et al., *J Clin Pathol* 2008;61(1):89.
2.7%	21.4%	36.1%	90.1%	**Weighted Average Percentage[d]**		
8.7%[e]		36.1%	90.1%	**16,142 Weighted Average Percentage[e]**		

Ab, antibody; IHC, immunohistochemistry.

[a]Inclusion in this tabular summary required a comparison of IHC scores to FISH status in at least 100 cases per study.

[b]The percentage of FISH-positive (ERBB2 gene amplified) cases within each IHC immunohistochemical category (0, 1+, 2+, 3+) is indicated.

[c]The total number of patients included in each study.

[d]The average percentage of patients in the 0/1+, 2+, and 3+ subcolumns is weighted for study number.

[e]Some studies reported low expression as pooled 0/1+ rather than separately as 0 and 1+.

with ERBB2-positive breast cancers (10,12,13,16). Although simultaneous targeting of ERBB1 and ERBB2 by lapatinib in model systems does result in a greater inhibition of cell growth compared with targeting either ERBB1 or ERBB2 independently (109,110), differential patient responsiveness to lapatinib is observed only in breast cancer patients whose tumors have ERBB2 amplification or overexpression (16). Expression of EGFR in the breast cancer tissue is not associated with lapatinib responsiveness (16). To determine if a patient is a candidate for treatment with these ERBB2 targeting drugs, it is critical to determine a patient's ERBB2 status accurately. Thus, the method utilized to determine ERBB2 status is important.

The discordance between the results of IHC and FISH assays for ERBB2 has been demonstrated in numerous published studies (Table 30.3). In these studies, patients with an IHC score of 0 or 1+ are considered to be ERBB2-negative, whereas those with a score of 3+ are interpreted as ERBB2-positive. Patients with an IHC score of 2+ are considered inconclusive or equivocal and are *reflexed* to FISH for assessment of gene amplification (56,57). The greatest discordance between IHC and FISH is observed in patients whose breast cancers are considered equivocal (Table 30.3). Large variations in ERBB2 amplification rates have been reported for patients in this group (Table 30.3). Indeed, ERBB2 gene amplification rates in the IHC 2+ group vary from 0% to 97%, although most report amplification rates between 15% and 50% (Table 30.3) (56,57,66,111). Because of the large variation in ERBB2 amplification rates reported for patients with inconclusive IHC results, the ASCO and CAP currently recommend that all patients with inconclusive ERBB2 IHC results (IHC 2+) undergo reflex re-evaluation with FISH for final determination of ERBB2 status before adjuvant therapy (56). The discordance in ERBB2 status as determined by FISH and IHC is not limited to the IHC 2+ group, although discordance in the 0, 1+, and 3+ IHC categories is more limited.

The percentages in the 0 and 1+ IHC categories shown in Table 30.3 represent the proportion of patients that is ERBB2-negative by IHC but ERBB2-amplified by FISH. Although an average of fewer than 10% of patients in the IHC 0 and 1+ categories exhibit amplification of the ERBB2 gene, this represents a significant proportion of patients with the ERBB2 alteration of gene amplification. Indeed, because the ERBB2 gene is amplified and overexpressed in only approximately 20% to 25% of human breast carcinomas (22,23), the 0 and 1+ IHC categories (ERBB2-negative) contain the most patients. Having as few as 4% of IHC 0/1+ patients with ERBB2 amplification still represents approximately 1 of every 10 women whose breast cancers have this alteration. The percentage of ERBB2 amplified breast cancers that has IHC 0 or 1+ immunostaining in FFPE samples ranges from approximately 3% to approximately 21%, depending on the study.

Those patients with ERBB2-negative breast carcinomas by IHC, but with ERBB2 amplication as determined by FISH, have tumors with biological phenotypes similar to other patients with ERBB2-amplified breast tumors. All women whose breast cancers have ERBB2 gene amplification, without exception in frozen tissue, have ERBB2 overexpression and this overexpression can be obscured by tissue fixation and processing as assessed by IHC staining in a variable proportion of these breast cancers (23). These false–negative IHC assessments, therefore, represent significant diagnostic problems especially because these women respond to ERBB2-targeted therapies (16).

Findings from the National Surgical Adjuvant Breast and Bowel Project (NSABP) B-31 (112), North Central Cancer Treatment Group (NCCTG) N9831 (112), and the European Breast International Group (BIG) Herceptin Adjuvant (HERA) (113) prospective randomized trials have shown trastuzumab to be efficacious in the adjuvant treatment of primary ERBB2-positive breast cancers. Similarly, the efficacy of lapatinib is restricted to ERBB2-positive patients (10,12,13,16). All patients enrolled in the EGF2002, EGF2008, and EGF103009 studies that responded to lapatinib therapy were ERBB2-positive (114,115). Women within the IHC 0 or 1+ groups with ERBB2-amplified tumors were excluded from all of these trials, since access to ERBB2 targeted therapies was based only on IHC ERBB2 test results (30). In these cases, the discordance between ERBB2 amplification and ERBB2 overexpression, as determined by FISH and IHC, respectively, results in denial of targeted therapy for patients with ERBB2-positive tumors that have been shown to respond to treatment (16).

In contrast, the percentage of ERBB2 not amplified or FISH-negative cases in the IHC 3+ category (Table 30.3) represents patients with strong immunostaining (IHC 3+) for the ERBB2 protein as shown by IHC in FFPE tissue, that lack amplification of the ERBB2 gene. The overall amplification rates for patients in the IHC 3+ group range from 49% to 100%, although most published amplification rates are above 85% with an average of 90% showing ERBB2 gene amplification (Table 30.3). Using an antibody that does not require antigen retrieval for IHC, most of these IHC3+, FISH-negative breast cancers have been shown to be IHC false–positive results (59). As shown in Table 30.3, these IHC3+/FISH-negative breast cancers represent approximately 10% of all IHC3+ cases. This false–positive rate is important because only women with ERBB2-amplified tumors respond to the ERBB2-targeted therapies, trastuzumab and lapatinib (14,16). Indeed, as shown by Mass et al. (14), clinical benefit from trastuzumab therapy in patients diagnosed with metastatic breast cancer is restricted to ERBB2 FISH-positive patients. Furthermore, inaccurate assessment of ERBB2 status can lead to the inap-

propriate treatment of breast cancer patients with trastuzumab, both in the adjuvant and metastatic settings and subject patients to unnecessary risk. Retrospective evaluation of outcome in the pivotal clinical trials of trastuzumab in women with metastatic breast cancer have shown that these IHC false–positive cases have an approximately 3% (or less) chance of responding to trastuzumab (14) and a similarly low probability of responding to lapatinib (16). Cardiac toxicity is a serious concern in patients with early-stage disease who are treated with both trastuzumab and anthracycline containing chemotherapy (112,113,117,118). Therefore, as with women diagnosed with 0 or 1+ ERBB2-negative tumors by IHC, the discordance between ERBB2 amplification and ERBB2 overexpression in women with IHC3+/ERBB2 not amplified tumors can result in inappropriate treatment of patients and, therefore, expose patients to unnecessary risk.

Regardless of the level of ERBB2 immunohistochemical staining as determined by IHC, a degree of discordance is found with ERBB2 gene amplification as determined by FISH and with overexpression as determined by other methods in frozen tissue. It has been apparent for many years that these IHC assays, performed on paraffin-embedded tissues, are associated with significant problems (23,58). There are problems with both false–positive (59) and false–negative (28) results as well as with the application of these techniques by different laboratories (64). Inaccurate assessment of ERBB2 status can lead to inappropriate treatment of breast cancer patients with trastuzumab in both the adjuvant and metastatic settings and with lapatinib in the metastatic setting. This exposes patients to unnecessary risk by either denying ERBB2-targeted therapies to patients who have a reasonable likelihood of responding to the drugs or by inclusion of patients in ERBB2-targeted treatment who do not exhibit ERBB2 amplification or overexpression. These concerns are especially relevant in countries, such as the United States, where most ERBB2 testing is performed with IHC assays (59).

ISSUES RELATED TO RESPONSE OF "ERBB2-NEGATIVE" BREAST CANCER PATIENTS TO ERBB2-TARGETED THERAPY

Although a recent report from the NSABP suggests that *ERBB2-negative* breast cancer patients in the B-31 trial respond to trastuzumab in the adjuvant setting (116), all of those patients were entered in the clinical trial based on their having *ERBB2-positive* breast cancer assessed in community laboratories. The NSABP central laboratory ERBB2-negative breast cancers represent 9.7% of women (174/1787) entered in the trial with follow-up data and this percentage is within the known range of testing variability between selected laboratories (16,55,57). Similar observations have been made for ERBB2-negative metastatic breast cancer patients and response to lapafinib therapy (14,16). A blinded reanalysis of the ERBB2-negative metastatic breast cancer patients from the latter clinical trial of lapatinib by a second central laboratory, eventually demonstrated that the apparent lapatinib responsiveness of ERBB2-negative breast cancer patients was due to testing errors in the original large, high-volume laboratory where a medical technician, rather than a board-certified pathologist, assessed ERBB2 status (16). Although the NSABP has not subjected their central laboratory ERBB2-negative breast cancers to independent assessment of ERBB2 status by FISH, these cases likely represent ERBB2 testing errors by FISH as has already been demonstrated for the EGF 100151 lapatinib clinical trial (16). Based on these findings, we strongly recommend assessment of ERBB2 status by FISH with interpretation by a board-certified pathologist.

CONCLUSIONS

Determination of a patient's ERBB2 status is critical for patients diagnosed with both primary and metastatic breast carcinoma. ERBB2 status is important for assessment of the patient's prognosis as well as a critically important factor in selecting the optimal chemotherapeutic or biologic treatment for a patient.

Although the ASCO-CAP guidelines indicate acceptance of primary assessment of ERBB2 status using IHC, followed by FISH for IHC 2+ cases, we disagree. Because of the IHC false–positive findings and IHC false–negative findings in FFPE tissues (summarized in this chapter), we strongly recommend primary FISH testing for all primary invasive breast cancers. IHC should be used for evaluation of ERBB2 status only in the approximately 1% to 5% of breast cancer cases where FISH fails to yield a result.

CLINICAL MANAGEMENT SUMMARY

Histologic diagnosis of invasive breast carcinoma:

- Assessment of ERBB2 status by FISH
  - ERBB2-amplified → ERBB2-targeted therapy (trastuzumab) in combination with chemotherapy (preferably a nonanthracycline chemotherapy regimen)
  - ERBB2 not amplified → nonanthracycline combination chemotherapy regimen with or without antiestrogen therapy, depending on estrogen receptor status
  - FISH failure (1% to 5% of cases) → IHC assessment of ERBB2 status (0/1+/2+, ERBB2 low expression; 3+, ERBB2 overexpression)

References

1. Jemal A, Siegel R, Ward E, et al. Cancer statistics, 2007. *CA Cancer J Clin* 2007; 57:43–66.
2. Hanahan D, Weinberg RA. The hallmarks of cancer. *Cell* 2000;100:57–70.
3. Oh J, Grosshans D, Wong S, Slamon D. Identification of differentially expressed genes associated with HER-2/neu overexpression in human breast cancer cells. *Nucl Acid Res* 1999;27(20):4008–4017.
4. Arboleda M, Lyons J, Kabbinavar F, et al. Overexpression of AKT2/protein kinase Bbeta leads to up-regulation of beta1 integrins, increased invasion, and metastasis of human breast and ovarian cancer cells. *Cancer Res* 2003;63(1):196–206.
5. Tommasi S, Paradiso A, Mangia A, et al. Biological correlation between HER-2/neu and proliferative activity in human breast cancer. *Anticancer Res* 1991; 11(4):1395–1400.
6. Chazin VR, Kaleko M, Miller AD, et al. Transformation mediated by the human HER-2 gene independent of the epidermal growth factor receptor. *Oncogene* 1992;7:1859–1866.
7. Witters L, Kumar R, Chinchilli V, et al. Enhanced anti-proliferative activity of the combination of tamoxifen plus HER-2-neu antibody *Breast Cancer Res Treat* 1997;42(1):1–5.
8. Kumar R, Yarmand-Bagheri R. The role of HER2 in angiogenesis. *Semin Oncol* 2001;28(5 Suppl 16):27–32.
9. Osborne C, Shou J, Massarweh S, et al. Crosstalk between estrogne receptor and growth factor receptor pathways as a cause for endocrine therapy resistance in breast cancer. *Clin Cancer Res* 2005;11:865s–870s.
10. Cameron D, Casey M, Press M, et al. A phase III randomized comparison of lapatinib plus capecitabine versus capecitabine alone in women with advanced breast cancer that has progressed on trastuzumab: updated efficacy and biomarker analyses. *Breast Cancer Res Treat* 2008;112:533–534.
11. Cobleigh MA, Vogel CL, Tripathy D, et al. Multinational study of the efficacy and safety of humanized anti-HER2 monoclonal antibody in women who have HER2-overexpressing metastatic breast cancer that has progressed after chemotherapy for metastatic disease. *J Clin Oncol* 1999;17:2639–2648.
12. Di Leo A, Gomez H, Aziz Z, et al. Lapatinib plus paclitaxel versus placebo plus paclitaxel as first-line treatment for patients with metastatic breast cancer: a phase III, double-blind, randomized study in 580 patients. *J Clin Oncol*, 2008, 26:5544–5552.
13. Geyer CE, Forster J, Lindquist D, et al. Lapatinib plus capecitabine for HER2-positive advanced breast cancer. *N Engl J Med* 2006;355:2733–2743.
14. Mass RD, Press MF, Anderson S, et al. Evaluation of clinical outcomes according to HER2 detection by fluorescence in situ hybridization in women with metastatic breast cancer treated with trastuzumab. *Clin Breast Cancer* 2005;6:240–246.
15. Pietras RJ, Poen JC, Gallardo D, et al. Monoclonal antibody to HER-2/neureceptor modulates repair of radiation-induced DNA damage and enhances radiosensitivity of human breast cancer cells overexpressing this oncogene. *Cancer Res* 1999;59:1347–1355.
16. Press M, Finn R, Cameron D, et al. HER2 gene amplification, HER2 and EGFR messenger RNA and protein expression and lapatinib efficacy in women with metastatic breast cancer. *Clin Cancer Res* 2008;14:7861–7870.
17. Slamon DJ, Leyland-Jones B, Shak S, et al. Use of chemotherapy plus a monoclonal antibody against HER2 for metastatic breast cancer that overexpresses HER2. *N Engl J Med* 2001;344:783–792.
18. Coussens L, Yang-Feng TL, Liao YC, et al. Tyrosine kinase receptor with extensive homology to EGF receptor shares chromosomal location with neu oncogene. *Science* 1985;230:1132–1139.
19. Tzahar E, Waterman H, Chen X, et al. A hierarchical network of interreceptor interactions determines signal transduction by Neu differentiation factor/neuregulin and epidermal growth factor. *Mol Cell Biol* 1996;16:5276–5287.
20. Prigent SA, Lemoine NR. The type 1 (EGFR-related) family of growth factor receptors and their ligands. *Prog Growth Factor Res* 1992;4:1–24.
21. Press MF, Cordon-Cardo C, Slamon DJ. Expression of the HER-2/neu proto-oncogene in normal human adult and fetal tissues. *Oncogene* 1990;5:953–962.
22. Slamon DJ, Clark GM, Wong SG, et al. Human breast cancer: correlation of relapse and survival with amplification of the HER-2/neu oncogene. *Science* 1987;235:177–182.
23. Slamon DJ, Godolphin W, Jones LA, et al. Studies of the HER-2/neu proto-oncogene in human breast and ovarian cancer. *Science* 1989;244:707–712.
24. Saffari B, Jones L, El-Naggar A, et al. Amplification and overexpression of HER-2/neu (c-erb B-2) in endometrial cancers: correlation with overall survival *Cancer Res* 1995;55:5693–5698.
25. Press M, Pike M, Hung G, et al. Amplification and overexpression of HER-2/neu in carcinomas of the salivary gland: correlation with poor prognosis *Cancer Res* 1994;54:5675–5682.
26. Prenzel N, Fischer OM, Streit S, et al. The epidermal growth factor receptor family as a central element for cellular signal transduction and diversification. *Endocr Relat Cancer* 2001;8:11–31.
27. Pauletti G, Godolphin W, Press, MF. Detection and quantitation of HER-2/neu gene amplification in human breast cancer archival material using fluorescence in situ hybridization. *Oncogene* 1996;13:63–72.
28. Press MF, Hung G, Godolphin W, et al. Sensitivity of HER-2/neu antibodies in archival tissue samples: potential source of error in immunohistochemical studies of oncogene expression. *Cancer Res* 1994;54:2771–2777.
29. Press MF, Slamon DJ, Flom KJ, et al. Evaluation of HER-2/neu gene amplification and overexpression: comparison of frequently used assay methods in a molecularly characterized cohort of breast cancer specimens. *J Clin Oncol* 2002;20:3095–3105.
30. Seidman A, Fornier M, Esteva F, et al. Weekly trastuzumab and paclitaxel therapy for metastatic breast cancer with analysis of efficacy by HER2 immunophenotype and gene amplification *J Clin Oncol* 2001;19:2587–2595.
31. Kallioniemi OP, Holli K, Visakorpi T, et al. Association of c-erbB-2 protein overexpression with high rate of cell proliferation, increased risk of visceral metastasis and poor long-term survival in breast cancer. *Int J Cancer* 1991;49:650–655.
32. Press MF, Bernstein L, Thomas PA, et al. HER-2/neu gene amplification characterized by fluorescence in situ hybridization: poor prognosis in node-negative breast carcinomas. *J Clin Oncol* 1997;15:2894–2904.
33. Muss HB, Thor AD, Berry DA, et al. c-erbB-2 expression and response to adjuvant therapy in women with node-positive early breast cancer. *N Engl J Med* 1994;330:1260–1266.
34. Hayes D, Thor A, Dressler L, et al. HER2 and response to paclitaxel in node-positive breast cancer. *N Engl J Med* 2007;357:1496–1506.
35. Drebin JA, Link VC, Greene MI. Monoclonal antibodies specific for the neu oncogene product directly mediate anti-tumor effects in vivo. *Oncogene* 1988; 2: 387–394.
36. Drebin JA, Link VC, Stern DF, et al. Down-modulation of an oncogene protein product and reversion of the transformed phenotype by monoclonal antibodies. *Cell* 1985;41:697–706.
37. Drebin JA, Link VC, Weinberg RA, et al. Inhibition of tumor growth by a monoclonal antibody reactive with an oncogene-encoded tumor antigen. *Proc Natl Acad Sci U S A* 1986;83:9129–9133.
38. Carter P, Presta L, Gorman C, et al. Humanization of an antip185HER2 antibody for human cancer therapy. *Proc Natl Acad Sci U S A* 1992;89:4285–4291.
39. Pietras R, Fendly B, Chazin V, et al. Antibody to HER-2/neu receptor blocks DNA repair after cisplatin in human breast and ovarian cancer cells. *Oncogene* 1994; 9:1829–1838.
40. Pietras R, Pegram M, Finn R, et al. Remission of human breast cancer xenografts on therapy with humanized monoclonal antibody to HER-2 receptor and DNA-reactive drugs. *Oncogene* 1998;17(17):2235–2249.
41. Hancock MC, Langton BC, Chan T, et al. A monoclonal antibody against the c-erbB-2 protein enhances the cytotoxicity of cis-diamminedichloroplatinum against human breast and ovarian tumor cell lines. *Cancer Res* 1991;51: 4575–4580.
42. McKenzie SJ, Marks PJ, Lam T, et al. Generation and characterization of monoclonal antibodies specific for the human neu oncogene product, p185. *Oncogene* 1989;4:543–548.
43. Stancovski I, Hurwitz E, Leitner O, et al. Mechanistic aspects of the opposing effects of monoclonal antibodies to the ERBB2 receptor on tumor growth. *Proc Natl Acad Sci U S A* 1991;88:8691–8695.
44. du Manoir JM, Francia G, Man S, et al. Strategies for delaying or treating in vivo acquired resistance to trastuzumab in human breast cancer xenografts. *Clin Cancer Res* 2006;12:904–916.
45. Hudziak RM, Lewis GD, Winget M, et al. p185HER2 monoclonal antibody has antiproliferative effects in vitro and sensitizes human breast tumor cells to tumor necrosis factor. *Mol Cell Biol* 1989;9:1165–1172.
46. Seidman A, Berry D, Cirrincione C, et al. Randomized Phase III Trial of Weekly Compared With Every-3-Weeks Paclitaxel for Metastatic Breast Cancer, With Trastuzumab for all HER2 Overexpressors and Random Assignment to Trastuzumab or Not in HER-2 Nonoverexpressors: Final Results of Cancer and Leukemia Group B Protocol 9840. *J Clin Oncol* 2008;26:1642–1649.
47. Vogel CL, Cobleigh MA, Tripathy D, et al. Efficacy and safety of trastuzumab as a single agent in first-line treatment of HER2-overexpressing metastatic breast cancer. *J Clin Oncol* 2002;20:719–726.
48. Bergqvist J, Ohd JF, Smeds J, et al. Quantitative real-time PCR analysis and microarray-based RNA expression of HER2 in relation to outcome. *Ann Oncol* 2007;18:845–850.
49. Ginestier C, Charafe-Jauffret E, Penault-Llorca F, et al. Comparative multimethodological measurement of ERBB2 status in breast cancer. *J Pathol* 2004; 202:286–298.
50. Gullick WJ, Love SB, Wright C, et al. c-erbB-2 protein overexpression in breast cancer is a risk factor in patients with involved and uninvolved lymph nodes. *Br J Cancer* 1991;63:434–438.

51. Rilke F, Colnaghi MI, Cascinelli N, et al. Prognostic significance of HER-2/neu expression in breast cancer and its relationship to other prognostic factors. *Int J Cancer* 1991;49:44–49.
52. Winstanley J, Cooke T, Murray GD, et al. The long term prognostic significance of c-erbB-2 in primary breast cancer. *Br J Cancer* 1991;63:447–450.
53. Gusterson BA, Gelber RD, Goldhirsch A, et al. Prognostic importance of c-erbB-2 expression in breast cancer. International (Ludwig) Breast Cancer Study Group. *J Clin Oncol* 1992;10:1049–1056.
54. Press M, Pike M, Chazin V, et al. Her-2/neu expression in node-negative breast cancer: direct tissue quantitation by computerized image analysis and association of overexpression with increased risk of recurrent disease. *Cancer Res* 1993; 53;4960–4970.
55. Dybdal N, Leiberman G, Anderson S, et al. Determination of HER2 gene amplification by fluorescence in situ hybridization and concordance with the clinical trials immunohistochemical assay in women with metastatic breast cancer evaluated for treatment with trastuzumab. *Breast Cancer Res Treat* 2005;93:3–11.
56. Wolff A, Hammond M, Schwartz J, et al. American Society of Clinical Oncology/College of American Pathologists guideline recommendations for human epidermal growth factor receptor 2 testing in breast cancer. *Arch Pathol Lab Med* 2007;131:18–43.
57. Wolff AC, Hammond ME, Schwartz JN, et al. American Society of Clinical Oncology/College of American Pathologists guideline recommendations for human epidermal growth factor receptor 2 testing in breast cancer. *J Clin Oncol* 2007;25:118–145.
58. Sauter G, Lee J, Bartlett J, et al. Guidelines for HER-2 Testing: Biologic and Methodologic Considerations. *J Clin Oncol* 2008; in press.
59. Press MF, Sauter G, Bernstein L, et al. Diagnostic evaluation of HER-2 as a molecular target: an assessment of accuracy and reproducibility of laboratory testing in large, prospective, randomized clinical trials. *Clin Cancer Res* 2005;11:6598–6607.
60. Penault-Llorca F, Adelaide J, Houvenaeghel G, et al. Optimization of immunohistochemical detection of ERBB2 in human breast cancer: impact of fixation. *J Pathol* 1994;173:65–75.
61. Carney WP, Leitzel K, Ali S, et al. HER-2/neu diagnostics in breast cancer. *Breast Cancer Res* 2007;9:207.
62. Fornier MN, Seidman AD, Schwartz MK, et al. Serum HER2 extracellular domain in metastatic breast cancer patients treated with weekly trastuzumab and paclitaxel: association with HER2 status by immunohistochemistry and fluorescence in situ hybridization and with response rate. *Ann Oncol* 2005;16:234–239.
63. Kay EW, Walsh CJ, Cassidy M, et al. C-erbB-2 immunostaining: problems with interpretation. *J Clin Pathol* 1994;47:816–822.
64. Paik S, Bryant J, Tan-Chiu E, et al. Real-world performance of HER2 testing—National Surgical Adjuvant Breast and Bowel Project experience. *J Natl Cancer Inst* 2002;94:852–854.
65. Perez E, Suman V, Davidson N, et al. HER2 testing by local, central, and reference laboratories in specimens from the North Central Cancer Treatment Group N9831 intergroup adjuvant trial. *J Clin Oncol* 2006;24:3032–3038.
66. Roche PC, Suman VJ, Jenkins RB, et al. Concordance between local and central laboratory HER2 testing in the breast intergroup trial N9831. *J Natl Cancer Inst* 2002;94:855–857.
67. Kumamoto H, Sasano H, Taniguchi T, et al. Chromogenic in situ hybridization analysis of HER-2/neu status in breast carcinoma: application in screening of patients for trastuzumab (Herceptin) therapy. *Pathol Int* 2001;51:579–584.
68. Tubbs R, Pettay J, Hicks D, et al. Novel bright field molecular morphology methods for detection of HER2 gene amplification. *J Mol Histol* 2004;35:589–594.
69. Tubbs R, Pettay J, Skacel M, et al. Gold-facilitated in situ hybridization: a bright-field autometallographic alternative to fluorescence in situ hybridization for detection of Her-2/neu gene amplification. *Am J Pathol* 2002;160:1589–1595.
70. Konecny G, Pauletti G, Pegram M, et al. Quantitative association between HER-2/neu and steroid hormone receptors in hormone receptor-positive primary breast cancer. *J Natl Cancer Inst* 2003;95:142–153.
71. Yeon CH, Pegram MD. Anti-erbB-2 antibody trastuzumab in the treatment of HER2-amplified breast cancer. *Invest New Drugs* 2005;23:391–409.
72. Cayre A, Mishellany F, Lagarde N, et al. Comparison of different commercial kits for HER2 testing in breast cancer: looking for the accurate cutoff for amplification. Breast *Cancer Res* 2007;9:R64.
73. Lal P, Salazar PA, Hudis CA, et al. HER-2 testing in breast cancer using immunohistochemical analysis and fluorescence in situ hybridization: a single-institution experience of 2,279 cases and comparison of dual-color and single-color scoring. *Am J Clin Pathol* 2004;121:631–636.
74. Ro JS, el-Naggar A, Ro JY, et al. c-erbB-2 amplification in node-negative human breast cancer. *Cancer Res* 1989;49:6941–6944.
75. Ross JS, Fletcher JA, Bloom KJ, et al. HER-2/neu testing in breast cancer. *Am J Clin Pathol* 2003;120 Suppl:S53–71.
76. Bartlett J, Going J, Mallon E, et al. Evaluating HER2 amplification and overexpression in breast cancer. *J Pathol* 2001;195:422–428.
77. Tubbs RR, Pettay JD, Roche PC, et al. Discrepancies in clinical laboratory testing of eligibility for trastuzumab therapy: apparent immunohistochemical false-positives do not get the message. *J Clin Oncol* 2001;19:2714–2721.
78. Perez EA, Roche PC, Jenkins RB, et al. HER2 testing in patients with breast cancer: poor correlation between weak positivity by immunohistochemistry and gene amplification by fluorescence in situ hybridization. *Mayo Clin Proc* 2002; 77:148–154.
79. Pauletti G, Dandekar S, Rong H, et al. Assessment of methods for tissue-based detection of the HER-2/neu alteration in human breast cancer: a direct comparison of fluorescence in situ hybridization and immunohistochemistry. *J Clin Oncol* 2000;18:3651–3664.
80. Cell Markers and Cytogenetics Committees, C. o. A. P. Clinical laboratory assays for HER-2/neu amplification and overexpression: quality assurance, standardization, and proficiency testing. *Arch Pathol Lab Med* 2002;126:803–808.
81. Arnould L, Denoux Y, MacGrogan G, et al. Agreement between chromogenic in situ hybridisation (CISH) and FISH in the determination of HER2 status in breast cancer. *Br J Cancer* 2003;88:1587–1591.
82. Dandachi N, Dietze O, Hauser-Kronberger C. Chromogenic *in situ* hybridization: a novel approach to a practical and sensitive method for the detection of HER2 oncogene in archival human breast carcinoma. *Lab Invest* 2002;82:1007–1014.
83. Tanner M, Gancberg D, Di Leo A, et al. Chromogenic in situ hybridization: a practical alternative for fluorescence in situ hybridization to detect HER-2/neu oncogene amplification in archival breast cancer samples. *Am J Pathol* 2000; 157: 1467–1472.
84. Tubbs R, Skacel M, Pettay J, et al. Interobserver interpretative reproducibility of GOLDFISH, a first generation gold-facilitated autometallographic bright field in situ hybridization assay for HER-2/neu amplification in invasive mammary carcinoma. *Am J Surg Pathol* 2002;26:908–913.
85. Zhao J, Wu R, Au A, et al. Determination of HER2 gene amplification by chromogenic *in situ* hybridization (CISH) in archival breast carcinoma. *Mod Pathol* 2002;15:657–665.
86. Lambros MB, Natrajan R, Reis-Filho JS. Chromogenic and fluorescent *in situ* hybridization in breast cancer. *Hum Pathol* 2007;38:1105–1122.
87. Hanna WM, Kwok K. Chromogenic *in-situ* hybridization: a viable alternative to fluorescence *in-situ* hybridization in the HER2 testing algorithm. *Mod Pathol* 2006;19:481–487.
88. Gupta D, Middleton LP, Whitaker MJ, et al. Comparison of fluorescence and chromogenic *in situ* hybridization for detection of HER-2/neu oncogene in breast cancer. *Am J Clin Pathol* 2003;119:381–387.
89. Isola J, Tanner M, Forsyth A, et al. Interlaboratory comparison of HER-2 oncogene amplification as detected by chromogenic and fluorescence *in situ* hybridization. *Clin Cancer Res* 2004;10:4793–4798.
90. Park K, Kim J, Lim S, et al. Comparing fluorescence in situ hybridization and chromogenic *in situ* hybridization methods to determine the HER2/neu status in primary breast carcinoma using tissue microarray. *Mod Pathol* 2003;16:937–943.
91. Vera-Roman JM, Rubio-Martinez LA. Comparative assays for the HER-2/neu oncogene status in breast cancer. *Arch Pathol Lab Med* 2004;128:627–633.
92. Hainfeld JF, Powell RD. New frontiers in gold labeling. *J Histochem Cytochem* 2000;48:471–480.
93. Zehbe I, Hacker GW, Su H, et al. Sensitive *in situ* hybridization with catalyzed reporter deposition, streptavidin–Nanogold, and silver acetate autometallography: detection of single–copy human papillomavirus. *Am J Pathol* 1997;150:1553–1561.
94. Mayer G, Leone RD, Hainfeld JF, et al. Introduction of a novel HRP substrate-Nanogold probe for signal amplification in immunocytochemistry. *J Histochem Cytochem* 2000;48:461–470.
95. Leitzel K, Teramoto Y, Sampson E, et al. Elevated soluble c-erbB-2 antigen levels in the serum and effusions of a proportion of breast cancer patients. *J Clin Oncol* 1992;10:1436–1443.
96. Carney WP, Hamer PJ, Petit D, et al. Detection and quantitation of the human neu oncoprotein. *J Tumor Marker Oncol* 1991;6:53–72.
97. Cook GB, Neaman IE, Goldblatt JL, et al. Clinical utility of serum HER-2/neu testing on the Bayer Immuno 1 automated system in breast cancer. *Anticancer Res* 2001;21:1465–1470.
98. Schwartz MK, Smith C, Schwartz DC, et al. Monitoring therapy by serum HER-2/neu. *Int J Biol Markers* 2000;15:324–329.
99. Payne RC, Allard JW, Anderson-Mauser L, et al. Automated assay for HER-2/neu in serum. *Clin Chem* 2000;46:175–182.
100. Carney WP, Neumann R, Lipton A, et al. Potential clinical utility of serum HER-2/neu oncoprotein concentrations in patients with breast cancer. *Clin Chem* 2003;49:1579–1598.
101. Pupa SM, Menard S, Morelli D, et al. The extracellular domain of the c-erbB-2 oncoprotein is released from tumor cells by proteolytic cleavage. *Oncogene* 1993;8:2917–2923.
102. Kong SY, Nam BH, Lee KS, et al. Predicting tissue HER2 status using serum HER2 levels in patients with metastatic breast cancer. *Clin Chem* 2006;52:1510–1515.
103. Beltran M, Colomer R. Does HER-2 status predict only a decreased response to hormone therapy in advanced breast cancer, or does it also predict the extent of metastatic disease? *J Clin Oncol* 2002;20:4605; author reply 4606.
104. Lipton A, Ali SM, Leitzel K, et al. Elevated serum Her-2/neu level predicts decreased response to hormone therapy in metastatic breast cancer. *J Clin Oncol* 2002;20:1467–1472.
105. Perez EA, Geeraerts L, Suman VJ, et al. A randomized phase II study of sequential docetaxel and doxorubicin/cyclophosphamide in patients with metastatic breast cancer. *Ann Oncol* 2002;13:1225–1235.
106. Colomer R, Llombart-Cussac A, Lluch A, et al. Biweekly paclitaxel plus gemcitabine in advanced breast cancer: phase II trial and predictive value of HER2 extracellular domain. *Ann Oncol* 2004;15:201–206.
107. Ludovini V, Gori S, Colozza M, et al. Evaluation of serum HER2 extracellular domain in early breast cancer patients: correlation with clinicopathological parameters and survival. *Ann Oncol* 2008;19:883–890.
108. Molina R, Filella X, Zanon G, et al. Prospective evaluation of tumor markers (c-erbB-2 oncoprotein, CEA and CA 15.3) in patients with locoregional breast cancer. *Anticancer Res* 2003;23:1043–1050.
109. Burris HA, 3rd. Dual kinase inhibition in the treatment of breast cancer: initial experience with the EGFR/ErbB-2 inhibitor lapatinib. *Oncologist* 2004;9 Suppl 3:10–15.
110. Rusnak DW, Affleck K, Cockerill SG, et al. The characterization of novel, dual ErbB-2/EGFR, tyrosine kinase inhibitors: potential therapy for cancer. *Cancer Res* 2001;61:7196–7203.
111. Simon R, Nocito A, Hubscher T, et al. Patterns of her-2/neu amplification and overexpression in primary and metastatic breast cancer. *J Natl Cancer Inst* 2001;93:1141–1146.
112. Romond EH, Perez EA, Bryant J, et al. Trastuzumab plus adjuvant chemotherapy for operable HER2-positive breast cancer. *N Engl J Med* 2005;353:1673–1684.
113. Piccart-Gebhart MJ, Procter M, Leyland-Jones B, et al. Trastuzumab after adjuvant chemotherapy in HER2-positive breast cancer. *N Engl J Med* 2005;353: 1659–1672.
114. Blackwell KL, Burstein H, Pegram M, et al. Determining relevant biomarkers from tissue and serum that may predict response to single agent lapatinib in trastuzumab refractory metastatic breast cancer. *J Clin Oncol* 2005;23:3004.
115. Ingle JN, Tu D, Pater JL, et al. Duration of letrozole treatment and outcomes in the placebo-controlled NCIC CTG MA.17 extended adjuvant therapy trial. *Breast Cancer Res Treat* 2006;99:295–300.
116. Paik S, Kim C, Wolmark N. HER2 Status and Benefit from Adjuvant Trastuzumab in Breast Cancer. *New England Journal of Medicine* 2008;358:1409–1411.
117. Levine MN. Trastuzumab cardiac side effects: only time will tell. *J Clin Oncol* 2005;23:7775–7776.
118. Tan-Chiu E, Yothers G, Romond E, et al. Assessment of cardiac dysfunction in a randomized trial comparing doxorubicin and cyclophosphamide followed by paclitaxel, with or without trastuzumab as adjuvant therapy in node-positive, human epidermal growth factor receptor 2-overexpressing breast cancer: NSABP B-31. *J Clin Oncol* 2005;23:7811–7819.
119. Hicks D, Tubbs R. Assessment of the HER2 status in breast cancer by fluorescence in situ hybridization: a technical review with interpretive guidelines. *Human Pathol* 2005;36:250–261.

Jenny C. Chang and Susan G. Hilsenbeck

Breast cancer is a clinically diverse disease, and this diversity is driven by multiple genetic alterations and molecular events. Some women with breast cancer, such as those with inflammatory breast cancer, have extremely poor prognosis, whereas others with tubular or mucinous subtypes have survival equivalent to the general population (1). Some women with breast cancer have a low likelihood of distant recurrence, whereas others are less fortunate. The factors that determine or correlate with the natural history of the disease, in the absence of intervening adjuvant systemic therapy and which are therefore reflective of the inherent aggressiveness of the cancer are termed *prognostic markers*. Prognostic markers include nodal status, tumor size, pathologic subtypes, demographic characteristics (age, ethnicity, menopausal status), and other molecular biomarkers purportedly involved in tumor metastases and disease progression. The relative effects of these factors are best assessed in systemically untreated patients. Generally, prognostic markers can be used to help determine a need to further systemic therapy, but not to discriminate relative benefits of particular therapies. Conversely, *predictive markers* are those associated with response or lack of response to a particular therapy. It is thus reasonable to expect a mechanistic linkage between the marker(s) and the therapy for which benefit is predicted. The most notable example of a predictive marker is the estrogen receptor (ER), which predicts for response to hormonal therapies in the adjuvant, neoadjuvant, and metastatic settings. In addition, some factors may share both *prognostic* and *predictive* properties. Indeed, ER expression is a weak prognostic factor for favorable outcome and a strong predictive factor for benefit from hormonal therapy. Expression of the growth factor receptor *cerb*B2 (ERBB2, formerly HER-2/*neu*), is a *prognostic* factor associated with poorer clinical outcome (2,3), and its amplification is also *predictive* of response to trastuzumab (trastuzumab [Herceptin, Genentech, Inc., CA], a humanized monoclonal antibody to ERBB2) and possibly *predictive* of a better response to anthracyclines or poorer response to hormonal agents such as tamoxifen (a selective ER modulator).

PURPOSE OF THE CHAPTER

This chapter describes the current standard prognostic and predictive factors for primary breast cancer. It is not intended to be an exhaustive list of all currently available biomarkers, but to describe individual factors that either are now or are likely to be of clinical utility and significance. We focus primarily on individual tumor associated markers and characteristics. Constitutional factors, such as P450 system genotype status, may have therapeutic implications related to the way in which drugs or prodrugs are processed. This important emerging topic is discussed in detail in Chapter 56. Finally, although still in their infancy in terms of clinical practice, array-based technologies have advanced substantially. At least two, so-called "multigene" assays are now commercially available (see Chapter 32 for a comprehensive discussion). Refinements of their use are being tested in large clinical trials.

HISTORICAL PERSPECTIVE

Historically, women estimated to have poor prognosis have been recommended systemic therapies, whereas others expected to have a better outcome have been spared the toxic side effects of such treatments. In the 1985 National Cancer Institute (NCI) consensus development conference, the panel of experts concluded that no standard therapy existed for node-negative patients (4). With the publication of the Oxford overview (5) in 1992 and results from several large randomized clinical trials showing benefit from adjuvant treatment in node-negative breast cancer, many clinicians, however, now prescribe systemic therapy for most women regardless of prognostic factors. The 1991 NCI consensus development conference recognized that clinical outcomes varied among women with primary breast cancer and concluded that nodal status, tumor size, and histologic subtype were of clinical significance but questioned the utility of the newer prognostic markers for breast cancer (6).

Nearly 10 years later, in their consensus statement, the College of American Pathologists (CAP) reviewed the evidence supporting a variety of prognostic factors in use in the United States (7). They divided factors into three categories, depending on the perceived degree of clinical utility (Table 31.1). The CAP reaffirmed the utility of nodal status, tumor size and histologic subtype, adding proliferation and grade as clinically useful markers. Interestingly, uPA and PAI-1 are not included, although strong evidence (see below) exists to support the likely clinical utility of these markers. The consensus panel also identified a number of methodologic and measurement issues associated with each marker. For example, interobserver variability in measurement of tumor size may arise owing to failure to determine the largest diameter, or to tumor multicentricity or presence of ductal carcinoma *in situ* (DCIS). Reported nodal status may depend on the extent of axillary dissection, or use of single or multilevel sectioning. The prognostic value of molecular markers may depend on the specific assay, methods of tissue fixation, or method of quantitation.

Concurrent with and largely in agreement with the CAP review, a consensus panel of the American Society of Clinical Oncology (ASCO) (8) updated earlier recommendations for tumor markers for breast and colorectal cancer. In late 2007, these recommendations were updated specifically for breast cancer, with careful review of the levels of evidence supporting clinical utility (9). Overall, few changes were made in recommendations, although the guidelines included discussion of several markers not previously discussed.

At present, the standard prognostic and predictive factors in primary breast cancers in clinical practice are as follows:

1. Axillary lymph node status, including micrometastasis (Nmic)
2. Tumor size
3. Histologic subtype
4. Nuclear or histologic grade
5. Proliferation indices, including mitotic index
6. Estrogen and progesterone receptor status (mainly as predictive markers of response to hormonal therapies) (see Chapter 29)
7. ERBB2 amplification or overexpression (mainly as a predictive marker of response to trastuzumab [Herceptin] and possibly as predictive of benefit from anthracyclines) (see Chapter 30)
8. Multiparameter-based markers (mainly as prognostic indicator of recurrence risk (see also Chapter 32)

The Human Genome Project has revealed information about the structure of all techniques have been developed for molecular analysis of gene and gene products. Validated results indicate

Table 31.1 SUMMARY OF PROGNOSTIC AND PREDICTIVE FACTORS IN BREAST CANCER

Factor or Marker	In Current Clinical Use?	College of American Pathologists Assessment Category (7)	ASCO Breast Tumor Markers Assessment Update 2007[c]	Level of Evidence[a] Prognostic	Predictive
Nodal status	Yes	I	NE	A	—
Sentinel lymphadenectomy	Increasing	I	NE	—	—
Tumor size	Yes	I	NE	A	—
Histologic and nuclear grade	Yes	I	NE	A	—
Histologic type	Yes	I	NE	A	—
Proliferation:	Yes	I	NE	B	—
Mitotic figure count					
MIB-1		II	NR	B	—
S-phase fraction		II	NR	A	—
Cyclin E		NE	NR	A	—
Steroid receptors:	Yes	I	R	—	A
Estrogen receptor					
Progesterone receptor	Yes	I	R	—	B
uPA/PAI-1	Yes[b]	NE	?	A	C
Growth Factors:					
EGFR		III	NE	C	C
C-erbB-2(Her2/neu)	Yes	II	R	—	A,C[d]
p53		II	NR	C	—
Lymphatic or vascular invasion		II	NE	—	—
Multiparameter gene expression	Yes	NE	?	B	C,D
Other factors, such as:					
Tumor angiogenesis					
TGFα		III	NR or NE	C,D	—
bcl-2					
pS2					
Cathepsin D					

ASCO , American Society of Clinical Oncology; EGFR, epidermal growth factor receptor; NE, not evaluated; TGFαm, tumor growth factor alpha; I, factors of proven value and clinical utility; I, factors extensively studied, but whose clinical utility remains to be validated; III, all other factors not sufficiently studied to demonstrate prognostic value.
[a]See Table 31.2 for definitions.
[b]Widely used in Europe, not generally used in the United States.
[c]R, recommended; ?, may be used; NR, not recommended (present data insufficient to recommend use).
[d]Evidence is strong for anti-Her2 therapy, but weaker for predictive effects for benefit from anthracyclin.

that these techniques, such as gene expression analysis, can accurately divide breast cancers at high versus low risk of recurrence. Recent advancements in microarray technology hold the promise of further increasing our understanding of the complexity and heterogeneity of this disease, and providing new avenues for the prognostication and prediction of breast cancer outcomes. These new technologies have many limitations, and have yet to be incorporated into routine clinical use, for both the diagnosis and the treatment of women with breast cancer (see Chapter 32). One interesting turn of events, however, is the potential utility of the individual components comprising multiparameter assays, such as Oncotype DX (Genomic Health, Inc., CA) or Mammaprint (Agendia Inc., CA) as an alternative method of assessment of single factors. For example, clinical reports from the Oncotype DX assay now include separate reporting of ER and progesterone receptor (PR), based on the quantified mRNA.

DISTINGUISHING BETWEEN PROGNOSTIC AND PREDICTIVE EFFECTS

As suggested by the definition above, some markers are thought to be purely prognostic, some are purely predictive, and some are both prognostic and predictive, providing insight into both natural history and likely benefit of specific therapy.

Although it may seem simple in concept to distinguish between prognostic, predictive, or mixed markers, the reality is more complex. It is important to distinguish markers of different types clearly, especially when attempting to use markers to optimize therapy. It is also important to recognize the difference between relative and absolute effects. Figure 31.1 illustrates some of the possible effects of a hypothetical new marker in node-negative breast cancer with or without adjuvant systemic therapy. On average, 10-year relapse-free survival (RFS) in node-negative breast cancer is about 70%. A purely predictive factor would separate treated cases, but not untreated cases (Fig. 31.1A). In a Cox regression, this is modeled as an interaction between marker and treatment, and is conceptualized as crossing or nonparallel lines in graphs such as those of Figure 31.1D, which shows the scale of measurement appropriate to Cox regression. Scale matters, and crossing or nonparallel lines on a graph of 10-year RFS do not necessarily imply a predictive effect (10,11).

In Figure 31.1B, the factor separates untreated patients into two groups: a *Good prognosis* group with a 10-year RFS of 85% and a *Poor prognosis* group with RFS of 55%. In this scenario, the prognostic effect of the factor can be detected by analysis (i.e., Cox proportional hazards regression) of untreated patients, because the factor separates untreated patients into groups with distinctly different 10-year RFS (untreated, Figs. 31.1B and C).

Figure 31.1B appears to represent a purely prognostic marker, because the separation between *Good* and *Poor* outcome

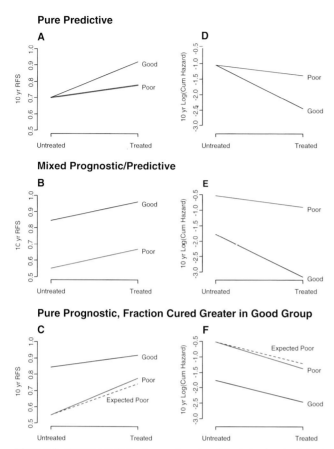

FIGURE 31.1. Illustration of effects of prognostic and predictive factors in untreated and treated patients.

is the same in the untreated and treated groups, but in fact, Figure 31.1B represents a factor with mixed effects, and Figure 31.1C represents a more nearly purely prognostic factor. This is more easily seen when the correct scale, relevant to the Cox proportional hazards regression used to test for interactions, is used to plot the data (Figs. 31.1D–F). Instead of plotting 10-year RFS, we plot the logarithm of the cumulative hazard at 10 years. High survival values correspond to low hazards. Now, Figure 31.1E clearly shows that treatment has a beneficial effect overall and that the separation between Good and Poor prognosis increases with treatment, indicating enhanced benefit in *Good* prognosis patients. When the treatment is tamoxifen, the ER exhibits just this type of pattern. Untreated ER-positive patients have a modestly better outcome than ER-negative patients, and with tamoxifen treatment, the outcome in ER-positive patients is considerably better than in ER-negative patients.

In addition, another, subtler problem exists that almost certainly plays a role in current analyses of putatively mixed prognostic and predictive factors. Figure 31.1F (and 31.1C) illustrates a factor that is purely prognostic but, in Cox regression analysis, also predicts for enhanced benefit from therapy in the poor prognosis group. The *dotted line* shows the RFS that would be seen if there is no statistical interaction between treatment and factor in the Cox model. The 10-year RFS would be 72% instead of 77%. With a sufficiently large sample size, modest interactive effects such as this will be detectable. A clinical trial would conclude that treatment offers especially enhanced benefit in the poor prognosis group. In this hypothetical example, however, the response rate in patients not "cured" by surgery alone is exactly the same (50%) in all patients. The apparent enhanced benefit arises because there are simply more patients, proportionately, in the *Poor prognosis*

group who are not "cured" by surgery and, therefore, remain at risk. This amounts to a violation of the assumption of proportional hazards, and typical Cox regression analysis fails to account for this. Factors that appear to exhibit enhanced benefit from chemotherapy in the adjuvant setting in a *Poor* prognosis group (i.e., ERB2/neu positivity and anthracycline response, or high uPA/PAI-1 and adjuvant chemotherapy) are potentially suspect and may be explained, at least in part, by this phenomenon. In contrast, factors that demonstrate enhanced benefit in a *Good prognosis* group (i.e., ER positivity and tamoxifen) provide clearer evidence of mixed prognostic and predictive effects. Obviously, great care is required in interpreting studies purporting to identify factors with prognostic or predictive effects, especially those with mixed effects. It should also be clear from this discussion that interpretation of uncontrolled marker studies of systemically treated cases is highly problematic.

Possible Levels of Evidence

Different molecular markers can be classified according to the available current evidence supporting its use as a predictive or prognostic marker. Table 31.2 outlines the criteria for recommendations using the principles of evidence-based medicine. Ideally, the prognostic effect of a factor should be established by studying patients not treated systemically to eliminate the confounding effects of therapy. With current trends toward adjuvant treatment of all but patients with the lowest risk of recurrence, prognostic factors usually have to be evaluated as retrospective studies of prospectively banked tumor samples with long-term follow-up, providing at best level III evidence. Studies of predictive markers have often been done in the context of a planned clinical trial, thereby ensuring uniformity in treatment. Such studies can provide level II evidence, although evaluation of the marker is often not the primary or even a secondary aim of the trial, and is conducted as a retrospective analysis, yielding level III evidence. Predictive factors are best studied in a setting that allows direct ascertainment of the patients at risk, and direct observation of the response to therapy, as for example in metastatic disease or neoadjuvant therapy. Indeed, ER was first identified as a predictive factor for response to endocrine therapy in the metastatic setting, and its predictive value is confirmed in more recent neoadjuvant studies (12).

Table 31.2	CRITERIA FOR RECOMMENDATIONS USING THE PRINCIPLES OF EVIDENCE-BASED MEDICINE
Level	Type of Evidence for Recommendation
I	Evidence obtained from meta-analysis of multiple well-designed controlled studies: randomized trials with low false–positives and low false–negative errors (high power)
II	Evidence obtained from at least one well-designed controlled study: randomized trials with low false–positives or low false–negative errors (low power)
III	Evidence obtained from well-designed quasi-experimental studies, such as nonrandomized controlled single-group, cohort, time or matched case-control studies
IV	Evidence obtained from well-designed nonexperimental studies, such as comparative and correlation descriptive and case studies
V	Evidence from case reports and clinical examples
Category	**Grade of Evidence**
A	Evidence of type I or consistent findings from multiple studies of types II, II, or IV
B	Evidence of type II, II, or IV and findings are generally consistent
C	Evidence of type II, II, or IV and findings are inconsistent
D	Little or no systematic evidence
NG	Grade not given

EVALUATION AND VALIDATION METHODOLOGIES

It is important to consider how to interpret the hundreds of biologic markers in the published literature to assess their importance as prognostic or predictive factors. In a review of molecular markers by McGuire (13), the minimal criteria for evaluating new prognostic markers were given as follows:

1. Prognostic factors should have biological relevance based on biological hypotheses
2. Methodologies for determining these markers should be validated and reproducible, with optimal cut-off values
3. Factors should be studied with adequate sample sizes without population bias

Others have expanded on these guidelines, suggesting issues that should be considered in the design of prognostic factor studies and offering guidelines for reporting of results (14–16). In their review of the many methodologic challenges in the evaluation of prognostic and predictive factors, Altman and Lyman (16) describe a progression of investigation much like that used in modern drug development. Phase I prognostic or predictive factor studies are exploratory, seeking associations between a marker and disease. Phase II studies may also be somewhat exploratory, but attempt to use marker values to predict outcome or response to treatment. Phase II studies might also refine assay methodology. In contrast, phase III studies are confirmatory, testing an *a priori* specified hypothesis to the value of a marker. Important recommendations for the design of late phase prognostic studies include *a priori* specification of hypotheses, specification of assay or measurement methodology and demonstration of reproducibility, blinded determination of marker with regard to outcome, planned sample size, and preplanned analysis. It is also important to consider whether new markers add to or can supersede older established or more easily assessed markers. Study designs should therefore account for associations between markers, both in the planning (17), and in the analysis.

In an effort to improve the quality of reporting of tumor marker studies, McShane et al. (18) proposed the REMARK (Reporting recommendations for tumor MARKer prognostic studies) guidelines. As with the highly successful Consolidated Standards for Reporting Trials (CONSORT) guidelines for reporting clinical trials, the guidelines were published in multiple journals simultaneously. Because of the diversity of studies for predictive markers, the guidelines focus on prognostic markers and build on and formalize many of the previous suggestions. They provide an excellent checklist for evidence-based review. Some of the key issues that should be described include the following: the target marker and hypotheses being tested; eligibility and patients included; methods of treatment assignment; handling of specimens assayed; specific assay; method of case selection; clinical end points; all candidate variables; rationale for sample size; statistical methods, including model building and assumption verification; distributions of patient demographics for each subgroup; standard prognostic factors and numbers of missing values; association of new marker to standard factors; univariate analyses of outcome; multivariate analyses, including models with standard factors; and interpretation in the context of prespecified hypotheses.

Despite the vast literature of prognostic and predictive factors, very few studies represent prospectively planned trials of marker efficacy, and indeed, such studies are extremely difficult to do. Simplistically, a definitive assessment of the utility of a marker to predict treatment benefit would randomize subjects to marker-guided treatment selection or standard treatment selection, with the aim of demonstrating that the marker-guided arm does better. Sargent et al. (19) call this the "marker-based strategy design." An alternative approach is the "marker by treatment interaction design," which can be conducted in the context of a traditional phase III trial, where subjects are stratified by marker, and a formal test of interaction is used to detect differential effects of treatment in marker groups. Such studies are becoming more common as correlative, secondary objectives in the context of targeted therapy trials. The *marker-based strategy* requires *a priori* knowledge of the marker and to date, no such studies have been done, in part because the interaction approach may be more efficient and require fewer subjects. A further complication in planning studies of new therapy and possible predictive markers is that the methods of marker measurement and interpretation may be under development concurrent with the study, and it may be unclear whether benefit is likely limited to marker positives, or whether a broader population might also derive benefit. A *biomarker-adaptive design* has recently been proposed that could allow evaluation of overall effects as well as assessment of specific benefit in marker-defined subgroups (20). No studies have utilized this approach as yet, although the approach seems promising.

The tremendous volume of prognostic and predictive literature necessitates the use of an evidence-based approach to integrating clinical experience with the best available scientific evidence derived from systematic research. In the 1970s, the Canadian Task Force on Periodic Health Examination developed a set of standardized criteria for evaluating and grading scientific evidence (21), and these criteria have been improved by the U.S. Preventive Services Task Force (22). For this review, the literature was reviewed to evaluate the status of validation of prognostic and predictive markers in breast cancer, and a grade of evidence has been assigned to these various markers using the criteria in Table 31.2.

PROGNOSTIC AND PREDICTIVE FACTORS

Axillary Lymph Nodes

The absence or presence of axillary lymph node metastasis is the single most powerful prognostic factor for primary breast cancer. Generally, a direct relationship exists between the number of lymph nodes and clinical outcome. Figure 31.2 demonstrates relapse-free survival as a function of number of positive lymph nodes for a group of patients from the tumor bank of the Breast Center at Baylor College of Medicine in Houston, Texas that were previously used in an evaluation of time-dependence of prognostic factors (23). Of note, the 5-year disease free

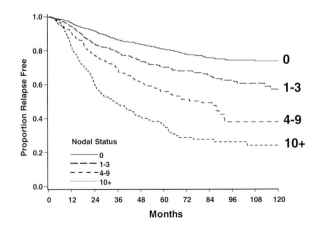

FIGURE 31.2. Relapse-free survival (RFS) by number of axillary lymph nodes (n = 2,873 patients, median follow-up of 37 months) (reanalysis of data presented in reference 23).

survival for node-negative patients is approximately 80%, that is 20% of patients in this low-risk group still experience relapse. Moreover, without adjuvant treatment, 20% of patients with 16 or more involved axillary nodes remain disease free at 5 years. As this suggests, despite a highly statistically significant relationship with outcome, even when combined with other clinical factors, sensitivity and specificity to predict outcome, such as 5- or 10-year survival is disappointingly low. In fact, for relapse at 5 years, we estimate from the data in Figure 31.2 that node positivity has a sensitivity of less than 63%.

Standard evaluation on routine axillary node dissection involves identification and pathologic examination of at least 6 to 10 nodes from levels I-II of the axilla. Axillary dissection can be associated with significant long-term morbidity. Therefore, several investigators have conducted studies to determine whether prognostic factors could predict axillary lymph node metastases in subsets of patients with primary breast cancer, so as to spare women with low risk of nodal disease the morbidity of axillary node dissection. Ravdin et al. (24) showed that age, S-phase fraction by flow cytometry, and ER concentration, could improve on tumor size for the prediction of nodal status. Nonetheless, these factors could not identify any subset of patients with at least a 95% chance of being node negative or positive. Suffice to say in clinical practice, surgical sampling of the axilla cannot be avoided except in patients with nonextensive, pure DCIS who derive little benefit from axillary surgery because of the very low incidence of nodal involvement. The evaluation of axillary lymph node status is an established parameter in breast cancer management (category A grade of evidence).

Because of the concerns of the morbidity of axillary node dissection, minimally invasive surgery, including sentinel lymph node (SLN) biopsies, has become commonplace in clinical practice (see Chapter 41). The use of SLN biopsies is an alternative to routine axillary dissection that provides more detailed histologic evaluation of the axilla without excessively increased cost or labor. Methods of SLN biopsies include radiocolloid injection and gamma probe localization (25,26), blue dye injection and visualization (27,28), or a combination of both (29). Because of the identification of a limited number of nodes by SLN biopsies (usually one to two, rarely, three), detailed pathologic evaluation of each node is possible, however, and consequently, up-staging of patients with node-positive disease can occur. Sentinel node evaluation usually includes intraoperative touch imprint cytology and postsurgery serial sectioning of paraffin blocks and may include immunohistochemical staining for epithelial cell markers. Such detailed evaluation could theoretically improve our ability to detect micrometastatic disease in these critical nodes. Regional lymph nodes may be divided into macrometastases (>2 mm), micrometastases (0.2 to 2 mm) and isolated tumor cells (<0.2 mm). Several retrospective studies have found that prognosis of patients with micrometastases (Nmi) in sentinel nodes with other axillary lymph nodes being negative is the same as that for patients with negative nodes (30,31), whereas others have suggested that such patients have worse prognosis (32,33). In general, in population-based studies, the prognosis of micrometastasis carries a prognosis intermediate to node-negative and N1 disease (34). Based on these studies, most practice guidelines consider Nmi as a stratification factor when deciding adjuvant therapy. The results of the large cooperative group studies prospectively evaluating SLN biopsies (ACSOG Z10/Z11 and NSABP B-31) are still awaited with anticipation. Nonetheless, these new techniques may help us refine the indications for adjuvant treatment to avoid both over- and undertreatment of women with early-stage breast cancer. The evaluation and possible clinical significance of micrometastatic involvement of lymph nodes is discussed in more detail in Chapters 41 and 42.

In a similar vein, detection of micrometastases in the bone marrow has been compared with axillary node status. Some investigators have found that immunocytochemical detection of micrometastatic cells in the bone marrow is an independent prognostic risk factor in patients with node-negative breast cancer (35,36). This observation has led to a multicenter study evaluating both the role of SLN biopsies and bone marrow (BM) aspiration in women with early stage breast cancer (ACSOG Z10/Z11). See Chapter 42 for more details.

Tumor Size

After nodal status, tumor size is one of the most consistent and powerful prognostic factor for distant relapse, especially in node-negative patients. Several large studies have examined the relationship between tumor size and survival (37–42). Disease recurrence generally increases as tumor size increases. Figure 31.3 displays RFS by tumor size for the same patients used in Figure 31.2, for all patients, and for node-negative patients. After 30 years, systemically untreated patients with tumor sizes under 2 cm have a risk of distant recurrence of approximately 25% (39). Risk increases to 35% with tumors 2 to 2.9 cm, 45% with tumors 3.0 to 3.9 cm, and to greater than 50% in tumors 4.0 to 4.9 cm. Consistent with the literature, very large tumors (i.e., >5 cm) actually have a better prognosis than those between 3 and 4.9 cm. It is possible that tumors that grow to very large sizes without nodal metastases may have a lower inherent ability to metastasize.

The consideration of both tumor size and nodal status further refines the estimation of the natural course of the disease,

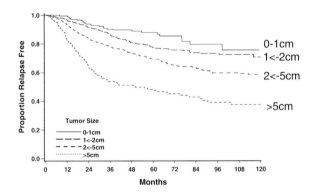

A All Patients

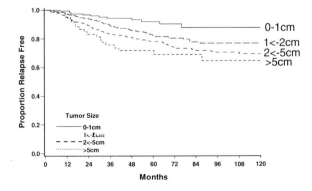

B Node-negative Patients

FIGURE 31.3. Relapse-free survival by tumor size for (**A**) both node-negative and node-positive patients (n = 2,873 patients, median follow-up of 37 months) and (**B**) node-negative patients (n = 1,613 node-negative patients, median follow-up of 43 months) (reanalysis of data presented in reference 23).

especially in node-negative breast cancer patients. To best define the category of patients who might be spared systemic treatments, studies have estimated the chance of recurrence in patients with small, node-negative tumors. Data from Memorial Sloan-Kettering Cancer Center indicate that patients with tumors less than 1 cm have a 20-year relapse rate of 12% (43). Data from large collaborative groups, such as the National Adjuvant Surgical Breast and Bowel Project (NSABP), indicate that the chance of distant metastases with tumors under 1 cm was approximately 10% (11). Even in those patients with favorable prognosis (postmenopausal, node negative disease, ER expression), several studies have shown benefit with the addition of adjuvant chemotherapy (45). The NSABP performed a retrospective analysis of more than 10,000 women, of whom 1,259 had tumors under 1 cm. The authors found that the addition of systemic therapy improved survival, regardless of ER status (44). Systemic therapy should be considered for patients with small, node-negative breast, based on the results of this study. Newer prognostic markers based on multigene assays may, however, better stratify those women with better prognosis to spare them toxic side effects of chemotherapy. In addition, as earlier detection of smaller cancers by mammography has decreased the distribution of tumor sizes at diagnosis, the natural history of these screen-detected lesions is unknown, and it is not clear that 1-cm lesions detected by imaging have the same clinical outcome as those detected by physical examination.

The evaluation of tumor size is an established parameter in breast cancer management (category A grade of evidence). In certain sized tumors (e.g., tumors <1 cm), other factors may need to be measured to refine the prognosis in these patients.

New Aspects of Tumor Staging

Because of the widespread use of screening mammography and the great heterogeneity in outcome in small cancers, new criteria apart from traditional TNM staging have been suggested. In addition, sentinel lymph node biopsies have become routine practice, and the relevance of regional lymph node metastases has fuelled the need for revision of the staging for breast cancer. Staging is presented in detail in Chapter 35. The major changes to the TNM staging are summarized below (46):

1. Micrometastases (0.2 to 2 mm) are distinguished from isolated tumor cells (<0.2 mm) on the basis of size.
2. Identifiers have been added to indicate the use of SLN dissection and immunohistochemical (IHC) or molecular techniques.
3. Major classifications of lymph node status are designated according to number of involved axillary nodes as determined by routine hematoxylin and eosin staining (preferred method) or by IHC.
4. The classification of infraclavicular node involvement has been added as N3.
5. Metastasis to internal mammary (IM) nodes has been reclassified, based on method of detection and presence or absence of axillary nodes. Microscopic involvement of IM nodes detected by SLN biopsy but not by imaging studies or clinical examination is classified as N1. Macroscopic involvement of IM nodes detected by SLN biopsy but not by imaging studies or clinical examination is classified as N2 in absence of axillary lymph node metastases, and N3 with axillary lymph node metastases.
6. Metastasis to supraclavicular nodes is classified as N3 rather than M1.

New Multiparameter Based Markers

Despite improvements in technology, complex mechanisms driving breast cancer evolution continue to present challenges

for the use of genomic approaches in the better understanding of breast and other cancers. This, combined with our use of different markers, methods, tumors (e.g., differing ER and ERBB2), and measurements of clinical outcomes impedes development of a consensus using these new technologies as predictive and prognostic markers for breast cancer. This will be discussed in greater detail in the following chapter.

Until recently, evaluations of *prognostic* and *predictive* factors have considered one factor at a time or have used small panels of markers. With the advent of new genomic technologies, such as microarrays capable of simultaneously measuring thousands of genes or gene products, we are beginning to construct molecular fingerprints of individual tumors so that accurate *prognostic* and *predictive* assessments of each cancer may be made. Clinicians may one day base clinical management on each woman's personal prognosis and predict the best individual therapies according to the genetic fingerprint of each individual cancer.

Microarrays can be used to measure the messenger RNA (mRNA) expression of thousands of genes at one time or survey genomic alterations that may distinguish molecular phenotypes associated with long-term recurrence-free survival or clinical response to treatment. These new technologies have been successfully applied to primary breast cancers, and may eventually outperform currently used clinical parameters in predicting disease outcome. At least 14 'multigene predictors' are under development for commercialization, although only 2 or 3 have reached regulatory approval or near approval (47). A study of sporadic breast tumor samples by Perou et al. (48,49) was the first to show that breast tumors could be classified into subtypes distinguished by differences in their expression profiles. Using 40 breast tumors and 20 matched pairs of samples before and after doxorubicin treatment, an "intrinsic gene set" of 476 genes were selected that were more variably expressed between the 40 sporadic tumors than between the paired samples. This intrinsic gene set was then used to cluster and segregate the tumors into four major subgroups: a "luminal cell-like" group expressing the ER, a "basal cell-like" group, an "Erb-B2 positive" group, and a "normal" epithelial group.

In a seminal study, van de Vijver et al. (50) used RNA expression microarray analyses to identify a 70-gene prognostic gene signature ("classifier") in young, untreated, axillary lymph node-negative patients using a training set of 44 good (disease-free >5 years) and 34 poor (distant relapse in <5 years) outcome tumors, and then tested the classifier in a validation set of 19 tumors. The prognostic classifier gene set correctly predicted outcome for 65 of the 78 (83%) patients, including 29 of 34 who experienced elapse, and therefore demonstrates the feasibility of using molecular profiling to predict patient outcomes. The same group (50) has now extended the study to a total of 295 young (<53 years), stage I-II breast cancer patients with both node-negative and node-positive disease, using the 70 genes classifier. The microarray-based predictions are consistent with, and perhaps better than, estimates that can be obtained with current prognostic indices. Using this 70-gene prognostic signature (Mammaprint assay) derived from frozen material, patients with early-stage, node-negative breast cancer could be segregated into groups with a different likelihood of developing distant metastasis. Gene expression profiling will be discussed in greater detail in the following chapter.

Other clinically available assays include the 21-gene Oncotype Recurrence Score (Genomic Health, Inc.). Recently, real-time reverse transcriptase-polymerase chain reaction (RT-PCR) has been shown to be able to quantify gene expression in formalin-fixed, paraffin-embedded (FFPE) tumor specimens with high reproducibility, specificity, and sensitivity. Using this technique to measure 250 candidate genes, three studies in a total of 447 patients were carried out to develop a recurrence score (RS) calculation based on a subset of 16 cancer-related and 5 reference genes. In a study conducted by the NSABP, the RS was clinically validated to prognosticate the risk of recurrence in 668 women with ER-positive, node-negative breast cancer treated with tamoxifen (51–53). A second study of 220 cases and 570 controls by others confirmed the findings of the NSABP (51–53).

Other studies indicate that patients with a high RS are most likely to derive benefit from chemotherapy (52,54,55). In one of these studies (NSABP B-20), patients (227 randomized to tamoxifen and 434 randomized to tamoxifen plus chemotherapy) were evaluated. Results demonstrated that patients with high RS and high risk of recurrence benefited most from chemotherapy, whereas patients with low RS had only minimal, if any, benefit from chemotherapy (52). Patients with intermediate scores were more problematic. Based on these and other studies, TAILORx (Trial Assigning Individualized Options for Treatment (Rx), a first-of-its-kind individualized treatment trial in the United States will utilize Oncotype DX to identify and assign treatment to more than 10,000 women from 900 sites in the United States and Canada, and will evaluate the significance of an intermediate score in more detail.

Histologic and Nuclear Grade

A number of histologic features of primary breast cancers have been shown to correlate with the risk of distant recurrence. Because of the somewhat subjective assessment, histologic grading has often been criticized for poor reproducibility and lack of agreement among different observers (56). This, together with a diversity of nonstandardized grading systems, has led to some of the difficulties in using grade as a prognostic tool. However, histologic grade when performed at single institutions by experienced pathologists does correlate well with clinical outcome (57–66). The two most widely used grading systems for breast cancer is the Scarff-Bloom-Richardson (SBR) classification (67,68), and Fisher's nuclear grading system (62), although both systems have since been modified.

The SBR grading system considers the degree of differentiation, the extent of pleomorphism, and the mitotic index, each scored from 1 to 3. *Differentiation* refers to the tumor's apparent similarity to differentiated tissues, such as tubular, glandular, and papillary formations. *Pleomorphism* refers to shape of the cell and nuclei, and higher scores are assigned to irregular cells distorted in size. The *mitotic index* assesses the number of mitoses (per high power field) in the tumor specimen, and is a reflection of the rate of proliferation of the cancer. Scores for each of these three components are summed and categorized as grade 1, grade 2, and grade 3. The Elston-Ellis–modified SBR system (MSBR) also referred to as the Nottingham Combined Histologic Grade (NCHG) omits the degree of differentiation and divides tumors into five groups according to their score. Higher grades are associated with higher rates of metastases, even at a short follow-up of 3.5 years (69).

Fisher's grading system assesses nuclear grade together with the presence of tubule or glandular formation. Nuclear grade includes nuclear size, shape, nucleolar component, chromatin pattern, and mitotic rate. After 8 years, patients who had good nuclear grade had a survival of 86% compared with those with the poorest grade who had 64% survival (70). A standardized grading system is therefore a powerful prognostic factor if reproducibility of these systems can be achieved by specific guidelines (68). Reproducibility remains a concern (71), and some evidence indicates that proliferation is the stronger of the components (72).

Several studies have also evaluated other histologic factors, such as the presence of extensive DCIS, lymphatic invasion, tumor necrosis, and inflammatory cells, and some have shown to be associated with clinical outcome. These factors have not as yet been validated. In a recent study, using paraffin sections from 177 patients, the presence of lymphovascular invasion (LVI) was significantly associated with the presence of lymph node metastasis, larger tumor size, development of distant metastasis, regional recurrence, worse disease-free interval, and overall survival. In multivariate analysis, LVI retained significant association with decreased disease-free interval and overall survival (73).

The most widely used grading system is the modified SBR or NCHG classification, which is also itself a component of the Nottingham prognostic index. The CAP recommends that all invasive breast cancers, except medullary carcinomas, be graded. The NCHG (74) is the grading system of choice, and recent publications have indeed confirmed that NCHG is an independent prognostic factor (75,76). Based on evidence, histologic grade and NCHG, in particular, is a category A factor, which should be documented in all breast cancers.

Histologic Subtypes

Most (80% to 90%) primary breast cancers are infiltrating ductal carcinoma of *no special type* (NST). Recognizable subtypes exist that carry different prognoses, however. Inflammatory breast cancer (see Chapter 62), a distinct form of invasive breast cancer, is a clinical entity characterized by rapid onset of skin edema and erythema, generalized breast enlargement typically without a dominant mass, and extremely poor prognosis as hallmarks of this disease (77). These cancers are uncommon, and account for approximately 2% of all breast cancers annually (78). Until the advent of systemic therapy, this disease was almost universally fatal. The median 5-year survival in most studies in patients with inflammatory breast cancer with local therapy alone was less than 5%, with a median survival of only 12 to 36 months (79).

Another distinct subtype of breast cancer is invasive lobular carcinoma (ILC), which comprises approximately 10% of breast cancers and appears to have a distinct biology. A large retrospective study of more than 4,000 patients with ILC identified that these tumors were more likely to occur in older patients; to be larger in size; to be ER or PR positive; to be associated with lower S-phase fraction; and to be ERBB2, p53, and epidermal growth factor receptor negative (80).

Conversely, "special" histologic types (pure papillary, tubular and mucinous) identify a small subset of patients who have a better prognosis compared with infiltrating ductal carcinomas of no special type (1,81). Node-negative tumors less than 3 cm that are pure papillary, mucinous, or tubular have a long-term risk of recurrence of under 10% (1). Medullary cancers have a better prognosis than other infiltrating ductal carcinomas (82), but may not have the same excellent prognosis as the other special type histologies. Despite some reproducibility issues, subtyping of invasive cancers is recommended as a category A factor.

Patient Characteristics

Age and Menopausal Status

Older postmenopausal women with cancer have increasing concentrations of ER in the tumor, and their cancers are generally better differentiated and with lower proliferation rates. As such, prognosis in these women is significantly improved. On the other hand, young onset breast cancers, in women under the age of 35 years, have worse clinical outcome compared with older women (83,84). In two separate studies (84,85), breast cancers in young women were associated with higher prevalence of adverse histologic features (e.g., poor differentiation, lymphatic invasion, extensive intraductal component). In addition, increasing tumor size, node involvement, ER negativity, high proliferation as measured by S-phase fraction, and p53 abnormalities were more common in women 30 to 35 years and younger. Following multivariate analysis to adjust for other prognostic factors, both studies concluded, however, that young age remained a significant predictor of recurrence and death. (See Chapters 91 and 92 for more detailed discussion s of breast cancers in younger and older women.)

Racial Background and Ethnicity

In the United States, survival is worse in black patients and, to a lesser extent, in Hispanic patients, compared with white patients (86). Patients who are black or Hispanic present with more advanced disease (larger tumors, node positivity), and their tumors display features of aggressive tumor biology (steroid hormone receptor negative, and higher proliferation indices) (86). Elledge et al. (86) compared several prognostic factors among 4,885 white, 1,016 black, and 777 Hispanic women. White women were older, presented with smaller tumors, had less lymph node involvement, had higher steroid hormone positivity, and lower S-phase fractions when compared with black or Hispanic women. No clinically significant differences were noted in histologic subtype, ploidy, HRBB2, and p53 expression. After adjustment for these other prognostic factors, being of black race or ethnicity independently predicted for poorer survival. More recently, a similar analysis using data from registries from six integrated health care system confirmed that adjustment for age at diagnosis, stage, grade, tumor size, receptor status, and treatment did not eliminate disparities in survival for black women with breast cancer, compared with white women (87). A pooled analysis of two metastatic CALGB studies, where treatment and eligibility are controlled, found that blacks had decreased overall survival, but no increase in time to treatment failure or overall response to therapy, suggesting that other factors, such as comorbid conditions or subsequent therapies also play a role (88). Although race and ethnicity, perhaps through socioeconomic disparities, is associated with differences in stage at presentation, and may also contribute to inherent differences in tumor biology.

Proliferation Indices

The ability of cancer cells to divide and replicate is the basis of the continued expansion of tumors. There are many different techniques for evaluating the rate of cell proliferation: mitotic index, thymidine labeling index (TLI), S-phase fraction (SPF) by flow cytometry, BrdU index, and immunohistochemistry using antibodies against specific cell cycle antigens (Ki67/Mib1, Ki-S5, Ki-S11), proliferating cell nuclear antigen (PCNA), topoisomerase II alpha (Ki-S1), various cyclins, and mitosin. Of these, mitotic index, SPF and IHC using Ki-67 and MIB-1 are the best characterized. The prognostic significance of cyclins has also been described in node-negative patients (89–91).

Mitotic Index

The oldest method for quantitating proliferation is by counting the number of mitotic bodies by light microscopy on hematoxylin and eosin (H&E) stained, paraffin-embedded tumor specimens. The mitotic index (MI) is generally expressed as the number of mitotic bodies per high-powered field. Few studies have validated this approach in assessing clinical outcome, and these indicate that higher mitotic rates are associated with increased mortality (92,93). Most of these studies report a 1.5- to 3-fold increased risk of recurrence with high MI. Other indices, such as the Nottingham prognostic index (94) and the Multivariate Prognostic Index (95), include the MI together with other prognostic factors (e.g., tumor size and axillary lymph node status). A prospective study on the reproducibility of the MI that included 2,469 patients and 14 pathology laboratories

throughout The Netherlands, found correlation coefficients ranging from 0.91 to 0.97 (mean 0.95), with consistency over time (96). The prognostic significance of MI was prospectively validated in a 516-patient study where high MI was associated with a 3- to 4-fold higher risk of recurrence and death (97). These results were confirmed in another large prospective study involving more than 800 patients (98). Although the methods of calculating MI and the cut-off to define high and low MI varies, MI appears to be a simple and cost effective method for measuring proliferation rate (75,99).

Thymidine Labeling Index

The TLI is assessed by counting the number of labeled nuclei on autoradiographed microsections after incubation of the fresh tumor specimen with tritiated thymidine. TLI measures the number of cells synthesizing DNA during the incubation and, therefore, provides an estimate of the proportion of cells in the S and G2/M phases of the cell cycle. TLI assays are not routinely available or standardized, and the counting of individualized labeled nuclei is labor intensive.

As a prognostic indicator, several studies have shown improved survival in node-negative breast cancer patients with slow proliferating tumors (100–106). In most of these studies on multivariate analysis, the relative risk of relapse in fast compared with slow proliferating tumors was approximately twofold.

S-Phase Fraction by Flow Cytometry

The SPF is a measure of cells in the S phase of the cell cycle, undergoing DNA synthesis. It is based on estimating the proportion of cells with partially replicated DNA (i.e., cells with more DNA than the normal amount in a cell in G_1 and less than double the normal amount, as is seen in G_2/M phases of the cell cycle). SPF is generally measured on fresh tissue or frozen samples by DNA flow cytometry. In addition to the measurements of the fraction of cells in the S-phase of the cell cycle, DNA flow cytometry also assesses the DNA content of cells. The cancer cells are defined as diploid if they have the same amount of DNA as normal cells, and aneuploid if the DNA content is greater or less than normal cells.

As a prognostic indicator, solid evidence exists for a positive correlation between poor outcome and high SPF in both node-positive and node-negative patients. Figure 31.4 displays relapse-free survival by S-phase fraction for the same patients used in Figure 31.2, for all patients, and for node-negative patients. A consensus panel in 1993 reviewed 43 of the published papers and concluded the utility of SPF in predicting recurrence and mortality (107).

Strong correlations between high SPF and other adverse prognostic factors have been reported. In a review of assay results from more than 127,000 patients, Wenger et al. (108) reported correlations between SPF and DNA ploidy, steroid hormone receptor status, number of positive axillary lymph nodes, tumor size, and age.

In a prospective clinical trial of node-negative breast cancer patients, the Intergroup Trial 0102 evaluated tumor size, receptor status, and SPF, and followed low-risk, node-negative patients (tumors <2 cm, receptor-positive, low SPF) without adjuvant treatment. These low-risk patients had good clinical outcome without systemic treatment, thus validating the use of these markers in evaluating prognosis in this small subset of patients (109).

The clinical use of SPF as a prognostic factor has been limited, however, because of the lack of standardization and quality control (108). Other limitations include the inclusion of stroma, which produces difficulty in interpretation if the tumor is diploid as both the normal and cancer cell populations overlap on the

A   All Patients

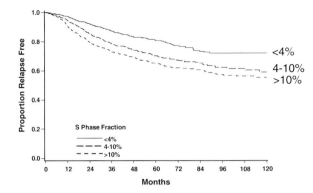

B   Node-negative Patients

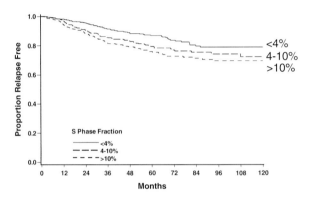

FIGURE 31.4.   Relapse-free survival by S phase fraction for (**A**) both node-negative and node-positive patients (n = 2,873 patients, median follow-up of 37 months) and (**B**) node-negative patients (n = 1,613 node-negative patients, median follow-up of 43 months) (reanalysis of data presented in reference 23).

DNA histogram (110). In addition, widespread routine clinical use has been limited by cost and the requirement for fresh or frozen tissue.

Ki67 (Mib1) by Immunohistochemistry

Monoclonal Ki67 is an antibody specific for a nuclear antigen expressed in proliferating cells (late G_1, S, M, G_2 phases of the cell cycle) (111). The function of the protein(s) detected by the Ki67 antibody remains unknown, although the gene (gene symbol = MKI67) is now known to be located on chromosome 10q25-qter (112). The original antibody was only useful on fresh or frozen tissue. Newer antibodies (Mib1 and polyclonal Ki67) have been developed that recognize peptides from recombinant fragments of the Ki67 antigen, and are effective in fixed, paraffin-embedded archival tissue (113,114). The distinction between low and high proliferation is subtle and assessment is generally quantitative rather than semiquantitative, requiring point counting to assess the percent of cells with nuclear staining for Ki67 or Mib1 (115).

Both Ki67 and Mib1 have been evaluated as a prognostic factor in several studies, and high proliferation, as measured by this methodology, is correlated with poor clinical outcome in most studies on univariate analysis (115–125). Conclusions in some studies, for both node-negative and node-positive patients, have been clouded by adjuvant treatments, and by

relatively short duration of follow-up. Brown et al. (115) examined 673 patients with a median follow-up of 52 months, and found, on multivariate analysis, that high Ki67 was an independent prognostic factor. High Ki67 is also correlated with other adverse prognostic factors, such as tumor size, node involvement, histologic grade, and vascular invasion, and it is inversely correlated with good factors such as steroid receptors (118,126,127). The advantages of this assay are lower cost, easy handling of fixed slides, and relative specificity for cells in S/G2/M phases of the cell cycle. A recent meta-analysis evaluating the impact of Ki-67/MIB-1 on survival was conducted. In a total of 12,000 patients assessed, Ki-67/MIB-1 positivity was associated with higher probability of relapse in all patients in both node-negative (hazard ratio [HR] = 1.93; $p < .001$), and node-positive patients (HR = 1.59; $p < .001$), and with worse survival in all patients (HR = 1.95; $p < .001$) (128).

In summary, proliferation indices are useful prognostic markers. SPF on frozen material is the most validated technique and is recommended as a category A factor. MI and Ki67/Mib1 by IHC are not as thoroughly validated, but can be performed on archival paraffin material and are classified as category B factors. The ASCO update did not find sufficient supportive data to recommend IHC-based markers of proliferation for use in determining prognosis in routine clinical practice (9).

Proliferation indices may also be helpful predictive markers of response to chemotherapy, possibly because DNA replication is the target of many chemotherapeutic agents. Remvikos et al. (129) reported higher tumor responsiveness to neoadjuvant chemotherapy in patients with high SPF. High SPF was not confirmed to be of predictive value for adjuvant cyclophosphamide, methotrexate, 5FU (CMF) in one study of node-negative patients (130), although two recent randomized, prospective studies do indicate the value of such measurements in prediction of response to adjuvant chemotherapy in node-negative breast cancer patients (131,132). Therefore, the utility of proliferative indices as predictive markers remain speculative, and are classified as category C.

Other Proliferation Markers: Cyclins

Each phase in the cell cycle is regulated by specific cyclin and cyclin-dependent kinase (Cdk) complexes. This is summarized in Figure 31.5. Intact cyclin E protein has been measured by IHC in formalin-fixed paraffin-embedded tissue, and mRNA for cyclin E has been quantitated by RT-PCR in fresh frozen specimens. Low molecular weight (LMW) forms of cyclin E have been measured by Western blot analysis of proteins in fresh frozen tissue. Discordance in the prognostic value of cyclin E between IHC and Western blot analysis may be related to the antibodies used for each assay, given that the reagents that detect intact cyclin E may not react with the LMW fragments. Even when antibodies recognize the intact protein and its fragments,

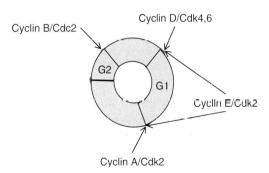

FIGURE 31.5. Regulation of cell cycle by cyclin-dependent kinases. Entry into mitosis is regulated by cyclin B/Cdc2 complex, passage through the restriction point is regulated by the cyclin D/Cdk4,6 complexes and cyclin E/Cdk2 complex. Both cyclin E/Cdk2 and cyclin A/Cdk2 regulate entry into S phase.

however, discordance between IHC and Western blot analysis has been observed in 37% of cases (89,90). In a single study, dramatic results regarding use of cyclin E and outcome were reported. In this single-institution, retrospective study using archived frozen specimens analyzed by Western blot assay, the hazard ratio for death from breast cancer for patients with high total cyclin E levels, as compared with those with low total cyclin E levels on Western blot analysis, was 13.3—about eight times as high as the hazard ratios associated with other independent clinical and pathologic risk factors. Although promising, these data are from a retrospective study, and additional properly designed studies are required to ascertain whether this marker has clinical utility, especially in the setting of no adjuvant chemotherapy.

In a recent meta-analysis of cyclin E overexpression of 2,534 patients in 12 published studies, overexpression of cyclin E was associated with a 2.32-fold (95% confidence interval [CI], 1.25- to 4.30-fold) increased risk of recurrence in univariate analysis and a 1.72 fold (95% CI, 0.95- to 3.10-fold) risk of recurrence in multivariate analysis (133). In addition, the combined hazard ratio estimate for overall survival and breast cancer-specific survival was 2.98 (95% CI, 1.85–4.78) and 2.86 (95% CI, 1.85 4.41) in univariate and multivariate analysis, respectively. In a recently published paper in which all patients received one of two regimens of adjuvant doxorubicin and cyclophosphamide in a prospective Southwest Oncology Group randomized clinical trial (SWOG 9313), cyclin E overexpression, as determined by IHC for the full-length protein, was not associated with a worse outcome (134). The negative results of this study must be considered carefully because all of these patients received chemotherapy and the assay was not specific for cyclin E fragments. Cyclin E might be correlated with response to chemotherapy, thereby obscuring its prognostic significance in treated patients.

Overall, the evidence for use of cyclins in clinical management is as yet limited. Cyclins may be important biologic factors, but these studies will require confirmation to whether they are prognostic of outcome, or predictive of response to adjuvant treatment in the clinic.

Steroid Hormone Receptors

The steroid receptors, estrogen receptor (ERα and ERβ, two distinct genes jointly referred as ER) and progesterone receptor (PRa and PRb, two isoforms jointly referred as PR) have established usefulness in the clinical management of women with breast cancer. The prognostic significance of ER was first reported in 1977, and larger studies have confirmed that patients with ER-positive disease have better disease-free survival than ER-negative patients, especially in the short term. As the time of follow-up increases, the prognostic advantage of ER positivity disappears (23,135,136), suggesting that ER expression may be a marker of slower growth rate rather than lower intrinsic metastatic potential. The main utility of these factors is in deciding who should receive hormonal therapy or not. Indeed, ER is the poster-child of predictive markers. Its absence predicts for lack of response to hormonal therapy in advanced breast cancer, as well as in the neoadjuvant and adjuvant settings. Most studies indicate a 50% to 60% response to first-line hormonal therapy in ER-positive tumors, whereas at most only 5% to 10% of ER-negative tumors benefit. Results are similar in neoadjuvant trials of letrozole (12). It is likely that the overall response of a tumor cell is the result of the combined interplay of signaling pathways mediated by both ER proteins, their isoforms, and their coactivators and corepressors (137). A variety of clinical assays are in common use, which may or may not distinguish among ER genes or PR isoforms, possibly accounting for some of the discrepancies between studies. The structure and function of these receptors,

assay methodology for assessing expression, and their clinical utility are discussed in detail in Chapter 29.

In summary, ER is a category B prognostic factor, and a category A predictive factor of response to endocrine therapy. The 2007 ASCO Update (9) continues to recommend that ER and PgR should be measured on every invasive breast cancer and may be remeasured on metastatic lesions if results will alter therapy. ER and probably PgR content are modestly associated with a favorable prognosis and, more importantly, highly predictive of benefit from endocrine treatment in both the adjuvant and metastatic settings. Deficiencies in standardization for ER and PgR reproducibility and accuracy for particular reagents as an important priority.

Growth Factor Receptors

The type I growth factor receptors include the Erb-B (HER) receptor family which consists of four transmembrane tyrosine kinases: Erb-B1 epidermal growth factor receptor (EGFR, HER1), Erb-B2/*neu* (HER2), Erb-B3 (HERBB3), and Erb-B4 (HERBB4). The extracellular domains of Erb-B1, Erb-B3, and Erb-B4 interact with a specific set of ligands, whereas no ligand has been identified thus far for the Erb-B2 receptor. Nonetheless, Erb-B2 can be activated by any of the other ligand activated Erb-B coreceptors. On ligand binding to the active domain of Erb-B1, Erb-B3, or Erb-B4, these receptors preferentially recruit Erb-B2 into a heterodimeric complex in which the Erb-B2 kinase can modulate receptor internalization and prolong signal transduction to potent cell proliferation and survival pathways.

Epidermal Growth Factor Receptor

Epidermal growth factor receptor (gene symbol = EGFR) is a 170-kDa transmembrane glycoprotein; it is expressed or overexpressed in many human solid tumors and plays an important role in progression to invasion and metastases. The tyrosine kinase function of the EGFR is activated by binding of a variety of ligands to the external domain. The ligand bound EGFR phosphorylates itself (autophosphorylation), initiating a signaling cascade that feeds downstream cell cycle control machinery regulating cell proliferation. These reactions are a major component in growth factor-induced proliferation of cancer cells.

The EGFR is expressed in normal ductal epithelium and other tissues, and is critical for normal breast development. It is expressed at low levels in 15% to 50% of human breast cancers, depending on assay sensitivity. A number of studies with varying sizes and patient characteristics have examined the prognostic significance of EGFR. These have been summarized in several reviews, with more than 3,000 patients (138,139). Most of these studies show a significant relationship between higher EGFR and poor clinical outcomes, with both shorter disease-free or overall survival on univariate analysis. Some of these studies have been confounded by intervening treatments, inclusion of both node-positive and node-negative patients, and lack of multivariate analysis. The prognostic and predictive value of EGFR is therefore unclear and this factor is considered category C at present.

A more exciting development for this biologic factor is its potential use as a target for new therapies. Several monoclonal antibodies and small molecules have been developed and are being tested for women with metastatic breast cancer (140–142). The utility of these targeted agents, either as single agents or in combination with hormonal therapies, is currently under investigation and is discussed in more detail in Chapter 79. If the therapies prove successful, measurement of this factor may be important in determining that the target is present and the patient is a candidate for therapy.

ERBB2

The proto-oncogene Erb-B2 (ERBB2, c-erbB-2, gene symbol= ERBB2) has been localized to chromosome 17q21.1 and encodes a 185 kDa transmembrane tyrosine kinase growth factor receptor. This important biologic marker is discussed in detail in Chapters 30, 51, and 75.

The greatest utility for ERBB2 testing is to predict the response to the recombinant DNA-derived humanized monoclonal antibody to the HRBB2 receptor, trastuzumab (Herceptin). Prospective randomized clinical trials have demonstrated that trastuzumab improves response rates, time to disease progression, and overall survival when combined with chemotherapy compared with chemotherapy alone in the metastatic setting (143). Eligibility for all of these trials was based on ERBB2 positivity, either by IHC or fluorescence *in situ* hybridization (FISH). In 2005, the results of five prospective adjuvant trials evaluating trastuzumab, involving more than 10,000 women, were presented (144,145). Despite differences in study design and short follow-ups of only 1 to 2 years, these studies show the same remarkable results—adjuvant trastuzumab therapy halves the recurrence rate and reduces mortality by 30% in patients whose tumors overexpress ERBB2. This benefit, on average, is greater than that of adjuvant chemotherapy and similar to that seen with adjuvant hormonal therapy.

ERBB2 is a category A predictive factor of response to ERBB2-targeted therapy and it should be measured on every invasive breast cancer and may be remeasured on metastatic lesions if results will alter therapy (9). Use for other clinical purposes is less clear. Despite attempts within the international pathology community to improve the status of ERBB2 testing in routine practice, testing inaccuracy remains a major issue with both IHC and FISH. Therefore, the ASCO and the CAP have established recommendations regarding ERBB2 testing in breast cancer as follows: a positive ERBB2 result is IHC staining of 3+ (uniform, intense membrane staining of >30% of invasive tumor cells), a FISH result of more than six gene copies per nucleus or a FISH ratio (*ERBB2* gene signals to chromosome 17 signals) of more than 2.2; a negative result is an IHC staining of 0 or 1+, a FISH result of less than 4.0 *ERBB2* gene copies per nucleus, or FISH ratio of less than 1.8 (146). Interpretation of equivocal ERBB2 test results remain problematic, however, and in these poorly studied subgroups, the value of trastuzumab is uncertain.

Topoisomerase IIα

Several groups have evaluated the abnormalities (amplification and deletion) of topoisomerase IIα (TOP2A), which is located on the same amplicon on chromosome 17 as ERBB2. Anthracyclines directly bind TOP2A and function, at least in part, by inhibiting its activity in DNA replication, therefore making it a potential marker for anthracycline activity. In preclinical studies, TOP2A may increase sensitivity to anthracyclines but relative resistance to alkylating agents (147,148). Some clinical cohorts have been evaluated for TOP2A amplification and the results generally support this explanation for altered sensitivity to anthracyclines in ERBB2-amplified breast tumors, but other studies do not confirm these findings (147,148).

In a recent paper, Slamon et al. (149) suggested that alteration of topo II was associated with responsiveness to anthracyclines. Retrospectively, two large adjuvant clinical trials, the BCIRG 005 (ERBB2-negative) and 006 (ERBB2-positive) trials, were evaluated for TOP2A amplification by FISH. None of these ERBB2-negative cancers in the BCIRG 005 trial involving more than 1,600 patients revealed TOP2A amplification. In contrast, BCIRG 006 which randomized 3,222 ERBB2-positive patients to doxorubicin or cyclophosphamide followed by docetaxel (AC-T), to AC-T plus trastuzumab (AC-TH), or to an experimental non–anthracycline-based regimen of docetaxel, carboplatin, and trastuzumab (TCH). Topo IIα was found to be coamplified with ERBB2 in 35% of cases. Preliminary results suggest patients with TOP2A overexpression had better disease-free survival after adjuvant therapy with trastuzumab and an anthracycline-containing combination (149). These studies are preliminary and would require further validation.

Plasminogen Activators and Inhibitors

Aside from the hormone receptors and growth factor receptors, molecular markers in the uPA system are perhaps the most extensively studied biologic markers in breast cancer. Urokinase plasminogen activator (uPA; gene symbol = PLAU), as with tissue plasminogen activator (tPA; gene symbol = PLAT), is a member of the serine protease family of proteins. When activated by plasmin, uPA can degrade various components of the extra-cellular matrix and is thus thought to promote tumor growth, invasion, and metastasis of breast cancer as well as other cancers (150). Other components of the system include the urokinase receptor, uPAR (gene symbol = PLAUR) and the inhibitors, PAI-1 and PAI-2. uPAR is a three-domain glycosylated cell surface protein that occurs on macrophages in tumor stroma as well as tumor cells, and is also found in plasma and tumor extracts as soluble full-length suPAR or as one or two domain fragments (151). PAI-1 (gene symbol = SERPINE1) and PAI-2 (gene symbol = SERPINB2) are members of a large family of serine protease inhibitors. PAI-1 is the primary inhibitor of both tPA and uPA and exists in several conformations, in which different epitopes are accessible to antibody-based detection systems. Activation of pro-uPA is rapidly followed by formation of the inactive uPA:PAI-1 complex. When complexed to receptor-bound uPA, the entire complex may be internalized and processed for degradation or recycling of components. PAI-2 is not detectable in normal plasma; it increases with pregnancy and is found in tumor extracts and plasma from cancer patients, although plasma and tumor levels of the various components are not correlated (152). PAI-2 reacts with, and inactivates, both free and receptor bound uPA. Quantitative characterization of the uPA system is thus complicated by the complex nature of the interplay of the components, by the interplay between tumor, stroma, and plasma, and by the diversity of accessible epitopes, which depend on activation state, binding to receptors or inhibitors, and cleavage products.

Most published studies of uPA and PAI-1 have used assay methods that require fresh frozen tissue. This is a significant logistic deterrent to use in the United States, now that frozen tissue is no longer required for assessment of hormone receptors. Attempts to use IHC methods to assess uPA and PAI-1 expression are qualitatively consistent with, but weaker than, results presented from enzyme-linked immunosorbent assay (ELISA), and the methods are not interchangeable (153). Results for uPAR and PAI-2 have been less clear cut and more dependent on the exact detection methods used. It has been suggested that mRNA levels of uPA system components are also associated with prognosis, although the relationship is weaker than that detected by protein assays and the correlation between mRNA and protein is weak (154–157).

Most retrospective studies of the prognostic value of the uPA system have used ELISA methods, in some cases focusing on detection of bound components of the uPA:PAI-1 complex. Despite differences in detection antibodies and extraction methods, most studies have consistently shown a strong relationship (hazard ratios range from 2 to 4) between high uPA and high PAI-1 expression in tumor extracts and poorer disease-free and overall survival. This result was confirmed in a pooled analysis of data on 8,377 breast cancers (158) from 17 different datasets. Figure 31.6 clearly shows that after accounting for other standard prognostic factors, patients in the highest

Node-negative

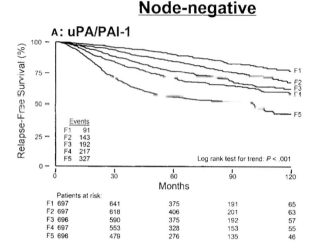

Node-positive

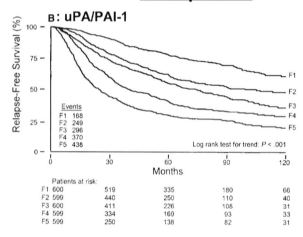

FIGURE 31.6. Relapse-free survival (**A** and **B**) probabilities as a function of categorized prognostic scores in lymph node-negative (**A**) and lymph node-positive (**B**) breast cancer patients. Groups (F1-F5) represent quintiles of prognostic scores owing to uPA and PAI-1 in a stratified multivariate model that included tumor size, nodes (in node-positive subset), estrogen receptor (ER), age, menopausal status, and grade. (From Look MP, van Putten WL, Duffy MJ, et al. Pooled analysis of prognostic impact of urokinase-type plasminogen activator and its inhibitor PAI-1 in 8377 breast cancer patients. *J Natl Cancer Inst* 2002;94: 116–128, with permission.)

quintiles of expression of uPA and PAI-1 have the poorest relapse-free and overall survival. A recent review confirms the clinical utility of the combination of high uPA and PAI-1 as a prognostic indicator of poor prognosis (159). The association with benefit from systemic therapy is less clear, but it is hoped will be better elucidated by ongoing studies in high risk node-negative breast cancer.

The combination of uPA and PAI-1 fulfill the criteria for a category A prognostic marker. Further, it is recommended that expression be assessed by a standardized ELISA kit. These ELISA techniques require fresh or frozen tissue, which has limited the utility of this prognostic marker.

Markers Regulating Cell Cycle and Cell Death

Tumor Suppressor Gene, p53

The p53 gene (gene symbol = TP53) is located on chromosome 17p13 and encodes a 53-kDa nuclear phosphoprotein that plays an essential role in regulation of the cell cycle, especially transition from resting G_0 to active proliferation in G_1 and in DNA repair. Lee and Bernstein (160) suggested that wild-type P53 may serve as a "guardian of the genome," preventing proliferation of a cell that has sustained genetic damage. Unphosphorylated p53 is thought to bind to DNA as a tetramer at p53-binding sites to upregulate genes that inhibit growth and invasion. Loss of functional p53 protein expression or phosphorylation and consequent increased degradation results in decreased expression of the growth inhibitory genes. Alterations in this gene are the most frequent genetic changes reported in many cancers, including breast cancer (161) with nearly a third of all breast cancers with mutation of the p53 gene (162,163).

Techniques to measure p53 overexpression or mutation include IHC, PCR-based amplification using single strand conformation polymorphism assays (SSCP), and sequencing, with IHC being the most commonly used. Wild-type p53 protein has a very short half-life and should, in theory, not be detected by IHC, whereas mutated p53 is stabilized and should be detectable. Nonetheless, IHC can also identify stabilized wild type, and point mutations in p53 detected by sequencing may not correlate with p53 protein accumulation.

As reviewed by Elledge and Allred (164), p53 overexpression is modestly associated with worse clinical outcome in node-negative patients who have not received systemic treatment. Differences in techniques with at least 13 different monoclonal antibodies available, study design, and a variety of treatments have resulted in inconsistent results on the prognostic significance of p53. p53 as a prognostic marker is therefore classified as category C.

As a predictive marker, p53 has been shown to predict for responsiveness to CMF-based chemotherapy in some studies (165,166), but not all (167). Thor et al. (168) reported that p53 and *cerb*B-2 overexpression might be associated with increased survival after high dose CAF chemotherapy. Overall, the lack of consensus on the best methodology to assess p53, conflicting or only modestly predictive effects, and the presence of other more useful prognostic and predictive markers has reduced interest in use of p53 in routine clinical practice.

BCL2 Family Members

A number of members of the BCL2 family such as BCL2, BAX, BAD, and BCL2L1 (also known as bclx$_s$ and bclx$_l$) form hetero- or homodimers and act in concert as anti- or proapoptotic regulators. BCL2 is a mitochondrial membrane protein that blocks the apoptotic death of some cells, whereas overexpression of BCL2 is associated with resistance to apoptosis (169). However, in breast cancer, BCL2 is regulated by ER. BCL2 overexpression is associated with markers of differentiation, such ER, low proliferation, and lack of p53 accumulation, and has been associated, at least weakly, with good prognosis and improved outcomes (170–172). Daidone et al. (170) have conducted a large review representing 5,000 patients of several different types. They found that the prognostic value of BCL2 in systemically untreated patients with early-stage disease was weakly positive but disappeared on multivariate analysis, whereas in about a third of studies of endocrine- or chemotherapy-treated patients, BCL2 overexpression remained weakly but significantly predictive of better outcome. Interestingly, low BCL2 expression or high BAX (a proapoptotic antagonist of BCL2) expression was predictive of longer local RFS following radiation therapy. Compared with BCL2, much less is known about the potential prognostic or predictive effects of overexpression of other BCL2 family members (171). Given the complexity of this family of genes and their protein products, it may be that the balance of their ratios, rather than absolute levels of expression, is important in prognosis and prediction of response, although studies to date have yielded conflicting results. The evaluation of these genes is currently considered investigational and should be classified as category C.

OTHER FACTORS

Many other biologic markers have been evaluated for potential clinical utility. These include many other markers of proliferation, such as proliferating cell nuclear antigen (PCNA) and mitosin (component of the nuclear matrix during the G_2 the may play a role in chromosome segregation), estrogen-regulated proteins like pS2 (trefoil factor 1) and several of the heat shock proteins (HSP), as well as markers of angiogenesis, apoptosis, and markers of invasiveness such as cathepsin D. Although hundreds of publications and reviews have been written on these factors, and there is no doubt important biologic insight to be gleaned, they have not emerged to be clinically useful.

SUMMARY OF BIOLOGIC FACTORS

The prognosis of women with breast cancer is currently estimated based on the established prognostic markers, in particular nodal status, tumor size, histologic grade and subtype, and the rate of proliferation. The promise of other molecular and biologic markers such as p53, cathepsin D, and angiogenic factors has yet to be fulfilled, however. Comprehensive, genomic-wide approaches are being used to identify clinically useful genetic profiles that will accurately predict outcome and prognosis of patients with breast cancer. Despite improvements in technology, complex mechanisms driving breast cancer evolution continue to present challenges for the use of genomic approaches in the better understanding of breast and other cancers. This, combined with our use of different markers, methods, tumors (i.e., differing ER, ERBB2, and p53 status), and measurements of clinical outcomes impedes development of a consensus regarding predictive and prognostic markers for breast cancer. Future research should incorporate rigorous analytic methods and, ideally, new markers should be tested in the context of prospective clinical trials.

References

1. Diab SG, Clark GM, Osborne CK, et al. Tumor characteristics and clinical outcome of tubular and mucinous breast carcinomas. *J Clin Oncol* 1999;17:1442–1448.
2. Allred DC, Clark GM, Tandon AK, et al. HER-2/neu in node-negative breast cancer: prognostic significance of overexpression influenced by the presence of in situ carcinoma. *J Clin Oncol* 1992;10:599–605.
3. Tandon AK, Clark GM, Chamness GC, et al. HER-2/neu oncogene protein and prognosis in breast cancer. *J Clin Oncol* 1989;7:1120–1128.
4. Consensus conference. Adjuvant chemotherapy for breast cancer. *JAMA* 1985; 254:3461–3463.
5. Systemic treatment of early breast cancer by hormonal, cytotoxic, or immune therapy. 133 randomised trials involving 31,000 recurrences and 24,000 deaths among 75,000 women. Early Breast Cancer Trialists' Collaborative Group. *Lancet* 1992;339:1–15.
6. NIH Consensus Development Conference on the Treatment of Early-Stage Breast Cancer. Bethesda, Maryland, June 18–21, 1990. *J Natl Cancer Inst Monogr* 1992: 1–187.
7. Hammond ME, Fitzgibbons PL, Compton CC, et al. College of American Pathologists Conference XXXV: solid tumor prognostic factors-which, how and so what? Summary document and recommendations for implementation. Cancer Committee and Conference Participants. *Arch Pathol Lab Med* 2000;124:958–965.
8. Bast RC, Jr., Ravdin P, Hayes DF, et al. 2000 update of recommendations for the use of tumor markers in breast and colorectal cancer: clinical practice guidelines of the American Society of Clinical Oncology. *J Clin Oncol* 2001;19:1865–1878.
9. Harris L, Fritsche H, Mennel R, et al. American Society of Clinical Oncology 2007 update of recommendations for the use of tumor markers in breast cancer. *J Clin Oncol* 2007;25:5287–5312.
10. Clark GM. Interpreting and integrating risk factors for patients with primary breast cancer. *J Natl Cancer Inst Monogr* 2001:17–21.
11. Hayes DF, Trock B, Harris AL. Assessing the clinical impact of prognostic factors: when is "statistically significant" clinically useful? *Breast Cancer Res Treat* 1998;52:305–319.
12. Ellis MJ, Coop A, Singh B, et al. Letrozole is more effective neoadjuvant endocrine therapy than tamoxifen for ErbB-1- and/or ErbB-2-positive, estrogen receptor-positive primary breast cancer: evidence from a phase III randomized trial. *J Clin Oncol* 2001;19:3808–3816.
13. McGuire WL. Breast cancer prognostic factors: evaluation guidelines. *J Natl Cancer Inst* 1991;83:154–155.
14. Simon R, Altman DG. Statistical aspects of prognostic factor studies in oncology. *Br J Cancer* 1994;69:979–985.
15. Hayes DF, Bast RC, Desch CE, et al. Tumor marker utility grading system: a framework to evaluate clinical utility of tumor markers. *J Natl Cancer Inst* 1996; 88:1456–1466.
16. Altman DG, Lyman GH. Methodological challenges in the evaluation of prognostic factors in breast cancer. *Breast Cancer Res Treat* 1998;52:289–303.
17. Schmoor C, Sauerbrei W, Schumacher M. Sample size considerations for the evaluation of prognostic factors in survival analysis. *Stat Med* 2000;19:441–452.
18. McShane LM, Altman DG, Sauerbrei W, et al. Reporting recommendations for tumor marker prognostic studies (REMARK). *J Natl Cancer Inst* 2005;97:1180–1184.
19. Sargent DJ, Conley BA, Allegra C, et al. Clinical trial designs for predictive marker validation in cancer treatment trials. *J Clin Oncol* 2005;23:2020–2027.
20. Jiang W, Freidlin B, Simon R. Biomarker-adaptive threshold design: a procedure for evaluating treatment with possible biomarker-defined subset effect. *J Natl Cancer Inst* 2007;99:1036–1043.
21. Goldbloom R, Battista WA. The periodic health examination:introduction. *CMAJ* 1986;134:721–723.
22. Harris RP, Helfand M, Woolf SH, et al. Current methods of the U.S. Preventive Services Task Force: a review of the process. *Am J Prev Med* 2001;20:21–35.
23. Hilsenbeck SG, Ravdin PM, de Moor CA, et al. Time-dependence of hazard ratios for prognostic factors in primary breast cancer. *Breast Cancer Res Treat* 1998; 52:227–237.
24. Ravdin PM, De Laurentiis M, Vendely T, et al. Prediction of axillary lymph node status in breast cancer patients by use of prognostic indicators. *J Natl Cancer Inst* 1994;86:1771–1775.
25. Krag D, Harlow S, Weaver D, et al. Technique of sentinel node resection in melanoma and breast cancer: probe-guided surgery and lymphatic mapping. *Eur J Surg Oncol* 1998;24:89–93.
26. Krag DN, Weaver DL, Alex JC, et al. Surgical resection and radiolocalization of the sentinel lymph node in breast cancer using a gamma probe. *Surg Oncol* 1993; 2:335–339; discussion 340.
27. Giuliano AE. Intradermal blue dye to identify sentinel lymph node in breast cancer. *Lancet* 1997;350:958.
28. Giuliano AE, Kirgan DM, Guenther JM, et al. Lymphatic mapping and sentinel lymphadenectomy for breast cancer. *Ann Surg* 1994;220:391–398; discussion 398–401.
29. Albertini JJ, Lyman GH, Cox C, et al. Lymphatic mapping and sentinel node biopsy in the patient with breast cancer. *JAMA* 1996;276:1818–1822.
30. Rosen PP, Saigo PE, Braun DW Jr., et al. Occult axillary lymph node metastases from breast cancers with intramammary lymphatic tumor emboli. *Am J Surg Pathol* 1982;6:639–641.
31. Clayton F, Hopkins CL. Pathologic correlates of prognosis in lymph node-positive breast carcinomas. *Cancer* 1993;71:1780–1790.
32. Cote RJ, Rosen PP, Lesser ML, et al. Prediction of early relapse in patients with operable breast cancer by detection of occult bone marrow micrometastases. *J Clin Oncol* 1991;9:1749–1756.
33. Cote RJ, Peterson HF, Chaiwun B, et al. Role of immunohistochemical detection of lymph-node metastases in management of breast cancer. International Breast Cancer Study Group. *Lancet* 1999;354:896–900.
34. Chen SL, Hoehne FM, Giuliano AE. The prognostic significance of micrometastases in breast cancer: a SEER population-based analysis. *Ann Surg Oncol* 2007; 14:3378–3384.
35. Braun S, Cevatli BS, Assemi C, et al. Comparative analysis of micrometastasis to the bone marrow and lymph nodes of node-negative breast cancer patients receiving no adjuvant therapy. *J Clin Oncol* 2001;19:1468–1475.
36. Braun S, Pantel K, Muller P, et al. Cytokeratin-positive cells in the bone marrow and survival of patients with stage I, II, or III breast cancer. *N Engl J Med* 2000; 342:525–533.
37. Carter CL, Allen C, Henson DE. Relation of tumor size, lymph node status, and survival in 24,740 breast cancer cases. *Cancer* 1989;63:181–187.
38. Fisher B, Slack NH, Bross ID. Cancer of the breast: size of neoplasm and prognosis. *Cancer* 1969;24:1071–1080.
39. Adair F, Berg J, Joubert L, et al. Long-term follow-up of breast cancer patients: the 30-year report. *Cancer* 1974;33:1145–1150.
40. Nemoto T, Vana J, Bedwani RN, et al. Management and survival of female breast cancer: results of a national survey by the American College of Surgeons. *Cancer* 1980;45:2917–2924.
41. Koscielny S, Tubiana M, Le MG, et al. Breast cancer: relationship between the size of the primary tumour and the probability of metastatic dissemination. *Br J Cancer* 1984;49:709–715.
42. Moon TE, Jones SE, Bonadonna G, et al. Development and use of a natural history data base of breast cancer studies. *Am J Clin Oncol* 1987;10:396–403.
43. Rosen PP, Groshen S, Saigo PE, et al. Pathological prognostic factors in stage I (T1N0M0) and stage II (T1N1M0) breast carcinoma: a study of 644 patients with median follow-up of 18 years. *J Clin Oncol* 1989;7:1239–1251.
44. Fisher B, Dignam J, Tan-Chiu E, et al. Prognosis and treatment of patients with breast tumors of one centimeter or less and negative axillary lymph nodes. *J Natl Cancer Inst* 2001;93:112–120.
45. Fisher B, Dignam J, Wolmark N, et al. Tamoxifen and chemotherapy for lymph node-negative, estrogen receptor-positive breast cancer. *J Natl Cancer Inst* 1997; 89:1673–1682.
46. Singletary SE, Allred C, Ashley P, et al. Revision of the American Joint Committee on Cancer staging system for breast cancer. *J Clin Oncol* 2002;20:3628–3636.
47. Ross JS, Hatzis C, Symmans WF, et al. Commercialized multigene predictors of clinical outcome for breast cancer. *Oncologist* 2008;13:477–493.
48. Perou CM, Sorlie T, Eisen MB, et al. Molecular portraits of human breast tumours. *Nature* 2000;406:747–752.
49. Sorlie T, Perou CM, Tibshirani R, et al. Gene expression patterns of breast carcinomas distinguish tumor subclasses with clinical implications. *Proc Natl Acad Sci U S A* 2001;98:10869–10874.
50. van de Vijver MJ, He YD, van't Veer LJ, et al. A gene-expression signature as a predictor of survival in breast cancer. *N Engl J Med* 2002;347:1999–2009.
51. Paik S. Development and clinical utility of a 21-gene recurrence score prognostic assay in patients with early breast cancer treated with tamoxifen. *Oncologist* 2007;12:631–635.

52. Paik S, Tang G, Shak S, et al. Gene expression and benefit of chemotherapy in women with node-negative, estrogen receptor-positive breast cancer. *J Clin Oncol* 2006;24:3726–3734.

53. Paik S, Shak S, Tang G, et al. A multigene assay to predict recurrence of tamoxifen-treated, node-negative breast cancer. *N Engl J Med* 2004;351:2817–2826.

54. Gianni L, Zambetti M, Clark K, et al. Gene expression profiles in paraffin-embedded core biopsy tissue predict response to chemotherapy in women with locally advanced breast cancer. *J Clin Oncol* 2005;23:7265–7277.

55. Chang JC, Makris A, Gutierrez MC, et al. Gene expression patterns in formalin-fixed, paraffin-embedded core biopsies predict docetaxel chemosensitivity in breast cancer patients. *Breast Cancer Res Treat* 2008;108:233–240.

56. Gilchrist KW, Kalish L, Gould VE, et al. Interobserver reproducibility of histopathological features in stage II breast cancer. An ECOG study. *Breast Cancer Res Treat* 1985;5:3–10.

57. Chevallier B, Mosseri V, Dauce JP, et al. A prognostic score in histological node-negative breast cancer. *Br J Cancer* 1990;61:436–440.

58. Contesso G, Mouriesse H, Friedman S, et al. The importance of histologic grade in long-term prognosis of breast cancer: a study of 1,010 patients, uniformly treated at the Institut Gustave-Roussy. *J Clin Oncol* 1987;5:1378–1386.

59. Davis BW, Gelber RD, Goldhirsch A, et al. Prognostic significance of tumor grade in clinical trials of adjuvant therapy for breast cancer with axillary lymph node metastasis. *Cancer* 1986:2662–2670.

60. Dawson AE, Austin RE, Jr., Weinberg DS. Nuclear grading of breast carcinoma by image analysis. Classification by multivariate and neural network analysis. *Am J Clin Pathol* 1991;95:S29–S37.

61. Elston CW, Ellis IO. Pathological prognostic factors in breast cancer. I. The value of histological grade in breast cancer: experience from a large study with long-term follow-up. *Histopathology* 1991;19:403–410.

62. Fisher ER, Redmond C, Fisher B. Histologic grading of breast cancer. *Pathol Annu* 1980;15:239–251.

63. Henson DE, Ries L, Freedman LS, et al. Relationship among outcome, stage of disease, and histologic grade for 22,616 cases of breast cancer. The basis for a prognostic index. *Cancer* 1991;68:2142–2149.

64. Le Doussal V, Tubiana-Hulin M, Friedman S, et al. Prognostic value of histologic grade nuclear components of Scarff-Bloom-Richardson (SBR). An improved score modification based on a multivariate analysis of 1,262 invasive ductal breast carcinomas. *Cancer* 1989;64:1914–1921.

65. Rank F, Dombernowsky P, Jespersen NC, et al. Histologic malignancy grading of invasive ductal breast carcinoma. A regression analysis of prognostic factors in low-risk carcinomas from a multicenter trial. *Cancer* 1987;60:1299–1305.

66. Schumacher M, Schmoor C, Sauerbrei W, et al. The prognostic effect of histological tumor grade in node-negative breast cancer patients. *Breast Cancer Res Treat* 1993;25:235–245.

67. Bloom HJG, Richardson WW. Histological grading and prognosis in breast cancer. *Br J Cancer* 1957;11:359–377.

68. Dalton LW, Page DL, Dupont WD. Histologic grading of breast carcinoma. A reproducibility study. *Cancer* 1994;73:2765–2770.

69. Le Doussal V, Tubiana-Hulin M, Hacene K, et al. Nuclear characteristics as indicators of prognosis in node negative breast cancer patients. *Breast Cancer Res Treat* 1989;14:207–216.

70. Fisher ER, Sass R, Fisher B. Pathologic findings from the National Surgical Adjuvant Project for Breast Cancers (protocol no. 4). X. Discriminants for tenth year treatment failure. *Cancer* 1984;53:712–723.

71. Tawfik O, Kimler BF, Davis M, et al. Grading invasive ductal carcinoma of the breast: advantages of using automated proliferation index instead of mitotic count. *Virchows Arch* 2007;450:627–636.

72. Meyer JS, Alvarez C, Milikowski C, et al. Breast carcinoma malignancy grading by Bloom-Richardson system vs proliferation index: reproducibility of grade and advantages of proliferation index. *Mod Pathol* 2005;18:1067–1078.

73. Mohammed RA, Martin SG, Gill MS, et al. Improved methods of detection of lymphovascular invasion demonstrate that it is the predominant method of vascular invasion in breast cancer and has important clinical consequences. *Am J Surg Pathol* 2007;31:1825–1833.

74. Fitzgibbons PL, Page DL, Weaver D, et al. Prognostic factors in breast cancer. College of American Pathologists Consensus Statement 1999. *Arch Pathol Lab Med* 2000;124:966–978.

75. Page DL, Gray R, Allred DC, et al. Prediction of node-negative breast cancer outcome by histologic grading and S-phase analysis by flow cytometry: an Eastern Cooperative Oncology Group Study (2192). *Am J Clin Oncol* 2001;24:10–18.

76. Simpson JF, Gray R, Dressler LG, et al. Prognostic value of histologic grade and proliferative activity in axillary node-positive breast cancer: results from the Eastern Cooperative Oncology Group Companion Study, EST 4189. *J Clin Oncol* 2000;18:2059–2069.

77. Lee B, Tannenbaum N. Inflammatory carcinoma of the breast: a report of twenty-eight cases from the breast clinic of memorial Hospital. *Surg Gynecol Obstet* 1924;39:580–585.

78. Levine PH, Steinhorn SC, Ries LG, et al. Inflammatory breast cancer: the experience of the surveillance, epidemiology, and end results (SEER) program. *J Natl Cancer Inst* 1985;74:291–297.

79. Jaiyesimi IA, Buzdar AU, Hortobagyi G. Inflammatory breast cancer: a review. *J Clin Oncol* 1992;10:1014–1024.

80. Arpino G, Bardou VJ, Clark GM, et al. Infiltrating lobular carcinoma of the breast: tumor characteristics and clinical outcome. *Breast Cancer Res* 2004;6:R149–R156.

81. Peters GN, Wolff M, Haagensen CD. Tubular carcinoma of the breast. Clinical pathologic correlations based on 100 cases. *Ann Surg* 1981;193:138–149.

82. Fisher ER, Kenny JP, Sass R, et al. Medullary cancer of the breast revisited. *Breast Cancer Res Treat* 1990;16:215–229.

83. Nixon AJ, Neuberg D, Hayes DF, et al. Relationship of patient age to pathologic features of the tumor and prognosis for patients with stage I or II breast cancer. *J Clin Oncol* 1994;12:888–894.

84. Albain KS, Allred DC, Clark GM. Breast cancer outcome and predictors of outcome: are there age differentials? *J Natl Cancer Inst Monogr* 1994:35–42.

85. Crowe JP, Jr., Gordon NH, Shenk RR, et al. Age does not predict breast cancer outcome. *Arch Surg* 1994;129:483–487; discussion 487–488.

86. Elledge RM, Clark GM, Chamness GC, et al. Tumor biologic factors and breast cancer prognosis among white, Hispanic, and black women in the United States. *J Natl Cancer Inst* 1994;86:705–712.

87. Field TS, Buist DS, Doubeni C, et al. Disparities and survival among breast cancer patients. *J Natl Cancer Inst Monogr* 2005:88–95.

88. Polite BN, Cirrincione C, Fleming GF, et al. Racial differences in clinical outcomes from metastatic breast cancer: a pooled analysis of CALGB 9342 and 9840—Cancer and Leukemia Group B. *J Clin Oncol* 2008;26:2659–2665.

89. Keyomarsi K, Tucker SL, Bedrosian I. Cyclin E is a more powerful predictor of breast cancer outcome than proliferation. *Nat Med* 2003;9:152.

90. Keyomarsi K, Tucker SL, Buchholz TA, et al. Cyclin E and survival in patients with breast cancer. *N Engl J Med* 2002;347:1566–1575.

91. Kuhling H, Alm P, Olsson H, et al. Expression of cyclins E, A, and B, and prognosis in lymph node-negative breast cancer. *J Pathol* 2003;199:424–431.

92. Russo J, Frederick J, Ownby HE, et al. Predictors of recurrence and survival of patients with breast cancer. *Am J Clin Pathol* 1987;88:123–131.

93. Clayton F. Pathologic correlates of survival in 378 lymph node negative infiltrating ductal breast carcinomas. Mitotic count is the best single predictor. *Cancer* 1991;68:1309–1317.

94. Galea MH, Blamey RW, Elston CE, et al. The Nottingham Prognostic Index in primary breast cancer. *Breast Cancer Res Treat* 1992;22:207–219.

95. van der Linden JC, Lindeman J, Baak JP, et al. The Multivariate Prognostic Index and nuclear DNA content are independent prognostic factors in primary breast cancer patients. *Cytometry* 1989;10:56–61.

96. van Diest PJ, Baak JP, Matze-Cok P, et al. Reproducibility of mitosis counting in 2,469 breast cancer specimens: results from the Multicenter Morphometric Mammary Carcinoma Project. *Hum Pathol* 1992;23:603–607.

97. Baak JP, van Diest PJ, Voorhorst FJ, et al. Prospective multicenter validation of the independent prognostic value of the mitotic activity index in lymph node-negative breast cancer patients younger than 55 years. *J Clin Oncol* 2005;23:5993–6001.

98. Baak JP, Gudlaugsson E, Skaland I, et al. Proliferation is the strongest prognosticator in node-negative breast cancer: significance, error sources, alternatives and comparison with molecular prognostic markers. *Breast Cancer Res Treat* 2008 (e-pub).

99. Thor AD, Liu S, Moore DH, 2nd, et al. Comparison of mitotic index, *in vitro* bromodeoxyuridine labeling, and MIB-1 assays to quantitate proliferation in breast cancer. *J Clin Oncol* 1999;17:470–477.

100. Silvestrini R, Daidone MG, Valagussa P, et al. Cell kinetics as a prognostic indicator in node-negative breast cancer. *Eur J Cancer Clin Oncol* 1989;25:1165–1171.

101. Meyer JS, Province M. Proliferative index of breast carcinoma by thymidine labeling: prognostic power independent of stage, estrogen and progesterone receptors. *Breast Cancer Res Treat* 1988;12:191–204.

102. Tubiana M, Pejovic MH, Koscielny S, et al. Growth rate, kinetics of tumor cell proliferation and long-term outcome in human breast cancer. *Int J Cancer* 1989;44:17–22.

103. Cooke TG, Stanton PD, Winstanley J, et al. Long-term prognostic significance of thymidine labelling index in primary breast cancer. *Eur J Cancer* 1992;28:424–426.

104. Courdi A, Hery M, Dahan E, et al. Factors affecting relapse in node-negative breast cancer. A multivariate analysis including the labeling index. *Eur J Cancer Clin Oncol* 1989;25:351–356.

105. Hery M, Gioanni J, Lalanne CM, et al. The DNA labelling index: a prognostic factor in node-negative breast cancer. *Breast Cancer Res Treat* 1987;9:207–211.

106. Silvestrini R. Feasibility and reproducibility of the [3H]-thymidine labelling index in breast cancer. The SICCAB Group for Quality Control of Cell Kinetic Determination. *Cell Prolif* 1991;24:437–445.

107. Hedley DW, Clark GM, Cornelisse CJ, et al. Consensus review of the clinical utility of DNA cytometry in carcinoma of the breast. Report of the DNA Cytometry Consensus Conference. *Cytometry* 1993;14:482–485.

108. Wenger CR, Beardslee S, Owens MA, et al. DNA ploidy, S-phase, and steroid receptors in more than 127,000 breast cancer patients. *Breast Cancer Res Treat* 1993;28:9–20.

109. Hutchins L, Green S, Ravdin P, et al. CMF vs CAF with and without tamoxifen in high-risk node-negative breast cancer patients and a natural history follow-up study in low-risk node-negative patients: First results of Intergroup Trial 0102. In: *Proc ASCO* 1998;17:19.

110. Herman CJ, Duque RE, Hedley D, et al. DNA cytometry in cancer prognosis. *Principles & Practice of Oncology PPO Updates* 1993;7:1–8.

111. Gerdes J, Schwab U, Lemke H, et al. Production of a mouse monoclonal antibody reactive with a human nuclear antigen associated with cell proliferation. *Int J Cancer* 1983;31:13–20.

112. Schluter C, Duchrow M, Wohlenberg C, et al. The cell proliferation-associated antigen of antibody Ki-67: a very large, ubiquitous nuclear protein with numerous repeated elements, representing a new kind of cell cycle-maintaining proteins. *J Cell Biol* 1993;123:513–522.

113. Cattoretti G, Becker MH, Key G, et al. Monoclonal antibodies against recombinant parts of the Ki-67 antigen (MIB 1 and MIB 3) detect proliferating cells in microwave-processed formalin-fixed paraffin sections. *J Pathol* 1992;168:357–363.

114. Key G, Petersen JL, Becker MH, et al. New antiserum against Ki-67 antigen suitable for double immunostaining of paraffin wax sections. *J Clin Pathol* 1993;46:1080–1084.

115. Brown RW, Allred CD, Clark GM, et al. Prognostic value of Ki-67 compared to S-phase fraction in axillary node-negative breast cancer. *Clin Cancer Res* 1996;2:585–592.

116. Bouzubar N, Walker KJ, Griffiths K, et al. Ki67 immunostaining in primary breast cancer: pathological and clinical associations. *Br J Cancer* 1989;59:943–947.

117. Weikel W, Beck T, Mitze M, et al. Immunohistochemical evaluation of growth fractions in human breast cancers using monoclonal antibody Ki-67. *Breast Cancer Res Treat* 1991;18:149–154.

118. Gasparini G, Dal Fior S, Pozza F, et al. Correlation of growth fraction by Ki-67 immunohistochemistry with histologic factors and hormone receptors in operable breast carcinoma. *Breast Cancer Res Treat* 1989;14:329–336.

119. Gasparini G, Pozza F, Bevilacqua P, et al. Growth fraction (Ki-67 antibody) determination in early-stage breast carcinoma: Histologic, clinical and prognostic correlations. *Breast* 1992;1:92–99.

120. Sahin AA, Ro J, Ro JY, et al. Ki-67 immunostaining in node-negative stage I/II breast carcinoma. Significant correlation with prognosis. *Cancer* 1991;68:549–557.

121. Wintzer HO, Zipfel I, Schulte-Monting J, et al. Ki-67 immunostaining in human breast tumors and its relationship to prognosis. *Cancer* 1991;67:421–428.

122. Gottardi O, Scanzi F, Zurrida S, et al. Clinical and prognostic usefulness of immunohistochemical determination of Ki-67 in early stage breast cancer. *Breast* 1993;2:33–36.

123. Railo M, Nordling S, von Boguslawsky K, et al. Prognostic value of Ki-67 immuno-labelling in primary operable breast cancer. *Br J Cancer* 1993;68:579–583.

124. Veronese SM, Gambacorta M, Gottardi O, et al. Proliferation index as a prognostic marker in breast cancer. *Cancer* 1993;71:3926–3931.
125. Gaglia P, Bernardi A, Venesio T, et al. Cell proliferation of breast cancer evaluated by anti-BrdU and anti-Ki-67 antibodies: its prognostic value on short-term recurrences. *Eur J Cancer* 1993;29A:1509–1513.
126. Charpin C, Andrac L, Vacheret H, et al. Multiparametric evaluation (SAMBA) of growth fraction (monoclonal Ki67) in breast carcinoma tissue sections. *Cancer Res* 1988;48:4368–4374.
127. Walker RA, Camplejohn RS. Comparison of monoclonal antibody Ki-67 reactivity with grade and DNA flow cytometry of breast carcinomas. *Br J Cancer* 1988;57:281–283.
128. de Azambuja E, Cardoso F, de Castro G, Jr, et al. Ki-67 as prognostic marker in early breast cancer: a meta-analysis of published studies involving 12,155 patients. *Br J Cancer* 2007;96:1504–1513.
129. Remvikos Y, Beuzeboc P, Zajdela A, et al. Correlation of pretreatment proliferative activity of breast cancer with the response to cytotoxic chemotherapy. *J Natl Cancer Inst* 1989;81:1383–1387.
130. Dressler LG, Eudey L, Gray R, et al. Prognostic potential of DNA flow cytometry measurements in node-negative breast cancer patients: preliminary analysis of an intergroup study (INT 0076). *J Natl Cancer Inst Monogr* 1992:167–172.
131. Amadori D, Nanni O, Marangolo M, et al. Disease-free survival advantage of adjuvant cyclophosphamide, methotrexate, and fluorouracil in patients with node-negative, rapidly proliferating breast cancer: a randomized multicenter study. *J Clin Oncol* 2000;18.3125–3134.
132. Paradiso A, Ranieri G, Silvestris N, et al. Failure of primary breast cancer neoangiogenesis to predict pattern of distant metastasis. *Clin Exp Med* 2001;1:127–132.
133. Wang L, Shao ZM. Cyclin e expression and prognosis in breast cancer patients: a meta-analysis of published studies. *Cancer Invest* 2006;24:581–587.
134. Porter PL, Barlow WE, Yeh IT, et al. p27(Kip1) and cyclin E expression and breast cancer survival after treatment with adjuvant chemotherapy. *J Natl Cancer Inst* 2006;98:1723–1731.
135. Adami HO, Graffman S, Lindgren A, et al. Prognostic implication of estrogen receptor content in breast cancer. *Breast Cancer Res Treat* 1985;5:293–300.
136. Schmitt M, Thomssen C, Ulm K, et al. Time-varying prognostic impact of tumour biological factors urokinase (uPA), PAI-1 and steroid hormone receptor status in primary breast cancer. *Br J Cancer* 1997;76:306–311.
137. Speirs V. Oestrogen receptor beta in breast cancer: good, bad or still too early to tell? *J Pathol* 2002;197:143–147.
138. Klijn JGM, Berns PMJJ, Schmitz PIM, et al. Epidermal growth factor receptor (EGF-R) in clinical breast cancer: Update 1993. *Endocr Rev* 1993;1:171–174.
139. Fox SB, Smith K, Hollyer J, et al. The epidermal growth factor receptor as a prognostic marker: results of 370 patients and review of 3009 patients. *Breast Cancer Res Treat* 1994;29:41–49.
140. Harris AL. What is the biological, prognostic, and therapeutic role of the EGF receptor in human breast cancer? *Breast Cancer Res Treat* 1994;29:1–2.
141. Baselga J. New therapeutic agents targeting the epidermal growth factor receptor. *J Clin Oncol* 2000;18:54S–59S.
142. Mendelsohn J, Baselga J. The EGF receptor family as targets for cancer therapy. *Oncogene* 2000;19:6550–6565.
143. Vogel CL, Cobleigh MA, Tripathy D, et al. Efficacy and safety of trastuzumab as a single agent in first-line treatment of HER2-overexpressing metastatic breast cancer. *J Clin Oncol* 2002;20:719–726.
144. Romond EH, Perez EA, Bryant J, et al. Trastuzumab plus adjuvant chemotherapy for operable HER2-positive breast cancer. *N Engl J Med* 2005;353:1673–1684.
145. Piccart-Gebhart MJ, Procter M, Leyland-Jones B, et al. Trastuzumab after adjuvant chemotherapy in HER2-positive breast cancer. *N Engl J Med* 2005;353:1659–1672.
146. Wolff AC, Hammond ME, Schwartz JN, et al. American Society of Clinical Oncology/College of American Pathologists Guideline Recommendations for Human Epidermal Growth Factor Receptor 2 Testing in Breast Cancer. *Arch Pathol Lab Med* 2007;131:18.
147. Pritchard KI, Messersmith H, Elavathil L, et al. HER-2 and topoisomerase II as predictors of response to chemotherapy. *J Clin Oncol* 2008;26:736–744.
148. Tanner M, Isola J, Wiklund T, et al. Topoisomerase IIalpha gene amplification predicts favorable treatment response to tailored and dose-escalated anthracycline-based adjuvant chemotherapy in HER-2/neu-amplified breast cancer: Scandinavian Breast Group Trial 9401. *J Clin Oncol* 2006;24:2428–2436.
149. Slamon D, Eiermann W, Robert N, et al. Phase III randomized trial comparing doxorubicin and cyclophosphamide followed by docetaxel (AC -> T) with doxorubicin and cyclophosphamide followed by docetaxel and trastuzumab (AC -> TH) with docetaxel, carboplatin and trastuzumab (TCH) in HER2 positive early breast cancer patients: BCIRG 006 study. *Breast Cancer Res Treat* 2005;94(Suppl 1):S5.
150. Guo Y, Pakneshan P, Gladu J, et al. Regulation of DNA methylation in human breast cancer. Effect on the urokinase-type plasminogen activator gene production and tumor invasion. *J Biol Chem* 2002;277:41571–41579.
151. Stephens RW, Brunner N, Janicke F, et al. The urokinase plasminogen activator system as a target for prognostic studies in breast cancer. *Breast Cancer Res Treat* 1998;52:99–111.
152. Grebenchtchikov N, Maguire TM, Riisbro R, et al. Measurement of plasminogen activator system components in plasma and tumor tissue extracts obtained from patients with breast cancer: an EORTC Receptor and Biomarker Group collaboration. *Oncol Rep* 2005;14:235–239.
153. Ferrier CM, de Witte HH, Straatman H, et al. Comparison of immunohistochemistry with immunoassay (ELISA) for the detection of components of the plasminogen activation system in human tumour tissue. *Br J Cancer* 1999;79:1534–1541.
154. Foekens JA, Buessecker F, Peters HA, et al. Plasminogen activator inhibitor-2: prognostic relevance in 1,012 patients with primary breast cancer. *Cancer Res* 1995;55:1423–1427.
155. Foekens JA, Look MP, Peters HA, et al. Urokinase-type plasminogen activator and its inhibitor PAI-1: predictors of poor response to tamoxifen therapy in recurrent breast cancer. *J Natl Cancer Inst* 1995;87:751–756.
156. Spyratos F, Bouchet C, Tozlu S, et al. Prognostic value of uPA, PAI-1 and PAI-2 mRNA expression in primary breast cancer. *Anticancer Res* 2002;22:2997–3003.
157. Sweep CG, Geurts-Moespot J, Grebenschikov N, et al. External quality assessment of trans-European multicentre antigen determinations (enzyme-linked immunosorbent assay) of urokinase-type plasminogen activator (uPA) and its type 1 inhibitor (PAI-1) in human breast cancer tissue extracts. *Br J Cancer* 1998;78:1434–1441.
158. Look MP, van Putten WL, Duffy MJ, et al. Pooled analysis of prognostic impact of urokinase-type plasminogen activator and its inhibitor PAI-1 in 8,377 breast cancer patients. *J Natl Cancer Inst* 2002;94:116–128.
159. Annecke K, Schmitt M, Euler U, et al. uPA and PAI-1 in breast cancer: review of their clinical utility and current validation in the prospective NNBC-3 trial. *Adv Clin Chem* 2008;45:31–45.
160. Lee JM, Bernstein A. p53 mutations increase resistance to ionizing radiation. *Proc Natl Acad Sci U S A* 1993;90:5742–5746.
161. Elledge RM, Allred DC. Prognostic and predictive value of p53 and p21 in breast cancer. *Breast Cancer Res Treat* 1998;52:79–98.
162. Barnes DM, Dublin EA, Fisher CJ, et al. Immunohistochemical detection of p53 protein in mammary carcinoma: an important new independent indicator of prognosis? *Hum Pathol* 1993;24:469–476.
163. Thor AD, Moore DH, II, Edgerton SM, et al. Accumulation of p53 tumor suppressor gene protein: an independent marker of prognosis in breast cancers. *J Natl Cancer Inst* 1992;84:845–555.
164. Elledge RM, Green S, Ciocca D, et al. HER-2 expression and response to tamoxifen in estrogen receptor-positive breast cancer: a Southwest Oncology Group Study. *Clin Cancer Res* 1998;4:7–12.
165. Elledge RM, Gray R, Mansour E, et al. Accumulation of p53 protein as a possible predictor of response to adjuvant combination chemotherapy with cyclophosphamide, methotrexate, fluorouracil, and prednisone for breast cancer. *J Natl Cancer Inst* 1995;87:1254–1256.
166. Stal O, Stenmark Askmalm M, Wingren S, et al. p53 expression and the result of adjuvant therapy of breast cancer. *Acta Oncol* 1995;34:767–770.
167. Degeorges A, de Roquancourt A, Extra JM, et al. Is p53 a protein that predicts the response to chemotherapy in node negative breast cancer? *Breast Cancer Res Treat* 1998;47:47–55.
168. Thor AD, Berry DA, Budman DR, et al. erbB-2, p53, and efficacy of adjuvant therapy in lymph node-positive breast cancer. *J Natl Cancer Inst* 1998;90:1346–1360.
169. Reed JC. Bcl-2 and the regulation of programmed cell death. *J Cell Biol* 1994;124:1–6.
170. Daidone MG, Luisi A, Veroneni S, et al. Clinical studies of Bcl-2 and treatment benefit in breast cancer patients. *Endocr Relat Cancer* 1999;6:61–68.
171. Krajewski S, Krajewska M, Turner BC, et al. Prognostic significance of apoptosis regulators in breast cancer. *Endocr Relat Cancer* 1999;6:29–40.
172. Krajewski S, Thor AD, Edgerton SM, et al. Analysis of Bax and Bcl-2 expression in p53-immunopositive breast cancers. *Clin Cancer Res* 1997;3:199–208.

Chapter 32
Gene Arrays, Prognosis, and Therapeutic Interventions

Lisa A. Carey and Charles M. Perou

Gene arrays, also termed *gene expression arrays* or DNA *microarrays*, is a method that examines the expression levels and patterns of up to all 25,000 human genes in a tumor or normal tissue simultaneously. In this chapter, we review how gene arrays have informed our understanding of the heterogeneity of breast cancer and how they are currently used for prognostication and therapeutic decision-making. The promise of gene array is that in the future we will be able to use the detailed tumor-specific and patient-specific information that they provide as a means to personalize therapy for cancer patients.

Breast cancer is a heterogeneous disease composed of a growing number of recognized biologic subtypes; however, recognition of this heterogeneity long predated the development of sophisticated technologies such as gene expression arrays. In particular, variations in risk factors (1,2), response to therapy (3), and clinical behavior (4) by hormone receptor status have been noted by clinicians and researchers for several decades. More recent data has implicated HER2 driven breast cancers as possessing unique characteristics such as responsiveness to anthracyclines (5).

Traditional single marker approaches to biomarker identification is limited because seldom is one gene or protein responsible for the entire action of a cellular pathway. Among the hallmarks of cancer is the redundancy of these pathways. Even more importantly, single marker studies do not address the important relationships among and within different pathways, which are increasingly becoming appreciated to define behavior and response to therapy. The explosion of 'omics'-type approaches, loosely defined as the comprehensive examination of a cellular characteristic such as genetic variation (single nucleotide polymorphism [SNP]), gene expression (genomics), protein expression (proteomics), or cellular metabolism (metabolomics), has allowed researchers to approach identification of risk factors, biologic characteristics, and drug targets in a far more robust and accurate manner. Moreover, these comprehensive portraits of malignant cells identify relationships between and among different genes and pathways in a specific tumor, and this information will likely dictate the way future therapy will be individualized.

GENE ARRAYS

Microarrays are a generalized approach that allows high throughput examination of a single protein expression in multiple tissues (tissue microarray) or multiple genes in a single tissue (gene expression array). The focus in this chapter is on gene expression arrays, which have been developed as means both to better define tumor biology and to predict outcome.

Gene expression arrays measure the level of expression of a particular gene by semiquantitatively determining the level of messenger RNA (mRNA) transcripts, which can be initially compared versus a reference sample (as in the case of two-color arrays, such as those produced by Agilent, Santa Clara, CA), or directly compared to other tumors or normal tissues (as in the case of one-color arrays like those produced by Affymetrix). The arrays themselves currently include essentially all human genes that are encompassed in tens of thousands of features or probes that are either oligonucleotides or polymerase chain reaction (PCR) amplified complementary DNA (cDNA) inserts. A tumor is processed for RNA, which is used to generate either cDNA or RNA, labeled with a fluorescent probe. These fluorescent probes that then either be directly applied to an array alone (one-color arrays) or combined with a second fluorescently labeled reference sample and then both are applied to an array (two-color array, in which by convention the color red is used for the sample of interest and the color green for the reference sample). From here on out, the experiment is basically a Southern blot with nucleic acid hybridization reactions occurring and binding, with the intensity(s) of the nucleic acids that hybridize to the individual gene probes reflecting the relative amounts of tumor versus reference RNA, which in the case of two-color arrays green predominance reflects low expression and red predominance reflects high expression of that gene in the tumor relative to the reference (Fig. 32.1). Thus, in a two-color array, it is not the value of the tumor versus the reference that is of greatest value, but the ratio of tumor or reference for each gene that is used as a quantitative measure of that gene in that sample. This value is then used to compare tumor to tumor, and tumor to normal; in this way, once a two-color array gives a tumor or reference value, it is used nearly identically to the one-color microarray intensity value, and thus, once the user gets past these initial different data normalization steps, all downstream analysis steps are very similar for one-color and two-color arrays.

Given the surfeit of data that microarrays provide, the challenge then becomes a meaningful analysis of such massive amounts of information with some large-scale microarray analyses generating millions of data points. Several kinds of analyses are relevant in cancer studies. In unsupervised cluster analysis, algorithms cluster genes together by finding genes with similar variations in expression across the set of selected samples, and then grouping them together regardless of other characteristics. The gene lists thus represent purely biologic differences among tumors, which makes this approach a favored one for scientists interested in discovery. In the case of breast cancer, a semiunsupervised approach (detailed in Intrinsic Subtypes below) contributed the breast cancer subtypes that many consider the new denominator for developing new prognostic or therapeutic advances. Complementary to unsupervised approaches are supervised analyses that are those in which the gene clusters represent those genes that differentiate tumors with a particular characteristic or end point, such as selecting the subset of genes that correlates with important clinical features, such as node positivity or relapse. These are more translational scientific approaches that are designed to be directly applied for patient benefit, and several are described further in the section Prognostic Arrays, that are in clinical use today.

MOLECULAR PROFILING OF BREAST CANCER

In molecular profiling experiments different tumors are compared at the molecular level (DNA, mRNA or protein) in a comprehensive manner, with hundreds to thousands of simultaneous evaluations performed on a single chip, or array. Most breast cancer molecular profiling studies have focused on gene expression profiling, which is performed on microscope slide-sized chips to which nucleic acid sequences (cDNA or oligonucleotides) are affixed. These sequences represent known, unknown but validated, and hypothetical genes, and all approximately 25,000 genes in the human genome can be included. Although this has been a very fruitful approach for improving

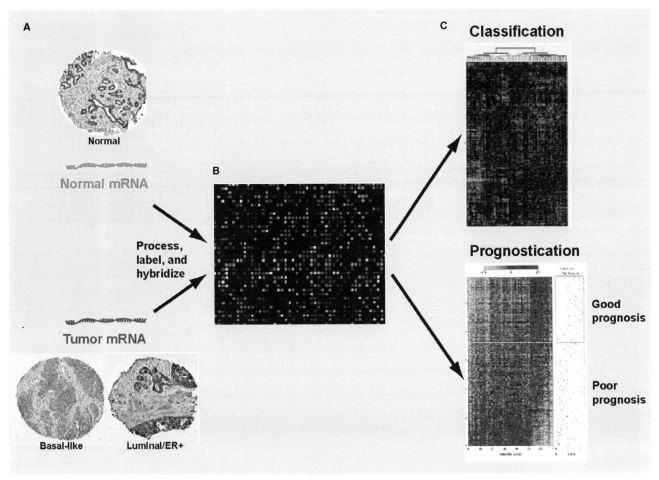

FIGURE 32.1. Illustration of gene expression array methodology and application. A: RNA from a tumor and reference sample is processed, fluorescently labeled, and hybridized to a microscope-sized chip to which probes for up to thousands of genes have been affixed. **B:** The red (relative overexpression in tumor) and green (relative underexpression in tumor) intensities can be simultaneously analyzed. **C:** Depending on the supervision of the analysis, tumors can be subtyped, or can be analyzed for gene sets associated with clinical outcome.

our understanding of breast cancer biology and for the development of gene sets related to prognosis, it is also true that this approach ignores processes such as post-translational modifications that can affect protein expression and does not provide information about the mechanism(s) responsible for altered gene expression.

Multiple approaches to analyzing gene expression arrays exist; it is self-evident that the answer acquired from genomic analysis depends on the question asked. For example, unsupervised analyses (analyzed regardless of any particular characteristic) can identify whether there are molecularly identifiable tumor subtypes, also called *class discovery*, whereas supervised analyses (analyzed with a particular clinical end point in mind) can identify if there are gene lists that can identify tumors that relapsed versus those that did not (prognostic profiles) or responded to a particular therapy versus did not (predictive profiles), also called *class comparison* (6,7). It is tempting to assume that the individual genes identified using these methods may themselves be causal in creating the subtype or the clinical characteristic; however, the identified genes themselves may be merely proxies for genetic events or pathway activation and may not themselves be the cause. A third category of analysis, *class prediction*, first uses a supervised analysis and a specific sample set to identify a gene list that is then used to assign a new individual tumor to a particular category such as a subtype or clinical class. This method refines the gene lists identified by discovery or comparison, and typically requires fewer genes.

The molecular profiling of breast cancer has provided important information for four major questions:

1. Are there subtypes of breast cancer based on intrinsic biologic differences?
2. Are there gene expression profiles that can distinguish patients with poor from those with good, thus allowing better informed decisions regarding adjuvant therapy?
3. Are there gene lists that can predict which tumor will respond to a specific therapy?
4. Can molecular profiling allow rational drug selection, or combinations of drugs, designed to exploit the particular weakness of an individual tumor?

BREAST CANCER INTRINSIC SUBTYPES

In 2000, Perou et al. (8) used a semiunsupervised approach to identify naturally occurring breast cancer subtypes in a population of 40 patients with locally advanced disease treated with neoadjuvant chemotherapy. They identified 496 genes termed the *intrinsic gene set* that showed little variance within repeated tumor sample, but high variance across different tumors, and then used this gene set for subtype discovery. Among these breast cancers they found that the patterns of expression of these genes segregated the tumors into five subtypes. The five intrinsic subtypes, so-called because the gene list that defines them reflects intrinsic properties of breast cancers rather than selected clinical behavior, have been consistently

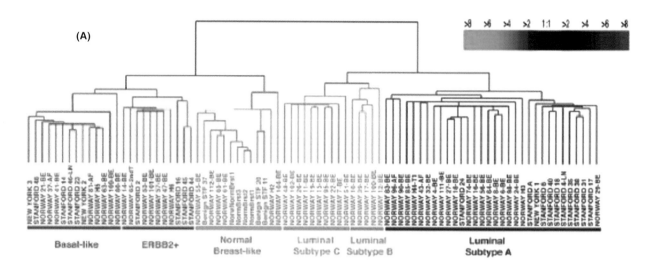

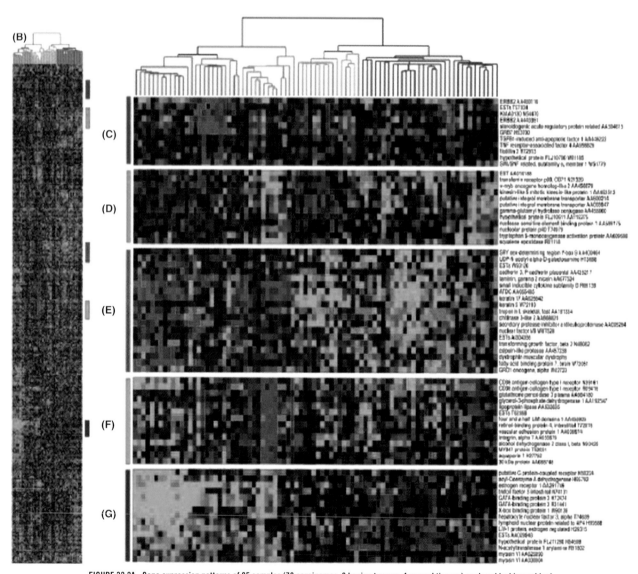

FIGURE 32.2A. Gene expression patterns of 85 samples (78 carcinomas, 3 benign tumors, 4 normal tissues) analyzed by hierarchical clustering using the 476 complementary DNA (cDNA) intrinsic clone set. (*A*) The tumor specimens were divided into subtypes based on differences in gene expression. The cluster dendrogram showing the subtypes of tumors are colored as luminal subtype A, dark blue; luminal subtype B, yellow; luminal subtype C, light blue; normal breast-like, green; basal-like, red; and ERBB2 + *, pink (* ERBB2 also known as HER2). (*B*) The full cluster diagram scaled down. The colored bars on the right represent the inserts presented in *C–G*. (*C*) *ERBB2* amplicon cluster. (*D*) Novel unknown cluster. (*E*) Basal epithelial cell-enriched cluster. (*F*) Normal breast-like cluster. (*G*) Luminal epithelial gene cluster containing *ER*. (From Sorlie T, Perou CM, Tibshirani R, et al. Gene expression patterns of breast carcinomas distinguish tumor subclasses with clinical implications. *Proc Natl Acad Sci U S A* 2001;98(19):10869–10874, with permission.)

(A) van't Veer data set

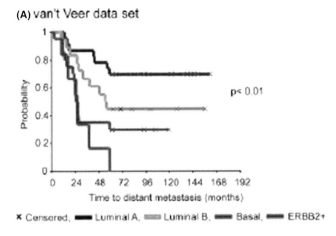

p< 0.01

✗ Censored, ▬▬ Luminal A, ▨▨ Luminal B, ▬▬ Basal, ▬▬ ERBB2+

(B) Norway/Stanford data set

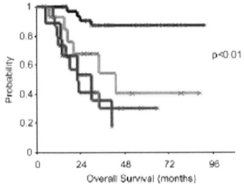

p <0.01

FIGURE 32.2B. Disease outcome in independent patient cohorts. (*A*) Time to development of distant metastasis in the 97 sporadic cases from van't Veer et al. (18). (*B*) Overall survival for 72 patients with locally advanced breast cancer in a cohort from Norway. (From Sorlie T, Tibshirani R, Parker J, et al. Repeated observation of breast tumor subtypes in independent gene expression data sets. *Proc Natl Acad Sci U S A* 2003;100(14):8418–8423, with permission.)

identified in independent datasets using multiple different methods (9–16), are conserved across ethic groups, and are present in preneoplasia (16,17). Reassuringly, the intrinsic subtypes are segregated by expression of hormone receptors and the genes they regulate, supporting earlier epidemiologic and biomarker studies suggesting that estrogen receptor (ER)-positive and ER-negative breast cancer are different. At least two hormone receptor-positive subtypes were identified, which are called *luminal A* and *luminal B*. Several subtypes are characterized by low expression of hormone receptor-related genes, one of which is called the HER2-positive/ER-negative subtype (HER2+/ER−) and another called the *basal-like subtype* (Fig. 32.2A). The fifth subtype, the normal-like, is less clearly a subtype rather than a technical artifact possibly caused by too much normal contaminating tissue. Ongoing studies are and will identify less frequent subtypes; for the time being, however, these five subtypes are consistently identified and commonly accepted. Although the intrinsic subtypes were identified heedless of outcome, these subtypes have strong prognostic implications (Fig. 32.2B); in particular, patients with basal-like or HER2+/ER− tumors demonstrate a significantly worse outcome compared with patients with luminal A tumors in datasets from patients treated homogenously (no systemic adjuvant treatment) and heterogeneously (9–14).

A critical aspect of biomarker biology is validation and the intrinsic subtypes have been validated on many independent datasets. For example, Sorlie et al. (14) examined the intrinsic gene classifications using the arrays from 295 patients that were used to develop the Amsterdam 70-gene prognostic profile described further below (18), and also included a second set of

49 tumors of mixed hormone receptor and nodal status (19). Using this method, the subtypes were represented with similar distributions in multiple datasets, despite differences in the populations—the original gene expression study was based on high-risk, more locally advanced tumors treated with chemotherapy or chemoendocrine therapy, whereas the Amsterdam 295-patient dataset included women under 55 years of age with lymph node-negative tumors that largely did not receive adjuvant systemic therapy (18), and the West et al. (19) dataset was a mixture of stages, nodal status, and hormone receptor status. An updated intrinsic gene list was also applied to the combined dataset from several of these and other sources (13–15,18), revealing persistence of the subtype signatures and prognostic predictions across different microarray platforms (11). Because the clustering methodology for identifying intrinsic subtypes is suboptimal for reproducible classifications, this is an area of active research. Several promising approaches in development are based on identifying the mean expression profiles, called *centroids*, for each subtype (11,12,20). Hu et al. (11) developed the Single Sample Predictor (SSP) tool to serve as an unchanging prognostic indicator for individual patient samples. The SSP compares the gene expression profile of an unknown sample with a prototypical profile of each intrinsic subtype and classifies the unknown sample according to the profile it most closely matches. A potential alternative to the SSP has also been recently described where, in these experiments, gene expression profiling using several different microarray platforms was used to group a set of patient tumor samples into the intrinsic subtype groups and identify signature genes associated with the luminal and basal-like subtypes (21). Fifty-four of these signature genes were identified as the minimal set needed to distinguish between luminal and basal-like subtypes. Whereas evaluation of the signature 54-gene set itself provokes interesting questions regarding the underlying biology of these two breast cancer subtypes, future directions may include its evaluation for clinical and clinical research applications. A similar approach was recently shown to be accurate in formalin-fixed tissue; this study was small but, if validated in a larger annotated dataset, would allow application to clinical specimens (22).

Luminal Subtypes

The most common subtypes of breast cancer are the luminal subtypes, so-called because they have a gene expression pattern reminiscent of the luminal epithelial component of the breast (8). These tumors are characterized by expression of the ER, progesterone receptor (PR), and genes associated with ER activation, such as *LIV1*, *GATA3*, and cyclin D1, as well as expression of luminal cytokeratins 8 and 18 (8,15,23). Luminal tumors are often low grade, and fewer than 20% have TP53 mutations (13,15). Within the luminal cluster are at least two subtypes, luminal A and luminal B, and there are many relevant differences between these two groups. For example, luminal A tumors generally have high expression of ER and ER-regulated genes, low expression of the HER2 cluster (which is variable in luminal B tumors), and low expression of proliferation-associated genes, including Ki-67 (13,14). Conversely, luminal B tumors tend to be highly proliferative, to be TP53 mutant, and to show lower expression (but some) of ER and ER-regulated genes.

In population-based studies, luminal A breast cancer is the most common, representing approximately 50% of tumors, whereas luminal B comprises approximately 10% (10,24,25); however, these numbers should be interpreted with caution because these studies differentiated luminal tumors using immunohistochemical proxies that misclassify many luminal B tumors. Expression array-based profiling studies, although not generalizable, suggest that luminal A comprises approximately 30% to 40% and luminal B approximately 20% of breast cancers (11,26). Luminal A breast cancers consistently have better prognosis than luminal B (13–15,27). Although risk factors for all of the subtypes remain enigmatic, it is increasingly clear that most traditional risk factors are primarily risk factors for luminal breast cancer (28). In addition, the population-based studies also show that premenopausal women and black women tend to develop fewer of the good-prognosis luminal A tumors and more of the poor-prognosis basal-like tumors (described further below), which may contribute to the poorer outcome associated with those groups (10,25). Although clinical assays to identify luminal A and B are not yet available, the Oncotype Recurrence Score (RS) assay includes many genes (*HER2*, *GRB7*, *ER*, *SCUBE2*, *Bcl2*, *Ki67*, *survivin*, *MYBL2*, *cyclin B1*) that are also used to define luminal A and luminal B tumors. To more directly compare intrinsic subtyping to the RS, Fan et al. (26) ran both classifiers on a single dataset of patients using a microarray surrogate for the RS and showed that 50% of 123 luminal A tumors had low RS (associated with good outcome), whereas only 2% of luminal B tumors had low RS (with almost all luminal B being called RS high). These findings have therapeutic implications because, as will be described below, a high RS is associated with a higher risk of relapse, despite tamoxifen (29) and a higher benefit of adjuvant chemotherapy (30).

HER2+/ER− Subtype

The hormone receptor-negative subtypes are comprised of the HER2+/ER− and basal-like subtypes. The HER2+/ER− subtype has elevated expression of HER2 and other genes that reside near HER2 in the genome including *GRB7* (see Recurrence Score below) because of HER2 genomic DNA amplification, and low expression of the luminal, hormone receptor-related gene cluster. It is important to note that some, but not all, HER2-driven breast cancers fall into this category; some HER2-driven breast cancers that have high expression of the luminal cluster and are ER+ fall into the luminal categories, not the HER2+/ER−, thus there exists at least two types of HER2-amplified tumors.

Another important feature of tumors in the HER2+/ER− gene expression-defined subtype is high expression of the proliferation cluster and, befitting this expression pattern, 75% are high-grade tumors and more than 40% have p53 mutations (10). This subtype is uncommon, comprising only 5% to 10% of all breast cancers in population-based studies (10). In the era before HER2-targeted therapy, the HER2+/ER− subtype carried a poor prognosis (13–15,27,31). Given that there is no apparent interaction between the benefit of HER2-targeted therapy, such as trastuzumab, and hormone receptor status, it is reasonable to presume that the HER2+/ER− subtype has benefited from the HER2-targeting revolution to the same degree as a HER2-positive luminal breast cancer (32). No specific risk factors are known for the HER2+/ER− subtype, and there is no apparent interaction with race or age (10,25). Although the SSP centroid-based approach shows promise (11), currently no accepted clinical test exists for molecular subtyping; however, approximately 90% of HER2+/ER− gene expression-defined tumor will have clinical assays negative for hormone receptors and positive for HER2 (31).

Basal-like Subtype

The basal-like subtype is characterized by low expression of the hormone receptor-related luminal genes, low expression of the HER2+ gene clusters, high expression of the proliferation cluster, and it shows high expression of a unique cluster of genes called the *basal cluster*. The basal gene cluster includes basal epithelial cytokeratins (CK), such as CK5, 14, and 17, epidermal growth factor receptor (EGFR), c-kit, vimentin, p-cadherin, fascin, caveolins 1 and 2, and αB-crystallin (8,15,23). Several risk factors for developing basal-like subtype have been identified. One of the most intriguing is the link between the basal-like breast cancer subtype and *BRCA1* mutation carriers (14,33–35).

When women who carry a deleterious mutation in *BRCA1* develop breast cancer, more than 80% of the time it is basal-like. Although *BRCA1* mutation carriers usually develop basal-like breast cancer, most basal-like breast cancers are sporadic and the *BRCA1* gene and protein appear intact in these tumors. A commonly held, but unproved, assumption is that the *BRCA1* pathway is somehow deranged in sporadic basal-like breast cancer, which if true, could have important therapeutic implications. The *BRCA1* and *2* pathways, which include a number of other genes, such as FANC family members, are involved in homologous recombination, which is a high fidelity DNA repair pathway. When the homologous pathway is lost or dysfunctional, DNA repair occurs by the more error-prone methods that involve poly(ADP-ribose) polymerase (PARP), which can be inhibited by a novel class of drugs that are being tested in clinical trials (36,37). Loss of normal DNA repair is also implicated in sensitivity to chemotherapy, particularly to DNA-damaging agents, such as platinum drugs (38), although recent studies suggest that basal-like breast cancers may have a general sensitivity to chemotherapy (31,39). Another notable association is between the basal-like subtype, race, and age. Several independent population-based studies have suggested that the basal-like subtype is overrepresented in breast cancer developing during the premenopausal years and in black women (10,24,25,40,41). In the Carolina Breast Cancer Study, basal-like breast cancer was the most common one among premenopausal black women (27%), and least common among postmenopausal women who were not black (9%) (25).

As might be expected by their ER-negative status and high proliferative capacity, basal-like breast cancer carries a poor prognosis in multiple datasets (10,11,14,42); this has raised the question of whether an excess of this subtype might contribute to the worse outcomes seen in black women with breast cancer. A variety of methods to identify basal-like breast cancer have been suggested, including reverse transcription (RT)-PCR–based methods, (11) IHC-based immunoprofiles (42,43), and the triple-negative (ER, PR, and HER2) phenotype that is already available in the clinic (31). Each approach has strengths and weaknesses; however, it is important to note that although most triple-negative tumors are basal-like and vice-versa, up to 30% of basal-like breast cancers identified by gene expression array will be misclassified by this method (44); thus, the addition of other markers to the triple-negative phenotype likely improves this classification (43).

BREAST CANCER SUBTYPES AND STEM CELLS

The categorization of breast cancers into luminal and basal-like subtypes arises from similarities of their gene expression patterns based on their inferred derivation from the expression patterns of normal breast epithelium. Luminal epithelial cells stain with antibodies against keratins 8 and 18, whereas basal epithelial cells stain with antibodies to keratin 5 and 17. These observations raise the question of whether these patterns arise from different progenitor cells rather than acquired variations during progression. Several lines of evidence support that breast cancer heterogeneity is an early phenomenon with distinct parallel lines of progression for each subtype. Basal-like, luminal, and HER2+/ER− subtypes are found in the preneoplastic, ductal carcinoma *in situ* stage (DCIS) (17,45,46). Gene copy number aberrations have characteristic patterns within invasive subtypes and in DCIS (47,48) and are more frequent in basal-like breast cancer even at diagnosis (49). A recent report focused on the genes associated with the putative cancer "stem cells" (50,51), which comprise less than 10% of the cells in breast cancer and are highly tumorigenic *in vivo*. These cells are characterized by high expression of the cell surface marker CD44, which is implicated in cell adhesion, migration, and proliferation, and low expression of the less well-characterized CD24. Comparison of CD44+ or CD24− cells with normal epithelial cells identified 186 genes associated with the tumorigenic cells, called the *invasiveness gene set* (IGS), which appeared prognostic in both breast and other tumor types. Examination of the 295-patient Amsterdam dataset revealed that the IGS is prognostic independent of clinical characteristics, and appears to be particularly so among ER+ or intermediate grade tumors. The IGS gene set overlapped little with other prognostic gene sets, and its impact was independent of the wound response signature described further below (52). Validation of the IGS and the stem cell component of breast cancer is an area of some controversy and intense research.

PROGNOSTIC APPLICATIONS OF ARRAYS

More than 90% of breast cancers are identified at a nonmetastatic, clinically curable stage; however, all are at risk of subsequent development of metastatic disease. Reduction in this risk requires medical therapy with chemotherapy, antiestrogen approaches, or one of an increasing number of targeted therapies discussed elsewhere. Identifying those at greatest risk of progression is crucial to limit the use of potentially toxic drugs to those most likely to benefit. This has been the purpose of prognostic indices in breast cancer.

Traditional prognosticators have been based on anatomic considerations, such as tumor size and locoregional extent, and involvement of axillary lymph nodes; often added to these are crude indicators of biology, such as grade and hormone receptor status. These traditional prognosticators include the Nottingham Prognostic Indicator (NPI), the St. Gallen criteria, the National Institutes of Health (NIH) consensus guidelines, and Adjuvant! Online, which use criteria, such tumor size, tumor grade, lymph node status, and hormone receptor status, to predict a patient's clinical outcome (53–56). The advent of genomics technology has allowed biology-based prognosticators to be developed (18,29,57–62), with the hope that these might add to, or replace, more traditional largely anatomy-based prognosticators. Only a handful of gene expression-based prognosticators, described below, have been validated and are in clinical use; in general, these complement, but do not replace, traditional prognostic factors.

A separate question is whether a study establishing prognostic relevance also establishes therapeutic relevance. In adjuvant therapy, prognostic relevance is often translated into therapeutic relevance simply because risk crosses a threshold for use of conventional adjuvant therapies to reduce risk. Two caveats should be kept in mind when considering gene array-based assays in this regard. First, unlike anatomic prognosticators, there may well be an interaction between the nature of the genes included in a particular profile and the benefit of systemic therapy. The most obvious analogy is the interaction between hormone receptor status and benefit of improved chemotherapy (3). This may mean that the interpretation of benefit may vary by profile, and should give warning to clinicians about excessive extrapolation. Second is that establishing therapeutic relevance is difficult to do. It requires either a prospective randomized clinical trial designed to test the therapeutic relevance of the marker (the holy grail of biomarker levels of evidence) or studies performed in a fairly homogeneous population with prospective ascertainment of clinical data, excellent representation of tumor samples, and *a priori*-defined profile definitions (63).

With these caveats in mind, the most clinically relevant scenario for prognostication by arrays is within node-negative breast cancer, because most of these patients do not relapse, yet most receive adjuvant therapy. Six prognostic profiles have shown promise in this arena and are relatively well characterized; of these, three have been validated and developed for clinical use in node-negative breast cancer: the Amsterdam 70-gene Mammaprint profile, the Recurrence Score, and the Rotterdam 76-gene signature. Several others, including the wound response signature and the invasiveness gene set, were developed from the same dataset as the 70-gene signature and appear to provide additional prognostic information within subsets. As mentioned above, another prognostic profile is the intrinsic subtypes, which were neither developed for prognostic purposes nor in node-negative disease, but have prognostic implications and can serve to identify relevant biologic pathways regardless of outcome (Table 32.1). Although the most clinically useful group for any prognostic profile are the node-negative population for chemotherapy decision-making, it is increasingly clear that the biologic pathways identified by these profiles are independent of anatomic extent of disease, and they may also provide useful information about identifying good-prognosis patients within the node-positive subset.

Recurrence Score

The 21-gene Recurrence Score assay (RS, Oncotype DX) was developed using unique methods and represents one of the most validated gene expression assays yet developed (29). Rather than supervised cluster analysis of genes related to outcome in frozen tissues, the investigators started with 250 candidate genes selected from the literature, genomic databases, and gene expression profiling experiments. Using 447 patients from three available datasets of mostly node-negative, hormone receptor-positive patients, and using a quantitative RT-PCR (qRT-PCR)-based approach that allows examination of limited number of genes in fixed tissue, they correlated gene expression with distant recurrence. From the 250 genes, 16 cancer-related and 5 reference genes were selected to be included in the RS assay. The RS is actually a score calculated using a published mathematical formula that assigns a weight to particular genes and groups of genes, which are then tabulated to give a single RS. This assay is unique in that it can be performed on fixed tumor samples and does not require frozen samples.

The RS was validated in an independent dataset derived from samples collected in the large cooperative group National Surgical Adjuvant Breast and Bowel Project (NSABP) B-14 trial, which examined the benefit of adjuvant tamoxifen in patients with hormone receptor-positive, lymph node-negative breast cancer. Of 2,617 tumors from the tamoxifen arm of the trial, 668 were available for assay and comparison with distant metastasis rates at approximately 10 years of follow-up (29). In those patients classified as low risk by the RS (RS <18) only 7% relapsed despite adjuvant tamoxifen, compared with high-risk patients (RS >31) among whom 31% relapsed (Fig. 32.3). In multivariate analysis including age, tumor size, tumor grade, ERBB2 status, and hormone receptor status, only the RS and grade 3 were significant predictors of clinical outcome. A topic of ongoing debate is how much of the prognostic value of the RS might be obtained by better pathologic grading and quantitative hormone receptor scoring as opposed to these biological properties being assayed by qRT-PCR. The main reclassification effect of the RS when compared with classic biomarkers is from high risk to low risk (64); befitting this effect, a recent report confirms that at least in largely academic practices the main clinical use of the RS is to change from planned chemoendocrine therapy to endocrine therapy alone (65). This study was a prospective cohort study, so is without many of the biases of a retrospective study, and can be considered level II evidence of the utility of the R.S.; based on these data, the RS has been accepted by many U.S. insurers and oncologists.

Table 32.1 | **PROGNOSTIC PROFILES**

Profile[a]	Training Population[a]	Validation Population[a]	End Point	Adjusted Hazard Ratio	Clinical Use and Notes
Recurrence Score (Oncotype DX) (29)	N = 447 N- or N+ ER+ and ER−, heterogeneous Rx	✓ Subset of prospective clinical trial (NSABP B14) N = 668 (of 2617) N0, ER+ Tamoxifen only Follow-up >10 yr	Distant metastasis at 10 yr	3.21 (2.23–4.61)	✓ Predictor of distant relapse in ER+ node-negative. ✓ Can be performed in fixed archival tissue.
Amsterdam 70-gene profile (Mammaprint) (18,61,72)	N = 78 N0, age <55yr, Follow-up >5 yr (18)	✓ Retrospective N = 295 (61 from training set) N− or N+, age <53 yr, T1-2, any ER Heterogeneous Rx Follow-up > 5 yr (61)	Distant metastasis first event	4.6 (2.3–9.2)	✓ Predictor of distant metastasis in Stage I-II. ✓ Frozen tissue required.
		✓ Retrospective N = 302 N0, age <61, T1-2, any ER No adjuvant systemic therapy Follow-up >10 yr (72)	Time to distant metastasis Overall survival Disease-free survival	2.13 (1.19–3.82) 2.63 (1.45–4.79) 1.36 (0.91–2.03)	
Rotterdam 76 gene signature (58,75)	N = 115 N0, No systemic Rx Followed >5 yr	✓ Retrospective N = 171 Mostly N0, 75% ER+ No systemic Rx Followed >5 yr (75)	Distant metastasis-free survival	5.55 (2.46–12.5)	✓ Predictor of distant metastasis-free survival in node-negative. ✓ Validated primarily in ER+. ✓ Requires frozen tissue.
		✓ Retrospective N = 180 N0, >90% ER+ Heterogeneous Rx Followed >5 yr (58)	Distant metastasis-free survival	11.36 (2.67–48.4)	
Two-gene signature (60,79,80)	N = 60 ER+ Adjuvant tamoxifen Follow-up >5 yr (60)	✓ Different methodology (not true validation) Subset of prospective clinical trial (NCCTG 89-30-52) N = 206 (of 256 in that arm) N0-1, ER+, T1-2 Tamoxifen Rx Follow-up 11 yr (78)	Relapse-free survival Disease-free survival Overall survival	1.63 (1.05–2.53) 1.75 (1.16–2.63) 1.63 (1.02–2.60)	✓ None at this time ✓ No consistent methodology so not yet validated ✓ Focus is on hormone receptor-positive ✓ Some methods use fixed tissue (78)
		✓ Different methodology (not true validation) Prospective tumor bank N = 225 N0, ER+ Untreated and tamoxifen Rx (from heterogeneous group of 852) Follow-up 6.8 yr (79)	Relapse-free survival	3.9 (1.5–10.3)	
		✓ Different methodology (not true validation) Retrospective N = 468 N0, ER+ No adjuvant Rx (from heterogeneous group of 1252) Follow-up 6 yr (80)	Disease-free survival	1.74 (1.17–2.59) method 1 1.61 (1.08–2.41) method 2	
Wound Response signature (71)	Core serum response genes in serum-stimulated fibroblasts	✓ Retrospective N = 295 (61) N0 and N+, age <53 yr, T1-2 Heterogeneous Rx Followed for >5 yr	Metastasis first event Overall survival	7.25 (1.75–30.0) 11.18 (2.52–49.6)	✓ None at this time ✓ Requires frozen tissue

Table 32.1	PROGNOSTIC PROFILES					
Invasiveness Gene Set (52)	186 genes differentiating CD44 +/CD24− cells from normal breast epithelium	✓ Retrospective N = 295 (61) N0 and N+, age <53 yr, T1-2 Heterogeneous Rx Followed for >5 yr	Metastasis-free survival	1.2 (1.1–1.4)	✓ None at this time ✓ Requires frozen tissue
			Overall survival	1.2 (1.0–1.4)	
Intrinsic Subtype (11,13,14)	N = 49 Before and after neoadjuvant doxorubicin (8)	✓ Retrospective N = 97 (Amsterdam training set+) Mostly N0, age <55 yr Follow-up >5 yr (14)	Time to distant metastasis	p <.01 across subtypes Not available	✓ None at this time ✓ Primary interest for stratification rather than prognostication
		✓ Retrospective N = 311 (multiple datasets, including training set) N0 and N+, ER any Heterogeneous Rx (11)	Relapse-free survival vs Luminal	2.02 (1.1–3.9) Basal-like 3.47 (1.8–6.8) HER2 +/ER 1.92 (1.1–3.5) Luminal B	✓ Requires frozen tissue

N0, lymph node negative; N+, lymph node positive; Rx, treatment.
^aNumbers in parentheses refer to references.

The RS was validated in a homogeneous patient population of node-negative, hormone receptor-positive and tamoxifen-treated women. For this reason, it was not clear if its prognostic ability reflected true prognosis, prediction of lack of tamoxifen benefit, or both. Moreover, the ability to intervene in the poor prognosis group with chemotherapy was at that time undocumented. Subsequent studies have illuminated the meaning and therapeutic role of the RS. In a population-based, case-control study, the RS provided independent prognostic information in tamoxifen-treated patients as expected; it also predicted outcome in untreated patients, suggesting a pure prognostic role in addition to the previously suggested predictive one for endocrine sensitivity (66). In addition to predicting worse outcome despite endocrine therapy, a high RS also predicts benefit of chemotherapy (30,67). Even more recently, the RS was examined in two datasets of node-positive breast cancer. In the Eastern Cooperative Oncology Group (ECOG) 2197, 2,603 women with node-negative or node-positive disease were randomized to receive Doxorubican plus docetaxel (AT) or Doxorubican plus cyclophosphamide (AC) adjuvant chemotherapy, with no significant differences seen (68). A subset of 465 underwent RS assay (69), which was a highly significant predictor of outcome despite chemoendocrine therapy in both node-negative and node-positive patients. In the Southwest Oncology Group (SWOG) 8814, 1,477 postmenopausal women with node-positive, hormone receptor-positive breast cancer were randomized to tamoxifen alone, cyclophosphamide, doxorubicin, plus fluorouracil (CAF) chemotherapy plus tamoxifen begun concurrently, or CAF chemotherapy followed by tamoxifen (70). The parent trial revealed a benefit of chemotherapy, particularly given sequentially with tamoxifen. The RS was performed in 367 tumors from the sequential CAF-tamoxifen arm of the study, and it revealed that in the node-positive population the RS was prognostic across nodal categories; moreover, that the benefit of the addition of CAF to tamoxifen was primarily seen in those with high RS. The caveat to clinical application of this finding to node-positive breast cancer is that this is an older regimen, and even in the "good risk" low RS group, the long term disease-free survival was only 60%.

Amsterdam 70-Gene Profile

The Amsterdam 70-gene prognostic profile (Mammaprint) was created by supervised analysis of gene expression arrays in frozen tumor samples from The Netherlands Cancer Institute. The 98 tumors included 78 from node-negative patients under the age of 55 at diagnosis, 34 of 78 (44%) had developed distant metastasis within 5 years of completing treatment and 44 of 78 (56%) had not developed any distant disease. As discussed above, included also were 20 tumors from hereditary breast cancers, 18 BRCA1 and 2 BRCA2 (18) By comparing the gene expression profile of the tumors with and without subsequent distant metastasis, a signature 70-gene set was identified. This 70-gene prognosticator was 83% accurate (65 of 78 patients) in predicting later distant metastasis among the patients used to generate the signature. Since the initial publication, there have been three external validation studies of the 70-gene prognostic profile. The first was a retrospective analysis of 295 patients from The Netherlands Cancer Institute who were under the age of 53 years at diagnosis with T1-2 tumors, either lymph node-negative (151 patients) or lymph node-positive (144 patients), heterogeneously treated with or without adjuvant therapy and

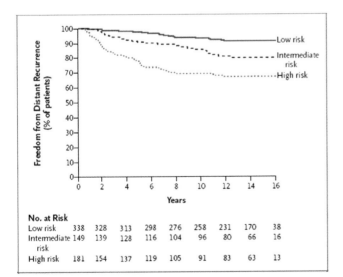

FIGURE 32.3. Likelihood of distant recurrence by Recurrence Score category in women with node-negative, hormone receptor-positive breast cancer treated with adjuvant tamoxifen on NSABP B-14. (From Paik S, Shak S, Tang G, et al. A multigene assay to predict recurrence of tamoxifen-treated, node-negative breast cancer. *N Engl J Med* 2004;351: 2817–2826, with permission.)

followed for nearly 7 years (61). Of the 295 patients, 180 of the patients were classified as having a poor 70-gene signature and 115 as having a good 70-gene signature. A strong correlation was found between signature status and likelihood of distant metastasis and death; the mean 5-year survival for the poor 70-gene signature group of patients was 74% versus 97% for the good 70-gene signature patients. This signature was able to predict prognosis regardless of lymph node status and remained significant in multivariate analysis of first event, as did the traditional prognostic criteria of tumor size, nodal involvement, and use of adjuvant chemotherapy. Among the criticisms of this 295-patient analysis was the inclusion of 61 tumors that had been in the original training set; however, the subsequent validation studies have not mixed training and test set samples and have proved value. Of note, the investigators have been strongly collaborative with this 295-patient array dataset, which has been used to develop or validate many other profiles, including the wound response signature (71), the invasiveness gene set (52), and the comparison of prognostic profiles (26).

A second, less heterogeneous, and truly independent retrospective external validation study of the 70-gene prognostic signature was performed in 302 women treated at several European institutions, who were under age 60 with node-negative T1-2 breast cancers and did not receive adjuvant systemic therapy, and who were followed for more than 10 years. Adjusted for clinical risk as assessed by Adjuvant! software, the 70-gene prognostic indicator effectively predicted time to distant metastasis (hazard ratio [HR] 2.13, 95% confidence intervals (CI) 1.19–3.82) and overall survival (HR 2.63, 95% CI 1.45–4.79); it did not significantly predict disease-free survival (HR 1.36, 95% CI 0.91–2.03) (Fig. 32.4) (72). There is a strong time dependence of the 70-gene profile, befitting the way it was developed because it far better predicts early (before 5 years) than later relapse (73). Notably, this profile is more useful in ER+ than ER− disease; among ER+ tumors, 50% had low profiles, whereas among ER− only 6% showed the favorable profile. This validation study provided the evidence needed for U.S. Food and Drug Administration (FDA) approval of the Mammaprint assay and implementation in the Microarray in Node-Negative Disease May Avoid Chemotherapy trial (MINDACT), which is described below.

One obstacle to large-scale use of the 70-gene signature has been the need for a significant amount of frozen tissue and the turnaround time of one-tumor-per-chip microarrays; a recent study employing a custom miniarray designed for high throughput processing found very good concordance with the earlier microarray data from the 295-patient validation series. This can help with the issue of how to manage large numbers of tumors simultaneously; however, it does not obviate the need for frozen tissue, a major impediment for use in the United States (74). The evidence to date supports a modest but real impact of the 70-gene prognosticator in predicting outcome independent of clinical variables. Level I evidence of its clinical utility awaits completion of the MINDACT trial, in which women with node-negative breast cancer will undergo clinical risk assessment via Adjuvant! Online and the 70-gene prognostic signature, and when these two tests disagree, patients will be randomized to be treated according to the predictions of one test alone.

The Rotterdam 76-gene Signature

The Rotterdam/Veridex 76-gene prognostic signature was developed in lymph node-negative breast cancer to identify those more or less likely to benefit from adjuvant systemic therapy, because most of these patients are cured with locoregional treatment alone (75). The test set included 286 node-negative breast cancers from patients who did not receive adjuvant therapy and had been followed more than 8 years, of which 93 patients developed distant metastases. These

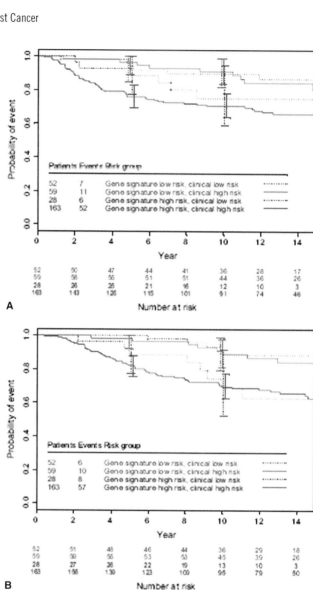

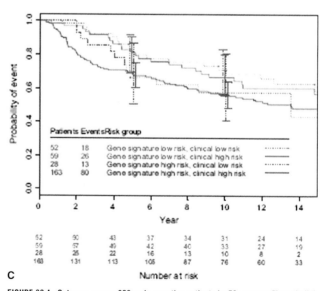

FIGURE 32.4. Outcome among 302 node-negative patients by 70-gene profile and clinical risk (with 95% confidence limits in bars). **A:** Time to distant metastasis. **B:** Overall survival. **C:** Disease-free survival. (From Buyse M, Loi S, van't Veer L, et al. Validation and clinical utility of a 70-gene prognostic signature for women with node-negative breast cancer. *J Natl Cancer Inst* 2006;98(17):1183–1192, with permission.)

tumors were divided into ER− and ER+ groups and subjected to gene expression profiling. Sixty genes were selected as prognostic for ER+ and 16 for ER− for a total of 76 prognostic genes. Of the 286 patients, 115 patients served as the training set, from which a prognostic model was created by combining the 76 selected genes selected from the profiling experiments and stratified by ER status data. The remaining 171 mixed ER+ (75%) and ER− (25%) tumors served as the validation set. The sensitivity of the 76-gene test in predicting distant metastasis was 93%, and the specificity was 48%. In multivariate analysis of distant metastasis-free survival, the 76-gene prognostic indicator outperformed clinical variables and was the only significant variable to contribute to prognosis prediction. In a subsequent independent validation study in 180 lymph node-negative patients who did not receive adjuvant systemic therapy the Rotterdam 76-gene signature was able to identify accurately poor prognosis patients (increased risk of distant metastasis within 5 years) versus good prognosis patients with a hazard ratio of 7.41 (95% CI

2.63–20.9) that remained significant in multivariate analysis (58). Notably, only 16 patients had ER-disease, making generalizations to this subset difficult. A second independent validation study was performed in a subset of 198 of the 302 node-negative patients earlier used in the 70-gene prognostic profile (72), chosen because of residual available tumor for analysis (76). The 76-gene prognosticator demonstrated an independent prognostic ability in time to distant metastasis that appeared stronger than the 70-gene profile in the same dataset (HR 5.78, 95% CI 1.78–18.80) and overall survival (2.87, 95% CI 1.21–6.82), although direct comparisons are limited by the subset nature of the analysis (Fig. 32.5). As with the 70-gene prognostic profile, the 76-gene profile had a clear time dependence and was more effective in predicting early relapse than later. Given that chemotherapy primarily affects early relapse, this interaction works in favor of the utility of these profiles in decision-making regarding adjuvant chemotherapy. As with the 70-gene prognosticator, the 76-gene Rotterdam assay also requires frozen samples.

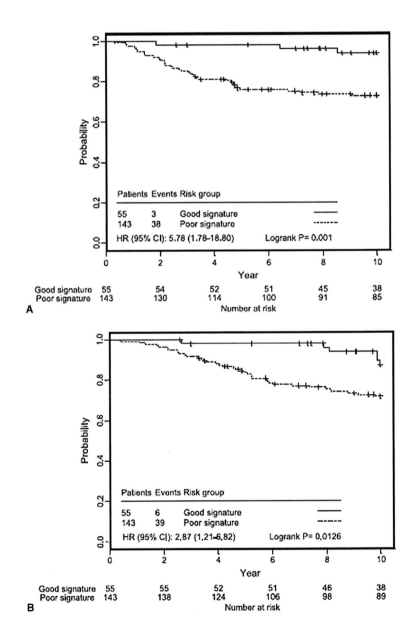

FIGURE 32.5. Outcome among a subset of 198 node-negative patients from the same population as in Figure 32.4 by 76-gene profile and clinical risk. **A:** Time to distant metastasis. **B:** Overall survival. (From Desmedt C, Piette F, Loi S, et al. Strong time dependence of the 76-gene prognostic signature for node-negative breast cancer patients in the TRANSBIG multicenter independent validation series. *Clin* Cancer Res 2007;13(11):3207–3214, with permission.)

A Two-Gene Signature for Outcome Predictions

The initial development of a two-gene signature (HOX13:IL17BR) was from 22,000-gene arrays performed in 60 node-positive women with hormone receptor-positive breast cancer treated with tamoxifen and followed for at least 5 years (60). HOXB13 was associated with recurrence, whereas IL17BR was associated with remaining disease free, making the ratio even more strongly associated with recurrence with an adjusted odds ratio of approximately 7. Using an adaptation of this assay to fixed tissue, however, failed to replicate the results (77). Another study using a 211-tumor subset of a prospective clinical trial (NCCTG 89-30-52) modified the methodology and also used fixed tissue, finding a significant association of HOXB13:IL17BR to relapse-free, disease-free, and overall survival in hormone receptor-positive, tamoxifen-treated women with mixed nodal status (78). Two larger studies have since been performed; however, both used slightly different methodologies from the original study and from each other; one included 852 patients with stage I-II tumors of mixed nodal and hormone receptor status followed for nearly 7 years (79); the two-gene signature was found to be prognostic among ER+ and node-negative patients in this dataset regardless of tamoxifen treatment. Another retrospective study (80) of 1252 heterogeneously treated patients found the two-gene ratio to be associated with grade and hormone receptor status. Among 468 mixed nodal status, ER+ untreated patients, the signature measured using two different methods yielded a significant association with relapse, with an HR of approximately 1.5 to 1.7. A study using tumors collected from patients treated on two different prospective studies of hormone receptor-positive breast cancer patients and using yet another methodology found that women with a low two-gene ratio appear to derive greater benefit of 5 compared with 2 years of adjuvant tamoxifen (81). This signature can be performed in fixed or frozen tissue, which makes it of considerable clinical interest; however, given the varying methodologies and cut points in the studies to date, it remains intriguing, but further implementation awaits ongoing validation studies.

Other Prognostic Signatures

A large number of prognostic signatures have been identified for breast cancer patients and all cannot be discussed here; however, several that are less clinically developed are of interest. The *wound response* gene expression signature is derived from a set of genes, termed *core serum response* (CSR) genes, which changed expression when cultured fibroblasts were activated with serum. Evaluation of the CSR genes suggested that they represented important processes in wound healing, such as matrix remodeling, cell motility, and angiogenesis, all of which are predicted to play a role in cancer invasion and metastasis (82). Subsequent evaluation of the CSR genes in the same 295-patient dataset used to validate the Amsterdam 70-gene profile suggested that an activated wound response signature was associated with decreased survival and increased probability of distant metastasis in both univariate and multivariate analyses (71). Thus, a conclusion from this profile is that genes and biology that come from nontumor cells can be an important determinant of patient outcomes.

Many signatures directly, or indirectly, contain genes indicative of cell proliferation rates (83). A proliferative gene profile was derived from the Amsterdam 70-gene dataset (18,61) that included 50 cell cycle-related genes, and provided additional prognostic information within the subset of patients with higher than expected ER expression (84). Given that one of the distinctions between luminal A and luminal B tumors is on the basis of the proliferation cluster, as is a large portion of the RS profile, this profile may in part differentiate these prognostically distinct groups also. Angiogenesis is an increasingly recognized component of tumor progression. Recent studies suggest that expression levels of hypoxia-induced genes are prognostic (85). Although the independent contribution of this signature is not yet clear, there are currently no markers effective in selecting patients for the antiangiogenic drugs being used in the metastatic setting and being tested in the adjuvant setting.

Although the intrinsic gene subtypes first described by Sorlie et al. (13) were not originally intended to function as prognostic indicators, the subtypes correlated with prognosis in the original population of patients with locally advanced tumors who had been treated with neoadjuvant doxorubicin (13). Patients with the luminal A subtype had the best prognosis as evaluated by overall survival (OS) and relapse-free survival (RFS) followed by luminal B. Both the basal-like and HER2+/ER− subtypes had the worst OS and RFS rates. Correlation of outcome with subtype in the independent van't Veer dataset revealed a significantly longer time to development of distant metastasis among patients with luminal A tumors compared with patients with luminal B, basal-like or HER2+/ER− tumors (14). Similarly, in both a far larger combined dataset of 311 frozen samples of heterogeneous breast cancers and a study using immunohistochemical proxies for the subtypes in a population-based study of nearly 500 tumors, the association of intrinsic subtype with prognosis remained, with the best outcome observed among patients with luminal A tumors compared with the other subtypes (10,11).

PROGNOSTIC PROFILES IN CONTEXT

A useful array-based prognostic profile must add independent information to more easily obtained clinical information, must be accurate, reproducible, and feasible using clinically available material. Many markers and profiles are prognostic and a few have met these criteria. Despite development and validation in relatively similar populations, in general, however, these profiles have shown little overlap in gene content. This is not only confusing, but raises the important question of validity and how the clinician chooses among potentially competing assays. Comparison of the Amsterdam 70-gene signature with the St. Gallen or NIH criteria reveals that the 70-gene signature assigns more patients to the low-risk group than the clinical factors: 40% versus 15% versus 7%, respectively (61). Comparison of the Amsterdam 70-gene signature to the Adjuvant! Online risk assessment also confirmed the added benefit of the 70-gene profile to clinical risk assessment. The additional benefit of this and similar genomic tools over clinical-pathologic criteria is still an area of some controversy (86). Similarly, the Rotterdam 76-gene signature also appears to provide independent prognostic information to the clinicopathologic St. Gallen and NIH consensus criteria (58,75). Using the 76-gene signature, approximately 40% of patients classified as average or high risk by the St. Gallen or NIH criteria would have been reclassified as low risk using the 76-gene signature (58). The independence of the genomic and the clinical prognosticators suggests that each will provide the best information when applied in concert with the other. In other words, both biology and anatomy are destiny and prognostication is best when both are used.

Comparison of the different prognostic profiles with one another is interesting. A recent study directly compared the Amsterdam 70-gene signature, the RS, the wound response profile, and the intrinsic subtypes in a single dataset, and found that all four models were highly concordant with respect to their ability to prognosticate (Table 32.2). Those tumors that classified into known biologically distinct intrinsic subtypes with poor prognosis, such as the basal-like, HER2+/ER−, or luminal B subtypes, typically also had poor prognostic signatures as assigned by the other three signatures (11,26,71). Conversely, comparison of several tamoxifen resistance profiles, including a 78-gene profile derived from a previously reported 81-gene profile (87), the RS

Table 32.2	PROGNOSTIC PROFILE BY INTRINSIC SUBTYPE (26)

Intrinsic Subtype	No. of Patients	Recurrence Score		70 Gene Profile		Wound Response	
		Classification	No. of Patients (%)	Classification	No. of Patients (%)	Classification	No. of Patients (%)
Basal-like	53	Low	0 (0)	Good	0 (0)	Quiescent	3 (6)
		Intermediate	0 (0)				
		High	53 (100)	Poor	53 (100)	Activated	50 (94)
Luminal A	123	Low	62 (50)	Good	87 (71)	Quiescent	45 (37)
		Intermediate	25 (20)				
		High	36 (29)	Poor	36 (29)	Activated	78 (63)
Luminal B	55	Low	1 (2)	Good	9 (16)	Quiescent	4 (7)
		Intermediate	4 (7)				
		High	50 (91)	Poor	46 (84)	Activated	51 (93)
HER2+/ER-	35	Low	0 (0)	Good	3 (9)	Quiescent	0 (0)
		Intermediate	0 (0)				
		High	35 (100)	Poor	32 (91)	Activated	35 (100)
Normal-like	29	Low	7 (24)	Good	16 (55)	Quiescent	15 (52)
		Intermediate	4 (14)				
		High	18 (62)	Poor	13 (45)	Activated	14 (48)

From Fan C, Oh DS, Wessels L, et al. Concordance among gene-expression-based predictors for breast cancer. *N Engl J Med* 2006;355:560–569, adapted with permission.

(29), and the two-gene profile (60) applied to a 246-patient dataset of ER+ metastatic tumors treated with tamoxifen revealed only 45% to 60% signature concordance; however, similar prognostic capabilities were noted (88). Although these profiles have few genes in common, these data suggest commonality of important pathways, including proliferation and ER status among disparate prognostic profiles (26) and argues that the ability to predict clinical outcome is not related to the expression of a specific few breast cancer-promoting genes but rather to large groups of genes that represent dominant biologic pathways that drive cancers (89).

PREDICTIVE ARRAY-BASED PROFILES

An area of great interest is the potential of gene expression arrays to identify gene lists that can predict response, or nonresponse, to particular regimens, with the hope for individualizing therapy by examining the tumor at the time of diagnosis. Predictive arrays are not as far along in development as prognostic arrays; however, a number of predictive profiles have been or are being developed that will be summarized here and in Table 32.1. These are often mindful of a particular indication, such as tamoxifen resistance, so are mentioned with predictive arrays, although in many cases these are developed as prognostic as well as predictive profiles.

Prediction of Endocrine Therapy Sensitivity

Because hormone receptor-positive breast cancer is virtually always treated with adjuvant endocrine therapy, identifying how much of an impact on outcome is prognostic versus predictive can be difficult. The RS is both prognostic in the untreated cohort and predictive of tamoxifen benefit in NSABP B-14, the randomized study examining tamoxifen versus placebo in node-negative, hormone receptor-positive patients (90). Other predictive profiles for endocrine therapy include the 81-gene tamoxifen resistance profile (87) and the two-gene signature, both of which predicted time to progression on tamoxifen in the first-line metastatic setting (88). The assumption is that predictive profiles developed on tamoxifen will equally predict response to aromatase inhibition; however, this may not be true and is currently untested. At this time, no predictive profile for endocrine sensitivity has been

validated, although several, such as the HOXB13:IL17BR two-gene test (Table 32.1) (60,78–80), may be predictive in addition to prognostic, and are in active development.

Prediction of Chemotherapy Sensitivity

Chemotherapy efficacy differs among different subtypes, in particular between ER− and ER+ subtypes (3), so multigene predictors must provide information beyond the available clinical assays. The most clearly developed predictive profile for chemotherapy sensitivity is the RS, which is also the only profile tested in the kind of prospectively annotated large datasets that provide reliable evidence of efficacy. In a subset of more than 600 tumors from ER+ node-negative patients in NSABP B-20, the RS predicted sensitivity to methotrexate plus fluorouracil with or without cyclophosphamide (MF/CMF) added to tamoxifen in hormone receptor-positive node-negative patients (30). Smaller neoadjuvant studies have correlated higher RS with pathologic complete response to doxorubicin plus paclitaxel (AT), although this particular end point was uncommon even in the highest RS tested (67), and another with clinical complete response to single agent doxorubicin (91). Finally, a study similar in design to the NSABP B20 study has been presented, which examined a subset of 367 tumors from postmenopausal women participating in SWOG 8814 and found that the benefit of CAF added to tamoxifen in hormone receptor-positive node-positive disease is primarily among high RS (70). These studies suggest that the RS predicts general sensitivity or resistance to chemotherapy, but cannot help select one agent or regimen over another. The clinical utility of the RS in adding chemotherapy to endocrine therapy in intermediate (11–25) RS scores is being prospectively examined in the TailoRx trial; however, recognizing the lack of regimen-specificity in the studies to date, the choice of chemotherapy is left to the discretion of the treating physician.

The area of greatest interest is in the development of chemotherapy regimen- or agent-specific predictive signatures. There have been several different predictive profiles for docetaxel sensitivity; an 85-gene signature (with cellular redox genes over-represented) that was approximately 80% accurate in predicting clinical response to the single agent in the neoadjuvant setting (92), a similarly derived 92-gene signature that was nearly 90% accurate (93), and a 50-gene signature derived from cell lines that was 92% accurate when applied to a small neoadjuvant dataset (94). An RT-PCR–based method for the 92-gene signature plus other candidate genes allowed testing in fixed tissue and found 14 genes predictive of clinical complete response to neoadjuvant docetaxel; however, the false discovery rate (likelihood of finding these genes by chance) was very high (91). All of these studies are limited by size, heterogeneity in tumor types, lack of independent validation, and the use of end points of unclear clinical significance.

A 74-gene predictor of an anthracycline and taxane-based regimen was developed from permutation modeling of a neoadjuvant dataset treated with paclitaxel, fluorouracil, doxorubicin, and cyclophosphamide (95). The investigators used a more rigorous end point, pathologic complete response, and permutation testing to develop the model, which required at least 70 genes to have a false discovery rate less than 10%. They expanded this dataset and modified the methodology to develop a 30-probe set predictor that was applied to an independent set of 51 patients. Interestingly, the best predictive model included both genomic and clinical data (96). The same group that identified the 92-gene signature also examined a cohort of patients treated neoadjuvantly with doxorubicin plus cyclophosphamide (AC), and identified 253 genes associated with clinical response (97). Interestingly, the 92-gene docetaxel signature did not predict response to AC, suggesting that regimen-specific signatures allowing selection of anthracycline- versus nonanthracycline-based chemotherapy may be feasible in the future. A similar comparison was made in a study involving a subset of 125 tumors from patients participating in a randomized neoadjuvant phase III trial of fluorouracil, epirubicin, and cyclophosphamide (FEC) versus a docetaxel and epirubicin regimen (TET) in ER− disease (98). The investigators used the same cell line-based approach as in an earlier docetaxel study (94) to derive regimen-specific signatures that were approximately 80% accurate. In a related effort, they found that signatures associated with oncogenic pathway activation and tumor microenvironment status was prognostic and may confer unique chemotherapy sensitivity (99); interpretation is limited by the retrospective and heterogeneous nature of the dataset and the need for analysis in light of other prognostic signatures. If validated, this approach is very intriguing in its ability to develop drug- and regimen-specific signatures *in vitro* that may show high accuracy *in vivo*.

As detailed above, multiple prior and ongoing efforts exist to develop gene expression signatures of chemotherapy response. It should be noted that most rely on the neoadjuvant setting for training and discovery, which assumes that the gene sets related to response will also relate to the development of distant disease. Given the tight association of pathologic response to outcome, this may be a reasonable assumption, however it is unproved. In addition, in assays used for decision-making regarding the use and selection of chemotherapeutic agents, even 10% to 20% inaccuracy may be unacceptable as even the slight benefit of a regimen is valuable.

Prediction of Response to HER2-targeted Agents

Most of the approaches to prediction of response to HER2-targeted agents, such as trastuzumab and lapatinib, have been single marker approaches and are discussed elsewhere. Only small hypothesis-generating studies have yet examined array-based approaches to identifying signatures of response to trastuzumab (100), although this is an area of great interest.

PITFALLS AND LIMITATIONS OF APPLIED ARRAY TECHNOLOGIES

The most important pitfall of array-based prognostic and predictive profiles has already been highlighted—namely that these are works in progress. Even the most validated assays have been studied in relatively small datasets or as subsets of larger clinical trials, and many have not been validated at all on independent test sets. None have met level I criteria for use in clinical decision-making, although both the RS and the Amsterdam 70-gene prognostic profile are in the midst of prospective trials that will define their clinical utility within defined populations. Of concern is that the field of breast cancer therapy is rapidly changing, and evidence of prognosis or efficacy of a particular approach can become obsolete during the performance of validation studies. For example, it may take 10 years to get the results of the MINDACT trial that is prospectively testing the value of the 70-gene assay in determining the benefit of chemotherapy, and so the difficult question is do we wait till this trial is completed to begin the everyday use of this assay? Approaches that will make development and validation of array-based signatures more nimble are crucial, and the treating oncologist must ask whether retrospective validation is sufficient evidence to support current clinical use.

Exceptional rigor—as always—is required in the tumor collection, processing, data management, and statistical methods used to analyze gene expression arrays, which are susceptible to overfitting owing to the very high number of genes analyzed, high false–negative rates because of the sheer volume and hypothesis-generating nature of arrays, and bias introduced by nonindependence of genes from one another and from clinical variables (101). Gene expression pattern reproducibility can also be an issue (102), as can data processing variability and tumor enrichment (33). In fact, one interpretation of the "normal-like" intrinsic subtype is that these are samples with an excess of stroma, and thus these assays may be more sensitive to tumor cell content versus other biomarker methods such IHC. Another methodologic issue is the generalizability and robustness of profiles developed in a certain population when applied to a different population. For example, the strength of the Amsterdam 70-gene prognosticator in predicting relapse was far higher in the original dataset (HR of relapse approximately 5) than in the independent validation studies, in which the HR was more modest (approximately 2). This may be owing to overfitting in the original series, which included some of the training set tumors in the validation set, or a more natural regression to the mean when a more heterogeneous population is studied. The importance of the studied population is also highlighted by RS studies demonstrating that, although the prognostic implication of the RS remains across tumor sizes and nodal categories, smaller tumors have lower risk even if the RS is high (66), whereas node-positive breast cancer carries a poor prognosis even if the profile is low (70). In other words, biology is not entirely destiny, which again suggests that a combination of genomic and classic biomarker assays is best.

FUTURE DIRECTIONS

The ongoing MINDACT and TailoRx trials will provide level I evidence of the clinical utility of the 70-gene prognosticator and the Recurrence Score assays, respectively; however, even these large-scale prognostic studies will have significant limitations. The 70-gene profile requires frozen tissue that is not conventionally available; large scale implementation would require a significant modification in the way that pathology is routinely handled in the United States or the profile would need to be developed and validated in fixed tissue. TailoRx is examining the benefit of chemotherapy added to endocrine therapy in a relatively restricted population of node-negative, hormone receptor-positive patients with low-intermediate (between 11 and 25) RS with the hope that an optimal cut point for the use of chemotherapy will be determined.

Although the Rotterdam 76-gene profile was developed in both ER+ and ER− disease, it is relatively invalidated in the ER− setting, and comparison of different profiles to intrinsic subtypes clearly suggests that current prognostic profiles largely detect biologic heterogeneity within ER+ disease (26). No prognostic profile has yet been developed for hormone receptor-negative breast cancer, because these tumors also have a heterogeneous prognosis, this would be a clinically valuable direction for researchers to take, as would efforts to define heterogeneity within intrinsic subtypes.

Although the technology for individualizing therapy on the basis of gene arrays for tumor characteristics has exploded, other facets have barely been explored. For example, the effectiveness of certain drugs, such as tamoxifen and the chemotherapy irinotecan, is mediated by metabolism by cytochrome p450 enzymes that have considerable variability based on genetic polymorphisms (103). Assays for clinically relevant individual cytochrome p450 genes already exist, and investigators and diagnostic companies are developing drug-metabolizing enzyme gene arrays that detect genetic variations in multiple genes. These single nucleotide polymorphism (SNP) chips, which detect actual gene variants (rather than gene expression variation), hold great promise for both individualizing medicine choices and detecting multiple gene interactions in risk of breast cancer. As stated, the future of prognostication and prediction lies in the integration of classic biomarkers, such as ER status and stage, with genomic biomarkers, with genetic biomarkers, which is occurring and resulting in more accurate outcome predictions for breast cancer patients.

References

1. Loman N, Johannsson O, Bendahl PO, et al. Steroid receptors in hereditary breast carcinomas associated with BRCA1 or BRCA2 mutations or unknown susceptibility genes. *Cancer* 1998;83:310–319.
2. Robson M, Rajan P, Rosen PP, et al. BRCA-associated breast cancer: absence of a characteristic immunophenotype. *Cancer Res* 1998;58:1839–1842.
3. Berry DA, Cirrincione C, Henderson IC, et al. Estrogen-receptor status and outcomes of modern chemotherapy for patients with node-positive breast cancer. *JAMA* 2006;295:1658–1667.
4. Hess KR, Pusztai L, Buzdar AU, et al. Estrogen receptors and distinct patterns of breast cancer relapse. *Breast Cancer Res Treat* 2003;78:105–118.
5. Gennari A, Sormani MP, Pronzato P, et al. HER2 status and efficacy of adjuvant anthracyclines in early breast cancer: a pooled analysis of randomized trials. *J Natl Cancer Inst* 2008;100:14–20.
6. Golub TR, Slonim DK, Tamayo P, et al. Molecular classification of cancer: class discovery and class prediction by gene expression monitoring. *Science* 1999;286: 531–537.
7. Simon R, Radmacher MD, Dobbin K. Design of studies using DNA microarrays. *Genet Epidemiol* 2002;23:21–36.
8. Perou CM, Sorlie T, Eisen MB, et al. Molecular portraits of human breast tumours. *Nature* 2000;406:747–752.
9. Abd El-Rehim DM, Pinder SE, Paish CE, et al. Expression of luminal and basal cytokeratins in human breast carcinoma. *J Pathol* 2004;203:661–671.
10. Carey LA, Perou CM, Livasy CA, et al. Race, breast cancer subtypes, and survival in the Carolina Breast Cancer Study. *JAMA* 2006;295:2492–2502.
11. Hu Z, Fan C, Oh DS, et al. The molecular portraits of breast tumors are conserved across microarray platforms. *BMC Genomics* 2006;7:96.
12. Perreard L, Fan C, Quackenbush JF, et al. Classification and risk stratification of invasive breast carcinomas using a real-time quantitative RT-PCR assay. *Breast Cancer Res* 2006;8:R23.
13. Sorlie T, Perou CM, Tibshirani R, et al. Gene expression patterns of breast carcinomas distinguish tumor subclasses with clinical implications. *Proc Natl Acad Sci U S A* 2001;98:10869–10874.
14. Sorlie T, Tibshirani R, Parker J, et al. Repeated observation of breast tumor subtypes in independent gene expression data sets. *Proc Natl Acad Sci U S A* 2003; 100:8418–8423.
15. Sotiriou C, Neo SY, McShane LM, et al. Breast cancer classification and prognosis based on gene expression profiles from a population-based study. *Proc Natl Acad Sci U S A* 2003;100:10393–10398.
16. Yu K, Lee CH, Tan PH, et al. Conservation of breast cancer molecular subtypes and transcriptional patterns of tumor progression across distinct ethnic populations. *Clin Cancer Res* 2004;10:5508–5517.
17. Livasy CA, Perou CM, Karaca G, et al. Identification of a basal-like subtype of breast ductal carcinoma *in situ*. *Hum Pathol* 2007;38:197–204.
18. van 't Veer LJ, Dai H, van de Vijver MJ, et al. Gene expression profiling predicts clinical outcome of breast cancer. *Nature* 2002;415:530–536.
19. West M, Blanchette C, Dressman H, et al. Predicting the clinical status of human breast cancer by using gene expression profiles. *Proc Natl Acad Sci U S A* 2001; 98:11462–11467.
20. Kapp AV, Jeffrey SS, Langerod A, et al. Discovery and validation of breast cancer subtypes. *BMC Genomics* 2006;7:231.
21. Sorlie T, Wang Y, Xiao C, et al. Distinct molecular mechanisms underlying clinically relevant subtypes of breast cancer: gene expression analyses across three different platforms. *BMC Genomics* 2006;7:127.
22. Mullins M, Perreard L, Quackenbush JF, et al. Agreement in breast cancer classification between microarray and quantitative reverse transcription PCR from fresh-frozen and formalin-fixed, paraffin-embedded tissues. *Clin Chem* 2007;53:1273–1279.
23. Oh DS, Troester MA, Usary J, et al. Estrogen-regulated genes predict survival in hormone receptor-positive breast cancers. *J Clin Oncol* 2006;24:1656–1664.
24. Morris GJ, Naidu S, Topham AK, et al. Differences in breast carcinoma characteristics in newly diagnosed African-American and Caucasian patients: a single-institution compilation compared with the National Cancer Institute's Surveillance, Epidemiology, and End Results database. *Cancer* 2007;110:876–884.
25. Millikan RC, Newman B, Tse CK, et al. Epidemiology of basal-like breast cancer. *Breast Cancer Res Treat* 2008 May;109(1):123–139.
26. Fan C, Oh DS, Wessels L, et al. Concordance among gene-expression-based predictors for breast cancer. *N Engl J Med* 2006;355:560–569.
27. Loi S, Haibe-Kains B, Desmedt C, et al. Definition of clinically distinct molecular subtypes in estrogen receptor-positive breast carcinomas through genomic grade. *J Clin Oncol* 2007;25:1239–1246.
28. Chen WY, Colditz GA. Risk factors and hormone-receptor status: epidemiology, risk-prediction models and treatment implications for breast cancer. *Nat Clin Pract Oncol* 2007;4:415–423.
29. Paik S, Shak S, Tang G, et al. A multigene assay to predict recurrence of tamoxifen-treated, node-negative breast cancer. *N Engl J Med* 2004;351:2817–2826.
30. Paik S, Tang G, Shak S, et al. Gene expression and benefit of chemotherapy in women with node-negative, estrogen receptor-positive breast cancer. *J Clin Oncol* 2006;24:3726–3734.
31. Carey LA, Dees EC, Sawyer L, et al. The triple negative paradox: primary tumor chemosensitivity of breast cancer subtypes. *Clin Cancer Res* 2007;13:2329–2334.
32. Piccart MJ, Loi S, Van't Veer L, et al. Multi-center external validation study of the Amsterdam 70-gene prognostic signature in node negative untreated breast cancer: are the results outperforming the clinical-pathological criteria? In: San Antonio Breast Cancer Symposium. San Antonio, Texas, December 11, 2004.
33. Foulkes WD, Brunet JS, Stefansson IM, et al. The prognostic implication of the basal-like (cyclin E high/p27 low/p53+/glomeruloid-microvascular-proliferation+) phenotype of BRCA1-related breast cancer. *Cancer Res* 2004;64:830–835.
34. Foulkes WD, Stefansson IM, Chappuis PO, et al. Germline BRCA1 mutations and a basal epithelial phenotype in breast cancer. *J Natl Cancer Inst* 2003;95: 1482–1485.
35. Olopade OI, Grushko T. Gene-expression profiles in hereditary breast cancer. *N Engl J Med* 2001;344:2028–2029.
36. Bryant HE, Schultz N, Thomas HD, et al. Specific killing of BRCA2-deficient tumours with inhibitors of poly(ADP-ribose) polymerase. *Nature* 2005;434:913–917.
37. Farmer H, McCabe N, Lord CJ, et al. Targeting the DNA repair defect in BRCA mutant cells as a therapeutic strategy. *Nature* 2005;434:917–921.
38. Kennedy RD, Quinn JE, Mullan PB, et al. The role of BRCA1 in the cellular response to chemotherapy. *J Natl Cancer Inst* 2004;96:1659–1668.
39. Rouzier R, Perou CM, Symmans WF, et al. Breast cancer molecular subtypes respond differently to preoperative chemotherapy. *Clin Cancer Res* 2005;11: 5678–5685.
40. Bauer KR, Brown M, Cress RD, et al. Descriptive analysis of estrogen receptor (ER)-negative, progesterone receptor (PR)-negative, and HER2-negative invasive breast cancer, the so-called triple-negative phenotype: a population-based study from the California cancer Registry. *Cancer* 2007;109:1721–1728.
41. Lund MJ, Trivers KF, Porter PL, et al. Race and triple negative threats to breast cancer survival: a population-based study in Atlanta, GA. *Breast Cancer Res Treat* 2009 Jan; 113(2):357–370.
42. Rakha EA, El-Rehim DA, Paish C, et al. Basal phenotype identifies a poor prognostic subgroup of breast cancer of clinical importance. *Eur J Cancer* 2006;42: 3149–3156.
43. Cheang MC, Voduc D, Bajdik C, et al. Basal-like breast cancer defined by five biomarkers has superior prognostic value than triple-negative phenotype. *Clin Cancer Res* 2008;14:1368–1376.
44. Bertucci F, Finetti P, Cervera N, et al. How basal are triple-negative breast cancers? *Int J Cancer* 2008;123:236–240.
45. Bryan BB, Schnitt SJ, Collins LC. Ductal carcinoma *in situ* with basal-like phenotype: a possible precursor to invasive basal-like breast cancer. *Mod Pathol* 2006;19:617–621.
46. Hannemann J, Velds A, Halfwerk JB, et al. Classification of ductal carcinoma *in situ* by gene expression profiling. *Breast Cancer Res* 2006;8:R61.
47. Buerger H, Otterbach F, Simon R, et al. Comparative genomic hybridization of ductal carcinoma *in situ* of the breast-evidence of multiple genetic pathways. *J Pathol* 1999;187:396–402.
48. Fridlyand J, Snijders AM, Ylstra B, et al. Breast tumor copy number aberration phenotypes and genomic instability. *BMC Cancer* 2006;6:96.
49. Bergamaschi A, Kim YH, Wang P, et al. Distinct patterns of DNA copy number alteration are associated with different clinicopathological features and gene-expression subtypes of breast cancer. *Genes Chromosomes Cancer* 2006;45: 1033–1040.
50. Al-Hajj M, Wicha MS, Benito-Hernandez A, et al. Prospective identification of tumorigenic breast cancer cells. *Proc Natl Acad Sci U S A* 2003;100:3983–3988.
51. Ponti D, Costa A, Zaffaroni N, et al. Isolation and *in vitro* propagation of tumorigenic breast cancer cells with stem/progenitor cell properties. *Cancer Res* 2005; 65:5506–5511.
52. Liu R, Wang X, Chen GY, et al. The prognostic role of a gene signature from tumorigenic breast-cancer cells. *N Engl J Med* 2007;356:217–226.
53. Olivotto IA, Bajdik CD, Ravdin PM, et al. Population-based validation of the prognostic model ADJUVANT! for early breast cancer. *J Clin Oncol* 2005;23: 2716–2725.
54. Galea MH, Blamey RW, Elston CE, et al. The Nottingham Prognostic Index in primary breast cancer. *Breast Cancer Res Treat* 1992;22:207–219.
55. Goldhirsch A, Wood WC, Gelber RD, et al. Meeting highlights: updated international expert consensus on the primary therapy of early breast cancer. *J Clin Oncol* 2003;21:3357–3365.
56. Eifel P, Axelson JA, Costa J, et al. National Institutes of Health Consensus Development Conference Statement: adjuvant therapy for breast cancer, November 1–3, 2000. *J Natl Cancer Inst* 2001;93:979–989.

57. Ahr A, Karn T, Solbach C, et al. Identification of high risk breast-cancer patients by gene expression profiling. *Lancet* 2002;359:131–132.
58. Foekens JA, Atkins D, Zhang Y, et al. Multicenter validation of a gene expression-based prognostic signature in lymph node-negative primary breast cancer. *J Clin Oncol* 2006;24:1665–1671.
59. Huang E, Cheng SH, Dressman H, et al. Gene expression predictors of breast cancer outcomes. *Lancet* 2003;361:1590–1596.
60. Ma XJ, Wang Z, Ryan PD, et al. A two-gene expression ratio predicts clinical outcome in breast cancer patients treated with tamoxifen. *Cancer Cell* 2004;5:607–616.
61. van de Vijver MJ, He YD, van't Veer LJ, et al. A gene-expression signature as a predictor of survival in breast cancer. *N Engl J Med* 2002;347:1999–2009.
62. Iwao K, Matoba R, Ueno N, et al. Molecular classification of primary breast tumors possessing distinct prognostic properties. *Hum Mol Genet* 2002;11:199–206.
63. Simon R. Development and validation of therapeutically relevant multi-gene biomarker classifiers. *J Natl Cancer Inst* 2005;97:866–867.
64. Paik S, Shak S, Tang G. Risk classification of breast cancer patients by the recurrence score assay: comparison to guidelines based on patient age, tumor size, and tumor grade [Abstract]. In: San Antonio Breast Cancer Symposium. San Antonio, Texas, December 11, 2004.
65. Lo SS, Norton L, Mumby PB, et al. Prospective multi-center study of the impact of the 21-gene Recurrence Score (RS) assay on medical oncologist (MO) and patient (pt) adjuvant breast cancer (BC) treatment selection. In: ASCO Annual Meeting, Chicago, Illinois, June 4, 2007.
66. Habel LA, Shak S, Jacobs MK, et al. A population-based study of tumor gene expression and risk of breast cancer death among lymph node-negative patients. *Breast Cancer Res* 2006;8:R25.
67. Gianni L, Zambetti M, Clark K, et al. Gene expression profiles in paraffin-embedded core biopsy tissue predict response to chemotherapy in women with locally advanced breast cancer. *J Clin Oncol* 2005;23:7265–7277.
68. Goldstein LJ, O'Neill A, Sparano JA, et al. E2197: Phase III AT (doxorubicin/docetaxel) vs. AC (doxorubicin/cyclophosphamide) in the adjuvant treatment of node positive and high risk node negative breast cancer. . In: ASCO; 2005; Orlando, FL, 2005.
69. Goldstein L, Ravdin P, Gray R, et al. Prognostic utility of the 21-gene assay compared with Adjuvant! in hormone receptor (HR) positive operable breast cancer with 0-3 positive axillary nodes treated with adjuvant chemohormonal therapy (CHT): an analysis of intergroup trial E2197. In: San Antonio Breast Cancer Symposium (SABCS). San Antonio, Texas, 2007.
70. Albain K, Barlow W, Shak S, et al. Prognostic and predictive value of the 21-gene recurrence score assay in postmenopausal, node-positive, ER-positive breast cancer (S8814,INT0100) [Abstract 10]. In: San Antonio Breast Cancer Symposium, San Antonio, Texas; 2007.
71. Chang HY, Nuyten DS, Sneddon JB, et al. Robustness, scalability, and integration of a wound-response gene expression signature in predicting breast cancer survival. *Proc Natl Acad Sci U S A* 2005;102:3738–3743.
72. Buyse M, Loi S, van't Veer L, et al. Validation and clinical utility of a 70-gene prognostic signature for women with node-negative breast cancer. *J Natl Cancer Inst* 2006;98:1183–1192.
73. Mook S, Van't Veer LJ, Rutgers EJ, et al. Individualization of therapy using Mammaprint: from development to the MINDACT Trial. *Cancer Genomics Proteomics* 2007;4:147–155.
74. Glas AM, Floore A, Delahaye LJ, et al. Converting a breast cancer microarray signature into a high-throughput diagnostic test. *BMC Genomics* 2006;7:278.
75. Wang Y, Klijn JG, Zhang Y, et al. Gene-expression profiles to predict distant metastasis of lymph-node-negative primary breast cancer. *Lancet* 2005;365:671–679.
76. Desmedt C, Piette F, Loi S, et al. Strong time dependence of the 76-gene prognostic signature for node-negative breast cancer patients in the TRANSBIG multicenter independent validation series. *Clin Cancer Res* 2007;13:3207–3214.
77. Reid JF, Lusa L, De Cecco L, et al. Limits of predictive models using microarray data for breast cancer clinical treatment outcome. *J Natl Cancer Inst* 2005;97:927–930.
78. Goetz MP, Suman VJ, Ingle JN, et al. A two-gene expression ratio of homeobox 13 and interleukin-17B receptor for prediction of recurrence and survival in women receiving adjuvant tamoxifen. *Clin Cancer Res* 2006;12:2080–2087.
79. Ma XJ, Hilsenbeck SG, Wang W, et al. The HOXB13:IL17BR expression index is a prognostic factor in early-stage breast cancer. *J Clin Oncol* 2006;24:4611–4619.
80. Jansen MP, Sieuwerts AM, Look MP, et al. HOXB13-to-IL17BR expression ratio is related with tumor aggressiveness and response to tamoxifen of recurrent breast cancer: a retrospective study. *J Clin Oncol* 2007;25:662–668.
81. Jerevall PL, Brommesson S, Strand C, et al. Exploring the two-gene ratio in breast cancer-independent roles for HOXB13 and IL17BR in prediction of clinical outcome. *Breast Cancer Res Treat* 2008;107:225–234.
82. Chang HY, Sneddon JB, Alizadeh AA, et al. Gene expression signature of fibroblast serum response predicts human cancer progression: similarities between tumors and wounds. *PLoS Biol* 2004;2:E7.
83. Whitfield ML, George LK, Grant GD, et al. Common markers of proliferation. *Nat Rev Cancer* 2006;6:99–106.
84. Dai H, van't Veer L, Lamb J, et al. A cell proliferation signature is a marker of extremely poor outcome in a subpopulation of breast cancer patients. *Cancer Res* 2005;65:4059–4066.
85. Chi JT, Wang Z, Nuyten DS, et al. Gene expression programs in response to hypoxia: cell type specificity and prognostic significance in human cancers. *PLoS Med* 2006;3:e47.
86. Eden P, Ritz C, Rose C, et al. "Good Old" clinical markers have similar power in breast cancer prognosis as microarray gene expression profilers. *Eur J Cancer* 2004;40:1837–1841.
87. Jansen MP, Foekens JA, van Staveren IL, et al. Molecular classification of tamoxifen-resistant breast carcinomas by gene expression profiling. *J Clin Oncol* 2005;23:732–740.
88. Kok M, Linn SC, Van Laar RK, et al. Comparison of gene expression profiles predicting progression in breast cancer patients treated with tamoxifen. *Breast Cancer Res Treat* 2009; Jan: 113(2):275–283.
89. Ein-Dor L, Kela I, Getz G, et al. Outcome signature genes in breast cancer: is there a unique set? *Bioinformatics* 2005;21:171–178.
90. Paik S, Shak S, Tang G, et al. Expression of the 21 genes in the Recurrence Score assay and tamoxifen clinical benefit in the NSABP study B-14 of node negative, estrogen receptor positive breast cancer. *J Clin Oncol* 2005;23:510a.
91. Chang JC, Makris A, Gutierrez MC, et al. Gene expression patterns in formalin-fixed, paraffin-embedded core biopsies predict docetaxel chemosensitivity in breast cancer patients. *Breast Cancer Res Treat* 2008;108:233–240.
92. Iwao-Koizumi K, Matoba R, Ueno N, et al. Prediction of docetaxel response in human breast cancer by gene expression profiling. *J Clin Oncol* 2005;23:422–431.
93. Chang JC, Wooten EC, Tsimelzon A, et al. Gene expression profiling for the prediction of therapeutic response to docetaxel in patients with breast cancer. *Lancet* 2003;362:362–369.
94. Potti A, Dressman HK, Bild A, et al. Genomic signatures to guide the use of chemotherapeutics. *Nat Med* 2006;12:1294–1300.
95. Ayers M, Symmans WF, Stec J, et al. Gene expression profiles predict complete pathologic response to neoadjuvant paclitaxel and fluorouracil, doxorubicin, and cyclophosphamide chemotherapy in breast cancer. *J Clin Oncol* 2004;22:2284–2293.
96. Hess KR, Anderson K, Symmans WF, et al. Pharmacogenomic predictor of sensitivity to preoperative chemotherapy with paclitaxel and fluorouracil, doxorubicin, and cyclophosphamide in breast cancer. *J Clin Oncol* 2006;24:4236–4244.
97. Cleator S, Tsimelzon A, Ashworth A, et al. Gene expression patterns for doxorubicin (Adriamycin) and cyclophosphamide (cytoxan) (AC) response and resistance. *Breast Cancer Res Treat* 2006;95:229–233.
98. Bonnefoi H, Potti A, Delorenzi M, et al. Validation of gene signatures that predict the response of breast cancer to neoadjuvant chemotherapy: a substudy of the EORTC 10994/BIG 00-01 clinical trial. *Lancet Oncol* 2007;8:1071–1078.
99. Acharya CR, Hsu DS, Anders CK, et al. Gene expression signatures, clinicopathological features, and individualized therapy in breast cancer. *JAMA* 2008;299:1574–1587.
100. Harris LN, You F, Schnitt SJ, et al. Predictors of resistance to preoperative trastuzumab and vinorelbine for HER2-positive early breast cancer. *Clin Cancer Res* 2007;13:11981–11207.
101. Simon R, Radmacher MD, Dobbin K, et al. Pitfalls in the use of DNA microarray data for diagnostic and prognostic classification. *J Natl Cancer Inst* 2003;95:14–18.
102. Reis-Filho JS, Westbury C, Pierga JY. The impact of expression profiling on prognostic and predictive testing in breast cancer. *J Clin Pathol* 2006;59:225–231.
103. Roden DM, Altman RB, Benowitz NL, et al. Pharmacogenomics: challenges and opportunities. *Ann Intern Med* 2006;145:749–757.

Jeffrey B. Smerage and Daniel F. Hayes

The development of distant metastases is the unfortunate result of spread of tumor cells through the lymphatic and vascular systems. In breast cancer, the most prominent example of this process is the identification of tumor cells in the axillary lymph nodes, and as discussed in Chapters 31 and 35, lymph node staging continues to be one of the most important prognostic variables in early stage breast cancer. Although axillary staging may be the strongest prognostic factor, it is far from definitive. Women with newly diagnosed breast cancer who have uninvolved axillary lymph nodes still have a 20% to 30% chance of recurrence and, conversely, even in the absence of adjuvant systemic therapy, approximately half of women with node-positive cancer will not have recurrence of their cancer (1). Thus, great interest continues in the development of new methods to detect micrometastatic disease in hope of improving the ability to make clinical treatment decisions. In addition, a better understanding of the biology of micrometastatic cells may allow the development of better strategies for the prevention and treatment of metastatic breast cancer. Advances in technology now allow the detection of micrometastatic disease, not just in the lymph nodes but also from bone marrow and peripheral blood. In the bone marrow they are commonly referred to as *disseminated tumor cells* (DTC), and in the peripheral blood they are commonly referred to as *circulating tumor cells* (CTC). Together, the detection of micrometastases in distant organs or blood has been designated *minimal residual disease* (MRD).

DETECTION OF MINIMAL RESIDUAL DISEASE

The greatest hurdle in detecting DTC and CTC is their rarity. For example, CTC occur at a frequency of approximately 1 tumor cell per $1 \times 10^{5-7}$ peripheral blood mononuclear cells (2). Multiple methods have been used to isolate and identify these cells based on their physical and biologic properties (Table 33.1). Older methods were based primarily on the differences in physical properties between cancer and normal hematopoietic cells, such as size and density. These methods have lacked sensitivity and specificity. Many protocols utilized density gradient centrifugation to isolate the mononuclear cell fraction, but this technique can result in decreased sensitivity because of loss of up to 35% to 90% of cells, if tested using cultured tumor cells spiked into whole blood (3–5). Morphologic methods of identification, such as light microscopy, have also proved to be insensitive, nonspecific, labor intensive, and complicated by a large number of false–positive events owing to preparation artifacts and misclassification of leukocytes (6). As a result of these limitations, research has mostly moved away from purely physical criteria and toward biologic markers, such as protein and messenger RNA (mRNA) expression, that either distinguishes epithelial from hematopoeitic cells, or malignant from nonmalignant cells, or both.

Biologic markers can be used for the isolation of DTC and CTC. The most prominent method currently in use is immunomagnetic selection, in which blood samples are incubated with ferromagnetic beads or ferrofluids coupled to antibodies against epithelial or tumor-associated antigens. Currently, the most frequently targeted epitope is the *epithelial cell adhesion molecule* (EpCAM) (7–12), although other epitopes have been targeted, including cytokeratin (13,14). Immunomagnetic separation techniques have been used extensively for CTC analysis (11,15), and are now being developed for DTC research (16). Recovery of EpCAM-expressing cells with these antibody-based methods is high. Using anti-EpCAM–bound ferrofluids, blood samples spiked with standardized numbers of cultured human breast cancer cells demonstrate a linear recovery over a range of 5 to 1,142 cells (correlation coefficient $R^2 = 0.99$), with an average recovery of greater than 85% at each level. There is also strong agreement between duplicate samples (correlation coefficient $R^2 = 0.975$) and between independent operators reviewing the same digital images (correlation coefficient $R^2 = 0.994$) (17).

After the cells are isolated they must be detected to identify, quantify, or verify their presence, most commonly by immunofluorescent microscopy (9) or reverse transcriptase-polymerase chain reaction (RT-PCR). Multiple epithelial or breast cancer markers have been used, including cytokeratins (CK), epidermal growth factor receptor (EGFR), mammoglobin, MUC-1, beta-human chorionic gonadotropin (beta-hCG), c-Met, GalNac-T, MAGE-3, and others (10,11). None of these markers is, however, completely sensitive or specific for CTC.

As with any diagnostic test, the challenge to increase sensitivity is burdened by the need to maintain specificity. Growing evidence indicates that the mainstay markers most commonly used to isolate these cells, EpCAM and cytokeratin, are only expressed in approximately 80% of epithelial tumor cells, and expression may decrease in those that have gained a foothold in potential metastatic sites (18,19). Several strategies have been used to increase sensitivity of detection of CTC. In general, it appears that RT-PCR techniques are more sensitive than immunoselection, especially if *positivity* is considered to be the presence of two or more markers when multiparameter testing is used (20).

Efforts to increase sensitivity often result in loss of specificity. Indeed, loss of specificity can be both technical and biological. Use of highly specific reagents (antibodies for immunologic approaches and nucleic acid probes for RT-PCR) for the presumed target are essential, and even if these reagents do not cross react with other molecular species, the target itself may be expressed by nonepithelial or nonmalignant cells. For example, many of the gene products exploited to identify epithelial and breast cancer cells, including EpCAM (4), cytokeratin (7), MUC-1 (21), and TAG-12 (22), are on occasion expressed by hematopoietic cells. Furthermore, the specificity of immunofluorescent or immunohistochemical microscopy methods are often lowered by the presence of contaminating white blood cells. Some of these false–positive findings are concentration-dependent, and can be minimized by simply reducing the antibody concentration (22). Others false–positive results are not so easily corrected.

Immunohistochemistry can stain plasma cells owing to nonspecific alkaline phosphatase reactions against the kappa and lambda light chains on the cell surface (23). The literature suggests that false–positive staining of plasma cells ranges from 22% to 61% and varies by the antibody and staining methods used. To circumvent these issues of specificity, most investigators are now using multiple markers for the positive identification of CTC, including at least one leukocyte marker to exclude contaminating and nonspecifically labeled white blood cells. Automation has also allowed increased reproducibility.

The RT-PCR methods have also been plagued by false positivity, ranging from 10% to 40% (10). These false–positive

	CELLULAR CHARACTERISTICS AND METHODOLOGIES USED TO ISOLATE AND IDENTIFY CIRCULATING TUMOR CELLS		
	Cellular Characteristic	**Technique(s)**	**Characteristics**
Physical			
	Size	Filtration	Tumor cells are 2–6 times larger in area than leukocytes (43,70)[a]
	Weight/mass	Density gradient centrifugation	Separates nucleated cells from red blood cells
	Morphology	Light microscopy	Larger cells with atypical nuclei, prominent nucleoli
Biologic			
	Membrane proteins	Immunomagnetic isolation Flow cytometry Immunofluorescent microscopy	EpCAM (7,9) Cytokeratins (71) ERBB2 (63–65)
	mRNA expression	RT-PCR	Cytokeratins (39) ERBB2 (20,72,73) Mammaglobin (74,75) MUC-1 (76)
	Gene mutation or duplication	PCR Comparative genomic hybridization (77) Microarray (67)	RASSF1A methylation (78) ERBB2 (64)
	Cytogenetic abnormalities	FISH	c-Myc (64) Chr 1,8,17 (64)

FISH, fluorescence *in situ* hybridization; mRNA, messenger RNA; PCR, polymerase chain reaction; RT-PCR, reverse transcription PCR.
[a]Numbers in parentheses are references.

results are attributed to issues with laboratory technique, primer selection, and illegitimate expression of the target genes in leukocytes. For example, cytokeratin 19 and carcinoembryonic antigen (CEA) overexpression can be induced in leukocytes by cytokines and growth factors (24–26). Many strategies have been used to increase the specificity, such as the use of quantitative RT-PCR (qRT-PCR), which increases specificity compared with nested RT-PCR. In normal control populations qRT-PCR had a false–positive rate of 2.2% and nested RT-PCR had a false–positive rate of 5.6% (27). The most common RT-PCR target is CK-19, which is a ubiquitous epithelial protein found on most epithelial tumor cells. RT-PCR of CK-19 has been complicated by the presence of two psuedogenes (28,29), which can cause false–positive amplification. Although new intron-spanning primers have been designed to prevent amplification of the pseudogene transcripts, the true advantage of such a strategy has not been clinically demonstrated (30). RT-PCR still has methodologic hurdles to overcome, but recognition of the causes of false–positive results has led to the development of newer, more specific methods. RT-PCR may ultimately prove be the best way to increase the sensitivity of CTC detection (31).

PREVALENCE, SENSITIVITY, AND SPECIFICITY OF TECHNIQUES TO DETECT MINIMAL RESIDUAL DISEASE

Disseminated Tumor Cells

Bone Marrow Biopsy

Almost all of the data regarding DTC have been generated in the setting of early-stage breast cancer and not in the metasta-

tic setting. This is largely because of the need to perform a bone marrow biopsy, which is most easily obtained during anesthesia at the time of surgery for early-stage breast cancer. In one widely publicized study, DTC were evaluated in bone marrow aspirates from 552 patients with stage I-III disease (32). Overall, 36% of patients had at least one detectable DTC at baseline before definitive surgery. The number of patients with detectable DTC was statistically higher in patients with clinical risk factors, such as increasing tumor size ($p <.001$), increasing tumor grade ($p = .017$), increasing number of axillary lymph nodes ($p <.001$), and inflammatory disease ($p < .001$). The same authors conducted a pooled analysis of the data from this trial and eight other qualitatively similar studies (33). A total of 4,703 patients with stage I-III breast cancer were included. When the patient data from all the trials were pooled, 30.6% of patients had identifiable DTC. It is notable that the fraction of patients found positive for cancer varied from study to study and ranged from 12% to 42%. The interstudy variability is believed to result from the differing isolation and staining techniques, differences in clinical stage distribution, and differences in adjuvant treatments. Attempts are now being made at standardizing the methods used for the detection of DTC (34). The false–positive rate for DTC is not well documented, but in one study bone marrow samples from 98 healthy donors were evaluated, and 4% were found to contain epithelial cells (35).

Following primary and adjuvant systemic therapy, it appears that the incidence of DTC is lower. In one study of high-risk stage IIIA and B patients, some patients receiving adjuvant therapy converted from positive to negative and others converted from negative to positive. Overall, the postadjuvant incidence of DTC was approximately 44% in this setting (36). In another study, 800 women with lower stage disease were followed serially over approximately 5 years. Only 13%

were found to have positive DTC at time points from 2 to 5 years after diagnosis (37). Little if any data are available to estimate the incidence of DTC in patients with metastatic breast cancer. In one study, approximately 18% of women with metastatic breast cancer but without clinical evidence of bone metastases were found to have DTC in their bone marrow (38).

Circulating Tumor Cells

Reverse Transcription-Polymerase Chain Reaction

Circulating tumor cells detected by RT-PCR have also been studied in both the early and metastatic breast cancer settings, although most of the data relate to early-stage breast cancer. In patients with early-stage breast cancer, detection of CTC by RT-PCR has ranged from 0% to 69% (10). The largest clinical database comes from studies that utilize CK-19 as the CTC marker. With older primers and using qRT-PCR for CK-19, CTC are detected in 30% to 41% of early-stage breast cancer patients before chemotherapy (27,39–41) and in 6.5% to 18% of patients after adjuvant systemic therapy (27,40). The studies varied in clinical stage distribution and in adjuvant treatments, and these variables may partly explain the variability in prevalence. False–positive rates in samples from healthy controls were 2.2% to 3.2% (30,41). As an attempt to increase the specificity of the cytokeratin RT-PCR, newer primers have been designed to eliminate amplification of the two known CK-19 pseudogenes (28–30). With these new primers, the assay was positive in 20% of early-stage breast cancer at baseline, and no apparent CTC were detected in 62 blood samples from healthy controls.

The prevalence of CTC detected in the metastatic setting is not as well understood because of the multiple methods and targets used for detection. Published data report that RT-PCR assays are positive in 21% to 100% of patients with metastatic disease (10). Interestingly, in one study, 40% of patients with metastatic breast cancer had detectable CTC at baseline, and the number of patients with detectable CTC was unchanged at 43% after three cycles of first-line chemotherapy (27). This suggests that RT-PCR may not be an ideal methodology for monitoring metastatic disease, although the data in the metastatic setting are so limited that it is probably premature to make this conclusion.

Immunomagnetic Isolation and Immunofluorescent Microscopy

Methods that isolate and then visually identify CTC from the peripheral blood have been primarily utilized in the metastatic setting. This is because of the low sensitivity in the early breast cancer setting, where larger volumes of blood (20–30 mL) are required for analysis, and despite larger volumes, only 10% of patients have CTC at baseline before the initiation of adjuvant systemic therapy (42). In the metastatic setting, the most highly validated cell detection system is known as CellSearch (Veridex LLC, Raritan, NJ). This system partially purifies CTC by immunomagnetic separation based on expression of EpCAM. The CTC are then visualized by immunofluorescent microscopy, utilizing an anticytokeratin antibody. Nonspecifically stained leukocytes are excluded from analysis via an antibody stain directed against the leukocyte marker CD45. The specificity of the CellSearch assay varies by the choice of threshold. For example, 60% of metastatic breast cancer patients have two or more "events" (presumed to be CTC) per 7.5 mL whole blood, compared with only 1% of normal healthy controls (9). Increasing the threshold to 5 or more CTC decreases the false–positive rate to 0% and only slightly decreases the prevalence to 50% (9). After one cycle of chemotherapy, the percentage of patients with 5 or more CTC decreases to 30% (9).

Other Methods

Recently several additional techniques have been published that show promise for future development. For example, a novel method was presented for a microfluidic *chip* platform (12). The technique utilizes the same immunoseparation strategy as CellSearch, but with anti-EpCAM–coated solid-state micropost capture strategy using microfluidics to isolate the CTC. The cells are then confirmed to be epithelial cells by fluorescent staining with DAPI (4′,6-diamidino-2-phenylindole), anti-cytokeratin, and anti-CD45. The microfluidic platform reported a 60% to 65% recovery of cells from spiked blood samples. Analysis of blood samples from 10 patients with metastatic breast cancer demonstrated 5 or more CTC in 100% of the patients. An additional 99 patients with either metastatic lung, prostate, pancreatic, or colon cancers were also evaluated, and 99% of the patients had 5 or more CTC. No correlation appeared to exist between the number of CTC captured and the total tumor volume, but an exploratory analysis found a correlation between changes in CTC number during therapy and change in tumor size using RECIST (Response Evaluation Criteria in Solid Tumors) criteria. In nine patients with measurable disease (three NSLC, two colon cancer, three pancreatic cancer, and one esophageal cancer), the percent change in CTC number correlated to the percent change in measurable disease with a Pearson's correlation coefficient of 0.68 ($p = .03$).

Another group of researchers, to avoid the inherent loss in sensitivity related to expression of biomarkers, has returned to microfiltration, albeit with a substantially more sophisticated technology (43). Using a microfabricated parylene membrane filter, they report an 89% recovery of tumor cells spiked into whole human blood. These investigators have not reported clinical results with this assay at this time.

Another recent report utilizes an assay based on the enzyme-linked immunosorbent spot test (ELISPOT) strategy of detecting secretion of soluble tumor-associated antigens, such as MUC-1 and CEA, from cells cultured on a membrane filter (44). The goal of the investigators was to differentiate between viable CTC, which secrete proteins, from dead or apoptotic CTC, which do not actively secrete proteins. In blood from 37 patients with stage I-III breast cancer, they found that 54% of the patients had cells that secreted either CK-19 or MUC-1 proteins (single-marker positive) and that 19% were dual positive. In patients with metastatic breast cancer, 90% had single-marker positive cells and 30% had dual positive cells. The study did not include a control population for this set of breast cancer markers. In an earlier study utilizing a similar assay, they found, however, that 30% of the healthy controls (n = 11) had cells that secreted MUC-1 (45). In another study, they utilized the same technology to detect prostate-specific antigen (PSA)-secreting cells, and no false–positives were found in 35 nonprostate cancer patients and in 8 healthy controls (46).

MINIMAL RESIDUAL DISEASE AND CLINICAL OUTCOMES

Over the last two decades, several studies have demonstrated that the presence of detectable DTC or CTC in patients with both primary and metastatic breast cancer is indicative of a worse prognosis. Only recently, however, have appropriately designed studies been reported that begin to provide insight into whether and how this information can be used in routine clinical care. Most research regarding detection and monitoring of MRD has focused on methodology development and sensitivity of detection in human samples. If clinical studies were performed, they were pilot in nature or correlative studies of convenience, in which the specimens happened to be

Table 33.2	TUMOR MARKER UTILITY GRADING SCALE (47)

Level	Type of Evidence
I	Evidence from a single, high-powered, prospective, controlled study that is specifically designed to test marker or evidence from meta-analysis, overview, or both of level II or III studies. In the former case, the study must be designed so that therapy and follow-up are dictated by protocol. Ideally, the study is a prospective, controlled, randomized trial in which diagnostic and therapeutic clinical decisions in one arm are determined at least in part on the basis of marker results, and diagnostic and therapeutic clinical decisions in the control arm are made independently of marker results. Study design may also include prospective but not randomized trials with marker data and clinical outcome as primary objective.
II	Evidence from a study in which marker data are determined in relationship to prospective therapeutic trial that is performed to test therapeutic hypothesis but not specifically designed to test marker utility (i.e., marker study is secondary objective of protocol). Specimen collection for marker study and statistical analysis are, however, prospectively determined in protocol as secondary objectives.
III	Evidence from large but retrospective studies from which variable numbers of samples are available or selected. Therapeutic aspects and follow-up of patient population may or may not have been prospectively dictated. Statistical analysis for tumor marker was not dictated prospectively at time of therapeutic trial design.
IV	Evidence from small retrospective studies that do not have prospectively dictated therapy, follow-up specimen selection, or statistical analysis. Study design may use matched case-controls, and so on.
V	Evidence from small pilot studies designed to determine or estimate distribution of marker levels in a sample population. Study design may include "correlation" with other known or investigational markers of outcome but is not designed to determine clinical utility.

available for a given assay. Most of these studies have significant limitations in their ability to assess the value of MRD as either a prognostic or predictive factor in breast cancer. These limitations are largely owing to the small size of studies, retrospective acquisition of samples, and wide variations in treatments received by the patients. Indeed, these types of limitations are not specific to MRD studies, but are generically problematic with tumor marker studies of all types. Therefore, a Tumor Marker Utility Grading System (TMUGS) has been developed (47), which classifies tumor marker studies into five level-of-evidence (LOE) categories (Table 33.2). Although most DTC and CTC studies have been LOE III or worse, several recent DTC and CTC studies have been published that are approaching level II-evidence, and prospective ongoing trials should provide LOE I results.

Prognosis in Early-stage Disease

Minimal residual disease data might be used in one or more of many circumstances in the breast cancer disease spectrum, ranging from screening to monitoring patients with metastatic disease. Currently, the low sensitivity and specificity for any technology to detect either DTC or CTC prevents the use of either of these to screen for previously undiagnosed primary breast cancers. Studies in the adjuvant setting have been limited primarily to analysis of bone marrow DTC and CTC detected by RT-PCR, because at least at present the sensitivity of immunologic-based assays appears quite low.

Several studies have been performed to evaluate the prognostic value of DTC in the early-stage breast cancer setting (32,37,48–52). The primary data from these studies have been combined to perform a meta-analysis (level III data) (33). Bone marrow biopsies were obtained for DTC analysis using a variety of techniques at the time of definitive breast surgery. The patients had stage I to III disease. Adjuvant treatments were variable, but represented the local standards of care. Data were available for a total of 4,703 patients, and bone marrow micrometastases were detectable in 30.6% of the patients. The presence of DTC was significantly associated with age, tumor size, tumor grade, and the number of axillary lymph nodes. In multivariate analysis, the presence of DTC was the strongest predictor of death (hazard ratio [HR] = 1.81), disease recurrence (HR = 1.85), and the development of distant metastases (HR = 2.03). All of these results had $p <.001$. On Kaplan-Meier analysis, the risk of both relapse (disease-free survival [DFS] HR = 2.13, $p <.01$) and death

(overall survival [OS] HR = 2.15, $p <.01$) were significantly higher for patients with detectable DTC (Fig. 33.1). These increased risks were seen in all treatment groups, including patients who only received hormonal therapy, received chemotherapy, and low-risk patients (TNM stage T1N0M0) who did not receive any adjuvant systemic therapy (33).

Accumulating evidence indicates that RT-PCR–based CTC assays may also provide strong prognostic information in the early breast cancer setting. A series of studies, principally but not exclusively performed in Greece, have been published in which blood samples were prospectively collected from patients being treated on a variety of clinical trials (level III evidence) (39,41). Peripheral blood mononuclear cells were isolated by density centrifugation followed by real-time RT-PCR for CK-19. The chemotherapies varied, but the criteria for hormonal therapy and for clinical follow-up were all identical. One study included 167 patients with node-negative breast cancer, with a median follow-up of 55 months. Patients who were CK-19 positive had a higher risk of recurrence (44% vs. 3%, $p = .000001$) and death (19% vs. 1%, $p = .00005$) (Fig. 33.2) (39). Most (75%) of all relapses were distant metastatic disease. In a second study, a higher risk population of 444 patients, spanning stages I-III was evaluated, with a median follow-up of 54 months (41). CK-19 positive patients were again found to be at significantly higher risk of relapse (30% vs. 15%, $p <.0001$) and death (15% vs. 6%; $p =.001$) compared with CK-19 negative patients. In multivariate analysis that included tumor size, lymph node status, and histologic grade, CK-19 positivity was the strongest independent predictor of DFS (HR = 2.4, $p <.001$) and OS (HR = 2.5, $p = .007$).

In the studies described above, DTC and CTC were obtained before adjuvant systemic therapy, but an alternative approach would be to monitor for evidence of MRD at the end of adjuvant chemotherapy or during follow-up when patients are ostensibly free of detectable metastases. For example, German investigators have reported that, in patients with stage IIIa or IIIb breast cancer, the presence of DTC after the completion of chemotherapy portends a much higher risk of relapse and death compared with women who were negative for DTC (36). Likewise, investigators from Germany and from Greece have reported that CTC during and after neoadjuvant chemotherapy are associated with worse prognosis (53,54). The presence of either DTC (35) or CTC (40) during long-term follow-up also appears to herald impending relapse, although only for a fraction of patients. For example, Wiedswang et al. (37) have reported that, in a study of 920 stage I and II patients followed for 0.5 to 85 months, 32% of patients with positive DTC at any

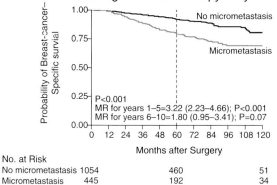

A. Patients Receiving Hormone Therapy Only

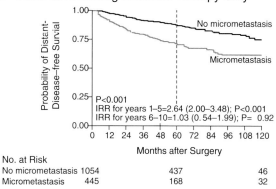

B. Patients Receiving Hormone Therapy Only

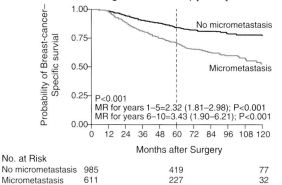

C. Patients Receiving Chemotherapy Only

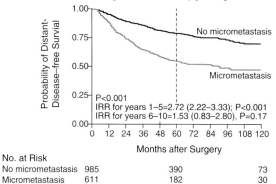

D. Patients Receiving Chemotherapy Only

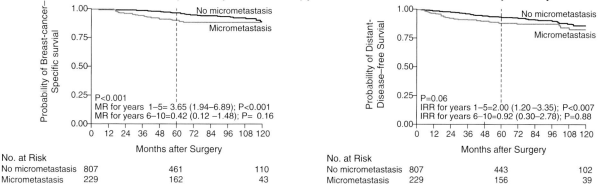

E. Low-Risk Patients with No Adjuvant Systemic Therapy **F.** Low-Risk Patients with No Adjuvant Systemic Therapy

FIGURE 33.1. Kaplan-Meier estimates of probabilities of progression-free survival and overall survival in patients early-stage breast cancer and disseminated tumor cells (DTC) detected in the bone marrow. Meta-analysis of 4,703 patients from 9 independent studies demonstrating prognostic value of DTC in estimating breast cancer-specific survival (**panels A, C, E**) and disease-free survival (**panels B, D, F**). DTC identified patients at higher risk of early mortality (hazard ratio [HR] = 2.32–3.65; p <.001) and earlier recurrence (HR = 2.00–2.72; p <.007). These increased risks were seen in all treatment groups, including patients who only received hormonal therapy (**panels A and B**), received chemotherapy (**panels C and D**), and low-risk patients (TNM stage T1N0M0) who did not receive any adjuvant systemic therapy (**panels E and F**). (From Braun S, Vogl FD, Naume B, et al. A pooled analysis of bone marrow micrometastasis in breast cancer. *N Engl J Med* 2005;353(8):793–802. Copyright © 2005 Massachusetts Medical Society. All rights reserved.)

time suffered relapse, compared with 14% of those who remained persistently negative. Likewise, the Greek investigators have reported that patients with CK-19 CTC at any time during adjuvant tamoxifen had a higher risk of recurrence compared with those who remained consistently CK-19 negative (32% to 50% vs. 9%) (40). Thus, CTC may represent a valuable prognostic factor in the postadjuvant therapy setting, but no current treatment strategy is known to improve outcomes for these higher risk women.

The examples above raise the interesting concept of a second type of "biological" false–positive finding, which is a potentially more perplexing problem than technological or assay-based false–positive findings. As noted, identification of lymph node involvement in early-stage breast cancer only portends a 50% risk of recurrence over the ensuing decade, even if the patient receives no adjuvant systemic therapy. Likewise, the recently reported pooled analysis of DTC demonstrates that, although the presence of bone marrow micrometastases was statistically significantly associated with worse prognosis, in patients who received no systemic therapy, only approximately 20% of these patients had a recurrence over 6 to 10 years (55). Although some of these patients may have had technical false–positive findings, as described above, these data suggest that not all peripherally detected cells that have apparent

A. Disease-free survival

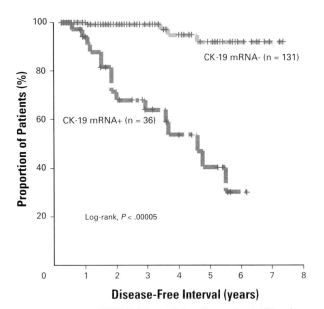

B. Overall survival

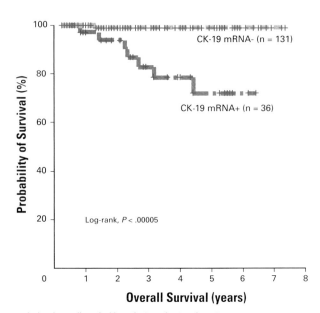

FIGURE 33.2. Kaplan-Meier estimates of probabilities of progression-free survival and overall survival in patients early-stage breast cancer and positive circulating tumor cells (CTC) by reverse transcription-polymerase chain reaction (RT-PCR) assay. A: Progression-free survival. **B:** Overall survival for 167 patients based on the presence or absence of cytokeratins–messenger RNA (CK-mRNA) by quantitative RT-PCR (qRT-PCR). (Adapted from Xenidis N, Perraki M, Kafousi M, et al. Predictive and prognostic value of peripheral blood cytokeratin-19 mRNA-positive cells detected by real-time polymerase chain reaction in node-negative breast cancer patients. *J Clin Oncol* 2006;24(23):3756–3762, with permission. Copyright © 2006 American Society of Clinical Oncology. All rights reserved.)

malignant characteristics are actually capable of growth into detectable and, therefore incurable, metastases. This issue will become an even greater concern as technologies evolve that detect putative cancer stem cells, because without better characterization, presumption that they are clinically important could lead to improper overtreatment.

Despite the current limitations of the existing technologies, taken together, these data suggest that patients who have detectable DTC or CTC, or both, have a high risk of recurrence and or death than those who do not. It is not presently clear, however, how assays for MRD might be used to make clinical decisions in the primary, adjuvant, or postadjuvant setting. Each of these studies has been conducted within patient cohorts in which therapy was not prospectively dictated, and no study has used either DTC or CTC results to direct therapy in comparison with a group of patients treated using standard prognostic and predictive criteria. Given the overall survival benefit, but annoying, and sometimes life-threatening, toxicities of adjuvant chemotherapy, use of any tumor marker, including assays for DTC or CTC, to make clinical decisions must be considered very carefully. The American Society of Clinical Oncology (ASCO) Tumor Marker Guidelines Panel has recommended that tissue levels of urokinase (uPA) and PAI-1 or values of the OncotypeDX 21-gene recurrence score may be used to identify patients whose prognosis is so favorable that they might forego adjuvant chemotherapy, especially for those patients who are node negative and have estrogen receptor-positive tumors and who will receive adjuvant endocrine therapy (56). The ASCO panel did not feel, however, that the currently available data support use of either DTC or CTC results to make clinical decisions about therapy in the early breast cancer setting.

 PROGNOSIS IN METASTATIC DISEASE

Although RT-PCR for CK-19 has been used to estimate risk of progression and death in breast cancer patients (10,27), most clinical outcomes data in the metastatic setting come from studies utilizing the CellSearch assay. The seminal study in this setting was a prospective, double-blind, multicenter trial in which CTC were assayed by CellSearch in 177 patients with metastatic breast cancer who were beginning a new therapy (9). Using a training set of 102 patient samples, a level of 5 or more CTC per 7.5 mL of whole blood was identified as the threshold that best distinguished progression-free survival (PFS) between the two groups. This threshold and its prognostic value were then confirmed in an independent, prospectively collected set of 75 patient samples. Elevated CTC at baseline predicted extremely short median PFS and OS of 3 and 10 months, respectively. This is in comparison with patients with low or negative CTC in whom PFS and OS were 7 and 22 months, respectively ($p = .005$). Thus, elevated CTC at baseline identify a group of high-risk patients.

Even more interesting, CTC values obtained after one cycle of therapy predicted which patients were likely on ineffective therapy. The frequency of elevated CTC ($\geq$5 CTC/7.5 mL whole blood) dropped from 50% at baseline to approximately 30% at first follow-up after initiation of therapy (3 to 5 weeks), suggesting beneficial response to the selected treatment. Confirming this suggestion, those patients with low CTC at this early time point, regardless of whether they did or did not have elevated CTC at baseline, had substantially shorter median PFS (2.1 vs. 7 months; $p <.001$) and OS (8.2 vs. >18, $p = .001$) than those who still had elevated CTC (Fig. 33.3).

Unplanned analyses of this study suggest that the assay may not be as robust for selected subsets. PFS and OS for patients initiating hormonal therapy were similar regardless of baseline CTC levels. However, CTC evaluated at first follow-up in this subset after initiating hormonal therapy did result in substantial differences in median PFS (2.3 vs. 8.3 months, $p = 0.15$) and median OS (10.9 vs. >18 months, $p = .002$). Although the PFS comparison was not statistically significant, it suggests that CTC may be able to distinguish patients who are on ineffective hormonal therapy. The subset of patients starting hormonal therapy was smaller (n = 53) than the group starting

A. Progression-free Survival

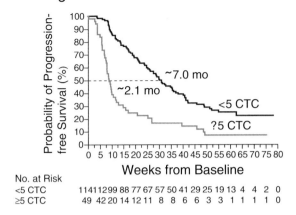

No. at Risk

<5 CTC	114	112	99	88	77	67	57	50	41	29	25	19	13	4	4	2	0
≥5 CTC	49	42	20	14	12	11	8	8	6	6	3	3	1	1	1	1	0

B. Overall Survival

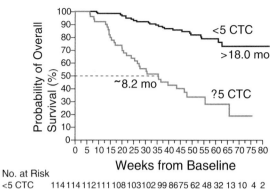

No. at Risk

<5 CTC	114	114	112	111	108	103	102	99	86	75	62	48	32	13	10	4	2
≥5 CTC	49	49	45	39	35	31	27	24	18	14	9	6	3	3	2	1	0

FIGURE 33.3. Kaplan-Meier estimates of probabilities of progression-free survival and overall survival in patients with metastatic breast cancer for those with fewer than 5 circulating tumor cells per 7.5 mL of whole blood and those in the group with 5 or more circulating tumor cells in 7.5 mL of whole blood at the first follow-up visit after initiation of a new line of therapy. All patients in the trial (n = 177) are included in these figures. **A:** Progression-free survival from baseline. **B:** Overall survival from baseline. (From Cristofanilli M, Budd GT, Ellis MJ, et al. Circulating tumor cells, disease progression, and survival in metastatic breast cancer. *N Engl J Med* 2004;351(8):781–791. Copyright © 2005 Massachusetts Medical Society. All rights reserved.)

chemotherapy (n = 109). So, the analysis in patients on hormonal therapy was likely underpowered and requires further investigation. Because of the lack of strong statistical significance in the hormonal therapy group, the U.S. Food and Drug Administration (FDA) cleared indication for the CTC assay is currently limited to women undergoing chemotherapy for metastatic breast cancer.

Further analysis of these data suggests that the prognostic value is independent of the line of chemotherapy. The original publication (9) presented combined data for all patients receiving any line of therapy. Approximately half of these patients were receiving first-line therapy, and a subsequent publication demonstrated that the prognostic information was the same in patients receiving first-line therapy. Subsequent reports have suggested that CTC levels at first follow-up may be more predictive of subsequent OS than classically used measures of response, such as history, physical examination, or staging radiographs, even when read by independent reviewers (57).

As in the early disease setting, even this prospective trial of the CellSearch technology remains correlative, and does not reach LOE I quality. The intriguing observation that CTC results very early in the course of therapy might be useful to direct a change to an alternative treatment plan is outside of the current standard of care paradigm (see Chapters 74, 75, and 77), which is to continue until evidence of clinical or radiographic progression. Therefore, a prospective randomized clinical trial is being conducted in the North American Breast Cancer Intergroup, led by the Southwest Oncology Group (SWOG S0500), to test whether women with metastatic breast cancer who have elevated CTC after one cycle of first-line chemotherapy have improved outcomes as a result of switching early to an alternate therapy (Fig. 33.4). By switching therapy before clinical progression, it is hypothesized that these patients will have improved outcomes by minimizing the time and toxicity spent on ineffective therapies and by spending more time on effective therapy.

Is there a role at all for monitoring CTC in the metastatic setting? Although the 2007 ASCO Tumor Marker Guidelines Committee did not recommend this utility, we believe that, as with standard circulating markers such as CA15-3, CA27.29, and CEA, CTC do provide some value in patients who have

been on a given therapy for some time and the clinician is having difficulty deciding if the patient's cancer is progressing. Thus CTC are another tool available to help determine whether to continue current therapy or to change to a different treatment strategy. From the primary CellSearch study described above, patients who had elevated CTC at any time point were very likely to exhibit classic evidence of progression within the next few weeks, whereas those who did not were likely to have a prolonged progression-free interval (58). CTC data may be of particular utility as an objective measure in patients with nonmeasurable forms of metastatic breast cancer. The determination of progression in nonmeasurable disease is often subjective, subtle, and difficult. In a preliminary study, 46 patients with nonmeasurable metastatic breast cancer underwent CTC evaluation at baseline and at first follow-up after initiating a new therapy. Patients with elevated CTC at baseline had trends toward worse median PFS at 4.4 versus 9.5 months, although this did not reach statistical significance ($p = .44$). Analysis of CTC at first follow-up demonstrated an even wider difference in median PFS (3.5 vs. 14.4 months, $p = .032$), which was statistically significant. Median OS had not been reached for either group at the time of presentation. These data suggest that patients with nonmeasurable disease who have elevated CTC at first follow-up are likely on ineffective therapy.

CIRCULATING TUMOR CELL PHENOTYPING AND FUTURE RESEARCH

The preceding discussions all point to the potential importance of enumerating DTC and CTC in patients with breast cancer. They also, however, highlight the concerns about sensitivity and, in particular, specificity. Indeed, the ability to do so may give insight into which detected cells have true malignant potential and which are more likely impotent, terminally differentiated cells that are detected but have no biological importance.

Furthermore, breast cancer, perhaps of all the known and treatable malignancies, is a disease for which targeted therapies have been most useful, in particular directed against the

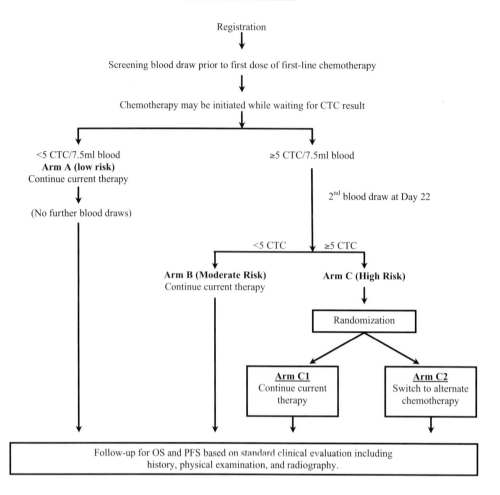

FIGURE 33.4. Schema for Southwest Oncology Group (SWOG) S0500.

estrogen receptor and ERBB2 (formerly HER2) (see Chapters 48, 50, 51, 73, and 75). Taken together, these considerations illustrate the need to not only count *events*, but to characterize better the genotype and phenotype of these cells.

Many investigators have developed methods to detect and monitor biologically important markers in CTC. Genetic changes can be detected in CTC, including abnormal telomerase activity (59), allelic loss, or amplification of multiple oncogenes not seen in normal control populations (60), and aneuploid changes in cellular chromosome content based on fluorescence *in situ* hybridization (FISH) analysis similar to those seen in the primary tumor (61). In addition, cancer-associated protein expression by DTC and CTC can be detected, such as ERBB2 (Fig. 33.5) (20,62–65). Interestingly, in one report, ERBB2 appears to have an inverse relationship with expression of cytokeratin, further raising the possibility that standard ways of isolating MRD may miss the very cells that are most important to monitor (63). Treatment-related markers, such as *bcl-2* and apoptosis can also be detected in CTC (66), and these phenotypic markers are now being investigated as possible biological indicators of target modulation and of response to treatment for the monitoring of target directed therapy. Investigators have also demonstrated early successes in gene expression profiling (67) and multiplex RT–PCR (68) from CTC. As each of these methodologies becomes more

sophisticated, the ability to isolate, detect, and phenotype these cells will continue to improve.

Dormancy and late relapse have presented a particularly enigmatic circumstance to clinicians caring for breast cancer patients. An interesting observation in several recent publications is the long-term persistence of DTC and CTC in patients previously treated for early-stage breast cancer, and who remain free of clinical recurrence. As already discussed, detection of DTC or CTC during 3 to 5 years of follow-up are associated with an increased risk of recurrence (35,40). These results have also led some authors to suggest that DTC in the bone marrow might serve as a reservoir of tumor cells that promotes eventual spread to other organs (44). A separate study measured CTC in women 7 or more years (range 7 to 22 years) after mastectomy (64). The CTC were isolated by immunomagnetic separation and immunofluorescently staining. Positive cells were defined as CK positive, DAPI positive, and CD45 negative. Of 36 patients, 13 (33%) had detectable CTC. These events were further characterized by FISH and found to be aneusomic for chromosomes 1, 3, 8, 11, or 17, ruling out contamination of normal epithelial cells. Furthermore, only 1 of 26 age-matched healthy control patients had a single CTC, which was not aneusomic. No clinical follow-up is yet reported for these patients. Taken together, these results further emphasize the importance of understanding the concept

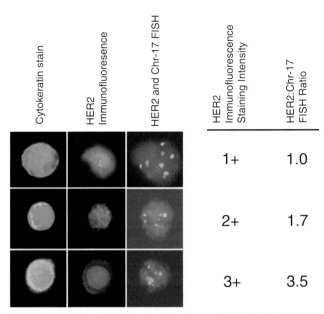

Cytokeratin stain	HER2 Immunofluoresence	HER2 and Chr-17 FISH	HER2 Immunofluorescence Staining Intensity	HER2:Chr-17 FISH Ratio
			1+	1.0
			2+	1.7
			3+	3.5

FIGURE 33.5. Detection of ERBB2 from circulating tumor cells (CTC) isolated by immuno-magnetic separation. Immunofluorescent staining of ERBB2 overexpression correlates with ERBB2 amplification, measured by the ERBB2:Chrom-17 ratio detected by fluorescence *in situ* hybridization (FISH). (Adapted from Meng S, Tripathy D, Shete S, et al. HER-2 gene amplification can be acquired a breast cancer progresses. *Proc Natl Acad Sci USA* 2004:101(25):9393–9398, with permission. Copyright © 2004 National Academy of Sciences, USA.)

of biological false–positive findings. In other words, these patients appear to have detectable CTC but no evidence of progressive disease. They may be living in symbiosis with apparently dormant metastatic cancers, although certainly concern is that subsequent changes either in the cancers cells themselves or surrounding microenvironment may be responsible for the late relapses not uncommonly observed in breast cancer survivors. These results also raise the issue of whether these cells represent cancer *stem* or *progenitor* cells that might be the long-term source of metastatic disease (69). Such issues are the focus of ongoing and future research.

SUMMARY

Modern biological techniques now allow the isolation and characterization of DTC and CTC with improved sensitivity and with high specificity and reproducibility; as a result, it has been possible to demonstrate that elevated DTC and CTC are a clinically significant and statistically significant prognostic factor in women with either early-stage or metastatic breast cancer. Of particular interest is the poor prognosis for patients who have completed one cycle of a new therapy. This observation suggests that these patients are on ineffective therapy and that their treatment should be changed even with no clinical evidence of disease progression. This theory is being tested in a prospective, randomized, blinded trial that is ongoing through SWOG and the North American Breast Cancer Intergroup. In addition, CTC represent a valuable source of tumor tissue that has potential in the monitoring of response. They are being approached as a minimally invasive biopsy that can be performed serially to monitor therapy through the assessment of drug targets and other biologically important cancer markers. With the evolving ability to detect protein expression with immunofluorescent microscopy, mRNA expression with RT–PCR, and gene amplification using FISH, it is expected that CTC will provide valuable insight into the biology of breast and other cancers, resulting in new treatment strategies and improved methods to monitor response to therapy.

References

1. Group EBCTC. Effects of chemotherapy and hormonal therapy for early breast cancer on recurrence and 15-year survival: an overview of the randomised trials. *Lancet* 2005;365(9472):1687–1717.
2. Ross AA, Cooper BW, Lazarus HM, et al. Detection and viability of tumor cells in peripheral blood stem cell collections from breast cancer patients using immuno-cytochemical and clonogenic assay techniques. *Blood* 1993;82(9):2605–2610.
3. Rolle A, Gunzel R, Pachmann U, et al. Increase in number of circulating disseminated epithelial cells after surgery for non-small cell lung cancer monitored by MAINTRAC(R) is a predictor for relapse: a preliminary report. *World J Surg Oncol* 2005;3(1):18.
4. Choesmel V, Pierga JY, Nos C, et al. Enrichment methods to detect bone marrow micrometastases in breast carcinoma patients: clinical relevance. *Breast Cancer Res* 2004;6(5):R556–R570.
5. Pachmann K, Clement JH, Schneider CP, et al. Standardized quantification of circulating peripheral tumor cells from lung and breast cancer. *Clin Chem Lab Med* 2005;43(6):617–627.
6. Christopherson WM. Cancer cells in the peripheral blood: a second look. *Acta Cytologica* 1965;9(2):169–174.
7. Racila E, Euhus D, Weiss AJ, et al. Detection and characterization of carcinoma cells in the blood. *Proc Natl Acad Sci U S A* 1998;95(8):4589–4594.
8. Witzig TE, Bossy B, Kimlinger T, et al. Detection of circulating cytokeratin-positive cells in the blood of breast cancer patients using immunomagnetic enrichment and digital microscopy. *Clin Cancer Res* 2002;8(5):1085–1091.
9. Cristofanilli M, Budd GT, Ellis MJ, et al. Circulating tumor cells, disease progression, and survival in metastatic breast cancer. *N Engl J Med* 2004;351(8):781–791.
10. Ring A, Smith IE, Dowsett M. Circulating tumour cells in breast cancer. *Lancet Oncol* 2004;5(2):79–88.
11. Lacroix M. Significance, detection and markers of disseminated breast cancer cells. *Endocr Relat Cancer* 2006;13(4):1033–1067.
12. Nagrath S, Sequist LV, Maheswaran S, et al. Isolation of rare circulating tumour cells in cancer patients by microchip technology. *Nature* 2007;450(7173):1235–1239.
13. Martin VM, Siewert C, Scharl A, et al. Immunomagnetic enrichment of disseminated epithelial tumor cells from peripheral blood by MACS. *Exp Hematol* 1998; 26(3):252–264.
14. Hu XC, Wang Y, Shi DR, et al. Immunomagnetic tumor cell enrichment is promising in detecting circulating breast cancer cells. *Oncology* 2003;64(2):160–165.
15. Smerage JB, Hayes DF. The measurement and therapeutic meaning of circulating tumour cells in breast cancer. *Br J Cancer* 2006;94(1):8–12.
16. Rao C, Herman ML, Doyle G, et al. Automated system to enumerate disseminated tumor cells in bone marrow. 5th International Symposium on Minimal Residual Cancer, San Francisco, California, September 11–14, 2005.
17. Allard WJ, Matera J, Miller MC, et al. Tumor cells circulate in the peripheral blood of all major carcinomas but not in healthy subjects or patients with nonmalignant diseases. *Clin Cancer Res* 2004;10(20):6897–6904.
18. Rao CG, Chianese D, Doyle GV, et al. Expression of epithelial cell adhesion molecule in carcinoma cells present in blood and primary and metastatic tumors. *Int J Oncol* 2005;27(1):49–57.
19. Woelfle U, Sauter G, Santjer S, et al. Down-regulated expression of cytokeratin 18 promotes progression of human breast cancer. *Clin Cancer Res* 2004;10(8):2670–2674.
20. Ignatiadis M, Kallergi G, Ntoulia M, et al. Prognostic value of the detection of circulating tumor cells using a multimarker RT-PCR (CK-19, mammaglobin A, HER2/neu) in early breast cancer. *Breast Cancer Res Treat* 2007;1006(S1):108.
21. Brugger W, Buhring HJ, Grunebach F, et al. Expression of MUC-1 epitopes on normal bone marrow: implications for the detection of micrometastatic tumor cells. *J Clin Oncol* 1999;17(5):1535–1544.
22. Ahr A, Scharl A, Muller M, et al. Cross-reactive staining of normal bone-marrow cells by monoclonal antibody 2E11. *Int J Cancer* 1999;84(5):502–505.
23. Borgen E, Beiske K, Trachsel S, et al. Immunocytochemical detection of isolated epithelial cells in bone marrow: non-specific staining and contribution by plasma cells directly reactive to alkaline phosphatase. *J Pathol* 1998;185(4):427–434.
24. Jung R, Kruger W, Hosch S, et al. Specificity of reverse transcriptase polymerase chain reaction assays designed for the detection of circulating cancer cells is influenced by cytokines *in vivo* and *in vitro. Br J Cancer* 1998;78(9):1194–1198.
25. Goeminne JC, Guillaume T, Salmon M, et al. Unreliability of carcinoembryonic antigen (CEA) reverse transcriptase-polymerase chain reaction (RT-PCR) in detecting contaminating breast cancer cells in peripheral blood stem cells due to induction of CEA by growth factors. *Bone Marrow Transplant* 1999;24(7):769–775.
26. de Graaf H, Maelandsmo GM, Ruud P, et al. Ectopic expression of target genes may represent an inherent limitation of RT-PCR assays used for micrometastasis detection: studies on the epithelial glycoprotein gene EGP-2. *Int J Cancer* 1997;72(1):191–196.
27. Stathopoulou A, Gizi A, Perraki M, et al. Real-time quantification of CK-19 mRNA-positive cells in peripheral blood of breast cancer patients using the lightcycler system. *Clin Cancer Res* 2003;9(14):5145–5151.
28. Savtchenko ES, Schiff TA, Jiang CK, et al. Embryonic expression of the human 40-kD keratin: evidence from a processed pseudogene sequence. *Am J Hum Genet* 1988;43(5):630–637.
29. Ruud P, Fodstad O, Hovig E. Identification of a novel cytokeratin 19 pseudogene that may interfere with reverse transcriptase-polymerase chain reaction assays used to detect micrometastatic tumor cells. *Int J Cancer* 1999;80(1):119–125.
30. Stathopoulou A, Ntoulia M, Perraki M, et al. A highly specific real-time RT-PCR method for the quantitative determination of CK-19 mRNA positive cells in peripheral blood of patients with operable breast cancer. *Int J Cancer* 2006;119(7):1654–1659.
31. Ring AE, Zabaglo L, Ormerod MG, et al. Detection of circulating epithelial cells in the blood of patients with breast cancer: comparison of three techniques. *Br J Cancer* 2005;92(5):906–912.
32. Braun S, Pantel K, Muller P, et al. Cytokeratin-positive cells in the bone marrow and survival of patients with stage I, II, or III breast cancer. *N Engl J Med* 2000;342(8):525–533.
33. Braun S, Vogl FD, Naume B, et al. A pooled analysis of bone marrow micrometastasis in breast cancer. *N Engl J Med* 2005;353(8):793–802.
34. Fehm T, Braun S, Muller V, et al. A concept for the standardized detection of disseminated tumor cells in bone marrow from patients with primary breast cancer and its clinical implementation. *Cancer* 2006;107(5):885–892.

35. Wiedswang G, Borgen E, Karesen R, et al. Isolated tumor cells in bone marrow three years after diagnosis in disease-free breast cancer patients predict unfavorable clinical outcome. *Clin Cancer Res* 2004;10(16):5342–5348.

36. Braun S, Kentenich C, Janni W, et al. Lack of effect of adjuvant chemotherapy on the elimination of single dormant tumor cells in bone marrow of high-risk breast cancer patients. *J Clin Oncol* 2000;18(1):80–86.

37. Wiedswang G, Borgen E, Karesen R, et al. Detection of isolated tumor cells in bone marrow is an independent prognostic factor in breast cancer. *J Clin Oncol* 2003;21(18):3469–3478.

38. Kamby C, Rasmussen BB, Kristensen B. Prognostic indicators of metastatic bone disease in human breast cancer. *Cancer* 1991;68(9):2045–2050.

39. Xenidis N, Perraki M, Kafousi M, et al. Predictive and prognostic value of peripheral blood cytokeratin-19 mRNA-positive cells detected by real-time polymerase chain reaction in node-negative breast cancer patients. *J Clin Oncol* 2006;24(23):3756–3762.

40. Xenidis N, Markos V, Apostolaki S, et al. Clinical relevance of circulating CK-19 mRNA-positive cells detected during the adjuvant tamoxifen treatment in patients with early breast cancer. *Ann Oncol* 2007;18(10):1623–1631.

41. Ignatiadis M, Xenidis N, Perraki M, et al. Different prognostic value of cytokeratin-19 mRNA positive circulating tumor cells according to estrogen receptor and HER2 status in early-stage breast cancer. *J Clin Oncol* 2007;25(33):5194–5202.

42. Rack BK, Schindlbeck C, Hofmann S, et al. Circulating tumor cells (CTCs) in peripheral blood of primary breast cancer patients. *J Clin Oncol* 2007;25(18S):10595.

43. Zheng S, Lin H, Liu JQ, et al. Membrane microfilter device for selective capture, electrolysis and genomic analysis of human circulating tumor cells. *J Chromatogr A* 2007;1162(2):154–161.

44. Alix-Panabieres C, Muller V, Pantel K. Current status in human breast cancer micrometastasis. *Curr Opin Oncol* 2007;19(6):558–563.

45. Alix-Panabieres C, Brouillet JP, Fabbro M, et al. Characterization and enumeration of cells secreting tumor markers in the peripheral blood of breast cancer patients. *J Immunol Methods* 2005;299(1–2):177–188.

46. Alix-Panabieres C, Rebillard X, Brouillet JP, et al. Detection of circulating prostate-specific antigen-secreting cells in prostate cancer patients. *Clin Chem* 2005;51(8):1538–1541.

47. Hayes DF, Bast R, Desch CE, et al. A tumor marker utility grading system (TMUGS): a framework to evaluate clinical utility of tumor markers. *J Natl Cancer Inst* 1996;88:1456–1466.

48. Gerber B, Krause A, Muller H, et al. Simultaneous immunohistochemical detection of tumor cells in lymph nodes and bone marrow aspirates in breast cancer and its correlation with other prognostic factors. *J Clin Oncol* 2001;19(4):960–971.

49. Pierga JY, Bonneton C, Vincent-Salomon A, et al. Clinical significance of immunocytochemical detection of tumor cells using digital microscopy in peripheral blood and bone marrow of breast cancer patients. *Clin Cancer Res* 2004;10(4):1392–1400.

50. Gebauer G, Fehm T, Merkle E, et al. Epithelial cells in bone marrow of breast cancer patients at time of primary surgery: clinical outcome during long-term follow-up. *J Clin Oncol* 2001;19(16):3669–3674.

51. Mansi JL, Gogas H, Bliss JM, et al. Outcome of primary-breast-cancer patients with micrometastases: a long-term follow-up study. *Lancet* 1999;354(9174):197–202.

52. Diel IJ, Kaufmann M, Costa SD, et al. Micrometastatic breast cancer cells in bone marrow at primary surgery: prognostic value in comparison with nodal status. *J Natl Cancer Inst* 1996;88(22):1652–1658.

53. Pachmann K, Dengler R, Lobodasch K, et al. An increase in cell number at completion of therapy may develop as an indicator of early relapse: quantification of circulating epithelial tumor cells (CETC) for monitoring of adjuvant therapy in breast cancer. *J Cancer Res Clin Oncol* 2008;134(1):59–65.

54. Xenidis N, Apostolaki S, Perraki M, et al. Circulating CK-19 mRNA (+) cells in patients with stage I and II breast cancer after the completion of adjuvant chemotherapy: evaluation of their prognostic relevance. *Breast Cancer Res Treat* 2007;106(S1):109.

55. Braun S, Naume B. Circulating and disseminated tumor cells. *J Clin Oncol* 2005;23:1623–1626.

56. Harris L, Fritsche H, Mennel R, et al. American Society of Clinical Oncology 2007 update of recommendations for the use of tumor markers in breast cancer. *J Clin Oncol* 2007;25(33):5287–5312.

57. Budd GT, Cristofanilli M, Ellis MJ, et al. Circulating tumor cells versus imaging—predicting overall survival in metastatic breast cancer. *Clin Cancer Res* 2006;12(21):6403–6409.

58. Hayes DF, Cristofanilli M, Budd GT, et al. Circulating tumor cells at each follow-up time point during therapy of metastatic breast cancer patients predict progression-free and overall survival. *Clin Cancer Res* 2006;12(14 Pt 1):4218–4224.

59. Soria JC, Gauthier LR, Raymond E, et al. Molecular detection of telomerase-positive circulating epithelial cells in metastatic breast cancer patients. *Clin Cancer Res* 1999;5(5):971–975.

60. Austrup F, Uciechowski P, Eder C, et al. Prognostic value of genomic alterations in minimal residual cancer cells purified from the blood of breast cancer patients. *Br J Cancer* 2000;83(12):1664–1673.

61. Fehm T, Sagalowsky A, Clifford E, et al. Cytogenetic evidence that circulating epithelial cells in patients with carcinoma are malignant. *Clin Cancer Res* 2002;8(7):2073–2084.

62. Meng S, Tripathy D, Shete S, et al. HER-2 gene amplification can be acquired as breast cancer progresses. *Proc Natl Acad Sci U S A* 2004;101(25):9393–9398.

63. Hayes DF, Walker TM, Singh B, et al. Monitoring expression of HER-2 on circulating epithelial cells in patients with advanced breast cancer. *Int J Oncol* 2002;21(5):1111–1117.

64. Meng S, Tripathy D, Frenkel EP, et al. Circulating tumor cells in patients with breast cancer dormancy. *Clin Cancer Res* 2004;10(24):8152–8162.

65. Braun S, Schlimok G, Heumos I, et al. ErbB2 overexpression on occult metastatic cells in bone marrow predicts poor clinical outcome of stage I-III breast cancer patients. *Cancer Res* 2001;61(5):1890–1895.

66. Smerage JB, Doyle GV, Budd GT, et al. The detection of apoptosis and Bcl-2 expression in circulating tumor cells (CTCs) from women being treated for metastatic breast cancer. *Proceedings of the American Association of Cancer Research* 2006;47:187a.

67. Smirnov DA, Zweitzig DR, Foulk BW, et al. Global gene expression profiling of circulating tumor cells. *Cancer Res* 2005;65(12):4993–4997.

68. O'Hara SM, Moreno JG, Zweitzig DR, et al. Multigene reverse transcription-PCR profiling of circulating tumor cells in hormone-refractory prostate cancer. *Clin Chem* 2004;50(5):826–835.

69. Wicha MS, Liu S, Dontu G. Cancer stem cells: an old idea—a paradigm shift. *Cancer Res* 2006;66(4):1883–1890; discussion 95–96.

70. Vona G, Sabile A, Louha M, et al. Isolation by size of epithelial tumor cells: a new method for the immunomorphological and molecular characterization of circulating tumor cells. *Am J Pathol* 2000;156(1):57–63.

71. Brandt B, Junker R, Griwatz C, et al. Isolation of prostate-derived single cells and cell clusters from human peripheral blood. *Cancer Res* 1996;56(20):4556–4561.

72. Ignatiadis M, Perraki M, Apostolaki S, et al. Molecular detection and prognostic value of circulating cytokeratin-19 messenger RNA-positive and HER2 messenger RNA-positive cells in the peripheral blood of women with early-stage breast cancer. *Clin Breast Cancer* 2007;7(11):883–889.

73. Fonseca FL, Soares HP, Manhani AR, et al. Peripheral blood c-erbB-2 expression by reverse transcriptase-polymerase chain reaction in breast cancer patients receiving chemotherapy. *Clin Breast Cancer* 2002;3(3):201–205.

74. Grunewald K, Haun M, Urbanek M, et al. Mammaglobin gene expression: a superior marker of breast cancer cells in peripheral blood in comparison to epidermal-growth-factor receptor and cytokeratin-19. *Lab Invest* 2000;80(7):1071–1077.

75. Zach O, Kasparu H, Wagner H, et al. Prognostic value of tumour cell detection in peripheral blood of breast cancer patients. *Acta Med Austriaca Suppl* 2002;59:32–34.

76. Aerts J, Wynendaele W, Paridaens R, et al. A real-time quantitative reverse transcriptase polymerase chain reaction (RT-PCR) to detect breast carcinoma cells in peripheral blood. *Ann Oncol* 2001;12(1):39–46.

77. Klein CA, Schmidt-Kittler O, Schardt JA, et al. Comparative genomic hybridization, loss of heterozygosity, and DNA sequence analysis of single cells. *Proc Natl Acad Sci U S A* 1999;96(8):4494–4499.

78. Fiegl H, Millinger S, Mueller-Holzner E, et al. Circulating tumor-specific DNA: a marker for monitoring efficacy of adjuvant therapy in cancer patients. *Cancer Res* 2005;65(4):1141–1145.

Chapter 34
Evaluation of Patients for Metastasis Prior to Primary Therapy

Yee Lu Tham, Rita Kramer, and C. Kent Osborne

The American Cancer Society estimates that 180,510 new cases of invasive breast cancer were diagnosed in the United States in 2007 (1). These individuals will question which laboratory and imaging studies are needed to ensure they receive optimal therapy. Patients may hope that careful staging will provide their physician information that will allow accurate prediction of their disease course. In reality, the primary goal of accurate staging is to exclude distant disease that would render the patient incurable. The patient seeking reassurance that her disease is confined to locoregional sites must be counseled that risk of relapse with systemic disease correlates with lymph node status, tumor size, and other tumor specific biomarkers (Chapter 31). Patients may believe that baseline studies improve the accuracy of surveillance. However, most of those who relapse with metastatic disease are diagnosed by symptoms rather than routine testing (Chapter 70). The physician must carefully consider which asymptomatic patients are at increased risk of having occult metastases that can be identified by staging procedures. These patients are then candidates for specific staging studies before systemic adjuvant therapy. Many patients are at low risk and extensive staging is inappropriate and wasteful for health care dollars and resources. Staging tests are expensive and many have high false-positive rates, leading to further testing. Unnecessary or low-yield testing financially burdens the already stressed health care system.

TIMING OF BASELINE STAGING TESTS

Presurgical Testing

Asymptomatic patients without locally advanced breast carcinoma should have limited staging performed before definitive surgery. History, physical examination, and routine chemistry testing should be performed before surgery.

Evaluation of the Ipsilateral and Contralateral Breasts

Patients should also have complete evaluation of the contralateral breast to exclude synchronous breast cancer and of the ipsilateral breast to exclude multifocal or multicentric disease. The prevalence of synchronous bilateral breast cancer is approximately 1% to 3% (2,3). Physical examination and mammography performed to screen for synchronous cancer in the contralateral breast detect disease in 0.2% to 1.0% and 1% to 3% of cases, respectively (4,5). Magnetic resonance imaging (MRI) has been investigated to determine whether it improves the detection rate of contralateral breast cancer. Studies in which patients were screened for contralateral breast cancer soon after the initial diagnosis of breast cancer have shown

that MRI can identify occult breast cancer in 3% to 5% of patients with a positive predictive value of 21% to 33% (6–9). The largest study conducted by the American College of Radiology Imaging Network included 969 women who underwent a contralateral breast MRI (9). Occult breast cancer was detected in the contralateral breast in 3.1% of patients. Approximately 12.5% of these women underwent biopsy and 30 cases of cancer were diagnosed (18 invasive and 12 *in situ*). The average tumor size was 10.9 mm and none had lymph node metastases. The positive predictive value for an abnormal MRI in this study was 21% and it was significantly higher in postmenopausal than in pre- or perimenopausal women (31% vs. 11%).

MRI has also been used to determine the extent of the tumor in the ipsilateral breast and to exclude multicentric lesions that would preclude breast-conservation surgery (Chapter 14). In view of the low risk of ipsilateral breast recurrence in patients treated by optimal local and systemic therapy, especially endocrine therapy when the tumor is estrogen-receptor (ER) positive, the value of identifying such lesions with MRI can be questioned. It can theoretically increase the number of mastectomies that are unnecessary since these occult multicentric lesions are eradicated by breast irradiation and systemic therapy. Therefore, the use of MRI routinely in all women recently diagnosed with unilateral breast cancer warrants further investigation in relation to the real benefits received and the costs and availability of MRI centers staffed with well-trained radiologists.

Screening for Occult Metastatic Disease

The risk that an asymptomatic patient may have occult bone, liver, brain, or lung metastasis is directly related to tumor size, the number of axillary lymph nodes involved with disease, and other tumor characteristics. Historically, patients often had baseline testing performed before surgery. The clinician was then hindered by lack of complete information regarding the primary tumor and the lymph node status. If careful preoperative history, physical examination, and routine chemistry testing reveal no evidence of locally advanced or distant disease, the authors advocate that decisions regarding additional staging be made after surgery. Those who are low risk of harboring identifiable distant metastases may then avoid unnecessary testing, whereas those at increased risk may be examined more carefully.

If chemistry testing reveals an abnormal alkaline phosphatase, a bone scan should be considered. In a series of 1,116 consecutive staging measurements of alkaline phosphatase, 1.5% of measurements were falsely positive and 96.6% of studies provided true-negative results (10). The sensitivity and specificity of alkaline phosphatase in this series was 0.8 and 0.98, respectively. Similarly, if staging chemistries reveal an

483

elevated gamma-glutamyl transferase, liver ultrasonography, or a computed tomography (CT) scan of the liver should be considered. Data from the same series of patients revealed a true-negative rate of 97.2% and a false-positive rate of 1.4% for this test. The sensitivity and specificity of gamma-glutamyl transferase in this series were 0.6 and 0.98, respectively.

An occasional patient staged after surgery is found to have occult metastatic disease and theoretically may have been "spared" surgery if preoperative staging had been performed. However, numerous retrospective analyses have shown that patients with stage IV disease at diagnosis who underwent definitive surgery of their primary breast tumor have longer survival than patients with metastatic disease who do not undergo surgery (Chapter 71) (11–14). The largest review conducted with the National Cancer Data Base identified 16,023 women presenting with stage IV disease (15). Local therapy was variable, with 57.2% of patients undergoing partial or total mastectomy and 42.8% either no surgery or one of several diagnostic or palliative procedures. Those with free margins after surgery had an improved 3-year survival (35% vs. 26%). A multivariate proportional hazards model identified the number of metastatic sites, the type of metastatic burden, and the extent of resection of the primary tumor as significant independent prognostic covariates. Women treated with surgical resection that resulted in free margins had a superior prognosis compared with those who did not (hazard ratio 0.61, 95% confidence interval [CI], 0.58–0.65). Optimal local control improves quality of life in all patients, even those with early metastatic disease. Thus, there is no compelling rational to perform staging procedures preoperatively in asymptomatic patients.

 ## ESTIMATING RISK OF OCCULT METASTATIC DISEASE

The risk of unsuspected metastasis in an asymptomatic woman with breast cancer correlates with disease stage. However, within a given stage, the risk may be quite variable. For example, the patient with stage II disease with four or more positive nodes is at substantially greater risk than the woman with a T2 primary and negative nodes. Most reports documenting the rate of detection of occult metastasis with staging provide results according to disease stage. The Cancer Care Ontario Practice Guideline Initiative performed a systematic review to determine the detection rate of commonly used staging studies in women with newly diagnosed breast cancer (16,17). Series were included if they reported the rates of abnormal tests indicative of metastasis and the total number of patients tested for each stage of disease. Data regarding bone scans were pooled from studies reported after 1980. Results from each study were summed and the detection rate (number of tests indicating metastasis divided by total number of tests) with a 95% CI was calculated for the pooled results for bone scan, chest radiography, and liver ultrasonography for stage I, II, and III disease (Table 34.1). Not surprisingly, occult metastasis was most frequently found in bone (3.1%) compared to lung (0.5%) or liver (0.6%). Patients with stage III disease were more likely than those with stage I or II to have asymptomatic metastasis detected by staging. Occult bone metastases were seen in 8.3% of patients with stage III disease, 2.4% with stage II, and 0.5% with stage I.

Fewer studies have correlated the detection rate of these tests with tumor size and number of involved axillary nodes, rather than just tumor stage. Ciatto et al. (18) retrospectively reviewed a series of 3,627 patients with newly diagnosed breast cancer undergoing staging. The sensitivity, specificity, and positive predictive value of bone scan, chest radiography, and liver ultrasonography were calculated. Asymptomatic distant metastases were detected by bone scan in 22 of 2,450

	DETECTION RATE OF BASELINE STAGING IN BREAST CANCER

Table 34.1

	Cancer Care Ontario Practice Guidelines		
Stage	Bone Scan	Liver Ultrasound	CXR
I	0.5% (0.1–0.9)	0% (0.0)	0.1% (0.0–0.3)
II	2.4% (1.8–3.0)	0.4% (0.0–0.8)	0.2% (0.0–0.4)
III	8.3% (6.7–9.9)	2.0% (0.4–3.6)	1.7% (0.8–2.6)
Total	3.1% (2.6–3.6)	0.6% (0.2–1.0)	0.5% (0.3–0.7)

CXR, chest x-ray.
Modified from www.ccopebc.ca/, with permission.

(0.90%), by chest radiography in 11 of 3,627 (0.30%), and by liver ultrasonography in 2 of 836 (0.24%). The risk of having occult metastasis increased with increasing T stage. Those with T3 and T4 primaries had a 0.79% and 1.33% risk, respectively, of having unsuspected bone metastasis. Detection rate also increased with increasing nodal involvement. Only 0.54% of node-negative patients had unsuspected bone metastasis compared with 1.23% of N1 and 2.58% of those with N2 disease. The authors did not report results according to the number of involved nodes. However, a smaller series (1,218 patients) reported by Ravaioli et al. (19) demonstrated that those with the fewest number of involved nodes have the lowest detection rate. Asymptomatic bone metastases were detected in 3 of 165 patients (1.82%) with one to three positive nodes, in 6 of 103 (5.82%) with four to six positive nodes, and in 9 of 126 (7.14%) with greater than six positive nodes. Few patients with T3 and T4 primaries were available for analysis, and when results for all nodal groups (negative and positive) with this T stage are summed, 1 of 30 (3.3%) patients with T3 and 5 of 43 (11.6%) of those with T4 primaries had unsuspected bone metastases. Thus, the detection rate of occult metastases with these diagnostic tests in asymptomatic patients is relatively low even in those with T3 lesions and multiple positive nodes. The value of these tests must also take into account specificity and the false-positive rate that can have disturbing psychological effects and lead to additional expensive or invasive procedures.

 ## SPECIFIC STAGING TESTS

Historically, the most commonly used techniques in breast cancer staging were bone scan, liver ultrasonography, chest radiography, alkaline phosphatase, alanine and aspartate aminotransferases, and gamma-glutamyl transferase. The false-positive rate, false-negative rate, sensitivity, and specificity of these tests are discussed later. Staging tools are constantly evolving, both because of technical improvements in previously used imaging tools and the development of newer tests. CT, MRI, positron emission tomography (PET), and tumor markers have also been studied as initial staging procedures.

Bone Scan

The sensitivity of staging bone scans ranges from 0.48 to 0.92 (18,19). The likelihood of having a false-positive study (2.9%) was nearly identical to the likelihood of having a true-positive study (3.1%) in a series of 1,193 patients reported by Ravaioli et al. (19). The specificity of staging bone scans ranges from

0.948 to 0.96 and varies with age (18,19). The incidence of false-positive scans is significantly greater in patients older than 50 years (18,20). Patients with one or two solitary abnormalities on bone scan should be carefully evaluated to exclude a nonmalignant etiology. In one series of follow-up scans performed in patients with breast cancer, 274 scans revealed one or two new abnormalities. Only 25 (9%) of these abnormalities were found to be due to malignancy (21). The positive predictive value of an initial bone scan for patients with stage I or II disease is approximately 11% (22,23). MRI and possibly bone biopsy should be performed to evaluate solitary abnormalities on bone scan before deeming a patient incurable.

Chest Radiograph

Staging chest radiography is less sensitive and specific for asymptomatic pulmonary metastasis. Sensitivity ranges from 0.31 to 0.75 and specificity from 0.996 to 0.99 in two large series (18,19).

The detection rate of pulmonary metastasis by chest radiography in a series of 1,003 patients with stage I and II disease reported by Chen et al. (24) was 0.099% (95% CI, 0.0%–0.6%). Five of the 1,003 procedures were abnormal, and the etiology of the abnormalities is instructive. Two of the five patients had primary lung cancers and three had benign lung disease; none had metastatic breast cancer.

Liver Ultrasonography or Radionucleotide Liver Scan

Ciatto et al. (18) evaluated staging liver ultrasonography and scintigraphy in 836 and 435 patients, respectively. Cases were evaluated retrospectively and were collected from 11 Italian centers. Different centers used different imaging tests. In this series, liver ultrasonography was more sensitive than scintigraphy (0.29 vs. 0.20) and more specific (0.995 vs. 0.972). Sensitivity of liver ultrasonography in the Ravaioli et al. (19) series (1,206 patients) was 0.62 and specificity was 0.99. The low detection rate of occult metastasis in liver (~1%) with both ultrasonography and scintigraphy led one author to suggest that a positive result on staging liver ultrasonography or scintigraphy is more likely to be a false-positive than a true-positive result (16–19,25). Obviously, before declaring a patient incurable on the basis of these tests, additional diagnostic evaluation, perhaps even a liver biopsy, is required.

Computed Tomography

There are few retrospective series analyzing the impact of CT staging in newly diagnosed breast cancer. The detection rate of occult metastasis is low, and evaluation with this modality often reveals nonmalignant abnormalities. Isaacs et al. (26) retrospectively determined the detection rate of CT in 117 patients undergoing staging CT of the head, chest, abdomen, and pelvis. Results were not reported by stage; however, 76% (89/117) of patients had either T1 or T2 primaries. Only 1 of these 89 (1.1%) was found to have metastasis. The overall detection rate of metastases was 4% (T1 to T4 primaries). There were 16 unrelated findings, two false-positive scans, and, surprisingly, a number of false-negative studies. Three patients had metastases detected on bone scan (one outside the CT field) and one hepatic metastasis detected by ultrasonography.

A small percentage of patients with very high-risk disease can be upstaged by CT. Crump et al. (27) reported the impact of CT scanning on stage in women with 10 or more involved axillary nodes thought to be free of metastatic disease and referred for high-dose chemotherapy and autologous transplantation. CT scans of the head, chest, abdomen, and pelvis were performed on 30 women between 1993 and 1995. Four

of the 30 women (13.3%) were upstaged. Three women were found to have disease in the chest (one internal mammary node, two with lung parenchymal disease). One patient was found to have unsuspected liver metastasis. The authors report that there was no obvious difference in either primary tumor size or the number of involved lymph nodes between those who had metastatic disease detected with CT scanning and those who did not. However, this study is too small to have detected any difference, and all patients had a minimum of 10 positive axillary nodes.

Many women treated with breast-conserving surgery undergo CT as planning for breast radiation therapy. Mehta and Goffinet (28) reported the results of careful reviews of 153 extended CT scans performed as part of radiation treatment planning. The extended pretreatment CTs included the breast, neck, thorax, and liver. Eleven percent of the studies revealed unsuspected abnormalities, but most of these were nonmalignant. Only four patients had unsuspected malignancy; two were already known to have stage IV disease. Therefore, only 2 of 153 scans revealed occult disease that resulted in stage change.

Three methods of hepatic screening for clinically occult metastasis are available: liver ultrasonography, liver scintigraphy, and CT. Liver ultrasonography is the least expensive of these modalities, although CT is the most accurate (29,30).

Positron Emission Tomography

PET using fluorine 18-fluorodeoxyglucose (FDG-PET) is an appealing imaging modality because it is hypothesized that it can detect increased glucose metabolism in primary tumors, involved axillary nodes, and distant sites, all in a single examination. The role of FDG-PET in detecting distant metastases in breast cancer has been investigated. A meta-analysis of the utility of FDG-PET for the evaluation of distant metastases reported a median sensitivity and specificity of 92.7% and 81.6%, respectively (31). However, when FDG-PET was compared with conventional imaging, FDG-PET provided little additional information as the number of women who had FDG-PET–detected metastases only was small (32–34). In a prospective trial of 200 women who underwent FDG-PET to detect distant metastases, six women were found to have distant metastases but only two who had FDG-PET detected metastases only (34). More disconcerting was the high false-positive rate of approximately 58%, which often resulted in additional work-up, including dangerous invasive procedures with a dramatic increase in costs. Therefore, FDG-PET is not yet recommended as a routine staging modality to detect distant metastases in women diagnosed with breast cancer (35). Future studies may be limited to specific populations, such as women with locally advanced breast cancer, or to the examination of specific sites, such as internal mammary or mediastinal nodes, or the primary breast tumor itself to determine early response to systemic therapy (Chapter 15). Today, most FDG-PET is performed in combination with conventional CT. Initial analysis of the use of FDG-PET with CT in detecting distant metastases showed that the integration of FDG-PET with CT may be more effective than CT or FDG-PET alone (36,37). However, due to the low detection rate of distant metastases and the high false-positive rate of FDG-PET, the integration of FDG-PET with CT did not provide additional improvement to conventional imaging (38,39).

Tumor Markers

Neither carcinoembryonic antigen, CA15-3, CA27.29, nor shed extracellular domain of HER2/(ERBB2) demonstrates sufficiently reliable performance characteristics to indicate that a patient at low risk should proceed to radiographic staging. Likewise,

Table 34.2	STAGING RECOMMENDATIONS FOR EARLY BREAST CANCER FROM NATIONAL COMPREHENSIVE CANCER NETWORK GUIDELINES		
	T0–2,N0–1; T3,N0	T3N1	Any T,N2; Any T,N3; T4,N0–1
Preoperative			
History and physical examination	+	+	+
Breast imaging	+	+	+
Routine chemistry testing	+	+	+
Postoperative[a]			
Bone scan	−	+	+
Liver ultrasound, CT, or MRI	−	+	+
Chest radiograph or CT	−	−	+

CT, computed tomography; MRI, magnetic resonance imaging.
[a]May be preoperative if locally advanced or inflammatory breast cancer or in early stage cancer with abnormal chemistries, history or physical examination, or receiving preoperative therapy.
From NCCN Breast Cancer Practice Guidelines. Practice guidelines in oncology v.2.2008. Available at http://www.nccn.org/professionals/physician_gls/PDF/breast.pdf, with permission.

none is sufficiently sensitive to exclude the presence of occult metastasis and preclude a patient with high-risk disease from undergoing appropriate imaging (40). These tumor markers are not recommended for initial staging (41).

Bone Marrow Aspirate and Biopsy and Circulating Tumor Cells

Bone marrow aspiration and biopsy are investigational staging studies. Crump et al. (27) report on the impact of bilateral bone marrow aspirate and biopsy on staging of 30 patients with high-risk breast cancer being evaluated for high-dose chemotherapy and autologous bone marrow transplantation as primary therapy. These patients had 10 or more positive axillary nodes and were evaluated for treatment according to clinical trial. The authors report that 3 of 30 patients were found to have bone marrow metastases by routine pathologic methods. Immunohistochemistry and flow cytometry were not performed on the samples. All three patients had negative bone scans and normal serum alkaline phosphatase levels.

Several investigators have identified occult bone marrow metastases in women newly diagnosed with breast cancer (42–44) (Chapter 33). A pooled analysis of data from nine studies involving 4,703 patients assessed the prognostic significance of the presence of micrometastases in the bone marrow at initial diagnosis (45). A surprisingly high percentage (30.6%) of patients had cytokeratin-positive cells. Patients with bone marrow micrometastases often had larger, higher grade and lymph node–positive tumors and they had an increased risk of relapsing with distant disease. Interestingly, 50% to 70% of women with marrow micrometastases do not develop clinically evident metastatic breast cancer (Chapter 33).

Presently, bone marrow assessment is not recommended as a baseline test due to lack of standardization of detection methods, and its contribution to clinical decisions regarding systemic therapy is unclear.

The ability to detect and measure circulating tumor cells in blood is a promising new technique. Tumor cells must enter the circulation to "seed" distant metastatic sites and quantifying them in peripheral blood is a less invasive procedure than bone marrow aspiration and biopsy. Early studies correlating circulating tumor cells with prognosis in early stage breast cancer suggested that the detection of circulating tumor cells is associated with poor survival (46,47). Additional studies will be needed to determine the role, if any, of circulating tumor cells in early stage breast cancer.

RECOMMENDATIONS

Recommendations for baseline staging tests in primary breast cancer have been published by a number of organizations, such as the National Comprehensive Cancer Network (NCCN), and authors (16–18,30,48,49) (Table 34.2). Preoperative evaluation with history, physical examination, bilateral mammography, and serum chemistry tests should be performed. Most recommend that baseline staging studies in women without locally advanced disease be performed after definitive surgery, when tumor size and number of involved axillary nodes and, thus, the risk of distant disease can be estimated (16–19). This sequence allows many women to avoid unnecessary testing.

The detection rate of baseline staging varies with nodal status, tumor size, clinical stage, and other patient and tumor characteristics. Those with a low risk of occult metastatic disease are more likely to experience a false-positive than a true-positive test when staged. The Breast Cancer Disease Site Group of the Cancer Care Ontario Practice Guideline reports that the detection rates for bone scan, chest radiography, and liver ultrasonography are less than 1% for patients with stage I disease (16,17). They and others recommend that women with stage I breast cancer be staged only with history, physical examination, and blood chemistry but not with bone scan, chest radiography, liver ultrasonography, or other studies. Patients with stage III disease have a higher risk of having occult disease that might be detected by staging, and more extensive evaluation of this group is recommended by the Cancer Care Ontario Practice Guideline (Table 34.1).

Only a few series specifically address staging for the heterogeneous risk population that comprises stage II disease, and recommendations for this group are more variable (16–19). The Cancer Care Ontario Practice Guideline group recommends bone scan but not chest radiography or liver ultrasonography for patients with stage II disease because the detection rate for bone scan was 2%, for chest radiography 0.2%, and for liver ultrasonography 0.4%. Ravaioli et al. (19) have also made staging recommendations for patients with stage II disease. These authors have subdivided patients with stage II disease based on tumor size and nodal involvement and recommend that patients with pathologic stage T1-3, N0-1 disease with no more than three involved nodes undergo staging by laboratory testing alone. Patients in their series with stage II disease with four or more involved nodes or N2 disease had a higher detection rate of occult metastatic disease, and

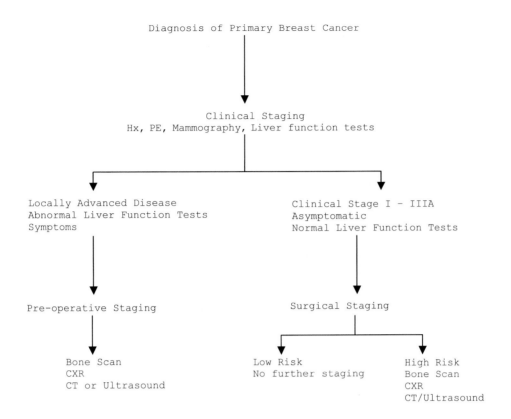

Diagnosis of Primary Breast Cancer

↓

Clinical Staging
Hx, PE, Mammography, Liver function tests

Locally Advanced Disease
Abnormal Liver Function Tests
Symptoms

↓

Pre-operative Staging

↓

Bone Scan
CXR
CT or Ultrasound

Clinical Stage I – IIIA
Asymptomatic
Normal Liver Function Tests

↓

Surgical Staging

Low Risk
No further staging

High Risk
Bone Scan
CXR
CT/Ultrasound

FIGURE 34.1. Staging recommendations prior to primary therapy. CT, computed tomography.

extensive staging with laboratory tests, bone scan, chest radiography, and liver ultrasonography after surgery was recommended (Table 34.1).

The authors recommend that evaluation of all patients be individualized. The risk of occult metastatic disease should be assessed on the basis of patient and tumor characteristics. Those who are low risk and have normal alkaline phosphatase and gamma-glutamyl transferase levels have a low likelihood of having occult metastases and need no further staging. Patients with large primary tumors or multiple involved nodes have a higher risk of having occult metastatic disease and may benefit from extensive staging. Based on the available data, suggested guidelines are shown in Figure 34.1. Molecular profiling of primary tumors is beginning to have a role in the clinic to estimate the risk of metastatic disease in conjunction with other features of the tumor and to estimate the likelihood of treatment benefits. The Oncotype DX (Genomic Health, Redwood City, California) and MammaPrint (Agendia, Huntington Beach, California) signature are reviewed in Chapter 57. In the future, the gene expression profile of an individual tumor may allow improved assessment of prognosis and refinement of recommendations regarding which individual patients should undergo extensive staging evaluation.

All staging studies are plagued by false-positive results, and the finding of an isolated abnormality on any study should be viewed with caution. Careful additional evaluation or biopsy to confirm the presence or absence of metastatic disease should be considered. MRI is frequently required to evaluate solitary abnormalities on bone scan. Similarly, CT is used further to define abnormalities found on staging liver ultrasonography and scintigraphy. Occasionally, MRI of the liver identifies an abdominal CT finding as a hemangioma. Those patients with a solitary abnormality suspicious for metastasis on any of these

studies should be considered for biopsy. PET scan, MRI of the chest and abdomen, tumor markers, bone marrow aspiration and biopsy and circulating tumor cells are not recommended routinely as baseline staging tests in primary breast cancer.

 MANAGEMENT SUMMARY

- All patients with early breast cancer should have baseline history, physical examination, bilateral mammography, and routine chemistry testing performed before definitive surgery.
- Patients with stage I disease do not require further staging tests postoperatively unless they have symptoms, abnormal examination, or chemistries.
- Patients with stage II or III disease may require further staging tests pre- or postoperatively as described in Table 39.2 and Figure 39.1.
- Staging tests include bone scan, liver ultrasound or CT, and chest radiograph or CT.
- PET or PET/CT, MRI of chest and abdomen, tumor markers, bone marrow aspiration or biopsy, and circulating tumor cells are not recommended as staging tests.

References

1. Jemal A, Siegel R, Ward E, et al. Cancer statistics, 2007. *CA Cancer J Clin* 2007; 57:43–66.
2. Donovan AJ. Bilateral breast cancer. *Surg Clin North Am* 1990;70:1141–1149.
3. Heron DE, Komarnicky LT, Hyslop T, et al. Bilateral breast carcinoma: risk factors and outcomes for patients with synchronous and metachronous disease. *Cancer* 2000;88:2739–2750.
4. Hungness ES, Safa M, Shaughnessy EA, et al. Bilateral synchronous breast cancer: mode of detection and comparison of histologic features between the 2 breasts. *Surgery* 2000;128:702–707.

5. Leis HP Jr. Managing the remaining breast. *Cancer* 1980;46:1026–1030.
6. Lehman CD, Blume JD, Thickman D, et al. Added cancer yield of MRI in screening the contralateral breast of women recently diagnosed with breast cancer: results from the International Breast Magnetic Resonance Consortium (IBMC) trial. *J Surg Oncol* 2005;92:9–16.
7. Liberman L, Morris EA, Kim CM, et al. MR imaging findings in the contralateral breast of women with recently diagnosed breast cancer. *AJR Am J Roentgenol* 2003;180:333–341.
8. Lee SG, Orel SG, Woo IJ, et al. MR imaging screening of the contralateral breast in patients with newly diagnosed breast cancer: preliminary results. *Radiology* 2003;226:773–738.
9. Lehman CD, Gatsonis C, Kuhl CK, et al. MRI evaluation of the contralateral breast in women with recently diagnosed breast cancer. *N Engl J Med* 2007;356:1295–1303.
10. Brar HS, Sisley JF, Johnson RH Jr. Value of preoperative bone and liver scans and alkaline phosphatase in the evaluation of breast cancer patients. *Am J Surg* 1993; 165:221–224.
11. Fields RC, Jeffe DB, Trinkaus K, et al. Surgical resection of the primary tumor is associated with increased long-term survival in patients with stage IV breast cancer after controlling for site of metastasis. *Ann Surg Oncol* 2007;14:3345–3351.
12. Babiera GV, Rao R, Feng L, et al. Effect of primary tumor extirpation in breast cancer patients who present with stage IV disease and an intact primary tumor. *Ann Surg Oncol* 2006;13:776–782.
13. Rapiti E, Verkooijen HM, Vlastos G, et al. Complete excision of primary breast tumor improves survival of patients with metastatic breast cancer at diagnosis. *J Clin Oncol* 2006;24:2743–2749.
14. Gnerlich J, Jeffe DB, Deshpande AD, et al. Surgical removal of the primary tumor increases overall survival in patients with metastatic breast cancer: analysis of the 1988–2003 SEER data. *Ann Surg Oncol* 2007;14:2187–2194.
15. Khan SA, Stewart AK, Morrow M. Does aggressive local therapy improve survival in metastatic breast cancer? *Surgery* 2002;132:620–627.
16. Myers RE, Johnston M, Pritchard K, et al. Baseline staging tests in primary breast cancer: a practice guideline. *Can Med Assoc J* 2001;164:1439–1444.
17. Baseline staging tests in primary breast cancer. Cancer Care Ontario PEBC evidence based reports 2003. Available at http://www.cancercare.on.ca/pdf/pebc1-14f.pdf.
18. Ciatto S, Pacini P, Azzini V, et al. Preoperative staging of primary breast cancer. A multicentric study. *Cancer* 1988;61:1038–1040.
19. Ravaioli A, Pasini G, Polselli A, et al. Staging of breast cancer: new recommended standard procedure. *Breast Cancer Res Treat* 2002;72:53–60.
20. Hadley D, Fowble B, Torosian MH. Evidence for selective use of bone scans in early stage breast cancer. *Oncol Rep* 1998;5:991–993.
21. Jacobson AF, Cronin EB, Stomper PC, et al. Bone scans with one or two new abnormalities in cancer patients with no known metastases: frequency and serial scintigraphic behavior of benign and malignant lesions. *Radiology* 1990;175: 229–232.
22. Yeh KA, Fortunato L, Ridge JA, et al. Routine bone scanning in patients with T1 and T2 breast cancer: a waste of money. *Ann Surg Oncol* 1995;2:319–324.
23. Burkett FE, Scanlon EF, Garces RM, et al. The value of bone scans in the management of patients with carcinoma of the breast. *Surg Gynecol Obstet* 1979;149:523–525.
24. Chen EA, Carlson GA, Coughlin BF, et al. Routine chest roentgenography is unnecessary in the work-up of stage I and II breast cancer. *J Clin Oncol* 2000;18: 3503–3506.
25. Wiener SN, Sachs SH. An assessment of routine liver scanning in patients with breast cancer. *Arch Surg* 1978;113:126–127.
26. Isaacs RJ, Ford JM, Allan SG, et al. Role of computed tomography in the staging of primary breast cancer. *Br J Surg* 1993;80:1137.
27. Crump M, Goss PE, Prince M, et al. Outcome of extensive evaluation before adjuvant therapy in women with breast cancer and 10 or more positive axillary lymph nodes. *J Clin Oncol* 1996;14:66–69.
28. Mehta VK, Goffinet DR. Unsuspected abnormalities noted on CT treatment-planning scans obtained for breast and chest wall irradiation. *Int J Radiat Oncol Biol Phys* 2001;49:723–725.
29. Alderson PO, Adams DF, McNeil BJ, et al. Computed tomography, ultrasound, and scintigraphy of the liver in patients with colon or breast carcinoma: a prospective comparison. *Radiology* 1983;149:225–230.
30. Baker RR. Preoperative assessment of the patient with breast cancer. *Surg Clin North Am* 1984;64:1039–1050.
31. Isasi CR, Moadel RM, Blaufox MD. A meta-analysis of FDG-PET for the evaluation of breast cancer recurrence and metastases. *Breast Cancer Res Treat* 2005;90:105–112.
32. Landheer ML, Steffens MG, Klinkenbijl JH, et al. Value of fluorodeoxyglucose positron emission tomography in women with breast cancer. *Br J Surg* 2005; 92:1363–1367.
33. van der Hoeven JJ, Krak NC, Hoekstra OS, et al. 18F-2-fluoro-2-deoxy-d-glucose positron emission tomography in staging of locally advanced breast cancer. *J Clin Oncol* 2004;22:1253–1259.
34. Carr CE, Conant MA, Rosen MA, et al. The impact of FDG PET in the staging of breast cancer. *J Clin Oncol* 2006;24:530.
35. Podoloff DA, Advani RH, Allred C, et al. NCCN task force report: positron emission tomography (PET)/computed tomography (CT) scanning in cancer. *J Natl Compr Cancer Netw* 2007;5[Suppl 1]:S1–S22.
36. Tatsumi M, Cohade C, Mourtzikos KA, et al. Initial experience with FDG-PET/CT in the evaluation of breast cancer. *Eur J Nucl Med Mol Imaging* 2006;33:254–262.
37. Tran A, Pio BS, Khatibi B, et al. 18F-FDG PET for staging breast cancer in patients with inner-quadrant versus outer-quadrant tumors: comparison with long-term clinical outcome. *J Nucl Med* 2005;46:1455–1459.
38. Fueger BJ, Weber WA, Quon A, et al. Performance of 2-deoxy-2-[F-18]fluoro-D-glucose positron emission tomography and integrated PET/CT in restaged breast cancer patients. *Mol Imaging Biol* 2005;7:369–376.
39. Khan QJ, O'Dea AP, Dusing RS, et al. Integrated FDG-PET/CT for initial staging of breast cancer. *J Clin Oncol* 2007;25:558.
40. Stearns V, Yamauchi H, Hayes DF. Circulating tumor markers in breast cancer: accepted utilities and novel prospects. *Breast Cancer Res Treat* 1998;52: 239–259.
41. Harris L, Fritsche H, Mennel R, et al. American Society of Clinical Oncology 2007 update of recommendations for the use of tumor markers in breast cancer. *J Clin Oncol* 2007;25:5287–5312.
42. Braun S, Pantel K, Muller P, et al. Cytokeratin-positive cells in the bone marrow and survival of patients with stage I, II, or III breast cancer. *N Engl J Med* 2000; 342:525–533.
43. Gebauer G, Fehm T, Merkle E, et al. Epithelial cells in bone marrow of breast cancer patients at time of primary surgery: clinical outcome during long-term follow-up. *J Clin Oncol* 2001;19:3669–3674.
44. Gerber B, Krause A, Muller H, et al. Simultaneous immunohistochemical detection of tumor cells in lymph nodes and bone marrow aspirates in breast cancer and its correlation with other prognostic factors. *J Clin Oncol* 2001;19:960–971.
45. Braun S, Vogl FD, Naume B, et al. A pooled analysis of bone marrow micrometastasis in breast cancer. *N Engl J Med* 2005;353:793–802.
46. Stathopoulou A, Vlachonikolis I, Mavroudis D, et al. Molecular detection of cytokeratin-19-positive cells in the peripheral blood of patients with operable breast cancer: evaluation of their prognostic significance. *J Clin Oncol* 2002;20:3404–3412.
47. Xenidis N, Perraki M, Kafousi M, et al. Predictive and prognostic value of peripheral blood cytokeratin-19 mRNA-positive cells detected by real-time polymerase chain reaction in node-negative breast cancer patients. *J Clin Oncol* 2006;24:3756–3762.
48. Feig SA. Imaging techniques and guidelines for evaluation and follow-up of breast cancer patients. *Crit Rev Diagn Imaging* 1987;27:1–16.
49. NCCN Breast Cancer Practice Guidelines. Practice guidelines in oncology v.2.2008. Available at http://www.nccn.org/professionals/physician_gls/PDF/breast.pdf.

Chapter 35
Staging of Breast Cancer

Jay R. Harris

Staging refers to the grouping of patients according to the extent of their disease. Staging is useful in (a) determining the choice of treatment for an individual patient, (b) estimating their prognosis, and (c) comparing the results of different treatment programs. Staging can be based on either clinical or pathologic findings. The staging of cancer is determined by the American Joint Committee on Cancer (AJCC). The AJCC comprises six founding organizations, four sponsoring organizations, and seven liaison organizations. Membership is reserved for those organizations whose missions or goals are consistent with or complementary to those of the AJCC. These organizations include the American Cancer Society, the American College of Surgeons, the American Society of Clinical Oncology, and the Centers for Disease Control and Prevention.

The AJCC system is both a clinical and pathologic staging system and is based on the TNM system, in which T refers to tumor, N to nodes, and M to metastasis. The sixth edition of the system is provided in this chapter (1). It details rules for classification, definition of the anatomy, and stage groups. It represents a significant change from the fifth edition, published in 1997. Sixth edition TNM staging is required for use with cases diagnosed as of January 1, 2003. As this fourth edition of *Diseases of the Breast* went to publication, a seventh edition of the TNM staging system was being developed. The latest edition of the staging system can be found at http://www.cancer-staging.org/education/smbreaststagingsystem.ppt#1.

A Breast Task Force was constituted to serve in an advisory role to the AJCC for this seventh edition. This task force is comprised of internationally recognized experts in the field of breast cancer management and is chaired by Dr. Daniel Hayes. The task force made some changes to the sixth edition (available at the URL given above), but also acknowledged that TNM staging, while still important, may be superseded by rapidly evolving molecular characterizations of breast cancers that more precisely define subgroups with different outcomes, both in terms of prognosis and response to specific treatments. A key specific issue addressed in the seventh edition was staging of patients treated with preoperative (or neoadjuvant) systemic therapy. In such patients, staging is needed both before and after preoperative systemic therapy. Although not finalized, the preliminary guidelines will include:

- A subscript will be added to the pretreatment N for both node-negative and node-positive patients to indicate whether the N was derived from clinical examination, fine-needle aspiration, core needle biopsy, or sentinel lymph node biopsy.
- The posttreatment T will be defined as the largest contiguous focus of tumor as defined histopathologically with a subscript to indicate the presence of single or multiple tumor foci.
- A description of the degree of response to preoperative systemic therapy (complete, partial, no response) will be collected for the National Cancer Database with the posttreatment TNM. A complete response is defined as the absence of invasive carcinoma in the breast and lymph nodes. Patients who have a positive node or nodes removed prior to preoperative systemic therapy should be designated CR* to indicate that this circumstance may not be reflective of the same prognosis as a patient who does not have nodes excised and has no residual disease.

- Posttreatment nodal metastasis less than 0.2 mm and detected by immunohistochemical (IHC) technique, while classified as pN0, do not constitute a complete response.
- Patients will be considered M1 (and therefore stage IV) if they have had clinically or radiographically detectable metastases prior to neoadjuvant systemic therapy, regardless of their status after neoadjuvant systemic therapy.

The Breast Task Force for the sixth edition, chaired by Dr. Eva Singletary, published an article outlining the new staging system and providing the justification for the revisions (2). Among the reasons cited for the major revisions were (a) the increased diagnosis of breast cancer at a very early stage based on the widespread use of screening mammography; (b) the increasing use of sentinel node procedure instead of axillary node dissection, accompanied by an increased use of more detailed sectioning of nodes and of immunochemical and molecular techniques for the detection of metastatic tumor deposits; and (c) increased knowledge about the prognostic significance of the location and extent of nodal involvement in the axillary, internal mammary, and supraclavicular lymph node (SCLN) areas. The task force used the following guidelines in deciding which changes should be made: (a) the revisions should be evidence-based; (b) the revisions should reflect a widespread clinical consensus about appropriate diagnostic and treatment standards; and (c) the revisions should support the uniform accrual of outcome information in national data banks.

The task force considered information on the use of serum or tumor markers and of histologic grade, but did not find that their use was sufficiently reliable to be incorporated into this revision. An editorial accompanying the task force article praised the advances in the revision, but pointed out that the new staging system is complicated and difficult to use (3). Both articles pointed out the need to develop new reliable markers of biologic aggressiveness of breast cancer to account better for the large inhomogeneity seen within each stage. It should be noted that stage reclassification using the new staging system results in significant changes in outcome by stage (4). Among the changes codified in the sixth edition were:

- Micrometastases are distinguished from isolated tumor cells on the basis of size and histologic evidence of malignant activity.
- Identifiers have been added to indicate the use of sentinel lymph node dissection and IHC or molecular techniques.
- Major classifications of lymph node status are designated according to the number of involved axillary lymph nodes as determined by routine hematoxylin-eosin (H&E) staining (preferred method) or by IHC staining.
- The classification of metastasis to the infraclavicular lymph nodes has been added as N3.
- Metastasis to the internal mammary nodes, based on the method of detection and the presence or absence of axillary nodal involvement, has been reclassified. Microscopic involvement of the internal mammary nodes detected by sentinel lymph node dissection using lymphoscintigraphy but not by imaging studies or clinical examination is classified as N1. Macroscopic involvement of the internal mammary nodes as detected by imaging studies (excluding lymphoscintigraphy) or by clinical examination is

classified as N2 if it occurs in the absence of metastases to the axillary lymph nodes or as N3 if it occurs in the presence of metastases to the axillary lymph nodes.
- Metastasis to the SCLNs has been reclassified as N3 rather than M1.

INTRODUCTION TO THE STAGING SYSTEM

This staging system for carcinoma of the breast applies to infiltrating (including microinvasive) and *in situ* carcinomas. Microscopic confirmation of the diagnosis is mandatory, and the histologic type and grade of carcinoma should be recorded.

Anatomy

Primary Site

The mammary gland, situated on the anterior chest wall, is composed of glandular tissue with a dense fibrous stroma. The glandular tissue consists of lobules that group together into 15 to 25 lobes arranged approximately in a spoke-like pattern. Multiple major and minor ducts connect the milk-secreting lobular units to the nipple. Small milk ducts course throughout the breast, converging into larger collecting ducts that open into the lactiferous sinus at the base of the nipple. Most cancers form initially in the terminal duct lobular units of the breast. Glandular tissue is more abundant in the upper outer portion of the breast; as a result, half of all breast cancers occur in this area.

Chest Wall

The chest wall includes ribs, intercostal muscles, and serratus anterior muscle, but not the pectoral muscles.

Regional Lymph Nodes

The breast lymphatics drain by way of three major routes: axillary, transpectoral, and internal mammary. Intramammary lymph nodes are coded as axillary lymph nodes for staging purposes. SCLNs are classified as regional lymph nodes for staging purposes. Metastasis to any other lymph node, including cervical or contralateral internal mammary lymph nodes, is classified as distant (M1).

The regional lymph nodes are as follows:

1. Axillary (ipsilateral): interpectoral (Rotter's) nodes and lymph nodes along the axillary vein and its tributaries that may be (but are not required to be) divided into the following levels:
   a. Level I (low-axilla): lymph nodes lateral to the lateral border of pectoralis minor muscle.
   b. Level II (mid-axilla): lymph nodes between the medial and lateral borders of the pectoralis minor muscle and the interpectoral (Rotter's) lymph nodes.
   c. Level III (apical axilla): lymph nodes medial to the medial margin of the pectoralis minor muscle, including those designated as apical.
2. Internal mammary (ipsilateral): lymph nodes in the intercostal spaces along the edge of the sternum in the endothoracic fascia.
3. Supraclavicular: lymph nodes in the supraclavicular fossa, a triangle defined by the omohyoid muscle and tendon (lateral and superior border), the internal jugular vein (medial border), and the clavicle and subclavian vein (lower border). Adjacent lymph nodes outside of this triangle are considered to be lower cervical nodes (M1) (1).

Metastatic Sites

Tumor cells may be disseminated by either the lymphatic or the blood vascular system. The four major sites of involvement are bone, lung, brain, and liver, but tumor cells are also capable of metastasizing to many other sites.

Rules for Classification

Clinical Staging

Clinical staging includes physical examination, with careful inspection and palpation of the skin, mammary gland, and lymph nodes (axillary, supraclavicular, and cervical), imaging, and pathologic examination of the breast or other tissues as appropriate to establish the diagnosis of breast carcinoma. The extent of tissue examined pathologically for clinical staging is not so great as that required for pathologic staging (see next section, Pathologic Staging). Imaging findings are considered elements of staging if they are collected within 4 months of diagnosis in the absence of disease progression or through completion of surgery (or surgeries), whichever is longer. Such imaging findings would include the size of the primary tumor and of chest wall invasion, and the presence or absence of regional or distant metastasis. Imaging findings and surgical findings obtained after a patient has been treated with neoadjuvant chemotherapy, hormonal therapy, immunotherapy, or radiation therapy are not considered elements of initial staging.

Pathologic Staging

Pathologic staging includes all data used for clinical staging, plus data from surgical exploration and resection as well as pathologic examination of the primary carcinoma, regional lymph nodes, and metastatic sites (if applicable), including not less than excision of the primary carcinoma with no macroscopic tumor in any margin of resection by pathologic examination. A cancer can be classified pT for pathologic stage grouping if there is only microscopic, but not macroscopic, involvement at the margin. If there is tumor in the margin of resection by macroscopic examination, the cancer is coded pTX because the total extent of the primary tumor cannot be assessed. If the primary tumor is invasive and not only microinvasive, resection of at least the low axillary lymph nodes (level I)—that is, those lymph nodes located lateral to the lateral border of the pectoralis minor muscle—should be performed for pathologic (pN) classification. Such a resection ordinarily includes six or more lymph nodes. Alternatively, one or more sentinel lymph nodes may be resected and examined for pathologic classification. Certain histologic tumor types (pure tubular carcinoma <1 cm, pure mucinous carcinoma <1 cm, and microinvasive carcinoma) have a very low incidence of axillary lymph node metastasis and do not usually require an axillary lymph node dissection. Cancerous nodules in the axillary fat adjacent to the breast, without histologic evidence of residual lymph node tissue, are classified as regional lymph node metastases (N). Pathologic stage grouping includes any of the following combinations of pathologic and clinical classifications: pT pN pM, or pT pN cM, or cT cN pM. If surgery occurs after the patient has received neoadjuvant chemotherapy, hormonal therapy, immunotherapy, or radiation therapy, the prefix "y" should be used with the TNM classification (e.g., ypTNM).

TNM CLASSIFICATION

Primary Tumor (T)

Determining Tumor Size

The clinical measurement used for classifying the primary tumor (T) is the one judged to be most accurate for that particular case (i.e., physical examination or imaging such as mammography or ultrasonography). The pathologic tumor size for the T classification is a measurement of the *invasive component only.* For example, if there is a 4.0-cm intraductal component and a 0.3-cm invasive component, the tumor is classified T1a. The size of the primary tumor is measured for T classification before any tissue is removed for special studies, such as for estrogen receptors. In patients who have received multiple core biopsies, measuring only the residual lesion may result in significantly underclassifying the T component and thus understaging the tumor. In such cases, original tumor size should be reconstructed on the basis of a combination of imaging and all histologic findings.

Tis Classification

Carcinoma *in situ*, with no evidence of an invasive component, is classified as Tis, with a subclassification indicating type. Cases of ductal carcinoma *in situ* (DCIS) and cases with both DCIS and lobular carcinoma *in situ* (LCIS) are classified Tis. LCIS is increasingly defined as a risk factor for subsequent breast cancer, although there is some evidence that it may occasionally be a precursor of invasive lobular carcinoma. For example, this may be the case with LCIS with more atypical cytology (pleomorphic), as well as more extensive and locally distorting examples of well-developed LCIS (5). Regardless of this controversy, LCIS is reported as a malignancy by national database registrars and should be designated as such in this classification system (e.g., Tis [LCIS]). Paget's disease of the nipple without an associated tumor mass (clinical) or invasive carcinoma (pathologic) is classified Tis (Paget's). Paget's disease with a demonstrable mass (clinical) anywhere in that breast or an invasive component (pathologic) is classified according to the size of the tumor mass or invasive component.

Microinvasion of Breast Carcinoma

Microinvasion is the extension of cancer cells beyond the basement membrane into the adjacent tissues with no focus more than 0.1 cm in greatest dimension. When there are multiple foci of microinvasion, the size of only the largest focus is used to classify the microinvasion. (Do not use the sum of all the individual foci.) The presence of multiple foci of microinvasion should be noted or quantified, as it is with multiple larger invasive carcinomas.

Multiple Simultaneous Ipsilateral Primary Carcinomas

The following guidelines are used in classifying multiple simultaneous ipsilateral primary (infiltrating, macroscopically measurable) carcinomas. These criteria do not apply to one macroscopic carcinoma associated with multiple separate microscopic foci. Most conservatively, tumors are defined as arising independently only if they occur in different quadrants of the breast.

1. Use the largest primary carcinoma to designate T classification. Do not assign a separate T classification for the smaller tumor(s).
2. Enter into the record that this is a case of multiple simultaneous ipsilateral primary carcinomas. The outcome of such cases should be analyzed separately.

Simultaneous Bilateral Breast Carcinomas

Each carcinoma is staged as a separate primary carcinoma in a separate organ.

Inflammatory Carcinoma

Inflammatory carcinoma is a clinicopathologic entity characterized by diffuse erythema and edema (*peau d'orange*) of the breast, often without an underlying palpable mass. These clinical findings should involve most of the skin of the breast.

Classically, the skin changes arise quickly in the affected breast. Thus, the term *inflammatory carcinoma* should not be applied to a patient with neglected locally advanced cancer of the breast presenting late in the course of her disease. On imaging, there may be a detectable mass and characteristic thickening of the skin over the breast. This clinical presentation is due to tumor emboli in dermal lymphatics, which may or may not be apparent on skin biopsy. The tumor of inflammatory carcinoma is classified T4d. It is important to remember that inflammatory carcinoma is primarily a clinical diagnosis. Involvement of the dermal lymphatics alone does not indicate inflammatory carcinoma in the absence of clinical findings. In addition to the clinical picture, however, a biopsy is still necessary to demonstrate cancer either in the dermal lymphatics or in the breast parenchyma itself.

Skin of Breast

Dimpling of the skin, nipple retraction, or any other skin change except those described under T4b and T4d may occur in T1, T2, or T3 without changing the classification.

Regional Lymph Nodes (N)

Macrometastasis

Cases in which regional lymph nodes cannot be assessed (previously removed or not removed for pathologic examination) are designated NX or pNX. Cases in which no regional lymph node metastasis is detected are designated N0 or pN0.

In patients who are clinically node positive, N1 designates metastasis to one or more movable ipsilateral axillary lymph nodes, N2a designates metastasis to axillary lymph nodes that are fixed to each other (matted) or to other structures, and N3a indicates metastasis to ipsilateral infraclavicular lymph nodes. Metastases to the ipsilateral internal mammary nodes are designated as N2b when they are detected by imaging studies (including computed tomography [CT] scan and ultrasonography, but excluding lymphoscintigraphy) or by clinical examination and when they do not occur in conjunction with metastasis to the axillary lymph nodes. Metastases to the ipsilateral internal mammary nodes are designated as N3b when they are detected by imaging studies or by clinical examination and when they occur in conjunction with metastasis to the axillary lymph nodes. Metastases to the ipsilateral SCLNs are designated as N3c regardless of the presence or absence of axillary or internal mammary nodal involvement.

In patients who are pathologically node positive with one or more tumor deposits greater than 2 mm, cases with 1 to 3 positive axillary lymph nodes are classified pN1a, cases with 4 to 9 positive axillary lymph nodes are classified pN2a, and cases with 10 or more positive axillary lymph nodes are classified pN3a. Cases with histologically confirmed metastasis to the internal mammary nodes, detected by sentinel lymph node dissection but not by imaging studies (excluding lymphoscintigraphy) or clinical examination, are classified as pN1b if occurring in the *absence* of metastasis to the axillary lymph nodes and as pN1c if occurring in the *presence* of metastases to one to three axillary lymph nodes. (If four or more axillary lymph nodes are involved, the classification pN3b is used.) Clinical involvement with histologic confirmation of the internal mammary nodes by imaging studies (excluding lymphoscintigraphy) in the absence or presence of axillary nodal metastases is classified as pN2b and pN3b, respectively. Histologic evidence of metastasis in ipsilateral SCLNs is classified as pN3c. A classification of pN3, regardless of primary tumor size or grade, is classified as stage IIIc. A case in which the classification is based only on sentinel lymph node dissection is given the additional designation (sn) for sentinel node—for example, pN1(sn). For a case in which an initial classification is based on a sentinel lymph node dissection but a standard axillary lymph node dissection is subsequently performed, the classification is based on the total results of the axillary lymph node dissection (i.e., including the sentinel node).

Isolated Tumor Cells and Micrometastases

Isolated tumor cells (ITCs) are defined as single cells or small clusters of cells not greater than 0.2 mm in largest dimension, usually with no histologic evidence of malignant activity (such as proliferation or stromal reaction). If an additional IHC examination was made for ITCs in a patient with histologically negative lymph nodes, the regional lymph nodes should be designated as pN0(i−) or pN0(i+), as appropriate.

Micrometastases are defined as tumor deposits greater than 0.2 mm but not greater than 2.0 mm in largest dimension that may have histologic evidence of malignant activity (such as proliferation or stromal reaction). Cases in which only micrometastases are detected (none >2 mm) are classified pN1mi. The classification is designated as (i+) for immunohistochemical if micrometastasis was detected only by IHC, for example, pN1mi (i+).

If histologically and immunohistochemically negative lymph nodes are examined for evidence of metastasis using molecular methods (reverse transcriptase polymerase chain reaction [RT-PCR]), the regional lymph nodes are classified as pN0(mol−) or pN0(mol+), as appropriate.

Distant Metastasis (M)

Cases in which distant metastasis cannot be assessed are designated MX, cases in which there is no distant metastasis are designated M0, and cases in which one or more distant metastases are identified are designated M1. A negative clinical history and examination are sufficient to designate a case as M0; extensive imaging or other testing is not required. Note that positive SCLNs are now classified as N3 rather than M1.

DEFINITION OF TNM

Primary Tumor (T)

Definitions for classifying the primary tumor (T) are the same for clinical and for pathologic classification. If the measurement is made by physical examination, the examiner will use the major headings (T1, T2, or T3). If other measurements, such as mammographic or pathologic measurements, are used, the subsets of T1 can be used. Tumors should be measured to the nearest 0.1-cm increment.

TX Primary tumor cannot be assessed
T0 No evidence of primary tumor
Tis Carcinoma *in situ*
Tis (DCIS) Ductal carcinoma *in situ*
Tis (LCIS) Lobular carcinoma *in situ*
Tis (Paget's) Paget's disease of the nipple with no tumor

Note: Paget's disease associated with a tumor is classified according to the size of the tumor.

T1 Tumor 2 cm or less in greatest dimension
T1mic Microinvasion 0.1 cm or less in greatest dimension
T1a Tumor more than 0.1 cm but not more than 0.5 cm in greatest dimension
T1b Tumor more than 0.5 cm but not more than 1 cm in greatest dimension
T1c Tumor more than 1 cm but not more than 2 cm in greatest dimension
T2 Tumor more than 2 cm but not more than 5 cm in greatest dimension
T3 Tumor more than 5 cm in greatest dimension
T4 Tumor of any size with direct extension to (a) chest wall or (b) skin, only as described below

T4a Extension to chest wall, not including pectoralis muscle
T4b Edema (including *peau d'orange*) or ulceration of the skin of the breast, or satellite skin nodules confined to the same breast
T4c Both T4a and T4b
T4d Inflammatory carcinoma

Regional Lymph Nodes (N)

Clinical

NX Regional lymph nodes cannot be assessed (e.g., previously removed)
N0 No regional lymph node metastasis
N1 Metastasis to movable ipsilateral axillary lymph node(s)
N2 Metastases in ipsilateral axillary lymph nodes fixed or matted, or in clinically apparent ipsilateral internal mammary nodes in the *absence* of clinically evident axillary lymph node metastasis
N2a Metastasis in ipsilateral axillary lymph nodes fixed to one another (matted) or to other structures
N2b Metastasis only in clinically apparent* ipsilateral internal mammary nodes and in the *absence* of clinically evident axillary lymph node metastasis
N3 Metastasis in ipsilateral infraclavicular lymph node(s) with or without axillary lymph node involvement, or in clinically apparent* ipsilateral internal mammary lymph node(s) and in the *presence* of clinically evident axillary lymph node metastasis; or metastasis in ipsilateral SCLNs with or without axillary or internal mammary lymph node involvement
N3a Metastasis in ipsilateral infraclavicular lymph node(s)
N3b Metastasis in ipsilateral internal mammary lymph node(s) and axillary lymph node(s)
N3c Metastasis in ipsilateral SCLNs

Pathologic (pN)[†]

pNX Regional lymph nodes cannot be assessed (e.g., previously removed, or not removed for pathologic study)
pN0 No regional lymph node metastasis histologically, no additional examination for ITC

Note: ITC are defined as single tumor cells or small cell clusters not greater than 0.2 mm, usually detected only by IHC or molecular methods but which may be verified on H&E stains. ITCs do not usually show evidence of malignant activity (e.g., proliferation or stromal reaction).

PN0(i−) No regional lymph node metastasis histologically, negative IHC
PN0(i+) No regional lymph node metastasis histologically, positive IHC, no IHC cluster greater than 0.2 mm
PN0(mol−) No regional lymph node metastasis histologically, negative molecular findings (RT-PCR)[‡]
PN0(mol+) No regional lymph node metastasis histologically, positive molecular findings (RT-PCR)[‡]
PN1 Metastasis in one to three axillary lymph nodes, or in internal mammary nodes with microscopic disease detected by sentinel lymph node dissection but not clinically apparent
PN1mi Micrometastasis (>0.2 mm, none >2.0 mm)
PN1a Metastasis in one to three axillary lymph nodes

Clinically apparent is defined as detected by imaging studies (excluding lymphoscintigraphy) or by clinical examination or grossly visible pathologically.
[†]Classification is based on axillary lymph node dissection with or without sentinel lymph node dissection. Classification based solely on sentinel lymph node dissection without subsequent axillary lymph node dissection is designated (sn) for "sentinel node," e.g., pN0(i+)(sn).
[‡]RT-PCR, reverse transcriptase/polymerase chain reaction.

PN1b Metastasis in internal mammary nodes with microscopic disease detected by sentinel lymph node dissection but not clinically apparent*

PN1c Metastasis in one to three axillary lymph nodes and in internal mammary lymph nodes with microscopic disease detected by sentinel lymph node dissection but not clinically apparent* (If associated with greater than three positive axillary lymph nodes, the internal mammary nodes are classified as pN3b to reflect increased tumor burden.)

pN2 Metastasis in four to nine axillary lymph nodes, or in clinically apparent internal mammary lymph nodes in the *absence* of axillary lymph node metastasis

pN2a Metastasis in four to nine axillary lymph nodes (at least one tumor deposit >2.0 mm)

pN2b Metastasis in clinically apparent[†] internal mammary lymph nodes in the absence of axillary lymph node metastasis

pN3 Metastasis in 10 or more axillary lymph nodes, or in infraclavicular lymph nodes, or in clinically apparent[†] ipsilateral internal mammary lymph nodes in the *presence* of 1 or more positive axillary lymph nodes; or in more than 3 axillary lymph nodes with clinically negative microscopic metastasis in internal mammary lymph nodes; or in ipsilateral SCLNs

pN3a Metastasis in 10 or more axillary lymph nodes (at least one tumor deposit >2.0 mm), or metastasis to the infraclavicular lymph nodes

pN3b Metastasis in clinically apparent[†] ipsilateral internal mammary lymph nodes in the presence of one or more positive axillary lymph nodes; or in more than three axillary lymph nodes and in internal mammary lymph nodes with microscopic disease detected by sentinel lymph node dissection but not clinically apparent*

pN3c Metastasis in ipsilateral SCLNs

Distant Metastasis (M)

MX Distant metastasis cannot be assessed
M0 No distant metastasis
M1 Distant metastasis

STAGE GROUPING

Stage 0	Tis	N0	M0
Stage I	T1[†]	N0	M0
Stage IIA	T0	N1	M0
	T1[†]	N1	M0
	T2	N0	M0
Stage IIB	T2	N1	M0
	T3	N0	M0
Stage IIIA	T0	N2	M0
	T1[†]	N2	M0
	T2	N2	M0
	T3	N1	M0
	T3	N2	M0
Stage IIIB	T4	N0	M0
	T4	N1	M0
	T4	N2	M0
Stage IIIC	Any T	N3	M0
Stage IV	Any T	Any N	M1

Note: Stage designation may be changed if postsurgical imaging studies reveal the presence of distant metastases, provided that the studies are carried out within 4 months of diagnosis in the absence of disease progression and provided that the patient has not received neoadjuvant therapy.

Clinically apparent is defined as detected by imaging studies (excluding lymphoscintigraphy) or by clinical examination.
[†]T1 includes T1mic.

HISTOPATHOLOGIC TYPE

The histopathologic types are the following:

In Situ Carcinomas

NOS (not otherwise specified)
Intraductal
Paget's disease and intraductal

Invasive Carcinomas

NOS
Ductal
Inflammatory
Medullary, NOS
Medullary with lymphoid stroma
Mucinous
Papillary (predominantly micropapillary pattern)
Tubular
Lobular
Paget's disease and infiltrating
Undifferentiated
Squamous cell
Adenoid cystic
Secretory
Cribriform

HISTOLOGIC GRADE (G) (NOTTINGHAM COMBINED HISTOLOGIC GRADE IS RECOMMENDED)

All invasive breast carcinomas with the exception of medullary carcinoma should be graded. The Nottingham combined histologic grade (Elston-Ellis modification of Scarff-Bloom-Richardson grading system) is recommended (6,7). The grade for a tumor is determined by assessing morphologic features (tubule formation, nuclear pleomorphism, and mitotic count), assigning a value of 1 (favorable) to 3 (unfavorable) for each feature, and adding together the scores for all three categories. A combined score of 3 to 5 points is designated as grade 1; a combined score of 6 or 7 points is grade 2; a combined score of 8 or 9 points is grade 3.

GX Grade cannot be assessed
G1 Low combined histologic grade (favorable)
G2 Intermediate combined histologic grade (moderately favorable)
G3 High combined histologic grade (unfavorable)

CONSIDERATIONS FOR EVIDENCE-BASED CHANGES TO THE *AJCC CANCER STAGING MANUAL*, SIXTH EDITION

Should Histologic Grade (Nottingham Combined Histologic Grade Recommended) Be Incorporated into the TNM Classification System?

It was first recognized by von Hansemann (8) in 1890 that the morphologic appearance of tumors was associated with the degree of malignancy, and the first formal grading of morphologic features in breast cancer occurred 35 years later (9). Since then, the histologic grading of invasive breast carcinoma has been clearly shown to provide significant prognostic information

(6,10–13). Different approaches to histologic grading have been described and used. Although all of these approaches offer some degree of prognostic information, there are varying levels of agreement among them, and this makes clinical studies difficult to compare. In addition, grading is by nature subjective, and there can be substantial differences in assessment even when the same grading system is used (14–17).

Several observers have pointed out that observer variation in estimating histologic grade may have only a small adverse effect in estimating prognosis, especially if the variation in outcome is greater than the variation among observers (12,18). This may be true in a general way, but it should be remembered that the inclusion of histologic grade in the AJCC staging system will affect data collection and coding for national cancer registrars. Institute-to-institute reproducibility will be an important requirement for data inclusion in these large databases. The modification of the Bloom and Richardson grading system by Elston and Ellis (the Nottingham combined histologic grade 6) was designed to make grading criteria more quantitative. Three morphologic features (percentage of tubule formation, degree of nuclear pleomorphism, and accurate mitotic count in a defined field area) are evaluated semiquantitatively, and a numeric score for each is used in calculating the overall grade. Elston and Ellis compiled long-term survival information from 1,831 patients for whom a Nottingham combined histologic grade was assessed, and they found a very strong correlation with prognosis ($p < .0001$). In subsequent studies, better inter-observer agreement was obtained with the Nottingham combined histologic grade than with previous systems (19–21), and it is recommended in the College of American Pathologists Consensus Statement (7). Thus, the Nottingham combined histologic grade is strongly recommended in this revision for the histologic grading of tumors.

Even with this more quantitative approach, significant variation in results can stem from technical variations in processing the tumor tissue. The time lag between surgical excision and fixation can vary greatly from one case to another (from 10 minutes to 4 hours in one published study) (22). A time lag of as little as 2 hours can result in mitotic rate decreases of 10% to 30% (23,24), and a delay of 24 hours can result in a striking decline of more than 75% (25). Even with fixation times standardized, the type of fixative used can also be an important element; some commonly used fixatives contribute to suboptimal cell morphology (21,22). Precise guidelines about these technical details will be important in ensuring data comparability across institutes.

Thus, histologic grading has prognostic value, and improved reproducibility is possible with the Nottingham combined histologic grade. The question of how to add grading to the existing TNM classification system remains. Because large tumors (T3, T4) nearly always carry a recommendation for adjuvant therapy, and because many such tumors tend to be high grade, the addition of grading information would not be expected to have a significant effect on treatment planning for this group. Most conservatively, grading should be considered in those cases in which it would influence treatment decisions most heavily, that is, for small (T1, T2) node-negative tumors. It is unfortunate, therefore, that available evidence about the interaction between tumor size and histologic grade as they relate to patient outcome is disappointingly meager for these small tumors. The results of a number of retrospective studies have analyzed outcome data on the basis of histologic grade in small tumors (12,18,22,26–30). Because of the variety of follow-up times, grading systems, patient samples, and measured outcomes, it is difficult to extract a consistent picture from these studies. All studies showed a difference between grade 1 and grade 3, but the positioning of the grade 2 intermediate tumors varied, sometimes clustering with grade 1 and at other times clustering with grade 3. In those studies that specifically

used the Nottingham combined histologic grade (22,28,30), grade 2 either clustered with grade 3 or else was intermediate between grades 1 and 3 for a variety of outcomes. Three studies specifically looked at T1a-b tumors (27–29). These studies used three different histologic grading systems and three different outcomes, but they nonetheless showed somewhat smaller outcome differences between grade 1 and grade 3 than other studies that included larger tumors.

These tentative observations, coupled with the overall sparseness and variability of the information, strongly suggest that the available data are not yet mature enough to offer guidance in incorporating histologic grade into the staging system for breast cancer. Because the evidence indicating that histologic grade is an important prognostic factor in breast cancer is so robust, it seems certain that emerging data will support the incorporation of grade into the AJCC staging system in the near future.

Should the Classification of Pathologic Lymph Node Status in Node-Negative Patients Be Amplified to Include Information about Isolated Tumor Cells Detected by Immunohistochemical Techniques?

ITCs are defined as single tumor cells or small clusters of cells that are not greater than 0.2 mm in size and that usually show no histologic evidence of malignant activity (e.g., proliferation or stromal reaction). Although there is a growing feeling that ITCs detected by IHC staining may be prognostically relevant, their clinical significance has not yet been demonstrated. Even with larger clusters of single cells, it is not clear whether a finding of ITC would justify an axillary lymph node dissection. This is especially true for ITCs found in sentinel lymph nodes in cases in which the primary tumor is very small and the probability of metastasis in a nonsentinel lymph node seems to be virtually zero (31).

Clearly, organized, large-scale data collection is essential for determining the clinical significance of ITCs. For this reason, a uniform shorthand is now suggested for describing pN0 patients where there has been IHC examination for ITCs. The added designation of "i+" or "i−" indicates that IHC staining was performed with positive or negative results.

Should Micrometastases (pN1mi) Detected by Immunohistochemical Staining and Not Verified by Hematoxylin and Eosin Staining Be Classified as pN1?

Micrometastases are defined as tumor deposits greater than 0.2 mm and no greater than 2.0 mm in size. Unlike isolated tumor cells, micrometastases may show histologic evidence of metastatic activity, such as proliferation or stromal reaction. The use of IHC techniques to detect occult micrometastases has increased dramatically with the growing acceptance of sentinel lymph node dissection. The reported incidence of nodal micrometastases detected by IHC in patients who are histologically node negative has ranged from 12% to 29% (32–36).

The unresolved issue is whether micrometastases detected by IHC and not verified by standard histologic staining have a significant impact on patient outcome. Retrospective studies have reported decreases in disease-free survival ranging from 10% to 22% in some subgroups of patients in whom micrometastatic axillary disease was detected by IHC techniques. A significant percentage of histologically node-negative patients ultimately experience distant recurrence and die of their disease, and it has been suggested that some of this subgroup of patients may be those with occult micrometastases in the axillary nodes, but bone marrow and other metastases may occur with no axillary involvement (34,35,37).

The premise that H&E verification is required to validate the metastatic potential of lesions detected by IHC is under increasing scrutiny. Cell deposits identified only by IHC are increasingly being used to make clinical recommendations without H&E verification. The size of the micrometastatic focus may prove to be critical; a 1-mm IHC-positive lesion may contain as many as 500,000 cells, and this would clearly meet the proliferation requirement for metastatic potential, regardless of H&E verification. Nonetheless, verification by H&E staining is recommended by the College of American Pathologists because it provides more definitive cytologic and histologic evidence of malignancy than is usually available from immunostained preparations and avoids overinterpretation of staining artifacts.

Should Size Criteria Be Used to Distinguish between Isolated Tumor Cells and Micrometastases?

Isolated tumor cells should theoretically be distinguishable from micrometastases on the basis of metastatic characteristics, such as proliferation or stromal reaction (38). This distinction can be highly subjective, however, and replication among pathologists and among institutions may be difficult. This revision incorporates size criteria to assist in making this distinction, with isolated tumor cell groups defined as not greater than 0.2 mm in diameter and micrometastases defined as greater than 0.2 mm and not greater than 2.0 mm in diameter. The use of 2.0 mm as an upper size limit for micrometastases, originally proposed by Huvos et al. (39) in 1971, is consistent with standards already used in the AJCC staging system. The use of 0.2 mm as a lower limit was selected because it significantly reduces the likelihood that ITCs will be recorded as micrometastases, without making it necessary to estimate actual cell number counts in ITCs. The resulting classification of patients with metastatic tumor deposits no greater than 0.2 mm as pN0 is consistent with the low recurrence rates typically seen in this patient group.

How Should Reverse Transcriptase Polymerase Chain Reaction Be Used in the Detection of Small Tumor Deposits?

An even finer level of resolution in the detection of isolated tumor cells and micrometastases is potentially available with the use of RT-PCR. Verbanac et al. (40) recently reported that this technique was able to identify a neoplastic marker in a significant percentage of sentinel nodes that were negative for disease by both histologic and IHC staining. This is not altogether surprising, given that RT-PCR is theoretically capable of identifying single cells. However, it seems unlikely that such cells would become clinically important. There is evidence that such highly sensitive tests produce false-positive results. Furthermore, because an entire block of lymph node tissue is digested in preparation for RT-PCR, it would be technically challenging to determine the exact size of the original lesion.

Pending further developments in this area, the latest edition of the *AJCC Cancer Staging Manual* will classify any lesion identified by RT-PCR alone as pN0 (the classification it would have had using standard histologic staining) for the purposes of staging. All cases that were histologically negative for regional lymph node metastasis and in which an additional examination for tumor cells was made with RT-PCR will have the appended designation (mol+) or (mol−), as appropriate.

Should the Classification of Pathologic Lymph Node Status in Node-Positive (All Nodes with Deposits >0.2 mm) Patients Be Changed to Reflect More Clearly the Prognostic Significance of Number of Affected Nodes?

In past editions of the *AJCC Cancer Staging Manual*, the TNM system has used similar definitions for clinical lymph node status and pathologic lymph node status. This has had the unfortunate result of assigning a number of affected lymph nodes to subcategories of the pN1 classification, effectively ignoring this important prognostic indicator.

In this revision, patients with 1 to 3 positive axillary lymph nodes (with at least one tumor deposit >2 mm and all tumor deposits >0.2 mm) are classified as pN1a, patients with 4 to 9 positive axillary lymph nodes are classified as pN2a, and patients with 10 or more positive axillary lymph nodes are classified as pN3a. This recognition of the prognostic importance of the absolute number of involved lymph nodes is in keeping with current clinical practice and is supported by a large body of clinical data. The decision to separate patients with one to three positive nodes from patients with four or more positive nodes is consistent with survival data reported by Carter et al. (41). These researchers examined 5-year survival rates by tumor size and lymph node status in 24,740 breast cancer cases recorded in the Surveillance, Epidemiology, and End Results (SEER) Program of the National Cancer Institute. In each size group of tumors (<2 cm, 2 to 5 cm, >5 cm), they found an inverse relationship between overall survival and number of positive nodes. In patients with tumors less than 2 cm in size, for example, the relative 5-year survival rate was 96.3% for patients with negative nodes, 87.4% for patients with one to three positive nodes, and 66.0% for patients with four or more positive nodes.

The decision to separate patients with 10 or more positive nodes into the N3a category, although somewhat more arbitrary, is based on the recognition that survival rates continue to decrease with increasing numbers of positive axillary lymph nodes. In a survey of 20,547 cases of breast carcinoma collected by the American College of Surgeons, Nemoto et al. (42) demonstrated that expected survival declined linearly with increasing number of axillary lymph nodes that were positive by histologic examination, up to a total of 21 positive nodes. The specific breakpoint used here (≥10) is in common use. See, for example, the report on the National Surgical Adjuvant Breast and Bowel Project [NSABP] B-11 protocol in Paik et al. [43] and various other clinical studies (44–46).

The change in classification of axillary lymph node–positive patients reorganizes the pathologic staging system to reflect more closely the current practice standards used by clinicians in stratifying patients for prognosis and treatment decisions.

Should a Finding of Positive Internal Mammary Lymph Nodes Retain a Current Classification of N3?

Data from the National Cancer Data Base (1985 to 1991) were analyzed to compare 5-year relative survival rates in all patients with stage IIIB breast cancer versus only patients with stage IIIB cancer with positive internal mammary nodes (N3) (JJ Douglas, personal communication). For all stage IIIB cancers (n = 9,775), the relative 5-year survival rate was 47.6%, with a 99% confidence interval (CI) of 45.7 to 49.5. For stage IIIB cases with N3 only (n = 717), the relative survival rate was 45.2% (99% CI, 38.6–51.9). This suggests no survival difference between patients with N3 disease and the stage IIIB group as a whole. In a separate report, Veronesi et al. (47) reported the results of a randomized trial carried out from 1964 to 1968 in which patients with T1-3, N0-1 breast cancer were treated with a Halsted mastectomy or with an extended mastectomy that included removal of the internal mammary nodes. In the 342 patients treated with extended mastectomy, the 5-year overall survival rate was 44% in patients with positive internal mammary nodes, compared with 78% in patients with negative internal mammary nodes. These survival rates are consistent with those taken from the National Cancer Data Base.

A problem with these reports is that neither one considers the independent survival effects of positive internal mammary lymph nodes (IM) in the absence of positive axillary lymph nodes (AX). Five studies have compared survival rates in patients who were IM−/AX+, IM+/AX−, and IM+/AX+ (48–52). Although the survival rates in the first two categories were similar, there was a significant decrease in survival in patients who were IM+ and AX+. On the basis of these findings, this revision classifies clinically positive internal mammary lymph nodes that are detected by imaging studies (including CT scan or ultrasonography, but excluding lymphoscintigraphy) or by clinical examination as N2b when they occur in the *absence* of positive axillary lymph nodes and as N3b when they occur in the *presence* of positive axillary lymph nodes. In cases in which proven microscopic disease is detected in the internal mammary lymph nodes, the classification is based on whether the disease was clinically occult. For positive internal mammary nodes with microscopic disease detected by sentinel lymph node dissection but not by imaging studies (excluding lymphoscintigraphy), the pathologic classification is pN1b in the *absence* of positive axillary lymph nodes and is pN1c in the *presence* of one to three positive axillary lymph nodes. Positive internal mammary nodes discovered by sentinel lymph node dissection but in the presence of four or more positive axillary lymph nodes are considered pN3b to reflect the increased tumor burden. For positive internal mammary nodes with histologic macroscopic disease detected by imaging studies (excluding lymphoscintigraphy) or by clinical examination, the classification is pN2b in the *absence* of positive axillary lymph nodes and is pN3b in the *presence* of positive axillary lymph nodes.

Should a Finding of Positive Supraclavicular Lymph Nodes Be Classified as N3 Rather than M1?

As early as 1907, it was recognized that clinically evident SCLNs conferred a poor prognosis for breast cancer patients (53). Clinical studies carried out from 1966 to 1995 reported 5-year survival rates ranging from 5% to 34% (median, 18%) (54). The bad prognosis led to the conclusion that SCLN metastasis qualified as distant metastasis (M1) rather than as an advanced regional lymph node metastasis (N3), and this change was incorporated into the 1997 revision of the *AJCC Cancer Staging Manual* (55).

An examination of these earlier studies reveals a bias against treating patients aggressively when a positive SCLN was treated as a distant metastasis. Because patients with distant metastases are considered incurable, most studies used only locoregional therapy (surgery, irradiation, or both) in the treatment of SCLN-positive patients, and such therapy was considered palliative.

A study by Brito et al. (56) provides evidence that aggressive treatment of SCLN-positive patients results in outcomes comparable with those in patients with locally advanced breast cancer (LABC, stage IIIB) without distant metastasis. In this study, 70 patients with SCLN-positive LABC received intensive treatment that included induction chemotherapy, surgery, postsurgical chemotherapy, and irradiation. At a median follow-up time of 8.5 years, there was no difference in disease-free survival or overall survival in patients with LABC with positive SCLN and no other sign of distant metastasis compared with patients with stage IIIB disease without distant metastasis. Both stage IIIB

and SCLN-positive patients differed significantly in overall survival compared with patients with stage IV disease. These findings indicate that classifying SCLN as a distant metastasis may be a disservice to patients because it implies incurability and may lead to suboptimal therapy. Patients with ipsilateral SCLN metastases and no other distant metastases should be classified as N3 rather than M1 because their clinical course and outcomes are similar to patients with stage IIIB LABC. To clarify the significance of N3 disease, the new category stage IIIC has been instituted for any T, N3 that includes pN3a, pN3b, or pN3c.

Are There Other Prognostic Factors that Are Powerful Enough to Consider for Inclusion in the TNM Grading System?

Prognostic factors provide information about potential patient outcome in the absence of systemic therapy. These factors tend to reflect biologic characteristics of the tumor, such as proliferation, invasiveness, and metastatic capacity. Prognostic factors must be carefully distinguished from predictive factors, which reflect response to a particular therapeutic agent or combination of agents.

A clinically useful prognostic factor is one that is statistically significant (its prognostic value only rarely occurs by chance), independent (it retains its prognostic value when combined with other factors), and clinically relevant (it has a major impact on prognostic accuracy). Axillary lymph node status has been shown definitively to be the single most important prognostic factor for disease-free and overall survival in patients with breast cancer (7).

The fifth edition of the *AJCC Cancer Staging Manual* reported that approximately 80 potential prognostic variables had been identified for human breast cancer. Since that time, additional factors have been suggested (various growth factors with their receptors and binding proteins; proteases, including cathepsin-D, urokinase-type plasminogen activator, and matrix metalloproteinases). Simultaneously, some factors that were once considered promising have yielded ambiguous or disappointing results in outcome studies (p53, *HER2/neu*), often because technical approaches have not been standardized and data are difficult to compare between studies.

In addition to axillary lymph node status, the College of American Pathologists Consensus Report 7 and the clinical practice guidelines from the American Society of Clinical Oncology (57,58) have identified tumor size, histopathologic grade, and mitotic index as clinically useful prognostic factors. (This revision recommends the routine use of the Nottingham combined histologic grading system, which incorporates mitotic index into the measurement of tumor grade.) DNA ploidy was reported to be an unreliable prognostic marker in both studies. Estrogen-receptor status, although a good predictive factor for response to hormonal therapy, is a relatively weak prognostic factor. Promising results have been reported in some cases for p53, but lack of standardization and data comparability are ongoing problems. Similar problems affect the use of *ERBB2* as a prognostic factor, although it should be routinely measured in patients to predict the likelihood of their response to trastuzumab (Herceptin) should they relapse after standard adjuvant therapy. Factors such as Ki-67 continue to have technical problems that limit interuser reproducibility.

It is expected that ongoing studies will provide more definitive evidence about the clinical usefulness of many of these factors. These studies should also contribute to the standardization of assay systems and analytic approaches that will be required to achieve reproducibility among different researchers and different institutions. Such studies of promising new prognostic factors should simultaneously measure and report proven factors—particularly size, nodal status, and histologic grade—to indicate how much the new factors reflect the classic ones.

BREAST

Hospital Name/Address	Patient Name/Information

Type of Specimen _____

Tumor Size _____

Histopathologic Type _____

Laterality: ☐ Bilateral   ☐ Left   ☐ Right

DEFINITIONS

Clinical	Pathologic		Primary Tumor (T)
☐	☐	TX	Primary tumor cannot be assessed
☐	☐	T0	No evidence of primary tumor
☐	☐	Tis	Carcinoma *in situ*
☐	☐	Tis	(DCIS) Ductal carcinoma *in situ*
☐	☐	Tis	(LCIS) Lobular carcinoma *in situ*
☐	☐	Tis	(Paget's) Paget's disease of the nipple with no tumor *Note:* Paget's disease associated with a tumor is classified according to the size of the tumor.
☐	☐	T1	Tumor 2 cm or less in greatest dimension
☐	☐	T1mic	Microinvasion 0.1 cm or less in greatest dimension
☐	☐	T1a	Tumor more than 0.1 cm but not more than 0.5 cm in greatest dimension
☐	☐	T1b	Tumor more than 0.5 cm but not more than 1 cm in greatest dimension

Clinical	Pathologic		Primary Tumor (T)
☐	☐	T1c	Tumor more than 1 cm but not more than 2 cm in greatest dimension
☐	☐	T2	Tumor more than 2 cm but not more than 5 cm in greatest dimension
☐	☐	T3	Tumor more than 5 cm in greatest dimension
☐	☐	T4	Tumor of any size with direct extension to (a) chest wall or (b) skin, only as described below.
☐	☐	T4a	Extension to chest wall, not including pectoralis muscle
☐	☐	T4b	Edema (including *peau d'orange*) or ulceration of the skin of the breast, or satellite skin nodules confined to the same breast
☐	☐	T4c	Both T4a and T4b
☐	☐	T4d	Inflammatory carcinoma

Clinical		Regional Lymph Nodes (N)
☐	NX	Regional lymph nodes cannot be assessed (e.g., previously removed)
☐	N0	No regional lymph node metastasis
☐	N1	Metastasis in movable ipsilateral axillary lymph node(s)
☐	N2	Metastases in ipsilateral axillary lymph nodes fixed or matted, or in clinically apparent[1] ipsilateral internal mammary nodes in the *absence* of clinically evident axillary lymph node metastasis
☐	N2a	Metastasis in ipsilateral axillary lymph nodes fixed to one another (matted) or to other structures
☐	N2b	Metastasis only in clinically apparent[1] ipsilateral internal mammary nodes and in the absence of clinically evident axillary lymph node metastasis
☐	N3	Metastasis in ipsilateral infraclavicular lymph node(s) with or without axillary lymph node involvement, or in clinically apparent[1] ipsilateral internal mammary lymph node(s) and in the presence of clinically evident axillary lymph node metastasis; or metastasis in ipsilateral supraclavicular lymph node(s) with or without axillary or internal mammary lymph node involvement

Pathologic		Regional Lymph Nodes (pN)[2]
☐	pNX	Regional lymph nodes cannot be assessed (e.g., previously removed, or not removed for pathologic study)
☐	pN0	No regional lymph node metastasis histologically, no additional examination for isolated tumor cells (ITC)[3]
☐	pN0(i−)	No regional lymph node metastasis histologically, negative IHC
☐	pN0(i+)	No regional lymph node metastasis histologically, positive IHC, no IHC cluster greater than 0.2 mm
☐	pN0(mol−)	No regional lymph node metastasis histologically, negative molecular findings (RT-PCR)[4]
☐	pN0(mol+)	No regional lymph node metastasis histologically, positive molecular findings (RT-PCR)[4]
☐	pN1	Metastasis in 1 to 3 axillary lymph nodes, and/or in internal mammary nodes with microscopic disease detected by sentinel lymph node dissection but not clinically apparent[5]
☐	pN1mic	Micrometastasis (>0.2 mm, none >2.0 mm)
☐	pN1a	Metastasis in 1 to 3 axillary lymph nodes
☐	pN1b	Metastasis in internal mammary nodes with microscopic disease detected by sentinel lymph node dissection but not clinically apparent[5]
☐	pN1c	Metastasis in 1 to 3 axillary lymph nodes and in internal mammary lymph nodes with microscopic disease detected by sentinel lymph node dissection but not clinically apparent[5,6]
☐	pN2	Metastasis in 4 to 9 axillary lymph nodes, or in clinically apparent 1 internal mammary lymph nodes in the absence of axillary lymph node metastasis

(continued)

BREAST *(continued)*

Clinical		Regional Lymph Nodes (N)	*Pathologic*		Regional Lymph Nodes (pN)[2]
			☐	pN2a	Metastasis in 4 to 9 axillary lymph nodes (at least one tumor deposit >2.0 mm)
			☐	pN2b	Metastasis in clinically apparent 1 internal mammary lymph nodes in the absence of axillary lymph node metastasis
			☐	pN3	Metastasis in 10 or more axillary lymph nodes, or infraclavicular lymph nodes, or in clinically apparent 1 ipsilateral internal mammary lymph nodes in the presence of 1 or more positive axillary lymph nodes; or in more than 3 axillary lymph nodes with clinically negative microscopic metastasis in internal mammary lymph nodes; or in ipsilateral supraclavicular lymph nodes
☐	N3a	Metastasis in ipsilateral infraclavicular lymph node(s) and axillary lymph node(s)	☐	pN3a	Metastasis in 10 or more axillary lymph nodes (at least one tumor deposit >2.0 mm), or metastasis to the infraclavicular lymph nodes
☐	N3b	Metastasis in ipsilateral internal mammary lymph node(s) and axillary lymph node(s)	☐	pN3b	Metastasis in clinically apparent[1] ipsilateral internal mammary lymph nodes in the presence of 1 or more positive axillary lymph nodes; or in more than 3 axillary lymph nodes and in internal mammary lymph nodes with microscopic disease detected by sentinel lymph node dissection but not clinically apparent[5]
☐	N3c	Metastasis in ipsilateral supraclavicular lymph node(s)	☐	pN3c	Metastasis in ipsilateral supraclavicular lymph nodes

Distant Metastasis (M)

Clinical	*Pathologic*	Distant Metastasis (M)	
☐	☐	MX	Distant metastasis cannot be assessed
☐	☐	M0	No distant metastasis
☐	☐	M1	Distant metastasis
			Biopsy of metastatic site performed ☐ Y ☐ N
			Source of pathologic metastatic specimen

Stage Grouping

Clinical	*Pathologic*				
☐	☐	0	Tis	N0	M0
☐	☐	I	T1[7]	N0	M0
☐	☐	IIA	T0	N1	M0
			T1[7]	N1	M0
			T2	N0	M0
☐	☐	IIB	T2	N1	M0
			T3	N0	M0
☐	☐	IIIA	T0	N2	M0
			T1[7]	N2	M0
			T2	N2	M0
			T3	N1	M0
			T3	N2	M0
☐	☐	IIIB	T4	N0	M0
			T4	N1	M0
			T4	N2	M0
☐	☐	IIIC	Any T	N3	M0
☐	☐	IV	Any T	Any N	M1

Notes

1. *Clinically apparent* is defined as detected by imaging studies (excluding lymphoscintigraphy) or by clinical examination.
2. Classification is based on axillary lymph node dissection with or without sentinel lymph node dissection. Classification based solely on sentinel lymph node dissection without subsequent axillary lymph node dissection is designated (sn) for "sentinel node," e.g., pN0(i +) (sn).
3. Isolated tumor cells (ITC) are defined as single tumor cells or small cell clusters not greater than 0.2 mm, usually detected only by immunohistochemical (IHC) or molecular methods but which may be verified on H&E stains. ITCs do not usually show evidence of metastatic activity (e.g., proliferation or stromal reaction.)
4. RT-PCR: reverse transcriptase/polymerase chain reaction.
5. *Not clinically apparent* is defined as not detected by imaging studies (excluding lymphoscintigraphy) or by clinical examination.
6. If associated with greater than 3 positive axillary lymph nodes, the internal mammary nodes are classified as pN3b to reflect increased tumor burden.
7. T1 includes T1mic

Note: Stage designation may be changed if post-surgical imaging studies reveal the presence of distant metastases, provided that the studies are carried out within 4 months of diagnosis in the absence of disease progression and provided that the patient has not received neoadjuvant therapy.

BREAST

Histologic Grade (G)

All invasive breast carcinomas with the exception of medullary carcinoma should be graded. The Nottingham combined histologic grade (Elston-Ellis modification of Scarff-Bloom-Richardson grading system) is recommended. The grade for a tumor is determined by assessing morphologic features (tubule formation, nuclear pleomorphism, and mitotic count), assigning a value of 1 (favorable) to 3 (unfavorable) for each feature, and adding together the scores for all three categories. A combined score of 3-5 points is designated as grade 1; a combined score of 6-7 points is grade 2; a combined score of 8-9 points is grade 3.

Histologic Grade *(Nottingham combined histologic grade is recommended)*

- ☐ GX Grade cannot be assessed
- ☐ GI Low combined histologic grade (favorable)
- ☐ G2 Intermediate combined histologic grade (moderately favorable)
- ☐ G3 High combined histologic grade (unfavorable)

Residual Tumor (R)

- ☐ RX Presence of residual tumor cannot be assessed
- ☐ R0 No residual tumor
- ☐ R1 Microscopic residual tumor
- ☐ R2 Macroscopic residual tumor

Additional Descriptors

For identification of special cases of TNM or pTNM classifications, the "m" suffix and "y," "r," and "a" prefixes are used. Although they do not affect the stage grouping, they indicate cases needing separate analysis.

m suffix indicates the presence of multiple primary tumors in a single site and is recorded in parentheses: pT(m)NM.

y prefix indicates those cases in which classification is performed during or following initial multi-modality therapy. The cTNM or pTNM category is identified by a "y" prefix. The ycTNM or ypTNM categorizes the extent of tumor actually present at the time of that examination. The "y" categorization is not an estimate of tumor prior to multimodality therapy.

r prefix indicates a recurrent tumor when staged after a disease-free interval, and is identified by the "r" prefix: rTNM.

a prefix designates the stage determined at autopsy: aTNM.

Prognostic Indicators (if applicable)

Physician's Signature _____ Date _____

Notes

Additional Descriptors

Lymphatic Vessel Invasion (L)

- LX   Lymphatic vessel invasion cannot be assessed.
- L0   No lymphatic vessel invasion
- L1   Lymphatic vessel invasion

Venous Invasion (V)

- VX   Venous invasion cannot be assessed
- V0   No venous invasion
- V1   Microscopic venous invasion
- V2   Macroscopic venous invasion

References

1. American Joint Committee on Cancer. *AJCC cancer staging manual.* 6th ed. New York: Springer-Verlag, 2002.
2. Singletary SE, Allred C, Ashley P, et al. Revision of the American Joint Committee on Cancer staging system for breast cancer. *J Clin Oncol* 2002;20:3628–3636.
3. Bunell CA, Winer EP. Lumping versus splitting: the splitters take this round. *J Clin Oncol* 2002;20:3576–3577.
4. Woodward WA, Strom EA, Tucker SL, et al. Changes in the 2003 American Joint Committee on Cancer staging for breast cancer dramatically affect stage-specific survival. *J Clin Oncol* 2003;21:3244.
5. Page DL, Kidd TE, Dupont WD, et al. Lobular neoplasia of the breast: higher risk for subsequent invasive cancer predicted by more extensive disease. *Hum Pathol* 1991;22:1232–1239.
6. Elston CW, Ellis IO. Pathological prognostic factors in breast cancer: I. The value of histologic grade in breast cancer: experience from a large study with long-term follow-up. *Histopathology* 1991;19:403–410.
7. Fitzgibbons PL, Page DL, Weaver D, et al. Prognostic factors in breast cancer. College of American pathologists consensus statement 1999. *Arch Pathol Lab Med* 2000;124:966–978.
8. von Hansemann D. Uber assymetrische Zelltheilung in Epithelkrebsen und deren biologische Bedeutung. *Virchows Arch Pathol Anat* 1890;119:299–326.
9. Greenough RB. Varying degrees of malignancy in cancer of the breast. *J Cancer Res* 1925;9:452–463.
10. Bloom HJG, Richardson WW. Histologic grading and prognosis in breast cancer. *Br J Cancer* 1957;9:359–377
11. Le Doussal V, Tubiana-Hulin M, Friedman S, et al. Prognostic value of histologic grade nuclear components of Scarff-Bloom-Richardson (SBR): an improved score modification based on multivariate analysis of 1,262 invasive ductal breast carcinomas. *Cancer* 1989;64:1914–1921.
12. Henson DE, Ries L, Freedman LS, et al. Relationship among outcome, stage of disease, and histologic grade for 22,616 cases of breast cancer. *Cancer* 1991;68:2142–2149.
13. Neville AM, Bettelheim R, Gelber RD, et al. Factors predicting treatment responsiveness and prognosis in node-negative breast cancer. *J Clin Oncol* 1992;10:696–705.
14. Delides GS, Garas G, Georgouli G, et al. Intralaboratory variations in the grading of breast carcinoma. *Arch Pathol Lab Med* 1982;106:126–128.
15. Stenkvist B, Bengtsson E, Eriksson O, et al. Histopathological systems of breast cancer classification: reproducibility and clinical significance. *J Clin Pathol* 1983;36:392–398.
16. Gilchrist KW, Kalish L, Gould VE, et al. Interobserver reproducibility of histopathological features in stage II breast cancer: an ECOG study. *Breast Cancer Res Treat* 1985;5:3–10.
17. Harvey JM, de Klerk NH, Sterrett GH. Histologic grading in breast cancer: interobserver agreement, and relation to other prognostic factors including ploidy. *Pathology* 1992;124:63–68.
18. Lundin J, Lundin M, Holli K, et al. Omission of histologic grading from clinical decision making may result in overuse of adjuvant therapies in breast cancer: results from a nationwide study. *J Clin Oncol* 2001;9:28–36.
19. Dalton LW, Page DL, Dupont WD. Histologic grading of breast carcinoma: a reproducibility study. *Cancer* 1994;73:2765–2770.
20. Frierson HF, Wolber RA, Berean KW, et al. Interobserver reproducibility of the Nottingham modification of the Bloom and Richardson histologic grading scheme for infiltrating ductal carcinoma. *Am J Clin Pathol* 1995;103:195–198.
21. Robbins P, Pinder S, de Klerk N, et al. Histologic grading of breast carcinomas: a study of interobserver agreement. *Hum Pathol* 1995;26:873–879.
22. Genestie C, Zafrani B, Asselain B, et al. Comparison of the prognostic value of Scarff-Bloom-Richardson and Nottingham histologic grades in a series of 825 cases of breast cancer: major importance of the mitotic count as a component of both grading systems. *Anticancer Res* 1998;18:571–576.
23. Donhuijsen K, Schmidt U, Hirche H, et al. Changes in mitotic rate and cell cycle fractions caused by delayed fixation. *Hum Pathol* 1990;21:709–714.
24. Cross SS, Start RD, Smith JHF. Does delay in fixation affect the number of mitotic figures in processed tissue? *J Clin Pathol* 1990;43:597–599.
25. Start RD, Flynn MS, Cross SS, et al. Is the grading of breast carcinomas affected by a delay in fixation? *Virchows Arch A Pathol Anat* 1991;419:475–477.
26. Rosen PP, Groshen S, Saigo PE, et al. Pathological prognostic factors in stage I (T1N0M0) and stage II (T1N1M0) breast carcinoma: a study of 644 patients with median follow-up of 18 years. *J Clin Oncol* 1989;7:1239–1251.
27. Rosner D, Lane WW. Should all patients with node-negative breast cancer receive adjuvant therapy? *Cancer* 1991;68:1482–1494.
28. Kollias J, Murphy CA, Elston CW, et al. The prognosis of small primary breast cancers. *Eur J Cancer* 1999;35:908–912.
29. Leitner SP, Swern AS, Weinberger D, et al. Predictors of recurrence for patients with small (one centimeter or less) localized breast cancer (T1a,bN0M0). *Cancer* 1995;76:2266–2274.
30. Reed W, Hannisdal E, Boehler PI, et al. The prognostic value of p53 and c-erb B-2 immunostaining is overrated for patients with lymph node negative breast cancer. *Cancer* 2000;88:804–813.
31. Czerniecki BH, Scheff AM, Callans LS, et al. Immunohistochemistry with pancytokeratins improves the sensitivity of sentinel lymph node biopsy in patients with breast carcinoma. *Cancer* 1999;85:1089–1103.
32. Trojani M, de Mascarel I, Bonichon F, et al. Micrometastases to axillary lymph nodes from carcinoma of breast: detection by immunohistochemistry and prognostic significance. *Br J Cancer* 1987;55:303–306.
33. Senmak DD, Meineke TA, Knechtges DS, et al. Prognostic significance of cytokeratin-positive breast cancer metastases. *Mod Pathol* 1989;2:516–520.
34. Chen ZL, Wen DR, Coulson WF, et al. Occult metastases in the axillary lymph nodes of patients with breast cancer node negative by clinical and histologic examination and conventional histology. *Dis Markers* 1991;9:238–248.
35. de Mascarel I, Bonichon F, Coindre JM, et al. Prognostic significance of breast cancer axillary lymph node micrometastases assessed by two special techniques: reevaluation with longer follow-up. *Br J Cancer* 1992;66:523–527.
36. Hainsworth PI, Tjandra JJ, Stillwell RG, et al. Detection and significance of occult metastases in node-negative breast cancer. *Br J Surg* 1993;80:459–463.
37. Clare SE, Sener SF, Wilkens W, et al. Prognostic significance of occult lymph node metastases in node-negative breast cancer. *Ann Surg Oncol* 1997;4:447–451.
38. Hermanek P, Hutter RVP, Sobin LH, et al. Classification of isolated tumor cells and micrometastasis. *Cancer* 1999;86:2668–2673.
39. Huvos AG, Hutter RVP, Berg JW. Significance of axillary macrometastases and micrometastases in mammary cancer. *Ann Surg* 1971;173:44–46.
40. Verbanac KM, Fleming TP, Min CH, et al. RT-PCR increases detection of breast cancer sentinel lymph node micrometastases. *Breast Cancer Res Treat* 1999;57:26(abst).
41. Carter CL, Allen C, Henson DE. Relation of tumor size, lymph node status, and survival in 24,740 breast cancer cases. *Cancer* 1989;63:181–187.
42. Nemoto T, Vana J, Bedwani RN, et al. Management and survival of female breast cancer: results of a national survey by the American College of Surgeons. *Cancer* 1980;45:2917–2924.
43. Paik S, Bryant J, Park C, et al. ERBB-2 and response to doxorubicin in patients with axillary lymph node-positive, hormone receptor-negative breast cancer. *J Natl Cancer Inst* 1998;90:1361–1370.
44. Crump M, Goss PE, Prince M, et al. Outcome of extensive evaluation before adjuvant therapy in women with breast cancer and 10 or more positive axillary lymph nodes. *J Clin Oncol* 1996;14:66–69.
45. Diab SG, Hilsenbeck SG, de Moor C, et al. Radiation therapy and survival in breast cancer patients with 10 or more positive axillary lymph nodes treated with mastectomy. *J Clin Oncol* 1998;16:1655–1660.
46. Fountzilas G, Nicolaides C, Aravantinos G, et al. Dose-dense adjuvant chemotherapy with epirubicin monotherapy in patients with operable breast cancer and >10 positive axillary lymph nodes: a feasibility study. *Oncology* 1998;55:508–512.
47. Veronesi U, Marubini E, Mariani L, et al. The dissection of internal mammary nodes does not improve the survival of breast cancer patients: 30-year results ora randomized trial. *Eur J Cancer* 1999;35.1320–1325.
48. Bucalossi P, Veronesi U, Zingo L, et al. Enlarged mastectomy for breast cancer: review of 1,213 cases. *AJR Am J Roentgenol* 1971;111:119–122.
49. Caceres E. An evaluation of radical mastectomy and extended radical mastectomy for cancer of the breast. *Surg Gynecol Obstet* 1967;123:337–341.
50. Li KYY, Shen Z-Z. An analysis of 1,242 cases of extended radical mastectomy. *Breast* 1984;10:10–19.
51. Urban JA, Marjani MA. Significance of internal mammary lymph node metastases in breast cancer. *AJR Am J Roentgenol* 1971;111:130–136.
52. Veronesi U, Cascinelli N, Bufalino R, et al. Risk of internal mammary lymph node metastases and its relevance on prognosis of breast cancer patients. *Ann Surg* 1983;198:681–684.
53. Halsted WS. The results of radical operations for the cure of cancer of the breast. *Ann Surg* 1907;46:1–5.
54. Debois JM. The significance of a supraclavicular node metastasis in patients with breast cancer: a literature review. *Strahlenther Onkol* 1997;173:1–12.
55. American Joint Committee on Cancer. *AJCC cancer staging manual.* 5th ed. Philadelphia: Lippincott-Raven, 1997.
56. Brito RA, Valero VV, Buzdar AU, et al. Long-term results of combined-modality therapy for locally advanced breast cancer with ipsilateral supraclavicular metastases: the University of Texas M. D. Anderson Cancer Center experience. *J Clin Oncol* 2001;19:628–633.
57. American Society of Clinical Oncology. Clinical practice guidelines for the use of tumor markers in breast and colorectal cancer. *J Clin Oncol* 1996;14:2843–2877.
58. American Society of Clinical Oncology. 1997 update of recommendations for the use of tumor markers in breast and colorectal cancer. *J Clin Oncol* 1998;16:793–795.

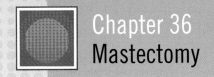

Chapter 36
Mastectomy

Mehra Golshan

Mehra Golshan

 HISTORY OF MASTECTOMY

The origin of the word mastectomy traces back to the Greek term *mastos*, meaning the breast. The advancement of mastectomy over the past century has evolved considerably from the description from Halsted and Meyer in the mid-1890s. Near the turn of the century, William Stewart Halsted published the Johns Hopkins Hospital experience and the standard of care became the radical mastectomy (1). Almost simultaneously, Willy Meyer in New York published his experience with the radical mastectomy (2). Halsted achieved a remarkable 3-year local recurrence rate of 3% and local regional control recurrence rate of 20% with no operative mortality. His actuarial survival was double those of untreated patients with 5-year survival at 40%, despite the lack of any further adjuvant therapy.

Prior to these remarkable descriptions, others had reported similar operative techniques in Great Britain and Germany. Charles Moore (3) in Liverpool in the late 1860s recommended intact removal of the breast and, if clinically involved, the lymph nodes, and in 1887 William Banks (4) removed the breast and lymph nodes as a routine. The Halsted theory held that cancer spread in an orderly fashion from breast to the lymph nodes, and the predominance of the radical mastectomy as the method of choice for the surgical extirpation of breast cancer remained dominant for nearly 80 years. The operation paid the price with high morbidity of large open wounds left to heal by granulation, near universal lymphedema, and overall disability.

Haagensen (5) helped develop the criteria for inoperability and was credited with the development of a physical examination–based staging of breast tumors, a forerunner to the TNM (tumor, node, metastasis) system developed in 1954. Several seminal changes in the practice of medicine allowed adjuvant treatment of breast cancer: the discovery of x-rays by Rontgen in 1895 and the hormonal treatment of breast cancer by Schinzinger and Beatson. Although these adjuvant efforts were under way, unfortunately surgical therapy took a step toward more extensive surgery. The extended radical mastectomy was described by Carey and Kirlin (6) in 1952 and was followed by descriptions from Urban (7) and Sugarbaker (8) advocating removal of the internal mammary nodes.

In contrast, during the same period, Patey and Dyson (9) described a conservative mastectomy allowing for preservation of the pectoralis major while resecting the pectoralis minor and complete axillary node dissection. The resection allowed for preservation of the medial and lateral pectoral nerves. Auchincloss's (10) modification of the surgery preserved both the pectoralis major and minor muscles with resection of the level I and II lymph nodes. The belief that cancer was spread by direct extension and that cancer cells did not spread through the blood stream was coming to an end.

The main challenge to this theory can be credited to Bernard Fisher et al. (11) and the multi-institutional National Surgery Adjuvant Breast and Bowel Project (NSABP). Fisher et al. asserted that breast cancer was a systemic disease and thus the orderly progression of breast cancer to lymph nodes and direct extension were not valid. The pivotal NSABP B-04 trial compared, in a randomized fashion, radical mastectomy to total mastectomy with or without radiation and the results failed to show a survival difference between the arms of this trial. Umberto Veronesi et al. (12), at the National Tumor Institute in Milan, randomized woman to radical mastectomy versus quadrentectomy, axillary dissection, and radiation and also failed to show a difference in breast cancer specific and overall survival. The NSABP B-06 trial and others have shown equivalent long-term survival between breast-conserving therapy and mastectomy (13–16). With these results breast-conserving therapy has become the favored treatment of women with early stage breast cancer. In 1990 a panel of the National Institutes of Health Consensus Development Conference indicated that breast-conserving therapy plus radiation is an appropriate and preferred method for the treatment of early stage breast cancer (17).

 ABSOLUTE AND RELATIVE CONTRAINDICATIONS

Despite these findings, many women choose or must undergo mastectomy. Absolute contraindications to breast-conserving therapy include multicentric breast cancer (tumors in more than one quadrant) or diffuse malignant appearing microcalcifications. Prior therapeutic radiation to the breast region, such as mantle radiation for Hodgkin's lymphoma, is considered an absolute contraindication. Pregnancy is an absolute contraindication to the use of radiation and thus the use of breast-conserving therapy; the caveat includes the possibility of breast-conserving therapy in the third trimester followed by radiation in the postpartum setting (18). Another option available during pregnancy is neoadjuvant therapy with specific agents that may be given during pregnancy and allow for breast-conserving therapy if appropriate in the postpartum setting. Persistently positive margins after multiple surgical attempts to achieve clear margins in relation to a cosmetically acceptable result are a final absolute contraindication to breast-conserving therapy.

Relative contraindications include history of collagen vascular disease, such as active scleroderma and active lupus, where radiation and healing are poorly tolerated in this population. The presence of diffuse indeterminate calcifications or multiple gross tumors within a single quadrant should be carefully assessed prior to offering breast-conserving therapy as the volume of resection may preclude clear margins or a cosmetically acceptable result. A large tumor size in relation to a small breast size, where cosmetic outcome would be significantly altered, should be considered a relative contraindication as the volume of resection may cause significant and unacceptable cosmetic deformity. In this case the consideration for preoperative therapy may be made where a percentage of patients may achieve a favorable response that allows for consideration of breast-conserving therapy. Other factors include patient preference or physician bias for mastectomy.

CURRENT TECHNIQUE

The modern technique of mastectomy includes the possibility of skin-sparing total mastectomy with immediate reconstruction, total or simple mastectomy without reconstruction, axillary staging with sentinel node biopsy, or axillary lymph node dissection when indicated. The operation, total or simple mastectomy, is the removal of the entire mammary gland and in general the nipple areolar complex along the anatomic boundaries of the breast superiorly to the clavicle, inferiorly to the rectus sheath insertion, medially to the sternal border, and laterally to the latissimus along with the pectoralis major fascia. The flap

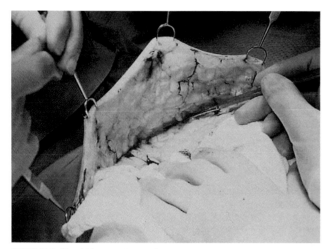

FIGURE 36.1. Flap thickness at the time of a modified radical mastectomy.

thickness should include all of the breast parenchyma while leaving a thin rim of subcutaneous fat and superficial vasculature to minimize the risk of necrosis (Fig. 36.1). The determination of flap thickness is left largely to the surgeon's preference and training, however, flaps thicker than 5 mm are associated with significant residual glandular breast tissue (19). Unfortunately, no reliable technique allows for intraoperative assessment of flap thickness. The choice of technique, knife, scissor, or electrocautery, is largely left to the individual surgeon. Some groups advocate the use of breast tumescence (a combination of lactated ringers and lidocaine with epinephrine) to help facilitate dissection, although data on its benefits and complications are sparse (Fig. 36.2). When reconstruction is not performed, the goal is to remove the breast and enough skin to leave the chest wall flat without redundancy as this surface helps facilitate the construction of an appropriate prosthesis. Redundant skin is difficult to care for and becomes scarred to the chest wall, making future reconstruction options compromised. The classic incisions include the Stewart elliptical incision across the chest wall from the sternum to the latissimus, a modified Stewart incision placed obliquely. Other less commonly used incisions include the Orr or modified Orr incision (a more vertically lined technique). At the time of a mastectomy, the pectoralis major fascia should be resected in all cases of invasive breast carcinoma, however, resection of muscle should be reserved for gross tumor invasion only. In general the pectoralis minor should be preserved and

resection reserved for cases of gross tumor invasion or facilitation of access to level III lymph nodes when clinically involved, an uncommon finding in the modern era. Cases of such locally advanced disease should be considered for neoadjuvant therapy to facilitate surgical resection and decrease morbidity. The outcomes from a mastectomy are in general favorable. A recent U.S. Department of Veterans Affairs study reported mortality rate and operation-related readmissions as less than 1% (20). The most common complications perioperatively were superficial wound infections at a 6% rate in this study. The National Surgical Quality Improvement Program Patient Safety in Surgery collected data from 14 university and four community centers on breast surgery. Mastectomy mortality rate was 0.24% and the 30-day mastectomy morbidity rate was 5.7%, of these the majority were wound related at 3.6% (21). The anticipated wound infection rate for a clean procedure ranges between 1% to 5% . The use of antibiotics varies by surgeon and center, and no standard has been obtained in the breast surgical oncology literature. A meta analysis by Platt et al. (22) suggests that antibiotics reduced infection by 38%, but this study was far from definitive. The formation of seroma is a universal by-product of mastectomy and should not be considered a complication. Drain placement after mastectomy remains a common part of the procedure and allows fusing of the dermal layer to the chest wall. Seroma aspiration rates vary in the literature and have been reported between 10% to 80% after mastectomy (23). Flap necrosis and hematoma rates are low and most report a number below 5% after mastectomy. Postoperative phantom and chronic pains are primarily neuropathic in etiology and can appear months to years after local therapy; unfortunately widespread studies have not been done on this finding. Smaller reviews suggest that these symptoms may occur in 20% to 30% of patients undergoing mastectomy (24,25). Management of these pains are difficult and often supportive only, and use of physical therapy and pharmacologic intervention may be considered with variable outcomes. Although overall complications rates remain low, a frank discussion about the risks associated with the mastectomy should be discussed with the patient in the preoperative setting.

RECONSTRUCTION AND SKIN-SPARING MASTECTOMY

When reconstruction is to be performed a skin-sparing incision is preferred. First described by Toth and Lappert (26) in 1991, this requires removing the nipple and areola and the breast parenchyma while maintaining as much of the natural skin as an envelope for the reconstruction surgeon. In general if a previous lumpectomy or excisional biopsy incision was performed the recommendation is to remove this ellipse of skin; some would also argue in favor of excising core biopsy tracts, although the literature is sparse and the reported frequency of breast carcinoma recurrences at core biopsy incision sites are few. Reconstruction techniques include expander and implant with or without AlloDerm (CellLife Corp, Branchburg, New Jersey) an acellular dermal matrix designed to re-create the inframammary crease) versus the use of muscle flap with or without implant and perforator flaps. The reconstruction techniques vary with each institution and the repertoire offered by the plastic surgery service. A detailed consultation is critical to the informed decision-making process. Close communication between the oncologic surgeon and reconstruction surgeon facilitates an improved outcome at the time of local therapy. Reviews by multiple groups have reported on the oncologic safety of the skin-sparing incision with local recurrences similar to those patients undergoing traditional non–skin-sparing mastectomies (27–29). The largest series with a medium range follow-up Carlson et al. (27) from Emory report a 5.5% rate of local recurrence with 78.1 month

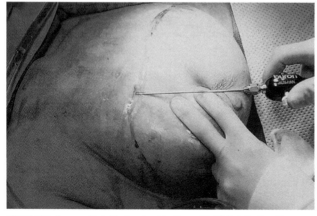

FIGURE 36.2. Tumescent injection to reduce bleeding and facilitate knife dissection.

follow-up. The importance of local control has been codified by the recent *Lancet* overview, which suggests that optimal locoregional control confers a survival benefit in early stage breast cancer (30). The addition of radiation therapy specifically in the node-positive population experienced statistically improved breast cancer–specific mortality and reduction in local recurrence, while the in node-negative population the small reduction in the local recurrence (from 6.3% to 2.3%) was outweighed by the risks of radiation therapy and a decrease in overall survival.

RADIATION THERAPY AND MASTECTOMY WITH RECONSTRUCTION

The use of radiation therapy and its effect on skin-sparing mastectomy and reconstruction continues to be a great source of debate among surgical oncologists, radiation oncologists, and reconstructive surgeons. No single answer can be used to determine the optimal decision for each patient. Information on the size of the tumor and lymph node status are often not known until during or after the operation. A frank discussion with the patient and discussion with the involved multidisciplinary team is crucial to the patient's outcome. Currently the American Society of Therapeutic Radiology and Oncology and the American Society of Clinical Oncology recommend postmastectomy radiation therapy for tumors greater than 5 cm and those with four or more positive lymph nodes (31,32). It should be noted that disagreement exists on whether postmastectomy radiation should be used with the current size criteria and those with one to three positive lymph nodes. Several models have been developed to help predict the possibility of having greater than four lymph nodes involved with metastatic disease and thus the need for postmastectomy radiation, although there widespread use has been limited (33,34). Of great concern to a reconstruction surgeon in respect to radiation is interstitial fibrosis and arteriolar damage, which increases the rate of capsular contracture and impaired skin healing with increased rates of infection when an expander or an implant is used (35). Studies on the use of implant and expander with postmastectomy radiation show a high rate of minor and major salvage procedures and failure rates. Wong et al. (36) had a 40% rate of major corrective surgery in the implant group as opposed to 9% in the flap cohort. The use of muscular or myocutaneous flaps tends to be better tolerated when radiation therapy is necessary, however, even in this group delayed reconstruction is often advantageous, allowing for the assessment and removal of radiation-damaged skin, although this clashes with the need for a larger skin flap, second prolonged anesthetic, and the psychological impact on the woman. One option suggested from the reconstruction surgeons is performing the sentinel node biopsy prior to the mastectomy and reconstruction; this leads to more than one anesthesia and a delay of several days to weeks before the second definitive surgery. Even if the sentinel node is positive, there is no guarantee that four total lymph nodes are involved with metastatic disease or that the tumor is greater than 5 cm, the criteria for postmastectomy radiation. Another option proposed is delayed immediate reconstruction, where an expander is left in place and definitive immediate reconstruction is delayed until final pathology becomes available (37). Again this requires a second surgical procedure. Other groups have reported low local recurrences (3%) and minimal morbidity (6%) without delay in further adjuvant therapy using a transverse rectus abdominis myocutaneous (TRAM) reconstruction (38). Unfortunately, recent data suggest that surgeons in general do a poor job of even allowing a patient to meet with a reconstruction surgeon to discuss her options. The recent Surveillance, Epidemiology, and End Results (SEER) review suggests that only a third of patients had reconstruction surgery mentioned to them during the surgical decision-making process for their cancer (39).

From the radiation oncologist standpoint, difficulty arises in optimizing delivery of postmastectomy radiation when the chest wall contour has been changed with the reconstruction. Specifically when a flap or implant is in place, the ability to radiate the internal mammary field and the chest wall comprehensively while protecting adjacent structures such as the heart and lung become compromised. A recent study from the M.D. Anderson group looked at postmastectomy radiation and reconstruction for those undergoing postmastectomy radiation without reconstruction. They found that over half of the former group had treatment compromised compared to 7% in the latter (40). With this in mind those patients who are known in advance to require postmastectomy radiation or who are at high risk of needing radiation should meet with a reconstruction surgeon and radiation oncologist prior to definitive local therapy to discuss the options and hopefully accept a delayed approach.

INOPERABILITY

Certain patients who present with breast cancer may not be even considered operable, and the criteria for this situation continue to be refined. Women who present with metastatic breast cancer in general are not offered local therapy. There have been recent published studies reviewing large databases and institutional data sets suggesting improved survival in women who undergo resection of the primary tumor site either by mastectomy or lumpectomy, however, this cannot be considered standard of care today (41). Women with inflammatory breast cancer are not candidates for immediate local therapy because of the aggressive nature of the disease and reliance on primary systemic therapy. Only those who show response undergo resection followed by radiation therapy. In the locally advanced setting, which constitutes, depending on the definition used, 15% to 20% of breast cancers in the United States, in general, preoperative or neoadjuvant therapy is given to down-size or debulk the tumor and facilitate surgical resection either by mastectomy or possibly by breast-conserving therapy. Tumors that remain large or fixed to the underlying chest wall can still be resected by radical mastectomy and en bloc resection of the underlying musculature or those with advanced disease and debilitating local wound issues may benefit from palliative toilet mastectomy (Fig. 36.3). Often primary closure is not possible, and the use of chest wall reconstruction techniques with skin-grafting, advancement flaps, omental flaps, or myocutaneous flaps are required to fill in the defect (Figs. 36.4 and 36.5).

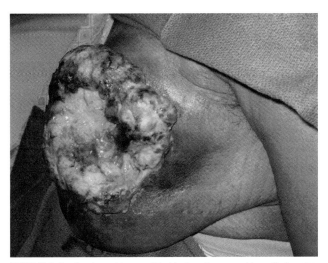

FIGURE 36.3. Locally advanced tumor resistant to chemotherapy requiring radical mastectomy and skin-grafting and omentum for closure.

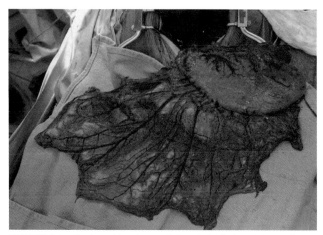

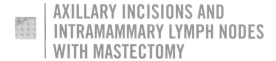

FIGURE 36.4. Locally advanced breast cancer that required radical mastectomy and reconstruction using a combination of omentum and skin-grafting to correct the chest wall deformity

AXILLARY INCISIONS AND INTRAMAMMARY LYMPH NODES WITH MASTECTOMY

The management of the axilla at the time of mastectomy has also evolved. In general those with node-positive disease undergo level I and II axillary node dissection, and the combination with a total mastectomy becomes the modified radical mastectomy. With the advent of the sentinel node procedure, mastectomy and lymphatic mapping and biopsy often occur at the same time, and the success rate is the same as those undergoing breast-conserving therapy. Some surgeons prefer to make a counter incision underneath the arm, while others perform the procedure through the same incision used for the mastectomy. In a recent review by Dominguez et al. (42), surgeons were split evenly between the sentinel node biopsy being performed via the mastectomy incision (52%) versus a separate axillary incision (48%). The use of sentinel node biopsy at the time of mastectomy is indicated for clinically node-negative invasive breast cancer and should be considered for ductal carcinoma *in situ* (DCIS). The caveat for DCIS is that when the breast is removed the ability to perform the sentinel node biopsy if an unsuspected invasive breast cancer is found will be lost. The use of the sentinel node in the prophylactic setting should be abandoned as the risk of finding invasive breast cancer in the appropriately screened patient is exceedingly low (1.1% to 1.9%) (43,44).

With the increased use of the sentinel node biopsy and scrutiny of the breast specimen, intramammary lymph node identification and involvement with carcinoma has increased and its clinical significance has been questioned. The probability of having additional axillary nodal disease varies between the studies, however, the total numbers in the series are small and whether completion axillary node dissection is required remains to be determined (45,46).

PROPHYLACTIC MASTECTOMY

Prophylactic mastectomy continues to be indicated as an option for patients at high risk of developing breast cancer, including known gene mutation carriers of *BRCA1* or *BRCA2*, strong family history of multiple first-degree relatives, or successive generation of breast or ovarian cancer and high-risk lesions such as atypical ductal hyperplasia and lobular carcinoma *in situ*. This decision should be made with the assistance of a multidisciplinary team and includes a thorough discussion of alternative such as close surveillance and risk-

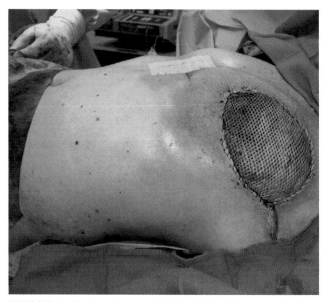

FIGURE 36.5. Locally advanced breast cancer that required radical mastectomy and reconstruction using a combination of omentum and skin grafting to correct the chest wall deformity.

reduction techniques (47). Many patients with unilateral breast cancer choose a prophylactic contralateral mastectomy to prevent breast cancer despite the availability of better imaging and chemoprevention strategies, and the reason behind this is not well known. A recent review of the SEER database showed that the contralateral prophylactic mastectomy rate increased from 4.2% in 1998 to 11.0% in 2003 (48).

NIPPLE- OR AREOLAR-SPARING MASTECTOMY

Nipple- and areolar-sparing mastectomy or total skin–sparing mastectomy have been increasingly used around the world in a subset of women. This is considered by many a natural extension from the skin-sparing mastectomy. The rate of occult nipple involvement varies between the studies, in older series the numbers ranged from 5% to 46%, and some groups evaluated the areola separately from the nipple and found only a 1% areolar involvement while 10.6% had nipple involved with cancer (49). Another study that excluded subareolar and multicentric tumors found a 3% nipple–areolar involvement in those undergoing skin-sparing mastectomy (50). With these findings many groups have embarked on the path of nipple- and/or areolar-sparing mastectomy with largely positive results being reported. Unfortunately, most of the data are single institution retrospective reviews and a randomized trial has not been performed. The incisions options include a periareolar incision with a lateral extension, transareolar with medial or lateral extensions, and mammary crease incisions. Criteria for ineligibility include retroareolar lesions within 1 cm of the nipple–areolar complex, segmental calcifications stretching from the nipple–areolar complex, tumors greater than 3 cm or a positive intraoperative biopsy of the nipple–areolar complex. To date most series report few if any nipple–areolar recurrences, however, necrosis rates of the nipple–areolar complex remain high (11%), and despite the preservation of the nipple–areolar complex, sensory loss remains a problem (51,52). The optimal patient selection and the ability to tailor a thin enough flap without necrosis of the nipple–areolar complex remains to be determined. Elegant studies of mastectomy specimens have tried to predict the optimal duct removal while not compromising vasculature and maybe useful in a future clinical trial determining the oncologic safety of a nipple-sparing mastectomy, while reducing nipple–areolar complication rates (53). Another method of preventing local recurrence at the nipple–areolar complex that has been reported by the Milan group is the delivery of intraoperative radiation to the nipple–areolar complex, and with a relatively short follow-up the cohort have had no local relapses at the nipple–areolar complex (54). Until long-term data or results from a randomized trial become available, careful consideration and scrutiny should be made before selecting patients for this procedure.

MARGIN STATUS AND PREDICTORS FOR LOCAL RECURRENCE

Locoregional recurrence after mastectomy is low and ranges between 3% to 5% for early stage breast cancer. Most local recurrences occur in the skin and subcutaneous tissue as opposed to the chest wall and muscle. Several studies have suggested that high tumor grade, advanced stage at presentation, and presence of lymphovascular invasion increase local recurrence after mastectomy. In one study, the quadrant of primary tumor predicted the site of recurrence, and high tumor grade indicated an increased risk of local recurrence (55). Many institutions' pathology departments report only posterior or deep margins with a mastectomy specimen, and gross involvement or multifocally close involvement with invasive carcinoma may necessitate the need for postmastectomy radiation especially in a younger population (56). In general and in the authors' institution, routine evaluation of the superficial margin is not performed. A recent study from Johns Hopkins Hospital suggests a significant rate of superficial margin involvement with carcinoma, and although long-term follow-up is not available, local recurrence seems to be higher (57). In their cohort additional superficial margins were important in achieving local control and microscopically clear margins. Surgical orientation of the pathology specimen and reviewing the tumor site with the pathologist will help in proper reporting of margin status in the mastectomy patient, especially when skin-sparing and nipple-sparing techniques are involved.

MANAGEMENT SUMMARY

- Mastectomy has historically been the primary mode of local therapy for breast cancer. Despite the increased use of breast-conserving therapy, mastectomy remains an option for women diagnosed with breast cancer.
- The technique of mastectomy has evolved from the radical mastectomy to the skin-sparing mastectomy with equivalent oncologic results and improved cosmetic outcome.
- The use of radiation therapy often compromises cosmetic results and often the delivery of therapy is severely challenged by the presence of reconstruction, therefore, delayed reconstruction should be considered.
- Mastectomy indications continue to be refined, and with the improvements in systemic therapy, most inoperable breast cancers can be converted to surgical candidates with appropriate neoadjuvant therapy. Surgery in the setting of metastatic disease should be considered in the trial setting.
- The management of the axilla at the time of mastectomy has also evolved from the routine dissection of level I, II, and III lymph nodes to the sentinel lymph node biopsy.
- The evolution from the skin-sparing to the nipple–areolar sparing mastectomy has begun, but long-term data are lacking and appropriate patient selection continues to be refined.

RELEVANT WEB SITES

National Comprehensive Cancer Network NCCN: www.nccn.org
Society of Surgical Oncology: www.surgonc.org
American Society of Breast Surgeons: www.breastsurgeons.org
American Society of Therapeutic Radiology and Oncology: www.astro.org

References

1. Halsted WS. The results of operations for the cure of cancer of the breast performed at the Johns Hopkins Hospital from June, 1889, to January, 1894. *Ann Surg* 1894;20(5):497–555.
2. Meyer W. An improved method of the radical operation for carcinoma of the breast. *Med Rec N Y* 1894;46;746–749.
3. Moore C. On the influence of inadequate operations on the theory of cancer. Royal Medical and Chirugical Society. London. *Med Chir Trans* 1867;32:245 280.
4. Banks WM. On free removal of mammary cancer with extirpation of the axillary glands as a necessary accompaniment. *Br Med J* 1882;2(1145):1138–1141.
5. Haagensen CD. In Harris JR, Lippman ME, Morrow M, et al., eds. *Diseases of the breast.* 2nd ed. Philadelphia: WB Saunders Co, 1971:394–395.
6. Carey JM, Kirlin JW. Extended radical mastectomy: a review of its concepts. *Proc Staff Meet Mayo Clin* 1952;27(22):436–440.
7. Urban JA. Extended radical mastectomy for breast cancer. *Am J Surg* 1963;106:399–404.
8. Sugarbaker ED. Extended radical mastectomy. Its superiority in treatment of breast cancer. *JAMA* 1964;187:96–99.
9. Patey DH, Dyson WH. The prognosis of carcinoma of the breast in relation to the type of mastectomy performed. *Br J Cancer* 1948;2:7–13.
10. Auchincloss H. Modified radical mastectomy: why not? *Am J Surg* 1970;119(5):506–509.
11. Fisher B, Redmond C, Fisher ER, et al. Ten-year results of a randomized clinical trial comparing radical mastectomy and total mastectomy with or without radiation. *N Engl J Med* 1985;312:674–681.
12. Veronesi U, Cascinelli N, Mariani L, et al. Twenty-year follow up of a randomized study comparing breast-conserving surgery with radical mastectomy for early breast cancer. *N Engl J Med* 2002;347:1227–1232.
13. Fisher B, Anderson S, Bryant J, et al. Twenty-year follow-up of a randomized trial comparing total mastectomy, lumpectomy, and lumpectomy plus irradiation for the treatment of invasive breast cancer. *N Engl J Med* 2002;347:1233–1241.
14. Sarrazin D, Le M, Rouesse J, et al. Conservative treatment versus mastectomy in breast cancer tumors with macroscopic diameter of 20 millimeters or less. The experience of the Institut Gustave-Roussy. *Cancer* 1984;53:1209–1213.
15. Van Dongen JA, Voogd AC, Fentiman IS, et al. Long-term results of a randomized trial comparing breast-conserving therapy with mastectomy: European Organization for Research and Treatment of Cancer 10801 trial. *J Natl Cancer Inst* 2000;92:1143–1150.
16. Jacobson JA, Danforth DN, Cowan KH, et al. Ten-year results of a comparison of conservation with mastectomy in the treatment of stage I and II breast cancer. *N Engl J Med* 1995;332:907–911.
17. Consensus statement: treatment of early-stage breast cancer. National Institutes of Health Consensus Development Panel. *J Natl Cancer Inst Monogr* 1992;11:1–5.
18. Morrow M, Strom EA, Bassett LW, et al. Standard of breast conserving therapy in the management of invasive breast cancer. *CA Cancer Clin J* 2002;52:277–300.
19. Torresan RZ, dos Santos CC, Okamura H, et al. Evaluation of residual glandular tissue after skin-sparing mastectomies. *Ann Surg Oncol* 2005;12:1037–1044.
20. Hynes DM, Weaver F, Morrow M, et al. Breast cancer surgery trends and outcomes: results from a National Department of Veterans Affairs study. *J Am Coll Surg* 2004;198:707–716.
21. El-Tamer MB, Ward BM, Schiffner T, et al. Morbidity and mortality following breast cancer surgery in women: national benchmarks for standard of care. *Ann Surg* 2007;245:665 671.
22. Platt R, Zucker JR, Zaleznik DF, et al. Perioperative antibiotic prophylaxis and wound infection following breast surgery. *J Antimicrob Chemother* 1993;31:43–48.
23. Pogson CJ, Adwani A, Ebbs SR. Seroma following breast cancer surgery. *Eur J Surg Oncol* 2003;29:711–717.
24. Stevens P, Dibble S, Miastowski C. Prevalence, characteristics, and impact of post-mastectomy pain syndrome: an investigation of women's experiences. *Pain* 1995;61:61–68.
25. Vitug AF, Newman LA. Complications in breast surgery. *Surg Clin North Am* 2007;87:431–451.
26. Toth BA, Lappert P. Modified skin incisions for mastectomy: the need for plastic surgical input in preoperative planning. *Plast Reconstr Surg* 1991;87:1048–1053.
27. Carlson GW, Styblo TM, Lyles RH, et al. The use of skin sparing mastectomy in the treatment of breast cancer: the Emory experience. *Surg Oncol* 2003;12:265–269.
28. Medina-Franco H, Vasconez LO, Fix RJ, et al. Factors associated with local recurrence after skin-sparing mastectomy and immediate breast reconstruction for invasive breast cancer. *Ann Surg* 2002;235:814–819.
29. Meretoja TJ, Rasia S, von Smitten KA, et al. Late results of skin-sparing mastectomy followed by immediate breast reconstruction. *Br J Surg* 2007;94:1220–1225.
30. Clarke M, Collins R, Darby S, et al. Early Breast Cancer Trialists' Collaborative Group (EBCTCG). Effects of radiotherapy and of differences in the extent of surgery for early breast cancer on local recurrence and 15-year survival: an overview of the randomized trials. *Lancet* 2005;366:2087–2106.
31. Recht A, Edge SB, Solin LJ, et al. Postmastectomy radiotherapy: guidelines of the American Society of Clinical Oncology. *J Clin Oncol* 2001;19:1539–1569.
32. Harris JR, Halpin-Murphy P, McNeese M, et al. Consensus statement on postmastectomy radiation therapy. *Int J Radiat Oncol Biol Phys* 1999;44:989–990.
33. Chagpar AB, Scoggins CR, Martin RC 2nd, et al. Predicting patients at low probability of requiring postmastectomy radiation therapy. *Ann Surg Oncol* 2007;14:670–677.

34. Katz A, Niemierko A, Gage I, et al. Factors associated with involvement of four or more axillary nodes for sentinel lymph node positive patients. *Int J Radiat Oncol Biol Phys* 2006;65:40–44.
35. Pomahac B, Recht A, May JW, et al. New trends in breast cancer: management: is the era of immediate breast reconstruction changing? *Ann Surg* 2006;244(2): 282–288.
36. Wong JS, Ho AY, Kaelin CM, et al. Incidence of major corrective surgery after post-mastectomy breast reconstruction and radiation therapy. *Breast J* 2008;14: 49–54.
37. Kronowitz SJ, Hunt KK, Kuerer HM, et al. Delayed-immediate breast reconstruction. *Plast Reconstr Surg* 2004;113:1617–1628.
38. Foster RD, Hansen SL, Esserman LJ, et al. Safety of immediate transverse rectus abdominis myocutaneous breast reconstruction for patients with locally advanced disease. *Arch Surg* 2005;140:196–200.
39. Alderman AK, Hawley ST, Waljee J, et al. Understanding the impact of breast reconstruction on the surgical decision-making process for breast cancer *Cancer* 2007;112:489–494.
40. Motwani SB, Strom EA, Schechter NR, et al. The impact of immediate reconstruction on the technical delivery of postmastectomy radiation. *Int J Radiat Oncol Biol Phys* 2006;66:76–82.
41. Khan SA. Does resection of an intact breast primary improve survival in metastatic breast cancer? *Oncology* 2007;21:924–931.
42. Dominguez FJ, Golshan M, Black DM, et al. Sentinel node biopsy is important in mastectomy for ductal carcinoma in situ. *Ann Surg Oncol* 2008;15:268–273.
43. Boughey JC, Cormier JN, Xing Y, et al. Decision analysis to assess the efficacy of routine sentinel lymphadenectomy in patients undergoing prophylactic mastectomy. *Cancer* 2007;110:2542–2550.
44. Wood WC. More answers about prophylactic mastectomy. *Ann Surg Oncol* 2007; 14:3283–3284.
45. Nassar A, Cohen C, Cotsonis G, et al. Significance of intramammary lymph nodes in the staging of breast cancer: correlation with tumor characteristics and outcome. *Breast J* 2008;14:22–27.
46. Intra M, Garcia-Etieene CA, Renne G, et al. When sentinel lymph node is intramammary. *Ann Surg Oncol* 2008;15:1304–1308.
47. Giuliano AE, Boolbol S, Degnim A, et al. Society of Surgical Oncology: position statement of prophylactic mastectomy. Approved by the Society of Surgical Oncology executive council, March 2007. *Ann Surg Oncol* 2007;14:2425–2427.
48. Tuttle TM, Habermann EB, Grund EH, et al. Increasing use of contralateral prophylactic mastectomy for breast cancer patients: a trend toward more aggressive surgical treatment. *J Clin Oncol* 2007;25:5203–5209.
49. Simmons RM, Brennan M, Christos P, et al. Analysis of nipple/areolar involvement with mastectomy: can the areola be preserved? *Ann Surg Oncol* 2002;9:165–168.
50. Laronga C, Kemp B, Johnston D, et al. The incidence of occult nipple-areola complex involvement in breast cancer patients receiving a skin-sparing mastectomy *Ann Surg Oncol* 1999;66:609–613.
51. Sacchini V, Pinotti JA, Barros AC, et al. Nipple-sparing mastectomy for breast cancer and risk reduction: oncologic or technical problem? *J Am Coll Surg* 2006;203: 704–714.
52. Crowe JP, Kim JA, Yetman R, et al. Nipple-sparing mastectomy: technique and results of 54 procedures. *Arch Surg* 2004;139:148–150.
53. Rusby JE, Brachterl EF, Taghian A, et al. George Peters award. Microscopic anatomy within the nipple: implication for nipple-sparing mastectomy. *Am J Surg* 2007;194:433–437.
54. Petit JY, Veronesi U, Rey P, et al. Nipple-sparing mastectomy: risk of nipple-areolar recurrences in a series of 578 cases. *Breast Cancer Res Treat* 2008. In press.
55. Vaughan A, Dietz JR, Aft R, et al. Scientific Presentation Award. Patterns of local breast cancer recurrence after skin-sparing mastectomy and immediate reconstruction. *Am J Surg* 2007;194:438–443.
56. Freedman GM, Fowble DL, Hanlon AL, et al. A close or positive margin after mastectomy is not an indication for chest wall irradiation except in women aged fifty or younger. *Int J Radiat Oncol Biol Phys* 1998;31:599–605.
57. Cao D, Tsangaris TN, Kouprina N, et al. The superficial margin of the skin-sparing mastectomy for breast carcinoma: factors predicting involvement and efficacy of additional margin sampling. *Ann Surg Oncol* 2008;15:1330–1340.

Chapter 37
Breast-Conserving Therapy: Conventional Whole Breast Irradiation

Thomas A. Buchholz and Kelly K. Hunt

Breast-conservation therapy is established as a standard-of-care locoregional treatment for early stage (stages I and II) breast cancer. The first clinical trials investigating breast conservation began over three decades ago, and the outcome data from these trials provided clear evidence that breast-conserving surgery followed by whole breast radiation achieved equivalent long-term survival as mastectomy. The adoption of breast conservation has benefited thousands of patients. Furthermore, the improved cure rates in breast cancer have increased the emphasis on maximizing the quality of life for breast cancer survivors. A major goal of breast cancer locoregional therapies should be organ preservation, which permits survivors to maintain normal breast anatomy and sensation. Studies have demonstrated that breast conservation positively impacts patient well-being and quality of life (1).

Currently, most patients with newly diagnosed breast cancer are candidates for breast-conservation therapy. The increased use of mammographic screening and improved public education about breast cancer has dramatically increased the percentage of cases that present with early stage disease (2). In addition, treatment advances have contributed to more favorable outcomes after breast-conservation therapy. Specifically, advances in surgery, radiation, and systemic treatments have reduced the risk of local recurrence for a patient with stage I disease to approximately 0.5% per year (3–5).

This chapter will review the progress that has been made in breast-conservation therapy. The data from randomized trials comparing breast-conservation therapy versus mastectomy will be reviewed, the importance of radiation as a component of treatment will be highlighted, the patient-, treatment-, and tumor-related factors that influence outcome will be discussed, and the technical details of optimizing both surgical and radiation treatment of early stage breast cancer will be summarized.

BREAST CONSERVATION AS AN ALTERNATIVE TO MASTECTOMY

After the advent of mammographic screening and increased public awareness, patients began presenting with early stage tumors and single institutions began pilot studies investigating breast-conserving surgery and radiation therapy as an alternative to mastectomy. Based on initial positive results, several phase III clinical trials were developed to directly compare these two approaches. One of the largest and most influential of these trials was conducted by the National Surgical Adjuvant Breast and Bowel Project (NSABP) between 1976 and 1984. The NSABP B-06 trial enrolled 1,600 women with primary tumors up to 4 cm and randomly assigned patients to one of three locoregional treatments: modified radical mastectomy, lumpectomy plus axillary dissection with breast irradiation, or lumpectomy plus axillary dissection alone (6). Twenty-year outcome data from this trial indicated that lumpectomy and whole breast radiation therapy provided equivalent long-term disease-free and overall survival compared with patients treated with a modified radical mastectomy. The 20-year probabilities of local or regional recurrence in the lumpectomy and radiation arm were 14.3% within the breast and 2.7% in the regional lymph nodes. Locoregional control was achieved with

a salvage mastectomy for the majority of patients who developed an in-breast recurrence. The 20-year locoregional recurrence rates for the patients treated with mastectomy were 10.2% for the chest wall and 4.6% for the regional lymph nodes (7).

A second important trial conducted at the Milan Cancer Institute during this same era also has reported 20-year outcome data comparing mastectomy and breast-conservation surgery with breast irradiation. In this study, 701 women with T1 primary tumors were randomized to radical mastectomy or a quadrantectomy, axillary dissection, plus whole breast radiation. After 20 years of follow-up there were no differences in the rates of distant metastases or overall survival. There was an increased risk of having an in-breast recurrence (8.8% at 20 years) compared to having a chest wall recurrence (2.3%) (8).

The Early Breast Cancer Trialists' Collaborative Group (EBCTCG) performed a meta-analysis using the raw data from the 4,125 women enrolled in randomized trials that compared mastectomy versus breast-conservation surgery and radiation. Their results confirmed equivalent rates of overall survival and rates of breast cancer mortality in patients treated with mastectomy and those treated with breast-conservation therapy (9). The rates of isolated local recurrences at 10 years (13% vs. 11%) and 15 years (17% vs. 12%) were slightly higher in the cohort of patients treated with breast-conservation surgery and radiation compared to those treated with mastectomy. One important aspect that needs to be considered when evaluating local recurrence data from these early trials is that major advances have occurred since that time in diagnostic imaging, image guidance of lesions for surgical resection, margin assessment, radiation treatment techniques, and systemic treatments, which have all served to significantly decreased the local recurrence rates with breast conservation. For example, investigators from the University of Texas M.D. Anderson Cancer Center reported their 27-year experience with treating 1,355 patients with breast-conservation therapy for invasive disease (3). Their analysis found that the 5-year rate of in-breast recurrence was significantly lower in the patients treated between 1994 to 1996 compared to the subgroup treated before 1994 (1.3% vs. 5.7%; $p = .0001$). In part, this was because the more recent patient cohort was less likely to have positive or unknown margin status and more likely to have received systemic treatments in addition to surgery and radiation.

For patients with lymph node–positive disease, breast-conservation therapy (which routinely involved radiation therapy) may offer an outcome advantage over treatment with mastectomy without radiation. A study using data from the Surveillance, Epidemiology, and End Results (SEER) compared the outcome of 12,693 patients with one to three positive lymph nodes treated with breast-conservation therapy with radiation to the outcome of 18,902 patients with one to three positive lymph nodes treated with mastectomy without radiation (10). The 15-year breast cancer–specific survival was 80% for breast conservation and 72% for mastectomy without radiation ($p < .001$). Cox regression analysis showed that mastectomy without radiation was associated with a 1.19 hazard ratio for breast cancer death ($p < .001$) and a 1.25 hazard ratio for overall death ($p < .001$).

ROLE OF RADIATION IN BREAST CONSERVATION

Radiation treatments play a critical role in successful breast-conservation therapy for patients with invasive breast cancer. It has been clearly demonstrated that radiation treatment of the ipsilateral breast reduces the probability of local recurrence after lumpectomy. More importantly, collective data from randomized prospective trials comparing surgery with or without postoperative radiation therapy indicate that by eradicating persistent local disease after surgery, radiation use reduces the risk of subsequent distant metastases and death.

Similar to the trials comparing mastectomy and breast conservation, the EBCTCG performed a meta-analysis of the data from 7,300 women who participated in randomized trials of breast-conserving surgery with or without radiation therapy. Their results indicated that breast irradiation reduced the 10-year rate of in-breast recurrence from 29% to 10% for patients with negative lymph nodes and from 47% to 13% for patients with positive lymph nodes (11). The more important finding from this meta-analysis concerned survival outcomes. For the first time, it was demonstrated that radiation use significantly decreased the 15-year risk of dying from breast cancer. As shown in Figure 37.1, in patients with negative lymph nodes the breast cancer mortality was

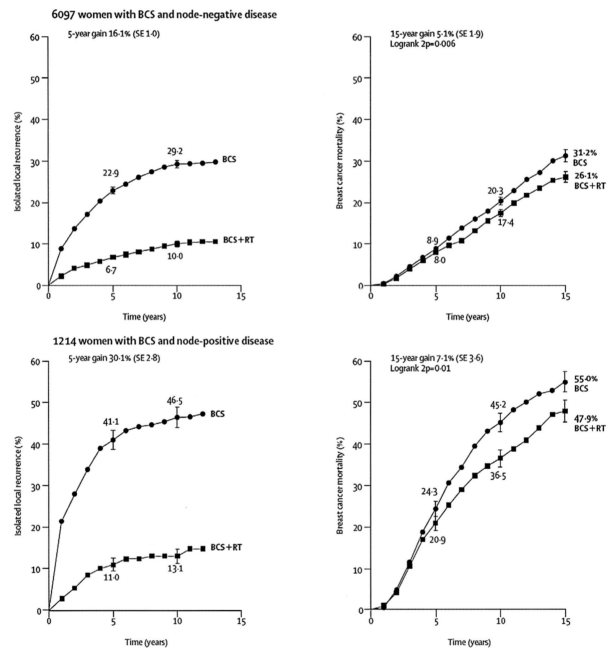

FIGURE 37.1. The data from the Early Breast Cancer Trialists' Collaborative Group (EBCTCG) meta-analysis of trials investigating breast-conservation therapy (BCT) with or without breast radiation. For both patients with lymph node–negative disease and those with lymph node–positive disease, radiation use significantly reduced isolated local recurrence and breast cancer mortality. (From Effects of radiotherapy and of differences in the extent of surgery for early breast cancer on local recurrence and 15-year survival: an overview of the randomised trials. Early Breast Cancer Trialists' Collaborative Group. *Lancet* 2005;366:2087–2106, with permission.)

reduced from 31% to 26% and for patients with positive lymph nodes and the breast cancer mortality was reduced from 55% to 48% (11). Finally, the 15-year overall death rates were also reduced (41% for breast-conservation surgery alone versus 35% for breast-conserving surgery plus radiation; $p = .005$). The EBCTCG recently updated these data to include more recent studies that predominantly focused on patients with more favorable disease characteristics. The most recent analysis included 9,000 patients and found very similar results: breast cancer mortality reduced from 26% to 23% ($p = .02$) for patients with negative lymph nodes and 51% to 43% ($p < .001$) for patients with positive lymph nodes (9).

These data conclusively demonstrate that radiation use after breast-conserving surgery eradicates disease within the breast in about 70% of patients who have persistent disease after surgery. Furthermore, one can conclude that foci of persistent disease, if not eradicated with radiation, can be a source of distant metastases and subsequent breast cancer–related death. These data suggest that one of four patients in whom radiation prevented a locoregional recurrence at 5 years avoided death due to breast cancer at 15 years of follow-up (11). The remaining patients were either successfully salvaged with additional treatments of their local recurrence or died from metastatic disease that was not prevented by eradicating persistent locoregional disease. The 5% to 7% absolute survival advantage associated with radiation is clinically significant and comparable to important advances in systemic treatments.

The EBCTCG meta-analysis provided a fundamental change in a thought paradigm that had been prevalent for many decades, namely that local recurrences were a marker of risk for distant metastases, but were not a source of distant metastases (12). This paradigm arose after individual trials failed to demonstrate survival differences despite improvements in local or regional control. There are two reasons why the EBCTCG meta-analysis was able to demonstrate a survival advantage whereas the individual trials did not. First, the meta-analysis had a much larger sample size and therefore was more adequately powered statistically to detect small but relevant survival differences. The second reason is that at the time the meta-analysis was conducted a number of trials had extended or mature follow-up. The survival curves in Figure 37.1 show that the survival advantages with radiation use were noted between 5 to 15 years of follow-up (11). This highlights the fact that the timing of realization of the survival benefits associated with improved locoregional treatment is fundamentally different from the timing of survival benefits associated with systemic treatments. Systemic treatments improve outcome by eradicating foci of micrometastatic disease foci that are present at the time of initial systemic treatment. When no systemic treatment is given, these foci progress, become clinically evident, and subsequently contribute to death. In contrast, locoregional treatments improve survival by eradicating persistent local disease in patients who may not have systemic micrometastatic disease (or who have micrometastatic disease eliminated by systemic treatments). In these situations, if adjuvant radiation is not used, the persistent local disease will progress, leading to 5-year differences in locoregional outcomes. However, for this persistent local disease to cause survival differences it must result in metastasis during the interval between the original local treatment and the salvage treatment for the local recurrence. The time needed for these new metastases to progress to the point where they are clinically meaningful likely takes many years, which accounts for the long delay before the survival advantage is seen in locoregional treatment trials.

Do All Patients Treated with Breast-Conservation Therapy Require Radiation?

The initial trials that demonstrated a clear benefit for radiation in breast-conservation therapy included populations that were heterogeneous with respect to risk factors associated with in-breast recurrence. Therefore, the second generation of clinical trials studying breast-conservation therapy investigated whether radiation could be safely omitted in favorable subgroups. Unfortunately, most of these studies were unsuccessful in answering the question. For example, a single arm, 82 patient prospective trial conducted at Harvard investigated whether breast radiation could be omitted in patients with pT1N0 breast cancer without an extensive intraductal component or lymphovascular space invasion that was excised with 1 cm or greater margins. Despite these favorable features, the trial needed to be closed early after the breast recurrence rate exceeded the predefined stopping rules. The local recurrence rate after a median follow-up of 86 months was 23% (13). These recurrence rates were similar to a trial from the Milan Cancer Institute that randomized women with tumors 2.5 cm or smaller to a quadrantectomy and axillary dissection without radiation or this same surgery followed by breast irradiation. Despite a more extensive surgical procedure than what is routinely utilized in most North American trials, the 10-year risk of in-breast recurrence was markedly higher in the absence of radiation therapy (24%) compared with patients who received radiation therapy (6%) ($p < .001$) (14). Randomized trials from Sweden and Finland have also attempted to specifically address whether patients with stage I disease require radiation therapy after breast-conserving surgery. As seen in the Harvard and the Milan trials, in both of these studies the rates of local recurrence without radiation remained clinically relevant such that and the use of radiation led to a highly significant improvement in local outcomes in those women randomized to receive radiation (15,16). Finally, it is also clear from several trials that the use of adjuvant chemotherapy does not obviate the need for breast irradiation. For example, in the NSABP B-06 trial, chemotherapy was used for patients with lymph node–positive disease and these patients had a 44% 20-year risk of in-breast recurrence without radiation compared to a rate of only 9% for those treated with lumpectomy, radiation, and chemotherapy (7).

The most recent randomized trials investigating whether a favorable cohort can be defined who have a low risk of in-breast recurrence without radiation have focused on postmenopausal women with hormone receptor–positive stage I disease treated with breast-conserving surgery and hormonal therapy. The data from these trials are shown in Table 37.1 and demonstrate that the combined modality treatment of breast-conserving surgery, radiation, and adjuvant hormonal therapy is associated with a very low 5-year risk of in-breast or locoregional recurrence. In contrast, data from the Scottish trial and the NSABP B-21 trial suggest that the risk of in-breast recurrence remains clinically relevant with breast-conserving surgery and hormonal therapy alone. The one cohort of patients for whom breast-conserving surgery without radiation might be considered as an appropriate option are elderly females with an estrogen receptor–positive stage I breast cancer who are treated with hormonal therapy. The Cancer and Leukemia Group-B (CALGB) Intergroup trial randomized women aged 70 and older with these disease characteristics to breast-conserving surgery plus tamoxifen or breast-conserving surgery, tamoxifen, and breast irradiation. The 5-year results of this trial noted a small but significant benefit for radiation, but the recurrence rate in the surgery and tamoxifen arm was only 4.4% (17). A 2006 update from this trial indicated that with a

Table 37.1	RANDOMIZED STUDIES COMPARING RADIATION USE AFTER BREAST-CONSERVING SURGERY IN PATIENTS WITH STAGE I DISEASE TREATED WITH HORMONAL THERAPY				
Trial (Reference)	No. Patients: Selection	Follow-Up (median mos)	Hormonal Therapy (%)	Hormonal Therapy + Radiation (%)	5-Yr End Point
NSABP B-21 (4)	1,009: ≤1 cm, pN0	87	8.4	1.1	LR
Scottish (78)	427: <70, T1,2, pN0	67	25.0	3.1	L-RR
Austrian (79)	869: ≤3 cm, grade 1, 2, pN0	54	5.1	0.4	LR
Canadian (80)	769: >50, T1/2, pN0	67	7.7	0.6	LR
			13.2	1.1	L-RR
CALGB (17,18)	636: >70, T1, c, pN0	95	7	1	Crude L-RR

LR, local recurrence; L-RR, local-regional recurrence.

median follow-up of 7.9 years, radiation reduced the locoregional recurrence from 7% to 1% (18). It should be noted that approximately one of six of these patients enrolled in this studied died of intercurrent disease by 5 years. Therefore, how these data should be applied to women over 70 who have a longer life-expectancy is less clear. To further study this question, investigators from Yale University reviewed the SEER-Medicare database and identified 8,724 patients who met the eligibility criteria for this trial. They found similar 5-year outcome rates as those reported in the Intergroup trial (19). However, these investigators also were able to analyze particular subsets and found that the benefits of radiation were of a clinically relevant magnitude for patients aged 70 to 79 who had no comorbidities. In contrast, those patients 80 years or older and those with multiple comorbidities had a higher risk of dying from nonbreast cancer–related causes within 5 years and therefore were not at high risk of developing an in-breast recurrence.

In conclusion, all of the clinical studies to date have indicated that without breast irradiation, the risk of local recurrences after breast-conserving surgery alone is too high, and, therefore, breast irradiation should be considered a standard component of treatment for all women with early stage invasive disease. Thus far, the attempts to define subsets of breast cancer patients with favorable early stage disease that may not require radiation by using standard clinical and pathologic criteria have been unsuccessful, with the possible exception of women over 70 with stage I, estrogen-receptor–positive disease who are willing to be treated with hormonal therapy. Studies are under way to find molecular markers that can reliably identify patients who may be adequately treated with breast-conserving surgery alone without the need for radiation.

SELECTION CRITERIA FOR BREAST-CONSERVATION THERAPY

Breast-conservation therapy is generally reserved for patients with tumors smaller than 4 cm. However, more important than absolute tumor size is the relationship between tumor size and breast size. The tumor must be small enough, in relation to the size of the breast, to permit the tumor to be resected with adequate margins and acceptable cosmesis.

In patients with invasive breast cancer in which the tumor to breast size ratio is unfavorable, the use of preoperative chemotherapy may decrease the tumor size sufficiently to permit breast-conservation therapy (discussed in Chapter 60). Another strategy for patients with large tumors is to use oncoplastic techniques such as local tissue rearrangement or pedicled myocutaneous flaps (e.g., a latissimus dorsi flap) to fill the defect resulting from breast-conservation therapy. For

patients requiring a large volume of breast to be resected, this approach can improve aesthetic outcomes. For patients with larger breasts, often the repair of the partial breast resection defect can be done with tissue rearrangement or reduction mammoplasty techniques. In contrast, smaller breasts may require an autologous tissue flap (20,21). Consulting with medical oncology and plastic surgery prior to the surgical intervention allows for a multidisciplinary approach and optimizes the chance of breast conservation in patients with larger tumors.

The success of breast-conservation therapy is dependent on the ability to surgically remove the gross volume of disease and achieve negative histological margins. Although this is a realistic goal for most patients with early stage breast cancer, there continue to be some subsets that are better suited for mastectomy. For example, some patients with early stage breast cancer present with diffuse ductal carcinoma *in situ* (DCIS) over a very large area of the breast, as determined by mammographically diffuse suspicious microcalcifications, and are better suited for mastectomy. In addition, mastectomy is appropriate when repeated attempts at breast-conserving surgery fail to achieve negative surgical margins. Patients with multicentric tumors are not considered to be good candidates for breast conservation since recurrence rates may be higher with such tumors and it is difficult to perform more than one breast-conserving surgery in the same breast with acceptable cosmesis.

There are also patient subsets that are at higher risk for a radiation-related complication that may benefit from undergoing mastectomy. For example, women who develop breast cancer during pregnancy should avoid radiation because the internal radiation scatter from treatment of the intact breast can reach lethal and teratogenic dose levels, particularly in the first trimester (22). For these reasons, it is critical that all women of child-bearing age be counseled against becoming pregnant during the course of radiation therapy. In addition, patients with specific connective tissue diseases are at increased risk for significant late radiation complications, including significant breast fibrosis and pain, chest wall necrosis, and brachial plexopathy. The collagen vascular diseases associated with the greatest risk for radiation injury are systemic scleroderma, systemic lupus erythematosus, polymyositis or dermatomyositis, and mixed connective tissue disorders (23,24). In a study from Massachusetts General Hospital in Boston, 131 patients with rheumatoid arthritis did not appear to have elevated rates of late toxic effects after breast irradiation (24).

Based on data such as those presented above, the American College of Surgeons, the American College of Radiology, the College of American Pathologists, and the Society of Surgical Oncology developed standards of care for breast-conservation therapy and published their most recent report in 2002 (25). Key portions of this report are summarized below.

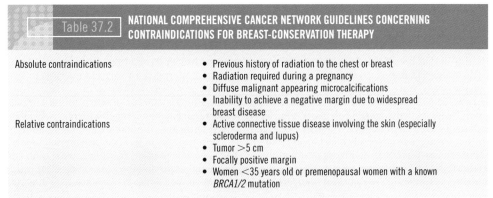

Table 37.2	NATIONAL COMPREHENSIVE CANCER NETWORK GUIDELINES CONCERNING CONTRAINDICATIONS FOR BREAST-CONSERVATION THERAPY
Absolute contraindications	• Previous history of radiation to the chest or breast • Radiation required during a pregnancy • Diffuse malignant appearing microcalcifications • Inability to achieve a negative margin due to widespread breast disease
Relative contraindications	• Active connective tissue disease involving the skin (especially scleroderma and lupus) • Tumor >5 cm • Focally positive margin • Women <35 years old or premenopausal women with a known *BRCA1/2* mutation

From Carlson RW, Anderson BO, Burstein HJ, et al. Invasive breast cancer. *J Natl Compr Canc Netw* 2007;5:246–312.

Because of the potential options for treatment of early stage breast cancer, careful patient selection and a multidisciplinary approach are necessary. The four critical elements in patient selection for breast-conservation therapy are: (a) history and physical examination, (b) mammographic evaluation, (c) histologic assessment of the resected breast specimen, and (d) assessment of the patient's needs and expectations.

Age, *per se*, whether young or old, is not a contraindication to breast conservation. In the elderly, physiologic age and the presence of comorbid conditions should be the primary determinants of local therapy. Retraction of the skin, nipple, and breast parenchyma are not necessarily signs of locally advanced breast cancer and are not contraindications to breast conservation.

The National Comprehensive Cancer Network has also published guidelines concerning the use of breast-conservation therapy (26). The contraindications for breast-conservation therapy according to NCCN guidelines are listed in Table 37.2. The NCCN also has provided guidelines for the use of radiation after breast-conserving surgery. The NCCN recommends whole breast irradiation for all patients with invasive disease treated with a lumpectomy, with the allowance for use of breast-conserving surgery with negative margins, plus hormonal therapy without breast irradiation for women aged 70 or older with negative lymph nodes and estrogen receptor-positive disease.

Patient-, Disease-, and Treatment-Related Factors Associated with Local Outcome after Breast-Conservation Therapy

Patients treated with breast-conservation therapy have excellent rates of local control. The EBCTCG meta-analysis of the first generation of clinical trials investigating breast conservation reported a 5-year in-breast recurrence rate of 6.7% for patients with node-negative disease and 11% for those with node-positive disease (11). The respective 10-year in-breast recurrence rates for these cohorts were 10% and 13.1%, respectively. As previously indicated, there have been a number of changes that occurred over the past few decades that have favorably affected these rates. In part these changes have come from a greater understanding of patient, disease, and treatment factors that are associated with local recurrences. Factors that are associated with local recurrences are highlighted in Table 37.3. The improved understanding of these factors that contribute to local recurrence has helped to refine the selection criteria for breast conservation and have led to changes in treatment techniques to improve outcomes.

Patient Factors

An important patient-related factor that affects in-breast recurrence rates is patient age. Several single-institution studies have reported that young patient age, usually defined as aged

Table 37.3	PATIENT-, DISEASE-, AND TREATMENT-RELATED FACTORS ASSOCIATED WITH LOCAL CONTROL AFTER BREAST-CONSERVATION THERAPY		
	Patient-Related Factors	**Disease-Related Factors**	**Treatment-Related Factors**
High risk for local recurrence— consider mastectomy	Pregnancy, scleroderma or active systemic lupus or other condition that precludes radiation treatments	Diffuse microcalcifications throughout the breast Gross multicentric disease Inflammatory breast cancer	Lack of radiation treatments Inability to obtain negative surgical margins despite re-excision
Intermediate risk—breast conservation still acceptable	Germline mutation in *BRCA1/2* Age 35 or less	High Onco*type* Dx score[a] Unfavorable molecular expression profile[a] Metaplastic histology	Lack of systemic therapy Lack of a tumor bed boost Margins under 2 mm or focally positive margins
Low risk—data are mixed, these factors should not affect decisions regarding breast conservation	Patient ethnicity Family history	Lobular histology Nuclear grade Estrogen/progesterone receptor status *HER2/neu* status	

[a] Additional data are needed to validate initial studies.

less than 30 to 40 years, is associated with an increased risk of local recurrence, distant metastasis, and reduced disease-specific survival (27–30). This finding was also noted in an European Organisation for Research and Treatment of Cancer (EORTC) randomized trial that investigated the use of a tumor bed boost after whole breast irradiation. Overall, when patients from both arms of the study were evaluated, the 5-year in-breast recurrence rate for patients aged 40 or less was 15%, compared to rates of 7% for patients aged 41 to 50, 4% for 51 to 60, and 3% for patients older than 60 (27). Younger age has also been shown in some studies to adversely affect local recurrence rates after mastectomy. A study from investigators at the M.D. Anderson Cancer Center retrospectively evaluated the locoregional treatment outcome of 668 breast cancers in patients 35 or less years of age (28). In this series, patients with stage I disease who were treated with chemotherapy had acceptable locoregional treatment outcomes with either breast-conservation therapy or mastectomy. However, the patients with stage II disease treated with breast conservation (18%) or mastectomy without radiation (23%) had higher 10-year locoregional recurrence rates than those treated with mastectomy and postmastectomy radiation (6%).

A second important patient-related factor that can influence rates of breast recurrence is the presence of a germline mutation in *BRCA1* or *BRCA2*. Investigators from Yale University sequenced the *BRCA* gene status in 127 patients aged 42 or younger who were treated with lumpectomy and radiation and found 22 with deleterious mutations. After 12 years, the rates of ipsilateral breast recurrence (49% vs. 21%; *p* = .007) and contralateral cancer s (42% vs. 9%; *p* = .001) were both significantly higher in the patients with *BRCA* mutations (31). Many of these ipsilateral breast "recurrences" may be second breast cancers. Also, these high rates of in-breast recurrence may be significantly less in carriers who have undergone a bilateral oophorectomy. This finding was noted in a multicenter retrospective study that did not find an overall difference in the 10-year rate of in-breast recurrence in mutation carriers (12%) versus matched controls (9%). However, mutation carriers who had not had a bilateral oophorectomy experienced increased rates of in-breast recurrence compared to controls (hazard ratio [HR] 1.99; *p* = .04) (32). Table 37.4 displays published studies that have evaluated the rates of ipsilateral tumor recurrences and of contralateral breast cancer in *BRCA* mutation carriers.

Disease-Related Factors

One of the most important pathologic factors that affect rates of local control after breast-conserving surgery and radiation therapy is surgical margins. When breast-conservation therapy was first introduced, the importance of achieving histologically negative margins was not recognized, and a number of patients in early breast-conservation therapy publications had either unknown margin status or positive surgical margins. Retrospective analyses indicated that such patients had higher

rates of in-breast recurrence, particularly if the disease had an extensive intraductal component (defined as tumors that are predominantly noninvasive or tumors with a DCIS component comprising at least 25% and with DCIS present in surrounding normal breast tissue) (33). A review of selected series evaluating the importance of surgical margins in breast-conservation therapy is shown in Table 37.5.

It is now standard practice to ink surgical specimens and report margin status quantitatively as the distance of tumor to inked surfaces. In addition, the recognition of the importance of margin status in local control has led to increased rates of re-excision. For patients in whom re-excision carries a significant aesthetic consequence, the degree of margin involvement should be considered. Specifically, some retrospective series have found that patients with a focally positive margin have better outcomes that those with margin involvement over a wider area. In one study, Vicini et al. (34) retrospectively reassessed margin status in 607 cases treated with breast conservation and reported a 12-year in-breast recurrence rate of 9% in patients with negative margins, 6% when a small amount of disease was close to the margin, 18% for those with an intermediate degree of disease close to the margin, 24% for those with a large volume of disease close to margin, and 30% for those with a positive margin. It is also useful to note that margins at the skin anteriorly or at the pectoral fascia posteriorly are not of concern since breast tissue does not extend beyond those margins. Good communication between the surgical and radiation oncologist is important in this regard.

Not surprising, the importance of margin status on in-breast recurrence is also affected by other factors, such as age, use of systemic therapy, and timing of radiation delivery. Park et al. (35) reported that the use of systemic treatments reduced the in-breast recurrence rates for patients with focally positive margins (8-year rate of 7%), whereas higher rates were seen in those with focally positive margins who did not receive systemic therapy and in all patients with more diffusely positive margins. Jobson et al. (36) showed that margin status was of particular importance in women aged 40 years old or less. In this younger cohort, the risk of in-breast recurrence according to margin status was 37% in those with positive margins compared with only 8% in those with negative margins. Finally, in a randomized prospective trial, investigators from Harvard found that patients with close or positive margins had a high rate of in-breast recurrence if radiation was delayed in order to first deliver adjuvant chemotherapy, but if negative margins were achieved, there was no adverse affect of radiation delay in local control (37).

Taken together, these data suggest that margin status correlates with long-term local control for patients treated with breast-conservation therapy. It is therefore reasonable to recommend re-excision for patients with positive margins and individualize treatment recommendations for patients with close margins. In general, re-excision should be performed for young patients with margins of less than 2 mm if it can be performed with an acceptable aesthetic outcome. In addition,

Table 37.4	RATES OF IPSILATERAL TUMOR RECURRENCES AND DEVELOPMENT OF CONTRALATERAL BREAST CANCER IN *BRCA* CARRIERS TREATED WITH BREAST-CONSERVATION THERAPY			
Study (Reference)	No. of Patients	Follow-Up (yrs)	Ipsilateral Breast Recurrence (%)	Contralateral Breast Cancer Development (%)
Pierce et al. (32)	160	15	24	39
Haffty et al. (31)	23	12	46	42
Robson et al. (81)	87	10	14	38
Seynaeve et al. (82)	87	10	30	14

| Table 37.5 | IPSILATERAL BREAST RECURRENCE RATES BY MARGIN STATUS (%) |

Author (Institution; Reference)	No. Patients (Median FU)	End Point	Negative	Close	Positive
Borger (The Netherlands; 83)	1,026 (6.5 yr)	5-yr actuarial	2	6	16
Dewar et al. (Gustave-Roussy; 84)	757 (9 yr)	10-yr actuarial	6	—	14
Freedman et al. (Fox Chase; 85)	1,262 (6.3 yr)	5-yr actuarial	4	7	5
		10-yr actuarial	7	14	12
Park et al. (JCRT; 35)	340 (10.8 yr)	8-yr crude rate	7	7	14[a]/27[b]
Anscher et al. (Duke; 86)	259 (3.8 yr)	5-yr actuarial	2	—	10
Smitt et al. (Stanford; 87)	289 (6 yr)	10-yr actuarial	2	16	0[a]/9[b]
Peterson et al. (U. Penn.; 88)	1,021 (6.1 yr)	8-yr actuarial	8	17	10
Wazer et al. (Tufts; 89)	498 (121 mos)	12-yr actuarial	5	9	17
Pittinger et al. (U. Rochester; 91)	211 (4.5 yr)	Crude rate (FU 54 mos)	3	2.9	25
Cowen et al. (Marseilles; 90)	152 (6 yr)	5-yr actuarial	—	—	20
Obedian and Haffty (Yale; 92)	984 (13 yr)	10-yr actuarial	2	2	18
Cabioglu et al (MDACC; 3)	1,043 (8.4 yr)	5-yr actuarial	4		8
Vicini et al. (William Beaumont; 34)	607 (8.5 yr)	12-yr actuarial	9	6	18[a]/24[b]

FU, follow-up; JCRT, Joint Center for Radiation Therapy; U. Penn, University of Pennsylvania; U. Rochester, University of Rochester; MDACC, M.D. Anderson Cancer Center.
[a]Focally positive.
[b]More than focally positive.

re-excision should be considered for patients with tumors that are triple negative (negative for estrogen receptor, progesterone receptor, and *HER2/neu*), whereas in older women with estrogen-receptor positive disease who are also going to receive hormonal therapy, treatment of a close margin with breast irradiation plus a boost is a reasonable alternative (35).

Other disease-related factors that have been correlated with local control rates include the presence of multicentric disease, histology of the tumor, lymphovascular space invasion, and the stage of disease. Limited data suggest that gross multicentric disease, defined as separate foci of disease in different quadrants of the breast, adversely affects local outcome (38). Most tumor histologies have similar local recurrence rates when all other factors are considered equal. For example, Salvadori et al. (39) reported that the in-breast tumor recurrence rate for 286 cases of lobular cancer was 7% and was equivalent to the rate for those patients with infiltrating ductal carcinoma. Similarly, investigators from the M.D. Anderson Cancer Center reported a 7% 10-year recurrence rate for patients with lobular carcinoma versus a 9% rate for those with invasive ductal carcinoma (40). One unusual histology that may be associated with higher rates of local recurrence after breast conservation and mastectomy is metaplastic carcinoma (41). Lymphovascular space invasion has also been noted by multiple authors to be associated with increased rates of in-breast recurrence after lumpectomy and radiation (16,42). Finally, stage of disease has a relatively minor influence on the likelihood of in-breast recurrence. In the EBCTCG meta-analysis of data from randomized trials, the 5-year risk of local recurrence was 11% in patients with positive lymph nodes versus 7% for those with negative lymph nodes (11). Investigators from the M.D. Anderson Cancer Center found that stage was an important factor in local recurrence rates for young breast cancer patients. The 10-year rate of local recurrence after breast-conserving surgery, radiation, and chemotherapy for patients aged 35 years or less was 12% for those with stage I disease and 18% for those with stage II disease (28).

Recently, there has been increasing interest in defining molecular features predictive of local recurrence after conservative surgery and radiation, but to date limited data are available. In the NSABP B-06 trial, grade and estrogen and progesterone-receptor status affected local recurrence rates for patients treated with lumpectomy alone but had no influence on recurrence patterns for patients treated with lumpectomy

and radiation therapy (43). Investigators from the University of Pennsylvania studied a cohort of patients treated with breast conservation and did not find a correlation between *HER2/neu* and in-breast recurrence (44). The more recent studies have focused on molecular subtyping breast cancer, based on either gene expression profiling or on the combination of the status of *HER2/neu* and estrogen receptor and progesterone receptor. One of the more aggressive subtypes is the category of triple negative disease, in which all three of these biomarkers (estrogen receptor, progesterone receptor,, and *HER2/neu*) are not expressed in the primary tumor. Haffty et al. (45) investigated the relationship of triple negative disease with outcome in 117 patients treated with breast conservation and reported a higher rate of distant recurrences with triple negative disease versus those with other subtypes but no differences in local control. In contrast, in a more contemporary series of patients treated with negative margins and common use of hormonal- and chemotherapy (but not trastuzumab), Nguyen et al. (46) noted an increased hazard ratio for local recurrence for patients with estrogen receptor–negative, *HER2/neu*-positive disease and for patients with a triple negative phenotype compared to patients with estrogen or progesterone receptor–positive disease. Although new therapies have yet to be established in the patients with triple negative disease, the relationship of *HER2/neu* and outcome will change with the routine use of trastuzumab, which has a significant positive effect in reducing recurrences in the *HER2/neu*-positive patient subset.

Preliminary data are also emerging from studies evaluating multigene predictors of local outcomes. Mamounas et al. (47) found that a 21-gene recurrence score (Onco*type* Dx, Genomic Health, Redwood City, California) could be used to predict for locoregional recurrence in tamoxifen-treated patients with estrogen receptor–positive, lymph node–negative breast cancer (47). Finally, investigators from The Netherlands have provided preliminary data characterizing a microarray-determined gene expression profile signature that predicted for local recurrence after breast-conservation therapy (48). These preliminary data will require validation in an independent set of patients.

Treatment Factors

Systemic treatments reduce the risk of recurrence in the ipsilateral breast in patients who are treated with whole breast

Table 37.6	EFFECT OF SYSTEMIC THERAPY ON IN-BREAST RECURRENCE RATES IN PATIENTS TREATED WITH BREAST-CONSERVING SURGERY AND RADIATION			
Study (Reference)	No. of Patients: Selection, Type of Systemic Treatment	Follow-Up (yrs)	Radiation (%)	Systemic Therapy + Radiation (%)
NSABP B-21 (4)	673: ≤1 cm, pN0, tamoxifen	8	9.3	2.8
NSABP B-13 (93)	760: pN0, chemotherapy	10	15.3	2.6
M.D. Anderson Cancer Center (94)	484: pN0, chemotherapy or tamoxifen	8	14.8	4.4
Yale (95)	548: chemotherapy or tamoxifen	7	12	6

irradiation. Table 37.6 shows data from prospective trials and single institution studies highlighting this benefit. In the NSABP B-21 trial, which enrolled patients with lymph node–negative breast tumors smaller than 1 cm, the crude rate of in-breast tumor recurrence was only 3% in patients treated with lumpectomy, radiation therapy, and tamoxifen compared with 7% in women treated with lumpectomy and radiation therapy without tamoxifen (4).

A tumor bed boost after whole breast irradiation is another treatment-related factor that can decrease the risk of in-breast recurrence. The first randomized trial investigating the impact of a 10-Gy boost after 50 Gy of breast irradiation was performed in Lyon, France. The use of a boost led to a small but statistically significant reduction in the rate of local recurrence at 5 years (3.6% vs. 4.5%; $p = .04$) (49). The EORTC has subsequently published a much larger trial that randomized patients to receive or not receive a 16 Gy boost after 50 Gy of whole breast radiation treatment. The use of a boost reduced the risk of an in-breast recurrence at 5 years by a factor of 2 ($p < .001$, the absolute reduction in risk at 5 years was ~4%) (27,50). All patient age subgroups appeared to achieve a benefit from the boost, but the absolute benefit was greatest in the younger patients. A recent update of this trial found that at 10-years, the risk of in-breast recurrence was reduced with a tumor bed boost from 10.2% to 6.2% (50). The 10-year results of the EORTC trial for patients divided according to age are shown in Table 37.7.

INTEGRATION OF RADIATION WITH SYSTEMIC TREATMENT

Most patients with early stage breast cancer are treated with surgery, systemic therapy, and radiation, and therefore the sequencing of radiation with systemic treatments remains an important clinical question. To determine the optimal sequencing schedule of chemotherapy and radiation, investigators from Harvard Dana Farber Cancer Center conducted a randomized trial that compared four cycles of doxorubicin-based combination chemotherapy followed by radiation therapy or radiation therapy followed by the same chemotherapy. The updated results showed no statistically significant differences in local recurrence, distant metastasis, or overall survival between the two groups (37). Patients with close surgical margins had an increased risk of local recurrence when sequenced with chemotherapy followed by radiation, suggesting that re-excision should be considered for such patients. A second important study from the CALGB addressed whether a more extended delay in radiation in order to treat with both anthracyclines and taxanes increased local recurrence risk. These investigators reported that those treated with paclitaxel after anthracyclines had lower risks of isolated locoregional recurrence than those treated with just four cycles of anthracyclines (3.7% vs. 9.7%, respectively; $p = .04$) (51). Given this information, it has become standard that patients receive initial chemotherapy followed by radiation therapy.

There are no randomized trials that directly compared concurrent tamoxifen and radiation versus radiation followed by tamoxifen. However, three recent retrospective reports reported no difference in outcome according to the sequencing of radiation and hormonal therapy. Pierce et al. (52) examined this question in 309 patients treated within the Southwest Oncology Group and found 10-year rates of recurrence of 7% with concurrent treatment versus 5% with sequential therapies ($p = .54$). Ahn et al. (53) from Yale University examined this issue in 495 patients treated with breast conservation and also found no difference in local control, development of distant metastases, and overall survival after 10 years. Finally, Harris et al. (54) from the University of Pennsylvania conducted a similar analysis and also found very similar results.

Finally, for patients receiving adjuvant trastuzumab, most have continued this therapy concurrently during the course of radiation and the data thus far suggest that this combination is not associated with increase rates of complications. Data from the NSABP B-31 trial showed a rate of congestive heart failure of 3.2% for patients treated with trastuzumab and left-sided

Table 37.7	TEN-YEAR IN-BREAST RECURRENCE RATES OF THE EUROPEAN ORGANISATION FOR RESEARCH AND TREATMENT OF CANCER BOOST VERSUS NO BOOST TRIAL FOR PATIENTS DIVIDED ACCORDING TO AGE	
	Boost (%)	No Boost (%)
Overall results	10.2	6.2
Age ≤40	23.9	13.5
Age 41–50	12.5	8.7
Age 51–60	7.8	4.9
Age ≥60	7.3	3.8

From Bartelink H, Horiot JC, Poortmans PM, et al. Impact of a higher radiation dose on local control and survival in breast-conserving therapy of early breast cancer: 10-year results of the randomized boost versus no boost EORTC 22881-10882 trial. *J Clin Oncol* 2007;25:3259–3265, with permission.

radiation compared to a rate of 4% for those treated with trastuzumab and no left-sided radiation ($p = .80$) (55). These data were supported by the North Central Cancer Treatment Group N9831 trial that compared the rate of cardiac events in patients treated with trastuzumab with (1.5%) or without (6.3%) radiation (56). Furthermore, none of the radiation-associated adverse events were increased in those treated concurrently with trastuzumab versus those who were not.

TREATMENT TECHNIQUES FOR BREAST-CONSERVATION THERAPY

Surgical Technique

The surgical incision should be placed as close to the primary tumor as possible. In the case of nonpalpable tumors that can be visualized with sonography, preoperative needle localization with sonographic guidance or intraoperative sonographic localization can be used to guide the surgical resection of the primary tumor. For nonpalpable lesions that cannot be visualized on sonography, mammographic needle localization is performed with a self-retaining hook wire that is placed under mammographic guidance. The tumor is resected with a margin of grossly normal tissue approximately 1-cm wide. The surgeon should orient the specimen anatomically for the pathologist. A specimen radiograph should be performed on all nonpalpable tumors to confirm resection of the index lesion. The pathologist or surgeon then should ink the margins and assess the microscopic margins histologically to confirm the adequacy of the excision. If the specimen is sectioned serially and repeat specimen radiographs are obtained, this can permit assessment of the relationship between the mammographic or sonographic abnormality and the margins of excision. A positive margin indicates that there is tumor at the inked margin of resection. A close margin is usually designated as tumor within 2 mm from the margin on final histologic analysis.

To optimize the cosmetic outcome, biopsy incisions in the upper breast are usually oriented in a curvilinear fashion, and biopsy incisions in the lower breast are oriented in a radial fashion. The incision is placed as close to the lesion being excised as possible, which results in less removal of uninvolved normal breast tissue. Once the lesion has been excised and the margins assessed, clips are placed to mark the extent of the resection cavity. Deep parenchymal sutures may be used for closing the defect, especially in patients who undergo large-volume excisions. If a large skin or parenchymal defect is anticipated before surgery, a plastic surgeon should be consulted or the surgeon should plan for the use of oncoplastic techniques. In patients with extensive calcifications, a postoperative mammogram is obtained before the initiation of radiation therapy. If the postoperative mammogram reveals residual calcifications in the breast, a re-excision should be performed to remove all suspicious microcalcifications.

In patients at risk for a suboptimal aesthetic outcome after partial mastectomy, oncoplastic breast surgery—that is, segmental or partial mastectomy to remove the tumor followed by plastic surgery to improve the aesthetic outcome—can potentially decrease the need and magnitude of surgery necessary for correction in the future. The need for oncoplastic breast surgery depends on several factors, including the extent of the planned resection, the tumor location, and the patient's breast size and body habitus. In general, oncoplastic techniques should be considered when (1) a significant area of skin needs to be resected with the specimen; (2) a large-volume defect is expected; (3) the tumor is located in an area associated with unfavorable cosmetic outcomes (e.g., the lower pole of the breast); or (4) excision may result in nipple malposition. The ratio of the volume of the defect to the volume of the remaining breast parenchyma will assist in determining the need for oncoplastic breast surgery.

Oncoplastic surgery has also raised new questions in the multidisciplinary management of breast cancer. To date, there are no long-term data regarding local recurrence risks with this approach. In addition, the tissue rearrangement frequently makes tumor bed localization for radiation boost treatment more difficult and can lead to difficulties with re-excisions should the final margin status return positive.

Radiation Treatments to the Whole Breast

Historically, radiation treatments have targeted the entire ipsilateral breast and treated this region to a dose of 45 to 50 Gy delivered in 25 to 28 daily fractions. Subsequently, a 1.5 to 2.0 cm volume around the surgical cavity is then treated as a tumor bed boost field with an additional 10 to 16 Gy in five to eight daily fractions, typically using electron beam. Treatments are given in an outpatient setting, and each daily treatment takes approximately 15 minutes in the treatment room. The entire course of therapy is typically 6 weeks.

The protracted nature of radiation treatments can place hardships on patients and medical systems. Accordingly, there has been an interest in studying whether the treatment course can be shortened without compromising the efficacy or increasing the toxicity of the therapy. The initial studies that investigated this question shortened the overall treatment course by giving a larger dose of radiation in each fraction. In a randomized prospective clinical trial, Whelan et al. (57) compared a 16-fraction course of whole breast radiation (42.5 Gy given over 22 days) to a 25-fraction course (50 Gy given over 35 days). All patients enrolled in this study had negative lymph nodes, 80% had T1N0 disease, and 75% were over age 50. Patients were treated without a boost to the primary site. After 5 years of follow-up, the 16-day hypofractionated schedule of radiation achieved equivalently low rates of in-breast recurrence and equivalently high rates of excellent to good aesthetic outcomes as the conventional 25-day schedule. A 2008 update of this trial with long-term results continued to show no difference between the two arms. Specifically, the 10-year risk of local recurrence was 6.2% (16 fraction course) versus 6.7% (25 fraction course), and the 10-year rates of good to excellent cosmetic outcome were 70% (16 fractions) versus 71% (25 fractions). For the 16 versus 25 fraction arms, the risk of moderate or severe late radiation effects for the skin was 6% versus 3% and for the subcutaneous tissue was 8% versus 4% respectively (58).

A similar prospective trial performed in the United Kingdom compared 50 Gy in 25 fractions (5 weeks) to 40 Gy in 15 fractions (3 weeks). The 5-year in-breast recurrence rate was 2.8%, and there were no significant differences in this end point between the two arms. The rate of change in the photographed appearance of the breast was also similar (58).

To date, implementation of these shorter fractionation schedules in the United States has been limited to postmenopausal patients with estrogen receptor–positive T1N0 disease who either have comorbid conditions or those for whom a 6-week course of therapy is a hardship. As discussed above, these patients are known to derive only a small absolute benefit from a boost. Treatment with larger fraction sizes has some theoretical disadvantages compared to the more protracted fractionation schedule. In addition, the significance of radiation fraction size may be different in different molecular classes of breast cancer. Specifically, it may be that lower dose per fraction schedules that are able to treat to high total doses may be very important in triple negative or "basal-type" cancers, whereas higher dose per fraction schedules may achieve equivalent outcome in estrogen receptor–positive disease or "luminal cancers." Additional research is needed to investigate such hypotheses.

Accelerated partial breast irradiation is also being investigated as a method to avoid the protracted course of whole breast treatment. This technique and the results are discussed in greater detail in Chapter 38. Briefly, the goal of this treatment is to complete radiation treatments in 1 week or less. To achieve this goal, the dose per fraction is significantly increased. Treatment of the entire breast volume with this fractionation scheme would be predicted to increase rates of complications. As complications are dependent on the relationship of dose and volume, these higher doses may be acceptable if treatment is limited to a much smaller treatment volume. The rationale for limiting the volume originated from the fact that the clinical trials investigating radiation in breast conservation demonstrated that the majority of in-breast recurrences develop at or near the tumor bed site when radiation is omitted. The absolute percentage of recurrences that develop in a location far away from the tumor bed is low, ranging from 3% to 5% (14,59,60), and some of these recurrences represent the development of new breast primaries that developed independent from the original cancer treatment.

There is a potential limitation in using data from studies that have investigated patterns of recurrence in patients treated with surgery alone to support the concept of treating only a small volume of breast tissue around the tumor bed. For patients with residual microscopic disease present after breast-conserving surgery, it is likely that the greatest disease burden will be located next to the tumor bed cavity, and, therefore, the first evidence of a recurrence would be predicted to be at the margin of the initial treatment. Partial breast radiation has the potential to extend this margin by 1 to 2 cm, but it is unclear whether the new margin of therapy will adequately capture the entire residual disease volume. Unfortunately, there are no tools with sufficient sophistication to accurately map out the area of potential residual disease. In many cases, the necessary target volume may be 0 cm beyond the surgical cavity in most of the areas, but 3 to 4 cm in another region of the tumor bed. Studies of mastectomy specimens support this. Faverly et al. (61) found that 28% of tumors measuring 2 cm or smaller had a focus of residual *in situ* or invasive carcinoma more than 2 cm from the primary tumor. Similarly, Vaidya et al. (62) performed a detailed three-dimensional pathologic analysis of whole-mount mastectomy specimens and found residual disease after lumpectomy in 63% of the cases, and in 79% of these cases, the disease extended beyond 25% of the breast volume surrounding the lumpectomy cavity.

Data from studies investigating the value of magnetic resonance imaging (MRI) in patients with early stage breast cancer also raise questions as to whether partial breast treatment covers the appropriate volume of tissue at risk for residual disease. An international collaborative study that examined MRI scanning in 417 patients with early stage breast cancer reported that 24% had incidental lesions detected away from the index site of disease (63). Seventy-one percent of these lesions were histologically confirmed to be cancer, and only 8% of these incidental lesions were detected by mammography. A second study investigating preoperative MRI scans in 267 breast-conservation surgery patients found that 18% of patients had foci of disease outside the index tumor bed (64). Such data suggest that a clinically relevant number of patients may have disease that extends beyond the partial breast treatment volume. In addition, these data may justify using breast MRI to help select optimal candidates for partial breast radiation.

The Milan III randomized trial that compared results using very wide excision (quadrantectomy) with and without whole breast radiation also provides some clinical insights about the potential value of whole breast treatment (14). In this trial, a larger volume of breast tissue surrounding the tumor was resected compared to a conventional lumpectomy, and despite a larger partial breast volume being treated, the 10-year rate of in-breast tumor recurrence rate in the quadrantectomy-only group was 24% versus 6% in the surgery plus whole breast irradiation arm.

The value and limitations of partial breast radiation will be defined by prospective clinical trials that are currently being conducted in the United States, Canada, and Europe. Until insights are available from the data of such studies, targeting the entire breast for patients treated with breast conservation is appropriate.

Indications for Targeting Lymph Nodes in the Radiation Treatment Volume

In addition to treatment of the breast, radiation treatments are highly effective in eradicating microscopic disease within regional lymph nodes. Accordingly, treatment of lymph node regions is indicated for appropriately selected patients. Patients with a negative sentinel lymph node dissection are at very low risk for residual nodal disease, and, therefore, radiation of lymphatics is not indicated. However, radiation of the lymphatics is indicated for selected patients with stage II disease and patients treated with breast conservation who are found to have four or more positive lymph nodes. Prospective clinical trials are currently being conducted to further define the risks, benefits, and indications for radiation of regional lymph nodes. Until such data are available, one reasonable approach for selection of lymphatic radiation treatment is shown in Table 37.8.

Technical Details of Radiation Treatments

A number of advances in radiation oncology technologies have significantly improved radiation treatments for breast cancer. Computed tomography (CT) simulation has replaced fluoroscopic guidance for delineation of treatment fields. The associated benefits of delineating and contouring three-dimensional target

Table 37.8	RADIATION TARGETING OF LYMPH NODES AS A COMPONENT OF BREAST-CONSERVING TREATMENT
Targeting of the breast only	Ductal carcinoma *in situ* Stage I disease with negative sentinel lymph node or axillary lymph node dissection
Targeting axillary levels I/II	Invasive breast cancer with unsuccessful or no sentinel lymph node dissection Positive sentinel lymph node without a completion level I/II axillary lymph node dissection
Targeting axillary level III and supraclavicular lymph nodes	Four or more positive lymph nodes found on sentinel and or axillary lymph node dissection Consider for 1–3 positive lymph nodes in the setting of: • young patient age • 20% or higher positive nodal ratio • extracapsular extension over 2 mm • extensive lymphovascular space invasion
Targeting the upper internal mammary lymph nodes	Positive internal mammary sentinel lymph nodes Consider when there is a positive axillary sentinel lymph node with dual drainage to the axilla and internal mammary chain on lymphoscintigraphy Consider when there is a positive axillary lymph node and the tumor is located in the medial, lower, or central breast

volumes and critical normal structures that are available with CT simulation have helped to improve the accuracy of treatment and potentially minimize risks of normal tissue injury.

The initial process in simulation is optimizing the patient positioning. Patients are typically treated supine with the arm abducted and externally rotated away from the breast. An immobilization cradle is created or a dedicated "breast" immobilization board is used to help ensure that the position is reproduced for the daily treatments. Subsequently, the patient undergoes a simulation CT scan and reference points within the required treatment fields are marked on the patient. The field length, width, angle of entrance and exit, and axial, sagittal, and coronal rotations are optimized on the CT data set. Targets and normal structures can be contoured to provide clear visualization of them within the beams-eye view of the treatment field. Typically, two opposed photon fields that tangentially cover the anterior chest and minimize the intrathoracic normal tissue are used to treat the breast. An example of such fields is shown in Figure 37.2. After 5 weeks of daily treatments to the breast, the irradiated volume is reduced to the area of the tumor bed with a 2-cm margin and treatment of this volume continues an additional 1 to 1.5 weeks. Typically, these tumor bed boost fields are treated with en face electron beam irradiation, which distributes its dose over a finite range that is determined by the energy of the beam. Three-dimensional treatment planning of these fields helps to select the appropriate energy to ensure optimal efficacy and safety. Figure 37.3 shows an example of a tumor bed boost field.

During simulation, it is helpful to contour the tumor bed and any targeted lymphatic regions that require treatment. This can ensure adequate dose coverage of these regions. For example, the depth of the level III and supraclavicular axillary nodes vary according to individual anatomy and patient weight. Historically, doses were empirically prescribed to a depth of 3 cm, which can significantly underdose contoured lymph node regions at risk in overweight and obese patients (65). Finally, for patients who require treatment to the low axilla, contouring the region at risk also helps to more precisely conform the dose distribution to the area in need of treatment. Many centers also routinely contour the heart and lung and typically add a heart block for left-sided cases where the heart is in the field and the block would not approach the primary tumor region. In some situations, a breath-hold technique can be used to avoid cardiac irradiation, which is discussed below.

A second major advance in breast cancer radiation treatments has been the development of computer algorithms that accurately calculate the distribution of radiation dose over the entire three-dimensional treatment volume. The goal of radia-

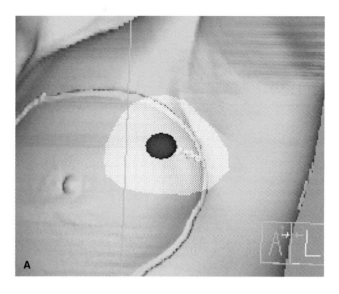

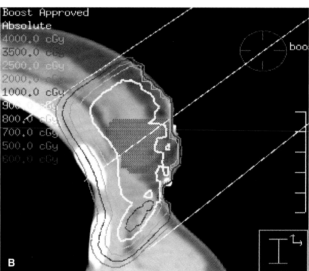

FIGURE 37.3. A skin rendering **(A)** and axial image **(B)** of a boost electron field to supplement the radiation dose to the tumor bed after completion of whole breast radiation treatment. The axial image shows the tumor bed contoured in pink with the isodose curves of the single electron beam. The selection of electron beam energy determines the penetration distance of the electron beam dose and allows the appropriate isodose curve to adequately encompass the target volume.

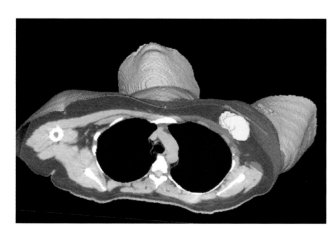

FIGURE 37.2. A skin rendering and axial image of medial and lateral tangential photon fields typically used to treat the breast. The two fields are opposed such that the dose-fall-off over depth is matched to provide a homogeneous distribution of dose. Angles of beam entrance and exit are selected to minimize dose to intrathoracic structures. In this figure, the tumor bed location within the breast has been contoured on sequential axial slices and reconstructed as a solid yellow contour.

tion treatment planning is to provide a uniform dose throughout the breast. After three-dimensional treatment planning systems were able to accurately calculate three-dimensional dose distributions, techniques were developed to modulate individual components of the beams to improve dose homogeneity within the treatment volume. This technique is often referred to as intensity modulated radiation therapy (IMRT) for breast cancer. An example of treatment fields used to modulate the intensity of the radiation therapy is shown in Figure 37.4.

Two recent prospective clinical trials have provided evidence that IMRT achieves improved clinical outcome compared to the historical two-dimensional dose compensation techniques. Pignol et al. (30) reported that IMRT reduced the volume of breast tissue receiving 105% or 110% of the prescribed dose. As a consequence, patients randomized to IMRT had lower rates of moist desquamation and less pain during this period of treatment. Donovan et al. (66) published a similar randomized trial but had longer follow-up to assess late radiation effects. In this randomized trial, IMRT dose compensation minimized the risk of a radiation-induced long-term cosmetic consequence, such as change in the photographic appearance of the breast. Patients with

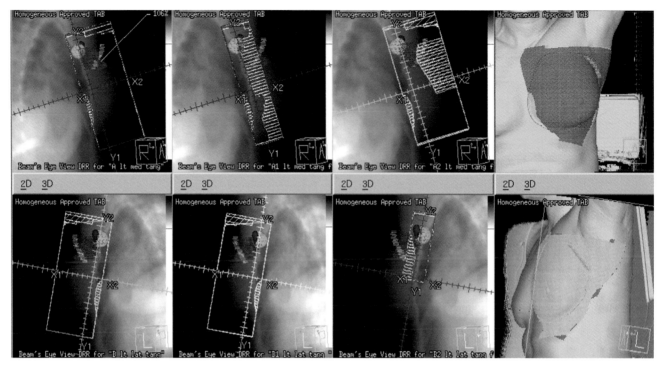

FIGURE 37.4.   An example of intensity modulated radiation treatment (IMRT) fields used to treat the breast.   Two opposed medial and lateral tangent fields generate a dose distribution in the breast that has excess dose in the thinner areas of the breast such as the apex where the distance traveled by the beam and resulting dose fall-off is less (relative to the base of the breast). Resulting "hot spots" are subsequently blocked by subfield created by inserting multileaf collimators located within the head of the linear accelerator and blocking dose to these regions. A multileaf collimator that shielded the heart was also used in the inferior portion of all of the fields in this particular case.

larger breast sizes achieve the greatest benefit from IMRT in that such patients have a greater degree of dose inhomogeneity with standard two-dimensional dose compensation techniques. In contrast, two-dimensional dose compensation techniques are highly effective for many patients with smaller breast sizes. It is also possible in some patients to substantially improve dose homogeneity with a small number of subfields, short of IMRT.

Morbidity of Whole Breast Irradiation

As a general rule, patients who receive radiation treatments as a component of breast-conservation therapy tolerate the course of treatment very well. Treatments require only 15 to 30 minutes each day, and most patients can continue their daily routines with minimal interruptions. Two short-term complications that occur in the majority of patients are fatigue and mild breast dermatitis or discomfort. The degree of fatigue varies across individuals and improves to baseline within a month after treatment. The skin reactions associated with radiation delivered with modern techniques are typically mild. Erythema, warmth, mild discomfort, and pruritis typically develop during the last week of treatment and improve shortly after treatment completion. Posttreatment skin edema and mild hyperpigmentation may persist many months.

Modern treatments are very safe with a very low likelihood of a permanent normal tissue injury. The most common complication after irradiation is subcutaneous fibrosis and atrophy of breast tissue. However, most series report that 80% to 95% of patients have good to excellent aesthetic outcomes after breast irradiation to total doses of 45 to 50.4 Gy in daily fractions of 1.8 to 2.0 Gy (67). The development of a second cancer induced by radiation treatments of the breast is a very unusual event. In an analysis based on the Connecticut cancer registry database of 41,109 breast cancer patients, Boice et al. (68) reported that breast irradiation may increase the incidence of contralateral breast cancer in women 45 years of age or younger who survived for at least 10 years after diagnosis (relative risk of a 1.33). The

EBCTCG meta-analysis of the data from all radiotherapy trials in breast cancer (including trials investigating postmastectomy radiation) reported a 1.18 ratio of rates for developing a second breast cancer for irradiated versus nonirradiated patients ($p = .002$) (11). Given these data, it is important to optimize techniques to minimize scatter radiation dose to the contralateral breast. The newer IMRT techniques that provide three-dimensional dose compensation with multileaf collimated subfields have the additional benefit of decreasing the dose to the contralateral breast by 65% to 82% (69). The EBCTCG meta-analysis also indicated an increased risk of lung cancer development in patients who received radiation (HR 1.61), although this included patients receiving older techniques of postmastectomy radiation therapy where the amount of lung irradiated is much greater than with currently used breast irradiation (11). Data from the NSABP indicated that this risk was in part dependent on the volume of lung included in the radiation fields. Specifically, an increased risk was found in patients treated in the NSABP B-04 trials where treatment included multiple fields to target the regional lymphatics in addition to the breast and chest wall, but not the B-06 trial where breast only treatment fields were used (70). Smoking is recognized as an important cofactor for the development of lung cancer after breast cancer radiation treatments. Kaufman et al. (71) conducted a population-based case-control study using the Connecticut Tumor Registry and reported that nonsmoking breast cancer patients who received radiation did not have a higher risk of lung cancer development, but irradiated breast cancer patients who were smokers did have a significantly increased risk. These data were similar to a case-control study published by the group from M.D. Anderson Cancer Center who also found that smoking was a significant independent risk factor for lung carcinoma after breast cancer and that smoking and radiation combined enhanced the effect of either alone (72).

One of the most significant potential serious injuries to normal tissue that can result from whole breast irradiation is cardiovascular disease and cardiac-related death. The meta-analysis from the EBCTCG indicated that patients treated with radiation had a 1.27 relative risk of death from heart disease compared to the patients who did not receive radiation (11). This result was predominantly seen in relatively older postmastectomy radiation studies that utilized treatment techniques and dose schedules no longer in use. With the advent of improved technologies, radiation treatments are much less likely to cause adverse cardiac events. For example, a study evaluating the SEER database suggested that radiation treatments increased cardiac-related deaths for patients treated in the 1970s, but there was no evidence for an increase in cardiac deaths in the patients treated in the 1980s (73). Similarly, a study that evaluated the SEER-Medicare database found no increase in cardiac events in patients over the age of 65 who were treated with radiation for a left-sided breast cancer (74). However, a recent study from the University of Pennsylvania indicated that patients treated with radiation as a component of breast-conservation therapy for a left-sided breast cancer had an increased risk of coronary artery disease compared to those treated for a right-sided breast cancer (75). Additionally, investigators from Duke

University have shown that inclusion of some of the left ventricle in tangential fields used to treat left-sided breast cancers can result in cardiac perfusion abnormalities (76).

Based on these data, it is very important that the risk of radiation-associated heart disease be minimized or completely avoided by ensuring that the heart is not within the treatment fields. For patients with upper outer quadrant tumors, a small heart block can be used, which may shield a small volume of the far medial and far lateral lower breast tissue. However, studies have reported that use of heart blocks do not increase the risk of in-breast recurrence (77). For tumors in the lower quadrants, new techniques are available to physically displace the heart from the tumor bed through breath-hold techniques. In this procedure, patients can monitor their respiratory cycle and hold their breath in a predefined volume that achieves cardiac displacement. The beam can then be turned only during the periods when the respiratory goals are reached. During deep inspiration, the diaphragm pulls the heart down and medial relative to the left breast. An example of this technique is shown in Figure 37.5. For

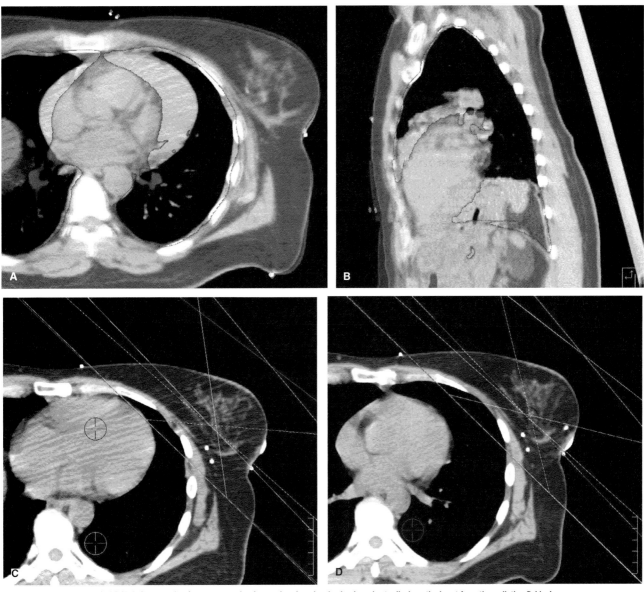

FIGURE 37.5. An example of a treatment that is gated to deep inspiration in order to displace the heart from the radiation field. As seen on the fused axial (**A**) coronal (**B**) image of a "free-breathing scan" and a "breath-hold scan," deep inspiration lowers the diaphragm and displaces the heart inferomedially. The next two axial images show the relationship of the heart to the radiation fields under free-breathing conditions (**C**) and breath-hold conditions (**D**). In this example, the treatment beam is only turned on during breath-hold periods to ensure that the heart is outside of the field.

patients with superficial tumors, another approach to avoiding cardiac irradiation is to use a prone, rather than supine, technique. Prone breast irradiation can also displace superficial breast tissue away from the heart. Prone technique can also be useful in patients with large and pendulous breasts.

 POSTOPERATIVE SURVEILLANCE

In patients who are treated with breast-conserving surgery and postoperative radiation therapy, a new baseline mammogram of the treated breast is obtained 4 to 6 months after the completion of radiation therapy. After all treatment is complete, patients have twice-yearly physical examinations and annual mammography for 5 years and annual physical examinations and mammography thereafter.

 MANAGEMENT SUMMARY

- Based on long-term results demonstrating both efficacy and safety, breast-conserving therapy consisting of breast-conserving surgery for removal of the primary with negative margins of resection followed by whole breast irradiation is an appropriate option for the majority of patients with early stage breast cancer.
- No patient subset based on clinical and pathology features has been identified that has a low risk of in-breast recurrence without radiation therapy. Breast-conserving surgery and hormonal therapy is an option in elderly women with small node-negative, hormone receptor–positive breast cancer, particularly if the patient has comorbid illnesses.
- Radiation therapy following breast-conserving surgery proportionally reduces local recurrence by about 70% and improves absolute long-term survival by approximately 5%.
- Following whole breast irradiation, a boost of additional irradiation is given to the primary site, particularly in younger patients.
- Absolute contraindications to breast-conservation therapy include previous radiation therapy to the chest or breast, radiation therapy required during a pregnancy, diffuse malignant appearing microcalcifications on mammography, and inability to achieve a negative margin of resection. The use of breast-conservation therapy is generally contraindicated in patients with multicentric cancer or with active connective tissue disease involving the skin.
- It is uncertain when a close margin (generally defined as tumor within 2 mm of an inked surface) requires re-excision. Other factors, such as patient age, tumor immunotype, amount of tumor close to the margin, and use of initial chemotherapy, need to be considered.
- The use of adjuvant systemic therapy developed to reduce distant metastasis has been demonstrated to substantially reduce in-breast recurrence when combined with breast irradiation.
- When a patient will receive both breast-conservation therapy and adjuvant chemotherapy, radiation therapy generally follows chemotherapy. Adjuvant hormonal therapy or trastuzumab can be given with or after radiation therapy.
- CT simulation with contouring of critical volumes is important and should be done for all patients with left-sided breast cancer. The treatment technique should exclude or minimize the heart from the treatment fields. Appropriate measures should be used to provide homogeneous irradiation.

References

1. Ganz PA, Kwan L, Stanton AL, et al. Quality of life at the end of primary treatment of breast cancer: first results from the moving beyond cancer randomized trial. *J Natl Cancer Inst* 2004;96:376–387.
2. American Cancer Society. *Breast cancer facts and figures 2007–2008*. Atlanta: American Cancer Society, 2008.
3. Cabioglu N, Hunt KK, Buchholz TA, et al. Improving local control with breast-conserving therapy: a 27-year single-institution experience. *Cancer* 2005;104:20–29.
4. Fisher B, Bryant J, Dignam JJ, et al. Tamoxifen, radiation therapy, or both for prevention of ipsilateral breast tumor recurrence after lumpectomy in women with invasive breast cancers of one centimeter or less. *J Clin Oncol* 2002;20:4141–4149.
5. Fisher B, Jeong JH, Dignam J, et al. Findings from recent National Surgical Adjuvant Breast and Bowel Project adjuvant studies in stage I breast cancer. *J Natl Cancer Inst Monogr* 2001;30:62–66.
6. Fisher B, Anderson S, Redmond CK, et al. Reanalysis and results after 12 years of follow-up in a randomized clinical trial comparing total mastectomy with lumpectomy with or without irradiation in the treatment of breast cancer. *N Engl J Med* 1995;333:1456–1461.
7. Fisher B, Anderson S, Bryant J, et al. Twenty-year follow-up of a randomized trial comparing total mastectomy, lumpectomy, and lumpectomy plus irradiation for the treatment of invasive breast cancer. *N Engl J Med* 2002;347:1233–1241.
8. Veronesi U, Cascinelli N, Mariani L, et al. Twenty-year follow-up of a randomized study comparing breast-conserving surgery with radical mastectomy for early breast cancer. *N Engl J Med* 2002;347:1227–1232.
9. Darby S. 2006 update from the Early Breast Cancer Trialists' Collaborative Group overview of radiation therapy for early breast cancer. Presentation at the 2007 ASCO annual meeting, Chicago, June 2007. Available at http://www.asco.org/ASCO/Abstracts+%26+Virtual+Meeting/Speaker?&spk=Darby%2C+Sarah+%5Bfau%5D.
10. Buchholz TA, Woodward WA, Duan Z, et al. Radiation use and long-term survival in breast cancer patients with T1, T2 primary tumors and one to three positive axillary lymph nodes. *Int J Radiat Oncol Biol Phys* 2008;71(4):1022–1027.
11. Effects of radiotherapy and of differences in the extent of surgery for early breast cancer on local recurrence and 15-year survival: an overview of the randomised trials. Early Breast Cancer Trialists' Collaborative Group. *Lancet* 2005;366:2087–2106.
12. Punglia RS, Morrow M, Winer EP, et al. Local therapy and survival in breast cancer. *N Engl J Med* 2007;356:2399–2405.
13. Lim M, Bellon JR, Gelman R, et al. A prospective study of conservative surgery without radiation therapy in select patients with stage I breast cancer. *Int J Radiat Oncol Biol Phys* 2006;65:1149–1154.
14. Veronesi U, Marubini E, Mariani L, et al. Radiotherapy after breast-conserving surgery in small breast carcinoma: long-term results of a randomized trial. *Ann Oncol* 2001;12:997–1003.
15. Holli K, Saaristo R, Isola J, et al. Lumpectomy with or without postoperative radiotherapy for breast cancer with favourable prognostic features: results of a randomized study. *Br J Cancer* 2001;84:164–169.
16. Liljegren G, Lindgren A, Bergh J, et al. Risk factors for local recurrence after conservative treatment in stage I breast cancer. Definition of a subgroup not requiring radiotherapy. *Ann Oncol* 1997;8:235–241.
17. Hughes KS, Schnaper LA, Berry D, et al. Lumpectomy plus tamoxifen with or without irradiation in women 70 years of age or older with early breast cancer. *N Engl J Med* 2004;351:971–977.
18. Hughes KS Schnaper LA, Berry D, et al. Lumpectomy plus tamoxifen with or without irradiation in women 70 years of age or older with early breast cancer: a report of further follow-up. *Breast Cancer Res Treat* 2006;100(abst11).
19. Smith BD, Gross CP, Smith GL, et al. Effectiveness of radiation therapy for older women with early breast cancer. *J Natl Cancer Inst* 2006;98:681–690.
20. Anderson BO, Masetti R, Silverstein MJ. Oncoplastic approaches to partial mastectomy: an overview of volume-displacement techniques. *Lancet Oncol* 2005;6:145–157.
21. Kronowitz SJ, Hunt KK, Kuerer HM, et al. Practical guidelines for repair of partial mastectomy defects using the breast reduction technique in patients undergoing breast conservation therapy. *Plast Reconstr Surg* 2007;120:1755–1768.
22. Stovall M, Blackwell CR, Cundiff J, et al. Fetal dose from radiotherapy with photon beams: report of AAPM Radiation Therapy Committee Task Group No. 36. *Med Phys* 1995;22:63–82.
23. Chen AM, Obedian E, Haffty BG. Breast-conserving therapy in the setting of collagen vascular disease. *Cancer J* 2001;7:480–491.
24. Morris MM, Powell SN. Irradiation in the setting of collagen vascular disease: acute and late complications. *J Clin Oncol* 1997;15:2728–2735.
25. Morrow M, Strom EA, Bassett LW, et al. Standard for breast conservation therapy in the management of invasive breast carcinoma. *CA Cancer J Clin* 2002;52:277–300.
26. Carlson RW, Anderson BO, Burstein HJ, et al. Invasive breast cancer. *J Natl Compr Canc Netw* 2007;5:246–312.
27. Antonini N, Jones H, Horiot JC, et al. Effect of age and radiation dose on local control after breast conserving treatment: EORTC trial 22881-10882. *Radiother Oncol* 2007;82(3):265–271.
28. Beadle BM, Woodward WA, Allen PK, et al. Locoregional recurrence rates in young women with breast cancer by treatment approach. *Int J Radiat Oncol Biol Phys* 2007;69:S212.
29. Oh JL, Bonnen M, Outlaw ED, et al. The impact of young age on locoregional recurrence after doxorubicin-based breast conservation therapy in patients 40 years old or younger: How young is "young?" *Int J Radiat Oncol Biol Phys* 2006;65:1345–1352.
30. Pignol J, Olivotto I, Rakovitch E, et al. A multicentre randomized trial of breast IMRT to reduce acute radiation dermatitis. *J Clin Oncol* 2008;26(13):2085–2092.
31. Haffty BG, Harrold E, Khan AJ, et al. Outcome of conservatively managed early-onset breast cancer by BRCA1/2 status. *Lancet* 2002;359:1471–1477.
32. Pierce LJ, Levin AM, Rebbeck TR, et al. Ten-year multi-institutional results of breast-conserving surgery and radiotherapy in BRCA1/2-associated stage I/II breast cancer. *J Clin Oncol* 2006;24:2437–2443.
33. Boyages J, Recht A, Connolly JL, et al. Early breast cancer: predictors of breast recurrence for patients treated with conservative surgery and radiation therapy. *Radiother Oncol* 1990;19:29–41.
34. Vicini FA, Goldstein NS, Pass H, et al. Use of pathologic factors to assist in establishing adequacy of excision before radiotherapy in patients treated with breast-conserving therapy. *Int J Radiat Oncol Biol Phys* 2004;60:86–94.

35. Park CC, Mitsumori M, Nixon A, et al. Outcome at 8 years after breast-conserving surgery and radiation therapy for invasive breast cancer: influence of margin status and systemic therapy on local recurrence. *J Clin Oncol* 2000;18:1668–1675.
36. Jobsen JJ, van der Palen J, Ong F, et al. The value of a positive margin for invasive carcinoma in breast-conservative treatment in relation to local recurrence is limited to young women only. *Int J Radiat Oncol Biol Phys* 2003;57:724–731.
37. Bellon JR, Come SE, Gelman RS, et al. Sequencing of chemotherapy and radiation therapy in early-stage breast cancer: updated results of a prospective randomized trial. *J Clin Oncol* 2005;23:1934–1940.
38. Leopold KA, Recht A, Schnitt SJ, et al. Results of conservative surgery and radiation therapy for multiple synchronous cancers of one breast. *Int J Radiat Oncol Biol Phys* 1989;16:11–16.
39. Salvadori B, Biganzoli E, Veronesi P, et al. Conservative surgery for infiltrating lobular breast carcinoma. *Br J Surg* 1997;84:106–109.
40. Vo TN, Meric-Bernstam F, Yi M, et al. Outcomes of breast-conservation therapy for invasive lobular carcinoma are equivalent to those for invasive ductal carcinoma. *Am J Surg* 2006;192:552–555.
41. Hennessy BT, Giordano S, Broglio K, et al. Biphasic metaplastic sarcomatoid carcinoma of the breast. *Ann Oncol* 2006;17:605–613.
42. Voogd AC, Nielsen M, Peterse JL, et al. Differences in risk factors for local and distant recurrence after breast-conserving therapy or mastectomy for stage I and II breast cancer: pooled results of two large European randomized trials. *J Clin Oncol* 2001;19:1688–1697.
43. Fisher ER. Lumpectomy margins and much more. *Cancer* 1997;79:1453–1460.
44. Harris EE, Hwang WT, Lee EA, et al. The impact of HER-2 status on local recurrence in women with stage I-II breast cancer treated with breast conserving therapy. *Breast J* 2006;12:431–436.
45. Haffty BG, Yang Q, Reiss M, et al. Locoregional relapse and distant metastasis in conservatively managed triple negative early-stage breast cancer. *J Clin Oncol* 2006;24:5652–5657.
46. Nguyen PL, Taghian AG, Katz MS, et al. Breast cancer subtype approximated by estrogen receptor, progesterone receptor, and HER-2 is associated with local and distant recurrence after breast-conserving therapy. *J Clin Oncol* 2008;26(14): 2373–2378.
47. Mamounas EP, Tang G, Bryant J, et al. Association between the 21-gene recurrence score assay (RS) and risk of locoregional failure in node-negative ER-positive breast cancer: results from NSABP B-14 and NSABP B-20. *Breast Cancer Res Treat* 2007;94:S16(abst29).
48. Nuyten DS, van de Vijver MJ. Gene expression signatures to predict the development of metastasis in breast cancer. *Breast Dis* 2006;26:149–156.
49. Romestaing P, Lehingue Y, Carrie C, et al. Role of a 10-Gy boost in the conservative treatment of early breast cancer. *J Clin Oncol* 1997;15:963–968.
50. Bartelink H, Horiot JC, Poortmans PM, et al. Impact of a higher radiation dose on local control and survival in breast-conserving therapy of early breast cancer: 10-year results of the randomized boost versus no boost EORTC 22881-10882 trial. *J Clin Oncol* 2007;25:3259–3265.
51. Sartor CI, Peterson BL, Woolf S, et al. Effect of addition of adjuvant paclitaxel on radiotherapy delivery and locoregional control of node-positive breast cancer: cancer and leukemia group B 9344. *J Clin Oncol* 2005;23:30–40.
52. Pierce LJ, Hutchins LF, Green SR, et al. Sequencing of tamoxifen and radiotherapy after breast-conserving surgery in early-stage breast cancer. *J Clin Oncol* 2005; 23:24–29.
53. Ahn PH, Vu HT, Lannin D, et al. Sequence of radiotherapy with tamoxifen in conservatively managed breast cancer does not affect local relapse rates. *J Clin Oncol* 2005;23:17–23.
54. Harris EE, Christensen VJ, Hwang WT, et al. Impact of concurrent versus sequential tamoxifen with radiation therapy in early-stage breast cancer patients undergoing breast conservation treatment. *J Clin Oncol* 2005;23:11–16.
55. Tan-Chiu E, Yothers G, Romond E, et al. Assessment of cardiac dysfunction in a randomized trial comparing doxorubicin and cyclophosphamide followed by paclitaxel, with or without trastuzumab as adjuvant therapy in node-positive, human epidermal growth factor receptor 2-overexpressing breast cancer: NSABP B-31. *J Clin Oncol* 2005;23:7811–7819.
56. Halyard MY, Pisansky TM, Solin LJ, et al. Adjuvant radiotherapy (RT) and trastuzumab in stage I-IIA breast cancer: toxicity data from North Central Cancer Treatment Group phase III trial N9831. ASCO annual meeting proceedings part I. *J Clin Oncol* 2006;24(18S):523.
57. Whelan T, MacKenzie R, Julian J, et al. Randomized trial of breast irradiation schedules after lumpectomy for women with lymph node-negative breast cancer. *J Natl Cancer Inst* 2002;94:1143–1150.
58. Whelan TJ, Pignol J, Julian J, et al. Long-term results of a randomized trial of accelerated hypofractionated whole breast irradiation following breast conserving surgery in women with node-negative breast cancer. *Int J Radiat Oncol Biol Phys* 2008;72:S28, abstract 60.
59. Clark RM, McCulloch PB, Levine MN, et al. Randomized clinical trial to assess the effectiveness of breast irradiation following lumpectomy and axillary dissection for node-negative breast cancer. *J Natl Cancer Inst* 1992;84:683–689.
60. Liljegren G, Holmberg L, Bergh J, et al. 10-Year results after sector resection with or without postoperative radiotherapy for stage I breast cancer: a randomized trial. *J Clin Oncol* 1999;17:2326–2333.
61. Faverly DR, Hendriks JH, Holland R. Breast carcinomas of limited extent: frequency, radiologic-pathologic characteristics, and surgical margin requirements. *Cancer* 2001;91:647--659.
62. Vaidya JS, Vyas JJ, Chinoy RF, et al. Multicentricity of breast cancer: whole-organ analysis and clinical implications. *Br J Cancer* 1996;74:820–824.
63. Bluemke DA, Gatsonis CA, Chen MH, et al. Magnetic resonance imaging of the breast prior to biopsy. *JAMA* 2004;292:2735–2742.
64. Bedrosian I, Mick R, Orel SG, et al. Changes in the surgical management of patients with breast carcinoma based on preoperative magnetic resonance imaging. *Cancer* 2003;98:468–473.
65. Liengsawangwong R, Yu TK, Sun TL, et al. Treatment optimization using computed tomography-delineated targets should be used for supraclavicular irradiation for breast cancer. *Int J Radiat Oncol Biol Phys* 2007;69:711–715.
66. Donovan E, Bleakley N, Denholm E, et al. Randomised trial of standard 2D radiotherapy (RT) versus intensity modulated radiotherapy (IMRT) in patients prescribed breast radiotherapy. *Radiother Oncol* 2007;82:254–264.
67. Taylor ME, Perez CA, Halverson KJ, et al. Factors influencing cosmetic results after conservation therapy for breast cancer. *Int J Radiat Oncol Biol Phys* 1995;31:753–764.
68. Boice JD, Jr., Harvey EB, Blettner M, et al. Cancer in the contralateral breast after radiotherapy for breast cancer. *N Engl J Med* 1992;326:781–785.
69. Borghero YO, Salehpour M, McNeese MD, et al. Multileaf field-in-field forward-planned intensity-modulated dose compensation for whole-breast irradiation is associated with reduced contralateral breast dose: a phantom model comparison. *Radiother Oncol* 2007;82:324–328.
70. Deutsch M, Land SR, Begovic M, et al. The incidence of lung carcinoma after surgery for breast carcinoma with and without postoperative radiotherapy. Results of National Surgical Adjuvant Breast and Bowel Project (NSABP) clinical trials B-04 and B-06. *Cancer* 2003;98:1362–1368.
71. Kaufman EL, Jacobson JS, Hershman DL, et al. Effect of breast cancer radiotherapy and cigarette smoking on risk of second primary lung cancer. *J Clin Oncol* 2008;26:392–398.
72. Ford MB, Sigurdson AJ, Petrulis ES, et al. Effects of smoking and radiotherapy on lung carcinoma in breast carcinoma survivors. *Cancer* 2003;98:1457–1464.
73. Giordano SH, Kuo YF, Freeman JL, et al. Risk of cardiac death after adjuvant radiotherapy for breast cancer. *J Natl Cancer Inst* 2005;97:419–424.
74. Patt DA, Goodwin JS, Kuo YF, et al. Cardiac morbidity of adjuvant radiotherapy for breast cancer. *J Clin Oncol* 2005;23:7475–7482.
75. Harris EE, Correa C, Hwang WT, et al. Late cardiac mortality and morbidity in early-stage breast cancer patients after breast-conservation treatment. *J Clin Oncol* 2006;24:4100–4106.
76. Prosnitz RG, Hubbs JL, Evans ES, et al. Prospective assessment of radiotherapy-associated cardiac toxicity in breast cancer patients: analysis of data 3 to 6 years after treatment. *Cancer* 2007;110:1840–1850.
77. Raj KA, Evans ES, Prosnitz RG, et al. Is there an increased risk of local recurrence under the heart block in patients with left-sided breast cancer? *Cancer J* 2006;12:309–317.
78. Forrest AP, Stewart HJ, Everington D, et al. Randomised controlled trial of conservation therapy for breast cancer: 6-year analysis of the Scottish trial. Scottish Cancer Trials Breast Group. *Lancet* 1996;348:708–713.
79. Potter R, Gnant M, Kwasny W, et al. Lumpectomy plus tamoxifen or anastrozole with or without whole breast irradiation in women with favorable early breast cancer. *Int J Radiat Oncol Biol Phys* 2007;68:334–340.
80. Fyles AW, McCready DR, Manchul LA, et al. Tamoxifen with or without breast irradiation in women 50 years of age or older with early breast cancer. *N Engl J Med* 2004;351:963–970.
81. Robson M, Svahn T, McCormick B, et al. Appropriateness of breast-conserving treatment of breast carcinoma in women with germline mutations in *BRCA1* or *BRCA2*: a clinic-based series. *Cancer* 2005;103:44–51.
82. Seynaeve C, Verhoog LC, van de Bosch LM, et al. Ipsilateral breast tumour recurrence in hereditary breast cancer following breast-conserving therapy. *Eur J Cancer* 2004;40:1150–1158.
83. Borger JH. The impact of surgical and pathological findings on radiotherapy on early breast cancer. *Radiother Oncol* 1991;22:230–236.
84. Dewar JA, Arriagada R, Benhamou S, et al. Local relapse and contralateral tumor rates in patients with breast cancer treated with conservative surgery and radiotherapy (Institut Gustave Roussy 1970–1982). IGR Breast Cancer Group. *Cancer* 1995;76:2260–2265.
85. Freedman G, Fowble B, Hanlon A, et al. Patients with early stage invasive cancer with close or positive margins treated with conservative surgery and radiation have an increased risk of breast recurrence that is delayed by adjuvant systemic therapy. *Int J Radiat Oncol Biol Phys* 1999;44:1005–1015.
86. Anscher MS, Jones P, Prosnitz LR, et al. Local failure and margin status in early-stage breast carcinoma treated with conservation surgery and radiation therapy. *Ann Surg* 1993;218:22–28.
87. Smitt MC, Nowels KW, Zdeblick MJ, et al. The importance of the lumpectomy surgical margin status in long-term results of breast conservation. *Cancer* 1995;76:259–267.
88. Peterson ME, Schultz DJ, Reynolds C, et al. Outcomes in breast cancer patients relative to margin status after treatment with breast-conserving surgery and radiation therapy: the University of Pennsylvania experience. *Int J Radiat Oncol Biol Phys* 1999;43:1029–1035.
89. Wazer DE, Jabro G, Ruthazer R, et al. Extent of margin positivity as a predictor for local recurrence after breast conserving irradiation. *Radiat Oncol Investig* 1999;7: 111–117.
90. Cowen D, Houvenaeghel G, Bardou V, et al. Local and distant failures after limited surgery with positive margins and radiotherapy for node-negative breast cancer. *Int J Radiat Oncol Biol Phys* 2000;47:305–312.
91. Pittinger TP, Maronian NC, Poulter CA, et al. Importance of margin status in outcome of breast-conserving surgery for carcinoma. *Surgery* 1994;116:605–608.
92. Obedian E, Haffty BG. Negative margin status improves local control in conservatively managed breast cancer patients. *Cancer J Sci Am* 2000;6:28–33.
93. Fisher B, Jeong JH, Anderson S, et al. Treatment of axillary lymph node-negative, estrogen receptor-negative breast cancer: updated findings from National Surgical Adjuvant Breast and Bowel Project clinical trials. *J Natl Cancer Inst* 2004;96: 1823–1831.
94. Buchholz TA, Tucker SL, Erwin J, et al. Impact of systemic treatment on local control for patients with lymph node-negative breast cancer treated with breast-conservation therapy. *J Clin Oncol* 2001;19:2240–2246.
95. Haffty BG, Fischer D, Rose M, et al. Prognostic factors for local recurrence in the conservatively treated breast cancer patient: a cautious interpretation of the data. *J Clin Oncol* 1991;9:997–1003.

Chapter 38
Breast-Conserving Therapy: Accelerated Partial Breast Irradiation

Douglas W. Arthur and Frank A. Vicini

The equivalence of breast-conserving therapy (BCT) to mastectomy in the treatment of women with early stage breast cancer has been demonstrated in several phase III trials (1,2) (see Chapter 37). Despite the undisputed efficacy of this treatment approach, recent investigations have explored methods to either reduce the time, inconvenience, or toxicity of its application. These approaches have included (a) accelerating the dose delivery scheme, (b) reducing the treatment target to less than whole breast, or (c) identifying subgroups of women in which adjuvant radiation therapy (RT) following lumpectomy can be safely omitted (3–7). Ultimately, it is anticipated that a spectrum of treatment approaches for early stage breast cancer will develop with the most appropriate technique selected based on the individual disease characteristics and technical specifics that present.

Currently, the requisite amount of clinically uninvolved breast tissue surrounding the lumpectomy cavity that needs to be irradiated after conservative surgery (CS) has yet to be definitively established. Standard RT after CS has included elective treatment of the whole breast for presumed occult disease. This is based on older pathologic data from mastectomy specimens demonstrating areas of occult disease in 30% to 40% of women undergoing treatment for early stage disease (8). However, review of both clinical and pathologic evidence finds that there are limited contemporary data supporting the concept that the entire breast requires treatment in all patients. More recent data suggest that the primary target requiring adjuvant treatment following CS (with negative surgical margins) is likely limited to a 1- to 2-cm boundary surrounding the lumpectomy cavity (9–15). The additional "prophylactic" treatment of the whole breast, including clinically uninvolved breast tissue with RT, is therefore generally considered responsible in part for the acute and chronic toxicity associated with standard CS and RT and for the protracted time commitment required for its completion. If it were possible to reduce this target to less than 40% of the whole breast, acceleration of the dose delivery and completion of treatment in less than 5 days becomes more feasible. Also, with the advent of new, widely available RT treatment techniques, the accurate delivery of a conformal, accelerated partial breast dose to a limited target in the breast becomes technically possible.

Accelerated partial breast irradiation (APBI) has been investigated as a possible option that incorporates both the quest to decrease the overall treatment time and to reduce the amount of normal tissue treated to a defined partial breast target (3). If proven efficacious, it is believed that such an approach could theoretically increase the frequency that BCT is chosen as a treatment option, offer the potential advantages of reduced treatment related toxicities, provide a logistically faster, convenient, and more accessible method for BCT, and potentially improve overall quality of life for early stage breast cancer patients (16).

For this new APBI treatment approach to become an accepted standard of care, data regarding appropriate application of proper patient selection criteria, treatment techniques, risk of toxicity, and long-term local control equivalence to traditional BCT incorporating whole breast irradiation must be obtained and analyzed. Considering that standard BCT data have consistently demonstrated excellent locoregional control rates, minimal acute and chronic morbidity, acceptable cosmetic results, and equivalent survival to mastectomy, the level of evidence needed to support this possible new paradigm shift is significant. In addition, recent data (meta-analyses) clearly demonstrate the importance of optimal local control on survival (17). Each of these critical issues will be addressed in this chapter.

 ## ACCELERATED PARTIAL BREAST IRRADIATION TREATMENT TECHNIQUES

Several treatment techniques have been developed for the delivery of APBI with many additional approaches and modifications emerging as technology and ideas are explored. There are four prevailing techniques that will be discussed here. Within the United States, three "classic" techniques dominate and include multicatheter interstitial brachytherapy, balloon catheter brachytherapy, and three-dimensional conformal external beam radiotherapy (3D-CRT). In Europe, in addition to multicatheter brachytherapy, intraoperative radiotherapy has been central to their APBI experience. Only recently have programs offered intraoperative radiotherapy in the United States. Each of these four techniques has unique advantages and disadvantages, but they all strive to satisfy the goals of comprehensively irradiating the treatment target volume, ensuring homogeneous dose coverage and minimizing the dose to nontarget tissues.

Multicatheter Interstitial Accelerated Partial Breast Irradiation

The APBI technique that has been in use the longest and has the most extensive follow-up is the multicatheter interstitial brachytherapy approach (18–20). With this technique, afterloading catheters are placed through the breast tissue to surround the lumpectomy cavity (Fig. 38.1). Catheters are generally positioned at 1- to 1.5-cm intervals to avoid hot and cold spots. These implants generally require 15 to 20 catheters to ensure proper dose coverage. The exact number of catheters used is determined by the size and shape of the target and the configuration of catheters by an understanding of brachytherapy dosimetric guidelines (21–24). Once the implant geometry is known (through mapping of catheter location), dosimetric planning is completed to determine how to optimally place the radioactive source within the catheters for dose delivery. The majority of patients undergoing this procedure tolerate the presence of these catheters well with minimal need for pain medication.

Recently, advances have been made to reduce the degree of operator dependence and improve the reproducibility of this procedure. With the incorporation of image-guided catheter placement techniques (stereotactic mammography, ultrasound, or computed tomography [CT] guided) and three-dimensional dosimetric planning, the multicatheter approach has evolved into a more reliable technique that can be used in a variety of treatment situations, regardless of lumpectomy cavity size, shape, or location within the breast (25,26). The interstitial catheter technique is the most versatile modality for APBI

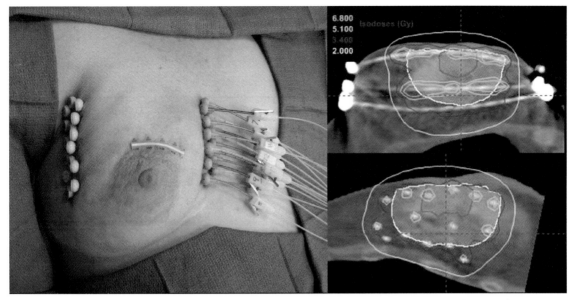

FIGURE 38.1. Multicatheter brachytherapy accelerated partial breast irradiation. External appearance as connected to remote after-loader with cross and sagittal sections of dosimetric coverage depicted on right. The lumpectomy cavity is outlined in red with the planning target volume, 1.5 cm expansion, in yellow.

because the catheter placement is individualized, allowing dose distributions to be tailored to the specific clinical scenario. This allows treatment delivery to a target surrounding a nonspherical cavity and relative dose sparing of the neighboring rib and skin. However, it should be noted that despite these recent image-guided technique improvements, interstitial brachytherapy remains a comparatively challenging treatment technique requiring a high level of attention to the details of catheter placement and dosimetric planning.

Several institutional series utilizing multicatheter brachytherapy have been reported with greater than 5-year follow-up (Table 38.1). The majority of these experiences have reported results in very favorable patients at low risk for local recurrence (Table 38.2). Vicini et al. (27) have reported on the largest series of

patients treated with interstitial brachytherapy as APBI for which long-term follow-up is available. One hundred and ninety-nine patients aged 40 or more years, the majority with invasive tumors less than 3 cm, excision margins greater than 2 mm, and negative axillary lymph nodes were implanted and treated with low-dose rate or high-dose rate (HDR) brachytherapy. Match-paired analysis of these patients at 5 years demonstrated an equivalent local recurrence rate of 1% compared with patients treated by whole breast irradiation (WBI). As well, this series has been extensively analyzed with respect to cosmesis, demonstrating good to excellent results in 95% to 99% of patients with only a 3.5% local recurrence rate at 10 years (28,29).

To date there has only been one prospective phase III trial for which mature results are available to evaluate APBI using

Table 38.1	ACCELERATED PARTIAL BREAST IRRADIATION INTERSTITIAL EXPERIENCE: STUDIES WITH GREATER THAN 5-YEAR FOLLOW-UP				
Institution (Reference)	No. of Cases	Median Follow-Up (mos)	5-Yr Actuarial Recurrence Rate Total (%)	5-Yr Elsewhere Failure Rate[a] (%)	Cosmesis Good/Excellent
William Beaumont Hospital (28)	199 LDR 120/HDR79	96	1.6	0.8	92
Tufts/Brown University (23)	33	83.9	6.1	6.1	88
RTOG 95-17 (58)	99	—	4	2	—
HDR	66	78	3	2	—
LDR	34	85	6	3	—
NIO, Hungary Phase I/II Trial (18)	45	80	6.7[b]	6.7[b]	84
NIO, Hungary Phase III Trial (30)	127	66	4.7	3.1	81
Ochsner Clinic (19)	51	74	3	0	75
Massachusetts General Hospital (20)	48	84	2 (8 yr)	2 (8 yr)	68
Guy's Hospital (31)	27	72	37	—	—
London Regional Cancer Center (32)	39	91	16.2	10	—

RTOG, Radiation therapy Oncology Group, HDR, high dose rate, LDR, low dose rate, NIO, National Institute of Oncology.
[a] Elsewhere failure rate is new ipsilateral breast cancer.
[b] Crude rate.

| Table 38.2 | ACCELERATED PARTIAL BREAST IRRADIATION INTERSTITIAL EXPERIENCE: PATIENT SELECTION CRITERIA |

Institution (Reference)	No. of Cases	Median Age	Size (Median)	Final Margin	ER (+) (%)	Lymph Node Negative (%)
William Beaumont Hospital (28)	199	65	11 mm	Negative	86	88
Tufts/Brown University (23)	33	63 (mean)	13 mm	Negative	79	91
RTOG 95-17 (58)	99					
HDR	66	62	88% T1	Negative	80	80
LDR	34	62	88% T1		64	79
NIO, Hungary Phase I/II Trial (18)	45	56	12 mm	Negative	84	80
NIO, Hungary Phase III Trial (30)	127	58	14 mm	Negative	91	90
Ochsner Clinic (19)	51	63	14 mm (mean)	Negative	64	77
Massachusetts General Hospital (20)	28	—	<20 mm	Negative	—	100
Guy's Hospital (31)	27	51 (mean)	30 mm (mean)	Unknown (gross tumor excision only)	—	66
London Regional Cancer Center (32)	39	59	15.6 mm	Negative	33	80

ER (+), estrogen receptor positive; RTOG, Radiation therapy Oncology Group, HDR, high dose rate, LDR, low dose rate, NIO, National Institute of Oncology.

primarily interstitial brachytherapy versus WBI. Polgar et al. (30) reported 5-year results on 258 randomized patients demonstrating similar rates of local recurrence (4.7% and 3.4%; p = .50), overall survival (94.6% vs. 91.8%), cancer-specific survival (98.3% vs. 96.0%), and disease-free survival (88.3% vs. 90.3%) for APBI versus WBI, respectively. In an earlier publication regarding this study, acute and long-term toxicities of APBI were reported and included a 20% rate of grade II or III breast fibrosis at the site of brachytherapy, a rate of grade II or III skin telangiectasia of 4.4%, a 20% rate of asymptomatic fat necrosis, and a 2.2% rate of symptomatic fat necrosis (18).

Despite the majority of studies demonstrating good results with APBI, there have been two published series describing suboptimal results using interstitial brachytherapy. In an early trial conducted at the Guy's Hospital in London, 27 patients were treated with HDR brachytherapy (31). With a median follow-up of 72 months, a local recurrence rate of 37% was noted. In this study, questions have been raised regarding the impact of only requiring grossly negative margins without microscopic margin assessment, the lack of target coverage confirmation, and the appropriateness of these patients for BCT with even standard techniques.

In a more contemporary multicatheter APBI experience in 39 patients from the London Regional Cancer Center in Canada, a local recurrence rate of 16.2% was noted with a median follow-up of 91 months (32). The target definition applied in this trial, restricting the target boundaries to the lumpectomy cavity alone and therefore excluding the high-risk area of adjacent breast tissue, has raised questions regarding the treatment of an appropriate target. After a thorough review of these investigations, it has been suggested that the negative results stem from both a lack of proper patient selection and acceptable dose delivery.

MammoSite Radiation Therapy System for Accelerated Partial Breast Irradiation

Alternative methods of dose delivery were created in an attempt to reduce the complexity and invasiveness of APBI. The first brachytherapy device designed with such a purpose was

the MammoSite (Hologic, Inc, Bedford, Massachusetts) breast brachytherapy applicator. Since receiving clearance by the U.S. Food and Drug Administration (FDA) in 2002, MammoSite has become the most widely used form of APBI, implanted in more than 40,000 women by early 2008 (33).

The MammoSite device consists of a single lumen catheter allowing the passage of a HDR afterloaded iridium-192 [^{192}Ir] source. The device can be implanted at the time of surgery (open technique) or under ultrasound guidance postoperatively through the same or alternative incision (closed technique). After insertion, the device is filled with radiographic contrast to allow evaluation of placement by CT scan. Device placement is assessed for the adequacy of skin spacing (optimally ≥7 mm) and conformality of the balloon surface to the lumpectomy cavity (>90%). The device is attached to an HDR afterloader for the delivery of 10 fractions of 3.4 Gy each, twice daily for 10 days with a minimum of 6 hours between treatments. This is the most common fractionation schedule used and is based on previous brachytherapy experience with interstitial catheters.

The initial experience with the MammoSite was published by Keisch et al. (33). This prospective, multi-institutional trial included 70 patients older than 45 years of age with invasive ductal carcinomas less than 2 cm, negative resection margins, and axillary node negative disease. The study demonstrated the feasibility of the technique and laid the framework for the regulatory clearance of the MammoSite device. Published 5-year data demonstrate no locoregional recurrences with 83.3% of these patients experiencing good to excellent cosmesis. Overall toxicity rates were reported and included an infection rate of 9.3%, seroma formation in 32.6% (12% were symptomatic), telangiectasias in 39.4%, and asymptomatic fat necrosis reported in 4 of 43 (34). This represents the earliest use of this brachytherapy device and there was a decrease in skin toxicity when the skin distance was 7 mm or more and a decrease in the rate of seroma formation when the device was placed postlumpectomy in a closed cavity.

Concurrently with FDA clearance of the device, the manufacturer initiated the MammoSite breast brachytherapy registry study. Control of this trial has subsequently been transferred to the American Society of Breast Surgeons (ASBrS). With more than 1,400 participants enrolled, the most recent report demonstrates a 3-year actuarial rate of local recurrence of 1.79% with similar rates of toxicity as reported in the original study used to obtain FDA clearance (35). Additionally, in a study of 483 patients contributed from multiple institutions, the local recurrence rate was 1.2% with a median follow-up of 24 months (36). Although significant acute and late treatment-related effects with the MammoSite have infrequently been reported with proper use, potential toxicities can include radiation dermatitis, breast hyperpigmentation, seroma formation, breast infection, fibrosis, telangiectasias, and persistent pigmentary changes (37). Skin spacing 7 mm or more, use of a closed cavity placement technique, use of prophylactic antibiotics, and the use of multiple dwell positions within the device during treatment have been associated with a decreased incidence of acute and late toxicities.

In some cases (up to 9% of patients in the ASBrS trial) the MammoSite device cannot meet specified criteria (dosimetric) and needs to be explanted (38). This has led to the development of other devices including the Contura (SenoRx, Aliso Viejo, California) multilumen radiation balloon (MLB) and intracavitary multicatheter devices including the Strut-Adjusted Volume Implant (Cianna Medical, Aliso Viejo, California) and the Clearpath Accelerated Partial Breast Irradiation System (North American Scientific, Chatsworth, California). Lastly, the Axxent Electronic Brachytherapy System (Xoft, Inc, Fremont, California) relies on a balloon-based catheter and a 50 keV x-ray source for afterloading instead of an HDR afterloader, thus significantly decreasing the need for shielding and making the delivery possible in a broader range of clinical settings. At the time of this publication, only minimal data were available using any of these modalities.

Finally, despite these good early results, concerns remain regarding (a) the long-term impact of this fractionation schedule both on local control and cosmesis, (b) the impact of the dosimetric characteristics of balloon brachytherapy on the development of late toxicities, and (c) the adequacy of the volume of uninvolved breast tissue surrounding the lumpectomy cavity that receives the full RT dose.

Three-Dimensional Conformal External Beam Radiation Therapy Accelerated Partial Breast Irradiation

The 3D-CRT technique employs a standard linear accelerator to deliver external beam radiation to a clinical target volume, usually the tumor bed plus a normal breast tissue margin of 10 to 15 mm, with an additional margin to account for breathing motion and setup uncertainties (generally 10 mm). Three to five beams are typically used to deliver the dose to patients in either the supine or prone position using photons alone or in combination with electrons (Fig. 38.2) (39).

APBI using 3D-CRT is less studied than brachytherapy techniques in terms of number of patients and length of follow-up. The initial experience using nonconformal, external beam partial breast irradiation in a phase III trial was discouraging with local failure in the partial breast irradiation arm nearly twice that of the WBI arm (20% vs. 11%) (40). The lack of pathologic microscopic margin assessment and confirmation of target coverage in this trial has been suggested as an explanation for these results. The concept was revived decades later by groups at William Beaumont Hospital, New York University, and the Massachusetts General Hospital using 3D-CRT (41,42). At these centers, much more stringent selection criteria were used, limiting patients to those 50 or more years of age, tumor size 3 cm or less, invasive ductal histology, negative surgical margins (>2 mm), and negative axillary nodes. The Massachusetts General Hospital experience has reported their initial experience with a combined photon-electron technique with only limited follow-up. Sixty-one patients were treated with 32 Gy delivered in eight 4 Gy fractions given twice a day (43). In the most recent analysis at William Beaumont Hospital, 91 consecutive patients were treated, using their previously reported 3D-CRT techniques (34 or 38.5 Gy in 10 fractions given over 5 consecutive days). With a median follow-up of 24 months, no local recurrences were reported and 91% of patients had good or excellent cosmesis (44).

At New York University, 78 patients were treated using a customized table top for prone treatment positioning to reduce

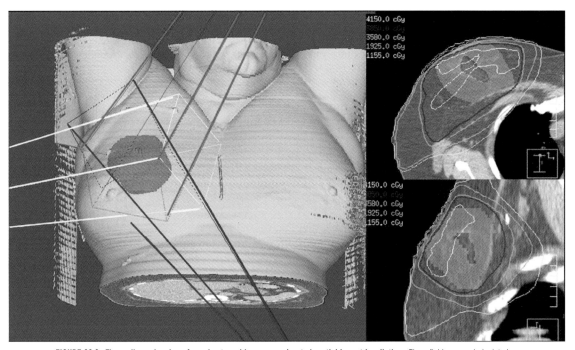

FIGURE 38.2. Three-dimensional conformal external bream accelerated partial breast irradiation. Three field approach depicted on left with planning target volume shown in red. Cross and sagittal sections of dosimetric coverage shown on the right. The lumpectomy cavity in red with planning target volume, a 2.5 cm expansion, in orange.

organ motion and to move target breast tissue away from the thoracic wall and associated critical structures (heart and lung) (45). They delivered a dose of 30 Gy in 6-Gy fractions over 10 days. With a follow-up of 28 months, no local recurrences were reported, and good or excellent cosmetic results were observed in 92% of cases (29).

A legitimate concern regarding the delivery of 3D-CRT utilizing photons or electrons is that the volume of nontarget tissue receiving 50% of the prescribed dose is typically 40%, which is much higher than with the brachytherapy techniques (46). Protons have dosimetric qualities that could limit the dose to nontarget tissue due to their sharp Bragg peak (47). Preliminary data in 20 patients with stage I breast cancer from Massachusetts General Hospital using proton 3D-CRT with a median follow-up of 12 months demonstrated no local recurrences, and good or excellent cosmesis was seen in 89% and 100%, at 6 months and 12 months, respectively.

The 3D-CRT offers several advantages over brachytherapy techniques. It is less invasive. Radiation oncologists are well versed in linear accelerator (LINAC)-based techniques. Treatments are likely to be delivered in a more consistent manner with better dose homogeneity. However, the need for additional margins to account for setup uncertainties can result in increased dose to critical structures, such as the heart, lung, and contralateral breast. The long-term effect of delivering these lower, but accelerated doses to an increased volume of normal tissue in patients with a long life expectancy is uncertain. In response to these concerns, investigators have set conservative normal tissue dose limitations to guide field orientation and design. These constraints limit the number of cases that can be treated with an external beam approach to those with small target sizes and specific locations within the breast. These dose restrictions are clearly outlined in the national phase III partial breast trial and state, in addition to dose restrictions to the lung, heart, and contralateral breast, that while delivering at least 90% of the prescribed dose to at least 90% of the treatment target, less than 60% of the whole breast reference volume should receive 50% or more of the prescribed dose and less than 35% of the whole breast reference volume should receive the prescribed dose (48).

Intraoperative Accelerated Partial Breast Irradiation

Outside the United States, intraoperative RT has been the primary focus of investigation for the delivery of APBI. The University College of London has investigated the use of low energy x-rays (maximum energy, 50 kv) delivered by a portable, spherical, radiation-generating device (Targeted Intraoperative Radiotherapy [TARGIT] trial) that is placed into the lumpectomy cavity following tumor resection (49). A dose of 20 Gy at 1 mm and 6 Gy at 10 mm from the applicator surface is delivered to the cavity. Although the lower energies delivered preclude the need for specially shielded operating rooms, there is concern that such low energies may be inadequate to "sterilize" the target volume of microscopic disease. Initial reports with this technique have reported acceptable cosmetic results, toxicity, and local control rates (50).

The European Institute of Oncology has used intraoperative electrons (generated by a mobile linear accelerator) delivering 21 Gy in one fraction (immediately following quadrantectomy). The breast is surgically manipulated to ensure that all targeted tissue is within the electron field boundaries and nontargeted normal tissue is either outside the electron field or shielded. The Milan group has published on a series of 590 patients using this technique with a median follow-up of 20 months demonstrating a local recurrence rate of 0.5%, with acceptable toxicities (51). Both institutions are presently conducting phase III randomized trials (see below).

Intraoperative treatment raises some important concerns. The treatment is completed before the availability of the final microscopic margin and axillary nodal status are known, information considered important in patient selection and in the determination of the target extent. Guidelines for target delineation and dose coverage using this approach are unclear. The late effects on breast tissue as a result of a very large single dose are uncertain.

 ## PATIENT SELECTION

One of the key components contributing to the successful early application of APBI is case selection. It should be emphasized that the concept of APBI demands the proper selection of patients with an anticipated low risk of harboring in-breast microscopic disease remote from the lumpectomy cavity. In response to the increased interest in APBI, two societies have endorsed conservative patient selection criteria. The American Brachytherapy Society patient selection criteria include patients 50 or more years of age, invasive ductal carcinoma only, tumor size of 3 cm or less, negative resection margins (defined as no tumor on ink), and a negative axillary nodal status (recent web-based update of American Brachytherapy Society guidelines changed the lowest age from 45 to 50) (52). The patient selection criteria endorsed by the ASBrS includes patients 45 or more years of age, invasive ductal carcinoma or ductal carcinoma *in situ*, tumor size of 3 cm or less, negative resection margins (defined as at least 2 mm in all directions), and a negative axillary nodal status. A third set of patient selection guidelines is forthcoming as a product of an American Society of Radiation Oncology (ASTRO) consensus panel (53) (see Management Summary). In reviewing the literature, requiring negative surgical margins and restricting treatment to patients with smaller tumors are the only two criteria that have been consistently applied within the successful APBI trials. However, the majority of the women included in the initial trials were older than 50 years old, estrogen receptor positive and axillary node negative. Additional criteria (extensive intraductal component, infiltrating lobular histology, and ductal carcinoma *in situ*) were inconsistently applied as exclusion criteria.

 ## PHASE III TRIALS

Continued studies are necessary to address questions regarding patient selection criteria, details of treatment technique, long-term efficacy and safety, and determining which APBI approach is best applied for each clinical setting. It is encouraging that there are six prospective randomized phase III trials currently enrolling patients comparing APBI and WBI (Table 38.3). These studies include the National Surgical Adjuvant Breast and Bowel Project (NSABP) B-39 Radiation Therapy Oncology Group (RTOG) 0413 (48). This protocol has an accrual goal of 4,300 patients. Patients are randomly assigned postoperatively to WBI or APBI and, if randomized to APBI, any of the three acceptable APBI techniques can be used; namely, multicatheter interstitial brachytherapy, MammoSite radiation therapy system brachytherapy, or 3D-CRT. The Canadian Randomized Trial of Accelerated Partial Breast Irradiation (RAPID) trial is focusing on conservatively selected patients and has an accrual goal of 2,128 patients (54). This trial randomizes patients between standard WBI and 3D-CRT APBI. The WBI fractionation can be either 50 Gy in 25 fractions or 42.5 Gy in 16 fractions and either with or without a boost of 10 Gy to the tumor bed. The 3D-CRT APBI fractionation is 38.5 Gy delivered in 10 twice daily fractions over 5 treatment days. In the United Kingdom, the Intensity Modulated and Partial Organ Radiotherapy, Low Risk (IMPORT LOW) trial has an accrual goal of 1,935 patients (55). Patients with tumors 2 cm or less will be randomized to WBI, 40 Gy in 15 fractions over 3 weeks, or to one of two test arms. Patients in test arm two receive 40 Gy to a partial breast target only while those patients in test arm one receive 40 Gy to the same partial breast target while simultaneously

| Table 38.3 | PHASE III TRIALS OF ACCELERATED PARTIAL BREAST IRRADIATION |||

Institution/Trial	No. of Cases	Control Arm	Experimental Arm
NSABP B-39/RTOG 0413	4,300	50–50.4 Gy WB +/− 10–16 Gy Boost	(1) Interstitial Brachytx, or (2) MammoSite, or (3) 3D Conformal EBRT
National Institute of Oncology Budapest, Hungary	258	50 Gy WB	(1) Interstitial Brachytx (5.2 Gy × 7) or (2) Electrons (50 Gy)
European Brachytherapy Breast Cancer GEC-ESTRO Working Group	1,170	50–50.4 Gy WB + 10 Gy Boost	Brachytherapy Only 32.0 Gy 8 fractions HDR 30.3 Gy 7 fractions HDR 50 Gy PDR
European Institute of Oncology ELIOT	1,200	50 Gy WB + 10 Gy Boost	Intra-operative Single fraction EBRT 21 Gy × 1
University College of London TARGIT	1,600	WB RT (per center) + Boost	Intra-operative Single fraction EBRT 5 Gy × 1
Canadian Trial RAPID	2,128	WB 42.5 Gy in 16 or 50 Gy in 25 +/− 10 Gy boost	3D CRT only 38.5 Gy in 10
Medical Research Council—UK IMPORT LOW	1,935	WB 2.67 Gy × 15	(1) WB 2.4 Gy × 15 PB 2.67 Gy × 15 (2) PB only 2.67 Gy × 15

NSABP, National Surgical Breast and Bowel Project; RTOG, Radiation Therapy Oncology Group; WB, whole breast, RT, radiation therapy; PB, partial breast; EBRT, external beam radiation therapy; GEC-ESTRO, Groupe Europeen de Curietherapie European Society for Therapeutic Radiology and Oncology; HDR, high dose rate; PDR, pulsed dose rate; TARGIT, Targeted Intraoperative Radiotherapy; ELIOT, Intraoperative Radiotherapy with Electrons; IMPORT LOW, Intensity Modulated and Partial Organ Radiotherapy, Low Risk; 3DCRT, three-dimensional conformal radiation therapy; RAPID, Randomized Trial of Accelerated Partial Breast Irradiation.

receiving a whole breast dose of 36 Gy in 15 fractions. The European Brachytherapy Breast Cancer (Groupe European de Curietherapie [European Society for Therapeutic Radiology and Oncology; GEC-ESTRO]) Working Group has initiated a multi-catheter interstitial based phase III trial with an accrual goal of 1,170 patients (56). The dose delivery schemes allow both HDR and pulsed dose rate brachytherapy. The fractionation for HDR will be 32 Gy in eight fractions over 4 days or 30.3 Gy in seven fractions and the fractionation for pulsed dose rate will be .6 to .8 Gy per hour to 50 Gy (1 pulse per hour, 24 hours per day). Two intraoperative phase III partial breast trials have also been initiated. The Intraoperative Radiotherapy with Electrons (ELIOT) trial from the European Institute of Oncology in Milan, Italy, compares standard WBI to intraoperative electrons delivering 21 Gy in one fraction following quadrantectomy (57). The accrual goal of 1,200 patients has been completed and outcome results are awaited. The TARGIT trial tests the use of an intraoperative kilovolt energy applicator (50). This trial is being conducted by the University College of London with several sites worldwide participating. The prescribed intraoperative treatment is 20 Gy to a 2-mm depth. There will be 1,600 patients accrued to this trial.

Treatment with APBI is increasingly being offered off protocol as the follow-up from the initial phase I and II trials increases with continued good results. This enthusiasm should be tempered with the understanding that most of these published 5-year data originate from single institutional phase I or II trials and included highly selected patients that were treated using meticulous quality. A conservative approach to off-protocol treatment is encouraged until additional data are available, and any patient seeking treatment with APBI needs to understand the limited present state of the supporting data. Participation in phase III trials is required to ensure that proper levels of supporting data are generated and that the optimal technique and patient selection criteria can be appropriately defined.

MANAGEMENT SUMMARY

- APBI is not presently accepted as a standard of care for early stage breast cancer by all physicians. The results from randomized clinical trials are needed.

- However, based on currently available treatment results, appropriately selected patients can be offered APBI off protocol using appropriate techniques and the following guidelines:
  - Inform patient of current status of APBI data
  - Selection of the optimal APBI technique to be used based upon the clinical situation, physician experience and patient preference. Technique selection will depend on lumpectomy cavity size and location in respect to breast size and shape. The technique chosen should easily comply with the dosimetric goals to assure optimal disease control while limiting toxicity.
- Incorporation of a thorough quality assurance program for APBI treatment delivery. Regardless of the treatment technique, the following should be incorporated:
  - careful attention to target definition and delineation
  - acceptable dosimetric coverage of the target
  - acceptable dose homogeneity
  - reduction of non-target breast and normal tissues dose
  - verification of treatment delivery
  - careful monitoring of acute and sub-acute toxicities based upon the APBI technique employed
- Adherence to conservative patient selection guidlines drafted by Task Force convened by the American Society of Therapeutic Radiology and Oncology (ASTRO) Health Services Research Committee is recommended. The final version of this cosensus statement is available in reference 53. Given that the information in reference 53. Given that the information in this field is rapidly evolving, please check for updated pulished versions of the ASTRO consensus statment.

Suitable conditates if all of the following criteria present:
- age ≥60 yo
- infiltrating ductal carcinoma and favorable subtypes
- ≤2 cm size
- lumpectomy achieving microscopically negative margins ≥2 mm
- negative axillary lymph nodes
- ER (+) tumors
- No extensive intraductal component
- No lymph vascular space invasion

Cautionary candidates: any of these criteria should invoke caution and concern when considering APBI:

- age 50–59 yo
- lesions 2.1 - 3.0 cm in size
- invasive Lobular
- pure DCIS ≤3cm
- lumpectomy achieving microscopically negative margins <2 mm
- extensive intraductal component <3cm
- limited/focal lymph vasular space invasion

Unsuitable candidates: outside of a clinical trial if any of these criteria are present

- age <50
- BRCA 1/2 mutation present
- lesion size >3cm
- axillary nodes positive
- lymph vascular space invasion present - extensive
- extensive intraductal component >3cm
- multicentric disease
- use of neoadjuvant therapy

References

1. Fisher B, Anderson S, Bryant J, et al. Twenty-year follow-up of a randomized trial comparing total mastectomy, lumpectomy, and lumpectomy plus irradiation for the treatment of invasive breast cancer. *N Engl J Med* 2002;347:1233–1241.
2. Veronesi U, Cascinelli N, Mariani L, et al. Twenty-year follow-up of a randomized study comparing breast-conserving surgery with radical mastectomy for early breast cancer. *N Engl J Med* 2002;347:1227–1232.
3. Arthur DW, Vicini FA. Accelerated partial breast irradiation as a part of breast conservation therapy. *J Clin Oncol* 2005;23:1726–1735.
4. Whelan T, MacKenzie R, Julian J, et al. Randomized trial of breast irradiation schedules after lumpectomy for women with lymph node-negative breast cancer. *J Natl Cancer Inst* 2002;94:1143–1150.
5. Bentzen SM, Agrawal RK, Aird EG, et al. The UK Standardisation of Breast Radiotherapy (START) Trial A of radiotherapy hypofractionation for treatment of early breast cancer: a randomised trial. *Lancet Oncol* 2008;9:331–341.
6. Bentzen SM, Agrawal RK, Aird EG, et al. The UK Standardisation of Breast Radiotherapy (START) Trial B of radiotherapy hypofractionation for treatment of early breast cancer: a randomised trial. *Lancet* 2008;371:1098–1107.
7. Hughes KS, Schnaper LA, Berry D, et al. Lumpectomy plus tamoxifen with or without irradiation in women 70 years of age or older with early breast cancer. *N Engl J Med* 2004;351:971–977.
8. Rosen PP, Fracchia AA, Urban JA, et al. "Residual" mammary carcinoma following simulated partial mastectomy. *Cancer* 1975;35:739–747.
9. Faverly D, Holland R, Burgers L. An original stereomicroscopic analysis of the mammary glandular tree. *Virchows Arch A Pathol Anat Histopathol* 1992;421:115–119.
10. Haffty BG, Carter D, Flynn SD, et al. Local recurrence versus new primary: clinical analysis of 82 breast relapses and potential applications for genetic fingerprinting. *Int J Radiat Oncol Biol Phys* 1993;27:575–583.
11. Imamura H, Haga S, Shimizu T, et al. Relationship between the morphological and biological characteristics of intraductal components accompanying invasive ductal breast carcinoma and patient age. *Breast Cancer Res Treat* 2000;62:177–184.
12. Ohtake T, Abe R, Kimijima I, et al. Intraductal extension of primary invasive breast carcinoma treated by breast-conserving surgery. Computer graphic three-dimensional reconstruction of the mammary duct-lobular systems. *Cancer* 1995;76:32–45.
13. Clark RM, Wilkinson RH, Miceli PN, et al. Breast cancer. Experiences with conservation therapy. *Am J Clin Oncol* 1987;10:461–468.
14. Veronesi U, Marubini E, Mariani L, et al. Radiotherapy after breast-conserving surgery in small breast carcinoma: long-term results of a randomized trial. *Ann Oncol* 2001;12:997–1003.
15. Sector resection with or without postoperative radiotherapy for stage I breast cancer: a randomized trial. The Uppsala-Orebro Breast Cancer Study Group. *J Natl Cancer Inst* 1990;82:1851.
16. Athas WF, Adams-Cameron M, Hunt WC, et al. Travel distance to radiation therapy and receipt of radiotherapy following breast-conserving surgery. *J Natl Cancer Inst* 2000;92:269–271.
17. Clarke M, Collins R, Darby S, et al. Effects of radiotherapy and of differences in the extent of surgery for early breast cancer on local recurrence and 15-year survival: an overview of the randomised trials. *Lancet* 2005;366:2087–2106.
18. Polgar C, Major T, Fodor J, et al. High-dose-rate brachytherapy alone versus whole breast radiotherapy with or without tumor bed boost after breast-conserving surgery: Seven-year results of a comparative study. *Int J Radiat Oncol Biol Phys* 2004;60:1173–1181.
19. King TA, Bolton JS, Kuske RR, et al. Long-term results of wide-field brachytherapy as the sole method of radiation therapy after segmental mastectomy for T(is,1,2) breast cancer. *Am J Surg* 2000;180:299–304.
20. MacDonald SM, Alm El-Din MA, Smith BL, et al. Low dose rate interstitial implants for early stage breast cancer: outcomes and late toxicity of a dose escalation trial. *Int J Radiat Oncol Biol Phys* 2007;69:(abst1016).
21. Kuske RR. Breast brachytherapy. *Hematol Oncol Clin North Am* 1999;13:543.
22. Kuske RR, Winter K, Arthur DW, et al. Phase II trial of brachytherapy alone after lumpectomy for select breast cancer: toxicity analysis of RTOG 95-17. *Int J Radiat Oncol Biol Phys* 2006;65:45–51.
23. Kaufman SA, DiPetrillo TA, Price LL, et al. Long-term outcome and toxicity in a phase I/II trial using high-dose-rate multicatheter interstitial brachytherapy for T1/T2 breast cancer. *Brachytherapy* 2007;6:286–292.
24. Zwicker RD, Arthur DW, Kavanagh BD, et al. Optimization of planar high-dose-rate implants. *Int J Radiat Oncol Biol Phys* 1999;44:1171–1177.
25. Das RK, Patel R, Shah H, et al. 3D CT-based high-dose-rate breast brachytherapy implants: treatment planning and quality assurance. *Int J Radiat Oncol Biol Phys* 2004;59:1224–1228.
26. Cuttino LW, Todor D, Arthur DW. CT-guided multi-catheter insertion technique for partial breast brachytherapy: reliable target coverage and dose homogeneity. *Brachytherapy* 2005;4:10–17.
27. Vicini FA, Kestin L, Chen P, et al. Limited-field radiation therapy in the management of early-stage breast cancer. *J Natl Cancer Inst* 2003;95:1205–1210.
28. Vicini FA, Antonucci JV, Wallace M, et al. Long-term efficacy and patterns of failure after accelerated partial breast irradiation: a molecular assay-based clonality evaluation. *Int J Radiat Oncol Biol Phys* 2007;68:341–346.
29. Chen PY, Vicini FA, Benitez P, et al. Long-term cosmetic results and toxicity after accelerated partial-breast irradiation. *Cancer* 2006;106(5):991–999.
30. Polgar C, Fodor J, Major T, et al. Breast-conserving treatment with partial or whole breast irradiation for low-risk invasive breast carcinoma: 5-year results of a randomized trial. *Int J Radiat Oncol Biol Phys* 2007;69(3):694–702.
31. Fentiman IS, Poole C, Tong D, et al. Inadequacy of iridium implant as sole radiation treatment for operable breast cancer. *Eur J Cancer* 1996;32A:608–611.
32. Perera F, Yu E, Engel J, et al. Patterns of breast recurrence in a pilot study of brachytherapy confined to the lumpectomy site for early breast cancer with six years' minimum follow-up. *Int J Radiat Oncol Biol Phys* 2003;57:1239–1246.
33. Keisch M, Vicini F, Kuske RR, et al. Initial clinical experience with the MammoSite breast brachytherapy applicator in women with early-stage breast cancer treated with breast-conserving therapy. *Int J Radiat Oncol Biol Phys* 2003;55:289–293.
34. Benitez PR, Keisch ME, Vicini F, et al. Five-year results: the initial clinical trial of MammoSite balloon brachytherapy for partial breast irradiation in early-stage breast cancer. *Am J Surg* 2007;194:456–462.
35. Vicini F, Beitsch PD, Quiet CA, et al. Three-year analysis of treatment efficacy, cosmesis, and toxicity by the American Society of Breast Surgeons MammoSite Breast Brachytherapy Registry Trial in patients treated with accelerated partial breast irradiation (APBI). *Cancer* 2008;112:758–766.
36. Cuttino LW, Keisch M, Jenrette JM, et al. Multi-institutional experience using the MammoSite radiation therapy system in the treatment of early-stage breast cancer: 2-year results. *Int J Radiat Oncol Biol Phys* 2008;71(1):107–114.
37. Chao KK, Vicini FA, Wallace M, et al. Analysis of treatment efficacy, cosmesis, and toxicity using the MammoSite breast brachytherapy catheter to deliver accelerated partial-breast irradiation: the William Beaumont Hospital experience. *Int J Radiat Oncol Biol Phys* 2007;69:32–40.
38. Vicini FA, Beitsch PD, Quiet CA, et al. First analysis of patient demographics, technical reproducibility, cosmesis, and early toxicity: results of the American Society of Breast Surgeons MammoSite breast brachytherapy trial. *Cancer* 2005;104:1138–1148.
39. Kozak KR, Doppke KP, Katz A, et al. Dosimetric comparison of two different three-dimensional conformal external beam accelerated partial breast irradiation techniques. *Int J Radiat Oncol Biol Phys* 2006;65:340–346.
40. Ribeiro GG, Magee B, Swindell R, et al. The Christie Hospital breast conservation trial: an update at 8 years from inception. *Clin Oncol (R Coll Radiol)* 1993;5:278–283.
41. Baglan KL, Sharpe MB, Jaffray D, et al. Accelerated partial breast irradiation using 3D conformal radiation therapy (3D-CRT). *Int J Radiat Oncol Biol Phys* 2003;55:302–311.
42. Formenti SC, Rosenstein B, Skinner KA, et al. T1 stage breast cancer: adjuvant hypofractionated conformal radiation therapy to tumor bed in selected postmenopausal breast cancer patients—pilot feasibility study. *Radiology* 2002;222:171–178.
43. Taghian AG, Kozak KR, Doppke KP, et al. Initial dosimetric experience using simple three-dimensional conformal external-beam accelerated partial-breast irradiation. *Int J Radiat Oncol Biol Phys* 2006;64:1092–1099.
44. Vicini FA, Chen P, Wallace M, et al. Interim cosmetic results and toxicity using 3D conformal external beam radiotherapy to deliver accelerated partial breast irradiation in patients with early-stage breast cancer treated with breast-conserving therapy. *Int J Radiat Oncol Biol Phys* 2007;69:1124–1130.
45. Wernicke AG, Gidea-Addeo D, Magnolfi C, et al. External beam partial breast irradiation following breast-conserving surgery: preliminary results of cosmetic outcome of NYU 00-23. *Int J Radiat Oncol Biol Phys* 2006;66:S32.
46. Weed DW, Edmundson GK, Vicini FA, et al. Accelerated partial breast irradiation: a dosimetric comparison of three different techniques. *Brachytherapy* 2005;4:121–129.
47. Kozak KR, Smith BL, Adams J, et al. Accelerated partial-breast irradiation using proton beams: initial clinical experience. *Int J Radiat Oncol Biol Phys* 2006;66:691–698.
48. Vicini F, White J, Arthur D, et al. NSABP protocol B39/RTOG protocol 0413: a randomized phase III study of conventional whole breast irradiation versus partial breast irradiation for women with stage 0,I, or II breast cancer, 2004. Website: http://www.rtog.org/members/protocols/0413/0413.pdf
49. Vaidya JS, Tobias JS, Baum M, et al. Intraoperative radiotherapy for breast cancer. *Lancet Oncol* 2004;5:165–173.
50. Vaidya JS. Partial breast irradiation using targeted intraoperative radiotherapy (TARGIT). *Natl Clin Pract Oncol* 2007;4:384–385.
51. Veronesi U, Orecchia R, Luini A, et al. Full-dose intraoperative radiotherapy with electrons during breast-conserving surgery: experience with 590 cases. *Ann Surg* 2005;242:101–106.
52. Arthur D, Vicini F, Kuske RR, et al. Accelerated partial breast irradiation: An updated report from the American Brachytherapy Society. *Brachytherapy* 2002;1:184–190.
53. Smith Bd, Arthur DW, Buchholz TA, et al. Accelerated partial breast irradiation consensus statement from the American Society of Therapeutic Radiology and Oncology. *Int J Radiat Oncol Biol Phys* 2009 (in press).
54. Whelan T. Olivotto I, Julian J. RAPID: Randomized trial of Accelerated Partial Breast Irradiation, 2006. Web site: http://www.clincaltrials.gov/ct/show/NCT00282035
55. Coles C, Yarnold J. The IMPORT trials are launched (September 2006). *Clin Oncol (R Coll Radiol)* 2006;18:587–590.
56. Polgar C, Strnaad V, Major T. Brachytherapy for partial breast irradiation: the European experience. *Semin Radiat Oncol* 2005;15:116–122.
57. Orrechia R, Ciocca M, Lazzari R, et al. Intraoperative radiation therapy with electrons (ELIOT) in early stage breast cancer. *Breast* 2003;12:483–490.
58. Arthur DW, Winter K, Kuske RR, et al. A phase II trial of brachytherapy alone after lumpectomy for select breast cancer: tumor control and survival outcomes of RTOG 95-17. *Int J Radiat Oncol Biol Phys* 2008;72(2):467–473.

Sameer A. Patel and Neal Stoddard Topham

Patients diagnosed with breast cancer who are offered unilateral or bilateral mastectomy or those who will undergo a lumpectomy affecting breast shape should be seen by a reconstructive plastic surgeon to discuss options for breast reconstruction regardless of age, body habitus, or cancer treatment. Table 39.1 lists the most common techniques of breast reconstruction employed by plastic and reconstructive surgeons. It is the role of the plastic surgeon to assess the patient to determine the best surgical option for breast reconstruction and the appropriate timing, then individually tailor these options to meet the goals of a well-informed patient. A complete evaluation includes consideration of patient expectations, body habitus, cancer treatment, patient habits such as smoking, and comorbidities. With these factors in mind, a reconstructive plan can be formulated and offered to patients that will maximize aesthetic outcome and patient satisfaction and minimize potential complications.

Figure 39.1 illustrates the factors involved in the process of selecting the best reconstructive option to match patient expectations, physical appearance, and cancer treatment. Once the factors for each patient are defined the best option becomes clear and an optimal aesthetic outcome is achieved. As an example, consider a thin patient with a "B" cup breast size undergoing bilateral mastectomies who will not require radiation and is willing to accept permanent breast prostheses. The best reconstructive option for this patient is immediate bilateral breast reconstruction with implants. In contrast, consider the use of breast implant reconstruction in a patient requiring unilateral reconstruction who is obese with a "D" cup ptotic breast. In this scenario the patient is a poor candidate for implant reconstruction but is a good candidate for immediate free transverse rectus abdominis myocutaneous (TRAM) flap reconstruction. Patients present with every conceivable clinical scenario. It is the responsibility of plastic surgeons to guide patients through the decision-making process to maximize their outcome. This chapter is intended to provide information regarding the full spectrum of options available for total breast reconstruction and provide insight into the process of selecting the best method of reconstruction for the individual patient. Careful attention to detail and disciplined decision making will minimize complications, maximize patient satisfaction, and restore the quality of life patients enjoyed in their pre-malignant condition.

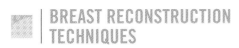

BREAST RECONSTRUCTION TECHNIQUES

Implant-Based Reconstruction

Despite the increasing popularity of autologous breast reconstruction, staged reconstruction using a tissue expander followed by exchange to a permanent implant remains the most common form of breast reconstructive procedure (Fig. 39.2). Almost all patients undergoing breast reconstruction are candidates for implant-based reconstruction. The only exceptions to this are in cases where there is a preexisting local infection or when there is an insufficient amount of skin to cover the tissue expander at the time of initial mastectomy. This latter scenario is exceedingly rare given the use of the skin-sparing

mastectomy. The following factors, although not absolute contraindications to implant-based reconstruction, increase the risk of failure and complication with this technique. First, patients with previous radiation therapy to the breast or patients who will require postexchange radiation therapy have been shown to have a worse aesthetic outcome (1) and increased rates of infection, extrusion, capsular contracture, and explantation of the implant as compared to patients without a history of radiation (2,3). Although the option of implant-based reconstruction should not be denied to women who have had or will require radiation therapy (1,4) and are strongly opposed to autologous reconstruction, every effort should be made to educate patients regarding these risks so they can formulate informed decisions. Furthermore, smokers undergoing two-staged reconstruction with tissue expander followed by implant placement have higher rates of overall complications, reconstructive failures, mastectomy flap necrosis, and infectious complications (5). Obesity is also a predictor of an increased risk of implant loss (6).

The ideal scenario for implant-based reconstruction is a patient undergoing bilateral skin-sparing mastectomies or, in the case of a unilateral mastectomy, one who has relatively small to moderate-sized breasts with minimal grade ptosis and who will not require radiation therapy. The use of bilateral implants makes the shape of the breasts more symmetric as opposed to having a unilateral implant. The asymmetry of a unilateral implant may be disguised with the use of a bra and clothing, but without clothes, the asymmetry is often readily apparent. For some, this may be acceptable, but many patients are much more critical, and in these patients, autologous reconstructive options should be encouraged. In addition, a breast reconstructed with an implant will not undergo ptosis as does a natural breast over time. Therefore, the asymmetry noticed in a unilateral breast reconstruction with an implant will worsen over time as the contralateral breast naturally becomes more ptotic.

This method of reconstruction can be performed either at the time of mastectomy (immediate) or in a delayed fashion and is generally performed in a minimum of two stages. Placement of a tissue expander at the time of mastectomy allows for preservation of the overlying skin and avoidance of the scarring and contracture of the skin that invariably occurs when reconstruction is delayed. However, this must be balanced against the increased risk of mastectomy skin flap necrosis, hematoma, and infection with immediate compared to delayed implant-based reconstruction (7,8).

At the first operation, a tissue expander is placed in a submuscular pocket (pectoralis, serratus anterior, rectus fascia) and the overlying skin then closed. Although some plastic surgeons advocate placement of the expander only partially in the submuscular position under the pectoralis or the pectoralis and serratus, leaving the inferior portion subcutaneous, the authors feel that total muscle coverage provides the most protection to the prosthesis in the event of mastectomy skin flap necrosis. Recently, the use of acellular dermis to obtain coverage of the inferolateral portion of the expander, where coverage is most difficult, as well as in cases where a portion of the pectoralis muscle is resected, has been increasingly popular (9,10). This technique provides total coverage of the expander with less pain by avoiding dissection of the serratus and rectus fascia. The pocket created by adding acellular dermis is larger than a purely

Table 39.1	OPTIONS FOR BREAST RECONSTRUCTION

Implant-Based Reconstruction
Saline-filled implant
Silicone-filled implant

Autologous Tissue Reconstruction
Latissimus dorsi myocutaneous flap with or without implant
Abdominal wall flaps:
   Pedicled TRAM (trans rectus abdominus myocutaneous) flap
   Free TRAM flap
   Muscle-sparing free TRAM flap
   DIEP (deep inferior epigastric perforator) flap
   SIEA (superficial inferior epigastric artery) flap
SGAP (superior gluteal artery perforator) flap
ALT (anterolateral thigh) flap
Gracilis myocutaneous flap

submuscular pocket, making it possible to inject more fluid into the tissue expander at the time of surgery. The availability of postmastectomy skin and the size of the pocket govern the volume of fluid injected intraoperatively into the tissue expander. The creation of a larger pocket reduces the number of postoperative visits required for tissue expansion and shortens the reconstructive process. The immediate insertion of a permanent implant has also been suggested with the use of acellular matrix. Using this method, a permanent implant is inserted into the pocket at the time of reconstruction, eliminating the tissue expansion process. Although this technique seems appealing, obtaining an optimal cosmetic outcome is difficult. The standard two-stage reconstructive technique allows for performing capsulotomy and reshaping of the breast pocket when the tissue expander is exchanged for the permanent implant.

This second surgery provides an opportunity to correct minor asymmetries and enhance the texture and appearance

of the reconstructed breast. Immediate implant placement procedures using acellular dermis are more appealing in elderly patients where one procedure can provide a breast mound that eliminates the need for a second surgery, but does not necessarily create a natural shape and appearance without a bra.

In the standard two-stage procedure, the tissue expander is serially expanded postoperatively in the office, usually in increments of 60 to 150 cc per expansion or as tolerated by the patient until the desired volume is reached. Most surgeons will allow the tissue expander to then remain at this volume from 6 weeks to 6 months before proceeding to the second stage of the reconstruction, which involves replacing the tissue expander with a permanent implant. Symmetry procedures on the contralateral breast can be performed in conjunction with the exchange of implants. Although some may perform the nipple reconstruction at this time, most surgeons defer the nipple reconstruction to a third stage to allow for more accurate nipple positioning.

The timing of adjuvant radiation therapy in relation to tissue expansion and exchange to permanent implant is often times difficult to predict. Ideally, tissue expansion should proceed during the course of adjuvant chemotherapy. After completion of chemotherapy and prior to the initiation of radiation therapy, the expander may be exchanged for a permanent implant. This eliminates the need to operate on irradiated breast skin, with its increased risk of wound healing problems and infection. Wright et al. (11) have reported a median interval of 8 weeks from completion of chemotherapy to initiation of radiation with acceptable 5 year locoregional control, distant metastasis-free survival, and overall survival using this sequence of expansion during chemotherapy followed by exchange to permanent implant and then initiation of radiation therapy. However, in some instances, expansion may not be complete by the time the patient is ready to begin radiation therapy. In these cases, the exchange to a permanent implant may be performed after the completion of radiation treatment, but consideration should be given to addition of a latissimus dorsi myocutaneous flap to provide healthy, vascularized coverage and to replace as much of the radiation damaged skin as possible.

The permanent implant can be either saline filled or a silicone cohesive gel. In the early to mid-1990s, silicone gel implants received much negative publicity due to the perception that these implants were associated with a risk of connective tissue disorders as well as a possible association with breast cancer secondary to their polyurethane shell. The U.S. Food and Drug Administration (FDA) subsequently placed a moratorium on the use of silicone implants and later allowed their use only in cases of reconstruction. Patients reconstructed with silicone implants were entered into an FDA-approved trial. Since that time, several large studies have failed to demonstrate any association of silicone gel implants with breast cancer or autoimmune disease (12–15). Because of this, the FDA has recently lifted the restriction on the use of silicone gel implants for both cosmetic augmentation and reconstruction.

With the issue of cancer and autoimmune risk with silicone gel implants resolved, the patient is now faced with the decision between silicone gel and saline-filled implants. The obvious advantage of silicone gel–filled prostheses is the much more natural feel of the device. In addition, prospective comparisons between saline and silicone gel–filled implants used for primary reconstruction, augmentation, and revision show similar rates of rupture or deflation, Baker grade III or IV contracture, reoperation rates, and explantation rates at 3 years (16).

Another concern many women have is the impact of breast implants on the detection of breast cancer. In reconstructive cases, this becomes an issue in patients with breast cancer who

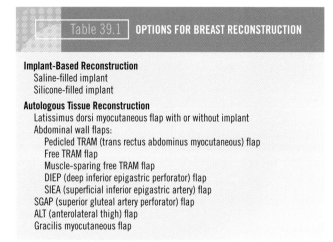

Selection of Reconstructive Method

Patient Expectations
No reconstruction
↓
Perfect Breast

Physical Appearance
Breast size/shape
Weight
Scars
Skin quality

Cancer Treatment
Chemotherapy
Radiation therapy
Unilateral vs bilateral

FIGURE 39.1. The choice of reconstructive technique should take into consideration patient expectations, physical appearance, and cancer treatment.

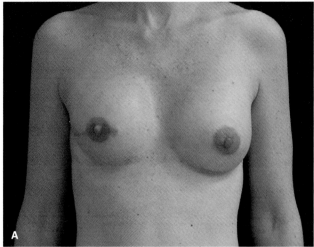

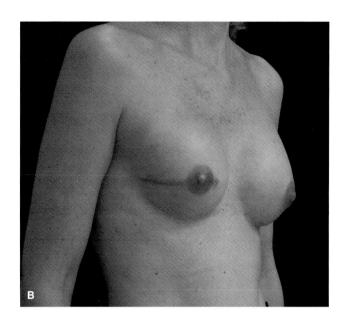

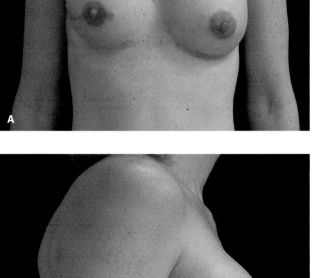

FIGURE 39.2. Implant-based right breast reconstruction with nipple reconstruction using a C-V flap and areolar tattooing. A: Frontal view. **B:** Oblique view. **C:** Lateral view.

have augmentation of the contralateral breast for symmetry as well as in surveillance for recurrence in the ipsilateral mastectomy site. The available literature indicates that cancer diagnosis is not delayed, and breast cancers diagnosed in patients with augmented breasts are not more advanced than those in patients without breast augmentation (17,18). In addition, breast cancer–related survival is not affected (17,18). Patients with implants should continue to have mammography as advised by their breast oncologist, but these studies should be performed in centers where there is expertise in special displacement techniques (19) that maximize the amount of breast parenchyma visualized compared to standard views. Ultrasonography is a useful adjunct in evaluation of mammographic findings as well as palpable abnormalities to differentiate implant irregularities from breast parenchymal abnormalities (20).

Autologous Tissue Reconstruction

Latissimus Dorsi Myocutaneous Flap

The use of the latissimus dorsi (LD) myocutaneous flap as a primary method of reconstruction has declined since the

1970s and has been replaced by implant-based reconstruction and TRAM-based reconstructions. However, it remains an important tool in the armamentarium of the reconstructive surgeon. Perhaps its most common use in breast reconstruction today is as a salvage procedure in failed reconstructions with other methods and in patients who are not candidates to undergo a TRAM-based reconstruction. This includes patients of a thin body habitus with insufficient abdominal pannus, as well as patients with previous abdominal surgery resulting in division of the inferior epigastric pedicle or the abdominal wall perforators (e.g., previous abdominoplasty). Absolute contraindications to use of the latissimus dorsi myocutaneous flap include previous posterior thoracotomy as well as injury to the thoracodorsal pedicle. The latter scenario may be seen in delayed reconstructions in patients who have had previous axillary dissection. The integrity of the pedicle can be tested by assessing the function of muscle contraction by having the patient actively flex the latissimus dorsi muscle. Because the nerve courses with the artery, an intact nerve implies an intact pedicle. The LD flap is useful in obese patients where pannus formation inhibits TRAM flap reconstruction and implants will not provide enough volume or definition. Postoperative seroma formation at the donor site can complicate LD flap reconstruction in obese patients. Bilateral breast reconstruction can be performed using LD flaps, but intraoperative patient repositioning is required. The procedure begins in supine position for bilateral mastectomies, then transitions to the prone position for bilateral flap harvest, then back to the supine position for the flap inset. For these reasons, in addition to the prominent back scars, LD flaps are primarily used in unilateral reconstruction. In patients with small breasts, the LD flap can also be used as a primary method of reconstruction without an implant. In most cases, where it is used in primary reconstruction, however, an implant is generally required to obtain the required volume for breast symmetry. The addition of the latissimus to an implant also provides some ptosis and additional coverage over the implant, providing a more natural appearance.

The latissimus dorsi myocutaneous flap harvest begins with positioning the patient (lateral decubitus or a prone position) and the design of an elliptical skin paddle overlying the muscle. This skin paddle can be oriented in either a transverse or an oblique direction, depending on the final position of the scar desired as well as the orientation of the skin paddle needed at the recipient site. A skin paddle with a width of up to 8 to 10 cm can be harvested and closed primarily depending on patient skin laxity.

The LD has a single dominant blood supply from the thoracodorsal artery and a segmental supply via perforators branching from the lumbar and posterior intercostal arteries. The thoracodorsal artery is the pedicle to this flap, and careful control of the segmental perforators during harvest is necessary to prevent postoperative hematoma. The innervation is supplied by the thoracodorsal nerve, and division of this nerve will prevent postoperative contraction of the muscle, which can be a source of much distress for the patient.

Once the flap is elevated, it is passed into the breast defect through a tunnel created high in the axilla, the donor site is closed in layers over drains, and the patient repositioned to a supine position. The pectoralis muscle can then be elevated to create a pocket for the implant or the pectoralis muscle is left intact and the implant is placed above the pectoralis muscle but underneath the latissimus flap. This creates a pocket for the prosthesis, and the latissimus dorsi is then sutured to the pectoralis muscle superiorly and the inframammary fold inferiorly. The lateral portion of the muscle is sutured to the chest wall to provide total muscle coverage of the prosthesis. The inset of the skin paddle is then performed based on the resulting mastectomy skin defect.

Flap loss with the LD flap is very rare given the excellent blood supply afforded by the thoracodorsal artery. Much more common is the formation of a seroma in the back donor site. For this reason, drains in the back are an absolute must if the LD flap is to be used. These drains may remain in place for several weeks before the drainage is adequately low to allow them to be removed.

Several modifications of the LD flap have been described. Perhaps one of the most useful is the extended LD flap, which incorporates the scapular, parascapular, and lumbar fat below the thoracodorsal facia to increase the volume of tissue (21–23). In many cases, this provides a totally autologous reconstruction without the use of implants. The reliability of this flap for totally autologous reconstruction of small to medium-sized breasts has been demonstrated (23).

For partial mastectomy defects not requiring skin replacement, the use of the latissimus muscle alone is an option. Latissimus dorsi miniflaps have been performed to restore breast volume in patients undergoing breast-conservation therapy (24–26). This technique allows for breast conservation in patients with larger breast tumors to breast volume ratios by immediately replacing the lost volume.

The thoracodorsal artery perforator (TDAP) flap has recently been described for application in reconstruction of partial mastectomy defects (27,28). This flap is based on perforating vessels off of the thoracodorsal artery, which are located preoperatively using a hand held Doppler, and preserves the integrity and innervation of the latissimus dorsi muscle. Only skin and subcutaneous tissue is harvested with this flap, leaving the latissimus dorsi muscle essentially undisturbed. The reliability of this flap is based on a large, pulsatile perforating vessel. If the perforator vessel is not of adequate caliber, a portion of the latissimus muscle may be taken to protect the perforator, leaving the majority of the muscle innervated and functional.

The latissimus dorsi myocutaneous flap and its variations provide a robust source of autologous tissue for reconstruction of the breast, either after total mastectomy or after breast-conservation therapy. The value of this flap for salvage of failed implant reconstructions in patients who are not candidates for other autologous tissue reconstructions cannot be overstated. Its use in primary reconstruction has decreased in recent years, but excellent aesthetic results can be obtained with use of the LD flap with implant in the primary setting as well.

Breast Reconstruction with Abdominal Donor Site

Breast reconstruction using autologous tissue provides the most natural texture and appearance. The results can be stunning when combined with skin-sparing mastectomy in the setting of immediate reconstruction (Fig. 39.3). The most common donor site is the abdominal wall. The pedicled TRAM flap was first described for breast reconstruction by Hartrampf et al. (29) in 1982. For many years the pedicled TRAM flap was the only technique available for reconstruction using abdominal tissue until the advent of microsurgery and techniques of free tissue transfer were introduced to reconstruct the breast. The pedicled TRAM flap performed well for the majority of patients, but as knowledge of both the abdominal wall anatomy and surgical experience increased, several limitations were identified in the use of the pedicled TRAM. Patients who underwent pedicled TRAM flaps had rates of clinically evident fat necrosis approaching 27%, and those who smoked, were obese, or had very large breasts developed postoperative fat necrosis, partial flap loss, and donor site complications at an even greater frequency, up to 37% in obese patients (30–33). There were also concerns regarding weakness and loss of function of the abdominal wall, especially in bilateral breast reconstruction, when it is necessary to divide and harvest the entire rectus muscle. The blood supply for the pedicled TRAM flap is the superior epigastric vessels. As the vessels descend through the rectus muscle, they branch and connect with branches of the deep inferior epigastric system. The inferior epigastric system has a direct route to the perforators in contrast to the superior system. These perforators typically pierce the fascia in two parallel rows called the medial and lateral row perforators. Because the inferior epigastric vessels have a direct route to the overlying tissue and are larger in diameter than the superior system, these vessels provide a more robust supply to the abdominal wall tissue. The perfusion limitations of the pedicled TRAM are manifested in patients who smoke or are obese, leading to increased fat necrosis and partial flap loss. Modifications have been introduced in pedicled TRAM flaps to overcome these limitations. Delay procedures require a first stage division of the inferior epigastric vessels in an effort to stimulate vasodilation and new vessel growth in the infraumbilical soft tissues (34–36). The second stage, flap elevation and reconstruction of the breast, is performed 2 weeks later, improving the performance of the pedicled TRAM. Another method to increase flap perfusion in patients is the bipedicled TRAM flap. This technique utilizes both rectus muscles to reconstruct one

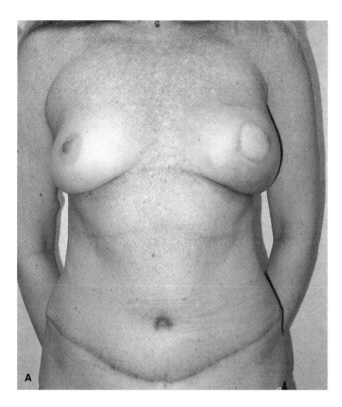

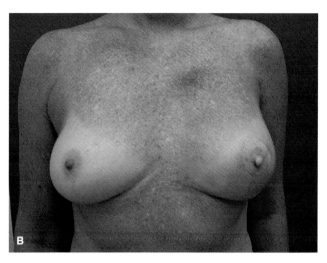

FIGURE 39.3. Autologous left breast reconstruction with muscle-sparing free muscle sparing transverse rectus abdominis myocutaneous flap. **A:** Before nipple-areolar reconstruction. **B:** After C-V flap nipple reconstruction with areolar tattooing.

side of the breast. Supercharging is a technique performed after a pedicle TRAM flap is raised and venous congestion or arterial insufficiency is encountered (37). The superficial inferior epigastric vein or deep inferior epigastric vessel remnant is attached to the thoracodorsal vessels or internal mammary vessels using microvascular techniques to salvage or support flap perfusion. Increasingly patients who smoke or are obese are referred to centers where microsurgery is performed.

Free tissue transfer allows for the movement of composite tissue such as skin, fat, and muscle from one area of the body to another based on a described vascular system. The artery and vein leading to the flap are divided at the donor site and reattached to vessels using microvascular techniques at the recipient site. In breast reconstruction these flaps are harvested from the abdominal wall and include the free TRAM, deep inferior epigastric perforator (DIEP) and superficial inferior epigastric artery (SIEA) flaps. Free flaps can also be harvested from the gluteal region or the leg and include the superior gluteal artery perforator (SGAP) flap, anterolateral thigh (ALT) flap, and the gracilis myocutaneous flap. Although described for breast reconstruction, these flaps are used infrequently and will be discussed later. The classic free TRAM flap, which includes harvest of the entire rectus abdominous muscle, has served as a springboard for a series of flaps based on the deep and superficial inferior epigastric blood vessels that perfuse the abdominal wall. In an effort to improve abdominal wall function and prevent abdominal bulge in the postoperative period, muscle-sparing free TRAM flaps were introduced that preserve up to two thirds of the rectus muscle but allow for harvesting the majority of the perforators leading from the inferior epigastric system to the overlying skin and fat (38,39). As a continuation of the same thought process, perforator flaps were designed so all of the rectus muscle was preserved, although muscle dissection was required to expose the blood vessels, leading to the skin and fat perforators (40,41). Typically one to three perforators are preserved during dissection, while four to eight perforators are preserved in muscle-sparing TRAM flaps. Flaps elevated in this

manner are referred to as DIEP flaps. The question remains whether abdominal wall function is improved when comparing the classic free TRAM, muscle-sparing free TRAM, and DIEP flaps. Current studies lack a prospective evaluation of abdominal wall function. Studies have compared these flaps and demonstrated no statistically significant differences (42,43). However, the absence of information on the preoperative functional status of the abdominal wall limits the conclusions that can be drawn from this data. The development of postoperative fat necrosis is another parameter that has been compared among flap techniques. It has been proposed that the DIEP flap may reduce morbidity to the abdominal wall by limiting muscle resection, but the tradeoff may be an increased incidence of fat necrosis due to the additional perforators that are divided during the flap harvest in comparison with the muscle-sparing TRAM flap (44). In patients requiring bilateral breast reconstruction the impact of dissection techniques may be greater when comparing abdominal wall flaps. In unilateral reconstruction the contralateral muscles compensate for loss of function from the resected or dissected muscle. The impact of muscle loss or loss of muscle innervation in bilateral TRAM flaps increases the likelihood of limiting abdominal wall function. Using DIEP flaps and preserving muscle likely have a greater impact in preserving function in this setting. In bilateral reconstruction the abdominal wall tissue is divided along the midline, creating a direct blood supply to the transferred tissue. The blood supply no longer crosses the midline, potentially reducing the risk of possible fat necrosis. For these reasons DIEP flaps rather than muscle-sparing or pedicled TRAM flaps appear more favorable in bilateral breast reconstruction.

The superficial epigastric system does not penetrate the abdominal wall fascia. It travels above the inguinal ligament to supply the abdominal wall fat and skin without traveling through muscle. The SIEA flap is based on this system. This flap is appealing because the flap can be raised without disruption of muscle or abdominal fascia, reducing the extent of dissection, decreasing postoperative pain, and maintaining abdominal wall function (45,46). The disadvantage of this flap is the variability in the anatomy of the superior epigastric vessels and the potential for fat necrosis. The pedicle supplying this flap can only be utilized 30% of the time (46); when present with an adequate diameter, operating time is reduced and patients enjoy the benefits listed above. If the pedicle is too small or absent, operative time is increased because of the need to elevate a standard TRAM flap. SIEA flaps should only be attempted by experienced microsurgeons and not promised to patients preoperatively.

Recovery after a TRAM flap is 6 to 8 weeks regardless of the type of flap used. During this time patients are asked not to perform repetitive movement such as vacuuming and not to lift more than 10 lb in an effort to allow the abdominal wall to heal so that the risk of bulge is reduced. The combination of a skin-sparing mastectomy with a TRAM flap reconstruction in the immediate setting, whether unilateral or bilateral, will produce the best outcome for the patient. Although, some minor surgeries may be required to shape the breast afterward, autologous tissue reconstruction is permanent, with a natural texture and shape. If it is certain that postoperative radiation is required, delayed reconstruction is offered to the patient until 6 months after radiation is completed.

Although TRAM flaps require a longer surgery time and involve a second surgical site (the abdomen), the success rate can be as high as 98% with less than 2% incidence of total and partial flap loss (47) and a more natural look and feel can be achieved than with implants. Immediate TRAM flap reconstruction with preservation of the patient's breast skin can produce the most stunning realistic reconstructive results. In the authors' practice all forms of abdominal flaps are offered to patients. Pedicled TRAM flaps are generally offered to patients who are of moderate weight, have a "B" cup breast, and do not smoke. Muscle-sparing free TRAM flaps are offered primarily to patients requiring unilateral breast reconstruction, who smoke, are of moderate weight or obese, but without a pannus. DIEP flaps are offered to patients undergoing bilateral breast reconstruction who are of moderate weight or obese. The authors do not offer DIEP flaps to patients with a history of smoking.

Statistically the number of patients reconstructed after the age of 70 drops off dramatically. As long as the patient has no significant coexisting disease processes that prohibit reconstruction, breast reconstruction can be offered (48). Age in and of its self is not a limiting factor to free tissue transfer (49). It is felt that breast reconstruction in older patients is underutilized. Many older patients are not given the opportunity to review their options with a plastic surgeon because they are simply not referred by their breast surgeon or medical oncologist.

Other Autologous Options for Breast Reconstruction

Generally speaking, reconstruction with autologous tissue results in the most aesthetic and natural feeling breast. In some patients, however, the abdominal donor site is not available, either because of an inadequate amount of tissue, previous surgery disrupting the blood supply, or because of patient preference. This has led to the development of other donor sites for purely autologous breast reconstruction.

The superior gluteal artery perforator flap for breast reconstruction was described by Allen and Tucker (50) in 1995. This flap utilizes the excess skin and fat in the upper gluteal region and in some patients may provide more volume than the abdominal donor site. For unilateral reconstruction, the flap is elevated with the patient in the lateral decubitus position. A line is drawn from the posterior superior iliac spine to the greater trochanter. Perforators can be Dopplered approximately a third of the distance from the posterior superior iliac spine along this line. An oblique elliptical skin paddle is

designed to encompass these perforators, and flap harvest is begun by incising around the ellipse. These perforators are identified in a subfacial plane and dissected to their origin off of the superior gluteal vessels. The harvest of the internal mammary (recipient) vessels is done concomitantly by a second surgical team, if available. The flap is then divided and the donor site closed in layers. The patient is then repositioned in the supine position for the microsurgery and insetting of the flap. Several reports in the literature attest to the safety, low flap loss rate, and aesthetic results with this flap, both in unilateral and bilateral reconstructions (51–54).

In some patients the gluteal excess is in the lower aspect of the gluteal region. In this case, an inferior gluteal artery perforator flap can be used for breast reconstruction (55,56). Again, with the patient in lateral decubitus position, an ellipse is marked out in the lower gluteal region with the inferior margin of the skin paddle in the gluteal crease. The dissection is similar to the SGAP flap elevation, although the perforator system and pedicle are the inferior gluteal vessels.

These flaps, although reasonable alternatives to TRAM-based reconstruction, do have some drawbacks that limit their popularity with many reconstructive surgeons. The need to reposition the patient adds some complexity to the case as well as lengthens the operative time. More importantly, however, the pedicle length is generally much shorter compared with the TRAM-based reconstructions, and this can make the microsurgery technically more challenging. Lastly, these procedures place a scar on another aesthetic unit of the female body, and many women object to such a scar.

Although these are the two most common donor sites for autologous breast reconstruction after the abdomen and the back, others have also been described, including the transverse gracilis myocutaneous free flap (57,58) and the anterolateral thigh free flap (59,60). These flaps can be employed in a few select cases where other donor sites are not available and the patient has enough excess tissue on the medial or anterolateral thigh. However, these options can leave unsightly scars on the thighs, and their applications are, at present, very limited.

Nipple and Areolar Reconstruction

The final stage of breast reconstruction is restoration of the nipple–areolar complex (NAC). Nipple reconstruction is usually performed as a minor procedure in the outpatient setting. Although some reconstructive surgeons will perform the nipple reconstruction at the same time as the breast mound reconstruction, most will perform this as a separate procedure once the reconstructed breast has healed and postoperative edema has resolved. The presence of a NAC on the reconstructed breast improves patient satisfaction as well as their own body image (61). The patient must understand that the nipple reconstruction will establish a small mound of tissue that looks like a nipple, but sensation and function will not be restored.

NAC reconstruction is indicated in almost every patient. However, in patients who have had radiation treatment, especially in cases of reconstructions with implants alone, the patient must be aware that there is a higher likelihood of tissue loss and delayed healing. NAC reconstruction in patients with implant reconstructions and a history of radiation should be considered if there are no acute or late sequela of radiation and if the mastectomy flaps are thick enough to allow such reconstruction (62).

The most important step in nipple reconstruction is determining the exact nipple position. This should be done with the patient in the standing position. For unilateral reconstructions, the nipple position should match the position of the contralateral nipple. In bilateral reconstructions, the nipple should be placed on the apex of the breast mound. The nipple position should be marked by the surgeon and inspected by the patient using a hand-held mirror to ensure that the position is acceptable to the patient. Minor changes in nipple position can then be made depending on patient preference.

Nipple reconstruction can be accomplished either with the use of a free nipple graft from the contralateral nipple, or more commonly, with a multitude of well-described local flaps. From an oncologic point of view, the use of tissue from the contralateral nipple has the potential to bring ductal tissue to the mastectomy site and carries with it a small risk of the development of a new primary cancer that would be manifest as a local recurrence. The "nipple sharing" technique can be used in patients who have a large contralateral nipple and are willing to accept a smaller nipple. Either the tip or the lower half of the contralateral nipple is harvested as a free graft and sewn onto a de-epithelialized portion of the reconstructed breast. The areola can then be created with a skin graft or tattooing (see below).

Several local flaps for nipple reconstruction have been described (63–67). Local flap options include the C-V flap (Figs. 39.2 and 39.3), bell flap, skate flap, double opposing tab flaps, modified fish-tail flap, and the modified star flap. Different techniques result in slightly different shapes and sizes of the reconstructed nipples, and the choice of flap should be determined accordingly. The greatest drawback to nipple reconstruction is the loss of long-term projection. At least a 40% loss in projection can be expected within 2 years, and with some techniques, over a 70% loss of projection can be seen (68). This loss of projection is the main cause of patient dissatisfaction with nipple reconstruction. To improve the long-term projection, reconstructions with local flaps augmented with various materials have been described. These include the use of costochondral rib grafts harvested at the time of mastectomy and breast mound reconstruction as well as acellular dermis (69–71).

Areolar reconstruction is generally done with either skin grafting or tattooing. The areolar perimeter is marked out with the patient in the standing position. Again, a unilateral areolar reconstruction should match the contralateral areola, while bilateral areola reconstructions should be appropriately sized to match the size of the breast. The average areolar diameter is 4.2 to 4.5 cm. If a skin graft is used, it can usually be taken from the inner thigh, inner gluteal crease, or the groin. The appropriate area on the breast mound is de-epithelialized and the graft sewn in place and "pie-crusted" to allow for egress of fluid. This yields acceptable results with an inconspicuous donor site. An equally acceptable technique involves intradermal deposition of pigment (tattooing) to the area to create the appearance of an areola. As the reconstructed breast skin is usually insensate, this can usually be done with little or no local anesthetic.

EFFECTS OF RADIATION THERAPY ON THE RECONSTRUCTED BREAST

The role of radiation therapy in improving locoregional control and overall survival in patients undergoing breast conservation or those with T3 lesions or involvement of four or more axillary lymph nodes is well established. However, radiation therapy has the potential to significantly affect the outcome of reconstruction.

Exposure of normal tissue to radiation results in both early and late changes. The early skin changes seen with radiation exposure include erythema, desquamation, and pruritus. Several mechanisms have been proposed in the development of the late skin changes seen after radiation exposure including indirect damage via free radicals, direct damage to DNA, and inflammatory pathways (72–74). Damage to small vessels lead-

ing to cell loss and fibrosis likely also contributes to the changes seen. These late changes include impaired collagen synthesis, angiogenesis, and ultimately, poor wound healing (75).

Generally speaking, radiation therapy negatively impacts on the results of breast reconstruction. However, the rates of complications as well as the aesthetic outcomes vary depending on the timing of the radiation therapy in relation to the reconstruction as well as on the type of reconstruction employed.

The optimal algorithm for the timing of radiation therapy in patients undergoing implant based reconstruction is still evolving. Tissue expander or implant reconstruction in patients previously treated with chest wall radiation (delayed reconstruction and those requiring salvage mastectomy following breast-conservation therapy) is associated with increased complication rates and inferior aesthetic outcomes. In one retrospective review expansion was difficult in 20% of patients undergoing reconstruction after salvage mastectomy, eventually resulting in underprojection of the final reconstructed breast (76). The expansion process is associated with more pain and less overexpansion, and the reconstructed breasts are harder with more irregularities and require significantly more capsulotomies for capsular contracture than in breasts not previously radiated, which results in lower patient satisfaction with the aesthetic result (77). A recent retrospective review of patients receiving radiation therapy prior to the completion of implant-based reconstruction demonstrated a higher incidence of complications requiring removal or replacement of the prosthetic device compared to those not receiving radiation therapy (18.5% vs. 4.2%) as well as higher incidence of overall complications compared to those not receiving radiation (40.7% vs. 16.7%) (2).

Immediate reconstruction with tissue expander/implant in patients requiring postmastectomy radiation can result in patients receiving radiation at various stages of the reconstructive process. Radiation therapy may be initiated prior to exchange to final prosthesis. This scenario is similar to operating on a previously radiated breast, as discussed above. An approach being more commonly employed involves rapid expansion during adjuvant chemotherapy followed by exchange to permanent implant prior to radiation therapy.

Using this approach, aesthetic results seem to be improved with greater patient satisfaction (4,78), although the incidence of capsular contractures remains higher than in the nonradiated control groups. This approach can be used with minimal delay in initiation of radiation therapy. A retrospective review from Memorial Sloan-Kettering Cancer Center demonstrated a median interval of 8 weeks from completion of chemotherapy to initiation of radiation therapy with acceptable 5-year locoregional control and overall survival (11).

Complications of infection of tissue expanders and implants in the setting of radiation can usually be salvaged by temporary removal of the implant followed by delayed reconstruction with an implant and a latissimus dorsi myocutaneous flap, which provides healthy, well-perfused tissue to cover the implant and replaces some of the radiation damaged skin. For further discussion on this topic, refer to the Latissimus Dorsi Myocutaneous Flap section of this chapter.

In general, autologous reconstruction improves aesthetic results and lowers the complication rate compared to implant based reconstruction in the setting of radiation. Again, as with implant reconstruction, autologous reconstruction may be performed in the setting of prior radiation therapy or may be performed before the initiation of postmastectomy radiation. The use of autologous tissue reconstruction in patients undergoing salvage mastectomy after initial breast conservation yields acceptable aesthetic results with minimal flap complications (79,80). The use of a free TRAM versus a pedicled TRAM reconstruction results in less fat necrosis and better aesthetic results in patients who have had previous radiation therapy

(32,80). Although a history of previous radiation therapy is not associated with a statistically significant higher flap failure rate (79), the aesthetic results are still inferior to those seen with autologous reconstruction in the absence of previous radiation therapy (81).

In patients who are known to require, or who have a high likelihood of needing postmastectomy radiation therapy, the issue of whether to perform immediate reconstruction or delay reconstruction remains debated. The theoretical advantage of performing immediate reconstruction relates to the greater pliability of the mastectomy flaps as well as a smaller requirement for external skin. Immediate reconstruction followed by radiation therapy can yield excellent results (82). On the other hand, radiation can have negative effects on an autologously reconstructed breast, including fibrosis, change in shape, and reduction in volume (83,84). The change in shape and volume can, in some cases, be so extreme so as to require additional tissue transfer to correct the deformity. It is difficult to predict which patients will experience this sequela of radiation therapy on the reconstructed breast. Therefore, it is important that the patient be well informed of these possible effects. Despite this, some patients are willing to accept these risks and proceed with autologous reconstruction prior to radiation so as to move on with their lives and avoid the interval of time in which they would otherwise have no breast.

The choice of donor site for autologous reconstruction in these patients also remains somewhat controversial. As stated above, free tissue transfer is generally less susceptible to fat necrosis and skin necrosis than the pedicled TRAM flap, likely because of the radiation-induced damage to the pedicle. However, at present, it is unclear whether there is any advantage among the free TRAM, muscle-sparing free TRAM, DIEP, or SIEA flap in terms of complications and aesthetic results in the setting of radiation therapy. Theoretically, the free TRAM and the muscle-sparing TRAM have a heartier blood supply than the DIEP or SIEA flap, and should be more resistant to the radiation-induced changes. However, this is a theoretical observation and is not proven.

MANAGEMENT OF THE CONTRALATERAL BREAST

Oftentimes the reconstructive algorithm involves modification of the shape or size of the contralateral breast to attain symmetry (85,86). The most common procedures necessary are reduction mammoplasty, mastopexy, or augmentation mammoplasty. This is largely determined by the patient's native breast size, type of reconstruction, and history of radiation. Before any surgery is performed on the contralateral breast, the surgeon should ensure the patient has had a recent normal mammogram of this breast. In addition, the possibilities of loss of nipple or areolar sensation, fat necrosis, delayed wound healing, seromas, and hematomas as well as the resulting scars should be extensively discussed with the patient. Smoking should be discontinued for at least 1 month prior to surgery.

Augmentation of the contralateral breast may be necessary in patients with relatively small breasts undergoing implant-based reconstruction after mastectomy. Reconstruction in a small-breasted woman who undergoes a unilateral mastectomy with implant-based reconstruction can leave the patient with a noticeable difference in both size and shape between the reconstructed breast and the native breast. In this patient population, augmentation of the contralateral breast helps in establishing symmetry between the two breasts. This can be done through a periareolar, inframammary, or axillary approach. The implant should be placed in a partially subpectoral position to minimize palpability of the implant in these patients, as there is only a small amount of breast

parenchyma to disguise the implant. In addition, subpectoral placement of the implant facilitates mammographic visualization of the breast tissue in this population at increased risk for the development of new primary cancers. The placement of an implant will generally also give a small lift to the breast, which is oftentimes necessary.

Mastopexy of the contralateral breast may be necessary in a number of scenarios. Some patients who have very ptotic native breasts know prior to mastectomy and reconstruction that they desire correction of the ptosis. This is important to know ahead of time so that the reconstructed breast can be positioned and shaped accordingly. The contralateral breast can then be lifted to match the reconstructed breast. This is particularly true in cases of implant-based reconstructions. Implant-based reconstructions cannot match the degree of ptosis seen in some patients, and therefore, the patients must understand that a mastopexy on the contralateral breast will be necessary for symmetry. A periareolar crescentic excision may be all that is necessary in cases where only a small lift is required. However, in most cases, either a vertical or an inverted T-shaped scar is necessary to obtain the amount of lift needed.

Reduction mammoplasty is a third balancing procedure that is oftentimes necessary to obtain symmetry. This may be necessary in patients who have large, ptotic breast and who are undergoing either mastectomy with reconstruction or breast conservation with lumpectomy. In the latter scenario, reduction techniques may be employed in both breasts to obtain symmetry in size and shape. This requires close coordination with the surgical oncologist performing the lumpectomy to plan the skin incisions so that they fall within the mammoplasty skin excision pattern. Another scenario in which reduction of the contralateral breast may be necessary is in the case of a patient who undergoes breast-conservation therapy and develops loss of breast volume and fibrosis as a sequela of radiation therapy. In this case, a reduction mammoplasty on the contralateral side may restore symmetry without additional surgery on the radiated breast.

There are several techniques of reduction mammoplasty described in the literature (87–91). The skin pattern excision, the parenchymal resection, and the pedicle to the NAC must be determined on an individual basis. However, the most commonly employed techniques use a wise pattern skin excision with an inferior pedicle or a vertical skin pattern excision with a superiorly based pedicle. In cases where a reduction pattern will be employed for breast conservation, it is important to consider the location of the tumor in developing the pedicle. The resulting scars as well as the risks should be discussed extensively with the patient prior to surgery.

The timing of contralateral breast surgery is surgeon dependent. Immediate reduction mammoplasty of the contralateral breast at the time of mastectomy and reconstruction has the advantages of eliminating a time period when the patient is left with asymmetric breasts and also may eliminate an additional surgery. However, the reconstructed breast will change in shape once it "settles," as well as in size once the swelling resolves, and therefore, the degree of symmetry between the breasts may change with time. Delaying surgery on the contralateral breast until completion of the reconstructive process leaves the patient with a period of asymmetric breasts, but the final symmetry obtained is generally better as the reconstructed breast has had a chance to "settle" and resolution of postoperative swelling has occurred.

IMMEDIATE VERSUS DELAYED RECONSTRUCTION

The decision of whether to proceed with immediate reconstruction versus delayed reconstruction is largely determined by the likelihood of the patient receiving postoperative radiation therapy. In cases where it is known that the patient will require postoperative radiation therapy, reconstruction should be delayed, and after completion of radiation therapy, an autologous reconstruction can be performed. When the patient has a diagnosis of ductal carcinoma *in situ* (DCIS) or early stage cancer (stage I and some stage II), the likelihood of needing postoperative radiation therapy is small, and immediate reconstruction is generally undertaken with the understanding that some of these patients will require postoperative radiation. Unfortunately, in the absence of a large tumor, involvement of the chest wall, or clinically positive axillary lymphadenopathy, it is not possible to definitely determine preoperatively which patients will need postoperative therapy.

The advantage of immediate reconstruction is primarily preservation of a pliable skin envelope. This advantage is lost in the delayed setting, in which case the skin becomes scarred and much less pliable. The results of immediate reconstruction are aesthetically more favorable compared to delayed reconstruction in the absence of postoperative radiation therapy (92). However, reconstruction by any technique in the immediate setting places the reconstruction at risk of exposure to radiation should final pathologic evaluation of the specimen indicate such treatment. With implant-based reconstructions, the risk of implant infection, extrusion, and capsular contracture all increase with exposure to radiation therapy (2,3,93). Similarly, radiation exposure to autologously reconstructed breasts also compromises the ultimate aesthetic result, secondary to loss of volume, contracture, and fat necrosis when compared to autologously reconstructed breasts not exposed to radiation (83,94,95).

The incidence of mastectomy skin flap necrosis is much higher in patients undergoing immediate breast reconstruction than in delayed reconstruction, with up to 16% of patients developing mastectomy skin flap necrosis in the immediate setting compared to nearly 0% in the delayed setting (96). For this reason, prosthesis-related complications are higher in the immediate setting (97). Furthermore, depending on the extent of the mastectomy flap necrosis, debridement and skin grafting may be necessary, compromising the overall aesthetic result.

In the absence of mastectomy flap necrosis, the aesthetic differences between immediate and delayed reconstructions can largely be attributed to the quality of the skin envelope. For this reason, delayed reconstructions in irradiated patients will require more donor skin and a larger visible skin paddle. Often, the chest wall skin inferior to the mastectomy scar is removed at the time of delayed reconstruction and replaced by the donor flap skin. This provides a more ptotic and natural appearing breast than would otherwise be possible if the inferior chest wall skin were left intact. Other differences in a delayed setting may include damage to the recipient vessels (either internal mammary or thoracodorsal), precluding their use in up to 20% to 25% of cases (98), and conversion to a pedicled flap may be necessary.

PARTIAL MASTECTOMY DEFECTS

Partial mastectomy defects (lumpectomy, segmentectomy, quadrantectomy) are in many ways more difficult to reconstruct than total mastectomy defects. With the demonstration that breast-conservation therapy for stage I and II cancer results in 20-year survival rates equal to those obtained with modified radical mastectomy and the decreasing rates of local recurrence after breast-conservation therapy (99,100), the number of patients opting to undergo breast conservation has increased steadily. From a reconstructive viewpoint, the advantages of preservation of native breast skin, parenchyma, and

the NAC come at the expense of the requirement for adjuvant radiation therapy. Although a partial mastectomy defect closed primarily may seemingly appear to have a good aesthetic result initially, the effects of radiation treatment can lead to compromise of the early result. These changes, which include nipple–areolar retraction and malposition, breast parenchyma retraction, and contour deformities, including concavity at the site of partial mastectomy, are secondary to the fibrosis, scarring, and loss of volume seen with radiation as well as resolution of edema and fluid collections, which initially "fill out" the partial mastectomy defect. The goals of reconstruction in the setting of breast conservation are to avoid these aesthetic deformities of the breast.

It is important to understand and identify the cause of these defects since the management may be different depending on the etiology. For instance, a concavity may represent loss of volume and the need to augment this area, whereas retraction of the NAC may be due to scarring and skin fibrosis, which may require excision of scar in addition to transferring skin and soft tissue. Likewise, a uniform reduction in volume with overall preservation of breast shape may be addressed with contralateral reduction mammoplasty.

Ideally, the goal should be to prevent such deformities through utilization of various oncoplastic techniques, which combine sound oncologic resection with immediate reconstruction of the resulting defect. In this setting, several parameters need to be considered, including native breast size, tumor size, and tumor location. Additionally, the patient's willingness to accept scars on the contralateral breast should be addressed. In general, if the tumor to native breast size is too large to allow any reconstructive option to provide an acceptable aesthetic result, than primary breast conservation should be reconsidered. Options in this circumstance include the use of neoadjuvant chemotherapy or endocrine therapy to shrink the tumor and allow a more cosmetic lumpectomy, or mastectomy. Likewise, in a large native breast with a small tumor, primary closure of the breast parenchyma and overlying skin may be all that is necessary. In between these two scenarios lies a wide spectrum of possible defects needing the attention of a reconstructive surgeon.

In patients with large native breast size and significant ptosis, partial mastectomy in conjunction with bilateral reduction mammoplasty provides tumor control with good aesthetic results and minimal complication rates (101,102). The skin pattern resection and choice of pedicle should take into account the location of the tumor. Patients with smaller native breasts may not be candidates for this type of reconstruction. In these patients, other techniques can be employed and include local tissue rearrangement, latissimus dorsi myocutaneous pedicled flap, thoracodorsal artery perforator flap, lateral thoracic flap, or a transverse thoracoepigastric flap. Again, the choice of flap depends on the location of the tumor and the defect. Lateral defects can be addressed with local tissue rearrangement, lateral thoracic flap, thoracodorsal artery perforator flap, or a LD myocutaneous flap. Medial defects may require local tissue rearrangement or a thoracoepigastric flap. Local tissue rearrangement should be attempted, if possible, in preference to these other flap options. Kronowitz et al. (103) report that the use of local tissue rearrangement yields better aesthetic results because of the better match in terms of skin color and parenchymal texture as well as lower complications over flap options in the immediate setting.

The issue of positive specimen margins needs special attention if immediate reconstruction is to be utilized for partial mastectomy defects. In one study 15.7% of partial mastectomy specimens in patients with invasive carcinoma and 18.5% in those with DCIS (104) had positive margins. This suggests that wider margins should be taken if immediate partial breast reconstruction is to be employed. If any doubt exists regarding the margin status at the time of partial mastectomy, the reconstruction may be delayed until final pathologic review of the specimen is available. If positive margins are found after immediate reconstruction, mastectomy may be necessary.

Although prevention of deformities secondary to partial mastectomies at the time of the initial surgery is ideal, the reconstructive surgeon may at times be faced with the challenge of reconstruction of a deformity after radiation. Correction of segmental deformities encountered in a delayed setting can be more problematic. Surgical manipulation of radiated breast tissue is associated with a complication rate as high as 50% (103). In this setting, a symmetry procedure on the contralateral breast may be a good option if the shape of the radiated breast is preserved and volume loss is the only sequela of the radiation. In cases where there are contour deformities or skin or nipple retraction, augmentation with autologous tissue is the best option. This should be done using tissue outside the field of radiation, and surgical options include latissimus dorsi myocutaneous flap, thoracodorsal artery perforator flap, pedicled TRAM, SIEA flap, free TRAM, or a DIEP flap. This decision is multifactorial and involves analysis of the cause of the deformity as well as patient preference.

SUMMARY

Advances in breast reconstruction techniques now allow the reconstructive surgeon to offer a wide array of reconstructive options to the breast cancer patient. The selection of the optimal reconstructive procedure shoud be based on an in-depth knowledge of the advantages and disadvantages of the various options, patient desires and expectations, and an appreciation of the impact of adjuvant therapies on the reconstructed breast. Communication is essential between all members of the breast cancer care team, including the surgical oncologist, medical oncologist, and radiation oncologist. Utilization of this approach optimizes patient satisfaction and outcome.

References

1. Cordeiro PG, McCarthy CM. A single surgeon's 12-year experience with tissue expander/implant breast reconstruction: part II. An analysis of long-term complications, aesthetic outcomes, and patient satisfaction. *Plast Reconstr Surg* 2006;118:832–839.
2. Ascherman JA, Hanasono MM, Newman MI, et al. Implant reconstruction in breast cancer patients treated with radiation therapy. *Plast Reconstr Surg* 2006;117.359–365.
3. Spear SL, Onyewu C. Staged breast reconstruction with saline-filled implants in the irradiated breast: recent trends and therapeutic implications. *Plast Reconstr Surg* 2000;105:930–942.
4. Cordeiro PG, Pusic AL, Disa JJ, et al. Irradiation after immediate tissue expander/implant breast reconstruction: outcomes, complications, aesthetic results, and satisfaction among 156 patients. *Plast Reconstr Surg* 2004;113:877–881.
5. Goodwin SJ, McCarthy CM, Pusic AL, et al. Complications in smokers after postmastectomy tissue expander/implant breast reconstruction. *Ann Plast Surg* 2005;55:16–20.
6. Woerdeman LA, Hage JJ, Hofland MM, et al. A prospective assessment of surgical risk factors in 400 cases of skin-sparing mastectomy and immediate breast reconstruction with implants to establish selection criteria. *Plast Reconstr Surg* 2007;119:455–463.
7. Alderman AK, Wilkins EG, Kim HM, et al. Complications in postmastectomy breast reconstruction: two-year results of the Michigan Breast Reconstruction Outcome Study. *Plast Reconstr Surg* 2002;109:2265–2274.
8. Holley DT, Toursarkissian B, Vasconez HC, et al. The ramifications of immediate reconstruction in the management of breast cancer. *Am Surg* 1995;61:60–65.
9. Gamboa-Bobadilla GM. Implant breast reconstruction using acellular dermal matrix. *Ann Plast Surg* 2006;56:22–25.
10. Breuing KH, Colwell AS. Inferolateral AlloDerm hammock for implant coverage in breast reconstruction. *Ann Plast Surg* 2007;59:250–255.
11. Wright JL, Cordeiro PG, Ben-Porat L, et al. Mastectomy with immediate expander-implant reconstruction, adjuvant chemotherapy, and radiation for stage II–III breast cancer: treatment intervals and clinical outcomes. *Int J Radiat Oncol Biol Phys* 2008;70:43–50.
12. Gabriel SE, O'Fallon WM, Kurland LT, et al. Risk of connective-tissue diseases and other disorders after breast implantation. *N Engl J Med* 1994;330: 1697–1702.
13. Deapen DM, Bernstein L, Brody GS. Are breast implants anticarcinogenic? A 14-year follow-up of the Los Angeles study. *Plast Reconstr Surg* 1997;99:1346–1353.
14. Janowsky EC, Kupper LL, Hulka BS. Meta-analyses of the relation between silicone breast implants and the risk of connective-tissue diseases. *N Engl J Med* 2000;342:781–790.
15. Brinton LA, Lubin JH, Burich MC, et al. Breast cancer following augmentation mammoplasty (United States). *Cancer Causes Control* 2000;11:819–827.
16. Bengtson BP, Van Natta BW, Murphy DK, et al. Style 410 highly cohesive silicone breast implant core study results at 3 years. *Plast Reconstr Surg* 2007;120: 40S–48S.
17. Birdsell DC, Jenkins H, Berkel H. Breast cancer diagnosis and survival in women with and without breast implants. *Plast Reconstr Surg* 1993;92:795–800.
18. Deapen D, Hamilton A, Bernstein L, et al. Breast cancer stage at diagnosis and survival among patients with prior breast implants. *Plast Reconstr Surg* 2000;105:535–540.
19. Eklund GW, Busby RC, Miller SH, et al. Improved imaging of the augmented breast. *AJR Am J Roentgenol* 1988;151:469–473.
20. Shestak KC, Ganott MA, Harris KM, et al. Breast masses in the augmentation mammaplasty patient: the role of ultrasound. *Plast Reconstr Surg* 1993;92: 209–216.
21. Hokin JA. Mastectomy reconstruction without a prosthetic implant. *Plast Reconstr Surg* 1983;72:810–818.
22. Germann G, Steinau HU. Breast reconstruction with the extended latissimus dorsi flap. *Plast Reconstr Surg* 1996;97:519–526.
23. Chang DW, Youssef A, Cha S, et al. Autologous breast reconstruction with the extended latissimus dorsi flap. *Plast Reconstr Surg* 2002;110:751–761.
24. Raja MA, Straker VF, Rainsbury RM. Extending the role of breast-conserving surgery by immediate volume replacement. *Br J Surg* 1997;84:101–105.
25. Rainsbury RM, Paramanathan N. Recent progress with breast-conserving volume replacement using latissimus dorsi miniflaps in UK patients. *Breast Cancer* 1998;5:139–147.
26. Navin C, Agrawal A, Kolar KM. The use of latissimus dorsi miniflap for reconstruction following breast-conserving surgery: experience of a small breast unit in a district hospital. *World J Surg* 2007;31:46–50.
27. Ortiz CL, Mendoza MM, Sempere LN, et al. Versatility of the pedicled thoracodorsal artery perforator (TDAP) flap in soft tissue reconstruction. *Ann Plast Surg* 2007;58:315–320.
28. Hamdi M, Van Landuyt K, Monstrey S, et al. Pedicled perforator flaps in breast reconstruction: a new concept. *Br J Plast Surg* 2004;57:531–539.
29. Hartrampf CR, Scheflan M, Black PW. Breast reconstruction with a transverse abdominal island flap. *Plast Reconstr Surg* 1982;69:216–225.
30. Ducic I, Spear SL, Cuoco F, et al. Safety and risk factors for breast reconstruction with pedicled transverse rectus abdominis musculocutaneous flaps: a 10-year analysis. *Ann Plast Surg* 2005;55:559–564.
31. Kroll SS. Necrosis of abdominoplasty and other secondary flaps after TRAM flap breast reconstruction. *Plast Reconstr Surg* 1994;94:637–643.
32. Kroll SS, Gherardini G, Martin JE, et al. Fat necrosis in free and pedicled TRAM flaps. *Plast Reconstr Surg* 1998;102:1502–1507.
33. Spear SL, Ducic I, Cuoco F, et al. Effect of obesity on flap and donor-site complications in pedicled TRAM flap breast reconstruction. *Plast Reconstr Surg* 2007;119:788–795.
34. Ozgentas HE, Shenaq S, Spira M. Study of the delay phenomenon in the rat TRAM flap model. *Plast Reconstr Surg* 1994;94:1018–1026.
35. Hudson DA. The surgically delayed unipedicled TRAM flap for breast reconstruction. *Ann Plast Surg* 1996;36:238–245.
36. Erdmann D, Sundin BM, Moquin KJ, et al. Delay in unipedicled TRAM flap reconstruction of the breast: a review of 76 consecutive cases. *Plast Reconstr Surg* 2002;110:762–767.
37. Marck KW, van der Biezen JJ, Dol JA. Internal mammary artery and vein supercharge in TRAM flap breast reconstruction. *Microsurgery* 1996;17:371–374.
38. Nahabedian MY, Dooley W, Singh N, et al. Contour abnormalities of the abdomen after breast reconstruction with abdominal flaps: the role of muscle preservation. *Plast Reconstr Surg* 2002;109:91–101.
39. Nahabedian MY, Momen B, Galdino G, et al. Breast reconstruction with the free TRAM or DIEP flap: patient selection, choice of flap, and outcome. *Plast Reconstr Surg* 2002;110:466–477.
40. Koshima I, Soeda S. Inferior epigastric artery skin flaps without rectus abdominis muscle. *Br J Plast Surg* 1989;42:645–648.
41. Allen RJ, Treece P. Deep inferior epigastric perforator flap for breast reconstruction. *Ann Plast Surg* 1994;32:32 38.
42. Nahabedian MY, Tsangaris T, Momen B. Breast reconstruction with the DIEP flap or the muscle-sparing (MS-2) free TRAM flap: is there a difference? *Plast Reconstr Surg* 2005;115:436–446.
43. Bajaj AK, Chevray PM, Chang DW. Comparison of donor-site complications and functional outcomes in free muscle-sparing TRAM flap and free DIEP flap breast reconstruction. *Plast Reconstr Surg* 2006;117:737–750.
44. Kroll SS. Fat necrosis in free transverse rectus abdominis myocutaneous and deep inferior epigastric perforator flaps. *Plast Reconstr Surg* 2000;106:576–583.
45. Arnez ZM, Khan U, Pogorelec D, et al. Breast reconstruction using the free superficial inferior epigastric artery (SIEA) flap. *Br J Plast Surg* 1999;52:276–279.
46. Chevray PM. Breast reconstruction with superficial inferior epigastric artery flaps: a prospective comparison with TRAM and DIEP flaps. *Plast Reconstr Surg* 2004;114:1077–1085.
47. Chen CM, Halvorson EG, Disa JJ, et al. Immediate postoperative complications in DIEP versus free/muscle-sparing TRAM flaps. *Plast Reconstr Surg* 2007;120: 1477–1482.
48. Lipa JE, Youssef AA, Kuerer HM, et al. Breast reconstruction in older women: advantages of autogenous tissue. *Plast Reconstr Surg* 2003;111:1110–1121.
49. Serletti JM, Higgins JP, Moran S, et al. Factors affecting outcome in free-tissue transfer in the elderly. *Plast Reconstr Surg* 2000;106:66–70.
50. Allen RJ, Tucker C Jr. Superior gluteal artery perforator free flap for breast reconstruction. *Plast Reconstr Surg* 1995;95:1207–1212.
51. Guerra AB, Metzinger SE, Bidros RS, et al. Breast reconstruction with gluteal artery perforator (GAP) flaps: a critical analysis of 142 cases. *Ann Plast Surg* 2004;52:118–125.
52. Granzow JW, Levine JL, Chiu ES, et al. Breast reconstruction with gluteal artery perforator flaps. *J Plast Reconstr Aesthet Surg* 2006;59:614–621.
53. Guerra AB, Soueid N, Metzinger SE, et al. Simultaneous bilateral breast reconstruction with superior gluteal artery perforator (SGAP) flaps. *Ann Plast Surg* 2004;53:305–310.
54. Hamdi M, Blondeel P, Van Landuyt K, et al. Bilateral autogenous breast reconstruction using perforator free flaps: a single center's experience. *Plast Reconstr Surg* 2004;114:83–92.

55. Allen RJ, Levine JL, Granzow JW. The in-the-crease inferior gluteal artery perforator flap for breast reconstruction. *Plast Reconstr Surg* 2006;118:333–339.
56. Allen R, Guarda H, Wall F, et al. Free flap breast reconstruction: the LSU experience (1984–1996). *J La State Med Soc* 1997;149:388–392.
57. Wechselberger G, Schoeller T. The transverse myocutaneous gracilis free flap: a valuable tissue source in autologous breast reconstruction. *Plast Reconstr Surg* 2004;114:69–73.
58. Arnez ZM, Pogorelec D, Planinsek F, et al. Breast reconstruction by the free transverse gracilis (TUG) flap. *Br J Plast Surg* 2004;57:20–26.
59. Rosenberg JJ, Chandawarkar R, Ross MI, et al. Bilateral anterolateral thigh flaps for large-volume breast reconstruction. *Microsurgery* 2004;24:281–284.
60. Wei FC, Suominen S, Cheng MH, et al. Anterolateral thigh flap for postmastectomy breast reconstruction. *Plast Reconstr Surg* 2002;110:82–88.
61. Wellisch DK, Schain WS, Noone RB, et al. The psychological contribution of nipple addition in breast reconstruction. *Plast Reconstr Surg* 1987;80:699–704.
62. Draper LB, Bui DT, Chiu ES, et al. Nipple-areola reconstruction following chest-wall irradiation for breast cancer: is it safe? *Ann Plast Surg* 2005;55:12–15.
63. Eng JS. Bell flap nipple reconstruction—a new wrinkle. *Ann Plast Surg* 1996;36:485–488.
64. Eskenazi L. A one-stage nipple reconstruction with the "modified star" flap and immediate tattoo: a review of 100 cases. *Plast Reconstr Surg* 1993;92:671–680.
65. Kroll SS, Hamilton S. Nipple reconstruction with the double-opposing-tab flap. *Plast Reconstr Surg* 1989;84:520–525.
66. Kroll SS. Nipple reconstruction with the double-opposing tab flap. *Plast Reconstr Surg* 1999;104:511–517.
67. Hartrampf CR Jr, Culbertson JH. A dermal-fat flap for nipple reconstruction. *Plast Reconstr Surg* 1984;73:982–986.
68. Shestak KC, Gabriel A, Landecker A, et al. Assessment of long-term nipple projection: a comparison of three techniques. *Plast Reconstr Surg* 2002;110:780–786.
69. Nahabedian MY. Secondary nipple reconstruction using local flaps and AlloDerm. *Plast Reconstr Surg* 2005;115:2056–2061.
70. Garramone CE, Lam B. Use of AlloDerm in primary nipple reconstruction to improve long-term nipple projection. *Plast Reconstr Surg* 2007;119:1663–1668.
71. Heitland A, Markowicz M, Koellensperger E, et al. Long-term nipple shrinkage following augmentation by an autologous rib cartilage transplant in free DIEP-flaps. *J Plast Reconstr Aesthet Surg* 2006;59:1063–1067.
72. Riley PA. Free radicals in biology: oxidative stress and the effects of ionizing radiation. *Int J Radiat Biol* 1994;65:27–33.
73. Rubin P, Johnston CJ, Williams JP, et al. A perpetual cascade of cytokines postirradiation leads to pulmonary fibrosis. *Int J Radiat Oncol Biol Phys* 1995;33:99–109.
74. Barcellos-Hoff MH. How do tissues respond to damage at the cellular level? The role of cytokines in irradiated tissues. *Radiat Res* 1998;150:S109–S120.
75. Tibbs MK. Wound healing following radiation therapy: a review. *Radiother Oncol* 1997;42:99–106.
76. Forman DL, Chiu J, Restifo RJ, et al. Breast reconstruction in previously irradiated patients using tissue expanders and implants: a potentially unfavorable result. *Ann Plast Surg* 1998;40:360–364.
77. Kraemer O, Andersen M, Siim E. Breast reconstruction and tissue expansion in irradiated versus not irradiated women after mastectomy. *Scand J Plast Reconstr Surg Hand Surg* 1996;30:201–206.
78. McCarthy CM, Pusic AL, Disa JJ, et al. Unilateral postoperative chest wall radiotherapy in bilateral tissue expander/implant reconstruction patients: a prospective outcomes analysis. *Plast Reconstr Surg* 2005;116:1642–1647.
79. Kroll SS, Robb GL, Reece GP, et al. Does prior irradiation increase the risk of total or partial free-flap loss? *J Reconstr Microsurg* 1998;14:263–268.
80. Moran SL, Serletti JM, Fox I. Immediate free TRAM reconstruction in lumpectomy and radiation failure patients. *Plast Reconstr Surg* 2000;106:1527–1531.
81. Kroll SS, Schusterman MA, Reece GP, et al. Breast reconstruction with myocutaneous flaps in previously irradiated patients. *Plast Reconstr Surg* 1994;93:460–471.
82. Anderson PR, Hanlon AL, Fowble BL, et al. Low complication rates are achievable after postmastectomy breast reconstruction and radiation therapy. *Int J Radiat Oncol Biol Phys* 2004;59:1080–1087.
83. Tran NV, Chang DW, Gupta A, et al. Comparison of immediate and delayed free TRAM flap breast reconstruction in patients receiving postmastectomy radiation therapy. *Plast Reconstr Surg* 2001;108:78–82.
84. Kronowitz SJ, Robb GL. Breast reconstruction with postmastectomy radiation therapy: current issues. *Plast Reconstr Surg* 2004;114:950–960.
85. Nahabedian MY. Symmetrical breast reconstruction: analysis of secondary procedures after reconstruction with implants and autologous tissue. *Plast Reconstr Surg* 2005;115:257–260.
86. Losken A, Carlson GW, Bostwick J 3rd, et al. Trends in unilateral breast reconstruction and management of the contralateral breast: the Emory experience. *Plast Reconstr Surg* 2002;110:89–97.
87. Courtiss EH, Goldwyn RM. Reduction mammaplasty by the inferior pedicle technique. An alternative to free nipple and areola grafting for severe macromastia or extreme ptosis. *Plast Reconstr Surg* 1977;59:500–507.
88. Benelli L. A new periareolar mammaplasty: the "round block" technique. *Aesthetic Plast Surg* 1990;14:93–100.
89. McKissock PK. Reduction mammaplasty by the vertical bipedicle flap technique. Rationale and results. *Clin Plast Surg* 1976;3:309–320.
90. Hall-Findlay EJ. A simplified vertical reduction mammaplasty: shortening the learning curve. *Plast Reconstr Surg* 1999;104:748–763.
91. Strombeck JO. Mammaplasty: report of a new technique based on the two-pedicle procedure. *Br J Plast Surg* 1960;13:79–90.
92. Kroll SS, Coffey JA Jr, Winn RJ, et al. A comparison of factors affecting aesthetic outcomes of TRAM flap breast reconstructions. *Plast Reconstr Surg* 1995;96:860–864.
93. Evans GR, Schusterman MA, Kroll SS, et al. Reconstruction and the radiated breast: is there a role for implants? *Plast Reconstr Surg* 1995;96:1111–1118.
94. Williams JK, Carlson GW, Bostwick J 3rd, et al. The effects of radiation treatment after TRAM flap breast reconstruction. *Plast Reconstr Surg* 1997;100:1153–1160.
95. Rogers NE, Allen RJ. Radiation effects on breast reconstruction with the deep inferior epigastric perforator flap. *Plast Reconstr Surg* 2002;109:1919–1926.
96. DeBono R, Thompson A, Stevenson JH. Immediate versus delayed free TRAM breast reconstruction: an analysis of perioperative factors and complications. *Br J Plast Surg* 2002;55:111–116.
97. Miller AP, Falcone RE. Breast reconstruction: systemic factors influencing local complications. *Ann Plast Surg* 1991;27:115–120.
98. Temple CL, Strom EA, Youssef A, et al. Choice of recipient vessels in delayed TRAM flap breast reconstruction after radiotherapy. *Plast Reconstr Surg* 2005;115:105–113.
99. Veronesi U, Cascinelli N, Mariani L, et al. Twenty-year follow-up of a randomized study comparing breast-conserving surgery with radical mastectomy for early breast cancer. *N Engl J Med* 2002;347:1227–1232.
100. Fisher B, Anderson S, Bryant J, et al. Twenty-year follow-up of a randomized trial comparing total mastectomy, lumpectomy, and lumpectomy plus irradiation for the treatment of invasive breast cancer. *N Engl J Med* 2002;347:1233–1241.
101. Spear SL, Pelletiere CV, Wolfe AJ, et al. Experience with reduction mammaplasty combined with breast conservation therapy in the treatment of breast cancer. *Plast Reconstr Surg* 2003;111:1102–1109.
102. Losken A, Elwood ET, Styblo TM, et al. The role of reduction mammaplasty in reconstructing partial mastectomy defects. *Plast Reconstr Surg* 2002;109:968–977.
103. Kronowitz SJ, Feledy JA, Hunt KK, et al. Determining the optimal approach to breast reconstruction after partial mastectomy. *Plast Reconstr Surg* 2006;117:1–14.
104. Pawlik TM, Perry A, Strom EA, et al. Potential applicability of balloon catheter-based accelerated partial breast irradiation after conservative surgery for breast carcinoma. *Cancer* 2004;100:490–498.

Chapter 40
Local Therapy for the Breast and Chest Wall

Monica Morrow and Jay R. Harris

The main options for cancer treatment for the breast and chest wall are breast-conserving therapy (BCT) or mastectomy, with or without immediate breast reconstruction. The results of individual trials comparing these options and a meta-analysis of all these trials have demonstrated equivalent survival with very long-term follow up. BCT in these trials involved whole breast irradiation given in conventional fractionation (180 to 200 cGy per day); more recently, there have been studies of BCT using accelerated partial breast irradiation (APBI), and this approach is discussed below.

A high percent of patients presenting with stage I or II breast cancer are suitable for BCT. The use of BCT is associated with improved body image and quality of life. Over time, the rates of local recurrence with BCT have decreased, and currently 10-year local (breast) recurrence (LR) rates of about 5% are typical. These very low rates of LR are due to three factors:

1. Detailed mammographic evaluation, particularly with regard to the detection of associated malignant-appearing microcalcifications and assurance of their removal,
2. Detailed pathologic analysis of the margins of the resected breast specimens to ensure negative margins, and
3. The increased use of adjuvant systemic therapy, which was developed to decrease distant metastases, but was found serendipitously to interact favorable with radiation therapy (RT) to substantially reduce LR.

It is uncertain how much of a margin is needed for BCT. The standard of care, at a minimum, is to ensure that there are no tumor cells at the inked margins of resection. (Note, however, that some margins, namely those at the pectoral fascia or at skin, are not relevant since there is no further breast tissue beyond the margin; the purpose of margin assessment is to ensure that the residual disease in the breast is limited so that it can be eradicated by the subsequent RT.) Margins of 2 mm are the conventional goal of breast-conserving surgery, but a less than 2-mm margin is not a routine indication for mastectomy or even re-excision. Margins of 1 cm or greater are excessive since the major factor determining the cosmetic outcome of BCT is the volume of resected breast tissue. It is reasonable to strive for clearly negative margins (2 mm) in young patients (aged 40 or less) and in patients whose cancers have an extensive intraductal component, two groups known to have a higher rate of LR compared to other patients when the margins of resection are not carefully assessed; however, young patients still have higher rates of LR that older patients even with negative margins (1).

The routine use of breast MRI in the evaluation of a patient with a newly diagnosed cancer who are being considered for BCT is controversial. It has been demonstrated that breast MRI in these patients finds additional foci of cancer in the ipsilateral breast in a substantial percentage of patients. However, there are three things to consider:

1. This percentage of additional cancers is much greater than the 10-year rate of LR seen in patients treated conventional BCT without MRI evaluation,
2. The high false-positive rate with breast MRI results in unnecessary biopsies, delays, and costs and
3. There are no clinical studies showing improved outcome, such as decreased LR or improved survival, decreased conversion from BCT to mastectomy, or a decrease in re-excision rate, with routine breast MRI. (The authors recommend against the routine use of breast MRI.)

Conventional whole breast irradiation involves 22 to 28 treatments given daily five times a week. In patients with a left-sided breast cancer, computed tomography (CT) simulation should be performed to contour the heart relative to the treatment fields. Given the known deleterious effects of RT on the heart, every reasonable effort should be made to exclude the heart from treatment fields. In nearly all patients, this can be accomplished if needed with the use of a block in the treatment fields to shield the heart. Additional dose to the primary site (a boost) further reduces the rate of LR beyond that seen with whole breast irradiation. However, the absolute benefit of a boost varies by patient age group; in younger patients, the benefit is substantial, while in older patients (aged 60 or greater), the benefit is small. Do we want to say that a boost should routinely be given in premenopausal women? Ten-year results from a Canadian trial comparing whole breast irradiation given at 180 cGy per day for 25 treatments and at 266 cGy per day for 16 treatments (both without a boost) demonstrated similar rates of LR and cosmetic results (2). Therefore, in patients aged 60 or greater with favorable pathology (e.g., clearly negative margins and hormone receptor–positive breast cancer) who need only tangential breast irradiation are reasonably treated with this accelerated whole breast irradiation, particularly if the patient has comorbid illnesses.

There is no subgroup based on clinical and pathologic features that has been established to have a low rate of LR in the absence of RT. It has now been established that the addition of RT after breast-conserving surgery is important not only to prevent LR, but also to maximize long-term survival. Patients older than 70, particularly with comorbid illness and hormone receptor–positive, node-negative breast cancer are reasonably treated with hormonal therapy in the absence of RT. However, the toxicity and benefits of adjuvant hormonal therapy and of adjuvant accelerated whole breast irradiation described above need to be compared in the individual patient.

In patients receiving adjuvant chemotherapy, RT typically follows chemotherapy. In patients receiving adjuvant hormonal therapy, this treatment can be given concurrently with RT or following RT.

The use of APBI as an alternative to conventional whole breast irradiation is controversial. APBI is typically given twice a day and completed in a week. APBI may be accomplished with interstitial irradiation, intracavitary irradiation, or by external beam irradiation with the longest follow-up available in patients treated with interstitial irradiation. (In Europe, there have been trials of APBI using a single large intraoperative dose of irradiation.) The technical requirements for high-quality APBI are greater than that for high-quality conventional whole breast irradiation. The amount of breast treated with external beam irradiation is substantially greater than the amount treated with interstitial or intracavitary irradiation; the implications of this on efficacy and toxicity are not known at this time. The vast majority of retrospective studies using APBI have been in patients aged 60 or greater with node-negative, hormone receptor–positive breast cancer. A large trial comparing APBI and conventional whole breast irradiation is being conducted jointly by the National Surgical Adjuvant Breast and Bowel Project and the Radiation Therapy Oncology Group, but the results will not be available for some time. In the interim, it seems prudent to restrict the use of APBI to patients aged 60 or greater with node-negative, hormone receptor–positive breast cancer. Patients should be informed that it has not been established that the results of APBI are equivalent to those seen with conventional whole breast irradiation and that the long-term toxicity of APBI has not been determined.

In patients treated with mastectomy, there is uncertainty regarding which patients should receive postmastectomy RT (PMRT) and, in patients to be treated with PMRT, what is the optimal integration of breast reconstruction and RT. Locoregional recurrence following mastectomy is predominantly seen on the chest wall. PMRT is indicated in patients with four or more positive nodes since the rate of LR following mastectomy and axillary node dissection is substantial in the absence of RT. The use of PMRT in patients with one to three positive nodes is controversial. Based on the results of the Oxford Overview, any patient anticipated to have a 10% or greater absolute reduction in LR with RT will have a significant reduction in long-term mortality with PMRT and should receive PMRT (3). (Since PMRT proportionally reduces LR by about 70%, this corresponds to patients with an anticipated LR rate of 15% in the absence of RT.) Unfortunately, there are no validated prognostic factors for LR following mastectomy in patients with one to three positive nodes. Several studies have identified the presence of lymphatic vessel invasion (LVI) as an important prognostic factor for LR, but there are questions regarding the reproducibility of diagnosing LVI. The Oxford Overview results identify tumor grade as a prognostic factor for LR (4). Likely, LR is more of a problem in patients with three positive nodes than in patients with a single positive node. The only established predictive factor for the use of PMRT is patient age. Data from the Oxford Overview demonstrate that younger patients are more likely than older patients to have a long-term mortality benefit from PMRT due to the absence of competing risks of mortality typically seen in younger patients and more commonly present in older patients.

Breast reconstruction is an important intervention for quality of life in patients treated with mastectomy. However, immediate breast reconstruction can limit the ability to deliver optimal PMRT in some patients. Therefore, coordination between the surgical oncologist, plastic surgeon, and radiation oncologist should occur prior to mastectomy to optimize cancer treatment and cosmetic results. In general, breast reconstruction and skin-sparing mastectomy have not been shown to increase the risk of local recurrence nor hinder its detection, and a discussion of the availability of both immediate and delayed reconstruction and the pros and cons of each approach should be a part of the initial consultation to discuss local therapy options for breast cancer treatment.

References

1. Antonini N, Jones H, Horiot JC, et al. Effects of age and radiation dose on local control after breast conserving treatment: EORTC trial 2281–10882. *Radiother Oncol* 2006.
2. Whelan T, Pignol JP, Julian J, et al. Long-term results of a randomized trial of accelerated hypofractionated whole breast irradiation following breast conserving surgery in women with negative node breast cancer. *Int J Radiat Oncol Biol Phys* 2008;72:S28.
3. Early Breast Cancer Trialists' Collaborative Group. Effects of radiotherapy and of differences in the extent of surgery for early breast cancer on local recurrence and 15-year survival: an overview of the randomised trials. *Lancet* 2005;366: 2087–2106.
4. Darby S. 2006 update from the Early Breast Cancer Trialists' Collaborative Group Overview of Radiation Therapy for Early Breast Cancer. *Presentation, at the 2007 ASCO Annual Meeting, Chicago, IL, June 2007.*

Chapter 41
Sentinel Lymph Node Dissection

Baiba J. Grube and Armando E. Giuliano

Axillary lymph node dissection (ALND) has been an integral component of the staging, prognosis, and treatment of invasive breast and is discussed in Chapter 42. For much of the 20th century, breast cancer was believed to spread in an orderly process from the primary tumor to the regional nodes. Radical *en bloc* Halstedian resection of the breast, adjacent tissues, and its draining lymphatics was the standard of surgical therapy. Surgical management of the axilla, however, has undergone a paradigm change since the concept of lymphatic mapping of the breast was introduced at the John Wayne Cancer Institute (JWCI) in 1991. The evolution of axillary staging with sentinel lymph node dissection (SLND) occurred through hypothesis-generated questions and systematic investigation.

The contemporary approach for detecting axillary metastases in clinically node negative patients with early stage breast cancer is intraoperative lymphatic mapping and SLND, a minimally invasive and a highly accurate staging procedure (1). This novel operative technique has lead to a re-examination of the role of ALND (2). The rationale and extent of axillary lymphadenectomy for early breast cancer is a topic of great interest and diverse views among clinicians treating breast carcinoma as a multidisciplinary team (3). Although tumor characteristics and molecular markers are increasingly contributing to the understanding of the biology of breast cancer, the status of the axilla remains the most important prognostic indicator for overall survival. The current algorithm for axillary management of invasive breast cancer incorporates outcomes information from SLND, ALND, and axillary irradiation as well as data from the effects of systemic therapies on axillary metastases. This chapter addresses the current understanding of the role of SLND in surgical management of the axilla for breast cancer.

SENTINEL NODE CONCEPT IN CANCER

The identification of regional lymph node metastases in breast cancer has been an active area of research. Historically, clinicians tried to identify axillary metastases through a variety of noninvasive technologies including radioactive and nonradioactive contrast materials. Newer technologies such as magnetic resonance imaging (MRI), positron emission tomography (PET), and ultrasound are also used to assess the axilla, but none of these methods can definitively evaluate the axilla and have not supplanted histologic examination (4–6).

In the early 1970s, Kett et al. (7,8) reported that the first regional lymph node, the "Sorgius node," could be identified in breast cancer using direct mammalymphography. This was a cumbersome technique that required a formal ALND to isolate the suspected lymph nodes, radiographic evaluation of the resected nodes to identify the suspicious ones, and determination of concordance through histopathologic confirmation.

Ramon Cabanas (9) coined the term *sentinel node* as a specific lymph center in penile carcinoma, located in a constant anatomic location. The sentinel node (SN) concept evolved from this observation and is based on the principle that a primary tumor is drained by an afferent lymphatic channel that courses to the first, "sentinel," lymph node in that specific regional lymphatic basin (10). Wong et al. (10) hypothesized that there is an SN that is the "gatekeeper" of the regional nodal basin. The SN concept postulates that there is an afferent lymphatic channel

that drains a primary tumor and travels to a specific SN in the regional lymphatic basin, and that the tumor status of the SN reflects the tumor status of the nodal basin (11). Wang et al. (10) and Morton et al. (12) tested the hypothesis that the SN in a given regional basin can be identified by an indicator dye in a feline model and then validated it in the clinical setting in a group of patients with melanoma.

Identification of a Sentinel Node in Breast Cancer

The feasibility of identifying an SN intraoperatively in breast cancer was first investigated at the JWCI by Giuliano et al. (13). In October 1991, the authors' group began to investigate the feasibility of lymphatic mapping and sentinel lymphadenectomy with isosulfan blue vital dye in breast cancer as a more accurate and less morbid approach to stage breast cancer. This pilot study demonstrated that SLND of the axilla is technically feasible, safe, and without added complications. With a defined technique and experience, a 100% accuracy to predict the status of the axilla was achieved (13,14). The probability of excising a tumor-bearing axillary lymph node is significantly greater with SLND (61.9%) than with random axillary node sampling (17.5%) (*p* <.0001) (13).

In addition to vital dye directed lymphatic mapping, three other technical approaches for SN identification in breast cancer have evolved: radioguided surgery, radioguided surgery with preoperative lymphoscintigraphy, and the combination of vital dye and isotope techniques (13,15–17). A smaller pilot study investigated the use of radioisotope as an indicator for the identification of the SN and also found 100% accuracy (15). In 1996 Albertini et al. (16) used the combination of blue dye and radioisotope techniques to localize the SN in 92% of patients with an accuracy of 100%. In 1997 Veronesi et al. (17) proposed the use of preoperative lymphoscintigraphy in conjunction with intraoperative radiolocalization to increase the accuracy and identify nonaxillary drainage preoperatively. The SN was identified in 98% of cases and accurately predicted the status of the axilla in 97.5%. Nonaxillary drainage, however, was not investigated. SN identification in breast cancer is technically feasible, safe, and an accurate predictor of the status of the axilla using several different technical approaches.

Proof of Principle

The SN hypothesis for breast cancer was initially disputed as an artifact of detailed histopathologic evaluation of the SN compared to non-SNs (18). In order to test the SN hypothesis in the clinical setting, the complete histopathologic evaluation of the SN and non-SNs was performed using the same pathologic processing with step sectioning, hematoxylin-eosin (H&E) and immunohistochemistry (IHC) for all H&E negative axillary lymph nodes (19). H&E staining identified 33 patients with a tumor-bearing SN (32%). IHC evaluation of 157 negative SNs upstaged 10 patients (14.3%). In 60 patients whose SNs were negative by H&E and IHC, 1,087 non-SNs were examined at two levels by IHC and only one additional tumor-positive node was identified. In 57.3% of patients the SN was negative. In the 44 patients with a tumor-positive SN, 56.8% had involvement of the SN alone. The SN hypothesis has been confirmed in two additional single institution studies that examined all non-SNs with the same rigorous histopathologic analysis (20,21). The NCI-sponsored multicenter trial reported similar findings for cases with a negative SN that had further evaluation with IHC (22). Occult metastases were found in 4.1% of the SNs and 0.35% of the non-SNs ($p < .001$). The odds of finding occult metastases in the SN compared to the non-SNs are 12.3 times greater. The SN concept has been validated by these studies.

LYMPHATIC ANATOMY OF THE BREAST AND IMPLICATIONS FOR SENTINEL NODE IDENTIFICATION

Patterns of Regional Nodal Drainage

The axilla is the primary site of drainage in 76% to 95% of breast cancer cases, with isolated internal mammary drainage seen in 1.3% to 9.9 % (23–27). Primary drainage to other nodal pathways is uncommon and seen in less than 0.3% to 3.2% of cases. Lymphoscintigrams can identify nodal uptake of radioisotope preoperatively in 64% to 99% of cases (Fig. 41.1) (23–26).

Although the axilla is the primary drainage site, with other regions receiving limited lymphatic flow, the prognostic value of the internal mammary nodal status is high, particularly when both axillary and internal mammary nodes are either negative with improved survival or positive, leading to a significantly decreased survival (28). In those rare cases, with small tumors and sole drainage to nodal stations other than the axilla, identification of tumor positive regional nodes may be important for adjuvant chemotherapy recommendations. In one study, internal mammary lymph node drainage was demonstrated in 22% of patients with 24% of them demonstrating metastases (29). Radiation fields were extended in 85% of these patients and systemic therapy was added in 30%.

Routine biopsy of internal mammary lymph nodes is not used in standard practice, but it does warrant further investigation to determine appropriateness for staging and identification of high-risk subgroups who may benefit from adjuvant treatment (30). The data from the National Surgical Adjuvant Breast and Bowel Project (NSABP) B-32 trial demonstrated that the majority of positive SNs came from levels I and II of the

ALND, and only 1.2% of the positive SN specimens came from nonaxillary locations (31).

Analysis of the superficial and deep lymphatic anatomy of the breast and upper torso from human cadaver studies supports the SN concept (32). Superficial lymphatic collectors drain into the same first-echelon node close to the lateral edge of the pectoralis minor muscle (Fig. 41.2). In most cases, the drainage was to only one SN. In several cases, however, there was at least one other first-echelon node from a collecting lymphatic that passed directly through the breast. The lymphatics of the nipple–areola complex are different from other areas of the breast and drain only into the first-echelon pectoral node shown in Fig. 41.2 in green, but not to the depicted orange node that receives lymphatic drainage that passes through the breast. This study did not identify any direct anastomosis between the superficial collecting system and the collectors associated with internal mammary vessels, an observation consistent with the findings of studies that have used lymphoscintigraphy to study patterns of lymphatic drainage by site of injection (33).

This anatomic study may explain the clinical experience with lymphatic mapping and the persistence of a false-negative (FN) rate of 8.4% to 11.8% (31,32,34,35). Dye injected deep into the parenchyma along the purple-colored track (depicted in Fig. 41.2) reaches both the depicted green and orange lymph nodes in the pectoral group, whereas dye injected into the subareolar or intradermal location reached only the depicted green node. SLND using the intraparenchymal injection technique would track to both nodes and suggests that the intraparenchymal route of injection may be more likely to track to both first-echelon nodes and result in a more accurate staging of the axilla. The proof of principle study discussed above was performed with the intraparenchymal injection method and had one FN node (19).

Cumulative Experience of Sentinel Node Identification for Staging

Investigators from academic centers and the surgical community worldwide have introduced SLND into clinical practice as a staging procedure (34). Several multicenter lymphatic mapping trials have confirmed the feasibility of SLND as a staging procedure and reported early data on identification and FN rate (Table 41.1) (31,35–44). The identification rate ranges from 86% to 97% with accuracy from 96% to 98% and a FN rate from 4% to 16.7%. Some data from the large, randomized prospective trials have not matured. Most of the multicenter trials required some formal instruction or validation prior to their participation.

National Surgical Adjuvant Breast and Bowel Project B-32 Trial

The NSABP B-32 trial was designed to address several goals. Subjects with clinically node negative invasive breast cancer were randomized to SLND followed by a level I or II ALND or to observation of the axilla if the SN was tumor free. The aim of this study was to determine success in identification, accuracy of SLND, long-term control of regional disease, disease-free survival, overall survival, and morbidity between these two arms. The study reported an SN identification rate of 97.2%, accuracy rate of 97.1%, and a FN rate of 9.8% (31). Long-term outcome data for disease-free survival and overall survival will be reported in the future.

Axillary Lymphatic Mapping Against Nodal Axillary Clearance Trial

The Axillary Lymphatic Mapping Against Nodal Axillary Clearance (ALMANAC) trial was a two-phase trial that

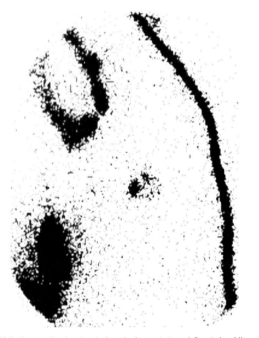

FIGURE 41.1. Preoperative lymphoscintigraphy demonstrates a left anterior oblique view of a sentinel node.

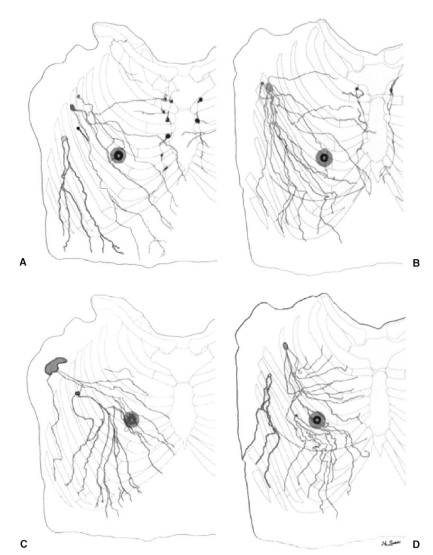

A

B

C

D

FIGURE 41.2. Tracing distally of lymphatics of both hemi upper torsos (male: **A** and **C**, female: **B** and **D**) from each first-tier lymph node color coded: pectoral node (green, orange, black, and yellow), subclavicular node (light blue), and internal mammary node (red). Note that the lymph collecting vessels from the nipple and areolar region on each specimen drain into the green-colored lymph node; the similar pattern of chest and breast drainage between the male and female studies; the breast lies in the pathway of collecting lymphatics that start peripherally; and although the majority of the breast drains to one sentinel node in **D**, every breast area is drained by more than one first-tier node in each study. (From Suami H, Pan W-R, Mann GB, et al. The lymphatic anatomy of the breast and its implications for sentinel lymph node biopsy: a human cadaver study. *Ann Surg Oncol* 2008;15:863–871, with permission.)

Table 41.1	IDENTIFICATION RATE AND FALSE-NEGATIVE RATE OF MULTICENTER SENTINEL LYMPH NODE TRIALS THAT EVALUATED THE STATUS OF THE AXILLA WITH SENTINEL LYMPH NODE DISSECTION FOLLOWED BY COMPLETION AXILLARY LYMPH NODE DISSECTION

Study (Reference)	No. of Surgeons	No. of Patients	Course	Academic Community	Identification Rate (%)	False Negative (%)
Krag et al. (36)	11	443	One-on-one training	Both	91	11
McMasters et al. (65)	99	806	No formal instruction	Mostly community	88	7
Tafra et al. (135)	48	529	Yes	Both	87	13
Bergkvist et al. (40)	28	498	Standard Protocol	—	90	11
Shivers et al. (38)	111	426	Yes	12 academic 30 community	86	4
Gill (41)	26 centers	150	Training workshop	Both	96 SLND 99 ALND	5
NSABP B-32 Training (44)	226	815	Training manual and trainer	Both	96.2	6.7
ALMANAC (42)	31	803	Validation phase	Both	96.1 97.6	6.7
NSABP B-32 (31)		5611	Validation phase	Both	97.1	9.8
Sentinella/GIVOM (43)	23	697	No formal instruction	Both	95	16.7

SLND, sentinel lymph node dissection; ALND, axillary lymph node dissection; NSABP, National Surgical Adjuvant Breast and Bowel Project; ALMANAC, Axillary Lymphatic Mapping Against Nodal Axillary Clearance.

required surgeons to demonstrate a 90% identification rate and a FN rate of less than 5% prior to proceeding to phase II, which was the two-armed prospective trial that randomized patients into SLND followed by ALND or to SLND alone if the SN was tumor free (45). If the SN was positive for tumor cells, the regional treatment was ALND or axillary irradiation. The primary aims of this study were to evaluate axillary morbidity, health economics, quality of life, and axillary recurrence. The secondary goal was to determine the incidence of long-term axillary recurrence rate with SLND alone compared to ALND. Performance evaluation of the first 13 surgeons completing 40 cases of SLND with ALND demonstrated a 96% success rate with the combination technique and a 5% FN rate (46). Axillary recurrence rate has not been reported yet.

Royal Australian College of Surgeons Sentinel Node versus Axillary Clearance Trial

The Royal Australian College of Surgeons (RACS) multicenter trial of SN versus Axillary Clearance (SNAC) multicenter randomized study was a phase III trial with a two stage design. Stage I tested performance measures for SLND. A sensitivity of 95%, FN rate of 5%, and a negative predictive value of 98% were reported for SN biopsy in stage I (41). Stage II was a randomized controlled trial of SLND alone versus axillary clearance. The study population for this trial included women with invasive breast cancer of less than 3 cm and clinically negative axillary nodes.

Sentinella/GIVOM Trial

The aim of the Italian Sentinella/Gruppo Interdisciplinare Veneto Oncologia Mammaria (GIVOM) study was to assess the efficacy and safety of SLND compared to ALND. The SN identification rate was 95%. Positive SNs were identified in 28% of patients. The FN rate was 16.7%. The trial did not include formal training or surgical quality control, but did require at least 15 cases of SLND followed by ALND with no false negatives before starting randomization (43). This trial was designed specifically to simulate the general clinical setting rather than the practice of highly selected, specialty focused surgeons.

HISTOPATHOLOGIC PROCESSING

When the authors' group at the JWCI compared ALND alone to SLND followed by completion ALND, axillary metastases were identified in 29.1% of the ALND-alone group compared to 42% in the SLND group (p <.03) (18). H&E analysis of multiple levels of the SN increased the sensitivity to detect micrometastases for SLND versus ALND (9.2% vs. 3.0%, respectively; p <.004), and when both H&E and IHC were used, there was increased sensitivity (16.0% vs. 3.0%, respectively; p <.0005) (Fig. 41.3). Focused histopathologic analysis of the SN is a more sensitive method to detect micrometastases by both H&E and IHC and leads to improved accuracy of axillary staging for a tumor-positive axillary lymph node.

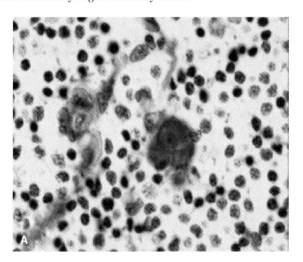
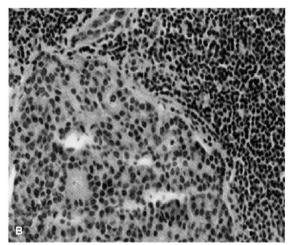
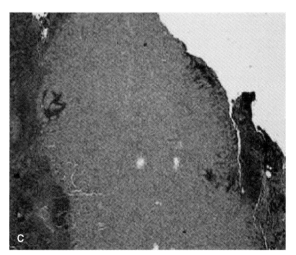
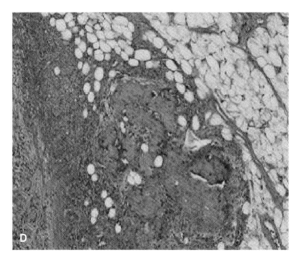

FIGURE 41.3. Sentinel node metastases. A: Demonstrates a single immunohistochemistry-positive cell. **B:** Demonstrates a high power view of an hematoxylin-eosin metastasis. **C:** Demonstrates a low power view of a macrometastasis. **D:** Demonstrates extracapsular extension of a sentinel node micrometastasis.

The American College of Pathologists has established guidelines to process the SN with frozen sections, imprint cytology, or permanent formalin processed specimens (47). The SN is bivalved along the longitudinal axis, serially sectioned at 1.5 to 2.0 mm thickness blocks and each block is sectioned at three levels. If metastases are identified in the SN (Fig. 41.3), the size of the metastasis is reported as macrometastases (>2.0 mm), micrometastases (>0.2 and ≤2.0 mm), or isolated tumor cells (≤0.2 mm), and the method of detection of the metastasis by H&E, IHC, or reverse transcription-polymerase chain reaction (RT-PCR) according to the new American Joint Committee on Cancer (AJCC) guidelines (48).

Molecular analysis of the SN is an area of emerging technology and interest. Some investigators feel that this is a more objective assessment of the tumor burden in the SN, is more reproducible, can be standardized, and evaluates more tissue in a shorter period of time (49). Quantitative RT-PCR evaluation demonstrates a 98% accuracy and can be performed in 40 minutes or less (50,51). A prospective trial to evaluate lymph node metastases with a multiplex RT-PCR-based assay detected 98% of metastases greater than 2 mm and 88% of those greater than 0.2 mm, and results were superior to frozen section histology or imprint cytology (49). RT-PCR has not been studied sufficiently to make treatment recommendations based on positive results.

The risks of completion ALND, axillary irradiation, or adjuvant chemotherapy for an IHC or RT-PCR tumor positive node must be weighed against the unknown significance of metastases detected through sophisticated technological methods without long-term, randomized trial data. In the absence of participation in a clinical trial, the reasonable management approach should be based on the H&E evaluation of axillary nodes; however, in clinical practice IHC is used in many centers for SNs that are found negative by H&E.

FACTORS INFLUENCING THE SUCCESS AND ACCURACY OF SENTINEL LYMPH NODE DISSECTION

In order to reduce the FN rate, causes of failure of SLND have been sought. Potential explanations for failure include surgical technique, surgeon and pathologist experience, lymphatic physiology, aberrant lymphatic patterns, and patient and tumor characteristics.

Effect of Sentinel Lymph Node Dissection Technique on Accuracy

A variety of technical factors, which include type of dye or radioisotope, filtered versus unfiltered isotope, timing of surgery after injection, and site of injection (peritumoral, subdermal, intradermal, subareolar), influence the performance of SLND. The success rate, sensitivity, negative predictive value, FN rate, and accuracy by method of detection and mean tumor size are shown in Table 41.2. A high degree of accuracy and a low FN rate with resection of only one or two lymph nodes is seen in most cases. Differences in the ability to find the SN are reflections of variations in methodology and experience (34,52). Internal mammary nodes are visualized less often with intradermal injection than with peritumoral injection (33,53–56). Subareolar injection of isotope offers some advantages over peritumoral injection, for example, when the tumor is nonpalpable, it increases the distance from the injection site of radioisotope to the axilla for upper outer quadrant lesions, reducing the shine through, and is a good choice for multicentric disease (57).

In the multi-institutional American College of Surgeons Z0010 trial 198 surgeons enrolled 5,237 patients and used blue dye with radiocolloid in 79.4% of cases, blue dye alone in 14.8%, and radiocolloid alone in 5.7% with a success rate of 98.7%, corresponding to a failure rate of 1.7% (58). The percent of failed SLND with blue dye was 1.4%, radiocolloid 2.3%, and the combination 1.2% (p = .2813). The number of cases (≤50 compared to >50) enrolled was associated with a statistically significant failure rate.

In a recent meta-analysis, the proportion of successful mapping with dye alone, radiocolloid alone, or the combination was 83.1%, 89.2%, and 91.9%, respectively (p = .007) (34). In the University of Louisville Breast Cancer Sentinel Lymph Node Study, 99 surgeons found that the SN identification rate with dye alone or dye plus isotope was the same (86% vs. 90%, respectively) in 806 patients (35).

Morrow et al. (59) evaluated isosulfan blue dye alone and compared it to dye with isotope. Surgeons achieved equal results with either method. A recent study from New Zealand confirms this work and reports that identification of the SN is similar with blue dye alone compared to triple modality approach (lymphoscintigraphy, intraoperative gamma probe, and intraoperative blue dye) (60). The blue dye had an accuracy of 98% and a sensitivity of 96% compared to the triple method accuracy of 95% and sensitivity of 91%. There has been a manufacturing shortage of isosulfan blue in the United States and methylene blue has been used as an alternative vital dye. The success rate of methylene blue with radioisotope is reported to be equivalent to isosulfan blue with isotope (61,62).

The site of injection of the tracer may influence the outcome of SLND. A prospective randomized trial compared intradermal, intraparenchymal, and subareolar routes of injection and demonstrated a significantly higher rate of localization, more rapid transit by lymphoscintigraphy, and shorter time to surgery with the intradermal injection (33). Another randomized multicenter trial compared periareolar and peritumoral injection of radiotracer and blue dye (53). The intraoperative success was similar for blue dye or gamma detection (99.1%). The detection rate was higher for the periareolar site for each tracer, but this was not statistically significant. The SN was blue in 94.7%, hot in 97.1%, and both in 92.6%. The concordance was 91.5% with the peritumoral injection and 95.6% with the periareolar injection. The blue dye and radiocolloid concordance for the positive SN patients was 94.5% and, when assessed by site of injection, 96.2% in the periareolar group and 92.9% in the peritumoral group.

The SLND procedure has been adopted by surgeons in both academic and community settings. National practice patterns from an American College of Surgeons survey conducted in 2001 indicated that 77% of U.S. surgeons perform SLND for breast cancer, 90% use the combination of blue dye and radioisotope, and 60% ordered preoperative lymphoscintigraphy (63). The efficacy of the method, dye, isotope or both is more likely a reflection of training and experience than variations in the success of the method itself. Each investigator should adhere to a defined method then collect data and analyze the outcome. The importance of quality control and appropriate training has been emphasized by groups evaluating this new technology (64).

Effect of Surgeon Experience: Training and Performance of Sentinel Lymph Node Dissection

A survey of U.S. surgeons reported that most learned SLND through courses (35%), surgical oncology fellowship training programs (26%), observation of colleagues (31%), or self-instruction (26%) (63). Although case number and volume contribute to successful lymphatic mapping (65), SLND alone was

| Table 41.2 | STUDIES WITH 100 OR MORE SUBJECTS REPORTING THE IDENTIFICATION AND ACCURACY OF SENTINEL LYMPH NODE DISSECTION FOLLOWED BY COMPLETION AXILLARY LYMPH NODE DISSECTION FOR INVASIVE BREAST CANCER ACCORDING TO TECHNIQUE |

Author (Reference)	Date	No. of Patients	Mean T (cm)	Success (%)	Sensitivity (%)	NPV (%)	False Negative (%)	Accuracy (%)	MEAN # SN	SN (+) ONLY
Vital Dye Method										
Giuliano et al. (13)	1994	174	—	66	88	94	4.3	96	1.8	38
Giuliano et al. (14)	1997	107	2.11	94	100	100	0.0	100	1.8	67
Guenther et al. (177)	1997	145	2.09	71	90	96	9.6	97	1.6	43
Ilum et al. (150)	2000	161	1.7	60	86	87	14.3	93	—	—
Nos et al. (178)	2003	324	—	86	89	95	11.1	96	—	—
Gamma Probe Guided Surgery										
No Lymphoscintigram										
Krag et al. (179)	1998	157	—	93	95	98	4.9	98		
Krag et al. (36)	1998	443	1.9	93	89	96	11.4	97		
Lymphoscintigram										
Veronesi et al. (17)	1997	163	—	98	95	95	4.7	98	1.4	38
Borgstein et al. (23)	1998	130	2.1	94	98	98	2.2	98	1.2	59
Veronesi et al. (154)	1999	376[a]	1.7	99	93	94	6.7	97	1.4	41
Zurrida et al. (180)	2000	376	—	99	93	94	6.7	97	—	39
Fraile et al. (181)	2000	132	1.9	96	96	97	4.0	98	2.0	46
Mariani et al. (182)	2000	197[b]	—	97	86	92	13.7	95	—	—
Rink et al. (183)	2001	123	—	94	92	96	7.7	97	2.6	38
Combined Technique with Dye and Isotope										
No Lymphoscintigram										
Morrow et al. (59)	1999	139[c]	1.7	86	97	—	—	96	1.9	43
Smillie et al. (184)	2001	106	—	84	95	96	6.0	98	—	53
Lymphoscintigram										
Kollias et al. (185)	1999	117	—	81	94	97	6.5	98	1.4	42
Hill et al. (133)	1999	104[d]	—	93	89	91	10.6	95	2.1	61
Doting et al. (186)	2000	136	1.9	93	95	96	5.1	98	1.7	39
Mariani et al. (182)	2000	197[b]	—	97	86	92	13.7	95	—	51
McMasters et al. (35)	2000	562	—	90	94	98	5.8	98	—	—
Motomura et al. (187)	2001	138[e]	—	95	100	100	0.0	100	—	—
Taffra et al. (37)	2001	529	—	87	87	95	13.0	96	—	—

Sensitivity, (true positive)/(true positive + false negative); NPV, negative predictive value (true negative)/(true negative + false negative); False negative, (false negative)/(true positive + false negative); Accuracy, (true positive + true negative)/(total number of patients).
[a]Includes subgroup of 54 patients who had patent blue dye and isotope.
[b]Analysis of 197 of 284 cases with axillary lymph node dissection.
[c]Analysis of 47 of 139 cases randomized.
[d]Subgroup of 104 of 500 cases with axillary lymph node dissection.
[e]Combine indigo-cyanine green and isotope arm.

performed after 10 or fewer cases of SLND followed by completion ALND by 28% of surgeons surveyed (63). Surgeon performance continues to improve beyond 20 to 30 cases (37,59). Formal lymphatic mapping instruction with hands-on experience leads to a 90% to 95% identification rate and a 3.8% to 4.3% FN rate when more than 30 cases are performed (37,66). The NSABP B-32 trial required a minimum of one to five prequalifying cases and reported a technical success rate of 97% (31). Surgical volume impacts identification rates (66,67). Surgeons who performed fewer than three cases per month had a success rate of 86.23% ± 8.30%, for three to six cases 88.73% ± 6.36%, and for six or more SN biopsies 97.81% ± 0.44% (66). Surgeon training and experience is important in determining SLND success and accuracy.

These studies describe above show individual variation in learning the skills and identify some of the pitfalls in learning the technique. Instruction in SLND is now part of surgical residency training in the United States. For those not trained in the technique during residency, formal instruction, use of dual agents, performance of approximately 20 SLND procedures with a backup ALND, and an adequate volume of cases to maintain skills are all factors that contribute to successful identification of SN and reduced FN rate. A consensus statement

from the American Society of Breast Surgeons suggests that prior to abandoning ALND for a negative SN, 20 cases of SLND be performed with an identification rate of 85% and a FN rate of 5% or less (68). The American Society of Breast Surgeons has provided updated guidelines (69). These should be adapted on an individual basis, with more cases performed by those with lower identification rates and higher FN rates and vice versa. One problem with their application is that most patients are SN negative, making the FN rate more difficult to determine with a high degree of certainty.

Effect of the Number of Sentinel Nodes Removed

Increasing the mean number of SNs removed may improve accuracy (31,70–72). The number of SNs removed statistically affected the FN rate in the NSABP B-32 trial (31). The FN rate was 17.7% when one node was removed, 10% for two, 6.9% for three, 5.5% for four, and 1% for five or more nodes removed. In the University of Louisville Breast Cancer Sentinel Lymph Node Study, 58% of the patients had multiple SNs removed (70). The overall SN identification rate was 90% with an 8.3% FN rate. If a single node was removed, the FN rate was 14.3% compared to 4.3% when multiple SNs were removed (p <.0004). The first two or three SNs removed predict the status of the axilla in about 98% of cases, but additional positive SNs will be identified when four or more nodes are removed, improving the FN rate (31,71,72). The removal of all blue or radioactive nodes with a count equal to or greater than 10% of the most radioactive node has been shown to decrease the FN rate in these studies. This increase in staging accuracy may be obtained at the cost of an increased rate of complications, especially lymphedema, but the goal is accurate staging for treatment decisions.

Effect of Patient and Tumor Characteristics

The data from the multi-institutional, randomized prospective NSABP B-32 trial reports a FN rate of 9.8% and an overall accuracy of 97.1% (31). Differences in tumor location (inner and central location vs. lateral and outer), no hot spot identified preoperatively, small tumor size, older age, and type of diagnostic biopsy (excision/incisional biopsy higher than fine-needle aspiration [FNA] or core needle biopsy [CNB]) increased the FN rate. In the ALMANAC study, increased body mass index (BMI), upper outer quadrant location, and nonvisualization on lymphoscintigraphy were significantly associated with failed identification ($p < .001$, $p = .008$, $p < .001$, respectively) (42). Neither age, tumor size, tumor histology, tumor grade, nor multifocality affected identification. In the American College of Surgical Oncology Group (ACOSOG) Z0010 trial, a higher failure to identify a SN occurred with increased BMI and age 70 or older (58).

Regional Control after Sentinel Lymph Node Dissection for Sentinel Node–Negative Patients

The first study to accept SLND as a staging procedure and a therapeutic procedure when the SN is free of tumor was initiated at the JWCI in 133 consecutive women with tumors 4 cm or less (73). SLND was the only axillary treatment if the SN contained no tumor cells. Completion ALND was performed when the SN contained metastases. No patient received axillary irradiation. SN identification was 99% with no locoregional recurrences at 39 months. There were fewer complications in the SLND group (3%) compared to ALND after SLND (35%) ($p = .001$). The complications in both groups were minimal, primarily wound seromas.

The FN rate for SLND ranges from 0.0% to 29.4% in the meta-analysis of single institution studies (average 8.4% across studies, median, 7%), raising concerns about the risk of axillary recurrence in patients with SLND alone (34).

There are two multicenter trials that have reported the outcome of SLND alone for a tumor-free SN (74,75). In one study, SLND was performed with subdermal injection of technetium Tc-99m-colloidal albumin in 479 patients (74). At a median follow-up of 35.8 months, there were no axillary recurrences. A mean number of 1.4 SNs were removed and 90.6% of patients were treated with adjuvant systemic therapy. The large, Swedish multicenter cohort study reported the axillary recurrence rate, disease-free survival, and overall survival in 2,246 SN-negative patients who underwent observation alone (75). The axilla was the only site of failure in 13 (0.6%), axilla and breast in 7 (0.3%), and axilla and distant disease in 7 (0.3%). The overall survival was 91.6%, disease-free survival 92.1%, and breast cancer–specific survival 94.7% at 5 years.

The largest single institution study is from the Memorial Sloan-Kettering Cancer Center, which reported an axillary failure rate of 0.12% in 2,340 patients (76). The single institution study with the longest follow-up is the European Institute of Oncology randomized trial with one (0.5%) failure in the axilla in the SLND-alone arm at 79 months (77). The Netherlands

Cancer Institute study reported an overall survival of 95.9% and the disease-free survival of 89.7% in 748 SN-negative patients at 5 years (78). Axillary failure occurred in two (0.25%) patients and supraclavicular failure in two (0.25%) patients.

Results from single institution studies examining local recurrence after SLND alone are summarized in Table 41.3 (79). A meta-analysis of 48 studies that included 14,959 SN-negative patients followed for a median of 34 months demonstrated an axillary failure in 67 patients (0.3%) (79). In the European Institute of Oncology Trial the predicted failure was eight cases, but only one case of overt axillary metastases has been diagnosed at 7.2 years of follow-up after surgery (Fig. 41.4). The possibility that the occult metastases in the FN nodes may never become overt has been observed from the single institution studies, the Swedish multicenter trial, and from the European Institute of Oncology trial at a relatively short follow-up. Although these results, showing low axillary relapse after a negative SN, are encouraging, the long-term follow-up data from the large multicenter randomized trials comparing axillary failure rates for SLND to ALND are essential for final confirmation. SLND appears to provide regional nodal control when the SN is negative at short-term follow-up. Standard tangent breast fields may contribute to axillary control in those who undergo breast conservation and receive whole breast irradiation, but several studies show that they do not encompass all the level I and II lymph nodes (80,81).

Reasons for a lower than expected axillary failure rate in the single institution and multicenter trials may be due to a relatively short follow-up, although historical information from the NSABP B-04 trials reported most axillary failures in the first 2 years. Alternatively, adjuvant systemic therapy may treat low-volume disease, and in cases of breast conservation postlumpectomy radiotherapy, tangents may treat the low axilla and some disease may lie dormant.

Summary

SLND has met with success in single institution studies and several multicenter trials with credentialed teams. There is a large body of evidence that suggests that SLND is an accurate staging procedure in expert hands. The greatest concern is that regional recurrence will be high and there may potentially be an adverse effect on regional and systemic control if the SN is falsely negative and appropriate treatment is not recommended.

Reliable staging with SLND depends on the success of SN identification, a low FN rate, and histopathologic accuracy. Guidelines for incorporating SLND into clinical practice, especially for SN-negative patients, were first put forth by experts in the field of breast cancer in the Philadelphia Consensus Conference of Sentinel Node in 2001 (82). More than a decade of experience with sentinel lymphadenectomy as the sole axillary treatment at a number of large single institution trials, limited national studies, the multicenter Swedish trial, and the randomized European Institute of Oncology trial suggests that this is a safe, reliable, and effective procedure for staging. Results from the randomized trials and long-term follow-up are awaited.

IMPACT OF SENTINEL LYMPH NODE DISSECTION ON SURVIVAL IN NODE-NEGATIVE PATIENTS

Definitive data on the impact of SLND on survival will only come from prospective, randomized trials. The NSABP B-32 prospective trial in the United States is designed to answer this question, as are the ALMANAC trial in the United Kingdom and

| Table 41.3 | PATTERNS OF RECURRENCE AFTER SENTINEL LYMPH NODE DISSECTION ALONE FOR TUMOR-FREE SENTINEL NODE |

Author	Year	No. of Patients	Recurrences	Interval (mos)	Follow-Up (mos)[a]	Sensitivity (%)[b]
Roumen	2001	100	1	14	24	—
Schrenk	2001	83	0	—	22	100
Guenther	2002	205	1	—	32	—
Bedrosian	2002	216	0	—	30	100
Chung	2002	206	3	4, 11, 40	26	97
Shivers	2002	309	0	—	16 M	100
Loza	2002	168	1	30	21	—
Roka	2002	383	2	7, 13	20	—
Blanchard	2003	685	1	41	29 M	—
Badgwell	2003	159	0	—	32	100
Ponzone	2003	150	0	—	15	100
Imoto	2004	112	4	—	52	—
Van Wessem	2004	59	1	24	28	—
Reitsamer	2004	200	0	—	36	100
Naik	2004	2340	3	—	31	—
Van der Vegt	2004	106	1	26	35	—
Torrenga	2004	104	1	24	57	—
Taback	2004	732	1	—	46	—
Khakpour	2005	192	0	—	26	100
Soni	2005	101	1	35	22	98
Veronesi	2005	953	3	26, 29, 37	38	—
Jeruss	2005	592	1	22	27 M	—
Kristen	2005	95	1	—	14 M	—
Snoj	2005	50	1	26	32	—
Zavagno	2005	479	0	—	36	100
Sanjuàn	2005	158	1	19	21	99
Swenson	2005	580	3	11, 13, 24	33	—
Langer	2005	122	1	14	42	—
Palesty	2006	335	2	5, 14	33	—
De Kanter	2006	149	4	10, 12, 14, 56	65	—
Pizzocaro	2006	257	0	—	26	100
Domenech	2006	97	0	—	49	100
Grigolato	2006	96	0	—	54	100
Sinko	2006	292	1	11	27 M	—
Van Wely	2006	387	9	4-63	52	—
Carcoforo	2006	566	3	17, 18, 24	26	98
Rosing	2006	89	1	37	26	—
Haid	2006	180	1	12	47	—
Kokke	2006	503	7	—	14-46	—
Susini	2006	165	0	—	46	100
Paajanen	2006	107	0	—	31	—
Pejavar	2006	110	1	—	—	—
Leikola	2006	183	2	24, 36	—	—
Snider	2006	242	0	—	25	100
Schulze	2006	26	0	—	47	100
Nagashima	2006	241	0	—	27	100
Marazzo	2006	233	0	—	33	100
Takei	2007	1,062	4	9, 18, 21, 29	34	—
Overall		14,959	67	—	34[c]	100

[a]Median duration of follow-up, except for the numbers followed by M (mean).
[b]Sensitivity calculated by dividing the number of patients with a tumor-positive sentinel node by the sum of all patients with a negative sentinel node who developed a recurrence and the number of patients with a positive sentinel node.
[c]Calculated from the studies that provided a median number of follow-up duration; –, unknown or not mentioned.
From van der Ploeg IM, Niewig OE, van Rijk MC, et al. Axillary recurrence after a tumour-negative sentinel node biopsy in breast cancer patients: a systematic review and meta-analysis of the literature. *Eur J Surg Oncol* 2008;34(12):1277–1284, with permission.

the RACS SNAC (Australian/New Zealand) trial, but data are not yet available (31,41,83).

In the absence of the data from these trials, some information can be gleaned from the single institution European Institute of Oncology randomized trial (84) and the small multicenter Sentinella/GIVOM trial (43). In the European Institute of Oncology randomized study, women with tumors less than 2 cm were randomized to SLND alone if the SN was tumor free or to SLND followed by ALND (77). In the ALND group, 32% had a positive SN and 8 of 174 SN-negative patients had a FN node. The SN was positive in 36% of the SLND-only

group with one axillary failure (eight expected) at a median follow-up of 79 months. Breast cancer–related events in the ALND and SN groups are shown in Figure 41.5 (77). The overall survival was the same for the ALND group compared to SLND alone (96.4% vs. 98.4%, respectively; *p* = .6) (77). The SLND-alone group had decreased morbidity and cost, with a lower than expected axillary failure rate at 79 months of follow-up.

The first multicenter trial to report results on patients randomized to SLND alone or SLND followed by ALND was the Sentinella/GIVOM trial (43). This study reported a FN rate of

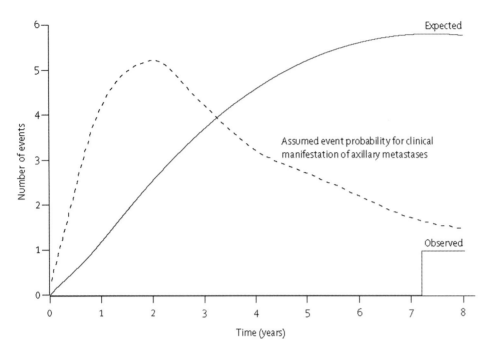

FIGURE 41.4. Observed and expected axillary metastases over time in sentinel lymph node group. (From Veronesi U, Paganellli G, Viale G, et al. Sentinel-lymph node biopsy as a staging procedure in breast cancer: update of a randomised controlled study. *Lancet Oncol* 2006;7:983–990, with permission.)

16.7%. Despite this high FN rate, there has only been one axillary failure in the SLND-alone group at 55.6 months. The overall survival was 95.5% in the ALND group and 94.8% in the SLND-alone group at 5 years of follow-up.

The data from the two small prospective SLND-only trials discussed above do not show any difference is disease-free or overall survival for the SN-negative patients treated with SLND alone when compared to SLND with ALND. This supports the findings of the older NSABP B-04 study (85), which found no significant difference in overall survival for patients treated with and without axillary dissection at 25 years, in spite of the fact that 38% of patients in the no axillary dissection arm had nodal disease (based on the findings in the dissection arm). The results of the NSABP B-04 trial, however, must be understood in context of a trial that was not powered to detect a small survival difference between groups. This is particularly relevant in light of the findings of the 15-year follow-up of the effect of radiotherapy and difference in the extent of surgery for early breast cancer on local recurrence and that local control improves disease-specific survival (86). Long-term results from large prospective randomized trials are necessary to determine the definitive regional failure rate and the impact on disease-free and overall survival, although it is unlikely that any single trial has sufficient statistical power to identify a small survival benefit for axillary dissection.

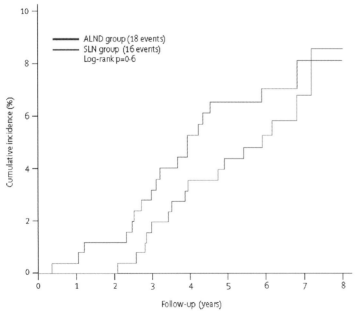

Patients at risk

ALND group	257	255	247	237	226	213	179	71	1
SLN group	259	259	258	249	241	228	190	78	0

FIGURE 41.5. Breast cancer related events in axillary lymph node dissection (ALND) group and sentinel lymph node (SLN) group. (From Veronesi U, Paganellli G, Viale G, et al. Sentinel-lymph node biopsy as a staging procedure in breast cancer: update of a randomised controlled study. *Lancet Oncol* 2006;7:983–990, with permission.)

MANAGEMENT OF THE AXILLA IN THE PATIENT WITH A POSITIVE SENTINEL NODE

ALND is the recommended treatment for a positive SN. The necessity of ALND for a positive SN is, however, an area of investigation. As tumor size has decreased, the nodal burden in patients with nodal metastases has also decreased (87). In the meta-analysis of 69 SN studies followed by ALND, the SN was positive in an average of 42% (median, 40%; mode, 50%) and ranged from 17% to 74% (34). Among those with a positive SN, 53% had additional nodes positive while 47% did not (34). The implication from these observations is that patients may be accurately staged and treated by removal of the SN alone, particularly if local axillary treatment of additional involved nodes does not impact survival.

The appropriate management of the axilla after a positive SN is being addressed in a number of prospective clinical trials. The ACOSOG Z0011 was a prospective clinical trial that randomized subjects with clinical T1 or T2N0M0 breast cancer with a tumor-positive SN to completion ALND or observation of the axilla. Treatment of the breast was breast conservation and whole breast radiotherapy. No third field was given to the axillary lymph nodes. The primary end point of this study was overall survival; morbidity and disease-free survival were secondary end points. A secondary aim was to evaluate surgical morbidity with SLND plus ALND versus SLND alone. The purpose of this study was to determine the therapeutic role of axillary dissection. Unfortunately, this study closed early due to poor accrual and a low event rate.

The After Mapping of the Axilla Radiotherapy or Surgery (AMAROS) study is a phase III international multicenter investigation to compare axillary irradiation to ALND for a tumor-positive SN for patients with tumors less than 3 cm in size (88). All patients had SLND and those with a tumor-free SN were observed, while those with nodal involvement were randomized to axillary irradiation or dissection. The main objective of the study is to prove equivalence of the two treatments for locoregional control. The second objective is to determine if SLND alone provides adequate axillary control when the SN is tumor free. Morbidity will also be compared. Results have not been reported.

A single institution prospective study examined the use of axillary irradiation instead of ALND to reduce the risks of lym-

phedema and chronic pain for SN positive patients (89). At a 32-month follow-up there was one axillary failure, which occurred in the ALND arm.

There are several studies that have reported the short-term outcomes in SN-positive patients who declined ALND and had no treatment of the axilla (76,90–93). In these studies the tumor size was small and the majority of patients had micrometastatic disease. There were no locoregional failures at short follow-up (29 to 32 months). A recent update from Memorial Sloan-Kettering Cancer Center on SN-positive patients who declined ALND investigated the clinical findings, pathologic features, nomogram scores, and axillary failure rate in 287 SN-positive patients (94). This group of patients was older, had more favorable tumors, a higher rate of breast conservation, and a lower estimate of residual nodal disease calculated by a nomogram than the group undergoing axillary dissection. The axillary relapse rate in the untreated group was 2% compared to 0.4% in the group who had a completion ALND ($p = .004$).

Although limited information is available from studies evaluating outcome in SN-positive patients who did not undergo standard axillary treatment, these small studies suggest that early isolated regional nodal failure is uncommon. Radiotherapy to the axilla may be an alternative treatment modality (Chapter 43).

The ability to predict the absence of additional positive nodes in the axilla when a tumor-positive SN is identified would be extremely useful, allowing avoidance of an ALND in those individuals at low risk of additional nodal disease. Tumor size, size of SN metastasis, extranodal tumor extension, and peritumoral lymphovascular invasion have been associated with non-SN metastases in some studies (95–98), while other studies were not able to define a subset of patients with a positive SN who were not at risk for addition positive axillary lymph nodes (99,100). Julian et al. (101) reported a higher incidence of positive non-SNs with increased number of positive SNs, lymphovascular invasion, clinical tumor size, and the number of hot spots. These authors concluded that while ALND may be helpful for prognosis and treatment planning, it may not be required in patients with small tumors, no lymphovascular invasion, and only a single positive SN out of multiple SNs (≥5).

Van Zee et al. (102) have developed a nomogram to help estimate the risk of additional nodal disease when the SN is positive (Fig. 41.6). The nomogram uses pathologic size, tumor type, nuclear grade, lymphovascular invasion, multifocality, estrogen-receptor status, histopathologic method used to detect a positive SN, and the ratio of the number of positive SN removed

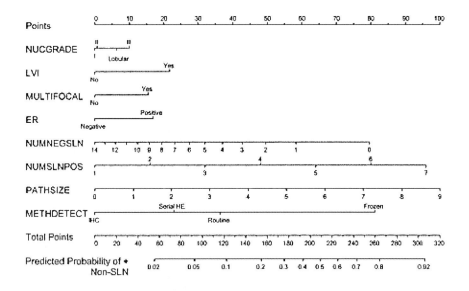

FIGURE 41.6. Nomogram to predict likelihood of additional, nonsentinel lymph node (non-SLN) metastases in a patient with a positive SLN. NUCGRADE, tumor type and nuclear grade (ductal, nuclear grade I; ductal, nuclear grade II; ductal, nuclear grade III; lobular); LVI, lymphovascular invasion; MULTIFOCAL, multifocality of primary tumor; ER, estrogen-receptor status; NUMNEGSLN, number of negative SLNs; NUMSLNPOS, number of positive SLNs; PATHSIZE, pathological size, defined in centimeters; and METHDETECT, method of detection of SLN metastases (frozen, routine hematoxylin-eosin [H&E], serial H&E, immunohistochemisty). The first row (POINTS) is the point assignment for each variable. Rows two through nine represent the variables included in the model. For an individual patient, each variable is assigned a point value (uppermost scale, POINTS) based on the histopathological characteristics. A vertical line is made between the appropriate variable value and the POINTS line. The assigned points for all eight variables are summed, and the total is found in row 10 (TOTAL POINTS). Once the total is located, a vertical line is made between TOTAL POINTS and the final row (predicted probability of +non-SLN). (From Van Zee KJ, Manasseh DM, Bevilacqua JLB, et al. A nomogram for predicting the likelihood of additional nodal metastases in breast cancer patients with a positive sentinel node biopsy. *Ann Surg Oncol* 2003;10:1140–1151, with permission.)

to the total number of SN removed to predict the likelihood of additional positive non-SNs. Retrospective data were used to create the model, which was tested prospectively at Memorial Sloan-Kettering Cancer Center and found to be predictive of metastases. The receiver operating characteristic (ROC) was 0.76 in the retrospective data set and 0.77 in the prospective group. Several groups have tested the nomogram and found fair to good reliability, but at the same time they have questioned the clinical usefulness (103). Others did not find good correlation, in particular with micrometastatic disease (104,105).

No study or predictive model has yet been able to identify the group of patients who are at no or very low risk of non-SN metastases to avoid ALND when the SN is positive. Further data from the large national trials may refine these risk categories, and some individuals may be considered for observation of the axilla in the future based on more clearly identified predictors of non-SN metastases. When the SN is positive, an ALND or axillary irradiation is standard of care.

 ## MANAGEMENT OF MICROMETASTATIC DISEASE IN THE SENTINEL NODE

Identification of micrometastases by IHC has resulted in a difficult management dilemma for surgeons, medical oncologists, and radiation oncologists. Historically adjuvant treatment recommendations have been made on the basis of H&E tissue examination. SN evaluation with IHC can upstage SN-negative patients, but the clinical implications of such upstaging are unknown (18).

Although lymph node metastases have been the strongest prognostic indicator for survival, 15% to 20% of node-negative patients recur by 5 years (106,107). One thought has been that this is due to missed nodal metastases. The 2002 AJCC Staging Manual identifies micrometastases by size: pN1mi >0.2 mm ≤2.0 mm and distinguishes isolated cells or clusters of cells; pN0(i+) ≤0.2 mm if identified by IHC or pN0(mol+) if identified by molecular findings (RT-PCR) (108).

Retrospective studies have tried to determine the prognostic significance of micrometastasis by re-examining axillary lymph node specimens initially processed with bisection of the nodes and H&E staining (107,109–122). A variety of methods have been used to detect occult metastases and correlate the findings to outcome: serial sectioning and H&E histology (107,114,115,117), serial sectioning and IHC (118), or a combination of serial sectioning, H&E, and IHC (109,110,113,120). Occult axillary metastases were found in 7% to 32% of cases with H&E and serial sections (107,114,115,123,124), in 7% to 23% with IHC and serial section (119–122,124), and in 17% to 25% with H&E, IHC, and serial section (110,113).

The disease-free or overall survival was not affected by identification of occult metastases in several single institution studies (107,113–115,122). Other single institution studies have reported a difference in disease-free or overall survival (113,119–125). Trojani et al. (119) demonstrated a decrease in disease-free and overall survival in patients with infiltrating ductal carcinoma, with too few cases of invasive lobular carcinoma to draw any meaningful conclusions with this histologic subtype at 10 years follow-up. Nasser et al. (113) found that disease recurrence at 14 years was statistically worse when nodal metastases were greater than 0.2 mm, located in the parenchyma, and had perinodal extension. Fisher et al. (107) also found that the location of the metastasis in the parenchyma of the node had an adverse outcome compared to the subcapsular location. Hainsworth et al. (120) identified the presence of micrometastases as a significant risk factor for disease recurrence by univariate, but not multivariate analysis. In the subgroup of patients who had two to four lymph nodes with

micrometastases, both a decrease in disease-free survival (p <.01) and overall survival (p <.05) were noted by univariate and multivariate analysis. DeMascarel et al. (121,122) defined micrometastases as tumor deposits less than 0.5 mm and reported survival data in 785 node negative patients. The 6-year follow-up study demonstrated a significant decrease in disease-free interval (p = .01) for invasive ductal carcinoma, but not for invasive lobular carcinoma, but no difference in overall survival for either. At 24-years of follow-up there was no difference in disease-free or overall survival for invasive ductal carcinoma or at 18 years for invasive lobular carcinoma (122). A complete histopathologic analysis of axillary lymph nodes from routine axillary dissections performed on 368 patients between 1976 and 1978, using the current standard processing of a SN with step sections and IHC, was performed by Tan et al. (125). They identified lymph node metastases in 23% of patients and 71% had only one node positive. None of these patients received systemic therapy. Among the nodal metastases, 73% were 0.2 mm or less, 20% were 0.3 to 2 mm, and 6% were larger than 2 mm. Disease-specific and disease-free survival were worse for the pN0(i+) and even poorer for the pN1mi group when compared to the pN0 patients with a 20-year follow-up by univariate and multivariate analysis.

The International Breast Cancer Study Group Ludwig V trial was a multicenter, prospective adjuvant chemotherapy trial that retrospectively analyzed prospectively collected archival tissue with serial step sections and H&E staining of axillary lymph nodes to identify metastases (123). Postoperative chemotherapy was given to the lymph node positive patients. Nine percent of the patients had micrometastases that were associated with a statistically significant reduction in survival. When disease-free survival was evaluated in patients who received no postoperative chemotherapy, there was a difference in survival between the group of patients who remained node negative after reexamination of the nodes compared to those who converted to node-positive status (76% vs. 61%, respectively; p = .006). A contemporary re-evaluation of the Ludwig V study confirmed a statistically significant difference in disease-free survival when micrometastases were detected by H&E (p = .001) but not by IHC (p = .09) (124). The data were not analyzed with respect to administration of postoperative adjuvant chemotherapy, and this may have confounded the results.

Prospective data using SLND to stage the axilla have been reported from the JWCI and showed no difference in disease-free or overall survival for patients with pN0(i+) or pN1mic at 8 years compared to pN0 (126). There was a significant decrease in disease-free and overall survival for the pN1 group. The majority of patients were treated with breast conservation and 76.5% received some form of systemic adjuvant therapy. Treatment recommendations were influenced by the status of the SN in this and other studies (126–128). No impact on disease-free survival was seen in several retrospective studies categorizing by pN0(i+) or pN1mic (129,130), while others report an impact on disease-free survival (125,127,128).

The ACOSOG Z0010 trial is a prospective observational study of subjects with stage I or II clinically node-negative invasive breast cancer treated with breast conservation, SLND, and bilateral iliac crest bone marrow aspirations. If the SN was free of tumor by H&E examination, no further ALND was undertaken. The aim of this study was to determine the prevalence and significance of IHC-positive micrometastases in lymph nodes, bone marrow metastases identified by immunocytochemistry (ICC), or both, and to determine the risk of regional recurrence. The secondary aim was to determine the morbidity associated with SLND. Blinded analysis of the SN by IHC and bone marrow by immunocytochemistry was performed in a central processing site on the SNs that were histologically negative by H&E. Adjuvant treatment recommendations were made on the basis of H&E examination of the axillary nodes. Results from this study are still maturing.

The International Breast Cancer Study Group (IBCSG) trial 23-01 randomizes patients with clinically node negative disease and tumors 5 cm or less who have micrometastases identified in the SN to ALND versus no ALND (131). The aim of this study is to determine the prognostic significance of minimal ($\leq$2 mm) nodal disease. No results for this trial have been reported.

The true significance of micrometastatic nodal deposits is unclear. The use of specialized techniques such as IHC and RT-PCR to identify ultramicrometastatic disease (i.e., individual tumor cells or isolated clusters of tumor cells) is even more problematic. There has been no multicenter prospective study to determine the importance of such findings as for prognosis or as a guide for adjuvant treatment recommendations. Before specialized techniques to identify micrometastatic nodal disease are incorporated into standard care, the results of the prospective multi-institutional ACOSOG Z0010, NSABP B-32, and IBCSG 23-01 trials should be awaited. Despite a lack of data, in a national survey IHC was performed at 80% of institutions and RT-PCR was performed in 15% (63). The American Society of Clinical Oncology (ASCO) guidelines recommend that ALND be performed for patients with micrometastases (>0.2 and 2 mm or less) independent of the method of detection (64).

 | ## SENTINEL LYMPH NODE DISSECTION

Anatomy

The axilla is bordered by the latissimus dorsi laterally, the axillary vein margin superiorly, and the pectoralis minor medially. Level I nodes are located inferior and lateral to the pectoralis minor muscle, level II nodes posterior to the pectoralis minor and below the axillary vein, and level III nodes are medial to the pectoralis minor and below the clavicle. Lymphatic drainage generally follows an orderly sequential pattern from level I to level II nodes and rarely to level III (132). SLND is a staging procedure that removes one or more lymph nodes from the axillary basin. The SN is found in level I in 83% of cases, level II in 15.6%, in level III in 0.5%, internal mammary in 0.5%, supraclavicular in 0.1%, and elsewhere in 0.3% (31).

Axillary Sentinel Lymph Node Dissection

When radioisotope is used, the incision is made directly over the location of a focal site of increased activity and dissection proceeds until the SN is identified by quantitative counts and resected (Fig. 41.7) (176). A radioactive node has been defined as a node with a cumulative 10-second count of greater than 25 (15), the hottest node by absolute counts, a 10 to 1 ratio of SN to background, or a fourfold reduction in counts after the SN is removed (17,23,133,134). Verification is done by *ex vivo* SN counts compared to residual *in vivo* background counts. Additional radioactive SNs are removed until the background is less than one-tenth the value of the hottest node. Lymph nodes with the highest radioactive uptake usually contain the greatest tumor burden, but on occasion tumor replaced nodes may have lymphatic obstruction, and if only the hottest node is removed, a positive SN with lower counts may be missed in 23% of cases (23,135). If blue dye is employed, a careful search for all blue nodes or lymphatics should be carried out. Palpation of the axillary space for any suspicious nodes will avoid missing a tumor-laden node that has occluded lymphatics and may not be blue. All suspicious palpable nodes must be removed at the time of SLND, regardless of technique—isotope or dye.

Complications of Sentinel Lymph Node Dissection

Dye Complications

Isolated case reports of adverse reactions with blue dye, including allergic urticaria and anaphylaxis, have been reported, but the rate is extremely low (136). Data from the NSABP B-32 trial shows 0.4% grade 1 and 2 allergic reactions and 0.2% grade 3 and 4 with no deaths (31). The data from ACOSOG Z0010 show 0.1% anaphylaxis with isosulfan blue alone or in combination with radiocolloid (137). Hives covering the trunk and upper extremities, not associated with hypotension, resolve within 24 to 48 hours after administration of methylprednisolone and diphenhydramine (136). Management of hypotensive anaphylaxis includes discontinuation of anesthetic agents, administration of fluids, epinephrine, diphenhydramine hydrochloride, and corticosteroids (136).

Isosulfan blue can affect pulse oximetry with a pseudodesaturation (138,139). Surgeons and anesthesiologists must investigate and verify that the partial pressure of oxygen, arterial (PaO_2) is normal (138). Isosulfan blue can cause transient staining of the epidermis, which can take several weeks to several months to completely fade. There is a transient change in color of the urine and stool to a greenish hue. Although these are temporary events, unless patients are forewarned about what to expect this can cause a great deal of unnecessary distress.

Methylene blue is associated with skin erythema, superficial ulceration, or necrosis with intradermal injections (136). Partial skin loss usually is treated with topical silver sulfadiazine (Silvadene) therapy and generally does not require surgical debridement (136).

Surgical Complications

Axillary complications and adverse side effects are reported with ALND, SLND, and axillary radiation, but to a lesser extent with SLND alone compared to ALND (Table 41.4). The incision is smaller with SLND with less tissue disruption and results in much less morbidity than complete ALND, as reported in the randomized studies (73,77,83,84,140). There is less pain, less limitation of motion, and fewer neurological sequela. In the randomized European Institute of Oncology trial, axillary pain, numbness and paresthesias, and arm swelling persisted to a significantly greater extent in the ALND than the SLND group (77).

SLND is associated with elimination of an axillary drain, less patient discomfort, and decreased incidence of lymphedema or neurovascular injury (68). Postmastectomy pain syndrome is significantly reduced with SLND compared to ALND (141). The risk of lymphedema after SLND ranges between 0% and 13% compared to 7% to 77% for ALND (142). Risk factors for developing lymphedema include upper outer quadrant lesions, postoperative trauma or infection, and previous axillary surgery (143,144).

Data from the multicenter trials, described above in the section Cumulative Experience of Sentinel Node Identification for Staging, are now available for morbidity and quality of life. The ACOSOG Z0010 trial, previously discussed, was a single arm SLND-only trial when the SN was negative. The secondary aim of the ACOSOG Z0010 trial was to determine morbidity of SLND (137). Anaphylaxis occurred in 0.1%, seroma in 7.1%, and wound infection in 1.4%. Younger age was associated with a higher incidence of paresthesias, while increased BMI was associated with lymphedema. The ACOSOG Z0011 trial randomized women with a positive SN to SLND alone or SLND plus ALND. Information on the differences in morbidity between SLND versus SLND plus ALND have been reported by Lucci et al. (140). Surgical complications were statistically greater in the SLND plus ALND arm than the SLND-alone arm of the

ACOSOG Z0011 trial: wound infections ($p \leq .016$), seromas ($p \leq .0001$), paresthesias ($p \leq .0001$), and subjective lymphedema at 1 year ($p \leq .0001$) (140). Overall quality of life and arm functioning scores were better in the SLND group in the ALMANAC trial (83). The quality of life was improved in the SLND group ($p < .003$) with less use of drains, less lymphedema, fewer days in the hospital, and earlier return to normal activities (83).

Variations in arm lymphatics contribute to the risk of developing lymphedema. A concept under study to attempt to reduce lymphedema is axillary reverse mapping (ARM) (142,145). This technique uses 2.5 to 5.0 cc of isosulfan blue injected intradermally or subcutaneously in the tissue of the upper inner arm to map the lymphatics draining the arm. Lymphatics draining the arm can be identified and preserved. At present this technique is experimental. The data comparing the morbidity of SLND to axillary dissection are summarized in Table 41.4.

INDICATIONS FOR SENTINEL LYMPH NODE DISSECTION

Guidelines for lymphatic mapping have been put forth by ASCO (64), National Comprehensive Cancer Network (NCCN) (146),

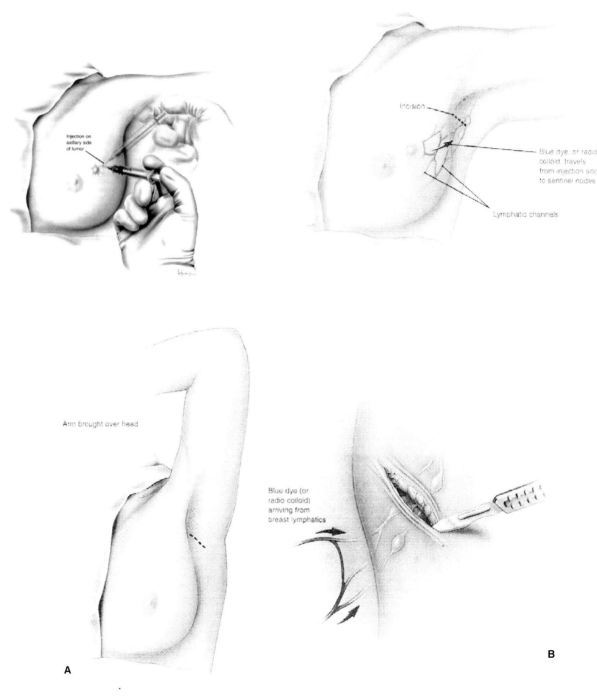

FIGURE 41.7. Intraoperative lymphatic mapping and sentinel lymphadenectomy for breast cancer. A. Location of incision 1 cm below hair-bearing area. **B.** Careful division of clavipectoral fascia exposes axillary contents and blue lymphatic channels that lead to SN. **C.** Identification of radioactive SN with gamma detection probe. (From Haigh PI, Giuliano AE. Intraoperative lymphatic mapping and sentinel lymphadenectomy for breast cancer. *Operative Techniques in General Surgery* 2000;2:161–165, with permission.) (*continued*)

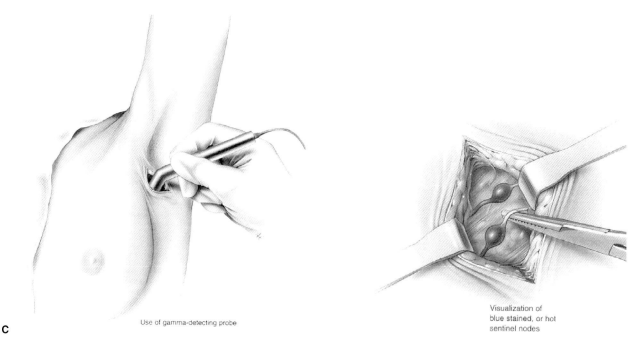

C

Use of gamma-detecting probe

Visualization of
blue stained, or hot
sentinel nodes

FIGURE 41.7. *Continued.*

American Society of Breast Surgeons (68,69), and single institution studies and are summarized in Table 41.5.

Acceptable Circumstances

Patient-Related Factors

A variety of factors contribute to the accuracy of SLND, including patient characteristics, tumor features, and technical expertise. SLND has been used successfully in both male and female patients (147,148) and in all age groups (13). The identification of the SN, however, has been less successful in older patients (58). The failed identification rate is 0.3% for age 39 or less and 2.7% for age 70 or older (58). Identification in older patients can be improved with isotope and dye combination (149). There is a progressive increase in failure rate as BMI increases above 26 (58,59).

Tumor-Related Factors

SLND has been performed for invasive ductal carcinoma, invasive lobular carcinoma, and other histologic subtypes (58,150,151). SLND for ductal carcinoma *in situ* (DCIS) is recommended for mastectomy patients (64). The routine use of SLND for patients with DCIS who are not undergoing mastectomy is not recommended and is discussed in detail in Chapter 26.

Multicentric Disease

Multifocality and multicentricity were initially considered relative contraindications to SLND, but this is no longer the case (64). A multi-institutional validation study of patients undergoing SLND followed by ALND included 125 of the patients with multicentric cancer and demonstrated a 91.5% identification rate and a 4% FN rate (152). The anatomic studies discussed in the section above on Lymphatic Anatomy also support the use of SLND in multifocal or multicentric cancers. There are a number of other studies evaluating SLND in multicentric disease using a variety of methods that report an identification rate

between 85.7% to 100%, FN rate of 0% to 33.3%, and an accuracy from 77.8% to 100% (57,153–155).

Type of Operative Procedure

The SN can be identified successfully when performing breast-conserving surgery, mastectomy, and skin-sparing mastectomy for unilateral disease or synchronous bilateral lesions (156,157). When mastectomy with immediate reconstruction is planned, staged SN biopsy before mastectomy facilitates surgical planning to avoid the complications of discovering a tumor-positive SN after reconstruction, especially when autologous tissue is used. This issue is discussed in detail in Chapter 36.

The performance of a diagnostic surgical biopsy was considered a contraindication to SLND in some early studies based on the hypothetical premise that the draining lymphatics were transected and mapping would be unreliable (16,17,23,154,158). This concern was refuted by Haigh et al. (159), who demonstrated that biopsy method (FNA, CNB, or excision), excision volume, time from initial biopsy to SLND, tumor size, and tumor location did not affect identification or accuracy by univariate and multivariate analysis. These findings have been confirmed by Wong et al. (157), who demonstrated no statistically significant difference in SN identification or false-negative rate for patients who had needle biopsy or excisional biopsy. The multicenter NSABP B-32 trial, however, does show a higher FN rate for excisional and incisional biopsy when compared to FNA or CNB, even with the use of both intraparenchymal and intradermal injection of technetium sulfur colloid and peritumoral injection of blue dye ($p = .0082$) (31).

The use of SLND in prophylactic mastectomy is controversial but is advocated by some because of a low but real incidence of identification of occult invasive carcinoma (5%) (160). In one study, 2 of 57 patients had a positive SN after four-quadrant periareolar dye and radioisotope injections prior to prophylactic mastectomy (160). No tumor was identified in the resected mastectomy specimens. All additional axillary nodes were negative. Two other patients had incidental invasive tumors; neither had metastases to the SN. In another study, the use of MRI was evaluated to determine if it was useful in

Table 41.4 A COMPARISON OF MORBIDITY FROM AXILLARY LYMPH NODE DISSECTION COMPARED TO SENTINEL LYMPH NODE DISSECTION

Study (Reference)	No. of Patients	ALND Morbidity	No. of Patients	SLND Morbidity	p-Value
Giuliano et al. (73)	67	35% overall 9 seroma 3 infection 4 hematoma 4 lymphedema	57	3% overall 1 infection 1 seroma	
Schrenk et al. (188)	35	15 seromas 9 subjective lymphedema 24 numbness 16 pain 6 arm mobility	35	0 0 0 2 pain 0	0.0001 0.0001 0.0001 0.01
Burak et al. (189)	48	Midbiceps circumference Antecubital fossa circumference 81.2% subjective numbness Drain days 13.2 Outpatient 14.6%	48	Lower Lower 16.7% numbness Drain 0.5 days Outpatient 87.5%	0.001 0.029 0.001 0.001 0.001
Temple et al. (190)	62	Higher discomfort Decreased mobility Paresthesias	171	Lower discomfort Increased mobility No paresthesias	0.001 0.001 0.001
Haid et al. (191)	85	Abduction 11.36[a] Arm volume 11.29[a] Strength 10.20[a] Sensitivity 1.80[a]	66	Abduction 11.5[a] Arm volume 11.95[a] Strength 11.45[a] Sensitivity 3.70[a]	0.8 0.016 0.025 0.0001
Swenson et al. (192)	78	78.8% pain 92.9% numbness 71.4% limited range of motion 17.1% swelling	169	56.5% pain 40.6% numbness 24.5% limited range of motion 9.4% swelling	0.002 0.001 0.001 0.005
Golshan et al. (193)	48	27% lymphedema	77	2.6% lymphedema	0.01
Schijven et al. (194)	213	23% pain 7.1% lymphedema 24.4% numbness 14.6% tingling 26.3% loss of strength 18.3% loss of range of motion	180	7.8% pain 1.1% lymphedema 3.9% numbness 3.9% tingling 3.9% loss of strength 6.0% loss of range of motion	0.00 0.00 0.00 0.00 0.00 0.02
Veronesi et al. (84)	257	Axillary pain 72% Paresthesias 85% 80%–100% mobility 73% Aesthetics 91% No arm swelling 31%	167	Axillary pain 14% Paresthesias 2% 80%–100% mobility 100% Aesthetics 98% No arm swelling 89%	
Mansel et al. (83)	476	No lymphedema 87% No nerve damage 69%	478	No lymphedema 95% No nerve damage 91%	<.001
Langer et al. (195)	210	No morbidity 31.4% Impaired range of motion 11.3% Lymphedema 19.1%	449	No morbidity 61% Impaired range of motion 3.5% Lymphedema 3.5%	<.0001 .0002 <.0001
Lucci et al. (140)	399	Wound infection 8% Axillary seromas 14% Axillary paresthesias 39% Lymphedema 11%	411	Wound infection 3% Axillary seromas 6% Axillary paresthesias 9% Lymphedema 6%	.0016 .0001 <.0001 .0786

[a]Summation scores, the lower the score the more severe the shoulder-arm syndrome.

Table 41.5 INDICATIONS AND CONTRAINDICATIONS TO SENTINEL LYMPH NODE DISSECTION

Routine SLND	Controversial Applications of SLND	Contraindications to SLND
Early stage invasive breast cancer Clinically node negative Unifocal or multicentric disease Either gender All ages Previous fine-needle aspiration, core biopsy, or excisional biopsy	Prophylactic mastectomy Previous SLND or ALND DCIS Suspicious axillary lymph nodes Preoperative chemotherapy	Inflammatory breast cancer Clinical N2 axillary disease Pregnancy

SLND, sentinel lymph node dissection; ALND, axillary lymph node dissection; DCIS, ductal carcinoma *in situ*.

identifying patients who would benefit from SLND (161). In 56 patients who underwent prophylactic mastectomy, 6 occult cancers, 5 DCIS, and 1 invasive ductal carcinoma were identified, all with negative SLNDs. The use of MRI in addition to SLND increases costs and, in this study, failed to identify a significant number of patients with occult malignancies.

In general, high-risk patients who undergo prophylactic mastectomy may be considered for SN biopsy at the time of surgery because identification of an unsuspected cancer in the mastectomy specimen could potentially require an ALND that could have been avoided by the minimally invasive SLND.

 ## CONTROVERSIAL APPLICATIONS OF SENTINEL LYMPH NODE DISSECTION

The greatest amount of information on SLND has been in patients with early stage disease that is clinically node negative and unifocal disease. These are the conditions under which the procedure has been validated. Attempts to incorporate this methodology for other clinical presentations, as listed below, have been reported in small single institution studies and should be considered as not having the same degree of validation.

Previous Breast or Axillary Surgery

SLND after prior breast conservation and axillary surgery has been successful at Memorial Sloan-Kettering Cancer Center (162). The SN was identified in 55% (64/117) of the cases that had had previous axillary surgery or a failed sentinel lymphadenectomy. Positive SNs were identified in 16% of the successful cases. The FN rate was 9% for reoperative SLND. The redo SLND was more likely to be successful after a previous SLND rather than an ALND. There was a higher rate of nonaxillary drainage with redo SLND than with primary SLND (30% vs. 6%; $p < .0001$). Reoperative SLND was feasible in this small series of patients, but more information is necessary before this can be recommended routinely. A smaller study reported an identification rate of 84% (163). Radioisotope alone identified 100% of the SNs, whereas isotope and blue dye failed to identify nodes in three cases.

Suspicious Axillary Lymph Nodes

Clinically suspicious axillary nodes have been considered a relative contraindication to SLND. Prior core or excisional breast biopsy for diagnosis can result in inflammatory changes in lymph nodes that are free of tumor. The correlation of clinical examination and pathologic nodal assessment indicates that the risk of lymph node metastasis is 40.4% if the clinical assessment is negative, 61.5% if the lymph nodes are palpable but not suspicious, and 84.4% if clinically suspicious (164). Clinical examination is subject to false-positive results in 53% of patients with moderately suspicious nodes and 23% of those with highly suspicious nodes (165). In one study from Denmark (150), enlarged axillary lymph nodes were not considered an exclusion criteria for SLND. Among the seven FN cases were two with clinically suspicious nodes. In another study, 11 patients with minor clinical involvement of the axilla demonstrated a tumor positive axilla in 9 cases (134). The SN predicted the status of the axilla in all cases. The clinically suspicious node however was not radioactive in two cases, but the SN procedure still identified additional radioactive metastatic nodes.

There is no reason to exclude such patients from SLND as long as the clinically suspicious node is resected and analyzed. Alternatively a suspicious node can be evaluated with FNA biopsy (4). The clinical assessment should take into account the inaccuracy of the clinical examination and dictate recommen-

dations for SLND in such circumstances on a selected basis, discussing the possible need for an ALND with the patient.

Preoperative Chemotherapy

The traditional approach to the management of the axilla in individuals who receive preoperative chemotherapy has been ALND. Increasingly preoperative chemotherapy is used for women who have smaller tumors and clinically negative nodes at the time of diagnosis, and there is a great deal of interest in avoiding an ALND in as many of these patients as possible (166). The clinical experience with lymphatic mapping, however, has largely been in patients who have not received preoperative chemotherapy, resulting in considerable debate about the timing of SLND in individuals undergoing induction chemotherapy. This issue is discussed in detail in Chapter 60.

The ASCO guidelines do not recommend SLND after preoperative chemotherapy, but consider it an option prior to preoperative chemotherapy (64). The recent National Cancer Institute conference on locoregional treatments after preoperative chemotherapy, however, concluded that SLND can be performed before or after preoperative chemotherapy with clinical N0 disease (167).

 ## CONTRAINDICATIONS TO SENTINEL LYMPH NODE DISSECTION

Pregnancy and Lactation

The safety of SLND with radioisotope in pregnancy has been studied by Pandit-Taskar et al. (168) at Memorial Sloan-Kettering Cancer Center. Retrospective data from nonpregnant women with breast cancer and SN biopsy was used in a phantom model calculation of the radiation-absorbed dose after a single intradermal dose of 99-mTc-sulfur colloid 0.1 mCi on the morning of surgery or 0.5 mCi on the afternoon before surgery. The highest estimated dose received by the fetus was seen with the two-day protocol, measured at 0.014 mGy, which is less than the National Council on Radiation Protection and Measurements limit to the pregnant woman (168). Two other theoretical studies have reached similar conclusions (169,170). The clinical application in pregnancy or lactation has been limited and questioned (171–173). Although radiolabeled technetium is probably safe in pregnancy, clinicians are reluctant to use it, and ASCO guidelines do not recommend it (64). ALND remains the standard of care for the pregnant patient diagnosed with breast cancer and in need of axillary staging. No data exist for dye usage in pregnancy, so dye should be avoided.

Advanced Disease

Grossly palpable, N2 lymph nodes have been a contraindication for SLND. Axillary evaluation with ultrasound and FNA of suspicious nodes can identify tumor-positive lymph nodes and avoid SLND. If the cytology or histology of the node is negative, staging with SLND is reasonable, as long as the palpable node is also removed. One contraindication to SLND after neoadjuvant chemotherapy is inflammatory breast cancer (174). Thirty-four patients with locally advanced breast cancer underwent neoadjuvant chemotherapy and SLND with a success rate of 85%. There were eight patients with inflammatory carcinoma in whom the success rate was 75% compared to 89% for other women with locally advanced, noninflammatory breast cancer.

Philadelphia Consensus Conference

The interest in sentinel lymphadenectomy has grown exponentially throughout the world. Because of the relative paucity of information from randomized clinical trials, a panel of experts in the field of breast surgery gathered in Philadelphia in April 2001 to discuss the role of sentinel lymphadenectomy for breast cancer and to suggest guidelines for its incorporation into the surgical management of early breast cancer (82,175). Many felt that a randomized trial was not necessary to validate a diagnostic test. The conference consensus statement concluded that:

1. SN biopsy is a technique that can accurately stage the axilla and replace traditional staging by ALND in experienced hands;
2. A negative SN is highly predictive of the status of the axilla and no further ALND is necessary in experienced hands; and
3. A tumor-positive SN requires further management of the axilla by either completion ALND, axillary radiation, or participation in ongoing clinical trials (175).

The *caveat* to these guidelines is a demonstration of technical skill and accuracy by the treating team. These guidelines are subject to modifications for unique clinical circumstances, and the decision to substitute SLND for ALND represents a cooperative understanding between patient and physician. There are several national and international clinical trials, some of which have completed accrual and are awaiting data analysis and others that are ongoing. Greater confidence in the integration of SLND into the armamentarium of surgical management of regional nodal disease for early breast cancer awaits these results. However, in practice SLND has replaced ALND for SN-negative patients at most centers in the United States.

CONCLUSION

Evaluation of the status of the axilla in invasive breast cancer is important for staging, prognosis, and perhaps survival. Although the status of the axilla was formerly the most important factor for adjuvant treatment recommendations, other factors related to tumor size, tumor features, molecular profiles, and patient age are increasingly entering the algorithm. Axillary treatment by ALND or axillary irradiation achieves excellent regional nodal control. Such treatment is associated with a potentially significant degree of chronic morbidity. The alternative for axillary staging, and perhaps treatment, is SLND. Single institution studies and small multicenter trials have validated this procedure as an acceptable method to stage the axilla and to be sufficient treatment in the SN-negative patient, and this approach has been widely adopted. Unanswered questions include the prognostic implications and appropriate local treatment of SN micrometastases, treatment of a tumor-positive SN, and the timing of SLND in the clinically node-negative patient receiving preoperative chemotherapy.

Future studies will provide further refinement in the understanding of the spread of tumor cells from the primary site to regional and systemic locations. Some of those answers will come from ongoing clinical trials of SLND in breast cancer.

MANAGEMENT SUMMARY

- SLND is a staging procedure that can be performed with vital dyes, radioactive tracers, or a combination of the two. The highest SN identification rates and the lowest FN rates are achieved with the combined technique.
- Expertise in the technique must be demonstrated by the procedure team through the collection and analysis of outcome data, and a multidisciplinary approach to management is essential.

- SLND alone for a negative SN accurately stages the axilla and is associated with isolated recurrence in the axilla in fewer than 1% of cases.
- ALND or axillary irradiation for a tumor positive SN is current standard care for macrometastases or micrometastases (>0.2 and ≤2 mm). The local and systemic management of isolated tumor cells and molecular tests that are positive for tumor are uncertain.
- The early and late postoperative morbidity of SLND is significantly lower than the morbidity of axillary dissection, but lymphedema occurs in about 5% of patients.
- SLND is contraindicated in pregnancy and inflammatory carcinoma.
- Age, tumor histology, tumor location, and biopsy type are not contraindications to the use of SLND.

References

1. Giuliano AE. Mapping a pathway for axillary staging: a personal perspective on the current status of sentinel lymph node dissection for breast cancer. *Arch Surg* 1999;134:195–199.
2. Cox CE, Salud CJ, Harrinton MA. The role of selective sentinel lymph node dissection in breast cancer. *Surg Clin North Am* 2000;80:1759–1777.
3. Robinson D, Senofsky GM, Ketcham AS. Role and extent of lymphadenectomy for early breast cancer. *Sem Surg Oncol* 1992;8:78–82.
4. Davis JT, Brill YM, Simmons S, et al. Ultrasound-guided fine-needle aspiration of clinically negative lymph nodes versus sentinel node mapping in patients at high risk for axillary metastases. *Ann Surg Oncol* 2006;13:1545–1552.
5. Veronesi U, De Cicco C, Galimberti VE, et al. A comparative study on the value of FDG-PET and sentinel node biopsy to identify occult axillary metastases. *Ann Oncol* 2007;18:473–478.
6. Wahl RL, Siegel BA, Coleman RE, et al. Prospective multicenter study of axillary nodal staging by positron emission tomography in breast cancer: a report of the staging breast cancer with PET study group. *J Clin Oncol* 2004;22:277–285.
7. Kett K, Varga G, Lukacs L. Direct lymphography of the breast. *Lymphology* 1970;1:3–12.
8. Kett K, Lukacs L. Diagnosis of regional lymph node metastases in cancer of the breast. A study of the lymphatic system of the diseased breast. *Am J Surg* 1974;128:398–401.
9. Cabanas RM. An approach for the treatment of penile carcinoma. *Cancer* 1977; 39:456–466.
10. Wong J, Cagle L, Morton D. Lymphatic drainage of the skin to a sentinel lymph node in a feline model. *Ann Surg* 1991;214:637–641.
11. Habal N, Giuliano AE, Morton DL. The use of sentinel lymphadenectomy to identify candidates for postoperative adjuvant therapy of melanoma and breast cancer. *Sem Oncol* 2001;28:41–52.
12. Morton D, Wen D-R, Cochran A. Management of early stage melanoma by intraoperative lymphatic mapping and selective lymphadenectomy: An alternative to routine elective lymphadenectomy or "watch and wait." *Surg Oncol Clin North Am* 1992;1:247–259.
13. Giuliano AE, Kirgan DM, Guenther JM, et al. Lymphatic mapping and sentinel lymphadenectomy for breast cancer. *Ann Surg* 1994;220:391–401.
14. Giuliano AE, Jones RC, Brennan MB, et al. Sentinel lymphadenectomy in breast cancer. *J Clin Oncol* 1997;15:2345–2350.
15. Krag DN, Weaver DL, Alex JC, et al. Surgical resection and radiolocalization of the sentinel lymph node in breast cancer using a gamma probe. *Surg Oncol* 1993;2:335–339.
16. Albertini JJ, Lyman GH, Cox C, et al. Lymphatic mapping and sentinel node biopsy in the patient with breast cancer. *JAMA* 1996;276:1818–1822.
17. Veronesi U, Paganelli G, Galimberti V, et al. Sentinel-node biopsy to avoid axillary dissection in breast cancer with clinically negative lymph-nodes. *Lancet* 1997;349:1864–1867.
18. Giuliano AE, Dale PS, Turner RR, et al. Improved axillary staging of breast cancer with sentinel lymphadenectomy. *Ann Surg* 1995;222:394–401.
19. Turner RR, Ollila DW, Krasne DL, et al. Histopathologic validation of the sentinel lymph node hypothesis for breast carcinoma. *Ann Surg* 1997;226:271–276.
20. Sabel M, Zhang P, Barnwell J, et al. Accuracy of sentinel node biopsy in predicting nodal status in patients with breast carcinoma. *J Surg Oncol* 2001;77:243–246.
21. Stitzenberg K, Calvo B, Iacocca M, et al. Cytokeratin immunohistochemical validation of the sentinel node hypothesis in patients with breast cancer. *Am J Clin Pathol* 2002;117:729–737.
22. Weaver D, Krag D, Harlow S, et al. Pathologic analysis of sentinel and nonsentinel lymph nodes in breast carcinoma. *Cancer* 2000;88:1099–1107.
23. Borgstein PJ, Pijpers R, Comans EF, et al. Sentinel lymph node biopsy in breast cancer: guidelines and pitfalls of lymphoscintigraphy and gamma probe detection. *J Am Coll Surg* 1998;186:275–283.
24. De Cicco C, Cremonesi M, Luini A, et al. Lymphoscintigraphy and radio-guided biopsy of the sentinel axillary node in breast cancer. *J Nucl Med* 1998;39: 2080–2084.
25. Haigh P, Hansen N, Giuliano A, et al. Factors affecting sentinel node localization during preoperative breast lymphoscintigraphy. *J Nucl Med* 2000;41:1682–1688.
26. McMasters K, Wong S, Tuttle T, et al. Preoperative lymphoscintigraphy for breast cancer does not improve the ability to identify axillary sentinel lymph nodes. *Ann Surg* 2000;231:724–731.
27. Morrow M, Foster RS Jr. Staging of breast cancer, a new rationale for internal mammary node biopsy. *Arch Surg* 1981;116:748–751.
28. Veronesi U, Marubini E, Mariani L, et al. The dissection of internal mammary nodes does not improve the survival of breast cancer patients: 30-year results of a randomised trial. *Eur J Cancer* 1999;35:1320–1325.

29. Madsen EVE, Gobardhan PD, Bongers V, et al. The impact on post-surgical treatment of sentinel lymph node biopsy of internal mammary lymph nodes in patients with breast cancer. *Ann Surg Oncol* 2007;14:1486–1492.
30. Klauber-DeMore N, Bevilacqua JLB, Van Zee KJ, et al. Comprehensive review of the management of internal mammary lymph node metastases in breast cancer. *J Am Coll Surg* 2001;193:547–555.
31. Krag DN, Anderson SJ, Julian TB, et al. Technical outcomes of sentinel-lymph-node resection and conventional axillary-lymph-node dissection in patients with clinically node-negative breast cancer: results from the NSABP B-32 randomised phase III trial. *Lancet Oncol* 2007;8:881–888.
32. Suami H, Pan W-R, Mann GB, et al. The lymphatic anatomy of the breast and its implications for sentinel lymph node biopsy: a human cadaver study. *Ann Surg Oncol* 2008;15:863–871.
33. Povoski SP, Olsen JO, Young DC, et al. Prospective randomized clinical trial comparing intradermal, intraparenchymal, and subareolar injection routes for sentinel lymph node mapping and biopsy in breast cancer. *Ann Surg Oncol* 2006;13:1412–1421.
34. Kim T, Giuliano AE, Lyman GH. Lymphatic mapping and sentinel lymph node biopsy in early-stage breast carcinoma. *Cancer* 2005;106:4–16.
35. McMasters K, Tuttle T, Carlson D, et al. Sentinel lymph node biopsy for breast cancer: a suitable alternative to routine axillary lymph node dissection in multi-institutional practice when optimal technique is used. *J Clin Oncol* 2000;18: 2560–2566.
36. Krag D, Weaver D, Ashikaga T, et al. The sentinel node in breast cancer—a multicenter validation study. *N Engl J Med* 1998;339:941–946.
37. Kersey T, Van Eyk J, Lannin D, et al. Comparison of intradermal and subcutaneous injection in lymphatic mapping. *J Surg Res* 2001;96:255–259.
38. Shivers S, Cox C, Leight G, et al. Final results of the Department of Defense multicenter breast lymphatic mapping trial. *Ann Surg Oncol* 2002;9:248–255.
39. Chua B, Olivotto I, Donald J, et al. Outcomes of sentinel node biopsy for breast cancer in British Columbia, 1996–2001. *Am J Surg* 2003;185:118–126.
40. Bergkvist L, Frisell J, Liljegren G, et al. Multicentre study of detection and false-negative rate in sentinel node biopsy for breast cancer. *Br J Surg* 2001;88: 1644–1648.
41. Gill PG. Sentinel lymph node biopsy versus axillary clearance in operable breast cancer. The RACS SNAC trial. A multicenter randomised trial of the Royal Australian College of Surgeons (RACS) section of breast surgery, in collaboration with the National Health and Medical Research Council Clinical Trials Center. *Ann Surg Oncol* 2004;11:216S–221S.
42. Goyal A, Newcombe R, Chhabra A, et al. Factors affecting failed localisation and false-negative rates of sentinel node biopsy in breast cancer—results of the ALMANAC validation phase. *Breast Cancer Res Treat* 2006;99:203–208.
43. Zavagno G, De Salvo GL, Scalco G, et al. A randomized clinical trial on sentinel lymph node biopsy versus axillary lymph node dissection in breast cancer. Results of the Sentinella/GIVOM trial. *Ann Surg* 2008;247:207–213.
44. Harlow SP, Krag DN, Julian TB, et al. Prerandomization surgical training for the National Surgical Adjuvant Breast and Bowel Project (NSABP) B-32 trial. *Ann Surg* 2005;241:48–54.
45. Clarke D, Khonji N, Mansel R. Sentinel node biopsy in breast cancer: ALMANAC trial. *World J Surg* 2001;25:819–822.
46. Clarke D. The learning curve in sentinel node biopsy in breast cancer: results from the ALMANAC trial. Presented at the 24th annual San Antonio Breast Cancer Symposium. San Antonio, Texas, 2001.
47. Fitzgibbons PL, Page DL, Weaver D, et al. Prognostic factor in breast cancer. College of American Pathologists Consensus Statement 1999. *Arch Pathol Lab Med* 2000;120:966–978.
48. Greene F. Breast cancer. In: Greene FL, Page DL, Fleming ID, et al., eds. *AJCC cancer staging manual*. New York: Springer-Verlag, 2002:221–240.
49. Blumencranz P, Whitworth PW, Deck K, et al. Sentinel node staging for breast cancer: intraoperative molecular pathology overcomes conventional histologic sampling errors. *Am J Surg* 2007;194:426–432.
50. Hughes SJ, Xi L, Raja S, et al. A rapid, fully automated, molecular-based assay accurately analyzes sentinel lymph nodes for the presence of metastatic breast cancer. *Ann Surg* 2006;243:389–398.
51. Viale G, Dell'Orto P, Biasi MO, et al. Comparative evaluation of an extensive histopathologic examination and a real-time reverse-transcription-polymerase chain reaction assay for mammoglobin and cytokeratin 19 on axillary sentinel lymph nodes of breast carcinoma patients. *Ann Surg* 2008;247:136–142.
52. Grube BJ, Giuliano AE. The current role of sentinel node biopsy in the treatment of breast cancer. *Adv Surg* 2004;38:121–166.
53. Rodier JF, Velten M, Martel P, et al. Prospective multicentric randomized study comparing periareolar and peritumoral injection of radiotracer and blue dye for the detection of sentinel lymph node in breast sparing procedures: FRASENODE trial. *J Clin Oncol* 2007;24:3664–3669.
54. McMasters K, Wong S, Martin II R, et al. Dermal injection of radioactive colloid is superior to peritumoral injection for breast cancer sentinel lymph node biopsy: results of the multi-institutional study. *Ann Surg* 2001;233:767–687.
55. Linehan DC, Hill ADK, Akhurst T, et al. Intradermal radiocolloid and intraparenchymal blue dye injection optimize sentinel node identification in breast cancer patients. *Ann Surg Oncol* 1999;6:450–454.
56. Martin R, Derossis A, Fey J, et al. Intradermal isotope injection is superior to intramammary in sentinel node biopsy for breast cancer. *Surgery* 2001;130: 432–438.
57. Schrenk P, Wayand W. Sentinel-node biopsy in axillary lymph-node staging for patients with multicentric breast cancer. *Lancet* 2001;357:122.
58. Posther K, McCall LM, Blumencranz PW, et al. Sentinel node skills verification and surgeon performance data from a multicenter clinical trial for early-stage breast cancer. *Ann Surg* 2005;242:593–602.
59. Morrow M, Rademaker AW, Bethke KP, et al. Learning sentinel node biopsy: results of a prospective randomized trial of two techniques. *Surgery* 1999;126: 714–720.
60. Meyer-Rochow GY, Martin RC, Harman CR. Sentinel node biopsy in breast cancer: validation study and comparison of blue dye alone with triple modality localization. *ANZ J Surg* 2003;73:815–818.
61. Eldrageely K, Vargas MP, Khalkhali I, et al. Sentinel lymph node mapping of breast cancer: a case-control study of methylene blue tracer compared to isosulfan. *Am Surg* 2004;70:872–875.
62. Blessing W, Stolier A, Teng S, et al. Comparison of methylene blue and isosulfan blue dyes for sentinel node mapping in breast cancer: a trial born out of necessity. *Am J Surg* 2002;184:341–345.
63. Lucci Jr A, Keleman P, Miller C, et al. National practice patterns of sentinel lymph node dissection for breast carcinoma. *J Am Coll Surg* 2001;192:453–458.
64. Lyman G, Giuliano AE, Somerfield M, et al. American Society of Clinical Oncology Guideline recommendations for sentinel lymph node biopsy in early-stage breast cancer. *J Clin Oncol* 2005;23:7703–7720.
65. McMasters KM, Wong SL, Chao C, et al. Defining the optimal surgeon experience for breast cancer sentinel lymph node biopsy: a model for implementation of new surgical techniques. *Ann Surg* 2001;234:292–300.
66. Cox CE, Salud CJ, Cantor A, et al. Learning curves for breast cancer sentinel lymph node mapping based on surgical volume analysis. *J Am Coll Surg* 2001; 193:593–600.
67. Johnson J, Orr R, Moline S. Institutional learning curve for sentinel node biopsy at a community teaching hospital. *Am Surg* 2001;67:1030–1033.
68. Simmons R. Review of sentinel lymph node credentialing: how many cases are enough? *J Am Coll Surg* 2001;193:206–209.
69. American Society of Breast Surgeons. Consensus statement of guidelines for performing sentinel lymph node dissection in breast cancer. 2005. Available at http://www.breastsurgeons.org/slnd.shtml.
70. Wong S, Edwards M, Chao C, et al. Sentinel lymph node biopsy for breast cancer: impact of the number of sentinel nodes removed on the false-negative rate. *J Am Coll Surg* 2001;192:684–691.
71. Zakaria S, Degnim AC, Kleer CG, et al. Sentinel lymph node biopsy for breast cancer: how many nodes are enough? *J Surg Oncol* 2007;96:554–559.
72. Chagpar AB, Scoggins CR, Martin RC 2nd, et al. Are 3 sentinel nodes sufficient? *Arch Surg* 2007;142:456–460.
73. Giuliano AE, Haigh PI, Brennan MB, et al. Prospective observational study of sentinel lymphadenectomy without further axillary dissection in patients with sentinel node-negative breast cancer. *J Clin Oncol* 2000;18:2553–2559.
74. Zavagno G, Carcoforo P, Franchini Z, et al. Axillary recurrence after negative sentinel lymph node biopsy without axillary dissection: a study on 479 breast cancer patients. *Eur J Surg Oncol* 2005;31:715–720.
75. Bergkvist L, de Boniface J, Jonsson P-E, et al. Axillary recurrence rate after negative sentinel node biopsy in breast cancer. Three-year follow-up of the Swedish multicenter cohort study. *Ann Surg* 2008;247(1):150–156.
76. Naik AM, Fey IV, Gemagnani M, et al. The risk of axillary relapse after sentinel lymph node biopsy for breast cancer is comparable with that of axillary lymph node dissection: a follow-up of 4,008 procedures. *Ann Surg* 2004;240:462–471.
77. Veronesi U, Paganellli G, Viale G, et al. Sentinel-lymph node biopsy as a staging procedure in breast cancer: update of a randomised controlled study. *Lancet Oncol* 2006;7:983–990.
78. van der Ploeg IM, Kroon BBR, Antonini N, et al. Axillary and extra-axillary lymph node recurrences after a tumor-negative sentinel node biopsy for breast cancer using intralesional tracer administration. *Ann Surg Oncol* 2008;15:1025–1031.
79. van der Ploeg IM, Niewig OE, van Rijk MC, et al. Axillary recurrence after a tumour-negative sentinel node biopsy in breast cancer patients: a systematic review and meta-analysis of the literature. *Eur J Surg Oncol* 2008;34(12): 1277–1284.
80. McCormick B, Botnick M, Hunt M, et al. Are the axillary lymph nodes treated by standard tangent breast fields? *J Surg Oncol* 2002;81:12–18.
81. Rabinovitch R, Ballonoff A, Newman F, et al. Evaluation of breast sentinel lymph node coverage by standard radiation therapy fields. *Int J Radiat Oncol Biol Phys* 2008;70:1468–1471.
82. Schwartz G, Giuliano A, Veronesi U, et al. Proceedings of the consensus conference on the role of sentinel lymph node biopsy in carcinoma of the breast, April 19 22, 2001, Philadelphia, Pennsylvania. *Cancer* 2002;94:2542–2551.
83. Mansel RE, Fallowfield L, Kissin M, et al. Randomized multicenter trial of sentinel node biopsy versus standard axillary treatment in operable breast cancer: the ALMANAC trial. *J Natl Cancer Inst* 2006;98:599–609.
84. Veronesi U, Paganelli G, Viale G, et al. A randomized comparison of sentinel-node biopsy with routine axillary dissection in breast cancer. *N Engl J Med* 2003;349: 546–553.
85. Fisher B, Jeong J-H, Anderson S, et al. Twenty-five year follow-up of a randomized trial comparing radical mastectomy, total mastectomy, and total mastectomy followed by irradiation. *N Engl J Med* 2002;347:567–575.
86. Clarke M, Collins R, Darby S, et al. Effects of radiotherapy and of differences in the extent of surgery for early breast cancer on local recurrence and 15-year survival: an overview of the randomised trials. *Lancet* 2005;366:2087–2106.
87. Coburn NG, Chung MA, Fulton J, et al. Decreased breast tumor size, stage, and mortality in Rhode Island: an example of a well-screened population. *Cancer Control* 2004;11:222–230.
88. Hurkmans CW, Beorger JH, Rutgers EJT, et al. Quality assurance of axillary radiotherapy in the EORTC AMAROS trial 10981/22023; the dummy run. *Radiother Oncol* 2003;68:233–240.
89. Gadd M, Harris JR, Taghian A, et al. Prospective study of axillary radiation without axillary dissection for breast cancer patients with a positive sentinel node. Presented at 28th San Antonio Breast Cancer Symposium. San Antonio, Texas, 2005.
90. Fant JS, Grant MD, Knox SM, et al. Preliminary outcome analysis in patients with breast cancer and a positive sentinel lymph node who declined axillary dissection. *Ann Surg Oncol* 2003;10:126–130.
91. Guenther JM, Hansen NM, DiFronzo LA, et al. Axillary dissection is not required for all patients with breast cancer and positive sentinel nodes. *Arch Surg* 2003;138:52–56.
92. Jeruss JS, Winchester DJ, Sener SF, et al. Axillary recurrence after sentinel node biopsy. *Ann Surg Oncol* 2005;12:34–40.
93. Hwang RF, Gonzalez-Angulo AM, Buchholz TA, et al. Low locoregional failure rates in selected breast cancer patients with tumor-positive sentinel lymph nodes who do not undergo completion axillary lymph node dissection. *Cancer* 2007;110:723–730.
94. Park J, Fey JV, Naik AM, et al. A declining rate of completion axillary dissection in sentinel lymph node-positive breast cancer patients is associated with the use of a multivariate nomogram. *Ann Surg* 2007;245:462–468.
95. Turner RR, Chu KU, Qi K, et al. Pathologic features associated with nonsentinel lymph node metastases in patients with metastatic breast carcinoma in a sentinel lymph node. *Cancer* 2000;89:574–581.

96. Chu K, Turner R, Hansen N, et al. Sentinel node metastasis in patients with breast carcinoma accurately predicts immunohistochemically detectable nonsentinel node metastasis. *Ann Surg Oncol* 1999;6:756–761.
97. Rahusen F, Torrenga H, van Diest P, et al. Predictive factors for metastatic involvement of nonsentinel nodes in patients with breast cancer. *Arch Surg* 2001;136:1059–1063.
98. Sachdev U, Murphy K, Derzie A, et al. Predictors of nonsentinel lymph node metastasis in breast cancer patients. *Am J Surg* 2002;183:213–217.
99. Mignotte H, Treilleux I, Faure C, et al. Axillary lymph-node dissection for positive sentinel nodes in breast cancer patients. *Eur J Surg Oncol* 2002;28:623–626.
100. Chua B, Ung O, Taylor R, et al. Treatment implications of a positive sentinel node biopsy for patients with early-stage breast carcinoma. *Cancer* 2001;92:1769–1774.
101. Julian TB, Anderson SJ, Fourchotte V, et al. Is completion axillary dissection always required after a positive sentinel node biopsy? NSABP B-32. Presented at the 30th annual Breast Cancer Symposium. December 13–16, 2007, San Antonio, Texas.
102. Van Zee KJ, Manasseh DM, Bevilacqua JLB, et al. A nomogram for predicting the likelihood of additional nodal metastases in breast cancer patients with a positive sentinel node biopsy. *Ann Surg Oncol* 2003;10:1140–1151.
103. Cserni G. Comparison of different validation studies on the use of the Memorial Sloan-Kettering Cancer Center nomogram predicting nonsentinel node involvement in sentinel node-positive breast cancer patients. *Am J Surg* 2007;194: 699–700.
104. Klar M, Jochmann A, Foeldi M, et al. The MSKCC nomogram for prediction the likelihood of non-sentinel node involvement in a German breast cancer population. *Breast Cancer Res Treat* 2008. In press.
105. Alaran S, De Rycke Y, Fourchotte V, et al. Validation and limitations of use of a breast cancer nomogram predicting the likelihood of non-sentinel node involvement after positive sentinel node biopsy. *Ann Surg Oncol* 2007;14:2195–2201.
106. Rosen P, Saigo P, Braun D, et al. Predictors of recurrence in Stage I (T1N0M0) breast carcinoma. *Ann Surg* 1980;193:15–25.
107. Fisher E, Swamidoss S, Lee C, et al. Detection and significance of occult axillary node metastases in patients with invasive breast cancer. *Cancer* 1978;42: 2025–2031.
108. Singletary SE, Allred C, Ashley P, et al. Revision of the American Joint Committee on Cancer staging system for breast cancer. *J Clin Oncol* 2002;20:3628–3636.
109. Bussolati G, Gugliotta P, Morra I, et al. The immunohistochemical detection of lymph node metastases from infiltrating lobular carcinoma. *Br J Cancer* 1986;54:631–636.
110. McGuckin M, Cummings M, Walsh M, et al. Occult axillary node metastases in breast cancer: their detection and prognostic significance. *Br J Cancer* 1996; 73:88–95.
111. Galea M, Athanassiou E, Bell J, et al. Occult regional lymph node metastases from breast carcinoma: immunohistological detection with antibodies CAM 5.2 and MCRC-11. *J Pathol* 1991;165:221–227.
112. Wilkinson E, Hause LL, Hoffman RG, et al. Occult axillary lymph node metastases in invasive breast carcinoma: characteristics of the primary tumor and significance of the metastases. *Path Ann* 1982;17:67–91.
113. Nasser I, Lee A, Bosari S, et al. Occult axillary lymph node metastases in "node negative" breast carcinoma. *Hum Pathol* 1993;24:950–957.
114. Pickren J. Significance of occult metastases: a study of breast cancer. *Cancer* 1961;14:1266–1271.
115. Rosen P, Saigo P, Braun D, et al. Axillary micro and macrometastases in breast cancer. *Ann Surg* 1981;194:585–591.
116. Huvos A, Hutter R, Berg J. Significance of axillary macrometastases and micrometastases in mammary carcinoma. *Ann Surg* 1971;173:44–46.
117. Saphir O, Amromin G. Obscure axillary lymph-node metastasis in carcinoma of the breast. *Cancer* 1947:238–241.
118. Wells C, Heryet A, Brochier J, et al. The immunohistochemical detection of axillary micrometastases in breast cancer. *Br J Cancer* 1984;50:193–197.
119. Trojani M, DeMarscel I, Coindre J, et al. Micrometastases to axillary lymph nodes from carcinoma of the breast: detection by immunohistochemistry and prognostic significance. *Br J Cancer* 1987;565:303–306.
120. Hainsworth P, Tlandra JJ, Stillwell RG, et al. Detection and significance of occult metastases in node-negative breast cancer. *Br J Surg* 1993;80:459–463.
121. De Mascarel I, Bonichon F, Coindre J, et al. Prognostic significance of breast cancer axillary lymph node micrometastases assessed by two special techniques: re-evaluation with longer follow-up. *Br J Cancer* 1992;66:523–527.
122. De Mascarel I, MacGrogan G, Soubeyran I, et al. Prognostic significance of breast axillary node metastases detected by immunohistochemical stainings (IHM) in 218 patients: re-evaluation with a longer follow-up and critical analysis. *Mod Pathol* 2001;14:24A.
123. Prognostic importance of occult axillary lymph node micrometastases from breast cancers. International (Ludwig) Breast Cancer Study Group. *Lancet* 1990;335:1565–1568.
124. Cote RJ, Peterson HF, Chaiwun B, et al. Role of immunohistochemical detection of lymph-node metastases in management of breast cancer. *Lancet* 1999;354: 896–900.
125. Tan LK, Hummer AJ, Panageas KS, et al. Occult axillary node metastases in breast cancer are prognostically significant: results in 368 node-negative patients with 20-year follow-up. *J Clin Oncol* 2008;26:1803–1809.
126. Hansen NM, Grube BJ, Ye X, et al. The impact of micrometastasis in the sentinel node of patients with invasive breast cancer. Presented at the 30th annual Breast Cancer Symposium. San Antonio, Texas, 2007.
127. Colleoni M, Rotmensz N, Peruzzotti G, et al. Size of breast cancer metastases in axillary lymph nodes: clinical relevance of minimal lymph node involvement. *J Clin Oncol* 2005;23:1379–1389.
128. Cox CE, Kiluk JV, Riker AI, et al. Significance of sentinel lymph node micrometastases in human breast cancer. *J Am Coll Surg* 2008;206:261–268.
129. Khan A, Sabel MS, Nees AV, et al. Comprehensive axillary evaluation in neoadjuvant chemotherapy patients with ultrasonography and sentinel lymph node biopsy. *Ann Surg Oncol* 2005;12:697–704.
130. Ryden L, Chebil G, Sjostrom L, et al. Determination of sentinel lymph node (SLN) status in primary breast cancer by prospective use of immunohistochemistry increases the rate of micrometastases and isolated tumour cells: analysis of 174 patients after SLN biopsy. *Eur J Surg Oncol* 2007;33:33–38.
131. Galimberti V. International breast cancer study group trial of sentinel node biopsy. *J Clin Oncol* 2005;24(1):210–211.
132. Veronesi U, Rilke F, Luimi A, et al. Distribution of axillary node metastases by level of invasion: an analysis of 539 cases. *Cancer* 1987;59:682–687.
133. Hill AD, Tran KN, Akhurst T, et al. Lessons learned from 500 cases of lymphatic mapping for breast cancer. *Ann Surg* 1999;229:528–535.
134. van der Ent F, Kengen R, van der Pol H, et al. Sentinel node biopsy in 70 unselected patients with breast cancer: increased feasibility by using 10 mCi radiocolloid in combination with a blue dye tracer. *Eur J Surg Oncol* 1999;25:24–29.
135. Tafra L, Lannin DR, Swanson MS, et al. Multicenter trial of sentinel node biopsy for breast cancer using both technetium sulfur colloid and isosulfan blue. *Ann Surg* 2001;233:51–59.
136. Thevarajah S, Huston TL, Simmons RM. A comparison of the adverse reaction associated with isosulfan blue versus methylene blue dye in sentinel lymph node biopsy. *Am J Surg* 2005;189:236–239.
137. Wilke LG, McCall LM, Posther KE, et al. Surgical complications associated with sentinel lymph node biopsy: results from a prospective international cooperative group trial. *Ann Surg Oncol* 2006;13:491–500.
138. Rizzi R, Thomas K, Pilnik S. Factious desaturation due to isosulfan dye injection. *Anesthesiology* 2000;93:1146–1147.
139. Vokach-Brodsky L, Jeffrey S, Lemmens H, et al. Isosulfan blue affects pulse oximetry. *Anesthesiology* 2000;93:1002–1003.
140. Lucci A, McCall LM, Beitsch PD, et al. Surgical complications associated with sentinel lymph node dissection (SLND) plus axillary lymph node dissection compared with SLND alone in the American College of Surgeons Oncology Group trial Z0011. *J Clin Oncol* 2007;25:3657–3663.
141. Miguel R, Kuhn A, Shons A, et al. The effect of sentinel node selective axillary lymphadenectomy on the incidence of postmastectomy pain syndrome. *Cancer Control* 2001,8.427–430.
142. Thompson M, Korourian S, Henry-Tillman R, et al. Axillary reverse mapping (ARM): a new concept to identify and enhance lymphatic preservation. *Ann Surg Oncol* 2007;14:1890–1895.
143. Sener S, Winchester D, Martz C, et al. Lymphedema after sentinel lymphadenectomy for breast carcinoma. *Cancer* 2001;92:748–752.
144. Hansen N, Grube B, Giuliano A. Is it time to change the algorithm for the surgical management of early breast cancer? *Arch Surg* 2002;184:1131–1135.
145. Nos C, Lesieur B, Clough KB, et al. Blue dye injection in the arm in order to conserve the lymphatic drainage of the arm in breast cancer patients requiring an axillary dissection. *Ann Surg Oncol* 2008;14:2490–2496.
146. National Comprehensive Cancer Network. NCCN clinical practice guidelines in oncology: breast cancer. V2.2008. Available at http://www.nccn.org/professionals/physician_gls/PDF/breast.pdf.
147. Boughey JC, Bedrosian I, Meric-Bernstam F, et al. Comparative analysis of sentinel lymph node operation in male and female breast cancer patients. *J Am Coll Surg* 2006;203:475–480.
148. Rusby JE, Smith BL, Dominguez FJ, et al. Sentinel lymph node biopsy in men with breast cancer: a report of 31 consecutive procedures and review of the literature. *Clin Breast Cancer* 2006;7:406–410.
149. Cody H, Fey J, Akhurst T, et al. Complementarity of blue dye and isotope in sentinel node localization for breast cancer: univariate and multivariate analysis of 966 procedures. *Ann Surg Oncol* 2001;8:13–19.
150. Ilum L, Bak M, Olsen K, et al. Sentinel node localization in breast cancer patients using intradermal dye injection. *Acta Oncol* 2000;39:423–428.
151. Grube B, Hansen N, Ye X, et al. Tumor characteristics predictive of sentinel node metastases in 105 consecutive patients with invasive lobular carcinoma. *Am J Surg* 2002;184:372–376.
152. Knauer M, Konstantiniuk P, Wenzel E, et al. Multicentric breast cancer: a new indication for sentinel node biopsy—a multi-institutional validation study. *J Clin Oncol* 2006;24:3374–3380.
153. Ferrari A, Dionigi P, Rovera F, et al. Multifocality and multicentricity are not contraindication for sentinel lymph node biopsy in breast cancer surgery. *World J Surg* 2006;4:79.
154. Veronesi U, Paganelli G, Viale G, et al. Sentinel lymph node biopsy and axillary dissection in breast cancer: results in a large series. *J Natl Cancer Inst* 1999;91:368–373.
155. Kumar R, Jana S, Heiba S, et al. Retrospective analysis of sentinel node localization in multifocal, multicentric, palpable or nonpalpable breast cancer. *J Nucl Med* 2002;44:7–10.
156. Stradling BL, Ahn M, Angelats J, et al. Skin-sparing mastectomy with sentinel lymph node dissection. *Arch Surg* 2001;136:1069–1075.
157. Wong SL, Edwards MJ, Chao C, et al. The effect of prior breast biopsy method and concurrent definitive breast procedure on success and accuracy of sentinel lymph node biopsy. *Ann Surg Oncol* 2002;9:272–277.
158. Feldman SM, Krag DN, McNally RK, et al. Limitation in gamma probe localization of the sentinel node in breast cancer patients with large excisional biopsy. *J Am Coll Surg* 1999;188:248–254.
159. Haigh P, Hansen N, Qi K, et al. Biopsy method and excision volume do not affect success rate of subsequent sentinel lymph node dissection in breast cancer. *Ann Surg Oncol* 2000;7:21–27.
160. Dupont E, Kuhn M, McCann C, et al. The role of sentinel lymph node biopsy in women undergoing prophylactic mastectomy. *Am J Surg* 2000;180:274–277.
161. Black DM, Specht M, Lee JM, et al. Detecting occult malignancy in prophylactic mastectomy: preoperative MRI versus sentinel lymph node biopsy. *Ann Surg Oncol* 2007;14:2477–2484.
162. Port ER, Garcia-Etienne CA, Park J, et al. Reoperative sentinel lymph node biopsy: a new frontier in the management of ipsilateral breast tumor recurrence. *Ann Surg Oncol* 2007;14:2209–2214.
163. Barone JL, Feldman SM, Estabrook A, et al. Reoperative sentinel lymph node biopsy in patients with locally recurrent breast cancer. *Am J Surg* 2007;194:491–493.
164. Lanng C, Hoffmann J, Galatius H, et al. Assessment of clinical palpation of the axilla as a criterion for performing the sentinel node procedure in breast cancer. *Eur J Surg Oncol* 2007;33:281–284.
165. Specht MC, Fey JV, Borgen PI, et al. Is the clinically positive axilla in breast cancer really a contraindication to sentinel lymph node biopsy. *Am J Surg* 2005;200:10–14.
166. Harris LN, Kaelin CM, Bellow JR, et al. Preoperative therapy for operable breast cancer. In: Harris JR, Lippman ME, Morrow M, eds. *Disease of the breast*. 3rd ed. Philadelphia: Lippincott Williams & Wilkins, 2004:929–943.
167. Buchholz TA, Lehman CD, Harris JR, et al. Statement of the science concerning locoregional treatments after preoperative chemotherapy for breast cancer: a National Cancer Institute conference. *J Clin Oncol* 2008;28:791–797.

168. Pandit-Taskar N, Dauer LT, St. Germain J, et al. Organ and fetal absorbed dose estimates from 99mTc-sulfur colloid lymphoscintigraphy and sentinel node localization in breast cancer patients. *J Nucl Med* 2006;47:1202–1208.
169. Keleher A, Wendt R 3rd, Delpassand ES, et al. The safety of lymphatic mapping in pregnant breast cancer patients using Tc-99m sulfur colloid. *Breast J* 2004;10:494–495.
170. Gentilini O, Cremonesi M, Trifiro G, et al. Safety of sentinel node biopsy in pregnant patients with breast cancer. *Ann Oncol* 2004;15:1348–1351.
171. Mondi MM, Cuenca RE, Ollila DW, et al. Sentinel lymph node biopsy during pregnancy: initial clinical experience. *Ann Surg Oncol* 2006;14:218–221.
172. Gentilini O, Masullo L, Rotmensz N, et al. Breast cancer diagnosed during pregnancy and lactation: biological features and treatment options. *Eur J Surg Oncol* 2005;31:232–236.
173. Dubermand G, Garbay JR, Rouzier R, et al. Safety of sentinel node biopsy in pregnant patients. *Ann Oncol* 2005;16:987.
174. Stearns V, Ewing CA, Slack R, et al. Sentinel lymphadenectomy after neoadjuvant chemotherapy for breast cancer may reliably represent the axilla for inflammatory breast cancer. *Ann Surg Oncol* 2002;9:235–242.
175. Giuliano AE, Schwartz GF. Summary of the proceedings of the Philadelphia Consensus conference on the role of sentinel lymph node biopsy in carcinoma of the breast. *Sem Breast Disease* 2002;5:110–113.
176. Haigh PI, Giuliano AE. Intraoperative lymphatic mapping and sentinel lymphadenectomy for breast cancer. *Oper Tech Gen Surg* 2000;2:161–165.
177. Guenther JM, Krishnamoorthy M, Tan LR. Sentinel lymphadenectomy for breast cancer in a community managed care setting. *Cancer J Sci Am* 1997;3:336–340.
178. Nos C, Freneaux P, Louis-Sylvestre C, et al. Macroscopic quality control improves the reliability of blue-dye-only sentinel lymph node biopsy in breast cancer. *Ann Surg Oncol* 2003;10:525–530.
179. Krag D, Ashikaga T, Harlow S, et al. Development of sentinel node targeting technique in breast cancer patients. *Breast J* 1998;2:67–74.
180. Zurrida S, Galimberti V, Orvieto E, et al. Radio-guided sentinel node biopsy to avoid axillary dissection in breast cancer. *Ann Surg Oncol* 2000;7:28–31.
181. Fraile M, Rull M, Julian F, et al. Sentinel node biopsy as a practical alternative to axillary lymph node dissection in breast cancer patients: an approach to it validity. *Ann Oncol* 2000;11:701–705.
182. Mariani G, Villa G, Gipponi M, et al. Mapping sentinel lymph node in breast cancer by combine lymphoscintigraphy, blue dye, and intraoperative gamma probe. *Cancer Biother Radiopharm* 2000;15:245–252.
183. Rink T, Heuser T, Fitz H, et al. Lymphoscintigraphic sentinel node imaging and gamma probe detection in breast cancer with Tc-99m nanocolloidal albumin: results of an optimized protocol. *Clin Nucl Med* 2001;26:293–298.
184. Smillie T, Hayashi A, Rusnak C, et al. Evaluation of feasibility and accuracy of sentinel node biopsy in early breast cancer. *Am J Surg* 2001;181:427–430.
185. Kollias J, Gill PG, Chatterton BE, et al. Reliability of sentinel node status in predicting axillary lymph node involvement in breast cancer. *Med J Aust* 1999;171:461–465.
186. Doting M, Jansen L, Niewig O, et al. Lymphatic mapping with intralesional tracer administration in breast carcinoma patients. *Cancer* 2000;88:2546–2552.
187. Motomura K, Inaji H, Komoike Y, et al. Combination technique is superior to dye alone in identification of the sentinel node in breast cancer patients. *J Surg Oncol* 2001;76:95–99.
188. Schrenk P, Rieger R, Shamiyeh A, et al. Morbidity following sentinel lymph node biopsy versus axillary lymph node dissection for patients with breast carcinoma. *Cancer* 2000;88:608–614.
189. Burak W, Hollenbeck S, Zervos E, et al. Sentinel lymph node biopsy result in less postoperative morbidity compared with axillary lymph node dissection for breast cancer. *Am J Surg* 2002;183:23–27.
190. Temple L, Baron R, Cody H, et al. Sensory morbidity after sentinel lymph node biopsy and axillary dissection: a prospective study of 233 women. *Ann Surg Oncol* 2002;9:654–662.
191. Haid A, Kuehn T, Konstantiniuk P, et al. Shoulder-arm morbidity following axillary dissection and sentinel node only biopsy for breast cancer. *Eur J Surg Oncol* 2002;28:705–710.
192. Swenson K, Nissen M, Ceronsky C, et al. Comparison of side effects between sentinel lymph node and axillary lymph node dissection for breast cancer. *Ann Surg Oncol* 2002;9:745–753.
193. Golshan M, Martin W, Dowlatshahi K. Sentinel lymph node biopsy lowers the rate of lymphedema when compared with standard axillary lymph node dissection. *Am Surg* 2003;69:209–212.
194. Schijven M, Vingerhoets A, Rutten H, et al. Comparison of morbidity between axillary lymph node dissection and sentinel node biopsy. *Eur J Surg Oncol* 2003;29:341–350.
195. Langer I, Guller U, Berclaz G, et al. Morbidity of sentinel lymph node biopsy (SLN) alone versus SLN and completion axillary lymph node dissection after breast cancer surgery. A prospective Swiss multicenter study on 659 patients. *Ann Surg* 2007;245:452–461.

Hiram S. Cody III

For patients with breast cancer, axillary node status remains the single most important prognostic factor. The primary goal of axillary surgery is staging to govern the use and type of systemic therapy; secondary goals include local control and the possibility of a small survival benefit. Axillary lymph node dissection (ALND) has been regarded for most of the 20th century as the gold standard operation to achieve these goals, but has largely been replaced over the past decade by sentinel lymph node (SLN) biopsy, first reported by Krag et al. (1) in 1993 and Giuliano et al. (2) in 1994. SLN biopsy can prevent ALND in SLN-negative patients, sparing them the morbidity of a larger operation and allowing the routine performance of additional pathologic studies, potentially increasing the accuracy of staging. Sixty-nine observational series (3) of SLN biopsy validated by a "backup" ALND and the early results of four randomized trials (4–7) comparing ALND with SLN biopsy confirm that the morbidity of SLN biopsy is less than ALND, that staging accuracy is at least equivalent, and, in the single randomized trial reporting long-term results (8), that survival and other disease-related adverse events are comparable at 7 years' follow-up. Although the role of ALND in the era of SLN biopsy has been reduced, it has not been eliminated, and this chapter surveys the historic evolution, current indications, operative technique, and morbidity of ALND. Looking ahead, prognostication through rapidly emerging genomic technologies may eventually rival (or even surpass) that of conventional histopathology, and the role of ALND will continue to change.

HISTORIC EVOLUTION OF AXILLARY LYMPH NODE DISSECTION

Jean Louis Petit (1674 to 1750), director of the French Surgical Academy, was probably the first surgeon to articulate a unified concept for breast cancer surgery (9). He emphasized the importance of a *en bloc* resection of the breast and axillary nodes, but his insight came too early: even by the mid-19th century, breast cancer was widely regarded as incurable by surgery. Halsted's landmark 1894 (10) and 1907 (11) reports of his meticulous technique for "radical mastectomy" (RM), which included removal of the breast and pectoral muscles with a complete ALND, were the first to demonstrate that coincident with a striking reduction in locoregional recurrence (LR) (from 51% to 82% reported by European center to 6%), 31% of patients (a significant proportion at that time) were disease free at 5 years. This intuitive concept relating local control and survival made RM the standard operation for breast cancer over the next 70 years, despite subsequent reports of techniques that were either more or less radical (12–14) including radical modified mastectomy (MRM). In the Halstedian era, the goal for ALND (as for mastectomy) was to maximize cure by minimizing local failure.

Coincident with the acceptance of MRM in the 1970s, Fisher (15) proposed that breast cancer survival was largely a function of tumor biology and not surgical technique. The Fisher hypothesis was tested in National Surgical Adjuvant Breast and Bowel Project (NSABP) B-04 (1971 to 1974) (16–18); patients with clinically node-positive breast cancer were randomized to RM versus total mastectomy with radiotherapy (RT), and patients with clinically node-negative breast cancer were randomized to RM versus total mastectomy with RT versus total mastectomy alone. At 25 years' follow-up there were no differ-

ences in any category of survival (overall, disease free, distant disease free) between the patients in the two node-positive arms or in the three node-negative arms of the trial. B-04 confirmed the overwhelming prognostic significance of axillary node metastasis, and for this reason, ALND was incorporated into all subsequent NSABP trials for invasive breast cancer. In the Fisherian era, the primary objective of ALND was prognostication to guide systemic therapy, the secondary objective was local control, and a survival benefit was unproved.

With a series of remarkable meta-analyses from the Early Breast Cancer Trialists Collaborative Group (EBCTCG), it has become clear that breast cancer is best viewed as a disease with a wide spectrum of behavior (19), rather than a predominantly local (Halsted) or systemic (Fisher) process. Separate EBCTCG overviews show that local control and survival are related (20), but that there is no survival advantage for more radical versus less radical versions of mastectomy (or for mastectomy versus breast conservation) (21), and that there is an incremental survival benefit from the addition of systemic adjuvant therapy to local treatment (22). At present, virtually all node-negative patients are staged by SLN biopsy alone, and the principal goal of ALND is to maximize local control in patients already proven by SLN biopsy to be node positive.

AXILLARY LYMPH NODE DISSECTION VERSUS OTHER METHODS OF STAGING

ALND can be compared with other methods of axillary staging: (a) no axillary surgery (with or without axillary RT), (b) axillary sampling, and (c) SLN biopsy.

Axillary Lymph Node Dissection or Axillary Radiotherapy versus No Axillary Surgery

The foremost trial comparing ALND with no axillary surgery is NSABP B-04 (Table 42.1), as described above (17). Among patients randomized to total mastectomy alone, 18% developed axillary LR as the first sign of treatment failure and required a delayed ALND; 79% of axillary LR occurred within 2 years and 95% within 5 years. Two more recent trials demonstrate far lower rates of axillary LR in older patients treated without ALND. Martelli et al. (23) randomized 219 patients (aged 65 to 80) with T1N0 disease to breast-conservation surgery with or without ALND, and all patients received 5 years of tamoxifen. At 5 years' follow-up there were no differences in disease-free or overall survival, and axillary LR in the no-ALND arm was 1%. Rudenstam et al. (24) randomized 473 patients (aged 60 or older) to breast surgery with or without ALND; all patients received 5 years of tamoxifen. At 6.6 years' follow-up there were no differences in disease-free or overall survival, and axillary LR in the ALND and no-ALND arms was 1% and 3%, respectively.

The addition of axillary RT improves local control in patients treated without axillary surgery (Table 42.1). In NSABP B-04 (17), LR at 10 years was lower with total mastectomy plus RT than with total mastectomy alone (5% vs. 31%), as was axillary LR (3% vs. 19%). In the Cancer Research Campaign King's Cambridge trial (25), 2,268 patients were randomized to total mastectomy with RT (to chest wall and axillary nodes) versus total mastectomy alone; again, crude LR

| | **Table 42.1** | **STUDIES OF AXILLARY TREATMENT VERSUS NO AXILLARY TREATMENT IN cN0 BREAST CANCER** | | | | | | | | |

	NSABP B-04 (17) (1971–1973)	Milan (23) (1996–2000)	SBCSG (24) (1993–2002)	King's-Cambridge (25) (1970–1975)	Curie (27) (1982–1987)	EIO (28) (1995–1998)	Baum and Coyle (29) (1973–1977)	Baxter et al. (30) (1977–1986)	Greco et al. (31) (1986–1994)
Design	RCT	RCT	RCT	RCT	RCT	RCT	Cohort	Cohort	Cohort
Breast treatment	Mastectomy	BCT	BCT or mastectomy	Mastectomy	Wide excision/RT	BCT	Mastectomy	Wide excision/RT	Wide excision/RT[a]
Axillary treatment	ALND vs. Ax RT vs. none	ALND vs. none	ALND vs. none	Ax RT vs. none	ALND vs. Ax RT	vs. Ax RT	none	none	none
No. of patients	1,079	219	473	2,268	658	435	48	112	401
Follow-up	10 yrs	5 yrs	6.6 yrs	1–5 yrs	15 yrs	5 yrs	1–4 yrs	10 yrs	5 yrs
Axillary local recurrence	ALND 1.4% Ax RT 3.1% none 19%	ALND 0% none 1%	ALND 1% none 3%	Ax RT 5% none 16%	ALND 1% Ax RT 3%	none 1.5% Ax RT 0.5%	21%	T1a,b 9% T1c 26% T2 33% Overall 28%	T1a 2.0% T1b 1.7% T1c 10% T2 18% Overall 7%
Overall survival	no difference	no difference	no difference	no difference	no difference	no difference	—	—	—
NED survival	no difference	no difference	no difference	no difference	no difference	no difference	—	—	—

SBCSG, Swedish Breast Cancer Study Group; EIO, European Institute of Oncology; ALND, axillary lymph node dissection; BCT, breast-conservation therapy; RCT, randomized controlled trial; RT, radiotherapy; NED, no evidence of disease; Wide excision/RT, RT to breast only; Ax RT, RT to axilla.
[a] In this study 96% had wide excision/RT and 4% had mastectomy.

was lower in the RT group (5% vs. 15%), as was axillary LR (2% vs. 13%). In a randomized trial from the Institut Curie, the authors compared the results of ALND and axillary RT in 658 patients; they observed a survival advantage for ALND at 5 years (26), but no survival differences between groups at 10 and 15 years (27). Axillary LR occurred slightly less often after ALND than after axillary RT (1% vs. 3%; $p = .04$). Finally, Veronesi et al. (28) randomized 435 patients, none of whom had ALND, to breast conservation with or without axillary RT. At 5 years' follow-up they found no differences in disease-free survival, and axillary LR in the axillary RT and no-ALND arms was 0.5% and 1.5%, respectively.

Three observational studies also report high rates of axillary LR in the untreated axilla for patients treated by mastectomy (29) or breast conservation (wide excision with breast RT) (30,31), but they also show that axillary LR is highly dependent on tumor size (Table 42.1). In the most recent of these studies, Greco et al. (31) report a 5-year axillary LR of 6.7%, ranging from 2% for T1a to 18% for T2 tumors.

Many studies have asked whether tumor characteristics alone can reliably predict axillary node status and collectively demonstrate that no combination of tumor and patient characteristics can predict a negative or a positive axilla with greater that 90% to 95% accuracy (32–38). Bevilacqua et al. (39) have recently developed a multivariate nomogram for the prediction of SLN metastases, using a sophisticated model based on 3,786 SLN biopsy procedures and prospectively validated in 1,545 subsequent procedures. They too found that the prediction of SLN status is imperfect, with only a 75% chance, between two randomly selected individuals (one of whom is node positive), of correctly identifying the node-positive patient.

Others have asked whether noninvasive imaging can replace surgical staging. Neither computed tomography (CT) nor magnetic resonance imaging (MRI) is adequate for lymph node staging. Positron emission tomography (PET) lacks the resolution to detect metastases smaller than 5 mm, so it is subject to false-negative and false-positive results; in five reports, sensitivity ranges from 27% to 94% and specificity from 43% to 97% (40–44). The results of axillary ultrasound with fine-needle aspiration (FNA) vary widely, reflecting differences in methodology and case selection (45–53); in a study of 726 *unselected* cN0 breast cancer patients, preoperative axillary ultrasound-guided

FNA identified node metastases in 8% of all patients and 21% of node positives. Ultrasound-guided FNA of axillary nodes can spare patients the added time and cost of SLN biopsy, but is insufficiently sensitive to replace surgical staging.

Axillary Lymph Node Dissection versus Axillary Sampling

As practiced in the United Kingdom, axillary sampling is a limited staging operation in which approximately four nodes are removed from the low axilla, guided by intraoperative palpation. Two randomized trials from Edinburgh have compared axillary sampling with ALND for patients having mastectomy (with 11 years' follow-up) (54) or breast conservation (wide excision with breast RT, with 4 years' follow-up) (55) (Table 42.2). Node-positive patients in each trial received axillary RT. Between sampling and ALND, the authors observed a comparable proportion of positive axillae, comparable rates of axillary LR (5.4% vs. 3%), and comparable survival between the two arms of each study, but greater long-term shoulder morbidity for patients who had sampling with RT compared to ALND. Since none of the U.K. axillary sampling data have been validated by a backup ALND (as has been done for SLN biopsy), one cannot calculate the performance characteristics of this method. In a separate Swedish study by Ahlgren et al. (56) axillary sampling (five-node biopsy) was validated by a planned backup ALND in 415 patients, and sensitivity for cN0 patients was 95.5%.

Axillary Lymph Node Dissection versus Sentinel Lymph Node Biopsy

Four randomized trials compare ALND and SLN biopsy (4–7), allocating patients to ALND versus SLN biopsy (plus ALND for SLN-positive patients), and collectively confirm that the staging accuracy of ALND and SLN biopsy is comparable, and that the morbidity of SLN biopsy is less. For two of the trials (4,6), patients in the ALND arm also had SLN biopsy, confirming false-negative rates for SLN biopsy of 8.8% and 9.7%, respectively. In the one trial reporting long-term follow-up, there were no differences in survival or in any other disease-related

Table 42.2	STUDIES OF AXILLARY LYMPH NODE DISSECTION VERSUS AXILLARY SAMPLING	
	Edinburgh I (54) (1980–1983) T1-3N0-1	Edinburgh II (55) (1987–1995) T1-3N01
Design	RCT Mastectomy: Randomized to ALND vs. sampling	RCT Lumpectomy/breast RT: Randomized to ALND vs. sampling
No. of Patients	417	466
Follow-up	11 yrs	4 yrs
Axillary local recurrence	ALND 3.0% Sampling[a] 5.4%	ALND 3.4% Sampling[b] 3.0%
Overall survival	no difference	no difference
NED survival	no difference	no difference

RCT, randomized controlled trial; RT, radiotherapy; NED, no evidence of disease; ALND, axillary lymph node dissection.
[a]All received axillary RT if node positive.
[b]All received axillary RT if node positive; 39 node-negative patients (1987–1990) also received axillary RT.

adverse events at 7 years, and there was a single case of axillary node recurrence following a negative SLN biopsy (8).

INDICATIONS FOR AXILLARY LYMPH NODE DISSECTION

In the simplest sense, ALND would seem to be indicated for any patient with a contraindication to SLN biopsy. In fact, most of the putative contraindications to SLN biopsy (including, among others, prior surgical biopsy, nonpalpable lesion, multicentric tumor, and T2 or T3 disease) have been disproved, and SLN biopsy is suitable for virtually all patients with clinical stage T1-3N0 invasive cancers (57). Although the role of ALND has diminished in the era of SLN biopsy, there are at least nine clear indications to perform it (Table 42.3).

Positive Axilla

Patients with proven axillary node metastases require ALND. However, since clinical axillary examination is equally subject to false-negative and false-positive results (58), the clinically positive axilla is not an absolute indication for ALND. In the author's experience, 25% of patients with highly suspicious axillary nodes on clinical assessment proved to be benign at the time of SLN biopsy (59). As noted above, there is a growing role for preoperative axillary ultrasound and ultrasound- or palpation-guided FNA, allowing patients with proven nodal metastases to avoid SLN biopsy and proceed directly to ALND.

Prior Inadequate Axillary Lymph Node Dissection

What constitutes an inadequate (or an adequate) ALND? In the NSABP B-04 trial, Fisher et al. (58) found that the proportion of cN0 patients with positive axillae was the same whether 3 to 5, 6 to 10, 11 to 15, or 16 to 20 nodes had been removed (i.e., the removal of relatively few nodes was sufficient to establish whether the axilla was positive or negative), but that the proportion with four or more positive nodes was highest when 26 or more nodes had been removed (i.e., a more complete node dissection was necessary to correctly determine the *degree* of node involvement). They also observed no cases of subsequent axillary LR when six or more nodes had been removed.

The apparent adequacy of ALND is multifactorial. First, while the operative technique is well defined, the performance of ALND in practice varies widely. Second, there is wide variation in the thoroughness with which pathologists examine the ALND specimen. Finally, in a small minority of patients very few nodes will be found, despite an anatomically correct ALND and a thorough pathologic assessment. For those patients who have had a recent ALND in which (a) the anatomic extent of surgery cannot be documented, (b) the gross specimen is not available for re-examination, (c) few nodes have been removed, and (d) most are positive (raising concern about residual gross axillary disease), it is quite reasonable to perform a completion ALND or to consider axillary RT.

Positive Sentinel Lymph Node

ALND is standard care for patients with a positive SLN, especially those detected on intraoperative assessment. Among patients whose SLN are negative on intraoperative examination but positive on permanent pathology, a majority have disease limited to the SLN, and there is debate over the role of ALND in this setting. The risk of non-SLN involvement is predicted by the same variables that predict lymph node involvement in general (especially tumor size, volume of SLN metastasis, and lymphovascular invasion) and a multivariate nomogram can estimate this risk (60). The rate of isolated axillary local recurrence in selected SLN-positive patients who do not have ALND is low, 1.9% in the study by Park et al. (61), and further study is required to identify subsets of SLN-positive patients who do not require ALND. Two prospective trials address this issue with randomization of SLN-positive patients to ALND versus observation (American College of Surgical Oncology Group [ACOSOG] Z0011) (62), or to ALND versus axillary RT (European Organisation for Research and Treatment of Cancer [EORTC] After Mapping of the Axilla Radiotherapy or Surgery [AMAROS]) (63).

Validation Trials of Sentinel Lymph Node Biopsy

SLN biopsy is a *diagnostic test* for the presence of axillary node metastases and is measured by standard test characteristics:

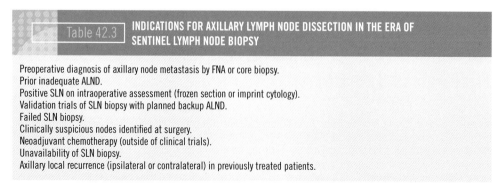

Table 42.3	INDICATIONS FOR AXILLARY LYMPH NODE DISSECTION IN THE ERA OF SENTINEL LYMPH NODE BIOPSY

Preoperative diagnosis of axillary node metastasis by FNA or core biopsy.
Prior inadequate ALND.
Positive SLN on intraoperative assessment (frozen section or imprint cytology).
Validation trials of SLN biopsy with planned backup ALND.
Failed SLN biopsy.
Clinically suspicious nodes identified at surgery.
Neoadjuvant chemotherapy (outside of clinical trials).
Unavailability of SLN biopsy.
Axillary local recurrence (ipsilateral or contralateral) in previously treated patients.

FNA, fine-needle aspiration; ALND, axillary lymph node dissection; SLN, sentinel lymph node.

sensitivity, specificity, positive predictive value, negative predictive value, and overall accuracy. These do not require a randomized trial, but do require that SLN biopsy be validated by an immediate planned "backup" ALND. In an overview of 69 observational (nonrandomized) studies of SLN biopsy with planned ALND (comprising 8,059 patients), the success and false-negative rates were 96% and 7%, respectively (3). The U.K. Axillary Lymphatic Mapping Against Nodal Axillary Clearance (ALMANAC) trial required each of its initial participant surgeons to do 40 SLN procedures validated by an ALND, with threshold success and false-negative rates of 95% and 5%, respectively, prior to entering the randomization phase; they observed a shorter "learning curve" than expected, with most failed and false-negative results occurring in the very first procedure (64). This observation is supported by the NASBP B-32 trial, in which a false-negative rate of 9.7% did not significantly decline with increasing surgeon experience (6).

Failed Sentinel Lymph Node Biopsy

With increasing experience, the success rate of SLN biopsy approaches but does not equal 100%. For that small fraction of failed SLN biopsy procedures, or for a SLN procedure that is technically unsatisfactory in any other way, it is reasonable to perform ALND (65).

Clinically Suspicious Nodes at Sentinel Lymph Node Biopsy

During SLN biopsy, a small proportion of patients will have a marked reactive adenopathy that is grossly indistinguishable from cancer. In this setting, benign intraoperative assessment (frozen section or imprint cytology) may not be completely reassuring, and it is reasonable on the basis of clinical suspicion alone to proceed with ALND (65).

Neoadjuvant Chemotherapy for Inflammatory Cancer

The suitability of SLN biopsy for T2 and T3 breast cancers is well established, but an overview of 21 small validation studies of SLN biopsy after neoadjuvant chemotherapy (given largely for noninflammatory cancers) observed success and false-negative rates (91% and 12%, respectively) somewhat inferior to those of SLN biopsy in general (66). In a separate study, 56 patients with axillary node metastases proven by FNA had neoadjuvant chemotherapy followed by SLN biopsy with a planned ALND; while 31% had a pathologic complete response, the false-negative rate of SLN biopsy in the remaining patients was unacceptably high (25%) (67). After neoadjuvant chemotherapy, SLN biopsy may be reasonable for patients with T2 and T3 tumors, but ALND should remain standard care for patients with T4 (inflammatory) cancers.

Unavailability of Sentinel Lymph Node Biopsy

SLN biopsy is not universally available, especially in developing nations where the added logistics and cost may prove to be excessive. Since the potential impact of SLN biopsy worldwide is substantial (a significant proportion of clinically diagnosed breast cancers are still node negative), the challenge will be to find ways to minimize the cost of SLN biopsy while maintaining accuracy. Where SLN biopsy is not available, ALND should remain standard care.

Isolated Locoregional Recurrence

Axillary local recurrence after a negative SLN biopsy is rare and comparable to that after ALND, occurring in less than 1% of patients (68). Most axillary masses that appear after SLN biopsy are benign, but for those that are proven malignant, ALND is indicated. ALND is also indicated for those patients who relapse in the contralateral axilla and do not have other distant sites of disease.

 AXILLARY ANATOMY

The axillary contents lie within a complex space best described as an eccentrically shaped pyramid. Viewed through a transverse section (Fig. 42.1), the axilla is a triangular space, bounded by the chest wall medially, the subscapularis posteriorly, the latissimus posterolaterally, and the pectoralis major and minor muscles anteriorly. Viewed from the front through a coronal section (Fig. 42.2), the triangle is bounded by the axillary vein superiorly, the latissimus laterally, and the chest wall medially.

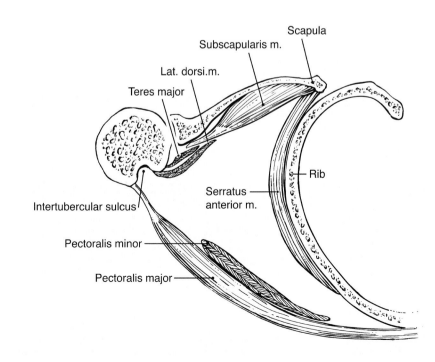

FIGURE. 42.1. The anatomic boundaries of axillary lymph node dissection, as seen in a transverse section through the midportion of the axilla, showing the pectoralis major and minor anteriorly, the serratus medially, and the latissimus and subscapularis posteriorly.

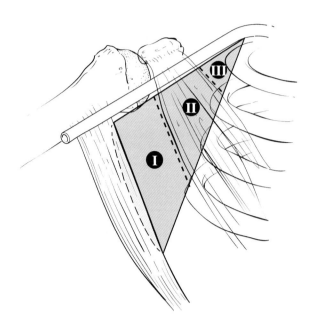

FIGURE. 42.2. The anatomic extent of axillary lymph node dissection, with levels I, II, and III designated as lying lateral to, behind, or medial to pectoralis minor muscle.

The axillary contents are arbitrarily divided into three levels: level I lying lateral to, level II lying posterior to, and level III lying medial to the pectoralis minor muscle (Fig. 42.2). Level I comprises the largest volume of axillary tissue and the largest proportion of the axillary nodes (perhaps two-thirds), with level II comprising most of the remainder, and level III 10% or less. The anatomic distinction between axillary levels I and II is somewhat arbitrary, while level III is more anatomically distinct. Historically, breast cancer prognosis was related to the *highest level* of axillary node involvement, but since about 1970 the *number* of positive nodes, and not the *level*, has emerged as the prognostically relevant variable.

The extent of ALND is formally classified as level I, level I and II, or level I to III (complete ALND); there is no evidence that the morbidity of ALND varies with the extent of the dissection. The historic justification for a complete ALND was the observation of *skip metastases* to levels II or III nodes, with level I negative (69–71). Since most skip metastases were found in level II (isolated level III disease is rare), many authorities recommended a level I and II ALND as standard care. At present, skip metastases are best viewed as level II or III SLN, which happen to receive lymphatic drainage *directly from the breast*. These nodes should be readily identified by lymphatic mapping and submitted for pathologic examination as SLN.

In the author's practice, ALND is usually a level I or II dissection, but the author performs a complete (level I to III) ALND in patients with high risk (T3 or T4) tumors or with grossly suspicious nodes identified at surgery.

Technique of Axillary Lymph Node Dissection

ALND is best done under general anesthesia, but for patients with comorbidity it is feasible under local anesthesia with sedation. The incision is either separate from or contiguous with the incision used for the breast operation. Separate axillary and breast incisions are cosmetically superior to contiguous ones, but a contiguous incision is reasonable for patients either having mastectomy without reconstruction or having breast conservation for tumors very high in the axillary tail.

The foremost technical element of ALND is to fully dissect the skin flaps to their anatomic limits (the axillary vein superiorly, the pectoralis major superomedially, the serratus inferiorly, and the latissimus laterally) *prior* to entering the axilla; virtually all technical difficulties with ALND stem from inadequate flap elevation at the outset of the procedure. The dissection is carried around the lateral border of the pectoralis major, taking care to avoid injury to the medial pectoral nerve.

The clavipectoral fascia is incised just anterior to the axillary vein and just lateral to the pectoralis minor, and with this step the axillary contents can be mobilized inferolaterally, completely exposing the axillary vein superiorly and the medial pectoral neurovascular bundle medially as it courses around the lateral border of the muscle. The arm is adducted and the major and minor are retracted medially, exposing level II. If gross axillary disease is palpable in levels II and III, the insertion of the pectoralis minor on the coracoid can be divided to fully expose level III.

The axillary contents are mobilized laterally off the chest wall, ligating side branches of the axillary vein as they are encountered. The long thoracic nerve (innervating the serratus anterior) and thoracodorsal nerve (innervating the latissimus dorsi) are identified and preserved, and the operation is completed by dissecting along the thoracodorsal neurovascular bundle and handing off the operative specimen. The axillary specimen is labeled with tags indicating levels I to III. A closed suction drain is placed and the skin incision is closed.

Patients having ALND with breast conservation are normally discharged the following day, and for those with mastectomy on the second postoperative day. All patients are instructed in wound care, given a log book to record their wound drainage (the drains are removed when 24-hour drainage is less than 30 cc), and given a program of postoperative shoulder exercises that they can usually begin immediately (except in the setting of breast reconstruction). Patients are encouraged to resume using their arm as soon, and as normally, as possible.

COMPLICATIONS OF AXILLARY LYMPH NODE DISSECTION

Lymphedema

Lymphedema is the single complication of greatest concern to patients and is the subject of an extensive but problematic literature. There are no large population-based studies that estimate the incidence of lymphedema, and across the literature there is wide variation in the definition of lymphedema, methods of assessment, patient characteristics, extent of surgery, extent of RT, and length of follow-up. In a classic 1986 report, Kissin et al. (72) found that (a) lymphedema was more frequent when measured by arm volume (25.5%) than by patient self-assessment (14%), (b) the frequency of subjective late lymphedema was similar for axillary RT alone (8.3%), axillary sampling plus RT (9.1%), and ALND (7.4%), and (c) lymphedema occurred far more often after ALND plus RT (38%; *p* <.001). In a comprehensive 2001 overview, Erickson et al. (73) cite 10 more recent studies (1991 to 2000) in which the incidence of lymphedema ranged from 2% to 43% and appeared to increase with patient age, body mass index, and length of follow-up.

The most useful current data regarding lymphedema will come from the four randomized trials that compare ALND with SLN biopsy, three of which report less arm swelling with SLN biopsy (4,5,7). In the ALMANAC trial, the patient-reported incidence at 12 months of moderate or severe lymphedema was less with SLN biopsy than with ALND (5% vs. 13%) and the relative risk of *any* lymphedema (for SLN biopsy relative to ALND) was 0.37 (95% confidence interval [CI], 0.23–0.60) (5). Regarding lymphedema and all of the other side effects of ALND, it is worth noting in the current era of SLN biopsy that the sequelae of ALND are not as severe as patients may expect, and that the sequelae of SLN biopsy may exceed expectations: in a recent report from the prospective ACOSOG Z0010 trial (comprising 5,327 patients), lymphedema developed following SLN biopsy in 6.9% of patients at 6 months (74).

Standard recommendations to patients for the prevention of lymphedema include the avoidance of (a) trauma or injury, (b) infection, (c) arm constriction (especially by blood pressure cuffs), and (d) heavy lifting or repetitive motions (73). These recommendations are deeply entrenched in the medical and nursing literature, but there is no evidence that any of them are effective in avoiding lymphedema, or that lymphedema *can* be avoided; they may even have the unintended consequence of making a patient feel that the lymphedema is *her fault*, rather than a known side effect of treatment.

Lymphedema cannot be cured but it can be treated. Using various combinations of elastic compression garments, compression pumps, bandaging, exercise, and complex physiotherapy, 15 studies (1989 to 1991) have reported reductions of 15% to 75% in arm volume or circumference (73). Large randomized studies are needed to determine the relative efficacy of these treatments and the natural history of lymphedema posttreatment.

Axillary Web Syndrome

Axillary web syndrome (AWS) has been long observed by surgeons but only recently named and described by Moskovitz et al. (75). AWS is characterized by the appearance 1 to 8 weeks after ALND (or SLN biopsy) of a network ("web") of tender subcutaneous cords running from the lateral axilla down the upper inner aspect of the arm, associated with pain and limitation of arm movement. Among 750 consecutive patients, they observed AWS in 6%. The presumed cause, surgical disruption of veins or lymphatics proximally at the level of the axilla, is supported by the observation of thrombosis in subcutaneous veins or lymphatics in four of their patients who underwent biopsy. AWS is a benign and self-limited condition that should not be confused with lymphedema and does not require treatment.

Sensory Morbidity

The sensory sequelae of ALND are largely related to the division of sensory nerves, most notably the intercostobrachial nerve (ICBN), a cutaneous sensory branch of T2 that innervates the upper inner arm, axilla, and superolateral breast. Technical modifications of ALND that allow preservation of the ICBN are the subject of an enthusiastic but anecdotal literature. In the single randomized trial comparing ICBN preservation versus division (76,77), ICBN preservation reduced the size of the sensory deficit, but there were otherwise no differences between groups in pain, shoulder movement, arm circumference, or presence of neuromas, either at 3 months or at 3 years of follow-up.

Of the four randomized trials, three report less sensory morbidity with SLN biopsy than with ALND (4,5,7). In the ALMANAC trial, the patient-reported incidence of sensory loss at 12 months was less with SLN biopsy than with ALND (11% vs. 31%) and the relative risk of sensory deficit (for SLN biopsy relative to ALND) was 0.37 (95% CI, 0.27–0.50) (5). This and other studies document that the sensory morbidity of ALND diminishes significantly over time and requires no treatment (78).

Shoulder Function

Restriction in shoulder range of motion (ROM) is a side effect of ALND, and of the four randomized trials, two report less limi-

tation in ROM after SLN biopsy than after ALND (4,5). In the ALMANAC trial, this difference was significant at 1 month, but shoulder ROM (flexion and abduction) improved rapidly in both groups, and at longer follow-up, the difference was no longer significant (5). Exercises to restore shoulder ROM are an essential element of postoperative care following ALND.

Infection

Cellulitis of the arm, chest wall, or breast is a well-recognized but relatively infrequent side effect of ALND and presumably reflects a localized immune impairment from the surgery. The incidence of cellulitis is unknown, but in a careful report by Roses et al. (79) of 200 patients followed 1 or more years after ALND, 5.5% developed cellulitis and 2% had multiple episodes. Cellulitis can arise following a nonsterile skin break (cut, abrasion, or burn) but often appears without an obvious cause. Patients are routinely advised following ALND to avoid injections, venipunctures, or an intravenous (IV) procedure in the ipsilateral arm, but there is no evidence whatsoever that *sterile* skin punctures cause cellulitis or that avoidance prevents either infection or lymphedema (73). Repeated episodes of infection are thought to increase the risk of lymphedema, although it remains unclear in this setting whether infection is a cause or an effect of lymphedema, and prompt treatment with oral or IV antibiotics is recommended.

 ## FUTURE DIRECTIONS

Clinical oncology has entered a dynamic new era in which genomic technologies (a) suggest a new classification of breast cancer (80), (b) appear to improve prognostication (81–83), (c) may better predict which patients will (or will not) benefit from adjuvant systemic therapy (84), and (d) promise the identification of new therapeutic targets and more effective drugs. If the prognostic and predictive power of gene expression profiling prove superior to that of conventional histopathology *and* if new classes of drugs with curative potential emerge, then ALND, lymph node staging, and breast cancer surgery, in general, could become obsolete. The present reality is that surgery remains the single most effective treatment for breast cancer, lymph node staging remains essential for prognostication, and ALND still has a role in achieving local control for most (if not all) node-positive patients.

 ## MANAGEMENT SUMMARY

- SLN biopsy has largely replaced ALND as the initial axillary staging procedure of choice for patients with cN0 breast cancers.
- Staging accuracy, local control, and survival appear to be comparable between SLN biopsy and ALND.
- ALND is indicated for:
  - a preoperative diagnosis of axillary node metastasis,
  - a positive SLN,
  - a recent inadequate ALND,
  - validation trials of SLN biopsy,
  - a failed SLN biopsy,
  - clinically suspicious nodes identified at surgery,
  - neoadjuvant chemotherapy (outside of clinical trials),
  - unavailability of SLN biopsy,
  - axillary local recurrence.
- A level I or II ALND is usually sufficient. A level I to III (complete) ALND is indicated for patients with gross axillary disease.
- Postoperative care after ALND should include shoulder exercises to maintain ROM.

- There is no evidence post-ALND that other standard recommendations (including the avoidance of trauma or injury, infection, blood pressure cuffs, heavy lifting, or repetitive motion) are effective in preventing lymphedema.
- There is no evidence post-ALND that the avoidance of venipuncture, injections, or IVs in the ipsilateral arm is effective in preventing either infection or lymphedema.

References

1. Krag DN, Weaver DL, Alex JC, et al. Surgical resection and radiolocalization of the sentinel lymph node in breast cancer using a gamma probe. *Surg Oncol* 1993;2:335–340.
2. Giuliano AE, Kirgan DM, Guenther JM, et al. Lymphatic mapping and sentinel lymphadenectomy for breast cancer. *Ann Surg* 1994;220:391–401.
3. Kim T, Giuliano AE, Lyman GH. Lymphatic mapping and sentinel lymph node biopsy in early-stage breast carcinoma. *Cancer* 2006;106:4–16.
4. Veronesi U, Paganelli G, Viale G, et al. A randomized comparison of sentinel-node biopsy with routine axillary dissection in breast cancer. *N Engl J Med* 2003;349:546–553.
5. Mansel RE, Fallowfield L, Kissin M, et al. Randomized multicenter trial of sentinel node biopsy versus standard axillary treatment in operable breast cancer: the ALMANAC Trial. *J Natl Cancer Inst* 2006;98:599–609.
6. Krag DN, Anderson SJ, Julian TB, et al. Technical outcomes of sentinel-lymph-node resection and conventional axillary-lymph-node dissection in patients with clinically node-negative breast cancer: results from the NSABP B-32 randomised phase III trial. *Lancet Oncol* 2007;8:881–888.
7. Purushotham AD, Upponi S, Klevesath MB, et al. Morbidity after sentinel lymph node biopsy in primary breast cancer: results from a randomized controlled trial. *J Clin Oncol* 2005;23:4312–4321.
8. Veronesi U, Paganelli G, Viale G, et al. Sentinel-lymph-node biopsy as a staging procedure in breast cancer: update of a randomised controlled study. *Lancet Oncol* 2006;7:983–990.
9. Power SD. The history of the amputation of the breast to 1904. *Liverpool Med Chirurigical J* 1934;42:29.
10. Halsted WS. The results of operations for the cure of cancer of the breast performed at the Johns Hopkins Hospital from June 1889 to January 1894. *Johns Hopkins Hosp Rep* 1894;4:297–350.
11. Halsted WS. The results of radical operations for the cure of carcinoma of the breast. *Ann Surg* 1907;46:1.
12. Urban JA. Radical excision of the chest wall for mammary cancer. *Cancer* 1951;4:1263–1285.
13. Patey DH, Dyson WH. The prognosis of carcinoma of the breast in relation to type of operation performed. *Br J Cancer* 1948;2:7–13.
14. Auchincloss H. Significance of location and number of axillary metastases in carcinoma of the breast: a justification for a conservative operation. *Ann Surg* 1963;158:37–46.
15. Fisher B. Laboratory and clinical research in breast cancer: a personal adventure: the David A. Karnofsky memorial lecture. *Cancer Res* 1980;40:3863–3874.
16. Fisher B, Montague E, Redmond C. Comparison of radical mastectomy with alternative treatments for primary breast cancer: a first report of results from a prospective randomized clinical trial. *Cancer* 1977;39[Suppl]:2827–2839.
17. Fisher B, Redmond C, Fisher E. Ten-year results of a randomized clinical trial comparing radical mastectomy and total mastectomy with or without radiation. *N Engl J Med* 1985;312:674–681.
18. Fisher B, Jeong JH, Anderson S, et al. Twenty-five-year follow-up of a randomized trial comparing radical mastectomy, total mastectomy, and total mastectomy followed by irradiation. *N Engl J Med* 2002;347:567–575.
19. Hellman S, Weichselbaum RR. Oligometastases. *J Clin Oncol* 1995;13:8–10.
20. Early Breast Cancer Trialists' Collaborative Group. Effects of radiotherapy and of differences in the extent of surgery for early breast cancer on local recurrence and 15-year survival: an overview of the randomised trials. *Lancet* 2005;366:2087–2106.
21. Early Breast Cancer Trialists' Collaborative Group. Effects of radiotherapy and surgery in early breast cancer—an overview of the randomized trials. *N Engl J Med* 1995;333:1444–1455.
22. Early Breast Cancer Trialists' Collaborative Group. Effects of chemotherapy and hormonal therapy for early breast cancer on recurrence and 15-year survival: an overview of the randomised trials. *Lancet* 2005;365:1687–1717.
23. Martelli G, Boracchi P, De Palo M, et al. A randomized trial comparing axillary dissection to no axillary dissection in older patients with T1N0 breast cancer: results after 5 years of follow-up. *Ann Surg* 2005;242:1–6.
24. Rudenstam CM, Zahrieh D, Forbes JF, et al. Randomized trial comparing axillary clearance versus no axillary clearance in older patients with breast cancer: first results of International Breast Cancer Study Group trial 10-93. *J Clin Oncol* 2006;24:337–344.
25. Cancer Research Campaign Working Party. Management of early cancer of the breast: report of an international multicentre trial supported by the Cancer Research Campaign. *BMJ* 1976;1:1035–1038.
26. Cabanes PA, Salmon RJ, Vilcoq JR, et al. Value of axillary dissection in addition to lumpectomy and radiotherapy in early breast cancer. The Breast Carcinoma Collaborative Group of the Institut Curie. *Lancet* 1992;339:1245–1248.
27. Louis-Sylvestre C, Clough K, Asselain B, et al. Axillary treatment in conservative management of operable breast cancer: dissection or radiotherapy? Results of a randomized study with 15 years of follow-up. *J Clin Oncol* 2004;22:97–101.
28. Veronesi U, Orecchia R, Zurrida S, et al. Avoiding axillary dissection in breast cancer surgery: a randomized trial to assess the role of axillary radiotherapy. *Ann Oncol* 2005;16:383–388.
29. Baum M, Coyle PJ. Simple mastectomy for early breast cancer and the behaviour of the untreated axillary nodes. *Bull Cancer* 1977;64:603–610.
30. Baxter N, McCready D, Chapman JA, et al. Clinical behavior of untreated axillary nodes after local treatment for primary breast cancer. *Ann Surg Oncol* 1996;3:235–240.
31. Greco M, Agresti R, Cascinelli N, et al. Breast cancer patients treated without axillary surgery: clinical implications and biologic analysis. *Ann Surg* 2000;232:1–7.
32. Ravdin PM, De Laurentiis M, Vendely T, et al. Prediction of axillary lymph node status in breast cancer patients by use of prognostic indicators. *J Natl Cancer Inst* 1994;86:1771–1775.
33. Chadha M, Chabon AB, Friedmann P, et al. Predictors of axillary lymph node metastases in patients with T1 breast cancer. A multivariate analysis. *Cancer* 1994;73:350–353.
34. Rivadeneira DE, Simmons RM, Christos PJ, et al. Predictive factors associated with axillary lymph node metastases in T1a and T1b breast carcinomas: analysis in more than 900 patients. *J Am Coll Surg* 2000;191:1–6.
35. Bader AA, Tio J, Petru E, et al. T1 breast cancer: identification of patients at low risk of axillary lymph node metastases. *Breast Cancer Res Treat* 2002;76:11–17.
36. Gann PH, Colilla SA, Gapstur SM, et al. Factors associated with axillary lymph node metastasis from breast carcinoma: descriptive and predictive analyses. *Cancer* 1999;86:1511–1519.
37. Marchevsky AM, Shah S, Patel S. Reasoning with uncertainty in pathology: artificial neural networks and logistic regression as tools for prediction of lymph node status in breast cancer patients. *Mod Pathol* 1999;12:505–513.
38. Silverstein MJ, Skinner KA, Lomis TJ. Predicting axillary nodal positivity in 2,282 patients with breast carcinoma. *World J Surg* 2001;25:767–772.
39. Bevilacqua JL, Kattan MW, Fey JV, et al. Doctor, what are my chances of having a positive sentinel node? A validated nomogram for risk estimation. *J Clin Oncol* 2007;25:3670–3679.
40. Greco M, Crippa F, Agresti R, et al. Axillary lymph node staging in breast cancer by 2-fluoro-2-deoxy-D-glucose-positron emission tomography: clinical evaluation and alternative management. *J Natl Cancer Inst* 2001;93:630–635.
41. Schirrmeister H, Kuhn T, Guhlmann A, et al. Fluorine-18 2-deoxy-2-fluoro-D-glucose PET in the preoperative staging of breast cancer: comparison with the standard staging procedures. *Eur J Nucl Med* 2001;28:351–358.
42. Wahl RL, Siegel BA, Coleman RE, et al. Prospective multicenter study of axillary nodal staging by positron emission tomography in breast cancer: a report of the staging breast cancer with PET study group. *J Clin Oncol* 2004;22:277–285.
43. Guller U, Nitzsche EU, Schirp U, et al. Selective axillary surgery in breast cancer patients based on positron emission tomography with 18F-fluoro-2-deoxy-D-glucose: not yet! *Breast Cancer Res Treat* 2002;71:171–173.
44. Lovrics PJ, Chen V, Coates G, et al. A prospective evaluation of positron emission tomography scanning, sentinel lymph node biopsy, and standard axillary dissection for axillary staging in patients with early stage breast cancer. *Ann Surg Oncol* 2004;11:846–853.
45. Bonnema J, van Geel AN, van Ooijen B, et al. Ultrasound-guided aspiration biopsy for detection of nonpalpable axillary node metastases in breast cancer patients: new diagnostic method. *World J Surg* 1997;21:270–274.
46. Damera A, Evans AJ, Cornford EJ, et al. Diagnosis of axillary nodal metastases by ultrasound-guided core biopsy in primary operable breast cancer. *Br J Cancer* 2003;89:1310–1313.
47. de Kanter AY, van Eijck CH, van Geel AN, et al. Multicentre study of ultrasonographically guided axillary node biopsy in patients with breast cancer. *Br J Surg* 1999;86:1459–1462.
48. Deurloo EE, Tanis PJ, Gilhuijs KG, et al. Reduction in the number of sentinel lymph node procedures by preoperative ultrasonography of the axilla in breast cancer. *Eur J Cancer* 2003;39:1068–1073.
49. Krishnamurthy S, Sneige N, Bedi DG, et al. Role of ultrasound-guided fine-needle aspiration of indeterminate and suspicious axillary lymph nodes in the initial staging of breast carcinoma. *Cancer* 2002;95:982–988.
50. Vaidya JS, Vyas JJ, Thakur MH, et al. Role of ultrasonography to detect axillary node involvement in operable breast cancer. *Eur J Surg Oncol* 1996;22:140–143.
51. Verbanck J, Vandewiele I, De Winter H, et al. Value of axillary ultrasonography and sonographically guided puncture of axillary nodes: a prospective study in 144 consecutive patients. *J Clin Ultrasound* 1997;25:53–56.
52. Yang WT, Ahuja A, Tang A, et al. High resolution sonographic detection of axillary lymph node metastases in breast cancer. *J Ultrasound Med* 1996;15:241–246.
53. van Rijk MC, Deurloo EE, Nieweg OE, et al. Ultrasonography and fine-needle aspiration cytology can spare breast cancer patients unnecessary sentinel lymph node biopsy. *Ann Surg Oncol* 2006;13:31–35.
54. Forrest AP, Everington D, McDonald CC, et al. The Edinburgh randomized trial of axillary sampling or clearance after mastectomy. *Br J Surg* 1995;82:1504–1508.
55. Chetty U, Jack W, Prescott RJ, et al. Management of the axilla in operable breast cancer treated by breast conservation: a randomized clinical trial. Edinburgh Breast Unit. *Br J Surg* 2000;87:163–169.
56. Ahlgren J, Holmberg L, Bergh J, et al. Five-node biopsy of the axilla: an alternative to axillary dissection of levels I-II in operable breast cancer. *Eur J Surg Oncol* 2002;28:97–102.
57. Cody HS 3rd. Sentinel lymph node biopsy for breast cancer: indications, contraindications, and new directions. *J Surg Oncol* 2007;95:440–442.
58. Fisher B, Wolmark N, Banes M. The accuracy of clinical nodal staging and of limited axillary dissection as a determinant of histologic nodal status in carcinoma of the breast. *Gynecol Obstet* 1981;152:765–772.
59. Specht MC, Fey JV, Borgen PI, et al. Is the clinically positive axilla in breast cancer really a contraindication to sentinel lymph node biopsy? *J Am Coll Surg* 2005;200:10–14.
60. Van Zee KJ, Manasseh DM, Bevilacqua JL, et al. A nomogram for predicting the likelihood of additional nodal metastases in breast cancer patients with a positive sentinel node biopsy. *Ann Surg Oncol* 2003;10:1140–1151.
61. Park J, Fey JV, Naik AM, et al. A declining rate of completion axillary dissection in sentinel lymph node-positive breast cancer patients is associated with the use of a multivariate nomogram. *Ann Surg* 2007;245:462–468.
62. Giuliano AE. Z0011: a randomized trial of axillary node dissection in women with clinical T1 or T2 N0 M0 breast cancer who have a positive sentinel node. Available at http://www.acosog.org/studies/synopses/Z0011_Synopsis pdf. 2003.
63. European Organisation for Research and Treatment of Cancer. EORTC 10981-22023 AMAROS trial. Available at http://www amaros nl. 2004.
64. Clarke D, Newcombe RG, Mansel RE. The learning curve in sentinel node biopsy: the ALMANAC experience. *Ann Surg Oncol* 2004;11:211S–215S.

65. Cody HS, Borgen PI. State-of-the-art approaches to sentinel node biopsy for breast cancer: study design, patient selection, technique, and quality control at Memorial Sloan-Kettering Cancer Center. *Surg Oncol* 1999;8:85–91.

66. Xing Y, Foy M, Cox DD, et al. Meta-analysis of sentinel lymph node biopsy after preoperative chemotherapy in patients with breast cancer. *Br J Surg* 2006;93: 539–546.

67. Shen J, Gilcrease MZ, Babiera GV, et al. Feasibility and accuracy of sentinel lymph node biopsy after preoperative chemotherapy in breast cancer patients with documented axillary metastases. *Cancer* 2007;109:1255–1263.

68. Naik AM, Fey J, Gemignani M, et al. The risk of axillary relapse after sentinel lymph node biopsy for breast cancer is comparable with that of axillary lymph node dissection: a follow-up study of 4,008 procedures. *Ann Surg* 2004;240:462–468.

69. Smith JA 3rd, Gamez-Araujo JJ, Gallager HS, et al. Carcinoma of the breast: analysis of total lymph node involvement versus level of metastasis. *Cancer* 1977;39:527–532.

70. Rosen PP, Lesser ML, Kinne DW, et al. Discontinuous or "skip" metastases in breast carcinoma. Analysis of 1,228 axillary dissections. *Ann Surg* 1983;197:276–283.

71. Veronesi U, Rilke F, Luini A, et al. Distribution of axillary node metastases by level of invasion. An analysis of 539 cases. *Cancer* 1987;59:682–687.

72. Kissin MW, Querci della RG, Easton D, et al. Risk of lymphoedema following the treatment of breast cancer. *Br J Surg* 1986;73:580–584.

73. Erickson VS, Pearson ML, Ganz PA, et al. Arm edema in breast cancer patients. *J Natl Cancer Inst* 2001;93:96–111.

74. Wilke LG, McCall LM, Posther KE, et al. Surgical complications associated with sentinel lymph node biopsy: results from a prospective international cooperative group trial. *Ann Surg Oncol* 2006;13:491–500.

75. Moskovitz AH, Anderson BO, Yeung RS, et al. Axillary web syndrome after axillary dissection. *Am J Surg* 2001;181:434–439.

76. Abdullah TI, Iddon J, Barr L, et al. Prospective randomized controlled trial of preservation of the intercostobrachial nerve during axillary node clearance for breast cancer. *Br J Surg* 1998;85:1443–1445.

77. Freeman SR, Washington SJ, Pritchard T, et al. Long term results of a randomised prospective study of preservation of the intercostobrachial nerve. *Eur J Surg Oncol* 2003;29:213–215.

78. Temple LK, Baron R, Cody HS 3rd, et al. Sensory morbidity after sentinel lymph node biopsy and axillary dissection: a prospective study of 233 women. *Ann Surg Oncol* 2002;9:654–662.

79. Roses DF, Brooks AD, Harris MN, et al. Complications of level I and II axillary dissection in the treatment of carcinoma of the breast. *Ann Surg* 1999;230: 194–201.

80. Perou CM, Sorlie T, Eisen MB, et al. Molecular portraits of human breast tumours. *Nature* 2000;406:747–752.

81. van't Veer LJ, Dai H, van de Vijver MJ, et al. Gene expression profiling predicts clinical outcome of breast cancer. *Nature* 2002;415:530–536.

82. van de Vijver MJ, He YD, van't Veer LJ, et al. A gene-expression signature as a predictor of survival in breast cancer. *N Engl J Med* 2002;347:1999–2009.

83. Wang Y, Klijn JG, Zhang Y, et al. Gene-expression profiles to predict distant metastasis of lymph-node-negative primary breast cancer. *Lancet* 2005;365: 671–679.

84. Paik S, Shak S, Tang G, et al. A multigene assay to predict recurrence of tamoxifen treated, node-negative breast cancer. *N Engl J Med* 2004;351:2817–2826.

Julia R. White

A major milestone in the management of early stage breast cancer over the past decade has been the transition from axillary lymph node dissection (ALND) to sentinel node biopsy (SNB) for the detection of axillary lymph node metastases (refer also to Chapters 41 and 42). This shift has triggered a reassessment of the goals, outcomes, morbidity, and alternatives to ALND. ALND has historically performed three important roles: (a) staging of the axilla by detection of nodal metastases; (b) risk stratification by identifying extent of nodal positivity (e.g., < or > than four axillary node metastases); and (c) tumor control in the axilla. The tumor control achieved by axillary node dissection can be an important element in patient prognosis. Meta-analyses have supported that the local control achieved by ALND can impact disease-free survival (DFS) (1,2), and salvage treatment of an axillary recurrence results in at best a 40% to 50% overall survival (OS) (3,4). In addition, axillary node dissection has been considered an important step in patient management by determining the type and extent of systemic therapy necessary. Despite these roles, axillary node dissection can significantly compromise patients' quality of life (QOL) by the occurrence of lymphedema, pain, restriction of shoulder movement, or anesthesia (5,6). The emergence of SNB has permitted reliable identification of axillary nodal metastases in a clinically negative axilla, therefore sparing 60% to 75% of patients the excess morbidity of ALND (7,8). Still, 25% to 40% of patients require completion ALND following positive SNB.

Axillary irradiation is a rational alternative to ALND. In a clinically negative axilla, irradiation achieves comparable local tumor control with less morbidity. In addition, there is now less reliance on the number of axillary lymph nodes with metastases as the primary indicator for systemic therapy. Other factors have emerged that may indicate the need for and the type of systemic therapy to be delivered including HER 2 neu overexpression, other gene expression, negative hormone receptors, and so forth. The combination of sentinel node biopsy to detect axillary metastases, other prognosticators as indicators for systemic therapy, and axillary irradiation for regional tumor control potentially fulfills the three primary goals of ALND.

In this chapter, the data from randomized control trials and single institution case studies evaluating the efficacy of axillary irradiation for primary management of the clinically negative axilla and in the setting of a positive sentinel node biopsy are reviewed. In addition, current methods for axillary irradiation are examined, and the implications for clinical practice are discussed.

 ## AXILLARY IRRADIATION INSTEAD OF AXILLARY LYMPH NODE DISSECTION

The National Surgical Adjuvant Breast and Bowel Project (NSABP) B-04 clinical trial provides data with very long follow-up, demonstrating that irradiation can achieve comparable tumor control in the axilla to dissection (9). This trial was designed to evaluate if total mastectomy alone or in combination with radiation therapy (RT) could yield outcomes comparable to radical mastectomy. In this study 1,079 patients with a clinically negative axilla (cN0) were randomized to one of three arms: (a) radical mastectomy (RM) with ALND, (b) total mastectomy (TM) with postoperative chest wall and regional RT, or (c) TM alone with subsequent ALND for axillary failures. The radiation dose employed was 50 Gy in 25 fractions to the axilla and chest wall and 45 Gy in 25 fractions to the supraclavicular (SCL) and internal mammary nodes. With 25 years of follow-up, the rate of nodal recurrence was the nearly same in the three treatment arms, 4%, 4%, and 6%, respectively, for RM, TM plus RT, and TM with ALND for salvage. The overall rate of locoregional recurrence was significantly lower with TM plus RT at 5% in comparison to 9% with RM, and 13% with TM with ALND salvage (p = .002). This reflects a significant benefit from radiation in reducing chest wall recurrence; 1% with RT versus 5% and 7%, respectively, with RM and TM alone. There was no difference in rate of distant metastases, DFS, or OS. The axillary tumor control achieved with RT is notable given that the rate of pathologically involved nodes for patients who had received RM with ALND was 40%, and 19% of women who underwent TM alone subsequently developed pathologically confirmed axillary nodes. The meta-analysis from the Early Breast Cancer Trialists Collaborative Group, which included NSABP B-04 and eight other trials, demonstrated no advantage of ALND compared to RT in terms of locoregional recurrences at 5 years (2).

Axillary irradiation has similarly demonstrated comparable local control when used instead of ALND in the setting of breast-conservation therapy (BCT) (Table 43.1) (10–12). A trial from the Institute Curie randomized 658 patients between 1982 and 1987 with tumors less than 3 cm in size and cN0 who underwent wide local excision of the breast disease to either axillary dissection or axillary irradiation (10). Those assigned to the radiation arm received treatment to the axillary and internal mammary nodes. Patients who had an ALND received RT to the internal mammary nodes if the tumor was medial or central in location. When positive nodes were found at ALND (21% of cases), RT was delivered to the supraclavicular and internal mammary nodes. All patients received whole breast irradiation to a dose of 55 Gy over 6 weeks followed by a 10 to 15 Gy boost to the surgical bed. A very low rate of isolated axillary recurrence was reported in both arms of the study. However, the 1% isolated axillary recurrence rate following dissection is statistically lower than the 3% reported after radiation at 15 years. By reviewing the distribution of isolated axillary recurrences in the dissection arm, there is a suggestion that this lower recurrence rate could be due to the addition of nodal radiation following ALND for node-positive patients. There were five axillary recurrences in the ALND arm; one in the node-positive group that was irradiated (~1.4% crude rate), and four in the 168 node-negative patients (~2.4% crude rate). The rates of in-breast recurrence, supraclavicular failures, and distant metastases were the same in the two groups. In addition, there was no difference in OS, DFS, and disease-specific survival between the two groups at 15 years.

A retrospective case study of 180 women 50 years and older with T1 or T2, cN0 tumors, treated with BCT, from the Netherlands Radiotherapeutic Institute likewise demonstrated a low regional relapse rate when axillary irradiation was used instead of ALND (Table 43.1) (11). Patients who had axillary RT were compared to a matched control group of 340 patients who had ALND and were treated over a similar time period (1991 to 2000). The rate of pathologically involved nodes in the ALND group was 23%. All patients underwent lumpectomy and whole breast irradiation plus boost. Patients without an ALND were irradiated to the axilla, supraclavicular, and ipsilateral internal mammary nodes. Axillary node dissection patients who had

| Table 43.1 | STUDIES DEMONSTRATING EFFICACY OF AXILLARY IRRADIATION IN COMPARISON TO DISSECTION IN BREAST-CONSERVATION THERAPY |

Institution, Author (Reference)	Year	Design	FU (yrs)	Chemo (%)	HT (%)	S	Breast RT	Axilla	n	pN+ (%)	Regional Recurrence (%)	P
Institute Curie, Louis-Sylvestre et al. (10)	2004	RCT	15	—	100	L	Y	ALND	326	21	1	0.04
								RT	332	—	3	
Radiotherapie Institute, Spruit et al. (11)	2007	Matched Case study	7.2	4	3	L	Y	ALND	340	23.2	1.5	NS
								RT	180	—	1.15	
Yale University, Pejavar et al. (12)	2006	Case study	13	29.6	34	T	Y	ALND	1330	26	2.3	NS
								RT	590	—	2.1	

FU, follow-up; Chemo, chemotherapy; HT, tamoxifen or other antiendocrine agent; S, breast surgery; pN+, pathologically positive axillary nodes; RCT, randomized control trial; ALND, axillary node dissection; RT, radiation therapy; T, tumorectomy; L, lumpectomy.

positive nodes or medial tumors received RT to the internal mammary nodes. With a median follow-up of 7.2 years, the number of regional recurrences was very low: two (1.1%) in the axillary RT group and five (1.5%) in the ALND group. Local recurrence (2.2% and 6.7%, respectively) and the distant metastatic rate (3.5% and 10.3%, respectively) were somewhat lower in the RT group compared to the ALND group, but OS was similar.

A large retrospective study of BCT patients from Yale University also reports a low regional relapse rate when the axilla is irradiated instead of dissected (Table 43.1) (12). This report examined 1,920 patients with stage I or II breast cancer treated with BCT from 1973 to 2003. All patients underwent tumorectomy, without a specific attempt to obtain or document free surgical margins, followed by whole breast irradiation plus a boost. For 590 patients, ALND was omitted and irradiation was delivered to the axillary and supraclavicular nodes with or without internal mammary nodal irradiation. Axillary node dissection was performed in 1,330 patients. Pathologically involved nodes were found in 26% and these patients also received supraclavicular nodal irradiation. The 10-year rate of nodal relapse was 2.1 % with axillary RT versus 2.6% for those who had ALND.

These very low nodal recurrence rates following axillary RT instead of ALND are corroborated by several other retrospective case studies in BCT patients (Table 43.2) (13–17). Patients in these studies were all clinically node negative and had breast-conserving surgery followed by whole breast irradiation plus boost. In nearly all cases, the axilla was irradiated by a separate radiation field that included the supraclavicular nodes (Table 43.2). There were no nodal recurrences in two studies (13,14) after axillary RT at 3.4 and 5 years follow-up, respectively. A total of three nodal recurrences (two axilla and one supraclavicular) were seen in a large cohort of patients (n = 292) from the Harvard Joint Center for Radiation Therapy (JCRT) after a median of 15 years of follow-up (15). In a series from Tufts University that focused on 73 elderly women (defined as age 65 or older), there was one axillary nodal recurrence (16). In an older study from Washington University, there were 2 axillary recurrences (2.7%) in 75 patients who had axillary RT instead of ALND (17). In this study, only a small percentage of patients received chemotherapy or hormonal therapy, which is known to enhance locoregional control. Aggregated data from these five studies give an average nodal recurrence rate of 0.9% with axillary RT instead of ALND in cN0 patients.

These retrospective studies also suggest that less arm morbidity is seen with axillary irradiation than ALND (Table 43.2) (13,15–17). The lymphedema rate reported in individual institutions is 1% to 5% after axillary irradiation without axillary dissection in patients who underwent breast-conserving surgery and breast irradiation (13,15–17). Likewise, the incidence of other arm morbidity, plexopathy, and impaired shoulder mobility after axillary irradiation is low.

| Table 43.2 | OUTCOMES FROM AXILLARY IRRADIATION INSTEAD OF AXILLARY NODE DISSECTION FOR BREAST CONSERVATION |

Institution, Author (Reference)	Year	N	Age (yrs)	RT AX/SCL	HT (%)	Chemo (%)	FU (yrs)	Nodal recurrence (%)	Arm edema (%)	Brach plex. (%)	RT pneum. (%)	Reduced ROM (%)
JCRT, Galper et al. (15)	2000	292	65▲	Y	2	2	15	1	1.4	1.4	0.7	—
The Netherlands Cancer Inst., Hoebers et al. (13)	1999	105	64▲	Y	71	—	3.4	0	5	0	0	6.6
Rush-St. Luke's, Kuznetsora et al. (14)	1995	36	70*	50%	30	—	5	0	—	—	—	—
Tufts University, Wazer et al. (16)	1994	73	74*	Y	90	—	4.5	1.4	0	0	0	—
Washington University, Halverson et al. (17)	1993	75	55▲	Y	10	20	4.6	2.6	1	—	2.7	—

JCRT, Joint Center for Radiation Therapy at Harvard Medical School; RT AX/SCL, separate field included axillary and supraclavicular nodes; HT, tamoxifen or other antiendocrine therapy; Chemo, chemotherapy; FU, follow-up; ROM, shoulder range of motion; *, median age; ▲, mean age; —, not reported.

USE OF TANGENTIAL BREAST IRRADIATION ALONE IN cN0 BREAST-CONSERVING THERAPY PATIENTS

Several studies have demonstrated low axillary recurrence rates in the setting of breast-conserving surgery and tangential breast irradiation (Table 43.3) without a specific axillary therapy in certain subsets of breast cancer patients (18–22). These results likely reflect that a substantial percentage of the lower axillary nodes are treated in the tangential breast irradiation fields.

The National Cancer Institute in Milan randomized 219 older women aged 65 to 80 with cN0 to ALND or to no ALND at the time of quadrantectomy (18). All patients underwent breast irradiation that did not intentionally target the axilla, but is described as typically including the lower portion of level I. In this population, 92% had T1 tumors, 87% had estrogen receptor–positive tumors, and all were prescribed tamoxifen for 5 years. There were two axillary failures in the no ALND arm (1.8%) and none in the ALND arm at 5 years' follow-up. The low axillary recurrence rate without ALND was probably impacted by the breast irradiation, sterilizing a portion of the low axilla. This concept is supported by another study from this institution in an even older population of breast cancer patients. This prospective trial examined 354 cN0 breast cancer patients 70 or more years of age that underwent quadrantectomy without axillary dissection and without breast irradiation (19). In this group, there was a somewhat higher crude rate of axillary failure: 4.2% at a median of 3 years and 4% in the 274 patients with T1 disease (Table 43.3). Certain subgroups had higher rates of axillary recurrence: 16.7% in the hormone receptor–negative group and 9.5% in the pT4b group (≤2.5 cm).

A prospective study from the Italian Oncology Senology Group randomized 435 women over the age of 45 with cN0 breast cancer 1.2 cm or less in size to quadrantectomy without ALND (observation of the axilla) versus quadrantectomy plus axillary RT (20). All patients received whole breast irradiation to 50 Gy in 25 treatments and a boost to the tumor bed of 10 Gy. Axillary RT was delivered through a separate field matched to the breast field. Approximately 74% of patients had tumors less than 1 cm in size, 84% were estrogen-receptor positive, 91%

received adjuvant tamoxifen, and 8% received CMF (cyclophosphamide, methotrexate, and 5-fluorouracil) chemotherapy. At a median of 5.2 years, there were three axillary recurrences in the observation arm (crude rate, 1.4%) versus one (crude rate, 0.45%) in the RT group. There were no significant differences between the treatment groups for in-breast recurrences, DFS, or OS. The investigators acknowledge that the low rate of axillary recurrences in the observation group is lower than expected and propose that this can be explained in part by their selection of a relatively low-risk breast cancer population and that the breast RT field encompassed the lower portion of the axilla (20).

Another prospective study from the National Cancer Institute in Milan of 401, T1 or T2, cN0 breast cancer patients who did not receive targeted axillary therapy reported somewhat higher rates of axillary failure (21). Ninety-five percent of patients underwent quadrantectomy (18 patients had total mastectomy), and breast irradiation was delivered to patients less than 70 years old (65%). Tamoxifen was administered to 34.4%, no patient received chemotherapy, 90.5% had T1 tumors, and 40% of the population was less than 60 years of age. At a median follow-up of 5 years, there were 27 pathologically documented axillary recurrences for a crude recurrence rate of 6.7%. The rate of axillary failures increased progressively with the size of the primary tumor: 2%, 15%, and 34%, respectively, for T1a-b, T1c, and T2 tumors.

Several case-control studies with relatively small patient numbers have similarly reported low axillary recurrence rates in patients who underwent breast irradiation after conserving surgery who did not have specific treatment directed to the axilla (14,17). In one of the larger studies, there were no axillary recurrences in 92 women who underwent lumpectomy without node dissection followed by standard breast irradiation at the JCRT with 4.2 years median follow-up (22). This population of patients had mostly T1 tumors (83%), 87% had estrogen receptor–positive tumors, 60% received adjuvant tamoxifen, and the median age was 69.

These studies demonstrate that certain subsets of cN0 breast cancer patients undergoing lumpectomy and standard whole breast irradiation will have very low rates of axillary recurrence without specific therapy (ALND or RT) directed to the axilla. These studies also show the lowest axillary recurrence rates were seen in those patients with T1a-b tumors (20,21), patients of older age (18,22), those with positive estro-

Table 43.3		AXILLARY RECURRENCES FOLLOWING BREAST-CONSERVING SURGERY AND RADIATION WITHOUT SPECIFIC THERAPY FOR THE AXILLA									
Institution, Author (Reference)	Year	Design	FU (yrs)	Age (yrs)	S	Breast RT	HT (%)	Chemo (%)	Axilla	n	Axillary Recurrence (%)
National Cancer Institue, Milan, Martelli et al. (18)	2005	RCT	5	70▲	Q[3]	Y	100	0	ALND	109	0
									OBS	110	1.8
Italian Oncology Senology Group, Veronesi et al. (20)	2005	RCT	5.25	57*	Q	Y	90	9	AxRT	214	0.04
									OBS	221	1.4
National Cancer Institute, Milan, Greco et al. (21)	2000	Prospective	5	—	Q[1]	65	34.4	0	OBS	401	6.7
National Cancer Institute , Milan, Martelli et al. (19)	2007	Prospective	15	77*	Q	N	100	0	OBS	354	4.2
JCRT, Wong et al. (22)	1997	Case study	4.24	69*	L[4]	Y	58	1	OBS	92	0

S, breast surgery; HT, tamoxifen or other antiendocrine agent; Chemo, chemotherapy; RCT, randomized control trial; ALND, axillary node dissection; AxRT, axillary radiation therapy; OBS, observation; Q, quadrantectomy; L, lumpectomy; *, median age; ▲, mean age.

gen receptors, or where tamoxifen was given (18–20), and when breast irradiation was delivered (18,20,22).

A negligible effect on arm morbidity is anticipated from breast irradiation alone after lumpectomy. This was demonstrated in a study evaluating arm morbidity in 381 patients from the Uppsala-Orebro trial that were randomized to either lumpectomy alone versus lumpectomy and whole breast irradiation. All patients had axillary node dissection. Complete arm circumference data were available from 273 patients (117 in the RT group and 155 in the non-RT group). There was no associated difference between arm edema or any of the other arm symptoms evaluated (pain, numbness, impaired shoulder mobility) with the addition of breast irradiation (23).

AXILLARY IRRADIATION AFTER SENTINEL NODE BIOPSY

Sentinel lymph node biopsy is now routinely used in women with early stage cN0 breast for staging of the axilla. Its use has been associated with reduced arm morbidity and better quality of life than with ALND (6,7,24). However, approximately 40% of breast cancer patients will still need completion ALND following a positive SNB. Based on the results given above from Fisher et al. (9) for mastectomy and BCT patients in other studies (10–17), axillary RT instead of ALND following a positive SNB might yield comparably low axillary recurrence rates and reduced arm morbidity. The use of axillary RT following a positive SNB has been reported in only a limited number of patients so far (12,25,26). The European Organisation for Research and Treatment of Cancer (EORTC) is addressing this question in the After Mapping of the Axilla Radiotherapy or Surgery (AMAROS) clinical trial (27). The AMAROS trial is a phase III study comparing ALND with axillary RT in sentinel node–positive patients. Patients enrolled in the trial must have an operable breast cancer greater than 5 mm and less than 3 cm without clinically suspect regional nodes. The main objective of the trial is to prove equivalent locoregional control and reduced morbidity for patients with proven axillary node metastases by SNB if treated with axillary RT instead of dissection. The trial opened in 2001 and has a targeted accrual of 3,485 patients. In this study, the axillary and supraclavicular nodes are treated with a separate RT field that matches to the breast or chest wall fields inferiorly (28).

Unlike the patients enrolled on the NSABP B-04 trial or even the earlier BCT experiences, most breast cancer patients are now diagnosed with smaller tumor burdens and less extensive nodal disease as a result of widespread and improved mammographic screening. Therefore, it is anticipated for a patient with T1cN0 disease who is found to have a positive sentinel node on biopsy that most of any additional lymph nodes containing disease will be within the low axilla (i.e, the volume typically removed with standard level I or II node dissection). The low axilla is partially included in standard breast irradiation fields, and this likely explains the low axillary recurrence rates seen following lumpectomy and breast irradiation when no specific axillary therapy is delivered (Table 43.3) (18,20,22). Breast tangential fields can be customized (see discussion above) to include most of level I and II of the axilla. This offers the advantage of a simplified radiation method and reduced radiation to the ipsilateral lung. However, the challenge exists to identify which patients with positive SNB require radiation to just the level I and II nodal regions to replace dissection and which would benefit from level III and supraclavicular nodal RT as well. Breast cancer patients with four or more axillary nodal metastases are recommended to receive radiation to the SCL and axillary nodes based on evidence that there is overall improvement in survival when radiation is added after mastectomy and chemotherapy in this population (2).

Multiple studies have reported primary tumor and sentinel node factors that are predictive for additional axillary metastasis at the time of completion ALND (29–34). (Refer also to Chapters 41 and 42.) These factors include more than one sentinel node with metastases (29,32), sentinel node metastases greater than 2 mm (29,31,32), extra nodal extension (ENE) (30,32), evidence of lymphatic or vascular invasion (LVI) in the primary tumor (29–32), and primary tumor size (29,32,33). Two studies in particular have sought to predict which patients with a positive SNB will have four or more positive nodes involved at the time of completion ALND (34,35). A University of Kentucky study reviewed 126 patients who had positive SNB to identify the variables that predicted for patients with N1 versus N2-3 stage disease at completion ALND (34). They found that three factors predicted for more than three positive axillary nodes: LVI in the primary tumor (p <.025), ENE in the sentinel node (p <.01), and sentinel node tumor deposit of more than 5 mm (p <.001). Patients with sentinel node tumor deposits measuring 5 mm or less all had a maximum of three positive nodes; with sentinel node only disease in 95%, and metastatic disease in a single node in 91% of them. A similar study from Brigham and Women's and the Massachusetts General Hospitals examined 402 breast cancer patients who had completion ALND for a positive SNB to identify factors predictive for four or more positive axillary nodal metastases (35). On multivariate analysis, increasing primary tumor size (p = .04), invasive lobular histology (p = .02), presence of LVI in the primary tumor (p = .003), ENE in the sentinel node (p = .001), increasing number on positive sentinel nodes (p = .001), macroscopic size of the sentinel node metastasis (p = .02), and decreasing number on uninvolved sentinel nodes (p = .01) correlated with an increased probability of having four or more axillary nodal metastases following completion of ALND. The authors developed a nomogram based on these seven pathologic factors from the primary tumor and SNB to calculate the probability of having four or more involved axillary nodes and demonstrated that is could predict those with three or less positive nodes in 94.7% of patients and those with four or more positive nodes in 97.5% of patients (35).

These data sets can help guide how to approach axillary irradiation for patients who have not undergone completion ALND for various reasons following a positive SNB. Patients with primary tumor and SNB pathologic features at high risk for N2 disease or four or more positive axillary nodal metastases should be considered for axillary and supraclavicular radiation using a separate field matched to the breast or chest wall fields. Other cases without these features could likely be treated with customized tangent breast radiation fields that include the level I and II axilla. Results of the AMAROS trial and others will be crucial to ensure that axillary RT can yield comparable local control and less morbidity compared to a completion axillary node dissection following a positive SNB. Until these results are known, completion ALND remains the standard of care.

METHODS FOR AXILLARY IRRADIATION

Axillary irradiation methods can be tailored to the clinical scenario and the goals for treatment. Typically, the dose for axillary irradiation is 45 to 50 Gy given with standard fractionation of 1.8 to 2.0 Gy daily. Treatment of the entire axilla is achieved with a separate radiation field that commonly also

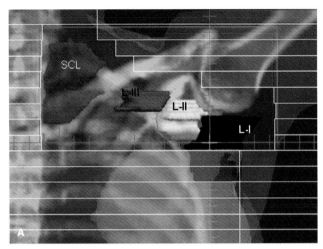 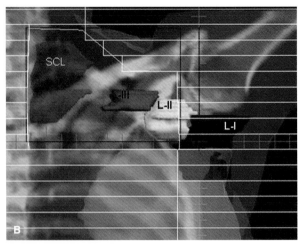

FIGURE 43.1. A: Radiation field for an undissected axilla that treats all three axillary levels (level I [L-I], level II [L-II], level III [L-III]) and the supraclavicular (SCL) nodes. **B:** Radiation field modified for treatment of a dissected axilla to exclude the lower axillary levels.

includes the supraclavicular nodes and is matched to the breast or chest wall fields caudally. This is the method of axillary irradiation used in the NSABP B-04 trial (9), all the studies listed in Tables 43.1 and 43.2 reporting on axillary RT instead of dissection for BCT (10–17), and is currently in use in the ongoing EORTC AMAROS clinical trial randomizing patients with a positive SNB to ALND versus axillary RT (28). Historically, this field has been delivered with two-dimensional radiation approaches that typically used 6 mega voltage (MV) photons through an anterior or 10- to 15-degree oblique field intended to include both the supraclavicular and axillary nodes with dose prescribed to a tissue depth between 3 to 5 cm. Generally, a supplemental posterior field (*posterior axillary boost*) is directed to the axilla as needed to ensure that a midaxilla calculation point receives the intended 45 to 50 Gy. Alternatively, this field can be treated with anterior- and posterior-opposed beam arrangements using various weighting to deliver the radiation dose to an appropriate calculation point. Currently, computed tomography (CT) planning is encouraged to ensure the delivery of 45 to 50 Gy to the targeted nodal volumes and to help minimize excessive dose heterogeneity or inadvertent normal tissue radiation. CT-based treatment planning permits the use of optimal beam energies, field shapes, and calculation points tailored to the anatomical position of the nodal volumes and the patient body habitus on CT. Figure 43.1A illustrates a field designed to treat the entire axilla that is a digitally reconstructed radiograph from a radiation planning CT with the anatomical nodal volumes delineated. A dose volume analysis (DVA) of the three-dimensional radiation plan that includes the breast treatment (XiO, CMS Software, St. Louis, Missouri) of this illustrated case confirms at least 95% of the SCL, level I to III (L-I, L-II, L-III) axilla volumes are covered by the prescribed 50 Gy, 95% of the breast volume receives 45 Gy, and 25% of the ipsilateral lung receives a dose of 20 Gy or more (V20). Note that the lower portion of the level I axilla is treated through the breast fields. In contrast, when the goal is to treat the residual undissected axilla and supraclavicular nodal regions following breast-conserving surgery or mastectomy with ALND, the field is modified with the lateral border moved medially to the coracoid process, as shown in Figure 43.1B. Commonly this is delivered through an anterior or slightly oblique field dosed to a depth of 3 to 5 cm, and there is no need for a posterior axillary boost. A DVA from a CT-based three-dimensional plan using this modified field reveals that

96% of the SCL and 100% L-III axilla receive the prescribed dose of 50 Gy; but only 29% L-II and 30% L-I axilla receives 50 Gy, 95% of the breast still receives 45 Gy, and the ipsilateral lung V20 is 18%.

For breast cancer patients with T1cN0 disease it is expected that most of any lymph nodes containing disease will be located within the low axilla (i.e., the volume typically removed with standard level I and II node dissection). Numerous studies have looked at the extent that the lower axilla is treated by radiation fields that are directed just at the breast (Table 43.4) (36–43). Multiple studies have looked at whether the ALND or SNB surgical clips can be seen within the confines of a standard two-dimensional breast tangent field radiograph (Table 43.4) (36–39). In two studies, all of the ALND surgical clips were included in the breast fields in only 38% and 43% of patients, respectively (36,37); but the SNB clips were included in 85% and 94% of the patients in two respective studies (37,38). A study from Perugia University looked at the inclusion of three surgical clips placed during dissection, the first at the start of level I, the second at the junction levels I and II, and the third at the end of level II. The level I axilla clips were included 65% of the time and the level II 50% of the time in the breast field radiograph (39). In each of these studies, the superior (cephalad) border of the radiation field was designed to include the clinical extent of the breast with a 1 to 2 cm margin and was typically located 1 to 3 cm inferior (caudal) to the humeral head on a simulation radiograph of the medial tangent field. A high tangent technique that places the superior border of the field at the humeral head has been shown to improve the inclusion of the ALND and SNB clips in the breast field (37). A modified high tangent technique, defined as the superior (cephalad) border at the humeral head and the deep border of the field to include 2 cm of lung, further improved the inclusion of the surgical clips to 95% and 80%, respectively, for SNB and ALND (37).

Numerous investigators have used three-dimensional CT volumes to evaluate the dose delivered to the axillary nodes with breast irradiation (Table 43.4) (40–43). For three of these studies (40–42), the levels of the axilla were delineated on the archived RT planning CT of patients previously treated with standard breast irradiation. The breast plans were then reconstructed and evaluated with regard to dose–volume coverage of the axilla. Although a somewhat diverse definition of the axillary volume was used, these studies demonstrated

Table 43.4	DEGREE OF AXILLARY NODE INCLUSION BY THE BREAST IRRADIATION FIELDS					
Institution, Author (Reference)	Year	N	RT Method	Measure	Inclusion (%)	
Memorial Sloan-Kettering CC, McCormick et al. (36)	2002	45	2-D	≥5 ALND clips in tangent	38	
MD Anderson CC, Schlembach et al. (37)	2001	65	2-D	SN clips in tangents	85	
		39	2-D	ALND clips in tangents	43	
Brown University, Chung et al. (38)	2002	36	2-D	SNB clips in tangents	94	
Perugia University, Aristei et al. (39)	2001	35	2-D	3 clips: L-I, L-II, L-III	L-I: 65 L-II: 50	
Universidad Nacional de Cordoba, Zunino et al. (40)	2007	31	3-D	SNB volume 95% included in: 50 Gy isodose line	23.5	
European Institute of Oncology, Orecchia et al. (41)	2005	15	3-D	Level I axillary volume included in: 80% prescribed dose 100% prescribed dose	30.7 2.7	
University of Washington, Reed et al. (42)	2005	50	3-D	LI-II axilla volume included in: 95% prescribed dose	55	
		18	3-D	ALND clip volume included in: 95% prescribed dose	80	
University of Massachusetts, Reznik et al. (43)	2005	35	3-D	L-I, L-II, L-III, Rotter's nodal Volumes included in: 95% prescribed dose	*ST* L-I 51 L-II 26 L-III 15 R 59	*HT* 79 51 49 96

CC, Cancer Center; 2-D, 2-dimensional; 3-D, 3-dimensionl; ALND, axillary node dissection; SNB, sentinel node; L-I, level I axilla; L-II, level II axilla; L-III, level III axilla; ST, standard tangential radiation field; HT, high tangential radiation field.

that only 23% to 55% of the nodal volume was receiving the prescribed radiation dose (Table 43.4). In a University of Massachusetts study, the levels of the axilla and Rotter's nodes were contoured onto 35 CT scans (43). Two plans were then developed; the first was a standard breast irradiation with the cephalad border placed below the humeral head at about the inferior aspect of the clavicular head, and the second was a high tangent such that the superior border was placed at the inferior aspect of the humeral head. A greater proportion of all of the delineated axillary nodal volumes received the prescribed dose with the use of the high tangent technique, as seen in Table 43.4.

The amount of axilla included in the breast radiation field is illustrated in Figure 43.2A–D with the same CT case utilized in Figure 43.1A–B. For comparison, the amount of the delineated axillary level receiving 45 Gy was assessed as well as the volume of the ipsilateral lung receiving 20 Gy or more (V20). In Figure 43.3A, a standard breast field without intent to treat any of the axilla delivered 45 Gy to 38% of level I, no dose to level II, and the V20 for the lung was 9.5%. When a high tangent technique is used (Fig. 43.3B) by placing the superior border at the humeral head, 45 Gy is delivered to 78% of level I, 1% of level II, and the V20 for the lung is 9.75%. A modified high tangent technique (Fig. 43.3C), as described by a M.D. Anderson Cancer Center study (37), resulted in 45 Gy delivered to 83% of level I, 3% of level II, with a V20 for the lung of 14.2%. Finally, a customized tangent designed to include the level I and II nodal volumes resulted in the best coverage, with 45 Gy delivered to 100% of level I, 95% of level II, and a V20 for lung of 13.2%. Smitt and Goffinet (44) previously described the advantage of customized breast tangent fields for improving the dose delivered to the low axilla volume in six cases by using CT-based three-dimensional treatment planning. It is of particular importance when the breast fields are modified that care is taken to minimize inadvertent dose to the ipsilateral lung and contralateral breast.

MANAGEMENT SUMMARY

- The available data suggest that axillary irradiation yields low rates of axillary recurrence in cN0 patients comparable to ALND, but with less morbidity.
- Axillary irradiation instead of a completion ALND following a positive SNB is under investigation in ongoing randomized clinical trials. Until these results are known, completion axillary dissection is the standard of care for a patient with a positive sentinel node.
- Axillary irradiation may prove to be a reasonable alternative to a completion ALND following a positive SNB when the findings from axillary dissection will not change the adjuvant systemic treatment plan.
- The most common method of axillary irradiation is separate field(s), which includes levels I through III of the axilla and supraclavicular nodes and is matched to the breast or chest wall radiation fields. Typically a posteroanterior field is used in addition to an anteroposterior field to provide better coverage of the level I and II nodes.
- A dose of 45 to 50 Gy with standard radiation fractionation of 1.8 to 2.0 Gy is recommended for axillary irradiation.
- Individualized chemotherapy-based radiation treatment planning is recommended to ensure adequate dose coverage of the targeted nodal volumes and to minimize excessive dose heterogeneity and inadvertent normal tissue radiation.
- For those patients who did not undergo completion ALND for a positive SNB and radiation is selected as treatment, a high tangent technique or a customized breast radiation field can be used to irradiate levels I and II of the axilla in selected favorable cases, such as patients with T1 tumors without LVI or extranodal extension and a micrometastases (≤2 mm) or a solitary positive sentinel node.

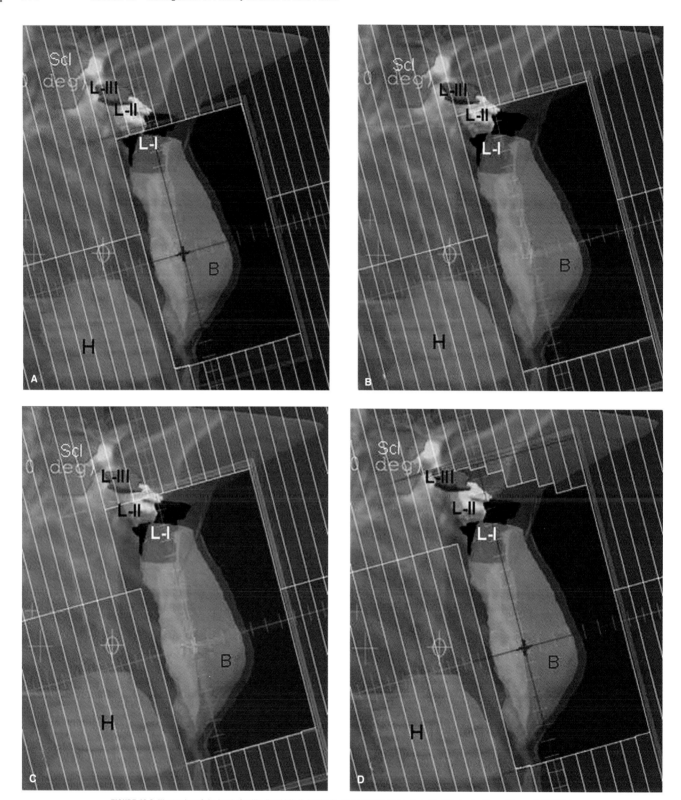

FIGURE 43.2. Illustration of the level of axilla (level I [L-I], level II [L-II], level III [L-III]) included in **(A)** standard breast tangent, **(B)** "high tangent" technique, **(C)** modified "high tangent" technique, and **(D)** customized breast tangent. B, breast; H, heart; Scl, supraclavicular.

REFERENCES

1. Orr R. The impact of prophylactic axillary node dissection on breast cancer survival: a Bayesian meta-analysis. *Ann Surg Oncol* 1999;6(1):109–116.
2. Clarke M, Collins R, Darby S, et al. Effects of radiotherapy and of differences in the extent of surgery for early breast cancer on local recurrence and 15-year survival: an overview of the randomised trials. *Lancet* 2005;366(9503):2087–2106.
3. Harris E, Hwang W, Seyednejad F, et al. Prognosis after regional lymph node recurrence in patients with stage I–II breast carcinoma treated with breast conservation therapy. *Cancer* 2003;98(10):481–488.
4. Konkin D, Tyldesley S, Kennecke H, et al. Management and outcomes of isolated axillary node recurrence in breast cancer. *Arch Surg* 2006;141:867–874.
5. Engel J, Kerr J, Schlesinger-Raab A, et al. Axilla surgery severely affects quality of life: results of a 5-year prospective study in breast cancer patients. *Breast Cancer Res Treat* 2003;79:47–57.
6. Langer I, Guller U, Berclaz G, et al. Morbidity of sentinel lymph node biopsy (SLN) alone versus SLN and completion axillary lymph node dissection after breast surgery. A prospective Swiss multicenter study on 659 patients. *Ann Surg* 2007;245:452–461.
7. Veronesi U, Paganelli G, Viale G, et al. A randomized comparison of sentinel node biopsy with routine axillary dissection in breast cancer. *N Engl J Med* 2003;349:546–553.

8. Kim T, Giuliano A, Lyman G. Lymphatic mapping and sentinel lymph node biopsy in early stage breast carcinoma. *Cancer* 2006;106:4–16.

9. Fisher B, Joeng J, Andersson S, et al. Twenty-five year follow-up of a randomized trial comparing radical mastectomy, total mastectomy, and total mastectomy followed by irradiation. *N Engl J Med* 2002;347(8):567–575.

10. Louis-Sylvestre C, Clough K, Asselain B, et al. Axillary treatment in conservative management of operable breast cancer: dissection or radiotherapy? Results of a randomized study with 15 years of follow-up. *J Clin Oncol* 2004;22:97–101.

11. Spruit P, Siesling S, Elferink M, et al. Regional radiotherapy versus an axillary lymph node dissection after lumpectomy: a safe alternative for an axillary lymph node dissection in a clinically uninvolved axilla in breast cancer. A case control study with 10 years follow-up. *Radiat Oncol* 2007;2:40.

12. Pejavar S, Wilson L, Haffty B. Regional nodal recurrence in breast cancer patients treated with conservative surgery and radiation therapy (BCS + RT). *Int J Radiat Oncol Biol Phys* 2006;66(5):1320–1327.

13. Hoebers F, Borer J, Hart A, et al. Primary axillary radiotherapy as axillary treatment in breast-conserving therapy for patients with breast carcinoma and clinically negative axillary lymph nodes. *Cancer* 2000;88(7):1633–1642.

14. Kuznetsova M, Graybill J, Zusag T, et al. Omission of axillary lymph node dissection in early stage breast cancer: effect on treatment outcome. *Radiology* 1995;197(2):507–510.

15. Galper S, Recht A, Silver B, et al. Is radiation alone adequate treatment to the axilla for patients with limited axillary surgery? Implications for treatment after a positive sentinel node biopsy. *Int J Radiat Oncol Biol Phys* 2000;48(1):125–132.

16. Wazer D, Erban J, Robert N, et al. Breast conservation in elderly women for clinically negative axillary lymph nodes without axillary dissection. *Cancer* 1994;74(3):878–883.

17. Halverson K, Taylor M, Perez C, et al. Regional node management and patterns of failure following conservative surgery and radiation therapy for stage I and II breast cancer. *Int J Radiat Oncol Biol Phys* 1993;26(4):593–599.

18. Martelli G, Boracchi P, De Palo M, et al. A randomized trial comparing axillary dissection to no axillary dissection in older patients with T1N0 breast cancer. Results after 5 years of follow-up. *Ann Surg* 2005;242(1):1–6.

19. Martelli G, Miceli R, Costa A, et al. Elderly breast cancer patients treated by conservative surgery alone plus adjuvant tamoxifen. Fifteen year results of a prospective trial. *Cancer* 2008;112(3):481–488.

20. Veronesi U, Orecchia R, Zurrida S, et al. Avoiding axillary dissection in breast cancer surgery: a randomized trial to assess the role of axillary radiotherapy. *Ann Oncol* 2005;16:383–388.

21. Greco M, Agresti R, Cascinelli N, et al. Breast cancer patients treated without axillary surgery. *Ann Surg* 2000;232(1):1–7.

22. Wong J, Recht A, Beard C, et al. Treatment outcome after tangential radiation therapy without axillary dissection in patients with early stage breast cancer and clinically negative axillary nodes. *Int J Radiat Oncol Biol Phys* 1997;39(4):915–920.

23. Liljegren G, Holmberg J, Bergh J, et al. 10-year results after sector resection with or without postoperative radiotherapy for stage I breast cancer: a randomized trial. *J Clin Oncol* 1999;17(8):2326–2333.

24. Mansel R, Fallowfield L, Kissin M, et al. Randomized multicenter trial of sentinel node biopsy versus standard axillary treatment in operable breast cancer: the ALMANAC trial. *J Natl Cancer Inst* 2006;98(9):599–609.

25. Hwang RF, Gonzalez-Angulo AM, Yi M, et al. Low locoregional failure rates in selected breast cancer patients with tumor-positive sentinel lymph nodes who do not undergo completion axillary node dissection. *Cancer* 2007;110:723–730.

26. Gadd M, Harris J, Taghian A, et al. Prospective study of axillary radiation without axillary dissection for breast cancer patients with a positive sentinel node. San Antonio Breast Conference (SABC) Proceedings, 2005 Abstract, 22.

27. Rutger E, Meijnen P, Bonnefoi H. Clinical trial update of the European Organization for Research and Treatment of Cancer Breast Cancer Group. *Breast Cancer Res* 2004;6:165–169.

28. Hurkmans C, Borger J, Rutgers E, et al. Quality assurance of axillary radiotherapy in the EORTC AMAROS trial 10981/22033: the dummy run. *Radiother Oncol* 2003;68:233–240.

29. Viale G, Maiorano E, Pruneri G, et al. Predicting the risk for additional axillary metastases in patients with breast carcinoma and positive sentinel lymph node biopsy. *Ann Surg* 2005;241(2):319–325.

30. Abdessalam S, Zervos E, Prasad M, et al. Predictors of positive axillary lymph nodes after sentinel lymph node biopsy in breast cancer. *Am J Surg* 2001;182(4):316–320.

31. Hwang R, Krishnamurthy S, Hunt K, et al. Clinicopathologic factors predicting involvement of nonsentinel axillary nodes in women with breast cancer. *Ann Surg Oncol* 2003;10(3):248–254.

32. Degnim A, Griffith K, Sabel M, et al. Clinicopathologic features of metastasis in nonsentinel lymph nodes of breast carcinoma patients. A meta-analysis. *Cancer* 2003;98:2307–2315.

33. Turner R, Chu K, Qi K, et al. Pathologic features associated with nonsentinel lymph node metastases in patients with metastatic breast carcinoma in a sentinel lymph node. *Cancer* 2000;89:574–581.

34. Samoilova E, Davis J, Hinson J, et al. Size of sentinel node tumor deposits and extent of axillary lymph node involvement: which breast cancer patients may benefit from less aggressive axillary dissections? *Ann Surg Oncol* 2007;14(8):2221–2227.

35. Katz A, Smith B, Golsham M, et al. Nomogram for the prediction of having four or more involved nodes for sentinel lymph node-positive breast cancer. *J Clin Oncol* 2008;26(13):2093–2098.

36. McCormick B, Botnick M, Hunt M, et al. Are the axillary lymph nodes treated by standard tangent breast fields? *J Surg Oncol* 2002;81:12–16.

37. Schlembach P, Buchholz T, Ross M, et al. Relationship of sentinel and axillary level I–II lymph nodes to tangential fields used in breast irradiation. *Int J Radiat Oncol Biol Phys* 2001;51(3):671–678.

38. Chung M, Dipetrillo, T, Hernandez S, et al. Treatment of the axilla by tangential breast radiotherapy in women with invasive breast cancer. *Am J Surg* 2002;184:401–402.

39. Aristei C, Chionne F, Marsella A, et al. Evaluation of level I and II axillary nodes included in the standard breast tangential fields and calculation of the administered dose: results of a prospective study. *Int J Radiat Oncol Biol Phys* 2001;51(1):69–73.

40. Zunino S, Garrigo E, Nestor C, et al. Dose received by the sentinel node volume during tangential radiation therapy to the breast. *Radiother Oncol* 2007;82:329–331.

41. Orecchia R, Huscher A, Leonardi M, et al. Irradiation with standard tangential breast fields in patients treated with conservative surgery and sentinel node biopsy: using a three-dimensional tool to evaluate the first level coverage of the axillary nodes. *Br J Surg* 2005;78:51–54.

42. Reed D, Lindsley S, Mann G, et al. Axillary lymph node dose with tangential breast irradiation. *Int J Radiat Oncol Biol Phys* 2005;61(2):358–364.

43. Reznik J, Cicchetti M, Degaspe B, et al. Analysis of axillary coverage during tangential radiation therapy to the breast. *Int J Radiat Oncol Biol Phys* 2005;26(13):163–168.

44. Smitt M, Goffinet D. Utility of three-dimensional planning for axillary node coverage with breast conserving radiation therapy: early experience. *Radiology* 1999;210(1):221–226.

Andrea L. Cheville and Nicole L. Stout

Primary breast cancer treatment is associated with long-term musculoskeletal problems in up to one third of patients. Problems arise secondary to normal tissue damage inflicted through cancer removal and staging procedures. Nerves, muscles, stroma, and lymphatics fall within surgical and radiation treatment fields, leaving them vulnerable to inadvertent injury. Musculoskeletal problems may develop within, adjacent to, or distant from treatment fields, manifesting as impairments in strength, flexibility, and integrated movement patterns (1). Table 44.1 lists impairments associated with breast cancer treatments, some of which may persist as many as 10 years following treatment. At all time points, impairments are associated with disability and diminished health-related quality of life (2–9). The likelihood of long-term disability correlates directly with the intensity of breast cancer treatment. More surgery (e.g., axillary lymph node dissection [ALND] vs. sentinel lymph node biopsy [SLNB]) and more radiation (e.g., four-field vs. tangent beam configurations) increase the probability that patients will develop musculoskeletal problems (2,4,10–14). Empirical data now reinforce theoretical concerns that musculoskeletal pathology at surgical and radiation sites will not spontaneously resolve independent of treatment (1,15).

Despite the clear correlation between breast cancer treatment and musculoskeletal problems, tissue-level changes remain ill defined. Radiation-induced fibrosis has been implicated on the basis of long-term follow-up studies (16,17). Additional radiation-related problems include shoulder capsule and epimysial contractures, compromised arterial perfusion with resultant muscle ischemia (18,19), lymphostasis, (20), and muscle hypertonicity secondary to neural irritation. Surgical procedures, even when limited to local tumor excision and SLNB, can produce maladaptive changes in posture and movement patterns. These changes are mediated through pain, scarring, and adaptive positioning in the postoperative period. Adjuvant chemotherapy may also contribute to musculoskeletal problems by reducing muscle mass (1) and oxidative capacity (21). The relative contributions of different cancer treatments and pathological processes to functional problems remain poorly characterized, despite growing understanding of treatment-related late toxicities. Fortunately, manual treatments and therapeutic exercises effectively address most problems.

Successful management of musculoskeletal problems depends on patients' willingness to perform therapeutic exercises. Because treatments are active and must often be continued indefinitely, their success requires a high level of commitment. Patient "buy in" can be substantially enhanced by the strong endorsement of the entire breast cancer treatment team. With increasing appreciation of latent treatment toxicities, the performance of prophylactic stretching and strengthening activities is now accepted as an integral component of comprehensive survivorship care (22). In the absence of such preventative activities, breast cancer survivors, treated years previously, may become uniquely vulnerable to delayed morbidities that manifest when the musculoskeletal and other systems senesce (23). This chapter outlines the evidence base regarding the epidemiology and management of breast cancer treatment–related musculoskeletal morbidity.

 EPIDEMIOLOGY

Functional disability following breast cancer treatment is primarily due to restricted range of motion (ROM), diminished strength, and persistent pain. Reported incidences of these problems vary widely depending on the type of breast cancer treatment, measurement technique, and duration of follow-up. Table 44.2 lists shoulder ROM deficits detected at different time points following surgery. Most patients experience an abrupt transient reduction in shoulder ROM after breast cancer surgeries (2,5). Two weeks postoperatively, incidences of restricted ROM as high as 86% have been reported following ALND and 45% following SLNB (24). At 6 weeks postoperatively the incidence of restricted shoulder abduction is substantially less, 26.5% after ALND and 24.8% after SLNB (25). Longitudinal studies suggest that restrictions in shoulder ROM gradually resolve and, in a majority of patients, ROM returns to baseline (7,26,27). Recovery may be gradual, requiring over 12 months for some patients. A significant minority of patients do not recover normal shoulder ROM in abduction, forward flexion, or external rotation. A history of ALND, modified radical mastectomy, and radiation therapy are associated with more significant and lasting limitations (6,7,25,27). Persistent deficits in ROM increase the likelihood that patients will report pain and difficulty performing activities of daily living that involve the shoulder (27).

Pain is a potentially disabling consequence of breast cancer treatment. Persistent shoulder pain 2 to 3 years following treatment is associated with poor mental and physical functioning (6). Pain is more common after ALND and axillary or supraclavicular radiation (4). Few studies differentiate musculoskeletal pain from neurogenic or lymphedema-related pain. As a consequence, the prevalence of posttreatment musculoskeletal pain is unknown. Table 44.3 lists reported pain prevalences. Reports do not specify pain etiologies nor do they report consistent outcome measures (e.g., presence or absence of pain vs. visual analog scores), making the data challenging to integrate. However, the table clearly demonstrates that a significant percentage of patients experience persistent pain in the shoulder or arm. In the authors' experience, symptomatic myofascial dysfunction and axillary webs are common primary sources of musculoskeletal pain following breast cancer treatment. The prevalence of myofascial dysfunction remains uncertain, however, axillary webs affect up to 72% of patients (24). Since breast cancer treatments may destabilize the balance of shoulder muscles, patients are placed at risk of secondary musculoskeletal problems (e.g., rotator cuff pathology and premature degenerative disease of the acromioclavicular and glenohumeral joints). However, the extent to which breast cancer treatment engenders these common problems has not been studied.

Strength deficits are less prevalent immediately following breast surgery but become increasingly problematic with time. This pattern has been appreciated for grip strength. In a longitudinal cohort, mean grip strength decreased by 16.9 nm at 6 weeks and by 41.3 nm at 24 months after ALND, relative to preoperative values (7,25). A similar pattern was noted after SLNB, although the reduction was less pronounced, 5.8 nm at 6 weeks and 17.2 nm at 24 months. These reductions agree with highly reported prevalences of impaired grip strength that range from 16% to 40% (3,13,27–30). The influence of lymphedema on grip strength remains inadequately characterized but may be an important mediating factor (31).

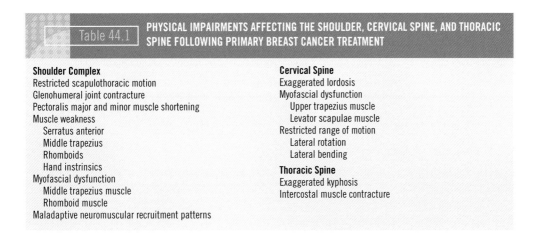

Table 44.1	**PHYSICAL IMPAIRMENTS AFFECTING THE SHOULDER, CERVICAL SPINE, AND THORACIC SPINE FOLLOWING PRIMARY BREAST CANCER TREATMENT**

Shoulder Complex
Restricted scapulothoracic motion
Glenohumeral joint contracture
Pectoralis major and minor muscle shortening
Muscle weakness
   Serratus anterior
   Middle trapezius
   Rhomboids
   Hand instrinsics
Myofascial dysfunction
   Middle trapezius muscle
   Rhomboid muscle
Maladaptive neuromuscular recruitment patterns

Cervical Spine
Exaggerated lordosis
Myofascial dysfunction
   Upper trapezius muscle
   Levator scapulae muscle
Restricted range of motion
   Lateral rotation
   Lateral bending

Thoracic Spine
Exaggerated kyphosis
Intercostal muscle contracture

Prevalences of reduced shoulder and arm strength are also high with self-reported limitations affecting up to 69% of patients (13). Objective reductions of 10 nm in shoulder abduction strength have been detected at 12 and 24 months following treatment (7,27). Shoulder strength deficits are more common following modified radical mastectomy (32). It has yet to be determined whether secondary musculoskeletal pain syndromes (e.g., rotator cuff tendinopathy) are responsible for shoulder strength deficits more than 2 years following treatment or if such deficits are confined to patients with reduced ROM. In the latter case, suboptimal muscle length–tension relationships could account for the finding.

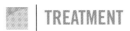

TREATMENT

Shoulder function depends on the coordinated recruitment of multiple muscles to perform even basic activities. For this reason, although deficits may initially be discreet, few problems remain isolated. The onset of secondary problems occurs commonly when patients lose flexibility in shoulder extension due to pectoral muscle tightness. Secondary strength and biomechanical deficits develop in uninvolved muscles. The anterior deltoid and coracobrachialis muscles, for example, may adopt dysfunctional length–tension relationships and firing patterns, which cause weakness

Table 44.2	**PREVALENCE AND SEVERITY OF SHOULDER RANGE OF MOTION DEFICITS AT DIFFERENT TIME POINTS FOLLOWING BREAST CANCER SURGERY**

Outcome Measure	Author (Reference)	6 wks ALND	6 wks SLNB	3 mos ALND	3 mos SLNB	6 mos ALND	6 mos SLNB	9–12 mos ALND	9–12 mos SLNB	24 mos ALND	24 mos SLNB	>2 yrs ALND	>2 yrs SLNB
Mean decrease from ipsilateral baseline AB	Rietman et al. 2003, 2006 (7,25)	26.4°	24.7°							21.0°	5.5°		
	Purushotham et al. 2005 (58)							6.3°	3.1°				
	Mansel et al. 2006 (26)			4.2°	1.9°	2.3°	1.5°	1.9°	2.5°				
Mean difference in AB relative to untreated shoulder	Hack et al. 1999 (3)											6.4°	
ROM <160° AB	Ernst et al. 2002 (32)							14.0%				8.0%	
ROM <20° normal value ≥1 plane	Langer et al. 2007 (51)											11.3%	3.5%
Self-reported limitation ROM	Leidenius et al. 2005 (52)											34.0%	16.0%
	Warmuth et al. 1998 (50)											8.0%	
	Veronesi et al. 2003 (49)					27.0%	0.0%			21.0%	0.0%		
ROM < normative values any plane	Lauridsen et al. 2008 (12)											35%	
Mean ROM (normal = 180°)	Rietman et al. 2004 (27)											156.6°AB	
	Gosselink et al. 2003 (2)			FF 126°	MRM 150°	BCT							
	Peintinger et al. 2003 (5)							143.8° AB		158.9° AB			

ALND, axillary lymph node dissection; SLNB, sentinel lymph node biopsy; FF, forward flexion; AB, abduction; BCT, breast-conservation therapy; MRM, modified radical mastectomy.
[a]For studies that did not collect data at specified intervals, the elapsed time after surgery is the cohort average.

Table 44.3	REPORTED PAIN PREVALENCES AND INTENSITIES FOLLOWING AT DIFFERENT TIME POINTS FOLLOWING BREAST CANCER SURGERIES										

		Elapsed Time after Breast Cancer Surgery[a]									
		≤6 wks		6 mos		9–12 mos		24 mos		>2 yrs	
Outcome Measure	Author (Reference)	ALND	SLNB	ALND	SLNB	ALND	SLNB	ALND	SLNB	ALND	SLNB
Mean change in EORTC QLQ-C30 Pain Scale Score	Peintinger et al. 2003 (5)	20.2	−2			7.2	0.1				
VAS (0–100) change from preoperative baseline	Rietman et al. 2003, 2006 (7,25)	1.3	1.1					8.7	0.6		
VAS > 0	Ernst et al. 2002 (32)									50.7%[b]	
	Peintinger et al. 2003 (5)					11.3	6.8				
Mean VAS score (0–100)	Hack et al. 1999 (3)									17.3	
	Rietman et al. 2004 (27)									25.0[b]	
Pain in neck, arm, or shoulder ≥2x/week	Lauridsen (2008)(12)									31.0%	
Severe or very severe axillary aching	Temple et al. 2002 (48)					19%	11%				
Sporadic or continuous axillary pain	Veronesi et al. 2003 (49)			91%	16%			39%	8%		
	Warmuth et al. 1998 (50)									30.0%	
	Hack et al. 1999 (3)									31.1%	
Shoulder/arm pain	Langer et al. 2007 (51)									21.2%	8.1%
	Voogd et al. 2003 (8)									28.3%[b]	
Arm pain	Leidenius et al. 2005 (52)									30.0%	12.0%

ALND, axillary lymph node dissection; SLNB, sentinel lymph node biopsy; EORTIC, European Organisation for Research and Treatment of Cancer; VAS, visual analog scale.
[a]For studies that did not collect data at specified intervals, the elapsed time after surgery is the cohort average.
[b]No distinction made between ALND and SLNB.

and further deviation from normal biomechanics (33). Over time clusters of related impairments may develop and produce global shoulder dysfunction. Addressing problems in isolation, whether primary or secondary will be limitedly successful at best. It is more clinically useful to treat generalized shoulder disability arising from multiple, interrelated impairments as an integrated whole.

Virtually all exercise and manual treatment-based approaches benefit musculoskeletal problems provided they are administered in a structured and monitored fashion (9–11,14,34–37). Regimens tested with randomized, controlled study designs are consistently superior to the common practice of providing patients with illustrated exercise sheets after surgery without formal follow-up. The fact that a variety of therapeutic techniques offer benefit reflects the straightforward treatment goals of restoring normal flexibility, strength, postural alignment, and biomechanics to the upper truncal quadrant. Positive results have been reported with therapist-directed programs emphasizing disparate approaches such as general kinesthetics (37) and pectoral muscle stretches (36). Although a wide range of structured regimens yield benefit, all therapy programs should have several essential elements, which are listed in Table 44.4 and described below.

Range of Motion Activities

ROM activities restore normal flexibility and influence scar formation to prevent restrictions. Distensive forces influence collagen deposition during scarring such that fibers align in an orderly fashion (38). With adequate traction, the resultant scar will be supple and distensible and will support normal musculoskeletal function. As mentioned previously, muscles within surgical and radiation fields are of greatest concern, however, adjacent and even remote muscle groups can also develop flexibility deficits. Therefore, comprehensive ROM activities should incorporate both treated and at-risk muscle groups.

Stretching can be performed in a variety of ways, and controlled studies have yet to shed light on which techniques are

most effective in breast cancer populations. Several general caveats apply:

1. ROM activities should never be pulsatile, painful, or overly aggressive.
2. Pain or swelling following ROM activities mandates revision of the program.
3. Patients should breath deeply and consciously during ROM activities to reduce sympathetic tone.
4. ROM activities should continue in an abbreviated fashion long after normal flexibility has been restored to prevent latent fascial contractures.

Active ROM activities can begin 7 days after breast cancer surgeries provided patients have not undergone breast reconstruction. In the latter case, patients should clear all physical rehabilitation activities with their plastic surgeons. Initial stretches include shoulder shrugs; shoulder retraction; wall walking; rowing motions; cervical rotation, extension, and lateral bending; and cane-based overhead stretches. Most institutions have printed sheets illustrating these activities, which are provided to patients on hospital dismissal.

Once patients' drains have been removed, a formal physical therapy evaluation will ensure that patients are performing ROM activities correctly and that their recovery is following a normal trajectory. This visit can be used to demonstrate how patients should advance their ROM activities, to educate patients in the long-term protective benefits of regular stretching, and to provide instruction in breathing techniques (e.g., breath stacking) (39). The latter will preserve intercostal muscle excursion. Patients should also be alerted to contact a health care provider if they have not recovered full, painless shoulder ROM 1 month prior to the start of radiation.

The major and minor pectoral muscles merit special attention as they are in proximity to breast surgeries, receive up to 60 Gy with conventional breast tangent beams (40), and may be affected by implant-based breast reconstruction. Pectoral

Table 44.4	**ESSENTIAL ELEMENTS OF ALL COMPREHENSIVE REHABILITATION PROGRAMS FOLLOWING PRIMARY BREAST CANCER TREATMENT**

Flexibility/Range of Motion Exercises

Shoulder:	Forward flexion
	Scaption (plane of the scapula; ~20 degrees of cross-abduction)
	Abduction
	Extension at 0 degrees and 90 degrees of abduction
	Internal/external rotation
Thorax:	Abdominal muscles: rectus and obliques
	Pectoral muscles
	Intercostal muscles
Cervical spine	Lateral rotation
	Lateral bending
	Extension

Progressive Resistive/Strengthening Exercises

Shoulder:	Scapular retractor muscles
Thorax:	Spinal extensor muscles
Cervical spine:	Spinal extensor muscles

Activities for Posture and Biomechanics

Education
Rationale for exercises (e.g., need for continued stretching activities)
Precautions (e.g., lymphedema)
Signs of complications (e.g., strain, infection, seroma)

Tailored Home Program
Instructions for tapering over time
Indefinite maintenance activities as needed
Emphasis on limited, "essential" exercises

stretching should be a central therapeutic focus since tightness produces well-characterized, maladaptive changes in shoulder biomechanics (33). Several approaches to pectoral stretching are illustrated in Figures 44.1 through 44.3. The standing corner stretch in Figure 44.1A and 44.1B should be held for at least five deep breaths, with the patient leaning forward and allowing her body weight to gently carry her into the stretch. The abdominal muscles should be lightly engaged, tilting the pelvis forward to protect the lower back, as illustrated by the curved arrow. The positions in Figures 44.2A–D should be passively maintained for as long as 15 minutes on a firm surface. The progression from 44.2A to 44.2D illustrates increasing shoulder external rotation, which places greater traction on the pectoral muscles and intensifies the stretch. At no time should patients experience discomfort. The pectoral stretch can also be increased by placing a pillow, rolled towel, or bolster between the scapulae (Fig. 44.3), ensuring that the head is adequately supported with a pillow to avoid anterior cervical muscle strain.

Strengthening

Resistive exercises normalize focal strength deficits, ensure adequate strength for normal biomechanics, and prevent periscapular muscle strain. Strength deficits are rarely immediately apparent after surgery in the absence of long thoracic nerve injury. More commonly, evaluations for pain reveal weakness or myofascial dysfunction of the muscles that act on the scapula and upper arm. Strength deficits generally respond to incremental, isotonic resistive activities in all but the rare cases of significant axonal damage. Muscle spasm and pain must be addressed before initiating strengthening exercise. A "no pain no gain" approach simply aggravates the problem and may aversively condition the patient. Resistance can be offered by Thera-Bands (Hygenic Corp, Akron, Ohio), light weights, circuit training equipment, or even soup cans. Activities should target the scapular retractor (middle trapez-

ius, rhomboids), scapular elevator (upper trapezius, levator scapulae), and thoracic spinal extensor muscles. The risk of inciting lymphedema mandates that resistive exercises be initiated at a low level and increased gradually with an emphasis on stamina rather than strength. Patients considered at

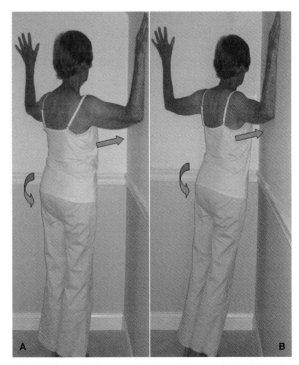

FIGURE 44.1. Wall stretches for pectoralis major and minor muscles should be performed with the abdominal muscles engaged to protect the low back as indicated by the arrow. Patients should allow their weight to gently carry them forward while focusing on breathing in a slow relaxed fashion. The stretch can be held for 5 to 10 breathes.

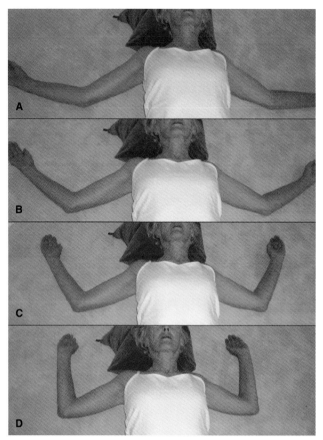

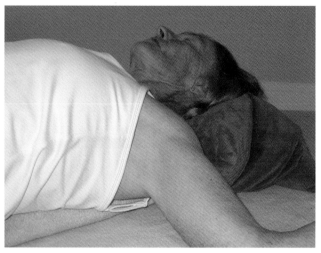

FIGURE 44.3. A rolled towel, pillow, or bolster can be placed between the shoulder blades to achieve greater pectoral extension. Patients should be encouraged to relax over the prop in a sustained, passive stretch.

FIGURE 44.2. Sustained anterior chest wall stretch which becomes more aggressive as shoulder external rotation increases from (A) through (D). The head should be supported to avoid strain of the anterior cervical muscles.

risk of developing lymphedema should inspect their arms following sessions and consider use of a prophylactic garment (http://www.lymphnet.org/pdfDocs/nlnexercise.pdf). The choice to use a garment should be discussed and supervised by a health care professional familiar with lymphedema.

Posture

Effective postural therapy requires restoration of adequate strength and flexibility. Once this essential foundation has been laid, patients can progress to activities designed to enhance truncal alignment. In the discussion that follows, posture and alignment are used interchangeably. Postural work following breast cancer treatment strives to eliminate exaggerated thoracic kyphosis, scapular protraction, compensatory cervical lordosis, and asymmetry in the shoulder girdle. Postural work can be deceptively subtle and, although not inherently difficult, may be more challenging than ROM and strength-building activities. Most patients recognize "good" posture and can adopt it with little concentrated effort provided they have the requisite strength and flexibility. However, many patients do not maintain "good" posture once their concentration drifts, as it eventually must, to an alternate focus. When no longer deliberately maintaining "good" posture, patients lapse gradually into their default alignment.

A host of factors operating within muscles and at different levels of the peripheral and central nervous systems determine patients' default posture. Several important factors may be influenced by breast cancer treatment: muscle length–tension relationships, muscle spindle and Golgi tendon organ sensitivity, and afferent proprioceptive input. The central nervous system responds to afferent proprioceptive input with efferent output that determines muscle tone and patients' default alignment (41,42). When an individual deviates too far from her default posture, afferent input triggers subconscious, autorighting mechanisms that restore her default.

Postural therapies refine patients' default alignment to avoid secondary musculoskeletal problems, reduce stress on osseous and articular structures, and support normal biomechanics. Effective therapies spare patients future difficulties, including premature osteoarthritis, neural impingement, and rotator cuff dysfunction. Fortunately, the physiological determinants of posture respond predictably to therapies. Once flexibility and strength have been normalized, postural work begins by bringing patients passively into proper alignment. Therapists then work through active assistive techniques to teach patients selective recruitment and relaxation of discrete muscles in order to maintain proper alignment. Work is ideally performed in front of mirrors that provide visual feedback from several planes (e.g., frontal, oblique, etc.). In this way patients can begin to appreciate when they are properly aligned and self-correct when out of alignment. Therapy's ultimate goal is automatic self-correction independent of visual feedback. With due diligence, patients develop a more functional default alignment and sustain it through subconscious, autorighting mechanisms. It should be noted that many patients have poor posture when diagnosed with breast cancer, and it is not the medical profession's responsibility to eradicate poor posture. However, attention to treatment-related problems that increase patients' vulnerability to future morbidities is an integral part of comprehensive cancer care.

Biomechanics

Biomechanics can be thought of as dynamic posture, or the interrelationship of body parts as patients engage in integrated, multiplanar movements. Restoration of normal upper quadrant biomechanics represents the culmination of successful therapy. Treatments attempt to preserve the optimized static relationships achieved through postural therapies. Initially therapists provide active assistance and tactile cuing to optimize patients' performance of simple motions such as shoulder abduction. Once patients can perform these motions with proper biomechanics, they are encouraged to do so repeatedly with visual feedback from mirrors and verbal cuing. Eventually patients are taught to self-correct independent of feedback while performing increasingly complex activities in several planes.

Timing

Much research to date has examined the timing of therapies following breast cancer surgeries. Precipitous and overly aggressive mobilization is associated with seroma formation, however, delayed therapy places patients at theoretical risk of shoulder contracture (43). A robust evidence base supports the safety and efficacy of gentle postoperative shoulder, neck, and truncal mobilization provided that shoulder forward flexion and abduction are restricted to 90 degrees for the first postoperative week (15,44,45). Thereafter, stretching and strengthening activities can be advanced as tolerated in the absence of breast reconstruction with autologous tissues.

The literature provides far less guidance in the optimal type, intensity, and timing of therapy after the subacute postoperative period. Continuous physiotherapy for 3 months following surgery is beneficial (10) but difficult to justify in the current era of medical cost containment. A majority of patients remain free of long-term musculoskeletal problems after limited physical therapy visits following removal of their surgical drains (15,44,45). This low musculoskeletal complication rate may reflect the current trend toward less anatomically disruptive treatments. Patients with advanced age or lymphedema and those who undergo ALND; chest wall, or supraclavicular radiation treatments; or breast reconstruction are at up to 10 times greater risk of developing shoulder disability (2,4,10–13,31). Anecdotal experience supports more extended physical therapy for these patients, with the goals of detecting incipient problems, education in self-diagnosis and referral, and provision with long-term prophylactic ROM and strengthening programs. When feasible, coordination of physical therapy visits with radiation treatments allows patients to minimize travel and time away from life responsibilities.

 ## POTENTIAL CONCERNS

Several clinical findings should alert physicians to the possibility that patients require additional attention and care. Lymphedema remains a concern when patients exercise, particularly if they have undergone ALND with or without axillary or supraclavicular irradiation. Patients who have undergone these treatments will generally benefit from a visit with a lymphedema therapist certified by the Lymphology Association of North America (LANA) to review precautions and formulate a safe yet effective rehabilitation program. (LANA-certified therapists can be located at http://www.clt-lana.org.)

Axillary web syndrome affects up to 72% of patients following breast cancer treatment (24). Affected patients develop palpable "cords" in their axillae (Fig. 44.4) that can extend distally as far as the wrist. These cords may or may not be painful. If painful, discomfort is triggered by shoulder abduction, which increases tension in the cords. Conjecture regarding the tissue composition of these cords persists despite a small case series that characterized resected cords as lymphatics or veins and fibrosed connective tissue (46). Longitudinal studies indicate that the cords resolve independent of treatment. However, their presence may be disturbing to patients and discourage them from performing shoulder ROM activities. Severely painful cords may warrant administration of as-needed anti-inflammatory or even opioid analgesics (20). If cords are painful or persist beyond 2 months after surgery, patients should be referred to a physical therapist familiar in treating breast cancer patients.

Added concern should always attend the rehabilitation of patients who have undergone breast reconstruction with autologous tissues. The range of harvesting and reconstruction techniques coupled with practitioner variability makes it difficult to accurately predict the locations and fragility of vascular anastomoses. Referral to a cancer rehabilitation physician specialist is

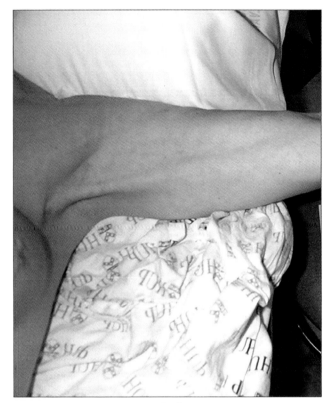

FIGURE 44.4. Axillary web syndrome or "cording."

advisable prior to initiating physical activity, particularly if reconstruction involved muscle tissue, as in transverse rectus abdominis or latissimus dorsi muscle flaps.

 ## INTEGRATED EXERCISE APPROACHES

An ever-expanding array of fitness approaches is available to breast cancer survivors at health clubs and, increasingly, cancer centers. Some approaches such as Feldenkrais movement therapy are long-established traditions utilized routinely by physical therapists (47). Other approaches have only become widely available within the past decade. To name but a few, patients may encounter Pilates, yoga, Alexander technique, Mensendieck exercise therapy, and tai chi. Each approach has unique emphases and most will benefit breast cancer survivors beyond enhancing general fitness and body awareness. For example, the Alexander technique focuses on craniocervical alignment, a critical dimension of postural therapy (47). Patients should be encouraged to explore different approaches with several caveats. First, most fitness instructors are unaware of lymphedema precautions, hence patients must function as their own self-advocates to protect against inadvertent lymphatic overload. Second, breast cancer patients' fitness regimens should include pectoral muscle stretching, strengthening of scapular retractors, and postural exercises, as discussed above. If an integrated exercise approach does not include these elements, patients will need to independently supplement with guidance from a health professional.

A number of exercise regimens have been tailored to breast cancer survivors and marketed through video classes, books, and weekend workshops. Table 44.5 lists several available resources. The developers of such approaches may or may not have formal clinical training and familiarity with the unique physical vulnerabilities associated with breast cancer treatment. No empiric data support the efficacy or safety of these tailored approaches. In the authors' opinion, the worth of such media derives from patients' enhanced comfort levels and enthusiasm.

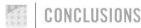

Medium	Author (Reference)	Title	Publisher	Year
Book	Kaelin (53)	The Breast Cancer Survivor's Fitness Plan	McGraw-Hill	2007
Compact disc	Cowden and Poppenberg (59)	Strength and Courage: Exercises for Breast Cancer Survivors	University of Pittsburgh Medical Center	2007
Book	Stumm (54)	Recovering from Breast Surgery: Exercises to Strengthen Your Body and Relieve Pain	Hunter House Inc.	1995
Book	Lebed Davis et al. (55)	Thriving After Breast Cancer: Essential Healing Exercises for Body and Mind	Broadway Books	2002
Book	Halverstadt and Leonard (56)	Essential Exercises for Breast Cancer Survivors	Harvard Common Press	2000
Book	Essert (57)	Breast Cancer WaterWork: Management Through Aquatic Exercise and Rehab Techniques	ECS Printing	2004

Table 44.5   **PATIENT-ORIENTED BREAST CANCER–SPECIFIC EXERCISE RESOURCES**

If patients feel more confident with breast cancer–oriented fitness materials, then they are unquestionably worthwhile.

CONCLUSIONS

Musculoskeletal problems involving the shoulder and upper truncal quadrant are common following primary breast cancer treatment, associated with disability, and a source of reduced health-related quality of life. A majority of patients recover normal strength and ROM after transient postoperative deficits resolve, however, a significant proportion develop chronic problems. Modified radical mastectomy, ALND, breast reconstruction, and axillary or supraclavicular irradiation increase the likelihood of chronicity.

All breast cancer patients should receive formal instruction in gentle progressive shoulder and arm ROM following surgery. Forward flexion and abduction should be restricted to 90 degrees until the seventh postoperative day and increased as tolerated thereafter. Patients at increased risk of long-term musculoskeletal problems should receive additional physical therapy with the goal of prevention and education in long-term risk reduction and self-advocacy. Irrespective of risk, all exercise programs should include several essential elements, including anterior chest wall stretching, strengthening of scapular retractor muscles, as well as activities to foster optimal posture and biomechanics. Patients treated with radiation therapy should indefinitely continue a limited ROM program targeting the anterior chest wall and shoulder muscles.

Empiric evidence suggests that musculoskeletal problems can be prevented with routine rehabilitative interventions after primary breast cancer treatment. Simple stretching, strengthening, and postural activities have the capacity to improve breast cancer survivors' health-related quality of life and represent an integral part of comprehensive care.

References

1. Shamley DR, Srinanaganathan R, Weatherall R, et al. Changes in shoulder muscle size and activity following treatment for breast cancer. *Breast Cancer Res Treat* 2007;106(1):19–27.
2. Gosselink R, Rouffaer L, Vanhelden P, et al. Recovery of upper limb function after axillary dissection. *J Surg Oncol* 2003;83(4):204–211.
3. Hack TF, Cohen L, Katz J, et al. Physical and psychological morbidity after axillary lymph node dissection for breast cancer. *J Clin Oncol* 1999;17(1):143–149.
4. Kwan W, Jackson J, Weir LM, et al. Chronic arm morbidity after curative breast cancer treatment: prevalence and impact on quality of life. *J Clin Oncol* 2002;20 (20):4242–4248.
5. Peintinger F, Reitsamer R, Stranzl H, et al. Comparison of quality of life and arm complaints after axillary lymph node dissection vs. sentinel lymph node biopsy in breast cancer patients. *Br J Cancer* 2003;89(4):648–652.
6. Rietman JS, Dijkstra PU, Hoekstra HJ, et al. Late morbidity after treatment of breast cancer in relation to daily activities and quality of life: a systematic review. *Eur J Surg Oncol* 2003;29(3):229–238.
7. Rietman JS, Geertzen JH, Hoekstra HJ, et al. Long term treatment related upper limb morbidity and quality of life after sentinel lymph node biopsy for stage I or II breast cancer. *Eur J Surg Oncol* 2006;32(2):148–152.
8. Voogd AC, Ververs JM, Vingerhoets AJ, et al. Lymphoedema and reduced shoulder function as indicators of quality of life after axillary lymph node dissection for invasive breast cancer. *Br J Surg* 2003;90(1):76–81.
9. Karki A, Simonen R, Malkia E, et al. Impairments, activity limitations and participation restrictions 6 and 12 months after breast cancer operation. *J Rehabil Med* 2005;37(3):180–188.
10. Beurskens CH, van Uden CJ, Strobbe LJ, et al. The efficacy of physiotherapy upon shoulder function following axillary dissection in breast cancer, a randomized controlled study. *BMC Cancer* 2007;7:166.
11. Lauridsen MC, Christiansen P, Hessov I. The effect of physiotherapy on shoulder function in patients surgically treated for breast cancer: a randomized study. *Acta Oncol* 2005;44(5):449–457.
12. Lauridsen MC, Overgaard M, Overgaard J, et al. Shoulder disability and late symptoms following surgery for early breast cancer. *Acta Oncol* 2008;47(4):569–575.
13. Ververs JM, Roumen RM, Vingerhoets AJ, et al. Risk, severity and predictors of physical and psychological morbidity after axillary lymph node dissection for breast cancer. *Eur J Cancer* 2001;37(8):991–999.
14. Cinar N, Seckin U, Keskin D, et al. The effectiveness of early rehabilitation in patients with modified radical mastectomy. *Cancer Nurs* 2008;31(2):160–165.
15. Shamley DR, Barker K, Simonite V, et al. Delayed versus immediate exercises following surgery for breast cancer: a systematic review. *Breast Cancer Res Treat* 2005;90(3):263–271.
16. Bentzen SM, Overgaard M, Thames HD. Fractionation sensitivity of a functional endpoint: impaired shoulder movement after post-mastectomy radiotherapy. *Int J Radiat Oncol Biol Phys* 1989;17(3):531–537.
17. Johansson S, Svensson H, Denekamp J. Timescale of evolution of late radiation injury after postoperative radiotherapy of breast cancer patients. *Int J Radiat Oncol Biol Phys* 2000;48(3):745–750.
18. Aitken RJ, Gaze MN, Rodger A, et al. Arm morbidity within a trial of mastectomy and either nodal sample with selective radiotherapy or axillary clearance. *Br J Surg* 1989;76(6):568–571.
19. Blomlie V, Rofstad EK, Skjonsberg A, et al. Female pelvic bone marrow: serial MR imaging before, during, and after radiation therapy. *Radiology* 1995;194(2): 537–543.
20. Cheville AL, Tchou J. Barriers to rehabilitation following surgery for primary breast cancer. *J Surg Oncol* 2007;95(5):409–418.
21. Demark-Wahnefried W, Peterson BL, Winer EP, et al. Changes in weight, body composition, and factors influencing energy balance among premenopausal breast cancer patients receiving adjuvant chemotherapy. *J Clin Oncol* 2001;19(9): 2381–2389.
22. Ganz PA, Hahn EE. Implementing a survivorship care plan for patients with breast cancer. *J Clin Oncol* 2008;26(5):759–767.
23. Rao AV, Demark-Wahnefried W. The older cancer survivor. *Crit Rev Oncol Hematol* 2006;60(2):131–143.
24. Leidenius M, Leppanen E, Krogerus L, et al. Motion restriction and axillary web syndrome after sentinel node biopsy and axillary clearance in breast cancer. *Am J Surg* 2003;185(2):127–130.
25. Rietman JS, Dijkstra PU, Geertzen JH, et al. Short-term morbidity of the upper limb after sentinel lymph node biopsy or axillary lymph node dissection for stage I or II breast carcinoma. *Cancer* 2003;98(4):690–696.
26. Mansel RE, Fallowfield L, Kissin M, et al. Randomized multicenter trial of sentinel node biopsy versus standard axillary treatment in operable breast cancer: the ALMANAC trial. *J Natl Cancer Inst* 2006;98(9):599–609.
27. Rietman JS, Dijkstra PU, Geertzen JH, et al. Treatment-related upper limb morbidity 1 year after sentinel lymph node biopsy or axillary lymph node dissection for stage I or II breast cancer. *Ann Surg Oncol* 2004;11(11):1018–1024.
28. Tasmuth T, von Smitten K, Kalso E. Pain and other symptoms during the first year after radical and conservative surgery for breast cancer. *Br J Cancer* 1996;74(12): 2024–2031.
29. Maunsell E, Brisson J, Deschenes L. Psychological distress after initial treatment of breast cancer. Assessment of potential risk factors. *Cancer* 1992;70(1):120–125.
30. Hladiuk M, Huchcroft S, Temple W, et al. Arm function after axillary dissection for breast cancer: a pilot study to provide parameter estimates. *J Surg Oncol* 1992; 50(1):47–52.
31. Balzarini A, Lualdi P, Lucarini C, et al. Biomechanical evaluation of scapular girdle in patients with chronic arm lymphedema. *Lymphology* 2006;39(3):132–140.
32. Ernst MF, Voogd AC, Balder W, et al. Early and late morbidity associated with axillary levels I-III dissection in breast cancer. *J Surg Oncol* 2002;79(3):151–156.

33. Smith J, Dietrich CT, Kotajarvi BR, et al. The effect of scapular protraction on isometric shoulder rotation strength in normal subjects. *J Shoulder Elbow Surg* 2006; 15(3):339–343.

34. Box RC, Reul-Hirche HM, Bullock-Saxton JE, et al. Shoulder movement after breast cancer surgery: results of a randomised controlled study of postoperative physiotherapy. *Breast Cancer Res Treat* 2002;75(1):35–50.

35. Wingate L, Croghan I, Natarajan N, et al. Rehabilitation of the mastectomy patient: a randomized, blind, prospective study. *Arch Phys Med Rehabil* 1989;70(1):21–24.

36. Lee TS, Kilbreath SL, Refshauge KM, et al. Pectoral stretching program for women undergoing radiotherapy for breast cancer. *Breast Cancer Res Treat* 2007;102(3): 313–321.

37. de Rezende LF, Franco RL, de Rezende MF, et al. Two exercise schemes in postoperative breast cancer: comparison of effects on shoulder movement and lymphatic disturbance. *Tumori* 2006;92(1):55–61.

38. Ramtani S, Fernandes-Morin E, Geiger D. Remodeled-matrix contraction by fibroblasts: numerical investigations. *Comput Biol Med* 2002;32(4):283–296.

39. Baker WL, Lamb VJ, Marini JJ. Breath-stacking increases the depth and duration of chest expansion by incentive spirometry. *Am Rev Respir Dis* 1990;141(2):343–346.

40. Cheville A, Das I, Scheuermann J, et al. SPECT/CT imaging to assess alterations in lymphatic function 12 months post-radiation in patients with breast cancer. *Radiother Oncol* 2007;84[Suppl 1]:S51.

41. Morton SM, Bastian AJ. Cerebellar control of balance and locomotion. *Neuroscientist* 2004;10(3):247–259.

42. Gilman SNS. *Manter and Gatz' essentials of clinical neuroanatomy and neurophysiology*. Philadelphia: FA Davis, 1987.

43. Dawson I, Stam L, Heslinga JM, et al. Effect of shoulder immobilization on wound seroma and shoulder dysfunction following modified radical mastectomy: a randomized prospective clinical trial. *Br J Surg* 1989;76(3):311–312.

44. Bendz I, Fagevik Olsen M. Evaluation of immediate versus delayed shoulder exercises after breast cancer surgery including lymph node dissection—a randomised controlled trial. *Breast* 2002;11(3):241–248.

45. Schultz I, Barholm M, Grondal S. Delayed shoulder exercises in reducing seroma frequency after modified radical mastectomy: a prospective randomized study. *Ann Surg Oncol* 1997;4(4):293–297.

46. Moskovitz AH, Anderson BO, Yeung RS, et al. Axillary web syndrome after axillary dissection. *Am J Surg* 2001;181(5):434–439.

47. Jain S, Janssen K, DeCelle S. Alexander technique and Feldenkrais method: a critical overview. *Phys Med Rehabil Clin North Am* 2004;15(4):811–825.

48. Temple LK, Baron R, Cody HS 3rd, et al. Sensory morbidity after sentinel lymph node biopsy and axillary dissection: a prospective study of 233 women. *Ann Surg Oncol* 2002;9(7):654–662.

49. Veronesi U, Paganelli G, Viale G, et al. A randomized comparison of sentinel-node biopsy with routine axillary dissection in breast cancer. *N Engl J Med* 2003;349(6): 546–553.

50. Warmuth MA, Bowen G, Prosnitz LR, et al. Complications of axillary lymph node dissection for carcinoma of the breast: a report based on a patient survey. *Cancer* 1998;83(7):1362–1368.

51. Langer I, Guller U, Berclaz G, et al. Morbidity of sentinel lymph node biopsy (SLN) alone versus SLN and completion axillary lymph node dissection after breast cancer surgery: a prospective Swiss multicenter study on 659 patients. *Ann Surg* 2007;245(3):452–461.

52. Leidenius M, Leivonen M, Vironen J, et al. The consequences of long-time arm morbidity in node-negative breast cancer patients with sentinel node biopsy or axillary clearance. *J Surg Oncol* 2005;92(1):23–31.

53. Kaelin C. *The breast cancer survivor's fitness plan*. New York: McGraw-Hill, 2007.

54. Stumm D. *Recovering from breast surgery: exercises to strengthen your body and relieve pain*. Alameda, CA: Hunter House, 1995.

55. Lebed Davis S, Gunning S, Campbell A, et al. *Thriving after breast cancer*. New York: Broadway Books, 2002.

56. Halverstadt A, Leonard A. *Essential exercises for breast cancer survivors*. Boston: Harvard Common Press, 2000.

57. Essert M. *Breast cancer waterwork: management through aquatic exercise and rehab techniques*. ECS Printing, 2004.

58. Purushotham AD, Upponi S, Klevesath MB, et al. Morbidity after sentinel lymph node biopsy in primary breast cancer: results from a randomized controlled trial. *J Clin Oncol* 2005;23(19):4312–4321.

59. Cowden S, Poppenberg J. Strength and courage: exercises for breast cancer survivors. DVD. Available at http://www.strengthandcourage.net/.

Chapter 45
Lymphedema

Sarah A. McLaughlin, Sara Cohen, and Kimberly J. Van Zee

In 2007 more than 2.2 million breast cancer survivors were living in the United States, according to the Centers for Disease Control and Prevention. Improvement in breast cancer survival rates is attributed to advances in imaging, allowing for earlier detection, and to advances in treatment, allowing for more targeted drug therapy. With the increasing number of breast cancer survivors, issues affecting survivorship have come to the forefront of breast cancer research.

Upper extremity lymphedema has been one of the most dreaded complications of breast cancer treatment. The reported incidence ranges from 6% to 70% (1–14), but it has been difficult to quantify due to the lack of standard diagnostic and universal assessment criteria and to delayed onset of symptoms up to 20 years after breast cancer surgery (8). Lymphedema is a chronic, disfiguring, and potentially disabling condition characterized by progressive interstitial accumulation of protein-rich fluid, resulting in significant edema, hypertrophy, and eventually fibrosis of the extremity tissues. Worrying about the future development of lymphedema represents a source of significant patient anxiety after surgery. This anxiety is heightened after diagnosis as these patients are frequently frustrated by the lack of presurgery education and postoperative support by health care providers (15,16), as well as by the paucity of effective clinical trials to prevent lymphedema.

The symptoms of lymphedema frequently result in significant lifestyle modifications as patients may experience physical impairment. The development of severe upper extremity or hand swelling can lead to musculoskeletal pain and loss of shoulder mobility. Upper extremity pain and swelling can impair one's ability to perform activities of daily living, which may become more dramatic if symptoms affect the dominant arm. Additionally, many patients consciously avoid recreational activities or carrying children, and practice additional precautionary behaviors to keep symptoms from worsening (17). Furthermore, the severely edematous arm may be difficult to conceal and may serve as a lifelong reminder of the struggle with breast cancer. Lymphedema places patients at higher risk for recurrent bouts of cellulitis or lymphangitis. Therefore, caring for a lymphedematous extremity requires methodical attention to cleanliness and wound care, as these women are subject to poor wound healing, skin breakdown, and skin necrosis. Failure to control lymphedema may lead to elephantine trophic changes of the skin and, in rare cases, lethal lymphangiosarcoma (Stewart-Treves's syndrome).

The diagnosis of lymphedema has been reported to negatively impact one's quality of life (18–20), as patients suffer not only physical, but also psychosocial and adverse sexual consequences. A recent review of 18 studies confirmed the psychological sequelae of lymphedema, including distress, frustration, depression, anxiety, and social morbidities, such as changes in role function, insomnia, decreased self-confidence and body image, lack of social support, feelings of isolation, and financial problems (21–23). Risk factors for poor adjustment to living with lymphedema include poor social support, use of avoidant and reclusive styles of coping, and the presence of pain of any intensity (24). Interestingly, in one study, the perception of one's limb size instead of the objective arm volume was more influential on physical, psychological, and social symptoms experienced by the patient (23).

Finally, patient frustration may be compounded by the medical community's slow dedication of financial resources to research focused on investigating the etiology, physiology, progression, and treatment of lymphedema. At present, only 6 of 166 National Institutes of Health grants for supportive care after the diagnosis of breast cancer address issues relating to lymphedema. Five focus on treatment (three phase II trials and two phase I trials); only one focuses on prophylaxis in patients categorized as high-risk status (25). Insurance and Medicare coverage of treatment expenses for patients with lymphedema has been variable. Although Medicare supports the evaluation and treatment of lymphedema by a trained specialist, Medicare limits coverage of treatment to only occupational or physical therapists, eliminating nearly 30% of other lymphedema care providers (nurses, and massage therapists). Additionally, the U.S. Congress has discussed imposing financial limits for therapy services provided. Finally, compression garments, which are a mainstay of lymphedema treatment, are coded as "surgical bandages" and therefore not considered reimbursable for in-home use under the Medicare program. These treatment limitations can result in burdensome financial constraints for patients who need these treatment services over their lifetimes (26).

ANATOMY AND PATHOPHYSIOLOGY

The lymphatic system is composed of lymphatic capillaries, transporting vessels, and lymph nodes. The lymphatic system has a low oncotic pressure, allowing diffusion of protein-rich interstitial fluid into lymphatic vessels and transport to the venous system. In the upper extremities, the superficial lymphatic system is composed of valveless capillaries located at the dermal–subcutaneous level that communicate directly with collecting lymphatic vessels coursing through subcutaneous tissues with the superficial veins. These collecting vessels, or secondary lymphatics, drain into tertiary lymphatics, which progressively network and ascend to the axilla. On the left, these lymphatic vessels join other thoracic and intercostal lymphatic channels, draining into the thoracic duct, which empties into the left subclavian vein. A smaller right lymphatic duct drains the right upper extremity and neck and enters the right subclavian vein. Secondary and tertiary lymphatic vessels have valves to aid in the unidirectional propulsion of lymph fluid. Lymphatic flow is encouraged by active skeletal muscle contraction, causing intermittent compression of the subcutaneous compartment and by nearby arterial pulsations. The lymph nodes act as points of filtration throughout the lymphatic drainage process and serve a primarily immunologic function.

The vessels of the deep lymphatic system run beneath the muscular fascia near neurovascular bundles. Little communication exists between the superficial and deep systems, and lymphedema generally spares the deep component. The etiology of lymphedema is incompletely understood, but it results from impaired lymphatic transport. The quantity of fluid within the interstitial space is determined by the delicate balance of hydrostatic and oncotic pressures between the vascular capillaries and the interstitial space. More than 90% of fluid within the interstitial space is removed by the venous capillaries; what remains is normally returned to the vascular system by lymphatics. The combination of the negative oncotic pressure of the lymphatic vessels and their indistinct, virtually nonexistent basement membranes allow larger proteins and macromolecules, such as bacteria and cellular debris, to passively diffuse from the interstitium into the lymphatic system. When the lymphatic system is dysfunctional, fluid transport is disrupted and interstitial protein accumulates, increasing its oncotic pressure. This draws more fluid into the interstitium (27–29). Excessive accumulation of interstitial fluid due to impaired lymphatic transport is called *lymphedema*.

The cycle of lymphedema self-perpetuates as increased lymphatic fluid volume causes stretch in lymphatic vessels, leading to incompetent valves and further failure of lymph transport. Additionally, the stagnant bacteria ignites a chronic inflammatory cascade, recruiting macrophages and neutrophils to the interstitium for wound healing, and leading to collagen deposition and fibrosis, hindering lymphatic contraction. Furthermore, the severity of edema can be exacerbated by episodes of lymphangitis, which destroy lymphatic vessels, by an increase in interstitial fluid production, as occurs with chronic inflammation or recurrent cellulitis, or by an increase in hydrostatic pressure, as occurs with venous flow alterations or obstruction (30,31).

Clinical Evaluation of Upper Extremity Lymphedema

The clinical appearance of lymphedema varies based on the severity of swelling and the duration of symptoms. Evaluation for asymmetry is performed by multipositional physical examination with arms outstretched and then fully flexed resting on the hips. In addition to edema, clinicians should evaluate for early signs of lymphedema, including loss of skin turgor or loss of bony prominences at the olecranon or ulnar styloid processes. Palpation for firmness or fibrosis is an essential part of the examination that may also detect early skin changes representative of lymphedema.

Historically, lymphedematous swelling was classified into three stages (stages I, II, and III). However, according to the most recent International Society of Lymphology consensus statement, most clinicians treating lymphedema also recognize the subclinical stage 0 (32). This clinical classification is defined in Table 45.1.

Metrics

In addition to physical examination, both subjective instruments and objective measurement techniques have been used to diagnose and quantify lymphedema. Multiple studies employ patient interviews or questionnaires assessing for symptoms of edema, upper extremity tightness, aching, tenderness, breast swelling, and differences in arm, neck, or shoulder sizes as a means of diagnosing lymphedema (17,33,34). Although these patient perceptions of arm swelling are important and impart significant influence on quality of life issues, there is little literature examining their correlation with arm measurement changes consistent with lymphedema. The authors' recent prospective study of 936 women 5 years after axillary surgery found that patients with sentinel lymph node (SLN) biopsy report less arm swelling than is measured (3% vs. 5%), whereas patients that underwent axillary lymph node dissection (ALND) report more arm swelling than is measured (27% vs. 16%) (17,35). It is well documented that up to 50% of patients having ALND and up to 20% of patients having SLN biopsy experience numbness and tingling 5 years after surgery (36). The presence of these symptoms may interfere with a woman's ability to subjectively assess the presence of lymphedema.

The objective measures of lymphedema generally attempt to quantify tissue volume differences between upper extremities. Volume displacement techniques are recognized as the gold standard in assessing lymphedema; however, this technique is cumbersome in a busy clinical setting. Other alternatives, including advanced calculations converting circumferential arm measurements into truncated cone volumes, infrared laser optoelectronic volumetry, and inverse volumetry methods, have been suggested but are similarly burdensome and difficult to reproduce across practices (37–40). A volume increase of less than 20% from baseline is considered minimal lymphedema, 20% to 40% is considered moderate, and greater than 40% is considered severe (41) (Figs. 45.1, 45.2, and 45.3). Circumferential arm measurements, used as a surrogate for volume change, have remained the most efficient way to objectively diagnose lymphedema. Validity as well as intra- and interrater reliability have been assessed; the most accurate results are obtained when the patient is measured by the same health care professional at each visit (38). For meaningful circumferential measurements, it is important to obtain baseline

Table 45.1	STAGES OF LYMPHEDEMA ACCORDING TO THE INTERNATIONAL SOCIETY OF LYMPHOLOGY

Stage	Signs and Symptoms
0	• Latent or subclinical. • Swelling absent despite impaired lymph transport. • May exist months or years before clinically apparent edema occurs.
I	• Early accumulation of protein rich fluid. • Edema resolves with limb elevation.
II	• More fluid accumulation not resolving with limb elevation. • Pitting, tissue fibrosis, woody texture.
III	• Lymphostatic elephantiasis without pitting. • Irreversible skin changes: acanthosis, fat deposits, warty growths, skin thickening, and hyperkeratosis.

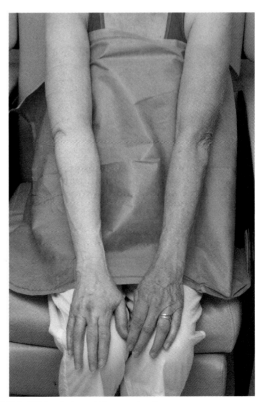

FIGURE 45.1. Mild lymphedema, right upper extremity.

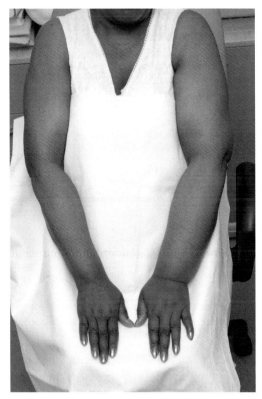

FIGURE 45.2. Moderate lymphedema.

measurements of both ipsilateral and contralateral arms prior to surgery and then at each postoperative visit. These checks help control for normal variations in arm diameter (42) that may be present at baseline, as well as for weight changes that may occur during follow-up. Unfortunately, the number of anatomic locations and the number of measurements obtained varies between studies. Although the measurement change that constitutes lymphedema is not defined, most investigators consider a 2-cm increase in circumference from baseline or as compared to the contralateral arm as being diagnostic of lymphedema (5,35,43,44). Although arm measurements are a simple and practical means of estimating volume change, they cannot determine the actual volume of extra lymphatic fluid.

The dilemma in diagnosing lymphedema remains that measurement changes alone may not capture all patients suffering

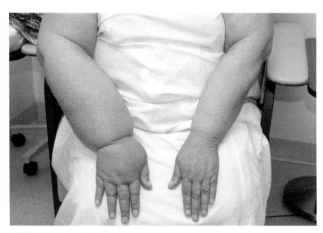

FIGURE 45.3. Severe lymphedema.

from clinically significant lymphedema and may overdiagnose those who are unaffected by their measurement change. A measurement change of less than 2 cm may be severely disfiguring for a thin woman and virtually unnoticeable in an obese woman. Also, subtle measurement changes less than 2 cm may be more symptomatic in women having axillary surgery in their dominant arm. The influence of patient perceptions of lymphedema cannot be underestimated, and it is likely that both objective and subjective parameters are needed to establish the true prevalence of lymphedema (17). This would allow patient classification as follows: symptomatic lymphedema (arm symptoms and measurement changes >2 cm), symptomatic nonlymphedema (arm symptoms with measurement changes <2 cm), nonsymptomatic lymphedema (no arm symptoms but measurement changes >2 cm), and no lymphedema (absence of arm symptoms and measurement changes).

A noninvasive measurement alternative to circumferential arm measurements is bioelectric impedance. This method passes electrical current through the extremity and measures electrical impedance. Reduction in impedance values, when compared with the control extremity, suggests an increase in extracellular fluid consistent with lymphedema (45). Bioelectric impedance may be helpful in risk assessment after breast cancer surgery or for diagnosing subclinical or latent lymphedema when measurement changes are equivocal (46). Its utility may also be found in monitoring treatment responses (47).

Imaging Techniques

In its advanced stages, lymphedema is diagnosed through history and clinical presentation. If clinical examination cannot definitively establish the diagnosis, several imaging techniques can be used. Historically, lymphangiography with slow injection of an oil emulsion directly into a surgically cannulated dermal lymphatic was performed. However, this technique has largely been abandoned due to the need for microsurgical skills and the risk of oil embolization; it has been replaced by the less invasive method of lymphoscintigraphy (48).

Lymphoscintigraphy requires hand or distal forearm injection of a radio-labeled tracer. The technique (type of radiotracer, dosage, imaging intervals) and injection sites are not standardized, but multiple static or dynamic images can demonstrate lymphatic dysfunction seen by pooling tracer, delayed transport times, or by measured tracer decay at the injection site. The images can also elucidate lymphatic obstruction secondary to extrinsic tumor compression (49,50). Unfortunately, radionuclide imaging is limited by poor image resolution (51). Some investigators have explored the use of lymphoscintigraphy to quantify treatment response using a ratio of radioactivity within the affected arm to that of the normal arm before and after therapy (52). Others have proposed the use of postoperative lymphoscintigraphy to identify those patients at risk for, or presenting with, latent edema (53). In experimental settings, lymphoscintigraphy has also demonstrated that patients with mild or no arm edema have a few remaining functional axillary lymph nodes, while those with severe edema do not (54). To date, none of these uses of lymphoscintigraphy have been adopted into routine clinical practice.

The role of computed tomography (CT) and magnetic resonance imaging (MRI) in diagnosis and treatment of lymphedema continues to evolve. High-resolution unenhanced CT demonstrates a sensitivity and specificity of 93% and 100%, respectively, for diagnosing lymphedema (55). MRI, however, offers higher-quality soft tissue imaging and may be better suited for lymphatic vasculature evaluation as MRI can differentiate lymphatic vessels from veins (56). CT and MRI findings, including skin thickening, subcutaneous edema, and honeycombing of the subcutaneous tissues due to fibrosis, are considered diagnostic of lymphedema. These modalities are infrequently required.

Causative Factors

Although many etiologic factors have been suggested, the development of upper extremity lymphedema after breast surgery is unpredictable. The most commonly cited contributing factors appear to be the extent of axillary surgery (SLN biopsy vs. ALND, or total number of nodes removed) and the use of axillary radiation.

Although some studies have found no relationship between the number of nodes removed and the risk of lymphedema (6,57), others have demonstrated an increasing risk of lymphedema as more nodes are removed (58–60). Kiel Rademacker (59) found that compared with patients who had no lymph nodes removed, the odds ratio for developing lymphedema was 7 (95% confidence interval [CI], 1–60) for patients with 1 to 10 nodes removed, 4 (95% CI, 0.5–37) for patients with 11 to 15 nodes removed, and 13 (95% CI, 2–103) for patients with 16 or more nodes removed. Similarly, Herd-Smith et al. (58) reported on 1,278 breast cancer patients and found the hazard ratio for lymphedema increased to 1.6 (95% CI, 1.0–2.7) when more than 30 lymph nodes were removed when compared with patients having less than 20 removed. Paskett et al. (60) showed that persistent swelling within the arm was significantly related to the number of nodes removed, and that for each additional node removed, the odds of persistent swelling increased by 3% (odds ratio [OR] = 1.03; $p = .01$). With the removal of fewer lymph nodes and less dissection within the axilla, rates of lymphedema are lower. Specifically, in randomized trials, SLN biopsy has been found to result in significantly lower rates of lymphedema than ALND (61–63).

Axillary radiation has also been used as a primary treatment modality instead of axillary node dissection. As demonstrated by 25 years of follow-up, the National Surgical Adjuvant Breast and Bowel Project (NSABP) B-04 trial failed to show a survival difference between the axillary treatment methods of radiation or lymph node dissection. However, axillary radiation alone is not without complication as these patients also demonstrate a two- to 4.5-fold increase in the risk of lymphedema (18). When compared with surgery, axillary radiation may be associated with less acute morbidity, but long-term complications, such as brachial plexopathy, may affect motor and sensory function of the upper extremity (64). The influence of such sensory changes after axillary radiation on one's perception of lymphedema is unknown.

The synergistic combination of axillary radiation and ALND is associated with significantly increased risk for the development of lymphedema (65–69). In one study, it was estimated that the combination of surgery and radiation to the axilla doubled the risk of lymphedema (66), while others have demonstrated that the combination results in a 3.5- to 10-fold higher risk of lymphedema when compared with surgery alone (6,42,69). With current breast cancer treatment strategies, direct axillary radiation is generally avoided unless more than 10 lymph nodes are involved by metastatic disease. However, even with prone patient positioning or CT planning for radiation simulation, scattered radiation tangents may still affect the lowest levels of the axilla during treatment, which may also lead to an increased risk of lymphedema (67).

Several studies have attempted to correlate clinicopathologic factors, such as age, extent of breast surgery, nodal positivity, body mass index (BMI), and injury or infection since axillary surgery, with the development of lymphedema. The majority of these studies are retrospective, and findings have been found to be contradictory. Older age at diagnosis has been associated with the development of lymphedema in some studies (59,70–72) and unrelated in others (8,17,35,60). The authors' personal experience suggests that age may not predispose to objectively measured lymphedema alone, but may influence patient perceptions of lymphedema. Younger patients seem to subjectively report lymphedema more than older patients (17), perhaps because they may be more sensitive to the discomfort caused by axillary surgery than older patients (73). Although this may be physiologic, it may also be due to age-related postoperative expectations or previous life experiences.

Extent of breast surgery may also influence the development of lymphedema. According to Horsley and Styblo (74), 40% of patients undergoing radical mastectomy developed lymphedema compared with 15% and 3% of those undergoing modified radical mastectomy or lumpectomy plus ALND, respectively. These findings concur with some reports (63,75), and are not supported by other reports (42,76).

It would seem intuitive that lymph node positivity would predispose to higher rates of lymphedema; this remains debatable, however, as conflicting data exist (6,42,58,68,77). In fact, Purushotham et al. (71) recently found that positive node status and the number of positive nodes were significantly inversely associated with arm volumes. These data were collected from prospectively followed patients, none of whom had received axillary radiation.

Greater body weight, weight gain since axillary surgery, and a higher BMI (>25) have been associated with a higher incidence of lymphedema (8,14,35,60,68). Patients suffering injury or infection to the ipsilateral upper extremity since axillary surgery are also at higher risk of developing lymphedema (8,44,68). However, rigorous evaluation of these two variables is difficult, as both are dependent upon patient recall. Although both appear to be significant risk factors, it is possible that women with lymphedema recall an inciting infection or injury more readily than a woman without lymphedema. Furthermore, it is possible that women with lymphedema are at higher risk of developing infection.

Incidence

The true incidence of lymphedema has been difficult to determine and is probably underestimated in most series due to relatively short follow-up periods. Historically, wide variations in the incidence of lymphedema, ranging from less than 10% to as high as 70%, are reported and attributed to the variety of measurement techniques, variability in surgical procedures both of the breast and axilla, and variations in use of postoperative radiation (1–14). In 1998 Petrek and Heelan (7) reviewed the published literature and identified seven studies since 1990 reporting the incidence of lymphedema after ALND as 6% to 30%. Petrek et al. (8), however, later documented that with 20-year follow-up this rate increased to nearly 50%. This finding suggests that lymphedema is more common than generally reported.

The adoption of SLN biopsy for axillary staging is credited with significantly decreasing the rate of lymphedema. Three prospective randomized trials and several prospective nonrandomized series have concluded that lymphedema by objective measurement after SLN biopsy is less common or severe than after ALND (5,10,43,44,78,79). These studies have limited follow-up of 6 to 36 months, and many do not report the actual incidence of lymphedema. Of those that do, the rates of lymphedema vary, from 7% to 77% after ALND, and from 0% to 7% after SLN biopsy.

Because lymphedema can occur years after surgery, it is possible that these estimates will rise with longer follow-up. A recent prospective study of nearly 1,000 women undergoing axillary staging for breast cancer assessed patients at a median of 5 years after their axillary surgery (17,35). Baseline and follow-up ipsilateral and contralateral arm circumferential measurements were taken of the upper arm and the forearm, and patients underwent a standardized interview.

Current arm swelling was reported by 3% of women undergoing SLN biopsy versus 27% of patients undergoing ALND ($p <.0001$), as compared with 5% and 16%, respectively, with lymphedema as defined by circumferential arm measurements.

Only 41% of patients reporting arm swelling had measured lymphedema, while 5% of patients reporting no arm swelling had measured lymphedema. Risk factors associated with reported arm swelling and measured lymphedema were greater body weight ($p < .0001$), higher BMI ($p < .0001$), infection ($p < .0001$), and injury ($p = .007$) in the ipsilateral arm since surgery. This study showed that ideally, both objective measurements and symptom assessment are needed to determine the prevalence of clinically significant lymphedema.

A new surgical technique called *axillary reverse mapping* (ARM) is currently being investigated as a way to further reduce the incidence of lymphedema resulting from breast cancer axillary surgery (80–82). ARM is based on the hypothesis that axillary lymphatic anatomy is virtually unknown, and that breast and arm lymphatic pathways to the axilla may be separate. Using this technique, blue dye is injected into the arm to map the lymphatic channels draining the upper extremity. The goal is to identify these blue lymphatics and protect them during axillary surgery. So far, upper extremity ARM identification rates are 61% to 71%, but preservation is only achieved in 47% (80–82).

In order to be truly successful, ARM must prove that efferent blue lymphatics from the upper extremity do not coalesce with the common lymphatic pathways draining the breast when exiting the axilla. Further study of ARM is needed before routine clinical use.

Treatment

The goals for treatment of lymphedema relate to the chronic nature of the disease (Table 45.2). Following implementation of an initial treatment program, successful management requires patients to adhere to a complex maintenance program for the rest of their lives. During this ongoing secondary phase of treatment, the challenge is to keep patients motivated in the absence of a cure (83). Receiving support and treatment early in the course of lymphedema is crucial to limiting its long-term effects, which include worsening of the edema, tissue fibrosis, pain or discomfort, recurrent cellulitis, and decreased function.

Risk-Reduction Strategies

Recommendations for hand and arm care following removal of axillary lymph nodes have traditionally included a long list of precautions. These are based on the theoretical risk of provoking fluid production in the affected quadrant and, due to compromised lymphatic outflow, resulting in the onset of lymphedema. Examples of situations involving increased lymphatic load include overuse or trauma of the at-risk limb, hot weather, high altitudes, application of external heat modalities, and vigorous massage.

Other areas for concern relate to skin care, air travel, and limb constriction. Patients have been cautioned to avoid venipuncture, injections, acupuncture, cuts, scrapes, and other arm traumas, and to avoid cutting cuticles in order to reduce

the risk of infection. Anecdotal reports of the onset of symptoms following air travel are the basis of a common recommendation for all patients at risk for lymphedema to use a compression garment prophylactically (84). Finally, some precautions relate to blocking lymphatic flow in an at-risk limb via blood pressure measurement, elastic at the distal portion of a sleeve, or tight jewelry. All of these situations are targets for risk-reduction strategies that have been recommended to patients in the past.

More recent studies have contradicted some of these older recommendations and added to physicians' understanding, as well as the controversy, surrounding risk-reduction strategies. Two studies address the precautions related to overuse of the involved extremity. In a retrospective study of 263 20-year breast cancer survivors, neither high-risk occupations (e.g., aerobic activity or heavy housework) nor moderate-risk occupations (e.g., walking or light housework) were associated with the development of lymphedema (8). In a 6-month randomized controlled trial of weight training following ALND or SLN biopsy with 78 women, there was no evidence of the onset of lymphedema following progressive resistive exercise in the intervention group (85). These studies contradict previous recommendations to limit arm use following ALND.

One study contradicts the recommendation that all at-risk patients wear a compression garment prophylactically (86). In this study of 287 breast cancer survivors, 145 were exposed to air travel. There was no difference in rates of lymphedema between those who had flown and those who had not, and no woman who had flown reported permanent new swelling or increased swelling after flying. The study also concluded that use of a compression garment preventively may have been counterproductive. This study is not the final word on prophylactic compression, and some lymphedema therapists continue to recommend prophylactic compression for all at-risk patients. Despite the controversy, most therapists agree that patients who already have a diagnosis of lymphedema or who exhibit subclinical symptoms should use arm and hand compression during air travel, whether in the form of compression garments or low-stretch bandages.

Other studies have confirmed earlier risk-reduction recommendations with regard to skin care and focused on a new area of concern: obesity. The suggestion that patients avoid skin punctures or injuries in order to reduce the risk of infection has been confirmed by two studies (8,87). Studies indicating that weight gain following treatment and a BMI greater than 26 kg/m^2 result in a higher incidence of lymphedema and support the results of a randomized controlled trial that followed 21 women for 12 weeks and indicated the benefit of weight reduction as a treatment for lymphedema (8,87,88).

Anecdotal reports of the onset or worsening of swelling following blood pressure measurement on the at-risk limb in hot or humid weather, after using heat modalities, or after receiving vigorous massage on the at-risk limb must be confirmed by research to more clearly guide patients in appropriate risk-reduction strategies.

The need for risk-reduction strategies following SLN biopsy continues to be controversial. Although SLN biopsy is associated with a lower risk of lymphedema and fewer sensory changes than ALND, more than 80% of SLN biopsy patients practice precautionary behaviors similar to those followed by patients undergoing ALND (17). Given the low incidence of lymphedema after SLN biopsy, the influence of these precautions on overall quality of life remains unclear and should be further studied. Furthermore, in the setting of SLN biopsy, it is possible that such lifestyle modifications may not be warranted for such little benefit.

Confounding elements in determining risk-reduction strategies include the unpredictability of onset of lymphedema and variation in patient factors, such as the extent of axillary surgery, radiotherapy, underlying medical conditions, and anatomic variation. Current risk reduction strategies are listed in Table 45.3.

Table 45.2	**GOALS FOR THE TREATMENT OF LYMPHEDEMA**

1. Educating the patient and patient's family and/or caregiver in the causes of lymphedema, risk reduction strategies, signs and symptoms of exacerbation, and treatment options.
2. Reducing edema and tissue fibrosis through stimulation of superficial and deep lymphatic vessels.
3. Promoting patient participation in a home management program.
4. Providing the patient with garments and supplies.
5. Reducing or preventing recurrence of infection.
6. Maximizing the return of the patient to prior functional roles.

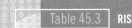

Table 45.3	RISK-REDUCTION STRATEGIES

1. Avoiding skin puncture, trauma, and injury to an at-risk limb to help prevent infection, and using appropriate first aid to care for all skin injuries.
2. Avoiding limb constriction, such as blood pressure measurements, on an at-risk limb.
3. Avoiding extremes of temperature, including prolonged exposure to cold or heat.
4. Encouraging exercise and activity in moderation, with more frequent rest periods and with knowledge of monitoring for precipitating symptoms.
5. Encouraging weight maintenance or weight reduction for those who are overweight.

Table 45.5	FACTORS THAT INFLUENCE THE ADHERENCE TO LYMPHEDEMA THERAPIES

1. Health care team and system-related factors, such as knowledge and training of the therapist, and the ability of the therapist to allow adequate time for consultation and follow-up.
2. Socioeconomic factors, such as insurance coverage of treatment and compression devices, and poverty or illiteracy of the patient.
3. Condition-related factors, such as severity of the lymphedema or coexisting medical conditions.
4. Therapy-related factors related to the complexity and duration of the therapy.
5. Patient-related factors, such as patient motivation, beliefs, cognitive skills, confidence in her ability to perform self-management tasks, and expectations for success.

Positioning

With postoperative edema or new onset lymphedema, patients are advised to elevate the affected extremity in a resting position above the level of the heart. Positioning may help temporarily reduce edema and discomfort in early lymphedema, but it is not a practical recommendation, since it interferes with normal daily activities. A more achievable solution is using nighttime elevation, and patients often report improvement in their lymphedema after resting their affected arm on a pillow overnight. This approach, however, will not be sufficient to prevent exacerbation of chronic lymphedema; therefore, intervention by a trained lymphedema therapist is necessary to individualize treatment for each patient.

TREATMENT COMPONENTS

The standard of care for treatment of lymphedema is a combination of treatments that together are referred to as complete or complex decongestive therapy (CDT) (Table 45.4).

An additional treatment component, intermittent pneumatic compression, is recommended by some therapists, particularly as an adjunct to CDT, and discouraged by others. Low-level laser therapy is a relatively new treatment modality that was developed in Australia. Currently, there are no medications or surgical procedures that are widely accepted as a treatment or cure for lymphedema.

Treatment Approaches

According to the International Society of Lymphology, CDT is provided in two phases. In phase I, patients are taught skin care and basic range-of-motion exercises, provided with manual lymph drainage (MLD), and wrapped in layers of short-stretch bandages. In phase II, patients are fitted with an elastic compression garment and are instructed to continue with basic skin care, exercises, and MLD self-massage (32).

In practice, many factors will influence the decision of the treating therapist on what course of therapy to recommend for

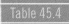

Table 45.4	COMPLETE DECONGESTIVE THERAPY

1. Skin care.
2. Manual lymphatic drainage.
3. Multilayer short-stretch compression bandaging.
4. Exercise.
5. Fitting for compression garments or alternative compression devices.
6. Instruction in a home management program.

each patient. A number of factors have been identified by the World Health Organization (89) as important in influencing the adherence to long-term therapies (83) (Table 45.5).

Therapy recommendations may range from simple to complex, depending on the factors described above. Therapists may utilize some or all of the components of traditional lymphedema therapy in order to realize the patient's goals.

Skin Care

A basic component of lymphedema therapy, education in skin care, promotes daily cleansing of the skin to reduce bacterial and fungal overgrowth, and hydration of the skin using a moisturizer to minimize dryness and cracking of the skin. Protection of the skin during daily activities (e.g., using gloves for washing dishes, cleaning, or gardening) also helps to minimize trauma and is recommended. Patients are instructed to be cautious when shaving and with nail and cuticle care, and to avoid sunburn and insect bites when possible. If a cut or burn does occur, patients are advised to clean the wound, apply antibiotic ointment for a cut or dry gauze for a burn, and monitor the area for evidence of infection. Patients are educated in symptoms of infection, including red blotches or streaks, pain, increased swelling, increased skin temperature, and fever or flu-like symptoms.

Manual Lymphatic Drainage

MLD is a gentle manual massage technique developed in Europe, popularized in Germany and Austria in the early 1970s, and first introduced in the United States by Robert Lerner in 1989 (90). It is designed to promote lymphatic transport and to reroute lymph flow away from the blocked drainage area of the involved axilla and toward a normally functioning adjacent lymph territory. This is accomplished by directing fluid across the trunk to the contralateral axilla or ipsilateral inguinal node basin. The massage strokes used in lymphatic massage are lighter than those employed in traditional massage and are applied in a particular order and duration. The various types of strokes apply tension to the skin, which in turn stretch the underlying superficial lymphatic vessels and promote contraction of deeper lying lymphangions. Stimulation of deeper lymphatic structures via abdominal pressure and breathing techniques support the locally applied therapy.

For treatment of upper-extremity lymphedema, MLD is provided by a specially trained therapist as a component of CDT. In the traditional approach to treatment, MLD is provided 5 days a week and is followed by application of moisturizing lotion, compression bandages, and other supplies. The patient then performs remedial exercises. The bandages are kept in place until the next treatment, at which point the bandages are removed, the patient cleanses the arm, and the cycle begins again. This intensive treatment phase, also called phase I, continues for 1 to 4 weeks. When the patient's measurements begin to plateau, phase II, or the maintenance phase, begins. During this secondary phase, the patient maintains the results achieved in the treatment phase by applying compression bandages at night, using fitted compression garments during the day, and continuing with skin care and remedial exercises.

A number of recent studies have demonstrated the efficacy of this treatment approach with breast cancer patients. In two prospective trials, Mondry et al. (91) demonstrated a median girth reduction of 1.5 cm and a median volume reduction of 138 mL following 2 to 4 weeks of standard CDT therapy in 20 outpatients, while Vignes et al. (92) followed a much larger sample of 537 patients with a mean absolute volume reduction of 407 mL following an 11-day course of inpatient intensive therapy. Koul et al. (93) reported a mean reduction of 188 mL in 138 patients, though not all patients were treated with all four components of CDT. In a retrospective review, Hamner et al. (94) showed an average of 237 mL reduction in 135 patients who received MLD twice per week, which was reported as a 41.7% decrease in the amount of lymphedema. Many of these studies conclude that effective maintenance therapy following the intensive phase is crucial to preserving the initial reduction.

In the years since its introduction, training programs for MLD have proliferated, each providing its own unique approach to MLD and CDT. In an effort to standardize treatment, the Lymphology Association of North America was created with the goal of establishing a standardized examination to certify lymphedema therapists. The first therapists were certified in 2001. The National Lymphedema Network has also recommended standards for training in CDT (95).

Despite these efforts at standardization, therapists continue to modify the traditional approach in order to better meet the needs of their clients. Consequently, MLD may initially be provided 5 days a week in some cases and not at all in other cases (especially patients who have very mild or subclinical lymphedema). In those situations, therapists often train patients, family members, or caretakers in a modified MLD-like massage technique as a component of the home management program.

Multilayer Short-Stretch Compression Bandaging

External arm compression in the form of short-stretch compression bandages is considered a mainstay of lymphedema therapy. These low-stretch bandages, in contrast to Ace, or high-stretch bandages, provide a low resting pressure and high working pressure. The effectiveness of the bandages is maximized during activity because they provide a strong counterpressure to contracting muscles. They are also safer to use at rest than high-stretch bandages because they are less likely to obstruct venous and lymphatic return (Fig. 45.4).

The bandages are applied in overlapping layers with more compression distally and less compression proximally. Because lymph stasis may result in tissue fibrosis, additional layers of foam or padding are added underneath the bandages to protect sensitive areas and to provide additional compression to fibrotic portions of the limb. The goal of bandaging is therefore to increase tissue pressure to promote the return of lymphatic and venous fluid and, ultimately, to reshape the limb and reduce tissue fibrosis.

Two studies demonstrated the beneficial effects of compression bandaging with a reported mean reduction of 26% and 36% following 2 to 4 weeks of therapy. Although both studies reported an added benefit of MLD, they also emphasized the value of compression bandaging as a time-efficient intervention compared with adding MLD to the treatment program (96, 112). Despite evidence of its effectiveness, the disadvantages of bandaging often lead to limited use by many patients. Proper application of bandages is challenging, and patients need training

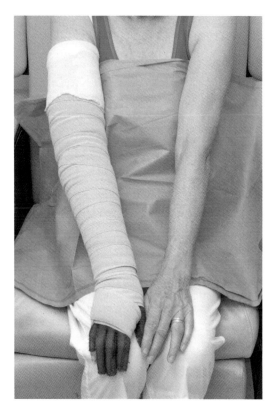

FIGURE 45.4. Multi-layer, short stretch compression bandaging.

and review of the technique. In addition, the bandages are time-consuming to apply and may be difficult to keep on, particularly in warm climates and weather. Patients often find bandages interfere with sleep and are cumbersome to use during daily activities. Finally, bandages and supplies must be replaced on a regular basis; costs that may not be covered by insurance. Because of their effectiveness, however, patients are often encouraged to use bandages intermittently, particularly after an episode of cellulitis or during periodic exacerbations of their condition.

Exercise

For many years, patients have been cautioned by their physicians to avoid lifting anything heavy with the affected arm following ALND in order to limit the risk of developing lymphedema or causing an exacerbation. A number of studies are beginning to refute this common advice. In addition to the study mentioned previously (85), others have demonstrated that exercise does not exacerbate existing symptoms of lymphedema (97), and that exercise increases quality of life in breast cancer survivors (98,99). Further investigation is needed to confirm the results and substantiate the hypothesis that progressive resistive exercise may be used as a treatment modality to reduce edema.

Whereas in the past only remedial active range-of-motion and flexibility exercises were recommended, therapists are now increasingly recommending strength, endurance, and aerobic exercises. For patients diagnosed with lymphedema or subclinical symptoms such as heaviness, aching, or fatigue with increased activity, any exercise program should be performed while using compression garments or bandages. Patients are instructed to begin a new exercise program slowly, monitor their swelling and symptoms, modify or reduce the exercise when symptoms worsen, and take more frequent rest breaks during exercise.

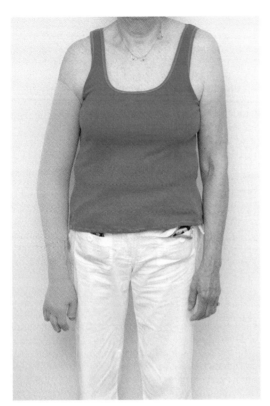

FIGURE 45.5. Compression garment.

For those patients at risk for lymphedema but with no sub-clinical symptoms, there continues to be controversy about using prophylactic compression during exercise. The lack of consensus on this issue is similar to the discussion about at-risk patients using prophylactic compression during air travel.

Compression Garments and Alternative Compression Devices

Compression garments are an essential component of lymphedema therapy and represent the most widely used form of compression (Fig. 45.5). Both garments and bandages have been shown to reduce edema, with one study showing a slight advantage of using bandages for a limited period prior to initiating use of a garment (100,101). Garments are simpler to apply than bandages and limit reaccumulation of edema following reduction with MLD and bandaging. Exactly how the garments work is unclear. One supposition relates to increased interstitial pressure in patients with lymphedema (102). Garments may help to maintain interstitial fluid homeostasis and prevent stretching of the patient's skin (103). As an added benefit, garments protect the arm against incidental trauma.

Both prefabricated and custom-made garments are available in a variety of fabrics, styles, and colors. Proper fitting of the garments is crucial to their efficacy and increases patient compliance with their use. One of the most problematic components of garment fitting is avoiding proximal constriction that limits distal return of lymph fluid. If not properly addressed, a worsening of the edema may occur, particularly in the hand and digits, although not all patients exhibit distal swelling.

Typical recommended pressures for upper extremity lymphedema garments are class I (20 to 30 mm Hg) and class II (30 to 40 mm Hg). Some patients may tolerate class III (40 to 50 mm Hg) garments. However, there is variation in the amount of pressure supplied by the numerous brands and fabrics within a particular compression class. Consequently, patients must experiment with different garments to determine which brand, fabric, and style is most comfortable and effective in controlling their edema.

Traditionally, compression garments are not recommended to be worn overnight because of their elasticity. Similar to high-stretch or Ace bandages, compression garments have a higher resting pressure than low-stretch bandages, thus creating the possibility of obstructing venous or lymphatic return, especially when patients are not activating the arm musculature at night. In addition, the pressure at the proximal or distal end of an elastic garment, or at a skin fold such as the elbow, may cause skin irritation, and patients might be unaware of a problem when they are asleep. To address the problem of low patient compliance with the safer alternative of nighttime bandaging, there are a number of products available as ready-made or custom-made compression devices that are designed to be used overnight (Fig. 45.6). The devices are made of foam covered by fabric, with additional compression supplied via Velcro straps or an outer sleeve. Unlike compression garments, these devices have properties similar to bandages and provide a low resting pressure, which is safer to use overnight.

Home Management Programs

Because lymphedema is a chronic condition, ongoing follow-up is the key to successful maintenance and avoidance of exacerbation or infection. Studies of other chronic conditions, such as hypertension and diabetes, show that nonadherence to the recommended therapy is common (83). Similarly, during the maintenance phase of lymphedema therapy, patients often become discouraged and frustrated with the complex and time-consuming regimens needed to control their swelling. At some point, either during active treatment or thereafter, reduction in swelling plateaus and patients may experience periods of exacerbation. Patients often lose motivation over

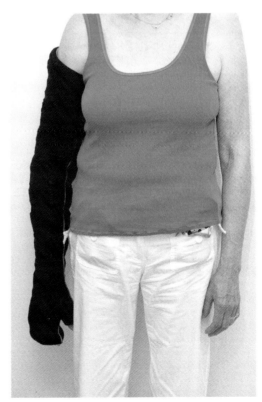

FIGURE 45.6. Alternative compression device.

time and discontinue their home management programs. In order to maximize adherence, patients must be monitored to review and modify their home management programs. Garments and supplies must be replaced regularly. If significant exacerbation occurs, more intensive therapy must be initiated.

Intermittent Pneumatic Compression

Use of intermittent pneumatic compression pumps for the treatment of lymphedema continues to be controversial. Prior to 1989 when MLD was first introduced in the United States, pneumatic compression was the most commonly prescribed treatment for lymphedema (52). Since then, some schools of lymphedema therapy have continued to advocate their use, while others are opposed.

The pneumatic pump attaches to a sleeve that covers the entire upper extremity. Newer devices have sleeves that extend over the adjacent trunk quadrants. The sleeve has multiple chambers that inflate and deflate in a particular order with varying amounts of compression for longer or shorter durations, depending on the type of pump.

Traditional schools of lymphedema therapy call attention to the ineffectiveness of pumps despite transient reductions in edema. They point out that pumps do not transport lymphatic fluid but rather the water component of the interstitial fluid, thus resulting in a later exacerbation of the swelling. In addition, they mention the possibility of damaging functioning lymph collectors with high pressures and increasing tissue edema or fibrosis proximally in the limb or in adjacent trunk quadrants (104). Other groups support the use of pumps with pressures up to 50 mm Hg, either in combination with MLD and CDT, or as a maintenance tool at the conclusion of intensive therapy. The benefits they report in one study include volume reduction, ease and independence of application, and lack of adverse effects (105).

In the latest consensus document of the International Society of Lymphology, pneumatic compression is listed as one of the treatment options for lymphedema. The recommendation is to apply compression garments following treatment in order to maintain edema reduction (96). It is important to relay to patients considering pneumatic compression that it does not take the place of utilizing external compression in the form of garments or bandages on a regular basis.

Surgical Treatment Options

Surgical interventions are not universally accepted treatments for lymphedema. The goals of surgical treatment are to reduce limb size, improve function, decrease frequency of infections, and improve quality of life. Proposed operations focus on either removal of excess tissue (excisional operations) or on improving lymphatic transport (lymphatic reconstructions). The operation proposed by Charles (106) is the most radical of the excisional techniques, removing skin and subcutaneous tissue occasionally with the deep fascia. Defects are closed by skin grafting. This procedure was popularized in the lower extremity. The most frequently used excisional operation has been the staged localized excision of fibrosed, edematous subcutaneous tissue beneath skin flaps (113). Although this appears to be the most reliable procedure, surgical complications and postoperative cosmetic appearance are dependent on flap thickness. Clinical benefit, however, is directly related to the amount of subcutaneous tissue excised. Liposuction as a means to reduce limb volume has been explored most recently. Brorson et al. (107) have demonstrated significant improvement in appearance and symptoms of the upper extremity after liposuction. Obtaining both pre- and postoperative volume displacement measurements, they demonstrated a return to arm volumes smaller than that at baseline. These results were sustained at 7 years.

Proposed lymphatic reconstructions include lymphovenous or lympholymphatic anastomoses. Both require microsurgical techniques and 11-0 monofilament nonabsorbable interrupted sutures. The largest series of lymphovenous anastomoses with 665 patients demonstrates successful arm volume reduction in 69% of patients (108). Lymphatic grafting (lympholymphatic anastomosis) may be more advantageous and less prone to thrombosis given the low pressure lymphatic system. With this technique, Baumeister and Siuda (109) reported a significant decrease in mean arm volume, with continued further reduction in volumes for up to 3 years postoperatively. Finally, microsurgical lymph node transplantation has been attempted and is credited with the resolution of lymphedema in 42% of patients with mean follow up of 8.3 years (110). Although encouraging, none of the three techniques is uniformly reproducible. Furthermore, direct benefit from surgical therapy is difficult to determine, as all patients are instructed to use compression garments postoperatively.

Other Treatment Options

Low-level laser therapy is a newly available treatment modality developed in Australia. In a double-blind, randomized, placebo-controlled trial with 64 participants, the therapy was shown to reduce tissue fibrosis and extracellular fluid levels, as measured by a bioimpedance device, in one third of the participants at 3 months following treatment. Further study of this modality is needed to verify the results and understand its mechanism of action (111).

No medications have been found to effectively treat lymphedema. Although diuretics temporarily reduce edema, they are not recommended for long-term management of lymphedema as they may lead to fluid and electrolyte imbalance (32). Benzopyrene and similar bioflavonoids that work to stimulate macrophage activity and theoretically reduce excess proteins in the tissue have been shown to be ineffective in treating upper extremity lymphedema and may have hepatotoxic effects (105).

MANAGEMENT SUMMARY

- Lymphedema is a complication of breast cancer surgery that occurs in 6% to 49% of patients undergoing ALND. With a median follow-up of 5 years or less, SLN biopsy demonstrates a significantly reduced rate of lymphedema, ranging from 0% to 7%.
- Lymphedema is categorized into four stages. The gold standard for diagnosis is water displacement, but in most cases diagnosis is made by physical examination and arm measurements; imaging modalities are generally not necessary.
- A combination of objective upper extremity measurements and subjective symptoms of arm swelling are important in defining lymphedema and in determining how patients perceive or are affected by their lymphedema.
- Common risk factors for lymphedema include ALND, axillary radiation, obesity or elevated BMI, weight gain since axillary surgery, and injury or infection in the ipsilateral arm since surgery. Factors such as age, extent of breast surgery, nodal involvement, and surgery ipsilateral to the dominant hand remain controversial risk factors.
- Treatment focuses on risk reduction, skin care, manual lymphatic drainage, compression garments and devices, and exercise. No medication has proven effective for the treatment of lymphedema.

- Compression garments are an essential component of lymphedema therapy and represent the most widely used form of compression. Both garments and bandages have been shown to reduce edema.

 RELEVANT WEB SITES

National Cancer Institute: www.cancer.gov
National Lymphedema Network: www.lymphnet.org
U.S. Centers for Disease Control and Prevention: www.cdc.gov/cancer/breast

References

1. Blanchard DK, Donohue JH, Reynolds C, et al. Relapse and morbidity in patients undergoing sentinel lymph node biopsy alone or with axillary dissection for breast cancer. *Arch Surg* 2003;138:482–488.
2. Haid A, Koberle-Wuhrer R, Knauer M, et al. Morbidity of breast cancer patients following complete axillary dissection or sentinel node biopsy only: a comparative evaluation. *Breast Cancer Res Treat* 2002;73:31–36.
3. Hoe AL, Iven D, Royle GT, et al. Incidence of arm swelling following axillary clearance for breast cancer. *Br J Surg* 1992;79:261–262.
4. Ivens D, Hoe AL, Podd TJ, et al. Assessment of morbidity from complete axillary dissection. *Br J Cancer* 1992;66:136–138.
5. Leidenius M, Leivonen M, Vironen J, et al. The consequences of long-time arm morbidity in node-negative breast cancer patients with sentinel node biopsy or axillary clearance. *J Surg Oncol* 2005;92:23–31.
6. Ozaslan C, Kuru B. Lymphedema after treatment of breast cancer. *Am J Surg* 2004;187:69–72.
7. Petrek JA, Heelan MC. Incidence of breast carcinoma-related lymphedema. *Cancer* 1998;83:2776–2781.
8. Petrek JA, Senie RT, Peters M, et al. Lymphedema in a cohort of breast carcinoma survivors 20 years after diagnosis. *Cancer* 2001;92:1368–1377.
9. Rockson SG. Lymphedema. *Am J Med* 2001;110:288–295.
10. Ronka R, von Smitten K, Tasmuth T, et al. One-year morbidity after sentinel node biopsy and breast surgery. *Breast* 2005;14:28–36.
11. Schijven MP, Vingerhoets AJ, Rutten HJ, et al. Comparison of morbidity between axillary lymph node dissection and sentinel node biopsy. *Eur J Surg Oncol* 2003;29:341–350.
12. Schrenk P, Rieger R, Shamiyeh A, et al. Morbidity following sentinel lymph node biopsy versus axillary lymph node dissection for patients with breast carcinoma. *Cancer* 2000;88:608–614.
13. Swenson KK, Nissen MJ, Ceronsky C, et al. Comparison of side effects between sentinel lymph node and axillary lymph node dissection for breast cancer. *Ann Surg Oncol* 2002;9:745–753.
14. Werner RS, McCormick B, Petrek J, et al. Arm edema in conservatively managed breast cancer: obesity is a major predictive factor. *Radiology* 1991;180:177–184.
15. Fu MR. Breast cancer survivors' intentions of managing lymphedema. *Cancer Nurs* 2005;28:446–457.
16. Greenslade MV, House CJ. Living with lymphedema: a qualitative study of women's perspectives on prevention and management following breast cancer-related treatment. *Can Oncol Nurs J* 2006;16:165–179.
17. McLaughlin SA, Wright MJ, Morris KT, et al. Prevalence of lymphedema in 936 women with breast cancer 5 years after sentinel lymph node biopsy or axillary dissection: patient perceptions and precautionary behaviors. *J Clin Oncol* 2008;26:5220–5226.
18. Kwan W, Jackson J, Weir LM, et al. Chronic arm morbidity after curative breast cancer treatment: prevalence and impact on quality of life. *J Clin Oncol* 2002;20:1212–1248.
19. Newman ML, Brennan M, Passik S. Lymphedema complicated by pain and psychological distress: a case with complex treatment needs. *J Pain Symptom Manage* 1996;12:376–379.
20. Voogd AC, Ververs JM, Vingerhoets AJ, et al. Lymphoedema and reduced shoulder function as indicators of quality of life after axillary lymph node dissection for invasive breast cancer. *Br J Surg* 2003;90:76–81.
21. McWayne J, Heiney SP. Psychologic and social sequelae of secondary lymphedema: a review. *Cancer* 2005;104:457–466.
22. Pyszel A, Malyszczak K, Pyszel K, et al. Disability, psychological distress and quality of life in breast cancer survivors with arm lymphedema. *Lymphology* 2006;39:185–192.
23. Ridner SH. Quality of life and a symptom cluster associated with breast cancer treatment-related lymphedema. *Support Care Cancer* 2005;13:904–911.
24. Passik SD. Predictors of psychological distress in lymphoedema related to breast cancer. *Psychooncology* 1995;4:255–263.
25. National Cancer Institute:www.cancer.gov.
26. National Lymphedema Network: www.lymphnet.org.
27. Clodius L. Lymphatics, lymphodynamics, lymphedema: an update. *Plast Surg Outlook* 1990;4:1.
28. Mortimer PS. The pathophysiology of lymphedema. *Cancer* 1998;83:2798–2802.
29. Pappenheimer JR. Effective osmotic pressure of the plasma proteins and other quantities associated with the capillary circulation in the hindlimbs of cats and dogs. *Am J Physiol* 1948;152:471–491.
30. Bennett Britton TM, Buczacki SJ, Turner CL, et al. Venous changes and lymphoedema 4 years after axillary surgery for breast cancer. *Br J Surg* 2007;94:833–834.
31. Pain SJ, Vowler S, Purushotham AD. Axillary vein abnormalities contribute to development of lymphoedema after surgery for breast cancer. *Br J Surg* 2005;92:311–315.
32. The diagnosis and treatment of peripheral lymphedema. Consensus document of the International Society of Lymphology. *Lymphology* 2003;36:84–91.
33. Armer JM, Radina ME, Porock D, et al. Predicting breast cancer-related lymphedema using self-reported symptoms. *Nurs Res* 2003;52:370–379.
34. Norman SA, Miller LT, Erikson HB, et al. Development and validation of a telephone questionnaire to characterize lymphedema in women treated for breast cancer. *Phys Ther* 2001;81:1192–1205.
35. McLaughlin SA, Wright MJ, Morris KT, et al. Prevalence of lymphedema in 936 women with breast cancer 5 years after sentinel lymph node biopsy or axillary dissection: objective measurements. *J Clin Oncol* 2008;26:5213–5219.
36. Baron RH, Fey JV, Borgen PI, et al. Eighteen sensations after breast cancer surgery: a 5-year comparison of sentinel lymph node biopsy and axillary lymph node dissection. *Ann Surg Oncol* 2007;14:1653–1661.
37. Damstra RJ, Glazenburg EJ, Hop WC. Validation of the inverse water volumetry method: a new gold standard for arm volume measurements. *Breast Cancer Res Treat* 2006;99:267–273.
38. Deltombe T, Jamart J, Recloux S, et al. Reliability and limits of agreement of circumferential, water displacement, and optoelectronic volumetry in the measurement of upper limb lymphedema. *Lymphology* 2007;40:26–34.
39. Meijer RS, Rietman JS, Geertzen JH, et al. Validity and intra- and interobserver reliability of an indirect volume measurements in patients with upper extremity lymphedema. *Lymphology* 2004;37:127–133.
40. Taylor R, Jayasinghe UW, Koelmeyer L, et al. Reliability and validity of arm volume measurements for assessment of lymphedema. *Phys Ther* 2006;86:205–214.
41. Stillwell GK. Treatment of postmastectomy lymphedema. *Mod Treat* 1969;6:396–412.
42. Kissin MW, Querci della Rovere G, Easton D, et al. Risk of lymphoedema following the treatment of breast cancer. *Br J Surg* 1986;73:580–584.
43. Langer I, Guller U, Berclaz G, et al. Morbidity of sentinel lymph node biopsy (SLN) alone versus SLN and completion axillary lymph node dissection after breast cancer surgery: a prospective Swiss multicenter study on 659 patients. *Ann Surg* 2007;245:452–461.
44. Wilke LG, McCall LM, Posther KE, et al. Surgical complications associated with sentinel lymph node biopsy: results from a prospective international cooperative group trial. *Ann Surg Oncol* 2006;13:491–500.
45. Warren AG, Janz BA, Slavin SA, et al. The use of bioimpedance analysis to evaluate lymphedema. *Ann Plast Surg* 2007;58:541–543.
46. Cornish BH, Chapman M, Hirst C, et al. Early diagnosis of lymphedema using multiple frequency bioimpedance. *Lymphology* 2001;34:2–11.
47. Ward LC. Bioelectrical impedance analysis: proven utility in lymphedema risk assessment and therapeutic monitoring. *Lymphat Res Biol* 2006;4:51–56.
48. Golueke PJ, Montgomery RA, Petronis JD, et al. Lymphoscintigraphy to confirm the clinical diagnosis of lymphedema. *J Vasc Surg* 1989;10:306–312.
49. Moshiri M, Katz DS, Boris M, et al. Using lymphoscintigraphy to evaluate suspected lymphedema of the extremities. *AJR Am J Roentgenol* 2002;178:405–412.
50. Yuan Z, Chen L, Luo Q, et al. The role of radionuclide lymphoscintigraphy in extremity lymphedema. *Ann Nucl Med* 2006;20:341–344.
51. Barrett T, Choyke PL, Kobayashi H. Imaging of the lymphatic system: new horizons. *Contrast Media Mol Imaging* 2006;1:230–245.
52. Szuba A, Achalu R, Rockson SG. Decongestive lymphatic therapy for patients with breast carcinoma-associated lymphedema. A randomized, prospective study of a role for adjunctive intermittent pneumatic compression. *Cancer* 2002;95:2260–2267.
53. Bourgeois P, Leduc O, Leduc A. Imaging techniques in the management and prevention of posttherapeutic upper limb edemas. *Cancer* 1998;83:2805–2813.
54. Szuba A, Pyszel A, Jedrzejuk D, et al. Presence of functional axillary lymph nodes and lymph drainage within arms in women with and without breast cancer-related lymphedema. *Lymphology* 2007;40:81–86.
55. Monnin-Delhom ED, Gallix BP, Achard C, et al. High resolution unenhanced computed tomography in patients with swollen legs. *Lymphology* 2002;35:121–128.
56. Lohrmann C, Foeldi E, Speck O, et al. High-resolution MR lymphangiography in patients with primary and secondary lymphedema. *AJR Am J Roentgenol* 2006;187:556–561.
57. Hinrichs CS, Watroba NL, Rezaishiraz H, et al. Lymphedema secondary to postmastectomy radiation: incidence and risk factors. *Ann Surg Oncol* 2004;11:573–580.
58. Herd-Smith A, Russo A, Muraca MG, et al. Prognostic factors for lymphedema after primary treatment of breast carcinoma. *Cancer* 2001;92:1783–1787.
59. Kiel KD, Rademacker AW. Early-stage breast cancer: arm edema after wide excision and breast irradiation. *Radiology* 1996;198:279–283.
60. Paskett ED, Naughton MJ, McCoy TP, et al. The epidemiology of arm and hand swelling in premenopausal breast cancer survivors. *Cancer Epidemiol Biomarkers Prev* 2007;16:775–782.
61. Mansel RE, Fallowfield L, Kissin M, et al. Randomized multicenter trial of sentinel node biopsy versus standard axillary treatment in operable breast cancer: the ALMANAC trial. *J Natl Cancer Inst* 2006;98:599–609.
62. Purushotham AD, Upponi S, Klevesath MB, et al. Morbidity after sentinel lymph node biopsy in primary breast cancer: results from a randomized controlled trial. *J Clin Oncol* 2005;23:4312–4321.
63. Veronesi U, Paganelli G, Viale G, et al. A randomized comparison of sentinel-node biopsy with routine axillary dissection in breast cancer. *N Engl J Med* 2003;349:546–553.
64. Pierquin B, Mazeron JJ, Glaubiger D. Conservative treatment of breast cancer in Europe: report of the Groupe Europeen de Curietherapie. *Radiother Oncol* 1986;6:187–198.
65. Bentzen SM, Dische S. Morbidity related to axillary irradiation in the treatment of breast cancer. *Acta Oncol* 2000;39:337–347.
66. Coen JJ, Taghian AG, Kachnic LA, et al. Risk of lymphedema after regional nodal irradiation with breast conservation therapy. *Int J Radiat Oncol Biol Phys* 2003;55:1209–1215.
67. Meek AG. Breast radiotherapy and lymphedema. *Cancer* 1998;83:2788–2797.
68. van der Veen P, De Voogdt N, Lievens P, et al. Lymphedema development following breast cancer surgery with full axillary resection. *Lymphology* 2004;37:206–208.
69. Vevers JM, Roumen RM, Vingerhoets AJ. Risk, severity and predictors of physical and psychological morbidity after axillary lymph node dissection for breast cancer. *Eur J Cancer* 2001;37:991–999.
70. Delouche G, Bachelot F, Premont M, et al. Conservation treatment of early breast cancer: long term results and complications. *Int J Radiat Oncol Biol Phys* 1987;13:29–34.

71. Purushotham AD, Bennett Britton TM, Klevesath MB, et al. Lymph node status and breast cancer-related lymphedema. *Ann Surg* 2007;246:42–45.

72. Starritt EC, Joseph D, McKinnon JG, et al. Lymphedema after complete axillary node dissection for melanoma: assessment using a new, objective definition. *Ann Surg* 2004;240:866–874.

73. Temple LK, Baron R, Cody HS 3rd, et al. Sensory morbidity after sentinel lymph node biopsy and axillary dissection: a prospective study of 233 women. *Ann Surg Oncol* 2002;9:654–662.

74. Horsley JS, Styblo T. Lymphedema in the postmastectomy patient. In: Bland KI, Copeland EM, eds. *The breast.* Philadelphia: WB Saunders, 1991:701–706.

75. Deutsch M, Flickinger JC. Shoulder and arm problems after radiotherapy for primary breast cancer. *Am J Clin Oncol* 2001;24:172–176.

76. Paci E, Cariddi A, Barchielli A, et al. Long-term sequelae of breast cancer surgery. *Tumori* 1996;82:321–324.

77. Querci della Rovere G, Ahmad I, Singh P, et al. An audit of the incidence of arm lymphoedema after prophylactic level I/II axillary dissection without division of the pectoralis minor muscle. *Ann R Coll Surg Engl* 2003;85:158–161.

78. Rietman JS, Dijkstra PU, Geertzen JH, et al. Treatment-related upper limb morbidity 1 year after sentinel lymph node biopsy or axillary lymph node dissection for stage I or II breast cancer. *Ann Surg Oncol* 2004;11:1018–1024.

79. Sener SF, Winchester DJ, Martz CH, et al. Lymphedema after sentinel lymphadenectomy for breast carcinoma. *Cancer* 2001;92:748–752.

80. Nos C, Lesieur B, Clough KB, et al. Comments to the letter to the editor by Dr. Ponzone. *Ann Surg Oncol* 2008;15:392–393.

81. Ponzone R, Mininanni P, Cassina E, et al. Axillary reverse mapping in breast cancer: can we spare what we find? *Ann Surg Oncol* 2008;15:390–391.

82. Thompson M, Korourian S, Henry-Tillman R, et al. Axillary reverse mapping (ARM): a new concept to identify and enhance lymphatic preservation. *Ann Surg Oncol* 2007;14:1890–1895.

83. Palmer SC. Barriers and facilitators to successful lymphedema therapy: the role of adherence. *Lymphlink* 2006;18:1.

84. Casley-Smith JR. Lymphedema initiated by aircraft flights. *Aviat Space Environ Med* 1996;67:52–56.

85. Ahmed RL, Thomas W, Yee D, et al. Randomized controlled trial of weight training and lymphedema in breast cancer survivors. *J Clin Oncol* 2006;24:2765–2772.

86. Graham PH. Compression prophylaxis may increase the potential for flight-associated lymphoedema after breast cancer treatment. *Breast* 2002;11:66–71.

87. Clark B, Sitzia J, Harlow W. Incidence and risk of arm oedema following treatment for breast cancer: a three-year follow-up study. *QJM* 2005;98:343–348.

88. Shaw C, Mortimer P, Judd PA. A randomized controlled trial of weight reduction as a treatment for breast cancer-related lymphedema. *Cancer* 2007;110:1868–1874.

89. World Health Organization. *Adherence to long-term therapies: evidence for action.* Geneva: World Health Organization, 2003.

90. Lerner R. Complete decongestive physiotherapy and the Lerner Lymphedema Services Academy of Lymphatic Studies (the Lerner School). *Cancer* 1998;83:2861–2863.

91. Mondry TE, Riffenburgh RH, Johnstone PA. Prospective trial of complete decongestive therapy for upper extremity lymphedema after breast cancer therapy. *Cancer J* 2004;10:42–49.

92. Vignes S, Porcher R, Arrault M, et al. Long-term management of breast cancer-related lymphedema after intensive decongestive physiotherapy. *Breast Cancer Res Treat* 2007;101:285–290.

93. Koul R, Dufan T, Russell C, et al. Efficacy of complete decongestive therapy and manual lymphatic drainage on treatment-related lymphedema in breast cancer. *Int J Radiat Oncol Biol Phys* 2007;67:841–846.

94. Hamner JB, Fleming MD. Lymphedema therapy reduces the volume of edema and pain in patients with breast cancer. *Ann Surg Oncol* 2007;14:1904–1908.

95. NLN Medical Advisory Committee: Training of lymphedema therapies. Position statement of the National Lymphedema Network 2005. www.lymphnet.org/pdfDocs/nlntraining.pdf.

96. Johansson K, Albertsson M, Ingvar C, et al. Effects of compression bandaging with or without manual lymph drainage treatment in patients with postoperative arm lymphedema. *Lymphology* 1999;32:103–110.

97. McKenzie DC, Kalda AL. Effect of upper extremity exercise on secondary lymphedema in breast cancer patients: a pilot study. *J Clin Oncol* 2003;21:463–466.

98. Harris SR, Niesen-Vertommen SL. Challenging the myth of exercise induced lymphedema following breast cancer: a series of case reports. *J Surg Oncol* 2000;74:95–99.

99. Turner J, Hayes S, Reul-Hirche H. Improving the physical status and quality of life of women treated for breast cancer: a pilot study of a structured exercise intervention. *J Surg Oncol* 2004;86:141–146.

100. Badger CM, Peacock JL, Mortimer PS. A randomized, controlled, parallel-group clinical trial comparing multilayer bandaging followed by hosiery versus hosiery alone in the treatment of patients with lymphedema of the limb. *Cancer* 2000;88:2832–2837.

101. Bertelli G, Venturini M, Forno G, et al. An analysis of prognostic factors in response to conservative treatment of postmastectomy lymphedema. *Surg Gynecol Obstet* 1992;175:455–460.

102. Bates DO, Levick JR, Mortimer PS. Subcutaneous interstitial fluid pressure and arm volume in lymphoedema. *Int J Microcirc Clin Exp* 1992;11:359–373.

103. Brennan MJ, Miller LT. Overview of treatment options and review of the current role and use of compression garments, intermittent pumps, and exercise in the management of lymphedema. *Cancer* 1998;83:2821–2827.

104. Zuther JE. *Lymphedema management: the comprehensive guide for practitioners.* New York: Thieme Medical Publishers, 2005.

105. Loprinzi CL, Kugler JW, Sloan JA, et al. Lack of effect of coumarin in women with lymphedema after treatment for breast cancer. *N Engl J Med* 1999;340:346–350.

106. Charles RH. Elephantiasis scroti. In: Latham AC, English TC, eds. *A system of treatment.* London: J&A Churchill, 1912:504.

107. Brorson H. Liposuction in arm lymphedema treatment. *Scand J Surg* 2003;92:287–295.

108. Campisi C, Boccardo F, Zilli A, et al. Long-term results after lymphatic-venous anastomoses for the treatment of obstructive lymphedema. *Microsurgery* 2001;21:135–139.

109. Baumeister RG, Siuda S. Treatment of lymphedemas by microsurgical lymphatic grafting: what is proved? *Plast Reconstr Surg* 1990;85:64–76.

110. Becker C, Assouad J, Riquet M, et al. Postmastectomy lymphedema: long-term results following microsurgical lymph node transplantation. *Ann Surg* 2006;243:313–315.

111. Carati CJ, Anderson SN, Gannon BJ, et al. Treatment of postmastectomy lymphedema with low-level laser therapy: a double blind, placebo-controlled trial. *Cancer* 2003;98:1114–1122.

112. McNeely ML, Magee DJ, Lees AW, et al. The addition of manual lymph drainage to compression therapy for breast cancer related lymphedema: a randomized controlled trial. *Breast Cancer Res Treat* 2004;86:95–106.

113. Miller TA, Wyatt LE, Rudkin GH. Staged skin and subcutaneous excision for lymphedema: a favorable report of long-term results. *Plast Reconstr Surg* 1998;102:1486–1501.

Chapter 46
Treatment of the Axilla and Other Regional Nodes

Monica Morrow and Jay R. Harris

Sentinel lymph node dissection (SLND) is a staging procedure that can be performed with vital dyes, radioactive tracers, or a combination of the two. SLND has rapidly replaced level I or II axillary lymph node dissection (ALND) as the standard procedure for staging a clinically axillary node-negative patient. Expertise in the technique must be demonstrated by the procedure team through the collection and analysis of outcome data. SLND is contraindicated in inflammatory carcinoma. Age, tumor histology, tumor location, biopsy type, and procedure on the breast are not contraindications to the use of SLND.

The American College of Pathologists has established guidelines to process the sentinel node. The sentinel node should be bivalved along the longitudinal axis, serially sectioned at 1.5- to 2.0-mm thickness blocks and each block sectioned at three levels and examined using routine hematoxylin-eosin stains. The routine use of immunohistochemical (IHC) staining or other molecular approaches is controversial; such approaches increase the likelihood of detecting isolated tumor cells, whose clinical significance is uncertain. (The authors recommend against the routine use of IHC.)

SLND alone for a negative sentinel node accurately stages the axilla and is associated with isolated recurrence in the axilla in less than 1% of cases. When the sentinel node shows either macro- or micrometastases, ALND has been the standard of care. There is growing evidence, however, that axillary irradiation is a reasonable alternative to ALND when there are no grossly abnormal nodes in the axilla and the findings from axillary dissection will not change the adjuvant systemic treatment plan. To date, this approach has primarily been applied in patients with low volume metastases in the sentinel node that are not detected intraoperatively. The most common method of axillary irradiation is separate field(s) that irradiate level I to III of the axilla and supraclavicular nodes and is matched to the breast or chest wall radiation fields. Typically a posteroanterior field is used in addition to an anteroposterior field to provide better coverage of the level I and II nodes. A dose of 45 to 50 Gy with standard radiation fractionation of 1.8 to 2.0 Gy is recommended for axillary irradiation. Individualized CT-based radiation treatment planning is recommended to ensure adequate dose coverage of the targeted nodal volumes and to minimize excessive dose heterogeneity and inadvertent normal tissue irradiation. A "high tangent" technique can be used to irradiate just level I or II of the axilla in selected favorable cases, such as patients with a lymphovascular invasion (LVI)-negative T1 tumor and a micrometastases on SLND.

The early and late postoperative morbidity of SLND is significantly lower than the morbidity of ALND. Lymphedema is reported to occur in about 5% of patients following SLND and in about 10% to 15% of patients following ALND. Lymphedema after axillary irradiation alone is seen in less than 5% of patients. The incidence of lymphedema after SNLD followed by full axillary irradiation is uncertain. Lymphedema can occur many years following surgery.

Axillary dissection remains the standard approach to the patient who presents with clinically evident nodal metastases. Histologic confirmation of disease should be obtained by needle biopsy since the positive predictive value of physical examination of nodes is surprisingly low. If metastases cannot be documented, SNLD, including the removal of clinically abnormal nodes, should be carried out prior to proceeding with axillary dissection.

Postoperative care after ALND should include shoulder exercises to maintain range of motion.

It is controversial whether common recommendations (including the avoidance of trauma or injury, infection, blood pressure cuffs, heavy lifting, or repetitive motion) are effective in preventing lymphedema. The gold standard for diagnosis of lymphedema is water displacement, but in most cases the diagnosis is made by arm measurements. Objective measurements and subjective symptoms of lymphedema are commonly not well correlated and both should be documented. The risk of lymphedema following ALND is increased in obese patients and in patients receiving full axillary irradiation. In patients requiring axillary irradiation after ALND, it is recommended that the surgical and radiation oncologist communicate regarding the extent of the dissection; in patients with an adequate dissection and no or limited extranodal extension, radiation therapy can be restricted to the axillary apex (level III) and supraclavicular nodes lessening the risk of lymphedema. (The coracoid process can be used as the lateral border of this field.) Treatment of lymphedema consists of manual lymphatic drainage, compression garments and devices, and exercise, but is typically only moderately successful.

The need to biopsy sentinel nodes in the internal mammary chain is controversial. Isolated internal mammary node (IMN) metastases are seen in fewer than 3% of patients and rarely occur in patients who are not candidates for systemic treatment based on features of the primary tumor. The inclusion of the IMNs either with breast-conserving therapy or postmastectomy radiation therapy is controversial. Microscopic involvement of IMNs can be high, especially in patients with positive axillary nodes and medial tumors; however, prior to the more recent use of positron emission tomography with computed tomography (PET-CT) for staging, recurrences in the IMNs have been rare. Until recently, the benefit of irradiating the IMNs has not been formally tested. Advocates of IMN irradiation point out that all of the positive postmastectomy radiation therapy trials included treatment of the IMNs. This issue will not likely be settled at least until the results of ongoing randomized trials of regional nodal irradiation are mature. The inclusion of the IMNs requires CT-based simulation and the use of techniques that avoid cardiac irradiation and minimize lung irradiation.

Atif J. Khan and Bruce G. Haffty

The use of postmastectomy radiation therapy (PMRT) is perhaps one of the most intensively studied topics in oncology and yet continues to be a cause of considerable debate. Indeed, some of the first ever prospective randomized trials to be conducted addressed the utility of PMRT (1). This area has attracted robust scientific inquiry since the initial efforts and has been the subject of over 20 randomized prospective trials. Despite the scientific scrutiny this area has attracted, important questions still remain to be answered.

This chapter will focus on the topic of PMRT and is divided into four sections: (a) a review of the data supporting the efficacy of PMRT as well as the risks and sequelae of PMRT, (b) criteria for patient selection, (c) reconstruction and PMRT, and (d) the technique of PMRT. The role of PMRT after neoadjuvant chemotherapy and in locally advanced and inflammatory breast cancer is discussed in Chapters 60, 61, and 62, respectively.

RATIONALE FOR POSTMASTECTOMY RADIATION THERAPY

The principle that irradiating the chest wall and regional lymph nodes after mastectomy can reduce subsequent locoregional recurrences has been well documented by multiple older trials comparing mastectomy alone to mastectomy with postoperative radiation (2–8). These trials typically used unsophisticated radiation techniques coupled with outdated radiation treatment machines that produced orthovoltage x-rays, resulting in less precise delivery of radiation to target tissues and increased doses to nontarget normal structures. Naturally, the relevance of these older trials is limited in the context of modern radiation therapy, but they adequately demonstrated two important facts: (a) PMRT can effectively reduce the burden of residual locoregional disease, and (b) radiation therapy is more comprehensive and more "radical," in terms of treatment volume, than even the most radical surgery. These trials did not demonstrate improvements in survival due to the beneficial effect with respect to breast cancer mortality being offset by the nonbreast cancer–related morbidity and mortality associated with the radiation techniques employed.

The Cuzick et al. (9,10) meta-analysis, published first in 1987 and then updated in 1994, pooled data from 10 early trials (all initiated before 1975 and all without chemotherapy) of mastectomy with or without PMRT, and, in the second report, attempted to define cause-specific mortality in over 4,000 patients who died at least 10 years after enrolling on study. In women who had a radical mastectomy, an 18% deficit in all-cause mortality was found in those who received radiation therapy compared to controls who were observed. There was no difference in the group that had either simple or modified radical mastectomy followed by RT versus those who were observed. When all trials were combined, a nonsignificant 7% decrement in survival was reported for patients who received RT (p = .21). Cause-specific mortality analysis revealed an excess of cardiac mortality in patients who received RT. At 10 years, an improvement in breast cancer mortality with RT tended to balance the cardiac-related mortality. The Cuzick et al. meta-analysis raised significant concerns in the oncology community about the safety of PMRT, especially given the emergence of and excitement surrounding systemic therapies.

The potential improvement in locoregional control that results from adjuvant systemic therapy alone can be studied through the numerous trials of systemic therapy versus nil that have reported patterns of failure (11–25) (Table 47.1). Data demonstrating a benefit of systemic cytotoxic chemotherapy on local-regional control are somewhat inconsistent, which may be related to confounding effects of patient selection, surgery, and radiation delivery. However, the most recent Early Breast Cancer Trialists' Collaborative Group (EBCTCG) meta-analysis of systemic therapy trials reported statistically fewer isolated local relapses in patients receiving polychemotherapy (recurrence rate ratio of 0.63 and 0.70 for women younger than 50 and 50 to 69, respectively) (26). Nonetheless, it appears that increasing the intensity or agents of chemotherapy does not improve locoregional control over standard chemotherapy (27–32). In contrast, adjuvant tamoxifen seems to improve locoregional control rather consistently, reducing the likelihood of recurrence on average by about half (11,13–15,24). This has been corroborated by the most recent EBCTCG meta-analysis, cited above, which showed an isolated local recurrence rate ratio of 0.47 with tamoxifen versus without (26). These observations, along with the demonstrable improvement in survival with systemic agents, raise the obvious question of the relative additional benefit of PMRT in patients receiving systemic therapy.

Several trials have studied the efficacy and added benefit of PMRT in the presence of systemic therapy (Table 47.2) (33–45). The most significant contributions have come from the Danish Breast Cancer Cooperative Group (41,42) and the British Columbia Cancer Agency (43). The trials conducted by these two groups, together with the updated findings of the EBCTCG meta-analysis of radiation trials, discussed later (46), have decisively altered practice and reaffirmed the role of PMRT in current breast oncology.

In protocol 82b, the Danish Breast Cancer Cooperative Group randomized premenopausal women with high-risk breast cancer after modified radical mastectomy (total mastectomy and level I and II axillary dissection) to either nine cycles of cyclophosphamide-methotrexate-fluorouracil (CMF) chemotherapy or to eight cycles of CMF chemotherapy and radiation therapy to the chest wall and regional nodes between the first and second cycles of chemotherapy (41). High-risk status was defined as positive lymph nodes, tumor size greater than 5 cm, or invasion of the skin or pectoralis fascia. Radiation therapy was delivered to a total dose of 50 Gy in 25 fractions or 48 Gy in 22 fractions using anterior electron fields to treat the chest wall and internal mammary (IM) nodes and a matched anterior photon field to treat the supraclavicular, infraclavicular, and axillary lymph nodes. A posterior axillary photon field was used in patients with a large anterior-posterior (AP) separation. Over 92% of all patients were treated with megavoltage equipment. The study enrolled 1,708 patients between 1982 to 1989. With a median follow-up of 114 months, the irradiated group demonstrated statistically significant improvements in locoregional recurrences (32% vs. 9%), disease-free survival (35% vs. 48% at 10 years), and overall survival (45% vs. 54% at 10 years). Over half of all locoregional recurrences were on the chest wall.

In the companion trial, protocol 82c (42), postmenopausal women younger than 70 with high-risk breast cancer (defined as in protocol 82b) were randomized after modified radical mastectomy to receive either 30 mg of tamoxifen daily for 1

| Table 47.1 | RANDOMIZED TRIALS OF ADJUVANT SYSTEMIC THERAPY VERSUS OBSERVATION FOLLOWING MASTECTOMY | | | | | |

				Locoregional Failure (%)		
Trial (Reference)	Study Years	No. of Patients	Systemic Treatment	Control	Systemic Therapy	Follow-Up (yrs)
Node Negative						
West Midlands Oncology Association (21)	1976–1984	543	LMF	19	10	8
Milan (25)	1980–1985	90	CMF	13[a]	4[a]	12
IBCSG V (18)	1981–1985	1,275	CMF	12	7	5
ECOG/Intergroup (19)	1981–1988	425	CMFP	9	3	4.5
NSABP B-13 (16)	1981–1988	760	MF	13	6	8
NSABP B-14 (15)	1982–1988	2,818	T	7	3	10
Node Positive						
NSABP B-05 (17)	1972–1974	380	L-PAM	24	14	11
Milan (12)	1973–1975	391	CMF	15	13	19
Guy's/Manchester (23)	1975–1979	370	L-PAM	27	18	_[a]
Guy's/Manchester (22)	1976–1985	391	CMF	44[b]	18[b]	8
West Midlands Oncology Association (20)	1976–1984	540	AVCMF	35	31	7
IBCSG III (13)	1978–1981	339	CMFPT	34	21	13
IBCSG IV (13,14)	1978–1981	349	pT	34	16	21
ECOG (24)	1978–1981	265	CMFP	13	CMFP 11 CMFPT 9	6
NCCTG (11)	1979–1985	234	CFP	19	CFP 8 CFPT 9	5

LMF, chlorambucil, methotrexate, and fluorouracil; CMF, cyclophosphamide, methotrexate, and fluorouracil; IBCSG, International Breast Cancer Study Group; ECOG, Eastern Cooperative Oncology Group; CMFP, cyclophosphamide, methotrexate, fluorouracil, and prednisone; NSABP, National Surgical Adjuvant Breast and Bowel Project; MF, methotrexate and fluorouracil; T, tamoxifen; L-PAM, L-phenylalanine mustard; AVCMF, doxorubicin, vincristine, cyclophosphamide, methotrexate, and fluorouracil; CMFPT, cyclophosphamide, methotrexate, fluorouracil, prednisone, and tamoxifen; pT, prednisone and tamoxifen; NCCTG, North Central Cancer Treatment Group; CFPT, cyclophosphamide, fluorouracil, prednisone, and tamoxifen.
[a]Includes breast-conservation failures.
[b]Premenopausal women.
Adapted from Pierce L. The use of postmastectomy radiotherapy after mastectomy: a review of the literature. *J Clin Oncol* 2005;23:1706–1717, with permission.

year beginning 2 to 4 weeks after surgery alone or with concurrent radiation therapy delivered to the chest wall and draining lymph nodes. A total of 1,375 patients were recruited between 1982 and 1990 and followed for a median time of 10 years. As in the protocol 82b study, the irradiated group demonstrated statistically significant improvements in locoregional recurrence (35% vs. 8%), disease-free survival (24% vs. 36%), and overall survival (36% vs. 45%). As in the protocol 82b study, recurrence at all locoregional subsites was lower with PMRT than without. Although these well-designed efforts by the Danish group are not without flaw (as discussed below), they nonetheless strengthened the theory that, in certain patient subsets, aggressive locoregional control could result in improvements in survival end points.

The smaller British Columbia trial enrolled 318 node-positive premenopausal breast cancer patients and randomized them after modified radical mastectomy to either radiation therapy or no additional locoregional therapy (43). Both groups received adjuvant CMF chemotherapy for 12 (first 80 patients) or 6 months. Radiation therapy was delivered to the chest wall to a dose of 37.5 Gy in 16 daily fractions through opposed tangential photon fields. The supraclavicular and axilla nodes were treated with an AP field and a posterior axillary field, with a target midaxilla dose of 35 Gy. Bilateral IM nodes were treated with an additional anterior field to a dose of 37.5 Gy in 16 fractions. All treatments were delivered with cobalt machines, between cycle four and five of chemotherapy. After a median follow-up of 20 years, the 20-year survival free of locoregional disease developing before systemic therapy was 61% in the chemotherapy alone arm and 87% in the irradiated group. The irradiated group had statistically significant improvements in 20-year event-free survival (25% vs. 38%), systemic disease-free survival (31% vs. 48%), breast–cancer–specific survival (38% vs.

53%), and overall survival (37% vs. 47%). There were slightly more nonbreast cancer deaths in the irradiated group (9% vs. 4%; $p = .11$). There were three cardiac deaths (2%) in the irradiated group versus one (0.6%) in the control group ($p = .62$), and 9% of patients in the irradiated group developed arm edema compared with 3% in the control group ($p = .035$). This study corroborated the Danish experience and again demonstrated some of the most remarkable improvements in survival end points ever reported for any adjuvant therapy.

Taken together, these studies demonstrated that certain patient cohorts have a high risk for locoregional recurrence that is inadequately addressed by systemic therapy alone. Furthermore, reducing the likelihood of locoregional recurrence can result in improved survival; presumably, persistent or recurrent locoregional disease can be a source of distant metastases and subsequent death. These studies imply that the benefit of systemic therapy is primarily to lower the competing risk of distant micrometastases, and that adjuvant locoregional therapy and adjuvant systemic therapy independently benefit these patients on the principle of spatial cooperation. There is no definitive randomized data supporting any specific sequencing of systemic therapy and radiation in the postmastectomy setting; for patients receiving both cytotoxic chemotherapy and PMRT, the prevailing practice typically sequences the cytotoxic chemotherapy first followed by radiation. Hormonal therapy, if indicated, may be given concurrently with radiation or following radiation, although some clinicians prefer to sequence tamoxifen after the radiation. Although there is little in the way of long-term follow-up data and additional studies will likely be forthcoming in the next few years, adjuvant systemic therapy with trastuzumab (typically administered for up to 1 year following chemotherapy) appears to be safe and effective given concurrently with radiation (47).

Table 47.2	RANDOMIZED TRIALS OF ADJUVANT SYSTEMIC THERAPY WITH/WITHOUT RADIOTHERAPY FOLLOWING MASTECTOMY

Trial (Reference)	Study Years	No. of Patients	Systemic Treatment	RT Dose Gy	RT Dose No. of Fractions	Locoregional Failure (%) No RT	Locoregional Failure (%) RT	Overall Survival (%) No RT	Overall Survival (%) RT	Follow-Up (yrs)
Mayo Clinic (37)	1973–1980	227	CFP	50	24[a]	30	10	66	68	5
Dana Farber (35)	1973–1984									
1–3 positive nodes		83	CMF	45	20	5	2	85	77	5
≥4 positive nodes		123	CA	45	20	20	6	63	59	5
Helsinki (Klefstrom et al. 36)	1976–1981	79	VAC ± L	45	15	45	10	65	90	5
Glasgow (38)	1976–1982	219	CMF	37.8	15	25	11			5
1–3 positive nodes								54	63	
≥4 positive nodes								22	33	
Piedmont (39)	1976–?	76	L-PAM	45–50	30	23	9	48	61	11
		83	CMF	45–50	30	14	5	58	46	11
SECSG (45)	1976–1983	270	CMF	50	25	20	10	35[b]	45[b]	10
M.D. Anderson (34)	1978–1980	97	FAC,BCG	Not Stated		Not Stated		69[c]	64[c]	3
SSBCG (44)	1978–1985	287	CMF	38–48	Unknown	17	6	Not Stated		8
	1978–1985	483	T	38–48	Unknown	18	6	Not Stated		8
British Columbia (43)	1978–1986	318	CMF	37.5	16	26	10	37	47	20
Helsinki (Blomqvist et al. 33)	1981–1984	99	CAFt	45	15	24	7	69	65	7.5
ECOG (40)	1982–1987	312	CAFTH	46	23	24	15	47	46	9
DBCCG 82b (41)	1982–1989	1708	CMF	48–50	25	32	9	45	54	10
DBCCG 82c (42)	1982–1990	1375	T	48–50	25	35	8	36	45	10

RT, radiotherapy; CFP, cyclophosphamide, fluorouracil, and prednisone; CMF, cyclophosphamide, methotrexate, and fluorouracil; CA, cyclophosphamide and doxorubicin; VAC ± L, vincristine, doxorubicin, cyclophosphamide ± levamisole; L-PAM, L-phenylalanine mustard; SECSG, Southeastern Cancer Study Group; FAC, fluorouracil, doxorubicin, and cyclophosphamide; BCG, Bacillus Calmette Guerin; SSBCG, South Swedish Breast Cancer Group; T, tamoxifen; CAFt, cyclophosphamide, doxorubicin, fluorouracil, and ftorafur; ECOG, Eastern Cooperative Oncology Group; CAFTH, cyclophosphamide, doxorubicin, fluorouracil, tamoxifen, and fluoxymesterone; DBCCG, Danish Breast Cancer Collaborative Group.

[a]Dose 25 Gy in 12 fractions delivered followed by 4-week break then additional 25 Gy in 12 fractions.
[b]Extrapolated from survival curves.
[c]Disease-free survival.
Adapted from Pierce L. The use of postmastectomy radiotherapy after mastectomy: a review of the literature. *J Clin Oncol* 2005;23:1706–1717, with permission.

The EBCTCG has collected primary data from every randomized trial of adjuvant radiotherapy in breast cancer and periodically reports the ongoing analyses on the benefits and risks of radiation therapy in these patients. The most recent report from 2005 reviewed data on 9,933 patients enrolled on 25 trials of PMRT, all of which were unconfounded by the use of systemic therapy (46). Node-positive patients who had axillary clearance and received radiation therapy after mastectomy had a 5-year locoregional recurrence rate of 6%, compared to 23% for unirradiated controls (15-year rates were 8% vs. 29%). In every large trial of PMRT in node-positive women, radiation therapy produced a similar proportional reduction in local recurrence, powerfully demonstrating the comparable efficacy of radiotherapy in achieving local control across all time periods. Even more significantly, PMRT also produced comparable proportional reductions in local recurrence in all women irrespective of age or tumor characteristics.

Absolute reductions in local recurrence were dependent on the absolute risk in the control arm (i.e., larger reductions were seen in subsets with greater risk). For patients with a control risk of local recurrence greater than 10%, the addition of RT improved local recurrence irrespective of systemic therapy. For women with node-positive disease who were irradiated after mastectomy and axillary clearance, a 17% absolute improvement in 5-year local control translated into a highly statistically significant 5.4% absolute improvement in 15-year breast cancer mortality (60.1% vs. 54.7%; $2p = .0002$) (46) (Fig. 47.1), and a 4.4% absolute improvement in 15-year all-cause mortality (64.2% vs. 59.8%; $2p = .0009$) over unirradiated controls.

In their review of the EBCTCG data, Punglia et al. (48) note that treatments that had little or no effect on decreasing the 5-year local recurrence rate produced no benefit in 15-year breast cancer mortality. Furthermore, the absolute reduction in 5-year local recurrence rates (by more extensive surgery or the addition of radiation) was proportional to the absolute reduction in 15-year breast cancer mortality in a 4:1 ratio, whereby a 20% absolute reduction in 5-year local recurrence resulted in a 5% absolute reduction in 15-year breast cancer mortality. The analysis by Punglia et al. also draws attention to a subgroup analysis in the EBCTCG report that showed that the use of radiation therapy after mastectomy in node-positive patients improved 15-year survival only in patients who also received adjuvant systemic therapy and not in patients who were treated with mastectomy alone. This certainly supports the concept of the independent yet cooperative effect of adjuvant locoregional and systemic therapy. Subgroup analysis also demonstrated that the benefit of irradiation was primarily significant in patients younger than 50, due perhaps to the competing risks for mortality present in the older populations. Alternatively, a larger control risk for recurrence in the younger population may lead to more significant improvements in the studied end points.

There was an excess cancer incidence in women studied on the updated EBCTCG report (including women treated with an intact breast), mainly in contralateral breast cancer and lung cancer, and an excess mortality from heart disease and lung cancer. The averaged detrimental effects were modest, with 15-year absolute loss of 1.8% for contralateral breast cancer and 1.3% for nonbreast cancer mortality. Importantly,

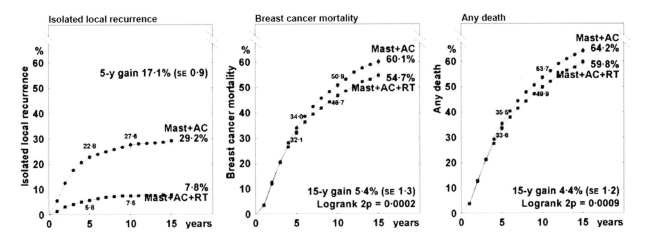

FIGURE 47.1. Probabilities for isolated local recurrence, breast cancer mortality, and any death in node-positive patients treated with postmastectomy radiation therapy after mastectomy and axillary clearance. Mast, mastectomy; AC, axillary clearance; RT, radiotherapy; SE, standard error. (From Early Breast Cancer Trialists' Collaborative Group. Effects of radiotherapy and differences in the extent of surgery for early breast cancer on local recurrence and 15-year survival: an overview of the randomized trials. *Lancet* 2005;366:2087–2106, with permission.)

the proportional excess of nonbreast cancer deaths was greatest at 5 to 14 years and more than 15 years after randomization, and the mean dates of randomization for these two groups was 1975 and 1970, respectively. The authors of the EBCTCG correctly point out that the late hazards evident in their report could well be substantially lower for modern radiation therapy technique and regimens.

The EBCTCG data was updated at the 2007 annual meeting of the American Society of Clinical Oncology (49). Although the data are still preliminary, several pertinent and new findings have been described. In contrast to the prior update, the subgroup of patients with one to three positive lymph nodes were reported to have statistically significant improvements in 15-year breast cancer mortality (50.9% vs. 43.3%; $2p$ = .002) and all-cause mortality (56.1% vs. 50.9%; $2p$ = .05) with PMRT. In addition, a study of prognostic factors for 5-year local recurrence risks identified tumor grade as a highly significant factor, even when controlling for other known risk factors.

The EBCTCG overview represents one of the most significant contributions to the study of PMRT. However, the relevance of its findings may be limited by the inclusion of older trials that used fractionation schemes, treatment machines, and treatment volumes that are antiquated by current standards, as well as by the usual limitations of meta-analyses. To address these issues, Van de Steene et al. (50) re-examined the EBCTCG data and identified four factors that selected for significant improvement in the odds ratio (OR) for survival in the irradiated versus control populations: start date of the trial (after 1970 [OR 0.935]), number of patients (>600 patients [OR 0.932]), fractionation (conventional [OR 0.896]), and crude survival on the trial (at least 80% [OR 0.799]). Excluding trials that began before 1970 and trials with small sample sizes produced a significant odds reduction of 12.3% ± 4.3% with irradiation. Gebski et al. (51) performed a meta-analysis in which they carefully attempted to control for the quality of radiation delivery in PMRT trials. The authors defined optimal dose as being between 40 and 60 Gy delivered in 2 Gy fractions (nonconventional fractionation schemes were converted to 2-Gy equivalents using bioeffective dose calculations) and appropriate treatment volumes as both chest wall and regional lymphatics. The authors reanalyzed data from the EBCTCG applying these criteria. The proportional reduction in locoregional recurrence was greater for trials with optimal dose and volume (80%), compared to those with suboptimal dose (70%) or field design

(64%). An improvement in breast cancer mortality was restricted to those trials that used appropriate doses and fields for irradiation (6.4% absolute increase in survival; p <.001).

The most concerning risk of PMRT for radiation oncologists is the risk of radiation-induced cardiac morbidity. As described above, the EBCTCG meta-analysis as well as other registry data have detected increased risks of cardiac mortality in irradiated patients (46,52,53). In contrast, an analysis of the Danish postmastectomy trials patients by Hojris et al. (54) found, using a technique of RT that avoided cardiac irradiation, equal rates of ischemic heart disease and acute myocardial infarction in the irradiated and unirradiated group. Approximately 3% of patients in both groups had ischemia-related morbidity at a median follow-up of 117 months, and less than 1% of patients in both arms had death due to cardiac causes. There was no difference in this study when comparing left- versus right-sided irradiation. However, these numbers may underestimate the true burden of radiation-related cardiac morbidity due to the competing risk of breast-cancer death in this high-risk population and also because this study was an unplanned retrospective report on a prospectively studied patient cohort.

Gyenes et al. (55) reviewed 960 patients treated on the first Stockholm Breast Cancer trial (modified radical mastectomy alone versus preoperative versus postoperative RT accrued 1971-1976) and reported 58 acute myocardial infarctions (MI) in the study population for a crude rate of 6%. There were no differences in acute MI or death due to cardiovascular disease (63/960) between irradiated and unirradiated patients. Importantly, the authors showed that only patients in the high-dose–volume group had an excess hazard ratio (HR) of cardiovascular death (HR = 2; 95% confidence interval [CI], 1.0–3.9; p = .04). A retrospective study by Harris et al. (56) examined cardiac events in a series of 961 women irradiated to the intact breast and reported no interaction between left- versus right-sided RT on cardiac mortality or congestive heart disease. A significant interaction was noted between left-sided RT in the subsequent development of coronary artery disease (20-year actuarial risk 25% vs. 10% for right-sided; p <.001) and MI (15% vs. 5%; p <.002). Coexistent hypertension was an independent hazard for the development of coronary artery disease.

A study of the Surveillance, Epidemiology, and End Results (SEER) database conducted by Giordano et al. (57) compared 15-year cardiac mortality rates in left- versus right-sided breast cancer as a function of the year of diagnosis in patients who received RT. Presumably, patients with left-sided lesions received more heart irradiation than those with right-sided lesions. Although the authors demonstrated excess cardiac mortality in left-sided breast cancer patients diagnosed between 1973 and 1979 (13% vs. 10%; $p = .02$), they found no significant difference in patients irradiated in the most recent time periods (~9% for both groups in the 1980 to 1984 cohort, and 5% to 6% in the 1985 to 1989 cohort). Beginning in 1979, the hazard of death from ischemic heart disease in left-sided breast cancer patients (vs. right-sided) declined by an average of 6% per year. Taken together, these data are reassuring and imply that improvements in image-based simulation and treatment delivery should further reduce morbidity associated with radiation therapy.

Few data exist on the cumulative effects of anthracyclines and radiation therapy on cardiac morbidity and function. Perhaps the best data on this topic comes from Fumoleau et al. (58) who reported long-term cardiac function in 3,577 assessable patients randomized on eight French trials of adjuvant therapy, 2,553 of whom received epirubicin-based chemotherapy. Ninety-seven percent of women on the epirubicin cohort had adjuvant radiation (to the intact breast or post-mastectomy) and 94% on the nonepirubicin cohort received RT (with about two thirds of these receiving RT to the IM nodes). The 7-year risk of *left-ventricular dysfunction* was 1.36% in the epirubicin arm and 0.2% in the nonanthracycline patients. Age 65 or greater and body mass index (BMI) greater than 27 kg/m^2 were additional significant risk factors.

Additional nonlife-threatening late risks of postmastectomy irradiation can include arm edema, fibrosis, shoulder stiffness, and brachial plexopathy. In an instructive report, the Danish postmastectomy investigators invited patients irradiated at Aarhus University Hospital who were alive and without evidence of disease to participate in a study of the late effects of PMRT (59). Eighty-four patients accepted the invitation and were eligible for analysis, and these patients were carefully assessed for late toxicity based primarily on LENT-SOMA (late effects of normal tissue-subjective, objective, management, and analytic) criteria. More women in the irradiated group had lymphedema (17% vs. 9%) and impaired shoulder movement (16% vs. 2%) that interfered with work or daily activities. Irradiated patients also had more arm paresthesias (21% vs. 7%) and more arm weakness (14% vs. 2%). Only the shoulder function comparison was statistically significant. Symptomatic pulmonary complications were equal in irradiated and unirradiated patients. In a separate report of 161 patients with neurological follow-up who were irradiated on the Danish 82 protocols, 5% of patients had disabling and 8% had mild radiation-induced brachial plexopathies (60). Kunht et al. (61) reported acute and chronic reactions in 194 patients receiving PMRT. Twenty-two percent of patients had any incidence of chronic effects, mostly from arm edema (28/43). Five patients had telangiectasia and one patient had plexopathy.

In conclusion, randomized trials as well as data from meta-analyses provide a strong rationale for PMRT in patients with a high likelihood of locoregional residual disease, despite the use of systemic therapy in these patients. Additional locoregional therapy in the form of RT reduces locoregional recurrence rates by a factor of approximately two-thirds, and one breast-cancer death is averted for every four locoregional recurrences prevented by RT. The risks of PMRT are modest but demonstrable, and cardiac effects may largely be attributable to older technique. The cardiac and pulmonary toxicities of modern day PMRT continue to be evaluated and are likely minimal with careful three-dimensional planning and treatment techniques.

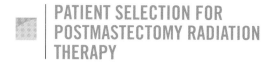

PATIENT SELECTION FOR POSTMASTECTOMY RADIATION THERAPY

Node Positive Patients

Node positivity in the axilla is the most significant predictor of locoregional recurrence after mastectomy. It should be borne in mind, however, that approximately two thirds of locoregional recurrences occur on the chest wall, and that axillary failures are far less common (62–65). Accordingly, the degree of node positivity should be viewed as an adverse feature that confers a higher risk for overall locoregional recurrence (i.e., not limited to failure at regional sites).

The Danish and Canadian PMRT trials demonstrated stable relative risk reductions for all events in all groups of node-positive patients. However, the conclusion that all node-positive patients warrant PMRT has been challenged. There are two general criticisms of these studies that limit the generalizing of these findings to all node-positive patients: (a) the adequacy of the systemic therapy in the control arms of these studies, and (b) the issue of the "background risk" in the relevant study populations.

The most recent EBCTCG meta-analysis of systemic therapy showed a significant but minor improvement for anthracycline containing polychemotherapy regimens over CMF regimens (26). Whether this incremental benefit improves locoregional control as well is unknown and is probably unlikely in patients with high risk for locoregional microscopic residual. Furthermore, neither the addition of taxanes nor increases in the intensity or density of chemotherapy have had demonstrable impacts on locoregional control in node-positive patients, although they do improve survival end points presumably by addressing micrometases (27–32). In sum, it seems unlikely that present-day chemotherapy regimens would significantly alter the findings of the postmastectomy trials. In contrast, the Danish protocol 82c trial treated postmenopausal patients (untested for estrogen/progesterone (ER/PR) status) with 1 year of tamoxifen (42), and it is unknown how a longer duration of hormonal therapy in a population known to be hormone-receptor positive would modulate the risk of locoregional recurrence and thus the benefit of PMRT.

A more significant factor that limits interpretation of the Danish and British Columbia trials is that node-positive patients on the control arm of these trials had higher locoregional recurrence rates than commonly reported for patients treated in the United States and elsewhere (41–43,62). This difference is especially obvious in patients with one to three positive lymph nodes, who represented about 60% of patients on these studies. In the unirradiated Danish population, the 18-year probability of locoregional recurrence (as first site of failure) was 59% for patients with four or more positive nodes, and 37% for those with one to three positive nodes (66). In the unirradiated Canadian population, the 20-year *isolated* locoregional recurrence rate was 41% for patients with four or more positive nodes, and 21% for patients with one to three positive nodes (43). Locoregional recurrence developing any time before distant failure (i.e., cumulative locoregional recurrence as first failure) was not reported as a function of the number of positive lymph nodes, but was 39% for the entire unirradiated group. In contrast, several large series of patients treated in the United States and elsewhere have reported locoregional recurrence rates in the range of 6% to 13% for patients with one to three positive nodes (63,64,67,68) (Table 47.3). This seems to indicate that the background risk for locoregional recurrence in the Danish and British Columbia trials was higher than average, and this may have exaggerated the benefit of PMRT in this population.

Table 47.3	LOCOREGIONAL RECURRENCE RATES IN PATIENTS NOT TREATED WITH RADIATION AFTER MASTECTOMY IN RANDOMIZED CLINICAL TRIALS	
Patterns-of-Failure Studies (Reference)	No. of Patients	Locoregional Recurrence Rates at 10 Years (%)
ECOG (64)		
1–3 +LN	1,018	13
≥4 +LN	998	29
M.D. Anderson (63)		
1–3 +LN	438	13
≥4 +LN	373	25
NSABP (67)		
1–3 +LN	2,957	13
≥4 +LN	2,784	27
IBCSG (70)		
1–3 +LN	2,402	17
≥4 +LN	1,659	31

+LN, positive lymph nodes; ECOG, Eastern Cooperative Oncology Group; NSABP, National Surgical Adjuvant Breast and Bowel Project; IBCSG, International Breast Cancer Study Group.

Differences in the extent of axillary surgery may partially explain the differences in the risk of locoregional recurrences in patients with one to three positive nodes. Full level I and II axillary dissections were not performed; a median of seven lymph nodes were removed in the Danish studies and a median of 11 lymph nodes were examined in patients on the Canadian trial (41–43). As such, many of the patients scored as having one to three positive lymph nodes may have actually had four or more positive nodes if full axillary dissections had been performed. Tellingly, failure in the axilla either alone or as a component of locoregional recurrence represented 43% of all locoregional recurrence in the Danish studies (62), compared to 14% in the data cited above (63).

However, it is important to note that the reports cited above and in Table 47.3 have reported 10-year locoregional control rates. The Danish studies report 18-year recurrence rates and also document a consistent locoregional recurrence of about 1% per year between follow-up years 10 and 25 (62). Similarly, in the British Columbia trial, which has reported 20-year recurrence rates, approximately 20% of locoregional recurrences occurred after follow-up year 10 (43). In addition, other identified and unidentified risk factors, such as T4 tumors or pectoral fascia invasion, may have been overrepresented in the postmastectomy trials (62), increasing the background risk for locoregional failure. For example, in a combined report of patients with one to three positive axillary nodes treated on the control arm of the British Columbia postmastectomy trial (n = 82) and similar patients treated on prospective systemic therapy trials at the M.D. Anderson Cancer Center (n = 462), statistically significant differences were detected in patients on the British Columbia trial who were younger (median age 43 vs. 48) and had more lymphovascular invasion (LVI) (52% vs. 33%), in addition to fewer examined nodes (median 10 vs. 16) (69). The resultant 10-year Kaplan-Meier estimates of locoregional recurrence were 21.5% and 12.6% for the British Columbia and M.D. Anderson Cancer Center patients, respectively.

Nonetheless, several reports have demonstrated the prognostic impact of total dissected nodes, nodal ratio (number of involved to uninvolved nodes), and number of total uninvolved nodes on locoregional recurrence and even overall survival (63,64,67–72). Attempts by Danish investigators to reanalyze their patients to include only those with adequate dissections are limited by the fact that these patients were not stratified by this important risk factor at randomization (73). This issue remains unclear and, because it has complicated the interpretation of the existing postmastectomy trials, can

only be addressed in the context of additional large, randomized trials.

Both the American Society of Therapeutic Radiology and Oncology (ASTRO) and the American Society of Clinical Oncology (ASCO) as well as other advisory organizations have endorsed the routine use of PMRT in women with four or more involved nodes and node-positive women with tumors greater than 5 cm, who have a high (>20% to 25%) risk of locoregional recurrence without RT. Both societies recognize the uncertain benefit of PMRT in patients with T1 or T2 primaries with one to three positive nodes (stage II) in whom the risk of locoregional recurrence is intermediate (around 10% to 20%) (74,75). The European SUPREMO trial (Selective Use of Postoperative Radiotherapy after Mastectomy) is currently open and will attempt to answer this question. This trial randomizes intermediate risk operable breast cancer (node-positive stage II tumors and node-negative tumors larger than 2 cm with adverse features [high grade or LVI]) to chest wall irradiation or observation after mastectomy.

Several groups have attempted to identify high-risk patients within the one to three positive lymph node group (Table 47.4). Clearly, this group of patients is heterogeneous in terms of various potential clinicopathological factors that may allow differentiation into low- and high-risk cohorts. One of the most significant efforts attempting to identify these risk factors comes from Wallgren et al. (68) who reviewed data on over 5,300 patients enrolled on the first seven trials of the International Breast Cancer Study Group (IBCSG). These trials of systemic therapy required a minimum of eight dissected lymph nodes and negative margins. In patients with one to three involved lymph nodes, premenopausal patients with LVI and grade 3 tumors had cumulative incidence functions (CIFs) exceeding 20% for any locoregional recurrence. Postmenopausal women with grade 3 tumors and tumors larger than 2 cm had correspondingly high risk. Collapsing this information, premenopausal women with one to three positive lymph nodes had locoregional recurrence risks ranging from 19% to 27% if they had grade 2 or 3 disease with vascular invasion, but that risk was less than 15% if they had grade 1 disease with no vascular invasion. In a subsequent report, the same group reported results from IBCSG trials one through nine and demonstrated the significant independent impact, in a multivariate model, of the number of uninvolved lymph nodes (70). More specifically, in the group of patients with one to three involved lymph nodes (n = 2,402), factors that independently predicted a CIF for locoregional recurrence exceeding 20%

Table 47.4	COFACTORS ASSOCIATED WITH A GREATER THAN 15% LOCOREGIONAL RECURRENCE AFTER MASTECTOMY AND CHEMOTHERAPY IN PATIENTS WITH ONE TO THREE POSITIVE LYMPH NODES		
Study (Reference)	No. of Patients	Cofactors	End Point
Wallgren et al. (68)	2,404	• Premenopausal, G2 or G3, LVSI • Postmenopausal, G3 • Postmenopausal, G2, T2 disease	• 10-yr LRF ± DF (isolated LRF or with simultaneous DF)
Taghian et al. (67)	2,403	• Age <50, T2 disease	• 10-yr LRF ± DF
Recht et al. (64)	1,018	• Premenopausal, T1 disease	• 10-yr LRF ± DF (isolated LRF or with simultaneous DF)
Truong et al. (72)	821	• Age<45[a] • 25% of lymph nodes involved[a] • ER-negative disease[a] • G3 disease • T2 disease • LVSI • Medial tumor location[a]	• 10-yr LRF ± DF (isolated LRF or with simultaneous DF)
Katz et al. (76)	466	• Tumor size >4 cm • Invasion of skin/nipple • Invasion of pectoralis fascia • Close or positive margins	• 10-yr LRF ± DF
Cheng et al. (78)	110	• Age <40 • Tumor size ≥3 cm • Presence of LVSI • Adjuvant hormonal therapy	• 4-yr LRF ± DF (isolated LRF or with simultaneous DF)

LRF, local-regional failure; DF, distant failure; LVSI, lymphovascular space invasion; ER, estrogen receptor; G2 or 3, grade 2 or 3.
[a]Retain significance on multivariate analysis.

included age younger than 40, fewer than 10 uninvolved lymph nodes, and LVI.

The investigators at M.D. Anderson Cancer Center have reported results from their cohort of 1,031 patients treated with mastectomy and doxorubicin-based chemotherapy without subsequent radiation therapy on five prospective trials between 1975 and 1994 (63,71,76). Three factors were significant for isolated and total locoregional recurrence on multivariate analysis of the entire group: T stage, number of involved nodes, and extranodal extension 2 mm or more. Restricting the analysis to patients with T1 or T2 disease and one to three axillary nodes (n = 404, overall isolated 10-year locoregional recurrence risk of 10%), multivariate predictors of locoregional recurrence were fewer examined nodes, higher T stage, and extracapsular extension (ECE), with isolated 10-year locoregional recurrence in excess of 25% for patients with gross ECE (33%) and tumor size greater than 4 cm (26%) (63). In a more detailed study of pathologic factors in the same group of patients, Katz et al. reported that close or positive margins and gross multicentric disease were also predictive of locoregional recurrence on multivariable analysis (76). However, in the subgroup of patients with one to three positive nodes, invasion of skin and nipple, pectoral fascia invasion, and close or positive margins, but not multicentricity, were significant predictors of higher locoregional recurrence. In a similar group of patients, Fowble et al. (77) reported that patients with multicentric disease without other strong risk factors for postmastectomy chest wall relapse had a 5-year actuarial risk of an isolated locoregional recurrence of only 8%.

Truong et al. (72) reported on 821 women with T1 and T2 primary lesions with one to three positive lymph nodes treated with mastectomy and systemic therapy (in 94%) within the British Columbia Cancer Agency. Twelve putative clinicopathologic factors were examined for their effect on locoregional recurrence in a multivariate model. Age less than 45, nodal ratio greater than 25%, ER-negative status, and medial location independently predicted for isolated and any locoregional recurrence, with age having the greatest effect (HR = 3.44).

The authors suggested using age and nodal ratio as first line discriminants of risk and medial location and ER-negative status as secondary factors.

Recht et al. (64) reported on the outcomes of over 2,000 patients enrolled in four randomized Eastern Cooperative Oncology Group (ECOG) studies of systemic therapy. Median follow-up of the entire group was 12 years and 983 patients had tumors 5 cm or less and one to three positive lymph nodes. In a multivariate analysis of all patients, increasing tumor size, increasing number of positive nodes, ER-negative status, and decreasing number of examined nodes were significant independent predictors of locoregional recurrence. Cheng et al. (78) identified 110 patients with one to three positive axillary nodes treated at their institution with modified radical mastectomy and systemic therapy but without radiation (median number of nodes examined, 17). Sixty-nine patients received adjuvant chemotherapy and 84 received adjuvant hormonal therapy with tamoxifen. On multivariate analysis, only tumor size (<3 cm vs. greater) was significant for locoregional recurrence. However, the authors found that the four most significant factors on univariate analysis (age <40 years, tumor ≥3 cm, ER-negative disease, and LVI) could segregate patients into a high-risk group (with three or four factors) and a low-risk group (with two or fewer factors). This report had relatively small numbers and short median follow-up (54 months). In a similar Hungarian study, the authors reported on 249 patients with T1 and T2 tumors with one to three positive axillary nodes, half of whom were treated with PMRT (79). Several putative risk factors for locoregional recurrence were examined in the unirradiated patients on multivariate analysis, and only age (≤45 years) and size (T2) emerged as independent predictors of locoregional recurrence. Finally, Cheng et al. (80) have reported on gene expression profiles that are predictive of locoregional recurrence after mastectomy, although the number of locoregional events in their patients with one to three positive nodes was small. This promising methodology may serve as a valuable tool of risk assessment in the future.

Node-Negative Patients

The most recent EBCTCG overview demonstrated a nominal 5-year local recurrence rate of 6% after mastectomy and axillary clearance in node-negative patients. The addition of PMRT reduced this rate to 2% (2*p* = .0002), producing a modest absolute 5-year gain of 4% (46). Given the low overall risk of locoregional recurrence in node-negative patients, several investigators have attempted to identify subsets within this group with locoregional recurrence risks high enough to warrant PMRT.

In a multivariate analysis of the IBCSG trial patients discussed above, LVI was a significant risk factor of locoregional recurrence in node-negative patients, as was size greater than 2 cm in premenopausal node-negative patients (68). Jagsi et al. (81) reported a retrospective analysis of a cohort of 870 node-negative patients (excluding T4 patients) treated with modified radical mastectomy without RT at the Massachusetts General Hospital between 1980 and 2000. A multivariate analysis of several potential risk factors for total locoregional recurrence revealed four significant independent predictors: margin status (<2 mm), premenopausal status, size (>2 cm), and LVI, with these latter two having the greater hazard ratios (3.8 and 3.2, respectively). Ten-year total locoregional recurrence rates were approximately 20% with two adverse factors and 40% with three adverse factors. Approximately two thirds of the patients in this cohort did not received systemic therapy.

Floyd et al. (82) published data on a multicenter effort of 70 patients treated with mastectomy, systemic therapy, and no radiation for patients with pathological T3N0 disease and reported a 5-year locoregional recurrence of only 8%. Those who had LVI had a 21% locoregional recurrence compared to a 4% rate for those without LVI. Taghian et al. (83) reported results on 313 patients with pathological stage T3N0 disease who were treated with mastectomy, systemic treatment, and no radiation on National Surgical Adjuvant Breast and Bowel Project (NSABP) clinical trials. The 10-year locoregional recurrence for this series was only 7%, with 24 of the 28 locoregional recurrences developing only on the chest wall.

Truong et al. (84) focused exclusively on patients with T1 or T2 node-negative breast cancer treated within the British Columbia Cancer Agency and extracted clinicopathological data on this cohort from their outcome database. They reported an actuarial 10-year locoregional recurrence risk of 8% in 1,505 women treated with mastectomy without RT. On logistic regression analysis, grade, LVI, T stage, and systemic therapy use were statistically significant independent predictors of locoregional recurrence. On recursive partitioning analysis, the first split occurred at histologic grade 3 (actuarial 10-year rate of locoregional recurrence 12% vs. 6%). The concomitant presence of LVI increased the Kaplan-Meier estimate for 10-year locoregional recurrence to 21% compared to 9% for grade 3 alone. Similarly, Yildirim and Berberoglu (85) reported on 502 patients treated with modified radical mastectomy for T1 or T2 node-negative disease in their retrospective study from Ankara Oncology Hospital. With a median follow-up of 77 months, only 3% of patients had locoregional recurrence. Within these small numbers, multivariate analysis revealed tumor size greater than 2 cm and LVI as predictors for high risk of locoregional recurrence in women 40 years or younger and tumor size greater than 3 cm, LVI, grade, and *ERBB2* (formerly *HER2*) status, and use of tamoxifen in the older women. Ten-year risks of locoregional recurrence exceeded 30% for younger women with both risk factors and older women with at least three risk factors.

Margin Status

Margin status is another potential risk factor for locoregional recurrence in postmastectomy patients. However, information documenting and quantifying the risk of locoregional

recurrence in these patients is scarce because margin issues are uncommon after mastectomy. Furthermore, interpreting the available data is difficult due to the variable definitions of close or positive margins and the small denominators in the handful of existing reports. Perhaps the best effort comes from British Columbia Cancer Agency who identified 94 women with tumor at the inked margin of resection after mastectomy in their outcomes database (86). Forty-one of these patients received PMRT, while 53 did not, and cumulative crude locoregional recurrence was 11.3% versus 4.9% in unirradiated and irradiated groups, respectively, with no significant difference between the two groups. Factors that resulted in a cumulative crude locoregional recurrence of approximately 20% (17% to 23%) without RT were age 50 or less, T2 tumor size, grade 3 histology, and LVI. The corresponding rates with RT were in the single digits (0% to 9%) but all comparisons were statistically nonsignificant. Also, with a median follow-up time of about 8 years, none of the 22 women with positive margins without these associated features had locoregional recurrence.

Freedman et al. (87) reviewed 34 patients with close or positive margins after mastectomy whose primary tumor was smaller than 5 cm with zero to three positive axillary nodes and who received no postoperative radiation. Five chest wall recurrences appeared at a median interval of 26 months (range, 7 to 127 months), resulting in an 8-year cumulative incidence of a chest wall recurrence of 18%. The authors reported a relatively high risk of local relapse among younger women (age 50 or younger) compared to older women (28% vs. 0 at 8 years; *p* = .04). In a multivariable analysis by Katz et al. (76) of factors predictive of locoregional recurrence in patients treated with mastectomy and chemotherapy without irradiation, close or positive margins were a significant independent predictor of locoregional recurrence. Although there were only 29 patients available for this analysis, their 10-year locoregional recurrence was 45%; the risk was 33% for those with pectoralis fascia invasion even when negative margins were achieved.

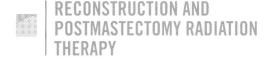

RECONSTRUCTION AND POSTMASTECTOMY RADIATION THERAPY

Many women desire breast reconstruction after mastectomy, and this presents a commonly encountered challenge in the management of these women should they also require radiation therapy. A multidisciplinary collaboration is warranted in which the surgical oncologist, reconstructive surgeon, and radiation oncologist confer with one another and with the patient to ensure an optimal aesthetic outcome without compromising the proven benefits of timely PMRT.

Breast reconstruction efforts can generally be categorized as either implant-based or autologous tissue reconstructions. In addition, reconstructions can occur at the time of the mastectomy (immediate reconstructions) or at some time after mastectomy, usually after the completion of radiotherapy (delayed reconstructions). Implant-based approaches are simpler to perform, avoid the potential morbidities associated with the donor site, and can be offered to thin women who do not have adequate autologous tissue in potential donor sites. A tissue expander is placed between the chest wall musculature and serially inflated until an appropriate tissue envelope is created, at which time the expander is replaced with a permanent prosthesis. Typically, implant-based reconstructions occur immediately after mastectomy because normal tissues can become less compliant after radiation, making tissue expansion problematic.

Autologous reconstructions are commonly performed using a transverse rectus abdominis myocutaneous (TRAM) flap. Alternatively, a latissimus dorsi flap or a flap based on the deep inferior epigastric perforator (DIEP) artery or gluteal arteries can be used for the reconstruction. These reconstructions can be immediate or delayed. In general, immediate reconstructions are accompanied by a skin-sparing mastectomy, thus preserving sensate skin and a natural inframammary sulcus for the reconstruction. The important advantages of an immediate reconstruction are offset by the potential adverse effects of radiation therapy on the reconstruction, and the negative impact the reconstruction can have on the design and delivery of PMRT.

PMRT can result in high rates of contracture, fibrosis, and poor cosmesis in patients who have immediate implant-based reconstructions. Spear et al. (88) reviewed the data on 40 consecutive patients who had undergone a two-stage saline implant reconstruction followed by RT and compared their outcomes to 40 controls[9]. Fifty-three percent of irradiated reconstructions had complications compared to 10% in controls, including a 33% capsular contracture rate in the irradiated patients compared to zero in the controls ($p <.00005$). Krueger et al. (89) reviewed data on 19 patients who had expander/implant reconstructions and radiation therapy and found that 13 (68%) had complications, compared to 19 of 62 (31%) in unirradiated controls ($p = .006$). In contrast, the group at Memorial Sloan-Kettering Cancer Center has reported results for their patients treated on an institutional algorithm of expander/implant reconstructions followed by PMRT and reported excellent disease control, no delays, and good to excellent aesthetic results in 80% of cases (90). For patients who have immediate autologous reconstructions, complications rates are generally lower (91).

Tran et al. (92) compared complication rates in immediate versus delayed TRAM reconstructions in patients who received PMRT. Twenty-four of 32 patients in the immediate reconstruction group had contracture, compared to 0 of 70 in the delayed reconstruction group ($p <.0001$). Furthermore, 28% of the patients with immediate reconstruction required an additional flap or prosthesis to improve cosmesis. In an attempt to reconcile the benefits of immediate and delayed reconstructions, Kronowitz et al. (93) have published on the "delayed-immediate" breast reconstruction wherein patients have a skin-sparing mastectomy, with preservation of sensate skin and subpectoral placement of a tissue expander. After final pathology is reviewed, those patients not requiring PMRT go on to have an "immediate" (within 2 weeks) autologous reconstruction, while the remainder have a delayed autologous reconstruction after RT. The expander is kept inflated throughout chemotherapy and then deflated before PMRT.

Breast reconstruction can alter the contour of the chest wall in a way that makes delivery of radiation to the necessary target volume much more challenging. In a recent report, Motwani et al. (94) reviewed 112 radiation plans designed to treat postmastectomy breast reconstructions and found that 52% of these required compromises in field design due to geometrical constraints imposed by the reconstruction (33% were scored as moderate compromises and 19% major compromises). Only 7% of similar plans in matched controls had compromises due to patient anatomy ($p <.0001$). In contrast, the group at Memorial Sloan-Kettering Cancer Center has demonstrated excellent coverage in a series of 40 patients with expander/implant reconstructions treated with intensity modulated radiation therapy (IMRT) (95).

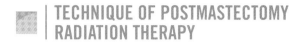

TECHNIQUE OF POSTMASTECTOMY RADIATION THERAPY

Treatment Volume, Dose, and Prescription

The volumes at greatest risk for recurrence, the chest wall and the supraclavicular lymph nodes, should always be included. However, a case can be made for omitting the supraclavicular/high axilla lymph nodes in patients with high-risk, node-negative breast cancer, due to the low risk of regional failure reported in these patients (81,83). The entire mastectomy flaps, inclusive of the mastectomy scar and drain sites, should be treated. Most commonly, a monoisocentric photon technique is used whereby opposed tangent split beams are employed for chest wall irradiation and are matched at isocenter to a superior AP supraclavicular field. The medial border is typically at midsternum and lateral border is at the mid- or posterior axillary line as clinically indicated. The inferior edge is 2 cm inferior to the level of where the inframammary fold existed. The contralateral breast (if it is intact) can be used to estimate the level of the inframammary fold. The superior border of the chest wall fields serves as the match plane and should be marked at the palpable inferior edge of the clavicular head. The gantry angles on the tangent fields are then designed as is done in conventional intact breast tangents, with half-beam or asymmetric jaws technique to limit posterior divergence into the lungs. Ultimately, the isocenter should be at midseparation (source to axis distance [SAD] technique) along a straight line connecting the medial and lateral wires through the central ray of the symmetrical tangents. Typically, 2 to 3 cm of lung in the tangents are required for adequate coverage of the chest wall. The isocenter is then translated cranially to the match plane, ensuring that the geometry of the tangents remains stable. Collimator rotations on the tangent fields (to correct for the slope of the chest wall) can be avoided by opening the jaws on the lung side of the tangents by 2 to 3 cm and adding a superior lung block to ensure 2 to 3 cm of lung throughout the long axis of the tangent beams-eye view. This eliminates the need to correct for the angulation of the cranial edge and simplifies the isocentric match with the supraclavicular field. If the length of a patient's torso makes coverage of the chest wall impossible with half of the available beam length, the tangent jaws can be opened (symmetrically or asymmetrically) and couch rotations can be performed for each tangent to create a straight nondivergent cranial edge for the tangent fields. Simple trigonometric calculations can be performed to calculate the required couch rotation, or the rod-and-chain technique can be used. All of these steps can be reproduced virtually on image data acquired at the time of a computed tomography (CT) simulation and fields designed as described above. Alternatively, the entire chest wall can be treated with electrons, but variations in patient thickness and slope can make optimal dosimetry difficult with this technique. In particular, transmission into lung has to be carefully accounted for. CT planning should be strongly considered for all left-sided lesions, and dose to the cardiac volume should be tracked and constrained. If the heart is placed anteriorly, the medial chest wall can be treated with an anterior electron field that is matched to shallower chest wall tangents. The target dose to the chest wall is 45 to 50 Gy in conventional 1.8- to 2-Gy fractions. Dose can be prescribed 1.5 cm from the posterior edge of the tangents at midseparation or at one third of the distance from this point to the anterior skin. Alternatively, dose can be normalized to a treatment isodose line covering the target volume. Ideally, the treatment volume should be homogenous for dose, with acceptable ranges within 95% to 107% of prescription dose. Contributions from 15 MV photons should be minimized and bolus placement should be considered to ensure superficial coverage. Forward-planned IMRT, electronic compensation, and inverse-planned IMRT can be important tools for the radiation oncologist to consider in meeting treatment objectives if the conventional techniques described above result in suboptimal dosimetry.

The supraclavicular field is typically an AP photon field with the upper border above the acromioclavicular joint (or just flashing the skin), medial border at the vertebral pedicles, and lateral border at the coracoid process in patients who have had complete axillary dissections. Alternatively, the lateral border can be placed to include the medial two thirds of the humeral head if the axilla is undissected or inadequately dissected. Strom et al. (96) found that in their population of well-dissected axillae (median, 17), failures in the low and midaxilla were uncommon (10-year actuarial rate 3%). The AP supraclavicular field is prescribed at a depth of 3 cm by convention, although in the age of the CT planning, an alternate anatomically defined depth can be used provided the superficial entrance dose remains acceptable. Six MV photons are typically used, although higher energies are reasonable to consider. A posterior axillary boost can be designed to supplement dose to the axillary apex if the contribution from the AP supraclavicular field to the midplane is inadequate. The depth of the supraclavicular prescription point can be altered to increase the midplane dose; the depth of the supraclavicular and high axilla nodes are often similar (97). Many centers are now routinely contouring axillary nodal stations as well as the supraclavicular nodal target, and this practice can be very helpful in treatment planning. Commonly, 50 Gy prescribed to the supraclavicular volume will result in 40 to 45 Gy to the axillary apex without need for a posterior axillary boost.

Inclusion of IM nodes is widely variable because of the conflicting data on the benefits and risks of irradiating these nodes. Although microscopic involvement of IM nodes can be high (98), especially in patients with positive axillary nodes and medial tumors, IM node failures are exceedingly unusual (0.1% in the ECOG experience) (64). Furthermore, the benefit of routinely irradiating (or dissecting) the IM nodes has never been proven, although it has not been tested in well-controlled studies. Advocates of IM node irradiation correctly point out that the postmastectomy radiation trials discussed earlier did include the IM nodes. This issue will not likely be settled at least until the results of ongoing randomized trials of regional nodal irradiation are mature. If the IM nodes are to be included, several techniques have been described, and these were compared by Arthur et al. (99) in a dosimetric study. The partially wide tangents technique, in which the tangents blocks are altered to deepen coverage in the upper three intercostal spaces (Fig. 47.2), resulted in the least amount of incidental heart and lung irradiation. A popular technique not compared in this study is a 5- to 6-cm wide electron patch matched to the entry point of the medial tangent and tilted to a gantry angle 5 to 15 degrees less than the medial tangent (Fig. 47.3). Nine or 12 MeV electrons can be employed to treat at the requisite CT defined depth. At 80% to 90% of prescribed dose, acute skin reactions may necessitate substituting the electron field with a photon field in the same geometry to allow skin sparing. The target dose is 45 to 50 Gy.

The area around the scar is commonly boosted with an additional 8 to 12 Gy with electrons. An electron "cut-out" can be created to treat a 2- to 3-cm margin around the mastectomy scar and drain sites. In patients with complex scar geometry or extensive chest wall curvature (especially after reconstruction), a creative way to avoid the uncertainty of matching electron fields is to create a customized thermoplastic surface applicator with embedded afterloading catheters for remote high-dose rate delivery of dose (100).

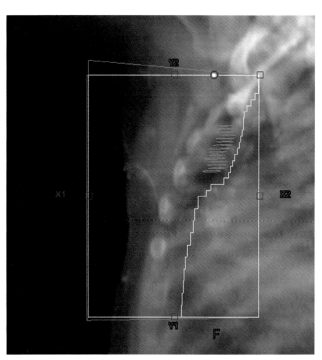

FIGURE 47.2. Beam's eye view reconstruction of a partially wide tangent field.

MANAGEMENT SUMMARY

- PMRT improves locoregional control, breast cancer–mortality, and all-cause mortality in appropriately selected patients and should be recommended for all patients who have a projected locoregional recurrence rate of 20% or greater. This includes patients with four or more involved axillary nodes, patients with one to three involved nodes and a primary tumor larger than 5 cm, and patients with T4 disease (skin involvement or involvement of the chest wall).
- Patients with T1 or T2 disease and one to three involved nodes have an intermediate risk of recurrence (10% to 20%) and should be considered for PMRT if they have less than 10 nodes removed, a nodal ratio greater than 0.20, age less than 45, positive margins, high-grade tumor, or LVI.
- Node-negative patients generally have low rates of locoregional recurrence, including those with T3N0 LVI-negative disease. PMRT can be considered in patients who

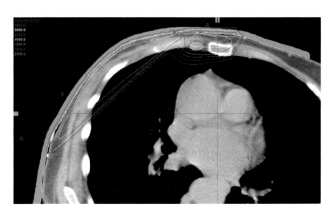

FIGURE 47.3. Axial view of isodose lines produced from a postmastectomy radiation treatment plan employing tangents and a matched electron strip angled toward the medial tangent.

have at least three of these additional adverse features: young age, histologic grade 3, LVI, T2 size, and absence of systemic therapy.

- In devising radiation fields, CT planning for left-sided cases is very important. The heart should be contoured and the cardiac volume limited.
- For patients desirous of reconstruction, a multidisciplinary collaboration is warranted in which the surgical oncologist, reconstructive surgeon, and radiation oncologist confer with one another and with the patient to ensure an optimal aesthetic outcome without compromising the proven benefits of timely PMRT.

References

1. Cole M. The place of radiotherapy in the management of early breast cancer. *Br J Cancer* 1964;51:216–220.
2. Early Breast Cancer Trialists' Collaborative Group. *Treatment of early breast cancer.* Vol 1. *Worldwide evidence, 1985–1990.* Oxford, Engl: Oxford University Press, 1990:111.
3. Haybittle J, Brinkley D, Houghton J, et al. Postoperative radiotherapy and late mortality: evidence from the Cancer Research Campaign trial for early breast cancer. *BMJ* 1989;298:1611–1614.
4. Host H, Brennhovd M, Loeb M. Postoperative radiotherapy in breast cancer: long term results from the Oslo study. *Int J Radiat Oncol Biol Phys* 1986;12: 727–732.
5. Jones J, Ribeiro G. Mortality patterns over 34 years of breast cancer patients in a clinical trial of postoperative radiotherapy. *Clin Radiol* 1989;40:204–208.
6. Lythgoe J, Palmer M. Manchester regional breast study—5 and 10 year results. *Br J Surg* 1982;69:693–696.
7. Rutqvist L, Lax I, Fornander M, et al. Cardiovascular mortality in a randomized trial of adjuvant radiation therapy versus surgery alone in primary breast cancer. *Int J Radiat Oncol Biol Phys* 1992;22:887–896.
8. Stewart H, Jack W, Everington D, et al. South-east Scottish trial of local therapy in node negative breast cancer. *Breast* 1994;3:31–39.
9. Cuzick J, Stewart H, Peto R, et al. Overview of randomized trials of postoperative adjuvant radiotherapy in breast cancer. *Cancer Treat Rep* 1987;71:15–29.
10. Cuzick J, Stewart H, Rutqvist L, et al. Cause-specific mortality in long-term survivors of breast cancer who participated in trials of radiotherapy. *J Clin Oncol* 1994;12:447–453.
11. Ingle J, Everson L, Wieand S, et al. Randomized trial of observation versus adjuvant therapy with cyclophosphamide, fluorouracil, prednisone with or without tamoxifen following mastectomy in postmenopausal women with node-positive breast cancer. *J Clin Oncol* 1988;6:1388–1396.
12. Bonadonna G, Valagussa P, Moliterni A, et al. Adjuvant cyclophosphamide, methotrexate, and fluorouracil in node-positive breast cancer. *N Engl J Med* 1995;332:901–906.
13. Castiglione-Gersch M, Johnsen C, Goldhirsh A, et al. The International (Ludwig) Breast Cancer Study Group trials I–IV: 5 years follow-up. *Ann Oncol* 1994;5: 717–724.
14. Crivellari D, Price K, Gelber R, et al. Adjuvant endocrine therapy compared with no systemic therapy for elderly women with early breast cancer: 21-year results of International Breast Cancer Study Group trial IV. *J Clin Oncol* 2003;21: 4517–4523.
15. Fisher B, Dignam J, Bryant J, et al. Five versus more than five years of tamoxifen therapy for breast cancer patients with negative lymph nodes and estrogen receptor-positive tumors. *J Natl Cancer Inst* 1996;88:1529–1542.
16. Fisher B, Dignam J, Eleftherios P, et al. Sequential methotrexate and fluorouracil for the treatment of node-negative breast cancer patients with estrogen receptor-negative tumors: eight-year results of from National Surgical Adjuvant Breast and Bowel Project (NSABP) B-13 and first report of findings from NSABP-B-19 comparing methotrexate and fluorouracil with conventional cyclophosphamide, methotrexate, and fluorouracil. *J Clin Oncol* 1996;14: 1982–1992.
17. Fisher B, Fisher E, Redmond C, et al. Ten-year results from the national surgical adjuvant breast and bowel project (NSABP) clinical trial evaluating *L*-phenylalanine mustard (L-PAM) in the management of primary breast cancer. *J Clin Oncol* 1985;4:929–941.
18. Goldhirsh A, Castiglione M, Gelber R, et al. A single perioperative adjuvant chemotherapy course for node-negative breast cancer: five-year results of trial V. International Breast Cancer Study Group (formerly Ludwig Group). *J Natl Cancer Inst Monogr* 1992;11:89–96.
19. Mansour E, Eudey L, Tormey D, et al. Chemotherapy versus observation in high-risk node-negative breast cancer patients. *J Natl Cancer Inst Monogr* 1992;11: 97–104.
20. Morrison J, Howell A, Kelly K, et al. West Midlands Oncology Association trials of adjuvant chemotherapy in operable breast cancer: results after a median follow-up of 7 years. I. Patients with involved axillary lymph nodes. *Br J Cancer* 1989;60:911–918.
21. Morrison J, Kelly K, Howell A, et al. West Midlands Oncology Association trial of adjuvant chemotherapy in node-negative breast cancer. *J Natl Cancer Inst Monogr* 1992;11:85–88.
22. Richards M, O'Reilly S, Howell A, et al. Adjuvant cyclophosphamide, methotrexate, and fluorouracil in patients with axillary node-positive breast cancer: an update of the Guy's Manchester trial. *J Clin Oncol* 1990;8:2032–2039.
23. Rubens R, Knight R, Fentiman I, et al. Controlled trial of adjuvant chemotherapy with melphalan for breast cancer. *Lancet* 1983;1:839–843.
24. Taylor S, Knuiman W, Sleeper L, et al. Six-year results of the Eastern Cooperative Oncology Group trial of observation versus CMFP versus CMFPT in postmenopausal patients with node-positive breast cancer. *J Clin Oncol* 1989;7(7):879–889.
25. Zambetti M, Valagussa P, Bonadonna G, et al. Adjuvant cyclophosphamide, methotrexate, and fluorouracil in node-negative and estrogen receptor negative breast cancer. *Ann Oncol* 1996;7:481–485.
26. Early Breast Cancer Trialists' Collaborative Group. Effects of chemotherapy and hormonal therapy for early breast cancer on recurrence and 15-year survival: an overview of the randomized trials. *Lancet* 2005;365:1687–1717.
27. Marks L, Halperin E, Prosnitz L, et al. Postmastectomy radiotherapy following adjuvant chemotherapy and autologous bone marrow transplantation for breast cancer patients with >10 positive axillary lymph nodes. *Int J Radiat Oncol Biol Phys* 1992;23:1021–1026.
28. Citron M, Berry D, Cirrincione C, et al. Randomized trial of dose-dense versus conventionally scheduled and sequential versus concurrent combination chemotherapy as postoperative adjuvant treatment of node-positive primary breast cancer: first report of Intergroup trial C9741/Cancer and Leukemia Group B trial 9741. *J Clin Oncol* 2003;21:1431–1439.
29. Fisher B, Anderson S, Wickerham D, et al. Increased intensification and total dose of cyclophosphamide in a doxorubicin-cyclophosphamide regimen for the treatment of primary breast cancer: findings of the National and Surgical Adjuvant Breast and Bowel Project B-22. *J Clin Oncol* 1997;15:1858–1869.
30. Hoeller U, Heide J, Kroeger N, et al. Radiotherapy after high-dose chemotherapy and peripheral blood stem cell support in high-risk breast cancer. *Int J Radiat Oncol Biol Phys* 2002;53:1234–1239.
31. Sartor C, Peterson B, Woolf S, et al. Effect of addition of adjuvant paclitaxel on radiotherapy delivery and locoregional control of node-positive breast cancer: Cancer and Leukemia Group B 9344. *J Clin Oncol* 2005;23:30–40.
32. Wood W, Budman D, Korzun A, et al. Dose and dose intensity of adjuvant chemotherapy for stage II, node-positive breast carcinoma. *N Engl J Med* 1994; 330:1253–1259.
33. Blomqvist C, Tiusanen K, Elomaa I, et al. The combination of radiotherapy, adjuvant chemotherapy (cyclophosphamide-doxorubicin-ftorafur) and tamoxifen in stage II breast cancer. Long-term follow-up results of a randomized trial. *Br J Cancer* 1992;66:1171–1176.
34. Buzdar A, Hortobagyi G, Kau S, et al. Breast cancer adjuvant therapy at the MD Anderson Cancer Center: results of four prospective studies. In: Salmon S, ed. *Adjuvant therapy of cancer.* Philadelphia: Lippincott, 1993:220–231.
35. Griem K, Henderson I, Gelman R, et al. The 5-year results of a randomized trial of adjuvant radiation therapy after chemotherapy in breast cancer patients treated with mastectomy. *J Clin Oncol* 1987;5:1546–1555.
36. Klefstrom P, Grohn P, Heinonen E, et al. Adjuvant postoperative radiotherapy, chemotherapy, and immunotherapy in stage III breast cancer. *Cancer* 1987;60: 936–942.
37. Martinez A, Ahmann D, O'Fallow J, et al. An interim analysis of the randomized surgical adjuvant trial for patients with unfavorable breast cancer. *Int J Radiat Oncol Biol Phys* 1984;10[Suppl 2]:106.
38. McArdle C, Crawford D, Dykes E, et al. Adjuvant radiotherapy and chemotherapy in breast cancer. *Br J Surg* 1986;73:264–266.
39. Muss H, Cooper M, Brockschmidt J, et al. A randomized trial of chemotherapy (L-PAM vs. CMF) and irradiation for node-positive breast cancer. Eleven year follow-up of Piedmont Oncology Association trial. *Breast Cancer Res Treat* 1991; 18:77–84.
40. Olson J, Neuberg D, Pandya K, et al. The role of radiotherapy in the management of operable locally advanced breast cancer: results of a randomized trial by the Eastern Cooperative Oncology Group. *Cancer* 1997;79:1138–1149.
41. Overgaard M, Hansen P, Overgaard J, et al. Postoperative radiotherapy in high-risk premenopausal women with breast cancer who receive adjuvant chemotherapy. *N Engl J Med* 1997;337:949–955.
42. Overgaard M, Jensen M, Overgaard J, et al. Postoperative radiotherapy in high-risk postmenopausal breast-cancer patients given adjuvant tamoxifen: Danish Breast Cancer Cooperative Group DBCG 82c randomized trial. *Lancet* 1999;353: 1641–1648.
43. Ragaz J, Olivotto I, Spinelli J, et al. Locoregional radiation therapy in patients with high-risk breast cancer receiving adjuvant chemotherapy: 20 year results of the British Columbia randomized trial. *J Natl Cancer Inst* 2005;97:116–126.
44. Tennvall-Nittby L, Tengrup I, Landberg T, et al. The total incidence of locoregional recurrence in a randomized trial of breast cancer TNM stage II. The South Sweden Breast Cancer trial. *Acta Oncol* 1993;32:641–646.
45. Velez-Garcia E, Carpenter J Jr, Moore M, et al. Postsurgical adjuvant chemotherapy with or without radiotherapy in women with breast cancer and positive axillary nodes: a Southeastern Cancer Study Group (SEG) trial. *Eur J Cancer* 1992; 28:1833–1837.
46. Early Breast Cancer Trialists' Collaborative Group. Effects of radiotherapy and of differences in the extent of surgery for early breast cancer on local recurrence and 15-year survival: an overview of the randomised trials. *Lancet* 2005;366: 2087–2106.
47. Bartelink H. Systemic adjuvant therapies and radiotherapy to the conserved breast: strategies revisited. *Breast* 2007;16[Suppl 2]:S84–S88.
48. Punglia R, Morrow M, Winer E, et al. Local therapy and survival in breast cancer. *N Engl J Med* 2007;356:2399–2405.
49. Darby S. New results from the worldwide overview of individual patient data from the randomised trials of radiotherapy. 2007 annual ASCO meeting. Available at http://www.asco.org/ASCO/Abstracts+%26+Virtual+Meeting/Virtual+Meeting?&vmview=vm_session_presentations_view&confID=47&trackID=1&sessionID=431.
50. Van de Steene J, Soete G, Storme G. Adjuvant radiotherapy for breast cancer significantly improves overall survival: the missing link. *Radiother Oncol* 2000;55:263–272.
51. Gebski V, Lagvela M, Keech A, et al. Survival effects of postmastectomy adjuvant radiation therapy using biologically equivalent doses: a clinical perspective. *J Natl Cancer Inst* 2006;98:26–38.
52. Early Breast Cancer Trialists' Collaborative Group. Favourable and unfavourable effects on long-term survival of radiotherapy for early breast cancer: an overview of the randomised trials. *Lancet* 2000;355:1757–1770.
53. Rutqvist L, Johansson H. Mortality by laterality of the primary tumor among 55,000 breast cancer patients from the Swedish Cancer Registry. *Br J Cancer* 1990;61:866–868.
54. Hojris I, Overgaard M, Christensen J, et al. Morbidity and mortality of ischaemic heart disease in high-risk breast-cancer patients after adjuvant postmastectomy systemic treatment with or without radiotherapy: analysis of DBCG 82b and 82c randomised trial. *Lancet* 1999;354:1425–1430.

55. Gyenes G, Rutqvist L, Liedberg A, et al. Long-term cardiac morbidity and mortality in a randomized trial of pre- and postoperative radiation therapy versus surgery alone in primary breast cancer. *Radiother Oncol* 1998;48:185–190.
56. Harris E, Correa C, Hwang W, et al. Late cardiac mortality and morbidity in early-stage breast cancer patients after breast-conservation treatment. *J Clin Oncol* 2006;24:4100–4106.
57. Giordano S, Kuo Y, Freeman J, et al. Risk of cardiac death after adjuvant radiotherapy for breast cancer. *J Natl Cancer Inst* 2005;97:419–424.
58. Fumoleau P, Roche H, Kerbat P, et al. Long-term cardiac toxicity after adjuvant epirubicin-based chemotherapy in early breast cancer: French Adjuvant Study Group Results. *Ann Oncol* 2006;17:85–92.
59. Hojris I, Andersen J, Overgaard M, et al. Late treatment-related morbidity in breast cancer patients randomized to postmastectomy radiotherapy and systemic treatment versus systemic treatment alone. *Acta Oncol* 2000;39:355–372.
60. Olsen N, Pfeiffer P, Johanssen L, et al. Radiation-induced brachial plexopathy: neurological follow-up in 161 recurrence-free breast cancer patients. *Int J Radiat Oncol Biol Phys* 1993;26:43–49.
61. Kuhnt T, Richter C, Enke H, et al. Acute radiation reaction and local control in breast cancer patients treated with postmastectomy radiotherapy. *Strahlenther Onkol* 1998;174:257–261.
62. Nielsen H, Overgaard M, Grau C, et al. Study of failure pattern among high-risk breast cancer patients with or without postmastectomy radiotherapy in addition to adjuvant systemic therapy: long-term results from the Danish Breast Cancer Cooperative Group (DBCG) 82b and 82c randomized studies. *J Clin Oncol* 2006; 24:2268–2275.
63. Katz A, Strom EA, Buchholz TA, et al. Locoregional recurrence patterns after mastectomy and doxorubicin-based chemotherapy: implications for postoperative irradiation. *J Clin Oncol* 2000;18:2817–2827.
64. Recht A, Gray R, Davidson NE, et al. Locoregional failure 10 years after mastectomy and adjuvant chemotherapy with or without tamoxifen without irradiation: experience of the Eastern Cooperative Oncology Group. *J Clin Oncol* 1999; 17:1689–1700.
65. Woodward W, Strom E, Tucker S, et al. Locoregional recurrence after doxorubicin-based chemotherapy and postmastectomy: implications for breast cancer patients with early-stage disease and predictors for recurrence after postmastectomy radiation. *Int J Radiat Oncol Biol Phys* 2003;57:336–344.
66. Nielsen H, Overgaard M, Grau C, et al. Locoregional recurrence after mastectomy in high-risk breast cancer—risk and prognosis. An analysis of patients from the DBCG 82 B&C randomization trials. *Radiother Oncol* 2006;79:147–155.
67. Taghian A, Jeong JH, Mamounas E, et al. Patterns of locoregional failure in patients with operable breast cancer treated by mastectomy and adjuvant chemotherapy with or without tamoxifen and without radiotherapy: results from five National Surgical Adjuvant Breast and Bowel Project randomized clinical trials. *J Clin Oncol* 2004;22:4247–4254.
68. Wallgren A, Bonetti M, Gelber R, et al. Risk factors for locoregional recurrence among breast cancer patients: results from International Breast Cancer Study Group trial I-VII. *J Clin Oncol* 2003;21:1205–1213.
69. Truong P, Woodward W, Thames H, et al. The ratio of positive to excised nodes identifies high-risk subsets and reduces inter-institutional differences in locoregional recurrence risk estimates in breast cancer patients with 1–3 positive nodes: an analysis of prospective data from British Columbia and the MD Anderson Cancer Center. *Int J Radiat Oncol Biol Phys* 2007;68:59–65.
70. Karlsson P, Cole B, Price K, et al. The role of number of uninvolved lymph nodes in predicting locoregional recurrence in breast cancer. *J Clin Oncol* 2007;25: 2019–2026.
71. Katz A, Buchholz TA, Thames H, et al. Recursive partitioning analysis of locoregional recurrence patterns following mastectomy: implications for adjuvant irradiation. *Int J Radiat Oncol Biol Phys* 2001;50:397–403.
72. Truong P, Olivotto I, Kader H, et al. Selecting breast cancer patients with T1–T2 tumors and one to three positive axillary nodes at high postmastectomy locoregional recurrence risk for adjuvant radiotherapy. *Int J Radiat Oncol Biol Phys* 2005;61:1337–1347.
73. Overgaard M, Nielsen H, Overgaard J. Is the benefit of postmastectomy irradiation limited to patients with four or more positive nodes, as recommended in the international consensus reports? A subgroup analysis of the DBCG 82 B&C randomized trials. *Radiother Oncol* 2007;82:247–253.
74. Harris J, Halpin-Murphy P, Mcneese M, et al. Consensus statement on postmastectomy radiation therapy. *Int J Radiat Oncol Biol Phys* 1999;44:989–990.
75. Recht A, Edge SB, Solin LJ, et al. Postmastectomy radiotherapy: clinical practice guidelines of the American Society of Clinical Oncology. *J Clin Oncol* 2001;19: 1539–1569.
76. Katz A, Strom EA, Buchholz TA, et al. The influence of pathologic tumor characteristics on locoregional recurrence rates following mastectomy. *Int J Radiat Oncol Biol Phys* 2001;50:735–742.
77. Fowble B, Yeh IT, Schultz DJ, et al. The role of mastectomy in patients with stage I–II breast cancer presenting with gross multifocal or multicentric disease or diffuse microcalcifications. *Int J Radiat Oncol Biol Phys* 1993;27:567–573.
78. Cheng J, Chen C, Liu M, et al. Locoregional failure of postmastectomy patients with 1–3 positive axillary lymph nodes without adjuvant radiotherapy. *Int J Radiat Oncol Biol Phys* 2002;52:980–988.
79. Fodor J, Polgar C, Major T, et al. Locoregional failure 15 years after mastectomy in women with one to three positive axillary nodes with or without irradiation. *Strahlenther Onkol* 2003;179:197–202.
80. Cheng S, Horng C, West M, et al. Genomic prediction of locoregional recurrence after mastectomy in breast cancer. *J Clin Oncol* 2006;24:4594–4602.
81. Jagsi R, Abi Raad R, Goldberg S, et al. Locoregional recurrence rates and prognostic factors for failure in node-negative patients treated with mastectomy: implications for postmastectomy radiation. *Int J Radiat Oncol Biol Phys* 2005;62: 1035–1039.
82. Floyd S, Buchholz T, Haffty B, et al. Low local recurrence rate without postmastectomy radiation in node-negative breast cancer patients with tumors 5 cm and larger. *Int J Radiat Oncol Biol Phys* 2006;66:358–364.
83. Taghian A, Jeong J, Mamounas E, et al. Low locoregional recurrence rate among node-negative breast cancer patients with tumors 5 cm or larger treated by mastectomy, with or without adjuvant systemic therapy and without radiotherapy: results from five National Surgical Adjuvant Breast and Bowel Project Randomized Clinical Trials. *J Clin Oncol* 2006;24:3927–2932.
84. Truong P, Lesperance M, Culhaci A, et al. Patient subsets with T1–T2, node-negative breast cancer at high locoregional recurrence risk after mastectomy. *Int J Radiat Oncol Biol Phys* 2005;62:175–182.
85. Yildirim E, Berberoglu U. Can a subgroup of node-negative breast carcinoma patients with T1–T2 tumor who may benefit from postmastectomy radiotherapy be identified? *Int J Radiat Oncol Biol Phys* 2007;68:1024–1029.
86. Truong P, Olivotto I, Speers C, et al. A positive margin is not always an indication for radiotherapy after mastectomy in early breast cancer. *Int J Radiat Oncol Biol Phys* 2004;58:797–804.
87. Freedman GM, Fowble BL, Hanlon AL, et al. A close or positive margin after mastectomy is not an indication for chest wall irradiation except in women aged fifty or younger. *Int J Radiat Oncol Biol Phys* 1998;41:599–605.
88. Spear S, Onyewu C. Staged breast reconstruction with saline-filled implants in the irradiated breast: recent trends and therapeutic implications. *Plast Reconstr Surg* 2000;105(3):930–942.
89. Krueger E, Wilkins E, Strawderman M, et al. Complications and patient satisfaction following expander/implant breast reconstruction with and without radiotherapy. *Int J Radiat Oncol Biol Phys* 2001;49:713–721.
90. Wright J, Cordeiro P, Ben-Porat L, et al. Mastectomy with immediate expander-implant reconstruction, adjuvant chemotherapy, and radiation for stage II-III breast cancer: treatment intervals and clinical outcomes. *Int J Radiat Oncol Biol Phys* 2008;70:43–50.
91. Chawla A, Kachnic L, Taghian A, et al. Radiotherapy and breast reconstruction: complications and cosmesis with TRAM versus tissue expander/implant. *Int J Radiat Oncol Biol Phys* 2002;54:520–526.
92. Tran N, Chang D, Gupta A, et al. Comparison of immediate and delayed free TRAM flap breast reconstruction in patients receiving postmastectomy radiation therapy. *Plast Reconstr Surg* 2001;108:78–82.
93. Kronowitz S, Hunt K, Kuerer H, et al. Delayed-immediate breast reconstruction. *Plast Reconstr Surg* 2004;113:1617–1628.
94. Motwani S, Strom E, Schechter N, et al. The impact of immediate breast reconstruction on the technical delivery of postmastectomy radiotherapy. *Int J Radiat Oncol Biol Phys* 2006;66:76–82.
95. Koutcher L, Rallangrud A, Cordeiro P, et al. Postmastectomy intensity modulated radiation therapy in women who undergo immediate breast reconstruction. *Int J Radiat Oncol Biol Phys* 2007;69:S222.
96. Strom E, Woodward W, Katz A, et al. Clinical investigation: regional nodal failure patterns in breast cancer patients treated with mastectomy without radiotherapy. *Int J Radiat Oncol Biol Phys* 2005;63:1508–1513.
97. Bentel G, Marks L, Hardenberg P, et al. Variability of the depth of supraclavicular and axillary lymph nodes in patients with breast cancer: is a posterior axillary boost field necessary? *Int J Radiat Oncol Biol Phys* 2000;47:755–758.
98. Freedman G, Fowble B, Nicolaou N, et al. Should the internal mammary lymph nodes in breast cancer be a target for the radiation oncologist? *Int J Radiat Oncol Biol Phys* 2000;46:805–814.
99. Arthur D, Arnfield M, Warwicke L, et al. Internal mammary node coverage: an investigation of presently accepted technique. *Int J Radiat Oncol Biol Phys* 2000; 48:139–146.
100. Stewart A, O'Farrell D, Bellon J, et al. CT computer-optimized high-dose-rate brachytherapy with surface applicator technique for scar boost radiation after breast reconstruction surgery. *Brachytherapy* 2005;4:224–229.

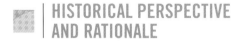

Chapter 48
Adjuvant Systemic Therapy: Endocrine Therapy

Mothaffar F. Rimawi and C. Kent Osborne

HISTORICAL PERSPECTIVE AND RATIONALE

Breast cancer causes death not because of the primary tumor in the breast but because of metastases in distant sites that gradually cause organ dysfunction. In the 1970s a major change in thinking about how breast cancer metastasizes was proposed and gradually accepted. Before that, breast cancer was thought to be a local-regional disease that remained confined to the breast and lymphatics for a relatively long time before eventually spreading to distant sites. The new concept held that the disease spread early in its course in some patients leading to death when local surgery was the only treatment, and it led to trials of breast preservation surgery rather than radical surgery and to trials of systemic therapy given after surgery, *adjuvant therapy*.

This conceptual change was not without controversy and it met considerable resistance. The long-term results of Halsted's innovation published 30 years later failed, however, to support his idea that distant metastases occurred late in the disease process (1). Only 12% of breast cancer patients treated by Halsted and his students survived 10 years despite radical surgery. More recent surgical studies, completed in an era when patients were diagnosed earlier with smaller tumors, provided more encouraging results from radical mastectomy with 50% of patients surviving 10 years (2). Still, 20% to 30% of patients with negative axillary nodes at diagnosis and 75% of those with nodal metastases have recurrence and die of their disease within 10 years when treated by local surgery alone (2). These data led to the seemingly obvious conclusion that distant metastases, although not evident clinically, must be present in many patients at the time of the initial diagnosis. These occult metastases have come to be called *micrometastases* because they are asymptomatic and cannot be identified by imaging studies; they can sometimes be found using special stains of bone marrow biopsies even in node-negative patients (see Chapter 33).

Adjuvant systemic therapy is defined as the administration of cytotoxic chemotherapy, targeted therapy such as endocrine treatment or treatment blocking the HER receptor pathway, or immunotherapy after primary surgery of breast cancer to kill or inhibit the growth of clinically occult micrometastases. *Neoadjuvant therapy* is similar except that the therapy is given before surgery to shrink the primary tumor as well as to kill micrometastases. The concept of adjuvant therapy received further support from preclinical animal models showing that early administration of chemotherapy, when the tumor burden was low and tumor growth kinetics most favorable, could eradicate tumors that become incurable when treatment is delayed (3). The first randomized trials of breast cancer adjuvant therapy involving ovarian ablation and short-term chemotherapy were initiated more than 50 years ago (4,5). Modern trials of prolonged postoperative treatment to kill micrometastases were begun in the late 1960s and early 1970s. First, single agent and combination chemotherapy trials were initiated in node-positive patients. Then, trials of the antiestrogen tamoxifen came along in the mid 1970s. The 1980s witnessed trials of doxorubicin-based chemotherapy and adjuvant therapy in node-negative patients. Trials of chemoendocrine therapy were also initiated during this decade. Chemotherapy dose intensity, including trials of high-dose chemotherapy with autologous bone marrow transplantation, was investigated in the 1990s. In addition, this decade saw the introduction of neoadjuvant chemotherapy and adjuvant trials evaluating taxane combinations. Later, newer forms of endocrine adjuvant therapy using aromatase inhibitors (AI) were initiated. The current decade will be recognized not only for trials of the aromatase inhibitors, but also trials of targeted therapy with the use of trastuzumab in HER2 (ERBB2)-positive patients. The cumulative result of all of these studies has been a steady decline in age-adjusted death rates of women with breast cancer, validating the hypothesis that micrometastases present at the time of initial diagnosis are the cause of treatment failure when therapy is directed only at the primary tumor in the breast.

INTERPRETATION OF ADJUVANT AND CLINICAL TRIALS

The meaning of various statistical end points is crucial for the interpretation of clinical trials. Disease-free survival (DFS) is defined as the time from randomization to first evidence of treatment failure or death, and overall survival (OS) is defined as the time from randomization to death from any cause. The definition of DFS varies somewhat from trial to trial. Some trials include contralateral breast cancer as an event whereas others do not. Time to treatment failure or time to recurrence (TTR) does not include death before recurrence as an end point. Other important end points include distant DFS, which is the time to first evidence of treatment failure outside of the primary disease site or death from any cause. Breast cancer specific DFS and OS are used less commonly because deaths from other causes may be related in some unknown way to the disease itself or its treatment. DFS focuses on the efficacy of the primary disease treatment, but it ignores what happens to the patient after disease recurrence. Survival after recurrence might be influenced by the adjuvant treatment received. Thus, although adjuvant treatments that prolong DFS might also be expected to prolong OS, this might not occur if the adjuvant treatment decreases response to treatments given after relapse, resulting in shorter postrelapse survival. The failure of AI when compared directly with tamoxifen to prolong OS despite significantly prolonging DFS may illustrate this phenomenon, although it is possible that prolongation of OS may eventually become evident with longer follow-up of existing trials.

The results of randomized clinical trials are frequently displayed by Kaplan-Meier survival curves in which the proportion of patients who remain disease free or alive is plotted against the time after randomization. Results are sometimes also presented as a hazard ratio which is the ratio of the hazard function of the experimental group to that of the control group. When the ratio is close to one, the hazards are the same and, therefore, no difference in efficacy exists. A hazard ratio less than one indicates a higher relapse or death rate in the control group, whereas a ratio greater than one indicates more events in the experimental group.

Physicians must understand the difference between absolute benefit and proportional benefit in discussing treatment options

Table 48.1	**ABSOLUTE REDUCTION IN MORTALITY AT 10 YEARS PER 100 TREATED**				
	Hypothetical Proportional Reduction in Mortality Owing to Treatment				
Estimated 10-year Death Rate with No Therapy	50%	40%	30%	20%	10%
70% (several positive nodes)	25	19	13	8	4
50% (5-cm tumor, negative nodes)	21	16	12	7	4
30% (average tumor diameter, negative nodes)	14	11	8	5	3
10% (≤1 cm tumor, negative nodes)	5	4	3	2	1

with patients (Table 48.1). The absolute benefit in a patient with a small node-negative tumor and an estimated 10-year death rate of 10% without treatment would only be 4% with treatment providing a 40% reduction in death, whereas a similar proportional reduction in a patient with several positive lymph nodes and a 70% 10-year death rate would be 19%.

Several caveats must be considered in the interpretation of randomized clinical trials. False–negative results can occur because of small patient populations with insufficient statistical power, but false–positive results may occur simply by the play of chance. Trials that produce positive results are more likely to be published, resulting in publication bias. Another hazard in the reporting of randomized trials is multiple subset analyses. Analysis of multiple subsets is bound to yield a misleadingly positive result simply by statistical chance. Thus, subset analyses, unless taken into consideration in the original statistical design of the study, should only be used to generate new hypotheses.

 ## META-ANALYSES

Given the large number of randomized adjuvant therapy trials, some of them are likely to be misleadingly promising, whereas others may be misleadingly negative, solely by the play of chance. Furthermore, some studies are far too small to detect modest but worthwhile treatment benefits. One method of overcoming these pitfalls is the overview or meta-analysis technique. To be valid, this approach uses information from all trials addressing the same question. The large numbers of patients contributed by all individual trials provide greater statistical power. This enables meta-analyses to detect reliably modest advantages for one treatment over another and then to correct false–negative results produced by small randomized trials. An important and unique aspect of the meta-analyses undertaken by the Early Breast Cancer Trialists' Collaborative Group (EBCTCG) is that it uses data from individual patients in all of the trials, whereas most meta-analyses typically rely only on published summary statistics. This allows detailed and comprehensive analyses.

Meta-analyses also have potential problems. For instance, the meta-analysis for adjuvant chemotherapy of breast cancer is likely to be an underestimate of the actual benefit achievable in a patient given the best drug regimen, because the analysis combines the results of studies using a variety drug doses and schedules. Similarly, the inclusion of estrogen receptor (ER)-unknown or ER-negative patients in meta-analyses of endocrine therapy will dilute the estimate of benefit for patients known to be ER-positive. Nevertheless, the meta-analysis of breast cancer adjuvant therapy has contributed substantially to

current medical practice patterns, by providing more certain evidence of the efficacy of adjuvant therapy, by resolving controversies originating in previously conflicting results, and by generating testable hypotheses for future studies.

 ## BIOLOGY OF ENDOCRINE THERAPY

Endocrine therapy of breast cancer represents the first molecularly targeted therapy for cancer. The success of this approach provided a strong rationale for the development and testing of other targeted therapies. All endocrine therapies target the ER protein, which is present in 70% to 80% of female breast cancers. The progesterone receptor (PR) has not been utilized as a treatment target itself, but its presence indicates a functioning ER pathway because it is an estrogen-induced gene, and, thereby, a tumor that is more likely to be inhibited by ER-targeted therapies. Additionally, a growing body of evidence suggests an important role for PR signaling in breast cancer development, implicating its potential as a therapeutic target.

Estrogen receptor is a nuclear transcription factor (see Chapter 29). After the binding of estrogen, ER is phosphorylated and its protein conformation is altered. Afterward, it dimerizes with another receptor monomer, recruits coregulatory proteins, and the receptor complex binds to target genes at specific estrogen response elements in their promoters (6–8). There are two estrogen receptors, alpha and beta (9,10). The function and role of ERβ in breast cancer is not totally defined, although several studies suggest that when it is present in abundance it may signal a tumor more likely to benefit from tamoxifen (11–13). When ERα (which will be called ER in this chapter) is bound by estrogen, it activates transcription of specific genes and inhibits transcription of others (genomic activity). Some of these induced genes encode proteins important for tumor cell growth and survival and, consequently, therapies designed to block this pathway have therapeutic benefit. Evidence also suggests that in some breast cancer cells, a small pool of ER is located outside the nucleus perhaps tethered to the cell membrane. This ER mediates the so-called nongenomic or rapid effects of estrogen to activate various growth factor pathways, among them epidermal growth factor receptor (EGFR), HER2, and insulin growth factor receptor (IGF1-R) (14–18).

All endocrine therapies target this pathway in one way or another. Ovarian ablation (surgical or medical) and AI lower the level of estrogen, thereby reducing the ligand-induced activation of ER signaling, both genomic and nongenomic. Selective ER modulators, such as tamoxifen and toremifene, bind ER just like estrogen, but they alter ER conformation in a slightly different way (19). These drugs demonstrate dual estrogen agonist and antagonist activity depending on the tissue, cell or gene context. Thus, tamoxifen behaves as an estrogen in the endometrium, bone, liver, and even on some genes in the breast, whereas for other genes in the breast, tamoxifen functions as an antagonist to inhibit estrogen-dependent transcription. Growing evidence suggests that this intrinsic agonist activity of tamoxifen and other selective estrogen receptor modulators (SERM) may be higher in some patient's tumors than in others owing to activation of the ER and its coactivators by growth factor and stress-response pathways, potentially causing loss of tamoxifen's antagonist activity and resulting, then, in *de novo* or acquired resistance (20–22). Additionally, tamoxifen acts as an agonist on nongenomic ER signaling, which may be a cause of tamoxifen resistance in some patients.

Pure antagonists or ER downregulators (e.g., fulvestrant) bind ER, but have no intrinsic agonist activity (15,23). Furthermore, they induce degradation of ER protein and one of them, fulvestrant, does not activate nongenomic ER (24–26). This class of agents has not yet been studied in the adjuvant setting, although the steroidal antiestrogen, fulvestrant, is as effective as the AI anastrozole in metastatic breast cancer (23). High doses of steroid hormones, including estrogens, progestins, and androgens, although effective in metastatic disease, are not used for adjuvant therapy because of their toxicity profiles. The mechanism of action of this class of agents remains unclear, although high-dose estrogen may induce apoptosis through its effects on Fas ligand (27).

ADJUVANT THERAPY WITH SELECTIVE ESTROGEN RECEPTOR MODULATORS

Tamoxifen is the most commonly prescribed SERM for the treatment of breast cancer. Toremifene, a drug with structural and functional similarities to tamoxifen, is also approved for adjuvant therapy and appears equally effective to tamoxifen (28), but is much less prescribed. Raloxifene is approved for prevention but not for treatment of breast cancer. These drugs are nonsteroidal compounds that bind to ER and display both estrogen antagonist and estrogen agonist properties. Although the agonist properties of this class of endocrine therapy may account for resistance in some patients (see above), they also account for the favorable effects in preserving bone mineral density in postmenopausal women and the favorable effect on blood lipid profiles (29,30), both attractive features in postmenopausal women for whom estrogen replacement therapy is inappropriate. The net result of the binding of tamoxifen to ER is a blockade of cell cycle transit in G1 phase, thereby inhibiting tumor growth (31). Some evidence suggests that programmed cell death (apoptosis) may also be induced to a slight degree by tamoxifen (32).

Because of its favorable toxicity profile and its activity in advanced breast cancer, tamoxifen entered clinical trials of adjuvant therapy in the middle to late 1970s. More than seventy randomized clinical trials of tamoxifen, some originating more than 30 years ago, were included in the latest Oxford meta-analysis and definitive conclusions about its effectiveness and its toxicity are clear (33).

More than 80,000 women from around the world have now been randomized in trials comparing at least 1 year of tamoxifen with a no tamoxifen arm (33–35). More than 48,000 of these patients were randomized to tamoxifen versus a no treatment control arm, whereas nearly 32,000 were randomized to different durations of tamoxifen (Table 48.2). The early trials focused on postmenopausal patients, although a few included some premenopausal patients. Most of these studies included both node-positive and node-negative patients, although a large trial from the National Surgical Adjuvant Breast and Bowel Project (NSABP) studied node-negative patients exclusively (36). Both ER-positive and ER-negative patients were included in many of the earlier studies because it was thought by some that tamoxifen might still have a beneficial effect even in tumors lacking ER expression. Nearly all of the early studies found a statistically significant DFS advantage for tamoxifen, but only two large studies, the North American Treaty Organization Trial and the Scottish Trial showed a significant OS advantage (37,38). A survival trend in favor of tamoxifen was found in most of the other trials.

The 2005 meta-analysis of tamoxifen confirms both a DFS and OS advantage for ER-positive patients treated with tamoxifen for 5 years (Table 48.3) (33). The reduction in the annual odds of recurrence during the first 5 years is approximately 40% to 50% (50% in trials of tamoxifen versus no tamoxifen in the absence of chemotherapy) and the reductions in the annual odds of death a little over 30%. This means that while the patients are on tamoxifen one of every two recurrences and approximately one of every three deaths are avoided by the tamoxifen therapy. Interestingly, tamoxifen continues to demonstrate further reductions in the odds of recurrence and death in years 5 through 9.

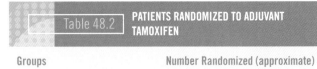

Table 48.2   PATIENTS RANDOMIZED TO ADJUVANT TAMOXIFEN

Groups	Number Randomized (approximate)
1–2 yr vs. nil	33,209
5 yr vs. nil	15,017
Longer vs. shorter tamoxifen	32,047
Total	80,237

Adapted from Early Breast Cancer Trialists' Collaborative Group. Effects of chemotherapy and hormonal therapy for early breast cancer on recurrence and 15-year survival: an overview of the randomised trials. *Lancet* 2005;365(9472):1687–1717, with permission.

Table 48.3   TAMOXIFEN RESULTS BY YEARS OF FOLLOW-UP; ESTROGEN RECEPTOR-POSITIVE OR UNKNOWN PATIENTS TREATED FOR 5 YEARS

	Reduction in Annual Odds ± Standard Error	
Years	Recurrence	Mortality
0–1	53 ± 5	29 ± 11
2–4	42 ± 5	32 ± 6
5–9	31 ± 6	35 ± 5
≥10	−1 ± 11	24 ± 9

Adapted from Early Breast Cancer Trialists' Collaborative Group. Effects of chemotherapy and hormonal therapy for early breast cancer on recurrence and 15-year survival: an overview of the randomised trials. *Lancet* 2005;365(9472):1687–1717, with permission.

For ER-positive tumors, the annual breast cancer mortality rates are similar during years 0 to 4 and 5 to 14, as are the proportional reductions in them by 5 years of tamoxifen, so the cumulative reduction in mortality is more than twice as big at 15 years as at 5 years after diagnosis (33). This *carry-over* effect of tamoxifen has not yet been explained but there continues to be significant reductions in recurrence and death for many years after the drug is stopped. It has also been reported in trials of AI as well and may be owing to a greater proportion of "cured" patients in the endocrine therapy groups.

Tamoxifen in Premenopausal and Postmenopausal Patients

Earlier meta-analyses suggested that tamoxifen had no benefit in women younger than age 50 (35,39). Because of the inclusion of women with ER-negative tumors, and because the duration of tamoxifen treatment was usually only 1 or 2 years in these early trials, definitive conclusions could not be drawn. Convincing evidence now indicates that more prolonged treatment (~5 years) results in a significant benefit in women younger than 50 years, as well as in older women, so long as their tumors are ER positive (33). In the previously mentioned NSABP node-negative adjuvant trial of tamoxifen versus placebo in ER-positive patients, tamoxifen was effective both in premenopausal and postmenopausal women (36,40). The recent meta-analyses confirm these results (Table 48.4) (33). Patients younger than 50 years of age, most of whom are premenopausal, benefit from 5 years of tamoxifen nearly as well as those 50 years of age and older. These reductions are just as impressive in young women less than 40 years of age who overall have a 44% reduction in recurrence and a 37% reduction in death from breast cancer (33). This analysis may represent an underestimate of the true benefit of 5 years of tamoxifen in ER-positive patients because it includes patients whose tumors were ER-unknown (about 20% of the total). Nevertheless, a sizable reduction in recurrence extends several years after completing tamoxifen therapy in both younger and older patients. The overall absolute reduction in recurrence at 15 years is 12% and the absolute reduction in deaths caused by breast cancer is 9%. The benefits found with 5 years of tamoxifen in younger women, along with the lack of benefit with the shorter durations used in earlier studies, strongly suggest that longer treatment is very important in this age group. These data also indicate that tamoxifen can inhibit the proliferation of breast cancer cells even in the presence of the high serum levels of estrogen typically found in these premenopausal patients taking the drug.

Whether tamoxifen is equivalent or even superior to chemotherapy in premenopausal women, as it appears to be in older women who have ER-positive tumors, remains a question. Although the data from the meta-analysis suggest that tamoxifen is at least as effective as adjuvant chemotherapy in women younger than age 50 with ER-positive tumors, few studies have directly addressed this question. In a single small trial of premenopausal women with ER-positive tumors, chemotherapy was superior to tamoxifen, but the duration of tamoxifen treatment was only 2 years (41). In a large randomized trial that compared chemotherapy plus tamoxifen with tamoxifen alone, the combination was more effective (42). However, this study did not have a chemotherapy-alone arm to assess the relative effectiveness of each single modality. Tamoxifen alone has not been compared with newer chemotherapy regimens, such as doxorubicin–taxane combinations, which may be superior to previous regimens. Interpretation of chemotherapy studies in young women is complicated by frequent ovarian ablative effects of the drugs resulting in a type of *endocrine therapy*.

In any event, with more than 25 years of follow-up from many studies, it is now certain that if tamoxifen is given for 5 years to patients selected on the basis of ER status, it is effective in both younger and older women. It is also important to note that the differences in outcome between tamoxifen and no tamoxifen observed after 5 years of follow-up grow even larger during the next 5 years, indicating that the benefits of tamoxifen are very durable over time (33).

Tamoxifen in Node-Negative and Node-Positive Patients

No biological reason exists for women with axillary node-negative breast cancer to respond differently to adjuvant systemic therapy compared with those with positive nodes, and many trials of adjuvant tamoxifen included both node-negative and node-positive patients. Fewer recurrences and deaths in the node-negative subset make it more difficult to show significant differences between tamoxifen and no treatment, but strong trends were evident early on in the larger studies (37,43). NSABP trial B-14 is by far the largest of the initial trials of adjuvant tamoxifen (2,644 patients), and it focused on patients with histologically negative axillary nodes (40,44,45). Both patients younger than 50 years of age (820 patients) and older patients (1,824 patients) were eligible, and all patients had ER-positive disease. Patients were randomly assigned to receive placebo or tamoxifen for 5 years, and those who received tamoxifen were reassigned at 5 years to stop therapy or to continue for 5 additional years.

Women who received tamoxifen had significantly higher probability of being free of local and distant recurrences (78% vs. 65%, $p < .0001$) and survival (71% vs. 65%, $p = .0008$) than with placebo. Tamoxifen-treated patients also had fewer

	EFFECT OF 5 YEARS OF TAMOXIFEN THERAPY BY AGE IN ESTROGEN RECEPTOR-POSITIVE AND UNKNOWN PATIENTS		

Table 48.4

	Reduction (±SE) in Annual Odds	
Age	Recurrence	Mortality
<40 yr	44 (±10%)	39 (±12%)
40–49 yr	29 (±7%)	24 (±9%)
50–59 yr	34 (±5%)	24 (±7%)
60–69 yr	45 (±5%)	35 (±6%)
≥70 yr	51 (±12%)	37 (±15%)

SE, standard error.
Adapted from Early Breast Cancer Trialists' Collaborative Group. Effects of chemotherapy and hormonal therapy for early breast cancer on recurrence and 15-year survival: an overview of the randomised trials. *Lancet* 2005;365(9472):1687–1717, with permission.

Table 48.5	BENEFITS OF TAMOXIFEN (5 YEARS) IN ESTROGEN RECEPTOR-POSITIVE OR UNKNOWN PATIENTS BY NODAL STATUS	
Reduction in Annual Odds (±SE)		
Nodes	Recurrence	Breast Cancer Mortality
Negative	39 (±4%)	31 (±5%)
Positive	39 (±4%)	31 (±5%)

SE, standard error.
Adapted from Early Breast Cancer Trialists' Collaborative Group. Effects of chemotherapy and hormonal therapy for early breast cancer on recurrence and 15-year survival: an overview of the randomised trials. *Lancet* 2005;365(9472):1687–1717, with permission.

Table 48.6	EFFECTS OF TAMOXIFEN FOR ABOUT 5 YEARS ACCORDING TO ESTROGEN RECEPTOR (ER) LEVEL	
Reduction (±SE) in Annual Odds		
ER Level	Recurrence	Breast Cancer Mortality
Poor (<10 fmol/mg)	−4 (±7%)	−4 (8%)
Positive (≥10 fmol/mg)	41 (±3)	34 (±5%)
Unknown	31 (±7%)	20 (±9%)

SE, standard error.
Adapted from Early Breast Cancer Trialists' Collaborative Group. Effects of chemotherapy and hormonal therapy for early breast cancer on recurrence and 15-year survival: an overview of the randomised trials. *Lancet* 2005;365(9472):1687–1717, with permission.

ipsilateral breast, local-regional, and distant recurrences than placebo-treated patients, and they had a substantial reduction (~50%) in contralateral breast cancer. These benefits persist beyond 15 years of follow-up (36,45).

The meta-analysis also suggests that the benefit with adjuvant tamoxifen is similar for node-negative and node-positive patients (33–35,39). The latest meta-analysis (Table 48.5) shows similar reductions in the annual odds of recurrence, and breast cancer mortality in node-negative and node-positive patients (33). These benefits are again an underestimate of the true benefit in ER-positive patients because these data include patients whose tumors were ER unknown and patients from trials confounded by chemotherapy. Breast cancer mortality is reduced by 33% to 40% in the first 4 years and this reduction continues in years 5 through 9 after tamoxifen is stopped. The 10-year absolute benefits are substantial for women with node-positive disease (12.6%) and for those with node-negative disease (5.3%). Because the overall recurrence rate is lower, the absolute benefit in lymph node-negative patients is somewhat less than in lymph node-positive patients although the relative benefits are similar. Thus, the cumulative data suggest that tamoxifen improves survival in both node-negative patients, who have a substantially lower baseline risk of recurrence and death, and in node-positive patients. Because of its favorable toxicity profile, tamoxifen (as part of an adjuvant hormonal therapy strategy) is especially attractive for treating women who have a lower risk of disease recurrence rather than exposing these women to the toxicity of chemotherapy.

Tamoxifen in Different Hormone Receptor Expression Subgroups

Many of the early tamoxifen adjuvant trials included patients with ER-negative or ER-poor as well as ER-positive and ER-unknown tumors. These studies helped to assess the potential benefits of tamoxifen in both subsets. The results are difficult to interpret, however, because of varying definitions of *ER-positive* and *ER-negative,* concerns about assay quality, and because only a fraction of the patients in some of these studies had ER assays performed.

Most studies of breast cancer cell lines or studies using animal models show little or no effects of tamoxifen in ER-negative cells at drug concentrations achieved in patients (46). Tamoxifen, however, has numerous effects on cells that are not mediated through the ER that could affect receptor-negative tumors. Alternatively, the effects of the drug on the few ER-positive cells present in an *ER-negative* tumor could indirectly inhibit cell populations that lack receptors through a paracrine mechanism. Finally, the drug has systemic effects, such as lowering serum IGF-I levels, that could inhibit growth of tumors regardless of ER content (47,48). Antitumor activity, even in ER-negative tumors, is therefore plausible. The low response

rates observed with tamoxifen in ER-negative metastatic disease (5% to 10%) argue, however, that these ancillary effects of tamoxifen are clinically unimportant and they suggest that the benefit is likely to be modest in the adjuvant setting. The few responses observed in such patients are consistent with false–negative ER assays.

Nevertheless, several European trials reported some advantage for tamoxifen in *ER-poor* patients in the trials of 1 to 2 years of tamoxifen, but no advantage was seen in the trials of approximately 5 years of treatment (33). Again, this apparent benefit might have been owing to false–negative ER measurements in some of the early trials of 1 to 2 years of tamoxifen.

Earlier meta-analyses suggested a small but statistically significant survival benefit in women with ER-poor tumors treated with adjuvant tamoxifen, but the most recent meta-analyses with longer follow-up and a larger sample size do not (34,35,39,49) (Table 48.6). Patients with ER-poor tumors, a subset that includes tumors with undetectable or borderline-positive ER (4 to 10 fmol/mg protein by ligand-binding assay), showed no reduction in the annual odds of recurrence or death. Women with tumors known to be definitely positive for ER had a 41% reduction in the annual odds of recurrence, a 34% reduction in breast cancer deaths, and a 27% reduction in the annual odds of death from any cause with 5 years of tamoxifen (not shown), and those with ER unknown tumors, about 30% of which should be ER-poor, had an intermediate benefit. Patients with very high tumor ER levels had a 49% reduction in the annual odds of recurrence and 33% reduction in deaths (not shown). This compares to a 36% reduction in recurrence and a 22% reduction in death for patients with tumors with low to moderate ER (10 to 100 fmol/mg protein). What the equivalent cutoffs are in various immunohistochemistry (IHC) assays done today is not clear.

Only two prospective, randomized trials designed to assess directly the value of 5 years of tamoxifen in ER-negative patients have been reported (50,51). These trials randomized either ER-positive and ER-negative node-negative patients (51), or only ER-negative patients (50) to chemotherapy alone, or chemotherapy plus tamoxifen. ER was measured by ligand-binding assay in laboratories with stringent quality control. Neither trial shows improved outcome in the ER-negative subset and one shows a trend for a detrimental effect on DFS and OS with tamoxifen in patients whose tumors have very low or undetectable ER (51). Neither of these two trials, nor the meta-analysis shows a reduction in contralateral breast cancer with tamoxifen in patients with ER-negative first primaries (see below).

Relatively few studies included measurements of PR. In the meta-analysis, among women with ER-positive tumors, the efficacy of tamoxifen was independent of the concentration of PR (33). Studies of patients with metastatic disease have shown consistently that patients with ER-negative, PR-positive tumors benefit from tamoxifen and other endocrine therapies and that those with ER-positive, PR-negative tumors respond less well than those positive for both receptors, but this has not been confirmed in the meta-analysis (33). Assay quality and standardization in these global studies are problematic, however. This issue is discussed in detail in Chapter 29.

A retrospective study of nearly 14,000 women whose tumors were assessed for ER and PR in an experienced central laboratory using ligand-binding assay suggested that PR is important in predicting tamoxifen benefit (52). In patients receiving tamoxifen adjuvant therapy, a multivariate analysis demonstrated that PR status was independently associated with both DFS and OS. The reduction in the relative risk of recurrence was 53% for ER-positive, PR-positive patients and only 25% for ER-positive, PR-negative tumors compared with those with tumors negative for both receptors. The reduction in the relative risk of death in patients with tumors positive for both receptors was approximately 50%.

These data suggest that when PR is measured accurately by ligand-binding assay, ER-positive, PR-positive patients derive more benefit from tamoxifen therapy than those positive for only ER. At the same time, this study found that PR was a weak prognostic factor in patients not receiving adjuvant therapy. This difference in benefit from tamoxifen therapy may be explained in part by the higher likelihood of these ER-positive, PR-negative tumors to be positive for EGFR expression or HER2 overexpression (53). Even in this large data set, patients with ER-negative, PR-positive tumors were too few for a meaningful conclusion, but trials in metastatic disease suggest that this subset does benefit from endocrine therapy.

More recent trials, in which ER and PR were measured by IHC, also show less benefit from tamoxifen and AI when PR is lost (54). The relatively greater advantage for anastrozole over tamoxifen originally reported in the Arimidex, Tamoxifen Alone or in Combination (ATAC) trial has not been confirmed in a later study (55). That study analyzed a subset of patients largely from the United Kingdom in which the assays were repeated in a central laboratory (56). Interestingly, this subset did not show a differential effect for anastrozole over tamoxifen, even when the original ER and PR assays performed locally were used. This suggests that the effect by PR status in the remaining patients, not reported in this study, might be even greater than the initial ATAC report (54,56).

Assays for PR are perhaps more problematic than those for ER and this issue is reviewed in detail in Chapter 29. PR has two isoforms (A and B) with apparently different functions (56–59). Tumors with a high ratio of the A to B isoforms have a more aggressive course (60). Many different antibodies now used for immunohistochemical assays have different specificities, with some recognizing one isoform or the other and some recognizing both (61). It is clear that more work is required to know the true value of PR determination in breast cancer.

It is now clear, however, that when the assays are done properly, patients with ER- and PR-negative tumors do not benefit from tamoxifen adjuvant therapy. Nor do they benefit with a reduction in contralateral breast cancer (see below). All of the data reviewed above were based, however, on receptor measurements derived from the ligand-binding assay, which had been rigidly standardized and quality controlled, at least in the United States. Laboratories have converted to immunohistochemical assays, which have not been standardized across laboratories. More importantly, rigorous determination and clinical validation of cutoff values for positive and negative receptor status in each laboratory have not been defined carefully. Data from experienced research laboratories suggest that the error rates in both the United Kingdom and the United States may be as high as 20% to 25% (62,63). This means that many patients today are not receiving a potentially life-saving therapy because of an incorrect test. Standardization and quality con-

trol of these relatively simple and inexpensive diagnostic tests are urgently needed, a process that would seem to be in the purview of national societies of pathology which represent the groups of physicians charged with providing responsible results. The College of American Pathologists and the American Society of Clinical Oncology are convening a committee to address the problems of ER and PR determination and to provide recommendations for their measurement.

Tamoxifen in Elderly Patients

Because it is generally well tolerated, tamoxifen has been used extensively to treat elderly patients with breast cancer. The meta-analysis demonstrates a significant mortality reduction in patients older than 70 years treated with adjuvant tamoxifen (Table 48.4) (33). Furthermore, some individual trials have specifically targeted this population. The Eastern Cooperative Oncology Group (ECOG) study randomized 181 patients 65 years of age or older to tamoxifen or placebo for 2 years (64). The drug was well tolerated, and significant reductions in recurrence and borderline significant reductions in mortality were observed. Tamoxifen also reduced the incidence of contralateral breast cancers. Most patients who died in this study (61%) succumbed to breast cancer, although, as anticipated, a significant number of these older women (22%) died of competing illnesses not related to cancer, a factor that must be considered when making adjuvant therapy decisions. Nonadherence to the prescribed dose and schedule of tamoxifen, which is surprisingly high overall, is even higher in elderly patients (65,66).

Several small, randomized trials have also evaluated the use of tamoxifen as sole treatment without surgery for operable primary breast cancer in elderly patients (67–69). These studies showed no survival advantage for the addition of surgery. Local control was poor in the tamoxifen alone group, however, and as a consequence, minimal surgery and hormonal therapy are still indicated in this group. Hormonal therapy as a single modality with tamoxifen or an aromatase inhibitor might be reserved for very old or frail patients for temporary disease control. Because these patients have a relatively high risk of thromboembolic complications, an AI is probably more preferable in elderly patients.

Delayed Adjuvant Tamoxifen

Although a rare situation today, the question whether patients could still benefit from adjuvant hormonal therapy, even if initiated years after their primary treatment, remains important for a small subset of patients. One study addressed this question and found that patients who had ER- or PR-positive tumors, and whose adjuvant therapy with tamoxifen was started 2 years or more after initial diagnosis, had improved DFS and OS, even when the delay in starting *adjuvant* tamoxifen was more than 5 years (70). Thus, those patients whose tumors are receptor positive and who, for whatever reason, were not started on adjuvant hormonal therapy at the time of diagnosis may still benefit from delayed treatment. It is likely that a similar benefit would be also seen with AI, although no studies have addressed this topic. However, the remaining risk of recurrence in such patients should be considered. Patients with a low risk at the time of diagnosis may have an extremely low risk of recurrence, not justifying the side effects of therapy if several years have elapsed since diagnosis. The cumulative risk of recurrence declines with each additional year of follow-up after diagnosis.

Tamoxifen Summary

Taking tamoxifen for 5 years prolongs DFS and OS in patients with ER-positive tumors regardless of axillary lymph node status. Equally beneficial effects are seen in premenopausal and postmenopausal women. With AI showing a small DFS benefit over tamoxifen, adjuvant hormonal therapy has shifted more toward the upfront or sequential use of these agents (see section on aromatase inhibitors). It is not yet certain that these agents should completely replace tamoxifen considering that no studies have shown superior OS. Until conclusive data are available, one may argue that tamoxifen still has an important role alone or in sequence with an AI. Tamoxifen should be avoided in women who have medical contraindications, such as a history of thromboembolic disease or blood-clotting disorders (see section Toxicity of Adjuvant Therapy). Aromatase inhibitors avoid these problems and may be preferred in these patients. Tamoxifen is certainly an acceptable alternative for women who cannot tolerate or afford an AI, and it is still the endocrine therapy of choice in premenopausal patients.

AROMATASE INHIBITORS

Adjuvant Therapy

Aromatase inhibitors block the synthesis of estrogen in tissues containing the enzyme. The enzyme is present in breast tumor tissue, fat, muscle, and brain, and it converts androgens of adrenal origin to estrogens. Two classes of aromatase inhibitors exist that have slightly different mechanisms of action and different mechanisms of resistance leading to incomplete cross-resistance. The nonsteroidal AI, including anastrozole and letrozole, bind aromatase in a reversible manner (71). Steroidal AI, such as exemestane, form an irreversible complex (71,72). Results from a phase III study confirmed earlier reports that patients with metastatic breast cancer progressing on a nonsteroidal aromatase inhibitor may respond occasionally to treatment with exemestane (72,73).

All of these drugs lower serum and tumor estrogen to very low levels. Although there are modest differences in the degree of aromatase inhibition among these agents, it is not clear whether they translate into differences in clinical benefit (74). Exemestane, with its steroidal structure, may have anabolic activity that could potentially provide a beneficial effect on bone density, but that has not been observed in clinical studies (75). Aromatase inhibitors have been shown to be modestly superior to tamoxifen in the first line treatment of patients with ER-positive metastatic breast cancer (76,77). Aromatase inhibitors are generally ineffective in premenopausal women. The reduced feedback of estrogen to the hypothalamus and pituitary increases gonadotropin secretion, which stimulates the ovary, leading to an increase in androgen substrate and aromatase (78). Therefore, it is imperative that women who receive AI are verifiably postmenopausal. Women who develop amenorrhea after adjuvant chemotherapy may still have premenopausal estradiol levels and others may start menstruating again when

therapy with an AI is initiated because of rising gonadotropin levels (follicle-stimulating hormone [FSH] and luteinizing hormone [LH]), which can stimulate the ovary. These women may be better off receiving tamoxifen at least initially while they are observed for resumption of menses. Gonadotropins and estradiol levels should be followed as well in such women.

Several large, randomized phase III clinical trials incorporating aromatase inhibitors in the adjuvant treatment of breast cancer have been completed. These studies generally followed one or more of three different strategies: upfront treatment with an AI compared with upfront tamoxifen; switching to an AI after initial tamoxifen treatment for 2 to 3 years; or using AI to extend adjuvant treatment after 5 years of tamoxifen.

Upfront Adjuvant Therapy

Arimidex, Tamoxifen, Alone or in Combination Trial

The ATAC trial was the first large, randomized trial to report on the use of an aromatase inhibitor in the adjuvant treatment of breast cancer (Table 48.7). In this trial, 9,366 patients were initially randomized after surgery to receive either anastrozole, tamoxifen, or a combination of the two. However, the combination arm was discontinued at 33 months of follow-up after this group was found to be equivalent to tamoxifen alone and inferior to anastrozole monotherapy (79). This trial first reported an advantage in DFS for the anastrozole-treated group over the tamoxifen-treated group in 2002 and several updates have confirmed this benefit (79,80). Despite long follow-up of patients on this study, no overall survival benefit has emerged (hazard ratio [HR] = 0.97, p = .70) (79).

At a median follow-up of 100 months, an updated analysis of the ATAC trial of the 6,241 patients randomized to anastrozole versus tamoxifen showed a continued DFS benefit for anastrozole (79). This advantage was observed in all randomized patients (intent-to-treat population) and in the clinically important hormone receptor-positive subgroup which comprised 84% of all patients on this study. In this subgroup the DFS (HR = 0.85, p = .003), time-to recurrence (TTR) (HR = 0.76, p = .0001), and time-to-distant-recurrence (TTDR) (HR = 0.84, p = .022) were superior for patients in the anastrozole-alone arm compared with tamoxifen alone. Anastrozole also showed a significantly lower ipsilateral and contralateral breast cancer recurrence rate (HR = 0.60, p = .004) (79).

In this study, the lower recurrence rate for anastrozole compared with tamoxifen was maintained after treatment was completed, especially for the hormone receptor-positive population where the absolute benefit of 2.8% (anastrozole, n = 245 events; tamoxifen, 312 events; HR 0.77, p = .002) at 5 years increased to 4.8% at 9 years (anastrozole, 391 events; tamoxifen, 494 events; HR 0.76, p = .0001). This finding suggests that the carryover benefit after treatment completion with anastrozole is greater than that known to exist after tamoxifen (33).

Table 48.7	EFFECTS OF UPFRONT THERAPY WITH AROMATASE INHIBITORS FOR 5 YEARS COMPARED WITH TAMOXIFEN				
Study	Experimental Arm	Patients (N)	Median Follow-up (Months)	DFS	OS
ATAC	Anastrozole for 5 yr	9,366	100	HR = 0.85 p = .003	HR = 0.97 p = .70
BIG 1-98[a]	Letrozole for 5 yr	8,028	51	HR = 0.83 p = .007	HR = 0.91 p = .35

[a]BIG 1-98 has two sequential therapy arms (tamoxifen → letrozole, letrozole → tamoxifen) that have not yet been reported.
ATAC, Arimidex, Tamoxifen, Alone or in Combination; BIG 1-98, Breast International Group; DFS, disease-free survival; HR, hazared ratio; OS, overall survival.

Subgroup analysis initially suggested a more pronounced DFS benefit for anastrozole in the ER-positive, PR-negative subgroup (HR = 0.42) than in the ER-positive, PR-positive subgroup (HR = 0.87) (54). This report considered the hormone receptor assays performed locally. To confirm these results, an attempt was made to obtain tumor blocks and repeat the receptor assays in an experienced central laboratory. Only one-third of these blocks were obtained and most came from patients in the United Kingdom. These central laboratory assay results failed to confirm the relationship between PR loss and greater benefit from anastrozole (56). Interestingly, the initial finding was not confirmed even when the local assay results were applied. These data suggest that the subset of patients comprising the smaller follow-up study is somehow different than other patients enrolled in ATAC, at least regarding measurement of PR. It is unfortunate that more blocks could not be obtained for this follow-up study, the results of which should be interpreted with caution. Another study, the Breast International Group (BIG) 1-98, comparing letrozole with tamoxifen also failed to show a relationship between PR loss and benefit from letrozole, although follow-up on this study is short (79,81). Until more data are available, PR status should not be used to select the type of adjuvant endocrine therapy.

Breast International Group 1-98 Trial

The Breast International Group 1-98 study is a large, randomized, phase III, double-blind trial comparing the following options: monotherapy with letrozole or with tamoxifen for 5 years, sequential administration of tamoxifen for 2 years followed by letrozole for 3 years, or sequential administration of letrozole for 2 years followed by tamoxifen for 3 years (Table 48.7). The trial was conducted in postmenopausal women with hormone receptor-positive operable invasive breast cancer. This trial was designed to address whether an aromatase inhibitor is more effective as initial adjuvant therapy or as therapy following a few years of adjuvant tamoxifen. This study randomized more than 8,000 women.

The BIG 1-98 trial used DFS as its primary end point, using a definition that included local recurrence after breast-conserving treatment, the appearance of metastatic disease, the development of a second primary tumor, or death from any cause. DFS in this trial included secondary nonbreast cancers, whereas DFS in the ATAC study did not. On the other hand, it did not include ductal carcinoma *in situ* (DCIS) in its DFS definition, whereas the ATAC study did (79,81).

Results from the primary core analysis (i.e., events from the two monotherapy arms as well as events occurring up to 30 days after switching in the sequential arms) at 25.8 months of median follow-up showed improved outcome in letrozole-treated patients compared with tamoxifen in DFS (HR = 0.81, p = .003), TTR (HR = 0.72, p <.001), and TTDR (HR = 0.73; p = .0012). An update of the letrozole and tamoxifen arms at a median follow-up of 51 months reported that the benefits in the primary core analysis were maintained (DFS, HR = 0.82, p = .007; TTR, HR = 0.78, p = 0.004; and TTDR, HR = 0.81, p = .03) (81).

Prospectively planned subgroup studies demonstrated that a significant benefit in DFS was observed in higher-risk patients (i.e., patients with tumors >2 cm [HR = 0.76, p = 0.004], those with node-positive disease [HR = 0.71, p <.001], and those who required chemotherapy [HR = 0.70, p = .01]) (81).

A planned central analysis of the ER, PR, and HER2 status in this trial was performed where these biomarkers were repeated centrally in 3,650 tumors (74% of the tamoxifen and letrozole patients) (81,82). Letrozole had the same small advantage over tamoxifen in all subgroups. The difference in benefit in the ER-positive, PR-negative subset reported in ATAC was not observed (81). Additionally, and although DFS was less favorable in patients with HER2-positive tumors, letrozole maintained its advantage over tamoxifen regardless of HER2 status (82).

Summary of Upfront Therapy with Aromatase Inhibitors

Upfront therapy with an aromatase inhibitor is beneficial, in terms of DFS, when compared with tamoxifen. Concerns with cross-trial comparisons do not allow a definite conclusion regarding the question of anastrozole versus letrozole, particularly because different methodologies were used and different subgroup analyses were performed. For example, the DFS advantage of letrozole over tamoxifen in the increased risk population, such as node-positive or chemotherapy-treated patients, was not seen with anastrozole in the ATAC trial. The Femara Anastrozole Clinical Evaluation (FACE) trial will determine if there are clinically important differences in safety or efficacy between these two agents. This study will randomize more 4,000 women with hormone receptor-positive, lymph node-positive breast cancer to either letrozole or anastrozole.

It is important to emphasize again that upfront aromatase inhibitors should be used only for women who are verifiably postmenopausal. It should probably be avoided in women with chemotherapy-induced amenorrhea because AI may promote recovery of ovarian function in some of them (83).

Sequential Adjuvant Therapy with Aromatase Inhibitors Following Tamoxifen

One of the problems that afflict switching trials is that the patients were not entered into the trial or randomized at the beginning of the adjuvant therapy. Rather, patients were randomized after they have been on tamoxifen for 2 to 3 years. Thus, patients who had an early recurrence while on tamoxifen were not included in these trials. Therefore, the risk reduction demonstrated in these switching trials should not be compared with that observed in the upfront adjuvant trials, in which all patients were randomized immediately after the diagnosis.

Intergroup Exemestane Study

The Intergroup Exemestane Study (IES) is the largest and most mature switching trial (Table 48.8). It tested the concept of whether switching to exemestane after 2 to 3 years of tamoxifen therapy is more effective than continuing tamoxifen therapy for the remainder of the 5 years of treatment. The primary end point was DFS defined as the time from randomization to recurrence of breast cancer at any site, diagnosis of a second primary breast cancer, or death from any cause. Similar to the ATAC trial, nonbreast primary cancers were not included in the definition of DFS. Of the 4,742 patients enrolled, 2,362 were randomized to switch to exemestane, and 2,380 to continue to receive tamoxifen (84).

The most recent published update on this study showed that at a median follow-up of 55.7 months, there were 809 events (354 exemestane, 455 tamoxifen). The hazard ratio was 0.76 (p = .0001) favoring exemestane, and the absolute benefit was 3.3% (85). Fewer deaths occurred in the exemestane group compared with the tamoxifen group (222 vs. 261, respectively; HR = 0.85, p = .08) that was statistically significant only after excluding 122 hormone receptor-negative patients (HR = 0.83, p = .05). In addition, switching from tamoxifen to exemestane demonstrated a significant reduction in contralateral breast cancer (HR = 0.56, p = .04) (85).

Arimidex-Nolvadex 95 Trial (ARNO 95)/Austrian Breast and Colorectal Cancer Study Group

The Austrian Breast and Colorectal Cancer Study Group (ABCSG) trial 8 and the Arimidex-Nolvadex 95 Trial (ARNO 95) by the German Adjuvant Breast Cancer Group (GABG) are both

			Median Follow-up		
Study	Experimental Arm	Patients (N)	(Months)	DFS	OS

Table 48.8 EFFECTS OF SEQUENTIAL THERAPY WITH TAMOXIFEN FOLLOWED BY AN AROMATASE INHIBITOR COMPARED TO 5 YEARS OF TAMOXIFEN[a]

Study	Experimental Arm	Patients (N)	Median Follow-up (Months)	DFS	OS
IES[b]	Tamoxifen for 2-3 yr → Exemestane for 2-3 yr	4,724	56	HR = 0.76 $p = .0001$	HR = 0.85 $p = .08$
ITA[b]	Tamoxifen for 2-3 yr → Anastrozole for 2-3 yr	448	64	HR = 0.57 $p = .005$	HR = 0.56 $p = .10$
ARNO95[b]/ABCSG8	Tamoxifen for 2 yr → Anastrozole for 3 yr	3,224	28	HR = 0.60 $p = .0009$	Not Reported
MA-17[a]	Tamoxifen for 5 yr → Letrozole for 5 yr	5,187	30	HR = 0.58 $p < .001$	HR = 0.82 $p = .30$

ABCSG8, Austrian Breast and Colorectal Cancer Study Group Trial-8; ARNO95, Arimidex-Nolvadex 95 Study; DFS, disease-free survival; IES, Intergroup Exemestane Study; ITA, Italian Tamoxifen/Arimidex Trial.
[a]In MA17 patients were randomized after 5 years of tamoxifen to letrozole versus placebo for 5 years.
[b]Patients were randomized after receiving 2 years of tamoxifen.

prospective, multicenter, randomized, open-label studies that had broadly similar inclusion criteria and outcome measures (Table 48.8) (86).

Eligible patients were postmenopausal women aged 80 years or younger (ABCSG trial 8) or 75 years or younger (ARNO 95) with surgically treated hormone receptor-positive breast cancer. No patients received prior chemotherapy. Eligibility criteria did differ slightly regarding tumor histologic features. ABCSG 8 included G1 and G2 ductal carcinomas and all lobular carcinomas, whereas ARNO 95 allowed all histologic types and all grades. Eligible patients underwent definitive surgery and radiotherapy, if indicated, followed by adjuvant tamoxifen therapy started within 6 weeks (ABCSG trial 8) or 4 weeks (ARNO 95).

In contrast to most switching trials, women were randomized before beginning treatment with tamoxifen in ABCSG trial 8 but not in the ARNO 95 trial. For both studies, patients had to complete 2 years of adjuvant tamoxifen therapy in accordance with local guidelines (20 mg daily in ABCSG 8 vs. 20 to 30 mg daily in ARNO 95). The analysis included 3,224 patients (86). After a median follow-up of 28 months, patients in the anastrozole group had a 40% decrease in the risk for an event compared with the tamoxifen group (67 events for anastrozole versus 110 events for tamoxifen, HR = 0.60; $p = .009$). (86).

A report of the ARNO 95 study (979 patients) with a median follow-up of 30 months showed that switching to anastrozole resulted in a significant reduction in the risk of disease recurrence (HR = 0.66, $p = .049$) with an absolute benefit of 4.2%. In this relatively small study, the anastrozole group also had a lower number of deaths (15 vs. 26 deaths), which resulted in improved overall survival (HR, 0.53, $p = .045$) compared with continuing tamoxifen (87).

Italian Tamoxifen/Arimidex Trial

The Italian Tamoxifen/Arimidex (ITA) trial also assessed switching patients from tamoxifen to anastrozole (Table 48.8). This small, open-label trial included ER-positive, lymph node-positive postmenopausal patients, approximately 67% of whom had previously received adjuvant chemotherapy. After 2 to 3 years of tamoxifen therapy, patients were randomized to receive either anastrozole (1 mg/day) or to continue tamoxifen (20 mg/day) for a total duration of 5 years. The primary end point was disease-free survival and secondary end points included safety and overall survival (88).

A total of 448 patients were enrolled. At a median follow-up of 64 months, 63 events had been reported in the tamoxifen group compared with 39 in the anastrozole group, resulting in

a significant difference in DFS (HR 0.57, $p = .005$). However, overall survival was not significantly different (88).

Combined Analysis of Sequential Trials Using Anastrozole

A combined analysis of the ARNO 95, ABCSG 8, and ITA trials was performed which included more than 4,000 patients (89). Patients who switched to anastrozole had fewer disease recurrences (92 vs. 159) and deaths (66 vs. 90) than did those who remained on tamoxifen, resulting in significant improvements in DFS (HR = 0.59, $p < .0001$), event-free survival (HR = 0.55, $p < .0001$), distant recurrence-free survival (HR = 0.61, $p = .002$), and overall survival (HR = 0.71, $p = .04$), suggesting that postmenopausal women receiving adjuvant tamoxifen should be switched to anastrozole after completing 2 to 3 years of treatment (89).

This report has the limitations of a meta-analysis, however. The three trials had different randomization schema; patients were randomized upfront in ABCSG 8, whereas they were randomized after 2 to 3 years of tamoxifen in the ARNO 95 and ITA trials. There were also differences in the definition of primary end points and in the entry criteria. It is worth noting that the survival advantage demonstrated in the pooled analysis may be driven by differences in deaths in the smaller studies because there was only a difference of two deaths between the anastrozole and tamoxifen arms in the ABCSG 8 trial (42 on anastrozole vs. 44 on tamoxifen), which was the largest trial in the analysis. Furthermore, the IES study which is individually larger than the pooled analysis, has not yet shown an overall survival advantage except in the subset of patients known to be ER-positive. It is interesting that the switching trials are now showing a survival advantage, whereas a trend is not even seen in the ATAC and BIG 1-98 studies directly comparing tamoxifen with an upfront AI. Longer follow-up of the BIG 1-98 trial with analysis of the switching arms to compare with the upfront arms is necessary to help resolve this issue.

Summary of Sequential Therapy with Aromatase Inhibitors

At the moment it is not clear whether initial treatment with an AI or a few years of tamoxifen followed by an AI is the superior strategy. Several investigators have used available published data and applied *in silico* computer modeling studies to compare the potential outcomes of each of these two strategies using various assumptions (90–92). Obviously, these studies cannot be used for clinical decision-making, but their results do provide a range of possible outcomes that are interesting to consider. Two of these studies used data from the original ATAC analysis, including the effect of ER and PR on the relative benefits of anastrozole and tamoxifen. They suggested that the switching strategy might be only marginally superior for patients whose tumors were ER-positive and PR-positive, whereas initial AI therapy was projected to be significantly better in patients with ER-positive but PR-negative tumors. The third study which incorporated receptor assessment and data from the BIG 1-98 study suggested that initial AI therapy would be superior regardless of the ER or PR status (81). Because the original ER and PR data from the ATAC trial have not been confirmed in subsequent analyses (55), any conclusions drawn from these studies become problematic and longer follow-up of BIG 1-98 is needed for more definitive conclusions.

EXTENDED ADJUVANT HORMONAL THERAPY

Theoretic reasons support a rationale for prolonged adjuvant hormonal therapy beyond the first 5 years. More prolonged therapy could prevent late recurrences in patients whose breast cancers would otherwise relapse. In addition, tumors resistant to SERM often respond to AI at least in the metastatic setting. On the other hand, side effects and cost of more prolonged therapy are important considerations. Extending tamoxifen, AI, or their sequence beyond 5 years is the subject of several completed and ongoing clinical trials.

EXTENDED ADJUVANT THERAPY WITH TAMOXIFEN

Several trials compared shorter versus longer tamoxifen adjuvant treatment directly. In two large European trials from Britain and Sweden, respectively, women treated with tamoxifen for 5 years had fewer recurrences and deaths than those treated for only 2 years (93,94). Two North American trials, the large trial from the NSABP and a much smaller trial, compared tamoxifen treatment for 5 years with treatment that lasted for approximately 10 years (44,45,95), and a trial from Scotland compared 5 years with indefinite tamoxifen treatment (96,97). Although the numbers of recurrences and deaths are few in these relatively small trials, they did not present any convincing evidence that treatment lasting longer than 5 years is beneficial. In fact, in two of these trials a trend, statistically significant in one, was seen toward a detrimental effect with treatment for more than 5 years (44,45,96,97). This lack of benefit for more prolonged tamoxifen in these two trials persisted at 14 and 15 years of follow-up, respectively. Nevertheless, the results of all of these relatively small trials with a paucity of events were not considered definitive.

Two large international twin trials (Adjuvant Tamoxifen, Longer Against Shorter [ATLAS] and Adjuvant Tamoxifen: to offer more? [aTTom]) are currently addressing the issue of very long-term tamoxifen. Preliminary data from the ATLAS trial were recently reported (98). ATLAS randomized 11,500 women in 38 countries who had completed about 5 years of adjuvant tamoxifen with an additional 5 years of tamoxifen (10 years total) or with stopping therapy. At a mean follow-up of 4.2 years, about 1,500 recurrences were reported, most of them in years 5 through 9. Overall, the recurrence rate was modestly, albeit statistically, significantly lower among those allocated to continue tamoxifen. Although breast cancer mortality and overall mortality were numerically lower among those allocated to continue the drug, these differences were not statistically significant. No significant differences in mortality before recurrence were seen, either overall or from particular causes (98). Its twin trial, aTTom, randomized 6,934 women with ER-positive or untested breast cancer who completed 5 years of adjuvant tamoxifen to 5 more years of

tamoxifen (10 years total) versus stopping (98). With a median follow-up of 4.2 years, there were fewer recurrences in the group randomized to more tamoxifen, but that was not statistically significant. Additionally seen was a doubling of the incidence of endometrial carcinoma in patients on longer tamoxifen (76 vs. 35 cases), although there was no difference in death from endometrial cancer, or any other cause (98). Further follow-up is needed to assess reliably the effects of prolonged tamoxifen on recurrence and toxicity and to evaluate its impact on survival, if any.

EXTENDED ADJUVANT THERAPY WITH AROMATASE INHIBITORS

Extending tamoxifen adjuvant therapy beyond 5 years using an aromatase inhibitor is the subject of three clinical trials. The National Cancer Institute of Canada (NCIC)-MA17 trial is the largest and most mature such trial (Table 48.8). More than 5,000 women who had completed 5 years of tamoxifen were randomly assigned to placebo versus letrozole. The study was terminated early after the first interim analysis demonstrated a significant improvement in DFS in the letrozole group, which was confirmed on longer follow-up (HR = 0.58; p <.0001) (99). Another analysis of MA.17 that pertains to the issue of duration of an aromatase inhibitor after tamoxifen demonstrated that the hazard ratio in favor of letrozole continued to improve each year throughout the first 4 years of treatment, suggesting that longer treatment might be better (100).

NSABP B-33, which had a similar design using exemestane, was closed to accrual when the results of MA.17 were made public, and patients assigned to placebo were given the option of crossing over to exemestane. At that time, only half of the planned 3,000 patients were enrolled, and more than 40% of patients initially assigned to placebo chose to cross over to receive exemestane. Despite these limitations, a similar trend for improved DFS was observed for the exemestane arm, although it did not reach statistical significance (HR = 0.68, p = .07) (101). ABCSG-6a study is a smaller study that randomized about 850 patients who completed 5 years of tamoxifen (with or without aminoglutethimide for the first 2 years) to anastrozole versus placebo for 3 more years (102). This study showed a significant improvement in DFS (HR = 0.64, p = .048). None of these three trials have shown an impact on overall survival.

It should be noted that studies of extended adjuvant therapy using tamoxifen or an aromatase inhibitor were performed in patients who received 5 years of initial tamoxifen therapy, a situation that is becoming increasingly less common in postmenopausal women in the era of AI therapy. Additionally, they all demonstrated an impact on DFS but not OS. However, they support the concept of prolonging endocrine therapy beyond 5 years to prevent late recurrences. The type of therapy (tamoxifen, AI, or their sequence) and the optimal duration remain unanswered questions. The NSABP is performing a study of extended adjuvant letrozole following 5 years of upfront AI or sequential therapy, a more modern adjuvant endocrine regimen. Additionally, patients who have completed 5 years of letrozole on the MA.17 study are being rerandomized to continue letrozole for 5 more years versus placebo (total 15 years of adjuvant endocrine therapy).

ADJUVANT OVARIAN ABLATION

Among the first randomized trials of adjuvant therapy in breast cancer were studies of adjuvant ovarian ablation, either by surgical oophorectomy or by irradiation (39,103). Some of these trials were not properly randomized by modern standards (5). Many were small, a few included both premenopausal and postmenopausal women, and none included ER analyses, which were not yet available. Most of these trials found a significant DFS advantage for ovarian ablation, and two reported a significant OS advantage (104,105).

The 1996 meta-analysis included data from 12 properly randomized trials of ovarian ablation involving 2,102 patients younger than 50 years of age; 7 of these trials compared ovarian ablation with no adjuvant therapy, and 5 compared ovarian ablation and chemotherapy with the same chemotherapy alone (103). As expected, no significant benefit was observed for oophorectomy among 1,354 women older than 50 years of age, most of whom were postmenopausal when randomized. Younger women had a significant DFS and OS advantage with ovarian ablation compared with no adjuvant therapy.

The EBCTCG 2005 meta-analysis analyzed almost 8,000 women younger than 50 years of age with ER-positive or ER-unknown disease randomized into trials of ovarian ablation by surgery or irradiation (4,317 women, 63% ER-untested) or of ovarian suppression by treatment with a luteinizing-hormone releasing-hormone (LHRH) inhibitor (3,408 women, 26% ER-untested).

Overall, a definite effect of ovarian ablation or suppression was evident on both recurrence and breast cancer mortality (Table 48.9). This effect, however, is not as large as it was reported in earlier meta-analyses of these trials, when ovarian ablation was not generally being tested against a background of effective systemic chemotherapy (33).

The absolute effect on 15-year outcomes showed that for recurrence, most of the advantage for ovarian ablation occurs during the first few years and seems to be maintained in later years. This early difference in recurrence translates into a later difference in mortality. However, the number of events in later years is too small for such results to be reliable. Nonetheless, for breast cancer mortality, a small difference was seen between treatment and control during the first few years, and a moderate difference at 10 years. The meta-analysis found no indication that the benefits that accrue during the first decade of follow-up are lost during the second decade (33).

All of these women were younger than 50 years of age when randomized and, therefore, there have been relatively few non-breast cancer-related deaths. These deaths do not appear, however, to be increased by treatment during either the first or the second decade (33). If estrogen is protective against cardiovascular disease, then the possibility of an increased risk of myocardial infarction and stroke years after ovarian ablation needs to be evaluated.

A recent meta-analysis of the role of medical ovarian suppression in early stage, hormone receptor-positive breast cancer was reported (106). The analysis included data from 11,906 premenopausal women with early breast cancer randomized in 16 trials. This report found that when used as the sole systemic adjuvant treatment, LHRH agonists did not significantly reduce recurrence or death after recurrence in hormone receptor-positive cancers. However, the number of patients may have been too small to elicit the benefit. When added to other systemic therapy (tamoxifen, chemotherapy, or both), LHRH reduced recurrence in women younger than 40 by 12.7% ($p = .02$), and death after recurrence by 15.1% ($p = .03$). When individual therapies were evaluated, adding LHRH agonists to tamoxifen alone did not result in significant benefit (106).

The numbers of patients included in these ovarian ablation studies is still relatively small, giving rise to high standard errors in some of the subgroups. These data are also underestimates of the true benefit, because they include a large percentage of patients from the early ovarian ablation trials who were ER-unknown. Nevertheless, patients younger than 40 years of age and those between 40 and 49 years of age (mostly premenopausal) benefit significantly from ovarian ablation. A benefit is not evident in patients receiving chemotherapy, probably because many of those patients already achieve ovarian ablation as a "side effect" of the chemotherapy. No major differences were found between LHRH agonists and other forms of ovarian ablation, although this question has not been well studied directly. Data are insufficient, in any trial or meta-analysis, to confirm whether, as with all other adjuvant endocrine therapies, ovarian ablation reduces the incidence of contralateral breast cancer.

The results with ovarian ablation or suppression are comparable to those achieved with chemotherapy or tamoxifen in women younger than 50 years of age. The relatively small number of patients precludes definitive statements about the benefits of ovarian ablation when combined with chemotherapy (chemoendocrine therapy is discussed in more detail in Chapter 50). One could argue that patients not achieving chemotherapy-induced ovarian ablation might benefit from the addition of ovarian ablation. Nor is it established whether ovarian ablation is equivalent to tamoxifen or whether the

Table 48.9	META-ANALYSIS OF THE EFFECTS OF OVARIAN ABLATION (OA), OVARIAN SUPPRESSION (LHRH), ESTROGEN RECEPTOR-POSITIVE OR UNKNOWN—OVERVIEW 2005	
	Reduction (±SE) in Annual Odds	
Group/Age	Recurrence (%)	Breast Cancer Mortality (%)
OA vs. nil		
<40	30 ± 17	29 ± 16
40–49	33 ± 8	32 ± 9
LHRH vs. nil		
<40	21 ± 16	27 ± 21
40–49	23 ± 9	21 ± 13
OA or LHRH vs. nil		
<40	25 ± 12	29 ± 13
40–49	29 ± 6	29 ± 7
OA or LHRH+ chemotherapy vs. chemotherapy		
<40	14 ± 9	4 ± 10
40–49	5 ± 7	−3 ± 8

LHRH, luteinizing hormone-releasing hormone; SE, standard error.
Adapted from Early Breast Cancer Trialists' Collaborative Group. Effects of chemotherapy and hormonal therapy for early breast cancer on recurrence and 15-year survival: an overview of the randomised trials. *Lancet* 2005;365(9472):1687–1717, with permission.

combination of the two modalities offers an advantage. Current trials are studying combining ovarian ablation with tamoxifen or an aromatase inhibitor.

Based on available data, ovarian ablation appears equivalent to chemotherapy alone in premenopausal ER-positive patients (106,107). However, a relatively small trial suggests that it might be better (108). More than 300 node-positive premenopausal patients were randomized to intravenous cyclophosphamide, methotrexate and 5-fluorouracil (CMF) or to ovarian ablation, each with or without prednisolone for 5 years. Prednisolone offered no advantage. At a median follow-up of approximately 14 years, no overall difference was noted between CMF and ovarian ablation. ER status was known for 81% of the patients in this trial, however, and analysis by ER status yielded interesting results. Patients with low ER (<20 fmol/mg protein, or ER negative by IHC) benefited more from chemotherapy, but those with high ER (20 fmol/mg protein or higher, or ER positive by IHC) benefited more from ovarian ablation. These results also suggest that chemotherapy works through a cytotoxic mechanism in addition to the endocrine effects achieved in patients who had chemical castration. Otherwise, the benefits of chemotherapy in the ER-negative subset would be more modest.

Results of several other trials shed additional light on the relative effectiveness of chemotherapy and ovarian ablation (109). Nearly all of these trials, however, used CMF-based chemotherapy, which is inferior to more contemporary regimens. A Swedish trial in patients with stage II, ER-positive disease randomized patients between ovarian ablation and CMF for nine cycles (110). The treatments were found to be equivalent. The Zoladex Early Breast Cancer Research Association (ZEBRA) trial directly compared goserelin monotherapy for 2 years with six cycles of a CMF-based chemotherapy regimen (111). In the ER-positive subgroup, goserelin was equivalent to chemotherapy, whereas in the ER-negative subgroup chemotherapy, as expected, was superior. Results of the German trial (Takeda Adjuvant Breast Cancer Study with Leuprorelin acetate (TABLE), which randomized 600 patients between leuprolide acetate for 2 years versus traditional CMF in ER-positive or unknown patients showed no difference between the treatments. An exploratory analysis of overall survival, however, favored the leuprolide arm (HR, 1.50; p = .005) (112,113).

Several other studies have compared ovarian ablation combined with tamoxifen versus chemotherapy (109). The largest trial, Trial 5 from the Austrian Breast Cancer Group, randomized 1,034 receptor-positive patients to 3 years of goserelin plus 5 years of tamoxifen or to six cycles of CMF (114). At 5 years of follow-up, there was a significant DFS advantage for the endocrine therapy and a trend for improved OS. Two smaller trials, a French trial comparing tamoxifen plus triptorelin for 3 years with an epirubicin-based chemotherapy regimen for six cycles, and an Italian trial comparing standard CMF with ovarian suppression by a variety of techniques combined with tamoxifen showed no difference in DFS and OS between the two groups (49,115). Finally, a trial in Vietnamese patients showed the superiority of oophorectomy combined with tamoxifen versus no treatment in ER-positive patients (116).

Therefore, most trials, most using CMF based chemotherapy, show equivalence between ovarian ablation and chemotherapy in ER-positive, premenopausal women. A suggestion is that the addition of tamoxifen to ovarian ablation may provide superior results. For the moment, ovarian ablation with or without tamoxifen is a reasonable alternative to chemotherapy in receptor-positive patients. The more important question of whether combinations of chemotherapy with endocrine therapy are superior to either one alone in specific subsets of patients is addressed in more detail in Chapter 50.

The database from which to draw definitive conclusions on the value of ovarian ablation is much less substantial than that for adjuvant tamoxifen or chemotherapy. Other current studies are comparing ovarian ablation with or without chemotherapy. More information on the long-term consequences of inducing ovarian failure in young women is also needed. Premature coronary artery disease and osteoporosis might be expected in some patients. Even short-term treatment with goserelin in premenopausal women with endometriosis was associated with bone loss (117). The meta-analysis does not yet show increased vascular deaths in women with breast cancer treated by ovarian ablation, but the database is small (33,39,103). Considering the relatively limited database, it is still difficult to know where ovarian ablation fits in our current armamentarium of adjuvant therapies for premenopausal patients. It might be considered in those who refuse other therapies, as an alternative to chemotherapy in certain patients, as an adjunct to chemotherapy in women not achieving chemical ovarian ablation, or for prevention in patients with a hereditary breast cancer syndrome who have a high risk of developing breast and ovarian cancer. Tamoxifen is the better choice in patients needing endocrine adjuvant therapy. The combination of tamoxifen plus ovarian ablation, and ovarian ablation combined with an aromatase inhibitor are currently being compared with tamoxifen in multiple studies. One of these studies, the ABCSG-12 randomized 1,801 patients according to a 2 × 2 design to the combination of the LHRH agonist goserelin with anastrozole, or to goserelin with tamoxifen, each with or without zoledronic acid every 6 months for 3 years. Preliminary results from this study showed no difference in DFS between the two endocrine therapy combinations (HR = 1.10, 95% CI = 0.79–1.54, p = .59). Interestingly, the study showed that the group that received zoledronic acid had a 35% reduction in the risk of recurrence. This benefit was observed in skeletal, visceral, and local recurrence rates (118) (see Chapter 52 for further review of the role of bisphosphonates in adjuvant therapy). No survival advantage was present for any of the groups yet. Further follow-up on this trial and results of other large trials, such the Suppression of Ovarian Function Trial (SOFT) trial, will provide further insight about the role of aromatase inhibitors with ovarian suppression as adjuvant therapy for premenopausal women.

LONG-TERM EFFECTS OF ADJUVANT ENDOCRINE THERAPY

Although we think of tamoxifen as an antiestrogen because of its antiproliferative properties in the breast, it is more appropriately classified as a SERM because it has estrogen agonist properties in many tissues and on certain genes, whereas it has estrogen antagonist properties on others. These unique dual activities of tamoxifen provide additional potential benefits for women taking the drug, although the agonist activity may cause other side effects and may also be a cause of resistance (22,119,120).

ANCILLARY BENEFITS OF TAMOXIFEN

Serum Lipids and Mortality from Cardiovascular Causes

In contrast to earlier meta-analyses, the 1998 and 2005 meta-analyses do not demonstrate a reduction in the incidence of non–cancer-related deaths (33,34). However, the meta-analyses include data from many different areas of the world, and accurate causes of death are difficult to ascertain in some countries. Individual trials of tamoxifen adjuvant therapy do suggest that the rate of nonbreast cancer-related deaths (deaths before relapse) may be reduced. This mortality reduction is largely because of a decrease in deaths from cardiovascular causes.

Data from the placebo-controlled NSABP tamoxifen prevention trial (Breast Cancer Prevention Trial [BCPT]) provides additional information regarding the cardiovascular effects of tamoxifen (121,122). Cardiovascular events were carefully assessed in this study and each event was adjudicated by a blinded panel. At 4 years of follow-up, this study found no differences between tamoxifen and placebo in fatal myocardial infarction, nonfatal myocardial infarction, unstable angina, or severe angina. Because the effects of tamoxifen on blood lipids and blood vessels are similar to those of estrogen, its favorable effects on serum lipoprotein may be obscured by an unfavorable impact on blood vessels. Nevertheless, the data from the meta-analysis, from individual trials, from the BCPT, and from trials in countries with excellent tumor registry information, strongly suggest that tamoxifen does not increase the risk of myocardial infarction.

Bone Mineral Density

Tamoxifen also has estrogen agonist properties in bone. In postmenopausal women, long-term tamoxifen treatment increases the bone density of the axial skeleton and stabilizes the bone density of the peripheral skeleton (29,123). In premenopausal women, however, tamoxifen may decrease bone mineral density by antagonizing the more potent activity of endogenous estrogen (124). Although evaluating osteoporotic fracture rates in patients with a diagnosis of breast cancer is problematic, prevention trials of tamoxifen do show a significant reduction in fractures with 5 years of treatment (121,125).

Contralateral Breast Cancer

Individual clinical trials in patients with invasive breast cancer, as well as the updated meta-analysis, indicate a nearly 50% reduction in the risk of contralateral breast cancer after approximately 5 years of tamoxifen treatment (33,126,127).

Some physicians have used tamoxifen adjuvant therapy in the past even if the primary breast tumor is ER-negative in the hope of reducing the incidence of contralateral breast cancer and maintaining bone density. Data from two prospective randomized trials assessing the value of tamoxifen in ER-negative patients and from the 2005 meta-analysis, however, do not support this strategy (33,50,128). These studies show impressive reductions in contralateral breast cancer with 5 years of tamoxifen in patients whose original primary tumors were ER-positive, but they show no reduction in contralateral breast cancer in patients whose original tumors were ER-negative. This intriguing result is difficult to explain because contralateral breast cancer is generally thought to be a second event independent of the first tumor, and it will require clarification by future studies.

TOXICITY OF TAMOXIFEN

In general, tamoxifen is well tolerated by most patients with breast cancer. In early trials of adjuvant therapy fewer than 5% of patients discontinued therapy early because of toxicity (129,130). In one of the largest randomized, placebo-controlled trials, 7% of tamoxifen-treated patients and 5% of placebo-treated patients withdrew from the study early for reasons that were possibly related to toxicity (40,44).

Menopausal Symptoms

The most frequently reported side effects in patients taking tamoxifen are menopausal symptoms (40,44,131). At least 50% to 60% of these women report some hot flashes, but 40% to 50% of placebo-treated patients report similar episodes. Tamoxifen may cause hot flashes more commonly in premenopausal women than in older women. Many postmenopausal patients have hot flashes before starting tamoxifen because of natural causes or because of the withdrawal of estrogen replacement therapy when breast cancer is diagnosed. Approximately 20% of patients report severe hot flashes while taking tamoxifen compared with 3% of patients on placebo. Vaginal discharge and irregular menses are also slightly more common in patients taking tamoxifen than in those receiving placebo. In one study, however, general quality of life scores were similar for tamoxifen and placebo (131). Headaches were reported less frequently with tamoxifen. The incidence of nausea, arthralgias, insomnia, restlessness, depression, and fatigue was similar with tamoxifen and placebo in this study.

Depression has not been reported to be increased in randomized, placebo-controlled trials, but this may reflect under reporting of symptoms that may be brought out by more careful and detailed questioning. A nonrandomized, single-institution study suggests that symptoms of depression can be identified in up to 10% of patients taking tamoxifen (132). Symptoms are occasionally severe and may require dose reduction, antidepressant medication, or even discontinuation of the drug. Failure to identify depression as a side effect in placebo-controlled trials suggests, however, that discontinuation of estrogen replacement therapy may be causally more important than tamoxifen itself.

The detailed analysis of depression in women on the BCPT adds additional insight on this topic (133), although the women in this trial may not accurately represent breast cancer patients who are diagnosed with a life-threatening disease and have more reason for depression. Nevertheless, no difference was seen in depression by treatment assignment (tamoxifen vs. placebo) in this study, suggesting that tamoxifen itself does not increase the risk of, or exacerbate, existing depression in women.

Although the diagnosis of depression may not be more common in women taking tamoxifen compared with other forms of treatment, depression is still a common and often overlooked condition in breast cancer patients, and the symptoms may be attributed to other causes. Women suffering from menopausal symptoms, whether related to tamoxifen or withdrawal of estrogen replacement therapy, may have depression together with hot flashes, loss of sleep, and gynecologic problems. Tamoxifen-induced hot flashes tend to be more severe in women who had hot flashes when they went through menopause and in women who were on estrogen replacement therapy at the time of diagnosis of breast cancer (134). Numerous remedies have been acclaimed for their ability to relieve menopausal symptoms in breast cancer survivors. Randomized, placebo-controlled trials of black cohosh and soy phytoestrogens showed no benefit for these popular remedies (135,136), although black cohosh was effective in another study in women without breast cancer (137). A similar trial of clonidine suggested that this drug is effective in some postmenopausal women (138). Megestrol acetate is effective in relieving hot flashes, but the effect of progestins on breast cancer recurrence is unknown (139). Selective serotonin reuptake inhibitors (SSRI) (e.g., paroxetine hydrochloride and venlafaxine) at relatively low doses may be the most useful agents in the treatment of vasomotor symptoms (140,141). These antidepressants have the added advantage of reducing symptoms of anxiety and depression that often accompany menopausal symptoms, although higher doses than those used initially for just hot flashes may be required.

Caution must be exercised when prescribing antidepressants to women on tamoxifen. These agents inhibit the cytochrome P450 CYP2D6 isoenzyme responsible for the metabolism of many drugs, including the conversion of tamoxifen to endoxifen, one of its important active metabolites, thus reducing the benefit from tamoxifen (142–144). Although this seems to be a class effect, different agents have variable inhibitory potency. Sertraline is a less potent inhibitor of this enzyme than paroxetine or fluoxetine (143) and venlafaxine may not interfere at all (143). Therefore, venlafaxine may be a better choice in women on tamoxifen therapy. Some women have a variant of CYP2D6 that results in less metabolism to endoxifen. Whether this genotype reduces the clinical benefit of adjuvant tamoxifen therapy is still somewhat controversial (144–148). This issue is discussed in greater detail in Chapter 55. Gabapentin may also be used in reducing hot flashes in some women (149).

Sexual Dysfunction

Sexual dysfunction is also common in breast cancer survivors, whether they are on endocrine therapy or not. Vaginal dryness, dyspareunia, and decreased sexual desire are common complaints. In addition to moisturizers, vaginal estrogen cream is often very helpful in women on tamoxifen in whom the systemic absorption of estrogen in these preparations is not of concern. This problem is more difficult to treat in women taking aromatase inhibitors. Even small amounts of estrogen absorbed systemically could bind ER and, then theoretically, counteract the beneficial effects of the treatment on breast cancer recurrence. Other vaginal estrogen preparations have less systemic absorption and may be helpful in selected patients (150–152). Clearly, more research is needed to evaluate the safety and efficacy of these or other strategies in patients receiving estrogen deprivation therapy. Until then, estrogens, whether plant-derived, natural, or synthetic, should be used sparingly or for short durations, if at all, in such patients. Management of menopausal and gynecologic problems in breast cancer patients is also discussed in Chapters 53 and 95.

Ocular Toxicity

Ocular toxicity has been reported with high tamoxifen doses (153). An uncontrolled study concluded that ocular toxicity in the form of retinopathy or keratopathy was a side effect of conventional doses of tamoxifen, a result not confirmed in a controlled study in which complete ophthalmologic examinations were performed in a blinded fashion (154,155). Other reports of ocular toxicity have been inconsistent (156–158). In the NSABP BCPT tamoxifen prevention trial, women with preexisting cataracts who were taking tamoxifen had a slightly increased risk of posterior subcapsular opacities and need for cataract surgery, but no vision-threatening ocular toxicity was found (121). Occasional ophthalmologic examination should be sufficient monitoring for patients with breast cancer who are receiving long-term tamoxifen or other endocrine therapies (159).

Thromboembolic and Hematologic Toxicities

An increased incidence of thromboembolic events has also been reported from studies of tamoxifen adjuvant therapy in patients with breast cancer as well as from tamoxifen prevention studies in high-risk women (37,40,121,160–163). This complication occurs more frequently when tamoxifen is combined with chemotherapy, although initiating tamoxifen after chemotherapy may decrease this problem. Most patients reported with this complication have superficial phlebitis and do not require hospitalization. Severe thromboembolic phenomena occur in less than 1% of patients given the drug. Deaths caused by thromboembolism have been reported, however, in patients with cancer and in healthy women in the prevention trials. The thromboembolic risk is especially high in women on tamoxifen having surgery for an unrelated prob-

lem (125). The risk of thromboembolism may vary with different SERM. In the Study of Tamoxifen and Raloxifene (STAR) (NSABP-P2) Prevention Trial, these events occurred less often with raloxifene than tamoxifen (relative risk [RR] = 0.70) (163). Raloxifene, however, is indicated only for breast cancer prevention and not treatment. Withdrawal of the drug and anticoagulation should be considered in such patients. Thrombocytopenia and leucopenia have also been reported with tamoxifen, but are unusual and rarely require cessation of therapy.

Endometrial and Other Cancers

Tamoxifen use, much as with estrogen therapy, is clearly related to an increased incidence of endometrial cancer (33,164–166). Even just 1 year of adjuvant tamoxifen is associated with a slightly increased incidence, but the risk rises with more prolonged treatment. Interpretation of these results is a problem, because many women taking tamoxifen were treated with estrogen replacement therapy before the diagnosis of breast cancer. Nevertheless, an 8-year follow-up of NSABP B-14, in which 2,843 patients were randomly assigned to receive at least 5 years of tamoxifen or placebo, indicates that tamoxifen was associated with an annual hazard rate of 1.7 per 1,000, a relative risk of 2.2 compared with population-based rates of endometrial cancer from Surveillance Epidemiology and End Results (SEER) program data (167). The type of endometrial cancer in patients taking tamoxifen is similar to that in patients not exposed to tamoxifen. Of the 23 cancers in NSABP B14, 18 were of low histologic grade, and most were stage I. Four patients died of uterine cancer, however, indicating the lethal potential of this complication and the need for early identification of symptoms, especially vaginal bleeding. The risk of endometrial cancer in tamoxifen users is related to the duration of therapy and is higher in obese women and women who have received prior hormone replacement therapy (168).

The role of endometrial cancer screening by vaginal ultrasound or endometrial biopsy and the role of progestins in reducing the risk of endometrial cancer have been reported (169–171). Routine transvaginal ultrasound did more harm than good in one study because of its false–positive rates, the requirement for additional tests, and increased iatrogenic morbidity. Neither transvaginal ultrasound nor regular screening endometrial biopsies at 6-month intervals were effective in diagnosing endometrial cancer. These procedures are not justified in asymptomatic patients, but should be considered in women presenting with abnormal bleeding. It is not yet clear whether systemic or intrauterine progestins are beneficial in this setting (172).

An increased incidence of endometrial cancer has also been observed in the BCPT prevention trial in women without breast cancer, but all of the cases reported have a very favorable histology (121). Increased endometrial thickness and the incidence of hyperplasia, polyps, and ovarian cysts can be increased by tamoxifen (120,173,174). In the STAR Prevention Trial, there were 36 cases of uterine cancers on tamoxifen and 23 on raloxifene (RR = 0.62) (163).

Tamoxifen is also a potent hepatocarcinogen in the rat, but not in the mouse (175,176). Although abnormal liver function tests, fatty liver, and massive liver steatohepatitis, rarely with cirrhosis, have been reported in patients receiving tamoxifen, only a few anecdotal cases of hepatoma have been reported thus far, and the incidence of hepatoma since the introduction of tamoxifen has not increased (177–180).

Data from the NSABP, the large Swedish randomized trials, and the meta-analysis indicate that tamoxifen adjuvant therapy has not yet resulted in an increased incidence of other solid tumors (33,120,127,167,177,181). Although these adverse effects of tamoxifen do not detract from the proven substantial survival benefits in patients with invasive breast cancer, they do raise caution for the use of tamoxifen in benign conditions or for breast cancer prevention. Raloxifene may be a better choice for breast cancer prevention in postmenopausal women (163).

 TOXICITY OF OVARIAN ABLATION

The side effects of ovarian ablation are caused by lowering the level of estrogen. Menopausal symptoms and gynecologic complaints are common and are similar to those observed with tamoxifen. An increase in the rate of cardiovascular disease has not been reported in the long-term follow-up of ovarian ablation trials, although the database is small (33). Bone loss and premature osteoporosis are likely to be significant in such patients who, therefore, demand close monitoring and the early institution of bisphosphonates when bone loss occurs. Zoledronic acid, administered every 6 months, has been shown to prevent treatment-related bone loss in premenopausal women receiving adjuvant endocrine therapy (182). Interestingly, a recent report also suggests that zoledronic acid reduces the risk for recurrence and distant metastasis (118). The use of bisphosphonates as adjuvant therapy is reviewed in Chapter 52.

 LONG-TERM EFFECTS AND TOXICITY OF AROMATASE INHIBITORS

By inhibiting the activity of the enzyme aromatase, aromatase inhibitors markedly suppress plasma estrogen levels in postmenopausal women. In contrast to tamoxifen, these compounds do not bind ER and therefore lack partial agonist activity and are not associated with the adverse effects of tamoxifen on the endometrium and blood vessel. However, they also lack the desirable effects of tamoxifen on bone and serum lipids. Several of the large trials that compared AI with tamoxifen (upfront or sequential strategy) reported on the quality of life and toxicity profile for these agents (80,81,99,183–186). They provide insight that needs to be considered in the decision to use aromatase inhibitors.

In general, and compared with tamoxifen, AI have a lower incidence of ischemic cerebrovascular events, venous thromboembolic events, hot flashes, and vaginal bleeding. However, lipid disorders, bone fractures, and musculoskeletal pain are more frequent with aromatase inhibitors. No significant difference was seen in the incidence of ischemic cardiovascular events (Tables 48.10 and 48.11).

Contralateral Breast Cancer and Second Primary Cancer

With 100-month follow up, the ATAC trial provides the most mature comparison between the side effects of an aromatase inhibitor and those of tamoxifen (79). It reported a 40% proportional risk reduction of contralateral breast cancers. Because tamoxifen reduces the risk of contralateral breast cancer by about 50%, anastrozole might prevent more than 70% of ER-positive contralateral breast tumors compared with no adjuvant treatment. Additionally, anastrozole had a significantly lower incidence of endometrial carcinoma. No significant difference was noted in the occurrence of any other cancer.

Musculoskeletal Symptoms and Effects on Bone

Musculoskeletal symptoms are significantly higher in patients on aromatase inhibitors compared with tamoxifen or no adjuvant therapy. Joint complaints have been reported to range from 20% to 50% in various trials of AI, depending on the definition of this side effect (79,81,85,99) (Tables 48.10 and 48.11). In the authors' experience, the incidence of arthralgias, joint stiffness, and musculoskeletal disorders in patients on AI may be more frequent than reported by some of the AI trials. When patients are questioned carefully, many of them complain of joint stiffness and pain that they attribute to "getting older" and not to the drug.

In contrast to tamoxifen, which has protective effects on bone density of postmenopausal women by virtue of its agonist activity, all aromatase inhibitors are associated with bone loss by lowering endogenous estrogen levels (79,81,85,99,187). In a report of 167 women who received serial bone mineral density (BMD) measurements on the ATAC trial, significant bone loss occurred at the lumbar spine and hip in the anastrozole group (median BMD decrease of 6.1% and 7.2%, respectively) compared with the tamoxifen group (median BMD increase of 2.8% and 0.7%, respectively) (188). Fracture rates were significantly higher in the anastrozole compared with the tamoxifen group (22.6 vs. 15.6/1,000 woman-years). Likewise, in the BIG 1-98 trial, fractures were more frequent with letrozole (5.7% vs. 4%) (189). In the MA.17 trial that compared letrozole with

Table 48.10   SIDE EFFECTS OF TAMOXIFEN AND ANASTROZOLE IN THE ATAC TRIAL

Side Effect	Anastrozole (%) (n = 3,092)	Tamoxifen (%) (n = 3,094)	p-value
Hot flashes	35.7	40.9	<.0001
Musculoskeletal	35.6	29.4	<.0001
Vaginal bleeding	5.4	10.2	<.0001
Vaginal discharge	3.5	13.2	<.0001
Endometrial cancer	0.2	0.8	.02
Fractures	11.0	7.7	<.0001
Ischemic heart disease	4.1	3.4	NS
Cerebrovascular events	2.0	2.8	.03
Venous thromboembolic event	2.8	4.5	.0004

NS, not significant.
Adapted from Forbes JF, Cuzick J, Buzdar A, et al. Effect of anastrozole and tamoxifen as adjuvant treatment for early-stage breast cancer: 100-month analysis of the ATAC trial. *Lancet Oncol* 2008;9(1):45–53; and Baum M, Buzdar A, Cuzick J, et al. Anastrozole alone or in combination with tamoxifen versus tamoxifen alone for adjuvant treatment of postmenopausal women with early breast cancer: first results of the ATAC randomised trial. *Lancet* 2002;359(9324):2131–2139, with permission.

Table 48.11	SIDE EFFECTS OF TAMOXIFEN AND LETROZOLE IN THE BIG 1-98 TRIAL

Side Effect	Letrozole (%) (n = 3,975)	Tamoxifen (%) (n = 3,988)	p-value
Hot flashes	33.5	38.0	<.001
Musculoskeletal	20.3	12.3	<.001
Vaginal bleeding	3.3	6.6	<.001
Fractures	5.7	4.0	<.001
Hyperlipidemia	43.6	19.2	N/A[a]
Cardiac disease	4.1	3.8	NS
Cerebrovascular events	1.0	1.0	NS
Venous thromboembolic event	1.5	3.5	<.001

BIG 1-98, Breast International Group1-98; NS, not significant.
[a]p-value not reported.
Adapted from Coates AS, Keshaviah A, Thürlimann B, et al. Five years of letrozole compared with tamoxifen as initial adjuvant therapy for postmenopausal women with endocrine-responsive early breast cancer: update of study BIG 1-98. *J Clin Oncol* 2007;25(5):486–492, with permission.

placebo after 5 years of tamoxifen, more modest reductions in BMD were observed (hip = −3.6%, lumbar spine = −5.35%) (187). In the IES trial, loss of bone mineral density also was observed during the 2 to 3 years of treatment with exemestane after initial tamoxifen therapy. However, no patient with a normal BMD at the start of therapy developed osteoporosis during treatment (190). Women receiving an AI should be assessed for other risk factors for osteoporosis, and bone density should be measured at baseline, and periodically during therapy.

Serum Lipids

All major aromatase inhibitor trials reported a higher incidence of hyperlipidemia in patients receiving AI. The BIG 1-98 trial showed a significantly higher incidence of hyperlipidemia in the letrozole arm compared with tamoxifen, although most cases were grade 1 (Table 48.11) (189). The ATAC trial reported a 6% incidence of hyperlipidemia in the anastrozole arm compared with 2.2% in the tamoxifen arm (p <.001) (79), and the ITA trial showed an 8% incidence of lipid disorders compared with 1.4% with tamoxifen (p = .01) at a median follow-up of 64 months.

This higher incidence can be attributed to a cholesterol-raising effect of aromatase inhibitors or to the cholesterol-lowering effects of tamoxifen. To that effect, the MA.17L substudy reported the effects of letrozole on lipid profile and showed no overall significant change from placebo (186).

However, treating physicians are generally aggressive in treating hyperlipidemia and the widespread use of lipid-lowering agents, such as statins, may mask the effects of AI on serum lipids. Women on AI should be followed with serial serum lipid measurements and appropriate therapy should be initiated when necessary.

Cardiac and Cerebrovascular Events

Compared with tamoxifen, aromatase inhibitors were associated with a lower risk of venous thromboembolic and ischemic cerebrovascular events in all AI trials. In some trials, however, AI were associated with an increase in the risk of ischemic cardiac disease, although the added risk appears to be small (79,84,99,191).

A recent meta-analysis addressed these issues in seven trials that compared tamoxifen with an aromatase inhibitor, either as initial therapy or in a sequential strategy (192). The absolute increase in the risk of a grade 3 and 4 cardiovascular adverse event (as defined by the NCIC common toxicity criteria, version 2) with an AI compared with tamoxifen alone was small, but statistically significant (RR = 1.31). It was estimated that between 160 and 180 patients would need to be treated (number needed to harm) to produce one event. On the other hand, thromboembolic events were significantly more frequent with tamoxifen (RR 0.53); with an absolute difference of 1.17% relative to aromatase inhibitor treatment, and the number needed to harm was 85 patients.

Table 48.12	TREATMENT GUIDELINES FOR ADJUVANT ENDOCRINE THERAPY

	NCCN	International Consensus
Premenopausal Women	Tamoxifen (Tam) for 5 yr ± ovarian suppression	Tamoxifen for 5 yr ± ovarian suppression OA alone in selected patients
Postmenopausal Women[a]	Upfront AI or Tam → AI If Tam for 5 yr → AI	Tam → AI for low risk patients Upfront AI if ERBB2+ or node positive. If Tam for 5 yr → AI

AI, aromatase inhibitor; NCCN, National Cancer Comprehensive Network.
[a]ASCO Technology Assessment in 2004 recommended incorporating AI in adjuvant endocrine therapy of postmenopausal women with breast cancer.

COGNITIVE FUNCTION IN PATIENTS ON ADJUVANT ENDOCRINE THERAPY

Estrogen regulates emotional responses and cortical activity during cognitive task performance in humans (193) and may have a protective effect on verbal memory (194). Despite widespread use of endocrine therapy for the treatment of breast cancer, few studies have examined the possible cognitive effects. In postmenopausal women, epidemiologic studies suggest that estrogen may have a beneficial effect on cognitive function or reduce the risk of age-related decline in cognitive function over time (195). These data raise the question of the effects of SERM or estrogen deprivation therapy, such as anastrozole or ovarian ablation, on cognitive function. Changes in cognitive function, which may be transient, are relatively common in women receiving adjuvant chemotherapy, but they are less well documented with endocrine therapies. Cognitive function was measured in the multiple outcomes of raloxifene evaluation trial in women with osteoporosis (196). Overall, no difference was found between placebo and raloxifene in several different tests of cognitive function, suggesting that it does not have an adverse effect worse than postmenopausal estrogen levels. A trend was found toward less decline with raloxifene on tests of verbal memory and attention. A clear beneficial effect to preserve cognitive function was not found. Whether tamoxifen would have a similar effect is not clear, although in a randomized study using magnetic resonance spectroscopy, both estrogen and tamoxifen had a favorable profile (197). Tamoxifen did not worsen the negative impact of chemotherapy (195). In other studies tamoxifen alone has been reported to improve or to worsen cognitive function, indicating the need for additional study (195).

Cognitive assessments that measured a range of memory and attention functions were reported on 94 patients from the ATAC trial and 35 noncancer controls (198). The patient group did not differ from controls on measures of working memory, attention, and visual memory, but was significantly impaired compared with the control group on measures of verbal memory ($p = .026$) and processing speed ($p = .032$). Cognitive performance in the patient group was not significantly related to length of time on trial or measures of psychological morbidity (198). Results from this small study suggest that anastrozole, as with tamoxifen, may cause a specific deficit in verbal memory. Aromatase is expressed in the brain, although its importance in cognitive function is not known (199). Larger studies with longer follow-up are needed to assess the long-term consequences of treatment with aromatase inhibitors. This topic is discussed at greater detail in Chapter 54.

FUTURE DIRECTIONS

Since its introduction 35 years ago, significant progress has been made in the field of systemic adjuvant therapy for breast cancer. The mortality reductions observed (25%) in most Western countries over the past 20 years have been attributed largely to the wide-spread use of adjuvant therapy, especially tamoxifen, and to a lesser extent chemotherapy (200). Patients are living longer and many can be considered cured by these treatments. Thus, the hypothesis that many breast cancer patients already have subclinical distant metastases at the time of diagnosis, and that these microscopic foci can be more effectively treated than gross metastatic disease, has been confirmed. Although earlier diagnosis in the future will no doubt identify more patients who do not yet have micrometastases, invasion and dissemination of tumor cells can occur very early in the disease process in some patients who will need effective systemic therapy. In the not too distant future we may be able to identify more accurately those patients harboring micrometastases and to select the most appropriate therapy based on the molecular profile of the tumor, just as we do today with ER, PR, and ERBB2.

In the meantime several questions regarding adjuvant endocrine therapy remain to be answered, and many of these are now being addressed in ongoing clinical trials.

- Does prolonging tamoxifen adjuvant therapy beyond 5 years benefit any subgroups of women with breast cancer?
- What is the optimal role of aromatase inhibitors in adjuvant therapy? Should they be used instead of or in sequence with tamoxifen? Are there groups of patients identified on the basis of predictive markers who are best treated with tamoxifen or best treated with aromatase inhibitors?
- Is ovarian ablation combined with tamoxifen or with an aromatase inhibitor, better than tamoxifen alone in premenopausal patients?
- What is the optimal duration of aromatase inhibition, and what are the possible long-term sequelae of treatment?
- Will low-dose aspirin or warfarin prevent the thromboembolic complications of SERM and chemotherapy?
- Are local slow release vaginal estrogen preparations safe to use with aromatase inhibitors?
- Do combinations of endocrine therapy and inhibitors of growth factor pathways improve outcome as they do in preclinical models?
- Do targeted therapies that inhibit growth factor receptors, insulin-like growth factor-1R, angiogenesis, mammalian target of rapamycin (mTOR), mitogen activated protein kinase pathway, or phosphoinositide-3 kinase (PI3K)/Akt pathway have a role in the adjuvant treatment of breast cancer?

MANAGEMENT SUMMARY

- Adjuvant endocrine therapy is the most effective systemic treatment modality for hormone receptor-positive breast cancer; it reduces the risk of recurrence by 50% or more across different tumor characteristics and clinical stages (Table 48.12).
- Optimal duration is not yet established. However, all patients should receive at least 5 years of therapy.

Premenopausal Women

- All premenopausal women should be encouraged to enroll in clinical trials of adjuvant hormone therapy.
- For women who do not have access to clinical trials, are not eligible, or choose not to participate, 5 years of tamoxifen is still the most appropriate treatment.
- Ovarian suppression or ablation (medical or surgical) may be appropriate in selected patients who have a contraindication or do not tolerate tamoxifen. Optimal duration of ovarian suppression (if done medically) is not established, but treating for 3 to 5 years is reasonable.
- Combining tamoxifen and ovarian suppression may be utilized in patients at high risk of recurrence. The International Consensus Panel guidelines suggest giving this combination to patients younger than 35 years or to patients with high risk disease (201).
- Aromatase inhibitors are indicated only for postmenopausal patients and should be avoided in women whose menopausal status is not established (83). Data on the use of aromatase inhibitors with ovarian suppression is promising but warrants validation and further follow-up before incorporating into clinical practice.

Postmenopausal Women

- Aromatase inhibitors offer a small advantage over tamoxifen and should be at least a part of the adjuvant endocrine therapy of most postmenopausal women with ER-positive breast cancer.

- Until more data are available from BIG 1-98 and other ongoing trials, upfront treatment with an aromatase inhibitor or sequencing with tamoxifen for 2 to 3 years followed by an aromatase inhibitor for 3 to 5 years are both considered acceptable options.

- The decision whether to use upfront aromatase inhibitor therapy or sequential therapy with tamoxifen followed by an aromatase inhibitor should take into consideration many factors, including patient age, years after menopause, risk of recurrence, bone health, history of thromboembolism, cardiac or cerebrovascular disease, menopausal symptoms, and sexual activity of the patient.

- Patients whose menopausal status is in question and those who develop amenorrhea after chemotherapy are best started on tamoxifen and hormone profiles followed. If they remain clinically amenorrheic and with postmenopausal hormone profiles for 2 years, they can be switched to an aromatase inhibitors.

- Postmenopausal women (or those who become postmenopausal) completing 5 years of tamoxifen should be considered for extended adjuvant therapy with an aromatase inhibitor. This group of patients may not be large because most postmenopausal women now receive aromatase inhibitors after 2 to 3 years of tamoxifen at the most.

- Patients on aromatase inhibitors should have serial monitoring of bone mineral density and serum lipids.

References

1. Lewis D, Rienhoff WF. Results of operations at the Johns Hopkins Hospital for Cancer of the Breast: performed at the Johns Hopkins Hospital from 1889 to 1931. *Ann Surg* 1932;95(3):336–400.
2. Fisher B, Gebhardt MC. The evolution of breast cancer surgery: past, present, and future. *Semin Oncol* 1978;5(4):385-394.
3. Skipper HE. Kinetics of mammary tumor cell growth and implications for therapy. *Cancer* 1971;28(6):1479–1499.
4. Fisher B et al. Surgical adjuvant chemotherapy in cancer of the breast: results of a decade of cooperative investigation. *Ann Surg* 1968;168(3):337–356.
5. Cole MP. A clinical trial of an artificial menopause in carcinoma of the breast. *Inserm* 1975;55:143.
6. Osborne CK et al. Estrogen receptor: current understanding of its activation and modulation. *Clin Cancer Res* 2001;7(12 Suppl):4338s–4342s; discussion 4411s–4412s.
7. Osborne CK, Schiff R. Estrogen-receptor biology: continuing progress and therapeutic implications. *J Clin Oncol* 2005;23(8):1616–1622.
8. Schiff R et al. Advanced concepts in estrogen receptor biology and breast cancer endocrine resistance: implicated role of growth factor signaling and estrogen receptor coregulators. *Cancer Chemother Pharmacol* 2005;56 Suppl 1:10–20.
9. Palmieri C et al. Estrogen receptor beta in breast cancer. *Endocr Relat Cancer* 2002;9(1):1–13.
10. Kumar R, Thompson EB. The structure of the nuclear hormone receptors. *Steroids* 1999;64(5):310–319.
11. Vinayagam R et al. Association of oestrogen receptor beta 2 (ER beta 2/ER beta cx) with outcome of adjuvant endocrine treatment for primary breast cancer—a retrospective study. *BMC Cancer* 2007;7:131.
12. Fuqua SA et al. Expression of wild-type estrogen receptor beta and variant isoforms in human breast cancer. *Cancer Res* 1999;59(21):5425–5428.
13. Fuqua SA et al. Estrogen receptor beta protein in human breast cancer: correlation with clinical tumor parameters. *Cancer Res* 2003;63(10):2434–2439.
14. Nemere I, Pietras RJ, Blackmore PF. Membrane receptors for steroid hormones: signal transduction and physiological significance. *J Cell Biochem* 2003;88(3):438–445.
15. Massarweh S et al. Tamoxifen resistance in breast tumors is driven by growth factor receptor signaling with repression of classic estrogen receptor genomic function. *Cancer Res* 2008;68(3):826–833.
16. Song RX et al. The role of Shc and insulin-like growth factor 1 receptor in mediating the translocation of estrogen receptor alpha to the plasma membrane. *Proc Natl Acad Sci U S A* 2004;101(7):2076–2081.
17. Marquez DC, Pietras RJ. Membrane-associated binding sites for estrogen contribute to growth regulation of human breast cancer cells. *Oncogene* 2001;20(39):5420–5430.
18. Pietras RJ et al. HER-2 tyrosine kinase pathway targets estrogen receptor and promotes hormone-independent growth in human breast cancer cells. *Oncogene* 1995;10(12):2435–2446.
19. McInerney EM, Katzenellenbogen BS. Different regions in activation function-1 of the human estrogen receptor required for antiestrogen- and estradiol-dependent transcription activation. *J Biol Chem* 1996;271(39):24172–24178.
20. Osborne CK et al. Role of the estrogen receptor coactivator AIB1 (SRC-3) and HER-2/neu in tamoxifen resistance in breast cancer. *J Natl Cancer Inst* 2003;95(5):353–361.
21. Schiff R et al. Breast cancer endocrine resistance: how growth factor signaling and estrogen receptor coregulators modulate response. *Clin Cancer Res* 2003;9(1 Pt 2):447S–454S.
22. Shou J et al. Mechanisms of tamoxifen resistance: increased estrogen receptor-HER2/neu cross-talk in ER/HER2-positive breast cancer. *J Natl Cancer Inst* 2004;96(12):926–935.
23. Osborne CK et al. Double-blind, randomized trial comparing the efficacy and tolerability of fulvestrant versus anastrozole in postmenopausal women with advanced breast cancer progressing on prior endocrine therapy: results of a North American trial. *J Clin Oncol* 2002;20(16):3386–3395.
24. Osborne CK. Aromatase inhibitors in relation to other forms of endocrine therapy for breast cancer. *Endocr Relat Cancer* 1999;6(2):271–276.
25. Morris C, Wakeling A. Fulvestrant ('Faslodex')—a new treatment option for patients progressing on prior endocrine therapy. *Endocr Relat Cancer* 2002;9(4):267–276.
26. Massarweh S et al. Mechanisms of tumor regression and resistance to estrogen deprivation and fulvestrant in a model of estrogen receptor-positive, HER-2/neu-positive breast cancer. *Cancer Res* 2006;66(16):8266–8273.
27. Song RX et al. Effect of long-term estrogen deprivation on apoptotic responses of breast cancer cells to 17beta-estradiol. *J Natl Cancer Inst* 2001;93(22):1714–1723.
28. Holli K et al. Safety and Efficacy Results of a Randomized Trial Comparing Adjuvant Toremifene and Tamoxifen in Postmenopausal Patients With Node-Positive Breast Cancer. *J Clin Oncol* 2000;18(20):3487–3494.
29. Love RR et al. Effects of tamoxifen on bone mineral density in postmenopausal women with breast cancer. *N Engl J Med* 1992;326(13):852–856.
30. Love RR et al. Effects of tamoxifen therapy on lipid and lipoprotein levels in postmenopausal patients with node-negative breast cancer. *J Natl Cancer Inst* 1990;82(16):1327–1332.
31. Osborne CK. Steroid hormone receptors in breast cancer management. *Breast Cancer Res Treat* 1998;51(3):227–238.
32. Ellis PA et al. Induction of apoptosis by tamoxifen and ICI 182780 in primary breast cancer. *Int J Cancer* 1997;72(4):608–613.
33. Early Breast Cancer Trialists' Collaborative Group, Effects of chemotherapy and hormonal therapy for early breast cancer on recurrence and 15-year survival. an overview of the randomised trials. *Lancet* 2005;365(9472):1687–1717.
34. Early Breast Cancer Trialists' Collaborative Group, Tamoxifen for early breast cancer: an overview of the randomised trials. *Lancet* 1998;351(9114):1451–1467.
35. Early Breast Cancer Trialists' Collaborative Group, Effects of adjuvant tamoxifen and of cytotoxic therapy on mortality in early breast cancer. An overview of 61 randomized trials among 28,896 women. *N Engl J Med* 1988;319(26):1681–1692.
36. Fisher B et al. Treatment of lymph-node-negative, oestrogen-receptor-positive breast cancer: long-term findings from National Surgical Adjuvant Breast and Bowel Project randomised clinical trials. *Lancet* 2004;364(9437):858–868.
37. NATO, Controlled trial of tamoxifen as a single adjuvant agent in the management of early breast cancer. 'Nolvadex' Adjuvant Trial Organisation. *Br J Cancer* 1988;57(6):608–611.
38. Breast Cancer Trials Committee, Adjuvant tamoxifen in the management of operable breast cancer: the Scottish Trial. Report from the Breast Cancer Trials Committee, Scottish Cancer Trials Office (MRC), Edinburgh. *Lancet* 1987;2(8552):171–175.
39. Early Breast Cancer Trialists' Collaborative Group, Systemic treatment of early breast cancer by hormonal, cytotoxic, or immune therapy. 133 randomised trials involving 31,000 recurrences and 24,000 deaths among 75,000 women. *Lancet* 1992;339(8785):71–85.
40. Fisher B et al. A randomized clinical trial evaluating tamoxifen in the treatment of patients with node-negative breast cancer who have estrogen-receptor-positive tumors. *N Engl J Med* 1989;320(8):479–484.
41. Kaufmann M et al. Adjuvant randomized trials of doxorubicin/cyclophosphamide versus doxorubicin/cyclophosphamide/tamoxifen and CMF chemotherapy versus tamoxifen in women with node-positive breast cancer. *J Clin Oncol* 1993;11(3):454–460.
42. Fisher B et al. Tamoxifen and chemotherapy for lymph node-negative, estrogen receptor-positive breast cancer. *J Natl Cancer Inst* 1997;89(22):1673–1682.
43. BCTC, Adjuvant tamoxifen in the management of operable breast cancer: the Scottish Trial. Report from the Breast Cancer Trials Committee, Scottish Cancer Trials Office (MRC), Edinburgh. *Lancet* 1987;2(8552):171–175.
44. Fisher B et al. Five versus more than five years of tamoxifen therapy for breast cancer patients with negative lymph nodes and estrogen receptor-positive tumors. *J Natl Cancer Inst* 1996;88(21):1529–1542.
45. Fisher B et al. Findings from recent National Surgical Adjuvant Breast and Bowel Project adjuvant studies in stage I breast cancer. *J Natl Cancer Inst Monogr* 2001(30):62–66.
46. Osborne CK, Hobbs K, Clark GM. Effect of estrogens and antiestrogens on growth of human breast cancer cells in athymic nude mice. *Cancer Res* 1985;45(2):584–590.
47. Lahti EI, Knip M, Laatikainen TJ. Plasma insulin-like growth factor I and its binding proteins 1 and 3 in postmenopausal patients with breast cancer receiving long term tamoxifen. *Cancer* 1994;74(2):618–624.
48. Pollak M et al. Effect of tamoxifen on serum insulinlike growth factor I levels in stage I breast cancer patients. *J Natl Cancer Inst* 1990;82(21):1693–1697.
49. Roche H et al. Complete hormonal blockade versus epirubicin-based chemotherapy in premenopausal, one to three node-positive, and hormone-receptor positive, early breast cancer patients: 7-year follow-up results of French Adjuvant Study Group 06 randomised trial. *Ann Oncol* 2006;17(8):1221–1227.
50. Fisher B et al. Tamoxifen and chemotherapy for axillary node-negative, estrogen receptor-negative breast cancer: findings from National Surgical Adjuvant Breast and Bowel Project B-23. *J Clin Oncol* 2001;19(4):931–942.
51. Hutchins LF et al. Randomized, controlled trial of cyclophosphamide, methotrexate, and fluorouracil versus cyclophosphamide, doxorubicin, and fluorouracil with and without tamoxifen for high-risk, node-negative breast cancer: treatment results of Intergroup Protocol INT-0102. *J Clin Oncol* 2005;23(33):8313–8321.
52. Bardou VJ et al. Progesterone receptor status significantly improves outcome prediction over estrogen receptor status alone for adjuvant endocrine therapy in two large breast cancer databases. *J Clin Oncol* 2003;21(10):1973–1979.
53. Arpino G et al. Estrogen receptor-positive, progesterone receptor-negative breast cancer: association with growth factor receptor expression and tamoxifen resistance. *J Natl Cancer Inst* 2005;97(17):1254–1261.

54. Dowsett M et al. Retrospective analysis of time to recurrence in the ATAC trial according to hormone receptor status: an hypothesis-generating study. *J Clin Oncol* 2005;23(30):7512–7517.
55. Dowsett M, AD. on Behalf of the TransATAC Investigators, Relationship between quantitative ER and PgR expression and HER2 status with recurrence in the ATAC trial. *Brease Cancer Research and Treatment* 2006;100(S1):S21.
56. Dowsett M et al. Relationship between quantitative estrogen and progesterone receptor expression and human epidermal growth factor receptor 2 (HER-2) status with recurrence in the Arimidex, Tamoxifen, Alone or in Combination trial. *J Clin Oncol* 2008;26(7):1059–1065.
57. Kraus WL, Montano MM, Katzenellenbogen BS. Cloning of the rat progesterone receptor gene 5′-region and identification of two functionally distinct promoters. *Mol Endocrinol* 1993;7(12):1603–1616.
58. Lydon JP et al. Reproductive phenotpes of the progesterone receptor null mutant mouse. *J Steroid Biochem Mol Biol* 1996;56(1–6 Spec No):67–77.
59. Shyamala G et al. Impact of progesterone receptor on cell-fate decisions during mammary gland development. *Proc Natl Acad Sci U S A* 2000;97(7):3044–3049.
60. Hopp TA et al. Breast cancer patients with progesterone receptor PR-A-rich tumors have poorer disease-free survival rates. *Clin Cancer Res* 2004;10(8):2751–2760.
61. Mote PA et al. Detection of progesterone receptor forms A and B by immunohistochemical analysis. *J Clin Pathol* 2001;54(8):624–630.
62. Rhodes A et al. Reliability of immunohistochemical demonstration of oestrogen receptors in routine practice: interlaboratory variance in the sensitivity of detection and evaluation of scoring systems. *J Clin Pathol* 2000;53(2):125–130.
63. Rhodes A et al. Study of interlaboratory reliability and reproducibility of estrogen and progesterone receptor assays in Europe. Documentation of poor reliability and identification of insufficient microwave antigen retrieval time as a major contributory element of unreliable assays. *Am J Clin Pathol* 2001;115(1):44–58.
64. Cummings FJ et al. Adjuvant tamoxifen versus placebo in elderly women with node-positive breast cancer: long-term follow-up and causes of death. *J Clin Oncol* 1993;11(1):29–35.
65. Demissie S, Silliman RA, Lash TL. Adjuvant tamoxifen: predictors of use, side effects, and discontinuation in older women. *J Clin Oncol* 2001;19(2):322–328.
66. Partridge AH et al. Nonadherence to adjuvant tamoxifen therapy in women with primary breast cancer. *J Clin Oncol* 2003;21(4):602–606.
67. Mustacchi G et al. Results of adjuvant treatment in breast cancer women aged more than 70: Italian cooperative group experience. *Tumori*, 2002;88(1 Suppl 1): S83–S85.
68. Horobin JM et al. Long-term follow-up of elderly patients with locoregional breast cancer treated with tamoxifen only. *Br J Surg* 1991;78(2):213–217.
69. Robertson JF et al. Comparison of mastectomy with tamoxifen for treating elderly patients with operable breast cancer. *BMJ* 1988;297(6647):511–514.
70. Delozier T et al. Delayed adjuvant tamoxifen: ten-year results of a collaborative randomized controlled trial in early breast cancer (TAM-02 trial). *Ann Oncol* 2000;11(5):515–519.
71. Smith IE, Dowsett M. Aromatase inhibitors in breast cancer. *N Engl J Med* 2003; 348(24):2431–2442.
72. Jones SA, Jones SE. Exemestane: a novel aromatase inactivator for breast cancer. *Clin Breast Cancer* 2000;1(3):211–216.
73. Gradishar W, Chia S, Piccart M. On behalf of the EFECT writing committee. *Fulvestrant versus exemestane following prior non-steroidal aromatase inhibitor therapy: first results from EFECT, a randomized, phase III trial in postmenopausal women with advanced breast cancer. in SABCS.* 2006. San Antonio, TX.
74. Geisler J et al. Influence of letrozole and anastrozole on total body aromatization and plasma estrogen levels in postmenopausal breast cancer patients evaluated in a randomized, cross-over study. *J Clin Oncol* 2002;20(3):751–757.
75. Goss P et al. The effects of exemestrane on bone and pilips in the ovariectomized rat. *Breast Cancer Res Treat* 2001;69:224.
76. Mouridsen H et al. Superior efficacy of letrozole versus tamoxifen as first-line therapy for postmenopausal women with advanced breast cancer: results of a phase III study of the International Letrozole Breast Cancer Group. *J Clin Oncol* 2001;19(10):2596–2606.
77. Nabholtz JM et al. Anastrozole is superior to tamoxifen as first-line therapy for advanced breast cancer in postmenopausal women: results of a North American multicenter randomized trial. Arimidex Study Group. *J Clin Oncol* 2000;18(22): 3758–3767.
78. Miller WR. Biological rationale for endocrine therapy in breast cancer. *Best Pract Res Clin Endocrinol Metab* 2004;18(1):1–32.
79. Forbes JF et al. Effect of anastrozole and tamoxifen as adjuvant treatment for early-stage breast cancer: 100-month analysis of the ATAC trial. *Lancet Oncol* 2008;9(1):45–53.
80. Baum M et al. Anastrozole alone or in combination with tamoxifen versus tamoxifen alone for adjuvant treatment of postmenopausal women with early breast cancer: first results of the ATAC randomised trial. *Lancet* 2002;359(9324): 2131–2139.
81. Coates AS et al. Five years of letrozole compared with tamoxifen as initial adjuvant therapy for postmenopausal women with endocrine-responsive early breast cancer: update of study BIG 1–98. *J Clin Oncol* 2007;25(5):486–492.
82. Rasmussen BB et al. Adjuvant letrozole versus tamoxifen according to centrally-assessed ERBB2 status for postmenopausal women with endocrine-responsive early breast cancer: supplementary results from the BIG 1–98 randomised trial. *Lancet Oncol* 2008;9(1):23–28.
83. Smith IE et al. Adjuvant aromatase inhibitors for early breast cancer after chemotherapy-induced amenorrhoea: caution and suggested guidelines. *J Clin Oncol* 2006;24(16):2444–2447.
84. Coombes RC et al. A randomized trial of exemestane after two to three years of tamoxifen therapy in postmenopausal women with primary breast cancer. *N Engl J Med* 2004;350(11):1081–1092.
85. Coombes RC et al. Survival and safety of exemestane versus tamoxifen after 2–3 years' tamoxifen treatment (Intergroup Exemestane Study): a randomised controlled trial. *Lancet* 2007;369(9561):559–570.
86. Jakesz R et al. Switching of postmenopausal women with endocrine-responsive early breast cancer to anastrozole after 2 years' adjuvant tamoxifen: combined results of ABCSG trial 8 and ARNO 95 trial. *Lancet* 2005;366(9484):455–462.
87. Kaufmann M et al. Improved overall survival in postmenopausal women with early breast cancer after anastrozole initiated after treatment with tamoxifen compared with continued tamoxifen: the ARNO 95 Study. *J Clin Oncol* 2007;25(19): 2664–2670.
88. Boccardo F et al. Switching to anastrozole versus continued tamoxifen treatment of early breast cancer. Updated results of the Italian tamoxifen anastrozole (ITA) trial. *Ann Oncol* 2006;17 Suppl 7:vii10–vii14.
89. Jonat W et al. Effectiveness of switching from adjuvant tamoxifen to anastrozole in postmenopausal women with hormone-sensitive early-stage breast cancer: a meta-analysis. *Lancet Oncol* 2006;7(12):991–996.
90. Cuzick J, Sasieni P, Howell A. Should aromatase inhibitors be used as initial adjuvant treatment or sequenced after tamoxifen? *Br J Cancer* 2006;94(4):460–464.
91. Hilsenbeck SG, Osborne CK. Is there a role for adjuvant tamoxifen in progesterone receptor-positive breast cancer? An in silico clinical trial. *Clin Cancer Res* 2006;12(3 Pt 2):1049s–1055s.
92. Punglia RS et al. Optimizing adjuvant endocrine therapy in postmenopausal women with early-stage breast cancer: a decision analysis. *J Clin Oncol* 2005; 23(22):5178–5187.
93. Swedish Breast Cancer Cooperative Group, Randomized trial of two versus five years of adjuvant tamoxifen for postmenopausal early stage breast cancer. Swedish Breast Cancer Cooperative Group. *J Natl Cancer Inst* 1996;88(21):1543–1549.
94. Current Trials Working Party of the Cancer Research Campaign Breast Cancer Trials Group, Preliminary results from the cancer research campaign trial evaluating tamoxifen duration in women aged fifty years or older with breast cancer. Current Trials working Party of the Cancer Research Campaign Breast Cancer Trials Group. *J Natl Cancer Inst* 1996;88(24):1834–1839.
95. Tormey DC, Gray R, Falkson HC. Postchemotherapy adjuvant tamoxifen therapy beyond five years in patients with lymph node-positive breast cancer. Eastern Cooperative Oncology Group. *J Natl Cancer Inst* 1996;88(24):1828–1833.
96. Stewart HJ et al. Randomised comparison of 5 years of adjuvant tamoxifen with continuous therapy for operable breast cancer. The Scottish Cancer Trials Breast Group. *Br J Cancer* 1996;74(2):297–299.
97. Stewart HJ, Prescott RJ, Forrest AP. Scottish adjuvant tamoxifen trial: a randomized study updated to 15 years. *J Natl Cancer Inst* 2001;93(6):456–462.
98. Peto R, Davies C. On Behalf of the ATLAS Collaboration. *ATLAS (Adjuvant Tamoxifen, Longer Against Shorter): international randomized trial of 10 versus 5 years of adjuvant tamoxifen among 11,500 women preliminary results. in San Antonio Breast Cancer Symposium.* San Antonio, 2007.
99. Goss PE et al. Randomized trial of letrozole following tamoxifen as extended adjuvant therapy in receptor-positive breast cancer: updated findings from NCIC CTG MA.17. *J Natl Cancer Inst* 2005;97(17):1262–1271.
100. Ingle JN et al. Duration of letrozole treatment and outcomes in the placebo-controlled NCIC CTG MA.17 extended adjuvant therapy trial. *Breast Cancer Res Treat* 2006;99(3):295–300.
101. Mamounas EP et al. Benefit from exemestane as extended adjuvant therapy after 5 years of adjuvant tamoxifen: intention-to-treat analysis of the National Surgical Adjuvant Breast And Bowel Project B-33 trial. *J Clin Oncol* 2008;26(12):1965–1971.
102. Jakesz R et al. Extended adjuvant therapy with anastrozole among postmenopausal breast cancer patients: results from the randomized Austrian Breast and Colorectal Cancer Study Group Trial 6a. *J Natl Cancer Inst* 2007;99(24): 1845–1853.
103. Early Breast Cancer Trialists' Collaborative Group, Ovarian ablation in early breast cancer: overview of the randomised trials. *Lancet* 1996;348(9036):1189–1196.
104. Bryant AJ, Weir JA. Prophylactic oophorectomy in operable instances of carcinoma of the breast. *Surg Gynecol Obstet* 1981;153(5):660–664.
105. Meakin JW et al. Ovarian irradiation and prednisone therapy following surgery and radiotherapy for carcinoma of the breast. *Can Med Assoc J* 1979;120(10): 1221–1229.
106. Cuzick J et al. Use of luteinising-hormone-releasing hormone agonists as adjuvant treatment in premenopausal patients with hormone-receptor-positive breast cancer: a meta-analysis of individual patient data from randomised adjuvant trials. *Lancet* 2007;369(9574):1711–1723.
107. Davidson NE et al. Chemoendocrine therapy for premenopausal women with axillary lymph node-positive, steroid hormone receptor-positive breast cancer: results from INT 0101 (E5188). *J Clin Oncol* 2005;23(25):5973–5982.
108. Thomson CS et al. Adjuvant ovarian ablation vs CMF chemotherapy in premenopausal breast cancer patients: trial update and impact of immunohistochemical assessment of ER status. *Breast* 2002;11(5):419–429.
109. Dees EC, Davidson NE. Ovarian ablation as adjuvant therapy for breast cancer. *Semin Oncol* 2001;28(4):322–331.
110. Ejlertsen B et al. Comparable effect of ovarian ablation and CMF chemotherapy in premenopausal hormone receptor positive breast cancer patients. *Program/Proceedings American Society of Clinical Oncology* 1999;18:66a.
111. Jonat W et al. Goserelin versus cyclophosphamide, methotrexate, and fluorouracil as adjuvant therapy in premenopausal patients with node-positive breast cancer: The Zoladex Early Breast Cancer Research Association Study. *J Clin Oncol* 2002;20(24):4628–4635.
112. Schmid P et al. Cyclophosphamide, methotrexate and fluorouracil (CMF) versus hormonal ablation with leuprorelin acetate as adjuvant treatment of node-positive, premenopausal breast cancer patients: preliminary results of the TABLE-study (Takeda Adjuvant Breast cancer study with Leuprorelin Acetate). *Anticancer Res* 2002;22(4):2325–2332.
113. Schmid P et al. Leuprorelin acetate every-3-months depot versus cyclophosphamide, methotrexate, and fluorouracil as adjuvant treatment in premenopausal patients with node-positive breast cancer: the TABLE study. *J Clin Oncol* 2007;25(18):2509–2515.
114. Jakesz R et al. Randomized adjuvant trial of tamoxifen and goserelin versus cyclophosphamide, methotrexate, and fluorouracil: evidence for the superiority of treatment with endocrine blockade in premenopausal patients with hormone-responsive breast cancer—Austrian Breast and Colorectal Cancer Study Group Trial 5. *J Clin Oncol* 2002;20(24):4621–4627.
115. Boccardo F et al. Cyclophosphamide, methotrexate, and fluorouracil versus tamoxifen plus ovarian suppression as adjuvant treatment of estrogen receptor-positive pre-/perimenopausal breast cancer patients: results of the Italian Breast Cancer Adjuvant Study Group 02 randomized trial. boccardo@hp380.ist.unige.it. *J Clin Oncol* 2000;18(14):2718–2727.
116. Love RR et al. Oophorectomy and tamoxifen adjuvant therapy in premenopausal Vietnamese and Chinese women with operable breast cancer. *J Clin Oncol* 2002;20(10):2559–2566.
117. Stevenson JC et al. A comparison of the skeletal effects of goserelin and danazol in premenopausal women with endometriosis. *Horm Res* 1989;32(Suppl 1):161–163; discussion 164.

118. Gnant M, Mlineritsch B, Schippinger W et al. On behalf of the ABCSG, Adjuvant ovarian suppression combined with tamoxifen or anastrozole, alone or in combination with zoledronic acid, in premenopausal women with hormone-responsive, stage I and II breast cancer: First efficacy results from ABCSG-12. *J Clin Oncol* 2008;26(May 20 suppl):LBA4.
119. Osborne CK et al. Comparison of the effects of a pure steroidal antiestrogen with those of tamoxifen in a model of human breast cancer. *J Natl Cancer Inst* 1995;87(10):746–750.
120. Osborne CK. Tamoxifen in the treatment of breast cancer. *N Engl J Med* 1998;339(22):1609–1618.
121. Fisher B et al. Tamoxifen for prevention of breast cancer: report of the National Surgical Adjuvant Breast and Bowel Project P-1 Study. *J Natl Cancer Inst* 1998; 90(18):1371–1388.
122. Reis SE et al. Cardiovascular effects of tamoxifen in women with and without heart disease: breast cancer prevention trial. National Surgical Adjuvant Breast and Bowel Project Breast Cancer Prevention Trial Investigators. *J Natl Cancer Inst* 2001;93(1):16–21.
123. Kristensen B et al. Tamoxifen and bone metabolism in postmenopausal low-risk breast cancer patients: a randomized study. *J Clin Oncol* 1994;12(5):992–997.
124. Powles TJ et al. Effect of tamoxifen on bone mineral density measured by dual-energy x-ray absorptiometry in healthy premenopausal and postmenopausal women. *J Clin Oncol* 1996;14(1):78–84.
125. IBIS, First results from the International Breast Cancer Intervention Study (IBIS-I): a randomised prevention trial. *Lancet* 2002;360(9336):817–824.
126. Rutqvist LE et al. Contralateral primary tumors in breast cancer patients in a randomized trial of adjuvant tamoxifen therapy. *J Natl Cancer Inst* 1991;83(18): 1299–1306.
127. Wilking N, Isaksson E, von Schoultz E. Tamoxifen and secondary tumours. An update. *Drug Saf* 1997;16(2):104–117.
128. Hutchins L et al. CMF versus CAF with and without tamoxifen in high-risk node-negative breast cancer patients and a natural history follow-up study in low-risk node-negative patients: first results of intergroup trial INT 0102. *Program/Proceedings American Society of Clinical Oncology* 1998;17:1A.
129. Scottish Cancer Trials Breast Group and ICRF Breast Unit, G.s.H., London, Adjuvant ovarian ablation versus CMF chemotherapy in premenopausal women with pathological stage II breast carcinoma: the Scottish trial. *Lancet* 1993; 341(8856):1293–1298.
130. Ribeiro G, Swindell R. The Christie Hospital adjuvant tamoxifen trial. *J Natl Cancer Inst Monogr* 1992(11):121–125.
131. Love RR et al. Symptoms associated with tamoxifen treatment in postmenopausal women. *Arch Intern Med* 1991;151(9):1842–1847.
132. Cathcart CK et al. Clinical recognition and management of depression in node negative breast cancer patients treated with tamoxifen. *Breast Cancer Res Treat* 1993;27(3):277–281.
133. Day R, Ganz PA, Costantino JP. Tamoxifen and depression: more evidence from the National Surgical Adjuvant Breast and Bowel Project's Breast Cancer Prevention (P-1) Randomized Study. *J Natl Cancer Inst* 2001;93(21):1615–1623.
134. Loprinzi CL et al. Tamoxifen-induced hot flashes. *Clin Breast Cancer* 2000;1(1): 52–56.
135. Jacobson JS et al. Randomized trial of black cohosh for the treatment of hot flashes among women with a history of breast cancer. *J Clin Oncol* 2001;19(10): 2739–2745.
136. Van Patten CL et al. Effect of soy phytoestrogens on hot flashes in postmenopausal women with breast cancer: a randomized, controlled clinical trial. *J Clin Oncol* 2002;20(6):1449–1455.
137. Liske E, Therapeutic efficacy and safety of Cimicifuga racemosa for gynecologic disorders. *Adv Ther* 1998;15(1):45–53.
138. Pandya KJ et al. Oral clonidine in postmenopausal patients with breast cancer experiencing tamoxifen-induced hot flashes: a University of Rochester Cancer Center Community Clinical Oncology Program study. *Ann Intern Med* 2000;132(10): 788–793.
139. Loprinzi CL et al. Megestrol acetate for the prevention of hot flashes. *N Engl J Med* 1994;331(6):347–352.
140. Loprinzi CL et al. Pilot evaluation of venlafaxine hydrochloride for the therapy of hot flashes in cancer survivors. *J Clin Oncol* 1998;16(7):2377–2381.
141. Stearns V et al. A pilot trial assessing the efficacy of paroxetine hydrochloride (Paxil) in controlling hot flashes in breast cancer survivors. *Ann Oncol* 2000; 11(1):17–22.
142. Stearns V et al. Active tamoxifen metabolite plasma concentrations after coadministration of tamoxifen and the selective serotonin reuptake inhibitor paroxetine. *J Natl Cancer Inst* 2003;95(23):1758–1764.
143. Jin Y et al. CYP2D6 genotype, antidepressant use, and tamoxifen metabolism during adjuvant breast cancer treatment. *J Natl Cancer Inst* 2005;97(1):30–39.
144. Goetz MP et al. The impact of cytochrome P450 2D6 metabolism in women receiving adjuvant tamoxifen. *Breast Cancer Res Treat* 2007;101(1):113–121.
145. Bernard S et al. Interethnic differences in genetic polymorphisms of CYP2D6 in the U.S. population: clinical implications. *Oncologist* 2006;11(2):126–135.
146. Borges S et al. Quantitative effect of CYP2D6 genotype and inhibitors on tamoxifen metabolism: implication for optimization of breast cancer treatment. *Clin Pharmacol Ther* 2006;80(1):61–74.
147. Goetz MP, Kamal A, Ames MM. Tamoxifen pharmacogenomics: the role of CYP2D6 as a predictor of drug response. *Clin Pharmacol Ther* 2008;83(1): 160–166.
148. Ingle JN. Pharmacogenomics of tamoxifen and aromatase inhibitors. *Cancer* 2008;112(3 Suppl):695–699.
149. Loprinzi L et al. Pilot evaluation of gabapentin for treating hot flashes. *Mayo Clin Proc* 2002;77(11):1159–1163.
150. Kendall A et al. Caution: Vaginal estradiol appears to be contraindicated in postmenopausal women on adjuvant aromatase inhibitors. *Ann Oncol* 2006;17(4): 584–587.
151. Henriksson L et al. A one-year multicenter study of efficacy and safety of a continuous, low-dose, estradiol-releasing vaginal ring (Estring) in postmenopausal women with symptoms and signs of urogenital aging. *Am J Obstet Gynecol* 1996;174(1 Pt 1):85–92.
152. Weisberg E et al. Endometrial and vaginal effects of low-dose estradiol delivered by vaginal ring or vaginal tablet. *Climacteric* 2005;8(1):83–92.
153. Kaiser-Kupfer MI, Lippman ME. Tamoxifen retinopathy. *Cancer Treat Rep* 1978; 62(3):315–320.
154. Pavlidis NA et al. Clear evidence that long-term, low-dose tamoxifen treatment can induce ocular toxicity. A prospective study of 63 patients. *Cancer* 1992; 69(12):2961–2964.
155. Longstaff S et al. A controlled study of the ocular effects of tamoxifen in conventional dosage in the treatment of breast carcinoma. *Eur J Cancer Clin Oncol* 1989;25(12):1805–1808.
156. Nayfield SG, Gorin MB. Tamoxifen-associated eye disease. A review. *J Clin Oncol* 1996;14(3):1018–1026.
157. Gorin MB et al. Long-term tamoxifen citrate use and potential ocular toxicity. *Am J Ophthalmol* 1998;125(4):493–501.
158. NIH/NCI, *Tamoxifen-associated eye toxicity*. Department of Health and Human Services, National Institutes of Health, National Cancer Institute: Bethesda, MD. 1997.
159. Gianni L et al. Ocular toxicity during adjuvant chemoendocrine therapy for early breast cancer: results from International Breast Cancer Study Group trials. *Cancer* 2006;106(3):505–513.
160. Rutqvist LE, Mattsson A. Cardiac and thromboembolic morbidity among postmenopausal women with early-stage breast cancer in a randomized trial of adjuvant tamoxifen. The Stockholm Breast Cancer Study Group. *J Natl Cancer Inst* 1993;85(17):1398–1406.
161. Pritchard KI et al. Increased thromboembolic complications with concurrent tamoxifen and chemotherapy in a randomized trial of adjuvant therapy for women with breast cancer. National Cancer Institute of Canada Clinical Trials Group Breast Cancer Site Group. *J Clin Oncol* 1996;14(10):2731–2737.
162. Levine MN. Prevention of thrombotic disorders in cancer patients undergoing chemotherapy. *Thromb Haemost* 1997;78(1):133–136.
163. Vogel VG et al. Effects of tamoxifen vs raloxifene on the risk of developing invasive breast cancer and other disease outcomes: the NSABP Study of Tamoxifen and Raloxifene (STAR) P-2 trial. *JAMA* 2006;295(23):2727–2741.
164. McDonald CC, Stewart HJ. Fatal myocardial infarction in the Scottish adjuvant tamoxifen trial. The Scottish Breast Cancer Committee. *BMJ* 1991;303(6800): 435–437.
165. Jordan VC, Morrow M. Should clinicians be concerned about the carcinogenic potential of tamoxifen? *Eur J Cancer* 1994;30A(11):1714–1721.
166. Assikis VJ, Jordan VC. Gynecologic effects of tamoxifen and the association with endometrial carcinoma. *Int J Gynaecol Obstet* 1995;49(3):241–257.
167. Fisher B et al. Endometrial cancer in tamoxifen-treated breast cancer patients: findings from the National Surgical Adjuvant Breast and Bowel Project (NSABP) B-14. *J Natl Cancer Inst* 1994;86(7):527–537.
168. Bernstein L et al. Tamoxifen therapy for breast cancer and endometrial cancer risk. *J Natl Cancer Inst* 1999;91(19):1654–1662.
169. Runowicz CD. Gynecologic surveillance of women on tamoxifen: first do no harm. *J Clin Oncol* 2000;18(20):3457–3458.
170. Gerber B et al. Effects of adjuvant tamoxifen on the endometrium in postmenopausal women with breast cancer: a prospective long-term study using transvaginal ultrasound. *J Clin Oncol* 2000;18(20):3464–3470.
171. Barakat RR et al. Effect of adjuvant tamoxifen on the endometrium in women with breast cancer: a prospective study using office endometrial biopsy. *J Clin Oncol* 2000;18(20):3459–3463.
172. Gardner FJE et al. Endometrial protection from tamoxifen-stimulated changes by a levonorgestrel-releasing intrauterine system: a randomised controlled trial. *Lancet* 2000;356:1711–1717.
173. Hann LE et al. Endometrial thickness in tamoxifen-treated patients: correlation with clinical and pathologic findings. *AJR Am J Roentgenol* 1997;168(3):657–661.
174. Shushan A et al. Ovarian cysts in premenopausal and postmenopausal tamoxifen-treated women with breast cancer. *Am J Obstet Gynecol* 1996;174(1 Pt 1):141–144.
175. Hard GC et al. Major difference in the hepatocarcinogenicity and DNA adduct forming ability between toremifene and tamoxifen in female Crl:CD(BR) rats. *Cancer Res* 1993;53(19):4534–4541.
176. Ahotupa M et al. Alterations of drug metabolizing and antioxidant enzyme activities during tamoxifen-induced hepatocarcinogenesis in the rat. *Carcinogenesis* 1994;15(5):863–868.
177. Fornander T et al. Adjuvant tamoxifen in early breast cancer: occurrence of new primary cancers. *Lancet* 1989;1(8630):117–120.
178. Muhlemann K, Cook LS, Weiss NS. The incidence of hepatocellular carcinoma in U.S. white women with breast cancer after the introduction of tamoxifen in 1977. *Breast Cancer Res Treat* 1994;30(2):201–204.
179. Oien KA et al. Cirrhosis with steatohepatitis after adjuvant tamoxifen. *Lancet* 1999;353(9146):36–37.
180. Nemoto Y et al. Tamoxifen-induced nonalcoholic steatohepatitis in breast cancer patients treated with adjuvant tamoxifen. *Intern Med* 2002;41(5):345–350.
181. Andersson M, Storm HH, Mouridsen HT. Incidence of new primary cancers after adjuvant tamoxifen therapy and radiotherapy for early breast cancer. *J Natl Cancer Inst* 1991;83(14):1013–1017.
182. Gnant MF et al. Zoledronic acid prevents cancer treatment-induced bone loss in premenopausal women receiving adjuvant endocrine therapy for hormone-responsive breast cancer: a report from the Austrian Breast and Colorectal Cancer Study Group. *J Clin Oncol* 2007;25(7):820–828.
183. Banerjee S et al. Comparative effects of anastrozole, tamoxifen alone and in combination on plasma lipids and bone-derived resorption during neoadjuvant therapy in the impact trial. *Ann Oncol* 2005;16(10):1632–1638.
184. Fallowfield LJ et al. Quality of life in the intergroup exemestane study: a randomized trial of exemestane versus continued tamoxifen after 2 to 3 years of tamoxifen in postmenopausal women with primary breast cancer. *J Clin Oncol* 2006; 24(6):910–917.
185. Mouridsen H et al. Cardiovascular adverse events during adjuvant endocrine therapy for early breast cancer using letrozole or tamoxifen: safety analysis of BIG 1–98 trial. *J Clin Oncol* 2007;25(36):5715–5722.
186. Wasan KM et al. The influence of letrozole on serum lipid concentrations in postmenopausal women with primary breast cancer who have completed 5 years of adjuvant tamoxifen (NCIC CTG MA.17L). *Ann Oncol* 2005;16(5):707–715.
187. Perez EA et al. Effect of letrozole versus placebo on bone mineral density in women with primary breast cancer completing 5 or more years of adjuvant tamoxifen: a companion study to NCIC CTG MA.17. *J Clin Oncol* 2006;24(22):3629–3635.
188. Eastell R et al. Effect of anastrozole on bone mineral density: 5-year results from the anastrozole, tamoxifen, alone or in combination trial 18233230. *J Clin Oncol* 2008;26(7):1051–1057.

189. Thurlimann B et al. A comparison of letrozole and tamoxifen in postmenopausal women with early breast cancer. *N Engl J Med* 2005;353(26):2747–2757.
190. Coleman RE et al. Skeletal effects of exemestane on bone-mineral density, bone biomarkers, and fracture incidence in postmenopausal women with early breast cancer participating in the Intergroup Exemestane Study (IES): a randomised controlled study. *Lancet Oncol* 2007;8(2):119–127.
191. Howell A et al. Results of the ATAC (Arimidex, Tamoxifen, Alone or in Combination) trial after completion of 5 years' adjuvant treatment for breast cancer. *Lancet* 2005;365(9453):60–62.
192. Cuppone F et al. Do adjuvant aromatase inhibitors increase the cardiovascular risk in postmenopausal women with early breast cancer? Meta-analysis of randomized trials. *Cancer* 2008;112(2):260–267.
193. Amin Z, Canli T, Epperson CN. Effect of estrogen-serotonin interactions on mood and cognition. *Behav Cogn Neurosci Rev* 2005;4(1):43–58.
194. Amin Z et al. Estradiol and tryptophan depletion interact to modulate cognition in menopausal women. *Neuropsychopharmacology* 2006;31(11):2489–2497.
195. Phillips KA, Bernhard J. Adjuvant breast cancer treatment and cognitive function: current knowledge and research directions. *J Natl Cancer Inst* 2003;95(3):190–197.
196. Yaffe K et al. Cognitive function in postmenopausal women treated with raloxifene. *N Engl J Med* 2001;344(16):1207–1213.
197. Chlebowski RT et al. *Tamoxifen and Estrogen Effects on Brain Chemistry Determined by MRI spectroscopy.* in *ASCO*. San Francisco: American Society of Clinical Oncology, 2001.
198. Shilling V et al. The effects of hormone therapy on cognition in breast cancer. *J Steroid Biochem Mol Biol* 2003;86(3–5):405–412.
199. Sasano H et al. Aromatase in the human central nervous system. *Clin Endocrinol (Oxf)* 1998;48(3):325–329.
200. Peto R et al. UK and USA breast cancer deaths down 25% in year 2000 at ages 20–69 years. *Lancet* 2000;355(9217):1822.
201. Goldhirsch A et al. Meeting highlights: international expert consensus on the primary therapy of early breast cancer 2005. *Ann Oncol* 2005;16(10):1569–1583.

Updates

At the 2008 San Antonio Breast Cancer Symposium, several studies were presented or updated. The BIG1-98 study presented the first results of its sequential therapeutic arms. More than three thousand patients who were randomized to tamoxifen for 2 years followed by letrozole 3 years or letrozole for 2 years followed by tamoxifen for 3 years were compared to patients in the upfront letrozole arm. With a median follow up of 71 months, the results showed that both sequential arms were similar to upfront letrozole and to each other in DFS, overall survival, and TTDR (Table 48.13) (1). Numerically there were a few more breast cancer events in the tamoxifen followed by letrozole arm compared to either opposite sequence or to letrozole alone.

An update of the ABCSG-8 trial showed a significant overall survival advantage in patients who were treated with a sequence of tamoxifen for 2 years then switched to anastrozole compared to patients who were treated with 5 years of tamoxifen (HR = 0.77, 95% CI 0.61–0.97, p = 0.025) (2). However, this analysis was for the actual treatment received and not an intent-to-treat analysis; it combined the patients who were originally randomized to the sequential treatment arm and patients who were crossed over after the initial positive results were presented in 2004. Therefore, this was a retrospective analysis. The trial also showed high levels of ER or PR were predictive of longer RFS, and overall survival (2).

Additionally, the Tamoxifen Exemestane Adjuvant Multinational (TEAM) trial reported its first results (3). This trial initially randomized close to 10 thousand patients to 5 years of tamoxifen or exemestane. When results from the IES study were announced, the study protocol was amended and the tamoxifen arm was changed to a sequential arm with initial tamoxifen for 2–3 years followed by exemestane. Results from the TEAM trial were analyzed at the switching point and therefore the data represented a comparison between upfront exemestane and tamoxifen. The study showed a numerical trend for improved DFS (its primary end point) for upfront exemestane that was not significant (HR = 0.85, p = 0.12) (3).

The Aromatase Inhibitor Overview Group (AIOG) presented a metanalysis that included data from all adjuvant aromatase inhibitor trials (4). However, the updated data from BIG1-98 and ABCSG-8 summarized above were not included. Results were presented from two cohorts: the first cohort consisted of patients who received upfront aromatase inhibitor compared to patients who received tamoxifen monotherapy. The second cohort consisted of patients who received sequential therapy with initial tamoxifen followed by an aromatase inhibitor compared to patients who received tamoxifen monotherapy.

This metanalysis showed that, compared to tamoxifen alone, upfront aromatase inhibitors reduce the risk of recurrence by 23% and the sequential approach by 29%. While upfront aromatase inhibitors did not have a breast cancer mortality or overall survival advantage, the cohort of sequential therapy showed a significant reduction in breast cancer mortality (0.7% at 3 years, and 1.6% at 6 years from treatment divergence from tamoxifen, p = 0.02) and a significant reduction in deaths from any cause (1.1% at 3 years and 2.2% at 6 years from treatment divergence, p = 0.004). Neither cohort showed a difference in non-breast cancer deaths, indicating the safety of aromatase inhibitors in general (4).

The Trans-ATAC study correlated Oncotype DX results with outcome of 1200 patients enrolled on the ATAC trial (5). The results confirmed the assay's ability to predict the risk of recurrence and showed a benefit for anastrozole across risk groups. But in patients with node negative cancers the only group to benefit from anastrozole compared to tamoxifen was the subset with a high risk Oncotype DX score (5). These intriguing results are hypothesis-generating and warrant further investigation. If validated, they may help identify patients who would derive the most benefit from aromatase inhibitors.

Another study reported on the CYP2D genotype in patients from the ABCSG-8 study (6). This study reported a 3.8 fold increase in the risk of recurrence in patients who were poor metabolizers compared to extensive metabolizers in patients in the tamoxifen monotherapy arm but not the arm that contained anastrozole (p = 0.017) (6). These results suggest that in postmenopausal women who have a poor metabolizer phenotype should be started on an aromatase inhibitor since they can not metabolize tamoxifen to its endoxifene, its most active metabolite. Not all studies have come to the same conclusion.

The above results still indicate that in postmenopausal women, aromatase inhibitors offer a small but significant disease-free survival advantage over tamoxifen alone. Aromatase inhibitors can be given upfront as monotherapy or in sequence after or before tamoxifen. Therefore, our recommendations are modified as follows:

1. For most postmenopausal women with breast cancer initial aromatase inhibitor for 5 years or the sequence of tamoxifen before or after an aromatase inhibitor are acceptable strategies.
2. For patients at high risk for early recurrence the BIG 1-98 and ATAC data support the initial use of an aromatase inhibitor.
3. While additional studies are needed to clarify several remaining issues regarding the role of CYP2D6 in the activity of tamoxifen, it seems prudent to use upfront aromatase inhibitor therapy instead of tamoxifen in patients who are poor metabolizers and to avoid concomitant use of drugs such as SSRIs that interfere with tamoxifen metabolism.

References

1. Mouridsen H, Giobbie-Hurder, A, Mauriac, L, Paridaens, R, Colleoni, M, Thürlimann, B, Forbes, JF, Gelber, RD, Wardley, A, Smith, I, Price, KN, Coates A, Goldhirsch, A. BIG 1-98: *A randomized double-blind phase III study evaluating letrozole and tamoxifen given in sequence as adjuvant endocrine therapy for postmenopausal women with receptor-positive breast cancer.* In *31st Annual San Antonio Breast Cancer Symposium* 2008. San Antonio, Texas.
2. Jakesz, R, Gnant, M, Griel, R, Tausch, C, Samonigg, H, Kwasny, W, Kubista, E, Stierer, M, Luschin, G, Rüecklinger, E, Mittlböck, M. *Tamoxifen and anastrozole as a sequencing strategy in postmenopausal women with hormone-responsive early breast cancer: updated data from the Austrian breast and colorectal cancer study group trial 8.* In *31st Annual San Antonio Breast Cancer Symposium* 2008. San Antonio, Texas.
3. Jones, S., Seynaeve, C, Hasenburg, A, Rae, D, Vannetzel, J-M, Paridaens, R, Markopoulos, C, Hozumi, Y, Putter, H, Hille, E, Kieback, D, Asmar, L, Smeets, J, Urbanski, R, Bartlett, JMS, van de Velde, CJH. *Results of the first planned analysis of the TEAM (tamoxifen exemestane adjuvant multinational) prospective randomized phase III trial in hormone sensitive postmenopausal early breast cancer.* In *31st Annual San Antonio Breast Cancer Symposium.* 2008. San Antonio, Texas.
4. Ingle, J.N., Dowsett, M., Cuzick, J., Davies, C. *Aromatase inhibitors versus tamoxifen as adjuvant therapy for postmenopausal women with estrogen receptor positive breast cancer: meta-analyses of randomized trials of monotherapy and switching strategies.* In *31st Annual San Antonio Breast Cancer Symposium.* 2008. San Antonio, Texas.
5. Dowsett, M., Cuzick, J, Wales, C, Forbes, J, Mallon, L, Salter, J, Quinn, E, Bugarini, R, Baehner, FL, Shak, S, on Behalf of the ATAC Trialists' Group. *Risk of distant recurrence using oncotype DX in postmenopausal primary breast cancer patients treated with anastrozole or tamoxifen: a TransATAC study.* In *31st Annual San Antonio Breast Cancer Symposium.* 2008. San Antonio, Texas.
6. Goetz, M., Ames, M, Gnant, M, Filpits, M, Jakesz, R, Greil, R, Marth, C, Samonigg, H, Suman, V, Safgren, S, Kuffel, M, Weinshilboum, R, Erlander, M, Ma, X-J, Ingle, J. *Pharmacogenetic (CYP2D6) and gene expression profiles (HOXB13/IL17BR and molecular grade index) for prediction of adjuvant endocrine therapy benefit in the ABCSG 8 trial.* in *31st Annual San Antonio Breast Cancer Symposium.* 2008. San Antonio, Texas.

Table 48.13 Results from BIG1-98 sequential treatment arms compared to upfront letrozole for disease-free survival (DFS), overall survival (OS), and time to distant recurrence (TTDR) with 99% confidence intervals.

Study Arm	DFS	OS	TTDR
Tamoxifen ♦ Letrozole	1.05 (0.84–1.32)	1.13 (0.83–1.53)	1.22 (0.88–1.69)
Letrozole ♦ Tamoxifen	0.96 (0.76–1.21)	0.90 (0.65–1.24)	1.05 (0.75–1.47)

Erica L. Mayer and Eric P. Winer

Despite optimal local therapy, a substantial number of women with breast cancer will develop a systemic recurrence of the disease. The initial rationale for adjuvant therapy grew out of several early observations and hypotheses. First, circulating tumor cells were observed in the blood of cancer patients at the time of surgical resection, sometimes distant from the site of surgery (1). Second, it was thought that hematogenous micrometastatic tumor dissemination might later develop into true metastatic disease, and that the administration of systemic therapy could eradicate occult cancer and improve survival. Third, the success with systemic chemotherapy in animal models led to early studies in solid tumor malignancies designed to further evaluate the role of adjuvant therapy as an adjunct to local treatment in solid tumors (2).

Over the past four decades, scores of clinical trials have investigated the role of cytotoxic chemotherapy to reduce the risk of disease recurrence and improve overall survival. Adjuvant treatment—chemotherapy, endocrine therapy, and targeted therapy—is a mainstay of clinical practice and has led to a substantial decline in breast cancer mortality in women with operable disease. As a result, we have a robust understanding of the benefits and risks of adjuvant chemotherapy for the overall population of women with operable breast cancer.

As described in this chapter, most clinical trials have enrolled patients based on eligibility criteria that focused on the anatomic extent of the disease. Without question, anatomic parameters (e.g., stage of disease) influence the absolute risk of disease recurrence. More recently, we have come to understand that breast cancer is a family of diseases. Although this understanding is still very much in evolution, it is clear that different subtypes of breast cancer, defined by hormone receptor status and ERBB2 (formerly HER), have different temporal patterns of recurrence and varying degrees of sensitivity to adjuvant chemotherapy. In simplest terms, the benefits from chemotherapy are not distributed equally across all patients with the disease. The challenge we face is of integrating our contemporary, and still changing, understanding of breast cancer with the results of clinical trials that were conducted at a time when the disease was viewed quite differently. Multiple unanswered questions remain, and future development of more effective agents and greater individualization of treatment based on disease heterogeneity may lead to substantial improvements in years ahead.

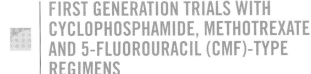

FIRST GENERATION TRIALS WITH CYCLOPHOSPHAMIDE, METHOTREXATE AND 5-FLUOROURACIL (CMF)-TYPE REGIMENS

Initial trials of adjuvant chemotherapy utilized single agents and included very brief preoperative exposures to treatments, such as thiotepa, melphalan, and cyclophosphamide (3–5). Subsequently, in a pivotal study from Milan, Bonadonna et al. (6) randomized 386 patients with axillary lymph node-positive disease after mastectomy to either CMF for 1 year (cyclophosphamide 100 mg/m^2 orally days 1 to 14, methotrexate 40 mg/m^2 intravenously [IV] day 1, and 8, and 5-fluorouracil 600

mg/m^2 IV days 1 and 8 every 28 days) versus observation alone. Treatment with this oral or *classic* CMF resulted in significant improvements in disease-free survival (DFS) and overall survival (OS) compared with observation (6). Similar beneficial results in DFS and OS were observed with use of L-phenylalanine mustard (melphalan) given orally for 2 years after surgery (7). Long-term follow-up has confirmed survival benefits from CMF, with a survival difference of 47% versus 22% (8). A subsequent trial from the Milan group demonstrated that 12 months of therapy offered no advantage over 6 months from the standpoint of efficacy, but did increase the overall toxicity burden (9,10). Based on the strength of these early trials, six cycles of CMF became the most frequently used systemic adjuvant therapy for breast cancer and remains a regimen still used with some frequency in the United States and around the world. The findings from the initial trials led to two types of clinical trials. First, studies sought to broaden the indication for adjuvant chemotherapy to include women with node-negative disease. Second, a series of clinical trials, including many that are ongoing today, have sought to develop more effective chemotherapy regimens.

Chemotherapy was initially not considered for node-negative breast cancer, because it was assumed that the absence of axillary nodal involvement predicted a favorable prognosis, and that adequate surgery was sufficient in management. Long-term follow-up from the original surgical trials suggested otherwise, as individuals with node negative disease not treated with adjuvant therapy had a significant chance of recurrence and death from disease in the years. In the late 1980s and early 1990s, numerous studies confirmed the benefits of chemotherapy in the node-negative population. Furthermore, these studies suggested that the reduction in hazards, or the relative risk reduction, did not seem to differ between node-positive and node-negative patients. This finding has been a cornerstone of breast cancer treatment and has had a profound influence on clinical trial design and clinical practice.

The primary trials in the node-negative setting have been performed in the cooperative group setting. The National Surgical Adjuvant Breast and Bowel Project (NSABP) evaluated the methotrexate/5-flourouracil (MF) regimen in patients with estrogen receptor (ER)-negative disease, and the Breast Cancer Intergroup of North America evaluated CMF-prednisone in those with ER-negative disease and in women with ER positive lesions that were 3 cm or larger (11,12). Both studies reported significant improvements in DFS for all subjects and in OS for either the entire study population (Intergroup trial) or the age 50 years or more subgroup (NSABP). A subsequent trial, NSABP B19, compared CMF × 6 versus MF × 6 in women with ER-negative tumors and demonstrated that the former was a superior regimen, at least in patients aged 49 years or younger (13). In NSABP B-20, it was also demonstrated that the addition of chemotherapy to tamoxifen in patients with ER-positive disease resulted in a small but statistically significant improvement in DFS (14). These node-negative trials formed the basis of the recommendation by the 2000 National Institutes of Health (NIH) Consensus Conference that all women with either tumors greater than 1 cm or positive lymph nodes be offered chemotherapy (15). These trials also led to the inclusion of patients with node-negative disease in many trials that might have otherwise restricted entry to those with node-positive breast cancer.

BETTER CHARACTERIZATION OF THE ROLE OF ADJUVANT CHEMOTHERAPY

The Early Breast Cancer Trialists' Collaborative Group (EBCTCG) was formed in the mid-1980s to perform a meta-analysis of randomized trials in the adjuvant setting, initially focusing on adjuvant chemotherapy and endocrine therapy for breast cancer. The *Overview Analysis* contains individual data from thousands of patients and has substantial power to detect relatively small differences in outcome. Since the EBCTCG was organized, an updated *Overview Analysis* has been published approximately every 5 years. Beyond the number of patients included in the *Overview*, the other major strength is the long-term follow-up that is available from many of the studies. The most recent *Overview* publication describing adjuvant chemotherapy was the *2000 Analysis*, published in 2005. The *Overview Analysis* has provided a rich source of data supporting contemporary treatment decisions, and has been critical in defining the benefit of chemotherapy regimens across patient populations defined by patient age and anatomic extent of disease. Many of the older studies did not routinely collect data on the hormone receptor status of the primary tumor, however, and most of the trials did not test for human epidermal growth factor receptor 2 (ERBB2). Both of these molecular markers play a critical role in decisions about adjuvant therapy in the current era.

The *2000 Overview Analysis* provides further support for the role of adjuvant chemotherapy in breast cancer treatment (16). Long-term follow-up of the 29,000 women who participated in early studies of polychemotherapy versus none continues to demonstrate significant improvements in both absolute risks of recurrence (relative risk [RR] 0.77) and breast cancer mortality (RR 0.83). At 15 years, these benefits remain significant across all age groups, although are more pronounced in women younger than 50 years (recurrence 12.4%, mortality 10%) compared with those age 50 to 69 years (recurrence 4.2%, mortality 3.0%). These proportional benefits are also evident in both node-negative and node-positive populations, regardless of age. The reduction in the risk of recurrence with chemotherapy is evident within the first 5 years after randomization; the absolute difference in the risk of recurrence seen at 5-year follow-up is maintained at the 10- and 15-year time points. In contrast, the improvement in survival gradually increases over time, with continued divergence of curves representing chemotherapy treated patients and controls. The absolute reduction in the risk of death doubles between 5 years and a 15-year follow-up. The first publication from the *2005 Overview Analysis* examines chemotherapy in ER-poor breast cancer. As described in Table 49.1 and discussed further later in this chapter (17), results continue to demonstrate consistent benefits in DFS and OS from the addition of chemotherapy for women of almost all ages (18).

Without question, results from the *Overview Analyses* confirm the essential role of adjuvant chemotherapy in breast cancer, and indicate that the absolute benefits may vary with the hormone receptor status of the tumor. As will be discussed later in this chapter, diversity within the ER-positive subgroup may lead to even further differential gains from chemotherapy treatment.

ROLE OF THE ANTHRACYCLINES

After demonstrating benefit in the metastatic setting, multiple randomized trials were initiated to evaluate the potential contribution of anthracyclines in adjuvant therapy. One of the first modifications of standard CMF-type chemotherapy involved either the substitution of methotrexate with an anthracycline (doxorubicin or epirubicin) or the addition of an anthracycline to the regimen, either concurrently or sequentially. In NSABP B-11, doxorubicin was introduced in a comparison of melphalan and fluorouracil versus doxorubicin, melphalan, and fluorouracil. The three-drug combination significantly improved DFS and OS compared with the two agents alone (19). The Cancer and Leukemia Group B (CALGB) investigated the addition of anthracyclines in CALGB 8082, which compared a prolonged regimen of cyclophosphamide, methotrexate, fluorouracil, vincristine, and prednisone (CMFVP) with CMFVP followed by anthracycline-based vinblastine, doxorubicin, thiotepa, and fluoxymesterone (VATH). At 11.5 years of follow-up, the incorporation of VATH resulted in significant improvements in DFS and OS (20). The Milan group approached the anthracycline question in a study randomizing 550 patients with limited nodal involvement to 12 months of IV CMF or 8 months CMF followed by four cycles of single agent doxorubicin. Results demonstrated no benefit in DFS or OS. The failure to observe a benefit in this study may have been a chance finding, or may relate to differences in the study population, such as the proportion of patients with ER-negative or ERBB2-positive disease (21).

Table 49.1	SUMMARY OF MAIN RESULTS FROM THE 2005 OXFORD OVERVIEW IN ER NEGATIVE DISEASE(18)		
	Reduction in Annual Odds (SE)		
	Breast Cancer Recurrence (%)	**Breast Cancer Mortality (%)**	**Any Death (%)**
Trials of Polychemotherapy Versus No Adjuvant			
<50	36 ± 7	25 ± 9	24 ± 9
50–59	28 ± 10	19 ± 11	17 ± 10
60–69	31 ± 69	24 ± 14	24 ± 12
Trials of Polychemotherapy Plus Tamoxifen Versus Tamoxifen Alone			
<50	60 ± 21	51 ± 25	51 ± 25
50–59	36 ± 8	28 ± 9	25 ± 9
60–69	13 ± 9	3 ± 9	3 ± 9
All Polychemotherapy Versus Not			
<50	39 ± 7	28 ± 8	26 ± 8
50–59	32 ± 6	25 ± 7	22 ± 7
60–69	18 ± 7	10 ± 8	9 ± 7

In study INT-0102, the US Intergroup evaluated the regimen of CAF (cyclophosphamide 100 mg/m^2 orally days 1 to 14, doxorubicin 30 mg/m^2 IV days 1 and 8, fluorouracil 500 mg/m^2 IV days 1 and 8) compared with classic CMF in a high-risk, node-negative population, with or without tamoxifen. Treatment in the anthracycline-based arm led to no difference in DFS, but a slight improvement in OS, which the investigators considered to be of marginal clinical significance (22). A similar European study comparing FAC (fluorouracil 500 mg/m^2 IV days 1 and 8, doxorubicin 50 mg/m^2 IV day 1, cyclophosphamide 500 mg/m^2 IV day 1) × 6 to IV CMF × 6 showed slight superiority of the anthracycline-containing regimen, particularly in the node-negative population (23). Epirubicin, an alternative anthracycline, has also been studied in the adjuvant setting. NCI-C MA.5 compared 6 months of CEF (cyclophosphamide 75 mg/m^2 orally days 1 to 14, epirubicin 60 mg/m^2 IV days 1 and 8, and fluorouracil 500 mg/m^2 IV days 1 and 8) or classic CMF as adjuvant therapy for node-positive breast cancer. Long-term results from this study have demonstrated superiority of the epirubicin-containing regimen (24).

The NSABP took a somewhat different approach. Rather than substituting an anthracycline for methotrexate or adding an anthracycline to CMF, they opted to include an anthracycline and design a shorter and more convenient regimen. NSABP B-15 compared 6 months of classic CMF with just four cycles of AC (doxorubicin 60 mg/m^2 IV and cyclophosphamide 600 mg/m^2 IV every 21 days), and demonstrated identical benefits in DFS, distant DFS, and OS with the anthracycline-based therapy (17). Building on these findings, in B-23 the NSABP subsequently randomized node-negative patients in a 2 × 2 distribution to classic CMF × 6 versus AC × 4, with or without tamoxifen. As in B-15, AC performed as well as the longer-duration, classic CMF (25). Finally, NSABP B-16 demonstrated benefit of a short regimen of AC with endocrine therapy over endocrine therapy alone (26). As a result of these trials, a regimen consisting of four cycles of AC chemotherapy became a standard adjuvant chemotherapy regimen in the United States. Unlike other anthracycline-containing regimens, AC × 4 has not been shown to be more effective than classic CMF for the overall study population in any of the NSABP trials. A number of reasons could explain the failure to see an improvement with AC over classic CMF, including the short duration of the regimen, the omission of 5-fluorouracil, and the use of intravenous cyclophosphamide. Its widespread use for many years was largely a consequence of the fact that it was shorter than many regimens and more convenient, making it appealing to both oncologists and patients alike. It remains in use today, and has also been incorporated into numerous sequential anthracycline-taxane regimens.

The *2000 Overview Analysis* evaluated the 14,000 women who participated in trials comparing CMF with an anthracycline-based regimen, and confirmed a modest but highly significant benefit favoring anthracyclines, with absolute benefits of 3.4% for recurrence and 3.3% for mortality at 15 years. The gains afforded by anthracycline-containing regimens appeared to be maintained in both younger and older women, and were independent of hormone receptor status (16). In general, epirubicin-containing regimens are favored in Europe and Canada, although no evidence exists favoring one agent over the other. Although epirubicin appears to have less direct cardiotoxicity than doxorubicin on a milligram by milligram basis, cumulative doses of epirubicin in the adjuvant setting are higher than those for doxorubicin, and much of the advantage from a cardiac toxicity standpoint is therefore lost. Table 49.2 delineates commonly used combination chemotherapy regimens for adjuvant therapy of breast cancer.

Although many questions exist about the use of anthracyclines and the need to include an anthracycline in current treatment regimens, doxorubicin and epirubicin have been a mainstay of breast cancer treatment for the past two decades. It is likely that anthracycline use will decline in the years ahead as we develop increasingly specific treatment approaches for subgroups of women with breast cancer. In particular, the role

of anthracyclines in the treatment of ERBB2-positive breast cancer is undergoing re-evaluation in the trastuzumab era, discussed further in Chapter 51. Given the established benefit of anthracyclines in adjuvant therapy, any decision to eliminate doxorubicin or epirubicin, particularly in patients who are at high risk of disease recurrence, should be based on the results of adequately powered prospective randomized trials.

ROLE OF TAXANES

The success of the microtubule-stabilizing taxane family of chemotherapies in the metastatic breast cancer setting led to multiple large randomized trials evaluating the role of taxanes, including paclitaxel and docetaxel, in adjuvant therapy. These trials fall into three main categories: sequential taxane after anthracycline exposure, concurrent taxane and anthracycline, or replacement of the anthracycline with a taxane. Taxanes currently have an established role in adjuvant therapy; however, review of the studies demonstrates some degree of heterogeneity in outcomes. Table 49.3 lists results from relevant trials discussed below evaluating the role of adjuvant taxane therapy.

The first study of sequential taxane therapy was CALGB 9344, which evaluated the addition of paclitaxel (175 mg/m^2 IV every 3 weeks) to four cycles of AC, with escalating doses of doxorubicin in patients with node positive disease. Significant improvements DFS and OS were observed; an unplanned subset analysis also identified a preferential benefit for ER-negative over ER-positive tumors (27). In a similar fashion, NSABP B-28 added four cycles of paclitaxel (225 mg/m^2 IV every 3 weeks) after AC × 4 in a node-positive cohort of 3,060 patients, leading to improvements in DFS but not OS at 5 years. In contrast to CALGB 9344, no differential benefit was observed by ER status (28). NSABP B-27 evaluated the addition of sequential docetaxel (100 mg/m^2) to four cycles of AC in the neoadjuvant setting; no significant improvements in DFS or OS were observed from the addition of the taxane, either preoperatively or postoperatively, despite achieving a doubling in the rate of pathologic complete response (29).

A number of studies have substituted a taxane in place of an anthracycline for a portion of the regimen. In the PACS 01 study, patients were randomized to six cycles of FEC (fluorouracil 500 mg/m^2, epirubicin 100 mg/m^2, and cyclophosphamide 500 mg/m^2, all IV on day 1) chemotherapy or three cycles of FEC followed by three cycles of docetaxel at a dose of 100 mg/m^2 IV every 3 weeks. The use of docetaxel resulted in improved DFS and OS (30). The GEICAM 9906 trial studied the addition of sequential paclitaxel to an anthracycline-based regimen. Node-positive patients were randomized to FEC × 6 or FEC × 4 followed by 8 consecutive weeks of paclitaxel (100 mg/m^2); the addition of the taxane resulted in a 23% reduction in risk of recurrence, without a significant increase in toxicity (31). The taxotere as adjuvant chemotherapy (TACT) study, which also evaluated the addition of docetaxel to an anthracycline regimen, was designed to offer the same duration of treatment in either arm. This study randomized 4,162 node-positive or high-risk node-negative women to a control arm, either FEC × 8 or E × 4 CMF × 4, or FEC × 4 followed by docetaxel (100 mg/m^2 every 3 weeks) × 4. At 5 years, no significant differences were seen in either DFS or OS, however there was increased toxicity seen in the taxane-containing arm (32).

Concurrent anthracycline and taxane therapy has been evaluated primarily in two large randomized studies. The Breast Cancer International Research Group (BCIRG) 001 compared FAC × 6 (5-flourouracil 500 mg/m^2 IV, doxorubicin 50 mg/m^2 IV, and cyclophosphamide 500 mg/m^2 IV every 3 weeks), to six cycles of TAC (docetaxel 75 mg/m^2 IV, doxorubicin 50 mg/m^2 IV and cyclophosphamide 500 mg/m^2 IV every 3 weeks). At 5 years, the substitution of docetaxel for 5-fluorouracil resulted in significant improvements in DFS and OS; subgroup analysis demonstrated equivalent benefits regardless

Table 49.2	COMMONLY USED COMBINATION CHEMOTHERAPY REGIMENS FOR ADJUVANT TREATMENT OF BREAST CANCER

Regimen	Agents, Dose (mg/m²) and Schedule	Frequency	Number of Cycles
Oral CMF ("classic")	Cyclophosphamide 100, PO days 1–14; Methotrexate 40, IV days 1 and 8 Fluorouracil 600, IV days 1 and 8	Every 28 days	6
IV CMF	Cyclophosphamide 600, IV day 1 Methotrexate 40, IV day 1; Fluorouracil 600, IV day 1	Every 21 days	9–12
AC × 4	Doxorubicin 60, IV day 1 Cyclophosphamide 600, IV day 1	Every 21 days	4
TC × 4	Docetaxel 75, IV day 1 Cyclophosphamide 600, IV day 1	Every 21 days	4
CAF × 6 (oral)	Cyclophosphamide 100, PO days 1–14 Doxorubicin 30, IV days 1 and 8; Fluorouracil 600, IV days 1 and 8	Every 28 days	6
CAF × 6 (FAC)	Cyclophosphamide 500, IV day 1 Doxorubicin 50, IV day 1 Fluorouracil 500, IV day 1 OR Cyclophosphamide 500, IV days 1 and 8 Doxorubicin 50, CI over 72 hours Fluorouracil 500, IV day 1	Every 21–28 days	6
CEF (Oral, Canadian)	Cyclophosphamide 75, PO days 1–14 Epirubicin 60, IV days 1 and 8 Fluorouracil 500, IV days 1 and 8	Every 28 days	6
CEF (FEC)	Cyclophosphamide 500, IV day 1 Epirubicin 100, IV day 1 Fluorouracil 500, IV day 1	Every 21 days	6
A ≥ CMF	Cycles 1–4: Doxorubicin 75, IV day 1, cycles 1–4 Cycles 5–12: Cyclophosphamide 600, IV day 1; Methotrexate 40, IV day 1; Fluorouracil 600, IV day 1	Every 21 days	8
AC ≥ P	Cycles 1–4: Doxorubicin 60, IV day 1 Cyclophosphamide 600, IV day 1 Cycles 5–8: Paclitaxel 175, IV day 1	Every 21 days	8
A ≥ P ≥ C	Cycles 1–4: Doxorubicin 60, IV day 1 Cycles 5–8: Paclitaxel 175, IV day 1 Cycles 9–12: Cyclophosphamide 600, IV day 1	21	12
Dose-dense AC ≥ P	Cycles 1–4: Doxorubicin 60, IV day 1 Cyclophosphamide 600, IV day 1 Cycles 5–8: Paclitaxel 175, IV day 1 GCSF days 3–10, or peg-filgrastim day 2, cycles 1–8	Every 14 days	
Dose-dense A ≥ P ≥ C	Cycles 1–4: Doxorubicin 60, IV day 1 Cycles 5–8: Paclitaxel 175, IV day 1 Cycles 9–12: Cyclophosphamide 600, IV day 1 GCSF days 3–10, or peg-filgrastim day 2, cycles 1–8		
TAC	Cyclophosphamide 500, IV day 1 Doxorubicin 50, IV day 1 Docetaxel 75, IV day 1 GCSF days 3–10, or peg-filgrastim day 2, cycles 1–8	Every 21 days	6

A, doxorubicin; C, cyclophosphamide; F, fluorouracil; E, epirubicin; P, paclitaxel; T, docetaxel; GCSF, granulocyte colony stimulating factor.

Table 49.3	SIGNIFICANT RESULTS FROM TRIALS EVALUATING THE ROLE OF ADJUVANT TAXANE THERAPY

Sequential with Anthracycline Therapy

Study	Patient Type	Number	Arms	Median Follow-up (Months)	Relative Risk (Taxane/No Taxane) DFS OS
CALBG 9344 (27)	N+	3,121	AC vs. AC-P	60	0.83[a] 0.82[a]
NSABP B-28 (28)	N+	3,060	AC vs. AC-P	60	0.83[a] 0.93
PACS01 (30)	N+	1,999	FEC vs. FEC-T	60	0.82[a] 0.73[a]
GEICAM 9906 (31)	N+	1,246	FEC vs. FEC-P	66	0.77[a] 0.78
TACT (32)	N+ or high risk N−	4,162	FEC vs. E-CMF vs. FEC-T	51.8	0.97 0.98

Concurrent with, or Replacing, Anthracycline Therapy

Study	Patient Type	Number	Arms	Median Follow-up (Months)	Relative Risk (Taxane/No Taxane)
BCIRG 001 (33)	N+	1,491	FAC vs. TAC	55	0.72[a] 0.70[a]
ECOG 2197 (34)	N+ or high risk N−	2,885	AC vs. AT	59	1.03 1.09
U.S. Oncology (35)	N+ or high risk N−	1,016	AC vs. TC	84	0.69[a] 0.73[a]

N+, node positive; N−, node negative; A, doxorubicin; C, cyclophosphamide; F, fluorouracil; E, epirubicin; P, paclitaxel; T, docetaxel.
[a]Statistically significant.

of hormone receptor subtype (33). Concurrent anthracycline and taxane therapy was also examined in ECOG 2197, in which 2,952 patients were randomized to AC × 4 versus AT (doxorubicin 60 mg/m² IV, doxetaxel, 60 mg/m² IV) × 4 (docetaxel 60 mg/m² IV). Results at 5 years demonstrated no difference in DFS or OS between the arms, with greater toxicity on at AT arm (34).

In the first trial to evaluate the replacement of an anthracycline with a taxane, the U.S. Oncology clinical trials group compared AC × 4 with TC (docetaxel 75 mg/m², cyclophosphamide 600 mg/m² every 3 weeks) × 4 in 1,016 women with predominantly stage I-II breast cancer. Analysis at 7 years of follow-up has demonstrated improvements in both DFS (85% vs. 79%, $p = .018$) and OS (88% vs. 84%, $p = .045$) for TC over AC (35). Toxicity analysis has highlighted the differential toxicity profile between these two regimens, with more febrile neutropenia, myalgia, and arthralgia with TC, and more nausea and risk of cardiac events or myeloid neoplasia with AC. TC is an important addition to the standard chemotherapy repertoire, but it is not clear how it will compare to third-generation regimens, such as dose-dense AC + T or TAC × 6. CALGB 40101, a 2 by 2 factorial randomization between dose dense AC × 4, AC × 6, paclitaxel × 4, and paclitaxel × 6 may provide yet another taxane-based alternative regimen for node-negative or low-risk node-positive disease.

Schedule of taxane administration appears to be relevant to both efficacy and toxicity. ECOG 1199 randomized 4,950 patients in a 2 by 2 fashion to four different schedules of adjuvant taxane therapy after completion of four cycles of standard AC for node-positive disease: paclitaxel 175 mg/m² every 3 weeks × 4, paclitaxel 80 mg/m² weekly for 12 weeks, docetaxel 100 mg/m² every 3 weeks × 4, or docetaxel 35 mg/m² weekly for 12 weeks. Results demonstrated 5-year DFS rates of 76.9% for paclitaxel every 3 weeks, 81.5% for weekly paclitaxel, 81.2% for docetaxel every 3 weeks, and 77.6% for weekly docetaxel. Both the weekly paclitaxel and the every-3-week docetaxel arms demonstrated statistically significant improvements in DFS compared with the every-3-week paclitaxel arm. Overall survival was significantly improved in only the weekly paclitaxel arm compared with the every-3-week paclitaxel arm. Toxicities were increased in the docetaxel arms, especially hematologic toxicity, leading to significantly fewer cycles of

therapy completed in the weekly docetaxel arm (36). These findings highlight the importance of the chemotherapy schedule and suggest weekly paclitaxel may be a desirable choice for future studies. The application of a dose-dense administration has also been favorable, discussed further below.

Meta-analyses have been performed to better define the role of the taxanes in adjuvant therapy. A contemporary meta-analysis of 14 randomized studies evaluating the addition of a taxane to an anthracycline-based adjuvant regimen has demonstrated a pooled highly significant reduction in both risk of recurrence (17% relative reduction) and OS (15% relative improvement) among the trials, regardless of taxane used (37). The EBCTCG has also evaluated the contribution of taxanes in the adjuvant setting. Data presented at the 2007 San Antonio Breast Cancer Symposium suggested highly significant improvements in both DFS and OS from the addition of taxane versus no chemotherapy, independent of hormone receptor status or age (38).

Despite the accumulation of data evaluating the role of taxanes in the management of early-stage breast cancer, many questions remain about their use in the adjuvant therapy. Protocol treatment with taxanes has been heterogeneous, because some trials have explored monotherapy, either before or after standard regimens, and others have incorporated the taxanes into new combinations. In addition, the duration of taxane exposure and dosing has varied across trials. At this time, no solid data suggest that one taxane is better than another from the standpoint of efficacy. There is the suggestion however, of differences in toxicity, as seen in ECOG 1199. Because most of the studies performed were conducted in individuals with positive axillary lymph nodes, questions have also focused on the role of the taxanes, and particularly regimens containing both anthracyclines and taxanes, in the node-negative or lower risk populations. Overall, the inclusion of a taxane in an adjuvant regimen appears to result in an improvement in outcomes in most studies; as described above, however, the results across studies are not entirely consistent. Although the taxanes are widely used and are incorporated into most adjuvant chemotherapy regimens, the incremental benefit associated with taxane use in unselected populations remains modest.

Multiple ongoing studies will continue to address the role of taxanes in adjuvant therapy. NSABP B-30 will compare sequential versus concurrent use of taxanes in a three-arm design: AC × 4 + T × 4 (docetaxel 100 mg/m² IV) every 3 weeks, versus AT (docetaxel 60 mg/m² IV) × 4 every 3 weeks, versus TAC × 4 every 3 weeks. In BCIRG 005, women with node-positive disease will be randomized to AC × 4 every 3 weeks + docetaxel × 4 every 3 weeks versus TAC × 6 every 3 weeks. The U.S. Oncology group is comparing the standard TAC regimen versus TC, with the goal of evaluating the role of doxorubicin in the context of modern chemotherapy with a taxane. In addition, multiple other studies continue to accrue or have recently completed accrual asking a range of questions. The role of the taxanes in the adjuvant setting will continue to evolve based on the results of the trials that will be reported in the next several years.

 ## CONSIDERATIONS RELATED TO DOSE AND SCHEDULING OF CHEMOTHERAPY

Dose Intensity

Initial observation from the early adjuvant trials suggested increased dose intensity, meaning provision of a higher dose of chemotherapy per dose or cycle, might provide additional benefit from a chemotherapy agent (39). Multiple trials were subsequently initiated evaluating outcomes with increased dose. CALGB 8541 evaluated three doses of CAF chemotherapy in 1,550 patients, randomized to three different levels of total dose and dose intensity of CAF chemotherapy. Results at 9 years demonstrated improvements in DFS and OS for the moderate and higher dose arms compared with the lower dose arm, and suggested, "more is better" (40). Similarly, FASG 05 demonstrated six cycles of FEC 100 to be better than six cycles of FEC 50 (41). Subsequently, NSABP B22 and B25 evaluated escalation of cyclophosphamide doses from the standard 600 mg/m² up to 2,400 mg/m². In neither trial was an improvement in outcomes observed, and a substantial increase in cases of myeloproliferative disorders, including acute leukemia, was observed in B25 (42,43). CALGB 9344 evaluated three doses of doxorubicin, 60 mg/m², 75 mg/m², and 90 mg/m² administered with a fixed dose of cyclophosphamide, and failed to demonstrate any improvement in outcome with higher doses, although there was a clear increase in toxicity (27). There has also been interest in establishing the appropriate duration of treatment. FASG 01 evaluated three different FEC-based regimens of different dose and duration; long-term follow-up of the 620 patients suggested six cycles, rather than three, was superior, regardless of epirubicin dose (44).

A number of trials have evaluated the role of myeloablative adjuvant regimens requiring autologous bone marrow or peripheral stem cell rescue. Despite promising phase II results, randomized trials have failed to demonstrate a clear benefit in disease-free or overall survival for the use of high-dose chemotherapy with stem cell support. A recent meta-analysis of 15 studies with more than 6,000 patients has demonstrated that, despite significant prolongation in DFS with myeloablative regimens, only minimal benefits in either breast cancer-specific or overall survival have been observed, with no specific benefits by age or hormone receptor subgroups (45). Given these findings, and the lack of comparison of high-dose regimens with contemporary taxane-containing regimens or trastuzumab-containing regimens (for those with ERBB2-positive tumors), high-dose myeloablative treatments do not have a role in adjuvant therapy for any patient subgroup.

Dose Density

Dose density refers to the administration of standard doses of chemotherapy with shorter intertreatment intervals, often with the use of growth factor support. The rationale for dose density is based on the concept of Gomperztian growth, which essentially suggests that small tumors grow more rapidly than larger tumors. Norton (46) and Simon hypothesized that if the cytotoxicity of chemotherapy depended on cell growth rates, then chemotherapy would be more effective for smaller rather than larger tumors. Thus, tumors given less chance to regrow between treatments will experience a greater fractional reduction in tumor cells with each chemotherapy dose, leading to a greater overall benefit (46). Early clinical evaluation of this concept, utilizing growth factor support to maintain scheduling, demonstrated that dose-dense therapy was clinically active and feasible. An Italian phase III study randomized 1,214 patients to six cycles of traditional FEC every 3 weeks versus FEC every 2 weeks. At a median follow-up of 10 years, although no statistically significant differences in progression free survival (PFS) or OS were observed, a suggestion of benefit was seen in ER-negative, ERBB2 positive, and younger age subgroups, with no sign of significant long-term adverse events (47). The result of an Italian study led by Bonadonna also supported the dose-dense hypothesis. In this trial, 400 node-positive women were randomized to either sequential A × 4 followed by CMF × 8 versus A and CMF given in alternating fashion. Although the same total dose of drug was given in each arm, the sequential arm, in which treatment was given in a more dose-dense fashion, demonstrated improved DFS and OS (39).

CALGB 9741 evaluated dose density within the context of a taxane-based treatment approach. In this trial, 2,005 node-positive patients were randomized in a 2 by 2 factorial design to concurrent arms of every-3-week AC and T versus every-2-week AC and T, and similar sequential arms with 3-week and 2-week intervals. Growth factor support was utilized to allow the more frequent administration of chemotherapy. The administration of every-2-week combination therapy was superior to standard every-3-week combination therapy, both in terms of DFS and OS. No differences in end points were observed between sequential and concurrent schedules (48). Based on the results of CALGB 9741, the dose-dense AC + T regimen has become commonly used in the United States, and is being compared with the TAC regimen as part of NSABP B38.

The NCIC MA.21 also evaluated a dose-dense, taxane-based regimen. In this three-arm trial, 2,104 patients were randomized to every-3-week AC + T, CEF × 6, or dose-dense EC + T. Analysis at a median follow-up of 30 months has suggested the AC + T regimen to be inferior to either CEF or dose dense EC + T. Although the study is not a pure test of the dose-dense hypothesis, it does confirm the inferiority of every-3-weeks AC followed by paclitaxel, and supports the concept that dose-dense regimens have a role in adjuvant treatment (49).

 ## WHICH PATIENTS BENEFIT FROM ADJUVANT CHEMOTHERAPY?

One of the greatest advances in the past decade in the understanding of breast cancer is the identification of distinct biologic tumor subgroups. Based on immunohistochemical techniques, breast cancers can be divided into essentially three subgroups: (a) ERBB2-positive disease, (b) so-called "triple negative disease" (ER, PR, ERBB2-negative); and (c) ER-positive, ERBB2-negative disease. The latter group is particularly heterogeneous and can be subdivided into two or more groups based on grade, markers of proliferation, and multigene assays. Although our understanding of these subgroups continues to evolve, the groups appear to be somewhat distinct biologic entities, both in terms of pattern of recurrence and response to treatment. The subgroups defined by immunohistochemical stains correlate closely with subgroups identified by microarray analyses. Such investigations have typically identified five distinct biologic subgroups: two hormone receptor-positive groups, designated luminal A and B; an ERBB2-positive group, typically hormone receptor-negative; a "basal-like" group, typically triple negative for all growth receptors; and a "normal-like" group (50,51). Relatively small studies have suggested that long-term outcomes, including risks of disease recurrence, appear to correlate with biologic subtype defined by microarray (50,51). Chapter 32 provides a more extended discussion of this topic.

Estrogen Receptor Status and Benefit from Chemotherapy

As demonstrated in the *Overview Analysis*, absolute benefits from chemotherapy for both younger and older women appear to be most significant in ER-negative populations (16). The first report from the *2005 Overview Analysis*, described in Table 49.1, has focused on the ER-negative group, now comprising 20,000 women (18). In the primary analysis of polychemotherapy versus no adjuvant treatment, a 33% relative reduction in risk of recurrence was observed at 10 years, corresponding to absolute reductions of 12.3% for those less than 50 years of age and 9.2% for those 50 to 69 years of age. Significant benefits in reduction of breast cancer-specific mortality were also observed in all age groups, with absolute benefits at 10 years of 8.6% for those less than 50 years and 6.1% for those 50 to 69 years. This recent analysis would argue that prior studies looking at benefit by age without adjustment for ER status may have erroneously suggested that age, in and of itself, plays an important role in determining the benefit from treatment. Increasingly, most breast cancer investigators believe that tumor biology, and not age, are most important in predicting benefit. Since the *Overview* data comparing chemotherapy with control reflects the use of older chemotherapy regimens, it is likely that more contemporary regimens provide even more significant benefits in reduction of recurrence and death in patient populations that are sensitive to chemotherapy.

Additional retrospective evaluations have attempted to better define the target population that receives the greatest benefit from chemotherapy. A review of three CALGB node-positive adjuvant studies has evaluated the selective benefits of escalating the dose of anthracycline, the addition of taxane, and the addition of dose density. As demonstrated in Figure 49.1, with each of these modern improvements, a significantly greater benefit was realized in the ER-negative subset compared with the ER-positive subset, with overall improvements in DFS and OS of 23% versus 7%, and 17% versus 4%, respectively. Importantly, much of the benefit from adjuvant chemotherapy in the ER-negative subset was realized in the first 2 to 3 years after treatment, an important observation given the propensity of these tumors to recur during that time period. Patients with ER-positive tumors received benefit in the first few years after diagnosis; however, the absolute benefit was substantially smaller.

In recent years, there has been considerable debate about the identification of appropriate populations for taxane treatment. The CALGB analysis identified the ER-negative subset as deriving substantially more benefit from adjuvant taxanes than the ER positive (52), whereas this relationship has not been consistent across trials. In contrast to the CALGB experience, a subset analysis from BCIRG 001, comparing FAC and TAC, showed the addition of the taxane to be of importance in both ER-positive and negative populations. No significant differences were found between the two arms in the proportion of patients with either ER-positive tumors or premenopausal status; however, it is possible that chemotherapy-induced premature ovarian failure occurred more frequently on the TAC arm, leading to improved outcomes in ER-positive patients. This potential outcome could confound comparisons by hormone receptor status, leading to difficulty in determining if observed benefits arose from the chemotherapy itself or its impact on ovarian function (33). Of interest, ECOG 1199 also failed to demonstrate a relationship between either ER or ERBB2 status and the benefits of weekly paclitaxel over every-3-week therapy (36). The *2005 Overview Analysis* demonstrates an overall

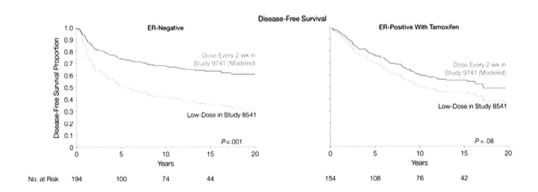

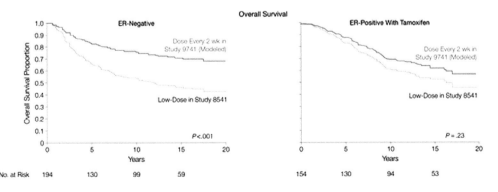

FIGURE 49.1. Comparison of disease-free and overall survival for patients in the National Surgical Adjuvant Breast and Bowel Project (NSABP) 8541 (low-dose cyclophosphamide, doxorubicin [Adriamycin], and fluorouracil [CAF]) versus Cancer and Leukemia Group B (CALGB) 9741 (dose-dense doxorubicin, cyclophosphamide, and paclitaxel) (52). Comparison by estrogen receptor (ER) status demonstrates the addition of dose density and taxanes to adjuvant regimens leads to significant benefit in the ER-negative subset. (Copyright © 2006, American Medical Association, all rights reserved.)

benefit from the addition of taxanes to an anthracycline regimen of any strength (RR 0.83). Comparison of taxane versus no chemotherapy suggests overall benefits for women younger than 50 years and those 50 to 60 years in risk of recurrence (RR 0.38 for <50 years of age, 0.52 for those 50 to 60 years) and in mortality for all ages (RR 0.46 for <50 years, 0.66 for 50 to 60 years); these benefits were significant in both ER-positive and ER-negative subsets (38). In the meta-analysis of the 14 randomized taxane trials, analysis by subgroup also has demonstrated equivalent benefits regardless of ER status, number of affected nodes, or age or menopausal status (37). Although the subgroup analyses based on hormone receptor status are inconsistent, overall the taxanes appear to provide benefit in patients with both ER-positive and negative disease.

Overall, although there is the strong suggestion of a differential benefit based on ER status, many women with ER-positive tumors derive benefit from adjuvant chemotherapy. The data suggest that a different threshold should be used when recommending adjuvant chemotherapy in *unselected patients* with ER-negative and positive tumors. Women with ER-positive tumors face a relatively constant risk of disease recurrence that extends beyond the first several years after a diagnosis, but chemotherapy has a relatively limited impact on these late recurrences. Instead, chemotherapy primarily decreases the risk of early relapse, which is often a lesser concern in many women with ER-positive disease. The differential benefit from chemotherapy (in absolute terms) in women with receptor-negative versus receptor-positive disease underscores the need to develop more robust predictors of chemotherapy benefit, particularly in patients with ER-positive breast cancer, a topic discussed further in Chapter 32. If a decision is made to administer chemotherapy, it does not appear that ER status can be used to select an optimal regimen and, in particular, should not be used in making a decision whether or not to include a taxane in the regimen.

ERBB2 Status and Benefit from Chemotherapy

Retrospective analysis of several large trials has suggested that patients whose tumors overexpress ERBB2 by immunohistochemistry or have ERBB2 gene amplification obtain greater benefit from anthracycline-containing adjuvant regimens. Analyses of data from both NSABP B-11 and B-15, which evaluated the introduction of anthracycline-based regimens, suggest that patients with ERBB2 overexpressing tumors potentially derive greater advantages in recurrence-free and overall survival with anthracycline-based therapy compared with those with ERBB2-negative tumors (53,54). Similarly, retrospective analysis of outcomes in CALGB 8541, a study of escalating doses of anthracyclines in the CAF regimen, has suggested that higher doses of anthracyclines were particularly beneficial in patients with ERBB2-positive tumors; the effect was seen whether ERBB2 was assessed by immunohistochemistry or gene amplication (55,56). Finally, analysis of the NCI-C MA.5 trial of CMF versus CEF by ERBB2 status has also demonstrated significantly improved benefits with the use of anthracyclines in patients with ERBB2-positive tumors (57). The biologic basis of increased anthracycline sensitivity in ERBB2-positive tumors may reflect coamplification of the topoisomerase 2 gene, which sits in close proximity to ERBB2 on chromosome 17q and is a target of anthracycline activity (58). Whether an anthracycline-based regimen is required for the management of ERBB2-positive disease is not confirmed by prospective studies (59); this topic is discussed further in Chapter 51.

The role of the taxanes in ERBB2-positive disease has also been the subject of several retrospective analyses. A secondary analysis of CALGB 9344 has evaluated the response to taxane therapy by ERBB2 status. Using a subgroup of 1,300 original samples from the study, ERBB2 status was determined and outcomes analyzed based on ER and ERBB2 status. In this analysis, as demonstrated in Figure 49.2, improved DFS and OS

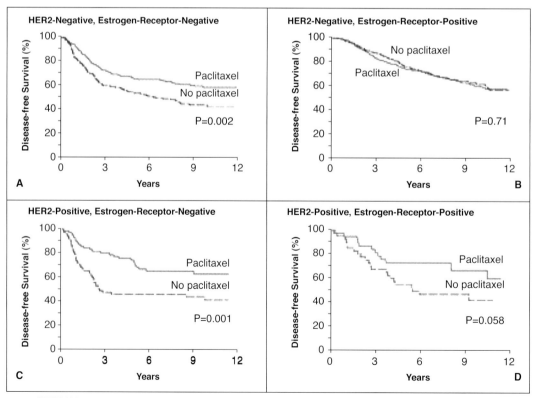

FIGURE 49.2. Disease-free survival among patients treated with or without paclitaxel according to estrogen receptor (ER) status and ERBB2 expression (60). Subgroup analysis of 1,322 patients participating in Cancer and Leukemia Group B (CALGB) 9344 by ER and ERBB2 status demonstrating significant benefits from the addition of paclitaxel in the ER-negative and ERBB2-positive populations. (Copyright © 2007, Massachusetts Medical Society, all rights reserved.)

were observed in the ERBB2 subset with the addition of the taxane, independent of ER status (60). Indeed, the benefit of taxane treatment was greater in patients with ERBB2-positive disease than other subsets. The BCIRG trial of TAC versus FAC also suggested a benefit for docetaxel in patients with ERBB2-positive disease, although a clear benefit was also seen in patients with ERBB2-negative disease (29). Subgroup analysis in GEICAM 9906 has demonstrated no interaction between benefit from the addition of the taxane and either ER or ERBB2 status (31). At this time, a decision to include or omit a taxane cannot be based on the ERBB2 status of the tumor. Furthermore, with the widespread use of trastuzumab in the adjuvant setting, retrospective studies examining the benefits of the taxanes without trastuzumab are of diminishing relevance to current clinical practice.

TREATMENT OF "LOWER RISK" DISEASE

Older studies of adjuvant therapy for breast cancer generally divided patient groups by anatomic features, including tumor size and, in particular, nodal status. More recently, boundaries have been less binary, with many studies including node-negative patients along with those who have one to three positive nodes. Other studies have combined patients with node-positive disease and so-called *high-risk* node-negative, a term that is used without uniform definition. Heterogeneity exists within the node-positive and negative populations, and subgroups of patients with node-positive breast cancer have a more favorable prognosis than many women with node-negative disease. As best we know, nodal status does not play a predictive role in identifying the most effective treatment, but it is clearly of prognostic significance, and several somewhat less-intensive regimens have been evaluated in patients with negative lymph nodes, or those with a small number of positive nodes. Because of the lower absolute risk of recurrence and death, the absolute benefits of chemotherapy are generally less in individuals with node-negative disease than node-positive disease as long as one controls for subtype (e.g., ERBB2 positive vs. not, ER-positive vs. not) and other biologic features, such as grade. Regimens studied in patients with node-positive disease may, in some cases, be appropriate in the node-negative setting, particularly if biologic features of the disease suggest a higher risk of disease recurrence or a greater potential benefit from treatment (as would be expected in the setting of patient with an ER-negative, ERBB2-positive tumor, or both).

Population-based studies have demonstrated the heterogeneity of outcomes in the node-negative population. Chia et al. (61) evaluated 10-year outcomes in a cohort of 1,187 patients with T1-T2, N0 tumors not treated with adjuvant therapy from 1989 to 1991. In their analysis, increasing tumor size was associated with increased risk of recurrence, as was higher tumor grade. Recurrence events continued through years 5 to 10, underscoring the need to obtain long-term follow-up of breast cancer patients. For very small tumors less than 1 cm, the rate of relapse at 10 years was 18%, and among those patients with grade 3 tumors, the risk of relapse was 26%, underscoring the more aggressive phenotype of this subset of small tumors. It must be pointed out, however, that a substantial number of the recurrences in the Chia cohort, as is the case in most clinical trials, were actually in-breast recurrences or new primaries in the contralateral breast. For example, among women with tumors less than 1 cm, greater than half of the first events were local, rather than distant (61). Because the goal of adjuvant therapy is largely to reduce the risk of life-threatening recurrence, it will be important for future trials to clearly delineate end points (62). Amar et al. (63) have also examined outcomes in small (≤1 cm) node-negative tumors, focusing on predictors of poor prognosis. In a cohort of 400

cases, ERBB2-positive or ER−/PR−/ERBB2− ("triple negative") tumors had a significantly higher rate of relapse, despite increased use of adjuvant chemotherapy in these patient subgroups. These data have been confirmed by a retrospective analysis of almost 1000 patients with stage 1 cancer which highlighted higher risks of recurrence in ERBB2 positive subsets (63a). These studies highlight the importance of identifying smaller tumors that are nevertheless biologically aggressive and place patients at higher risk of disease recurrence. A major research priority in the next decade is to optimize the treatment of these patients without routinely over-treating all women with small tumors.

Several regimens are often used in the management of patients who are considered to be at lower absolute risk of disease recurrence, including AC × 4, TC × 4, and traditional CMF. These regimens are not intended for patients who are thought to have chemotherapy-unresponsive disease (see Chapters 48 and 50 on endocrine therapy and chemoendocrine therapy), but are intended for those likely to benefit from chemotherapy but with a relatively low absolute risk of disease recurrence, particularly if there is a desire to limit the duration of treatment and the toxicity of the chemotherapy program. Although the regimens mentioned above are not without side effects and risks, they are generally less toxic than the third-generation treatment programs that contain both a taxane and an anthracycline.

DECISION-MAKING WITH ADJUVANT CHEMOTHERAPY

Given the extraordinary recent advances in the understanding of breast cancer classification and biology, decision-making about adjuvant chemotherapy must consider both anatomic features, such as size and lymph node status, and biologic features, including ER status, ERBB2 status, and pathologic grade. Decisions regarding use of adjuvant chemotherapy are based both on the estimated risk of recurrence, and the benefit of adjuvant therapy. Multiple published guidelines exist, including those from the National Comprehensive Care Network (NCCN) (64) and the St. Gallen Consensus (65). Although the guidelines are updated regularly, recommendations are sometimes conflicting. Furthermore, guidelines cannot account for all tumor and patient variables. An analysis of treatment patterns in the recent past at participating NCCN sites demonstrated that only slightly more than half of patients received treatment that was in keeping with published guidelines at the time, and significant heterogeneity existed across institutions (66). More recently, many published guidelines have sought to include greater flexibility to account for the evolving understanding of breast cancer biology. If anything, however, this change places greater responsibility on the physician who must consider a range of factors in developing a recommendation for adjuvant chemotherapy.

Patient preferences are central to decisions about adjuvant therapy. Communication regarding the benefits of adjuvant therapy can be complex. Patient preferences may differ from what oncologists might expect, and are also highly variable. In general, surveys of breast cancer survivors have demonstrated not only overestimation of the value of adjuvant chemotherapy, but also acceptance of adjuvant chemotherapy for very small benefits in reduction of recurrence or death from disease (67–69). Such studies highlight the need for clear patient–physician communication in making choices about adjuvant therapy. Figure 49.3 graphically demonstrates the need to balance risks of recurrence, potential tumor sensitivity to treatment, and patient preferences in making individualized decisions about adjuvant chemotherapy.

Computerized modeling has improved the ability to predict risks of future breast cancer events and to provide more accurate and personalized estimates of benefit from therapy.

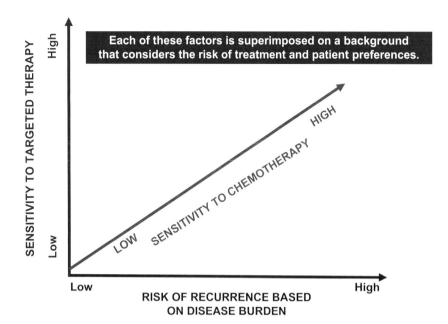

FIGURE 49.3. Factors to consider when individualizing chemotherapy decisions. (Adapted with permission from HJ Burstein.)

Adjuvant! is an online decision tool that uses information-derived from Surveillance, Epidemiology and End Results (SEER) databases, meta-analyses, and individual studies to calculate the risks of disease recurrence and death for patients both with and without adjuvant therapies. The estimates incorporate both the specific characteristics of the tumor and competing health risks of the patient (70). Population-based validation has confirmed the value of this tool in general practice, although the inability to adjust estimates based on additional risk factors, such as lymphovascular invasion and ERBB2 status, limits its use in some situations (71). Continuous updating of the web application has allowed Adjuvant! to remain a valuable tool for many practicing clinicians.

The availability of individualized genomic analysis of tumors has opened new opportunities to individualize adjuvant therapy, but has also added new complexities to the process of decision-making. Analysis and quantification of gene expression appear to predict outcome and, in some cases, the potential benefit of adjuvant chemotherapy. These types of analyses are reviewed as well in Chapter 32. The Oncotype DX™ assay is a 21-gene panel performed on paraffin-fixed tissue by reverse transcription-polymerase chain reaction (RT-PCR) analysis; a complex algorithm is utilized to derive the Recurrence Score. The test was validated using the tumor materials from the node-negative, ER-positive breast cancer population treated with tamoxifen in NSABP B14. This analysis demonstrated that the Recurrence Score was an independent and continuous predictor of both disease recurrence and survival (72). Further analysis using tumor materials from NSABP B20, which randomized patients with node negative, ER-positive disease to tamoxifen alone or tamoxifen plus chemotherapy, demonstrates that Oncotype DX may be predictive of chemotherapy benefit, as demonstrated graphically in Figure 49.4 (73). In patients with node-negative disease whose tumors have low Recurrence Scores, chemotherapy appears to add little, if any, benefit. For these women, many believe that the toxicities of chemotherapy can now be avoided and the focus can turn to the optimization of endocrine treatment. Individuals with intermediate Recurrence Scores derive unknown benefits from chemotherapy, and the prospective Trial Assigning IndividuaLized Options for Treatment (Rx) (TAILORX) study will attempt to better define populations of patients with inter-mediate scores who may or may not need adjuvant chemotherapy treatment. In contrast, women who have tumors with a high score appear to derive substantial benefit from a course of chemotherapy. Analysis of tumor tissue from node-positive studies indicates Oncotype DX testing may be of value in these populations as well (74,75).

Other genomic analyses are in more limited use because of the need for fresh frozen tumor tissue for analysis. The Mammoprint™ assay is a 70-gene expression profile analysis able to dichotomize stage I and II breast cancer into low- and high-risk signatures. Analysis of a cohort of frozen tumor samples has demonstrated the Mammoprint profile to be an independent predictor of disease outcome and survival (76,77). Although the requirement for fresh tissue limits the clinical utility of this test, a potential advantage is the lack of an intermediate category of unclear clinical significance. Although most tumors that were considered to have a good signature were ER-positive, a small number of ER-negative tumors did fall within this category. The initial work with 70-gene signature also included both node-negative and node-positive tumors. The Mammoprint assay has been approved by the U.S. Food and Drug Administration (FDA), and the Microarray in Node Negative Disease may Avoid ChemoTherapy (MINDACT) study will prospectively evaluate the utility of the Mammoprint assay in determining suitability for adjuvant chemotherapy. Other independent genomic predictors of outcome have also been identified (78,79).

An analysis of the performance of the available genomic tools using a single set of tumor samples has demonstrated remarkable concordance in their ability to identify higher risks of recurrence, suggesting despite their disparate individual genes, these tools can consistently identify biologic pathways leading to differential growth patterns. Multivariate analysis from this study suggests these tools provide prognostic information independent of standard pathologic factors, including tumor grade (80). It is still not clear to what extent the results of genomic assays add to the deliberations of a thoughtful clinician who has access to high-quality interpretation of ER, PR, ERBB2, and tumor grade. In all likelihood, genomic predictors add another dimension and enhance decision-making about adjuvant therapy, but ongoing studies continue to evaluate the utility of these tests in clinical practice.

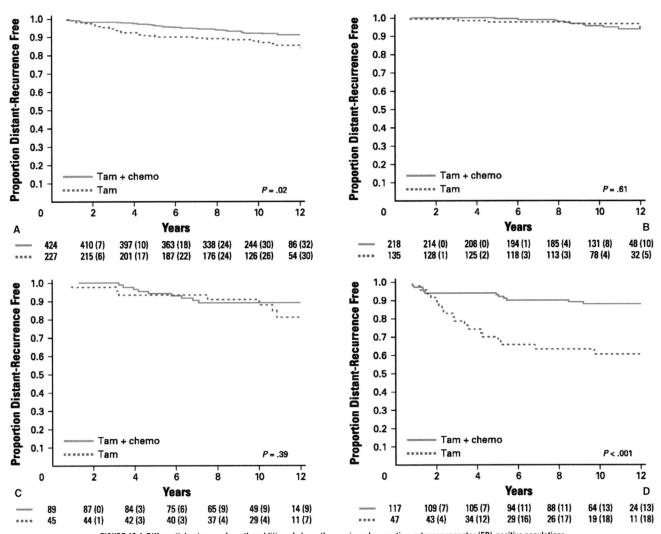

FIGURE 49.4. Differential outcomes from the addition of chemotherapy in node-negative, estrogen receptor (ER)-positive populations segregated by Recurrence Score (RS) category. Distant recurrence comparing treatment with tamoxifen (Tam) alone versus treatment with tamoxifen plus chemotherapy (Tam + chemo). **A**: All patients. **B**: Low risk (RS < 8). **C**: Intermediate risk (RS 18–30). **D**: High risk (RS ≥31) (73). (Reprinted with permission from the American Society of Clinical Oncology.)

SPECIAL POPULATIONS

Certain special populations are not well represented in most large clinical trials, leading to additional challenges in defining treatment plans. Very young breast cancer patients, defined as age less than 35 years, more commonly present with aggressive, ER-negative tumors (81). Although age under 35 has been considered an independent predictor of poor outcome (82), it is unclear if young age would remain an important predictor of outcome if an analysis accurately controlled for tumor biology and physiologic response to treatment. Because most young women have tumors that are either ER-negative, ERBB2-positive, or high-grade, adjuvant chemotherapy is generally an integral part of the treatment program. In support of this approach, a Danish analysis of outcomes in younger women suggests in women not receiving adjuvant chemotherapy, risk of relapse increases with decreasing age; this effect was not observed in cohorts receiving adjuvant chemotherapy (83). Further evaluation of chemotherapy effects by ER status suggests differential survival outcomes for ER-positive and ER-negative patients, perhaps because very young women with ER-positive cancers do not experience the ovarian suppression from chemotherapy that

is commonly seen in older premenopausal women. Future studies should focus more specifically on the interactions between young age, ER positivity, and response to treatment (84).

In contrast, there is a tendency among oncologists toward undertreatment of older women (>70 years) (85–87) Few older women have been evaluated in the context of adjuvant clinical trials, therefore little is known about our ability to extrapolate results from the *Overview Analysis* to the population of women in their 70s and 80s. Review of data from four CALGB studies has demonstrated clear benefits from the use of adjuvant chemotherapy in reducing risk of relapse in older populations (88). The toxicity profile of chemotherapy differs by age, with more hematologic toxicity in older patients, and greater risk of treatment-related death (89). Treatment decisions in older woman must be individualized, and consider not only tumor characteristics but also comorbid conditions and potential life expectancy. Given the aging of the U.S. population, prospective clinical trials targeting the older population, such as CALGB 49907, are certainly needed. In this study, 633 women older than 65 years were randomized to standard chemotherapy with either AC × 4 or CMF × 6 (at the discretion of the physician and patient) versus oral capecitabine therapy. The investigational arm in CALGB 49907 was thought to be a better-tolerated regimen and many investigators hypothesized that it would be as efficacious as standard therapy. Contrary to this hypothesis, the study demonstrated that capecitabine was relatively toxic in this setting, and, more importantly, led to statistically significantly worse outcome in terms of DFS and OS. The inferior outcome with capecitabine was particularly dramatic in patients with ER-negative disease (90). Further information on the treatment of younger and older patients with breast cancer is available in Chapters 91–92.

TOXICITY OF TREATMENT

With the advent of superior antiemetic therapy and growth factor support, the experience of receiving adjuvant chemotherapy has improved substantially over the past decades. Potential toxicities of adjuvant chemotherapy can be acute, occurring during the time of administration of agents, or long term, appearing months to years after treatment is completed. Overall, the decision to provide adjuvant therapy needs to be balanced against any potential short- or long-term risks incurred by the treatment. Potential toxicities are discussed here briefly; for further discussion of long-term toxicity, please refer to Chapter 55.

Most chemotherapy-related toxicities depend on the chemotherapy agents used, and tend to be of moderate severity. Only in rare instances are there severe or life-threatening problems. Characteristic side effects include nausea, alopecia, fatigue, myelosuppression, and anemia. Hematologic toxicity tends to be more pronounced with the use of dose-dense regimens and frequently requires the concomitant use of growth factors (91). Anthracycline-based therapy is more often associated with mucositis, rash, or gastrointestinal disturbance, whereas taxane treatment can be accompanied by neuropathy, myalgias, and hypersensitivity reactions. Most acute chemotherapy-related toxicity resolves within the weeks to months following completion of the regimen.

Other adverse effects of chemotherapy linger for months to years after treatment is complete. Weight gain has been commonly reported during adjuvant chemotherapy and following its completion; the cause of this finding is likely multifactorial, including changes in activity level and metabolic rate, the use of glucocorticoid therapy, and flux in hormonal levels (92–94). Many women also experience fatigue, with 20% reporting symptoms persistent for years after completion of treatment (95). Several factors appear to contribute to fatigue, including longer treatments, comorbid conditions, and depression; more recent work has also suggested elevations in proinflammatory cytokines and disorder of the hypothalamic-pituitary axis may contribute to the symptomatology (96). Other long-term toxicities, including cardiac dysfunction, neurocognitive changes, and secondary cancers, are discussed further in Chapter 55, and the effect of adjuvant chemotherapy on ovarian function and fertility is discussed in Chapter 96. Individual variation in drug metabolism can alter the risk of toxicity, and evolving pharmacogenetic research may soon assist in identification of those at risk of chemotherapy-related toxicity, discussed further in Chapter 56. It is hoped that improved future understanding of the mechanisms and etiology of chemotherapy-related toxicity may enhance individual tailoring of adjuvant therapy as well as supportive care.

NOVEL TREATMENT APPROACHES

In addition to the standard chemotherapy-based regimens discussed above, the advent of targeted therapy has heralded the entry of these biologic agents into the adjuvant setting. One of the most significant advances in the past decade in the adjuvant treatment of breast cancer has been the addition of adjuvant trastuzumab into adjuvant regimens for ERBB2-positive patients. Adjuvant treatment of ERBB2-positive disease is discussed further

in Chapter 51. Bevacizumab (B), a humanized monoclonal antibody against vascular endothelial growth factor (VEGF) has an established role in the treatment of metastatic breast cancer, and is discussed further in Chapter 78 (97). A pilot study has demonstrated that the administration of bevacizumab is feasible in the adjuvant setting (98). ECOG 5103 is a three-arm, phase III, placebo-controlled, double-blinded trial that will randomize 5,000 node-positive or high-risk, node-negative women to either AC and placebo plus weekly T and placebo, AC and placebo plus weekly TB, or ACB plus weekly TB. After treatment is completed, the arms will be unblinded and the third arm will receive an additional 30 weeks of single agent bevacizumab every 3 weeks. Multiple other novel biologic agents, including VEGF receptor antagonists (e.g., sunitinib) and new chemotherapy agents (e.g., ixabepilone), are in testing in the metastatic breast cancer setting, and will likely be evaluated as part of future adjuvant chemotherapy trials.

Considerable interest also is seen in improving the treatment of triple negative breast cancers, which often possess an aggressive phenotype and poor prognosis (50). Preclinical data have suggested a potential role for platinum chemotherapy for this subset of tumors (99), and platinum agents may be examined in future adjuvant studies. It is hoped that identification of new therapeutic targets in triple negative breast cancers may improve the ability to treat this aggressive disease.

FUTURE DIRECTIONS

Over the past 40 years, substantial advances have been made in the treatment of patients with early-stage breast cancer. Adjuvant treatment and, in particular, adjuvant chemotherapy, have led to clinically significant reductions in disease recurrence and mortality. This progress reflects work from multiple randomized trials involving tens of thousands of patients. Over time, these trials have built on one another and there have been incremental improvements in adjuvant therapy over the past four decades, but the work has been largely empiric.

Advances in our understanding of the biologic complexity of breast cancer have created new opportunities for research in the adjuvant setting. Increasingly, it is apparent that breast cancer is a family of diseases and that the benefits of adjuvant chemotherapy are not distributed equally across all patients. In the years ahead, we must exploit our evolving understanding of breast cancer biology to improve outcomes for women with early-stage breast cancer in at least two ways. First, we need to understand which patients benefit from our available treatments, both to reduce the risk of disease recurrence in those who benefit, and to avoid the toxicity of therapy in those who are unlikely to realize a reduction in disease recurrence. Second, we need to identify new therapeutic targets, particularly in those who remain at highest risk of breast cancer recurrence and death. Increasingly, adjuvant trials will focus on distinct biologic subtypes with careful attention to both clinical and correlative end points. With this approach, it is hoped that there will be a substantial decline in breast cancer mortality in the next decade and an improvement in the overall therapeutic index.

MANAGEMENT SUMMARY

- A wealth of clinical trial information reflecting more than 30 years of investigation has demonstrated substantial improvements in long-term survival from the use of adjuvant chemotherapy for operable breast cancer.
- Both retrospective analyses of trial results and clinical studies using molecular techniques highlight the heterogeneity of breast cancer and the differential benefits from chemotherapy across patient subsets.

- Anatomic designations of node-positive and node-negative, historically used in adjuvant chemotherapy decisions, may no longer be as relevant today as in the past. Decisions regarding adjuvant chemotherapy should take into account the biologic features of the disease as well as the stage. In general, adjuvant chemotherapy has greater absolute benefits in high-grade versus low-grade cancers, hormone receptor-negative versus hormone receptor-positive cancers, and node-positive versus node-negative patients. Ongoing research continues to explore and identify subsets of patients defined by tumor characteristics who derive greater or lesser absolute benefit from chemotherapy. It is likely that biologic features other than those described above will play an expanding role in adjuvant chemotherapy decisions in the years ahead.
- A variety of chemotherapy regimens have confirmed benefit in the adjuvant setting (Table 49.2), and the use of contemporary supportive care medications allows manageable toxicity. In general, shorter duration chemotherapy regimens, such as AC × 4 or TC × 4, are acceptable standard therapy for lower risk patients, including those with relatively small, node-negative disease or selected patients with limited nodal involvement. More complex, longer, and generally more toxic regimens containing both anthracyclines and taxanes, such as dose dense AC + T or TAC, are typically selected for patients with higher risk disease, such as those with larger tumors or significant lymph node involvement. These regimens are often used in patients with a limited disease burden, but who have tumors with biologic features that predict a greater benefit from chemotherapy.
- Molecular genomic testing can provide both more precise prognostic information and tailored predictive information which may guide treatment decisions. One such test, Oncotype DX™, has been validated in node-negative hormone receptor-positive patients treated with tamoxifen, and may have utility as well in selected hormone receptor-positive patients with positive nodes. An alternative test, Mammoprint™, has been approved by the FDA and may have a role as well in guiding adjuvant treatment decisions. A major benefit of these types of evaluations is the ability to identify good-prognosis patients with biologically more indolent tumors less likely to benefit from chemotherapy, who can then be spared exposure to the physical, emotional, and economic expense of adjuvant treatment.
- Ideally, the treating clinician needs to carefully consider in the patient both the biologic features of the tumor and the disease burden, as well as comorbid conditions and preferences in (a) deciding to proceed with chemotherapy and (b) selecting the appropriate adjuvant regimen.

References

1. Fisher ER, Turnbull RB Jr. The cytologic demonstration and significance of tumor cells in the mesenteric venous blood in patients with colorectal carcinoma. *Surg Gynecol Obstet* 1955;100(1):102–108.
2. Shapiro DM, Fugmann RA. A role for chemotherapy as an adjunct to surgery. *Cancer Res* 1957;17(11):1098–1101.
3. Fisher B, Ravdin RG, Ausman RK, et al. Surgical adjuvant chemotherapy in cancer of the breast: results of a decade of cooperative investigation. *Ann Surg* 1968;168(3):337–356.
4. Fisher B, Redmond C, Fisher ER, et al. Systemic adjuvant therapy in treatment of primary operable breast cancer: National Surgical Adjuvant Breast and Bowel Project experience. *NCI Monogr* 1986(1):35–43.
5. Kjellgren K, Nissen-Meyer R, Norin T. Perioperative adjuvant chemotherapy in breast cancer. The Scandinavian Adjuvant Chemotherapy Study 1. *Acta Oncol* 1989;28(6):899–901.
6. Bonadonna G, Brusamolino E, Valagussa P, et al. Combination chemotherapy as an adjuvant treatment in operable breast cancer. *N Engl J Med* 1976;294(8):405–410.
7. Fisher B, Fisher ER, Redmond C. Ten-year results from the National Surgical Adjuvant Breast and Bowel Project (NSABP) clinical trial evaluating the use of L-phenylalanine mustard (L-PAM) in the management of primary breast cancer. *J Clin Oncol* 1986;4(6):929–941.
8. Bonadonna G, Valagussa P, Moliterni A, et al. Adjuvant cyclophosphamide, methotrexate, and fluorouracil in node-positive breast cancer: the results of 20 years of follow-up. *N Engl J Med* 1995;332(14):901–906.
9. Tancini G, Bonadonna G, Valagussa P, et al. Adjuvant CMF in breast cancer: comparative 5-year results of 12 versus 6 cycles. *J Clin Oncol* 1983;1(1):2–10.
10. Bonadonna G, Moliterni A, Zambetti M, et al. 30 years' follow-up of randomised studies of adjuvant CMF in operable breast cancer: cohort study. *BMJ* 2005;330(7485):217.
11. Fisher B, Dignam J, Mamounas EP, et al. Sequential methotrexate and fluorouracil for the treatment of node-negative breast cancer patients with estrogen receptor-negative tumors: eight-year results from National Surgical Adjuvant Breast and Bowel Project (NSABP) B-13 and first report of findings from NSABP B-19 comparing methotrexate and fluorouracil with conventional cyclophosphamide, methotrexate, and fluorouracil. *J Clin Oncol* 1996;14(7):1982–1992.
12. Mansour EG, Gray R, Shatila AH, et al. Survival advantage of adjuvant chemotherapy in high-risk node-positive breast cancer: ten-year analysis—an intergroup study. *J Clin Oncol* 1998;16(11):3486–3492.
13. Fisher B, Jeong JH, Dignam J, et al. Findings from recent National Surgical Adjuvant Breast and Bowel Project adjuvant studies in stage I breast cancer. *J Natl Cancer Inst Monogr* 2001(30):62–66.
14. Fisher B, Dignam J, Wolmark N, et al. Tamoxifen and chemotherapy for lymph node-negative, estrogen receptor-positive breast cancer. *J Natl Cancer Inst* 1997;89(22):1673–1682.
15. Adjuvant Therapy for Breast Cancer. NIH Consensus Statement 2000;17(4):1–23.
16. Effects of chemotherapy and hormonal therapy for early breast cancer on recurrence and 15-year survival: an overview of the randomised trials. *Lancet* 2005;365(9472):1687–1717.
17. Fisher B, Brown AM, Dimitrov NV, et al. Two months of doxorubicin-cyclophosphamide with and without interval reinduction therapy compared with 6 months of cyclophosphamide, methotrexate, and fluorouracil in positive-node breast cancer patients with tamoxifen-nonresponsive tumors: results from the National Surgical Adjuvant Breast and Bowel Project B-15. *J Clin Oncol* 1990;8(9):1483–1496.
18. Clarke M, Coates AS, Darby SC, et al. Adjuvant chemotherapy in oestrogen-receptor-poor breast cancer: patient-level meta-analysis of randomised trials. *Lancet* 2008;371(9606):29–40.
19. Fisher B, Redmond C, Wickerham DL, et al. Doxorubicin-containing regimens for the treatment of stage II breast cancer: The National Surgical Adjuvant Breast and Bowel Project experience. *J Clin Oncol* 1989;7(5):572–582.
20. Perloff M, Norton L, Korzun AH, et al. Postsurgical adjuvant chemotherapy of stage II breast carcinoma with or without crossover to a non-cross-resistant regimen: a Cancer and Leukemia Group B study. *J Clin Oncol* 1996;14(5):1589–1598.
21. Bonadonna G, Zambetti M, Moliterni A, et al. Clinical relevance of different sequencing of doxorubicin and cyclophosphamide, methotrexate, and Fluorouracil in operable breast cancer. *J Clin Oncol* 2004;22(9):1614–1620.
22. Hutchins LF, Green SJ, Ravdin PM, et al. Randomized, controlled trial of cyclophosphamide, methotrexate, and fluorouracil versus cyclophosphamide, doxorubicin, and fluorouracil with and without tamoxifen for high-risk, node-negative breast cancer: treatment results of Intergroup Protocol INT-0102. *J Clin Oncol* 2005;23(33):8313–8321.
23. Martin M, Villar A, Sole-Calvo A, et al. Doxorubicin in combination with fluorouracil and cyclophosphamide (i.v. FAC regimen, day 1, 21) versus methotrexate in combination with fluorouracil and cyclophosphamide (i.v. CMF regimen, day 1, 21) as adjuvant chemotherapy for operable breast cancer: a study by the GEICAM group. *Ann Oncol* 2003;14(6):833–842.
24. Levine MN, Pritchard KI, Bramwell VH, et al. Randomized trial comparing cyclophosphamide, epirubicin, and fluorouracil with cyclophosphamide, methotrexate, and fluorouracil in premenopausal women with node-positive breast cancer: update of National Cancer Institute of Canada Clinical Trials Group Trial MA5. *J Clin Oncol* 2005;23(22):5166–5170.
25. Fisher B, Anderson S, Tan-Chiu E, et al. Tamoxifen and chemotherapy for axillary node-negative, estrogen receptor-negative breast cancer: findings from National Surgical Adjuvant Breast and Bowel Project B-23. *J Clin Oncol* 2001;19(4).931–942.
26. Fisher B, Redmond C, Legault-Poisson S, et al. Postoperative chemotherapy and tamoxifen compared with tamoxifen alone in the treatment of positive-node breast cancer patients aged 50 years and older with tumors responsive to tamoxifen: results from the National Surgical Adjuvant Breast and Bowel Project B-16. *J Clin Oncol* 1990;8(6):1005–1018.
27. Henderson IC, Berry DA, Demetri GD, et al. Improved outcomes from adding sequential Paclitaxel but not from escalating Doxorubicin dose in an adjuvant chemotherapy regimen for patients with node-positive primary breast cancer. *J Clin Oncol* 2003;21(6):976–983.
28. Mamounas EP, Bryant J, Lembersky B, et al. Paclitaxel after doxorubicin plus cyclophosphamide as adjuvant chemotherapy for node-positive breast cancer: results from NSABP B-28. *J Clin Oncol* 2005;23(16):3686–3696.
29. Bear HD, Anderson S, Smith RE, et al. Sequential preoperative or postoperative docetaxel added to preoperative doxorubicin plus cyclophosphamide for operable breast cancer: National Surgical Adjuvant Breast and Bowel Project Protocol B-27. *J Clin Oncol* 2006;24(13):2019–2027.
30. Roche H, Fumoleau P, Spielmann M, et al. Sequential adjuvant epirubicin-based and docetaxel chemotherapy for node-positive breast cancer patients: the FNCLCC PACS 01 Trial. *J Clin Oncol* 2006;24(36):5664–5671.
31. Martin M, Rodriguez-Lescure A, Ruiz A, al. E. Randomized phase 3 trial of fluorouracil, epirubicin, and cyclophosphamide alone or followed by paclitaxel for early breast cancer. *J Natl Cancer Inst* 2008;100(11):805–815.
32. Ellis P, Barrett-Lee P, Bloomfield D, et al. Preliminary results of the UK Taxotere as Adjuvant Chemotherapy (TACT) Trial. *Breast Cancer Res Treat* 2007;106(S1):A78.
33. Martin M, Pienkowski T, Mackey J, et al. Adjuvant docetaxel for node-positive breast cancer. *N Engl J Med* 2005;352(22):2302–2313.
34. Goldstein L, O'Neill A, Sparano J, et al. E2197: Phase III AT (doxorubicin/docetaxel) vs. AC (doxorubicin/cyclophosphamide) in the adjuvant treatment of node positive and high risk node negative breast cancer. *J Clin Oncol* 2005;23(16S):A512.
35. Jones S, Holmes F, O'Shaughnessy J, et al. Extended follow-up and analysis by age of the U.S. Oncology Adjuvant trial 9735: docetaxel/cyclophosphamide is associated with an overall survival benefit compared to doxorubicin/cyclophosphamide and is well-tolerated in women 65 or older. *Breast Cancer Res Treat* 2007;106(S1):A12.

36. Sparano JA, Wang M, Martino S, et al. Weekly paclitaxel in the adjuvant treatment of breast cancer. *N Engl J Med* 2008;358(16):1663–1671.
37. De Laurentiis M, Cancello G, D'Agostino D, et al. Taxane-based combinations as adjuvant chemotherapy of early breast cancer: a meta-analysis of randomized trials. *J Clin Oncol* 2008;26(1):44–53.
38. Peto R. The worldwide overview: provisional results of updated (2005–2006) meta-analyses of trials. *Breast Cancer Res Treat* 2007;106(S1).
39. Bonadonna G, Zambetti M, Valagussa P. Sequential or alternating doxorubicin and CMF regimens in breast cancer with more than three positive nodes. Ten-year results. *JAMA* 1995;273(7):542–547.
40. Budman DR, Berry DA, Cirrincione CT, et al. Dose and dose intensity as determinants of outcome in the adjuvant treatment of breast cancer. The Cancer and Leukemia Group B. *J Natl Cancer Inst* 1998;90(16):1205–1211.
41. Benefit of a high-dose epirubicin regimen in adjuvant chemotherapy for node-positive breast cancer patients with poor prognostic factors: 5-year follow-up results of French Adjuvant Study Group 05 randomized trial. *J Clin Oncol* 2001;19(3):602–611.
42. Fisher B, Anderson S, Wickerham DL, et al. Increased intensification and total dose of cyclophosphamide in a doxorubicin-cyclophosphamide regimen for the treatment of primary breast cancer: findings from National Surgical Adjuvant Breast and Bowel Project B-22. *J Clin Oncol* 1997;15(5):1858–1869.
43. Fisher B, Anderson S, DeCillis A, et al. Further evaluation of intensified and increased total dose of cyclophosphamide for the treatment of primary breast cancer: findings from National Surgical Adjuvant Breast and Bowel Project B-25. *J Clin Oncol* 1999;17(11):3374–3388.
44. Fumoleau P, Bremond A, Kerbrat P, et al. Better outcome of premenopausal node-positive (N+) breast cancer patients (pts) treated with 6 cycles vs. 3 cycles of adjuvant chemotherapy: eight year follow-up results of FASG 01. *Proc Am Soc Clin Oncol* 1999;18(67a):A252.
45. Berry D, Ueno N, Johnson M, et al. High-dose chemotherapy with autologous stem-cell support versus standard-dose chemotherapy: meta-analysis of individual patient data from 15 randomized adjuvant breast cancer trials. *Breast Cancer Res Treat* 2007;106(S1):A11.
46. Norton L. Theoretical concepts and the emerging role of taxanes in adjuvant therapy. *Oncologist* 2001;6(Suppl 3):30–35.
47. Venturini M, Del Mastro L, Aitini E, et al. Dose-dense adjuvant chemotherapy in early breast cancer patients: results from a randomized trial. *J Natl Cancer Inst* 2005;97(23):1724–1733.
48. Citron ML, Berry DA, Cirrincione C, et al. Randomized trial of dose-dense versus conventionally scheduled and sequential versus concurrent combination chemotherapy as postoperative adjuvant treatment of node-positive primary breast cancer: first report of Intergroup Trial C9741/Cancer and Leukemia Group B Trial 9741. *J Clin Oncol* 2003;21(8):1431–1439.
49. Burnell M, Levine M, Chapman J, et al. A phase III adjuvant trial of sequenced EC + filgrastim + epoetin-alpha followed by paclitaxel compared to sequenced AC followed by paclitaxel compared to CEF in women with node-positive or high-risk node-negative breast cancer (NCIC CTG MA.21). *J Clin Oncol* 2007; 25(18S):A550.
50. Sorlie T, Perou CM, Tibshirani R, et al. Gene expression patterns of breast carcinomas distinguish tumor subclasses with clinical implications. *Proc Natl Acad Sci U S A* 2001;98(19):10869–10874.
51. Sorlie T, Tibshirani R, Parker J, et al. Repeated observation of breast tumor subtypes in independent gene expression data sets. *Proc Natl Acad Sci U S A* 2003; 100(14):8418–8423.
52. Berry DA, Cirrincione C, Henderson IC, et al. Estrogen-receptor status and outcomes of modern chemotherapy for patients with node-positive breast cancer. *JAMA* 2006;295(14):1658–1667.
53. Paik S, Bryant J, Park C, et al. erbB-2 and response to doxorubicin in patients with axillary lymph node-positive, hormone receptor-negative breast cancer. *J Natl Cancer Inst* 1998;90(18):1361–1370.
54. Paik S, Bryant J, Tan-Chiu E, et al. HER2 and choice of adjuvant chemotherapy for invasive breast cancer: National Surgical Adjuvant Breast and Bowel Project Protocol B-15. *J Natl Cancer Inst* 2000;92(24):1991–1998.
55. Muss HB, Thor AD, Berry DA, et al. c-erbB-2 expression and response to adjuvant therapy in women with node-positive early breast cancer. *N Engl J Med* 1994;330(18):1260–1266.
56. Thor AD, Berry DA, Budman DR, et al. erbB-2, p53, and efficacy of adjuvant therapy in lymph node-positive breast cancer. *J Natl Cancer Inst* 1998;90(18): 1346–1360.
57. Pritchard KI, Shepherd LE, O'Malley FP, et al. HER2 and responsiveness of breast cancer to adjuvant chemotherapy. *N Engl J Med* 2006;354(20):2103–2111.
58. Pritchard KI, Messersmith H, Elavathil L, et al. HER-2 and topoisomerase II as predictors of response to chemotherapy. *J Clin Oncol* 2008;26(5):736–744.
59. Slamon DJ, Eiermann W, Robert NJ, et al. Phase III randomized trial comparing doxorubicin and cyclophosphamide followed by docetaxel (ACT) with doxorubicin and cyclophosphamide followed by docetaxel and trastuzumab (ACTH) with docetaxel, carboplatin and trastuzumab (TCH) in HER2 positive early breast cancer patients: BCIRG 006 study. *Breast Cancer Res Treat* 2005;94:S5.
60. Hayes DF, Thor AD, Dressler LG, et al. HER2 and response to paclitaxel in node-positive breast cancer. *N Engl J Med* 2007;357(15):1496–1506.
61. Chia SK, Speers CH, Bryce CJ, et al. Ten-year outcomes in a population-based cohort of node-negative, lymphatic, and vascular invasion-negative early breast cancers without adjuvant systemic therapies. *J Clin Oncol* 2004;22(9): 1630–1637.
62. Hudis CA, Barlow WE, Costantino JP, et al. Proposal for standardized definitions for efficacy end points in adjuvant breast cancer trials: the STEEP system. *J Clin Oncol* 2007;25(15):2127–2132.
63. Amar S, Ann M, Geiger X, et al. Prognosis and clinical outcome of patients with node negative 1cm breast cancer. *Breast Cancer Res Treat* 2007;106(S1):A6024.
63a. Rakkhit R, Broglio K, Peintinger F, et al. Significant increased recurrence rates among breast cancer patients with HER2-positive, T1abNOMO tumors. *Cancer Res* 2009;69(52):A701.
64. National Cancer Comprehensive Network (NCCN), Breast Cancer Panel (BCP). *NCCN Practice Guidelines in Oncology—Breast Cancer*, 2008.
65. Goldhirsch A, Wood WC, Gelber RD, et al. Progress and promise: highlights of the international expert consensus on the primary therapy of early breast cancer 2007. *Ann Oncol* 2007;18(7):1133–1144.
66. Hassett M, Hughes M, Niland J, et al. Chemotherapy use for hormone receptor-positive, lymph node-negative breast cancer. *J Clin Oncol* 2008;26(34):5553–5560.
67. Lindley C, Vasa S, Sawyer WT, et al. Quality of life and preferences for treatment following systemic adjuvant therapy for early-stage breast cancer. *J Clin Oncol* 1998;16(4):1380–1387.
68. Ravdin PM, Siminoff IA, Harvey JA. Survey of breast cancer patients concerning their knowledge and expectations of adjuvant therapy. *J Clin Oncol* 1998;16(2): 515–521.
69. Simes RJ, Coates AS. Patient preferences for adjuvant chemotherapy of early breast cancer: how much benefit is needed? *J Natl Cancer Inst Monogr* 2001(30): 146–152.
70. Ravdin PM, Siminoff LA, Davis GJ, et al. Computer program to assist in making decisions about adjuvant therapy for women with early breast cancer. *J Clin Oncol* 2001;19(4):980–991.
71. Olivotto IA, Bajdik CD, Ravdin PM, et al. Population-based validation of the prognostic model ADJUVANT! for early breast cancer. *J Clin Oncol* 2005;23(12):2716–2725.
72. Paik S, Shak S, Tang G, et al. A multigene assay to predict recurrence of tamoxifen-treated, node-negative breast cancer. *N Engl J Med* 2004;351(27):2817–2826.
73. Paik S, Tang G, Shak S, et al. Gene expression and benefit of chemotherapy in women with node-negative, estrogen receptor-positive breast cancer. *J Clin Oncol* 2006;24(23):3726–3734.
74. Albain K, Barlow W, Shak S, et al. Prognostic and predictive value of the 21-gene recurrence score assay in postmenopausal, node-positive, ER-positive breast cancer (S8814,INT0100). *Breast Cancer Res Treat* 2007;106(S1):A10.
75. Goldstein L, Ravdin P, Gray R, et al. Prognostic utility of the 21-gene assay compared with Adjuvant! in hormone receptor (HR) positive operable breast cancer with 0-3 positive axillary nodes treated with adjuvant chemohormonal therapy (CHT): an analysis of intergroup trial E2197. *Breast Cancer Res Treat* 2007; 106(S1):A63.
76. van 't Veer LJ, Dai H, van de Vijver MJ, et al. Gene expression profiling predicts clinical outcome of breast cancer. *Nature* 2002;415(6871):530–536.
77. van de Vijver MJ, He YD, van't Veer LJ, et al. A gene-expression signature as a predictor of survival in breast cancer. *N Engl J Med* 2002;347(25):1999–2009.
78. Chang HY, Nuyten DS, Sneddon JB, et al. Robustness, scalability, and integration of a wound-response gene expression signature in predicting breast cancer survival. *Proc Natl Acad Sci U S A* 2005;102(10):3738–3743.
79. Ma XJ, Wang Z, Ryan PD, et al. A two-gene expression ratio predicts clinical outcome in breast cancer patients treated with tamoxifen. *Cancer Cell* 2004;5(6):607–616.
80. Fan C, Oh DS, Wessels L, et al. Concordance among gene-expression-based predictors for breast cancer. *N Engl J Med* 2006;355(6):560–569.
81. Colleoni M, Rotmensz N, Robertson C, et al. Very young women (<35 years) with operable breast cancer: features of disease at presentation. *Ann Oncol* 2002; 13(2):273–279.
82. Chung M, Chang HR, Bland KI, et al. Younger women with breast carcinoma have a poorer prognosis than older women. *Cancer* 1996;77(1):97–103.
83. Kroman N, Jensen MB, Wohlfahrt J, et al. Factors influencing the effect of age on prognosis in breast cancer: population based study. *BMJ* 2000;320(7233):474–478.
84. Goldhirsch A, Gelber RD, Yothers G, et al. Adjuvant therapy for very young women with breast cancer: need for tailored treatments. *J Natl Cancer Inst Monogr* 2001(30):44–51.
85. Greenfield S, Blanco DM, Elashoff RM, et al. Patterns of care related to age of breast cancer patients. *JAMA* 1987;257(20):2766–2770.
86. Newschaffer CJ, Penberthy L, Desch CE, et al. The effect of age and comorbidity in the treatment of elderly women with nonmetastatic breast cancer. *Arch Intern Med* 1996;156(1):85–90.
87. Silliman RA, Guadagnoli E, Weitberg AB, et al. Age as a predictor of diagnostic and initial treatment intensity in newly diagnosed breast cancer patients. *J Gerontol* 1989;44(2):M46–M50.
88. Muss HB, Woolf S, Berry D, et al. Adjuvant chemotherapy in older and younger women with lymph node-positive breast cancer. *JAMA* 2005;293(9):1073–1081.
89. Muss HB, Berry DA, Cirrincione C, et al. Toxicity of older and younger patients treated with adjuvant chemotherapy for node-positive breast cancer: the Cancer and Leukemia Group B Experience. *J Clin Oncol* 2007;25(24):3699–3704.
90. Muss H, Berry D, Cirrincione C, et al. Standard chemotherapy (CMF or AC) versus capecitabine in early-stage breast cancer (BC) patients aged 65 and older: results of CALCB/CTSU 49907. *J Clin Oncol* 2008;26(15S):A507.
91. Burstein HJ, Parker LM, Keshaviah A, et al. Efficacy of pegfilgrastim and darbepoetin alfa as hematopoietic support for dose-dense every-2-week adjuvant breast cancer chemotherapy. *J Clin Oncol* 2005;23(33):8340–8347.
92. Demark-Wahnefried W, Winer EP, et al. Why women gain weight with adjuvant chemotherapy for breast cancer. *J Clin Oncol* 1993;11(7):1418–1429.
93. Goodwin PJ, Ennis M, Pritchard KI, et al. Adjuvant treatment and onset of menopause predict weight gain after breast cancer diagnosis. *J Clin Oncol* 1999;17(1):120–129.
94. Camoriano JK, Loprinzi CL, Ingle JN, et al. Weight change in women treated with adjuvant therapy or observed following mastectomy for node-positive breast cancer. *J Clin Oncol* 1990;8(8):1327–1334.
95. Bower JE, Ganz PA, Desmond KA, et al. Fatigue in long-term breast carcinoma survivors: a longitudinal investigation. *Cancer* 2006;106(4):751–758.
96. Ganz PA, Bower JE. Cancer related fatigue: a focus on breast cancer and Hodgkin's disease survivors. *Acta Oncol* 2007;46(4):474–479.
97. Miller K, Wang M, Gralow J, et al. Paclitaxel plus bevacizumab versus paclitaxel alone for metastatic breast cancer. *N Engl J Med* 2007;357(26):2666–2676.
98. Miller K, O'Neill A, Perez E, et al. Phase II feasibility trial incorporating bevacizumab into dose dense doxorubicin and cyclophosphamide followed by paclitaxel in patients with lymph node positive breast cancer: a trial of the Eastern Cooperative Oncology Group (E2104). *Breast Cancer Res Treat* 2007;106(S1):A3063.
99. Tassone P, Tagliaferri P, Perricelli A, et al. BRCA1 expression modulates chemosensitivity of BRCA1-defective HCC1937 human breast cancer cells. *Br J Cancer* 2003;88(8):1285–1291.

Vered Stearns and Nancy E. Davidson

Adjuvant systemic therapy will be recommended to many women with a newly diagnosed breast cancer following definitive breast surgery to decrease the risk of cancer recurrence or death. It may consist of endocrine therapy, chemotherapy, a biologic agent, or a combination of one or more of these treatment modalities. The observed benefit with each of these treatments alone is discussed in detail in other chapters of this textbook. Currently, endocrine therapy is considered for almost every woman whose tumor expresses the estrogen receptor α (ER) or progesterone receptor (PR) proteins. The key question that a woman with early hormone receptor-positive breast cancer and her health care professional face is whether to add adjuvant chemotherapy to the endocrine manipulation. Secondary considerations include type, duration, and sequence of each treatment. Finally, additional research is required to identify women whose tumors express hormone receptors, but who may not benefit from endocrine therapies. In this chapter, we discuss considerations for administration of endocrine manipulations and chemotherapy, designated *chemoendocrine therapy*, in properly selected women.

WHO IS A CANDIDATE FOR ENDOCRINE MANIPULATION AND CHEMOTHERAPY?

Over the past two decades it has been conclusively demonstrated that only women whose tumors express ER or PR respond to endocrine therapies. Overall, 5 years of adjuvant tamoxifen therapy administered to women with ER-positive disease is expected to reduce annual recurrence rate by 41% and breast cancer mortality by 34% (1). Therefore, every woman with a primary tumor that expresses ER or PR should be considered for endocrine manipulations. Selection of the type of endocrine manipulation varies by menopausal status and is discussed in detail in Chapter 48. Postmenopausal women may be recommended 5 years of an aromatase inhibitor (AI), 2 to 3 years of tamoxifen followed by an AI for a total of 5 years, or 5 years of tamoxifen with or without 5 additional years of an AI (2,3). The standard endocrine treatment for premenopausal women remains tamoxifen for 5 years (4). Ovarian suppression or ablation alone or in combination with tamoxifen or an AI for premenopausal women is under study and may be appropriate for women with contraindications to tamoxifen or those participating in clinical trials.

The decision to give endocrine therapy should be made regardless of the decision whether or not to administer chemotherapy because very few data are currently available to recommend withholding endocrine therapy from any woman whose tumor expresses hormone receptors. Depending on the stage of the disease and tumor and host characteristics, clinicians should consider whether the woman is expected to derive additional benefit from adjuvant chemotherapy. The *Oxford Overview*, other retrospective analyses, and large single prospective clinical trials, have addressed some key questions regarding chemoendocrine therapy.

Summary of Results from the 2000 Oxford Overview

Until recently, clinicians utilized only age, stage, comorbid conditions, and single molecular characteristics to determine who should be offered chemotherapy in addition to endocrine therapy. Guidance was derived from the Early Breast Cancer Trialists' Cooperative Group (EBCTCG) systematic overview, also designated the *Oxford Overview*. The EBCTCG has met every 5 years since 1985 to perform a systematic review of all randomized clinical trials (published and unpublished) that have been performed in early breast cancer to maximize statistical power and minimize the biases that may lead to differences in results in individual trials. The most recent EBCTCG overview of adjuvant therapy for early breast cancer was performed in 2005 to 2006, but results have not yet been published.

The *2000 Overview* included data from approximately 200 randomized trials of adjuvant chemotherapy or hormonal therapy that began by 1995. Individual data were available from about 150,000 participants. Tamoxifen for 5 years reduces annual breast cancer recurrence and mortality rates by 41% and 34 %, respectively, in women with ER-positive breast cancer (Table 50.1) (1). In total, the Overview investigators reported that any chemotherapy (single-agent or multiagent) reduced annual event rates of breast cancer recurrence and mortality compared with no chemotherapy by 23% and 17%, respectively (1). Polychemotherapy provides greater benefits than single agent chemotherapy. Moreover, anthracycline or taxane-based therapy is preferable as long as contraindications do not exist. Based on individual studies and the cumulative data presented in the *Overview*, polychemotherapy has become the mainstay of adjuvant chemotherapy for breast cancer. A more detailed discussion of specific chemotherapy regimens is included in Chapter 49.

The *Overview* suggests that the benefits from chemotherapy may vary by age and menopausal status. Although adjuvant chemotherapy provides benefit to women of all age groups and any menopausal status, use of chemotherapy is associated with a greater proportional benefit in women under age 50 years. The *Overview* did not consider other individual tumor characteristics for each age group. Therefore, it is possible that age is a surrogate not only for menopausal status but also for a different tumor biology in cancers in younger versus older women. Indeed, cancer in older women is more likely to contain ER/PR, lack ERBB2 (formerly HER2/neu) overexpression or amplification, and display low grade, all factors that may be predictive of endocrine responsiveness and relative chemotherapy resistance. Older women are also more likely to have comorbid conditions or a lower life expectancy, and the benefits of chemotherapy may not outweigh the risks associated with the treatment. These *Overview* data were supported by a recent report from Cancer and Acute Leukemia Group B (CALGB) investigators who evaluated outcomes for 542 women (8%) aged 65 years or older and 159 women (2%) who were 70 years or older who were included in one of four studies evaluating chemotherapy questions in node-positive breast cancer between 1975 and 1999. No association was found between age and disease-free survival (DFS), but overall survival (OS) was significantly worse (*p* <.001) for patients aged 65 or older owing to death from causes other than breast cancer (5).

The *Overview* also considered node status, tumor size, and tumor differentiation. In sum, it suggests that women derive similar proportional benefit from chemotherapy regardless of nodal status or tumor size. Women younger than 50 years gain similar benefit from chemotherapy regardless of tumor differentiation. In contrast, women who were 50 to 59 years of age

Table 50.1	CHEMOENDOCRINE THERAPY: SUMMARY RESULTS FROM THE 2000 OXFORD OVERVIEW

| Treatment | Age (years) | Ratio of Annual Event Rates Therapy: Control (SE) | |
		Breast Cancer Mortality	Breast Cancer Recurrence
Polychemotherapy	<40	0·60 (0·06)	0·71 (0·07)
	40–49	0·64 (0·04)	0·70 (0·05)
	50–59	0·77 (0·03)	0·85 (0·04)
	60–69	0·87 (0·03)	0·91 (0·04)
	≥70	0·88 (0·11)	0·87 (0·12)
Chemotherapy Type			
CMF-based	<50	0·59 (0·04)	0·66 (0·05)
Anthracycline-based		0·67 (0·08)	0·74 (0·09)
Other polychemotherapy		0·68 (0·07)	0·79 (0·08)
CMF-based	50–69	0·81 (0·03)	0·90 (0·03)
Anthracycline-based		0·79 (0·04)	0·83 (0·05)
Other polychemotherapy		0·89 (0·06)	0·93 (0·07)
Presence or Absence of Tamoxifen			
CT with Tam vs. Tam alone	<50	0·65 (0·07)	0·66 (0·09)
CT then Tam vs. Tam alone		NA	NA
CT alone vs. Nil (no adjuvant)		0·62 (0·04)	0·71 (0·05)
CT with Tam vs. Tam alone	50–69	0·84 (0·03)	0·90 (0·03)
CT then Tam vs. Tam alone		0·77 (0·08)	0·80 (0·10)
CT alone vs. Nil (no adjuvant)		0·78 (0·04)	0·87 (0·04)
ER Status and Tamoxifen (ER-positive)			
PolyCT alone vs. nil	<50	0·56 (0·07)	0·69 (0·10)
PolyCT+ Tam vs. Tam only		0·64 (0·08)	0·65 (0·10)
PolyCT alone vs. nil	50–69	0·84 (0·07)	0·95 (0·08)
PolyCT+ Tam vs. Tam only		0·85 (0·04)	0·89 (0·04)
About 5 Years of Tamoxifen (ER-positive)			
Tam alone vs. Nil (no adjuvant)		0·59 (0·03)	0·66 (0·04)
Presence or absence of cytotoxics			
CT with Tam vs. CT alone		0·60 (0·08)	0·61 (0·09)
CT then Tam vs. CT alone		0·69 (0·07)	0·76 (0·10)
Entry age	<40	0·56 (0·10)	0·61 (0·12)
	40–49	0·71 (0·07)	0·76 (0·09)
	50–59	0·66 (0·05)	0·76 (0·07)
	60–69	0·55 (0·05)	0·65 (0·06)
	≥70	0·49 (0·12)	0·63 (0·15)
Ovarian Ablation (OA)			
OA vs. nil	<40	0·70 (0·17)	0·71 (0·16)
	40–49	0·67 (0·08)	0·68 (0·09)
OA+CT vs. CT	<40	0·96 (0·11)	1·04 (0·13)
	40–49	0·90 (0·08)	0·98 (0·09)
Ovarian Suppression (LHRH)			
LHRH vs. nil	<40	0·79 (0·16)	0·73 (0·21)
	40–49	0·77 (0·09)	0·79 (0·13)
LHRH+CT vs. CT	<40	070 (0·13)	0·80 (0·17)
	40–49	1·08 (0·13)	NA
Ovarian Ablation or Suppression (OAS)			
OAS vs. nil	<40	0·75 (0·12)	0·71 (0·13)
	40–49	0·71 (0·06)	0·71 (0·07)
OAS+CT vs. CT	<40	0·86 (0·09)	0·96 (0·10)
	40–49	0·95 (0·07)	1·03 (0·08)

CMF, cyclophosphamide, methotrexate, 5 fluorouracil, CT, chemotherapy; LHRH, luteinizing hormone-releasing hormone; NA, nonapplicable; OA, ovarian ablation; OAS, ovarian ablation or suppression; SE, standard error; Tam, tamoxifen; vs., versus.
Adapted from Effects of chemotherapy and hormonal therapy for early breast cancer on recurrence and 15-year survival: an overview of the randomised trials. *Lancet* 2005;365(9472): 1687–1717.

had more substantial benefit when the tumor was poorly differentiated. The observation in younger women may reflect the direct effects of chemotherapy and the indirect endocrine effects of chemotherapy-induced ovarian failure.

In aggregate, published data suggest that decisions regarding treatment should not be based solely on nodal status or tumor size; rather a more comprehensive evaluation of additional prognostic factors to determine magnitude of benefit from different modalities of treatment is required. This may help select the women who are more likely to benefit from endocrine therapy alone or chemoendocrine therapy, or who may not derive benefit from endocrine therapy despite the presence of hormone receptors and should be considered for chemotherapy alone or other treatment modalities.

Prognostic and Predictive Factors

Although results from the *Oxford Overview* have suggested that almost every woman would derive some benefit from adjuvant systemic chemotherapy, recommendations about treatment of the individual have been at the discretion of the patient and her physician. Biologic factors can assist in determining with a better accuracy the absolute benefit an individual woman may derive from specific treatment and have already revolutionized decision-making. Two types of biologic factors help in decision-making. *Prognostic factors* reflect the underlying natural history of the cancer in the absence of therapy and are used to estimate risk of recurrence (6–8). *Predictive factors* may be used to determine whether a woman with specific tumor characteristics is likely to respond to a specific treatment or agent. Most factors are both prognostic and predictive, and are reviewed in Chapter 31.

Hundreds of prognostic markers have been investigated in breast cancer, but only a few have been accepted for clinical use to determine whether to recommend adjuvant systemic therapy, and if so, what type. Traditional markers that help select who is at a high risk of recurrence and who should be considered for chemotherapy in addition to endocrine therapy include axillary lymph node status, tumor size, histologic grade, and steroid receptor status. More recently, with the advent of new high throughput technologies, breast cancers have been divided into specific subtypes. These newer classifications may provide both prognostic and predictive information and assist in differentiating the women whose tumors are associated with excellent prognosis and need not receive adjuvant therapy from those who should receive specific modalities of adjuvant systemic therapy.

In the interim, models such as Adjuvant! (9) estimate a woman's risk of relapse based on data from the *Oxford Overview* and from recent large individual clinical trials and the absolute benefit that specific therapy would provide. Endocrine manipulations are offered to most women with hormone receptor-positive breast cancer because the ratio of risk to benefit is generally favorable. But no one marker can be used to predict response to chemotherapy, and chemotherapy-associated side effects are more substantial. Based on risk and benefit estimates, chemotherapy was recommended to otherwise healthy women with node-positive disease of any size or node-negative disease with tumor size greater than 1 cm (4,10). Women with specific histologic subtypes, such as node-negative tubular and mucinous carcinoma up to 3 cm in size, have an excellent prognosis and adjuvant chemotherapy may not provide additional benefit. Nonetheless up to 20% of women with stage I breast cancer may have a recurrence, and it would be desirable to identify prognostic factors that could distinguish women with these seemingly favorable tumors that are more or less likely to recur. Factors that may predict sensitivity or resistance to endocrine therapy and can help select women for chemoendocrine therapy include ER, PR, epidermal growth factor receptors (EGFR or ERBB1 and 2), tumor grade, multigene assays, and other tumor and host characteristics.

Estrogen Receptor

Clearly, the presence of hormone receptors is essential for benefit from endocrine therapy (discussed in more detail in Chapter 29). Other data suggest that hormone receptors may also predict reduced response to chemotherapy, perhaps owing to lower proliferation. Indeed, recent studies suggest that, although women with ER-positive tumors gain additional benefit from chemotherapy, the proportional benefit may be smaller than observed in ER-negative women.

For example, National Surgical Adjuvant Breast and Bowel Project (NSABP) investigators evaluated more than 10,000 women whose tumors were 1 cm or smaller in size from five prospective, randomized clinical trials of adjuvant chemotherapy versus no adjuvant chemotherapy (11). Of 1,259 node-negative breast cancer patients, 235 women were ER-positive and 1,024 were ER-negative. Recurrence-free survival (RFS) and OS were improved for both ER-positive and ER-negative patients when chemotherapy was added, but the absolute benefit from chemotherapy added to tamoxifen was statistically significant but clinically small.

The CALGB investigators have recently reviewed outcomes of node-positive women who were enrolled in one of three trials of chemoendocrine therapy. Study C8541 compared three regimens of cyclophosphamide, doxorubicin, and 5-fluorouracil (CAF), whereas C9344 included three doses of doxorubicin concurrent with cyclophosphamide (AC), with or without sequential paclitaxel, and C9741 compared sequential doxorubicin, paclitaxel, and cyclophosphamide with concurrent doxorubicin and cyclophosphamide followed by paclitaxel, administered every 3 or every 2 weeks. In each of the studies, endocrine therapy was recommended, but not assigned, for hormone receptor-positive women. A total of 6,644 women were included in the three studies and outcomes in each of the studies were reported by ER status. Absolute benefits owing to chemotherapy were greater for patients with ER-negative compared with ER-positive tumors (Table 50.2). Overall, when the most intense regimen in C9741 (i.e., chemotherapy administered every 2 weeks) was compared with the low-dose CAF in C8541, 22.8% more ER-negative patients were disease-free at 5 years compared with 7.0% for ER-positive patients (12). Five year OS in ER-negative and positive patients was improved by 16.7% and 4.0%, respectively. The authors noted that biweekly AC plus

	ABSOLUTE DIFFERENCE (%) IN 5-YEAR DISEASE-FREE AND OVERALL SURVIVAL ACCORDING TO ESTROGEN RECEPTOR STATUS IN CALGB TRIALS				

Table 50.2

	Absolute Difference (%) in 5-Year Survival				
	ER-Negative		ER-Positive	
CALGB Study Comparison	Disease-Free	Overall	Disease-Free	Overall
8541 (high dose vs. low dose)	13.9	6.6	6.6	4.0
9344 (paclitaxel vs. no paclitaxel)	8.2	7.4	2.1	0
9741 (every 2 wk vs. every 3 wk)	9.1	7.4	2.8	−0.2
Overall (low dose in 8,541 vs. every 2 wk in 9,741)	22.8	16.7	7.0	4.0

CALGB, Cancer and Leukemia Group B; ER, estrogen receptor; vs., versus; wk, week.
From Berry DA, Cirrincione C, Henderson IC, et al. Estrogen-receptor status and outcomes of modern chemotherapy for patients with node-positive breast cancer. *JAMA* 2006;295(14):1658–1667. Copyright © 2006 American Medical Association. All rights reserved.

paclitaxel in C9741 lowered the rate of recurrence and death in ER-negative breast cancer by more than 50% in comparison with low-dose CAF used in C8541. Although patients with ER-positive breast tumors have also derived some benefit from chemotherapy, the magnitude of benefit was smaller (26% and 23% reduction in recurrence and death, respectively) compared with the observed benefits for patients with ER-negative disease.

The magnitude of hormone receptor positivity and expression patterns of PR and growth factor receptors are not known in the *Overview*, NSABP, and CALGB analyses. More recently, diagnostic tools that provide better quantitative ER data suggest that the strength of the expression may predict likelihood of sensitivity to the hormone therapy. Harvey et al. have reported that a scale that incorporates both the estimated proportion and intensity of steroid receptor positive-staining tumor cells (range, 0 to 8) was predictive of DFS in patients who received endocrine therapy alone (13). Using the scale, it is expected that women with tumors with ER score of 7 or 8 will greatly benefit from endocrine therapy. In contrast, women with a score of 3 to 6 may be only partially responsive to endocrine therapy, and those with a score of 0 or 2 have a high chance of recurrence with endocrine therapy alone and are good candidates for adjuvant chemotherapy (13). Other methods to determine quantitative ER expression are under study. In addition, functional status of the ER, impaired balance of coactivators and corepressors, and crosstalk between ER and growth factor signaling may also predict response to endocrine therapy and are discussed in Chapter 29.

Progesterone Receptor and Growth Factor Receptors

Others examined the role of PR in determining response to endocrine therapy alone. The cumulative data suggest that tumors that express ER but lack PR have reduced sensitivity to tamoxifen and aromatase inhibitors compared with tumors that express both steroid hormone receptors (14). ER-positive, PR-negative tumors may also express ERBB1 and overexpress ERBB2 and be associated with a more aggressive phenotype. Therefore, women with PR-negative tumors may be candidates for chemoendocrine therapy.

This is best shown in a report of about 45,000 breast cancer patients wherein DFS and OS were significantly improved in the 31,415 patients with tumors that expressed both ER and PR compared with outcomes of 13,404 patients with ER-positive and PR-negative tumors. Furthermore, among all tamoxifen-treated women, recurrence was higher among women with ERBB1-expressing tumors than with ERBB1-negative tumors (hazard ratios [HR] 1.9, 95% confidence interval [CI] 1.0–3.5, $p = .05$), and those with ERBB2 overexpression versus not (HR 2.3, 95% CI 1.2–4.3, $p = .006$) (15). Importantly, in women with ER- and PR-positive tumors, neither ERBB1 nor ERBB2 status was associated with worse DFS. Among women with ER-positive but PR-negative tumors, both ERBB1 expression (HR 2.4, 95% CI 1.0–5.4, $p = .036$) and ERBB2 overexpression (HR 2.6, 95% CI 1.1–6.0, $p = .022$) were associated with a higher likelihood of recurrence (15).

Finally, other studies have evaluated ERBB2 status regardless of PR status. Overall, tumors that express both ER and ERBB2 derive reduced benefit from endocrine therapy alone (16). Because ERBB2 expression is clearly predictive for improved outcome with the humanized monoclonal antibody, trastuzumab, women with tumors that are ERBB2-positive are candidates for chemoendocrine therapy plus trastuzumab and recommended regimens are included in Chapter 51. Studies evaluating endocrine therapies and anti-ERBB2 agents are currently underway. Whether trastuzumab provides additional benefit to endocrine therapy alone in the adjuvant setting is not known, and the combination should not be used outside of clinical trials.

Other Markers that May Predict Sensitivity or Response to Endocrine Therapy

Higher tumor grade or proliferative index or poor differentiation predicts worse prognosis in the absence of treatment and an improved response to cytotoxic therapy. Few prospective data are available to determine whether chemoendocrine therapy is better than endocrine therapy alone in these settings. In the *Overview*, information regarding tumor differentiation was available from 44% of all tumors; they were divided into 16% good, 53% moderately, and 31% poorly differentiated tumors. The proportional risk reductions produced by chemotherapy were statistically similar in all differentiation groups (1). Data were not available on most of the specimens, however, and central review was not conducted.

With the recent understanding of human genetics and the availability of high throughput technologies, other tools have become available that can be used both to estimate prognosis and to predict response to endocrine therapy, chemotherapy, or both. Some assays include a combination of known and novel markers whereas others utilize genes that are novel.

Oncotype DX and other emerging multigene assays may help select women whose tumors are endocrine-sensitive and who do not require chemotherapy. Developed for use in women with node-negative hormone receptor-positive breast cancer, Oncotype DX is a reverse transcriptase-polymerase chain reaction (RT-PCR) assay of 21 prospectively selected genes that can be performed on paraffin-embedded tumor tissue. The levels of expression of 16 cancer-related genes and 5 reference genes are evaluated and a predefined algorithm is used to calculate a recurrence score. Women are then categorized into low, intermediate, or high recurrence score groups. The score can be used to inform the woman of her individual risk of recurrence if she receives tamoxifen alone, and what additional benefit she will gain from chemotherapy (Fig. 50.1A) (17,18). Studies to date suggest that women with node-negative receptor-positive breast cancer with a low recurrence score do not benefit from the addition of chemotherapy to tamoxifen whereas those with a high recurrence score have substantial chemotherapy benefit.

The utility of this assay is being assessed by The North American Breast Cancer Intergroup through a prospective randomized trial, designated **T**rial **A**ssigning **I**ndividuaLized **O**ptions for Treatment (**Rx**), or TAILORx. In this study, tumors from approximately 10,000 node-negative hormone receptor-positive women will be analyzed by the Oncotype Dx test. Women with a low recurrence score tumor will receive endocrine therapy alone, whereas those with a high score tumor will receive chemoendocrine therapy, and those in the intermediate group will be randomized to endocrine versus chemoendocrine therapy. The samples obtained through TAILORx will be available for future studies of new and emerging technologies and hypotheses.

Recent preliminary data suggest that the predictive utility of the Oncotype DX assay can be also extended to node-positive women. Southwest Oncology Group (SWOG) investigators evaluated samples from patients enrolled in study S8814 (Intergroup 0100). In S8814, node-positive, hormone receptor-positive, postmenopausal women were randomly assigned to tamoxifen alone or to cyclophosphamide, doxorubicin, and 5-fluorouracil (CAF) with concurrent or sequential tamoxifen (CAF-T). In the parent trial, women who received chemoendocrine therapy had a significant improvement in DFS and OS compared with those treated with tamoxifen alone (19). Overall, 45% of the study participants provided tumor specimens, and RNA was sufficient for RT-PCR on 367 patients (tamoxifen, 148; CAF-T, 219). The recurrence score was prognostic for DFS in the tamoxifen-alone arm ($p = .006$) (20). Observed effects were similar in women with one to three and four or more involved nodes. For women with a low recurrence score, there was no

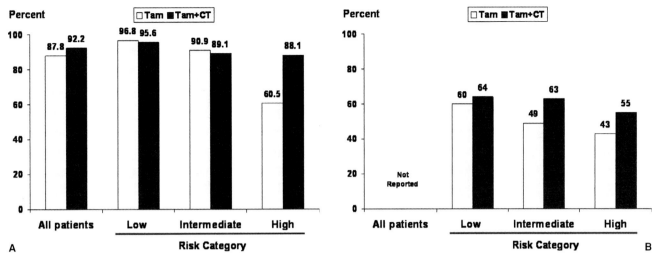

FIGURE 50.1. Estimates of the proportion of patients free of distant recurrence at 10 years of tamoxifen-treated patients and tamoxifen plus chemotherapy-treated patients using the Oncotype DX Recurrence Score in node-negative women (**A**) (17) and in node-positive women (**B**) (20). CT, chemotherapy (includes the methotrexate and 5-fluorouracil with or without cyclophosphamide regimen in node-negative women and the cyclophosphamide, doxorubicin, and 5-fluorouracil regimen in node-positive women); Tam, tamoxifen. Risk category reflects the recurrence score (RS): Low: RS <18, Intermediate: RS 18–30, High: RS >30.

benefit from CAF-T compared with tamoxifen for either DFS or OS (Fig. 50.1B). In contrast, a large benefit was observed for women with high recurrence score tumors in the CAF-T group compared to those on tamoxifen alone.

The role of Oncotype DX was also evaluated in women with zero to three axillary nodes who received chemotherapy with combination AC or doxorubicin and docetaxel (AT) in the Eastern Cooperative Oncology Group (ECOG) Trial E2197. No difference was seen between the two arms for DFS or OS (21). The investigators determined recurrence score of 99 participants with hormone receptor-positive disease who received chemoendocrine therapy and had a recurrence and of 366 women who did not suffer a recurrence. Recurrence score was a significant predictor of recurrence both in node-negative (p = .0007) and node-positive (p = .0004) patients (22). Low recurrence score predicted a less than 5% risk of recurrence regardless of nodal status, although it is noted that all E2197 participants received chemotherapy. In aggregate, these three reports suggest that multiplex biologic measures of the tumors may predict the sensitivity to endocrine interventions with better accuracy regardless of nodal status and, importantly, may also help to identify chemotherapy-sensitive subgroups.

Other multigene assays are being introduced commercially. The MammaPrint assay includes a panel of 70 genes that predicts prognosis of primary breast cancer and may help select patients who should receive adjuvant therapy. Currently, no data suggest that this signature can help predict relative benefit from individual modalities of treatment or specific agents (23). Another RT-PCR-based assay that has been developed and validated includes a ratio of two genes (*HOXB13* and *IL17BR*)

and is designated H/I (24). It is suggested that H/I ratio may also predict outcomes in tamoxifen-treated women (25).

Finally, host factors may modulate benefit from endocrine therapy. Emerging data suggest that pharmacogenetics of drug target or metabolizing enzymes may influence efficacy and safety. For example, the presence of variant alleles in the cytochrome P450 2D6 gene (*CYP2D6*) is associated with perturbed metabolism of tamoxifen and reduced concentrations of the active metabolite endoxifen (26–28) and may predict reduced benefit from the drug (29). These individuals may therefore be candidates for alternative endocrine strategies or for the addition of chemotherapy. Potential implications of these factors on endocrine treatment decisions are discussed in more detail in Chapter 56.

Work on elucidating the host and tumor features that might predict for benefit from endocrine versus chemoendocrine therapy continues. In the interim, panelists at the 2007 St. Gallen conference provided expert opinion about key adjuvant systemic therapy questions and attempted to incorporate some prognostic factor information into treatment selection. The consensus panel defined three endocrine responsiveness categories for ERBB2-negative tumors (Table 50.3) (10). A *highly endocrine responsive* group includes those with tumors that express high levels of both ER and PR in a majority of cells, whereas an *incompletely endocrine responsive* group includes women whose tumors demonstrate some expression of steroid hormone receptors but at lower levels or lack either ER or PR. A third group is *endocrine nonresponsive* and includes tumors with no detectable expression of steroid hormone receptors. The panel recommended that the women in the incompletely

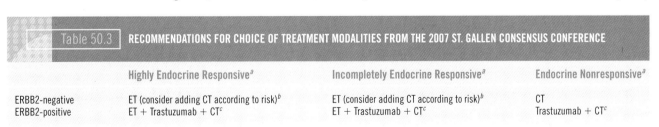

Table 50.3 | **RECOMMENDATIONS FOR CHOICE OF TREATMENT MODALITIES FROM THE 2007 ST. GALLEN CONSENSUS CONFERENCE**

	Highly Endocrine Responsive[a]	Incompletely Endocrine Responsive[a]	Endocrine Nonresponsive[a]
ERBB2-negative	ET (consider adding CT according to risk)[b]	ET (consider adding CT according to risk)[b]	CT
ERBB2-positive	ET + Trastuzumab + CT[c]	ET + Trastuzumab + CT[c]	Trastuzumab + CT[c]

CT, chemotherapy; ET, endocrine therapy.
[a]Responsiveness to endocrine therapies is defined in the text.
[b]Within the highly and incompletely endocrine responsive categories, addition of chemotherapy may be based on degree of steroid hormone receptor expression and level of risk.
[c]Trastuzumab should be used as discussed in Chapter 51.
From Goldhirsch A, Wood WC, Gelber RD, et al. Progress and promise: highlights of the international expert consensus on the primary therapy of early breast cancer 2007. *Ann Oncol* 2007;18(7):1133–1144, by permission of Oxford University Press.

endocrine responsive group receive chemoendocrine therapy. Other known and emerging tumor and host characteristics that may influence endocrine responsiveness in both the first and second groups were not, however, felt to be sufficiently validated to use in routine clinical decision-making.

CHEMOENDOCRINE THERAPY: SELECTION OF ENDOCRINE TREATMENT

Until conclusive evidence is available to select tumors that are resistant to endocrine therapy despite the expression of hormone receptors, every woman whose breast cancer contains ER, PR, or both should be considered for adjuvant endocrine manipulations because of demonstrated efficacy and relatively low toxicity profile. Considerations regarding endocrine recommendations are described in detail in Chapter 48. The decision regarding endocrine therapy should be made irrespective of the decision whether or not to administer chemotherapy. Here evidence to guide selection of endocrine therapy in the setting of a plan of chemoendocrine therapy is summarized.

Tamoxifen

The *Overview* suggested that chemoendocrine therapy is better than either modality alone. The investigators examined the additional benefits observed when chemotherapy is added to tamoxifen or when tamoxifen is added to chemotherapy. Most of the studies included in the *Overview* used the cyclophosphamide, methotrexate, and 5-fluorouracil (CMF) combination. In ER-positive women age 50 to 69, polychemotherapy and tamoxifen reduces annual recurrence and mortality event rates by 15% and 11%, respectively, compared with tamoxifen alone. In women younger than 50, the addition of chemotherapy to tamoxifen is associated with additional reductions of 36% and 35% in recurrence and mortality rates, respectively, compared with tamoxifen alone (Table 50.1) (1). Tamoxifen combined with chemotherapy results in a 40% and 39% additional reduction in recurrence and mortality rates, respectively, compared with chemotherapy alone. Similarly, tamoxifen administered sequentially following chemotherapy results in a 31% and 24% additional reduction in recurrence and mortality rates, respectively, compared with chemotherapy alone.

Several individual studies have addressed the value of chemotherapy in addition to tamoxifen in women by age or menopausal status. NSABP investigators reevaluated the outcomes of node-negative hormone receptor-positive women who were included in studies B-14 and B-20 by age (<50 years, 50–59 years, ≥60 years) and menopausal status. In NSABP B-14, a total of 2,892 women were randomly assigned to placebo or tamoxifen. RFS was significantly improved among women treated with tamoxifen compared with those assigned placebo, irrespective of age, menopausal status, or tumor estrogen-receptor concentration (HR for RFS 0.58, 95% CI 0.50–0.67, p <.0001; HR for OS 0.80, 95% CI 0.71–0.91, p = .0008) (30,31). In NSABP B-20, 2,363 women were randomly assigned to tamoxifen and six cycles of CMF (CMFT), tamoxifen and six cycles of MF, or tamoxifen only. Overall, the women who received CMFT had improved 5-year DFS and OS compared with women who received tamoxifen alone (HR for RFS 0.52, 95% CI 0.39–0.68, p <.0001; HR for OS 0.78, 95% CI 0.60–1.01, p = .063) (31,32). Importantly, in B-20, RFS and OS were significantly improved in the CMFT-treated women aged 49 years or younger compared with women who received tamoxifen alone. In women aged 50 to 59 years, the advantage of CMFT over tamoxifen was significant for RFS, but borderline for OS. Finally, for women 60 years of age or older, no difference was found in outcomes between the treatment groups (Table 50.4) (31). A significant interaction was observed for effectiveness of chemotherapy between age groups in OS (p = .027), and a trend for RFS (p = .17).

Notably, in both NSABP studies, RFS and OS benefit was more significant in women whose tumors had higher concentrations of ER (≥50 vs. 10 to 49 fmol/mg) (31). Because older women tend to have higher tumor ER concentrations and are more likely to benefit from tamoxifen than from chemotherapy compared with younger women, likely the use of tamoxifen or chemoendocrine therapy should be based more on biological features than age alone. Other large studies have enrolled only postmenopausal or only premenopausal women and are described below.

In International Breast Cancer Study Group (IBCSG) Trial IX, 1,669 postmenopausal node-negative women received three cycles of classic CMF and tamoxifen (CMFT) or tamoxifen alone. With a 71-month follow-up, 5-year DFS and OS were improved only for women with ER-negative disease who received combination therapy (33). In women with ER-positive tumors, no statistically significant difference was seen between the CMFT and

	Tamoxifen (n = 770)			CMFT (n = 766)			
	Patients	Events	12 years[a]	Patients	Events	12 years[a]	Hazard Ratio (95% CI)
Recurrence-Free Survival							
Age (years)							
≤49	345	76	76%	354	38	89%	0·46 (0·31–0·68)[b]
50–59	215	42	78%	208	19	88%	0·44 (0·25–0·75)[b]
≥60	210	26	85%	204	20	89%	0·80 (0·45–1·44)
Overall Survival							
Age (years)							
≤49	345	53	84%	354	34	90%	0·61 (0·40–0·95)[b]
50–59	215	32	84%	208	18	90%	0·57 (0·32–1·01)
≥60	210	39	81%	204	45	77%	1·21 (0·79–1·85)

Table 50.4   **OUTCOME ACCORDING TO TREATMENT GROUP AND AGE IN NSABP TRIAL B-20**

CI, confidence interval; CMFT, cyclophosphamide, methotrexate, 5-fluorouracil, and tamoxifen; NSABP, National Surgical Adjuvant Breast and Bowel Project.
[a]Percent event-free at 12 years after surgery.
[b]Statistically significant.
Reprinted from Fisher B, Jeong JH Bryant J, *et al.* Treatment of lymph-node-negative, oestrogen-receptor-positive breast cancer: long-term findings from National Surgical Adjuvant Breast and Bowel Project randomised clinical trials. *Lancet* 2004;364(9437):858–868. Copyright 2004, with permission from Elsevier. Reprinted from The Lancet, Copyright 2004, with permission from Elsevier.

tamoxifen only groups for DFS (84% vs. 85% for CMFT and tamoxifen alone, respectively, $p = .92$) or OS (95% vs. 93% for CMFT and tamoxifen alone, respectively, $p = .80$). These data suggest that chemotherapy that would be considered suboptimal by today's standard (i.e., three instead of six cycles of classic CMF) did not provide additional benefit in postmenopausal women with ER-positive breast cancer who received tamoxifen. However, these results cannot exclude the possibility that CMF chemotherapy of longer duration or an anthracycline- or taxane-based regimen may further improve outcomes for tamoxifen-treated women with ER-positive disease.

Preliminary results from Intergroup Trial 0100 (SWOG 8814) demonstrated that six cycles of CAF chemotherapy followed by 5 years of tamoxifen (CAFT) was associated with substantial improvement in DFS and OS for postmenopausal women with node-positive, steroid receptor-positive breast cancer compared with tamoxifen. In Intergroup Trial 0100, 1,477 participants were randomly assigned to tamoxifen alone, CAF followed by tamoxifen (CAF-T) or concurrent CAF and tamoxifen (CAFT-T). At 5 years, the addition of CAFT improved DFS by 9% (76% vs. 67%) and OS by 5% (84% vs. 79%) (19). The possibility that further testing with assays, such as Oncotype DX, could refine selection of chemotherapy beneficiaries was discussed earlier.

Taken together, the results of the *Overview* and several prospective trials demonstrate that the addition of chemotherapy to tamoxifen may be associated with gain in DFS and OS for postmenopausal women with receptor-positive disease. The benefit appears to be greatest for women with node-positive disease who receive an anthracycline or those younger than 60 years of age who receive CMF. The value of CMF may be less substantial or nonexistent for women older than age 60, especially those with node-negative disease. The magnitude of benefit associated with the addition of adjuvant chemotherapy to tamoxifen in older women has been uncertain, partly because of the small number of such women who have been included in prospective, randomized clinical trials. It is also possible that older women are more likely to receive suboptimal regimens and to experience dose delays or reductions, and less likely to receive anthracycline-based regimens. As noted earlier, it is not clear whether the age-associated differences in the benefits of adjuvant chemotherapy are owing to the differences in age or tumor biology.

Other studies have more specifically addressed the use of tamoxifen in premenopausal women. For decades chemotherapy was considered the adjuvant treatment of choice for premenopausal women with node-positive breast cancer regardless of hormone receptor status. However, the 1995 *Overview* analysis demonstrated unequivocally that receptor-positive women younger than 50 years old (and presumably mostly premenopausal) had a substantial reduction in breast cancer recurrence and death with the use of tamoxifen regardless of the use of chemotherapy. The report led to a change in practice. Adjuvant tamoxifen is currently offered to women with hormone receptor-positive disease regardless of age or menopausal status. The 2000 Oxford Overview has confirmed that tamoxifen's benefits were similar in woman age 40 or younger and those aged 40 to 49 years (1).

Because tamoxifen use in premenopausal women became standard only a little over a decade ago, few mature studies that investigated the role of chemotherapy and tamoxifen in premenopausal women have been reported. In Trial 13-93, IBCSG investigators treated node-positive premenopausal women with three cycles of anthracycline-based chemotherapy followed by three cycles of CMF with or without 5 years of tamoxifen (34). A significant improvement was observed in DFS (HR 0.59, 95% CI 0.46–0.75, $p < .0001$) but not in OS (HR 0.86, 95% CI 0.62–1.19, $p = .36$) with combined therapy. The DFS benefit of tamoxifen was observed both in women 40 or

older (HR 0.60, 95% CI, 0.44–0.81, $p = .0009$) and in those younger than 40 (HR 0.57, 95% CI, 0.38–0.86, $p = .008$).

Taken together, the existing data suggest that chemotherapy and tamoxifen are appropriate for premenopausal women with high-risk hormone receptor-positive disease. Further investigation is required, however, to separate the groups of women with endocrine-responsive disease for whom chemotherapy may provide little benefit, if any. New prognostic and predictive factors may help further inform decision-making.

Aromatase Inhibitors

During the last decade, several clinical trials have demonstrated the superiority of aromatase inhibitors over single agent tamoxifen in the adjuvant treatment of postmenopausal women. Three approaches have been investigated in adjuvant clinical trials: 5 years of tamoxifen versus 5 years of an AI (upfront); 2 to 3 years of tamoxifen followed by an AI for a total of 5 years (sequential) versus 5 years of tamoxifen; and 5 years of tamoxifen followed by 5 years of an AI (extended) versus placebo. Most studies allowed adjuvant chemotherapy before initiating endocrine therapy, thereby permitting an assessment of chemoendocrine approaches.

Approximately 20% of women included in the Arimidex, Tamoxifen, Alone or in Combination trial (ATAC) received chemotherapy before the assigned endocrine therapy. Women who did not receive chemotherapy had an improved time to recurrence with 5 years of anastrozole compared with 5 years of tamoxifen (HR 0.71, 95% CI 0.61–0.83) (35). No difference was found in outcome with tamoxifen or anastrozole in women who received prior chemotherapy (HR 0.89, 95% CI 0.70–1.13), but the number of events was small (35,36).

In the Breast International Group (BIG) 1-98 trial, 5 years of letrozole were superior to 5 years of tamoxifen and approximately 25% of participants (n = 1,232) received chemotherapy. DFS was superior in the letrozole-compared with the tamoxifen-treated group, both in women who received chemotherapy (HR 0.74, 95% CI 0.56–0.97, $p = .03$) and those who did not (HR 0.86, 95% CI 0.73–1.01, $p = .07$) (37). Thus, in contrast to the ATAC trial, women in BIG 1-98 had improved benefit with an AI even if they had received prior chemotherapy.

The largest trial of the sequential approach was the Intergroup Exemestane Study (IES) of 4,724 postmenopausal patients with ER-positive or unknown breast cancer who were disease-free after 2 to 3 years of tamoxifen, of whom 32% received adjuvant chemotherapy. The women were randomly assigned to switch to exemestane or to continue tamoxifen for a total of 5 years of endocrine therapy. Exemestane-treated women enjoyed a superior DFS and a trend for improved OS. Improved DFS was observed both in women who received adjuvant chemotherapy (HR 0.78, 95% CI 0.63–0.98) and in those who did not receive the treatment (HR 0.75, 95% CI 0.62–0.89) (38). Three additional studies investigated the role of anastrozole following 2 to 3 years of tamoxifen treatment versus a continuation of tamoxifen for a total of 5 years, including the Austrian Breast and Colorectal Cancer Study Group (ABCSG 8), the Arimidex-Nolvadex (ARNO 95), and the Italian Tamoxifen Anastrozole (ITA) trials. A recent meta-analysis included data from the 1,997 participants in the three trials. Because neither ABCSG 8 nor ARNO 95 allowed adjuvant chemotherapy, only 8% of the patients in this meta-analysis received adjuvant chemotherapy. Anastrozole was superior to tamoxifen irrespective of adjuvant chemotherapy (HR 0.67, 95% CI 0.53–0.85 in women who did not receive chemotherapy and HR 0.33, 95% CI 0.18–0.61 in women who received the prior treatment) (39).

Finally, in the extended setting, the National Cancer Institute of Canada (NCIC) Trial MA.17 investigators compared outcomes in 5,187 women who were randomly assigned to 5 years of letrozole or placebo following 5 years of tamoxifen of whom 45% received adjuvant chemotherapy. DFS was identical regardless of chemotherapy use (HR 0.58, 95% CI, 0.40–0.83 in women who received chemotherapy and HR 0.58, 95% CI 0.40–0.84 in women without prior chemotherapy) (40).

In summary, initial results from the large studies that compared aromatase inhibitors with tamoxifen in the upfront, sequential, or extended setting in postmenopausal women suggest that the benefits observed with an AI over tamoxifen are irrespective of adjuvant chemotherapy use. Additional analyses may help further evaluate which women do not need chemotherapy and other studies will examine the utility of new prognostic and predictive factors specifically for this group of agents.

Because aromatase inhibitors are an integral part of the adjuvant treatment of postmenopausal women with hormone receptor-positive breast cancer, there has been great interest in incorporating the agents in younger women. However, aromatase inhibitors should not be used as monotherapy in premenopausal women because suppression of peripheral aromatase may result in a reduced feedback to the hypothalamus and an increase in ovarian stimulation (41). Aromatase inhibitors may be used with ovarian ablation or suppression in women for whom tamoxifen is contraindicated or in clinical trials.

Importantly, many premenopausal women with hormone receptor-positive breast cancer receive chemotherapy, and a large proportion of these women may experience chemotherapy-induced amenorrhea or ovarian failure. Because women who received chemotherapy are likely at high risk for disease recurrence, AI use would theoretically be especially desirable for these women. Current predictors for chemotherapy-induced ovarian failure are crude, however, and depend on patient age, type and duration of chemotherapy, and definition of chemotherapy-induced menopause or chemotherapy-induced ovarian failure (42). Because hormone concentrations immediately following chemotherapy may not provide an accurate prediction of ovarian function, caution should be used when considering the use of an AI in women who are premenopausal before adjuvant chemotherapy. Recent reports suggest that AI increase circulating estrogens in younger women and may stimulate ovarian function; indeed, pregnancies have been reported (43,44).

Given the uncertainty about whether chemotherapy-induced ovarian failure is permanent in women who were premenopausal before the treatment, initiation of tamoxifen with consideration of a sequential transition to an AI with close monitoring of circulating estrogens is recommended. If the clinician believes a woman is likely menopausal and prefers the use of an AI, estradiol concentrations should be measured with a high sensitivity assay (43).

Whether aromatase inhibitors and ovarian suppression are superior to tamoxifen in premenopausal women is still under investigation. The question will be answered in part by the ongoing Suppression of Ovarian Function Trial (SOFT), in which women are randomized to tamoxifen alone, tamoxifen and ovarian suppression, or exemestane and ovarian suppression.

Ovarian Ablation and Suppression

Ovarian ablation has been used for hormone receptor-positive premenopausal women for many more decades than tamoxifen. Several studies evaluated the role of ovarian ablation by surgery or radiotherapy or suppression with luteinizing hormone-releasing hormone (LHRH) agonists and chemotherapy. Interpretation of trials of chemotherapy with or without ovarian ablation is confounded by a high incidence of chemotherapy-induced ovarian failure in premenopausal women.

The *2000 Overview* reported that ovarian ablation or suppression alone in women younger than 50 is associated with a 30% reduction in recurrence and mortality rates (1). The addition of ovarian suppression to chemotherapy results in minimal

additional benefits. When the two modalities are used, the annual recurrence risk is reduced by 5% in women aged 40 to 49 years, and by 14% in those younger than 40 (Table 50.1) (1). A recent separate meta-analysis that included 16 trials and 9,002 premenopausal women with hormone receptor-positive disease who have received adjuvant LHRH agonists reported similar results (45). In 2,376 women who were included in the comparison of LHRH agonists and chemotherapy versus chemotherapy alone, percentage change in hazard ratios for outcomes in women with hormone receptor-positive cancer was -11.7 (95% CI $-22.8-1.0$, $p = .07$) for recurrence and -11.5 (95% CI $-24.8-4.2$, $p = .14$) for death. When further evaluated by age group, women 40 or younger (n = 714) had a significant reduction in percentage change in hazard ratios of recurrence (-24.7, 95% CI $-39.5 - -6.2$, $p = .01$) and death (-27.5, 95% CI $-44.2 - -5.7$, $p = .02$). In contrast, those older than 40 (n = 1,662) did not benefit from the addition of LHRH agonists to chemotherapy (HR for recurrence -5.1, 95% CI $-20.1-12.7$, $p = .55$, and death -2.2, 95% CI $-20.9-20.8$, $p = .83$).

In particular, results from E5188/Intergroup 0101 suggest that ovarian suppression in addition to chemotherapy benefits younger women. In this study, 1,503 premenopausal hormone receptor-positive, node-positive women were randomized to CAF chemotherapy alone or CAF followed by goserelin or CAF followed by goserelin, and tamoxifen. Overall, the addition of 5 years of goserelin to CAF did not provide significant additional benefits compared with chemotherapy alone. However, women younger than 40 derived benefit from the combination (46). In IBCSG Trial 13-93, women with ER-positive tumors who achieved chemotherapy-induced amenorrhea had a significantly improved outcome (HR for amenorrhea vs. no amenorrhea = 0.61; 95% CI, 0.44–0.86, $p = .004$) (34). These reports indirectly support the hypothesis that women who resume menstruation following chemotherapy may have worse outcomes compared with women with chemotherapy-induced ovarian failure and that the addition of ovarian suppression may provide survival benefit.

In the LHRH agonist meta-analysis, outcomes of women who received chemotherapy and tamoxifen, with or without ovarian suppression, were not statistically different regardless of the age group. In Intergroup 0101, women randomized to chemotherapy, goserelin, and tamoxifen had improved outcomes compared with women in the other two groups. The combination of chemotherapy, goserelin, and tamoxifen was significantly more effective than chemotherapy and goserelin improving time to recurrence by 26% (95% CI, 0.60–0.91, $p <.01$). However, OS was not statistically different among the groups.

The Adjuvant Breast Cancer Trials Collaborative Group Ovarian Ablation Or Suppression Trial included 2,144 pre- or perimenopausal women with tumors that were ER-positive or unknown who received tamoxifen for 5 years with or without ovarian suppression; chemotherapy was not assigned but was administered to those at high risk. Overall, 942 women received ovarian suppression and no benefit was observed from the addition of ovarian suppression to tamoxifen (HR for recurrence 0.95, 95% CI 0.81–1.12; HR for OS 0.94, 95% CI 0.78–1.13) (47). In IBCSG Trial 11-93, 174 node-positive, hormone-receptor positive premenopausal women were randomly assigned to 5 years of ovarian suppression and tamoxifen, with or without four cycles of adjuvant anthracycline-based chemotherapy. DFS and OS were identical in the two arms, but this underpowered trial was closed early because of low accrual rate (48).

Taken together, additional benefits from ovarian ablation are likely small in women who received chemotherapy, especially in women older than 40. Several explanations have been proposed, including the possibility that concurrent use in some studies may have interfered with the cytotoxic effects of chemotherapy or that ovarian ablation is not efficacious in the setting of chemotherapy-induced ovarian failure. With the documented efficacy of tamoxifen in premenopausal women and the unknown additional benefits of ovarian suppression to tamoxifen in women who received chemotherapy, ovarian suppression has not been recommended to most women. However, availability of LHRH agonists and the important role of AI in postmenopausal women have led to a renewed interest in ovarian suppression. The SOFT trial may help not only to further define the role of ovarian suppression plus tamoxifen to tamoxifen alone with or without prior chemotherapy, but will also identify the effectiveness of ovarian suppression and AI compared with tamoxifen. Other information will be gleaned from the Tamoxifen and Exemestane Trial (TEXT) and ABCSG 12 that are randomizing women to ovarian suppression and tamoxifen or ovarian suppression and AI. Indeed, preliminary data from ABCSG 12 suggest that there is no difference in outcome between ovarian suppression plus tamoxifen and ovarian suppression plus anastrozole (49). Finally two studies aimed at evaluating the role of chemotherapy in premenopausal women who were receiving endocrine therapy, Premenopausal Endocrine Responsive Chemotherapy Trial (PERCHE) and Premenopausal Optimal Management IS Endocrine therapy (PROMISE), were closed prematurely because of poor accrual. Until further data are available, tamoxifen remains standard, but it is reasonable to discuss the controversial role of ovarian suppression with individual women with high-risk hormone receptor-positive breast cancer who retain or regain ovarian function after chemotherapy. The possible marginal benefit of the treatment must be weighed against the menopausal symptoms and bone loss that the women may incur. It is hoped that predictive factors, such as circulating hormone concentrations, may ultimately help identify women who are likely to derive benefit from the addition of ovary-targeted therapy to chemotherapy and tamoxifen.

CHEMOENDOCRINE THERAPY: CHEMOTHERAPY CONSIDERATIONS

If chemoendocrine therapy is selected, then major questions about what type of chemotherapy to use and how to sequence treatments must be considered. The *Oxford Overview* and prospective clinical trials evaluated CMF-based regimens, anthracycline-containing regimens, and anthracycline-taxane combinations.

The *Overview* suggested that polychemotherapy was better than single agent therapy and that anthracycline-based therapy was superior to CMF-based regimens, reducing both annual event and death rates, but did not consider the contribution of specific regimens to the benefits observed with tamoxifen. Anthracycline-based regimens reduce the annual breast cancer death rate by about 38% and 20% for women younger than 50 years and for those of age 50 to 69 years, respectively (Table 50.1) (1). The benefit was similar whether or not endocrine therapy was administered. Similarly, the 31% reduction in annual breast cancer death rate observed with tamoxifen is seen regardless of the use of chemotherapy. Together, chemoendocrine therapy reduces average annual death rate from breast cancer by approximately 50%.

These results have been confirmed in a large randomized trial, Intergroup Trial 0102. In this study, 3,965 node-negative women were assigned to low-risk versus high-risk groups using tumor size, hormone receptor status, and proliferation index. High-risk patients (n = 2,690) were randomized to CMF or CAF with or without tamoxifen. Overall, outcomes were similar in both chemotherapy treatment groups. The addition of tamoxifen to CMF or CAF was associated with significant improvement in DFS and OS for ER-positive women, but not for ER-negative women (50). Women in the low-risk group did not receive adjuvant therapy and most had favorable long-term outcomes.

Most studies that compared different doses, schedules, or regimens that have been reported in recent years included subgroup analyses by hormone receptor status. Two recent studies compared an anthracycline-based regimen with a regimen that contained both anthracycline and taxanes. In E2197, DFS and OS were identical in women treated with AC or AT combination. In an exploratory analysis, a small improvement was seen in 5-year DFS for women with hormone receptor-negative tumors who were treated with AT compared with AC (19% and 6%, respectively) (21). However, a pivotal study demonstrated that the docetaxel, doxorubicin, and cyclophosphamide (TAC) regimen was superior to FAC, both in hormone receptor negative (DFS HR 0.69, 95% CI, 0.49–0.97) and hormone receptor-positive women (DFS HR 0.72, 95% CI, 0.56–0.92) with a hazard ratio of 1.08 (p = .72) (51).

In addition, ERBB2-positive tumors may be associated with higher sensitively to anthracycline- or taxane-based chemotherapy compared with other regimens. CALGB investigators evaluated whether hormone receptor status and ERBB2 status predicted benefit from adjuvant doxorubicin doses above standard levels, or from the addition of paclitaxel following AC combination, or from both. The investigators randomly selected 1,500 women from 3,121 women with node-positive breast cancer who were previously enrolled in C9344. Tissue blocks were available from 1,322 of the women. No interaction was seen between ERBB2 positivity and doxorubicin doses above 60 mg/m^2 but ERBB2 overexpression was associated with a significant benefit from paclitaxel (HR for recurrence of 0.59, p = .01) (52). Although patients with ERBB2-positive breast cancer benefited from paclitaxel regardless of ER status, paclitaxel did not improve outcome for patients with ERBB2-negative, ER-positive tumors. The authors concluded that patients with ERBB2-negative, ER-positive, node-positive breast cancer may gain little benefit from the administration of paclitaxel following combination AC.

Two additional studies asked questions regarding optimal dose and schedule of anthracycline and taxanes. In ECOG Trial 1199, 4,950 eligible women with node-positive or high-risk node-negative breast cancer received 4 cycles of AC every 3 weeks, followed by either paclitaxel or docetaxel administered either every 3 weeks for 4 cycles or weekly for 12 cycles. Compared with paclitaxel every 3 weeks, weekly paclitaxel was associated with improved DFS (HR 1.27, p = .006) and OS (HR 1.32, p = .01). Every-3-week docetaxel was also associated with improved DFS (HR 1.23, p = .015) compared with every-3-week paclitaxel, but not OS. In an exploratory subset analysis in ERBB2-negative patients (as determined by local laboratories), improvement in DFS and OS was comparable for hormone receptor-positive and negative disease. In particular for women with ERBB2-negative disease, weekly paclitaxel was associated with improvement in DFS (HR 1.33, p = .009) and OS (HR 1.34, p = .03). Subset analysis showed that weekly paclitaxel was associated with similar improvement in DFS in women with ERBB2-negative and hormone receptor-positive disease (HR 1.31, p = .05) and in ERBB2-negative and hormone receptor-negative disease (HR 1.37, p = .07). Trends for improved OS were likewise similar in ERBB2-negative patients regardless of hormone receptor status (21,53). In contrast in C9741, an exploratory analysis suggested that women with hormone receptor-positive disease did not benefit from a dose-dense schedule compared with women who received the same regimen on an every-3-week schedule (54). Finally in a study that compared outcomes of node negative women who received four cycles of AC or docetaxel and cyclophosphamide (TC), TC was slightly better than AC both in women with hormone receptor-positive and negative tumors (55).

Although not completely consistent, taken together, the data presented to date support the use of the same regimens for women at high risk regardless of hormone receptor status. Decisions about type of chemotherapy should be made based on estimates of risk of recurrence and death without consideration of steroid receptor-status.

DOSE, SCHEDULE, AND DURATION OF CHEMOENDOCRINE THERAPY

Decisions regarding dose, schedule, and duration of specific endocrine and chemotherapy therapies should be made based on the principles presented in Chapters 48 and 49, respectively. Only a few studies attempted to investigate these considerations specifically for women treated with chemoendocrine therapy. They have largely addressed the question of sequential versus concurrent administration of chemotherapy and tamoxifen.

In the *Overview*, both concurrent and sequential administration of chemotherapy and tamoxifen were associated with substantial benefit compared with use of tamoxifen alone. Compared with women who received tamoxifen alone, women aged 50 to 59 years who received chemotherapy and tamoxifen *concurrently* had a 16% reduction in the annual odds of recurrence, whereas women who received chemotherapy and tamoxifen *sequentially* had a 23% reduction (Table 50.1) (1).

Three clinical trials have prospectively tested this question. In the largest study, Intergroup Trial 0100, concurrent use of CAF chemotherapy and tamoxifen (CAFT-T) was associated with a worse outcome compared with the sequential use of chemotherapy followed by tamoxifen (CAF-T). Eight-year DFS rates were 67% for CAF-T and 62% for CAFT-T, compared with 55% for tamoxifen alone (19). Two smaller trials did not show a significant difference, but they were not powered to identify small but real differences. Based on these results, a reasonable approach is to administer tamoxifen after completion of adjuvant chemotherapy. Whether the sequential administration of chemotherapy and hormone therapy should be extended to other therapies, such as ovarian ablation or AI, is not known. It is unlikely that data about chemotherapy and aromatase inhibitors will emerge as the large randomized studies that included AI mandated sequential chemoendocrine administration. It is possible that some insight about this question will emerge from ongoing clinical trials in which concurrent chemoendocrine therapy is administered in the neoadjuvant setting. Currently in the absence of randomized data, sequential administration appears to be the most prudent strategy.

For women who are recommended chemoendocrine therapy, is there an optimal duration for each of the treatment modalities? Data presented to date cannot answer whether women prescribed both modalities should receive a different duration than the duration recommended for each treatment alone. In the absence of such information, endocrine therapy should be prescribed to the woman based on her risk of recurrence and the considerations discussed elsewhere. Likewise, duration of chemotherapy should be prescribed based on baseline risk and not hormone receptor status.

TOXICITY OF ADJUVANT CHEMOENDOCRINE THERAPY

Each adjuvant modality is associated with toxicities which are described in more detail in other chapters. Women receiving chemoendocrine therapy are at risk for both chemotherapy- and endocrine therapy-associated side effects. It is possible that some toxicities will be greater when both chemotherapy and endocrine therapy are administered, but few data are available. In particular, many premenopausal women who are treated with chemotherapy will have ovarian failure. Prevalence and severity of menopausal symptoms in these women is higher compared with other subgroups. Those women may also encounter greater

bone loss. Further, whether chemoendocrine therapy will have a greater effect on cognitive function than either approach alone is not known. In addition, women treated with anthracycline- or trastuzumab-based therapy are at risk for cardiac toxicities and it appears that aromatase inhibitors may be associated with a slight increase in cardiac events. Whether chemoendocrine therapy that incorporates AI and trastuzumab is associated with an increased susceptibility for cardiac disease is simply not known.

Concurrent therapy may also place women at higher risk for specific toxicities. For example, the combination of chemotherapy and tamoxifen may be associated with a greater risk of thromboembolic disease compared with each modality given alone. Women who receive CAF chemotherapy followed by ovarian suppression are at a slightly higher risk for weight gain, hypertension, diabetes, anemia, and hot flashes, and the addition of tamoxifen to CAF-Z slightly increases the incidence of diabetes, hot flashes, and anemia (46).

SUMMARY AND FUTURE DIRECTIONS

Decades of randomized clinical trials have firmly established a role for adjuvant chemoendocrine therapy in the management of early-stage breast cancer. In the next decade, it is expected that clinical trials will lead to the identification of more powerful prognostic and predictive factors that will help to match the most suitable treatment with characteristics of the individual woman and her specific tumor type. Currently, nodal status, tumor size, hormone receptor status, age, and tumor differentiation are imperfect gauges of prognosis. Established predictive markers can partially predict for endocrine responsiveness and new multigene assays are being tested as markers for chemotherapy response or resistance. It is hoped that new genomic, proteomic, and pharmacogenetic tools will lead to even better understanding of tumor and host biology and eventually to individualization of treatment.

It appears unlikely at this time that one type of endocrine or cytotoxic therapy will be suitable for all women who are recommended chemoendocrine therapy. Prospective investigations may help clarify whether specific chemotherapies are more appropriate for hormone receptor-positive women who will also be receiving endocrine therapy and to identify optimal combinations, sequence, and duration of treatment. It is hoped that the future generation of clinical trials will also include women who are likely to benefit from endocrine therapy but for whom chemotherapy may add little benefit.

Both chemotherapy and endocrine therapy provide substantial benefit to women with primary breast cancer and are likely to continue to be the mainstay of adjuvant treatment in the next decade. But it is certain that other targeted treatments will also become part of the spectrum. Studies in the adjuvant setting will attempt to integrate new targeted therapies or agents that enhance sensitivity or reverse resistance. Importantly, combinations of endocrine treatment and novel therapies, with or without chemotherapy, should be studied prospectively. It is likely that studies in the next decade will be conducted not exclusively by age or tumor stage, but preferentially according to tumor subtypes. Although many ongoing studies incorporate these novel strategies with chemotherapy, there is also a desire and need to study combinations of endocrine interventions with promising agents. Finally, a better understanding of host characteristics will help assure that the right treatment is administered to the woman who is most likely to derive benefit.

MANAGEMENT SUMMARY

- Every woman with a primary tumor that expresses estrogen or progesterone receptor protein should be considered for endocrine treatment.

- Selection of the type of endocrine manipulation varies by menopausal status and is discussed in detail in Chapter 48.
  - Postmenopausal women may be recommended 5 years of an aromatase inhibitor, 2 to 3 years of tamoxifen followed by aromatase inhibitor for total of 5 years, or 5 years of tamoxifen with or without 5 additional years of an aromatase inhibitor.
  - The standard endocrine treatment for premenopausal women remains tamoxifen for 5 years.
  - Ovarian suppression or ablation alone or in combination with tamoxifen or an aromatase inhibitor for premenopausal women is under study and may be appropriate for select women.
- The recommendation for endocrine therapy should be made regardless of the decision about whether or not to administer chemotherapy. Use of chemotherapy should follow the guidelines in Chapter 49.
  - Data to date suggest that the addition of chemotherapy should not be solely based on nodal status or tumor size, but should be considered for women with specific tumor characteristics. For example, the absence of the progesterone receptor, the overexpression of the ERBB2 receptor, or both may indicate a relative endocrine resistance. In addition, newer methods such as Oncotype DX can be used to determine magnitude of benefit from tamoxifen alone or with the addition of chemotherapy.
  - The decision regarding type and duration of chemotherapy should be independent of the hormone receptor status. Data today suggest that polychemotherapy with anthracycline, a taxane-based regimen, or both is superior to other therapies. Currently, data support the use of the same regimen for women at high risk for a systemic recurrence regardless of hormone receptor status.
- When chemoendocrine therapy is recommended, sequential rather than concurrent administration appears to be the most prudent strategy.

ACKNOWLEDGMENTS

Supported by National Institutes of Health (NIH) CA88843.

References

1. Effects of chemotherapy and hormonal therapy for early breast cancer on recurrence and 15-year survival: an overview of the randomised trials. *Lancet* 2005; 365(9472):1687–1717.
2. Winer EP, Hudis C, Burstein HJ, et al. American Society of Clinical Oncology technology assessment on the use of aromatase inhibitors as adjuvant therapy for postmenopausal women with hormone receptor-positive breast cancer: status report 2004. *J Clin Oncol* 2005;23(3):619–629.
3. Carlson RW, Hudis CA, Pritchard KI. Adjuvant endocrine therapy in hormone receptor-positive postmenopausal breast cancer: evolution of NCCN, ASCO, and St Gallen recommendations. *J Natl Compr Canc Netw* 2006;4(10):971–979.
4. Carlson RW, Brown E, Burstein HJ, et al. NCCN Task Force Report: Adjuvant Therapy for Breast Cancer. *J Natl Compr Canc Netw* 2006;4(Suppl 1):S1–S26.
5. Muss HB, Woolf S, Berry D, et al. Adjuvant chemotherapy in older and younger women with lymph node-positive breast cancer. *JAMA* 2005;293(9):1073–1081.
6. McGuire WL, Clark GM. Prognostic factors and treatment decisions in axillary-node-negative breast cancer. *N Engl J Med* 1992;326(26):1756–1761.
7. Gasparini G. Prognostic variables in node-negative and node-positive breast cancer [editorial]. *Breast Cancer Res Treat* 1998;52(1–3):321–331.
8. Hayes DF, Trock B, Harris A. Assessing the clinical impact of prognostic factors: When is "statistically significant" clinically useful? *Breast Cancer Res Treat* 1998; 52:305–319.
9. Ravdin PM, Siminoff LA, Davis GJ, et al. Computer program to assist in making decisions about adjuvant therapy for women with early breast cancer. *J Clin Oncol* 2001;19(4):980–991.
10. Goldhirsch A, Wood WC, Gelber RD, et al. Progress and promise: highlights of the international expert consensus on the primary therapy of early breast cancer 2007. *Ann Oncol* 2007;18(7):1133–1144.
11. Fisher B, Dignam J, Tan-Chiu E, et al. Prognosis and treatment of patients with breast tumors of one centimeter or less and negative axillary lymph nodes. *J Natl Cancer Inst* 2001;93(2):112–120.
12. Berry DA, Cirrincione C, Henderson IC, et al. Estrogen-receptor status and outcomes of modern chemotherapy for patients with node-positive breast cancer. *JAMA* 2006;295(14):1658–1667.
13. Harvey JM, Clark GM, Osborne CK, et al. Estrogen receptor status by immunohistochemistry is superior to the ligand-binding assay for predicting response to adjuvant endocrine therapy in breast cancer. *J Clin Oncol* 1999;17(5):1474–1481.
14. Bardou VJ, Arpino G, Elledge RM, et al. Progesterone receptor status significantly improves outcome prediction over estrogen receptor status alone for adjuvant endocrine therapy in two large breast cancer databases. *J Clin Oncol* 2003;21(10):1973–1979.
15. Arpino G, Weiss H, Lee AV, et al. Estrogen receptor-positive, progesterone receptor-negative breast cancer: association with growth factor receptor expression and tamoxifen resistance. *J Natl Cancer Inst* 2005;97(17):1254–1261.
16. Yamauchi H, Stearns V, Hayes DF. When is a tumor marker ready for prime time? A case study of c-erbB-2 as a predictive factor in breast cancer. *J Clin Oncol* 2001;19(9):2334–2356.
17. Paik S, Shak S, Tang G, et al. A multigene assay to predict recurrence of tamoxifen-treated, node-negative breast cancer. *N Engl J Med* 2004;351(27):2817–2826.
18. Paik S, Tang G, Shak S, et al. Gene expression and benefit of chemotherapy in women with node-negative, estrogen receptor-positive breast cancer. *J Clin Oncol* 2006;24(23):3726–3734.
19. Albain K, Green S, Ravdin P, et al. Overall survival after cyclophosphamide, adriamycin, 5-FU, and tamoxifen (CAFT) is superior to T alone in postmenopausal, receptor(+), node(+) breast cancer: new findings from phase III Southwest Oncology Group Intergroup Trial S8814 (INT-0100). *Proc Am Society Clin Oncol* 2001;20:(abstract 94).
20. Albain K, Barlow W, Shak S, et al. Prognostic and predictive value of the 21-gene recurrence score assay in postmenopausal, node-positive, ER-positive breast cancer (S8814,INT0100). *Breast Cancer Res Treat* 2007;108(abstract 10).
21. Goldstein L, O'Neill A, Sparano J, et al. E2197: Phase III AT (doxorubicin/docetaxel) *vs.* AC (doxorubicin/cyclophosphamide) in the adjuvant treatment of node positive and high risk node negative breast cancer. *J Clin Oncol* 2008;26: 4092–4099.
22. Goldstein L, Ravdin P, Gray R, et al. Prognostic utility of the 21-gene assay compared with Adjuvant! in hormone receptor (HR) positive operable breast cancer with 0-3 positive axillary nodes treated with adjuvant chemohormonal therapy (CHT): an analysis of intergroup trial E2197. *J Clin Oncol* 2008;26:4063–4071.
23. van de Vijver MJ, He YD, van't Veer LJ, et al. A gene-expression signature as a predictor of survival in breast cancer. *N Engl J Med* 2002;347(25):1999–2009.
24. Ma XJ, Wang Z, Ryan PD, et al. A two-gene expression ratio predicts clinical outcome in breast cancer patients treated with tamoxifen. *Cancer Cell* 2004;5(6): 607–616.
25. Goetz MP, Suman VJ, Ingle JN, et al. A two-gene expression ratio of homeobox 13 and interleukin-17B receptor for prediction of recurrence and survival in women receiving adjuvant tamoxifen. *Clin Cancer Res* 2006;12(7 Pt 1):2080–2087.
26. Stearns V, Johnson MD, Rae JM, et al. Active tamoxifen metabolite plasma concentrations after coadministration of tamoxifen and the selective serotonin reuptake inhibitor paroxetine. *J Natl Cancer Inst* 2003;95(23):1758–1764.
27. Jin Y, Desta Z, Stearns V, et al. CYP2D6 genotype, antidepressant use, and tamoxifen metabolism during adjuvant breast cancer treatment. *J Natl Cancer Inst* 2005;97(1):30–39.
28. Borges S, Desta Z, Li L, et al. Quantitative effect of CYP2D6 genotype and inhibitors on tamoxifen metabolism: implication for optimization of breast cancer treatment. *Clin Pharmacol Ther* 2006;80(1):61–74.
29. Goetz MP, Rae JM, Suman VJ, et al. Pharmacogenetics of tamoxifen biotransformation is associated with clinical outcomes of efficacy and hot flashes. *J Clin Oncol* 2005;23(36):9312–9318.
30. Fisher B, Costantino J, Redmond C, et al. A randomized clinical trial evaluating tamoxifen in the treatment of patients with node-negative breast cancer who have estrogen-receptor-positive tumors. *N Engl J Med* 1989;320:479–484.
31. Fisher B, Jeong JH, Bryant J, et al. Treatment of lymph-node-negative, oestrogen-receptor-positive breast cancer: long-term findings from National Surgical Adjuvant Breast and Bowel Project randomised clinical trials. *Lancet* 2004;364(9437):858–868.
32. Fisher B, Dignam J, Wolmark N, et al. Tamoxifen and chemotherapy for node-negative, estrogen receptor-positive breast cancer. *J Natl Cancer Inst* 1997;89:1673–1682.
33. International Breast Cancer Study Group. Endocrine responsiveness and tailoring adjuvant therapy for postmenopausal lymph node-negative breast cancer: a randomized trial. *J Natl Cancer Inst* 2002;94(14):1054–1065.
34. Colleoni M, Gelber S, Goldhirsch A, et al. Tamoxifen after adjuvant chemotherapy for premenopausal women with lymph node-positive breast cancer: International Breast Cancer Study Group Trial 13-93. *J Clin Oncol* 2006;24(9):1332–1341.
35. Forbes JF, Cuzick J, Buzdar A, et al. Effect of anastrozole and tamoxifen as adjuvant treatment for early-stage breast cancer: 100-month analysis of the ATAC trial. *Lancet Oncol* 2008;9(1):45–53.
36. Baum M, Buzdar A, Cuzick J, et al. Anastrozole alone or in combination with tamoxifen versus tamoxifen alone for adjuvant treatment of postmenopausal women with early-stage breast cancer: results of the ATAC (Arimidex, Tamoxifen Alone or in Combination) trial efficacy and safety update analyses. *Cancer* 2003;98(9):1802–1810.
37. Coates AS, Keshaviah A, Thurlimann B, et al. Five years of letrozole compared with tamoxifen as initial adjuvant therapy for postmenopausal women with endocrine-responsive early breast cancer: update of study BIG 1-98. *J Clin Oncol* 2007;25(5):486–492.
38. Coombes RC, Hall E, Gibson LJ, et al. A randomized trial of exemestane after two to three years of tamoxifen therapy in postmenopausal women with primary breast cancer. *N Engl J Med* 2004;350(11):1081–1092.
39. Jonat W, Gnant M, Boccardo F, et al. Effectiveness of switching from adjuvant tamoxifen to anastrozole in postmenopausal women with hormone-sensitive early-stage breast cancer: a meta-analysis. *Lancet Oncol* 2006;7(12):991–996.
40. Goss PE, Ingle JN, Martino S, et al. Randomized trial of letrozole following tamoxifen as extended adjuvant therapy in receptor-positive breast cancer: updated findings from NCIC CTG MA.17. *J Natl Cancer Inst* 2005;97(17):1262–1271.
41. Smith IE, Dowsett M. Aromatase inhibitors in breast cancer. *N Engl J Med* 2003; 348(24):2431–2442.
42. Stearns V, Schneider B, Henry NL, et al. Breast cancer treatment and ovarian failure: risk factors and emerging genetic determinants. *Nat Rev Cancer* 2006;6(11): 886–893.
43. Smith IE, Dowsett M, Yap YS, et al. Adjuvant aromatase inhibitors for early breast cancer after chemotherapy-induced amenorrhoea: caution and suggested guidelines. *J Clin Oncol* 2006;24(16):2444–2447.

44. Burstein HJ, Mayer E, Patridge AH, et al. Inadvertent use of aromatase inhibitors in patients with breast cancer with residual ovarian function: cases and lessons. *Clin Breast Cancer* 2006;7(2):158–161.

45. Cuzick J, Ambroisine L, Davidson N, et al. Use of luteinising-hormone-releasing hormone agonists as adjuvant treatment in premenopausal patients with hormone-receptor-positive breast cancer: a meta-analysis of individual patient data from randomised adjuvant trials. *Lancet* 2007;369(9574):1711–1723.

46. Davidson NE, O'Neill AM, Vukov AM, et al. Chemoendocrine therapy for premenopausal women with axillary lymph node-positive, steroid hormone receptor-positive breast cancer: results from INT 0101 (E5188). *J Clin Oncol* 2005;23(25):5973–5982.

47. Adjuvant Breast Cancer Trials Collaborative Group. Ovarian ablation or suppression in premenopausal early breast cancer: results from the international adjuvant breast cancer ovarian ablation or suppression randomized trial. *J Natl Cancer Inst* 2007;99(7):516–525.

48. Thurlimann B, Price KN, Gelber RD, et al. Is chemotherapy necessary for premenopausal women with lower-risk node-positive, endocrine responsive breast cancer? 10-year update of International Breast Cancer Study Group Trial 11-93. *Breast Cancer Res Treat* 2009;113:137–144.

49. Gnant M, Mlineritsch B, Schippinger W, et al. Adjuvant ovarian suppression combined with tamoxifen or anastrozole, alone or in combination with zoledronic acid, in premenopausal women with hormone-responsive, stage I and II breast cancer: first efficacy results from ABCSG-12 [Abstract LBA4]. *J Clin Oncol* 2008;26.

50. Hutchins LF, Green SJ, Ravdin PM, et al. Randomized, controlled trial of cyclophosphamide, methotrexate, and fluorouracil versus cyclophosphamide, doxorubicin, and fluorouracil with and without tamoxifen for high-risk, node-negative breast cancer: treatment results of Intergroup Protocol INT-0102. *J Clin Oncol* 2005;23(33):8313–8321.

51. Martin M, Pienkowski T, Mackey J, et al. Adjuvant docetaxel for node-positive breast cancer. *N Engl J Med* 2005;352(22):2302–2313.

52. Hayes DF, Thor AD, Dressler LG, et al. HER2 and response to paclitaxel in node-positive breast cancer. *N Engl J Med* 2007;357(15):1496–1506.

53. Sparano JA, Wang M, Martino S, et al. Weekly paclitaxel in the adjuvant treatment of breast cancer. *N Engl J Med* 2008;358(16):1663–1671.

54. Hudis C, Citron M, Berry D, et al. Five year follow-up of INT C9741: dose-dense (DD) chemotherapy (CRx) is safe and effective [Abstract 41]. *Proc San Antonio Breast Cancer Symposium* 2005.

55. Jones SE, Savin MA, Holmes FA, et al. Phase III trial comparing doxorubicin plus cyclophosphamide with docetaxel plus cyclophosphamide as adjuvant therapy for operable breast cancer. *J Clin Oncol* 2006;24(34):5381–5387.

Chapter 51
Adjuvant Treatment of ERBB2 Positive Breast Cancer

Evandro de Azambuja and Martine Piccart-Gebhart

Breast cancer is the most common cause of malignancy among women. The human epidermal growth factor receptor 2 (ERBB2, formerly HER2) is a tyrosine kinase receptor that is overexpressed in approximately 20% to 25% of patients with breast cancer (1,2). It belongs to a family of four members, EGFR (ErbB1), HER-2 (ErbB2), HER-3 (ErbB3) and HER-4 (ErbB4), which form homo- or heterodimers and share a common structure, namely an extracellular ligand-binding region, a single membrane-spanning region, and a cytoplasmic tyrosine-kinase-containing domain (the latter being absent for ERBB3) (3). ERBB2-positive status is well recognized as an adverse prognostic marker in breast cancer as well as a positive predictive marker of response to anti-ERBB2 therapies, such as trastuzumab or lapatinib (4). Because of its extreme importance, the American Society of Clinical Oncology (ASCO) recommends evaluation of ERBB2 status for all primary breast tumors, and has recently issued specific guidelines for its measurements and reporting (5). More information on the clinical aspects of ERBB2 is provided in Chapter 30.

Because ERBB2 overexpression has an impact on both prognosis and treatment, it is of paramount importance to determine its presence accurately. Currently, two different methods are used worldwide, immunohistochemistry (IHC) assessing ERBB2 protein overexpression and fluorescence *in situ* hybridization (FISH) assessing ERBB2 gene amplification (6). Alternative methods, such as real time-polymerase chain reaction (RT-PCR) (7) and chromogen *in situ* hybridization (CISH), are being developed, but experience in using them is more limited (8).

Histochemistry is a semiquantitative method that evaluates ERBB2 receptor expression on the cell surface using a grading scale (0, 1+, 2+, and 3+). IHC is performed on paraffin tumor blocks; it is not time-consuming and relatively low in cost. However, this method is highly operator-dependent and the result can be influenced by different factors, such as the use of different fixation protocols, assay methods, selected antibodies, and scoring systems. In contrast, FISH is a quantitative method that measures the number of ERBB2 gene copies present in each tumor cell, either in isolation or in comparison with the number of centromeres of chromosome 17. The results are reported as positive or negative (meaning amplification or noamplification, respectively). Although FISH is believed to be somewhat more reproducible than IHC, it is more time-consuming and expensive than IHC.

According to the new ASCO guidelines, ERBB2 status should be reported as an algorithm defining positive, equivocal, and negative values as follow (5):

- **ERBB2 positive:** IHC staining of 3+ (uniform, intense membrane staining of >30% of invasive tumor cells); a FISH result >6.0 ERBB2 gene copies per nucleus; or a FISH ratio (ERBB2 gene signals to chromosome 17 signals) >2.2.
- **ERBB2 negative:** IHC staining of 0 or 1+; a FISH result of <4.0 ERBB2 gene copies per nucleus; or a FISH ratio of <1.8.
- **ERBB2 equivocal:** IHC 3+ staining of 30% or less of invasive tumor cells or 2+ staining; a FISH result of 4 to 6 ERBB2 gene copies per nucleus; or a FISH ratio between 1.8 and 2.2.

Trastuzumab is a recombinant humanized monoclonal antibody (mAb) directed against the extracellular domain (ECD) of the ERBB2 receptor. Based on results demonstrating a significant survival benefit when used in combination with chemotherapy (CT), the U.S. Food and Drug Administration (FDA) approved trastuzumab in 1998 for the treatment of metastatic breast cancer (MBC) patients whose tumors overexpress ERBB2 (9). In the adjuvant setting, the combination or sequential use of trastuzumab with different CT regimens demonstrated a striking benefit in reducing breast cancer recurrences as well as in improving patient survival (10–14).

Nonetheless, there is a proportion of patients who do not benefit from trastuzumab (*de novo* resistance) and, in those who respond well initially, resistance to trastuzumab can often develop within 9 to 12 months of treatment initiation (acquired resistance). The mechanisms underlying acquired resistance to trastuzumab, although not completely defined, include the existence of compensatory pathways and downstream signaling aberrations, such as loss of phosphatase and tensin homolog (PTEN) function; absence or loss of the external domain of the receptor leading to the truncated form of the receptor known as p95ERBB2; modulation of p27kip1; and increased insulin-like growth factor I receptor (IGF-IR) signaling (15). Consequently, a clear need exists for new drugs, such as lapatinib, a tyrosine kinase inhibitor (TKI) currently being tested in the adjuvant setting. For complete information on the treatment of ERBB2-positive MBC.

In that chapter, the authors describe the five landmark trastuzumab adjuvant trials, as well as the recent French adjuvant trial, providing an update on the efficacy, safety, and limitations of this drug in early-stage breast cancer. The future role of lapatinib in the adjuvant treatment of ERBB2 positive breast cancer patients is also discussed.

ADJUVANT TRASTUZUMAB IN EARLY BREAST CANCER

In all six adjuvant trials described in Table 51.1, patients with ERBB2-positive invasive breast cancer were enrolled after surgery (lumpectomy or mastectomy). Patients with node-positive or high-risk node-negative disease were eligible; they were to receive adjuvant CT and, when indicated, radiotherapy (RT) and endocrine therapy. ERBB2 positivity was defined as IHC 3+ or FISH positive in all except in the Finnish Herceptin (FinHer) study, in which CISH was used. The main characteristics and results of these adjuvant trials are discussed below.

The HERceptin Adjuvant (HERA) trial was an international, multicenter, randomized, controlled trial comparing 1-year or 2-years of 3 weekly of trastuzumab with observation. To be eligible, patients had to have completed locoregional therapy and a minimum of four courses of any acceptable neo- or adjuvant CT. HERA's primary end point was disease-free survival (DFS), defined as time from randomization to the occurrence of any of the following events: local, regional, or distant recurrence; contralateral breast cancer, including ductal carcinoma *in situ* (DCIS); secondary nonbreast malignancy; or death without evidence of recurrence. Secondary end points included cardiac safety, overall survival (OS), and time to distant recurrence (12).

Of the 5,102 patients enrolled, 3,401 had data available for analysis, 1,703 in the 1-year trastuzumab arm and 1,698 in the observation arm. At the latest update and with 23.5 months of median follow-up, there were 539 DFS events and 149 deaths. The unadjusted hazard ratio (HR) for the risk of death with

Table 51.1 MAIN RESULTS OF TRASTUZUMAB IN ERBB2-POSITIVE EARLY BREAST CANCER

Trial (Reference)	Patients (N)	Patient Characteristics	Treatment Regimens	Primary End Point	Median Follow-up	DFS HR (CI; p value)	OS HR (CI; p value)
NSABP B-31 (16)	2,043	Node-positive	AC × 4 → P × 4 / AC × 4 → P × 4 + T (P given 3 weekly)				
Intergroup N9831 (16)	2,766	Node-positive	AC × 4 → P × 4 / AC × 4 → P × 4 + T starting concurrently with P / AC × 4 → P × 4 + T starting after P (P given weekly)	DFS	2.9 yr	Pooled analysis: 0.48 (CI 0.41–0.57; $p <.00001$)	Pooled analysis: 0.65 (CI 0.51–0.84; $p = .0007$)
HERA (11)	5,102	All except small (<1 cm) node-negative	Any accepted CT alone (observation) / T for 1 yr after completion of CT / T for 2 yr after completion of CT	DFS	2 yr	0.64 (CI 0.54–0.76; $p <.0001$)	0.66 (CI 0.47–0.91; $p <.015$)
BCIRG 006 (14)	3,222	Node-positive or high risk node-negative	AC × 4 → D × 4 (I) / AC × 4 → D × 4 + T starting concurrently with D (II) / D + Cb × 6 + T (D given 3 weekly) (III)	DFS	3 yr	0.61 (II vs. I) (CI 0.48–0.76; $p <.0001$) / 0.67 (III vs. I) (CI 0.54–0.83; $p = .0003$)	0.59 (II vs. I) (CI 0.42–0.85; $p = .004$) / 0.66 (III vs. I) (CI 0.47–0.93; $p = .0017$)
FinHer (13)	232	Node-positive or high risk node-negative	V or D × 3 with or without T 9 wk followed by FEC × 3	RFS	38 mo	0.42 (CI 0.21–0.83) ($p = .0078$)	0.41 (CI 0.47–1.08) ($p = .07$)
PACS-04 (17)	528	Node-positive	FEC × 6 or ET × 6	DFS	48 mo	0.86 (0.61–1.22) ($p = .41$)	1.27 (0.68–2.38) p not provided

AC, doxorubicin, cyclophosphamide; BCIRG, Breast Cancer International Research Group; Cb, carboplatin; CI, confidence interval; D, docetaxel; DFS, disease-free survival; ET, epirubicin, docetaxel; FEC, 5-fluorouracil, epirubicin, cyclophosphamide; HERA, HERceptin Adjuvant; HR, hazard ratio; NSABP, National Surgical Adjuvant Breast and Bowel Project; PACS, Protocole Adjuvant dans le cancer du sein; OS, overall survival; P, paclitaxel; RFS, relapse-free survival; T, trastuzumab; V, vinorelbine.

trastuzumab compared with observation was 0.66 (0.47-0.91; $p = .0115$), corresponding to an absolute OS benefit of 2.7%. The unadjusted HR for the risk of an event with trastuzumab was 0.64 (0.54–0.76; p <.0001), corresponding to an absolute DFS benefit of 6.3% (11).

The National Surgical Adjuvant Breast and Bowel Project (NSABP B-31) trial compared four cycles of doxorubicin and cyclophosphamide (AC) followed by four cycles of 3 weekly of paclitaxel (arm 1) with the same regimen plus 52 weeks of trastuzumab beginning with the first cycle of paclitaxel (arm 2). The Intergroup N9831 trial randomized patients in 1 of three regimens: four cycles of AC followed by 12 cycles of weekly paclitaxel (arm A); the same regimen followed by 52 weekly of trastuzumab (arm B); or the same regimen plus 52 weekly doses of trastuzumab initiated concomitantly with paclitaxel (arm C). Because of similarities between arms 1 and 2 of NSABP B-31 and arms A and C of N9831, the National Cancer Institute (NCI) and the FDA approved a joint analysis of both trials with the exclusion of arm B of the N9831 trial (10). The primary end point for this combined analysis was DFS, and secondary end points included OS, time to distant relapse, death from breast cancer, contralateral breast cancer, and second primary cancers.

In the second combined analysis including 3,968 patients (1,989 in the trastuzumab arm and 1,979 in the control arm)—with a median follow-up of 2.9 years, 619 DFS events and 258 deaths—patients treated with trastuzumab experienced a longer DFS with a 52% lower risk of an event (HR 0.48; 95% confidence interval [CI] 0.41–0.57; p <.00001). This corresponded to an absolute difference in DFS of 13% at 4 years. In patients receiving trastuzumab, the risk of death was 35% lower (HR 0.65; 95% CI 0.51–0.84; $p = .0007$), reflecting an absolute difference in OS of 3.2% at 4 years (16).

The Breast Cancer International Research Group (BCIRG) 006 trial evaluated the benefit of adding trastuzumab to two CT regimens, one with and one without anthracyclines, with the intention of maximizing efficacy and minimizing cardiotoxicity. The regimens were four cycles of AC followed by four cycles of 3 weekly of docetaxel (AC-D); four cycles of AC-D combined with 1-year of trastuzumab (AC-DH); or six cycles of docetaxel and carboplatin with 1-year of trastuzumab (DCbH) (14). The primary end point was DFS, and secondary end points included OS, toxicity, and the evaluation of pathologic and molecular markers for predicting efficacy in these patients.

At the second interim efficacy analysis, with a median follow-up of 36 months, there were 462 DFS events and 185 deaths among 3,222 enrolled patients. The HR for DFS was 0.61 (95% CI 0.48–0.76; p <.0001) for the AC-DH arm, and 0.67 (0.54–0.83; $p = .00003$) for the DCbH arm, compared with the AC-D arm, translating into absolute benefits of 6% and 5%, respectively. The HR for OS was 0.59 (0.42–0.85; $p = .004$) for AC-DH and 0.66 (0.47–0.93; $p = .017$) for DCbH over AC-D.

In the FinHer trial, 1,010 patients were randomized to three cycles of 3 weekly docetaxel or 8 weekly cycles of vinorelbine followed by three cycles of fluorouracil, epirubicin, and cyclophosphamide (FEC). ERBB2-positive patients (n = 232) were further randomized to either receive (n = 116) or not receive (n = 116) 9 weeks of trastuzumab, given concomitantly with the first three cycles of docetaxel or vinorelbine (13). The primary end point was recurrence-free survival (RFS), and secondary end points included adverse events (AE), cardiac safety, time to distant recurrence, and OS.

Results presented at a 3-year median follow-up showed a significant reduction in distant recurrence (HR 0.29; 95% CI 0.13–0.64; $p = .002$), an improved 3-year DFS (HR 0.42; 95% CI 0.21–0.83; $p = .01$) and a nonstatistically significant trend toward improved OS (HR 0.41; 95% CI 0.16–1.08; $p = .07$) favoring the patients treated with trastuzumab.

Presented at the 2007 San Antonio Breast Cancer Symposium (SABCS), the French Protocole Adjuvant dans le Cancer du Sein (PACS) 04 failed to show any benefit of adding trastuzumab to the adjuvant treatment of node-positive early breast cancer. In this trial, 3,010 patients were randomized to receive six cycles of FEC (100 mg/m^2) or docetaxel plus epirubicin (75 mg/m^2 of each drug) and, in the subset of ERBB2-positive tumors, patients were randomized to receive either 1 year of adjuvant trastuzumab (260 patients) or none (268 patients). ERBB2 status was assessed using IHC 3+ ($\sim$87%) or FISH + if IHC 2+ ($\sim$13%). The primary end point for this second randomization was 3-year DFS. With a median follow-up of 48 months and 70 events in the observation arm and 59 in the trastuzumab arm, this trial failed to show a clear benefit in terms of DFS (HR 0.86; 95% CI 0.61–1.22; $p = .41$) and OS (HR 1.27; 95% CI 0.68–2.38; p-value not provided). The 4-year DFS was 72.7% in the trastuzumab arm versus 73.2% in the observation arm, and the 4-year OS was 91.5% in the trastuzumab arm versus 93.0% in the observation arm (17).

SIMILARITIES AND DIFFERENCES AMONG ALL TRIALS

Some similarities in patient populations were seen across all studies and they include the following:

- Young age, with approximately 50% of enrolled patients being younger than 50 years;
- A high proportion of histologic grade 3 tumors (60% to 69%); and
- Estrogen receptor (ER), progesterone receptor (PR), or both positivity in 46% to 61% of patients (Table 51.2)

Nevertheless, there are several important differences between the trials. The first concerns the variation to be found regarding the inclusion of patients with node-negative breast cancer, which was considered high risk: 32% in HERA (only in case of tumor size >1 cm), 29% in BCIRG 006 (only if hormone receptor-negative tumors), 7% in the combined analysis of NSABP B-31 and N9831, and 16% in FinHer (only if tumor size was >2 cm and PR negative). Of note, no node-negative patients were included in the PACS-04 study.

A second difference is to be found was with respect to the use of taxanes: all patients in BCIRG 006 and the combined U.S. trials (NSABP B-31 and N9831) received taxanes (docetaxel and paclitaxel, respectively), compared with 26% in HERA (docetaxel or paclitaxel) and 50% in the FinHer and PACS-04 trials (docetaxel in both). Notably, because HERA allowed several types of CT regimens, its results apply to women with ERBB2-positive breast cancer worldwide, more accurately reflecting the reality of daily clinical practice. Interestingly, the BCIRG 006 trial compared anthracycline-based versus non–anthracycline-based (docetaxel plus carboplatin) regimens. Although no difference in efficacy between the two regimens was seen, cardiac safety data were better for the nonanthracycline arm. These results are provocative and suggest that the risk of cardiotoxicity may be minimized without compromising efficacy by using trastuzumab with a nonanthracycline regimen. Although this would seem to provide an attractive option for many patients, it should be considered with great caution owing to the short follow-up of the trial and the lack of full published data at this writing (only abstract and oral presentation available). It should be noted that all trials have excluded patients with previous cardiac disease.

The time elapsed between surgery and the start of trastuzumab also varied considerably among the six trials.

Table 51.2	SIMILARITIES AND DIFFERENCES AMONG THE ADJUVANT TRIALS				
	HERA (11)[a]	NSABP B-31/N9831 (16)	BCIRG 006 (14)	FinHer (13)	PACS-04 (17)
Trastuzumab schedule	Every 3 weeks	Weekly/weekly	Weekly with CT, then every 3 weeks	Weekly	Every 3 weeks
ERBB2 testing	Centralized IHC ± FISH	IHC a/o FISH in "approved" laboratories	Centralized FISH	Centralized CISH	NA
Age <50 years (%)	51	50	52	NA	NA
Node-negative (%)	32[b]	7	29[c]	16[d]	0
Grade 3 tumors	60	69	NA	64	66
Taxane-based CT	26	100	100	50	50
ER+ a/o PR+	47	58	54	46[e]	58
Baseline LVEF assessment	At completion of CT and RT	At completion of 4 AC	After surgery	After surgery	At completion of CT and RT
Cross-over to trastuzumab after first analysis (%)	50	20.9	1.6	NA	NA
Participating countries	39	1	40	1	2

AC, doxorubicin, cyclophosphamide; CISH, chromogenic *in situ* hybridization; CT, chemotherapy; ER, estrogen receptor; FISH, fluorescence *in situ* hybridization; IHC, immunohistochemistry; LVEF, left ventricular ejection function; NA, not available; PACS, Protocole Adjuvant dans le cancer du sein; PR, progesterone receptor; RT: radiotherapy.
[a]Reference numbers in parentheses.
[b]Only if tumor size >1 cm.
[c]Only if other concomitant risk factors (grade >1, hormone receptors negative).
[d]Only if size >20 mm and PR negative.
[e]ER positive only.

The design of the HERA trial delayed the start of trastuzumab for a median of 8 months after surgery (patients completed all CT and RT); this contrasts with a median time of 4 months in the combined NSABP B-31 and N9831 group (at completion of AC); 2.6 months in PACS-04 (time elapsed between first and second randomization); 1 month in the FinHer trial; and 1 month also in the platinum-taxane arm of BCIRG 006 (upfront with CT).

Another variation across the trials is the way trastuzumab was administered, with the 3-week schedule used in HERA and PACS-04, the weekly schedule used in NSABP B-31/N9831/FinHer, and both schedules in BCIRG 006. Whether the weekly or the 3-week schedule is the best is still unknown, but both schedules have been tested in the metastatic setting, where they have shown comparable efficacy (18).

Similarly, RT was administered differently in the trials: before randomization in the HERA and PACS-04 trials, after completion of CT and trastuzumab in the FinHer trial, and after CT and concomitantly with trastuzumab in the BCIRG 006, N9831 and NSABP B-31 trials

A key difference for the FinHer trial should be noted with respect to treatment duration. Although trastuzumab was given empirically for 1 year in the HERA, NSABP B-31, N9831, BCIRG 006, and PACS-04 trials, the small FinHer trial was particularly provocative in having reduced the duration of trastuzumab administration to only 9 weeks. Although this trial is clearly a positive trial, the confidence intervals for the treatment effects are wide and its small sample size (232 patients) limits confidence in safety. Therefore, 9 weeks of trastuzumab should not be considered as standard of care, but rather a hypotheses generator for the design of future studies.

Finally, differences among these adjuvant trials also concern percentages of crossover to trastuzumab in the *control* arms. After the results of the trials had been presented or published, patients enrolled in the observation arms were offered to cross over to trastuzumab therapy, and this occurred in approximately 50% of patients in the HERA trial, which contrasts with low rate of crossover in the combined N9831 and NSABP B-31 trials (20.9%) and in the BCIRG 006 trial (1.6%).

CONGESTIVE HEART FAILURE WITH TRASTUZUMAB

Cardiac safety was very closely monitored in all trials (Table 51.3). In the HERA trial, severe congestive heart failure (CHF; New York Heart Association [NYHA] class III-IV) occurred in 0.6% of patients treated with trastuzumab. Symptomatic CHF was seen in 1.7% and 0.06% of patients in the trastuzumab and observation arms, respectively; 51 patients experienced a confirmed left ventricle ejection fraction (LVEF) decrease (defined as an EF decrease of >10 points from baseline and to below 50%) with trastuzumab. Most of the patients with cardiac dysfunction recovered in fewer than 6 months (11,19), and the risk factors for cardiac dysfunction were higher cumulative doses of anthracyclines, lower screening LVEF, and higher body mass index (19).

In the NSABP B-31 trial, the 5-year cumulative incidence of cardiac events for trastuzumab-treated patients was 3.9%, compared with 1.3% in the control group. An asymptomatic decline in LVEF (defined as >10% decline or to 55%) occurred in 17% of patients enrolled in arm 1 and 34% in arm 2, with a HR of 2.1 (1.7–2.6; *p* <.0001). The difference in cumulative incidence at 5 years was 2.7%. Risk factors for CHF were age 50 years or more (5.2% to 5.3%), treatment with hypertension medication (7.7%), and post–AC-LVEF values of 50% to 54% (13.0%) (20). In the N9831 trial, the 3-year cumulative incidence of cardiac events in arm A (AC → T) was 0.3%, in arm B (AC → T → H) was 2.8%, and in arm C 3.3% (AC → TH) (21).

In the BCIRG 006 trial, clinically symptomatic cardiac events were detected in 0.38% of patients in the AC-D arm, 1.87% in the AC-DH arm, and 0.37% in the DCbH arm. A statistically significant higher incidence was seen of both asymptomatic LVEF and persistent decrease in LVEF in the AC-DH arm than in either the AC-D or DCbH arms. Although promising, the results of a nonanthracycline regimen in this trial must be carefully interpreted owing to the relatively short follow-up at the time of reporting.

In the FinHer trial, none of the patients who received trastuzumab experienced clinically significant cardiac events (CHF) and, in fact, LVEF was preserved in all women (13). In the PACS-04 trial, CHF was seen in 1.7% of patients receiving trastuzumab and 0.4% of patients in the observation arm (17).

| Table 51.3 | CARDIAC SAFETY RESULTS IN ADJUVANT TRASTUZUMAB TRIALS |

	HERA (11,19)[a]		NSABP B-31 (20)			N9831 (21)		BCIRG 006 (14)			PACS-04 (17)	
Treatment arms	Obs	1-yr H	AC→P	AC→PH	AC→P	AC→P→H	AC→PH	AC→D	AC→DH	DCb+H	Obs	1-yr H
Women at risk (n)	1,708	1,678	872	932	767	718	875	1,050	1,068	1,056	268	260
Cardiac deaths	1	0	1	0	1	1	0	0	0	0	0	0
CHF NYHA class 3–4 (%)	0	10 (0.6)	9 (1)	35 (3.9)	2 (0.3)	18 (2.5)	19 (2.2)	4 (0.38)	20 (1.87)	4 (0.37)	1 (0.4)	4 (1.7)

AC, doxorubicin and cyclophosphamide; BCIRG, Breast Cancer International Research Group; Cb, carboplatin; CHF, congestive heart failure; D, docetaxel; H: Herceptin (trastuzumab); HERA, HERceptin Adjuvant; NSABP, National Surgical Adjuvant Breast and Bowel Project; NYHA, New York Heart Association; Obs, observation; P, paclitaxel; PACS, Protocole Adjuvant dans le cancer du sein.
[a]Reference numbers in parentheses.
Note: NSABP B-31: cumulative incidence at 5 years; N9831: cumulative incidence at 3 years; No CHF class 3-4 and no cardiac death reported in the FinHer trial.

The low incidence of cardiac events in the HERA trial may be explained by several factors:

- A required baseline LVEF of greater than or equal to 55%, which was higher than in the other trials.
- Similar to PACS-04, the timing of the first protocol-mandated LVEF assessment after completion of all CT and RT, which may have selected patients with better cardiac function; this contrasts with the other trials in which some of the CT or RT was given after the patient had been randomized.
- The much longer time interval between the administration of the anthracycline and the onset of trastuzumab treatment. Additional information on the side effects of systemic therapy, including cardiac dysfunction, is provided in Chapter 55.

The assessment of LVEF before the initiation of treatment with trastuzumab, and at regular intervals during treatment, is crucial. A thorough cardiac assessment at initiation includes history, physical examination, and determination of LVEF by echocardiogram or Multiple Gated Acquisition (MUGA) scan. Beyond this thorough baseline examination, the following schedule is to be used to monitor cardiac function in clinical studies and in daily practice (22):

- LVEF measurements every 3 months during and on completion of treatment with trastuzumab
- LVEF measurements every 6 months for at least 2 years following completion of treatment
- Repeat LVEF measurements at 4-week intervals if trastuzumab is withheld for significant LVEF dysfunction

Trastuzumab administration should be withheld for at least 4 weeks in the following two scenarios:

1. Greater than equal to 16% absolute decrease in LVEF from pretreatment values
2. LVEF below institutional limits of normal and greater than equal to 10% absolute decrease in LVEF from pretreatment values

Trastuzumab may be resumed if the LVEF returns to normal limits and the absolute decrease from baseline is 15% or less within 4 to 8 weeks after withholding it. Permanent discontinuation of trastuzumab is recommended in case of persistent (>8 weeks) LVEF decrease or in case of suspension of trastuzumab administration on more than three occasions because of cardiomyopathy (22).

INCIDENCE OF BRAIN METASTASES

ERBB2-positive breast cancer patients present a high incidence of central nervous system (CNS) metastases (up to 50% in MBC patients treated with trastuzumab). Interestingly, the survival time after the diagnosis of brain metastases is longer than the one seen in patients with ERBB2-negative tumors and brain metastases (22.4 vs. 9.4 months; $p = .0002$). This difference is most probably because of better systemic disease control with trastuzumab (23,24). A retrospective analysis of a cohort of 9,524 women with early breast cancer who were randomized to several trials between 1978 and 1999 showed a 10-year cumulative incidence of CNS as site of first relapse in 2.7% of ERBB2-positive patients compared with 1.0% in ERBB2-negative ones ($p < .01$) (25). It is generally thought that trastuzumab does not cross the intact blood–brain barrier owing to its large molecular size, yet very recent data seem to suggest that it may cross an impaired blood–brain barrier (26).

The first results of the combined NSABP B-31 and N9831 analysis revealed that the incidence of isolated brain metastases as first event was higher in the trastuzumab group than in the control group (21 vs. 11 in NSABP B-31 and 12 vs. 4 in N9831), although this was not reported during the second analysis presented at ASCO 2007 (10,16). Similarly, in the first analysis of HERA, CNS metastases were more frequent in the trastuzumab group than in the control group (21 vs. 15, respectively), but CNS relapses were not reported during the second analysis (11,12). The HERA team is now studying patients with CNS relapse to better understand this event in both groups (trastuzumab vs. observation). No information about brain metastases is currently available for the BCIRG 006, FinHer, and PACS-04 trials.

TRASTUZUMAB PLUS BEVACIZUMAB IN THE ADJUVANT SETTING

In a randomized phase III trial in MBC patients, the combination of paclitaxel plus bevacizumab significantly prolonged progression-free survival (11.8 months vs. 5.9 months; $p < .001$) and increased the objective response rate (36.9% vs. 21.2%; $p < .001$) compared with paclitaxel alone (27). In addition, a phase II trial of trastuzumab plus bevacizumab showed partial response in 13 of 28 (46%) evaluable patients. An additional 9 of 28 patients had stable disease at week 8. However, a possible increased cardiotoxic signal in this trial calls for very close cardiac monitoring with this double antibody therapy in the adjuvant setting (28). The combination of bevacizumab with trastuzumab is now being investigated in the adjuvant setting in the BETH (A Multicenter Phase III Randomized Trial of Adjuvant Therapy for Patients with HER2-Positive Node-Positive or High Risk Node-Negative Breast Cancer Comparing Chemotherapy Plus Trastuzumab with Chemotherapy Plus Trastuzumab Plus Bevacizumab) trial (NSABP B-44-I). This phase III, randomized, open-label trial will investigate whether CT plus trastuzumab and bevacizumab improves invasive DFS relative to CT plus trastuzumab alone. Central ERBB2 status determination will be performed (either positive by FISH or IHC 3+). Patients in this trial will be enrolled in one of two CT regimen cohorts: (a) six cycles of docetaxel, carboplatin, and trastuzumab (TCH) with or without bevacizumab; or (b) three cycles of docetaxel plus trastuzumab given with or without bevacizumab followed by three cycles of 5-fluorouracil, epirubicin, cyclophosphamide (TH-FEC). With both regimens, patients will continue trastuzumab with or without bevacizumab following CT for 1 year of targeted therapy. Following completion of CT, patients will also receive adjuvant radiotherapy and endocrine therapy as clinically indicated. The secondary end points of this study include DFS, OS, recurrence-free interval (RFI), and distant recurrence-free interval (DRFI). The planned sample size for the trial is 3,000 patients randomized in the faster accruing cohort and a minimum of 3,500 patients overall (29).

QUESTIONS UNANSWERED BY THE ADJUVANT TRASTUZUMAB TRIALS CONDUCTED SO FAR

Despite treatment with trastuzumab demonstrating a significant reduction in the number of relapses and deaths in women with ERBB2-positive breast cancer, some questions about how best to use adjuvant trastuzumab remain unanswered. These are summarized below.

Optimal Duration of Trastuzumab Therapy

The question of the optimal duration of trastuzumab therapy remains controversial when examining the results available to date. With the exception of FinHer (13), in all adjuvant trials the duration of trastuzumab therapy was empirically set at 1 year (13). As previously described, the outcome of the 9-week course of trastuzumab used in the FinHer trial was particularly provocative and led to the hypothesis that a short duration of treatment could be as efficacious as an extended one. Interestingly, the shorter trastuzumab treatment was able to produce comparable hazard ratios for DFS (0.42) and OS (0.41), although the confidence intervals were wide for both (95% CI 0.21–0.83, $p = .001$ and 95% CI 0.16–1.08, $p = .07$, respectively). These striking results may be partially explained by the upfront use of trastuzumab within a synergistic CT combination (vinorelbine or docetaxel) or by its concomitant use with an anthracycline regimen (FEC). Indeed, is important to consider that this second synergy (trastuzumab plus FEC) may have played a role, given the long half-life of trastuzumab, which continues to exert its action for a few weeks after it has last been administered (30).

In contrast to the FinHer trial, HERA will evaluate duration from the opposite perspective: this trial randomized patients to 2 years versus 1 year of trastuzumab treatment, with the intention of determining whether efficacy could be improved with longer rather than shorter therapy. The results of the 2-year arm have not yet been released and, thus, they are eagerly awaited.

To better elucidate the trastuzumab duration issue, two important trials have been initiated more recently and are currently recruiting patients. The first is the Protocol Herceptin Adjuvant with Reduced Exposure (PHARE) study, which is a noninferiority French phase III trial comparing 6 months versus 1 year of trastuzumab in 3,400 ERBB2-positive early breast cancer patients (31). The primary end point is DFS and 1,040 events are required to establish noninferiority with an absolute difference between the two treatment durations of less than 2%. Notably, randomization will occur when patients have received between 3 and 6 months of trastuzumab therapy. In other words, contrary to the other

trials, this approach does not involve upfront randomization and it may select more trastuzumab-sensitive patients (32). The second trial is the Synergism Or Long Duration (SOLD) trial, which compares 9 weeks versus 1 year of trastuzumab. In this trial, 3,000 patients will be randomized to receive docetaxel concomitantly with trastuzumab (9 weeks of treatment) followed by three cycles of FEC. Half of the patients will complete 1 year of trastuzumab therapy after terminating treatment with FEC. The primary end point is DFS, and 600 events are required in this superiority study. Interestingly, ERBB2 positivity will be confirmed using CISH, FISH, or IHC, and node-negative patients with tumors greater than 5 mm will be included (33).

Needless to say, answering the trastuzumab duration question depends largely on the results of HERA, PHARE, and SOLD. Until then, 1-year of trastuzumab therapy will continue to be the empiric standard-of-care for ERBB2-positive early breast cancer patients.

Use of Trastuzumab in Small (<1 cm) Node-negative ERBB2-Positive Tumors

Small (<1 cm) node-negative ERBB2-positive breast cancer patients have a moderate risk of locoregional and distant recurrence. Five-year DFS is 90.5% for T1a-b tumors, 89.5% for T1c tumors, and 79.5% for patients with T2 tumors (34). Information on tumors smaller than 1 cm is rather scarce in almost all trastuzumab adjuvant trials. In the FinHer trial, approximately 7% of patients had tumors smaller than 1 cm, but no final efficacy results have been reported on this subgroup of patients because of the small sample size. In the BCIRG 006 trial, these patients were included in the subgroup of tumors 2 cm or less (range 38% to 41%), which is similar to the combined analysis of the N9831 and NSABP B-31 trials (38% to 40%), HERA (39% to 40%), and PACS-04 (30% to 34%). Therefore, it is difficult to draw any conclusions based on the available data for patients with small tumors.

Additionally, node-negative disease and small tumor size (<1 cm) remains a subject of constant debate among oncologists. According to the 10th St. Gallen consensus meeting held in 2007, most experts shared the opinion that trastuzumab should not be regarded as a standard treatment for women with node-negative tumors less than 1 cm, mainly because of the lack of relevant trial data (35). In each of the five adjuvant trials reported to date, the inclusion of node-negative patients (Table 51.2) was low: 7% in NSABP B-31 and N9831; 32% in HERA, where tumors were greater than 1 cm; 29% in BCIRG 006 in the presence of other concomitant risks such as high grade or hormone receptor negativity; and 16% in FinHer (if tumors were >2 cm and PR negative).

Subgroup analyses may be informative, although they are often confounded by the increased likelihood of false–positive or negative results. They should therefore always be interpreted with caution (36). In the trastuzumab trials presented here, a significant benefit of adjuvant trastuzumab was seen in the subgroup of node-negative tumors in HERA (HR 0.59; 95% CI 0.39–0.91) and in BCIRG 006 (no HR provided); in contrast, a nonsignificant reduction in the risk of an event was observed in the combined analysis of NSABP B-31 and N9831 (HR 0.80; 95% CI 0.28–2.23), but the number of patients included in this analysis was very small (n = 281).

With respect to the HERA subgroup analysis in the node-negative cohort (all eligible tumor sizes), it was shown that the magnitude of absolute improvement in 3-year DFS for trastuzumab compared with observation ranged from 0.6% for hormone-receptor negative patients (HR = 0.68) and 11.3% for hormone receptor-positive patients (HR = 0.46) (37).

Table 51.4	BENEFIT OF TRASTUZUMAB IN DFS ACCORDING TO IHC/FISH POSITIVITY			
		Patients (N)	HR	95% CI
N9831 (16)				
IHC 3 +	FISH ≥2.0	1,405	**0.47**	0.34–0.66
	FISH <2.0	53	0.61	0.11–3.29
IHC 0, 1, 2 +	FISH ≥2.0	218	0.98	0.33–2.91
	FISH <2.0	103	0.51	0.21–1.2
NSABP B-31 (39)				
	FISH ≥2.0	1,588	**0.47**	0.36–0.61
	FISH <2.0	207	**0.40**	0.18–0.89
	IHC 3 +	1,407	**0.45**	0.34–0.59
	IHC 0, 1, 2 +	255	**0.28**	0.12–0.66
IHC 0, 1, 2 +	FISH ≥2.0	125	0.30	0.08–1.07
	FISH <2.0	161	**0.36**	0.14–0.92
HERA (40)				
Local IHC 3+	No central FISH	1,264	**0.60**	0.46–0.80
Local IHC 3+	Central FISH +	1,628	**0.73**	0.57–0.94
Local IHC 2+	Central FISH +	340	**0.56**	0.32–0.99

CI, confidence interval; FISH, fluorescence *in situ* hybridization; HERA, HERceptin Adjuvant; HR, hazard ratio; IHC, immunohistochemistry; NSABP, National Surgical Adjuvant Breast and Bowel Project.
Note: HR in bold are statistically significant; reference numbers in parentheses.

Finally, the SOLD trial, as described above, will include node-negative patients with tumors greater than 5 mm, but these results are unlikely to shed more light on the benefit of trastuzumab in this patient population given the lack of an observation arm (33).

Therefore, in patients with node-negative disease, trastuzumab is only recommended when tumors are a minimum of 1 cm or greater, unless contraindications exist to its use, such as previous cardiac disease or cardiac dysfunction.

Use of Trastuzumab in Elderly Patients

Worldwide, nearly a third of breast cancer cases occurs in patients over the age of 65 years, and this proportion rises to more than 40% in more developed countries. The International Society of Geriatric Oncology (SIOG) has recently created a taskforce to review the published literature and to provide evidence-based recommendations for the diagnosis and treatment of breast cancer in older individuals. Regarding the use of trastuzumab in this age group, SIOG recommends the following: "In the absence of cardiac contraindications, adjuvant trastuzumab should be offered to older patients with HER-2 (ERBB2) positive breast cancer when CT is indicated, but cardiac monitoring is essential" (38).

Indeed, the elderly population appears to be underrepresented in all six adjuvant trials: approximately 16% of patients were 60 or more years of age in HERA and 17.5% in the NSABP B-31 and N9831 trials (between 60 and 69 years). Beyond that, information is lacking in BCIRG 006 (patients were characterized as more or <50 years), and in the FinHer and PACS-04 trials in which patients included in the ERBB2 analysis were aged 65 years and older.

Despite the small numbers, however, this older population clearly benefited from the addition of trastuzumab in the NSABP B-31 and N9831 combined analysis (DFS: 665 patients ≥60 years; HR 0.40; 95% CI 0.26–0.59) and demonstrated a nonsignificant improvement in the HERA trial (DFS: 544 patients ≥60 years; HR 091; 95% CI 0.59–1.41. Therefore, the decision to give adjuvant trastuzumab to elderly patients should not be based on age, but rather on several other characteristics, such as cardiac function, risk of relapse, and comorbid conditions.

Benefit of Trastuzumab According to Immunohistochemistry, Fluorescence *In Situ* Hybridization, or Other Molecular Markers

Interesting results have been presented regarding level of IHC and FISH positivity and benefit from trastuzumab (Table 51.4). Although only IHC 3+ and FISH + patients benefited significantly from the addition of 1 year of trastuzumab in the N9831 trial, a similar analysis in HERA and NSABP B-31 revealed positive results in several subgroups (16,39,40). Contrary to N9831 and NSABP B-31, the HERA trial was the only study to show a significant benefit for the subgroup of IHC 2+ and FISH + (HR 0.56) (16,39,40). Although noteworthy, all these results should be interpreted cautiously because they were not prospectively dictated in the trials and the numbers are small, with wide confidence intervals.

Several publications have suggested that ERBB2 positivity is associated with an incremental benefit from anthracycline-containing regimens compared with non–anthracycline-containing ones. However, the mechanism of action by which ERBB2 is associated with increased sensitivity to anthracyclines remains unclear. It is believed that this may relate to the physical proximity on chromosome 17q of the ERBB2 gene to the topoisomerase-II alpha (TOP2A) gene, given that topoisomerase II is integrally involved in the mechanism of action of anthracyclines. Some studies and meta-analyses have suggested that ERBB2 positivity predicts better response to higher-dose anthracycline-containing regimens and predicts a differential benefit from the addition of taxanes, such as paclitaxel or docetaxel. For more details on ERBB2 and TOP2A as predictors of response to CT, the authors highly recommend a recently published review (41).

Although these studies have reached level 2 evidence (prospective therapeutic trials in which marker utility is a secondary study objective), given the uncertainty regarding the biologic relationship between TOP2 expression, copy number, proliferation, and benefit from anthracyclines, ASCO guideline recommendations view TOP2A assessment as unreliable at this time (42).

At present, the BCIRG 006 trial is the only trial to retrospectively demonstrate the impact of coamplification of TOP2A in patients receiving adjuvant trastuzumab. TOP2A coamplification was detected in 1,057 (35%) of 2,990 patient tumor blocks screened. Patients whose tumors showed coamplification of the two genes had a statistically significant improvement in DFS compared with patients with nonamplified tumors (HR 1.44; 95% CI 1.16–1.78; p <.001). Importantly, when the first trial results were presented, the DCbH arm seemed to be as efficacious as the AC-DH arm, and both clearly superior to the AC-D arm (p <.001), for patients without coamplification of ERBB2 and TOP2A, whereas for patients with this coamplification, the AC-DH arm was superior to the other two arms; however, in the latest update of the trial results, these differences were no longer significant (14). Furthermore, women whose breast cancers showed TOP2A gene coamplification had a significantly longer DFS (p <.001), RFS (p <.001), and OS (p = .01) compared with women whose breast cancers lacked this amplification. Unexpectedly, the added beneficial effect of trastuzumab was not seen in patients with TOP2A coamplified breast cancer in the larger BCIRG 006 trial (43). Therefore, the assessment of TOP2A is not yet recommended as standard of care, and more data are required before the performance of this predictive marker reaches level 1 evidence.

In NSABP B-31, using FISH analysis in 1,549 available cases, c-MYC was found to be amplified in 432 cases (30%). Patients with this amplification had worse outcome when they were treated with CT alone (HR 0.63), but showed a 4-year RFS rate of 90% if treated with CT and trastuzumab (HR 0.24; p = .007). These results suggest exquisite sensitivity to trastuzumab, as well as the drug's possible role in reversing the antiapoptotic function of dysregulated c-MYC (44). These data, however, require independent validation.

Trastuzumab Concomitant with or in Sequence to Taxanes

With the exception of the HERA and PACS-04 trials, and arm B of N9831, all other adjuvant trastuzumab trials have given trastuzumab concurrently with CT. At the time of the first interim combined analysis of the NSABP B31 and N9831 trials, an unplanned analysis of arms B (sequential) and C (concurrent) of N9831 was requested by the overseeing data monitoring committee despite the short follow-up period and the small number of events. Based on the 1,682 patients randomized to either arm B or C, a significant benefit in DFS (HR 0.64; 95% CI 0.46–0.91; p = .00114) and a nonsignificant benefit in OS (HR 0.74; 95% CI 0.43–1.26; p = .2696) favoring concurrent over sequential taxane plus trastuzumab treatment (45). Although these results seem interesting, this comparison should be interpreted very cautiously given the unplanned and premature nature of the results and the wide confidence intervals. Furthermore, these efficacy data should not be interpreted in isolation, but must also take into account the cardiotoxicity reported with the combination of trastuzumab and CT.

The controversy of how to use trastuzumab and taxanes remains largely unresolved with the data currently available. Until the results of the N9831 trial are updated, the scheduling of taxanes and trastuzumab will depend on a variety of factors, such as clinician preferences, patient cardiac risk, and the rules applying across different health care systems.

Lapatinib in Early Breast Cancer

Lapatinib is a small tyrosine kinase inhibitor molecule that has the potential of dual inhibition of EGFR and ERBB2, resulting in potent inhibition of signaling (46). Although TKI targeting the ERBB family are described in Chapter 79, some key information is briefly summarized below.

In some tumors ERBB2 lacks its extracellular domain (truncated form), compromising the activity of antibodies such as trastuzumab, which binds to this extracellular domain. The truncated form of ERBB2, called p95, has greater kinase activity than the wild-type ERBB2, and lapatinib has been shown to inhibit baseline p95 phosphorylation in BT474 cells and in tumor xenografts. This is not seen with trastuzumab (47), although some data show that trastuzumab prevents the formation of p95 (4,48).

Lapatinib has other potential advantages in comparison to trastuzumab. The antitumor activity of trastuzumab in ERBB2 overexpressing breast cancer seems to be dependent on the presence of phosphatase and tensin homologue deleted on chromosome 10 (PTEN), a phosphatase that reduces phosphatidylinositol 3-kinase-Akt signaling. PTEN deficiency has been demonstrated in approximately 50% of breast cancer and predicts for resistance to trastuzumab monotherapy. Another advantage of lapatinib over trastuzumab is that lapatinib seems to exert its antitumor activity in a PTEN-independent manner (49).

Recent data suggest that lapatinib is a potent eradicator of "tumorigenic stem cells" present in the primary tumor; if such cells do exist and explain late relapses from breast cancer despite neoadjuvant CT, lapatinib could represent a very effective new weapon against the disease (50).

In single agent studies, objective responses with lapatinib given to patients whose cancers had progressed on multiple trastuzumab-containing regimens were observed in approximately 4.3% to 7.8% of patients. Despite a low level of overall objective tumor responses, a substantial number of subjects with ERBB2 overexpressing tumors had stable disease at 4 months (34% to 41%) and 6 months (18% to 21%) while on lapatinib (51).

The first interim analysis of the phase III EGF100151 trial reported on 324 patients with ERBB2-positive locally advanced or metastatic breast cancer whose disease progressed on anthracyclines, taxanes, and trastuzumab and who were randomized to capecitabine treatment, with or without lapatinib. The results showed significant improvement in median time-to-progression (TTP) for patients receiving lapatinib and capecitabine compared with patients treated with capecitabine alone (8.4 vs. 4.4 months; p <.0001, HR = 0.49; 95% CI 0.34–0.71; p <.001). A similar improvement was obtained in median progression-free-survival (PFS) as well (8.4 vs. 4.1 months; p <.0001, HR = 0.47; 95% CI 0.33–0.67; p <.001). By the closure of randomization, a total of 399 women had been enrolled in the study. The updated results confirm an improvement in median TTP from 19 weeks to 27 weeks (HR 0.57; 95% CI, 0.43–0.77; p <.001), and continue to show significant reduction in the relative risk of progression when lapatinib is added to capecitabine therapy (52–54). Diarrhea, dyspepsia, and rash of any grade were more commonly seen in the lapatinib plus capecitabine group, whereas a trend to more fatigue was seen in the capecitabine alone group. Adverse events led to the discontinuation of treatment in 22 women in the combination group (13%) and in 18 women in the monotherapy group (12%) (52). Based on these results, the FDA and the European Medicine Agency (EMEA) approved the use of lapatinib plus capecitabine in MBC patients whose breast cancer had progressed despite treatment with anthracyclines, taxanes, and trastuzumab.

Some indirect data suggest that lapatinib may be able to cross the intact blood–brain barrier. In the EGF100151 study, for example, CNS relapse was significantly greater in the capecitabine alone arm (11%) than in the capecitabine plus lapatinib arm (2%) (p = .0445) (53). In addition, lapatinib monotherapy was given to 241 heavily pretreated and trastuzumab-exposed ERBB2-positive breast cancer patients with CNS involvement in the EGF105084 trial (phase II). In an exploratory analysis, 19 patients (7%) experienced a volumetric tumor reduction of 50% or greater, and 46 patients (19%) a 20% or greater reduction. In an exploratory analysis of extension of capecitabine plus lapatinib in 40 patients, 8 patients (20%) experienced a volumetric tumor reduction of 50% or greater, and 16 patients (40%) a 20% or greater reduction (55). A recent update presented at the SABCS showed that in 242 patients with CNS involvement, 15 patients (6%) experienced a volumetric tumor reduction of 50% or greater, and 41 patients (17%) a 20% or greater reduction. Again, in the exploratory analysis of the extension of capecitabine plus lapatinib in 51 patients, 10 patients (20%) experienced a volumetric tumor reduction of 50% or greater, and 18 patients (37%) a 20% or greater reduction (56).

Another advantage of lapatinib over trastuzumab is the lower incidence of cardiac toxicity. Albeit low, the incidence of CHF with trastuzumab may jeopardize the treatment and long-term safety of patients treated in the adjuvant setting. In an important review of the cardiotoxicity data of lapatinib in 43 studies involving 3,558 patients enrolled who were already treated with lapatinib, either as a single-agent or in combination, encouraging results have been shown. An asymptomatic decrease in LVEF was observed in only 1.6% of patients, whereas 0.2% experienced a symptomatic decrease of LVEF. In general, these cardiac events were reversible and of short duration, the average being an LVEF decrease of 4.8 weeks (57). Nonetheless, these data must be interpreted cautiously: many patients included in this lapatinib meta-analysis had not been previously exposed to anthracyclines, and some had received prior trastuzumab; therefore, the available figures pertain to selected populations (46).

Lastly, with lapatinib most of the associated adverse events are generally mild to moderate (grade 1 or 2), whereas severe (grades 3 or 4) toxicities are uncommon. Diarrhea and cutaneous rash, apart from the cardiac events described above, remain the most common toxicities of lapatinib, but rarely impact on treatment delivery or compliance (46).

Because of the potential advantages described above, lapatinib is currently being tested in the adjuvant setting. The Adjuvant Lapatinib and/or Trastuzumab Treatment Optimisation (ALTTO) trial is a global collaboration between the Breast International Group (BIG) and the Breast Cancer Intergroup of North America (TBCI). ALTTO is a four-arm phase III trial evaluating the efficacy of lapatinib, either given alone, sequentially, or in combination with trastuzumab. Eight thousand patients with ERBB2-positive early breast cancer will be randomly assigned to one of the following treatment arms: lapatinib for 52 weeks; trastuzumab for 52 weeks; trastuzumab for 12 weeks followed by a wash-out period of 6 weeks and then treatment for 34 weeks with lapatinib; or lapatinib in combination with trastuzumab for 52 weeks. This trial has two designs, one with and one without paclitaxel concomitantly with target therapy (12 weeks). The first patient was recruited in Europe in June 2007 (58).

The ALTTO has been designed with a number of important quality controls in place, as well as a view to the future. In contrast to most studies to date, all patients enrolled in this trial will have their ERBB2 status centrally assessed using both IHC and FISH techniques to maximize the reliability of results. The central testing of estrogen and progesterone receptors is also mandatory before randomization. Moreover, in all 8,000 patients, PTEN, *c-MYC*, p95, and TOP2A will be prospectively evaluated using tissue microarray. This will contribute to the central tumor bank foreseen for future research that will lead to a better understanding of the mechanisms of sensitivity or resistance to both drugs. Finally, ALTTO anticipates an important additional translational research program with the collection of blood samples for pharmacogenomics, proteomics, and circulating tumor cells together with frozen tumor samples in a subset of its patients.

Following these same principles, there is an ALTTO "sister" trial being conducted in parallel: the Neo–Adjuvant Lapatinib and/or Trastuzumab Treatment Optimisation (NEO-ALTTO) trial will randomly assign women with ERBB2-positive tumors larger than 2 cm to one of the following three treatment arms: lapatinib for 6 weeks followed by the addition of weekly paclitaxel for an additional 12 weeks; trastuzumab for 6 weeks followed by the addition of weekly paclitaxel for an additional 12 weeks; trastuzumab plus lapatinib for 6 weeks followed by the addition of weekly paclitaxel for an additional 12 weeks. Definitive surgery is performed within 4 weeks of the last dose of paclitaxel. After surgery, patients will receive three cycles of adjuvant CT (FEC) followed by the same assigned preoperative targeted therapy for 34 weeks, with the intention to complete 1 year of anti-ERBB2 therapy (59). This trial started recruiting patients in early 2008.

The Tykerb Evaluation After Chemotherapy (TEACH) trial is chronologically the first trial evaluating lapatinib in the adjuvant setting. Because of complete recruitment of 3,000 women in early 2008, it will evaluate the effectiveness of lapatinib given both as immediate or delayed therapy in early ERBB2-positive breast cancer. TEACH is a phase III randomized, double-blind, multicenter, placebo-controlled trial of lapatinib and its primary objective is to determine whether adjuvant therapy with lapatinib for 1 year will improve DFS. Eligible women must have completed adjuvant CT; be free of disease at entry; have either a new diagnosis and be unable or unwilling to receive trastuzumab; or have a previous diagnosis of ERBB2-positive breast cancer and not have received prior adjuvant trastuzumab (60).

To return to the neoadjuvant setting, two American trials are, as is NEO-ALTTO, evaluating lapatinib in early breast cancer: NSABP B-41 and Cancer and Leukemia Group B (CALGB) 40601. The NSABP B-41 is a phase III study, the primary purpose of which is to determine whether breast cancer tumors respond (as measured by pathologic complete response, the absence of microscopic evidence of invasive tumor cells in the breast) to combined doxorubicin plus cyclophosphamide (four cycles) followed by paclitaxel plus trastuzumab (12 weeks) or lapatinib (12 weeks) or both (12 weeks) in 522 patients with operable ERBB2-positive breast cancer. Trastuzumab will also be given to all patients after surgery. In addition, the study will look at whether there are gene expression profiles in the tumor tissue that can predict pathologic complete response (61). The CALGB 40601 is a phase III study, in which the primary end point is also pathologic complete response. The trial will randomize 400 patients with operable ERBB2-positive breast cancer to paclitaxel plus trastuzumab (12 weeks) or lapatinib (12 weeks) or both (12 weeks). After surgery, patients are to receive dose-dense AC (recommended) followed by 40 weeks of trastuzumab given every 3 weeks. An important part of this trial will be obtaining samples of tumor tissue at diagnosis and during surgery to evaluate potential biomarkers that may be helpful in predicting response to therapy (62).

These five trials (ALTTO, Neo-ALTTO, TEACH, NSABP B-41, and CALGB 40601) will help us elucidate the role of (neo)-adjuvant lapatinib and better understand the sensitivity or resistance to lapatinib and trastuzumab in ERBB2-positive breast cancer patients.

CONCLUSIONS

The use of trastuzumab in the adjuvant setting has proved to be highly effective in reducing the number of recurrences and improving overall survival in women with ERBB2-positive early breast cancer. Results as striking as those for trastuzumab had not been reported since the benefit of adjuvant tamoxifen was determined 30 years ago. Importantly, the benefit of adding trastuzumab to the adjuvant armamentarium against breast cancer was consistently demonstrated across five of six adjuvant trials, leading therefore to a fundamental change in clinical practice.

Despite the impressive reduction in the risk of relapse and death for women with ERBB2-positive breast cancer, the reality is that not all patients will respond to trastuzumab and, in those who do, trastuzumab resistance may appear later on. Therefore, a need exists to identify accurately from among the whole population of ERBB2-positive breast cancer those patients most likely to benefit from adjuvant trastuzumab. This approach will minimize long-term toxicities, such as the incidence of cardiotoxicity, as well as reduce overall health care costs.

Alternative and efficacious therapeutic solutions for patients who develop resistance to trastuzumab are being sought through the use of new anti-ERBB2 therapies, such as lapatinib, as well as through ambitious translational research programs being incorporated into the clinical trials testing the development of these novel treatments. Specifically, Neo ALTTO and ALTTO, testing lapatinib as either neo- or adjuvant therapy, respectively, will incorporate an extensive translational research program designed to answer a number of clearly defined scientific questions. The knowledge gained from this research will contribute to the improved tailoring of anti-ERBB2 treatment. It is only the common efforts between clinicians and scientists that will ultimately help us unravel the complexities of ERBB2 breast cancer, which is well on the way to changing its status from being a "poor prognosis" disease to one with multiple, effective treatment options and good prognosis.

Management Summary for Adjuvant Treatment of ERBB2-Positive Breast Cancer

- The tumors of all newly diagnosed breast cancer patients should be tested for ERBB2 overexpression or amplification in an accredited laboratory.
- ERBB2 equivocal results (IHC 3+ staining of ≤30% of invasive tumour cells or 2+ staining, FISH result of 4 to 6 ERBB2 gene copies per nucleus, or FISH ratio between 1.8 and 2.2) require additional testing for final determination. ERBB2 testing should be performed in an accredited laboratory or in a laboratory that meets the accreditation and proficiency testing requirements as per ASCO/CAP guidelines.
- One year of adjuvant trastuzumab remains the standard of care in ERBB2-positive breast cancer patients (node-negative and tumour size ≥1 cm or node-positive) unless there is a contraindication, such as previous cardiac disease.
- Trastuzumab can be administered either weekly or every 3 weeks.
- Thorough cardiac assessment (MUGA or ECHO) should be performed in all patients receiving adjuvant trastuzumab.
- LVEF assessment should be performed before initiation of trastuzumab, every 3 months during trastuzumab therapy, and every 6 months for at least 2 years following completion of trastuzumab (if no cardiac dysfunction has been observed).
- Trastuzumab administration should be withheld for at least 4 weeks in the following circumstances: greater than or equal to 16% absolute decrease in LVEF from pretreatment values; LVEF below institutional limits of normal, and greater than or equal to 10% absolute decrease in LVEF from pretreatment values. Trastuzumab may be resumed if the LVEF returns to normal limits and the absolute decrease from baseline is less than or equal to 15% within 4 to 8 weeks after withholding it.

- Permanent discontinuation of trastuzumab is recommended in case of persistent (>8 weeks) LVEF decrease or in case of suspension of trastuzumab administration on more than three occasions because of cardiomyopathy.
- Trastuzumab should not be used with concomitant adjuvant anthracycline chemotherapy.
- Because the results for concomitant taxane and trastuzumab relative to the sequential use of chemotherapy and trastuzumab are not conclusive, treatment with concomitant taxanes and trastuzumab will depend on clinician and patient preferences as well as patient risk of relapse or cardiotoxicity.
- At this moment (2008), adjuvant lapatinib remains investigational and should not be used outside clinical trials.

References

1. Slamon DJ, Clark GM, Wong SG, et al. Human breast cancer: correlation of relapse and survival with amplification of the HER-2/neu oncogene. *Science* 1987;235 (4785):177–182.
2. Slamon DJ, Godolphin W, Jones LA, et al. Studies of the HER-2/neu proto-oncogene in human breast and ovarian cancer. *Science* 1989;244(4905):707–712.
3. Yarden Y, Sliwkowski MX. Untangling the ErbB signalling network. *Nat Rev Mol Cell Biol* 2001;2(2):127–137.
4. Nahta R, Esteva FJ. Herceptin: mechanisms of action and resistance. *Cancer Lett* 2006;232(2):123–138.
5. Wolff AC, Hammond ME, Schwartz JN, et al. American Society of Clinical Oncology/College of American Pathologists guideline recommendations for human epidermal growth factor receptor 2 testing in breast cancer. *J Clin Oncol* 20071;25(1):118–145.
6. Pauletti G, Dandekar S, Rong H, et al. Assessment of methods for tissue-based detection of the HER-2/neu alteration in human breast cancer: a direct comparison of fluorescence in situ hybridization and immunohistochemistry. *J Clin Oncol* 20001;18(21):3651–3664.
7. Suo Z, Daehli KU, Lindboe CF, et al. Real-time PCR quantification of c-erbB-2 gene is an alternative for FISH in the clinical management of breast carcinoma patients. *Int J Surg Pathol* 2004;12(4):311–318.
8. Denoux Y, Arnould L, Fiche M, et al. [HER2 gene amplification assay: is CISH an alternative to FISH?]. *Ann Pathol* 2003;23(6):617–622.
9. Slamon DJ, Leyland-Jones B, Shak S, et al. Use of chemotherapy plus a monoclonal antibody against HER2 for metastatic breast cancer that overexpresses HER2. *N Engl J Med* 2001;344(11):783–792.
10. Romond EH, Perez EA, Bryant J, et al. Trastuzumab plus adjuvant chemotherapy for operable HER2-positive breast cancer. *N Engl J Med* 2005;353(16): 1673–1684.
11. Smith I, Procter M, Gelber RD, et al. 2-year follow-up of trastuzumab after adjuvant chemotherapy in HER2-positive breast cancer: a randomised controlled trial. *Lancet* 2007;369(9555):29–36.
12. Piccart-Gebhart MJ, Procter M, Leyland-Jones B, et al. Trastuzumab after adjuvant chemotherapy in HER2-positive breast cancer. *N Engl J Med* 200520; 353(16):1659–1672.
13. Joensuu H, Kellokumpu-Lehtinen PL, Bono P, et al. Adjuvant docetaxel or vinorelbine with or without trastuzumab for breast cancer. *N Engl J Med* 200623; 354(8):809–820.
14. Slamon D, Eiermann W, Robert N, et al. BCIRG 006 : 2nd interim analysis phase III randomized trial phase III comparing doxorubicin and cyclophosphamide followed by docetaxel (AC-T) with doxorubicin and cyclophosphamide followed by docetaxel and trastuzumab (AC-TH) with docetaxel, carboplatin and trastuzumab (TCH) in HER2 positive early breast cancer patients [Abstract]. *Breast Cancer Res Treat* 2006;100(Suppl 1):General Session 2.
15. Hynes NE, Lane HA. ERBB receptors and cancer: the complexity of targeted inhibitors. *Nat Rev Cancer* 2005;5(5):341–354.
16. Perez EA, Romond EH, Suman VJ, et al. Updated results of the combined analysis of NCCTG N9831 and NSABP B-31 adjuvant chemotherapy with/without trastuzumab in patients with HER2-positive breast cancer [Abstract 512]. *J Clin Oncol* 2007;25(18S).
17. Spielman M, Roché H, Humblet Y, et al. 3-year follow-up of trastuzumab following adjuvant chemotherapy in node positive HER2-positive breast cancer patients: results of the PACS-04 trial [Abstract 72]. *Breast Cancer Res Treat* 2007;106(Suppl 1):S19.
18. Baselga J, Carbonell X, Castaneda-Soto NJ, et al. Phase II study of efficacy, safety, and pharmacokinetics of trastuzumab monotherapy administered on a 3-weekly schedule. *J Clin Oncol* 2005;23(10):2162–2171.
19. Suter TM, Procter M, van Veldhuisen DJ, et al. Trastuzumab-Associated Cardiac Adverse Effects in the Herceptin Adjuvant Trial. *J Clin Oncol* 2007;25(25): 3859–3865.
20. Rastogi P, Jeong J, Geyer CE, et al. Five year update of cardiac dysfunction on NSABP B-31, a randomized trial of sequential doxorubicin/cyclophosphamide (AC)→paclitaxel (T) vs. AC→T with trastuzumab (H) [Abstract LBA513]. *J Clin Oncol* 2007;25(18S).
21. Perez EA, Suman VJ, Davidson NE, et al. Cardiac Safety Analysis of Doxorubicin and Cyclophosphamide Followed by Paclitaxel With or Without Trastuzumab in the North Central Cancer Treatment Group N9831 Adjuvant Breast Cancer Trial. *J Clin Oncol* 2008;26(8):1231–1238.
22. 2008 [cited 2008 May 07]; Available from: http://www.gene.com/gene/products/information/pdf/herceptin-prescribing.pdf.
23. Gori S, Rimondini S, De Angelis V, et al. Central nervous system metastases in HER-2 positive metastatic breast cancer patients treated with trastuzumab: incidence, survival, and risk factors. *Oncologist* 2007;12(7):766–773.

24. Kirsch DG, Ledezma CJ, Mathews CS, et al. Survival after brain metastases from breast cancer in the trastuzumab era. *J Clin Oncol* 2005;23(9):2114–2116; author reply 6–7.

25. Pestalozzi BC, Zahrieh D, Price KN, et al. Identifying breast cancer patients at risk for central nervous system (CNS) metastases in trials of the International Breast Cancer Study Group (IBCSG). *Ann Oncol* 2006;17(6):935–944.

26. Stemmler HJ, Schmitt M, Willems A, et al. Ratio of trastuzumab levels in serum and cerebrospinal fluid is altered in HER2-positive breast cancer patients with brain metastases and impairment of blood–brain barrier. *Anticancer Drugs* 2007;18(1):23–28.

27. Miller K, Wang M, Gralow J, et al. Paclitaxel plus bevacizumab versus paclitaxel alone for metastatic breast cancer. *N Engl J Med* 2007;357(26):2666–2676.

28. Pegram M, Chan D, Dichmann RA, et al. Phase II combined biological therapy targeting the HER2 proto-oncogene and the vascular endothelial growth factor using trastuzumab (T) and bevacizumab (B) as first line treatment of HER2-amplified breast cancer [Abstract 301]. *Breast Cancer Res Treat* 2006;100(Suppl1):S28–S29.

29. Treatment of HER2 positive breast cancer with chemotherapy plus trastuzumab vs. chemotherapy plus trastuzumab plus bevacizumab (BETH). 2008 February 28, 2008 [cited 2008 April 21]; Available from: http://clinicaltrials.gov/ct2/show/record/NCT00625898.

30. Leyland-Jones B, Gelmon K, Ayoub JP, et al. Pharmacokinetics, safety, and efficacy of trastuzumab administered every three weeks in combination with paclitaxel. *J Clin Oncol* 2003;21(21):3965–3971.

31. Trastuzumab for 6 months or 1 year in treating women with nonmetastatic breast cancer that can be removed by surgery. 2007 July 30, 2007 [cited 2007 August 22]; Available from: http://clinicaltrials.gov/ct/show/NCT00381901.

32. Phase III randomized study of adjuvant trastuzumab (Herceptin) administered for 6 months versus 12 months in women with nonmetastatic, resectable breast cancer. 2007 [cited 2007 December, 26]; Available from: http://www.cancer.gov/clinicaltrials/INCA-PHARE.

33. The Synergism Or Long Duration (SOLD) Study. 2008 22 January, 2008 [cited 2008 31 January]; Available from: http://clinicaltrials.gov/ct2/show/NCT00593697.

34. Black D, Younger J, Martei Y, et al. Recurrence risk in T1a-b, node negative, HER2 positive breast cancer [Abstract 2037]. *Breast Cancer Res Treat* 2006;100(Suppl 1):S92.

35. Goldhirsch A, Wood WC, Gelber RD, et al. Progress and promise: highlights of the international expert consensus on the primary therapy of early breast cancer 2007. *Ann Oncol* 2007;18(7):1133–1144.

36. Lagakos SW. The challenge of subgroup analyses—reporting without distorting. *N Engl J Med* 2006;354(16):1667–1669.

37. Untch M, Gelber RD, Jackisch C, et al. Estimating the Magnitude of Trastuzumab Effects Within Patient Subgroups in the HERA Trial. *Ann Oncol* 2008;19(6):1090–1096.

38. Wildiers H, Kunkler I, Biganzoli L, et al. Management of breast cancer in elderly individuals: recommendations of the International Society of Geriatric Oncology. *Lancet Oncol* 2007;8(12):1101–1115.

39. Paik S, Kim C, Jeong J, et al. Benefit from adjuvant trastuzumab may not be confined to patients with IHC 3+ and/or FISH-positive tumors: central testing results from SABP B-31 [Abstract 511]. *J Clin Oncol* 2007;25(18S):5S (abstract 511).

40. McCaskill-Stevens W, Procter M, Goodbrand J, et al. Disease-free survival according to local immunohistochemistry for HER2 and central fluorescence in situ hybridization for patients treated with adjuvant chemotherapy with and without trastuzumab in the HERA (BIG 01-01) trial [Abstract 71]. *Breast Cancer Res Treat* 2007;106(Suppl 1):S18.

41. Pritchard KI, Messersmith H, Elavathil L, et al. HER-2 and topoisomerase II as predictors of response to chemotherapy. *J Clin Oncol* 2008;26(5):736–744.

42. Harris L, Fritsche H, Mennel R, et al. American Society of Clinical Oncology 2007 update of recommendations for the use of tumor markers in breast cancer. *J Clin Oncol* 2007;25(33):5287–5312.

43. Press MF, Sauter G, Buyse M, et al. Alteration of topoisomerase II-alpha gene in human breast cancer and its association with responsiveness to anthracycline-based chemotherapy [Abstract 524]. *J Clin Oncol* 2007;25(18S):8S.

44. Kim C, Bryant J, Horne Z, et al. Trastuzumab sensitivity of breast cancer with co-amplification of HER2 and cMYC suggests pro-apoptotic function of dysregulated cMYC in vivo [Abstract 46]. *Breast Cancer Res Treat* 2005;94(Suppl 1):S6.

45. Perez EA, Suman VG, Davidson NE, et al. May 2005 Update. Slide presentation at the 41st American Society of Clinical Oncology Annual Meeting, Orlando, Florida, May 13–17, 2005. 2005 [cited 2008 May 5]; Available from: www.asco.org.

46. Moy B, Goss PE. Lapatinib-associated toxicity and practical management recommendations. *Oncologist* 2007;12(7):756–765.

47. Xia W, Liu LH, Ho P, et al. Truncated ErbB2 receptor (p95ErbB2) is regulated by heregulin through heterodimer formation with ErbB3 yet remains sensitive to the dual EGFR/ErbB2 kinase inhibitor GW572016. *Oncogene* 2004;23(3):646–653.

48. Molina MA, Codony-Servat J, Albanell J, et al. Trastuzumab (herceptin), a humanized anti-Her2 receptor monoclonal antibody, inhibits basal and activated Her2 ectodomain cleavage in breast cancer cells. *Cancer Res* 2001; 61(12):4744–4749.

49. Xia W, Husain I, Liu L, et al. Lapatinib antitumor activity is not dependent upon phosphatase and tensin homologue deleted on chromosome 10 in ErbB2-overexpressing breast cancers. *Cancer Res* 2007;67(3):1170–1175.

50. Li X, Creighton C, Wong H, et al. Decrease in tumorigenic breast cancer stem cells in primary breast cancers with neoadjuvant lapatinib [Abstract 82]. *Breast Cancer Res Treat* 2007;106(Suppl 1):S22.

51. Howard A, Burris I. Dual kinase inhibition in the treatment of breast cancer: initial experience with the EGFR/ErbB-2 inhibitor lapatinib. *Oncologist* 2004;9(Suppl 3):10–15.

52. Geyer CE, Forster J, Lindquist D, et al. Lapatinib plus capecitabine for HER2-positive advanced breast cancer. *N Engl J Med* 2006;355(26):2733–2743.

53. Geyer CE, Martin A, Newstat B, et al. Lapatinib (L) plus capecitabine (C) in HER2+ advanced breast cancer (ABC): genomic and updated efficacy data [Abstract 1035]. *J Clin Oncol* 2007;25(18S).

54. Cameron D, Casey M, Press M, et al. A phase III randomized comparison of lapatinib plus capecitabine versus capecitabine alone in women with advanced breast cancer that has progressed on trastuzumab: updated efficacy and biomarker analyses. *Breast Cancer Res Treat* 2009;113(2):207–209.

55. Lin NU, Dieras V, Paul D, et al. GF105084, a phase II study of lapatinib for brain metastases in patients (pts) with HER2+ breast cancer following trastuzumab (H) based systemic therapy and cranial radiotherapy (RT) [Abstract 1012]. *J Clin Oncol* 2007;25(18S).

56. Lin NU, Paul D, Dieras V, et al. Lapatinib and capecitabine for the treatment of brain metastases in patients with HER2+ breast cancer an updated analysis from EGF105084 [Abstract 6076]. *Breast Cancer Res Treat* 2007;106(Suppl 1):S72.

57. Perez EA, Byrne JA, Isaac W, et al. Cardiac safety experience in 3,127 patients treated with lapatinib [Abstract 1420]. *Ann Oncol* 2006;17(Suppl 9):ix70.

58. Piccart-Gebhart MJ, Perez EA, Baselga J, et al. ALTTO (adjuvant lapatinib and/or trastuzumab treatment optimization) study [BIG 02-06/N063D/EGF106708]: a phase III study for HER-2 overexpressing early breast cancer (BC) [Abstract P118]. *Breast* 2007;16(Suppl 1):S46.

59. Eidtmann H, Di Cosimo S, Gelber R, et al. Neo-ALTTO: neo-adjuvant lapatinib and/or trastuzumab treatment optimisation study—BIG 1-06/EGF106903. *Breast International Group Newsletter* 2007;9(1):11–12.

60. Moy B, Goss PE. Lapatinib: current status and future directions in breast cancer. *Oncologist* 2006;11(10):1047–1057.

61. Study of AC Followed by a Combination of Paclitaxel Plus Trastuzumab or Lapatinib or Both Given Before Surgery to Patients With Operable HER2 Positive Invasive Breast Cancer. 2008 December 13, 2007 [cited 2008 May 07]; Available from: http://clinicaltrials.gov/ct2/show/NCT00486668.

62. Kulkarni S, Hicks DG. HER2-positive early breast cancer and trastuzumab: a surgeon's perspective. *Ann Surg Oncol* 2008;15(6):1677–1688.

Chapter 52

Adjuvant Systemic Therapy: Bisphosphonates

Julie R. Gralow

Bone is the most common site of distant recurrence in breast cancer. The development of skeletal metastases involves complex interactions between cancer cells and the bone microenvironment. The presence of tumor in bone is associated with activation of osteoclasts, resulting in excessive bone resorption. Bisphosphonates are potent inhibitors of osteoclastic bone resorption, with proved efficacy in reducing tumor-associated skeletal complications. Studies are investigating the adjuvant use of these drugs in breast cancer, with evaluation of their impact on bone density, bone metastases, and survival. Preclinical experiments have shown that the development of bone metastases can be inhibited by bisphosphonates, through both bone-mediated and possible direct antitumor mechanisms. Three randomized, controlled clinical trials in early-stage breast cancer of the addition of the oral bisphosphonate clodronate yielded promising yet conflicting results with respect to the development of bone metastases and survival. A recent study investigating the adjuvant use of zoledronic acid in premenopausal, estrogen receptor (ER)-positive breast cancer reported an improvement in disease-free survival (DFS) in addition to favorable effects on bone mineral density. Ongoing studies will further define the role of bisphosphonates in the adjuvant treatment of breast cancer, including determining optimal drugs, dosing, schedules, and patient and tumor populations. The data available to date suggest an increasing role for adjuvant bisphosphonates in the treatment of early-stage breast cancer. A strong need exists for continued clinical and laboratory investigation of these drugs in the adjuvant breast cancer setting.

RATIONALE: THE BIOLOGY OF BONE METASTASES

Metastases involving the skeleton are common in patients with advanced breast cancer. Circulating breast cancer cells have affinity for bone, which may serve as a reservoir for malignant cells early in the metastatic process. Bone is the first site of distant disease in 25% to 40% of breast cancer recurrences (1). The incidence of eventual development of skeletal metastases in metastatic breast cancer is as high as 60% to 80%. Understanding the biology of bone and bone metastases, and exploring methods of interrupting the metastatic process early in development through adjuvant therapy, has the potential to improve outcome in early-stage breast cancer.

Healthy bone is in a constant state of remodeling. Bone-derived osteoblasts and osteoclasts work together through the influence of cytokines and other humoral factors to balance mineralization and resorption. Osteoblasts, derived from hematogenous precursors, produce collagen matrix and contribute to bone formation. Osteoclasts, multinucleated giant cells related to macrophages, are the major mediator of bone degradation. In normal bone remodeling, the relationship between osteoblastic bone mineralization and osteoclastic bone resorption is balanced. When malignant cells infiltrate bone spaces, the balance of new bone formation and bone destruction is disturbed. Interactions between metastatic tumor cells and the bone microenvironment contribute to the development of skeletal metastases.

The process of breast cancer metastasis includes tumor cell seeding, tumor dormancy, and metastatic growth. The primary tumor releases cells that pass through the extracellular matrix,

penetrate the basement membrane of angiolymphatic vessels, and then are transported to distant organs via the circulatory system. These circulating cells can adhere to the vessels and sinusoids of the bone marrow, invading into the marrow and intertrabecular spaces with the help of adhesion molecules. Tumor cells have been shown to exhibit chemotactic responses to areas of bone undergoing resorption (2). Most disseminated tumor cells die, but some are capable of micrometastatic proliferation or remain dormant, only to grow later. Disseminated tumor cells have been reported in the bone marrow of 30% to 40% of early-stage breast cancer patients at the time of diagnosis (3).

Mundy (4) has described a "vicious cycle" that occurs when cancer cells arrive within the bone matrix (Fig. 52.1). Products produced by the tumor induce breakdown of bone, causing release of factors that cause stimulation and further growth of malignant cells, which in turn leads to further bone resorption. At the microscopic level, osteoclasts are visible between cancer cells and the bone surface that is being destroyed (5,6). Osteoclasts are activated by cytokines produced directly or indirectly by the tumor cell, including parathyroid hormone related peptide (PTHrP), prostaglandins, and interleukins (7). In response to cancer-derived cytokines, osteoblasts secrete factors such as receptor activator of NF-κB ligand (RANKL) and macrophage colony-stimulating factor (M-CSF) which increase osteoclast activation and bone resorption (8–10). As bone matrix is broken down, a rich supply of mitogenic factors is released, including insulin-like growth factor (IGF-1), platelet-derived growth factor (PDGF), and transforming growth factor β (TGFβ). These factors can lead to increased growth and proliferation of the breast cancer metastases (11). The overall effect is the creation of a self-sustaining *vicious cycle* with multidirectional interactions between cancer cells, osteoclasts, osteoblasts, and the bone microenvironment.

BISPHOSPHONATES: AGENTS AND MECHANISM OF ACTION

Bisphosphonates are effective in treating conditions in which there is excessive bone resorption and osteoclast activity, including Paget disease of bone, osteoporosis, fibrous dysplasia, and hypercalcemia of malignancy. Bisphosphonates have a proven role in reducing skeletal complications in breast cancer patients with bone involvement, and a potential emerging role in the prevention of breast cancer metastases.

Within the family of bisphosphonates are more similarities in pharmacologic effects than differences, although side effect profiles, rates of oral absorption, and potency differ. Although some differences in their exact mechanism of action exist, all bisphosphonates have a final inhibitory effect on osteoclast function. Bisphosphonates have an affinity for bone and are preferentially delivered to sites of increased bone formation or resorption. Once deposited on the bone surface, bisphosphonates are ingested by osteoclasts engaged in bone resorption. These agents interfere with bone resorption by producing a direct toxic apoptotic effect on osteoclasts, and by inhibiting their differentiation and maturation. Bisphosphonates are analogs of endogenous pyrophosphate, in which a carbon atom replaces the central oxygen atom (Fig. 52.2). As with pyrophosphate, they strongly bind to hydroxyapatite on the bone surface.

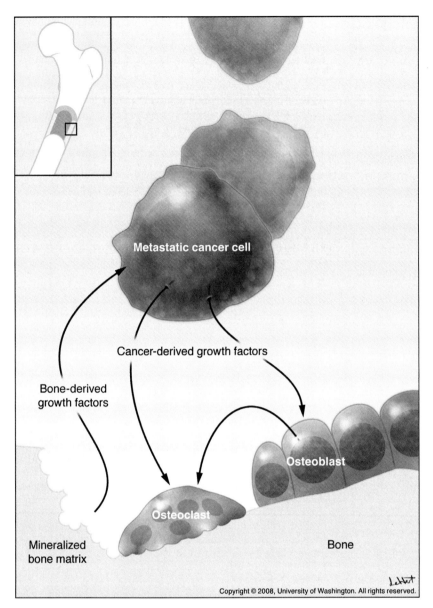

FIGURE 52.1. This illustration highlights the interaction between breast cancer cells and the bone microenvironment. A variety of cancer-derived growth factors, including parathyroid hormone-related protein (PTHrP), prostaglandins, and interleukins, stimulate osteoclastic activity. Other osteoclast-stimulating cytokines, such as receptor activator of NF-κB ligand (RANKL) and macrophage colony-stimulating factor (M-CSF), are indirectly released through interactions between cancer cells and osteoblasts, macrophages, and other cells within the bone environment. Bone provides a favorable niche for the cancer cell because it is a repository for tumor-stimulating growth factors, such as transforming growth factor β (TGFβ) and insulin-like growth factor (IGF-1), which are released with bone resorption.

Unlike pyrophosphate, which is rapidly split by the hydrolytic enzymes of osteoclasts, bisphosphonates are stable owing to the central carbon substitution that makes them resistant to hydrolysis. This substitution also allows two additional side chains of variable structure that affect the pharmacologic properties of these agents. One of the side chains usually contains a hydroxyl moiety, which allows high affinity for calcium and bone mineral. The structural variation in the other side chain produces differences in the antiresorptive properties and toxicities. Bisphosphonates fall into two classes, based on whether this second side chain is nitrogen-containing or not. First-generation bisphosphonates, such as clodronate and etidronate, do not contain nitrogen. These agents substitute into the production of adenosine triphosphate, which then becomes a toxic adenosine triphosphate analogue that poisons the osteoclast (12,13). Nitrogen-containing bisphosphonates, such as pamidronate, alendronate, risedronate, ibandronate, and zoledronic acid, interfere with cell signaling and block the prenylation of small signaling proteins that are essential for osteoclast function and survival (13–15). Evidence suggests that bisphosphonates may also exert influences on macrophages, osteoblasts, and tumor cells (16,17).

Several bisphosphonates are available worldwide for various conditions, with variable antiresorptive potency and route of administration (Table 52.1). The clinical impact of the differences in relative potency between bisphosphonates is not well documented, because few direct clinical trial comparisons have been conducted. Although all bisphosphonates can theoretically be administered either orally or intravenously, the oral bioavailability of any bisphosphonate is extremely limited. The dose and frequency of administration varies depending on the clinical

$$
\begin{array}{ccc}
\text{OH} & \text{R} & \text{OH} \\
| & | & | \\
\text{O} = \text{P} - \text{C} - \text{P} = \text{O} \\
| & | & | \\
\text{OH} & \text{R} & \text{OH}
\end{array}
$$

FIGURE 52.2. The basic chemical structure of bisphosphonates includes a central carbon and two variable side chains (*R*). Variations in the side chains alter the potency and side effects of the drugs.

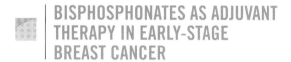

| Table 52.1 | BISPHOSPHONATES: ANTIRESORPTIVE POTENCY AND ROUTE OF ADMINISTRATION | |

Bisphosphonate	Relative Antiresorptive Potency	Route of Administration
Etidronate	1	Oral, IV
Clodronate	10	Oral
Tiludronate	10	Oral
Pamidronate	100	IV
Alendronate	1,000	Oral
Risedronate	5,000	Oral
Ibandronate	10,000	Oral, IV
Zoledronic acid	100,000	IV

IV, intravenously.

indication, with doses used to treat bone metastases being about 10-fold higher than doses used to treat osteoporosis. The zoledronic acid dose approved for treating bone metastases is 4 mg intravenously every 3 to 4 weeks. When used in the treatment of osteoporosis, it is approved as a 5 mg dose once yearly. Ibandronate, available in both oral and intravenous forms, is given 50 mg orally daily or 6 mg intravenously monthly for bone metastases, compared with 150 mg orally monthly or 3 mg intravenously every 3 months for osteoporosis. In the United States, ibandronate is only approved for the osteoporosis indication. Doses of bisphosphonates under investigation in the adjuvant breast cancer setting for prevention of metastases have ranged from full bone metastasis treatment doses to somewhat lower doses or less frequent administrations.

BISPHOSPHONATES AS ADJUVANT THERAPY IN EARLY-STAGE BREAST CANCER

Preclinical data provide biologic plausibility for a role of bisphosphonates in inhibiting the development of bone metastases. *In vitro* studies have demonstrated that bisphosphonates can inhibit critical steps in development of metastases in the bone, including adhesion and invasion (18–20). Animal models have shown that bisphosphonates can inhibit development of bone metastases, reduce tumor burden in the bones, and improve survival in nude mice injected with a human breast cancer cell line (21). Although most animal models suggest that the primary antitumor effect of bisphosphonates is manifested in the bone, some data indicate an effect of bisphosphonates on extraskeletal metastases. Laboratory experiments have shown that bisphosphonates can have an impact on cancer cells through antiangiogenic, anti-invasive, and immunomodulatory mechanisms (22–26). Nitrogen-containing bisphosphonates can directly induce tumor cell apoptosis and inhibit tumor cell proliferation, and laboratory studies suggest that they may act synergistically with cytotoxic chemotherapy agents commonly used in breast cancer treatment (27). The high doses of bisphosphonates that have been used in most laboratory studies are incompatible with the clinical doses approved for the treatment of cancer patients. Whether a direct antitumor effect of bisphosphonates plays a clinically significant role in the treatment or prevention of cancer in humans remains unproved.

Clinical trials showing benefit of bisphosphonates in patients with bone metastases, along with supportive preclinical data, provide the basis for studying these drugs in early-stage breast cancer. A summary of reported and ongoing randomized trials of adjuvant bisphosphonates with DFS end points is included in

Table 52.2. Three adjuvant trials evaluating oral clodronate in early-stage breast cancer patients have been reported, with promising but conflicting results (28–33). A recent study investigating the adjuvant use of zoledronic acid in premenopausal, ER-positive breast cancer reported an improvement in DFS in this specific patient population (34). Results are anxiously anticipated from several additional large, randomized adjuvant bisphosphonate trials in early-stage breast cancer patients.

In a small, randomized, open-label study, 302 women with breast cancer and micometastases detected in a bone marrow aspirate at the time of diagnosis were randomized to receive either clodronate (1,600 mg/day) or no bisphosphonate for 2 years. Additionally, patients received standard adjuvant systemic therapy (28). Patients who received clodronate had a 50% reduction in the incidence of bone metastases ($p = .003$), and a significantly longer bone metastasis-free survival ($p < .001$). A later analysis at 8.5 years of follow-up continued to confirm a significant improvement in overall survival for patients given clodronate, although the significance in DFS no longer persisted (29).

A larger, randomized, placebo-controlled, multinational trial was conducted in which 1,079 patients with early-stage breast cancer were randomized to receive either clodronate (1,600 mg/day) or placebo for 2 years in addition to standard systemic therapy (30). Patients were assessed for bone metastases at 2 and 5 years, and as clinically indicated. The final analysis showed that oral clodronate significantly reduced the risk of bone metastases at 2 years (hazard ratio [HR] 0.546; $p = .03$) and 5 years (HR 0.692; $p = .04$). This reduction was predominantly seen in patients with stage II-III breast cancer. A significant reduction was also seen in mortality (HR 0.768, $p = .048$). Follow-up showed a continued separation of the survival curves between years 5 and 10 (31).

The results of the two previous studies are in conflict with a third small, randomized, open-label study investigating 3 years of adjuvant clodronate therapy (1,600 mg/day) in 299 patients with lymph node-positive breast cancer (32). This study showed no reduction in bone metastases in the clodronate treated arm, although bone as a first site of relapse was less frequent in the clodronate group than in the controls (14% vs. 30%). There was, however, a worrisome increase in visceral metastases and a reduction in overall survival at 5 years for patients receiving clodronate. A possible explanation for these adverse outcomes is an imbalance in hormone receptor-negative cases between the arms of the study, with significantly more progesterone (PR)-negative (45% vs. 31%; $p = .03$) and a trend toward more ER-negative (35% vs. 23%) tumors in the clodronate group. This difference was potentially exacerbated by the practice in this trial of assigning endocrine therapy alone to all postmenopausal women and chemotherapy alone to all premenopausal women, regardless of ER or PR status. The negative impact of clodronate on overall survival appears to be neutralized when the imbalance in hormone receptor negativity is corrected. Even without correction, the survival detriment no longer showed significance at 10 years (33). A meta-analysis using the 5-year data from these three adjuvant clodronate trials did not show a statistically significant difference in overall or bone metastasis-free survival when the data were pooled (34) Noted was marked heterogeneity among the trials that in part explains the wide confidence interval (CI) around their hazard ratio (HR 0.75, 95% CI 0.31, 1.82).

A recent study investigating the adjuvant use of zoledronic acid reported an improvement in disease-free survival, in addition to favorable effects on bone mineral density (35,36). The Austrian Breast and Colorectal Cancer Study Group (ABCSG) 12 trial enrolled 1,800 premenopausal women with ER-positive breast cancer. All patients received ovarian suppression for 3 years with a leutinizing hormone-releasing hormone (LHRH) analogue, goserelin. Patients were randomized in a 2 × 2

Table 52.2 | BISPHOSPHONATES AS ADJUVANT BREAST CANCER THERAPY

Study/ (Reference)	Patients	Therapy	Follow-up (mo)	Population	Results
Powles (30,31)	1,079	Clodronate 1,600 mg/day for 2 yr vs. placebo	66 (final analysis)	Stage I-III breast cancer	Bone metastases significantly reduced at 2 and 5 yr; survival improved on clodronate arm (HR 0.77, $p = .048$)
Diel (28,29)	302	Clodronate 1,600 mg/day for 2 yr vs. no therapy	103	Primary breast cancer and tumor cells in bone marrow aspirate	Both bone and visceral metastases significantly lower on clodronate; survival improved on clodronate arm ($p = .001$)
Saarto (32,33)	299	Clodronate 1,600 mg/day for 3 yr vs. no therapy	120	Node-positive breast cancer; significantly more HR-negative patients on clodronate arm	No difference in bone metastases; visceral metastases increased on clodronate arm; no difference in overall survival at 10 yr
ABCSG-12 (35,36)	1,803	Zoledronic acid 4 mg every 6 mo × 3 yr	60	ER/PR+, premenopausal breast cancer, <10+ nodes; receiving ovarian suppression and tamoxifen or anastrozole	Disease-free survival improved on zoledronic acid arm (HR 0.643, $p = .011$)
NSABP B-34	3,200	Clodronate 1,600 mg/day for 3 yr vs. placebo		Stage I-II breast cancer, treated with standard systemic adjuvant chemotherapy and/or endocrine therapy	Accrual completed 2004
SWOG S0307	4,500	Clodronate 1,600 mg/day vs. ibandronate 50 mg/day vs. zoledronic acid 4 mg monthly × 6, then every 3 mo; 3 yr total		Stage I-III breast cancer, treated with standard systemic adjuvant chemotherapy and/or endocrine therapy	Accrual ongoing
AZURE	3,304	Zoledronic acid 4 mg monthly × 6, then every 3 mo × 8, then every 6 mo to complete 5 yr vs. no treatment		Stage II-III breast cancer, treated with standard systemic adjuvant chemotherapy and/or endocrine therapy	Accrual completed 2006. 6-mo safety data presented (62)

ABCSG, Austrian Breast and Colorectal Cancer Study Group; AZURE, Adjuvant Zoledronic acid redUce REcurrence trial; ER, estrogen receptor; HR, hazard ratio; NSABP, National Surgical Adjuvant Breast and Bowel Project; PR, progesterone receptor; SWOG, Southwest Oncology Group.

design to receive tamoxifen versus anastrozole, and zoledronic acid (4 mg every 6 months) or not. At the first efficacy analysis, reported after 137 events (70 distant relapses) with approximately 60 months of follow-up, no difference was seen in outcome with respect to the endocrine therapy randomization. There was, however, a statistically significant improvement in DFS for the patients who received zoledronic acid (HR 0.64; $p = .01$), with a similar trend toward improved overall survival (HR 0.60, $p = .10$). Although ABCSG-12 clearly provides additional support for the metastasis-suppressing potential of adjuvant bisphosphonates, this study enrolled only a narrow subset of breast cancer patients: premenopausal women with ER-positive tumors who did not receive adjuvant chemotherapy. Although promising, caution must be taken not to over extrapolate these findings, or this dose schedule, to all breast cancer patients.

The Zometa-Femara Adjuvant Synergy Trials (Z-FAST and ZO-FAST) enrolled ER-positive, postmenopausal women receiving letrozole and randomized them to *upfront* versus *delayed* zoledronic acid therapy (every 6 months for 5 years) in an attempt to reduce bone loss-related morbidity (37,38). Time to recurrence was a secondary end point. A recent combined analysis of these trials showed lower recurrence rates in the group receiving upfront zoledronic acid therapy (1.1% vs. 2.3%, $p = .04$) (39). Additionally, several small trials have evaluated the impact of monthly dosing of zoledronic acid in early-stage breast cancer patients by evaluating disseminated tumor cells in serial bone marrow aspirates, as a surrogate for response (40–42). All have shown some degree of reduction in bone marrow micrometastases in patients receiving zoledronic acid.

Two additional large trials of adjuvant bisphosphonates have met their targeted accrual goals with efficacy analysis pending.

The National Surgical Adjuvant Breast and Bowel Project (NSABP) B-34 trial enrolled women with stage I-II breast cancer and compared 3 years of daily oral clodronate (1,600 mg/day) with placebo. The primary end point of this trial is disease-free survival. B-34 closed to accrual in 2004, and is expected to report its first efficacy analysis in late 2009. The trial asking "does Adjuvant Zoledronic acid redUce REcurrence in patients with high-risk localized breast cancer?" (AZURE) enrolled stage II-III breast cancer patients, comparing standard adjuvant cancer therapy alone or given with *intensive* zoledronic acid for 5 years (4 mg monthly for 6 months, followed by every 3 months for 2 years, then every 6 months through year 5). This trial closed to accrual in 2006 and is expected to report in late 2008. The North American Breast Cancer Intergroup, in combination with the NSABP, is conducting Southwest Oncology Group (SWOG) S0307, a comparison of three different bisphosphonates in the adjuvant breast cancer setting. This trial is randomizing 4,500 stage I-III breast cancer patients receiving standard adjuvant therapy to oral clodronate (1,600 mg daily) versus oral ibandronate (50 mg daily) versus zoledronic acid (4 mg intravenously monthly for 6 months, then every 3 months), all for 3 years. These unreported trials include all patient and tumor subsets, including both pre- and postmenopausal women, ER-positive and negative tumors, and patients who received a range of standard systemic therapy, including chemotherapy. The results of these trials will be critical in determining how broadly applicable bisphosphonates are across the spectrum of breast cancer patients. Several additional ongoing early-stage bisphosphonate trials are evaluating various agents, doses, schedules, and adjuvant settings, including residual disease after preoperative chemotherapy and in elderly populations.

The adjuvant bisphosphonate trials reported to date support the potential role of these drugs on having an impact on recurrence and survival in early-stage breast cancer. The data do not yet support the addition of adjuvant bisphosphonates as standard of care for all patients. The promising, yet somewhat contradictory, results of the three reported adjuvant clodronate studies suggest that bisphosphonates can have an impact on disease recurrence, but highlight the need for further investigation. Based on recent reports of an adjuvant trial of zoledronic acid, use of bisphosphonates in women with early-stage breast cancer is currently supported in premenopausal women with ER-positive cancers receiving ovarian suppression. Extrapolation of these findings to postmenopausal women, ER-negative tumors, and women receiving chemotherapy will require data which will be supplied by ongoing clinical trials. These studies will aid in defining the optimal patient and tumor populations for the addition of adjuvant bisphosphonates, as well as optimal doses and schedules of administration, and long-term toxicities. Whether doses used in metastatic disease are required for prevention or whether lower doses will suffice is unknown. It is unclear whether adjuvant bisphosphonates should be given continuously and orally, whether intravenous therapy is preferable, and whether *less intensive* intravenous regimens will turn out to be as effective as *more intensive* regimens. The optimal duration of adjuvant bisphosphonate therapy is also unknown.

BONE HEALTH IN PATIENTS WITH BREAST CANCER

Most women with breast cancer are at risk for osteoporosis, owing to either their breast cancer therapy or their age (43). The optimal role of bisphosphonates in preventing bone density loss is a subject of increasing clinical importance in breast cancer patients. Aromatase inhibitors, increasingly used in postmenopausal breast cancer patients, have a detrimental impact on bone mineral density and fracture rates (44). In the premenopausal setting, ovarian suppression and chemotherapy-induced ovarian failure can lead to rapid, profound loss of bone density (45). Accelerated bone loss brings with it an increased fracture risk, and affects quality of life, costs, and survival (46). The American Society of Clinical Oncology (ASCO) 2003 update on the role of bisphosphonates and bone health issues in women with breast cancer stated that oncology specialists need to take an expanded role in managing bone health in breast cancer patients (47).

Women with early-stage breast cancer should be evaluated for fracture risk. Counseling on nutrition and lifestyle for bone health is advised for all patients, and appropriate calcium and vitamin D supplementation is recommended. Bisphosphonate therapy should be considered on an individualized basis based on bone mineral density and other fracture risk factors (including body mass index, personal and family history of fracture, smoking, and corticosteroid use). Evidence from randomized trials indicates that several intravenous and oral bisphosphonates can be effective in preventing bone loss and accelerated bone turnover in breast cancer patients receiving endocrine or chemotherapy (36,37,38,48–55). The comparative efficacy of these bisphosphonates has not been defined.

In premenopausal women, studies have shown that clodronate, risedronate, alendronate, and zoledronic acid prevent and reduce bone loss caused by chemotherapy-induced menopause, ovarian suppression with LHRH analogues, and tamoxifen (which has a net negative effect on bone in the premenopausal setting in contrast to its positive effect in the postmenopausal setting) (35,48–51,54). The ABCSG-12 study prospectively examined the effects on bone density caused by ovarian suppression combined with tamoxifen or anastrozole, with or without zoledronic acid (4 mg every 6 months) in premenopausal women (36). In addition to the improvement in DFS described above, the addition of zoledronic acid inhibited loss of bone mineral density in both the tamoxifen and anastrozole arms and stabilized it at baseline levels. Without zoledronic acid, significant bone loss occurred; the mean reductions in bone mineral density at 3 years were 8% and 16%, with tamoxifen and anastrozole, respectively. The Cancer and Leukemia Group B (CALGB) recently reported first results of C79809, a randomized trial of zoledronic acid (4 mg every 3 months) in premenopausal women who developed ovarian failure owing to adjuvant chemotherapy (54). The mean percent change in lumbar spine bone mineral density at 12 months was +2.6% in the group receiving zoledronic acid, and −6.4% in the control group ($p <.0001$). Zoledronic acid added minimal toxicity and prevented the accelerated bone loss occurring in young women who developed ovarian failure from adjuvant chemotherapy.

In postmenopausal women receiving aromatase inhibitor therapy, studies have evaluated the impact of risedronate and zoledronic acid on bone density (37,38,52,53,55). In the Z-FAST and ZO-FAST studies, postmenopausal women with early-stage breast cancer starting letrozole were randomized to receive upfront intravenous zoledronic acid (4 mg every 6 months) versus a delayed treatment in which zoledronic acid was initiated based on changes in bone mineral density (37,38). At 36 months, upfront administration of zoledronic acid was effective at preventing bone loss, with increased lumbar spine and total hip bone mineral density. Less than 10% of patients on the delayed treatment arm met the protocol-specified criteria for starting zoledronic acid for T-score changes or fractures, however, and no differences in fracture rates were seen. Early reports of smaller randomized trials of risedronate and ibandronate in postmenopausal women receiving aromatase inhibitor therapy have also shown favorable impacts on bone mineral density (53,55). A recent trial reported results for the RANK ligand inhibitor denosumab (60 mg subcutaneously every 6 months) versus placebo given to women receiving aromatase inhibitors in early-stage breast cancer (56). The study showed increased bone mineral density over 24 months in the denosumab arm.

Bisphosphonates are effective in preventing cancer treatment-associated loss of bone mineral density. Many issues need to be clarified to determine optimal management of bone loss in women with breast cancer. Whether early implementation of bisphosphonates will have an impact on long-term fracture rates remains a critical question. Is there harm incurred in delaying therapy until patients meet criteria for significant increased fracture risk? To date we have no direct comparison of agents or delivery routes to guide in drug selection. We need to determine which early-stage breast cancer patients are at most risk of clinically significant bone loss, and who will benefit most from early addition of bisphosphonates for preservation of bone mineral density.

SAFETY AND ADVERSE EFFECTS OF BISPHOSPHONATES

As a group, bisphosphonates are generally well tolerated at both osteoporosis and bone metastases treatment doses. Few serious adverse effects have been reported in clinical trials when given either orally or intravenously. Gastrointestinal toxicity in the form of dyspepsia is the most common side effect for oral agents. Esophageal inflammation and ulceration are described as a rare but serious adverse effect (57). The efficacy of oral bisphosphonates is compromised by poor absorption.

Generally, only a few percent of an oral dose is absorbed from the gastrointestinal tract and intake of any food or beverage further diminishes absorption to negligible levels. Patients are therefore advised to take their oral medication in the morning on an empty stomach and wait 30 to 60 minutes before eating to maximize absorption.

Intravenous bisphosphonate administration can be associated with acute-phase reactions, which include flu-like symptoms, such as bone pain, transient arthralgias and myalgias, nausea, and fever. These reactions typically occur only after the first or second infusion, and symptoms usually resolve in 48 hours. The symptoms respond well to antipyretic and non-steroidal anti-inflammatory drugs, and are not an indication to discontinue treatment. Hypocalcemia is another reported complication of bisphosphonate therapy. Clinically relevant hypocalcemia is rare, and generally may be prevented with the addition of supplemental calcium and vitamin D. FDA-approved labeling for pamidronate and zoledronic acid recommends periodic monitoring of serum calcium, electrolytes, phosphate, and magnesium.

Bisphosphonates have a potential for renal toxicity. The pharmacokinetics vary from agent to agent, and between oral and intravenous formulations, but all bisphosphonates are primarily renally excreted. Clinical trials with pamidronate and zoledronic acid have shown renal toxicity, especially in patients with pre-existing renal impairment (58). The dose, frequency, and speed of infusion have been found to be related to renal toxicity; reducing the dose and slowing the infusion decrease toxicity. It is recommended that serum creatinine be monitored before each dose of these drugs. For patients with renal impairment or reduced creatinine clearance, it is recommended that the dose be reduced.

Osteonecrosis of the jaw (ONJ) has been reported to occur in cancer patients treated with intravenous bisphosphonates (59,60). This entity is defined as an area of exposed, nonhealing bone in the maxillofacial region. The most common predisposing factors appear to be the type and total dose of bisphosphonate, a history of dental surgery (such as tooth extraction), and dental trauma. The true incidence of this problem is still not known. It appears to be most commonly associated with zoledronic acid when used at bone metastasis treatment doses, and is rarely seen with oral bisphosphonates used at osteoporosis treatment doses. It is recommended that before initiating bisphosphonate therapy, particularly intravenous administration, patients should receive a dental examination and appropriate preventive dentistry (61). While on therapy, patients should maintain excellent oral hygiene and avoid, if possible, invasive dental procedures. Recently reported safety data from the AZURE adjuvant breast cancer trial identified seven cases of presumptive ONJ, all in the zoledronic acid arm (0.4% of patients) occurring after a median of eight doses (62).

CONCLUSIONS

Bisphosphonates are a promising group of compounds in the adjuvant breast cancer setting. This class of drugs has two potential roles in the treatment of early-stage breast cancer patients: prevention of metastasis with resultant improved disease-free and overall survival, and prevention and treatment of osteoporosis.

Preclinical studies provide good proof of principle for the role of bisphosphonates in preventing the growth and development of bone metastases. The promising, yet somewhat contradictory, results of the three reported adjuvant clodronate studies in breast cancer patients suggest a possible role for adjuvant use of bisphosphonates to reduce recurrence. Based on recent reports of an adjuvant trial of zoledronic acid, use of bisphosphonates in women with early-stage breast cancer with the intention of reducing recurrence is currently supported in premenopausal women with ER-positive cancers receiving ovarian suppression. Extrapolation of these findings to postmenopausal women, ER-negative tumors, and women receiving chemotherapy will require data which will be supplied by several recently closed or ongoing clinical trials. These studies will aid in defining the optimal patient and tumor populations for the addition of adjuvant bisphosphonates, as well as optimal doses and schedules of administration, and long-term toxicities. Ultimately, we would like to determine which adjuvant breast cancer patients might benefit most from the addition of bisphosphonates to maximize benefit and minimize costs and risk. Tumor or patient characteristics, urine or serum markers of bone turnover, and bone marrow micrometastases may predict who is at highest risk for bone recurrence.

Breast cancer patients can have an added benefit from bisphosphonates, unrelated to the reduction of bone metastases, in the form of preservation of bone density. Several recent trials in early-stage breast cancer patients have demonstrated that bisphosphonates are effective in treating and preventing bone loss associated with cancer treatment. Optimal timing of initiation of bisphosphonates to suppress loss of bone density, whether early in the treatment course or after bone loss has occurred, has not been established. The major studies of bisphosphonates in cancer treatment-induced bone loss have not yet shown difference in fracture rates.

In addition to bisphosphonates, several new classes of agents with antiosteoclastic activity are in various stages of investigation for treatment of bone metastases, prevention of bone metastases, and prevention and treatment of osteoporosis. These include RANK-ligand inhibitors, src kinase inhibitors, and cathepsin-k inhibitors. The relative efficacy and toxicity profiles of these agents compared with bisphosphonates will be of great interest. Whether these agents will be optimally used as an alternative for or in combination or sequence with bisphosphonates remains to be studied. The role of bisphosphonates and other antiosteoclast agents in the adjuvant breast cancer setting will be further defined in the near future, through randomized, large-scale, multicenter clinical trials.

MANAGEMENT SUMMARY

- Use of bisphosphonates in women with early-stage breast cancer with the intention of reducing bone metastases is currently supported in premenopausal women with ER-positive cancers receiving ovarian suppression. Extrapolation of these findings to postmenopausal women, ER-negative tumors, and women receiving chemotherapy will require data which will be supplied by several recently closed or ongoing clinical trials. Before the release of these trial results, it may be reasonable to consider the adjuvant use of bisphosphonates in a broader group of patients (particularly those at high risk of bone relapse), a recommendation which can be additionally supported by the favorable impact of bisphosphonates on preserving bone density in the setting of cancer treatment-related bone loss.
- Before initiating bisphosphonates, baseline dental examinations should be performed, to identify and treat oral problems that could lead to the need for dental surgery. It is important that patients maintain good oral hygiene, undergo regular dental examination, and be advised on appropriate measures for reducing the risk of osteonecrosis of the jaw.
- When giving intravenous bisphosphonates, it is advised that serum creatinine be checked before infusion. The dose of bisphosphonate may need to be adapted to renal function.

- All breast cancer patients on high-dose bisphosphonates should be advised to take calcium and vitamin D supplementation to avoid the risk of hypocalcemia. Periodic monitoring of serum calcium, electrolytes, phosphate, and magnesium should be performed.
- Women with early-stage breast cancer should be evaluated for their bone density and risk of fracture. Nutrition and lifestyle interventions should be advised for all women. Early-stage cancer patients at risk of developing cancer treatment-induced bone loss should be monitored by bone mineral density and considered for bisphosphonate treatment.

DISCLOSURES

Julie Gralow has received research funding from Novartis, Roche, sanofi-aventis, and Amgen.

ACKNOWLEDGMENTS

The author would like to acknowledge the significant contributions of Aparna Jotwani, M.D in the writing of this manuscript. Appreciation is also extended to Erin Pearson for help in manuscript preparation.

RELEVANT WEBSITE TABLE

Website	URL	Description
ASCO Clinical Practice Guidelines	http://www.asco.org/ASCO/Quality+Care+%26+Guidelines	2003 Update on the Role of Bisphosphonates and Bone Health Issues in Women With Breast Cancer
National Cancer Institute Clinical Trials	http://www.cancer.gov/clinicaltrials/ft-SWOG-S0307	Information summary for SWOG S0307 adjuvant bisphosphonate trial
NIH Office of Dietary Supplements	http://ods.od.nih.gov/	Vitamin and Mineral Supplement Fact Sheets
U.S. Department of Health and Human Services	http://www.surgeongeneral.gov/library/bonehealth/	Bone Health and Osteoporosis: A Report of the Surgeon General
National Institute of Arthritis and Musculoskeletal and Skin Diseases	http://www.niams.nih.gov/Health_Info/Bone/	The NIH Osteoporosis and Related Bone Diseases National Resource Center

References

1. Coleman RE, Smith P, Rubens RD. Clinical course and prognostic factors following bone recurrence from breast cancer. *Br J Cancer* 1998;77:336–340.
2. Orr FW, Varani J, Gondetz MD, et al. Chemotactic responses of tumor cells to products of resorbing bone. *Science* 1979;203:176–179.
3. Diel IJ, Kaufmann M, Costa SD, et al. Micrometastatic breast cancer cells in bone marrow at primary surgery: prognostic value in comparison to nodal status. *J Natl Cancer Inst* 1996;88:1652–1658.
4. Mundy GR. Bone resorption and turnover in health and disease. *Bone* 1987;8: S9–S16.
5. Hiraga T, Whilliams PI, Mundy GR, et al. The bisphosphonate ibandronate promotes apoptosis in MDA-231 human breast cancer cells in bone metastases. *Cancer Res* 2001;61:4418–4424.
6. Shimamura T, Amizuka N, Li M, et al. Histological observations on the microenvironment of osteolytic bone metastasis by breast carcinoma cell line. *Biomed Res* 2005;26:159–179.
7. Hauschka PV, Chen TL, Mavrakos AE. Polypeptide growth factors in bone matrix. *Ciba Found Symp* 1988;136:207–225.
8. Siwek B, Lacroix M, DePollak C, et al. Secretory products of breast cancer cells specifically affect human osteoblastic cells: partial characterization of active factors. *J Bone Miner Res* 1997;12:552–560.

9. Aktari M, Mansuri J, Newman KA, et al. Biology of breast cancer bone metastases. *Cancer Biol Ther* 2007;7:1–7.
10. Kakonen SM, Mundy GR. Mechanisms of osteolytic bone metastases in breast carcinoma. *Cancer* 2003;97:834–839.
11. van der Pluijm G, Lowik C, Papapoulos S, et al. Tumor progression and angiogenesis in bone metastases from breast cancer: new approaches to an old problem. *Cancer Treat Rev* 2000;26:11–27.
12. Frith J, Monkkonen J, Auriola S, et al. Clodronate and liposome-encapsulated clodronate are metabolized to a toxic ATP analog, adenosine 5'- (beta, gamma-dichloromethylene) triphosphate, by mammalian cells *in vitro. J Bone Miner Res* 1997;12:1358.
13. Rogers MJ, Gordon S, Benford HL, et al. Cellular and molecular mechanisms of action of bisphosphonates. *Cancer* 2000;88:2961–2978.
14. Luckman SP, Hughes DE, Coxon FP, et al. Nitrogen-containing bisphosphonates inhibit the mevalonate pathway and prevent post-translational prenylation of GTP-binding proteins, including Ras. *J Bone Miner Res* 1998;13:581–589.
15. Goffinet M, Thoulouzan M, Pradines A, et al. Zoledronic acid treatment impairs protein geranyl-geranylation for biological effects in prostatic cells. *BMC Cancer* 2006;6:60.
16. Selander KS, Monkkonen J, Karhukorpi EK, et al. Characteristics of clodronate-induced apoptosis in osteoclasts and macrophages. *Mol Pharmacol* 1996;50: 1127–1138.
17. Vitte C, Fleisch H, Guenther HL, et al. Bisphosphonates induce osteoblasts to secrete an inhibitor of osteoclast-mediated resorption. *Endocrinology* 1996;137: 2324–2333.
18. van der Pluijm G, Vloedgraven H, van Beek E, et al. Bisphosphonates inhibit the adhesion of breast cancer cells to bone matrices *in vitro. J Clin Invest* 1996;98: 698–705.
19. Boissier S, Magnetto S, Frappart L, et al. Bisphosphonates inhibit prostate and breast cancer cell adhesion to unmineralized and mineralized bone extracellular matrices. *Cancer Res* 1997;57:3890–3894.
20. Teronen O, Heillila P, Konttinen YT, et al. MMP inhibition and down regulation by bisphosphonates. *Ann N Y Acad Sci* 1999;878:453–465.
21. Sasaki A, Boyce BF, Story B, et al. Bisphosphonate risedronate reduces metastatic human breast cancer burden in bone in nude mice. *Cancer Res* 1995;55:3551–3557.
22. Daubine F, Le Gall C, Gasser J, et al. Antitumor effects of clinical dosing regimens of bisphosphonates in experimental breast cancer bone metastasis. *J Natl Cancer Inst* 2007;99:322–330.
23. Clezardin P. Anti-tumour activity of zoledronic acid. *Cancer Treat Rev* 2005;31:1–8.
24. Santini D, Martini F, Fratto ME, et al. *In vivo* effects of zoledronic acid on peripheral gammadelta T lymphocytes in early breast cancer patients. *Cancer Immunol Immunother* 2009;58:31–38.
25. Santini D, Vincenzi B, Galluzzo S, et al. Repeated intermittent low-dose therapy with zoledronic acid induces an early, sustained, and long-lasting decrease of peripheral vascular endothelial growth factor levels in cancer patients. *Clin Cancer Res* 2007;13:4482–4486.
26. Kunzmann V, Bauer E, Feurle J, et al. Stimulation of gammadelta T cells by amino-bisphosphonates and induction of antiplasma cell activity in multiple myeloma. *Blood* 2000;96:384–392.
27. Winter MC, Holen I, Coleman RE. Exploring the anti-tumor activity of bisphosphonates in early breast cancer. *Cancer Treat Rev* 2008. Epub ahead of print.
28. Diel IJ, Solomayer EF, Costa SD, et al. Reduction in new metastases in breast cancer with adjuvant clodronate treatment. *N Engl J Med* 1998;339:357–363.
29. Jaschke A, Bastert G, Slolmayer EF, et al. Adjuvant clodronate treatment improves the overall survival of primary breast cancer patients with micrometastases to bone marrow-longtime follow-up [Abstract 529]. *Proc Am Soc Clin Oncol* 2004;22:9s.
30. Powles T, Paterson S, Kanis JA, et al. Randomized, placebo-controlled trial of clodronate in patients with primary operable breast cancer. *J Clin Oncol* 2002;20: 3219–3224.
31. Powles T, Paterson A, McCloskey E, et al. Reduction in bone relapse and improved survival with oral clodronate for adjuvant treatment of operable breast cancer. *Breast Cancer Res* 2006;8:R13.
32. Saarto T, Blomqvist C, Virkkunen P, et al. Adjuvant clodronate treatment does not reduce the frequency of skeletal metastases in node-positive breast cancer patients: 5-year results of a randomized controlled trial. *J Clin Oncol* 2001;19:10–17.
33. Saarto T, Vehmanen L, Virkkunen P, et al. Ten-year follow-up of a randomized controlled trial of adjuvant clodronate treatment in node-positive breast cancer patients. *Acta Oncol* 2004;43:650–656.
34. Ha TC, Li H. Meta-analysis of clodronate and breast cancer survival. *Br J Cancer* 2007;96:1796–1801.
35. Gnant M, Mlineritsch B, Schippinger W, et al. Adjuvant ovarian suppression combined with tamoxifen or anastrozole, alone or in combination with zoledronic acid, in premenopausal women with endocrine-responsive, stage I and II breast cancer: first efficacy results from ABCSG-12 [Abstract LBA4]. *Proc Am Soc Clin Oncol* 2008;26:1006S.
36. Gnant MFX, Mlineritsch B, Luschin-Ebengreuth G, et al: Zoledronic acid prevents cancer treatment-induced bone loss in premenopausal women receiving adjuvant endocrine therapy for hormone-responsive breast cancer: a report from the Austrian Breast and Colorectal Cancer Study Group. *J Clin Oncol* 2007;25:820–828.
37. Brufsky A, Harker GJ, Beck T, et al: Zoledronic acid inhibits adjuvant letrozole-induced bone loss in postmenopausal women with early breast cancer. *J Clin Oncol* 2007;25:829–836.
38. Bundred NJ, Campbell ID, Davidson N, et al. Effective inhibition of aromatase inhibitor-associated bone loss by zoledronic acid in postmenopausal women with early breast cancer receiving adjuvant letrozole: ZO-FAST Study results. *Cancer* 2008;112:1001–1010.
39. Brufsky A, Bundred N, Coleman R, et al. Integrated analysis of zoledronic acid for prevention of aromatase inhibitor-associated bone loss in postmenopausal women with early breast cancer receiving adjuvant letrozole. *Oncologist* 2008;13:503–514.
40. Aft R, Watson M, Ylagan L, et al. Effect of zoledronic acid on bone marrow micrometastases in women undergoing neoadjuvant chemotherapy for breast cancer [Abstract 1021]. *Proc Am Soc Clin Oncol* 2008;26:46S.
41. Lin AY, Park JW, Scott J, et al. Zoledronic acid as adjuvant therapy for women with early stage breast cancer and disseminated tumor cells in bone marrow [Abstract 559]. *Proc Am Soc Clin Oncol* 2008;26:20S.
42. Rack BK, Jueckstock J, Genss E-M, et al. Effect of zoledronate on persisting isolated tumor cells in the bone marrow of patients without recurrence of early breast cancer [Abstract 511]. *Breast Cancer Res Treat* 2007;106:S40.

43. Pfeilschifter J, Diel IJ. Osteoporosis due to cancer treatment: pathogenesis and management. *J Clin Oncol* 2000;18:1570–1593.

44. Eastell R, Hannon RA, Cuzick J, et al. Effect of an aromatase inhibitor on BMD and bone turnover markers: 2-year results of the Anastrozole, Tamoxifen, Alone or in Combination (ATAC) trial. *J Bone Miner Res* 2006;21:1215–1223.

45. Shapiro CL, Manola J, Leboff M. Ovarian failure after adjuvant chemotherapy is associated with rapid bone loss in women with early-stage breast cancer. *J Clin Oncol* 2001;19;3306–3311.

46. Hoff AO, Gagel RF. Osteoporosis in breast and prostate cancer survivors. *Oncology* 2005;19:651–658.

47. Hillner BE, Ingle JN, Cheblowski RT, et al. American Society of Clinical Oncology 2003 update on the role of bisphosphonates and bone health issues in women with breast cancer. *J Clin Oncol* 2003;21:4042–4057.

48. Saarto T, Blomqvist C, Valimaki M, et al. Clodronate improves bone mineral density in post-menopausal breast cancer patients treated with adjuvant antioestrogens. *Br J Cancer* 1997;75:602–605.

49. Saarto T, Blomqvist C, Valimaki M, et al. Chemical castration induced by adjuvant cyclophosphamide, methotrexate, and fluorouracil chemotherapy causes rapid bone loss that is reduced by clodronate: a randomized study in premenopausal breast cancer patients. *J Clin Oncol* 1997;15:1341–1347.

50. Delmas PD, Balena R, Confravreux E, et al. Bisphosphonate risedronate prevents bone loss in women with artificial menopause due to chemotherapy of breast cancer: a double-blind, placebo-controlled study. *J Clin Oncol* 1997;15:955–962.

51. Ripps BA, VanGilder K, Minhas B, et al. Alendronate for the prevention of bone mineral loss during gonadotropin-releasing hormone agonist therapy. *J Reprod Med* 2003;48:761–766.

52. Greenspan SL, Brufsky A, Lembersky BC, et al. Risedronate prevents bone loss in breast cancer survivors: a 2-year, randomized, double-blind, placebo-controlled clinical trial. *J Clin Oncol* 2008;26:2644–2652.

53. Van Poznak C, Hannon RA, Clack G, et al. The SABRE (Study of Anastrozole with the Bisphosphonate RisedronatE) study: 12-month analysis [Abstract 502]. *Breast Cancer Res Treat* 2007;106:S37.

54. Shapiro CL, Halabi S, Gibson G, et al. Effect of zoledronic acid on bone mineral density in premenopausal women who develop ovarian failure due to adjuvant chemotherapy: first results from CALGB trial 79809 [Abstract 512]. *Proc Am Soc Clin Oncol* 2008;26:9S.

55. Lester JE, Gutcher SA, Ellis SP, et al. Effect of monthly oral ibandronate on anastrozole-induced bone loss during adjuvant treatment for breast cancer: one-year results from the ARIBON study [Abstract 553]. *Proc Am Soc Clin Oncol* 2007;25:16S.

56. Ellis G, Bone HG, Chlebowski R, et al. A Phase 3 study of the effect of denosumab therapy on bone mineral density in women receiving aromatase inhibitors for non-metastatic breast cancer [Abstract 47]. *Breast Cancer Res Treat* 2007:106.

57. De Groen PC, Lubbe DF, Hirsch LJ, et al. Esophagitis associated with the use of alendronate. *N Engl J Med* 1966;335:1015–1021.

58. Rosen LS, Gordon D, Kaminski M, et al. Long-term efficacy and safety of zoledronate compared with pamidronate disodium in the treatment of skeletal complications in patients with advanced multiple myeloma or breast carcinoma: a randomized, double-blind, multicenter, comparative trial. *Cancer* 2003;98:1735–1744.

59. Marx RE. Pamidronate and zoledronate induced avascular necrosis of the jaws: a growing epidemic. *J Oral Maxillofac Surg* 2003;61:1115–1117.

60. Ruggiero SL, Mehrotra B, Rosenberg TJ, et al. Osteonecrosis of the jaws associated with the use of bisphosphonates: a review of 63 cases. *J Oral Maxillofac Surg* 2004;62:527–534.

61. Woo SB, Hellstein JW, Kalmar JR. Systemic review: bisphosphonates and osteonecrosis of the jaws. *Ann Intern Med* 2006;144:753–761.

62. Coleman R, Thorpe H, Cameron D, et al. Zoledronic acid is well tolerated and can be safely administered with adjuvant chemotherapy—first safety data from the AZURE trial [Abstract 2080]. *Breast Cancer Res Treat* 2006;100:S107.

Rowan T. Chlebowski and Jennifer A. Ligibel

Observational studies suggest that lifestyle factors, including obesity, low physical activity, and differences in dietary intake may influence breast cancer prognosis (1–3). Recently, two full-scale, randomized clinical trials have evaluated lifestyle interventions in women with early-stage, resected breast cancer (4,5). This chapter outlines the observational study evidence regarding lifestyle and breast cancer outcomes, with emphasis on recent reports, and presents and contrasts the design and findings from the two randomized trials.

 ## BODY WEIGHT AND BREAST CANCER OUTCOME

Observational studies of the influence of obesity on clinical outcome in breast cancer patients have provided mixed results (1,6,7). In 36 of 51 studies, a significant adverse effect of higher body weight on breast cancer prognosis was seen, but few studies have adequately controlled for systemic adjuvant therapy use (6).

Several recent reports may be of more relevance. The influence of excess weight on breast cancer outcomes was recently examined in a cohort of 14,709 patients with localized disease. A consistent negative effect of obesity on clinical outcomes was seen: metastatic recurrence (hazard ratio [HR] 1.32, 95% confidence interval [CI] 1.19–1.48); overall survival (HR 1.43, 95% CI 1.28–1.60) and second primary cancer (HR 1.57, 95% CI 1.19–2.07) (8). In the Nurse's Health Study (NHS) cohort, higher body weight at diagnosis was associated with decreased survival in 5,204 women with localized breast cancer, but the relationship was statistically significant only in those who never smoked (9). Holick et al. (10) reported on a cohort of 3,924 women with localized breast cancer where obese women with a body mass index (BMI) 30 kg/m^2 or greater were more likely then lean women (BMI <23 kg/m^2) to die of breast cancer (HR 1.34, 95% CI 1.09–1.65). In a population-based cohort of 1,360 Australian women with early-stage breast cancer, a BMI 30 kg/m^2 or greater was associated with increased breast cancer recurrence (HR 1.57, 95% CI 1.11–2.22) and all cause mortality (HR 1.56, 95% CI 1.01–2.40) (11). Finally, in a similarly sized population of 1,376 breast cancer patients with stage I to II disease, significantly increased mortality was seen in the highest weight category, with greatest effects on hormone receptor-negative subgroups (12).

Potential Confounding Factors

To account for factors potentially confounding lifestyle and breast cancer associations, further study in populations receiving contemporary systemic treatment is needed. Estrogen modulation has been proposed as a potential mediator of the influence of obesity on prognosis (13,14). Current pharmacologic strategies effectively reduce estrogen levels, however, and no studies have reported on the influence of obesity on breast cancer outcome in postmenopausal women treated with aromatase inhibitors in the adjuvant setting. Race or ethnicity differences also can influence findings in this area. Black women are commonly heavier than white women and their breast cancers carry a worse prognosis (15,16). However, the prognosis has been more strongly associated with genetic factors rather than body weight or lifestyle differences (15). Another potential confounder is differential chemotherapy use. In population

studies, obese women often received less than full dose chemotherapy, with consequent adverse impact on recurrence rates (17–19). Evidence from multicenter breast cancer adjuvant trials that control systemic therapy dose and schedule address, to some degree, these issues.

Body Weight and Breast Cancer Outcome (in Cooperative Group Trials)

The National Surgical Breast and Bowel Project (NSABP) examined associations among obesity, tamoxifen use, and clinical outcome in receptor-positive, early-stage breast cancer in 3,385 participants in a randomized trial comparing tamoxifen with placebo. With more than 166 months of follow-up, tamoxifen efficacy was not influenced by obesity, and both contralateral breast cancer risk and all cause mortality were significantly greater in obese women (HR 1.59, 95% CI 1.10–2.25 and HR 1.31, 95% CI 1.12–1.5, respectively) (20).

The International Breast Cancer Study Group combined several randomized adjuvant trials into a cohort of 6,792 early-stage breast cancer patients and related clinical outcomes to BMI in analyses incorporating conventional prognostic factors (21). Higher BMI at diagnosis was associated with decreased overall survival, with a suggestion of greater effect in pre- and perimenopausal women (comparing obese with not obese women, HR 1.22, 95% CI 1.05–1.42 and HR 1.11, 95% CI 0.97–1.24, respectively) (Table 53.1). More recently, a report from M.D. Anderson described negative effects of obesity on outcome of 606 women with advanced but not metastatic breast cancer. All received similar anthracycline chemotherapy and doses were not adjusted for weight. Obesity was associated with significantly lower 10-year survival for both locally advanced disease (57.3% vs. 42.4%, for obese women versus not, respectively $p < .05$) and inflammatory breast cancer (50.9% vs. 43.7, respectively, $p < .05$) (22). These reports provide provocative information regarding the potential role of obesity in altering breast cancer clinical outcome even in patients receiving contemporary anticancer adjuvant treatment.

Weight Gain after Diagnosis and Breast Cancer Outcome

The association between obesity and poor prognosis in early-stage breast cancer is especially worrisome given the weight gain seen in many women following diagnosis (23) where, even with anthracycline-based adjuvant regimens, weight gain of 2 to 6 kg is commonly reported (24,25). Four of five studies which looked at the impact of weight gain after diagnosis on recurrence reported an increased risk associated with weight gain (26–29). In a NHS report in 2,206 nonsmoking women with early-stage breast cancer, women who gained 2.0 kg/m^2 or more (median weight gain of 17 pounds) had higher risk of breast cancer recurrence, breast cancer death, and all-cause mortality than did women who did not gain weight (30).

Obesity and Breast Cancer Outcome: Summary

Obesity has been associated with increased dietary fat intake and decreased physical activity, and all these factors have all been related to adverse breast cancer outcome in at least some reports (3,31,32). Given the common association of these factors, it is unlikely that retrospective analyses of existing patient

Table 53.1 CLINICAL OUTCOMES COMPARING OBESE WITH NONOBESE WOMEN IN ADJUVANT BREAST CANCER MULTICENTER CLINICAL TRIAL GROUPS

	Obese (BMI >30) versus not		
Outcome	NSABP HR (95% CI)	IBCSG HR (95% CI)	
	Premenopausal and Postmenopausal	Premenopausal and Perimenopausal	Postmenopausal
Breast Cancer Recurrence[a]	0.98 (0.80, 1.18)	1.16 (1.02, 1.33)	1.06 (0.96–1.17)
Overall survival	1.31 (1.12, 1.54)	1.22 (1.05, 1.42)	1.11 (0.97–1.24)

BMI, body mass index; CI, confidence interval; HR, hazard ratio; IBCSG, International Breast Cancer Study Group; NSABP, National Surgical Adjuvant Breast Cancer Project.
[a]As disease-free survival, which includes recurrence rates, second nonbreast invasive cancer or death from any cause.

populations will provide definitive information regarding a role for weight loss or weight maintenance as a breast cancer management strategy. A few small pilot studies have looked at weight loss and weight maintenance interventions in breast cancer survivors and have demonstrated that increased physical activity and mild calorie restriction can help prevent weight gain during and after breast cancer treatment (6,33). An ongoing randomized trial (described below) will help determine whether losing weight after breast cancer diagnosis will help prevent recurrence and improve overall survival.

 ## PHYSICAL ACTIVITY AND BREAST CANCER OUTCOME

Although the preponderance of observational studies suggest increased physical activity may modulate breast cancer incidence, until recently the effects of physical activity on breast cancer prognosis was largely unexamined. Three observational studies now suggest that women who engage in modest amounts of physical activity after breast cancer diagnosis have a better prognosis than more sedentary women, and another study demonstrates improved prognosis in premenopausal women who were physically active in the year before breast cancer diagnosis (Table 53.2).

The NHS investigators prospectively examined relationships among physical activity and clinical outcomes in a cohort of 2,987 women diagnosed with stage I-IIIA breast cancer. Questionnaire information on physical activity was collected 2 or more years after initial cancer diagnosis to generate a metabolic equivalent (MET) hr/wk score for duration and intensity of physical activity. Compared with women with less than 3 MET hr/wk of physical activity (equivalent to walking at a moderate pace for less than 1 hr/wk), the adjusted relative risk (RR) of breast cancer mortality was 0.80 95% CI, 0.60–1.06 for 3–8.9 MET hr/wk of activity and 0.50 (95% CI 0.31–0.82) for 9–14.9 MET hr/wk. Breast cancer recurrence and all-cause mortality demonstrated similar favorable associations with

Table 53.2 OBSERVATIONAL STUDIES EVALUATING PHYSICAL ACTIVITY ASSOCIATION WITH CLINICAL OUTCOME IN EARLY STAGE, RESECTED BREAST CANCER

						Clinical Outcome		
Author	Study Population	Age (y)	Total	Follow-up	Follow-up	Breast Cancer Death	Total Death	Results
Holick et al. *Cancer Epidemiol Biomarkers Prev* 2008;17:379–386	Breast cancer patients in Collaborative Women's Longevity Study (CWLS) identified <2 yr after diagnosis	20–79 yr	4,482	5.6 yr (median)	—	109	412	Versus <2.8 MET-h/wk for breast cancer death: for 2.8–7.9, HR 0.58 (0.45–0.75); for 8.0–20.9, HR 0.52 (0.40–0.68)
Abrahamson et al. *Cancer* 2006;107: 1777–1785	Population-based cohort with diagnosed breast cancer	20–54 yr	1,264	8–10 yr	—	—	290	Total mortality lowest in highest quartile of physical activity (for obese/overweight) HR 0.70 (0.49–0.99)
Holmes et al. *JAMA* 2005;293:2479–2486	Participants in Nurse's Health Study (NHS) who developed breast cancer	30–55 yr at entry in NHS	2,987		370	280	463	Versus <3 MET-h/wk for total mortality: for 3.0–8.9, HR 0.71 for (0.56–0.80); for 9.0–14.9, HR 0.57 (0.38–0.85)
Pierce et al. *J Clin Oncol* 2007;25: 2345–2351	Breast cancer patients participating as controls in randomized trial, entered <2 yr after diagnosis	<70 yr	1,490	6.7 yr (mean)	236	135	118	Combination of ≥5 vegetable/fruit servings/day plus physical activity equivalent to walking 30 min, 6 days/wk, for total mortality vs. not: HR 0.56 (0.31–0.98)

HR, hazard ratio; MET, metabolic equivalent.

physical activity and benefit, seen in both pre- and post-menopausal women, was independent of BMI (3).

Holick et al. (10) prospectively studied associations between postdiagnosis physical activity and breast cancer mortality in 4,482 women with localized disease. Questionnaires on physical activity were used to calculate MET hr/wk and patients were subsequently followed for recurrence. Women expending more than 2.8 MET hr/wk had lower breast cancer mortality when compared with women with lower levels of activity (HR 0.65, 95% CI 0.39–1.08 for 2.8–7.9 MET hr/wk; and HR 0.59, 95% CI 0.35–1.01 for 8.0–20.9 MET hr/wk). A 15% decrease in breast cancer mortality for each additional 5 MET hr/wk was calculated (p for trend = 0.03) with associations independent of age, BMI, or disease stage.

Using a somewhat different study design, Abrahamson et al. (34) examined the association of prediagnosis physical activity and survival in 1,264 premenopausal women with early-stage breast cancer. A nonsignificant trend for reduced mortality (HR 0.78, 95% CI 0.56–1.08) was seen in favor of the quartile reporting more physical activity. Finally, the Women's Healthy Eating and Living Study (WHEL) examined the association between survival and physical activity, body weight, and dietary pattern in early-stage breast cancer patients randomized to the control group in a clinical trial evaluating a dietary lifestyle change (35). After 8.7 years median follow-up, a linear trend between mortality and physical activity was seen. Compared with inactive participants, those who performed 636 to 1,320 MET-minutes of activity per week and those who performed more than 1,320 MET-minutes of activity per week had 24% and 42% lower mortality, respectively (p for trend = 0.02). However, composite measures suggested the association was also dependent on dietary fruit and vegetable intake.

Taken together, the results are consistent with a modest increase in physical activity being associated with substantial improvement in clinical outcome for patients with early-stage breast cancer. No randomized trial has reported on an intervention designed to increase physical activity in breast cancer patients in this setting.

Observational studies have demonstrated that a breast cancer diagnosis often is associated with a substantial decrease in physical activity (36). Intervention trials of physical activity in women with localized breast cancer have been largely limited to relatively short duration trials with end points including quality of life (37), fitness, weight change (38–40), and potential biomarkers of breast cancer risk and prognosis, such as estrogen (41) and insulin (42). These trials have demonstrated that physical activity is both feasible during and after breast cancer therapy, and is associated with improved quality of life and decreased fatigue (43,44), and fewer treatment-related side effects. Large-scale, randomized clinical trials are needed to determine whether increasing physical activity after breast cancer diagnosis will not only help women feel better, but also lead to improvements in prognosis.

DIETARY INTAKES AND BREAST CANCER OUTCOME

Studying the relationship between postdiagnosis dietary intakes and breast cancer prognosis represents an especially challenging area for observational studies, with methodologic issues related to the optimal timing of data collection, difficulty in accurately measuring the dietary exposure, and the modest range of intake for nutrients of interest in a general population (2).

The relationship between dietary fat intake and breast cancer outcome has been examined in 14 observational studies. Although recent analyses suggest that commonly used instruments may have difficulty in accurately measuring this parameter (44,45), 7 reports demonstrated a significant association between lower fat intakes and lower recurrence risk (1,4). These reports did not adjust for BMI or total energy intake, however, making interpretation problematic. Reports relating vegetable and related nutrient intake to breast cancer prognosis presents a similarly mixed picture with three of eight reports describing significant associations between higher intake and lower recurrence risk (5,46). Recently, two randomized clinical trials have provided a higher level of evidence on the question of the influence of nutrient intake on breast cancer outcomes.

POTENTIAL MEDIATORS OF LIFESTYLE CHANGE

At present, while estrogen, leptin, and inflammatory factors are of interest, no mediator of lifestyle influence on breast cancer outcome has been definitively identified. However, an emerging body of preclinical and observational study evidence suggests that insulin may play a substantial role in the process (47). Higher fasting insulin levels have been associated with obesity and also with increased recurrence risk and death in early-stage breast cancer patients, with greatest influence seen on hormone receptor-negative cancers (48). In a similar study, women with either high insulin levels or the insulin resistance syndrome had significantly more beast cancer mortality. In this cohort of 603 early-stage breast cancer patients, high insulin levels were significantly associated with mortality risk as well (RR 1.9 95% CI 0.7–6.6) (49). Finally, in an adjuvant study in hormone receptor-positive postmenopausal women receiving tamoxifen, high levels of c-peptide (a break down product of proinsulin cleavage) were significantly associated with worse breast cancer outcomes (50).

Cross sectional analyses in postmenopausal women without cancer suggest both low physical activity and high caloric intake are related to higher fasting insulin levels (51). Ligibel et al. (42) has examined the impact of increasing physical activity on insulin levels, in a randomized trial evaluating a mixed strength and endurance exercise intervention in 82 overweight, sedentary women with early-stage breast cancer. The 16-week intervention reduced circulating insulin levels by 28% (p = .03) with a trend toward improvement in insulin sensitivity. Although further study is needed, insulin remains a potential mediator of lifestyle influence on breast cancer outcome (42).

ADJUVANT BREAST CANCER RANDOMIZED TRIALS EVALUATING LIFESTYLE CHANGE

Two recently reported full-scale, randomized clinical trials have evaluated lifestyle interventions targeting dietary change in the adjuvant breast cancer setting. The Women's Intervention Nutrition Study (WINS) and WHEL study enrolled different populations and studied different dietary patterns, but both aimed to reduce dietary fat intake. These trials are compared and contrasted below (Table 53.2).

The WINS is a randomized, prospective multicenter clinical trial evaluating the impact of a dietary intervention on disease-free survival (DFS) in women with resected, early-stage breast cancer receiving conventional cancer management (4). Participants were required to have histologically confirmed, resected early-stage, invasive breast cancer, be between 49 and 79 years of age, and receive acceptable adjuvant therapy. The dietary intervention was designed to reduce fat intake with eight every-other-week visits during the intensive intervention period followed by every-3-month contacts during the maintenance period, implemented by centrally trained, registered dietitians using a previously developed low-fat eating plan (52). Nutrient intake information was collected annually using unannounced telephone recalls and patients were followed for recurrence and survival.

After 5.6 years median follow-up, a sustained statistically significant reduction in dietary fat intake, in terms of both fat grams and percent calories from fat, was seen reduced in intervention participants (Table 53.3). Although weight loss was not a specific intervention target, significantly lower body weight was also seen in the intervention group throughout. More relapse events occurred in the control (181 of 1,462, 12.4%) compared with the intervention group (96 of 975, 9.8%, HR 0.76, 95% CI 0.60–0.98, $p = .034$). Preliminary analyses from an additional 3 years of follow-up provide similar results (relapse-free survival HR 0.79, 95% CI 0.62–1.00), but the difference is no longer statistically significant (53). Continued nonintervention follow-up of these patients is ongoing. In exploratory subgroup analyses, substantially greater influence was seen in women with ER-negative, PR-negative breast cancer (overall survival HR 0.34, 95% CI 0.16–0.70) (53). The WINS results suggest a hypothesis that a lifestyle intervention reducing dietary fat intake and associated with modest weight

loss may improve outcome of breast cancer patients receiving conventional cancer management.

Although a primary prevention trial, results from the Women's Health Initiative Dietary Modification trial (WHI DM) may inform the WINS results. In the WHI DM 48,832, postmenopausal women without a breast cancer history were randomized to a dietary intervention program largely targeting dietary fat intake reduction (54). Statistically significant dietary fat intake reduction was achieved and fewer breast cancer diagnoses were made in the dietary intervention group, but the differences did not achieve statistical significance (HR 0.91, 95% CI 0.83–1.01). However, as in WINS, greater evidence of dietary effect was seen in risk of hormone receptor-negative breast cancer (54).

The Women's Healthy Eating and Living Randomized Trial

The WHEL is a multicenter, randomized prospective trial of a dietary intervention program being evaluated in 3,088 women with early-stage, resected breast cancer with an objective to determine whether a dietary pattern, including an increase in vegetable, fruit, and fiber intake and a decrease in fat intake, would influence breast cancer recurrence risk and all-cause mor-

Table 53.3	RANDOMIZED CLINICAL TRIALS EVALUATING LIFESTYLE CHANGE IN EARLY STAGE, RESECTED BREAST CANCER: STUDY DESIGNS AND REPORTED OUTCOME		
	WINS	**WHEL**	**LISA**
Eligibility			
Stage	I–III A	I– II A	I–III A
Time from surgery	≤12 mo	≤48 mo	≤15 mo
Chemotherapy	AC, CMF, FAC, or AC → Paclitaxel	Any (before randomization)	Any (before randomization)
Hormonal therapy	Tamoxifen	Any	Letrozole
Receptor status	Any	Any	Receptor positive
Age	48–79 yr	18–70 yr	Any postmenopausal (life expectancy >5 yr)
Weight/BMI	Any	Any	BMI ≥21 <40 kg/m^2
Diet at baseline	≥20% caloric from fat	Any	Any
Dietary Intervention			
Intervention phase	Eight individual dietitian visit over 16 wk	Eighteen telephone calls over 12 mo, 4 cooking classes (average attended)	Telephone calls (19–22) over 6 mo
Maintenance phase	Individual dietitian visits every 3 mo	Telephone calls every 3 mo	Telephone calls (19) over 2 yr
Number of patients (randomization type)	2,437 (3:2 randomization)	3,088 (1:1 randomization)	2,150 (1:1 randomization)
Intervention target			
Fat	↓ to 15% calories from fat	↓ to <20% calories from fat	↓ to 20% calories from fat
Calories			Decrease 500–1000 calories/day
Vegetable	Increase (no target)	Increase to 5 serving/day and 16 oz vegetable juice/day	Increase (no target)
Fruit	Increase (no target)	Increase to 3 servings/day	Increase (no target)
Body weight	N/A	N/A	10% loss to BMI ≥21 kg/m^2
Physical activity	N/A	N/A	Increase to 150–200 min/wk walking plus resistance/flexibility
Follow-up Interval	5 yr	7.3 yr	0 (Entering patients)
End point	Relapse-free survival	Breast cancer event free-survival	Disease-free survival
Self-monitoring	Daily "keeping score" book	No	Daily log books for diet and physical activity
Dietary assessment	Two 24-hr unannounced telephone calls/yr	Four prescheduled 24-hr telephone calls at 1, 4, and 6 yr	N/A
Endpoint events (n)	277	518	N/A
Primary breast cancer outcome	HR 0.76 (95% CI 0.60–0.98, $p = .034$)[a]	0.96 (95% CI 0.80–1.14, $p = .63$)[b]	N/A

AC, doxorubicin (adriamycin) and cyclophosphamide (Cytoxan); BMI, body mass index; CMF, cyclophosphamide, methotrexate and 5-fluorouracil; FAC, Fluorouracil (5-FU), doxorubicin and cyclophosphamide; LISA, Lifestyle Intervention Study in Adjuvant Treatment of Early Breast Cancer; WHEL, Women's Healthy Eating and Living Study; WINS, Women's Intervention Nutrition Study.
[a]Chlebowski RT, Blackburn G, Thomson CA, et al. *J Natl Cancer Inst* 2006;98(24):1767–1776.
[b]Pierce JP, Natarajan L, Caan BJ, et al. *JAMA* 2007;298:289–298.

tality (5). Intervention participants received a telephone counseling program involving 18 calls during the first year with a subsequent decrease in intensity (55) (Table 53.3). Significant changes were achieved in the nutrition targets: vegetables plus 65%, fruit plus 25%, fiber plus 30%, and energy intake from fat minus 13%. Over the 7.3-year mean follow-up, no difference emerged in invasive breast cancer events (HR 0.96, 95% CI 0.80–1.14, $p = .63$) or overall (HR 0.91, 95% CI 0.72–1.15; $p = .43$) (5).

Although both WINS and WHEL included dietary fat intake reduction as an objective and entered early-stage breast cancer patients, substantial differences between these trials exist (Table 53.3) (56). The WHEL intervention resulted in a substantial and sustained increase in vegetable, fruit, and fiber intake and a relatively short duration, moderate reduction in fat intake. The WINS intervention did not report increased vegetable, fruit, or fiber intake, but resulted in a substantial, sustained reduction in fat intake, which was associated with significant weight loss (Table 53.4), which may account for the apparent differences in influence on clinical outcome seen.

The Lifestyle Intervention Study in Adjuvant Treatment of Early Breast Cancer

One adjuvant breast cancer trial is currently evaluating an intervention designed to reduce weight through increased physical activity and dietary modification. The Lifestyle Intervention Study in Adjuvant treatment of early breast cancer (LISA) of the Ontario Clinical Oncology Group is an ongoing

trial that will evaluate the impact of an individualized weight loss intervention (telephone and mail-based) on DFS in postmenopausal women with recently diagnosed, hormone receptor-positive breast cancer (47). In this multicenter, randomized clinical trial involving 2,150 women, intervention group participants will receive a program targeting individual weight loss, dietary fat reduction, and increased physical activity. Participants will be postmenopausal women with stage I-II A, resected breast cancer who have a BMI between 24 and 40 kd/m^2, have completed chemotherapy, and are on letrozole adjuvant hormone therapy. The WINS, WHEL, and LISA trials are compared in Table 53.2.

 CONCLUSIONS

As the evidence linking lifestyle factors and breast cancer outcomes mounts, there is a growing desire on the part of many patients to make lifestyle changes after breast cancer diagnosis. However, given the relative paucity of available randomized data, and that most medical oncologists lack expertise in this area, many breast cancer patients do not receive any guidance to help make these changes.

Observational evidence suggests that women who are overweight or obese at the time of breast cancer diagnosis, and those who gain weight during and after cancer treatment, appear to have a worse prognosis as compared with leaner women. Similar evidence suggests that women who are inactive after breast cancer diagnosis also have a poor prognosis compared with women who engage in modest amounts of physical activity. Randomized data suggest that lowering fat intake, or modest weight loss, is associated with a modest decrease in breast cancer recurrence, whereas increasing fruit, vegetable, and fiber intake does not appear to have an impact on breast cancer outcomes. The LISA trial will help determine whether weight loss decreases the risk of cancer recurrence in breast cancer survivors, but it will be several years until the results of this study will be available and further work is clearly needed to help define the role of lifestyle change in breast cancer patients.

MANAGEMENT SUMMARY

- Advocating weight maintenance for women with a BMI less than 25, and moderate weight loss for overweight and obese women, are reasonable goals for most breast cancer patients.
- Reduction in caloric intake is essential for weight loss, whereas exercise has been demonstrated to be a key component of maintaining weight in a target range.
- Specific recommendations for individual patients will depend on the goals of the treatment plan (weight maintenance vs. weight loss), as well as the presence of comorbid conditions that could influence diet or activity level.
- For weigh loss, a diet emphasizing complex carbohydrates and limiting refined sugars and fats could be recommended for most breast cancer patients.
- The U.S. Surgeon General recommends 30 minutes of moderate exercise five times per week as a general health measure, and this level of physical activity may be associated with improved survival in breast cancer patients.

Table 53.4	DIETARY INTAKE AND BODY WEIGHT CHANGE DURING WINS AND WHEL INTERVENTION	
	WHEL	**WINS**
%Energy from fat		
Baseline	28.5 ± 0.18	29.6 ± 7.1
1 yr	22.7 ± 0.20	20.3 ± 7.8
4 yr	27.1 ± 0.24	22.6 ± 8.5
6 yr	28.9 ± 0.25	23.0 ± 9.2
Body weight (kg)		
Baseline	73.5 ± 0.42	72.7 ± 15.9
1 yr	73.0 ± 0.45	70.6 ± 15.2
4 yr	74.2 ± 0.51	71.2 ± 14.9
6 yr	74.1 ± 0.54	69.4 ± 13.9
Fiber g/d		
Baseline	21.1 ± 0.21	18.4 ± 4.1
1 yr	29.0 ± 0.28	19.5 ± 4.7
Vegetable Servings/d		
Baseline	3.9 ± 0.06	Not reported
1 yr	7.8 ± 0.09	—
Fruit Servings/d		
Baseline	3.5 ± 0.05	Not reported
1 yr	4.2 ± 0.06	—

WHEL, Lifestyle Intervention Study in Adjuvant Treatment of Early Breast Cancer; WINS, Lifestyle Intervention Study in Adjuvant Treatment of Early Breast Cancer.
WINS values, all mean ⊥ standard deviation (SD); WHEL values, all mean ± standard error (SE).
In WINS, dietary fat intake difference comparing both intervention with control groups and baseline with each time period value in the intervention group was substantially significant ($p <.0001$). In WHEL, dietary fat intake differences comparing intervention with control groups was statistically significant ($p <.001$). In WHEL, the baseline to each time period value in the intervention group was not tested for significance.
In WINS, body weight difference comparing intervention with control groups and baseline with each time period value in the intervention group were statistically significant ($p <.005$) at all intervals. In WHEL, no significant body weight differences were seen.
In WINS, fiber, vegetable, and fruit intake were either not reported or not significantly different. In WHEL, vegetables, fruit, and fiber intake comparing intervention with control groups were statistically significant ($p <.001$) for each dietary target across the control intervention period.

References

1. Chlebowski RT, Aiello E, McTiernan A. Weight loss in breast cancer patient management. *J Clin Oncol* 2002;20:1128–1143.
2. Kushi LH, Kwan ML, Lee MM, Ambrosome CB. Lifestyle factors and survival in women with breast cancer. *J Nutr* 2007;137:236S–242S.
3. Holmes MD, Chen WY, Feskanich D, et al. Physical activity ad survival after breast cancer diagnosis. *JAMA* 2005;293(20):2479–2486.

4. Chlebowski RT, Blackburn G, Thomson CA, et al. Dietary fat reduction and breast cancer outcome: Interim efficacy results from the Women's Intervention Nutrition Study (WINS). *J Natl Cancer Inst* 2006;98(24):1767–1776.
5. Pierce JP, Natarajan L, Caan BJ, et al. Influence of a diet very high in vegetables, fruit, and fiber and low in fat on prognosis following treatment for breast cancer: The Women's Healthy Eating and Living (WHEL) Randomized Trial. *JAMA* 2007; 98:289–298.
6. Goodwin PJ, Esplen MJ, Wincour J, et al. Development of a weight management program in women with newly diagnosed locoregional breast cancer. In: Bitzer J, Stauber M, eds. *Pschosomatic obstetrics and gynecology*. Bologna: Moduzzi Editore, International Proceedings Division, 1995:491–496.
7. Carmichael AR. Obesity and prognosis of breast cancer. *Obesity* 2006;7:333–340.
8. Majed B, Moreau T, Senouci K, et al. Is obesity an independent prognosis factor in women breast cancer? *Breast Cancer Res Treat* 2008;111(2):329–342.
9. Kroenke CH, Chen WY, Rosner B, et al. Weight, weight gain and survival after breast cancer diagnosis. *J Clin Oncol* 2005;23(7):683–694.
10. Holick CN, Newcomb PA, Trentham-Dietz A, et al. Physical activity and survival after diagnosis of invasive breast cancer. *Cancer Epidemiol Biomarkers Prev* 2008;17(2):379–386.
11. Loi S, Milne RL, Friedlander ML, et al. Obesity and outcomes in premenopausal and postmenopausal breast cancer. *Cancer Epidemiol Biomarkers Prev* 2005;14(7):1686–1691.
12. Enger SM, Greif JM, Polikoff J, et al. Body weight correlates with mortality in early stage breast cancer. *Arch Surg* 2004;139:954–960.
13. Key TJ, Appleby PN, Reeves GK, et al. Body mass index, serum sex hormones, and breast cancer risk in postmenopausal women. *J Natl Cancer Inst* 2003;95(16): 1218–1226.
14. McTiernan A, Rajan KB, Tworoger SS, et al. Adiposity and sex hormones in post-menopausal breast cancer survivors. *J Clin Oncol* 2003;21(10):1961–1966.
15. Chlebowski RT, Chen Z, Anderson GL, et al. Ethnicity and breast cancer: factors influencing differences in incidence and outcome. *J Natl Cancer Inst* 2005; 97(6):439–447.
16. Carey LA, Perou CM, Livasy CA, et al. Race, breast cancer subtypes, and survival in the Carolina Breast Cancer Study. *JAMA* 2006;295(21):2492–2502.
17. Griggs JJ, Sorbero ME, Lyman GH. Undertreatment of obese women receiving breast cancer chemotherapy. *Arch Intern Med* 2005;165(11):1267–1273.
18. Jenkins P, Elyan S, Freeman S. Obesity is not associated with increased myelosuppression in patients receiving chemotherapy for breast cancer. *Eur J Cancer* 2007;43(3):544–548.
19. Rosner GL, Hargis JB, Hollis DR, et al. Relationship between toxicity and obesity in women receiving adjuvant chemotherapy for breast cancer: results from cancer and leukemia group B study 8541. *J Clin Oncol* 1996;14(11):3000–3008.
20. Dignam JJ, Wieand K, Johnson K, et al. Obesity, tamoxifen use, and outcomes in women with estrogen receptor-positive early stage breast cancer. *J Natl Cancer Inst* 2003;95:1467–1476.
21. Berclaz G, Li S, Price KN, et al. Body mass index as a prognostic feature in operable breast cancer: the International Breast Cancer Study Group experience. *Ann Oncol* 2004;15:875–884.
22. Dawood S, Broglio K, Gonzalez-Angulo AM, et al. Prognostic value of body mass index in locally advanced breast cancer. *Clin Cancer Res* 2008;14:1718–1725.
23. Goodwin P, Ennis M, Pritchard K, et al. Adjuvant treatment and the onset of menopause predict weight gain after breast cancer diagnosis. *J Clin Oncol* 1999; 17:120–129.
24. Shepherd L, Parulekar W, Day A, et al. Weight gain during adjuvant therapy in high risk pre/perimenopausal breast cancer patients: analysis of a National Cancer Institute of Canada Clinical Trials Groups (NCIC CTG) phase III study. *Proceedings of the American Society of Clinical Oncology* 2001;20:36a.
25. Makari-Judson G, Judson C, Mertens W. Breast cancer patient weight gain in the adjuvant era: defining groups at risk [Abstract 2920] *Proceedings of the American Society of Clinical Oncology* 2003;22.
26. Camoriano J, Loprinzi C, Ingle J, et al. Weight change in women treated with adjuvant therapy or observed following mastectomy for node-positive breast cancer. *J Clin Oncol* 1990;8:1327–1334.
27. Bonomi P, Bunting N, Fishman D, et al. Weight gain during adjuvant chemotherapy or hormono-chemotherapy for stage II breast cancer in relation to disease free survival [Abstract]. *Breast Cancer Res Treat* 1984;4:339.
28. Chlebowski R, Weiner J, Reynolds R, et al. Long-term survival following relapse after 5-FU but not CMF chemotherapy. *Breast Cancer Res Treat* 1986;7:23–29.
29. Levine E, Raczynski J, Carpenter J, et al. Weight gain with breast cancer adjuvant treatment. *Cancer* 1991;67:1954–1959.
30. Kroenke CH, Chen WY, Rosner B, et al. Weight, weight gain, and survival after breast cancer diagnosis. *J Clin Oncol* 2005;23(7):1370–1378.
31. Zhang S, Folsom AR, Sellers TA, et al. Better breast cancer survival for post-menopausal women who are less overweight and eat less fat. The Iowa Women's Health Study. *Cancer* 1995;76:275–283.
32. Holmes MD, Stampfer MJ, Colditz GA, et al. Dietary factors and the survival of women with breast carcinoma. *Cancer* 1999;86:826–835.
33. Dujuric Z, Dilaura NM, Jenkins I, et al. Combining weight-loss counseling with the Weight Watchers plan for obese breast cancer survivors. *Obes Res* 2002;10:657–665.
34. Abrahamson PE, Gammon MD, Lund MJ, et al. Recreational physical activity and survival among young women with breast cancer. *Cancer* 2006;107(8): 1777–1785.
35. Courneya KS, Segal RJ, Mackey JR, et al. Effects of aerobic and resistance exercise in breast cancer patients receiving adjuvant chemotherapy: a multicenter randomized controlled trial. *J Clin Oncol* 2007;28:4396–4404.
36. Irwin ML, McTiernan A, Bernstein L, et al. Physical activity levels among breast cancer survivors. *Med Sci Sports Exerc* 2004;36(9):1484–1491.
37. Vallance JKH, Courneya KS, Plotnikoff RC, et al. Randomized controlled trial of the effects of print materials and step pedometers on physical activity and quality of life in breast cancer survivors. *J Clin Oncol* 2007;25(17):2352–2359.
38. Courneya K, Mackey J, Bell G, et al. Randomized controlled trial of exercise training in postmenopausal breast cancer survivors. Cardiopulmonary and quality of life outcomes. *J Clin Oncol* 2003;21:1660–1668.
39. Knols R, Aaronson NK, Uebelhart D, et al. Physical exercise in cancer patients during and after medical treatment: a systemic review of randomized and controlled clinical trials. *J Clin Oncol* 2005;23:3830–3842.
40. McNeely ML, Campbell KL, Rowe BH, et al. A meta-analysis of exercise interventions in breast cancer patients and survivors. *CMAJ* 2006;175:34–41.
41. Campbell KL, Westerland KC, Harber VJ, et al. Effects of aerobic exercise training on estrogen metabolism in premenopausal women: a randomized controlled trial. *Cancer Epidemiol Prev* 2007;16(4):731–739.
42. Ligibel JA, Campbell N, Partridge A, et al. Impact of a mixed strength and endurance exercise intervention on insulin levels in breast cancer survivors. *J Clin Oncol* 2008;26(6):907–912.
43. Mock V, Frangakis C, Davidson NE, et al. Exercise manages fatigue during breast cancer treatment: a randomized controlled trial. *Psychooncology* 2005;14(6):464–477.
44. Segal R, Evans W, Johnson D, et al. Structured exercise improves physical functioning in women with stages I and II breast cancer: results of a randomized controlled trial. *J Clin Oncol* 2001;19(3):657–665.
45. Freedman LS, Potischman N, Kipnis V, et al. A comparison of two dietary instruments for evaluating the fat breast cancer relationship. *Int J Epidemiol* 2006;35: 1101–1121.
46. Rock C, Demark-Wahnerfried W. Nutrition and survival after the diagnosis of breast cancer: a review of the evidence. *J Clin Oncol* 2002;20:3302–3316.
47. Goodwin PJ. Insulin in the adjuvant breast cancer setting: a novel therapeutic target for lifestyle and pharmacologic interventions? *J Clin Oncol* 2008;26(6): 833–834.
48. Goodwin PJ, Ennis M, Pritchard KI, et al. Fasting insulin and outcome in early-stage breast cancer: results of a prospective cohort study. *J Clin Oncol* 2002;20: 42–51.
49. Pasanisi P, Berrino F, De Petris M, et al. Metabolic syndrome as a prognostic factor for breast cancer recurrences. *Int J Cancer* 2006;119:236–238.
50. Pollak MN, Chapman JW, Shepherd L, et al. Insulin resistance, estimated by serum C-peptide level, is associated with reduced event-free survival for postmenopausal women in NCIC CTG MA.14 adjuvant breast cancer trial. *Proceedings of the American Society of Clinical Oncology* 2006;24:524.
51. Chlebowski RT, Pettinger M, Stefanick M, et al. Insulin levels, physical activity and energy intake in postmenopausal women: Implications for breast cancer. *J Clin Oncol* 2004;22(22):4518–4521.
52. Chlebowski RT, Blackburn GL, Buzzard IM, et al. Adherence to a dietary fat intake reduction program in postmenopausal women receiving therapy for early breast cancer. *J Clin Oncol* 1993;11:2072–2080.
53. Chlebowski RT, Blackburn GL, Elashoff RM, et al. Mature analysis from the women's intervention nutrition study (WINS) evaluating dietary fat reduction and breast cancer outcome [Abstract 32]. San Antonio Breast Cancer Symposium (SABCS) 2006.
54. Prentice RL, Cann B, Chlebowski RT, et al. Women's Health Initiative trial of a low-fat dietary pattern and breast cancer. *JAMA* 2006;295:629–642.
55. Pierce JP, Newman VA, Flatt SW, et al. Telephone counseling intervention increases intakes of micronutrient and phytochemical-rich vegetable, fruit and fiber in breast cancer survivors. *J Nutr* 2004;134(2):452–458.
56. Chlebowski RT, Blackburn G. Response: Re: Dietary fat reduction and breast cancer outcome. Interim efficacy results from the women's intervention nutrition study. *J Natl Cancer Inst* 2007;99(11):900–901.

Chapter 54
Management of Menopausal Symptoms in Breast Cancer Survivors

Dawn Hershman and Charles L. Loprinzi

In the United States today, more than 2 million women live as breast cancer survivors (1). Because the number of women diagnosed with invasive and noninvasive breast cancer is increasing (in large part because of screening programs), and the number of women who die from breast cancer has decreased (2), the number of breast cancer survivors is likely to continue increasing (2). This is particularly true for women diagnosed with early-stage breast cancer, who have a life expectancy similar to age-matched controls (2). The issues facing cancer survivors are unique. As the number of cancer survivors grows, the long-term side effects of cancer treatment and of aging play an increasingly prominent role in the routine care of these patients. Of special concern are the short- and long-term effects of sex hormone deprivation; currently, several trials are investigating ways to counteract these effects.

The average age of onset of natural menopause is 51 years. However, breast cancer therapy often leads to both an earlier onset of menopause and the exacerbation of existing menopausal symptoms. In premenopausal women with breast cancer, adjuvant chemotherapy is frequently associated with temporary or permanent amenorrhea, owing to chemotherapy-induced toxicity to the ovary (3). The incidence of chemotherapy-induced ovarian failure depends on the regimen used, the cumulative drug doses, and the age of the patient. Chemotherapy-induced ovarian failure causes symptoms similar to natural menopause and is associated with decreased circulating levels of estrogen and progesterone and increased levels of follicle-stimulating hormone and luteinizing hormone. The rapid changes in hormone concentrations associated with chemotherapy can lead to more severe symptoms than those associated with the more gradual decline in estrogen concentrations during normal aging (4,5). Women who are closer to the age of natural menopause often experience more severe symptoms when treated for breast cancer, suggesting that the natural, age-related symptoms are exacerbated by adjuvant therapy or tamoxifen, a commonly prescribed hormonal medication for breast cancer.

Estrogen (alone or combined with a progestational agent) therapy is frequently used to treat these problems in the general population, but concerns about the potential of this approach to increase the risk of breast cancer in high-risk women, or to increase the risk of recurrence in breast cancer survivors, have forced physicians to utilize alternative treatments. Although long-term hormone replacement therapy has beneficial effects on women's bones, this is more than offset by an increased risk of venous thromboembolic disease, breast cancer, stroke, cognitive decline, and coronary artery disease. In addition, the routine use of hormone replacement therapy in women does not appear to increase quality of life (6,7). These results support that long-term combination therapy with estrogen and progesterone cannot be recommended to most women at this time (8).

This chapter reviews current issues surrounding the acute and late effects associated with hormone deprivation in breast cancer survivors, and summarizes the scientific and therapeutic discoveries to date to identify optimal nonestrogenic treatments for individual patients.

 ## VASOMOTOR INSTABILITY

Vasomotor instability usually begins 1 to 2 years before menopause and often persists for 6 months to 5 years after menopause. It is characterized by the sudden onset of a sensation of intense warmth that typically begins in the chest and progresses to the neck and face. It is often accompanied by anxiety, palpitations, profuse sweating, and red blotching of the skin. Hot flash symptoms can affect a woman's ability to work, her social life, her sleep pattern, and her general perception of health (9–13). When it occurs in breast cancer patients, these symptoms can also affect their quality of life, as well as compliance with therapy and satisfaction with treatment decisions. The cause of vasomotor symptoms in breast cancer patients can be the result of abrupt estrogen loss owing to surgery, chemotherapy, hormonal therapy, discontinuation of hormone replacement therapy, or from natural menopause. Hot flashes affect about three-fourths of all postmenopausal women and are the most commonly described health problem among this age group (14).

Changes in circulating estrogen levels can induce abnormalities of the central thermoregulatory centers, resulting in hot flashes (15). Perspiration and vasodilation, classic mechanisms of heat loss controlled by the hypothalamus, are activated during a hot flash (15). In normal homeostasis, these mechanisms are activated to maintain core body temperature in a regulated range termed, the *thermoregulatory zone*. Complex neuroendocrine pathways that involve norepinephrine, estrogen, testosterone, and endorphins appear to govern regulation in the thermoregulatory nucleus and are possible sites where dysfunction may occur (15–17). Recent studies show that, in up to 60% of hot flash episodes, small changes in core body temperatures occur before hot flashes. These studies suggest that subtle increases in temperature before a hot flash, coupled with a narrow homeostatic temperature zone, may trigger the heat loss mechanisms that lead to hot flash symptoms.

Hot flashes are the most common reason women seek estrogen replacement therapy and, although estrogen effectively relieves symptoms for 80% to 90% of women who initiate treatment (18–20), women with a history of breast, ovarian, or uterine cancer, venous thromboembolism, or a family history of breast cancer comprise large populations for whom estrogen therapy may be contraindicated (21–33). Increasing evidence also suggests that women with a recent myocardial infarction or established coronary artery disease may be poor candidates for estrogen therapy (34–38). In addition, results from the Women's Health Initiative (WHI), in combination with other reports, suggest that long-term combined estrogen and progesterone therapy may not be as beneficial for women as was once believed (7,30–32,39,40). Similarly, a WHI trial investigating estrogen alone compared with a placebo, was also closed early because interim results indicated no reasonable chance existed for it to demonstrate long-term benefit (41). For these reasons, many women assume that hot flashes are an inevitable symptom of being a breast cancer survivor.

Tamoxifen, the most commonly prescribed pharmacologic treatment for breast cancer over the past decade, is associated with hot flashes in more than 50% of users (42–45).

Tamoxifen-associated hot flashes increase over the first several months of treatment and then gradually resolve (42). Postmenopausal women with a history of hot flashes before tamoxifen use are likely to experience more severe hot flashes with tamoxifen therapy (46).

Investigators have identified predictors of subsequent hot flash problems. Hot flashes in women undergoing natural menopause are associated with a maternal history of hot flashes as well as with cigarette smoking (47), whereas prior history of moderate to severe hot flashes with menopause and a history of prior estrogen therapy use are predictive for subsequent hot flash problems in breast cancer survivors (42).

It is difficult to evaluate the efficacy of pharmacologic therapy for hot flashes with anecdotal reports alone because of placebo affects. Multiple placebo-controlled trials demonstrate a 20% to 35% reduction in hot flashes with 4 weeks of placebo treatment (48–53). These studies suggest that one in five women will have at least a 50% reduction in hot flashes with placebo alone, and one in ten women at least a 75% reduction.

A randomized, placebo-controlled, crossover trial in 120 women found that vitamin E therapy decreased the average hot flash frequency by one episode per day (50). The low cost and minimal side effects of vitamin E make a trial of this agent (800 IU every day) one approach for individuals with mild symptoms that do not interfere with sleep or daily function, although newer information that suggests that vitamin E can increase morbidity tempers previous enthusiasm regarding this (54).

Several clinical trials have investigated soy protein, a prominent source of phytoestrogen, for the treatment of hot flashes. The results are mixed, but suggest that soy protein (90–400 mg/day) and isolated isoflavones do not reduce hot flashes (51,55–60). Furthermore, the long-term safety of pharmacologic doses of soy in patients with a history of breast or uterine cancer is not established. To explore the systemic hormonal effects of soy, several trials evaluated endometrial thickness, vaginal cytology, and uterine artery pulsatile index (57,58,61). No differences between soy- and placebo-treated patients are reported. Although reassuring, these surrogate end points and the short follow-up period cannot establish the safety of soy use in women with a history of breast cancer.

Other nonhormonal treatments for hot flashes are available and under study, most notably the newer antidepressant agents. Venlafaxine is thought to inhibit serotonin reuptake at lower doses and to induce a more profound inhibition of norepinephrine reuptake at higher doses. A double-blind, placebo-controlled trial with 191 breast cancer survivors randomized subjects to placebo or to one of three venlafaxine doses (37.5, 75, or 150 mg daily) (53). After 4 weeks of treatment, the placebo groups had a 27% reduction in symptoms versus 40%, 61%, and 61% reductions in the three venlafaxine groups, respectively. The side effects observed with venlafaxine include dry mouth, decreased appetite, nausea, and constipation (the latter only at doses of 150 mg/day). If venlafaxine is used, it should be started at a low dose (i.e., 37.5 mg/day) and increased to 75 mg/day after 1 week in patients who do not get adequate benefit at lower doses. When the drug is to be stopped, it should be slowly weaned down.

Selective serotonin reuptake inhibitors (SSRI) are also effective for the treatment of hot flashes. A double-blind, randomized, placebo-controlled, cross-over clinical trial demonstrated that fluoxetine reduces the incidence of hot flashes, although the reduction does not appear to be as great as that observed with venlafaxine (52,53). No significant toxicity was observed. A pilot study of open-label paroxetine, another SSRI, suggested a similar degree of efficacy; however, 4 of 30 women in the paroxetine trial experienced somnolence necessitating dose reduction in 2 patients and discontinuation of treatment in the other 2 patients (62). Two subsequent placebo-controlled, double-

blinded, randomized trials confirmed that paroxetine decreased hot flashes significantly more than did a placebo (63–65). However, both paroxetine and fluoxetine inhibit P450 (CYP) 2D6, an enzyme that is important for the metabolism of tamoxifen (66). Concerns have been raised about the coadministration of these drugs with tamoxifen, because they may lower the mean endoxifen level, the active metabolite of tamoxifen (67). Venlafaxine, however, does not appear to inhibit CYP 2D6 to any appreciable degree (67). Further information regarding tamoxifen metabolism can be found in Chapter 56. Along this line, it is of interest that information indicates that it is endoxifen, not the parent molecule, tamoxifen, that causes hot flashes. This is based on at least two pieces of information. First, patients with decreased CYP 2D6 activity are less likely to have prominent hot flashes after starting tamoxifen (68). Secondly, patients who take tamoxifen and do not suffer from hot flashes appear to have less efficacy from tamoxifen (69). This is hypothesized to be because such women are poor metabolizers of tamoxifen, which results in both decreased benefit and fewer complaints of hot flashes.

Three randomized, placebo-controlled trials have evaluated sertraline (50–100 mg/day) but the results with sertraline appear to be much less effective against hot flashes than are venlafaxine or paroxetine. There are two other reported randomized, placebo-controlled clinical trials of newer antidepressants (70,71) in the literature that have been interpreted to be negative studies (72). Nonetheless, neither of these trials had hot flash diary data from a baseline period before the initiation of the study agents, making it impossible to determine to what degree hot flash reduction occurred. An individual patient-pooled analysis of all the randomized trials looking at newer antidepressants that had baseline data available (73) demonstrates that they significantly decrease hot flashes ($p < .0001$).

In a small case series and in pilot trials, gabapentin, a γ-aminobutyric acid (GABA) analogue that has most commonly been used to treat a variety of neurologic disorders, appeared to be a promising new therapy for relief of hot flashes in patients unable to use hormone replacement therapy (74,75). Three placebo-controlled trials have confirmed the ability of gabapentin to decrease hot flashes (74,76,77). Side effects included lightheadedness and sleepiness early on, which generally resolve with continued treatment. Some women also developed a rash and edema, the latter of which appears to be related to decreased serum albumin concentrations (63).

Veralipride, a benzamide derivative with antidopaminergic effects, is also effective against menopausal symptoms, but this drug is not available in the United States and it can cause dystonic reactions (78–80). Clonidine decreases hot flashes to a moderate degree, but is associated with side effects that limit its utility (76,81). Methyldopa and belladonna alkaloids do not appear to be very useful for hot flashes because of modest efficacy and unpleasant side effects (48). Despite anecdotal reports, the benefits of herbal therapies in clinical trials have been disappointing to date. Herbal treatments, such as black cohosh (82,83) (*Cimicifuga racemosa*), and a standardized blend of 12 Chinese herbs (84) have been prospectively evaluated, with minimal activity observed. Acupuncture has also been evaluated for the treatment of hot flashes (85,86). Although uncontrolled studies suggest a benefit, when compared with sham acupuncture, there was not a significant reduction in symptoms (87,88).

For individuals with severe symptoms that are not responsive to nonhormonal drugs, progestational agents represent a reasonable alternative for the treatment of hot flash symptoms. A double-blind, placebo-controlled, crossover trial among breast and prostate cancer survivors found a 75% to 80% reduction in hot flashes with megestrol acetate compared with a 20% to 25% reduction in the placebo group (49). Lower doses (20 mg) are as effective as the 40-mg dose, with an improved side effect profile (89). Although minimal side effects are described during the treatment period, some women experienced withdrawal bleeding 1 to 4 weeks after discontinuation of treatment (48). A 3-year follow-up of the patients in the above study suggests that the benefits of megestrol acetate may be long-lasting (90). An alternative progestational agent approach is to use medroxyprogesterone acetate (91). In a randomized trial comparing a single intramuscular dose of medroxyprogesterone acetate with venlafaxine, medroxyprogesterone acetate was more effective and appeared to have fewer short-term toxicities (92). It should be noted, however, that no long-term prospective data have yet established the safety of progesterone analogs agents for women with hormone-sensitive breast cancer.

What about using estrogen therapy for treating hot flashes in breast cancer survivors? There have been pilot studies (93–97) where no increased breast cancer recurrence risk was observed in women who chose to take hormone therapy versus those who did not take hormone therapy. Also, two of the studies reported a lower risk of death when hormone therapy was used (96,97). Since the above studies were not prospective randomized, controlled trials, they are not very definitive.

There was a randomized clinical trial of hormone replacement in breast cancer survivors (98) that involved more than 400 patients, but it was stopped early for safety reasons, after a higher risk of breast cancer recurrences were seen in the treated arm (hazard ratio [HR] 3.5; 95% confidence interval [CI] 1.5–8.1). In another randomized clinical trial, where there was an attempt to limit the use of progesterone therapy, the risk of breast cancer recurrence was numerically decreased in the group that received hormone replacement therapy (HR 0.82; 95% CI, 0.35–1.9) (99). Nonetheless, given the current thoughts about hormone replacement therapy in healthy women, the enthusiasm about using it in breast cancer survivors is likely to continue to wane.

These data underscore the importance of identifying the cause of hot flashes as a step to developing effective nonestrogenic treatments for the treatment of this problem. Other comprehensive reviews of the pathogenesis and treatment of hot flashes in breast cancer survivors are available (100–102). Table 54.1 provides a summary of the most active available therapies for hot flashes.

OSTEOPOROSIS

Osteoporosis is a metabolic bone disease characterized by low bone mass and microarchitectural deterioration of bone tissue, leading to enhanced bone fragility and a consequent increase in fracture risk (103). Decreased bone mass is the most important known risk factor for fracture (104). A bone mineral

density (BMD) that is 2.5 standard deviations below the young adult female mean value is used to diagnose osteoporosis (105). Peak bone mass among women occurs at 20 to 30 years of age and begins to decline at about age 40 in women. During the 4- to 5-year period around menopause, declining serum estrogen levels are associated with an increase in osteoclast-mediated bone reabsorption and subsequent bone loss (106). Although osteoblast activity also increases, the amount of bone reabsorbed is greater than that formed at each remodeling site. At menopause, women enter a 10-year period of accelerated bone loss responsible for a 20% to 30% loss of cancellous bone and a 5% to 10% loss of cortical bone. This decade is followed by an indefinite period of slower bone loss. The rapid bone loss following menopause is thought to represent 50% of lifetime spinal bone loss in women (106). Estrogen and testosterone play important roles in the regulation of BMD and bone health. In postmenopausal women (107), the conversion of adrenal androgens to estrogen by the enzyme, aromatase, leads to continued low levels of circulating estrogen these may play an important role in calcium homeostasis through their effects on renal and gastrointestinal (GI) absorption of calcium (108). In addition to menopause, other risk factors associated with osteoporosis in the general population include older age, Northern European ethnicity, white race, low body weight, family history, dietary calcium deficiency, lack of weight-bearing physical activity, certain medications, cigarette smoking, heavy alcohol use, trauma, and some chronic diseases (103,109).

Women with premenopausal breast cancer have higher than average rates of bone loss and fracture, with nonmetastatic breast cancer patients having a risk of vertebral fractures nearly five times that of the general population (110,111). Bone loss is greatest in women who become amenorrheic as a result of chemotherapy, suggesting that estrogen deficiency is an important etiologic factor (110). Premature ovarian failure owing to chemotherapy, estrogen blocking therapies, aromatase inhibition, or ovarian ablation therapy, as well as direct effects of chemotherapy on bone, inactivity, use of corticosteroids, and inadequate intake of calcium and vitamin D can all contribute to the increased osteoporosis risk in breast cancer survivors (110,112–116).

The effects of adjuvant tamoxifen therapy, a selective estrogen receptor inhibitor with both agonist and antagonist activity (117), which reduces breast cancer recurrence in hormone receptor-positive women (118,119), on BMD differ depending on the menopausal status of the patient at the time of treatment (114,120–124). Tamoxifen preserves bone density in postmenopausal women; reabsorption of bone is lower in women treated with tamoxifen compared with those who receive placebo. However, in premenopausal women tamoxifen therapy is associated with varying levels of bone loss. Powles et al. (114) evaluated BMD in 179 pre- and postmenopausal women treated with either tamoxifen or placebo for chemoprevention of breast cancer. Premenopausal women treated with tamoxifen experienced a 1.4% decrease in BMD per year over the 3-year study compared with placebo-treated premenopausal women (114,125).

In contrast, postmenopausal women receiving tamoxifen experience an increase in BMD compared to postmenopausal women receiving placebo (114,123). Presumably, the partial agonist activity confers a net benefit in postmenopausal women with minimal circulating estrogen, whereas the partial agonist effect of tamoxifen is not as strong as natural estrogen and thus it blunts estrogenic activity on bone in premenopausal women with high circulating estrogen levels. Treatment with tamoxifen also reduces bone turnover marker levels in postmenopausal women (126).

Another selective estrogen receptor inhibitor, raloxifene, also reduces the risk of fractures from osteoporosis in postmenopausal

Table 54.1	HOT FLASH TREATMENT OPTIONS	
Treatment Option	Efficacy[a] (%)	Comment
Estrogen	85	Breast cancer concern
Progesterone[b]	85	Breast cancer concern
Antidepressants (e.g., venlafaxine and paroxetine)	50–60	Do not use paroxetine with tamoxifen
Gabapentin	50–60	

[a]Percent reduction from baseline after about 4 weeks, noting that a placebo decreases hot flashes about 20% to 30%
[b]Megestrol acetate (20–40 mg/day) orally or medroxyprogesterone acetate 400 mg intramuscularly once.

women (127). The effects of this agent in premenopausal women are currently unknown. It is not clear what effect raloxifen will have on breast cancer cells that have been exposed to 5 years of tomoxifen; therefore, raloxifene may not be an appropriate preventive agent for osteoporosis in women previously treated with tamoxifen (128–131).

Antiaromatase agents play a central role in the management of postmenopausal breast cancer (132,133). They almost completely eliminate endogenous estrogen production, affecting bone metabolism in breast cancer patients (134,135). This abrupt decline in serum estradiol and estrogen in both postmenopausal healthy women and postmenopausal patients with breast cancer may dramatically affect bone turnover and loss (136).

To evaluate this issue, BMD and bone turnover were measured in a subgroup of 308 postmenopausal women from an adjuvant study comparing tamoxifen and anastrozole (the Arimidex, Tamoxifen Alone or in Combination [ATAC] trial) and 46 control patients with breast cancer who did not receive hormone therapy. Bone resorption was measured with urinary *N*-telopeptide (NTX) and free deoxypyridinoline (DPD), and bone formation was measured by bone alkaline phosphatase. At 1 year, therapy with anastrozole was associated with bone loss at the spine and hip, most notably at the spine where the BMD was reduced from baseline by 2.6%, compared with a 0.4% reduction in healthy controls. Tamoxifen therapy, on the other hand, increased the BMD and decreased the markers of bone turnover. The ATAC researchers concluded that treatment with anastrozole increased bone remodeling, bone loss, and subsequent fracture risk (137). The other aromatase inhibitors (AI), letrozole and exemestane, have similar effects on bone density.

Estrogen administration reduces bone turnover and the rate of bone loss, and thereby increases BMD substantially in postmenopausal women (138,139). It is associated with a reduced risk of vertebral and possibly hip fractures (140). As soon as estrogen therapy is discontinued, however, BMD begins to decline at a rate similar to that observed before initiation of estrogen therapy (141). For women with a history of breast cancer, the use of estrogen to prevent bone loss has classically been considered contraindicated (142–144). Other pharmacologic agents used to prevent and treat bone loss include calcium, vitamin D supplements, bisphosphonates, and calcitonin. Increased intake of calcium with vitamin D is associated with a 20% to 25% reduction in the risk of fractures among elderly women (109). Calcium is also of critical importance as cotherapy in the prevention and treatment of established osteoporosis. Four bisphosphonates (alendronate, risedronate, ibandronate, and zoledronate) are approved for both the treatment and prevention of osteoporosis (145,146). Salmon calcitonin is approved for the treatment of osteoporosis, but is less efficacious than the bisphosphonates, with respect to improvement of BMD and the reduction of fracture rates (147).

Bisphosphonates are pyrophosphate analogues that are avidly adsorbed to bone surfaces (148,149). They reduce bone turnover by specifically inhibiting osteoclastic bone reabsorption and have demonstrated therapeutic efficacy in the treatment of hypercalcemia of malignancy, lytic bone disease associated with multiple myeloma, and mixed lytic and blastic bone metastases associated with breast cancer (150–153). The precise mechanism by which bisphosphonates inhibit osteoclast function is not fully understood, but may include a direct toxic effect on mature osteoclasts, an inhibition of osteoclast production from precursor cells, and an impairment of osteoclast chemotaxis to sites of active bone (154–158).

Alendronate and risedronate, the most extensively studied bisphosphonates, reduce vertebral and hip fractures by 50% in women with osteoporosis, and prevent bone loss in perimenopausal and postmenopausal women without osteoporosis at baseline (159–162). Clinical trials suggest that these drugs

prevent bone loss as effectively as the recommended dose of estrogen in standard hormone replacement therapy regimens (163). In addition, unlike estrogen, these drugs can be discontinued without causing rapidly accelerated bone loss (164). They, however, can trigger erosive esophagitis. Newer, more potent bisphosphonates include zoledronate and ibandronate. The preclinical safety (toxicology) profile of zoledronate is, in general, similar to that of other bisphosphonates, but this compound appears to produce fewer and less-severe adverse events at what are considered to be pharmacologically effective doses (165,166). In addition, the intravenous second- and third-generation bisphosphonates can be given every 6 to 12 months, to achieve appropriate effects on bone loss (167).

The ability of intravenous bisphosphonates to restore bone in patients with osteolytic lesions associated with breast cancer or multiple myeloma is established. An 11% increase in lumbar spine BMD was noted in patients receiving zoledronic acid at 2 mg or 4 mg; with the 4 mg/month dose being more effective (168).

Oral clodronate has been evaluated in two British studies of early-stage breast cancer (169,170). Among these patients, most of whom also received chemotherapy, hormonal therapy, or both, a randomized, placebo-controlled trial found that oral clodronate, taken for 2 years, was efficacious in preventing bone loss. By 1 year, BMD had fallen by 2.2% in the placebo group and had risen by 0.2% in the clodronate group (mean difference of 2.4%). In a second trial in premenopausal women receiving chemotherapy with cyclophosphamide, methotrexate and 5-fluorouracil (CMF), the clodronate and placebo groups differed in lumbar spine BMD by 3% at 1 year and by 3.7% at 2 years ($p < .01$). Among patients who developed ovarian failure, the lumbar spine bone loss in the clodronate group was 5.9%, versus 9.5% in the placebo group ($p < .001$). In both groups, the treatment was well tolerated, with no differences in adverse events (113).

Prevention is probably the most important strategy to combat osteoporosis. It can be argued that all women who experience ovarian failure as a result of chemotherapy should undergo BMD testing, and many experts advocate such testing for women who are postmenopausal at the time of diagnosis (171). The World Health Organization (WHO) criteria for the diagnosis of osteopenia by dual isotope x-ray absorption (DEXA) is a T-score 1 to 2.5 standard deviations below the mean for young adult women, whereas the criteria for osteoporosis is 2.5 or more standard deviations below the mean (105). Women with normal BMD or who meet the criteria for osteopenia on DEXA should receive prophylactic treatment to prevent osteoporosis. This includes calcium (total daily dose 1,000–1,500 mg, including dietary intake) and vitamin D ($\geq 1,000$ IU/day), which have been shown to reduce hip and vertebral fractures by 43% and 32%, respectively (172–175). Smoking cessation and weight-bearing physical activity should also be recommended to all women for osteoporosis prevention.

The use of bisphosphonates for primary prevention has recently undergone evaluation in premenopausal women without osteoporosis, as they initiate adjuvant systemic breast cancer treatment. Several studies have evaluated bisphosphonates for the prevention of bone loss during and following chemotherapy. Delmas et al. (176) evaluated an unconventional cyclic regimen of risedronate in women who had entered an early menopause secondary to chemotherapy and who had completed chemotherapy an average of 15 months before randomization. Greenspan et al. (177) evaluated weekly oral risedronate in patients who had completed chemotherapy an average of 3 years before randomization, and who were receiving other medications known to affect bone metabolism, such as tamoxifen and AI. In both studies, BMD remained stable or increased in the risedronate-treated groups.

In addition, premenopausal women were randomized before initiation of chemotherapy in several studies. Saarto et al. (113) randomized women to 1,600 mg of clodronate or placebo. At 1 year, the women in the placebo group sustained 4% bone loss at the lumbar spine, whereas BMD declined by only 1% in the clodronate-treated women. Clodronate, however, is not available in the United States and is associated with GI side effects. A second study randomized 40 premenopausal Lebanese women to pamidronate (60 mg every 3 months) or placebo before initiating chemotherapy (178). In the placebo arm, lumbar spine BMD declined by approximately 3.2% by 12 months, and by 4% in the group that became amenorrheic. This loss was prevented with pamidronate. Similar results have also been reported with the use of zoledronate (4 mg every 3 months) (179). However, initiating bisphosphonate therapy in young women who are at low risk of fractures with the goal of preventing short-term bone loss that may result in future fractures may not be necessary, beneficial or cost-effective, and from this perspective, it remains unclear when to intervene (180).

The timing of treatment initiation with bisphosphonates has been evaluated in postmenopausal women initiating AI therapy; less bone loss was observed at 12 months in patients treated with upfront zoledronate than in patients in whom zoledronate was initiated when the T-score declined to less than −2.0 (181). However, fracture rate did not differ between the groups. As a result, the optimal timing for the initiation of bisphosphonate therapy in postmenopausal women on AI therapy also remains unclear (180). Regular monitoring with BMD testing is recommended, with treatment initiation based on standard osteoporosis treatment guidelines (105). Table 54.2 reviews common therapeutic options for preventing and treating osteoporosis.

SEXUAL DYSFUNCTION

Sexual dysfunction occurs in up to 60% of breast cancer survivors, which may be owing to the effects of surgery, radiation therapy, or chemotherapy (182). Many women are hesitant to discuss sexual dysfunction with their health care providers (183); however, when questioned, 96% of women report at least one problem (182,184,185), including problems with desire (libido), lubrication, anorgasmy, dyspareunia, and satisfaction. In one study of breast cancer survivors, 64% of women reported decreased libido, 38% reported dyspareunia, 44% anorgasmy, and 42% lubrication problems (182). Sexual dysfunction tends to worsen over the first several years of treatment, but improve with longer follow-up (186,187).

Although breast-conserving surgical procedures have shown benefits over mastectomy with regard to body image (188,189), most studies find no difference between lumpectomy and mastectomy in regard to sexual functioning (185,190). A prospective evaluation of women during the first year after mastectomy or lumpectomy failed to show a difference in sexual function or quality of life between groups (189). Studies of survivors evaluated 4 to 8 years after treatment also found no differences in sexual function between patients treated with mastectomy or breast conservation surgery (191,192). The effect of mastectomy or breast conservation surgery on feelings of sexuality may depend on patient age; age may be a significant factor in a patient's self-image and thus lumpectomy may have a different effect on quality of life for younger women (189,192–194). In these studies, however, the relationship of self-image to sexual function is not entirely clear (192).

Sexual dysfunction is increased in women who have been treated with adjuvant chemotherapy (184,191,195,196). Such women are 5.7 times more likely to report vaginal dryness, 5.5 times more likely to report dyspareunia, 3 times more likely to report decreased libido, and 7.1 times more likely to report difficulty achieving orgasm (196). Younger women appear to be at increased risk of sexual dysfunction after receiving chemotherapy (184,197). The effect of chemotherapy on sexual dysfunction, nonetheless, appears to diminish over time. Cancer survivors more than 10 years out from treatment report similar levels of sexual functioning, regardless of whether they had received prior chemotherapy (187).

In contrast to chemotherapy, hormonal therapy with tamoxifen does not appear to cause sexual dysfunction (184,196, 198,199), despite tamoxifen being associated with symptoms such as vaginal discharge. Ganz et al. (199) surveyed 1,098 breast cancer survivors 1 to 5 years after primary breast cancer treatment. The women who had been treated with tamoxifen (n = 305) did not, after controlling for adjuvant chemotherapy, report more sexual function troubles. Comparing women on tamoxifen with a group of noncancer controls, Mortimer et al. (199) likewise found no differences in sexual desire, sexual arousal, or the ability to achieve orgasm (199). Treatment of breast cancer using the gonadotropin-releasing hormone (GnRH) agonist Zoladex in combination with tamoxifen was associated with increased sexual dysfunction, in comparison to patients treated with Zoladex alone; the reason for this is not clear. Interestingly, in this same study, tamoxifen as a single agent did not produce sexual dysfunction (200). Thus, these investigations suggest that chemotherapy is the therapy most strongly linked to sexual dysfunction after treatment, and that women treated with chemotherapy are at highest risk for dissatisfaction with their sex lives (184).

Treatment of sexual dysfunction requires comprehensive assessment and intervention. Ganz et al. (201) found a significant decrease in sexual dysfunction in women randomized to undergo a comprehensive assessment of menopausal symptoms by a nurse practitioner who screened for symptoms of vaginal dryness. If symptoms of sexual dysfunction were identified, recommendations for vaginal lubricants were provided along with individualized counseling and referral as indicated (201). Other data also suggest that vaginal dryness may play a significant, if not central, role in sexual dysfunction after chemotherapy (185,195,201–204). Vaginal lubricants (Astroglide) and vaginal moisturizers (KY Jelly, Replens) can be used to treat symptoms of dryness or for lubrication, and may indirectly improve other sexual problems as well (185,201,203,205). A prospective study in breast cancer survivors reported that women using Replens had decreased vaginal dryness equal to that of women using a water-soluble lubricating placebo (203); however, a decrease in dyspareunia was significantly better with Replens than with the placebo lubricant (203).

Topical estrogen preparations appear to alleviate vaginal dryness more effectively than do nonestrogenic vaginal preparations.

Table 54.2	MANAGEMENT OPTIONS FOR PREVENTION AND TREATMENT OF OSTEOPOROSIS
Lifestyle Recommendations	Weight-bearing exercise Maintenance of ideal body weight No smoking Moderation of alcohol use
Dietary Nutrients	Calcium (1,200–1,500 mg/day, including dietary intake) Vitamin D (800–1,000 IU/day)
Bisphosphonates	Such as zoledronate, alendronate, risedronate, or clodronate
Selective Estrogen Receptor Modifiers (SERM)	Raloxifene or tamoxifen
Thyroid-derived Hormone	Calcitonin

At least three formulations exist which are associated with decreased systemic absorption: Estring is an estrogen-impregnated ring that is inserted into the vagina, where it releases small amounts of estrogen over a 12-week period (206). Another is a vaginal estrogen tablet called Vagifem (207). This tablet is inserted into the vagina with an applicator (207). Lastly, a small dose of Premarin vaginal cream can be helpful. Nonetheless, there is evidence of some absorption of virtually all vaginal estrogen products and newer data, showing that decreasing postmenopausal estrogen levels lower by AI leads to improved breast cancer outcomes, makes clinicians concerned about the use of any vaginal estrogen products.

Testosterone improves sexual desire and the frequency of sexual activity in women after surgical menopause or with sexual arousal disorders (208). A phase III randomized, placebo-controlled, crossover clinical trial evaluated this issue further by studying postmenopausal women with a history of cancer, who had no current evidence of disease, had a reported a decrease in sexual desire, and had a sexual partner. Eligible women were randomly assigned to receive 2% testosterone in Vanicream, for a testosterone dose of 10 mg daily, or placebo Vanicream for 4 weeks and were then crossed over to the opposite treatment for an additional 4 weeks. The primary end point was sexual desire or libido. Women who were on active testosterone cream had higher serum levels of bioavailable testosterone than women on placebo. The mean intrapatient libido change from baseline to weeks 4 and 8 was, however, similar on both arms (209). The reason that the findings in this study were negative, whereas in other similar studies they were positive, may be because all of the other positive study findings involved women who were premenopausal or were receiving ongoing estrogen therapy, whereas the current study did not include women receiving concurrent estrogen therapy. Thus, it appears that testosterone, when used without concurrent estrogen, does not improve libido.

ARTHRALGIAS

Aromatase inhibitor therapy is the standard of care for postmenopausal women with both early and late stage hormone-sensitive breast tumors (210–212). In large adjuvant trials involving AI, the incidence of musculoskeletal disorders was 20% to 40%, and nearly 5% of patients discontinued therapy in the AI group because of toxic effects (210,212,213). The exact mechanism of AI-related arthralgia is unclear, but is thought to be related to estrogen deprivation. Osteoarthritis (OA) is a disease of joints, resulting in progressive and permanent articular cartilage degeneration (214). More than 80 years ago, Cecil and Archer (215) first described "arthritis of the menopause" as the rapid development of hand and knee osteoarthritis coinciding with cessation of menses. Furthermore, observational studies of the incidence and prevalence of osteoarthritis in postmenopausal women with and without hormone therapy has provided strong support for a protective effect of estrogens in osteoarthritis (216–218).

Recent studies have shown that AI arthralgias are more prevalent than originally reported from clinical trials. In a cross-sectional survey of 200 consecutive postmenopausal women receiving adjuvant AI therapy for early-stage, hormone-sensitive breast cancer, 94 (47%) reported having AI-related joint pain and 88 (44%) reported AI-related joint stiffness. In multiple logistic regression analysis, being overweight (body mass index [BMI] of 25–30 kg/m^2) and prior tamoxifen therapy were inversely associated with AI-related joint symptoms. Patients who received taxane chemotherapy were more than four times more likely than other patients to have AI-related joint pain and stiffness (219).

Prospective evaluations of interventions to treat and prevent AI-related joint symptoms are in progress. In a nonrandom-ized, pilot study, 21 patients with moderate to severe AI-related joint symptoms were treated with acupuncture. These women reported that acupuncture relieved their AI-related joint symptoms, reduced the severity of their symptoms, and improved their functional ability. In addition, no adverse outcomes were reported; many patients reported that acupuncture was effective and relaxing and that they would recommend it to others (220). Understanding the potential large placebo effect in such a pilot trial, ongoing randomized trials of acupuncture and vitamin D are in progress. Exercise has also been suggested as a remedy but needs to be tested.

WEIGHT GAIN

Weight gain is a common side effect for women who receive adjuvant chemotherapy. Gains in weight can be up to 50 pounds or more, and may be influenced by menopausal status; nodal status; and the type, duration, and intensity of treatment. Weight gain appears to be greater among premenopausal women; in those who are node-positive; those receiving higher dose, longer duration, multiagent regimens; and those who enter into menopause (221,222). Psychosocial research suggests that weight gain has a profoundly negative impact on the quality of life for patients with breast cancer (221,223). Although there is some variability in the literature, in one study, the mean change in weight of 100 women treated with chemotherapy was +3.68 kg ($p <$.001); 64% of patients gained more than 2 kg in weight, approximately one-third of patients gained more than 5 kg, and 6 patients gained more than 10 kg. Most of these patients (85%) received steroids as antiemetics, but no effect of steroid dose was seen on the level of weight change (224).

Limited research has been conducted to investigate the underlying mechanisms that contribute to weight gain in this population. Changes in rates of metabolism, physical activity, and dietary intake are all plausible mechanisms. Mean body weight increases significantly during chemotherapy, primarily because of an increase in mean total body and mean fat mass (225). Factors related to energy balance, including body composition, resting energy expenditure, dietary intake, percentage of body fat, fat mass, lean body mass, and leg lean mass have been reported. Chemotherapy-induced weight gain appears to be distinctive. The available data do not support overeating as a major cause of weight gain among breast cancer patients. Weight gain in the presence of lean tissue loss or the absence of lean tissue gain supports the need for interventions focused on exercise, especially resistance training in the lower body, to prevent undesirable weight gain (226).

Use of a dietitian to prevent weight gain was evaluated in a prospective randomized trial. Premenopausal women starting adjuvant chemotherapy for breast cancer were randomized to a control group, or to receive monthly counseling by a dietitian aimed at weight maintenance. The median weight changes at 6 months after the start of chemotherapy, were gains of 2.0 kg in the dietitian counseling group versus 3.5 kg in the control group (statistically insignificant differences). The median changes in average caloric consumption were reductions of 120 versus 46 cal/day on weekdays and 196 versus 20 cal/day on weekends for the counseling and control groups, respectively. Routine prospective dietitian counseling aimed at weight maintenance, thus appeared to produce small but statistically insignificant reductions in both caloric consumption and weight gain in this group of patients (227).

Other data also suggest that exercise may be an effective intervention to minimize weight gain in women with breast cancer receiving adjuvant chemotherapy. Seventy-eight women who had recently received a diagnosis of breast cancer and who were beginning adjuvant chemotherapy were enrolled in a home-based exercise study during the first four cycles of chemotherapy. Women who adhered to the exercise program maintained their body weight, whereas nonexercisers steadily gained weight ($p < .05$) (228). Additional exercise intervention studies are in progress.

CONCLUSION

As the population of breast cancer survivors grows, it has become increasingly important to develop strategies to prevent and treat both short-term, and long-term, complications from breast cancer treatment. Advances in this area may improve the quality of life of the more than 3 million breast cancer survivors in the United States alone.

MANAGEMENT SUMMARY

- Nonhormonal means of treating hot flashes are available, including the use of antidepressants (e.g., venlafaxine and paroxetine) and gabapentin.
- Paroxetine should not be used in patients taking tamoxifen.
- Osteoporosis is a common problem in women with a history of breast cancer, primarily related to estrogen deprivation.
- Standard measures for preventing and treating osteoporosis should include adequate calcium and vitamin D intake and weight-bearing exercise.
- Bisphosphonates should be used in patients with substantial osteopenia and osteoporosis.
- Although bisphosphonates can attenuate bone loss from chemotherapy-induced ovarian suppression or aromatase inhibitors, routine use of these in clinical practice is not yet recommended. Although some clinicians use bisphosphonates in selected patients, most would recommend routine surveillance with bone mineral density testing.
- Although sexual dysfunction is common in women with breast cancer, testosterone, in the absence of estrogen, does not alleviate this problem.
- Vaginal dryness can be treated with nonestrogenic vaginal lubricants or local estrogen therapy, although there are some safety concerns regarding the latter.
- Aromatase inhibitor induced arthralgias are common, but no good established therapy for this problem exists.
- Weight gain is common after a diagnosis of breast cancer treatment. Therapy to prevent this primarily resolves around decreasing caloric intake and increasing caloric output (i.e., exercise).

References

1. Hewitt M, Breen N, Devesa S. Cancer prevalence and survivorship issues: analyses of the 1992 National Health Interview Survey. *J Natl Cancer Inst* 1999; 91(17)1480–1486.
2. Wingo PA, et al. Long-term cancer patient survival in the United States. *Cancer Epidemiol Biomarkers Prev* 1998;7(4):271–282.
3. Bines J, Oleske DM, Cobleigh MA. Ovarian function in premenopausal women treated with adjuvant chemotherapy for breast cancer. *J Clin Oncol* 1996;14(5): 1718–1729.
4. Berg G, et al. Climacteric symptoms among women aged 60–62 in Linkoping, Sweden, in 1986. *Maturitas* 1988;10(3):193–199.
5. Carpenter JS, et al. Hot flashes in postmenopausal women treated for breast carcinoma: prevalence, severity, correlates, management, and relation to quality of life. *Cancer* 1998;82(9):1682–1691.
6. Rossouw JE. Effect of postmenopausal hormone therapy on cardiovascular risk. *J Hypertens* 2002;20 Suppl 2:S62–S65.
7. Rossouw JE, et al. Risks and benefits of estrogen plus progestin in healthy postmenopausal women: principal results From the Women's Health Initiative randomized controlled trial. *JAMA* 2002;288(3):321–333.
8. Stephenson J. FDA orders estrogen safety warnings: agency offers guidance for HRT use. *JAMA* 2003;289(5):537–538.
9. Stein KD, et al. Impact of hot flashes on quality of life among postmenopausal women being treated for breast cancer. *J Pain Symptom Manage* 2000;19(6): 436–445.
10. Finck G, et al. Definitions of hot flashes in breast cancer survivors. *J Pain Symptom Manage* 1998;16(5):327–333.
11. Roberts J, et al. Psychosocial adjustment in post-menopausal women. *Can J Nurs Res* 1992;24(4):29–46.
12. Daly E, et al. Measuring the impact of menopausal symptoms on quality of life. *BMJ* 1993;307(6908):836–840.
13. Greendale GA, Lee NP, Arriola ER. The menopause. *Lancet* 1999;353(9152): 571–580.
14. McKinlay SM, Jefferys M. The menopausal syndrome. *Br J Prev Soc Med* 1974; 28(2):108–115.
15. Casper RF, Yen SS. Neuroendocrinology of menopausal flushes: an hypothesis of flush mechanism. *Clin Endocrinol (Oxf)* 1985;22(3):293–312.
16. Rodenberg H, et al. Left upper-extremity weakness in an 18-year-old man. *Ann Emerg Med* 1991;20(6):672–679.
17. Kronenberg F, Downey JA. Thermoregulatory physiology of menopausal hot flashes: a review. *Can J Physiol Pharmacol* 1987;65(6):1312–1324.
18. Rabin DS, et al. Why menopausal women do not want to take hormone replacement therapy. *Menopause* 1999;6(1):61–67.
19. Notelovitz M, et al. Initial 17beta-estradiol dose for treating vasomotor symptoms. *Obstet Gynecol* 2000;95(5):726–731.
20. Lobo RA, et al. Depo-medroxyprogesterone acetate compared with conjugated estrogens for the treatment of postmenopausal women. *Obstet Gynecol* 1984; 63(1):1–5.
21. Garg PP, et al. Hormone replacement therapy and the risk of epithelial ovarian carcinoma: a meta-analysis. *Obstet Gynecol* 1998;92(3):472–479.
22. Coughlin SS, et al. A meta-analysis of estrogen replacement therapy and risk of epithelial ovarian cancer. *J Clin Epidemiol* 2000;53(4):367–375.
23. Riman T, et al. Hormone replacement therapy and the risk of invasive epithelial ovarian cancer in Swedish women. *J Natl Cancer Inst* 2002;94(7):497–504.
24. Smith DC, et al. Association of exogenous estrogen and endometrial carcinoma. *N Engl J Med* 1975;293(23):1164–1167.
25. McDonald TW, Malkasian GD, Gaffey TA. Endometrial cancer associated with feminizing ovarian tumor and polycystic ovarian disease. *Obstet Gynecol* 1977; 49(6):654–658.
26. Hoibraaten E, et al. Increased risk of recurrent venous thromboembolism during hormone replacement therapy—results of the randomized, double-blind, placebo-controlled estrogen in venous thromboembolism trial (EVTET). *Thromb Haemost* 2000;84(6):961–967.
27. Grady D, et al. Postmenopausal hormone therapy increases risk for venous thromboembolic disease. The Heart and Estrogen/progestin Replacement Study. *Ann Intern Med* 2000;132(9):689–696.
28. Barrett-Connor E, Grady D. Hormone replacement therapy, heart disease, and other considerations. *Annu Rev Public Health* 1998;19:55–72.
29. Hulley S, et al. Noncardiovascular disease outcomes during 6.8 years of hormone therapy: Heart and Estrogen/progestin Replacement Study follow-up (HERS II). *JAMA* 2002;288(1):58–66.
30. Chen CL, et al. Hormone replacement therapy in relation to breast cancer. *JAMA* 2002;287(6):734–741.
31. Lacey JV, Jr, et al. Menopausal hormone replacement therapy and risk of ovarian cancer. *JAMA* 2002;288(3):334–341.
32. Vastag B. Hormone replacement therapy falls out of favor with expert committee. *JAMA* 2002;287(15):1923–1924.
33. Creasman WT. Estrogen and cancer. *Gynecol Oncol* 2002;86(1):1–9.
34. Tanis BC, et al. Oral contraceptives and the risk of myocardial infarction. *N Engl J Med* 2001;345(25):1787–1793.
35. Heckbert SR, et al. Risk of recurrent coronary events in relation to use and recent initiation of postmenopausal hormone therapy. *Arch Intern Med* 2001;161(14): 1709–1713.
36. Alexander KP, et al. Initiation of hormone replacement therapy after acute myocardial infarction is associated with more cardiac events during follow-up. *J Am Coll Cardiol* 2001;38(1):1–7.
37. Hulley S, et al. Randomized trial of estrogen plus progestin for secondary prevention of coronary heart disease in postmenopausal women. Heart and Estrogen/progestin Replacement Study (HERS) Research Group. *JAMA* 1998;280(7):605–613.
38. Grady D, et al. Cardiovascular disease outcomes during 6.8 years of hormone therapy: Heart and Estrogen/progestin Replacement Study follow-up (HERS II). *JAMA* 2002;288(1):49–57.
39. Weiss LK, et al. Hormone replacement therapy regimens and breast cancer risk(1). *Obstet Gynecol* 2002;100(6):1148–1158.
40. Hlatky MA, et al. Quality-of-life and depressive symptoms in postmenopausal women after receiving hormone therapy: results from the Heart and Estrogen/Progestin Replacement Study (HERS) trial. *JAMA* 2002;287(5): 591–597.
41. Anderson GL, et al. Effects of conjugated equine estrogen in postmenopausal women with hysterectomy: the Women's Health Initiative randomized controlled trial. *JAMA* 2004;291(14):1701–1712.
42. Loprinzi CL, et al. Tamoxifen-induced hot flashes. *Clin Breast Cancer* 2000;1(1): 52–56.
43. Ganz PA. Impact of tamoxifen adjuvant therapy on symptoms, functioning, and quality of life. *J Natl Cancer Inst Monogr* 2001;(30):130–134.
44. Ganz PA, et al. Quality of life in long-term, disease-free survivors of breast cancer: a follow-up study. *J Natl Cancer Inst* 2002;94(1):39–49.
45. Mourits MJ, et al. Tamoxifen treatment and gynecologic side effects: a review. *Obstet Gynecol* 2001;97(5 Pt 2):855–866.
46. Love RR, et al. Symptoms associated with tamoxifen treatment in postmenopausal women. *Arch Intern Med* 1991;151(9):1842–1847.
47. Staropoli CA, et al. Predictors of menopausal hot flashes. *J Womens Health* 1998;7(9):1149–1155.
48. Loprinzi CL, et al. Transdermal clonidine for ameliorating post-orchiectomy hot flashes. *J Urol* 1994;151(3):634–636.
49. Loprinzi CL, et al. Megestrol acetate for the prevention of hot flashes. *N Engl J Med* 1994;331(6):347–352.
50. Barton DL, et al. Prospective evaluation of vitamin E for hot flashes in breast cancer survivors. *J Clin Oncol* 1998;16(2):495–500.
51. Quella SK, et al. Evaluation of soy phytoestrogens for the treatment of hot flashes in breast cancer survivors: a North Central Cancer Treatment Group Trial. *J Clin Oncol* 2000;18(5):1068–1074.

52. Loprinzi CL, et al. Phase III evaluation of fluoxetine for treatment of hot flashes. *J Clin Oncol* 2002;20(6):1578–1583.
53. Loprinzi CL, et al. Venlafaxine in management of hot flashes in survivors of breast cancer: a randomised controlled trial. *Lancet* 2000;356(9247):2059–2063.
54. Lonn E, et al. Effects of long-term vitamin E supplementation on cardiovascular events and cancer: a randomized controlled trial. *JAMA* 2005;293(11):1338–1347.
55. Van Patten CL, et al. Effect of soy phytoestrogens on hot flashes in postmenopausal women with breast cancer: a randomized, controlled clinical trial. *J Clin Oncol* 2002;20(6):1449–1455.
56. Vincent A, Fitzpatrick LA. Soy isoflavones: are they useful in menopause? *Mayo Clin Proc* 2000;75(11):1174–1184.
57. Upmalis DH, et al. Vasomotor symptom relief by soy isoflavone extract tablets in postmenopausal women: a multicenter, double-blind, randomized, placebo-controlled study. *Menopause* 2000;7(4):236–242.
58. Scambia G, et al. Clinical effects of a standardized soy extract in postmenopausal women: a pilot study. *Menopause* 2000;7(2):105–111.
59. Albertazzi P, et al. Dietary soy supplementation and phytoestrogen levels. *Obstet Gynecol* 1999;94(2):229–231.
60. Albertazzi P, et al. The effect of dietary soy supplementation on hot flushes. *Obstet Gynecol* 1998;91(1):6–11.
61. Han KK, et al. Benefits of soy isoflavone therapeutic regimen on menopausal symptoms. *Obstet Gynecol* 2002;99(3):389–394.
62. Stearns V, et al. A pilot trial assessing the efficacy of paroxetine hydrochloride (Paxil) in controlling hot flashes in breast cancer survivors. *Ann Oncol* 2000;11(1):17–22.
63. Stearns V, et al. Paroxetine is an effective therapy for hot flashes: results from a prospective randomized clinical trial. *J Clin Oncol* 2005;23:6919–6930.
64. Beebe K, Stearns V, Iyengar M. A randomized, double-blind study assessing controlled-release paroxetine (Paroxetine CR, Paxil) in the treatment of hot flashes associated with menopause. in The U.S. Psychiatric & Mental Health Congress. 2002. Las Vegas, Nevada.
65. Stearns V, et al. Paroxetine is an effective treatment for hot flashes: results from a prospective randomized clinical trial. *J Clin Oncol* 2005;23(28):6919–6930.
66. Otton SV, et al. Venlafaxine oxidation *in vitro* is catalysed by CYP2D6. *Br J Clin Pharmacol* 1996;41(2):149–156.
67. Jin Y, et al. CYP2D6 genotype, antidepressant use, and tamoxifen metabolism during adjuvant breast cancer treatment. *J Natl Cancer Inst* 2005;97(1):30–39.
68. Goetz MP, et al. Pharmacogenetics of tamoxifen biotransformation is associated with clinical outcomes of efficacy and hot flashes. *J Clin Oncol* 2005;23(36):9312–9318.
69. Mortimer JE, et al. Tamoxifen, hot flashes and recurrence in breast cancer. *Breast Cancer Res Treat* 2008;108(3):421–426.
70. Evans ML, et al. Management of postmenopausal hot flushes with venlafaxine hydrochloride: a randomized, controlled trial. *Obstet Gynecol* 2005;105(1):161–166.
71. Suvanto-Luukkonen E, et al. Citalopram and fluoxetine in the treatment of postmenopausal symptoms: a prospective, randomized, 9-month, placebo-controlled, double-blind study. *Menopause* 2005;12(1):18–26.
72. Nelson HD, et al. Nonhormonal therapies for menopausal hot flashes: systematic review and meta-analysis. *JAMA* 2006;295(17):2057–2071.
73. Loprinzi C, et al. Newer antidepressants and gabapentin for hot flashes: an individual subject pooled analysis. *J Clin Oncol* 2009, in press.
74. Guttuso T, et al. Gabapentin's effects on hot flashes in postmenopausal women: a randomized controlled trial. *Obstet Gynecol* 2003;101(2):337–345.
75. Loprinzi L, et al. Pilot evaluation of gabapentin for treating hot flashes. *Mayo Clin Proc* 2002;77:1159–1163.
76. Pandya KJ, et al. Gabapentin for hot flashes in 420 women with breast cancer: a randomised double-blind placebo-controlled trial. *Lancet* 2005;366(9488):818–824.
77. Reddy SY, et al. Gabapentin, estrogen, and placebo for treating hot flushes: a randomized controlled trial. *Obstet Gynecol* 2006;108(1):41–48.
78. David A, et al. Veralipride: alternative antidopaminergic treatment for menopausal symptoms. *Am J Obstet Gynecol* 1988;158(5):1107–1115.
79. Vercellini P, et al. Veralipride for hot flushes during gonadotropin-releasing hormone agonist treatment. *Gynecol Obstet Invest* 1992;34(2):102–104.
80. Wesel S, Bourguignon RP, Bosuma WB. Veralipride versus conjugated oestrogens: a double-blind study in the management of menopausal hot flushes. *Curr Med Res Opin* 1984;8(10):696–700.
81. Goldberg RM, et al. Transdermal clonidine for ameliorating tamoxifen-induced hot flashes. *J Clin Oncol* 1994;12(1):155–158.
82. Jacobson JS, et al. Randomized trial of black cohosh for the treatment of hot flashes among women with a history of breast cancer. *J Clin Oncol* 2001;19(10):2739–2745.
83. Pockaj BA, et al. Phase III double-blind, randomized, placebo-controlled crossover trial of black cohosh in the management of hot flashes: NCCTG Trial N01CC1. *J Clin Oncol* 2006;24(18):2836–2841.
84. Davis SR, et al. The effects of Chinese medicinal herbs on postmenopausal vasomotor symptoms of Australian women. A randomised controlled trial. *Med J Aust* 2001;174(2):68–71.
85. Porzio G, et al. Acupuncture in the treatment of menopause-related symptoms in women taking tamoxifen. *Tumori* 2002;88(2):128–130.
86. Dong H, et al. An exploratory pilot study of acupuncture on the quality of life and reproductive hormone secretion in menopausal women. *J Altern Complement Med* 2001;7(6):651–658.
87. Deng G, et al. Randomized, controlled trial of acupuncture for the treatment of hot flashes in breast cancer patients. *J Clin Oncol* 2007;25(35):5584–5590.
88. Vincent A, et al. Acupuncture for hot flashes: a randomized, sham-controlled clinical study. *Menopause* 2007;14(1):45–52.
89. Goodwin J, et al. Double blind phase III trial of placebo (P) vs. megestrol acetate (MA) 20 mg vs. MA 40 mg as treatment for symptoms of ovarian failure in breast cancer survivors: initial results of Southwest Oncology Group S9626. in *San Antonio Breast Cancer Symposium*. 2001.
90. Quella SK, et al. Long term use of megestrol acetate by cancer survivors for the treatment of hot flashes. *Cancer* 1998;82(9):1784–1788.
91. Barton D, et al. Depomedroxyprogesterone acetate for hot flashes. *J Pain Symptom Manage* 2002;24(6):603–607.
92. Loprinzi CL, et al. Phase III comparison of depomedroxyprogesterone acetate to venlafaxine for managing hot flashes: North Central Cancer Treatment Group Trial N99C7. *J Clin Oncol* 2006;24(9):1409–1414.
93. DiSaia PJ, et al. Hormone replacement therapy in breast cancer survivors: a cohort study. *Am J Obstet Gynecol* 1996;174(5):1494–1498.
94. Powles TJ, et al. Hormone replacement after breast cancer. *Lancet* 1993;342(8862):60–61.
95. Wile AG, Opfell RW, Margileth DA. Hormone replacement therapy in previously treated breast cancer patients. *Am J Surg* 1993;165(3):372–375.
96. Eden JA, Wren BG. Hormone replacement therapy after breast cancer: a review. *Cancer Treat Rev* 1996;22(5):335–343.
97. O'Meara ES, et al. Hormone replacement therapy after a diagnosis of breast cancer in relation to recurrence and mortality. *J Natl Cancer Inst* 2001;93(10):754–762.
98. Holmberg L, Anderson H. HABITS (hormonal replacement therapy after breast cancer—is it safe?), a randomised comparison: trial stopped. *Lancet* 2004;363(9407):453–455.
99. von Schoultz E, Rutqvist LE. Menopausal hormone therapy after breast cancer: the Stockholm randomized trial. *J Natl Cancer Inst* 2005;97(7):533–535.
100. Shanafelt TD, et al. Pathophysiology and treatment of hot flashes. *Mayo Clin Proc* 2002;77(11):1207–1218.
101. Stearns V, Hayes DF. Approach to menopausal symptoms in women with breast cancer. *Curr Treat Options Oncol* 2002;3(2):179–190.
102. Berendsen HH. The role of serotonin in hot flushes. *Maturitas* 2000;36(3):155–164.
103. Consensus development conference: prophylaxis and treatment of osteoporosis. *Osteoporos Int* 1991;1(2):114–117.
104. van der Voort DJ, Geusens PP, Dinant GJ. Risk factors for osteoporosis related to their outcome: fractures. *Osteoporos Int* 2001;12(8):630–638.
105. Kanis JA. Assessment of fracture risk and its application to screening for postmenopausal osteoporosis: synopsis of a WHO report. WHO Study Group. *Osteoporos Int* 1994;4(6):368–381.
106. *Primer on Metebolic Bone Diseases and Disorders of Mineral Metabolism*. 4th ed, ed. M.J. Favus. 1999, Philadelphia: Lippincott. 502.
107. The Writing Group for the PEPI. Effects of hormone therapy on bone mineral density: results from the postmenopausal estrogen/progestin interventions (PEPI) trial. *JAMA* 1996;276(17):1389–1396.
108. Prince RL. Counterpoint: estrogen effects on calcitropic hormones and calcium homeostasis. *Endocr Rev* 1994;15(3):301–309.
109. NIH Consensus, Development Panel on Osteoporosis Prevention, Diagnosis, and Therapy. *JAMA* 2001;285(6):785–795.
110. Bruning PF, et al. Bone mineral density after adjuvant chemotherapy for premenopausal breast cancer. *Br J Cancer* 1990;61(2):308–310.
111. Kanis JA, et al. A high incidence of vertebral fracture in women with breast cancer. *Br J Cancer* 1999;79(7–8):1179–1181.
112. Delmas PD, Fontana A. Bone loss induced by cancer treatment and its management. *Eur J Cancer* 1998;34(2):260–262.
113. Saarto T, et al. Clodronate improves bone mineral density in post-menopausal breast cancer patients treated with adjuvant antioestrogens. *Br J Cancer* 1997;75(4):602–605.
114. Powles TJ, et al. Effect of tamoxifen on bone mineral density measured by dual-energy x-ray absorptiometry in healthy premenopausal and postmenopausal women. *J Clin Oncol* 1996;14(1):78–84.
115. Friedlaender GE, et al. Effects of chemotherapeutic agents on bone. I. Short-term methotrexate and doxorubicin (adriamycin) treatment in a rat model. *J Bone Joint Surg Am* 1984;66(4):602–607.
116. Wang TM, Shih C. Study of histomorphometric changes of the mandibular condyles in neonatal and juvenile rats after administration of cyclophosphamide. *Acta Anat (Basel)* 1986;127(2):93–99.
117. Riggs BL, Hartmann LC. Selective estrogen-receptor modulators—mechanisms of action and application to clinical practice. *N Engl J Med* 2003;348(7):618–629.
118. Benson JR, Pitsinis V. Update on clinical role of tamoxifen. *Curr Opin Obstet Gynecol* 2003;15(1):13–23.
119. Tamoxifen for early breast cancer: an overview of the randomised trials. Early Breast Cancer Trialists' Collaborative Group. *Lancet* 1998;351(9114): 1451–1467.
120. Grey AB, et al. The effect of the antiestrogen tamoxifen on bone mineral density in normal late postmenopausal women. *Am J Med* 1995;99(6):636–641.
121. Love RR, et al. Effects of tamoxifen on bone mineral density in postmenopausal women with breast cancer. *N Engl J Med* 1992;326(13):852–856.
122. Resch A, et al. Evidence that tamoxifen preserves bone density in late postmenopausal women with breast cancer. *Acta Oncol* 1998;37(7–8):661–664.
123. Fisher B, et al. Tamoxifen for prevention of breast cancer: report of the National Surgical Adjuvant Breast and Bowel Project P-1 Study. *J Natl Cancer Inst* 1998;90(18):1371–1388.
124. Love RR, et al. Bone mineral density in women with breast cancer treated with adjuvant tamoxifen for at least two years. *Breast Cancer Res Treat* 1988;12(3):297–302.
125. Vogel VG. Follow-up of the breast cancer prevention trial and the future of breast cancer prevention efforts. *Clin Cancer Res* 2001;7(12 Suppl):4413s–4418s; discussion 4411s–4412s.
126. Yoneda K, et al. Influence of adjuvant tamoxifen treatment on bone mineral density and bone turnover markers in postmenopausal breast cancer patients in Japan. *Cancer Lett* 2002;186(2):223–230.
127. Ettinger B, et al. Reduction of vertebral fracture risk in postmenopausal women with osteoporosis treated with raloxifene: results from a 3-year randomized clinical trial. Multiple Outcomes of Raloxifene Evaluation (MORE) Investigators. *JAMA* 1999;282(7):637–645.
128. O'Regan RM, et al. Effect of Raloxifene after Tamoxifen on breast and endometrial cancer growth in athymic mice. *J Natl Cancer Inst* 2002;94(4):274–283.
129. Delmas PD, et al. Effects of raloxifene on bone mineral density, serum cholesterol concentrations, and uterine endometrium in postmenopausal women. *N Engl J Med* 1997;337(23):1641–1647.
130. Chlebowski RT, et al. American Society of Clinical Oncology technology assessment on breast cancer risk reduction strategies: tamoxifen and raloxifene. *J Clin Oncol* 1999;17(6):1939–1955.
131. Ettinger B, et al. Reduction of vertebral fracture risk in postmenopausal women with osteoporosis treated with raloxifene: results from a 3-year randomized clinical trial. Multiple Outcomes of Raloxifene Evaluation (MORE) Investigators. *JAMA* 1999;282(7):637–645.
132. Anastrozole alone or in combination with tamoxifen versus tamoxifen alone for adjuvant treatment of postmenopausal women with early breast cancer: first results of the ATAC randomised trial. *Lancet* 2002;359(9324):2131–2139.

133. Cohen MH, et al. Approval summary: letrozole in the treatment of postmenopausal women with advanced breast cancer. *Clin Cancer Res* 2002;8(3):665–669.
134. Harper-Wynne CL, et al. Comparison of the systemic and intratumoral effects of tamoxifen and the aromatase inhibitor vorozole in postmenopausal patients with primary breast cancer. *J Clin Oncol* 2002;20(4):1026–1035.
135. Bajetta E, et al. The aromatase inhibitor letrozole in advanced breast cancer: effects on serum insulin-like growth factor (IGF)-I and IGF-binding protein-3 levels. *J Steroid Biochem Mol Biol* 1997;63(4–6):261–267.
136. Heshmati HM, et al. Role of low levels of endogenous estrogen in regulation of bone resorption in late postmenopausal women. *J Bone Miner Res* 2002;17(1):172–178.
137. Eastell R, HR, et al. Effect of anastrozole on bone density and bone turnover: results of the arimidex (anastrozole), tamoxifen, alone or in combination (ATAC) study. In *Programs and Proceedings of the 24th Annual Meeting of the American Society for Bone and Mineral Research*. 2002. San Antonio, TX.
138. Lindsay R, Cosman F. Estrogen in prevention and treatment of osteoporosis. *Ann N Y Acad Sci* 1990;592:326–333.
139. Riis BJ, Overgaard K, Christiansen C. Biochemical markers of bone turnover to monitor the bone response to postmenopausal hormone replacement therapy. *Osteoporos Int* 1995;5(4):276–280.
140. Cauley JA, et al. Estrogen replacement therapy and fractures in older women. Study of Osteoporotic Fractures Research Group. *Ann Intern Med* 1995;122(1):9–16.
141. Lindsay R, et al. Bone response to termination of oestrogen treatment. *Lancet* 1978;1(8078):1325–1327.
142. Natrajan PK, Gambrell RD, Jr. Estrogen replacement therapy in patients with early breast cancer. *Am J Obstet Gynecol* 2002;187(2):289–294; discussion 294–295.
143. Hormone replacement therapy and cancer. *Gynecol Endocrinol* 2001;15(6):453–465.
144. Genazzani AR, Gadducci A, Gambacciani M. Controversial issues in climacteric medicine II. Hormone replacement therapy and cancer. International Menopause Society Expert Workshop. 9–12 June 2001, Opera del Duomo, Pisa, Italy. *Climacteric* 2001;4(3):181–193.
145. Cranney A, et al. Meta-analyses of therapies for postmenopausal osteoporosis. II. Meta-analysis of alendronate for the treatment of postmenopausal women. *Endocr Rev* 2002;23(4):508–516.
146. Harris ST, et al. Effects of risedronate treatment on vertebral and nonvertebral fractures in women with postmenopausal osteoporosis: a randomized controlled trial. Vertebral Efficacy With Risedronate Therapy (VERT) Study Group. *JAMA* 1999;282(14):1344–1352.
147. Downs RW, Jr, et al. Comparison of alendronate and intranasal calcitonin for treatment of osteoporosis in postmenopausal women. *J Clin Endocrinol Metab* 2000;85(5):1783–1788.
148. Licata AA. Bisphosphonate therapy. *Am J Med Sci* 1997;313(1):17–22.
149. Reszka AA, Rodan GA. Bisphosphonate mechanism of action. *Curr Rheumatol Rep* 2003;5(1):65–74.
150. Berenson JR, et al. Efficacy of pamidronate in reducing skeletal events in patients with advanced multiple myeloma. Myeloma Aredia Study Group. *N Engl J Med* 1996;334(8):488–493.
151. Body JJ. Clinical research update: zoledronate. *Cancer* 1997;80(8 Suppl):1699–1701.
152. Lipton A. Zoledronate in the treatment of osteolytic bone metastases. *Br J Clin Pract Suppl* 1996;87:21; discussion 22.
153. Lipton A, et al. Pamidronate prevents skeletal complications and is effective palliative treatment in women with breast carcinoma and osteolytic bone metastases: long term follow-up of two randomized, placebo-controlled trials. *Cancer* 2000;88(5):1082–1090.
154. Flanagan AM, Chambers TJ. Inhibition of bone resorption by bisphosphonates: interactions between bisphosphonates, osteoclasts, and bone. *Calcif Tissue Int* 1991;49(6):407–415.
155. Pataki A, et al. Effects of short-term treatment with the bisphosphonates zoledronate and pamidronate on rat bone: a comparative histomorphometric study on the cancellous bone formed before, during, and after treatment. *Anat Rec* 1997;249(4):458–468.
156. Rogers MJ, et al. Molecular mechanisms of action of bisphosphonates. *Bone* 1999;24(5 Suppl):73S–79S.
157. Tumber A, et al. Human breast-cancer cells stimulate the fusion, migration and resorptive activity of osteoclasts in bone explants. *Int J Cancer* 2001;91(5):665–672.
158. Hall DG, Stoica G. Effect of the bisphosphonate risedronate on bone metastases in a rat mammary adenocarcinoma model system. *J Bone Miner Res* 1994;9(2):221–230.
159. Cummings SR, et al. Effect of alendronate on risk of fracture in women with low bone density but without vertebral fractures: results from the Fracture Intervention Trial. *JAMA* 1998;280(24):2077–2082.
160. Karpf DB, et al. Prevention of nonvertebral fractures by alendronate. A meta-analysis. Alendronate Osteoporosis Treatment Study Groups. *JAMA* 1997;277(14):1159–1164.
161. Black DM, et al. Randomised trial of effect of alendronate on risk of fracture in women with existing vertebral fractures. Fracture Intervention Trial Research Group. *Lancet* 1996;348(9041):1535–1541.
162. Hosking D, et al. Prevention of bone loss with alendronate in postmenopausal women under 60 years of age. Early Postmenopausal Intervention Cohort Study Group. *N Engl J Med* 1998;338(8):485–492.
163. Liberman UA, et al. Effect of oral alendronate on bone mineral density and the incidence of fractures in postmenopausal osteoporosis. The Alendronate Phase III Osteoporosis Treatment Study Group. *N Engl J Med* 1995;333(22):1437–1443.
164. Stock JL, et al. Increments in bone mineral density of the lumbar spine and hip and suppression of bone turnover are maintained after discontinuation of alendronate in postmenopausal women. *Am J Med* 1997;103(4):291–297.
165. Pavlakis N, Stockler M. Bisphosphonates for breast cancer. *Cochrane Database Syst Rev* 2002;(1):CD003474.
166. Zolendronate (zometa). *Med Lett Drugs Ther* 2001;43(1120):110–111.
167. CGP 42446 Protocol 007 (data on file). *Novartis Pharmaceuticals* 1998.
168. Berenson J. Phase II trial of Zoledronate vs Pamidronate in Multiple Myeloma and Breast Cancer Patients with Osteolytic Lesions. in Second North American Symposium on Skeletal Complications of Malignancy. 1999. Montreal, Canada.
169. Kanis JA, et al. Clodronate decreases the frequency of skeletal metastases in women with breast cancer. *Bone* 1996;19(6):663–667.
170. Powles TJ, et al. Oral clodronate and reduction in loss of bone mineral density in women with operable primary breast cancer. *J Natl Cancer Inst* 1998;90(9):704–708.
171. Pfeilschifter J, Diel IJ. Osteoporosis due to cancer treatment: pathogenesis and management. *J Clin Oncol* 2000;18(7):1570–1593.
172. Reid IR, et al. Long-term effects of calcium supplementation on bone loss and fractures in postmenopausal women: a randomized controlled trial. *Am J Med* 1995;98(4):331–335.
173. Chapuy MC, et al. Vitamin D3 and calcium to prevent hip fractures in the elderly women. *N Engl J Med* 1992;327(23):1637–1642.
174. Dawson-Hughes B, et al. Effect of calcium and vitamin D supplementation on bone density in men and women 65 years of age or older. *N Engl J Med* 1997;337(10):670–676.
175. Tang BM, et al. Use of calcium or calcium in combination with vitamin D supplementation to prevent fractures and bone loss in people aged 50 years and older: a meta-analysis. *Lancet* 2007;370(9588):657–666.
176. Delmas PD, et al. Bisphosphonate risedronate prevents bone loss in women with artificial menopause due to chemotherapy of breast cancer: a double-blind, placebo-controlled study. *J Clin Oncol* 1997;15(3):955–962.
177. Greenspan SL, et al. Prevention of bone loss in survivors of breast cancer: a randomized, double-blind, placebo-controlled clinical trial. *J Clin Endocrinol Metab* 2007;92(1):131–136.
178. Fuleihan Gel H, et al. Pamidronate in the prevention of chemotherapy-induced bone loss in premenopausal women with breast cancer: a randomized controlled trial. *J Clin Endocrinol Metab* 2005;90(6):3209–3214.
179. Hershman DL, et al. Zoledronic acid prevents bone loss in premenopausal women undergoing adjuvant chemotherapy for early stage breast cancer. *Breast Cancer Res Treat*. 2007;106(S38), San Antonio Breast Conference.
180. Gralow JR. Bone density in breast cancer: when to intervene? *J Clin Oncol* 2007;25(22):3194–3197.
181. Brufsky A, et al. Zoledronic acid inhibits adjuvant letrozole-induced bone loss in postmenopausal women with early breast cancer. *J Clin Oncol* 2007;25(7):829–836.
182. Barni S, Mondin R. Sexual dysfunction in treated breast cancer patients. *Ann Oncol* 1997;8(2):149–153.
183. Katz A. The sounds of silence: sexuality information for cancer patients. *J Clin Oncol* 2005;23(1):238–241.
184. Ganz PA, et al. Impact of different adjuvant therapy strategies on quality of life in breast cancer survivors. *Recent Results Cancer Res* 1998;152:396–411.
185. Thors CL, Broeckel JA, Jacobsen PB. Sexual functioning in breast cancer survivors. *Cancer Control* 2001;8(5):442–448.
186. Ganz PA, et al. Breast cancer survivors: psychosocial concerns and quality of life. *Breast Cancer Res Treat* 1996;38(2):183–199.
187. Joly F, et al. Long-term quality of life in premenopausal women with node-negative localized breast cancer treated with or without adjuvant chemotherapy. *Br J Cancer* 2000;83(5):577–582.
188. Wapnir IL, Cody RP, Greco RS. Subtle differences in quality of life after breast cancer surgery. *Ann Surg Oncol* 1999;6(4):359–366.
189. Ganz PA, et al. Breast conservation versus mastectomy. Is there a difference in psychological adjustment or quality of life in the year after surgery? *Cancer* 1992;69(7):1729–1738.
190. Fallowfield LJ, et al. Psychological outcomes of different treatment policies in women with early breast cancer outside a clinical trial. *BMJ* 1990;301(6752):575–580.
191. Schover LR, et al. Partial mastectomy and breast reconstruction. A comparison of their effects on psychosocial adjustment, body image, and sexuality. *Cancer* 1995;75(1):54–64.
192. Dorval M, et al. Type of mastectomy and quality of life for long term breast carcinoma survivors. *Cancer* 1998;83(10):2130–2138.
193. Kiebert GM, de Haes JC, van de Velde CJ. The impact of breast-conserving treatment and mastectomy on the quality of life of early-stage breast cancer patients: a review. *J Clin Oncol* 1991;9(6):1059–1070.
194. Moyer A. Psychosocial outcomes of breast-conserving surgery versus mastectomy: a meta-analytic review. *Health Psychol* 1997;16(3):284–298.
195. Ganz PA, et al. Predictors of sexual health in women after a breast cancer diagnosis. *J Clin Oncol* 1999;17(8):2371–2380.
196. Young-McCaughan S. Sexual functioning in women with breast cancer after treatment with adjuvant therapy. *Cancer Nurs* 1996;19(4):308–319.
197. Lindley C, et al. Quality of life and preferences for treatment following systemic adjuvant therapy for early-stage breast cancer. *J Clin Oncol* 1998;16(4):1380–1387.
198. Mortimer JE, et al. Effect of tamoxifen on sexual functioning in patients with breast cancer. *J Clin Oncol* 1999;17(5):1488–1492.
199. Ganz PA, et al. Life after breast cancer: understanding women's health-related quality of life and sexual functioning. *J Clin Oncol* 1998;16(2):501–514.
200. Berglund G, et al. Effect of endocrine treatment on sexuality in premenopausal breast cancer patients: a prospective randomized study. *J Clin Oncol* 2001;19(11):2788–2796.
201. Ganz PA, et al. Managing menopausal symptoms in breast cancer survivors: results of a randomized controlled trial. *J Natl Cancer Inst* 2000;92(13):1054–1064.
202. Nachtigall LE. Comparative study: Replens versus local estrogen in menopausal women. *Fertil Steril* 1994;61(1):178–180.
203. Loprinzi CL, et al. Phase III randomized double-blind study to evaluate the efficacy of a polycarbophil-based vaginal moisturizer in women with breast cancer. *J Clin Oncol* 1997;15(3):969–973.
204. Greendale GA, et al. Symptom relief and side effects of postmenopausal hormones: results from the Postmenopausal Estrogen/Progestin Interventions Trial. *Obstet Gynecol* 1998;92(6):982–988.
205. Phillips SM, Sherwin BB. Effects of estrogen on memory function in surgically menopausal women. *Psychoneuroendocrinology* 1992;17(5):485–495.
206. Nash HA, et al. Estradiol-delivering vaginal rings for hormone replacement therapy. *Am J Obstet Gynecol* 1999;181(6):1400–1406.
207. Rioux JE, et al. 17beta-estradiol vaginal tablet versus conjugated equine estrogen vaginal cream to relieve menopausal atrophic vaginitis. *Menopause* 2000;7(3):156–161.
208. Davis SR, Tran J. Testosterone influences libido and well being in women. *Trends Endocrinol Metab* 2001;12(1):33–37.

209. Barton DL, et al. Randomized controlled trial to evaluate transdermal testosterone in female cancer survivors with decreased libido; North Central Cancer Treatment Group protocol N02C3. *J Natl Cancer Inst* 2007;99(9):672–679.

210. Baum M, et al. Anastrozole alone or in combination with tamoxifen versus tamoxifen alone for adjuvant treatment of postmenopausal women with early breast cancer: first results of the ATAC randomised trial. [see comment] [erratum appears in *Lancet* 2002 Nov 9;360(9344):1520]. *Lancet* 2002;359(9324):2131–2139.

211. Goss PE, et al. A randomized trial of letrozole in postmenopausal women after five years of tamoxifen therapy for early-stage breast cancer. [see comment]. *New England Journal of Medicine* 2003;349(19):1793–1802.

212. Howell A, et al. Results of the ATAC (Arimidex, Tamoxifen, Alone or in Combination) trial after completion of 5 years' adjuvant treatment for breast cancer. *Lancet* 2005;365(9453):60–62.

213. Forbes JF, et al. Effect of anastrozole and tamoxifen as adjuvant treatment for early-stage breast cancer: 100-month analysis of the ATAC trial. *Lancet Oncol* 2008;9(1):45–53.

214. Cicuttini FM, et al. Comparison of tibial cartilage volume and radiologic grade of the tibiofemoral joint. *Arthritis Rheum* 2003;48(3):682–688.

215. Cecil RL, Archer BH. Arthritis of the menopause. *JAMA* 1925;84:75–79.

216. Nevitt MC, et al. Association of estrogen replacement therapy with the risk of osteoarthritis of the hip in elderly white women. Study of Osteoporotic Fractures Research Group. *Arch Intern Med* 1996;156(18):2073–2080.

217. Hannan MT, et al. Estrogen use and radiographic osteoarthritis of the knee in women. The Framingham Osteoarthritis Study. *Arthritis Rheum* 1990;33(4):525–532.

218. Spector TD, et al. Is hormone replacement therapy protective for hand and knee osteoarthritis in women? The Chingford Study. *Ann Rheum Dis* 1997;56(7):432–434.

219. Crew KD, et al. Prevalence of joint symptoms in postmenopausal women taking aromatase inhibitors for early-stage breast cancer. *J Clin Oncol* 2007;25(25):3877–3883.

220. Crew KD, et al. Pilot Study of Acupuncture for the Treatment of Joint Symptoms Related to Adjuvant Aromatase Inhibitor Therapy in Postmenopausal Breast Cancer Patients. *Journal of Cancer Survivorshp* 2007;1(4).

221. Demark-Wahnefried W, Winer EP, Rimer BK. Why women gain weight with adjuvant chemotherapy for breast cancer. *J Clin Oncol* 1993;11(7):1418–1429.

222. Goodwin PJ, et al. Adjuvant treatment and onset of menopause predict weight gain after breast cancer diagnosis. *J Clin Oncol* 1999;17(1):120–129.

223. McInnes JA, Knobf MT. Weight gain and quality of life in women treated with adjuvant chemotherapy for early-stage breast cancer. *Oncol Nurs Forum* 2001;28(4):675–684.

224. Lankester KJ, Phillips JE, Lawton PA. Weight gain during adjuvant and neoadjuvant chemotherapy for breast cancer: an audit of 100 women receiving FEC or CMF chemotherapy. *Clin Oncol (R Coll Radiol)* 2002;14(1):64–67.

225. Aslani A, et al. Changes in body composition during breast cancer chemotherapy with the CMF-regimen. *Breast Cancer Res Treat* 1999;57(3):285–290.

226. Demark-Wahnefried W, et al. Changes in weight, body composition, and factors influencing energy balance among premenopausal breast cancer patients receiving adjuvant chemotherapy. *J Clin Oncol* 2001;19(9):2381–2389.

227. Loprinzi CL, et al. Randomized trial of dietician counseling to try to prevent weight gain associated with breast cancer adjuvant chemotherapy. *Oncology* 1996;53(3):228–232.

228. Schwartz AL. Exercise and weight gain in breast cancer patients receiving chemotherapy. *Cancer Pract* 2000;8(5):231–237.

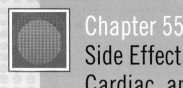

Chapter 55
Side Effects of Systemic Therapy: Neurocognitive, Cardiac, and Secondary Malignancies

Alvaro Moreno Aspitia and Edith A. Perez

The National Cancer Institute estimates that more than 2.4 million women with a history of breast cancer are alive in the United States (1). In 2007, an estimated 180,510 new cases of invasive breast cancer and an estimated 62,030 additional cases of *in situ* breast cancer were diagnosed (2). At the time of diagnosis, 92% of these patients have stage I-III disease, making many of them eligible to receive adjuvant or neoadjuvant systemic chemotherapy. This treatment modality is well recognized to increase their disease-free and overall survival. However, these systemic therapies, which typically involve chemotherapy, have been associated with several potentially important adverse effects including, although not limited to, neurocognitive dysfunction, cardiac toxicity, and even secondary malignancies. Careful data analysis is important to dispel misconceptions, and to determine risk reduction strategies and interventions to optimize patient outcome.

 ## EFFECTS OF ADJUVANT CHEMOTHERAPY ON NEUROCOGNITIVE FUNCTIONS OF PATIENTS WITH BREAST CANCER

Potential neurocognitive dysfunction, sometimes labeled *chemobrain*, is one of the growing concerns related to long-term effects of chemotherapy. Symptoms are often described as a lack of concentration, inability to think clearly, and short-term memory loss. Current literature suggests that approximately 15% to 50% of breast cancer patients receiving adjuvant chemotherapy describe some degree of cognitive dysfunction, although determining a potential causal relationship has been difficult at best (3–9). A limitation of the published literature is that most of the information is derived from small cross-sectional studies lacking appropriately selected control patients. An additional hurdle in the interpretation of the current body of research is that researchers use different neuropsychological tests, inclusion and exclusion criteria, definitions of cognitive impairment, and statistical analysis plans, making standard comparisons across studies difficult. However, it is worth reviewing the available data.

Cross-sectional Studies

The studies reviewed in this chapter are summarized in Table 55.1. Eight cross-sectional studies have been conducted, evaluating neurocognitive function in a total of approximately 729 breast cancer survivors. A total of 425 were exposed to chemotherapy, 304 underwent surgery alone, and 155 were healthy individuals who served as controls. Arguably, Wieneke and Dienst (9) conducted the first study to associate cognitive dysfunction and chemotherapy. In the study, 28 patients with a history of breast cancer who had received adjuvant chemotherapy consisting of either cyclophosphamide, methotrexate, and 5-fluorouracil (CMF), cyclophosphamide, doxorubicin, and 5-fluorouracil (CAF), or a combination, were subjected to a battery of neuropsychological testing. Mild cognitive impairment represented a score greater than or equal to 1 standard deviations (SD) below the normative data on two or more neuropsychological domains, and moderate cognitive impairment was

defined as a greater than or equal to 2 SD below the normative data on at least one neuropsychological measure. Of participants, 75% were found to have moderate cognitive impairment based on the above criterion and the two areas most affected were memory and concentration. An additional study (8) of 104 breast cancer patients who were treated with either high-dose chemotherapy (n = 34), standard-dose chemotherapy (n = 36), or no systemic therapy (n = 34), suggested an association between the chemotherapy dose received and the degree of cognitive impairment. Of these patients, 32% who received high-dose chemotherapy, 17% who received standard-dose chemotherapy, and 9% of the control group had cognitive deficits defined as scoring greater than or equal to 2 SD below the mean score of the control group on three or more neuropsychological tests. However, such association between dosing of the chemotherapy and degree of impairment was not observed on a more recent study where the degree of global cognitive deficit was 8% in patients receiving high-dose chemotherapy with stem cell support, 13% for patients treated with standard-dose chemotherapy, and 3% in patients with early breast cancer not treated with chemotherapy. All patients were at least 5 years after completion of the chemotherapy (10). A fourth small cross-sectional study was conducted on patients with a history of breast cancer who received either CMF (n = 39) or no systemic treatment (n = 34). It showed that 28% of patients who received chemotherapy and 12% of patients in the control group (p = .013) had cognitive impairment defined as a score of greater than or equal to 2 SD below the mean of the control group on three or more neuropsychological tests (6).

Four additional studies evaluated breast cancer survivors who did or did not receive chemotherapy, and compared them with a group of healthy individuals. The first of such study reported on 71 breast cancer patients (31 receiving active chemotherapy and 40 who already completed adjuvant chemotherapy), and 36 individuals who represented a healthy control group. The study demonstrated moderate or severe *impairment* among 48% of patients receiving chemotherapy, 50% who completed chemotherapy, and 11% of controls (p ≥.002) (4). Most patients had received either CMF or CEF (cyclophosphamide, epirubicin, and 5-fluorouracil). Castellon et al. (11) evaluated 53 breast cancer survivors who were 2 to 5 years from diagnosis and had received either CMF or a doxorubicin-based adjuvant chemotherapy (n = 36) or surgery alone (n = 17); 19 individuals served as the healthy control. Patients who received adjuvant chemotherapy had a significantly lower Global Neurocognitive Performance score than those who did not receive adjuvant chemotherapy (p = .01); however, neither group had scores significantly different from the healthy control group. This study did not demonstrate any association between subjective cognitive complaints and objective findings on neuropsychological tests. Ahles et al. (3) reported a cross-sectional neuropsychological study of patients who were survivors of either breast cancer or lymphoma. In the breast cancer survivors, 35 had received chemotherapy and 35 had been treated with local therapy alone. At 10 years median follow-up, cognitive impairment was described in 39% of patients who received chemotherapy and 14% of those treated with surgery alone (p <.01), suggesting that the deficit associated with the chemotherapy may be durable. The largest

Table 55.1   **BREAST CANCER PATIENTS AND COGNITIVE DYSFUNCTION SUMMARY OF STUDIES REVIEWED IN THIS CHAPTER**

Study/(Reference)	Sample Size (n)	Patients ± Control	Impairment (%)	Cognitive Comments Groups (n)
Cross-sectional Studies				
Wieneke (9) 1995	28	All received CT	75	First study to associate cognitive impairment and CT
Van Dam (8) 1998	104	34: high-dose CT 36: standard CT 34-no CT	32 17 9	First study to associate dose of CT and degree of cognitive impairment
Scherwath (10) 2006	76	24: high-dose CT 23: standard CT 29: no CT	8 13 3	Contrary to the above, this study found no association between dosing of CT and degree of deficit
Schagen (6) 1999	73	39: CT 34: no CT	28 12	
Brezden (4) 2000	106	31: on active CT 40: post CT 36: healthy controls	48 50 11	First study to compare cognitive impairment on patients receiving CT with healthy noncancer patients
Castellon (11) 2004	72	53: CT 17: surgery alone N/A 19: healthy controls		Lower cognitive performance score. but not significantly different from the healthy group
Ahles (3) 2002	70	35: CT 35: surgery alone	39 14	Cognitive deficit associated to CT seems durable (10 yr)
Tchen (7) 2003	200	100: CT 100: healthy controls	16 4	Largest cross-sectional study. Difference is significant ($p = .008$)
Prospective Longitudinal Studies				
Wefel (12) 2004	25	All received CT	33 before CT 61 at 6-mo follow-up	Stabilization (50%) or improvement (50%) noted at 1-yr post-CT
Bender (13) 2006	46	19: CT 15: CT plus tamoxifen 12: surgery alone (DCIS)	 N/A	High attrition rate (common in longitudinal studies)
Shilling (14) 2005	93	50: CT 43: healthy controls	34 19	No correlation between self-reported memory problems and objective performance in tests
Hurria (15) 2006	31	28: evaluable patients, all received CT		Study in patients ≥65 yr 25% decline in cognition but not in functional status or depression
Schagen (16) 2006	184	28: high-dose CT 39: standard dose CT 57: no CT 60: healthy controls	25 13 18 7	Higher dose of CT associated with greater changes in cognitive function but not with degree of fatigue, depression, or anxiety
Meta-analysis				
Falleti (19) 2005	372	Ahles (3), Schagen (6), Van Dam (8), Wieneke (9), Castellon (11), Wefel (12)		Concluded that magnitude of impairment depends on the type of study design used
Stewart (20) 2006	478	Ahles (3), Brezden (4), Schagen (6), Van Dam (8), Wieneke (9), Castellon (11), Wefel (12)		Reported subtle yet consequential cognitive decline

CT, chemotherapy; DCIS, ductal carcinoma *in situ*.

cross-sectional study evaluated cognitive function (High Sensitivity Cognitive Screen), fatigue, and menopausal symptoms in 100 patients (who were receiving different type of chemotherapy regimens), and in 100 healthy controls (7). Of the chemotherapy patients, 16% were categorized as having

moderate to severe cognitive impairment compared to 4% of the control group ($p = .008$).

The above cross-sectional studies suggest the presence of neurocognitive deficits in breast cancer survivors after being treated with chemotherapy in the adjuvant setting. Such impairment seems to affect only a subset of patients; to potentially negatively affect a variety of cognitive domains including memory, language, and spatial abilities; that such effects may be durable and observed many years after therapy, in some (but not all) patients; that depression, anxiety, and fatigue are associated with self-perceived but not objective deficits; and that the effects of chemotherapy might be dose-dependent and associated more with some agents than others. Many methodologic limitations exist, however, confounding factors and caveats associated with these cross-sectional studies. Specifically, there is heterogeneity in the types of chemotherapy given, limited control for the potential effects of menopausal status or hormonal therapy, use of different control groups and possible selection bias for this cohort, variable length of time between the completion of chemotherapy and the delivery of the neuropsychological testing, and the relatively small sample sizes of these studies. Larger prospective, long-term longitudinal studies, using patients as their own control and utilizing standard validated neuropsychiatric testing at various time points are necessary to better understand these potential adverse events in the setting of adjuvant or neoadjuvant chemotherapy.

Prospective Longitudinal Studies

Five prospective, longitudinal trials evaluating cognitive function have been reported and several others are ongoing. The first one was conducted by investigators at M.D. Anderson Cancer Center (12), where 25 women with breast carcinoma consented to undergo a comprehensive neuropsychological evaluation before treatment at baseline, at short-term, defined as approximately 6 months after baseline, and long-term intervals after chemotherapy, defined as 18 months after baseline or 12 months after completion of the chemotherapy. Chemotherapy consisted of six cycles of 5-fluorouracil, doxorubicin, and cyclophosphamide (FAC). Patients were evaluated with a comprehensive battery of cognitive tests, self-report questionnaires regarding their personality traits and affective status, and a breast carcinoma-specific self-report survey of quality of life (QOL). Before the start of systemic therapy, 33% of women exhibited cognitive impairment. At the 6 months follow-up time point, 61% of the patients exhibited a decline relative to baseline in one or more domains of cognitive functioning and reported greater difficulty in maintaining their ability to work. The most common domains of cognitive dysfunction were related to attention, learning, and processing speed. Approximately 1 year from completion of the chemotherapy, however, 50% of patients who experienced declines in cognitive function demonstrated improvement, and the other 50% remained stable. Self-reported ability to perform work-related activities also improved over this interval. Neither impairment at baseline nor subsequent treatment-related cognitive decline exhibited any statistically significant correlation with affective well-being or with demographic or clinical characteristics.

A second multicenter trial reported by Bender et al. (13), included three groups of women (n = 46); groups 1 (n = 19; chemotherapy) and 2 (n = 15; chemotherapy plus tamoxifen) consisted of women with stage I or II breast cancer, group 3 (n = 12) consisted of women with ductal carcinoma *in situ* (DCIS) who had not received chemotherapy or tamoxifen. Cognitive function was measured with neuropsychological tests aimed to assess attention, learning and memory, psychomotor speed, mental flexibility, visuoconstructional ability, executive function, and general intelligence, which was administered at three time points: after surgery but before chemotherapy, 1

week and 1 year after completion of the chemotherapy. Of these patients, 52% dropped off the study before completion, and 20% had progression of disease during the evaluation period. The attrition rate noted in this study is a problem common in the longitudinal studies assessing cognitive impairment in breast cancer survivors. Results showed that, with the exception of performances on specific objective memory measures, there was no significant group with demonstratable interactions of time on measures of any other cognitive domains. The performance of subjects in groups 1 and 2 on memory measures, including Four Word Short Term Memory Test 5-s, 15-s, and 30-s, and the delayed recall Rey Complex Figure Test, deteriorated over time compared with women who received no adjuvant therapy. Women who received chemotherapy plus tamoxifen exhibited the largest deteriorations in memory, with declines in visual memory and verbal. An additional study reported the preliminary results of an observational longitudinal study of 50 patients with early-stage breast cancer who had received chemotherapy and 43 healthy controls (14). Patients who received chemotherapy were tested before chemotherapy and 4 weeks after completion of chemotherapy; the healthy control group was tested at baseline and 6 months later. Meaningful cognitive decline in the Reliable Change Index, defined as a reliable decline in at least 2 of 14 measures of cognitive function, was observed in 34% of patients who received chemotherapy, but only in 18.6% of the control group (p = .0475). As noted on the cross-sectional studies conducted by Ahles et al. (3) and Schagen et al. (6), no significant correlation was found between self-reported memory problems and objective performance on the neuropsychological tests.

The role of cognitive dysfunction in older women was studied by investigators at Memorial Sloan-Kettering Cancer Center (15), in a small trial of 31 patients, aged 65 and older with stage I to III breast cancer. Of these 31 patients, 3 refused post-testing and 28 were evaluable. In this trial, 71% (n = 20) of patients received CMF; 7% (n = 2) received doxorubicin plus cyclophosphamide (AC); 18% (n = 5) received ACT (AC followed by paclitaxel); and 4% (n = 1) received ACT followed by trastuzumab. Neuropsychological testing in the domains of cognitive function, including attention; verbal memory; visual memory; and verbal, spatial, psychomotor, and executive functions, and a geriatric assessment, including evaluation of activities of daily living, Karnofsky performance status, comorbid medical conditions, cognition per Mini-Mental State Examination, depression, and quality of life, were performed before chemotherapy and 6 months after chemotherapy. The number of scores 2 SD below the norm for neuropsychological tests were calculated for each patient before and after 6 months of chemotherapy: 14 (50%) had no change, 11 (39%) worsened, and 3 (11%) improved (p = .05). Seven patients (25%) experienced a decline in cognitive function. No significant difference was seen in functional status, comorbidity, or depression scores before and 6 months after chemotherapy for the group as whole. The authors concluded that a subset of older patients receiving adjuvant chemotherapy for breast cancer experience a decline in cognitive function from before to 6 months after chemotherapy. As noted in some of the cross-sectional studies, the domains of neuropsychological functioning most affected included visual memory, spatial function, psychomotor function, and attention. As in many other published studies, however, there was not a control group of similar patients who did not receive chemotherapy, making it impossible to evaluate what degree of cognitive decline was caused by normal aging in this group of older individuals. It is important to note that the intense 2-hour of neuropsychological testing was poorly tolerated by these patients; the investigators had to modify the battery of tests to allow compliance and to let the patients complete them in a reasonable amount of time (45 minutes).

A more recent study (16) prospectively examined changes in cognitive performance among three groups of breast cancer patients, including 28 high-risk breast cancer patients who had received high-dose chemotherapy; 39 patients who received standard-dose chemotherapy; 57 patients with stage I breast cancer who had received no systemic chemotherapy, and a control group of healthy women without cancer (n = 60). All patients underwent neuropsychological testing before and 6 months after treatment (12-month interval); control subjects underwent repeated testing over a 6-month interval. No differences in cognitive functioning between the four groups were observed at the first assessment. More of the high-dose chemotherapy group than the control subjects experienced a deterioration in cognitive performance over time (25% vs. 6.7%; odds ratio [OR] = 5.3, 95% confidence interval [CI] = 1.3–21.2, p = .02). No such difference was observed for the standard-dose chemotherapy or the no-chemotherapy groups. Cognitive performance at baseline and follow-up was not associated with subjects' reports of anxiety, depression, fatigue, or menopausal status.

Despite the evidence of potential association between chemotherapy and neurocognitive impairment in some of the studies, at least two other studies failed to find any significant association between the use of chemotherapy and cognitive changes (17,18). A prospective longitudinal study of 177 women divided in three groups, including 85 patients who had early-stage breast cancer and were scheduled to receive adjuvant chemotherapy, 43 patients scheduled for endocrine therapy or radiotherapy only, and 49 healthy controls, found no statistically significant difference in the neuropsychological functioning between the three groups (17). A battery of neuropsychological tests were performed at baseline (T1), after chemotherapy (T2 = 4 weeks after chemotherapy, or 6 months for the other two groups), and at 18 months (T3 = 12 months after chemotherapy or 18 months in the other groups). Reliable decline on multiple tasks was seen in 20% of chemotherapy patients, 26% of nonchemotherapy patients, 18% of controls at T2; and in 18%, 14%, and 11%, respectively, at T3. As noted in other studies, psychological distress, QOL measures, and self-reported cognitive failures did not have an impact on the objective tests of cognitive function. The other study was a cross sectional study performed in 143 women, 6 months at completion of chemotherapy plus radiotherapy (n = 60) or radiotherapy alone (n = 83), for treatment of stage 0 to II breast cancer (18). No statistically significant differences were found between the two groups with regard to their average performance on tests of episodic memory, attention, complex cognition, motor performance, or language.

The above prospective longitudinal studies overcome some of the methodologic problems associated with cross-sectional studies, but much room for improvement is needed. These studies were still small, had a high attrition rate, lacked an appropriate control group, and there was no uniformity in the battery of testing performed. They support the hypothesis that a subset of breast cancer patients exposed to chemotherapy experience subtle but diffuse neurocognitive impairment affecting the domains of verbal and visual memory, attention, and concentration, and such deficits are more noticeable in the few months following treatment but might improve over time. Despite the results of the above studies, the current knowledge of the exact prevalence, pathophysiologic mechanisms of disease, and characterization of the cognitive impairment is quite limited. We hope that the ongoing longitudinal studies will shed more light on the above questions and that clinical investigators will invest as much time and interest in this disorder as given to the study of bone health in breast cancer survivors.

Meta-analysis

Two meta-analyses regarding the neuropsychological effects of adjuvant chemotherapy in patients with breast cancer have been published. In the first study by Falleti et al. (19), five of the above cross-sectional studies (3,6,8,9,11) and one prospective study (12) were analyzed. This study reviewed data on a total of 233 breast cancer patients treated with chemotherapy and 139 control participants (120 breast cancer patients who did not received chemotherapy and 19 healthy controls). Conclusions included that cognitive impairment occurs reliably in women with breast cancer undergoing adjuvant chemotherapy, that deficit is global but small in the attention domain and unreliable in the spatial function, and that the effects appear to diminish as the time from chemotherapy increases. The magnitude of the neurocognitive impairment depends on the type of design that was used in each independent study. The meta-analysis by Stewart et al. (20) reviewed data from seven studies, all of them previously reviewed in this chapter (3,4,6,8–11). Similar conclusions were reached, that adjuvant chemotherapy results in a small but significant decline in global cognitive functioning, and that no association exists between cognitive performance and age, education, affective well-being, fatigue, and menopausal status. It was noted by the authors that, although the findings offered evidence for cognitive decline related to the use of chemotherapy, none of the findings reached clinically significant levels.

THE ETIOLOGY OF CHEMOTHERAPY-INDUCED NEUROCOGNITIVE DEFICITS

It is critical not only to have a better understanding of the potential relation between chemotherapy and cognitive functioning, but also to identify an etiology (if it exists). The etiology of this perceived disorder is not well understood and the presence of multiple confounding factors, such as fatigue (7,21–24), anemia, stress, depression, and availability of coping skills (24–27), level of intelligence and education, hormonal status (28–35), use of concomitant medications that affect the central nervous system (e.g., antiemetics, anxiolytics, and opioid analgesics) among others, make the research of this topic much more problematic.

Other hypotheses regarding the mechanisms of cognitive dysfunction caused by chemotherapy include host susceptibility or genetic predisposition, such as polymorphisms of the gene multidrug resistance 1 (MDR1) that encodes the protein P-glycoprotein (P-gp), which in turn has been reported to be expressed in the capillary endothelial cells of the brain. A higher concentration of the cytotoxic drug may reach the brain of patients with lower levels of P-gp (36–38), which may overwhelm the mechanisms of cellular repair of cells in the central nervous system (CNS), leading to decreased metabolism, demyelination, or cell death (39–41). By the same token, similar effects might be observed even at physiologic levels of the cytotoxic agents if there are intrinsic defects in the mechanisms of DNA repair. Additionally, changes in the gene that encodes apolipoprotein E (APOE), a glycolipoprotein that seems to have an important role in neuronal repair and plasticity after injury, might lead to impaired neuronal healing after chemotherapy-induced trauma. A study by Ahles et al. (42) demonstrated an association between APOE genotype and cognitive functioning in long-term cancer survivors. This study showed that breast cancer and lymphoma survivors with at least one E4 allele scored significantly lower in the visual memory and spatial ability domains compared with survivors who did not carry an E4 allele. It is also well known that some chemotherapy agents or their metabolites are able to cross the blood–brain barrier and cause neurotoxicity (43–49). The mechanisms of damage may be caused by direct cellular toxicity from the chemotherapy, or be sequelae of microvascular injury (50), tissue hypoxia (51–53), altered cerebral metabolism (54), or release of inflammatory cytokines caused by any of the above pathways (55–60).

A recent study explored the relationship of regional cerebral blood flow and metabolism with cognitive function and past exposure to chemotherapy for breast cancer using F-18 fluorodeoxyglucose positron-emitting tomography (FDG PET) scan technology (54). Sixteen women with history of breast cancer, who had been treated with adjuvant chemotherapy 5 to 10 years before enrollment in the study, including 11 who had also undergone tamoxifen therapy, were compared with a control group of 8 women, who had never received chemotherapy. During performance of a short-term recall task, including Rey–Osterreith Complex Figure (ROCF) Delayed Recall Test, the modulation of cerebral blood flow in specific regions of frontal cortex and cerebellum was significantly altered in chemotherapy-treated subjects. Those who had received chemotherapy had a lower resting brain metabolism, and the questions activated a larger portion of their frontal cortex compared with the brain of untreated women, suggesting that to perform the same cognitive task, they had to work that part of the brain much harder to get up to the level that they would have had if it had not been impaired. Peak cerebral activation in chemotherapy-treated subjects differed most significantly from untreated subjects in the inferior frontal gyrus ($p < .0005$). Resting metabolism in this area correlated with performance on a short-term memory task previously found to be particularly impaired in chemotherapy-treated subjects. Performance on the ROCF Delayed Recall test of the chemotherapy-treated group averaged 3.2 points (13%) lower than the performance of the control group. Additionally, metabolism of the basal ganglia was significantly decreased in patients treated with tamoxifen plus chemotherapy compared with chemotherapy-only breast cancer subjects, or with subjects who had not received chemotherapy. Chemotherapy alone was not associated with decreased basal ganglia activity relative to untreated subjects. This finding is comparable to another study that demonstrated decreased metabolism in certain parts of the forebrain of women who had received tamoxifen without previous chemotherapy (61). This study by Silverman et al. (54) is the first to show specific alterations in functional activity of frontal cortex, cerebellum, and basal ganglia in breast cancer survivors, 5 to 10 years after completion of chemotherapy. An additional study is prospectively analyzing the metabolic activity of the brain in breast cancer patients before, 1 month, and 1 year after chemotherapy and comparing findings with breast cancer patients who did not receive chemotherapy and healthy control subjects (62). Preliminary results have suggested a pattern of reduced activation in frontal areas during a working memory task.

Summary

Overall, current data suggest that the neurocognitive difficulties observed in breast cancer patients receiving adjuvant or neoadjuvant chemotherapy appear real, but subtle and mostly limited to memory deficits. Patients do not appear to experience a clinically significant difference that limits their ability to function in the real world, unless confronted with cognitively challenging situations. Prospective, randomized long-term longitudinal studies (including breast cancer patients with or without treatment, as well as matched age control patients), utilizing validated neuropsychiatric testing sufficiently sensitive to provide detailed information on the different domains of cognitive function, are necessary to determine accurately the significance of the preliminary data reported to date.

Cardiotoxicity of Systemic Chemotherapy

Similar to the neurocognitive deficits related to chemotherapy, cardiotoxicity in breast cancer survivors is another important topic. Although anthracycline-related acute and chronic cardiotoxicity were identified decades ago (63), good data of potential cardiotoxic effects of current doses and types of chemotherapy and the newer nonchemotherapy agents, such as the monoclonal antibodies and tyrosine kinase inhibitors (TKI), have brought renewed interest in this topic (64). Cardiac events are broad and can vary from asymptomatic electrocardiographic changes all the way to cardiac arrest and death. Such events include changes in cardiac function, especially left ventricular failure and congestive heart failure (CHF); dilated cardiomyopathy; symptomatic arrhythmias; myocarditis; pericarditis; and thrombotic events, such as myocardial infarction.

THE EFFECT OF ANTINEOPLASTIC AGENTS ON CARDIAC FUNCTION

Anthracyclines

Interpretation of data related to anthracyclines relies on understanding the mechanism of action, impact of dose and schedules, and the extent of short- or long-term patient follow-up. Potential conclusions related to reliability of data also need to be placed in the context, whether they were obtained as part of population-based epidemiologic studies or as part of prospective studies in which cardiac effects are part of the primary study end points. Anthracyclines are antineoplastic antibiotics with activity in solid and hematologic malignancies, and among the most frequent chemotherapeutic agents used in breast cancer. Doxorubicin and epirubicin are the two most commonly used for breast cancer management. They are believed to cause damage to the myocardium by forming free reactive oxygen radicals, direct DNA damage, or interference with DNA repair, and the induction of immune reactions leading to cardiomyocyte apoptosis (65–67). Anthracyclines can lead to impaired left ventricular function, including systolic, diastolic, or a combination of both. Most institutions define systolic dysfunction as having a left ventricular ejection fraction (LVEF) of less than 50%. LVEF lower than 40% is often associated with symptoms of CHF. One retrospective analysis of 4,018 patient records showed that the overall incidence of doxorubicin-induced CHF was 2.2%. Risk factors for anthracycline cardiotoxicity included age older than 70 years, hypertension, preexisting coronary artery disease, female sex, and previous cardiac irradiation or previous anthracycline exposure (63). Another retrospective review of three trials (n = 630 patients; two breast cancer trials and one with patients with small-cell lung cancer), has indicated that the incidence of doxorubicin-induced CHF can be as high as 5.1% (n = 32) and the estimated cumulative incidence of CHF as high as 26% after a cumulative dose of 400 mg/m², with older patients (age >65 years) showing a greater incidence of events (68). However, interpretation of these data is confounded by multiple variables, because the results were derived before the current standard adjuvant regimens, which typically utilize doxorubicin at cumulative doses of 240 to 300 mg/m² or up to 720 mg/m² for epirubicin.

A population-based study of the Surveillance, Epidemiology, and End Results (SEER) Medicare database of 43,338 women with no history of CHF, ages 66 to 80 years and diagnosed with stage I to III breast cancer between 1992 and 2002 was recently reported (69). The data demonstrated that the adjusted hazard ratio (HR) for CHF was 1.26 (95% CI, 1.12–1.42) for women aged 66 to 70 who were treated with an anthracycline-based regimen compared with other chemotherapy. However, an increased risk of CHF was not observed in women aged 71 to 80, a finding which was contrary to the commonly held notion that these older women would also be found to be at higher risk. Age, black race, trastuzumab treatment, hypertension, diabetes, and coronary artery disease, were found to be significant predictors of CHF. Left-sided chest wall radiotherapy was not found to be associated with risk of CHF. The significantly higher rates of CHF continued to increase through more than 10 years of follow-up. The caveats of these SEER analyses are many, including the lack of information related to cumulative dose of anthracyclines or other treatments. So, although interesting, this report cannot be considered to be conclusive related to the isolated effect of adjuvant anthracyclines (at currently recommended doses) on long-term cardiac morbidity.

The recently reported study by Ganz et al. (70) did not detect differences in LVEF levels that were below normal when comparing long-term effects of either six cycles of CAF and CMF adjuvant chemotherapy. This is an important longitudinal study, which also demonstrated a lack of difference of median LVEF after 10 years of treatment for the anthracycline versus nonanthracycline adjuvant treatments. These data on the lack of significant clinical differences between anthracycline versus nonanthracycline were also reported in the comparative National Cancer Institute of Canada (NCIC) trial comparing six cycles of CEF versus CMF as adjuvant therapy for breast cancer. Despite these reassuring data, theoretical concerns still exist, and further studies are needed. Important facts include a balance of efficacy versus potential long-term effects.

The probability of doxorubicin-induced congestive heart failure has been directly related to the total dose of doxorubicin administered, with the risk being significantly increased with a cumulative dose greater than 450 to 550 mg/m^2. For epirubicin, such risk is usually observed with a dose twice of that of doxorubicin (>950 to 1,100 mg/m^2), which might be owing to a reduction in the formation of cardiotoxic alcoholic metabolites (71). Although continuous infusion or weekly dose schedule of doxorubicin were noted to be associated with a lower incidence of CHF (72–75), asymptomatic decline of LVEF as well as symptomatic congestive heart failure can be observed in patients receiving a lifetime dose of anthracyclines much lower than the above conventional limits, so there is not a *safe dose* of these agents, under which no patients would sustain any cardiac event. Additionally, the concomitant or sequential use of mediastinal irradiation, even if given many years later, has also been associated with increased cardiac sensitivity to anthracycline damage (76); although mainly utilizing radiation techniques and ports no longer in use today.

Pegylated liposomal doxorubicin is a novel formulation that has shown some potential for reduced cardiotoxicity (77). In a phase III clinical trial conducted in 509 women with metastatic breast cancer, this agent offered equivalent efficacy (progression free-survival [PFS] = 6.9 vs. 7.8 months) but a significantly lower risk of cardiotoxicity (HR = 3.16, 95% CI 1.58–6.31, p <.001), compared with conventional doxorubicin (78). Similarly, in a retrospective analysis of eight phase I and II protocol studies where 42 patients were treated with doses of liposomal doxorubicin exceeding 500 mg/m^2 (range 500 to 1500 mg/m^2), a low incidence of cardiotoxicity was observed (79). However, very limited data are currently available regarding the use of this agent in the adjuvant setting, where the long-term impact of cardioprotection is most important. So, at this time, it is not possible to determine if there might be long-term differences in cardiac safety between standard or pegylated liposomal doxorubicin.

Prevention of Anthracycline-induced Cardiotoxicity

No single strategy has been successful to prevent or delay cumulative anthracycline-induced cardiotoxicity and so limitation of cumulative dose and early detection remain the most effective method to deter a potentially clinical evident adverse event. Dexrazoxane, a derivative of EDTA capable of chelating intracellular iron, is used to prevent the formation of toxic iron-mediated free radicals, but the precise cardioprotective mechanism of this agent is not well known. It is indicated to reduce the incidence and severity of doxorubicin-induced cardiomyopathy in patients with metastatic breast cancer who have received a cumulative doxorubicin dose of 300 mg/m^2, and who, in the opinion of the treating physician, would benefit from continuing such treatment (80). It is not recommended to be used with the initiation of anthracycline-based chemotherapy because of the lower response rate (48% vs. 63%; p = .007) and shorter time to progression observed in a prospective placebo-controlled, randomized clinical trial where patients with advanced cancer received dexrazoxane starting with their first cycle of FAC chemotherapy (81). Although the overall survival of these patients was similar to the group of patients who received FAC plus placebo, these findings raised concerns regarding its use in adjuvant therapy.

A multicenter phase III trial has also demonstrated the efficacy of dexrazoxane in patients with advanced breast cancer treated with an epirubicin-containing regimen (82). Cardiotoxicity, defined as clinical signs of congestive heart failure, a decrease in resting LVEF to 45% or less, or a decrease from baseline resting LVEF of 20 or more EF units, was recorded in 23.1% of patients (18 of 78) in the control arm, but only in 7.3% in the dexrazoxane arm (6 of 82). The cumulative probability of developing cardiotoxicity was significantly lower in dexrazoxane-treated patients than in control patients (p = .006; odds ratio, 0.29; 95% confidence limit [CL], 0.09–0.78). Although the optimal cumulative dose of epirubicin at which dexrazoxane should be instituted is not known, some have suggested to use this agent when the cumulative dose of epirubicin reaches 550 mg/m^2 (83).

A meta-analysis of six randomized controlled trials (n = 1070) (83) indicated that the risk of experiencing clinical cardiotoxicity was significantly reduced by dexrazoxane (risk ratio [RR] 0.24, 95% CI 0.11–0.52; p = .00031). No significant benefit was shown in individual trials for objective response or survival except for the above-mentioned trial that showed a significantly lower objective response rate in the dexrazoxane arm. A meta-analysis of objective response across five different trials of breast cancer patients (n = 818) did not confirm this effect (odds ratio 0.85, 95% CI 0.61–1.18, p = .33). However, the use of dexrazoxane has been associated to an increased incidence of myelosuppression and other mild noncardiac toxicities.

The recommended dosage ratio of dexrazoxane for doxorubicin is 10:1 (e.g., 100 mg/m^2 of dexrazoxane to each 10 mg/m^2 of doxorubicin). However, dose should be adjusted in patients with renal insufficiency (creatine clearance <40 mL/min) to a 5:1 ratio.

Concurrent use of angiotensin-converting enzyme inhibitors (ACE-inhibitors), beta-blockers, or both may be able to prevent, delay, or slow the onset of clinically significant LEVF dysfunction. No large prospective, randomized clinical trial has been reported. A small randomized, single-blind, placebo-controlled trial of patients (n = 25) with different malignancies who were to receive an anthracycline-containing regimen (doxorubicin or epirubicin), demonstrated that carvedilol (12.5 mg once a day started before chemotherapy and maintained for 6 months during chemotherapy) had cardioprotective properties in this patient population (84). The 6-month follow-up mean LVEF of the carvedilol group was significantly higher (68.9% vs. 52.3%; p <.001) than the control group. A prospective study of 473 patients with different malignances who underwent high-dose chemotherapy and were evaluated for elevation of troponin I at baseline, immediately after, and 12, 24, 36, and 72 hours after the end of chemotherapy infusion identified 114 patients who showed an increase in troponin I level soon after high-dose chemotherapy (85). These patients were then randomized to receive 1 year of prophylactic enalapril (n = 56) or not (open-label control; n = 58). The primary end point was an absolute decrease more than 10% units in LVEF, with a decline below the normal limit value. The enalapril-treated group had significantly lower declines in LEVF and suffered fewer cardiac events (1 of 56 vs. 30 of 58, p <.001). This approach might be beneficial for those patients in whom an asymptomatic systolic dysfunction is detected early on during their adjuvant treatment, especially for those receiving adjuvant anti-ERBB2 (formerly HER2) therapies. Although the reduction in cardiac events from the above trials are impressive, larger multi-institutional, prospective, randomized, placebo-control trials are necessary before wide-spread use of ACE inhibitors for the prevention and treatment of chemotherapy-induced cardiomyopathy in at-risk population of breast cancer patients. Similarly, there is currently a need for data on the use of beta-blockers for the prevention and treatment of chemotherapy-induced cardiomyopathy.

Taxane Cardiotoxicity

Single-agent taxanes, in general, have not been associated with events such as cardiomyopathy or CHF except in conjunction with anti-ERBB2 therapy or concurrent anthracyclines use. Other cardiac events have been noted, however. Chest pain, myocardial infarction, hypotension, bradyarrhythmia, ventricular arrhythmia, and atrioventricular block have been reported with the infusion of paclitaxel (86–89). Docetaxel have been associated with similar adverse events, but with a much higher incidence of severe peripheral edema and fluid retention (90). Cardiac event related to albumin-bound paclitaxel have been similar to conventional paclitaxel (91).

Cardiotoxicity of Targeted Drugs (Trastuzumab, Lapatinib, Bevacizumab)

Trastuzumab is a recombinant DNA-derived humanized monoclonal antibody that selectively binds to the extracellular domain of the ERBB2 protein (92,93). Trastuzumab is indicated in combination with paclitaxel for first-line treatment and as a single agent for second- or third-line treatment of metastatic breast cancer as well as in the adjuvant setting in patients whose tumor overexpress the ERBB2 receptor (92). When used in combination with chemotherapy in the first-line treatment of metastatic breast cancer, trastuzumab improves response rate, response duration, time to progression, time to treatment failure, and median overall survival compared with treatment with chemotherapy alone (94–96). An unexpected adverse event observed during the pivotal trials of trastuzumab for advanced breast cancer was cardiac dysfunction (left ventricular systolic dysfunction and CHF) (96,98,99). A retrospective analysis of all data collected from seven of the most relevant phase II and III clinical trials using trastuzumab for metastatic breast cancer demonstrated that the incidence of cardiac dysfunction was greatest in patients receiving concomitant trastuzumab and anthracycline plus cyclophosphamide (27%) and it was substantially lower in patients receiving paclitaxel and trastuzumab (13%) or trastuzumab alone (3% to 7%) (98). The incidence of class III or IV cardiac dysfunction (New York Heart Association [NYHA] criteria for diagnosis of diseases of the heart) was 2% for patients receiving first-line trastuzumab, 4% for patients receiving trastuzumab in the refractory setting, 2% for those receiving concurrent paclitaxel plus trastuzumab, 1% for those receiving paclitaxel alone, 16% for patients receiving concurrent doxorubicin and cyclophosphamide (AC) plus

trastuzumab, and 4% for those receiving AC alone. The relative increased incidence of clinically evident cardiac events for patents randomized to the AC plus trastuzumab arm occurred after a cumulative dose of doxorubicin was greater than 300 mg/m². Most trastuzumab-treated patients developing cardiac dysfunction were symptomatic (75%), and most improved with standard treatment for CHF (79%). Because cardiac toxicity was not anticipated, cardiac monitoring was not performed in earlier clinical trials. Since the above data emerged, the monitoring of left ventricular function in all patients before and during trastuzumab treatment is now recommended, however, and the cardiac safety is currently being prospectively evaluated in several clinical trials using trastuzumab as well other targeted agents, such as lapatinib, bevacizumab, and other anti- vascular endothelial growth factor (VEGF) therapies.

As with the effects of chemotherapy in the neurocognitive function of breast cancer survivors, understanding the risks of cardiotoxicity with trastuzumab in the adjuvant setting is of critical importance. More than 13,000 patients with ERBB2-positive breast cancer have enrolled in trastuzumab adjuvant trials. Four large-scale, multicenter, randomized adjuvant trials of trastuzumab are being conducted: the North Central Cancer Treatment Group (NCCTG) Intergroup trial N9831, National Surgical Adjuvant Breast and Bowel Project (NSABP) trial B-31, Breast Cancer International Research Group trial (BCIRG) 006, and the HERA (Herceptin Adjuvant) trial. In the North American adjuvant trials N9831 and B-31, the use of trastuzumab in combination with paclitaxel led to a 52% reduction in the risk of breast cancer relapse and a 33% reduction in the risk of death (p = .015) (97).

The joint efficacy analysis of the N9831 and NSABP B-31 trials demonstrated that trastuzumab therapy was associated with a 3-year cumulative incidence of class III or IV CHF or death from cardiac causes of 4.1% in trial B-31 and 2.9% in trial N9831. A more recent detailed analysis of the 3,505 patients who participated in N9831 has been recently published by Perez et al. (100–102). Of those patients, 2,992 completed all four initial cycles of doxorubicin and cyclophosphamide. Of these, 5% (n = 151) had LVEF decreases disallowing trastuzumab-based therapy (decrease below normal: 2.4%, decrease >15%:2.6%). LVEF was measured at 6, 9, and 18 to 21 months postregistration. A total of 1,944 patients proceeded to post-AC therapy. Cardiac events (CHF or cardiac death [CD]) were noted in three patients (2 CHF, 1 CD) in arm A (AC followed by weekly paclitaxel × 12; control arm); 19 patients (18 CHF, 1 CD) in arm B (AC followed by weekly paclitaxel × 12 followed by trastuzumab for 52 weeks; sequential arm); and a similar number (all 19 CHF) in arm C (AC followed by weekly paclitaxel plus trastuzumab × 12 followed by trastuzumab alone × 40 weeks; concurrent arm). The 3-year cumulative incidence of cardiac events was 0.3%, 2.8%, and 3.3%, respectively. Cardiac function improved in most CHF cases following trastuzumab discontinuation and cardiac medication. Factors associated with increased risk of a cardiac event in arms B and C were older age (p <.003), prior or current antihypertensive agents (p = .005), and lower registration LVEF (p = .033). The incidence of asymptomatic LVEF decreases requiring holding trastuzumab was 8% to 10%; however, LVEF recovered and trastuzumab was restarted in approximately 50% of these patients.

A detailed analysis of the cardiotoxicity observed in the NSABP B-31 trial is also available (103). This trial compared standard AC followed by every-3-week paclitaxel with the same regimen plus 52 weekly infusions of trastuzumab beginning concurrently with paclitaxel in patients with node-positive, ERBB2-positive breast cancer. Initiation of trastuzumab required normal post-AC LVEF. Multi-gated acquisition (MUGA) scans were required in both treatment arms before entry, after AC, and at 6, 9, and 18 months. Of the 2,043 patients enrolled in the trial, 1,664 patients (81%) were included in this analysis. Among patients with normal post-AC LVEF who began post-AC treatment, 5 of 814 control patients subsequently had confirmed cardiac events (four CHF and one cardiac death) compared with 31 of 850 trastuzumab-treated patients (31 CHF and no cardiac deaths). Of these 31 patients, 26 were asymptomatic at the time of last assessment (6 months after diagnosis of CHF), and 18 remained on cardiac medication. The 3-year cumulative incidence of cardiac events was 0.8% (95% CI, 0.3%–1.9%) in the control arm compared with 4.1% (95% CI, 2.9%–5.8%) in the trastuzumab-treated evaluable patients. Congestive heart failures were more frequent in older patients and patients with marginal post-AC and LVEF. Fourteen percent of patients discontinued trastuzumab because of asymptomatic decreases in LVEF and 4% discontinued trastuzumab because of symptomatic cardiotoxicity.

The Breast Cancer International Research Group trial (BCIRG) 006 compared adjuvant standard AC chemotherapy for four cycles followed by a taxane (docetaxel every-3-week × 4 cycles) versus a similar regimen with concurrent taxane-trastuzumab versus a nonanthracycline regimen (docetaxel plus carboplatin with concurrent trastuzumab). Total length of anti-ERBB2 therapy is 52 weeks for both arms. In this trial, baseline LVEF was required to be 50% or greater after surgery and cardiac events were defined as cardiac death, CHF, grade 3 or 4 arrhythmias, or grade 3 or 4 cardiac ischemia or infarction. Different than the other studies, the BCIRG 006 had an upper age limits of 70 years, which may be an important issue related to cardiac safety of trastuzumab. The final analyses of the BCIRG 006 is not yet available, but preliminary results show that at a 2-year median follow-up, both experimental trastuzumab-containing arms showed significantly longer disease-free survival (DFS) compared with the nontrastuzumab control arm. Ten (0.95%) patients who received AC followed by docetaxel experienced clinically significant cardiac events compared with 25 (2.3%) who received AC followed by docetaxel and trastuzumab and 14 (1.3%) who received docetaxel in combination with carboplatin and trastuzumab (125). Three (0.3%) patients in the control arm experienced grade 3 or 4 CHF, compared with 17 (1.6%) in the AC followed by docetaxel plus trastuzumab arm and 4 (0.4%) in the docetaxel, carboplatin, and trastuzumab arm. No cardiac deaths occurred in any of the treatment arms, but four (0.4%) patients in the AC followed by docetaxel plus trastuzumab arm and one (0.1%) in the docetaxel, carboplatin and trastuzumab arm sustained grade 3 or 4 cardiac ischemia or infarction compared with no patients in the control arm. The above data suggest that the nonanthracycline regimen might be as effective but less cardiotoxic than treatment containing anthracycline-taxane-trastuzumab. More mature data are needed, however, to assess the long-term efficacy and safety of these regimens.

The HERA trial is a three-arm, multicenter, open-label randomized trial that compares 1 or 2 years of trastuzumab given once every 3 weeks with observation in patients with ERBB2–positive breast cancer who have completed at least four cycles of (neo)adjuvant chemotherapy (126). To be eligible, patients were required to have a LVEF 55% or greater after completion of chemotherapy and radiotherapy. LVEF was evaluated at baseline and at 3, 6, 12, 18, 24, 30, 36, and 60 months after randomization with either MUGA or echocardiography. All chemotherapy (and radiotherapy when appropriate) had to be completed before the initiation of trastuzumab. The mean time between completion of the chemotherapy and initiation of trastuzumab in this study was 89 days. Cardiac safety data were recently reported for 1,693 patients randomly assigned to 1 year trastuzumab and 1,693 patients randomly assigned to observation (127). The incidence of trastuzumab discontinuation owing to cardiac events was low (4.3%). The incidence of

severe CHF (0.60% vs. 0.00%; 95% CI for difference in incidence, 0.20%–0.99%), symptomatic CHF (2.15% vs. 0.12%; 95% CI for difference in incidence, 1.29%–2.77%), and confirmed significant LVEF drop (3.04% vs. 0.53%; 95% CI for difference in incidence, 1.59%–3.43%) was significantly higher in the trastuzumab group compared with observation. These patients who developed a trastuzumab-associated cardiac event had received a significantly higher mean cumulative dose of anthracycline (287 mg/m^2 vs. 257 mg/m^2 for doxorubicin and 480 mg/m^2 vs. 422 mg/m^2 for epirubicin), had a lower baseline LVEF, and a higher body mass index than those who did not. Most patients with cardiac dysfunction recovered in fewer than 6 months. Specifically, 6 of 10 patients with severe CHF recovered their LVEF at a median of 124 days (range, 36 to 409 days); 24 of 36 patients with symptomatic CHF recovered their LVEF at a median of 151 days (range, 26 to 831 days), and 35 of 51 patients with a confirmed significant LVEF drop recovered at a median of 191 days (range, 13 to 831 days). Although cross-study impressions are fraught with confounding factors, it appears that the incidence of cardiac events may be a bit lower in the HERA trial (1-year arm) than in the trastuzumab containing arms of NSABP B-31, N9831 (arm C), or BCIRG trials (severe CHF = 0.6% vs. 3.6% vs. 3.3% vs. 2.2% or 1.3%, respectively). This lower incidence of cardiotoxicity may be owing to the longer interval between the administration of chemotherapy and trastuzumab or to the difference in required baseline entry level of LVEF (55% of HERA vs. "normal" in the other trials) (128). The efficacy and safety data from the 2-year arm of the HERA trial and of arm B (sequential treatment arm) of the N9831 are eagerly awaited.

The use of trastuzumab before an anthracycline regimen in the adjuvant setting was investigated in two clinical trials, the Eastern Cooperative Oncology Group study 2198 (E2198) (129) and the FinHer trial (130). In E2198, 234 patients with stage II breast cancer were randomized either to paclitaxel (175 mg/m^2 every 3 weeks × 4 cycles) plus weekly trastuzumab for 10 cycles (4 mg/kg loading dose followed by 2 mg/kg × 9 weeks) followed by standard dose AC chemotherapy every 3 weeks for four cycles (arm A), or to the same regimen followed by trastuzumab for 52 weeks (arm B). At a median follow-up of 64 months, the DFS at 5 years was equivalent for arms A and B (76% vs. 73%, p = .55 log rank test). Overall survival at 5 years was also equivalent in the two arms (88% vs. 83%, p = 0.29 log rank test). Congestive heart failure was reported in seven patients, occurring at 2, 4, 9, 10, 14, 20, and 36 months following initiation of therapy (three in arm A, four in arm B). As noted in the previous larger adjuvant trials of trastuzumab, most CHF events occurred at an early point in time (4 of 7 within the first year, and none after 3 years), and the overall incidence was similar to N9831 and NSABP B-31. No cardiac-related deaths occurred. This trial did not show a significant advantage for prolonged trastuzumab administration. It was not designed to test this question, however. In the FinHer trial 1,010 women with axillary-node-positive or high-risk node-negative cancer were assigned to receive three cycles of docetaxel or vinorelbine, followed by (in both groups) three cycles of fluorouracil, epirubicin, and cyclophosphamide. There were 232 women whose tumors had an amplified ERBB2 gene and these patients were further assigned to receive or not to receive 9 weekly trastuzumab infusions along with docetaxel or vinorelbine. Within this subgroup of patients, those who received trastuzumab had better 3-year recurrence-free survival than those who did not receive the antibody (89% vs. 78%; HR for recurrence or death, 0.42; 95% CI, 0.21–0.83, p = 0.01) and did not have an increase of adverse cardiac events. On the contrary, patients receiving trastuzumab had a slightly better ejection fraction than those who did not receive trastuzumab. A decrease by more than 10 percentage points, resulting in an ejection fraction of less than 50%, occurred in only three patients, none of whom had received trastuzumab. The results of these two trials suggest that the combination of a taxane or vinorelbine and trastuzumab for 9 to 10 weeks followed by an anthracycline-based regimen were associated with a lower incidence of cardiac events (CHF) and similar risk reduction of relapse rate as observed in some of the larger trastuzumab-based adjuvant breast cancer trials. The main critique to the E2198 and the FinHer trials has been their small sample size, resulting in larger confidence intervals. Whether providing shorter-term trastuzumab before an anthracycline-based regimen is a strategy that can lead to less immediate and long-term cardiotoxicity, without sacrificing efficacy, is an approach that will require larger prospective, randomized trials.

An important area of research is to investigate potential mechanisms for trastuzumab-related cardiac toxicity, which has been summarized by Perez et al. and other investigators (100–103). Data from both *in vitro* and *in vivo* studies suggest that ERBB2 signaling is important in embryonic cardiac development and may be important in repair mechanisms after cardiac injury. Studies evaluating whether clinical parameters, genetic polymorphisms, and interaction with other comarked conditions, whether surrogates of toxicity (including functional magnetic resonance imaging [MRI] or blood test), may help with early identification, and allow for consideration of introduction of preventive strategies for those selected patients.

A compelling need exists to find reliable biochemical markers for the early detection of anthracyclines- and trastuzumab-induced cardiotoxicity. The use of cardiac biomarkers, such as brain natriuretic peptide (BNP), atrial natriuretic peptide, N-terminal proB-type natriuretic peptide, cardiac troponin I and T, creatinine kinase MB, heart-type fatty acid binding protein, glycogen phosphorylase BB, and carnitine, have been partially studied in pediatric and adult patients receiving an anthracycline- or trastuzumab-containing regimens (104–122). Some of these studies have shown that anthracycline and trastuzumab treatment is associated with acute and chronic neurohumoral activation of cardiac dysfunction that is manifested by an increase of some of these cardiac biomarkers. Such studies have failed, however, to consistently demonstrate their clinical utility in asymptomatic patients with early cardiac dysfunction. An analysis of cardiac biomarkers and LVEF indicated that BNP may be a predictive marker for early detection of cardiotoxicity associated to trastuzumab use, as demonstrated in the context of a subset of patients in the N9831 adjuvant study (123). For those patients who developed cardiotoxicity, defined as a drop in LVEF of 10% to 15% to less than the institutional lower limit of normal or a greater than 15% decline in LVEF, pretreatment BNP more than 40 mg/mL was seen in 21% of patients versus 8% of controls ($p = .18$), and subsequent doubling of BNP was seen in 27% of patients with cardiotoxicity versus 7% of controls ($p = .09$). These data can only be considered exploratory, however, because the study had several limitations, including a very small patient population (only 67 patients were able to be studied). That BNP concentrations are found to be positively correlated to cumulative dose of anthracyclines and negatively correlated to LVEF values was suggested in a small study of 70 patients treated with anthracyclines, trastuzumab, or both (124). Further prospective studies using more sensitive markers of cardiac damage are needed. Ongoing breast cancer adjuvant clinical trials using anthracyclines plus antivascular endothelial growth factor agents, trastuzumab or lapatinib are ideal settings to study potential predictive markers of early cardiotoxicity.

Lapatinib is an oral dual tyrosine kinase inhibitor targeting *EGFR1* and *EGFR2* (ERBB2). It has demonstrated to be active in trastuzumab-pretreated ERBB2-positive metastatic and inflammatory breast cancer as well as in brain metastases (131–134). It is indicated in combination with capecitabine for the treatment of ERBB2-overexpressing, advanced, or metastatic breast cancer in patients who have previously received an anthracycline, a taxane, and trastuzumab. The combination use of lapatinib and capecitabine significantly prolonged the time to disease progression (TTP) among patients with ERBB2-positive, locally advanced, or metastatic breast cancer who had progressed after prior treatments compared with capecitabine alone in a phase III, open-label, randomized trial (131,135). The potential benefits of this agent are both the convenience of oral administration and a possible lower incidence of cardiac toxicity compared with trastuzumab. Perez et al. (136) reviewed the cardiotoxicity data of lapatinib in 3,689 patients, including 2,275 breast cancer patients, treated with the drug alone or in combination with other agents. Evaluation of LVEF was done every 8 weeks while patients were receiving therapy. A total of 784 patients (21.3%) had more than 3 months exposure to lapatinib, 598 patients (16.8%) were previously treated with an anthracyclines, and 759 patients (21.3%) received prior trastuzumab therapy. Of these patients, 5% (n = 196) received lapatinib concurrently with trastuzumab and 60 patients (1.6%) developed a cardiac event. Asymptomatic cardiac events were reported in 53 patients (1.4%) and symptomatic cardiac events in 7 (0.2%). None of the 53 asymptomatic patients received any cardiac-related treatment. The other seven patients developed signs and symptoms of CHF that responded promptly to standard therapy with furosemide, corticosteroids, and diuretics, or diuretics and nitroglycerin. The mean baseline LVEF for the 60 patients who sustained a cardiac event was 61.6% ± 8.4% (range, 37% to 78%), the mean absolute LVEF decrease from baseline was 18.8% ± 5.2% (range, 11% to 32%), and mean nadir LVEF at the time of the event was 43% ± 6.7% (range, 20% to 54.5%). The mean time to onset of the event was 13 weeks ± 9 weeks (range, 2 to 54 weeks), and the mean duration of LVEF decrease was 7.6 weeks ± 10.4 weeks (range, 0.3 to 46 weeks). The mean absolute LVEF decrease from baseline for the symptomatic patients was 23.7% ± 5.2% (range, 14.5% to 32%) and the mean decrease relative to baseline was 35.5% ± 8.6% (range, 25% to 51.6%). Follow-up data were available in 35 of those 60 patients. All recovered from the cardiac event (full = 19; partial = 16). A relationship between lapatinib use and prior anthracyclines use and cardiac events was not established, although this may be related to the low incidence of cardiac events observed.

Considering the potential advantages of lapatinib over trastuzumab and to maximize anti-ERBB2 therapy in the adjuvant setting, a global four-arm, multicenter, open-label randomized trial that compares standard 1 year of trastuzumab versus lapatinib, trastuzumab plus sequential lapatinib, or the combination of both agents, is currently undergoing. The Adjuvant Lapatinib and/or Trastuzumab Treatment Optimisation (ALTTO) trial (also known as N063D and BIG2-06 trial) aims to accrue 8,000 patients who will receive adjuvant anthracycline treatment followed by anti-ERBB2 therapy, with or without paclitaxel. Special emphasis has been put in place for the long-term evaluation of cardiac safety in these patients. LVEF assessment will be performed at baseline and every 3 months for the first year, every 6 months during the second and third year, and yearly thereafter up to year 10 after randomization. It will be the largest and probably most comprehensive study of cardiotoxicity of any adjuvant chemotherapy trial (www.alltotrials.com).

Bevacizumab is a humanized monoclonal antibody directed against all isoforms of the vascular endothelial growth factor (VEGF) (137). It is active in combination with standard chemotherapy in the treatment of advanced colon, lung, brain, and breast cancers (138–143) and as a single agent in renal cell cancer (144). Pooled data from randomized, controlled clinical trials have shown an overall increased risk of arterial hypertension (12% to 34% for all grades), arterial thromboembolic events (4.4% to 8.5%), congestive heart failure (1.7% to 4%), and deep vein thrombosis (6% to 9%) in patients receiving bevacizumab plus chemotherapy compared with patients receiving chemotherapy alone (137). Its efficacy and tolerability in breast cancer was demonstrated in the E2100 trial, a randomized phase III trial of bevacizumab plus paclitaxel versus paclitaxel alone as first-line therapy in metastatic breast cancer (140). A total of 722 patients were enrolled. Paclitaxel plus bevacizumab significantly prolonged progression-free survival as compared with paclitaxel alone (median, 11.8 vs. 5.9 months; HR for progression, 0.60; $p <$.001) and increased the objective response rate (36.9% vs. 21.2%, $p <$.001). The overall survival rate, however, was similar in the two groups (median, 26.7 vs. 25.2 months; HR, 0.88; $p = $.16). Hypertension and thromboembolic events were more common in patients receiving bevacizumab. A significant increase was seen in cerebrovascular ischemia among patients receiving bevacizumab-based therapy (1.9% vs. 0.0%, $p = $.02).

A pilot study was recently conducted to assess the safety and feasibility of combining bevacizumab and anthracyclines in the adjuvant setting. E2104 was a two-arm, nonrandomized phase II trial where 226 patients were sequentially assigned to one of two treatment arms (145). All patients received doxorubicin and cyclophosphamide followed by paclitaxel, with bevacizumab (10 mg/kg every 2 weeks × 26) being initiated concurrently with AC (arm A; n = 103) and concurrently with paclitaxel (arm B; n = 120). The primary end point was the incidence of clinically apparent cardiac dysfunction (CHF). Median follow-up was 9.1 months for arm A and 5.3 months for arm B. Episodes of CHF occurred in both arms of the study, but patients who initiated bevacizumab concurrently with AC had the highest incidence of clinical CHF (4 vs. 2 patients), LVEF decline 10% or more (26 vs. 19 patients), and LVEF below 50% (11 vs. 6 patients). This proof of concept trial led the way to a large prospective phase III adjuvant clinical trial, E5103, which plans to randomize 4,950 patients in one of three arms that use a sequential anthracycline (AC every 2 or 3 weeks) and taxane (weekly paclitaxel × 12) chemotherapy backbone with or without concurrent bevacizumab (every 2 to 3 weeks). Some patients subsequently are going to be randomized to observation versus maintenance bevacizumab (every 3 weeks × 10). Only a large trial such as this can fully define the safety and feasibility of bevacizumab in the adjuvant setting.

Other Cardiotoxic Effects of Anti-neoplastic Agents

Several other nonanthracycline agents have been linked to cardiotoxic events, but in very few of them can the mechanisms of cardiotoxicity be firmly established. The agents with relevance in the treatment of breast cancer include fluorouracil (5FU) and capecitabine (CHF, arrhythmias, coronary spasm, ischemia or myocardial infarction, and sudden death) (146–153), methotrexate (pericarditis, CHF, arrhythmias, thrombosis, and ischemia or myocardial infarction) (154), high-dose cyclophosphamide (heart block, tachyarrhythmia, hemorrhagic myopericarditis, and CHF) (155), cisplatin (bradyarrhythmia, cardiomyopathy, and myocardial infarction) (156–160), and vinorelbine (myocardial infarction) (161–164).

SUMMARY

The cardiac safety data of different adjuvant agents continues to be explored, but long-term follow-up studies are necessary to understand the potential causal effects of therapy accurately, in the context of aging of the population and other confounding factors. Some of the newer trials incorporate evaluating potential predictive serum markers and studies of single nucleotide polymorphisms that may shed light into this issue.

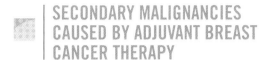

SECONDARY MALIGNANCIES CAUSED BY ADJUVANT BREAST CANCER THERAPY

Although the long-term risk of secondary malignancies after adjuvant therapy for early breast cancer remains much lower than the previously discussed side effects, it is often a devastating outcome for those afflicted by them. By far the most common events are the onset of myelodysplastic syndrome (MDS), characterized by abnormal marrow cytogenetics and an almost inevitably evolution into acute myelogenous leukemia (AML), and secondary acute leukemia with poor prognosis and characterized by refractoriness to standard induction therapy. Such leukemogenic potential is caused by the use of alkylating agents (cyclophosphamide) and topoisomerase II inhibitors (anthracyclines). In general, such risk is approximately 1% or less and seems directly related to the chemotherapy agent being used, its dose, and length of therapy (165,166). A retrospective review of 8,563 women who participated in six of the adjuvant NSABP breast cancer trials (B-15, B-16, B-18, B-22, B-23, and B-25) (167) that tested regimens containing both doxorubicin and cyclophosphamide (AC) showed that in patients receiving two or four cycles of cyclophosphamide at 2,400 mg/m^2 with granulocyte colony-stimulating factor (G-CSF) support, the cumulative incidence of AML or MDS at 5 years was 1.01% (95% CI, 0.63%–1.62%), compared with 0.21% (95% CI, 0.11%–0.41%) for patients treated with standard AC. Similar findings were observed in a French study of 9,796 patients randomized into 19 trials of adjuvant chemotherapy (166). Most patients received an epirubicin- (n = 7,110) and cyclophosphamide- (n = 6541) based regimen. The risk of developing AML or MDS increased in relation to planned epirubicin dose per cycle, planned epirubicin dose intensity, and administered cumulative doses of epirubicin and cyclophosphamide. Patients with administered cumulative doses of both epirubicin and cyclophosphamide not exceeding those used in standard regimens (≤720 mg/m^2 and ≤6,300 mg/m^2, respectively) had an 8-year cumulative probability of developing AML or MDS of 0.37% (95% CI, 0.13%–0.61%) compared with 4.97% (95% CI, 2.06%–7.87%) for patients administered higher cumulative doses of both epirubicin and cyclophosphamide. A retrospective analysis of 2,638 patients with previously untreated primary operable breast cancer who were treated in six clinical trials conducted by the ECOG between 1978 and 1987 demonstrated, however, that the estimated incidence rate for MDS and acute leukemia was 26 per 100,000 person-years of follow-up study (95% CI, 8–61 per 100,000 person-years) (168). The authors concluded that the risk of secondary AML or MDS among these patients with early breast cancer who received standard-dose cyclophosphamide-containing adjuvant chemotherapy was not much higher than in the general population.

Older chemotherapeutic agents, such as melphalan and mitoxantrone, used in breast cancer treatment were associated with an increased risk of developing MDS or AML (165,169–171). However, no data exist of an increased risk of MDS or AML with taxanes, but we hope the current CALGB 40101 trial, comparing standard dose AC regimen versus single agent paclitaxel in the adjuvant setting, will help answer such question. The leukemogenic effect of other agents, such as growth factors (G-CSF, or granulocyte monocyte colony stimulating factor, GM-CSF) is controversial. A study from

SEER Medicare database of 5,510 women age 65 years or older with stages I-III breast cancer who received G-CSF or GM-CSF concurrently with chemotherapy demonstrated that 16 (1.77%) of the 906 patients who were treated with G-CSF developed MDS or AML compared with 48 (1.04%) of 4,604 patients who did not (HR 2.14) (172). In the NSABP B-25 adjuvant trial (173), which accrued 2,545 node-positive women who were randomized to receive standard doxorubicin (60 mg/m^2) with escalated or intensified doses of cyclophosphamide (1,200 mg/m^2 plus G-CSF for four cycles, cyclophosphamide 2,400 mg/m^2 plus G-CSF for two cycles, or cyclophosphamide 2,400 mg/m^2 plus G-CSF for four cycles), it was suggested that G-CSF may possibly be independently correlated with an increased risk of MDS or AML, especially when a higher dose of this drug was administered. Of the patients diagnosed with AML or MDS, 72% (n = 25) had received cumulative G-CSF doses higher than the median dose (167). However, such findings might be more a reflection of the higher dose of chemotherapy used than an effect of the growth factor support *per se*. An increased risk of MDS or AML was not observed in the intergroup trial C9741 (adjuvant standard vs. dose-dense chemotherapy in node-positive breast cancer) among women who received prophylactic G-CSF in the dose-dense arm and those who did not in the standard every-3-weeks arms (174).

The risk of MDS and acute leukemia are increased if adjuvant radiation therapy is utilized (167,175). A retrospective study of 1,474 patients with stage II or III breast cancer who participated in six prospective trials of adjuvant, or neoadjuvant chemotherapy with fluorouracil, doxorubicin, and cyclophosphamide, with or without other drugs, demonstrated that the 10-year estimated leukemia rate was 1.5% (95% CI, 0.7%–2.9%) for all patients treated, 2.5% (95% CI, 1.0%–5.1%) for the radiotherapy-plus-chemotherapy group, and 0.5% (95% CI, 0.1%–2.4%) for the chemotherapy-only group ($p = .01$). The use of radiation therapy for breast cancer has also been associated with a slight increased risk of contralateral breast cancer (RR, 1.18–1.33) (176,177), soft tissue sarcomas (15-year cumulative incidence rate of 3.2 per 1,000) (178), lung (especially in smokers; 10- and 15-year RR was 2.0 and 2.8, respectively) (179–181) and esophageal cancer (standardized incidence ratio of 1.1–2.0) (182,183).

SUMMARY

Data to date demonstrate a very modest potential risk of secondary malignancies related to currently used doses of adjuvant therapies for breast cancer.

CONCLUSIONS

The beneficial effects of early detection and use of adjuvant therapies for cancer have allowed for an increased number of survivors, and has enhanced our ability to identify potential long-term effects. Proper methodology to quantify those effects has not been easy to utilize, because of the changing nature of the treatments, the fact that just a few patients have been invited or have elected to participate in studies of long-term, noncancer outcomes, and the many confounding factors, including aging, other medications, and even cancer recurrence, which may impair understanding of the true effects of systemic anticancer treatments. At least we can confirm that newer studies are attempting to individualize treatments (to avoid unnecessary drug exposures), minimizing doses that may adversely affect persons, and trying to use proper methodology to minimize acute and long-term adverse effects of treatment.

References

1. Ries L, Melbert D, Krapcho M, et al. SEER Cancer Statistics Review. *National Cancer Institute* 2008;(11):1975–2005.
2. Surveillance E. End Results (SEER) Program. SEER* Stat Database: incidence—SEER 17 Regs Limited Use. *National Cancer Institute*, 2006. DCCPS (Surveillance Research Program).
3. Ahles TA, Saykin AJ, Furstenberg CT, et al. Neuropsychologic impact of standard-dose systemic chemotherapy in long-term survivors of breast cancer and lymphoma. *J Clin Oncol* 2002;20(2):485–493.
4. Brezden CB, Phillips KA, Abdolell M, et al. Cognitive function in breast cancer patients receiving adjuvant chemotherapy. *J Clin Oncol*, 2000;18(14):2695–2701.
5. Schagen SB, Muller MJ, Boogerd W, et al. Late effects of adjuvant chemotherapy on cognitive function: a follow-up study in breast cancer patients. *Ann Oncol* 2002;13(9):1387–1397.
6. Schagen SB, van Dam FS, Muller MJ, et al. Cognitive deficits after postoperative adjuvant chemotherapy for breast carcinoma. *Cancer* 1999;85(3):640–650.
7. Tchen N, Juffs HG, Downie FP, et al. Cognitive function, fatigue, and menopausal symptoms in women receiving adjuvant chemotherapy for breast cancer. *J Clin Oncol* 2003;21(22):4175–4183.
8. van Dam FS, Schagen SB, Muller MJ, et al. Impairment of cognitive function in women receiving adjuvant treatment for high-risk breast cancer: high-dose versus standard-dose chemotherapy. *J Natl Cancer Inst* 1998;90(3):210–218.
9. Wieneke M, Dienst E. Neuropsychological Assessment of Cognitive Functioning Following Chemotherapy for Breast Cancer. *Psycho-Oncology*, 1995;4:61–66.
10. Scherwath A, Mehnert A, Schleimer B, et al. Neuropsychological function in high-risk breast cancer survivors after stem-cell supported high-dose therapy versus standard-dose chemotherapy: evaluation of long-term treatment effects. *Ann Oncol* 2006;17(3):415–423.
11. Castellon SA, Ganz PA, Bower JE, et al. Neurocognitive performance in breast cancer survivors exposed to adjuvant chemotherapy and tamoxifen. *J Clin Exp Neuropsychol* 2004;26(7):955–969.
12. Wefel JS, Lenzi R, Theriault RL, et al. The cognitive sequelae of standard-dose adjuvant chemotherapy in women with breast carcinoma: results of a prospective, randomized, longitudinal trial. *Cancer* 2004;100(11):2292–2299.
13. Bender C, Sereika S, Berga S, et al. Cognitive Impairment Associated with Adjuvant Therapy in Breast Cancer. *Psycho-Oncology* 2006;5:422–430.
14. Shilling V, Jenkins V, Morris R, et al. The effects of adjuvant chemotherapy on cognition in women with breast cancer—preliminary results of an observational longitudinal study. *Breast* 2005;14(2):142–150.
15. Hurria A, Rosen C, Hudis C, et al. Cognitive function of older patients receiving adjuvant chemotherapy for breast cancer: a pilot prospective longitudinal study. *J Am Geriatr Soc* 2006;54(6):925–931.
16. Schagen SB, Muller MJ, Boogerd W, et al. Change in cognitive function after chemotherapy: a prospective longitudinal study in breast cancer patients. *J Natl Cancer Inst* 2006;98(23):1742–1745.
17. Jenkins V, Shilling V, Deutsch G, et al. A 3-year prospective study of the effects of adjuvant treatments on cognition in women with early stage breast cancer. *Br J Cancer* 2006;94(6):828–834.
18. Donovan KA, Small BJ, Andrykowski MA, et al. Cognitive functioning after adjuvant chemotherapy and/or radiotherapy for early-stage breast carcinoma. *Cancer* 2005;104(11):2499–2507.
19. Falleti MG, Sanfilippo A, Maruff P, et al. The nature and severity of cognitive impairment associated with adjuvant chemotherapy in women with breast cancer: a meta-analysis of the current literature. *Brain Cogn* 2005;59(1):60–70.
20. Stewart A, Bielajew C, Collins B, et al. A meta-analysis of the neuropsychological effects of adjuvant chemotherapy treatment in women treated for breast cancer. *Clin Neuropsychol* 2006;20(1):76–89.
21. Bower JE, Ganz PA, Desmond KA, et al. Fatigue in breast cancer survivors: occurrence, correlates, and impact on quality of life. *J Clin Oncol* 2000;18(4):743–753.
22. Broeckel JA, Jacobsen PB, Horton J, et al. Characteristics and correlates of fatigue after adjuvant chemotherapy for breast cancer. *J Clin Oncol* 1998;16(5):1689–1696.
23. de Jong N, Candel MJ, Schouten HC, et al. Prevalence and course of fatigue in breast cancer patients receiving adjuvant chemotherapy. *Ann Oncol* 2004;15(6):896–905.
24. Valentine AD, Meyers CA. Cognitive and mood disturbance as causes and symptoms of fatigue in cancer patients. *Cancer* 2001;92(6 Suppl):1694–1698.
25. Knobf MT. Physical and psychologic distress associated with adjuvant chemotherapy in women with breast cancer. *J Clin Oncol* 1986;4(5):678–684.
26. Lee-Jones C, Humphris G, Dixon R, et al. Fear of Cancer Recurrence—A Literature Review and Proposed Cognitive Formulation to Explain Exacerbation fo Recurrence Fears. *Psycho-Oncology* 1997;6:95–105.
27. Schmidt JE, Andrykowski MA. The role of social and dispositional variables associated with emotional processing in adjustment to breast cancer: an internet-based study. *Health Psychol* 2004;23(3):259–266.
28. Bender CM, Paraska KK, Sereika SM, et al. Cognitive function and reproductive hormones in adjuvant therapy for breast cancer: a critical review. *J Pain Symptom Manage* 2001;21(5):407–424.
29. Bender CM, Sereika SM, Brufsky AM, et al. Memory impairments with adjuvant anastrozole versus tamoxifen in women with early-stage breast cancer. *Menopause* 2007;14(6):995–998.
30. Drew SV. Cognitive function after HRT. *Lancet* 2001;357(9256):641.
31. Jenkins V, Atkins L, Fallowfield L. Does endocrine therapy for the treatment and prevention of breast cancer affect memory and cognition? *Eur J Cancer* 2007;43(9):1342–1347.
32. Jenkins V, Shilling V, Fallowfield L, et al. Does hormone therapy for the treatment of breast cancer have a detrimental effect on memory and cognition? A pilot study. *Psycho-Oncology* 2004;13:61–66.
33. LeBlanc ES, Janowsky J, Chan BK, et al. Hormone replacement therapy and cognition: systematic review and meta-analysis. *JAMA* 2001;285(11):1489–1499.
34. Shilling V, Jenkins V, Fallowfield L, et al. The effects of oestrogens and anti-oestrogens on cognition. *Breast* 2001;10(6):484–491.
35. Yaffe K, Lui LY, Grady D, et al. Cognitive decline in women in relation to non-protein-bound oestradiol concentrations. *Lancet* 2000;356(9231):708–712.

36. Dietrich J, Han R, Yang Y, et al. CNS progenitor cells and oligodendrocytes are targets of chemotherapeutic agents *in vitro* and *in vivo*. *J Biol* 2006;5(7):22.

37. Hoffmeyer S, Burk O, von Richter O, et al. Functional polymorphisms of the human multidrug-resistance gene: multiple sequence variations and correlation of one allele with P-glycoprotein expression and activity in vivo. *Proc Natl Acad Sci U S A* 2000;97(7):3473–3478.

38. Kreb R. Implications of genetic polymorphisms in drug transporters for pharmacotherapy. *Cancer Letter* 2006;234:4–33.

39. Blasiak J, Arabski M, Krupa R, et al. Basal, oxidative and alkylative DNA damage, DNA repair efficacy and mutagen sensitivity in breast cancer. *Mutat Res* 2004;554(1–2):139–148.

40. Fishel ML, Vasko MR, Kelley MR. DNA repair in neurons: so if they don't divide what's to repair? *Mutat Res* 2007;614(1–2):24–36.

41. Rolig R, McKinnon P. Linking DNA damage and neurodegeneration. *Trends Neurosci* 2005;23:417–424.

42. Ahles T, Saykin A, Noll W, et al. The relationship of APOE genotype to neuropsychological performance in long-term cancer survivors treated with standard dose chemotherapy. *Psycho-Oncology* 2003;12:612–619.

43. Alici-Evcimen Y, Breitbart W. Ifosfamide neuropsychiatric toxicity in patients with cancer. *Psycho-Oncology* 2007;16:956–960.

44. Brunello A, Basso U, Rossi E, et al. Ifosfamide-related encephalopathy in elderly patients:report of five cases and review of the literature. *Drugs Aging* 2007; 24(11):967–973.

45. Choi SM, Lee SH, Yang YS, et al. Cho, 5-fluorouracil-induced leukoencephalopathy in patients with breast cancer. *J Korean Med Sci* 2001;16(3):328–334.

46. Jansen C, Miaskowski C, Dodd M, et al. Potential mechanisms for chemotherapy-induced impairments in cognitive function. *Oncol Nurs Forum* 2005;32(6): 1151–1163.

47. Lopes MA, Meisel A, Dirnagl U, et al. Doxorubicin induces biphasic neurotoxicity to rat cortical neurons. *Neurotoxicology* 2008;29(2):286–293.

48. Tuxen MK, Hansen SW. Neurotoxicity secondary to antineoplastic drugs. *Cancer Treat Rev* 1994;20(2):191–214.

49. Verstappen CC, Heimans JJ, Hoekman K, et al. Neurotoxic complications of chemotherapy in patients with cancer: clinical signs and optimal management. *Drugs* 2003;63(15):1549–1563.

50. Farkas E, De Jong GI, de Vos RA, et al. Pathological features of cerebral cortical capillaries are doubled in Alzheimer's disease and Parkinson's disease. *Acta Neuropathol* 2000;100(4):395–402.

51. Cerami A, Brines M, Ghezzi P, et al. Effects of epoetin alfa on the central nervous system. Seminars in Oncology 2001;28(Supplement 8 Number 2):66–70.

52. Fernando MS, Simpson JE, Matthews F, et al. White matter lesions in an unselected cohort of the elderly: molecular pathology suggests origin from chronic hypoperfusion injury. *Stroke* 2006;37(6):1391–1398.

53. Hare G. Anemia and the Brain. *Current Opinion in Anaesthesiology* 2004; 17(5):363–369.

54. Silverman DH, Dy CJ, Castellon SA, et al. Altered frontocortical, cerebellar, and basal ganglia activity in adjuvant-treated breast cancer survivors 5–10 years after chemotherapy. *Breast Cancer Res Treat* 2007;103(3):303–311.

55. Bower JE, Ganz PA, Aziz N, et al. Fatigue and proinflammatory cytokine activity in breast cancer survivors. *Psychosom Med* 2002;64(4):604–611.

56. Collado-Hidalgo A, Bower JE, Ganz PA, et al. Inflammatory biomarkers for persistent fatigue in breast cancer survivors. *Clin Cancer Res* 2006;12(9): 2759–2766.

57. Lee BN, Dantzer R, Langley KE, et al. A cytokine based neuroimmunologic mechanism of cancer-related symptoms. *Neuroimmunomodulation* 2004;11(5): 279–292.

58. Minghetti L. Role of COX-2 in inflammatory and degenerative brain diseases. *Subcell Biochem* 2007;42:127–141.

59. Reichenberg A, Yirmiya R, Schuld A, et al. Cytokine-associated emotional and cognitive disturbances in humans. *Arch Gen Psychiatry* 2001;58(5):445–452.

60. Wilson CJ, Finch CE, Cohen HJ. Cytokines and cognition—the case for a head-to-toe inflammatory paradigm. *J Am Geriatr Soc* 2002;50(12):2041–2056.

61. Eberling JL, Wu C, Tong-Turnbeaugh R, et al. Estrogen- and tamoxifen-associated effects on brain structure and function. *Neuroimage* 2004;21(1):364–371.

62. Saykin A. Altered brain activation following systemic chemotherapy for breast cancer: interim analysis from a prospective study. *Journal of the International Neuropsychological Society* 2006;12:131.

63. Hoff V, Layard M, Basa P. Risk factors for doxorubicin-induced congestive heart failure. *Ann Int Med* 1979;91:710–717.

64. Steinherz LJ, Steinherz PG, Tan CT, et al. Cardiac toxicity 4 to 20 years after completing anthracycline therapy. *JAMA* 1991;266(12):1672–1677.

65. Arola OJ, Saraste A, Pulkki K, et al. Voipio-Pulkki, Acute doxorubicin cardiotoxicity involves cardiomyocyte apoptosis. *Cancer Res* 2000;60(7):1789–1792.

66. Gianni L, Myers C. The role of free radical formation in teh cardiotoxicity of anthracycline Muggia F. M. Green M.D. Speyer J. L eds. *Cancer Treat Heart* 1992:9–46.

67. Saraste A, Pulkki K, Kallajoki M, et al. Apoptosis in human acute myocardial infarction. *Circulation* 1997;95(2):320–323.

68. Swain SM, Whaley FS, Ewer MS. Congestive heart failure in patients treated with doxorubicin: a retrospective analysis of three trials. *Cancer* 2003;97(11): 2869–2879.

69. Pinder MC, Duan Z, Goodwin JS, et al. Congestive heart failure in older women treated with adjuvant anthracycline chemotherapy for breast cancer. *J Clin Oncol* 2007;25(25):3808–3815.

70. Ganz PA, Hussey MA, Moinpour CM, et al. Late cardiac effects of adjuvant chemotherapy in breast cancer survivors treated on Southwest Oncology Group protocol s8897. *J Clin Oncol* 2008;26(8):1223–1230.

71. Minotti G, Licata S, Saponiero A, et al. Anthracycline metabolism and toxicity in human myocardium: comparisons between doxorubicin, epirubicin, and a novel disaccharide analogue with a reduced level of formation and [4Fe-4S] reactivity of its secondary alcohol metabolite. *Chem Res Toxicol* 2000;13(12): 1336–1341.

72. Gasparini G, Dal Fior S, Panizzoni GA, et al. Weekly epirubicin versus doxorubicin as second line therapy in advanced breast cancer. A randomized clinical trial. *Am J Clin Oncol* 1991;14(1):38–44.

73. Hortobagyi GN, Frye D, Buzdar AU, et al. Decreased cardiac toxicity of doxorubicin administered by continuous intravenous infusion in combination chemotherapy for metastatic breast carcinoma. *Cancer* 1989;63(1):37–45.

74. Kimmick G, Shelton B, Case L, et al. Long-term follow-up of a phase II trial studying a weekly doxorubicin-based multiple drug adjuvant therapy for stage II node-positive carcinoma of the breast. *Breast Cancer Res Treat* 2002;72(3):233–243.

75. Umsawasdi T, Valdivieso M, Booser DJ, et al. Weekly doxorubicin versus doxorubicin every 3 weeks in cyclophosphamide, doxorubicin, and cisplatin chemotherapy for non-small cell lung cancer. *Cancer* 1989;64(10):1995–2000.

76. Billingham ME, Bristow MR, Glatstein E, et al. Adriamycin cardiotoxicity: endomyocardial biopsy evidence of enhancement by irradiation. *Am J Surg Pathol* 1977;1(1):17–23.

77. Batist G. Cardiac safety of liposomal anthracyclines. *Cardiovasc Toxicol* 2007; 7(2):72–74.

78. O'Brien ME, Wigler N, Inbar M, et al. Reduced cardiotoxicity and comparable efficacy in a phase III trial of pegylated liposomal doxorubicin HCl (CAELYX/Doxil) versus conventional doxorubicin for first-line treatment of metastatic breast cancer. *Ann Oncol* 2004;15(3):440–449.

79. Safra T, Muggia F, Jeffers S, et al. Pegylated liposomal doxorubicin (doxil): reduced clinical cardiotoxicity in patients reaching or exceeding cumulative doses of 500 mg/m^2. *Ann Oncol* 2000;11(8):1029–1033.

80. Zinecard$^®$, [Prescribing Information]. Pharmacia & Upjohn Company, 2005.

81. Swain SM, Whaley FS, Gerber MC, et al. Delayed administration of dexrazoxane provides cardioprotection for patients with advanced breast cancer treated with doxorubicin-containing therapy. *J Clin Oncol* 1997;15(4):1333–1340.

82. Venturini M, Michelotti A, Del Mastro L, et al. Multicenter randomized controlled clinical trial to evaluate cardioprotection of dexrazoxane versus no cardioprotection in women receiving epirubicin chemotherapy for advanced breast cancer. *J Clin Oncol* 1996;14(12):3112–3120.

83. Seymour L, Bramwell V, Moran LA. Use of dexrazoxane as a cardioprotectant in patients receiving doxorubicin or epirubicin chemotherapy for the treatment of cancer. The Provincial Systemic Treatment Disease Site Group. *Cancer Prev Control* 1999;3(2):145–159.

84. Kalay N, Basar E, Ozdogru I, et al. Protective effects of carvedilol against anthracycline-induced cardiomyopathy. *J Am Coll Cardiol* 2006;48(11):2258–2262.

85. Cardinale D, Colombo A, Sandri MT, et al. Prevention of high-dose chemotherapy-induced cardiotoxicity in high-risk patients by angiotensin-converting enzyme inhibition. *Circulation* 2006;114(23):2474–2481.

86. Taxol$^®$, Paclitaxel [Prescribing Information]. Bristol-Myers Squibb Company, 2003.

87. Hekmat E. Fatal myocardial infarction potentially induced by paclitaxel. *Ann Pharmacother* 1996;30(10):1110–1112.

88. McGuire WP, Rowinsky EK, Rosenshein NB, et al. Taxol: a unique antineoplastic agent with significant activity in advanced ovarian epithelial neoplasms. *Ann Intern Med* 1989;111(4):273–279.

89. Rowinsky EK, Cazenave LA, Donehower RC. Taxol: a novel investigational antimicrotubule agent. *J Natl Cancer Inst* 1990;82(15):1247–1259.

90. Taxotere$^®$ [Prescribing Information]. Aventis Pharmaceuticals Inc., 2006.

91. Abraxane$^®$ [Prescribing Information]. American Pharmaceutical Partners, Inc., 2005.

92. Herceptin$^®$ [Prescribing Information]. Genentech, Inc., 2006.

93. Coussens L, Yang-Feng TL, Liao YC, et al. Tyrosine kinase receptor with extensive homology to EGF receptor shares chromosomal location with neu oncogene. *Science* 1985;230(4730):1132–1139.

94. Cobleigh MA, Vogel CL, Tripathy D, et al. Multinational study of the efficacy and safety of humanized anti-HER2 monoclonal antibody in women who have HER2-overexpressing metastatic breast cancer that has progressed after chemotherapy for metastatic disease. *J Clin Oncol* 1999;17(9):2639–2648.

95. Norton L, Slamon D, Leyland-Jones B, et al. Overall survival (OS) advantage to simultaneous chemotherapy (CRx) plus the humanized anti-HER2 monoclonal antibody Herceptin (H) in HER2-overexpressing (HER2+) metastatic breast cancer (MBC). *Proc Am Soc Clin Oncol* 1999;18:127a.

96. Slamon DJ, Leyland-Jones B, Shak S, et al. Use of chemotherapy plus a monoclonal antibody against HER2 for metastatic breast cancer that overexpresses HER2. *N Engl J Med* 2001;344(11):783–792.

97. Romond EH, Perez EA, Bryant J, et al. Trastuzumab plus adjuvant chemotherapy for operable HER2-positive breast cancer. *N Engl J Med* 2005;353(16): 1673–1684.

98. Seidman A, Hudis C, Pierri MK, et al. Cardiac dysfunction in the trastuzumab clinical trials experience. *J Clin Oncol* 2002;20(5):1215–1221.

99. Vogel CL, Cobleigh MA, Tripathy D, et al. Efficacy and safety of trastuzumab as a single agent in first-line treatment of HER2-overexpressing metastatic breast cancer. *J Clin Oncol* 2002;20(3):719–726.

100. Perez E, Morgan J. Cardiotoxicity of Trastuzumab. *UpToDate* 2008;16.1(January 31):1–22.

101. Perez EA. Cardiac Toxicity of ErbB2-targeted therapies: What do we know? *Clin Breast Cancer* 2008;8(Supplement 3):S114–S120.

102. Perez EA, Suman VJ, Davidson NE, et al. Cardiac safety analysis of doxorubicin and cyclophosphamide followed by paclitaxel with or without trastuzumab in the North Central Cancer Treatment Group N9831 adjuvant breast cancer trial. *J Clin Oncol* 2008;26(8):1231–1238.

103. Tan-Chiu E, Yothers G, Romond E, et al. Assessment of cardiac dysfunction in a randomized trial comparing doxorubicin and cyclophosphamide followed by paclitaxel, with or without trastuzumab as adjuvant therapy in node-positive, human epidermal growth factor receptor 2-overexpressing breast cancer: NSABP B-31. *J Clin Oncol* 2005;23(31):7811–7819.

104. Auner HW, Tinchon C, Linkesch W, et al. Prolonged monitoring of troponin T for the detection of anthracycline cardiotoxicity in adults with hematological malignancies. *Ann Hematol* 2003;82(4):218–222.

105. Bryant J, Picot J, Baxter L, et al. Use of cardiac markers to assess the toxic effects of anthracyclines given to children with cancer: a systematic review. *Eur J Cancer* 2007;43(13):1959–1966.

106. Cardinale D, Sandri MT, Martinoni A, et al. Myocardial injury revealed by plasma troponin I in breast cancer treated with high-dose chemotherapy. *Ann Oncol* 2002;13(5):710–715.

107. Cardinale D, Sandri MT, Martinoni A, et al. Left ventricular dysfunction predicted by early troponin I release after high-dose chemotherapy. *J Am Coll Cardiol* 2000;36(2):517–522.

108. Ekstein S, Nir A, Rein AJ, et al. N-terminal-proB-type natriuretic peptide as a marker for acute anthracycline cardiotoxicity in children. *J Pediatr Hematol Oncol* 2007;29(7):440–444.

109. Fink FM, Genser N, Fink C, et al. Cardiac troponin T and creatine kinase MB mass concentrations in children receiving anthracycline chemotherapy. *Med Pediatr Oncol* 1995;25(3):185–189.
110. Germanakis I, Anagnostatou N, Kalmanti M. Troponins and natriuretic peptides in the monitoring of anthracycline cardiotoxicity. *Pediatr Blood Cancer* 2008;51(3):327–333.
111. Horacek JM, Pudil R, Jebavy L, et al. Assessment of anthracycline-induced cardiotoxicity with biochemical markers. *Exp Oncol* 2007;29(4):309–313.
112. Horacek JM, Tichy M, Jebavy L, et al. Use of multiple biomarkers for evaluation of anthracycline-induced cardiotoxicity in patients with acute myeloid leukemia. *Exp Oncol* 2008;30(2):157–159.
113. Kilickap S, Barista I, Akgul E, et al. cTnT can be a useful marker for early detection of anthracycline cardiotoxicity. *Ann Oncol* 2005;16(5):798–804.
114. Kremer LC, Bastiaansen BA, Offringa M, et al. Troponin T in the first 24 hours after the administration of chemotherapy and the detection of myocardial damage in children. *Eur J Cancer* 2002;38(5):686–689.
115. Mathew P, Suarez W, Kip K, et al. Is there a potential role for serum cardiac troponin I as a marker for myocardial dysfunction in pediatric patients receiving anthracycline-based therapy? A pilot study. *Cancer Invest* 2001;19(4):352–359.
116. Nousiainen T, Vanninen E, Jantunen E, et al. Natriuretic peptides during the development of doxorubicin-induced left ventricular diastolic dysfunction. *J Intern Med* 2002;251(3):228–234.
117. Okumura H, Iuchi K, Yoshida T, et al. Brain natriuretic peptide is a predictor of anthracycline-induced cardiotoxicity. *Acta Haematol* 2000;104(4):158–163.
118. Raderer M, Kornek G, Weinlander G, et al. Serum troponin T levels in adults undergoing anthracycline therapy. *J Natl Cancer Inst* 1997;89(2):171.
119. Soker M, Kervancioglu M. Plasma concentrations of NT-pro-BNP and cardiac troponin-I in relation to doxorubicin-induced cardiomyopathy and cardiac function in childhood malignancy. *Saudi Med J* 2005;26(8):1197–1202.
120. Sparano JA, Brown DA, Wolff AC. Predicting cancer therapy-induced cardiotoxicity: the role of troponins and other markers. *Drug Saf* 2002;25(5):301–311.
121. Suzuki T, Hayashi D, Yamazaki T, et al. Elevated B-type natriuretic peptide levels after anthracycline administration. *Am Heart J* 1998;136(2):362–363.
122. Vogelsang TW, Jensen RJ, Hesse B, et al. BNP cannot replace gated equilibrium radionuclide ventriculography in monitoring of anthracycline-induced cardiotoxicity. *Int J Cardiol* 2008;124(2):193–197.
123. Kutteh L, Hobday T, Jaffe A, et al. A correlative study of cardiac biomarkers and left ventricular ejection fraction (LVEF) from N9831, a phase III randomized trial of chemotherapy and trastuzumab as adjuvant therapy for HEr2-positive breast cancer. *J Clin Oncol* 2007;25(18S Part I):22s.
124. Pichon MF, Cvitkovic F, Hacene K, et al. Drug-induced cardiotoxicity studied by longitudinal B type natriuretic peptide assays and radionuclide ventriculography. *In Vivo* 2005;19(3):567–576.
125. Slamon D, Eiermann W, Robert NJ. Phase III randomized trial comparing doxorubicin and cyclophosphamide followed by docetaxel (AC-T) with doxorubicin and cyclophosphamide followed by docetaxel and trastuzumab (AC-TH) with docetaxel, carboplatin and trastuzumab (TCH) in HER2 positive early breast cancer patients: BCIRG 006 study. *Breast Cancer Res Treat* 2005;94(Suppl 1):S5.
126. Piccart-Gebhart MJ, Procter M, Leyland-Jones B, et al. Trastuzumab after adjuvant chemotherapy in HER2-positive breast cancer. *N Engl J Med* 2005; 353(16):1659–1672.
127. Suter TM, Procter M, van Veldhuisen DJ, et al. Trastuzumab-associated cardiac adverse effects in the herceptin adjuvant trial. *J Clin Oncol* 2007;25(25):3859–3865.
128. Ewer MS, Lenihan DJ. Is trastuzumab associated with adverse cardiac effects in patients with breast cancer? *Nat Clin Pract Oncol* 2008;5(4):192–193.
129. Sledge G, O'Neill A, Thor A, et al. Adjuvant trastuzumab: long-term results of E2198. *Breast Cancer Res Treat*, 2006;S106(Supp 11).
130. Joensuu H, Kellokumpu-Lehtinen PL, Bono P, et al. Adjuvant docetaxel or vinorelbine with or without trastuzumab for breast cancer. *N Engl J Med* 2006;354(8): 809–820.
131. Geyer C, Forster J, Lindquist D, et al. Lapatinib plus Capecitabine for HER2-Positive Advanced Breast Cancer. *N Engl J Med* 2006;355(26):2733–2744.
132. Gomez H, Chavez M, Doval D, et al. A phase II, radomized trial using the small molecule tyrosine kinase inhibitor lapatinib as a first-line treatment in patients with FISH positive advanced or metastatic breast cancer. *J Clin Oncol* 2005; 23(16S):3046.
133. Lin NU, Carey LA, Liu MC, et al. Phase II trial of lapatinib for brain metastases in patients with human epidermal growth factor receptor 2-positive breast cancer. *J Clin Oncol* 2008;26(12):1993–1999.
134. Spector N, Blackwell K, Hurley J, et al. EGF103009, a phase II trial of lapatinib monotherapy in patients with relapsed/refractory inflammatory breast cancer (IBC): clinical activity and biologic predictors of response. *J Clin Oncol* 2006; 24(18S):502.
135. Tykerb® [Prescribing Information]. GlaxoSmithKline, 2007.
136. Perez EA, Koehler M, Byrne J, et al. Cardiac safety of lapatinib: pooled analysis of 3,689 patients enrolled in clinical trials. *Mayo Clin Proc* 2008;83(6):679–686.
137. Avastin® [Prescribing Information]. Genentech, Inc., 2006.
138. Hurwitz H, Fehrenbacher L, Novotny W, et al. Bevacizumab plus irinotecan, fluorouracil, and leucovorin for metastatic colorectal cancer. *N Engl J Med* 2004;350(23):2335–2342.
139. Johnson DH, Fehrenbacher L, Novotny WF, et al. Randomized phase II trial comparing bevacizumab plus carboplatin and paclitaxel with carboplatin and paclitaxel alone in previously untreated locally advanced or metastatic non-small-cell lung cancer. *J Clin Oncol* 2004;22(11):2184–2191.
140. Miller K, Wang M, Gralow J, et al. Paclitaxel plus bevacizumab versus paclitaxel alone for metastatic breast cancer. *N Engl J Med* 2007;357(26):2666–2676.
141. Norden AD, Young GS, Setayesh K, et al. Bevacizumab for recurrent malignant gliomas: efficacy, toxicity, and patterns of recurrence. *Neurology* 2008;70(10): 779–787.
142. Saltz LB, Clarke S, Diaz-Rubio E, et al. Bevacizumab in combination with oxaliplatin-based chemotherapy as first-line therapy in metastatic colorectal cancer: a randomized phase III study. *J Clin Oncol* 2008;26(12):2013–2019.
143. Sandler A, Gray R, Perry MC, et al. Paclitaxel-carboplatin alone or with bevacizumab for non-small-cell lung cancer. *N Engl J Med* 2006;355(24):2542–2550.
144. Yang J, Haworth L, Sherry M, et al. A Randomized Trial of Bevacizumab, and Anti-Vascular Endothelial Growth Factor Antibody, for Metastatic Renal Cancer. *N Engl J Med* 2003;349(5):427–434.
145. Miller K, O'Neill A, Perez E, et al. Phase II feasiblity trial incorporating bevacizumab into dose dense doxorubicin and cyclophosphamide followed by paclitaxel in patients with lymph node positive breast cancer: a trial of the Eastern Cooperative Oncology Group (E2104). San Antonio Breast Cancer Symposium, 2007.
146. Adrucil® [Prescribing Information]. Sicor Pharmaceuticals, Inc., 2003.
147. Xeloda® [Prescribing Information]. Roche Laboratories Inc., 2005.
148. Becker K, Erckenbrecht JF, Haussinger D, et al. Cardiotoxicity of the antiproliferative compound fluorouracil. *Drugs* 1999;57(4):475–484.
149. Coronel B, Madonna O, Mercatello A, et al. Myocardiotoxicity of 5 fluorouracil. *Intensive Care Med* 1988;14(4):429–430.
150. Dent RG, McColl I. Letter: 5-Fluorouracil and angina. *Lancet* 1975;1(7902): 347–348.
151. Freeman NJ, Costanza ME. 5-Fluorouracil-associated cardiotoxicity. *Cancer* 1988;61(1):36–45.
152. Gradishar W, Vokes E, Schilsky R, et al. Vascular events in patients receiving high-dose infusional 5-fluorouracil-based chemotherapy: the University of Chicago experience. *Med Pediatr Oncol* 1991;19(1):8–15.
153. Kleiman NS, Lehane DE, Geyer CE Jr, et al. Prinzmetal's angina during 5-fluorouracil chemotherapy. *Am J Med* 1987;82(3):566–568.
154. Methotrexate LPF® [Prescribing Infromation]. Mayne Pharma, 2003.
155. Cytoxan® [Prescribing Information]. Bristol-Myers Squibb Company, 2005.
156. Platinol® [Prescribing Information]. Bristol-Myers Squibb Company, 2002.
157. Altundag O, Celik I, Kars A. Recurrent asymptomatic bradycardia episodes after cisplatin infusion. *Ann Pharmacother* 2001;35(5):641–642.
158. Doll DC, List AF, Greco FA, et al. Acute vascular ischemic events after cisplatin-based combination chemotherapy for germ-cell tumors of the testis. *Ann Intern Med* 1986;105(1):48–51.
159. Meinardi MT, Gietema JA, van der Graaf WT, et al. Cardiovascular morbidity in long-term survivors of metastatic testicular cancer. *J Clin Oncol* 2000;18(8): 1725–1732.
160. Nieto Y, Cagnoni PJ, Bearman SI, et al. Cardiac toxicity following high-dose cyclophosphamide, cisplatin, and BCNU (STAMP-I) for breast cancer. *Biol Blood Marrow Transplant* 2000;6(2A):198–203.
161. Vinorelbine® [Prescribing Information]. 2000.
162. Bergeron A, Raffy O, Vannetzel JM. Myocardial ischemia and infarction associated with vinorelbine. *J Clin Oncol* 1995;13(2):531–532.
163. Dubos C, Prevost JN, Brun J, et al. [Myocardial infarction and vinorelbine. Report of a case]. *Rev Mal Respir* 1991;8(3):299–300.
164. Zabernigg A, Gattringer C. Myocardial infarction associated with vinorelbine (Navelbine). *Eur J Cancer* 1996;32A(9):1618–1619.
165. Curtis RE, Boice JD Jr, Stovall M, et al. Risk of leukemia after chemotherapy and radiation treatment for breast cancer. *N Engl J Med* 1992;326(26):1745–1751.
166. Praga C, Bergh J, Bliss J, et al. Risk of acute myeloid leukemia and myelodysplastic syndrome in trials of adjuvant epirubicin for early breast cancer: correlation with doses of epirubicin and cyclophosphamide. *J Clin Oncol* 2005;23(18): 4179–4191.
167. Smith RE, Bryant J, DeCillis A, et al. Acute myeloid leukemia and myelodysplastic syndrome after doxorubicin-cyclophosphamide adjuvant therapy for operable breast cancer: the National Surgical Adjuvant Breast and Bowel Project Experience. *J Clin Oncol* 2003;21(7):1195–1204.
168. Tallman MS, Gray R, Bennett JM, et al. Leukemogenic potential of adjuvant chemotherapy for early-stage breast cancer: the Eastern Cooperative Oncology Group experience. *J Clin Oncol* 1995;13(7):1557–1563.
169. Le Deley MC, Suzan F, Cutuli B, et al. Anthracyclines, mitoxantrone, radiotherapy, and granulocyte colony-stimulating factor: risk factors for leukemia and myelodysplastic syndrome after breast cancer. *J Clin Oncol* 2007;25(3):292–300.
170. Linassier C, Barin C, Calais G, et al. Early secondary acute myelogenous leukemia in breast cancer patients after treatment with mitoxantrone, cyclophosphamide, fluorouracil and radiation therapy. *Ann Oncol* 2000;11(10):1289–1294.
171. Saso R, Kulkarni S, Mitchell P, et al. Secondary myelodysplastic syndrome/acute myeloid leukaemia following mitoxantrone-based therapy for breast carcinoma. *Br J Cancer* 2000;83(1):91–94.
172. Hershman D, Neugut AI, Jacobson JS, et al. Acute myeloid leukemia or myelodysplastic syndrome following use of granulocyte colony-stimulating factors during breast cancer adjuvant chemotherapy. *J Natl Cancer Inst* 2007;99(3):196–205.
173. Fisher B, Anderson S, DeCillis A, et al. Further evaluation of intensified and increased total dose of cyclophosphamide for the treatment of primary breast cancer: findings from National Surgical Adjuvant Breast and Bowel Project B-25. *J Clin Oncol* 1999;17(11):3374–3388.
174. Citron ML, Berry DA, Cirrincione C, et al. Randomized trial of dose-dense versus conventionally scheduled and sequential versus concurrent combination chemotherapy as postoperative adjuvant treatment of node-positive primary breast cancer: first report of Intergroup Trial C9741/Cancer and Leukemia Group B Trial 9741. *J Clin Oncol* 2003;21(8):1431–1439.
175. Diamandidou E, Buzdar AU, Smith TL, et al. Treatment-related leukemia in breast cancer patients treated with fluorouracil-doxorubicin-cyclophosphamide combination adjuvant chemotherapy: the University of Texas M.D. Anderson Cancer Center experience. *J Clin Oncol* 1996;14(10):2722–2730.
176. Boice JD Jr, Harvey EB, Blettner M, et al. Cancer in the contralateral breast after radiotherapy for breast cancer. *N Engl J Med* 1992;326(12):781–785.
177. Clarke M, Collins R, Darby S, et al. Effects of radiotherapy and of differences in the extent of surgery for early breast cancer on local recurrence and 15-year survival: an overview of the randomised trials. *Lancet* 2005;366(9503):2087–2106.
178. Yap J, Chuba PJ, Thomas R, et al. Sarcoma as a second malignancy after treatment for breast cancer. *Int J Radiat Oncol Biol Phys* 2002;52(5):1231–1237.
179. Inskip PD, Stovall M, Flannery JT. Lung cancer risk and radiation dose among women treated for breast cancer. *J Natl Cancer Inst* 1994;86(13):983–988.
180. Neugut AI, Robinson E, Lee WC, et al. Lung cancer after radiation therapy for breast cancer. *Cancer* 1993;71(10):3054–3057.
181. Prochazka M, Granath F, Ekbom A, et al. Lung cancer risks in women with previous breast cancer. *Eur J Cancer* 2002;38(11):1520–1525.
182. Levi F, Randimbison L, Te VC, et al. Increased risk of esophageal cancer after breast cancer. *Ann Oncol* 2005;16(11):1829–1831.
183. Salminen EK, Pukkala E, Kiel KD, et al. Impact of radiotherapy in the risk of esophageal cancer as subsequent primary cancer after breast cancer. *Int J Radiat Oncol Biol Phys* 2006;65(3):699–704.

Chapter 56
Pharmacogenomics of Systemic Therapy of Breast Cancer

David A. Flockhart and James Michael Rae

Many predictors of the efficacy of treatments for breast cancer now exist. A superior understanding of the estrogen-sensitive biology of the tumor (1) has meant that the treatment of breast cancer has led the treatment of many other cancers. The use of tumor-based markers, such as the estrogen and progesterone receptors, to guide endocrine therapy, first with tamoxifen, worldwide (2) and now with the aromatase inhibitor class of drugs, is the standard of care worldwide (3). These advances have been supplemented in the last 5 years by the advent of ERBB2 (previously HER2)-based therapy in the form of trastuzumab aimed at tumors that express the ERBB2 receptor (4). Most recently, the targeting of therapy based on tumor estrogen, progesterone, and human epidermal growth factor receptor 2 expression has recently been supplemented by the use of RNA-based arrays that allow prediction of the benefits of chemotherapy. These have been made possible by the introduction of multiplex profiling technologies, in turn made possible by the unprecedented availability of genomic data. Of the 14 multigene arrays that have become available, the Oncotype DX 21 gene array and the MammaPrint array have become widely used (5).

Although approaches based on tumor biology have clearly resulted in improvements in recurrence-free survival, the morbidity and mortality associated with breast cancer remain unacceptably high, and the toxicity of current therapies results in unacceptably low levels of compliance (6). As a result, the need for further improvements in targeting and treatment remains high, and the possibility that inherited variants in genes that control the metabolism, distribution and elimination of drugs, and that code for their targeted receptors and signaling pathways might be important predictors of drug effects and toxicity in breast cancer. The availability of high throughput genomic technologies that can screen for hundreds of thousands of individual variants at once has provided insights into the pathogenesis of breast cancer (7), and is now poised to identify inherited genetic associations with responses to specific therapies. In approaching questions that involve more than one genetic variant or one gene it is important to appreciate that a hierarchy of clinically relevant pharmacogenomics data and different challenges arise at different points in the continuum (Fig. 56.1).

It seems particularly important to explore the inherited germ line for clues to therapeutic response, when it is clear that the treatments now available have been tested and validated in primarily white populations. Our ability to treat breast cancer in black patients, in whom the incidence of breast cancer is 20% lower than that in whites, but the mortality is 20% higher, would appear more limited. Similarly, the notably increasing rates of increasingly lethal breast cancer in Asian populations (8) demand serious attention to the question of whether we can ignore differences in response to therapy that might be based not on tumor biology, but on the inheritance of factors that might alter drug efficacy and toxicity. There is widespread precedent for the concept of pharmacogenomics in other fields of medicine where, for example, it is recognized that 7% of the population experience little analgesic benefit from codeine because they lack the ability to metabolize codeine to morphine via thee CYP2D6 enzyme (9), or experience an increased risk of intracranial bleeding while being treated with warfarin because of variants in the CYP2C9 or VKCOR genes (10).

In addition, a number of pharmacogenomic tests are already available in other areas of cancer treatment.

PHARMACOGENOMICS IN CANCER

Thiopurine S-methyltransferase and Mercaptopurine

Perhaps one of the best studied examples for the application of pharmacogenomic strategies to prevent adverse drug reactions is the polymorphism of the thiopurine S-methyltransferase (TPMT) gene. TPMT catalyses the S-methylation of thiopurine drugs, such as mercaptopurine and its prodrug azathioprine. These drugs are successfully used to treat acute lymphoblastic leukemia (ALL), and gastroenterologists prescribe thiopurine drugs as second-line (off-label) therapy for Crohn disease and ulcerative colitis. Because methylation by TPMT is the predominant pathway for inactivation of thiopurines, patients with a TPMT deficiency accumulate active thioguanine nucleotides and this can lead to severe and life-threatening hematologic toxicity. TPMT activity in erythrocytes is trimodally distributed among Europeans, European Americans, and African Americans and this distribution corresponds well to the genotypes or the respective presence of 2, 1, or 0 functional TPMT alleles. Twenty mutant alleles of TPMT have been associated with low TPMT activity and three of these variants (TPMT*2, TPMT*3A, and TPMT*3C) account for approximately 95% of low TPMT activity phenotypes (11). Approximately 1 of 150 to 300 individuals is homozygous for inactive TPMT alleles, approximately 10% of patients are heterozygous and have intermediate activity, and approximately 90% are normal or high methylators in a Northern European Caucasian population (11).

Because of the strong genotype-phenotype concordance and the severe toxicity associated with high concentrations of thioguanine nucleotides, several cancer centers routinely genotype patients for TPMT mutant alleles and use genotype-derived algorithms for dosing. Intermediate metabolizers receive approximately 65% and poor metabolizers 5% to 10% of standard doses of mercaptopurine (12). Dose reductions in patients with variant TPMT alleles lead to similar or superior survival compared to patients with wild-type alleles.

Of major concern is a report of an increased incidence of secondary brain tumors after radiotherapy in children with decreased TPMT activity phenotypes or high concentrations of thioguanine nucleotides in blood cells (13). The implications for therapeutic decisions regarding prophylactic radiotherapy in ALL therefore, must be further investigated.

UDP-Glucuronosyltransferase (UGT) 1A1 and Irinotecan

Results from several recently published trials suggest that patients who are homozygous for a UGT gene variant known as UGT1A1*28 (the "7/7" genotype) are at greater risk for irinotecan-induced severe diarrhea or neutropenia (14). Irinotecan is a camptothecin analogue that acts on cancer via inhibition of topoisomerase. The disposition of irinotecan is complex and involves numerous metabolic enzymes and transport proteins. SN-38 is the active metabolite of irinotecan and is eliminated via UGT1A1 conversion to SN-38G, an inactive glucuronide cleared via biliary excretion.

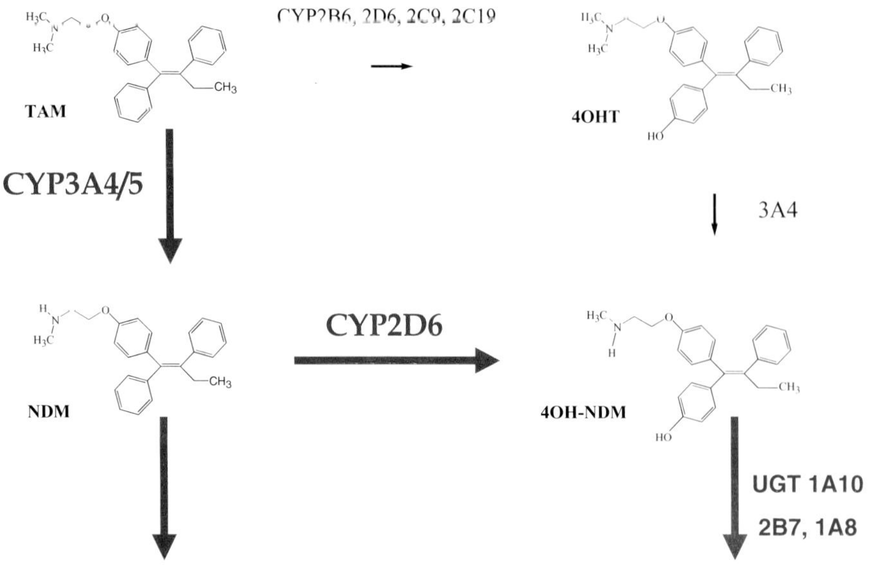

FIGURE 56.1. Metabolism of Tamoxifen. Most of the parent drug (TAMOXIFEN) is metabolized via the CYP3A4/5 cytochrome P450 enzymes to N-desmethyl-tamoxifen (NDM), and then to endoxifen (4OH-NDM) via CYP2D6. The route via 4-hydroxy-tamoxifen (4OHT) is relatively minor.

Reduced activity of *UGT1A1* is linked to an approximately fourfold increased risk of severe toxicity, including dose-limiting diarrhea and neutropenia. Significant correlations between patients carrying one or two copies of the *UGT1A1*28* allele and reduced *UGT1A1* expression and reduced SW38 glucuronidation are now been well documented.

More than 50 mutations in *UGT1A1* have been reported, many of which are found in patients with Gilbert syndrome, a form of mild nonhemolytic unconjugated hyperbilirubinemia. The most common mutant gene is *UGT1A1*28*, which contains seven dinucleotide repeats in the *TATA* box of the promoter (A(TA)$_7$TAA) instead of the normal six repeats, and leads to approximately 70% reduction of transcriptional activity. Many rare mutations also lead to Gilbert syndrome, and individuals with this syndrome are predisposed to SN-38 initiated toxicity. Although, as always, a number of additional factors influence the toxicity of SN-38 in the intestine and bone narrow, assessment of the presence of the *UGT1A1*28* allele in patients before irinotecan treatment may allow lower starting doses or a change to alternative therapies. Although four pharmacogenetic studies support this position, it is also clear the association of this toxicity with *UGT1A1* genotype is irinotecan dose-dependant (15). As a result, many oncologists prefer to simply adjust the irinotecan dose and avoid *UGT1A1* genotyping.

PHARMACOGENOMICS IN BREAST CANCER

The study of pharmacogenomics in breast and other cancers has been impaired in part by the lack of availability of germ line DNA in most cancer trials until very recently. This is in contrast to other medical disciplines, where the collection of blood, buccal swabs, or saliva to allow extraction of germ line DNA has been routine for many years. This obstacle has been overcome in part by the recent and key demonstration that effective germ-line genotyping can be carried out on DNA extracted from paraffin blocks (16,17). The technical ability to genotype germ line DNA from paraffin opens up the possibility of addressing pharmacogenomic questions in a large range of studies that have been completed, but for which archived paraffin blocks are available. As a result, significant progress has been made in studies designed to examine germ-line genetic associations with both the efficacy and toxicity of treatments for breast cancer.

Genetic Variants Associated with Toxicity of Agents Used To Treat Breast Cancer

Cyclophosphamide

Most chemotherapeutic regimens that have been used to treat all stages of breast cancer have used cyclophosphamide as an integral component. Cyclophosphamide is a prodrug that requires metabolic activation by cytochrome P450 (CYP) enzymes to 4-hydroxycyclophosphamide. Multiple CYP have been implicated in this activation, including CYP2A6, 2B6, 2C19, 2C9, 3A4, and 3A5, but CYP2C19 appears to be a key enzyme particularly at low cyclophosphamide concentrations. CYP2C19 is a genetically polymorphic enzyme that is expressed primarily in the liver and that has been shown to be responsible for the metabolism of a wide range of important therapeutic agents (18). This genetic polymorphism, now studied in a wide range of human populations (18), results in complete absence of enzyme activity in 3% to 5% of white and in 15% to 25% of Asian populations (18). In addition, the *CYP2C19*17* allele, which is present in 18% of whites and blacks, and in 4% of Asian, codes for a more active enzyme (19), and has been associated with a decreased risk for breast cancer (20). It is reasonable to hypothesize that the large number of individuals who do not carry active *CYP2C19* alleles may experience less cyclophosphamide activation and effects, and that those who carry the *CYP2C10*17* allele may experience more.

Thus, in a recent study conducted in lupus nephritis patients taking cyclophosphamide monotherapy, it was found that *CYP2C19*2* is a predictor of premature ovarian failure and progression to end-stage renal disease (21). These findings have now been validated by other investigators (22). Although the precise mechanism of this effect is unclear, these observations suggest that *in vitro* and clinical investigations are necessary to determine the cause of ovarian toxicity, and thus to prevent it in women at risk, an example of *reverse* translational research. Although these studies suggest that there is clinical relevance to the role of *CYP2C19* in the use of cyclophosphamide in other settings, studies to test whether these variants in *CYP2C19* or variants in other candidate genes are associated with cyclophosphamide outcomes in breast cancer are not available at present.

Vincristine

Although cyclophosphamide is used in many adjuvant regimens for treatment of breast cancer, the use of vincristine is confined to the metastatic setting. After many years during which the metabolism of vincristine was poorly understood (23), it has recently been shown that vincristine is primarily metabolized by a highly genetically polymorphic enzyme: CYP3A5 (23,24). This enzyme has been shown to be coded by a gene containing single-nucleotide polymorphisms (SNP) in *CYP3A5*3* and *CYP3A5*6* that cause alternative splicing, and protein truncation results in the absence of *CYP3A5* in some people. Of note, *CYP3A5* was more frequently expressed in livers of blacks (60%) than in those of whites (33%) (25). In a clear demonstration of the potential clinical relevance of this variability, whites have recently been shown to be notably more vulnerable to vincristine-related neurotoxicity than blacks (26). Of total doses administered to white patients, 4% were reduced owing to vincristine-related neurotoxicity compared with 0.1% given to blacks (*p* <.0001), and 1.2% of all protocol-indicated doses for whites were held owing to severe vincristine-associated toxicity compared with 0.1% of doses for blacks (*p* <.01) (26). These data suggest that the unpredictable neurotoxicity that patients experience with vincristine may actually be predictable, and that *CYP3A5* genotype may contribute. Although it is reasonable to test whether the *CYP3A5* genotype is a valuable predictor of the efficacy of vincristine, no trials yet have been reported that test this hypothesis.

Tamoxifen

The selective estrogen modulator tamoxifen is an essential part of standard adjuvant and palliative systemic therapy for patients with steroid hormone receptor-positive breast tumors. Adjuvant tamoxifen significantly decreases relapse rates and mortality in pre- and postmenopausal patients, and the therapeutic benefit resulting from 5 years of adjuvant tamoxifen is maintained for more than 10 years after diagnosis (27,28). Tamoxifen is a valid therapy option next to aromatase inhibitors (AI) in postmenopausal patients with endocrine-responsive disease (29); it is considered the standard care for premenopausal patients, for prevention of invasive breast cancer in women at high risk, including those who have had ductal carcinoma *in situ* (DCIS), and for the treatment of male breast cancer (29). It is important to note that, although the clinical benefit of tamoxifen has been evident for more than three decades, up to 50% of patients receiving adjuvant tamoxifen relapse or die because of tumor resistance or lack of response to the drug (30). In addition, although tamoxifen is a very effective drug, as with all potent medications, it also has side effects.

Studies over many years in many populations made clear that the most common of these were vasomotor symptoms, or hot flashes, similar to those experienced by women undergoing natural menopause. Tamoxifen has also been associated with an increased incidence of thromboses when it is used to treat (31) or even to prevent breast cancer (32), and a small but significant increase in the incidence of endometrial cancer (32). These side effects seem to be less common when the AI class of drugs are used in place of tamoxifen (33), but these drugs also have side effects, including debilitating musculoskeletal symptoms (34), that compromise compliance with treatment. Because the difference in efficacy between tamoxifen and the AI class of drugs is in the 2% to 4% range, we are in great need of biomarkers that can predict the efficacy of specific endocrine treatments, and that help identify individual patients who are most likely to experience specific side effects that are not predictable *a priori*.

Efforts to identify genomic biomarkers for tamoxifen effects have been significantly aided by an improved understanding of tamoxifen metabolism in recent years that has helped identify candidate genes involved in the actions of the drug. Because tamoxifen is a prodrug that is converted to active metabolites, the idea that inherited variations in human drug metabolism might alter the activity and toxicity of tamoxifen has recently been proposed (35,36).

Data on the metabolism of tamoxifen carried out in the 1980s in rats indicated that the drug is extensively metabolized by the cytochrome P450 system and that it is primarily demethylated to N-desmethyl tamoxifen or hydroxylated (37). Jordan (38) showed the 4-hydroxylated metabolite was approximately 100 times more potent as a ligand at the estrogen receptor (ER) than other metabolites, and it was subsequently believed by many that 4-hydroxy-tamoxifen was *the* active metabolite. As a result, this metabolite was synthesized by a number of companies and remains the most widely used substitute for tamoxifen in many laboratory studies. Another hydroxylated metabolite, 4-hydroxy-N-desmethyl tamoxifen is created in humans (39), but not in mice (37), by the hydroxylation of N-desmethyl tamoxifen, and this has more recently been clearly documented to be the most abundant species in human serum at steady state (35,36,40,41). Stearns et al. reported in 2003 that the serum concentrations of this metabolite, now designated endoxifen, were notably lower in patients who were coprescribed paroxetine, and in patients who carried a single variant of the *CYP2D6* gene.

This genetically polymorphic gene has been intensively studied over the last 50 years, and is the subject of numerous reviews (42,43). It is a key metabolic route for many drugs, including many antidepressants, neuroleptics, antiarrhythmics, and other commonly used drugs. It is absent in 7% of white populations as the result of genetic variants that code or do not code for active enzyme. A high prevalence of reduced function alleles in Asian populations results in lower average activity in this population (42), and the presence of multiple copies of the gene results in high or "ultrarapid" activity in 5% of whites, but in more than 20% of East African populations in Ethiopia and Saudi Arabia (43).

To confirm a clinically important involvement of this enzyme in tamoxifen metabolism, Desta et al. (44), subsequently conducted a comprehensive evaluation of the metabolism by the cytochrome P450 system, and demonstrated that the metabolism of N-desmethyl to endoxifen is carried out almost exclusively by the genetically polymorphic *CYP2D6*. The human metabolism of tamoxifen is now well understood (Fig. 56.2). It

Hierarchy of Pharmacogenetic Information

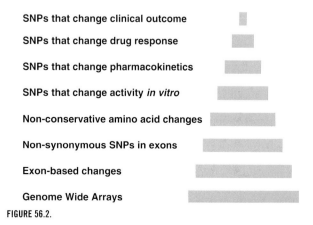

SNPs that change clinical outcome

SNPs that change drug response

SNPs that change pharmacokinetics

SNPs that change activity *in vitro*

Non-conservative amino acid changes

Non-synonymous SNPs in exons

Exon-based changes

Genome Wide Arrays

FIGURE 56.2.

involves the conversion of the parent drug to two well-documented active metabolites: 4-hydroxy tamoxifen, which is formed directly from tamoxifen by 4-hydroxylation catalyzed by at least three enzymes, and the independent conversion of tamoxifen to N-desmethyl tamoxifen by cytochrome P450 3A, followed by secondary metabolism to endoxifen catalyzed exclusively by CYP2D6 (44).

The observation that endoxifen is present at concentrations in the serum of women with breast cancer that are five- to ten-fold higher than those of 4-hydroxy tamoxifen (36,40,41) led to the hypothesis that *CYP2D6* genotype might be associated with breast cancer outcomes, and this idea has now been tested in a number of trials. In an examination of a randomized, controlled, prospective trial, Goetz et al. (45) successfully isolated intact DNA from paraffin blocks from 223 of 256 eligible patients, and found that women with the *CYP2D6 *4/*4* genotype had worse relapse-free time (p = .023) and disease-free survival (DFS) (p = .012), but not overall survival (p = .169), and did not experience moderate to severe hot flashes relative to women heterozygous or homozygous for the wild-type allele. In the multivariate analysis, women with the *CYP2D6 *4/*4* genotype still tended to have worse RFS (hazard ratio [HR], 1.85, p = .176) and DFS (HR, 1.86, p = .089). Of note, the *CYP3A5*3* variant was not associated with any of these clinical outcomes. They concluded that women with the *CYP2D6*4/*4* genotype tend to have a higher risk of disease relapse and a lower incidence of hot flashes, consistent with the previous observation that *CYP2D6* is responsible for the metabolic activation of tamoxifen to endoxifen.

Several subsequent investigations have addressed the interaction between *CYP2D6* genotype and outcomes in women who were treated with tamoxifen in the prevention (46), adjuvant (47), and metastatic settings. The results of three adjuvant studies (45,47,48) showed a two- to fivefold increased risk of recurrence in women who carried variant alleles, as did a metastatic trial and a study in the prevention setting study (46). These studies are consistent with the hypothesis that women with variant *CYP2D6* genotype have worse outcomes. However, two studies in the adjuvant setting (49,50) provided statistically significant evidence of exactly the opposite effect—women with homozygous *CYP2D6* variants have better outcomes than those who have wild type alleles when treated with tamoxifen. The differences in these results may result from different patient populations, different genotyping approaches, or tamoxifen compliance.

Punglia et al. (51) used assumptions drawn from the Mayo–Consortium on Breast Cancer Pharmacogenics (COBRA) study (45) to build a model to estimate whether women with wild-type *CYP2D6* might have superior outcomes if they take tamoxifen rather than an AI. Applying this model to results produced from the Breast International Group 1-98 trial, they concluded that women who have the wild-type *CYP2D6* genotype would actually have lower rates of relapse when treated with tamoxifen. This approach is illustrated in Figure 56.3. If this model is correct, the role of *CYP2D6* genotype testing would be critical for selecting the optimal adjuvant endocrine treatment for women with ER-positive breast cancer because it makes clear that more than 90% of women (those who are wild type for *CYP2D6*) would actually have better outcomes if they received tamoxifen instead of an AI and that those who are homozygous for inactivating variant alleles should take an AI.

The interaction between antidepressants and tamoxifen has also received considerable attention as a result of this work, because it is clear that *CYP2D6*-inhibiting selective serotonin reuptake inhibitors (SSRI), such as paroxetine and fluoxetine, lower endoxifen concentrations (36,41,52). The demonstration by Jin et al. (36) that venlafaxine, a weak inhibitor of *CYP2D6*, does not appreciably lower the concentrations of active tamoxifen metabolites, afforded women with breast

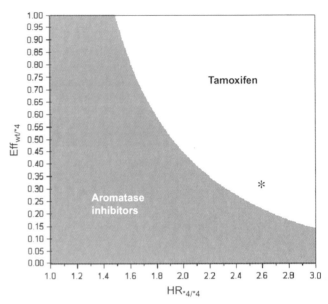

FIGURE 56.3. A two-way sensitivity analysis comparing the hazard ratios for response to treatment with estimates of the effect of a CYP2D6 *4 variant allel on outcome. The hazard ratio of recurrence among the homozygous mutation carriers (HR *4/*4) is plotted on the x-axis, and proportion of HR *4/*4 attributed to heterozygotes (Eff wt/*4) is plotted on the y-axis. The gray zone represents the combinations of Eff wt/*4 and HR *4/*4 for which aromatase inhibitors optimize 5-year disease-free survival for wt/wt patients. The white zone represents the combinations of Eff wt/*4 and HR *4/*4 for which tamoxifen optimizes 5-year disease-free survival for these patients. The asterisk marks the combination of HR *4/*4 and calculated Eff wt/*4—2.6 and 0.316, respectively—that corresponds to updated but unadjusted estimates from the North Central Cancer Treatment Group trial data(45). Adapted from Punglia et al. (51).

cancer the possibility of taking an effective antidepressant that is also able to treat hot flashes, and has little risk of altering the risk of recurrence.

Postmenopausal women being treated with endocrine therapy for breast cancer clearly now have a number of alternative therapies available to them. These include tamoxifen, and the AI anastrozole, letrozole, and exemestane. The choice of which therapy should be used in which woman should obviously be guided by the potential benefits for each woman and the attendant risks of specific therapies in each woman, but also by the tolerability of specific therapies, because it is clear that compliance with tamoxifen or the AI class of drugs can influence outcomes. Although we do not believe that all such women should be tested, we do believe that specific women may benefit from testing, in circumstances where alternative therapy is available to them. We also believe that women taking tamoxifen should avoid *CYP2D6*-inhibiting drugs *if possible*. In situations where women are committed to a *CYP2D6*-inhibiting antidepressant by years of effective treatment that is not easily substituted for by another drug, we would recommend using an AI if possible. Of note, these recommendations do *not* apply to women in the premenopausal setting, in whom the AI are not effective alternatives to tamoxifen, and for whom there is only limited data on the clinical consequences of *CYP2D6* genomics.

Pharmacogenomics in the Use of Antiangiogenic Agents in Breast Cancer

The possibility that host genomics might influence outcome is perhaps greatest in situations where the host response to the tumor might be modified. This is obviously the case in the physiology of tumor angiogenesis, where the host's ability to confer a sustaining blood supply to a solid tumor is widely recognized as variable, and a target of therapy. This has most recently been made clear by the approval of bevacizumab, an antivascular endothelia growth factor antibody used to treat breast cancer. Bevacizumab was approved because of the results from a number of trials, including a trial designated as E-2100, in which women with metastatic breast cancer were treated with either paclitaxel alone, or paclitaxel with bevacizumab. The results of this trial indicated that bevacizumab prolonged DFS from 5.9 to 11.8 months, but did not alter overall survival. Using techniques similar to those developed by Rae et al. (16) for CYP pharmacogenetics testing, Schneider et al. (17) were able to obtain sufficient high-quality DNA to conduct germ-line genetic testing from paraffin blocks to allow genotyping for candidate genes that are in the angiogenesis response pathway. When these techniques were applied to paraffin blocks obtained during the E2100 trial, they were able to show that women who carried either of two promoter single nucleotide polymorphisms in the *VEGF* gene experienced notably longer overall survival (Schneider et al. *J Clin Oncol* 2008; *In Press*). Women who carried the -2578 AA variant experienced a 10-month increase in median overall survival ($p = .023$), relative to the control arm, whereas women who carried the -1154 AA variant survived for 20 months longer ($p = .001$) than those in the control, paclitaxel alone arm (Schneider et al. *J Clin Oncol* 2008; *In Press*). Although these data require validation, the size of the effects is large, and the cost of bevacizumab therapy argues that it may make both clinical and economic sense to conduct pharmacogenetics testing before treatment with bevacizumab in this setting and in many others.

FUTURE IMPACT OF PHARMACOGENOMICS IN BREAST CANCER

Although the science of pharmacogenetics is 50 or more years old, only recently have pharmacogenetics tests been tested as possible biomarkers of response to therapy in breast cancer. Women with breast cancer have benefited tremendously from improved understanding of tumor biology and we now routinely stratify therapy based on the presence of estrogen, progesterone, ERBB2, and expression array data. Great potential exists for similar stratification of therapy using germ-line pharmacogenomics, and ongoing studies in the areas of chemotherapy, endocrine therapy, and antiangiogenic therapy make clear that this is now both an active area of investigation and one in which a great potential exists to identify women most likely to respond to very expensive biologic therapies as well as treatment that have become more routine. This is now clear to many investigators, and so the pace of pharmacogenetic studies in breast cancer is accelerating rapidly.

MANAGEMENT SUMMARY

At present, pharmacogenomic testing is most valuable in breast cancer as a tool for deciding WHICH therapy should be administered and not as a tool that is useful in decisions about dose. It follows that such testing is of most value when more than one therapeutic alternative is available.

- In the premenopausal setting, women with hormone receptor-positive breast cancer do not have multiple alternative therapies for endocrine therapy beyond tamoxifen because neither raloxifene nor the aromatase inhibitors are effective in this context. We would *not* recommend pharmacogenomic testing for *CYP2D6* in this context. Similarly, in the prevention setting, there are currently insufficient data to guide pharmacogenetic recommendations.

- In the postmenopausal setting, women with hormone receptor-positive breast cancer have multiple potential alternative therapies that include tamoxifen and three aromatase inhibitors. Although the ideal sequence of these therapies in individual women is still a subject of intense research, we do not believe that all women in this context should be subjected to pharmacogenomic testing. Women who are eligible would be those who could be prescribed tamoxifen, but who could also tolerate an aromatase inhibitor. In this context, women who are poor metabolizers of *CYP2D6* might most reasonably be prescribed an aromatase inhibitor, whereas women who are extensive metabolizers would most likely benefit most from tamoxifen.

- In the metastatic setting, one study exists on which to base any pharmacogenomic recommendations, but sparse data from others settings would suggest that tamoxifen could be reasonably considered as an alternative to aromatase inhibitor therapy. It follows that all other things being equal, a poor metabolizer might most reasonably be prescribed an aromatase inhibitor if the side effects of aromatase inhibitors are tolerable.

- In terms of antiangiogenic therapy, we have one large prospective trial in women with metastatic breast cancer (E2100) to rely on for pharmacogenomic data, so it remains premature to make firm recommendations at this time. If data from this trial are validated, then we will be able to identify quickly a group of women who stand to derive considerable benefit from this effective but expensive treatment, and another group who do not and who should therefore not be so treated.

References

1. Lippman ME, Bolan G. Oestrogen-responsive human breast cancer in long term tissue culture. *Nature* 1975;256(5518):592–593.
2. Early Breast Cancer Trialists Collaborative Group. Effects of chemotherapy and hormonal therapy for early breast cancer on recurrence and 15-year survival: an overview of the randomised trials. *Lancet* 2005;365(9472):1687–1717.
3. Harris L, Fritsche H, Mennel R, et al. American Society of Clinical Oncology 2007 update of recommendations for the use of tumor markers in breast cancer. *J Clin Oncol* 2007;25(33):5287–5312.
4. Wolff AC, Hammond ME, Schwartz JN, et al. American Society of Clinical Oncology/College of American Pathologists Guideline Recommendations for Human Epidermal Growth Factor Receptor 2 Testing in Breast Cancer. *Arch Pathol Lab Med* 2007;131(1):18.
5. Ross JS, Hatzis C, Symmans WF, et al. Commercialized multigene predictors of clinical outcome for breast cancer. *Oncologist* 2008;13(5):477–493.
6. Owusu C, Buist DS, Field TS, et al. Predictors of tamoxifen discontinuation among older women with estrogen receptor-positive breast cancer. *J Clin Oncol* 2008; 26(4):549–555.
7. Easton DF, Pooley KA, Dunning AM, et al. Genome-wide association study identifies novel breast cancer susceptibility loci. *Nature* 2007;447(7148): 1087–1093.
8. Deapen D, Liu L, Perkins C, et al. Rapidly rising breast cancer incidence rates among Asian-American women. *Int J Cancer* 2002;99(5):747–750.
9. Caraco Y, Sheller J, Wood AJ. Pharmacogenetic determination of the effects of codeine and prediction of drug interactions. *J Pharmacol Exp Ther* 1996;278(3): 1165–1174.
10. Rieder MJ, Reiner AP, Gage BF, et al. Effect of VKORC1 haplotypes on transcriptional regulation and warfarin dose. *N Engl J Med* 2005;352(22): 2285–2293.
11. Shaeffeler E, Fischer C, Brockmeier D, et al. Comprehensive analysis of thiopurine S-methyltransferase phenotype-genotype correlation in a large population of German-Caucasians and identification of novel TPMT variants. *Pharmacogenetics* 2004;14(7):407–417.
12. Evans WE, Relling MV. Moving towards individualized medicine with pharmacogenomics. *Nature* 2004;429(6990):464–468.
13. Relling MV, Rubnitz JE, Rivera GK, et al. High incidence of secondary brain tumours after radiotherapy and antimetabolites [see comments]. *Lancet* 1999;354 (9172):34–39.
14. Innocenti F, Undevia SD, Iyer L, et al. Genetic variants in the UDP-glucuronosyltransferase 1A1 gene predict the risk of severe neutropenia of irinotecan. *J Clin Oncol* 2004;22(8):1382–1388.
15. Hoskins JM, Marcuello E, Altes A, et al. Irinotecan pharmacogenetics: influence of pharmacodynamic genes. *Clin Cancer Res* 2008;14(6):1788–1796.
16. Rae JM, Cordero KE, Scheys JO, et al. Genotyping for polymorphic drug metabolizing enzymes from paraffin-embedded and immunohistochemically stained tumor samples. *Pharmacogenetics* 2003;13(8):501–507.
17. Schneider BP, Skaar TC, Sledge GW, et al. Analysis of angiogenesis genes from paraffin-embedded breast tumor and lymph nodes. *Breast Cancer Res Treat* 2006; 96(3):209–215.

18. Desta Z, Zhao X, Shin JG, et al. Clinical significance of the cytochrome P450 2C19 genetic polymorphism. *Clin Pharmacokinet* 2002;41(12):913–958.
19. Sim SC, Risinger C, Dahl ML, et al. A common novel CYP2C19 gene variant causes ultrarapid drug metabolism relevant for the drug response to proton pump inhibitors and antidepressants. *Clin Pharmacol Ther* 2006;79(1):103–113.
20. Justenhoven C, Hamann U, Pierl CB, et al. CYP2C19*17 is associated with decreased breast cancer risk. *Breast Cancer Res Treat* 2008; June 3 (Epub ahead of print).
21. Takada K, Arefayene M, Desta Z, et al. Cytochrome P450 pharmacogenetics as a predictor of toxicity and clinical response to pulse cyclophosphamide in lupus nephritis. *Arthritis Rheum* 2004;50(7):2202–2210.
22. Singh G, Saxena N, Aggarwal A, et al. Cytochrome P450 polymorphism as a predictor of ovarian toxicity to pulse cyclophosphamide in systemic lupus erythematous. *J Rheumatol* 2007;34(4):731–733.
23. Dennison JB, Kulanthaivel P, Barbuch RJ, et al. Selective metabolism of vincristine *in vitro* by CYP3A5. *Drug Metab Dispos* 2006;34(8):1317–1327.
24. Dennison JB, Jones DR, Renbarger JL, et al. Effect of CYP3A5 expression on vincristine metabolism with human liver microsomes. *J Pharmacol Exp Ther* 2007; 321(2):553–563.
25. Kuehl P, Zhang J, Lin Y, et al. Sequence diversity in CYP3A promoters and characterization of the genetic basis of polymorphic CYP3A5 expression. *Nat Genet* 2001; 27(4):383–391.
26. Renbarger JL, McCammack KC, Rouse CE, et al. Effect of race on vincristine-associated neurotoxicity in pediatric acute lymphoblastic leukemia patients. *Pediatr Blood Cancer* 2008;50(4):769–771.
27. Fisher B, Costantino J, Redmond C, et al. A randomized clinical trial evaluating tamoxifen in the treatment of patients with node-negative breast cancer who have estrogen-receptor-positive tumors. *N Engl J Med* 1989;320(8):479–484.
28. Belfiglio M, Valentini M, Pellegrini F, et al. Twelve-year mortality results of a randomized trial of 2 versus 5 years of adjuvant tamoxifen for postmenopausal early-stage breast carcinoma patients (SITAM 01). *Cancer* 2005;104(11):2334–2339.
29. Lin NU, Winer EP. Advances in adjuvant endocrine therapy for postmenopausal women. *J Clin Oncol* 2008;26(5):798–805.
30. Jordan VC, O'Malley BW. Selective estrogen-receptor modulators and antihormonal resistance in breast cancer. *J Clin Oncol* 2007;25(36):5815–5824.
31. Tamoxifen for early breast cancer: an overview of the randomised trials. Early Breast Cancer Trialists' Collaborative Group. *Lancet* 1998;351(9114):1451–1467.
32. Fisher B, Costantino JP, Wickerham DL, et al. Tamoxifen for prevention of breast cancer: report of the National Surgical Adjuvant Breast and Bowel Project P-1 Study. *J Natl Cancer Inst* 2001;90(18):1371–1388.
33. Baum M, Budzar AU, Cuzick J, et al. Anastrozole alone or in combination with tamoxifen versus tamoxifen alone for adjuvant treatment of postmenopausal women with early breast cancer: first results of the ATAC randomised trial. *Lancet* 2002;359(9324):2131–2139.
34. Henry NL, Giles JT, Ang D, et al. Prospective characterization of musculoskeletal symptoms in early stage breast cancer patients treated with aromatase inhibitors. *Breast Cancer Res Treat* 2007;111(2):365–372.
35. Stearns V, Johnson MD, Rae JM, et al. Active tamoxifen metabolite plasma concentrations after coadministration of tamoxifen and the selective serotonin reuptake inhibitor paroxetine. *J Natl Cancer Inst* 2003;95(23):1758–1764.
36. Jin Y, Desta Z, Stearns V, et al. CYP2D6 genotype, antidepressant use, and tamoxifen metabolism during adjuvant breast cancer treatment. *J Natl Cancer Inst* 2005; 97(1):30–39.
37. Jordan VC, Collins MM, Rowsby L, et al. A monohydroxylated metabolite of tamoxifen with potent antioestrogenic activity. *J Endocrinol* 1977;75(2):305–316.
38. Jordan VC. Metabolites of tamoxifen in animal and man: identification, pharmacology, and significance. *Breast Cancer Res Treat* 1982;2:123–138.
39. Lien EA, Solheim E, Lea OA, et al. Distribution of 4-hydroxy-N-desmethyltamoxifen and other tamoxifen metabolites in human biological fluids during tamoxifen treatment. *Cancer Res* 1989;49(8):2175–2183.
40. Lien EA, Anker G, Lonning PE, et al. Decreased serum concentrations of tamoxifen and its metabolites induced by aminoglutethimide. *Cancer Res* 1990;50(18): 5851–5857.
41. Borges S, Desta Z, Li L, et al. Quantitative effect of CYP2D6 genotype and inhibitors on tamoxifen metabolism: implication for optimization of breast cancer treatment. *Clin Pharmacol Ther* 2006;80(1):61–74.
42. Meyer UA. Pharmacogenetics—five decades of therapeutic lessons from genetic diversity. *Nat Rev Genet* 2004;5(9):669–676.
43. Zanger UM, Raimundo S, Eichelbaum M. Cytochrome P450 2D6: overview and update on pharmacology, genetics, biochemistry. *Naunyn Schmiedebergs Arch Pharmacol* 2004;369(1):23–37.
44. Desta Z, Ward BA, Soukhova NV, et al. Comprehensive evaluation of tamoxifen sequential biotransformation by the human cytochrome P450 system *in vitro*: prominent roles for CYP3A and CYP2D6. *J Pharmacol Exp Ther* 2004;310(3): 1062–1075.
45. Goetz MP, Rae JM, Suman VJ, et al. Pharmacogenetics of tamoxifen biotransformation is associated with clinical outcomes of efficacy and hot flashes. *J Clin Oncol* 2005;23(36):9312–9318.
46. Bonanni B, Macis D, Maisonneuve P, et al. Polymorphism in the CYP2D6 tamoxifen-metabolizing gene influences clinical effect but not hot flashes: data from the Italian Tamoxifen Trial. *J Clin Oncol* 2006;24(22):3708–3709.
47. Kiyotani K, Mushiroda T, Sasa M, et al. Impact of CYP2D6*10 on recurrence-free survival in breast cancer patients receiving adjuvant tamoxifen therapy. *Cancer Sci* 2008;99(5):995–999.
48. Schroth W, Antoniadou L, Fritz P, et al. Breast cancer treatment outcome with adjuvant tamoxifen relative to patient CYP2D6 and CYP2C19 genotypes. *J Clin Oncol* 2007;25(33):5187–5193.
49. Wegman P, Elingarami S, Carstensen J, et al. Genetic variants of CYP3A5, CYP2D6, SULT1A1, UGT2B15 and tamoxifen response in postmenopausal patients with breast cancer. *Breast Cancer Res* 2007;9(1):R7.
50. Wegman P, Vainikka L, Stal O, et al. Genotype of metabolic enzymes and the benefit of tamoxifen in postmenopausal breast cancer patients. *Breast Cancer Res* 2005;7(3):R284–R290.
51. Punglia RS, Burstein HJ, Winer EP, et al. Pharmacogenomic variation of CYP2D6 and the choice of optimal adjuvant endocrine therapy for postmenopausal breast cancer: a modeling analysis. *J Natl Cancer Inst* 2008;100(9):642–648.
52. Stearns V, Johnson MD, Rae JM, et al. Active tamoxifen metabolite plasma concentrations after coadministration of tamoxifen and the selective serotonin reuptake inhibitor paroxetine. *J Natl Cancer Inst* 2003;95(23):1758–1764.

Nancy E. Davidson, Eric P. Winer, and C. Kent Osborne

The first step in adjuvant therapy decision-making involves an assessment of risk of distant recurrence using known prognostic factors. The second and equally important step is to estimate the benefit of treatment using the available predictive factors. Therapy of some type should be considered for most women with invasive breast cancer. Individual patients and their physicians should take into account prognosis, potential treatment benefit, and the patient's health and preferences to make a final decision.

Established prognostic factors include nodal status, pathologic tumor size, histologic grade and subtype, measures of proliferation, and steroid receptor and ERBB2 (formerly HER-2) expression. Steroid receptor and ERBB2 expression are the best validated predictive markers at present because absence of steroid receptor expression predicts for lack of response to endocrine therapy and normal ERBB2 expression (as judged by the absence of ERBB2 gene amplification or low ERBB2 protein expression by immunohistochemistry) predicts for lack of response to anti-ERBB2 therapy, such as with trastuzumab or lapatinib. Uncertainty remains about the role of steroid receptors or ERBB2 protein expression as predictors for response to chemotherapy. In some studies, tumors that lack estrogen receptor (ER) and progesterone receptor (PR) expression appear to be more responsive to chemotherapy than those that express either or both receptors. Indeed, physicians and patients are increasingly more selective about the use of chemotherapy in patients whose tumors are both steroid receptor-positive and ERBB2 normal, especially if the patient has a low risk of recurrence. Recent studies suggest that a low recurrence score using the Oncotype DX assay may help to select women with receptor-positive breast cancer who do not benefit from the addition of chemotherapy to tamoxifen, especially those with node-negative breast cancer. Another recently approved multigene test (Mammaprint) provides information about prognosis and long-term risk of recurrence, but does not shed light on what type of treatment is useful. Finally, in some trials ERBB2-positive tumors appear to be less responsive to endocrine therapy and perhaps more responsive to doxorubicin hydrochloride- or taxane-based chemotherapy. These results are not definitive and neither steroid receptor status nor ERBB2 expression should be used to select for the type of chemotherapy.

A critical component of the decision-making process is an accurate assessment of the likelihood of benefit that can be expected from therapy. Several tools can help guide this discussion (1). For most patients, an estimation of absolute rather than relative risk and benefit is more likely to be informative. Physicians have frequently used a threshold of greater than 90% disease-free survival at 10 years with local therapy alone to define a group of women whose outcome is so good that they may not benefit sufficiently to warrant use of adjuvant systemic chemotherapy, especially if the characteristics of the tumor suggest that the potential benefit from chemotherapy is small. Limited life expectancy because of other health problems clearly represents a contraindication to adjuvant systemic therapy. In addition, some adjuvant endocrine therapies are associated with rare potentially severe side effects such as thromboembolism or stroke that will be more common in older patients and in those with comorbid conditions or conditions that limit ambulation.

ADJUVANT ENDOCRINE THERAPY

Endocrine therapy is the cornerstone of adjuvant therapy for women with tumor that expresses ER, PR, or both. Five years of adjuvant tamoxifen citrate is a standard endocrine therapy for women of any age whose tumor expresses ER or PR (2). A large study evaluating immunohistochemical assessment of ER suggested that women whose tumors express ER in as few as 1% of cells benefit from tamoxifen (3). However, randomized trials and the Early Breast Cancer Trialists' Collaborative Group meta-analysis show in aggregate that women whose tumor is completely devoid of ER and PR expression do not benefit from endocrine therapy. All others should be counseled about the potential benefits and risks of hormonal approaches. ER and PR immunohistochemical assays still, however, have not been standardized despite their critical importance, and errors, most commonly false–negative findings, occur.

Aromatase inhibitors offer a small advantage over tamoxifen and should be considered as part of the adjuvant endocrine therapy for most postmenopausal women with steroid receptor-positive breast cancer (4). Randomized trials suggest that initial treatment with an aromatase inhibitor or the sequence of tamoxifen before or after an aromatase inhibitor are acceptable strategies. The decision about which approach to use should take into account a number of factors, including patient age, years after menopause, risk of recurrence, bone and cardiac health, and menopausal symptoms. Patients on aromatase inhibitors should have serial monitoring of bone mineral density and serum lipids. No information exists currently about the relative efficacy of the three commercially available aromatase inhibitors, anastrozole, letrozole, and exemestane; a prudent strategy is to prescribe their use according to the reported adjuvant trials. Optimal duration of aromatase inhibitor is not yet established. Given their mechanisms of action, aromatase inhibitors should not be used for the management of premenopausal women, including those who have become amenorrheic with chemotherapy because some of these women still have ovarian production of estrogen or their ovarian function can recover over time (5).

For premenopausal women with steroid receptor-positive breast cancer, 5 years of tamoxifen is standard. Temporary ovarian suppression by luteinizing hormone-releasing hormone (LHRH) analogs or ovarian ablation by surgery may be used as an alternative to (or in combination with) tamoxifen citrate under selected circumstances (2,6). The use of LHRH analog with aromatase inhibitor is an investigational approach. Optimal duration of ovarian suppression is not known; most trials supporting this approach have used at least 2 years.

ADJUVANT CHEMOTHERAPY

Adjuvant chemotherapy is generally considered for healthy women with moderate to high risk breast cancer. It represents the only viable strategy for women with *triple negative* breast cancer, that is, breast cancer that lacks expression of ER, PR, and ERBB2 protein. A number of adjuvant regimens have been studied

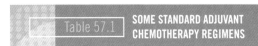

Table 57.1   SOME STANDARD ADJUVANT CHEMOTHERAPY REGIMENS

Non–trastuzumab-Containing Regimens
- FAC/CAF (fluorouracil/doxorubicin/cyclophosphamide)
- FEC/CEF (fluorouracil/epirubicin/cyclophosphamide)
- AC (doxorubicin/cyclophosphamide) ± sequential paclitaxel at 2- or 3-week intervals
- EC (epirubicin/cyclophosphamide)
- TAC (docetaxel/doxorubicin/cyclophosphamide)
- A → CMF (doxorubicin followed by cyclophosphamide/methotrexate/fluorouracil)
- E → CMF (epirubicin followed by cyclophosphamide/methotrexate/fluorouracil)
- CMF (cyclophosphamide/methotrexate/fluorouracil)
- A → T → C (doxorubicin followed by paclitaxel followed by cyclophosphamide)
- FEC → T (fluorouracil/epirubicin/cyclophosphamide followed by docetaxel)
- TC (docetaxel and cyclophosphamide)

Trastuzumab-containing Regimens
- AC → T + concurrent trastuzumab (doxorubicin/cyclophosphamide followed by paclitaxel plus trastuzumab)
- TCH (docetaxel, carboplatin, trastuzumab)
- AC → docetaxel + trastuzumab

Adapted from the National Comprehensive Cancer Network (www.nccn.org), with permission.

and represent valid choices (Table 57.1). Chemotherapy generally includes more than one agent and is given over a period of 3 to 6 months. Anthracycline-containing regimens appear to be more effective than CMF-type therapies (cyclophosphamide, methotrexate, 5-fluorouracil), but the degree of added benefit must be balanced against the extra toxicity (2). Several studies suggest a benefit from the addition of taxane to anthracycline (7). Trials suggest that either sequential use of single agents or combination regimens is an acceptable approach. Maintenance of dose is important to ensure optimal outcome. Many randomized trials have failed, however, to show any advantage for the routine use of doses above the standard range, including regimens requiring autologous bone marrow or stem cell support. Results from trials of a dose-dense approach (increasing the frequency of chemotherapy through use of colony-stimulating factors) suggest a benefit over more conventional schedules (8). Although older trials suggest that the benefits of adjuvant chemotherapy are most prominent in women younger than 50 years of age, recent analyses suggest that the biological characteristics of the tumor are more important that patient age. Thus, chronologic age should generally not be used as a selection criterion for use of adjuvant chemotherapy (9). Appropriate use of antiemetics and colony-stimulating factors will help to minimize the acute toxicity of chemotherapy; current information suggests that it may be

prudent to avoid the use of erythroid-stimulating agents in women receiving adjuvant chemotherapy (10).

CHEMOENDOCRINE THERAPY

For women with steroid receptor-positive breast cancer, use of both endocrine therapy and chemotherapy may be considered. Selection of women with steroid receptor-positive breast cancer who might benefit most from chemotherapy should not be based solely on nodal status or tumor size. Rather, chemotherapy could be considered for women with specific tumor characteristics, such as low, albeit positive ER levels, absence of PR, overexpression of ERBB2 protein, or a high recurrence score with the Oncotype DX multigene assay (11). For women who will receive chemoendocrine therapy, the tenets that guide selection of each type of therapy individually should be applied to considerations for combination therapy. When chemoendocrine therapy is recommended, sequential rather than concurrent administration appears to be the most prudent strategy.

ADJUVANT THERAPY FOR ERBB2-POSITIVE BREAST CANCER

For women with tumors that overexpress the ERBB2 protein, use of the monoclonal anti-ERBB2 antibody, trastuzumab, should be considered in addition to adjuvant chemotherapy and adjuvant endocrine therapy if the tumor is ER-positive (12). One year of trastuzumab is regarded as the standard of care in women with node-negative tumors 1 cm or greater or node-positive breast cancers of any size unless there is a contraindication, such as cardiac disease. Ongoing studies are evaluating shorter and longer durations of therapy. Clinical trials support the administration of trastuzumab on either a weekly or an every 3-weekly schedule. Use of trastuzumab with concurrent taxane or after completion of adjuvant chemotherapy represents an evidence-based strategy; trastuzumab should not be used with concomitant anthracycline chemotherapy. Careful assessment of ERBB2 status in a reliable laboratory using well-validated assays is critical to guide use of anti-ERBB2 therapy. Further, meticulous assessment of cardiac function before and during trastuzumab use and adherence to published guidelines for modification of a schedule based on cardiac function are vital. The adjuvant application of lapatinib alone or in conjunction with trastuzumab is under evaluation; lapatinib should not be prescribed as part of standard adjuvant practice at present.

Table 57.2   ALGORITHM FOR ADJUVANT SYSTEMIC THERAPY FOR BREAST CANCER

	ER- and/or PR-Positive	ER- and PR-Negative
ERBB2 negative[a]	Endocrine therapy ± chemotherapy depending on risk	Chemotherapy
ERBB2 positive	Endocrine therapy + chemotherapy + trastuzumab	Chemotherapy + trastuzumab

ER, estrogen receptor; PR, progesterone receptor.
[a]Formerly HER-2.
Adapted from Goldhirsch A, Wood WC, Gelber RD, et al. Progress and promise: highlights of the international expert consensus on the primary therapy of early breast cancer 2007. *Ann Oncol* 2007;18:1133–1144, with permission.

ADJUVANT BISPHOSPHONATES

Promising results have been reported from trials assessing the antineoplastic effects of bisphosphonates in addition to adjuvant systemic chemotherapy or endocrine therapy. At present, however, the indication for their use should be restricted to maintenance of bone health (13).

 ## SUMMARY

Several groups have provided evidence-based or expert opinion-derived guidelines for adjuvant therapy of breast cancer. Among them the recommendations of the 2007 St. Gallen Consensus Conference and National Comprehensive Cancer Network (NCCN) may be particularly useful to clinicians (14,15). These recommendations should be viewed as guidelines rather than mandates for management of the individual patient. A proposed algorithm for use of adjuvant systemic therapy is provided in Table 57.2. Finally, the central importance of clinical trials in patient management cannot be overemphasized. Indeed, participation in a clinical trial often provides optimal management for the individual patient.

References

1. Ravdin PM, Siminoff LA, Davis GJ, et al. Computer program to assist in making decisions about adjuvant therapy for women with breast cancer. *J Clin Oncol* 2001;19:980–991 and www.adjuvantonline.org.

2. Early Breast Cancer Trialists' Collaborative Group (EBCTCG). Effects of chemotherapy and hormonal therapy for early breast cancer on recurrence and 15-year survival: an overview of the randomized trials. *Lancet* 2005;365:1687–1717.

3. Harvey JM, Clark GM, Osborne CK, et al. Estrogen receptor status by immunochemistry is superior to the ligand-binding assay for predicting response to adjuvant endocrine therapy in breast cancer. *J Clin Oncol* 1999;17:1471–1781.

4. Winer EP, Hudis C Burstein HJ, et al. American Society of Clinical Oncology technology assessment on the use of aromatase inhibitors as adjuvant therapy for postmenopausal women with hormone receptor-positive breast cancer: status report 2004. *J Clin Oncol* 2005;23:619–629.

5. Smith IE, Dowsett M, Yap YS, et al. Adjuvant aromatase inhibitors for early breast cancer after chemotherapy-induced amenorrhoea: caution and suggested guidelines. *J Clin Oncol* 2006;24:2444–2447.

6. LHRH agonists in Early Breast Cancer Overview Group Cuzick J, Ambroisine L, Davidson N et al. Use of luteinising-hormone-releasing agonists as adjuvant treatment in premenopausal patients with hormone-receptor-positive breast cancer: a meta-analysis of individual patient data from randomized adjuvant trials. *Lancet* 2007;369:1711–1723.

7. DeLaurentiis M, Cancello G, D'Agostino D, et al. Taxane-based combinations as adjuvant chemotherapy of early breast cancer: a meta-analysis of randomized trials. *J Clin Oncol* 2008;26:44–53.

8. Citron ML, Berry DA, Cirrincione C, et al. Randomized trial of dose-dense versus conventionally scheduled and sequential versus concurrent combination chemotherapy as postoperative adjuvant treatment of node-positive primary breast cancer: first report of Intergroup Trial C9741/Cancer and Leukemia Group B Trial C9741. *J Clin Oncol* 2003;21:1431–1439. Erratum in *J Clin Oncol* 2003;21:2226.

9. Early Breast Cancer Trialists' Collaborative Group (EBCTCG) Clarke M, Coates AS, Darby SC, et al. Adjuvant chemotherapy in oestrogen-receptor-poor breast cancer: patient-level meta-analysis of randomized trials. *Lancet* 2008;371:29–40.

10. http://www.fda.gov/cder/drug/infopage. Accessed September 28, 2008.

11. Paik S, Tang G, Shak S, et al. Gene expression and benefit of chemotherapy in women with node-negative, estrogen receptor-positive breast cancer. *J Clin Oncol* 2006;24:3726–3734.

12. Hudis CA. Trastuzumab—mechanism of action and use in clinical practice. *N Engl J Med* 2007;357:39–51.

13. Hillner BE, Ingle JN, Chlebowski RT, et al. American Society of Clinical Oncology 2003 update on the role of bisphosphonate and bone health issues in women with breast cancer. *J Clin Oncol* 2003;21:4042–4057.

14. Goldhirsch A, Wood WC, Gelber RD, et al. Progress and promise: highlights of the international expert consensus on the primary therapy of early breast cancer 2007. *Ann Oncol* 2007;18:1133–1144.

15. http://www.nccn.org.

Section VIII | Preoperative Systemic Therapy

Chapter 58
Preoperative Therapy for Operable Breast Cancer

Chau T. Dang and Clifford Hudis

Although postoperative systemic (adjuvant) therapy has improved disease-free and overall survival, it is not always the optimal approach (1). For some patient cohorts, preoperative (neoadjuvant) therapy is preferred because it can offer specific advantages. Historically preoperative therapy was used in women with locally advanced breast cancer (LABC) to improve local control by increasing operability. As is true in the adjuvant setting, this use of systemic chemotherapy also offered an overall survival. More recently, the reach of preoperative therapy has been extended because it has been demonstrated to down-stage breast cancers, allowing some patients to opt for breast conservation instead of mastectomy. Finally, there is an increasing number of preoperative research trials in which in-breast response or specimen studies are the primary end points. This chapter will review some of the key preoperative systemic chemotherapy studies and consider how this approach should be incorporated into the standard treatment of patients outside of clinical trials. The chapter will review preoperative chemotherapy and biologic therapies and discuss their integration into the overall treatment approach for patients with operable breast cancer.

PREOPERATIVE CHEMOTHERAPY FOR LOCALLY ADVANCED BREAST CANCER

Neoadjuvant chemotherapy was pioneered in the setting of LABC as first reported in the 1970s (2). At that time several trials assessed the benefit of chemotherapy in women with LABC and in addition to improving the rates of operability, most suggested a survival benefit as well (3–9). Based on these results and the lack of effective alternative strategies, the administration of preoperative chemotherapy prior to local therapy became standard in cases of initially inoperable, nonmetastatic breast cancer.

The next generation of trials essentially extends the observations made in inoperable breast cancer to the larger group of patients with large, but resectable, disease. In this setting preoperative therapy can render more patients candidates for breast conservation. Most patients who are treated with preoperative chemotherapy experience a clinical (and pathologic) response. The clinical response rate is typically 49% to 93% and the pathologic complete response (pCR) rate is usually in the range of 4% to 30% (Table 58.1). With such responses breast conservation is made more likely. In addition to facilitating breast conservation, preoperative therapy allows for an *in vivo* treatment sensitivity assessment, although the interpretation and utility of this activity is not yet clear. How response is assessed becomes especially important because clinical complete response (cCR) does not always correlate with the pCR, as about one third of patients with a cCR have pathologic disease

at the time of surgery (5–6). It is important to note that despite difficulties in accurately assessing clinical response, patients who have a cCR or a pCR have better outcomes than those who do not achieve these end points (5).

PREOPERATIVE CHEMOTHERAPY FOR OPERABLE BREAST CANCER

A series of trials have evaluated the results of administering preoperative versus postoperative chemotherapy for women with operable breast cancer. Because earlier systemic therapy was postulated to be superior, it was hypothesized that preoperative chemotherapy would improve disease-free survival (DFS) and overall survival (OS) while also possibly improving the rate of breast conservation. The earliest nonrandomized trials in women with operable breast cancer showed a response rate of 67% to 85% with a cCR rate of 30% to 58% (10–13). However, DFS and OS appeared to be similar to patients who historically received chemotherapy postoperatively. Bonadonna et al. (12) reported results from two prospective nonrandomized trials in 536 patients with tumors greater than 2.5 cm. In these two studies, three to four cycles of cyclophosphamide, methotrexate, and fluorouracil (CMF)-based or anthracycline-based regimens were delivered preoperatively and additional postoperative chemotherapy was given to those with high-risk disease. Following the so-called primary chemotherapy, the breast conservation rate was 85% and it was noted that there was a pCR rate of 3%. In a multivariate analysis, the pathologic response in the breast ($p = .034$) as well in the nodes ($p < .001$) correlated significantly with relapse-free survival (RFS). These results supported several randomized studies designed to assess the benefit of preoperative chemotherapy associated with tumor down-staging.

DOWN-STAGING OF TUMORS WITH PREOPERATIVE CHEMOTHERAPY

United Kingdom Trial

The first-generation trials showed that most tumors responded to induction chemotherapy. A response to preoperative chemotherapy may typically down-stage breast tumors at the time of surgery. In most trials this rendered the primary tumors smaller and facilitated a higher rate of node-negative disease and improved the rate of breast conservation. However, this did not necessarily always result in improved DFS or OS. More consistently, patients who achieved a pCR, compared with those who did not, had improved outcomes. This suggests that

| Table 58.1 | CHEMOTHERAPY FOR LOCALLY ADVANCED BREAST CANCER |

Study (Reference)	No. of Patients	Clinical PR (%)	Clinical CR (%)	PCR (%)
Swain et al. (3)	76	44	49	30
Perloff et al. (4)	113	55	22	NR
Hortobagyi et al. (5)	174	71	17	8
Bonadonna et al. (6)	165	60	17	4
Jacquillat et al. (7)	98	45	30	NR
Pierce et al. (8)	107	NR	49	29
Schwartz et al. (9)	189	NR	85 (CR + PR)	10

CR, complete response; PR, partial response; pCR, pathologic complete response; NR, not reported.

response *per se* is not sufficient to change the natural history of systemic disease, but that complete response is, or that complete response is a marker of particularly chemosensitive systemic disease.

One of the first randomized trials of chemoendocrine therapy was conducted by Powles et al. (13) (Table 58.2). In this study, 212 patients with operable breast cancer were randomized to four cycles of methotrexate, mitoxantrone with or without mitomycin (MMM) followed by surgery followed by four more cycles of MMM versus all eight cycles of MMM postoperatively. Tamoxifen was given concurrently with chemotherapy. In the preoperative group, the clinical response was 85%. On pathologic examination more patients in the preoperative group had tumors less than 2 cm (86% vs. 43%; p <.001). In the preoperative group the pCR rate was 10%. There was a higher breast conservation rate (87% vs. 72%; p <.005) in the preoperative group. At a median follow-up of 28 months, the ipsilateral breast tumor recurrence (IBTR) was 1% in preoperative and 2% in postoperative groups. Despite down-staging of the tumors in the preoperative group (smaller tumor sizes at the time of surgical resection and a higher breast conservation rate), there was no difference in DFS or OS.

National Surgical Adjuvant Breast and Bowel Project B-18

In 1998 the National Surgical Adjuvant Breast and Bowel Project (NSABP) conducted a large phase III study (NSABP B-18) to compare pre- and postoperative chemotherapy (Table 58.2)

(14). In this trial 1,523 women with operable breast cancer were randomly assigned to pre- or postoperative doxorubicin and cyclophosphamide (AC; at 60/600 mg/mg^2) for four cycles. Tamoxifen was administered to women 50 years of age or older after the completion of chemotherapy. The clinical size of the breast and axillary tumors were determined before each cycle of AC and before surgery. Breast tumor sizes were reduced in 79% of patients after preoperative AC, with a 36% cCR rate, 43% clinical partial response, and a 13% pCR rate. Clinical nodal response was observed in 89% of patients with node-positive disease; 73% had a nodal cCR, and 44% of these patients had pCR. In terms of the pathologic node status, 42% of postoperative patients versus 58% of preoperative patients had node-negative disease (p <.0001). Overall, 12% more lumpectomies were performed in the preoperative group (68% vs. 60%; p = .001). However, in contrast to the hypothesis that early is better, there continue to be no statistically significant differences in outcomes. Again, despite the down-staging of tumors in the preoperative group (79% clinical response rate, a higher rate of node-negative disease, and breast conservation), there was no difference in DFS or OS between the two groups (15). The 5-, 8-, and 16-year DFS estimates were 67%, 58%, and 42% for the preoperative group and 67%, 55%, and 39% for the postoperative group, respectively (p = .27). The 5-, 8- and 16- survival estimates were 80%, 72%, and 55% for the preoperative group and 81%, 72%, and 55% for the postoperative group, respectively (p = .90) (15). There was a numerically higher rate of IBTR in the preoperative group (13% vs. 10%), but this difference was not statistically significant (p = .21). At 16 years of follow-up, in patients less than 50 years of age, there was a trend favoring preoperative over postoperative chemotherapy for DFS (44% vs. 38%; hazard ratio [HR] = 0.85; p = .09) and OS (61% vs. 55%; HR = 0.81; p = .06). In patients 50 years of age or older, there was a trend favoring postoperative over preoperative chemotherapy for OS (55% vs. 50%; HR = 1.23; p = .07). The DFS was not statistically different between treatment groups in this older population. It is possible that younger patients have more ER-negative tumors that are more sensitive to chemotherapy up front, but data on the hormone-receptor status of these younger patients are limited in NSABP B-18. Because this is a retrospective analysis and subject to the usual limitations, for now age should not be used to determine if a patient should or should not receive preoperative chemotherapy.

At the same time it is noted that women who had a pCR had a statistically significant increased DFS (HR = 0.47; p <.0001) and OS (HR = 0.32; p <.0001) compared with those who had residual tumor in the breast (15). In a multivariate model that

| Table 58.2 | FIRST-GENERATIONS PREOPERATIVE CHEMOTHERAPY TRIALS |

Study (Reference)	No. of Patients	Stage	Treatment	Objective Response Rate (CR + PR) (%)	PCR (%)	Breast Conservation	DFS	OS
Powles et al. (13)	212	T1–T3	MMM → S → MMM vs. S → MMM	85	10	87% vs. 72% (p <.005)	Med FU of 28 mos 91% vs. 90% (p = NR)	Med FU of 28 mos (NR)
NSABP B-18 (14,15)	1,523	Operable breast cancer	AC → S vs. S → AC	80	9	67% vs. 60% p = .002	Med FU of 9 yrs 55% vs. 53% (p = 0.50)	Med FU of 9 yrs 69% vs. 70% (p = 0.80)
EORTC 10902 (16)	698	T1–T4 N0–N1	FEC → S vs. S → FEC	49	2	23% vs. 18% p = NR	Med FU of 56 mos 65% vs. 70% (p = 0.27)	Med FU of 5 yrs 82% vs. 84% (p = 0.38)

Med, median; FU, follow-up; CR, complete response; PR, partial response, pCR, pathologic complete response; DFS, disease-free survival; OS, overall survival; S, surgery MMM = methotrexate, mitoxantrone +/− mitomycin; AC, doxorubicin, cyclophosphamide; FEC, fluorouracil, epirubicin, cyclophosphamide; NR, not reported.

included known predictors of outcome, achieving a pCR was an independent predictor of survival. This is consistent with other data associating complete response with improved overall outcomes.

European Organisation for Research and Treatment of Cancer 10902

The European Organisation for Research and Treatment of Cancer (EORTC) conducted a trial, 10902 (Table 58.2), which was similar to NSABP B-18 (16). In this study 698 patients with breast cancer (T1c, T2, T3, T4b, N0-1) were randomly assigned to four cycles of fluorouracil, epirubicin, and cyclophosphamide (FEC; at 600/60/600 mg/m^2) given preoperatively (350 patients) or postoperatively (348 patients). The overall clinical response rate was 49% with a 6.6% cCR. Overall, 13 of 350 patients (4%) in the preoperative group had a pCR. There was a higher rate of tumors, with sizes <2 cm in the preoperative versus postoperative groups (47% vs. 26%; p value not reported). Pathologic examination after surgery showed a numerically higher rate of node-negative disease in the preoperative versus postoperative groups (38% vs. 35%; p value not reported). In the preoperative group 23% of patients underwent breast conservation (instead of the planned mastectomy). Despite the down-staging of tumors in the preoperative group (a higher rate of tumors <2 cm, numerically more patients with node-negative disease, and a 23% of patients converted to receiving breast conservation), at a median follow-up of 56 months, there was no significant difference in terms of progression-free survival (PFS) (65% vs. 70%; $p = .27$) or OS (82% vs. 84%; $p = .38$) for pre- and postoperative groups, respectively. Time to locoregional recurrence was the same for both arms. Of note, the 4% of patients who had a pCR after preoperative therapy had a significant advantage in terms of OS over those who had residual disease (HR = 0.86; $p = .008$).

National Surgical Adjuvant Breast and Bowel Project B-27

NSABP B-27 was a randomized trial designed to evaluate the benefits of adding four cycles of docetaxel preoperatively or postoperatively to four cycles of preoperative AC (Table 58.3) (17). In this study more than 2,400 patients were randomly assigned to receive neoadjuvant AC → surgery or AC → docetaxel → surgery or AC → surgery → docetaxel. The doses of AC (60/600 mg/m^2) and docetaxel (100 mg/m^2) were standard (15,17). Four cycles of AC as well as four cycles of docetaxel were given. All cycles were given every 3 weeks. Preoperative AC → docetaxel modestly increased the overall clinical response rate (90.7% vs. 85.5%; $p <.001$) and the cCR rate (63.6% vs. 40.1%; $p <.001$) when compared to AC alone. There was a doubling of the pCR in those who received preoperative AC → docetaxel versus AC (26.1% vs. 13.7%; $p <.001$). Furthermore, more patients who had AC → docetaxel versus AC had negative axillary nodes at the time of surgery (58.2% vs. 50.8%; $p <.001$). However, the rate of breast conservation was similar in all arms, suggesting that four cycles of preoperative AC may convert as many patients to lumpectomy as does AC → docetaxel. Based on the results of NSABP B-18 (14–15), it was anticipated that patients with a pCR would have improved outcomes when compared to those who did not, and this was seen in NSABP B-27 as well. However, in NSABP B-27, when looking at all three groups, and despite a doubling of the pCR rates in patients who received AC → docetaxel when compared to those treated with AC alone preoperatively, there was no statistically significant difference in DFS or OS at 5 or 8 years of follow-up (15,17). The 5- and 8-year DFS rates were 68% and 59% for AC → surgery group, 71% and 62% for AC → docetaxel → surgery group, and 70% and 62% in AC → surgery → docetaxel group. The 5- and 8-year OS rates were 82% and 74% for AC → surgery group, 83% and 75% for AC → docetaxel → surgery group, and 82% and 75% in AC → surgery → docetaxel group. Thus, despite the down-staging of tumors in the preoperative group receiving AC → docetaxel versus AC (a doubling of

---

Table 58.3   **SECOND-GENERATIONS PREOPERATIVE CHEMOTHERAPY TRIALS**

Study (Reference)	No. of Patients	Stage	Treatment	Objective Response (CR + PR)	pCR	Breast Conservation
NSABP B-27 (17)	2,411	Operable breast cancer	AC → S vs. AC → D → S vs. AC → S → D	90.7% vs. 85.5% favoring AC → D over AC ($p <.001$)	26.1% vs. 13.7% favoring AC → D over AC ($p <.001$)	Same
Aberdeen Trial (20)	162	T3–T4, N2	CVAP (non-resp)→ D vs. CVAP (resp) → CVAP vs. CVAP (resp)→ D	94% vs. 66% in favor of CVAP → D over CVAP → CVAP ($p = .001$)	31% vs. 15% in favor of CVAP → D over CVAP → CVAP ($p = .06$)	67% vs. 48% in favor of CVAP → D over CVAP → CVAP ($p <.01$)
Gerpar-DUO (23)	913	T2–T3 N0–N2	dd AD → vs. AC → D	85% vs. 75% in favor of AC → D ($p <.001$)	14% vs. 7% in favor of AC → D ($p <.001$)	63% vs. 58% in favor of AC → D ($p = .05$)
Hoosier Trial (24)	40	Stage II–III	dd A → D vs. AD	89% vs. 81% in favor of dd A → D ($p = NR$)	16% vs. 10% in favor of dd A → D ($p = NR$)	39% vs. 19% in favor of dd A → D ($p = NR$)
MDACC (26)	258	Stage I–IIIA	w P → FAC vs. 3w P → FAC	Same ($p = .25$)	28% vs. 16% in favor of w P → FAC ($p = .02$)	47% vs. 38% in favor of w P → FAC ($p = .05$)
ECTO Trial (19)	1,355	T2–T3 N0–N1	S → A → CMF vs. S → AP → CMF vs. AP → CMF→ S	78% in preoperative AP → CMF→ S	17% in preoperative AP → CMF → S	65% vs. 34% in favor of AP → CMF → S ($p <.001$)
AGO Study (29)	631	T >3 cm	dd E → P vs. EP	NR	18% vs. 10% in favor of dd E → P ($p = .03$)	66% vs. 55% in favor of dd E → P ($p = .016$)

CR, complete response; PR, partial response; pCR, pathologic complete response; S, surgery; Non-resp, non-responders; Resp, responders; AC, doxorubicin, cyclophosphamide; D, docetaxel; CVAP = cyclophosphamide, vincristine, doxorubicin, prednisolone; AD, doxorubicin, docetaxel; P, paclitaxel; FAC, fluorouracil, doxorubicin, cyclophosphamide; AP, doxorubicin, paclitaxel; CMF, cyclophosphamide, methotrexate, fluorouracil; E, epirubicin; EP, epirubicin, paclitaxel; w, weekly, 3 w, every 3-weekly.

the pCR and a higher rate of node-negative disease), the breast conservation rate was the same across all three groups as well as DFS and OS. However, there was a trend toward increased RFS in those who received neoadjuvant docetaxel in AC → docetaxel when compared with AC alone (5-year RFS 74% vs. 69.6%; HR = 0.85; p = .08). Taken together, this study (at least in isolation) calls into question the assumptions that in-breast response can serve as a simple surrogate for longer-term outcomes, including DFS and OS.

In NASBP B-27, events for DFS included all local, regional, or distant recurrences, all clinically inoperable and residual disease at surgery, all deaths, and all second and contralateral cancers. Events for calculation of RFS included the first breast cancer recurrence, clinically inoperable and residual disease at surgery, and any death. To facilitate comparisons with other trials in using a standard definition for DFS, a *post hoc* end point of RFS was created in which the difference between RFS and DFS was that second cancers and contralateral breast cancers were not considered to be events for RFS. In the future, reliance on standard definitions for end point collections in adjuvant therapy trials may ease cross-study comparisons (18). This possible advantage for the all preoperative delivery in NSABP B-27 is consistent with other evidence that chemotherapy dose-density is an important variable predicting treatment outcomes. Here, the delivery of uninterrupted chemotherapy maximized dose-density (AC → docetaxel → surgery) compared to the arm in which there was a split in the chemotherapy regimen (AC → surgery → docetaxel). Like the NSABP B-18, through 8 years of follow-up posttreatment, the pCR was a significant predictor of DFS (HR = 0.49; p <.0001) and OS regardless of treatment (HR = 0.36; p <.0001) (15).

European Cooperative Trial in Operable Breast Cancer

The European Cooperative Trial in Operable (ECTO) Breast Cancer randomly tested the efficacy of postoperative chemotherapy doxorubicin (75 mg/m²) followed by CMF (600/40/600 mg/m² days 1 and 8 every 4 weeks) or doxorubicin and paclitaxel (AP; at 60/200 mg/m²) followed by CMF versus preoperative chemotherapy (AP followed by CMF) (19) (Table 58.3). A total of 1,355 patients entered the study. Overall, preoperative chemotherapy induced a clinical response in 78% of the patients and the pCR rate was 23%. The axillary down-staging occurred in a significant proportion of patients (60% vs. 39% were node-negative in preoperative and postoperative groups, respectively, p <.0001), and breast conservation was higher in the preoperative group (65% vs. 34%; p <.001). Survival data were not reported. This is another study demonstrating that a higher breast conservation rate can be achieved with preoperative chemotherapy.

Conclusions on the Benefit of Down-Staging of Tumors with Preoperative Chemotherapy

Overall, the clearest potential gain of preoperative chemotherapy in these trials is the achievement of a higher breast conservation rate when mastectomy may have been initially indicated based on clinical presentation (U.K. trial, NSABP B-18, EORTC 10902, ECTO) (13,15,16,19). Other benefits include smaller tumors found at the time of surgery (U.K. trial, EORTC 10902) (13,16) and a higher rate of node-negative disease (NSABP B-18, EORTC 10902, NSABP B-27, ECTO) (15–19). However, DFS and OS were the same despite the down-staging of these tumors. Of note, when considering patients who achieved a pCR versus those who did not, there was a statistically significant improvement in outcomes in multiple trials (NSABP B-18, EORTC 10902, NSABP B-27) (15–17).

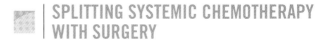

SPLITTING SYSTEMIC CHEMOTHERAPY WITH SURGERY

It is unknown whether there is a true advantage to delivering all intended chemotherapy without interruption before surgery or is there a disadvantage if the same chemotherapy is split with half of the regimen given before and half given after surgery. The NSABP B-27 addressed this because, as described above, half of the docetaxel-treated patients had surgery before receiving this chemotherapy and half had the surgery only after completing all systemic treatment. The patients with all eight cycles of chemotherapy administered preoperatively had a trend toward improvement in RFS (17). One caveat with this study is that at the time it was conducted, all patients received tamoxifen, which was initiated concurrently with chemotherapy, regardless of hormone-receptor status. The simultaneous administration of tamoxifen with chemotherapy may have diluted some benefit from chemotherapy. In other words, the true potential magnitude of the improvement in RFS may not be seen with concurrent tamoxifen.

UTILITY OF IN-BREAST RESPONSE TO TAILOR THERAPY

The administration of preoperative chemotherapy provides a unique opportunity to assess for tumor response to treatment and potentially to allow the physician to tailor therapy based on this response. However, to date there is no evidence to support the routine use of midcourse chemotherapy regimen changes, based on the initial response or lack of in-breast response as a means of improving overall outcomes. Below are the results of two key trials that suggest that in-breast response should not be used to tailor therapy, except when there is progression of disease.

Aberdeen Trial

The Aberdeen trial addressed the important question of whether clinicians can or should use in-breast response as a guide to switching chemotherapy agents (Table 58.3). In this study 162 patients with large operable tumors or LABC received four cycles of cyclophosphamide (1,000 mg/m²), vincristine 1.5 (mg/m²), doxorubicin (50 mg/m²), and prednisolone (40 mg orally per day for 5 days) (CVAP) (20). Patients who had a response to CVAP were then randomized to four more cycles of CVAP (the drugs to which their tumors were demonstrably sensitive) or to docetaxel in four cycles at 100 mg/m², all given at 21-day intervals. Those who did not have a response to CVAP were assigned to receive docetaxel in four cycles as "rescue" therapy. Patients then underwent surgery at the completion of eight cycles of therapy. After four cycles of CVAP, the overall clinical response rate was 66%. In the responding patients, four additional cycles of docetaxel resulted in a significantly higher clinical response rate compared with those who continued on four cycles of CVAP (94% vs. 66%; p = .001). Patients who received docetaxel had a pCR rate of 31%, which was more than double the response rate of 15% for those who continued on CVAP (p = .06). Patients who received docetaxel had an increase in the breast conservation rate (67% vs. 48%; p <.01). There was also a survival gain in those who received docetaxel. At a median follow-up of 65 months, 93% of patients received docetaxel after a response to CVAP were alive versus 78% of those who had eight cycles of CVAP (p = .04). Of those who had stable or progressive disease after CVAP in four cycles and were assigned to docetaxel, 47% had a clinical response with docetaxel. This trial provides evidence that it is the addition of a noncross resistant drug (i.e., taxane after CVAP), rather than the continuation of more cycles of the same regimen, regardless of tumor response, that seemingly offers benefit. This strongly suggests that in-breast response cannot be used to tailor conventional chemotherapy in the preoperative setting: essentially all patients potentially benefited from the switch and even those with sensitive tumors did *not* benefit from more of what was known to be effective therapy for them.

Gepar-TRIO Trial

The German Breast Group Gepar-TRIO study assessed the response to preoperative docetaxel, doxorubicin, and cyclophosphamide (TAC) after two cycles (21,22). In this study patients received two cycles of TAC (75 mg/m^2, 50 mg/m^2, 500 mg/m^2) 3 weeks apart. In the initial phase of the study patients whose tumors responded to TAC for two cycles received four more cycles of TAC. Those whose tumors did not respond were instead randomized to four more cycles of TAC or four cycles of vinorelbine/capecitabine (N at 25 mg/m^2 days 1 and 8 and X at 2,000 mg/m^2 daily days 1 through 4) every 3 weeks. Prior to surgery, in the responders to TAC for two cycles (who received further TAC in four cycles), the cCR rate was 50.5% and the pCR rate was 22.9%. In the nonresponders to TAC for two cycles (who were randomized to TAC for four cycles or NX in four cycles), the cCR rates were the same (22.5% for TAC vs. 21.9% for NX) and the pCR rates were statistically the same (7.3% for TAC vs. 3.1% for NX). This led to a larger study in which patients with tumors that responded to TAC for two cycles were then randomized to more TAC for four cycles versus six cycles (21). Overall, the pathologic responses were the same whether patients received six versus eight cycles of preoperative TAC. The Gepar-TRIO trial is consistent with and complementary to the Aberdeen trial described above. Again, knowledge of chemotherapy resistance does not appear to allow clinicians to select a more effective crossover therapy based on in-breast response nor does sensitivity predict a greater benefit for more of what was already proven effective (TAC in this case).

▓ OTHER SECOND-GENERATION PREOPERATIVE TRIALS

German Preoperative Adriamycin Docetaxel Trial

The German Preoperative Adriamycin Docetaxel Trial (Gepar-DUO) from the German Breast Group evaluated 913 women with operable breast cancer and compared responses between preoperative dose-dense every 2–weekly doxorubicin/docetaxel (AD; at 50/75 mg/m^2) for four cycles versus AC (60/600 mg/m^2) for four cycles → D (100 mg/m^2) for four cycles (23) (Table 58.3). Clinical responses (85% vs. 75.2%; p <.001) and radiographic responses (78.6% vs. 68.6%; p <.001) were higher in the AC → D group. Like the NSABP B-27 and the Aberdeen trial, the pCR was higher with sequential use of docetaxel (14.3% for AC → D vs. 7% for AD; p <.001). The rate of breast conservation was also in favor of the AC → D group (63.4% vs. 58.1%; p = .05). The reasons that AC → D was superior to AD could be that higher doses of doxorubicin and docetaxel were used when given sequentially, more cycles were delivered (eight vs. four cycles), or a greater number of drugs (three vs. two drugs) were administered. Survival data were not reported.

Hoosier Oncology Group trial (Dose-Dense Sequential Anthracycline followed by Docetaxel Chemotherapy vs. Combination)

Similarly, the Hoosier Oncology Group trial showed superiority with sequential docetaxel (Table 58.3). This study involved a small group of patients (N = 40) with stage II or noninflammatory stage III breast cancer who were assigned to dose-dense every 2-weekly A (75 mg/m^2) for three cycles → D (100 mg/m^2) for three cycles versus AD (56/75 mg/m^2) every 3 weeks for four cycles (24). Granulocyte-colony stimulating factor was given on days 2 to 12 to both groups. Overall, clinical responses were similar in both groups (89% vs. 81%; p value not reported) and the pCR rate was higher in the sequential docetaxel group (16% vs. 10%; p value not reported). Patients who received sequential docetaxel also had fewer positive nodes (mean, 2.17 vs. 4.8; p <.037) and were more likely to have breast conservation (37% vs. 19%; p value not reported). Although the total cumulative doses of doxorubicin and docetaxel were the same in the two arms, the superior results achieved with sequential A → D could be due to the higher dose-density of this dose-dense every 2-weekly schedule. Of note, there was a higher incidence of grade 3or 4 hand-foot syndrome with the dose-dense A → D arm (42% vs. 0%). Survival data were not reported.

M.D. Anderson Cancer Center Trials

Although many trials studied docetaxel in the preoperative setting (NSABP B-27, Aberdeen, Gepar-TRIO, Gepar-DUO), there were others that similarly evaluated paclitaxel. M.D. Anderson Cancer Center (MDACC) conducted an adjuvant and neoadjuvant trial that tested the sequential use of paclitaxel and FAC (25). In this study 524 patients with operable breast cancer were randomly assigned to receive FAC (500 mg/m^2 on days 1 and 4, 50 mg/m^2 on days 1 to 3, 500 mg/m^2 on day 1) for eight cycles versus paclitaxel (P) (250 mg/m^2) for four cycles as a 24-hour continuous infusion followed by FAC for four cycles (paclitaxel → FAC). In this study, 174 patients received chemotherapy preoperatively either as FAC → surgery → FAC or paclitaxel → surgery → FAC. Patients who were 50 years of age or older with hormone-receptor (HR)-positive disease received tamoxifen for 5 years. Clinical responses and breast conservation rates were similar in both arms, suggesting that single agent paclitaxel had comparable antitumor activity as FAC. However, at a median follow-up of 60 months, the 4-year DFS of all patients collectively was not statistically different between the two groups (83% for FAC → FAC and 86% for P → FAC; p = .09) (24). Overall survival data are pending. Because of its modest size, this trial cannot demonstrate statistical significance for any modest benefit by crossing over to a noncross resistant regimen (i.e., P → FAC).

The MDACC also reported another trial evaluating paclitaxel given at two different schedules in the preoperative setting (26) (Table 58.3). In this study 258 patients were randomly assigned to receive weekly paclitaxel or standard every 3-weekly paclitaxel to determine if different schedules or dose densities of paclitaxel would achieve improved pCR rates. The doses of weekly paclitaxel varied based on clinical status of axillary nodes. Weekly paclitaxel was given at a dose of 80 mg/m^2 for 12 weeks to those with clinically node-negative disease or 150 mg/m^2 (3 weeks on and 1 week off) for four cycles to those with clinically node-positive disease. Standard paclitaxel was administered as 24-hour infusion at 225 mg/m^2 every 3 weeks for four cycles. After completion of paclitaxel, all patients received FAC. Clinical responses were similar in both groups (p = .25). The pCR rates were higher in those who received weekly paclitaxel (28.2%) than those who received standard paclitaxel (15.7%; p = .02) with an improved breast conservation rate (47% vs. 38%; $p = .05$). Whether this will translate to better outcomes will require longer follow-up. However, there are already data supporting the superiority of weekly paclitaxel over every 3-weekly paclitaxel in the metastatic setting as reported by Seidman et al. (27) for the Cancer and Leukemia Group B (CALGB) 9840 and in the adjuvant setting with the Eastern Cooperative Oncology Group (ECOG) 1199 by Sparano et al. (28). Thus, when paclitaxel is used in the preoperative setting, the weekly appears to be superior to the every 3-weekly schedule as is true in other settings.

Dose-Dense Anthracycline Followed by Paclitaxel Study versus Combination

Like the Hoosier Oncology study (24), Untch et al. (29) conducted a preoperative study Arbeitsgemein Schaft [A]GO study [Gynaekologische Onkologie]) comparing dose-dense sequential anthracycline followed by a taxane versus combination chemotherapy (Table 58.3). In this study 631 patients were randomized to dose-dense sequential epirubicin followed by paclitaxel (E → P) versus combination E + P every 3 weeks. Both regimens were given for a total of 12 weeks. Preliminary data on 475 patients showed a higher breast conservation rate (66% vs. 55%; $p = .016$) and pCR rate (18% vs. 10%; $p = .03$) with the dose-dense E → P arm. Although the total cumulative doses of each chemotherapy agent was slightly higher in the sequential arm, the superior results could also be due to the dose-density of this regimen, which would be consistent with the findings of the CALGB trial 9741 (30).

Role of Additional Chemotherapy in Patients with Residual Disease?

After preoperative chemotherapy, patients with operable disease generally proceed with definitive breast surgery and biologic therapy if appropriate (i.e., trastuzumab in *ERBB2* [formerly *HER2*]-positive disease), radiation therapy, and hormonal therapy. Clinicians, aware of the unfavorable prognosis for patients with less than complete responses, often wonder if more chemotherapy should be given postoperatively. To date, there is no trial showing that additional postoperative chemotherapy after a standard preoperative chemotherapy improves outcome, but this is an appropriate area for research. Both hypotheses are tenable based on the data presented: the poor prognosis of such patients makes them good candidates for more treatment or the demonstration of chemotherapy resistance means that they are unlikely to reap a benefit from more therapy. Outside of a clinical trial, the use of additional chemotherapy after a full regimen of preoperative chemotherapy is not recommended, but it is important to stress that a standard adjuvant chemotherapy regimen should be fully delivered in all patients either pre-, peri-, or postoperatively.

Preoperative Chemotherapy in Practice

In operable breast cancer, there is no survival advantage for chemotherapy delivered before surgery nor is there a disadvantage. Patients with a pCR have an OS advantage. The first-generation trials show that DFS and OS are the same when the same chemotherapy is given pre- or postoperatively, and that more breast conservation may be achieved with preoperative therapy. The second generation trials focused on the addition of the taxanes and alternative and dose-dense schedules. Consistent with the adjuvant trials, adding a taxane improves outcomes (31), and in the preoperative setting, this resulted in increased clinical and pathologic responses. Because these drugs are being added, perhaps rendering these regimens inherently more active than those of the first generation of studies, the increased antitumor

effects of the taxanes do not always translate into a higher breast conservation rate or overall survival (NSABP B-27). Importantly, and frustratingly, the early improvements in the pCR rates do not reliably predict improved DFS or OS in these studies. This means that small trials testing of in-breast responses cannot be used as replacements for larger conventional adjuvant trials. It is possible that better outcomes may be achieved if all chemotherapy is given up front before definitive surgery, rather than splitting the regimen, because of the maintenance of dose density (NSABP B-27). Of critical importance to clinicians, it must be recognized that in-breast response cannot be used to tailor therapy in the preoperative setting (Aberdeen, Gerpa-TRIO). This observation should save patients and their clinicians tremendous amounts of uncertainty and stress. Similarly, knowledge of chemotherapy resistance does not allow physicians to select a more effective crossover treatment based on in-breast response (Gepar-TRIO). Both these trials show that treatments should be planned at the outset to include full delivery of a standard adjuvant regimen already associated (from adjuvant trials) with improved DFS and OS, and these should not be altered unless there is disease progression. Specific regimens can include docetaxel given in a every 3-weekly schedule (NSABP B-27, Aberdeen, Gepar-TRIO, Gepar-DUO) while caution should be used with dose-dense every 2-weekly docetaxel as it may cause more toxicities, such as hand-foot syndrome (Hoosier Oncology trial). When using paclitaxel, both dose-dense every 2-weekly and weekly schedules improve outcomes compared to the every 3-weekly schedule (AGO, MDACC). Finally, if there is residual disease at surgery, there is no proven role for additional postoperative chemotherapy after a full adjuvant regimen has been delivered preoperatively.

PREOPERATIVE BIOLOGIC THERAPY WITH CHEMOTHERAPY

The use of newly available biologic agents in combination with standard chemotherapy may improve response rates and outcomes, and the in-breast response may, within clinical trials, provide important leads as drugs are developed. Buzdar et al. (32,33) tested trastuzumab (Herceptin) in a group of patients with *ERBB2*-positive tumors (Table 58.4). These data predicted the subsequent reports of benefit for this monoclonal antibody in the adjuvant setting (34–37). Here, among 42 patients with

Table 58.4	PREOPERATIVE TRASTUZUMAB TRIALS			
Study (Reference)	No. of Patients	Stage	Treatment	pCR
Buzdar et al. (32)	42	Operable	P → FEC +/–Phase I dose-escalation and pharmacokinetic study of lapatinib in combination with trastuzumab Tras → S	65% vs. 26% ($p = .016$)
Gianni et al. (38)	228	LABC	AP → P → CMF +/– Tras → S	43% vs. 23% ($p = .002$)
Fenton et al. (39)	55	Operable LABC	P+ Carbo +/– Tras → S	78% vs. 29% (NR)
Chang et al. (40)	28	LABC	D+ Carbo +/– Tras → S	36% vs. 9% (NR)

P, paclitaxel; FEC, 5-fluorouracil, epirubicin, cyclophosphamide; AP, doxorubicin, paclitaxel; CMF, = cyclophosphamide, methotrexate, 5-fluorouracil; Tras, trastuzumab; Carbo, carboplatin; LABC, locally advanced breast cancer; S, surgery; pCR, pathologic complete response; NR, not reported.

operable *ERBB2*-positive breast cancer who were randomized to paclitaxel (225 mg/m²) for four cycles followed by FEC (for 500 mg/m² days 1 and 4, 75 mg/m² day 1, 500 mg/m² day 1) in four cycles or the same chemotherapy with concurrent weekly trastuzumab (2 mg/kg weekly) for 24 weeks. Overall, the cCR rate was superior in the trastuzumab containing arm (86.9% vs. 47.4%). Similarly the pCR rate was increased with the addition of trastuzumab (65.2% vs. 26%; *p* = .016) (32). When this difference in response rate was recognized, the study was modified to include an additional 22 patients on the trastuzumab arm (33). In the additional cohort, the pCR rate was 54.5%, and when combining all patients on trastuzumab containing regimen, the pCR rate was 60%. It is noteworthy that while three patients have experienced recurrence in the chemotherapy alone arm, no patient has recurred in the trastuzumab arm, thus giving a DFS at 1 and 3 years of 100% (*p* = .041).

Similar results were reported by Gianni et al. (38) using neoadjuvant trastuzumab in locally advanced breast cancer in the NOAH (neoadjuvant Herceptin) study. In this study 228 patients with *ERBB2*-positive disease were randomized to chemotherapy with or without trastuzumab before surgery. The chemotherapy regimen was doxorubicin/paclitaxel (60 mg/m² and 150 mg/m²) for three cycles followed by paclitaxel (175 mg/m²) for four cycles followed by CMF for three cycles. Overall, the response rate was superior in the trastuzumab containing arm (80.9% vs. 73.4%) as well as the pCR rate (43% vs. 23%; *p* = .002). Although this study shows the benefit of trastuzumab, clinicians should be cautious regarding the concurrent use of trastuzumab with an anthracycline. The safety of concurrent versus sequential trastuzumab with epirubicin is being evaluated by the American College of Surgery Oncology Group.

Fenton et al. (39) reported the results of preoperative paclitaxel (80 mg/m² weekly in 16 cycles) plus carboplatin (AUC; 6 every 4 weeks) plus trastuzumab (in *ERBB2*-positive) versus paclitaxel/carboplatin (in *ERBB2*-negative) in a group of 55 breast cancer patients (Table 58.4). In this study the pCR rate was nearly triple in the trastuzumab group (78% vs. 29%; *p* value not reported). Chang et al. (40) reported the results of neoadjuvant docetaxel plus carboplatin plus trastuzumab versus docetaxel plus carboplatin (Table 58.4). In this group of 28 *ERBB2*-positive patients, the pCR rate was much higher with the addition of trastuzumab (36.4% vs. 9%). Thus, these studies confirm the benefit of trastuzumab in the treatment of *ERBB2*-positive breast cancer.

Another anti-*ERBB2* targeted agent is now ready to be studied in the preoperative setting. Lapatinib (Tykerb), a dual inhibitor of both EGFR and *ERBB2* tyrosine kinase activity, has demonstrated activity as a single agent, combined with trastuzumab, as well as with chemotherapy (41–43). Lapatinib is now being evaluated in the adjuvant setting and naturally should be studied in the neoadjuvant setting. The CALGB, NSABP, and others will be conducting randomized trials to evaluate trastuzumab and lapatinib in the preoperative setting. Several other trials are ongoing to evaluate these two drugs in the neoadjuvant setting, including neo-ALTTO (Neoadjuvant Lapatinib and/or Trastuzumab Treatment Optimization). This trial will compare three treatments: lapatinib, trastuzumab, or the combination of both with weekly paclitaxel before surgery.

In the *ERBB2*-normal (nonoverexpressed) group bevacizumab (Avastin) is being evaluated preoperatively. Bevacizumab is an antiangiogenic antibody that binds to human vascular endothelial growth factor (VEGF). Bevacizumab improves progression-free survival when combined with paclitaxel versus paclitaxel alone as front-line treatment of metastatic *ERBB2*-normal breast cancer (44). Bevacizumab is now being studied in a large phase III study in the adjuvant setting (ECOG 5103). In terms of neoadjuvant treatment, Wedan et al. (45) reported the result of preoperative doxorubicin plus docetaxel plus bevacizumab in 21 patients with inflammatory or LABC, showing a clinical response

rate of 67%, a cCR rate of 0%, and a pCR rate of 5%. Other groups are also evaluating preoperative chemotherapy with or without bevacizumab (46). Other targeted antiangiogenic agents will also likely be studied neoadjuvantly.

With the emergence of novel and targeted agents that have shown clinical benefit in the metastatic setting, it is appropriate to study them in the adjuvant and neoadjuvant settings where they offer the promise of increased cure. Trastuzumab has demonstrated a significant benefit in all three settings (metastatic, adjuvant, neoadjuvant), and the results are awaited that will allow similar evaluation of lapatinib, bevacizumab, and other targeted agents. As an important aside, a critical potential advantage of the preoperative setting is the potential for the collection of matched pairs of tissue samples. These can inform drug development, patient selection, and the overall biology of breast cancer and should be carefully considered in the design of all preoperative treatment trials.

 ## PATHOLOGIC ASSESSMENT

The delivery of preoperative systemic therapy depends on accurate baseline tumor assessments using all standard pathologic and imaging tools. It is critical to obtain adequate tissue by a core needle biopsy before preoperative therapy to allow not only confirmation of invasiveness, but also testing for estrogen-receptor, progesterone-receptor, and *ERBB2* status. In clinical trials tissue is usually required at baseline for research purposes (i.e., biomarker research) as well. It is helpful to place clips to mark the tumor location before instituting therapy. This will aid the radiologist, surgeon, and pathologist in providing posttreatment assessment. The sixth edition of American Joint Committee on Cancer Staging manual uses the "y" to indicate pathologic staging after neoadjuvant therapy (47).

As described above, the achievement of a pCR has emerged as an important surrogate end point to determine the efficacy of preoperative chemotherapy and has correlated in some studies with improved overall outcomes. The definition for pCR has, however, varied throughout the various clinical trials. Thus, cross-study comparisons are difficult and the authors join the call for a uniformed agreement on the definition of pCR. Because the presence of residual ductal carcinoma *in situ* (DCIS) after preoperative therapy does not impact DFS or OS (48), pCR may not require the absence of DCIS. Clinicians should be careful to understand the CR definition used in the individual trials reported to date and going forward.

WHAT ARE THE POTENTIAL PITFALLS OF PREOPERATIVE CHEMOTHERAPY?

One of the unresolved issues is the timing of the sentinel lymph node biopsy (SLNB). Lymphatic mapping with SLNB is a well-established alternative to axillary lymph node dissection in women with clinically node-negative disease. False-negative rates for SLNB range from 1% to 10% (49). In patients with LABC or inflammatory breast cancer, the likelihood of node-positive disease is high, so SLNB is not generally performed. However, in those with operable breast cancer who receive preoperative chemotherapy, an accurate assessment of the axilla can be a dilemma. Both SLNB and ultrasound-guided fine-needle aspiration (FNA) have been used to detect axillary metastasis for preoperative chemotherapy. However, axillary ultrasound has a reported false-negative rate of 15% to 20% because of the limited ability to detect metastatic foci less than 5 to 10 mm (50). Thus, SLNB has been routinely performed in many centers prior to preoperative chemotherapy. Follow-up of patients who were node-negative before chemotherapy in general has not revealed node-positive disease after chemotherapy. Ollila et al. (51) reported the result of the completion of axillary lymph node dissection (ALND) after preoperative chemotherapy on a group of patients, regardless of whether they were node-negative or node-positive on SLNB prior to chemotherapy. This study showed that patients who were node-negative with SLNB preoperatively remained node-negative. Other studies have confirmed these data and suggest patients who are node-negative by preoperative SLNB may not require further ALND (52,53). However, long-term follow-up of these patients is needed. Currently, patients who have SLNB before preoperative chemotherapy may be treated in several ways. Some attempt another SLNB after chemotherapy, some have no further surgery, and some undergo axillary lymph node dissection.

An alternative approach is to perform the SLNB after preoperative chemotherapy. However, SLNB following preoperative therapy is similarly fraught with controversy. The lymphatic flow may be altered by chemotherapy or may be blocked by necrotic tumor cells from chemotherapy, and, thus, the flow of dye or tracer to the sentinel node may be impaired (54). The false-negative rate for SLNB after preoperative chemotherapy is reported as high as 11% and this could lead to undertreatment for a subset of patients (55).

Another pitfall lies in the area of chest wall radiation (56,57). If a patient still requires a mastectomy after preoperative chemotherapy and is found to have three or fewer lymph nodes involved with metastasis at the time of surgery, it will not be clear whether she should receive postmastectomy radiation therapy based on the American Society of Clinical Oncology (ASCO) guidelines (58) or not as the true number of involved nodes will not be accurately known after preoperative chemotherapy. This is yet another argument in favor of the generation of a clear treatment plan before therapy commences.

CONCLUSION

Preoperative systemic therapy is effective for patients with inoperable and operable breast cancer. All else being equal, it currently appears that the delivery of a full course of standard treatment delivers the same OS and DFS regardless of whether it precedes or follows surgery. There is some suggestion that interrupting a standard treatment to perform surgery could be less effective. For patients with inoperable breast cancer, preoperative (neoadjuvant) therapy is the only option. For patients with operable disease that requires mastectomy, preoperative therapy is a reasonable option if the patient desires breast conservation and the surgeon believes it could be feasible following a response. For patients who present as candidates for breast conservation, there is no evidence that preoperative therapy offers any advantage.

When patients are treated with preoperative therapy, the in-breast response can provide an indication of the overall outcome with pathologic complete response associated with a greater chance of DFS and OS. However, assessment of the in-breast response has not been successfully used to tailor therapy and improve overall outcomes. Participation in one of the increasing number of available preoperative trials should be the goal of patients and clinicians seeking to answer these unresolved questions.

References

1. Early Breast Cancer Trialists' Collaborative Group (EBCTCG). Effects of chemotherapy and hormonal therapy for early breast cancer on recurrence and 15-year survival. *Lancet* 2005;365(9472):1687–1717.
2. De Lena M, Zucali R, Viganotti G, et al. Combined chemotherapy radiotherapy approach in locally advanced (T3b-T4) breast cancer. *Cancer Chemother Pharmacol* 1978;1:53–59.
3. Swain SM, Sorace RA, Bagley CS, et al. Neoadjuvant chemotherapy in the combined modality approach of locally advanced nonmetastatic breast cancer. *Cancer Res* 1987;47:3889–3894.
4. Perloff M, Lesnick GJ, Korzun A, et al. Combination chemotherapy with mastectomy or radiotherapy for stage III breast carcinoma: a Cancer and Leukemia Group B study. *J Clin Oncol* 1988;6:261–269.
5. Hortobagyi GN, Ames FC, Buzdar AU, et al. Management of stage III primary breast cancer with primary chemotherapy, surgery, and radiation therapy. *Cancer* 1988;62:2507–2516.
6. Bonadonna G, Veronesi U, Bramdilla C, et al. Primary chemotherapy to avoid mastectomy in tumors with diameters of three centimeters or more. *J Natl Cancer Inst* 1990;82:1539–1545.
7. Jacquillat C, Baillet F, Weil M, et al. Results of a conservative treatment combining induction (neoadjuvant) and consolidation chemotherapy, hormonotherapy, and external and interstitial irradiation in 98 patients with locally advanced breast cancer (IIIA-IIIB). *Cancer* 1988;61:1877–1982.
8. Pierce LJ, Lippman M, Ben-Baruch N, et al. The effect of systemic therapy on local-regional control in locally advanced breast cancer. *Int J Radiat Oncol Biol Phys* 1992;23:949–960.
9. Schwartz GF, Birchansky CA, Komarnicky LT, et al. Induction chemotherapy followed by breast conservation for locally advanced carcinoma of the breast. *Cancer* 1994;73:362–369.
10. Jacquillat C, Weil M, Baillet F, et al. Results of neoadjuvant chemotherapy and radiation therapy in the breast-conserving treatment of 250 patients with all stages of infiltrative breast cancer. *Cancer* 1990;66:119–129.
11. Smith IE, Jones AL, O'Brien ME, et al. Primary medical (neo-adjuvant) chemotherapy for operable breast cancer. *Eur J Cancer* 1993;29:1796–1799.
12. Bonadonna G, Valagussa P, Brambilla C, et al. Primary chemotherapy in operable breast cancer: eight-year experience at the Milan cancer Institute. *J Clin Oncol* 1998;16(1):93–100.
13. Powles TJ, Hickish TF, Makris A, et al. Randomized trial of chemoendocrine therapy started before or after surgery for treatment of primary breast cancer. *J Clin Oncol* 1995;13:547–552.
14. Fisher B, Brown A, Mamounas E, et al. Effect of preoperative chemotherapy on local-regional disease in women with operable breast cancer: findings from the National Surgical Adjuvant Breast and Bowel Project B-18. *J Clin Oncol* 1997;15(7):2483–2493.
15. Rastogi P, Anderson SJ, Bear H, et al. Preoperative chemotherapy: updates of National Surgical Adjuvant Breast and Bowel Project B-18 and B-27. *J Clin Oncol* 2008;26:778–785.
16. van der Hage JA, van de Velde CJ, Julien JP, et al. Preoperative chemotherapy in primary operable breast cancer: results from the European Organization for Research and Treatment of Cancer trial 10902. *J Clin Oncol* 2001;19(22):4224–4237.
17. Bear HD, Anderson S, Smith RE, et al. Sequential preoperative or postoperative docetaxel added to preoperative doxorubicin plus cyclophosphamide for operable breast cancer: National Surgical Adjuvant Breast and Bowel Project Protocol B-27. *J Clin Oncol* 2006;24:2019–2027.
18. Hudis CA, William BE, Constantino JP, et al. Proposal for standardized definitions for efficacy end points in adjuvant breast cancer trials: the STEEP system. *J Clin Oncol* 2007;25:2127–2132.
19. Gianni L, Baselga J, Eiermann W, et al. Feasibility and tolerability of sequential doxorubicin/paclitaxel followed by cyclophosphamide, methotrexate, and fluorouracil and its effects on tumor response as preoperative therapy. *Clin Cancer Res* 2005;11(24):8715–8721.
20. Heys SD, Hutcheon AW, Sarkar TK, et al. Neoadjuvant docetaxel in breast cancer: 3-year survival results from the Aberdeen trial. *Clin Breast Cancer* 2002;3[Suppl 2]:S69–S74.
21. von Minckwitz G, Blohmner JU, Raab G, et al. *In vivo* chemosensitivity-adapted preoperative chemotherapy in patients with early-stage breast cancer: the GEPAR-TRIO pilot study. *Ann Oncol* 2005;16:56–63.
22. von Minckwitz G, Blohmer J, Vogel P, et al. Comparisons of neoadjuvant 6 vs. 8 cycles of docetaxel/doxorubicin/cyclophosphamide (TAC) in patients early responding to TACx2-the GEPARTRIO study. *Proc Am Soc Clin Oncol* 2006;24:18S(abst 576).
23. von Minckwitz G, Raab G, Caputo A, et al. Doxorubicin with cyclophosphamide followed by docetaxel every 21 days compared with doxorubicin and docetaxel every 14 days as preoperative treatment in operable breast cancer: the GEPARDUO study of the German Breast Group. *J Clin Oncol* 2005;23(12):2676–2685.
24. Miller K, Mc-Caskill-Stevens W, Sisk J, et al. Combination versus sequential doxorubicin and docetaxel as primary chemotherapy for breast cancer: a randomized pilot trial of the Hoosier Oncology Group. *J Clin Oncol* 1999;17:3033–3037.
25. Buzdar AU, Singletary SE, Valero V, et al. Evaluation of paclitaxel in adjuvant chemotherapy for patients with operable breast cancer: preliminary data of a prospective randomized trial. *Clin Cancer Res* 2002;8:1073–1079.
26. Green MC, Buzdar AU, Smith T, et al. Weekly paclitaxel improves pathologic complete remission in operable breast cancer when compared with paclitaxel once every 3 weeks. *J Clin Oncol* 2005;23:5983–5992.
27. Seidman AD, Berry D, Cirrincione C, et al. CALGB 9840: phase II study of weekly (W) paclitaxel (P) via 1-hour (h) infusion versus standard (S) 3 h infusion every third week in the treatment of metastatic breast cancer (MBC), with trastuzumab (T) for HER2 positive MBC and randomized for T in HER2 normal MBC. *Proc Am Soc Clin Oncol* 2004;23:6S(abst 512).
28. Sparano JA, Wang M, Martino S, et al. Phase III study of doxorubicin–cyclophosphamide followed by paclitaxel or docetaxel given every 3 weeks or weekly in patients with axillary node-positive or high-risk node-negative breast cancer: results of North American Breast Cancer Intergroup Trial E1199. *Proc Am Soc Clin Oncol* 2007;25(18S)[Suppl]:516.
29. Untch M, Konecny G, Ditsch N, et al. Dose-dense sequential epirubicin-paclitaxel as preoperative treatment of breast cancer: results of a randomized AGO study. *Proc Am Clin Oncol* 2002;21:34a.
30. Hudis C, Citron M, Berry D, et al. Five year follow-up of INT C9741: dose-dense chemotherapy is safe and effective. *Breast Cancer Res Treat* 2005;94[Suppl 1]:S20(abst 49).
31. De Laurentis M, Cancello G, D'Agostino D, et al. Taxane-based combinations as adjuvant chemotherapy of early breast cancer: a meta-analysis of randomized trials. *J Clin Oncol* 2008;26:44–53.
32. Buzdar AU, Ibrahim NK, Francis D, et al. Significantly higher pathologic complete remission rate after neoadjuvant therapy with trastuzumab, paclitaxel, and epirubicin chemotherapy: results of a randomized trial in human epidermal growth factor receptor 2-positive operable breast cancer. *J Clin Oncol* 2005;23:3676–3685.

33. Buzdar AU, Valero V, Ibrahim NK, et al. Neoadjuvant chemotherapy with paclitaxel followed by 5-fluorouracil, epirubicin, and cyclophosphamide chemotherapy and concurrent trastuzumab in human epidermal growth factor receptor 2-positive operable breast cancer: an update of the initial randomized study population and data of additional patients treated with the same regimen. *Clin Cancer Res* 2007;13(1):228–233.

34. Romond EH, Perez EA, Bryant J, et al: Trastuzumab plus adjuvant chemotherapy for operable HER2-positive breast cancer. *N Engl J Med* 2005;353(16):1673–1684.

35. Piccart-Gebhart MJ, Procter M, Leyland-Jones B, et al: Trastuzumab after adjuvant chemotherapy in HER2-positive breast cancer. *N Engl J Med* 2005;353(16):1659–1672.

36. Slamon DJ, Eiermann W, Robert NJ, et al. Phase III randomized trial comparing doxorubicin and cyclophosphamide followed by docetaxel and trastuzumab with docetaxel, carboplatin and trastuzumab in the adjuvant treatment of HER2 positive early breast cancer patients: second interim efficacy analysis. *Breast Cancer Res* 2006. Oral presentation at San Antonio Breast Cancer Symposium 2006.

37. Smith I, Procter M, Gelber RD, et al. 2-year follow-up of trastuzumab after adjuvant chemotherapy in HER2-positive breast cancer: a randomized controlled trial. *Lancet* 2007;369(9555):29–36.

38. Gianni L, Semiglazov V, Manikhas GM, et al. Neoadjuvant trastuzumab plus doxorubicin, paclitaxel, and CMF in locally advanced breast cancer (NOAH) trial: feasibility, safety, and anti-tumor effects. *Proc Am Soc Clin Oncol* 2007;10S(abst 532).

39. Fenton M, Ries L, Strenger RS, et al. Frequent pathologic complete responses seen with neoadjuvant q4week carboplatin and weekly paclitaxel ± weekly trastuzumab in resectable and locally advanced breast cancer: a Brown University Oncology Group (BrUOG) study. *Breast Cancer Res Treat* 2005;94[Suppl 1](abst 5054).

40. Chang H, Slamon D, Prati R, et al. A phase II study of neoadjuvant docetaxel/carboplatin with or without trastuzumab in locally advanced breast cancer: response and cardiotoxicity. *Proc Am Soc Clin Oncol* 2006;24:18S(abst 845).

41. Gomez HL, Doval DC, Chavez MA, et al. Efficacy and safety of lapatinib as first-line therapy for ERBB2 amplified locally advanced or metastatic breast cancer. *J Clin Oncol* 2008;26(18):2999–3005.

42. Storniolo AM, Pegram MD, Overmoyer B, et al. Phase I dose-escalation and pharmacokinetic study of lapatinib in combination with trastuzumab in patients with advanced ErbB 2-positive breast cancer. *J Clin Oncol* 2008;26(20):3317–3323.

43. Geyer CE, Forster J, Lindquist D, et al. Lapatinib plus capecitabine for HER2-positive advanced breast cancer. *N Engl J Med* 2006;355(26):2733–2743.

44. Miller K, Wang M, Gralaw J, et al: Paclitaxel plus bevacizumab versus paclitaxel alone for metastatic breast cancer. *N Engl J Med* 2007;357:2666–2676.

45. Wedam SB, Low JA, Yang JA, et al. Antiangiogenic and antitumor effects of bevacizumab in patients with inflammatory and locally advanced breast cancer. *J Clin Oncol* 2006;24:769–777.

46. Lyons J, Silverman P, Remick S, et al. Toxicity results and early outcome data on a randomized phase II study of docetaxel ± bevacizumab for locally advanced, unresectable breast cancer. *Proc Am Soc Clin Oncol* 2006;24:18S(abst 3049).

47. Greene FL, Page DL, Fleming ID, et al. *American Joint Committee on Cancer staging manual.* 6th ed. Philadelphia: Springer, 2002.

48. Mazouni C, Peintinger F, Wan-Kau s, et al. Residual ductal carcinoma *in situ* in patients with complete eradication of invasive breast cancer after neoadjuvant chemotherapy dose not adversely affect patient outcome. *J Clin Oncol* 2007;25:2650–2655.

49. Waljee JF, Newman LA. Neoadjuvant systemic therapy and the surgical management of breast cancer. *Surg Clin North Am* 2007;87:399–415.

50. Krishnamurthy S, Sneige N, Bedi DG, et al. Role of ultrasound-guided fine-needle aspiration of indeterminate and suspicious axillary lymph nodes in the initial staging of breast carcinoma. *Cancer* 2002;95(5):982–988.

51. Ollila DW, Neuman HB, Sartor C, et al. Lymphatic mapping and sentinel lymphadenectomy prior to neoadjuvant chemotherapy in patients with large breast cancers. *Am J Surg* 2005;190:371–375.

52. Sabel MS, Schott AF, Kleer CG, et al. Sentinel node biopsy prior to neoadjuvant chemotherapy. *Am J Surg* 2003;186(2):102–105.

53. Schrenk P, Hochreiner G, Fridrik M, et al. Sentinel node biopsy performed before preoperative chemotherapy for axillary node staging in breast cancer. *Breast J* 2003;9(4):282–287.

54. Kuerer HM, Hunt KK. The rationale for integration of lymphatic mapping and sentinel node biopsy in the management of breast cancer patients receiving neoadjuvant chemotherapy. *Semin Breast Dis* 2002;5:80–87.

55. Jones JL, Zabicki K, Christian RL, et al. A comparison of sentinel node biopsy before and after neoadjuvant chemotherapy: timing is important. *Am J Surg* 2005;190(4):517–520.

56. Bunchholz TA, Katz A, Strom EA, et al. Pathologic tumor size and lymph node status predict for different rates of locoregional recurrence after mastectomy for breast cancer patients treated with neoadjuvant versus adjuvant chemotherapy. *Int J Radiat Oncol Biol Phys* 2002;53(4):880–888.

57. Bunchholz TA, Tucker SL, Masullo L, et al. Predictors of local-regional recurrence after neoadjuvant chemotherapy and mastectomy without radiation. *J Clin Oncol* 2002;20(1):17–23.

58. Recht A, Edge SB, Solin LJ, et al. Postmastectomy radiotherapy: guidelines of the American Society of Clinical Oncology. *J Clin Oncol* 2001;19:1539–1569.

Ian E. Smith

Preoperative endocrine therapy is not as commonly used as preoperative chemotherapy, particularly in the United States, and has been less widely studied. Nevertheless its origins go back more than 50 years. In 1957 Kennedy et al. (1) reported on 27 postmenopausal women whose large and sometimes locally advanced breast cancers were treated with hormone therapy prior to surgery, mainly using estrogen, which was novel at the time; they described tumor softening and shrinking, with some tumors becoming "more difficult or impossible to palpate."

Since then there have been occasional reports of premenopausal women treated with preoperative oophorectomy or leuprorelin and responses have been described (2,3), but the data are insufficient to allow meaningful conclusions, and preoperative chemotherapy is much more widely used for younger women. This chapter will therefore focus on patients who are postmenopausal.

There are both clinical and research-directed reasons to use preoperative endocrine therapy in women with hormone receptor–positive breast cancer. Clinically this approach might be considered as an alternative to surgery, particularly in women unfit for this procedure through age or medical infirmity. This approach has obvious short-term attractions but also important limitations, as described below. The main clinical indication is to down-stage large breast cancers, so that mastectomy might be avoided or to achieve operability in previously inoperable cancers (4).

In parallel to its clinical role, a key research aim for preoperative endocrine therapy is to develop short-term surrogate molecular end points that might predict for long-term outcome in adjuvant trials. Such trials are large, expensive to run, and take years to achieve their outcome. For example the adjuvant ATAC (anastrozole, tamoxifen alone or in combination) trial, which started in 1996, involved 9,366 patients and reported its first results 6 years later (5), while the similarly designed Breast International Group (BIG) 1-98 compared adjuvant letrozole with tamoxifen, involving over 8,000 patients, ran to a similar timescale (6). The option of a rapid preoperative alternative involving a relatively small number of patients could improve significantly the rate at which novel therapies in early breast cancer could be investigated. A further research aim would be to develop predictive short-term end points for long-term outcome in the individual patient and to allow individualized adjuvant therapy rather than the current blind approach based on probabilities derived from adjuvant trials' data. A key factor underlying this type of research is the anatomic accessibility of the breast, allowing serial biopsies to investigate molecular changes during treatment and providing research opportunities that are unrivaled elsewhere in cancer medicine.

PREOPERATIVE ENDOCRINE THERAPY AS AN ALTERNATIVE TO SURGERY

Tamoxifen was first evaluated as an alternative to surgery in early breast cancer in a series of small studies in the 1980s. In an early study, it was reported to achieve tumor responses sufficient to continue treatment beyond the first follow-up visit in 73% of elderly women over 75 years of age (7). Eighteen percent took more than 12 months to achieve maximum response. In a subsequent small randomized trial involving 116 patients

aged 70 or over comparing tamoxifen alone with surgery alone, no difference was found in either time to progression or survival between the two treatments (8). Indeed, there was a nonsignificant trend toward a decreased risk of local recurrence and a delay in the development of distant metastases in patients on primary tamoxifen. This trial had a large number of patients with T3 or T4 cancers. In a similar trial involving 135 patients over 70, no survival difference was found between the two groups, but here there was a 43% local failure rate in the tamoxifen alone arm at 3 years follow-up (9). In a larger Cancer Research Campaign UK trial comparing tamoxifen alone or surgery and tamoxifen in 381 women aged 70 or over, no significant differences in survival or quality of life were found between the two approaches at 34 months' follow-up, but a significantly higher locoregional relapse rate was seen in the tamoxifen alone arm (23% vs. 8%) (10). In a subsequent analysis, however, both overall mortality and breast cancer mortality were worse with tamoxifen alone (hazard ratio [HR] 1.29 and 1.68, respectively), although these differences did not emerge for 3 years (11).

In contrast, in an Italian multicenter trial in which 474 patients over 70 years with operable breast cancer were randomized to receive tamoxifen alone versus surgery followed by tamoxifen, long-term follow-up with a median 80 months did not show any difference in overall survival or breast cancer survival (12). There was, however, a significantly higher incidence of local recurrences in the tamoxifen alone group (106 vs. 27; $p = .0001$).

These trials in elderly patients therefore urged caution in using preoperative endocrine therapy as a substitute for surgery in most patients, but show that this approach is a reasonable one for patients who are frail or otherwise unfit for surgery.

PREOPERATIVE ENDOCRINE THERAPY BEFORE SURGERY

There are numerous small studies of preoperative endocrine therapy before surgery in the literature, starting with the preoperative estrogen report described above (1). Response rates vary and are often loosely defined, but they are generally higher than in the more rigorous randomized trials described below. In two of the tamoxifen versus surgery trials described above, response to tamoxifen was 55% at 6 months and 63% best ever in one (9), and 25% at 6 months followed by 47% best ever in the other (10).

EMERGENCE OF THE AROMATASE INHIBITORS

In recent years the so-called third-generation aromatase inhibitors including in particular anastrozole, letrozole, and exemestane, have challenged the role of tamoxifen as first-line endocrine therapy in postmenopausal women with both advanced and early breast cancer (6,13,14).

Initial small nonrandomized studies suggested that these agents might also be more effective than tamoxifen as preoperative therapy in older women with locally advanced or large operable cancers, in terms of tumor regressions and the possibility of breast-conserving surgery (15–19). These studies have now been superseded by a series of randomized comparative preoperative trials comparing the aromatase inhibitors with tamoxifen.

COMPARATIVE TRIALS OF PREOPERATIVE ENDOCRINE THERAPY

Vorozole versus Tamoxifen

Vorozole, a nonsteroidal third-generation inhibitor similar in structure to anastrozole and letrozole, has now been discontinued from clinical study but was the first to be compared to tamoxifen in a preoperative randomized trial for 12 weeks prior to surgery in a small series of 53 postmenopausal patients with estrogen-receptor–positive (ER+) tumors (20). Nine patients (39%) had a clinical response to tamoxifen compared with 5 (22%) with vorozole (no significant difference); 3 patients had progressive disease (1 on tamoxifen and 2 on vorozole). An important aim of this small trial was to determine biological changes within the tumor during treatment, and these are described below.

Letrozole versus Tamoxifen

There has been one multinational double-blind randomized trial (PO24) comparing preoperative letrozole 2.5 mg with tamoxifen for 4 months prior to surgery (21). This involved 337 postmenopausal women with ER or progesterone receptor–positive (PR+) tumors, defined by at least 10% nuclear staining and assayed locally. All patients would have otherwise required mastectomy at entry to the trial or were considered inoperable (14%). Diagnosis was established by core needle biopsy. Overall clinical objective response rate, the primary end point, was significantly higher for letrozole than for tamoxifen (55% vs. 36%; p <.001). The median time to response was 66 days for letrozole and 70 days for tamoxifen. Progressive disease during treatment was seen with 12% of patients treated with letrozole and 17% with tamoxifen. Letrozole was also more effective than tamoxifen when the response rate was determined by ultrasound (35% vs. 25%; p = .0042) and by mammography (34% vs. 16%; p <.001).

The main secondary end point of the trial was breast conservation, and significantly more breast-conserving surgery was achieved with letrozole than with tamoxifen (45% vs. 35%; p = .022). Pathological complete remission in the primary breast lesion was seen in only two patients treated with letrozole and three with tamoxifen. Only two of these five patients with path complete remissions had no involved nodes at surgery.

In a further analysis of the same study ER and PR expression were reassessed in a central laboratory and 12% of patients were found to have tumors that were both ER and PR negative (22). In patients whose tumors were confirmed ER or PR+, the response rate to letrozole was 60% compared with 41% for tamoxifen (p = .004) and 48% versus 36%, respectively, underwent successful breast conserving surgery (p = .036).

In this analysis ER and PR were quantified using the Allred scoring system in which an intensity score (range, 1 to 3) is added to a frequency score (range, 1 to 5) (23). Letrozole response rates were numerically superior to tamoxifen for all ER Allred scores from 3 to 8; furthermore responses to letrozole were seen in all Allred scores between 3 to 8, whereas responses were only seen in tamoxifen for scores 6 to 8. Based on this, the authors suggest that letrozole might be more effective than tamoxifen in patients whose tumors show relatively low ER expression, but is important to note that the numbers were small in each of these Allred groupings and no definite conclusions should be drawn.

Anastrozole versus Tamoxifen

There have been two multinational double-blind trials comparing preoperative anastrozole 1 mg daily with tamoxifen for 12 weeks prior to surgery in postmenopausal women with hormone receptor–positive breast cancer: IMPACT (*IM*mediate *P*reoperative *A*nastrozole tamoxifen or *C*ombined with *T*amoxifen) and PROACT (*PR*e*O*perative *A*nastrozole *C*ompared with *T*amoxifen). The IMPACT trial compared anastrozole with tamoxifen or with both in combination given for only 12 weeks (in contrast to 16 for PO24 above) (24); the trial was designed to be the preoperative equivalent of ATAC. The main clinical aim was to compare the efficacies of these treatments in terms of response and more particularly in down-staging to avoid mastectomy. An important further aim, however, was to determine whether short-term surrogate end points of response could be identified to predict for long-term outcome in the adjuvant ATAC trial; these included clinical changes after 12 weeks or biological change in proliferation assessed by Ki-67 after 2 and 12 weeks. For this reason, postmenopausal patients with smaller breast cancers not necessarily requiring mastectomy were also included, and in this important respect the IMPACT trial differs from the preoperative letrozole trial described above.

This study was comprised of 330 patients with confirmed invasive histology and ER positivity on core needle biopsy. Median age was 73 years, median tumor size was 4 cm for each of the three groups, and tumors were confirmed in a central reference laboratory as ER+ in 98% of cases. Objective clinical response rates by caliper measurement for anastrozole, tamoxifen, and the combination were 37%, 36%, and 39%, respectively, on an intent-to-treat basis, and none of these differences was significant. Ultrasound response rates were 24%, 20%, and 28%, respectively; again, none of these differences was significant. Progressive disease during treatment occurred in 9%, 5%, and 5% of patients, respectively.

A subgroup of 124 patients was assessed by the surgeon as requiring mastectomy at baseline. In these, 46%, 22%, and 26% were deemed to have achieved tumor regression sufficient to allow breast-conserving surgery after treatment with anastrozole, tamoxifen, and combination therapy, respectively. The improvement with anastrozole compared with tamoxifen was statistically significant with an odds ratio (OR) of 2.94 (p = .03). There was no significant difference between the tamoxifen and combination groups.

In the second preoperative anastrozole trial, PROACT, also multicenter and double-blind, 451 postmenopausal women with operable or locally advanced but potentially operable (T2-4b) hormone receptor–positive breast cancer were randomized to anastrozole 1 mg or tamoxifen 20 mg for 12 weeks prior to surgery (25). As in the IMPACT trial, patients with small breast cancers appropriate for breast-conserving surgery were eligible for entry. In contrast to other trials concomitant chemotherapy was also allowed and was given to 29% of patients on anastrozole and 32% on tamoxifen. Mean age was 67 in both groups and mean ultrasound tumor diameter 3.6 cm. Overall ultrasound response, the primary end point, was 40% for anastrozole and 35% for tamoxifen (p = .29). Clinical response by caliper measurement was 50% and 46%, respectively. (p = .37). In the 314 patients treated with endocrine therapy alone without chemotherapy, ultrasound and clinical response rates for anastrozole and tamoxifen, respectively, were 36% versus 27% (p = .07) and 50% versus 40% (p = .08).

In the 262 patients treated with endocrine therapy alone without chemotherapy who would have required mastectomy or had locally advanced disease at baseline, as in the letrozole trial, ultrasound and clinical response rates were significantly better for anastrozole than tamoxifen and were, respectively, 37% versus 25% (OR 1.81; p = .03) and 49% versus 36% (OR 1.69; p = .04). In this subgroup surgical improvement (inoperable to mastectomy or mastectomy to breast-conserving surgery) was deemed feasible in 47% after anastrozole compared with 38% after tamoxifen ($p = .15$) and actually occurred in 43% versus 31% ($p = .04$).

Combined IMPACT and PROACT Results

A common population of 535 patients treated with anastrozole or tamoxifen alone was derived from the combined results of the IMPACT and PROACT trials, with respective caliper-measured response rates of 45% for anastrozole and 36% for tamoxifen ($p = .052$) (26). Of these 344 were deemed to require mastectomy or had inoperable cancer at baseline, representing a comparable group to the PO24 letrozole trial (21), and in this subgroup the clinical response rate was significantly higher for anastrozole than for tamoxifen (47% vs. 35%; OR 1.65; $p = .026$). In this group, improvement in feasible surgery was 47% and 35% (OR 1.67; $p = .021$) and in actual surgery 43% and 31% (OR 1.70; $p = .019$), respectively.

Exemestane versus Tamoxifen

Only one small trial comparing preoperative exemestane with tamoxifen has been reported. Seventy-three postmenopausal women with hormone receptor–positive status were randomized to receive exemestane 25 mg or tamoxifen 20 mg daily for 3 months before surgery (27). Clinical objective response rates were reported as 89% for exemestane compared with 57% for tamoxifen ($p < .05$), including complete clinical remission rates of 14% and 11%, respectively (ns). Ultrasound response rates were 70% and 41% (ns), and breast conservation rates 39% versus 11%, respectively ($p < .05$). Two pathological complete remissions were found with exemestane and one with tamoxifen. The authors reported without details that responses were more likely with higher levels of estrogen-receptor expression.

 ## CLINICAL MEASUREMENT OF SMALLER CANCERS IN NEOADJUVANT ENDOCRINE THERAPY

At first sight the IMPACT and PROACT data appear paradoxical, with the suggestion in both trials of significantly greater efficacy for anastrozole over tamoxifen in larger than in smaller cancers. Biologically this would be unlikely, and indeed in the IMPACT trial no biological differences were detected between larger and smaller cancers as assessed by mean ER, mean PR, mean Ki-67, or in the proportion with *ERBB2* (formerly *HER2* positive cancers) (unpublished data). A more plausible explanation is that serial clinical measurements in smaller cancers during preoperative endocrine therapy where response may be slow are likely to be exposed to larger errors; this problem could be compounded by follow-up core biopsies for biological studies after 2 weeks of treatment and the associated risk of subsequent hematoma and tissue edema. It may be that preoperative endocrine therapy trials with primary clinical end points should therefore be restricted to patients with larger cancers, although patients with smaller breast cancers could still be appropriate for trials with a biological end point.

 ## OPTIMAL DURATION OF PREOPERATIVE ENDOCRINE THERAPY

The optimal duration of preoperative endocrine therapy is uncertain and has not been addressed formally in comparative trials. Eighteen percent of elderly women treated with preoperative tamoxifen were reported in an early study to take more than 12

months to achieve maximum response, as described above (7). In the IMPACT trial the clinical response rate to anastrozole given for 12 weeks was 37% (24), and it was 61% in a subsequent trial by the same investigators also involving gefitinib, described below, where treatment was given for the longer period of 16 weeks (28). In another study involving 63 patients treated with extended duration preoperative letrozole, tumor volume continued to decrease for over 12 months in some patients with very few initial responders relapsing during this period (29). Clinically it would seem sensible to continue preoperative endocrine therapy for a minimum period of 4 months providing the tumor is responding and to continue beyond that until the point is reached when conservative surgery becomes feasible.

 ## PREOPERATIVE ENDOCRINE THERAPY VERSUS CHEMOTHERAPY

Only one trial to this point has directly compared preoperative chemotherapy (doxorubicin 60 mg/m^2 and paclitaxel 200 mg/m^2 every 3 weeks in four courses) against aromatase-inhibitor endocrine therapy (exemestane or anastrozole for 3 months) in 239 postmenopausal women with hormone receptor–positive cancer (30). The primary end point, overall clinical response rate, was very similar for each treatment (63% for chemotherapy, 67% for exemestane, and 62% for anastrozole). Rates of breast-conserving surgery were higher in the endocrine therapy group (33% vs. 24%; $p = .058$). The authors concluded that neoadjuvant endocrine therapy, with its low toxicity, was a reasonable alternative to chemotherapy in this elderly population. It is important to consider that for some patients preoperative endocrine therapy may have as high a chance of achieving a response as preoperative endocrine therapy, but in the current era, when increasing emphasis is being placed on molecular markers including gene expression assays to select appropriate adjuvant therapies, the value of direct comparative one size fits all trials of this type is doubtful.

 ## PREOPERATIVE ENDOCRINE THERAPY IN TUMORS OVEREXPRESSING *ERBB1* OR *ERBB2*

In the PO24 letrozole neoadjuvant trial 15 of 17 patients whose tumors overexpressed *ERBB2* or *ERBB1* responded to letrozole (88%) compared with only 4 of 19 patients to tamoxifen (21%) (OR 28; $p = .004$). In contrast, the respective response rates for the majority of patients whose tumors did not over express either of these receptors was 54% versus 42%, which was not statistically significant ($p = 0.078$) (22).

Likewise in the IMPACT trial, 239 patients had tumors that were assessable for *ERBB2*, of whom 34 (14%) were *ERBB2* positive, as assessed in a central reference laboratory by immunohistochemistry or fluorescence *in situ* hybridization (FISH). (Only two tumors overexpressed *ERBB1*, including one also overexpressing *ERBB2*.) In this small subgroup, objective responses were seen in 7 of 12 patients with anastrozole (58%), 2 of 9 patients with tamoxifen (22%), and 4 of 13 patients (31%) with the combination treatment (24). This difference between anastrozole and tamoxifen was not quite significant ($p = .09$), and because of small numbers, the analysis was underpowered.

Initially, these results strongly supported the hypothesis that aromatase inhibitors might be selectively more effective than tamoxifen in the treatment of ER-positive early breast cancer that also overexpresses *ERBB2*. They were supported by experimental data suggesting that *ERBB2* overexpression may be associated with tamoxifen resistance (31,32). More recently, however, data from both the ATAC and the BIG 1-98 adjuvant trials have shown that aromatase inhibitors are more effective than tamoxifen against *ERBB2* positive cancer, but there is no evidence of an increased effect of either anastrozole or letrozole over tamoxifen compared with cancers not overexpressing *ERBB2* (33,34). These contradictory results emphasize the pitfall of using preoperative response rates as a surrogate for long-term outcome in adjuvant trials.

PREOPERATIVE AROMATASE INHIBITORS WITH SIGNAL TRANSDUCTION AGENTS

There are compelling preclinical data to suggest that cross-talk occurs between growth factor receptor pathways, including epidermal growth factor receptor (EGFR), and estrogen receptors (35). Concurrent blockade of both oestrogen receptor and EGFR signaling pathways might therefore enhance response to endocrine therapy. Gefitinib is an orally active EGF tyrosine kinase inhibitor shown to suppress the growth of MCF7 cells otherwise resistant to estrogen withdrawal (36). This hypothesis was tested in a preoperative endocrine therapy trial in which 206 postmenopausal women with hormone–receptor–positive early breast cancer received anastrozole daily for 16 weeks and were randomized in a 2:5:5 ratio to receive in addition gefitinib 250 mg daily orally for 16 weeks versus placebo orally for 2 weeks and then gefitinib for 14 weeks versus placebo for 16 weeks (28). Based on the IMPACT trial results (37), the primary end point was biological change in proliferation as measured by Ki-67 at 2 and 16 weeks, and the main secondary end point was objective clinical response. The trial was designed to see whether tumors that did not show significant Ki-67 suppression after 2 weeks (and by implication were relatively resistant to endocrine therapy) could have this resistance reversed by the addition of gefitinib.

There was no significant difference on the mean change in Ki-67 with anastrozole and gefitinib versus anastrozole alone between baseline and 16 weeks, baseline and 2 weeks, or between 2 and 16 weeks. Forty-eight percent achieved clinical response with anastrozole and gefitinib versus 61% on anastrozole alone, and this nonsignificant trend in favor of anastrozole alone was reflected in the Ki-67 change at 16 weeks with reductions of 77.4% and 83.6%, respectively. In the progesterone receptor–positive subgroup there was a significant difference in favor of anastrozole alone versus the combination (72% vs. 48%; *p* = .03), and this was consistent with the Ki-67 changes in this subgroup. This trial, using biological as well as clinical end points, therefore failed to demonstrate a benefit from the addition of gefitinib to anastrozole and indeed suggested the possibility of an adverse interaction.

PREOPERATIVE VERSUS ADJUVANT ENDOCRINE THERAPY

Thus far there have been no published trials comparing preoperative with adjuvant endocrine therapy, by analogy with the National Surgical Adjuvant Breast and Bowel Project (NSABP) B-14 and other chemotherapy trials. Experimental data suggest that a benefit in favor of the preoperative approach might exist. Many years ago it was shown that noncurative surgery in a murine model was associated with serum growth factor stimulation of residual metastases that could be blocked by tamoxifen (38). Recently it has been shown that very short-term preoperative endocrine therapy for 2 weeks prior to surgery significantly reduces tumor cell proliferation (37) (see below). The hypothe-

sis that there may be a clinical advantage in short-duration preoperative endocrine therapy before surgery is therefore about to be tested clinically in the UK POETIC (*P*re-*O*perative *E*ndocrine *T*herapy: *I*ndividualising *C*are) trial, in which postmenopausal women with hormone receptor–positive breast cancer were randomized to 2 weeks of preoperative aromatase inhibitor or not before surgery.

PROLIFERATION EFFECT IN PREOPERATIVE ENDOCRINE THERAPY TRIALS

The nuclear nonhistone protein Ki-67 is widely used as a marker of proliferation and is suppressed in hormone receptor–positive cancers with different forms of preoperative endocrine therapy including tamoxifen (39,40) other selective estrogen-receptor modulators (41,42) the so-called pure antiestrogen fulvestrant (43), aromatase inhibitors (44–46), and even by withdrawal of hormone-replacement therapy (47). Some of these studies have also suggested that early changes in Ki-67 following endocrine therapy correlate positively with clinical response (39,44,45,48,49).

In the IMPACT trial (discussed above), proliferation measured by Ki-67 staining using MIB1 antibody was significantly reduced by all three treatments after 2 and 12 weeks, anastrozole by 76% and 82%, tamoxifen by 60% and 64%, and the combination by 65% and 64%. Change after 2 weeks correlated with the change after 12 weeks. The decrease with anastrozole was significantly greater than that with tamoxifen, as assessed by geometric mean ratios of the changes in Ki-67 after 2 weeks treatment (*p* = .04) and again after 12 weeks (*p* <.001), but there were no significant differences between tamoxifen and the combination (50). The changes in Ki-67 after only 2 weeks of treatment therefore predicted for long-term differences in relapse-free survival in the adjuvant ATAC trial. The IMPACT trial results therefore suggested that change in proliferation as measured by Ki-67 might be a short-term surrogate for predicting differences in long-term outcome between different endocrine therapies in adjuvant trials.

This possibility is reinforced in an earlier and much smaller preoperative trial comparing vorozole with tamoxifen, which found a similar but nonsignificant trend in favor of an aromatase inhibitor, with mean drops in Ki-67 of 58% and 43% for vorozole and tamoxifen, respectively, after 2 weeks treatment (20).

A statistically significant correlation was found between Ki-67 reduction after 2 weeks and response in the IMPACT trial, but this was not seen with Ki-67 reduction at 12 weeks: a weakly significant relationship was seen between the percentage of tumor shrinkage and change in Ki-67 (50).

APOPTOSIS IN PREOPERATIVE ENDOCRINE THERAPY

A positive correlation between Ki-67 and apoptosis at baseline was found in the IMPACT trial (50). A significant drop in apoptotic index was seen between baseline and 2 weeks and to a lesser extent 12 weeks for anastrozole but not for tamoxifen or the combination.

SURROGATE MARKERS FOR LONG-TERM OUTCOME IN THE INDIVIDUAL PATIENT

Further follow-up in the IMPACT trial (median, 37 months) showed that expression of Ki-67 after 2 weeks of endocrine therapy was significantly associated with recurrence-free survival ($p = .004$), the highest tertile of Ki-67 expression carrying an excellent prognosis and the lowest tertile a poor one (37). The predictive significance of 2-week Ki-67 was sustained in a multivariate analysis. In contrast, baseline Ki-67 was only just significant in univariate analysis and dropped out in multivariate analysis. The authors postulated that tumor Ki-67 after 2 weeks may improve the prediction of recurrence-free survival by integrating both the prognostic value of Ki-67 levels at baseline with changes in Ki-67 associated with sensitivity or not to therapy. In the same study, the 2-week estrogen-receptor level was also significantly associated with recurrence-free survival. These findings, if validated, could provide the basis for predicting which patients might require additional chemotherapy based on 2 weeks pretreatment with an aromatase inhibitor.

This search for short-term surrogate markers predicting for long-term outcome in the individual patient has been further developed from the P024 trial (neoadjuvant letrozole versus tamoxifen). With a median follow-up of 61 months, patients whose tumors were down-staged to stage 1 or 0 at surgery after 4 months of preoperative therapy had a 100% relapse-free survival, which was significantly different from higher stages ($p = .006$) (51). A minority of tumors confirmed estrogen-receptor positive at baseline converted to estrogen-receptor negative following treatment, and in a multivariate analysis these also had a worse relapse-free survival and breast cancer–specific survival. Finally, Ki-67 level at the time of surgery after 4 months treatment likewise predicted for the same outcome end point in a multivariate analysis.

This has allowed the development of a multivariate model based on pathological stage at surgery, posttreatment estrogen-receptor status, and Ki-67 to distinguish subgroups at high, intermediate, and low-risk for late relapse. This predictive model has been independently validated in the IMPACT trial. As suggested above, these results may prove useful in determining which patients continue to be at significant risk of relapse following preoperative endocrine therapy and might therefore benefit from further intervention including in particular chemotherapy.

CONCLUSION

Preoperative endocrine therapy is effective in down-staging to avoid mastectomy in 30% to 40% of older women with hormone receptor–positive disease, and it can also be used to achieve operability in cancers deemed inoperable at presentation. Both letrozole and anastrozole are significantly superior to tamoxifen in achieving this. No direct comparison between the two aromatase inhibitors as preoperative therapy has been made, but indirect comparisons on similar groups of patients suggest that their efficacies are similar.

Preoperative aromatase inhibitors appear to be markedly more active than tamoxifen against tumors overexpressing *ERBB2* in terms of short-term tumor regression, but adjuvant therapy trials have not shown any selective long-term benefit for this subgroup compared with tumors not overexpressing *ERBB2*.

Short-term changes in the proliferation factor Ki-67 after 2 weeks of treatment predicted long-term disease-free survival in the adjuvant ATAC trial, and further work is now required to determine whether this short-term surrogate marker might be a more general predictive marker for long-term outcome in trials of novel therapies for early breast cancer. In addition, Ki-67 levels after 2 weeks, 12 weeks, and 16 weeks of preoperative aromatase inhibitor therapy have all been shown to predict for long-term outcome in the individual patient. Preoperative endocrine therapy therefore remains an important research tool with the potential for Ki-67 and other molecular markers

after short-term treatment to provide important predictive information on planning further adjuvant treatment.

References

1. Kennedy BJ, Kelley RM, White G, et al. Surgery as an adjunct to hormone therapy of breast cancer. *Cancer* 1957;10:1055–1075.
2. Mansi JL, Smith IE, Walsh G, et al. Primary medical therapy for operable breast cancer. *Eur J Cancer Clin Oncol* 1989;25:1623–1627.
3. Anderson ED, Forrest AP, Hawkins RA, et al. Primary systemic therapy for operable breast cancer. *Br J Cancer* 1991;63:561–566.
4. Dixon JM, Anderson TJ, Miller WR. Neoadjuvant endocrine therapy of breast cancer: a surgical perspective. *Eur J Cancer* 2002;38:2214–2221.
5. ATAC Trialists' Group. Anastrozole alone or in combination with tamoxifen versus tamoxifen alone for adjuvant treatment of postmenopausal women with early breast cancer: first results of the ATAC randomised trial. *Lancet* 2002;359:2131–2139.
6. BIG 1-98 Collaborative Group. A comparison of letrozole and tamoxifen in postmenopausal women with early breast cancer. *N Engl J Med* 2005;353:2747–2757.
7. Preece PE, Wood RAB, Mackie CR, et al. Tamoxifen as initial sole treatment of localised breast cancer in elderly women: a pilot study. *BMJ* 1982;284:869–870.
8. Gazet J-C, Markopoulos CH, Ford HT, et al. Prospective randomised trial of tamoxifen versus surgery in elderly patients with breast cancer. *Lancet* 1988;1:679–681.
9. Robertson JFR, Todd JH, Ellis IO, et al. Comparison of mastectomy with tamoxifen for treating elderly patients with operable breast cancer. *BMJ* 1988;297:511–514.
10. Bates T, Riley DL, Houghton J, et al. Breast cancer in elderly women: a Cancer Research Campaign trial comparing treatment with tamoxifen and optimal surgery with tamoxifen alone. *Br J Surg* 1991;78:591–594.
11. Fennessy M, Bates T, MacRae K, et al. Late follow-up of a randomized trial of surgery plus tamoxifen versus tamoxifen alone in women aged over 70 years with operable breast cancer. *Br J Surg* 2004;91(6):699–704.
12. Mustacchi G, Ceccherini R, Milani S, et al. Tamoxifen alone versus adjuvant tamoxifen for operable breast cancer of the elderly: long-term results of the phase III randomized controlled multicenter GRETA trial. *Ann Oncol* 2003;14(3):414–420.
13. Smith IE, Dowsett MD. Aromatase inhibitors in breast cancer. *N Engl J Med* 2003;348:2431–2442.
14. Howell A, Cuzick J, Baum M, et al. Results of the ATAC (Arimidex, Tamoxifen, Alone or in Combination) trial after completion of 5 years adjuvant treatment for breast cancer. *Lancet* 2005;365:60–62.
15. Dixon JM, Renshaw L, Bellamy C, et al. The effects of neoadjuvant anastrozole (Arimidex) on tumor volume in postmenopausal women with breast cancer: a randomized, double-blind, single-center study. *Clin Cancer Res* 2000;6:2229–2235.
16. Miller WR, Dixon JM. Endocrine and clinical endpoints of exemestane as neoadjuvant therapy. *Cancer Control* 2002;9:9–15.
17. Dixon JM, Jackson J, Renshaw L, et al. Neoadjuvant tamoxifen and aromatase inhibitors: comparisons and clinical outcomes. *J Steroid Biochem Mol Biol* 2003;86:295–299.
18. Milla-Santos A, Milla L, Rallo L, et al. Anastrozole as neoadjuvant therapy for hormone-dependent locally advanced breast cancer in postmenopausal patients. *Proc Am Soc Clin Oncol* 2002;21:40a(abst).
19. Anderson TJ, Dixon JM, Stuart M, et al. Effect of neoadjuvant treatment with anastrozole on tumour histology in postmenopausal women with large inoperable breast cancer. *Br J Cancer* 2002;87:334–338.
20. Harper-Wynne CL, Sacks NPM, Shenton K, et al. Comparison of the systemic and intratumoral effects of tamoxifen and the aromatase inhibitor vorozole in postmenopausal patients with primary breast cancer. *J Clin Oncol* 2002;20:1026–1035.
21. Eiermann W, Paepke S, Appfelstaedt J, et al. Preoperative treatment of postmenopausal breast cancer patients with letrozole: a randomized double-blind multicentre study. *Ann Oncol* 2001;12:1527–1532.
22. Ellis MJ, Coop A, Singh B, et al. Letrozole is more effective neoadjuvant endocrine therapy than tamoxifen for ERBB-1- and/or ERBB2-positive, estrogen receptor-positive primary breast cancer: evidence from a phase III randomized trial. *J Clin Oncol* 2001;19:3808–3816.
23. Allred DC, Harvey JM, Derardo M et al. Prognostic and predictive factors in breast cancer by immunocytochemical analysis. *Mod Pathol* 1998;11:155–168.
24. Smith IE, Dowsett M, Ebbs SR, et al. Neoadjuvant treatment of postmenopausal breast cancer with anastrozole, tamoxifen, or both in combination: the Immediate Preoperative Anastrozole, Tamoxifen, or Combined with Tamoxifen (IMPACT) multicenter double-blind randomized trial. *J Clin Oncol* 2005;23(22):5108–5116.
25. Cataliotti L, Buzdar AU, Noguchi S, et al. Comparison of anastrozole versus tamoxifen as preoperative therapy in postmenopausal women with hormone receptor-positive breast cancer: the Pre-Operative "Arimidex" Compared to Tamoxifen (PROACT) trial. *Cancer* 2006;106(10):2095–2103.
26. Smith I, Cataliotti L, on behalf of the IMPACT and PROACT Trialists. Anastrozole versus tamoxifen as neoadjuvant therapy for oestrogen receptor-positive breast cancer in postmenopausal women: the IMPACT and PROACT trials. Presented at fourth European Breast Cancer Conference. Hamburg, Germany. March 16–20, 2004.
27. Semiglazov VF, Kletsel A, Zhiltzova E, et al. Exemestane (E) vs tamoxifen (T) as neoadjuvant endocrine therapy for postmenopausal women with ER+ breast cancer (T2N1-2, T3N0-1, T4N0M0). American Society of Clinical Oncology annual meeting (abst 530). 2005.
28. Smith IE, Walsh G, Skene A, et al. A phase II placebo-controlled trial of neoadjuvant Anastrozole alone or with gefitinib in early breast cancer. *J Clin Oncol* 2007;25:3816–3822.
29. Macaskill EJ, Dixon JM. Neoadjuvant use of endocrine therapy in breast cancer. *Breast J* 2007;13(3):243–250.
30. Semiglazov VV, Semiglazov VG, Dashyan G, et al. Phase 2 randomised trial of primary endocrine therapy versus chemotherapy in postmenopausal patients with ER-positive breast cancer. *Cancer* 2007;110:244–254.
31. Benz CC, Scott GK, Sarup JC, et al. Estrogen dependent tamoxifen resistant tumorigenic growth of MCF-7 cells transfected with HER2/neu. *Breast Cancer Res Treat* 1993;24:85–95.
32. Osborne CK, Bardou V, Hopp TA, et al. Role of the estrogen receptor coactivator AIB1 (SRC-3) and HER2/neu resistance in breast cancer. *J Natl Cancer Inst* 2003;95:353–361.

33. Dowsett M, Allred C, Knox J, et al. Relationship between quantitative estrogen and progesterone receptor expression and human epidermal growth factor receptor 2 (HER-2) status with recurrence in the Arimidex, Tamoxifen, Alone or in Combination Trial. *J Clin Oncol* 2008;26(7):1059–1065.

34. Rasmussen B, Regan MM, Lykkesfeldt AE, et al. Adjuvant letrozole versus tamoxifen according to centrally-assessed ERBB2 status for postmenopausal women with endocrine-responsive early breast cancer: supplementary results from the BIG 1-98 randomised trial. *Lancet Oncol* 2008;9:23–28.

35. Johnston SR, Head J, Pancholi S, et al. Integration of signal transduction inhibitors with endocrine therapy: an approach to overcoming hormone resistance in breast cancer. *Clin Cancer Res* 2003;9:524S–532S.

36. Martin LA, Farmer I, Johnston SR, et al. Enhanced estrogen receptor (ER) alpha, ERBB2, and MAPK signal transduction pathways operate during the adaptation of MCF-7 cells to long-term oestrogen deprivation. *J Biol Chem* 2003;287:30458–30468.

37. Dowsett M, Smith IE, Ebbs SR, et al. Prognostic value of Ki-67 expression after short-term presurgical endocrine therapy for primary breast cancer. *J Natl Cancer Inst* 2007;99(2):167–170.

38. Fisher B, Saffer EA, Rudock C, et al. Effect of local or systemic treatment prior to primary tumour removal on the production and response to a serum growth-stimulating factor in mice. *Cancer Res* 1989;49:2002–2004.

39. Chang J, Powles TJ, Allred DC, et al. Prediction of clinical outcome from primary tamoxifen by expression of biologic markers in breast cancer patients. *Clin Cancer Res* 2000;6:616–621.

40. Parton M, Krajewski S, Smith I, et al. Coordinate expression of apoptosis-associated proteins in human breast cancer before and during chemotherapy. *Clin Cancer Res* 2002;8:2100–2108.

41. Johnston SR, Boeddinghaus IM, Riddler S, et al. Idoxifene antagonizes estradiol-dependent MCF-7 breast cancer xenograft growth through sustained induction of apoptosis. *Cancer Res* 1999;59:3646–3651.

42. Dowsett M, Bundred NJ, Decensi A, et al. Effect of raloxifene on breast cancer cell Ki-67 and apoptosis: a double-blind, placebo-controlled, randomized clinical trial in postmenopausal patients. *Cancer Epidemiol Biomark Prev* 2001;10:961–966.

43. Robertson JF, Nicholson RI, Bundred NJ, et al. Comparison of the short-term biological effects of 7alpha-[9-(4,4,5,5,5-pentafluoropentylsulfinyl)-nonyl]estra-1,3,5,(10)-triene-3,17beta-diol (Faslodex) versus tamoxifen in postmenopausal women with primary breast cancer. *Cancer Res* 2001;61:6739–6746.

44. Geisler J, Detre S, Berntsen H, et al. Influence of neoadjuvant anastrozole (Arimidex) on intratumoral estrogen levels and proliferation markers in patients with locally advanced breast cancer. *Clin Cancer Res* 2001;7:1230–1236.

45. Ellis MJ, Coop A, Singh B, et al. Letrozole inhibits tumor proliferation more effectively than tamoxifen independent of HER1/2 expression status. *Cancer Res* 2003;63:6523–6531.

46. Cleator S, Parton M, Dowsett M. The biology of neoadjuvant chemotherapy for breast cancer. *Endocr Relat Cancer* 2002;9:183–195.

47. Prasad R, Boland GP, Cramer A, et al. Short-term biologic response to withdrawal of hormone replacement therapy in patients with invasive breast carcinoma. *Cancer* 2003;98:2539–2546.

48. Makris A, Powles TJ, Allred DC, et al. Changes in hormone receptors and proliferation markers in tamoxifen treated breast cancer patients and the relationship with response. *Breast Cancer Res Treat* 1998;48:11–20.

49. Kenny FS, Willsher PC, Gee JM, et al. Change in expression of ER, bcl-2 and MIB1 on primary tamoxifen and relation to response in ER positive breast cancer. *Breast Cancer Res Treat* 2001;65:135–144.

50. Dowsett M, Smith IE, Ebbs SR, et al. Proliferation and apoptosis as markers of benefit in neoadjuvant endocrine therapy of breast cancer. *Clin Cancer Res* 2006;12:1024s–1030s.

51. Ellis M, Ma C. Letrozole in the neoadjuvant setting: the PO24 trial. *Breast Cancer Res Treat* 2007;105:33–43.

Chapter 60
Local-Regional Therapy Considerations in Patients Receiving Preoperative Chemotherapy

Eleftherios P. Mamounas and Jennifer R. Bellon

The establishment of adjuvant chemotherapy as a valid option for the majority of patients with early stage breast cancer led to considerable interest in the evaluation of preoperative (neoadjuvant) chemotherapy for this cohort of patients. The clinical rationale for preoperative chemotherapy originated from studies in patients with locally advanced breast cancer, in whom this approach was used to successfully render them operable candidates. The rationale was further expanded to include patients with operable disease, when lumpectomy was established as the surgical treatment of choice in the majority of such patients and when adjuvant chemotherapy was found to significantly improve outcomes not only in node-positive patients but also in those with negative nodes.

Several large, well-designed, randomized clinical trials compared preoperative with postoperative (adjuvant) chemotherapy and eventually demonstrated the equivalence between these two approaches in their ability to prolong disease-free and overall survival (1–3). In addition, these trials identified several potential advantages with the preoperative approach. Compared to patients treated with surgery first, those treated with preoperative chemotherapy were significantly more likely to undergo breast-conserving surgery without significant increase in local recurrence (1–3). Furthermore, preoperative chemotherapy was found to downstage the disease in axillary lymph nodes in a considerable proportion of patients (up to 40% with anthracycline- and taxane-containing regimens) (1,2,4,5). Although this observation had limited clinical significance when axillary dissection was the only surgical method for staging the axilla, the development and validation of sentinel node biopsy (SNB) provided an additional potential advantage for preoperative chemotherapy, that is, the possibility of decreasing the extent and morbidity of axillary surgery. This approach is naturally predicated on the premise that SNB is feasible and accurate following preoperative chemotherapy. Lastly, several of the randomized (as well as nonrandomized) trials of preoperative chemotherapy have demonstrated a significant correlation between the achievement of pathologic complete response in the breast and axillary nodes and improved outcome, raising the possibility that pathologic tumor response can be used as an intermediate marker of chemotherapy efficacy and as a guide for further local-regional and systemic therapy decisions. Based on the above findings, preoperative chemotherapy has become the standard of care for patients with locally advanced breast cancer and a reasonable alternative for those with large, operable tumors.

Several unique local-regional therapy issues have emerged in patients who are candidates for preoperative chemotherapy. These relate to the appropriate surgical management of primary breast tumors and axillary lymph nodes as well as the optimal use of radiotherapy in this setting. Additional important issues in this group of patients surround the accurate assessment of the location and extent of the tumor in the breast and axillary nodes before, during, and after preoperative chemotherapy since this directly impacts the execution and outcomes of local-regional therapy.

 ## ASSESSMENT OF PRIMARY BREAST TUMOR BEFORE, DURING, AND AFTER PREOPERATIVE CHEMOTHERAPY

Core Needle Biopsy versus Fine-Needle Aspiration of the Primary Breast Tumor for Initial Diagnosis and Biomarker Assessment

Although, for breast cancer diagnosis, the rate of a false-positive fine-needle aspiration (FNA) is very low (6), this technique cannot readily differentiate invasive from noninvasive carcinoma. This is a potentially significant weakness when one considers using FNA in patients who are candidates for preoperative chemotherapy. On the other hand, core needle biopsy results in minimal tumor perturbation while providing important diagnostic information, including the identification of tumors that are predominantly or completely *in situ* (7). This approach has essentially eliminated the problem of a false-positive diagnosis in patients who are candidates for preoperative chemotherapy and has become the diagnostic method of choice in this setting. An additional advantage of core needle biopsy is that it provides adequate material for the evaluation of the necessary prognostic and predictive tumor biomarkers (e.g., estrogen/progesterone receptors (ER/PR), *ERBB2* [formerly *HER2/neu*], grade, and Ki-67) (8,9). Assessment of at least ER/PR and *ERBB2* status before the administration of preoperative chemotherapy is paramount for selecting the most appropriate preoperative regimen and for optimizing adjuvant therapy after surgery, particularly in cases of pathologic complete response in the breast and axillary nodes. Furthermore, from a research standpoint, core needle biopsy usually provides adequate material for some of the new promising molecular studies (10,11), although some of these studies can also be successfully performed from FNA material (11–14).

Clinical and Radiologic Assessment of the Extent of Primary Breast Tumor before and after Preoperative Chemotherapy

One of the most important benefits of preoperative chemotherapy is the potential for converting patients, who, based on large tumor size, require mastectomy, to candidates for breast-conserving surgery. Thus, accurate assessment of the location and extent of the primary tumor in the breast before, during, and after preoperative chemotherapy is crucial. Careful physical examination and a prechemotherapy mammogram are essential to delineate the extent of the primary tumor and to rule out the presence of diffuse malignant microcalcifications potentially indicative of an extensive intraductal component (15). In cases in which breast density interferes with appropriate mammographic assessment of the extent of primary tumor, ultrasound can provide an accurate assessment of the size of the invasive tumor and can also be used for tumor monitoring during preoperative chemotherapy (16). Although mammography is generally superior to clinical examination in predicting clinical complete response, it is not very accurate in predicting pathologic complete response (17).

Recently, several newer imaging modalities have been employed in an effort to more accurately define the extent and growth patterns of primary breast tumors as well as their response to preoperative chemotherapy. Magnetic resonance imaging (MRI) has emerged as a very useful tool for defining the extent and patterns of growth of primary breast tumors (18), particularly in high-risk patients (19,20) and in patients with increased mammographic density (21). MRI has also proven valuable in assessing tumor response to preoperative chemotherapy (22,23) and has shown superior accuracy when compared to mammography (18). The size of residual tumor by MRI correlates well with microscopic findings on pathologic examination (24,25), although MRI is less predictive of the true residual tumor size when there is substantial clinical response (but not a pathologic complete response) (26,27). Furthermore, since MRI is less sensitive in detecting ductal carcinoma *in situ* (DCIS) (28), it may underestimate the amount of residual non-invasive disease in the breast following preoperative chemotherapy. MRI before and after preoperative chemotherapy can identify distinct patterns of tumor growth and shrinkage (concentric vs. dendritic) (29), and thus can be useful in identifying appropriate candidates for breast-conserving surgery after preoperative chemotherapy (30). Other investigators have identified five distinct patterns of tumor growth in the breast that are associated with varying response rates (21) and are predictive of the ability to perform breast-conserving surgery in this setting (Fig. 60.1) (31). On the other hand, the high sensitivity but generally low specificity of MRI has raised concerns regarding the potential of decreasing the pool of candidates for breast-conserving surgery whether patients receive preoperative chemotherapy or not (28). Thus, for patients who are not good candidates for breast-conserving surgery based on the presence of multicentric lesions on the original or postchemotherapy MRI, consideration should be given to obtaining histologic confirmation of these additional MRI abnormalities before the decision to proceed with mastectomy (28).

Contrast-enhanced computed tomography (CE-CT) has also shown high sensitivity and specificity in determining the extent of disease in the breast before and after preoperative chemotherapy and in identifying appropriate candidates for breast-conserving surgery (32). Similar to MRI, CE-CT classifies breast tumors into localized and diffuse patterns of growth (33). Tumors exhibiting localized pattern of growth generally shrink concentrically, have higher rates of pathologic complete response, and are often appropriate candidates for breast-conserving surgery. On the other hand, tumors exhibiting a diffuse type of growth shrink in a mosaic pattern, have lower rates of pathologic complete response, and are not generally suitable

for breast-conserving surgery (33). Thus, CE-CT may offer a lower cost alternative to MRI in assessing primary breast tumors in patients who undergo preoperative chemotherapy, but studies comparing these two modalities are needed.

Finally, recent results with 18-fluoro-deoxy-glucose positron emission tomography (^{18}FDG-PET) and technetium-99 sestamibi scintimammography have also shown that these imaging modalities can be of potential value in patients who undergo preoperative chemotherapy. Changes in ^{18}FDG uptake have shown strong correlation with clinical response (34–36). However, its value in identifying pathologic complete responders among clinical complete responders is variable (34,35).

Identifying the Exact Tumor Bed Location in Cases of Clinical or Pathologic Complete Response

As the efficacy of preoperative chemotherapy regimens continues to increase, an issue that requires careful consideration before and during preoperative chemotherapy is the ability to identify the exact tumor location in cases of complete clinical response (or tumor bed location in cases of pathologic complete response). In most cases of clinical complete response, residual mammographic abnormalities remain, making wire localization and tumor removal fairly straightforward. However, in some patients with clinical complete response (and in most of those with a pathologic complete response), there is no residual abnormality on mammography or other imaging studies (including MRI). Therefore, it is always prudent in a patient who is about to receive preoperative chemotherapy to consider marking the exact tumor location by inserting a radiopaque marker under mammographic or sonographic guidance (titanium clip, metallic harpoon, embolization coils) (Fig. 60.2) (37,38). This can be performed either at the time of the initial core biopsy or at a subsequent time when there is clinical evidence of response. In the latter situation, the patient should be monitored closely by physical examination, and the corresponding mammographic or sonographic abnormality should be promptly marked when clinical response first becomes evident. In cases where the primary tumor is poorly visible mammographically because of dense breast parenchyma, the placement of the radiopaque marker should precede initiation of preoperative chemotherapy and in such cases the marker can usually be placed under sonographic guidance. Marker placement is crucial in cases where pathologic complete response has occurred because it allows the pathologist to focus on that particular area in search of residual tumor. If radiopaque marker placement is neither available nor feasible, tattooing the skin of the breast in four quadrants around the edge of the tumor before initiating preoperative chemotherapy is an easy, but not as accurate, alternative.

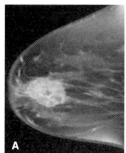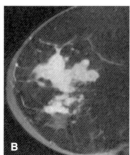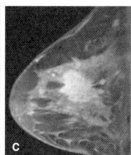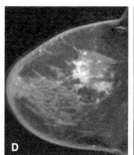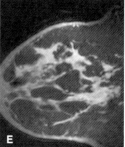

FIGURE 60.1. Magnetic resonance imaging phenotypes of patterns of growth of primary breast tumors. A: Single predominant mass with identifiable rim, displacing. **B:** Nodular pattern, irregular borders. **C:** Diffuse infiltrative pattern. **D:** Patchy enhancement. **E:** Septal spread. (Courtesy of Dr. Esserman, personal communication.)

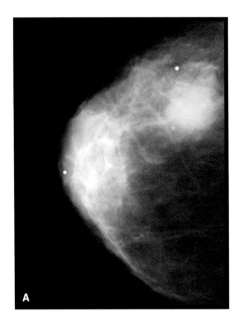
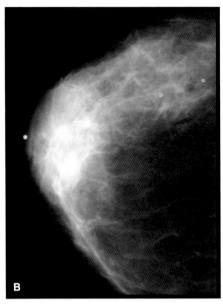

FIGURE 60.2. Titanium clip placement for tumor bed localization. A: Mammogram depicting a large mammographic (and palpable) tumor in the outer portion of the breast before preoperative chemotherapy. **B:** Radiopaque clip placement marking the area of the tumor bed following preoperative chemotherapy. The patient had a clinical and mammographic complete response, which eventually was confirmed as a pathologic complete response on surgical excision.

ASSESSMENT OF AXILLARY NODAL STATUS BEFORE PREOPERATIVE CHEMOTHERAPY

One of the concerns surrounding the use of preoperative chemotherapy relates to the lack of knowledge of the initial pathologic axillary nodal status (before preoperative chemotherapy), as this may impact further patient management, both local regional and systemic. Thus, assessment of the axillary nodal status with noninvasive or minimally invasive techniques should be attempted before preoperative chemotherapy. This assessment can be performed by imaging modalities, by FNA of radiologically enlarged nodes, or by SNB.

Radiologic Assessment of Axillary Nodal Status before Preoperative Chemotherapy

Despite the development of several innovative noninvasive, imaging modalities such as MRI, CE-CT scan, PET scan, and sestamibi scan, none so far has been shown to be of significant value in predicting the subclinical involvement of axillary nodes. The sensitivity of these methods ranges from 70% to 90% (32,34,39), but it is considerably lower when the involvement of axillary lymph nodes is limited to micrometastases or small macrometastases (34). A recent promising approach is to use ultrasound of the axilla to identify any pathologically enlarged lymph nodes and then to biopsy these lymph nodes by FNA (40,41). This is a simple, minimally invasive, and reliable technique for the initial determination of axillary lymph node status in experienced hands. However, common causes of decreased sensitivity with this approach include failure to visualize all lymph nodes by ultrasound and the small size of axillary metastases in some patients (41). Although this method has not become widely used, it can provide meaningful information for making subsequent therapeutic decisions and can provide, in some cases, direct evidence of chemosensitivity of axillary metastases to preoperative chemotherapy.

Sentinel Node Biopsy before Preoperative Chemotherapy

SNB is another approach for establishing the status of axillary nodes before preoperative chemotherapy (42–44). The major advantage of this approach is that information on the status of the axillary nodes can be obtained without the potential confounding effects of preoperative chemotherapy. This, in turn, can provide an advantage regarding the subsequent local-regional treatment of the patient and can help in the selection of optimal preoperative chemotherapy regimens as well as in the identification of optimal candidates for adjuvant chemotherapy after the preoperative regimen.

The feasibility and accuracy of SNB in patients with large operable breast cancer who are the typical candidates for preoperative chemotherapy has been demonstrated in several single institution series (42–46). Furthermore, patients with large operable breast cancer have been included in several of the multicenter and randomized trials, and so far, none of these trials has shown decreased feasibility or accuracy of SNB according to tumor size (47–50). However, by definition, SNB before systemic therapy has only been studied in patients who have clinically negative axillary nodes at the time of presentation, since those with clinically positive axillary nodes would have been excluded from these studies.

SURGICAL MANAGEMENT OF THE PRIMARY BREAST TUMOR AFTER PREOPERATIVE CHEMOTHERAPY

One clear clinical advantage of preoperative chemotherapy in women with large primary tumors, or in those with moderate size tumors but large tumor size to breast size ratio, is the potential for tumor shrinkage in order to facilitate breast-conserving surgery (51–53). Bonadonna et al. (52), reporting the 8-year results of two prospective trials from the Milan Cancer Institute in women with primary tumors larger than 2.5 cm, found that 85% could undergo breast-conserving surgery following a variety of preoperative chemotherapy regimens. In addition, breast conservation was possible in 62% of patients who presented with primary tumors larger than 5.0 cm. Vlastos et al. (53) reported on the M.D. Anderson Cancer Center experience and found significant downsizing in 129 patients treated with preoperative chemotherapy (either paclitaxel or FAC [fluorouracil, doxorubicin, and cyclophosphamide]). Although the number of patients eligible for breast conservation was not defined preoperatively, 26% of tumors initially T2 were down-staged to less than 1.0 cm, and 11% had a pathologic complete response in the breast. In addition, in tumors clinically greater than 5 cm, 29% decreased to less than 1.0 cm and 9% had no residual disease at surgery. Overall, 34% underwent breast conservation. In contrast, in the National Surgical Adjuvant Breast and Bowel Project (NSABP) B-18 trial (54), in which patients were randomized to preoperative versus adjuvant chemotherapy and surgeons were required to state beforehand whether a patient was a candidate for breast conservation, breast-conservation rates improved significantly but only from 60% to 67%. Similarly, in the Royal Marsden randomized trial of preoperative plus adjuvant chemotherapy (mitoxantrone/methotrexate with or without mitomycin) versus the same chemotherapy given all in the adjuvant setting, breast conservation was increased from 13% to 28% (55). In addition, 23% of patients in the European Organisation for Research and Treatment of Cancer (EORTC) randomized trial of preoperative fluorouracil, epirubicin, and cyclophosphamide (FEC) underwent breast conservation instead of a planned mastectomy (2). Criteria for breast conservation both before and after chemotherapy, however, are often dependent on the individual surgeon or institution, making it difficult to extrapolate from these randomized trials, and making comparisons of breast-conservation rates across trials problematic.

Another important, but difficult to objectively evaluate, contribution of preoperative chemotherapy is its potential to reduce the amount of breast tissue that needs to be removed during lumpectomy, even if the patient is already a candidate for breast-conserving surgery. For this approach to be successful, the surgeon should take into account the original tumor configuration, the pattern of tumor shrinkage, and the presence or absence of suspicious microcalcifications (indicating an extensive intraductal component). It is generally reasonable for the surgeon to plan the extent of lumpectomy on the basis of the residual tumor size after chemotherapy as identified by clinical and imaging assessment; however, the status of the surgical margins must be carefully assessed, and the surgeon must be prepared to perform additional resection if on pathologic evaluation the lumpectomy margins are found to be compromised or if there is evidence of "honeycomb" tumor regression.

Particular attention needs to be paid when planning the extent of lumpectomy in patients who present with invasive lobular carcinoma. Invasive lobular carcinoma is often multicentric, can extensively involve the breast without significant clinical or imaging findings of a defined mass (28,56,57), and is associated with lower rates of clinical response when compared to invasive ductal carcinoma (58,59). More importantly, among patients with lobular invasive histology, the rate of pathologic complete response is low (59–61), and, in one series, lobular histology was identified as one of the independent predictors of ineligibility for breast-conserving surgery after preoperative chemotherapy (62). Thus, for patients who present with extensive lobular invasive carcinoma requiring mastectomy, it is unlikely that preoperative chemotherapy will convert them to lumpectomy candidates.

Ipsilateral Breast Tumor Recurrence Following Preoperative Chemotherapy and Lumpectomy

One of the concerns with converting patients who are mastectomy candidates to candidates for breast-conserving surgery with preoperative chemotherapy is that this approach may lead to significantly higher rates of local recurrence (or ipsilateral breast tumor recurrence). However, results from studies in patients with operable breast cancer and in those with locally advanced disease have demonstrated that breast-conserving surgery can be safely performed in patients who respond to preoperative chemotherapy without compromising local control (1,2,5,63). The evidence is stronger in patients with operable breast cancer where large randomized trials have shown no statistically significant increase in local recurrence between the preoperative and adjuvant chemotherapy arms of the trial (1,2,5). In the NSABP B-18 trial, in which 1,523 women were randomized to preoperative versus postoperative doxorubicin and cyclophosphamide chemotherapy, there was a small difference in local recurrence rates favoring the adjuvant chemotherapy arm, but this was not significantly significant. At 9 years, the risk of local recurrence among the patients undergoing lumpectomy was 10.7% with preoperative chemotherapy versus 7.6% with adjuvant chemotherapy (1). Similarly, no significant difference in local-regional recurrence (LRR) was observed in the EORTC trial that compared preoperative versus postoperative 5-fluorouracil, epirubicin, and cyclophosphamide chemotherapy in 689 patients (2).

Two recently published meta-analyses of randomized trials of preoperative versus adjuvant chemotherapy have demonstrated a small but statistically significant difference in local recurrence with the preoperative approach (64,65). In the first meta-analysis of nine randomized trials that included 3,946 patients, preoperative chemotherapy was statistically significantly associated with an increased risk of LRR compared with adjuvant chemotherapy (risk ratio [RR] = 1.22; 95% confidence interval [CI], 1.04–1.43), although in-breast and postmastectomy recurrences were not examined separately. Furthermore, this increased risk was especially observed in trials where more patients in the preoperative, than the adjuvant, arm received radiation therapy (RT) without surgery (RR = 1.53; 95% CI, 1.11–2.10) (64). In the second and most recent meta-analysis of 14 trials, preoperative chemotherapy was also found to increase LRR rates, but again this was not the case in studies in which surgery remained part of the treatment even after complete tumor regression (hazard ratio [HR] 1.12; 95% CI, 0.92–1.37; $p = .25$) (65). Thus, if surgery is included in the local-regional management following preoperative chemotherapy, there is no convincing evidence that LRR rates are significantly increased with preoperative versus adjuvant chemotherapy.

One issue of potential concern is the observation from the largest randomized trial (NSABP B-18) that patients who were mastectomy candidates and were converted to lumpectomy by preoperative chemotherapy had significantly higher ipsilateral breast tumor recurrence rates when compared to those who were lumpectomy candidates from the beginning (15.9% vs. 9.9% at 9 years) (1). Although this subset of patients was small ($n = 69$), the difference was statistically significant ($p = .04$). However, this type of comparison has associated bias since patients with large tumors who are initially mastectomy candidates but are converted to candidates for breast-conserving surgery have inherently higher propensity for local failure whether they are treated with mastectomy (as originally planned) or with breast-conserving surgery (after down-staging). Careful assessment of the tumor shrinkage patterns and the amount of residual tumor after preoperative chemotherapy as well as meticulous margin assessment are paramount for this group of patients.

It is also useful to attempt to identify factors that define optimal candidates for breast-conserving surgery after preoperative chemotherapy. Rouzier et al. (66) reported on factors that predicted for breast conservation after three or four cycles of anthracycline-based preoperative chemotherapy in 594 patients with invasive T2 or T3 breast carcinoma (49 mm mean diameter) who were ineligible for breast-conserving surgery. After preoperative chemotherapy, 48% became eligible for breast-conserving surgery. Initial tumor diameter greater than 5 cm, low histologic grade, lobular histology, and multicentricity were independent predictive factors of breast conservation ineligibility in multivariate analysis. Local recurrence rates were similar in patients treated with lumpectomy and those treated with mastectomy (66).

Whether established risk factors for local recurrence after adjuvant chemotherapy are applicable to breast conservation after preoperative chemotherapy also remains to be determined. Rouzier et al. (67) from the Institute Curie retrospectively analyzed the results of 257 women with clinical T1 to T3 (6% T1; 84% T2; 10% T3) invasive carcinomas treated with a variety of preoperative chemotherapy regimens followed by breast-conserving surgery. The 5- and 10-year actuarial local recurrence rates were 16% and 21.5%, respectively. On univariate analysis, age 40 or less, S-phase fraction greater than 4%, and margins 2 mm or less were associated with local recurrence. On multivariate analysis, age, S-phase fraction, and margin status remained independent predictors of local recurrence, as did tumor size greater than 2 cm at the time of surgery. Risk of local recurrence at 5 years was 29% in women with margins 2 mm or less compared with 13% in women with margins greater than 2 mm. These rates are somewhat higher than those seen in other retrospective studies of local recurrence according to margin status in patients treated without preoperative chemotherapy (68,69). In contrast, the Milan group reported on 536 patients with primary tumors larger than 2.5 cm who underwent preoperative chemotherapy with the goal of breast conservation (52). Breast-conserving surgery was feasible in 85%. At a median follow-up of 8 years local recurrence was 6.8% (95% CI, 3.9%–8.8%). The lower rate of local recurrence in the Italian series compared to the French series may be related to the standard use of quadrantectomy in the former, which may *de facto* result in larger surgical margins compared to lumpectomy in the French series. In the adjuvant setting, margin status remains the most important risk factor for local recurrence.

Whether the same criteria for acceptable margins after lumpectomy also apply to patients who have been treated with preoperative chemotherapy also remains to be determined. Because of the above mentioned slight increase in local recurrence in patients treated with breast-conserving surgery after preoperative chemotherapy, perhaps close margins are of even greater importance in this setting. Another potential reason for the slight increase in local recurrence after breast-conserving surgery is the observation that some breast cancers regress in response to preoperative chemotherapy in a "honeycomb" pattern rather than in a "concentric" pattern. In an update of the M.D. Anderson Cancer Center experience, Chen et al. (70) reported on 340 patients who underwent breast-conserving surgery following preoperative chemotherapy. With a median follow-up of 5 years, ipsilateral breast recurrence rate was 4%, although the number of patients who did not become eligible for breast conservation was not stated. On multivariate analysis, a multifocal pattern of disease (along with residual disease >2 cm, clinical N2 or N3 nodal disease, and lymphovascular space invasion) predicted for LRR. It seems prudent, therefore, to take a more conservative stance with eligibility for breast conservation after preoperative chemotherapy and to attempt to identify the pattern of tumor spread and tumor shrinkage by imaging studies (particularly MRI) before and after chemotherapy. Breast conservation may even be possible in carefully selected women with T4 disease, classically thought to be candidates for mastectomy (71). This is discussed in Chapter 61 on Locally Advanced Breast Cancer.

Breast Reconstruction after Preoperative Chemotherapy and Mastectomy

The administration of preoperative chemotherapy should not constitute a contraindication for performing immediate breast reconstruction following mastectomy in patients who were not converted to lumpectomy candidates (72). Several studies have shown that in patients who have received prior preoperative chemotherapy, immediate breast reconstruction with autologous tissue is safe (73–75) does not delay further adjuvant therapy (73,76) and is not associated with an increase in local recurrence (73,77) or with a delay in detecting such a recurrence (78). However, there is evidence that immediate reconstruction can compromise the quality of RT, which can lead to radiating more heart and lung (79). The optimal type of reconstruction (autologous tissue reconstruction vs. implant reconstruction) is still the subject of debate since the effect of RT (which is likely to be needed in patients with large operable and locally advanced breast cancer) on breast implants or on autologous tissue is unpredictable and may lead to increase in capsular contraction or flap contraction, respectively (75,77,80). Given this concern, some investigators have recently adopted the so-called immediate-delayed or delayed-delayed reconstruction approach in patients who are likely to require postmastectomy radiotherapy (81). According to this approach, following a skin-sparing mastectomy, a submuscular expander is placed and is partially inflated. Following the final pathology report, if it is determined that the patient needs adjuvant RT, the expander is deflated so RT can be adequately delivered to the skin or chest wall and ipsilateral regional nodes and flap reconstruction follows at a later time. If RT is not required, expansion continues and the expander is replaced by the permanent implant at a later time.

 ## SURGICAL MANAGEMENT OF THE AXILLARY NODES AFTER PREOPERATIVE CHEMOTHERAPY

As SNB has been established as the procedure of choice for staging patients with operable breast cancer and as preoperative chemotherapy continues to be increasingly employed in this setting, the question of whether SNB is feasible and accurate following preoperative chemotherapy has become one of significant importance. As mentioned earlier, preoperative chemotherapy has been shown to downstage axillary lymph nodes in a considerable proportion of patients (up to 40% with anthracycline- and taxane-containing regimens). Thus, if SNB is accurate following preoperative chemotherapy, patients who present with involved axillary nodes at the time of diagnosis may potentially be spared from axillary dissection if, following preoperative chemotherapy, the sentinel node is found to be negative. However, there are theoretical reasons for questioning whether the performance characteristics of SNB after preoperative chemotherapy may differ from those of SNB at the time of diagnosis and before systemic therapy. Does tumor response to chemotherapy cause tissue scarring, affecting the lymphatic drainage pattern? Does preoperative chemotherapy have the same effect on involved nonsentinel nodes as it does on involved sentinel nodes? Lastly, even if SNB after preoperative chemotherapy accurately reflects the status of the axilla at that time, the implications for LRR are still unclear. That is, it is still unclear to what degree the initial extent of disease and the response to preoperative chemotherapy combine to determine the risk of axillary recurrence if previously involved axillary lymph nodes are not surgically removed.

Sentinel Node Biopsy after Preoperative Chemotherapy

Initially, small, single-institution studies have examined the efficacy of lymphatic mapping and the accuracy of SNB after preoperative chemotherapy with significant variability in the rate of sentinel node identification and in the rate of false-negative sentinel node (82–99). More recently, larger single institution studies were reported, including some in which the axillary nodes were documented to be involved prior to preoperative chemotherapy (100–105). When these studies are examined collectively (106,107), or when larger, multicenter data sets are analyzed (108,109), SNB after preoperative chemotherapy appears to have similar performance characteristics to those of SNB before systemic therapy (47,48,50,109, 110).

Single Institution Studies of Sentinel Node Biopsy after Preoperative Chemotherapy

Single-institution studies of SNB after preoperative chemotherapy are summarized in Table 60.1 (82–105). These studies generally included patients with operable as well as locally advanced breast cancer (58% had histologically positive nodes after preoperative chemotherapy) and have reported significant variability in the success rate of sentinel node identification (72% to 100%) and in the rate of false-negative sentinel node (0% to 39%). This variability is primarily due to the small size of the earlier studies (2000 to 2004) with numbers of patients ranging between 14 to 55 and, more importantly, with numbers of patients with positive nodes after preoperative chemotherapy ranging between 9 and 33. The significant variability in the rates of a false-negative sentinel node led to

Table 60.1   SINGLE INSTITUTION SERIES EVALUATING SENTINEL NODE BIOPSY AFTER PREOPERATIVE CHEMOTHERAPY

Author (Reference)	Year	Stage/ Eligibility	Method of Lymphatic Mapping	No. of Patients	No. of Node (+) Patients[a]	No. with SN Identified	ID Rate (%)	No. with FN SN	FN Rate (%)	Conclusion
Breslin et al. (82)	2000	T1-3N0-1M0	BD +/– RC	51	25	43	84.3	3	12	Accurate
Nason et al. (83)	2000	T2-4N0-1M0	BD + RC	15	9	13	86.7	3	33	Inaccurate
Fernandez et al. (84)	2001	T1-4N0-1M0	RC	40	20	34	85	4	20	Inaccurate
Haid et al. (85)	2001	T1-3 Operable	BD + RC	33	18	29	87.9	0	0	Accurate
Stearns et al. (86)	2002	T3-4N0-3M0	BD	34	21	29	85.3	3	14	Accurate[b]
Miller et al. (87)	2002	T1-3 Operable	BC, RC, Both	35	9	30	85.7	0	0	Accurate
Brady (88)	2002	Stage I-IIIB	BD (RC:1 pt)	14	10	13	92.8	0	0	Accurate
Reitsamer et al. (89)	2003	T2-3N0-1M0	BD + RC	30	15	26	86.7	1	6.7	Accurate
Schwartz and Meltzer (90)	2003	T1-3N0-1M0	BD	21	11	21	100	1	9.1	Accurate
Balch et al. (91)	2003	T-2-4N0-1M0	BD + RC	32	19	31	96.9	1	5.3	Accurate
Piato et al. (92)	2003	T1-2N0M0	RC	42	18	41	97.6	3	16.7	Accurate
Vigario et al. (93)	2003	T1-2N0M0	RC	37	18	36	97.3	7	38.9	Inaccurate
Aihara et al. (94)	2004	T2-4N0M0	Indigo carmine	20	12	17	85	1	8.3	Accurate
Kang et al. (95)	2004	T1-4 NxM0	BD, RC , Both	54	27	39	72.2	3	11.1	Accurate[c]
Shimazu et al. (96)	2004	T2-4N0-2M0	BD + RC	47	33	44	93.6	4	12.1	Accurate
Patel et al. (97)	2004	T2-4N0-1M0	BC, RC , Both	42	19	40	95	0	0	Accurate
Lang et al. (98)	2004	Stage II-III (N0-3)	BC, RC , Both	53	24	50	94.3	1	4.1	Accurate
All Studies 2000–2004				600	308	536	89.3	35	11.4	
Jones et al. (99)	2005	T2-4N0-1M0	BD + RC	36	18	29	80.6	2	11.1	Accurate
Tanaka et al. (100)	2005	T1-3N0-2M0	BD	70	20	63	90	1	5	Accurate
Yu et al. (101)	2006	T3N0M0	BD	127	69	116	91.3	5	7.2	Accurate
Shen et al. (103)	2006	T1-T4, N1-N3[d]	BD, RC , Both	69	40	64	92.8	10	25	Inaccurate
Lee et al. (105)	2006	T1-T4, Node (+)[e]	BD, RC , Both	219	124	170	77.6	7	5.6	Accurate[c]
Newman et al. (104)	2007	T1-3N1M0[d]	BD, RC , Both	40	28	40	100	3	10.7	Accurate
Kinoshita (102)	2007	T2-4N0-2M0	BD + RC	104	40	97	93.3	4	10	Accurate
All Studies 2005–2007				665	339	579	87.1	32	9	
All Studies 2000–2007				1,265	647	1,115	88.1	67	10.4	

SN, sentinel node; ID, identification rate; FN, false negative; BD, blue dye; RC, radiocolloid.
[a]After preoperative chemotherapy.
[b]Excluding inflammatory breast cancer.
[c]low identification rate.
[d]Fine-needle aspiration by ultrasound.
[e]Palpable and (+) on fine-needle aspiration or greater than 1-cm thick with loss of fat hilum on ultrasound and standardized uptake value greater than 2.5 on positron emission tomography.

different conclusions regarding the accuracy of the procedure in this setting. When one examines the earlier studies (2000 to 2004) collectively (600 patients, 308 node-positive patients), the average identification rate was 89.3% and the average false-negative rate was 11.4% (Table 60.1). Although the sentinel node identification rate after preoperative chemotherapy is somewhat lower compared to those observed in studies of SNB before systemic therapy, the false-negative rates between the two approaches are comparable (50,111–113). Sentinel node identification rates in these studies were generally higher when radiocolloid was used for lymphatic mapping compared to when blue dye alone was used.

The more recently reported single institution studies of SNB after preoperative chemotherapy (2005 to present) were generally larger (36 to 219 patients, 18 to 124 node-positive patients) and also included patients with operable as well as locally advanced breast cancer (59% had histologically positive nodes after preoperative chemotherapy). Included in this group were three studies in which all patients had documented axillary involvement before preoperative chemotherapy (Table 60.1) (103–105). As with the earlier reported single institution studies of SNB after preoperative chemotherapy, the more recently published studies have also reported considerable variability in the success rate of sentinel node identification (77.6% to 100%) and in the rate of false-negative sentinel node (5% to 25%). When the more recent studies are examined collectively (665 patients, 339 node-positive patients), the identification rate (87.1%) remains somewhat lower than in studies of SNB before systemic therapy, but the false-negative rate (9%) is again comparable to that reported in studies of SNB before systemic therapy (see discussion below) (50,111–113).

Sentinel Node Biopsy after Preoperative Chemotherapy in Patients with Known Axillary Involvement at Diagnosis

The three studies of SNB after preoperative chemotherapy in patients who were known to be node positive before preoperative chemotherapy deserve a more detailed discussion.

Shen et al. (103) reported on 69 patients with clinical T1-4, N1-3 disease who had axillary metastases identified by ultrasound-guided FNA and then underwent SNB following preoperative chemotherapy on prospective, institutional protocols. All but eight patients underwent axillary lymph node dissection. The sentinel node identification rate was 92.8%. In the 56 patients in whom a sentinel node was identified and an axillary dissection was performed, 10 patients had a false-negative sentinel node (false-negative rate 25%). Based on these results, the authors concluded that SNB is feasible after preoperative chemotherapy, even in patients who initially presented with cytologically involved axillary nodes, but that the false-negative rate of SNB in this group of patients is much higher than those observed in clinically node-negative patients. However, the relatively small number of patients with positive nodes after preoperative chemotherapy and the inclusion of patients with T4 tumors and N2-3 disease make the results of this study less representative to the general population of patients with large operable breast cancer and clinically N1 disease, in which SNB after preoperative chemotherapy is considered.

More recently, Lee et al. (105) reported on 238 patients who were found to have positive axillary nodes at presentation and underwent SNB and axillary dissection following preoperative chemotherapy. The definition of axillary nodal positivity in that study included lymph nodes that were palpable and positive by FNA or nodes that were more than 1-cm thick with loss of fat hilum on ultrasound *and* had a standardized uptake value greater than 2.5 on PET scan. The identification rate was significantly lower in patients who received preoperative

chemotherapy (77.6%) when compared to patients from the same institution who did not (97.0%; $p < .001$). However, the false-negative rate was 5.6%, similar to that observed in patients who did not receive preoperative chemotherapy (7.4%; p not significant). Based on these results, the authors concluded that for patients who present with involved axillary nodes and who achieve complete clinical axillary response with preoperative chemotherapy, SNB could replace axillary node dissection.

Finally, Newman et al. (104) reported their institutional findings using a novel comprehensive approach to axillary management of node-positive patients receiving preoperative chemotherapy. From 2001 to 2005, they evaluated 54 consecutive breast cancer patients with biopsy-proven (in some with SNB) axillary nodal metastases at diagnosis who underwent SNB and axillary lymph node dissection after receiving preoperative chemotherapy. The sentinel node identification rate was 98% (100% in patients who did not also undergo a SNB before preoperative chemotherapy). Thirty-six patients (66%) had residual axillary metastases (including 8 patients who had also undergone SNB before preoperative chemotherapy). Of the 28 patients with positive nodes after preoperative chemotherapy and no prior SNB before preoperative chemotherapy, the false-negative rate was 10.7% (3 patients). Based on their results, the authors concluded that SNB after preoperative chemotherapy in patients with documented nodal disease at presentation accurately identified cases that were down-staged and commented that this approach can potentially spare this subset of patients (32%) the morbidity of an axillary dissection.

Multicenter Studies of Sentinel Node Biopsy after Preoperative Chemotherapy

The variability in the efficacy and accuracy of SNB after preoperative chemotherapy, as documented in the small, single institution series, underscores the importance of evaluating this approach in larger cohorts of patients from multicenter studies. The largest report to date comes from the NSABP B-27 trial (108), in which 428 of the 2,411 patients treated with preoperative chemotherapy underwent lymphatic mapping and an attempt for SNB prior to the required axillary node dissection (Table 60.2). Since performance of SNB was not mandated in the trial, there was no predefined protocol dictating the method of lymphatic mapping or the approach to SNB. Despite that, the identification rate was 85% and was significantly higher when radiocolloid (with or without Lymphazurin [isosulfan blue; TYCO Healthcare Group, North Haven, Connecticut]) was used for lymphatic mapping (88% to 89%) compared to when Lymphazurin alone was used (78%). The false-negative rate was 11% and again was lower when radiocolloid (with or without Lymphazurin) was used for lymphatic mapping (8%) compared to when Lymphazurin alone was used (14%). Interestingly, there were no significant differences in the false-negative rates of patients who presented with clinically negative versus clinically positive axillary nodes (12.4% vs. 7.0%, respectively; $p = .51$).

A smaller experience with SNB after preoperative chemotherapy was reported as part of a larger multicenter trial that was initiated in 1997 to evaluate the diagnostic accuracy of SNB in patients with breast cancer (109). Of 968 patients enrolled into the trial, 29 were treated with preoperative chemotherapy. The sentinel node identification rate for the preoperative chemotherapy group was 93% compared to 88% for the group that had surgery first. No false negatives were reported in patients receiving preoperative chemotherapy compared to a 13% false-negative rate in those who had surgery first (Table 60.2).

Table 60.2	MULTICENTER SERIES EVALUATING SENTINEL NODE BIOPSY AFTER PREOPERATIVE CHEMOTHERAPY									

Author (Reference)	Year	Stage/ Eligibility	Method of Lymphatic Mapping	No. of Patients	No. of Node (+) Patients	No. with SN Identified	ID Rate (%)	No. with FN SN	FN Rate (%)	Conclusion
Mamounas et al. (108)	2005	T1-3, N0-1 No predefined protocol for SNB	BD, RC, Both	428	140	363	85 BD: 77 RC: 90 Both: 88	15	11 BD:14 RC: 5 Both: 9	Accurate
Tafra et al. (109)	2001	Based on predefined protocol for SNB, investigators recruited after attending a course on the technique	BD + RC	29	15	27	93	0	0	Accurate

SNB, sentinel node biopsy; ID, identification rate; FN, false negative; BD, blue dye; RC, radiocolloid.

Meta-Analysis of Studies Evaluating Sentinel Node Biopsy after Preoperative Chemotherapy

Xing et al. (106) recently published a meta-analysis of 21 studies of SNB after preoperative chemotherapy. Studies were eligible for inclusion if they evaluated patients with operable breast cancer who had undergone SNB after preoperative chemotherapy followed by an axillary dissection. A total of 1,273 patients were included in the 21 studies. The reported identification rates ranged from 72% to 100%, with a pooled estimate of 90%. The sensitivity of SNB ranged from 67% to 100% with a pooled estimate of 88% (95% CI, 85%–90%). Thus the false-negative rate ranged from 0% to 33% with a pooled estimate of 12%. Based on their results, the authors concluded that SNB is a reliable tool for planning treatment after preoperative chemotherapy.

When one compares the identification rates and false-negative rates of SNB after preoperative chemotherapy observed in multicenter studies and in the meta-analysis to those from other multicenter and randomized trials of SNB before systemic therapy, the identification rates are somewhat lower after preoperative chemotherapy, but the false-negative rates are similar (Table 60.3) (47,48,50,110). Furthermore, when one compares the confidence intervals around the false-negative rates between studies evaluating SNB before systemic therapy with those of SNB after preoperative chemotherapy, there is considerable overlap (Fig. 60.3).

Optimal Candidates for Sentinel Node Biopsy after Preoperative Chemotherapy

If one were to start performing SNB without completion axillary dissection in patients who have received preoperative chemotherapy, it would make intuitive sense to first do so in patients who have the least likelihood of having positive axillary lymph nodes after the preoperative regimen in order to minimize the rate of leaving behind positive nonsentinel nodes. This rate is a factor of the sentinel node false-negative rate as well as the rate of axillary node positivity. In NSABP B-27 (4) as well as in other large preoperative chemotherapy trials (5,54,114), patients achieving a pathologic complete response in the breast have the lowest rate of having involved axillary nodes (13% to 15%). On the other hand, in the NSABP B-27 SNB experience, there were no significant differences in the sentinel node false-negative rates according to clinical or pathologic breast tumor response. Thus, as expected, in the NSABP B-27 trial the rate of leaving behind positive nonsentinel nodes was lowest among patients with pathologic complete response (1.7%) compared to those with clinical complete response but residual invasive cancer in the breast (4.0%) and those with any other type of clinical response (5.5%), although these differences did not reach statistical significance.

Thus, as surgeons start to utilize SNB after preoperative chemotherapy without completion axillary dissection, patients achieving a clinical complete response (and more importantly a

Table 60.3	COMPARISON OF FALSE-NEGATIVE RATES BETWEEN MULTICENTER STUDIES/RANDOMIZED TRIALS EVALUATING SENTINEL NODE BIOPSY BEFORE SYSTEMIC THERAPY AND MULTICENTER STUDIES/META-ANALYSES EVALUATING SENTINEL NODE BIOPSY AFTER PREOPERATIVE CHEMOTHERAPY		

Study/Clinical Trial (Reference)	False-Negative Rate (%)	No. of SN (−)/Axillary Node (+)
SNB before Systemic Therapy		
Multicenter SB-2 Trial (110)	11	13/114
Italian Randomized Trial (48)	9	8/91
Ann Arundel Multicenter Trial (49)	13	25/193
University of Louisville Multicenter Trial (50)	7	24/333
NSABP B-32 Randomized Trial (47)	10	75/766
SNB after Preoperative Chemotherapy		
NSABP B-27 Trial (108)	11	15/140
Meta-Analysis of SNB after Preoperative Chemotherapy) (106)	12	65/540

SN, sentinel node; SNB, sentinel node biopsy; NSABP, National Surgical Adjuvant Breast and Bowel Project.

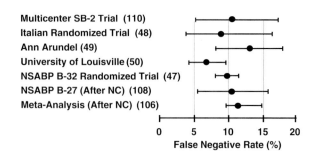

FIGURE 60.3. Comparison of false-negative rates and 95% confidence intervals (*indicated by the horizontal line width*) between studies (reference numbers given in parentheses) evaluating sentinel node biopsy before systemic therapy and those evaluating sentinel node biopsy after preoperative chemotherapy. NSABP, National Surgical Adjuvant Breast and Bowel Project; NC, neoadjuvant chemotherapy.

pathologic complete response) are the best candidates for this approach if the sentinel node is negative. Touch imprint cytology is reliable for intraoperative detection of nodal metastases after preoperative chemotherapy (115), and preoperative imaging studies as well as traditional frozen section can be used for preoperative and intraoperative assessment of pathologic complete response in the breast, respectively. As more data and clinical experience accumulate with SNB after preoperative chemotherapy, this approach could be expanded to patients with lesser clinical and pathologic response.

Pros and Cons of Sentinel Node Biopsy before versus after Preoperative Chemotherapy

The timing of SNB in patients treated with preoperative chemotherapy has been the subject of considerable controversy (Table 60.4). This is because there are several advantages as well as limitations with each approach. The main advantage with SNB *before* preoperative chemotherapy is that it provides information on the status of axillary nodes without the potential confounding effects of chemotherapy. This information can be used for selecting optimal candidates for preoperative chemotherapy and appropriate preoperative chemotherapy regimens and for deciding on the subsequent local-regional management of the patient. Particularly, if the sentinel node is negative, the patient is spared an axillary dissection and possibly will generally not require local-regional radiation other than breast radiation after lumpectomy. The main limitation of SNB before preoperative chemotherapy is that it does not take advantage of the potential down-staging effect of preoperative chemotherapy on the axillary nodes, since patients with a positive sentinel node (typically 50% to 70% of the patients with large operable breast cancer) will generally require an axillary node dissection either before or after preoperative chemotherapy (47–50,106,108,110). In addition, SNB before preoperative chemotherapy requires two surgical procedures for patient management, whether the sentinel node is negative or positive. Furthermore, although upfront knowledge of the status of the sentinel node is useful in some low-risk patients who will not need chemotherapy if the sentinel node is negative, this is not generally required for the majority of typical candidates for preoperative chemotherapy. For most of such patients, little if anything is to be gained by knowing the pathologic nodal status at presentation, since clinical tumor size and biomarkers from the primary tumor, such as ER/PR and *ERBB2* (obtained by core biopsy), are usually sufficient to quantify risk for recurrence and benefit from adjuvant or preoperative chemotherapy. Recently published data with genomic profiling indicate that patients with ER-positive,

node-negative breast cancer and a low recurrence score by Onco*type* DX (Genomic Health, Redwood City, California) have a good prognosis and receive minimal to no benefit from the addition of adjuvant chemotherapy to hormonal therapy (116,117). These data have strengthened the rationale for proceeding with SNB before preoperative chemotherapy in ER-positive patients. However, more recently reported preliminary data suggest that patients with ER-positive disease and a low recurrence score by Onco*type* DX may not benefit from adjuvant chemotherapy even if they are node positive (118,119). Thus, it is possible that in the future, genomic profiling will be obtained on core biopsy material from the primary breast tumor and patients with low risk would not be candidates for preoperative chemotherapy, whether they are ultimately node negative or node positive. This would further diminish the value of SNB before preoperative chemotherapy.

Knowledge of the sentinel node status before preoperative chemotherapy has a generally minimal impact on deciding which preoperative chemotherapy regimen to use or whether to add adjuvant chemotherapy after surgery. For the majority of the typical preoperative chemotherapy candidates, an anthracycline- and taxane-based regimen is used (with the addition of trastuzumab if the tumor is *ERBB2* positive). Following preoperative chemotherapy, the presence and the amount of residual disease in the breast or axillary nodes is a good correlate of long-term outcome (120,121), but benefit from additional chemotherapy has not been demonstrated (once an anthracycline and a taxane have already been used in the preoperative setting). Furthermore, although it is well documented that residual involvement of axillary nodes after preoperative chemotherapy generally predicts poor outcome (120,122–124) and that negative nodes after preoperative chemotherapy or documented eradication of disease in the lymph nodes predict good outcome (123,125), the prognostic significance of negative axillary nodes after preoperative chemotherapy *and prior positive SNB* is uncertain since axillary node negativity in this setting may reflect axillary nodal down-staging from preoperative chemotherapy or merely the removal of all positive nodes by the sentinel node procedure.

Perhaps the more important argument for performing SNB before preoperative chemotherapy is that knowledge of sentinel node status before chemotherapy can help identify optimal candidates for local-regional RT to the chest wall (after mastectomy) or to regional lymph nodes (irrespective of surgical procedure). This is because most of the available information on the rates and patterns of LRR and the need for adjuvant RT is based on the pathologic status of the axillary nodes at presentation (as determined at surgery). Little information exists on the rates and patterns of LRR in patients with operable breast cancer who have received prior preoperative chemotherapy, and the effect of clinical and pathologic tumor response on the rates and patterns of LRR has not been well studied. Since in most series of preoperative chemotherapy patients who have residual positive nodes are offered breast and regional nodal RT after lumpectomy and chest wall and regional nodal RT after mastectomy, few data sets are available that can address this question. These studies will be reviewed in detail in the following section discussing local-regional radiation issues in patients treated with preoperative chemotherapy.

Finally, besides the loss of prognostic information (discussed above), the main limitation of SNB *after* preoperative chemotherapy is the concern over its performance characteristics, when compared with up-front SNB. As described earlier, there is much less information regarding the performance characteristics of SNB after preoperative chemotherapy compared to the up-front setting. Moreover, there is practically no information on axillary recurrence rates with SNB alone after

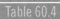

	Table 60.4	ADVANTAGES AND LIMITATIONS OF SENTINEL NODE BIOPSY BEFORE VERSUS AFTER PREOPERATIVE CHEMOTHERAPY

	SNB before Preoperative Chemotherapy	SNB after Preoperative Chemotherapy
Advantages	• Provides information on the status of axillary nodes without the confounding effects of preoperative chemotherapy • Helps with the selection of optimal candidates of preoperative chemotherapy and the use of appropriate preoperative chemotherapy regimens • Helps with decisions regarding further local-regional management with surgery and radiation therapy	• Takes advantage of the down-staging effects of preoperative chemotherapy (with modern active chemotherapy regimens, up to 40% of node-positive patients are converted to node-negative with preoperative chemotherapy) • Generally requires one surgical procedure for the management of the primary breast tumor and axillary nodes • Provides direct evidence of chemosensitivity if the axillary nodes were cytologically positive before preoperative chemotherapy and the SNB is negative afterward
Limitations	• Does not take advantage of the down-staging effect of preoperative chemotherapy and generally commits patients with positive SN to axillary dissection or axillary radiation • Requires two surgical procedures for patient management whether the SN is positive or negative • The prognostic significance of negative axillary nodes after preoperative chemotherapy and prior SNB is uncertain • Knowledge of SN status before preoperative chemotherapy has generally minimal impact in selecting appropriate candidates for preoperative chemotherapy and in deciding which preoperative and adjuvant chemotherapy regimens to use	• There is considerably less information regarding the performance characteristics of SNB after preoperative chemotherapy compared to the up-front setting • SN identification rates are lower after preoperative chemotherapy when compared to the up-front setting • No information on axillary recurrence rates with SNB alone after preoperative chemotherapy • Complicates the decision on whether to use adjuvant radiation if the SN is negative, particularly if the axillary nodes were clinically or cytologically positive before preoperative chemotherapy

SNB, sentinel node biopsy; SN, sentinel node.

preoperative chemotherapy. Thus, some surgeons may want to wait for more data before implementing SNB alone after preoperative chemotherapy. Others, however, may feel comfortable with this approach based on the existing data. After all, up-front SNB alone was widely adopted before data on axillary recurrence were available and, to this date, data from large randomized trials on axillary recurrence, disease-free and overall survival between SNB alone and SNB followed by axillary dissection are still not available.

LOCAL-REGIONAL RADIATION THERAPY ISSUES IN PATIENTS TREATED WITH PREOPERATIVE CHEMOTHERAPY

Although the use of breast radiation after breast-conserving surgery in patients who receive preoperative chemotherapy is well established, there is still considerable debate on the use of postmastectomy chest wall RT and the use of regional nodal RT in patients treated with preoperative systemic therapy. The optimal use of RT following initial surgery has been fairly well defined. In the postmastectomy setting, large randomized trials have shown a benefit to postmastectomy RT in both premenopausal (126,127) and postmenopausal (126) women with node-positive breast cancer. Not only did RT decrease the risk of LRR, but the improvement in local control also translated into an improvement in overall survival (126–129). The magnitude of the survival benefit is directly correlated with the absolute reduction in LRR, with the greatest benefit observed in patients with the highest rate of LRR. Large retrospective series of the risk of LRR stratified by clinical and pathologic risk factors in patients treated with adjuvant chemotherapy and mastectomy serve as a guide for recommendations for adjuvant RT (130–133). In these studies, LRR is substantial when four or more nodes are involved, and postmastectomy radiation is routinely indicated in these patients. Controversy still remains in the subset of women with one to three involved lymph nodes, particularly those treated with full axillary dissection

and anthracycline-based chemotherapy. (See Chapter 47 on Postmastectomy Radiation Therapy.)

Following preoperative chemotherapy, the risk of LRR and therefore the optimal use of local-regional RT have not been fully elucidated. It remains to be determined how the initial clinical stage and the final pathologic stage combine to determine the risk of LRR. Buchholz et al. (134) retrospectively reviewed the outcome of 150 patients who had been treated on five prospective preoperative chemotherapy protocols at the M.D. Anderson Cancer Center. Clinical stage at diagnosis was I in 1%, II in 43%, IIIA in 23%, IIIB in 25%, and IV in 7%. No patient had inflammatory breast cancer. All patients received either a doxorubicin-containing regimen (n = 121) or single-agent paclitaxel (n = 29) followed by mastectomy without adjuvant RT. Patients receiving preoperative chemotherapy were compared to a group of 1,031 patients treated with mastectomy and adjuvant chemotherapy. The preoperative group had a more advanced clinical stage, but a lower pathologic stage, and a higher rate of LRR (27% vs. 15% actuarial LRR at 5 years). When grouping patients by pathologic tumor size and number of involved lymph nodes, again the preoperative group had consistently higher rates of LRR (Table 60.5), indicating that both the initial clinical stage as well as the final pathologic stage contribute to the risk of LRR. Buchholz et al. also compared rates of LRR in patients matched by clinical stage at diagnosis (Table 60.5). There was no statistical difference among the matched subgroups in 5-year LRR for any pathologic tumor size or nodal status comparison, although among patients with four or more nodes, the risk of LRR was 31% in the preoperative group compared with 21% in the adjuvant group. Despite pathologic down-staging, the risk of LRR was not lower among patients with similar clinical stage who received preoperative therapy, and this was especially true for those with more advanced disease.

Other efforts from M.D. Anderson Cancer Center have attempted to identify subsets of patients at low risk for LRR without RT. In a retrospective review of 132 patients with clinical stage I or II disease treated with a preoperative doxorubicin-based regimen or paclitaxel, mastectomy, but without RT, the 5-year LRR rate was 10% (median follow-up,

| Table 60.5 | FIVE-YEAR LOCAL-REGIONAL RECURRENCE AS A FUNCTION OF PRIMARY TUMOR PATHOLOGIC SIZE AND NUMBER OF INVOLVED LYMPH NODES FOR PATIENTS RECEIVING ADJUVANT VERSUS PREOPERATIVE CHEMOTHERAPY, OVERALL AND MATCHED BY INITIAL CLINICAL STAGE |

	Overall Group		Subgroup Matched by Clinical Stage	
	Adjuvant (%)	Preoperative (%)	Adjuvant (%)	Preoperative (%)
Pathologic tumor size (cm)				
0–2.0	9	12[a]	7	8
2.1–5.0	15	36[a]	12	17
>5.0	28	46[a]		
Number of involved axillary nodes				
0	7	12	0	5
1–3	10	18	12	14
≥4	23	53[a]	21	31

[a]$p < .05$ comparing the preoperative versus adjuvant groups.
From Buchholz TA, Katz A, Strom EA, et al. Pathologic tumor size and lymph node status predict for different rates of locoregional recurrence after mastectomy for breast cancer patients treated with neoadjuvant versus adjuvant chemotherapy. *Int J Radiat Oncol Biol Phys* 2002;53:880–888, with permission.

46 months) (135). Multiple clinical and pathologic factors were found to predict 5-year LRR, including: clinical stage T3N0 (LRR 29% compared with 2% for T1-2N0; $p = .0057$), four or more positive lymph nodes (LRR 67%; $p < .0001$ for comparison with node negative and one to three positive node groups), age less than or equal to 40 years (LRR 31% compared with 4% for older patients; $p = .0001$), and no use of tamoxifen (LRR 2% for ER-positive patients receiving tamoxifen, 9% for patients with ER-negative disease who did not receive tamoxifen, and 27% for those with ER-positive disease who did not receive tamoxifen; $p = .0067$). Among 42 patients with clinical T1 to T2 disease and one to three pathologically positive nodes, the risk of LRR was only 5% (135). However, these very small numbers, particularly in the subset analysis, limits the generalizability of these findings. In addition, M.D. Anderson Cancer Center utilizes careful ultrasound evaluation of the axilla with FNA of clinically suspicious axillary nodes at presentation (41), which is not widely used elsewhere. Prior identification of clinically occult axillary disease by ultrasound and FNA favorably biases the remaining node-negative patients who may not be comparable to clinically node-negative patients at other institutions.

The NSABP preoperative trials in patients with operable breast cancer (B-18 and B-27) provide an important data set to address some of the above raised questions. In both trials, regional nodal RT after lumpectomy or chest wall and regional nodal RT after mastectomy were not allowed per protocol guidelines, avoiding the confounding effects of selective use of

RT in patients with positive nodes or other high-risk features. A combined preliminary analysis of LRR rates from NSABP B-18 and B-27 included 2,192 patients with 229 events. In multivariate analysis, predictors of LRR included clinical tumor size and nodal status (before preoperative chemotherapy) and pathologic breast or nodal tumor response (after preoperative chemotherapy). By using these independent predictors, rates of LRR in different patient subsets can be defined without the knowledge of pathologic axillary nodal status before preoperative chemotherapy. Similar to the M.D. Anderson Cancer Center data, patients with node-negative disease after preoperative chemotherapy had a less than 10% rate of LRR at 8 years. However, among 447 patients with positive nodes after preoperative chemotherapy, the 8-year risk of LRR was 15%. Tables 60.6 and 60.7 include data from patients treated with either breast-conserving therapy (including breast RT) or mastectomy, stratified by pathologic response in the breast and pathologic status of axillary lymph nodes. Whether a subset of patients with a small number of positive nodes or a combination of other pathologic or clinical factors could be identified with a lower risk of LRR remains to be determined. Of note, patients in the NSABP as well as the M.D. Anderson Cancer Center series all underwent axillary dissection following chemotherapy. Whether these results can be generalized to patients who have negative SNB after preoperative chemotherapy remains to be determined.

In contrast to patients with operable breast cancer, such as those included in the NSABP trials, patients with locally

| Table 60.6 | EIGHT-YEAR CUMULATIVE INCIDENCE RATES OF LOCAL-REGIONAL RECURRENCE AFTER PREOPERATIVE CHEMOTHERAPY AND LUMPECTOMY PLUS BREAST RADIATION IN THE NSABP B-18/B-27 TRIALS ACCORDING TO PATHOLOGIC RESPONSE IN THE BREAST AND PATHOLOGIC AXILLARY NODAL STATUS AT SURGERY |

	Pathologic Breast Response/Pathologic Nodal Status					
Type of Surgery/Radiation	Node-Negative/pCR (n = 245)		Node-Negative/No pCR (n = 644)		Node-Positive (n = 518)	
	8-Year Cumulative Incidence of Recurrence (%)					
Breast-conserving surgery/breast radiation	In-Breast	Regional	In-Breast	Regional	In-Breast	Regional
	5.6	1.2	5.9	1.1	6.4	3.4

NSABP, National Surgical Adjuvant Breast and Bowel Project; pCR, pathologic complete response.
From Mamounas E, et al. State of the Science Conference on Preoperative Chemotherapy. Bethesda, MD. 2007.

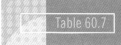

| Table 60.7 | EIGHT-YEAR CUMULATIVE INCIDENCE RATES OF LOCAL-REGIONAL RECURRENCE AFTER PREOPERATIVE CHEMOTHERAPY AND MASTECTOMY IN THE NSABP B-18/B-27 TRIALS ACCORDING TO PATHOLOGIC RESPONSE IN THE BREAST AND PATHOLOGIC AXILLARY NODAL STATUS AT SURGERY | | | | | |

	Pathologic Breast Response/Pathologic Nodal Status					
Type of Surgery/Radiation	Node-Negative/pCR (n = 68)		Node-Negative/No pCR (n = 270)		Node-Positive (n = 447)	
	8-Year Cumulative Incidence of Recurrence (%)					
Mastectomy/no radiation[a]	Chest Wall	Regional	Chest Wall	Regional	Chest Wall	Regional
	1.5	4.4	5.0	3.0	11.2	3.7

NSABP, National Surgical Adjuvant Breast and Bowel Project; pCR, pathologic complete response.
[a]No chest wall or regional nodal radiation was allowed per protocol.
From Mamounas E, et al. State of the Science Conference on Preoperative Chemotherapy. Bethesda, MD. 2007.

advanced disease have a high rate of LRR in the absence of RT, independent of their response to preoperative chemotherapy. McGuire et al. (136), also from M.D. Anderson Cancer Center, reported on 106 patients who achieved a pathologic complete response to preoperative chemotherapy (92% anthracycline based). Median follow-up was 62 months among surviving patients. Among 32 patients with clinical stage I and II disease, no patients experienced an LRR (including those who did and did not receive RT). Among 74 patients with clinical stage III disease (2003 American Joint Committee on Cancer criteria), however, the LRR rate was 7.3% with RT compared to 33.3% without RT ($p = .040$), despite having achieved a pathologic complete response. Disease-free and overall survival rates were also improved with the addition of RT for clinical stage III patients. Although these results are limited by their retrospective nature, they support the hypothesis that patients with locally advanced breast cancer require RT independent of their response to preoperative chemotherapy.

At the present time, there are no data from randomized trials examining the benefit of postmastectomy RT in patients receiving preoperative chemotherapy, and, therefore, the potential benefit at this time must be based on the retrospective studies and extrapolated from the adjuvant chemotherapy setting. It seems reasonable to offer postmastectomy RT to all patients with stage III disease, independent of their response to chemotherapy. In patients with clinical stage II disease and positive axillary nodes following preoperative chemotherapy, postmastectomy RT should also be considered. In patients with clinical stage II disease with no axillary involvement after preoperative chemotherapy, it seems reasonable to not recommend RT. As discussed previously, in some institutions, a SNB is performed at diagnosis, so that postmastectomy RT can be omitted in women with node-negative disease. However, this approach has the disadvantage that it generally commits women with a positive sentinel node to undergo a completion dissection.

CURRENT AND FUTURE DIRECTIONS IN LOCAL-REGIONAL MANAGEMENT AFTER PREOPERATIVE CHEMOTHERAPY

Relative to the effects of preoperative chemotherapy on the primary breast tumor, a remaining important question is whether the use of more effective preoperative chemotherapy regimens (with or without incorporation of biologics) will lead to further increases in the rates of breast-conserving surgery. Although in the NSABP B-27 trial the addition of preoperative docetaxel to preoperative doxorubicin and cyclophosphamide

did not significantly improve the rate of breast-conserving surgery (despite doubling the rate of pathologic complete response from 14% to 26%) (4), it is hoped that more effective regimens and more appropriate selection of subgroups of patients (leading to pathologic complete response rates of 45% to 65%) (137,138) will still result in further reduction in mastectomy rates. With more active chemotherapy regimens, future studies should attempt to further tailor the extent of, or even the need for, surgical resection in the breast following complete clinical and radiologic response to preoperative chemotherapy. Although previous studies of preoperative chemotherapy followed by breast irradiation and then surgical resection have shown high rates of pathologic complete response (over 40%) (139,140), similar studies in which breast irradiation was not followed by surgical resection have shown high rates of local recurrence (51,141,142). If in future studies elimination of surgical resection is to be evaluated (either before or after breast RT), one needs to at least attempt to demonstrate an absence of residual tumor either by sensitive imaging studies or by percutaneous biopsy of the tumor bed area. Newer percutaneous tumor ablation techniques (such as radiofrequency ablation or cryoablation) (143) may become a substitute for surgical excision (either before or after breast irradiation) in selected patients with complete clinical and radiologic response. However, before widespread adoption, the safety and efficacy of these newer techniques need to be documented in large clinical trials. Finally, genomic technology is starting to be utilized for identification of molecular signatures predictive of high likelihood of pathologic complete response in the breast (144). This new technology could have a tremendous impact on the selection of appropriate candidates for exploring some of the above questions.

Similar strategies need to be explored relative to the surgical management of the axilla. It is likely that the results of large randomized trials comparing SNB alone with SNB followed by axillary dissection will confirm those from an already reported smaller randomized trial (48) and demonstrate equivalence in local-regional failure, disease-free survival, and overall survival between the two procedures. Similar trials are not available for patients who have received SNB following preoperative chemotherapy. Thus, unless a randomized trial comparing SNB alone with SNB followed by axillary dissection demonstrates equivalence between the two approaches, the future adoption of SNB after preoperative chemotherapy will depend on the continuous demonstration of the feasibility and accuracy of this procedure in retrospective reviews of single-institution and multicenter experiences in which SNB is followed by completion axillary dissection, such as the ones reviewed in this chapter. In addition, further validation for this approach will have to be provided by future reports demonstrating low rates of axillary recurrence in patients who receive preoperative chemotherapy and undergo SNB alone without completion axillary dissection or axillary radiotherapy. At this time, such reports are lacking.

With the development of more active chemotherapy regimens and the increasing utilization of genomic profiling as a tool for predicting pathologic complete response in the breast and axillary nodes, future studies should attempt to further individualize the extent of, or even the need for, axillary surgery after preoperative chemotherapy. By identifying patients at high likelihood of having negative axillary nodes (based on molecular or genomic markers and the achievement of pathologic complete response in the breast), axillary surgery (including SNB) may be avoided altogether. By identifying patients at high likelihood of having positive sentinel nodes but negative nonsentinel nodes, completion axillary dissection can be avoided in an additional subset of sentinel node–positive patients. For those sentinel node–positive patients at high likelihood of having residual positive nonsentinel nodes, the most appropriate therapeutic strategy (completion axillary dissection vs. axillary radiotherapy) will have to be determined, and this question is currently being addressed in randomized clinical trials (145) and other clinical studies (146).

 ## CONCLUSION

Preoperative chemotherapy represents a valid approach by which local-regional therapy can be tailored based on clinical and pathologic response of the primary breast tumor and axillary lymph nodes. Although several areas of controversy still exist regarding the optimal local-regional management of patients treated with preoperative chemotherapy, this approach holds great promise for the future. As more active preoperative chemotherapy regimens (with or without the addition of biologics) are being developed and as novel molecular and imaging techniques allow better identification of pathologic complete responders, further individualization of local-regional management is expected to occur, resulting in increased efficacy while minimizing morbidity.

 ## MANAGEMENT SUMMARY

- Preoperative systemic therapy has been shown to increase the use of breast-conserving therapy and has the potential to decrease the use of axillary dissection. In the United States, preoperative chemotherapy is typically used.
- The use of preoperative systemic therapy in patients with operable breast cancer has created new challenges for breast surgeons and radiation oncologists.
- Clinical and radiological assessment of the extent of primary cancer before and after preoperative chemotherapy is important. Physical examination, mammography, and ultrasonography are the standard methods of assessment, but their performance characteristics in predicting a pathologic complete response are not optimal.
- MRI can demonstrate the pattern of cancer growth in the breast, which may be prognostic of response to preoperative chemotherapy. In addition, MRI may provide a better means to assess response. Studies are under way to tests these hypotheses. Other newer imaging methods are being tested as well.
- It is critical that a core needle biopsy be performed on all suspicious abnormalities found in the ipsilateral and contralateral breasts before chemotherapy. Radiopaque clips should be placed within all malignant tumors to provide localization for subsequent surgical removal.

- Surgical resection of the tumor bed to confirm the clinical or radiographic impression of complete response is an essential part of management.
- SNB can be performed either before or after preoperative chemotherapy. There are potential advantages and limitations with each approach. Studies are under way to confirm the preliminary data that a negative SNB after preoperative chemotherapy can obviate the need for axillary dissection.
- In patients treated with breast-conserving surgery, clearly negative margins of resection should be obtained. Even in patients with a pathological complete response in the breast, breast RT should be used.
- For patients treated with mastectomy, chest wall and regional nodal RT should be considered for patients who present with clinical stage III disease or have histologically positive axillary nodes after preoperative chemotherapy. Additional prospective studies are needed to determine the need for RT in patients with clinical stage I or II disease at presentation who are node negative after preoperative chemotherapy.

References

1. Wolmark N, Wang J, Mamounas E, et al. Preoperative chemotherapy in patients with operable breast cancer: nine-year results from National Surgical Adjuvant Breast and Bowel Project B-18. *J Natl Cancer Inst Monogr* 2001;30:96–102.
2. van der Hage JA, van de Velde CJ, Julien JP, et al. Preoperative chemotherapy in primary operable breast cancer: results from the European Organization for Research and Treatment of Cancer trial 10902. *J Clin Oncol* 2001;19: 4224–4237.
3. Gianni L, Baselga J, Eirmann W, et al. European Cooperative Trial in Operable Breast Cancer (ECTO): improved freedom from progression (FFP) from adding paclitaxel (T) to doxorubicin (A) followed by cyclophosphamide methotrexate and fluorouracil (CMF). *J Clin Oncol* 2005;23:7S(abst 513).
4. Bear HD, Anderson S, Brown A, et al. The effect on tumor response of adding sequential preoperative docetaxel to preoperative doxorubicin and cyclophosphamide: preliminary results from National Surgical Adjuvant Breast and Bowel Project Protocol B-27. *J Clin Oncol* 2003;21:4165–4174.
5. Gianni L, Baselga J, Eiermann W, et al. First report of the European Cooperative Trial in operable breast cancer (ECTO): effect of primary systemic therapy. *Proc Am Soc Clin Oncol* 2002;21:34A(abst 132).
6. Chaiwun B, Settakorn J, Ya-In C, et al. Effectiveness of fine-needle aspiration cytology of breast: analysis of 2,375 cases from northern Thailand. *Diagn Cytopathol* 2002;26:201–205.
7. El-Tamer M, Axiotis C, Kim E, et al. Accurate prediction of the amount of *in situ* tumor in palpable breast cancers by core needle biopsy: implications for neoadjuvant therapy. *Ann Surg Oncol* 1999;6:461–466.
8. Kaneko S, Gerasimova T, Butler WM, et al. The use of FISH on breast core needle samples for the presurgical assessment of HER-2 oncogene status. *Exp Mol Pathol* 2002;73:61–66.
9. Taucher S, Rudas M, Gnant M, et al. Sequential steroid hormone receptor measurements in primary breast cancer with and without intervening primary chemotherapy. *Endocr Relat Cancer* 2003;10:91–98.
10. Ellis M, Davis N, Coop A, et al. Development and validation of a method for using breast core needle biopsies for gene expression microarray analyses. *Clin Cancer Res* 2002;8:1155–1166.
11. Symmans WF, Ayers M, Clark EA, et al. Total RNA yield and microarray gene expression profiles from fine-needle aspiration biopsy and core-needle biopsy samples of breast carcinoma. *Cancer* 2003;97:2960–2971.
12. Sotiriou C, Powles TJ, Dowsett M, et al. Gene expression profiles derived from fine needle aspiration correlate with response to systemic chemotherapy in breast cancer. *Breast Cancer Res* 2002;4:R3.
13. Nizzoli R, Bozzetti C, Naldi N, et al. Comparison of the results of immunocytochemical assays for biologic variables on preoperative fine-needle aspirates and on surgical specimens of primary breast carcinomas. *Cancer* 2000;90:61–66.
14. Marrazzo A, Taormina P, Leonardi P, et al. Immunocytochemical determination of estrogen and progesterone receptors on 219 fine-needle aspirates of breast cancer. A prospective study. *Anticancer Res* 1995;15:521–526.
15. Herrada J, Iyer RB, Atkinson EN, et al. Relative value of physical examination, mammography, and breast sonography in evaluating the size of the primary tumor and regional lymph node metastases in women receiving neoadjuvant chemotherapy for locally advanced breast carcinoma. *Clin Cancer Res* 1997;3: 1565–1569.
16. Kuerer HM, Singletary SE, Buzdar AU, et al. Surgical conservation planning after neoadjuvant chemotherapy for stage II and operable stage III breast carcinoma. *Am J Surg* 2001;182:601–608.
17. Vinnicombe SJ, MacVicar AD, Guy RL, et al. Primary breast cancer: mammographic changes after neoadjuvant chemotherapy, with pathologic correlation. *Radiology* 1996;198:333–340.
18. Esserman L, Hylton N, Yassa L, et al. Utility of magnetic resonance imaging in the management of breast cancer: evidence for improved preoperative staging. *J Clin Oncol* 1999;17:110–119.
19. Stoutjesdijk MJ, Boetes C, Jager GJ, et al. Magnetic resonance imaging and mammography in women with a hereditary risk of breast cancer. *J Natl Cancer Inst* 2001;93:1095–1102.

20. Kriege M, Brekelmans CT, Boetes C, et al. Efficacy of MRI and mammography for breast-cancer screening in women with a familial or genetic predisposition. *N Engl J Med* 2004;351:427–437.
21. Esserman L, Kaplan E, Partridge S, et al. MRI phenotype is associated with response to doxorubicin and cyclophosphamide neoadjuvant chemotherapy in stage III breast cancer. *Ann Surg Oncol* 2001;8:549–559.
22. Drew PJ, Kerin MJ, Mahapatra T, et al. Evaluation of response to neoadjuvant chemoradiotherapy for locally advanced breast cancer with dynamic contrast-enhanced MRI of the breast. *Eur J Surg Oncol* 2001;27:617–620.
23. Balu-Maestro C, Chapellier C, Bleuse A, et al. Imaging in evaluation of response to neoadjuvant breast cancer treatment benefits of MRI. *Breast Cancer Res Treat* 2002;72:145–152.
24. Cheung YC, Chen SC, Su MY, et al. Monitoring the size and response of locally advanced breast cancers to neoadjuvant chemotherapy (weekly paclitaxel and epirubicin) with serial enhanced MRI. *Breast Cancer Res Treat* 2003;78: 51–58.
25. Partridge SC, Gibbs JE, Lu Y, et al. Accuracy of MR imaging for revealing residual breast cancer in patients who have undergone neoadjuvant chemotherapy. *AJR Am J Roentgenol* 2002;179:1193–1199.
26. Wasser K, Sinn HP, Fink C, et al. Accuracy of tumor size measurement in breast cancer using MRI is influenced by histological regression induced by neoadjuvant chemotherapy. *Eur Radiol* 2003;13:1213–1223.
27. Rosen EL, Blackwell KL, Baker JA, et al. Accuracy of MRI in the detection of residual breast cancer after neoadjuvant chemotherapy. *AJR Am J Roentgenol* 2003;181:1275–1282.
28. Morris EA. Review of breast MRI: indications and limitations. *Semin Roentgenol* 2001;36:226–237.
29. Nakamura S, Kenjo H, Nishio T, et al. Efficacy of 3D-MR mammography for breast conserving surgery after neoadjuvant chemotherapy. *Breast Cancer* 2002;9:15–19.
30. Nakamura S, Kenjo H, Nishio T, et al. 3D-MR mammography-guided breast conserving surgery after neoadjuvant chemotherapy: clinical results and future perspectives with reference to FDG-PET. *Breast Cancer* 2001;8:351–354.
31. Kaplan E, Yu E, Tripathy D, et al. MRI patterns predict the ability to perform breast conservation following neoadjuvant chemotherapy for locally advanced breast cancer. *Br Cancer Res Treat* 2003;82:S19(abst 101).
32. Akashi-Tanaka S, Fukutomi T, Sato N, et al. The role of computed tomography in the selection of breast cancer treatment. *Breast Cancer* 2003;10:198–203.
33. Akashi-Tanaka S, Fukutomi T, Sato N, et al. The use of contrast-enhanced computed tomography before neoadjuvant chemotherapy to identify patients likely to be treated safely with breast-conserving surgery. *Ann Surg* 2004;239:238–243.
34. Danforth DN Jr, Aloj L, Carrasquillo JA, et al. The role of 18F-FDG-PET in the local/regional evaluation of women with breast cancer. *Breast Cancer Res Treat* 2002;75:135–146.
35. Burcombe RJ, Makris A, Pittam M, et al. Evaluation of good clinical response to neoadjuvant chemotherapy in primary breast cancer using [18F]-fluorodeoxyglucose positron emission tomography. *Eur J Cancer* 2002;38:375–379.
36. Mankoff DA, Dunnwald LK, Gralow JR, et al. Changes in blood flow and metabolism in locally advanced breast cancer treated with neoadjuvant chemotherapy. *J Nucl Med* 2003;44:1806–1814.
37. Baron LF, Baron PL, Ackerman SJ, et al. Sonographically guided clip placement facilitates localization of breast cancer after neoadjuvant chemotherapy. *AJR Am J Roentgenol* 2000;174:539–540.
38. Alonso-Bartolome P, Ortega Garcia E, Garijo Ayensa F, et al. Utility of the tumor bed marker in patients with breast cancer receiving induction chemotherapy. *Acta Radiol* 2002;43:29–33.
39. Mankoff DA, Dunnwald LK, Gralow JR, et al. Monitoring the response of patients with locally advanced breast carcinoma to neoadjuvant chemotherapy using [technetium 99m]-sestamibi scintimammography. *Cancer* 1999;85:2410–2423.
40. Oruwari JU, Chung MA, Koelliker S, et al. Axillary staging using ultrasound-guided fine needle aspiration biopsy in locally advanced breast cancer. *Am J Surg* 2002;184:307–309.
41. Krishnamurthy S, Sneige N, Bedi DG, et al. Role of ultrasound-guided fine-needle aspiration of indeterminate and suspicious axillary lymph nodes in the initial staging of breast carcinoma. *Cancer* 2002;95:982–988.
42. Bedrosian I, Reynolds C, Mick R, et al. Accuracy of sentinel lymph node biopsy in patients with large primary breast tumors. *Cancer* 2000;88:2540–2545.
43. Schrenk P, Hochreiner G, Fridrik M, et al. Sentinel node biopsy performed before preoperative chemotherapy for axillary lymph node staging in breast cancer. *Breast J* 2003;9:282–287.
44. Sabel MS, Schott AF, Kleer CG, et al. Sentinel node biopsy prior to neoadjuvant chemotherapy. *Am J Surg* 2003;186:102–105.
45. Ollila DW, Neuman HB, Sartor C, et al. Lymphatic mapping and sentinel lymphadenectomy prior to neoadjuvant chemotherapy in patients with large breast cancers. *Am J Surg* 2005;190:371–375.
46. Chung MH, Ye W, Giuliano AE. Role for sentinel lymph node dissection in the management of large (> or = 5 cm) invasive breast cancer. *Ann Surg Oncol* 2001;8:688–692.
47. Krag DN, Anderson SJ, Julian TB, et al. Technical outcomes of sentinel-lymph-node resection and conventional axillary-lymph-node dissection in patients with clinically node-negative breast cancer: results from the NSABP B-32 randomised phase III trial. *Lancet Oncol* 2007;8:881–888.
48. Veronesi U, Paganelli G, Viale G, et al. A randomized comparison of sentinel-node biopsy with routine axillary dissection in breast cancer. *N Engl J Med* 2003;349: 546–553.
49. Tafra L, Lannin DR, Swanson MS, et al. Multicenter trial of sentinel node biopsy for breast cancer using both technetium sulfur colloid and isosulfan blue dye. *Ann Surg* 2001;233:51–59.
50. McMasters KM, Tuttle TM, Carlson DJ, et al. Sentinel lymph node biopsy for breast cancer: a suitable alternative to routine axillary dissection in multi-institutional practice when optimal technique is used. *J Clin Oncol* 2000;18:2560–2566.
51. Mauriac L, MacGrogan G, Avril A, et al. Neoadjuvant chemotherapy for operable breast carcinoma larger than 3 cm: a unicentre randomized trial with a 124-month median follow-up. Institut Bergonie Bordeaux Groupe Sein (IBBGS). *Ann Oncol* 1999;10:47–52.
52. Bonadonna G, Valagussa P, Brambilla C, et al. Primary chemotherapy in operable breast cancer: eight-year experience at the Milan Cancer Institute. *J Clin Oncol* 1998;16:93–100.
53. Vlastos G, Mirza NQ, Lenert JT, et al. The feasibility of minimally invasive surgery for stage IIA, IIB, and IIIA breast carcinoma patients after tumor downstaging with induction chemotherapy. *Cancer* 2000;88:1417–1424.
54. Fisher B, Brown A, Mamounas E, et al. Effect of preoperative chemotherapy on local-regional disease in women with operable breast cancer: findings from National Surgical Adjuvant Breast and Bowel Project B-18. *J Clin Oncol* 1997;15: 2483–2493.
55. Powles TJ, Hickish TF, Makris A, et al. Randomized trial of chemoendocrine therapy started before or after surgery for treatment of primary breast cancer. *J Clin Oncol* 1995;13:547–552.
56. Bazzocchi M, Facecchia I, Zuiani C, et al. [Diagnostic imaging of lobular carcinoma of the breast: mammographic, ultrasonographic and MR findings]. *Radiol Med (Torino)* 2000;100:436–443.
57. Lesser ML, Rosen PP, Kinne DW. Multicentricity and bilaterality in invasive breast carcinoma. *Surgery* 1982;91:234–240.
58. Sinn HP, Schmid H, Junkermann H, et al. [Histologic regression of breast cancer after primary (neoadjuvant) chemotherapy]. *Geburtshilfe Frauenheilkd* 1994;54: 552–558.
59. Cocquyt VF, Blondeel PN, Depypere HT, et al. Different responses to preoperative chemotherapy for invasive lobular and invasive ductal breast carcinoma. *Eur J Surg Oncol* 2003;29:361–367.
60. Cristofanilli M, Gonzalez-Angulo A, Sneige N, et al. Invasive lobular carcinoma classic type: response to primary chemotherapy and survival outcomes. *J Clin Oncol* 2005;23:41–48.
61. Julian TB, Anderson S, Fourchotte V, et al. Is invasive lobular breast cancer a prognostic factor for neoadjuvant chemotherapy response and long term outcomes? *Br Cancer Res Treat* 2006;100:S146(abst 3065).
62. Newman LA, Buzdar AU, Singletary SE, et al. A prospective trial of preoperative chemotherapy in resectable breast cancer: predictors of breast-conservation therapy feasibility. *Ann Surg Oncol* 2002;9:228–234.
63. Kuerer HM, Hunt KK, Newman LA, et al. Neoadjuvant chemotherapy in women with invasive breast carcinoma: conceptual basis and fundamental surgical issues. *J Am Coll Surg* 2002;190:350–363.
64. Mauri D, Pavlidis N, Ioannidis JP. Neoadjuvant versus adjuvant systemic treatment in breast cancer: a meta-analysis. *J Natl Cancer Inst* 2005;97:188–194.
65. Mieog JS, van der Hage JA, van de Velde CJ. Preoperative chemotherapy for women with operable breast cancer. *Cochrane Database Syst Rev* 2007; CD005002.
66. Rouzier R, Mathieu MC, Sideris L, et al. Breast-conserving surgery after neoadjuvant anthracycline-based chemotherapy for large breast tumors. *Cancer* 2004; 101:918–925.
67. Rouzier R, Extra JM, Carton M, et al. Primary chemotherapy for operable breast cancer: incidence and prognostic significance of ipsilateral breast tumor recurrence after breast-conserving surgery. *J Clin Oncol* 2001;19:3828–3835.
68. Solin LJ, Fowble BL, Schultz DJ, et al. The significance of the pathology margins of the tumor excision on the outcome of patients treated with definitive irradiation for early stage breast cancer. *Int J Radiat Oncol Biol Phys* 1991;21: 279–287.
69. Park CC, Mitsumori M, Nixon A, et al. Outcome at 8 years after breast-conserving surgery and radiation therapy for invasive breast cancer: influence of margin status and systemic therapy on local recurrence. *J Clin Oncol* 2000;18:1668–1675.
70. Chen AM, Meric-Bernstam F, Hunt KK, et al. Breast conservation after neoadjuvant chemotherapy: the M.D. Anderson Cancer Center experience. *J Clin Oncol* 2004;22:2303–2312.
71. Shen J, Valero V, Buchholz TA, et al. Effective local control and long-term survival in patients with T4 locally advanced breast cancer treated with breast conservation therapy. *Ann Surg Oncol* 2004;11:854–860.
72. McMasters KM, Hunt KK. Neoadjuvant chemotherapy, locally advanced breast cancer, and quality of life. *J Clin Oncol* 1999;17:441–444.
73. Styblo TM, Lewis MM, Carlson GW, et al. Immediate breast reconstruction for stage III breast cancer using transverse rectus abdominis musculocutaneous (TRAM) flap. *Ann Surg Oncol* 1996;3:375–380.
74. Deutsch MF, Smith M, Wang B, et al. Immediate breast reconstruction with the TRAM flap after neoadjuvant therapy. *Ann Plast Surg* 1999;42:240–244.
75. Newman LA, Kuerer HM, Hunt KK, et al. Feasibility of immediate breast reconstruction for locally advanced breast cancer. *Ann Surg Oncol* 1999;6:671–675.
76. Sultan MR, Smith ML, Estabrook A, et al. Immediate breast reconstruction in patients with locally advanced disease. *Ann Plast Surg* 1997;38:345–351.
77. Hunt KK, Baldwin BJ, Strom EA, et al. Feasibility of postmastectomy radiation therapy after TRAM flap breast reconstruction. *Ann Surg Oncol* 1997;4:377–384.
78. Slavin SA, Love SM, Goldwyn RM. Recurrent breast cancer following immediate reconstruction with myocutaneous flaps. *Plast Reconstr Surg* 1994;93:1191–1207.
79. Motwani SB, Strom EA, Schechter NR, et al. The impact of immediate breast reconstruction on the technical delivery of postmastectomy radiotherapy. *Int J Radiat Oncol Biol Phys* 2006;66:76–82.
80. McKeown DJ, Hogg FJ, Brown IM, et al. The timing of autologous latissimus dorsi breast reconstruction and effect of radiotherapy on outcome. *J Plast Reconstr Aesthet Surg* 2008. In press.
81. Kronowitz SJ. Immediate versus delayed reconstruction. *Clin Plast Surg* 2007; 34:39–50(abst 6).
82. Breslin TM, Cohen L, Sahin A, et al. Sentinel lymph node biopsy is accurate after neoadjuvant chemotherapy for breast cancer. *J Clin Oncol* 2000;18:3480–3486.
83. Nason KS, Anderson BO, Byrd DR, et al. Increased false negative sentinel node biopsy rates after preoperative chemotherapy for invasive breast carcinoma. *Cancer* 2000;89:2187–2194.
84. Fernandez A, Cortes M, Benito E, et al. Gamma probe sentinel node localization and biopsy in breast cancer patients treated with a neoadjuvant chemotherapy scheme. *Nucl Med Commun* 2001;22:361–366.
85. Haid A, Tausch C, Lang A, et al. Is sentinel lymph node biopsy reliable and indicated after preoperative chemotherapy in patients with breast carcinoma? *Cancer* 2001;92:1080–1084.
86. Stearns V, Ewing CA, Slack R, et al. Sentinel lymphadenectomy after neoadjuvant chemotherapy for breast cancer may reliably represent the axilla except for inflammatory breast cancer. *Ann Surg Oncol* 2002;9:235–242.
87. Miller AR, Thomason VE, Yeh IT, et al. Analysis of sentinel lymph node mapping with immediate pathologic review in patients receiving preoperative chemotherapy for breast carcinoma. *Ann Surg Oncol* 2002;9:243–247.

88. Brady EW. Sentinel lymph node mapping following neoadjuvant chemotherapy for breast cancer. *Breast J* 2002;8:97–100.

89. Reitsamer R, Peintinger F, Rettenbacher L, et al. Sentinel lymph node biopsy in breast cancer patients after neoadjuvant chemotherapy. *J Surg Oncol* 2003;84: 63–67.

90. Schwartz GF, Meltzer AJ. Accuracy of axillary sentinel lymph node biopsy following neoadjuvant (induction) chemotherapy for carcinoma of the breast. *Breast J* 2003;9:374–379.

91. Balch GC, Mithani SK, Richards KR, et al. Lymphatic mapping and sentinel lymphadenectomy after preoperative therapy for stage II and III breast cancer. *Ann Surg Oncol* 2003;10:616–621.

92. Piato JR, Barros AC, Pincerato KM, et al. Sentinel lymph node biopsy in breast cancer after neoadjuvant chemotherapy. A pilot study. *Eur J Surg Oncol* 2003; 29:118–120.

93. Vigario A, Sapienza MT, Sampaio AP, et al. Primary chemotherapy effect in sentinel node detection in breast cancer. *Clin Nucl Med* 2003;28:553–557.

94. Aihara T, Munakata S, Morino H, et al. Feasibility of sentinel node biopsy for breast cancer after neoadjuvant endocrine therapy: a pilot study. *J Surg Oncol* 2004;85:77–81.

95. Kang SH, Kang JH, Choi EA, et al. Sentinel lymph node biopsy after neoadjuvant chemotherapy. *Breast Cancer* 2004;11:233–241.

96. Shimazu K, Tamaki Y, Taguchi T, et al. Sentinel lymph node biopsy using periareolar injection of radiocolloid for patients with neoadjuvant chemotherapy-treated breast carcinoma. *Cancer* 2004;100:2555–2561.

97. Patel NA, Piper G, Patel JA, et al. Accurate axillary nodal staging can be achieved after neoadjuvant therapy for locally advanced breast cancer. *Am Surg* 2004; 70:696–700.

98. Lang JE, Esserman LJ, Ewing CA, et al. Accuracy of selective sentinel lymphadenectomy after neoadjuvant chemotherapy: effect of clinical node status at presentation. *J Am Coll Surg* 2004;199:856–862.

99. Jones JL, Zabicki K, Christian RL, et al. A comparison of sentinel node biopsy before and after neoadjuvant chemotherapy: timing is important. *Am J Surg* 2005;190:517–520.

100. Tanaka Y, Maeda H, Ogawa Y, et al. Sentinel node biopsy in breast cancer patients treated with neoadjuvant chemotherapy. *Oncol Rep* 2006;15:927–931.

101. Yu JC, Hsu GC, Hsieh CB, et al. Role of sentinel lymphadenectomy combined with intraoperative ultrasound in the assessment of locally advanced breast cancer after neoadjuvant chemotherapy. *Ann Surg Oncol* 2007;14:174–180.

102. Kinoshita T. Sentinel lymph node biopsy is feasible for breast cancer patients after neoadjuvant chemotherapy. *Breast Cancer* 2007;14:10–15.

103. Shen J, Gilcrease MZ, Babiera GV, et al. Feasibility and accuracy of sentinel lymph node biopsy after preoperative chemotherapy in breast cancer patients with documented axillary metastases. *Cancer* 2007;109:1255–1263.

104. Newman EA, Sabel MS, Nees AV, et al. Sentinel lymph node biopsy performed after neoadjuvant chemotherapy is accurate in patients with documented node-positive breast cancer at presentation. *Ann Surg Oncol* 2007;14(10):2946– 2952.

105. Lee S, Kim EY, Kang SH, et al. Sentinel node identification rate, but not accuracy, is significantly decreased after pre-operative chemotherapy in axillary node-positive breast cancer patients. *Breast Cancer Res Treat* 2007;102:283–288.

106. Xing Y, Foy M, Cox DD. Meta-analysis of sentinel lymph node biopsy after preoperative chemotherapy in patients with breast cancer. *Br J Surg* 2006;93: 539–546.

107. Mamounas EP. Sentinel lymph node biopsy after neoadjuvant systemic therapy. *Surg Clin North Am* 2003;83:931–942.

108. Mamounas EP, Brown A, Anderson S, et al. Sentinel node biopsy after neoadjuvant chemotherapy in breast cancer: results from National Surgical Adjuvant Breast and Bowel Project Protocol B-27. *J Clin Oncol* 2005;23:2694–2702.

109. Tafra L, Verbanac KM, Lannin DR. Preoperative chemotherapy and sentinel lymphadenectomy for breast cancer. *Am J Surg* 2001;182:312–315.

110. Krag D, Weaver D, Ashikaga T, et al. The sentinel node in breast cancer—a multicenter validation study. *N Engl J Med* 1998;339:941–946.

111. O'Hea BJ, Hill AD, El-Shirbiny AM, et al. Sentinel lymph node biopsy in breast cancer: initial experience at Memorial Sloan-Kettering Cancer Center. *J Am Coll Surg* 1998;186:423–427.

112. Krag DN, Weaver DL, Alex JC, et al. Surgical resection and radiolocalization of the sentinel lymph node in breast cancer using a gamma probe. *Surg Oncol* 1993;2:335–340.

113. Giuliano AE, Kirgan DM, Guenther JM, et al. Lymphatic mapping and sentinel lymphadenectomy for breast cancer. *Ann Surg* 1994;220:391–401.

114. Kuerer HM, Newman LA, Buzdar AU, et al. Pathologic tumor response in the breast following neoadjuvant chemotherapy predicts axillary lymph node status. *Cancer J Sci Am* 1998;4:230–236.

115. Jain P, Kumar R, Anand M, et al. Touch imprint cytology of axillary lymph nodes after neoadjuvant chemotherapy in patients with breast carcinoma. *Cancer* 2003;99:346–351.

116. Paik S, Shak S, Tang G, et al. A multigene assay to predict recurrence of tamoxifen-treated, node-negative breast cancer. *N Engl J Med* 2004;351:2817– 2826.

117. Paik S, Tang G, Shak S, et al. Gene expression and benefit of chemotherapy in women with node-negative, estrogen receptor-positive breast cancer. *J Clin Oncol* 2006;24:3726–3734.

118. Hayes DF, Thor AD, Dressler LG, et al. HER2 and response to paclitaxel in node-positive breast cancer. *N Engl J Med* 2007;357:1496–1506.

119. Albain KS, Barlow W, Shak S, et al. Prognostic and predictive value of the 21-gene recurrence score assay in postmenopausal, node-positive, ER-positive breast cancer (S8814, INT0100). *Br Cancer Res Treat* 2007;106[Suppl 1]:(abst10).

120. Fisher B, Bryant J, Wolmark N, et al. Effect of preoperative chemotherapy on the outcome of women with operable breast cancer. *J Clin Oncol* 1998;16: 2672–2685.

121. Symmans WF, Peintinger F, Hatzis C, et al. Measurement of residual breast cancer burden to predict survival after neoadjuvant chemotherapy. *J Clin Oncol* 2007;25:4414–4422.

122. Cure H, Amat S, Penault-Llorca F, et al. Prognostic value of residual node involvement in operable breast cancer after induction chemotherapy. *Breast Cancer Res Treat* 2002;76:37–45.

123. Pierga JY, Mouret E, Laurence V, et al. Prognostic factors for survival after neoadjuvant chemotherapy in operable breast cancer. the role of clinical response. *Eur J Cancer* 2003;39:1089–1096.

124. Kuerer HM, Newman LA, Buzdar AU, et al. Residual metastatic axillary lymph nodes following neoadjuvant chemotherapy predict disease-free survival in patients with locally advanced breast cancer. *Am J Surg* 1998;176:502–509.

125. Kuerer HM, Sahin AA, Hunt KK, et al. Incidence and impact of documented eradication of breast cancer axillary lymph node metastases before surgery in patients treated with neoadjuvant chemotherapy. *Ann Surg* 1999;230:72–78.

126. Overgaard M, Hansen PS, Overgaard J, et al. Postoperative radiotherapy in high-risk premenopausal women with breast cancer who receive adjuvant chemotherapy. Danish Breast Cancer Cooperative Group 82b Trial. *N Engl J Med* 1997;337: 949–955.

127. Ragaz J, Jackson SM, Le N, et al. Adjuvant radiotherapy and chemotherapy in node-positive premenopausal women with breast cancer. *N Engl J Med* 1997; 337:956–962.

128. Overgaard M, Jensen MB, Overgaard J, et al. Postoperative radiotherapy in high-risk postmenopausal breast-cancer patients given adjuvant tamoxifen: Danish Breast Cancer Cooperative Group DBCG 82c randomised trial. *Lancet* 1999;353: 1641–1648.

129. Clarke M, Collins R, Darby S, et al. Effects of radiotherapy and of differences in the extent of surgery for early breast cancer on local recurrence and 15-year survival: an overview of the randomised trials. *Lancet* 2005;366:2087–2106.

130. Fowble B, Gray R, Gilchrist K, et al. Identification of a subgroup of patients with breast cancer and histologically positive axillary nodes receiving adjuvant chemotherapy who may benefit from postoperative radiotherapy. *J Clin Oncol* 1988;6:1107–1117.

131. Recht A, Gray R, Davidson NE, et al. Locoregional failure 10 years after mastectomy and adjuvant chemotherapy with or without tamoxifen without irradiation: experience of the Eastern Cooperative Oncology Group. *J Clin Oncol* 1999;17: 1689–1700.

132. Katz A, Strom EA, Buchholz TA, et al. Locoregional recurrence patterns after mastectomy and doxorubicin-based chemotherapy: implications for postoperative irradiation. *J Clin Oncol* 2000;18:2817–2827.

133. Wallgren A, Bonetti M, Gelber RD, et al. Risk factors for locoregional recurrence among breast cancer patients: results from International Breast Cancer Study Group Trials I through VII. *J Clin Oncol* 2003;21:1205–1213.

134. Buchholz TA, Katz A, Strom EA, et al. Pathologic tumor size and lymph node status predict for different rates of locoregional recurrence after mastectomy for breast cancer patients treated with neoadjuvant versus adjuvant chemotherapy. *Int J Radiat Oncol Biol Phys* 2002;53:880–888.

135. Garg AK, Strom EA, McNeese MD, et al. T3 disease at presentation or pathologic involvement of four or more lymph nodes predict for locoregional recurrence in stage II breast cancer treated with neoadjuvant chemotherapy and mastectomy without irradiation. *Int J Radiat Oncol Biol Phys* 2004;59:138–145.

136. McGuire SE, Gonzalez-Angulo AM, Huang EH, et al. Postmastectomy radiation improves the outcome of patients with locally advanced breast cancer who achieve a pathologic complete response to neoadjuvant chemotherapy. *Int J Radiat Oncol Biol Phys* 2007;68:1004–1009.

137. Buzdar AU, Ibrahim NK, Francis D, et al. Significantly higher pathologic complete remission rate after neoadjuvant therapy with trastuzumab, paclitaxel, and epirubicin chemotherapy: results of a randomized trial in human epidermal growth factor receptor 2–positive operable breast cancer. *J Clin Oncol* 2005;23:3676–3685.

138. Rouzier R, Pusztai L, Delaloge S, et al. Nomograms to predict pathologic complete response and metastasis-free survival after preoperative chemotherapy for breast cancer. *J Clin Oncol* 2005;23:8331–8339.

139. Aryus B, Audretsch W, Gogolin F, et al. Remission rates following preoperative chemotherapy and radiation therapy in patients with breast cancer. *Strahlenther Onkol* 2000;176:411–415.

140. Gerlach B, Audretsch W, Gogolin F, et al. Remission rates in breast cancer treated with preoperative chemotherapy and radiotherapy. *Strahlenther Onkol* 2003; 179:306–311.

141. Jacquillat C, Weil M, Baillet F, et al. Results of neoadjuvant chemotherapy and radiation therapy in the breast-conserving treatment of 250 patients with all stages of infiltrative breast cancer. *Cancer* 1990;66:119–129.

142. Scholl SM, Fourquet A, Asselain B, et al. Neoadjuvant versus adjuvant chemotherapy in premenopausal patients with tumours considered too large for breast conserving surgery: preliminary results of a randomised trial: S6. *Eur J Cancer* 1994;30A:645–652.

143. Singletary SE. Minimally invasive surgery in breast cancer treatment. *Biomed Pharmacother* 2001;55:510–514.

144. Pusztai L, Ayers M, Simman FW, et al. Emerging science: prospective validation of gene expression profiling-based prediction of complete pathologic response to neoadjuvant paclitaxel/FAC chemotherapy in breast cancer. *Proc Am Soc Clin Oncol* 2003;22:1(abst 1).

145. Hurkmans CW, Borger JH, Rutgers EJ, et al. Quality assurance of axillary radiotherapy in the EORTC AMAROS trial 10981/22023: the dummy run. *Radiother Oncol* 2003;68:233–240.

146. Buchholz TA, Strom EA, McNeese MD, et al. Radiation therapy as an adjuvant treatment after sentinel lymph node surgery for breast cancer. *Surg Clin North Am* 2003;83:911–930.

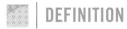

Chapter 61
Locally Advanced Breast Cancer

Gabriel N. Hortobagyi, Sonja Eva Singletary, and Eric A. Strom

DEFINITION

Locally advanced breast cancer (LABC) remains an important public health problem and a challenging management problem around the world (1). In groups of women who participate in periodic screening programs, the incidence of LABC is lower than 5%, whereas in medically underserved areas of the United States and in many developing countries, LABC represents 40% to 60% of newly found malignant breast neoplasms (2–4). It can be estimated that between 300,000 and 450,000 new cases of LABC are diagnosed around the world every year.

LABC includes large primary tumors (>5 cm, T3 in the American Joint Committee on Cancer [AJCC] cancer staging system), tumors of any size associated with skin or chest wall involvement (T4), tumors with fixed or matted axillary lymph nodes (N2), and those with involvement of the ipsilateral subclavicular and supraclavicular lymph nodes (N3) (5). Operationally, even moderate-sized tumors, 3 to 5 cm in size, located in a small breast behave like LABC and are best treated with similar combined-modality approaches. The management of patients with LABC has evolved substantially over the past three decades, and this chapter will summarize current therapeutic options.

HISTORICAL PERSPECTIVE

Adjuvant systemic treatments have become integral components of the curative management of primary breast cancer (6,7). Postoperative adjuvant chemotherapy, hormone therapy, and trastuzumab produce highly significant reductions in odds of recurrence and death from breast cancer for patients of any age, with node-negative or node-positive tumors. Although the great majority of clinical trials on which the value of adjuvant chemotherapy is based included predominantly patients with stages I and II primary breast cancer, many of these trials also included patients with stage III operable breast cancer (8). The Oxford overview indicated that the proportional reduction in odds of recurrence and death was similar in all prognostic subgroups, whether based on stage, number of lymph nodes, or tumor size. The effectiveness of systemic therapy varied markedly, however, based on predictors of therapeutic benefit. Thus, only patients with estrogen receptor– or progesterone receptor–positive breast cancer benefit from endocrine therapy; only patients with overexpression or amplification of *ERBB2* (formerly *HER2*) benefit from trastuzumab. In addition, the efficacy of chemotherapy is several fold greater in patients with negative hormone receptors than in patients with positive hormone receptors.

Randomized trials designed for stage III breast cancer suggested that adjuvant systemic therapies also decreased the probability of recurrence and death in this group of patients (7,9–11). Although questions related to adjuvant systemic therapy have been tested in multiple randomized trials, most of the information about the management of LABC is based on phase II trials or single institution experiences. Therefore, the levels of evidence on which many of the recommendations made in this chapter are based are lower than the levels of evidence that support adjuvant systemic therapy.

Historically, patients with LABC treated with surgery only fared poorly: although surgical resection was technically possible in most patients with LABC, 10 years after diagnosis more than 80% of patients had succumbed to the disease (12). On the basis of this experience, Haagensen and Stout (13) defined the concepts of operable and inoperable breast cancer. Skin ulceration, edema, and fixation, as well as fixation of the tumor to the chest wall, were all correlated with almost universal treatment failure and became, therefore, markers of inoperability.

Subsequent to Haagensen and Stout's landmark publication, patients with inoperable tumors were treated with radiation therapy (RT) alone or associated with surgical resection (12,14,15). However, the large doses of radiation necessary to optimize local control were often associated with long-term complications, including skin and chest wall fibrosis, skin ulceration, pulmonary fibrosis, rib necrosis or resorption, brachial plexopathy, and lymphedema of the arm (16–18). The combination of surgery and radiotherapy improved significantly the local control rates, but the overall cure rate and duration of survival remained unchanged (12).

It was on this background that the initial combined modality treatment approaches were developed, in parallel with the postoperative adjuvant chemotherapy programs. However, because LABC is far less frequent in North America and Europe, where the bulk of clinical research in breast cancer has been performed, most of the clinical information about LABC was derived from single-arm phase II studies or from retrospective reviews of single institution experiences with a treatment strategy. Despite these limitations, combinations of systemic and local-regional therapies represent the standard of care for all patients with LABC.

DIAGNOSIS AND STAGING

Most LABCs are easily palpable and even visible. Most represent neglected primaries present for months or sometimes years before the initial consultation. Patients are usually aware of the breast or lymph node abnormality, but because of fear, denial, or lack of access to appropriate health care, they delay seeking medical attention. However, some LABCs present with diffuse infiltration of the breast and without a dominant mass. These require mammographic or sonographic assessment, and they often appear as large areas of calcification or parenchymal distortion; sometimes skin thickening is also present. Occasionally, even large lesions are mammographically and sonographically silent and magnetic resonance imaging (MRI) is needed for definitive imaging.

A core needle biopsy usually establishes the histologic diagnosis; incisional biopsies are seldom required, although some recommend a full-thickness skin biopsy when inflammatory breast cancer is suspected. If an experienced cytopathologist is available, the diagnosis of malignancy can be confirmed by fine-needle aspiration cytology (FNAC); nuclear grade, flow cytometry, estrogen (ER)- and progesterone-receptor (PR) status and *ERBB2* can all be assayed on FNAC samples, and so can most other proposed prognostic indicators (PCNA [proliferating cell nuclear antigen], Ki-67, p53, etc.). It has also been reported that gene expression profiling can be accomplished using a FNAC sample (19). However, FNAC cannot differentiate invasive from noninvasive tumors. If palpable regional nodes exist, a positive fine-needle aspirate of a node confirms the presence of invasive breast cancer.

Once the diagnosis is established, the extent of tumor involvement is ascertained. The extent of obvious tumor can sometimes mask the importance of obtaining a detailed understanding of the locoregional extent of tumor. Bilateral mammogram serves to assess the known primary tumor and to rule out the presence of synchronous bilateral cancer or contralateral metastases. Sonography serves to further define tumor dimensions and to detail any regional lymph node involvement. The authors' sonographic examination includes, in addition to the breast and axillary area, the infraclavicular, supraclavicular, and internal mammary lymph node chains. Lymph nodes in these chains are involved in the majority of cases of LABC. Nearly one third of advanced breast cancers at M.D. Anderson Cancer Center have radiographic involvement of the internal mammary, infraclavicular, or supraclavicular nodal basins. For lesions poorly defined by mammography or sonography, MRI can be helpful. Bilateral MR mammography is increasingly used for baseline assessment of the extent of tumor involvement, additional foci of cancer, and following neoadjuvant systemic therapy to assess response to therapy. This is particularly true of some subtypes of breast cancer that are frequently mammographically silent, such as invasive lobular cancer or inflammatory breast cancer. Accurate imaging evaluation at baseline and following systemic therapy are critical to guide optimal local-regional therapy planning and for assessment of response. A biochemical survey, tumor markers, and chest radiograph and bone scan complement a complete physical examination, with quantitative documentation of all palpable abnormalities. Abdominal imaging (computerized tomography [CT] or sonography) is recommended to rule out intra-abdominal metastases. Areas of increased radionuclide uptake on bone scan are assessed by radiographs, MRI, or CT scanning. Other tests are indicated only by specific symptoms or for investigational purposes. Increasingly, positron emission tomography (PET) is also being employed to rule out metastatic deposits at the time of diagnosis.

DEVELOPMENT OF COMBINED MODALITY STRATEGIES

Systemic therapy was introduced in the management of inoperable breast cancers more than 40 years ago (20). Surgery or radiotherapy, or both, followed systemic therapy in these trials. For optimal utilization of all treatment modalities, all interested specialists (radiologist, pathologist, and surgical, radiation, and medical oncologists) should review the diagnostic data, examine the patient, and determine the optimal type and sequence of therapies before any treatment is implemented. Treatment strategies that include induction systemic therapy have several potential advantages: early initiation of systemic therapy, *in vivo* assessment of response, and reduction in the extent of primary tumor and regional lymphatic metastases. The potential (theoretical) shortcomings include delay in local treatment, induction of drug resistance, and unreliability of clinical staging. The practical advantages have exceeded, by far, the disadvantages. The ability to monitor response to therapy by serial measurements of the primary tumor and the reduction in tumor volume that often permits breast conservation are the two major clinical advantages of these treatment strategies.

Neoadjuvant Chemotherapy

The first clinical trials with neoadjuvant chemotherapy (NACT) (also called induction chemotherapy, primary chemotherapy, or preoperative chemotherapy) started in the late 1960s, but the earliest reports of its use were published in the 1970s (21,22). Since then, multiple reports have documented the

effectiveness of primary systemic therapy in patients with LABC (12,23–29). Most reports of combined modality therapy of locally advanced breast cancer are based on anthracycline-containing combination chemotherapy regimens (see also Chapter 58). Administration of combination chemotherapy produces major reductions in tumor volume in 60% to 90% of patients. Tumor reduction has been consistently documented in both the primary tumor and the enlarged regional lymph nodes (18,23,27–38). Although mixed responses (response in the primary tumor and no response in the regional lymph nodes, or vice versa) have been reported, they are uncommon (35, 39–41). Clinical complete remissions have been reported in 10% to 20% of patients with LABC treated with anthracycline-containing combination chemotherapy regimens (27,30,35, 36,42). Response rates, and especially complete response rates, improve if a taxane is added, especially in sequential regimens. The median number of cycles required to achieve a partial remission was reported to be four, and for a complete remission, five (41). Pathological complete remission is uncommonly obtained with chemotherapy in ER+ tumors and is rare after neoadjuvant endocrine therapy. Since the introduction of trastuzumab, a number of reports indicated that in combination with chemotherapy, trastuzumab produces pathological complete remission rates ranging from 20% to 70% in *ERBB2*-amplified or overexpressing breast cancers (43).

Clinical measurements of breast masses are often inaccurate, and there is substantial interindividual variation among examiners (44). Therefore, imaging methods are often used to more reliably document extent of disease (44–46). The combination of physical examination with either mammography or ultrasound gives measurements that closely approach those achieved by histopathology, and it reduces error rates in serial monitoring of response to systemic therapy (46). MRI is also frequently used to determine extent of disease, especially in the preoperative setting to help define optimal surgical therapy (47). The determination of clinical complete remission requires that no residual disease be present by physical examination and by imaging (mammography or ultrasound) in the breast or regional lymph nodes (35). Even following these criteria, only half to two thirds of patients thought to have a clinical complete remission are found to have a pathologic complete remission (i.e., no residual disease) (10,27,30,35,41,46). Furthermore, a third of patients with no residual disease by histologic examination will have residual clinical or imaging abnormalities that preclude the diagnosis of clinical complete remission. Patients who achieve a histologically documented complete remission have a markedly improved long-term prognosis compared with patients who achieve incomplete or no responses (29,48). Furthermore, these patients are often excellent candidates for breast-conserving strategies, with or without surgical intervention. In recent years, in addition to refinements to the sequential evaluation of extent of disease during therapy utilizing mammography, sonography, and MRI, PET has been evaluated. Several authors have reported that not only does PET identify metastatic lesions not found by other imaging modalities but it is also a very sensitive tool to monitor the functional status of the tumor. Thus, changes in PET imaging, such as marked reductions in standardized uptake values, are under evaluation for early determination of response to neoadjuvant systemic therapy (49).

Most initial reports of combined-modality treatment of LABC were based on anthracycline-containing combination chemotherapy regimens, such as doxorubicin and cyclophosphamide (AC) or fluorouracil, doxorubicin, and cyclophosphamide (FAC) or FEC when the anthracycline used was epirubicin. Since the introduction of the taxanes over the past two decades, there have been multiple reports based on the use of an anthracycline and taxane combination (epirubicin/paclitaxel or doxorubicin/docetaxel, with or without the addition of

Table 61.1	TAXANE-CONTAINING NEOADJUVANT CHEMOTHERAPY REGIMENS FOR OPERABLE AND LOCALLY ADVANCED BREAST CANCER

Neoadjuvant Docetaxel-Containing Regimens

Author (Reference)	n	Drug(s)	Clinical Stage	cCR (%)	cPR (%)	ORR (%)	pCR (%)
Gradishar et al. (50)	30	docetaxel	III	18	67	85	1
von Minckwitz et al. (51)	42	docetaxel + doxorubicin	II, IIIA, IIIB	33	60	93	5
Miller et al. (52)	19	docetaxel + doxorubicin	III	6	11	17	3
Miller et al. (52)	21	docetaxel + doxorubicin	III	2	15	17	1
Valero et al. (53)	50	docetaxel + doxorubicin	IIIB	6	82	88	12
Luporsi et al. (54)	90	docetaxel + epirubicin	II/III	84	NA	NA	24
Malhotra et al. (56)	38	docetaxel + doxorubicin	III	NA	NA	90	14
Von Minckwitz et al. (57)	126	docetaxel + doxorubicin +	II, III	13	65	78	10
Von Minckwitz et al. (57)	121	docetaxel + doxorubicin + tamoxifen	II, III	6	62	68	9
Ardavanis et al. (58)	28	docetaxel + epirubicin	III	57	NA	89	18
Borrega et al. (59)	22	docetaxel + epirubicin	IIIA, IIIB	NA	NA	95	32
Hurley et al. (60)	16	docetaxel + cisplatin + trastuzumab	IIIA, IIIB, IV	56	44	100	25
Bines et al. (61)	36	docetaxel	IIIA, IIIB	3	NA	54	NA
Estevez et al. (62)	56	docetaxel	II, III	25	46	72	18
Vinholes et al. (63)	210	docetaxel + doxorubicin	III	NA	NA	72	16
Evans et al. (64)	183	docetaxel + epirubicin	II/III	NA	NA	88	8
Ganem et al. (65)	20	docetaxel + doxorubicin	35	45	80	12	
Baltali et al. (66)	63	docetaxel + epirubicin + fluorouracil	III	25	70	95	NA
Limentani et al. (55)	19	docetaxel + doxorubicin	IIB-III	26	NA	89	NA

Neoadjuvant Paclitaxel-Containing Regimens

Author (Reference)	n	Drug(s)	Clinical Stage	cCR (%)	cPR (%)	ORR (%)	pCR (%)
Moliterni et al. (67)	38	Paclitaxel + doxorubicin	IIIB	31	NA	NA	NA
Moliterni et al. (67)	41	Paclitaxel + doxorubicin	II, IIIA	20	NA	NA	NA
Gogas et al. (77)	35	Paclitaxel + pegylated liposomal doxorubicin	III	17	54	71	9
Ezzat et al. (71)	72	paclitaxel + cisplatin	III	18	72	90	22
Taillilbert et al. (72)	21	Paclitaxel + epirubicin + cyclophosphamide	II, III	21	63	NA	21
Goubely-Brewer et al. (73)	23	Paclitaxel + epirubicin + 5-fluorouracil	NA	NA	NA	83	52
Cristofanilli et al. (74)	20	Paclitaxel	III	40	NA	NA	25
Burstein et al. (75)	25	Paclitaxel + trastuzumab	II, III	NA	NA	64	20
Buzdar et al. (69)	87	Paclitaxel	IIA, IIB, IIIA	27	53	80	18
Dieras et al. (70)	180	Paclitaxel + doxorubicin	III	NA	NA	83	16
Fumoleau et al. (76)	99	Paclitaxel + doxorubicin	II, IIIA	NA	NA	NA	5
Fumoleau et al. (76)	92	Paclitaxel + doxorubicin	II, IIIA	NA	NA	NA	17
Green et al. (78)	127	Paclitaxel	II, III	NA	NA	NA	31
Untch et al. (79)	475	Paclitaxel + epirubicin	III	NA	NA	NA	18
Untch et al. (79)	475	Paclitaxel + epirubicin	III	NA	NA	NA	10

cCR, clinical complete remission; cPR, clinical partial response; ORR, overall response rate; pCR, pathologic complete response; NA, not available.

other agents) (50–79) (Table 61.1). These newer regimens were reported to have marked antitumor activity, with overall response rates in the 80% to 95% range. Unfortunately, the reported clinical and pathologic complete remission rates were only modestly higher than those reported with older combinations. Table 61.2 summarizes prospective randomized trials that compare anthracycline- and taxane-containing regimens with anthracycline-containing combinations without a taxane (54,63,64,69,70,78–82). In several randomized trials in which a taxane was administered sequentially, after the initial four cycles of an anthracycline/cyclophosphamide-containing neoadjuvant regimen, a significant increase in pathologic complete remission was reported (81,82). In a small, multicenter trial conducted on patients with LABC, the increase in clinical and pathologic complete response rate was associated with improved disease-free and overall survival rates (81,83). Of note, both responders and nonresponders to the initial anthracycline-containing combination benefited from crossover to docetaxel. The National Surgical Adjuvant Breast and Bowel Project (NSABP) protocol B-27 included a crossover to docetaxel after four cycles of neoadjuvant AC; the addition of docetaxel resulted in significant increases in overall and complete response rates, pathologic complete response rates, and increased breast-

conserving surgery rates (82). However, while there was a borderline improvement in relapse-free survival, the primary end point of the study, improved disease-free survival, was not significantly altered. Other drugs under investigation in the neoadjuvant setting are gemcitabine, vinorelbine, platinum analogs, ixabepilone, trastuzumab, bevacizumab, and lapatinib. Single-agent trastuzumab was reported to achieve a 23% partial response rate after 3 weeks of treatment in patients with LABC in one study and a 45% response rate in another (84,85). In combination with a taxane or vinorelbine, or two-drug combination chemotherapy regimens, clinical complete remission rates of 24% to 59% were reported (43,86–88). The corresponding pathological complete remission rates ranged from 18% to 45%. In a small randomized trial of sequential paclitaxel followed by fluorouracil, epirubicin, and cyclophosphamide, with or without trastuzumab, pathological complete remission rate increased from 26% to 65% with the addition of trastuzumab (87). These results were confirmed by a larger randomized trial that included 235 patients with *ERBB2*-positive primary breast cancer (89). A large, multicenter confirmatory study is currently accruing patients with T2 and T3, *ERBB2*-positive breast cancer (American College of Surgery Oncology Group [ACOSOG] protocol Z1041).

Table 61.2	RANDOMIZED PHASE III STUDIES COMPARING ANTHRACYCLINE AND TAXANE-CONTAINING REGIMENS WITH ANTHRACYCLINE-CONTAINING COMBINATIONS WITHOUT TAXANES				
Author (Reference)	n	Clinical Stage	Treatment	ORR (%)	pCR (%)
Smith et al. (81)	162	IIB, III	CVAP	64	15
			vs.		
			CVAP + docetaxel	85 (p = .03)	31 (p = .06)
Vinholes et al. (63)	407	IIIA, IIIB	Docetaxel + doxorubicin	72	16
			vs.		
			FAC	63 (p = .0056)	11
Luporsi et al. (54)	90	II, III	FEC	72	24
			vs.		
			ET	84	24
NSABP B-27 (82)	2,411	II	AC	85	14
			vs.		
			AC + T + surgery	91	25
			vs.		
			AC + surgery + T	85	14
Evans et al. (64)	365	II, III	AC	78	12
			vs.		
			AT	88	8
Buzdar et al. (69)	174	II-IIIA	Paclitaxel	80	8
			vs.		
			FAC	79	14
Pouillart et al. (115)	247	IIA, IIB, IIA	AC	10	66
			vs.		
			AT	16	83
Green et al. (78)	127	I, II, IIIA	T q 3 weeks	18	NA
			vs.		
			weekly T	31	N/A
Untch et al. (79)	475	II, IIIA+B	Dose-dense sequential E to T,	18	NA
			vs.		
			standard ET	10	NA

ORR, overall response rate; pCR, pathologic complete response; CVAP, cyclophosphamide, vincristine, doxorubicin, prednisolone; FAC, 5-fluorouracil, doxorubicin, cyclophosphamide; FEC, fluorouracil, epirubicin, cyclophosphamide; ET, epirubicin, paclitaxel; AC, Adriamycin (doxorubicin) and cyclophosphamide; AT, doxorubicin, docetaxel; T, paclitaxel; NA, not available.

 ## NEOADJUVANT ENDOCRINE THERAPY

Most of the clinical investigation with neoadjuvant systemic therapy was conducted with cytotoxic therapy. More limited information is available about neoadjuvant endocrine therapy (90) (see also Chapter 59). For patients with ER+ breast cancer, neoadjuvant endocrine therapy is an appropriate option. The initial trials used tamoxifen and included patients selected on the basis of older age or comorbidity that precluded chemotherapy (91–93). The results suggested that neoadjuvant endocrine therapy was therapeutically effective and produced marked reduction in tumor volume in 40% to 60% of patients. A significant minority of tumors progressed during neoadjuvant endocrine therapy; thus, close monitoring is required so that early progressors are identified promptly and appropriate regional therapy (or crossover to chemotherapy) can be implemented. Several studies also concluded that tamoxifen alone was insufficient therapy for patients with primary and locally advanced breast cancer, and that appropriate surgery or RT was needed for optimal local and systemic control (94,95). Endocrine therapy should be restricted to patients with hormone receptor–positive breast cancer. More recent trials compared selective aromatase inhibitors with drugs in the same family or with tamoxifen (96,97). In these studies, greater antitumor efficacy was observed with aromatase inhibitors compared to tamoxifen (97). In general, response to neoadjuvant endocrine

therapy occurs in 35% to 50% of patients with hormone receptor–positive breast cancer, but fewer than 5% achieve pathological complete remission. Response rates to neoadjuvant endocrine therapies in this setting are lower than response rates to anthracycline- or taxane-based chemotherapy in unselected patients with LABC (95); pathological complete remission rates with NACT for patients with ER+ breast cancer are observed in 5% to 14%, several fold lower than for patients with ER– breast cancer. Early progression is observed more frequently after neoadjuvant endocrine therapy (12% to 17%) (98) than after NACT (5% to 10%) (12). The poor prognosis of patients with LABC indicates that all treatment modalities are needed for optimal results, so all patients with ER+ or progesterone receptor assays should receive adjuvant endocrine treatment as part of their multidisciplinary therapy. The authors' preference is to initiate adjuvant endocrine treatment after the completion of NACT, surgical resection, and radiotherapy. Whether there is a subset of patients with hormone receptor–positive LABC that does not benefit from and therefore does not require NACT remains to be established.

Considerations for Imaging

A common denominator underlying clinical decisions about appropriate surgical treatment for LABC is the importance of accurate imaging. It is important at initial presentation to estimate tumor size and determine if the patient is a good candidate for NACT. During and after NACT, imaging of the primary tumor and the axillary lymph nodes is used to assess treatment response and aid in surgical planning.

Standard Imaging Modalities after Neoadjuvant Chemotherapy

Mammography and ultrasound have been shown to offer accurate predictions of pathologic tumor size in patients with small invasive ductal carcinomas without an extensive intraductal component, provided the patients have not received NACT (99) (see Chapters 12 and 13). In patients who have received NACT, however, there have been widely disparate reports on the accuracy of these imaging approaches for predicting residual pathologic tumor size. Even in two reports from the same institution (98,99), substantially dissimilar results were obtained, reflecting a different (although overlapping) patient population and a different statistical approach for the assessment of predictive power (one using raw data and the other using logarithmically transformed data). Overall, as reviewed in the report from Chagpar et al. (98), physical examination appears to be at least as accurate as mammography or ultrasound in estimating residual tumor size, with correlation coefficients ranging from 0.42 to 0.73, compared to a range of 0.33 to 0.65 for mammography and 0.29 to 0.60 for ultrasound. However, the false-negative rate associated with physical examination has been reported to be almost 60% (98), indicating that many small tumors might be missed using this approach. Similarly, the false-positive rates from ultrasound and mammography may be 50% or higher (98), suggesting that these imaging approaches may pick up inflammatory or fibrotic changes induced by the chemotherapy. The mixed reports about the usefulness of ultrasound and mammography in assessing residual tumor size have driven the search for more accurate imaging modalities. Currently, there is growing interest in the possibility of using MRI, but other researchers are exploring new approaches involving functional imaging and the tools of nanotechnology as well as additional refinements to mammography and ultrasound (see Chapters 14 and 15).

Magnetic Resonance Imaging for the Assessment of Neoadjuvant Chemotherapy Response

MRI of breast lesions is captured before and after the injection of a gadolinium-based contrast agent. Because malignant lesions are typically more vascular than benign lesions, they tend to take up the contrast agent faster. They can also be distinguished from benign lesions by having spiculated rather than smooth edges. MRI originally suffered from an unacceptably high rate of false positives, but improved algorithms for combining morphologic and kinetic data have greatly improved this picture, with specificity now ranging from 81% to 99% (100–103) (see Chapter 14).

At the authors' institution, other indications for MRI include cancer that is occult on standard imaging, unknown primary tumor in patients with axillary node metastases, multifocal or multicentric disease in patients with a known primary tumor, residual disease in patients with positive margins after breast-conserving surgery, recurrence in patients after completion of RT, and evaluation of the response to NACT.

Although the results of trials assessing the accuracy of MRI after NACT are varied, overall, MRI appears to allow a more precise estimation of residual tumor than mammography or ultrasound (104–106). Despite its sensitivity, however, the ability of MRI to detect a complete pathologic response has shown great variability in different series, presumably because the limits of detection for MRI do not allow the identification of very small foci of *in situ* or invasive disease. For this reason, a negative report on MRI should be evaluated conservatively and

Table 61.3	**NEW APPROACHES TO BREAST IMAGING**
Technique	Rationale
Breast tomosynthesis	Uses a standard mammography x-ray tube, but moves in a 50 degree arc about the breast, taking 11 low-dose pictures from various angles that are pieced together by a computer.
Color Doppler ultrasonography	Ultrasound waves register the change in pitch caused by moving blood cells and convert it into an array of colors that depict the speed and direction of blood flow.
Ultrasound tomography	Ultrasound waves are launched from a variety of angles, resulting in a scattered field of reflected and refracted sound waves that are sampled by collectors completely surrounding the target.
Nanoshells	Nanoshell bioconjugates can be constructed to scatter incident near-infrared light that can be collected for imaging. The shells can be loaded with specific antibodies that react with tumor cell-surface antigens.

properly used only to assess a patient's candidacy for breast-conserving therapy.

Other Approaches to Breast Imaging

PET produces images that reflect metabolic and physiologic functions occurring in living cells. A positron-emitting radionuclide is attached to a molecule (typically a sugar) that is ingested or metabolized at a high rate in the rapidly growing cancer cells. PET is very specific for the detection of malignant breast tumors, and problems with spatial resolution and "noise" from normal tissue can be reduced by using a small parallel pair of detector heads placed directly above and below the breast (107,108). A general problem with PET is the lack of anatomical specificity. This problem can be resolved by running the scan concurrently or sequentially with an alternate anatomical imaging modality. Li et al. (109) used hybrid PET-CT imaging to assess the response to NACT in 45 patients with primary breast cancer. They were able to demonstrate a sensitivity of 90.9% and a specificity of 83.3% for the prediction of clinical response by PET-CT. Mammography can also be used as an anatomical imaging adjunct for PET; using the small parallel detector heads, the scan can be run concurrently or sequentially with mammography without releasing the breast compression (107,108) (see Chapter 15).

Table 61.3 lists additional approaches to breast imaging that are in an earlier stage of development but that show promise for increased accuracy in assessing tumor size before and after NACT.

APPROACHES TO LOCAL THERAPY

For patients with operable (stage IIIA) LABC, a modified radical mastectomy, followed by systemic adjuvant therapy, represents an effective treatment option (110). Selected patients with small T4 tumors may also be approached with surgery as their initial treatment modality (111). However, the administration of NACT as the first modality of treatment, before surgical therapy is instituted, is favored by most expert groups for the management of stage III and most large stage II breast cancers (29,31,36,37,41,42,112). NACT results in major objective responses and down-staging for approximately 70% to 95% of patients (12,29,35,42,112). After NACT, surgery alone (21,32, 113,114), radiotherapy alone (21,23,29,34,112,113,115,116), or a combination of both (21,28,113,114) has been used in the context of multidisciplinary management. Surgical therapy may require a total mastectomy or only a wide excision (lumpectomy or quadrantectomy), both with an axillary dissection, especially in the presence of palpable axillary lymph nodes (see also Chapter 60). Multiple reports have indicated that breast-conserving therapy for locally advanced breast cancers after NACT is feasible and, if appropriate selection criteria are applied, safe and associated with high local control rates (29,117–121).

Considerations for Breast-Conserving Surgery

The use of NACT has become standard management for patients with LABC, in part because it frequently reduces the size of the primary tumor enough to allow previously inoperable tumors to become operable. For selected patients (i.e., complete resolution of skin edema [*peau d'orange*], adequate reduction in the tumor size, no extensive intramammary lymphatic invasion, absence of extensive suspicious microcalcifications, and no evidence of multicentricity), breast-conserving therapy can be an appropriate local treatment option. In patients meeting these criteria, the local recurrence rate and 10-year overall survival after breast-conserving therapy are equivalent to those seen in early stage breast cancer patients (122).

As with any curative breast cancer surgery, the primary goal is to completely remove the tumor with negative margins. This is a potential problem in LABC patients treated with NACT because approximately 30% of these patients (and up to 60% of those treated with trastuzumab) will achieve a clinical complete response, making it difficult to locate the tumor site during surgery (123). In addition, nearly two thirds of patients with a clinical complete response will prove to have residual tumor on final pathology, so it is critically important to be able to precisely localize and remove the original tumor site and ensure that the surgical specimen has clean margins (123). This can be accomplished by the placement of a metallic marker in the tumor during the course of the chemotherapy. Studies have shown that identification of the tumor site would be difficult or impossible in as many as half of patients receiving NACT without the placement of such a marker (124,125).

The Significance of Skin Involvement in the Clinical Diagnosis of Locally Advanced Breast Cancer

The clinical definition of LABC has traditionally included tumors of any size that are associated with skin or chest wall involvement, classified as T4 in the AJCC cancer staging system (5). Classification of a tumor as T4b indicates the presence of noninflammatory skin changes, including edema, ulceration of the skin of the breast, or presence of satellite skin nodules confined to the same breast. Such skin involvement has been associated with a poor prognosis, and these patients are usually recommended for mastectomy, under the assumption that local failure rates would be unacceptably high with breast-conserving therapy. Evidence from the authors' institution and others suggests that this generalized approach to T4b tumors may be too simplistic.

A 2004 study by Shen et al. (124) looked at local control and long-term survival in 33 patients with noninflammatory T4b disease treated with breast-conserving therapy. The median tumor size at study entry was 7 cm (range, 2 to 12 cm), and all patients had one or more types of skin involvement. After a median of four cycles of NACT, 28 patients had a complete or partial clinical response, and 28 patients showed a complete resolution of skin changes. Patients were chosen for breast-conserving therapy on the basis of resolution of skin edema; residual tumor less than 5 cm; no skin or chest wall fixation; no

contraindication for RT; no extensive suspicious microcalcifications; no evidence of multicentricity; and no extensive intra-mammary lymphatic invasion. At a median follow-up time of 91 months, only five patients (6%) had developed a locoregional recurrence, similar to rates observed in patients without noninflammatory skin involvement who received breast-conserving therapy after NACT. The 5-year overall survival rate was 78%, superior to most published survival data for patient with noninflammatory T4b disease, likely reflecting the careful selection criteria that were used.

Few series have examined patients with noninflammatory skin changes independently from those with large tumors or with bulky nodal disease. A 2005 study by Guth et al. (125) proposed that the adverse outcome typically linked with skin involvement might instead be attributed to the large tumor size that is frequently associated with T4b disease. They examined the effect of tumor size on outcome in 119 patients with noninflammatory skin involvement compared with a control group of patients matched by tumor size without skin involvement. They found that for the greater than 50% of patients with T4b carcinomas who had primary tumors less than 5 cm in size, there was no difference in long-term survival compared with patients from the control group with similarly sized tumors. Based on these findings, they suggested that patients with noninflammatory skin involvement should be classified according to tumor size and lymph node status, and that the T4 category of the AJCC staging system should be revised to include only inflammatory breast carcinoma. This distinctive clinicopathologic entity, characterized by diffuse skin changes that involve the majority of the skin on the breast, always carries a very grave prognosis.

Although the report by Guth et al. awaits independent confirmation, clinicians should be aware that the presence of skin involvement at presentation is not an absolute contraindication for breast-conserving therapy, especially when found in combination with smaller tumors and if negative margins can be achieved. This is true even for selected patients with skin ulceration, among the most alarming of symptoms and one that is usually associated with long-neglected locally advanced disease. For example, tumors of the inframammary fold can be quite small (<1 cm) and present with skin ulceration. The direct skin involvement might occur as a result of the tumor's location very close to the skin surface. These patients can be treated conservatively for an early stage cancer, and their prognosis is similar to other small tumors without skin involvement.

The physicians at M.D. Anderson Cancer Center monitor tumor response to NACT after every cycle of chemotherapy. The marker is placed under ultrasound or mammographic guidance when the tumor has shrunk to less than 2 cm in size (126,127). If it is placed before the initiation of NACT, the tumor may shrink eccentrically, leaving the marker on the edge of the residual tumor, rather than in the epicenter. a Cook coil (Cook, Inc., Bloomington, Indiana) is sometimes used, which is a small platinum marker with a coiled diameter of 2 mm and an extended length of 1 cm (Fig. 61.1). Platinum is preferable to the stainless steel rods that were originally used because it is more compatible with MRI. The marker is inserted with a 15 gauge 8-cm long needle and a blunt stylet under ultrasound guidance (Fig. 61.1). Alternatively, the authors' may use stereotactic clips, which are much smaller in size. Mammography is performed immediately after marker implantation to precisely document the position of the marker in relation to the tumor.

At the beginning of surgery a guide wire is inserted by the radiologist under ultrasound or mammographic guidance to indicate the location of the marker. Surgical excision does *not* attempt to remove the prechemotherapy volume of tumor. Rather, the goal is to remove any residual lesion with 1 cm of clear margins or, if there is no detectable residual lesion, a 2-cm

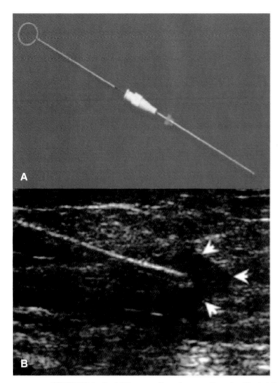

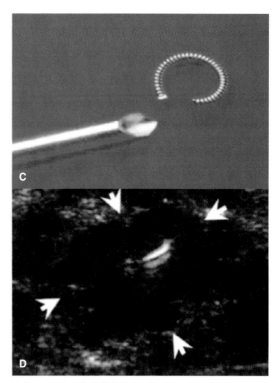

FIGURE 61.1. **A:** A 15-gauge, 8-cm long needle and a blunt stylet used to insert metal marker to indicate the site of the primary tumor during and after neoadjuvant chemotherapy. **B:** Sonogram showing placement of needle in center of tumor. **C:** Cook coil (Cook, Inc., Bloomington, Indiana) used for marking tumor site. **D:** sonogram showing Cook coil placed in epicenter of tumor. (Photographs courtesy of Dr. Henry Kuerer and Dr. Peter Dempsey.)

specimen with the metal coil in the center. When the specimen is removed, the orientation is designated prior to leaving surgery. A multicolor inking system is used to identify the superior, inferior, lateral, medial, anterior, and posterior surfaces. In pathology, a specimen radiograph is taken to verify the presence of the marker within the excised specimen (Fig. 61.2). While the patient is still in surgery, the specimen is then sectioned, with the order of all sections maintained so that the site of any positive or close margin can be identified and the surgeon can remove additional tissue from this area to obtain a negative margin. At M.D. Anderson Cancer Center, the reexcision rate is only about 4% because great care is taken to make sure margins are clear during the initial surgery.

Sentinel lymph node biopsy has become widely accepted and used because it offers accurate assessment with a substantially

reduced occurrence of the morbidities usually associated with complete axillary lymph node dissection (e.g., edema, reduced mobility, pain, etc.). However, there is a small but significant probability that patients receiving sentinel lymph node biopsy using blue dye may suffer from a serious anaphylactic reaction to the dye. In addition, if final pathology of the sentinel node(s) shows the presence of metastasis, a second surgery may be required, with its associated risks and costs. To reduce this risk, ultrasound-guided fine-needle aspiration can be used after NACT to up front screen out patients with positive nodes. Ultrasound is routinely used after NACT to assess response to the chemotherapy. Nodes that are indeterminate or suspicious as defined by size, morphology, internal echogenicity, shape, or cortical thickening are further assessed with FNA. Ultrasound-guided fine-needle aspiration in patients with ultrasound

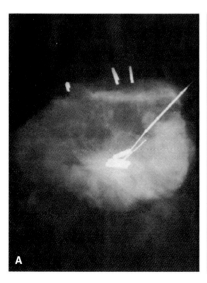

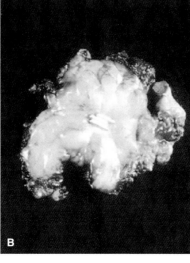

FIGURE 61.2. **A:** Specimen radiograph showing position of metal markers and guide wire inside the excised specimen. **B:** Metal markers in the sectioned specimen. (Photographs courtesy of Dr. Henry Kuerer and Dr. Peter Dempsey.)

suspicious nodes has been reported to have 89% sensitivity, 100% specificity, and 100% positive predictive value (128). Patients who are node positive on FNA proceed directly to complete axillary lymph node dissection without an intervening sentinel lymph node biopsy.

Considerations for Reconstructive Surgery

Many patients with LABC will become good candidates for breast-conserving therapy after NACT, but some will still need or prefer to receive a mastectomy. Current reconstructive techniques using autologous tissue flaps offer excellent cosmetic results without compromising long-term outcomes (see Chapter 39). Ideally, breast reconstruction can be carried out during the same surgery as the mastectomy, lessening the cost and the risk of multiple surgeries. However, there are potential restrictions to immediate reconstructions in patients with LABC that both physician and patient need to understand and discuss.

Patients with LABC are known to have a high risk of chest wall recurrences following mastectomy alone (129). For this reason, most are recommended for RT of the chest wall and the axilla following surgery. The optimal sequencing of RT and reconstruction is controversial. Immediate breast reconstruction can be an important factor in recovery, contributing to a more positive body image. On the other hand, there has been concern that a reconstructed chest mound might interfere with the delivery of the proper radiation dose, especially to the internal mammary nodes, or that there might be volume loss and asymmetry in the flap as a side effect of the RT.

A report by Tran et al. (130) examined both early and late complications from RT in patients with a free transverse rectus abdominis myocutaneous (TRAM) flap breast reconstruction. Of 102 patients in the study, 32 had immediate TRAM flap reconstruction before RT and 70 had RT before delayed TRAM flap reconstruction. Mean follow-up times for the immediate reconstruction and delayed reconstruction groups were 3 and 5 years, respectively. There was a slightly higher rate of early complications from RT in patients who received delayed reconstruction, but the differences were not significant. Late complications, including fat necrosis, volume loss in the flap, and contracture in the flap, were significantly more common in patients with immediate reconstruction. Fat necrosis occurred in 44% of patients with immediate reconstruction compared with 9% of patients with delayed reconstruction. No patients with delayed reconstruction experienced volume loss or contracture, versus 88% and 75%, respectively, of patients receiving immediate reconstruction.

A more recent study by Foster et al. (131) argues that immediate breast reconstruction has minimal morbidity and that complications tend to be minor. This study involved 35 patients who received immediate TRAM flap reconstruction followed by RT. At a minimum follow-up time of 1 year, they reported fat necrosis in three patients, two of whom developed volume loss of the flap and required additional surgery. Two patients had cellulitis, one developed a periumbilical hernia, and one experienced fascial laxity of the lower abdomen. Although the median follow-up time was 48 months, no data were presented about long-term cosmetic outcomes. In addition, there was no comparison group of patients who received RT prior to a delayed reconstruction, as in the Tran et al. study.

Although most authors acknowledge that radiotherapy to an immediate reconstruction may impair the final cosmetic outcome for some patients, until recently there was no information about the impact of immediate reconstruction on radiotherapy planning. A recent M.D. Anderson Cancer Center study of 110 patients who had mastectomy with immediate reconstruction and postoperative radiotherapy were compared with contemporaneous stage-matched patients who had undergone mastectomy without intervening reconstruction (132). Each of the radiotherapy plans were assessed for completeness of coverage and avoidance of adjacent critical structures. Of the radiotherapy plans scored after reconstruction, 52% had compromises compared with 7% of matched controls ($p < .0001$). Left-sided radiotherapy plans had larger compromises after immediate reconstruction than right-sided ones. Because of this, the potential for compromised postmastectomy radiation therapy planning should be considered when deciding between immediate versus delayed reconstruction.

Physicians at M.D. Anderson Cancer Center generally defer reconstruction until after the completion of RT in patients with LABC who receive a mastectomy. The exception would be the case of the patient who required flap coverage because of a chest wall defect after the completion of primary surgery. The authors' technique of choice is a free TRAM flap for breast reconstruction or a latissimus dorsi flap to repair a chest wall defect.

 ## ROLE OF RADIATION THERAPY IN LOCALLY ADVANCED BREAST CANCER

Comprehensive irradiation is an effective therapy to eliminate occult deposits of tumor in local and regional tissues after surgical removal of macroscopic tumor. Patients with stage III breast cancer have a 30% to 50% risk of local-regional recurrence when surgery or radiation is used as the sole local treatment (21,24,32,34,133,134). This level of risk indicates the need to administer radiation therapy after a total mastectomy and certainly after breast-preserving surgery (see also Chapters 37 and 47). For operable stage III breast cancer, the postoperative administration of chemotherapy and radiotherapy resulted in improved local control and overall survival rates, compared to the use of either adjuvant treatment alone (9). Advanced regional nodal involvement, poor response to chemotherapy, ER-negative tumors, extracapsular tumor, and involvement of the skin or nipple are associated with particularly high locoregional recurrence rates (135). For local-regional treatment to be effective, it must encompass all the volumes at risk, and it must eliminate any tumor cells therein. For LABC, this means treating the entire soft tissue of the chest wall, including any residual breast tissue, the surrounding skin, the connective tissue, and the regional lymphatics. Most local recurrences occur on the chest wall, followed in order of frequency by the axillary and supraclavicular chain and, infrequently, the internal mammary chain. Failure in the dissected axilla is unusual, provided no gross disease remains (136). In the presence of known residual disease, higher doses of RT are required, with the consequent increase in acute and long-term complications. For this reason, if there is residual disease after induction chemotherapy, the authors prefer a surgical excision, particularly for disease that is larger than 1 cm, followed by radiotherapy.

Usually, at the M.D. Anderson Cancer Center the chest wall is treated with tangential fields of 6-MeV photons, although electrons may be used for treatment of patients with favorable anatomic configurations. CT planning is highly desired, but intensity modulated radiation therapy should be used only with caution because of the limitations of current planning software to accurately model the dose in thin chest walls. In locally advanced breast cancers the internal mammary chain will contain tumor in more than 25% of patients subjected to internal mammary chain dissection (137). Thus, an adjacent, matching electron beam field is typically used to treat the lymph nodes of the internal mammary chain. With this technique, the left ventricle can be completely excluded from the irradiated volume, and a maximum of 2 to 3 cm of lung is treated (Fig. 61.3). Alternatively, a series of electron beam fields can be used to

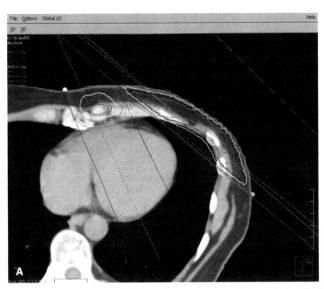
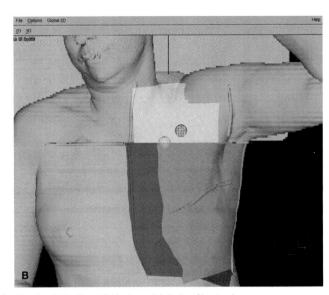

FIGURE 61.3.   A: Left postmastectomy radiotherapy isodose distribution. Use of multiple adjacent fields allows minimization of heart and lung volume. **B:** Left postmastecomy radiotherapy field projections.

treat the chest wall and internal mammary nodes. The undissected lymphatics of the axillary apex and supraclavicular fossa are treated with low-energy photons or electrons. This field may frequently need to be expanded in patients with advanced presentations (especially if known supraclavicular adenopathy has been documented) to cover all regions at risk (138). A 50 Gy dose is delivered in 25 fractions, followed by a boost to the chest wall, to a total dose of at least 60 Gy. Areas of initial nodal involvement not removed at surgery are also treated to 50 Gy followed by electron boosts to the site of original disease to achieve a total dose of 60 Gy for a complete response and 66 Gy for minimal residual disease. At these higher doses, care should be employed to avoid sensitive structures like spinal cord or brachial plexus. Combined-modality therapy offers excellent local control to 90% or more of those with stage IIIB or IIIC breast cancer who have no gross residual disease, and an even higher proportion of those with stage IIIA disease (35). However, if any part of the multidisciplinary treatment strategy is suboptimal, it compromises the efficacy of the entire program. Patients with clinical stage II breast cancer at the time of diagnosis and four or more positive lymph nodes after NACT should also receive postmastectomy RT; however, it is uncertain whether patients with three or fewer positive nodes after chemotherapy need RT.

Unfortunately, a small minority of patients with advanced breast cancer will not respond to initial therapy. These patients present a difficult management problem because of tumor ulceration, necrosis and superinfection, or regional consequences in the neck or brachial plexus. Radiotherapy, with or without concurrent chemotherapy, is an important tool to provide local symptom palliation for these individuals.

SEQUENCING TREATMENT MODALITIES

There are many possible ways to combine or sequence the therapeutic modalities used for breast cancer. The high incidence of distant metastases in patients with LABC makes the early introduction of systemic therapy imperative. Whether simultaneous chemotherapy and radiotherapy result in improved local and distant control compared to sequential administration of chemotherapy and radiotherapy remains to be established (139,140). Therefore, most combined-modality strategies for inoperable LABC start with induction chemotherapy, usually

with an anthracycline- and taxane-containing multidrug regimen. The extensive experience the authors' group has acquired over the past three decades suggests that induction chemotherapy followed by surgical resection, adjuvant chemotherapy, and consolidation radiotherapy is a well tolerated, safe, and effective sequence of therapies for patients with LABC (35). In recent years, the authors have modified this sequence slightly on the basis of two important observations: the first, that the ability to monitor response (or lack of response) to systemic chemotherapy helps guide treatment. If there is no response, or progression of the tumor is demonstrated, the treatment being used can be stopped so that additional toxicity can be avoided and another non–cross-resistant chemotherapy regimen can be introduced. The second observation indicates that both responders and nonresponders to NACT benefit from a fixed crossover to another non–cross-resistant regimen (81). Therefore, the authors now administer all chemotherapy before surgical resection and consistently use two chemotherapy regimens in sequence: FAC and a taxane-containing regimen. The authors and others have documented an increase in overall and pathologic complete response rates with this approach and have reduced the percentage of patients with primary resistance to NACT (53,78,81,82). Whether this increase in response is related to longer duration of chemotherapy or to the introduction of a second chemotherapy regimen has not been fully defined, although the limited data that exist seem to support the second explanation. Increased frequency and quality of objective responses is usually associated with down-staging, thus facilitating the surgical procedure and sometimes allowing breast-conserving surgery, even in patients with LABC. Whether administering all chemotherapy before surgery is better than administering some before and some after surgery has not been definitely established. The only large, prospective trial where these two approaches could be compared was NSABP B-27. In this study there was a trend favoring giving all chemotherapy up front, although this difference was not definitive. Since B-27 included only operable breast cancer, the relevance of these results to LABC is uncertain. It can also be stated that there is no apparent superiority (be it conceptual or empirical) to administering some chemotherapy before and reserving some for postoperative administration.

The addition of trastuzumab to the preoperative treatment of patients with *ERBB2*-positive breast cancer has further increased overall and complete response rates (43). The contribution of

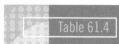

| Table 61.4 | SELECTION CRITERIA FOR BREAST-PRESERVING SURGERY AFTER NEOADJUVANT CHEMOTHERAPY |

Patient desires breast-conserving therapy
Availability of radiotherapy
Family and/or social support systems available
Resolution of skin edema
Healing of skin ulceration
Residual solitary tumor size of <5 cm
No skin or chest-wall fixation
No collagen vascular disease
No extensive intra-mammary lymphatic invasion
Absence of extensive suspicious microcalcifications
No known evidence of multicentricity
Clear surgical margins

trastuzumab to locoregional control remains to be fully assessed after ongoing studies mature. Adjuvant endocrine therapy should be administered to all patients with hormone receptor–positive breast cancer.

There are multiple patient and tumor characteristics that must be considered in the process of selecting candidates for breast-conserving therapy (Table 61.4). Age, histologic type, tumor differentiation, surgical margins, and availability of familial and social support systems are other factors variously considered for this purpose. There are very few absolute contraindications to breast-conserving therapy, although each of the factors listed may increase moderately the risk of recurrence within the breast. Although these criteria can be used for patients treated with induction chemotherapy, they were originally derived from patients with early (stages I and II) breast cancer. Selection of patients with LABC for breast-conserving therapy should be done with caution and implemented only by groups with experience in combined-modality therapy. The authors' institutional criteria to select patients for breast-conserving surgery after NACT or endocrine therapy are listed on Table 61.4. All criteria must be fulfilled before breast-conserving surgery is offered.

The radiotherapeutic technique for breast conservation in patients with LABC is particularly challenging because the target volume extends beyond the intact breast to include the regional lymphatics. This involves the use of multiple adjacent fields. Ideally, the use of noncoplanar beams with precise matching techniques is used when photon fields abut one another. Typically, the breast and undissected lymphatics will be treated to a dose of 50 Gy in 25 fractions over 5 weeks' time, followed by a 10-Gy boost to the tumor bed, which had been marked intraoperatively with clips. In patients with LABC down-staged with systemic therapy, the authors' current practice is to design treatment fields on the basis of the original extent of disease.

 ## TOLERANCE AND TOXICITY

Combined modality regimens have been well tolerated, and no increase in surgical complications has been reported (141). Over the past decade the authors have elected to administer all chemotherapy (usually eight to nine cycles, or 24 to 27 weeks) before the surgical intervention. The expected acute toxic effects of combination chemotherapy are observed with the same frequency and intensity as in the postoperative adjuvant setting (40,82). In studies with simultaneous radiotherapy and chemotherapy, a slight increase in hematologic toxicity and enhancement of acute radiation effects (erythema, moist desquamation) have been reported (140). Simultaneous administration of chemotherapy (especially anthracycline-containing

regimens) and radiotherapy impairs to some extent the cosmetic results of breast-conserving therapy. Although some impairment of cosmesis is also observed with the sequential use of chemotherapy and radiotherapy, this effect is not clinically important for most patients (142). For patients with left breast cancer, synergistic cardiac toxicity is a danger with simultaneous anthracycline and RT (143,144). Sequential administration of chemotherapy and radiotherapy, a modification in radiotherapy techniques, and careful attention to the total dose of anthracycline minimize the risk of cardiac toxicity. The administration of doxorubicin by 48- or 96-hour continuous infusion schedules, the use of a cardiac protector (such as dexrazoxane), or use of a less cardiotoxic anthracycline (epirubicin or a liposome-encapsulated anthracycline) also reduces the risk of cardiac toxicity substantially (145).

 ## SURVIVAL EFFECTS OF COMBINED MODALITY STRATEGIES

The bulk of the information regarding the multidisciplinary treatment of stage III and LABC was obtained from open (uncontrolled) phase II trials; therefore, the effects of the various components of these treatments on survival are tentative at best, and definitive conclusions might not be reached. For patients with inoperable stage III or inflammatory breast cancer, it is highly unlikely that randomized trials including a control arm without systemic therapy will ever be conducted. The results of phase II trials compare favorably to the outcomes of historical control series, or literature controls, suggesting higher 5- and 10-year survival rates, especially for the worst prognostic subgroups (12,140) or for patients with supraclavicular lymph node involvement (35,146), and patients with T4 primary lesions. Figure 61.4A shows the disease-free survival of patients with stages II, IIIA, and IIIB treated at this institution with induction chemotherapy followed by surgery, radiotherapy, and adjuvant chemotherapy, with a maximum follow-up now exceeding 20 years. Figure 61.4B shows the overall survival curves from the same three groups of patients. The median relapse-free and overall survival times for patients with stages II and IIIA breast cancer treated with combined-modality therapy at the authors' institution have not been reached at 240 months. This is in contrast with a median relapse-free survival of 102 months for similar stage IIIA patients treated with surgery and radiotherapy at the authors' institution in earlier years. Similarly, the median overall survival has not been reached for patients with stages II and IIIA breast cancer treated with chemotherapy, surgery, and radiotherapy, whereas it was 140 months for patients treated without systemic therapy. It is generally accepted that patients with stage III breast cancer treated with local therapy followed by postoperative adjuvant chemotherapy have a significant relapse-free (6,7,9,10,147) and overall survival advantage over those treated with only local therapy. The results of randomized trials comparing induction (or preoperative) chemotherapy with postoperative chemotherapy suggest that the two approaches are therapeutically equivalent (40,148–152) (Table 61.5).

No randomized trials comparing preoperative to postoperative systemic therapy have been conducted in patients with LABC. However, two large randomized clinical trials have compared neoadjuvant and postoperative adjuvant chemotherapy in patients with operable breast cancer (40,151,152) (Table 61.5). In both studies, the chemotherapy regimen given before or after surgery was the same. In both studies, the relapse-free and overall survival curves of the neoadjuvant and adjuvant chemotherapy–treated groups were superimposable. Since both these studies included patients with T3 lesions, it is

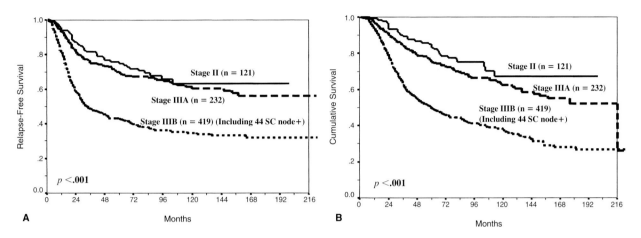

FIGURE 61.4. Patients with stages II, IIIA, and IIIB breast cancer were treated with three to four cycles of induction chemotherapy (FAC; fluorouracil, doxorubicin, and cyclophosphamide), followed by surgical resection, radiotherapy, and adjuvant chemotherapy between 1973 and 1995 on four consecutive prospective clinical trials (n = 772 [including 44 patients with supraclavicular [SC] or infraclavicular lymph node involvement at the time of diagnosis]). **A:** Relapse-free survival curves. **B:** Overall survival curves.

unlikely that the results of similar trials conducted in patients with LABC would be any different.

For decades it was believed that patients with ipsilateral supraclavicular or infraclavicular lymph node involvement at presentation had overt metastatic disease and were incurable. Brito et al. (146) reported in 2001 that such patients treated with combined modality treatments, such as those described for LABC in this chapter, have outcomes similar to other patients with LABC, and that 32% survive without evidence of recurrence or progression for 10 years or longer. As a result of that observation and confirmation from other studies, patients with supraclavicular involvement at presentation, but no other evidence of distant metastases, were moved to the stage III category, following the most recent edition of the AJCC staging manual (5).

PROGNOSTIC FACTORS

The ability to predict outcome will change with the efficacy of the treatments used. For LABC treated with regional therapies only, large tumor size, presence of involved axillary lymph nodes, involved supraclavicular lymph nodes, skin edema, inflammatory breast cancer, diffuse primary tumor, and short duration of symptoms were predictive of decreased relapse-free and overall survival rates (13,153,154). Evaluation of the prognostic value of axillary lymph node involvement after induction chemotherapy showed that the number of involved nodes was the best predictor for both relapse and death in a multivariate analysis (155,156). The pathologic nodal subgroups of 0, 1 to 3, 4 to 10, and greater than 10 positive lymph

					Survival (%)	
Author (Reference)	Treatment Program	No. of Patients	Rendered Disease-Free (%)	Median Survival (mos)	3 Yrs	5 Yrs
Rubens et al. (11)	CT → RT[a] → CT	12	67	36	50	NR
	RT[a] → CT	12	75	36	50	NR
McCready et al. (155), Kuerer et al. (156)	S → CT	134	99	NR	87	80
	CT → S	138	99	NR	94	80
Vilcoq et al. (154)	RT → S → CT	190	NA	NR	87	78
	CT → RT → S	200	NA	NR	92	86
Merajver et al. (119)	RT[a]	45	75	42	59	37
	RT[a] → CT	71	50	45	59	37
	CT → RT[a] → CT	3,971	50	61	37	
Balawajder et al. (26)	CT → RT[a] → CT	59	51	34	NA	33
	RT[a] → CT	60	42	24	NA	32
Jacquillat et al. (157)	CT → S	760	100	NR	90	80
	S → CT	763	100	NR	90	80
Jacquillat et al. (158)	CT → S	350	100	NR	90	85
	S → CT	348	100	NR	87	82

Table 61.5 SURVIVAL OF PATIENTS WITH STAGE II OR III BREAST CANCER AFTER COMBINED MODALITY PROGRAMS BASED ON INDUCTION CHEMOTHERAPY FOLLOWED BY LOCAL TREATMENT. RESULTS OF RANDOMIZED TRIALS

NR, not reached; NA, not available; S, surgery; RT, radiotherapy; CT, chemotherapy; H, hormone therapy.
[a]Low-dose radiotherapy, probably inadequate for optimal local control.

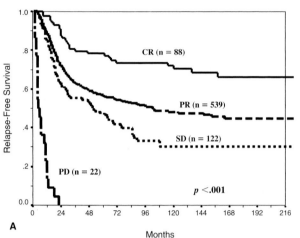
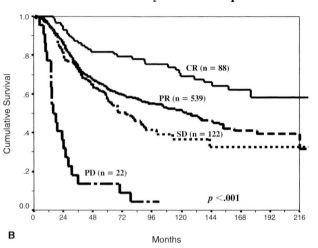

FIGURE 61.5. Clinical response to induction chemotherapy (n = 771; response could not be evaluated in one patient). **A:** Correlation with relapse-free survival. **B:** Correlation with overall survival. CR, complete response; PR, partial response; SD, stable disease; PD, progressive disease.

nodes after induction chemotherapy predicted a prognostic distribution similar to that found in previously untreated patients. Other important and independent factors found in this study by multivariate analysis were clinical tumor stage at presentation, clinical response to induction chemotherapy (Fig. 61.5), and menopausal status. Other investigators have reported clinical response to induction chemotherapy, or its surrogate, histologically detected extent of residual disease, as an important prognostic indicator (157,158).

Response (and especially complete response) to induction chemotherapy was reported to occur significantly more often in patients with poorly differentiated tumors in some (39,157,159) but not all (37,160) reported series. Response rates were also higher in patients with hormone receptor–negative tumors (161,162). Provocative data from pilot studies suggested that responses were more common in patients with aneuploid tumors and in those with high proliferative fraction (163,164). The results of retrospective analyses of randomized clinical trials have suggested that tumors that overexpress the Erbb2 oncoprotein might be relatively resistant to the CMF (cyclophosphamide, methotrexate, and 5-fluorouracil) combination and to hormonal therapy with tamoxifen (165). Another analysis suggested that higher doses of doxorubicin might be more effective in this same group (166). Preliminary reports suggest that p53 overexpression is associated with poorer prognosis and relative resistance to chemotherapy, whereas bcl2 overexpression would be a predictor of good prognosis but resistance to chemotherapy (167). The results of all these studies should be confirmed prospectively before these molecular markers are adopted to select optimal systemic therapy.

Other studies have assessed the prognostic importance of various factors in terms of relapse-free and overall survival. Initial TNM stage, clinical tumor size, clinical nodal stage, and histologic grade have been shown to correlate with both end points in univariate analyses (28,30,35,37,149). In multivariate analyses, histologic or nuclear grade, both clinical and surgical nodal stages, initial tumor size, and response to induction chemotherapy were significant predictors of disease-free survival (35,153,155), whereas tumor size, nodal status, grade, and response to induction chemotherapy correlated with overall survival (35,153,155). The most important predictor of

outcome in the authors' institutional experience is pathologic complete response, defined as complete absence of residual invasive cancer in the surgical specimen, including the axillary lymph nodes (Fig. 61.6).

Local control is related to response to NACT and to initial stage of the disease (Fig. 61.7). Although the authors' initial clinical trials dictated that a mastectomy should be performed if the tumor was (or became) operable, their more recent clinical trials offered the option of breast-conserving surgery if down-staging was of sufficient magnitude. The authors' experience confirms that if selection criteria are strictly followed, optimal local control can be obtained after NACT and breast-conserving surgery.

PROSPECTS FOR THE FUTURE

Much progress has been made in the management of locally advanced breast cancer, but much remains to be accomplished. The taxanes (paclitaxel, nab-paclitaxel, and docetaxel) have been effectively incorporated into the management of metastatic breast cancer, and multiple reports suggest that they contribute to the curative regimens in locally advanced and early breast cancer. Anthracycline–taxane combinations are effective in locally advanced breast cancer. Vinorelbine is highly effective and an accepted part of the management of metastatic breast cancer. New cytotoxic agents, with demonstrated antitumor efficacy against metastatic breast cancer, were developed recently: gemcitabine, capecitabine, liposomal doxorubicin preparations, and several antifols have also shown modest activity, in the 20% to 45% range (168), in metastatic breast cancer, and clinical investigation is ongoing in the neoadjuvant and adjuvant setting. Ixabepilone, the first agent of the epothilone family, was recently approved by the U.S. Food and Drug Administration in view of substantial antitumor activity in metastatic breast cancer, including taxane-resistant tumors, and the epothilones are being tested in the neoadjuvant setting (169).

Although progress in the development of cytotoxic agents continues, there is increased emphasis on the development of molecularly targeted therapy. Trastuzumab (Herceptin), a

Relapse-Free Survival by Pathologic Response

Overall Survival by Pathologic Response

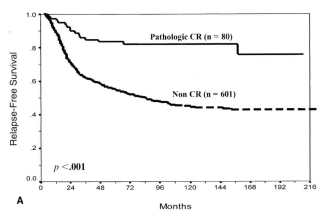
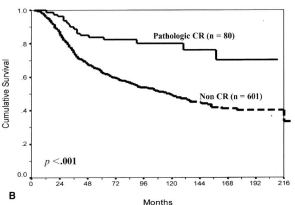

FIGURE 61.6. Pathologic complete response (CR) (n = 681; 91 patients did not have surgical resection). A: Correlation with relapse-free survival. **B:** Correlation with overall survival.

monoclonal antibody against the extracellular domain of the Erbb2 oncoprotein, demonstrated clear-cut antitumor activity in patients with *ERBB2*-amplified (or overexpressed) metastatic breast cancer (170) and resulted in significant prolongation of overall survival in combination with chemotherapy in randomized clinical trials (171,172). The results of six multicenter, randomized clinical trials of trastuzumab used in the adjuvant setting have been reported or published (173–177). In patients with *ERBB2*-positive primary breast cancer, the addition of trastuzumab to chemotherapy reduces the annual odds of recurrence by about 50% and the annual odds of death by one-third. The addition of trastuzumab to NACT of patients with *ERBB2*-positive operable or locally advanced breast cancer led

to significant increases in the proportion of patients achieving a pathological complete remission, in some cases as high as 65%. Another *ERBB2*-directed agent, lapatinib (a small molecule tyrosine kinase inhibitor), was also reported to have important clinical activity in metastatic and locally advanced breast cancer (178). This drug is active in trastuzumab-resistant metastatic breast cancer and improved the activity of capecitabine in a randomized trial. Additional studies testing lapatinib in the neoadjuvant and adjuvant settings are ongoing. Progress in antiangiogenic treatment indicates that bevacizumab (a monoclonal antibody that targets vascular endothelial growth factor) and sunitinib (a small molecule tyrosine kinase inhibitor) have single-agent activity in breast cancer,

Local Failure by Clinical Staging Censored at Recurrence

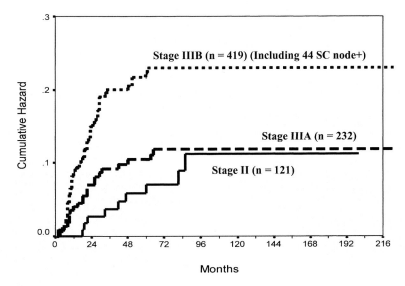

IIIB & II Hazard Ratio = 0.354   *p* =.004

IIIB & III A Hazard Ratio = 0.492   *p* =.003

FIGURE 61.7. Cumulative rate of local-regional recurrence as first event by clinical stage (n = 772). Patients who developed distant metastases without local-regional recurrence were censored at the time of the metastases.

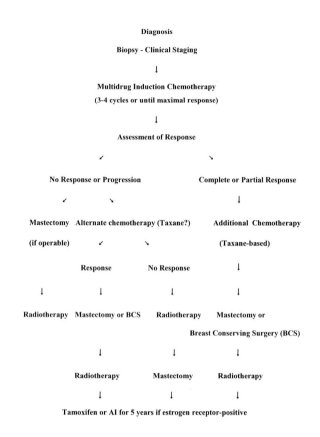

Diagnosis

Biopsy - Clinical Staging

↓

Multidrug Induction Chemotherapy
(3-4 cycles or until maximal response)

↓

Assessment of Response

No Response or Progression   Complete or Partial Response

↓

Mastectomy   Alternate chemotherapy (Taxane?)   Additional Chemotherapy

(if operable)   (Taxane-based)

Response   No Response   ↓

↓   ↓   ↓   ↓

Radiotherapy   Mastectomy or BCS   Radiotherapy   Mastectomy or

                                          Breast Conserving Surgery (BCS)

↓   ↓   ↓

Radiotherapy   Mastectomy   Radiotherapy

↓   ↓   ↓

Tamoxifen or AI for 5 years if estrogen receptor-positive

FIGURE 61.8. Flow diagram for the treatment of patients with locally advanced breast cancer. AI, avomatose inhibitor.

and both are under evaluation in adjuvant and neoadjuvant studies in association with chemotherapy. As molecular therapeutics develops, further multiple new agents are expected to be incorporated into the management strategy of primary breast cancer (179).

The efficacy of sequential local and systemic treatments in combined modality therapy for locally advanced breast cancer makes these approaches the standard of care for these high-risk groups of patients (Fig. 61.8). Using these approaches as a platform, ongoing trials assess the efficacy of limited surgery, both breast-conserving surgery and sentinel lymph node biopsy, in patients with LABC. Ongoing work is testing several modifications of radiotherapy technique to minimize toxicity without compromising outcome. There is renewed interest in assessing the contribution of neoadjuvant endocrine therapy in the multidisciplinary approach to LABC. There is need for developing more effective predictive markers for response to systemic therapy. Candidate approaches under investigation include genomics and proteomics.

The prevention of LABC might be the most effective treatment. Since the end of the 19th century, the frequency of LABC decreased from almost 100% of newly diagnosed breast cancer to less than 5% today in populations with access to mammographic screening. Public and professional education emphasizing the importance of early diagnosis, the identification of women at high risk, and the systematic use of screening mammography might further decrease the frequency with which this high-risk lesion is found and contribute to the cure of breast cancer.

Combined-modality therapy that includes induction chemotherapy permits optimal local control with less radical surgical and radiotherapeutic intervention. By down-staging

primary and regional tumors, breast conservation becomes an option for some patients. In addition, the multidisciplinary management of stage III and locally advanced breast cancer provides an excellent biologic model to assess the effects of systemic therapy on the primary tumor. On the clinical side, this provides *in vivo* assessment of response and the possibility of modifying subsequent therapy on the basis of this evaluation of response.

These successful strategies, developed for the management of LABC, are being successfully applied to earlier primary breast cancer.

MANAGEMENT SUMMARY

- Combined-modality treatment, starting with neoadjuvant or induction chemotherapy, represents the treatment of choice for patients with stage IIIB breast cancer. Effective and well-tolerated induction chemotherapy regimens are shown in Tables 61.1 and 61.2. A similar approach is feasible in lower stage LABC.
- Patients who receive neoadjuvant systemic therapy should be closely monitored. Repeat imaging after the final dose of chemotherapy is indicated to assess response and determine appropriate surgical therapy. During treatment, if there is clinical uncertainty regarding disease progression, imaging may aid in the evaluation. The authors' institution's policy is to use a detailed physical examination and the imaging modality that most clearly demonstrates the extent of disease at baseline for monitoring every 6 to 12 weeks of therapy.
- Close and continued interaction between all therapeutic and diagnostic specialists is needed to deliver optimal therapy.
- In the authors' experience, mammography combined with physical examination is optimal for monitoring breast masses for the majority of patients. Physical examination combined with sonography is appropriate to monitor the axilla and the supraclavicular and internal mammary chains. At many centers, MRI is becoming increasingly helpful to monitor response to therapy.
- Any third-generation chemotherapy regimen that has been validated in the adjuvant setting can be appropriately used in the neoadjuvant setting.
- Treatment must be individualized depending on the response to (and the tolerance for) therapy.
- Trastuzumab (or lapatinib) should be administered to all patients with *ERBB2*-positive cancers.
- Endocrine therapy should be administered to all patients with estrogen or progesterone receptor–positive cancers.
- Carefully selected patients with LABC can undergo breast-conserving therapy.
- Patients with LABC treated with mastectomy should receive postmastectomy radiation therapy, regardless of response.
- The use and type of immediate breast reconstruction should involve consideration of whether it might compromise subsequent radiation therapy.

References

1. Hortobagyi GN, de la Garza Salazar J, Pritchard K, et al. The global breast cancer burden: variations in epidemiology and survival. *Clin Breast Cancer* 2005; 6(5):391–401.
2. Seidman H, Gelb SK, Silverberg E, et al. Survival experience in the Breast Cancer Detection Demonstration Project. *CA Cancer J Clin* 1987;37:258–290.
3. Zeichner GI, Mohar BA, Ramirez UMT. Epidemiologia del Cancer de Mama en el Instituto Nacional de Cancerologia (1989–1990). *Cancerologia* 1993;39:1825–1830.
4. Moisa FC, Lopez J, Raymundo C. Epidemiologia del carcinoma del seno mamario en Latino America. *Cancerologia* 1989;35:810–814.

5. Anonymous. Part VII. Breast. In: Green FL, Page DL, Fleming ID, et al., eds. *AJCC cancer staging handbook*. 6th ed. New York: Springer, 2002:255–281.
6. Effects of adjuvant tamoxifen and of cytotoxic therapy on mortality in early breast cancer: an overview of 61 randomized trials among 28,896 women. Early Breast Cancer Trialists' Collaborative Group. *N Engl J Med* 1988;319:1681–1692.
7. Polychemotherapy for early breast cancer: an overview of the randomised trials. Early Breast Cancer Trialists' Collaborative Group. *Lancet* 1998;352:930–942.
8. Rivkin SE, Green S, Metch B, et al. Adjuvant CMFVP versus melphalan for operable breast cancer with positive axillary nodes: 10-year results of a Southwest Oncology Group Study. *J Clin Oncol* 1989;7:1229–1238.
9. Grohn P, Heinonen E, Klefstrom P, et al. Adjuvant postoperative radiotherapy, chemotherapy, and immunotherapy in stage III breast cancer. *Cancer* 1984;54: 670–674.
10. Bartelink H, Rubens RD, van der Schueren E, et al. Hormonal therapy prolongs survival in irradiated locally advanced breast cancer: a European Organization for Research and Treatment of Cancer phase III trial. *J Clin Oncol* 1997;15: 207–215.
11. Rubens RD, Bartelink H, Engelsman E, et al. Locally advanced breast cancer: the contribution of cytotoxic and endocrine treatment to radiotherapy. *Eur J Cancer* 1989;25:667–678.
12. Hortobagyi GN, Buzdar AU. Locally advanced breast cancer: a review including the M.D. Anderson experience. In: Ragaz J, Ariel IM, eds. *High-risk breast cancer*. Berlin: Springer-Verlag, 1991:382–415.
13. Haagensen CD, Stout AP. Carcinoma of the breast: criteria of inoperability. *Am Surg* 1943;118:859–866.
14. Zucali R, Uslenghi C, Kenda R, et al. Natural history and survival of inoperable breast cancer treated with radiotherapy and radiotherapy followed by radical mastectomy. *Cancer* 1976;37:1422–1431.
15. Harris JR, Sawicka J, Gelman R, et al. Management of locally advanced carcinoma of the breast by primary radiation therapy. *Int J Radiat Oncol Biol Phys* 1983;9:345–349.
16. Baclesse F. Roentgen therapy as the sole method of treatment of cancer of the breast. *Am J Roentgenol* 1949;62:311–319.
17. Fletcher GH, Montague ED. Radical irradiation of advanced breast cancer. *Am J Roentgenol* 1965;93:573–584.
18. Spanos WJ, Montague ED, Fletcher FH. Late complications of radiation only for advanced breast cancer. *Int J Radiat Oncol Biol Phys* 1980;6:1473–1476.
19. Symmans WF, Ayers M, Clark EA, et al. Total RNA yield and microarray gene expression profiles from fine needle aspiration biopsy and core needle biopsy samples of breast carcinoma. *Cancer* 2003;97(12):2960–2971.
20. Fisher B, Ravdin RD, Ausman RK, et al. Surgical adjuvant chemotherapy in cancer of the breast: results of a decade of cooperative investigation. *Ann Surg* 1968;168:337–356.
21. DeLena M, Zucali R, Viganotti G, et al. Combined chemotherapy-radiotherapy approach in locally advanced (T3b-T4) breast cancer. *Cancer Chemother Pharmacol* 1978;1:53–59.
22. Hortobagyi GN, Blumenschein GR, Tashima CK, et al. Multidisciplinary treatment of locally advanced (stage III) breast cancer. *Proc Am Soc Clin Oncol* 1978;19: 361(abst C-219).
23. Rubens RD, Sexton S, Tong D, et al. Combined chemotherapy and radiotherapy for locally advanced breast cancer. *Eur J Cancer* 1980;16:351–356.
24. Valagussa P, Zambetti M, Bignami PD, et al. T3b-T4 breast cancer: factors affecting results in combined modality treatment. *Clin Exp Metastasis* 1983;1: 191–202.
25. Pawlicki M, Skolyszewski J, Brandys A. Results of combined treatment of patients with locally advanced breast cancer. *Tumori* 1983;69:249–253.
26. Balawajder I, Antich PP, Boland J. An analysis of the role of radiotherapy alone and in combination with chemotherapy and surgery in the management of advanced breast cancer. *Cancer* 1983;51:574–580.
27. Conte PF, Alama A, Bertelli G, et al. Chemotherapy with estrogenic recruitment and surgery in locally advanced breast cancer: clinical and cytokinetic results. *Int J Cancer* 1987;40:490–494.
28. Swain SM, Sorace RA, Bagley CS, et al. Neoadjuvant chemotherapy in the combined modality approach of locally advanced nonmetastatic breast cancer. *Cancer Res* 1987;47:3889–3894.
29. Jacquillat C, Baillet F, Weil M, et al. Results of a conservative treatment combining induction (neoadjuvant) and consolidation chemotherapy, hormonotherapy, and external and interstitial irradiation in 98 patients with locally advanced breast cancer (IIIA-IIIB). *Cancer* 1988;61:1977–1982.
30. Burn I. Primary endocrine therapy of advanced local breast cancer. *Rev Endocr Relat Cancer* 1985;16:5–8.
31. DeLena M, Varini M, Zucali R, et al. Multimodal treatment for locally advanced breast cancer: results of chemotherapy-radiotherapy versus chemotherapy-surgery. *Cancer Clin Trials* 1981;4:229–236.
32. Hortobagyi GN, Blumenschein GR, Spanos W, et al. Multimodal treatment of locoregionally advanced breast cancer. *Cancer* 1983;51:763–768.
33. Hobar PC, Jones RC, Schouten J, et al. Multimodality treatment of locally advanced breast carcinoma. *Arch Surg* 1988;123:951–955.
34. Perloff M, Lesnick GJ, Korzun A, et al. Combination chemotherapy with mastectomy or radiotherapy for stage III breast carcinoma: a cancer and leukemia group B study. *J Clin Oncol* 1988;6:261–269.
35. Hortobagyi GN, Ames FC, Buzdar AU, et al. Management of stage III primary breast cancer with primary chemotherapy, surgery, and radiation therapy. *Cancer* 1988;62:2507–2516.
36. Cocconi G, di Blasio B, Bisagni G, et al. Neoadjuvant chemotherapy or chemotherapy and endocrine therapy in locally advanced breast carcinoma. *Am J Clin Oncol* 1990;13:226–232.
37. Touboul E, Lefranc JP, Blondon J, et al. Multidisciplinary treatment approach to locally advanced non-inflammatory breast cancer using chemotherapy and radiotherapy with or without surgery. *Radiother Oncol* 1992;25:167–175.
38. Gardin G, Rosso R, Campora E, et al. Locally advanced non-metastatic breast cancer: analysis of prognostic factors in 125 patients homogeneously treated with a combined modality approach. *Eur J Cancer* 1995;31A:1428–1433.
39. Kemeny F, Vadrot J, d'Hubert E, et al. Evaluation histologique e radioclinique de l'effet de la chimiotherapie premiere sur les cancers non inflammatoires du sein. *Cahiers Cancer* 1991;3:705–714.
40. Fisher B, Brown A, Mamounas E, et al. Effect of preoperative chemotherapy on local-regional disease in women with operable breast cancer: findings from National Surgical Adjuvant Breast and Bowel Project B-18. *J Clin Oncol* 1997; 15:2483–2493.
41. Lippman ME, Sorace RA, Bagley CS, et al. Treatment of locally advanced breast cancer using primary induction chemotherapy with hormonal synchronization followed by radiation therapy with or without debulking surgery. *NCI Monogr* 1986;1:153–159.
42. Schwartz GF, Cantor RI, Biermann WA. Neoadjuvant chemotherapy before definitive treatment for stage III carcinoma of the breast. *Arch Surg* 1987;122: 1430–1434.
43. Mehra R, Burtness B. Antibody therapy for early-stage breast cancer: trastuzumab adjuvant and neoadjuvant trials. *Expert Opin Biol Ther* 2006;6: 951–962.
44. Cocconi G, di Blasio B, Alberti G, et al. Problems in evaluating response of primary breast cancer to systemic therapy. *Breast Cancer Res Treat* 1984;4: 309–313.
45. Fornage BD, Toubas O, Morel M. Clinical, mammographic, and sonographic determination of preoperative breast cancer size. *Cancer* 1987;60:765–771.
46. Herrada J, Iyer RB, Atkinson EN, et al. Relative value of physical examination, mammography, and breast sonography in evaluating the size of the primary tumor and regional lymph node metastases in women receiving neoadjuvant chemotherapy for locally advanced breast carcinoma. *Clin Cancer Res* 1997;3: 1565–1569.
47. Drew PJ, Kerin MJ, Mahapatra T, et al. Evaluation of response to neoadjuvant chemoradiotherapy for locally advanced breast cancer with dynamic contrast-enhanced MRI of the breast. *Eur J Surg Oncol* 2001;27:617–620.
48. Feldman LD, Hortobagyi GN, Buzdar AU, et al. Pathological assessment of response to induction chemotherapy in breast cancer. *Cancer Res* 1986;46: 2578–2581.
49. Mankoff DA, Dunnwald LK, Gralow JR, et al. Blood flow and metabolism in locally advanced breast cancer: relationship to response to therapy. *J Nucl Med* 2002;43:500–509.
50. Gradishar WJ, Wedam SB, Jahanzeb M, et al. Neoadjuvant docetaxel followed by adjuvant doxorubicin and cyclophosphamide in patients with stage III breast cancer. *Ann Oncol* 2005;16(8):1297–1304.
51. von Minckwitz G, Costa SD, Eiermann W, et al. Maximized reduction of primary breast tumor size using preoperative chemotherapy with doxorubicin and docetaxel. *J Clin Oncol* 1999;17:1999–2005.
52. Miller KD, McCaskill-Stevens W, Sisk J, et al. Combination versus sequential doxorubicin and docetaxel as primary chemotherapy for breast cancer: a randomized pilot trial of the Hoosier Oncology Group. *J Clin Oncol* 1999;17:3033–3037.
53. Valero V, Esteva FJ, Sahin AA, et al. Phase II trial of neoadjuvant chemotherapy with docetaxel and doxorubicin, surgery, adjuvant CMF, and radiotherapy +/– tamoxifen in locally advanced breast cancer. *Breast Cancer Res Treat* 2000; 64(1):69(abst 253).
54. Luporsi E, Vanlemmens L, Coudert B. 6 cycles of FEC 100 vs. 6 cycles of epirubicin-docetaxel as neoadjuvant chemotherapy in operable breast cancer patients: preliminary results of a randomized phase II trial of GIREC S01. *Proc Am Soc Clin Oncol* 2000;19:92a(abst 355).
55. Limentani SA, Erban JK, Sprague KA, et al. Phase II study of doxorubicin and docetaxel as neoadjuvant therapy for women with stage IIB or III breast cancer. *Proc Am Soc Clin Oncol* 2000;19:131a(abst 511).
56. Malhotra V, Dorr VJ, Lyss AP, et al. Neoadjuvant and adjuvant chemotherapy with doxorubicin and docetaxel in locally advanced breast cancer. *Clin Breast Cancer* 2004;5(5):377–384.
57. von Minckwitz G, Costa SD, Raab G, et al. Dose-dense doxorubicin, docetaxel, and granulocyte colony-stimulating factor support with or without tamoxifen as preoperative therapy in patients with operable carcinoma of the breast: a randomized, controlled, open phase IIb study. *J Clin Oncol* 2001;19:3506–3515.
58. Ardavanis A, Pateras C, Pissakas G, et al. A. Sequential epirubicin and docetaxel followed by surgery and postoperative chemo-radiotherapy for locally advanced breast cancer. *Proc Am Soc Clin Oncol* 2001;20:8b(abst 1779).
59. Espinosa, E, Morales S, Borrega P, et al. Docetaxel and high-dose epirubicin as neoadjuvant chemotherapy in locally advanced breast cancer. *Cancer Chemother Pharmacol* 2004;54(6):546–552.
60. Hurley J, Doliny P, Reis I, et al. Docetaxel, cisplatin, and trastuzumab as primary systemic therapy for human epidermal growth factor receptor 2-positive locally advanced breast cancer. *J Clin Oncol* 2006;24(12):1831–1838.
61. Bines J, Vinholes J, del Giglio A, et al. Induction chemotherapy with weekly docetaxel (Taxotere) in unfavorable locally advanced breast cancer. *Proc Am Soc Clin Oncol* 2001;20:33b(abst 1881).
62. Estevez LG, Cuevas JM, Anton A, et al. Weekly docetaxel as neoadjuvant chemotherapy for stage II and III breast cancer: efficacy and correlation with biological markers in a phase II, multicenter study. *Clin Cancer Res* 2003;9(2): 686–692.
63. Vinholes J, Bouzid K, Salas F, et al. Preliminary results of a multicentre phase III trial of Taxotere and doxorubicin versus 5-fluorouracil, doxorubicin and cyclophosphamide in patients with unresectable locally advanced breast cancer. *Proc Am Soc Clin Oncol* 2001;20:26a(abst 101).
64. Evans T, Gould A, Foster E, et al. Phase III randomised trial of Adriamycin (A) and docetaxel (D) versus A and cyclophosphamide (C) as primary medical therapy in women with breast cancer: an ACCOG study. *Proc Am Soc Clin Oncol* 2002;21:35a(abst 136).
65. Ganem G, Tubiana-Hulin M, Fumoleau P, et al. Phase II trial combining docetaxel and doxorubicin as neoadjuvant chemotherapy in patients with operable breast cancer. *Ann Oncol* 2003;14(11):1623–1628.
66. Baltali E, Altundag MK, Onat DA, et al. Neoadjuvant chemotherapy with Taxotere-epirubicin-5-fluorouracil (TEF) in local-regionally advanced breast cancer: a preliminary report. *Tumori* 2002;88:474–477.
67. Moliterni A, Tarenzi E, Capri G, et al. Pilot study of primary chemotherapy with doxorubicin plus paclitaxel in women with locally advanced or operable breast cancer. *Semin Oncol* 1997;24[Suppl 17]:10–14.
68. Akerley W, Sikov WM, Cummings F, et al. Weekly high-dose paclitaxel in metastatic and locally advanced breast cancer: a preliminary report. *Semin Oncol* 1997; 24:87–90.
69. Buzdar AU, Singletary SE, Theriault RL, et al. Prospective evaluation of paclitaxel versus combination chemotherapy with fluorouracil, doxorubicin, and cyclophosphamide as neoadjuvant therapy in patients with operable breast cancer. *J Clin Oncol* 1999;17:3412–3417.

70. Dieras V, Fumoleau P, Romieu G, et al. Randomized parallel study of doxorubicin plus paclitaxel and doxorubicin plus cyclophosphamide as neoadjuvant treatment of patients with breast cancer. *J Clin Oncol* 2004;22(24):4958–4965.
71. Ezzat AA, Ibrahim EM, Ajarim DS, et al. Phase II study of neoadjuvant paclitaxel and cisplatin for operable and locally advanced breast cancer: analysis of 126 patients. *Br J Cancer* 2004;90(5):968–974.
72. Taillibert S, Antoine E, Mousseau M, et al. Preliminary results of a multicenter clinicobiological phase II study combining epirubicin, cyclophosphamide and paclitaxel as induction chemotherapy for women with stage II and III breast cancer. *Proc Am Soc Clin Oncol* 2001;20:15b(abst 1809).
73. Goubely-Brewer YP, Serin D, Kirscher S, et al. C. Neoadjuvant concurrent chemoradiotherapy with paclitaxel (Taxol) and 5-fluorouracil (5-FU) followed by 5-FU-epirubicin-cyclophosphamide (FEC) and surgery in patients with locally advanced breast cancer (LABC). *Proc Am Soc Clin Oncol* 2001;20:17b(abst 1815).
74. Cristofanilli M, Gonzalez-Angulo AM, Buzdar AU, et al. Paclitaxel improves the prognosis in estrogen receptor negative inflammatory breast cancer: the M.D. Anderson Cancer Center experience. *Clin Breast Cancer* 2004;4(6):415–419.
75. Burstein HJ, Harris LN, Gelman R, et al. Preoperative therapy with trastuzumab and paclitaxel followed by sequential adjuvant doxorubicin/cyclophosphamide for HER2 overexpressing stage II or III breast cancer: a pilot study. *J Clin Oncol* 2003;21(1):46–53.
76. Fumoleau P, Tubiana-Hulin M, Romieu G, et al. A randomized phase II study of 4 or 6 cycles of Adriamycin/Taxol (paclitaxel) as neoadjuvant treatment of breast cancer. *Breast Cancer Res Treat* 2001;69(3):298(abst 508).
77. Gogas H, Papadimitriou C, Kalofonos HP, et al. Neoadjuvant chemotherapy with a combination of pegylated liposomal doxorubicin (Caelyx) and paclitaxel in locally advanced breast cancer: a phase II study by the Hellenic Cooperative Oncology Group. *Ann Oncol* 2002;13:1737–1742.
78. Green MC, Buzdar AU, Smith T, et al. Weekly paclitaxel improves pathologic complete remission in operable breast cancer when compared with paclitaxel every-3-week. *J Clin Oncol* 2005;23(25):5983–5992.
79. Untch M, Konecny G, Ditsch N, et al. Dose-dense sequential epirubicin-paclitaxel as preoperative treatment of breast cancer: results of a randomised AGO study. *Proc Am Soc Clin Oncol* 2002;21:34a(abst 133).
80. Gianni L, Baselga J, Eiermann W, et al. Feasibility and tolerability of sequential doxorubicin/paclitaxel followed by cyclophosphamide, methotrexate, and fluorouracil and its effects on tumor response as preoperative therapy. *Clin Cancer Res* 2005;11(24 Pt 1):8715–8721.
81. Smith IC, Heys SD, Hutcheon AW, et al. Neoadjuvant chemotherapy in breast cancer: significantly enhanced response with docetaxel. *J Clin Oncol* 2002;20:1456–1466.
82. Rastogi P, Anderson SJ, Bear HD, et al. Preoperative chemotherapy: updates of National Surgical Adjuvant Breast and Bowel Project Protocols B-18 and B-27. *J Clin Oncol* 2008;26(5):778–785.
83. Hutcheon AW, Heys SD, Miller ID, et al. Improvements in survival in patients receiving primary chemotherapy with docetaxel for breast cancer: a randomised controlled trial. *Breast Cancer Res Treat* 2001;69(3):298(abst 506).
84. Mohsin SK, Weiss HL, Gutierrez MC, et al. Neoadjuvant trastuzumab induces apoptosis in primary breast cancers. *J Clin Oncol* 2005;23(11):2460–2468.
85. Gennari R, Menard S, Fagnoni F, et al. Pilot study of the mechanism of action of preoperative trastuzumab in patients with primary operable breast tumors overexpressing HER2. *Clin Cancer Res* 2004;10(17):5650–5655.
86. Limentani SA, Brufsky AM, Erban JK, et al. Phase II study of neoadjuvant docetaxel, vinorelbine, and trastuzumab followed by surgery and adjuvant doxorubicin plus cyclophosphamide in women with human epidermal growth factor receptor 2–overexpressing locally advanced breast cancer. *J Clin Oncol* 2007;25(10):1232–1238.
87. Buzdar AU, Valero V, Ibrahim NK, et al. Neoadjuvant therapy with paclitaxel followed by 5-fluorouracil, epirubicin, and cyclophosphamide chemotherapy and concurrent trastuzumab in human epidermal growth factor receptor 2–positive operable breast cancer: an update of the initial randomized study population and data of additional patients treated with the same regimen. *Clin Cancer Res* 2007;13(1):228–233.
88. Wenzel C, Hussian D, Bartsch R, et al. Preoperative therapy with epidoxorubicin and docetaxel plus trastuzumab in patients with primary breast cancer: a pilot study. *J Cancer Res Clin Oncol* 2004;130(7):400–404.
89. Gianni L, Semiglazov V, Manikhas GM, et al. Neoadjuvant trastuzumab plus doxorubicin, paclitaxel and CMF in locally advanced breast cancer (NOAH trial): feasibility, safety and antitumor effects. Proceedings of the 2007 Breast Cancer Symposium, September 7–8, 2007, San Francisco, California, p. 131 (abst 144).
90. Kennedy BJ, Kelley RM, White G, et al. Surgery as an adjunct to hormone therapy of breast cancer. *Cancer* 1957;10:1055–1075.
91. Preece PE, Wood RA, Mackie CR, et al. Tamoxifen as initial sole treatment of localised breast cancer in elderly women: a pilot study. *Br Med J Clin Res Educ* 1982;284:869–870.
92. Bradbeer JW, Kyngdon J. Primary treatment of breast cancer in elderly women with tamoxifen. *Clin Oncol* 1983;9:31–34.
93. Bergman L, van Dongen JA, van Ooijen B, et al. Should tamoxifen be a primary treatment choice for elderly breast cancer patients with locoregional disease? *Breast Cancer Res Treat* 1995;34:77–83.
94. Bates T, Riley DL, Houghton J, et al. Breast cancer in elderly women: a Cancer Research Campaign Trial comparing treatment with tamoxifen and optimal surgery with tamoxifen alone. *Br J Surg* 1991;78:591–594.
95. Kenny FS, Robertson JFR, Ellis IO, et al. Long-term follow-up of elderly patients randomized to primary tamoxifen or wedge mastectomy as initial therapy for operable breast cancer. *Breast* 1998;7:335–339.
96. Goss PE, Strasser K. Aromatase inhibitors in the treatment and prevention of breast cancer. *J Clin Oncol* 2001;19:881–894.
97. Ellis MJ, Coop A, Singh B, et al. Letrozole is more effective neoadjuvant endocrine therapy than tamoxifen for ErbB-1– and/or ErbB-2–positive, estrogen receptor-positive primary breast cancer: evidence from a phase III randomized trial. *J Clin Oncol* 2001;19:3808–3816.
98. Sperber F, Weinstein Y, Sarid D, et al. Preoperative clinical, mammographic and sonographic assessment of neoadjuvant chemotherapy response in breast cancer. *Israel Med Assoc J* 2006;8:342–346.
99. Chagpar AB, Middleton LP, Sahin AA, et al. Accuracy of physical examination, ultrasonography, and mammography in predicting residual pathologic tumor size in patients treated with neoadjuvant chemotherapy. *Ann Surg* 2006;243:257–264.
100. Kriege M, Brekelmans CTM, Boetes C, et al. Efficacy of MRI and mammography for breast-cancer screening in women with a familial or genetic predisposition. *N Engl J Med* 2004;351:427–437.
101. Warner E, Plewes DB, Hill KA, et al. Surveillance of BRCA1 and BRCA2 mutation carriers with magnetic resonance imaging, ultrasound, mammography and clinical breast examination. *JAMA* 2004;292:1317–1325.
102. MARIBS study group. Screening with magnetic resonance imaging and mammography of a UK population at high familial risk of breast cancer: a prospective multicenter cohort study. *Lancet* 2005;365:1769–1778.
103. Kuhl CK, Schmutzler RK, Leutner CC, et al. Breast MRI imaging screening in 192 women proved or suspected to be carriers of a breast cancer susceptibility gene. Preliminary results. *Radiology* 2000;215:267–279.
104. Esserman L, Hylton N, Yassa L, et al. Utility of magnetic resonance imaging in the management of breast cancer: evidence for improved preoperative staging. *J Clin Oncol* 1999;17:110–119.
105. Julius T, Kemp SE, Kneeshaw PJ, et al. MRI and conservative treatment of locally advanced breast cancer. *Eur J Surg Oncol* 2005;31:1129–1134.
106. Bleicher RJ, Morrow M. MRI and breast cancer: role in detection, diagnosis, and staging. *Oncology* 2007;21:1521–1528.
107. Levine EA, Freimanis RI, Perrier NC, et al. Positron emission mammography: initial clinical results. *Ann Surg Oncol* 2003;10:86–91.
108. Rosen EL, Turkington TG, Soo MS, et al. Detection of primary breast carcinoma with a dedicated large-field-of-view FDG PET mammography device: initial experience. *Radiology* 2005;234:527–534.
109. Li D, Yao Q, Li L, et al. Correlation between hybrid 18F-FDG PET/CT and apoptosis induced by neoadjuvant chemotherapy in breast cancer. *Cancer Biol Ther* 2007;6(9):1442–1448.
110. Hortobagyi GN. Drug therapy: treatment of breast cancer. *N Engl J Med* 1998;339(14):974–984.
111. Zucali R, Kenda R. Small size T4 breast cancer: natural history and prognosis. *Tumori* 1981;67:225–230.
112. Bonadonna G, Veronesi U, Brambilla C, et al. Primary chemotherapy to avoid mastectomy in tumors with diameters of three centimeters or more. *J Natl Cancer Inst* 1990;82:1539–1545.
113. Olson JE, Gray R, Sponzo R, et al. Primary chemotherapy for nonresectable locally advanced breast cancer: 8 year results of an ECOG trial. *Breast Cancer Res Treat* 1990;16:148(abst 15).
114. Papaioannou A, Lissaios B, Vasilaros S, et al. Pre- and postoperative chemoendocrine treatment with or without postoperative radiotherapy for locally advanced breast cancer. *Cancer* 1983;51:1284–1290.
115. Pouillart P, Palangie T, Jouve M, et al. Essai pilote de chimiotherapie neo-adjuvante dans le cancer du sein. In: Jacquillat C, Weil M, Khayat D, eds. *Neo-adjuvant chemotherapy*. Paris: Libbey, 1986:257–267.
116. Schaake-Koning C, van der Linden EH, Hart G, et al. Adjuvant chemo- and hormonal therapy in locally advanced breast cancer: a randomized clinical study. *Int J Radiat Oncol Biol Phys* 1985;11:1759–1763.
117. Cance WG, Carey LA, Calvo BF, et al. Long-term outcome of neoadjuvant therapy for locally advanced breast carcinoma: effective clinical downstaging allows breast preservation and predicts outstanding local control and survival. *Ann Surg* 2002;236:295–302.
118. Clark J, Rosenman J, Cance W, et al. Extending the indications for breast-conserving treatment to patients with locally advanced breast cancer. *Int J Radiat Oncol Biol Phys* 1998;42:345–350.
119. Merajver SD, Weber BL, Cody R, et al. Breast conservation and prolonged chemotherapy for locally advanced breast cancer: the University of Michigan experience. *J Clin Oncol* 1997;15:2873–2881.
120. Schwartz GF. Breast conservation following induction chemotherapy for locally advanced breast cancer: a personal experience. *Breast J* 1996;2:78–82.
121. Kuerer HM, Singletary SE, Buzdar AU, et al. Surgical conservation planning after neoadjuvant chemotherapy for stage II and operable stage III breast carcinoma. *Am J Surg* 2001;182:601–608.
122. Chen AM, Meric-Bernstam F, Hunt KK, et al. Breast conservation after neoadjuvant chemotherapy. *Cancer* 2005;103(4):689–695.
123. Nadeem R, Chagla LS, Harris O, et al. Tumour localization with a metal coil before the administration of neo-adjuvant chemotherapy. *Breast* 2005;14:403–407.
124. Shen J, Valero V, Buchholz TA, et al. Effective local control and long-term survival in patients with T4 locally advanced breast cancer treated with breast conservation therapy. *Ann Surg Oncol* 2004;11:854–860.
125. Guth U, Wight E, Schotzau A, et al. Breast carcinoma with noninflammatory skin involvement (T4b). *Cancer* 2005;104:1862–1870.
126. Dash N, Chafin S, Johnson R, et al. Usefulness of tissue marker clips in patients undergoing neoadjuvant chemotherapy for breast cancer. *AJR Am J Roentgenol* 1999;173:911–917.
127. Eideken BS, Fornage BD, Bedi DG, et al. U.S.-guided implantation of metallic markers for permanent localization of the tumor bed in patients with breast cancer who undergo preoperative chemotherapy. *Radiology* 1999;213:895–900.
128. Jain A, Haisfield-Wolfe ME, Lange J, et al. The role of ultrasound-guided fine-needle aspiration of axillary nodes in the staging of breast cancer. *Ann Surg Oncol* 2007;15(2):462–471.
129. Fowble B, Gray R, Gilchrest K, et al. Identification of a subgroup of patients with breast cancer and histologically positive axillary nodes receiving adjuvant chemotherapy who may benefit from postoperative radiotherapy. *J Clin Oncol* 1988;6:107–117.
130. Tran NV, Chang DW, Gupta A, et al. Comparison of immediate and delayed free TRAM flap breast reconstruction in patients receiving postmastectomy radiation therapy. *Plast Reconstr Surg* 2001;108:78–82.
131. Foster RD, Hansen SL, Esserman LJ, et al. Safety of immediate transverse rectus abdominis myocutaneous breast reconstruction for patients with locally advanced disease. *Arch Surg* 2005;140:196–200.
132. Motwani SB, Strom EA, Schechter NR, et al. The impact of immediate breast reconstruction on the technical delivery of postmastectomy radiotherapy. *Int J Radiat Oncol Biol Phys* 2006;66(1):76–82.
133. Aisner J, Morris D, Elias G, et al. Mastectomy as an adjuvant to chemotherapy for locally advanced or metastatic breast cancer. *Arch Surg* 1982;117:882–887.
134. Buchholz TA, Tucker SL, Masullo L, et al. Predictors of local-regional recurrence after neoadjuvant chemotherapy and mastectomy without radiation. *J Clin Oncol* 2002;20(1):17–23.

135. Huang EH, Tucker SL, Strom EA, et al. Predictors of locoregional recurrence in patients with locally advanced breast cancer treated with neoadjuvant chemotherapy, mastectomy, and radiotherapy. *Int J Radiat Oncol Biol Phys* 2005; 62(2):351–357.

136. Strom EA, Woodward WA, Katz A, et al. Clinical investigation: regional nodal failure patterns in breast cancer patients treated with mastectomy without radiotherapy. *Int J Radiat Oncol Biol Phys* 2005;63(5):1508–1513.

137. Huang O, Wang L, Shen K, et al. Breast cancer subpopulation with high risk of internal mammary lymph nodes metastasis: analysis of 2,269 Chinese breast cancer patients treated with extended radical mastectomy. *Breast Cancer Res Treat* 2008;107(3):379–387.

138. Reed VK, Cavalcanti JL, Strom EA, et al. Risk of subclinical micrometastatic disease in the supraclavicular nodal bed according to the anatomic distribution in patients with advanced breast cancer. *Int J Radiat Oncol Biol Phys* 2008;71(2): 435–440.

139. Piccart MJ, de Valeriola D, Paridaens R, et al. Six-year results of a multimodality treatment strategy for locally advanced breast cancer. *Cancer* 1988;62: 2501–2506.

140. Bedwinek JM, Ratkin GA, Philpott GW, et al. Concurrent chemotherapy and radiotherapy for nonmetastatic, stage IV breast cancer. *Am J Clin Oncol* 1983;6: 159–165.

141. Broadwater JR, Edwards MJ, Kuglen C, et al. Mastectomy following preoperative chemotherapy. *Ann Surg* 1991;213:126–129.

142. Recht A, Come SE. Sequencing of irradiation and chemotherapy for early-stage breast cancer. *Oncology* 1994;8:19–37.

143. Buzzoni R, Bonadonna G, Valagussa P, et al. Adjuvant chemotherapy with doxorubicin plus cyclophosphamide, methotrexate, and fluorouracil in the treatment of resectable breast cancer with more than three positive nodes. *J Clin Oncol* 1991;9:2134–2140.

144. Valagussa P, Moliterni A, Zambetti M, et al. Long-term sequelae from adjuvant chemotherapy. In: Senn HJ, Goldhirsch A, Gelber RD, Thurlimann B, eds. *Adjuvant therapy of breast cancer: IV. Recent results cancer research*. 127th ed. Berlin: Springer, 1993:248–255.

145. Hortobagyi GN, Frye D, Buzdar AU, et al. Decreased cardiac toxicity of doxorubicin administered by continuous intravenous infusion in combination chemotherapy for metastatic breast cancer. *Cancer* 1989;63:37–45.

146. Brito RA, Valero V, Buzdar AU, et al. Long-term results of combined-modality therapy for locally advanced breast cancer with ipsilateral supraclavicular metastases: the University of Texas M.D. Anderson Cancer Center experience. *J Clin Oncol* 2001;19:628–633.

147. Rainer H, Arbeitskreis fur Perioperative Chemotherapie. Prospective randomized clinical trial of primary therapy in breast cancer stages T3/4, N+/–, M0: chemo- vs. radiotherapy. In: Salmon SE, ed. *Adjuvant therapy of cancer VI*. Philadelphia: WB Saunders, 1990:232–239.

148. Scholl SM, Fourquet A, Asselain B, et al. Neoadjuvant versus adjuvant chemotherapy in premenopausal patients with tumors considered too large for breast conserving surgery: preliminary results of a randomised trial: S6. *Eur J Cancer* 1994;30A:645–652.

149. Mauriac L, Durand M, Avril A, et al. Effects of primary chemotherapy in conservative treatment of breast cancer patients with operative tumors larger than 3 centimeters: results of a randomized trial in a single center. *Ann Oncol* 1991; 2:347–354.

150. Mauriac L, MacGrogan G, Avril A, et al. Neoadjuvant chemotherapy for operable breast carcinoma larger than 3 cm: a unicentre randomized trial with a 124-month median follow-up. Institut Bergonie Bordeaux Groupe Sein (IBBGS). *Ann Oncol* 1999;10:47–52.

151. Fisher B, Bryant J, Wolmark N, et al. Effect of preoperative chemotherapy on the outcome of women with operable breast cancer. *J Clin Oncol* 1998;16:2672–2685.

152. van der Hage JA, van de Velde CJ, Julien JP, et al. Preoperative chemotherapy in primary operable breast cancer: results from the European Organization for Research and Treatment of Cancer trial 10902. *J Clin Oncol* 2001;19:4224–4237.

153. Stewart JH, King RJB, Winter PJ, et al. Oestrogen receptors, clinical features and prognosis in stage III breast cancer. *Eur J Cancer Clin Oncol* 1982;18:1315–1320.

154. Vilcoq JR, Fourquet A, Jullien D, et al. Prognostic significance of clinical nodal involvement in patients treated by radical radiotherapy for a locally advanced breast cancer. *Am J Clin Oncol* 1984;7:625–628.

155. McCready DR, Hortobagyi GN, Kau SW, et al. The prognostic significance of lymph node metastases after preoperative chemotherapy for locally advanced breast cancer. *Arch Surg* 1989;124:21–25.

156. Kuerer HM, Newman LA, Fornage BD, et al. Role of axillary lymph node dissection after tumor downstaging with induction chemotherapy for locally advanced breast cancer. *Ann Surg Oncol* 1998;5(8):673–680.

157. Jacquillat C, Weil M, Baillet F, et al. Results of neoadjuvant chemotherapy and radiation therapy in the breast-conserving treatment of 250 patients with all stages of infiltrative breast cancer. *Cancer* 1990;66:119–129.

158. Jacquillat C, Weil M, Auclerc G, et al. Neo-adjuvant chemotherapy in the conservative management of breast cancers—study on 205 patients. In: Jacquillat C, Weil M, Khayat D, eds. *Neo-adjuvant chemotherapy*. London: John Libbey, 1986:197–206.

159. Abu-Farsakh H, Sneige N, Atkinson N, et al. Pathologic predictors of tumor response to preoperative chemotherapy in patients with locally advanced breast carcinoma. *Breast J* 1995;1:96–101.

160. Belembaogo E, Feillel V, Chollet P, et al. Neoadjuvant chemotherapy in 126 operable breast cancers. *Eur J Cancer* 1992;28A:896–900.

161. Colleoni M, Minchella I, Mazzarol G, et al. Response to primary chemotherapy in breast cancer patients with tumors not expressing estrogen and progesterone receptors. *Ann Oncol* 2000;11:1057–1059.

162. Colleoni M, Gelber S, Coates AS, et al. Influence of endocrine-related factors on response to perioperative chemotherapy for patients with node-negative breast cancer. *J Clin Oncol* 2001;19:4141–4149.

163. Spyratos F, Brifford M, Tubiana-Hulin M, et al. Sequential cytopunctures during preoperative chemotherapy for primary breast carcinoma. *Cancer* 1992;69: 470–475.

164. Remvikos Y, Jouve M, Beuzeboc P, et al. Cell cycle modifications of breast cancers during neoadjuvant chemotherapy: a flow cytometry study on fine needle aspirates. *Eur J Cancer* 1995;29A:1843–1848.

165. Yamauchi H, Stearns V, Hayes DF. When is a tumor marker ready for prime time? a case study of c-erbB-2 as a predictive factor in breast cancer. *J Clin Oncol* 2001;19:2334–2356.

166. Muss HB, Thor AD, Berry DA, et al. c-erbB-2 expression and response to adjuvant therapy in women with node-positive early breast cancer. *N Engl J Med* 1994;330:1260–1266.

167. Hortobagyi GN, Hayes DF, Pusztai L. Integrating newer science into breast cancer prognosis and treatment: a review of current molecular predictors and profiles. ASCO 2002 Annual Meeting Summaries, 2002;192–201.

168. Hamilton A, Hortobagyi G. Chemotherapy: what progress in the last 5 years? *J Clin Oncol* 2005;23(8):1760–1775.

169. Hussar DA. New drugs: doripenem, raltegravir, and ixabepilone. *J Am Pharm Assoc* 2008;48(1):108–111.

170. Baselga J, Tripathy D, Mendelsohn J, et al. Phase II study of weekly intravenous recombinant humanized anti-p185 HER2 monoclonal antibody in patients with HER2/neu-overexpressing metastatic breast cancer. *J Clin Oncol* 1996;14: 737–744.

171. Slamon DJ, Leyland-Jones B, Shak S, et al. Use of chemotherapy plus a monoclonal antibody against HER2 for metastatic breast cancer that overexpresses HER2. *N Engl J Med* 2001;344:783–792.

172. Marty M, Cognetti F, Maraninchi D, et al. Randomized phase II trial of the efficacy and safety of trastuzumab combined with docetaxel in patients with human epidermal growth factor receptor 2–positive metastatic breast cancer administered as first-line treatment: the M77001 study group. *J Clin Oncol* 2005;23(19): 4265–4274.

173. Perez EA, Hortobagyi GN. Ongoing and planned adjuvant trials with trastuzumab. *Semin Oncol* 2000;27:26–32.

174. Piccart-Gebhart MJ, Procter M, Leyland-Jones B, et al. Trastuzumab after adjuvant chemotherapy in HER2-positive breast cancer. *N Engl J Med* 2005;353(16): 1659–1672.

175. Romond EH, Perez EA, Bryant J, et al. Trastuzumab plus adjuvant chemotherapy for operable HER2-positive breast cancer. *N Engl J Med* 2005;353(16): 1673–1684.

176. Smith I, Procter M, Gelber RD, et al. 2-year follow-up of trastuzumab after adjuvant chemotherapy in HER2-positive breast cancer: a randomised controlled trial. *Lancet* 2007;369(9555):29–36.

177. Joensuu H, Kellokumpu-Lehtinen PL, Bono P, et al. Adjuvant docetaxel or vinorelbine with or without trastuzumab for breast cancer. *N Engl J Med* 2006;354(8): 809–820.

178. Dhillon S, Wagstaff AJ. Lapatinib. *Drugs* 2007;67(14):2101–2108.

179. Craft BS, Hortobagyi GN, Moulder SL. Adjuvant biologic therapy for breast cancer. *Cancer J* 2007;13(3):156–161.

Sofia D. Merajver, Maria D. Iniesta, and Michael S. Sabel

Inflammatory breast cancer (IBC) is a rapidly progressive and distinct form of breast cancer that warrants special clinical (1–3) and scientific consideration (4). It must be diagnosed aggressively and promptly to avert progression and death. Although relatively rare in incidence, accounting for 1% to 5% of breast cancers in the United States, it represents a much larger burden of morbidity and mortality (5). The clinical presentation of IBC is characterized by a profound dermatotropism, which is manifested by erythema, *peau d'orange*, or fine dimpling of the skin, and warmth. This chapter will review the definition of IBC, its diagnosis and treatment, and major efforts under way to understand the genetic basis for this particularly aggressive phenotype of breast cancer.

DEFINITION

IBC is a form of locally advanced breast cancer characterized by the following clinical features, which arise rapidly, typically over weeks, less than 6 months, not years: discoloration ranging from red to purple and affecting at least one third of the breast, thickening or fine dimpling (*peau d'orange*), edema or warmth, and a palpable ridge present at the margin of induration (2) (Fig. 62.1). Other features that may accompany IBC, but are not part of its definition, include scattered erythematous, nonblanchable nodules over the chest, breast pain, and ecchymoses; a distinct mass cannot be palpated in 50% of the cases (6). Biopsy of the affected skin may reveal clusters of tumor cells within dermal lymphatics, but this helpful pathologic feature is neither required nor sufficient for a diagnosis of IBC, which is made so far on physical examination. Tumor emboli within dermal lymphatics may be observed, albeit rarely, in non-IBC breast cancers of any stage, so these are not sufficient for a diagnosis of IBC, but they are a helpful feature.

IBC accounts for 1% to 5% of all breast cancer cases in the United States (5,7), for 10% in Pakistan (8), and, surprisingly, for 17% of cases in the Gharbeia province (in the Nile delta) in Egypt (9). Among patients selected for presenting with locally advanced disease, IBC is far more prevalent. In studies of locally advanced breast cancer (LABC) at the University of Michigan and at the M.D. Anderson Cancer Center, the rates of IBC were 40% (10) and 24% (11) of LABC cases, respectively. Therefore, IBC should be considered as a distinct epidemiologic entity within LABC.

The average age at diagnosis of IBC in the United States is younger for both white (57 years for IBC, compared with 62 years for non-IBC) and African American women (52 years for IBC, compared with 57 years for non-IBC). Surveillance, Epidemiology, and End Results (SEER) data indicate an improvement in 3-year survival for white patients with IBC (from 32% to 42%) between the periods 1975 to 1979 and 1988 to 1992, a greater increase in survival than that for non-IBC, which was observed to improve from 80% to 85% in the same period (5). Review of SEER data between 1992 and 1999 clearly reaffirmed IBC as a distinct epidemiologic entity, separate from non-IBC stage III breast cancer (12). In addition to finding worse survival rates for IBC, a higher proportion of estrogen receptor (ER)–negative tumors, and a younger age of onset, this study found that the age-specific incidence rates of IBC flattened after age 50, in contrast to those of non-IBC stage III, which continued to increase after age 50 (12). This difference in age-specific incidence trends suggests that early premenopausal

hormonal status or environmental exposures in early life may play an important role in IBC. Pregnancy and lactation do not appear to increase the risk of IBC versus non-IBC, and IBC does not occur commonly in families, although anecdotal reports of familial aggregation exist.

DIAGNOSIS, DIFFERENTIAL DIAGNOSIS, AND STAGING

The diagnosis of IBC is made when the history and physical examination document the rapid onset (within 6 months, not years) of the characteristic skin features, and a biopsy of the breast or of the affected skin shows adenocarcinoma of the breast, most commonly invasive ductal carcinoma. Physical examination often reveals palpable or matted axillary lymph nodes, as nearly all women with IBC have nodal involvement. IBC-like features render a tumor T-stage T4d, one of the subcategories of stage IIIB.

Evaluation of the patient with IBC involves a diagnostic mammogram, which is nearly always abnormal (6), and breast ultrasound to help define in detail the disease-associated features that may be followed to assess response during subsequent therapy. In addition, it is imperative that the original tumor bed be adequately marked with a radio-opaque clip or marker, to guide access to it in the future, in case the patient achieves complete clinical or radiologic response.

Mammographic findings associated with a mass or dominant opacity are present in 80% to 90% of patients, whereas 10% to 15% present with only mammographic signs of inflammation, such as skin thickening, stromal coarsening, increased vascularity, or diffuse opacity. These data refute the misconception that IBC does not present with an abnormal mammogram or that mammographic abnormalities in the setting of locally advanced breast cancer favor non-IBC stage III breast cancer. However, the radiographic evaluation of the breast in IBC can be challenging; because of the diffuse increase in density often observed in patients with IBC, the initial evaluation of calcifications may be difficult (13,14). Ultrasonography can be very helpful in the evaluation of regional nodal status. In a recent study regional axillary nodal disease was diagnosed in 93% of IBC patients by this modality (15), while previous series have reported lower detection rates (16). Moreover, the proportion of patients with metastasis in infraclavicular, supraclavicular, and internal mammary nodes was 50%, 33%, and 13%, respectively. The most common findings with sonography are skin thickening, the presence of axillary adenopathies, increased vascularity, and architectural distortion. In some cases, ultrasonography plays an important role in the localization of masses prior to biopsy. The role of magnetic resonance imaging (MRI) in IBC is currently being studied. Its potential roles are in diagnosis, staging, and monitoring response to treatment. Yang et al. (15) have reported that MRI revealed a primary breast lesion in 100% of the cases as compared to 96% with combined positron emission tomography and computed tomography (PET-CT), 95% with ultrasonography, and 80% with mammography. Although those results are promising, the utility of MRI is not yet firmly established. It is important to mention that among the technical limitations of MRI, difficulties on patient positioning and long duration of the study may cause unacceptable levels of discomfort for some patients;

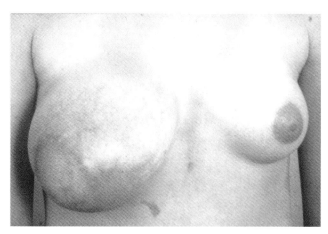

FIGURE 62.1. Clinical presentation of inflammatory breast cancer, characterized by early presentation and a rapid evolution. This image shows a case of 6 weeks of evolution.

analgesia may be required if the potential advantages of the study outweigh the drawbacks. PET has the advantage of identifying the local extent of metabolically active carcinomas, as well as lymph node and distance metastases, all in one procedure. PET appears to be more sensitive than other imaging techniques in the detection of metastasis, but it has a lower specificity, so it is not routinely used but can be helpful in certain situations, such as in establishing eligibility for clinical trials. Currently, the role of PET in breast cancer is complementary to well-established techniques, such as mammography, in difficult cases (17). PET-CT is an emerging technique with the advantage of contributing both anatomic and functional information in the same image (18). Preliminary results (15) suggest that PET-CT is accurate at demonstrating locoregional disease and distant metastases.

At diagnosis approximately 25% of patients with IBC will have distant metastases (19), so that radiologic examinations aimed at detecting the presence of distant metastatic disease should be performed as indicated by history or physical examination findings; in the patient who is asymptomatic outside of the breast, these studies should include bone scan and computer-assisted tomography of the chest, abdomen, and head, with contrast. Blood samples with liver enzymes and alkaline phosphatase could be used to guide detection of liver or bone metastases.

Patients with infection, trauma, and, rarely, other neoplastic diseases may present with features similar to those of IBC. Infectious mastitis is most common in lactating women or in the immediate postweaning period. In contrast to IBC, mastitis often presents with fever, leukocytosis, and systemic malaise. Most importantly, antibiotics tend to be of immediate benefit in mastitis and breast abscess, but not in IBC. Ductal ectasia, trauma, or venous stasis (20) may be accompanied by a self-limited and localized inflammation, which can be very similar to early IBC, but these conditions improve in a period of days to 1 to 2 weeks, whereas IBC does not. Leukemia, small cell carcinoma of the breast, and metastatic cancer can affect the skin overlying the breast. In these cases, histologic evaluation and immunohistochemistry of a skin or breast biopsy lead to the correct diagnosis.

Inflammatory noninfectious diseases such as atopic dermatitis, psoriasis, eczema, idiopathic granulomatous mastitis (21), systemic lupus erythematosus, and vasculitis may also mimic IBC, but they seldom involve just the breast, and a skin biopsy is usually diagnostic. When the clinical diagnosis is in doubt, treatment with steroids for conditions affecting only or primarily the breast should not be undertaken without first obtaining a biopsy, as the clinical manifestations of IBC may temporarily improve slightly with steroids, thereby delaying appropriate antineoplastic treatment, with possible dire consequences to the patient.

Recurrent breast cancer can present in the remaining or contralateral breast, on the mastectomy or lumpectomy scar, or on the chest wall with IBC-like features, and a biopsy often reveals widespread invasion of the cancer in an infiltrative pattern into the dermis and epidermis, a feature that is relatively rare in primary IBC. These cases are termed IBC-like recurrences or secondary IBC, but they do not constitute true IBC, which is a designation that applies only to a primary lesion. It is important to emphasize that locally advanced breast cancers neglected for years may have features in common with IBC, but they should not be classified as IBC. In contrast to true IBC, many of these tumors have a large palpable mass, have been growing slowly over many years, and are continuing to progress at a very slow rate.

Although the traditional clinical definition of IBC does not specify a fast rate of progression, epidemiologic studies, clinical research, and molecular markers indicate that IBC, more narrowly defined by the rapidly appearing skin changes, is a distinct subset of LABC. Henceforth, the time course of symptoms to have occurred in a period under 6 months would be part of the definition of IBC. In contrast to non-IBC LABC, IBC has younger age of onset, a worse prognosis, more ER-negative tumors, and concordant overexpression of the RhoC-GTPase oncogene and loss of expression of the *WISP3* gene, increased lymphangiogenesis and angiogenesis, increased expression of chemokines and persistent expression of E-cadherin, among other molecular characteristics (22). Nonetheless, from a practical standpoint, however, given the present state of knowledge, a slow-growing LABC with the characteristic skin changes of IBC may be treated following the guidelines of treatment for IBC. It would be very informative to understand the molecular bases of IBC-like recurrences in comparison to primary IBC.

HISTORICAL PERSPECTIVE ON THE ORIGINS OF COMBINATION THERAPY IN INFLAMMATORY BREAST CANCER

Nearly 100 years after Bell (1) initially described inflammatory breast cancer, the role of surgery in the treatment of this disease remained ill defined. In 1916 Learmonth (23) reviewed 45 cases reported in the literature and could identify only one patient that was disease free after 5 years. On this basis, it was surmised that the best chance for a cure lay with the most radical operation possible, the Halsted radical mastectomy, which included radical removal of the axillary and supraclavicular nodes. However, review of Halsted's (24) experience with radical mastectomy shows that although the majority of cases (>75%) were locally advanced, none fit the description of inflammatory breast cancer. Subsequent reports of attempts to treat IBC by radical mastectomy demonstrated extremely poor results. Each series described the rapid recurrence of disease and a poor outcome. For example, Haagensen (2) reported that of 30 patients with IBC treated by radical mastectomy, the mean survival was only 19 months. There was only one 5-year survivor, who died 68 months after surgery. Treves (25) reported the largest series of patients with IBC of the time who were treated by radical mastectomy (114 patients), with only four patients (3.5%) alive at 5 years. On the basis of these discouraging results and the previous reports in the literature, Treves insightfully concluded that in most patients the disease was disseminated at the time of diagnosis, and that radical mastectomy was contraindicated in the treatment of IBC.

In 1942, when Haagensen and Stout (26) defined the concepts of operable and inoperable breast cancer, they included classic clinical findings of IBC in their criteria of inoperable tumors. Radiotherapy, which to that point had been used primarily for patients who were not candidates for a radical mastectomy, became the primary modality of treatment. Local control rates ranged from 10% to 46% (27,28). Mean survival remained dismal, between 4 and 20 months, with practically no one surviving 5 years (29). In addition, large doses of radiation were necessary to optimize local control. At these dosages, the complications were significant, including skin and chest wall ulceration and fibrosis, rib necrosis or resorption, brachial plexopathy, and lymphedema of the arm (30–32). To improve local control and minimize toxicity, several researchers looked at the combination of surgery and radiotherapy, thereby initiating the modern era of combination therapy for IBC (28,29).

LOCOREGIONAL THERAPY FOR INFLAMMATORY BREAST CANCER

The Role of Surgery in Inflammatory Breast Cancer

Several groups attempted to examine the impact of mastectomy on locoregional control and overall survival, with mixed results. Fields et al. (33) reported on 107 patients with nonmetastatic IBC who were treated with either radiotherapy alone, surgery and radiotherapy, chemotherapy and radiotherapy, or combined modality (chemotherapy, surgery, and radiotherapy). With a median follow-up of 30 months, the group who received chemotherapy, surgery, and radiotherapy, followed by maintenance chemotherapy, had significantly better disease-free and overall survival (37% and 48%, respectively) at 5 years than the other groups. Perez et al. (34) found a significant advantage to the addition of mastectomy to chemotherapy and radiation in local recurrence, disease-free survival (6% vs. 40%), and overall survival (16% vs. 38%). Chevallier et al. (35) reported on combined-modality treatment in 178 patients. In patients who had no supraclavicular lymph node involvement and at least a partial response after chemotherapy, surgery alone compared with radiation alone resulted in an improved median disease-free survival (37.8 months vs. 19 months; $p <.05$). They also noted a trend toward improved overall survival and locoregional recurrence, although these were not statistically significant. In a report of 178 women with IBC treated at the M.D. Anderson Cancer Center, the addition of mastectomy after doxorubicin-based chemotherapy and radiotherapy improved the local recurrence rates from 16% to 36% ($p = .015$) (36). The authors concluded that there is no reason to exclude surgery as locoregional treatment for IBC patients who are suitable candidates. Other studies have failed to demonstrate a disease-free or overall survival advantage to the addition of mastectomy to chemotherapy and radiation.

De Boer et al. (37) reviewed 54 patients at the Royal Marsden Hospital who had responsive or stable disease after chemotherapy. Patients went on to have radiotherapy alone (n = 35) or surgery plus radiotherapy (n = 19). There were no statistically significant differences in disease-free survival, overall survival, or local recurrence rates among the groups. In a randomized trial addressing this question, published with a long-term follow-up analysis, 83 patients with IBC treated with primary chemotherapy were then randomized to radiation alone or surgery alone, and Mourali et al. (38) found no significant differences between the treatment groups after chemotherapy. The authors concluded that the two modalities are complementary and can be used together for local and regional control, but the trial did not specifically address the combination of surgery and radiation therapy as an independent arm.

The majority of the data on locoregional treatment of IBC is retrospective and has several inherent biases. In particular, the selection of radiation, surgery, or both was based primarily on physician preference and rarely on tumor response to chemotherapy. In some cases, patients with a complete clinical response to primary chemotherapy were encouraged to have radiation alone. In other cases the opposite is true, and patients with bulky local-regional disease are selected for radiation only, reserving surgery for patients with less extensive disease. An appropriately designed, prospective, randomized trial would adequately answer the question of the survival value of surgery added to radiotherapy and chemotherapy in IBC.

Although it is not definitely known whether surgery improves disease-free survival and overall survival compared with radiation therapy alone, surgery offers several advantages. Surgery provides important prognostic information regarding the pathologic effectiveness of chemotherapy. The clinical and mammographic evaluation of response to induction chemotherapy for IBC correlates poorly with the amount of residual disease found on pathologic examination of the mastectomy specimen (39–42). There is considerable variability in tumor persistence after initial chemotherapy, and physical examination and imaging methods do not accurately predict the amount of residual tumor (43). The full extent of residual disease evaluated by a mastectomy performed after induction therapy is a useful biologic marker to gauge the extent and aggressiveness of further chemotherapy (41). Surgery results in prompt local tumor control and healing, thereby interrupting chemotherapy only minimally, and the cytoreductive effect of surgery on persisting tumor burden (e.g., for patients who experience a partial response to neoadjuvant chemotherapy) may allow a slightly lower dose of radiation to be delivered to the chest wall.

Although the survival value of surgery in IBC cannot be addressed without a prospective randomized clinical trial, which would be very difficult to carry out, a rational approach to the locoregional control of the patient with IBC can be reached from the available data. At the completion of chemotherapy, patients are considered candidates for modified radical mastectomy based on tumor response and resectability. Complete resolution of the skin inflammation is crucial. Local control is poor following mastectomy in the presence of persistent skin involvement and recurrence can occur rapidly. In a study of mastectomy following chemotherapy by Thoms et al. (40), the local control rate was 33% among nonresponders compared with 68% for partial responders and 89% for patients with a complete clinical response. Other contraindications to surgery include persistent fixed axillary adenopathy or chest wall involvement beyond the pectoralis major muscle. For IBC patients deemed poor candidates for surgery following chemotherapy, radiation should be the next step. If feasible, patients who become resectable following radiation therapy should proceed with mastectomy. In a retrospective analysis of 485 patients with IBC, mastectomy was associated with superior local control following chemotherapy and radiation therapy than among patients treated by chemotherapy and radiation therapy alone (44). However, because this is a retrospective study, selection bias cannot be ruled out, and breast cancer–specific survival was not significantly different. Therefore, the decision to proceed with surgery in this setting should be individualized based on response to chemotherapy, response to radiation, repeat staging for distant metastases, patient comorbidities, and the relative benefits of local control. When a mastectomy is performed after radiation, wound healing is poor and soft tissue coverage of the chest wall using a rotational flap will be necessary.

For patients with IBC who experience a satisfactory response to neoadjuvant chemotherapy and are good candidates for surgery, the next step is typically a modified radical mastectomy. IBC is generally accepted to be a contraindication to breast-conservation therapy, although rare cases of breast conservation for complete pathologic responders have been reported (10,45,46). In spite of the increasing body of evidence on the favorable rates of local control with breast-conservation surgery after neoadjuvant chemotherapy for T1 to T3 tumors (46–49), these series did not include patients with IBC, so the data may not apply to them. Immediate breast reconstruction following a modified radical mastectomy for IBC is controversial but should generally be avoided. Postmastectomy radiation is routine in IBC and can have deleterious effects on both an implant or expander and an autologous flap (50–52). Although some authors have reported the use of immediate reconstruction in IBC, the local recurrence rate was high, particularly in the presence of positive mastectomy margins (53,54). A safer approach is to delay reconstruction until after the completion of therapy. If immediate reconstruction is considered, the use of skin-sparing mastectomies in IBC is absolutely contraindicated.

Another trend in the locoregional management of breast cancer has been the use of sentinel lymph node (SLN) biopsy after neoadjuvant chemotherapy to stage the axilla. Advantages include a more accurate assessment of the response to chemotherapy in the regional nodes and the avoidance of a complete node dissection among patients whose nodal disease has been sterilized. However, concerns have been raised regarding the accuracy of the procedure following chemotherapy. This is particularly true in IBC, where lymphatics blocked by tumor cells would prevent the accurate uptake of either blue dye or radiocolloid in the SLN. In the only study to examine SLN following chemotherapy for IBC, of eight patients undergoing the procedure, two patients (25%) failed to map and two patients (25%) had a false-negative finding (55). In summary, taken together, these data suggest that it is appropriate to offer the IBC patient with a good response to chemotherapy a modified radical mastectomy plus radiotherapy to enhance locoregional control.

The Role of Radiotherapy in Inflammatory Breast Cancer

The use of radiotherapy has been consistently studied in many nonrandomized series in locally advanced breast cancer with IBC patients being included in the cohort. Not all of those studies stratified the patients with regard to IBC status, but overall there is a strong trend toward improved local control rates with radiotherapy (56–58).

A particularly noteworthy trial conducted by the Eastern Cooperative Oncology Group studied 332 women with locally advanced breast cancer who had no progression after six courses of neoadjuvant chemohormonal therapy (58). The women were randomized to receive either surgery alone or surgery plus radiotherapy. After 9 years of follow-up, there were no differences in overall survival between the two treatment arms. However, when analyzing the locoregional failure rates alone, it appeared that those patients who received radiotherapy had a significantly lower local failure rate than those who did not (4% vs. 27%). These data, coupled to randomized trials showing the overall survival advantages of postmastectomy radiotherapy in high-risk breast cancer (59,60), clearly support the use of radiotherapy in IBC based on the high-risk initial stage of the disease.

Although the exact radiotherapy protocol to be used after neoadjuvant therapy in general, and for IBC in particular, is still somewhat variable across institutions, some general recommendations and guidelines can be suggested. IBC patients presenting with a complete pathologic response assessed surgically (i.e., by mastectomy) or by biopsy and axillary lymph node dissection after neoadjuvant chemotherapy should receive radiation to the breast and/or chest wall, supraclavicular area, and/or internal mammary nodes. On the other hand, patients with a partial response to neoadjuvant chemotherapy and no prior staging of the lymph nodes should receive a modified radical mastectomy and comprehensive chest irradiation, which includes radiation to the axillary fields. It is important to emphasize that the patient with IBC should receive radiotherapy, regardless of whether a pathologic complete response to neoadjuvant chemotherapy is achieved.

SYSTEMIC THERAPY FOR INFLAMMATORY BREAST CANCER

Neoadjuvant Therapy for Inflammatory Breast Cancer

Rationale

Given the propensity of IBC to rapidly establish distant metastases, it is clear that metastases are the major determinant of survival in patients with IBC. Moreover, historically local therapies such as surgery or radiation used alone or in combination have proven inadequate in increasing survival presumably because of the great metastatic potential of IBC from its inception. "The hypothesis that micrometastatic systemic disease present at diagnosis in IBC is responsible for the poor survival of these patients led to the use of neoadjuvant chemotherapy with two distinct but related goals: control of growth of metastatic disease and downstaging of the breast and nodal disease to achieve operability or breast conservation" (10).

A prospective, randomized trial performed by investigators from the National Cancer Institute of Milan, Italy, first demonstrated the efficacy of giving chemotherapy up front in the treatment of noninflammatory, locally advanced breast cancer (61). DeLena et al. (49) then applied this approach to 36 patients with IBC. Treatment consisted of chemotherapy, followed by local therapy, with or without maintenance chemotherapy. Maintenance therapy improved disease-free but not overall survival. This work encouraged many investigators to take a more aggressive systemic approach to inflammatory breast cancer, following the pioneering work of the M.D. Anderson Cancer Center group led by G. Hortobagyi (10,11,35,62–68). Overall, the use of anthracycline-based chemotherapy in both the neoadjuvant and consolidation modes resulted in improved local control rates and clinical complete response rates of 70% to 76% and a 5-year overall survival rate of 40%. Because this constitutes a definite improvement, anthracyclines-containing combination regimens are the standard of care for neoadjuvant chemotherapy in IBC.

Neoadjuvant chemotherapy enables the use of the clinical tumor response to guide systemic and local therapy and to estimate prognosis. Because tissue is relatively easily accessible, the potential exists during neoadjuvant chemotherapy to investigate molecular hypotheses that may lead to improved therapies. For the small proportion of patients who will progress during therapy (between 5% and 20%), a more suitable alternative systemic treatment or locoregional therapy can be undertaken promptly, thus avoiding prolonged administration of ineffective therapy. For this distinct advantage of neoadjuvant chemotherapy to be realized, however, it is important that the patient be carefully evaluated by a consistent observer at all sites of known disease, prior to initiating each cycle of chemotherapy. Although neoadjuvant chemotherapy may theoretically promote drug resistance early in treatment, the small proportion of nonresponders in most regimens suggests that

Table 62.1 SUMMARY OF SELECTED STUDIES OF NEOADJUVANT CHEMOTHERAPY FOR INFLAMMATORY BREAST CANCER

Author (Reference)	No. of Patients	Response			Survival %		Median		Survival	
		CCR	CPR	PD + Minor	PCR	PPR	3 yr	5 yr	OS (mos)	DFS (mos)
DeLena et al. (49)	110	15.5	54.5	NA	NA	NA	52.8	NA	NA	NA
Pawlicki et al. (81)	72	1.2	41	15	NA	NA	61.5	NA	NA	NA
Keiling et al. (70)	41	NA	NA	26.8	24.4	48.8	73	NA	NA	44
Fastenberg et al. (62)	63	NA	NA	NA	NA	NA	58	31	43	24
Rouesse et al. (68)	91 (Group A)	41	27	32	NA	NA	NA	(4-yr) 44	38	19
Rouesse et al. (68)	79 (Group B)	54	26	20	NA	NA	NA	(4-yr) 66	NA	43
Jacquillat et al. (82)	66	NA	NA	NA	NA	NA	NA	(4-yr) 62	NA	NA
Maloisel et al. (66)	43	CCR + CPR = 38		12	NA	NA	NA	75	46	NA
Koh et al. (83)	106 (A/B/C)	80/36/72	20/44/28	0/20/0	NA	NA	NA	37/30/48	142	76
Chevallier et al. (71)	45	91	9	0	25.6	NA	NA	NA	NA	NA
Noguchi et al. (84)	28	25	64.3	74.4	NA	NA	NA	59	NA	NA
Swain et al. (67)	56	56	41	0	NA	NA	NA	~20	35.3	23.2
Perloff and Lesnick (85)	14	CCR + PCR = 7	NA	NA		NA	NA	NA	26.9	23.3
Palangie et al. (86)	223	CCR + PCR = 67		7	NA	NA	NA	(5-, 10-yr) 41,32	41	19
Schwartz et al. (45)	30	14	33	33	14	NA	NA	51	NA	NA
Perez et al. (34)	36	61	36	3	28	NA	NA	40 DFS	NA	NA
Merajver et al. (10)	89	52	CPR + PD + minor = 48		30	72	NA	54	NA	29
Harris et al. (72)	54	NA	NA	NA	NA	NA	NA	56	62	NA
Iino et al. (87)	22	NA	NA	NA	NA	NA	NA	35	NA	NA
Cristofanilli et al. (78)	42	7	74	19	14	NA	NA	NA	46	22

CCR, clinical complete response; CPR, clinical partial response; PD, progressive disease; PCR, pathologic complete response; PPR, pathologic partial response; OS, overall survival; DFS, disease-free survival; A, B, or C, groups with different chemotherapy regimens within a study; NA, not available.

this is not a major problem with the use of combination chemotherapy regimens.

Neoadjuvant Regimens for Inflammatory Breast Cancer

The majority of studies of neoadjuvant chemotherapy in stage III breast cancer utilized an anthracycline-based combination regimen anchored by either doxorubicin or epirubicin. Most of the studies are nonrandomized, with a highly variable preponderance of IBC cases. Table 62.1 presents important selected studies, some of which are exclusively or mainly devoted to IBC, and in others, IBC cases are analyzed as a group. Early on it was shown that an anthracycline-containing regimen was superior in response and disease-free survival to nonanthracycline regimens containing antimetabolites such as methotrexate [69].

The response rates to doxorubicin-based neoadjuvant chemotherapy are listed in Table 62.1 for a selection of studies that used different regimens and different lengths of treatment. Across studies, the major predictor of disease-free survival is pathologic complete response [10,67,70–74] assessed at mastectomy immediately after neoadjuvant chemotherapy. In some studies, a group of patients received radiotherapy prior to mastectomy, so the pathologic complete response to chemotherapy alone is not known. Prolonged chemotherapy (four or more cycles) [10,67,74] was better at eliciting a complete response than three or fewer cycles. The rates of clinical complete response, with very few exceptions, are highly discordant with the rates of pathologic complete response; pathologic complete responses vary between 13% and 30% for most anthracycline-based regimens, whereas clinical complete response is much higher, 70% to 90% in most recent studies using four or more cycles of combination chemotherapy. Because pathologic complete response is the most predictive factor in survival from IBC, it is important that clinical trials of IBC evaluate this variable as part of the protocol.

In the past decade attempts have been made to achieve better complete response rates with high-dose chemotherapy and a stem cell or other form of bone marrow progenitor transplantation approach [75–77]. Unfortunately, to date, none of the high-dose regimens appears superior to standard anthracycline-based prolonged neoadjuvant chemotherapy, and other regimens typically exhibit much greater toxicity. A salvage approach for nonresponders that is being employed with some success is the use of taxanes, if they were not included in the induction regimen [78]. Most studies under way utilize a combination of anthracycline and a taxane as the initial induction regimen, and several studies are also investigating the use of dose-dense induction in IBC. At this time, combination chemotherapy employing an anthracycline and a taxane, together or sequentially, is the standard of care for neoadjuvant treatment of IBC, outside of clinical trials.

Among the early successes of molecular targeted therapies in combination with chemotherapy to report in IBC is the combination trastuzumab, paclitaxel, and epirubicin in the treatment of *ERBB2* (formerly *HER2*)-positive disease. Early results demonstrate a significant improvement with respect to historic controls of the rate of pathological complete response from the addition of trastuzumab [79]. Other molecular targeted therapies are being investigated in IBC, especially antiangiogenic therapies, the rationale of which is predicated on the profuse angiogenesis of IBC. The understanding of the molecular basis of IBC is progressing at a fast pace, making IBC an appealing form of breast cancer on which to try newer therapies. However, the authors caution that, in spite of the possibly strong justification to try new therapies in IBC, trials in IBC must be designed carefully and cleverly to not compromise the patient's chance of a cure, which albeit more rare than in non-IBC, is not impossible. Unexpected severe toxicities from novel combination therapies that possibly may compromise the delivery of effective cytotoxics are clearly not going to have long-term effectiveness in IBC [80]. Thus, because of the tendency to rapid progression in IBC, it is imperative to have clinical trials designed to adjust the therapeutic strategy in the face of even mild progression. Of the current designs, there is enormous excitement about the potential for circulating tumor cells and stem cell therapies to be helpful in IBC. Other approaches directed against oncogenes, such as RhoC, also hold considerable hope but still await testing in patients.

Hormonal Therapy in Inflammatory Breast Cancer

IBCs are predominantly estrogen- and progesterone-receptor negative [88]. However, in the small subset of IBC patients with estrogen or progesterone receptor–positive tumors, adjuvant hormonal therapy with either tamoxifen or aromatase inhibitors, depending on the menopausal status, should be added [89].

In summary, urgent and prolonged or dose-dense neoadjuvant anthracycline-based chemotherapy is the current standard for initial treatment of IBC, after an appropriate and thorough diagnostic work-up that must include marking the original tumor bed for future radiotherapy planning and other evaluations. Locoregional surgical therapy consists of modified radical mastectomy or, if breast conservation is considered, this should be approached under controlled protocols where there has been very careful mapping of the original lesions. All patients with IBC should receive radiotherapy regardless of the down-staging of the disease achieved with chemotherapy. The exact fields depend on whether the initial axillary extent of disease was sampled prior to chemotherapy. If there has been no prior sampling, these patients should undergo comprehensive breast radiotherapy that includes axillary fields.

An algorithm for diagnosis and treatment of IBC is shown in Figure 62.2.

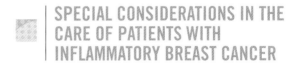

SPECIAL CONSIDERATIONS IN THE CARE OF PATIENTS WITH INFLAMMATORY BREAST CANCER

The rapidity of onset and the severity of the symptoms of IBC may be very frightening to the patient and give rise to special challenges faced by the physician and health care providers caring for patients with IBC. The drastic lack of local control in the chest of patients with untreated IBC causes a major reduction in quality of life. Unlike most other patients with breast cancer who have many reasons to be optimistic, patients with IBC encounter overwhelmingly negative messages in the lay press and in medical textbooks with regard to their prognosis. Because they have a relatively rare form of breast cancer, they are unlikely to have peer cancer patients who have had similar experiences. The patient with IBC may, in addition, have undergone one or more ineffective treatments for her worsening condition, adding to the anxiety and despair. For all of these reasons, the following clinical pearls are put forth to assist health care providers in the care of patients of IBC.

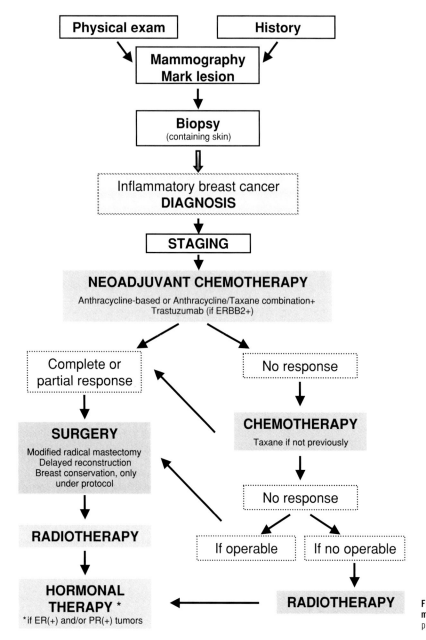

FIGURE 62.2. Algorithm for the diagnosis and treatment of inflammatory breast cancer. ER(+), estrogen-receptor positive; PR(+), progesterone-receptor positive.

1. Convey a sense of calm and exercise enhanced patience and understanding toward the anxious patient with IBC. Explain the seriousness of the diagnosis in the context of the positive advances that make IBC a lot more treatable and survivable in the long term than it is often conveyed in outdated publications.
2. Explain the biologic basis of IBC to the patient and her family. This explanation will naturally lend itself to an understanding by the patient of why initiation of chemotherapy is urgent.
3. If an IBC support group is available, refer the patient to it.
4. Encourage communication with IBC patient advocates; for example, review with the patient lay support resources available through the Internet, such as the web sites www.ibcresearch.org and www.ibcsupport.org.
5. Explain to the patient how her multidisciplinary therapy will be carried out at your institution or office.
6. Involve support health care personnel, such as nurses and social workers, to ensure that the patient always has someone to turn to for reassurance during treatment.
7. Maintain an optimistic attitude yourself.
8. Initiate therapy urgently.

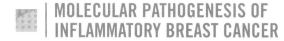

MOLECULAR PATHOGENESIS OF INFLAMMATORY BREAST CANCER

Almost all women with primary IBC have lymph node involvement, and approximately one third have distant metastases at the time of diagnosis (10,90). Primary IBC has several salient biologic features that have helped guide molecular research aimed at uncovering the pathogenetic basis of this disease.

Rapid Progression

Patients with IBC report that new skin lesions arise within a period of a few hours to a few days, suggesting a highly invasive and motile phenotype, as such rates of progression are generally not compatible with the typical growth rates of solid tumors.

Angiogenicity and Angioinvasiveness

Examination of histologic sections of IBC specimens reveals a high degree of neovascularization and angiolymphatic invasion (91), which may be responsible for the high metastatic rate for IBC, even at the time of diagnosis.

The classic histologic finding in IBC on biopsy of affected skin is dermal lymphatic invasion by tumor cells; this change can also be seen in areas of skin that appear clinically normal. These tumor emboli interfere with lymphatic drainage, thereby contributing to the clinical symptoms of IBC (92,93) and presumably to its high rate of lymph node metastasis. The term inflammatory breast cancer does not refer to infiltration of inflammatory cells into the tumor, which is not a prominent IBC feature, but to the erythema and warmth present in the skin of patients affected with IBC.

As noted earlier, the angioinvasive nature of primary IBC is an intrinsic characteristic of this tumor type from its inception; it is not a progressive event in a clinical sense (94). By the time IBC has become a clinical entity, it exhibits all the aggressive characteristics of tumors with full metastatic potential. These characteristic features of IBC were approximately recapitulated in a novel human xenograft model. Implantation of noninflammatory human tumors into the mammary fat pad in mice resulted in the growth of isolated subcutaneous nodules (94). In contrast, implantation of an IBC resulted in exclusive growth within lymphatic and blood vessels, with marked erythema of the overlying skin.

Several experimental studies have undertaken investigation of molecular markers that may correlate with this phenotype (4,91,95). Among the most important molecular markers that have been evaluated in IBC tissues are hormone receptor status, the *erb-2* oncogene, and the p53 gene and protein status. This chapter summarizes the most important recent studies on molecular markers of IBC. This work is being pursued intensively at several laboratories, where it is hypothesized that understanding the key pathogenetic markers will lead to improved treatments.

HORMONAL RECEPTORS, C-MYB, AND ERB2

IBCs are overwhelmingly hormone receptor–negative (83,88,94). A study that compared the hormone receptor status and cell kinetics in 28 IBC patients and 50 noninflammatory LABC patients showed that IBC more often lacked expression of cytosolic estrogen receptor (ER) (44% vs. 64%) and progesterone receptor (PR) (30% vs. 51%) (88). In addition, cell kinetics revealed a twofold higher thymidine labeling index in IBC patients, and among IBC patients, the highest proliferation rates were, not surprisingly, in premenopausal women. Importantly, this study also investigated these markers as predictors of survival. Whereas the labeling index was not significantly associated with survival, those patients with IBC whose tumors had a lower labeling index and were PR positive had a longer survival (31 vs. 18 months for tumors that lacked these characteristics). Another study evaluated the association between the expression of ERs and the proto-oncogene *c-myb* in 57 IBC patients and 112 non-IBC patients (96). C-myb expression was associated only with ER positivity in both groups. Approximately 60% of IBC patients expressed or overexpressed the epidermal growth factor receptor (EGFR) and c-erb-B2; expression of c-myb correlated inversely with c-erb-B2 expression.

In summary, the majority of IBC patients are ER and PR negative but EGFR and c-erb-B2 positive, and they have a high thymidine labeling index. Unfortunately, however, this set of markers is not specific for IBC and indeed, many non-IBC tumors with better prognosis exhibit these changes as well. At the pres-

Table 62.2	MOLECULAR MARKERS IN INFLAMMATORY BREAST CANCER	
	IBC	Non-IBC
ER (−)	56% (88)	36% (88)
PR (−)	70% (88)	49% (88)
ERBB2 (↑)	52% (118)	25%–30% (119)
p53 (↑)	57% (95)	37% (95)
E-cadherin (↑)	100% (120)	68% (120)
RhoC (↑)	90% (101)	38% (101)
WISP3 (−)	80% (101)	21% (101)

IBC, inflammatory breast cancer; ER, estrogen receptor; PR, progesterone receptor; (−), lack of expression; (↑), overexpression.

ent time, in spite of the studies described here, there is no reliable method for discerning prognostic groups within IBC patient groups with the standard markers used for breast cancer in general. Table 62.2 summarizes the molecular markers of IBC.

P53 TUMOR SUPPRESSOR GENE

Mutations in the *p53* tumor suppressor gene and abnormal accumulation of p53 protein have been reported in 20% to 50% of human breast cancers (97,98). These abnormalities are more often seen in patients with familial or hereditary breast cancer syndromes (such as hereditary breast and ovarian cancer and Li-Fraumeni's syndrome) than in those with sporadic breast cancer.

The p53 status in IBC was evaluated by immunohistochemistry in a series of 27 patients (97). Three groups of patients with tumors of almost equal size were identified: tumors with high levels of p53 in the nucleus, tumors with no detectable p53 in the cells, and tumors with p53 in the cytoplasm. The latter two groups had only wild type *p53,* whereas the samples with intense nuclear staining had a variety of missense mutations. These findings suggested that at least two of the known mechanisms of *p53* inactivation—direct mutation and cytoplasmic sequestration of wild type protein—can interfere with the normal function of p53 in IBC.

In a subsequent study, the same group evaluated 24 additional patients with IBC in an attempt to determine the prognostic significance of p53 (99). Those patients with a *p53* gene mutation and nuclear overexpression of p53 protein had an 8.6-fold higher risk of death than patients who had neither mutation nor protein overexpression; in addition, there appeared to be an important prognostic interaction between p53 and ER expression. The subset of patients who were ER negative and also had nuclear p53 overexpression had a 17.9-fold higher risk of death, compared with a 2.8-fold higher risk for women with tumors that had p53 nuclear overexpression alone.

Similar findings were noted in a study of locally advanced breast cancers, 32 of which were confirmed as IBC by clinical and pathologic criteria (100). Mutations in *p53* were detected in 41% of the tumors analyzed, all but three of which had intense p53 nuclear staining. Consistent with the results of previous studies on the p53 expression in stage II breast cancers, the presence of *p53* mutations in IBC was also significantly associated with large tumor size and disseminated disease at diagnosis. There was also a nonsignificant trend toward an association between *p53* mutation, negative ER status, and a lower rate of response to therapy.

In summary, studies of conventional clinical markers and of EGFR and *p53* yield interesting and consistent information with regard to IBC prognosis, but they lack sufficient sensitivity and specificity to stratify IBC patients for treatment purposes.

TOWARD SPECIFIC DETERMINANTS OF INFLAMMATORY BREAST CANCER: RHOC AND WISP3

The rapidity with which IBC spreads is a striking feature of its clinical presentation. As IBC arises over a very short period of time compared with breast cancer in general and other adenocarcinomas, van Golen et al. (101) hypothesized that a limited number of genetic alterations occurring early in carcinogenesis result in this aggressive phenotype. In an effort to identify new genes that may contribute to the specific phenotypic features of IBCs, genome-wide expression differences between an IBC cell line (SUM149) and normal mammary epithelial cell lines (HME) were assessed. Seventeen distinct transcripts were identified as being differentially expressed: eight were up-regulated by the normal cell lines relative to the tumor cells, and nine were up-regulated by the tumor cell line. Subsequently, a blinded analysis of the 17 transcripts by *in situ* hybridization on 20 archival IBC and 30 stage-matched non-IBC patients revealed that only two genes were significantly altered in IBC compared with non-IBC cells. RhoC GTPase and a novel gene (*LIBC*: "lost in inflammatory breast cancer"), later termed *WISP3*, were concordantly altered in 91% of the IBC specimens compared with none of the controls. The putative RhoC GTPase oncogene was more often overexpressed (90% vs. 38%) and *WISP3* was commonly lost in IBC (80% vs. 21%). Work was subsequently undertaken to understand the biologic role of these genes in breast cancer.

RHOC GTPASE: INVASION, MOTILITY, AND ANGIOGENESIS IN INFLAMMATORY BREAST CANCER

RhoC GTPase is a member of the Ras superfamily of small GTP-binding proteins (102,103). It is involved in cytoskeletal reorganization, via regulation of the actin cytoskeleton (104), and the formation of focal adhesions required for polarization and movement. Transfection of a homologous gene or the RhoC GTPase gene leads to malignant transformation and the inception of a highly angiogenic phenotype characterized by the abundant release of angiogenic cytokines such as vascular endothelial growth factor (VEGF) (105). The additional observation that overexpression of RhoC GTPase correlates with tumor progression in aggressive ductal pancreatic cancer (106) is consistent with the hypothesis that RhoC GTPase is an important contributor to the IBC metastatic phenotype. Overexpression of RhoC GTPase in previously immortalized mammary epithelial cells resulted in a fully invasive and metastatic phenotype, signaling RhoC to be a transforming oncogene of breast cells. The phenotype of the transformed cells strongly resembled the known biologic features of IBC, further supporting an important pathogenetic role for RhoC in IBC (101,105,107).

In preclinical models, IBC tumor cell lines and tumor specimens release increased amounts of VEGF, basic fibroblast growth factor (bFGF), and interleukin (IL)-6 and IL-8, and increased release of these cytokines is also known to occur, as mentioned previously, in human mammary epithelial cells that are transfected with and overexpressed the RhoC GTPase gene. The VEGF receptor-3 (VEGFR-3) is expressed in the lymphatic endothelium, plays an important role in lymphatic development, and is activated after binding to VEGF-C and VEGF-D. The VEGFR-3 pathway may play an important role in breast tumor lymphangiogenesis and subsequent metastasis (108,109). As an example, VEGF-C is overexpressed in some breast cancer cells, promoting both intratumoral lymphangiogenesis and

metastases to the regional lymph nodes and lungs (108). In contrast, overexpression of VEGF ligands to VEGFR-2 does not stimulate lymphangiogenesis (109). These observations could potentially be applicable to human disease. A study in which breast cancer cell lines were screened for expression the VEGF family members revealed that expression of VEGF-A and VEGF-B was seen in both node-positive and node-negative tumors, expression of VEGF-C (a ligand for VEGFR-3) was detectable in some node-positive breast cancers but not in node-negative tumors, and, more importantly, expression of VEGF-D (another ligand for VEGFR-3) was detected only in an IBC cell line and in a tumor cell line that was developed from an inflammatory skin metastasis (110). Thus, it appears reasonable to postulate that activation of VEGFR-3, particularly by the VEGF-D ligand in IBC, may be involved in the lymphotactic process through the development of new lymphatic vessels near the IBC tumor.

Although RhoC GTPase was not commonly overexpressed in non-IBC tumors, Merajver's group (111) hypothesized that very small breast tumors that overexpressed RhoC may show nodal metastasis as a result of the highly metastatic potential conferred to breast cells by RhoC overexpression. Indeed, this study (111) showed that RhoC overexpression had 82% sensitivity and 46% specificity as a marker of breast cancers of less than 1 cm that have metastases to the lymph nodes. This work suggests that RhoC overexpression may be a unique and useful marker, not only in advancing the understanding of IBC but also in discerning which T1 tumors have a high metastatic potential.

WISP3

The product of the *WISP3* (*LIBC*) gene is an insulin-like growth factor binding protein–related protein (IGFBP-rP) termed IGFBPrP-9 (112). It has been suggested that both the high-affinity IGF binding proteins (IGFBPs) and the IGFBPrPs modulate the availability of insulin-like growth factor to the cell surface IGF receptors (113). If so, they could either potentiate or inhibit IGF-mediated functions or, alternatively, they may also promote or inhibit tumor cell growth by IGF-independent effects (114).

There is suggestive evidence that at least some IGFBPrPs play a role in tumor progression. Down-regulation or loss of IGFBPrP-1 expression has been associated with progression of breast cancer and prostate cancer (115,116), and transfection of IGFBPrP-1 in prostate cancer cells results in a less malignant phenotype that is dose dependent (116). Of note, restoration of *WISP3* function to IBC cells that had lost expression of *WISP3* resulted in a significant attenuation of the phenotype, strongly supporting a tumor suppressor role for *WISP3* in IBC (117).

TOWARD A MOLECULAR SIGNATURE OF INFLAMMATORY BREAST CANCER

A goal of the international research community in IBC is to achieve two major goals. First, it would be extremely helpful to arrive at a set of drivers of the IBC phenotype in human tumors. Although the data indicate that RhoC and loss of *WISP3* may be salient driver events, it is expected that at least several other genetic or expression changes will be important. Of course, some of these changes may not be independent of one another, such as the link already known between RhoC and *WISP3* (121), as well as the relationship between NFκB expression and IBC (122–124). Second, it would be of great interest to have a highly specific and predictive molecular bar code for IBC to facilitate diagnosis and stratification of patients.

More recently, specific NFκB regulated genes such as chemokine receptors CXCR4 and CCR7 have been corroborated to be expressed in IBC (125). Likewise, for VEGF (107) it could lead to the identification of one or more important targets to attack IBC. Moreover, although IBC remains a unique entity it shares many characteristics with non IBC, such as increased proliferation (127). From these preliminary findings it follows that, in spite of some progress, researchers are still a long way away from knowing how to inhibit recurrences of IBC effectively. In fact, all of the evidence seems to indicate that long-term therapy for micrometastasis or against cancer stem cells may be what is needed for IBC.

CONCLUSION

IBC is a distinct clinical entity within breast cancer that warrants urgent and aggressive treatment with neoadjuvant chemotherapy followed by multimodality locoregional therapy. With a 5-year survival of approximately 50%, it is clear that although strides have been made in IBC, novel treatment approaches are needed to improve outcomes. Following the success of therapeutic drugs aimed at important molecular targets, it seems appropriate to hypothesize that a deeper understanding of the molecular determinants of IBC will facilitate the development of new drugs against it.

IBC has some unique phenotypic and genetic changes that set it apart from slowly progressive, locally advanced breast cancer. The development of IBC cell lines and xenograft models (94,101,105) provide suitable substrates for hypothesis testing and therapeutic preclinical development. Taken together, the molecular data on the specific alterations present in IBC at diagnosis suggest potential new targets for therapeutic development, with RhoC and *WISP3* as well as NFκB, and some of its dependent genes appear to be involved either as causal events or as crucial epigenetic determinants of the pathogenesis of IBC.

MANAGEMENT SUMMARY

Diagnosis

- Physical examination and history of present illness are crucial for the diagnosis of IBC. Observation revealed the presence of an enlarged breast with skin alterations such as edema, erythema, and *peau d'orange*. Signs and symptoms have progressed rapidly.
- Differential diagnosis includes mastitis, trauma, and inflammatory noninfectious connective tissue diseases. Set a course of antibiotics (7 to 10 days); if condition does not resolve completely, mammogram and biopsy should be performed urgently.
- If IBC, biopsy is likely to reveal the presence of tumor clusters of cells penetrating tubular structures presumed to be dermal lymphatics.
- Mammography is nearly always abnormal. The mammographic pattern is characterized by increased density, skin thickening, and stromal coarsening. Nipple inversion and focal opacities are present in more than half of patients. Insertion of markers to delineate tumor bed is required.
- Ultrasonography plays an important role in the evaluation of regional nodes.
- Magnetic resonance imaging is useful in diagnosis and staging and can also provide important information during the monitoring of treatment response.
- Systemic staging to detect distant metastasis should be tailored to the physical examination findings. In asymptomatic patients work-up should include a bone scan and computer-assisted tomography of the chest, abdomen, and head with contrast. The role of PET on the staging of patients with IBC is under investigation, but results are promising.
- Serum markers (CA 15.3 and CEA) have a limited role in breast cancer in general, but may prove useful to detect late recurrences.

Treatment

- The recommended treatment for IBC is based on multimodality therapy involving a systemic approach (neoadjuvant chemotherapy) followed by a locoregional approach (surgery and radiotherapy), and further systemic hormonal therapy, if indicated.
- The standard chemotherapy regimens in IBC are based on anthracyclines and taxanes. Clinical trials are encouraged. Participation in tissue collections and registries is important to increase knowledge about this relatively rare condition.
- Modified radical mastectomy is the recommended surgery. Breast-conservation surgery can be considered for patients with a pathological complete response, under protocol.
- Breast reconstruction surgery is delayed until completion of therapy.
- Sentinel lymph node biopsy is not recommended in patients with IBC, due to its low level of accuracy and the high probability of significant axillary lymph node involvement.
- All patients with IBC should receive radiotherapy.
- Trastuzumab should be given as part of systemic therapy to patients with *ERBB2*-positive tumors.
- The role of other targeted therapies, such as lapatinib or bevacizumab, is under investigation in clinical trials.
- For IBC patients with ER- or PR-positive tumors, hormonal treatment with tamoxifen for 2 years followed by and aromatase inhibitors for 5 years should be added.

ACKNOWLEDGMENTS

This work was supported in part by the Breast Cancer Research Foundation (SDM), the Burroughs Wellcome Fund (SDM). MDI was supported by a grant from Alfonso Martin Escudero Foundation, Spain.

References

1. Bell CA. A system of operative surgery. *Surgery* 1814;11:136.
2. Haagensen CD. *Diseases of the breast*. 2nd ed. Philadelphia: WB Saunders, 1971.
3. Green FL, Page DL, Fleming ID, et al. Breast. In: Green FL, ed. *AJCC cancer staging handbook*. 6th ed. New York: Springer-Verlag, 2002:255–281.
4. Kleer CG, van Golen KL, Merajver SD. Molecular biology of breast cancer metastasis. Inflammatory breast cancer: clinical syndrome and molecular determinants. *Breast Cancer Res* 2000;2(6):423–429.
5. Chang S, Parker SL, Pham T, et al. Inflammatory breast carcinoma incidence and survival: the Surveillance, Epidemiology, and End Results program of the National Cancer Institute, 1975–1992. *Cancer* 1998;82(12):2366–2372.
6. Tardivon AA, Viala J, Corvellec Rudelli A, et al. Mammographic patterns of inflammatory breast carcinoma: a retrospective study of 92 cases. *Eur J Radiol* 1997;24(2):124–130.
7. Berg JW, Hutter RV. Breast cancer. *Cancer* 1995;75[1 Suppl]:257–269.
8. Aziz SA, Pervez S, Khan S, et al. Case control study of prognostic markers and disease outcome in inflammatory carcinoma breast: a unique clinical experience. *Breast J* 2003;7(6):398–404.
9. Soliman A, Banerjee M, Lo A, et al. High proportion of inflammatory breast cancer in the population-based cancer registry of Gharbiah, Egypt. *Breast* 2008. In press.
10. Merajver SD, Weber BL, Cody R, et al. Breast conservation and prolonged chemotherapy for locally advanced breast cancer: the University of Michigan experience. *J Clin Oncol* 1997;15:2873–2881.
11. Buzdar AU, Singletary SE, Booser DJ, et al. Combined modality treatment of stage III and inflammatory breast cancer. M.D. Anderson Cancer Center experience. *Surg Oncol Clin North Am* 1995;4(4):715–734.
12. Anderson WF, Chu KC, Chang S. Inflammatory breast carcinoma and noninflammatory locally advanced breast carcinoma: distinct clinicopathologic entities? *J Clin Oncol* 2003;21(12):2254–2259.

13. Dershaw DD, Moore MP, Liberman L, et al. Inflammatory breast carcinoma: mammographic findings. *Radiology* 1994;190(3):831–834.
14. Droulias CA, Sewell CW, Mcsweeney MB, et al. Inflammatory carcinoma of the breast: a correlation of clinical, radiologic and pathologic findings. *Ann Surg* 1976;184(2):217–222.
15. Yang WT, Le-Petross HT, Macapinlac H, et al. Inflammatory breast cancer: PET/CT, MRI, mammography, and sonography findings. *Breast Cancer Res Treat* 2008;109(3):417–426.
16. Gunhan-Bilgen I, Ustun EE, Memis A. Inflammatory breast carcinoma: mammographic, ultrasonographic, clinical, and pathologic findings in 142 cases. *Radiology* 2002;223(3):829–838.
17. Baslaim MM, Bakheet SM, Bakheet R, et al. 18-Fluorodeoxyglucose-positron emission tomography in inflammatory breast cancer. *World J Surg* 2003;27(10): 1099–1104.
18. Beyer T, Townsend DW, Brun T, et al. A combined PET/CT scanner for clinical oncology. *J Nucl Med* 2000;41(8):1369–1379.
19. Wingo PA, Jamison PM, Young JL, et al. Population-based statistics for women diagnosed with inflammatory breast cancer (United States). *Cancer Causes Control* 2004;15(3):321–328.
20. Blum C, Baker M. Venous congestion of the breast mimicking inflammatory breast cancer: case report and review of literature. *Breast J* 2008;14(1):97–101.
21. Aktories K, Braun U, Rosener S, et al. The Rho gene product expressed in *E. coli* is a substrate of botulinum ADP-ribosyltransferase C3. *Biochem Biophys Res Commun* 1989;158(1):209–213.
22. Dirix LY, van DP, Prove A, et al. Inflammatory breast cancer: current understanding. *Curr Opin Oncol* 2006;18(6):563–571.
23. Learmonth GE. Acute mammary carcinoma (Volmann's mastitis carcinomatosa). *Can Med Assoc J* 1916;6(499):511.
24. Halsted WS. The results of operations for the cure of cancer of the breast performed at the Johns Hopkins Hospital from June 1889–January, 1894. *Johns Hopkins Hosp Bull* 1894;4:1111.
25. Treves N. The inoperability of inflammatory carcinoma of the breast. *Surg Gynecol Obstet* 1959;109:240–242.
26. Haagensen CD, Stout AP. Carcinoma of the breast II—criteria of operability. *Ann Surg* 1942;118:859–870.
27. Barker JL, Nelson AJ, Montague ED. Inflammatory carcinoma of the breast. *Radiology* 1976;121(1):173–176.
28. Zucali R, Uslenghi C, Kenda R, et al. Natural history of survival of inoperable breast cancer treated with radiotherapy and radiotherapy followed by radical mastectomy. *Cancer* 1976;37:1422–1431.
29. Lopez MJ, Porter KA. Inflammatory breast cancer. *Surg Clin North Am* 1996; 76(2):411–429.
30. Baclesse F. Roentgen therapy alone as the method of treatment of cancer of the breast. *AJR Am J Roentgenol* 1949;62:311–319.
31. Fletcher GH, Montague ED. Radical irradiation of advanced breast cancer. *Am J Roentgenol Radium Ther Nucl Med* 1965;93:573–584.
32. Spanos WJ, Montague ED, Fletcher GH. Late complications of radiation only for advanced breast cancer. *Int J Radiat Oncol Biol Phys* 1980;6:1473–1476.
33. Fields JN, Perez CA, Kuske RR, et al. Inflammatory carcinoma of the breast: treatment results on 107 patients. *Int J Radiat Oncol Biol Phys* 1989;17(2):249–255.
34. Perez CA, Fields JN, Fracasso PM, et al. Management of locally advanced carcinoma of the breast. II. Inflammatory carcinoma. *Cancer* 1994;74[1 Suppl]:466–476.
35. Chevallier B, Bastit P, Graic Y, et al. The Centre H. Becquerel studies in inflammatory non metastatic breast cancer. Combined modality approach in 178 patients. *Br J Cancer* 1993;67(3):594–601.
36. Fleming RY, Asmar L, Buzdar AU, et al. Effectiveness of mastectomy by response to induction chemotherapy for control in inflammatory breast carcinoma. *Ann Surg Oncol* 1997;4(6):452–461.
37. de Boer RH, Allum WH, Ebbs SR, et al. Multimodality therapy in inflammatory breast cancer: is there a place for surgery? *Ann Oncol* 2000;11(9):1147–1153.
38. Mourali N, Tabbane F, Muenz LR, et al. Ten-year results utilizing chemotherapy as primary treatment in nonmetastatic, rapidly progressing breast cancer. *Cancer Invest* 1993;11(4):363–370.
39. Declan Fleming RY, Singletary SE. Inflammatory breast cancer. In: Singletary SE, ed. *Breast cancer*. New York: Springer-Verlag, 1999;18:365.
40. Thoms WW Jr, McNeese MD, Fletcher GH, et al. Multimodal treatment for inflammatory breast cancer. *Int J Radiat Oncol Biol Phys* 1989;17(4):739–745.
41. Curcio LD, Rupp E, Williams WL, et al. Beyond palliative mastectomy in inflammatory breast cancer—a reassessment of margin status. *Ann Surg Oncol* 1999;6(3):249–254.
42. Akashi-Tanaka S, Fukutomi T, Watanabe T, et al. Accuracy of contrast-enhanced computed tomography in the prediction of residual breast cancer after neoadjuvant chemotherapy. *Int J Cancer* 2001;96(1):66–73.
43. Schafer P, Alberto P, Forni M, et al. Surgery as part of a combined modality approach for inflammatory breast carcinoma. *Cancer* 1987;59(6):1063–1067.
44. Panades M, Olivotto IA, Speers CH, et al. Evolving treatment strategies for inflammatory breast cancer: a population-based survival analysis. *J Clin Oncol* 2005;23(9):1941–1950.
45. Schwartz GF, Birchansky CA, Komarnicky LT, et al. Induction chemotherapy followed by breast conservation for locally advanced carcinoma of the breast. *Cancer* 1994;73:362–369.
46. Calais G, Berger C, Descamps P, et al. Conservative treatment feasibility with induction chemotherapy, surgery, and radiotherapy for patients with breast carcinoma larger than 3 cm. *Cancer* 1994;74(4):1283–1288.
47. Veronesi U, Bonadonna G, Zurrida S, et al. Conservation surgery after primary chemotherapy in large carcinomas of the breast. *Ann Surg* 1995;222:612–618.
48. Schaake-Koning C, van der Linden EH, Hart G, et al. Adjuvant chemo- and hormonal therapy in locally advanced breast cancer: a randomized clinical study. *Int J Radiat Oncol Biol Phys* 1985;11(10):1759–1763.
49. DeLena M, Zucali R, Viganotti G. Combined chemotherapy-radiotherapy approach in locally advanced (T3b-T4) breast cancer. *Cancer Chemother Pharmacol* 1978;1:53–59.
50. Chawla AK, Kachnic LA, Taghian AG, et al. Radiotherapy and breast reconstruction: complications and cosmesis with TRAM versus tissue expander/implant. *Int J Radiat Oncol Biol Phys* 2002;54(2):520–526.
51. Javaid M, Song F, Leinster S, et al. Radiation effects on the cosmetic outcomes of immediate and delayed autologous breast reconstruction: an argument about timing. *J Plast Reconstr Aesthet Surg* 2006;59(1):16–26.
52. Senkus-Konefka E, Welnicka-Jaskiewicz M, et al. Radiotherapy for breast cancer in patients undergoing breast reconstruction or augmentation. *Cancer Treat Rev* 2004;30(8):671–682.
53. Slavin SA, Love SM, Goldwyn RM. Recurrent breast cancer following immediate reconstruction with myocutaneous flaps. *Plast Reconstr Surg* 1994;93(6): 1191–1204.
54. Chin PL, Andersen JS, Somlo G, et al. Esthetic reconstruction after mastectomy for inflammatory breast cancer: is it worthwhile? *J Am Coll Surg* 2000;190(3): 304–309.
55. Stearns V, Ewing CA, Slack R, et al. Sentinel lymphadenectomy after neoadjuvant chemotherapy for breast cancer may reliably represent the axilla except for inflammatory breast cancer. *Ann Surg Oncol* 2002;9(3):235–242.
56. Buchholz TA, Tucker SL, Moore RA, et al. Importance of radiation therapy for breast cancer patients treated with high-dose chemotherapy and stem cell transplant. *Int J Radiat Oncol Biol Phys* 2000;46(2):337–343.
57. Abdel-Wahab M, Wolfson A, Raub W, et al. The importance of postoperative radiation therapy in multimodality management of locally advanced breast cancer: a phase II trial of neoadjuvant MVAC, surgery, and radiation. *Int J Radiat Oncol Biol Phys* 1998;40(4):875–880.
58. Olson JE, Neuberg D, Pandya KJ, et al. The role of radiotherapy in the management of operable locally advanced breast carcinoma: results of a randomized trial by the Eastern Cooperative Oncology Group. *Cancer* 1997;79(6):1138–1149.
59. Overgaard M, Hansen PS, Overgaard J, et al. Postoperative radiotherapy in high-risk premenopausal women with breast cancer who receive adjuvant chemotherapy. *N Engl J Med* 1997;337:949–955.
60. Ragaz J, Jackson SM, Le N, et al. Adjuvant radiotherapy and chemotherapy in node-positive premenopausal women with breast cancer. *N Engl J Med* 1997; 337:956–962.
61. DeLena M, Varini M, Zucali R, et al. Multimodal treatment for locally advanced breast cancer: results of chemotherapy-radiotherapy versus chemotherapy-surgery. *Cancer Clin Trials* 1981;4:229–236.
62. Fastenberg NA, Martin RG, Buzdar AU, et al. Management of inflammatory carcinoma of the breast. A combined modality approach. *Am J Clin Oncol* 1985;8(2): 134–141.
63. Perloff M, Lesnick GJ, Korzun A, et al. Combination chemotherapy with mastectomy or radiotherapy for stage III breast carcinoma: a cancer and leukemia group b study. *J Clin Oncol* 1988;6:261–269.
64. Bozzetti F, Saccozzi R, De Lena M, et al. Inflammatory cancer of the breast: analysis of 114 cases. *J Surg Oncol* 1981;18(4):355–361.
65. Delarue JC, May-Levin F, Mouriesse H, et al. Oestrogen and progesterone cytosolic receptors in clinically inflammatory tumors of the human breast. *Br J Cancer* 1981;44:911–916.
66. Maloisel F, Dufour P, Bergerat JP, et al. Results of initial doxorubicin, 5-fluorouracil and cyclophosphamide combination chemotherapy for inflammatory carcinoma of the breast. *Cancer* 1990;65(4):851–855.
67. Swain SM, Sorace RA, Bagley CS, et al. Neoadjuvant chemotherapy in the combined modality approach of locally advanced nonmetastatic breast cancer. *Cancer Res* 1987;47:3889–3894.
68. Rouesse S, Sarrazin D, Mouriesse H. Primary chemotherapy in the treatment of inflammatory breast carcinoma: a study of 230 cases from the Institut Gustave-Roussy. *J Clin Oncol* 1986;4(1765):1771.
69. Casper ES, Guidera CA, Bosl GJ, et al. Combined modality treatment of locally advanced breast cancer: adjuvant combination chemotherapy with and without doxorubicin. *Breast Cancer Res Treat* 1987;9:39–44.
70. Keiling R, Guiochet N, Calderoli H, et al. Preoperative chemotherapy in the treatment of inflammatory breast cancer. In: Wagener DJT, Blijham GH, Smeets JBE, et al., eds. *Primary chemotherapy in cancer medicine*. New York: Liss, 1985: 95–104.
71. Chevallier B, Roche H, Olivier JP, et al. Inflammatory breast cancer. Pilot study of intensive induction chemotherapy (FEC-HD) results in a high histologic response rate. *Am J Clin Oncol* 1993;16(3):223–228.
72. Harris EE, Schultz D, Bertsch H, et al. Ten-year outcome after combined modality therapy for inflammatory breast cancer. *Int J Radiat Oncol Biol Phys* 2003;55(5): 1200–1208.
73. Wahl RL, Zasadny K, Helvie M, et al. Metabolic monitoring of breast cancer chemohormonotherapy using positron emission tomography: initial evaluation. *J Clin Oncol* 1993;11(11):2101–2111.
74. Hortobagyi GN, Ames FC, Buzdar AU, et al. Management of stage III primary breast cancer with primary chemotherapy, surgery, and radiation therapy. *Cancer* 1988;62:2507–2516.
75. Fields KK, Elfenbein GJ, Perkins JB, et al. Defining the role of novel high-dose chemotherapy regimens for the treatment of high-risk breast cancer. *Semin Oncol* 1998;25(2)[Suppl 4]:1–6.
76. Dazzi C, Cariello A, Rosti G, et al. Neoadjuvant high dose chemotherapy plus peripheral blood progenitor cells in inflammatory breast cancer: a multicenter phase II pilot study. *Haematologica* 2001;86(5):523–529.
77. Schwartzberg L, Weaver C, Lewkow L, et al. High-dose chemotherapy with peripheral blood stem cell support for stage IIIB inflammatory carcinoma of the breast. *Bone Marrow Transplant* 1999;24(9):981–987.
78. Cristofanilli M, Buzdar AU, Sneige N, et al. Paclitaxel in the multimodality treatment for inflammatory breast carcinoma. *Cancer* 2001;92(7):1775–1782.
79. Gonzalez-Angulo AM, Hennessy BT, Broglio K, et al. Trends for inflammatory breast cancer: is survival improving? *Oncologist* 2007;12(8):904–912.
80. Overmoyer B, Fu P, Hoppel C, et al. Inflammatory breast cancer as a model disease to study tumor angiogenesis: results of a phase IB trial of combination SU5416 and doxorubicin. *Clin Cancer Res* 2007;13(19):5862–5868.
81. Pawlicki M, Skolyszewski J, Brandys A. Results of combined treatment of patients with locally advanced breast cancer. *Tumori* 1983;69(3):249–253.
82. Jacquillat C, Weil M, Auclerc G. Neoadjuvant chemotherapy in the conservative management of breast cancer: a study of 205 patients. In: Salmon SE, ed. *Adjuvant therapy of cancer V*. Philadelphia: JB Lippincott, 1987:403–409.
83. Koh EH, Buzdar A, Ames FC, et al. Inflammatory carcinoma of the breast: results of a combined-modality approach—M.D. Anderson Cancer Center Experience. *Cancer Chemother Pharmacol* 1990;27(2):94–100.
84. Noguchi S, Miyauchi K, Nishizawa Y, et al. Management of inflammatory carcinoma of the breast with combined modality therapy including intraarterial infusion chemotherapy as an induction therapy. Long-term follow-up results of 28 patients. *Cancer* 1988;61(8):1483–1491.

85. Perloff M, Lesnick GJ. Chemotherapy before and after mastectomy in stage III breast cancer. *Arch Surg* 1982;117:879–881.

86. Palangie T, Mosseri V, Mihura J, et al. Prognostic factors in inflammatory breast cancer and therapeutic implications. *Eur J Cancer* 1994,30A(7).921–927.

87. Iino Y, Takei H, Maemura M, et al. Multidisciplinary treatment with anthracyclines in inflammatory breast cancer. *Anticancer Res* 1996;16(5B):3111–3115.

88. Paradiso A, Tommasi S, Brandi M, et al. Cell kinetics and hormonal receptor status in inflammatory breast carcinoma. Comparison with locally advanced disease. *Cancer* 1989;64(9):1922–1927.

89. Giordano SH, Hortobagyi GN. Inflammatory breast cancer: clinical progress and the main problems that must be addressed. *Breast Cancer Res* 2003;5(6):284–288.

90. Jaiyesimi IA, Buzdar AU, Hortobagyi G. Inflammatory breast cancer: a review. *J Clin Oncol* 1992;10(6):1014–1024.

91. McCarthy N, Linnoila IR, Merino M, et al. Microvessel density, expression of estrogen receptor alpha, MIB-1, p53, and c-erbB-2 in inflammatory breast cancer. *Clin Cancer Res* 2002;8(12):3857–3862.

92. Rosen PP. *Rosen's breast pathology*. Philadelphia: Lippincott-Raven, 1996.

93. Robbins GF, Shah J, Rosen P, et al. Inflammatory carcinoma of the breast. *Surg Clin North Am* 1974;54:801–810.

94. Alpaugh ML, Tomlinson JS, Shao Z-M, et al. A novel human xenograft model of inflammatory breast cancer. *Cancer Res* 1999;59:5079–5084.

95. Turpin E, Bieche I, Bertheau P, et al. Increased incidence of ERBB2 overexpression and TP53 mutation in inflammatory breast cancer. *Oncogene* 2002;21(49):7593–7597.

96. Guerin M, Sheng ZM, Andrieu N, et al. Strong association between c-*myb* and oestrogen-receptor expression in human breast cancer. *Oncogene* 1990;5(1):131–135.

97. Moll UM, Riou G, Levine AJ. Two distinct mechanisms alter p53 in breast cancer: mutation and nuclear exclusion. *Proc Natl Acad Sci U S A* 1992;89(15):7262–7266.

98. Davidoff AM, Humphrey PA, Iglehart JD, et al. Genetic basis for p53 overexpression in human breast cancer. *Proc Natl Acad Sci U S A* 1991;88(11):5006–5010.

99. Riou G, Le M, Travagli JP, et al. Poor prognosis of p53 gene mutation and nuclear overexpression of p53 protein in inflammatory breast carcinoma. *J Natl Cancer Inst* 1993;85(21):1765–1767.

100. Faille A, DeCremoux P, Extra JM, et al. p53 mutations and overexpression in locally advanced breast cancers. *Br J Cancer* 1994;69(6):1145–1150.

101. van Golen KL, Davies S, Wu ZF, et al. A novel putative low-affinity insulin-like growth factor-binding protein, LIBC (lost in inflammatory breast cancer), and RhoC GTPase correlate with the inflammatory breast cancer phenotype. *Clin Cancer Res* 1999;5(9):2511–2519.

102. Ridley AJ. The GTP-binding protein Rho. *Int J Biochem Cell Biol* 1997;29:1225–1229.

103. Nobes CD, Hall A. Rho GTPases control polarity, protrusion, and adhesion during cell movement. *J Cell Biol* 1999;144(6):1235–1244.

104. Hall A. Rho GTPases and the actin cytoskeleton. *Science* 1998;279:509–514.

105. van Golen KL, Wu ZF, Qiao XT, et al. RhoC GTPase overexpression modulates induction of angiogenic factors in breast cells. *Neoplasia* 2000;2(5):418–425.

106. Suwa H, Ohshio G, Imamura T, et al. Overexpression of the RhoC gene correlates with progression of ductal adenocarcinoma of the pancreas. *Br J Cancer* 1998;77(1):147–152.

107. van Golen KL, Bao L, Pan Q, et al. Mitogen activated protein kinase pathway is involved in RhoC GTPase induced motility, invasion and angiogenesis in inflammatory breast cancer. *Clin Exp Metastasis* 2002;19:301–311.

108. Skobe M, Hawighorst T, Jackson DG, et al. Induction of tumor lymphangiogenesis by VEGF-C promotes breast cancer metastasis. *Nat Med* 2001;7(2):192–198.

109. Stacker SA, Caesar C, Baldwin ME, et al. VEGF-D promotes the metastatic spread of tumor cells via the lymphatics. *Nat Med* 2001;7(2):186–191.

110. Kurebayashi J, Ostuski T, Kunisue H, et al. Expression of vascular endothelial growth factor (VEGF) family members in breast cancer. *Jpn J Cancer Res* 1999;90(9):977–981.

111. Kleer CG, van Golen KL, Zhang Y, et al. Characterization of RhoC expression in benign and malignant breast disease: a potential new marker for small breast carcinomas with metastatic ability. *Am J Pathol* 2002;160(2):579–584.

112. Hwa V, Oh Y, Rosenfeld RG. The IGFBP superfamily. *Endocr Rev* 1999;20(6):761–787.

113. Clemons DR. Role of insulin-like growth factor binding proteins in controlling IGF actions. *Mol Cell Endocrinol* 1998;140:19–24.

114. Oh Y. IGF-independent regulation of breast cancer growth by IGF binding proteins. *Breast Cancer Res Treat* 1998;47:283–293.

115. Burger A, Zhang X, Li H, et al. Down-regulation of T1A12/mac25, a novel insulin-like growth factor binding protein related gene, is associated with disease progression in breast carcinomas. *Oncogene* 1998;16:2459–2467.

116. Sprenger CC, Damon SE, Hwa V, et al. Insulin-like growth factor binding protein-related protein 1 (IGFBP-rP1) is a potential tumor suppressor for prostate cancer. *Cancer Res* 1999;59(10):2370–2375.

117. Kleer CG, Zhang Y, Pan Q, et al. WISP3 is a novel tumor suppressor gene of inflammatory breast cancer. *Oncogene* 2002;21(20):3172–3180.

118. Parton M, Dowsett M, Ashley S, et al. High incidence of HER-2 positivity in inflammatory breast cancer. *Breast* 2004;13(2):97–103.

119. Slamon DJ, Godolphin W, Jones LA, et al. Studies of the HER-2/neu proto-oncogene in human breast and ovarian cancer. *Science* 1989;244:707–712.

120. Di Palma F, Holme RH, Bryda EC, et al. Mutations in Cdh23, encoding a new type of cadherin, cause stereocilia disorganization in waltzer, the mouse model for Usher syndrome type 1D. *Nat Genet* 2001;27(1):103–107.

121. Kleer CG, Zhang Y, Merajver SD. CCN6 (WISP3) as a new regulator of the epithelial phenotype in breast cancer. *Cells Tissues Organs* 2007;185(1–3):95–99.

122. Pan Q, Bao LW, Kleer CG, et al. Antiangiogenic tetrathiomolybdate enhances the efficacy of doxorubicin against breast carcinoma. *Mol Cancer Ther* 2003;2(7):617–622.

123. Pan Q, Bao LW, Merajver SD. Tetrathiomolybdate inhibits angiogenesis and metastasis through suppression of the NFκB signaling cascade. *Mol Cancer Res* 2003;1(10):701–706.

124. Van Laere SJ, Van DA, I, Van Den Eynden GG, et al. NF-κB activation in inflammatory breast cancer is associated with oestrogen receptor downregulation, secondary to EGFR and/or ErbB2 overexpression and MAPK hyperactivation. *Br J Cancer* 2007;97(5):659–669.

125. Cabioglu N, Gong Y, Islam R, et al. Expression of growth factor and chemokine receptors: new insights in the biology of inflammatory breast cancer. *Ann Oncol* 2007;18(6):1021–1029.

126. Al-Mowallad A, Kirwan C, Byrne G, et al. Vascular endothelial growth factor-C in patients with breast cancer. *In Vivo* 2007;21(3):549–551.

127. Nguyen DM, Sam K, Tsimelzon A, et al. Molecular heterogeneity of inflammatory breast cancer: a hyperproliferative phenotype. *Clin Cancer Res* 2006;12(17):5047–5054.

Chapter 63
Management Summary on Preoperative Systemic Therapy

C. Kent Osborne and Jay R. Harris

Established indications for preoperative (also known as neoadjuvant) systemic therapy are (a) in patients with locally advanced and inoperable (stage IIIB) breast cancer and (b) in stage I or II patients with an unfavorable tumor to breast size ratio to facilitate breast-conserving therapy (BCT). In the United States, preoperative chemotherapy is typically used. The pathological response to preoperative chemotherapy is an established major prognostic factor, and patients with a pathologic complete response (pCR) have excellent long-term disease-free and overall survival. It should be stressed, however, that in patients with estrogen-receptor (ER)–positive cancers, pCR is uncommon with chemotherapy (about 5%), and adjuvant endocrine therapy reduces distant recurrence and prolongs survival more than adjuvant chemotherapy in this subset of patients; therefore, endocrine therapy is increasingly being used in the preoperative setting. Preoperative chemotherapy is typically given for 3 to 4 months prior to definitive surgery. Preoperative endocrine therapy may require longer treatment durations for optimal down-staging because it tends to work more slowly. The direct relationship between degree of response (pCR) and survival seen with preoperative chemotherapy has not been demonstrated for preoperative endocrine therapy. With preoperative endocrine therapy for only 3 to 4 months, pCR is uncommon, yet long-term survival benefits (with continued adjuvant therapy) are substantial.

The use of preoperative systemic therapy is a fertile area for clinical trials offering the possibility of hastened results compared with adjuvant systemic therapy trials and the opportunity for correlative biologic studies. In particular, short-term "presurgical" therapy is usually reserved for investigation of new drugs in which the duration of therapy is limited to days or weeks. A key research aim for preoperative systemic therapy is to develop short-term intermediate or surrogate molecular end points that predict for long-term outcome in adjuvant trials. As an example, reduction in Ki-67 by preoperative endocrine therapy correlates with better long-term outcome than reduction in tumor size. The use of preoperative systemic therapy has the potential to allow for modification of systemic therapy based on response and to decrease the need for axillary dissection, but neither of these uses has been established.

It is highly recommended that patients treated with preoperative systemic therapy be seen by a surgical and a radiation oncologist at or near the start of treatment. Response is typically assessed by physical examination, mammography, and ultrasonography; however, these tests do not reliably predict pathologic response. Breast magnetic resonance imaging (MRI) can demonstrate the pattern of cancer growth in the breast, which may be predictive of response to preoperative chemotherapy. In addition, MRI may provide a better means to assess response, although its impact on treatment selection remains to be demonstrated.

Combined-modality treatment (consisting of chemotherapy, surgery, and radiation therapy), starting with preoperative chemotherapy, represents the treatment of choice for patients with stage IIIB breast cancer. Any chemotherapy regimen that has been validated in the adjuvant setting can be used in the preoperative setting. Long-term survival rates in stage IIIB patients treated with combined-modality treatment are considerably higher than those seen in historical controls. This approach is also commonly used in patients with stage IIIA breast cancer. Appropriate anti-*ERBB2* (formerly *HER2*) therapy should be administered to all patients with *ERBB2*-positive cancers along with chemotherapy, and endocrine therapy should be administered to all patients with ER or progesterone-receptor (PR)–positive cancers following completion of chemotherapy and surgery. In patients with locally advanced ER- or PR-positive breast cancer, preoperative endocrine therapy is a reasonable option, especially in older patients. Aromatase inhibitors are more effective in this setting than is tamoxifen. Given the proven survival benefits of adjuvant endocrine therapy, some experts are using it in the neoadjuvant setting in other patients with endocrine-responsive disease (high ER and PR, low *ERBB2*). Patients with locally advanced breast cancer treated with mastectomy should receive postmastectomy radiation therapy, regardless of response. Carefully selected patients with locally advanced breast cancer can undergo BCT, although precise guidelines for BCT in this setting have not been established.

In patients with stage I or II breast cancer, preoperative systemic therapy has been shown to increase the use of BCT but has not been shown to improve survival compared to the use of adjuvant systemic therapy. As in stage III patients, appropriate anti-*ERBB2* therapy should be administered to all patients with *ERBB2*-positive cancers along with chemotherapy, and endocrine therapy should be administered to all patients with ER- or PR-positive cancers following completion of chemotherapy and surgery. In patients with an ER-positive cancer, about 50% treated with a preoperative aromatase inhibitor for 3 to 4 months can be successfully down-staged to avoid mastectomy, a rate similar to that seen with preoperative chemotherapy. No studies have directly compared these two modalities in patients with ER-positive cancers in the preoperative setting.

The use of preoperative chemotherapy in patients with operable breast cancer has created new challenges for breast surgeons and radiation oncologists since the rules regarding the use of surgery and radiation therapy following preoperative systemic therapy are not well established. A core needle biopsy should be performed on all suspicious abnormalities found in the ipsilateral and contralateral breast before the start of chemotherapy. It is critical that radiopaque clips be placed within all cancers at the time of biopsy or early in the course of preoperative treatment to provide localization for surgical removal in the event a complete clinical response occurs. Surgical resection of a portion of the tumor bed, even in the setting of a complete clinical response, is an essential part of management. Sentinel node biopsy (SNB) can be performed either before or after preoperative chemotherapy. There are potential advantages and limitations with each approach. Studies are under way to determine whether a negative SNB after preoperative chemotherapy can obviate the need for axillary dissection. In patients treated with breast-conserving surgery, clearly negative margins of resection should be obtained. Even in patients with a pCR in the breast, breast irradiation should be used. For patients treated with mastectomy, chest wall and regional nodal irradiation should be given for patients with histologically positive axillary nodes after preoperative systemic therapy. Additional studies are needed to determine the need for such irradiation in patients with clinical stage I or II or cTN0 disease at presentation who are node negative after preoperative chemotherapy.

Chapter 64
Male Breast Cancer

Kari B. Wisinski and William J. Gradishar

 EPIDEMIOLOGY

Male breast cancer (MBC) is a rare disease worldwide. In the United States, it is estimated that 2,030 men will be diagnosed with breast cancer and 450 will have died from this disease in 2007 (1). MBC accounts for approximately 1% of all breast cancers and less than 0.5% of all male cancer deaths in the United States.

The ratio of female–to-MBC in white Western populations is 100:1; however, in the black population in the United States, the female-to-male ratio of breast cancer is 100:1.4 (2). Limited registry data from black African populations also suggest a lower female-to-male ratio of 100:6 in a narrow geographic band stretching across Africa from Angola to Tanzania (3). Worldwide, the highest incidence of MBC reported was 3.4 cases per 100,000 human-years in Recife, Brazil (4), whereas the lowest incidence rates of 0.1 cases per 100,000 have been reported in parts of Columbia, Singapore, Hungary, and Japan. The best estimate for the incidence rate for MBC in all populations where data are available is 1 case per 100,000 human-years or less (4).

According to the Surveillance, Epidemiology and End Results (SEER) Registry database, the incidence rates of breast cancer among men in the United States have slightly increased from 1975 to 2004 (from 0.9 to 1.2 cases per 100,000 men at risk) (5). However, an analysis of death certificates for MBC in the United States and Europe suggested no increase in the disease from the 1960s through the 1980s (6,7). From the mid-1970s to mid-1990s, there was also an increase in the incidence rates of female breast cancer in both the United States and European countries. This may reflect the introduction of mammographic screening in these countries or a change in risk factors that are specific to women, or both. The most recent SEER data show a decline in the incidence of female breast cancer since 1998 (5).

In the United States, MBC is predominately a disease of older men, with median age at diagnosis between 65 and 67 years (5,8). The median age of diagnosis for female breast cancer is 61 years (9). In a meta-analysis of case-control studies, the risk of developing MBC was positively associated with the following characteristics: never married, Jewish descent, previous benign breast disease, gynecomastia, history of testicular pathology, prior liver disease, and first-degree relative with breast cancer (2) (Table 64.1). Prior exposure to radiation may also increase the risk of MBC (10–12). In addition, a retrospective study from the California Cancer Registry found that 11.5% of men with a diagnosis of breast cancer developed a second primary cancer, with a significantly elevated risk of a second breast cancer (13).

Several of these risk factors suggest that conditions leading to estrogen excess or lack of androgens may be associated with MBC (2,14). Cases of MBC have been described in patients with a personal history of orchitis, undescended testes, and testicu-lar injury (8,14–16). Although the association between MBC and these disorders suggests that hormonal imbalances may play a causative role in MBC, no data yet support abnormal testosterone levels at the time of diagnosis.

The strongest risk factor for MBC is Klinefelter syndrome (14,17–19). This rare condition results from the inheritance of an additional X chromosome (XXY). Men with this condition have atrophic testes, gynecomastia, high levels of gonadotropins (follicle-stimulating hormone, luteinizing hormone), and low plasma levels of testosterone. Thus, the estrogen-to-testosterone ratio in these individuals is elevated compared with the XY male. The risk of MBC in these individuals is 20 to 50 times higher than that for men with a normal genotype (14,20).

Chronic liver disorders, including cirrhosis (21–23), chronic alcoholic injury (15), and shistosomiasis (24,25), have been associated with an increased risk of MBC. Cirrhosis limits the liver's ability to metabolize endogenously produced estrogen, leading to a relative hyperestrogenic state with an increased estrogen-to-testosterone ratio. In addition, several studies suggest that women who consume more than moderate amounts of alcohol may be at increased risk for developing breast cancer (26). Ethanol is a metabolic modifier for mammary epithelium and may promote the most carcinogenic pathway of estradiol metabolism to catechol estrogen. Despite the increased risk of breast cancer in men with cirrhosis or chronic alcoholism, few cases of MBC have been reported, perhaps owing to the shortened lifespan associated with these disorders.

Gynecomastia, when related to states of estrogen excess, has been associated with MBC (2). Gynecomastia can result from certain medications that cause an increased estrogen-to-testosterone ratio. In addition, several medications that cause gynecomastia have been associated with an increased risk of MBC (14,16,27). MBC has been described in three men who were prescribed finasteride, a drug approved for treatment of prostatic hyperplasia (28). Cases of MBC have also been reported with digoxin, thioridazine, and spironolactone (14,16,27). Other conditions, including obesity, thyroid disease, use of marijuana, and exogenous estrogen ingestion, are also associated with an increased estrogen-to-testosterone ratio and sometimes, gynecomastia, but a clear association with MBC has not been established (14,16).

Prolactin can act as an initiator and promoter of cancer in animals; however, physiologic states of prolactin excess in humans (e.g., multiple pregnancies) do not increase the risk of breast cancer in women and may be protective. Several case reports have described the development of MBC in association with a prolactinoma, a setting in which low plasma testosterone levels are often observed (29–31). The association between prolactin excess and MBC remains unclear.

Androgens may convey a protective effect on breast tissue by inhibiting cell proliferation. Mutations in the androgen receptor (AR) gene have been implicated in the development of MBC in two reports (32,33). These mutations occurred in the DNA-binding domain, in two adjacent amino acid positions in

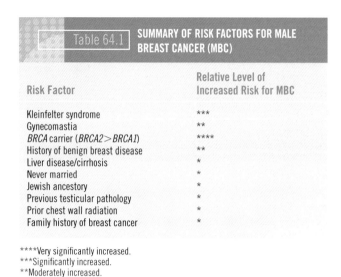

Table 64.1   SUMMARY OF RISK FACTORS FOR MALE BREAST CANCER (MBC)

Risk Factor	Relative Level of Increased Risk for MBC
Kleinfelter syndrome	***
Gynecomastia	**
BRCA carrier (BRCA2>BRCA1)	****
History of benign breast disease	**
Liver disease/cirrhosis	*
Never married	*
Jewish ancestry	*
Previous testicular pathology	*
Prior chest wall radiation	*
Family history of breast cancer	*

****Very significantly increased.
***Significantly increased.
**Moderately increased.
*Mildly increased.

the second zinc finger, believed to be an area responsible for transcriptional control (32,33). A pathologic case study that analyzed tumor material from two series of patients with MBC without clinical evidence of androgen insensitivity reported no AR gene mutations (34,35), however.

In the female population, approximately 5% to 10% of all breast cancer cases are thought to be hereditary (Section IV: Chapter 18). The breast/ovarian cancer genes BRCA1 and BRCA2, which account for most of these cases, have an autosomal-dominant pattern of inheritance (36–38). In women who carry a BRCA1 or BRCA2 mutation, the lifetime risk of developing breast cancer ranges from 50% to 85% (36,39). Limited evidence exists supporting the risk for MBC in BRCA1 carriers. One Dutch and one American family have been described with a BRCA1 mutation; each had one case of male breast cancer, as well as multiple associated female breast cancer cases (40,41). A recent report from the National Cancer Institute Cancer Genetics Network suggests that the cumulative risk of breast cancer by age 70 in men carrying a BRCA1 mutation is 1.2% (95% confidence interval [CI], 0.22%–2.8%) (42).

In contrast, men who carry a BRCA2 mutation have an approximate 6.5% cumulative risk for breast cancer by age 70 (42,43), which is a 100-fold higher risk than the general male population. Germline mutations in the BRCA2 gene have been identified in men with MBC and a founder mutation, BRCA22999del5, has been reported to account for nearly 44% of MBC cases in Iceland (44,45). In another study of 50 patients with MBC, BRCA2 germline mutations were detected in 14% of patients, 85% of whom (6 of 7) had a family history of male or female breast cancer (46). Similarly, a study reported on a population-based series of 54 patients with MBC showed that 17% had at least one first-degree family member with breast or ovarian cancer (47). No BRCA1 mutations were found and only two patients (4%) had BRCA2 germline mutations. Only one of the two patients with a BRCA2 mutation had a family history of cancer. Another population-based series of 25 patients with MBC in Italy found four mutations, one in BRCA1 and three in BRCA2 (48). Interestingly, those with the germline BRCA2 mutations had tumors with markers of aggressive behavior, including high-grade and c-erb-2 expression. The possibility that BRCA2 mutation carriers may not manifest the cancer phenotype (e.g., variable penetrance) is also suggested from the report on Icelandic populations, in which 3 of 12 patients with MBC who carry the same BRCA2 mutations have no family history of breast cancer (45). Alternatively, the MBC cases with an associated family history of breast cancer, ovarian cancer, or both that

do not carry a BRCA2 mutation may be explained by insensitive mutation screening techniques, chance clustering owing to the high frequency of sporadic female breast cancer in the general population, or other inherited breast cancer susceptibility genes that have yet to be characterized (49).

Guidelines from the National Comprehensive Cancer Network (NCCN) recommend that BRCA mutation testing be offered to men who develop breast cancer as well as to those from families that have a known BRCA mutation, a case of male breast cancer, or the presence of female relatives with a history of breast or ovarian cancer that suggests the presence of an inherited breast or ovarian cancer syndrome (50). Male carriers of BRCA genes should be trained in breast self-examination, undergo a clinical breast examination every 6 months, and have baseline mammogram with annual reimaging if there is gynecomastia or parenchymal glandular breast tissue on the baseline study. Furthermore, adherence to recommended screening guidelines for prostate cancer is advised.

Cowden syndrome is an autosomal-dominant cancer susceptibility syndrome characterized by multiple hamartomas (51). This syndrome is associated with germline mutations in the tumor suppressor gene PTEN located on chromosome 10 (52). The most common malignancies associated with Cowden syndrome are female breast cancer and thyroid malignancies (53). Two cases of MBC have been reported with germline PTEN mutations and the Cowden syndrome phenotype (54).

CLINICAL FEATURES

Most breast tissue in males is located in the subareolar area. Therefore, MBC typically presents as a painless, firm subareolar mass (55). A mass in the upper outer quadrant is the second most common presentation. A slight predilection exists for the left breast in multiple series. Bilateral breast cancer in males is very unusual (<1%) (56). Nipple discharge is a rare presentation of the disease. If serosanguineous or bloody nipple discharge is noted, malignancy should be suspected. Other findings on examination for malignancy include nipple retraction, ulceration of the nipple or skin, fixation to skin or muscle, tumor tenderness, enlarged axillary lymph nodes, or Paget disease (55).

The differential diagnosis of a male breast mass includes gynecomastia, breast abscess, metastasis to the breast, and other primary malignancies, including sarcomas (57). Gynecomastia is common, occurring in up to 40% of men without MBC and is seen in an equal proportion of MBC tumor samples (58). Gynecomastia can be unilateral or bilateral symmetric enlargement of the breast with poorly defined borders. On mammography, MBC is usually subareolar and eccentric to the nipple. The lesion is frequently well defined, and calcifications are rarer and coarser than those occurring in female breast cancer (59). In contrast, gynecomastia appears as a round or triangular area of increased density positioned symmetrically in the retroareolar region on mammography. Because of the low incidence of MBC in the general population, there is no role for screening mammography in men.

DIAGNOSIS

Although mammography can usually distinguish between malignancy and gynecomastia, its benefit in MBC remains uncertain. A recent retrospective analysis of 198 men undergoing mammography at a single institution showed that only 9 men (4%) had suspicious findings. Eight of these men had biopsies, with only two having invasive breast cancer. Both of these men had clinical findings consistent with breast cancer, which would have prompted evaluation without the mammographic findings. Overall, 96% of the mammograms showed benign findings, with 62% having findings consistent with gynecomastia. Most of the men (83%) with gynecomastia were taking medications or had underlying medical disorders related to this condition (60). Another study has also suggested that mammography added no diagnostic information to the combination of physical examination and pathologic evaluation (61). Therefore, mammography may add little to the management of clinical breast abnormalities in men. Although evidence suggests that the criteria used to characterize female breast tumors on magnetic resonance imaging (MRI) also applies to male breast cancers, no prospective data exist regarding MRI use in screening, diagnosis, or treatment of MBC (62).

Once a suspicious breast mass is identified, pathologic confirmation with either core needle biopsy or fine-needle aspiration (FNA) should be performed to obtain the diagnosis. The combination of physical examination and FNA has been shown to avoid surgical biopsy in 59% of patients (61). The efficacy of FNA in diagnosis of MBC is difficult to establish, however, given the small number of cases reported in various series and limited cytopathology resources in many centers. Adequate tissue sampling is critical for establishing the diagnosis and for performing estrogen receptor (ER), progesterone receptor (PR), and ERBB2 (formerly HER2) analysis.

PATHOLOGY

The most common histopathologic type of MBC is invasive ductal carcinoma, accounting for 85% of all cases (57,63–66). In most series of MBC, lobular carcinoma is rare or has not been reported (56,67,68), whereas lobular carcinoma accounts for approximately 10% of all female breast cancers (69). The rarity of lobular carcinoma in males is thought to be owing to the lack of acini and lobules in normal male breast tissue. Ductal carcinoma *in situ* (DCIS) accounts for 20% to 25% of all cases of female breast cancer (70). In contrast, the frequency of DCIS in men ranges from 0% to 17%, with an average of 7% (71). Few cases reports of lobular carcinoma *in situ* (LCIS) are found in the literature (72). Paget disease of the breast accounts for 1% to 5% of all female breast tumors. The frequency of Paget disease in MBC is unknown, but it appears to be associated with a worse 5-year survival in men (73). All other subtypes of breast cancer, including inflammatory breast cancer, have been reported in men (74).

In females with breast cancer, tumors are ER-positive, PR-positive, or both in 60% to 70% of patients. In contrast, series of MBC in the literature suggest that up to 91% are ER-positive and 75% to 96% are PR-positive (56,75).

Limited information is available regarding other molecular markers in MBC. In a series of 111 patients with MBC from the Mayo Clinic, tumor samples were analyzed for AR, the proto-oncogene p53, and ERBB2, the cell cycle regulatory proteins cyclin D1 and MIB1, and *bcl-2*, a marker of apoptosis (75). AR was positive in 95% of patients with MBC, which was consistent with other reports. *Bcl-2*, which in female breast cancer has been associated with expression of ER, was expressed in 95% of male breast tumors. In this series, ERBB2 was overexpressed in 29% of patients, comparable to the 30% of female breast tumors with this finding. Cyclin D1 is important in cell cycle regulation. It forms complexes with the cyclin-dependent kinases, which then phosphorylate the retinoblastoma gene protein. In both female and male breast cancer, approximately 50% of tumors overexpress cyclin D1. MIB1 is an antibody directed against Ki-67, an antigen associated with tumor cell proliferation. In MBC, 38% of tumors are MIB1-positive. In this case series, p53 was positive in 21%

of patients with MBC, somewhat lower than other reports in which up to 54% of samples were p53-positive (Section VI: Chapter 32).

TREATMENT: SURGICAL MANAGEMENT

The current operative procedure of choice for localized breast cancer in men is a total mastectomy with sentinel node (SLN) biopsy (Section 7: Chapter 36). Until relatively recently modified radical mastectomy (MRM) was the preferred operation. Although randomized studies have not been conducted in men, retrospective data suggest the equivalence of radical mastectomy and MRM in terms of local recurrence and survival (64,76,77) and randomized studies in women also support the therapeutic equivalence of these two surgical procedures. The only exception is that men who have extensive chest wall muscle involvement or Rotter node involvement may benefit from a radical mastectomy if neoadjuvant chemotherapy does not sufficiently reduce the tumor. Although breast conservation therapy with lumpectomy followed by breast irradiation has been shown to have equivalent outcomes as mastectomy in women with early-stage breast cancer (78), breast-conserving therapy is generally not an option for men because of the lack of adequate surrounding breast tissue and the central location of most tumors.

In early-stage breast cancer in women, SLN biopsy has emerged as an alternative to axillary lymph node dissection (ALND) and is associated with less morbidity (79). In an effort to understand the best technique for SLN biopsy in men, Albo et al. (80) reported on seven patients with MBC and clinically negative axillary lymph nodes who underwent preoperative and intraoperative lymphoscintography, followed by SLN biopsy. SLN biopsy was performed using a combination of isosulfan blue dye and technetium 99m (^{99m}Tc). Preoperative lymphoscintigraphy identified SLN in five of seven patients. Intraoperatively, SLN were identified in all seven patients. Six SLN were found with the γ-probe and seven with blue dye, indicating that these techniques are complementary. Several small series have evaluated outcomes with SLN biopsy in men with breast cancer. In one series of 16 men with localized breast cancer, one or more sentinel nodes were identified in 15 subjects by the combined use of radiocolloid and blue dye (81). Of the 10 men with a negative SLN biopsy, 6 had full ALND, and no further positive lymph nodes were identified. A retrospective study of 32 men with clinically negative lymph nodes evaluated preoperative lymphoscintigraphy with colloid particles of human serum albumin labeled with ^{99m}Tc (82). In this analysis, one or more SLN were identified in all of the subjects. Twenty-six patients had negative SLN and did not have an ALND. After a median follow-up of 30 months, no axillary recurrence of disease was seen. A recent report by Rusby et al. (83) summarized the data on SLN biopsy from the 110 patients with MBC reported in the literature. The results showed that a sentinel node was identified in 96% of cases. Of the 13 cases where a negative SLN biopsy was followed by ALND, no false–negative findings were seen. Memorial Sloan-Kettering Cancer Center also recently reported their experience with SLN biopsy in MBC (84). Of the 78 subjects with MBC, SLN biopsy was successful in 76 (97%). Negative SLN were found in 39 of 76 (51%) patients. Of these, three (8%) were found to have a positive non-SLN during intraoperative palpation. Positive SLN were found in 37 of 76 (49%) patients. The two patients with failed SLN biopsy underwent ALND with positive nodes. At a median follow-up of 28 months, there were no axillary recurrences in the axillary nodes. These experiences with SLN biopsy in men are comparable to those in women and SLN biopsy is now the standard of care for clinically axillary node-negative MBC.

PROGNOSTIC FACTORS

Male and female breast cancers are staged according to the American Joint Committee on Cancer (AJCC) Staging System (Section 7: Chapter 35). Similar to women with breast cancer, stage, tumor size, and axillary lymph node status appear to be the most important factors influencing outcome. Guinee et al. (85) confirmed the importance of nodal status as a predictor of survival in MBC. The 335 patients were registered over a 20-year period. The survival rate at 10 years was 84% for patients with histologically negative nodes, 44% for those with one to three positive nodes, and 14% for the group with four or more histologically positive nodes. Another analysis on 42 well-characterized patients with MBC revealed a 5-year survival of 100% for patients with stage I disease, 83% for those with stage II disease, 60% for those with stage III disease, and 25% for those with stage IV disease (86). Patients with axillary lymph node involvement had a decreased 10-year adjusted overall survival (36 vs. 58%) and disease-free survival (18% vs. 44%) compared with patients without axillary nodal involvement. Donegan et al. (65) confirmed the prognostic value of tumor stage by reporting data on 217 patients with MBC accessed from tumor registries at 18 institutions in Wisconsin between 1953 and 1995. Consistent with other reports, 5-year survival declined with increasing stage of disease and increasing number of involved axillary lymph nodes. This analysis also found that since 1986, patients presented with earlier stage disease and were more likely to be treated with modified radical mastectomy followed by adjuvant systemic therapy. Likely related to these differences, when outcomes after 1986 were compared with the preceding years, improved 5-year survival was noted. Other series have reported similar findings (63,64,87–92).

Because MBC is rare and prospective, large studies have not been performed, the prognostic value of other molecular and pathologic markers has not been well validated. Although many reports describe various molecular markers in MBC (e.g., DNA ploidy, nuclear differentiation, MIB1 positivity, cathepsin D, and ERBB2), their correlation with prognosis has not been confirmed (75,93,94).

Some reports have also suggested that MBC has a worse prognosis than female breast cancer. The most recent analyses which carefully matched subjects by stage, do not, however, substantiate a difference in outcomes between genders (95,96). Retrospective data do suggest that adjuvant treatment was significantly different in age, ethnicity, and stage-matched female and male breast cancer patients (97). Ethnicity may also influence breast cancer prognosis and treatment. It is known that black women with breast cancer have poorer survival than white women (98). In an analysis of 510 MBC cases (456 white, 34 black), black men were approximately 50% less likely to undergo consultation with an oncologist and subsequently receive chemotherapy (99). After multivariate analysis, breast cancer-specific mortality hazard ratio was shown to be more than triple for black versus white men.

TREATMENT OF METASTATIC DISEASE

Hormonal manipulation has played a central role in the management of metastatic MBC since bilateral orchiectomy was reported to have an impact on disease progression in 1942 (100). Multiple reports of orchiectomy as treatment of metastatic MBC indicate response rates between 32% and 67%, with a median survival of 56 months in responding patients versus 38 months in nonresponding patients (55). Other ablative surgical procedures have been evaluated in metastatic MBC, either as primary treatment or at the time of disease progression after orchiectomy. Adrenalectomy and hypophysectomy are associated with response rates of 76% and 58%, respectively (55). These surgical interventions are rarely used today, however, for various reasons, including the unwillingness of many men to accept orchiectomy for psychological reasons, the morbidity associated with ablative surgical procedures, and the introduction of medical management of metastatic disease.

Because most MBC express the ER, tamoxifen is the endocrine treatment of choice for metastatic disease. Objective response rates as high as 81% have been reported in ER-positive MBC with tamoxifen treatment (101). Other endocrine therapies, including aminoglutethimide, estrogen, megestrol acetate, androgens, steroids, and luteinizing hormone-releasing hormone analogs, have also been used for metastatic MBC. Although clinical information in these studies is limited, the response rates with these interventions are usually greater than 40% for ER-positive tumors (101).

The new selective aromatase inhibitors (anastrozole, letrozole, and exemestane) are also very active agents for the treatment of advanced disease in postmenopausal women with hormone receptor-positive breast cancer (102). In ER-positive MBC, there is one report with anastrozole in which no objective responses were observed in five men with metastatic disease, four of whom had progressive disease on tamoxifen therapy (103). In men with normal testes, aromatase inhibitors only block approximately 80% of estrogen production, which may explain these lower objective response rates when compared with tamoxifen. Of the five cases, however, three had disease stabilization with anastrozole and two patients showed significant clinical benefit, which was defined as stable disease for longer than 24 weeks. Two case reports are found in the literature of clinical responses to aromatase inhibitors in MBC (104,105). This limited experience suggests that the aromatase inhibitors may provide clinical benefit to patients with MBC, but more data are needed with these agents. The Southwestern Oncology Group is investigating the combination of aromatase inhibitor and goserelin in hormone-responsive metastatic male breast cancer.

In advanced MBC, treatment with chemotherapy should be considered for patients with ER-negative tumors, for those with rapidly progressing disease, and in patients who are refractory to endocrine manipulations. Numerous anecdotal reports have described the activity of single-agent and combination chemotherapy regimens in MBC (101). Although the optimal chemotherapy regimen has not been defined for MBC, treatment guidelines used for women are reasonable considerations in men.

Adjuvant Systemic Therapy

Recommendations for adjuvant endocrine, chemotherapy, or both after surgical resection of the tumor in MBC are based largely on the benefits derived from these interventions in clinical trials for women with early-stage breast cancer. The low incidence of MBC precludes the development and timely completion of clinical trials to assess the efficacy of adjuvant therapy.

Because most patients with MBC have ER-positive tumors, adjuvant tamoxifen therapy for 5 year is often recommended. Ribeiro and Swindell (106) reported improved 5-year actuarial survival and disease-free survival in 39 patients who received tamoxifen compared with a historical control group (61% vs. 44% and 56% vs. 28%, respectively). Tamoxifen is generally well tolerated in men, but a 1994 report described frequent side effects in 24 male patients undergoing adjuvant tamoxifen therapy (107). The most common side effects were decreased libido (29%), weight gain (25%), hot flashes (21%), mood alteration (21%), and depression (17%). Overall, 21% of the men in this study discontinued tamoxifen because of side effects; the attrition was 4% in women who received adjuvant tamoxifen.

The role of adjuvant chemotherapy in MBC has also not been rigorously studied. One report on 11 patients with stage II or stage III MBC treated with adjuvant cyclophosphamide, methotrexate, and 5-fluorouracil (CMF) showed favorable outcomes compared with historical controls (108). At the National Cancer Institute, 31 patients with axillary node-positive, stage II MBC were treated with adjuvant CMF chemotherapy for up to 12 cycles. The initial report on 24 of theses patients showed a 5-year survival of more than 80% and median overall survival of 98 months (109). This was an improvement compared with historical controls. A recent update on the 20-year follow-up from all 31 of these patients treated with adjuvant CMF showed the overall survival at 10, 15, and 20 years was 64.5%, 51.6%, and 42.4%, respectively (110). It is rational that current recommendations for adjuvant therapy in MBC should be adopted from those for women with early-stage breast cancer (Section VII, Chapter 49).

Adjuvant Radiation Therapy

No prospective, randomized clinical trials are available that evaluate the clinical impact of adjuvant radiation therapy. In several series, postoperative radiation therapy was administered to some patients, but the technical aspects of radiotherapy varied between series and over time, making any assessment of clinical impact difficult. Postmastectomy radiation therapy for MBC appears to reduce locoregional recurrence, but has had no apparent impact on overall survival (65,111,112). The publications of two clinical trials showing a survival advantage for women with stage II breast cancer who received postmastectomy radiation therapy may, however, be applicable for similar patients with MBC (113,114). A retrospective study from Johns Hopkins University suggested that the same indications for postmastectomy radiation that apply to female breast cancer should be used in men (115) (Section VII, Chapter 47).

MANAGEMENT SUMMARY

A suspicious breast mass in a man must be evaluated by tissue sampling. Needle biopsy is the preferred method of diagnosis. Total mastectomy is the treatment of choice for most male cancers. Sentinel node biopsy is an accurate technique for axillary staging. Chest wall and regional lymph node irradiation should be given using the criteria developed for use in women.

Adjuvant systemic therapy recommendations are similar to those for women with the same stage of disease. For patients with tumors which express steroid hormone receptors, adjuvant tamoxifen with or without chemotherapy should be recommended. For patients with hormone receptor-negative disease, chemotherapy should be recommended. In patients with metastatic disease, chemotherapy should be recommended for rapidly progressing disease, or hormone receptor-negative disease. Antiestrogens, progestins, and perhaps aromatase inhibitors should be considered for patients with indolent hormone receptor-positive disease.

References

1. Jemal A, Siegel R, Ward E, et al. Cancer Statistics, 2007. *CA Cancer J Clin* 2007; 57(1):43–66.
2. Sasco AJ, Lowenfels AB, Pasker-de Jong P. Review Article: Epidemiology of male breast cancer. A meta-analysis of published case-control studies and discussion of selected aetiological factors. *Int J Cancer* 1993;53(4):538–549.
3. Parkin D. *Cancer occurrence in developing countries*. IARC Scientific Publications 75. Lyon: International Agency for Research on Cancer, 1986.
4. Muir C, Waterhouse J, Mack T, et al. *Cancer incidence in five continents* 1987. IARC Scientific Publications, Lyon.
5. Breast cancer (invasive): Age adjusted SEER incidence rates by year. *Surveillance Epidemiology and End Results (SEER)*; 1975–2004.
6. La Vecchia C, Levi F, Lucchini F. Descriptive epidemiology of male breast cancer in Europe. *Int J Cancer* 1992;51(1):62–66.
7. La Vecchia C, Lucchini F, Negri E, et al. Trends of cancer mortality in Europe, 1955–1989: Respiratory tract, bone, connective and soft tissue sarcomas, and skin. *Eur J Cancer* 1992;28(2–3):514–599.
8. Mabuchi K, Bross DS, Kessler, II. Risk factors for male breast cancer. *J Natl Cancer Inst* 1985;74(2):371–375.
9. SEER*Stat Database: Populations—Total U.S. (1969–2004) NCI, DCCPS, Surveillance Research Program, Cancer Statistics Branch, released April 2007. Surveillance Epidemiology and End Results (SEER) Program (www.seer.cancer.gov); 1975–2004.
10. Cohen R, Schauer PK. Male breast cancer following repeated fluoroscopy. *Am J Med* 1984;76(5):929–930.
11. Curtin CT, McHeffy B, Kolarsick AJ. Thyroid and breast cancer following childhood radiation. *Cancer* 1977;40(6):2911–2913.
12. Thompson DK, Li FP, Cassady JR. Breast cancer in a man 30 years after radiation for metastatic osteogenic sarcoma. *Cancer* 1979;44(6):2362–2365.
13. Satram-Hoang S, Ziogas A, Anton-Culver H. Risk of second primary cancer in men with breast cancer. *Breast Cancer Res* 2007;9(1):R10.
14. Thomas DB. Breast cancer in men. *Epidemiol Rev* 1993;15(1):220–231.
15. Olsson H, Ranstam J. Head trauma and exposure to prolactin-elevating drugs as risk factors for male breast cancer. *J Natl Cancer Inst* 1988;80(9):679–683.
16. Thomas DB, Jimenez LM, McTiernan A, et al. Breast cancer in men: risk factors with hormonal implications. *Am J Epidemiol* 1992;135(7):734–748.
17. Harnden DG, Maclean N, Langlands AO. Carcinoma of the breast and Klinefelter's syndrome. *J Med Genet* 1971;8(4):460–461.
18. Hultborn R, Hanson C, Kopf I, et al. Prevalence of Klinefelter's syndrome in male breast cancer patients. *Anticancer Res* 1997;17(6D):4293–4297.
19. Scheike O, Visfeldt J, Petersen B. Male breast cancer. 3. Breast carcinoma in association with the Klinefelter syndrome. *Acta Pathol Microbiol Scand [A]* 1973; 81(3):352–358.
20. Swerdlow AJ, Schoemaker MJ, Higgins CD, et al. Cancer incidence and mortality in men with Klinefelter syndrome: a cohort study. *J Natl Cancer Inst* 2005;97(16): 1204–1210.
21. Lenfant-Pejovic MH, Mlika-Cabanne N, Bouchardy C, et al. Risk factors for male breast cancer: a Franco-Swiss Case-Control Study. *Int J Cancer* 1990;45(4): 661–665.
22. Misra SP, Misra V, Dwivedi M. Cancer of the breast in a male cirrhotic. Is there an association between the two? *Am J Gastroenterol* 1996;91(2):380–382.
23. Sorensen HT, Friis S, Olsen JH, et al. Risk of breast cancer in men with liver cirrhosis. *Am J Gastroenterol* 1998;93(2):231–233.
24. Bhagwandeen SB. Carcinoma of the male breast in Zambia. *East Afr Med J* 1972; 49(2):89–93.
25. El-Gazayerli MM, Abdel-Aziz AS. Salivary gland tumours in Egypt and non-Western countries. *Br J Cancer* 1964;18:649–654.
26. Smith-Warner SA, Spiegelman D, Yaun SS, et al. Alcohol and breast cancer in women: a pooled analysis of cohort studies. *JAMA* 1998;279(7):535–540.
27. Lamy O, Elmiger H, Fiche M, et al. Acquired hemophilia as first manifestation of breast carcinoma in a man under long-term spironolactone therapy. *Int J Clin Oncol* 2004;9(2):130–133.
28. Green L, Wysowski DK, Fourcroy JL. Gynecomastia and breast cancer during finasteride therapy. *N Engl J Med* 1996;335(11):823.
29. Haga S, Watanabe O, Shimizu T, et al. Breast cancer in a male patient with prolactinoma. *Surg Today* 1993;23(3):251–255.
30. Olsson H, Alm P, Aspegren K, et al. Increased plasma prolactin levels in a group of men with breast cancer—a preliminary study. *Anticancer Res* 1990;10(1): 59–62.
31. Volm MD, Talamonti MS, Thangavelu M, et al. Pituitary adenoma and bilateral male breast cancer: an unusual association. *J Surg Oncol* 1997;64(1):74–78.
32. Lobaccaro JM, Lumbroso S, Ktari R, et al. An exonic point mutation creates a maeiii site in the androgen receptor gene of a family with complete androgen insensitivity syndrome. *Hum Mol Genet* 1993;2(7):1041–1043.
33. Wooster R, Mangion J, Eeles R, et al. A germline mutation in the androgen receptor gene in two brothers with breast cancer and reifenstein syndrome. *Nat Genet* 1992;2(2):132–134.
34. Hiort O, Naber SP, Lehners A, et al. The role of androgen receptor gene mutations in male breast carcinoma. *J Clin Endocrinol Metab* 1996;81(9):3404–3407.
35. Syrjakoski K, Hyytinen ER, Kuukasjarvi T, et al. Androgen receptor gene alterations in finnish male breast cancer. *Breast Cancer Res Treat* 2003;77(2): 167–170.
36. Easton DF, Bishop DT, Ford D, et al. Genetic linkage analysis in familial breast and ovarian cancer: results from 214 families. The Breast Cancer Linkage Consortium. *Am J Hum Genet* 1993;52(4):678–701.
37. Hall JM, Lee MK, Newman B, et al. Linkage of early-onset familial breast cancer to chromosome 17q21. *Science* 1990;250(4988):1684–1689.
38. Miki Y, Swensen J, Shattuck-Eidens D, et al. A strong candidate for the breast and ovarian cancer susceptibility gene BRCA1. *Science* 1994;266(5182):66–71.
39. Wooster R, Bignell G, Lancaster J, et al. Identification of the breast cancer susceptibility gene BRCA2. *Nature* 1995;378(6559):789–792.
40. Hogervorst FB, Cornelis RS, Bout M, et al. Rapid detection of BRCA1 mutations by the protein truncation test. *Nat Genet* 1995;10(2):208–212.
41. Struewing JP, Brody LC, Erdos MR, et al. Detection of eight BRCA1 mutations in 10 breast/ovarian cancer families, including 1 family with male breast cancer. *Am J Hum Genet* 1995;57(1):1–7.
42. Tai YC, Domchek S, Parmigiani G, et al. Breast cancer risk among male BRCA1 and BRCA2 mutation carriers. *J Natl Cancer Inst* 2007;99(23):1811–1814.
43. Easton DF, Steele L, Fields P, et al. Cancer risks in two large breast cancer families linked to BRCA2 on chromosome 13q12-13. *Am J Hum Genet* 1997;61(1): 120–128.
44. Thorlacius S, Olafsdottir G, Tryggvadottir L, et al. A single BRCA2 mutation in male and female breast cancer families from iceland with varied cancer phenotypes. *Nat Genet* 1996;13(1):117–119.
45. Thorlacius S, Sigurdsson S, Bjarnadottir H, et al. Study of a single BRCA2 mutation with high carrier frequency in a small population. *Am J Hum Genet* 1997;60(5): 1079–1084.
46. Couch FJ, Farid LM, DeShano ML, et al. BRCA2 germline mutations in male breast cancer cases and breast cancer families. *Nat Genet* 1996;13(1):123–125.
47. Friedman LS, Gayther SA, Kurosaki T, et al. Mutation analysis of BRCA1 and BRCA2 in a male breast cancer population. *Am J Hum Genet* 1997;60(2):313–319.
48. Ottini L, Masala G, D'Amico C, et al. BRCA1 and BRCA2 mutation status and tumor characteristics in male breast cancer: a population-based study in Italy. *Cancer Res* 2003;63(2):342–347.

49. Basham VM, Lipscombe JM, Ward JM, et al. BRCA1 and BRCA2 mutations in a population-based study of male breast cancer. *Breast Cancer Res* 2002; 4(1):R2.

50. National Comprehensive Cancer Network (NCCN) Guidelines Available Online at www.Nccn.Org/Professionals/Physician_Gls/Default.Asp.

51. Thyresson HN, Doyle JA. Cowden's disease (multiple hamartoma syndrome). *Mayo Clin Proc.* 1981;56(3):179–184.

52. Liaw D, Marsh DJ, Li J, et al. Germline Mutations of the pten gene in Cowden disease, an inherited breast and thyroid cancer syndrome. *Nat Genet* 1997; 16(1):64–67.

53. Starink TM, van der Veen JP, Arwert F, et al. The Cowden syndrome: a clinical and genetic study in 21 patients. *Clin Genet* 1986;29(3):222–233.

54. Fackenthal JD, Marsh DJ, Richardson AL, et al. Male breast cancer in Cowden syndrome patients with germline pten mutations. *J Med Genet* 2001;38(3): 159–164.

55. Donegan WL, Redlich PN. Breast cancer in men. *Surg Clin North Am* 1996;76(2). 343–363.

56. Goss PE, Reid C, Pintilie M, et al. Male breast carcinoma: a review of 229 patients who presented to the Princess Margaret Hospital during 40 Years: 1955–1996. *Cancer* 1999;85(3):629–639.

57. Burga AM, Fadare O, Lininger RA, et al. Invasive carcinomas of the male breast: a morphologic study of the distribution of histologic subtypes and metastatic patterns in 778 Cases. *Virchows Arch* 2006;449(5):507–512.

58. Heller KS, Rosen PP, Schottenfeld D, et al. Male breast cancer: a clinicopathologic study of 97 cases. *Ann Surg* 1978;188(1):60–65.

59. Appelbaum AH, Evans GF, Levy KR, et al. Mammographic appearances of male breast disease. *Radiographics* 1999;19(3):559–568.

60. Hines SL, Tan WW, Yasrebi M, et al. The role of mammography in male patients with breast symptoms. *Mayo Clin Proc* 2007;82(3):297–300.

61. Vetto J, Schmidt W, Pommier R, et al. Accurate and cost-effective evaluation of breast masses in males. *Am J Surg* 1998;175(5):383–387.

62. Morakkabati-Spitz N, Schild HH, Leutner CC, et al. Dynamic contrast-enhanced breast mr imaging in men: preliminary results. *Radiology* 2006;238(2):438–445.

63. Ciatto S, Iossa A, Bonardi R, et al. Male breast carcinoma: review of a multicenter series of 150 cases. Coordinating Center and Writing Committee of Foncam (National Task Force for Breast Cancer), Italy. *Tumori* 1990;76(6):555–558.

64. Cutuli B, Lacroze M, Dilhuydy JM, et al. Male breast cancer: results of the treatments and prognostic factors in 397 cases. *Eur J Cancer* 1995;31A(12):1960–1964.

65. Donegan WL, Redlich PN, Lang PJ, et al. Carcinoma of the breast in males: a multiinstitutional survey. *Cancer* 1998;83(3):498–509.

66. Joshi N, Pande C. Papillary carcinoma of the male breast diagnosed by fine needle aspiration cytology. *Indian J Pathol Microbiol* 1998;41(1):103–106.

67. Michaels BM, Nunn CR, Roses DF. Lobular carcinoma of the male breast. *Surgery* 1994;115(3):402–405.

68. San Miguel P, Sancho M, Enriquez JL, et al. Lobular carcinoma of the male breast associated with the use of cimetidine. *Virchows Arch* 1997;430(3):261–263.

69. Arpino G, Bardou VJ, Clark GM, et al. Infiltrating lobular carcinoma of the breast: tumor characteristics and clinical outcome. *Breast Cancer Res* 2004;6(3): R149–156.

70. Erbas B, Provenzano E, Armes J, et al. The natural history of ductal carcinoma in situ of the breast: a review. *Breast Cancer Res Treat* 2006;97(2):135–144.

71. Camus MG, Joshi MG, Mackarem G, et al. Ductal carcinoma in situ of the male breast. *cancer.* 1994;74(4):1289–1293.

72. Nance KV, Reddick RL. In situ and infiltrating lobular carcinoma of the male breast. *Hum Pathol* 1989;20(12):1220–1222.

73. Desai DC, Brennan EJ, Jr., Carp NZ. Paget's disease of the male breast. *Am Surg* 1996;62(12):1068–1072.

74. Spigel JJ, Evans WP, Grant MD, et al. Male inflammatory breast cancer. *Clin Breast Cancer* 2001;2(2):153–155.

75. Rayson D, Erlichman C, Suman VJ, et al. Molecular markers in male breast carcinoma. *Cancer* 1998;83(9):1947–1955.

76. Borgen PI, Wong GY, Vlamis V, et al. Current management of male breast cancer. a review of 104 cases. *Ann Surg* 1992;215(5):451–457; discussion 457–459.

77. Gough DB, Donohue JH, Evans MM, et al. A 50-year experience of male breast cancer: is outcome changing? *Surg Oncol* 1993;2(6):325–333.

78. Fisher B, Redmond C, Poisson R, et al. Eight-year results of a randomized clinical trial comparing total mastectomy and lumpectomy with or without irradiation in the treatment of breast cancer. *N Engl J Med* 1989;320(13):822–828.

79. Veronesi U, Paganelli G, Viale G, et al. A randomized comparison of sentinel-node biopsy with routine axillary dissection in breast cancer. *N Engl J Med* 2003; 349(6):546–553.

80. Albo D, Ames FC, Hunt KK, et al. Evaluation of lymph node status in male breast cancer patients: a role for sentinel lymph node biopsy. *Breast Cancer Res Treat* 2003;77(1):9–14.

81. Port ER, Fey JV, Cody HS, 3rd, et al. Sentinel lymph node biopsy in patients with male breast carcinoma. *Cancer* 2001;91(2):319–323.

82. Gentilini O, Chagas E, Zurrida S, et al. Sentinel lymph node biopsy in male patients with early breast cancer. *Oncologist* 2007;12(5):512–515.

83. Rusby JE, Smith BL, Dominguez FJ, et al. Sentinel lymph node biopsy in men with breast cancer: a report of 31 consecutive procedures and review of the literature. *Clin Breast Cancer* 2006;7(5):406–410.

84. Flynn LW, Park J, Patil SM, et al. Sentinel lymph node biopsy is successful and accurate in male breast carcinoma. *J Am Coll Surg* 2008;206(4):616–621.

85. Guinee VF, Olsson H, Moller T, et al. The prognosis of breast cancer in males: a report of 335 cases. *Cancer* 1993;71(1):154–161.

86. Joshi MG, Lee AK, Loda M, et al. Male breast carcinoma: an evaluation of prognostic factors contributing to a poorer outcome. *Cancer* 1996;77(3):490–498.

87. Crocetti E, Buiatti E. Male breast cancer: incidence, mortality and survival rates from an Italian population-based series. *Eur J Cancer* 1994;30A(11):1732–1733.

88. Izquierdo MA, Alonso C, De Andres I, et al. Male breast cancer. report of a series of 50 cases. *Acta Oncol* 1994;33(7):767–771.

89. Kinne DW. Management of male breast cancer. *Oncology (Williston Park)* 1991;5(3):45–47; discussion 47–48.

90. Salvadori B, Saccozzi R, Manzari A, et al. Prognosis of breast cancer in males: an analysis of 170 cases. *Eur J Cancer* 1994;30A(7):930–935.

91. Stierer M, Rosen H, Weitensfelder W, et al. Male breast cancer: austrian experience. *World J Surg.* 1995;19(5):687–692; discussion 692–683.

92. Williams WL, Jr, Powers M, Wagman LD. Cancer of the male breast: a review. *J Natl Med Assoc* 1996;88(7):439–443.

93. Hecht JR, Winchester DJ. Male breast cancer. *Am J Clin Pathol* 1994;102(4 Suppl 1):S25–30.

94. Weber-Chappuis K, Bieri-Burger S, Hurlimann J. Comparison of prognostic markers detected by immunohistochemistry in male and female breast carcinomas. *Eur J Cancer* 1996;32A(10):1686–1692.

95. Borgen PI, Senie RT, McKinnon WM, et al. Carcinoma of the male breast: analysis of prognosis compared with matched female patients. *Ann Surg Oncol* 1997; 4(5):385–388.

96. Willsher PC, Leach IH, Ellis IO, et al. A comparison outcome of male breast cancer with female breast cancer. *Am J Surg* 1997;173(3):185–188.

97. Scott-Conner CE, Jochimsen PR, Menck HR, et al. An analysis of male and female breast cancer treatment and survival among demographically identical pairs of patients. *Surgery* 1999;126(4):775–780; discussion 780–771.

98. Joslyn SA, West MM. Racial differences in breast carcinoma survival. *Cancer* 2000;88(1):114–123.

99. Crew KD, Neugut AI, Wang X, et al. Racial disparities in treatment and survival of male breast cancer. *J Clin Oncol* 2007;25(9):1089–1098.

100. Farrow JH, Adair FE. Effect of orchidectomy on skeletal metastases from cancer of the male breast. *Science* 1942;95(2478):654.

101. Jaiyesimi IA, Buzdar AU, Sahin AA, et al. Carcinoma of the male breast. *Ann Intern Med* 1992;117(9):771–777.

102. Smith IE, Dowsett M. Aromatase inhibitors in breast cancer. *N Engl J Med* 2003; 348(24):2431–2442.

103. Giordano SH, Valero V, Buzdar AU, et al. Efficacy of anastrozole in male breast cancer. *Am J Clin Oncol* 2002;25(3):235–237.

104. Italiano A, Largillier R, Marcy PY, et al. [Complete remission obtained with letrozole in a man with metastatic breast cancer]. *Rev Med Interne* 2004;25(4): 323–324.

105. Zabolotny BP, Zalai CV, Meterissian SH. Successful use of letrozole in male breast cancer: a case report and review of hormonal therapy for male breast cancer. *J Surg Oncol* 2005;90(1):26–30.

106. Ribeiro G, Swindell R. Adjuvant tamoxifen for male breast cancer (Mbc). *Br J Cancer* 1992;65(2):252–254.

107. Anelli TF, Anelli A, Tran KN, et al. Tamoxifen administration is associated with a high rate of treatment-limiting symptoms in male breast cancer patients. *Cancer* 1994;74(1):74–77.

108. Patel HZ, 2nd, Buzdar AU, Hortobagyi GN. Role of adjuvant chemotherapy in male breast cancer. *Cancer* 1989;64(8):1583–1585.

109. Bagley CS, Wesley MN, Young RC, et al. Adjuvant chemotherapy in males with cancer of the breast. *Am J Clin Oncol* 1987;10(1):55–60.

110. Walshe JM, Berman AW, Vatas U, et al. A prospective study of adjuvant cmf in males with node positive breast cancer: 20-year follow-up. *Breast Cancer Res Treat* 2004;103(2):177–183.

111. Erlichman C, Murphy KC, Elhakim T. Male breast cancer: a 13-year review of 89 patients. *J Clin Oncol* 1984;2(8):903–909.

112. Schuchardt U, Seegenschmiedt MH, Kirschner MJ, et al. Adjuvant radiotherapy for breast carcinoma in men: a 20-year clinical experience. *Am J Clin Oncol* 1996;19(4):330–336.

113. Overgaard M, Hansen PS, Overgaard J, et al. Postoperative radiotherapy in high-risk premenopausal women with breast cancer who receive adjuvant chemotherapy. Danish Breast Cancer Cooperative Group 82b Trial. *N Engl J Med* 1997;337(14):949–955.

114. Ragaz J, Jackson SM, Le N, et al. Adjuvant radiotherapy and chemotherapy in node-positive premenopausal women with breast cancer. *N Engl J Med* 1997; 337(14):956–962.

115. Chakravarthy A, Kim CR. Post-mastectomy radiation in male breast cancer. *Radiother Oncol.* 2002;65(2):99–103.

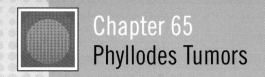

Chapter 65
Phyllodes Tumors

Kristine Elizabeth Calhoun, Thomas J. Lawton, Janice Nam Kim, Constance D. Lehman, and Benjamin Olney Anderson

HISTORICAL AND EPIDEMIOLOGICAL PERSPECTIVE

Phyllodes tumors are fibroepithelial breast tumors capable of a diverse range of biological behavior. Also termed *phylloides tumors* or *cystosarcoma phyllodes*, these lesions are similar to benign fibroadenomas in their least aggressive form, albeit with a propensity for local recurrence following excision. Although the original term *cystosarcoma phylloides* coined by Johannes Muller in 1838 was used to describe the tumor's grossly fleshy physical appearance, it was not intended to indicate metastatic potential as is typically implied by the term *sarcoma* (1). Phyllodes tumors in their most aggressive form, however, can recur with distant metastases, histologically degenerating into a sarcomatous lesion lacking an epithelial component (2). This metastatic variant is uncommon, however, with fewer than 5% of phyllodes tumors ever developing distant metastases (3). The first such case of a metastatic phyllodes tumor, in fact, was not reported until 1931 (4). Given a lack of uniformity in nomenclature, the World Health Organization recommended in 1982 that all such lesions be referred to as *phyllodes tumors*, which has now been widely accepted.

TUMOR CHARACTERISTICS

Macroscopic Appearance

The gross appearance of most phyllodes tumors is that of a circumscribed, round to oval multinodular mass that lacks a true histologic capsule. Phyllodes tumor size is variable, with reports in the literature ranging from less than 1 cm up to 40 cm (5). Most tumors have a grayish-white appearance and frequently bulge from the surrounding breast tissue when cut. Necrosis and hemorrhage can occur, particularly in larger tumors. Most phyllodes tumors, particularly those that are histologically benign, are very similar to fibroadenomas on gross examination.

Microscopic Appearance

Histologically, phyllodes tumors have a broad range of appearances, covering the spectrum from those that resemble fibroadenomas to others that appear as outright sarcomatous lesions. As with the fibroadenoma, phyllodes tumors contain a blend of stroma and epithelium, with both layers capable of manifesting a range of histopathologic changes. The characteristic *leaf-like architecture* of phyllodes tumors contains changes in both, where elongated cleft-like spaces as well as papillary projections of epithelial-lined stroma extend into cystic spaces (Fig. 65.1). This leaf-like intracanalicular growth pattern may not be present in all tumors, particularly those toward the malignant end of the spectrum, where the epithelial component is typically minimal or absent (Fig. 65.2). The epithelium is generally single layered, but hyperplasia, atypical hyperplasia, *in situ* carcinoma, or epithelial metaplasia may be seen (6–13). It is the stromal characteristics rather than the epithelial features, however, which determine subclassification and clinical behavior of phyllodes tumors, with stromal overgrowth linked to both local recurrence and distant disease development. Although the degree of stromal cellularity can vary, a consistent characteristic of phyllodes tumors is the presence of increased cellularity in the immediate subepithelial zone.

Histologic Classification

Numerous studies have attempted to determine which histologic features of phyllodes tumors are useful in predicting clinical behavior (5,14–18). Most pathologists use a combination of several histologic features to subclassify phyllodes tumors. The four most widely accepted classification features include (a) degree of stromal cellular atypia, (b) mitotic activity per 10 high-power fields (hpfs), (c) presence or absence of stromal overgrowth, defined as a single 40× field of pure stroma devoid of epithelium, and (d) infiltrative versus circumscribed tumor margins.

Based on the above four features, phyllodes tumors can generally be subclassified as benign, borderline, or malignant (Table 65.1). *Benign phyllodes tumors* (low-grade lesions) are characterized by increased stromal cellularity with no more than mild to moderate cellular atypia, circumscribed tumor margins, low mitotic rates, (generally <4/10 hpf), and a lack of stromal overgrowth. *Borderline phyllodes tumors* are characterized by a greater degree of stromal cellularity and atypia, microscopically infiltrative borders, and mitotic rates in the 4 to 9/10 hpf range, but a lack of stromal overgrowth (Fig. 65.3). *Malignant phyllodes tumors* (high-grade lesions) are characterized by marked stromal cellularity and atypia, infiltrative borders, high mitotic rates, generally greater than 10/10 hpf, and most importantly, areas of stromal overgrowth, a finding not seen in borderline or benign tumors (Fig. 65.2). More than 50% of lesions are classified as benign in most large series. Alternatively, some authors continue to refer to tumors as low-, intermediate-, or high-grade lesions (19,20).

Many tumors do not fit neatly into one of these three categories, however. Because these are uncommon lesions, most pathologists diagnose few cases, resulting in a wide range of percentages representing the individual subtypes that may unduly influence outcome data with respect to individual subtypes. In addition, tumors have a range of behaviors within each category, causing some authors to suggest that histology is not particularly useful in predicting behavior in phyllodes tumors (21). Nonetheless, the presence of *stromal overgrowth* (Fig. 65.2B) appears to be one criterion that consistently has been associated with aggressive, metastatic behavior (5,15–16,22). Stromal overgrowth, occurring in 29% of cases in the M.D. Anderson series reported by Chaney et al. (2) in 2000, was the only predictor of distant failure in multivariate analysis. The highest rate of distant failure occurred in patients who had large (>5 cm) tumors exhibiting stromal overgrowth. Multiple series since that time have demonstrated that such overgrowth correlates with development of distant metastatic disease (23–27).

Sarcomatous Differentiation

Phyllodes tumors can have sarcoma-like areas of differentiation, particularly if the lesion recurs and loses its epithelial component (28). The stroma can vary from slightly more cellular than fibroadenomas on the benign end of the spectrum, to

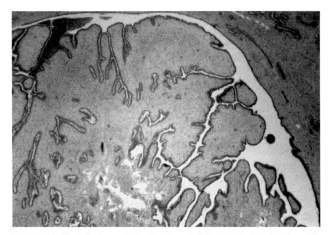

FIGURE 65.1. Phyllodes tumor illustrating characteristic "leaf-like" architecture. This histopathology image is from the borderline phyllodes tumor surgical case shown in Figure 65.5.

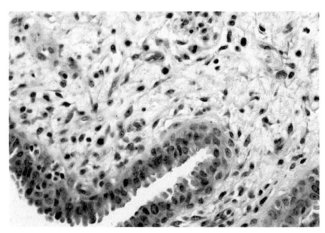

FIGURE 65.3. Borderline phyllodes tumor demonstrating intermediate level of mitotic activity and lacking stromal overgrowth. This histopathology image is from the surgical case illustrated in Figure 65.5.

fully sarcomatous in malignant varieties. Heterologous stromal elements have been reported in malignant phyllodes tumors, including liposarcoma, osteosarcoma, leiomyosarcoma, chrondrosarcoma, and angiosarcoma (29–35), but this finding does not appear to represent an independent prognostic feature of metastatic behavior.

Differential Diagnosis

The differential diagnosis for benign phyllodes tumors includes juvenile fibroadenoma and fibroadenoma with increased stromal cellularity. Juvenile fibroadenomas tend to have pronounced epithelial hyperplasia and lack noticeable mitotic activity, rarely up to 3/10 hpf. So called *cellular fibroadenomas* contain increased stromal cellularity, generally lack the prominent intracanalicular growth pattern of phyllodes tumors (leaf-like pattern), and have a negligible mitotic rate. Unlike the juvenile fibroadenoma, they do not share the trait of epithelial hyperplasia. Data are conflicting regarding the usefulness of MIB1 staining in distinguishing fibroadenomas from benign phyllodes tumors (36,37). Other ancillary tests, including hormone receptor status (38), electron microscopy (39), and clonality studies (40), have also not proved particularly helpful in this distinction.

On the malignant end of the spectrum, the main differential diagnosis includes metaplastic carcinoma and primary breast sarcoma. In many recurrent or metastatic lesions, stromal proliferation may predominate without identifiable epithelial elements. Usually, with careful sampling, identification of a typical infiltrating ductal carcinoma or residual phyllodes tumor architecture can distinguish between metaplastic carcinoma and phyllodes tumor. For cases in which only a malignant stroma is present, cytokeratin immunostaining for an epithelial marker will help. The histologic features of breast sarcomas are similar to those presenting in other parts of the body. The differential diagnosis of metastatic phyllodes tumor should be considered in the appropriate clinical setting when examining any pleomorphic spindle cell tumor.

Histogenesis and Genetic Evidence of Clonal Progression

Because of their similarity to fibroadenomas, and the heterogeneity of the stroma that can exist in any given phyllodes tumor, many theorize that phyllodes tumors arise from preexisting fibroadenomas (41). Two studies have suggested phyllodes tumors can progress from fibroadenomas based on clonal

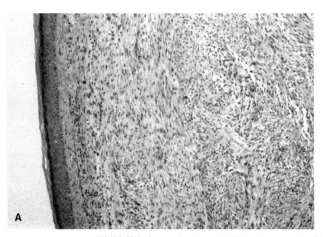

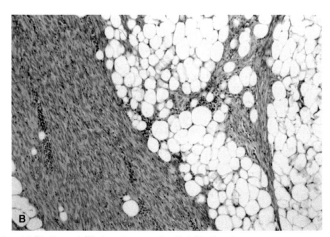

FIGURE 65.2. Recurrent malignant phyllodes tumor showing **(A)** dermal infiltration and **(B)** stromal overgrowth with infiltration of surrounding fatty breast tissue. Note the loss of epithelial elements from this recurrent tumor. These histopathology images are from the surgical case illustrated in Figure 65.8.

Table 65.1	HISTOLOGIC FEATURES USED IN CLASSIFICATION OF PHYLLODES TUMOR SUBTYPES		
Histologic Features	Benign	Borderline	Malignant
Stromal cellular atypia	Mild	Marked	Marked
Mitotic activity	<4 per 10 hpf	4–9 per 10 hpf	≥10 per 10 hpf
Stromal overgrowth	Absent	Absent	Present
Tumor margins	Circumscribed	Circumscribed or infiltrative	Infiltrative

hpf, high power field.

analysis of the stroma using the X-linked human androgen receptor gene as a target (42,43). Whether all phyllodes tumors originate as fibroadenomas or conversely start *de novo* is a matter of debate. Interestingly, in the recent MSKCC series of 293 patients, 37% (109 patients) reported a history of fibroadenoma diagnosed before identification of their phyllodes tumor (26).

Kuijper et al. (43) studied clonal progression in fibroadenomas and phyllodes tumors and concluded that fibroadenomas can progress in an epithelial direction to carcinoma *in situ* or in a stromal direction to phyllodes tumors. Chromosomal changes in phyllodes tumors have also been identified, with allelic imbalance (AI) on chromosomes 3p and 1q occurring in phyllodes tumors. Sawyer et al. (44) identified AI in 10 of 42 phyllodes tumors (24%) and observed that it can occur in both the stroma and epithelium, sometimes as independent genetic events, throwing into doubt the classic view that phyllodes tumors are simply stromal neoplasms. Finally, Sawyer et al. (45) studied stromal–epithelial interactions in phyllodes tumors. They suggested that abnormalities in the Wnt-APC-beta-catenin pathway, which has been implicated as a mediator of cellular proliferation, occur in the epithelium rather than the stroma of phyllodes tumors. During progression toward malignancy, the stromal proliferation appears to become independent of the Wnt pathway and, presumably, of the epithelial component of these tumors (45).

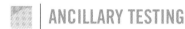 ANCILLARY TESTING

Tumor Marker Expression

Given the difficulty of the aforementioned histologic classification in predicting clinical behavior, concentration has turned to studying the usefulness of immunohistochemical testing of recognized tumor markers. Some studies have shown a correlation between MIB1 (Ki-67) positivity and histologic grade (36,46–49). Others have found that p53 expression in phyllodes tumors correlates with increasing tumor grade (48–52), suggesting possible prognostic significance (53).

Other markers studied with phyllodes tumors are oncogene epidermal growth factor receptor (EGFR) family members such as c-erbB-2 (52,54), tumor markers including CD34 and CD117 (55), actin (55), BM28 (54), and growth factors such as platelet-derived growth factor (PDGF) and PDGF-β receptor (PDGFR-β) (56). No marker has been found to predict conclusively and reproducibly recurrence or metastasis. Telomerase activity has been observed in recurrent phyllodes tumors, but it is unclear whether this finding in primary lesions is an adverse prognostic finding predicting recurrence (57). To date, none of these markers add substantially to information provided by standard histopathologic analysis.

The results of flow cytometric experiments have been mixed, but cytometry alone does not appear to be a useful independent prognostic feature distinct from histologic features in the diagnosis of phyllodes tumors (58,59). Only one study suggests

DNA content of phyllodes tumors is a significant predictor of outcome in a multivariate analysis (60).

Although the findings from these and other studies have been consistent with the hypothesis that these different tumor markers could play a role in the development of phyllodes tumors, they appear to have limited clinical relevance. The association between increased tumor marker expression and worsened outcome has not been reproducibly shown to predict outcome independently and no specific therapeutic implications exist for most of these finding.

Steroid Receptors

Estrogen receptor (ER), progesterone receptor (PR), and androgen receptor (AR) protein expression differs between the epithelial and stromal components of phyllodes tumors (61). Epithelial ER and PR protein expression is common, occurring in 43% to 84% of phyllodes tumors. By contrast, the expression of epithelial AR protein and stromal ER, PR, and AR proteins is uncommon, occurring 5% or less of the time. Given this general lack of stromal ER or PR expression, both of which are the components most likely involved in metastatic spread, there is no role for routine measuring of these receptors, because the information will have no impact on therapy decisions.

Circulating Tumor Markers

No circulating factors have been found to correlate with histologic diagnosis or outcome. Serum prolactin levels have been evaluated and they are not helpful in distinguishing benign from malignant phyllodes tumors (62).

CLINICAL CHARACTERISTICS

Incidence

Phyllodes tumors are uncommon breast masses, accounting for 0.3% to 0.5% of breast tumors in females (16). In one review of 8,567 patients with breast cancer treated between 1969 and 1993, only 32 cases of phyllodes tumors (0.37%) were identified among 31 patients (63). More recent series have reported numbers ranging from 33 to 821 patients (23–26,64–66). A population-based study from California noted a higher risk in Latino than in white or Asian women, with an overall risk of malignant phyllodes tumors of 2.1 per 1 million women (67). Phyllodes tumors have been reported in males, but are extremely rare, occurring in conjunction with gynecomastia and lobular development in male breast tissue (68,69).

Most patients with phyllodes tumors tend to be in their 40s, a decade or so older than that for women diagnosed with palpable fibroadenomas. Although those with benign phyllodes lesions are younger than those with malignant tumors by a decade, on average (41), the age distribution is broad and can

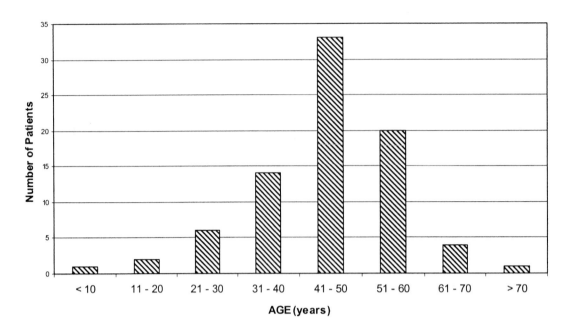

FIGURE 65.4. Age distribution of women diagnosed with phyllodes tumors. (Modified from Salvadori B, Cusumano F, Del Bo R, et al. Surgical treatment of phyllodes tumors of the breast. *Cancer* 1989;63(12):2532–2536, with permission.)

include girls under the age of 10 as well as women over the age of 70 (Fig. 65.4). Phyllodes tumors have been reported in prepubertal females (70–72), but overall they are quite rare among adolescents (73).

Clinical Presentation

Phyllodes tumors most commonly present as unilateral, single, painless, palpable breast masses in women typically in their 30s or 40s at initial presentation. These women may report that the mass suddenly "appeared," they may say that the mass has been growing continuously, or they may describe a mass that previously seemed stable recently started growing to relatively large size in a matter of a few months (3). On clinical breast examination, the phyllodes tumors feel firm and well circumscribed, similar to common fibroadenomas, but are often of larger size (>2–3 cm) at the point at which they are first detected.

The mass may produce visible bulging when it expands quickly (Fig. 65.5A). Although large tumors may grow quickly, rapid growth does not necessarily indicate malignancy. Shiny, stretched, and attenuated skin with varicose veins can overlie a phyllodes tumor as it pushes against the skin. In neglected cases, skin ulceration can develop from ischemia secondary to stretching and pressure. Such skin changes can occur with benign, borderline, or malignant lesions, so although ulceration associated with carcinoma is an indication of malignant behavior (T4 lesion), it is not necessarily an indication of metastatic potential with phyllodes tumors. The nipple may be effaced, but invasion or retraction is unusual (3). Bloody nipple discharge has been reported in a single case report.

Risk Factors

No clear risk factors for the development of phyllodes tumors have been identified. Patients with germline p53 mutations (Li-Fraumeni syndrome) are at increased risk for developing these lesions, but this represents only a small portion of diagnosed tumors (74).

Phyllodes Tumor in Ectopic Breast Tissue

Phyllodes tumors arising from ectopic breast tissue of the vulva, although an extremely rare occurrence, has been reported (75), whereas a tumor similar to phyllodes tumor of the breast can occur in the male prostate gland (76).

Associated Tumors and Bilaterality

Bilateral phyllodes tumors (synchronous or metachronous) have been reported, but are most uncommon. The Memorial Sloan-Kettering Cancer Center (MSKCC) series of 293 found only 10 individuals (3.4%) with bilateral lesions (26). Typically, concurrent tumors have similar histology, but in at least one documented case, a patient presented with a benign phyllodes tumor in one breast and a synchronous malignant phyllodes tumor in the other (77).

Patients can present with phyllodes tumors as well as separate noninvasive (78) or invasive breast carcinoma lesions (79,80). One case of synchronous recurrent phyllodes tumor with coexisting inflammatory breast cancer has also been described (81). Because phyllodes tumors are so uncommon, it is unclear if there is any physiologic connection between phyllodes and other breast tumors when they occur in the same patient, such as a familial genetic abnormality predisposing to both lesions.

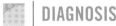 ## DIAGNOSIS

Clinical Features

Preoperative clinical suspicion of a phyllodes tumor is important but, because the lesions resemble fibroadenomas both on imaging and tissue sampling, this can be a challenging diagnosis. Features that should heighten the clinician's suspicion include older patient age, larger tumor size, and history of rapid growth. In practice, most phyllodes tumors will not be diagnosed preoperatively. In an individual series of 21 cases, only 6 (29%) were successfully identified before surgery on the basis of clinical features or preoperative diagnostic investigations (82).

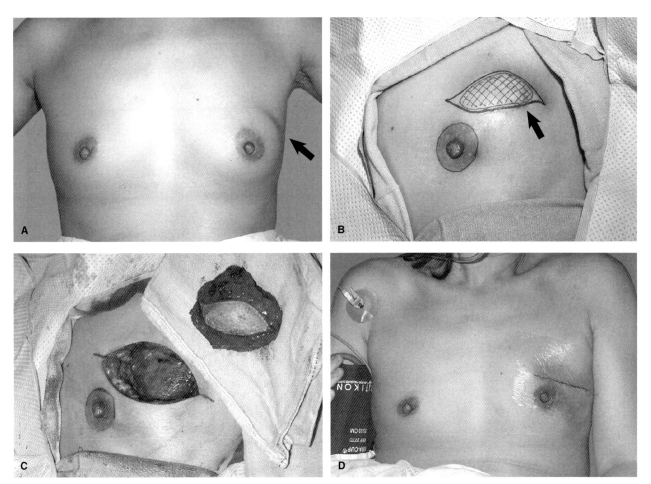

FIGURE 65.5. Presentation and excision of a primary phyllodes tumor. A 44-year-old woman presented with a palpable mass in the left upper outer quadrant, which had grown from 2.4 to 5.2 cm over 6 months. Imaging and core needle sampling at first presentation were interpreted as "fibroadenoma." The final pathology on excision was a borderline phyllodes tumor. **A:** Preoperative presentation with bulging mass apparent on inspection. The mass is located in the upper outer quadrant (*arrow*). **B:** Operative preparation showing the borders of palpable tumor (*hatch marks*) and planned skin excision (*outer line*), which is located immediately superficial to the mass. **C:** Operative excision down to level of pectoral fascia. **D:** Postoperative closure with flap advancement mastopexy closure.

Most phyllodes tumors, therefore, are surgically "shelled out" (enucleated) at initial intervention, resulting in inadequate surgical margins which are associated with an increased risk of local recurrence in the absence of additional surgery.

Imaging Features

No distinct imaging characteristics can reliably distinguish between a fibroadenoma, benign phyllodes tumor, or malignant phyllodes tumor. On imaging studies, phyllodes tumors commonly resemble large fibroadenomas (Fig. 65.6A) (83). They tend to present as large round, oval, or lobulated circumscribed masses on mammography (Fig. 65.6B), which may be associated with calcifications (83,84). On ultrasound, phyllodes tumors present as hypoechoic, well-circumscribed masses that may contain scattered cystic regions (Fig. 65.6C) (83–85). Although large size (>3 cm) and intramural cystic regions or clefts make the diagnosis of phyllodes tumor more likely, significant overlap is seen between fibroadenoma and both benign and malignant phyllodes tumors. For these reasons, large initial size or significant interval growth of circumscribed solid masses warrants excision to rule out phyllodes tumor. On magnetic resonance imaging (MRI), phyllodes tumors present as oval, round, or lobulated circumscribed masses with high signal intensity on T-2 weighted images (Fig. 65.7). On contrast-enhanced images, they tend to show rapid,

progressive enhancement that becomes more significant on delayed postcontrast images (Fig. 65.7B and C). Although MRI may more accurately delineate the true extent of disease before surgery, few data support the routine use of MRI in imaging phyllodes tumors at this time (86). MRI may be most helpful when mastectomy is being considered secondary to margin excisions, but the actual extent of the tumor is difficult to determine from standard imaging.

Technetium (^{99m}Tc)-MIBI (Sestamibi) nuclear medicine imaging has been shown to identify phyllodes tumor in the breast (87), but it has not been found to be useful in distinguishing benign from malignant lesions (88).

Fine Needle Aspiration and Core Needle Biopsy

Phyllodes tumors can be difficult to distinguish from fibroadenomas on both find needle aspiration (FNA) and core biopsy. Many studies have evaluated the efficacy of FNA in diagnosis of phyllodes tumors. Although cytologic criteria have been described to help stratify phyllodes tumors into benign, borderline, and malignant categories (89), the practical value of these studies is limited.

Most cytologic features fail to distinguish fibroadenoma and phyllodes tumors (90). Hypercellular stromal fragments occur in both lesions and cannot be used as the sole criterion for making a diagnosis of phyllodes tumor on FNA. Multinucleated

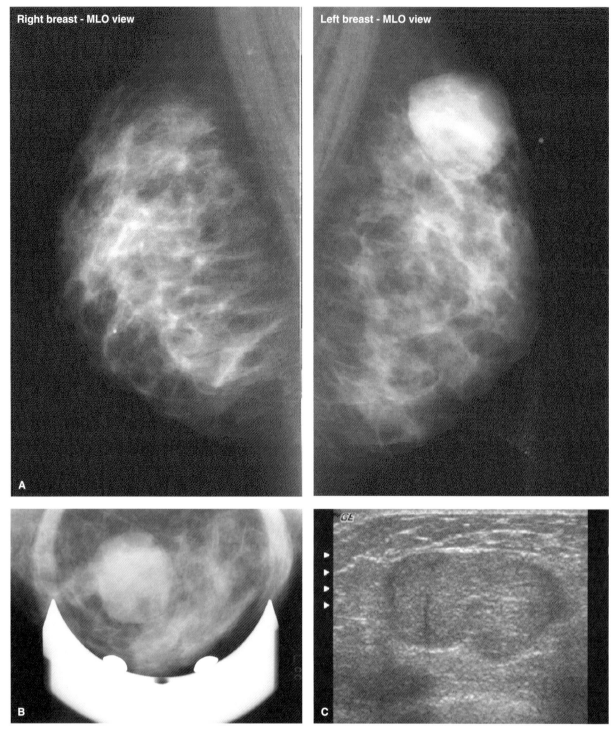

Right breast - MLO view

Left breast - MLO view

A

B

C

FIGURE 65.6.   Standard imaging studies of a phyllodes tumor. A: Bilateral mammogram, mediolateral oblique (MLO) view, demonstrating circumscribed round mass at 12 o'clock in left breast, biopsy proven phyllodes tumor. **B:** Spot compression view and of phyllodes tumor from Figure 65.5A. **C:** Ultrasound image of 2.4 cm phyllodes tumor, showing ultrasonographic characteristics included lobulated circumscribed solid mass with tiny cystic components.

stromal giant cells are rarely identified in FNA biopsies of fibroadenoma and may be indicative of more sinister conditions, such as phyllodes tumor or metaplastic carcinoma. This finding is not specific, however, and cannot be used as a sole diagnostic criterion in making this distinction (91). Because cytology of tumors with cystic degeneration shows thick fluid in the background, foamy macrophages, and apocrine cells, aspirates from these are commonly labeled "fibrocystic change" on cytology and as such can be a source of diagnostic error on FNA (92).

Similarly, the histologic features of benign phyllodes tumors can be difficult to distinguish from fibroadenoma on core needle sampling. It is common for needle sampling of a phyllodes tumor to be interpreted as "fibroepithelial tumor, phyllodes tumor cannot be ruled out." As a result, if a patient presents clinically with findings that are suggestive of phyllodes tumor, the clinician is advised to alert the pathologist interpreting the needle sample so that the unique features of these lesions can be specifically sought on core needle specimen.

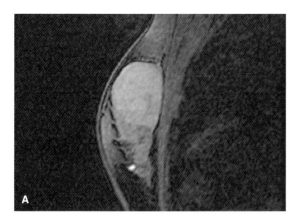

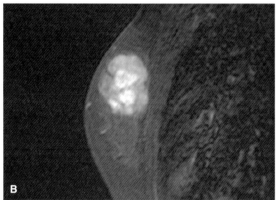

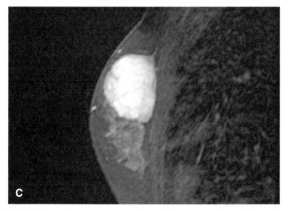

FIGURE 65.7. Magnetic resonance imaging (MRI) images of a phyllodes tumor. **A:** Precontrast. **B:** 2 minutes postcontrast. **C:** 5 minutes postcontrast. Note the progressive enhancement of the phyllodes tumor on the delayed postcontrast images. These MRI images are from the surgical case illustrated in Figure 65.5.

Although FNA and core needle biopsy may be helpful, ultimately, the final assessment will likely depend on the pathology results from complete surgical excision. The clinical challenge for the surgeon will be to decide whether to enucleate the lesion for diagnosis, as is done for a typical fibroadenoma, or to excise the lesion with wide margins, as is therapeutically indicated for phyllodes tumors.

TREATMENT

Surgical Excision and Margins

The core principle of local therapy for phyllodes tumors, whether benign or malignant, is local excision to negative margins to achieve definitive local control. Most studies advocate for at least a 1-cm margin, which has traditionally been accepted as an adequate resection (16,93–95). Negative surgical margins independently predicted improved disease-free survival and decreased local tumor recurrence in multiple retrospective national and international series (Table 65.2) (96). Mangi et al. (94) found that recurrence correlated with excision margin, but not with tumor grade or size. Of 40 patients, local recurrence occurred in 5, each who had margins less than 1 cm on initial excision or reexcision. These 5 patients remained free of disease after reexcision with a 1-cm margin.

The desired at least 1-cm margin width is based on retrospective analysis. Because these lesions are rare, any trial to study optimal margin width is impractical. A pseudocapsule of dense, compressed, normal tissue containing microscopic projections of the lesion commonly surrounds phyllodes tumors. As a result, more tissue typically needs to be removed to achieve the desired histologic 1-cm margin than might be predicted on the basis of preoperative physical examination or imaging findings (97). Some authors actually argue that 2 cm should be considered the standard of care for desired surgical margin for excision of phyllodes tumors, with a 2- to 3-cm margin desired if a phyllodes tumor locally recurs (Table 65.2) (3). A recent investigation from Germany identified 8 of 33 patients with local recurrence, with 7 of the 8 having less than a 2-cm margin at initial resection (64). In practice, margins of 2 to 3 cm can be difficult to achieve with good cosmesis, except when the breast is quite large.

Breast Conservation versus Mastectomy

In the M.D. Anderson experience of 101 patients with phyllodes tumors (2), surgery included local excision with breast conservation (47%) or mastectomy (53%). Microscopic surgical margins were negative in 99% of cases. Six patients received adjuvant radiotherapy. Four patients had local recurrence, with an

| Table 65.2 | **FACTORS ASSOCIATED WITH RISK OF LOCAL RECURRENCE** |

Study (Reference)	Stromal Atypia	Positive Margins (Definition of Positive Margin)	Necrosis	Fibroproliferation	Other
Asoglu, 2004 (23)	No	Yes (<1 cm)	No	No	Size
Chen, 2005 (24)	No	Yes (<1 cm)	No	No	Age >40 yr Mitosis
Fou, 2006 (25)	Yes	No (None given)	No	No	N/A
Barrio, 2007 (26)	No	Yes (<1 mm)	Yes	Yes	N/A
Lenhard, 2007 (64)	No	Yes (<2 cm)	No	No	N/A
Telli, 2007 (27)	Yes	Yes (<1 cm)	No	No	N/A
Belkacemi, 2008 (65)	Yes	Yes (<1 cm)	Yes	No	1N/A

N/A, not applicable.

actuarial 10-year rate of 8%. The investigators concluded that local failure was low, showing that breast-conserving surgery with negative margins is the preferred primary therapy.

Some investigators instead recommend mastectomy for histologically aggressive lesions. Kok et al. (98) endorse breast-conserving surgery with adequate resection margin for benign and borderline lesions, but recommend simple mastectomy without axillary dissection for malignant lesions. This distinction is based on clinical rationale rather than objective data and should not be considered standard of care. In contrast, Kleer et al. (47) found that histologically high-grade malignant phyllodes tumors have a favorable prognosis if widely excised without mastectomy. Multiple recent series have also failed to show a benefit to mastectomy over lumpectomy in patients who are otherwise good breast-conserving therapy candidates, regardless of tumor histology, provided negative surgical margins can be achieved with lumpectomy (23,26).

Reexcision Following Narrow Margin Excision

Approximately 20% of phyllodes tumors recur locally if excised with inadequate margins (99). The proportion of recurrences is likely to be somewhat higher with borderline or malignant varieties and lower with benign phyllodes tumors. Nonetheless, authors differ to whether immediate reexcision is necessarily required when an unsuspected phyllodes is diagnosed on permanent section after narrow or no margin excision. In a review of 106 benign phyllodes tumor patients, Chua et al. (100) concluded that because only 16% of patients presumptively operated on for fibroadenoma developed a local recurrence, a policy of close follow-up may be acceptable. Zurrida et al. (101) from Milan similarly argued based on their series of 216 patients. With a mean period of follow-up of 118 months, they found that only 8% of benign lesions recurred (vs. 20% to 23% for borderline or malignant phyllodes tumors) and that these recurrences occurred significantly later following initial diagnosis (32 months vs. 18 to 22 months on average). On this basis, these authors suggest that a "wait-and-watch" policy for benign phyllodes tumors may be considered as an alternative to mandatory surgical reexcision (101). Other authors, however, have demonstrated a benefit to negative margin resection for all histologic types secondary to all lesions having a propensity to recur with anything short of wide local excision (Table 65.2).

Technical Considerations in Lumpectomy

To achieve 1-cm or greater surgical margins with lumpectomy, special approaches may be necessary, particularly when a phyllodes tumor develops in a smaller breast. Tunneling through the fibroglandular tissue from a periareolar incision, although appropriate for a fibroadenoma biopsy, is contraindicated with phyllodes tumor excisions because of the potential for tumor seeding. Even a standard curvilinear circumareolar incision directly over the mass without removal of skin may be too small to obtain adequate surgical margins, or may leave excessive redundant skin behind when a large section of fibroglandular tissue is removed (Fig. 65.5A). Full-thickness excisions from skin to chest wall muscle can be very helpful in achieving the 1-cm desired surgical margins. This approach allows en bloc removal of skin, tumor, and surrounding fibroglandular tissue in an oncoplastic fashion (Fig. 65.5B). The excision is then carried out full thickness from the skin island, widely around the mass and down to and including the pectoral muscle fascia (Fig. 65.5C).

The remaining tissue defect typically requires a mastopexy flap advancement closure, where fibroglandular breast tissue on each side of the residual tumor bed is widely mobilized and advanced across the tumor bed to close the tissue deficit, both at the level of the pectoral muscle and at the level just deep to

the skin. This will improve the cosmetic outcome, with the added benefit of achieving more uniformly negative margins, and prevent adhesion between the skin and muscle surface (Fig. 65.5D).

Axillary Staging

Phyllodes tumors, like soft tissue sarcomas, are unlikely to have nodal metastases, making routine axillary dissection unnecessary in patients with phyllodes tumors (63,102). Although axillary nodes are palpable in 20%, fewer than 5% will actually have histologic nodal involvement (94). More recent studies continue to demonstrate a near uniform lack of nodal involvement, even with malignant lesions. In a series of 45 patients with phyllodes tumors who underwent axillary staging, none were found to have axillary metastases (103). Isolated cases of patients with gross nodal disease have been reported, albeit in association with locally advanced, histologically aggressive disease (104). Axillary dissection can, therefore, be considered in the exceptional situation wherein there are clinically suspicious axillary nodes.

If suspicious lymph nodes are identified clinically or on imaging studies, directed axillary ultrasound with core needle sampling (if indicated) can be performed. If the workup finding is negative, sentinel lymph node biopsy can be considered with belief that the axillary nodes are involved. In the absence of such suspicion, sentinel node biopsy is not indicated in the surgical management of phyllodes tumors.

Adjuvant Radiotherapy

Overall, the role of radiation therapy for phyllodes tumors is unclear (105). Clinical data supporting the use of adjuvant or neoadjuvant radiation are based on case reports and not large patient series. No series has shown radiation therapy to be of benefit in the primary treatment of phyllodes tumors. Although some have considered adjuvant therapy when the primary tumor is greater than 5 cm, has stromal overgrowth, a high mitotic index, or infiltrating border, the M.D. Anderson series did not support the use of adjuvant radiotherapy for patients with adequately resected disease (2). Information reported in a recent Surveillance, Epidemiology and End Results (SEER) database analysis suggested worsened outcomes when adjuvant radiotherapy was administered (106). In contrast, a recent European study demonstrated improved local control, but no survival benefit, when radiation therapy was used following surgery for either borderline or malignant lesions (65).

Based on anecdotal experience, adjuvant radiation therapy may be considered appropriate treatment for selected locally recurrent phyllodes tumors (96,104). Phyllodes tumors are so uncommon and biologically heterogeneous, that no large series of locally recurrent phyllodes tumors is ever likely to be collected. Radiation therapy may be considered when phyllodes tumors recur following mastectomy (Fig. 65.8). Adjuvant radiation therapy may be justified after reexcision despite the absence of definitive proof of efficacy, because any further local recurrence could be debilitating and difficult to treat. Chest wall recurrence following mastectomy may demand extensive surgery, such as multiple partial rib resections with rigid chest wall methylmethacrylate reconstruction and myocutaneous flap coverage, which is best avoided if possible.

Adjuvant Chemoradiation Therapy

Some reports have supported the use of combined chemoradiation following phyllodes tumor recurrence. In a case study of a locally recurrent malignant phyllodes tumor, neoadjuvant hyperfractionated radiotherapy, superficial hyperthermia, and ifosfamide were administered after the second local recurrence

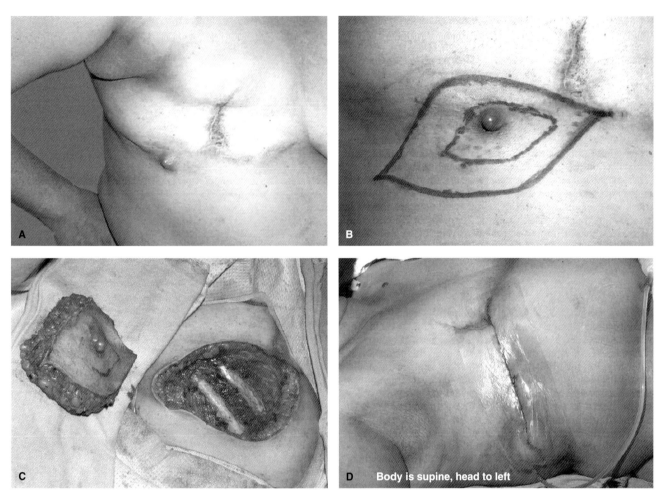

FIGURE 65.8. Presentation and excision of a malignant phyllodes tumor that recurred locally following mastectomy. At age 37, this patient had a palpable breast mass surgically shelled out. The mass proved to be a malignant phyllodes tumor and was reexcised with a partial mastectomy. The mass recurred in the lumpectomy site 15 months later. A subsequent mastectomy was performed using a three-sided incision to facilitate wide excision down to the level of skeletal muscle. Despite this second reexcision, the mass recurred again within 23 months, this time adjacent to the mastectomy incision. **A:** Recurrent nipple-like mass growing inferior to lateral limb of mastectomy incision. In addition to the protuberant mass, the tumor extends under the skin into the surround soft tissue and fat. **B:** Operative preparation showing palpable edge of subcutaneous tumor (*inner ring*) and planned skin excision (*outer ring*). **C:** Full-thickness operative excision, including skin, soft tissue, and skeletal muscle, excised down to the level of the ribs. **D:** Soft-tissue advancement flap closure with subcutaneous drain.

of this tumor. Toxicity was reportedly mild. Resection of the tumor bed revealed a pathologically complete response with an actual disease-free follow-up of 48 months (107).

Adjuvant Endocrine Therapy

Although phyllodes tumors have been shown to variably express steroid receptors, no value to adjuvant endocrine therapy with tamoxifen or aromatase inhibitors is known (108). Little rationale would exist for using these drugs; because steroid receptor protein expression decreases with increasing malignancy, they are primarily expressed by the epithelial component of phyllodes tumors, and only the stromal component of phyllodes tumors metastasizes (61). Overall, the systemic treatment principles of phyllodes tumors are driven by similar principles to those governing the management of soft tissue sarcoma.

Cytotoxic Chemotherapy

Chaney et al. (2) observed that patients with stromal overgrowth, particularly when the tumor size was greater than 5 cm, were found to have high rates of distant failure. These authors sug-

gested that such patients merit consideration of a trial that examines the efficacy of systemic therapy, even in the absence of metastatic involvement (2). Burton et al. (108) found that two of three patients with metastases achieved effective palliation when treated with cisplatin and etoposide combination chemotherapy. The current National Cancer Comprehensive Network (NCCN) guidelines suggest that patients with metastases be managed according to the Soft Tissue Sarcoma Clinical Practice Guidelines in Oncology (27).

RECURRENCE AND PROGNOSIS

Local Recurrence Following Resection

Local recurrence rates of up to 46% have been reported for phyllodes tumors (104). A retrospective study on the treatment and outcome of 27 women diagnosed with phyllodes tumors between 1986 and 1998 identified 19 (73%) histologically benign lesions, 3 (12%) borderline lesions, and 4 (15%) malignant lesions. Complete follow-up was available in 26 cases with a mean period of 37 months. Four patients (16%) had recurrences after surgery, occurring among all histologic subtypes (one benign, one borderline, and two malignant lesions). Mean time to recurrence was 9 months (98). In another small series, local recurrence developed in 3 of 21 cases (15%) and was not associated with patient age, tumor size, or histologic subtype (82). Time to recurrence seems to correspond best to the degree of histologic differentiation. In a Milan series of 216 patients operated on between 1970 and 1989, the average disease-free interval was 32 months for benign phyllodes tumors, 22 months for malignant, and 18 months for borderline phyllodes tumors (101). The recent MSKCC series revealed local recurrences among patients with both benign and malignant lesions, as did a smaller series from Germany (26,64).

When a phyllodes tumor recurrence occurs following partial mastectomy, wide reexcision must be performed and sometimes mastectomy is required. If recurrence occurs following mastectomy, full-thickness excision from skin to rib cage may be necessary to achieve 1-cm margins (Fig. 65.8). Soft tissue advancement flap closure is typically necessary to close the defect (Fig. 65.8D).

Predictive Factors of Recurrence

Surgical margins are the best predictor of phyllodes tumor local recurrence, with wide margins (typically >1 cm and potentially >2 cm) associated with the lowest risk of recurrence (Table 65.2). *Stromal overgrowth* is the most important histologic criterion for predicting the metastatic behavior of malignant phyllodes tumor (Table 65.2) (2,23–26,112). Two studies, from Europe and MSKCC, have suggested that tumor necrosis is also linked to an increased risk of local recurrence (Table 65.2). Although many markers have been studied and evaluated, no individual or combination of markers has been found to be more predictive than standard histologic analysis.

Barrio et al. (26) from MSKCC defined "fibroproliferation" as the presence of coexisting fibroadenoma or fibroadenomatoid change in the breast tissue surround the phyllodes tumor (26). In their series of 293 patients with median follow-up of 42 months, fibroproliferation was found to be significantly associated with a higher actuarial local recurrence rate. Although no other series have described fibroproliferation as a local recurrence risk factor, this histologic feature was not specifically analyzed or referenced in prior studies (Table 65.2).

Little difference exists in the tendency for benign versus malignant tumors to recur locally (3). A series of malignant phyllodes tumors at Memorial Sloan-Kettering Cancer Center found a low 8% local recurrence rate (99). In their series from Oklahoma, Geisler et al. (63) observed a tendency toward a higher rate of locoregional recurrences and metastases existed with high-grade lesions, but neither high-grade nor large tumor size was a statistically significant predictor of recurrence or survival (63).

Multifactor scoring systems have been proposed to better predict recurrence risk for phyllodes tumors. Meneses et al. (103) developed a system for assessing the degree of histologic aggressiveness based on specific histologic parameters, including stromal-to-gland ratio, tumor margins, mitotic index, and degree of stromal pleomorphism (103). The relative risk for recurrence was 6.0 for intermediate (borderline) lesions and 11.4 for malignant lesions when compared with the benign category. Although this system may be useful for predicting likelihood of recurrence, it is unclear to what degree this system actually changes clinical management, where the principles remain those of wide surgical excision without axillary sampling or dissection.

Distant Metastases

In the M.D. Anderson series of 101 patients, 8 patients developed distant metastases, with an actuarial 10-year rate of 13%. Overall survival in the series was 88%, 79%, and 62% at 5, 10, and 15

Table 65.3	FACTORS ASSOCIATED WITH RISK OF METASTATIC RECURRENCE			
Study (Reference)	Mitotic Index	Stromal Overgrowth	Tumor Size	Other
Asoglu, 2004 (23)	No	Yes	No	N/A
Chen, 2005 (24)	Yes	Yes	No	Margins
Fou, 2006 (25)	Yes	Yes	Yes	N/A
Barrio, 2007 (26)	Yes	Yes	Yes	Necrosis Cellularity
Telli, 2007 (27)	No	Yes	Yes	N/A

N/A, not applicable.

years, respectively. For patients with nonmalignant (benign or borderline) and malignant phyllodes tumors, the overall survival was 91% and 82%, respectively, at 5 years, and 79% and 42%, respectively, at 10 years. Multivariate analysis using Cox proportional hazards regression revealed stromal overgrowth to be the only independent predictor of distant failure in this series. Other factors implicated as having an increased risk of metastatic development include large tumor size, infiltrative borders, necrosis, and increased mitotic index (Table 65.3).

In a review of 67 reported cases of metastatic phyllodes tumors, Kessinger et al. (113) reported that the average survival time after diagnosis of metastasis was 30 months. Metastatic lesions have been reported as early as initial presentation of the primary tumor and as late as 12 years after diagnosis. The longest reported survival time after development of metastatic disease is 14.5 years (113). Prognosis is uniformly poor if metastatic disease develops.

The lung is the most common site of phyllodes tumor metastases. Pulmonary disease can present on computed tomography (CT) scan as multiple thin-walled cavities and nodules (114). Although thin-walled cavitary lesions from malignant phyllodes tumor are rare, pulmonary metastasis of malignant phyllodes tumor should be considered with disease that exhibits thin-walled cavities as a radiographic manifestation. As with sarcomas, distant pulmonary metastases may be resectable for cure in selected cases (22).

Other metastatic sites can include bone, liver, heart, distant lymph nodes (113,115), and distant soft tissue locations, such as the forearm (112), the thyroid (116), and the pancreas (117). Although these lesions rarely metastasize to the brain or central nervous system (CNS), such occurrences are refractory to therapy, and carry a dismal prognosis (118).

Patient Follow-up

After resection of a phyllodes tumor, a clinical breast examination should be performed within 4 to 6 months, with new baseline imaging at 6 months. Breast ultrasound should be included if that modality showed the mass initially. August and Kearney (97) recommend physical examinations and breast imaging studies twice per year for the first 5 years, then on an annual basis for patients after a phyllodes tumor resection. Routine breast ultrasound examination of the lumpectomy site should be considered, because if there is recurrence, it will most likely develop in the excision bed. If the breast is dense and ample in volume such that ultrasound might not be able to identify a mass, our institutional preference is to consider performing breast MRI at 1 year following excision, or sooner if the tumor grew rapidly or might be malignant. We have not found CT useful for imaging the breast.

August and Kearney also suggest obtaining routine chest and abdomen CT scans for 2 to 5 years for high-risk lesions

(>5cm, stromal overgrowth present, >10 mitoses/hpf, or infiltrating margins). The benefits of routine imaging of the lung and liver are unproved.

 MANAGEMENT SUMMARY

- Suspicion of phyllodes tumor is typically based on clinical criteria, including older patient age, rapid growth, or large tumor size.
- Mammogram and ultrasound evaluations are advised, although imaging studies may fail to distinguish the phyllodes tumor from a fibroadenoma.
- When preoperative tissue sampling is warranted, core needle sampling is preferable to fine needle aspiration for preoperative tissue sampling, because fibroadenomas and phyllodes tumors have similar cytologic features.
- Surgical management consists of excision to achieve surgical margins to decrease the likelihood of local breast recurrence. Most studies indicate a margin of greater than 1 cm is preferable, with some actually advocating for greater than 2 cm.
- When phyllodes tumors are excised with narrow or no margin, reexcision should be performed.
- The role of adjuvant radiation is controversial, with some studies indicating improved local control, but no increased survival, when used in patients with borderline or malignant lesions.
- Locally recurrent tumors may warrant adjuvant chest wall radiation following reexcision, because the high morbidity of second or third local recurrences from these locally aggressive lesions could be devastating.
- Routine adjuvant systemic therapy following initial excision is not recommended. Chemotherapy for locally recurrent tumors remains questionable. When used for treatment of metastatic disease, guidelines for treating sarcoma, rather than breast carcinoma, should be followed.

References

1. Muller J. *Uber den feineran Bau und die Forman der krankhaften Geschwilste.* Berlin: G Reimer, 1838.
2. Chaney AW, Pollack A, McNeese MD, et al. Primary treatment of cystosarcoma phyllodes of the breast. *Cancer* 2000;89(7):1502–1511.
3. Petrek J. Phyllodes tumors. In: Harris JR, Lippman ME, Morrow M, et al., eds. *Diseases of the breast.* 2nd ed. Philadelphia: Lippincott-Raven, 2000:669–675.
4. Lee B, Pack G. Giant intracanalicular fibroadenomyxoma of the breast. *Am J Cancer* 1931;15:2583.
5. Hawkins RE, Schofield JB, Fisher C, et al. The clinical and histologic criteria that predict metastases from cystosarcoma phyllodes. *Cancer* 1992;69(1):141–147.
6. Yamaguchi R, Tanaka M, Kishimoto Y, et al. Ductal carcinoma in situ arising in a benign phyllodes tumor: report of a case. *Surg Today* 2008;38(1):42–45.
7. Sugie T, Takeuchi E, Kunishima F, et al. A case of ductal carcinoma with squamous differentiation in malignant phyllodes tumor. *Breast Cancer* 2007;14(3): 327–332.
8. Ramdass MJ, Dindyal S. Phyllodes breast tumour showing invasive squamous-cell carcinoma with invasive ductal, clear-cell, secretory, and squamous components. *Lancet Oncol* 2006;7(10):880.
9. Lim SM, Tan PH. Ductal carcinoma in situ within phyllodes tumour: a rare occurrence. *Pathology* 2005;37(5):393–396.
10. Nomura M, Inoue Y, Fujita S, et al. A case of noninvasive ductal carcinoma arising in malignant phyllodes tumor. *Breast Cancer* 2006;13(1):89–94.
11. Parfitt JR, Armstrong C, O'Malley F, et al. *In-situ* and invasive carcinoma within a phyllodes tumor associated with lymph node metastases. *World J Surg Oncol* 2004;2:46.
12. Kodama T, Kameyama K, Mukai M, et al. Invasive lobular carcinoma arising in phyllodes tumor of the breast. *Virchows Arch* 2003;442(6):614–616.
13. Haagensen CD. Cystosarcoma phyllodes. In: Haagensen CD, ed. *Diseases of the breast.* 3rd ed. Philadelphia: WB Saunders, 1986:284–312.
14. Treves N, Sunderland DA. Cystosarcoma phyllodes of the breast: a malignant and a benign tumor. A clinicopathological study of seventy-seven cases. *Cancer* 1951; 4:1286–1332.
15. Cohn-Cedermark G, Rutqvist LE, Rosendahl I, et al. Prognostic factors in cystosarcoma phyllodes. A clinicopathologic study of 77 patients. *Cancer* 1991; 68(9):2017–2022.
16. Reinfuss M, Mitus J, Duda K, et al. The treatment and prognosis of patients with phyllodes tumor of the breast: an analysis of 170 cases. *Cancer* 1996;77(5): 910–916.
17. McKenna AM, Pintilie M, Youngson B, et al. Quantification of the morphologic features of fibroepithelial tumors of the breast. *Arch Pathol Lab Med* 2007; 131(10):1568–1573.
18. Fajdic J, Gotovac N, Hrgovic Z, et al. Phyllodes tumors of the breast diagnostic and therapeutic dilemmas. *Onkologie* 2007;30(3):113–118.
19. Morales-Vasquez F, Gonzalez-Angulo AM, Broglio K, et al. Adjuvant chemotherapy with doxorubicin and dacarbazine has no effect in recurrence-free survival of malignant phyllodes tumors of the breast. *Breast J* 2007;13(6):551–556.
20. Azzopardi JG, Ahmed A, Millis RR. Problems in breast pathology. *Major Problems in Pathology* 1979;11:1–466.
21. Salvadori B, Cusumano F, Del Bo R, et al. Surgical treatment of phyllodes tumors of the breast. *Cancer* 1989;63(12):2532–2536.
22. Hart WR, Bauer RC, Oberman HA. Cystosarcoma phyllodes. A clinicopathologic study of twenty-six hypercellular periductal stromal tumors of the breast. *Am J Clin Pathol* 1978;70(2):211–216.
23. Asoglu O, Ugurlu MM, Blanchard K, et al. Risk factors for recurrence and death after primary surgical treatment of malignant phyllodes tumors. *Ann Surg Oncol* 2004;11(11):1011–1017.
24. Chen WH, Cheng SP, Tzen CY, et al. Surgical treatment of phyllodes tumors of the breast: retrospective review of 172 cases. *J Surg Oncol* 2005;91(3):185–194.
25. Fou A, Schnabel FR, Hamele-Bena D, et al. Long-term outcomes of malignant phyllodes tumors patients: an institutional experience. *Am J Surg* 2006;192(4).492–495.
26. Barrio AV, Clark BD, Goldberg JI, et al. Clinicopathologic features and long-term outcomes of 293 phyllodes tumors of the breast. *Ann Surg Oncol* 2007;14(10): 2961–2970.
27. Telli ML, Horst KC, Guardino AE, et al. Phyllodes tumors of the breast: natural history, diagnosis, and treatment. *J Natl Compr Canc Netw* 2007;5(3):324–330.
28. Satou T, Matsunami N, Fujiki C, et al. Malignant phyllodes tumor with liposarcomatous components: a case report with cytological presentation. *Diagn Cytopathol* 2000;22(6):364–369.
29. Anani PA, Baumann RP. Osteosarcoma of the breast. *Virchows Arch A Pathol Anat* 1972;357(3):213–218.
30. Lubin J, Rywlin AM. Cystosarcoma phyllodes metastasizing as a mixed mesenchymal sarcoma. *South Med J* 1972;65(5):636–637.
31. Powell CM, Rosen PP. Adipose differentiation in cystosarcoma phyllodes. A study of 14 cases. *Am J Surg Pathol* 1994;18(7):720–727.
32. Kracht J, Sapino A, Bussolati G. Malignant phyllodes tumor of breast with lung metastases mimicking the primary. *Am J Surg Pathol* 1998;22(10):1284–1290.
33. Vera-Alvarez J, Marigil-Gomez M, Abascal-Agorreta M, et al. Malignant phyllodes tumor with pleomorphic liposarcomatous stroma diagnosed by fine needle aspiration cytology: a case report. *Acta Cytol* 2002;46(1):50–56.
34. McKenzie CA, Philips J. Malignant phyllodes tumor metastatic to the lung with osteogenic differentiation diagnosed on fine needle aspiration biopsy. A case report. *Acta Cytol* 2002;46(4):718–722.
35. Tomas D, Bujas T, Stajduhar E, et al. Malignant phyllodes tumor with associated osteosarcomatous, chondrosarcomatous, and liposarcomatous overgrowth. *APMIS* 2007;115(4):367–370.
36. Kocova L, Skalova A, Fakan F, et al. Phyllodes tumour of the breast: immunohistochemical study of 37 tumours using MIB1 antibody. *Pathol Res Pract* 1998; 194(2):97–104.
37. Kaya R, Pestereli HE, Erdogan G, et al. Proliferating activity in differential diagnosis of benign phyllodes tumor and cellular fibroadenomas: is it helpful? *Pathol Oncol Res* 2001;7(3):213–216.
38. Umekita Y, Yoshida H. Immunohistochemical study of hormone receptor and hormone-regulated protein expression in phyllodes tumour: comparison with fibroadenoma. *Virchows Arch* 1998;433(4):311–314.
39. Yeh IT, Francis DJ, Orenstein JM, et al. Ultrastructure of cystosarcoma phyllodes and fibroadenoma. A comparative study. *Am J Clin Pathol* 1985;84(2):131–136.
40. Kasami M, Vnencak-Jones CL, Manning S, et al. Monoclonality in fibroadenomas with complex histology and phyllodal features. *Breast Cancer Res Treat* 1998; 50(2):185–191.
41. McDivitt RW, Urban JA, Farrow JH. Cystosarcoma phyllodes. *Johns Hopkins Med J* 1967;120(1):33–45.
42. Noguchi S, Aihara T, Koyama H, et al. Clonal analysis of benign and malignant human breast tumors by means of polymerase chain reaction. *Cancer Lett* 1995;90(1):57–63.
43. Kuijper A, Buerger H, Simon R, et al. Analysis of the progression of fibroepithelial tumours of the breast by PCR-based clonality assay. *J Pathol* 2002;197(5): 575–581.
44. Sawyer EJ, Hanby AM, Ellis P, et al. Molecular analysis of phyllodes tumors reveals distinct changes in the epithelial and stromal components. *Am J Pathol* 2000;156(3):1093–1098.
45. Sawyer EJ, Hanby AM, Rowan AJ, et al. The Wnt pathway, epithelial-stromal interactions, and malignant progression in phyllodes tumours. *J Pathol* 2002; 196(4):437–444.
46. Umekita Y, Yoshida H. Immunohistochemical study of MIB1 expression in phyllodes tumor and fibroadenoma. *Pathol Int* 1999;49(9):807–810.
47. Kleer CG, Giordano TJ, Braun T, et al. Pathologic, immunohistochemical, and molecular features of benign and malignant phyllodes tumors of the breast. *Mod Pathol* 2001;14(3):185–190.
48. Niezabitowski A, Lackowska B, Rys J, et al. Prognostic evaluation of proliferative activity and DNA content in the phyllodes tumor of the breast: immunohistochemical and flow cytometric study of 118 cases. *Breast Cancer Res Treat* 2001; 65(1):77–85.
49. Dacic S, Kounelis S, Kouri E, et al. Immunohistochemical profile of cystosarcoma phyllodes of the breast: a study of 23 cases. *Breast J* 2002;8(6):376–381.
50. Millar EK, Beretov J, Marr P, et al. Malignant phyllodes tumours of the breast display increased stromal p53 protein expression. *Histopathology* 1999;34(6): 491–496.
51. Gatalica Z, Finkelstein S, Lucio E, et al. p53 protein expression and gene mutation in phyllodes tumors of the breast. *Pathol Res Pract* 2001;197(3):183–187.
52. Shpitz B, Bomstein Y, Sternberg A, et al. Immunoreactivity of p53, Ki-67, and c-erbB-2 in phyllodes tumors of the breast in correlation with clinical and morphologic features. *J Surg Oncol* 2002;79(2):86–92.
53. Kuenen-Boumeester V, Henzen-Logmans SC, Timmermans MM, et al. Altered expression of p53 and its regulated proteins in phyllodes tumours of the breast. *J Pathol* 1999;189(2):169–175.
54. Suo Z, Nesland JM. Phyllodes tumor of the breast: EGFR family expression and relation to clinicopathological features. *Ultrastruct Pathol* 2000;24(6):371–381.
55. Chen CM, Chen CJ, Chang CL, et al. CD34, CD117, and actin expression in phyllodes tumor of the breast. *J Surg Res* 2000;94(2):84–91.

56. Feakins RM, Wells CA, Young KA, et al. Platelet-derived growth factor expression in phyllodes tumors and fibroadenomas of the breast. *Hum Pathol* 2000;31(10):1214–1222.
57. Mokbel K, Ghilchik M, Parris CN, et al. Telomerase activity in phyllodes tumours. *Eur J Surg Oncol* 1999;25(4):352–355.
58. Layfield LJ, Hart J, Neuwirth H, et al. Relation between DNA ploidy and the clinical behavior of phyllodes tumors. *Cancer* 1989;64(7):1486–1489.
59. Keelan PA, Myers JL, Wold LE, et al. Phyllodes tumor: clinicopathologic review of 60 patients and flow cytometric analysis in 30 patients. *Hum Pathol* 1992;23(9):1048–1054.
60. El-Naggar AK, Ro JY, McLemore D, et al. DNA content and proliferative activity of cystosarcoma phyllodes of the breast. Potential prognostic significance. *Am J Clin Pathol* 1990;93(4):480–485.
61. Tse GM, Lee CS, Kung FY, et al. Hormonal receptors expression in epithelial cells of mammary phyllodes tumors correlates with pathologic grade of the tumor: a multicenter study of 143 cases. *Am J Clin Pathol* 2002;118(4):522–526.
62. Nicol M, Willis C, Yiangou C, et al. Relationship between serum prolactin levels and histology of benign and malignant breast lesions: a detailed study of 153 consecutive cases. *Breast J* 2002;8(5):281–285.
63. Geisler DP, Boyle MJ, Malnar KF, et al. Phyllodes tumors of the breast: a review of 32 cases. *Am Surg* 2000;66(4):360–366.
64. Lenhard MS, Kahlert S, Himsl I, et al. Phyllodes tumour of the breast: clinical follow-up of 33 cases of this rare disease. *Eur J Obstet Gynecol Reprod Biol* 2008;138(2):217–221.
65. Belkacemi Y, Bousquet G, Marsiglia H, et al. Phyllodes tumor of the breast. *Int J Radiat Oncol Biol Phys* 2008;70(2):492–500.
66. Grabowski J, Salzstein SL, Sadler GR, et al. Malignant phyllodes tumors: a review of 752 cases. *Am Surg* 2007;73(10):967–969.
67. Bernstein L, Deapen D, Ross RK. The descriptive epidemiology of malignant cystosarcoma phyllodes of the breast. *Cancer* 1993;71(10):3020–3024.
68. Ansah-Boateng Y, Tavassoli FA. Fibroadenoma and cystosarcoma phyllodes of the male breast. *Mod Pathol* 1992;5(2):114–116.
69. Bapat K, Oropeza R, Sahoo S. Benign phyllodes tumor of the male breast. *Breast J* 2002;8(2):115–116.
70. Martino A, Zamparelli M, Santinelli A, et al. Unusual clinical presentation of a rare case of phyllodes tumor of the breast in an adolescent girl. *J Pediatr Surg* 2001;36(6):941–943.
71. Pasqualini M, Misericordia M, Russo M, et al. Philloides tumor of the breast detected by US in an 11 years old patients. A case report. *Radiol Med (Torino)* 2002;103(5–6):537–539.
72. Tagaya N, Kodaira H, Kogure H, et al. A case of phyllodes tumor with bloody nipple discharge in juvenile patient. *Breast Cancer* 1999;6(3):207–210.
73. Elsheikh A, Keramopoulos A, Lazaris D, et al. Breast tumors during adolescence. *Eur J Gynaecol Oncol* 2000;21(4):408–410.
74. Birch JM, Alston RD, McNally RJ, et al. Relative frequency and morphology of cancers in carriers of germline TP53 mutations. *Oncogene* 2001;20(34):4621–4628.
75. Chulia MT, Paya A, Niveiro M, et al. Phyllodes tumor in ectopic breast tissue of the vulva. *Int J Surg Pathol* 2001;9(1):81–83.
76. Schapmans S, Van Leuven L, Cortvriend J, et al. Phyllodes tumor of the prostate. A case report and review of the literature. *Eur Urol* 2000;38(5):649–653.
77. Mrad K, Driss M, Maalej M, et al. Bilateral cystosarcoma phyllodes of the breast: a case report of malignant form with contralateral benign form. *Ann Diagn Pathol* 2000;4(6):370–372.
78. Villanueva MJ, Navarro F, Sanchez A, et al. [Coexistence of breast cystosarcoma phyllodes and bilateral in situ lobular carcinoma]. *Rev Clin Esp* 1999;199(11):776.
79. Alo PL, Andreano T, Monaco S, et al. [Malignant phyllodes tumor of the breast with features of intraductal carcinoma]. *Pathologica* 2001;93(2):124–127.
80. Gebrim LH, Bernardes Junior JR, et al. Malignant phyllodes tumor in the right breast and invasive lobular carcinoma within fibroadenoma in the other: case report. *Sao Paulo Med J* 2000;118(2):46–48.
81. Garbely J, Kukora J, Auerback H, et al. Synchronous recurrent phyllodes tumor (PT) and occult inflammatory ductal breast carcinoma. *Breast Dis* 1995;8:19–23.
82. Gabriele R, Borghese M, Corigliano N, et al. [Phyllodes tumor of the breast. Personal contribution of 21 cases]. *G Chir* 2000;21(11–12):453–456.
83. Yilmaz E, Sal S, Lebe B. Differentiation of phyllodes tumors versus fibroadenomas. *Acta Radiol* 2002;43(1):34–39.
84. Liberman L, Bonaccio E, Hamele-Bena D, et al. Benign and malignant phyllodes tumors: mammographic and sonographic findings. *Radiology* 1996;198(1):121–124.
85. Chao TC, Lo YF, Chen SC, et al. Sonographic features of phyllodes tumors of the breast. *Ultrasound Obstet Gynecol* 2002;20(1):64–71.
86. Farria DM, Gorczyca DP, Barsky SH, et al. Benign phyllodes tumor of the breast: MR imaging features. *AJR Am J Roentgenol* 1996;167(1):187–189.

87. Katayama N, Inoue Y, Ichikawa T, et al. Increased activity in benign phyllodes tumor on Tc-99m MDP scintimammography. *Clin Nucl Med* 2000;25(7):551–552.
88. Pappo I, Horne T, Merdad H, et al. [Primary breast tumor and malignant phyllodes tumor of the breast—two rare cases demonstrated by technetium 99m scintimammography]. *Harefuah* 2000;138(11):932–935, 1007.
89. Bhattarai S, Kapila K, Verma K. Phyllodes tumor of the breast. A cytohistologic study of 80 cases. *Acta Cytol* 2000;44(5):790–796.
90. Krishnamurthy S, Ashfaq R, Shin HJ, et al. Distinction of phyllodes tumor from fibroadenoma: a reappraisal of an old problem. *Cancer* 2000;90(6):342–349.
91. Ng WK. Fine needle aspiration cytology of fibroadenoma with multinucleated stromal giant cells. A review of cases in a six-year period. *Acta Cytol* 2002;46(3):535–539.
92. Shet T, Rege J. Cystic degeneration in phyllodes tumor. A source of error in cytologic interpretation. *Acta Cytol* 2000;44(2):163–168.
93. Rowell MD, Perry RR, Hsiu JG, et al. Phyllodes tumors. *Am J Surg* 1993;165(3):376–379.
94. Mangi AA, Smith BL, Gadd MA, et al. Surgical management of phyllodes tumors. *Arch Surg* 1999;134(5):487–492; discussion 492–493.
95. de Roos WK, Kaye P, Dent DM. Factors leading to local recurrence or death after surgical resection of phyllodes tumours of the breast. *Br J Surg* 1999;86(3):396–399.
96. Pandey M, Mathew A, Kattoor J, et al. Malignant phyllodes tumor. *Breast J* 2001;7(6):411–416.
97. August DA, Kearney T. Cystosarcoma phyllodes: mastectomy, lumpectomy, or lumpectomy plus irradiation. *Surg Oncol* 2000;9(2):49–52.
98. Kok KY, Telesinghe PU, Yapp SK. Treatment and outcome of cystosarcoma phyllodes in Brunei: a 13-year experience. *J R Coll Surg Edinb* 2001;46(4):198–201.
99. Hajdu SI, Espinosa MH, Robbins GF. Recurrent cystosarcoma phyllodes: a clinicopathologic study of 32 cases. *Cancer* 1976;38(3):1402–1406.
100. Chua CL, Thomas A, Ng BK. Cystosarcoma phyllodes: a review of surgical options. *Surgery* 1989;105(2 Pt 1):141–147.
101. Zurrida S, Bartoli C, Galimberti V, et al. Which therapy for unexpected phyllode tumour of the breast? *Eur J Cancer* 1992;28(2–3):654–657.
102. Shabahang M, Franceschi D, Sundaram M, et al. Surgical management of primary breast sarcoma. *Am Surg* 2002;68(8):673–677; discussion 677.
103. Meneses A, Mohar A, de la Garza-Salazar J, et al. Prognostic factors on 45 cases of phyllodes tumors. *J Exp Clin Cancer Res* 2000;19(1):69–73.
104. Eich PD, Diederich S, Eich HT, et al. Diagnostic radiation oncology: malignant cystosarcoma phylloides. *Strahlenther Onkol* 2000;176(4):192–195.
105. Hopkins ML, McGowan TS, Rawlings G, et al. Phyllodes tumor of the breast: a report of 14 cases. *J Surg Oncol* 1994;56(2):108–112.
106. Macdonald OK, Lee CM, Tward JD, et al. Malignant phyllodes tumor of the female breast: association of primary therapy with cause-specific survival from the Surveillance, Epidemiology, and End Results (SEER) program. *Cancer* 2006;107(9):2127–2133.
107. Paulsen F, Belka C, Gromoll C, et al. Cystosarcoma phyllodes malignum: a case report of a successive triple modality treatment. *Int J Hyperthermia* 2000;16(4):319–324.
108. Burton GV, Hart LL, Leight GS Jr., et al. Cystosarcoma phyllodes. Effective therapy with cisplatin and etoposide chemotherapy. *Cancer* 1989;63(11):2088–2092.
109. Ueyama Y, Abe Y, Ohnishi Y, et al. In vivo chemosensitivity of human malignant cystosarcoma phyllodes xenografts. *Oncol Rep* 2000;7(2):257–260.
110. Hawkins RE, Schofield JB, Wiltshaw E, et al. Ifosfamide is an active drug for chemotherapy of metastatic cystosarcoma phyllodes. *Cancer* 1992;69(9):2271–2275.
111. Moffat CJ, Pinder SE, Dixon AR, et al. Phyllodes tumours of the breast: a clinicopathological review of thirty-two cases. *Histopathology* 1995;27(3):205–218.
112. Rocha PS, Pinto RG, Nadkarni NS, et al. Malignant phyllodes tumor metastatic to the forearm: a case report. *Diagn Cytopathol* 2000;22(4):243–245.
113. Kessinger A, Foley JF, Lemon HM, et al. Metastatic cystosarcoma phyllodes: a case report and review of the literature. *J Surg Oncol* 1972;4(2):131–147.
114. Yagishita M, Nambu Y, Ishigaki M, et al. [Pulmonary metastatic malignant phyllodes tumor showing multiple thin walled cavities]. *Nihon Kokyuki Gakkai Zasshi* 1999;37(1):61–66.
115. Reinfuss M, Mitus J, Smolak K, et al. Malignant phyllodes tumours of the breast. A clinical and pathological analysis of 55 cases. *Eur J Cancer* 1993;29A(9):1252–1256.
116. Giorgadze T, Ward RM, Baloch ZW, et al. Phyllodes tumor metastatic to thyroid Hurthle cell adenoma. *Arch Pathol Lab Med* 2002;126(10):1233–1236.
117. Yu PC, Lin YC, Chen HM, et al. Malignant phyllodes tumor of the breast metastasizing to the pancreas: case report. *Changgeng Yi Xue Za Zhi* 2000;23(8):503–507.
118. Hlavin ML, Kaminski HJ, Cohen M, et al. Central nervous system complications of cystosarcoma phyllodes. *Cancer* 1993;72(1):126–130.

Nora M. Hansen

Paget's disease, a rare presentation of breast cancer accounts for 1% to 3% of all breast cancers (1–3). Most cases are associated with an underlying malignancy and prognosis depends on the stage of the underlying cancer (4). In a recent review of the Surveillance, Epidemiology and End Results (SEER) data by Chen et al. (5), it was reported that the incidence of Paget's disease has decreased between 1988 and 2002. The age-adjusted incidence rates decreased by 49% for Paget's disease associated with invasive ductal cancer and by 44% for Paget's disease associated with ductal carcinoma *in situ* (DCIS).

The first description of Paget-like features was in 1307 by John of Arderne who recorded the several-year evolution of nipple ulceration in a male priest, with the subsequent development of a breast cancer (6). Velpeau (7) is typically credited with the first clinical description of Paget's disease when in 1840 he described the visual surface lesion of Paget's disease in two patients. It was in 1874 that Sir James Paget (8) recorded the association of the clinical findings with an underlying breast cancer in 15 patients, although he speculated that the chronic skin condition was benign. It was Thin (9), in 1881, who concluded that the nipple lesion was not a benign entity, but a malignant one. He postulated that the nipple lesion contained cells that were related to the underlying cancer which had extended to the nipple through the major lactiferous sinuses which we refer to today as Pagetoid spread.

PATHOGENESIS

The pathogenesis of Paget's disease is an interesting one because there are two main theories for the origin of Paget's disease. The most widely accepted one is the epidermotropic theory, first described by Jacobeus (10), which suggests that the Paget cells arise in breast ducts and spread through the lactiferous sinuses to the nipple epidermis. This view is supported by several observations. First, it is well documented that most patients with Paget's disease have an underlying breast carcinoma that is ductal in origin and that the immunohistochemical profile and pattern of gene expression in the Paget cell and the underlying cancer are similar (11–13). In addition, heregulin alpha, a motility factor released by normal epidermal keratinocytes can induce chemotaxis of the Paget cells to migrate into the overlying nipple epidermis (14).

Because not all Paget's disease is associated with an underlying carcinoma, another theory, the intraepidermal transformation theory (*in situ* transformation theory) proposes that the Paget cells arise either in the terminal portion of the lactiferous duct at its junction with the epidermis or from multipotential cells in the epidermal basal layer. Support for this theory is found in the rare cases of Paget's disease without an underlying breast carcinoma or cases in which the Paget's disease and the underlying carcinoma appear to be separate tumors (15–19). Other studies have identified desmosomal attachments between the Paget cells and adjacent keratinocytes supporting the *in situ* development of the Paget cell (20).

Histologically, Paget's disease is characterized by the infiltration of the nipple epidermis by Paget cells described as large, pale-staining cell with round or oval nuclei and prominent nucleoli. The cells are between the normal keratinocytes of the nipple epidermis, occurring singly in the superficial layers, and in clusters toward the basement membrane. Serous fluid can seep through the disrupted keratinocyte layer, result-

ing in the crusting and scaling of the nipple skin. Paget cells can traverse the epithelium and thus sometimes are found in the superficial layers. The basement membrane of the lactiferous sinuses is in continuity with the basement membrane of the skin. Paget cells do not invade through the dermal basement membrane and therefore are a form of carcinoma *in situ*. Paget's disease is often associated with a chronic inflammatory infiltrate in the dermis (21) (Figs. 66.1 and 66.2).

INCIDENCE

The incidence of Paget's disease varies whether referring to the pathologic or clinical entity. Paget's disease is a more common pathologic than clinical entity (1,22–25). Its clinical incidence ranges from 0.5% to 2.8%, with a mean of 1.3% in more than 50,900 patients combined from nine studies (1,22–29). Histologic evidence of Paget's disease is present in 0.5% to 4.7% of nipples from breast cancer specimens (1,22,23). In a series by Lagios et al. (25), of 3,000 consecutive breast cancer mastectomy specimens, 21 (0.7%) had clinical evidence of Paget's disease and 147 (4.9%) had Paget cells histologically, thus yielding a sevenfold difference.

Of the 158,621 microscopically confirmed female and male breast cancer registrants from the SEER registry of the National Cancer Institute (NCI), 1,775 (1.1%) had histologic Paget's disease (30). Of patients with breast cancer from this database, Paget's disease was histologically identified in 1.1% of white female patients, 1.3% of black female patients, 1.1% of white male patients, and no black male patients. Clinical Paget's disease has been reported in patients ranging in age from 23 to 90 years, with mean ranging from 53 to 65 years (1,3,21–23,29,31–39). In a further analysis of the SEER data, the mean age of women with Paget's disease was 62 years and that of the men was 69 years. This was not significantly different from female (61 years) and male (67 years) patients with ductal breast cancer. In an update of the SEER data Paget's disease associated with both invasive and DCIS has decreased from 1988 to 2002 by 49% and 44%, respectively (5). This may have been accounted for by the increased use of mammography and finding cancers at an earlier stage before they develop Pagetoid features.

CLINICAL PRESENTATION AND DIAGNOSIS

Most patients with Paget's disease present with eczema or ulceration of the nipple and many have a prolonged period of symptoms before diagnosis. It is therefore important to have a high index of suspicion for Paget's when a patient presents with nipple complaints. The most common initial presentation is erythema and mild eczematous scaling, which progresses to crusting, skin erosion, and ulceration, with exudation or frank discharge (Figs. 66.3, 66.4, 66.5).

The clinical differential diagnosis of scaling skin and erythema of the nipple–areola complex (NAC), in addition to Paget's includes eczema, contact dermatitis, and postradiation dermatitis. Although bilateral Paget's has been reported, bilateral symptoms are most consistent with eczema or contact dermatitis (40,41). Skin changes that are confined to the areola

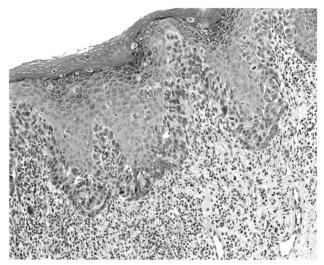

FIGURE 66.1. Section through the nipple epidermis demonstrating Paget's cells. Hematoxylin and eosin stain. Large, pale staining Paget's cells are more densely concentrated toward the basement membrane. (Courtesy of Barbara Susnik MD, Department of Pathology, Northwestern Memorial Hospital, Feinberg School of Medicine, Northwestern University.)

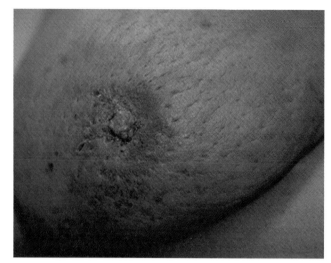

FIGURE 66.4. Photograph of Paget's nipple. Ulceration of nipple with progression onto areola.

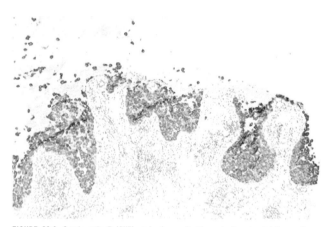

FIGURE 66.2. Cytokeratin 7 (CK7) stain demonstrating cytoplasmic staining pattern, which differentiates Paget's disease from melanoma or squamous cell carcinoma. (Courtesy of Barbara Susnik MD, Department of Pathology, Northwestern Memorial Hospital, Feinberg School of Medicine, Northwestern University.)

and spare the nipple are typically attributed to eczema, although they can occur rarely in Paget's disease (21,33). The clinical differential diagnosis has prompted initial topical steroid treatment, often with transient improvement of symptoms (3). Other patients have been treated with antibiotics (23). In patients who have been previously treated with breast conservation, Paget's disease may mimic postradiation scaling. Given the infrequency of Paget's disease in this setting, the diagnosis of Paget's disease may be delayed. Symptom duration preceding the diagnosis of Paget's disease is variable and averages 9.5 weeks to 27 months, with a range of 1 week to 20 years (31,42–45). In a study from the Mayo Clinic, the median duration of symptoms was 6 days with a range of 1 to 80 days, clearly a unique patient population (14).

Less common diagnoses in the clinical differential of mammary Paget's disease include nipple adenoma (46), papillomatosis (47,48), melanoma (49), Bowen disease (50), and rarely basal cell carcinoma (51), squamous carcinoma, sebaceous carcinoma, Merkel cell carcinoma, infiltrating lobular carcinoma, cutaneous T-cell lymphoma, Spitz nevus, and epidermotropic metastases (52), alteration of keratinocytes present in 10% of normal nipples. Toker cells can be distinguished from Paget cells by their lack of nuclear pleomorphism or cytologic atypia and their absence of mucin (21,53,54).

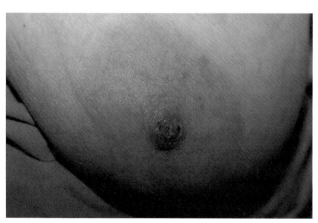

FIGURE 66.3. Photograph of Paget's nipple. Erythema and crusting of nipple occupy most of the nipple surface.

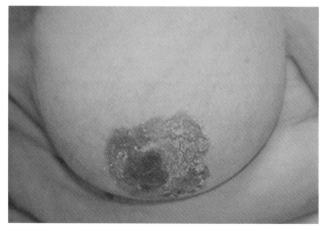

FIGURE 66.5. Photograph of Paget's nipple. Advanced Paget's with crusting and ulceration extending from nipple and encompassing areola.

Although most patients with Paget's disease present with nipple changes,up to 50% will present with a palpable mass. Most patients who present with a palpable mass have an underlying invasive cancer and thus have a worse prognosis. Patients who present with a palpable mass also have a higher rate of nodal positivity (4,55,56).

The diagnosis can be obtained by scrape cytology (49), a superficial epidermal shave biopsy, a punch biopsy, a wedge incision biopsy, or nipple excision (21). The ideal specimen contains adequate epidermis to provide Paget cells and a lactiferous duct. Paget cells may be distributed in a patchy fashion throughout the nipple, so additional specimen sampling may be required to secure the diagnosis (55).

The histologic differential diagnosis of Paget's disease includes superficial spreading melanoma, squamous cell carcinoma in situ (Bowen's disease), and clear-cell changes of squamous cells of the epidermis (Toker cells). The cell type can be determined by immunohistochemical studies, including low-molecular-weight keratins (CK7, cellular adhesion molecule 5.2[CAM-5.2]), broad-spectrum keratins, melanoma antibodies, and mucin stains (21).

Paget cells are immunoreactive for keratins (CK7, CAM-5.2, and AE1/AE3) (57), occasionally are immunoreactive to S100 (58), and are not immunoreactive for Human Melanoma Black (HMB) 45 or high-molecular-weight keratins (59). In one study, mucin was present in 55% of 20 patients and, thus, was not informative in 45% of patients (21,59). Paget cells can phagocytose melanin from adjacent epidermal melanocytes and may be mistaken for melanoma if immunohistochemistry is not performed (59,60). Melanomas are immunoreactive for S100; they are often immunoreactive for HMB45 and are only very rarely immunoreactive for low–molecular-weight (CAM-5.2), broad-spectrum keratins (AE1/AE3), or mucin stains (57,59,61–65). Squamous cells are immunoreactive for low-molecular-weight keratins and broad-spectrum keratins (AE1/AE3) are infrequently immunoreactive for S100 and are not immunoreactive for CAM-5.2, HMB45 or mucin stains (54,65,66). Toker cells or clear-cell changes of the epidermal squamous cells are a nonneoplastic DCIS, and 1% had Paget's disease only (21,52).

RADIOGRAPHIC EVALUATION

In patients with clinical Paget's disease, the reported incidence of mammographic findings varies in the literature. For those patients with Paget's disease without a palpable breast mass, mammography has been reported as normal in 2.5% to 100% of patients. Of the 324 patients in these 11 series, 174 (54%) had normal mammograms (3,21,31,32,35,37,38,67–71). In 9 series, breast histology was evaluated for 144 patients with clinical Paget's disease and normal mammograms, with 29 patients (20%) found to have an associated invasive breast cancer, 111 patients (77%) found to have DCIS, and 4 patients (3%) found to have Paget's disease of the nipple without an associated invasive cancer or DCIS (21,31,35,37,67–71). These retrospective studies included patients accrued in the late 1970s, when xeromammography was still in use and retroareolar spot compression views were not routine (21,70,71).

Mammographic findings include skin, nipple, and areolar thickening; nipple retraction; subareolar or more diffuse malignant microcalcifications; and a discrete mass or architectural distortion (72). Mammography inadequately determines the existence of underlying disease in patients with Paget's disease. In addition, it cannot map the true distribution of the underlying pathology and, therefore, has limited value in determining the appropriate surgical procedure (72).

Ultrasound may be a useful tool in evaluating the patient with Paget's disease, especially if the mammogram does not demonstrate any abnormalities. Günhan-Bilgen and Oktay (72)

confirmed the presence of tumor in 67% of patients with Paget's disease using ultrasound in their study of which 2% of patients had a normal mammogram. However in 13% of patients the mammogram did not demonstrate the mass seen on ultrasound and only documented microcalcifications. Because Paget's disease has been associated with multifocal and multicentric cancers in 42% to 63% of patients, it is important to evaluate the entire breast (2,3,69).

Magnetic resonance imaging (MRI) of the breast is an effective diagnostic tool to identify clinically and mammographically occult tumors and some evidence suggests that it may be beneficial in the evaluation of patients with Paget's disease. Recent studies have demonstrated the sensitivity of MRI in detecting breast cancer ranging from 88% to 100% (73,74). In cases of DCIS, contrast-enhanced MRI has a sensitivity of 95% compared with 70% on mammography alone (75). Several small series and case reports have evaluated the use of MRI in patients with Paget's disease. The combined series evaluated 27 patients and MRI detected the cancer in 20 of these patients of which 15 were mammographically occult (76–81). MRI failed to identify one invasive cancer and four cases of DCIS. MRI was able to determine accurately the extent of disease and, therefore, may be able to help determine which patients are best suited for breast conservation, particularly in the subset of patients with mammographically occult cancers.

Technetium 99 methoxyisobutylisonitrite (MIBI) uptake is increased in breast cancer, which is thought to be owing to the increased blood flow from angiogenesis and increased cellular metabolism. Several case reports have demonstrated the usefulness of ^{99m}Tc-MIBI scans in evaluating the extent of disease in patients with Paget's disease; however, this technique has not been widely adapted to date (82).

TREATMENT OPTIONS

Various treatment options have been described in the literature for the management of patients with Paget's disease, including nipple excision alone, radiotherapy alone, central lumpectomy or quadrantectomy, with or without the addition of radiation therapy, and mastectomy. Treatment options have followed the evolution of surgical options for patients with an invasive breast cancer. For years mastectomy with or without axillary lymph node dissection has been the standard of care for patients with Paget's disease; however, multiple randomized trials have demonstrated that breast conservation is equal in terms of survival to mastectomy and, therefore, the role breast conservation in patients with Paget's disease has been evaluated (83,84).

Although no randomized trials exist that relate specifically to Paget's disease, the use of breast conservation should be acceptable as long as negative margins are achieved and the patient has an acceptable cosmetic result. Several studies have shown that 20% to 40% of mastectomy specimens have multicentric or multifocal cancers that were underestimated in the mammogram, which potentially would mandate a mastectomy in this subgroup of patients (2,3,68). In addition, although most cancers associated with Paget's disease are centrally located, there are multiple reports depicting the variability of tumor location despite negative mammograms. Paone and Baker (85) reported 12% of cases in which the underlying cancer was 2 cm or more from the nipple, whereas Ikeda et al. (69) reported that in 55% of patients the DCIS was located far from the nipple and in 40% of patient's multicentric disease was identified. Others have reported a 50% incidence of peripherally located tumors, most of whom had a negative mammogram (38). Wertheim and Ozzello (86a) reported a 22% incidence of peripherally located invasive tumors in 18 patients with Paget's disease undergoing a mastectomy. Kothari et al. (32) reported a 75% rate of tumor extension beyond the central quadrant. Failure to identify peripheral cancers when patients are treated with breast-conservation surgery without irradiation may yield increased local failure rates.

BREAST CONSERVATION WITHOUT RADIATION

Breast conservation alone leads to a high local failure rate and is not recommended. Several series published have reported high local recurrence rates with central lumpectomy alone. Polgar et al. (39) reported a 33% rate of local recurrence in 33 patients with Paget's disease of the nipple undergoing conservation; 30 patients had an underlying DCIS and 3 patients had Paget's disease of the nipple without an underlying malignancy. With a median 6-year follow-up, 11 patients (33%) experience a local recurrence, of which 10 were invasive with 6 developing metastatic disease. Dixon et al. (3) evaluated 10 patients with Paget's disease without any documented underlying disease on imaging. The NAC was excised with an underlying cone biopsy. All patients were found to have underlying DCIS and one patient had an invasive cancer. Despite negative margins on pathologic examination, at a median follow-up of 56 months, 40% of patients had a local recurrence. Zurrida et al. (86b) treated 31 patients with wide excision alone and 29% developed a local recurrence with a median follow up of 60 months. Other studies have reported low recurrence rates; however, there were limited number of patients and the length of follow-up was not specified (19,85).

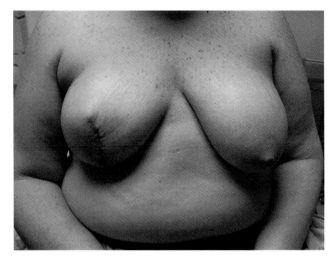

FIGURE 66.6. Photograph of patient with Paget's disease who underwent central lumpectomy with removal of the nipple–areola complex.

RADIATION WITHOUT SURGERY

Radiation treatment alone for patients with Paget's disease without a palpable mass or abnormal mammogram has been reported; however, widespread experience with such conservative treatment remains limited. Although the numbers are small, the local recurrence rates range from 0 to 17%. Bulens et al. (45) treated 13 patients with radiotherapy alone and reported no recurrence with a median follow-up of 52 months. Christiaens et al. (87) reported a 14.8% local recurrence rate in 27 patients at a median follow-up of 79 months, whereas Fourquet (88) with the longest follow-up of 90 months reported a 17.6% local recurrence rate. Stockdale et al. (89) treated 19 patients; of these 3 patients experienced recurrence, 1 with invasive cancer and 2 with microinvasive cancer. Clearly, this approach should be limited to patients with minimal disease, which is difficult to evaluate without surgical intervention.

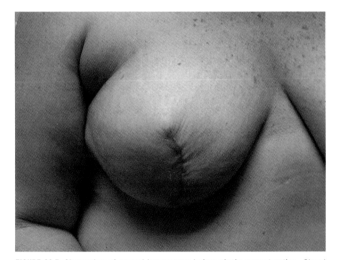

FIGURE 66.7. Closer view of central lumpectomy before nipple reconstruction. Closed with vertical incision because the patient plans on proceeding with left mastopexy after radiation treatment and nipple reconstruction to right breast.

BREAST CONSERVATION WITH RADIATION

If breast conservation is to be considered, the gold standard should be a central lumpectomy with postoperative radiation therapy (Figs. 66.6, 66.7, 66.8). The addition of radiotherapy has improved the efficacy of breast-conserving surgery for patients with Paget's disease. Several recent retrospective nonrandomized studies have compared breast conservation with mastectomy in patients with Paget's disease. The studies are difficult to compare, however, owing to the varying presentations of the disease and the varied treatment algorhythms. Initial studies only offered breast conservation to patients without a palpable mass or mammographic finding, whereas more recent studies included all types of disease presentation. In a prospective single-arm trial by the European Organization for Research and Treatment of Cancer, Bijker et al. (37) evaluated

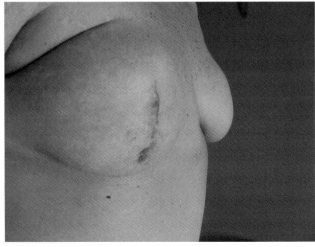

FIGURE 66.8. Patient with Paget's disease who had a central lumpectomy with removal of the nipple–areola complex, side view demonstrating shape of breast is intact.

61 patients with Paget's disease. Most (93%) had an underlying DCIS and were treated with excision of the NAC and underlying breast tissue to tumor-free margins followed by whole-breast radiation (50 gy in 25 fractions). Most patients did not have an underlying mass (97%) or mammographic abnormality (84%). With 6.4 years of follow-up, the 5-year local recurrence rate was 5.2%. Marshall et al. (36), in an update of a previous study, reported the 10- and 15-year results for 36 cases of Paget's disease, none of which had a palpable mass or mammographic abnormality from seven institutions. Of the 36 patients, 69% had a complete excision of the NAC, 25% had a partial resection and 6% had a biopsy alone. Final margins were negative in 56% of cases. All patients received whole breast irradiation to a median dose of 50 Gy with a boost to the tumor bed in 97% of cases for a total medial dose of 61.5 Gy. 83% of patients had a documented underlying malignancy, the majority were DCIS. At a median follow-up of 113 months, 11% were found to have a local recurrence, all of whom had a complete resection of the NAC. No clinical factors were identified as a significant predictor of local recurrence. Actuarial local control rates for breast recurrence were 91%, 83%, and 76% at 5, 10, and 15 years, respectively. Actuarial rates for disease-free survival (DFS) were 97% for 5, 10, and 15 years. Overall survival rates were 93% at 5 years and 90% at 10 and 15 years. These findings confirm that, for selected patients without a palpable mass or mammagraphic abnormality, breast conservation affords excellent rates of local control, DFS and overall survival for patients with Paget's disease. In a study by Dalberg et al. (55), 223 patients at 13 Swedish hospitals were diagnosed with Paget's disease. Most (79%) had an underlying malignancy diagnosed before surgery, 30% were invasive cancers. Of patients, 19% underwent breast conservation, whereas 75% had a mastectomy and only 19% of patients had radiation treatment. Eleven elderly patients had no surgical intervention. At 10 years, the local recurrence rate for the mastectomy patients was 8%, whereas the patients who had breast conservation had a local recurrence rate of 16%, which may be partly owing to the low rate of postoperative radiation therapy. Risk factors associated with breast cancer recurrence and death were presence of invasive cancer and a palpable mass. Lymph node metastasis was a risk factor for recurrence, but not cancer death. In the largest series from the SEER data base Chen et al. (5) reported on 1,642 patients with Paget's disease diagnosed between 1973 and 1987. The 15-year breast cancer-specific survival for patients with DCIS who had breast conservation treatment, was 92% compared with 94% for patients who had a mastectomy. For patients with invasive cancer, there was an 87% 15-year breast cancer-specific survival and only a 60% survival for patients who underwent a mastectomy. No difference, however, was seen between the groups after adjusting for tumor size and lymph node status. Only tumor size and lymph node status were significant prognostic indicators of disease-specific mortality. The group from M.D. Anderson Cancer Center (56) reported on 104 patients with Paget's disease and demonstrated that breast-conserving approaches had local control and survival rates similar to those achieved with mastectomy and a positive nodal status was the only significant predictor of disease-free and relapse-free survival with a disease-specific survival of 47% in node-positive patients and 93% in node-negative patients. The local recurrence rate with breast conservation was 8% at a median follow-up of 7 years and all patients had postoperative radiation. Zakaria et al. (4) also demonstrated no difference in survival based on the surgical procedure, but the presence of a palpable mass, suspicious mammogram, advanced tumor stage, invasive cancer, and axillary metastases were all associated with a worse outcome. Disease-free survival decreased from 90% to 60% and 86% to 30% at 5 and 10 years, respectively, for patients who presented with a palpable mass and suspicious mammogram compared

with those patients without a palpable mass and a benign mammogram.

The European Institute of Oncology of Milan (90) reported their experience with Paget's disease in women from May 1996 to February 2003. Most patients presented with typical nipple changes and 77% were associated with suspicious x-ray findings. Of patients, 94% had an underlying malignancy identified. Of the 114 patients, 71 were treated with mastectomy and 43 with breast conservation. More loco regional recurrences were seen in the conservation group, but this did not have an impact on survival. Vascular invasion was the only statistically significant prognostic factor for DFS and cancer-specific survival; however, tumor size greater than 2 cm and nodal involvement were associated with a worse outcome. Joseph et al. (91) reported that younger patients in their study were more commonly offered mastectomy compared to conservation and that the use of radiation therapy (RT) also appeared to be based on age. They reported similar local recurrence rates and survival rates with a median follow-up of 82.5 months for patients treated with either breast-conservation treatment or mastectomy.

Several studies have demonstrated that patients with Paget's disease were more likely to be estrogen receptor (ER) negative, progesterone receptor (PR) negative with a high histologic grade and an overexpression of *c-erb* B2 oncoprotein was found in up to 88% of cases (5,55,90).

Breast conservation has become an alternative to mastectomy for patients with Paget's disease with acceptable local recurrence rates and similar survival rates. With better reconstructive options available to patients, the loss of the NAC can be corrected and patients can have an excellent cosmetic outcome. In a study by Chung et al. (91), an immediate reconstructive technique was used in 29 women with Paget's disease or a subareolar cancer that necessitated the removal of the NAC along with a central lumpectomy. Using a standard Wise pattern incision for reduction mammoplasty, a central lumpectomy with removal of the NAC was performed. The inferior pedicle was de-epitheliealized and rotated or advanced to fill the central defect. The breast and skin flaps were then mobilized to the midline and inframammary fold and closed. The nipple reconstruction was performed after the completion of the radiation. In all 29 cases, the NAC felt to be well centered without central depression deformities and there were no local recurrences at a mean follow-up of 3.5 years.

NODAL EVALUATION: SENTINEL NODE BIOPSY AND AXILLARY LYMPH NODE DISSECTION

Paget's disease is associated with an underlying malignancy in most cases and, although many patients have an underlying DCIS, a substantial portion may have an invasive cancer. Lymph node metastasis is considered the most important prognostic indicator for patients with invasive breast cancer and all patients with invasive cancer should be offered axillary staging. Sentinel node biopsy (SNB) has now replaced axillary lymph node dissection (ALND) as a less-invasive procedure to stage patients with invasive breast cancer. It has been shown to be effective and accurate in detecting the presence of metastases in many single and multicenter studies (92–94).

Several investigators have evaluated the role of SNB in patients with Paget's disease. In the three reported series, a total of 105 patients have been evaluated (90,95,96). The SN identification rate ranged from 97% to 100%. An invasive cancer was identified in 45 of 105 patients and a positive SN was identified in 20 of the 105 patients. None of the patients with DCIS were found to have nodal disease and 44% of the patients

Table 66.1	SENTINEL NODE (SN) STUDIES IN PAGET'S DISEASE			
Author (Reference)	Number	ID Rate (%)	SN + Rate	+NSN (%)
Sukumvanich et al. (95)	39 (16 invasive, 23 DCIS)	98	11/39 (28.2%)	45
Laronga et al. (96)	36 (10 invasive, 36 Paget's ± DCIS)	97	4/36 (11.1%) All 4 invasive cancer	25
Caliskan et al. (90)	30 (19 invasive, 11 DCIS)	100	5/19 (26.3%) invasive 0/11 DCIS	Not reported

DCIS, ductal carcinoma *in situ*; ID, SN Identification Rate; NSN, Non Sentinel Node.

with invasive cancer were found to have a positive SN. In a study by Sukumvanich et al. (95) from Memorial Sloan-Kettering Cancer Center of the patients with a positive SN, 45% had additional positive nonsentinel nodes, whereas in the study by Laronga et al. (96), the SN was the only positive node in 75% of cases (Table 66.1).

Patients with Paget's disease and a known invasive cancer should be offered an SNB to evaluate their nodal status. If breast conservation is to be performed, a sentinel node biopsy could be done at a later date only if invasive disease was identified. If a mastectomy is to be performed, a sentinel node biopsy should be done at the time of surgery due to the possibility that invasive cancer may be identified in the mastectomy specimen. The role of SNB in DCIS is controversial and, therefore, patients undergoing breast conservation for Paget's disease without a known invasive cancer is unknown. Some clinicians may await the final pathologic evaluation and only proceed with an SNB if invasive disease is documented, whereas others will offer an SNB at the time of breast conservation. The final decision should be made by the treating clinician and the patient.

MANAGEMENT SUMMARY FOR PAGET'S DISEASE

- Paget's disease, a rare presentation of breast cancer, accounts for 1% to 3% of all breast cancers.
- Most patients present with erythema or ulceration of the nipple.
- Diagnosis is made by either a scrape cytology or nipple biopsy.
- Radiologic workup should include mammogram with retroareolar spot compression views and ultrasound and, if negative, consider MRI to evaluate occult cancer and to rule out multicentric disease.
- Most underlying tumors are DCIS and located centrally.
- Breast conservation in appropriately selected patients has similar outcome to mastectomy in nonrandomized trials.
- Radiation therapy is important in reducing local recurrence risk in patients having breast conserving treatment.
- Patients with multicentric disease or disease extending beyond the central portion of the breast should be offered mastectomy.
- Patients with known invasive cancer should be offered axillary nodal evaluation with sentinel node biopsy.

References

1. Ashikari R, Park K, Huvos AG, et al. Paget's disease of the breast. *Cancer* 1970; 26:680–685.
2. Chaudary MA, Millis RR, Lane EB, et al. Paget disease of the nipple: a ten year review including clinical, pathological, and immunohistochemical findings. *Breast Cancer Res Treat* 1986;8:139–146.
3. Dixon AR, Galea MH, Ellis IO, et al. Paget's disease of the nipple. *Br J Surg* 1991; 78:722–723.
4. Zakaria S, Pantvaidya G, Ghosh K, et al. Paget's disease of the breast: accuracy of preoperative assessment. *Breast Cancer Res Treat* 2007;102(2):137–142.
5. Chen CY, Sun LM, Anderson BO. Paget disease of the breast: changing patterns of incidence, clinical presentation, and treatment in the U.S. *Cancer.* 2006;107(7): 1448–1458.
6. Graham H. *The story of surgery,* 1st ed. New York: Doubleday, Doran & Company, 1939.
7. Velpeau A. *Lecons orales de clinique chirurgicale faites a l'hospital de la charite,* vol 2. Paris: G. Bailliere, 1840.
8. Paget J. On disease of the mammary areola preceding cancer of the mammary gland. *St Barts Hospital Rep* 1874;10:87.
9. Thin G. On the connection between diseases of the nipple and areola and tumors of the breast. *Trans Pathol Soc London* 1881;32:218.
10. Jacobeus HC. Paget's disease und sein verhaltnis zum milchdrusenkarzinom. *Virchows Arch Pathol Anat* 1904;178:124.
11. Jahn H, Osther PJ, Nielsen EH, et al. An electron microscopic study of clinical Paget's disease of the nipple. *APMIS* 1995;103:628–634.
12. Cohen C, Guarner J, DeRose PB. Mammary Paget's disease and associated carcinoma. An immunohistochemical study. *Arch Pathol Lab Med* 1993;117:291–294.
13. Wood WS, Hegedus C. Mammary Paget's disease and intraductal carcinoma. Histologic, histochemical, and immunocytochemical comparison. *Am J Dermapathol* 1988;10:183–188.
14. Schelfhout VR, Coene ED, Delaey B, et al. Pathogenesis of Paget's disease: epidermal heregulin-alpha, motility factor, and the HER receptor family. *J Natl Cancer Inst* 2000;92:622–628.
15. Sagebiel RW. Ultrastructural observations on epidermal cells in Paget's disease of the breast. *Am J Pathol* 1969;57:49–64.
16. Rosen PP, Oberman HA. *Atlas of tumor pathology: tumors of the mammary gland,* 3rd series, Vol. 7. Armed Forces Institute of Pathology. Washington: Fasciclez, 1993.
17. Nance FC, DeLoach DH, Welsh RA, et al. Paget's disease of the breast. *Ann Surg* 1970;171:864–874.
18. Jones RE Jr. Mammary Paget's disease without underlying carcinoma. *Am J Dermapathol* 1985;7:361–365.
19. Lagios MD, Westdahl PR, Rose MR, et al. Paget's disease of the nipple. Alternative management in cases without or with minimal extent of underlying breast carcinoma. *Cancer* 1984;54:545–551.
20. Mai KT. Morphological evidence for field effect as a mechanism for tumor spread in mammary Paget's disease. *Histopathology* 1999;35:567–566.
21. Kaelin CK. Paget's disease. In Harris J, Lippman ME, Morrow M, Osborne CK, eds. *Diseases of the breast,* 2nd ed. Philadelphia: Lippincott Williams & Wilkins, 2000:1007–1013.
22. Kister SJ, Haagensen CD. Paget's disease of the breast. *Am J Surg* 1970;119: 606–609.
23. Freund H, Maydovnik M, Laufer N, et al. Paget's disease of the breast. *J Surg Oncol* 1977;9:93–98.
24. Kay S. Paget's disease of the nipple. *Surg Gynecol Obstet* 1966;123:1010.
25. Lagios MD, Gates EA, Westdahl PR, et al. A guide to the frequency of nipple involvement in breast cancer. A study of 149 consecutive mastectomies using a serial subgross and correlated radiographic technique. *Am J Surg* 1979;138: 135–142.
26. Chaudary MA, Millis RR, Lane EB, et al. Paget's disease of the nipple: a ten year review including clinical, pathological, and immunohistochemical findings. *Breast Cancer Res Treat* 1986;8:139–146.
27. Rissanen PM, Holsti P. Paget's disease of the breast: the influence of the presence or absence of an underlying palpable tumor on the prognosis and on the choice of treatment. *Oncology* 1969;23:209–216.
28. Ascenso AC, Marques MS, Capitao-Mor M. Paget's disease of the nipple. Clinical and pathological review of 109 female patients. *Dermatologica* 1985;170:170–179.

29. Maier WP, Rosemond GP, Harasym EL Jr, et al. Paget's disease in the female breast. *Surg Gynecol Obstet* 1969;128:1253–1263.
30. Berg JW, Hutter RV. Breast cancer. *Cancer* 1995;75:257–269.
31. Fu W, Mittel VK, Young SC. Paget disease of the breast: analysis of 41 patients. *Am J Clin Oncol* 2001;24:397–400.
32. Kothari AS, Beechey-Newman N, Hamed H, et al. Paget disease of the nipple: a multifocal manifestation of higher-risk disease. *Cancer* 2002;95:1–7.
33. Colcock BP, Sommers SC. Prognosis in Paget's disease of the breast. *Surg Clin North Am* 1954;35:773.
34. Sheen-Chen SM, Chen HS, Chen WJ, et al. Paget disease of the breast—an easily overlooked disease? *J Surg Oncol* 2001;76:261–265.
35. Yim JH, Wick MR, Philpott GW, et al. Underlying pathology in mammary Paget's disease. *Ann Surg Oncol* 1997;4:287–292.
36. Marshall JK, Griffith KA, Haffty BG, et al. The conservative management of Paget's disease of the breast with radiotherapy: 10- and 15-year results. *Cancer* 2003;97(9):2142–2149.
37. Bijker N, Rutgers EJ, Duchateau L, et al. Breast-conserving therapy for Paget's disease of the nipple: a prospective European Organization for Research and Treatment of Cancer study of 61 patients. *Cancer* 2001;91:472–477.
38. Kollmorgen DR, Varanasi JS, Edge SB, et al. Paget's disease of the breast: a 33-year experience. *J Am Coll Surg* 1998;187:171–177.
39. Polgar C, Orosz Z, Kovacs T, et al. Breast-conserving therapy for Paget disease of the nipple: a prospective European Organization for Research and Treatment of Cancer study of 61 patients. *Cancer* 2002;94:1904–1905.
40. Anderson WR. Bilateral Paget's disease of the nipple: case report. *Am J Obstet Gynecol* 1979;134:877–878.
41. Fernandes FJ, Costa MM, Bernardo M. Rarities in breast pathology. Bilateral Paget's disease of the breast—a case report. *Eur J Surg Oncol* 1990;16:172–174.
42. Menzies D, Barr L, Ellis H. Paget's disease of the nipple occurring after wide local excision and radiotherapy for carcinoma of the breast. *Eur J Surg Oncol* 1989;15:271–273.
43. Markopoulos C, Gazet JC. Paget's disease of the nipple occurring after conservative management of early breast cancer. *J Surg Oncol* 1988;14:77–78.
44. Plowman PN, Gilmore OJ, Curling M, et al. Paget's disease of the nipple occurring after conservation management of early infiltrating breast cancer. *Br J Surg* 1986;73:45.
45. Bulens P, Vanuytsel L, Rijnders A, et al. Breast conserving treatment of Paget's disease. *Radiother Oncol* 1990;17:305–309.
46. Perzin KH, Lattes R. Papillary adenoma of the nipple (florid papillomatosis, adenoma, adenomatosis). A clinicopathologic study. *Cancer* 1972;29:996–1009.
47. Rosen PP, Caicco JA. Florid papillomatosis of the nipple. A study of 51 patients, including nine with mammary carcinoma. *Am J Surg Pathol* 1986;10:87–101.
48. Scott P, Kissin MW, Collins C, et al. Florid papillomatosis of the nipple: a clinico-pathological surgical problem. *Eur J Surg Oncol* 1991;17:211–213.
49. Culberson JD, Horn RCJ. Paget's disease of the nipple: a review of 25 cases with special reference to melanin pigmentation of Paget's cells. *Arch Surg* 1956;72:224.
50. Venkataseshan VS, Budd DC, Un Kim D, et al. Intraepidermal squamous carcinoma (Bowen's disease) of the nipple. *Hum Pathol* 1994;25:1371–1374.
51. Sauven P, Roberts A. Basal cell carcinoma of the nipple. *J R Soc Med* 1983;76:699–701.
52. Kohler S, Rouse RV, Smoller BR. The differential diagnosis of pagetoid cells in the epidermis. *Mod Pathol* 1998;11:79–92.
53. Park BW, Kim SI, Lee KS, et al. Ductal eccrine carcinoma presenting as a Paget's disease–like lesion of the breast. *Breast J* 2001;7:358–362.
54. Rosen PP. Syringomatous adenoma of the nipple. *Am J Surg Pathol* 1983;7:739–745.
55. Dalberg K, Hellborg H, Wärnberg F.. Paget's disease of the nipple in a population based cohort. *Breast Cancer Res Treat* 2008;111:313–319.
56. Kawase K, Dimaio DJ, Tucker SL, et al. Paget's disease of the breast: there is a role for breast-conserving therapy. *Ann Surg Oncol* ;2005;12(5):391–397. Epub 2005 March 29. PMID: 15915373.
57. Smith KJ, Tuur S, Corvette D, et al. Cytokeratin 7 staining in mammary and extra-mammary Paget's disease. *Mod Pathol* 1997;10:1069–1074.
58. Gillett CE, Bobrow LG, Millis RR. S100 protein in human mammary tissue—immunoreactivity in breast carcinoma, including Paget's disease of the nipple, and value as a marker of myoepithelial cells. *J Pathol* 1990;160:19–24.
59. Ramachandra S, Gillett CE, Millis RR. A comparative immunohistochemical study of mammary and extramammary Paget's disease and superficial spreading melanoma, with particular emphasis on melanocytic markers. *Virchows Arch* 1996;429:371–376.
60. Requena L, Sanchez Yus E, Nunez C, et al. Epidermotropically metastatic breast carcinomas. Rare histopathologic variants mimicking melanoma and Paget's disease. *Am J Dermapathol* 1996;18:385–395.
61. Ben-Izhak O, Stark P, Levy R, et al. Epithelial markers in malignant melanoma. A study of primary lesions and their metastases. *Am J Dermapathol* 1994;16:241–246.
62. Gown AM, Vogel AM, Hoak D, et al. Monoclonal antibodies specific for melanocytic tumors distinguish subpopulations of melanocytes. *Am J Pathol* 1986;123:195–203.
63. Bishop PW, Menasce LP, Yates AJ, et al. An immunophenotypic survey of malignant melanomas. *Histopathology* 1993;23:159–166.
64. Wick MR, Swanson PE, Rocamora A. Recognition of malignant melanoma by monoclonal antibody HMB-45. An immunohistochemical study of 200 paraffin-embedded cutaneous tumors. *J Cutan Pathol* 1988;15:201–207.
65. Shah KD, Tabibzadeh SS, Gerber MA. Immunohistochemical distinction of Paget's disease from Bowen's disease and superficial spreading melanoma with the use of monoclonal cytokeratin antibodies [published erratum in *Am J Clin Pathol* 1988;89(4):572]. *Am J Clin Pathol* 1987;88:689–695.
66. Hitchcock A, Topham S, Bell J, et al. Routine diagnosis of mammary Paget's disease. A modern approach. *Am J Surg Pathol* 1992;16:58–61.
67. Ceccherini AF, Evans AJ, Pinder SE, et al. Is ipsilateral mammography worthwhile in Paget's disease of the breast? *Clin Radiol* 1996;51:35–38.
68. Stomper P, Penetrante R, Carson W. Sensitivity of mammography on patients with Paget's disease of the nipple. *Breast Dis* 1995;8:173.
69. Ikeda DM, Helvie MA, Frank TS, et al. Paget disease of the nipple: radiologic-pathologic correlation. *Radiology* 1993;189:89–94.
70. Sawyer RH, Asbury DL. Mammographic appearances in Paget's disease of the breast. *Clin Radiol* 1994;49:185–188.
71. Edeiken S. Mammography in the symptomatic woman. *Cancer* 1989;63:1412–1414.
72. Günhan-Bilgen I, Oktay A. Paget's disease of the breast: clinical, mammographic, sonographic and pathologic findings in 52 cases. *Eur J Radiol* 2006;60(2):256–263.
73. Gundry KR. The application of breast MRI in staging and screening for breast cancer. *Oncology* 2005 19(2):159–169.
74. Teifke A, Hlawatsch A, Beier T, et al. Undetected malignancies of the breast: dynamic contrast-enhanced MR imaging at 1.0T *Radiology* 2002;224:881–888.
75. Soderstrom CE, Copit DS, et al. 3D RO-DEO breast MRI of lesions containing ductal carcinoma in situ. *Radiology* 1996;201:427–432.
76. Morrogh M, Morris EA, Liberman L, et al. MRI identifies otherwise occult disease in select patients with Paget disease of the nipple. *J Am Coll Surg* 2008;206(2):316–321.
77. Capobianco G, Spaliviero B, Dessole S, et al.Paget's disease of the nipple diagnosed by MRI. *Arch Gynecol Obstet* 2006;274:316–318.
78. Frei KA, Bonel HM, Pelte MF, et al. Paget disease of the breast: findings at magnetic resonance imaging and histopathologic correlation. *Invest Radiol* 2005;40:363–367.
79. Amano G, Yajima M, Morobashi Y, et al. MRI accurately depicts underying DCIS in a patient with Paget's disease of the breast without palpable mass and mammography findings. *Jpn J Clin Oncol* 2005;35:149–153.
80. Mitchell ML, Napoletano J, Penman EJ. The MRI appearance of Paget's disease of the nipple: images from a single case. *Del Med J* 2006;78:105–106.
81. Kollmorgan DR, Varanasi JS, Edge SB, et al. Paget's disease of the breast. *Am Coll Surg* 1998;187:171–177.
82. Han S, Kim JS, Kim BS, et al. 99mTc-MIBI Scan in mammary Paget's disease: a case report. *J Korean Med Sci* 1999;14:675–678.
83. Fisher B, Anderson S, Bryant J, et al. Twenty-year follow-up of a randomized trial comparing total mastectomy, lumpectomy, and lumpectomy plus irradiation for the treatment of invasive breast cancer. *N Engl J Med* 2002;347:1233–1241.
84. Veronesi U, Cascinelli N, Mariani L, et al. Twenty-year follow-up of a randomized study comparing breast-conserving surgery with radical mastectomy for early breast cancer. *N Engl J Med* 2002;347:1227–1232.
85. Paone JF, Baker RR. Pathogenesis and treatment of Paget's disease of the breast. *Cancer* 1981;48:825–829.
86a. Wertheim U, Ozzello L. Neoplastic involvement of nipple and skin flap in carcinoma of the breast. *Am J Surg Pathol* 1980;4:543–549.
86b. Zurrida S, Squiccarini P, Bartoli C, et al. Treatment of Paget's disease of the breast without an underlying mass lesion: an unresolved problem. *The Breast* 1993;2:248–249.
87. Christiaens MR, Knol J, Van den Bogaert R, et al. Treatment of Paget's disease of the breast with radiotherapy only [Abstract 259]. *Proceeding of the Annual Meeting of the American Society of Clinical Oncology* 1998.
88. Fourquet A, Campana F, Vielh P, et al. Paget's disease of the nipple without detectable tumor: conservative management with radiation therapy. *Int J Radiat Oncol Biol Physics* 1987;13:1463–1465.
89. Stockdale AD, Brierley JD, White WF, et al. Radiotherapy for Paget's disease of the nipple: a conservative alternative. *Lancet* 1989;2:664–666.
90. Caliskan M, Gatti G, Sosnovskikh I, et al. Paget's disease of the breast: the experience of the European institute of oncology and review of the literature. *Breast Cancer Res Treat* 2008. Epub ahead of print; PMID: 18240020.
91. Joseph KA, Ditkoff BA, Estabrook A, et al. Therapeutic options for Paget's disease: A single institution long-term follow-up study. *Breast J* 2007;13:110–111.
92. Giuliano AE, Dale PS, Turner RR, Morton DL, et al. Improved axillary staging of breast cancer with sentinel lymphadenectomy. *Ann Surg* 197;225.126–127.
93. Lyman GH, Giuliano AE, Somerfield MR, et al. American Society of Clinical Oncology guideline recommendations for sentinel lymph node biopsy in early-stage breast cancer. *J Clin Oncol* 2005;23;7703–7720.
94. Krag D, Harlow S, Julian T. Breast cancer and the NSABP-B32 sentinel node trial. *Breast Cancer* 2004;11:221–224.
95. Sukumvanich P, Bentrem DJ, Cody HS 3rd, et al. The role of sentinel lymph node biopsy in Paget's disease of the breast. *Ann Surg Oncol* 2007;14(3):1020–1023.
96. Laronga C, Hasson D, Hoover S, et al. Paget's disease in the era of sentinel lymph node biopsy. *Am J Surg* 2006;192(4):481–483.

Francisco J. Esteva and Carolina Gutierrez

Nonepithelial malignancies of the breast account for less than 1% of breast tumors. The most common primary nonepithelial breast cancers are sarcomas and lymphomas. Young et al. (1) evaluated the demographic and tumor characteristics of all malignant noncarcinomas of the breast using 26 population-based registries in the United States and found that of 363,801 women with malignant breast tumors diagnosed between 1994 and 1998, only 1,401 (0.4%) women had tumors that were nonepithelial in origin. All but nine of the nonepithelial breast cancers in that study were some form of soft tissue sarcoma. The most common nonepithelial cancer was malignant phyllodes tumor, which accounted for 61% of these diagnoses. In addition to the 363,801 malignant cancers classified as breast tumors, another 613 tumors in Young's study arose in the breast, but were classified as myelomas or lymphomas; two as solitary myelomas, two as Hodgkin's lymphoma, and the remaining 609 as non-Hodgkin's lymphoma (1). Cutaneous melanomas arising in the breast or the skin over the breast have been reported. Despite the infrequent presentation of these nonepithelial breast malignancies, knowledge of their unique features, clinical characteristics, pathology, molecular biology, appropriate diagnostic evaluation, proper staging, and treatment is important to provide optimal patient care. Metastasis to the breast from other organs is another presentation of nonepithelial cancers. When the primary site is unknown, establishing this diagnosis requires extensive pathologic examination using conventional histology, special immunohistochemistry, flow cytometry, cytogenetics, and electron microscopy. Limited data are available regarding the molecular biology of most nonepithelial malignancies of the breast.

PRIMARY SARCOMAS OF THE BREAST

Primary sarcomas of the breast are malignant tumors arising from the connective tissue within the breast and account for less than 1% of all breast malignancies. According to the Surveillance, Epidemiology, and End Results (SEER) Program of the National Cancer Institute (NCI), the annual incidence of breast sarcomas is 4.5 cases per million women (2,3). Sarcomas can arise de novo (primary) or as a consequence of treatment of an epithelial breast cancer (secondary) (4–7). Radiation therapy for breast carcinoma can lead to the development of secondary sarcomas with a latency of up to 20 years (8).

Malignant mesenchymal tumors of the breast are broadly composed of cystosarcoma phyllodes (or malignant phyllodes tumor) and soft tissue sarcoma. The stroma of cystosarcoma phyllodes develops from the hormonally sensitive periductal and intralobular stroma of the mammary gland that undergoes malignant change. Primary soft tissue sarcomas of the breast arise from interlobular mesenchymal elements that comprise the supporting mammary stroma and exhibit histologic subtypes that do not differ from sarcomas seen in other sites in the body. In general, fibrosarcoma, angiosarcoma, malignant fibrous histiocytoma (MFH), liposarcoma, osteosarcoma, and stromal sarcoma comprise the major histologic subtypes (7,9). The histologic distinction is still important as new molecular classification and targeted therapies are developed. Although the etiology of most soft tissue sarcomas remains unknown, angiosarcoma of the breast has increasingly been associated with prior external beam radiation therapy of the breast and with lymphedema

that occurs after radical surgery, with or without radiation, for primary breast cancer (5,10–12). Because of the rarity of breast angiosarcoma, only small series of patients have been reported (10,11,13,14).

Primary breast sarcomas typically clinically present with a unilateral mass with a growth rate that often is rapid when compared with epithelial breast cancer. The size of these tumors is variable, ranging from 1 to 40 cm in most studies, with an average median size of 5 to 6 cm (15–18). The gross appearance of these tumors is influenced in part by the specific histologic features, but, in general, they consist of firm, fleshy, tan to gray tissue with variable soft, cystic, and hemorrhagic areas.

Pathologic grading plays a critical role in the prognosis of mammary sarcomas (19). The tumors vary from hypercellular, fairly uniform spindle cell fibroblastic proliferations to atypical, highly anaplastic cells (16), and most tumors are intermediate to high grade. Increased mitotic activity (>10/10 high power field [hpf], range 0 to 43) and necrosis are additional findings. A diagnosis of primary breast sarcoma must be established only after a range of benign and malignant spindle cell lesions have been excluded, such as fibromatosis, nodular fasciitis, fibrous histiocytoma, sarcomatoid carcinoma, and metaplastic carcinoma. The distinction is important for treatment and for prognosis. The pathologic evaluation of primary breast sarcomas must include extensive sampling and, in some instances, markers of differentiation, cell surface markers, immunohistochemical studies, cytogenetics, and in some cases, electron microscopy (18,20–22).

Breast sarcomas differ clinically from primary breast epithelial tumors. The most common mode of spread is hematogenous, and axillary lymph node involvement is not as frequent as it is seen with epithelial breast tumors (2,17,18). The most frequent sites of initial metastases are the lungs, bone marrow, and the liver (23–25). Breast imaging studies are nonspecific except that microcalcifications are rare, the mass is often well circumscribed, and tumors tend to be heterogeneous because of the presence of necrosis within the tumor (26–28). Diagnosis of a primary breast sarcoma requires a core, incisional, or excisional biopsy. A fine needle aspiration is not adequate. Excisional biopsy is preferred, with attention to negative surgical margins. Tumor size, the presence of regional or distant metastases and the tumor grade are important factors to determine the stage and prognosis (19,24).

The treatment for primary breast sarcomas is wide excision that allows adequate margins free of cancer cells (2,3,7,29,30). Axillary lymph node dissection is not recommended unless there are enlarged lymph nodes or lymph nodes that appear suspicious under ultrasound or magnetic resonance imaging (MRI). Radiation therapy and chemotherapy may be considered in patients with angiosarcomas and high-grade sarcomas because these lesions have a tendency to recur locally, and can also metastasize. The role of adjuvant therapy in this setting is, however, controversial (2,7,30). A retrospective review of 55 patients with primary breast sarcoma treated at the Mayo Clinic between 1975 and 2001, reported that adjuvant chemotherapy and radiation therapy did not improve survival, although an advantage could easily be missed in such a small study (7). The treatment regimen should be individualized and a multidisciplinary approach involving a collaboration among the surgeon, radiation oncologist, and medical oncologist is mandatory.

Angiosarcoma of the Breast

Angiosarcoma arises in the breast more often than in any other organ and it is also the most common soft tissue sarcoma involving the breast (11,31). Angiosarcoma of the breast tends to occur in younger women at a median of 38 years (32). Because the disease affects younger women, an association with pregnancy has been observed; however, no evidence is found for a hormonal basis for breast angiosarcoma. A correlation has also been suggested between prior radiation therapy in the setting of breast-conserving surgery and the development of angiosarcomas (9–14). The SEER program data compiled by the NCI included more than 194,000 women who were treated for breast carcinoma. Among patients in the radiotherapy cohort, the relative risk of developing angiosarcoma was 15.9 (5). The median latency period between radiation for breast cancer and the diagnosis of angiosarcoma has been estimated to be about 6 years. One study failed to confirm the observation that prior radiation increased the risk of developing angiosarcoma (33). A study of women treated with prior breast-conserving surgery and radiation for breast cancer showed an incidence of angiosarcomas similar to what would be expected in healthy women without a history of breast cancer. In that series, only nine cases of angiosarcoma were documented, which represents a prevalence of 5 per 10,000 (33). Cutaneous angiosarcoma of the chest wall after mastectomy and radiation therapy may also occur (8,10).

Typically, patients present with a rapidly growing painless breast mass. The overlying skin may have blue or purple discoloration (31,32,34). In the largest series containing 69 patients with breast angiosarcoma, size varied between 1 and 14 cm with a median of 5.5 cm (13). In most cases, the angiosarcoma forms a friable, firm, or spongy hemorrhagic tumor. In high-grade lesions, cystic, hemorrhagic necrosis is usually present. Hemorrhagic discoloration in the surrounding breast tissue may indicate tumor extending beyond the evident mass. In some cases, the tumors have been described as poorly defined areas of thickening or induration.

Microscopically three distinct patterns of growth have been described; they reflect the degree of differentiation and were thought to correlate with prognosis, although a recent report did not find a relationship between grade and patient outcome (33,35,36). Low-grade or type I tumors (Fig. 67.1A) are composed of open, anatomizing vascular channels that invade mammary glandular tissue and fat-producing atrophy of the terminal duct lobular units. Some prominent hyperchromatic endothelial nuclei may be found, but most often they have inconspicuous nuclei. The endothelial cells are distributed in a flat monolayer around the vascular spaces without papillary endothelial proliferation and rare mitoses are seen. Intermediate grade or type II (Fig. 67.1B) shows scattered focal areas of more cellular proliferation consisting of well-developed papillary endothelial proliferation that may combine polygonal or spindle cells. Infrequent mitoses may be found in cellular or

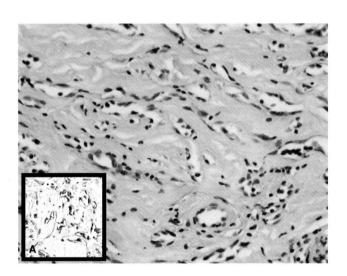

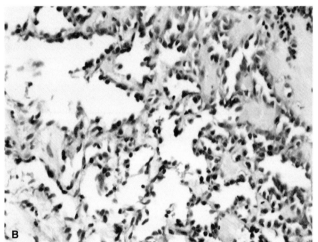

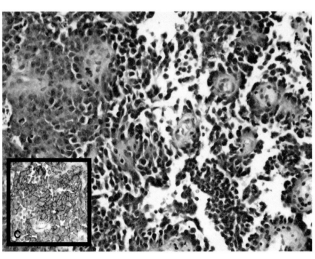

FIGURE 67.1. A: Low-grade or type I angiosarcoma. Open, anatomizing vascular channels with prominent endothelial nuclei are evident. *Insert* shows positive staining for CD31. **B:** Intermediate-grade or type II angiosarcoma. More cellular than low-grade with small buds of endothelial cells projecting into the vascular lumen are observed. **C:** High-grade or type III angiosarcoma. Solid papillary formations and prominent endothelial tufting containing cytologically malignant cells are evident. *Insert* shows marked positivity for CD31.

spindle areas. Type III or high-grade angiosarcoma (Fig. 67.1C) exhibits highly malignant features that comprise more than 50% of the tumor (37). These tumors consist of prominent epithelial tufting and solid papillary formations with cytologically malignant endothelial cells. Mitoses are readily found. Areas of necrosis and hemorrhage, so called "blood" lakes are only found in high-grade angiosarcomas. The high-grade tumors have infiltrative borders that feature low-grade vascular channels which may lead to the erroneous diagnosis of a low-grade lesion on a core biopsy. High-grade tumors tend to occur in young women (median 29 years) compared with intermediate grade (median 34 years) and low-grade (median 43 years) (17). Immunohistochemically, angiosarcomas are positive for factor VIII related antigen, thrombomodulin, B72.3, CD31, and CD34. These reagents are useful for distinguishing angiosarcomas from carcinoma and other neoplasms. A recent report suggests that the level of the cell cycle protein SKp2 and the Ki67 index as a measure of proliferation can be used to distinguish benign vascular lesions, such as hemangiomas, from malignant low-grade angiosarcomas (38).

Postirradiation Angiosarcomas of the Skin

The histologic features of postradiation angiosarcomas of the skin, subcutaneous tissue, and breast differ from primary breast angiosarcomas not associated with radiotherapy (39). High-grade areas are solid epithelioid or spindle cell foci with slit-like spaces with intraluminal or extravasated red blood cells. In addition, regardless of the microscopic pattern, malignant cells in postradiation angiosarcoma have poorly differentiated nuclei with prominent nucleoli and mitotic activity. Angiosarcoma in the skin and breast after radiotherapy must be distinguished from benign vascular lesions that arise in the same clinical setting—called *atypical vascular lesions* (AVL) (39). These lesions appear 2 to 5 years after radiotherapy as single or multiple skin nodules measuring 5 mm or less in diameter. Histologically, a focal proliferation of anastomizing vascular channels lined by a single layer of endothelial cells with occasional hyperchromatic nuclei is seen. The vascular spaces are usually empty and are limited to the superficial and mid dermal areas (40). Insufficient information exists to determine definitively whether AVL can progress to sarcomas. One report suggests that AVL may be precursors of angiosarcomas (41).

Treatment of Angiosarcomas of the Breast

Because breast angiosarcoma of one breast can occur synchronously or asynchronously in the contralateral breast, MRI screening at diagnosis and during follow-up has been suggested (42). Given the rarity of these lesions, it is not known if this approach is really cost-effective. The optimal surgical treatment of breast angiosarcoma is segmental mastectomy if negative margins can be achieved, or total mastectomy if the former is not possible. Axillary dissection is not recommended. Patients with angiosarcomas have a worse prognosis than patients with other types of sarcoma (7). The most important prognostic markers are histologic grade (subtype) and tumor size, although histologic grade was not prognostic in a recent study. However, the roles of adjuvant chemotherapy and radiation therapy are unclear. Several series suggest that adjuvant therapies do not improve disease-free or overall survival (7). A review of 69 patients with angiosarcoma of the breast treated at the M.D. Anderson Cancer Center found no improvement in survival of patients with angiosarcoma of the breast treated with neoadjuvant chemotherapy or radiation therapy. However, the response rate to anthracycline- and gemcitabine-based chemotherapy in the metastatic setting was 48%, suggesting that breast angiosarcoma is potentially a chemosensitive disease (13).

Osteogenic Sarcoma of the Breast

Extraskeletal osteosarcoma of the breast is an extremely rare tumor, accounting for 12.5% of mammary sarcomas (43,44). Primary breast osteosarcomas are considered highly aggressive tumors with early local recurrence and hematogenous spread most commonly to the lungs. The most common presentation is a circumscribed and movable mass that on mammography may show osseous trabeculae or coarse calcifications (45). Silver and Tavassoli (46) reported a series of 50 patients with osteogenic sarcoma of the breast diagnosed at the Armed Forces Institute of Pathology(AFIP) between 1957 and 1995. The median patient age at presentation in that study was 64.5 years and the tumor size varied from 1.4 to 13 cm at the time of diagnosis. The histologic features are similar to other extraskeletal osteosarcomas. The most common variants observed are fibroblastic, osteoblastic, and osteoclastic (46). In the osteoblastic osteosarcoma, the osteoid is deposited in a fine, ramifying, lace-like or coarsely trabecular pattern and sometimes in sheaths of osteoid or bone. Atypical cartilage has been reported in 36% of primary breast osteosarcomas. Necrotic foci can be identified in 30% of the cases. Multinucleated osteoclastic giant cells are usually present in areas of bone formation. Immunohistochemistry is helpful in ruling out a metaplastic carcinoma with heterologous elements which expresses CAM 5.2, pancytokeratin, and high molecular weight keratin (Fig. 67.2).

The relationship between prior breast or chest wall irradiation and breast osteosarcoma is not clear. One of the patients in the AFIP series had received radiotherapy for ipsilateral breast carcinoma 9 years before presentation, but none of the other patients had been exposed to radiation therapy. As with other sarcomas, spread to regional lymph nodes is uncommon with breast osteosarcoma. No axillary lymph node involvement was noted in 20 patients who underwent axillary lymph node dissection (46). Of 39 patients with follow-up, locally recurrent (n = 11) or metastatic disease (n = 15) was documented at a mean of 10.5 and 14.5 months from diagnosis, respectively. Adjuvant radiation therapy and chemotherapy are not recommended.

Embryonal Rhabdomyosarcoma of the Breast

Primary embryonal rhabdomyosarcomas of the breast are rare tumors that typically occur in adolescents and young women. Of the 3,500 cases of rhabdomyosarcoma registered between 1972 and 1992 with the Intergroup Rhabdomyosarcoma Group of the United States only 7 (0.2%) originated in the breast.

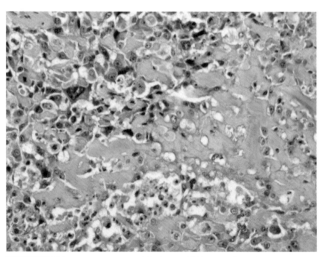

FIGURE 67.2. Primary osteosarcoma of the breast. Malignant cells with round nuclei and prominent nucleoli with lace-like osteoid are seen.

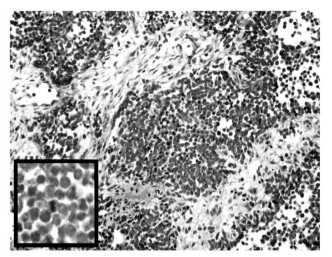

FIGURE 67.3. Alveolar rhabdomyosarcoma of the breast in a 16-year-old girl. The tumor is composed of a proliferation of small round cells mimicking a lymphoma. Molecular diagnostic pathology testing by reverse-transcription-polymerase chain reaction (RT-PCR) showed PAX3-FKHR translocation [t (2; 13)].

When the data were confined to the 423 women aged between 10 and 21 years, only 1.6% had rhabdomyosarcoma of breast origin. The median age was 15 years in a series of 26 patients with primary or secondary rhabdomyosarcomas of the breast (47). Ultrasound may aid in the diagnosis of breast rhabdomyosarcomas in children (48). The most common histologic subtype is alveolar rhabdomyosarcoma (49,50).

Histologically, alveolar rhabdomyosarcoma is composed of small, round cells that make poorly defined aggregates (Fig. 67.3). Mitoses are easily identified. The differential diagnosis, which includes malignant lymphoma and invasive lobular carcinoma, can be resolved by using immunostains for myoid, epithelial, and lymphoid markers. Cytogenetic studies may show the characteristic translocations t (2;13) (q35;q14) or t (1;13) (p36;q14). Most of these tumors are metastatic from nonmammary primary sites, although they can be primary in the breast.

The treatment of choice for embryonal rhabdomyosarcomas of the breast is surgical resection with wide tumor-free margins. Total mastectomy may provide a better outcome in some patients (50). Limited data exist regarding the role of lymphatic mapping and sentinel node (SLN) biopsy in the management of sarcomas because most sarcomas rarely metastasize to regional nodes. Rhabdomyosarcomas, however, are usually high-grade tumors that do have a propensity for regional lymph node metastases, and it has been suggested that these patients may benefit from SLN biopsy (51). Treatment of rhabdomyosarcomas is multidisciplinary and may include radiation and chemotherapy in addition to surgery. Excellent survival rates are observed in children with this disease. A 5-year survival rate of 43% was reported in patients with breast rhabdomyosarcomas who tend to be slightly older and to have the alveolar subtype (47).

Miscellaneous Breast Sarcomas

A variety of other soft tissue sarcomas can originate in the breast. They should be described, classified, and treated in a manner similar to sarcomas originating in other sites. These tumors include stromal sarcoma, leiomysarcoma, liposarcoma, malignant fibrous histiocytoma, and fibrosarcoma (2,9). These tumors are rare. Some, such as malignant fibrous histiocytoma and fibrosarcoma, are sequelae of prior postmastectomy irradiation (4–8). These tumors can occur in all age groups, but tend to be found more frequently in women above age 40 to 50. They present clinically as a mass, although they can be found by breast imaging. Treatment of these lesions is surgical. Wide excision or total mastectomy has been performed, with the decision based on the characteristics of the tumor and the

patient. The rather high local recurrence rate after wide excision in some studies suggests that total mastectomy might be preferred (30). Axillary dissection is not indicated because these tumors spread hematogenously.

Other mesenchymal tumors have been observed rarely in the breast. These include hemangiopericytoma, which has an excellent prognosis and can be treated by wide excision (52); dermatofibrosarcoma protuberans (53,54), which arises in the skin of the breast and can be confused with locally advanced breast cancer clinically (7,53,55); Kaposi's sarcoma, and tumors of the peripheral nerve sheath (17,56). These rare lesions are described in detail elsewhere (15).

Lymphedema-Associated Lymphangiosarcoma

Lymphedema-associated lymphangiosarcoma, also known as Stewart-Treves syndrome, has been reported in women treated typically with radical mastectomy and chest wall irradiation who have chronic upper extremity edema (57). The incidence of lymphedema-associated lymphangiosarcoma in the United States is 1.6 per 100,000 persons (58). The pathogenic mechanism of this syndrome is unknown, but several hypotheses have been postulated. Proliferation of lymphatic vessels is often seen in areas of chronically edematous tissue (59). It has been suggested that the block of the lymphatics increases the expression of growth factors and cytokines, which stimulates proliferation of blood vessels and lymphatics (60). The association between radiotherapy and chest wall sarcomas is well known, but it is unclear whether radiation therapy contributes to this entity, because most reported postradiation sarcomas are not lymphangiosarcomas (61). Although postmastectomy radiation is a major predisposing factor for the development of lymphedema, other factors (e.g., hypertension and cardiovascular disease) have also been described as risk factors (62). With multimodality therapy, the 5-year survival rate for lymphedema-associated lymphangiosarcoma is less than 5% (63–66). The incidence of this complication of extensive surgery and radiation is on the decline with the increasing use of breast conservation, limited radiation, and SLN biopsy.

PRIMARY LYMPHOMAS OF THE BREAST

Primary breast lymphomas (PBL) account for 1.7% to 2.2% of extranodal lymphomas, 0.04% to 1.1% of breast neoplasms, and 0.38% to 0.7% of non-Hodgkin's lymphomas (NHL) (67–69). Wiseman and Liao (70) used the following criteria to define PBL: (a) no prior diagnosis of extramammary lymphoma and the breast is the primary site of disease; (b) mammary tissue and lymphomatous infiltrate are in close association with no evidence of concurrent widespread disease; and (c) pathology is confirmed by technically adequate specimens.

The predominant pathologic type of PBL is diffuse large B-cell lymphoma (DLBCL) (Fig. 67.4A), but other types can be found (Fig. 67.4B) (68,71,72). Most B-cell lymphomas of the breast present as a palpable breast mass with or without enlarged axillary nodes (69,72,73). Typically, the mass is not painful and it is not fixed to the chest wall or skin (74,75). Skin ulceration, erythema, or erosion suggests extension into the skin. When the skin is involved, a T-lymphocyte phenotype should be suspected. Other primary lymphomas that may involve the skin overlying the breasts include epidermotropic mycosis fungoides, peripheral T-cell lymphomas, or cutaneous B-cell lymphomas. It has been suggested that the monocytoid B-cell lymphomas of the breast are the equivalent of the malignant lymphomas of the mucosa-associated lymphoid tissues (MALT) (76). Primary Hodgkin lymphoma of the breast has also been reported (77). Although extremely rare, a Burkitt-type lymphoma has been reported in pregnant or lactating women with bilateral, diffuse, and rapidly fatal disease (71,76,78).

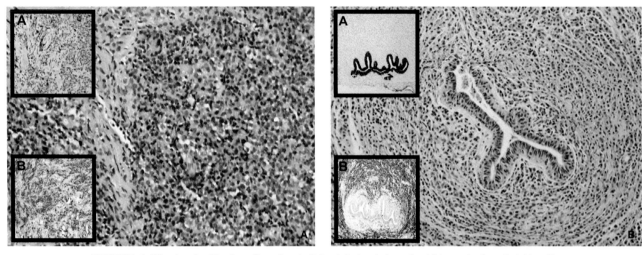

FIGURE 67.4. **A:** Diffuse large B-cell lymphoma. The malignant cells invade the breast stroma. *Insert A* shows only a few cells staining with CD3. *Insert B* shows the majority of cells staining for CD20. **B:** Lymphoma mimicking invasive lobular carcinoma. *Insert A* shows positive staining for AE1/AE3 in the normal breast duct, whereas the neoplastic cells are negative. *Insert B* shows intense staining of the malignant cells with CD45, confirming the lymphoid lineage.

Radiographic imaging features of PBL are nonspecific, with the exception that calcifications are rare (79,80). Positron emission tomography (PET) and computed tomography (CT) scanning may be of some use in distinguishing breast lymphomas from other breast neoplasms after response to therapy and in determining remission status in the presence of minimal residual masses determined by physical examination or other imaging methods (81,82). Diagnosis is typically made by core biopsy of a palpable breast mass. High-grade lymphoma must be distinguished from melanoma and poorly differentiated carcinoma because curative treatment differs radically among these tumor types. Immunostaining with a broad panel of markers, including epithelial markers (cytokeratins), melanoma (S-100, human melanoma, black-45 (HMB-45) and Melan A), and lymphoid markers (CD45, CD3, CD20) usually leads to the correct diagnosis. After diagnosis, the disease should be fully staged to determine extent of disease using the World Health Organization (WHO) classification of lymphoma (83). The WHO classification subdivides tumors into those of B-cell or T/Natural Killer (T/NK)-cell origin and into tumors with an immature or blastic appearance versus those developing from more mature stages of lymphoid development. The latter tumors, in the case of T-cell lymphomas, are referred to as *peripheral* T-cell lymphomas. The diagnostic evaluation should include immunophenotyping and might require cytogenetics, fluorescent *in situ* hybridization (FISH), antigen receptor gene rearrangement studies, and other investigations (84). Clinical staging procedures include CT scans of the chest, abdomen, and pelvis; a PET scan; and bilateral bone marrow biopsies and aspirates. Other staging studies may include head CT of the brain, MRI scans, lumbar puncture with evaluation of cerebrospinal fluid chemistry, and cytology, depending on the clinical presentation and histologic subtype of lymphoma. A variety of biopsy techniques, including gastrointestinal endoscopy, bronchoscopy, mediastinoscopy, thoracoscopy, laparoscopy, thoracotomy, or laparotomy, may be indicated in the process of diagnosis and staging (84,85).

The role of surgery in PBL should be limited to acquisition of adequate material for diagnosis, typically with a biopsy either from the breast mass or from an involved lymph node. Treatment by mastectomy offers no survival benefit or protection from recurrence (68). Rituximab plus anthracycline-based chemotherapy and involved field radiation therapy are the mainstays of treatment for PBL (68,86). It should be noted that most PBL reports describe patients treated in the pre-rituximab era. Systemic chemotherapy with rituximab, cyclophosphamide,

doxorubicin, vincristine, and prednisone (RCHOP) is currently the standard of care for patients with DLBCL, and this regimen should be used in patients with PBL as well (87–89). Although some studies reported a high recurrence rate in the central nervous system (CNS) (71,90–94), other studies reported low CNS involvement (71,72,95). Currently, prophylactic whole-brain irradiation is not recommended for patients with PBL.

MELANOMA OF THE BREAST

Although melanoma can metastasize to the breast, primary cutaneous melanomas of the breast tissue or skin can also rarely occur (96–98). When melanomas occur in the nipple–areolar area, phagocytosis of melanin by Paget's cells distinguishes the melanomas from Paget's disease of the breast (99–101). The clinical presentation of melanoma involving the skin of the breast includes changes in size, pigmentation, ulceration, and bleeding of a pre-existing mole (96–98). The most important prognostic factors are the presence of regional lymph node metastases, the thickness of the primary tumor,

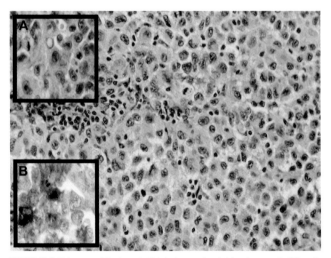

FIGURE 67.5. Melanoma of the breast. This lesion can be mistaken for a poorly differentiated carcinoma or a large-cell lymphoma when melanin pigment is not readily seen. *Insert A* shows a characteristic intranuclear inclusion in a malignant cell. *Insert B* shows intense staining for human melanoma, black-45 (HMB-45) confirming the diagnosis of melanoma.

Table 67.1	**RECOMMENDED EXCISION MARGINS FOR PRIMARY CUTANEOUS MELANOMA**			
Tumor Thickness	UK Trial (137)[a]	WHO Trial (138)[a]	Australian Trial (139)[a]	Dutch Trial (110)[a]
In situ	2–5 mm	5 mm	5 mm	5 mm
<1 mm	1 cm	1 cm	1 cm	1 cm
1–2 mm	1–2 cm	1 cm[b]	1 cm	1 cm
2.1–4 mm	2–3 cm; 2 cm preferred	2 cm	1 cm	2 cm
>4 mm	2–3 cm	2 cm	2 cm	2 cm

UK, United Kingdom; WHO, World Health Organization.
[a]Reference numbers.
[b]For melanomas thicker than 1.5 mm, recommended excision margin is 2 cm.
Adapted from Lens MB, Nathan P, Bataille V. Excision margins for primary cutaneous melanoma: updated pooled analysis of randomized controlled trials. *Arch Surg* 2007;142:885–891, with permission.

and the presence of ulceration (102–105). As described above, melanoma and high-grade lymphoma can be confused with a poorly differentiated carcinoma. These tumors must be distinguished from one another to provide appropriate curative treatment. Staining with HMB-45, S-100, or Melan-A is helpful to confirm the diagnosis of melanoma (Fig. 67.5).

Treatment of cutaneous melanoma of the breast involves *en bloc* excision of the tumor or biopsy site, with a margin containing normal-appearing skin and underlying subcutaneous tissue (Table 67.1) (106). Randomized clinical trials have shown that a 1- to 2-cm margin of excision is adequate (103). Wider margins have not translated to improvement in survival. The recommended excision margins for primary melanoma of the breast are similar to other cutaneous melanomas (Table 67.1) (106–110). All patients with melanoma of the breast should undergo SLN biopsy because involvement of the axillary lymph node basin is the most important prognostic factor. Histopathologic and molecular assessment of the SLN improve the detection of clinically occult nodal metastases, thereby distinguishing patients who might benefit from immediate lymphadenectomy from those for whom this procedure is unlikely to be helpful. This procedure also identifies patients who might be candidates for clinical trials of adjuvant systemic therapy. Clinical trials are ongoing to determine the clinical value of a variety of molecular prognostic markers in patients with melanoma undergoing SLN assessment (111).

 ## METASTASES TO THE BREAST

The incidence rate of metastases to the breast from extramammary sites ranges from 1.7% to 6.6% in autopsy series and 1.2% to 2% in clinical reports (112). The most common presentation is the development of metastasis from the contralateral breast by a cross-lymphatic route, especially in premenopausal women (113). Other malignancies that can metastasize to the breast include non-Hodgkin lymphomas (114), leukemias (115), melanomas (116), lung cancer (115), gastric cancer (117–119), and ovarian cancer (120). Rarely, metastases from fallopian tube cancer (121), ovarian disgerminoma (122), renal cancer (123), medullary thyroid cancer (124), carcinoid (121,125), medulloblastoma (126), malignant schwannoma (127), and pharyngeal carcinoma (128) have been reported.

Radiographic imaging using mammography and ultrasonography are not sufficient to determine whether a tumor is primary or metastatic. Skin thickening and axillary lymph node involvement may be apparent. A fine-needle aspiration, a core needle biopsy, or both are needed to make the diagnosis. Pathologic assessment for metastases to the breast includes conventional histology, immunohistochemistry, cytogenetics, flow cytometry, and electron microscopy analysis (113–115).

Clinically, it is important to differentiate bilateral primary tumors from metastatic tumors that coexist with a primary breast cancer. All suspicious lesions should be biopsied to clarify the overall diagnosis and treatment approach (129–131). Factors suggesting contralateral metastatic breast cancer include short disease-free interval, multiple breast lesions, and known metastatic breast cancer at other distant sites (130,132,133). Factors suggesting nonbreast metastatic disease include location in fat or subcutaneous tissue as opposed to breast parenchyma, lack of *in situ* disease histologically, and lack of microcalcifications on mammography (129–136).

Metastatic breast cancer to the contralateral breast is treated with systemic therapy directed to the primary tumor. Palliative surgery, radiation therapy, or both are often used for local control. If it is not clear whether the tumor is a primary breast cancer versus a metastasis, it should be treated with curative intent as a primary breast cancer. If the tumor is clearly metastatic but its origin is uncertain, treatment planning should take into account the most probable histologic diagnosis and primary site of the tumor as well as the potential efficacy of systemic treatments available for the presumed primary tumor.

References

1. Young JL Jr., Ward KC, Wingo PA, et al. The incidence of malignant non-carcinomas of the female breast. *Cancer Causes Control* 2004;15:313–319.
2. Zelek L, Llombart-Cussac A, Terrier P, et al. Prognostic factors in primary breast sarcomas: a series of patients with long-term follow-up. *J Clin Oncol* 2003;212:583–2588.
3. McGowan TS, Cummings BJ, O'Sullivan B, et al. An analysis of 78 breast sarcoma patients without distant metastases at presentation. *Int J Radiat Oncol Biol Phys* 2000;46:383–390.
4. Karlsson P, Holmberg E, Samuelsson A, et al. Soft tissue sarcoma after treatment for breast cancer—a Swedish population-based study. *Eur J Cancer* 1998;34:2068–2075.
5. Huang J, Mackillop WJ. Increased risk of soft tissue sarcoma after radiotherapy in women with breast carcinoma. *Cancer* 2001;92:172–180.
6. Brady MS, Garfein CF, Petrek JA, et al. Post-treatment sarcoma in breast cancer patients. *Ann Surg Oncol* 1994;1:66–72.
7. Blanchard DK, Reynolds CA, Grant CS, et al. Primary nonphylloides breast sarcomas. *Am J Surg* 2003;186:359–361.
8. Kirova YM, Vilcoq JR, Asselain B, et al. Radiation-induced sarcomas after radiotherapy for breast carcinoma: a large-scale single-institution review. *Cancer* 2005;104:856–863.
9. Adem C, Reynolds C, Ingle JN, et al. Primary breast sarcoma: clinicopathologic series from the Mayo Clinic and review of the literature. *Br J Cancer* 2004;91:237–241.
10. Vorburger SA, Xing Y, Hunt KK, et al. Angiosarcoma of the breast. *Cancer* 2005;104:2682–2688.
11. Fayette J, Martin E, Piperno-Neumann S, et al. Angiosarcomas, a heterogeneous group of sarcomas with specific behavior depending on primary site: a retrospective study of 161 cases. *Ann Oncol* 2007;18:2030–2036.
12. Cha C, Antonescu CR, Quan ML, et al. Long-term results with resection of radiation-induced soft tissue sarcomas. *Ann Surg* 2004;239:903–909.
13. Sher T, Hennessy BT, Valero V, et al. Primary angiosarcomas of the breast. *Cancer* 2007;110:173–178.
14. Luini A, Gatti G, Diaz J, et al. Angiosarcoma of the breast: the experience of the European Institute of Oncology and a review of the literature. *Breast Cancer Res Treat* 2007;105:81–85.

15. Callery CD, Rosen PP, Kinne DW. Sarcoma of the breast. A study of 32 patients with reappraisal of classification and therapy. *Ann Surg* 1985;201:527–532.
16. Norris HJ, Taylor HB. Sarcomas and related mesenchymal tumors of the breast. *Cancer* 1968;22:22–28.
17. Pollard SG, Marks PV, Temple LN, et al. Breast sarcoma. A clinicopathologic review of 25 cases. *Cancer* 1990;66:941–944.
18. Terrier P, Terrier-Lacombe MJ, Mouriesse H, et al. Primary breast sarcoma: a review of 33 cases with immunohistochemistry and prognostic factors. *Breast Cancer Res Treat* 1989;13:39–48.
19. Greene FL, Fritz AG, Balch CM. Soft tissue sarcoma: . In: *Cancer* AJCo, eds. Greene FL, Page DL, Fleming ID, et al. *AJCC cancer staging manual*, 6th ed. New York: Springer, 2002:193–197.
20. Antonescu CR, Baren A. Spectrum of low-grade fibrosarcomas: a comparative ultrastructural analysis of low-grade myxofibrosarcoma and fibromyxoid sarcoma. *Ultrastruct Pathol* 2004;28:321–332.
21. Rubin BP, Goldblum JR. Pathology of soft tissue sarcoma. *J Natl Compr Canc Netw* 2007;5:411–418.
22. Skubitz KM, D'Adamo DR. Sarcoma. *Mayo Clin Proc* 2007;821:409–1432.
23. Barnes L, Pietruszka M. Sarcomas of the breast: a clinicopathologic analysis of ten cases. *Cancer* 1977;40:1577–1585.
24. Costa J, Wesley RA, Glatstein E, et al. The grading of soft tissue sarcomas. Results of a clinicohistopathologic correlation in a series of 163 cases. *Cancer* 1984;53:530–541.
25. Khanna S, Gupta S, Khanna NN. Sarcomas of the breast: homogenous or heterogenous? *J Surg Oncol* 1981;18:119–128.
26. D'Orsi CJ, Feldhaus L, Sonnenfeld M. Unusual lesions of the breast. *Radiol Clin North Am* 1983;21:67–80.
27. Langham MR Jr, Mills AS, DeMay RM, et al. Malignant fibrous histiocytoma of the breast. A case report and review of the literature. *Cancer* 1984;54:558–563.
28. Yang WT, Hennessy BT, Dryden MJ, et al. Mammary angiosarcomas: imaging findings in 24 patients. *Radiology* 2007;242:725–734.
29. Shabahang M, Franceschi D, Sundaram M, et al. Surgical management of primary breast sarcoma. *Am Surg* 2002;68:673–677.
30. Gutman H, Pollock RE, Ross MI, et al. Sarcoma of the breast: implications for extent of therapy. The M.D. Anderson experience. *Surgery* 1994;116:505–509.
31. Abraham JA, Hornicek FJ, Kaufman AM, et al. Treatment and outcome of 82 patients with angiosarcoma. *Ann Surg Oncol* 2007;141:953–1967.
32. Rosen PP, Kimmel M, Ernsberger D. Mammary angiosarcoma. The prognostic significance of tumor differentiation. *Cancer* 1988;62:2145–2151.
33. Marchal C, Weber B, de Lafontan B, et al. Nine breast angiosarcomas after conservative treatment for breast carcinoma: a survey from French Comprehensive Cancer Centers. *Int J Radiat Oncol Biol Phys* 1999;44:113–119.
34. Chen KT, Kirkegaard DD, Bocian JJ. Angiosarcoma of the breast. *Cancer* 1980;46:368–371.
35. Merino MJ, Carter D, Berman M. Angiosarcoma of the breast. *Am J Surg Pathol* 1983;7:53–60.
36. Nascimento AF, Raut CP, Fletcher CD. Primary angiosarcoma of the breast. *Am J Surg Pathol* 2008;32:1896–1904.
37. Merino MJ, Carter D, Berman M. Angiosarcoma of the breast. *Am J Surg Pathol* 1983;7:53–60.
38. Shin SJ, Lesser M, Rosen PP. Hemangiomas and angiosarcomas of the breast: diagnostic utility of cell cycle markers with emphasis on Ki-67. *Arch Pathol Lab Med* 2007;131:538–544.
39. Deutsch M, Rosenstein MM. Angiosarcoma of the breast mimicking radiation dermatitis arising after lumpectomy and breast irradiation: a case report. *Am J Clin Oncol* 1998;21:608–609.
40. Fineberg S, Rosen, P.P. Cutaneous angiosarcoma and atypical vascular lesions of the skin and breast after radiation therapy for breast carcinoma. *Am J Clin Pathol* 1994;102:757–763.
41. Patton KT, Deyrup AT, Weiss SW. Atypical vascular lesions after surgery and radiation of the breast: a clinicopathologic study of 32 cases analyzing histologic heterogeneity and association with angiosarcoma. *Am J Sur Pathol* 2008;32:943–950.
42. Marchant LK, Orel SG, Perez-Jaffe LA, et al. Bilateral angiosarcoma of the breast on MR imaging. *AJR Am J Roentgenol* 1997;169:1009–1010.
43. Jernstrom P, Lindberg AL, Meland ON. Osteogenic sarcoma of the mammary gland. *Am J Clin Pathol* 1963;40:521–526.
44. Bahrami A, Resetkova E, Ro JY, et al. Primary osteosarcoma of the breast: report of 2 cases. *Arch Pathol Lab Med* 2007;131:792–795.
45. Roditi G, Prasad S. Case report: radiology of stromal sarcoma of the breast with ossifying pleural metastases. *Br J Radiol* 1994;67:212–214.
46. Silver SA, Tavassoli FA. Primary osteogenic sarcoma of the breast: a clinicopathologic analysis of 50 cases. *Am J Surg Pathol* 1998;22:925–933.
47. Hays DM, Donaldson SS, Shimada H, et al. Primary and metastatic rhabdomyosarcoma in the breast: neoplasms of adolescent females, a report from the Intergroup Rhabdomyosarcoma Study. *Med Pediatr Oncol* 1997;29:181–189.
48. Garcia CJ, Espinoza A, Dinamarca V, et al. Breast US in children and adolescents. *Radiographics* 2000;20:1605–1612.
49. Binokay F, Soyupak SK, Inal M, et al. Primary and metastatic rhabdomyosarcoma in the breast: report of two pediatric cases. *Eur J Radiol* 2003;48:282–284.
50. Nogi H, Kobayashi T, Kawase K, et al. Primary rhabdomyosarcoma of the breast in a 13-year-old girl: report of a case. *Surg Today* 200;737:38–42. Epub 2007 January 2001.
51. Blazer DG, III, Sabel MS, Sondak VK. Is there a role for sentinel lymph node biopsy in the management of sarcoma? *Surg Oncol* 2003;12:201–206.
52. Brodie C, Provenzano E. Vascular proliferations of the breast. *Histopathology* 2008;52:30–44.
53. Karcnik TJ, Miller JA, Fromowitz F, et al. Dermatofibrosarcoma protuberans of the breast: a rare malignant tumor simulating benign disease. *Breast J* 1999;5:262–263.
54. Chargui R, Damak T, Khomsi F, et al. [Dermatofibrosarcoma protuberans of the breast]. *Tunis Med* 2006;84:122–124.
55. Bulliard C, Murali R, Chang LY, et al. Subcutaneous dermatofibrosarcoma protuberans in skin of the breast: may mimic a primary breast lesion. *Pathology* 2007;39:446–448.
56. Woo OH, Yong HS, Lee JB, et al. A giant malignant peripheral nerve sheath tumour of the breast: CT and pathological findings. *Br J Radiol* 2007;80:e44–47.
57. Ocana A, Delgado C, Rodriguez CA, et al. Case 3. Upper limb lymphangiosarcoma following breast cancer therapy. *J Clin Oncol* 2006;24:1477–1478.
58. Mack TM. Sarcomas and other malignancies of soft tissue, retroperitoneum, peritoneum, pleura, heart, mediastinum, and spleen. *Cancer* 1995;75:211–244.
59. Woodward AH, Ivins JC, Soule EH. Lymphangiosarcoma arising in chronic lymphedematous extremities. *Cancer* 1972;30:562–572.
60. Ocana A, Hortobagyi GN, Esteva FJ. Concomitant versus sequential chemotherapy in the treatment of early-stage and metastatic breast cancer. *Clin Breast Cancer* 2006;6:495–504.
61. Wiklund TA, Blomqvist CP, Raty J, et al. Postirradiation sarcoma. Analysis of a nationwide cancer registry material. *Cancer* 1991;68:524–531.
62. Bohler FK, Rhomberg W, Doringer W. [Hypertension as risk factor for increased rate of side effects in the framework of breast carcinoma irradiation]. *StrahlentherOnkol* 1992;168:344–349.
63. Kuten A, Sapir D, Cohen Y, et al. Postirradiation soft tissue sarcoma occurring in breast cancer patients: report of seven cases and results of combination chemotherapy. *J Surg Oncol* 1985;28:168–171.
64. Clements WD, Kirk SJ, Spence RA. A rare late complication of breast cancer treatment. *Br J Clin Pract* 1993;47:219–220.
65. Clark MA, Thomas JM. Amputation for soft-tissue sarcoma. *Lancet Oncol* 2003;4:335–342.
66. Aygit AC, Yildirim AM, Dervisoglu S. Lymphangiosarcoma in chronic lymphoedema. Stewart-Treves syndrome. *J Hand Surg [Br]* 1999;24:135–137.
67. Topalovski M, Crisan D, Mattson JC. Lymphoma of the breast. A clinicopathologic study of primary and secondary cases. *Arch Pathol Lab Med* 1999;123:1208–1218.
68. Jennings WC, Baker RS, Murray SS, et al. Primary breast lymphoma: the role of mastectomy and the importance of lymph node status. *Ann Surg* 2007;245:784–789.
69. Domchek SM, Hecht JL, Fleming MD, et al. Lymphomas of the breast: primary and secondary involvement. *Cancer* 2002;94:6–13.
70. Wiseman C, Liao KT. Primary lymphoma of the breast. *Cancer* 1972;29:1705–1712.
71. Ryan G, Martinelli G, Kuper-Hommel M, et al. Primary diffuse large B-cell lymphoma of the breast: prognostic factors and outcomes of a study by the International Extranodal Lymphoma Study Group. *Ann Oncol* 2008;19:233–241.
72. Ganjoo K, Advani R, Mariappan MR, et al. Non-Hodgkin lymphoma of the breast. *Cancer* 2007;110:25–30.
73. Lin Y, Guo XM, Shen KW, et al. Primary breast lymphoma: long-term treatment outcome and prognosis. *Leuk Lymphoma* 2006;47:2102–2109.
74. Bobrow LG, Richards MA, Happerfield LC, et al. Breast lymphomas: a clinicopathologic review [Review]. *Hum Pathol* 1993;24:274–278.
75. Abbondanzo SL, Seidman JD, Lefkowitz M, et al. Primary diffuse large B-cell lymphoma of the breast. A clinicopathologic study of 31 cases. *Pathol Res Pract* 1996;192:37–43.
76. Hugh JC, Jackson FI, Hanson J, et al. Primary breast lymphoma. An immunohistologic study of 20 new cases. *Cancer* 1990;66:2602–2611.
77. Dao AH, Adkins RB Jr, Glick AD. Malignant lymphoma of the breast: a review of 13 cases. *Am Surg* 1992;58:792–796.
78. Giardini R, Piccolo C, Rilke F. Primary non-Hodgkin's lymphomas of the female breast. *Cancer* 1992;69:725–735.
79. Mussurakis S, Carleton PJ, Turnbull LW. MR imaging of primary non-Hodgkin's breast lymphoma. A case report. *Acta Radiol* 1997;38:104–107.
80. Liberman L, Giess CS, Dershaw DD, et al. Non-Hodgkin lymphoma of the breast: imaging characteristics and correlation with histopathologic findings. *Radiology* 1994;192:157–160.
81. Smith IC, Welch AE, Hutcheon AW, et al. Positron emission tomography using [F-18]-fluorodeoxy-D-glucose to predict the pathologic response of breast cancer to primary chemotherapy. *J Clin Oncol* 2000;18:1676–1688.
82. Schelling M, Avril N, Nahrig J, et al. Positron emission tomography using [F-18] fluorodeoxyglucose for monitoring primary chemotherapy in breast cancer. *J Clin Oncol* 2000;18:1689–1695.
83. Jaffe E, Harris N, Stein H, et al. Pathology and genetics of tumours of haematopoietic and lymphoid tissues. World Health Organization Classification of Tumors. Lyon: IARC Press, 2001.
84. Armitage JO. Staging non-Hodgkin lymphoma. *CA Cancer J Clin* 2005;55:368–376.
85. Freter C. Other cancers of the breast. In: Harris JR ed. *Disease of the breast*, 2nd ed. Philadelphia: Lippincott Williams & Wilkins, 2000:683–689.
86. Miller TP, Dahlberg S, Cassady JR, et al. Chemotherapy alone compared with chemotherapy plus radiotherapy for localized intermediate- and high-grade non-Hodgkin's lymphoma. *N Engl J Med* 1998;339:21–26.
87. Coiffier B, Lepage E, Briere J, et al. CHOP chemotherapy plus rituximab compared with CHOP alone in elderly patients with diffuse large-B-cell lymphoma. *N Engl J Med* 2002;346:235–242.
88. Habermann TM, Weller EA, Morrison VA, et al. Rituximab-CHOP versus CHOP alone or with maintenance rituximab in older patients with diffuse large B-cell lymphoma. *J Clin Oncol* 2006;24:3121–3127.
89. Pfreundschuh M, Trumper L, Osterborg A, et al. CHOP-like chemotherapy plus rituximab versus CHOP-like chemotherapy alone in young patients with good-prognosis diffuse large-B-cell lymphoma: a randomised controlled trial by the MabThera International Trial (MInT) Group. *Lancet Oncol* 2006;7:379–391.
90. Aviles A, Delgado S, Nambo MJ, et al. Primary breast lymphoma: results of a controlled clinical trial. *Oncology* 2005;69:256–260.
91. Fruchart C, Denoux Y, Chasle J, et al. High grade primary breast lymphoma: is it a different clinical entity? *Breast Cancer Res Treat* 2005;93:191–198.
92. Gholam D, Bibeau F, El Weshi A, et al. Primary breast lymphoma. *Leuk Lymphoma* 2003;44:1173–1178.
93. Hill QA, Owen RG. CNS prophylaxis in lymphoma: who to target and what therapy to use. *Blood Rev* 2006;20:319–332.
94. Wong WW, Schild SE, Halyard MY, et al. Primary non-Hodgkin lymphoma of the breast: the Mayo Clinic experience. *J Surg Oncol* 200280:19–25.
95. Bierman PJ, Villanueva ML, Armitage JO. Diffuse large B-cell lymphoma of the breast: a distinct entity? *Ann Oncol* 2008;19:201–202.
96. Ariel IM, Caron AS. Diagnosis and treatment of malignant melanoma arising from the skin of the female breast. *Am J Surg* 1972;124:384–390.
97. Papachristou DN, Kinne DW, Rosen PP, et al. Cutaneous melanoma of the breast. *Surgery* 1979;85:322–328.
98. Roses DF, Harris MN, Stern JS, et al. Cutaneous melanoma of the breast. *Ann Surg* 1979;189:112–115.

99. Culberson JD, Horn RC. Paget's disease of the nipple; review of twenty-five cases with special reference to melanin pigmentation of Paget cells. *AMA Arch Surg* 1956;72:224–231.

100. Peison B, Benisch B. Paget's disease of the nipple simulating malignant melanoma in a black woman. *Am J Dermatopathol* 1985;7:165–169.

101. Sau P, Solis J, Lupton GP, et al. Pigmented breast carcinoma. A clinical and histopathologic simulator of malignant melanoma. *Arch Dermatol* 1989;125: 536–539.

102. Balch CM, Buzaid AC, Soong SJ, et al. Final version of the American Joint Committee on Cancer staging system for cutaneous melanoma. *J Clin Oncol* 2001;19:3635–3648.

103. Balch CM, Soong SJ, Gershenwald JE, et al. Prognostic factors analysis of 17,600 melanoma patients: validation of the American Joint Committee on Cancer melanoma staging system. *J Clin Oncol* 2001;19:3622–3634.

104. Breslow A. Thickness, cross-sectional areas and depth of invasion in the prognosis of cutaneous melanoma. *Ann Surg* 1970;172:902–908.

105. Clark WH Jr, From L, Bernardino EA, et al. The histogenesis and biologic behavior of primary human malignant melanomas of the skin. *Cancer Res* 1969;29:705–727.

106. Essner R. Surgical treatment of malignant melanoma. *Surg Clin North Am* 2003;83:109–156.

107. Bishop JA, Corrie PG, Evans J, et al. UK guidelines for the management of cutaneous melanoma. *Br J Plast Surg* 2002;55:46–54.

108. Kelly JW, Henderson MA, Thursfield VJ, et al. The management of primary cutaneous melanoma in Victoria in 1996 and 2000. *Med J Aust* 2007;187:511–514.

109. Lens MB, Nathan P, Bataille V. Excision margins for primary cutaneous melanoma: updated pooled analysis of randomized controlled trials. *Arch Surg* 2007;142:885–891.

110. van Everdingen JJ, van der Rhee HJ, Koning CC, et al. Guideline 'Melanoma' (3rd revision). *Ned Tijdschr Geneeskd* 2005;149:1839–1843.

111. Amersi F, Morton DL. The role of sentinel lymph node biopsy in the management of melanoma. *Adv Surg* 2007;41:241–256.

112. Alva S, Shetty-Alva N. An update of tumor metastasis to the breast data. *Arch Surg* 1999;134:450.

113. Hajdu SI, Urban JA. Cancers metastatic to the breast. *Cancer* 1972;29:1691–1696.

114. Gorczyca W, Olszewski W, Tuziak T, et al. Fine needle aspiration cytology of rare malignant tumors of the breast. *Acta Cytol* 1992;36:918–926.

115. Sneige N, Zachariah S, Fanning TV, et al. Fine-needle aspiration cytology of metastatic neoplasms in the breast. *Am J Clin Pathol* 1989;92:27–35.

116. Arora R, Robinson WA. Breast metastases from malignant melanoma. *J Surg Oncol* 1992;50:27–29.

117. Hamby LS, McGrath PC, Cibull ML, et al. Gastric carcinoma metastatic to the breast. *J Surg Oncol* 1991;48:117–121.

118. Qureshi SS, Shrikhande SV, Tanuja S, et al. Breast metastases of gastric signet ring cell carcinoma: a differential diagnosis with primary breast signet ring cell carcinoma. *J Postgrad Med* 2005;51:125–127.

119. Di Cosimo S, Ferretti G, Fazio N, et al. Breast and ovarian metastatic localization of signet-ring cell gastric carcinoma. *Ann Oncol* 2003;14:803–804.

120. Moore DH, Wilson DK, Hurteau JA, et al. Gynecologic cancers metastatic to the breast. *J Am Coll Surg* 1998;187:178–181.

121. Fishman A, Steel BL, Girtanner RE, et al. Fallopian tube cancer metastatic to the breast. *Eur J Gynaecol Oncol* 1994;15:101–104.

122. Kattan J, Droz JP, Charpentier P, et al. Ovarian disgerminoma metastatic to the breast. *Gynecol Oncol* 1992;46:104–106.

123. Lesho EP. Metastatic renal cell carcinoma presenting as a breast mass. *Postgrad Med* 1992;91:145–146.

124. Soo MS, Williford ME, Elenberger CD. Medullary thyroid carcinoma metastatic to the breast: mammographic appearance. *AJR Am J Roentgenol* 1995;165: 65–66.

125. Upalakalin JN, Collins LC, Tawa N, et al. Carcinoid tumors in the breast. *Am J Surg* 2006;191:799–805.

126. Baliga M, Holmquist ND, Espinoza CG. Medulloblastoma metastatic to breast, diagnosed by fine-needle aspiration biopsy. *Diagn Cytopathol* 1994;10:33–36.

127. Matsuda M, Sone H, Ishiguro S, et al. Fine needle aspiration cytology of malignant schwannoma metastatic to the breast. *Acta Cytol* 1989;33:372–376.

128. Nunez DA, Sutherland CG, Sood RK. Breast metastasis from a pharyngeal carcinoma. *J Laryngol Otol* 1989;103:227–228.

129. Harvey EB, Brinton LA. Second cancer following cancer of the breast in Connecticut, 1935–82. *Natl Cancer Inst Monogr* 1985;68:99–112.

130. Leis HP Jr. Managing the remaining breast. *Cancer* 1980;46:1026–1030.

131. Lewison EF. The follow-up examination of the contralateral breast: from the viewpoint of the surgeon. *Cancer* 1969;23:809–810.

132. Finney GG Jr, Finney GG, Montague AC, et al. Bilateral breast cancer, clinical and pathological review. *Ann Surg* 1972;175:635–646.

133. Fisher ER, Fisher B, Sass R, et al. Pathologic findings from the National Surgical Adjuvant Breast Project (Protocol No. 4). XI. Bilateral breast cancer. *Cancer* 1984; 54:3002–3011.

134. Chaudary MA, Millis RR, Hoskins EO, et al. Bilateral primary breast cancer: a prospective study of disease incidence. *Br J Surg* 1984;71:711–714.

135. Egan RL. Bilateral breast carcinomas: role of mammography. *Cancer* 1976;38: 931–938.

136. Lewison EF, Neto AS. Bilateral breast cancer at the Johns Hopkins Hospital. A discussion of the dilemma of contralateral breast cancer. *Cancer* 1971;28: 1297–1301.

137. Thomas JM, Newton-Bishop J, A'Hern R, et al. Excision margins in high-risk malignant melanoma. *N Engl J Med* 2004;350:757–766.

138. Veronesi U, Cascinelli N. Narrow excision (1-cm margin). A safe procedure for thin cutaneous melanoma. *Arch Surg* 1991;126:438–441.

139. *NHMRC and Australian Cancer Network clinical practice guidelines.* The management of cutaneous melanoma. Canberra: NHMRC and Australian Cancer Network. Commonwealth of Australia, 1999.

Chapter 68
Breast Cancer during Pregnancy and Subsequent Pregnancy in Breast Cancer Survivors

Jennifer Keating Litton and Richard Lee Theriault

Pregnancy and fertility issues surrounding the diagnosis of breast cancer have become a significant concern for younger breast cancer patients. Young breast cancer patients can be faced not only with the diagnosis and treatment of their breast cancer, but also with issues surrounding fertility, future pregnancies, and, in some cases, diagnosis and treatment during pregnancy. Gestational or pregnancy-associated breast cancer is defined as breast cancer that is either diagnosed during pregnancy or within 1 year postpartum. As women are delaying childbirth, the incidence of breast cancer and pregnancy, as well as the issue of future pregnancies after treatment for breast cancer, must be considered when discussing treatment of breast cancer in younger women. We review the treatment and diagnosis of breast cancer concurrent with pregnancy, and the prognosis, effects on the children exposed to treatments *in utero*, and the potential for future pregnancies.

EPIDEMIOLOGY

Breast cancer and cervical cancer are the most commonly diagnosed malignancies during pregnancy. In a large retrospective population-based study in California between 1991 and 1997, there were 1.3 cases of breast cancer per 10,000 live births (1). In women under the age of 50 who are diagnosed with breast cancer, approximately 0.2 to 3.8% are diagnosed during pregnancy (2,3). When breast cancer is diagnosed in women 30 years of age or younger, 10% to 20% of cancers are detected during pregnancy or within the first postpartum year (4,5). As women delay childbearing, the incidence of breast cancer coinciding with pregnancy is likely to increase because the risk of breast cancer increases with age (6).

Recent Prior Pregnancy

Evidence indicates that pregnancy itself may increase a woman's risk of developing breast cancer in the 3 to 10 years after pregnancy despite the long-term protective effects of pregnancy. Because the definition of pregnancy-associated breast cancer often encompasses the year after breast cancer diagnosis, women may have had a subclinical breast cancer during pregnancy. Concern also exists that pregnancy itself may contribute to the risk for subsequent breast cancer to develop or worsen the prognosis of a subsequent breast cancer.

Three population-based series have described this phenomenon (7–10). Interestingly, Wohlfahrt et al. (10) looked at family history as a prognostic factor. Women with a strong family history had a significantly higher risk of postpartum breast cancers. Given this strong correlation, a substantial percentage of the increased postpartum risk may be influenced by hereditary factors (10). Therefore, genetic predispositions, including *BRCA1* or *BRCA2* mutations, may play a role in this transient increase in postpartum breast cancer risk.

In patients with breast cancer with a recent past pregnancy, some retrospective analyses have shown a worse prognosis. In a multi-institutional, retrospective case-control study, Guinee, et al. (11) examined the impact of recent prior pregnancy on breast cancer outcome in a group of 407 women, ages 20 to 29, with breast cancer. The women were

matched for age and stage of disease and had never been pregnant. For each 1-year increment in the time between the latest previous pregnancy and breast cancer diagnosis, the risk of dying decreased by 15% (relative risk [RR] 0.85, *p* = .011) (11). In a study of 540 patients from Memorial Sloan-Kettering Cancer Center, patients with previous childbirth within 2 years of the diagnosis of breast cancer also were shown to have a worse prognosis with an adjusted relative risk of dying from the cancer of 3.1 (12). Kroman, et al. (13) from Denmark noted an increased RR of dying from breast cancer for those women who had childbirth within 2 years of diagnosis. After adjusting for age, cancer characteristics, and stage, a breast cancer diagnosis within 2 years of childbirth was significantly associated with death (RR = 1.58, 95% confidence interval [CI], 1.24–2.02) compared with patients who gave birth more than 5 years before their breast cancer diagnosis (13). These studies were unable to control for delay in diagnosis, treatment, or treatment modalities of the breast cancer. Future translational research may help identify if a true biologic difference exists in breast cancers diagnosed soon after pregnancy to account for these differences.

BRCA1 and *BRCA2* Mutation Carriers and Pregnancy

Women who are more susceptible to breast cancers at younger ages, such as those with deleterious mutations in the *BRCA1* or *BRCA2* genes, may be over-represented in this population. Few studies, with small numbers of patients, have evaluated the potential increased risk in hereditary breast cancer patients (14,15). Women with genetic predispositions to cancer, such as *BRCA1* and *BRCA2* deleterious mutations, tend to develop breast cancers at earlier ages and, therefore, may have more cancers diagnosed during childbearing years.

Additionally the relationship of number of pregnancies and age of parity may be significant in *BRCA1* and *BRCA2* mutation carriers. In a recent study, Antoniou et al. (16) evaluated 457 mutation carriers who developed breast cancer and 332 mutation carriers without a history of cancer. Parous *BRCA1* and *BRCA2* mutation carriers had a lower risk of developing cancer, but only among carriers who were older than 40 years of age (hazard ratio [HR] 0.54, 95% CI, 0.37–0.81). Patients with an increased age at first parity had an increased breast cancer risk in *BRCA2* mutation carriers, but not *BRCA1* mutation carriers (16). Kotsopoulos et al. (17) performed a matched case-control study on 1,816 pairs of *BRCA1* and *BRCA2* mutation carriers, and showed that age at first parity did not influence the development of breast cancers in mutation carriers. Also, they did not show a difference between *BRCA1* and *BRCA2* mutation carriers in univariate or multivariable models. An Icelandic study examining 100 *BRCA2* mutation carriers showed no decrease in risk of breast cancer in *BRCA2* mutation carriers with an increased number of births as is seen in nonmutation carriers (18). Not only was the protective effect of parity modulated in these patients, but in a large matched case-control study comparing 1,260 pairs of women with known *BRCA* mutations, increased parity was associated with an increased risk of breast cancer in *BRCA2* mutation carriers when compared with nulliparous women (odds ration [OR] 1.53, 95% CI, 1.01–2.32, p = .05). *BRCA2* mutation carriers who were under the age of 50 had a 17% increase in adjusted risk of breast cancer with each additional birth versus nulliparous *BRCA2* mutation carriers (OR 1.17, 85% CI, 1.01–1.36, p = .03) (19).

Given the risk of a deleterious mutation in women who develop breast cancer at an early age, genetic counseling should be considered for all such patients. Having children early does not provide the same protection in patients with deleterious *BRCA1* or *BRCA2* genes as those without mutations. In fact, recent parity may increase the risk of developing a breast cancer more notably in BRCA2 mutation carriers.

 ## DIAGNOSIS OF BREAST CANCER DURING PREGNANCY

Pregnant women with breast cancer tend to present with similar physical examination findings as their nonpregnant counterparts, including a palpable mass or breast thickening. Other diagnoses to consider include a lactating adenoma, fibroadenoma, cystic disease, lobular hyperplasia, galactocele, lipoma, abscess, or hamartoma. Other very rare diagnoses include lymphoma, leukemia, sarcoma, phyllodes tumor, neuroma, or tuberculosis (20). Owing to the physiologic changes in the breast during pregnancy and subsequent lactation, including increased size and density of the breast tissue, diagnosis may be delayed because of these factors obscuring detection (14). These physiologic changes may be even more pronounced in patients under the age of 30 (4). Therefore, women diagnosed with breast cancer during pregnancy often present with an advanced tumor stage and axillary lymph node involvement. Given the concern for delay of diagnosis, palpable masses persisting more than 2 weeks should be investigated, although approximately 80% of breast biopsies during pregnancy will be benign (21,22).

 ## EVALUATION OF BREAST MASSES DURING PREGNANCY

Imaging of the Breast during Pregnancy

Mammography

Mammography should be ordered in pregnancy with proper abdominal shielding. Exposure to the fetus is estimated at 0.4 mrad (23). This level is well below the level of 5 rad, a level at which multiple studies have shown no known increase in congenital malformations or growth retardation (24–25). Because of the increased water content in the pregnant breast and loss of contrasting fat, sensitivity of mammography may be decreased. Sensitivity for detecting masses in the pregnant breast ranges from 63% to 90% (14,26–28).

Ultrasonography

Ultrasound (US) can distinguish between cystic and solid breast masses in approximately 97% of cases without risk of fetal radiation exposure. Most breast cancers diagnosed during pregnancy are found to be a solid mass, although one report described two of four malignant tumors having benign characteristics (14,26,29). One study diagnosed 100% of the masses as well as axillary metastases in 18 of 20 women (28). US was also shown to be effective for restaging to evaluate response to preoperative chemotherapy in the pregnant breast (28).

Table 68.1	U.S. FOOD AND DRUG ADMINISTRATION PREGNANCY CATEGORY DEFINITIONS

A   Controlled studies in women who fail to demonstrate a risk to the fetus in the first trimester, and the possibility of fetal harm appears remote.

B   Animal studies do not indicate a risk to the fetus and there are no controlled human studies, or animal studies to show an adverse effect on the fetus, but well-controlled studies in pregnant women have failed to demonstrate a risk to the fetus.

C   Studies have shown that the drug exerts animal teratogenic or embryocidal effects, but there are no controlled studies in women, or no studies are available in either animals or women.

D   Positive evidence of human fetal risk exists, but benefits in certain situations (e.g., life-threatening situations or serious diseases for which safer drugs cannot be used or are ineffective) may make use of the drug acceptable despite its risks.

X   Studies in animal or humans have demonstrated fetal abnormalities or there is evidence of fetal risk based on human experience, or both, and the risk clearly outweighs any positive benefit.

Breast Magnetic Resonance Imaging

Magnetic resonance imaging (MRI) has not been prospectively studied for the diagnosis of a breast mass in pregnant or lactating women. Gadolinium-enhanced MRI may be more sensitive than conventional mammography, however, data regarding the safety of gadolinium during pregnancy is limited. Gadolinium has been shown to cross the placenta and be associated with fetal abnormalities in animal models (30,31).

Animal studies have shown diverse fetal effects and gadolinium is considered a pregnancy category C drug (Table 68.1). There have been no controlled human studies to date. However, several studies have observed no significant toxicity when gadolinium has been given during human pregnancy. De Santis et al. (32) enrolled 26 patients who were exposed to gadolinium contrast either periconception or during the first trimester. None of these were breast MRI. One fetus was terminated, one spontaneously miscarried, and one child was born with two hemangiomas. Birchard et al. (33) described seven cases of women who received gadolinium during pregnancy who had no adverse events. Marcos et al. (34) described 11 patients who were exposed to gadolinium agents to evaluate the placenta and no adverse events were seen. When assessing gadolinium exposure in neonates and infants less than 6 months of age, Marti-Bonmati (35) conducted a phase II study in 59 children (20 received no gadolinium based contrast). There were three serious adverse events including increased transaminases, bilirubin and vomiting (35). Traditionally, gadolinium-enhanced MRI should be reserved for detection in women postpartum for whom the mammogram or ultrasound is nondiagnostic (36). As more data evolve regarding the safety of gadolinium-based agents in pregnancy, the use of gadolinium in routine screening and staging for breast cancer during pregnancy may be readdressed as a standard procedure. Data on tumor characteristics and MRI interpretation will need to be rigorously assessed.

Staging and Diagnosis of Breast Cancer during Pregnancy

Biopsy

Any clinically suspicious mass should be biopsied, even if the ultrasound and mammogram are equivocal or nondiagnostic. Fine needle aspirate (FNA) in the pregnant breast is well established. However, it is important for the pathologist to be aware that the specimen is from the breast of a pregnant patient because there are some descriptions that cytology of the breast may show increased cellularity, anisonucleosis, variable granular chromatin with proteinaceous background, and lipid secretion that may increase the chance of a false–positive interpretation (37–39). Additionally, core and excisional biopsies can be performed safely under local anesthesia, with only one report of the development of a milk-fistula after a core needle biopsy (40).

Pathology of Breast Cancer Diagnosed during Pregnancy

Most breast cancer cases are infiltrating ductal adenocarcinomas with one prospective cohort showing 84% with poorly differentiated tumors (41). When compared with nonpregnant premenopausal women, pregnant patients are reported to have a lower frequency of estrogen receptor (ER), progesterone (PR), or both expression (41–44). Amplification of ERBB2 (formerly (HER-2/neu) is seen in approximately 20% to 30 percent of breast cancers. In some series, ERBB2 amplification has been reported to be disproportionately amplified in pregnant patients (up to 58% vs. 16 % in nonpregnant counterparts) (45); however, other series show similar ERBB2 amplification (28%) in pregnant and nonpregnant patients (41).

Staging Evaluations during Pregnancy

The American Joint Committee on Cancer (AJCC) TNM staging system is used and, along with tumor biologic characteristics, forms the basis for treatment decisions. Staging procedures need to be modified for the pregnant breast cancer patient with safety considerations for both the patient and the fetus. The staging is important, however, for better understanding of the full extent of treatment recommendations, the influence of the treatment on cancer outcome, and the potential impact of the cancer treatment on pregnancy. Radiation exposure for the fetus and outcomes regarding different imaging modalities are available (24).

Some guidelines have been established regarding imaging and staging during pregnancy (36,46). Recommended initial staging should include the following: complete history and physical examination, comprehensive metabolic panel, and complete blood count with differential. It is important to note that pregnant patients can have anemia because of the increase in circulating plasma volume as well as increases in serum alkaline phosphatase level, which can be doubled or tripled because of the pregnancy itself. A thorough physical examination of the breast and nodal basins needs to include tumor measurements, when possible, and extent of clinical nodal involvement. Given the sites of breast cancer, metastases are most commonly bone, liver, and lung, these areas should be evaluated in the pregnant breast cancer patient who has a clinical stage II or higher breast cancer as is done in nonpregnant patients (See Chapter 34 for further details). These staging evaluations can include chest x-ray with proper abdominal shielding; echocardiogram before the use of an anthracycline-based chemotherapy regimen; ultrasound of the liver; and a screening noncontrast MRI of the thoracic and lumbar spine to exclude bone metastases. With further concerns of liver metastases after ultrasound, an abdominal non–gadolinium-enhanced MRI can be considered, especially because the liver may tend to have fatty replacement during pregnancy. Noncontrast MRI is used routinely and safely in the pregnant patient. Computed tomography (CT) scans and bone scans are not recommended owing to concerns over fetal radiation exposures (36). Radionuclide scanning, including bone scanning, has very limited data, but can be considered if the diagnosis of bone metastases would change the decision for treatment or continuation of the pregnancy. To decrease the potential toxicity from the radionuclide agent, maternal oral and intravenous hydration with frequent voiding can be used to decrease radiation exposure (23,47,48).

Locoregional Therapy

Surgery and Anesthesia

Breast surgery can be safely performed in all trimesters of pregnancy, however, many patients and surgeons will choose to wait until after the 12th week of gestation when the risk of spontaneous abortion may be lower (36). Multiple studies evaluating the use of anesthesia have not shown an increase in fetal abnormalities (48,49). Mazze and Kallen (50) reported on a registry of 5,405 pregnant patients who had any kind of surgery during pregnancy. They observed no difference in the risk of fetal malformation when they compared this group with 720,000 women who did not have a surgical procedure during pregnancy. No difference in outcomes was found in women who had their surgeries in the first trimester. There was, however, an increase in the frequency of low and very low birth weight infants. This was attributed to the underlying illness or trauma necessitating the surgery (50). In a Canadian report of 2,565 pregnant women who underwent surgery, Duncan et al. (49) reported no increase in fetal abnormalities compared with a control population of pregnant women who did not have an operation.

Although in most published reports, patients opt for mastectomies because of concerns regarding radiation therapy; breast-conserving surgery is also an option, especially for women in their third trimesters who can receive radiation therapy after delivery. With the addition of preoperative chemotherapy during pregnancy, breast-conserving surgery can be done later in the pregnancy or after delivery (51).

Safety and efficacy of sentinel lymph node biopsies is currently under investigation. The sensitivity and specificity of sentinel lymph node biopsies in the pregnant woman with breast cancer has not been well established. Estimated radiation exposure to the fetus is low and calculated to a maximum of 4.3 mGy (52). Isosulfan blue dye mapping is not recommended, however, because of concerns of unknown effects to the fetus as well as risk of anaphylaxis. Sensitivity of sentinel lymph node mapping may therefore be significantly decreased without using isosulfan blue.

Radiation Therapy

Completion of appropriate locoregional therapy should be obtained despite the diagnosis during pregnancy. Should the patient meet criteria for postmastectomy radiation therapy or have breast-conserving surgery, radiation therapy should be administered and, currently, this is recommended only after delivery of the fetus. Although actual radiation exposure per treatment unit can be limited, a significant portion of exposure can occur from internal scatter from the mother, for which shielding would be ineffective. Radiation exposure to the fetus is dependent on the energy source, field size, and distance of the fetus from the field center (53). The fetus is at the highest risk of damage to organogenesis in the first trimester and with each successive trimester would sustain a higher proportion of the standard 50 to 60 Gy used (25).

Information regarding radiation during pregnancy is limited to small series of patients treated for hematologic malignancies. Woo et al. from M.D. Anderson reported on 16 patients with Hodgkin's disease treated with 3,500 to 4,000 cGy while in the second and third trimesters. This is approximately three-fourths of the total breast cancer treatment dose (54). All 16 of these women delivered normal full-term infants. There is also a case report of a patient from Greece who underwent whole-breast radiation during pregnancy and delivered a healthy neonate (55). Additionally, Antolak and Strom (56) reported a case of locally recurrent breast cancer treated with electron-beam radiation to the chest wall during pregnancy with a simulated fetal dose exposure with abdominal shielding to be less than 1.5 cGy.

Systemic Therapy

Chemotherapy

Systemic chemotherapeutic agents are designed as antiprolifative drugs. The U.S. Food and Drug Administration (FDA) categorize drugs into pregnancy categories describing safety to mother and fetus. Category A and B are felt to be generally safe for use in pregnant patients with category C describing some teratogenic or embryocidal effects in animal studies, but no information in humans. Category D describes positive evidence of human fetal risks (Table 68.1). Although most chemotherapeutic agents are category D, data exist demonstrating that systemic chemotherapy can be given safely during pregnancy during the second and third trimester. Consideration of the use of systemic therapies should be similar in pregnant and nonpregnant patients. Although little is known regarding pharmacokinetics of chemotherapeutic agents in breast cancer owing to physiologic changes (increased plasma volume, impaired renal and hepatic function, and third spacing potential), several published patient cohorts have described successful administration of chemotherapies to pregnant breast cancer patients. Published reports demonstrate that first trimester chemotherapy exposure is associated with a 14% to 19% (57) risk of fetal malformations, whereas second and third trimester exposure is significantly safer, with a fetal malformation risk of 1.3%. It is not recommended that chemotherapy be administered during the first trimester (57). Additionally, antifolates, such as methotrexate, have been shown to carry higher risks of teratogenesis and methotrexate is a known abortifactant (57). Therefore, methotrexate and methotrexate-containing regimens, such as cyclophosphamide, methotrexate and 5-fluorouracil (CMF), are not given during pregnancy.

Drug Pharmacokinetcs during Pregnancy

Generally, pregnant women receive similar weight-based chemotherapy as nonpregnant breast cancer patients. The chemotherapy doses are weight adjusted for continued weight gain and typically administered without dose modifications in pregnant women (58). Little pharmacokinetic information for chemotherapeutic agents during pregnancy exists, but some effects on drug metabolism may occur owing to the physiologic changes of pregnancy. These physiologic changes may include increases in blood volume, alterations in renal and hepatic clearance of drugs, and increased cardiac output, which could result in a decrease in an effective dose. However, there may also be diminished gastric motility for orally available drugs, or increased amounts of unbound active drugs as plasma albumin concentrations decrease (59).

Anthracycline-Based Chemotherapy

Numerous case reports and case series exist regarding different chemotherapeutic agents given during pregnancy, mostly with anthracycline-based regimens. M.D. Anderson Cancer Center has the largest prospective cohort of pregnant breast cancer patients treated on a standardized protocol, with the last published update of this ongoing prospective trial in 2006 (60). A total of 57 women were treated with 5-fluorouracil 500 mg/m^2 intravenously on days 1 and 4, doxorubicin 50 mg/m^2 given by continuous infusion over 72 hours and cyclophosphamide 500 mg/m^2 given intravenously on day 1 (FAC). A median of four cycles were adminis-

tered during pregnancy. Patients were given doses on actual weight at each visit and not dose adjusted from baseline (early pregnancy or nonpregnant) weight. Premedications included standard doses of dexamethasone, lorazepam, and ondansetron. Depending on the week of gestation at the time of delivery, most women receive four to six cycles of FAC chemotherapy during pregnancy. Chemotherapy should be held after the 35th week of pregnancy to avoid the potential for neutropenia at the time of delivery. Of the 57 women at the time of the last published update, 40 are alive and disease-free, 3 have recurrent breast cancer, 12 died from breast cancer, 1 died from other causes, and 1 was lost to follow-up. Mean gestational age at delivery was 37 weeks. Of the 25 patients who received preoperative FAC, 6 had a pathologic complete response, 4 had no tumor response to chemotherapy and eventually died from their disease. All women who delivered had live births. One child has Down syndrome and 2 have congenital anomalies (club foot; congenital bilateral ureteral reflux). The children are healthy and those in school are doing well, although 2 children, including the child with Down syndrome, have special educational needs. One mother died from a pulmonary embolus after a cesarean delivery (60).

Multiple retrospective case reports and series consisting of less than 10 reported patients are in the literature. The larger reports of patients treated with chemotherapy during pregnancy are highlighted (Table 68.2).

A French National survey retrospectively identified 20 women treated for breast cancer with chemotherapy during pregnancy. Of note, only 7 of the 30 obstetric or oncologic units responded to this query. Two of the women received chemotherapy during the first trimester and both of these patients experienced a spontaneous abortion. One woman, who was treated at week 23, experienced an intrauterine death and delivered a stillborn fetus. The remaining 17 women went on to deliver with a mean week of delivery of 34.7 ± 2.2 weeks. Of note, there was no consistent dosing or chemotherapeutic agents used among these 20 cases. Chemotherapy complications in the newborn included transient leucopenia, transient anemia, respiratory distress syndrome, and intrauterine growth retardation (IUGR). Of the 17 children born, 16 were alive and well at a median follow-up of 3.5 years. One of the children died at age 8 days without the cause of death being determined (61).

A retrospective analysis of 28 women who were evaluated for breast cancer during pregnancy described 24 women who received chemotherapy for early breast cancer and 4 women who received chemotherapy for metastatic disease. Sixteen women received anthracyclines-based chemotherapy and 12 received cyclophosphamide, methotrexate and 5-fluourouracil. One spontaneous abortion occurred in the woman treated with methotrexate-based chemotherapy during her first trimester. The median gestational age at delivery was 37 weeks. One child had IUGR caused by placental insufficiency, none had birth weight less than the tenth percentile for gestational age, and 2 newborns experienced respiratory distress for a total of 5 newborns requiring transfer to neonatal high dependency units. With a median follow-up of 40.5 months, the combined survival rate for stage I to IIIB was 67% and the disease-free survival rate was 63%. Four of the women were stage IV at diagnosis and 2 of these women died within 3 years of diagnosis (62).

An Irish study described 12 cases of chemotherapy administered during pregnancy, one of which was diagnosed 5 weeks postpartum. Three of the patients were metastatic at the time of diagnosis. One pregnancy was terminated and there were two fetal deaths. The authors state that these were after anthracycline exposure; however, drug, dosing, route, and rate of administration and other concomitant chemotherapeutic agents are not described (63).

No data describe the safety or use of dose-dense anthracyclines-based regimens, with or without taxanes, during pregnancy.

Table 68.2	BREAST CANCER AND PREGNANCY. TUMOR STAGE, NUMBER NODES, HISTOLOGY, DIFFERENTIATION, AND RECEPTOR STATUS					
Reference	T Stage (%)	Nodes (N) (%)	Differentiation (N) (%)	Histology (%)	Receptor Status (%)	HER2
Giacalone et al., (61) N = 20	I 5 II 40 III 30 IV 25	0 25 1-3 15 ≥4 15 Unknown 45	Grade 3 15 Grade 2 5 Grade 1	Ductal 100	ER + 30 ER − 45 ER unknown 25	Not given
Healy et al., (63) N = 11	I — II 36 III 45 IV 18	N+ 9 N1	Not given	Ductal 90	Not given/ assessed	Not given
Ring et al., (62) N = 24 7 patients with NC 17 patients No NC	NC: mean tumor size 6 cm No NC: mean tumor size 3.6 cm	NC: (43% node +, 4 unknown) No NC (88% node +, 2 unknown)	Grade 3 (71%) Grade 2 (25%)	Ductal 79	ER + 11 ER − 8 ER unknown 5	5 amplified, 7 not amplified and 12 not known
Hahn et al., (60) N = 57	Clinical Stage[a] I II 53% III 38% IV	70% node positive disease	Grade 3 (82%) Grade 2 (16%)	Ductal 85% Other 15%	ER− PR− 69%	10 amplified out of 35 evaluated

ER, estrogen receptor; NC, neoadjuvant chemotherapy; PR, progesterone receptor.
[a]Of the 32 patients who received surgery before chemotherapy. An additional 25 patients received neoadjuvant chemotherapy and were more likely (56% vs. 38%) to have a stage III disease at diagnosis.

Taxane Therapy

Case reports describe the use of taxanes (paclitaxel and docetaxel) during pregnancy. The use of taxanes is often delayed, however, until after delivery because of the paucity of safety data during pregnancy. Multiple case reports in the literature describe the use of taxanes during breast cancer with no apparent deleterious effects on the fetus. Also, multiple reports of taxane use with and without platinum compounds have been described in gynecologic cancers with no short-term deleterious effects described in the fetus (64–71). As the data continue to increase regarding the use of taxanes during pregnancy, taxanes may become used more frequently in the second and third trimesters. Current use appears to be confined to patients whose disease has failed to respond to anthracycline therapy and are inoperable during pregnancy.

Other Systemic Chemotherapy Agents

Other agents have been described in the literature, including vinorelbine, carboplatin, and cisplatin (72). Multiple case reports of platinum-based compounds have been reported to treat ovarian, cervical, and even small cell lung cancer during pregnancy, however, only one report could be found for cisplatin therapy for a squamous cell breast cancer (73). Vinorelbine has been reported at least six times, administered in the adjuvant and the metastatic settings, with five of the six children reported healthy at 6 to 35 months of follow-up (follow-up of one child has not yet been reported). Neonatal complications included grade 4 neutropenia in one infant and transient cytopenia at day 6 of life (74–77).

Biologic Agents

At least seven reports have appeared of trastuzumab administered during pregnancy. No fetal abnormalities have been reported, however, anhydramnios with its use was described in six of the case reports (74,78–83). One of the children born developed respiratory failure, capillary leak syndrome, infections, and necrotizing enterocolitis and died from multiple organ failure 21 weeks after delivery (82). One report describes reversible heart failure in the mother but no anhydramnios in the fetus (80). Bader et al. (83) described reversible renal failure in the fetus. Another biologic agent, lapatinib, was also recently described in a patient who conceived while on lapatinib and despite approximately 11 weeks' exposure, the pregnancy was otherwise uncomplicated with delivery of a healthy baby (84). Given the very limited data of use of biologic agents during pregnancy, they are not recommended for routine administration.

Endocrine Therapy

Endocrine therapy, if indicated, should be initiated after delivery and completion of chemotherapy. Although there are some case reports of fetal exposure to tamoxifen without damage to the child, there are other reports including Goldenhar syndrome (microtia, preauricular skin tags and hemifacial microsomia) (85), ambiguous genitalia and other birth defects as well as reports of vaginal bleeding and spontaneous abortion (36,85–88). Aromatase inhibitors are not indicated in premenopausal women.

Other Systemic Agents

Commonly used antiemetics are rated as pregnancy risk category C. Newer agents, such as ondansetron and granisetron, are rated as pregnancy risk category B and are used to manage nausea in pregnant women receiving chemotherapy. Dexamethasone also can be used short term for nausea prophylaxis but long-term exposure is not recommended. For neutropenia prophylaxis, no randomized trials have yet evaluated the us of granulocyte colony-stimulating factor (G-CSF) (filgastrim) or granulocyte-macrophage colony-stimulating factor (GM-CSF) in pregnant breast cancer patients, but G-CSF has been used in neonatal neutropenia and sepsis (89,90) and safe usage in pregnancy has been reported (91). There are no data regarding pegfilgastrim use in pregnancy.

Table 68.3	RECENT STUDIES ON PREGNANCY FOLLOWING BREAST CANCER WITH RISK OF DEATH COMPARED WITH CONTROL PATIENTS WITH NO SUBSEQUENT PREGNANCY			
Reference	Study	Patients in Study Group (N)	Year	RR of Death[a]
Harvey et al., (111)	Case series	41	1981	
Ribeiro et al., (93)	Case series	57	1986	
Ariel et al., (112)	Case series	47	1989	
Von Schoultz et al., (107)	Case comparison clinical trial registrants	50	1995	No difference
Gelber et al., (113)	Case comparison	94	2001	Decreased
Mueller et al., (105)	Cohort study	438	2003	Decreased
Kroman et al., (114)	Multiple registries/ comparative	371	2008	Decreased

RR, relative risk.
[a]When compared with control patients.

 ## MONITORING THE PREGNANCY

Patients should be referred directly to an obstetrician specializing in high risk pregnancies. Evaluation of fetal viability before the initiation of therapy and confirmation of the age of fetus must be determined before administering any systemic therapy. Frequent visits with well-coordinated communication among the patient, medical oncologist, surgical oncologist, and obstetrician are warranted. Obstetric monitoring can include frequent ultrasonography, fetal nonstress testing and biophysical profiles. When clinically appropriate, amniocentesis can be performed. Consideration of the time of delivery is also important with the last administration of chemotherapy to be administered no less than 2 weeks from estimated date of delivery. This may minimize the risk of neutropenia in both the mother and the infant. Pregnancy-related complications including pre-ecclampsia and preterm labor should be treated according to standard care guidelines. Planned induction or cesarean deliveries are often performed to avoid these hematologic complications (36). Of note, the M.D. Anderson case series had 51% vaginal deliveries (60).

 ## BREAST-FEEDING

Many chemotherapeutic agents are excreted in breast milk and neutropenia in an infant breastfed during maternal treatment with cyclophosphamide has been described (91,92). Therefore, breast-feeding during administration of chemotherapy, biologic therapy, endocrine therapy, and radiation therapy should be avoided.

PROGNOSIS

Many series describe advanced stage at diagnosis for their pregnant versus nonpregnant patients. The advanced stage at diagnosis, as well as delays of diagnosis and initiation of treatment, may account for the apparently worse prognosis. There are, however, some mixed results comparing pregnant and nonpregnant patients.

Ribeiro et al. (93) reported on a series of 178 patients with pregnancy-associated breast cancer. A total of 121 women had breast cancer during pregnancy and there was a significant decrease in survival. These women with pregnancy-associated breast cancer presented with more advanced disease, including 72% with node-positive disease. Per the authors, most patients received treatment postpartum, but did not describe any chemotherapy given during pregnancy (93).

Tretli et al. (94) describe 35 patients from 1954 to 1981 and matched the patients for age and stage at diagnosis. Of these, 20 were diagnosed during pregnancy and 15 during lactation. The median diagnosis delay during pregnancy was estimated at 2.5 months and 6 months in the lactating group with a relative risk of death for breast cancer patients diagnosed during pregnancy of 3.1 ($p < .05$). However, treatment and delay of treatment is not described in this case-control study (94). An additional retrospective multi-institutional study by Bonnier et al. (43) evaluated 154 patients diagnosed with breast cancer between 1960 and 1993, either during pregnancy or within the first 6 months postpartum, and also found that breast cancer during pregnancy was an independent and significant worse prognostic factor. Chemotherapy was administered to some of these women; however, chemotherapies used and the delay in starting chemotherapy were not addressed.

Other recent case-control studies cannot confirm a difference in prognosis. A case-control study from Saudi Arabia matched 28 pregnant women by age and stage of disease with 84 nonpregnant women. Adjuvant chemotherapy was given to 23 of the pregnant patients. No difference in overall or relapse-free survival was found (95). Several other studies also have shown pregnancy at the time of diagnosis is not an independent worse prognostic factor. In a Toronto-based study, no statistically significant difference was seen in survival between these groups when matched for age, stage, and year of diagnosis (96). Several other studies, including one from Japan (14) and New Zealand (97), show similar results.

Although many of these studies show a worse prognosis for pregnancy-associated breast cancer, those studies in which breast cancer was diagnosed and treated during pregnancy with local and systemic therapy did not show the same dramatically worse survival as the older studies in which treatment often was not given until after delivery. Although many of the studies describe a worse prognosis for those women diagnosed with breast cancer in the first few months and years after a pregnancy, the grouping of women diagnosed during and after pregnancy may confound these overall results.

 ## CONSIDERATION OF PREGNANCY TERMINATION

The decision to terminate a pregnancy is a highly personal decision that a fully informed woman should make in conjunction with her physician. Early data suggested that the combination of breast cancer and pregnancy was nearly lethal and that termination of pregnancy was warranted and even showed some possible improvement in patient survival (98). Gradually, the data that have emerged regarding termination in this group of women have shown that early termination of pregnancy does not improve the outcome of pregnancy-associated breast cancer (99). Two reports suggest that early termination may have decreased patient survival (100,101). Although termination does not appear to improve survival or response to anthracycline-based therapy, some women may choose termination when diagnosed with an advanced cancer in the early weeks of pregnancy, depending on their symptoms and ability to delay systemic treatment until the second trimester.

SHORT- AND LONG-TERM COMPLICATIONS FOR THE CHILD

There is a paucity of data regarding the short-term and long-term effects of treatment for children exposed to chemotherapy for breast cancer *in utero*. The largest single prospective data set reported for breast cancer during pregnancy is from the M.D. Anderson Cancer Center. Immediately after delivery, there may be some early and reversible fetal toxicity from the chemotherapy, which can include anemia, neutropenia, and alopecia. In the prospective series from M.D. Anderson Cancer Center, there were no miscarriages, stillbirths, or perinatal deaths. Most of the children did not have significant neonatal complications and appeared to be similar to the general population of neonates. The most common complication was difficulty breathing in 10% and one child born at 38 weeks' gestation had a subarachnoid hemorrhage 2 days postpartum. The age of children at the time of the health survey ranged from 2 to 157 months. One child had Down syndrome and 2 children had congenital abnormalities (club foot, bilateral ureteral reflux). Overall, the children were healthy with 2 of the 40 children described having special educational needs (60).

Much of the children's health and outcomes data are derived from case reports of children exposed to different chemotherapeutic agents for hematologic malignancies in the mother. A large study from Mexico described 84 children with follow-up of 18.7 years born to women who received chemotherapy *in utero* for hematologic malignancies. This review did not report any significant physical, neurologic, or psychological abnormalities (102,103). Reynoso et al. (104) describe seven cases of eight children exposed *in utero* to chemotherapy for acute leukemia with follow-up ranging from 1 to 17 years. One of the children in a twin pregnancy was born with multiple congenital malformations and eventually developed a neuroblastoma and thyroid cancer. The other seven children have had normal growth and development and no malignant diagnoses (104).

Further evaluations of neurocognitive and cardiac function, as well as prospective evaluation for future malignancies and reproductive history, will need to be continued for children have been exposed to chemotherapy *in utero*.

FUTURE PREGNANCIES AFTER TREATMENT FOR BREAST CANCER

Future pregnancies are often a very important concern for young breast cancer survivors. Most studies, including four large registry-based series, conclude that women who become pregnant after successful treatment for breast cancer do not have a worse prognosis than those women who do not have subsequent pregnancies. In some studies, it appears that future pregnancies may have a protective effect with a decreased risk ratio for recurrence and death from breast cancer. In the largest study (105) of 438 women with postcancer pregnancies and 2,775 controls the relative risk of dying was estimated at 0.54 (95% CI, 0.41–0.71) for women who gave birth within 10 months of a diagnosis of breast cancer compared with women with breast cancer who did not have a subsequent pregnancy (Table 68.3) (13,105–108).

These data may reflect a selection bias, referred to as the "healthy mother effect." That is, those women who are healthier will tend to become pregnant, whereas women whose disease is relapsing or who are being treated for other medical problems may not go on to conceive future pregnancies. Often, physicians will advise patients to wait a period of time, commonly 2 to 3 years, before contemplating pregnancy because breast cancer recurrences occur most often in the first two to three years after initial diagnosis. During that time, a new pregnancy may interfere with therapy to treat recurrences. Also, given the safety profile of tamoxifen and biologic agents, such as trastuzumab, it is advised not to conceive while taking these agents. Women receiving these agents are advised to use barrier or other non–hormone-based contraception.

ETHICAL ISSUES OF TREATING BREAST CANCER DURING PREGNANCY

Multiple articles have been written to discuss the rights of the cancer patient as well as rights of the fetus (109,110). The breast cancer patient should be aware of the risks and benefits of treatment and nontreatment for her malignancy as well as risks to the fetus. As the information regarding the efficacy of treating women during pregnancy for their cancer continues to emerge and the risk to the fetus of iatrogenic morbidity and mortality appears to be minimal, albeit from only very small case series, there appears to be increasing congruence between the physician's obligation to treat the cancer patient and the welfare of the fetus (109,110). As these data continue to emerge, the importance of informed consent should direct the clinical care. The physician needs to provide a clear description of the options, the data available, the areas where data are lacking, as well as descriptions of safety measures to be provided (i.e., close maternal and fetal monitoring). The physician must describe the patient's option to discontinue therapy should her condition or the condition of the fetus change (110). As the decision to proceed with pregnancy during systemic treatment for breast cancer is a highly personal one for the patient, full support for her to make these decisions for herself and her unborn fetus should be respected.

MANAGEMENT SUMMARY

The treatment of pregnancy and breast cancer should include a multidisciplinary approach with active communication among the patient, obstetrician, medical, surgical, and radiation oncologists. Appropriate diagnosis, biopsy, and imaging direct this multidisciplinary approach, which can include surgery as well as preoperative or adjuvant systemic chemotherapy (Fig. 68.1). Radiation therapy, and several chemotherapeutic, biologic, and endocrine therapies should be postponed until after delivery. Continued evaluation of the children exposed to chemotherapeutic agents *in utero* is also warranted. Recommendations include the following:

- Breast imaging, including mammography, breast ultrasound
- Staging can include nongadolinium MRI- and ultrasound-based imaging.

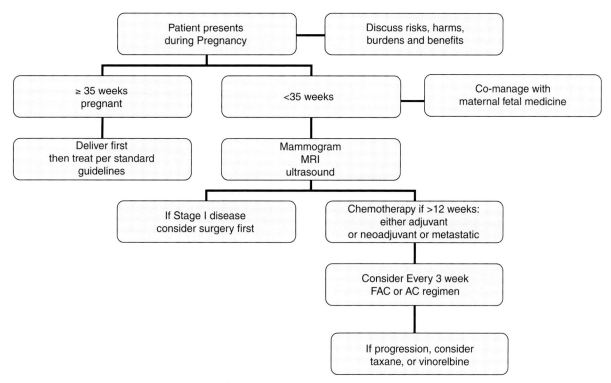

FIGURE 68.1. Management of the pregnant breast cancer patient.

- Appropriate local management for breast cancer, either with mastectomy or lumpectomy
- As for the nonpregnant patient, chemotherapy with an anthracycline-based regimen should be considered after the first trimester and before the 35th week of pregnancy. Most of the data reported are with every-3-week doxorubicin given over a 72-hour infusion, such as in the FAC regimen. Taxanes have limited safety data but can be considered on a case-by-case basis. Trastuzumab has been associated with anhydramnios and should be avoided during pregnancy.
- Radiation therapy should be completed after delivery, per standard guideline recommendations.
- A multidisciplinary approach emphasizing communication among the medical oncologist, surgical oncologist, radiation oncologist, and maternal-fetal specialist.

References

1. Smith L, Dalrymple J, Leiserowitz G, et al: Obstetrical deliveries associated with maternal malignancy in California, 1992 through 1997. *Am J Obstet Gynecol* 2001;184:1504–12.
2. Wallack M, Wolf J, Bedwinek J, et al: Gestational carcinoma of the female breast. *Curr Probl Cancer* 1983;7:1–58.
3. Crosby C, Barclay T: Carcinoma of the breast:surgical management of patients with special conditions. *Cancer* 1971;28:1628–36.
4. Anderson B, Petrek J, Byrd D, et al: Pregnancy influences breast cancer stage at diagnosis in women 30 years of age or younger. *Ann Surg Oncol* 1996;3:204–211.
5. Noyes R, Spanos W, Montague E: Breast cancer in women aged 30 and under. *Cancer* 1982;49:1302–7.
6. Ventura S, Martin J, Curtin S, et al: Births: Final Data for 1997. *Natl Vital Stat Rep* 1999;47:1–96.
7. Albrektsen G, Heuch I, Kvale G: Further evidence of a dual effect of a completed pregnancy on breast cancer risk. *Cancer Causes Control* 1996;7:487–488.
8. Lambe M, Hsieh C, Trichopoulos D, et al: Transient increase in the risk of breast cancer after giving birth. *N Engl J Med* 1994;331:5–9.
9. Wohlfahrt J, Andersen PK, Mouridsen HT, et al: Risk of Late-stage Breast Cancer after a Childbirth. *Am. J. Epidemiol.* 2001;153:1079–1084.
10. Wohlfahrt J, Olsen JH, Melbye M: Breast cancer risk after childbirth in young women with family history (Denmark). *Cancer Causes and Control* 2002; 13:169–174,
11. Guinee V, Olsson H, Moller T, et al: Effect of pregnancy on prognosis for young women with breast cancer. *Lancet* 1994;343:1587–9.
12. Olson S, Zauber A, Tang J, et al: Relation of time since last birth and parity to survival of young women with breast cancer. *Epidemiology* 1998;9:669.
13. Kroman N, Jensen M-B, Melbye M, et al: Should women be advised against pregnancy after breast-cancer treatment? *The Lancet* 1997;350:319–322.
14. Ishida T, Yokoe T, Kasmu F, et al: Clinicopathologic characteristics and prognosis of breast cancer patients associated with pregnancy and lactation: analysis of case control study in Japan. *Jpn J Cancer Res* 1992;83:1143–1149.
15. Johannsson O, Loman N, Borg A, et al: Pregnancy-associated breast cancer in BRCA1 and BRCA2 germline mutation carriers. *Lancet* 1998;352:1359–60.
16. Antoniou A, Shenton A, Maher E, et al: Parity and breast cancer risk among BRCA1 and BRCA2 mutation carriers. *Breast Cancer Research* 2006;8:R72.
17. Kotsopoulos J, Lubinski J, Lynch H, et al: Age at first birth and the risk of breast cancer in BRCA1 and BRCA2 mutation carriers. *Breast Cancer Research and Treatment* 2007;105:221–228.
18. Tryggvadottir L, Olafsdottir E, Gudlaugsdottir S, et al: BRCA2 mutation carriers, reproductive factors and breast cancer risk. *Breast Cancer Research* 2003;5: R121–125.
19. CA Cullinane, Lubinski J, Neuhausen S, et al: Effect of pregnancy as a risk factor for breast cancer in BRCA1/BRCA2 mutation carriers. *International Journal of Cancer* 2005;117:988–991.
20. Woo JC, Yu T, Hurd TC: Breast Cancer in Pregnancy: A Literature Review. *Arch Surg* 2003;138:91–98.
21. Byrd B, Bayer D, Robertson J, et al: Treatment of breast tumors associated with pregnancy and lactation. *Ann Surg* 1962;155:940–947.
22. Collins J, Liao S, Wile A: Surgical management of breast masses associated with pregnancy and lactation. *J Reprod Med* 1995;40:785–8.
23. Nicklas A, Baker M: Imaging strategies in the pregnant breast cancer patient. *Semin Oncol* 2000;27:623–32.
24. Brent R: The effect of embryonic and fetal exposure to x-ray, microwaves and ultrasound: Counseling the pregnant and non-pregnant patient about these risks. *Seminars in Oncology* 1989;16:347–368.
25. Mazonakis M, Varveris H, Damilakis J, et al: Radiation dose to conceptus resulting from tangential breast irradiation. *International Journal of Radiation Oncology*Biology*Physics* 2003;55:386–391.
26. Liberman L, Giess C, Dershaw D, et al: Imaging of pregnancy associated breast cancer. *Radiology* 1994;191:245–248.
27. Samuels T, Liu F, Yaffe M, et al: Gestational breast cancer. *Can Assoc Radiol J* 1998;49:172–180.
28. Yang WT, Dryden MJ, Gwyn K, et al: Imaging of Breast Cancer Diagnosed and Treated with Chemotherapy during Pregnancy. *Radiology* 2006;239:52–60.
29. Ahn B, Kim H, Moon W, et al: Pregnancy and lactation-associated breast cancer: mammographic and sonnographic findings. *J Ultrasound Med* 2003;22:491–497.
30. Novak Z, Thurmond A, Ross P, et al: Gadolinium DTPA transplacental transfer and distribution in rabbits. *Invest Radiol* 1993;28:828–30.
31. Webb JAW, Thomsen HS, Morcos SK: The use of iodinated and gadolinium contrast media during pregnancy and lactation. *European Radiology* 2005; 15:1234–1240.
32. De Santis M, Straface G, Cavaliere AF, et al: Gadolinium periconceptional exposure: pregnancy and neonatal outcome. *Acta Obstetricia & Gynecologica Scandinavica* 2007;86:99–101.
33. Birchard KR, Brown MA, Hyslop WB, et al: MRI of Acute Abdominal and Pelvic Pain in Pregnant Patients. *Am. J. Roentgenol.* 2005;184:452–458.

34. Marcos HB, Semelka RC, Worawattanakul S: Normal placenta: gadolinium-enhanced dynamic MR imaging. *Radiology* 1997;205:493–496.
35. Marti-Bonmati L, Vega T, Benito C, et al: Safety and efficacy of Omniscan (gadodiamide injection) at 0.1 mmol/kg for MRI in infants younger than 6 months of age: phase III open multicenter study. *Invest Radiol* 2000;35:141–7.
36. Loibl S, Minckwitz Gv, Gwyn K, et al: Breast carcinoma during pregnancy. *Cancer* 2006;106:237–246.
37. Gupta R, McHutchison A, Dowle C, et al: Fine-needle aspiration cytodiagnosis of breast masses in pregnant and lactating women and its impact on management. *Diagn Cytopathol* 1993;9:156–9.
38. Bottles K, Taylor R: Diagnosis of breast masses in pregnant and lactating women by aspiration cytology. *Obstet Gynecol* 1985;66:76S–78S.
39. Novotny D, Maygarden S, Shermer R, et al: Fine needle aspiration of benign and malignanct breast masses associated with pregnancy. *Acta Cytol* 1991;25:676–86.
40. Schackmuth E, Harlow C, Norton L: Milk fistula: a complication after core breast biopsy. *AJR Am J Roentgenol* 1993;161:961–2.
41. Middleton L, Amin M, Gwyn K, et al: Breast carcinoma in pregnant women. *Cancer* 2003;98:1055–1060.
42. Reed W, Hannisdal E, Skovlund E, et al: Pregnancy and breast cancer: a population-based study. *Virchows Archiv* 2003;443:44–50.
43. Bonnier P, Romain S, Dilhuydy J, et al: Influence of pregnancy on the outcome of breast cancer: A case-control study. *International Journal of Cancer* 1997; 72:720–727.
44. Berry DL, Theriault RL, Holmes FA, et al: Management of Breast Cancer During Pregnancy Using a Standardized Protocol. *J Clin Oncol* 1999;17:855-.
45. Elledge R, Ciocca D, Langone G, et al: Estrogen receptor, progesterone receptor, and HER-2/neu protein in breast cancers from pregnant patients. *Cancer* 1993;71:2499–2506.
46. National Comprehensive Cancer Network: Breast Cancer During Pregnancy. *NCCN Guidelines* 2008;v2.2008:55.
47. Baker J, Ali A, Groch M, et al: Bone scanning in pregnant patients with breast carcinoma. *Clin Nuc Med* 1987;12:519–524.
48. Ertl-Wagner B, Lienemann A, Strauss A, et al: Fetal magnetic resonance imaging: indications, technique, anatomical considerations and a review of fatal abnormalities. *European Radiology* 2002;12:1931–1940.
49. Duncan P, Pope W, Cohen M, et al: Fetal risk of anesthesia and surgery during pregnancy. *Anesthesiology* 1986;64:790.
50. Mazze R, Kallen B: Reproductive outcome after anesthesia and operation during pregnancy: a registry study of 5405 cases. *J Obstet Gynecol* 1989;161:1178.
51. Kuerer HM, Gwyn K, Ames FC, et al: Conservative surgery and chemotherapy for breast carcinoma during pregnancy. *Surgery* 2002;131:108–110.
52. Keleher A, Wendt R, Delpassand E, et al: The Safety of Lymphatic Mapping in Pregnant Breast Cancer Patients Using Tc-99m Sulfur Colloid. *The Breast Journal* 2004;10:492–495.
53. Mayr N, Wen B, Saw C: Radiation therapy during pregnancy. *Obstet Gynecol Clin North Am* 1998;25:301–321.
54. Woo SY, Fuller LM, Cundiff JH, et al: Radiotherapy during pregnancy for clinical stages IA-IIA Hodgkin's disease. *Int J Radiat oncol Biol Phys* 1992;23:407.
55. Kouvaris JR, Antypas CE, Sandilos PH, et al: Postoperative tailored radiotherapy for locally advanced breast carcinoma during pregnancy: A therapeutic dilemma. *American Journal of Obstetrics and Gynecology* 2000;183:498–499.
56. Antolak J, Strom E: Fetal dose estimates for electron-beam treatment to the chest wall of a pregnant patient. *Med Phys* 1998;25:2388–91.
57. Doll D, Ringenberg Q, Yarbro J: Antineoplastic agents in pregnancy. *Semin Oncol* 1989;16:337–346.
58. Cardonick E, Iacobucci A: Use of chemotherapy during human pregnancy. *The Lancet Oncology* 2004;5:283–291.
59. Wiebe V, Sipila P: Pharmacology of antineoplastic agents in pregnancy. *Critical Reviews in Oncology/Hematology* 1994;12:123–8.
60. Hahn K, Johnson P, Gordon N, et al: Treatment of pregnant breast cancer patients and outcomes of children exposed to chemotherapy in utero. *Cancer* 2006;107: 1219–1226.
61. Giacalone P, Laffargue F, Bénos P: Chemotherapy for breast carcinoma during pregnancy. *Cancer* 1999;86:2266–2272.
62. Ring AE, Smith IE, Jones A, et al: Chemotherapy for Breast Cancer During Pregnancy: An 18-Year Experience From Five London Teaching Hospitals. *J Clin Oncol* 2005;23:4192–4197.
63. Healy C, Dijkstra B, Kelly L, et al: Pregnancy-associtaed breast cancer. *Irish Medical Journal* 2002;95:51–53.
64. Palaia I, Pernice M, Graziano M, et al: Neoadjuvant chemotherapy plus radical surgery in locally advanced cervical cancer during pregnancy: a case report. *American Journal of Obstetrics and Gynecology* 2007;197:e5-e6.
65. Gonzalez-Angulo A, Walters R, Carpenter R, et al: Paclitaxel chemotherapy in a pregnant patient with bilateral breast cancer. *Clin Breast Cancer* 2004;5:317–9.
66. Modares Gilani M, Karimi Zarchi M, Behtash N, et al: Preservation of pregnancy in a patient with advanced ovarian cancer at 20 weeks of gestation: case report and literature review. *International Journal of Gynecological Cancer* 2007;17: 1140–1143.
67. Hubalek M, Smekal-Schindelwig C, Zeimet A, et al: Chemotherapeutic treatment of a pregnant patient with ovarian dysgerminoma. *Archives of Gynecology and Obstetrics* 2007;276:179–183.
68. Potluri V, lewis D, Burton G: Chemotherapy with taxanes in breast cancer during pregnancy: case report and review of the literature. *Clin Breast Cancer* 2006;7:167–70.
69. Sood A, Shahin M, Sorosky J: Paclitaxel and Platinum chemotherapy for ovarian carcinoma during pregnancy. *Gynecologic Oncology* 2001;83:599–600.
70. DeSantis M, Lucchese A, DeCarolis S, et al: Metastatic breast cancer in pregnancy: first case of chemotherapy with docetaxel. *European journal of Cancer Care* 2000;9:235–237.
71. Gadducci A, Cosio S, Fanucchi A, et al: Chemotherapy with epirubicin and paclitaxel for breast cancer during pregnancy: case report and review of the literature. *Anticancer Research* 2003;23:5225–5230.
72. Mir O, Berveiller P, Ropert S, et al: Emerging therapeutic options for breast cancer chemotherapy during pregnancy. *Ann Oncol* 2008;19:607–613.
73. Zanconati F, Zanella M, Falconieri G, et al: Gestational squamous cell carcinoma of the breast: an unusual mammary tumor associated with aggressive clinical course. *Pathol Res Pract.* 1997;193:783–7.
74. Fanale M, Uyei A, Theriault R, et al: Treatment of metastatic breast cancer with trastuzumab and vinorelbine during pregnancy. *Clin Breast Cancer* 2005; 6:354–6.
75. Jänne PA, Rodriguez-Thompson D, Metcalf DR, et al: Chemotherapy for a Patient with Advanced Non-Small-Cell Lung Cancer during Pregnancy: A Case Report and a Review of Chemotherapy Treatment during Pregnancy. *Oncology* 2001;61: 175–183.
76. De Santis M, Lucchese A, De Carolis S, et al: Metastatic breast cancer in pregnancy: first case of chemotherapy with docetaxel. *European Journal of Cancer Care* 2000;9:235–237.
77. Cuvier C, Espie M, Extra JM, et al: Vinorelbine in pregnancy. *European Journal of Cancer* 1997;33:168–169.
78. Watson WJ: Herceptin (Trastuzumab) Therapy During Pregnancy: Association With Reversible Anhydramnios. *Obstet Gynecol* 2005;105:642–643.
79. Pant S, Landon MB, Blumenfeld M, et al: Treatment of Breast Cancer With Trastuzumab During Pregnancy. *J Clin Oncol* 2008;26:1567–1569.
80. Shrim A, Garcia-Bournissen F, Maxwell C, et al: Favorable pregnancy outcome following Trastuzumab (Herceptin(R)) use during pregnancy—Case report and updated literature review. *Reproductive Toxicology* 2007;23:611–613.
81. Shrim A, Garcia-Bournissen F, Maxwell C, et al: Trastuzumab treatment for breast cancer during pregnancy. *Can Fam Physician* 2008;54:31–32.
82. Witzel ID, Muller V, Harps E, et al: Trastuzumab in pregnancy associated with poor fetal outcome. *Ann Oncol* 2008;19:191-a-192.
83. Bader AA, Schlembach D, Tamussino KF, et al: Anhydramnios associated with administration of trastuzumab and paclitaxel for metastatic breast cancer during pregnancy. *The Lancet Oncology* 2007;8:79–81.
84. Kelly H, Graham M, Humes E, et al: Delivery of a healthy baby after first-trimester maternal exposure to lapatinib. *Clin Breast Cancer* 2006;7:339–341.
85. Cullins S, Pridjian G, Sutherland C: Goldenhar syndrome associated with tamoxifen given to the mother during gestation. *JAMA* 1994;271:1905–6.
86. Cunha G, Taguchi O, Namikawa R, et al: Teratogenic effects of clomiphene, tamoxifen and diethylstilbestrol on the developing human female genital tract. *Hum Pathol* 1987;18:1132–1143.
87. Isaacs RJ, Hunter W, Clark K: Tamoxifen as Systemic Treatment of Advanced Breast Cancer during Pregnancy—Case Report and Literature Review. *Gynecologic Oncology* 2001;80:405–408.
88. Tewari K, Bonebrake RG, Asrat T, et al: Ambiguous genitalia in infant exposed to tamoxifen *in utero*. *The Lancet* 1997;350:183.
89. Bilgin K, Yaramis A, Haspolat K, et al: A Randomized Trial of Granulocyte-Macrophage Colony-Stimulating Factor in Neonates With Sepsis and Neutropenia. *Pediatrics* 2001;107:36–41.
90. Schibler KR, Osborne KA, Leung LY, et al: A Randomized, Placebo-Controlled Trial of Granulocyte Colony-stimulating Factor Administration to Newborn Infants With Neutropenia and Clinical Signs of Early-onset Sepsis. *Pediatrics* 1998;102:6–13.
91. Briggs G, Freeman R, Yaffee S: A reference guide to fetal and neonatal risk: drugs in pregnancy and lactation. Philadelphia: Lippincott Williams & Wilkins, 1998.
92. Durodola J: Administration of cyclophosphamide during late pregnancy and early lactation: a case report. *J Natl Med Assoc* 1979;71:165–6.
93. Ribeiro G, Jones D, Jones M: Carcinoma of the breast associated with pregnancy. *Br J Surg* 1986;73:607–609.
94. Tretli S, Kvalheim G, Thoresen S, et al: Survival of breast canecr patients diagnosed during pregnancy or lactation. *Br J Cancer* 1988;58:382–384.
95. Ezzat A, Raja A, Berry J, et al: Impact of pregnancy on non-metastatic breast cancer: a case control study. *Clinical Oncology* 1996;8:367–370.
96. Zemlickis D, Lishner M, Degendorfer P, et al: Maternal and fetal outcome after breast cancer in pregnancy. *Am J Obstet Gynecol* 1992;166:781–7.
97. Lethaby A, O'Neill M, Mason B, et al: Overall survival from breast cancer in women pregnant or lactating at or after diagnosis. Auckland Breast Cancer Study group. *Int J Cancer* 1996;67:751.
98. Adair F: Cancer of the breast. *Surg clin North Am* 1953;33:313.
99. Nugent P, O'Connell T: Breast Cancer and Pregnancy. *Arch Surg* 1985;120:1221–4.
100. Clark R, Chua T: Breast cancer and pregnancy: the ultimate challenge. *Clin Oncol* 1989;1:11.
101. Deemarsky L, Neishtadt E: Breast cancer and pregnancy. *Breast* 1981;7:17.
102. Aviles A, Neri N: Hematologic malignancies and pregnancy: a final report of 84 children who received chemotherapy in utero. *Clin Lymphoma* 2001;2:173–7.
103. Aviles A, Neri N, Nambo MJ: Long-term evaluation of cardiac function in children who received anthracyclines during pregnancy. *Ann Oncol* 2006;17:286–288.
104. Reynoso EE, Shepherd FA, Messner HA, et al: Acute leukemia during pregnancy: the Toronto Leukemia Study Group experience with long-term follow-up of children exposed in utero to chemotherapeutic agents. *J Clin Oncol* 1987; 5:1098–1106.
105. Mueller B, Simon M, Deapen D, et al: Childbearing and survival after breast carcinoma in young women. *Cancer* 2003;98:1131–1140.
106. Velentgas P, Daling J, Malone K, et al: Pregnancy after breast carcinoma. *Cancer* 1999;85:2424–2432.
107. von Schoultz E, Johansson H, Wilking N, et al: Influence of prior and subsequent pregnancy on breast cancer prognosis. *J Clin Oncol* 13:430–434, 1995.
108. Ives A, Saunders C, Bulsara M, et al: Pregnancy after breast cancer: population based study. *BMJ* 2007;334:194-.
109. Minkoff H PL: The rights of "Unborn children" and the value of pregnant women. *Hastings Cent Rep* 2006;36:26–8.
110. Chervenak F, McCullough L, Knapp R, et al: A clinically comprehensive ethical framework for offering and recommending cancer treatment before and during pregnancy. *Cancer* 2004;100:215–222.
111. Harvey J, Rosen P, Ashikari R, et al: The effect of pregnancy on the prognosis of carcinoma of the breast following radical mastectomy. *Surg Gynecol Obstet* 1981;153:723–5.
112. Ariel I, Kempner R: The prognosis of patients who become pregnant after mastectomy for breast cancer. *Int Surg* 1989;74:185–7.
113. Gelber S, Coates AS, Goldhirsch A, et al: Effect of Pregnancy on Overall Survival After the Diagnosis of Early-Stage Breast Cancer. *J Clin Oncol* 2001;19: 1671–1675.
114. Kroman N, Jensen MB, Wohlfahrt J, et al: Pregnancy after treatment of breast cancer—a population-based study on behalf of Danish Breast Cancer Cooperative Group. *Acta Oncol* 2008;47:545–9.

Alain Fourquet, Youlia M. Kirova, and François Campana

Breast cancer can sometimes present as an isolated axillary adenopathy without any detectable breast tumor by palpation or radiologic examination. These occult primary cancers are staged as T0, N1 (stage II in the Union Internationale Contre le Cancer/American Joint Committee classification). This staging requires that proper clinical *and* mammographic investigations be done to rule out the presence of small breast tumor. If this is accomplished, axillary metastases of occult breast primary cancer represent a rare clinical entity first described by Halsted in 1907 (1).

FREQUENCY

The incidence of an occult primary tumor with axillary metastases is low. Incidence rates ranged from 0.3% to 1.0% of operable breast cancers in the largest reported series (2–6). More than 350 cases have been reported in the literature since the 1950s. Because these series are limited and management policies have varied widely during this period, comparing characteristics of the patients, management, and results of treatment is difficult. Many of these patients had suspicious mammograms (2,7–9). Presumably, the constant improvement of the quality of mammography and ultrasonography as well as the use of magnetic resonance imaging (MRI) has decreased the rate of occult primary tumor with axillary metastases. Interpretation of these comparisons should only be done with caution.

The characteristics of the patients with T0, N1 breast cancer are similar to those of patients with typical stage II disease. The series from the Institut Curie included 59 patients treated between 1960 and 1997. The median patient age was 57 years (range, 36 to 79 years). Thirty-four patients (58%) were postmenopausal, including two patients under hormone replacement therapy. Fifteen patients (25%) had family histories of breast cancer. Twenty-eight (47.5%) had left axillary nodes, and 31 (52.5%) had right axillary nodes.

DIAGNOSIS

Axillary Adenopathy

Isolated axillary adenopathy is a benign condition in most patients. Lymphomas are the most frequently occurring malignant tumors (10).

Adenocarcinoma in areas other than the breast may include thyroid, lung, gastric, pancreatic, and colorectal cancer (11). These tumors, however, rarely have isolated axillary metastases as the only presentation of disease. Although in the past an extensive search for primary adenocarcinoma other than breast cancer was not recommended (4,9,12), these patients, nowadays, usually have computed tomography (CT) scans of the chest and abdomen for evaluation of metastases. In addition, tumor markers may help in the diagnosis of metastatic colon or pancreatic cancers.

Axillary adenopathy usually consists of one or two involved nodes, sometimes with large diameters. The median axillary node size at presentation in the patients treated at the Institut Curie was 30 mm (range, 10 to 70 mm). The initial diagnosis of

malignancy was achieved by node excision in 25 of 59 patients, by fine-needle aspiration in 26 patients, and by core-needle biopsy (drill biopsy) in 8 patients.

A primary breast cancer located in the axillary tail of the breast may be confounded with an axillary node. The presence of normal lymph node structure surrounding foci of carcinoma on the pathologic sample usually leads to the diagnosis of metastasis to a lymph node. The recognition of a metastatic lymph node can, however, be difficult because of massive involvement, with extension of the tumor into the axillary fat and disappearance of the lymphoid patterns. The rapid development of molecular biology techniques would possibly in the future help to identify a genetic breast origin.

Breast Cancer

Bilateral mammography should always be performed in the presence of metastatic adenocarcinoma in an axillary lymph node. Baron et al. (2) report an overall 44% accuracy in the diagnosis of occult breast cancer in a series of 34 patients, in which only nine mammographies were considered suspicious. Many of these tumors are missed owing to their relative small size and the fact that they are obscured on the mammogram by dense fibroglandular tissue (13). Nonetheless, any suspicious image should be removed for pathologic analysis.

Traditional imaging for the diagnosis and staging of breast cancer has relied on the tissue morphology of cancers in the background of normal patterns of fibroglandular breast tissue. X-ray mammography and ultrasound have been the primary modalities for the diagnosis and the workup of breast cancer (13,14). New modalities have been validated, including MRI. Promising results were published of the use of MRI in characterizing nonpalpable, but radiologically detectable, breast lesions in patients (14,15, and *Diseases of the Breast*, Current edition, Chapter 14). In patients with T0, N1 breast cancer, studies have shown that MRI could detect early contrast-enhanced images in the breast. Morris et al. (16) report on 12 patients with axillary node metastases without clinically or mammographically detectable breast tumor. Breast MRI detected early contrast-enhanced foci in 9 of the 12 patients (75%). Breast cancer was found in all but one of the nine patients who subsequently had surgery. Buchanan et al. (17) used MRI to identify a suspicious lesion in 76% (42 of 55) stage II patients. Of these 42 suspicious MRI lesions, 26 proved to be the primary breast carcinoma, 12 were false–positive findings, and 4 patients were lost to follow-up. Brenner and Rothman (18) performed MRI of the breast on four patients with occult carcinoma metastatic to the axilla: Foci of enhancement were detected in all patients, and ultrasound-guided surgical biopsies could be performed in all cases. Breast carcinoma was identified in all four patients. Similarly, Tilanus-Linthorst et al. (19) detected enhancing lesions with MRI in four patients: MRI-directed, ultrasound-guided fine-needle aspiration cytology found carcinoma cells in all four patients. Olson et al. (20) identified the primary breast lesion with MRI in 28 of 40 patients (70%) with occult breast cancer. Breast cancer was found in 21 of the 22 patients (95%) who had surgery. At the Institut Curie, 15 patients with metastatic axillary nodes, negative breast clinical examination, and without any mammographic target had breast MRI between 1997 and 2000. Early contrast-enhanced images were detected in 14 of the 15 patients

(93%). A surgical excision was performed in 11 patients: In four patients, a second MRI-guided ultrasound examination was able to disclose and localize the breast lesion; in 3 patients localization was achieved with an orthogonal mammogram, because of the superficial localization of the lesion and the small size of the breast; and finally in 4 patients the lesion was localized using CT-scan with bolus injection. Invasive breast cancer was found in 9 of the 11 patients (82%) who underwent surgery.

The high sensitivity of breast MRI suggests that it could be used systematically in searching for a breast primary tumor. However, because of its low specificity and the difficulties in localizing small, early contrast-enhancing foci in some instances, difficult management problems may occur. The use of MRI-directed sonographic, mammographic, or scanographic guidance (21,22) can help to localize the breast tumor in most patients. Other breast imaging procedures are under investigation, such as color Doppler sonography and positron emission tomography (PET) (23–25). Some new intraoperative techniques of detection as sonography and F-18 fluorodeoxyglucose positron-emitting tomography (FDG PET)/CT imaging and handheld gamma probe detection, as well as using an intraoperative portable gamma camera, showed promising results in the last years (25–27). The detection of occult lesions during the surgical procedure is an interesting option for patients with nonpalpable breast lesions (26,27). It was shown that the 18F-FDG PET/CT imaging has a place in the detection of primary site in patients with metastases from adenocarcinoma of unknown primary (28). This represents an interesting option for T0, N1 breast cancer patients. New modalities on the horizon include optical imaging, exploiting again the differential perfusion properties of cancers in a background of normal glandular tissue. Even more specificity can be achieved with the addition of ductal or intravenous introduction of optical probes specific to tumor-associated antigens, such as the ERBB2 (formerly HER-2/neu) receptor in aggressive breast cancers. Quantum dots and other fluorescent dyes coupled to peptides or other probes will greatly enhance our ability to detect cancers earlier and without ionizing radiation (29).

In patients who have nonpalpable breast masses and normal imaging workup, the mammary origin of a metastatic adenocarcinoma to an axillary lymph node cannot be established with certainty. Therefore, the diagnosis of occult breast cancer can only be highly presumed based on many elements, including sex, age, isolated adenopathy, and histologic diagnosis of adenocarcinoma.

High estrogen or progesterone receptors levels found in the metastatic axillary nodes can help to confirm a primary breast tumor (30); however, three series (2,3,31) reported that 50% to 86% of occult breast cancer cases were found to be negative for estrogen receptors. Because surgical excision of the palpable node was often the first diagnostic procedure, rarely was an attempt made to analyze the receptors by biochemical methods. In the Institut Curie series, receptor analysis was done in only 14 of the 59 tumors (24%) and was positive in 6 of 14. Immunohistochemical detection of hormone receptors can now be done in paraffin-embedded tissue (32), and should therefore be carried out systematically.

Natural History

After removal of an axillary adenopathy, a breast cancer eventually developed in the untreated breast in 32 of 76 patients (42%) described in the literature, with recurrence intervals ranging from 5 months to 67 months (Table 69.1). Patients samples were limited in these series, however, and follow-up periods varied widely. In addition, these data were obtained before the systematic use of breast MRI.

| Table 69.1 | OCCURRENCE OF BREAST CANCER IN THE NONTREATED BREAST |

Investigators (Reference)	Breast Failures/ Nontreated Breasts	Delay (mo)
Atkins and Wolff (33)	5/9	9–17
Ellerbroek et al., (3)	7/13	11–47
Feigenberg et al., (8)	0/4	—
Feuerman et al., (34)	0/1	—
Haagensen (5)	3/5	5–64
Halsted (1)	2/3	NA
Kemeny et al., (12)	0/7	—
Klopp (35)	1/1	48
Merson et al., (31)	9/17	2–34
Van Ooijen et al., (36)	3/14	16–56
Institut Curie, present series	2/2	9, 67

NA, not available.

The number of pathologically involved lymph nodes seen after axillary dissection is high. Rosen and Kimmel (37) report a median of three involved nodes (range, 1 to 65 nodes) in 48 patients. Merson et al. (31) reported that more than three nodes were involved in 23 of 46 patients who underwent axillary dissections. Forty patients in the Institut Curie series had an axillary dissection as initial treatment. The median number of involved nodes was 3 (range, 1 to 20). During follow-up, 16 of the 59 patients in the series had distant metastases: 4 (25%) in the brain, 5 (31%) in the liver, 3 (19%) as cervical nodes, and 3 in multiple sites. One patient had isolated bone metastases. Ten patients had contralateral disease, which occurred in the contralateral breast alone in 6 patients. Of note, 4 patients had isolated contralateral axillary node metastases.

Treatment and Results

Mastectomy with axillary node dissection has been the most commonly used treatment in patients with occult primary tumors. The combined analysis of 13 published series has shown that breast cancer was found in the mastectomy specimen in 156 of 221 patients (71%) (Table 69.2). Invasive tumors were found in 145 of 221 patients (66%). These data, along with the fact that nearly 50% of the patients who received no form of breast treatment will eventually have disease recurrence in the breast, support the recommendation that the breast be treated when no tumor can be detected clinically or mammographically.

Three studies reported the results of breast-conserving treatment of T0, N1 cancer. The group from M.D. Anderson Cancer Center in Houston (3) treated 29 of 42 patients with breast preservation; the breast was irradiated in 16, and no breast treatment was given to 13. Breast cancer recurrences occurred in 18 % of the irradiated breast group and in 54% of the nonirradiated breast group. Survival did not differ between those who had mastectomy and those who did not. In the Memorial Sloan-Kettering series (2), 7 of 35 patients had a breast-conserving treatment, with radiotherapy in 6. Five-year survival rates were similar between this group and patients who had a mastectomy. Merson et al. (31) reported on 29 patients who had breast conservation treatment. Of 17 patients who did not receive breast irradiation, 9 had breast cancer recurrence as did 2 of 6 patients who had breast irradiation. Of the 59 patients treated between 1960 and 1997 at the Institut Curie, 3 had mastectomies. Two patients had neither mastectomy nor breast irradiation. Both eventually had breast cancer at 9 months and 67 months, respectively. Fifty-four patients

Table 69.2	**PATHOLOGIC REPORT AFTER MASTECTOMY**				
Investigators (Reference)	Years	Patients with Mastectomy	*In Situ* Carcinoma	Invasive Carcinoma	Carcinoma (%)
Ashikari et al., (7)	1946–1975	34	3	20	67
Bhatia et al., (30)	1977–1985	11	2	9	100
Baron et al., (2)	1975–1978	28	4	16	71
Ellerbroek et al., (3)	1944–1987	13	0	1	8
Feigenberg et al., (8)	1971–1974	4	0	3	80
Feuerman et al., (34)	1949–1961	2	0	1	50
Fitts et al., (4)	1948–1963	11	0	7	70
Haagensen (5)	1916–1966	13	0	12	92
Kemeny et al., (12)	1973–1985	11	2	3	45
Merson et al., (31)	1945–1987	33[a]	0	27	82
Owen et al., (6)	1907–1950	27	0	25	92
Patel et al., (9)	1952–1979	29	0	16	60
Weigenberg and Stetten (38)	1937–1948	5	0	5	100

[a]Includes six patients with superolateral quadrantectomy.

received whole-breast irradiation (median dose, 59 Gy; range, 50 to 70 Gy). Of 54 patients, 13 had breast tumor recurrence: The 5 and 10-year risks of ipsilateral breast recurrence were 7.5 % and 20%, respectively. In comparison, the 10-year rate of contralateral breast cancer in these 54 patients was 15%. All patients who had recurrences were treated by mastectomy. The 10-year breast-preservation rate for all 59 patients was 85%. The results of these studies therefore support the use of breast irradiation as an alternative to mastectomy (39).

After axillary node dissection, should irradiation be delivered to the remaining lymph nodes? Few data are available in the literature to support any treatment options. A substantial risk for nodal involvement of the upper axilla can be suspected, however, based on the fact that three involved nodes are expected to be found in one-half of the patients. In patients with axillary node involvement associated with an invasive breast cancer, irradiation of the upper axilla is typically delivered when four or more nodes are involved (40). Studies (41–44 and *Diseases of the Breast*, current edition, Chapters 43 and 47) have shown that, in patients with axillary node involvement, postmastectomy irradiation of the chest wall and regional nodes decreased the rate of long-term distant metastases and improved survival, even in patients who received adjuvant chemotherapy or hormone therapy. Therefore, by analogy with other stage II tumors, irradiation of the upper axilla can be recommended in these instances, providing that axillary dissection was performed. Of 59 patients treated at the Institut Curie, 58 received nodal irradiation. In most instances, only the upper axilla and supraclavicular nodes were treated after complete axillary nodal dissection, whereas the whole axilla was treated when a simple adenectomy had been performed. There were four axillary node recurrences: One was isolated, but three were associated with a breast recurrence. The indications for internal mammary node irradiation are currently much debated in patients with a breast mass and central or medial tumor or axillary involvement. Recommendations about treatment of the internal mammary nodes in patients with occult primaries and axillary adenopathy are difficult to formulate, because the evaluation of internal mammary node irradiation in this rare form of breast cancer is impossible on the basis of limited retrospective series. Because the location of the primary tumor is unknown, the Institut Curie policy supports the irradiation of the internal mammary nodes in all patients.

The reported 5-year actuarial survival rates after treatment of occult breast cancer with axillary metastases range from 36% to 79% (Table 69.3). The 5- and 10-year survival estimates in the 59 patients treated at the Institut Curie were 84.5% and 74% with a median follow-up of 151 months (range, 22 to 458 months). These figures seem higher than those observed after treatment of patients with stage II disease and detectable breast tumor. This has been emphasized by several authors (4,6,12,31,34). These survival rate estimates are, however, derived from small series of patients with various durations of follow-up and heterogeneous treatment modalities. Rosen and Kimmel (37) attempted to evaluate the results more precisely by matching a series of 48 patients with occult breast primary and axillary node metastases with a series of patients with stage II breast cancer who presented with palpable breast tumor (T1, N1 and T2, N1). Although the difference was not statistically significant, higher overall survival and size- or node status–adjusted survival rates were observed in the group of patients with occult primary tumors.

Reliable prognostic analyses are difficult to perform because of the multiple selection biases in the retrospective series and the small sample size. Rosen and Kimmel (37) showed that survival was determined by the number of axillary nodes involved; patients with fewer than four nodes involved did better than those with more than four nodes involved. Baron et al. (2) showed that estrogen receptor-positive patients fared better than estrogen receptor-negative patients. Our findings corroborated those indicating that survival was longer in patients with less than four involved axillary nodes: The 10-year survival rates were 88% and 60%, respectively ($p = .04$).

Table 69.3	**FIVE-YEAR SURVIVAL RATES FOR PATIENTS WITH OCCULT BREAST CARCINOMA**		
Investigators	Patients	Follow-up (mo)	Actuarial Survival Rate (%)
Ashikari et al., (7)	42	NA	79
Baron et al., (2)	35	58 (mean)	75
Ellerbroek et al., (3)	42	131 (median)	72
Feuerman et al., (34)	47	NA	36[a]
Kemeny et al., (12)	18	NA	57
Merson et al., (31)	56	123 (median)	76.5
Institut Curie, present series	59	151 (median)	84.5[b]

NA, not available.
[a]Crude survival rate.
[b]10-year rate: 74%.

Is there a role for adjuvant systemic treatment in patients with occult primary breast cancer? As mentioned previously, because of the rarity of this disease and the multiple selection biases, the efficacy of systemic therapy in patients with T0, N1 breast cancer is impossible to ascertain. By analogy with stage II node-positive breast cancer, the general tendency is to use the same criteria (i.e., axillary node involvement) to prescribe systemic chemotherapy or hormone therapy. Of the 59 patients treated at Institut Curie, 27 received adjuvant chemotherapy, with a regimen of cyclophosphamide, doxorubicin, and 5 fluorouracil. Patients who received chemotherapy were slightly younger and had more involved nodes than those who did not, but these differences were not statistically significant. Survival and metastases-free interval rates were not statistically different in the 27 patients who received chemotherapy and in the 32 patients who did not. This apparent lack of benefit from chemotherapy may be explained by the fact that in this particular group of patients, chemotherapy did not reverse the adverse prognostic influence of massive nodal involvement. Little is known about the effect of hormone therapy in these patients. Of 13 patients who received tamoxifen for at least 2 years in the Institut Curie series, only 1 developed distant metastases, 7 years after diagnosis. The numbers are too small to make significant statistical comparisons, but these results suggest that hormone treatment may be very effective and support its use, at least in patients who have high hormone receptor levels.

The common policy in most institutions is to give adjuvant systemic therapy to patients with involved axillary nodes. Although the outcome of patients with occult primary and axillary metastases seems slightly better than that of patients with stage II node-positive breast cancer, these findings need to be confirmed by larger series. Therefore, adjuvant systemic treatment should be given to such patients.

MANAGEMENT SUMMARY

- Occult primary breast cancer presenting as an axillary lymph node is rare and represents a clinical entity with an outcome better than in patients with a clinically detectable mass and axillary involvement.
- The heterogeneity of treatment and the limited number of patients studied in the published literature make it difficult to standardize treatment options.
- After the diagnosis of adenocarcinoma has been established by surgical removal of an isolated axillary mass, extensive workup evaluation is not necessary. A thorough clinical examination, chest radiographs, bilateral mammograms, and tumor markers are sufficient to establish a high presumption of axillary metastases of mammary origin.
- Breast MRI should be used in all cases. If MRI localization is not available, the additional use of ultrasound or CT scan can help to localize an early contrast-enhancing image, which can be then biopsied or surgically excised.
- An axillary dissection is generally performed to provide additional prognostic information and to provide local control in the axilla.
- The breast should be treated. Breast-conserving therapy in patients with an occult breast primary tumor by whole breast irradiation to a dose of 50 to 55 Gy limits the risk for disease recurrence and is an alternative to mastectomy.
- Irradiation of the upper axilla and supraclavicular area, to a minimum dose of 45 Gy, is recommended in patients with more than three involved axillary nodes. In case of patients with one to three nodes, the value of this irradiation is debated. The whole axilla should be irradiated in patients who did not undergo axillary node dissection.

- Recommendations for adjuvant systemic therapy based on estrogen receptor, progesterone receptor, and ERBB2 in patients with an occult primary should be similar to that for other patients with node-positive breast cancer, even though their outcome appears to be slightly better.

References

1. Halsted W. The results of radical operations for the cure of carcinoma of the breast. *Ann Surg* 1907;46:1.
2. Baron PL, Moore MP, Kinne DW, et al. Occult breast cancer presenting with axillary metastases: updated management. *Arch Surg* 1990;125:210.
3. Ellerbroek N, Holmes F, Singletary T, et al. Treatment of patients with isolated axillary nodal metastases from an occult primary carcinoma consistent with breast origin. *Cancer* 1990;66:1461.
4. Fitts WT, Steiner GC, Enterline HT. Prognosis of occult carcinoma of the breast. *Am J Surg* 1963;106:460.
5. Haagensen CD. The diagnosis of breast carcinoma. In: Haagensen CD, ed. *Diseases of the breast*. Philadelphia: WB Saunders, 1971:486.
6. Owen HW, Dockerty MB, Gray HK. Occult carcinoma of the breast. *Surg Gynecol Obstet* 1954;98:302.
7. Ashikari R, Rosen PP, Urban JA, et al. Breast cancer presenting as an axillary mass. *Ann Surg* 1976;183:415.
8. Feigenberg Z, Zer M, Dinstman M. Axillary metastases from an unknown primary source: a diagnostic and therapeutic approach. *Isr J Med Sci* 1976;12:1153.
9. Patel J, Nemoto T, Rosner D, et al. Axillary lymph node metastasis from an occult breast cancer. *Cancer* 1981;47:2923.
10. Pierce EH, Gray HK, Dockerty MB. Surgical significance of isolated axillary adenopathy. *Ann Surg* 1957;145:104.
11. Copeland EM, McBride CM. Axillary metastases from unknown primary sites. *Ann Surg* 1973;178:25.
12. Kemeny MM, Rivera DE, Teri JJ, et al. Occult primary adenocarcinoma with axillary metastases. *Am J Surg* 1986;152:43.
13. Kolb TM, Lichy J, Newhouse JH. Occult cancer in women with dense breasts: detection with screening US—diagnostic yield and tumor characteristics. *Radiology* 1998;207:191.
14. Orel SG, Mendonca MH, Reynolds C, et al. MR imaging of ductal carcinoma *in situ*. *Radiology* 1997;202:413.
15. Gilles R, Meunier M, Trouffleau P, et al. Diagnosis of infraclinical lesions of the breast with dynamic MRI: results of a prospective and multicenter study. *J Radiol* 1997;78:293.
16. Morris EA, Schwarz LH, Dershaw DD. Imaging of the breast in patients with occult primary breast carcinoma. *Radiology* 1997;205:437.
17. Buchanan CL, Morris EA, Dorn PL, et al. Utility of breast magnetic resonance imaging in patients with occult primary breast cancer. *Ann Surg Oncol* 2005;12:1045.
18. Brenner RJ, Rothman BJ. Detection of primary breast cancer in women with known adenocarcinoma metastatic to the axilla: use of MRI after negative clinical and mammographic examination. *J Magn Reson Imaging* 1997;7:1153.
19. Tilanus-Linthorst MMA, Obdeijn AIM, Botenbal M, et al. MRI in patients with axillary metastases of occult breast carcinoma. *Breast Cancer Res Treat* 1997;44:179.
20. Olson JA Jr, Morris EA, Van Zee KJ, et al. Magnetic resonance imaging facilitates breast conservation for occult breast cancer. *Ann Surg Oncol* 2000;7:411.
21. Obdeijn IM, Brouwers-Kuyper EM, Tilanus-Linthorst MM, et al. MR imaging-guided sonography followed by fine-needle aspiration cytology in occult carcinoma of the breast. *AJR Am J Roentgenol* 2000;174:1079.
22. Lee WJ, Chu JS, Chang KJ, et al. Occult breast carcinoma. Use of color Doppler in localization. *Breast Cancer Res Treat* 1996;37(3):299.
23. Block EF, Meyer MA. Positron emission tomography in diagnosis of occult adenocarcinoma of the breast. *Am Surg* 1998;64 (9):906.
24. Scoggins CR, Vitola JV, Sandler MP, et al. Occult breast carcinoma presenting as an axillary mass. *Am Surg* 1999;65:1.
25. Haid A, Knauer M, Dunzinger S, et al. Intra-operative sonography: a valuable aid during breast-conserving surgery for occult breast cancer. *Ann Surg Oncol* 2007;14:3090.
26. Hall NC, Povoski SP, Murrey DA, et al. Combined approach of perioperative 18F-FDG PET/CT imaging and intraoperative 18F-FDG handheld gamma probe detection for tumor localization and verification of complete tumor resection in breast cancer. *World J Surg Oncol* 2007;5:143.
27. Paredes P, Vidal-Sicart S, Zanón G, et al. Radioguided occult lesion localisation in breast cancer using an intraoperative portable gamma camera: first results. *Eur J Nucl Med Mol Imaging* 2008;35(2):230.
28. Kolesnikov-Gauthier H, Levy E, Merlet P, et al. FDG PET in patients with cancer of an unknown primary. *Nucl Med Commun* 2005;26(12):1059–1066.
29. Park JM, Ikeda DM. Promising techniques for breast cancer detection, diagnosis, and staging using non-ionizing radiation imaging techniques. *Phys Med* 2006;21(Suppl 1):7.
30. Bhatia SK, Saclarides TJ, Witt TR, et al. Hormone receptor studies in axillary metastases from occult metastases. *Cancer* 1987;59:1170.
31. Merson M, Andreola S, Galimberti V, et al. Breast carcinoma presenting as axillary metastases without evidence of a primary tumor. *Cancer* 1992;70 (2):504.
32. Pertschuk LP, Kim DS, Nayer K, et al. Immunocytochemical estrogen and progestin receptor assays in breast cancer with monoclonal antibodies. Histopathologic, demographic and biochemical correlations and relationship to endocrine response and survival. *Cancer* 1990;66:1663.
33. Atkins H., Wolff B. The malignant gland in the axilla. *Guys Hosp Rep* 1960;109:1.
34. Feuerman L, Attie JN, Rosenberg B. Carcinoma in axillary lymph nodes as an indicator of breast cancer. *Surg Gynecol Obstet* 1962;114:5.
35. Klopp CT. Metastatic cancer of axillary lymph node without a demonstrable primary lesion. *Ann Surg* 1950;131:437.
36. Van Ooijen B Bontenbal M, Henzen-Logmans, et al. Axillary nodal metastases from an occult primary consistent with breast carcinoma. *Br J Surg* 1993;80 (10):1299.
37. Rosen PP, Kimmel M. Occult breast carcinoma presenting with axillary lymph node metastases: A follow-up study of 48 patients. *Human Pathol* 1990;21:518.

38. Weigenberg HA, Stetten D. Extensive secondary axillary lymph node carcinoma without clinical evidence of primary breast lesion. *Surgery* 1951;29:217.

39. Vlastos G, Jean MF, Mirza AN, et al. Feasibility of breast preservation in the treatment of occult primary carcinoma presenting with axillary metastases. *Ann Surg Oncol* 2001;8:425.

40. Harris JR, Recht A. Conservative surgery and radiotherapy. In: Harris JR, Hellman S, Henderson CI, et al., eds. *Breast diseases*, 2nd ed. Philadelphia: JB Lippincott, 1991:413.

41. Overgaard M, Hansen PS, Overgaard J et al. Postoperative radiotherapy in high-risk premenopausal women with breast cancer who receive adjuvant chemotherapy. Danish Breast cancer Cooperative Group 82b Trial. *N Engl J Med* 1997;337(14):949.

42. Overgaard M, Nielsen HM, Overgaard J. Is the benefit of postmastectomy irradiation limited to patients with four or more positive nodes, as recommended in international consensus reports? A subgroup analysis of the DBCG 82 b&c randomized trials. *Radiother Oncol* 2007;82(3):247–253.

43. Early Breast Cancer Trialists' Collaborative Group (EBCTCG). Effects of radiotherapy and of differences in the extent of surgery for early breast cancer on local recurrence and 15-year survival: an overview of the randomized trials. *Lancet* 2005;366:2087–2106.

44. Ragaz J, Olivotto IA, Spinelli JJ, et al. Locoregional radiation therapy in patients with high-risk breast cancer receiving adjuvant chemotherapy: 20-year results of the British Columbia Randomized Trial. *J Natl Cancer Inst* 2005;97(2):116–126.

Chapter 70
Surveillance of Patients Following Primary Therapy

Robert W. Carlson

The increasing success of therapy for breast cancer results in an increasing number of breast cancer survivors being monitored for the development of recurrent disease. It is estimated that there are over 2.4 million breast cancer survivors in the United States alone (1). The magnitude of the follow-up of this large population requires efficient, timely, and cost-effective monitoring. The optimal monitoring for recurrence of disease requires knowledge of the risk for recurrence, common sites of recurrence, accuracy of methods of detection of recurrence, and potential benefits and risks of detection of early disease recurrence.

ASSESSMENT FOR RISK OF RECURRENCE OF DISEASE

Assessment for risk of recurrence of disease may be performed by the integration of the anticipated natural history of a breast cancer based on anatomic and biologic prognostic factors and the anticancer treatment delivered. The hazard rates for recurrence of disease have been studied retrospectively among 3,585 patients enrolled in seven large clinical trials (2). The peak for annual hazard for recurrence occurred in years 1 to 2 and then decreased consistently to 5 years, and then declined slowly through year 12. The hazard for recurrence was especially high for those with four or more involved axillary lymph nodes during the first 5 to 6 years of follow-up, but thereafter was similar to those with fewer nodes involved. The hazard rate for recurrence was higher in those women with estrogen receptor–negative versus receptor positive–breast cancer during the first 3 years of follow-up, and then similar or lower thereafter.

Long-term follow-up studies have documented that the most common sites of recurrent disease are local soft tissue, bone, lung, liver, and brain. Multiple sites are often involved at the time of detection of first recurrence and almost always during the course of the metastatic disease. Tumors that are estrogen receptor positive, progesterone receptor positive, low or intermediate grade, and with low mitotic rate are more likely to metastasize to bone rather than viscera than tumors without those features (Table 70.1) (3,4). In contrast, menopausal status, tumor size, and nodal status do not impact the frequency of bone versus visceral site of metastatic disease. Further, many factors associated with overall prognosis at diagnosis of early breast cancer retain prognostic significance for survival following first diagnosis of metastatic breast cancer (5–7). Long-term survival after recurrent breast cancer is relatively unusual, and apparent cures of disease are uncommon except for patients with ipsilateral breast tumor recurrences (8).

A number of methodological biases including lead-time bias and length time bias confound many breast cancer surveillance studies. Lead time bias represents the diagnosis of disease earlier in its natural history, even though the outcome, such as date of death, is not impacted. Length time bias represents the greater likelihood that a slow growing tumor will be detected by routine surveillance studies, while a rapidly growing tumor is more likely to present during the interval between routine screening evaluations. These biases may be substantially overcome in surveillance studies by the performance of randomized trials using survival from date of diagnosis of the initial, not recurrent, disease as the primary end point. The goals of surveillance are primarily to detect recurrences at an early time point so as to initiate therapy to improve survival and to maintain a high quality of life. As will be discussed below, there is little high-level evidence that these goals are achieved by any surveillance program.

CONTRALATERAL BREAST

Frequency of Contralateral Disease

The occurrence of breast cancer in the contralateral breast of women with a known history of breast cancer may represent either a new primary tumor or a metastasis from the originally diagnosed breast cancer. Although the determination of a new primary versus a metastasis may be difficult, a contralateral breast cancer clearly represents a new primary if the cancer is of a different histology (e.g., ductal vs. lobular) or is associated with an *in situ* component. Multigene array technology likely will allow the more precise classification of contralateral breast metastasis versus second primary breast cancer in the future. Metachronous second primary breast cancers are more likely to be *in situ* cancer, small size, and node negative (9,10). The risk of a metachronous, contralateral, second primary breast cancer is generally estimated at 0.5% to 1.0% per year (10–14). Factors that increase the risk include a known *BRCA1* or *BRCA2* mutation, young age at first primary, family history of breast cancer, lobular histology for first primary breast cancer, and prior radiation exposure (11–13,15–18). Factors that decrease the risk include prior chemotherapy or endocrine therapy (13,17,19,20). Although there are no randomized studies of screening mammography of the contralateral breast, contralateral second primary breast cancer in women undergoing routine screening mammography is smaller and more likely to be *in situ* and node negative than those in women not undergoing routine mammography (9,21). The occurrence of metachronous contralateral breast cancer has a modest impact on overall survival (14,21).

Table 70.1	SITE OF RECURRENCE BY ESTROGEN RECEPTOR STATUS		
Site	ER Negative (%) (N = 333)	ER Positive (%) (N = 682)	*p*-Value
Brain	9	5	.0025
Liver	17	10	.0007
Lung	28	15	.0001
Other viscera	9	9	.98
Bone	33	44	.0008
Soft tissue	51	41	.0036
Contralateral breast	6	12	.0071
Multiple sites	44	31	.001

ER, estrogen receptor.
From Clark GM, Sledge GW Jr, Osborne CK, et al. Survival from first recurrence: relative importance of prognostic factors in 1,015 breast cancer patients. *J Clin Oncol* 1987;5(1):55–61, with permission.

Screening for Contralateral Disease

Conceptually, the monitoring for a new primary breast cancer in the contralateral breast may be viewed as monitoring a high risk for breast cancer population with an increased risk of competing mortality secondary to the initial primary breast cancer. In the general population of women aged 40 and older, the use of screening mammography has been demonstrated to decrease breast cancer mortality. It is thus likely that routine screening mammography would decrease breast mortality from a second primary tumor, although the mortality rate for second primary breast cancers is low.

Breast magnetic resonance imaging (MRI) screening has high sensitivity, low to moderate specificity, and high cost as an adjunct to the performance of diagnostic or screening mammography. No randomized clinical trials of breast MRI scanning are available in any clinical setting. Nonrandomized trials in women without known breast cancer but at a high genetic risk of breast cancer document a higher detection rate of breast cancer with the use of breast MRI scanning (22). To date, no similar trial has been reported in the follow-up of women following diagnosis of breast cancer (23–26). The American Cancer Society currently recommends screening MRI as an adjunct to screening mammography based on nonrandomized screening trials and observational studies in women with known *BRCA* mutation, those who have a first-degree relative with a known *BRCA* mutation, those who have a lifetime risk greater than 20% to 25% based on family history, those who have had radiation exposure to the chest between age 10 to 30 years, and those who have known Li-Fraumeni's syndrome (or in first-degree relatives) or Cowden's and Bannayan-Riley-Ruvalcaba's syndromes (or in first-degree relatives) (27). The American Cancer Society currently recommends annual MRI screening in such individuals and makes no recommendation for or against screening MRI in women with a personal history of breast cancer. A study of breast MRI screening in women at risk of breast cancer and with negative mammograms included 245 subjects with a personal history of breast cancer (23). Breast cancers were documented in 4% of the subjects with a prior history of breast cancer, and the positive predictive value of MRI recommended biopsy was 33%. The nonrandomized nature of all of these studies prohibits assessment of the impact of breast MRI screening on breast cancer mortality.

The value of clinical breast examination has never been adequately studied, although the performance of clinical breast examination is a generally accepted part of routine health care of the adult female. Breast self-examination was found to be of no advantage in early detection or mortality reduction in a large randomized clinical trial in a population of factory workers in China (28).

Based on the increased risk of a second primary breast cancer in the contralateral breast, it appears prudent to perform regular clinical breast examinations and screening mammography as a routine part of surveillance programs. The role of breast MRI screening is yet to be fully defined but would appear reasonable in those with very high contralateral risk. Such high risk patients are those with a known or a high risk for a genetic mutation conferring risk for breast cancer or a prior history of thoracic radiation. For other populations, insufficient information exists to allow for specific recommendations regarding the use of screening MRI. The value of breast self-examination has not been demonstrated.

LOCOREGIONAL RECURRENCES

Most patients with a locoregional recurrence of breast cancer following either breast-conserving therapy or mastectomy present with symptoms. Approximately 40% of isolated locoregional recurrences are detected during routine examinations in asymptomatic patients and approximately 18% in symptomatic patients, and approximately 41% of locoregional recurrences are diagnosed outside routine follow-up visits (29,30).

Ipsilateral Breast Tumor Recurrence

Ipsilateral breast tumor recurrence following breast-conserving surgery is experienced by 5 years in approximately 7% of patients with whole breast irradiation and 26% of patients without whole breast irradiation (31). The addition of a radiation boost to the tumor bed decreases in breast recurrence rates by approximately 41% compared with whole breast irradiation alone (32). Most recurrences occur in the prior tumor bed, and positive pathologic margins, younger age, higher grade tumor, larger tumor size, negative estrogen receptor status, and involvement of axillary lymph nodes have all been reported to increase the risk of ipsilateral breast tumor recurrence (31–35). Approximately 70% of ipsilateral breast tumor recurrences occur within the first 5 years of primary diagnosis (31,33,36). Breast recurrence during the first 5 years of follow-up is associated with a substantially worse overall prognosis than in breast recurrences that manifest later (34,36).

Detection of ipsilateral breast tumor recurrence is often difficult because of postsurgical, postradiotherapy changes in the breast. The sensitivity of mammography for ipsilateral breast tumor recurrences is approximately 50% to 70% and ultrasonography 80% to 85%. Overall, approximately 33% to 85% of local recurrences are first detected by the patient or on clinical examination (37–44). Breast MRI scanning has high sensitivity for detecting in-breast recurrences, but is expensive and is associated with highly variable specificity (37,45–47).

Locoregional Recurrence Postmastectomy

Locoregional recurrence following mastectomy is experienced within 5 years in approximately 6% of patients with postmastectomy regional irradiation and 23% of patients without postmastectomy irradiation (48). In the overview analysis, axillary lymph node status strongly predicted for absolute risk for locoregional recurrence (48). In women with axillary lymph node–negative disease, the 5-year local recurrence risk following surgery alone was 6%, and this was reduced to 2% with the use of locoregional irradiation. In women with axillary lymph node–positive disease, the 5-year local recurrence risk following surgery alone was 23%, and this was reduced to 6% with the addition of locoregional irradiation. Increasing tumor grade, tumor size, and number of involved axillary lymph nodes increases the risk of locoregional recurrence.

Detection of locoregional recurrences following mastectomy with or without radiation is typically the result of either patient identification or of a routine clinical examination. Locoregional recurrences are rarely detected by radiographs or other screening studies.

Distant Recurrences

Well-established prognostic factors allow the estimation of risk for development of systemic disease following treatment for stages 0, I, II, and III breast cancer. Known prognostic factors include histologic subtype of breast cancer, tumor grade, tumor size, involvement of skin or chest wall, extent of involvement of regional lymph nodes, hormone receptor status, *ERBB2* (formerly *HER2*) level of expression or amplification, and perhaps multigene array expression profile.

Breast cancer metastases occur in a generally predictable pattern, with synchronous multiple sites of recurrence being common. Bone is the most common site of disseminated disease, and it represents approximately 40% of first recurrences. The most commonly involved bones are the spine, ribs, pelvis, skull, femur, and humerus. Breast cancer metastasis to bone distal to the elbow or knee is rare. Other common sites for metastatic disease include lung, liver, lymph nodes, and soft tissue. The site of first metastasis from breast cancer is influenced by estrogen receptor status (Table 70.1). Estrogen receptor–positive breast cancer is more likely to spread to bone, while receptor negative breast cancer is more likely to spread to viscera and soft tissues and is associated with a higher rate of early recurrence (Table 70.1) (4,6). Even in those patients undergoing routine surveillance during follow-up, most recurrent disease is symptomatic at time of diagnosis (30,49) (Table 70.2).

Infiltrating lobular breast cancer has a propensity for recurrences in intra-abdominal and retroperitoneal sites. Common sites include stomach, intestine, peritoneum, and ureter (often bilateral) (50–52).

Currently available treatment of recurrent or metastatic breast cancer is rarely curative, even when the recurrence is limited (8). Furthermore, the amount of tumor burden in asymptomatic or minimally symptomatic patients does not predict disease response to systemic treatment, ability to palliate symptoms, or overall survival. Thus, there is little advantage to diagnosing asymptomatic, early, subclinical disease.

Routine Blood Tests

The routine performance of blood tests for alkaline phosphatase, aspartate aminotransferase, γ-glutamyl transferase, bilirubin, calcium, and creatinine was studied by the International Breast Cancer Study Group in 4,105 women with invasive breast cancer (53). At the time of analysis, 2,140 patients had experienced a relapse, 93 had a second nonbreast primary tumor, and 111 had died without relapse during a 10-year median follow-up period. In this analysis, only alkaline phosphatase was abnormal in at least 20% of patients with recurrent disease and was abnormal in 32% of patients with bone metastasis and 71% of patients with liver metastasis. Aspartate aminotransferase and γ-glutamyl transferase were elevated in 62% and 75% of patients with liver metastasis. Bilirubin, calcium, and creatinine were of no value in detecting recurrent disease. Thus, while alkaline phosphatase was the most reliable of the blood tests, it was of low sensitivity for bone or liver disease. In another study of 1,371 patients with node-positive breast cancer, serial alkaline phosphatase determinations were found to have low sensitivity and specificity for bone recurrence (54). Thus monitoring of routine blood tests as a part of breast cancer surveillance is not recommended.

Circulating Tumor Markers

Tests of serum carcinoembryonic antigen (CEA) and MUC-1 antigen (CA 15-3, CA 27.29) have been proposed as tumor markers for the surveillance of breast cancer recurrence. Elevations in these antigens are common in patients with newly diagnosed breast cancer, and their levels are prognostic in some studies (55–59). Prospective and retrospective studies using these markers in breast cancer surveillance following primary treatment demonstrate that recurrences of breast cancer may be detected with low to modest sensitivity approximately 5 to 6 months prior to the detection of metastatic or recurrent disease by other methods (60–65). However, false-positive elevations in these markers are not uncommon with associated risk of incorrectly diagnosing recurrence of disease, and no advantage in overall survival or quality of life has been demonstrated with the use of these markers. Guidelines generated by expert panels consistently recommend specifically against or do not recommend surveillance using any serum tumor marker test (66–69). Thus, the monitoring of circulating tumor markers, including those measuring CEA or MUC-1 antigen, appears to be of no value and is not recommended in the surveillance of women following treatment for early stage breast cancer.

Bone-Specific Monitoring

Bone pain is a common symptom of bone metastasis from breast cancer. However, many patients with bone pain do not have recurrent cancer, and up to 32% of patients with bone metastasis do not have pain (70,71).

Radionuclide bone scanning is in general a sensitive and moderately specific imaging modality for breast cancer metastatic to bone. The National Surgical Adjuvant Breast and Bowel Project (NSABP) has reported on the benefit of 7,984 routine follow-up bone scans in 2,697 patients with node-positive breast

Table 70.2	RESULTS OF A RETROSPECTIVE ANALYSIS OF PRESENCE OR ABSENCE OF SYMPTOMS AT TIME OF DIAGNOSIS OF FIRST RECURRENCE BY SITE OF RECURRENT DISEASE		
Site	Asymptomatic	Symptomatic	Total Number
Bone	22 (31%)	49 (69%)	71
Local	16 (34%)	31 (66%)	47
Multiple	11 (26%)	32 (74%)	43
Pulmonary	23 (58%)	17 (42%)	40
Regional	17 (50%)	17 (50%)	43
Visceral	0 (0%)	13 (100%)	13
Total	89 (36%)	159 (64%)	248

From Tomin R, Donegan WL. Screening for recurrent breast cancer—its effectiveness and prognostic value. *J Clin Oncol* 1987;5(1):62–67, with permission.

cancer as a part of NSABP B-09 (72). Scans were obtained at baseline, every 6 months for 3 years, and then annually. At the time of the analysis, 779 patients had experienced a recurrence, and 163 of these were in bone only. In 146 of the patients with bone recurrence, information about the presence or absence of symptoms was available. Ninety-five patients had the bone recurrence detected by routine scheduled bone scans, and 35 of these patients were asymptomatic. All 51 patients who had the bone recurrence documented by a nonroutine bone scan were symptomatic. At most, only 0.6% of the total number of bone scans were positive in the absence of symptoms.

In a study of 241 patients with node-positive breast cancer, the use of serial bone scans detected 25 patients with bone metastasis, only 13 of whom were asymptomatic (73). In a study of 1,601 women with node-positive breast cancer, 1,441 had a baseline and repeat bone scan at 1 year of follow-up (54). This study documented the inability of the 1-year bone scan to predict for the eventual development of bone recurrence. With a median of 4 years of follow-up, those women with a normal 1-year bone scan had a 6.9% risk for development of first relapse in bone, while those with a doubtful 1-year bone scan had an 11.2% chance of first relapse in bone. Abnormal, radiologically confirmed, 1-year bone scans were present in only 1.2% of all patients.

Recent studies have suggested that the use of whole body MRI scanning may be more sensitive and specific for the early detection of bone recurrence (74). However, the routine use of whole body MRI scanning is currently too cost-prohibitive to consider.

There is thus no evidence supporting the use of routine surveillance for bone recurrences in women with a history of early stage breast cancer.

Liver-Specific Monitoring

Prospective study of intensive surveillance including liver ultrasonography and liver function tests versus minimal testing have found no difference in the cumulative rate of detection of breast cancer hepatic metastasis during any time interval up to 5 years (49).

No prospective studies testing the value of computed tomography of the liver as surveillance have been reported. Existing data from other surveillance studies predict that computed tomography surveillance would be neither efficacious nor cost-effective. Thus, there is no evidence supporting the performance of liver-specific monitoring in the surveillance of women with a history of early stage breast cancer.

Lung-Specific Monitoring

Most patients with pulmonary recurrences of breast cancer present with symptoms referable to the chest. Studies addressing the use of routine screening chest radiographs have demonstrated very low rates of metastases detection in the asymptomatic patient. In a study of 241 patients with node-positive breast cancer who had undergone serial chest radiography during the first 2 years following diagnosis, 3.4% were found to have asymptomatic pulmonary metastasis (73). In a prospective randomized trial or intensive versus spontaneous surveillance, the utility of chest radiographs was specifically assessed (75). Neither disease-free nor overall survival was improved with the routine performance of chest radiographs. Thus, the use of chest radiography in the surveillance of women with early stage breast cancer is discouraged.

SECOND NONBREAST CANCERS

Individuals with breast cancer have a risk of developing second malignancies from a variety of potential causes including those associated with genetic mutations such as the *BRCA1* and *BRCA2* mutations, secondary cancer related to treatment with chemotherapy, radiation, and endocrine agents, and the usual wide variety of other cancers unrelated to breast cancer and its treatment. A population-based study of 525,527 women with primary breast cancer reported an increased incidence following breast cancer diagnosis of stomach, colorectal, nonmelanoma skin, endometrial, ovarian, kidney, and thyroid cancers, melanoma, soft tissue sarcoma, and leukemia (76). Whether these increased risks were attributable to underlying susceptibility, treatment, surveillance, or other factors could not be assessed within the cohort.

Radiation Therapy-Treated Patients

In the Early Breast Cancer Trialists' Collaborative Group analysis of patients with early breast cancer treated with radiation therapy, the occurrence of second malignancies, including lung cancer, esophageal cancer, leukemia, and soft tissue sarcomas, was found to be increased, although the absolute risk was small (31). The impact of radiation postmastectomy or breast-conserving therapy on second cancers was the subject of a single institution study of 16,705 women with breast cancer. At 10 years of follow-up, an excess of sarcomas (relative risk [RR] 7.46; 95% confidence interval [CI], 1.02–54.52; $p = .02$.) and lung cancers (RR 3.09; 95% CI, 1.12–8.53; $p = .022$) was observed. The absolute risk of a second primary sarcoma or lung cancer was, however, extremely low with 35 of 13,472 patients treated with radiation therapy experiencing a sarcoma and 58 experiencing lung cancer. Of the patients experiencing lung cancer, 52 occurred in patients with a history of tobacco use. There was no difference in other tumor types in this institutional experience.

Chemotherapy-Treated Patients

An analysis of 2,465 patients studied in consecutive adjuvant programs utilizing CMF (cyclophosphamide, methotrexate, and 5-fluorouracil) chemotherapy with or without doxorubicin found no excess second cancer risk at 15 years of follow-up (77). The Early Breast Cancer Trialists' Collaborative Group analysis of second cancers in patients with early breast cancer treated with polychemotherapy documented a decreased risk of contralateral breast cancer in women under the age of 50 years but no statistically significant difference in risk of any other second cancer (31). In an analysis of AC (doxorubicin and cyclophosphamide)-based NSABP trials, the cumulative incidence of acute myeloid leukemia and myelodysplastic syndrome at 5 years was 0.21% (95% CI, 0.11%–0.41%) with standard AC and increased to 1.01% (95% CI, 0.63%–1.62%) with intensification of the cyclophosphamide (78).

Endocrine-Treated Patients

The Early Breast Cancer Trialists' Collaborative Group analysis of second cancers in patients with early breast cancer treated with tamoxifen documented a decreased risk in contralateral breast cancer in women with a first breast cancer that was estrogen-receptor positive or estrogen-receptor unknown and an increased risk of cancer of the uterus (31). The incidence of uterine cancer with tamoxifen was approximately 1.9 per 1,000 per year versus 0.6 per 1,000 per year without tamoxifen. There was no difference in second cancers at any other site. Similar rates of tamoxifen-associated endometrial cancer have been documented by the NSABP (79). The increased risk of endometrial cancer associated with tamoxifen is limited to postmenopausal women, and no additional monitoring beyond routine gynecologic care is recommended (80). The vast majority of tamoxifen-associated endometrial cancers are associated with symptoms of vaginal bleeding, bloody vaginal discharge, staining, or spotting. In the absence of these symptoms, routine gynecologic care is appropriate. In the presence of these symptoms, gynecologic evaluation to exclude the presence of benign or malignant endometrial pathology is appropriate.

Analysis of adjuvant endocrine therapy trials incorporating an aromatase inhibitor document a greater risk reduction for contralateral breast cancer than is achieved with tamoxifen alone. In the ATAC (anastrozole, tamoxifen alone or in combination) trial, anastrozole compared to tamoxifen reduced the occurrence of contralateral breast cancer by 42% (95% CI, 12%–62%; $p = .01$) and in the patients with receptor-positive disease by 53% (95% CI, 25%–71%; $p = .001$) (81). Because the use of tamoxifen decreases the occurrence of contralateral breast cancer by approximately 50%, the use of an aromatase inhibitor would appear to decrease overall contralateral breast cancer by 70% to 80% to contralateral rates of breast cancer not dissimilar to those of women without a history of breast cancer. Similar reductions in contralateral breast cancer have been observed in trials switching to an aromatase inhibitor after 2 to 3 years of tamoxifen or as extended adjuvant therapy (82,83).

There is thus no evidence that screening studies other than those recommended for general health maintenance (such as routine screening colonoscopy according to published guidelines) should be performed to detect second primary nonbreast cancers in women under surveillance for recurrence breast cancer, other than routine gynecologic evaluation in women receiving endocrine therapy with tamoxifen.

PROSPECTIVE TRIALS OF SURVEILLANCE FOLLOWING BREAST CANCER TREATMENT

Several high-quality, multicenter, randomized trials of follow-up strategies have been reported. The Gruppo Interdisciplinare perla Valutazione degli Interventi in Oncologia (GIVIO) investigators randomized 1,320 women with stage I, II, and III primary breast cancer to an intensive surveillance program, including physician visits; annual radionuclide bone scan, liver echography and mammography; every 6 months chest radiographs; and every 3 months alkaline phosphatase and γ-glutamyl transferase versus the same frequency of physician visits and annual mammography alone (49). Quality of life assessments were also performed. At a median follow-up of 71 months, there were no differences in deaths between the two groups (odds ratio = 1.12; 95% CI, 0.87–1.43) or in number of distant metastasis. The intense surveillance resulted in a less than 1-month difference in mean time to detection of a distant metastasis. Patterns of site of first recurrence were also similar between the two treatment groups (Table 70.3). Even in the intense follow-up group, only 31% of recurrences were found in asymptomatic patients. Assessment of quality of life did not differ across multiple dimensions between the two treatment groups.

In another randomized trial preformed by the National Research Council Project on Breast Cancer, 1,243 patients with nonmetastatic invasive breast cancer were randomized to intensive surveillance with physical examination; radionuclide bone scan and chest radiography every 6 months; and mammography every year versus the control group who underwent physical examinations and mammography at the same intervals (84). Relapse-free survival was inferior in the intensive follow-up group, presumably because of earlier diagnosis of recurrent disease, but there was no difference in overall survival (5-year mortality 18.6% in the intensive follow-up group vs. 19.5% in the clinical follow-up group). Sites of recurrent disease were similar between the two groups (Table 70.3). A more recent follow-up of this trial reported 10-year mortality of 34.8% with intensive follow-up compared with 31.5% in the control group (85). Survival analysis revealed a hazard ratio of 1.05 (95% CI, 0.87–1.26).

In a smaller study, 472 patients with localized breast cancer following primary treatment were randomized to receive follow-up visits either every 3 or 6 months and also randomized to receive routine blood counts, calcium, sedimentation rate, liver enzymes, and CA 15-3 at every visit, chest x-ray every 6 months, and liver ultrasound and bone scan every second year, or to no routine testing (75,86). At a median follow-up of

	GIVIO Trial[a]		National Research Council Project on Breast Cancer[b]	
Type of Recurrence	Intensive Monitoring (n = 201 recurrences or deaths)	Control (n = 196 recurrences or deaths)	Intensive Monitoring (n = 219 recurrences)	Control (n = 174 recurrences)
Local regional recurrence alone	32 (15.9%)	36 (18.4%)	55 (25.1%)	49 (28.2%)
Contralateral breast alone	12 (11.4%)	13 (6.6%)	Not stated	Not stated
Distant metastases	127 (63.1%)	127 (64.8)	164 (75.9%)	125 (71.8%)
Bone	52 (25.9%)	55 (28.1%)	84 (38.3%)	53 (30.5%)
Liver	13 (6.5%)	12 (6.1%)	—	—
Lung/pleura	24 (11.9%)	21 (10.7%)	28 (12.8%)	18 (10.3%)
Other sites	19 (9.4%)	27 (13.8%)	22 (10.0%)	21 (12.1%)
Multiple sites	19 (9.4%)	12 (6.1%)	30 (13.7%)	33 (19.0%)
Second primary (not breast)	8 (4.0%)	11 (5.6%)	—	—
Death without recurrence	11 (5.5%)	9 (4.6%)	—	—

Table 70.3 LOCATION OF FIRST RECURRENCE IN RANDOMIZED TRIALS OF INTENSIVE VERSUS ROUTINE SURVEILLANCE

GIVIO, Gruppo Interdisciplinare perla Valutazione degli Interventi in Oncologia.
[a]From Impact of follow-up testing on survival and health-related quality of life in breast cancer patients. A multicenter randomized controlled trial. The GIVIO investigators. *JAMA* 1994;271(20):1587–1592, with permission.
[b]From Rosselli Del Turco M, Palli D, Cariddi A, et al. Intensive diagnostic follow-up after treatment of primary breast cancer. A randomized trial. National Research Council Project on Breast Cancer follow-up. *JAMA* 1994;271(20):1593–1597, with permission.

4.2 years, there was no significant difference in number of recurrences detected, disease-free survival, overall survival, number of patient initiated phone calls concerning breast cancer, or extra medical visits. Costs of care were specifically assessed, and the intensive surveillance increased follow-up costs by more than twofold.

In a trial of 196 women with breast cancer, the subjects were randomized to regular follow-up surveillance visits or to yearly visits at the time of mammography (87). The number of recurrences was too low at the time of the report for assessment. However, the vast majority of participants found their clinic visits reassuring and the majority wished to continue their follow-up with the specialist clinic. However, 25% of the regular follow-up group and 35% of the annual follow-up group preferred less frequent follow-up evaluations in the future.

A study randomized 296 women with breast cancer to specialist follow-up or to follow-up in generalist practices (88). No difference was observed for time to diagnosis of recurrence by practice setting, and most recurrences (69%) presented as interval events between scheduled visits. A separate study randomized 968 patients who were 9 to 15 months following diagnosis and at least 3 months following completion of adjuvant chemotherapy and radiotherapy to follow-up through a tertiary care cancer center or to follow-up with their own primary care physician (89). The primary care physicians were provided with a one-page guideline that outlined recommended follow-up and diagnostic tests to investigate signs or symptoms suggestive of recurrent or new primary cancer. Patients were to be referred back to the cancer center if recurrence or new primary tumor developed. The primary end point of the study was recurrence-related serious clinical events such as spinal cord compression, pathologic fracture, and hypercalcemia. Health-related quality of life was a secondary end point. The results document equivalent rates of serious clinical events between cancer center versus primary care physician follow-up groups (Table 70.4). Health-related quality of life did not differ between the two treatment groups throughout the study period.

Studies using the Surveillance, Epidemiology, and End Results (SEER) Medicare databases have evaluated the use of routine testing, including mammography, bone scans, tumor antigen tests, chest radiographs, and other chest or abdominal imaging (90,91). These analyses demonstrate that women seeing medical oncologists, radiation oncologists, or surgeons are more likely to undergo routine mammography than women seeing other specialists. Women with breast cancer being followed by medical oncologists are also more likely than those followed by other specialists to undergo testing including tumor antigen testing, chest radiographs, and chest or abdominal imaging, although the rates of utilization are falling most rapidly among medical oncologists. To what extent the differing utilization of testing among specialists reflects differing risk populations versus inappropriate routine testing could not be determined from the SEER Medicare database. There is evidence that medical oncologists are more likely to follow young and high-risk patients longer than patients who are older or lower risk (92).

Thus, the optimal surveillance of women following treatment for breast cancer requires relatively little testing and can be performed equivalently by an interested, informed primary care physician. As the long-term treatment of women with breast cancer occurs, such as with the extended adjuvant therapies of hormone receptor–positive disease, one of the major challenges of primary care follow-up is the need to keep the primary care provider up to date regarding changes in optimal practice.

Patient Expectations of Surveillance

Despite the extensive data demonstrating limited value of routine testing, many patients expect routine follow-up from their physicians (93). To a substantial degree this is because patients have unrealistic expectations of tests and their health care provider to detect recurrent breast cancer and to implement treatment so that it impacts overall survival substantially. During the follow-up period, patients require education about

Table 70.4	**RECURRENCE, DEATH, AND SERIOUS ADVERSE EVENTS COMPARING FAMILY PRACTICE VERSUS SPECIALIST SURVEILLANCE**					
	Family Practice Group (n = 483)		Cancer Center Group (n = 485)		Risk	
Outcome Event	No. of Patients	%	No.	%	Difference, CC-FP (%)	95% CI (%)
Recurrence[a]	54	11.2	64	13.2	2.02	−2.13 to 6.16
Distant	36	—	38	—	—	—
Local	10	—	12	—	—	—
Contralateral	11	—	15	—	—	—
Death (all causes)	29	6.0	30	6.2	0.18	−2.90–3.26
Serious clinical event[b]	17	3.5	18	3.7	0.19	−2.26–2.65
Spinal cord compression	0	—	1	—	—	—
Pathologic fracture	3	—	8	—	—	—
Uncontrolled recurrence	2	—	0	—	—	—
KPS ≤70	14	—	18	—	—	—
Brachial plexopathy	0	—	0	—	—	—
Hypercalcemia	2	—	2	—	—	—

CC-FP, cancer center-family practice; CI, confidence interval; KPS, Karnofsky performance status.
[a]Four patients had more than one recurrence.
[b]Thirteen patients had more than one serious adverse event.
From Grunfeld E, Levine MN, Julian JA, et al. Randomized trial of long-term follow-up for early-stage breast cancer: a comparison of family physician versus specialist care. *J Clin Oncol* 2006;24(6):848–855, with permission.

Table 70.5	**COMPARISON OF GUIDELINE RECOMMENDATIONS FOR SURVEILLANCE OF WOMEN FOLLOWING PRIMARY THERAPY OF BREAST CANCER**			
	National Comprehensive Cancer Network[a]	American Society of Clinical Oncology[b]	European Society of Medical Oncology[c]	Canadian Breast Cancer Initiative[d]
History and physical examination	Every 4–6 mos for 5 yrs, then annually	Every 3–6 mos for 3 yrs, then every 6–12 mos for 2 yrs, then annually	Every 3–6 mos for 3 yrs, then every 6–12 mos for 3 yrs, then annually	According to individual patient's needs
Mammography	Every 12 mos	Every 12 mos	Every 12–24 mos	Every 12 mos
Breast self-examination	—	Monthly	—	If a woman wishes
Gynecologic assessment	Every 12 mos for women on tamoxifen if uterus present	Regular gynecologic follow-up	—	For women taking tamoxifen, important to ask about vaginal bleeding
Bone health assessment	Ongoing monitoring of bone health	Routine and regular assessment	—	Postmenopausal, premenopausal with risk factors for osteoporosis, or taking an aromatase inhibitor should have screening bone mineral density test Patients should be counseled on exercise and adequate intake of calcium and vitamin D Osteoporosis treatment should include a bisphosphonate
Encourage adherence to endocrine therapy	Ongoing	—	—	—

[a]From Carlson RW, Anderson BO, Burstein HJ, et al. The NCCN invasive breast cancer clinical practice guidelines in oncology. *J Natl Compr Cancer Netw* 2007(5):246–312.
[b]From Khatcheressian JL, Wolff AC, Smith TJ, et al. American Society of Clinical Oncology 2006 update of the breast cancer follow-up and management guidelines in the adjuvant setting. *J Clin Oncol* 2006;24(31):5091–5097.
[c]From Pestalozzi B. Primary breast cancer: ESMO clinical recommendations for diagnosis, treatment and follow-up. *Ann Oncol* 2007;18[Suppl 2]:ii5–ii8.
[d]From Grunfeld E, Dhesy-Thind S, Levine M. Clinical practice guidelines for the care and treatment of breast cancer: follow-up after treatment for breast cancer (summary of the 2005 update). *Can Med Assoc J* 2005;172(10):1319–1320.

the importance of self-reporting symptoms and the limited value of routine blood tests and radiographic studies other than annual mammography.

RECOMMENDED SURVEILLANCE

The large number of patients alive without recurrence of disease following treatment of early stage breast cancer and the availability of multiple studies addressing surveillance for recurrence of disease present an opportunity for the widespread application of evidence-based surveillance. Given the large number of women alive with a history of breast cancer, the use of evidence-based surveillance monitoring has a large economic impact. A number of professional organizations have evaluated the evidence relating to surveillance of breast cancer and issued recommendations for evidence-based follow-up. Recommendations from representative major organizations are outlined on Table 70.5. As can be seen, there is remarkable consistency among the recommendations.

The optimal surveillance for breast cancer recurrence involves routine follow-up history taking and physical examination, yearly mammography of any retained breast, and monitoring for treatment-related endometrial carcinoma in patients treated with tamoxifen and bone health in women experiencing a treatment-related menopause or receiving an aromatase inhibitor. The guidelines are very consistent in not recommending surveillance radiographs, blood counts, blood chemistries, tumor markers, radionuclide scans, and so forth in the asymptomatic patient. Patients with symptoms, physical findings, or concerning abnormalities on follow-up mammography warrant a full, expeditious symptom or finding directed evaluation.

 MANAGEMENT SUMMARY

- Breast cancer recurrences are most common in soft tissues, bone, lung, liver, and brain.
- Second primary breast cancers are common in women with a history of early breast cancer, and yearly mammography of the contralateral breast and the ipsilateral breast if conserved is appropriate.
- Ipsilateral breast recurrences following breast-conserving therapy are usually found by the patient, on clinical examination or mammography.
- Periodic follow-up visits should include the performance of history taking and focused physical examination.
- Distant recurrences are uncommonly detected by routine surveillance studies in asymptomatic patients without physical findings.
- No high-level evidence supports the surveillance for breast cancer recurrence with routine chest x-rays, computed tomography, ultrasounds, MRI scans, bone scans, liver function tests, alkaline phosphatase, tumor markers, or blood counts. The use of any or all of these tests is therefore discouraged in surveillance for breast cancer recurrence. Patients who have symptoms or physical findings concerning for recurrent disease should have a focused, expeditious evaluation appropriate for the organ system of concern.
- Women treated with tamoxifen should have a yearly gynecologic assessment, and postmenopausal women with vaginal spotting should be promptly evaluated for the presence of endometrial carcinoma.
- Women experiencing treatment-related ovarian failure or who are treated with an aromatase inhibitor should have monitoring of bone health.

References

1. Ries LAG, Melbert D, Krapcho M, et al. SEER cancer statistics review, 1975–2004. Available at http://seer.cancer.gov/csr/1975_2004/. Bethesda, MD: National Cancer Institute, 2007.
2. Saphner T, Tormey DC, Gray R. Annual hazard rates of recurrence for breast cancer after primary therapy. *J Clin Oncol* 1996;14(10):2738–2746.
3. Solomayer EF, Diel IJ, Meyberg GC, et al. Metastatic breast cancer: clinical course, prognosis and therapy related to the first site of metastasis. *Breast Cancer Res Treat* 2000;59(3):271–278.
4. Hess KR, Pusztai L, Buzdar AU, et al. Estrogen receptors and distinct patterns of breast cancer relapse. *Breast Cancer Res Treat* 2003;78(1):105–118.
5. Chang J, Clark GM, Allred DC, et al. Survival of patients with metastatic breast carcinoma: importance of prognostic markers of the primary tumor. *Cancer* 2003; 97(3):545–553.
6. Clark GM, Sledge GW Jr, Osborne CK, et al. Survival from first recurrence: relative importance of prognostic factors in 1,015 breast cancer patients. *J Clin Oncol* 1987; 5(1):55–61.
7. Howell A, Barnes DM, Harland RN, et al. Steroid-hormone receptors and survival after first relapse in breast cancer. *Lancet* 1984;1(8377):588–591.
8. Greenberg PA, Hortobagyi GN, Smith TL, et al. Long-term follow-up of patients with complete remission following combination chemotherapy for metastatic breast cancer. *J Clin Oncol* 1996;14(8):2197–2205.
9. Mellink WA, Holland R, Hendriks JH, et al. The contribution of routine follow-up mammography to an early detection of asynchronous contralateral breast cancer. *Cancer* 1991;67(7):1844–1848.
10. Samant RS, Olivotto IA, Jackson JS, et al. Diagnosis of metachronous contralateral breast cancer. *Breast J* 2001;7(6):405–410.
11. Chaudary MA, Millis RR, Hoskins EO, et al. Bilateral primary breast cancer: a prospective study of disease incidence. *Br J Surg* 1984;71(9):711–714.
12. Chen Y, Thompson W, Semenciw R, et al. Epidemiology of contralateral breast cancer. *Cancer Epidemiol Biomarkers Prev* 1999;8(10):855–861.
13. Broet P, de la Rochefordiere A, Scholl SM, et al. Contralateral breast cancer: annual incidence and risk parameters. *J Clin Oncol* 1995;13(7):1578–1583.
14. Rosen PP, Groshen S, Kinne DW, et al. Contralateral breast carcinoma: an assessment of risk and prognosis in stage I (T1N0M0) and stage II (T1N1M0) patients with 20-year follow-up. *Surgery* 1989;106(5):904–910.
15. Bernstein JL, Thompson WD, Risch N, et al. Risk factors predicting the incidence of second primary breast cancer among women diagnosed with a first primary breast cancer. *Am J Epidemiol* 1992;136(8):925–936.
16. Hislop TG, Elwood JM, Coldman AJ, et al. Second primary cancers of the breast: incidence and risk factors. *Br J Cancer* 1984;49(1):79–85.
17. Horn PL, Thompson WD. Risk of contralateral breast cancer. Associations with histologic, clinical, and therapeutic factors. *Cancer* 1988;62(2):412–424.
18. Dawson LA, Chow E, Goss PE. Evolving perspectives in contralateral breast cancer. *Eur J Cancer* 1998;34(13):2000–2009.
19. Healey EA, Cook EF, Orav EJ, et al. Contralateral breast cancer: clinical characteristics and impact on prognosis. *J Clin Oncol* 1993;11(8):1545–1552.
20. Early Breast Cancer Trialists' Collaborative Group. Systemic treatment of early breast cancer by hormonal, cytotoxic, or immune therapy. *Lancet* 1992;339(8784):1–15.
21. Kollias J, Evans AJ, Wilson AR, et al. Value of contralateral surveillance mammography for primary breast cancer follow-up. *World J Surg* 2000;24(8):983–989.
22. Lehman CD, Blume JD, Weatherall P, et al. Screening women at high risk for breast cancer with mammography and magnetic resonance imaging. *Cancer* 2005;103(9): 1898–1905.
23. Morris EA, Liberman L, Ballon DJ, et al. MRI of occult breast carcinoma in a high-risk population. *AJR Am J Roentgenol* 2003;181(3):619–626.
24. Kriege M, Brekelmans CT, Boetes C, et al. Efficacy of MRI and mammography for breast-cancer screening in women with a familial or genetic predisposition. *N Engl J Med* 2004;351(5):427–437.
25. Leach MO, Boggis CR, Dixon AK, et al. Screening with magnetic resonance imaging and mammography of a UK population at high familial risk of breast cancer: a prospective multicentre cohort study (MARIBS). *Lancet* 2005;365(9473):1769–1778.
26. Liberman L. The high risk patient and magnetic resonance imaging. In: Morris EA, Liberman L, eds. *Breast MRI diagnosis and intervention.* New York: Springer, 2005:184–199.
27. Saslow D, Boetes C, Burke W, et al. American Cancer Society guidelines for breast screening with MRI as an adjunct to mammography. *CA Cancer J Clin* 2007; 57(2):75–89.
28. Thomas DB, Gao DL, Ray RM, et al. Randomized trial of breast self-examination in Shanghai: final results. *JNCI Cancer Spectrum* 2002;94(19):1445–1457.
29. de Bock GH, Bonnema J, van Der Hage J, et al. Effectiveness of routine visits and routine tests in detecting isolated locoregional recurrences after treatment for early-stage invasive breast cancer: a meta-analysis and systematic review. *J Clin Oncol* 2004;22(19):4010–4018.
30. Tomin R, Donegan WL. Screening for recurrent breast cancer—its effectiveness and prognostic value. *J Clin Oncol* 1987;5(1):62–67.
31. Early Breast Cancer Trialists' Collaborative Group. Effects of chemotherapy and hormonal therapy for early breast cancer on recurrence and 15-year survival: an overview of the randomised trials. *Lancet* 2005;365(9472):1687–1717.
32. Bartelink H, Horiot JC, Poortmans PM, et al. Impact of a higher radiation dose on local control and survival in breast-conserving therapy of early breast cancer: 10-year results of the randomized boost versus no boost EORTC 22881-10882 trial. *J Clin Oncol* 2007;25(22):3259–3265.
33. Wapnir IL, Anderson SJ, Mamounas EP, et al. Prognosis after ipsilateral breast tumor recurrence and locoregional recurrences in five National Surgical Adjuvant Breast and Bowel Project node-positive adjuvant breast cancer trials. *J Clin Oncol* 2006;24(13):2028–2037.
34. Komoike Y, Akiyama F, Iino Y, et al. Ipsilateral breast tumor recurrence (IBTR) after breast-conserving treatment for early breast cancer: risk factors and impact on distant metastases. *Cancer* 2006;106(1):35–41.
35. Horst KC, Smitt MC, Goffinet DR, et al. Predictors of local recurrence after breast-conservation therapy. *Clin Breast Cancer* 2005;5(6):425–438.
36. Kurtz JM, Spitalier JM, Amalric R, et al. The prognostic significance of late local recurrence after breast-conserving therapy. *Int J Radiat Oncol Biol Phys* 1990;18(1):87–93.
37. Belli P, Costantini M, Romani M, et al. Magnetic resonance imaging in breast cancer recurrence. *Breast Cancer Res Treat* 2002;73(3):223–235.
38. Dershaw DD. Mammography in patients with breast cancer treated by breast conservation (lumpectomy with or without radiation). *AJR Am J Roentgenol* 1995; 164(2):309–316.
39. Dershaw DD, McCormick B, Osborne MP. Detection of local recurrence after conservative therapy for breast carcinoma. *Cancer* 1992;70(2):493–496.
40. Fowble B, Solin LJ, Schultz DJ, et al. Breast recurrence following conservative surgery and radiation: patterns of failure, prognosis, and pathologic findings from mastectomy specimens with implications for treatment. *Int J Radiat Oncol Biol Phys* 1990;19(4):833–842.
41. Hartsell WF, Recine DC, Griem KL, et al. Delaying the initiation of intact breast irradiation for patients with lymph node positive breast cancer increases the risk of local recurrence. *Cancer* 1995;76(12):2497–2503.
42. Orel SG, Fowble BL, Solin LJ, et al. Breast cancer recurrence after lumpectomy and radiation therapy for early-stage disease: prognostic significance of detection method. *Radiology* 1993;188(1):189–194.
43. Orel SG, Troupin RH, Patterson EA, et al. Breast cancer recurrence after lumpectomy and irradiation: role of mammography in detection. *Radiology* 1992;183(1): 201–206.
44. Stomper PC, Recht A, Berenberg AL, et al. Mammographic detection of recurrent cancer in the irradiated breast. *AJR Am J Roentgenol* 1987;148(1):39–43.
45. Gilles R, Guinebretiere JM, Shapeero LG, et al. Assessment of breast cancer recurrence with contrast-enhanced subtraction MR imaging: preliminary results in 26 patients. *Radiology* 1993;188(2):473–478.
46. Mussurakis S, Buckley DL, Bowsley SJ, et al. Dynamic contrast-enhanced magnetic resonance imaging of the breast combined with pharmacokinetic analysis of gadolinium-DTPA uptake in the diagnosis of local recurrence of early stage breast carcinoma. *Invest Radiol* 1995;30(11):650–662.
47. Dao TH, Rahmouni A, Campana F, et al. Tumor recurrence versus fibrosis in the irradiated breast: differentiation with dynamic gadolinium-enhanced MR imaging. *Radiology* 1993;187(3):751–755.
48. Clarke M, Collins R, Darby S, et al. Effects of radiotherapy and of differences in the extent of surgery for early breast cancer on local recurrence and 15-year survival: an overview of the randomised trials. *Lancet* 2005;366(9503):2087–2106.
49. Impact of follow-up testing on survival and health-related quality of life in breast cancer patients. A multicenter randomized controlled trial. The GIVIO investigators. *JAMA* 1994;271(20):1587–1592.
50. Borst MJ, Ingold JA. Metastatic patterns of invasive lobular versus invasive ductal carcinoma of the breast. *Surgery* 1993;114(4):637–642.
51. McLemore EC, Pockaj BA, Reynolds C, et al. Breast cancer: presentation and intervention in women with gastrointestinal metastasis and carcinomatosis. *Ann Surg Oncol* 2005;12(11):886–894.
52. Taal BG, Peterse H, Boot H. Clinical presentation, endoscopic features, and treatment of gastric metastases from breast carcinoma. *Cancer* 2000;89(11):2214–2221.
53. Crivellari D, Price KN, Hagen M, et al. Routine tests during follow-up of patients after primary treatment for operable breast cancer. International (Ludwig) Breast Cancer Study Group (IBCSG). *Ann Oncol* 1995;6(8):769–776.
54. Pedrazzini A, Gelber R, Isley M, et al. First repeated bone scan in the observation of patients with operable breast cancer. *J Clin Oncol* 1986;4(3):389–394.
55. Ebeling FG, Stieber P, Untch M, et al. Serum CEA and CA 15.3 as prognostic factors in primary breast cancer. *Br J Cancer* 2002;86:1217–1222.
56. Gion M, Boracchi P, Dittadi R, et al. Prognostic role of serum CA 15.3 in 362 node-negative breast cancers. An old player for a new game. *Eur J Cancer* 2002;38(9): 1181–1188.
57. Kumpulainen EJ, Keskikuru RJ, Johansson RT. Serum tumor marker CA 15.3 and stage are the two most powerful predictors of survival in primary breast cancer. *Breast Cancer Res Treat* 2002;76(2):95–102.
58. Martin A, Corte MD, Alvarez AM, et al. Prognostic value of pre-operative serum CA 15.3 levels in breast cancer. *Anticancer Res* 2006;26(5B):3965–3971.
59. Molina R, Filella X, Alicarte J, et al. Prospective evaluation of CEA and CA 15.3 in patients with locoregional breast cancer. *Anticancer Res* 2003;23(2A):1035–1041.
60. Chan DW, Beveridge RA, Muss H, et al. Use of Truquant BR radioimmunoassay for early detection of breast cancer recurrence in patients with stage II and stage III disease. *J Clin Oncol* 1997;15(6):2322–2328.
61. Guadagni F, Ferroni P, Carlini S, et al. A re-evaluation of carcinoembryonic antigen (CEA) as a serum marker for breast cancer: a prospective longitudinal study. *Clin Cancer Res* 2001;7(8):2357–2362.
62. De La Lande B, Hacene K, Floiras JL, et al. Prognostic value of CA 15.3 kinetics for metastatic breast cancer. *Int J Biol Markers* 2002;17(4):231–238.
63. Valenzuela P, Mateos S, Tello E, et al. The contribution of the CEA marker to CA 15.3 in the follow-up of breast cancer. *Eur J Gynaecol Oncol* 2003;24(1):60–62.
64. Kokko R, Holli K, Hakama M. CA 15.3 in the follow-up of localised breast cancer: a prospective study. *Eur J Cancer* 2002;38(9):1189–1193.
65. Nicolini A, Tartarelli G, Carpi A, et al. Intensive post-operative follow-up of breast cancer patients with tumour markers: CEA, TPA or CA 15.3 vs. MCA and MCA-CA 15.3 vs CEA-TPA-CA 15.3 panel in the early detection of distant metastases. *BMC Cancer* 2006;6:269.
66. Carlson RW, Anderson BO, Burstein HJ, et al. The NCCN invasive breast cancer clinical practice guidelines in oncology. *J Natl Compr Cancer Netw* 2007(5):246–312.
67. Grunfeld E, Dhesy-Thind S, Levine M. Clinical practice guidelines for the care and treatment of breast cancer: follow-up after treatment for breast cancer (summary of the 2005 update). *Can Med Assoc J* 2005;172(10):1319–1320.
68. Harris L, Fritsche H, Mennel R, et al. American Society of Clinical Oncology 2007 update of recommendations for the use of tumor markers in breast cancer. *J Clin Oncol* 2007;25(33):5287–5312.
69. Pestalozzi B. Primary breast cancer: ESMO clinical recommendations for diagnosis, treatment and follow-up. *Ann Oncol* 2007;18[Suppl 2]:ii5–ii8.
70. Front D, Schneck SO, Frankel A, et al. Bone metastases and bone pain in breast cancer. Are they closely associated? *JAMA* 1979;242(16):1747–1748.
71. Schutte HE. The influence of bone pain on the results of bone scans. *Cancer* 1979; 44(6):2039–2043.
72. Wickerham L, Fisher B, Cronin W, et al. The efficacy of bone scanning in the follow-up of patients with operable breast cancer. *Breast Cancer Res Treat* 1984;4:303–307.
73. Chaudary MA, Maisey MN, Shaw PJ, et al. Sequential bone scans and chest radiographs in the postoperative management of early breast cancer. *Br J Surg* 1983; 70(9):517–518.
74. Engelhard K, Hollenbach HP, Wohlfart K, et al. Comparison of whole-body MRI with automatic moving table technique and bone scintigraphy for screening for bone metastases in patients with breast cancer. *Eur Radiol* 2004;14(1):99–105.

75. Kokko R, Hakama M, Holli K. Role of chest x-ray in diagnosis of the first breast cancer relapse: a randomized trial. *Breast Cancer Res Treat* 2003;81(1):33–39.

76. Mellemkjaer L, Friis S, Olsen JH, et al. Risk of second cancer among women with breast cancer. *Int J Cancer* 2006;118(9):2285–2292.

77. Valagussa P, Moliterni A, Terenziani M, et al. Second malignancies following CMF-based adjuvant chemotherapy in resectable breast cancer. *Ann Oncol* 1994;5(9):803–808.

78. Smith RE, Bryant J, DeCillis A, et al. Acute myeloid leukemia and myelodysplastic syndrome after doxorubicin-cyclophosphamide adjuvant therapy for operable breast cancer: the National Surgical Adjuvant Breast and Bowel Project experience. *J Clin Oncol* 2003;21(7):1195–1204.

79. Fisher B, Costantino JP, Redmond CK, et al. Endometrial cancer in tamoxifen-treated breast cancer patients: findings from the National Surgical Adjuvant Breast and Bowel Project (NSABP) B-14. *J Natl Cancer Inst* 1994;86(7):527–537.

80. ACOG committee opinion. No. 336: tamoxifen and uterine cancer. *Obstet Gynecol* 2006;107(6):1475–1478.

81. Howell A, Cuzick J, Baum M, et al. Results of the ATAC (Arimidex, tamoxifen, alone or in combination) trial after completion of 5 years' adjuvant treatment for breast cancer. *Lancet* 2005;365(9453):60–62.

82. Coombes RC, Hall E, Gibson LJ, et al. A randomized trial of exemestane after two to three years of tamoxifen therapy in postmenopausal women with primary breast cancer. *N Engl J Med* 2004;350(11):1081–1092.

83. Goss PE, Ingle JN, Martino S, et al. Randomized trial of letrozole following tamoxifen as extended adjuvant therapy in receptor-positive breast cancer: updated findings from NCIC CTG MA.17. *J Natl Cancer Inst* 2005;97(17):1262–1271.

84. Rosselli Del Turco M, Palli D, Cariddi A, et al. Intensive diagnostic follow-up after treatment of primary breast cancer. A randomized trial. National Research Council Project on Breast Cancer follow-up. *JAMA* 1994;271(20):1593–1597.

85. Palli D, Russo A, Saieva C, et al. Intensive vs clinical follow-up after treatment of primary breast cancer: 10-year update of a randomized trial. National Research Council Project on Breast Cancer Follow-up. *JAMA* 1999;281(17):1586.

86. Kokko R, Hakama M, Holli K. Follow-up cost of breast cancer patients with localized disease after primary treatment: a randomized trial. *Breast Cancer Res Treat* 2005;93(3):255–260.

87. Gulliford T, Opomu M, Wilson E, et al. Popularity of less frequent follow-up for breast cancer in randomised study: initial findings from the hotline study. *BMJ* 1997;314(7075):174–177.

88. Grunfeld E, Mant D, Yudkin P, et al. Routine follow-up of breast cancer in primary care: randomised trial. *BMJ* 1996;313(7058):665–669.

89. Grunfeld E, Levine MN, Julian JA, et al. Randomized trial of long-term follow-up for early-stage breast cancer: a comparison of family physician versus specialist care. *J Clin Oncol* 2006;24(6):848–855.

90. Keating NL, Landrum MB, Guadagnoli E, et al. Factors related to underuse of surveillance mammography among breast cancer survivors. *J Clin Oncol* 2006;24(1):85–94.

91. Keating NL, Landrum MB, Guadagnoli E, et al. Surveillance testing among survivors of early-stage breast cancer. *J Clin Oncol* 2007;25(9):1074–1081.

92. Donnelly P, Hiller L, Bathers S, et al. Questioning specialists' attitudes to breast cancer follow-up in primary care. *Ann Oncol* 2007;18(9):1467–1476.

93. Muss HB, Tell GS, Case LD, et al. Perceptions of follow-up care in women with breast cancer. *Am J Clin Oncol* 1991;14(1):55–59.

Tari A. King

The traditional dogma that surgery is reserved for the palliation of symptoms in stage IV breast cancer is being challenged by advances in breast cancer diagnosis and treatment. Widespread mammographic screening and increased awareness have resulted in fewer patients presenting with inoperable disease, improved imaging technologies have resulted in the detection of low-volume metastatic disease in patients who would have previously been classified as having earlier stage disease, and improved efficacy of modern chemotherapy regimens, including the use of targeted hormonal and biologic therapies, has resulted in prolonged survival for women with metastatic disease. Thus, in modern breast cancer treatment, the goals of therapy for patients with metastatic disease often extend beyond palliation; however, the role of local treatment in this setting remains untested.

Although the mean survival for patients with metastatic breast cancer remains 18 to 24 months, the range of survival extends from a few months to many years, and recent reports of improved survival in the more recent decades of treatment raises the possibility of cure for a select group of patients in the future. Andre et al. (1) reported survival rates over two time periods for 724 consecutive breast cancer patients presenting with metastatic disease at diagnosis; overall 3-year survival for patients treated from 1987 to 1993 was 27%, which increased to 44% for those treated from 1994 to 2000. Patient age, sites of metastases, number of organs involved, and hormone receptor status were similar in the two time periods, suggesting that the survival trend was related to treatment advances that occurred after 1993. Notably, 76% of patients diagnosed during the later time period and living at least 3 years received either a taxane (46%) or an aromatase inhibitor (63%). Giordano et al. (2) also demonstrated a trend toward improved survival with more recent year of recurrence and treatment in a multivariate analysis of 834 women who developed recurrent breast cancer between 1974 and 2000. Each more recent year of recurrence was associated with a 1% per year reduction in the risk of death. Neither of these two data sets included the benefits obtained from newer therapies such as trastuzumab and bevacizumab, yet both demonstrate that improvements in systemic therapy have resulted in demonstrable improvements in survival for patients with metastatic disease.

Targeted therapy with the monoclonal antibody trastuzumab has further improved both survival and quality of life in patients with ERBB2 (formerly HER-2/neu) positive metastatic breast cancer (3). The randomized trial that clearly confirmed the activity of trastuzumab in the metastatic setting (4) represents the value of translational science in the modern era. The combined efforts from the laboratory to elucidate the biologic role of ERBB2, and the early clinical trials, which demonstrated the importance of patient selection based on amplification of the ERBB2 gene, were critical to the success of this therapy and highlight the need to address breast cancer in biologically meaningful subtypes (see Chapters 30 and 51 for a detailed discussion). Whether or not this rationale can be applied to the role of local surgery in the setting of metastatic disease is now a matter of great interest and debate.

HISTORICAL PERSPECTIVE

Conventional wisdom suggests that surgical excision of the primary tumor is unlikely to offer the patient any survival advantage and therefore should be reserved for the palliation of symptoms. However, this approach stems from a time before modern advances in systemic treatments and supportive care. Patients with metastatic cancer were often debilitated, not considered fit for general anesthesia, and often had bulky tumors in the breast and axilla that required extensive surgical procedures for complete extirpation. Survival after the diagnosis of metastatic disease was often brief, leading to the desire to avoid unnecessary morbidity from surgery during the remaining year of life. In the modern era this concern is largely outdated, as many patients will experience a significant interval of remission with initiation of therapy (5), with far fewer side effects from therapy, and the morbidity of common surgical procedures for breast cancer remains exceedingly low (6).

Other historical arguments against surgery have included the desire to follow easily measurable disease for response to therapy, and the fear that removal of the primary tumor would result in increased angiogenesis and growth of otherwise dormant metastatic disease (7,8). Animal models suggests that resection of the primary tumor may be accompanied by release of growth-enhancing factors and induction of temporary immunosuppression (9,10). Further, circulating antiangiogenic factors such as angiostatin and endostatin are felt to result directly or indirectly from the presence of the primary tumor, and function to at least partially control angiogenesis of existing dormant micrometastatic tumors (11). According to the angiogenesis concept, upon removal of the primary tumor, angiogenesis is switched on and dormant cells begin to grow. Although this has been documented in the Lewis lung animal model (8), there are few data to support a negative impact of surgery-induced tumor growth changes in humans. Therefore, surgery has maintained a primary role in the treatment of most neoplasms, and its effect on residual tumor growth dynamics remains an area of investigation.

CURRENT PERSPECTIVE

It is now quite clear that local control does impact survival in stage I to III breast cancer, and this is particularly evident in patients with positive nodes and those at higher risk of local relapse (12). If preventing local recurrence decreases the incidence of distant relapse in earlier-stage disease, a natural extension of this argument is to consider whether optimizing local control, by removal of the intact primary tumor, may benefit select patients with metastatic disease. In 2002 Khan et al. (13) first challenged the traditional thinking with a report of 16,023 patients presenting between 1990 and 1993 with stage IV disease as captured by the National Cancer Database (NCDB) of the American College of Surgeons. Surprisingly, this database, which reflects a cross-section of cancer treatment around the country, revealed that 9,162 (57.2%) patients underwent either partial (3,513) or total mastectomy (5,649) in the setting of stage IV disease, and surgical removal of the primary tumor was associated with a 39% reduction in the risk of death. Adding further support to the argument for local control, women treated surgically with clear margins had a 3-year survival of 35%, as compared to 26% for those with positive margins, and 17% for those not having surgery ($p < .0001$). Additional studies, both population-based and single-institution series, examining survival outcomes relative to surgical resection of the intact primary tumor, have reported remarkably similar results (Table 71.1).

A population-based study was published in 2006 from the Geneva Cancer Registry by Rapiti et al. (14). The authors measured the impact of surgical therapy of the primary tumor on survival in 300 women with metastatic breast cancer at the time of initial diagnosis. Women having surgery with negative margins had a 50% reduction in breast cancer mortality compared to women who did not undergo surgery (5-year breast cancer specific survival, 27% vs. 12%; $p = .0002$). Interestingly, the survival benefit was not seen for women with positive or unknown margins (5-year breast cancer specific survival: 16% and 12%, respectively). The authors also stratified by site of metastasis and found that the positive effect of surgery with negative margins was particularly evident for women with bone-only metastases (multiadjusted hazard ratio, 0.2; 95% confidence interval [CI], 0.1–0.4; $p = .001$). In both the Rapiti et al. publication and the Khan et al. series, the survival benefit for surgery with negative margins persisted after adjusting for confounding factors such as number of metastatic sites, location of metastases (visceral vs. bone and soft tissue), and type of systemic therapy; however, neither series was able to demonstrate a survival benefit for axillary surgery. Rapiti et al. also observed improved survival in patients diagnosed in more recent time periods. The hazard ratio for death was 0.6 (95% CI, 0.4–0.9; $p < .01$) for those diagnosed between 1992 and 1996, as compared with those diagnosed between 1977 and 1981 (15).

Similarly, Gnerlich et al. (16) examined 1988 to 2003 National Cancer Institute Surveillance, Epidemiology, and End Results (SEER) program data and also found a survival advantage for surgical removal of the primary tumor. In this study, median survival was significantly longer for those women having surgery who were still alive at the end of the study period (36 vs. 21 months; $p < .001$) and for those who died during the study period (18 vs. 7 months; $p < .001$). Controlling for demographic and clinical factors associated with survival on univariate analysis (age, race, marital status, tumor size, tumor grade, estrogen/progesterone [ER/PR] status, year of diagnosis, and receipt of radiation treatment) and for propensity scores, which described the predicted probability of having surgery, women with metastatic breast cancer having surgery were 37% less likely to die during the study period than women who did not undergo surgery.

Acknowledging the well-known limitations of a population database such as SEER, the authors of this series also conducted a single institution retrospective review of 409 patients with stage IV breast cancer treated at the Washington University Medical Center from 1996 to 2005 (17). This single institution series again confirmed the findings from the two previously published population-based series and the multi-institutional convenience sample NCDB, demonstrating that surgical resection was performed in about half the women presenting with stage IV disease and was associated with an approximate halving of the hazard ratio (aHR) of death during the follow-up period in multivariate analyses (aHR, 0.53; 95% CI, 0.42–0.67).

Although all retrospective studies are subject to patient selection bias, an advantage of single institution series is their ability to provide greater detail regarding the specifics of treatment, the course of the disease, and other patient factors. The Washington University series included an adult comorbidity evaluation

(ACE-27) score that categorizes comorbid conditions as none, mild, moderate, and severe; and they found that this score was not significantly predictive of survival in patients with metastatic breast cancer (17). They also included patients who underwent surgery at any point in their disease course, and in about half of the cases (53%), surgery was undertaken to palliate symptoms associated with the primary lesion. In contrast, 43% of patients were believed to undergo surgery in the setting of unknown metastatic disease, which was then discovered on subsequent staging examination performed within 1 month of surgery. In a related report of 111 women with stage IV breast cancer treated at Northwestern Memorial Hospital (1995 to 2005), 47 (42%) patients underwent surgery for the primary tumor, 26 of whom (55%) underwent surgery prior to staging (18). Unfortunately, the frequency with which unsuspected metastatic disease is diagnosed after surgery is not ascertainable from population-based registries, yet this may partially account for the finding that younger patients with smaller tumors were more likely to undergo surgical resection in all reported series. Alternatively, surgery may be a surrogate for more aggressive therapy overall in select patients with metastatic disease.

Data from single institution series can also be used to generate hypotheses about which subsets of patients may benefit from more aggressive local therapy. Fields et al. (17) found that women with bone-only metastatic disease lived longer than those with metastases at other sites, regardless of whether surgical resection was performed (aHR 0.76; 95% CI, 0.58–0.98). This is consistent with the known indolent course of osseous metastases and supports the findings from the stratified analysis of the Geneva Cancer Registry (14). In a retrospective analysis of 224 patients presenting to the M.D. Anderson Cancer Center (MDACC) with stage IV disease and an intact primary tumor or following recent (within 3 months) removal of the primary tumor with stage IV disease, Babiera et al. (19) identified 82 patients (37%) who underwent primary tumor removal in addition to systemic treatments. In this series, surgery was associated with a trend toward improvement in overall survival (risk ratio [RR] 0.50; 95% CI, 0.21–1.19) and a significant improvement in metastatic progression-free survival (RR 0.54; 95% CI, 0.38–0.77). Independent predictors of survival included the presence of only one metastatic site and *ERBB2* amplification. Surgical indications included excision for diagnosis in 29 patients, definitive treatment to the breast in 41, palliation in 7, and other reasons in 5. Of the 41 patients who underwent definitive surgery, 11 (27%) underwent surgery with curative intent, including treatment of metastatic sites with surgery, systemic therapy, or both. To eliminate potential bias associated with inclusion of these 11 aggressively treated patients, they were excluded in a second analysis of survival, and the benefit of surgery in prolonging metastatic progression-free survival persisted, prompting these authors to suggest that surgically achieved local control can lead to improved survival as part of multimodality therapy in select patients.

Similarly, Blanchard et al. (20) reported on 395 women with stage IV breast cancer from an existing database at the Baylor College of Medicine. Of these, 242 (61%) underwent surgical resection of the primary tumor as part of their initial therapy. The interval from diagnosis to death was 27.1 months for the surgical group and 16.8 months for the nonsurgical group ($p < .0001$). Other factors that were also significant in their final multivariate model included surgical therapy (HR = 0.7; 95% CI, 0.56–0.91; $p = .006$), ER positivity (HR = 0.6; 95% CI, 0.45–0.81; $p = .001$), PR positivity (HR = 0.7; 95% CI, 0.53–0.86; $p = .002$), and the number of metastatic sites (HR = 1.3; 95% CI, 1.07–1.51; $p = .006$) (18,20,21).

In total, these studies consistently demonstrate that about half of women presenting with *de novo* metastatic breast cancer undergo resection of the primary tumor and suggest that

Table 71.1 RESULTS OF STUDIES EXAMINING SURVIVAL OUTCOMES RELATIVE TO SURGICAL RESECTION OF THE PRIMARY TUMOR IN STAGE IV BREAST CANCER

Study (Reference)	Years	Source	n	No. of Patients Who Had Surgery	Tumor Size[a] T1/2 (%)	T3/4 (%)	Type of Surgery Mastectomy[b] (%)	Partial Mastectomy (%)	Free Margins (%)	Follow-Up Duration	Primary End Point	Findings Adjusted HR in Surgical Group (95% CI)	Risk ratio Surgical Group (95% CI)
Khan et al., 2002 (13)	1990–1993	NCDB	16,024	9,162 (57.2%)	45.7	43.1	61.7	38.3	37[c]	—	OS	0.6 (0.58–0.65)	—
Rapiti et al., 2006 (14)	1976–1996	Geneva Cancer Registry	300	127 (42.3%)	31.0	53.7	68.5	31.5	48	—	5-yr DSS[d]	0.6 (0.4–1.0)	—
Babiera et al., 2006 (19)	1997–2002	MDACC	244	82 (33.6%)	38.4	49.5	52.4	47.6	62	32.1 mos	OS PFS	—	0.5 (0.21–1.19) 0.54 (0.38–0.77)
Blanchard et al., 2008 (20)	1973–1991	Baylor College of Medicine	395	242 (61.3%)	22	78[e]	77.8	22.3	—	—	OS	0.71 (0.56–0.91)	—
Gnerlich et al., 2007 (16)	1988–2003	SEER	9,734	4,578 (47.0%)	58	28.1	54.3	40.3	NR	—	OS	0.63 (0.60–0.66)	—
Fields et al., 2007 (17)	1996–2005	Washington University	409	187 (45.7%)	43.9	47.1	55.1	32.6	49	142 mos	OS	0.53 (0.42–0.67)	—

HR, hazard ratio; CI, confidence interval; NCBD, National Cancer Database Study; OS, overall survival; DSS, disease-specific survival; MDACC, M.D. Anderson Cancer Center; PFS, progression-free survival; SEER, National Cancer Institute Surveillance, Epidemiology, and End Results; NR, not reported.

[a] Tumor size data reported for patients undergoing surgery.
[b] Includes total mastectomy, modified radical mastectomy and radical mastectomy.
[c] Data available for 5,957 (69.5%) of surgery group.
[d] Breast-cancer specific.
[e] Reported as tumors >2 cm and tumors ≤2 cm.

women undergoing surgery survive longer than those treated without resection. Although all available studies are retrospective and therefore inherently biased by the inability to control for patient selection and other treatment factors, they provide evidence that the dogma to reserve surgery only for the palliation of symptoms in stage IV disease has been largely ignored and may be outdated. However, with the limited data that exist, it is not clear whether it is extent of metastatic disease, the sensitivity to chemotherapy, or some combination of these factors that may predict which patients are most likely to benefit from surgical resection of the primary tumor (15). It is clear, however, that critical evaluation of whether surgically achieved local control can lead to improved survival in this setting deserves consideration.

RATIONALE FOR RESECTION OF THE PRIMARY

Why was surgical resection performed in nearly 50% of patients with stage IV breast cancer in all reported series? There are few available data documenting physician or patient behavior in this setting, yet it is not unreasonable to assume that "fear of advanced local-regional disease" or perhaps patient preference to "get rid of the cancer" would be cited as possible indications for surgery. Combined with the rationale that major complications from breast surgery are infrequent, the risk compares favorably with toxicity profiles of many systemic therapy agents used in the metastatic setting, perhaps adding to the appeal of surgical local control. In a retrospective review of surgical practice patterns over a 15-year period at Memorial Sloan-Kettering Cancer Center (MSKCC) (22), the frequency of mastectomy in the setting of any stage IV disease remained stable at 1.7% of all mastectomies performed, yet the indication for mastectomy as cited by the treating surgeon changed over time. The rate of traditional "toilet" mastectomy or mastectomy performed for "symptoms" of local disease decreased from 41% to 25% between the two time periods analyzed (1990 to 1995 and 2000 to 2005), while rates of "local control" mastectomy increased from 34% to 66%. These time trend data included patients with recurrent and *de novo* stage IV disease and did not include information pertaining to other treatment modalities. Among 84 patients presenting with *de novo* stage IV disease from the same study, a more detailed review of treatment data demonstrated that the most frequent indication for surgery of the primary tumor was to "optimize local control" in the setting of a complete, good, or stable response of distant disease to systemic therapy. Surgery was performed for symptom control in 30 of 84 (36%) patients in this series presenting with *de novo* stage IV disease.

It is well documented that overall survival after a diagnosis of stage IV breast cancer is largely determined by the site of metastases (i.e., less than 6 months for visceral disease, approximately 18 months for regional-nodal disease, and 3 to 4 years for bony metastases) (23). Although these time periods may shift toward longer intervals with improvements in systemic therapy, one cannot assume that the primary tumor will respond to systemic therapy in parallel with metastatic sites of disease, and progressive local disease may lead to impaired quality of life and the need for palliation. The true frequency with which unresected local disease becomes a "local control" problem or "symptom control" problem requiring surgery in the modern era is difficult to ascertain without prospective collection of patient information. Single-institution series are biased by the treatment culture of the institution, and detailed indications for surgery are not available from population-based databases. Hazard et al. have suggested that it may be reasonable to assume that complete resection of the primary tumor would be protective against uncontrolled chest wall disease, but data are limited. In their report from Northwestern they found that surgery was strongly protective against symptomatic chest wall disease in 47 patients with stage IV breast cancer undergoing surgery either at diagnosis or following response to systemic therapy, as compared to 64 patients managed either nonoperatively or with delayed (palliative) surgery (odds ratio [OR] 0.14; 95% CI, 0.04–0.5; $p = .002$) (18). Ultimately, 23 of 64 patients (36%) required delayed local palliation. Further adjusting for survival by chest wall status, with or without the use of surgery, and controlling for other potential confounding factors, they found that a control of disease on the chest wall mediated the survival benefit of surgical resection in this patient cohort. This again supports the hypothesis that optimizing local control may impact survival in patients with distant disease.

Other reports also suggest that when surgery is performed for local control, the results are generally favorable. In the MSKCC series, among 256 patients with *de novo* or recurrent stage IV breast cancer undergoing a local surgical procedure (1995 to 2005), 128 procedures were performed to optimize local control in the setting of favorable or stable response to systemic therapy (22). The median time from stage IV diagnosis to surgery for this group of patients was 11.7 months (range, 0 to 75.2) and at a median follow-up of 35 months, 73 patients (57%) remained alive, 11 of whom had evidence of recurrent local disease. Among the 55 patients who died during the follow-up period, 14 died with recurrent local disease. Carmichael et al. (24) also reported good control of local disease in 20 patients with metastatic disease undergoing breast surgery following or immediately prior to systemic therapy. In this series, only 3 of 10 patients who died had local disease at the time of death.

The consistent benefit for surgery demonstrated in all reports of *de novo* stage IV breast cancer is also consistent with an increasing body of evidence that local therapy impacts on survival for breast cancer patients with stage I to III disease. This relationship was first suspected from analyses of the patterns of local and distant recurrence in the early breast conservation trials, which suggested that local recurrences were predictive of distant metastases (25,26). Prospective randomized trials of postmastectomy radiotherapy followed, demonstrating that local therapy in the form of chest wall and node field irradiation prolonged survival in node-positive women receiving tamoxifen or chemotherapy (27–29). Finally, in the Oxford Overview Analysis, the use of radiotherapy after lumpectomy or after mastectomy in node-positive women significantly reduced the risk of local recurrence, which translated into improved survival after 15 years of follow-up (12). Although concerns have been raised regarding the extent of surgery and chemotherapy regimens used in some of these studies, when viewed in total, these data suggest that uncontrolled local disease may act as a source of tumor reseeding, diminishing the effectiveness of systemic therapy.

Additional support for the rationale of optimizing local control includes the identification of a larger population of patients with oligometastatic or low volume metastatic disease, many of whom would have been treated aggressively for cure in the era before widespread magnetic resonance imaging (MRI) and positron emission tomography (PET) (30,31). The natural history of this category of stage IV breast cancer is largely unknown, yet conceptually they may not be very different from patients with earlier stage disease who are found to harbor occult bone marrow micrometastases (32). Studies suggest that bone marrow micrometastases are present in up to 30% of stages I to III patients at the time of diagnosis and are associated with a poor overall survival and breast cancer disease-free survival (33), yet surgical treatment and adjuvant therapy are routinely performed in these patients, resulting in a significant number of long-term survivors.

Hortobagyi (34) has also suggested that an aggressive multimodal approach that includes surgery produces long-term, disease-free survival or cure in a subset of patients with limited metastatic breast cancer. These long-term survivors with stage IV disease are typically young, with limited metastatic disease and excellent performance status (34,35). Holmes et al. (36) reported a 15-year disease-free survival rate of 24% in 134 patients with solitary locoregional recurrences or metastases treated with surgical resection, with or without radiation therapy, followed by systemic chemotherapy and hormonal therapy. At a maximum follow-up of 26 years, only two additional breast cancer events had occurred (37). Related reports from Borner et al. (38) and from Nieto et al. (39) provide additional evidence that an aggressive multimodality approach can significantly increase disease-free survival in selected patients with limited metastatic breast cancer. Nieto et al. reported the outcome of 60 patients with minimal recurrent or metastatic disease treated with surgery and/or radiation therapy, high-dose chemotherapy, and autologous hematopoietic stem cell support. Among this group were 17 patients with distant metastatic disease at the time of diagnosis. At a median follow-up of 62 months, 51.6% of the entire patient group (95% CI, 39%–64%) remained alive and free of disease. In the patients with metastatic disease at presentation, 46% were alive and free of disease. Although limited, these data support the validity of testing an aggressive multimodality approach in the more modern era of breast cancer treatment in select patients with *de novo* stage IV disease.

An analogous situation is the breast cancer patient with a solitary recurrence or metastatic lesion that is resected surgically or treated with radiotherapy at curative doses, rendering them stage IV NED (no evidence of disease). Although this again represents a minority of patients with metastatic disease, a review by Singletary et al. (40) demonstrates that surgery combined with adjuvant therapy, compared with radiation or systemic therapy alone, can result in significantly better survival in select patients with metastatic disease to the lung, liver, brain, or sternum. Across the four disease sites (lung, liver, brain, bone), better patient outcomes after surgery were associated with good performance status, long disease-free interval after treatment of the primary tumor, complete resection of the tumor, and restriction of metastasis to single tumors or to a single site. Given the improved efficacy of modern chemotherapy and the benefits gained from locoregional treatment with surgery, now demonstrated in a variety of settings in both early and late-stage disease, many authors agree that it is time to re-evaluate the role of surgical excision of the intact primary in select patients with stage IV disease (13–17,19,22,32).

Additional theoretical advantages for removing the primary tumor include cessation of tumor cell seeding into the circulation and decreasing the overall tumor burden. The level of circulating tumor cells (CTC) before treatment is an independent predictor of progression-free survival and overall survival in patients with metastatic breast cancer, and patients who experience a decrease in the level of CTC after the initiation of therapy have a better prognosis than those who do not (41). New concepts of metastases also suggest that ongoing seeding from both the primary tumor and distant sites may be an important mechanism of continued tumor growth and metastases (42). Further, support for decreasing tumor burden or debulking in other malignancies, including ovarian (43), colorectal (44), melanoma (45), gastric (46), and renal cell cancer (47), continues to emerge. Whether or not these theories are valid in the setting of metastatic breast cancer with an intact primary is uncertain and await further investigation into the biology of metastases and the relation to the primary tumor.

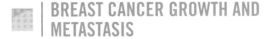

BREAST CANCER GROWTH AND METASTASIS

The growth mechanisms of breast cancer have important implications both biologically and clinically. The fundamental question that has been debated over the past century is whether breast cancer is a *local* disease that spreads in an orderly fashion and becomes systemic, or whether breast cancer is a *systemic* disease at its inception. These two opposing theories, classically referred to as the Halstead and Fisher paradigms, formed the basis for breast cancer treatment in the 20th century. The increasing acceptance of the Fisher paradigm over Halstead's theory resulted in a shift away from more radical surgery to increasing use of systemic therapies in recent decades; however, the increasing body of evidence demonstrating that local control does impact survival suggests that the truth is likely in the middle. Breast cancer may be, but is not universally, systemic at its inception, and local-regional treatments are important.

At present, metastatic disease is largely incurable and remains so due to a limited understanding of the molecular mechanisms of metastasis. The conventional model teaches that most primary tumor cells have a low metastatic potential; however, during later stages of tumorigenesis, rare subpopulations of cells within the primary tumor may acquire advantageous genetic alterations, which enable these cells to metastasize and form new solid tumors at distant sites (48). Yet experimental findings do not always support this conventional model. For example, tumor cells derived from metastases do not always have greater metastatic potential than those isolated from the corresponding tumor (49–51), and there is no consistent relationship between metastatic potential and tumor size (52). As a result, different hypotheses have been put forward to reconcile these discrepancies, such as the *dynamic heterogeneity model*, which proposes that metastatic subpopulations are generated at high rates in a primary tumor, but that these variants are relatively unstable, resulting in a dynamic equilibrium between the generation and the loss of metastatic variants (53,54), and the *clonal dominance theory*, which proposes that once a metastatic subclone emerges within a primary tumor, the progeny of this subclone overgrows and dominates the tumor mass itself (55,56). But no direct evidence of these models have been documented in human tumors, leading one to question whether findings made in animals and *in vitro* models can be compared to metastasis of breast tumors in patients (57).

In the genomic era, new concepts of metastatic dissemination have been proposed. The ability of gene-expression profiles of human primary breast cancers to predict metastatic potential (58,59) suggests that the ability to metastasize is an early and perhaps inherent, genetically predetermined property of the primary tumor cell. Support for this concept includes the finding of similar gene expression profiles from pairs of human primary breast tumors and their distant metastases (60), as well as similar gene expression patterns between premalignant, preinvasive, and invasive breast cancers (61). Kang et al. (62) have further proposed a variation of this model, which states that within the population of tumor cells with metastatic capacity, as defined by a poor prognosis signature, subpopulations of cells also have a superimposed tissue-specific gene-expression profile that predicts the site of metastasis. Mathematical models have expanded this theory, suggesting that not only does this "escapee" cell have the capacity to seed distant sites, but it may also metastasize back to the primary tumor (self-seed), thereby contributing both to the ongoing growth and destruction at the site of primary disease, as well as to an ever-growing source of disseminating tumor cells (42). Within the context of metastatic breast cancer, this theory of self-seeding would strongly support complete excision of the primary tumor.

The analysis of human disseminated cancer cells has led to another model, termed the *parallel evolution model*, which proposes that the dissemination of metastatic cancer cells occurs early and is independent from tumor cells at the primary site (63). This theory is based on the finding that disseminated tumor cells in the bone marrow of patients without metastatic disease do not share the same genomic abnormalities as cells from the primary tumor; however, in patients with known metastatic disease, these cells are similar to the primary tumor. This theory challenges the concept of clonal genomic evolution, yet the true biologic potential, and therefore clinical significance, of disseminated cells found in the bone marrow of patients with early stage disease is unknown, and multimodal therapy, including surgery, remains standard care for these patients (57).

Finally, there is an emerging body of evidence supporting the *cancer stem cell theory*. This theory proposes that rare cells with indefinite proliferative potential are responsible for the formation and growth of tumors (64). Further, these specialized tumor-initiating stem cells have the exclusive potential to proliferate and form new sites of tumor metastasis (65), perhaps providing an explanation for the so-called tumor dormancy phenomenon (57). Experimentally, these cells represent only a minority of human breast cancer cells, and recent advances that allow them to be identified with immunohistochemistry-based assays for cell surface marker expression promise to provide greater detail regarding their true role in tumorigenesis (66).

In contrast to the conventional model, the newer concepts of metastases all support removal of the primary tumor to reduce either self-seeding, tumor cell dissemination, or the population of native cancer stem cells, followed by effective systemic therapy. Clinical trials to validate these models will require a shift in physicians' approach to the stage IV patient. Other areas of investigation that may contribute to the understanding of the role of local treatment in metastatic disease include the study of the tumor microenvironment and the immune system. Primary tumors frequently express genes whose products alter the microenvironment, such as extracellular matrix proteases, glycosylases, proangiogenesis factors, regulators of cell adhesion, and mediators of inflammation and angiogenesis (42). Gene expression signatures that include these genes predict for poor survival and have led investigators to evaluate therapeutic targets other than those involved with cell proliferation, such as trials combining chemotherapy with antiangiogenic agents. Data regarding the role of the immune system in the development or progression of breast cancer remain limited and largely unclear (67).

 ## FUTURE DIRECTIONS AND QUESTIONS

There is a biologic rationale that supports a proper evaluation of the role of surgery for the primary tumor in stage IV disease, and given the documentation of improved survival for women with stage IV breast cancer and the anticipation that survival for this group will continue to improve with newer targeted systemic agents, the question of whether or not improved local control impacts survival in this setting is increasingly important. The question also has wider implications than the specific population of women who present with *de novo* metastases, such as for those women who present with a synchronous in-breast recurrence and distant metastases. Critics of the available data point to the inherent selection bias of retrospective analysis, and in current practice clinicians are left with many unanswered questions regarding

the who, what, and when of local treatment in the metastatic setting.

The importance of patient selection is evident in all aspects of breast cancer treatment, from choosing appropriate candidates for breast conservation, postmastectomy radiation therapy, hormonal therapy, and trastuzumab; hence future studies are needed to identify those patients most likely to benefit from surgery for the intact primary in stage IV disease. Traditional criteria for analysis include extent and type of metastatic disease, sensitivity to chemotherapy, and size of primary tumor. Published data suggest that women with bone-only disease may benefit the most from surgical resection of the primary, but in the absence of randomized data, physicians cannot distinguish if these women derive a survival benefit from surgery or if their improved outcomes are a reflection of the indolent course of their disease. Published data also identify smaller tumor size as a selection factor for surgical therapy, yet this may be a reflection of patient or physician bias toward more aggressive therapy overall in what appears to be a smaller burden of disease. Recent data from MDACC also suggest that response to neoadjuvant chemotherapy may predict improved survival with local therapy (68). Ongoing studies with the benefit of trastuzumab and continued research into the biology of metastases may identify new criteria for analyses, ultimately allowing for the identification of distinct biologic subtypes of stage IV disease most likely to benefit from local therapy.

What type of operation should be performed? Historically, surgery in stage IV disease was limited to palliation, hence the term *toilet mastectomy*; however, in the series from Rapiti et al. (14) and Khan et al. (13), 31% and 46% of all patients, respectively, had T1 and T2 tumors. Only 12% and 16% of all patients had T3 tumors (Table 71.1), suggesting that many primary tumors in patients with metastatic disease are amenable to treatment with lumpectomy, a procedure with very low morbidity. In breast conservation, published data provide consistent evidence that negative margins *plus* radiation therapy are important in local control. In the metastatic setting, data regarding regional radiotherapy are limited to the study by Rapiti et al. (14); however, in this series the lack of radiotherapy in women treated with lumpectomy was also independently associated with an increased hazard of death. Unfortunately, the use of local radiation cannot be distinguished from radiation to metastatic sites in the National Cancer Database Study or the SEER database study to further investigate this finding.

If removal of the primary tumor improves survival by reducing tumor burden, one might also assume that reduction of the tumor burden in the axillary nodes would be beneficial, yet it remains controversial as to whether there is a survival benefit for any patient with breast cancer who undergoes axillary dissection. This procedure continues to be performed, however, in stages I to III breast cancer, primarily for local control, and to obtain prognostic information and guide treatment. Available data in the metastatic setting are limited; in the Khan et al. (13) and the Rapiti et al. (14) series, neither were able to demonstrate a benefit for axillary dissection. It has been suggested that this was likely due to the small number of axillary dissections performed and their correlation with excision to negative margins (15). In a subsequent report from MDACC (69), among the 82 patients who underwent surgical intervention at the primary site in combination with appropriate systemic therapy, including trastuzumab, patients who underwent axillary lymph node dissection demonstrated a trend toward improved overall survival on univariate analysis compared to patients who underwent sentinel lymph node biopsy alone or no axillary surgery (log rank test, $p = .051$). Further study is needed to elucidate potential confounding factors and the value of axillary surgery in this setting.

The timing of surgery is also relevant to the hypothesis that local therapy of the primary tumor is beneficial. If the tumor functions as a source of new metastatic deposits, treating it early in the course would intuitively seem to have greater benefit. Here the data are also limited to the report from MDACC (69) where among the 82 patients who underwent surgical intervention at the primary site, patients having surgery 3 to 8.9 months after diagnosis or greater than 9 months after diagnosis had a longer metastatic progression-free survival that those having surgery within 3 months of diagnosis. However, there were several other significant differences between these surgical groups, such as use of chemotherapy or hormonal therapy alone, margin status, type of surgery, and indication for surgery, making it difficult to draw any meaningful conclusions. Thus second report of this patient population had a median follow-up of 36.1 months and also included ethnicity data. Multivariate analysis again confirmed that patients with fewer metastatic sites and those with negative margins had improved metastatic progression-free survival, as did patients of Caucasian ethnicity (69).

Whether or not surgery ultimately impacts survival in stage IV breast cancer, one cannot ignore its role in controlling symptomatic local disease. Limited data exist to describe the frequency with which surgical palliation is undertaken in the modern era, and published data range from a low of 9% (7 of 82 patients) undergoing palliation in the MDACC series (19) to 36% in both the MSKCC data set (22) and the Northwestern series (18), to 50% and 53% reported in the Edinburgh (24) and Washington University series (17), respectively. All of these figures are likely biased by the culture of the individual institution and the inherent inaccuracy of abstracting "subjective" information by retrospective chart review. Data regarding the frequency of recurrent local disease at time of death is limited to the Edinburgh report and the MSKCC report, both of which suggest that following surgical intervention, death with local disease is uncommon. In the MSKCC series, patients undergoing surgery for local control (n = 128) had an 11% incidence of death with recurrent local disease (median follow-up, 35 months), and patients undergoing surgery for palliation of symptoms (n = 49) had a 10% incidence of death with recurrent local disease (median follow-up, 29 months). Perhaps the strongest evidence to date in favor of surgery for local control is that from Hazard et al. (18) who reported that surgery is strongly protective against uncontrolled chest-wall disease, and further that a controlled chest wall mediates the survival benefit of surgical resection. These data await prospective validation.

 ## CLOSING REMARKS

As new insights into cancer biology are achieved in the laboratory, there has been a shift in our approach to systemic treatment for breast cancer with an increased focus on targeted therapy. Yet in the current era of improving survival with targeted systemic therapy, the role of local treatment in metastatic breast cancer remains untested. Recent observations suggest that local treatment may have a greater influence on breast cancer survival than previously thought. Emerging evidence suggests that for patients with limited metastatic disease, combining surgery, radiotherapy, and systemic therapy may provide a survival benefit. These data are also complimented by recent publications that suggest a potential survival benefit from complete excision of the primary tumor in select patients with metastatic breast cancer. These observations raise intriguing questions, and when viewed in parallel with the new biological concepts of breast cancer metastasis, they challenge the traditional surgical approach to stage IV disease.

MANAGEMENT SUMMARY

- Survival in patients with metastatic breast cancer is improving due to more sensitive imaging modalities, resulting in an increased rate of diagnosis in asymptomatic patients with a low disease burden, and to improvements in systemic therapy.
- The role of surgery of the intact primary tumor on survival in patients with metastatic disease is uncertain. Multiple retrospective studies suggest a survival benefit, but selection bias in these studies prohibits firm conclusions. Surgery is an effective means of maintaining local control on the chest wall during the patient's lifetime. Either mastectomy or lumpectomy are appropriate approaches when surgery is chosen. The data on axillary surgery are extremely limited, but if surgery is undertaken, removal of all gross disease seems prudent.
- The benefit of radiation therapy following surgery is also uncertain, and decisions regarding its use should be made on a case-by-case basis.
- Formal trials of this approach are urgently needed.

References

1. Andre F, Slimane K, Bachelot T, et al. Breast cancer with synchronous metastases: trends in survival during a 14-year period. *J Clin Oncol* 2004;22:3302–3308.
2. Giordano SH, Buzdar AU, Kau SW. Improvement in breast cancer survival: results from M.D. Anderson Cancer Center Protocols from 1975–2000. *Proc Am Soc Clin Oncol* 2002:54a.
3. Slamon DJ, Clark GM, Wong SG, et al. Human breast cancer: correlation of relapse and survival with amplification of the *HER-2/neu* oncogene. *Science* 1987;235:177–182.
4. Slamon DJ, Leyland-Jones B, Shak S, et al. Use of chemotherapy plus a monoclonal antibody against HER2 for metastatic breast cancer that overexpresses *HER2*. *N Engl J Med* 2001;344:783–792.
5. Ellis NJ, Hayes DF, Lippman ME. Treatment of metastatic breast cancer. In: Harris JR, Lippman ME, Morrow M, et al., eds. *Diseases of the breast*. 3rd ed. Baltimore: Lippincott Williams & Wilkins, 2004:1101–1159.
6. El-Tamer MB, Ward BM, Schifftner T, et al. Morbidity and mortality following breast cancer surgery in women: national benchmarks for standards of care. *Ann Surg* 2007;245:665–671.
7. Fisher B, Fisher ER. Experimental evidence in support of the dormant tumor cell. *Science* 1959;130:918–919.
8. O'Reilly MS, Holmgren L, Shing Y, et al. Angiostatin: a novel angiogenesis inhibitor that mediates the suppression of metastases by a Lewis lung carcinoma. *Cell* 1994; 79:315–328.
9. Fisher B, Gunduz N, Coyle J, et al. Presence of a growth-stimulating factor in serum following primary tumor removal in mice. *Cancer Res* 1989;49:1996–2001.
10. Pollock RE, Lotzova E, Stanford SD. Effect of surgical stress on murine natural killer cell cytotoxicity. *J Immunol* 1987;138:171–178.
11. Folkman J. Angiogenesis in cancer, vascular, rheumatoid and other disease. *Nat Med* 1995;1:27–31.
12. Clarke M, Collins R, Darby S, et al. Effects of radiotherapy and of differences in the extent of surgery for early breast cancer on local recurrence and 15-year survival: an overview of the randomised trials. *Lancet* 2005;366:2087–2106.
13. Khan SA, Stewart AK, Morrow M. Does aggressive local therapy improve survival in metastatic breast cancer? *Surgery* 2002;132:620–627.
14. Rapiti E, Verkooijen HM, Vlastos G, et al. Complete excision of primary breast tumor improves survival of patients with metastatic breast cancer at diagnosis. *J Clin Oncol* 2006;24:2743–2749.
15. Morrow M, Goldstein L. Surgery of the primary tumor in metastatic breast cancer: closing the barn door after the horse has bolted? *J Clin Oncol* 2006;24:2694–2696.
16. Gnerlich J, Jeffe DB, Deshpande AD, et al. Surgical removal of the primary tumor increases overall survival in patients with metastatic breast cancer: analysis of the 1988–2003 SEER data. *Ann Surg Oncol* 2007;14:2187–2194.
17. Fields RC, Jeffe DB, Trinkaus K, et al. Surgical resection of the primary tumor is associated with increased long-term survival in patients with stage IV breast cancer after controlling for site of metastasis. *Ann Surg Oncol* 2007;14:3345–3351.
18. Hazard HW, Gorla SR, Scholtens D, Kiel K, Gradishar WJ, Khan SA. Surgical resection of the primary tumor, chest wall control, and survival in women with metastatic breast cancer. *Cancer* 2008;113(8):2011–2019.
19. Babiera GV, Rao R, Feng L, et al. Effect of primary tumor extirpation in breast cancer patients who present with stage IV disease and an intact primary tumor. *Ann Surg Oncol* 2006;13:776–782.
20. Blanchard DK, Shetty PB, Hilsenbeck SG, et al. Association of surgery with improved survival in stage IV breast cancer patients. *Ann Surg* 2008;247:732–738.
21. Khan SA. Does resection of an intact breast primary improve survival in metastatic breast cancer? *Oncology (Williston Park)* 2007;21:924–931.
22. Morrogh M, Park A, Norton L, et al. Changing indications for surgery in patients with stage IV breast cancer: a current perspective. *Cancer* 2008;112:1445–1454.
23. Esteva FJ, Valero V, Pusztai L, et al. Chemotherapy of metastatic breast cancer: what to expect in 2001 and beyond. *Oncologist* 2001;6:133–146.
24. Carmichael AR, Anderson ED, Chetty U, et al. Does local surgery have a role in the management of stage IV breast cancer? *Eur J Surg Oncol* 2003;29:17–19.
25. Fisher B, Anderson S, Fisher ER, et al. Significance of ipsilateral breast tumour recurrence after lumpectomy. *Lancet* 1991;338:327–331.

26. Veronesi U, Luini A, Del Vecchio M, et al. Radiotherapy after breast-preserving surgery in women with localized cancer of the breast. *N Engl J Med* 1993;328: 1587–1591.

27. Overgaard M, Hansen PS, Overgaard J, et al. Postoperative radiotherapy in high-risk premenopausal women with breast cancer who receive adjuvant chemotherapy. Danish Breast Cancer Cooperative Group 82b trial. *N Engl J Med* 1997;337: 949–955.

28. Overgaard M, Jensen MB, Overgaard J, et al. Postoperative radiotherapy in high-risk postmenopausal breast-cancer patients given adjuvant tamoxifen: Danish Breast Cancer Cooperative Group DBCG 82c randomised trial. *Lancet* 1999;353: 1641–1648.

29. Ragaz J, Jackson SM, Le N, et al. Adjuvant radiotherapy and chemotherapy in node-positive premenopausal women with breast cancer. *N Engl J Med* 1997;337: 956–962.

30. Pocard M, Pouillart P, Asselain B, et al. [Hepatic resection for breast cancer metastases: results and prognosis (65 cases)]. *Ann Chir* 2001;126:413–420.

31. Vlastos G, Smith DL, Singletary SE, et al. Long-term survival after an aggressive surgical approach in patients with breast cancer hepatic metastases. *Ann Surg Oncol* 2004;11:869–874.

32. Lang JE, Babiera GV. Locoregional resection in stage IV breast cancer: tumor biology, molecular and clinical perspectives. *Surg Clin North Am* 2007;87:527–538.

33. Braun S, Vogl FD, Naume B, et al. A pooled analysis of bone marrow micrometastasis in breast cancer. *N Engl J Med* 2005;353:793–802.

34. Hortobagyi GN. Can we cure limited metastatic breast cancer? *J Clin Oncol* 2002; 20:620–623.

35. Greenberg PA, Hortobagyi GN, Smith TL, et al. Long-term follow-up of patients with complete remission following combination chemotherapy for metastatic breast cancer. *J Clin Oncol* 1996;14:2197–2205.

36. Holmes FA, Buzdar AU, Kau SW, et al. Combined-modality approach for patients with isolated recurrences of breast cancer (IV-NED): the M.D. Anderson experience. *Breast Dis* 1994;7:7–20.

37. Rivera E, Holmes FA, Buzdar AU, et al. Fluorouracil, doxorubicin, and cyclophosphamide followed by tamoxifen as adjuvant treatment for patients with stage IV breast cancer with no evidence of disease. *Breast J* 2002;8:2–9.

38. Borner M, Bacchi M, Goldhirsch A, et al. First isolated locoregional recurrence following mastectomy for breast cancer: results of a phase III multicenter study comparing systemic treatment with observation after excision and radiation. Swiss Group for Clinical Cancer Research. *J Clin Oncol* 1994;12:2071–2077.

39. Nieto Y, Nawaz S, Jones RB, et al. Prognostic model for relapse after high-dose chemotherapy with autologous stem-cell transplantation for stage IV oligometastatic breast cancer. *J Clin Oncol* 2002;20:707–718.

40. Singletary SE, Walsh G, Vauthey JN, et al. A role for curative surgery in the treatment of selected patients with metastatic breast cancer. *Oncologist* 2003;8:241–251.

41. Cristofanilli M, Budd GT, Ellis MJ, et al. Circulating tumor cells, disease progression, and survival in metastatic breast cancer. *N Engl J Med* 2004;351:781–791.

42. Norton I, Massague J. Is cancer a disease of self-seeding? *Nat Med* 2006;12: 875–878.

43. Dauplat J, Le Bouedec G, Pomel C, et al. Cytoreductive surgery for advanced stages of ovarian cancer. *Semin Surg Oncol* 2000;19:42–48.

44. Hotta T, Takifuji K, Arii K, et al. Potential predictors of long-term survival after surgery for patients with stage IV colorectal cancer. *Anticancer Res* 2006;26:1377–1383.

45. Young SE, Martinez SR, Essner R. The role of surgery in treatment of stage IV melanoma. *J Surg Oncol* 2006;94:344–351.

46. Doglietto GB, Pacelli F, Caprino P, et al. Palliative surgery for far-advanced gastric cancer: a retrospective study on 305 consecutive patients. *Am Surg* 1999;65:352–355.

47. Flanigan RC, Salmon SE, Blumenstein BA, et al. Nephrectomy followed by interferon alfa-2b compared with interferon alfa-2b alone for metastatic renal-cell cancer. *N Engl J Med* 2001;345:1655–1659.

48. Fidler IJ, Kripke ML. Metastasis results from preexisting variant cells within a malignant tumor. *Science* 1977;197:893–895.

49. Giavazzi R, Alessandri G, Spreafico F, et al. Metastasizing capacity of tumour cells from spontaneous metastases of transplanted murine tumours. *Br J Cancer* 1980;42:462–472.

50. Mantovani A, Giavazzi R, Alessandri G, et al. Characterization of tumor lines derived from spontaneous metastases of a transplanted murine sarcoma. *Eur J Cancer* 1981; 17:71–76.

51. Milas L, Peters LJ, Ito H. Spontaneous metastasis: random or selective? *Clin Exp Metastasis* 1983;1:309–315.

52. Weiss L, Holmes JC, Ward PM. Do metastases arise from pre-existing subpopulations of cancer cells? *Br J Cancer* 1983;47:81–89.

53. Hill RP, Chambers AF, Ling V, et al. Dynamic heterogeneity: rapid generation of metastatic variants in mouse B16 melanoma cells. *Science* 1984;224:998–1001.

54. Ling V, Chambers AF, Harris JF, et al. Quantitative genetic analysis of tumor progression. *Cancer Metastasis Rev* 1985;4:173–192.

55. Kerbel RS, Waghorne C, Korczak B, et al. Clonal dominance of primary tumours by metastatic cells: genetic analysis and biological implications. *Cancer Surv* 1988;7:597–629.

56. Kerbel RS, Waghorne C, Man MS, et al. Alteration of the tumorigenic and metastatic properties of neoplastic cells is associated with the process of calcium phosphate-mediated DNA transfection. *Proc Natl Acad Sci U S A* 1987;84: 1263–1267.

57. Weigelt B, Peterse JL, van't Veer LJ. Breast cancer metastasis: markers and models. *Nat Rev Cancer* 2005;5:591–602.

58. van de Vijver MJ, He YD, van't Veer LJ, et al. A gene-expression signature as a predictor of survival in breast cancer. *N Engl J Med* 2002;347:1999–2009.

59. van't Veer LJ, Dai H, van de Vijver MJ, et al. Gene expression profiling predicts clinical outcome of breast cancer. *Nature* 2002:530–536.

60. Weigelt B, Glas AM, Wessels LF, et al. Gene expression profiles of primary breast tumors maintained in distant metastases. *Proc Natl Acad Sci U S A* 2003;100: 15901–15905.

61. Ma XJ, Salunga R, Tuggle JT, et al. Gene expression profiles of human breast cancer progression. *Proc Natl Acad Sci U S A* 2003;100:5974–5979.

62. Kang Y, Siegel PM, Shu W, et al. A multigenic program mediating breast cancer metastasis to bone. *Cancer Cell* 2003;3:537–549.

63. Schmidt-Kittler O, Ragg T, Daskalakis A, et al. From latent disseminated cells to overt metastasis: genetic analysis of systemic breast cancer progression. *Proc Natl Acad Sci U S A* 2003;100:7737–7742.

64. Reya T, Morrison SJ, Clarke MF, et al. Stem cells, cancer, and cancer stem cells. *Nature* 2001;414:105–111.

65. Al-Hajj M, Clarke MF. Self-renewal and solid tumor stem cells. *Oncogene* 2004; 23:7274–7282.

66. Al-Hajj M, Wicha MS, Benito-Hernandez A, et al. Prospective identification of tumorigenic breast cancer cells. *Proc Natl Acad Sci U S A* 2003;100:3983–3988.

67. Sabel MS, Nehs MA. Immunologic approaches to breast cancer treatment. *Surg Oncol Clin North Am* 2005;14:1–31.

68. Lang JE, Tereffe W, Rao R, et al. Use of neoadjuvant chemotherapy prior to resection of the primary tumor in stage iv breast cancer may predict for improved survival. *Official Proceedings of the 9th Annual ASBS Meeting* 2008;9:60.

69. Rao R, Feng L, H.M. K, et al. Timing of surgical intervention for the intact primary in stage IV breast cancer patients. *Ann Surg Oncol* 2008;15:15:1696–1702.

Chapter 72
Local-Regional Recurrence after Breast-Conservation Treatment or Mastectomy

Lawrence J. Solin, Eleanor E. R. Harris, Susan P. Weinstein, Angela DeMichele, and Julia Tchou

After the definitive local treatment of breast cancer using mastectomy or breast-conservation treatment (generally defined as lumpectomy [with or without axillary staging] followed by definitive radiation treatment), a tumor can recur in the local or regional lymph node areas. Local recurrence after breast-conservation treatment is defined as the reappearance of cancer in the ipsilateral treated breast, including breast parenchyma or breast skin. Local recurrence after mastectomy is defined as the reappearance of cancer in the ipsilateral chest wall, including skin. For either breast-conservation treatment or mastectomy, regional recurrence is defined as the reappearance of cancer involving the ipsilateral axillary, supraclavicular, infraclavicular, or internal mammary lymph nodes.

Local recurrence can be the first manifestation of disease (isolated or solitary recurrence), or can occur simultaneously with or after regional or distant metastatic disease. Comparison between studies is somewhat problematic because of the differences in definitions of local recurrence between studies. In addition, the assessment of local-regional recurrence after the development of distant metastatic disease is often poorly evaluated clinically.

 ## LOCAL RECURRENCE AFTER BREAST CONSERVATION TREATMENT

Presenting Symptoms and Signs

Approximately one fourth to one half of local recurrences after initial treatment of invasive cancers with breast-conservation surgery and radiation treatment are detected solely by routine mammography (Table 72.1). This variability in detecting local recurrences emphasizes the need for following patients with both mammography and physical examination. In general, the clinical and radiologic characteristics of recurrent lesions are similar to those of the initially presenting tumors.

The physical examination following breast-conservation treatment often shows only mild thickening without a mass effect. Changes in the physical examination that occur more than 1 to 2 years following the completion of radiation treatment must be viewed as suspicious. Either surgery or radiation treatment may cause a change in physical examination, such as a mass-like region of fibrosis that may occasionally be difficult clinically to distinguish from a local recurrence. The findings associated with a local recurrence may be subtle, especially when the primary tumor was infiltrating lobular carcinoma. Recurrences of these lesions can produce only minimal thickening or retraction at the biopsy site without a mass.

The clinical classification of the location of local recurrence is determined by the relationship of the location of the local recurrence to the location of the primary tumor (1). Local recurrences are classified as (a) true recurrence, defined as being within the primary tumor site or the boost volume of the treated breast; (b) marginal miss, defined as being near the boost volume; or (c) elsewhere. True recur-

rence and marginal miss are often combined since the distinction between these two can be somewhat difficult on clinical grounds and has little treatment or prognostic value. Some authors also score various less common manifestations of local recurrence, such as diffuse disease, multifocal disease, skin recurrence, or inflammatory recurrence. Paget's disease of the nipple as the presentation of local recurrence has been reported, but is rare (2). Various authors have evaluated the location of local recurrence (Table 72.2). In general, the largest fraction of local recurrences is scored as a true recurrence or marginal miss (46% to 91%). Elsewhere recurrences tend to occur later compared to true recurrences or marginal misses, with the reported median time to local recurrence of 3.1 to 5.8 years compared to 3.0 to 3.8 years, respectively (3–7).

Another method of classifying local recurrence is according to whether the local recurrence represents a true recurrence of the initially treated primary breast carcinoma versus the development of a new primary breast carcinoma. This distinction is commonly made by comparing the initial tumor versus the local recurrence for such characteristics as location, pathologic features, and interval to local recurrence. Small studies have recently been reported that demonstrate the value of molecular characteristics to distinguish a true recurrence from a new primary carcinoma, and this distinction may have prognostic value (8,9).

The Role of Breast Imaging in the Detection of Local Recurrence

The role of mammography after breast-conservation treatment is close surveillance of the treated breast for clinically occult recurrent breast cancer as well as screening of the contralateral breast (4,10–12). Patients typically obtain their first posttreatment mammogram 6 to 12 months after completion of radiation treatment. The delay after completion of radiation treatment serves a twofold purpose. First, this delay allows for stabilization of the posttreatment changes, and second, it allows the patients to better tolerate the mammogram. The first mammogram after completion of radiation treatment serves as the new baseline mammogram for the patient. The posttreatment baseline mammogram is obtained at a time when a local recurrence is highly unlikely.

The degree of edema and distortion that is seen on the mammogram can vary significantly from one patient to another. At the time of the baseline mammogram after completion of treatment, some patients will have extensive edema, trabecular thickening, and architectural distortion, while other patients will have minimal mammographic changes. These posttreatment changes tend to be maximal at about 6 months after treatment and may pose a challenge to the breast imager in detecting recurrent disease. On subsequent mammograms, the posttreatment changes may remain stable but usually decrease in prominence over time. Therefore, any new or worsening finding on subsequent screening mammography, such as new calcifications, new mass, or increasing architectural distortion, needs to be

Table 72.1   METHOD OF DETECTION OF LOCAL RECURRENCE AFTER BREAST-CONSERVATION TREATMENT

Study (Reference)	No. of Patients	Method of Detection of Local Recurrence		
		Mammography No. (%)	Physical Examination No. (%)	Both No. (%)
Ashkanani et al., 2001 (45)	21	8 (38)	8 (38)	5 (24)
Chaudary et al., 1998 (3)	45	21 (47)	—	24 (53)
Chen et al., 2003 (171)	125	48 (38)	46 (37)	31 (25)
Dalberg et al., 1998 (36)	85	25 (29)	60 (71)	
Dershaw et al., 1992 (4)	43	18 (42)	14 (33)	11 (26)
Doyle et al., 2001 (49)	112	47 (42)	42 (37)	23 (21)
Fowble et al., 1990 (37)	66	19 (29)	33 (50)	14 (21)
Galper et al., 2005 (50)	247[a]	124 (50)	47 (19)	76 (31)
Haffty et al., 1991 (38)	50	14 (28)	22 (44)	14 (28)
Haffty et al., 1993 (51)	82	25 (30)	34 (41)	23 (28)
Hassell et al., 1990 (10)	48	13 (27)	29 (60)	6 (13)
Kurtz et al., 1989 (39)	161	22 (14)	139 (86)	
Orel et al., 1993 (52)	72	34 (47)	24 (33)	14 (19)
Stotter et al., 1989 (5)	51	9 (18)	42 (82)	
Voogd et al., 2005 (47)	189[a]	47 (25)	102 (54)	40 (21)

[a]Excludes patients with incomplete or unknown information.

Table 72.2   LOCATION OF LOCAL RECURRENCE AFTER BREAST-CONSERVATION TREATMENT

Study (Reference)	No. of Patients	Location of Local Recurrence		
		True Recurrence or Marginal Miss No. (%)	Elsewhere No. (%)	Diffuse or Multifocal No. (%)
Chaudary et al., 1998 (3)	45	34 (76)	5 (11)	6 (13)
Clark et al., 1992 (174)	23	19 (83)	4 (17)	
Dalberg et al., 1998 (36)	85	61 (72)	14 (16)	10 (12)
Dershaw et al., 1992 (4)	43	25 (58)	18 (42)	—
Dershaw et al., 1997 (173)	22[a]	20 (91)	2 (9)	—
Fourquet et al., 1989 (40)	56	26 (46)	30 (54)	—
Fowble et al., 1990 (37)	66	43 (65)	17 (26)	6 (9)
Freedman et al., 2005 (172)	105	63 (60)	28 (27)	14 (13)[b]
Galper et al., 2005 (50)	303[c]	220 (73)	70 (23)	13 (43)
Geiss et al., 1999 (11)	27	19 (70)	8 (30)	—
Haffty et al., 1991 (38)	50	36 (72)	14 (28)	—
Haffty et al., 1993 (51)	79	48 (61)	31 (39)	—
Kurtz et al., 1989 (39)	178	140 (79)	38 (21)	—
Leung et al., 1986 (41)	44[c]	32 (73)	12 (27)	—
Orel et al., 1993 (52)	72	50 (69)	20 (28)	2 (31)
Osborne et al., 1992 (53)	42[c]	37 (88)	4 (10)	1 (2)
Recht et al., 1988 (6)	66[c]	48 (73)	12 (18)	6 (8)[b]
Stotter et al., 1989 (5)	51	29 (57)	11 (22)	11 (22)
Voogd et al., 1999 (7)	253[c]	164 (65)	37 (15)	52 (21)

[a]Mammographically detected local recurrences only.
[b]Includes skin local recurrences.
[c]Excludes patients with incomplete or unknown information.

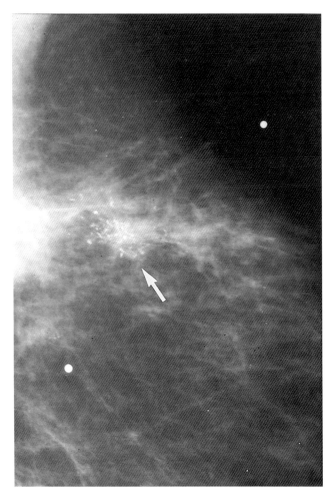

FIGURE 72.1. Mammographically detected local breast cancer recurrence. Spot magnification view of the lumpectomy bed (marked by skin *bb*s at the ends of the lumpectomy surgical scar) demonstrates a cluster of pleomorphic calcifications (*arrow*). Pathology showed ductal carcinoma *in situ*.

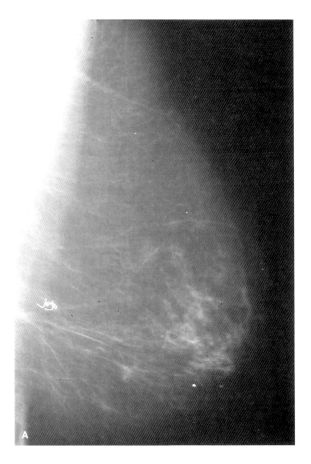

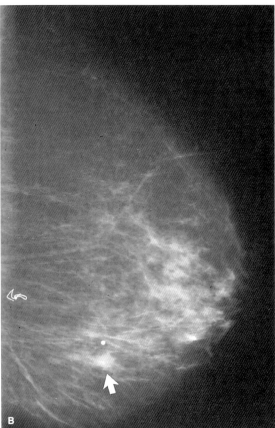

FIGURE 72.2 A, B: Mammographically detected local breast cancer recurrence. Mediolateral oblique view mammograms obtained 12 months apart reveal (**B**) a developing mass (*arrow*). Ultrasound-guided core biopsy showed invasive ductal carcinoma.

viewed cautiously, and evaluated carefully for recurrent disease (Figs. 72.1 and 72.2).

Routine yearly mammograms are typically obtained after breast-conservation treatment. There is, however, literature advocating obtaining biannual mammograms of the treated breast for the first 3 years, but no prospective controlled studies have validated this recommendation (10,11,13). In addition, the likelihood of recurrence after breast-conservation treatment within the first 2 to 3 years is low. Therefore, given the lack of scientific evidence, short-term 6 month follow-up mammography is not routinely obtained for screening.

The mammographic appearance of the recurrent cancer may appear different from the appearance of the primary cancer. Burrell et al. (14) looked at 31 patients who recurred after breast conservation treatment. The authors found that 78% of primary breast cancers that presented as masses also recurred as masses. Similarly, 83% of primary breast cancers that presented as malignant calcifications also recurred as microcalcifications. In the study by Burrell et al., the cancers that were originally mammographically occult also recurred as mammographically occult cancers. In another series of 26 patients with 27 recurrent breast cancers, Giess et al. (11) found that the mammographic findings of the recurrent cancers were usually similar to the primary carcinoma. However, in a recent series from the University of Pennsylvania of 95 patients that recurred after breast-conservation treatment, Weinstein et al. (15) reported that the mammographic appearance of the local

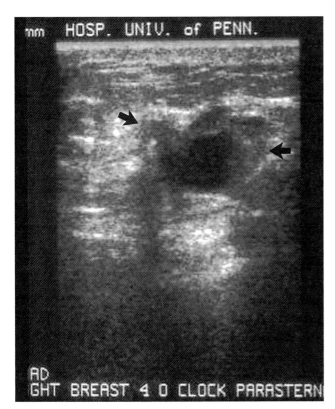

FIGURE 72.3. Ultrasound demonstrating local breast cancer recurrence. The patient presented with a mass in the treated breast several years after breast-conservation treatment. Mammograms (not shown) revealed no suspicious abnormality. Directed ultrasound showed an ill-defined hypoechoic mass (*arrows*) corresponding to the palpable mass. Ultrasound-guided core biopsy showed invasive ductal carcinoma.

62 patients underwent short-term follow-up examinations. Limitations of screening ultrasound examinations include the high false-positive rate and a high rate of interventional recommendations (21). Therefore, screening sonographic examinations need to be balanced by the costs of additional false positives in terms of emotional stress and inconvenience to the patient as well as financial costs of benign biopsies and follow-up evaluations (22–24).

In the American College of Radiology Imaging Network (ACRIN) 666 trial, the largest prospective ultrasound screening trial with 2,504 patients, preliminary results showed that the addition of ultrasound to mammography can yield 1.2 to 7.6 cancers per 1,000 patients (22). However, the ultrasound examination resulted in biopsy recommendations in 6.7% of the participants, with a cancer yield of only 7.1%. An additional 8% of the patients were prompted to have a short interval follow-up (22,23). The majority of the patients (53%) enrolled in the ACRIN screening ultrasound trial were patients with a personal history of breast cancer.

Breast magnetic resonance imaging (MRI) is well known to be able to detect mammographically occult breast cancer (25–27). Unlike mammography and sonography, MRI dynamically evaluates the breast tissue. In addition to assessing the morphology of the breast lesions, the vascularity of any lesions may be evaluated after intravenous contrast enhancement. Lesion enhancement is based on the number and the permeability of the blood vessels. There is however, some overlap in enhancement characteristics seen in benign and malignant lesions.

In women with equivocal mammographic findings after breast-conservation treatment, the enhancement pattern on contrast-enhanced MRI can be helpful in differentiating posttreatment scar from recurrent cancer (28–32). Breast MRI can also detect mammographically occult local recurrence in the breast after breast-conservation treatment (Fig. 72.4). Mature scarring in the lumpectomy site would be expected to enhance minimally or not at all. In the early posttreatment period, false-positive enhancement may occur due to fat necrosis and inflammatory changes. Contrast enhancement secondary to posttreatment changes may be seen up to 18 months (28,31,33). However, reports of false-positive enhancement have been described as far out as 32 months (34). Although MRI may be helpful in problem solving, there are few published data on the utility of screening patients with MRI after breast-conservation treatment (30,31,33). American Cancer Society guidelines do not recommend routine MRI screening for women after breast-conservation treatment (35).

Compared with conventional film mammography, digital mammography has greater accuracy in women with dense breast tissue, which is often seen as a component of posttreatment changes. Therefore, digital mammography could potentially have a role in screening patients after lumpectomy and radiation treatment. Another advantage of digital mammography is that it may serve as a platform for other advanced applications. One such application is digital breast tomosynthesis (DBT). One of the limitations of digital or film screen mammography is that a three-dimensional structure, the breast, is imaged in two-dimensional planes. The two-dimensional imaging and the subsequent superimposition of normal fibroglandular tissue can limit visualization of an underlying cancer. Further, overlapping of the normal breast tissue may also mimic false-positive "pseudolesions," which may require additional imaging evaluation. Tomosynthesis imaging is a novel approach to breast imaging during which the breast tissue is imaged in three-dimensional planes, acquired at different angles. The images are subsequently reconstructed using a mathematical algorithm similar to a computed tomography (CT) scan. Future studies may address the potential for three-dimensional imaging to improve the

recurrence often varied from the appearance of the original breast cancer. In women who presented with mammographically occult primary breast cancer, the recurrence was detected mammographically 77% of the time.

For the evaluation of new or suspicious mammographic masses as well as clinically palpable findings, breast sonography is an essential tool that plays a complementary role to mammography and physical examination (Fig. 72.3). Sonography can characterize the mammographic or palpable masses as cystic or solid. In the evaluation of palpable breast masses, sonography is particularly helpful in patients who are status post–breast-conservation treatment, since the mammographic evaluation can be limited due to the posttreatment changes. In patients presenting with palpable breast masses, prospective and retrospective studies have reported the negative predictive value of combined mammography and sonography to be very high, approaching 100% (16,17). In addition, if a lesion is visible on sonography, a minimally invasive core needle biopsy or fine-needle aspiration can be performed under sonographic guidance.

Given the limitations of mammography, particularly in dense breasts, there has been interest in detecting cancers on screening sonography. In contrast to mammography, the sensitivity of sonography increases with increasing breast density (18,19). Screening sonography can detect cancers that are mammographically and clinically occult (18–21). Crystal et al. (20) performed 1,517 screening ultrasound examinations in asymptomatic women with dense breasts with negative mammograms and negative physical examinations. Seven cancers were found, resulting in a cancer detection rate of 0.46%. Complex cystic lesions or solid masses were detected in 90 women (5.9%), resulting in 38 biopsy procedures. The remaining

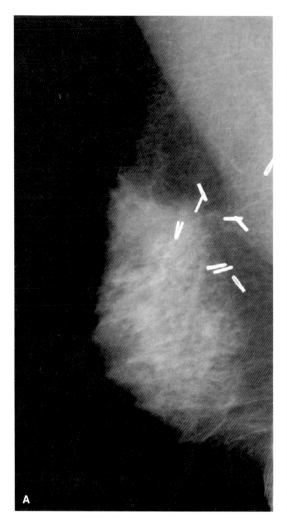
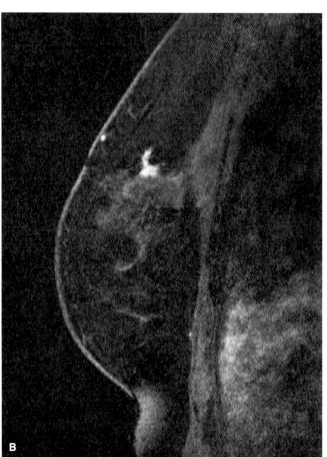

FIGURE 72.4. Magnetic resonance imaging (MRI) detected local recurrence. A: Routine screening mammogram performed after breast-conservation treatment showed dense breast tissue with stable posttreatment changes. **B:** Contrast-enhanced MRI of the breast in the sagittal plane demonstrated an area of enhancement in the superior breast adjacent to the patient's lumpectomy bed. Pathology from biopsy showed invasive ductal carcinoma.

sensitivity of mammography in patients after breast-conservation treatment, where the posttreatment changes limit the interpretation of the two-dimensional images.

Treatment Results

Mastectomy

The vast majority of patients with local recurrence after breast-conservation treatment are treated with salvage mastectomy. Most series report an operability rate of 75% to 100%, although exceptions have been reported (3,4,11,36–44). Factors that traditionally render a patient inoperable include local-regionally advanced disease or concurrent distant metastases. Approximately 5% to 10% of patients with local recurrence will present with concurrent distant metastases (5,36–41,43), although in one series, one third of patients had distant failure at presentation (45). Another 5% to 10% will have locally extensive recurrences or inoperable regional nodal recurrences that preclude surgery (37,41,43,46). Patients who recur in the skin alone or with an inflammatory-type picture have a poor prognosis (46–48).

After salvage surgery, overall survival rates have been reported as 34% to 88% at 5 years and 57% to 69% at 10 years (5,7,37–40,42,47,49–54). Five-year relapse-free or disease-free survival rates have been reported as 55% to 73% (37,52,53).

These high rates of salvage contribute to the safety of initial breast-conservation treatment for women with early stage breast carcinoma.

Subsequent chest wall recurrences occur in fewer than 10% of patients treated with mastectomy in most series (55–57), although chest wall failure rates of approximately 50% have been reported in two series of salvage mastectomy following initial treatment with breast-conservation surgery without radiation treatment (58,59) and a rate of 18% in a series that did not separate those patients who had or had not had radiation treatment as part of their initial treatment (36). Most patients who develop further local failure following mastectomy will have progressive local-regional disease despite further treatment (36,57).

Factors that influence prognosis in operable patients are not well established. A number of studies have looked at potential prognostic factors for outcome after local recurrence (Table 72.3). The factor that appears most reproducibly correlated with prognosis after local recurrence is the interval to local recurrence. The large majority of studies have shown that patients with a shorter interval to local recurrence have a significantly worse prognosis compared to patients with a longer interval to local recurrence. Various authors have used different cutoffs to measure this effect, and the most commonly used cutoffs to separate prognostic groups are 2 years or 5 years. Although many other patient, tumor, and treatment factors

| Table 72.3 | POTENTIAL PROGNOSTIC FACTORS FOR OUTCOME AFTER LOCAL RECURRENCE FOLLOWING BREAST-CONSERVATION TREATMENT |

Factor	Favorable Characteristic	Positive Study[a]	Negative Study[a]
Patient			
Age	Older age		Abner et al., 1993 (55), Doyle et al., 2001 (49), Fowble et al., 1990 (37), Galper et al., 2005 (50), Komoike et al., 2006 (176), Kurtz et al., 1989 (39), Orel et al., 1993 (52), Recht et al., 1989 (43), Voogd et al., 1999[b] (7), Voogd et al., 2005[b] (47)
Tumor			
Tumor size	Smaller size	Cajucom et al., 1993 (58), Chaudary et al., 1998 (3), Voogd et al., 1999[b] (7), Voogd et al., 2005[b] (47)	Abner et al., 1993 (55), Doyle et al., 2001 (49), Komoike et al., 2006 (176), Le et al., 2002 (54)
Axillary lymph nodes	Node negative	Cajucom et al., 1993 (58), Komoike et al., 2006[b] (176), Voogd et al., 1999[b] (7), Voogd et al., 2005[b] (47)	Doyle et al., 2001 (49), Le et al., 2002 (54)
Initial stage	Lower stage		Cajucom et al., 1993 (58)
Site of local recurrence	In field or marginal miss	Haffty et al., 1991 (38), Haffty et al., 1993 (51), Voogd et al., 2005[b] (47)	Abner et al., 1993 (55), Doyle et al., 2001 (49), Fowble et al., 1990 (37), Kurtz et al., 1989 (39), Recht et al., 1989 (43)
Extent of disease	Localized	Haffty et al., 1991 (38), Kurtz et al., 1989 (39), Kurtz et al., 1991 (46), Stotter et al., 1989 (5)	Fowble et al., 1990 (37)
Estrogen receptor status	Positive	Haffty et al., 1991 (38)	Komoike et al., 2006 (176), Kurtz et al., 1989 (39)
Grade	Lower grade	Kurtz et al., 1989 (39), Voogd et al., 1999[b] (7)	Le et al., 2002 (54)
Histology	Non-invasive	Abner et al., 1993 (55), Galper et al., 2005 (50), Recht et al., 1989 (43), Voogd et al., 1999[b] (7), Voogd et al., 2005[b] (47)	Doyle et al., 2001 (49), Fowble et al., 1990 (37), Orel et al., 1993 (52)
Method of detection	Mammography only	Doyle et al., 2001 (49)	Abner et al., 1993 (55), Fowble et al., 1990 (37), Orel et al., 1993 (52)
Treatment			
Type of surgery	Excision		Galper et al., 2005 (50), Kurtz et al., 1989 (39), Orel et al., 1993 (52)
Systemic treatment	Hormones	Kurtz et al., 1989 (39)	Doyle et al., 2001 (49)
Systemic treatment	Chemotherapy		Doyle et al., 2001 (49), Fowble et al., 1990 (37), Orel et al., 1993 (52)
Other			
Interval to local recurrence	Longer interval	Chaudary et al., 1998 (3), Doyle et al., 2001 (49), Fourquet et al., 1989 (40), Fowble et al., 1990 (37), Galper et al., 2005 (50), Haffty et al., 1991 (38), Haffty et al., 1996 (175), Komoike et al., 2006[b] (176), Kurtz et al., 1989 (39), Kurtz et al., 1990 (56), Orel et al., 1993 (52), Osborne et al., 1992 (53), van der Sangen et al., 2006 (177), Veronesi et al., 1995 (178)	Abner et al., 1993 (55), Recht et al., 1989 (43), Voogd et al., 1999[b] (7), Voogd et al., 2005[b] (47)

[a]Positive study indicates improved outcome associated with favorable characteristic, and negative study indicates either no improved outcome or worse outcome associated with favorable characteristic.
[b]Multivariate Cox regression analysis.

have been evaluated for prognostic importance, consistent findings between studies have not been observed.

Doyle et al. (49) from the University of Pennsylvania reported on the outcome of 112 patients after local recurrence. The 10-year rates of overall survival were 69% for the overall group and 64% for the patients with invasive local recurrences. The 10-year rates of freedom from distant metastases were 47% for the overall group and 44% for patients with invasive local recurrences. On multivariable analysis, interval from initial diagnosis to local recurrence of 2 years or less proved to be an independent predictor for worse outcome after local recurrence. The 5-year overall survival rates were 65% for an interval to local recurrence of 2 years or less, 84% for an interval of 2.1 to 5 years, and 89% for an interval greater than 5 years.

In one of the largest studies of local recurrence, Voogd et al. (7,47) analyzed the outcome for 266 patients with local recurrence after breast-conservation treatment. For the patients with invasive local recurrence, the 10-year rate of overall survival was 39%, the distant recurrence-free survival rate was 36%, and the local control rate was 68% (47). On Cox regression analysis, factors associated with overall survival, distant

recurrence-free survival, and local control were lymph node status of the primary tumor, skin involvement, and combined tumor size plus location of the local recurrence.

Few patients with a known *BRCA* mutation and with local recurrence after breast-conservation treatment have been reported. In a report of the Yale University experience, Turner et al. (60) reported that all eight patients identified as having a germline mutation for the *BRCA1* or *BRCA2* gene who developed a local failure underwent salvage mastectomy and were alive without recurrence at a median follow-up of 7.7 years. In a multi-institutional study, Pierce et al. (61) reported on three patients with *BRCA1* or *BRCA2* mutations treated successfully at the time of local recurrence with salvage mastectomy. In an updated report, the median time to local recurrence was 8.7 years for mutation carriers compared to 4.7 years for controls ($p = .01$) (62).

Re-exploration of the previously dissected axilla does not appear warranted for all patients in the absence of suspicious lymphadenopathy (43). However, selected re-exploration may be indicated. In a subset of patients, Doyle et al. (49) reported that the incidence of positive axillary lymphadenopathy at the time of local recurrence was 39% (12/31); however, this represented only 13% (12/93) of the overall group. Complications after re-exploration surgery of the axilla have been reported (57). In one series, 3 of 19 patients treated initially with axillary irradiation only developed a lymphocele after complete axillary dissection performed at the time of mastectomy (63). Repeat sentinel lymph node biopsy at the time of local recurrence has been described for patients who had undergone sentinel lymph node biopsy as a component of primary breast-conservation surgical treatment (64).

Postoperative complications following salvage mastectomy were rare in two series (43,53). However, slow wound healing, wound breakdown, and infections have been noted (57,63).

Many patients treated with mastectomy for local failure desire breast reconstruction. Immediate reconstruction with a myocutaneous flap at the time of mastectomy is psychologically advantageous and also promotes tissue healing. Myocutaneous flap reconstructions are the preferred method of reconstruction and show improved cosmetic results and lower complication rates compared to implant reconstructions.

Breast-Conservation Surgery

Whether salvage mastectomy results in superior long-term survival rates for patients with local failure following initial breast-conservation treatment compared to treatment with lesser surgical procedures is unclear. However, salvage mastectomy specimens frequently reveal substantial residual disease outside the biopsy cavity. In two series, 22% and 29% of evaluated specimens, respectively, had residual tumor located in two or more quadrants of the breast (37,65). Experience using breast-conservation surgery for the salvage treatment of local recurrence shows that patients have a substantial risk of further (second) local breast recurrence of 14% to 48% (Table 72.4), consistent with these pathologic data.

There are few data available regarding the chances of preserving the breast in patients who fail initial treatment with breast-conservation surgery alone without initial radiation. Rates of performing salvage breast-conservation surgery in such patients have ranged from 30% to 100% (66–69). It is not clear what the risk of a second local recurrence is for such individuals. In one series, the 5-year actuarial second local recurrence rate was 69% for patients treated with further breast-conservation surgery alone and 11% for 14 patients treated with breast-conservation surgery and radiation treatment (70).

Reirradiation

Small cohorts of patients have been described who have been retreated with wide excision and interstitial implantation or external beam irradiation to a small volume of the breast (71–76). Deutsch (73) reported on 39 patients who received initial radiation doses of 45 to 50 Gy to the breast (with or without a boost) and who were treated for local recurrence with repeat lumpectomy and re-irradiation. The prescribed re-irradiation dose was 50 Gy in 25 fractions using electrons. The rate of second local recurrence was 29% (8/39). Overall cosmetic outcome was excellent or good for 75% (27/36) of the evaluable patients. Trombetta et al. (74) reported on 21 patients treated for local recurrence using excision plus interstitial brachytherapy to a dose of 45 to 50 Gy. The rate of second local recurrence was 5% (1/21), and 10% (2/21) of the patients developed metastatic disease. Treatment using salvage mastectomy plus re-irradiation of the chest wall has been described, but appears to be associated with an increased risk of complications (76).

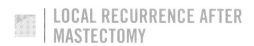

LOCAL RECURRENCE AFTER MASTECTOMY

Presentation

Local recurrence after initial treatment with mastectomy most often presents as one or more asymptomatic, palpable nodules in or near the scar of the mastectomy or on or under the skin of the chest wall (77). Occasionally local recurrence presents as an erythematous, pruritic skin rash. Recurrence in the pectoralis muscle alone has been described (78). Asymptomatic gross and microscopic recurrences have been documented at the time of delayed reconstruction (79). Recurrences can develop at the suture lines or remaining skin of the chest wall following reconstruction with a myocutaneous flap and rarely are found posterior to the flap itself (80–82). Chest wall recurrence accounts for approximately 40% to 60% of local-regional recurrences (82–84). Carcinoma *en cuirasse* is a distinct form of diffuse infiltration of the skin or subcutaneous tissues of the chest wall, with woody induration and spread of tumor often beyond the limits of standard surgical or radiation treatment boundaries. Nodules and ulceration are often present. The skin of the chest wall can also be diffusely involved with inflammatory changes without a mass. The rate of local recurrence does not appear to be different for skin sparing mastectomy versus non–skin-sparing mastectomy (85,86). After mastectomy and reconstruction, local recurrence presents predominantly as a subcutaneous mass and, less commonly, in the chest wall (87,88).

Regional recurrence in the axillary, supraclavicular, or internal mammary nodes occurs in about 30% to 40% of mastectomy patients with a local recurrence (77,82,89). The supraclavicular nodes are the most common site of regional

Table 72.4	OUTCOME AFTER LOCAL EXCISION FOR THE TREATMENT OF FIRST LOCAL RECURRENCE AFTER BREAST-CONSERVATION TREATMENT

Study (Reference)	No. of Patients	Second Local Recurrence	Overall Survival At 5 yrs	At 10 yrs	Median Follow-Up (yrs)
Galper et al., 2005 (50)	27	48% (13/27)	—	—	7.1
Kurtz et al., 1988 (179)	52	23% (12/52)	79%	64%	6.0
Leung et al., 1986 (41)	6	33% (2/6)	—	—	—
Salvadori et al., 1999 (44)	57	14% (8/57)	85%	—	6.1
Voogd et al., 1999 (7)	20	40% (8/20)	—	—	4.3

recurrence, occurring in 11% to 35% of patients (83,90). As is found after breast-conservation treatment, recurrence in the axillary lymph nodes is more favorable than in the supraclavicular nodes, with 5-year survival rates of approximately 37% to 50% versus 16% to 28%, respectively (82–84).

Local-regional recurrences after mastectomy tend to occur earlier than in-breast recurrences after breast-conservation treatment (91). Up to 90% of local recurrences will appear by 5 years after mastectomy, with a median interval to local-regional recurrence of about 3 years (92,93). However, local recurrences have been reported even decades after initial surgery. These late recurrences may be new primary tumors arising in breast tissue not removed by mastectomy, rather than true recurrences of the prior cancer.

Approximately 20% to 30% of patients with local or regional recurrence will have had preceding distant metastases (93–95). A similar percentage of patients will be diagnosed as having simultaneous local and distant failure or will develop distant metastases within a few months of the discovery of local recurrence (77,89,95).

Breast Imaging following Mastectomy

Radiologic imaging after initial treatment using mastectomy rarely demonstrates recurrences that were not suspected clinically, and therefore, routine imaging of the mastectomy site is not recommended. Fajardo et al. (96) looked at 827 post mastectomy patients with or without reconstruction and found that mammography demonstrated recurrences that were already clinically suspected based on physical examination findings. Similarly, Propeck and Scanlan (97) studied a group of 185 postmastectomy patients and concluded that routine imaging of this population was not helpful in detecting recurrent disease. However, the contralateral breast, if present, should be imaged in the routine fashion.

Imaging of the reconstructed breast after a transverse rectus abdominis myocutaneous (TRAM) reconstruction is controversial. Recurrent breast cancer after reconstruction, although uncommon, may occur (96,98,99). Surveillance of the reconstructed breast is usually performed clinically using physical examination, and routine mammography has not been advocated (96,100,101). Helvie et al. (100) retrospectively looked at 214 consecutive screening mammograms in asymptomatic 113 women with TRAM flaps. Six patients underwent surgery, and two cases (1.9%) were biopsy proven cancers. Although some retrospective data have demonstrated a small number of recurrences detected in asymptomatic women, no large-scale studies have been performed to demonstrate the utility of imaging these patients. However, once an abnormality is palpated, a diagnostic imaging evaluation using sonography and mammography may be performed, as necessary, as with any patient presenting with a palpable breast mass. MRI may also provide additional information when the conventional imaging methods yield equivocal results.

Pretreatment Evaluation

Other conditions may resemble a local recurrence, such as a foreign body cyst around suture material or a bony nodule that develops on a rib or costal cartilage as a result of surgical trauma. Patients who undergo reconstruction with a myocutaneous flap can develop areas of fat necrosis that may clinically or radiologically mimic recurrent disease. Radiation-induced sarcomas of the bone or soft tissues of the chest wall can appear 5 to 10 years after postoperative treatment (102,103). Therefore, a biopsy should be obtained in all cases of suspected local recurrence to establish the diagnosis and to obtain tissue for estrogen- and progesterone-receptor assays. The estrogen-receptor status of the primary tumor and that of the subsequent recurrence will be the same in about 75% to 85% of patients.

The patient should have a restaging work-up to rule out distant metastases. CT scan of the chest is useful for differentiating sites of recurrence in the skin, subcutaneous fat, pectoralis muscles, and brachial plexus from postoperative and postradiation changes. In addition, patients with chest wall or nodal recurrences may have additional sites of involvement discovered only on a CT scan of the chest (104–106). Such findings appear to be more common in patients with a short disease-free interval or multiple sites of disease. One site of unsuspected disease is in the internal mammary lymph nodes, usually located under or near the second and third intercostal spaces (106). Other evidence of disease that can be detected on CT scan includes sternal erosion, mediastinal lymphadenopathy, ipsilateral and contralateral axillary lymphadenopathy, rib metastases, involvement of the brachial plexus, nonpalpable tumor in the chest wall, and lung metastases. Lymphatic drainage patterns may be substantially altered following primary treatment (107). MRI of the chest and nodal regions may also delineate fibrosis from recurrent tumor after prior surgery or irradiation and may be useful for evaluation of patients with a reconstructed breast. As of yet, no study has compared the effectiveness of MRI to CT in this context, and in practice, the two are often used interchangeably. Whole-body positron emission tomography (PET) using fluorine-18-deoxyglucose appears to detect some sites of recurrence, particularly small lymph nodes, not seen on CT or MRI (108). However, PET scan also may result in both false-positive and false-negative results (108,109).

Prognosis

Despite aggressive local treatment, the large majority of patients with an isolated local recurrence following mastectomy will eventually develop distant metastases. Numerous factors have been proposed as influencing the disease-free interval and length of survival after the discovery and treatment of an isolated local or regional recurrence. Such factors include the interval between mastectomy and local recurrence; initial surgical stage; lymph node status at the time of mastectomy; the number of sites of recurrence; the location of recurrence (i.e., in the chest wall alone, lymph nodes alone, or a combination of sites); tumor grade; patient age; extent of disease at recurrence; estrogen- and progesterone-receptor status; and prior treatment.

Several institutional series have analyzed the impact of these potential prognostic factors (83,88,110–117). Although not all possible factors were examined in each of these studies, factors that consistently appear to predict for better outcomes are longer disease-free interval, limited chest wall involvement, and surgical excision of disease. Haffty et al. (113) reported that positive *HER-2/neu* status was associated with an increased rate of local-regional disease progression compared to negative *HER-2/neu* (41% vs. 8%, respectively; *p* = .007) (113).

In a cohort of 128 patients reported by Schwaibold et al. (116), a disease-free interval of 2 years or longer, ability to excise the recurrence and the initial axillary lymph nodal status were predictive of disease-free survival. Prolonged disease-free interval, tumor excision, and achieving subsequent local control were statistically significant predictors of overall survival. When all three factors were favorable, the 5-year rates of relapse-free survival and overall survival were 59% and 61%, respectively. In a separate study, the subset of favorable patients presenting with a disease-free interval after mastectomy of 2 or more years, isolated chest wall recurrence of 3 cm or less, and completely excised had a better outcome (117). For this favorable subset, the 10-year overall survival was 72%, cause specific survival 77%, and local control 86%.

There is limited information about whether patients who develop a local recurrence despite adjuvant postmastectomy radiation treatment have a different prognosis after local recurrence than patients who were never irradiated (82,83,88,93, 118–120). In a report of 535 patients with local-regional recurrence from the randomized DBCG (Danish Breast Cancer Group) 82b and 82c trials, Nielsen et al. (82) reported that there was no difference in the 10-year rate of developing distant metastatic disease based on original randomization to postmastectomy radiation treatment versus not (80% vs. 81%, respectively; $p = .96$). In a report of 39 patients with local-regional recurrence from the randomized British Columbia trial, Ragaz et al. (118) also reported no difference in the rate of developing distant metastatic disease (relative risk = 1.02; $p = .96$).

Treatment Results

Radiation Treatment

The outcomes after radiation treatment for isolated local-regional recurrence after mastectomy are shown in Table 72.5. The 5-year overall survival ranges from 35% to 82%, and the 10-year overall survival ranges from 26% to 62%.

Comprehensive irradiation to the chest wall and regional nodes provides the best chance of local-regional control and minimizes the risk of subsequent recurrence (83,121,122). In the Mallinckrodt series reported by Halverson et al. (121), the 5-year and 10-year subsequent chest wall failure rates were 25% and 37%, respectively, when "adequate" volumes were treated, compared to 64% and 82%, respectively, when small fields were treated.

Even when comprehensive chest wall and regional nodal irradiation fields are used, subsequent local failures can occur at the original sites of disease. The volume of disease remaining at the time of irradiation is a critical determinant of the likelihood of achieving long-term local control. However, gross tumor excision is not possible in all patients (116,120,121). In the University of Pennsylvania series reported by Schwaibold et al. (116), after radiation with or without gross excision, most subsequent failures (94%) had chest wall recurrence as a component. The subsequent chest wall failure rate was 61% when there was gross residual disease and 20% when complete excision was first performed. The 5-year local-regional control rate for these patients was 48%, compared to 34% for patients who had biopsy only prior to irradiation. Increasing the dose of radiation after excision from 45 to 50 Gy to more than 50 Gy did not improve local control. For patients with gross disease, the size and dose of radiation were important factors in local control. If the gross disease measured 4 cm or less and a dose of 60 Gy or more was used, local control was 57%, compared to 15% if less than 60 Gy was delivered.

After comprehensive irradiation, failures in the adjacent chest wall or other areas at the edges of the fields may still occur. These "marginal misses" appear to be more likely in patients with large tumor size or multiple sites of recurrence. Patients with chest wall recurrences may subsequently fail in regional lymph nodes when only the chest wall is irradiated. The risk of recurrence in untreated supraclavicular lymph nodes has been reported as 5% to 16% (116,121). The risk of clinically evident recurrence in untreated axillary or internal mammary lymph nodes is low. Therefore, routine or prophylactic treatment of the internal mammary lymph nodes in patients with local-regional recurrence, particularly those who have previously received systemic therapies associated with cardiac toxicity such as doxorubicin or trastuzumab, does not appear to be warranted.

The ability to achieve local control with radiation treatment is also related to the specific sites involved. Most series show higher local control rates when either the chest wall or lymph

Table 72.5 | **RESULTS OF SALVAGE RADIATION TREATMENT FOR ISOLATED LOCAL REGIONAL RECURRENCE AFTER MASTECTOMY**

Author (Reference)	No. of Patients	Years	Median Follow-Up (mos)	Local Control	Freedom from Distant Metastases		Overall Survival	
					At 5 yrs (%)	At 10 yrs (%)	At 5 yrs (%)	At 10 yrs (%)
Aberizk et al., 1986 (120)	90	1968–1978	81	35% (10 yr)	30	7	50	26
Chagpar et al., 2003 (114)	130	1988–1998	68.5	78% (crude)	—	—	48	29
Deutsch et al., 1986 (84)	107	1970–1979	NS	45% (5 yrs)	35 (RFS)	—	35	—
Haffty et al., 2004 (113)	113	1975–1999	122	79% (10 yrs)	49	40	46	28
Halverson et al., 1990 (121)	224	1964–1986	46	57% (5 yrs)	25	15 (RFS)	43	26
Haylock et al., 2000 (119)	120	1979–1989	24	RT only: 66% (10 yrs)	60	45	74	50
				RT+Chemo: 58% (10 yrs)	75	49	82	62
Mendenhall et al., 1988 (123)	47	1964–1983	24 (min)	61% (10 yrs)	41	17	50	34
Nielsen et al., 2006 (82)	535	1982–1990	216	47% (5 yrs)	27	20	36	—
Ragaz et al., 2005 (118)	39	1979–1986	249	—	58[a]	35[a]	—	—
Schwaibold et al., 1991 (116)	128	1967–1988	33	43% (5 yrs)	24	—	49	—
van Tienhoven et al., 1999 (91)	67	1980–1989	74	62% (5 yrs)	—	—	58	—

NS, not stated; RFS, relapse-free survival; RT, radiation treatment; Chemo, chemotherapy; min, minimum.
[a]Estimated from curve.

nodes are involved, rather than both (120,122,123). Control of inflammatory-type skin recurrences is especially difficult. However, it is not clear to what degree these results are governed by the volume or resectability of disease, rather than the specific site. In the University of Pennsylvania series reported by Schwaibold et al. (116), 76% of patients who had gross excision had disease 4 cm or less, compared to 51% of those who were not excised, although in the patients undergoing excision, the size did not affect the subsequent local recurrence rates. Patients who suffer a local failure following mastectomy and reconstruction have local control rates and outcomes similar to those of patients who had not had a reconstruction (124).

The technique used for radiation treatment of chest wall recurrence, with or without regional lymph nodal recurrence, is similar to that used for postmastectomy radiation treatment. Tangential chest wall beams are matched to an anterior supraclavicular field, with or without a posterior axillary boost, depending on the presentation of recurrence, and comprise the typical field arrangements for the majority of patients. The lateral border of the tangential fields is usually placed at the midaxillary line, or 2 cm beyond the lateral extent of mastectomy incision or gross disease. Supplementary electron beam fields matched to the edge of the photon fields are sometimes necessary in order to cover adequately the target volume laterally or medially. The match line between the tangential and supraclavicular fields should be placed in a location that avoids overlapping any area of gross disease. The optimal frequency with which to apply bolus is not known. At a minimum, gross surface lesions and biopsy scars should be covered with bolus daily. The remainder of the chest wall is treated with bolus in place generally every other day to minimize excessive skin toxicity requiring a treatment break. When patients have had prior reconstruction with a myocutaneous flap, bolus needs to be applied to at least the mastectomy scar, although whether to use the bolus on the entire reconstructed breast is uncertain. In general, daily 1.8 to 2.0 Gy fractions are delivered five times weekly. Initial doses of 45 to 50 Gy are used, with a boost of 10 to 20 Gy to areas of gross disease and biopsy scars, yielding a minimum total dose of 60 Gy or higher. Boosts are usually done with electrons. Radiation treatment is given without a planned break.

In a randomized study from the M.D. Anderson Cancer Center reported by Buchholz et al. (125), hyperfractionated twice daily radiation treatment was compared to conventional once daily radiation treatment. The 15-year results showed no difference in local-regional control between the two arms, but the incidence of acute skin toxicity of moist desquamation was higher in the hyperfractionated arm.

Treatment can be given with electron beams alone or with mixed photon-electron beams. Techniques using electron arcs or rotational motions have also been described (126). A "reverse hockey stick" technique may be useful for patients with extensive chest wall and nodal involvement (127). Other radiation treatment techniques have also been used either in conjunction with conventional external beam treatments or by themselves, such as low- or high-dose rate surface molds and interstitial implantation (128,129). There are no clear differences in local control between the different megavoltage photon or electron treatment techniques, and the selection of these is dictated by institutional practice.

Complication rates of contemporary radiation treatment techniques are low. Acute erythema and skin desquamation are nearly universal but self-limited. Telangiectasias and mild subcutaneous fibrosis commonly develop with time, but serious subacute or chronic complications are uncommon. In one series of 224 patients with prior axillary dissection, 3% developed radiation pneumonitis, 4% soft tissue necrosis or ulceration, 3% bone necrosis, and 1% neuropathy (121). The risk of arm lymphedema was reported as 11% when elective axillary irradiation was given compared to 1% when not used. All soft tissue complications

occurred among patients who received a dose of 60 Gy or higher, except one patient who received 50 Gy, and for whom doxorubicin was given concurrently with radiation treatment. Chest wall ulceration or soft tissue necrosis occurred in approximately 5% of patients treated to doses above 60 Gy (130). Concurrent administration of chemotherapy may also increase the risk of complications (123). Both the chemotherapy program and the details of radiation treatment administration may be important relative to the development of complications.

The results of most series suggest that patients who achieve a complete response or maintain local control after aggressive radiation treatment for an isolated local recurrence have longer survival times than patients who do not (112,116,121–123). This may reflect the effects of treatment or a less aggressive natural history. Nonetheless, most patients who achieve local control eventually develop distant metastases and subsequently die of breast cancer. However, even if only rarely curative, effective local treatment and local control certainly have an important impact on the overall quality of life.

Reirradiation

Limited data exist on retreatment of patients after adjuvant postmastectomy irradiation or previous radiation treatment given for recurrence (71,83,122,128,131–133). In a multi-institutional, retrospective study of 53 patients reported by Wahl et al. (71), the rate of acute toxicity was 35%, and the rate of severe late toxicity (grade 3 or 4) was 4%. Although the radiation treatment technique was variable, no radiation dose response was seen, even for radiation doses greater than 110 Gy, for acute toxicity, severe late toxicity, complete response rate, or local control at 1 year. In a series reported by Willner et al. (83), limited re-irradiation fields were used in 40 patients at the time of recurrence. A lower local-regional control after recurrence was noted in re-irradiated patients compared to patients without preceding radiation (79% vs. 91%). Patients who received radiation to the total site of recurrence had a higher 5-year survival rate than those who had small local fields only (47% vs. 31%). However, prior postmastectomy irradiation was not a significant prognostic factor for survival. In a series reported by Toonkel et al. (131), 36 previously irradiated patients had lower rates of local control (36% vs. 68%) and survival at 10 years (20% vs. 35%) than 88 previously unirradiated patients. Chen et al. (122) reported on 60 patients who received reirradiation to only the site of recurrent disease, and their local-regional control rate was 73%.

A small series reported on 13 patients who received 40 to 60 Gy in 4 to 6 weeks using electrons, after previous treatment of 40 to 50 Gy to the entire chest wall, with a 70% local-regional control rate and no evidence of soft-tissue necrosis (132). A small group of nine patients who had received postmastectomy radiation treatment were retreated with electrons to small fields, giving a dose of 40 to 50 Gy, with or without a 10 to 15 Gy boost (133). Complete durable response or stable disease after treatment with full healing of the chest wall was achieved in 89% (8/9), with one instance of osteomyelitis. Local control was achieved in 9 of 11 patients retreated with a surface mold to doses of 60 Gy in two to three applications (128). Thus, retreatment of at least limited volumes with limited radiation doses can result in meaningful palliation in selected patients.

Surgery

Subsequent local failure occurs in 60% to 75% of patients after limited local excision only (134,135). For selected patients, high local control rates have been obtained with very wide local excision of skin and subcutaneous tissue or with partial or full-thickness chest wall resection, with some patients surviving 5 years or more (115,136–138). The likelihood of further local recurrence is higher for patients presenting with multiple nodules on the chest wall than for those with a single nodule.

Some authors have advocated using chest wall resection as the initial treatment of isolated local failure. However, the local and distant relapse rates after this approach are high, and the treatment-related morbidity may be substantial. In a series by Dahlstrøm et al. (139), 69 patients underwent wide local excision for local recurrences, and the 5-year actuarial local control rate was 50%, with 5-year overall survival of 62%. Among 23 patients reported by Miyauchi et al. (140) treated with full thickness chest wall resection, 48% had further local-regional recurrence. The 5-year relapse-free and overall survival rates were 26% and 48%, respectively.

Complications after chest wall resection are not well documented but may be substantial. Approximately 40% of patients with breast cancer undergoing partial or full-thickness chest wall resection at the M.D. Anderson Cancer Center reported by Kroll et al. (137) developed significant complications, although most of these did not require major interventions. In a series of 18 patients treated in Milan reported by Muscolino et al. (138), only one patient required reoperation for repair of flap necrosis.

Hyperthermia

Six randomized trials have compared the results of radiation treatment with or without hyperthermia (141–143). Four of these trials showed no difference in complete response rates between the comparison arms, while in two trials (including the largest, which included only 149 patients), there was a benefit to hyperthermia. A meta-analysis that included five of these studies showed a complete response rate of 49% to radiation treatment alone, compared to 59% for hyperthermia plus radiation treatment (143). However, there was substantial heterogeneity among the patient populations, treatment parameters, and response rates among these five trials. In an update of a randomized trial of 122 patients from Duke University, reported by Jones et al. (141), the complete response rate was higher after hyperthermia plus radiation treatment compared to radiation treatment alone (66% vs. 42%; $p = .02$). In a multi-institutional, retrospective study, Wahl et al. (71) reported a trend toward an increased complete response rate associated with hyperthermia (67% vs. 39%, respectively; $p = .08$).

Hyperthermia may increase the risk of complications, including thermal blisters, ulcerations, and necrosis (144,145). Most of these complications heal slowly with conservative management, although surgery is occasionally required in some cases.

Overall, the value of hyperthermia in combination with irradiation in the management of patients with locally recurrent breast cancer is uncertain. Tumor size and technical factors may play substantial roles in the likelihood of benefit from hyperthermia (142,146,147).

Other Local Therapies

Photodynamic treatment (PDT) uses laser light in combination with a photosensitizing drug (a hematoporphyrin derivative) for the treatment of cancer (148). PDT for cutaneous chest wall recurrence has variable complete response rates ranging from in small series (149–151). Most patients included in these series were heavily pretreated and often had extensive disease, although better results were noted for smaller nodular tumors or limited sites. PDT can cause pain and prolonged superficial skin necrosis, although surgical repair is rarely needed (150).

Other local therapies that have been reported in small studies include intra-arterial regional chemotherapy, topical injection of chemotherapy, biologic response modifiers, or interferon (152–155).

Subsequent Local-Regional Recurrence

After salvage radiation treatment to the chest wall or regional nodes, subsequent local control is achieved in about two thirds of patients, and the use of tamoxifen may further improve these results (156). Subsequent local or regional recurrence after salvage treatment occurs in 25% to 35% of treated patients, usually within 5 years of salvage treatment (91). Factors related to local outcome after salvage treatment include the extent of local-regional failure, the interval to first local-regional failure, and the pathologic nodal stage. About 30% of patients with chest wall failure suffer significant morbidity due to their local recurrence (93,157). In a series of patients with uncontrolled local-regional disease, 62% had one or more significant symptoms before death (94). Local recurrence in itself may directly be a cause of death due to infection or pulmonary compromise (89,157). Treatment at the time of local-regional rerecurrence must be individualized, depending on respectability, prior radiation received, and prior systemic treatment.

 ## REGIONAL LYMPH NODE RECURRENCE

Regional lymph node recurrence can occur after mastectomy or breast-conservation treatment. Regional lymph node recurrence can occur in the axillary, supraclavicular, infraclavicular, or internal mammary lymph node region. Regional lymph node recurrence can occur as an isolated event or concurrently with local or distant disease.

The first manifestation of regional lymph node recurrence is usually an asymptomatic mass in the axilla or in the supraclavicular fossa (Table 72.6). Nodal failures may occur more than 5 years, and even 10 years, after primary treatment (157–161). Isolated internal mammary lymph node recurrence can occasionally be misinterpreted as a solitary "sternal" metastasis (162).

Table 72.6   SITE(S) OF REGIONAL LYMPH NODE RECURRENCE(S) AFTER BREAST-CONSERVATION TREATMENT

		Isolated Lymph Node Recurrence			
Study (Reference)	No. of Patients	Axillary	Supraclavicular	Internal Mammary	Multiple Sites
Fourquet et al., 1989 (40)	9	8 (89%)	1 (11%)	—	—
Harris et al., 2003 (158)	39	21 (54%)	8 (20%)	3 (8%)	7 (18%)
Kemperman et al., 1995 (42)	26	11 (42%)	13 (50%)	1 (4%)	1 (4%)
Recht et al., 1989 (43)	10	5 (50%)	3 (30%)	1 (10%)	1 (10%)
Recht et al., 1991 (159)	38	22 (58%)	11[a] (29%)	2 (5%)	3 (8%)
Stotter et al., 1991 (57)	4	3 (75%)	—	—	1 (25%)

[a]Includes one patient with infraclavicular failure.

Only a minority of patients present with symptoms referable to regional failure, for example, arm edema, neurologic impairment, or pain. In the JCRT (Joint Center for Radiation Therapy) series of patients with nodal recurrence without simultaneous breast failure, such symptoms were found at presentation in 32% (12/38) of patients (159). These included 23% of patients (5/22) with isolated axillary failure and 44% of patients (7/16) with other sites of nodal failure. Significant pain or other distressing symptoms at last follow-up or death were present in 32% of patients with regional failure (12/38). In another series, 24% of patients who developed regional nodal failure following mastectomy had at least one significant symptom during follow-up (93). Pain or arm edema may be more common among patients with supraclavicular recurrence.

Harris et al. (158) reported the results of treatment of 39 patients with regional lymph node recurrence. Prognosis was related to the site of disease, and only those patients with axillary only nodal failure were salvaged, whereas patients with supraclavicular, internal mammary node, or multiple sites of nodal disease were not salvaged. The overall survival rate for patients with regional recurrence only was 67% at 5 years and 44% at 10 years. Galper et al. (160) reported the outcome of 28 patients with isolated axillary nodal recurrence. The 5-year overall survival after treatment was 70%, and the median survival time was 9.5 years.

For the patient presenting with regional lymph node recurrence, careful evaluation for local, other nodal, and distant sites of failure should be conducted prior to treatment. In patients with regional lymph node failure after breast-conservation treatment, the presence of a simultaneous breast recurrence should be ruled out by physical examination, mammography, and other imaging studies, as indicated. In one series, 27% of patients (7/26) with nodal failure after mastectomy who did not undergo elective chest wall irradiation were subsequently found to have local recurrence on the chest wall (121). Concurrent distant metastases are especially common in patients with supraclavicular disease (42). In patients with symptoms suggestive of brachial plexopathy or arm edema without obvious lymphadenopathy, it may be difficult to distinguish clinically between tumor recurrence in the axilla and the effects of postoperative radiation treatment. The use of MRI may be helpful in this regard, as local enhancement with gadolinium suggests the presence of tumor, rather than radiation related fibrosis.

Prognosis after nodal recurrence is related to which site is involved, and an isolated axillary recurrence generally has the most favorable prognosis (83,84,110,121–123,158–161). Gross surgical excision is associated with improved regional control (121,159,161).

SYSTEMIC THERAPY

There are few data on the role of systemic therapy after local recurrence. Studies examining survival outcomes after local-regional recurrence typically have not considered the role of subsequent systemic therapy in modifying the risk of subsequent local-regional relapse, distant metastatic disease, or survival. Adjuvant systemic therapy is now commonly used following initial diagnosis of the primary tumor. Therefore, for many patients who suffer local recurrence, questions of drug resistance and tolerance to further systemic treatment must be considered, similar to those facing patients with overt systemic relapse.

Systemic therapy alone, without surgery or radiation, is of questionable long-term efficacy (77,163). Some individuals with chest wall fixation may respond sufficiently to chemotherapy or hormonal therapy to allow mastectomy. However, systemic therapy alone is not effective in obtaining permanent local control of inoperable disease (57). The value of adjuvant systemic therapy after regional lymph node recurrence is difficult to assess (158–160).

Retrospective series of patients with local-regional recurrence have failed to show improvement in outcome in patients treated with systematic therapy in addition to radiotherapy or resection (37,49,52,55), but those patients who received systemic therapy likely had poorer prognoses than those who did not. For example, Doyle et al. (49) from the University of Pennsylvania reported that the 5-year rate of overall survival was 72% for patients receiving chemotherapy and 88% for patients not receiving chemotherapy ($p = .13$). A small number of patients have been reported using high-dose chemotherapy and autologous bone marrow transplantation (164,165).

Few prospective trials of systemic therapy for local-regional relapse have been published. An Italian multicenter phase II trial reported by Pergolizzi et al. (166) enrolled 44 patients with isolated ipsilateral supraclavicular lymph node metastases at least 6 months after treatment for primary operable breast cancer into a phase II study of six cycles of either anthracycline-based combination chemotherapy or paclitaxel monotherapy. Radiotherapy was given after the third cycle of chemotherapy. The 5-year actuarial disease-free and overall survival rates were 20% and 35%, respectively. A German phase II study reported by Semrau et al. (167) of 36 patients with local-regional recurrence, the majority of which were inoperable, were given concurrent radiotherapy and taxane, with or without cisplatin. Small numbers per group and the mix of resected and unresected patients preclude definitive conclusions regarding response; however, toxicity, including dermatitis and leukopenia, was substantial.

Three randomized trials have been published addressing the role of systemic therapy after local-regional recurrence (156,168–170). During the 1970s, Olson et al. (169) randomized 32 women to actinomycin-D or control after radiotherapy. Chemotherapy improved the local control rate, but had no apparent effect on overall survival. During the 1980s, Fentiman et al. (170) randomized 32 patients to either α-interferon or observation after radiotherapy. α-Interferon had no apparent effect on the further course of the disease. Finally, the largest randomized trial to date, conducted by the Swiss Group for Clinical Cancer Research, addressed the use of systemic therapy (either chemotherapy or tamoxifen) at the time of local recurrence after mastectomy (156). For 167 good risk patients (defined as positive or undetermined estrogen receptors, disease-free interval greater than 1 year, and three or fewer nodules measuring 3 cm or smaller), treatment included complete gross tumor resection and 50 Gy to the involved region. Patients were randomized to receive tamoxifen until relapse or observation. With a median follow-up of 11.6 years, the addition of tamoxifen improved the 5-year rates of disease-free survival (61% vs. 40%, respectively; $p = .053$), and local control (8% vs. 25%, respectively; $p = .011$), but not overall survival (73% vs. 79%, respectively; $p = .79$).

Because of the scarcity of existing data and lack of a recognized standard for the optimal systemic treatment after local-regional relapse, participation in ongoing multicenter clinical trials should be encouraged. The International Breast Cancer Study Group and National Surgical Adjuvant Breast and Bowel Project are jointly conducting an international study that randomizes women to chemotherapy or not after local-regional resection. Two trials currently under way in Europe include the German Adjuvant Breast Cancer Group GABG-6 trial, which randomizes patients to doxorubicin or docetaxel versus control, and the Federation Nationale des Centres de Lutte Contre le Cancer PACS-03 that randomizes patients to FEC (5-fluorouracil, epirubicin, and cyclophosphamide) followed by docetaxel versus control. All three trials include quality of life evaluation as a primary end point. In the absence of a clinical trial, considerations for systemic therapy in the management of local-regional recurrence are individualized to the patient and must include considerations regarding risk of subsequent distant recurrence, toxicity, and quality of life.

MANAGEMENT SUMMARY

Local Recurrence after Breast-Conservation Treatment

- Local recurrence after breast-conservation treatment is detected by mammography or physical examination. The diagnosis can be established by core biopsy or excisional biopsy. Patients with an invasive local recurrence should be considered for a work-up for metastatic disease based on the characteristics of the recurrence.
- Mastectomy is the standard treatment for local recurrence after breast-conservation treatment.
- There is limited experience with excision with or without reirradiation, and the available results suggest a substantially higher rate of subsequent local recurrence than with mastectomy. Experimental trials of accelerated partial breast irradiation are under way.
- The role of systemic therapy is undefined in patients with an isolated local recurrence. In a patient with an ER/PR-positive local recurrence, hormonal therapy seems reasonable.

Local Recurrence after Mastectomy

- Local recurrence after mastectomy is most commonly detected on physical examination.
- The diagnosis can be established on surgical biopsy.
- Metastatic work-up is indicated.
- If the local recurrence is operable, surgical excision followed by radiation therapy is the standard treatment. The volume of radiation treatment should include the entire chest wall and appropriate nodal regions (depending on prior axillary surgery). A boost to the area of recurrence to a total dose of at least 60 Gy should be given.
- After surgical excision and radiation therapy, the role of systemic treatment is not defined. In a patient with an ER/PR-positive local recurrence, hormonal therapy seems reasonable.
- If the local recurrence is not operable, consider systemic treatment to render the recurrence operable.
- For patients with a local recurrence after mastectomy and postmastectomy radiation therapy, there is no standard treatment. Full chest wall reirradiation is associated with a substantial risk of complications. Systemic therapy and limited volume reirradiation are often used. Novel local modalities, such as hyperthermia or photodynamic treatment, can be considered.

Regional Lymph Node Recurrence

- Regional lymph node recurrence is most commonly detected on physical examination.
- The diagnosis can be established by fine-needle aspiration, core biopsy, or surgical biopsy.
- Metastatic work-up is indicated.
- If the regional recurrence is operable, surgical excision is indicated.
- After surgical excision, the role of systemic treatment is not defined.

- In view of the wide variation in presentations of regional lymph node recurrence, the overall treatment program must be individualized based on site(s) of recurrence and prior treatment.

References

1. Recht A, Silver B, Schnitt S, et al. Breast relapse following primary radiation therapy for early breast cancer. I. Classification, frequency and salvage. *Int J Radiat Oncol Biol Phys* 1985;11:1271–1276.
2. Plastaras JP, Harris EE, Solin LJ. Paget's disease of the nipple as local recurrence after breast-conservation treatment for early-stage breast cancer. *Clin Breast Cancer* 2005;6:349–353.
3. Chaudary MA, Nagadowska M, Smith P, et al. Local recurrence after breast conservation treatment: outcome following salvage mastectomy. *Breast* 1998;7:33–38.
4. Dershaw DD, McCormick B, Osborne MP. Detection of local recurrence after conservative therapy for breast carcinoma. *Cancer* 1992;70:493–496.
5. Stotter AT, McNeese MD, Ames FC, et al. Predicting the rate and extent of locoregional failure after breast conservation therapy for early breast cancer. *Cancer* 1989;64:2217–2225.
6. Recht A, Silen W, Schnitt SJ, et al. Time-course of local recurrence following conservative surgery and radiotherapy for early stage breast cancer. *Int J Radiat Oncol Biol Phys* 1988;15:255–261.
7. Voogd AC, van Tienhoven G, Peterse HL, et al. Local recurrence after breast conservation therapy for early stage breast carcinoma: detection, treatment and outcome in 266 patients. Dutch Study Group on Local Recurrence after Breast Conservation (BORST). *Cancer* 1999;85:437–446.
8. Vicini FA, Antonucci JV, Goldstein N, et al. The use of molecular assays to establish definitively the clonality of ipsilateral breast tumor recurrences and patterns of in-breast failure in patients with early-stage breast cancer treated with breast-conserving therapy. *Cancer* 2007;109:1264–1272.
9. Bollet MA, Servant N, Neuvial P, et al. High-resolution mapping of DNA breakpoints to define true recurrences among ipsilateral breast cancers. *J Natl Cancer Inst* 2008;100:48–58.
10. Hassell PR, Olivotto IA, Mueller HA, et al. Early breast cancer: detection of recurrence after conservative surgery and radiation therapy. *Radiology* 1990;176:731–735.
11. Giess CS, Keating DM, Osborne MP, et al. Local tumor recurrence following breast-conserving therapy: correlation of histopathologic findings with detection method and mammographic findings. *Radiology* 1999;212:829–835.
12. Orel SG, Troupin RH, Patterson EA, et al. Breast cancer recurrence after lumpectomy and irradiation: role of mammography in detection. *Radiology* 1992;183:201–206.
13. Mendelson EB. Imaging of the post-surgical breast. *Semin Ultrasound CT MR* 1989;2:154–170.
14. Burrell HC, Sibbering DM, Evans AJ, et al. Do mammographic features of locally recurrent breast cancer mimic those of the original tumor? *Breast* 1996;5:233–236.
15. Weinstein SP, Orel SG, Pinnamaneni P, et al. Mammographic appearance of recurrent breast cancer after breast conservation therapy. *Acad Radiol* 2008;15:240–244.
16. Moy L, Slanetz PJ, Moore R, et al. Specificity of mammography and US in the evaluation of a palpable abnormality: retrospective review. *Radiology* 2002;225:176–181.
17. Soo MS, Rosen EL, Baker JA, et al. Negative predictive value of sonography with mammography in patients with palpable breast lesions. *AJR Am J Roentgenol* 2001;177:1167–1170.
18. Kolb TM, Lichy J, Newhouse JH. Comparison of the performance of screening mammography, physical examination, and breast US and evaluation of factors that influence them: an analysis of 27,825 patient evaluations. *Radiology* 2002;225:165–175.
19. Leconte I, Feger C, Galant C, et al. Mammography and subsequent whole-breast sonography of nonpalpable breast cancers: the importance of radiologic breast density. *AJR Am J Roentgenol* 2003;180:1675–1679.
20. Crystal P, Strano SD, Shcharynski S, Koretz MJ. Using sonography to screen women with mammographically dense breasts. *AJR Am J Roentgenol* 2003;181:177–182.
21. Kaplan SS. Clinical utility of bilateral whole-breast US in the evaluation of women with dense breast tissue. *Radiology* 2001;221:641–649.
22. Berg WA, Blume JD, Cormack JB, et al. Yield of screening breast ultrasound and mammography compared to mammography alone: results of first screen in ACRIN (American College of Radiology Imaging Network). *RSNA* 2007;SSC01-02(abst).
23. Berg WA, Blume JD, Cormack JB, et al. Risk of false positives with supplemental screening breast: results from the first screen in ACRIN (American College of Radiology Imaging Network). *RSNA* 2007;SSC01-03(abst).
24. Lehman CD, Isaacs C, Schnall MD, et al. Cancer yield of mammography, MR, and US in high-risk women: prospective multi-institution breast cancer screening study. *Radiology* 2007;244:381–388.
25. Lehman CD, Blume JD, Weatherall P, et al. International Breast MRI Consortium Working Group. Screening women at high risk for breast cancer with mammography and magnetic resonance imaging. *Cancer* 2005;103:1898–1905.
26. Lehman CD, Blume JD, Thickman D, et al. Added cancer yield of MRI in screening the contralateral breast of women recently diagnosed with breast cancer: results from the International Breast Magnetic Resonance Consortium (IBMC) trial. *J Surg Oncol* 2005;92:9–15.
27. Morris EA, Liberman L, Ballon DJ, et al. MRI of occult breast carcinoma in a high-risk population. *AJR Am J Roentgenol* 2003;181:619–626.
28. Dao TH, Rahmouni A, Campana F, et al. Tumor recurrence versus fibrosis in the irradiated breast: differentiation with dynamic gadolinium-enhanced MR imaging. *Radiology* 1993;187:751–755.
29. Viehweg P, Heinig A, Lampe D, et al. Retrospective analysis for evaluation of the value of contrast-enhanced MRI in patients treated with breast conservative therapy. *MAGMA* 1998;7:141–152.
30. Belli P, Pastore G, Romani M, et al. Role of magnetic resonance imaging in the diagnosis of recurrence after breast conserving therapy. *Rays* 2002;27:241–257.

31. Lewis-Jones HG, Whitehouse GH, Leinster SJ. The role of magnetic resonance imaging in the assessment of local recurrent breast carcinoma. *Clin Radiol* 1991;43:197–204.

32. Preda L, Villa G, Rizzo S, et al. Magnetic resonance mammography in the evaluation of recurrence at the prior lumpectomy site after conservative surgery and radiotherapy. *Breast Cancer Res* 2006;8:R53.

33. Gilles R, Guinebretiere JM, Shapeero LG, et al. Assessment of breast cancer recurrence with contrast-enhanced subtraction MR imaging: preliminary results in 26 patients. *Radiology* 1993;188:473–478.

34. Solomon B, Orel SG, Reynolds C, et al. Delayed development of enhancement in fat necrosis after breast conservation therapy: a potential pitfall of MR imaging of the breast. *AJR Am J Roentgenol* 1998;170:966–968.

35. Saslow D, Boetes C, Burke W, et al. American Cancer Society guidelines for breast screening with MRI as an adjunct to mammography. *CA Cancer J Clin* 2007;57:75–89.

36. Dalberg K, Mattsson A, Sandelin K, et al. Outcome of treatment for ipsilateral breast tumor recurrence in early-stage breast cancer. *Breast Cancer Res Treat* 1998;49:69–78.

37. Fowble B, Solin L, Schultz D, et al. Breast recurrence following conservative surgery and radiation: patterns of failure, prognosis, and pathologic findings from mastectomy specimens with implications for treatment. *Int J Radiat Oncol Biol Phys* 1990;19:833–842.

38. Haffty BG, Fischer D, Beinfield M, et al. Prognosis following local recurrence in the conservatively treated breast cancer patient. *Int J Radiat Oncol Biol Phys* 1991;21:293–298.

39. Kurtz JM, Amalric R, Brandone H, et al. Local recurrence after breast-conserving surgery and radiotherapy. Frequency, time course, and prognosis. *Cancer* 1989;63:1912–1917.

40. Fourquet A, Campana F, Zafrani B, et al. Prognostic factors of breast recurrence in the conservative management of early breast cancer: a 25-year follow-up. *Int J Radiat Oncol Biol Phys* 1989;17:719–725.

41. Leung S, Otmezguine Y, Calitchi E, et al. Locoregional recurrences following radical external beam irradiation and interstitial implantation for operable breast cancer: a twenty-three year experience. *Radiother Oncol* 1986;5:1–10.

42. Kemperman H, Borger J, Hart A, et al. Prognostic factors for survival after breast conserving therapy for stage I and II breast cancer. The role of local recurrence. *Eur J Cancer* 1995;31A:690–698.

43. Recht A, Schnitt SJ, Connolly JL, et al. Prognosis following local or regional recurrence after conservative surgery and radiotherapy for early stage breast carcinoma. *Int J Radiat Oncol Biol Phys* 1989;16:3–9.

44. Salvadori B, Marubini E, Miceli R, et al. Reoperation for locally recurrent breast cancer in patients previously treated with conservative surgery. *Br J Surg* 1999;86:84–87.

45. Ashkanani F, Sarkar T, Needham G, et al. What is achieved by mammographic surveillance after breast conservation treatment for breast cancer? *Am J Surg* 2001;182:207–210.

46. Kurtz JM, Jacquemier J, Brandone H, et al. Inoperable recurrence after breast conserving surgical treatment and radiotherapy. *Surg Gynecol Obstet* 1991;172:357–361.

47. Voogd AC, van Oost FJ, Rutgers EJT, et al. Long-term prognosis of patients with local recurrence after conservative surgery and radiotherapy for early breast cancer. *Eur J Cancer* 2005;41:2637–2644.

48. Gage I, Schnitt SJ, Recht A, et al. Skin recurrences after breast-conserving therapy for early stage breast cancer. *J Clin Oncol* 1998;16:480–486.

49. Doyle T, Schultz DJ, Peters C, et al. Long-term results of local recurrence after breast conservation treatment for invasive breast cancer. *Int J Radiat Oncol Biol Phys* 2001;51:74–80.

50. Galper S, Blood E, Gelman R, et al. Prognosis after local recurrence after conservative surgery and radiation for early-stage breast cancer. *Int J Radiat Oncol Biol Phys* 2005;61:348–357.

51. Haffty BG, Carter D, Flynn SD, et al. Local recurrence versus new primary: clinical analysis of 82 breast relapses and potential applications for genetic fingerprinting. *Int J Radiat Oncol Biol Phys* 1993;27:575–583.

52. Orel SG, Fowble BL, Solin LJ, et al. Breast cancer recurrence after lumpectomy and radiation therapy for early-stage disease: prognostic significance of detection method. *Radiology* 1993;188:189–194.

53. Osborne MP, Borgen PI, Wong GY, et al. Salvage mastectomy for local and regional recurrence after breast-conserving operation and radiation therapy. *Surg Gynecol Obstet* 1992;174:189–194.

54. Le MG, Arriagada R, Spielmann M, et al. Prognostic factors for death after an isolated local recurrence in patients with early-stage breast carcinoma. *Cancer* 2002;94:2813–2820.

55. Abner AL, Recht A, Eberlein T, et al. Prognosis following salvage mastectomy for recurrence in the breast after conservative surgery and radiation therapy for early-stage breast cancer. *J Clin Oncol* 1993;11:44–48.

56. Kurtz JM, Spitalier J-M, Amalric R, et al. The prognostic significance of late local recurrence after breast-conserving therapy. *Int J Radiat Oncol Biol Phys* 1990;18:87–93.

57. Stotter A, Kroll S, McNeese M, et al. Salvage treatment for loco-regional recurrence following breast conservation therapy for early breast cancer. *Eur J Surg Oncol* 1991;17:231–236.

58. Cajucom CC, Tsangaris TN, Nemoto T, et al. Results of salvage mastectomy for local recurrence after breast-conserving surgery without radiation therapy. *Cancer* 1993;71:1774–1779.

59. McReady DR, Fish EB, Hiraki GY, et al. Total mastectomy is not always mandatory for the treatment of recurrent breast cancer after lumpectomy alone. *Can J Surg* 1992;35:485–488.

60. Turner BC, Harrold E, Matloff E, et al. *BRCA1/BRCA2* germline mutations in locally recurrent breast cancer patients after lumpectomy and radiation therapy: implications for breast-conserving management in patients with *BRCA1/BRCA2* mutations. *J Clin Oncol* 1999;17:3017–3024.

61. Pierce LJ, Strawderman M, Narod SA, et al. Effect of radiotherapy after breast-conserving treatment in women with breast cancer and germline *BRCA1/2* mutations. *J Clin Oncol* 2000;18:3360–3369.

62. Pierce LJ, Levin AM, Rebbeck TR, et al. Ten-year multi-institutional results of breast-conserving surgery and radiotherapy in *BRCA1/2*-associated stage I/II breast cancer. *J Clin Oncol* 2006;24:2437–2443.

63. Barr LC, Phillips RH, Brunt AM, et al. Salvage mastectomy after failed breast-conserving therapy for carcinoma of the breast. *Ann R Coll Surg (Engl)* 1991;73:126–129.

64. Port ER, Fey J, Gemignani ML, et al. Reoperative sentinel lymph node biopsy: a new option for patients with primary or locally recurrent breast carcinoma. *J Am Coll Surg* 2002;195:167–172.

65. Schnitt SJ, Connolly JL, Recht A, et al. Breast relapse following primary radiation therapy for early breast cancer. II. Detection, pathologic features and prognostic significance. *Int J Radiat Oncol Biol Phys* 1985;11:1277–1284.

66. Martelli G, DePalo G, Rossi N, et al. Long-term follow-up of elderly patients with operable breast cancer treated with surgery without axillary dissection plus adjuvant tamoxifen. *Br J Cancer* 1995;72:1251–1255.

67. Schnitt SJ, Hayman J, Gelman R, et al. A prospective study of conservative surgery alone in the treatment of selected patients with stage I breast cancer. *Cancer* 1996;77:1094–1100.

68. Clark RM, Whelan T, Levine M, et al. Randomized clinical trial of breast irradiation following lumpectomy and axillary dissection for node-negative breast cancer: an update. *J Natl Cancer Inst* 1996;88:1659–1664.

69. Liljegren G, Holmberg L, Adami H-O, et al. Sector resection with or without postoperative radiotherapy for stage I breast cancer: five-year results of a randomized trial. *J Natl Cancer Inst* 1994;86:717–722.

70. McCready DR, Chapman J-A, Wall JL, et al. Characteristics of local recurrences following lumpectomy for breast cancer. *Cancer Invest* 1994;12:568–573.

71. Wahl AO, Rademaker A, Kiel KD, et al. Multi-institutional review of repeat irradiation of chest wall and breast for recurrent breast cancer. *Int J Radiat Oncol Biol Phys* 2008;70:477–484.

72. Kuerer HM, Arthur DW, Haffty BG. Repeat breast-conserving surgery for in-breast local breast carcinoma recurrence: the potential role of partial breast irradiation. *Cancer* 2004;100:2269–2280.

73. Deutsch M. Repeat high-dose external beam radiation for in-breast tumor recurrence after previous lumpectomy and whole breast irradiation. *Int J Radiat Oncol Biol Phys* 2002;53:687–691.

74. Trombetta M, Julian T, Bhandari T, et al. Breast conservation surgery and interstitial brachytherapy in the management of locally recurrent carcinoma of the breast: the Allegheny General Hospital experience. *Brachytherapy* 2008;7:29–36.

75. Resch A, Fellner C, Mock U, et al. Locally recurrent breast cancer: pulse dose rate brachytherapy for repeat irradiation following lumpectomy—a second chance to preserve the breast. *Radiology* 2002;225:713–718.

76. Racadot S, Marchal C, Charra-Brunaud C, et al. Re-irradiation after salvage mastectomy for local recurrence after a conservative treatment: a retrospective analysis of twenty patients. *Cancer Radiother* 2003;7:369–379.

77. Gilliland MD, Barton RM, Copeland EM. The implications of local recurrence of breast cancer as the first site of therapeutic failure. *Ann Surg* 1983;197:284–287.

78. Scanlon EF. Local recurrence in the pectoralis muscles following modified radical mastectomy for carcinoma. *J Surg Oncol* 1985;30:149–151.

79. Granik MS, Bragdon RW, Hanna DC. Recurrent breast cancer at the time of breast reconstruction. *Ann Plast Surg* 1987;18:69–70.

80. Salas AP, Helvie MA, Wilkins EG, et al. Is mammography useful in screening for local recurrences in patients with TRAM flap breast reconstruction after mastectomy for multifocal DCIS? *Ann Surg Oncol* 1998;5:456–463.

81. Mund DF, Wolfson P, Gorczyca DP, et al. Mammographically detected recurrent nonpalpable carcinoma developing in a transverse rectus abdominis myocutaneous flap. A case report. *Cancer* 1994;74:2804–2807.

82. Nielsen HM, Overgaard M, Grau C, et al. Loco-regional recurrence after mastectomy in high-risk breast cancer—risk and prognosis. An analysis of patients from the DBCG 82b & c randomization trials. *Radiother Oncol* 2006;79:147–155.

83. Willner J, Kiricuta IC, Kolbl O. Locoregional recurrence of breast cancer following mastectomy: always a fatal event? Results of univariate and multivariate analysis. *Int J Radiat Oncol Biol Phys* 1997;37:853–863.

84. Deutsch M, Parsons J, Mittal BB. Radiation therapy for local-regional recurrent breast cancer. *Int J Radiat Oncol Biol Phys* 1986;12:2061–2065.

85. Carlson GW, Bostwick J III, Styblo TM, et al. Skin-sparing mastectomy: oncologic and reconstructive considerations. *Ann Surg* 1997;225:570–575.

86. Kroll SS, Khoo A, Singletary SE, et al. Local recurrence risk after skin-sparing and conventional mastectomy: a 6-year follow-up. *Plast Reconstr Surg* 1999;104:421–425.

87. Langstein HN, Chang MH, Singletary SE, et al. Breast cancer recurrence after immediate reconstruction: patterns and significance. *Plast Reconstr Surg* 2003;111:712–720.

88. Chagpar A, Langstein HN, Kronowitz SJ, et al. Treatment and outcome of patients with chestwall recurrence after mastectomy and breast reconstruction. *Am J Surg* 2004;187:164–169.

89. Andry G, Suciu S, Vico P, et al. Locoregional recurrences after 649 modified radical mastectomies: incidence and significance. *Eur J Surg Oncol* 1989;15:476–485.

90. Rangan AM, Ahern V, Yip D, Boyages J. Local recurrence after mastectomy and adjuvant CMF: implications for adjuvant radiation therapy. *Aust N Z J Surg* 2000;70:649–655.

91. van Tienhoven G, Voogd AC, Peterse JL, et al. Prognosis after treatment for loco-regional recurrence after mastectomy or breast conserving therapy in two randomised trials (EORTC 10801 and DBCG-82TM). EORTC Breast Cancer Cooperative Group and the Danish Breast Cancer Cooperative Group. *Eur J Cancer* 1999;35:32–38.

92. Janni W, Dimpfl T, Braun S, et al. Radiotherapy of the chest wall following mastectomy for early-stage breast cancer: impact on local recurrence and overall survival. *Int J Radiat Oncol Biol Phys* 2000;48:967–975.

93. Tennvall-Nittby L, Tenegrup I, Landberg T. The total incidence of loco-regional recurrence in a randomized trial of breast cancer TNM stage II: the South Sweden Breast Cancer Trial. *Acta Oncol* 1993;32:641–646.

94. Bedwinek JM, Lee J, Fineberg B, Ocwieza M. Analysis of failures following local treatment of isolated local-regional recurrence of breast cancer. *Int J Radiat Oncol Biol Phys* 1981;7:581–585.

95. Katz A, Strom EA, Buchholz TA, et al. The influence of pathologic tumor characteristics on locoregional recurrence rates following mastectomy. *Int J Radiol Oncol Biol Phys* 2001;50:735–742.

96. Fajardo LL, Roberts CC, Hunt KR. Mammographic surveillance of breast cancer patients: should the mastectomy site be imaged? *AJR Am J Roentgenol* 1993;161:953–955.

97. Propeck PA, Scanlan KA. Utility of axillary views in postmastectomy patients. *Radiology* 1993;187:769–771.

98. Noone RB, Frazier TG, Noone GC, et al. Recurrence of breast carcinoma following immediate reconstruction: a 13-year review. *Plast Reconstr Surg* 1994;93:96–106.

99. Howard MA, Polo K, Pusic AL, et al. Breast cancer local recurrence after mastectomy and TRAM flap reconstruction: incidence and treatment options. *Plast Reconstr Surg* 2006;117:1381–1386.
100. Helvie MA, Bailey JE, Roubidoux MA, et al. Mammographic screening of TRAM flap breast reconstructions for detection of nonpalpable recurrent cancer. *Radiology* 2002;224:211–215.
101. Helvie MA, Wilson TE, Roubidoux MA, et al. Mammographic appearance of recurrent breast carcinoma in six patients with TRAM flap breast reconstructions. *Radiology* 1998;209:711–715.
102. Monroe AT, Feigenberg SJ, Mendenhall NP. Angiosarcoma after breast-conserving therapy. *Cancer* 2003;97:1832–1840.
103. Brady MS, Gaynor JJ, Brennan MF. Radiation-associated sarcoma of bone and soft tissue. *Arch Surg* 1992;127:1379–1385.
104. Lindfors KK, Meyer JE, Busse PM, et al. CT evaluation of local and regional breast cancer recurrence. *AJR Am J Roentgenol* 1985;145:833–837.
105. Rosenman J, Churchill CA, Mauro MA, et al. The role of computed tomography in the evaluation of post-mastectomy locally recurrent breast cancer. *Int J Radiat Oncol Biol Phys* 1988;14:57–62.
106. Scatarige JC, Fishman EK, Zinreich ES, et al. Internal mammary lymphadenopathy in breast carcinoma: CT appraisal of anatomic distribution. *Radiology* 1988;167:89–91.
107. Perre CI, Hoefnagel CA, Kroon BBR, et al. Altered lymphatic drainage after lymphadenectomy or radiotherapy of the axilla in patients with breast cancer. *Br J Surg* 1996;83:1258.
108. Bender H, Kirst J, Palmedo H, et al. Value of ^{18}fluoro-deoxyglucose positron emission tomography in the staging of recurrent breast carcinoma. *Anticancer Res* 1997;17:1687–1692.
109. Moon DH, Maddahi J, Silverman DHS, et al. Accuracy of whole-body fluorine-18-FDG PET for the detection of recurrent or metastatic breast carcinoma. *J Nucl Med* 1998;39:431–435.
110. Halverson KJ, Perez CA, Kuske RR, et al. Locoregional recurrence of breast cancer: a retrospective comparison of irradiation alone versus irradiation and systemic therapy. *Am J Clin Oncol* 1992;15:93–101.
111. Kamby C, Senegeløv L. Pattern of dissemination and survival following isolated locoregional recurrence of breast cancer. A prospective study with more than 10 years of follow-up. *Breast Cancer Res Treat* 1997;45:181–192.
112. Mora EM, Singletary SE, Buzdar AU, et al. Aggressive therapy for locoregional recurrence after mastectomy in stage II and III breast cancer patients. *Ann Surg Oncol* 1996;3:162–168.
113. Haffty BG, Hauser A, Choi DH, et al. Molecular markers for prognosis after isolated postmastectomy chest wall recurrence. *Cancer* 2004;100:252–263.
114. Chagpar A, Meric-Bernstam F, Hunt KK, et al. Chest wall recurrence after mastectomy does not always portend a dismal outcome. *Ann Surg Oncol* 2003;10:628–634.
115. Faneyte IF, Rutgers EJT, Zoetmulder FAN. Chest wall resection in the treatment of locally recurrent breast carcinoma: indications and outcome for 44 patients. *Cancer* 1997;80:886–891.
116. Schwaibold F, Fowble BL, Solin LJ, et al. The results of radiation therapy for isolated local regional recurrence after mastectomy. *Int J Radiat Oncol Biol Phys* 1991;21:299–310.
117. Hsi RA, Antell A, Schultz DJ, et al. Radiation therapy for chest wall recurrence of breast cancer after mastectomy in a favorable subgroup of patients. *Int J Radiat Oncol Biol Phys* 1998;42:495–499.
118. Ragaz J, Olivotto IA, Spinelli JJ, et al. Locoregional radiation therapy in patients with high-risk breast cancer receiving adjuvant chemotherapy: 20-year results of the British Columbia randomized trial. *J Natl Cancer Inst* 2005;97:116–126.
119. Haylock BJ, Coppin CM, Jackson J, et al. Locoregional first recurrence after mastectomy: prospective cohort studies with and without immediate chemotherapy. *Int J Radiat Oncol Biol Phys* 2000;46:355–362.
120. Aberizk WJ, Silver B, Henderson IC, et al. The use of radiotherapy for treatment of isolated locoregional recurrence of breast carcinoma after mastectomy. *Cancer* 1986;58:1214–1218.
121. Halverson KJ, Perez CA, Kuske RR, et al. Isolated local regional recurrence of breast cancer following mastectomy: radiotherapeutic management. *Int J Radiat Oncol Biol Phys* 1990;19:851–858.
122. Chen KK-Y, Montague E, Oswald M. Results of irradiation in the treatment of locoregional breast cancer recurrence. *Cancer* 1985;56:1269–1273.
123. Mendenhall NP, Devine JW, Mendenhall WM, et al. Isolated local-regional recurrence following mastectomy for adenocarcinoma of the breast treated with radiation therapy alone or combined with surgery and/or chemotherapy. *Radiother Oncol* 1988;12:177–185.
124. Chu FCH, Kaufmann TP, Dawson GA, et al. Radiation therapy of cancer in prosthetically augmented or reconstructed breasts. *Radiology* 1992;185:429–433.
125. Buchholz TA, Strom EA, Oswald MJ, et al. Fifteen-year results of a randomized prospective trial of hyperfractionated chest wall irradiation versus once-daily chest wall irradiation after chemotherapy and mastectomy for patients with locally advanced noninflammatory breast cancer. *Int J Radiat Oncol Biol Phys* 2006;65:1155–1160.
126. Gaffney DK, Lee CM, Leavitt DD, et al. Electron arc irradiation of the postmastectomy chest wall in locally recurrent and metastatic breast cancer. *Am J Clin Oncol* 2003;26:241–246.
127. Pezner RD, Lipsett JA, Forell B, et al. The reverse hockey stick technique: postmastectomy radiation therapy for breast cancer patients with locally advanced tumor presentation or extensive loco-regional recurrence. *Int J Radiat Oncol Biol Phys* 1989;17:191–197.
128. Delanian S, Housset M, Brunel P, et al. Iridium 192 plesiocurietherapy using silicone elastomer plates for extensive locally recurrent breast cancer following chest wall irradiation. *Int J Radiat Oncol Biol Phys* 1992;22:1099–1104.
129. Fritz P, Hensley FW, Berns C, et al. First experiences with superfractionated skin irradiation using large afterloading molds. *Int J Radiat Oncol Biol Phys* 1996;36:147–157.
130. Madoc-Jones H, Nelson AJ, Montague ED. Evaluation of the effectiveness of radiotherapy in the management of early nodal recurrences from adenocarcinoma of the breast. *Breast* 1976;2:31.
131. Toonkel LM, Fix I, Jacobson LH, Wallach CB. The significance of local recurrence of carcinoma of the breast. *Int J Radiat Oncol Biol Phys* 1983;9:33–39.
132. Laramore GE, Griffin TW, Parker RG, et al. The use of electron beams in treating local recurrence of breast cancer in previously irradiated fields. *Cancer* 1978;41:991–995.
133. Elkort RJ, Kelly W, Mozden PJ, et al. A combined treatment program for the management of locally recurrent breast cancer following chest wall irradiation. *Cancer* 1980;46:647–653.
134. Bedwinek JM, Lee J, Fineberg B, et al. Prognostic indicators in patients with isolated local-regional recurrence of breast cancer. *Cancer* 1981;47:2232–2235.
135. Probstfeld MR, O'Connell TX. Treatment of locally recurrent breast carcinoma. *Arch Surg* 1989;124:1127–1129.
136. Salvadori B, Rovini D, Squicciarini P, et al. Surgery for local recurrences following deficient radical mastectomy for breast cancer: a selected series of 39 cases. *Eur J Surg Oncol* 1992;18:438–441.
137. Kroll SS, Schusterman MA, Larson DL, et al. Long-term survival after chest-wall reconstruction with musculocutaneous flaps. *Plast Reconstr Surg* 1990;86:697–701.
138. Muscolino G, Valente M, Lequaglie C, et al. Correlation between first disease-free interval from mastectomy to second disease-free interval from chest wall resection. *Eur J Surg Oncol* 1992;18:49–52.
139. Dahlstrøm KK, Andersson AP, Andersen M, et al. Wide local excision of recurrent breast cancer in the thoracic wall. *Cancer* 1993;72:774–777.
140. Miyauchi K, Koyama H, Noguchi S, et al. Surgical treatment for chest wall recurrence of breast cancer. *Eur J Cancer* 1992;28A:1059–1062.
141. Jones EL, Oleson JR, Prosnitz LR, et al. Randomized trial of hyperthermia and radiation for superficial tumors. *J Clin Oncol* 2005;23:3079–3085.
142. Perez CA, Pajak T, Emami B, et al. Randomized phase III study comparing irradiation and hyperthermia with irradiation alone in superficial measurable tumors. *Am J Clin Oncol* 1991;14:133–141.
143. International Collaborative Hyperthermia Group. Radiotherapy with or without hyperthermia in the treatment of superficial localized breast cancer: results from five randomized controlled trials. *Int J Radiat Oncol Biol Phys* 1996;35:731–744.
144. Scott R, Gillespie B, Perez CA, et al. Hyperthermia in combination with definitive radiation therapy: results of a phase I/II RTOG study. *Int J Radiat Oncol Biol Phys* 1988;15:711–716.
145. Kapp DS, Barnett TA, Cox RS, et al. Hyperthermia and radiation therapy of local-regional recurrent breast cancer: prognostic factors for response and local control of diffuse or nodular tumors. *Int J Radiat Oncol Biol Phys* 1991;20:1147–1164.
146. Sherar M, Liu F-F, Pintilie M, et al. Relationship between thermal dose and outcome in thermoradiotherapy treatments for superficial recurrences of breast cancer: data from a phase III trial. *Int J Radiat Oncol Biol Phys* 1997;39:371–380.
147. Lee HK, Antell AG, Perez CA, et al. Superficial hyperthermia and irradiation for recurrent breast carcinoma of the chest wall: prognostic factors in 196 tumors. *Int J Radiat Oncol Biol Phys* 1998;40:365–375.
148. Dougherty TJ, Gomer CJ, Henderson BW, et al. Photodynamic therapy. *J Natl Cancer Inst* 1998;90:889–905.
149. Schuh M, Nseyo UO, Potter WR, et al. Photodynamic therapy for palliation of locally recurrent breast carcinoma. *J Clin Oncol* 1987;5:1766–1770.
150. Sperduto PW, DeLaney TF, Thomas G, et al. Photodynamic therapy for chest wall recurrence in breast cancer. *Int J Radiat Oncol Biol Phys* 1991;21:441–446.
151. Khan SA, Dougherty TJ, Mang TS. An evaluation of photodynamic therapy in the management of cutaneous metastases of breast cancer. *Eur J Cancer* 1993;29A:1686–1690.
152. Lewis WG, Walker VA, Ali HH, et al. Intra-arterial chemotherapy in patients with breast cancer: a feasibility study. *Br J Cancer* 1995;71:605–609.
153. David M, Sindermann H, Junge K, et al. Topical treatment of skin metastases with 6% miltefosine solution (Miltex) in patients with breast cancer. A meta-analysis of 443 patients. *Proc Am Soc Clin Oncol* 1997;16:150(abst).
154. Fernando I, Eisenberg PD, Roshon S, et al. Evaluation of intratumoral cisplatin/epinephrine injectable gel for palliative treatment of metastatic breast cancer. *Ann Oncol* 1998;9[Suppl 2]:181(abst).
155. Habif DV, Ozzello L, De Rosa CM, et al. Regression of skin recurrences of breast carcinomas treated with intralesional injections of natural interferons alpha and gamma. *Cancer Invest* 1995;13:165–172.
156. Waeber M, Castiglione-Gertsch M, Dietrich D, et al. Adjuvant therapy after excision and radiation of isolated postmastectomy locoregional breast cancer recurrence: definitive results of a phase III randomized trial (SAKK 23/82) comparing tamoxifen with observation. *Ann Oncol* 2003;14:1215–1221.
157. Marshall K, Redfern A, Cady B. Local recurrences of carcinoma of the breast. *Surg Gynecol Obstet* 1974;139:406–408.
158. Harris EER, Hwang W-T, Seyednajad F, et al. Prognosis after regional lymph node recurrence in patients with stage I–II breast carcinoma treated with breast conservation therapy. *Cancer* 2003;98:2144–2151.
159. Recht A, Pierce SM, Abner A, et al. Regional nodal failure after conservative surgery and radiotherapy for early-stage breast carcinoma. *J Clin Oncol* 1991;9:988–996.
160. Galper S, Blood E, Gelman R, et al. Prognosis after isolated axillary nodal recurrence following conservative surgery and radiotherapy for early-stage breast carcinoma. *Int J Radiat Oncol Biol Phys* 2002;54[Suppl 2]:56(abst).
161. Newman LA, Hunt KK, Buchholz T, et al. Presentation, management and outcome of axillary recurrence from breast cancer. *Am J Surg* 2000;180:252–256.
162. Kwai AH, Stomper PC, Kaplan WD. Clinical significance of isolated scintigraphic sternal lesions in patients with breast cancer. *J Nucl Med* 1988;29:324–328.
163. Hoogstraten B, Gad-el-Mawla N, Maloney TR, et al. Combined modality therapy for first recurrence of breast cancer: a Southwest Oncology Group study. *Cancer* 1984;54:2248–2256.
164. Mundt AJ, Sibley GS, Williams S, et al. Patterns of failure of complete responders following high dose chemotherapy and autologous bone marrow transplantation for metastatic breast cancer: implications for the use of adjuvant radiation therapy. *Int J Radiat Oncol Biol Phys* 1994;30:151–160.
165. Overmoyer BA, Carinder J, Andresen S, et al. The efficacy of high dose chemotherapy with autologous bone marrow transplantation for the treatment of osseous metastasis from breast cancer. *Breast Cancer Res Treat* 1997;46:72(abst).
166. Pergolizzi S, Adamo V, Russi E, et al. Prospective multicenter study of combined treatment with chemotherapy and radiotherapy in breast cancer women with the rare clinical scenario of ipsilateral supraclavicular node recurrence without distant metastases. *Int J Radiat Oncol Biol Phys* 2006;65:25–32.
167. Semrau S, Gerber B, Reimer T, et al. Concurrent radiotherapy and taxane chemotherapy in patients with locoregional recurrence of breast cancer: a retrospective analysis. *Strahlenther Onkol* 2006;182:596–603.
168. Rauschecker H, Clarke M, Gatzemeier W, et al. Systemic therapy for treating locoregional recurrence in women with breast cancer. *Cochrane Database Syst Rev* 2004:CD002195.

169. Olson CE, Ansfield FJ, Richards MJ, et al. Review of local soft tissue recurrence of breast cancer irradiated with and without actinomycin-D. *Cancer* 1977;39: 1981–1983.

170. Fentiman IS, Balkwill FR, Cuzick J, et al. A trial of human alpha interferon as an adjuvant agent in breast cancer after loco-regional recurrence. *Eur J Surg Oncol* 1987;13:425–428.

171. Chen C, Orel SG, Harris EER, et al. Relation between the method of detection of initial breast carcinoma and the method of detection of subsequent ipsilateral local recurrence and contralateral breast carcinoma. *Cancer* 2003;98:1596–1602.

172. Freedman GM, Anderson PR, Hanlon AL, et al. Pattern of local recurrence after conservative surgery and whole-breast irradiation. *Int J Radiat Oncol Biol Phys* 2005;61:1328–1336.

173. Dershaw DD, Geiss CS, McCormick B, et al. Patterns of mammographically detected calcifications after breast conserving therapy associated with tumor recurrence. *Cancer* 1997;79:1355–1361.

174. Clark RM, McCulloch PB, Levine MN, et al. Randomized clinical trial to assess the effectiveness of breast irradiation following lumpectomy and axillary dissection for node-negative breast cancer. *J Natl Cancer Inst* 1992;84: 683–689.

175. Haffty BG, Reiss M, Beinfield M, et al. Ipsilateral breast tumor recurrence as a predictor of distant disease: implications for systemic therapy at the time of local relapse. *J Clin Oncol* 1996;14:52–57.

176. Komoike Y, Akiyama F, Iino Y, et al. Ipsilateral breast tumor recurrence (IBTR) after breast-conserving treatment for early breast cancer: risk factors and impact on distant metastases. *Cancer* 2006;106:35–41.

177. van der Sangen MJC, van de Poll-Franse LV, Roumen RMH, et al. The prognosis of patients with local recurrence more than five years after breast conservation therapy for invasive breast carcinoma. *Eur J Surg Oncol* 2006;32: 34–38.

178. Veronesi U, Marubini E, Del Vecchio M, et al. Local recurrences and distant metastases after conservative breast cancer treatments: partly independent events. *J Natl Cancer Inst* 1995;87:19–27.

179. Kurtz JM, Amalric R, Brandone H, et al. Results of wide excision for mammary recurrence after breast conserving therapy. *Cancer* 1988;61:1969–1972.

Sacha J. Howell and Anthony Howell

The outlook of patients with primary breast cancer has improved in many countries related to earlier diagnosis and the widespread use of adjuvant therapy. Nonetheless, tumor relapse continues to occur and remains almost uniformly fatal. The clinician's role in this situation is to try to enhance both the length and quality of life by the judicious use of the therapeutic modalities available. Historically, endocrine therapy was the first systemic therapy used before chemotherapy became available. In patients with estrogen receptor (ER)–positive tumors, studies have shown little difference in outcome between initial endocrine and chemotherapy (1,2). It is customary, therefore, to treat these patients with the less toxic endocrine therapy first except in patients with rapidly progressive disease. This chapter will discuss patient selection for and monitoring during endocrine therapy, the endocrine treatments available for pre- and postmenopausal women, and the mechanisms of resistance to endocrine therapy and how these can be circumvented. The historical development of therapies in use today is outlined in Table 73.1.

PATIENT SELECTION

The ideal for patients with recurrent breast cancer is to select treatment most likely to be effective and with the least negative impact on their quality of life. Traditional predictors of responsiveness to endocrine therapy have been clinical factors such as long disease-free interval after adjuvant therapy, patients who are more than 5 years postmenopause and those who have nonvisceral disease and a well-differentiated primary tumor. Because the ER is the primary target of endocrine therapies, it has become mandatory to measure receptor expression in the primary tumor (3). Negative ER in the primary tumor is rarely associated with response, in particular in the absence of progesterone receptor (PR), and is an indicator for alternative systemic therapies. The response rate to first-line endocrine therapy is positively associated with quantitative ER expression and is increased in tumors that express both ER and PR. However, only 50% to 70% of tumors judged as ER positive on analysis of the primary tumor respond to first-line endocrine therapy for advanced disease. Thus ER expression has greater negative than positive predictive value.

Recent data have suggested that one reason for the poor positive predictive value of receptor measurements is a change in receptor phenotype between primary tumor and metastases (4). In a study of 200 patients in whom ER was measured in the primary tumor and a metastasis (mainly lymph node, bone, lung, and liver), Lower et al. (4) demonstrated that in 39 patients (19.5%), the ER was positive in the primary and negative in the metastasis, with the reverse situation seen in a further 21 patients (10.5%). Loss of ER in metastases predicted for inferior response to endocrine therapy and a shorter overall survival compared to tumors that retained or gained ER expression during metastasis. A number of smaller studies show similar changes in receptor phenotype, highlighting the importance of the biopsy in metastatic breast cancer (MBC) to accurately define the phenotype and treatment modality of recurrent cancers (4,5).

An approach to avoid biopsy is to measure the presence of ER in metastases *in vivo* by imaging uptake of ^{18}F-fluoroestra-diol (FES) by positron emission tomography (PET). However, studies have shown that whereas lack of uptake is associated with no responses to endocrine therapy, uptake itself has relatively poor positive predictive value (6,7). However, studies using ^{18}F-fluorodeoxyglucose (FDG) PET seem more promising. It is well known that endocrine agents can temporarily stimulate tumor activity soon after the initiation of treatment. This is known as *tumor flare* and usually indicates a subsequent response to treatment following achievement of steady state therapeutic concentrations (8,9). Clinical flare reactions, such as increased bone pain or lesion size, occur infrequently. However, metabolic flare can be detected if FDG-PET scans are performed before and shortly after the initiation of treatment. Such studies, using tamoxifen (20 mg) or estradiol (30 mg), have shown that measured FDG uptake has positive and negative predictive value for subsequent response to endocrine therapy of over 90% (6,10). If confirmed this technique may be the optimal method for determination of suitability for endocrine therapy.

ASSESSMENT OF RESPONSE TO ENDOCRINE THERAPY

The primary roles of endocrine therapy in MBC are to prolong life and to prevent or palliate cancer-related symptoms (2,11). As is the case for the majority of solid tumors, assessment of efficacy of endocrine therapy in MBC is primarily based on clinical examination, cross-sectional imaging, and in some cases serial tumor markers measured in blood or urine (3). Response is assessed according to criteria such as those devised by the World Health Organization (WHO) and the Response Evaluation Criteria in Solid Tumors (RECIST) authors (12). These criteria primarily help to define the limits for stable disease by giving the percentage increase in tumor burden above which the cancer is said to be progressing (PD) and the percentage shrinkage, below which the cancer is said to be objectively responding (OR). Complete disappearance of the cancer by clinicoradiological assessment is termed complete response (CR) and all other ORs are termed partial responses (PR).

However, in the age of novel agents that target tumor vasculature and in tumors that produce large amounts of extracellular matrix or connective tissue, it is increasingly argued that objective shrinkage of a tumor may not be required for maximum tumor control in the metastatic setting (13). In fact this phenomenon has long been recognized in the treatment of MBC and the term *clinical benefit* has been used to include patients whose cancers achieve OR and stable disease (SD), the latter for at least 24 weeks. The equivalence of OR and SD for more than 24 weeks has been demonstrated in large phase III trials of endocrine therapy and highlights the importance of the cytostatic effects of endocrine therapy (14–16). Although the quality of life of women with SD on second-line endocrine therapy has been shown to be inferior to those with OR, time to treatment failure was similar (17). Communication of the fact that SD equates to a response to therapy to these patients is essential to avoid unnecessary anxiety.

Table 73.1	**TIME LINE OF THE INTRODUCTION OF ENDOCRINE THERAPIES IN USE TODAY**	
Therapy	**Author (Ref)**	**Date**
Ovarian ablation	Beatson (19)	1896
Ovarian irradiation	DeCourmelles (22)	1922
Androgens	Ulrich (63)	1938
Estrogens	Haddow et al. (72)	1944
Progestins	Escher et al. (276)	1951
Hypophysectomy	Perrault et al. (277)	1952
Adrenalectomy	Huggins and Dao (44)	1953
Tamoxifen	Cole et al. (90)	1971
Aminoglutethimide	Griffiths et al. (46)	1973
LHRH analogs	Klijn and de Jong (33)	1982
Raloxifene	Buzdar et al. (100)	1988
Letrozole	Iveson et al. (278)	1993
Exemestane	Zilembo et al. (279)	1995
Pure antiestrogens	Howell and Robertson (113)	1995
Anastrazole	Jonat et al. (280)	1996

LHRH, luteinizing hormone-releasing hormone.

THERAPEUTIC OPTIONS

Ovarian Ablation

Oophorectomy is the oldest successful systemic treatment for breast cancer. The operation was first suggested by the German clinician A. Schinzinger (18), on the basis of his observation that younger women had more aggressive breast cancer. However, it was not until 1896 that Beatson (19) reported the first results of therapeutic oophorectomy in women with recurrent and locally advanced breast cancer. His first operation was performed on June 15, 1895, at the Glasgow Cancer Hospital. The patient was a 33-year-old premenopausal woman with recurrent breast cancer on the chest wall that had developed 6 months postmastectomy. The chest wall disease completely resolved for 49 months, but she died

2 years after this progression. Two of the six patients treated by Beatson responded and the one-third response rate was confirmed in two large series of 54 (20) and 99 (21) patients. These studies indicated that women aged 40 to 50 without visceral disease were most likely to respond (21).

Ovarian irradiation has also been shown to be effective (22). No formal comparison of the two types of ovarian ablation has been performed, but they were considered equivalent in the Oxford Overview (23). It is possible that irradiation may be less effective, since estrogen secretion may continue for some time after treatment, and in a small number of cases menses may resume (24). It would be of interest to perform a comparative analysis of the two techniques as a survey in the United Kingdom indicated that ovarian irradiation was the most common form of ovarian ablation used (radiotherapy 60%, surgery 30%, and luteinizing hormone-releasing hormone [LHRH] analogs 9%) (25).

More modern series of patients treated by oophorectomy are shown in Table 73.2. Objective response rates vary between 22.5% and 51.0%, with a median duration of remission of about 16 months (26–28). When tamoxifen was shown to be active in premenopausal women, the question of how it compared with ovarian ablation was asked. A meta-analysis of four studies showed no significant difference in response rate, time to progression, and survival between the two approaches, although there was a nonsignificant trend in favor of tamoxifen (29–32). However, 6 of 25 (24%) of patients initially treated by tamoxifen responded to subsequent oophorectomy, whereas 4 of 47 (8.5%) responded to tamoxifen after oophorectomy, suggesting that tamoxifen should be used first in the sequence.

LHRH analogs were first used to treat advanced premenopausal breast cancer in 1982 (33–35). Ovarian estrogen production is controlled by the hypothalamic pituitary ovarian axis. The hypothalamus releases LHRH in a pulsatile fashion under normal physiological conditions. LHRH regulates the pituitary release of gonadotrophin, which, in turn, stimulates ovarian estrogen production LHRH analogs (buserelin, goserelin, leuprorelin, triptorelin), which have higher binding affinities to pituitary gonadotrophin-releasing hormone (GnRH) receptors and greater resistance to degradation than endogenous LHRH. Chronic administration of LHRH analogs causes internalization of pituitary GnRH receptors, thus rendering the

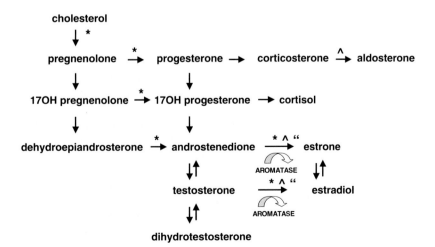

FIGURE 73.1. Steroid biosynthetic pathways showing the sites of inhibition of the first-generation aromatase inhibitor aminoglutethimide (*), the second-generation inhibitor fadrozole (^) and of the modern third-generation inhibitors ("), which do not appreciably affect adrenal steroid biosynthesis and inhibit peripheral aromatase.

Table 73.2	OVARIAN ABLATION ALONE AND COMPARATIVE TRIALS WITH OTHER APPROACHES IN PREMENOPAUSAL WOMEN WITH ADVANCED BREAST CANCER					
Author (Reference)	Treatment	n	ORR (%)	ORR ER + (%)	ORR ER − (%)	MDR (mos)
Veronesi et al. (28)	Oophorectomy	639	29.5	—	—	16
Conte et al. (26)	Oophorectomy	105	51.0	71	21	16
Oriana et al. (27)	Oophorectomy	71	50.7	67	17	—
Crump et al. (30)	Ovarian ablation[a]	111	22.5	—	—	4[b]
	vs. tamoxifen	109	22.9	—	—	6[b]
Blamey et al. (37)	Goserelin	228	36.4	44	31	11
Taylor et al. (281)	Goserelin	69	31	—	—	4[b]
	vs. oophorectomy	67	27	—	—	6[b]
Klijn et al. (39)	Buserelin	54	34	—	—	6.3[b]
	vs. tamoxifen	54	28	—	—	5.6[b]
	vs. both	53	48	—	—	9.7[b]
Klijn et al. (40)	LHRH + tamoxifen	250	39	42	—	602[c]
	vs. tamoxifen	256	30	33	—	350[c]

ORR, objective response rate; MDR, median duration of response; ER +, estrogen receptor positive; ER−, estrogen receptor negative; LHRH, luteinizing hormone-releasing hormone.
[a]Some oophorectomy and other irradiation.
[b]Progression-free survival.
[c]Days.

gonadotrophic cells refractory to endogenous LHRH. LHRH analog administration causes an initial rise in serum estrogen concentrations, which may lead to a tumor flare before a decline in estrogen concentrations to postmenopausal levels after 2 to 3 weeks (34). Although several LHRH analogs are available, over 90% of reported patients have been treated with goserelin, the only analog accepted by the U.S. Food and Drug Administration (FDA) (35,36). Goserelin is administered as a subcutaneous injection in a depot formulation once every 28 days. In an overview of all studies, 36.4% of patients had an objective response with a median duration of response of 11 months (37,38). A higher response rate was seen in patients with ER-positive tumors but 31% of women with ER-negative–disease responded, leading the authors to suggest that the ER assays used were inaccurate (38). Response rates to the other less commonly used LHRH analogs have also been reported (buserelin 14% to 41%, leuprorelin 34% to 44%, and triptorelin 30% to 70%) (35) (Table 73.2). The only randomized trial of oophorectomy versus an LHRH agonist (goserelin) showed no statistically significant difference between the two treatments for response, failure-free, or overall survival, although the study was underpowered (281) (Table 73.2). The question of whether the combination of an LHRH agonist with tamoxifen is superior to either drug used alone was investigated by the European Organisation for Research and Treatment of Cancer (EORTC) (39). The combination of buserelin with tamoxifen was associated with a greater response rate, median progression-free survival (9.7 months for the combination, 6.3 months buserelin alone, 5.6 months tamoxifen alone, $p = .03$), and overall survival (Table 73.2). In an overview analysis of four trials of the combination of LHRH agonist with tamoxifen versus an LHRH agonist alone, the combination was associated with a greater response rate, progression-free, and overall survival (40). Finally, the question arises whether aromatase inhibitors (AI) should be used before or after tamoxifen in goserelin-treated patients. Responses have been reported to goserelin and anastrozole (41) and goserelin and 4-hydroxyandrostenedione (42) after failure of goserelin and tamoxifen, but data are not available for the reverse treatment (i.e., AI followed by tamoxifen). In a relatively small adjuvant study, the combination of goserelin and anastrozole was not shown to be superior to goserelin plus tamoxifen (43).

Thus the treatment of premenopausal women with endocrine therapy is associated with a relative paucity of data since many of the trials have relatively few patients due to poor accrual. Although ovarian irradiation is widely used (at least in the United Kingdom), it is not known whether this is equivalent to oophorectomy and LHRH agonist. The series of oophorectomy alone studies suggest the possibility of a longer response duration than with an LHRH agonist (16 months vs. 11 months), and in the small trial comparing the two approaches there was a nonsignificant trend in favor of the operative technique. The combination of an LHRH agonist with tamoxifen is superior to either alone, and since there is a survival advantage in these studies, combination ovarian suppression, by surgical or pharmacological means, plus tamoxifen is considered the first-line treatment of choice.

Aromatase Inhibitors

The observations that adrenal hyperplasia occurred after oophorectomy in rodents and that estrogen and estradiol could still be detected in oophorectomized women, suggesting an extraovarian source of estrogens, led to the introduction of adrenalectomy by Huggins and Dao (44) and Nathanson and Towne (45) for treatment of women with breast cancer. This approach produced responses in postmenopausal women as frequently and with similar durations as oophorectomy in premenopausal women. Although corticosteroids showed some adrenal suppressive effects, the era of systemic inhibitors of estrogen biosynthesis was initiated with the use of the antiepileptic drug aminoglutethimide. This was later shown to be as effective as adrenalectomy with respect to tumor response and duration of response (46,47). The demonstration by Santen et al. (48) that aminoglutethimide inhibited the peripheral conversion of adrenal androgens to estrogens by the enzyme aromatase led to the search for and development of specific and progressively more potent inhibitors of the aromatase enzyme (49–51).

Aromatase is an enzyme of the cytochrome P450 super family and is highly expressed in the placenta and the granulosa cells of the ovary, where its expression depends on cyclical gonadotrophin stimulation. Aromatase is found at low levels in subcutaneous fat, liver, muscle, brain, normal breast, and

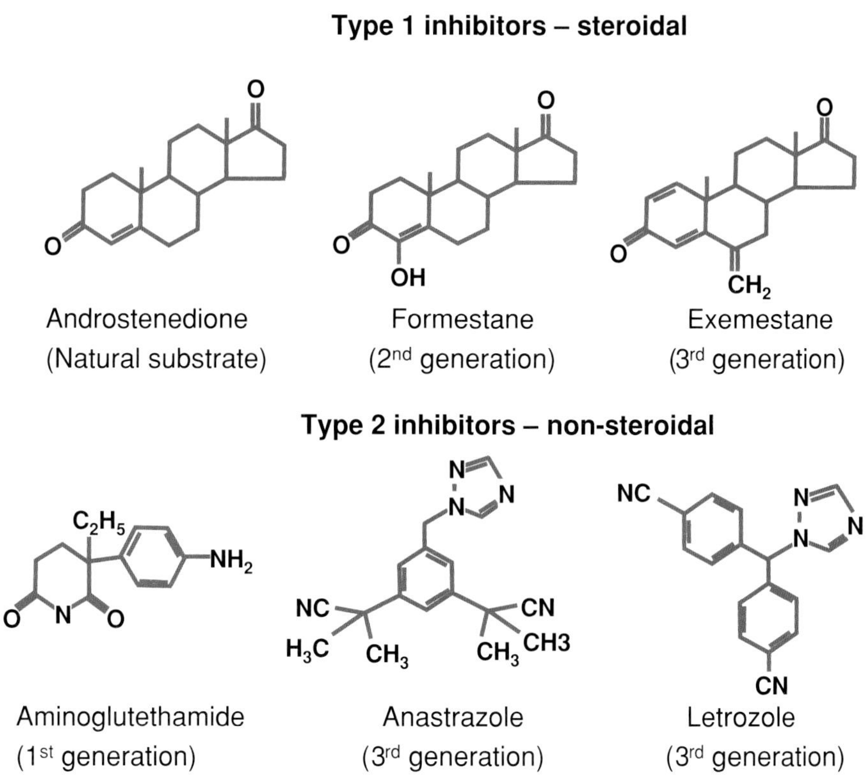

Type 1 inhibitors – steroidal

Androstenedione	Formestane	Exemestane
(Natural substrate)	(2nd generation)	(3rd generation)

Type 2 inhibitors – non-steroidal

Aminoglutethamide	Anastrazole	Letrozole
(1st generation)	(3rd generation)	(3rd generation)

FIGURE 73.2. Chemical structure of the substrate of the aromatase enzyme, androstenedione, and first-, second-, and third-generation inhibitors of type 1 and type 2.

breast cancer tissue including the epithelial cells in some but not all cancers (52,53). The AIs were developed in the 1980s and 1990s and have been termed first-, second-, and third-generation inhibitors in chronological order of their development (Fig. 73.2). They are further classified as type 1 or type 2 inhibitors according to their mechanisms of action. Type 1 inhibitors are steroidal analogs of androstenedione, which bind irreversibly to the aromatase enzyme and inactivate it. Type 2 inhibitors such as anastrazole and letrozole bind reversibly to the haem group of the enzyme via the nitrogen atom. Several techniques have been used to develop progressively more potent inhibitors. These include *in vitro* assays using placental or ovarian aromatase (54), ovarectomized male nude mice xenografted with MCF cells transduced by the aromatase enzyme (55), and studies in volunteers and patients using estimation of whole body aromatase (after injection of labelled androgens) and plasma and tissue estrogens by highly sensitive assays, which are required to assess low steroid concentrations (49).

These studies have demonstrated that the third-generation AIs (anastrozole, letrozole, and exemestane) inhibit total body and tumor aromatization by over 95% and consequently reduce concentrations of postmenopausal estradiol by over 95% (Table 73.3). Crossover studies have demonstrated that letrozole is slightly more active than anastrozole as an inhibitor of whole body aromatase, but whether this is clinically significant is not clear (56). In a study comparing the effectiveness of letrozole with anastrozole in advanced breast cancer no significant differences were seen in response rate, time to progression, or survival in the ER-positive population, suggesting the two AIs are clinically equivalent. However, more data are required, particularly from ongoing studies comparing the efficacy of the third-generation AIs head to head in the adjuvant setting (57). Studies also demonstrate that the third-generation aromatase inhibitors have no appre-

ciable effect on adrenal cortisol or aldosterone biosynthesis, whereas aminoglutethimide suppressed the synthesis of both steroids and fadrozole suppressed aldosterone biosynthesis (Fig. 73.1) (49).

The third-generation AIs were first assessed as second-line agents against the then standard treatment, megestrol acetate. Thereafter, in a series of important large phase III randomized trials, they were compared with tamoxifen in the first-line

| Table 73.3 | EFFECTS OF AROMATASE INHIBITORS ON PLASMA ESTROGEN CONCENTRATIONS AND WHOLE BODY AROMATIZATION (% SUPPRESSED FROM BASELINE) |

Aromatase Inhibitors	Dose	Plasma Estrogen (%)	Whole Body Aromatization (%)
First generation			
Aminoglutethimide	250 mg qid	81.4	90.6
Second generation			
Fadrozole[a]	2 bd	nd	92.6
Formestane[b]	250 mg, 2 weekly	51.8	84.8
Third generation			
Anastrozole[a]	1 mg od	93.5	97.3
Letrozole[a]	25 mg od	98.0	98.9
Exemestane[b]	25 mg od	93.2	97.9

nd, not done.
[a]Inhibitors.
[b]Inactivators.
After Geisler J. Aromatase inhibitors: from bench to bedside and back. *Breast Cancer* 2008;15:17–26.

Table 73.4	TRIALS OF AROMATASE INHIBITORS COMPARED WITH MEGESTROL ACETATE AS SECOND-LINE THERAPY FOR ADVANCED DISEASE					
Author (Reference)	AIs	n	ORR (%)	CBR	Median TTP	Median OS
Buzdar et al. (282)	Anastrozole	263	10	35	4.8	Not given
	MA 160 mg	253	8	34	4.8	Not given
Dombernowsky et al. (283)	Letrozole	174	24[a]	35	5.6	25
	MA 160 mg	189	16	32	5.5	22
Buzdar et al. (284)	Letrozole	199	16	27	3	29
	MA 160 mg	201	15	24	3	26
Kaufmann et al. (285)	Exemestane	366	15	37	4.7[a]	NR[a]
	MA 160 mg	403	12	35	3.8	28

AI, aromatase inhibitor; ORR, objective response rate; CBR, clinical, benefit rate; TTP, time to progression; OS, overall survival; MA, megestrol acetate; NR, not reached.
[a]Significant difference from the result with megestrol acetate.

setting (Tables 73.4 and 73.5). These studies first established that third-generation AIs were superior to megestrol acetate and then that they were superior to tamoxifen. These results differed from previous studies with first- and second-generation compounds where, in general, no advantage in efficacy was established (58,59). An overview demonstrated a survival advantage in trials of third- but not first- and second-generation AIs (60). Recent trials indicate no therapeutic advantage to adding celecoxib 400 mg twice a day to exemestane compared to exemestane alone (61) and that the newer third-generation AI, atamestane combined with toremifene was not superior to letrozole alone (62).

Estrogens

Apart from testosterone (63), high-dose estrogens were the first additive systemic treatment for breast cancer. Their development is of interest since they introduced the concept of high-dose inhibition of growth and one of the first used synthetic estrogens, triphenylchloroethylene was the base molecule for the development of the antiestrogens. Haddow (64) was the first to point out that many polycyclic hydrocarbons that induce cancer inhibit cell growth when used at higher concentrations. This concept applies to estrogen and synthetic compounds with estrogenic activity. Evidence that estrogens could cause cancer came from experiments in which murine ovaries, transplanted into male mice of a strain susceptible to breast cancer, induced mammary cancers (65). After purification of

estrone by Allen and Doisy (66), Lacassagne (67) demonstrated that injection of estrone induced tumors in the mouse. Synthetic estrogens such as triphenylethylene and stilbestrol were also shown to be carcinogenic on repeated injections in rodents (67–69), whereas high doses inhibited growth of the normal gland (70) and tumors (71). These considerations led Haddow et al. (72) to assess the effect of high doses of the synthetic estrogens trichlorophenylethylene and diethylstilbestrol in women with advanced breast cancer and demonstrated that they could induce tumor regressions. Other estrogens including dienestrol, tribromophenylethylene (73), and ethinylestradiol and Premarin (74) were also shown to be effective. Also it was demonstrated that stilbestrol, ethinylestradiol and Premarin had relatively shallow dose response curves (74,75). In a study of 523 postmenopausal women, response rates to 1.5, 15, 150, or 1,500 mg per day of diethylstilbestrol were 10%, 15%, 17%, and 21%, respectively, with a concomitant increase in toxicity but very similar response durations (75).

The introduction of antiestrogens into the clinic in the late 1960s and early 1970s led to them being assessed against diethylstilbestrol and ethinylestradiol (Table 73.6). Overall there were no significant differences in effectiveness of the two approaches. However, there were fewer side effects in most studies in women taking tamoxifen. The overall objective response rate to tamoxifen in the six reported trials was 28.5% and for estrogens (diethylstilbestrol or ethinylestradiol) was 25.1%. The median durations of response were 9.9 and 9.4 months, respectively. In trials where withdrawal responses were assessed after high-dose estrogens there was an objective response in 11 of 42 (26%) patients, whereas 0 of 23 responded to withdrawal of tamoxifen (76–81) (Table 73.6). In the only trial to report survival there was an advantage for diethylstilbestrol (36 months vs. 28.8 months), which was thought to be related to withdrawal responses seen after stilboestrol in 5 of 18 (28%) of patients in whom it was assessed (82). More recent studies have shown high response rates to ethinylestradiol and diethylstilbestrol in heavily pretreated patients, leading to a re-evaluation of this approach (83–85) (Table 73.7).

Selective Estrogen Receptor Modulators

Tamoxifen

Knowledge of the structure of trichlorophenylethylene led to the development of a number of triphenylethylene-like compounds such as clomiphene, MER 25, nafoxidine, and tamoxifen (275) (Fig. 73.3). Clomiphene and MER 25 proved too toxic for treatment of breast cancer (86,87). Nafoxidine showed

Table 73.5	TRIALS OF AROMATASE INHIBITORS COMPARED WITH TAMOXIFEN AS FIRST-LINE THERAPY FOR ADVANCED DISEASE				
Author (Reference)	AI Studied	n	ORR (%)	CBR (%)	Median TTP (mos)
Mouridsen et al. (286)	Letrozole	453	30[a]	49[a]	9.4[a]
	Tamoxifen	454	20	38	6.0
Nabholtz et al. (287)	Anastrozole	171	21	59[a]	11.1[a]
	Tamoxifen	182	17	46	5.6
Bonneterre et al. (288)	Anastrozole	340	33	56	8.2
	Tamoxifen	328	33	56	8.3
Paridaens et al. (289)	Exemestane	61	41	57	Not given
	Tamoxifen	59	17	42	Not given

AI, aromatase inhibitor; ORR, objective response rate; CBR, clinical benefit rate; TTP, time to progression.
[a]Significant difference from the result with tamoxifen.

Table 73.6	COMPARATIVE TRIALS OF ANTIESTROGENS AND ESTROGENS

			OR (%)		MDR (mos)		WR	
Treatment	Author (Reference)	n	AE	E	AE	E	AE	E
Nafoxidine vs. EE$_2$	Heuson et al. (78)	98	15/49 (31%)	7/49 (14%)	11	12	NA	NA
Tamoxifen vs. DES	Stewart et al. (81)	56	9/29 (31%)	6/27 (22%)	9.5	8	NA	NA
Tamoxifen vs. EE$_2$	Beex et al. (76)	59	10/30 (33%)	9/29 (31%)	12	11	0/13 (0%)	4/18 (22)
Tamoxifen vs. DES	Ingle et al. (79)	143	23/69 (33%)	30/74 (41%)	11.8	9.9	NA	5/18 (28%)
Tamoxifen vs. EE$_2$	Matelski et al. (80)	43	10/19 (53%)	6/24 (25%)	NA	NA	0/10 (0%)	2/6 (33%)
Tamoxifen vs. DES	Gockerman et al. (77)	90	3/46 (6%)	4/44 (9%)	5	6	NA	NA
Overall			69/242 (28.5%)	62/247 (25.1%)	9.9	9.4	0/23 (0%)	11/42 (26.2%)

EE, ethinylestradiol; DES, diethylstilbestrol; AE, antiestrogen; E, estrogen; OR, objective response, MDR, median duration of response months; WR, withdrawal response; NA, not assessed.

activity in advanced breast cancer, but because of marked skin photo toxicity and hair loss it was not developed further (78) (Table 73.6). Tamoxifen was initially developed as a contraceptive but was shown to induce ovulation (88,89). The trans isomer of tamoxifen was shown to be predominantly antiestrogenic, whereas the cis isomer was estrogenic (88). In the immature rat uterus assay tamoxifen inhibited the action of estrogen, whereas it was a partial agonist on the uterus in the absence of estrogen. In a phase II trial tamoxifen was shown to be active to about the same extent as estrogens and androgens (90). The initial dose used was 20 mg per day, which showed greater clinical activity than 10 mg per day (91). Increasing the dose to 40 mg after progression on 20 mg produced a small number of additional responses, however, the standard dose of tamoxifen remains at 20 mg per day (92).

The first clinical study with tamoxifen in breast cancer began in 1969 (90). Forty-six postmenopausal patients were treated with 10 to 20 mg of tamoxifen daily for 3 months. An objective remission rate of 22% was seen, comparable with stilboestrol but with reduced toxicity. Subsequent studies using the 20-mg dose have confirmed an overall objective response rate (CR+PR) of 34%. If patients with disease stabilization for 6 months or more are included, the clinical benefit of tamoxifen increases to 53% (93). Fossati et al. (58) reviewed all comparative trials of tamoxifen with other agents up until that time. This overview of 35 randomized trials involving 5,160 patients produced 38 comparisons with other endocrine therapies. Overall the objective response rate for tamoxifen was 29% and for other therapies combined 30%. In addition, survival data were available from 24 of these studies (n = 4,126) and showed no significant differences between therapies. It is important to note that these analyses did not include modern AIs. These tend to show higher response rates and the modern AIs confer survival advantages over tamoxifen (60).

A number of studies have investigated whether a combination of tamoxifen with other endocrine therapies is superior to tamoxifen alone. A higher objective response rate was seen for combinations of tamoxifen with aminoglutethimide, fluoxymesterone, and corticosteroids but not with bromocriptine, estrogen, nandrolone, and progestins (22 randomized studies, 2,949 patients). Overall the hazard ratio for combination versus single-agent therapy was 1.34 but monotherapy was better tolerated and there was no significant survival advantage for combinations (12 studies with 1,819 patients).

Table 73.7	RECENT STUDIES OF HIGH-DOSE ESTROGENS

Author (Reference)	Treatment/ Dose	n	Line of Therapy	OR (%)	CB (%)	MDCB (mos)
Boyer and Tattersall (84)	Diethylstilbestrol 10–20 mg/day	11	—	4 (36%)	9 (82%)	—
Lonning et al. (85)	Diethylstilbestrol 15 mg/day	32	2–10	10 (31%)	12 (37.5%)	12
Agrawal et al. (83)	Ethinylestradiol 1 mg/day	12	3–7	3 (25%)	4 (33%)	10

OR, objective response; CB, clinical benefit; MDCB, median duration of clinical benefit.

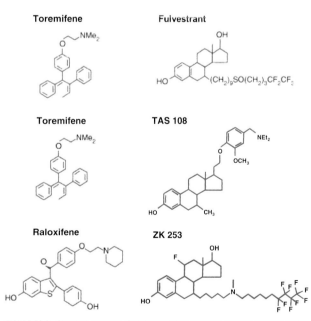

FIGURE 73.3. Chemical structure of triphenylethylene selective estrogen receptor modulators tamoxifen and toremifene and the benzopyrene derivative "fixed ring" compound raloxifene (*left panel*). Also shown are the selective estrogen receptor down-regulator fulvestrant and estrogen receptor destabilizers TAS-108 and ZK-253. (Adapted from Hoffmann J, Bohlmann R, Heinrich N, et al. Characterization of new estrogen receptor destabilizing compounds: effects on estrogen-sensitive and tamoxifen-resistant breast cancer. *J Natl Cancer Inst* 2004;96:210–218; Yamaya H, Yoshida K, Kuritani J, et al. Safety, tolerability, and pharmacokinetics of TAS-108 in normal healthy post-menopausal female subjects: a phase I study on single oral dose. *J Clin Pharm Ther* 2005;30:459–470; Howell SJ, Johnston SR, Howell A. The use of selective estrogen receptor modulators and selective estrogen receptor down-regulators in breast cancer. *Best Pract Res Clin Endocrinol Metab* 2004;18:47–66.)

Other Selective Estrogen-Receptor Modulators

The term *selective estrogen-receptor modulator* (SERM) implies compounds have alternative agonist or antagonist effects on different target organs. Several approaches have been used to improve on tamoxifen by attempting to increase antitumor activity, maintaining a positive effect on bone and lipids, and reducing gynecologic toxicity, particularly endometrial cancer. Two basic approaches have been taken in chemical modifications of tamoxifen: by altering its side chains to produce toremifene, idoxifene, and droloxifene, or by altering the triphenylethylene ring structure of tamoxifen to produce nonsteroidal "fixed ring" compounds such as the benzothiophene derivatives raloxifene and arzoxifene and benzopyran derivatives such as acolbifene and its prodrug EM800 (Fig. 73.3) (94–96).

Tamoxifen-Like Triphenylethylene Selective Estrogen-Receptor Modulators

For each of the triphenylethylene-like SERMs preclinical data suggested improved activity over tamoxifen, which led to their clinical development. Examples of differential activity compared with tamoxifen include the reduction of liver DNA adducts with toremifene and the higher binding activity and reduced estrogenicity in the rat uterus of droloxifene and idoxifene (96). However, in five phase III trials toremifene had exactly the same activity as tamoxifen and the potential reduction in carcinogenity was not investigated (and is probably unimportant clinically) (97). Despite the potential favorable activity of droloxifene it was shown to be inferior in a phase III trial and its development was stopped (98). Idoxifene was compared with tamoxifen in two phase III trials that showed almost no difference in efficacy between the two agents, but because of potentially increased gynecological toxicity idoxifene development was also stopped (96,99).

Fixed-Ring Selective Estrogen-Receptor Modulators

Interest in fixed-ring SERMs was founded on their lack of agonist activity on the endometrium while maintaining agonist activity on bone. Although raloxifene binds to the ER with similar affinity to tamoxifen, its activity is not superior to tamoxifen in advanced breast cancer. In a study of 14 patients failing tamoxifen there was only one minor response to raloxifene 200 mg per day (100). As first-line therapy in 21 patients with ER-positive metastatic disease, raloxifene 150 mg twice a day resulted in 4 (19%) partial responses with an additional 3 (14%) showing stable disease (101). Given these data raloxifene has not been developed for advanced breast cancer. Arzoxifene, another benzothiophene analog related to raloxifene, showed good efficacy in phase II trials in tamoxifen pretreated patients. However, in a recently reported phase III trial versus tamoxifen, enrollment was stopped after an interim analysis of the first 200 patients suggesting arzoxifene was significantly inferior to tamoxifen (102).

Acolbifene (EM-652) is a benzopyrene derivative of an orally active pro-drug EM-800 (SCH-57050). It has significantly higher ER binding and was more effective than fulvestrant (see below) at inhibiting estradiol-induced breast cancer cell proliferation *in vitro* and in the MCF-7 nude mouse model. Again phase II studies showed promising activity in tamoxifen pretreated patients, but acolbifene appeared to have lower activity than anastrozole in a phase III randomized trial and development was attenuated, although further development is planned (103).

Fulvestrant (Faslodex ICI 182,780)

The data outlined above indicate that neither the many analogs of the triphenylethylene tamoxifen nor the fixed-ring compounds have shown superior efficacy to tamoxifen. The search for novel agents that would completely block ER signaling led to the synthesis of a series of steroidal 7α alkylamide analogs of estradiol. Of these ICI 164,384 was the first "pure" antiestrogen to be described, completely blocking the uterotropic action of both estradiol and tamoxifen in rats (104). Following this, a far more potent "pure" estrogen antagonist, fulvestrant, was developed and entered clinical evaluation (105). Fulvestrant is a 7α alkylsulfonate analog of estradiol that is structurally distinct from the nonsteroidal estrogen antagonists (Fig. 73.3). The side chain is responsible for the inhibitory action through its effect on the ER. Fulvestrant inhibits dimerization and nucleocytoplasmic shutting of the ER and reduces its half life secondary to an increase in ubiquitination. *In vitro* fulvestrant showed no evidence of the low-dose stimulation of MCF-7 cell proliferation that is secondary to the partial agonist activity of tamoxifen. Fulvestrant also inhibited colony formation in semisolid media of pleural effusion cells taken from patients resistant to tamoxifen. In this assay tamoxifen was shown to stimulate growth, and this could also be inhibited by additional fulvestrant (106). *In vivo*, fulvestrant, at the doses used clinically, inhibited growth of MCF-7 cells in the nude mouse model to the same extent as tamoxifen but acted for twice as long (105,107).

The first human study in cancer patients was a presurgical trial in 56 women with breast cancer who were randomized to receive no preoperative treatment (n = 16) or daily intramuscular (IM) fulvestrant (6 mg, n = 21; 18 mg, n = 16) for 7 days prior to surgery (106). There was no evidence of agonist activity of fulvestrant, it inhibited ER and PR expression almost completely and reduced proliferation by approximately two-thirds. In a more recent study, fulvestrant at 50, 125, or 250 mg doses given as a single IM injection 14 to 21 days prior to surgery reduced ER and Ki-67 expression in a dose-dependent manner to a greater extent than tamoxifen (at 20 mg per day). Whereas the agonist effect of tamoxifen increased PR, fulvestrant significantly reduced PR, demonstrating pure antagonist effects on the ER (108). The fulvestrant-induced reduction of ER expression in primary breast cancers is dose dependent. A single IM dose of 250 mg gives mean plasma concentrations of 5 ng/mL and reduces ER expression by approximately 70% (108), whereas the 18 mg per day dosage produced a plasma concentration of 23 ng/mL and near complete suppression of ER (106). Although the steady state plasma concentration are similar with the approved dose (AD; 250 mg every 4 weeks) and loading dose (LD; 500 mg on day 0, 250 mg on day 14, 250 mg on day 28 and every 4 weeks thereafter), steady state is achieved in 1 month with the LD compared to 4 to 6 months with the AD (109). Preliminary data also suggest that a high-dose regimen (HD; 500 mg on day 0, 500 mg on day 14, 500 mg on day 28 and every 4 weeks thereafter) has greater efficacy in the reduction of primary breast cancer mean Ki-67 percentage at 4 and 16 weeks (*p* <.001 for both) compared with the AD (110). Thus higher dosing may translate into greater antitumor effects than the standard dose schedule in MBC (111).

Preclinical data suggesting that fulvestrant may be beneficial in the treatment of tamoxifen-resistant tumors were supported by the first phase II clinical study of fulvestrant. Over two thirds (13/19, 69%) of postmenopausal women with tamoxifen-resistant disease treated with fulvestrant experienced clinical benefit (112,113). Moreover, a long duration of response was observed in these women (median duration 25 months) supporting preclinical evidence that fulvestrant suppressed tumor growth for longer than tamoxifen (107). Thus, fulvestrant was shown not to be cross-resistant with tamoxifen in the clinical setting.

Fulvestrant at the AD was tested in two phase III trials, against the then standard second-line agent anastrozole, in postmenopausal women with advanced breast cancer whose cancers had progressed after receiving antiestrogen treatment (114,115). Both studies had a similar design in which fulvestrant

(250 mg per month IM, n = 428) was compared with the AI anastrozole (1 mg per day orally, n = 423). In one study, fulvestrant was administered as a single 5-mL injection in an open-label comparison (international) whereas in the other study fulvestrant was administered as two separate 2.5-mL injections in a double-blind comparison (North American). At median follow-up of 15.1 months the median time to progression (TTP) was comparable in both groups (5.5 months vs 4.1 months for fulvestrant and anastrozole, respectively) and the OR rate was not significantly different between the two groups (19.2% in the fulvestrant group compared with 16.5% in the anastrozole group; $p = .31$). In addition, there were no differences in OR rates between fulvestrant and anastrozole in the subgroup of patients who had any visceral metastases (15.7% vs. 13.2%, respectively; $p = .49$) or those with visceral metastases only (18.8% vs. 14.0%, respectively; $p = .43$) (116).

In patients who had an OR further follow-up was performed at a median of 22.1 months (35). The median duration of response was 16.7 and 13.7 months in patients who responded to fulvestrant (n = 84) and anastrozole (n = 73), respectively; mean duration of response was significantly greater for fulvestrant than anastrozole (hazard ratio [HR] 1.30; 95% confidence interval [CI], 1.13–1.50; $p < .01$). A similar proportion of patients experienced clinical benefit (43.5% patients receiving fulvestrant and 40.9% patients receiving anastrozole) and the median duration of clinical benefit was also similar between the groups (11.8 months vs. 11.2 months, respectively). A survival analysis conducted at a median follow-up of 27 months showed that overall survival was very similar with fulvestrant and anastrozole (median 27.4 months vs. 27.7 months, respectively; HR 0.98; 95% CI, 0.84–1.15; $p = .809$) and that three fourths of patients had died in each group (74.5% vs. 76.1%, respectively) (117).

The efficacy of first-line fulvestrant versus tamoxifen has been investigated in postmenopausal women with metastatic or locally advanced breast cancer. In a phase III study endocrine-naive patients, or patients who had completed endocrine therapy 1 year or more previously, were treated with either fulvestrant (250 mg per month IM injection with placebo tamoxifen, n = 313) or tamoxifen (20 mg per day orally with placebo fulvestrant, n = 274) (95). Approximately 20% to 25% of patients had received prior adjuvant treatment therapy for their primary breast cancer. In the intent-to-treat (ITT) population fulvestrant did not meet the criteria for noninferiority to tamoxifen (upper 95% CI, <1.25) for the TTP end point (median 6.8 months vs. 8.3 months respectively; HR 1.18; 95% CI, 0.98–1.44; $p = .088$). OR rates were similar between the two arms (31.6% for fulvestrant vs. 33.9% for tamoxifen). However, clinical benefit rates were significantly higher in the tamoxifen group (54.3% for fulvestrant vs. 62.0% for tamoxifen; $p = .026$). In patients experiencing an OR, the median duration of response was similar (17.3 months vs. 19.8 months with fulvestrant and tamoxifen, respectively). In a *post hoc* analysis of patients with breast tumors that were positive for both ER and PR (42% of patients), the findings for median TTP were again shown to be comparable in the two groups (11.4 months vs. 8.5 months for fulvestrant and tamoxifen, respectively; HR 0.85%; 95% CI, 0.63–1.15; $p = .31$).

In the combined analysis of the two phase III trials of patients undergoing second-line treatment with fulvestrant and anastrozole, the safety population comprised 423 patients in each group (118). Adverse events (AEs) were generally mild to moderate in intensity. The most commonly reported AEs with fulvestrant and anastrozole, respectively, were nausea (26.0% vs. 25.3%), asthenia (22.7% vs. 27.0%), pain (18.9% vs. 20.3%), vasodilation (17.7% vs. 17.3%), and headache (15.4% vs. 16.8%). Joint disorders was the only AE that was significantly different between the groups, experienced by fewer patients receiving fulvestrant versus anastrozole (5.4% vs. 10.6%, respectively; $p = .0036$). Local injection site reactions occurred in 1.1% of courses in patients given a single 5-mL injection and

in 4.6% and 4.4% of courses in patients given two 2.5-mL fulvestrant or placebo injections, respectively.

In the study comparing fulvestrant and tamoxifen, the safety population comprised 310 and 271 patients, respectively, and the median follow-up was 14.5 months (95). The most commonly reported AEs in the fulvestrant and tamoxifen groups, respectively, were nausea (20.3% vs. 22.5%), asthenia (19.4% vs. 20.3%), vasodilation (14.8% vs. 21.4%), pain (13.9% vs. 19.2%), and bone pain (13.9% vs. 17.0%). There were fewer patients treated with fulvestrant with hot flashes (17.7% vs. 24.7%) compared with tamoxifen ($p = .05$).

Data were collected on 338 patients with advanced breast cancer treated in 10 specialist centers in order to determine the effectiveness of fulvestrant after previous endocrine therapy and chemotherapy and in tumors with various ER and PR expression patterns (Fig. 73.4). The clinical benefit rate was approximately 40% whether fulvestrant was used first, second, or third line (Fig. 73.4A); however, in common with other endocrine therapies the response rate declined when used fourth line and beyond. Fulvestrant also gives a clinical benefit rate of approximately 40% after first- or second-line chemotherapy (Fig. 73.4B) and gives similar clinical benefit rates in the ER/PR subtypes and whether tumors were *ERBB2* (formerly *HER2*) positive or not (Fig. 73.4C). These results were similar to the data from the clinical trials outlined above (119).

Other Pure Estrogen Antagonists in Development

Although fulvestrant is the first pure estrogen antagonist, several other pure estrogen antagonists are undergoing preclinical development. Two new pure estrogen antagonists, ZK-703 and ZK-253, which destabilize the ER, have been investigated using the MCF-7 xenograft model. Both agents were more effective than either tamoxifen or fulvestrant at inhibiting the growth of ER-positive xenografts, and they also showed highly potent activity in tamoxifen-resistant xenografts (120). These agents are beginning clinical development. Another compound with pure antiestrogenic activity (TAS-108 SR 16234) has completed phase I and II trials and is now being evaluated in a multicenter phase III study (121–123).

Progestins and Antiprogestins

Progesterone was synthesized in the 1930s and shown to inhibit estrogen-stimulated tumor growth in rats (124). After the first clinical use (125), a large number of progesterone analogs were tested, most of which had clinical activity (126,127). The precise mechanisms of antitumor action are unclear. In some human tumor cell lines progestins are antiproliferative and can abolish the proliferative effects of estrogens. They may act by suppression of ER in addition to PR and also bind to androgen and glucocorticoid receptors, thus suggesting alternative mechanisms of action. Progestins may also act through suppression of pituitary corticotropin secretion and secondary reduction of adrenal androgens and serum estrogens or they may be converted to estrogens and exert their suppressive effects due to high dose inhibition (128,129).

Similar to high-dose estrogens, the highest response rates to progestins are more likely to be seen in patients with ER- and PR-positive tumors, treated more than 10 years after the menopause, with a long disease-free interval (more than 2 years) and soft tissue disease, although acceptable response rates have been reported for visceral disease (130). In the United States most trials of therapy have used the oral progestin megestrol acetate (MA), whereas in Europe both MA and medroxyprogesterone acetate (MPA) have been investigated. The standard dose of MA is 160 mg, which may be given as a single or divided dose. Trials suggest that this dose gives equivalent responses to tamoxifen but with considerably greater toxicity including weight gain,

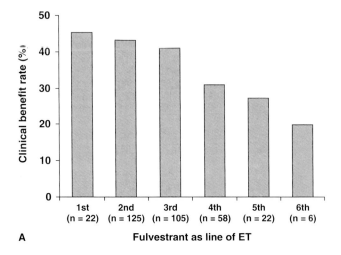

A   Fulvestrant as line of ET

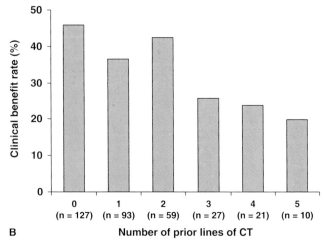

B   Number of prior lines of CT

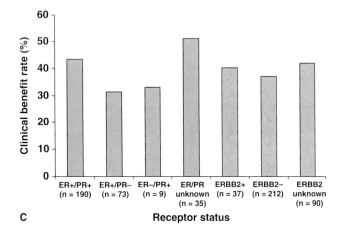

C   Receptor status

FIGURE 73.4. Data from 338 patients treated with fulvestrant at various stages of advanced disease. A: Clinical benefit rate related to number of previous endocrine therapies (ET). **B:** Clinical benefit rate related to number of previous chemotherapies (CT). **C:** Clinical benefit rate related to estrogen receptor (ER) and progesterone receptor (PR) status and *ERBB2* subtype.

hypertension, and edema (58). In a large randomized trial including 341 patients comparing 160, 800, and 1,600 mg of MA per day, there were no significant differences in response rates (131). MPA, when used at conventional doses (less than 500 mg daily), has been found to be less effective than MA probably related to its poor bioavailability. Trials comparing conventional with high oral doses of MPA have in general shown similar effects, and no significant differences in response rates or response durations were seen with IM doses of 500 mg, 1,000 mg, or 1,500 mg daily (132). MA has been shown in large randomized studies to be inferior to treatment with third-generation AIs as second-line therapy, and its use is generally confined to at least fourth-line therapy and often in end stage disease (Table 73.4).

Antiprogestins

In principle, pure progesterone-receptor antagonists (PRAs) and progesterone-receptor modulators (PRMs, mixed agonist/antagonists) form a new category of hormonal agents for breast cancer, but their development has been delayed because of efficacy and toxicity problems (133). The first agent to be used, mifepristone (RU38486) showed growth inhibitory effects in human tumor cell lines and decrease PR expression almost to zero. A second-generation pure PRA, onapristone (ZK98299), was more potent than mifepristone both *in vitro* and in animal models and was shown to induce tumor differentiation and apoptosis. Also there was increased activity when PRAs/PRMs were combined with tamoxifen or fulvestrant. Two phase II studies of mifepristone (second and third line) showed 4 PRs in 33 patients (133,134) and in a second-line study of onapristone there were

10 objective remissions in 101 evaluable patients (135). As first-line agents mifepristone showed 11% objective remissions (3/28), (136) and onapristone 56% PR (10/18) (137), with a median duration of remission of 70 weeks. Onapristone is well tolerated symptomatically, but the majority of patients treated developed liver function test abnormalities and a phase III study versus megestrol acetate was stopped. A new PRA without liver toxicity is now in phase II clinical trial (Lonaprisan, ZK230211) and PRAs may well prove to be an important new endocrine therapy.

Androgens and Antiandrogens

Androgens were the first systemic therapy to be used to treat metastatic breast cancer (63). With high-dose estrogens they were the treatment of choice until the development of the antiestrogens in the 1970s. Understandably their use waned, primarily because of the associated toxicities, particularly virilization, but also because, in general, they were found to be less effective than estrogens and antiestrogens. The androgens testosterone, fluoxymesterone, testolactose danazol, and calusterone are associated with objective response rates of approximately 20%, which is lower than other available additive endocrine therapies (138). Antiandrogens such as flutamide have received only limited evaluation. In one trial a single partial response was seen in 29 evaluable patients given flutamide 750 mg daily (139). However, the recent demonstration, using RNA microarrays, of a group of ER-negative but androgen receptor–positive apocrine tumors has led to renewed interest in the assessment of antiandrogen therapy in this restricted group of tumors (140).

TUMOR FLARE AND WITHDRAWAL RESPONSES

Tumor flair and withdrawal responses noted during endocrine treatment give some insight into the mechanisms of response and resistance to endocrine therapy. The flare is an increase in tumor activity seen usually with additive endocrine therapies, such as tamoxifen or estrogens. It is seen in a small number of cases (<5% clinically) presumed to be caused by the initial low "physiological" serum concentrations of drug causing tumor growth or activity before the agents attain steady state therapeutic concentrations. The flare is characterized by bone pain, occasional hypercalcaemia, diffuse increased uptake on the bone scan, and increase in size and redness of skin nodules. Symptoms occur 2 to 21 days after initiation of therapy and subside spontaneously. It is important to realize that a flare usually indicates an endocrine-sensitive tumor since such tumors usually go on to respond (8,9,141,142). The increased metabolic activity of the tumor in response to initiating endocrine therapy can be detected as increased uptake of FDG by PET scan. Indeed Dehdashti et al. (10) used estrogen (30 mg) immediately before a scan in 51 patients due to start subsequent endocrine therapy with anastrozole or fulvestrant (both of which are highly unlikely to cause a flare). An increase in FDG uptake was seen in 15 of 17 responders, whereas none of the 34 nonresponders had a flare reaction. This important study indicates that the metabolic flare may be used to determine therapy, whereas a clinical flare is insufficiently frequent to be useful.

A withdrawal response (WR) is a response after stopping therapy. WRs, like clinical flares, are relatively uncommon (<10% patients) but also give an indication of one mechanism of resistance, since their existence presumably indicates that the tumor is being stimulated to grow at therapeutic concentrations of drug. WRs usually occur after cessation of androgens (first report of a WR) (125), estrogens (143), and tamoxifen (144) but have been reported after cessation of progestins (144) and aromatase inhibitors (145,146). WR may be a useful additional therapy for the patient. Howell et al. (144) assessed 65 patients for a WR after stopping tamoxifen. The patients were selected to have relatively slow growing soft tissue, lung, and bone disease. There were 5 partial responses (8%) and 14 (22%) stabilization with a median duration of WR of 10 months (range, 3 to 40 months). WR were also seen in 4 of 21 (19%) patients stopping norethisterone acetate used as a second-line endocrine therapy. In order to obtain a clear indication of the incidence of WR, Canney et al. (147) looked for a WR on 61 *consecutive* patients stopping tamoxifen and saw 6 (9.8%) examples of WR, which may represent the true incidence. Although WR usually occurs after previous response, this need not necessarily be the case since 3 PRs were seen in 12 women who had stopped tamoxifen after failing to respond (144).

SEQUENCING OF ENDOCRINE THERAPIES

Because it is possible to keep patients in remission for many months or years using a sequence of endocrine therapies, the question of which is the optimal sequence for a particular patient arises. Although there is a large amount of clinical trial data indicating the responsiveness of tumors to the available endocrine therapies, there are no formal trials of one sequence versus an alternative sequence. In general, there was no survival advantage of one endocrine treatment compared with another in the older literature, so agents were selected on the basis of toxicity (58). However, this situation is altered because of the overview of Mauri et al. (60),

End Point	RANDOMISED CONTROLLED TRIAL OF FULVESTRANT VERSUS EXEMESTANE (EFECT TRIAL)		
	Fulvestrant (n = 351)	Exemestane (n = 342)	*p* Value
TTP (mos)	3.7	3.7	0.65
OR (%)	7.4	6.7	0.74
CB (%)	32.2	31.5	0.85
MDCB (mos)	9.3	8.3	—

TTP, time to progression; OR, objective response; CB, clinical benefit; MDCB, median duration of clinical benefit.
From Chia S, Gradishar W, Mauriac L, et al. Double-blind, randomized placebo controlled trial of fulvestrant compared with exemestane after prior nonsteroidal aromatase inhibitor therapy in postmenopausal women with hormone receptor-positive, advanced breast cancer: results from EFECT. *J Clin Oncol* 2008;26:1664–1670.

in which the third-generation AIs were associated with a survival advantage when compared with standard therapies such as tamoxifen, progestins, and second-generation AIs. These data indicate that a third-generation AI should be considered as the treatment of first choice. After an AI the next therapy depends on available clinical trial data. Information concerning the optimal second-line therapy comes from the recently reported Evaluation of Fulvestrant versus Exemestane (EFECT) trial showing that after failure on a nonsteroidal AI, the steroidal AI exemestane was equivalent to fulvestrant in terms of TTP, OR, and clinical benefit rates in a randomized phase III study (Table 73.8) (148). This study indicates that fulvestrant and exemestane are equally active as second- or third-line agents after an AI, so other consideration such as route of administration may influence treatment decisions. Another consideration may be how active one treatment is after another. AIs should be used first line if there was no adjuvant therapy or if the adjuvant therapy was tamoxifen (whether relapse occurred during or after completion of tamoxifen treatment or not). There are few data concerning the response to AIs in advanced disease in women who relapsed during or after adjuvant AI. The most appropriate action may be to use a steroidal AI or fulvestrant after previous adjuvant nonsteroidal AI, and nonsteroidal AI after adjuvant steroidal AI (Fig. 73.5). The combination of fulvestrant with an AI to

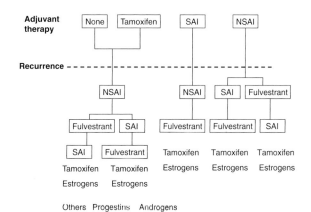

FIGURE 73.5. Potential sequence of endocrine therapy for advanced disease according to previous endocrine therapy. NSAI, nonsteroidal aromatase inhibitor; SAI, steroidal aromatase inhibitor.

Table 73.9	CURRENT AND FUTURE TRIALS INVOLVING FULVESTRANT IN POSTMENOPAUSAL WOMEN	
Trial	**Disease Setting**	**Details**
EFECT	HR+ ABC, recurrence or progression on a nonsteroidal AI	Fulvestrant (LD) vs. exemestane
SOFEA	HR+ ABC, recurrence or progression on a nonsteroidal AI	Fulvestrant (LD) vs. fulvestrant (LD) + anastrozole v exemestane
SWOG S0226	First-line HR+ ABC	Anastrozole vs. fulvestrant (LD) + anastrozole
FACT	HR+ first-line ABC in postmenopausal women or premenopausal women on goserelin	Fulvestrant (LD) + anastrozole vs. anastrozole
ECOG 4101	First/second-line ABC	Fulvestrant + gefitinib vs. anastrozole + gefitinib
Fulvestrant/trastuzumab	HR+ and HER2/neu+ ABC	Fulvestrant (HD) vs. trastuzumab vs. fulvestrant (HD) + trastuzumab
CALGB 40302	HR+ and HER2/neu+ and/or EGFR+ ABC	Fulvestrant + lapatinib vs. fulvestrant

HR+, hormone receptor positive; ABC, advanced breast cancer; LD, loading dose; HR, high dose; AI, aromatase inhibitor; HER2, human epidermal growth factor receptor 2; EGFR, epidermal growth factor receptor.

maintain low estrogen conditions is also being tested in randomized studies (Table 73.9). Subsequent treatments will depend on data from previous studies as to whether an endocrine agent is active after the previous treatment. Although estrogens have been reported to have high toxicity, this is by no means always the case, and there are arguments for using lower doses after failure of an AI (149). Three recent studies have demonstrated high response rates to diethylstilbestrol and ethinylestradiol after several previous endocrine therapies (Table 73.7) (83–85).

Pharmacogenomics may also impact on the relative efficacy of the endocrine agents used in metastatic breast cancer. This topic is covered in detail in Chapter 56 and the majority of data are derived from studies in healthy volunteers and in the adjuvant treatment setting. There is a relative paucity of data on the efficacy of endocrine agents in metastatic breast cancer related to drug metabolism or target polymorphisms. In a Korean study of 202 patients on 20 mg per day tamoxifen, those homozygous for the cytochrome P450 (CYP) 2D6*10 allele demonstrated significantly lower concentrations of the active metabolites of tamoxifen: 4-hydroxy-N-desmethyltamoxifen and 4-hydroxytamoxifen than those with other genotypes. Of the 23 patients in the study with MBC the 12 carrying the CYP2D6*10/*10 genotype had a significantly shorter median TTP than those with other genotypes (5.0 months vs. 21.8 months; $p = .0032$), which persisted in multivariate analysis (150). The *10 allele occurs in as few as 2% of indigenous Western populations however, and prospective testing of the more common variant alleles for particular populations will be required to investigate the impact of tamoxifen pharmacogenomics on outcome in patients with MBC.

In a study of single nucleotide polymorphisms (SNP) in the aromatase gene (CYP19), a SNP in the 3′ untranslated region of the gene (rs4646 variant) predicted for improved TTP with letrozole (17.2 months vs. 6.4 months; $p = .02$) compared with the wild type gene (151). Preliminary data from a second study suggest that allelic variants of common CYP enzymes involved in aromatase inhibitor metabolism do not influence outcome in MBC (152). Thus routine pharmacogenomic testing of patients prior to initiation of endocrine therapy cannot be recommended. The majority of women will be treated with an AI as first-line therapy for MBC, and the only clinical data to date suggest an improved rather than deleterious outcome with variant alleles in the aromatase enzyme. As tamoxifen is used later in the treatment sequence (Fig. 73.5), the worth of genotyping seems low, although prospective evaluation of the relative efficacy of tamoxifen versus AI, based on SNP analysis of drug metabolism or target enzymes, may help to refine treatment strategies in the future.

 MANAGEMENT SUMMARY

General Points

- Endocrine therapy should only be employed in patients with tumors that express ER or PR (or in combination with agents to induce ER expression in ER-negative tumors).
- Most ER-positive patients are suitable for first-line endocrine therapy unless they have rapidly progressive visceral metastases, when chemotherapy is preferred.
- When possible, biopsy of metastases should be performed to re-evaluate for ER and PR expression, and patient management should be based on these results.
- *In situ* assessment of ER expression or functionality may be feasible using modalities such as FDG-PET.

Premenopausal Women

- In endocrine therapy–naive patients, the combination of tamoxifen and ovarian suppression (OS), by oophorectomy or LHRH analog, should be used as first-line therapy.
- In women who relapse on adjuvant tamoxifen or progress on first-line therapy and are still suitable for endocrine therapy, combination OS and a third-generation AI should be considered.
- There are few data to guide endocrine therapy decisions in the third-line setting and beyond.
- Withdrawal response to combination LHRH analog and AI treatment has been observed.
- Switching class of third-generation AI while maintaining OS or fulvestrant plus OS needs to be tested in clinical trials before it can be recommended.

Postmenopausal Women

- In endocrine therapy–naive patients or those relapsing on or following adjuvant tamoxifen, first-line therapy for metastatic breast cancer should be with a nonsteroidal third-generation AI.

- Following relapse on a nonsteroidal AI, second-line therapy is equally efficacious with a steroidal AI or fulvestrant. Route of administration and toxicity profile may influence treatment choice.
- Whether an AI should be continued with fulvestrant, to maintain low estrogen levels, and the most efficacious dose of fulvestrant are the subjects of several large randomized studies.
- There is probably little to choose between tamoxifen, the alternative class of AI, or fulvestrant in third-line therapy.
- Low-dose estrogen may have a role in restoring endocrine sensitivity following treatment with an AI.
- Progestins and androgens are generally used in end-stage disease, after treatment with all other agents has been explored.

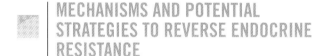

MECHANISMS AND POTENTIAL STRATEGIES TO REVERSE ENDOCRINE RESISTANCE

Endocrine resistance is commonly defined as either intrinsic or acquired. Intrinsic resistance refers to tumors that do not respond to any endocrine therapy, whereas acquired resistance occurs after initial benefit from at least one endocrine agent. The primary tumor is usually the site for determination of ER and PR expression. The negative predictive value of ER, in particular in the absence of PR expression, infers intrinsic endocrine resistance in ER-negative tumors and endocrine therapy is highly unlikely to be of benefit (153,154). There are two important caveats to this statement. The first is the need for biopsy of metastases wherever possible to reassess expression of ER and PR. Approximately 5% to 10% of tumors classified as ER-negative at primary diagnosis will show ER expression in their metastases. Such cancers are of better prognosis than those that lose the ER during metastasis or maintain an ER-negative phenotype from primary to metastasis, and endocrine therapy may be effective in such patients (5,154). The second caveat is the potential to induce the expression of the ER in previously ER poor tumors with reversion of epigenetically silenced ER or the inhibition of ER suppressing growth factor pathways.

For those tumors that retain ER expression upon relapse, approximately half will exhibit intrinsic resistance and not respond to first or subsequent lines of endocrine therapy. In contrast the other half will respond to at least one line of therapy, before the near universal emergence of acquired resistance. Although this dichotomous definition provides a convenient way to classify experimental and clinical observations, the mechanisms underlying intrinsic and acquired resistance overlap considerably. In addition, resistance is often agent specific, exemplified by the different response and TTP rates seen with antiestrogenic agents with diverse mechanisms of action in phase III studies of first-line therapy and by the occurrence of second or third responses to endocrine agents upon progression on first-line therapy. In the following sections the current understanding of the known mechanisms of resistance to the different endocrine agents used to treat breast cancer will be discussed.

Estrogen Receptor Induction, Mutation, and Amplification and Estrogen Receptor β

Estrogen Receptor Induction

The lack of expression of the ER and hence an active ER pathway precludes the use of antiestrogens and is considered to represent intrinsic resistance. However, aberrant methylation of CpG islands in the promoters of the ER and PR genes has been observed in 25% to 40% of ER- and PR-negative breast cancers, respectively (155,156). More recently histone deacetylation has also been recognized as a potential mechanism to reverse ER suppression, and hence receptor negativity, in breast cancer cell lines (157). The combination of histone deacetylase (HDAC) inhibitors and DNA methyltransferase 1 (DNMT1) inhibitors results in a more open chromatin structure necessary for reactivation of silenced ER transcription and has been shown to induce ERα and ERβ expression in ER-negative cell lines and, importantly, to sensitize them to the effects of antiestrogens such as tamoxifen (158–161). The HDAC inhibitor suberoylanilide hydroxamic acid (SAHA, vorinostat) has recently entered early phase studies to examine its efficacy in combination with tamoxifen in aromatase inhibitor resistant MBC (162). Outside phase I and presurgical window studies, these drugs are yet to be employed in ER-negative MBC, a potentially fruitful avenue of investigation in view of the preclinical data outlined above.

A second encouraging approach to induce expression of functional ER in tumors negative for ER at the mRNA and protein level has been to inhibit mitogen activated protein kinase (MAPK) activity. In both cell lines and primary breast cancer samples cultured *in vitro*, pharmacological inhibition of MAPK with the small molecule inhibitor U0126 induced expression of ER and restored sensitivity to tamoxifen and fulvestrant (163,164). The reverse situation has also been demonstrated in which hyperactivation of MAPK by multiple experimental techniques, including growth factor pathway overexpression, directly represses ER expression. Such ER repression was also reversible using U0126 and may be clinically relevant in re-establishing functional ER expression to be targeted by endocrine therapy (163).

Estrogen Receptor Mutation and Amplification

In prostate cancer 50% to 60% of tumors develop androgen resistance secondary to inactivating androgen receptor (AR) mutations or amplification (165). In contrast, inactivating ER mutations or splice variants are rarely seen in breast cancer and do not appear to be induced by endocrine therapy (166,167). Only one study has demonstrated ER amplification in a significant proportion (20%) of breast cancers (168). These data are in conflict with previously published literature and yet to be confirmed independently but suggest improved endocrine sensitivity in patients with tumors harboring ER amplification compared to tumors without (169). Thus genetic aberrations in the ER appear to fail to explain the emergence of the majority of endocrine-resistant phenotypes.

Estrogen Receptor β

The second ER gene, known as ERβ, has also been investigated for its role in endocrine resistance (170,171). There is currently no consensus on the relationship between the expression of ERβ or its variants on the endocrine sensitivity of breast tumors. At least two major questions remain unanswered. The first is whether coexpression of ERβ, or its putative dominant negative variant ERβcx, with ERα has any independent prognostic value or capacity to predict response to endocrine therapy. The data to date are conflicting, although intriguingly a recent small study suggests that ERβcx, which does not bind estradiol, may act as a dominant negative regulator of ERα function and confer increased responsiveness to endocrine therapy; however, larger studies are required to validate this finding (172). The second question is whether there may be a role for endocrine therapy in ERβ positive but ERα negative breast cancers. Prospective studies will be required to elucidate the answer to this question, and as yet treatment decisions cannot be made on the basis of ERβ expression levels (170).

Enhanced Growth Factor Pathway Activity

Epidermal Growth Factor Receptor

Epidermal growth factor receptor (EGFR) belongs to a family of transmembrane tyrosine kinase receptors including EGFR, *ERBB2* (formerly *HER2*, human epidermal growth factor receptor 2), *ERBB3*, and *ERBB4*. Stromal EGFR is required for normal mammary gland development, and its overexpression in murine mammary glands induces epithelial cell transformation to carcinoma (173,174). However, the expression of EGFR is inversely related to that of the ER in human breast carcinomas, potentially as a result of a direct effect of the ER on EGFR gene expression (175–178). Retrospective analysis of adjuvant studies demonstrates intrinsic resistance to tamoxifen in tumors that coexpress EGFR and ER (177,179,180). The ER continues to be expressed and functional in most breast cancers after the development of tamoxifen resistance (181). Compelling *in vitro* data show that EGFR activation contributes to tumor growth in this situation, in part by EGF-stimulated ligand independent activation of the ER, and antagonism of EGFR activity with the tyrosine kinase inhibitor (TKI) gefitinib can delay the onset of tamoxifen resistance (182–184).

These encouraging results have led to the investigation of the EGFR TKIs gefitinib and erlotinib in presurgical studies in early breast cancer and in combination with endocrine therapies in MBC (Table 73.10) (185–190). Single-agent erlotinib given for 6 to 14 days preoperatively reduced tumor cell proliferation (Ki-67) and Akt, MAPK, and ribosomal protein S6 phosphorylation

to a significant level in ER-positive tumors, although numerical decreases were seen in *ERBB2*-positive and triple-negative cancers also (189). Similarly in a double-blind, placebo-controlled randomized trial of gefitinib with or without anastrazole given for 4 to 6 weeks preoperatively in ER- and EGFR-positive primary breast cancers, single-agent gefitinib reduced Ki-67 by a mean of 92.4% (95% CI, 85.1–96.1) and induced objective tumor responses in 50% of patients (186). Combination treatment significantly increased the magnitude of mean Ki-67 reduction to 98.0% (95% CI, 96.1–98.9) without increasing objective responses. In both groups, abolition of ER phosphorylation at Ser118 correlated with objective response. The patient selection for this study is noteworthy in that only women with tumors that coexpressed ER and EGFR were included. Despite prior observations that tumors that coexpress EGFR and ER tend to have weaker ER expression than those without EGFR, 49 of 56 (87.5%) of the patients in this study exhibited strong (3+) ER expression by immunohistochemistry (178,186). In contrast Smith et al. (187) conducted a phase II, placebo-controlled trial of neoadjuvant anastrazole alone or with gefitinib in early breast cancer. In their study of 206 postmenopausal women with ER-positive tumors, only one coexpressed EGFR. The combination of anastrazole and gefitinib was inferior to anastrazole alone in terms of the primary end point of reduction in Ki-67 and in OR rate, which both reached statistical significance in tumors coexpressing PR. Thus patient selection appears to be of utmost importance in these short-term treatment studies.

In the metastatic setting the combination of anastrazole and gefitinib showed no activity in 15 patients progressing on an aromatase inhibitor (185). However, more recent randomized placebo-controlled, phase II data from 93 women with newly

| Table 73.10 | REPORTED TRIALS OF EPIDERMAL GROWTH FACTOR RECEPTOR TKI AND ENDOCRINE THERAPY IN ESTROGEN AND/OR PROGESTERONE RECEPTOR POSITIVE BREAST CANCER |

Author (Reference)	Disease Setting	Trial Design	EGFR+ Selection	Agents	Primary End Point	Secondary End Point
Polychronis et al. (186)	Pre-op 4–6 weeks N = 56	Randomized DB placebo phase II	Yes	G + A/plac	Mean Ki-67 reduction (p = .005) G + A = 98% G + plac = 92%	OR (p >.05) 14/28 (50%) 12/22 (55%)
Smith et al. (187)	Neoadjuvant N = 188	Randomized DB placebo phase II (3 arm[b])	No (n = 1 EGFR+)	A + G/plac	Mean Ki-67 reduction at 16 weeks[a] (p = 0.26) A + plac = 83.6% A + G = 77.4%	OR (p = .08) 61% 48%
Mita et al. (185)	Advanced N = 15	Phase II single arm after AI failure	No	G + A	OR 0%	CBR 0%
Cristofannilli et al. (188)	Advanced N = 93	Randomized DB placebo phase II (2 arm)	No	A + G/plac	PFS (mos) A + G = 14.5 A + P = 8.2	CBR A + G = 21/43 (49%) A + plac = 17/50 (34%)
Osborne et al. (290)	Advanced N = 290	Randomized DB placebo phase II (2 arm in 2 strata[b])	No	T + G/plac	PFS (mos) Stratum 1 T + plac = 8.8 T + G = 10.9 (p = 0.31) Stratum 2 T + plac = 7.0 T + G = 5.7 (p = 0.58)	CBR 45.5% 50.5% (p = 0.07) 31% 29% (p = 0.05)

Pre-op, preoperative; DB, double blind; G, gefitinib; A, anastrazole; plac, placebo; EGFR, epidermal growth factor receptor; AI, aromatase inhibitor; CBR clinical benefit rate; PFS, progression-free survival; T, tamoxifen.
[a]Two weeks also reported and no significant difference (p = .22).
[b]See text.

diagnosed MBC demonstrate superior progression-free survival (PFS) with combination gefitinib and anastrazole compared to anastrazole alone (HR for progression 0.55; 95% CI, 0.32–0.94; median, 14.5 months vs. 8.2 months, respectively) (188). Objective responses were numerically greater in the anastrazole alone arm (12% vs. 2%), but clinical benefit rate was superior with the combination (21/43 [49%] vs. 17/50 [34%]). EGFR expression in these tumors is yet to be reported. Arpino et al. (190) have reported data from a similar randomized study using tamoxifen as the endocrine agent with or without gefitinib. Again this was a randomized, placebo-controlled, phase II study in ER- and/or PR-positive MBC, but importantly the 290 patients were stratified according to prior endocrine responsiveness. Stratum 1 consisted of patients with newly diagnosed MBC or those who completed adjuvant tamoxifen 1 year or more prior to presentation, whereas patients in stratum 2 had developed MBC while taking adjuvant AI or had progressed on first-line AI for MBC. EGFR expression was not reported but *ERBB2* was positive in 43 of 290 (14.8%) patients. The addition of gefitinib to tamoxifen in stratum 1 resulted in a nonsignificant improvement in PFS (hazard ratio of gefitinib to placebo was 0.84; 95% CI, 0.59–1.18; $p = .31$; median PFS 10.9 months vs. 8.8 months). OR and clinical benefit rates were 12.4% (13/108) and 50.5% (53/105) with combination therapy and 14.9% (15/101) and 45.5% (46/101) with tamoxifen alone ($p > .3$ for both). In stratum 2, there were no significant differences in clinical benefit rates between the groups (no ORs were seen) but PFS favored monotherapy with tamoxifen (HR for gefitinib to placebo of 1.16; 95% CI, 0.69–1.93; $p - .58$; median PFS 5.7 months vs. 7.0 months). Taken together the data from these two studies suggest that if there is a role for EGFR antagonism in ER-positive MBC it is likely to be in the prevention or delay of acquired endocrine therapy resistance (188,190). There is a clear difference between the endocrine agents used in these studies (i.e., SERM vs. AI) and preclinical data suggest that the resistance mechanisms to these agents may also be different (191). This has been confirmed in clinical studies of endocrine therapy sequencing in which responses to second-line agents are seen following progression on first-line therapy (192). The study of Osborne et al. (290) also highlights the importance of careful study design and patient stratification to help rationalize the use of increasing numbers of targeted therapies to the subpopulations of patients most likely to gain clinical benefit. Despite the inference from presurgical studies that EGFR expression *may* identify subpopulations more likely to benefit from combined EGFR and ER targeted therapy, this has not been validated and it must be remembered that EGFR expression alone is a poor predictor of EGFR TKI activity in other solid tumors (193).

ERBB2

ERBB2 (formerly *HER2*, also known as cerbB2) is the second of the EGFR family of transmembrane tyrosine kinase receptors and the target of multiple novel therapies entering or already in clinical use, including trastuzumab, pertuzumab, and lapatinib, the latter of which is a dual targeted TKI against EGFR and *ERBB2*. *ERBB2* is expressed in the normal mammary epithelium and is overexpressed in 20% to 25% of breast carcinomas as a result of gene amplification. Half of *ERBB2*-positive breast cancers coexpress the ER, and multiple studies have confirmed that patients with such tumors derive less clinical benefit from endocrine therapy than their ER-positive *ERBB2*-negative counterparts. Twelve of these studies (published from 1990 to 2003) have been subjected to meta-analyses that demonstrated a relative risk of failure of any endocrine therapy of 1.42 (95% CI, 1.32–1.52; $p < .00001$; test for heterogeneity = 0.380) for *ERBB2*-positive versus -negative tumors, independent of type of endocrine therapy used (tamoxifen vs. any other)

(194). As with the EGFR the inverse relationship between *ERBB2* and ER appears to be a result of crosstalk between the receptors. Transfection of ER-positive cell lines with *ERBB2* results in down-regulation of both the ER and PR and subsequent resistance to endocrine therapy both *in vitro* and *in vivo* (195–197). In the clinical setting several studies have demonstrated that the majority of cancers positive for both *ERBB2* and ER have reduced or absent PR (198–200). The reduced expression of PR is secondary to relative inactivity of the ER pathway and also to direct suppression by growth factor pathway activation of Akt (200–202). Importantly, treatment of *ERBB2* positive cell lines and xenograft tumors with the *ERBB2* directed monoclonal antibody trastuzumab, and other *ERBB2* targeted agents, can at least partially restore endocrine therapy sensitivity (190,203,204). In a single arm, phase II study, the combination of the aromatase inhibitor letrozole with trastuzumab, as first- or second-line therapy, was well tolerated and resulted in objective responses in 8 of 31 (26%) patients and clinical benefit in 16 of 31 (52%) (205). However, these rates are no different from the single-agent response and clinical benefit rates to trastuzumab in populations not selected for ER expression, and it is not possible to define the role of the endocrine agent in this study (206,207). To answer this question the TAnDEM study randomized patients with *ERBB2* and ER- or PR- positive MBC to anastrazole or combination anastrazole and trastuzumab (208). The relative resistance to endocrine therapy of tumors coexpressing *ERBB2* was evident from the objective response and PFS rates in the anastrazole alone group of only 6.8% and 2.4 months, respectively. The addition of trastuzumab significantly improved these rates to 20.3% and 4.8 months, but again these do not differ from the results seen with single-agent trastuzumab cited above. Three-arm studies are required, comparing each agent alone versus the combination, to adequately address the efficacy of *ERBB2*-targeted therapy on reversion of endocrine resistance.

In preclinical studies Arpino et al. (190) employed two xenograft models to better define the roles of the ER and *ERBB* family pathways in resistance to tamoxifen and estrogen deprivation therapy. The MCF-7 breast cancer cell line, transfected with the *ERBB2* gene (MCF/ERBB2-18), expressed ER and *ERBB2* at high levels compared to the BT474 cell line, which has naturally amplified *ERBB2* and lower ER expression. In MCF/ERBB2-18 tumors, endocrine sensitivity to tamoxifen or estrogen deprivation was maintained despite pharmacological *ERBB* family blockade, enhancing the effects of the *ERBB1* and *ERBB2* targeted agents. In contrast BT474 xenografts, which may be a more representative model of human (nontransfected) breast cancer, lost sensitivity to estrogen and tamoxifen after short-term growth *in vivo* while retaining sensitivity to the *ERBB* family targeted agents. Thus the combination of ER and *ERBB* family targeted agents may be beneficial in only a subset of patients, potentially those with high levels of receptor expression for both families, although this remains to be demonstrated in clinical studies. More than half of the patients treated with the combination of anastrazole and trastuzumab in the TANDEM study derived no clinical benefit. Inadequate targeting of one or both pathways, or heterodimerization between the *ERBB* family receptors, may be responsible for this observation (208). Studies employing agents such as lapatinib, a dual target TKI against EGFR and *ERBB2*, and pertuzumab, a monoclonal antibody preventing dimerization of *ERBB2* and *ERBB3*, are ongoing in combination with endocrine agents including tamoxifen, letrozole, and fulvestrant to investigate this hypothesis (190,209,210).

It is important to note that following the initial increase in *ERBB* family dependence with tamoxifen resistance, the ER is still functional and ER down-regulation with drugs such as fulvestrant is effective in reducing tumor growth (183,211). However, both *de novo* resistance to fulvestrant and resistance developing after tamoxifen are characterized by exaggerated *ERBB* family activity and growth inhibition with *ERBB* targeted therapies (183). Thus *ERBB* family receptor expression appears to be an important mechanism of adaptive resistance in preclinical studies to the three major classes of endocrine therapy, SERMS, ER down-regulators, and AIs.

Steroid Receptor Coactivators or Corepressors

The transcriptional regulatory activity of the ER is under tight control by nuclear receptor coactivators and corepressors (212). Only one coactivator, amplified in breast cancer 1 (AIB1)/steroid receptor coactivator 3 (SRC3), a member of the p160/steroid receptor coactivator family, has been shown to be overexpressed or amplified in breast cancer (213,214). AIB1 overexpression reduces the antagonist effects of tamoxifen in preclinical studies, however, expression levels in ER-positive primary breast cancers show no consistent prognostic or predictive readout in treatment-naive or tamoxifen-treated patients (211,215–218). In contrast three of these studies have demonstrated that tumors with high levels of both AIB1 and *ERBB* family expression have worse outcomes with adjuvant tamoxifen treatment than those without (211,217,218). These studies augment preclinical observations that mediators downstream of EGFR and *ERBB2* pathways activate AIB1 by phosphorylation and that phosphorylated AIB1 enhances the activation of the *ERBB* family in both tumorigenesis and cancer progression (219–221). Thus AIB1 may be a valuable biomarker in endocrine therapy selection, in particular in *ERBB* family overexpressing tumors. Nuclear corepressors also represent potential biomarkers of outcome on endocrine therapy. The nuclear corepressor NCOR binds to the tamoxifen bound ER, suppressing its transcriptional activity (222–224). Low NCOR expression (vs. intermediate and high) is associated with significantly shorter relapse-free survival on tamoxifen, and its interaction with the ER is disrupted in the presence of high level *ERBB2* signaling via MAPK (203,223).

Activation of Downstream Signal Transduction Intermediates

In addition to members of the *ERBB* family, many other diverse membrane-bound receptors, such as insulin-like growth factor receptor-1 (IGF1R) (225), c-met (226), and β4 integrin (227), have been identified as markers of adaptive endocrine resistance in preclinical studies. In addition, gene expression studies and siRNA screens now raise the prospect that many other receptor targets will be identified as regulators of endocrine resistance (228,229). Antagonism of common intracellular signaling pathways may be a more successful approach, given both the divergence of targets identified between studies and the apparent commonality of effector pathways downstream of many of these receptors. The two most common effectors studied to date are the Raf/MAPK and PI3K/Akt/mTOR pathways. Increasing evidence suggests that these pathways play critical roles in *de novo* and acquired resistance to multiple types of endocrine therapy.

Raf/MAPK Pathway

Constitutive MAPK activation in endocrine sensitive cells leads to p27(Kip1) deregulation and antiestrogen resistance in human breast cancer cells (230). Multiple preclinical models of resistance to tamoxifen, fulvestrant, estrogen deprivation, and aromatase inhibition have demonstrated increased MAPK activity in the resistant compared to sensitive cells and resensitization to endocrine therapy upon MAPK inhibition (163,164,191,203,231–236). As discussed above, the majority of ER-positive breast cancers retain ER expression following the development of endocrine resistance. Activated MAPK has

been shown to induce phosphorylation of the ER at multiple serine residues in the AF1 domain, inducing ligand independent ER activation, a potential mechanism of endocrine resistance (237,238). Serine 118 phosphorylation in pretreatment biopsies correlates with more differentiated tumors and better prognosis, presumably as an indicator of ER pathway activity (182,239). However, Ser118 is elevated in tumor biopsies taken from patients who have relapsed following tamoxifen treatment compared to pretreatment biopsies, suggesting that it is also involved in the resistance process (182,183,240). Other signaling intermediates can also activate the ER at Ser118 and one study, demonstrating increased Ser118 phosphorylation following relapse on tamoxifen, did not show a corresponding increase in MAPK activation. Thus other intracellular pathways may be mediating ER phosphorylation and endocrine resistance in these tumors (240).

These observations have led to the combination of endocrine agents with MAPK targeted agents in MBC. However, targeting the Raf/MAPK pathway itself (rather than signal initiating growth factor receptor pathways) is far from simple and has largely met with negative outcomes clinically. The primary focus of pathway inhibition to date has been on farnesyltransferase inhibitors that inhibit Ras activation. Ras proteins are mitogenic switches between growth factor receptors and the Raf/MAPK cascade and are frequently aberrantly expressed in breast cancer (241). The farnesyltransferase inhibitor R115777 (tipifarnib) in combination with tamoxifen, fulvestrant, or estrogen deprivation was shown to act synergistically to inhibit MCF-7 breast cancer cell proliferation *in vitro* and *in vivo* (242,243). However, in a randomized phase II study of letrozole with or without tipifarnib in MBC no difference was seen in any efficacy end point between the two treatment groups (244). Further studies of farnesyltransferase inhibitors in combination with endocrine agents are ongoing, which may identify subgroups of patients that benefit from such therapy, although incomplete understanding of their mechanism of action and relatively "upstream" site of pathway inhibition may limit their therapeutic utility. Whether inhibition of the "nodal point" of this signaling cascade (i.e., MAPK) is feasible clinically remains to be seen. Such an agent would be of great potential interest in the therapy of tumors with either acquired or intrinsic endocrine resistance, including those with absent baseline ER expression.

PI3K/Akt/mTOR

The phosphoinositide-3-kinase (PI3K)/protein kinase B (PKB/Akt)/mammalian target of rapamycin (mTOR) pathway is a critical regulator of multiple cellular processes, most notably apoptosis. Activating mutations of PI3K can be found in 20% to 40% of breast cancers and a further 20% to 40% demonstrate reduced or absent expression of protein tyrosine phosphatase (PTEN), the primary negative regulator of PI3K activity (245–247). Transfection of such constitutively active PI3K mutants into breast epithelial cells results in their oncogenic transformation (248). Activation of PI3K phosphorylates Akt resulting in ligand-independent activation of the ER secondary to its phosphorylation at serine 167 (249). Tumors with an activated PI3K pathway, either as a result of PI3K activation or PTEN suppression, do poorly on adjuvant tamoxifen therapy compared to those without, demonstrating intrinsic resistance (250–253). Multiple preclinical models have demonstrated increased PI3K/Akt pathway activation upon the development of acquired endocrine therapy resistance to tamoxifen (254), long-term estrogen deprivation (255,256), and fulvestrant (226,254). Many of the studies cited above have demonstrated that the AKT activation seen in the resistant state is a result of up-regulated *ERBB* family expression signaling through the PI3K pathway. Inhibition of this signaling in model systems either delays the development of resistance or restores sensitivity to endocrine agents once acquired resistance has developed. However, inhibition is often incomplete, and resistance to the inhibitors themselves develops universally over time. Combinations of receptor inhibitors may improve this situation, although direct blockade of the PI3K pathway downstream of such receptors shows promise in preclinical studies, as discussed below (190).

Rapamycin analogs such as everolimus (RAD-001) and temsirolimus (CCI-779) inhibit mTOR, a key target protein of Akt. These analogs demonstrate synergistic increase in cell cycle arrest and apoptosis, in combination with letrozole, in MCF-7 cells transfected with aromatase (257). Similarly, MCF-7 cells resistant to tamoxifen, letrozole, or fulvestrant, secondary to expression of constitutively active Akt, revert to an endocrine sensitive phenotype with mTOR inhibition (258,259). In a phase I study, everolimus given to 18 patients with SD or PD after 4 months of letrozole induced a CR in one, reduction of liver metastases by 28% in another, and SD longer than 6 months in another five (260). In phase II studies, single-agent temsirolimus induced objective responses in 10 of 109 (9%) patients with MBC but did not demonstrate superiority over letrozole alone (207,261). A randomized phase III study of letrozole with or without temsirolimus was stopped early due to lack of benefit of the combination over letrozole alone (262). Although a minority of ER-positive breast tumors are clearly sensitive to the effects of mTOR inhibition, the majority are resistant. This is likely due to the demonstration that RAD-001 induces insulin receptor substrate-1 expression and disinhibits a negative feedback loop, resulting in activation of IGF-1R and Akt in both cell lines and tumor samples (263,264). The development of potent and specific PI3K inhibitors is an exciting development in the field of endocrine resistance, although at the time of writing these are only just entering phase I clinical studies (265).

Estrogen Deprivation, Hypersensitivity, and Fulvestrant Resistance

Because oophorectomy and modern AIs effectively deprive tumor cells of estrogens, a surrogate method for studying the mechanism of resistance to estrogen deprivation is to grow ER-positive human mammary tumors in estrogen-depleted culture medium. When ER-positive cells are placed in such media they are growth arrested for 3 to 6 months and then begin to regrow. When their response to estradiol at the time of regrowth is retested, it is found that the dose–response curve is shifted to the left and maximal proliferation occurs at approximately 10^{-14} mol/L, instead of 10^{-9} mol/L in wild-type cells (Fig. 73.6) (266,267). Proliferation at such low levels of estradiol can be inhibited by fulvestrant, indicating that hypersensitivity occurs via an ER-dependent mechanism (266,267). Resistance in this setting is associated with several cellular changes, including enhanced *ERBB* family, IGF-1R, and ER expression, and increased signal transduction via the MAPK and PI3K pathways (255,267,268). Nongenomic actions of estrogen, through membrane-associated ER, have also been proposed to contribute to endocrine resistance in long-term estrogen deprivation, although the precise mechanisms of estrogen-induced activation of downstream signaling events, which occur too rapidly to be transcription dependent, are still to be determined (269). Under conditions of estradiol hypersensitivity and indeed long-term tamoxifen treatment, physiological levels of estradiol become growth inhibitory and have been shown to induce apoptosis via the mitochondrial pathway (149,266,267,270). At least two groups have demonstrated that, in the context of estradiol-induced growth suppression in long-term estrogen deprivation cells, the ER down-regulator fulvestrant stimulates growth (270,271). This has important implications for the treatment of postmenopausal women with cancer that has progressed through therapy with

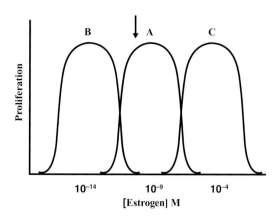

FIGURE 73.6. **Hypothetical dose response curves for MCF-7 cells. A:** Wild-type cells with maximal proliferation at "physiological" estrogen concentrations seen in premenopausal women. **B:** Shift of the dose–response curve to the left when MCF-7 cells are grown under estrogen-free conditions. Maximal proliferation occurs at 10^{-14} M estradiol. In these cells, "physiological" concentrations of estradiol cause growth inhibition (*down arrow*). (Adapted from Masamura S, Santner SJ, Heitjan DF, et al. Estrogen deprivation causes estradiol hypersensitivity in human breast cancer cells. *J Clin Endocrinol Metab* 1995;80:2918–2925.) **C:** Dose–response curve that might be seen after response, but then progression on additive estrogens.

a potent third-generation aromatase inhibitor. Furthermore, in a xenograft model using MCF-7 cells stably transfected with the human aromatase gene (MCF-7ca) the combination of fulvestrant and letrozole or anastrazole significantly delayed the onset of resistance to both drugs, whereas the combination of letrozole and tamoxifen reduced the efficacy of letrozole alone in line with results from the ATAC (anastrozole, tamoxifen alone or in combination) study (55,231,272). Although the EFECT study demonstrated equivalent efficacy between fulvestrant and exemestane as second-line therapy after the failure of a nonsteroidal AI, these preclinical models suggest that fulvestrant could be more appropriately combined with an AI to maintain maximal suppression of estradiol, and this is currently being tested in randomized phase II studies (Table 73.9) (148,273).

These observations may also facilitate the use of lower, better tolerated doses of estrogen to treat MBC in postmenopausal women following response then progression on a third-generation AI. In early studies of estrogen therapy in MBC, lower doses, such as those used in oral contraceptives and hormone replacement therapy (HRT), were somewhat less effective but better tolerated than supraphysiological doses (75,274). Stoll (74) demonstrated that the greater the time between menopause and estrogen treatment, the greater chance of obtaining a tumor response, suggesting that tumors developing or growing in a low-estrogen environment have increased sensitivity to growth inhibition by estrogen. Thus in the face of profound suppression of estradiol levels, as seen with third-generation AIs, physiological (premenopausal) doses of estrogen may be as effective and less toxic than higher doses (149). This hypothesis is currently being tested in clinical studies in MBC.

SUMMARY OF POTENTIAL STRATEGIES TO REVERT KEY MECHANISMS OF ENDOCRINE RESISTANCE

- Induction of ER expression in epigenetically silenced ER negative tumors using HDAC and DNMT1 inhibitors.
- Inhibition of growth factor receptor activity using tyrosine kinase inhibitors, monoclonal antibodies, and so forth.

- Inhibition of downstream signaling cascade "nodes" such as MAPK or PI3K.
- Induction of apoptosis and "resetting" to a sensitive phenotype with estradiol following resistance to aromatase inhibition.

References

1. Beslija S, Bonneterre J, Burstein H, et al. Second consensus on medical treatment of metastatic breast cancer. *Ann Oncol* 2007;18:215–225.
2. Wilcken N, Hornbuckle J, Ghersi D. Chemotherapy alone versus endocrine therapy alone for metastatic breast cancer. *Cochrane Database Syst Rev* 2003;CD002747.
3. Harris L, Fritsche H, Mennel R, et al. American Society of Clinical Oncology 2007 update of recommendations for the use of tumor markers in breast cancer. *J Clin Oncol* 2007;25:5287–5312.
4. Lower EE, Glass EL, Bradley DA, et al. Impact of metastatic estrogen receptor and progesterone receptor status on survival. *Breast Cancer Res Treat* 2005;90:65–70.
5. Kuukasjarvi T, Kononen J, Helin H, et al. Loss of estrogen receptor in recurrent breast cancer is associated with poor response to endocrine therapy. *J Clin Oncol* 1996;14:2584–2589.
6. Mortimer JE, Dehdashti F, Siegel BA, et al. Metabolic flare: indicator of hormone responsiveness in advanced breast cancer. *J Clin Oncol* 2001;19:2797–2803.
7. Linden HM, Stekhova SA, Link JM, et al. Quantitative fluoroestradiol positron emission tomography imaging predicts response to endocrine treatment in breast cancer. *J Clin Oncol* 2006;24:2793–2799.
8. Clarysse A. Hormone-induced tumor flare. *Eur J Cancer Clin Oncol* 1985;21:545–547.
9. Coleman RE, Mashiter G, Whitaker KB, et al. Bone scan flare predicts successful systemic therapy for bone metastases. *J Nucl Med* 1988;29:1354–1359.
10. Dehdashti F, Mortimer JE, Trinkaus K, et al. PET-based estradiol challenge as a predictive biomarker of response to endocrine therapy in women with estrogen-receptor-positive breast cancer. *Breast Cancer Res Treat* 2008. In press.
11. Semiglazov VF, Semiglazov VV, Dashyan GA, et al. Phase II randomized trial of primary endocrine therapy versus chemotherapy in postmenopausal patients with estrogen receptor-positive breast cancer. *Cancer* 2007;110:244–254.
12. Therasse P, Arbuck SG, Eisenhauer EA, et al. New guidelines to evaluate the response to treatment in solid tumors. European Organization for Research and Treatment of Cancer, National Cancer Institute of the United States, National Cancer Institute of Canada. *J Natl Cancer Inst* 2000;92:205–216.
13. Michaelis LC, Ratain MJ. Measuring response in a post-RECIST world: from black and white to shades of grey. *Nat Rev Cancer* 2006;6:409–414.
14. Howell A, Mackintosh J, Jones M, et al. The definition of the "no change" category in patients treated with endocrine therapy and chemotherapy for advanced carcinoma of the breast. *Eur J Cancer Clin Oncol* 1988;24:1567–1572.
15. Robertson JF, Howell A, Buzdar A, et al. Static disease on anastrozole provides similar benefit as objective response in patients with advanced breast cancer. *Breast Cancer Res Treat* 1999;58:157–162.
16. Robertson JF, Willsher PC, Cheung KL, et al. The clinical relevance of static disease (no change) category for 6 months on endocrine therapy in patients with breast cancer. *Eur J Cancer* 1997;33:1774–1779.
17. Bernhard J, Thurlimann B, Schmitz SF, et al. Defining clinical benefit in postmenopausal patients with breast cancer under second-line endocrine treatment: does quality of life matter? *J Clin Oncol* 1999;17:1672–1679.
18. Schinzinger A. Ueber carcinoma mammae. 18th Congress of the German Society for Surgery. *Beilage Centralblatt Chirurgie* 1889;16:55–56.
19. Beatson G. On the treatment of inoperable cases of carcinoma of the mamma. Suggestions for a new method for treatment with illustrative cases. *Lancet* 1896;2:162–165.
20. Boyd S. On oophorectomy in cancer of the breast. *BMJ* 1900;2:1161–1167.
21. Lett H. An analysis of 99 cases of inoperable carcinoma of the breast treated by oophorectomy. *Lancet* 1908;1:227.
22. DeCourmelles F. La radiotherapie indirecte, ou dirigee par les correlations organiques. *Arch Elect Med* 1922;32:264.
23. Early Breast Cancer Trialists' Collaborative Group (EBCTCG). Ovarian ablation for early breast cancer. *Cochrane Database Syst Rev* 2000;CD000485.
24. Block G, Vial A, Pullen F. Estrogen secretion following operative and irradiation castration in cases of mammary cancer. *Surgery* 1958;43:415.
25. Featherstone CJ, Harnett AN, Brunt AM, et al. Methods of ovarian suppression used in the UK. *Breast* 2002;11:23–29.
26. Conte CC, Nemoto T, Rosner D, et al. Therapeutic oophorectomy in metastatic breast cancer. *Cancer* 1989;64:150–153.
27. Oriana S, Bohm S, Baeli A, et al. Clinical response and survival according to estrogen receptor levels after bilateral ovariectomy in advanced breast cancer. *Eur J Surg Oncol* 1989;15:39–42.
28. Veronesi U, Pizzocaro G, Rossi A. Oophorectomy for advanced carcinoma of the breast. *Surg Gynecol Obstet* 1975;141:569–570.
29. Buchanan RB, Blamey RW, Durrant KR, et al. A randomized comparison of tamoxifen with surgical oophorectomy in premenopausal patients with advanced breast cancer. *J Clin Oncol* 1986;4:1326–1330.
30. Crump M, Sawka CA, DeBoer G, et al. An individual patient-based meta-analysis of tamoxifen versus ovarian ablation as first line endocrine therapy for premenopausal women with metastatic breast cancer. *Breast Cancer Res Treat* 1997;44:201–210.
31. Ingle JN, Krook JE, Green SJ, et al. Randomized trial of bilateral oophorectomy versus tamoxifen in premenopausal women with metastatic breast cancer. *J Clin Oncol* 1986;4:178–185.
32. Sawka CA, Pritchard KI, Shelley W, et al. A randomized crossover trial of tamoxifen versus ovarian ablation for metastatic breast cancer in premenopausal women: a report of the National Cancer Institute of Canada Clinical Trials Group (NCIC CTG) trial MA.1. *Breast Cancer Res Treat* 1997;44:211–215.
33. Klijn JG, de Jong FH. Treatment with a luteinising-hormone-releasing-hormone analogue (buserelin) in premenopausal patients with metastatic breast cancer. *Lancet* 1982;1:1213–1216.
34. Prowell TM, Davidson NE. What is the role of ovarian ablation in the management of primary and metastatic breast cancer today? *Oncologist* 2004;9:507–517.
35. Robertson JF, Blamey RW. The use of gonadotrophin-releasing hormone (GnRH) agonists in early and advanced breast cancer in pre- and perimenopausal women. *Eur J Cancer* 2003;39:861–869.
36. Williams MR, Walker KJ, Turkes A, et al. The use of an LH-RH agonist (ICI 118630, Zoladex) in advanced premenopausal breast cancer. *Br J Cancer* 1986;53:629–636.
37. Blamey RW, Jonat W, Kaufmann M, et al. Goserelin depot in the treatment of premenopausal advanced breast cancer. *Eur J Cancer* 1992;28A:810–814
38. Blamey RW, Jonat W, Kaufmann M, et al. Survival data relating to the use of goserelin depot in the treatment of premenopausal advanced breast cancer. *Eur J Cancer* 1993;29A:1498.
39. Klijn JG, Beex LV, Mauriac L, et al. Combined treatment with buserelin and tamoxifen in premenopausal metastatic breast cancer: a randomized study. *J Natl Cancer Inst* 2000;92:903–911.
40. Klijn JG, Blamey RW, Boccardo F, et al. Combined tamoxifen and luteinizing hormone-releasing hormone (LHRH) agonist versus LHRH agonist alone in premenopausal advanced breast cancer: a meta-analysis of four randomized trials. *J Clin Oncol* 2001;19:343–353.
41. Forward DP, Cheung KL, Jackson L, et al. Clinical and endocrine data for goserelin plus anastrozole as second-line endocrine therapy for premenopausal advanced breast cancer. *Br J Cancer* 2004;90:590–594.
42. Stein RC, Dowsett M, Hedley A, et al. The clinical and endocrine effects of 4-hydroxyandrostenedione alone and in combination with goserelin in premenopausal women with advanced breast cancer. *Br J Cancer* 1990;62:679–683.
43. Gnant M, Mlineritsch B, Schippinger W, et al. Adjuvant ovarian suppression combined with tamoxifen or anastrozole, alone or in combination with zoledronic acid, in premenopausal women with hormone-responsive, stage I and II breast cancer: first efficacy results from ABCSG-12. *J Clin Oncol* 2008;26:LBA4.
44. Huggins C, Dao TL. Adrenalectomy and oophorectomy in treatment of advanced carcinoma of the breast. *J Am Med Assoc* 1953;151:1388–1394.
45. Nathanson I, Towne L. The urinary excretion of estrogen and androgen and FSH following administration of testosterone to human female castrates. *Endocrinology* 1939;25:754.
46. Griffiths CT, Hall TC, Saba Z, et al. Preliminary trial of aminoglutethimide in breast cancer. *Cancer* 1973;32:31–37.
47. Wells SA Jr, Worgul TJ, Samojlik E, et al. Comparison of surgical adrenalectomy to medical adrenalectomy in patients with metastatic carcinoma of the breast. *Cancer Res* 1982;42:3454s–3457s.
48. Santen RJ, Santner S, Davis B, et al. Aminoglutethimide inhibits extraglandular estrogen production in postmenopausal women with breast carcinoma. *J Clin Endocrinol Metab* 1978;47:1257–1265.
49. Geisler J. Aromatase inhibitors: from bench to bedside and back. *Breast Cancer* 2008;15:17–26.
50. Geisler J, Lonning PE. Aromatase inhibition: translation into a successful therapeutic approach. *Clin Cancer Res* 2005;11:2809–2821.
51. Smith IE, Dowsett M. Aromatase inhibitors in breast cancer. *N Engl J Med* 2003;348:2431–2442.
52. Miller WR, Forrest AP. Oestradiol synthesis by a human breast carcinoma. *Lancet* 1974;2:866–868.
53. Miki Y, Suzuki T, Sasano H. Controversies of aromatase localization in human breast cancer—stromal versus parenchymal cells. *J Steroid Biochem Mol Biol* 2007;106:97–101.
54. Brodie A, Lu Q, Liu Y, et al. Aromatase inhibitors and their antitumor effects in model systems. *Endocr Relat Cancer* 1999;6:205–210.
55. Macedo LF, Sabnis GJ, Goloubeva OG, et al. Combination of anastrozole with fulvestrant in the intratumoral aromatase xenograft model. *Cancer Res* 2008;68:3516–3522.
56. Geisler J, Haynes B, Anker G, et al. Influence of letrozole and anastrozole on total body aromatization and plasma estrogen levels in postmenopausal breast cancer patients evaluated in a randomized, cross-over study. *J Clin Oncol* 2002;20:751–757.
57. Rose C, Vtoraya O, Pluzanska A, et al. An open randomised trial of second-line endocrine therapy in advanced breast cancer. Comparison of the aromatase inhibitors letrozole and anastrozole. *Eur J Cancer* 2003;39:2318–2327.
58. Fossati R, Confalonieri C, Torri V, et al. Cytotoxic and hormonal treatment for metastatic breast cancer: a systematic review of published randomized trials involving 31,510 women. *J Clin Oncol* 1998;16:3439–3460.
59. Gibson LJ, Dawson CK, Lawrence DH, et al. Aromatase inhibitors for treatment of advanced breast cancer in postmenopausal women. *Cochrane Database Syst Rev* 2007;CD003370.
60. Mauri D, Pavlidis N, Polyzos NP, et al. Survival with aromatase inhibitors and inactivators versus standard hormonal therapy in advanced breast cancer: meta-analysis. *J Natl Cancer Inst* 2006;98:1285–1291.
61. Dirix LY, Ignacio J, Nag S, et al. Treatment of advanced hormone-sensitive breast cancer in postmenopausal women with exemestane alone or in combination with celecoxib. *J Clin Oncol* 2008;26:1253–1259.
62. Goss P, Bondarenko IN, Manikhas GN, et al. Phase III, double-blind, controlled trial of atamestane plus toremifene compared with letrozole in postmenopausal women with advanced receptor-positive breast cancer. *J Clin Oncol* 2007;25:4961–4966.
63. Ulrich P. Testosterone et son role possible dans le traitment de certains cancers du sein. *Int Union Against Cancer* 1939;4:377.
64. Haddow A. Influence of certain polycyclic hydrocarbons on the growth of the Jensen rat sarcoma. *Nature* 1935;136:868.
65. Murray W. Transplantation of ovaries in inbred strains of mice causes or promotes cancer. *J Cancer Res* 1928;12:8.
66. Allen E, Doisy E. An ovarian hormone. Preliminary report on its localisation, extraction and partial purification, and action in test animals. *J Am Med Assoc* 1923;81:819–821.
67. Lacassagne A. Apparition de cancers de la mamelle chez lar souris male, soumise a des injections de folliculurie. *C R Acad Sci* 1932;195:630.
68. Dodds E, Goldberg L, Lawson W, et al. Oestrogenic activity of certain synthetic compounds. *Nature* 1938;141:247–248.
69. Robson J, Bonser G. Triphenylethylene causes cancer. *Nature* 1938;142:836.
70. Gardner W, Smith G, Strong L. 1935 Inhibition of normal gland. *Proc Soc Exper Biol Med* 1935;33:138.
71. Lacassagne A. Apparition d'adenocarcinomes mammaires chez des souris males traits pare une substance oestrogene synthetique. *C R Soc Biol Paris* 1938;129:64.

72. Haddow A, Watkinson J, Paterson E. Influence of synthetic oestrogens upon advanced malignant diseases. *BMJ* 1944;2:393–398.
73. Walpole AL, Paterson E. Synthetic oestrogens in mammary cancer. *Lancet* 1949; 2:783–786.
74. Stoll BA. Hypothesis: breast cancer regression under oestrogen therapy. *BMJ* 1973;3:446–450.
75. Carter AC, Sedransk N, Kelley RM, et al. Diethylstilbestrol: recommended dosages for different categories of breast cancer patients. Report of the Cooperative Breast Cancer Group. *JAMA* 1977;237:2079–2078.
76. Beex L, Pieters G, Smals A, et al. Tamoxifen versus ethinyl estradiol in the treatment of postmenopausal women with advanced breast cancer. *Cancer Treat Rep* 1981;65:179–185.
77. Gockerman JP, Spremulli EN, Raney M, et al. Randomized comparison of tamoxifen versus diethylstilbestrol in estrogen receptor-positive or -unknown metastatic breast cancer: a Southeastern Cancer Study Group trial. *Cancer Treat Rep* 1986;70:1199–1203.
78. Heuson JC, Engelsman E, Blonk-Van Der Wijst J, et al. Comparative trial of nafoxidine and ethinyloestradiol in advanced breast cancer: an E.O.R.T.C. study. *BMJ* 1975;2:711–713.
79. Ingle JN, Ahmann DL, Green SJ, et al. Randomized clinical trial of diethylstilbestrol versus tamoxifen in postmenopausal women with advanced breast cancer. *N Engl J Med* 1981;304:16–21.
80. Matelski H, Greene R, Huberman M, et al. Randomized trial of estrogen vs. tamoxifen therapy for advanced breast cancer. *Am J Clin Oncol* 1985;8: 128–133.
81. Stewart HJ, Forrest AP, Gunn JM, et al. The tamoxifen trial—a double-blind comparison with stilboestrol in postmenopausal women with advanced breast cancer. *Eur J Cancer Suppl* 1980;1:83–88.
82. Peethambaram PP, Ingle JN, Suman VJ, et al. Randomized trial of diethylstilbestrol vs. tamoxifen in postmenopausal women with metastatic breast cancer. An updated analysis. *Breast Cancer Res Treat* 1999;54:117–122.
83. Agrawal A, Robertson JF, Cheung KL. Efficacy and tolerability of high dose "ethinylestradiol" in post-menopausal advanced breast cancer patients heavily pre-treated with endocrine agents. *World J Surg Oncol* 2006;4:44.
84. Boyer MJ, Tattersall MH. Diethylstilbestrol revisited in advanced breast cancer management. *Med Pediatr Oncol* 1990;18:317–320.
85. Lonning PE, Taylor PD, Anker G, et al. High-dose estrogen treatment in postmenopausal breast cancer patients heavily exposed to endocrine therapy. *Breast Cancer Res Treat* 2001;67:111–116.
86. Clemons M, Danson S, Howell A. Tamoxifen ("Nolvadex"): a review. *Cancer Treat Rev* 2002;28:165–180.
87. Osborne CK. Tamoxifen in the treatment of breast cancer. *N Engl J Med* 1998; 339:1609–1618.
88. Harper MJ, Walpole AL. Contrasting endocrine activities of cis and trans isomers in a series of substituted triphenylethylenes. *Nature* 1966;212:87.
89. Harper MJ, Walpole AL. A new derivative of triphenylethylene: effect on implantation and mode of action in rats. *J Reprod Fertil* 1967;13:101–119.
90. Cole MP, Jones CT, Todd ID. A new anti-oestrogenic agent in late breast cancer. An early clinical appraisal of ICI46474. *Br J Cancer* 1971;25:270–275.
91. Ward HW. Anti-oestrogen therapy for breast cancer: a trial of tamoxifen at two dose levels. *BMJ* 1973;1:13–14.
92. Watkins SM. The value of high dose tamoxifen in postmenopausal breast cancer patients progressing on standard doses: a pilot study. *Br J Cancer* 1988;57:320–321.
93. Litherland S, Jackson IM. Antioestrogens in the management of hormone-dependent cancer. *Cancer Treat Rev* 1988;15:183–194.
94. Baumann CK, Castiglione-Gertsch M. Estrogen receptor modulators and down regulators: optimal use in postmenopausal women with breast cancer. *Drugs* 2007;67:2335–2353.
95. Howell A, Robertson JF, Abram P, et al. Comparison of fulvestrant versus tamoxifen for the treatment of advanced breast cancer in postmenopausal women previously untreated with endocrine therapy: a multinational, double-blind, randomized trial. *J Clin Oncol* 2004;22:1605–1613.
96. Johnston SR. Endocrinology and hormone therapy in breast cancer: selective oestrogen receptor modulators and downregulators for breast cancer—have they lost their way? *Breast Cancer Res* 2005;7:119–130.
97. Pyrhonen S, Ellmen J, Vuorinen J, et al. Meta-analysis of trials comparing toremifene with tamoxifen and factors predicting outcome of antiestrogen therapy in postmenopausal women with breast cancer. *Breast Cancer Res Treat* 1999;56:133–143.
98. Buzdar A, Hayes D, El-Khoudary A, et al. Phase III randomized trial of droloxifene and tamoxifen as first-line endocrine treatment of ER/PgR-positive advanced breast cancer. *Breast Cancer Res Treat* 2002;73:161–175.
99. Arpino G, Nair Krishnan M, Doval Dinesh C, et al. Idoxifene versus tamoxifen: a randomized comparison in postmenopausal patients with metastatic breast cancer. *Ann Oncol* 2003;14:233–241.
100. Buzdar AU, Marcus C, Holmes F, et al. Phase II evaluation of Ly156758 in metastatic breast cancer. *Oncology* 1988;45:344–345.
101. Gradishar W, Glusman J, Lu Y, et al. Effects of high dose raloxifene in selected patients with advanced breast carcinoma. *Cancer* 2000;88:2047–2053.
102. Deshmane V, Krishnamurthy S, Melemed AS, et al. Phase III double-blind trial of arzoxifene compared with tamoxifen for locally advanced or metastatic breast cancer. *J Clin Oncol* 2007;25:4967–4973.
103. Labrie F. Future perspectives of selective estrogen receptor modulators used alone and in combination with DHEA. *Endocr Relat Cancer* 2006;13:335–355.
104. Wakeling AE, Bowler J. Steroidal pure antioestrogens. *J Endocrinol* 1987;112: R7–R10.
105. Wakeling AE, Dukes M, Bowler J. A potent specific pure antiestrogen with clinical potential. *Cancer Res* 1991;51:3867–3873.
106. DeFriend DJ, Howell A, Nicholson RI, et al. Investigation of a new pure antiestrogen (ICI 182780) in women with primary breast cancer. *Cancer Res* 1994; 54:408–414.
107. Osborne CK, Coronado-Heinsohn EB, Hilsenbeck SG, et al. Comparison of the effects of a pure steroidal antiestrogen with those of tamoxifen in a model of human breast cancer. *J Natl Cancer Inst* 1995;87:746–750.
108. Robertson JF, Nicholson RI, Bundred NJ, et al. Comparison of the short-term biological effects of 7alpha-[9-(4,4,5,5,5-pentafluoropentylsulfinyl)-nonyl]estra-1,3,5, (10)-triene-3,17beta-diol (Faslodex) versus tamoxifen in postmenopausal women with primary breast cancer. *Cancer Res* 2001;61:6739–6746.
109. McCormack P, Sapunar F. Pharmacokinetic profile of the fulvestrant (Fasolodex) loading-dose regimen in postmenopausal women with hormone receptor-positive advanced breast cancer. *Breast Cancer Res Treat* 2007;106[Suppl]:S115.
110. Kuter I HR, Singer CF, Badwe R, et al. Fulvestrant 500 mg vs. 250 mg: first results from NEWEST, a randomized, phase II neoadjuvant trial in postmenopausal women with locally advanced, estrogen receptor-positive breast cancer. *Breast Cancer Res Treat* 2007;6[Suppl].
111. Robertson JF. Fulvestrant (Faslodex)—how to make a good drug better. Oncologist 2007;12:774–784.
112. Howell A, DeFriend DJ, Robertson JF, et al. Pharmacokinetics, pharmacological and anti-tumour effects of the specific anti-oestrogen ICI 182780 in women with advanced breast cancer. *Br J Cancer* 1996;74:300–308.
113. Howell A, Robertson J. Response to a specific antioestrogen (ICI 182780) in tamoxifen-resistant breast cancer. *Lancet* 1995;345:989–990.
114. Osborne CK, Pippen J, Jones SE, et al. Double-blind, randomized trial comparing the efficacy and tolerability of fulvestrant versus anastrozole in postmenopausal women with advanced breast cancer progressing on prior endocrine therapy: results of a North American trial. *J Clin Oncol* 2002;20:3386–3395.
115. Howell A, Robertson JF, Quaresma Albano J, et al. Fulvestrant, formerly ICI 182,780, is as effective as anastrozole in postmenopausal women with advanced breast cancer progressing after prior endocrine treatment. *J Clin Oncol* 2002;20: 3396–3403.
116. Mauriac L, Pippen JE, Quaresma Albano J, et al. Fulvestrant (Faslodex) versus anastrozole for the second-line treatment of advanced breast cancer in subgroups of postmenopausal women with visceral and non-visceral metastases: combined results from two multicentre trials. *Eur J Cancer* 2003;39:1228–1233.
117. Howell A, Pippen J, Elledge RM, et al. Fulvestrant versus anastrozole for the treatment of advanced breast carcinoma: a prospectively planned combined survival analysis of two multicenter trials. *Cancer* 2005;104:236–239.
118. Robertson JF, Osborne CK, Howell A, et al. Fulvestrant versus anastrozole for the treatment of advanced breast carcinoma in postmenopausal women: a prospective combined analysis of two multicenter trials. *Cancer* 2003;98:229–238.
119. Howell A, Abram P. Clinical development of fulvestrant ("Faslodex"). *Cancer Treat Rev* 2005;31[Suppl 2]:S3–S9.
120. Hoffmann J, Bohlmann R, Heinrich N, et al. Characterization of new estrogen receptor destabilizing compounds: effects on estrogen-sensitive and tamoxifen-resistant breast cancer. *J Natl Cancer Inst* 2004;96:210–218.
121. Yamaya H, Yoshida K, Kuritani J, et al. Safety, tolerability, and pharmacokinetics of TAS-108 in normal healthy post-menopausal female subjects: a phase I study on single oral dose. *J Clin Pharm Ther* 2005;30:459–470.
122. Blakely LJ, Buzdar A, Chang HY, et al. A phase I and pharmacokinetic study of TAS-108 in postmenopausal female patients with locally advanced, locally recurrent inoperable, or progressive metastatic breast cancer. *Clin Cancer Res* 2004; 10:5425–5431.
123. Buzdar AU. TAS-108: a novel steroidal antiestrogen. *Clin Cancer Res* 2005;11: 906s–908s.
124. Noble R, Collip J. Regression of estrogen-induced mammary tumours in female rats following removal of the stimulus. *Can Med Assoc J* 1941;44:1–5.
125. Escher G. Clinical improvement of inoperable breast carcinoma under steroid treatment. Proceedings of the 1st Conference on Steroid Hormones and Mammary Carcinoma. The Therapeutic Trials Committee of the Council on Pharmacy and Chemistry of the American Medical Association. Chicago. 1949:92–99.
126. Segaloff A, Ochsner A. Progress report: results of studies by the Cooperative Breast Cancer Group. *Cancer Chemother Rep* 1960;11:109–141.
127. Stoll BA. Progestin therapy of breast cancer: comparison of agents. *BMJ* 1967;3: 338–341.
128. Lundgren S, Lonning PE, Utaaker E, et al. Influence of progestins on serum hormone levels in postmenopausal women with advanced breast cancer I. General findings. *J Steroid Biochem* 1990;36:99–104.
129. Santen RJ, Manni A, Harvey H, et al. Endocrine treatment of breast cancer in women. *Endocr Rev* 1990;11:221–265.
130. Haller DG, Glick JH. Progestational agents in advanced breast cancer: an overview. *Semin Oncol* 1986;13:2–8.
131. Abrams J, Aisner J, Cirrincione C, et al. Dose-response trial of megestrol acetate in advanced breast cancer: cancer and leukemia group B phase III study 8741. *J Clin Oncol* 1999;17:64–73.
132. Pannuti F, Martoni A, Di Marco AR, et al. Prospective, randomized clinical trial of two different high dosages of medroxyprogesterone acetate (MAP) in the treatment of metastatic breast cancer. *Eur J Cancer* 1979;15:593–601.
133. Klijn JG, Setyono-Han B, Foekens JA. Progesterone antagonists and progesterone receptor modulators in the treatment of breast cancer. *Steroids* 2000;65:825–830.
134. Romieu G, Maudelonde T, Ulmann A, et al. The antiprogestin RU486 in advanced breast cancer: preliminary clinical trial. *Bull Cancer* 1987;74:455–461.
135. Jonat W, Giurescu M, Robertson J. The clinical efficacy of progesterone antagonists in breast cancer. In: Robertson J, Nicholson R, Hayes D, eds. *Endocrine therapy of breast cancer*. London: Martin Dunitz, 2002:118–124.
136. Perrault D, Eisenhauer EA, Pritchard KI, et al. Phase II study of the progesterone antagonist mifepristone in patients with untreated metastatic breast carcinoma: a National Cancer Institute of Canada Clinical Trials group study. *J Clin Oncol* 1996;14:2709–2712.
137. Robertson JF, Willsher PC, Winterbottom L, et al. Onapristone, a progesterone receptor antagonist, as first-line therapy in primary breast cancer. *Eur J Cancer* 1999;35:214–218.
138. Muss HB. Endocrine therapy for advanced breast cancer: a review. *Breast Cancer Res Treat* 1992;21:15–26.
139. Perrault DJ, Logan DM, Stewart DJ, et al. Phase II study of flutamide in patients with metastatic breast cancer. A National Cancer Institute of Canada Clinical Trials group study. *Invest New Drugs* 1988;6:207–210.
140. Farmer P, Bonnefoi H, Becette V, et al. Identification of molecular apocrine breast tumours by microarray analysis. *Oncogene* 2005;24:4660–4671.
141. Berruti A, Osella G, Raucci CA, et al. Transient increase in total serum alkaline phosphatase predicts radiological response to systemic therapy in breast cancer patients with osteolytic and mixed bone metastases. *Oncology* 1993;50: 218–221.
142. Coleman RE, Whitaker KB, Moss DW, et al. Biochemical prediction of response of bone metastases to treatment. *Br J Cancer* 1988;58:205–210.
143. Huseby RA. Estrogen therapy in the management of advanced breast cancer. *Am Surg* 1954;20:112–124.

144. Howell A, Dodwell DJ, Anderson H, et al. Response after withdrawal of tamoxifen and progestogens in advanced breast cancer. *Ann Oncol* 1992;3:611–617.
145. Bhide SA, Rea DW. Metastatic breast cancer response after Exemestane withdrawal: a case report. *Breast* 2004;13:66–68.
146. Cigler T, Goss PE. Aromatase inhibitor withdrawal response in metastatic breast cancer. *J Clin Oncol* 2006;24:1955–1956.
147. Canney PA, Griffiths T, Latief TN, et al. Clinical significance of tamoxifen withdrawal response. *Lancet* 1987;1:36.
148. Chia S, Gradishar W, Mauriac L, et al. Double-blind, randomized placebo controlled trial of fulvestrant compared with exemestane after prior nonsteroidal aromatase inhibitor therapy in postmenopausal women with hormone receptor-positive, advanced breast cancer: results from EFECT. *J Clin Oncol* 2008;26:1664–1670.
149. Lewis JS, Meeke K, Osipo C, et al. Intrinsic mechanism of estradiol-induced apoptosis in breast cancer cells resistant to estrogen deprivation. *J Natl Cancer Inst* 2005;97:1746–1759.
150. Lim HS, Ju Lee H, Seok Lee K, et al. Clinical implications of CYP2D6 genotypes predictive of tamoxifen pharmacokinetics in metastatic breast cancer. *J Clin Oncol* 2007;25:3837–3845.
151. Colomer R, Monzo M, Tusquets I, et al. A single-nucleotide polymorphism in the aromatase gene is associated with the efficacy of the aromatase inhibitor letrozole in advanced breast carcinoma. *Clin Cancer Res* 2008;14:811–816.
152. Minami H, Ohsumi S, Nakamura S, et al. Impact of CYP2A6 genotype on pharmacokinetics, safety and efficacy of letrozole treatment in Japanese postmenopausal women with metastatic breast cancer. *Breast Cancer Res Treat* 2007;106[Suppl].
153. Early Breast Cancer Trialists' Collaborative Group (EBCTCG). Effects of chemotherapy and hormonal therapy for early breast cancer on recurrence and 15-year survival: an overview of the randomised trials. *Lancet* 2005;365:1687–1717.
154. Osborne CK, Yochmowitz MG, Knight WA 3rd, et al. The value of estrogen and progesterone receptors in the treatment of breast cancer. *Cancer* 1980;46:2884–2888.
155. Lapidus RG, Ferguson AT, Ottaviano YL, et al. Methylation of estrogen and progesterone receptor gene 5' CpG islands correlates with lack of estrogen and progesterone receptor gene expression in breast tumors. *Clin Cancer Res* 1996;2:805–810.
156. Ottaviano YL, Issa JP, Parl FF, et al. Methylation of the estrogen receptor gene CpG island marks loss of estrogen receptor expression in human breast cancer cells. *Cancer Res* 1994;54:2552–2555.
157. Normanno N, Di Maio M, De Maio E, et al. Mechanisms of endocrine resistance and novel therapeutic strategies in breast cancer. *Endocr Relat Cancer* 2005;12:721–747.
158. Zhou Q, Atadja P, Davidson NE. Histone deacetylase inhibitor LBH589 reactivates silenced estrogen receptor alpha (ER) gene expression without loss of DNA hypermethylation. *Cancer Biol Ther* 2007;6:64–69.
159. Sharma D, Saxena NK, Davidson NE, et al. Restoration of tamoxifen sensitivity in estrogen receptor-negative breast cancer cells: tamoxifen-bound reactivated ER recruits distinctive corepressor complexes. *Cancer Res* 2006;66:6370–6378.
160. Sharma D, Blum J, Yang X, et al. Release of methyl CpG binding proteins and histone deacetylase 1 from the Estrogen receptor alpha (ER) promoter upon reactivation in ER-negative human breast cancer cells. *Mol Endocrinol* 2005;19:1740–1751.
161. Jang ER, Lim SJ, Lee ES, et al. The histone deacetylase inhibitor trichostatin A sensitizes estrogen receptor alpha-negative breast cancer cells to tamoxifen. *Oncogene* 2004;23:1724–1736.
162. Stearns V, Zhou Q, Davidson NE. Epigenetic regulation as a new target for breast cancer therapy. *Cancer Invest* 2007;25:659–665.
163. Creighton CJ, Hilger AM, Murthy S, et al. Activation of mitogen-activated protein kinase in estrogen receptor alpha-positive breast cancer cells in vitro induces an in vivo molecular phenotype of estrogen receptor alpha-negative human breast tumors. *Cancer Res* 2006;66:3903–3911.
164. Bayliss J, Hilger A, Vishnu P, et al. Reversal of the estrogen receptor negative phenotype in breast cancer and restoration of antiestrogen response. *Clin Cancer Res* 2007;13:7029–7036.
165. Linja MJ, Visakorpi T. Alterations of androgen receptor in prostate cancer. *J Steroid Biochem Mol Biol* 2004;92:255–264.
166. Karnik PS, Kulkarni S, Liu XP, et al. Estrogen receptor mutations in tamoxifen-resistant breast cancer. *Cancer Res* 1994;54:349–353.
167. Hopp TA, Fuqua SA. Estrogen receptor variants. *J Mammary Gland Biol Neoplasia* 1998;3:73–83.
168. Holst F, Stahl PR, Ruiz C, et al. Estrogen receptor alpha (ESR1) gene amplification is frequent in breast cancer. *Nat Genet* 2007;39:655–660.
169. Watts CK, Handel ML, King RJ, et al. Oestrogen receptor gene structure and function in breast cancer. *J Steroid Biochem Mol Biol* 1992;41:529–536.
170. Murphy LC, Watson PH. Is oestrogen receptor-beta a predictor of endocrine therapy responsiveness in human breast cancer? *Endocr Relat Cancer* 2006;13:327–334.
171. McDonnell DP, Norris JD. Connections and regulation of the human estrogen receptor. *Science* 2002;296:1642–1644.
172. Palmieri C, Lam EW, Mansi J, et al. The expression of ER beta cx in human breast cancer and the relationship to endocrine therapy and survival. *Clin Cancer Res* 2004;10:2421–2428.
173. Brandt R, Eisenbrandt R, Leenders F, et al. Mammary gland specific hEGF receptor transgene expression induces neoplasia and inhibits differentiation. *Oncogene* 2000;19:2129–2137.
174. Sternlicht MD, Sunnarborg SW, Kouros-Mehr H, et al. Mammary ductal morphogenesis requires paracrine activation of stromal EGFR via ADAM17-dependent shedding of epithelial amphiregulin. *Development* 2005;132:3923–3933.
175. deFazio A, Chiew YE, McEvoy M, et al. Antisense estrogen receptor RNA expression increases epidermal growth factor receptor gene expression in breast cancer cells. *Cell Growth Differ* 1997;8:903–911.
176. Yarden RI, Lauber AH, El-Ashry D, et al. Bimodal regulation of epidermal growth factor receptor by estrogen in breast cancer cells. *Endocrinology* 1996;137: 2739–2747.
177. Dowsett M, Houghton J, Iden C, et al. Benefit from adjuvant tamoxifen therapy in primary breast cancer patients according oestrogen receptor, progesterone receptor, EGF receptor and HER2 status. *Ann Oncol* 2006;17:818–826.
178. Klijn JG, Berns PM, Schmitz PI, et al. The clinical significance of epidermal growth factor receptor (EGF-R) in human breast cancer: a review on 5,232 patients. *Endocr Rev* 1992;13:3–17.
179. Giltnane JM, Ryden L, Cregger M, et al. Quantitative measurement of epidermal growth factor receptor is a negative predictive factor for tamoxifen response in hormone receptor positive premenopausal breast cancer. *J Clin Oncol* 2007;25: 3007–3014.
180. Knoop AS, Bentzen SM, Nielsen MM, et al. Value of epidermal growth factor receptor, HER2, p53, and steroid receptors in predicting the efficacy of tamoxifen in high-risk postmenopausal breast cancer patients. *J Clin Oncol* 2001;19:3376–3384.
181. Johnston SR, Lu B, Dowsett M, et al. Comparison of estrogen receptor DNA binding in untreated and acquired antiestrogen-resistant human breast tumors. *Cancer Res* 1997;57:3723–3727.
182. Chen D, Washbrook E, Sarwar N, et al. Phosphorylation of human estrogen receptor alpha at serine 118 by two distinct signal transduction pathways revealed by phosphorylation-specific antisera. *Oncogene* 2002;21:4921–4931.
183. Gee JM, Robertson JF, Gutteridge E, et al. Epidermal growth factor receptor/HER2/insulin-like growth factor receptor signalling and oestrogen receptor activity in clinical breast cancer. *Endocr Relat Cancer* 2005;12[Suppl 1]:S99–S111.
184. Massarweh S, Osborne CK, Creighton CJ, et al. Tamoxifen resistance in breast tumors is driven by growth factor receptor signaling with repression of classic estrogen receptor genomic function. *Cancer Res* 2008;68:826–833.
185. Mita M, de Bono J, Mita A, et al. A phase II and biologic correlative study investigating anastrozole (A) in combination with geftinib (G) in post menopausal patients with estrogen receptor positive (ER) metastatic breast carcinoma (MBC) who have previously failed hormonal therapy. *Breast Cancer Res Treat* 2005; 94[Suppl 1]:A1117.
186. Polychronis A, Sinnett HD, Hadjiminas D, et al. Preoperative gefitinib versus gefitinib and anastrozole in postmenopausal patients with oestrogen-receptor positive and epidermal-growth-factor-receptor-positive primary breast cancer: a double-blind placebo-controlled phase II randomised trial. *Lancet Oncol* 2005;6: 383–391.
187. Smith IE, Walsh G, Skene A, et al. A phase II placebo-controlled trial of neoadjuvant anastrozole alone or with gefitinib in early breast cancer. *J Clin Oncol* 2007; 25:3816–3822.
188. Cristofanilli M, Valero V, Mangalik A, et al. A phase II multicenter, double-blind, randomized trial to compare anastrozole plus gefitinib with anastrozole plus placebo in postmenopausal women with hormone receptor-positive (HR+) metastatic breast cancer (MBC). *J Clin Oncol* 2008;26[Suppl]:(abst 1012).
189. Guix M, Granja Nde M, Meszoely I, et al. Short preoperative treatment with erlotinib inhibits tumor cell proliferation in hormone receptor-positive breast cancers. *J Clin Oncol* 2008;26:897–906.
190. Arpino G, Gutierrez C, Weiss H, et al. Treatment of human epidermal growth factor receptor 2-overexpressing breast cancer xenografts with multiagent HER-targeted therapy. *J Natl Cancer Inst* 2007;99:694–705.
191. Kurokawa H, Arteaga CL. ErbB (HER) receptors can abrogate antiestrogen action in human breast cancer by multiple signaling mechanisms. *Clin Cancer Res* 2003;9:511S–515S.
192. Howell A, Howell SJ, Clarke R, et al. Where do selective estrogen receptor modulators (SERMs) and aromatase inhibitors (AIs) now fit into breast cancer treatment algorithms? *J Steroid Biochem Mol Biol* 2001;79:227–237.
193. Tsao MS, Sakurada A, Cutz JC, et al. Erlotinib in lung cancer—molecular and clinical predictors of outcome. *N Engl J Med* 2005;353:133–144.
194. De Laurentiis M, Arpino G, Massarelli E, et al. A meta-analysis on the interaction between HER-2 expression and response to endocrine treatment in advanced breast cancer. *Clin Cancer Res* 2005;11:4741–4748.
195. Benz CC, Scott GK, Sarup JC, et al. Estrogen-dependent, tamoxifen-resistant tumorigenic growth of MCF-7 cells transfected with HER2/neu. *Breast Cancer Res Treat* 1992;24:85–95.
196. Pietras RJ, Arboleda J, Reese DM, et al. HER-2 tyrosine kinase pathway targets estrogen receptor and promotes hormone-independent growth in human breast cancer cells. *Oncogene* 1995;10:2435–2446.
197. Liu Y, el-Ashry D, Chen D, et al. MCF-7 breast cancer cells overexpressing transfected c-erbB-2 have an in vitro growth advantage in estrogen-depleted conditions and reduced estrogen-dependence and tamoxifen-sensitivity in vivo. *Breast Cancer Res Treat* 1995;34:97–117.
198. Arpino G, Weiss H, Lee AV, et al. Estrogen receptor-positive, progesterone receptor-negative breast cancer: association with growth factor receptor expression and tamoxifen resistance. *J Natl Cancer Inst* 2005;97:1254–1261.
199. Huang HJ, Neven P, Drijkoningen M, et al. Association between HER-2/neu and the progesterone receptor in oestrogen-dependent breast cancer is age-related. *Breast Cancer Res Treat* 2005;91:81–87.
200. Kim HJ, Cui X, Hilsenbeck SG, et al. Progesterone receptor loss correlates with human epidermal growth factor receptor 2 overexpression in estrogen receptor-positive breast cancer. *Clin Cancer Res* 2006;12:1013s–1018s.
201. Konecny G, Pauletti G, Pegram M, et al. Quantitative association between HER-2/neu and steroid hormone receptors in hormone receptor-positive primary breast cancer. *J Natl Cancer Inst* 2003;95:142–153.
202. Cui X, Zhang P, Deng W, et al. Insulin-like growth factor-I inhibits progesterone receptor expression in breast cancer cells via the phosphatidylinositol 3-kinase/Akt/mammalian target of rapamycin pathway: progesterone receptor as a potential indicator of growth factor activity in breast cancer. *Mol Endocrinol* 2003;17:575–588.
203. Kurokawa H, Lenferink AE, Simpson JF, et al. Inhibition of HER2/neu (erbB-2) and mitogen-activated protein kinases enhances tamoxifen action against HER2-overexpressing, tamoxifen-resistant breast cancer cells. *Cancer Res* 2000;60:5887–5894.
204. Witters L, Engle L, Lipton A. Restoration of estrogen responsiveness by blocking the HER-2/neu pathway. *Oncol Rep* 2002;9:1163–1166.
205. Marcom PK, Isaacs C, Harris L, et al. The combination of letrozole and trastuzumab as first or second-line biological therapy produces durable responses in a subset of HER2 positive and ER positive advanced breast cancers. *Breast Cancer Res Treat* 2007;102:43–49.
206. Vogel CL, Cobleigh MA, Tripathy D, et al. 2002 Efficacy and safety of trastuzumab as a single agent in first-line treatment of HER2-overexpressing metastatic breast cancer. *J Clin Oncol* 2002;20:719–726.
207. Baselga J, Roché H, Fumoleau P, et al. Treatment of postmenopausal women with locally advanced or metastatic breast cancer with letrozole alone or in combination with temsirolimus: a randomized, 3-arm, phase 2 study. *Breast Cancer Res Treat* 2005;94(1):(abst 1068).
208. Mackey J, Kaufman B, Clemens M, et al. Trastuzumab prolongs progression-free survival in hormone-dependent and HER2-positive metastatic breast cancer. *Breast Cancer Res Treat* 2006;100[[Suppl 1]:(abst 3).
209. Leary AF, Sirohi B, Johnston SR. Clinical trials update: endocrine and biological therapy combinations in the treatment of breast cancer. *Breast Cancer Res* 2007; 9:112.

210. Chu I, Blackwell K, Chen S, et al. The dual ErbB1/ErbB2 inhibitor, lapatinib (GW572016), cooperates with tamoxifen to inhibit both cell proliferation- and estrogen-dependent gene expression in antiestrogen-resistant breast cancer. *Cancer Res* 2005;65:18–25.
211. Osborne CK, Bardou V, Hopp TA, et al. Role of the estrogen receptor coactivator AIB1 (SRC-3) and HER-2/neu in tamoxifen resistance in breast cancer. *J Natl Cancer Inst* 2003;95:353–361.
212. Lonard DM, O'Malley BW. Nuclear receptor coregulators: judges, juries, and executioners of cellular regulation. *Mol Cell* 2007;27:691–700.
213. List HJ, Reiter R, Singh B, et al. Expression of the nuclear coactivator AIB1 in normal and malignant breast tissue. *Breast Cancer Res Treat* 2001;68:21–28.
214. Anzick SL, Kononen J, Walker RL, et al. AIB1, a steroid receptor coactivator amplified in breast and ovarian cancer. *Science* 1997;277:965–968.
215. Smith CL, Nawaz Z, O'Malley BW. Coactivator and corepressor regulation of the agonist/antagonist activity of the mixed antiestrogen, 4-hydroxytamoxifen. *Mol Endocrinol* 1997;11:657–666.
216. Harigopal M, Heymann J, Ghosh S, et al. Estrogen receptor co-activator (AIB1) protein expression by automated quantitative analysis (AQUA) in a breast cancer tissue microarray and association with patient outcome. *Breast Cancer Res Treat* 2008. In press.
217. Kirkegaard T, McGlynn LM, Campbell FM, et al. Amplified in breast cancer 1 in human epidermal growth factor receptor–positive tumors of tamoxifen-treated breast cancer patients. *Clin Cancer Res* 2007;13:1405–1411.
218. Dihge L, Bendahl PO, Grabau D, et al. Epidermal growth factor receptor (EGFR) and the estrogen receptor modulator amplified in breast cancer (AIB1) for predicting clinical outcome after adjuvant tamoxifen in breast cancer. *Breast Cancer Res Treat* 2008;109:255–262.
219. Font de Mora J, Brown M. AIB1 is a conduit for kinase-mediated growth factor signaling to the estrogen receptor. *Mol Cell Biol* 2000;20:5041–5047.
220. Fereshteh MP, Tilli MT, Kim SE, et al. The nuclear receptor coactivator amplified in breast cancer-1 is required for Neu (ErbB2/HER2) activation, signaling, and mammary tumorigenesis in mice. *Cancer Res* 2008;68:3697–3706.
221. Lahusen T, Fereshteh M, Oh A, et al. Epidermal growth factor receptor tyrosine phosphorylation and signaling controlled by a nuclear receptor coactivator, amplified in breast cancer 1. *Cancer Res* 2007;67:7256–7265.
222. Girault I, Lerebours F, Amarir S, et al. Expression analysis of estrogen receptor alpha coregulators in breast carcinoma: evidence that NCOR1 expression is predictive of the response to tamoxifen. *Clin Cancer Res* 2003;9:1259–1266.
223. Shou J, Massarweh S, Osborne CK, et al. Mechanisms of tamoxifen resistance: increased estrogen receptor-HER2/neu cross-talk in ER/HER2-positive breast cancer. *J Natl Cancer Inst* 2004;96:926–935.
224. Wang LH, Yang XY, Zhang X, et al. Disruption of estrogen receptor DNA-binding domain and related intramolecular communication restores tamoxifen sensitivity in resistant breast cancer. *Cancer Cell* 2006;10:487–499.
225. Jones HE, Goddard L, Gee JM, et al. Insulin-like growth factor-I receptor signalling and acquired resistance to gefitinib (ZD1839; Iressa) in human breast and prostate cancer cells. *Endocr Relat Cancer* 2004;11:793–814.
226. Hiscox S, Jordan NJ, Jiang W, et al. Chronic exposure to fulvestrant promotes overexpression of the c-Met receptor in breast cancer cells: implications for tumour-stroma interactions. *Endocr Relat Cancer* 2006;13:1085–1099.
227. Bon G, Folgiero V, Bossi G, et al. Loss of beta4 integrin subunit reduces the tumorigenicity of MCF7 mammary cells and causes apoptosis upon hormone deprivation. *Clin Cancer Res* 2006;12:3280–3287.
228. Chanrion M, Negre V, Fontaine H, et al. A gene expression signature that can predict the recurrence of tamoxifen-treated primary breast cancer. *Clin Cancer Res* 2008;14:1744–1752.
229. Iorns E, Turner NC, Elliott R, et al. Identification of CDK10 as an important determinant of resistance to endocrine therapy for breast cancer. *Cancer Cell* 2008; 13:91–104.
230. Donovan JC, Milic A, Slingerland JM. Constitutive MEK/MAPK activation leads to p27(Kip1) deregulation and antiestrogen resistance in human breast cancer cells. *J Biol Chem* 2001;276:40888–40895.
231. Brodie A, Jelovac D, Macedo L, et al. Therapeutic observations in MCF-7 aromatase xenografts. *Clin Cancer Res* 2005;11:884s–888s.
232. Gee JM, Robertson JF, Ellis IO, et al. Phosphorylation of ERK1/2 mitogen-activated protein kinase is associated with poor response to anti-hormonal therapy and decreased patient survival in clinical breast cancer. *Int J Cancer* 2001; 95:247–254.
233. Jelovac D, Sabnis G, Long BJ, et al. Activation of mitogen-activated protein kinase in xenografts and cells during prolonged treatment with aromatase inhibitor letrozole. *Cancer Res* 2005;65:5380–5389.
234. Wang X, Masri S, Phung S, et al. The role of amphiregulin in exemestane-resistant breast cancer cells: evidence of an autocrine loop. *Cancer Res* 2008;68: 2259–2265.
235. Santen RJ, Song RX, McPherson R, et al. The role of mitogen-activated protein (MAP) kinase in breast cancer. *J Steroid Biochem Mol Biol* 2002;80:239–256.
236. Massarweh S, Osborne CK, Jiang S, et al. Mechanisms of tumor regression and resistance to estrogen deprivation and fulvestrant in a model of estrogen receptor-positive, HER-2/neu-positive breast cancer. *Cancer Res* 2006;66: 8266–8273.
237. Thomas RS, Sarwar N, Phoenix F, et al. Phosphorylation at serines 104 and 106 by MAPK is important for estrogen receptor-alpha activity. *J Mol Endocrinol* 2008;40:173–184.
238. Kato S, Endoh H, Masuhiro Y, et al. Activation of the estrogen receptor through phosphorylation by mitogen-activated protein kinase. *Science* 1995;270:1491–1494.
239. Murphy LC, Niu Y, Snell L, et al. Phospho-serine-118 estrogen receptor-alpha expression is associated with better disease outcome in women treated with tamoxifen. *Clin Cancer Res* 2004;10:5902–5906.
240. Sarwar N, Kim JS, Jiang J, et al. Phosphorylation of ERalpha at serine 118 in primary breast cancer and in tamoxifen-resistant tumours is indicative of a complex role for ERalpha phosphorylation in breast cancer progression. *Endocr Relat Cancer* 2006;13:851–861.
241. Clark GJ, Der CJ. Aberrant function of the Ras signal transduction pathway in human breast cancer. *Breast Cancer Res Treat* 1995;35:133–144.
242. Martin LA, Head JE, Pancholi S, et al. The farnesyltransferase inhibitor R115777 (tipifarnib) in combination with tamoxifen acts synergistically to inhibit MCF-7 breast cancer cell proliferation and cell cycle progression *in vitro* and *in vivo*. *Mol Cancer Ther* 2007;6:2458–2467.
243. Dalenc F, Giamarchi C, Petit M, et al. Farnesyl-transferase inhibitor R115,777 enhances tamoxifen inhibition of MCF-7 cell growth through estrogen receptor dependent and independent pathways. *Breast Cancer Res* 2005;7:R1159–R1167.
244. Johnston SR, Semiglazov VF, Manikhas GM, et al. A phase II, randomized, blinded study of the farnesyltransferase inhibitor tipifarnib combined with letrozole in the treatment of advanced breast cancer after antiestrogen therapy. *Breast Cancer Res Treat* 2008;110:327–335.
245. Bachman KE, Argani P, Samuels Y, et al. The PIK3CA gene is mutated with high frequency in human breast cancers. *Cancer Biol Ther* 2004;3:772–775.
246. Saal LH, Holm K, Maurer M, et al. PIK3CA mutations correlate with hormone receptors, node metastasis, and ERBB2, and are mutually exclusive with PTEN loss in human breast carcinoma. *Cancer Res* 2005;65:2554–2559.
247. Perez-Tenorio G, Alkhori L, Olsson B, et al. PIK3CA mutations and PTEN loss correlate with similar prognostic factors and are not mutually exclusive in breast cancer. *Clin Cancer Res* 2007;13:3577–3584.
248. Isakoff SJ, Engelman JA, Irie HY, et al. Breast cancer-associated PIK3CA mutations are oncogenic in mammary epithelial cells. *Cancer Res* 2005;65:10992–11000.
249. Campbell RA, Bhat-Nakshatri P, Patel NM, et al. Phosphatidylinositol 3-kinase/AKT-mediated activation of estrogen receptor alpha: a new model for anti-estrogen resistance. *J Biol Chem* 2001;276:9817–9824.
250. Perez-Tenorio G, Stal O. Activation of AKT/PKB in breast cancer predicts a worse outcome among endocrine treated patients. *Br J Cancer* 2002;86:540–545.
251. Kirkegaard T, Witton CJ, McGlynn LM, et al. AKT activation predicts outcome in breast cancer patients treated with tamoxifen. *J Pathol* 2005;207:139–146.
252. Tokunaga E, Kimura Y, Oki E, et al. Akt is frequently activated in HER2/neu-positive breast cancers and associated with poor prognosis among hormone-treated patients. *Int J Cancer* 2006;118:284–289.
253. Shoman N, Klassen S, McFadden A, et al. Reduced PTEN expression predicts relapse in patients with breast carcinoma treated by tamoxifen. *Mod Pathol* 2005;18:250–259.
254. Frogne T, Jepsen JS, Larsen SS, et al. Antiestrogen-resistant human breast cancer cells require activated protein kinase B/Akt for growth. *Endocr Relat Cancer* 2005;12:599–614.
255. Santen RJ, Song RX, Zhang Z, et al. Long-term estradiol deprivation in breast cancer cells up-regulates growth factor signaling and enhances estrogen sensitivity. *Endocr Relat Cancer* 2005;12[Suppl 1]:S61–S73.
256. Sabnis GJ, Jelovac D, Long B, et al. The role of growth factor receptor pathways in human breast cancer cells adapted to long-term estrogen deprivation. *Cancer Res* 2005;65:3903–3910.
257. Boulay A, Rudloff J, Ye J, et al. Dual inhibition of mTOR and estrogen receptor signaling *in vitro* induces cell death in models of breast cancer. *Clin Cancer Res* 2005;11:5319–5328.
258. deGraffenried LA, Friedrichs WE, Russell DH, et al. Inhibition of mTOR activity restores tamoxifen response in breast cancer cells with aberrant Akt activity. *Clin Cancer Res* 2004;10:8059–8067.
259. Beeram M, Tan QT, Tekmal RR, et al. Akt-induced endocrine therapy resistance is reversed by inhibition of mTOR signaling. *Ann Oncol* 2007;18:1323–1328.
260. Awada A, Cardoso F, Fontaine C, et al. The oral mTOR inhibitor RAD001 (everolimus) in combination with letrozole in patients with advanced breast cancer: results of a phase I study with pharmacokinetics. *Eur J Cancer* 2008;44:84–91.
261. Chan S, Scheulen ME, Johnston S, et al. Phase II study of temsirolimus (CCI-779), a novel inhibitor of mTOR, in heavily pretreated patients with locally advanced or metastatic breast cancer. *J Clin Oncol* 2005;23:5314–5322.
262. Chow L, Sun Y, Jassem J, et al. Phase 3 study of temsirolimus with letrozole or letrozole alone in postmenopausal women with locally advanced or metastatic breast cancer. *Breast Cancer Res Treat* 2006;100[Suppl 1]:S286(abst 6091).
263. O'Reilly KE, Rojo F, She QB, et al. mTOR inhibition induces upstream receptor tyrosine kinase signaling and activates Akt. *Cancer Res* 2006;66:1500–1508.
264. Tabernero J, Rojo F, Calvo E, et al. Dose- and schedule-dependent inhibition of the mammalian target of rapamycin pathway with everolimus: a phase I tumor pharmacodynamic study in patients with advanced solid tumors. *J Clin Oncol* 2008;26:1603–1610.
265. Raynaud FI, Eccles S, Clarke PA, et al. Pharmacologic characterization of a potent inhibitor of class I phosphatidylinositide 3-kinases. *Cancer Res* 2007;67:5840–5850.
266. Masamura S, Santner SJ, Heitjan DF, et al. Estrogen deprivation causes estradiol hypersensitivity in human breast cancer cells. *J Clin Endocrinol Metab* 1995;80: 2918–2925.
267. Martin LA, Farmer I, Johnston SR, et al. Elevated ERK1/ERK2/estrogen receptor cross-talk enhances estrogen-mediated signaling during long-term estrogen deprivation. *Endocr Relat Cancer* 2005;12[Suppl 1]:S75–S84.
268. Berstein LM, Zheng H, Yue W, et al. New approaches to the understanding of tamoxifen action and resistance. *Endocr Relat Cancer* 2003;10:267–277.
269. Arpino G, Wiechmann L, Osborne CK, et al. Crosstalk between the estrogen receptor and the HER tyrosine kinase receptor family: molecular mechanism and clinical implications for endocrine therapy resistance. *Endocr Rev* 2008;29: 217–233.
270. Ariazi EA, Lewis-Wambi JS, Gill SD, et al. Emerging principles for the development of resistance to antihormonal therapy: implications for the clinical utility of fulvestrant. *J Steroid Biochem Mol Biol* 2006;102:128–138.
271. Martin LA, Pancholi S, Chan CM, et al. The anti-oestrogen ICI 182,780, but not tamoxifen, inhibits the growth of MCF-7 breast cancer cells refractory to long-term oestrogen deprivation through down-regulation of oestrogen receptor and IGF signalling. *Endocr Relat Cancer* 2005;12:1017–1036.
272. Baum M, Budzar AU, Cuzick J, et al. Anastrozole alone or in combination with tamoxifen versus tamoxifen alone for adjuvant treatment of postmenopausal women with early breast cancer: first results of the ATAC randomised trial. *Lancet* 2002;359:2131–2139.
273. Dodwell D, Coombes G, Bliss JM, et al. Combining fulvestrant (Faslodex) with continued oestrogen suppression in endocrine-sensitive advanced breast cancer: the SoFEA trial. *Clin Oncol (R Coll Radiol)* 2008;20:321–324.
274. Stoll BA. Effect of Lyndiol, an oral contraceptive, on breast cancer. *BMJ* 1967;1: 150–153.
275. Howell SJ, Johnston SR, Howell A. The use of selective estrogen receptor modulators and selective estrogen receptor down-regulators in breast cancer. *Best Pract Res Clin Endocrinol Metab* 2004;18:47–66.
276. Escher G, Heber J, Woodward H, et al. Newer steroids in the treatment of advanced mammary carcinoma. Symposium on Steroids in experimental and Clinical Practice. Philadelphia, 1951:375–378.

277. Perrault M, Le Beau J, Klotz B, et al. [Total hypophysectomy in the treatment of breast cancer; first French case; future of the method]. *Therapie* 1952;7: 290–300.

278. Iveson TJ, Smith IE, Ahern J, et al. Phase I study of the oral nonsteroidal aromatase inhibitor CGS 20267 in postmenopausal patients with advanced breast cancer. *Cancer Res* 1993;53:266–270.

279. Zilembo N, Noberasco C, Bajetta E, et al. Endocrinological and clinical evaluation of exemestane, a new steroidal aromatase inhibitor. *Br J Cancer* 1995;72: 1007–1012.

280. Jonat W, Howell A, Blomqvist C, et al. A randomised trial comparing two doses of the new selective aromatase inhibitor anastrozole (Arimidex) with megestrol acetate in postmenopausal patients with advanced breast cancer. *Eur J Cancer* 1996;32A:404–412.

281. Taylor CW, Green S, Dalton WS, et al. Multicenter randomized clinical trial of goserelin versus surgical ovariectomy in premenopausal patients with receptor-positive metastatic breast cancer: an intergroup study. *J Clin Oncol* 1998;16: 994–999.

282. Buzdar A, Jonat W, Howell A, et al. Anastrozole, a potent and selective aromatase inhibitor, versus megestrol acetate in postmenopausal women with advanced breast cancer: results of overview analysis of two phase III trials. Arimidex Study Group. *J Clin Oncol* 1996;14:2000–2011.

283. Dombernowsky P, Smith I, Falkson G, et al. Letrozole, a new oral aromatase inhibitor for advanced breast cancer: double-blind randomized trial showing a dose effect and improved efficacy and tolerability compared with megestrol acetate. *J Clin Oncol* 1998;16:453–461.

284. Buzdar A, Douma J, Davidson N, et al. Phase III, multicenter, double-blind, randomized study of letrozole, an aromatase inhibitor, for advanced breast cancer versus megestrol acetate. *J Clin Oncol* 2001;19:3357–3366.

285. Kaufmann M, Bajetta E, Dirix LY, et al. Exemestane is superior to megestrol acetate after tamoxifen failure in postmenopausal women with advanced breast cancer: results of a phase III randomized double-blind trial. The Exemestane Study Group. *J Clin Oncol* 2000;18:1399–1411.

286. Mouridsen H, Gershanovich M, Sun Y, et al. Superior efficacy of letrozole versus tamoxifen as first-line therapy for postmenopausal women with advanced breast cancer: results of a phase III study of the International Letrozole Breast Cancer Group. *J Clin Oncol* 2001;19:2596–2606.

287. Nabholtz JM, Buzdar A, Pollak M, et al. Anastrozole is superior to tamoxifen as first-line therapy for advanced breast cancer in postmenopausal women: results of a North American multicenter randomized trial. Arimidex Study Group. *J Clin Oncol* 2000;18:3758–3767.

288. Bonneterre J, Buzdar A, Nabholtz JM, et al. Anastrozole is superior to tamoxifen as first-line therapy in hormone receptor positive advanced breast carcinoma. *Cancer* 2001;92:2247–2258.

289. Paridaens R, Dirix L, Lohrisch C, et al. Mature results of a randomized phase II multicenter study of exemestane versus tamoxifen as first-line hormone therapy for postmenopausal women with metastatic breast cancer. *Ann Oncol* 2003;14:1391–1398.

290. Osborne C, Neven P, Dirix L, et al. Randomized phase II study of gefitinib (IRESSA) or placebo in combination with tamoxifen in patients with hormone receptor positive metastatic breast cancer. *Breast Cancer Res Treat* 2007; 106[Suppl].

Chapter 74

Treatment of Metastatic Breast Cancer: Chemotherapy

Sing-Huang Tan and Antonio C. Wolff

Breast cancer has become a burgeoning global health problem resulting in an estimated 1.3 million women diagnosed with the disease in 2007 and over 465,000 deaths (1). In the United States, breast cancer is the most prevalent cancer and the second most common cause of cancer death in women (2). In 2008 an estimated 182,460 new cases of invasive breast cancer and 40,480 breast cancer–related deaths were expected to occur in women (2), and its incidence in developing nations has increased as much as 5% per year (3,4). The lower availability of screening in these countries is frequently associated with a higher stage at presentation and greater mortality risk. Consequently, although only half of breast cancers are diagnosed in the developing world, those countries account for three fourths of total deaths from advanced disease (3). In contrast to the treatment of early breast cancer, the treatment of advanced breast cancer is more resource intensive and associated with worse outcomes, further taxing countries with scarce resources that could greatly benefit from early detection strategies (5). In addition, women of Asian and African origin are at a higher risk for developing estrogen receptor (ER)–negative tumors and are not amenable to more tolerable and affordable endocrine interventions.

In the United States 75% to 80% of breast cancers are hormone-receptor positive (ER or progesterone receptor [PR]) (6). About 20% to 25% of tumors overexpress the human epidermal growth factor receptor 2 (*HER2*, more currently *ERBB2*) and half of them are hormone-receptor positive (7), while the remaining 10% to 15% lack expression of these markers (triple negative) (6). Triple-negative tumors have a higher risk of leading to visceral metastases and local recurrence (8). They are also more frequent in younger women (6). This tumor subtype is particularly common among premenopausal African American women (9).

Access to screening programs resulted in a greater proportion of women now diagnosed with earlier and more curable stages of disease. Still, many patients are at risk for developing metastatic disease and approximately 3% to 5% of new patients in the United States present with stage IV disease (10). Traditionally, the median survival of metastatic breast cancer (MBC) is 18 to 24 months (11,12), with barely 2% still alive 20 years after initial diagnosis (Fig. 74.1A,B) (13). Encouragingly, institutional databases show an improvement of survival of MBC over the past quarter century, likely because of improving therapies and earlier diagnosis (14,15). Similar findings were reported by the British Columbia Cancer Agency (16) among women aged 75 and younger since 1991, which reflects the gradual introduction of new therapies such as paclitaxel and vinorelbine in the early 1990s, docetaxel and aromatase inhibitors in the mid-1990s, and capecitabine and trastuzumab in the late 1990s. Unfortunately, cure is a rare event in metastatic breast cancer, and the ultimate goals of treatment of MBC are to prolong survival, prevent and palliate symptoms, improve or maintain quality of life (QOL), and delay disease progression (17).

PRINCIPLES OF CHEMOTHERAPY

Over the past two decades, meaningful improvements in survival have resulted from the introduction of newer and more effective systemic agents, especially endocrine and antibody-targeted therapies (Fig. 74.2) (16,18). ER and *ERBB2* are the most useful predictive markers of response available in clinical practice, and their presence identifies those likely to benefit from endocrine therapy and trastuzumab, respectively (19). Patients with MBC that are most likely to have a longer survival include those with ER-positive disease, longer disease-free interval (>2 years), limited metastatic burden with soft tissue or bone involvement, and no impairment of vital organ function (20). Although a poor prognostic marker, *ERBB2*-positive disease is now associated with an improved outcome in the setting of anti-*ERBB2* therapy.

Breast cancer is among the most chemosensitive of the solid tumors. Although studies comparing chemotherapy to no chemotherapy historical controls show contradictory results (21–25), an overview by A'Hern et al. (26) suggested a positive correlation between improved response rates and median survival. Prospective randomized clinical trials comparing chemotherapy to best supportive care in women with MBC are not available, and such trials are unlikely to be done in view of the survival benefit seen with adjuvant therapy (27) and the frequent responses observed in patients with advanced disease (28). Various trials have also shown survival benefits when comparing different chemotherapy regimens (29–34), therefore suggesting a similar benefit when compared to no therapy (17).

Chemotherapy agents interfere with various aspects of the cell cycle machinery, especially DNA and RNA synthesis. The most active classes of drugs include anthracyclines, taxanes, vinca alkaloids, alkylating agents, and antimetabolites. Although effective, they are often more toxic than endocrine therapy. As monotherapy, they produce response rates of 25% to 60%, with a median time to progression of approximately 6 months (35). Combination regimens lead to higher response rates but not more complete responders. Unfortunately, most responses are transient, few achieve a complete response (13), and disease progresses on average within 12 to 24 months of initiating treatment (36,37). Complete responses may be more common in patients with a better performance status (13) and may predict a longer progression-free survival (38). The clinical significance of stable disease in chemotherapy-treated patients is less clear, but this group appears to have intermediate outcomes (13).

Endocrine therapy is the preferred option for women with hormone receptor–positive MBC who are not at risk for a visceral crisis. In contrast, systemic chemotherapy is typically reserved for women with hormone-refractory disease, hormone receptor–negative disease, and selected women with rapidly progressive or symptomatic visceral metastases (39). Randomized trials of sequential endocrine therapy followed by chemotherapy (or vice versa) versus combined chemoendocrine therapy as treatment for MBC demonstrated that the initiation of endocrine therapy up front yielded comparable long-term results without the toxicities of chemotherapy (40). In addition, chemoendocrine therapy compared to chemotherapy may prolong time to treatment failure in ER-positive patients with no apparent survival benefit. However, data from the adjuvant setting suggest a negative interaction between endocrine therapy and cytotoxic chemotherapy and discourage their use in combination (41).

Optimal timing of treatment initiation and continuation has to be individualized. Generally, treatment choices are guided by the tumor, patient, and treatment-related factors. These include hormone receptor status of the primary tumor or metastatic site,

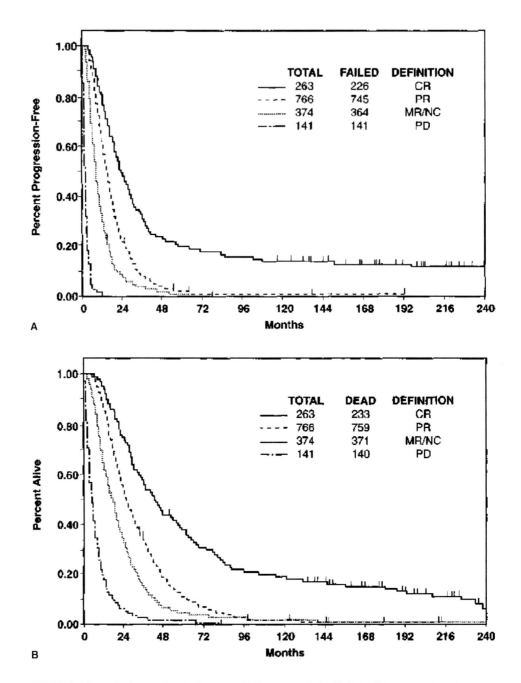

FIGURE 74.1. A: Progression-free survival Kaplan-Meier curves of 1,544 patients (excluding 37 with insufficient response data) with metastatic breast cancer according to maximum response achieved with the predominant regimen of FAC (5-fluorouracil, doxorubicin, cyclophosphamide) induction therapy followed by maintenance CMF (cyclophosphamide, methotrexate, 5-fluorouracil). **B:** Overall survival Kaplan-Meier curves of 1,544 patients (excluding 37 with insufficient response data) with metastatic breast cancer according to maximum response achieved with the predominant regimen of FAC induction therapy followed by maintenance CMF : the M.D. Anderson Cancer Center experience. CR, complete response; MR, marginal response; NC, no change; PD, progressive disease; PR, partial response. (From Greenberg PAC, Hortobagyi GN, Smith TL, et al. Long-term follow-up of patients with complete remission following combination chemotherapy for metastatic breast cancer. *J Clin Oncol* 1996;14:2197, with permission.)

ERBB2 status, length of relapse-free interval since the primary diagnosis of breast cancer, the presence of visceral metastases, patient age, performance status, comorbidities, symptoms, preferences, previous treatment and outcome, anticipated side effects, and access to therapy (41). Although chemotherapy regimens have undergone several modifications related to drug combinations, scheduling, formulations, and delivery platforms, these general principles still apply. This chapter reviews pharmacologic principles and factors that influence decisions about the use of various chemotherapy options for the treatment of MBC.

USE OF CHEMOTHERAPY IN CLINICAL PRACTICE

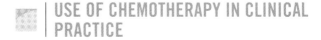

Sequential Single versus Combination Chemotherapy

An ideal combination regimen would employ active, non-cross-resistant single agents with preclinical evidence of synergy with non-overlapping safety profiles (Table 74.1). However, this is a difficult standard to meet. Although randomized trials of

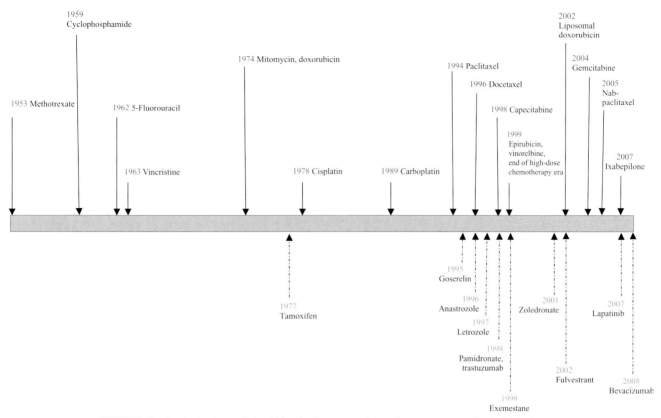

FIGURE 74.2. Time line showing the years during which various breast cancer therapeutic agents were approved by the U.S. Food and Drug Administration (FDA).

combination chemotherapy versus sequential single agents may have shown an improvement in response rates and time to disease progression, only a marginal survival benefit has been observed with taxane-free (42–47) or taxane-containing regimens (29,34,48–53).

Sequential single agents allow the administration of each drug at the maximum tolerated dose while avoiding overlapping toxicities. In an early systemic review of 15 early trials consisting of 2,442 patients treated in the pretaxane era, the complete remission (CR) and partial remission rates observed with multiple-drug chemotherapy were significantly better than with single-agent chemotherapy among other comparisons, as shown in Table 74.2 (28). A 2005 Cochrane meta-analysis of 37 published trials (including trials of newer drugs) comparing combination versus single agents showed that the former was favorably associated with higher response rates (RRs) (odds ratio [OR] 1.28; 95% confidence interval [CI], 1.15–1.42; $p < .00001$) and improved time to progression (TTP) (hazard ratio [HR] 0.78; 95% CI, 0.73–0.83; $p < .00001$), with a small significant or nonsignificant 12% survival advantage (22% if analysis is limited to trials of first-line therapy) (54). Not surprisingly, toxicities such as leukopenia, alopecia, nausea, and vomiting were significantly higher with combination regimens.

A few basic study designs have been used in the investigation of the efficacy of single versus combination chemotherapy. One is a single-agent drug A versus a combination regimen using drugs B and C. Another is a single-agent drug A versus a combination regimen using drugs A and B.

With the advent of newer drugs such as taxanes, superiority in terms of survival of single-agent paclitaxel or docetaxel over older nonanthracycline or taxane regimens such as CMFP, mitomycin/vinblastine and intravenous (IV) CMF (cyclophosphamide, methotrexate [MTX], and 5-fluorouracil [5-FU]), respectively, have been proven in several randomized trials (32,33). Another newer chemotherapeutic agent capecitabine

was shown to have comparable TTP and overall survival (OS) outcomes compared with the older regimen IV CMF (55) Several trials in the second type of clinical trial design comparing single agents to combination regimens containing that agent also do not support a survival benefit for polychemotherapy (50,56,57). The Eastern Cooperative Oncology Group (ECOG) trial 1193 comparing doxorubicin versus paclitaxel versus the combination with a crossover design built in the monotherapy arms showed equivalent overall survival (50).

Other trials comparing anthracycline-taxane combination such as epirubicin/paclitaxel or doxorubicin/docetaxel versus sequential administration of each agent have also reported similar RRs, TTP, and OS rates in the various arms (51–53,57,58). A trial reported in abstract form by the Mexican Oncology Study Group at the annual meeting of the American Society of Clinical Oncology (ASCO) in 2006 did not show a benefit from the capecitabine/docetaxel combination in anthracycline pretreated MBC (56). Their study design was single-agent capecitabine followed at progression by either docetaxel or paclitaxel, compared with the combination regimens of capecitabine and paclitaxel or docetaxel.

Furthermore, myriad trials have shown a more favorable toxicity profile and presumably a better QOL for the monotherapy arm without compromise on important clinical end points such as TTP and OS. These trials include those comparing paclitaxel versus CMFP (32), epirubicin versus epirubicin/cisplatin (59), mitoxantrone versus CEF (cyclophosphamide, epirubicin, 5-FU) (60), epirubicin followed by mitomycin as second-line versus CEF followed by second-line mitomycin/vinblastine (44), doxorubicin versus doxorubicin/vinorelbine (42), dose sequential epirubicin/paclitaxel versus the combination (52), and alternating or sequential doxorubicin/docetaxel regimens versus the combination (51).

Aside from the two earlier trials previously mentioned that demonstrated a survival benefit for taxanes over older

Table 74.1   CLINICAL TRIAL SUMMARY OF SINGLE VERSUS COMBINATION THERAPY

Author (Reference)	Regimen	Sample No. Evaluable (n)	Median Follow-Up (mos)	RR	TTP/PFS (mos)	OS (mos)
Martin et al., 2007 (49)	VNB vs. VNB/Gem	251	not stated	26% vs. 36% ($p = 0.093$)	4 vs. 6 ($p = .0028$)	16.4 vs. 15.9 ($p = .805$)
Soto et al., 2006 (56)	Cap → Pac/Doc vs. Cap + Pac vs. Cap + Doc	277	15.5	46% vs. 65% vs. 74%	6.3 vs. 6.5 vs. 8.5	31.5 vs. 33.1 vs. 28.6
Beslija et al., 2006 (63)	Doc → Cap after progression vs. Cap + Doc	100	not stated	40% vs. 68% ($p = .004$)	7.7 vs. 9.3 ($p = .001$)	19 vs. 22 ($p = .006$)
Cresta et al., 2004 (51)	Dox alt with Doc vs. Dox → Doc vs. Dox comb Doc	121	22	52% vs. 61% vs. 63% ($p = ns$)	34 wks vs. 33 wks vs. 36 wks ($p = ns$)	34 all 3 groups
Conte et al., 2004 (57)	Epi + Pac vs. Epi × 4 cycles → Pac × 4 cycles	198	not stated	62% vs. 53% ($p = .23$)	11 vs. 10.8 ($p = ns$)	20 vs. 26 ($p = ns$)
Albain et al., 2008 (34)	Pac vs. Pac/Gem	529	not stated	26.2% vs. 41.4% ($p = 0.0002$)	3.98 vs. 6.94 ($p = 0.0002$)	15.8 vs. 18.6 ($p = 0.0489$)
Alba et al., 2004 (58)	Dox × 3 cycles → Doc × 3 cycles vs. Dox + Doc	144	17.5	61% vs. 51% ($p = ns$)	10.5 vs. 9.2 ($p = ns$)	22.3 vs. 21.8 ($p = ns$)
Sledge et al., 2003 (50)	Dox vs. Pac vs. Dox + Pac	731	not stated	36% vs. 34% vs. 47% ($p = 0.84$, Dox vs. pac; $p = 0.007$, Dox vs. Dox/Pac; $p = 0.004$, Pac vs. Dox/Pac)	5.8 vs. 6 vs. 8 ($p = 0.68$, Dox vs. Pac; $p = .003$, Dox vs. Dox/Pac; $p = .009$, Pac vs. Dox/Pac)	18.9 vs. 22.2 vs. 22 ($p = ns$)
O'Shaugnessy et al., 2002 (29)	Doc/Cap vs. Doc	511	15 (minimal follow-up)	42% vs.30% ($p = .006$)	6.1 vs. 4.2 ($p = .0001$)	14.5 vs. 11.5 ($p = .0126$)
Heidemann et al., 2002 (60)	Mitoxantrone vs. FEC	238	17.4	57% vs. 66% ($p = ns$)	4.4 vs. 6.15 ($p = ns$)	14.1 vs. 15.8 ($p = ns$)
O'Shaugnessy et al., 2001 (55)	Cap vs. IV CMF	93	not stated	30% vs. 16% (trial not designed to determine statistical difference)	4.1 vs. 3	19.6 vs. 17.2
Koroleva et al., 2001 (53)	A: Doc 75 mg/m² + Dox 50 mg/m² B: Doc 60 mg/m² + Dox 60 mg/m² C: Doc 100 mg/m² × 4 cycles → Dox 75 mg/m² × 4 cycles	131	not stated	49% vs. 59% vs. 56%	6.7 vs. 8.3 vs. 6.9	11.9 vs. 14.5 vs. 13.8
Fountzilas et al., 2001 (52)	Dose dense Epi × 4 cycles → Pac × 4 cycles q 2 weeks vs. Epi + Pac	183	16.5	55% vs. 42% ($p = .10$)	10 vs. 8.5 ($p = 0.27$)	21.5 vs. 20 ($p = .17$)
Norris et al., 2000 (42)	Dox vs. Dox/VNB	289	29	30% vs. 38% ($p = .2$)	6.1 vs. 6.2 ($p = 0.5$)	14.4 vs. 13.8 ($p = .4$)
Nielsen et al., 2000 (59)	Epi vs. Epi + cisplatin	139	not stated	61% vs. 66% ($p = ns$)	8.4 vs. 15.3 ($p = .045$)	15.1 vs. 21.5 ($p = .41$)
Nabholtz et al., 1999 (33)	Doc vs. Mitomycin + vinblastine	392	19	30% vs. 11.6% ($p < .0001$)	19 wks vs. 11 wks ($p = .001$)	11.4 vs. 8.7 ($p = .0097$)
Bishop et al., 1999 (32)	Pac vs. CMFP	209	26	29% vs. 35% ($p = .37$)	5.3 vs. 6.4 ($p = .25$)	17.3 vs. 13.9 ($p = .068$)
Joensuu et al., 1998 (44)	Epi (weekly until PD or 1,000 mg/m²) → mitomycin vs. CEF (3-weekly until PD or Epi 1,000 mg/m²) → mitomycin/ vinblastine	303	not stated	48% (Epi) vs. 55% (CEF) ($p = .21$) 16% (mitomycin) vs. 7% (mitomycin vinblastine) ($p = .12$)	8 vs. 10 ($p = .19$)	16 vs. 18 ($p = .62$)
French Epirubicin Study Group, 1991 (47)	Epirubicin vs. FEC 50 vs. FEC 75	365	not stated	30.6% vs. 44.6% vs. 44.7% ($p = .04$, FEC50 vs. Epi; $p = .0006$, FEC75 vs. Epi)	no difference ($p = .47$)	no difference ($p = .46$)

Cap, capecitabine; CEF, cyclophosphamide, epirubicin, 5-fluorouracil; CMF, cyclophosphamide, methotrexate, 5-fluorouracil; CMFP, cyclophosphamide, methotrexate, 5-fluorouracil, prednisone; Doc, docetaxel; Dox, doxorubicin; Epi, epirubicin; FEC, 5-fluorouracil, epirubicin, cyclophosphamide; Gem, gemcitabine; IV, intravenous; OS, overall survival; Pac, paclitaxel; PFS, progression-free survival; RR, response rates; TTP, time to progression; VNB, vinorelbine.

Table 74.2	OVERALL RESPONSES (COMPLETE PLUS PARTIAL) IN PUBLISHED RANDOMIZED CONTROLLED CHEMOTHERAPY TRIALS BY TREATMENT COMPARISONS		
	Response		
Comparisons	%	OR	95% CI
Polychemotherapy vs. single agent	48 vs. 34	1.79	1.51–2.12
Anthracycline vs. non anthracycline-containing regimens	51 vs. 45	1.30	1.16–1.46
Other chemotherapy vs. CMF	49 vs. 44	1.22	1.05–1.42
Epirubicin vs. doxorubicin	44 vs. 47	0.87	0.71–1.08
High- vs. low-intensity (lower doses or shorter duration) chemotherapy	44 vs. 33	1.67	1.43–1.95

CI, confidence interval; CMF, cyclophosphamide, methotrexate, 5-fluorouracil; OR, odds ratio.
Modified from Fossati R. Cytotoxic and hormonal treatment for metastatic breast cancer: a systematic review of published randomized trials involving 31,510 women. *J Clin Oncol* 1998;16:3439.

regimens (32,33), two other important trials compared taxane-containing combinations versus the taxane itself and showed a significant survival benefit (29,34,48). Preclinical data suggesting a synergy of the docetaxel-induced thymidine phosphorylase up-regulation and the capecitabine-induced Bcl-2 downregulation (61,62) led to a trial by O'Shaughnessy et al. (29) showing that the docetaxel/capecitabine combination had significantly superior response rates, TTP, and survival over single-agent docetaxel with a manageable toxicity profile. However, 65% of patients in the combination arm required dose reduction in one or both drugs as opposed to only 36% in the docetaxel monotherapy arm. Also, this was not designed as a crossover study, and only 17% of patients on the docetaxel alone arm used capecitabine on progression. Given the known activity of capecitabine in anthracycline and taxane pretreated patients, this may have contributed to the observed survival benefit. A separate abstract at ASCO 2006 reported a similar survival advantage of 3 months with the combination of capecitabine and docetaxel versus docetaxel followed by capecitabine on progression (22 months vs. 19 months; $p - .006$) (63). A separate gemcitabine/paclitaxel versus paclitaxel trial showed superior RRs, TTP, and OS compared to single-agent paclitaxel, and once again the results may have been biased by lack of a planned crossover design (34,48). Therefore, the real question being addressed by some of these trials was investigational drug "now" versus investigational drug "never," and therapy with combination chemotherapy may give a higher response rate or TTP without conferring a survival advantage over serial single-agent therapy (Table 74.3). Polychemotherapy regimens are also more toxic and may impair QOL.

Hence, sequential single agents are useful in the metastatic setting where efficacy must be balanced with maintenance of a good QOL. They are also particularly appropriate for patients with slowly progressing tumors, or in frail, elderly patients who may not be able to tolerate excessive toxicity. However, in special cases of a need for rapid shrinkage of tumor due to an impending visceral crisis or for fast relief of symptoms, combination chemotherapy is a necessary option. Nonetheless, treatment decisions on the use of sequential single or combination chemotherapy must be made based on tumor-associated symptoms, extent of visceral disease, age, comorbidities, and performance status and balanced with treatment-related toxicities and patient preferences.

Chemotherapy Dosing

Understanding the different ways in which dose can be increased is critical to interpreting data from clinical trials. Dose can be escalated by an increase in cumulative dose, dose

intensity (i.e., dose of effective drug administered per unit time such as mg/m^2 per week), or through changes in drug scheduling, for example, by increasing dose density (i.e., frequency of effective drug dose administered) (64). The issue of drug scheduling will be covered in the next section. This section will concentrate mainly on trials that alter dose size and dose intensity.

The goal of chemotherapy in the metastatic setting is to use the dose that produces the maximal effect without having untoward toxicity. This fine balance has been the subject of trials focusing on the dose that gives the best efficacy. Hryniuk et al. (65,66) have studied retrospectively the effect of dose intensity and concluded that it was a major determinant of breast cancer outcomes in the metastatic and adjuvant settings. The dose-response curve of most anticancer drugs is poorly characterized as the objective of most phase I studies is to concentrate mainly on the drug toxicity, maximum tolerated dose, and pharmacokinetics (67). Furthermore, the precise effects of dose are difficult to determine because body surface area dosing does not account for the complex processes of drug elimination. Hence, it is possible that unrecognized underdosing may occur in 30% or more of patients receiving standard regimens, leading to significantly reduced anticancer effect (68).

The relation between dose and outcome can also be difficult to determine because of the intrinsic antiangiogenic effect of chemotherapy agents at lower than usual doses needed for their cytotoxic effects (69,70). For example, a drop in vascular endothelial growth factor (VEGF) was associated with low-dose oral MTX and CTX (melphalan, chlorambucil, cyclophosphamide), suggesting an additional antiangiogenic effect other than that of direct toxicity on tumor cells (71).

Phase II studies typically have not investigated dose–response relations in breast cancer, but a clear dose–response effect has been shown with some agents in the metastatic setting, as illustrated below, and has been proposed for most cytotoxic agents (72).

Doses Below Standard Levels

Suboptimal chemotherapy doses for MBC result in inferior outcomes. A meta-analysis of 189 clinical trials consisting of 31,510 patients with MBC has reported a modest effect on outcome with chemotherapy doses in the upper range of conventional dosing (28). Several individual trials examining taxanes and anthracyclines have also observed a dose–response relationship. A multicenter study evaluated two doses of paclitaxel of 175 mg/m^2 or 135 mg/m^2 as a 3-hour infusion every 3 weeks in MBC patients who had failed to respond to previous chemotherapy (including prior anthracyclines in most). A dose effect was observed in favor of the high-dose arm for response rate (RR) (29% vs. 22%; $p = .108$), median TTP (4.2 months vs. 3 months; $p = .027$), and median survival (11.7 months vs. 10.5 months; $p = .321$) (73). Similarly, a phase III study of three doses of docetaxel (100 vs. 75 vs. 60 mg/m²) showed a better cancer outcome with the higher-dose arm (74).

Tannock et al. (75) stratified 133 patients to either 3-weekly IV CMF 600/40/600 mg/m² or 300/20/300 mg/m², and the higher dose regimen resulted in a significantly longer RR (30% vs. 11%; $p = .03$) and marginally improved survival (15.6 months vs. 12.8 months; $p = .026$) (75). Although greater toxicity such as vomiting and myelosuppression was experienced in the short term, there was an improvement in general health and some breast cancer–related indices such as pain for the higher-dose therapy in a subset of 26 patients who completed a QOL assessment.

Dose-intensified weekly epirubicin (50 mg/m² on days 1 and 8) in combination with CTX and 5-FU has also shown significantly better RRs (69% vs. 41%; $p < .001$) and TTP (19 months vs. 8 months; $p < .02$) compared to the 3-weekly regime where epirubicin 50 mg/m² was only delivered on day 1 (76). A phase III study of 456 MBC patients randomized to receive either epirubicin 100 mg/m² (FEC 100) or 50 mg/m² (FEC 50) in combination with 5-FU 500 mg/m² and cyclophosphamide 500 mg/m² IV every 21 days for a maximum of six cycles (eight in cases of CR) revealed a significantly higher objective response rate for FEC 100 versus FEC 50 (57% vs. 41%; $p = .003$) with a higher CR rate in the FEC 100 arm (12% vs. 7%; $p = .07$). Median time to progression (7.6 months vs. 7 months) and overall survival (18 vs. 17 months) were similar. Grade 4 infection and febrile neutropenia was observed in 8% of the patients treated with FEC 100 versus 0.4% of those on FEC 50, but cardiotoxicity was similar (77).

Another trial comparing FEC 120 to FEC 60 revealed a significantly longer time to progression (19.2 vs. 13.1 months; $p = .04$) for the FEC 120 regimen, although both regimens showed the same RR and improvement in overall baseline QOL (78).

Doses Above Standard Levels that May Require Growth Factor Support

Randomized trials evaluating higher than standard drug doses of epirubicin (>90 mg/m²) (64,79), paclitaxel (>175 mg/m²) (80,81), CAF (escalating doses of doxorubicin to 100 mg/m² and CTX to 1,800 mg/m²) (82), CEF (1,000/80/600 mg/m² every 2 weeks with GCSF [granulocyte colony stimulating factor]) (83), and epirubicin plus paclitaxel (epirubicin 110 mg/m² in four cycles followed by paclitaxel 225 mg/m² in four cycles every 2 weeks with G-CSF) (52) did not show any survival benefit over conventional dosing.

High-Dose Therapy with Autologous Marrow Support

High-dose chemotherapy (HDC) requiring hematopoietic stem cell support has not been shown to confer survival benefit in various randomized studies (84–86), including a Cochrane meta-analysis (87). Given its increased toxicity and costs without additional benefit, the time of high-dose therapy and autologous stem cell transplant for breast cancer has passed, at least for now (88).

Chemotherapy Scheduling

The impact of chemotherapy scheduling in the metastatic setting has been less well studied compared to that of increasing doses. In a large randomized trial comparing "classical" oral CMF (CTX for 14 days; MTX and 5-FU on days 1 and 8) every 28 days with modified IV CMF 3 weekly, RR (48% vs. 29%; $p = .003$) and OS (17 vs. 12 months; $p = .016$) favored the oral CMF regimen possibly due to scheduling (89). Weekly therapy has been utilized to maximize frequency of drug exposure and cumulative doses achieved with a more favorable toxicity profile. In the adjuvant setting, dose density has been shown to confer a survival benefit in operable node-positive breast cancer (90). Several small trials of taxanes, anthracyclines, and 5-FU in MBC exploring weekly scheduling instead of 3-4 weekly have shown that this is a feasible option with reasonable toxicity (91–97). Data from Cancer and Leukemia Group-B (CALGB) 9840 showed a higher RR and TTP favoring paclitaxel given weekly instead of 3-weekly (98).

Trials evaluating 5-FU scheduling have studied weekly continuous 24- or 48-hour infusions of 5-FU and leucovorin or alternating weekly doxorubicin and 5-FU/leucovorin with encouraging results (96,97,99).

The Norton-Simon hypothesis is derived from clinical and laboratory observations and states that chemotherapy results in a rate of tumor volume regression proportional to the rate of growth for an unperturbed tumor of that size (100–102). This is in contradistinction to the "log kill" theory by Skipper (103), stating that a given dose of chemotherapy would kill a constant fraction of tumor cells, regardless of tumor size. According to the Norton-Simon theory, the chances of tumor eradication would be maximized by delivering the most effective drug doses over as short a time as possible. This theory was certainly well illustrated from the results of the CALGB 9741 adjuvant trial (90), which confirmed the superiority of dose-dense 2-weekly doxorubicin/cyclophosphamide in four cycles → paclitaxel in four cycles with growth factor support over 3-weekly doxorubicin/cyclophosphamide in four cycles → paclitaxel in four cycles in terms of disease recurrence and death. The latter trial also evaluated whether doxorubicin/cyclophosphamide in four cycles → paclitaxel in four cycles was better than doxorubicin in four cycles → paclitaxel in four cycles → cyclophosphamide in four cycles and found no difference. Another trial by Venturini et al. (104) comparing 5-FU/epirubicin/cyclophosphamide in 6 cycles every 3 versus every 2 weeks with filgrastim support did not show a statistical difference in outcomes, although in an exploratory subgroup analysis, the dose-dense regimen did show substantially better outcomes for patients less than 50 years old and those who had hormone– receptor–negative or *ERBB2*-positive tumors. Given this evidence in the adjuvant setting, perhaps a similar advantage may be present in the metastatic setting although this is an area that needs further study.

Another scheduling approach designed to exploit the full efficacy of agents that are theoretically noncrossresistant has been to utilize them in a sequential fashion, crossing over to the other agent or adding on additional agents after the initial fixed number of cycles. So far, as with studies of dose density, the results of these trials using mainly anthracyclines and taxanes have not shown any remarkable clinical significance (52,105–107).

In summary, the randomized trials conducted in MBC do not report any major benefit from using doses over and above that of standard conventional doses, dose-densified chemotherapy, and sequential non-crossresistant regimens. However, randomized trials have indicated that using suboptimal dose levels below that recommended for standard regimens or employing accelerated chemotherapy with reduced doses per cycles results in poorer outcomes and should not be recommended (108).

Chemotherapy Duration (Intermittent vs. Maintenance Therapy)

When to stop chemotherapy in the absence of progressive disease or excessive toxicity remains an unsettled issue that must also take into account quality of life, personal preferences, and costs concerns. Several randomized trials have tried to address

Table 74.3	IMPACT OF CROSS-OVER TO INVESTIGATIONAL REGIMENS IN METASTATIC BREAST CANCER TRIALS

| Study (Reference) | Regimen | | | Crossover | | |
	Standard	vs	Investigational	Agent	Frequency	Survival Benefit
Sledge et al., 2003 (50)	Dox or Pac		Dox/Pac	Pac or Dox	57%	No
Paridaens et al., 2000 (175)	Dox		Pac	Pac	47%	No
Nabholtz et al., 1999 (33)	MV		Doc	Doc	24%	Yes
O'Shaughnessy et al., 2002 (29)	Doc		Cap/Doc	Cap	17%	Yes
Albain et al., 2008 (34)	Pac		Gem/Pac	Gem	15.6%	Yes
Bishop et al., 1999 (32)	CMFP		Pac	Taxane	6%	Yes

Cap, capecitabine; CMFP, cyclophosphamide, methotrexate, 5-fluorouracil, prednisone; Doc, docetaxel; Dox, doxorubicin; Gem, gemcitabine; MV, mitomycin,vinblastine; Pac, paclitaxel.

the potential benefits of continuous chemotherapy versus induction chemotherapy for a fixed number of cycles, then resumption only at progression of disease (Table 74.4) (79,105, 109–117).

A meta-analysis (118) of three trials (109–111) comparing shorter with longer durations of chemotherapy in 666 women with advanced breast cancer indicated a 23% increase in median survival favoring longer durations of chemotherapy ($p = .01$ for weighted combination of log-rank tests). A fourth trial compared a conventional six-course regimen of VAC (vincristine, doxorubicin, cyclophosphamide), VEC (vincristine, epirubicin, cyclophosphamide), or MMM (mitoxantrone, MTX, mitomycin C) followed (if stable disease or response) by a randomization to stopping therapy or continuing with an additional six cycles of the same regimen, and showed a significant advantage for the maintenance arm in terms of duration of response ($p < .02$) and progression-free survival (PFS) ($p < .01$) (112). However, there was no survival difference between the two groups, and treatment toxicity (similar in both groups) persisted longer in the maintenance arm. Although the benefit for continuous therapy seems modest, most women consider small survival gains valuable (119). In these four trials, only one had a QOL assessment and showed better scores favoring continuous chemotherapy (109).

A trial by the European Organisation for Research and Treatment of Cancer (EORTC) Breast Cancer Group comparing six cycles of CMF followed by continued CMF until disease progression or by no further treatment with reintroduction of CMF upon progression had a significant albeit small increase in time-to-treatment failure (TTF) favoring continuous therapy without an OS difference (113). Mean quality-adjusted survival time favored slightly the intermittent treatment group (8.4 months vs. 7.9 months; 95% CI of difference, 0.5 ± 2.5 months). A similar trial by the Piedmont Oncology Association randomly assigned 250 women with MBC who had stable or responsive disease after six cycles of CAF to further CMF maintenance therapy or no further treatment (114). While median TTP was significantly better for the maintenance arm (9.4 vs. 3.2 months; $p < .001$), there was no significant difference in OS (21.1 vs. 19.6 months; $p = .67$). Although QOL was not formally assessed, both groups maintained similar changes in performance status, although continuous therapy led to significantly more frequent toxicities such as mucositis, nausea, and vomiting. A German phase II trial (115) randomized patients with MBC to treatment interruption after an initial response epirubicin/ifosfamide had superior QOL parameters compared to those given continuous therapy, similar to the EORTC study mentioned above. A modest relapse-free survival (RFS) advantage of over 2 months was observed in the continuous treatment arm, but without a survival benefit.

Falkson et al. (117) randomly assigned 195 (141 eligible) patients with MBC who experienced a complete response with

six cycles of doxorubicin-based induction chemotherapy to more chemotherapy with CTX, MTX, 5-FU, prednisone, tamoxifen, and halotestin versus observation. Despite the longer median time to relapse in the maintenance chemohormonal therapy arm (18.6 vs. 7.8 months; $p < .0001$), OS was similar.

It is important to notice that all studies mentioned thus far were conducted in the pretaxane era. A more recent study by Gennari et al. (116) studied 459 MBC patients who had no evidence of disease progression after six to eight courses of first-line epirubicin 90 mg/m^2 day 1 plus paclitaxel 200 mg/m^2 over 3 hours on day 1 (or doxorubicin 50 mg/m^2 day 1 plus paclitaxel 200 mg/m^2 over 3 hours on day 2) every 3 weeks and who were then randomized to receive paclitaxel 175 mg/m^2 over 3 hours every 3 weeks for eight courses or no additional chemotherapy. Both groups had a similar median PFS (8 months vs. 9 months; $p = .817$) and median OS (28 vs. 29 months; $p = .547$).

In summary, there has been no clear significant survival advantage for continuous chemotherapy in the majority of randomized studies so far. Intermittent therapy consisting of an optimal number of cycles of standard chemotherapy (six to eight cycles), followed by a "drug holiday," then resumption of chemotherapy with new agents once the disease has progressed is a reasonable treatment strategy. However, decisions need to be individualized and balanced against QOL issues. Strategies such as endocrine therapy, metronomic chemotherapy, and the newer biological targeted agents need to be evaluated in this setting.

Is Metastatic Breast Cancer Ever Curable?

Unlike early stage breast cancer, MBC is generally considered incurable. Complete remissions are uncommon in this setting and usually limited in duration (8 to 14 months) (120,121). However, a small percentage of patients can remain free of disease for extended periods of time (21,120–122), and available data from the literature have reported that women who achieve a CR following chemotherapy have better disease-free survival (DFS) and OS rates (13,123). A CR is more likely to occur in patients with a good performance status and a low tumor burden (121,124) and in patients with predominant soft tissue disease, while less likely to occur in patients with visceral disease (121).

Older reports from the 1970s and 1980s have also reported on complete responders to conventional chemotherapy with CR rates ranging from 4% to 18% at varying periods of follow-up from about 2 to 13 years (120–123,125,126). More recently, Greenberg et al. (13) reviewed their experience of 1,581 MBC patients treated at M.D. Anderson Cancer Center between 1973 and 1982 with front-line regimens that included doxorubicin and an alkylating agent. Two hundred and sixty-three women from this group (16.6%) achieved a CR and 49 women

| Table 74.4 | SUMMARY OF CLINICAL TRIAL RESULTS THAT EXAMINED THE EFFICACY OF MAINTENANCE VERSUS INTERMITTENT CHEMOTHERAPY |

Author (Reference)	N Evaluable	Experimental (Exp) arm	Control Arm	Median TTP/ PFS (mos) Exp Arm	Median TTP/ PFS (mos) Control Arm	Median Survival (mos) Exp Arm	Median Survival (mos) Control Arm	Median Follow-Up
Coates et al., 1987 (109)	305	Continuous AC or oral CMFP	AC or oral CMFP × 3 cycles → AC or CMFP × 3 cycles on disease progression	6	4 p = sig	10.7	9.4 p = 0.19	Not stated
Ejlertsen et al., 1993 (110)	318	Tamoxifen + CEF × 24 cycles or until PD	Tamoxifen + CEF × 8 cycles or until PD → CEF × 16 cycles or until subsequent PD	14	10 p = .00003	23	18 p = .03	Not stated
Harris et al., 1990 (111)	43	Continuous mitoxantrone	Mitoxantrone × 4 cycles	5.5	6.5 p = ns	12	13 p = ns	Not stated
Gregory et al., 1997 (112)	100	VAC, VEC or MMM × 12 cycles	VAC, VEC or MMM × 6 cycles	10	7 p = .01	13	10.5 p = .3	Not stated
Nooij et al., 2003 (113)	196	Continuous oral CMF	Oral CMF × 6 cycles → CMF on disease progression	5.2	3.5 p = .011	14	14.4 p = .77	Not stated
Muss et al., 1991 (114)	145	CAF × 6 cycles → oral CMF × 12 cycles or 1 year	CAF × 6 cycles → oral CMF × 12 cycles or 1 year on disease progression	9.4	3.2 p <.001	21.1	19.6 p = .67	36.1 mos
Becher et al., 1996 (115) (randomized phase II trial)	331	Epirubicin and ifosfamide × 6–8 cycles → epirubicin and ifosfamide × 8 cycles	Epirubicin and ifosfamide × 6–8 cycles → epirubicin and ifosfamide on progression	5.4	3.2 p <.01	13.5	13.2 p = ns	Not stated
Gennari et al., 2006 (116)	238	Epirubicin or doxorubicin + paclitaxel × 6–8 cycles → paclitaxel × 8 cycles	Epirubicin or doxorubicin + paclitaxel × 6–8 cycles	8	9 p = 0.817	28	29 p = 0.547	Not stated
Falkson et al., 1998 (117)	141	Doxorubicin-containing chemotherapy × 6 cycles → CMF(P)TH	Doxorubicin-containing chemotherapy × 6 cycles	18.7	7.8 p <.0001	32.2	28.7 p = .74	50 mos
French Epirubicin Study Group, 2000 (79)	392	A: FEC75 × 11 cycles B: FEC100 × 4 cycles → FEC50 × 8 cycles	C: FEC100 × 4 cycles → FEC100 × 4 cycles on disease progression	10.3 8.3 p = .38 (A vs. B)	6.2 p <.001 (A + B vs. C)	17.9 18.9	16.3 p = .49	41 mos
Cocconi et al., 1990 (105)	95	CMF × 6 cycles → CMF until disease progression	CMF × 6 cycles → CMAV, CFAV, MFAV × 2 cycles each for a total of 6 cycles	16.25	16.75 p = .47	37	35.5 p = .55	5.5 yrs

AC, doxorubicin, cyclophosphamide; AV, doxorubicin, vincristine; CAF, cyclophosphamide, doxorubicin, 5-fluorouracil; CEF, cyclophosphamide, epirubicin, 5-fluorouracil; CFAV, cyclophosphamide, 5-fluorouracil, doxorubicin, vincristine; CMAV, cyclophosphamide, methotrexate, doxorubicin, vincristine; CMF, cyclophosphamide, methotrexate, 5-fluorouracil; CMFP, cyclophosphamide, methotrexate, 5-fluorouracil, prednisone; CMF(P)TH, cyclophosphamide, methotrexate, 5-fluorouracil, prednisone, tamoxifen, halotestin; FEC, 5-fluorouracil, epirubicin, cyclophosphamide; MFAV, methotrexate, 5-fluorouracil, doxorubicin, vincristine; MMM, mitoxantrone, mitomycin C, methotrexate; PD, progressive disease; PFS, progression-free survival; TTP, time to progression; VAC, vincristine, doxorubicin, cyclophosphamide; VEC, vincristine, epirubicin, cyclophosphamide.

(18.6% of all complete responders and 3.1% of the total patient population) remained in CR for more than 5 years. At a median follow-up of approximately 16 years, 26 patients (1.6%) remained in first CR, and a few remained disease-free for more than 20 years. Those who had achieved long-term CR in this group were found to be younger, premenopausal, have a lower tumor burden, and a better performance status.

A retrospective study by the EORTC (127) with 1,045 MBC patients enrolled in one of five EORTC trials for women with no prior chemotherapy for advanced disease (89,128–132) identified 75 patients who had a CR and 21 patients (28%) were still alive and 18 (24%) showing no evidence of disease at a median follow-up of 6 years. The median TTP was 19.5 months and

median OS was 32.5 months for the overall group. Multivariate analysis identified use of anthracyclines and a good performance status as significant predictors of favorable long-term outcome.

A certain subgroup of MBC manifesting as "oligometastatic disease" may be more amenable to long-term CRs or even cure using multimodality therapy. This term was initially used by Hellman (133) in 1994 to describe a restricted locoregional tumor load for which he advocated "aggressive" chemotherapy and radiotherapy. This term has now become synonymous with isolated distant metastases, limited to a single organ, and mostly to a single lesion (134). Patients with a solitary metastasis represent 1% to 3% of patients (134), and it is thought that these lesions arise from dormant micrometastases (135,136).

Surgical resection is often used for diagnosis, and some remain free of recurrence thereafter (stage IV NED [no evidence of disease]) (137–139). Patients with isolated locoregional or distant recurrences are amenable to surgical resection or irradiation with curative intent in only 1% to 10% of patients (140). After local treatment for locoregional recurrence, 30% to 40% develop widespread metastatic disease within 3 months, and 50% to 80% develop metastatic disease within 2 years (140–147). The 5-year survival rate reported retrospectively ranges from 4% to 36% (141,143,146,148).

Several small retrospective or single-arm studies have evaluated the treatment of oligometastatic disease in various visceral or bony sites. The surgical resection of isolated liver metastases followed subsequently by regional hepatic artery or portal vein (149,150) or systemic chemotherapy (151) have shown mixed results. Most of these data come from small heterogenous, single institution series, and these observations are not easily translated for routine clinical practice.

Pulmonary "metastectomy" in breast cancer may lead to a better outcome than those in lung cancer or melanoma, but not as favorable an outcome compared with other malignancies such as renal, colorectal, or head and neck carcinomas (152). Surgical resection of pulmonary metastases with or without subsequent adjuvant systemic therapy or radiation therapy (RT) was compared with primary systemic chemotherapy/hormonal therapy with or without local RT in a selected patient population, and found to result in a better outcome in terms of 5-year survival (36% vs. 11%) (153). Resection of pulmonary metastasis followed by adjuvant systemic therapy in the majority was reported to show a 5-year survival of 49.5% in a single-institution study (154). An older series by Mountain et al. (155) suggests a 5-year survival rate of 14% likely due to patient selection and a difference in systemic agents. Borner et al. (156) reported data from a randomized trial showing a beneficial DFS benefit of tamoxifen over observation in patients with locoregional recurrence after excision and RT (82 vs. 26 months; $p = .007$). These data support the use of endocrine therapy in patients with stage IV NED disease. The role of chemotherapy was evaluated by Blumenschein et al. (157) in 45 patients with limited stage IV breast cancer who underwent surgical excision of all evaluable disease between 1985 and 1996. Surgery was followed by a doxorubicin-containing regimen and late-consolidation with a non-crossresistant regimen (methotrexate, 5-FU, cisplatin, and cyclophosphamide or 5-FU, mitomycin, etoposide, and cisplatin); 53% of patients were alive and free of disease after a median follow-up of 44 months.

A series from the M.D. Anderson Cancer Center updates experience spanning 30 years for combined-modality treatment of stage IV NED breast cancer (158). Between 1974 to 2004, 285 patients with stage IV NED disease were treated on one of four consecutive phase II protocols; 259 were on one of the three doxorubicin-based trials: study 1 in 1974 to 1982 (140,159,160), study 2 in 1982 to 1988 (160), study 3 in 1988 to 1992 (161), and 26 in a docetaxel-based trial in 1998 to 2004 (158). Study 1 treated stage IV NED patients with FAC (5-FU, doxorubicin, cyclophosphamide) until a cumulative doxorubicin dose of 450 mg/m^2, followed by maintenance CMF for a total chemotherapy duration (FAC plus CMF) of 2 years. Study 2 used a combination of vincristine, doxorubicin, CTX, and prednisone (VACP) until a cumulative doxorubicin dose of 450 mg/m^2 followed by a shorter and potentially non-crossresistant maintenance regimen of sequential MTX and 5-FU for a total chemotherapy duration of 1 year from the time of commencement of VACP. Those with hormone-receptor unknown or positive status had tamoxifen for 1 year. Study 3 scheduled patients to receive six cycles of standard FAC every 21 days followed by tamoxifen for 5 years if hormone receptor positive or unknown. The patients on the doxorubicin-based studies had previously been compared with 62 historical controls with solitary recur-

rence or metastasis treated with surgery, with or without radiotherapy, between 1967 and 1976. Study 4 evaluated six cycles of docetaxel 100 mg/m^2 every 21 days followed by hormonal therapy for 5 years (tamoxifen or aromatase inhibitors) in those with hormone receptor-positive or unknown tumors for stage IV NED women who had recurred after adjuvant anthracycline-based chemotherapy.

In doxorubicin trial series, the ER status was known only for 125 patients, but endocrine therapy was used only in studies 2 and 3. Patients in study 4 had 5-year DFS and OS rates of 34% and 59%, respectively, after a median follow-up of 45 months. In the three doxorubicin studies, the estimated DFS was 41% and 34% and estimated OS was 56% and 42% after 5 and 10 years, respectively, after a median follow-up for all living patients of 212.5 months (range, 76 to 352 months). Despite the historical biases associated with the use of historical controls such as more patients with ER-status unknown, no *ERBB2* testing, and more locoregional first recurrences in studies 1, 2, and 3, and the higher use of endocrine therapy in study 4, this is the largest series to date of stage IV NED patients with the longest follow-up, and the 5-year DFS and OS rates on the docetaxel study were similar to those on the doxorubicin-based trials.

The role of HDC with stem cell rescue was also prospectively studied in this setting, albeit without a control arm. Investigators at the University of Colorado treated 60 patients with minimal metastatic disease (18 had locoregional recurrence) with surgical resection or radiation therapy followed by HDC with autologous stem cell transplant (162,163). After a median follow-up of 62 months, there were four treatment-related deaths (6.6%) and the reported 5-year RFS was 52% (95% CI, 39%–64%) and OS 62% (95% CI, 49%–74%). Multivariate analysis suggested that *ERBB2* overexpression and more than one tumor site were independent risk factors for recurrence-free survival and *ERBB2* overexpression and axillary nodal ratio were independent predictors of OS (163). A caveat was the small number of relapses and deaths due to lack of a negative impact from bone marrow involvement (only 10% of patients had marrow involvement), in addition to inherent patient selection bias in single-arm studies of HDC.

A randomized trial for patients with oligometastatic disease rendered NED with local therapy or systemic therapy versus observation is a difficult task. For now, various issues remain unresolved, such as:

1. How should the subset of stage IV NED patients most likely to benefit from systemic therapy be selected?
2. In addition to endocrine or targeted therapy, is chemotherapy needed and what drugs?
3. How long should patients be treated?
4. If multimodality therapy is found useful in patients with oligometastatic disease, should the role of surveillance be revisited in patients with early stage breast cancer and how can issues of lead-time bias be avoided?
5. Are there prognostic markers based on clinical or molecular that would be useful in this setting?

These limited data suggest a good outcome in patients with limited metastatic disease receiving aggressive multimodality treatment. It is, however, not clear if this represents a subset of patients with indolent disease who would have done relatively well regardless of more intensive therapy. The available data are retrospective in nature, limited by small sample sizes and patient selection bias, and without proper controls. In the absence of prospective randomized data, it is appropriate to consider some form of systemic therapy in carefully selected patients, for instance, using anti-estrogens and anti-*ERBB2* in patients with marker-positive disease. Although a benefit might exist for a subset of patients with stage 4 NED, HDC remains investigational and should not be used off study in this setting.

The optimal role of standard chemotherapy (regimen and duration) in this setting remains unsettled.

CHEMOTHERAPY APPROACHES AND BREAST CANCER PHENOTYPES

MBC is a heterogeneous disease, with substantial variations in biological behavior and responsiveness to therapy (164), hence its clinical outcome does not always conform to published data based on population averages. Furthermore, a higher RR and

TTP do not always translate into significant survival benefits. However, over the past two decades, with the introduction of newer, more effective therapeutic agents, improved outcomes have been observed (Fig. 74.3).

Hormone-positive disease that is relatively asymptomatic and indolent, with a long disease-free interval and mainly bone and soft tissue involvement, may benefit from endocrine therapy initially, regardless of whether the disease is *ERBB2* positive or negative. This mode of therapy also confers a more favorable side effect profile and a resulting better QOL. Based on data from early and MBC, concurrent use of endocrine therapy and cytotoxic agents should not be encouraged (165).

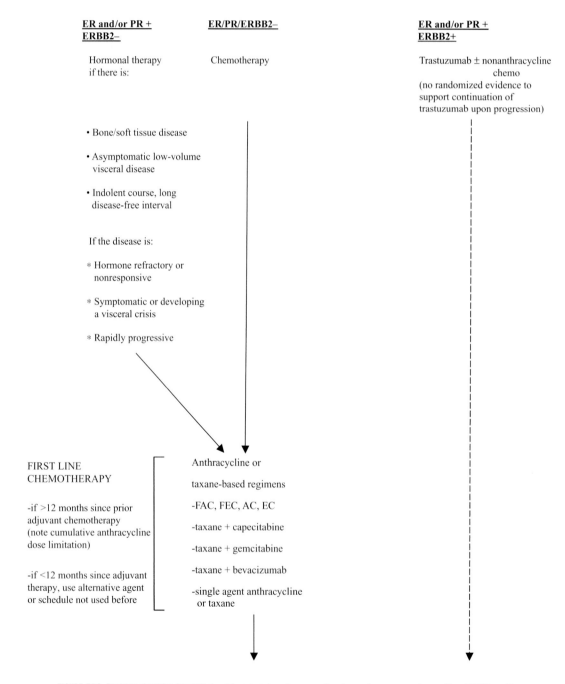

FIGURE 74.3. Decision algorithm for patients with various breast cancer phenotypes: hormone receptor positive, *ERBB2* negative; hormone-receptor negative, *ERBB2* negative; hormone-receptor positive or negative, *ERBB2* positive. FAC, 5-fluorouracil, doxorubicin, cyclophosphamide; FEC, 5-fluorouracil, epirubicin, cyclophosphamide; AC, doxorubicin, cyclophosphamide; EC, epirubicin, cyclophosphamide; CMF, cyclophosphamide, methotrexate, 5-fluorouracil.

However, in a clinical crisis, if the patient is relatively sympto-matic or if the disease is no longer hormone responsive, then chemotherapy with or without targeted therapy should be con-sidered. Hormone therapy can then be continued once a fixed number of cycles of chemotherapy have palliated the acute episode. The response rates to first-line chemotherapy for MBC are approximately 30% to 60% depending on the regimen used, which also provides successful palliation of symptoms and improvement of QOL.

ERBB2-Positive Disease

When trastuzumab became commercially available in the late 1990s, the treatment of *ERBB2*-positive MBC changed dramat-ically. Because of the relative importance of this new drug,

ERBB2 testing should be done for all patients, including in the metastatic site if tissue is available (166). The use of anti-*ERBB2* therapies in MBC is further discussed in depth else-where in this book.

Although there have been no randomized comparisons between the trastuzumab and paclitaxel combination versus trastuzumab alone, many consider the combination to be a superior option for the first-line treatment of women with hor-mone-refractory or unresponsive *ERBB2*-positive MBC. On the other hand, a randomized trial comparing the combination of paclitaxel and trastuzumab with paclitaxel alone appears to improve response, TTP, and OS (167). This landmark finding will be discussed in detail in a separate chapter, but these data suggest that when chemotherapy is appropriate in *ERBB2*-positive patients, this combination of trastuzumab with paclitaxel

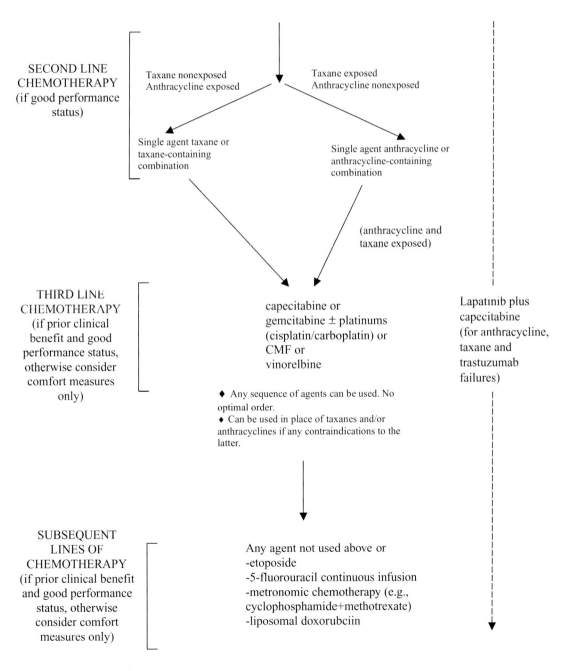

FIGURE 74.3. *Continued*.

or docetaxel (168,169) should be strongly considered, particularly in the setting of rapidly progressive symptomatic visceral disease. However, there is no obvious survival benefit to this approach as opposed to sequential monotherapy. In indolent and relatively asymptomatic disease, the authors would recommend the serial administration of trastuzumab, followed by a taxane after progression. An anthracycline and trastuzumab combination should not be used due to the high risk of cardiac dysfunction. Caution should also be exercised in patients who have previously been exposed to an anthracycline, although this is not a contraindication to the use of trastuzumab.

In second-line therapy, the benefit of continuing trastuzumab after failure of initial trastuzumab-containing therapy is uncertain. Preclinical studies have suggested trastuzumab can enhance the efficacy or can be additive to certain chemotherapy agents, although these have not been proven clinically (170). The decision must be made on an individual patient basis, weighing the costs and toxicity (which is relatively low) of continuing trastuzumab with the potential benefit.

Lapatinib (Tykerb) is an orally administered small molecule tyrosine kinase inhibitor associated with the epidermal growth factor receptor (EGFR, also called *ERBB1*) and *ERBB2* approved in combination with capecitabine for the treatment of patients with advanced or metastatic breast cancer whose tumors overexpress *ERBB2* and who have received prior therapy including an anthracycline, a taxane, and trastuzumab. This will be discussed in further detail in a separate chapter.

Although it has recently been shown that *ERBB2* positivity may be associated with a benefit from adding paclitaxel in the adjuvant setting (171), reports on a similar interaction with *ERBB2* status and paclitaxel in the metastatic setting have been conflicting (172–174).

ERBB2-Negative Disease

In *ERBB2*-negative disease, chemotherapy is used for those who are hormone-receptor negative (ER/PR/*ERBB2* negative) and those who are hormone-receptor positive (ER and/or PR positive, *ERBB2* negative) but unresponsive or refractory to hormone therapy or symptomatic. First-line chemotherapy options in these groups of patients include anthracyclines or taxanes as single agents, or combination regimens such as FAC, CEF, AC (adriamycin and cyclophosphamide), EC (epirubicin and cyclophosphamide), taxanes plus capecitabine or gemcitabine, and (most recently) first-line paclitaxel with bevacizumab.

There is no evidence to support the preferential use of a doxorubicin over a taxane as first-line treatment. Either paclitaxel or docetaxel compared with doxorubicin has not shown a marked benefit of one arm over the other (50,175,176). The type of adjuvant chemotherapy is probably the most important determinant as to the choice of subsequent chemotherapy agents used. Generally, patients should not be retreated with regimens that they have displayed resistance to in the past. However, one can retreat using the same agents if there has been a long disease-free period (>12 months) between completion of adjuvant therapy and relapse (177), provided one has not reached the cumulative dose for unacceptable toxicity, for example, in the case of anthracyclines. Data have shown that taxanes may be superior to nonanthracycline regimens (32,33).

Combinations of anthracyclines and taxanes may result in high response rates but are very toxic without clear impact on survival, as discussed in the previous section. Hence, their use should only be reserved for situations in which there is rapidly progressive visceral metastases with limited survival duration in which failure of an initial regimen may not leave sufficient time for trial of another subsequent line of therapy.

Bevacizumab with paclitaxel could be considered in those who have not received prior chemotherapy for MBC and who do not have clotting or bleeding problems or brain metastases. Bevacizumab used in combination with paclitaxel has recently been shown to prolong RR (36.9% vs. 21.2%; $p < .001$) and PFS (11.8 months vs. 5.9 months; HR 0.6; $p < .001$) but not OS (26.7 vs. 25.2 months; HR 0.88; $p = .16$) in a phase III E2100 study (178). Similarly, the combination of bevacizumab and capecitabine increased the RR but did not significantly increase the OS rate compared with capecitabine alone (179). Based on the E2100 study, bevacizumab received accelerated U.S. Food and Drug Administration (FDA) approval in February 2008 in combination with paclitaxel for first-line treatment of locally recurrent or metastatic *ERBB2*-negative breast cancer, although the toxicities and costs in relation to the PFS benefit must be discussed. A phase III study in MBC investigating two doses of bevacizumab (7.5 or 15 mg/kg) in combination with docetaxel compared to docetaxel alone has met its primary end point of PFS in a preliminary report, although overall survival data are not mature yet (180).

Triple-Negative Disease

Breast cancer is a far more heterogeneous disease than anticipated, as evidenced by landmark findings in this decade of five distinct molecular portraits revealed by gene expression profiling; namely, luminal A and luminal B, erbB2 positive subtype, basal subtype, and normal breast-like subtype (181,182). DNA microarray and immunohistochemical analyses have shown that 80% to 90% of triple-negative breast cancers are basal-like in morphology and clinical behavior (183). Historically, hormone receptor–negative tumors are known to have a generally poorer outcome with a lack of hormone responsiveness, higher recurrence rates, and inferior survival. Furthermore, they are more likely to possess unfavorable histological characteristics such as poor differentiation and a higher histological grade (183). Despite *ERBB2*-negative disease having a more favorable prognosis compared to *ERBB2*-positive tumors, it lacks the responsiveness to targeted agents such as trastuzumab that appears to have changed the natural history of patients with this tumor subtype. Taken in aggregate, this confers limited therapeutic choices in triple-negative disease; a disease that already has an intrinsic aggressive clinical behavior.

Triple-negative breast cancers account for 15% of all types of breast cancers and are more prevalent in premenopausal women (6), those of African American descent (9), and *BRCA1* mutation carriers (184). They have a poor prognosis, likely a combination of limited treatment options and inherent aggressiveness, and are characterized by shorter relapse-free survival times and a tendency to develop visceral metastases (8,181,185). A Canadian study of 180 women with triple-negative breast cancer (median follow-up 8.1 years) revealed that these cancers had an increased likelihood of distant recurrence (HR 2.6; 95% CI, 2.0–3.5; $p < .0001$) and death (HR 3.2; 95% CI, 2.3–4.5; $p < .001$) within 5 years of diagnosis but not thereafter compared to women with other subtypes of breast cancer (186). The mean time to distant recurrence was also shorter (2.6 years vs. 5 years; $p < .0001$). The risk of distant recurrence peaked at approximately 3 years for triple-negative patients and declined rapidly thereafter, whereas those in the other cohort had distant recurrences even up to 17 years after diagnosis. Few (15 of 59 women treated with breast-conserving surgery; 25%) women with triple-negative breast cancer experienced a local recurrence before a distant recurrence. In addition, although patients in the triple-negative group had relatively larger tumors (two thirds >2 cm) and a high rate of node involvement (54%), there appeared to be no correlation between tumor size and lymph node positivity (55% with tumors 1 cm or less had at least one positive node).

There are currently no specific recommendations for the type of chemotherapy regimen to be used in this setting and no hard data to base choices on. In general, evidence points to an inherent responsiveness of triple-negative cancers to chemotherapy (187,188), due perhaps to their ER-negativity (189) and high Ki-67 expression (190), although data on which specific agents to use are less clear. Bevacizumab with chemotherapy-like taxanes could be a therapeutic option in this group of patients. In the recent trial by Miller et al. (178) comparing bevacizumab and paclitaxel with paclitaxel alone in first-line treatment of MBC both ER-positive and ER-negative subgroups equally benefit, but there appeared to be a significant interaction between the combination arm and age ($p = .04$) in the planned subgroup analyses, suggesting that the effect of bevacizumab declined with age. This could thus be a suitable chemotherapy regimen in triple-negative patients who are usually younger at presentation.

The *BRCA1* pathway may be impaired in triple-negative cancers, and since it functions in DNA repair, cytotoxic agents that cause interstrand breaks (such as platinums) and double-stranded breaks may be effective, as opposed to spindle poisons such as vinca alkaloids and taxanes (191). However, it has been shown in a study by Hayes et al. (171) that evaluated *ERBB2* and responsiveness to paclitaxel in node-positive early breast cancer that the subgroup of patients who had estrogen and *ERBB2*-negative breast cancers benefited from paclitaxel significantly. Whether this translates into the metastatic setting is not established at present. Overexpression of EGFR occurs in triple-negative breast cancers and EGFR-targeted therapy could be an option, although data show that 73% of basal-like tumors are considered EGFR negative using criteria that has not been properly validated (192). Nevertheless, occasional responses have been reported using anti-EGFR agents such as cetuximab (193), and clinical trials are still ongoing. Early trials of PARP1 inhibitors, c-KIT tyrosine kinase inhibitors (e.g., imatinib), multikinase inhibitors (e.g., lapatinib and pertuzumab), and downstream messenger inhibition (e.g., Ras farnesylation, Raf, MEK, MTOR, Src, HSP90) are being carried out, although there is no concrete evidence of activity to date (6). Some suggest that HDC should remain the subject of clinical studies in this patient group, although adequate patient identification is the main challenge to support this assertion (194).

STANDARD CHEMOTHERAPY

Alkylating Agents

Background and Structure

The use of mustard gas in World War I dramatically demonstrated the biological potential of alkylating agents (195). The first nitrogen mustard to be used extensively in the clinic was mechlorethamine. Subsequent alterations in drug formulation by replacing the methyl group of mechlorethamine with a variety of chemical groups gave rise to the development of four drug derivatives; namely, melphalan (L-phenylalanine mustard), chlorambucil, cyclophosphamide (CTX) and ifosfamide. The latter two agents are unique in possessing no alkylating activity, requiring *in vivo* metabolic activation to produce active alkylating compounds (196). Of these four agents, CTX has established itself as a cornerstone in chemotherapy regimens in both adjuvant and metastatic breast cancer settings.

Preclinical studies revealed the excellent antitumor activity of CTX against transplanted rat tumors (197–199) and murine leukemia (200). Since the first clinical trial in the 1958 (201), the usefulness of cyclophosphamide has been demonstrated in autoimmune diseases (202,203) and a wide-ranging spectrum of malignancies including breast cancer.

Mechanism of Action

CTX is a cell cycle phase, nonspecific alkylating agent. It is extensively metabolized *in vivo* to active and inactive metabolites (204). The drug is biotransformed to alkylating and cytotoxic metabolites by specific hepatic cytochrome P450 mixed-function oxidase enzymes to its two tautomer forms: hydroxycyclophosphamide and aldophosphamide (205). These noncytotoxic transport forms may readily enter cells where they are oxidized by aldehyde dehydrogenase (aldehyde oxygenase) into inactive metabolites (comprising 80% of a dose of administered CTX) (206,207), or are spontaneously converted to the cytotoxic metabolites acrolein and phosphoramide mustard (208). Most of the production of the cytotoxic metabolites occurs within hepatic cells and within the collecting system of the genitourinary tract. Metabolism of CTX to its active metabolites may also occur in the lungs, initiating peroxidative injury, which may be linked to CTX-induced pulmonary toxicity (209). The intracellular concentrations of aldehyde dehydrogenase in many tumor cells are much lower than in the liver and most other normal cells, hence decreasing the tumor cells' ability to inactivate the tautomer forms of CTX. Activation of CTX may also occur via co-oxidation, which form oxygen radicals and acrolein via prostaglandin H synthetase, although metabolism by this pathway is several-fold lower (210). Phosphoramide mustard is responsible for nearly all of the cytotoxic activity of CTX (211), and conversely, acrolein accounts for the bladder and possibly pulmonary toxicity (209,212).

Drug Resistance

Drug resistance is mediated primarily by DNA repair enzymes like O^6-methylguanine-DNA methyltransferase (MGMT), with an inverse relationship between MGMT activity and the growth-inhibiting effect of CTX (213). Other postulated mechanisms of resistance include increased expression of the glutathione S transferase group of enzymes, resulting in increased deactivation of potentially damaging metabolites of cyclophosphamide (214) and depletion of cellular glutathione (215). Decreased expression or mutation of p53 has also been associated with chemoresistance and a poor prognosis (216). In addition, high intracellular aldehyde dehydrogenase activity has been reported to be an important determinant of cyclophosphamide sensitivity in leukemia cell lines (217).

Pharmacokinetics

CTX is available as oral or IV preparations. D'Incalci et al. (218) reported the systemic availability of the unchanged drug after oral administration of 100-mg doses to be 97% of that after IV injection of the same dose. For breast cancer, the oral formulation of CTX together with methotrexate and 5-FU appears to be superior to its intravenous counterpart in metastatic disease (89,219). Elimination takes place primarily via the kidneys where approximately 70% of a dose of CTX undergoes urinary excretion as inactive carboxyifosfamide (207,220). Dosing recommendations for renal impaired patients are: CrCl greater than 10 mL/min, administer 100% of dose; CrCl less than 10 mL/min, 75% of dose. As the pharmacokinetics of CTX are not significantly altered in hepatic dysfunction, no dose adjustments are recommended in this case.

Drug Interactions

As CTX is a major substrate of CYP2B6 and CYP3A4, respective inducers or inhibitors of these pathways can decrease or increase the levels and subsequent effects of its active metabolites accordingly. Examples of the CYP2B6 inducers include carbamazepine, phenobarbital, phenytoin, and rifampicin.

Examples of inhibitors of CYP2B6 include desipramine, paroxetine, and sertraline. Examples of CYP3A4 inducers are aminoglutethimide, carbamazepine, phenobarbital, phenytoin, and rifamycin, and the inhibitors include azole antifungals, ciprofloxacin, clarithromycin, diclofenac, doxycycline, erythromycin, imatinib, isoniazid, quinidine, and verapamil. Allopurinol may cause increased bone marrow suppression and elevations of CTX cytotoxic metabolites. CTX reduces serum pseudocholinesterase concentrations and prolongs the neuromuscular blocking activity of succinylcholine, hence it should be used with caution in this situation due to the increased risk of apnea (221). Caution should also be exercised when used with other anesthetic agents such as halothanes and nitrous oxide. The reports on the risk of cardiomyopathy in patients treated with CTX in combination anthracyclines are conflicting, although CTX probably does not augment doxorubicin-induced cardiac damage (222).

Toxicity

Myelosuppression is a major dose-limiting toxicity for cyclophosphamide. Neutrophils reach a nadir at about 8 to 14 days, recovering 1 to 2 weeks later. The other dose-limiting side effect is hemorrhagic cystitis (223) due to acrolein (212) and possibly others metabolites such as phosphoramide mustard, which can be fatal but unlikely to occur in doses conventionally used in breast cancer. It varies in severity, although uncommon with the doses routinely used in breast cancer. Adequate hydration and care to ensure frequent voiding is recommended to avoid this toxicity. Other side effects include nausea and vomiting, alopecia, hyperpigmentation of the skin or fingernails, rarely mucositis, diaphoresis, facial flushing, nasal congestion, a metallic taste in the mouth, anaphylaxis, pulmonary fibrosis, transient myopia (224), or electrocardiographic changes. Syndrome of inappropriate antidiuretic hormone (SIADH) has also been reported with high doses with large fluid loads (225). CTX can be carcinogenic, not only for the bladder but also for bone marrow (226). Alkylating agents such as CTX cause an increased risk of secondary acute myelocytic leukemia (AML) and the risk is clearly dose dependent (227–230).

Clinical Trials

Alkylating agents have become an integral component of chemotherapy regimens in the adjuvant and metastatic settings since their use first began in the 1950s and 1960s (231). Cyclophosphamide is the most widely used drug, with response rates of 10% to 60% in patients with previously untreated MBC (232,233). Ifosfamide is an undesirable choice for breast cancer due to its low activity as monotherapy in breast cancer (234–237).

Antimetabolites

Background

An antimetabolite is defined as a drug that interferes with the normal metabolic processes within cells (238). Antimetabolites have been in use for the treatment of malignant disease for close to 60 years, since the discovery by Farber et al. (239) that aminopterin could cause remission of leukemia. Although their main application is in cancer therapy, antimetabolites have found use in a variety in other settings as antibiotics and immune modulators. Methotrexate and 5-FU have been the mainstay of antimetabolite treatment in solid tumors for several decades, with the emergence of newer agents such as capecitabine and gemcitabine in recent years.

Two important complex metabolic pathways exist in cells that give rise to the synthesis of purines and pyrimidines, involving many different enzymes and folate-derived cofactors. Antimetabolites are designed to affect various processes in this pathway, for example inhibitors of vital enzymes such as dihydrofolate reductase (DHFR), thymidylate synthase (TS), and glycineamide ribonucleotide formyltransferase (GAFRT). Other pharmacological amtimetabolite targets have included transport mechanisms such as the reduced folate carrier (RFC) and the membrane-associated folate-binding protein (mFBP); the drugs either bypassing the transport mechanisms or acting as better substrates than their *in vivo* counterparts. Nucleoside analogues, which exert their effect after incorporation into DNA or RNA, giving rise to chain termination and cell death or stasis, are the most widely used of the antimetabolites. This section will discuss the chemotherapy agents most commonly used for breast cancer, such as the antifolate antimetabolite methotrexate; the pyrimidine analogs 5-FU and its oral systemic pro-drug formulation capecitabine, and gemcitabine, which is also a pyrimidine analog.

Structure

MTX is a 4-amino, 10-methyl analog of folic acid (240). 5-FU is a nucleoside analog of uracil and has a fluorine atom substituted in place of hydrogen at the C5 position of the pyrimidine ring (241). Capecitabine, the first oral 5-FU prodrug is a N^4-pentoxycarbonyl-5′-deoxy-5-fluorocytidine. Gemcitabine (2′, 2′-difluorodeoxycytidine, dFdC) is a difluorinated nucleoside analog with structural similarity to deoxycytidine.

Mechanism of Action

Inhibition of DNA biosynthesis by MTX is a multifactorial process consisting both of partial depletion of reduced-folate substrates and direct inhibition of folate-dependent enzymes (242). MTX and its polyglutamate metabolites compete for the folate-binding site of DHFR (243,244). Inhibition of DHFR results in depletion of intracellular reduced folate pools and ultimately in reduced synthesis of purines and pyrimidines (238). Metabolism of the parent MTX to polyglutamated derivatives and accumulation of the metabolites of MTX, dihydrofolate and 10-formyldihydrofolate polyglutamates as a consequence of DHFR inhibition may also contribute to cytotoxicity (245–249).

The precise mechanism of action of 5-FU is unclear and is partly dose and schedule dependent. 5-FU is a proliferation-dependent agent and has effects on progression of cells through the G1 and S phases of the cell cycle, although it kills cells in both S and non-S phases.

The most important mechanism of cytotoxicity is the metabolite 5-fluorodeoxyuridylate (5dUMP) competing with the natural substrate deoxyuridine monophosphate (dUMP) for the catalytic site on TS (250,251), with incorporation of the folate cofactor; 5, 10-methylenetetrahydrofolate (MTHF), forming a covalent ternary complex, causing an inability of dUMP to be converted by TS to thymidine (238). 5dUMP itself may also be incorporated into DNA with subsequent effects on DNA repair. Another important metabolite is fluorouridine triphosphate (FUTP), which acts by inhibiting RNA metabolism.

The 5-FU pro-drug capecitabine is a cytidine analog (252) and is administered via the oral route, passing unchanged through the intestinal mucosa. It is activated through a three-step series of enzymatic conversions in the liver and tumor cells. It is hydrolyzed in the liver via hepatic carboxylesterase yielding 5′-deoxy-5′-fluorocytidine (5′-dFCyd). Cytidine deaminase, a widely distributed enzyme, then converts 5′-dFCyd to 5′-deoxy-5-fluorouridine (5′-dFUrd). Finally, thymidine phosphorylase, which is an enzyme with higher activity in tumor tissue, hydrolyzes 5′-dFUrd to active 5-FU (241).

Gemcitabine is a potent inhibitor of DNA synthesis. Its killing effects are not confined to the S phase of the cell cycle but is as effective against confluent cells as it is against cells in the log-phase of growth (253). It requires intracellular phosphorylation using deoxycytidine kinase (dCk) resulting in gemcitabine triphosphate (dFdCTP) subsequently affecting DNA synthesis though inhibition of DNA polymerases (254). This drug exerts its maximal effect on cells undergoing DNA synthesis (S phases) and on cells between the G1 and S phases (255).

Drug Resistance

MTX resistance is multifactorial and may involve:

1. Reduced influx or increased efflux of MTX;
2. Impaired polyglutamation of MTX (256,257);
3. Altered amounts of DHFR through gene amplification (258,259), changes of the affinity of DHFR for MTX (260), nonactive site DHFR mutations (261), or naturally occurring differing DHFR alleles (262);
4. Reduction of TS activity (263); or
5. Reduced cell proliferation as MTX appears to select for tumors with a high growth fraction (264).

Resistance to 5-FU (and capecitabine) is complex. It is mediated by several mechanisms, the most important being alterations in the target enzyme thymidylate synthase (TS). Other mechanisms include deletion or decreased activity of other enzymes in the metabolic pathway, such as thymidine or uridine kinase, thymidine or uridine phosphorylase, and orotate phosphoribosyl transferase. Alternatively, decreased activity of catabolic enzymes, or decreased incorporation of 5-FU into RNA and DNA, may also contribute to drug resistance. Interestingly, there is a lack of cross-resistance between bolus 5-FU and subsequent continuous infusion of 5-FU (265).

Gemcitabine mechanisms of resistance include:

1. Cells lacking in nucleoside transporters (266);
2. Deoxycytidine kinase deficiency (240);
3. Overexpression of ribonucleotide reductase (267); or
4. Induction of heat-shock proteins and cytidine deaminase (268,269).

Interestingly, P-glycoprotein has not been associated with gemcitabine resistance.

Pharmacokinetics

MTX is albumin bound and has a wide distribution in all body compartments except the central nervous system (CNS). MTX is eliminated primarily by the kidneys, but 10% of it undergoes biliary excretion (240). Patients with renal dysfunction, third-space fluid collections, or cystectomies with ileal conduit loop diversions have a potentially increased risk for drug toxicity (242,270). Dose adjustments for renal impairment begin when creatinine clearance (CrCl) drops below 80 mL/min and MTX must be avoided if CrCl is less than 10 mL/min. MTX dose is also reduced if bilirubin is greater than 3.1 and not given if it is greater than 5 mg/dL.

5-FU is erratically absorbed orally because of the high levels of dihydropyrimidine dehydrogenase (DPD), its metabolizing enzyme, present in the gastrointestinal tract. It is given parenterally and is rapidly distributed to all sites of the body, including the CNS and third-space accumulations such as pleural effusions and ascitic collections (271). Eighty percent of 5-FU is primarily metabolized by the hepatic route, with less than 10% of unchanged drug excreted by the kidney. Due to the relatively minor role of elimination by the kidneys, no dose adjustment is recommended in renal impairment. It is recommended to omit use of 5-FU if the bilirubin is greater than 5 mg/dL.

Capecitabine is a rationally designed chemotherapy agent because it is a tumor-selective and tumor-activated oral fluoropyrimidine carbamate (272). Its pharmacokinetics, once it is converted to 5-FU, is similar to intravenous 5-FU itself. Capecitabine can theoretically provide significant tumor selectivity through its activation by enzymes that are expressed at higher levels in many tumor cells, thereby reducing systemic toxicity and maintaining high intratumoral 5-FU concentrations (272). It attains peak blood levels 1.5 hours after ingestion and peak 5-FU levels at 2 hours. Although capecitabine is recommended to be taken with water within 30 minutes after eating a meal, food reduces the speed of quantity of drug absorbed. Capecitabine is primarily albumin-bound and is excreted by the kidneys. If the CrCl is 30 to 50 mL/min, 75% of the normal dose is recommended and if CrCl is less than 30 mL/min, its use is contraindicated. No dose adjustment is needed if mild to moderate liver impairment is present, and there are insufficient data on its use with severe hepatic impairment.

The principal metabolite of gemcitabine is difluorodeoxyuridine (dFdU). Gemcitabine is excreted almost completely in the urine as the parent compound and primary metabolite (dFdU), but no specific dose adjustments are recommended for those with renal or hepatic impairment. The CALGB 9565 tried to ascertain if hepatic or renal dysfunction led to increased toxicity (273). Based on their data, patients with elevated transaminases but normal bilirubin and creatinine levels did not require dose reductions. The dosing of gemcitabine in patients with renal dysfunction should be done cautiously, but because of the varied toxicities observed, their data did not support specific dosing recommendations.

Drug Interactions

MTX, when used with hepatotoxic agents such as azathioprine, retinoids, or sulfasalazine, may increase the risk of hepatotoxic reactions. Drugs that can impair renal function can increase MTX toxicity, such as aminoglycoside antibiotics and cisplatin-based chemotherapy. Corticosteroids (except dexamethasone) may decrease uptake of MTX into cells. Severe bone marrow suppression, aplastic anemia, and gastrointestinal toxicity have been reported with concomitant nonsteroidal anti-inflammatory drugs (NSAIDs). Data have been reported on the interaction between ketoprofen, ibuprofen, piroxicam, and flurbiprofen (274,275). Salicylates and NSAIDs can increase MTX toxicity by inhibiting renal excretion (276,277). Several drug interactions with antibiotics may occur. Penicillins and cephalosporins may increase MTX concentrations due to a reduction in renal elimination. Sulfonamides may displace MTX from albumin, causing increased toxicity. Trimethoprim is an inhibitor of DHFR, and its concurrent use with MTX can lead to enhanced MTX toxicity and pancytopenia (278,279). Macrolides can prolong plasma clearance of MTX, leading to increased toxicity (280). Tetracyclines can also increase MTX toxicity. Conversely, MTX may increase theophylline levels. Live virus vaccines, when used with MTX, may result in vaccinia infections.

Concomitant use of 5-FU and warfarin may increase activated partial thromboplastin time (aPTT) and bleeding time. Cimetidine can increase 5-FU levels (281). Allopurinol allows a reduction in 5-FU toxicity (282). Capecitabine may increase the levels and hence effects of both phenytoin and warfarin, therefore, close monitoring is required.

Bleomycin, when used concurrently with gemcitabine, may lead to severe pulmonary toxicity. Gemcitabine may also increase the levels and concomitant effects of 5-FU.

Toxicity

The main side effects of MTX are myelosuppression and gastrointestinal toxicity, such as mucositis (usually 3 to 7 days after therapy) or hepatotoxicity. These side effects are completely reversed within 14 days unless elimination mechanisms are impaired. For intrathecal MTX used to treat leptomeningeal disease, three distinct CNS effects have been observed: most commonly an acute arachnoiditis; a subacute form in 10% of patients in week 2 or 3 of therapy, consisting of motor paralysis of extremities, cranial nerve palsies, seizure, or coma; lastly a demyelinating encephalopathy seen months or years later, usually in association with cranial irradiation or other systemic chemotherapy.

Although the spectrum of side effects for 5-FU vary according to its dose, schedule, and route of administration, its two primary toxicities are specifically gastrointestinal and bone marrow related. Although 5-FU has less emetogenic potential than other agents such as anthracyclines, the epithelial ulceration from 5-FU can lead to mucositis and diarrhea. Coupled with nausea and vomiting, the patient can experience severe dehydration and hypotension if inadequately treated. Treatment consists of supportive measures such as rehydration, antiemetics, antidiarrheal agents, such as diphenoxylate and loperamide, and in persistent diarrhea, even subcutaneous octreotide. In severe cases, the dose of 5-FU may have to be reduced or even withheld. Myelosuppression tends to be more pronounced for the bolus scheduling. It occurs usually in 7 to 10 days with a nadir at 14 days and recovery at 21 days for the bolus 5-day schedule of 5-FU, whereas it usually occurs after week 4 with the weekly schedule. Other side effects include dermatologic toxicities such as alopecia, fingernail changes, dermatitis, photosensitivity reactions, increased pigmentation over infused veins, hand-foot syndrome (usually in the continuous infusion regimens), ocular toxicities such as blepharitis, conjunctivitis, epiphora, and tear duct stenosis, neurologic symptoms such as cerebellar ataxia (283), and myocardial ischemia-like symptoms such as angina, cardiac enzyme elevations, and electrocardiographic changes coupled with arrhythmias and sudden death (284). The oral pro-drug capecitabine has also been reported to cause an acute coronary syndrome and should be used with caution in patients previously reported to have 5-FU induced cardiotoxicity (285). 5-FU does not induce alopecia to the same extent as anthracyclines and taxanes. People with DPD deficiency are susceptible to life-threatening 5-FU toxicity (286–288). In humans, more than 85% of 5-FU is degraded through the catabolic pathway, with DPD being the initial rate-limiting step (289). Although DPD is widely distributed in human tissues, including in peripheral blood mononuclear cells (PBMNCs), the liver is the major source of this enzyme (290,291). However, there is variable correlation between PBMNC DPD activity and toxicity due to large interpatient variability in DPD content in PBMNCs and changes in leukocyte populations, influencing enzyme activity due to differences in DPD activity among monocytes, lymphocytes, and neutrophils (292,293). Hence, systemic DPD levels are not measured routinely before administering 5-FU. Testing of DPD-deficient patients has revealed an autosomal recessive pattern of inheritance (287,294,295). It is estimated that as high as 3% of adult cancer patients may have significantly decreased DPD activity (286).

Capecitabine, unlike IV 5-FU, does not cause myelosuppression in most cases. Its more common side effects include lymphopenia, anemia, fatigue, hyperbilirubinemia, dermatitis, nausea, vomiting, diarrhea, and hand-foot syndrome (about 54% to 60%; grade 3: 11% to 17%) (296). Hand-foot syndrome is often a function of cumulative dose and prolonged high plasma levels, with grade 2 or 3 symptoms necessitating interruption of dosing until it improves in intensity to grade 1. Dose reduction may be necessary in grade 3 or recurrent grade 2 hand-foot syndrome. Treatment also involves supportive measures, and prevention is usually not possible. Oral pyridoxine was demonstrated to be ineffective in prevention of hand-foot syndrome associated with capecitabine (297).

Gemcitabine is usually well tolerated, although myelosuppression is a main side effect in heavily pretreated patients (298). Nausea, vomiting, or hair loss is minimal. Other potential side effects include a flu-like syndrome in about 45% of patients, transient transaminitis, and asthenia. Uncommon and possibly fatal pulmonary symptoms can occur 2 to 40 days after administration of gemcitabine, including pulmonary infiltrates, acute respiratory distress, and hypoxemia (299), and may be more common when gemcitabine is used in combination with radiation or taxanes (299–303). A rare occurrence of hemolytic-uremic syndrome has been reported in 0.015% (range, 0.008% to 0.078%) of patients at a median duration of gemcitabine therapy of 5.8 months (range, 3.8 to 13.1 months) and therapy should be discontinued (304).

Clinical Trials

MTX is a widely used antifolate that is administered intravenously. MTX has limited activity when used as a single agent. However, it is often a component of effective combination regimens such as oral or intravenous CMF (89). Small studies of high-dose MTX at 2 to 3 g/m^2 do not indicate an increased benefit at present, and this is not recommended for the conventional treatment of metastatic cancer because of the potential for toxicity and the fact that the response rates cited are probably not superior to those that can be achieved by conventional doses of MTX (305,306).

5-FU is widely used in MBC either as a single agent or combined with other active chemotherapeutic regimens. As a single agent, bolus 5-FU has a response rate of around 25%; this includes many patients in older series who were chemotherapy naive (307). It can be administered using varying dose schedules, but its activity is higher with prolonged or frequent infusions compared to bolus regimens (308). The possible active regimens include (a) a daily bolus regimen using 5-FU (400 to 600 mg/m^2 daily for 5 days every 4 weeks) or (b) low-dose prolonged continuous infusion of 5-FU (175 to 250 mg/m^2 daily). The overall response rate across all the studies with continuously infused 5-FU is about 30% (307,309). However, the majority of these patients were heavily pretreated, and response rates of up to 54% have been reported at doses ranging from 175 to 250 mg/m^2 per day (307,310). Furthermore, rechallenge with 5-FU infusion in patients who have progressed on previous 5-FU containing regimens have proven to be encouraging (311).

Fluoropyrimidines have been studied in combination with other active agents such as mitoxantrone (312) and taxanes. In a randomized phase II study comparing 5-FU combinations of NFL (mitoxantrone, 5-FU, leucovorin [LV]) with IV CMF as first-line treatment for MBC, NFL produced higher response rates (45% vs. 26%) and longer remission (9 vs. 6 months) but no difference in OS (19 vs. 16 months) (313). Both regimens were well tolerated. Adding paclitaxel to NFL did not improve its efficacy (313). NFL has also proven active in advanced breast cancer following anthracycline-containing chemotherapy (314).

Nonrandomized trials have shown benefit when LV is added to 5-FU (315), even when patients have progressed on previous 5-FU containing adjuvant or metastatic regimens due to stabilization of the FdUMP-TS-folate ternary complex *in vivo* (316). This regimen has also shown activity for heavily pretreated patients who have a primary resistance to doxorubicin (96). However, a CALGB trial reported that modulation of CAF with LV improved neither response rates nor survival among women with metastatic breast cancer compared with CAF alone (317), even in the subset with visceral crisis. From its limited activity as a single agent, it is reasonable to conclude that 5-FU should be used in combination therapy for the early treatment of MBC. Single-agent IV 5-FU, preferably as a prolonged continuous infusion, should be reserved for refractory disease after more active agents have been utilized.

Capecitabine was, in 1998, the first oral fluoropyrimidine to be FDA approved for MBC in anthracycline and taxane refractory patients. The overall response rates to capecitabine monotherapy in patients pretreated. with anthracyclines and taxanes range from 15% to 28% (318–323). Capecitabine is approved to be used at a dose of 2,500 mg/m^2 per day. However, this dose often leads to drug-related toxicities such as palmar-plantar erythrodysesthesias, diarrhea, stomatitis, and nausea and vomiting. Dose reductions anecdotally improve tolerability without compromising efficacy (324,325). Hence, lower doses should be considered especially in patients older than 65 years and those with renal dysfunction, especially since maintenance of QOL is an important aspect of treatment in the metastatic setting. Capecitabine has been compared with IV CMF in older patients (≥55 years) as first-line treatment for MBC in a randomized phase II trial and found to have similar survival outcomes (median, 19.6 vs. 17.2 months) (55).

Capecitabine has been combined with paclitaxel (326,327) and vinorelbine (328) in phase II trials with promising results. More recently, the capecitabine and docetaxel combination have shown to significantly improve time-to-progression, response rates, and survival when compared with docetaxel alone in anthracycline pretreated patients with advanced MBC (29), as discussed in detail in a later section.

Tegafur (Ftorafur), like capecitabine, is a pro-drug metabolized *in vivo* to 5-FU and is active in heavily pretreated metastatic breast cancer, even after previous 5-FU therapy (329). It is usually combined with uracil (UPT) to decrease 5-FU degradation, though not available in the United States. Single agent response rates with LV or without range from 14% to 32% (329–332).

Gemcitabine is an antimetabolite drug with proven antitumor activity and tolerability in metastatic breast cancer (333). Gemcitabine as a single agent has response rates of approximately 15% to 40% in either first-line or refractory settings (334–337). As a single agent, gemcitabine is usually delivered intravenously at a dose of between 800 to 1,200 mg/m^2 weekly (336–338), using lower doses in heavily pretreated patients or in combination with other agents. Gemcitabine has been combined with doxorubicin (339), epirubicin (340,341), liposomal doxorubicin (342), capecitabine or IV 5-FU (343–345), mitoxantrone (346,347), cisplatin (348–350), carboplatin (351), vinorelbine (49,352–356), paclitaxel (34,48), and docetaxel (357–360), with response rates ranging from 30% to 79%, even in those who have been pretreated. Of interest, gemcitabine/taxane combinations have been evaluated in a number of phase III clinical trials. The gemcitabine/paclitaxel combination was compared with paclitaxel alone as first-line treatment of MBC and found to be significantly better in terms of OS, overall response rate [ORR], TTP, and PFS (see the section Taxanes as Combination Therapy below) (34). Gemcitabine/docetaxel was also compared with capecitabine/docetaxel in anthracycline pretreated MBC patients and found to have similar efficacies (361). The gemcitabine/platinum combination is a particularly well-tolerated regimen suitable for use as third- or fourth-line therapy. Gemcitabine used as triplet therapy (gemcitabine-epirubicin-paclitaxel) was compared with 5-FU-epirubicin-CTX as first-line therapy in MBC and found to have no difference in ORR or TTP at a median follow-up of 20.4 months (341).

Anthracyclines and Anthraquinones

Background

Doxorubicin and epirubicin have remained the cornerstone of adjuvant and metastatic regimens. Anthracyclines changed the face of cancer treatment immeasurably more than 40 years ago with the independent discoveries by Grein et al. (362), Dubost et al. (363) of an anthracycline antibiotic, derived from a *Streptomyces* soil mold. This red-pigmented compound, which had significant activity against leukemias, was known as daunorubicin. In 1969 a closely related analog known as doxorubicin was reported to have a broader preclinical activity against both hematologic and solid tumors (364). Other anthracyclines such as epirubicin (a semisynthetic stereoisomer analog of doxorubicin with identical molecular weight and formula) were soon formulated (365).

Structure

Anthracyclines share a quinone-containing rigid planar aromatic ring structure bound by a glycosidic bond to an amino sugar, daunosamine (366). Doxorubicin differs from daunorubicin by an additional hydroxyl group at the C14 position, hence it is sometimes referred to as hydroxydaunorubicin. Epirubicin is an epimer of doxorubicin with a reversed orientation of the C4 hydroxyl group on the sugar, and it is this simple structural modification that confers its relatively lower cardiotoxicity on a milligram-per-milligram basis.

Mechanism of Action

Anthracyclines have a diverse molecular effect and their cytotoxic effect occurs in various ways. They can induce direct cytotoxicity to the cell membrane, intercalate with and alkylate DNA through covalent binding, resulting in DNA cross-linking, and inhibit DNA synthesis. A seminal discovery of the molecular mechanism of anthracyclines recognized their ability to inhibit the religation reaction of topoisomerase II, causing accumulation of covalently protein-bound double- and single-strand DNA breaks (cleavable complexes) (367). However, the mechanism of stabilization of DNA topoisomerase IIα cleavable complexes is not well defined and may be independent of DNA intercalation. Some drugs such as doxorubicin or daunorubicin act as true topoisomerase enzyme inhibitors by directly inhibiting topoisomerase IIα independent of cleavable complex stabilization) or they may inhibit other enzymes such as cellular helicases, among other mechanisms (368). Ultimately, these effects culminate in the induction of apoptosis.

Drug Resistance

There are two major mechanisms for resistance. One is classic multidrug resistance related to expression of P-glycoprotein. The other is a variety of P-glycoprotein-independent mechanisms such as increased glutathione transferase activity, increased DNA repair through the induction of DNA mismatch repair proteins (369), and altered topoisomerase II activity.

Pharmacokinetics

Anthracyclines are poorly absorbed by the oral route. They undergo predominantly hepatic metabolism to several metabolites, including doxorubicinol. It is widely distributed in the body including breast milk but does not penetrate the CNS. They undergo primarily hepatic and biliary excretion, with 4% to 5% eliminated via urinary excretion, thus causing a reddish hue in the urine. Epirubicin similarly is widely distributed in tissues and excreted primarily via the biliary route with approximately 10% eliminated in the urine.

Both doxorubicin and epirubicin should be dose reduced in hepatic impairment and their use is contraindicated in severe liver dysfunction. Doxorubicin dose should be reduced by half if the bilirubin level is 1.2 to 3 mg/dL, by 75% if bilirubin is

3.1–5 mg/dL and withheld if bilirubin above 5 mg/dL. Its use is contraindicated in severe hepatic impairment. Care should be taken when administering anthracyclines in women older than 70 due to clearance and toxicity issues. Renal adjustments are not required for doxorubicin, but lower epirubicin doses should be considered in renal impairment, although precise guidelines do not exist (370).

Drug Interactions

Doxorubicin is a major substrate of CYP2D6 and CYP3A4. Hence CYP2D6 inhibitors such as chlorpromazine, fluoxetine, and paroxetine may increase the levels of doxorubicin. Similarly, CYP3A4 inhibitors, including azole antifungals, clarithromycin, erythromycin, diclofenac, doxycycline, isoniazid, and verapamil, may increase the levels and concomitant effects of doxorubicin. Conversely, CYP3A4 inducers such as carbamazepine, and phenytoin may decrease the levels of doxorubicin. Doxorubicin itself may decrease plasma levels of phenytoin and digoxin. Doxorubicin inhibits CYP2B6 moderately; hence levels of substrates of this enzyme such as bupropion, promethazine, propofol, selegiline, and sertraline may be increased when administered concurrently with doxorubicin. Epirubicin administered concomitantly with cimetidine can increase the serum concentrations of epirubicin and increase the risk of toxicity. Trastuzumab enhances the cardiotoxicity of anthracyclines, but the data are less clear with bevacizumab. The pharmacokinetic interactions between anthracyclines and taxanes will be discussed in detail in a later section.

Toxicity

The dose-limiting acute toxicity is myelosuppression with neutrophil nadirs occurring 10 to 14 days after injection and recovery at 21 to 28 days posttreatment (11). Other side effects include nausea, vomiting, diarrhea, mucositis, alopecia, and hyperpigmentation of the nail beds (371). Radiation sensitization of normal tissues can occur after doxorubicin administration even many years after radiation exposure (368). Rarely, secondary myelogenous leukemia may occur (371).

The cardiotoxicity manifests as acute and chronic forms (11). Several distinct early electrocardiogram changes have been described. Rare cases of subacute cardiotoxicity, resulting in acute failure of the left ventricle, pericarditis, or a fatal pericarditis myocarditis syndrome characterized by fever, pain, and congestive heart failure (CHF), have been reported (372). The chronic form is a dose-dependent cardiomyopathy. Although the risk of CHF was at first felt to be increased at doses above 450 mg/m^2, it is now recognized that asymptomatic drops in left ventricle ejection fraction (LVEF) can be seen with doses as low as 240 mg/m^2 (373,374). Although reports conflict, proposed risk factors for chronic anthracycline cardiotoxicity include higher rates of drug administration (375), mediastinal radiation (376,377), advanced age (378–380), very young age (381,382), female sex (383), pre-existing heart disease, and hypertension (380). The equitoxic dose ratio of doxorubicin/epirubicin is 1:1.2 for hematologic toxicity, 1:1.5 for nonhematologic toxicity, and 1:18 for cardiac toxicity (384). The hematological and cardiotoxic effects are less severe after epirubicin administration than after equimolar doses of doxorubicin (385), although it is less potent than doxorubicin at identical doses.

Various approaches have been adopted to reduce the risk of anthracycline-induced toxicity, including altered administration schedules, liposome formulations of the anthracycline molecule, and the use of adjunctive cardioprotectants. Lower single doses of doxorubicin or prolonged infusions of 6 to 96 hours may lower the incidence of cardiotoxicity compared to bolus therapy with equivalent efficacy (375,386, 387).

The primary aim of doxorubicin encapsulation in liposomes has been to decrease nonspecific organ toxicity. Various liposomal formulations of doxorubicin have been developed and evaluated in clinical trials, including a pegylated formulation (Doxil in the United States or Caelyx elsewhere) and a nonpegylated version (Myocet). The carrier for nonpegylated doxorubicin is composed of egg phosphatidylcholine and cholesterol, while pegylated liposomal doxorubicin utilizes a pegylated lipid formulation that is comprised of hydrogenated soya phosphatidylcholine, cholesterol, and PEG-modified phosphatidylethanolamine (388). The nonpegylated formulation releases more than half of its associated doxorubicin within 1 hour of IV administration and more than 90% of its entrapped contents within 24 hours (388). In contrast, pegylated liposomal doxorubicin releases less than 10% of its excapsulated doxorubicin 24 hours after IV administration (389). As anticipated, these variations in drug release are reflected in the toxicity profile, with the nonpegylated formulation being more acutely toxic than the pegylated formulation (388). The more common adverse reactions (>20%) are asthenia, fever, fatigue, anorexia, nausea, vomiting, stomatitis, constipation, diarrhea, hand-foot syndrome, rash, neutropenia, thrombocytopenia, and anemia (390).

Palmar-plantar erythrodysesthesia (PPE) is more frequently observed with the pegylated formulation. This syndrome was observed after multiple dosing (388). Treatment involves dose reduction or withholding the drug, supportive measures such as cold compresses, emollients, analgesia, elevation of limbs, and oral or topical corticosteroids. The pegylated liposomal doxorubicin formulation has also been associated with a higher degree of mucositis than conventional doxorubicin (388). However, the nonpegylated formulation is comparable to free doxorubicin with respect to toxicities such as alopecia and neutropenia (388).

Incorporation of doxorubicin into liposomes was discovered to permit substantially higher cumulative doses with less concomitant cardiac side effects (391,392). This has been evaluated via small trials using endomyocardial biopsies and proven to be true even at doses of pegylated liposomal doxorubicin above 500 mg/m^2 (393,394). Despite the reduced toxicities associated with the use of liposomal doxorubicin, clinical trials to date have not identified a clear survival advantage for these formulations over the use of free doxorubicin. Several trials have shown promising results with equivalent outcomes for both liposomal and conventional formulations of doxorubicin whether used as single agents (395–397) or in combination with cyclophosphamide as first-line treatment for MBC (398). Liposomal doxorubicin has also demonstrated efficacy comparable to that of certain salvage regimens such as vinorelbine and mitomycin C/vinblastine in taxane-refractory MBC with a significantly longer progression-free survival time relative to the comparator regimens (399). However, a lack of activity has been observed in patients refractory to the free drug (400).

In an EORTC retrospective analysis of elderly patients a higher toxicity was observed in those given liposome doxorubicin 60 mg/m^2 every 6 weeks compared to those given the same drug at a dose of 50 mg/m^2 every 4 weeks, making the latter a preferred regimen (401). In a retrospective analysis on pooled data from two prospective phase III randomized clinical trials comparing liposome doxorubicin versus conventional doxorubicin in combination with cyclophosphamide and as single agents for MBC treatment for patients who had previously received adjuvant doxorubicin, the former demonstrated significantly reduced cardiotoxicity (22% for liposomal doxorubicin/CTX vs. 39% for conventional doxorubicin/CTX, with significantly improved tumor response rates (31% vs. 11%; $p = .04$), time to treatment failure (4.2 vs. 2.1 months; $p = .01$), and similar median survival (16 vs. 15 months, $p = 0.71$) (402).

Several studies have demonstrated the potential benefits and safety of combining liposomal doxorubicin with various chemotherapy agents such as vinorelbine (403), paclitaxel (404), gemcitabine (342), and cyclophosphamide with or without 5-FU (402,405).

Dexrazoxane

Dexrazoxane is the first chemical cardioprotectant used successfully with anthracyclines. It has been shown in several randomized trials to confer protection by decreasing the incidence and severity of CHF without affecting clinical activity or noncardiac toxicities (406,407). The recommendations for use of dexrazoxane states that given the potential for increased expense and possibly increased toxicity, it continues to be reasonable to recommend against the use of dexrazoxane at the initiation of doxorubicin-based chemotherapy in patients with MBC, unless a cumulative dose of 300 mg/m^2 is reached (408,409). Similarly, the use of dexrazoxane may be considered for patients responding to epirubicin-based therapy for MBC for whom continued therapy may be indicated (408). A meta-analysis indicated that dexrazoxane was associated with decreased risk of clinical cardiotoxicity (OR 0.24; 95% CI, 0.11–0.52; $p = .00031$) with no compromise in objective response (410). A pharmacoeconomic evaluation found that this drug required a cost of $5,661.77 per cardiac event prevented (411). There is insufficient evidence to recommend the use of dexrazoxane in patients with cardiac risk factors or underlying cardiac disease (408). Cardiac monitoring is recommended to be repeated after 500 mg/m^2 and subsequently after every 50 mg/m^2 (408). Termination of therapy should be considered once there is a decline in LVEF to below institutional limits of normal or when clinical CHF develops (408). The dose of dexrazoxane should be at a ratio of 10:1 with doxorubicin or epirubicin administered 15 to 30 minutes before anthracycline administration (408).

In clinical practice, the costs of liposomal doxorubicin and dexrazoxane are limiting factors, and longer or more frequent infusions of free doxorubicin may be inconvenient. In most cases, resistance to the anthracycline would have set in before the cardiotoxic level of drug had been reached, thus negating the need for these therapeutic maneuvers. However, dexrazoxane can be considered in patients who continue to respond to the anthracycline as delayed administration has been shown to be effective (409).

Clinical Trials

Response rates to monotherapy are 35% to 50% in anthracycline-naive patients or those who develop metastases more than 12 months after adjuvant anthracycline-based therapy (42,50,175,412–414). The efficacy in those who were treated with anthracyclines less than 12 months ago is less certain. This group of drugs is a major component of combination therapies such as doxorubicin or epirubicin with cyclophosphamide and 5-fluorouracil (FAC or FEC) (82,95, 415–417) or doxorubicin with cyclophosphamide (AC) (418). These regimens produce responses in 20% to 60% of patients as first-line treatment in MBC.

These combined regimens are more active but also more toxic than nonanthracycline-containing regimens such as CMF (419,420). The value of inclusion of doxorubicin in combination-type regimens was examined in an overview of published studies of randomized clinical trials comparing Cooper type regimens that contain doxorubicin with regimens in which doxorubicin was replaced by one or more compounds. Only trials that published data on survival, time to treatment failure, and response rate were chosen. This study suggests that doxorubicin conferred advantages on all of these end points (421).

Epirubicin, at equivalent doses to doxorubicin, has been shown to be equally efficacious and less toxic than doxorubicin in several reports, including a review of 13 randomized controlled trials (422,423).

In contrast, mitoxantrone (an anthracenedione derivative) is generally less efficacious than doxorubicin and epirubicin, whether used as a single agent (412,414) or in combination (415,424), although the data are not consistent (425). It also appears to have a more favorable toxicity profile particularly in contrast to doxorubicin with respect to nausea, stomatitis, alopecia, and cardiotoxicity (412,414,424), although its dose-limiting toxicity is potent myelosuppression, particularly leukopenia. Its narrow spectrum of antitumor activity has limited its ability to replace doxorubicin in clinical practice.

Platinums

Background

Platinum compounds are active in a wide range of solid tumors (426). Although platinum complexes have shown activity in MBC, the toxicity of cisplatin in particular has limited their widespread use. Cisplatin was discovered serendipitously in the 1960s by Barnett Rosenberg while studying the effects of electromagnetic radiation on *Escherichia coli* in a chamber containing platinum electrodes (427) and the first clinical studies were carried out in the 1970s (427–429). Carboplatin was developed as a cisplatin analog, and from clinical trials in the early 1980s, it was clear that while retaining the activity of cisplatin, it was substantially less toxic.

Mechanism of Action

Platinum agents are non–cell cycle specific. Their major mechanism of action is inhibiting DNA synthesis causing interstrand DNA cross-linking, leading to cessation of DNA synthesis and, ultimately, apoptosis.

Drug Resistance

Drug resistance for the platinums can occur by the following mechanisms: decreased drug entry into the cell (430), increased glutathione synthesis (431), increased nuclear excision repair ability (432), increased tolerance for the unrepaired DNA lesions (433), and resistance to apoptosis through loss of mismatch-repair (432).

Pharmacokinetics

Platinum agents are extensively bound to plasma proteins and are metabolized in the liver, although the kidney is the principal excretory organ. No guidelines are available for hepatic dysfunction. In renal impairment the following guidelines have been suggested: (cisplatin) CrCl 46 to 60 mL/minute, reduce dose by 25%; CrCl 31 to 45 mL/minute, reduce dose by 50%; CrCl, less than 30 mL/minute, consider use of alternative drug (434). Carboplatin dosage is calculated from sex, age, weight, serum creatinine and AUC (area under the curve) of carboplatin using formulas such as the Cockroft-Gault, Jelliffe, Modified-Jelliffe, Wright, or Chatelut (435).

Drug Interactions

Cisplatin does not generally demonstrate cross-resistance with other alkylating agents. Aminoglycosides may enhance the nephrotoxic or ototoxic effects of platinums. Phenytoin levels may be decreased by cisplatin, so levels should be monitored closely when used concurrently. It is important to note that when administered as sequential infusions, taxanes should be administered before platinum derivatives to limit myelosuppression and enhance efficacy.

Toxicities

More common adverse reactions of cisplatin include neurotoxicity, nausea and vomiting, nephrotoxicity, ototoxicity, and myelosuppression (nadir at about 2 weeks) (436). Carboplatin has the dose-limiting toxicity of myelosuppression, with the thrombocytopenia nadir occurring about 2 to 3 weeks after treatment followed a few days later by leukopenia. The other side effects are similar to cisplatin, albeit milder.

Clinical Trials

Studies of single-agent cisplatin in the 1980s showed a mean RR of 50% in previously untreated MBC and <10% in pretreated patients (437). Later studies on single-agent carboplatin showed mean RRs of 32% and <10% in previously untreated and treated MBC patients, respectively (437). Cisplatin and carboplatin have been combined with other chemotherapy agents such as taxanes (438), capecitabine (439), etoposide (440), vinorelbine (441), and gemcitabine (351,442) with promising results. Cisplatin and trastuzumab achieved higher response rates than would be expected with either agent alone in heavily pretreated MBC patients (443). In the first-line setting, high response rates have been observed in combination with taxanes or vinorelbine (RR about 60%) (444–448). These regimens appear superior to older combinations such as with etoposide (RR 30% to 50%) (449,450) and 5-FU (RR 30% to 60%) (451,452). Although triple-therapy combinations achieve high RR of around 60% to 80%, these regimens are difficult to administer and are more toxic (453,454). However, in view of the availability of less toxic agents and lack of a demonstrable progression or survival benefit of platinum-containing regimens, it is difficult to justify their use, especially as first-line therapy in routine clinical practice (455,456).

Oxaliplatin is also a platinum compound, but breast cancer data are not established for other platinums like oxaliplatin and ZD0473. A prospective phase II trial of ZD0473 given every 3 weekly proved disappointing with a RR of only 3.8% (457). Other oxaliplatin combinations are still under study (458–460).

Taxanes

Background

Taxanes are a novel family of structurally related compounds that share a core ring structure known as baccatin III. Among them, paclitaxel and docetaxel have emerged in the past two decades as effective antitumor agents, possessing a wide spectrum of activity in a variety of malignancies.

Paclitaxel is a natural product originally extracted in the early 1960s from the bark of the Pacific Yew, *Taxus brevifolia*, although it is now chemically synthesized. Clinical phase I trials commenced in 1983, although initial progress was hampered by hypersensitivity reactions. Despite this, drug development continued, culminating in the FDA approval of paclitaxel in 1992 for the treatment of advanced, drug-refractory ovarian carcinoma (461) and in 1994 for MBC.

Docetaxel was originally obtained in the 1980s by hemisynthesis, using the starting material, 10-deacetyl baccatin III extracted from the needles of the European Yew tree, *Taxus baccata* (462). Its successful broad spectrum of activity has resulted in its approval in more than 30 countries worldwide. It was first FDA approved in the United States for the treatment of locally advanced or MBC in May 1996.

Structure

Paclitaxel is a complex alkaloid ester consisting of a taxane ring with four-member oxetan ring attachments at positions C4 and C5 and a bulky ester side chain at C13 (463,464). The configuration of this ester side chain determines the antitumor activity. Docetaxel structure differs from paclitaxel by the loss of the acetyl group esterified to the C10 hydroxyl on the baccatin ring and by the attachment structure linked to the 3′ position in the C13 side chain (465).

Mechanism of Action

Both paclitaxel and docetaxel have similar mechanisms of action. They enhance microtubule assembly and inhibit depolymerization of tubulin (462). As a result, the cells become blocked during the G2 and M phases of the cell cycle and are unable to form a normal mitotic spindle for cell division (466). This also disrupts many essential cellular functions, such as transport between organelles, signal transmission, motility, and maintenance cell shape (467). Paclitaxel binds to high-affinity binding sites in a specific, reversible and saturable manner (462). Docetaxel apparently competes with paclitaxel for the same binding site, with an approximately 1.9-fold larger effective affinity (468).

The link between microtubule stabilization and cell death affected by taxanes is unclear. It is proposed that the taxanes cause activation of apoptosis and hence cytotoxicity (469,470). Other mechanisms of action include bcl-2 phosphorylation, p53 modulation, and the resulting apoptotic effect related or unrelated to these mechanisms (471–474). Paclitaxel can also induce transcription factors and enzymes that are involved with proliferation, apoptosis, and inflammation, and also the induction of tumor necrosis factor-α (475,476). Paclitaxel has also been shown to have strong antiangiogenic activity at doses below those that induce cytotoxicity (477). This contribution to its antitumor effect is unclear. Taxanes have a radiosensitizing effect that could be related to the similar radiosensitivity of the G2 and M cell cycle phases on which it acts (478,479).

Of interest are the results of several preclinical and clinical studies suggesting that paclitaxel and docetaxel may not be totally cross-resistant, due to the relative differences in drug resistance mechanisms, potency, and efficacy of the two agents (480–483).

Drug Resistance

Resistance to taxanes has been attributed to the multidrug resistance phenotype (484) or to the development of altered microtubule structure or function (475,485,486). Animal studies have shown that the MDR protein may be less involved with docetaxel compared with paclitaxel resistance, hence conferring incomplete cross-resistance between the two drugs (480).

Pharmacokinetics

Taxane metabolism is primarily hepatic and renal clearance is minimal (<10% in the urine) (467,487). Both taxanes are metabolized by hepatic cytochrome P450 enzyme systems and eliminated by biliary excretion (487,488). Because of their hepatobiliary clearance, taxanes are the drug of choice for patients with renal disease and older patients with impaired creatinine clearance (489,490).

Paclitaxel should be dose reduced if there is hepatic impairment but avoided if the transaminase levels are 10 times or more upper limit of normal and bilirubin level greater than five times upper limit of normal.

Docetaxel should generally not be administered if the total bilirubin is greater than ULN (upper limit of normal) or the AST/ALT (aspartate aminotransferase/alanine aminotransferase) is greater than 1.5 times ULN concomitant with an ALP (alkaline phosphatase) greater than 2.5 times ULN (491).

Weekly taxanes that are delivered at lower doses may be ideal for patients with hepatic dysfunction, and this schedule being less myelosuppressive can be titrated closely against white blood cell counts. Dose adjustments have not been studied in docetaxel given weekly as compared with the traditional 3-weekly regimen (492).

Drug Interactions

Paclitaxel is a major substrate of CYP2C8. Hence, inducers of CYP2C8 such as carbamazepine, phenobarbital, phenytoin, and rifampicin may decrease the levels and effects of paclitaxel. Conversely, inhibitors of CYP2C8 such as gemfibrozil, ketoconazole, and montelukast may increase the levels and effects of paclitaxel. Paclitaxel is also a major substrate of CYP3A4; hence inducers or inhibitors may decrease or increase the levels of paclitaxel respectively when administered concurrently. Interaction of paclitaxel with warfarin (a CYP2C8, CYP2C9 inhibitor) exists. Docetaxel is a also major substrate of CYP3A4 and consequently drugs that are inducers or inhibitors of this enzyme can decrease or increase the levels and hence effects of docetaxel when administered concurrently.

Several important sequence-dependent effects and toxicological interactions between the taxanes and other chemotherapy agents have been described. These will be described in detail in the section Taxanes as Combination Therapy below.

Toxicity

Paclitaxel and docetaxel each possess unique chemical and pharmacologic characteristics that account for significant differences in their toxicological profiles. In general, paclitaxel is associated with a higher incidence of neurotoxicity, cardiac conduction effects, arthralgias, and myalgias, whereas fluid retention and skin and nail side effects are features of docetaxel toxicity.

Paclitaxel
The important toxicities are listed in the sections that follow.

Myelosuppression. Neutropenia is the principal toxicity of 3-weekly paclitaxel, and although transient and noncumulative, it can be dose-limiting. Neutropenia occurs in 78% to 98% of people and can be severe at times. Its onset is usually on days 8 to 10, median nadir being 11 days with recovery in 15 to 21 days. The severity of neutropenia is related to the duration of paclitaxel infusion (465). Paclitaxel alone rarely causes severe thrombocytopenia and anemia. However, weekly paclitaxel can be administered continuously for several weeks with a remarkable lack of myelosuppression.

Hypersensitivity Reactions. At first, 25% to 30% of patients experienced histamine-related hypersensitivity reactions (HSRs), manifesting as flushing, hypotension, bronchospasm, and bradycardia, but premedication and longer administration schedules

have reduced the incidence of major reaction to 1% to 3% (493,494). Anaphylaxis has only rarely been reported (495). The majority of HSRs occur after the first or second dose (467). HSRs commonly occur within the first 2 to 3 minutes of therapy, with the majority occurring within 10 minutes (467). Recovery usually follows discontinuation of therapy and necessary supportive measures such as fluids, antihistamines, steroids, and occasionally vasopressors. Minor HSRs have not been associated with subsequent development of a major reaction (467). The duration of infusion and dose appears to be unrelated to the risk of a major HSR (467,494). Premedication with an H2 receptor antagonist, diphenhydramine, and dexamethasone or slowing the infusion rate is recommended to minimize HSRs (496). With weekly paclitaxel infused over 1 hour at moderate doses, oral dexamethasone premedication requirements are reduced.

The mechanism of paclitaxel-related HSRs is unclear but may be multifaceted. It is also not clear if the drug itself or its solvent (the polyoxyethylated castor oil vehicle Cremophor EL) is responsible for this reaction due to its ability to induce histamine release (497). Half of the reactions occur from the first administration of paclitaxel, which suggests that HSRs are unlikely solely due to IgE-mediated responses (494). Similar reactions are induced by other polyoxyethylated castor oil formulated drugs (494,498). Cremophor EL can also activate complement via the classical pathway in *in vitro* studies (499). Although successful rechallenging of paclitaxel after a major hypersensitivity reaction has been reported (500,501), caution must be used as the reaction may reoccur (502,503). Rechallenge is discouraged in grade 3/4 HSRs (496). A switch to docetaxel is possible in some cases (504,505) but reportedly has a high rate of cross-sensitivity, and Cremophor EL-free formulations of paclitaxel are now commercially available in some countries.

Neurological Side Effects. Neurotoxicity manifested primarily by a motor and sensory polyneuropathy is the principal nonhematological side effect of paclitaxel. Paclitaxel produces a toxic effect involving either axons or ganglion cell bodies, or both, rather than a myelinopathy (506). Peripheral neuropathy occurs in 40% to 70% of patients, usually after multiple courses at conventional doses (135 to 250 mg/m^2) with severe neurotoxicities occurring rarely (<10%) at doses less than 200 mg/m^2 (467). As with other toxic polyneuropathies, patients with preexisting peripheral neuropathies, such as those caused by other chemotherapy agents, diabetes mellitus, or alcoholism, appear to be at a higher risk. Although weekly paclitaxel, despite its larger cumulative dose, appear to carry less risk of neuropathy in certain phase II studies (93); this has been proven otherwise in the CALGB 9840 study (98). The incidence and severity of the neuropathic manifestations also appear to be related to the paclitaxel dose level, the cumulative dose of paclitaxel, shorter infusion times, and possibly to the use of paclitaxel in combination with cisplatin. To date, amifostine has not been proven to definitely decrease the rate of neuropathy (507). Motor and autonomic dysfunction can also manifest especially at high paclitaxel doses and in patients with a predisposition caused by conditions such as diabetes mellitus and ethanol ingestion (467). Rarely, transient encephalopathy or visual disturbances such as scintillating scotoma can occur (508,509).

Cardiovascular Side Effects. A diverse spectrum of cardiac disturbances have been observed during paclitaxel administration. Sinus bradycardia has been observed in 3% of patients. However, isolated asymptomatic bradycardia is not an indication to discontinue paclitaxel (467). Nevertheless, it should be noted that bradycardia can progress to higher grades of atrioventricular conduction delays such as Mobitz type I, Mobitz type II, atrioventricular 2:1 conduction blocks, and complete heart blocks (510), although the incidence of these is low (<1%) and often reversible. Atrial and ventricular arrhythmias including bigeminy, trigeminy, increased premature ventricular contractions, and cardiac ischemia have also been observed (510). It is unclear whether paclitaxel or its excipient is responsible for these cardiac disturbances (510). The presence of a preexisting cardiac conduction defect may be a relative contraindication to paclitaxel (465). Infusion-related hypotension or hypertension may also occur.

Musculoskeletal. Transient dose-related myalgia and arthralgia is a common occurrence in about two thirds of cases, usually noted 1 to 3 days after therapy and resolving after about 3 to 5 days. The symptoms differ in severity among patients but can frequently require use of analgesics. A low-dose prednisone regimen for 5 days starting 24 hours after completion of chemotherapy in patients who had arthralgias or myalgias uncontrolled by NSAIDs has been reported to offer improvement (511,512), although many patients do not tolerate steroids very well.

Other Side Effects. Include infrequent vomiting, diarrhea, mucositis, or reversible alopecia in almost all patients especially with the 3-weekly dose schedule. Radiation-recall dermatitis is possible (513) and, rarely, interstitial pneumonitis (514,515), lung fibrosis (516), and pulmonary lipid embolism (517) can occur. Rare cases of neutropenic enterocolitis have also been reported when paclitaxel is used in combination with doxorubicin or cyclophosphamide (467,518).

Docetaxel
Some important toxicities are listed in the sections that follow.

Myelosuppression. Dose-dependent neutropenia affects the majority of patients on 3-weekly docetaxel (grade 4 severity ranging from 75% to 86%), with febrile neutropenia affecting one eighth of cases (519). It is transient and noncumulative. The onset is at 4 to 7 days with a nadir at 5 to 9 days and recovery at 21 days. In contrast to paclitaxel, even a 1 hour infusion of docetaxel can produce severe neutropenia (465). The weekly docetaxel schedule is less myelosuppressive (94) but associated with more epiphora due to canalicular stenosis and skin and nail toxicities (520,521).

Hypersensitivity Reactions. Although docetaxel is formulated in Tween 80 (ICI Americas Inc.) and not the Cremophor EL vehicle, HSRs can still occur, albeit less frequently compared with paclitaxel, especially during the first two infusions. This usually occurs within the first few minutes following the initiation of docetaxel and most reactions are minor, consisting of flushing or localized skin reactions. However, severe HSRs have been reported such as generalized rash or erythema, hypotension or bronchospasm, or rarely, fatal anaphylaxis. Those with a history of severe HSRs should not be rechallenged with docetaxel (496).

Fluid Retention. A dose-cumulative fluid retention syndrome has been observed in about half of patients who receive a cumulative dose of 400 mg/m^2 (522), manifesting as pleural effusions, ascites, peripheral edema, and weight gain. Corticosteroids are of benefit in fluid retention (523), and premedication with a 3-day course of dexamethasone starting 1 day prior to docetaxel has been recommended (491). The symptoms generally resolve once therapy is discontinued. This syndrome has been attributed to capillary leakage rather than a true HSR.

Other Side Effects. Include severe cumulative neurosensory symptoms (20–60%; grade 3/4 in 5.5%) of patients (519). Like paclitaxel, docetaxel commonly causes reversible alopecia gastrointestinal toxicity (nausea, vomiting, diarrhea, stomatitis) (524). Unlike paclitaxel, single-agent docetaxel has fewer cardiac effects, and dose-related myalgia and arthralgia are less common with docetaxel therapy (465). Other side effects include nail changes (525,526), severe fever in the absence of infection, and skin toxicities (519).

Clinical Trials

Taxanes as Monotherapy
Paclitaxel as a single agent has significant activity in doxorubicin-naive (RR 25%–55%) (32,50,175,527) and refractory (RR 20%–30%) MBC (73,528–531). In an overview of 18 randomized phase II (n = 1) or III (n = 17) trials, the dose and schedule associated with the most favorable therapeutic index for paclitaxel was 175 mg/m^2 given as a 3-hour infusion every 3 weeks (532).

Weekly administration of paclitaxel has been postulated to increase efficacy or decrease toxicities (533). Weekly paclitaxel 80 to 100 mg/m^2 is also a reasonable treatment approach with a remarkable lack of hematologic or neurotoxicity (93,534). The efficacy and toxicity of weekly versus 3-weekly regimens of paclitaxel were compared in several randomized clinical trials. In the CALGB 9840 study (91), 735 women with MBC (158 patients "borrowed" from the 175 mg/m^2 arm of CALGB 9342) (80) were randomized to receive weekly (80 mg/m^2) or 3-weekly (175 mg/m^2) paclitaxel either as first- or second-line treatment (plus a second randomization of trastuzumab versus not if *ERBB2*-non-overexpressing disease). In this study, the weekly paclitaxel schedule was found to be superior in terms of response rates (42% vs. 29%; unadjusted odds ratio (OR) = 1.75; p = .0004) and TTP (9 vs. 5 months; adjusted HR = 1.43; p <.0001), with significant difference in overall survival (24 months vs. 12 months; adjusted HR = 1.28; p = .0092). This trial demonstrated the importance of frequency over dose intensity in this case (Table 74.5). Neurotoxicity was significantly higher in the weekly arm and granulocytopenia in the 3-weekly arm. Another phase III trial (the Anglo-Celtic IV trial) (535), comparing weekly (90 mg/m^2 for 12 weeks) to 3-weekly (175 mg/m^2 for 6 cycles) paclitaxel also showed higher response rates for the weekly schedule (42% vs. 27%; p = .002), although its primary end point TTP was not significantly different, possibly due to mismatched treatment duration.

Several studies have attempted to elucidate the superiority of either anthracyclines or taxanes in MBC treatment. An EORTC study compared paclitaxel 200 mg/m^2 over 3 hours to doxorubicin 75 mg/m^2 bolus every 3-weekly as first-line single-agent therapy in MBC, which included crossover on progression (175). Doxorubicin was significantly better than paclitaxel

Table 74.5	CALGB 9342 VERSUS CALGB 9840: WHY DIFFERENT RESULTS IF DOSE INTENSITY IS THE SAME?

CALGB 9342	Dose (mg/m^2) Every 21 days		
Study arms	175	210	250
Dose intensity (mg/m^2/week)	58.3	70	83.3
			CALGB 9840

CALGB, Cancer and Leukemia Group-B.
In CALGB 9342, higher 3-weekly paclitaxel doses (210 mg/m^2 or 250 mg/m^2) were not superior to the 175 mg/m^2 dose. The 250 mg/m^2 dose approximated to 80 mg/m^2/week which was the weekly dose used in CALGB 9840. Hence, frequency mattered, dose intensity did not.

for response rate (41% vs. 25%; p = .003) and PFS (7.5 vs. 3.9 months; p <.001) but median survival was similar (18.3 vs. 15.6 months; p = .38). In second-line therapy, crossover to doxorubicin (91 patients) and to paclitaxel (77 patients) gave response rates of 30% and 16%, respectively. In the doxorubicin arm, hematological, gastrointestinal and cardiac toxicities were more frequently observed, but this was counterbalanced by better symptom control. There was no difference in global health status or QOL after the 3rd cycle of first-line treatment.

In a three-armed Intergroup trial (E1193), 3-weekly doxorubicin 60 mg/m^2 intravenously versus paclitaxel 175 mg/m^2 over 24 hours versus the combination of doxorubicin 50 mg/m^2 followed 3 hours later by paclitaxel 150 mg/m^2 over 24 hours was compared as first-line therapy for MBC (50). Doxorubicin was administered for a maximum of eight cycles and paclitaxel was administered until disease progression. Crossover to the other drug was allowed for patients on the single-drug arms. The combination resulted in significantly superior response rates (36% for doxorubicin, 34% for paclitaxel, and 47% for AP [doxorubicin plus paclitaxel] patients; p = .84 for doxorubicin vs. paclitaxel, p = .007 for doxorubicin vs. AP, p = .004 for paclitaxel vs. AP) and TTF (5.8 months for doxorubicin, 6.0 months for paclitaxel, and 8.0 months for AP; p = .68 for doxorubicin vs. paclitaxel, p = .003 for doxorubicin vs. AP, p = .009 for paclitaxel vs. AP) but did not improve either survival or QOL compared to sequential therapy. Responses were seen in 28 of 129 (22%) of patients crossed over to paclitaxel and in 25 of 128 (20%) of patients crossed over to doxorubicin. The median TTF for crossover paclitaxel was 4.5 months and the median TTF for crossover doxorubicin was 4.2 months. Median survival for patients taking paclitaxel after entry to crossover is 14.9 months, whereas median survival for doxorubicin is 12.7 months (p = .11). Interestingly, cardiotoxicity was similar in the combination arm compared to the doxorubicin only arm (about 9%) due to the dose and schedule of administration of the two drugs together.

Possible reasons for the failure to demonstrate a benefit for the combination arm may be due to the composite response rate to sequential therapy approximating the response rate to combination therapy, the OS rate being more closely related to the underlying biology of the disease and finally, the doses and frequency of chemotherapy administration being limited when delivered in combination thus negating optimal synergism (50). Furthermore, combination therapy with its attendant increased toxicities may not deliver an improved QOL as hoped for in spite of improved TTF or response rates. Hence, there does not seem to be a "better" agent with respect to anthracyclines or taxanes and either agent can be used as up front therapy.

Because of similar survival or response duration benefits observed between anthracycline and nonanthracycline regimens in advanced breast cancer (28,536,537), this provided the rationale for the use of CMFP as a control arm for comparison with paclitaxel (32). This study compared paclitaxel 200 mg/m^2 over 3 hours every 3 weeks for eight cycles with oral cyclophosphamide 100 mg/mg^2 per day on days 1 through 14, or methotrexate 40 mg/m^2 on days 1 and 8, 5-FU 600 mg/m^2 on days 1 and 8, and oral prednisolone 40 mg/m^2 per day on days 1 through 14 (CMFP) every 28 days for six cycles as first-line therapy for MBC. The two groups had nearly identical response rates and PFS rates. However, the median survival duration was 17.3 months for paclitaxel and 13.9 months for CMFP with a 19% survival improvement at 2 years in favor of paclitaxel. This benefit may simply reflect a more optimal sequence of therapy because approximately 40% of patients in each arm received second-line anthracyclines at progression.

Docetaxel is highly active as first-line therapy or even in doxorubicin pretreated patients with overall RRs of 20% to 60% (538–545). Response to docetaxel has also been observed in

approximately 25% of MBC patients who have become resistant to paclitaxel (482). The usual IV doses range from 60 to 100 mg/m^2 every 3 weeks or 30 to 40 mg/m^2 weekly (74,92,94,532,546,547), with a lower initial dosing used for elderly, heavily pretreated patients or those with hepatic dysfunction (548,549). The optimal schedule of administration of docetaxel (weekly vs. 3-weekly) is unresolved (550). So far, weekly docetaxel has only been shown to decrease myelosuppression but does not increase efficacy.

Docetaxel has been compared with various nonanthracycline regimens in order to determine its comparative efficacy. Docetaxel 100 mg/m^2 every 3 weeks was compared with mitomycin C and vinblastine (MV) in MBC after anthracycline failure either in the metastatic setting or less than 12 months after adjuvant anthracyclines (33). This study was not designed for a crossover. At a median follow-up of 19 months, docetaxel was significantly superior to MV in terms of response (30.0% vs. 11.6%; p <.0001), TTP (19 weeks vs. 11 weeks; p = .001), and survival (11.4 months vs. 8.7 months; p =.0097). Similarly, docetaxel 100 mg/m^2 every 3 weeks compared with 5-FU 750 mg/m^2 per day continuous infusion (CI) plus vinorelbine 25 mg/m^2 days 1 and 5 every 3 weeks in anthracycline-refractory (neo/adjuvant or one line of palliative anthracycline-based chemotherapy) patients did not show any significant difference in TTP or OS (551). Docetaxel was less toxic in general except for neutropenia (82% vs. 67%; p = .02), although febrile neutropenia was less frequent (13% vs. 22%; p = .1).

Docetaxel 100 mg/m^2 every 3 weeks was also compared with sequential methotrexate and 5-FU at days 1 and 8 every 3 weeks in MBC after anthracycline failure either as first-line therapy or within 12 months of adjuvant treatment (552). Crossover was recommended in this study. There was significant difference in favor of docetaxel for RR (42% vs. 21%; p <.001), which was maintained on crossover, TTP (6.3 vs. 3 months; p <.001), but not OS at a median follow-up of 11 months. The QOL differences were minor in the two groups, hence single-agent taxane for most patients with MBC is an appropriate strategy (553).

A European study compared docetaxel 100 mg/m^2 to doxorubicin 75 mg/m^2 every 3 weeks for a maximum of seven cycles in MBC patients who have failed either adjuvant or palliative alkylating chemotherapy (176). No crossover was planned, although 26% of patients in the doxorubicin group received taxoid-containing therapy, and 28% of patients in the docetaxel group received anthracycline-containing therapy on progression. At a median follow-up of 23 months the RR rate was significantly higher with docetaxel (47.8% vs. 33.3%; p =.008), although there were similar TTP and OS rates. The difference between treatment groups remained not significant when OS was adjusted for the crossover treatment as a time-dependent covariate. The incidence of toxic deaths was higher in the doxorubicin group with increased febrile neutropenia and severe infection. Cardiac toxicities, nausea, vomiting, and stomatitis were more frequent for doxorubicin, while diarrhea, neuropathy, fluid retention, and skin or nail changes were higher for docetaxel. However, QOL scores between the two groups were not significantly different.

The value of dose escalation has been evaluated using 3-weekly docetaxel (60 mg/m^2, 75 mg/m^2 or 100 mg/m^2) for at least six cycles in women with pretreated MBC, the majority of whom had progressed after an anthracycline (74). A significant dose–response was observed for response rates (22.1% vs. 23.3% vs. 36%; p =.007) but not for TTP or survival in the intent-to-treat analysis at a median follow-up of 30 months. Most hematologic and nonhematologic toxicities were dose related, with grade 3 or 4 neutropenia and febrile neutropenia rates expectedly more frequent with higher doses of therapy.

A single randomized trial has compared 3-weekly docetaxel (100 mg/m^2) directly with paclitaxel (175 mg/m^2) in women with MBC who have failed with anthracyclines (554). The median number of cycles administered was higher in the docetaxel arm (6 cycles vs. 4 cycles), and this arm was also superior in terms of response rates (32% vs. 25%; p = .1), TTP (5.7 vs. 3.6 months; p = <0.0001) and overall survival (15.4 vs. 12.7 months; p = .03) compared to paclitaxel at a median follow-up of 5.1 years. Although both hematologic and nonhematologic toxicities were more frequent with docetaxel, with four treatment-related docetaxel deaths versus none in the paclitaxel arm, there was no statistical difference in QOL between both treatment groups over time. At present, either drug is a reasonable treatment option for MBC.

A meta-analysis using individualized patient data to detect any advantages of taxanes in first-line treatment of patients with metastatic breast cancer showed that single-agent anthracyclines were significantly better than single-agent taxanes with respect to PFS (HR 1.19; 95% CI, 1.04–1.36; p = .01), marginally better in response rate (38% vs. 33%; p =.08) but not OS (HR 1.01; 95% CI, 0.88–1.16; p = 0.90 [three trials; n = 919]). However, anthracycline taxane-based combinations resulted in significantly better response rates than anthracycline combinations (56% vs. 45%; p <.001) but were only marginally better in terms of PFS (HR 0.93; 95% CI, 0.87–1.00; p = .06) but not OS (HR 0.95; 95% CI, 0.88–1.03; p = 0.23 [nine trials; n = 3,337]) (555). The following sections will review the different taxane-based combinations and some of their pharmacological interactions.

Taxanes as Combination Therapy

AnthracyclineTaxane Combinations. The rationale for combining anthracyclines with taxanes include different mechanisms of action (topoisomerase II inhibition vs. microtubular assembly disturbance), lack of a complete cross-resistance, different dose-limiting toxicities, and a similar high efficacy in breast tumors. Pharmacokinetic studies in conjunction with clinical investigations of paclitaxel/doxorubicin and docetaxel/doxorubicin combinations have elucidated differences in their drug interactions, which may account in part for their differing clinical toxicity profiles. This section will review the pharmacology and relevant clinical trials of this drug combination.

Doxorubicin/Taxane Combinations. Clinical development of the paclitaxel/doxorubicin combination was first undertaken in 1992, but at that time investigations were hampered by a paucity of data on the optimal dose and schedule for paclitaxel itself and the best sequence and schedule for combination with doxorubicin. Initial phase I trials conducted by Holmes et al. (556) studied the sequential administration of paclitaxel 125 mg/m^2 over 24 hours before or after doxorubicin 48 mg/m^2 over 48 hours in MBC patients. Those receiving the paclitaxel → doxorubicin sequence showed an approximately one-third reduction in the clearance rate of doxorubicin and its metabolites such as doxorubicinol, resulting in greater hematological and mucosal toxicities. Reversing the sequence to doxorubicin → paclitaxel resulted in less mucositis, neutropenia, and fever (557). This was confirmed by Sledge et al. (557a) when they compared a 24-hour paclitaxel infusion before or after bolus doxorubicin separated by a 4-hour interval in MBC cases. In the first phase II trial by Gianni et al. (558), they evaluated incremental doses (by 25 mg/m^2) of paclitaxel from 125 to 200 mg/m^2 as a 3-hour infusion 15 minutes before or after bolus doxorubicin 60 mg/m^2 every 3 weeks to a maximum of eight cycles in chemonaive MBC women. Patients responding to therapy could receive subsequent paclitaxel (175 to 200 mg/m^2) every 3 weeks. The overall response rate was 94% with 41% having a complete response. Although the incidence of CHF was about 20%, it was found that the risk of cardiotoxicity

could be minimized to less than 5% if the cumulative dose of doxorubicin could be kept below 360 mg/m^2. In another well-designed pharmacological trial, Gianni et al. (559) reported that paclitaxel formulated in Cremophor EL enhanced the non-linearity of doxorubicin pharmacokinetics (PKs) and increased the concentrations of plasma doxorubicin and doxorubicinol. These effects were paclitaxel dose-dependent, doxorubicin concentration-dependent, and likely a result of competition for biliary and hepatic transporter proteins such as P-glycoprotein (Pgp). In this landmark study, the inhibition of doxorubicin clearance by the Cremophor EL vehicle, possibly due to PK interference and competition for Pgp, was demonstrated using *in vitro* cell studies. Competition for biliary excretion mediated by Pgp concerning the anthracyclines with paclitaxel or its castor oil vehicle Cremophor EL or both has also been suggested in other studies (465,560). Similar phase II evaluations of the doxorubicin/paclitaxel combination have shown similar CHF rates of about 20% but were unfortunately unable to replicate the high RRs and CR rates of the Milan trial (558) partly because of the better performance status and lack of prior chemotherapy in that study (561,562).

Available studies point to a PK interaction between doxorubicin and paclitaxel that is schedule dependent, which includes factors such as infusion duration, sequencing, and interval between administration. It is important to note that sequence-dependent interactions have been noted only with prolonged 24-hour infusions of paclitaxel and less with the more commonly used 3-hour ones. However, pharmacological interactions occur even with the 3-hour infusional schedule, and combination treatment of this with doxorubicin is associated with a higher incidence of congestive cardiotoxicity (558–560). So far this combination appears to require certain restrictions for safe use. Studies have shown that CHF is minimized if the maximum single dose of doxorubicin is 50 mg/m^2 or less, the maximum cumulative dose of doxorubicin is 360 mg/m^2 or less (563–565), the interval between drugs is at least 4 to 24 hours, liposomal doxorubicin or dexrazoxane is used, or doxorubicin is administered before paclitaxel, with paclitaxel being administered over 24 hours separated by at least a 4-hour interval after doxorubicin (566,567).

The doxorubicin/paclitaxel combination has been evaluated in several phase III trials. In the ECOG 1193 trial (50), 739 women with previously untreated MBC received doxorubicin 60 mg/m^2 or paclitaxel 175 mg/m^2 over 24 hours or the combination of doxorubicin 50 mg/m^2 followed in 4 hours by paclitaxel 150 mg/m^2 over 24 hours. At time of progression, crossover was allowed in the monotherapy arms. Tumor responses (36% vs. 34% vs. 47%) and median time-to-treatment failure (5.8 months vs. 6 months vs. 8 months) were higher in the combination group, although median survival was not significantly different (18.9 vs. 22.2 vs. 22 months) and QOL was also similar. The further response rates for both the crossover arms were approximately 20%, TTF was about 4 months, and median survival about 12 to 15 months. Moderate to severe cardiac complications were seen in 8.7% of doxorubicin, 3.7% of paclitaxel and 8.6% of combination arm patients. It appears that the combination arm did not result in a greater degree of cardiotoxicity compared to single-agent doxorubicin perhaps due to its administration schedule and dose.

An EORTC phase III trial (568) evaluated doxorubicin 60 mg/m^2 as an intravenous bolus plus paclitaxel 175 mg/m^2 as a 3-hour infusion or doxorubicin 60 mg/m^2 plus cyclophosphamide 600 mg/m^2 every 3 weeks for a maximum of six cycles. Response rates, PFS, and OS were similar. The incidence of CHF was 2% and 1%, respectively.

Another European trial (30) studied the regimen doxorubicin 50 mg/m^2 followed 24 hours later by paclitaxel 220 mg/m^2 (AT) or IV 5-FU 500 mg/m^2, doxorubicin 50 mg/m^2, cyclophosphamide 500 mg/m^2 (FAC), each administered every 3 weeks for up to eight cycles. Overall response rates were significantly higher for AT compared to FAC (68% vs. 55%, $p = .032$). Median time to progression (8.3 vs. 6.2 months; $p = .034$); and OS (23.3 vs. 18.3 months; $p = .013$) at a median follow-up of 29 months were also significantly longer for AT compared with FAC. About 25% of patients on FAC received taxanes on progression. Neutropenia was the most frequently encountered toxicity, with grade 3 or 4 toxicity observed in 89% of patients receiving AT and in 65% of patients receiving FAC ($p < .001$), although there was no difference in the incidence of febrile neutropenia between the AT and FAC arms (8% and 5% of patients, respectively; $p = .339$). The incidence of cardiotoxicity (LVEF $< 50\%$) was similarly low (about 6%) in both arms. Baseline QOL scores were similar between the two treatment groups. In summary, combination anthracycline/taxane therapy does not result in notable increases in response rates compared to sequential single-agent therapy, or standard regimens such as AC or FAC.

The docetaxel/doxorubicin combination possesses notable activity, but interestingly, clinically significant cardiac toxicity does not appear to exceed the incidence expected with doxorubicin alone (569–571). Schuller et al. (572) investigated the sequence of doxorubicin 50 mg/m² followed by docetaxel 75 mg/m² over 1 hour separated by an hour versus not and found the clearance of doxorubicin did not change for both regimens. However, doxorubicin significantly increased the AUC for docetaxel in both schedules. Another similarly designed study by Bellot et al. (573) did not reveal any significant PK interactions of doxorubicin and docetaxel or their metabolites, and the safety profile was similar in the two groups. It is of interest that PK-induced toxic effects have not been noted with docetaxel, which does not possess the castor oil vehicle Cremophor EL. The lack of cardiac conduction disturbances, its linear pharmacokinetics, and its short infusion time enable it to be given on an outpatient basis, make the doxorubicin/docetaxel regimen an attractive combination (566). Phase II studies of TAC (doxorubicin 50 mg/m² bolus followed by cyclophosphamide 500 mg/m² bolus, then docetaxel 75 mg/m², 1-hour infusion an hour after completion of doxorubicin infusion for a maximum of eight 3-week cycles have shown high response rates of 77% (6% complete response), with the incidence of anthracycline-induced cardiomyopathy at a similar rate to single-agent doxorubicin (574).

Randomized phase III trials comparing doxorubicin 50 mg/m² plus docetaxel 75 mg/m² (AT) to doxorubicin 60 mg/m² plus cyclophosphamide 600 mg/m² (AC) have shown significantly superior outcomes for AT in terms of response rates (59% vs. 47%; $p = .009$) and TTP (median, 37.3 vs. 31.9 weeks; $p = 0.014$), although 4-year survival was essentially similar (418). Low rates of CHF occurred in 3% of patients receiving AT and 4% receiving AC, although the cumulative dose of doxorubicin was greater than 360 mg/m² in more than half of the patients in each group.

A Dutch clinical trial comparing doxorubicin 50 mg/m² and docetaxel 75 mg/m² to 5-FU 500 mg/m², doxorubicin 50 mg/m², cyclophosphamide 500 mg/m² (FAC) as first-line therapy in MBC showed a significantly higher RR (58% vs. 37%; $p = .003$), longer TTP (8 vs. 6.6 months; $p = .004$) and OS (22.6 vs. 16.2 months; $p = .019$) for the doxorubicin/docetaxel arm, demonstrating that this combination was a valid treatment option for MBC (575). Neutropenic fever and grade 3 to 4 infections were more frequently observed in patients treated with doxorubicin/docetaxel with two toxic deaths in this group. A phase III study evaluated TAC (75/50/500 mg/m²) with FAC (500/50/500 mg/m²) as first-line treatment for metastatic disease and found the former to have a significantly higher response rate (55% vs. 44%; $p = .02$) with equivalent TTP and OS rates (576). A higher incidence of grade 3 and 4 hematological and nonhematological toxicities were reported with TAC, including more cardiotoxicity (clinical CHF 2.4% vs. 0.4%).

In a randomized phase III study by the Spanish Breast Cancer Research Group (GEICAM 9903), doxorubicin and docetaxel administered in sequence were found to have equivalent outcomes to being administered concurrently with significantly less febrile neutropenia rates (58). An additional trial, the ERASME 3 French study, which was recently published, compared doxorubicin/docetaxel to doxorubicin/paclitaxel every 3 weeks for a maximum of four cycles, then four cycles of single-agent docetaxel or paclitaxel respectively for first-line therapy in MBC and found no difference in RR, median PFS, OS, and QOL (577).

Epirubicin/Taxane Combinations. Esposito et al. (578) examined the comparative effects of paclitaxel or docetaxel on the PK of epirubicin in breast cancer patients. Chemotherapy consisted of epirubicin alone 90 mg/m² given as an IV bolus; epirubicin 90 mg/m² given as an IV bolus followed immediately by paclitaxel 175 mg/m² in a 3-hour infusion; epirubicin 90 mg/m² given as an IV bolus followed by docetaxel 70 mg/m² in a 1-hour infusion every 3 weeks. No change in the PK of epirubicin was found when it was administered before the taxanes. However, there were differences in its metabolism with a statistically significant increase in plasma epirubinol (EOL) with subsequent paclitaxel but not with docetaxel. This may be due to the different vehicle formulations (Cremophor EL for paclitaxel vs. Tween 80 for docetaxel) as the former is also known to increase the bioavailability of doxorubicin and its major metabolite, doxorubicinol (579). Both taxanes cause a significant increase in the plasma levels of the aglycone metabolite 7d-Aone as well as the glucuronidase-sensitive metabolites of epirubicin (578). It has been suggested that an inverse relationship may exist between the 7-deoxy-aglycones from epirubicin and the generation of cardiotoxic free radicals (580). Hence, the differing mechanisms of epirubicin metabolism induced by paclitaxel (increased plasma levels of EOL, 7d-Aone, and glucuronide metabolites) in contrast to docetaxel (increased plasma levels of 7d-Aone and glucuronide metabolites) may account for a resulting difference in cardiotoxicity. Phase I and II studies suggest a similar high level of activity and a low cardiac toxicity incidence for the epirubicin/docetaxel and doxorubicin/docetaxel regimens (579). In conclusion, both the differing vehicle formulations as well as the intrinsic properties of the taxanes themselves play a role in epirubicin metabolism. The absence of significant cardiotoxicity and the limited severity of other nonhematologic toxicities make the epirubicin/ taxane combination highly attractive.

The epirubicin/paclitaxel combination, although active and well tolerated, had an apparently lower activity than that reported with the doxorubicin/paclitaxel combination although differences in pre-treatment chemotherapy exposure could explain this disparity (580a). The dose-limiting factor of the epirubicin/paclitaxel combination is grade 3 or 4 hematologic toxicities (579).

Phase III studies, such as the U.K. National Cancer Research Institute trial AB01 (581) and a study by the Ago Breast Cancer Group (582), have directly compared epirubicin/paclitaxel to epirubicin/cyclophosphamide in first-line treatment af MBC and have shown equivalent outcomes in terms of PFS for both studies and OS for the former.

A meta-analysis was published in 2005 to determine whether the anthracycline/taxane combination provided an advantage over standard anthracycline-based regimens (583). Seven phase III trials (three published original articles and four abstracts) were collected up to October 2003. Significant differences in favor of the anthracycline-taxane combination were observed for ORR (RR 1.21; 95% CI, 1.10–1.32; $p < 0.001$) in the pooled analysis; translating into a 21% benefit, with the anthracycline/taxane group twice as likely to achieve a CR. A borderline significance for anthracycline/taxane therapy was also observed for TTP (RR 1.1, 95% CI, 1.00–1.21; p = .05); translating into a 6% to 10% benefit, as well as a nonsignificant trend for OS. However, there were significantly increased rates of neutropenia and febrile neutropenia with anthracycline/taxane combinations compared to nontaxane containing regimens. However, the results of this meta-analysis are hampered by incomplete information based only on abstracts, substantial variation of follow-up durations, and a lack of analysis based on individualized patient data.

In general, most of these trials are underpowered and they lack a preplanned crossover design in their monotherapy arms. Hence, there is no clear benefit of the anthracycline/taxane combination over sequential single agents. One instance in which this combination could be used is in patients with symptomatic rapidly progressive visceral metastases in whom expected survival would be limited in the absence of effective therapy. Such a regimen may be needed as first-line treatment as the patient may deteriorate too quickly for a later alternative regimen to be tested.

Platinum/Taxane Combinations. Taxane/platinum combinations have been studied in the hopes of developing an effective nonanthracycline-based regimen. Like the anthracycline/taxane combinations, there have been pharmacological interactions in the form of sequence-dependent interactions observed when paclitaxel was administered over 24 hours or longer with cisplatin. It was demonstrated that when cisplatin was administered prior to paclitaxel (over 24 hours), it caused a more profound neutropenia possibly due to 25% lower paclitaxel clearance rates (584). *In vitro* studies have shown a suboptimal cytotoxic effect when cisplatin was administered before paclitaxel (585,586). Although the mechanisms of this is unclear at present, several postulations have been made such as (a) the depression of the cytochrome P450 enzymes by cisplatin, causing inadequate metabolism of paclitaxel by this pathway (587) or (b) cisplatin being able to inhibit cells in the G2 phase, thereby preventing progression to the M phase; a phase in which cells are known to be sensitive to taxanes (588), or (c) paclitaxel can inhibit cisplatin-DNA adducts (588).

Carboplatin, in contrast, does not seem capable of significantly modulating the enzymes of the cytochrome P450 system and does not affect the pharmacokinetics of paclitaxel (587,589). Paclitaxel and carboplatin in combination cause less severe thrombocytopenia compared with carboplatin alone, which is not explained by pharmacokinetic interactions (590,591).

Unlike paclitaxel, sequence-dependent effects have not been observed with docetaxel/cisplatin combinations in which docetaxel is administered over 1 hour (592).

The combination of platinums and taxanes is ideal as both are active agents in breast cancer and both have nonoverlapping toxicities (except for neurotoxicity) and are non–cross-resistant. Furthermore, these agents are not used as frequently as anthracyclines in the adjuvant setting.

The cisplatin/paclitaxel regimen can be administered weekly, biweekly, or 3-weekly (444,446,437,445). Cisplatin plus paclitaxel 3-weekly has been administered with paclitaxel given as 24-hour continuous infusions or 3-hour infusions with the absence of a significant benefit for the former (527,593). Hence, every 3 weeks paclitaxel is administered over 3 hours. The response rates for cisplatin/paclitaxel range from about 45% to 80%, with an average response rate of about 60% in the first-line setting (437,594–596). Responses have been confirmed even when used beyond first-line therapy (mean RR 47%) (437,595,596). Weekly cisplatin/paclitaxel (cisplatin 40 mg/m^2 and paclitaxel 75 to 85 mg/m^2 on day 1 with granulocyte cell stimulating factor) has shown good RRs of 81% as first-line and 37% as subsequent line treatment, respectively (597). There is no established data on whether the weekly or 2–3

weekly schedules are superior, but the latter may be preferred in terms of patient convenience.

Cisplatin/docetaxel has shown RRs ranging from 55% to 60% (mean, 58%) as first-line treatment (598,599). Cisplatin and docetaxel doublets have RRs of 36% to 56% (average 47%) and RRs of about 50% when docetaxel is used at doses of 80 and 100 mg/m^2, respectively (437,438,600–602). A randomized phase II trial comparing docetaxel 60 mg/m^2/cisplatin 50 mg/m^2 with paclitaxel 175 mg/m^2/cisplatin 50 mg/m^2 every 3 weeks in 101 patients with advanced breast cancer showed a nonsignificant difference in favor of the docetaxel-containing combination in terms of overall RR (62.5% vs. 42.6%) and TTP (9.8 vs. 6.5 months), although OS was similar (22.7 vs. 22.4 months) (603).

Carboplatin/paclitaxel doublets have been shown in various studies to have a RR of approximately 39% to 62% (mean, 51%) (437,531,604–607). The average RR is higher than one would expect for each individual agent alone, hence the effect of this combination appears to be additive. In a phase III study by the Hellenic Cooperation Oncology Group, 327 women with advanced breast cancer were randomized to first-line paclitaxel 175 mg/m^2 over 3 hours followed by epirubicin 80 mg/m^2 or paclitaxel at the same dose followed by carboplatin AUC 6 mg × minute/mL every 3 weeks for six cycles (605). Previous anthracycline adjuvant therapy had been received in 28% and 24% of each arm, respectively. Median TTF (8.1 vs. 10.8 months; p = .04) was significantly better for the carboplatin/paclitaxel arm, although RR (47% vs. 41%; p = .32) and median survival (22.4 vs. 27.8 months; p = .25) was similar. Both regimens were well tolerated with no significant differences in the QOL analysis. Studies have also examined the carboplatin/docetaxel combination and have shown RRs of about 40% to 60% (608–610). In view of its shorter infusion time and its comparable RRs to the carboplatin/paclitaxel combination, the carboplatin/docetaxel regimen warrants further study.

Hence, the taxane/platinum combination can be incorporated into first-line regimens for MBC particularly if higher response rates are needed and if anthracyclines are contraindicated. Given its more favorable toxicity profile, carboplatin may be preferred over cisplatin. In the setting of MBC, it is not common for a combination regimen to demonstrate a survival benefit compared to single-agent therapy. The following two sections will illustrate two taxane-containing combinations that show a benefit over taxane monotherapy.

Capecitabine/Taxane Combinations. The capecitabine/taxane combination has been found to be active in phase II studies (326,327,611), even in anthracycline pretreated patients, and this regimen has progressed to phase III trials with encouraging results. In a phase III trial of 511 women with anthracycline-refractory MBC, where capecitabine 1,250 mg/m^2 twice daily from days 1 to 14 and docetaxel 75 mg/m^2 on day 1 every 21 days was compared with docetaxel 100 mg/m^2 every 3 weeks in patients with MBC, there were significantly superior tumor response rates (42% vs. 30%; p = .006), TTP (median, 6.1 vs. 4.2 months; p = .0001) and OS (median, 14.5 vs. 11.5 months; p = .0126) (29). Gastrointestinal side effects and hand-foot syndrome were more pronounced with combination therapy, whereas myalgia, arthralgia, and neutropenic fever were more common with docetaxel, although QOL was similar. However, this study did not mandate a crossover and only 17% of patients on docetaxel received the new investigational drug capecitabine on progression, raising a doubt on the magnitude of benefit the combination provided over single-agent docetaxel (612). An interesting aspect of this study is the synergy between docetaxel and capecitabine, even if the nature of this interaction has yet to be fully defined (61,613). The FDA has since approved the capecitabine/docetaxel combination for first-line treatment of MBC patients pretreated with anthracyclines.

Interestingly, a lack of PFS or survival benefit was shown for the sequential single-agent capecitabine followed by paclitaxel or docetaxel on progression or combined capecitabine with either of the taxanes, although response rates were higher for the combination arms (56).

Although not as widely accepted as the capecitabine/docetaxel regimen, capecitabine combined with paclitaxel has been studied in various small MBC phase I and II studies in Europe and the United States as first-line therapy or after an anthracycline (326,327,611,614–616). Capecitabine plus paclitaxel administered weekly or 3-weekly revealed response rates ranging from 40% to 73%, with an OS of up to 30 months (617). The combination had a fairly tolerable safety profile with the most common grade 3 or 4 adverse events for the 3-weekly paclitaxel schedule being alopecia, hand-foot syndrome, and neutropenia (617). Nail toxicity, hand-foot syndrome, and neutropenia were the common grade 3 or 4 toxicities for the weekly paclitaxel regimen (617).

The combination of capecitabine and paclitaxel was found to have a comparable efficacy to epirubicin and paclitaxel in first-line treatment of MBC (618).

Gemcitabine/Taxane Combinations. The gemcitabine/taxane combination is another regimen evaluated for its efficacy in the metastatic setting. A phase III trial compared gemcitabine 1,250 mg/m^2 on days 1 and 8 with paclitaxel 175 mg/m^2 on day 1 versus paclitaxel 175 mg/m^2 alone on day 1 every 21 days in 529 women with MBC (34). Almost all (96%) had prior adjuvant/neoadjuvant anthracycline treatment. The gemcitabine group had a significantly better response rate (41.4% vs. 26.2%; $p = .0002$), TTP (6.14 vs. 3.98 months; $p = .0002$), and median survival (18.6 vs. 15.8 mths; $p = .0489$). The lack of a planned crossover did not allow for analysis of a combination versus sequential approach. As expected, gemcitabine/paclitaxel had higher rates of grade 3/4 neutropenia (47.9% vs. 11.5%) and febrile neutropenia (5% vs. 1.2%). Based on the data, gemcitabine combined with paclitaxel was approved by the FDA in May 2004 for the first-line treatment of patients previously treated with neo/adjuvant anthracyclines. To date, it remains unclear if this combination is better than each agent used in succession since toxicities for the combined regimen are greater and survival benefits modest.

Gemcitabine/docetaxel as first or subsequent line therapy has been examined in phase II trials and found to have a response rate of about 50% to 80% (357–360). Both regimens were found to have equivalent outcomes in a randomized trial comparing gemcitabine/docetaxel versus capecitabine/docetaxel as first or second-line therapy in women with MBC who had relapsed after an anthracycline-based regimen, although more treatment toxicity-related discontinuations were present in the latter arm (27% vs. 14%) (619).

5FU/Taxane Combinations. Paclitaxel with 5-FU and leucovorin have been studied in the phase II setting both as first-line or in pretreated patients and found to be active (RR approximately 50%) and well tolerated particularly in those who are not candidates for anthracycline-based therapy, even in the elderly (≥65 years) and those with hepatic dysfunction (620,621).

Docetaxel/Paclitaxel Combinations. The low dose combination arm of paclitaxel 40 mg/m^2 and docetaxel 25 mg/m^2 administered on days 1 and 8, 3-weekly in previously treated patients with MBC, all of whom had received prior anthracyclines and majority of whom had received prior taxanes, showed an overall response rate of 68% and a median duration of response of 10 months (622). Myelosuppression was rare and grade 3 cutaneous toxicity was observed in only two patients, but this approach is hard to justify clinically.

In summary, taxanes have established themselves as cornerstones of first-line therapy for nonendocrine-response and hormone-refractory MBC, particularly as anthracyclines are commonly used in the adjuvant setting. They have an abundance of clinical data and have demonstrated a small but potentially important survival advantage compared to nonanthracycline regimens (32,33). Furthermore, if used judiciously, they are reasonably well tolerated, although questions remain pertaining to their optimal use in terms of combination with other chemotherapy and targeted agents.

Nanoparticle Formulations

ABI-007 or nab-paclitaxel (Abraxane; Abraxis Bioscience, Los Angeles, California) is a Cremophor-free formulation of paclitaxel prepared by its homogenization with human-albumin with resultant particle size approximately 130 nm (623). This nanometer particle albumin-bound paclitaxel was designed to avoid the toxicities associated with polyethylated castor oil. It does not require steroid premedication and it permits a higher paclitaxel concentration in solution that is delivered as a decreased infusion volume over 30 minutes without the need for special administration sets.

Several studies have proven that the use of nab-paclitaxel, both as weekly or 3 weekly infusion, is active and well tolerated with minimal HSRs (624–627). The objective response is higher for patients undergoing first-line as opposed to beyond first-line therapy (64% vs. 21%) (624). The recommended dose is 260 mg/m^2 every 3 weeks. Superiority of nab-paclitaxel relative to conventional paclitaxel was suggested in a phase III multicentered trial of 460 patients with MBC randomly assigned to either ABI-007 (260 mg/m^2 IV over 30 minutes) or standard paclitaxel (175 mg/m^2 IV over 3 hours) both on day 1 every 21 days (625). Eighty-eight percent of the study population had prior chemotherapy and 41% had experienced progression after first-line therapy for metastatic disease. In addition, 50% of patients had previously received anthracycline-based therapy for metastatic disease. Nab-paclitaxel demonstrated a higher ORR than for standard paclitaxel (33% vs. 19%, respectively; $p = .001$), even in those who had received prior anthracycline therapy in either the adjuvant/metastatic setting (34% vs. 18%, respectively; $p = .002$) or the metastatic setting only (27% vs. 14%, respectively; $p = .010$). Median TTP was also significantly longer with nab-paclitaxel than with standard paclitaxel (23.0 weeks vs. 16.9 weeks, respectively; HR = 0.75; $p = .006$). There was a trend for greater median survival for all patients treated with nab-paclitaxel than with standard paclitaxel (65.0 vs. 55.7 weeks, respectively; $p = .374$). Although the nab-paclitaxel group received an average paclitaxel dose-intensity 49% greater than that received in the standard paclitaxel group, no differences in QOL were noted between the two treatment groups. The incidence of treatment-related grade 4 neutropenia was significantly lower in the nab-paclitaxel group than in the standard paclitaxel group (9% vs. 22%; $p < .001$), although febrile neutropenia was low (<2%) in both groups. However, grade 3 sensory neuropathy occurred more frequently in the nab-paclitaxel arm (10% vs. 2%; $p < .001$). No grade 3 or 4 HSRs occurred with nab-paclitaxel despite the absence of premedication and shorter infusion time.

The albumin-bound nanoparticle nab-paclitaxel was designed to preferentially deliver paclitaxel to tumors by biologically interacting with albumin receptors that mediate drug transport. *In vitro* studies have demonstrated a 4.2-fold increase in paclitaxel transport across endothelial cells for nab-paclitaxel compared with standard paclitaxel (628), possibly due to inhibition of this transport mechanism by the polyethylated castor oil (629). An overexpression of SPARC (secreted protein, acidic and rich in cysteine), an albumin-binding protein expressed by breast tumor cells may account for increased tumor accumulation of nab-paclitaxel (630).

Nab-paclitaxel as a single agent is approved in the United States for relapsed or refractory MBC for which prior therapy should have included an anthracycline unless clinically contraindicated. Both myelosuppression and sensory neuropathy are dose-limiting toxicities. The appropriate dose of nab-paclitaxel for those with bilirubin greater than 1.5 mg/dL or creatinine greater than 2 mg/dL is not known (Lexi-Comp, Inc, Copyright 1978–2009). Despite certain advantages over conventional paclitaxel, especially the lack of premedication, it is more costly and its role in the treatment of MBC relative to unbound paclitaxel or docetaxel is not established. Nab-paclitaxel is currently under study in combination with other agents in the metastatic setting (631).

Epothilones

The epothilones and their analogs are a new class of chemotherapeutic agents. These compounds, structurally homologous to a family of 16-membered macrolide antibiotics, were initially discovered as cytotoxic metabolites from the mycobacterium *Sorangium cellulosum* (632). They represent the first class of compounds to be described in two decades following the original discovery of paclitaxel, and their microtubule-stabilizing action is similar to taxanes. They share the same microtubule-binding site and similar microtubule affinity as paclitaxel and result in cell cycle arrest at the G2-M transition, leading to apoptotic cell death (633). However, they are structurally distinct. Unlike taxanes and anthracyclines, epothilones have a low susceptibility to multiple mechanisms of drug resistance such as efflux transporters (P-glycoprotein and MDR protein-1) and class III isoform of β-tubulin (634–637). Ixabepilone (Ixempra; BMS-247550; Bristol-Meyers Squibb, New York) is a semisynthetic analog of epothilone B and was the first approved agent in this class.

Single-Agent Ixabepilone

Ixabepilone is FDA approved for use as monotherapy in the treatment of locally advanced or metastatic breast cancer after failure of anthracyclines, taxanes, and capecitabine (638). The recommended dose of ixabepilone is 40 mg/m^2 IV over a 3-hour infusion every 21 days as determined in phase I studies (639), with premedication consisting of an H1 antagonist and an H2 antagonist approximately 1 hour before. Additional premedication with dexamethasone is only required in patients who experienced an HSR to ixabepilone (638). Ixabepilone is extensively metabolized by the liver; hence dose reduction is necessary in liver impairment. Ixabepilone in combination with capecitabine must not be administered when the AST or ALT is greater than 2.5 times ULN or bilirubin greater than 1 times ULN due to increased toxicity and neutropenia-related deaths (638). Inhibitors or inducers of CYP3A4 may increase or decrease plasma concentrations of ixabepilone, respectively.

The most common adverse reactions include peripheral sensory neuropathy, fatigue, asthenia, myalgia, arthralgia, nausea and vomiting, mucositis, stomatitis, diarrhea, and musculoskeletal pain (638). In general, the rate of ixabepilone-associated neurotoxicity appears to be comparable to that observed in weekly paclitaxel (640). As with taxanes, the formulation of ixabepilone in polyoxyethylated castor oil may be partly responsible for its neurotoxicity (641). Myelosuppression is also quite common.

Ixabepilone (40 mg/m^2 over 3 hours every 21 days) evaluated in a phase II study of MBC or locally advanced breast cancer resistant to anthracyclines, taxanes, and capecitabine showed a RR of 18.3% (95% CI, 11.9%–26.1%), while 50% of patients had stable disease (14.3% remained free of progression for 6 months or more) (642). Median duration of response was 5.7 months and median OS was 8.6 months. Grade 3 or 4 sensory neuropathy occurred in 14%. Comparable results were noted in taxane-resistant MBC given in 1- or 3-hour infusions of ixabepilone 50 mg/m^2, but the dose was subsequently modified to 40 mg/m^2 over 3 hours every 3 weeks (643). The RR at 40 mg/m^2 was 12% (95% CI, 4.7%–26.5%), median duration of response was 10.4 months, and median survival 7.9 months.

Two small phase II studies examined ixabepilone in taxane-naive or minimally exposed patients. Roche et al. (644) noted an overall response rate of about 41% after ixabepilone 40 mg/m^2 over 3 hours every 3 weeks in MBC patients (n = 65) who had received a prior anthracycline-based adjuvant regimen. Denduluri et al. (645) examined a different schedule of ixabepilone 6 mg/m^2 per day IV on days 1 to 5 every 3 weeks in MBC patients (n = 23) who were taxane naive and noted a 57% partial response rate. Median time to progression and duration of response were 5.5 and 5.6 months, respectively, and 52% experienced grade 1 or 2 sensory neurotoxicity (none grade 3 or 4). Another phase II study (n = 37) used an identical ixabepilone schedule over 5 days every 3 weeks in taxane-exposed patients and revealed a low risk of grade 3/4 sensory neuropathy (3%) (646). There were 13 with stable disease (35%), 7 with partial response (19%) and 1 with complete response (3%). Weekly schedules are being further explored.

Ixabepilone as Combination Therapy

Ixabepilone was also FDA approved in combination with capecitabine in the treatment of metastatic or locally advanced breast cancer after failure of anthracyclines and taxanes (638). Ixabepilone has also been investigated in combination with other chemotherapeutic agents. A phase III study compared ixabepilone 40 mg/m^2 on day 1 plus capecitabine 2,000 mg/m^2 on days 1 to 14 versus capecitabine 2,500 mg/m^2 on days 1 to 14 every 21 days in 752 patients with anthracycline-pretreated or -resistant and taxane-resistant locally advanced or metastatic breast cancer (647). Fifteen percent of patients were *ERBB2* positive; 8% had progressed within 1 year of prior adjuvant anthracycline/taxane therapy, and 92% received ixabepilone as second- or third-line therapy. The combination was superior to single-agent capecitabine regarding the primary endpoint of PFS (5.8 vs. 4.2 months) with an HR of 0.75 (95% CI, 0.64–0.88) and RR (35% vs. 14%; *p* <.0001). Clinical benefit in favor of combination therapy was maintained across subgroups, including patients aged 65 years or older with ERBB2-positive disease.

The magnitude of this benefit after anthracycline and taxane exposure in progression-free survival is comparable with that observed after first-line capecitabine/docetaxel chemotherapy in taxane-naive patients and is clinically meaningful (29). However, peripheral sensory neuropathy occurred in 65% of patients treated with the combination (16% in the capecitabine-only arm) with fatigue and neutropenia (68% vs. 11%) also more frequent in the combination arm (647). Risk of death was high (31%) among those with grade 2 or higher liver function tests (AST or ALT 2.5 or greater times ULN or bilirubin 1.5 or greater times ULN) (647). Studies evaluating the role of ixabepilone in combination with trastuzumab, bevacizumab, or liposomal doxorubicin in advanced breast cancer are ongoing (639).

Vinca Alkaloids

Background

Vinca derivatives were the first in a new class of drugs now known as "spindle poisons," and only two vinca alkaloids, vincristine and vinblastine, were approved for use in the United States until 1994. Vinblastine is derived from the Madagascar periwinkle plant (*Vinca rosea*, now called *Catharanthis rosea*) (648). Vinorelbine (VNB) is a semisynthetic derivative of vinblastine with broad antitumor activity and was FDA approved for the treatment of non–small cell lung cancer in 1994 and registered for advanced breast cancer in many countries (649,650). This following sections will focus on this drug.

Structure

The vinca alkaloids are large dimeric asymmetrical molecules composed of two multiringed units; an indole nucleus (catharanthine) linked to a dihydroindole nucleus (vindoline) (588). The semisynthetic vinblastine derivative vinorelbine has been structurally modified on its catharanthine nucleus.

Mechanism of Action

The principal mechanism of action is to prevent assembly of microtubules, inhibiting DNA replication (651). However, they are capable of many other disruptive biologic activities that may or may not be related to their effects on microtubules, including competition for amino acid transport into cells, inhibition of purine, RNA, DNA, and protein biosynthesis, disruption of lipid metabolism, elevation of oxidized glutathione, alterations in release of antidiuretic hormone, inhibition of histamine release, enhanced epinephrine release, inhibition of calcium-calmodulin–regulated cyclic adenosine monophosphate phosphodiesterase, and disruption in the cell membrane and membrane function (588). Vinca alkaloids induce cytotoxicity in the G1, S, and mitotic phases of the cell cycle (588).

Drug Resistance

Two basic mechanisms of drug resistance to the vinca alkaloids have been described. The first is resistance by the P-glycoprotein mediated multidrug resistance (MDR) system which can be innate or acquired (652). The second is due to structural and functional alterations in the α- or β-tubulin, perhaps from mechanisms such as genetic mutations or posttranslational modifications (653–655).

Pharmacokinetics

VNB is widely distributed and high levels are found in all tissue except the brain (650,656–658). The liver plays a major role in drug metabolism (659), with the principal route of excretion in the feces (33% to 80%), whereas urinary excretion represents only 16% to 30% of drug elimination (660,661). The majority of VNB excreted in the urine is in the form of unchanged drug (659). No dose adjustments are required for renal insufficiency, but dose reduction is needed in patients with hepatic dysfunction.

Drug Interactions

VNB is a major substrate of the cytochrome P450 CYP3A4 isoenzyme (649,662), hence drugs that induce or inhibit the CYP3A4 pathway will decrease or increase the levels of VNB, respectively.

Toxicities

The dose-limiting toxicity of VNB is neutropenia, occurring in almost 90% of patients at some point, with nadirs occurring within 7 to 10 days and resolving within 2 to 3 weeks. It can also cause peripheral neuropathy principally sensory in nature in 20% to 25% of patients. Although it can cause mild to moderate nausea and vomiting, other gastrointestinal symptoms such as constipation, diarrhea, or stomatitis although frequent are usually mild. Pancreatitis has been reported with VNB (663). Mild and reversible alopecia occurs in about 10–30% of patients. Rash, dermatitis, and photosensitivity are rare. Hand-foot syndrome was described in patients who had been given a prolonged 96-hour infusion of VNB (664). Discomfort and phlebitis may also occur, especially if following administration of the drug the vein is not adequately flushed. Vinca alkaloids are vesicants and care must be taken during administration to avoid extravasation and resulting local tissue damage. Dyspnea has been rarely observed in patients after the first or subsequent cycles of VNB due to postulated allergic or endothelium-alveolar damage mechanisms (665). An acute respiratory distress syndrome can also occur. Liver toxicity manifesting as an increased aspartate transaminase (67%) and increased total bilirubin (5–13%) may occur. SIADH is a rare side effect of VNB and the hyponatremia generally responds to fluid restriction (666,667). VNB can rarely induce acute severe peritumoral pain during or immediately after the infusion (668). This reaction, although occasionally recurrent, is self-limiting with no residual long-term effects.

Clinical Trials

Vincristine is more commonly used in pediatric rather than adult malignancies due to their better tolerance to this agent and greater tumor sensitivity. In small phase II studies of breast cancer, response rates to single-agent vincristine are usually low (about 10% or less) (669,670). Vincristine's side effect is dose-limiting neurotoxicity, which has limited its use compared to less toxic options such as vinorelbine, vindesine and vinblastine (671–676). VNB is often used in older women concerned about the subjective side effects of chemotherapy (677). It is a reasonably active monotherapy given at doses of 20 to 30 mg/m² weekly with acceptable neurotoxicity, hematological, and gastrointestinal toxicity profiles. Other schedules of VNB (continuous 96-hour infusions or day 1 to 3 dose escalation schedules every 3 weeks) have been tested and found to have increased toxicity without improved efficacy (678,679).

Intravenous VNB has been studied in combination with anthracyclines such as epirubicin, doxorubicin, and mitoxantrone (42,680–682), antimetabolites such as 5-FU (683,684), capecitabine (685) and methotrexate (686), alkylating agents such as CTX (687), cisplatin (688) and carboplatin (689), and taxanes such as docetaxel (690) and paclitaxel (691). Although combination regimens may achieve a higher response rate, the risk of toxicity is higher and overall survival is not improved. Mitomycin/vinblastine was frequently used in the pretaxane era (692). When compared to docetaxel in a large phase III trial, this combination offers a worse survival, TTP, and overall response along with a higher risk for hemolytic-uremic syndrome and thrombocytopenia (33).

An oral formulation of VNB (about 40% bioavailable) is approved outside the United States at doses of 60 to 80 mg/m² per week (693,694). Although no head-to-head studies have directly compared the efficacy of the oral and IV formulations, data from patients with non–small cell lung cancer have shown that both have comparable activity (695), and two phase II studies have demonstrated the efficacy of oral VNB as first-line, single-agent therapy (696,697) with RR approximately 30%. Combinations with other chemotherapy drugs like capecitabine and trastuzumab are being tested (698–702).

Topoisomerase Inhibitors

Etoposide (VP-16)

Etoposide is a semisynthetic epipodophyllotoxin derived from the root of the plant *Podophyllum peltatum*, commonly known as the mandrake. It is a topoisomerase II inhibitor that causes DNA damage via at least two mechanisms (703), one by blocking the religation reaction of topoisomerase IIα and the other causing DNA strand breaks and formation of crosslinks with resulting secondary DNA fragmentation and cell death by apoptosis

(704–706). Etoposide has predominant effects on the late S and G2 phases, and resistance is due to diverse mechanisms such as low levels of topoisomerase II gene expression and possibly mutations or overexpression of the MDR phenotype (707–709).

Despite extensive use in other malignancies, etoposide has played a minor role in the treatment of patients with breast cancer, and most studies tested it using the oral formulation. Its oral absorption is erratic with approximately 50% bioavailability and not improved by food intake or fasting (710). The drug undergoes hepatic metabolism to a variable extent, with the major excretory route being renal (about 35% excreted as parent drug) (711). Etoposide should be used with caution and dosage adjusted in hepatic and renal impairment. Although there is no FDA-approved hepatic dosing adjustment guideline, it has been recommended by some to reduce the dose by 50% if the bilirubin is 1.5 to 3.0 mg/dL or the AST is more than 3 times upper limit of normal (712). Etoposide is metabolized mostly via CYP3A4; hence inducers of this pathway may decrease the levels of etoposide. Conversely, CYP3A4 inhibitors may increase the levels and side effects of etoposide. Etoposide used concurrently with warfarin may elevate prothrombin time.

The main toxicities are myelosuppression (especially leucopenia) and gastrointestinal (especially nausea and vomiting, anorexia, and diarrhea). Mucositis and alopecia are usually mild and anaphylaxis may occur in 1% to 2% of patients (713). Phase II trials showed that etoposide has objective response or stable disease rates of 20% to 50%, even in heavily pretreated patients (714–721). Oral etoposide is a reasonable salvage regimen because of its ease of administration, relatively low toxicity profile, and reasonable activity rate. Small phase II studies have studied the role of oral or IV VP-16 in combination with platinum agents as first-line or beyond first-line therapy with encouraging results (450,722–727). Cisplatin/VP-16 was compared to CMF and found to have a trend toward better response rates of borderline significance (63% vs. 48%; p = .08) but with more hematological and frequent gastrointestinal toxicities (728). Of interest, cisplatin plus oral VP-16 was found to be superior to paclitaxel with respect to response rates and survival in anthracycline resistant MBC (440).

Irinotecan/Topotecan

Irinotecan (a topoisomerase I inhibitor) weekly or 3 weekly has activity in previously treated patients with MBC, but the observed response rates thus far have not been encouraging (729). Similarly, the observed rate with topotecan in the first-line setting were not encouraging (730).

Metronomic Chemotherapy

The concept of "metronomic" chemotherapy delivered so as to maximize potential antiangiogenic properties involves more frequent, regular scheduling using doses well below the maximum tolerated dose (MTD) for extended periods (731). In fact, continuous infusion of 5-FU, which has been reported to be successful in the treatment of MBC, appears to be an early example of "metronomically" delivered chemotherapy. Studies of oral CTX (50 mg daily) and MTX (2.5 mg twice daily on days 1 and 4) in advanced breast cancer either as first-line or beyond suggest that this is a well-tolerated regimen with some degree of activity (732). In one study, the RR was 21% (41% clinical benefit), median TTP 3.8 months, and the most frequent toxicity was transaminitis in 56% of subjects (733). Combination oral UFT and CTX have also been explored (734), and there is interest in testing these chemotherapy approaches combined with antiangiogenesis-targeted antibodies and tyrosine kinase inhibitors. If proven effective, metronomic schedules may offer improve QOL and potentially be more cost-effective, especially if using older, less costly drugs (735).

 ## NOVEL STRATEGIES

Vaccine Studies

There have been major technological advances in the search for a breast cancer therapeutic or preventive vaccine, but their role in this disease remains investigational at present. Tumor vaccines offer the potential for cancer prevention in high-risk individuals, preventing relapse after adjuvant treatment for early breast cancer and treating advanced disease in tumors resistant to standard cytotoxic regimens (736,737). Most therapeutic vaccines developed to date have not yet advanced beyond preclinical testing or else have achieved promising, albeit limited results in clinical studies. Several approaches have been attempted including tumor cell/dendritic cell fusion (738) and DNA vaccines based on single purified antigens (739) or DNA fragments from whole cells (740). Strategies involving host factors that mitigate immune response against tumors have also been tested with promising results (741).

Treatment of mice bearing tumors derived from melanoma, sarcoma, colon cancer, breast cancer, and glioma with OX40 MAb can result in prolonged survival that is dependent on both CD4+ and CD8+ T cells (742). ONTAK (denileukin diftitox), a recombinant DNA-derived cytotoxic protein FDA approved for CD25+ cutaneous T-cell leukemia and lymphoma, was found to deplete CD4+CD25+ regulatory T cells and markedly inhibit tumor growth tested in a *neu* transgenic mouse model of spontaneous breast cancer (743). ONTAK has been tested as a single agent in one study involving eight patients with lung, breast, or ovarian cancers with promising results (744). A pilot study of timed sequential therapy with CTX, doxorubicin, and a GM-CSF–secreting allogeneic breast tumor vaccine in metastatic breast cancer has recently been completed in 2008 (745). Recently, Manning et al. (746) reported that combining multitargeted cancer therapy consisting of immune-based and antiangiogenic agents (DC101, a rat monoclonal antibody specific for mouse VEGF-R2 and *ERBB2*-targeted vaccination) was found to induce T cell–mediated antitumor immune responses greater than either therapy alone in the preclinical setting. Preventive vaccination, targeting known tumor-associated antigens in patients with high-risk disease, has also shown encouraging preliminary results (747,748). This strategy could well be a reality in the near future, implemented in patients rendered disease free by standard therapies such as surgery, chemotherapy, and radiotherapy.

 ## QUALITY OF LIFE AND COSTS

The goals of treatment for patients with MBC are to (a) prolong survival; (b) relieve symptoms; (c) maintain and possibly improve QOL; and (d) delay disease progression (17). The treatment of breast cancer requires an integrated multidisciplinary approach utilizing multiple resources in a focused, disease-oriented manner (5). At present, MBC is virtually incurable and most successive lines of chemotherapy with their attendant lower response rates have not shown a consistent improvement in median survival (749). Therefore, it is important to assess the impact of treatment on symptom control, toxicity, socioeconomic factors, and QOL, aside from its gains in response rates and TTP, before deciding on the type of therapy. However, patients are frequently willing to trade quality for quantity of life (750). It has been shown that approximately 15% of patients would receive high-risk treatment for as little as 1 month of additional life expectancy, although younger patients were more willing to assume the risks involved (751). In addition, patients were observed to be more likely to accept radical treatment for minimal benefit compared to the level of acceptance from health care workers (752).

Cancer-related QOL has been defined as a multidimensional concept that encompasses the impact of cancer and its treatment on the physical, psychological, and social components of the patients' lives (753–755). QOL has been shown to be an independent and strong prognostic factor for survival in several types of advanced cancers including MBC (756–758), although the association is still not completely clear at present. Gains in survival must be considered in relation to the quality of survival and the costs required to achieve them. Hence, cost-effectiveness is an increasingly important outcome in clinical trials (759) and is often reported in terms of cost per year of life saved (LY) or cost per quality-adjusted year of life saved (QALY) (760). A Working Group of the Health Services Committee of the American Society of Clinical Oncology (ASCO) further agreed that prolongation in survival is not an absolute prerequisite to justify recommending treatment for MBC, QOL improvement also being an important criteria (760). Patient outcomes such as survival, toxicity, and QOL should receive higher priority than cancer outcomes such as response rates and response durations for guideline development and technology assessment (760). However, it is important to note that there is no minimum QOL benefit above which treatments are justified. Rather, benefits should be weighed against toxicity and costs (760). In the past, QOL was evaluated through limited surrogates, such as toxicity measures, performance status, decrease in analgesic requirements, or antitumor activity (761). Over the years, more objective health-related QOL measurement instruments have been developed in North America and Europe and are now widely used in breast cancer clinical trials (762,763). The inclusion of these measurements often adds to the complexity of the trial and increases time consumption and costs. Moreover, the extent of their additional contribution is currently not firmly established.

Cancer has a major financial impact on a country's health budget. The U.S. National Institutes of Health estimated the overall costs for cancer in 2007 at $219.2 billion, with breast cancer projected to account for 20% to 25% of the total costs (2,764). Costs of breast cancer treatment, especially in limited-resource countries, have always been a critical deciding factor for the kind of breast cancer treatment received. Unfortunately, it is precisely in these economically disadvantaged countries where advanced initial disease presentations are found, with high fatality rates, compounded by inadequate resources to provide standard cancer therapy. Even in the best of circumstances, it is difficult and far more costly to treat women with late-stage breast cancer, who are likely to have a poor outcome regardless of therapy (765). It has been estimated that the least cost-effective option was treating stage IV disease with stage I treatment being the most cost-effective. Hence, implementing successful early detection programs and treatments for early stage breast cancer may ultimately prove more resource effective.

CONCLUSIONS

Chemotherapy in MBC has been shown to provide palliation in symptoms, improvement in QOL, and a modest prolongation of survival. Various classes of drugs such as anthracyclines, alkylating agents, antimetabolites, taxanes, topoisomerase inhibitors, vinca alkaloids, and platinums appear to be active in this disease. However, anthracyclines and taxanes are known to be the two most active groups of agents in breast cancer and should be used as first-line therapy in this setting if there are no contraindications and chemotherapy is needed.

Treatment for each individual patient should be tailored according to the extent of disease, performance status, comor-

bidities, and the biological characteristics of the tumor such as hormone receptor and *ERBB2* status. Generally, given its minimal toxicity profile, endocrine therapy is favored over chemotherapy if the disease is hormone-receptor positive, limited to the bone and soft tissue, if there is a long disease-free interval, and there appears to be an indolent clinical course, even if there is visceral involvement. In clinical scenarios where the patient would require rapid relief of her symptoms, if there is significant visceral involvement or in triple-negative breast cancer, chemotherapy is likely to be the best course of action. In *ERBB2*-positive disease, trastuzumab, possibly as a single-agent or with chemotherapy, should be considered, although up front endocrine therapy alone should still be considered in patients with ER-positive disease.

If a rapid response is needed, combination therapy would be preferred despite its attendant greater toxicity rate. However, there has been no consistent evidence of a survival benefit of combination as opposed to sequential single-agent monotherapy in MBC treatment. The optimal dosing of cytotoxic drugs is also important as suboptimal drug doses can impact negatively on disease recurrence and survival. There is a prolongation of response but no survival benefit from maintenance chemotherapy after a standard number of six to eight cycles, and one should consider a "drug holiday" after that. Historically, the high rates of clinical response observed in single-institutional phase II studies of single-agent or combination chemotherapy have not been reproduced in subsequent multicenter or randomized studies.

A new class of chemotherapy agents known as epothilones have recently emerged as an active and promising new alternative, albeit rather toxic when given in combination regimens. A large number of novel formulations such as nab-paclitaxel and liposomal doxorubicin also serve to improve drug delivery and the therapeutic-to-toxic ratio, respectively. Preliminary studies are still ongoing for breast cancer vaccines. Currently, the monitoring of treatment response is limited to careful history taking, physical examination, radiological investigations, and sometimes, tumor marker assessments. The clinical utility of circulating tumor cells as a marker for prognosis and treatment response (766–768), although appearing promising, is at present not recommended for routine use for lack of a predictive utility for therapy selection at present (19). The role of pharmacogenomics and gene expression profiling as predictive tools is the subject of ongoing clinical investigations. Taken in total, these new developments in the treatment of advanced breast cancer are a step in the right direction in improving the treatment outcomes in metastatic breast cancer.

MANAGEMENT SUMMARY

- On the suspicion of recurrent or metastatic breast cancer, full restaging is required to evaluate the extent of disease.
- Tissue acquisition from a recurrent or metastatic disease should be obtained whenever possible with evaluation of ER/PR and *ERBB2* status, preferably from a core biopsy specimen for proper histologic evaluation and immunostains. It should be noted that ER positive or PR positive tumors have been observed to become negative in metastatic sites with some variability across sites of disease (769,770). The discrepancy rate between primary and metastatic sites appears to be less in regard to *ERBB2*.
- The goal of treatment of MBC should be prolongation of life and improvement of symptoms and QOL. Systemic therapy forms the therapeutic backbone, but some patients may benefit from combined multimodality therapy that includes surgery or radiation therapy. Individual characteristics such as comorbid conditions, performance status, age, and support network should help inform this decision.

- Patient preferences, goals, and expectations must also be considered and openly discussed to ensure that all involved have a general understanding and agreement on expected objectives of any proposed treatment.
- Tumor characteristics such as disease-free interval since any previous diagnosis of early stage disease, any prior adjuvant therapy, extent of disease, pace of progression, and receptor marker status (preferably in a metastatic site) should guide therapy decisions.
- Endocrine therapy should always be considered, preferably without chemotherapy and possibly without anti-*ERBB2* therapy, in patients with ER- or PR-positive disease, especially if minimally symptomatic.
- There is no apparent benefit from combination over single-agent chemotherapy, except perhaps in patients with more symptomatic disease where an earlier initial response is of interest.
- Bevacizumab in combination with paclitaxel is a reasonable option when considering first-line chemotherapy. Its use beyond the first-line setting remains investigational.
- Single-agent trastuzumab is a reasonable option in patients with *ERBB2*-positive disease. Chemotherapy may be added upon progression, and the role of further trastuzumab with subsequent chemotherapy regimens is unclear.
- Lapatinib has activity as first-line therapy or in patients with progressive disease after trastuzumab. It may also have activity in metastatic sites in the CNS.
- There is no role for trastuzumab or lapatinib as anti-*ERBB2* therapies in patients with *ERBB2* negative disease (immunohistochemistry [IHC] and fluorescence *in situ* hybridization [FISH]). The role of measures of *ERBB2* in serum remain investigational.
- There is a lack of a standard approach for second and subsequent lines of treatment and this should be made on the basis of the chemotherapeutic drug's efficacy accompanied with the least toxic profile.
- Monitor the response each time using history and physical examination, tumor markers (if necessary), and imaging studies, and assess the drug toxicity to decide whether to continue a particular therapy or switch agents.
- Although most patients will remain on some therapy, there is no established role for maintenance therapy after an initial response or a period of stable disease, and drug holidays should be considered especially in patients developing therapy-related toxicities.

References

1. Garcia M, Jemal A, Ward EM, et al. *Global cancer facts and figures 2007.* Atlanta: American Cancer Society, 2007.
2. American Cancer Society. *Cancer facts and figures 2008.* Atlanta: American Cancer Society, 2008.
3. Stewart BW, Kleihues PE. World cancer report. Lyon, France: IARC Press, 2003.
4. International Agency for Research on Cancer Working Group on the evaluation of cancer-preventive strategies. *Handbooks of cancer prevention,* vol. 7, *breast cancer screening.* Lyon, France: IARC Press, 2003.
5. Eniu A, Carlson RW, Aziz Z, et al. Breast cancer in limited-resource countries: treatment and allocation of resources. *Breast J* 2006;12[Suppl 1]:S38–S53.
6. Cleator S, Heller W, Coombes RC. Triple-negative breast cancer: therapeutic options. *Lancet Oncol* 2007;8:235–244.
7. Konecny G, Pauletti G, Pegram M, et al. Quantitative association between HER-2/neu and steroid hormone receptors in hormone receptor-positive primary breast cancer. *J Natl Cancer Inst* 2003;95:142–153.
8. Rodriguez-Pinilla SM, Sarrio D, Honrado E, et al. Prognostic significance of basal-like phenotype and fascin expression in node-negative invasive breast carcinomas. *Clin Cancer Res* 2006;12:1533–1539.
9. Carey LA, Perou CM, Livasy CA, et al. Race, breast cancer subtypes, and survival in the Carolina Breast Cancer Study. *JAMA* 2006;295:2492–2502.
10. Ries LAG, Eisner MP. Cancer of the female breast. In: Ries LAG, Young JL, Keel GE, et al., eds. *SEER survival monograph: cancer survival among adults: U.S. SEER Program, 1988–2001, patient and tumor characteristics.* NIH Pub. No. 07-6215. Bethesda, MD: National Cancer Institute, SEER Program, 2007:chap 13.
11. Miller KD, Sledge GW Jr. The role of chemotherapy for metastatic breast cancer. *Hematol Oncol Clin North Am* 1999;13:415–434.

12. Stockler M, Wilcken NR, Ghersi D, et al. Systematic reviews of chemotherapy and endocrine therapy in metastatic breast cancer. *Cancer Treat Rev* 2000;26:151–168.
13. Greenberg PA, Hortobagyi GN, Smith TL, et al. Long-term follow-up of patients with complete remission following combination chemotherapy for metastatic breast cancer. *J Clin Oncol* 1996;14:2197–2205.
14. Giordano SH, Buzdar AU, Kau SC, et al. Improvement in breast cancer survival: results from M.D. Anderson Cancer Center protocols from 1975–2000. *Proc Am Soc Clin Oncol* 2002;21:54a(abst 212).
15. Wolff AC. Systemic therapy. *Curr Opin Oncol* 2002;14:600–608.
16. Chia SKL, Speers C, Kang A, et al. The impact of new chemotherapeutic and hormonal agents on the survival of women with metastatic breast cancer (MBC) in a population based cohort. *Proc Am Soc Clin Oncol* 2003;22:6(abst 22).
17. Smith I. Goals of treatment for patients with metastatic breast cancer. *Semin Oncol* 2006;33:S2–S5.
18. Giordano SH, Buzdar AU, Smith TL, et al. Is breast cancer survival improving? *Cancer* 2004;100:44–52.
19. Harris L, Fritsche H, Mennel R, et al. American Society of Clinical Oncology 2007 update of recommendations for the use of tumor markers in breast cancer. *J Clin Oncol* 2007;25:5287–5312.
20. Colozza M, de Azambuja E, Personeni N, et al. Achievements in systemic therapies in the pregenomic era in metastatic breast cancer. *Oncologist* 2007;12:253–270.
21. Ross MB, Buzdar AU, Smith TL, et al. Improved survival of patients with metastatic breast cancer receiving combination chemotherapy. *Cancer* 1985;55:341–346.
22. Patel JK, Nemoto T, Vezeridis M, et al. Does more intense palliative treatment improve overall survival in metastatic breast cancer patients? *Cancer* 1986;57:567–570.
23. Powles TJ, Coombes RC, Smith IE, et al. Failure of chemotherapy to prolong survival in a group of patients with metastatic breast cancer. *Lancet* 1980;1:580–582.
24. Todd M, Shoag M, Cadman E. Survival of women with metastatic breast cancer at Yale from 1920 to 1980. *J Clin Oncol* 1983;1:406–408.
25. Brincker H. Distant recurrence in breast cancer. Survival expectations and first choice of chemotherapy regimen. *Acta Oncol* 1988;27:729–732.
26. A'Hern RP, Ebbs SR, Baum MB. Does chemotherapy improve survival in advanced breast cancer? A statistical overview. *Br J Cancer* 1988;57:615–618.
27. Polychemotherapy for early breast cancer: an overview of the randomised trials. Early Breast Cancer Trialists' Collaborative Group. *Lancet* 1998;352:930–942.
28. Fossati R, Confalonieri C, Torri V, et al. Cytotoxic and hormonal treatment for metastatic breast cancer: a systematic review of published randomized trials involving 31,510 women. *J Clin Oncol* 1998;16:3439–3460.
29. O'Shaughnessy J, Miles D, Vukelja S, et al. Superior survival with capecitabine plus docetaxel combination therapy in anthracycline-pretreated patients with advanced breast cancer: phase III trial results. *J Clin Oncol* 2002;20:2812–2823.
30. Jassem J, Pienkowski T, Pluzanska A, et al. Doxorubicin and paclitaxel versus fluorouracil, doxorubicin, and cyclophosphamide as first-line therapy for women with metastatic breast cancer: final results of a randomized phase III multicenter trial. *J Clin Oncol* 2001;19:1707–1715.
31. Stewart DJ, Evans WK, Shepherd FA, et al. Cyclophosphamide and fluorouracil combined with mitoxantrone versus doxorubicin for breast cancer: superiority of doxorubicin. *J Clin Oncol* 1997;15:1897–1905.
32. Bishop JF, Dewar J, Toner GC, et al. Initial paclitaxel improves outcome compared with CMFP combination chemotherapy as front-line therapy in untreated metastatic breast cancer. *J Clin Oncol* 1999;17:2355–2364.
33. Nabholtz JM, Senn HJ, Bezwoda WR, et al. Prospective randomized trial of docetaxel versus mitomycin plus vinblastine in patients with metastatic breast cancer progressing despite previous anthracycline-containing chemotherapy. 304 Study Group. *J Clin Oncol* 1999;17:1413–1424.
34. Albain KS, Nag SM, Calderillo-Ruiz G, et al. Gemcitabine plus paclitaxel versus paclitaxel monotherapy in patients with metastatic breast cancer and prior anthracycline treatment. *J Clin Oncol* 2008;26:3950–3957.
35. Wood WC, Muss HB, Solin LJ, et al., eds. Cancer. Principles and practice of oncology. 7th ed. Philadelphia: Lippincott Williams & Wilkins, 2005:1415–1477.
36. Diaz-Canton EA, Valero V, Rahman Z, et al. Clinical course of breast cancer patients with metastases confined to the lungs treated with chemotherapy. The University of Texas M.D. Anderson Cancer Center experience and review of the literature. *Ann Oncol* 1998;9:413–418.
37. Rahman ZU, Frye DK, Smith TL, et al. Results and long term follow-up for 1,581 patients with metastatic breast carcinoma treated with standard dose doxorubicin-containing chemotherapy: a reference. *Cancer* 1999;85:104–111.
38. Bruzzi P, Del Mastro L, Sormani MP, et al. Objective response to chemotherapy as a potential surrogate end point of survival in metastatic breast cancer patients. *J Clin Oncol* 2005;23:5117–5125.
39. Mayer EL, Burstein HJ. Chemotherapy for metastatic breast cancer. *Hematol Oncol Clin North Am* 2007;21:257–272.
40. A randomized trial in postmenopausal patients with advanced breast cancer comparing endocrine and cytotoxic therapy given sequentially or in combination. The Australian and New Zealand Breast Cancer Trials group, Clinical Oncological Society of Australia. *J Clin Oncol* 1986;4:186–193.
41. Sledge GW Jr, Hu P, Falkson G, et al. Comparison of chemotherapy with chemohormonal therapy as first-line therapy for metastatic, hormone-sensitive breast cancer: an Eastern Cooperative Oncology Group study. *J Clin Oncol* 2000;18:262–266.
42. Norris B, Pritchard KI, James K, et al. Phase III comparative study of vinorelbine combined with doxorubicin versus doxorubicin alone in disseminated metastatic/recurrent breast cancer: National Cancer Institute of Canada Clinical Trials Group Study MA8. *J Clin Oncol* 2000;18:2385–2394.
43. Chlebowski RT, Smalley RV, Weiner JM, et al. Combination versus sequential single agent chemotherapy in advanced breast cancer: associations with metastatic sites and long-term survival. The Western Cancer Study Group and the Southeastern Cancer Study Group. *Br J Cancer* 1989;59:227–230.
44. Joensuu H, Holli K, Heikkinen M, et al. Combination chemotherapy versus single-agent therapy as first- and second-line treatment in metastatic breast cancer: a prospective randomized trial. *J Clin Oncol* 1998;16:3720–3730.
45. Andersson M, Daugaard S, von der Maase H, et al. Doxorubicin versus mitomycin versus doxorubicin plus mitomycin in advanced breast cancer: a randomized study. *Cancer Treat Rep* 1986;70:1181–1186.

46. Gundersen S, Kvinnsland S, Klepp O, et al. Weekly adriamycin versus VAC in advanced breast cancer. A randomized trial. *Eur J Cancer Clin Oncol* 1986;22:1431–1434.
47. A prospective randomized trial comparing epirubicin monochemotherapy to two fluorouracil, cyclophosphamide, and epirubicin regimens differing in epirubicin dose in advanced breast cancer patients. The French Epirubicin Study Group. *J Clin Oncol* 1991;9:305–312.
48. O'Shaughnessy J, Nag S, Calderillo-Ruiz G, et al. Gemcitabine plus paclitaxel versus paclitaxel as first-line treatment for anthracycline-pretreated metastatic breast cancer: interim results of a global phase III study. *Proc Am Soc Clin Oncol* 2003;22:7a(abst).
49. Martin M, Ruiz A, Munoz M, et al. Gemcitabine plus vinorelbine versus vinorelbine monotherapy in patients with metastatic breast cancer previously treated with anthracyclines and taxanes: final results of the phase III Spanish Breast Cancer Research Group (GEICAM) trial. *Lancet Oncol* 2007;8:219–225.
50. Sledge GW, Neuberg D, Bernardo P, et al. Phase III trial of doxorubicin, paclitaxel, and the combination of doxorubicin and paclitaxel as front-line chemotherapy for metastatic breast cancer: an intergroup trial (E1193). *J Clin Oncol* 2003;21:588–592.
51. Cresta S, Grasselli G, Mansutti M, et al. A randomized phase II study of combination, alternating and sequential regimens of doxorubicin and docetaxel as first-line chemotherapy for women with metastatic breast cancer. *Ann Oncol* 2004;15:433–439.
52. Fountzilas G, Papadimitriou C, Dafni U, et al. Dose-dense sequential chemotherapy with epirubicin and paclitaxel versus the combination, as first-line chemotherapy, in advanced breast cancer: a randomized study conducted by the Hellenic Cooperative Oncology Group. *J Clin Oncol* 2001;19:2232–2239.
53. Koroleva I, Wojtukiewicz M, Zaluski J, et al. Preliminary results of a phase ii randomized trial of Taxotere (T) and doxorubicin (A) given in combination or sequentially as first line chemotherapy (CT) for metastatic breast cancer (MBC). *Proc Am Soc Clin Oncol* 2001;20:(abst 117).
54. Carrick S, Parker S, Wilcken N, et al. Single agent versus combination chemotherapy for metastatic breast cancer. *Cochrane Database Syst Rev* 2005;2:CD003372.
55. O'Shaughnessy JA, Blum J, Moiseyenko V, et al. Randomized, open-label, phase II trial of oral capecitabine (Xeloda) vs. a reference arm of intravenous CMF (cyclophosphamide, methotrexate and 5-fluorouracil) as first-line therapy for advanced/metastatic breast cancer. *Ann Oncol* 2001;12:1247–1254.
56. Soto C, Torrecillas L, Reyes S, et al. Capecitabine (X) and taxanes in patients (pts) with anthracycline-pretreated metastatic breast cancer (MBC): Sequential vs. combined therapy results from a MOSG randomized phase III trial. ASCO annual meeting proceedings Part I. *J Clin Oncol* 2006;24(18S)[Suppl]:570.
57. Conte PF, Guarneri V, Bruzzi P, et al. Concomitant versus sequential administration of epirubicin and paclitaxel as first-line therapy in metastatic breast carcinoma: results for the Gruppo Oncologico Nord Ovest randomized trial. *Cancer* 2004;101:704–712.
58. Alba E, Martin M, Ramos M, et al. Multicenter randomized trial comparing sequential with concomitant administration of doxorubicin and docetaxel as first-line treatment of metastatic breast cancer: a Spanish Breast Cancer Research Group (GEICAM-9903) phase III study. *J Clin Oncol* 2004;22:2587–2593.
59. Nielsen D, Dombernowsky P, Larsen SK, et al. Epirubicin or epirubicin and cisplatin as first-line therapy in advanced breast cancer. A phase III study. *Cancer Chemother Pharmacol* 2000;46:459–466.
60. Heidemann E, Stoeger H, Souchon R, et al. Is first-line single-agent mitoxantrone in the treatment of high-risk metastatic breast cancer patients as effective as combination chemotherapy? No difference in survival but higher quality of life were found in a multicenter randomized trial. *Ann Oncol* 2002;13:1717–1729.
61. Sawada N, Ishikawa T, Fukase Y, et al. Induction of thymidine phosphorylase activity and enhancement of capecitabine efficacy by Taxol/Taxotere in human cancer xenografts. *Clin Cancer Res* 1998;4:1013–1019.
62. Fujimoto-Ouchi K, Tanaka Y, Tominaga T. Schedule dependency of antitumor activity in combination therapy with capecitabine/5'-deoxy-5-fluorouridine and docetaxel in breast cancer models. *Clin Cancer Res* 2001;7:1079–1086.
63. Beslija S, Obralic N, Basic H, et al. Randomized trial of sequence vs. combination of capecitabine (X) and docetaxel (T): XT vs. T followed by X after progression as first-line therapy for patients (pts) with metastatic breast cancer (MBC). ASCO annual meeting proceedings Part I. *J Clin Oncol* 2006;24(18S)[Suppl]:571.
64. Bastholt L, Dalmark M, Gjedde SB, et al. Dose-response relationship of epirubicin in the treatment of postmenopausal patients with metastatic breast cancer: a randomized study of epirubicin at four different dose levels performed by the Danish Breast Cancer Cooperative Group. *J Clin Oncol* 1996;14:1146–1155.
65. Hryniuk W, Bush H. The importance of dose intensity in chemotherapy of metastatic breast cancer. *J Clin Oncol* 1984;2:1281–1288.
66. Hryniuk W, Levine MN. Analysis of dose intensity for adjuvant chemotherapy trials in stage II breast cancer. *J Clin Oncol* 1986;4:1162–1170.
67. Budman DR. Dose and schedule as determinants of outcomes in chemotherapy for breast cancer. *Semin Oncol* 2004;31:3–9.
68. Gurney H. How to calculate the dose of chemotherapy. *Br J Cancer* 2002;86:1297–1302.
69. Gately S, Kerbel R. Antiangiogenic scheduling of lower dose cancer chemotherapy. *Cancer J* 2001;7:427–436.
70. Miller KD, Sweeney CJ, Sledge GW Jr. Redefining the target: chemotherapeutics as antiangiogenics. *J Clin Oncol* 2001;19:1195–1206.
71. Colleoni M, Rocca A, Sandri MT, et al. Low-dose oral methotrexate and cyclophosphamide in metastatic breast cancer: antitumor activity and correlation with vascular endothelial growth factor levels. *Ann Oncol* 2002;13:73–80.
72. Evans WE, Relling MV. Clinical pharmacokinetics-pharmacodynamics of anticancer drugs. *Clin Pharmacokinet* 1989;16:327–336.
73. Nabholtz JM, Gelmon K, Bontenbal M, et al. Multicenter, randomized comparative study of two doses of paclitaxel in patients with metastatic breast cancer. *J Clin Oncol* 1996;14:1858–1867.
74. Harvey V, Mouridsen H, Semiglazov V, et al. Phase III trial comparing three doses of docetaxel for second-line treatment of advanced breast cancer. *J Clin Oncol* 2006;24:4963–4970.
75. Tannock IF, Boyd NF, DeBoer G, et al. A randomized trial of two dose levels of cyclophosphamide, methotrexate, and fluorouracil chemotherapy for patients with metastatic breast cancer. *J Clin Oncol* 1988;6:1377–1387.
76. Focan C, Andrien JM, Closon MT, et al. Dose-response relationship of epirubicin-based first-line chemotherapy for advanced breast cancer: a prospective randomized trial. *J Clin Oncol* 1993;11:1253–1263.
77. Brufman G, Colajori E, Ghilezan N, et al. Doubling epirubicin dose intensity (100 mg/m^2 versus 50 mg/m^2) in the FEC regimen significantly increases response rates. An international randomised phase III study in metastatic breast cancer. The Epirubicin High Dose (HEPI 010) Study Group. *Ann Oncol* 1997;8:155–162.
78. Riccardi A, Tinelli C, Brugnatelli S, et al. Doubling of the epirubicin dosage within the 5-fluorouracil, epirubicin and cyclophosphamide regimen: a prospective, randomized, multicentric study on antitumor effect and quality of life in advanced breast cancer. *Int J Oncol* 2000;16:769–776.
79. Epirubicin-based chemotherapy in metastatic breast cancer patients: role of dose-intensity and duration of treatment. *J Clin Oncol* 2000;18:3115–3124.
80. Winer EP, Berry DA, Woolf S, et al. Failure of higher-dose paclitaxel to improve outcome in patients with metastatic breast cancer: cancer and leukemia group B trial 9342. *J Clin Oncol* 2004;22:2061–2068.
81. Di Leo A, Piccart MJ. Paclitaxel activity, dose, and schedule: data from phase III trials in metastatic breast cancer. *Semin Oncol* 1999;26:27–32.
82. Hortobagyi GN, Bodey GP, Buzdar AU, et al. Evaluation of high-dose versus standard FAC chemotherapy for advanced breast cancer in protected environment units: a prospective randomized study. *J Clin Oncol* 1987;5:354–364.
83. Del Mastro L, Venturini M, Lionetto R, et al. Accelerated-intensified cyclophosphamide, epirubicin, and fluorouracil (CEF) compared with standard CEF in metastatic breast cancer patients: results of a multicenter, randomized phase III study of the Italian Gruppo Oncologico Nord-Ouest-Mammella Inter Gruppo Group. *J Clin Oncol* 2001;19:2213–2221.
84. Stadtmauer EA, O'Neill A, Goldstein LJ, et al. Conventional-dose chemotherapy compared with high-dose chemotherapy plus autologous hematopoietic stem-cell transplantation for metastatic breast cancer. Philadelphia Bone Marrow Transplant Group. *N Engl J Med* 2000;342:1069–1076.
85. Schmid P, Schippinger W, Nitsch T, et al. Up-front tandem high-dose chemotherapy compared with standard chemotherapy with doxorubicin and paclitaxel in metastatic breast cancer: results of a randomized trial. *J Clin Oncol* 2005;23:432–440.
86. Crump M, Gluck S, Tu D, et al. Randomized trial of high-dose chemotherapy with autologous peripheral-blood stem-cell support compared with standard-dose chemotherapy in women with metastatic breast cancer: NCIC MA.16. *J Clin Oncol* 2008;26:37–43.
87. Farquhar C, Basser R, Hetrick S, et al. High dose chemotherapy and autologous bone marrow or stem cell transplantation versus conventional chemotherapy for women with metastatic breast cancer. *Cochrane Database Syst Rev* 2003:CD003142.
88. Vogl DT, Stadtmauer EA. High-dose chemotherapy and autologous hematopoietic stem cell transplantation for metastatic breast cancer: a therapy whose time has passed. *Bone Marrow Transplant* 2006;37:985–987.
89. Engelsman E, Klijn JC, Rubens RD, et al. "Classical" CMF versus a 3-weekly intravenous CMF schedule in postmenopausal patients with advanced breast cancer. An EORTC Breast Cancer Co-operative Group Phase III Trial (10808). *Eur J Cancer* 1991;27:966–970.
90. Citron ML, Berry DA, Cirrincione C, et al. Randomized trial of dose-dense versus conventionally scheduled and sequential versus concurrent combination chemotherapy as postoperative adjuvant treatment of node-positive primary breast cancer: first report of Intergroup trial C9741/Cancer and Leukemia Group B trial 9741. *J Clin Oncol* 2003;21:1431–1439.
91. Seidman AD, Berry D, Cirrincione C, et al. Randomized phase III trial of weekly compared with every-3-weeks paclitaxel for metastatic breast cancer, with trastuzumab for all HER2 overexpressors and random assignment to trastuzumab or not in HER-2 non-overexpressors: final results of cancer and leukemia Group B protocol 9840. *J Clin Oncol* 2008;26:1642–1649.
92. Hainsworth JD, Burris HA 3rd, Erland JB, et al. Phase I trial of docetaxel administered by weekly infusion in patients with advanced refractory cancer. *J Clin Oncol* 1998;16:2164–2168.
93. Seidman AD, Hudis CA, Albanell J, et al. Dose-dense therapy with weekly 1-hour paclitaxel infusions in the treatment of metastatic breast cancer. *J Clin Oncol* 1998;16:3353–3361.
94. Burstein HJ, Manola J, Younger J, et al. Docetaxel administered on a weekly basis for metastatic breast cancer. *J Clin Oncol* 2000;18:1212–1219.
95. Blomqvist C, Elomaa I, Rissanen P, et al. Influence of treatment schedule on toxicity and efficacy of cyclophosphamide, epirubicin, and fluorouracil in metastatic breast cancer: a randomized trial comparing weekly and every-4-week administration. *J Clin Oncol* 1993;11:467–473.
96. Nieto Y, Martin M, Alonso JL, et al. Weekly continuous infusion of 5-fluorouracil with oral leucovorin in metastatic breast cancer patients with primary resistance to doxorubicin. *Breast Cancer Res Treat* 1998;50:167–174.
97. Ellis GK, Green S, Schulman S, et al. Alternating weekly doxorubicin and 5-fluorouracil/leucovorin followed by weekly doxorubicin and daily cyclophosphamide in stage IV breast cancer. A Southwest Oncology Group study. *Cancer* 1991;68: 934–939.
98. Seidman AD, Berry D, Cirrincione C, et al. Randomized phase III trial of weekly compared with every-3-weeks paclitaxel for metastatic breast cancer, with trastuzumab for all HER-2 overexpressors and random assignment to trastuzumab or not in HER-2 nonoverexpressors: final results of Cancer and Leukemia Group B protocol 9840. *J Clin Oncol* 2008;26:1642–1649.
99. Wilke H, Klaassen U, Achterrath W, et al. Phase I/II study with a weekly 24-hour infusion of 5-fluorouracil plus high-dose folinic acid (HD-FU/FA) in intensively pretreated patients with metastatic breast cancer. *Ann Oncol* 1996;7:55–58.
100. Norton L, Simon R. Tumor size, sensitivity to therapy, and design of treatment schedules. *Cancer Treat Rep* 1977;61:1307–1317.
101. Norton L, Simon R. Growth curve of an experimental solid tumor following radiotherapy. *J Natl Cancer Inst* 1977;58:1735–1741.
102. Norton L, Simon R. The Norton-Simon hypothesis revisited. *Cancer Treat Rep* 1986;70:163–169.
103. Skipper HE. Laboratory models: some historical perspective. *Cancer Treat Rep* 1986;70:3–7.
104. Venturini M, Del Mastro L, Aitini E, et al. Dose-dense adjuvant chemotherapy in early breast cancer patients: results from a randomized trial. *J Natl Cancer Inst* 2005;97:1724–1733.

105. Cocconi G, Bisagni G, Bacchi M, et al. A comparison of continuation versus late intensification followed by discontinuation of chemotherapy in advanced breast cancer. A prospective randomized trial of the Italian Oncology Group for Clinical Research (G.O.I.R.C.). *Ann Oncol* 1990;1:36–44.
106. Perez EA, Geeraerts L, Suman VJ, et al. A randomized phase II study of sequential docetaxel and doxorubicin/cyclophosphamide in patients with metastatic breast cancer. *Ann Oncol* 2002;13:1225–1235.
107. Paridaens R, Van Aelst F, Georgoulias V, et al. A randomized phase II study of alternating and sequential regimens of docetaxel and doxorubicin as first-line chemotherapy for metastatic breast cancer. *Ann Oncol* 2003;14:433–440.
108. Fizazi K, Zelek L. Is one cycle every three or four weeks obsolete? A critical review of dose-dense chemotherapy in solid neoplasms. *Ann Oncol* 2000;11: 133–149.
109. Coates A, Gebski V, Bishop JF, et al. Improving the quality of life during chemotherapy for advanced breast cancer. A comparison of intermittent and continuous treatment strategies. *N Engl J Med* 1987;317:1490–1495.
110. Ejlertsen B, Pfeiffer P, Pedersen D, et al. Decreased efficacy of cyclophosphamide, epirubicin and 5-fluorouracil in metastatic breast cancer when reducing treatment duration from 18 to 6 months. *Eur J Cancer* 1993;29A:527–531.
111. Harris AL, Cantwell BM, Carmichael J, et al. Comparison of short-term and continuous chemotherapy (mitoxantrone) for advanced breast cancer. *Lancet* 1990; 335:186–190.
112. Gregory RK, Powles TJ, Chang JC, et al. A randomised trial of six versus twelve courses of chemotherapy in metastatic carcinoma of the breast. *Eur J Cancer* 1997;33:2194–2197.
113. Nooij MA, de Haes JC, Beex LV, et al. Continuing chemotherapy or not after the induction treatment in advanced breast cancer patients. clinical outcomes and oncologists' preferences. *Eur J Cancer* 2003;39:614–621.
114. Muss HB, Case LD, Richards F 2nd, et al. Interrupted versus continuous chemotherapy in patients with metastatic breast cancer. The Piedmont Oncology Association. *N Engl J Med* 1991;325:1342–1348.
115. Becher R, Kloke O, Hayungs J, et al. Epirubicin and ifosfamide in metastatic breast cancer. *Semin Oncol* 1996;23:28–33.
116. Gennari A, Amadori D, De Lena M, et al. Lack of benefit of maintenance paclitaxel in first-line chemotherapy in metastatic breast cancer. *J Clin Oncol* 2006;24: 3912–3918.
117. Falkson G, Gelman RS, Pandya KJ, et al. Eastern Cooperative Oncology Group randomized trials of observation versus maintenance therapy for patients with metastatic breast cancer in complete remission following induction treatment. *J Clin Oncol* 1998;16:1669–1676.
118. Stockler M, Wilcken N, Coates A. Chemotherapy for metastatic breast cancer—when is enough enough? *Eur J Cancer* 1997;33:2147–2148.
119. Simes RJ, Coates AS. Patient preferences for adjuvant chemotherapy of early breast cancer: how much benefit is needed? *J Natl Cancer Inst Monogr* 2001;30: 146–152.
120. Legha SS, Buzdar AU, Smith TL, et al. Complete remissions in metastatic breast cancer treated with combination drug therapy. *Ann Intern Med* 1979;91: 847–852.
121. Pedrazzini A, Cavalli F, Brunner KW, et al. Complete remission following endocrine or combined cytotoxic and hormonal treatment in advanced breast cancer. A retrospective analysis. *Oncology* 1987;44:51–59.
122. Decker DA, Ahmann DL, Bisel HF, et al. Complete responders to chemotherapy in metastatic breast cancer. Characterization and analysis. *JAMA* 1979;242: 2075–2079.
123. Shinagawa K, Ogawa M, Horikoshi N, et al. [A study of complete responders in cases of metastatic breast cancer treated with combination chemotherapy]. *Gan No Rinsho* 1989;35:581–586.
124. Swenerton KD, Legha SS, Smith T, et al. Prognostic factors in metastatic breast cancer treated with combination chemotherapy. *Cancer Res* 1979;39:1552–1562.
125. Fischer J, Rose CJ, Rubens RD. Duration of complete response to chemotherapy in advanced breast cancer. *Eur J Cancer Clin Oncol* 1982;18:747–754.
126. Hortobagyi GN, Frye D, Buzdar AU, et al. Complete remissions (CR) in metastatic breast cancer (MBC): a thirteen year (YR) follow-up report. *Proc Am Soc Clin Oncol* 1988;7:A143.
127. Tomiak E, Piccart M, Mignolet F, et al. Characterisation of complete responders to combination chemotherapy for advanced breast cancer: a retrospective EORTC Breast Group study. *Eur J Cancer* 1996;32A:1876–1887.
128. Paridaens R, Van der Wijst JB, Julien JP, et al. Aminoglutethimide and estrogenic stimulation before chemotherapy for treatment of advanced breast cancer. Preliminary results of a phase II study conducted by the E.O.R.T.C. Breast Cancer Cooperative Group. *J Steroid Biochem* 1985;23:1181–1813.
129. Paridaens R, Heuson JC, Julien JP, et al. Assessment of estrogenic recruitment before chemotherapy in advanced breast cancer: preliminary results of a double-blind randomized study of the EORTC Breast Cancer Cooperative Group. *J Steroid Biochem Mol Biol* 1990;37:1109–1113.
130. Paridaens R, Heuson JC, Julien JP, et al. Assessment of estrogenic recruitment before chemotherapy in advanced breast cancer: a double-blind randomized study. European Organization for Research and Treatment of Cancer Breast Cancer Cooperative Group. *J Clin Oncol* 1993;11:1723–1728.
131. Paridaens R, Van Zijl J, Van der Merwe J, et al. Comparison between the alternating and sequential administration of three different chemotherapy regimens in advanced breast cancer. A randomized study of the EORTC Breast Cancer Cooperative Group. Presented at the 5th EORTC Breast Cancer Working Conference. September 3–6, 1991.
132. Nooy MA, Beex LVAM, JM DeHaas JC, et al.Short versus long term treatment with CMF in postmenopausal patients with advanced breast cancer; an EORTC Breast Cancer Cooperative Group phase III trial (10852). Presented at the 7th European Conference on Clinical Oncology and Cancer Nursing (ECCO 7). November 1993.
133. Hellman S, Weichselbaum RR. Oligometastases. *J Clin Oncol* 1995;13:8–10.
134. Hortobagyi GN. Can we cure limited metastatic breast cancer? *J Clin Oncol* 2002; 20:620–623.
135. Demicheli R. Tumour dormancy: findings and hypotheses from clinical research on breast cancer. *Semin Cancer Biol* 2001;11:297–306.
136. Holmgren L, O'Reilly MS, Folkman J. Dormancy of micrometastases: balanced proliferation and apoptosis in the presence of angiogenesis suppression. *Nat Med* 1995;1:149–153.
137. Girard P, Baldeyrou P, Le Chevalier T, et al. Surgery for pulmonary metastases. Who are the 10-year survivors? *Cancer* 1994;74:2791–2797.
138. McKenna RJ Jr, McMurtrey MJ, Larson DL, et al. A perspective on chest wall resection in patients with breast cancer. *Ann Thorac Surg* 1984;38:482–487.
139. Temple WJ, Ketcham AS. Surgical management of isolated systemic metastases. *Semin Oncol* 1980;7:468–480.
140. Buzdar AU, Blumenschein GR, Montague ED, et al. Combined modality approach in breast cancer with isolated or multiple metastases. *Am J Clin Oncol* 1984;7: 45–50.
141. Donegan WL, Perez-Mesa CM, Watson FR. A biostatistical study of locally recurrent breast carcinoma. *Surg Gynecol Obstet* 1966;122:529–540.
142. Valagussa P, Bonadonna G, Veronesi U. Patterns of relapse and survival following radical mastectomy. Analysis of 716 consecutive patients. *Cancer* 1978;41: 1170–1178.
143. Di Pietro S, Bertario L, Piva L. Prognosis and treatment of loco-regional breast cancer recurrences: critical considerations on 120 cases. *Tumori* 1980;66: 331–338.
144. Gilliland MD, Barton RM, Copeland EM 3rd. The implications of local recurrence of breast cancer as the first site of therapeutic failure. *Ann Surg* 1983;197: 284–287.
145. Toonkel LM, Fix I, Jacobson LH, et al. The significance of local recurrence of carcinoma of the breast. *Int J Radiat Oncol Biol Phys* 1983;9:33–39.
146. Bedwinek JM, Fineberg B, Lee J, et al. Analysis of failures following local treatment of isolated local-regional recurrence of breast cancer. *Int J Radiat Oncol Biol Phys* 1981;7:581–585.
147. Fentiman IS, Lavelle MA, Caplan D, et al. The significance of supraclavicular fossa node recurrence after radical mastectomy. *Cancer* 1986;57:908–910.
148. Beck TM, Hart NE, Woodard DA, et al. Local or regionally recurrent carcinoma of the breast: results of therapy in 121 patients. *J Clin Oncol* 1983;1:400–405.
149. Schneebaum S, Walker MJ, Young D, et al. The regional treatment of liver metastases from breast cancer. *J Surg Oncol* 1994;55:26–32.
150. Tekin K, Kocaoglu H, Bayar S. Long-term survival after regional chemotherapy for liver metastases from breast cancer. A case report. *Tumori* 2002;88:167–169.
151. Elias D, Lasser PH, Montrucolli D, et al. Hepatectomy for liver metastases from breast cancer. *Eur J Surg Oncol* 1995;21:510–513.
152. Long-term results of lung metastasectomy: prognostic analyses based on 5,206 cases. The International Registry of Lung Metastases. *J Thorac Cardiovasc Surg* 1997;113:37–49.
153. Staren ED, Salerno C, Rongione A, et al. Pulmonary resection for metastatic breast cancer. *Arch Surg* 1992;127:1282–1284.
154. Lanza LA, Natarajan G, Roth JA, et al. Long-term survival after resection of pulmonary metastases from carcinoma of the breast. *Ann Thorac Surg* 1992;54: 244–248.
155. Mountain CF, Khalil KG, Hermes KE, et al. The contribution of surgery to the management of carcinomatous pulmonary metastases. *Cancer* 1978;41:833–840.
156. Borner M, Bacchi M, Goldhirsch A, et al. First isolated locoregional recurrence following mastectomy for breast cancer: results of a phase III multicenter study comparing systemic treatment with observation after excision and radiation. Swiss Group for Clinical Cancer Research. *J Clin Oncol* 1994;12:2071–2077.
157. Blumenschein GR, DiStefano A, Caderao J, et al. Multimodality therapy for locally advanced and limited stage IV breast cancer: the impact of effective non-cross-resistance late-consolidation chemotherapy. *Clin Cancer Res* 1997;3:2633–2637.
158. Hanrahan EO, Broglio KR, Buzdar AU, et al. Combined-modality treatment for isolated recurrences of breast carcinoma: update on 30 years of experience at the University of Texas M.D. Anderson Cancer Center and assessment of prognostic factors. *Cancer* 2005;104:1158–1171.
159. Buzdar AU, Blumenschein GR, Smith TL, et al. Adjuvant chemoimmunotherapy following regional therapy for isolated recurrences of breast cancer (stage IV NED). *J Surg Oncol* 1979;12:27–40.
160. Holmes FA, Buzdar AU, Kau S-W, et al. Combined modality approach for patients with isolated recurrences of breast cancer (IV-NED): the M.D. Anderson Cancer Center experience. *Breast Dis* 1994;7:7–20.
161. Rivera E, Holmes FA, Buzdar AU, et al. Fluorouracil, doxorubicin, and cyclophosphamide followed by tamoxifen as adjuvant treatment for patients with stage IV breast cancer with no evidence of disease. *Breast J* 2002;8:2–9.
162. Nieto Y, Cagnoni PJ, Shpall EJ, et al. Phase II trial of high-dose chemotherapy with autologous stem cell transplant for stage IV breast cancer with minimal metastatic disease. *Clin Cancer Res* 1999;5:1731–1737.
163. Nieto Y, Nawaz S, Jones RB, et al. Prognostic model for relapse after high-dose chemotherapy with autologous stem-cell transplantation for stage IV oligometastatic breast cancer. *J Clin Oncol* 2002;20:707–718.
164. Hortobagyi GN. Treatment of breast cancer. *N Engl J Med* 1998;339:974–984.
165. Beslija S, Bonneterre J, Burstein H, et al. Second consensus on medical treatment of metastatic breast cancer. *Ann Oncol* 2007;18:215–225.
166. Wolff AC, Hammond ME, Schwartz JN, et al. American Society of Clinical Oncology/College of American Pathologists guideline recommendations for human epidermal growth factor receptor 2 testing in breast cancer. *J Clin Oncol* 2007;25:118–145.
167. Slamon DJ, Leyland-Jones B, Shak S, et al. Use of chemotherapy plus a monoclonal antibody against HER2 for metastatic breast cancer that overexpresses HER2. *N Engl J Med* 2001;344:783–792.
168. Sato N, Sano M, Tabei T, et al. Combination docetaxel and trastuzumab treatment for patients with HER-2-overexpressing metastatic breast cancer: a multicenter, phase-II study. *Breast Cancer* 2006;13:166–171.
169. Marty M, Cognetti F, Maraninchi D, et al. Randomized phase II trial of the efficacy and safety of trastuzumab combined with docetaxel in patients with human epidermal growth factor receptor 2-positive metastatic breast cancer administered as first-line treatment: the M77001 study group. *J Clin Oncol* 2005;23: 4265–4274.
170. Pegram M, Hsu S, Lewis G, et al. Inhibitory effects of combinations of HER-2/neu antibody and chemotherapeutic agents used for treatment of human breast cancers. *Oncogene* 1999;18:2241–2251.
171. Hayes DF, Thor AD, Dressler LG, et al. HER2 and response to paclitaxel in node-positive breast cancer. *N Engl J Med* 2007;357:1496–1506.
172. Konecny GE, Thomssen C, Luck HJ, et al. Her-2/neu gene amplification and response to paclitaxel in patients with metastatic breast cancer. *J Natl Cancer Inst* 2004;96:1141–1151.
173. Schmidt M, Bachhuber A, Victor A, et al. p53 expression and resistance against paclitaxel in patients with metastatic breast cancer. *J Cancer Res Clin Oncol* 2003;129:295–302.

174. Sezgin C, Karabulut B, Uslu R, et al. Potential predictive factors for response to weekly paclitaxel treatment in patients with metastatic breast cancer. *J Chemother* 2005;17:96–103.

175. Paridaens R, Biganzoli L, Bruning P, et al. Paclitaxel versus doxorubicin as first-line single-agent chemotherapy for metastatic breast cancer: a European Organization for Research and Treatment of Cancer randomized study with cross-over. *J Clin Oncol* 2000;18:724–733.

176. Chan S, Friedrichs K, Noel D, et al. Prospective randomized trial of docetaxel versus doxorubicin in patients with metastatic breast cancer. *J Clin Oncol* 1999; 17:2341–2354.

177. Crown J, Dieras V, Kaufmann M, et al. Chemotherapy for metastatic breast cancer—report of a European expert panel. *Lancet Oncol* 2002;3:719–727.

178. Miller K, Wang M, Gralow J, et al. Paclitaxel plus bevacizumab versus paclitaxel alone for metastatic breast cancer. *N Engl J Med* 2007;357:2666–2676.

179. Miller KD, Chap LI, Holmes FA, et al. Randomized phase III trial of capecitabine compared with bevacizumab plus capecitabine in patients with previously treated metastatic breast cancer. *J Clin Oncol* 2005;23:792–799.

180. Miles D, Chan A, Romieu G, et al. Randomized, double-blind, placebo-controlled, phase III study of bevacizumab with docetaxel or docetaxel with placebo as first-line therapy for patients with locally recurrent or metastatic breast cancer (mBC): AVADO. *J Clin Oncol* 2008;26[Suppl]:(abst LBA1011).

181. Perou CM, Sorlie T, Eisen MB, et al. Molecular portraits of human breast tumours. *Nature* 2000;406:747–752.

182. Sorlie T, Perou CM, Tibshirani R, et al. Gene expression patterns of breast carcinomas distinguish tumor subclasses with clinical implications. *Proc Natl Acad Sci U S A* 2001;98:10869–10874.

183. Rakha EA, El-Sayed ME, Green AR, et al. Prognostic markers in triple-negative breast cancer. *Cancer* 2007;109:25–32.

184. Foulkes WD, Stefansson IM, Chappuis PO, et al. Germline BRCA1 mutations and a basal epithelial phenotype in breast cancer. *J Natl Cancer Inst* 2003;95: 1482–1485.

185. Minn AJ, Gupta GP, Siegel PM, et al. Genes that mediate breast cancer metastasis to lung. *Nature* 2005;436:518–524.

186. Dent R, Trudeau M, Pritchard KI, et al. Triple-negative breast cancer: clinical features and patterns of recurrence. *Clin Cancer Res* 2007;13:4429–4434.

187. Carey LA, Dees EC, Sawyer L, et al. The triple negative paradox: primary tumor chemosensitivity of breast cancer subtypes. *Clin Cancer Res* 2007;13:2329–2334.

188. Rouzier R, Perou CM, Symmans WF, et al. Breast cancer molecular subtypes respond differently to preoperative chemotherapy. *Clin Cancer Res* 2005;11: 5678–5685.

189. Guarneri V, Broglio K, Kau SW, et al. Prognostic value of pathologic complete response after primary chemotherapy in relation to hormone receptor status and other factors. *J Clin Oncol* 2006;24:1037–1044.

190. Urruticoechea A, Smith IE, Dowsett M. Proliferation marker Ki-67 in early breast cancer. *J Clin Oncol* 2005;23:7212–7220.

191. Altundag K, Harputluoglu H, Aksoy S, et al. Potential chemotherapy options in the triple negative subtype of breast cancer. *J Clin Oncol* 2007;25:1294–1296.

192. Kreike B, van Kouwenhove M, Horlings H, et al. Gene expression profiling and histopathological characterization of triple-negative/basal-like breast carcinomas. *Breast Cancer Res* 2007;9:R65.

193. Gholam D, Chebib A, Hauteville D, et al. Combined paclitaxel and cetuximab achieved a major response on the skin metastases of a patient with epidermal growth factor receptor-positive, estrogen receptor-negative, progesterone receptor-negative and human epidermal growth factor receptor-2-negative (triple-negative) breast cancer. *Anticancer Drugs* 2007;18:835–837.

194. Rodenhuis S, Bontenbal M, van Hoesel QG, et al. Efficacy of high-dose alkylating chemotherapy in HER2/neu-negative breast cancer. *Ann Oncol* 2006;17:588–596.

195. Goldenberg GJ, Moore MJ. Nitrogen mustards. In: Teicher BA, ed. *Cancer therapeutics: experimental and clinical agents (Cancer Drug Discovery and Development)*. 1st ed. Totowa, NJ: Humana Press, 1997:3.

196. Tew KD, Colvin OM, Jones RB. Clinical and high dose alkylating agents. In: Chabner, BA, Longo DL, eds. *Cancer chemotherapy and biotherapy: principles and practice*. 4th ed. Philadelphia: Lippincott Williams & Wilkins, 2005:283–309.

197. Brock N, Wilmanns H. [Effect of a cyclic nitrogen mustard-phosphamidester on experimentally induced tumors in rats; chemotherapeutic effect and pharmacological properties of B518 ASTA]. *Dtsch Med Wochenschr* 1958;83:453–458.

198. Brock N. [Pharmacological characterization of cyclic nitrogen mustard phosphamide esters as cancer therapeutic agents]. *Arzneimittelforschung* 1958;8: 1–9.

199. Arnold H, Bourseaux F, Brock N. Chemotherapeutic action of a cyclic nitrogen mustard phosphamide ester (B518-ASTA) in experimental tumours of the rat. *Nature* 1958;181:931.

200. Lane M. Some effects of cyclophosphamide (cytoxan) on normal mice and mice with L1210 leukemia. *J Natl Cancer Inst* 1959;23:1347–1359.

201. Gross R, Lambers K. [First experience in treating malignant tumors with a new nitrogen mustard-phosphamidester.]. *Dtsch Med Wochenschr* 1958;83:458–462.

202. Diamanti AP, Rosado MM, Carsetti R, et al. B cells in SLE: different biological drugs for different pathogenic mechanisms. *Autoimmun Rev* 2007;7:143–148.

203. Deegens JK, Wetzels JF. Membranous nephropathy in the older adult: epidemiology, diagnosis and management. *Drugs Aging* 2007;24:717–732.

204. Sladek NE. Metabolism of oxazaphosphorines. *Pharmacol Ther* 1988;37: 301–355.

205. Chang TK, Weber GF, Crespi CL, et al. Differential activation of cyclophosphamide and ifosfamide by cytochromes P-450 2B and 3A in human liver microsomes. *Cancer Res* 1993;53:5629–5637.

206. Struck RF, Kirk MC, Mellett LB, et al. Urinary metabolites of the antitumor agent cyclophosphamide. *Mol Pharmacol* 1971;7:519–529.

207. Bakke JE, Feil VJ, Fjelstul CE, et al. Metabolism of cyclophosphamide by sheep. *J Agric Food Chem* 1972;20:384–388.

208. Colvin M, Padgett CA, Fenselau C. A biologically active metabolite of cyclophosphamide. *Cancer Res* 1973;33:915–918.

209. Patel JM. Metabolism and pulmonary toxicity of cyclophosphamide. *Pharmacol Ther* 1990;47:137–146.

210. Kanekal S, Kehrer JP. Evidence for peroxidase-mediated metabolism of cyclophosphamide. *Drug Metab Dispos* 1993;21:37–42.

211. Friedman OM, Myles A, Colvin M. Cyclophosphamide and related phosphoramide mustards: current status and future prospects. In: Rosowsky A, ed. *Advances in cancer chemotherapy*. New York: Marcel Dekker, 1979:159.

212. Cox PJ. Cyclophosphamide cystitis—identification of acrolein as the causative agent. *Biochem Pharmacol* 1979;28:2045–2049.

213. Mattern J, Eichhorn U, Kaina B, et al. O6-methylguanine-DNA methyltransferase activity and sensitivity to cyclophosphamide and cisplatin in human lung tumor xenografts. *Int J Cancer* 1998;77:919–922.

214. McGown AT, Fox BW. A proposed mechanism of resistance to cyclophosphamide and phosphoramide mustard in a Yoshida cell line *in vitro*. *Cancer Chemother Pharmacol* 1986;17:223–226.

215. Crook TR, Souhami RL, Whyman GD, et al. Glutathione depletion as a determinant of sensitivity of human leukemia cells to cyclophosphamide. *Cancer Res* 1986;46:5035–5038.

216. Kirsch DG, Kastan MB. Tumor-suppressor p53: implications for tumor development and prognosis. *J Clin Oncol* 1998;16:3158–3168.

217. Hilton J. Role of aldehyde dehydrogenase in cyclophosphamide-resistant L1210 leukemia. *Cancer Res* 1984;44:5156–5160.

218. D'Incalci M, Bolis G, Facchinetti T, et al. Decreased half life of cyclophosphamide in patients under continual treatment. *Eur J Cancer* 1979;15:7–10.

219. Stuart-Harris R, Odell H, Sturgiss E. Adjuvant chemotherapy for early breast cancer: is cyclophosphamide, methotrexate and 5-fluorouracil still the standard? *Asia-Pacific J Clin Oncol* 2005;1:13–24.

220. Jardine I, Fenselau C, Appler M, et al. Quantitation by gas chromatography-chemical ionization mass spectrometry of cyclophosphamide, phosphoramide mustard, and nornitrogen mustard in the plasma and urine of patients receiving cyclophosphamide therapy. *Cancer Res* 1978;38:408–415.

221. Dillman JB. Safe use of succinylcholine during repeated anesthetics in a patient treated with cyclophosphamide. *Anesth Analg* 1987;66:351–353.

222. Torti FM, Bristow MR, Howes AE, et al. Reduced cardiotoxicity of doxorubicin delivered on a weekly schedule. Assessment by endomyocardial biopsy. *Ann Intern Med* 1983;99:745–749.

223. Stillwell TJ, Benson RC Jr. Cyclophosphamide-induced hemorrhagic cystitis. A review of 100 patients. *Cancer* 1988;61:451–457.

224. Arranz JA, Jimenez R, Alvarez-Mon M. Cyclophosphamide-induced myopia. *Ann Intern Med* 1992;116:92–93.

225. DeFronzo RA, Braine H, Colvin M, et al. Water intoxication in man after cyclophosphamide therapy. Time course and relation to drug activation. *Ann Intern Med* 1973;78:861–869.

226. Levine EG, Bloomfield CD. Leukemias and myelodysplastic syndromes secondary to drug, radiation, and environmental exposure. *Semin Oncol* 1992;19:47–84.

227. Greene MH, Harris EL, Gershenson DM, et al. Melphalan may be a more potent leukemogen than cyclophosphamide. *Ann Intern Med* 1986;105:360–367.

228. Curtis RE, Boice JD Jr, Moloney WC, et al. Leukemia following chemotherapy for breast cancer. *Cancer Res* 1990;50:2741–2746.

229. Valagussa P, Moliterni A, Terenziani M, et al. Second malignancies following CMF-based adjuvant chemotherapy in resectable breast cancer. *Ann Oncol* 1994; 5:803–808.

230. Curtis RE, Boice JD Jr, Stovall M, et al. Risk of leukemia after chemotherapy and radiation treatment for breast cancer. *N Engl J Med* 1992;326:1745–1751.

231. Hortobagyi GN. Developments in chemotherapy of breast cancer. *Cancer* 2000;88.3073–3079.

232. Mouridsen HT, Palshof T, Brahm M, et al. Evaluation of single-drug versus multiple-drug chemotherapy in the treatment of advanced breast cancer. *Cancer Treat Rep* 1977;61:47–50.

233. Miller JJ 3rd, Williams GF, Leissring JC. Multiple late complications of therapy with cyclophosphamide, including ovarian destruction. *Am J Med* 1971;50: 530–535.

234. Sorio R, Lombardi D, Spazzapan S, et al. Ifosfamide in advanced/disseminated breast cancer. *Oncology* 2003;65[Suppl 2]:55–58.

235. Bisagni G, Boni C, Manenti AL, et al. Ifosfamide bolus followed by five days continuous infusion in extensively pretreated patients with advanced breast cancer: a phase II study. *Tumori* 1998;84:659–661.

236. Walters RS, Holmes FA, Valero V, et al. Phase II study of ifosfamide and mesna in patients with metastatic breast cancer. *Am J Clin Oncol* 1998;21:413–415.

237. Lauro VD, Spazzapan S, Lombardi D, et al. Fourteen-day infusion of ifosfamide in the management of advanced breast cancer refractory to protracted continuous infusion of 5-fluorouracil. *Tumori* 2001;87:27–29.

238. Kaye SB. New antimetabolites in cancer chemotherapy and their clinical impact. *Br J Cancer* 1998;78[Suppl 3]:1–7.

239. Farber S, Diamond LK, Mercer RD, et al. Temporary remissions in acute leukemia in children produced by folic acid antagonist, 4-aminopteroyl-glutamic acid (aminopterin). *N Engl J Med* 1948;238:787–793.

240. Kummar S, Noronha V, Chu E. Antimetabolites. In: DeVita VT Jr, Hellman S, Rosenberg SA, eds. *Cancer: principles and practice of oncology*. 7th ed. Philadelphia: Lippincott Williams & Wilkins, 2005:358–374.

241. Grem JL. 5-Fluoropymidines. In: Chabner BA, Longo DL, eds. *Cancer chemotherapy and biotherapy: principles and practice*. 4th ed. Philadelphia: Lippincott Williams & Wilkins, 2005:125–182.

242. Monahan BP, Allegra CJ. Antifolates. In: Chabner BA, Longo DL, eds. *Cancer chemotherapy and biotherapy: principles and practice*. 4th ed. Philadelphia: Lippincott Williams & Wilkins, 2005:91–124.

243. Waltham MC, Holland JW, Robinson SC, et al. Direct experimental evidence for competitive inhibition of dihydrofolate reductase by methotrexate. *Biochem Pharmacol* 1988;37:535–539.

244. Bertino JR. Karnofsky memorial lecture. Ode to methotrexate. *J Clin Oncol* 1993; 11:5–14.

245. Allegra CJ, Fine RL, Drake JC, et al. The effect of methotrexate on intracellular folate pools in human MCF-7 breast cancer cells. Evidence for direct inhibition of purine synthesis. *J Biol Chem* 1986;261:6478–6485.

246. Matherly LH, Barlowe CK, Phillips VM, et al. The effects on 4-aminoantifolates on 5-formyltetrahydrofolate metabolism in L1210 cells. A biochemical basis of the selectivity of leucovorin rescue. *J Biol Chem* 1987;262:710–717.

247. Allegra CJ, Hoang K, Yeh GC, et al. Evidence for direct inhibition of de novo purine synthesis in human MCF-7 breast cells as a principal mode of metabolic inhibition by methotrexate. *J Biol Chem* 1987;262:13520–13526.

248. Baram J, Chabner BA, Drake JC, et al. Identification and biochemical properties of 10-formyldihydrofolate, a novel folate found in methotrexate-treated cells. *J Biol Chem* 1988;263:7105–7111.

249. Kumar P, Kisliuk RL, Gaumont Y, et al. Inhibition of human dihydrofolate reductase by antifolyl polyglutamates. *Biochem Pharmacol* 1989;38:541–543.

250. Santi DV, McHenry CS, Sommer H. Mechanism of interaction of thymidylate synthetase with 5-fluorodeoxyuridylate. *Biochemistry* 1974;13:471–481.
251. Sommer H, Santi DV. Purification and amino acid analysis of an active site peptide from thymidylate synthetase containing covalently bound 5-fluoro-2'-deoxyuridylate and methylenetetrahydrofolate. *Biochem Biophys Res Commun* 1974;57:689–695.
252. Miwa M, Ishikawa T, Eda H, et al. Comparative studies on the antitumor and immunosuppressive effects of the new fluorouracil derivative N4-trimethoxybenzoyl-5'-deoxy-5-fluorocytidine and its parent drug 5'-deoxy-5-fluorouridine. *Chem Pharm Bull (Tokyo)* 1990;38:998–1003.
253. Rockwell S, Grindey GB. Effect of 2',2'-difluorodeoxycytidine on the viability and radiosensitivity of EMT6 cells in vitro. *Oncol Res* 1992;4:151–155.
254. Guchelaar HJ, Richel DJ, van Knapen A. Clinical, toxicological and pharmacological aspects of gemcitabine. *Cancer Treat Rev* 1996;22:15–31.
255. Huang P, Plunkett W. Fludarabine- and gemcitabine-induced apoptosis: incorporation of analogs into DNA is a critical event. *Cancer Chemother Pharmacol* 1995;36:181–188.
256. Pizzorno G, Mini E, Coronnello M, et al. Impaired polyglutamylation of methotrexate as a cause of resistance in CCRF-CEM cells after short-term, high-dose treatment with this drug. *Cancer Res* 1988;48:2149–2155.
257. Galpin AJ, Schuetz JD, Masson E, et al. Differences in folylpolyglutamate synthetase and dihydrofolate reductase expression in human B-lineage versus T-lineage leukemic lymphoblasts: mechanisms for lineage differences in methotrexate polyglutamylation and cytotoxicity. *Mol Pharmacol* 1997;52:155–163.
258. Schimke RT. Methotrexate resistance and gene amplification. Mechanisms and implications. *Cancer* 1986;57:1912–1917.
259. Haber DA, Schimke RT. Unstable amplification of an altered dihydrofolate reductase gene associated with double-minute chromosomes. *Cell* 1981;26:355–362.
260. Bertino JR. Clinical pharmacology of methotrexate. *Med Pediatr Oncol* 1982;10:401–411.
261. Dicker AP, Waltham MC, Volkenandt M, et al. Methotrexate resistance in an in vivo mouse tumor due to a non-active-site dihydrofolate reductase mutation. *Proc Natl Acad Sci U S A* 1993;90:11797–11801.
262. Chu E, Takimoto CH, Voeller D, et al. Specific binding of human dihydrofolate reductase protein to dihydrofolate reductase messenger RNA in vitro. *Biochemistry* 1993;32:4756–4760.
263. Curt GA, Jolivet J, Carney DN, et al. Determinants of the sensitivity of human small-cell lung cancer cell lines to methotrexate. *J Clin Invest* 1985;76:1323–1329.
264. Fernandes DJ, Sur P, Kute TE, et al. Proliferation-dependent cytotoxicity of methotrexate in murine L5178Y leukemia. *Cancer Res* 1988;48:5638–5644.
265. Sobrero AF, Aschele C, Guglielmi AP, et al. Synergism and lack of cross-resistance between short-term and continuous exposure to fluorouracil in human colon adenocarcinoma cells. *J Natl Cancer Inst* 1993;85:1937–1944.
266. Mackey JR, Mani RS, Selner M, et al. Functional nucleoside transporters are required for gemcitabine influx and manifestation of toxicity in cancer cell lines. *Cancer Res* 1998;58:4349–4357.
267. Goan YG, Zhou B, Hu E, et al. Overexpression of ribonucleotide reductase as a mechanism of resistance to 2,2-difluorodeoxycytidine in the human KB cancer cell line. *Cancer Res* 1999;59:4204–4207.
268. Sliutz G, Karlseder J, Tempfer C, et al. Drug resistance against gemcitabine and topotecan mediated by constitutive hsp70 overexpression in vitro: implication of quercetin as sensitiser in chemotherapy. *Br J Cancer* 1996;74:172–177.
269. Neff T, Blau CA. Forced expression of cytidine deaminase confers resistance to cytosine arabinoside and gemcitabine. *Exp Hematol* 1996;24:1340–1346.
270. Fossa SD, Heilo A, Bormer O. Unexpectedly high serum methotrexate levels in cystectomized bladder cancer patients with an ileal conduit treated with intermediate doses of the drug. *J Urol* 1990;143:498–501.
271. Myers CE, Diasio R, Eliot HM, et al. Pharmacokinetics of the fluoropyrimidines: implications for their clinical use. *Cancer Treat Rev* 1976;3:175–183.
272. Mackean M, Planting A, Twelves C, et al. Phase I and pharmacologic study of intermittent twice-daily oral therapy with capecitabine in patients with advanced and/or metastatic cancer. *J Clin Oncol* 1998;16:2977–2985.
273. Venook AP, Egorin MJ, Rosner GL, et al. Phase I and pharmacokinetic trial of gemcitabine in patients with hepatic or renal dysfunction: Cancer and Leukemia Group B 9565. *J Clin Oncol* 2000;18:2780–2787.
274. Thyss A, Milano G, Kubar J, et al. Clinical and pharmacokinetic evidence of a life-threatening interaction between methotrexate and ketoprofen. *Lancet* 1986;1:256–258.
275. Tracy TS, Worster T, Bradley JD, et al. Methotrexate disposition following concomitant administration of ketoprofen, piroxicam and flurbiprofen in patients with rheumatoid arthritis. *Br J Clin Pharmacol* 1994;37:453–456.
276. Mandel MA. The synergistic effect of salicylates on methotrexate toxicity. *Plast Reconstr Surg* 1976;57:733–737.
277. Paxton JW. Protein binding of methotrexate in sera from normal human beings: effect of drug concentration, pH, temperature, and storage. *J Pharmacol Meth* 1981;5:203–213.
278. Jeurissen ME, Boerbooms AM, van de Putte LB. Pancytopenia and methotrexate with trimethoprim-sulfamethoxazole. *Ann Intern Med* 1989;111:261.
279. Govert JA, Patton S, Fine RL. Pancytopenia from using trimethoprim and methotrexate. *Ann Intern Med* 1992;117:877–878.
280. Thyss A, Milano G, Renee N, et al. Severe interaction between methotrexate and a macrolide-like antibiotic. *J Natl Cancer Inst* 1993;85:582–583.
281. Harvey VJ, Slevin ML, Dilloway MR, et al. The influence of cimetidine on the pharmacokinetics of 5-fluorouracil. *Br J Clin Pharmacol* 1984;18:421–430.
282. Howell SB, Wung WE, Taetle R, et al. Modulation of 5-fluorouracil toxicity by allopurinol in man. *Cancer* 1981;48:1281–1289.
283. Koenig H, Patel A. The acute cerebellar syndrome in 5-fluorouracil chemotherapy: a manifestation of fluoroacetate intoxication. *Neurology* 1970;20:416.
284. Wacker A, Lersch C, Scherpinski U, et al. High incidence of angina pectoris in patients treated with 5-fluorouracil. A planned surveillance study with 102 patients. *Oncology* 2003;65:108–112.
285. Frickhofen N, Beck FJ, Jung B, et al. Capecitabine can induce acute coronary syndrome similar to 5-fluorouracil. *Ann Oncol* 2002;13:797–801.
286. Takimoto CH, Lu ZH, Zhang R, et al. Severe neurotoxicity following 5-fluorouracil-based chemotherapy in a patient with dihydropyrimidine dehydrogenase deficiency. *Clin Cancer Res* 1996;2:477–481.
287. Harris BE, Carpenter JT, Diasio RB. Severe 5-fluorouracil toxicity secondary to dihydropyrimidine dehydrogenase deficiency. A potentially more common pharmacogenetic syndrome. *Cancer* 1991;68:499–501.
288. Houyau P, Gay C, Chatelut E, et al. Severe fluorouracil toxicity in a patient with dihydropyrimidine dehydrogenase deficiency. *J Natl Cancer Inst* 1993;85:1602–1603.
289. Diasio RB, Lu Z. Dihydropyrimidine dehydrogenase activity and fluorouracil chemotherapy. *J Clin Oncol* 1994;12:2239–2242.
290. Di Paolo A, Danesi R, Falcone A, et al. Relationship between 5-fluorouracil disposition, toxicity and dihydropyrimidine dehydrogenase activity in cancer patients. *Ann Oncol* 2001;12:1301–1306.
291. Ho DH, Townsend L, Luna MA, et al. Distribution and inhibition of dihydrouracil dehydrogenase activities in human tissues using 5-fluorouracil as a substrate. *Anticancer Res* 1986;6:781–784.
292. Grem JL, Yee LK, Venzon DJ, et al. Inter- and intraindividual variation in dihydropyrimidine dehydrogenase activity in peripheral blood mononuclear cells. *Cancer Chemother Pharmacol* 1997;40:117–125.
293. Van Kuilenburg AB, van Lenthe H, Blom MJ, et al. Profound variation in dihydropyrimidine dehydrogenase activity in human blood cells: major implications for the detection of partly deficient patients. *Br J Cancer* 1999;79:620–626.
294. Diasio RB, Beavers TL, Carpenter JT. Familial deficiency of dihydropyrimidine dehydrogenase. Biochemical basis for familial pyrimidinemia and severe 5-fluorouracil-induced toxicity. *J Clin Invest* 1988;81:47–51.
295. Lu Z, Zhang R, Diasio RB. Dihydropyrimidine dehydrogenase activity in human peripheral blood mononuclear cells and liver: population characteristics, newly identified deficient patients, and clinical implication in 5-fluorouracil chemotherapy. *Cancer Res* 1993;53:5433–5438.
296. Wagstaff AJ, Ibbotson T, Goa KL. Capecitabine: a review of its pharmacology and therapeutic efficacy in the management of advanced breast cancer. *Drugs* 2003;63:217–236.
297. Lee S, Lee S, Chun Y, et al. Pyridoxine is not effective for the prevention of hand foot syndrome (HFS) associated with capecitabine therapy: results of a randomized double-blind placebo-controlled study. ASCO annual meeting proceedings Part I. *J Clin Oncol* 2007;25(18S)[Suppl]:9007.
298. Locker GJ, Wenzel C, Schmidinger M, et al. Unexpected severe myelotoxicity of gemcitabine in pretreated breast cancer patients. *Anticancer Drugs* 2001;12:209–212.
299. Pavlakis N, Bell DR, Millward MJ, et al. Fatal pulmonary toxicity resulting from treatment with gemcitabine. *Cancer* 1997;80:286–291.
300. Sauer-Heilborn A, Kath R, Schneider CP, et al. Severe non-haematological toxicity after treatment with gemcitabine. *J Cancer Res Clin Oncol* 1999;125:637–640.
301. Bhatia S, Hanna N, Ansari R, et al. A phase II study of weekly gemcitabine and paclitaxel in patients with previously untreated stage IIIb and IV non-small cell lung cancer. *Lung Cancer* 2002;38:73–77.
302. Harries M, Moss C, Perren T, et al. A phase II feasibility study of carboplatin followed by sequential weekly paclitaxel and gemcitabine as first-line treatment for ovarian cancer. *Br J Cancer* 2004;91:627–632.
303. Thomas AL, Cox G, Sharma RA, et al. Gemcitabine and paclitaxel associated pneumonitis in non-small cell lung cancer: report of a phase I/II dose-escalating study. *Eur J Cancer* 2000;36:2329–2334.
304. Fung MC, Storniolo AM, Nguyen B, et al. A review of hemolytic uremic syndrome in patients treated with gemcitabine therapy. *Cancer* 1999;85:2023–2032.
305. Frei E 3rd, Blum RH, Pitman SW, et al. High dose methotrexate with leucovorin rescue. Rationale and spectrum of antitumor activity. *Am J Med* 1980;68:370–376.
306. Benz C, Silverberg M, Cadman E. Use of high-dose oral methotrexate sequenced at 24 hours with 5-FU: a clinical toxicity study. *Cancer Treat Rep* 1983;67:297–299.
307. Cameron DA, Gabra H, Leonard RC. Continuous 5-fluorouracil in the treatment of breast cancer. *Br J Cancer* 1994;70:120–124.
308. Lokich JJ, Ahlgren JD, Gullo JJ, et al. A prospective randomized comparison of continuous infusion fluorouracil with a conventional bolus schedule in metastatic colorectal carcinoma: a Mid-Atlantic Oncology Program Study. *J Clin Oncol* 1989;7:425–432.
309. Hansen RM. 5-Fluorouracil by protracted venous infusion: a review of recent clinical studies. *Cancer Invest* 1991;9:637–642.
310. Huan S, Pazdur R, Singhakowinta A, et al. Low-dose continuous infusion 5-fluorouracil. Evaluation in advanced breast carcinoma. *Cancer* 1989;63:419–422.
311. Jabboury K, Holmes FA, Hortobagyi G. 5-Fluorouracil rechallenge by protracted infusion in refractory breast cancer. *Cancer* 1989;64:793–797.
312. Hainsworth JD, Andrews MB, Johnson DH, et al. Mitoxantrone, fluorouracil, and high-dose leucovorin: an effective, well-tolerated regimen for metastatic breast cancer. *J Clin Oncol* 1991;9:1731–1735.
313. Hainsworth JD. Mitoxantrone, 5-fluorouracil and high-dose leucovorin (NFL) in the treatment of metastatic breast cancer: randomized comparison to cyclophosphamide, methotrexate and 5-fluorouracil (CMF) and attempts to improve efficacy by adding paclitaxel. *Eur J Cancer Care (Engl)* 1997;6:4–9.
314. Bascioni R, Giorgi F, Silva RR, et al. Mitoxantrone, fluorouracil, and L-folinic acid in anthracycline-pretreated metastatic breast cancer patients. *Breast Cancer Res Treat* 1997;45:205–210.
315. Loprinzi CL. 5-Fluorouracil with leucovorin in breast cancer. *Cancer* 1989;63:1045–1047.
316. Doroshow JH, Leong L, Margolin K, et al. Refractory metastatic breast cancer: salvage therapy with fluorouracil and high-dose continuous infusion leucovorin calcium. *J Clin Oncol* 1989;7:439–444.
317. Parnes HL, Cirrincione C, Aisner J, et al. Phase III study of cyclophosphamide, doxorubicin, and fluorouracil (CAF) plus leucovorin versus CAF for metastatic breast cancer: Cancer and Leukemia Group B 9140. *J Clin Oncol* 2003;21:1819–1824.
318. Blum JL, Jones SE, Buzdar AU, et al. Multicenter phase II study of capecitabine in paclitaxel-refractory metastatic breast cancer. *J Clin Oncol* 1999;17:485–493.
319. Wist EA, Sommer HH, Ostenstad B, et al. Oral capecitabine in anthracycline- and taxane-pretreated advanced/metastatic breast cancer. *Acta Oncol* 2004;43:186–189.
320. Blum JL, Dieras V, Lo Russo PM, et al. Multicenter, phase II study of capecitabine in taxane-pretreated metastatic breast carcinoma patients. *Cancer* 2001;92:1759–1768.

321. Fumoleau P, Largillier R, Clippe C, et al. Multicentre, phase II study evaluating capecitabine monotherapy in patients with anthracycline- and taxane-pretreated metastatic breast cancer. *Eur J Cancer* 2004;40:536–542.
322. Reichardt P, Von Minckwitz G, Thuss-Patience PC, et al. Multicenter phase II study of oral capecitabine (Xeloda) in patients with metastatic breast cancer relapsing after treatment with a taxane-containing therapy. *Ann Oncol* 2003;14: 1227–1233.
323. Pierga JY, Fumoleau P, Brewer Y, et al. Efficacy and safety of single agent capecitabine in pretreated metastatic breast cancer patients from the French compassionate use program. *Breast Cancer Res Treat* 2004;88:117–129.
324. O'Shaughnessy JA. The evolving role of capecitabine in breast cancer. *Clin Breast Cancer* 2003;4[Suppl 1]:S20–S25.
325. Hennessy BT, Gauthier AM, Michaud LB, et al. Lower dose capecitabine has a more favorable therapeutic index in metastatic breast cancer: retrospective analysis of patients treated at M.D. Anderson Cancer Center and a review of capecitabine toxicity in the literature. *Ann Oncol* 2005;16:1289–1296.
326. Batista N, Perez-Manga G, Constenla M, et al. Phase II study of capecitabine in combination with paclitaxel in patients with anthracycline-pretreated advanced/metastatic breast cancer. *Br J Cancer* 2004;90:1740–1746.
327. Gradishar WJ, Meza LA, Amin B, et al. Capecitabine plus paclitaxel as front-line combination therapy for metastatic breast cancer: a multicenter phase II study. *J Clin Oncol* 2004;22:2321–2327.
328. Ghosn M, Farhat F, Kattan J, et al. Final results of a phase II study of vinorelbine in combination with capecitabine as first line chemotherapy for metastatic breast cancer (MBC). *Proc Am Soc Clin Oncol* 2003;22:(abst 270).
329. Kajanti MJ, Pyrhonen SO, Maiche AG. Oral tegafur in the treatment of metastatic breast cancer: a phase II study. *Eur J Cancer* 1993;29A:863–866.
330. Sole LA, Albanell J, Bellmunt J, et al. Phase II trial of an all-oral regimen of tegafur and folinic acid in patients with previously treated metastatic breast cancer. *Cancer* 1995;75:831–835.
331. Yardley DA, Jones SF, Greco FA, et al. A phase II trial of Orzel (UFT + leucovorin) in women with previously treated metastatic breast cancer. *Proc Am Soc Clin Oncol* 2001;20:(abst 2031).
332. Schwartzberg L, Irwin D, Havlin K, et al. Phase II study of a novel, fixed-dose schedule of UFT plus leucovorin (UFT/L) for patients (pts) with progressive, metastatic breast cancer after prior chemotherapy. *Proc Am Soc Clin Oncol* 2002;21:(abst 240).
333. Heinemann V. Role of gemcitabine in the treatment of advanced and metastatic breast cancer. *Oncology* 2003;64:191–206.
334. Qu G, Perez EA. Gemcitabine and targeted therapy in metastatic breast cancer. *Semin Oncol* 2002;29:44–52.
335. Rha SY, Moon YH, Jeung HC, et al. Gemcitabine monotherapy as salvage chemotherapy in heavily pretreated metastatic breast cancer. *Breast Cancer Res Treat* 2005;90:215–221.
336. Carmichael J, Possinger K, Phillip P, et al. Advanced breast cancer: a phase II trial with gemcitabine. *J Clin Oncol* 1995;13:2731–2736.
337. Blackstein M, Vogel CL, Ambinder R, et al. Gemcitabine as first-line therapy in patients with metastatic breast cancer: a phase II trial. *Oncology* 2002;62:2–8.
338. Possinger K, Kaufmann M, Coleman R, et al. Phase II study of gemcitabine as first-line chemotherapy in patients with advanced or metastatic breast cancer. *Anticancer Drugs* 1999;10:155–162.
339. El Serafi MM, El Khodary AI, El Zawahry HR, et al. Gemcitabine plus doxorubicin as first-line treatment in advanced or metastatic breast cancer (MBC), a phase II study. *J Egypt Natl Cancer Inst* 2006;18:209–215.
340. Campone M, Fumoleau P, Viens P, et al. Gemcitabine and epirubicin in patients with metastatic breast cancer: a phase I/II study. *Breast* 2006;15:601–609.
341. Zielinski C, Beslija S, Mrsic-Krmpotic Z, et al. Gemcitabine, epirubicin, and paclitaxel versus fluorouracil, epirubicin, and cyclophosphamide as first-line chemotherapy in metastatic breast cancer: a Central European Cooperative Oncology Group International, multicenter, prospective, randomized phase III trial. *J Clin Oncol* 2005;23:1401–1408.
342. Ulrich-Pur H, Kornek GV, Haider K, et al. Phase II trial of pegylated liposomal doxorubicin (Caelyx) plus gemcitabine in chemotherapeutically pretreated patients with advanced breast cancer. *Acta Oncol* 2007;46:208–213.
343. Andres R, Mayordomo JI, Lara R, et al. Gemcitabine/capecitabine in patients with metastatic breast cancer pretreated with anthracyclines and taxanes. *Clin Breast Cancer* 2005;6:158–162.
344. Awada A, Biganzoli L, Cufer T, et al. An EORTC-IDBBC phase I study of gemcitabine and continuous infusion 5-fluorouracil in patients with metastatic breast cancer resistant to anthracyclines or pre-treated with both anthracyclines and taxanes. *Eur J Cancer* 2002;38:773–778.
345. Frasci G, D'Aiuto G, Comella P, et al. A phase I-II study on a gemcitabine-cyclophosphamide-fluorouracil/folinic acid triplet combination in anthracycline- and taxane-refractory breast cancer patients. *Oncology* 2002;62:25–32.
346. Onyenadum A, Gogas H, Kosmidis P, et al. Mitoxantrone plus gemcitabine in pretreated patients with metastatic breast cancer. *J Chemother* 2006;18:192–198.
347. Lorusso V, Crucitta E, Silvestris N, et al. Phase I/II study of gemcitabine plus mitoxantrone as salvage chemotherapy in metastatic breast cancer. *Br J Cancer* 2003;88:491–495.
348. Nagourney RA, Link JS, Blitzer JB, et al. Gemcitabine plus cisplatin repeating doublet therapy in previously treated, relapsed breast cancer patients. *J Clin Oncol* 2000;18:2245–2249.
349. Seo JH, Oh SC, Choi CW, et al. Phase II study of a gemcitabine and cisplatin combination regimen in taxane resistant metastatic breast cancer. *Cancer Chemother Pharmacol* 2007;59:269–274.
350. Burch PA, Mailliard JA, Hillman DW, et al. Phase II study of gemcitabine plus cisplatin in patients with metastatic breast cancer: a North Central Cancer Treatment Group trial. *Am J Clin Oncol* 2005;28:195–200.
351. Nasr FL, Chahine GY, Kattan JG, et al. Gemcitabine plus carboplatin combination therapy as second-line treatment in patients with relapsed breast cancer. *Clin Breast Cancer* 2004;5:117–124.
352. Stathopoulos GP, Rigatos SK, Pergantas N, et al. Phase II trial of biweekly administration of vinorelbine and gemcitabine in pretreated advanced breast cancer. *J Clin Oncol* 2002;20:37–41.
353. Morabito A, Filippelli G, Palmeri S, et al. The combination of gemcitabine and vinorelbine is an active regimen as second-line therapy in patients with metastatic breast cancer pretreated with taxanes and/or anthracyclines: a phase I-II study. *Breast Cancer Res Treat* 2003;78:29–36.
354. Sanal SM, Gokmen E, Karabulut B, et al. Gemcitabine and vinorelbine combination in patients with metastatic breast cancer. *Breast J* 2002;8:171–176.
355. Ardavanis A, Kountourakis P, Maliou S, et al. Gemcitabine and oral vinorelbine as salvage treatment in patients with advanced anthracycline- and taxane-pretreated breast cancer. *Anticancer Res* 2007;27:2989–2992.
356. Gennatas C, Michalaki V, Mouratidou D, et al. Gemcitabine in combination with vinorelbine for heavily pretreated advanced breast cancer. *Anticancer Res* 2006; 26:549–552.
357. Palmeri S, Vaglica M, Spada S, et al. Weekly docetaxel and gemcitabine as first-line treatment for metastatic breast cancer: results of a multicenter phase II study. *Oncology* 2005;68:438–445.
358. Laufman LR, Spiridonidis CH, Pritchard J, et al. Monthly docetaxel and weekly gemcitabine in metastatic breast cancer: a phase II trial. *Ann Oncol* 2001;12: 1259–1264.
359. Mavroudis D, Malamos N, Alexopoulos A, et al. Salvage chemotherapy in anthracycline-pretreated metastatic breast cancer patients with docetaxel and gemcitabine: a multicenter phase II trial. Greek Breast Cancer Cooperative Group. *Ann Oncol* 1999;10:211–215.
360. Kornek GV, Haider K, Kwasny W, et al. Treatment of advanced breast cancer with docetaxel and gemcitabine with and without human granulocyte colony-stimulating factor. *Clin Cancer Res* 2002;8:1051–1056.
361. Levy C, Fumoleau P. Gemcitabine plus docetaxel: a new treatment option for anthracycline pretreated metastatic breast cancer patients? *Cancer Treat Rev* 2005;31[Suppl 4]:S17–S22.
362. Grein A, Spella C, DiMarco A, et al. [Descrizione e classificazione di un attionamicette (*Streptomyces peucetius* sp novo) produltore di un sostanza ad attivite antitumorale; la daunomicina]. *Giorn Microbiol* 1963;11:109–118.
363. Dubost M, Gauter P, Maral R. [Un novel antibiotique a proprietes cytostatiques; la rubidomycine]. *C R Acad Sci Paris* 1963;257:1813–1815.
364. Di Marco A, Gaetani M, Scarpinato B. Adriamycin (NSC-123,127): a new antibiotic with antitumor activity. *Cancer Chemother Rep* 1969;53:33–37.
365. Launchbury AP, Habboubi N. Epirubicin and doxorubicin: a comparison of their characteristics, therapeutic activity and toxicity. *Cancer Treat Rev* 1993;19: 197–228.
366. Doroshow JH. Anthracyclines and anthracenediones. In: Grochow LB, Ames MM, eds. *A clinician's guide to chemotherapy pharmacokinetics and pharmacodynamics*. 1st ed. Baltimore: Lippincott Williams & Wilkins, 1998:93.
367. Tewey KM, Rowe TC, Yang L, et al. Adriamycin-induced DNA damage mediated by mammalian DNA topoisomerase II. *Science* 1984;226:466–468.
368. Doroshow JH. Anthracyclines and anthracenediones. In: Chabner BA, Longo DL, eds. *Cancer chemotherapy and biotherapy: principles and practice*. 4th ed. Philadelphia: Lippincott Williams & Wilkins, 2005:414–450.
369. Belloni M, Uberti D, Rizzini C, et al. Induction of two DNA mismatch repair proteins, MSH2 and MSH6, in differentiated human neuroblastoma SH-SY5Y cells exposed to doxorubicin. *J Neurochem* 1999;72:974–979.
370. Takimoto CH. Topoisomerase interactive agents. In: DeVita VT Jr, Hellman S, Rosenberg SA, eds. *Cancer: principles and practice of oncology*. 7th ed. Philadelphia: Lippincott Williams & Wilkins, 2005:375–390.
371. Doxorubicin hydrochloride for injection, USP [package insert]. New York: Pfizer Labs, 2006.
372. Bristow MR, Billingham ME, Mason JW, et al. Clinical spectrum of anthracycline antibiotic cardiotoxicity. *Cancer Treat Rep* 1978;62:873–879.
373. Perez EA, Suman VJ, Davidson NE, et al. Effect of doxorubicin plus cyclophosphamide on left ventricular ejection fraction in patients with breast cancer in the North Central Cancer Treatment Group N9831 Intergroup adjuvant trial. *J Clin Oncol* 2004;22:3700–3704.
374. Perez EA, Suman VJ, Davidson NE, et al. Cardiac safety analysis of doxorubicin and cyclophosphamide followed by paclitaxel with or without trastuzumab in the North Central Cancer Treatment Group N9831 adjuvant breast cancer trial. *J Clin Oncol* 2008;26:1231–1238.
375. Legha SS, Benjamin RS, Mackay B, et al. Reduction of doxorubicin cardiotoxicity by prolonged continuous intravenous infusion. *Ann Intern Med* 1982;96: 133–139.
376. Ferrans VJ. Overview of cardiac pathology in relation to anthracycline cardiotoxicity. *Cancer Treat Rep* 1978;62:955–961.
377. Bristow MR, Mason JW, Billingham ME, et al. Doxorubicin cardiomyopathy: evaluation by phonocardiography, endomyocardial biopsy, and cardiac catheterization. *Ann Intern Med* 1978;88:168–175.
378. Li J, Gwilt PR. The effect of age on the early disposition of doxorubicin. *Cancer Chemother Pharmacol* 2003;51:395–402.
379. Fisher B, Redmond C, Wickerham DL, et al. Doxorubicin-containing regimens for the treatment of stage II breast cancer: the National Surgical Adjuvant Breast and Bowel Project experience. *J Clin Oncol* 1989;7:572–582.
380. Von Hoff DD, Layard MW, Basa P, et al. Risk factors for doxorubicin-induced congestive heart failure. *Ann Intern Med* 1979;91:710–717.
381. Steinherz LJ, Steinherz PG, Tan CT, et al. Cardiac toxicity 4 to 20 years after completing anthracycline therapy. *JAMA* 1991;266:1672–1677.
382. Pratt CB, Ransom JL, Evans WE. Age-related adriamycin cardiotoxicity in children. *Cancer Treat Rep* 1978;62:1381–1385.
383. Silber JH, Jakacki RI, Larsen RL, et al. Increased risk of cardiac dysfunction after anthracyclines in girls. *Med Pediatr Oncol* 1993;21:477–479.
384. Mouridsen HT. New cytotoxic drugs in treatment of breast cancer. *Acta Oncol* 1990;29:343–347.
385. Coukell AJ, Faulds D. Epirubicin. An updated review of its pharmacodynamic and pharmacokinetic properties and therapeutic efficacy in the management of breast cancer. *Drugs* 1997;53:453–482.
386. Bielack SS, Erttmann R, Winkler K, et al. Doxorubicin: effect of different schedules on toxicity and anti-tumor efficacy. *Eur J Cancer Clin Oncol* 1989;25: 873–882.
387. Speyer JL, Green MD, Dubin N, et al. Prospective evaluation of cardiotoxicity during a six-hour doxorubicin infusion regimen in women with adenocarcinoma of the breast. *Am J Med* 1985;78:555–563.
388. Waterhouse DN, Tardi PG, Mayer LD, et al. A comparison of liposomal formulations of doxorubicin with drug administered in free form: changing toxicity profiles. *Drug Saf* 2001;24:903–920.
389. Gabizon A, Catane R, Uziely B, et al. Prolonged circulation time and enhanced accumulation in malignant exudates of doxorubicin encapsulated in polyethylene-glycol coated liposomes. *Cancer Res* 1994;54:987–992.

390. DOXIL (doxorubicin HCL liposome injection) for intravenous infusion [package insert]. Bedford, OH: Alza Stealth, 2007.
391. Rahman A, White G, More N, et al. Pharmacological, toxicological, and therapeutic evaluation in mice of doxorubicin entrapped in cardiolipin liposomes. *Cancer Res* 1985;45:796–803.
392. Cowens JW, Creaven PJ, Greco WR, et al. Initial clinical (phase I) trial of TLC D-99 (doxorubicin encapsulated in liposomes). *Cancer Res* 1993;53:2796–2802.
393. Berry G, Billingham M, Alderman E, et al. The use of cardiac biopsy to demonstrate reduced cardiotoxicity in AIDS Kaposi's sarcoma patients treated with pegylated liposomal doxorubicin. *Ann Oncol* 1998;9:711–716.
394. Safra T, Muggia F, Jeffers S, et al. Pegylated liposomal doxorubicin (Doxil): reduced clinical cardiotoxicity in patients reaching or exceeding cumulative doses of 500 mg/m^2. *Ann Oncol* 2000;11:1029–1033.
395. Harris L, Batist G, Belt R, et al. Liposome-encapsulated doxorubicin compared with conventional doxorubicin in a randomized multicenter trial as first-line therapy of metastatic breast carcinoma. *Cancer* 2002;94:25–36.
396. O'Brien ME, Wigler N, Inbar M, et al. Reduced cardiotoxicity and comparable efficacy in a phase III trial of pegylated liposomal doxorubicin HCl (Caelyx/Doxil) versus conventional doxorubicin for first-line treatment of metastatic breast cancer. *Ann Oncol* 2004;15:440–449.
397. Wigler N, Inbar M, O'Brien M, et al. Reduced cardiac toxicity and comparable efficacy in a phase III trial of pegylated liposomal doxorubicin (Caelyx/Doxil) vs. doxorubicin for first-line treatment of metastatic breast cancer. *Proc Am Soc Clin Oncol* 2002;21:(abst 177).
398. Batist G, Ramakrishnan G, Rao CS, et al. Reduced cardiotoxicity and preserved antitumor efficacy of liposome-encapsulated doxorubicin and cyclophosphamide compared with conventional doxorubicin and cyclophosphamide in a randomized, multicenter trial of metastatic breast cancer. *J Clin Oncol* 2001;19: 1444–1454.
399. Keller AM, Mennel RG, Georgoulias VA, et al. Randomized phase III trial of pegylated liposomal doxorubicin versus vinorelbine or mitomycin C plus vinblastine in women with taxane-refractory advanced breast cancer. *J Clin Oncol* 2004;22: 3893–3901.
400. Rivera E, Valero V, Esteva FJ, et al. Lack of activity of stealth liposomal doxorubicin in the treatment of patients with anthracycline-resistant breast cancer. *Cancer Chemother Pharmacol* 2002;49:299–302.
401. Biganzoli L, Coleman R, Minisini A, et al. A joined analysis of two European Organization for the Research and Treatment of Cancer (EORTC) studies to evaluate the role of pegylated liposomal doxorubicin (Caelyx) in the treatment of elderly patients with metastatic breast cancer. *Crit Rev Oncol Hematol* 2007;61:84–89.
402. Batist G, Harris L, Azarnia N, et al. Improved anti-tumor response rate with decreased cardiotoxicity of non-pegylated liposomal doxorubicin compared with conventional doxorubicin in first-line treatment of metastatic breast cancer in patients who had received prior adjuvant doxorubicin: results of a retrospective analysis. *Anticancer Drugs* 2006;17:587–595.
403. Addeo R, Faiola V, Guarrasi R, et al. Liposomal pegylated doxorubicin plus vinorelbine combination as first-line chemotherapy for metastatic breast cancer in elderly women > or =65 years of age. *Cancer Chemother Pharmacol* 2008; 62(2):285–292.
404. Moore MR, Srinivasiah J, Feinberg BA, et al. Phase II randomized trial of doxorubicin plus paclitaxel (AT) versus doxorubicin HCl liposome injection (Doxil) plus paclitaxel (DT) in metastatic breast cancer. *Proc Am Soc Clin Oncol* 1998;17:160a(abst 614).
405. Valero V, Buzdar AU, Theriault RL, et al. Phase II trial of liposome-encapsulated doxorubicin, cyclophosphamide, and fluorouracil as first-line therapy in patients with metastatic breast cancer. *J Clin Oncol* 1999;17:1425–1434.
406. Swain SM, Whaley FS, Gerber MC, et al. Cardioprotection with dexrazoxane for doxorubicin-containing therapy in advanced breast cancer. *J Clin Oncol* 1997; 15:1318–1332.
407. Venturini M, Michelotti A, Del Mastro L, et al. Multicenter randomized controlled clinical trial to evaluate cardioprotection of dexrazoxane versus no cardioprotection in women receiving epirubicin chemotherapy for advanced breast cancer. *J Clin Oncol* 1996;14:3112–3120.
408. Schuchter LM, Hensley ML, Meropol NJ, et al. 2002 update of recommendations for the use of chemotherapy and radiotherapy protectants: clinical practice guidelines of the American Society of Clinical Oncology. *J Clin Oncol* 2002;20: 2895–2903.
409. Swain SM, Whaley FS, Gerber MC, et al. Delayed administration of dexrazoxane provides cardioprotection for patients with advanced breast cancer treated with doxorubicin-containing therapy. *J Clin Oncol* 1997;15:1333–1340.
410. Seymour L, Bramwell V, Moran LA. Use of dexrazoxane as a cardioprotectant in patients receiving doxorubicin or epirubicin chemotherapy for the treatment of cancer. The Provincial Systemic Treatment Disease Site group. *Cancer Prev Control* 1999;3:145–159.
411. Bates M, Lieu D, Zagari M, et al. A pharmacoeconomic evaluation of the use of dexrazoxane in preventing anthracycline-induced cardiotoxicity in patients with stage IIIB or IV metastatic breast cancer. *Clin Ther* 1997;19:167–184.
412. Neidhart JA, Gochnour D, Roach R, et al. A comparison of mitoxantrone and doxorubicin in breast cancer. *J Clin Oncol* 1986;4:672–677.
413. Hortobagyi GN, Yap HY, Kau SW, et al. A comparative study of doxorubicin and epirubicin in patients with metastatic breast cancer. *Am J Clin Oncol* 1989; 12:57–62.
414. Henderson IC, Allegra JC, Woodcock T, et al. Randomized clinical trial comparing mitoxantrone with doxorubicin in previously treated patients with metastatic breast cancer. *J Clin Oncol* 1989;7:560–571.
415. Pavesi L, Preti P, Da Prada G, et al. Epirubicin versus mitoxantrone in combination chemotherapy for metastatic breast cancer. *Anticancer Res* 1995;15: 495–501.
416. Falkson G, Tormey DC, Carey P, et al. Long-term survival of patients treated with combination chemotherapy for metastatic breast cancer. *Eur J Cancer* 1991;27: 973–977.
417. Coombes RC, Bliss JM, Wils J, et al. Adjuvant cyclophosphamide, methotrexate, and fluorouracil versus fluorouracil, epirubicin, and cyclophosphamide chemotherapy in premenopausal women with axillary node-positive operable breast cancer: results of a randomized trial. The International Collaborative Cancer group. *J Clin Oncol* 1996;14:35–45.
418. Nabholtz JM, Falkson C, Campos D, et al. Docetaxel and doxorubicin compared with doxorubicin and cyclophosphamide as first-line chemotherapy for metastatic breast cancer: results of a randomized, multicenter, phase III trial. *J Clin Oncol* 2003;21:968–975.
419. Aisner J, Weinberg V, Perloff M, et al. Chemotherapy versus chemoimmunotherapy (CAF v CAFVP v CMF each +/– MER) for metastatic carcinoma of the breast: a CALGB study. Cancer and Leukemia Group B. *J Clin Oncol* 1987;5:1523–1533.
420. Ackland SP, Anton A, Breitbach GP, et al. Dose-intensive epirubicin-based chemotherapy is superior to an intensive intravenous cyclophosphamide, methotrexate, and fluorouracil regimen in metastatic breast cancer: a randomized multinational study. *J Clin Oncol* 2001;19:943–953.
421. A'Hern RP, Smith IE, Ebbs SR. Chemotherapy and survival in advanced breast cancer: the inclusion of doxorubicin in Cooper type regimens. *Br J Cancer* 1993; 67:801–805.
422. Perez DJ, Harvey VJ, Robinson BA, et al. A randomized comparison of single-agent doxorubicin and epirubicin as first-line cytotoxic therapy in advanced breast cancer. *J Clin Oncol* 1991;9:2148–2152.
423. Findlay BP, Walker-Dilks C. Epirubicin, alone or in combination chemotherapy, for metastatic breast cancer. Provincial Breast Cancer Disease Site group and the Provincial Systemic Treatment Disease Site group. *Cancer Prev Control* 1998;2: 140–146.
424. Bennett JM, Muss HB, Doroshow JH, et al. A randomized multicenter trial comparing mitoxantrone, cyclophosphamide, and fluorouracil with doxorubicin, cyclophosphamide, and fluorouracil in the therapy of metastatic breast carcinoma. *J Clin Oncol* 1988;6:1611–1620.
425. Heidemann E, Steinke B, Hartlapp J, et al. Randomized clinical trial comparing mitoxantrone with epirubicin and with doxorubicin, each combined with cyclophosphamide in the first-line treatment of patients with metastatic breast cancer. *Onkologie* 1990;13:24–27.
426. Go RS, Adjei AA. Review of the comparative pharmacology and clinical activity of cisplatin and carboplatin. *J Clin Oncol* 1999;17:409–422.
427. Higby DJ, Wallace HJ Jr, Holland JF. Cis-diamminedichloroplatinum (NSC-119875): a phase I study. *Cancer Chemother Rep* 1973;57:459–463.
428. Wiltshaw E, Carr B. Cis-platinumdiamminedichloride. In: Connors TA, Robert JJ, eds. *Platinum coordination complexes in cancer chemotherapy*. Heidelberg: Springer-Verlag, 1974:178–182.
429. Wiltshaw E, Kroner T. Phase II study of cis-dichlorodiammineplatinum (II) (NSC-119875) in advanced adenocarcinoma of the ovary. *Cancer Treat Rep* 1976;60: 55–60.
430. Schmidt W, Chaney SG. Role of carrier ligand in platinum resistance of human carcinoma cell lines. *Cancer Res* 1993;53:799–805.
431. Godwin AK, Meister A, O'Dwyer PJ, et al. High resistance to cisplatin in human ovarian cancer cell lines is associated with marked increase of glutathione synthesis. *Proc Natl Acad Sci U S A* 1992;89:3070–3074.
432. Reed E. Cisplatin, carboplatin and oxaliplatin. In: Chabner BA, Longo DL, eds. *Cancer chemotherapy and biotherapy: principles and practice*. 4th ed. Philadelphia: Lippincott Williams & Wilkins, 2005;332–343.
433. de Graeff A, Slebos RJ, Rodenhuis S. Resistance to cisplatin and analogues: mechanisms and potential clinical implications. *Cancer Chemother Pharmacol* 1988;22:325–332.
434. Kintzel PE, Dorr RT. Anticancer drug renal toxicity and elimination: dosing guidelines for altered renal function. *Cancer Treat Rev* 1995;21:33–64.
435. Nagao S, Fujiwara K, Imafuku N, et al. Difference of carboplatin clearance estimated by the Cockroft-Gault, Jelliffe, Modified-Jelliffe, Wright or Chatelut formula. *Gynecol Oncol* 2005;99:327–333.
436. Loehrer PJ, Einhorn LH. Drugs five years later. Cisplatin. *Ann Intern Med* 1984; 100:704–713.
437. Decatris MP, Sundar S, O'Byrne KJ. Platinum-based chemotherapy in metastatic breast cancer: current status. *Cancer Treat Rev* 2004;30:53–81.
438. Spielmann M, Llombart A, Zelek L, et al. Docetaxel-cisplatin combination (DC) chemotherapy in patients with anthracycline-resistant advanced breast cancer. *Ann Oncol* 1999;10:1457–1460.
439. Donadio M, Ardine M, Berruti A, et al. Weekly cisplatin plus capecitabine in metastatic breast cancer patients heavily pretreated with both anthracycline and taxanes. *Oncology* 2005;69:408–413.
440. Icli F, Akbulut H, Uner A, et al. Cisplatin plus oral etoposide (EoP) combination is more effective than paclitaxel in patients with advanced breast cancer pretreated with anthracyclines: a randomised phase III trial of Turkish Oncology Group. *Br J Cancer* 2005;92:639–644.
441. Vassilomanolakis M, Koumakis G, Demiri M, et al. Vinorelbine and cisplatin for metastatic breast cancer: a salvage regimen in patients progressing after docetaxel and anthracycline treatment. *Cancer Invest* 2003;21:497–504.
442. Sanchez-Escribano Morcuende R, Ales-Martinez JE, Aramburo Gonzalez PM. Low dose gemcitabine plus cisplatin in a weekly-based regimen as salvage therapy for relapsed breast cancer after taxane-anthracycline-containing regimens. *Clin Transl Oncol* 2007;9:459–464.
443. Pegram MD, Lipton A, Hayes DF, et al. Phase II study of receptor-enhanced chemosensitivity using recombinant humanized anti-p185 HER2/neu monoclonal antibody plus cisplatin in patients with HER2/neu-overexpressing metastatic breast cancer refractory to chemotherapy treatment. *J Clin Oncol* 1998; 16:2659–2671.
444. Sparano JA, Neuberg D, Glick JH, et al. Phase II trial of biweekly paclitaxel and cisplatin in advanced breast carcinoma: an Eastern Cooperative Oncology Group study. *J Clin Oncol* 1997;15:1880–1884.
445. Gelmon KA, O'Reilly SE, Tolcher AW, et al. Phase I/II trial of biweekly paclitaxel and cisplatin in the treatment of metastatic breast cancer. *J Clin Oncol* 1996;14:1185–1191.
446. McCaskill-Stevens W, Ansari R, Fisher W, et al. Phase II study of biweekly cisplatin (C) and paclitaxel (P) in the treatment of metastatic breast cancer. *Proc Am Soc Clin Oncol* 1996;15:120(abst).
447. Mustacchi G, Muggia M, Milani S, et al. A phase II study of cisplatin and vinorelbine in patients with metastatic breast cancer. *Ann Oncol* 2002;13:1730–1736.
448. Hochster H, Wasserheit C, Siddiqui N, et al. Vinorelbine/cislpatin therapy of locally advanced and metastatic breast cancer: an active regimen. *Proc Am Soc Clin Oncol* 1997;16:173a.
449. Deltetto F, Durando A, Camanni M, et al. Carboplatin plus etoposide regimen in advanced breast cancer. A phase II study. *Eur J Gynaecol Oncol* 1997;18: 185–187.
450. Crown J, Hakes T, Reichman B, et al. Phase II trial of carboplatin and etoposide in metastatic breast cancer. *Cancer* 1993;71:1254–1257.

451. Fernandez Hidalgo O, Gonzalez F, Gil A, et al. 120 hours simultaneous infusion of cisplatin and fluorouracil in metastatic breast cancer. *Am J Clin Oncol* 1989;12:397–401.

452. Chauvergne J, Mauriac L, Durand M, et al. [Relay chemotherapy using continuous perfusion of cisplatin and fluoro-uracil in advanced cancer of the breast. Analysis of a series of 50 cases]. *Rev Fr Gynecol Obstet* 1990;85:211–219.

453. Kourousis C, Kakolyris S, Androulakis N, et al. Salvage chemotherapy with paclitaxel, vinorelbine, and cisplatin (PVC) in anthracycline-resistant advanced breast cancer. *Am J Clin Oncol* 1998;21:226–232.

454. Jones AL, Smith IE, O'Brien ME, et al. Phase II study of continuous infusion fluorouracil with epirubicin and cisplatin in patients with metastatic and locally advanced breast cancer: an active new regimen. *J Clin Oncol* 1994;12:1259–1265.

455. Carrick S, Ghersi D, Wilcken N, et al. Platinum containing regimens for metastatic breast cancer. *Cochrane Database Syst Rev* 2004:CD003374.

456. Berruti A, Bitossi R, Gorzegno G, et al. Time to progression in metastatic breast cancer patients treated with epirubicin is not improved by the addition of either cisplatin or lonidamine: final results of a phase III study with a factorial design. *J Clin Oncol* 2002;20:4150–4159.

457. Gelmon KA, Vandenberg TA, Panasci L, et al. A phase II study of ZD0473 given as a short infusion every 3 weeks to patients with advanced or metastatic breast cancer: a National Cancer Institute of Canada Clinical Trials Group trial, IND 129. *Ann Oncol* 2003;14:543–548.

458. Caruba T, Cottu PH, Madelaine-Chambrin I, et al. Gemcitabine-oxaliplatin combination in heavily pretreated metastatic breast cancer: a pilot study on 43 patients. *Breast J* 2007;13:165–171.

459. Airoldi M, Cattel L, Passera R, et al. Gemcitabine and oxaliplatin in patients with metastatic breast cancer resistant to or pretreated with both anthracyclines and taxanes: clinical and pharmacokinetic data. *Am J Clin Oncol* 2006;29:490–494.

460. Petit T, Benider A, Yovine A, et al. Phase II study of an oxaliplatin/vinorelbine combination in patients with anthracycline- and taxane-pretreated metastatic breast cancer. *Anticancer Drugs* 2006;17:337–343.

461. McGuire WP, Rowinsky EK, Rosenshein NB, et al. Taxol: a unique antineoplastic agent with significant activity in advanced ovarian epithelial neoplasms. *Ann Intern Med* 1989;111:273–279.

462. Gelmon K. The taxoids: paclitaxel and docetaxel. *Lancet* 1994;344:1267–1272.

463. Wani MC, Taylor HL, Wall ME, et al. Plant antitumor agents. VI. The isolation and structure of Taxol, a novel antileukemic and antitumor agent from *Taxus brevifolia*. *J Am Chem Soc* 1971;93:2325–2327.

464. Kearns CM. Pharmacokinetics of the taxanes. *Pharmacotherapy* 1997;17:105S–109S.

465. Eisenhauer EA, Vermorken JB. The taxoids. Comparative clinical pharmacology and therapeutic potential. *Drugs* 1998;55:5–30.

466. Horwitz SB. Mechanism of action of Taxol. *Trends Pharmacol Sci* 1992;13:134–136.

467. Rowinsky EK, Donehower RC. Paclitaxel (Taxol). *N Engl J Med* 1995;332:1004–1014.

468. Diaz JF, Andreu JM. Assembly of purified GDP tubulin into microtubules induced by Taxol and Taxotere: reversibility, ligand stoichiometry, and competition. *Biochemistry* 1993;32:2747–2455.

469. Milross CG, Mason KA, Hunter NR, et al. Relationship of mitotic arrest and apoptosis to antitumor effect of paclitaxel. *J Natl Cancer Inst* 1996;88:1308–1314.

470. Ireland CM, Pittman SM. Tubulin alterations in Taxol-induced apoptosis parallel those observed with other drugs. *Biochem Pharmacol* 1995;49:1491–1499.

471. Wahl AF, Donaldson KL, Fairchild C, et al. Loss of normal p53 function confers sensitization to Taxol by increasing G2/M arrest and apoptosis. *Nat Med* 1996;2:72–79.

472. Haldar S, Jena N, Croce CM. Inactivation of Bcl-2 by phosphorylation. *Proc Natl Acad Sci U S A* 1995;92:4507–4511.

473. Blagosklonny MV, Schulte T, Nguyen P, et al. Taxol-induced apoptosis and phosphorylation of Bcl-2 protein involves c-Raf-1 and represents a novel c-Raf-1 signal transduction pathway. *Cancer Res* 1996;56:1851–1854.

474. Ganansia-Leymarie V, Bischoff P, Bergerat JP, et al. Signal transduction pathways of taxanes-induced apoptosis. *Curr Med Chem Anticancer Agents* 2003;3:291–306.

475. Dumontet C, Sikic BI. Mechanisms of action of and resistance to antitubulin agents: microtubule dynamics, drug transport, and cell death. *J Clin Oncol* 1999;17:1061–1070.

476. Burkhart CA, Berman JW, Swindell CS, et al. Relationship between the structure of Taxol and other taxanes on induction of tumor necrosis factor-alpha gene expression and cytotoxicity. *Cancer Res* 1994;54:5779–5782.

477. Belotti D, Vergani V, Drudis T, et al. The microtubule-affecting drug paclitaxel has antiangiogenic activity. *Clin Cancer Res* 1996;2:1843–1849.

478. Tishler RB, Geard CR, Hall EJ, et al. Taxol sensitizes human astrocytoma cells to radiation. *Cancer Res* 1992;52:3495–3497.

479. Creane M, Seymour CB, Colucci S, et al. Radiobiological effects of docetaxel (Taxotere): a potential radiation sensitizer. *Int J Radiat Biol* 1999;75:731–737.

480. Vanhoefer U, Cao S, Harstrick A, et al. Comparative antitumor efficacy of docetaxel and paclitaxel in nude mice bearing human tumor xenografts that overexpress the multidrug resistance protein (MRP). *Ann Oncol* 1997;8:1221–1228.

481. Bissery MC, Vrignaud P, Lavelle F. Preclinical profile of docetaxel (Taxotere): efficacy as a single agent and in combination. *Semin Oncol* 1995;22:3–16.

482. Valero V, Jones SE, Von Hoff DD, et al. A phase II study of docetaxel in patients with paclitaxel-resistant metastatic breast cancer. *J Clin Oncol* 1998;16:3362–3368.

483. Ishitobi M, Shin E, Kikkawa N. Metastatic breast cancer with resistance to both anthracycline and docetaxel successfully treated with weekly paclitaxel. *Int J Clin Oncol* 2001;6:55–58.

484. Greenberger LM, Williams SS, Horwitz SB. Biosynthesis of heterogeneous forms of multidrug resistance-associated glycoproteins. *J Biol Chem* 1987;262:13685–143689.

485. Cabral FR. Isolation of Chinese hamster ovary cell mutants requiring the continuous presence of Taxol for cell division. *J Cell Biol* 1983;97:22–29.

486. Kavallaris M, Kuo DY, Burkhart CA, et al. Taxol-resistant epithelial ovarian tumors are associated with altered expression of specific beta-tubulin isotypes. *J Clin Invest* 1997;100:1282–1293.

487. Cortes JE, Pazdur R. Docetaxel. *J Clin Oncol* 1995;13:2643–2655.

488. Cresteil T, Monsarrat B, Alvinerie P, et al. Taxol metabolism by human liver microsomes: identification of cytochrome P450 isozymes involved in its biotransformation. *Cancer Res* 1994;54:386–392.

489. Dreicer R, Gustin DM, See WA, et al. Paclitaxel in advanced urothelial carcinoma: its role in patients with renal insufficiency and as salvage therapy. *J Urol* 1996;156:1606–1608.

490. Woo MH, Gregornik D, Shearer PD, et al. Pharmacokinetics of paclitaxel in an anephric patient. *Cancer Chemother Pharmacol* 1999;43:92–96.

491. Taxotere (Docetaxel) injection concentrate, intravenous infusion [package insert]. Bridgewater, NJ: Sanofi-Aventis U.S. LLC, 2007.

492. Superfin D, Iannucci AA, Davies AM. Commentary: oncologic drugs in patients with organ dysfunction: a summary. *Oncologist* 2007;12:1070–1083.

493. Rowinsky EK, Eisenhauer EA, Chaudhry V, et al. Clinical toxicities encountered with paclitaxel (Taxol). *Semin Oncol* 1993;20:1–15.

494. Weiss RB, Donehower RC, Wiernik PH, et al. Hypersensitivity reactions from Taxol. *J Clin Oncol* 1990;8:1263–1268.

495. Ciesielski-Carlucci C, Leong P, Jacobs C. Case report of anaphylaxis from cisplatin/paclitaxel and a review of their hypersensitivity reaction profiles. *Am J Clin Oncol* 1997;20:373–375.

496. Lenz HJ. Management and preparedness for infusion and hypersensitivity reactions. *Oncologist* 2007;12:601–609.

497. Lorenz W, Reimann HJ, Schmal A, et al. Histamine release in dogs by Cremophor EL and its derivatives: oxethylated oleic acid is the most effective constituent. *Agents Actions* 1977;7:63–67.

498. Lassus M, Scott D, Leyland-Jones B. Allergic reactions associated with Cremophor containing antineoplastics. *Proc Am Soc Clin Oncol* 1985;4:268.

499. Szebeni J, Muggia FM, Alving CR. Complement activation by Cremophor EL as a possible contributor to hypersensitivity to paclitaxel: an in vitro study. *J Natl Cancer Inst* 1998;90:300–306.

500. Peereboom DM, Donehower RC, Eisenhauer EA, et al. Successful re-treatment with Taxol after major hypersensitivity reactions. *J Clin Oncol* 1993;11:885–890.

501. Olson JK, Sood AK, Sorosky JI, et al. Taxol hypersensitivity: rapid retreatment is safe and cost effective. *Gynecol Oncol* 1998;68:25–28.

502. Taxol (Paclitaxel) injection [package insert]. Princeton, NJ: Bristol-Meyers-Squibb Company, 2007.

503. Laskin MS, Lucchesi KJ, Morgan M. Paclitaxel rechallenge failure after a major hypersensitivity reaction. *J Clin Oncol* 1993;11:2456–2457.

504. Dizon DS, Schwartz J, Rojan A, et al. Cross-sensitivity between paclitaxel and docetaxel in a women's cancers program. *Gynecol Oncol* 2006;100:149–151.

505. Bernstein BJ. Docetaxel as an alternative to paclitaxel after acute hypersensitivity reactions. *Ann Pharmacother* 2000;34:1332–1335.

506. Rowinsky EK, Chaudhry V, Cornblath DR, et al. Neurotoxicity of Taxol. *J Natl Cancer Inst Monogr* 1993;15:107–115.

507. Gelmon K, Eisenhauer E, Bryce C, et al. Randomized phase II study of high-dose paclitaxel with or without amifostine in patients with metastatic breast cancer. *J Clin Oncol* 1999;17:3038–3047.

508. Perry JR, Warner E. Transient encephalopathy after paclitaxel (Taxol) infusion. *Neurology* 1996;46:1596–1599.

509. Capri G, Munzone E, Tarenzi E, et al. Optic nerve disturbances: a new form of paclitaxel neurotoxicity. *J Natl Cancer Inst* 1994;86:1099–1101.

510. Rowinsky EK, McGuire WP, Guarnieri T, et al. Cardiac disturbances during the administration of Taxol. *J Clin Oncol* 1991;9:1704–1712.

511. Markman M, Kennedy A, Webster K, et al. Use of low-dose oral prednisone to prevent paclitaxel-induced arthralgias and myalgias. *Gynecol Oncol* 1999;72:100–101.

512. Garrison JA, McCune JS, Livingston RB, et al. Myalgias and arthralgias associated with paclitaxel. *Oncology* (Williston Park) 2003;17:271–277.

513. Raghavan VT, Bloomer WD, Merkel DE. Taxol and radiation recall dermatitis. *Lancet* 1993;341:1354.

514. Fujimori K, Yokoyama A, Kurita Y, et al. Paclitaxel-induced cell-mediated hypersensitivity pneumonitis. Diagnosis using leukocyte migration test, bronchoalveolar lavage and transbronchial lung biopsy. *Oncology* 1998;55:340–344.

515. Khan A, McNally D, Tutschka PJ, et al. Paclitaxel-induced acute bilateral pneumonitis. *Ann Pharmacother* 1997;31:1471–1474.

516. Sotiriou C, van Houtte P, Klastersky J. Lung fibrosis induced by paclitaxel. *Support Care Cancer* 1998;6:68–71.

517. Brandwein MS, Rosen M, Harpaz N, et al. Fatal pulmonary lipid embolism associated with Taxol therapy. *Mt Sinai J Med* 1988;55:187–189.

518. Pestalozzi BC, Sotos GA, Choyke PL, et al. Typhlitis resulting from treatment with Taxol and doxorubicin in patients with metastatic breast cancer. *Cancer* 1993;71:1797–1800.

519. Lyseng-Williamson KA, Fenton C. Docetaxel: a review of its use in metastatic breast cancer. *Drugs* 2005;65:2513–2531.

520. Engels FK, Verweij J. Docetaxel administration schedule: from fever to tears? A review of randomised studies. *Eur J Cancer* 2005;41:1117–1126.

521. Esmaeli B, Amin S, Valero V, et al. Prospective study of incidence and severity of epiphora and canalicular stenosis in patients with metastatic breast cancer receiving docetaxel. *J Clin Oncol* 2006;24:3619–3622.

522. Trudeau ME, Eisenhauer EA, Higgins BP, et al. Docetaxel in patients with metastatic breast cancer: a phase II study of the National Cancer Institute of Canada Clinical Trials group. *J Clin Oncol* 1996;14:422–428.

523. Piccart MJ, Klijn J, Paridaens R, et al. Corticosteroids significantly delay the onset of docetaxel-induced fluid retention: final results of a randomized study of the European Organization for Research and Treatment of Cancer investigational drug branch for breast cancer. *J Clin Oncol* 1997;15:3149–3155.

524. Vaishampayan U, Parchment RE, Jasti BR, et al. Taxanes: an overview of the pharmacokinetics and pharmacodynamics. *Urology* 1999;54:22–29.

525. Llombart-Cussac A, Pivot X, Spielmann M. Docetaxel chemotherapy induces transverse superficial loss of the nail plate. *Arch Dermatol* 1997;133:1466–1467.

526. Obermair A, Binder M, Barrada M, et al. Onycholysis in patients treated with docetaxel. *Ann Oncol* 1998;9:230–231.

527. Smith RE, Brown AM, Mamounas EP, et al. Randomized trial of 3-hour versus 24-hour infusion of high-dose paclitaxel in patients with metastatic or locally advanced breast cancer: National Surgical Adjuvant Breast and Bowel Project Protocol B-26. *J Clin Oncol* 1999;17:3403–3411.

528. Rivera E, Holmes FA, Frye D, et al. Phase II study of paclitaxel in patients with metastatic breast carcinoma refractory to standard chemotherapy. *Cancer* 2000;89:2195–2201.

529. Geyer CE Jr, Green SJ, Moinpour CM, et al. Expanded phase II trial of paclitaxel in metastatic breast cancer: a Southwest Oncology Group study. *Breast Cancer Res Treat* 1998;51:169–181.
530. Gianni L, Munzone E, Capri G, et al. Paclitaxel in metastatic breast cancer: a trial of two doses by a 3-hour infusion in patients with disease recurrence after prior therapy with anthracyclines. *J Natl Cancer Inst* 1995;87:1169–1175.
531. Fountzilas G, Athanassiadis A, Kalogera-Fountzila A, et al. Paclitaxel by 3-h infusion and carboplatin in anthracycline-resistant advanced breast cancer. A phase II study conducted by the Hellenic Cooperative Oncology Group. *Eur J Cancer* 1997;33:1893–1895.
532. Sparano JA. Taxanes for breast cancer: an evidence-based review of randomized phase II and phase III trials. *Clin Breast Cancer* 2000;1:32–42.
533. Marchetti P, Urien S, Cappellini GA, et al. Weekly administration of paclitaxel: theoretical and clinical basis. *Crit Rev Oncol Hematol* 2002;44[Suppl]:S3–S13.
534. Perez EA, Vogel CL, Irwin DH, et al. Multicenter phase II trial of weekly paclitaxel in women with metastatic breast cancer. *J Clin Oncol* 2001;19: 4216–4223.
535. Verrill MW, Lee J, Cameron DA, et al. Anglo-Celtic IV: First results of a UK National Cancer Research Network randomised phase 3 pharmacogenetic trial of weekly versus 3 weekly paclitaxel in patients with locally advanced or metastatic breast cancer (ABC). ASCO annual meeting proceedings. Part I. *J Clin Oncol* 2007;25(18S)[Suppl]:LBA1005.
536. Muss HB, White DR, Richards F 2nd, et al. Adriamycin versus methotrexate in five-drug combination chemotherapy for advanced breast cancer: a randomized trial. *Cancer* 1978;42:2141–2148.
537. Bull JM, Tormey DC, Li SH, et al. A randomized comparative trial of adriamycin versus methotrexate in combination drug therapy. *Cancer* 1978;41:1649–1657.
538. Dieras V, Chevallier B, Kerbrat P, et al. A multicentre phase II study of docetaxel 75 mg m^2 as first-line chemotherapy for patients with advanced breast cancer: report of the Clinical Screening Group of the EORTC. European Organization for Research and Treatment of Cancer. *Br J Cancer* 1996;74:650–656.
539. Ravdin PM, Burris HA 3rd, Cook G, et al. Phase II trial of docetaxel in advanced anthracycline-resistant or anthracenedione-resistant breast cancer. *J Clin Oncol* 1995;13:2879–2885.
540. Valero V, Holmes FA, Walters RS, et al. Phase II trial of docetaxel: a new, highly effective antineoplastic agent in the management of patients with anthracycline-resistant metastatic breast cancer. *J Clin Oncol* 1995;13:2886–2894.
541. Alexandre J, Bleuzen P, Bonneterre J, et al. Factors predicting for efficacy and safety of docetaxel in a compassionate-use cohort of 825 heavily pretreated advanced breast cancer patients. *J Clin Oncol* 2000;18:562–573.
542. Adachi I, Watanabe T, Takashima S, et al. A late phase II study of RP56976 (Docetaxel) in patients with advanced or recurrent breast cancer. *Br J Cancer* 1996;73:210–216.
543. O'Brien ME, Leonard RC, Barrett-Lee PJ, et al. Docetaxel in the community setting: an analysis of 377 breast cancer patients treated with docetaxel (Taxotere) in the UK. UK Study Group. *Ann Oncol* 1999;10:205–210.
544. Chevallier B, Fumoleau P, Kerbrat P, et al. Docetaxel is a major cytotoxic drug for the treatment of advanced breast cancer: a phase II trial of the Clinical Screening Cooperative Group of the European Organization for Research and Treatment of Cancer. *J Clin Oncol* 1995;13:314–322.
545. ten Bokkel Huinink WW, Prove AM, Piccart M, et al. A phase II trial with docetaxel (Taxotere) in second line treatment with chemotherapy for advanced breast cancer. A study of the EORTC Early Clinical Trials Group. *Ann Oncol* 1994;5: 527–532.
546. Hainsworth JD, Burris HA 3rd, Yardley DA, et al. Weekly docetaxel in the treatment of elderly patients with advanced breast cancer: a Minnie Pearl Cancer Research Network phase II trial. *J Clin Oncol* 2001;19:3500–3505.
547. Tomiak E, Piccart MJ, Kerger J, et al. Phase I study of docetaxel administered as a 1-hour intravenous infusion on a weekly basis. *J Clin Oncol* 1994;12: 1458–1467.
548. Salminen E, Bergman M, Huhtala S, et al. Docetaxel: standard recommended dose of 100 mg/m^2 is effective but not feasible for some metastatic breast cancer patients heavily pretreated with chemotherapy—a phase II single-center study. *J Clin Oncol* 1999;17:1127.
549. Salminen E, Bergman M, Huhtala S, et al. Docetaxel, a promising novel chemotherapeutic agent in advanced breast cancer. *Anticancer Res* 2000;20: 3663–3668.
550. Hainsworth JD. Practical aspects of weekly docetaxel administration schedules. *Oncologist* 2004;9:538–545.
551. Bonneterre J, Roche H, Monnier A, et al. Docetaxel vs 5-fluorouracil plus vinorelbine in metastatic breast cancer after anthracycline therapy failure. *Br J Cancer* 2002;87:1210–1215.
552. Sjostrom J, Blomqvist C, Mouridsen H, et al. Docetaxel compared with sequential methotrexate and 5-fluorouracil in patients with advanced breast cancer after anthracycline failure: a randomised phase III study with crossover on progression by the Scandinavian Breast group. *Eur J Cancer* 1999;35:1194–1201.
553. Hakamies-Blomqvist L, Luoma M, Sjostrom J, et al. Quality of life in patients with metastatic breast cancer receiving either docetaxel or sequential methotrexate and 5-fluorouracil. A multicentre randomised phase III trial by the Scandinavian breast group. *Eur J Cancer* 2000;36:1411–1417.
554. Jones SE, Erban J, Overmoyer B, et al. Randomized phase III study of docetaxel compared with paclitaxel in metastatic breast cancer. *J Clin Oncol* 2005;23: 5542–5551.
555. Piccart MJ, Burzykowski T, Sledge GW, et al. Effects of taxanes alone or in combination with anthracyclines on tumor response, progression-free survival and overall survival in first-line chemotherapy of patients with metastatic breast cancer: an analysis of 4,256 patients randomized in 12 trials. *Breast Cancer Res Treat* 2005;94:S278.
556. Holmes FA, Madden T, Newman RA, et al. Sequence-dependent alteration of doxorubicin pharmacokinetics by paclitaxel in a phase I study of paclitaxel and doxorubicin in patients with metastatic breast cancer. *J Clin Oncol* 1996;14: 2713–2721.
557. Holmes FA, Valero V, Walters RS, et al. Paclitaxel by 24-hour infusion with doxorubicin by 48-hour infusion as initial therapy for metastatic breast cancer: pphase I results. *Ann Oncol* 1999;10:403–411.
557a. Sledge GW, Goldstein RN, Cpavano J, et al. Phase I trial of Adriamycin (A)+ Taxol (T) in metastatic breast cancer. *Eur J Cancer* 29A:S81, 1993 (suppl 6) (abstr 421).
558. Gianni L, Munzone E, Capri G, et al. Paclitaxel by 3-hour infusion in combination with bolus doxorubicin in women with untreated metastatic breast cancer: high antitumor efficacy and cardiac effects in a dose-finding and sequence-finding study. *J Clin Oncol* 1995;13:2688–2699.
559. Gianni L, Vigano L, Locatelli A, et al. Human pharmacokinetic characterization and in vitro study of the interaction between doxorubicin and paclitaxel in patients with breast cancer. *J Clin Oncol* 1997;15:1906–1915.
560. Vigano L, Locatelli A, Grasselli G, et al. Drug interactions of paclitaxel and docetaxel and their relevance for the design of combination therapy. *Invest New Drugs* 2001;19:179–196.
561. Dombernowsky P, Gehl J, Boesgaard M, et al. Doxorubicin and paclitaxel, a highly active combination in the treatment of metastatic breast cancer. *Semin Oncol* 1996;23:23–27.
562. Gehl J, Boesgaard M, Paaske T, et al. Combined doxorubicin and paclitaxel in advanced breast cancer: effective and cardiotoxic. *Ann Oncol* 1996;7:687–693.
563. Holmes FA, Rowinsky EK. Pharmacokinetic profiles of doxorubicin in combination with taxanes. *Semin Oncol* 2001;28:8–14.
564. Giordano SH, Booser DJ, Murray JL, et al. A detailed evaluation of cardiac toxicity: a phase II study of doxorubicin and one- or three-hour-infusion paclitaxel in patients with metastatic breast cancer. *Clin Cancer Res* 2002;8:3360–3368.
565. Hortobagyi GN, Willey J, Rahman Z, et al. Prospective assessment of cardiac toxicity during a randomized phase II trial of doxorubicin and paclitaxel in metastatic breast cancer. *Semin Oncol* 1997;24:S17-65–S17-68.
566. Valero V, Perez E, Dieras V. Doxorubicin and taxane combination regimens for metastatic breast cancer: focus on cardiac effects. *Semin Oncol* 2001;28: 15–23.
567. Hortobagyi GN, Holmes FA. Optimal dosing of paclitaxel and doxorubicin in metastatic breast cancer. *Semin Oncol* 1997;24:S4–S7.
568. Biganzoli L, Cufer T, Bruning P, et al. Doxorubicin and paclitaxel versus doxorubicin and cyclophosphamide as first-line chemotherapy in metastatic breast cancer: the European Organization for Research and Treatment of Cancer 10961 multicenter phase III trial. *J Clin Oncol* 2002;20:3114–3121.
569. Misset JL, Dieras V, Gruia G, et al. Dose-finding study of docetaxel and doxorubicin in first-line treatment of patients with metastatic breast cancer. *Ann Oncol* 1999;10:553–560.
570. Sparano JA, O'Neill A, Schaefer PL, et al. Phase II trial of doxorubicin and docetaxel plus granulocyte colony-stimulating factor in metastatic breast cancer: Eastern Cooperative Oncology Group Study E1196. *J Clin Oncol* 2000;18: 2369–2377.
571. Dieras V, Barthier S, Beuzeboc P, et al. Phase II study of docetaxel in combination with doxorubicin as 1st line chemotherapy of metastatic breast cancer. *Breast Cancer Res Treat* 1998;50:262(abst).
572. Schuller I, Czejka M, Kletzl H, et al. Doxorubicin and Taxotere: a pharmacolinetic study of the combination in advanced breast cancer. *Proc Am Soc Clin Oncol* 1998;17:205a(abst 790).
573. Bellot R, Robert J, Dieras V, et al. Taxotere does not change the pharmacokinetic profile of doxorubicin and doxorubicinol. *Proc Am Soc Clin Oncol* 1998;17:221a.
574. Nabholtz JM, Mackey JR, Smylie M, et al. Phase II study of docetaxel, doxorubicin, and cyclophosphamide as first-line chemotherapy for metastatic breast cancer. *J Clin Oncol* 2001;19:314–321.
575. Bontenbal M, Creemers GJ, Braun HJ, et al. Phase II to III study comparing doxorubicin and docetaxel with fluorouracil, doxorubicin, and cyclophosphamide as first-line chemotherapy in patients with metastatic breast cancer: results of a Dutch Community Setting Trial for the Clinical Trial Group of the Comprehensive Cancer Centre. *J Clin Oncol* 2005;23:7081–7088.
576. Mackey JR, Paterson A, Dirix LY, et al. Final results of the phase III randomized trial comparing docetaxel (T), doxorubicin (A) and cyclophosphamide (C) to FAC as first line chemotherapy (CT) for patients (pts) with metastatic breast cancer (MBC). *Proc Am Soc Clin Oncol* 2002;21:(abst 137).
577. Cassier PA, Chabaud S, Trillet-Lenoir V, et al. A phase-III trial of doxorubicin and docetaxel versus doxorubicin and paclitaxel in metastatic breast cancer: results of the ERASME 3 study. *Breast Cancer Res Treat* 2008;109(2):343–350.
578. Esposito M, Venturini M, Vannozzi MO, et al. Comparative effects of paclitaxel and docetaxel on the metabolism and pharmacokinetics of epirubicin in breast cancer patients. *J Clin Oncol* 1999;17:1132.
579. Trudeau M, Pagani O. Epirubicin in combination with the taxanes. *Semin Oncol* 2001;28:41–50.
580a. Conte FP, Baldini E, Gennari A, et al. Dose-finding study and pharmacokinetics of epirubicin and paclitaxel over 3 hours: a regimen with high activity and low cardiotoxicity in advanced breast cancer. *J Clin Oncol* 1997;15:2510–2517.
580. Mross K, Maessen P, van der Vijgh WJ, et al. Pharmacokinetics and metabolism of epidoxorubicin and doxorubicin in humans. *J Clin Oncol* 1988;6:517–526.
581. Langley RE, Carmichael J, Jones AL, et al. Phase III trial of epirubicin plus paclitaxel compared with epirubicin plus cyclophosphamide as first-line chemotherapy for metastatic breast cancer: United Kingdom National Cancer Research Institute trial AB01. *J Clin Oncol* 2005;23:8322–8330.
582. Luck H, Thomssen C, Untch M, et al. Multicentric phase III study in first line treatment of advanced metastatic breast cancer (ABC). Epirubicin/paclitaxel (ET) vs epirubicin/cyclophosphamide (EC). A study of the AGO Breast Cancer Group. *Proc Am Soc Clin Oncol* 2000;19:(abst 280).
583. Bria E, Giannarelli D, Felici A, et al. Taxanes with anthracyclines as first-line chemotherapy for metastatic breast carcinoma. *Cancer* 2005;103:672–679.
584. Rowinsky EK, Gilbert MR, McGuire WP, et al. Sequences of taxol and cisplatin: a phase I and pharmacologic study. *J Clin Oncol* 1991;9:1692–1703.
585. Rowinsky EK, Citardi MJ, Noe DA, et al. Sequence-dependent cytotoxic effects due to combinations of cisplatin and the antimicrotubule agents taxol and vincristine. *J Cancer Res Clin Oncol* 1993;119:727–733.
586. Parker RJ, Dabholkar MD, Lee KB, et al. Taxol effect on cisplatin sensitivity and cisplatin cellular accumulation in human ovarian cancer cells. *J Natl Cancer Inst Monogr* 1993:83–88.
587. LeBlanc GA, Sundseth SS, Weber GF, et al. Platinum anticancer drugs modulate P-450 mRNA levels and differentially alter hepatic drug and steroid hormone metabolism in male and female rats. *Cancer Res* 1992;52:540–547.
588. Rowinsky EK. Donehower RC. Antimicrotubule agents. In: Chabner BA, Longo DL, eds. Cancer chemotherapy and biotherapy 3rd ed. Philadelphia: Lippincott Williams & Wilkins, 2001:329–372.
589. Huizing MT, Giaccone G, van Warmerdam LJ, et al. Pharmacokinetics of paclitaxel and carboplatin in a dose-escalating and dose-sequencing study in patients with non-small-cell lung cancer. The European Cancer Centre. *J Clin Oncol* 1997;15:317–329.

590. Obasaju CK, Johnson SW, Rogatko A, et al. Evaluation of carboplatin pharmacokinetics in the absence and presence of paclitaxel. *Clin Cancer Res* 1996;2:549–552.
591. Belani CP, Kearns CM, Zuhowski EG, et al. Phase I trial, including pharmacokinetic and pharmacodynamic correlations, of combination paclitaxel and carboplatin in patients with metastatic non-small-cell lung cancer. *J Clin Oncol* 1999;17:676–684.
592. Pronk LC, Schellens JH, Planting AS, et al. Phase I and pharmacologic study of docetaxel and cisplatin in patients with advanced solid tumors. *J Clin Oncol* 1997;15:1071–1079.
593. Peretz T, Sulkes A, Chollet P. A multicenter randomized study of two schedules of paclitaxel (PTX) in patients with advanced breast cancer (ABC). *Eur J Cancer* 1995;31A:S75[Suppl 5]:(abst 345).
594. Ezzat A, Raja MA, Berry J, et al. A phase II trial of circadian-timed paclitaxel and cisplatin therapy in metastatic breast cancer. *Ann Oncol* 1997;8:663–667.
595. Maiche AG, Jekunen AP, Kaleva-Kerola J, et al. High response rate with a lower dose of paclitaxel in combination with cisplatin in heavily pretreated patients with advanced breast carcinoma. *Cancer* 2000;88:1863–1868.
596. Rosati G, Riccardi F, Tucci A, et al. A phase II study of paclitaxel/cisplatin combination in patients with metastatic breast cancer refractory to anthracycline-based chemotherapy. *Tumori* 2000;86:207–210.
597. Frasci G, Comella P, D'Aiuto G, et al. Weekly paclitaxel-cisplatin administration with G-CSF support in advanced breast cancer. A phase II study. *Breast Cancer Res Treat* 1998;49:13–26.
598. Gainford C, O'Leary M, El-Fiki T, et al. Phase I trial of docetaxel (T) and cisplatin (P) as first-line chemotherapy for metastatic breast cancer (MBC). *Proc Am Soc Clin Oncol* 2000;19:113a(abst 439).
599. Crown J, Fumoleau P, Kerbrat K, et al. Phase I trial of docetaxel (D) with cisplatin (P) as first-line chemotherapy of metastatic breast cancer (MBC). *Proc Am Soc Clin Oncol* 1997;16:233a (abst 821).
600. Llombart-Cussac A, Spielmann M, Dohollou N, et al. Cisplatin-Taxotere phase I/II trial in patients with anthracycline-resistant advanced breast cancer (ABC). *Proc Am Soc Clin Oncol* 1997;16:551(abst 629).
601. Antoine E, Meric JB, Coeffic D, et al. Anthracycline-primary resistant breast cancer (APRBC): confirmatory results of the high level of activity of the docetaxel (D)-cisplatin (C) regimen. *Proc Am Soc Clin Oncol* 1999;18:129a(abst 491).
602. Bernard A, Antoine EC, Gozy M, et al. Docetaxel (T) and cisplatin (P) in anthracycline pretreated advanced breast cancer (ABC): results of a phase II pilot study. *Proc Am Soc Clin Oncol* 1998;17:128a(abst 491).
603. Lin YC, Chang HK, Chen JS, et al. A phase II randomized study of two taxanes and cisplatin for metastatic breast cancer after anthracycline: a final analysis. *Jpn J Clin Oncol* 2007;37:23–29.
604. Fountzilas G, Dimopoulos AM, Papadimitriou C, et al. First-line chemotherapy with paclitaxel by three hour infusion and carboplatin in advanced breast cancer (final report): a phase II study conducted by the Hellenic Cooperative Oncology Group. *Ann Oncol* 1998;9:1031–1034.
605. Fountzilas G, Kalofonos HP, Dafni U, et al. Paclitaxel and epirubicin versus paclitaxel and carboplatin as first-line chemotherapy in patients with advanced breast cancer: a phase III study conducted by the Hellenic Cooperative Oncology Group. *Ann Oncol* 2004;15:1517–1526.
606. Perez EA, Hillman DW, Stella PJ, et al. A phase II study of paclitaxel plus carboplatin as first-line chemotherapy for women with metastatic breast carcinoma. *Cancer* 2000;88:124–131.
607. Loesch D, Robert N, Asmar L, et al. Phase II multicenter trial of a weekly paclitaxel and carboplatin regimen in patients with advanced breast cancer. *J Clin Oncol* 2002;20:3857–3864.
608. Alberti AM. A phase II study of docetaxel (T) and carboplatin (CBP) as second line chemotherapy in metastatic breast cancer. *Proc Am Soc Clin Oncol* 2000;19:113a(abst 438).
609. Fitch TR, Suman VJ, Malliard JA, et al. N9932: phase II cooperative group trial of docetaxel (D) and carboplatin (CBDCA) as first-line chemotherapy for metastatic breast cancer (MBC). *Proc Am Soc Clin Oncol* 2003;22:23(abst 90).
610. Brufsky AM, Matin K, Cleary D, et al. A phase II study of carboplatin and docetaxel as first line chemotherapy for metastatic breast cancer. *Proc Am Soc Clin Oncol* 2002;21:52b(abst 2020).
611. Blum JL, Dees EC, Chacko A, et al. Phase II trial of capecitabine and weekly paclitaxel as first-line therapy for metastatic breast cancer. *J Clin Oncol* 2006;24:4384–4390.
612. Miles D, Ayoub J-P, O'Shaugnessy JA. Survival benefit with Xeloda (capecitabine)/Taxotere(docetaxel) (XT) versus Taxotere: analysis of post-study therapy. *Breast Cancer Res Treat* 2001;69:287.
613. Kurosumi M, Tabei T, Suemasu K, et al. Enhancement of immunohistochemical reactivity for thymidine phosphorylase in breast carcinoma cells after administration of docetaxel as a neoadjuvant chemotherapy in advanced breast cancer patients. *Oncol Rep* 2000;7:945–948.
614. Susnjar S, Bosnjak S, Radulovic S, et al. Dose-finding study of capecitabine in combination with weekly paclitaxel for patients with anthracycline-pretreated metastatic breast cancer. *J BUON* 2007;12:189–196.
615. Uhlmann C, Ballabeni P, Rijken N, et al. Capecitabine with weekly paclitaxel for advanced breast cancer: a phase I dose-finding trial. *Oncology* 2004;67: 117–122.
616. Gick U, Rochlitz C, Mingrone W, et al. Efficacy and tolerability of capecitabine with weekly paclitaxel for patients with metastatic breast cancer: a phase II report of the SAKK. *Oncology* 2006;71:54–60.
617. Gelmon K, Chan A, Harbeck N. The role of capecitabine in first-line treatment for patients with metastatic breast cancer. *Oncologist* 2006;11[Suppl 1]:42–51.
618. Lueck H, Minckwitz GV, Du Bois A, et al. Epirubicin/paclitaxel (EP) vs. capecitabine/paclitaxel (XP) in first-line metastatic breast cancer (MBC): A prospective, randomized multicentre phase III study of the AGO Breast Cancer Study group. ASCO Annual Meeting Proceedings Part I. *J Clin Oncol* 2006;24(18S) [Suppl]:517.
619. Chan S, Romieu G, Huober J, et al. Gemcitabine plus docetaxel (GD) versus capecitabine plus docetaxel (CD) for anthracycline-pretreated metastatic breast cancer (MBC) patients (pts): results of a European phase III study. ASCO Annual Meeting Proceedings. *J Clin Oncol* 2005;23(16S, Pt I of II)[Suppl]:581.
620. Loesch DM, Asmar L, Canfield VA, et al. A phase II trial of weekly paclitaxel, 5-fluorouracil, and leucovorin as first-line treatment for metastatic breast cancer. *Breast Cancer Res Treat* 2003;77:115–123.
621. Nicholson BP, Paul DM, Hande KR, et al. Paclitaxel, 5-fluorouracil, and leucovorin (TFL) in the treatment of metastatic breast cancer. *Clin Breast Cancer* 2000;1:136–144.
622. Gennari A, Guarneri V, Landucci E, et al. Weekly docetaxel/paclitaxel in pretreated metastatic breast cancer. *Clin Breast Cancer* 2002;3:346–352.
623. Ibrahim NK, Desai N, Legha S, et al. Phase I and pharmacokinetic study of ABI-007, a Cremophor-free, protein-stabilized, nanoparticle formulation of paclitaxel. *Clin Cancer Res* 2002;8:1038–1044.
624. Ibrahim NK, Samuels B, Page R, et al. Multicenter phase II trial of ABI-007, an albumin-bound paclitaxel, in women with metastatic breast cancer. *J Clin Oncol* 2005;23:6019–6026.
625. Gradishar WJ, Tjulandin S, Davidson N, et al. Phase III trial of nanoparticle albumin-bound paclitaxel compared with polyethylated castor oil-based paclitaxel in women with breast cancer. *J Clin Oncol* 2005;23:7794–7803.
626. Nyman DW, Campbell KJ, Hersh E, et al. Phase I and pharmacokinetics trial of ABI-007, a novel nanoparticle formulation of paclitaxel in patients with advanced nonhematologic malignancies. *J Clin Oncol* 2005;23:7785–7793.
627. O'Shaughnessy JA, Blum JL, Sandbach JF, et al. Weekly nanoparticle albumin paclitaxel (Abraxane) results in long-term disease control in patients with taxane-refractory metastatic breast cancer (abstract). Presented at the 27th annual San Antonio Breast Cancer Symposium, December 4–8, 2005.
628. Desai N, Trieu V, Yao Z, et al. Increased antitumor activity, intratumor paclitaxel concentrations, and endothelial cell transport of cremophor-free, albumin-bound paclitaxel, ABI-007, compared with cremophor-based paclitaxel. *Clin Cancer Res* 2006;12:1317–1324.
629. Desai N, Trieu V, Yao R, et al. Increased transport of nanoparticle albumin-bound paclitaxel (ABI-007) by endothelial gp60-mediated caveolar transcytosis: a pathway inhibited by Taxol. Presented at the 16th annual meeting of the European Organisation for Research and Treatment of Cancer–National Cancer Institute–American Association for Cancer Research, Geneva, Switzerland. September 28–October 1, 2004.
630. Desai N, Trieu V, Yao R, et al. SPARC expression in breast tumors may correlate to increased tumor distribution of nanoparticle albumin-bound paclitaxel (ABI-007) vs Taxol. Presented at the 27th annual San Antonio Breast Cancer Symposium, San Antonio, Texas. December 8–11, 2004.
631. Lobo C, Lopes G, Silva O, et al. Paclitaxel albumin-bound particles (Abraxane) in combination with bevacizumab with or without gemcitabine: early experience at the University of Miami/Braman Family Breast Cancer Institute. *Biomed Pharmacother* 2007;61:531–533.
632. Gerth K, Bedorf N, Hofle G, et al. Epothilons A and B: antifungal and cytotoxic compounds from *Sorangium cellulosum* (Myxobacteria). Production, physico-chemical and biological properties. *J Antibiot (Tokyo)* 1996;49:560–563.
633. Bollag DM, McQueney PA, Zhu J, et al. Epothilones, a new class of microtubule-stabilizing agents with a Taxol-like mechanism of action. *Cancer Res* 1995;55:2325–2333.
634. Wartmann M, Altmann KH. The biology and medicinal chemistry of epothilones. *Curr Med Chem Anticancer Agents* 2002;2:123–148.
635. Lee FY, Borzilleri R, Fairchild CR, et al. BMS-247550: a novel epothilone analog with a mode of action similar to paclitaxel but possessing superior antitumor efficacy. *Clin Cancer Res* 2001;7:1429–1437.
636. Jordan MA, Miller H, Ray A, et al. The Pat-21 breast cancer model derived from a patient with primary Taxol resistance recapitulates the phenotype of its origin, has altered β-tubulin expression and is sensitive to ixabepilone. *Proc Am Assoc Cancer Res* 2006;47:(abst LB-280).
637. Lee FYF, Carmuso A, Castenada S, et al. Preclinical studies of ixabepilone (BMS-247550) demonstrate optimal antitumor activity against both chemotherapy-sensitive and -resistant tumor types. *Proc Am Assoc Cancer Res* 2006;47:119 (abst 503).
638. Ixempra kit (ixabepilone) for injection [package insert]. Princeton, NJ: Bristol-Meyers Squibb Company, 2007.
639. Fornier MN. Epothilones in breast cancer: review of clinical experience. *Ann Oncol* 2007;18[Suppl 5]:v16–v21.
640. Mielke S, Sparreboom A, Mross K. Peripheral neuropathy: a persisting challenge in paclitaxel-based regimes. *Eur J Cancer* 2006;42:24–30.
641. ten Tije AJ, Verweij J, Loos WJ, et al. Pharmacological effects of formulation vehicles: implications for cancer chemotherapy. *Clin Pharmacokinet* 2003;42: 665–685.
642. Perez EA, Lerzo G, Pivot X, et al. Efficacy and safety of ixabepilone (BMS-247550) in a phase II study of patients with advanced breast cancer resistant to an anthracycline, a taxane, and capecitabine. *J Clin Oncol* 2007;25:3407–3414.
643. Thomas E, Tabernero J, Fornier M, et al. Phase II clinical trial of ixabepilone (BMS-247550), an epothilone B analog, in patients with taxane-resistant metastatic breast cancer. *J Clin Oncol* 2007;25:3399–3406.
644. Roche H, Yelle L, Cognetti F, et al. Phase II clinical trial of ixabepilone (BMS-247550), an epothilone B analog, as first-line therapy in patients with metastatic breast cancer previously treated with anthracycline chemotherapy. *J Clin Oncol* 2007;25:3415–3420.
645. Denduluri N, Low JA, Lee JJ, et al. Phase II trial of ixabepilone, an epothilone B analog, in patients with metastatic breast cancer previously untreated with taxanes. *J Clin Oncol* 2007;25:3421–3427.
646. Low JA, Wedam SB, Lee JJ, et al. Phase II clinical trial of ixabepilone (BMS-247550), an epothilone B analog, in metastatic and locally advanced breast cancer. *J Clin Oncol* 2005;23:2726–2734.
647. Thomas ES, Gomez HL, Li RK, et al. Ixabepilone plus capecitabine for metastatic breast cancer progressing after anthracycline and taxane treatment. *J Clin Oncol* 2007;25:5210–5217.
648. Duffin J. Poisoning the spindle: serendipity and discovery of the anti-tumor properties of the Vinca alkaloids (Part II). *Pharm Hist* 2002;44:105–119.
649. Budman DR. Vinorelbine (Navelbine): a third-generation vinca alkaloid. *Cancer Invest* 1997;15:475–90.
650. Johnson SA, Harper P, Hortobagyi GN, et al. Vinorelbine: an overview. *Cancer Treat Rev* 1996;22:127–142.
651. Correia JJ. Effects of antimitotic agents on tubulin-nucleotide interactions. *Pharmacol Ther* 1991;52:127–147.
652. Adams DJ, Knick VC. P-glycoprotein mediated resistance to 5′-nor-anhydro-vinblastine (Navelbine). *Invest New Drugs* 1995;13:13–21.
653. Drukman S, Kavallaris M. Microtubule alterations and resistance to tubulin-binding agents (review). *Int J Oncol* 2002; 21:621–628.
654. Cabral F, Barlow SB. Resistance to antimitotic agents as genetic probes of microtubule structure and function. *Pharmacol Ther* 1991;52:159–171.
655. Hari M, Wang Y, Veeraraghavan S, et al. Mutations in alpha- and beta-tubulin that stabilize microtubules and confer resistance to colcemid and vinblastine. *Mol Cancer Ther* 2003;2:597–605.

656. Himes RH. Interactions of the catharanthus (vinca) alkaloids with tubulin and microtubules. *Pharmacol Ther* 1991;51:257–267.
657. Rahmani R, Gueritte F, Martin M, et al. Comparative pharmacokinetics of antitumor vinca alkaloids: intravenous bolus injections of navelbine and related alkaloids to cancer patients and rats. *Cancer Chemother Pharmacol* 1986;16:223–228.
658. Rahmani R, Zhou XJ. Pharmacokinetics and metabolism of vinca alkaloids. In: Workman P, Graham M, eds. *Cancer surveys*, vol 17: *pharmacokinatics and cancer chemotherapy*. Plainview, NY: Cold Spring Harbor Laboratory Press, 1993:269.
659. Jehl F, Quoix E, Leveque D, et al. Pharmacokinetic and preliminary metabolic fate of navelbine in humans as determined by high performance liquid chromatography. *Cancer Res* 1991;51:2073–2076.
660. Krikorian A, Rahmani R, Bromet M, et al. Pharmacokinetics and metabolism of Navelbine. *Semin Oncol* 1989;16:21–25.
661. Bore P, Rahmani R, van Cantfort J, et al. Pharmacokinetics of a new anticancer drug, navelbine, in patients. Comparative study of radioimmunologic and radioactive determination methods. *Cancer Chemother Pharmacol* 1989;23:247–251.
662. Gebbia V, Puozzo C. Oral versus intravenous vinorelbine: clinical safety profile. *Expert Opin Drug Saf* 2005;4:915–928.
663. Tester W, Forbes W, Leighton J. Vinorelbine-induced pancreatitis: a case report. *J Natl Cancer Inst* 1997;89:1631.
664. Hoff PM, Valero V, Ibrahim N, et al. Hand-foot syndrome following prolonged infusion of high doses of vinorelbine. *Cancer* 1998;82:965–969.
665. Tassinari D, Sartori S, Gianni L, et al. Is acute dyspnoea a rare side effect of vinorelbine? *Ann Oncol* 1997;8:503–504.
666. Canzler U, Schmidt-Gohrich UK, Bergmann S, et al. Syndrome of inappropriate antidiuretic hormone secretion (SIADH) induced by vinorelbine treatment of metastatic breast cancer. *Onkologie* 2007;30:455–456.
667. Garrett CA, Simpson TA Jr. Syndrome of inappropriate antidiuretic hormone associated with vinorelbine therapy. *Ann Pharmacother* 1998;32:1306–1309.
668. Long TD, Twillman RK, Cathers-Schiffman TA, et al. Treatment of vinorelbine-associated tumor pain. *Am J Clin Oncol* 2001;24:414–415.
669. Jackson DV, White DR, Spurr CL, et al. Moderate-dose vincristine infusion in refractory breast cancer. *Am J Clin Oncol* 1986;9:376–378.
670. Hopkins JO, Jackson DV Jr, White DR, et al. Vincristine by continuous infusion in refractory breast cancer: a phase II study. *Am J Clin Oncol* 1983;6:529–532.
671. Smith IE, Coombes RC, Evans BD, et al. Vindesine as a single agent and in combination with adriamycin in the treatment of metastatic breast carcinoma. *Eur J Cancer* 1980;[Suppl 1]:271–273.
672. Robins HI, Tormey DC, Skelley MJ, et al. Vindesine. A phase II trial in advanced breast cancer patients. *Cancer Clin Trials* 1981;4:371–375.
673. DiBella NJ, Berris R, Garfield D, et al. Vindesine in advanced breast cancer, lymphoma and melanoma. A Colorado Clinical Oncology Group study. *Invest New Drugs* 1984;2:323–328.
674. Cobleigh MA, Williams SD, Einhorn LH. Phase II study of vindesine in patients with metastatic breast cancer. *Cancer Treat Rep* 1981;65:659–663.
675. Bezwoda WR, de Moor NG, Derman D, et al. Combination chemotherapy of metastatic breast cancer: a randomized trial comparing the use of adriamycin to that of vinblastine. *Cancer* 1979;44:392–397.
676. Yap HY, Blumenschein GR, Keating MJ, et al. Vinblastine given as a continuous 5-day infusion in the treatment of refractory advanced breast cancer. *Cancer Treat Rep* 1980;64:279–283.
677. Vogel C, O'Rourke M, Winer E, et al. Vinorelbine as first-line chemotherapy for advanced breast cancer in women 60 years of age or older. *Ann Oncol* 1999;10:397–402.
678. Havlin KA, Ramirez MJ, Legler CM, et al. Inability to escalate vinorelbine dose intensity using a daily x3 schedule with and without filgrastim in patients with metastatic breast cancer. *Cancer Chemother Pharmacol* 1999;43:68–72.
679. Ibrahim NK, Rahman Z, Valero V, et al. Phase II study of vinorelbine administered by 96-hour infusion in patients with advanced breast carcinoma. *Cancer* 1999;86:1251–1257.
680. Ejlertsen B, Mouridsen HT, Langkjer ST, et al. Phase III study of intravenous vinorelbine in combination with epirubicin versus epirubicin alone in patients with advanced breast cancer: a Scandinavian Breast Group Trial (SBG9403). *J Clin Oncol* 2004;22:2313–2320.
681. Blajman C, Balbiani L, Block J, et al. A prospective, randomized phase III trial comparing combination chemotherapy with cyclophosphamide, doxorubicin, and 5-fluorouracil with vinorelbine plus doxorubicin in the treatment of advanced breast carcinoma. *Cancer* 1999;85:1091–1097.
682. Namer M, Soler-Michel P, Turpin F, et al. Results of a phase III prospective, randomised trial, comparing mitoxantrone and vinorelbine (MV) in combination with standard FAC/FEC in front-line therapy of metastatic breast cancer. *Eur J Cancer* 2001;37:1132–1140.
683. Dieras V, Extra JM, Bellissant E, et al. Efficacy and tolerance of vinorelbine and fluorouracil combination as first-line chemotherapy of advanced breast cancer: results of a phase II study using a sequential group method. *J Clin Oncol* 1996;14:3097–3104.
684. Gonzalez Vela JL, Sanchez Guillen JM, et al. [Effectiveness of 5-fluoruracil and vinorelbine in patients who had received multi-treatments for metastatic breast cancer]. *Clin Transl Oncol* 2005;7:441–446.
685. Ghosn M, Kattan J, Farhat F, et al. Phase II trial of capecitabine and vinorelbine as first-line chemotherapy for metastatic breast cancer patients. *Anticancer Res* 2006;26:2451–2456.
686. Isik B, Altundag K. Vinorelbine, methotrexate and fluorouracil (VMF) as first-line therapy in metastatic breast cancer: significance of the time between initiation of adjuvant therapy and of therapy for metastatic breast cancer. *Ann Oncol* 2004;15:175.
687. Ardavanis A, Extra JM, Espie M, et al. Phase II trial of a combination of vinorelbine, cyclophosphamide and 5-fluorouracil in the treatment of advanced breast cancer. *In Vivo* 1998;12:559–562.
688. Shamseddine AI, Otrock ZK, Khalifeh MJ, et al. A clinical phase II study of a non-anthracycline sequential combination of cisplatin-vinorelbine followed by docetaxel as first-line treatment in metastatic breast cancer. *Oncology* 2006;70:330–338.
689. Kosmas C, Agelaki S, Giannakakis T, et al. Phase I study of vinorelbine and carboplatin combination in patients with taxane and anthracycline pretreated advanced breast cancer. *Oncology* 2002;62:103–109.
690. Bonneterre J, Campone M, Koralewski P, et al. Vinorelbine/docetaxel combination treatment of metastatic breast cancer: a phase I study. *Cancer Chemother Pharmacol* 2007;60:365–373.
691. Berruti A, Bitossi R, Gorzegno G, et al. Paclitaxel, vinorelbine and 5-fluorouracil in breast cancer patients pretreated with adjuvant anthracyclines. *Br J Cancer* 2005;92:634–638.
692. Perrone F, De Placido S, Carlomagno C, et al. Chemotherapy with mitomycin C and vinblastine in pretreated metastatic breast cancer. *Tumori* 1993;79:254–257.
693. Aapro MS, Conte P, Esteban González E, Trillet-Lenoir V. Oral vinorelbine: role in the management of metastatic breast cancer. *Drugs* 2007;67:657–667.
694. Oral Navelbine (package insert) Pierre Fabre Medicament; April 2004.
695. Jassem J, Kosmidis P, Ramlau R, et al. Oral vinorelbine in combination with cisplatin: a novel active regimen in advanced non-small-cell lung cancer. *Ann Oncol* 2003;14:1634–1639.
696. Freyer G, Delozier T, Lichinister M, et al. Phase II study of oral vinorelbine in first-line advanced breast cancer chemotherapy. *J Clin Oncol* 2003;21:35–40.
697. Amadori D, Koralewski P, Tekiela A, et al. Efficacy and safety of navelbine oral (VNBO) in first line metastatic breast cancer (MBC). *Eur J Cancer* 2001;37[Suppl 6]:195(asbt).
698. Nole F, Catania C, Sanna G, et al. Dose-finding and pharmacokinetic study of an all-oral combination regimen of oral vinorelbine and capecitabine for patients with metastatic breast cancer. *Ann Oncol* 2006;17:322–329.
699. Nole F, Catania C, Sanna G, et al. Phase II study with dose finding of oral vinorelbine in combination with capecitabine as first line chemotherapy of metastatic breast cancer (MBC): preliminary results of the phase II part of the study. *Eur J Cancer* 2006;[Suppl 4]:(abst 408).
700. Finek J, Holubec L, Elgrova L, et al. The effect of oral vinorelbine and capecitabine in patients with metastatic breast cancer. ASCO annual meeting proceedings Part I. *J Clin Oncol* 2006;24(18S)[Suppl]:10605.
701. Delacambre C, Veyret C, Levy C, et al. A phase I/II study of capecitabine combined with oral vinorelbine as first- or second-line therapy in locally advanced or metastatic breast cancer. *Breast Cancer Res Treat* 2005;94[Suppl 1]:P1081.
702. Chan A, Tubiana N, Ganju V, et al. Optimal tolerance of an all-oral combination chemotherapy (CT) of oral vinorelbine (NVBo), capecitabine (C) with/without trastuzumab (T) in metastatic breast cancer (MBC) patients (pts): safety results of two international multicenter studies. ASCO annual meeting proceedings Part I. *J Clin Oncol* 2006;24(18S)[Suppl]:10607.
703. van Maanen JM, Retel J, de Vries J, et al. Mechanism of action of antitumor drug etoposide: a review. *J Natl Cancer Inst* 1988;80:1526–1533.
704. Kamesaki S, Kamesaki H, Jorgensen TJ, et al. Bcl-2 protein inhibits etoposide-induced apoptosis through its effects on events subsequent to topoisomerase II-induced DNA strand breaks and their repair. *Cancer Res* 1993;53:4251–4256.
705. Okamoto-Kubo S, Nishio K, Heike Y, Yoshida M, et al. Apoptosis induced by etoposide in small-cell lung cancer cell lines. *Cancer Chemother Pharmacol* 1994;33:385–390.
706. Sun XM, Snowden RT, Dinsdale D, et al. Changes in nuclear chromatin precede internucleosomal DNA cleavage in the induction of apoptosis by etoposide. *Biochem Pharmacol* 1994;47:187–195.
707. Ferguson PJ, Fisher MH, Stephenson J, et al. Combined modalities of resistance in etoposide-resistant human KB cell lines. *Cancer Res* 1988;48:5956–5964.
708. Giaccone G, Gazdar AF, Beck H, et al. Multidrug sensitivity phenotype of human lung cancer cells associated with topoisomerase II expression. *Cancer Res* 1992;52:1666–1674.
709. Takigawa N, Ohnoshi T, Ueoka H, et al. Establishment and characterization of an etoposide-resistant human small cell lung cancer cell line. *Acta Med Okayama* 1992;46:203–212.
710. Harvey VJ, Slevin ML, Joel SP, et al. The effect of food and concurrent chemotherapy on the bioavailability of oral etoposide. *Br J Cancer* 1985;52:363–367.
711. Hande K, Bennett R, Hamilton R, Grote T, Branch R. Metabolism and excretion of etoposide in isolated, perfused rat liver models. *Cancer Res* 1988;48:5692–5695.
712. Floyd J, Mirza I, Sachs B, Perry MC. Hepatotoxicity of chemotherapy. *Semin Oncol* 2006;33:50–67.
713. Friedland D, Gorman G, Treat J. Hypersensitivity reactions from taxol and etoposide. *J Natl Cancer Inst* 1993;85:2036.
714. Pusztai L, Walters RS, Valero V, et al. Daily oral etoposide in patients with heavily pretreated metastatic breast cancer. *Am J Clin Oncol* 1998;21:442–446.
715. Martin M, Lluch A, Casado A, et al. Clinical activity of chronic oral etoposide in previously treated metastatic breast cancer. *J Clin Oncol* 1994;12:986–991.
716. Bezwoda WR, Seymour L, Ariad S. High-dose etoposide in treatment of metastatic breast cancer. *Oncology* 1992;49:104–107.
717. Atienza DM, Vogel CL, Trock B, et al. Phase II study of oral etoposide for patients with advanced breast cancer. *Cancer* 1995;76:2485–2490.
718. Calvert AH, Lind MJ, Millward MM, et al. Long-term oral etoposide in metastatic breast cancer: clinical and pharmacokinetic results. *Cancer Treat Rev* 1993;19[Suppl C]:27–33.
719. Neskovic-Konstantinovic ZB, Bosnjak SM, Radulovic SS, et al. Daily oral etoposide in metastatic breast cancer. *Anticancer Drugs* 1996;7:543–547.
720. Saphner T, Weller EA, Tormey DC, et al. 21-day oral etoposide for metastatic breast cancer: a phase II study and review of the literature. *Am J Clin Oncol* 2000;23:258–262.
721. Jagodic M, Cufer T, Zakotnik B, et al. Selection of candidates for oral etoposide salvage chemotherapy in heavily pretreated breast cancer patients. *Anticancer Drugs* 2001;12:199–204.
722. Icli F, Gunel N, Dincol D, et al. Cisplatin plus VP-16 combination chemotherapy in advanced refractory breast cancer. *J Surg Oncol* 1992;50:251–253.
723. Cox EB, Burton GV, Olsen GA, et al. Cisplatin and etoposide: an effective treatment for refractory breast carcinoma. *Am J Clin Oncol* 1989;12:53–56.
724. Krook JE, Loprinzi CL, Schaid DJ, et al. Evaluation of the continuous infusion of etoposide plus cisplatin in metastatic breast cancer. A collaborative North Central Cancer Treatment Group/Mayo Clinic phase II study. *Cancer* 1990;65:418–421.
725. Vinolas N, Daniels M, Estape J, et al. Phase II trial of carboplatin and etoposide activity in pretreated breast cancer patients. *Am J Clin Oncol* 1992;15:160–162.
726. Barker LJ, Jones SE, Savin MA, et al. Phase II evaluation of carboplatin and VP-16 for patients with metastatic breast cancer and only one prior chemotherapy regimen. *Cancer* 1993;72:771–773.

727. van der Gaast A, Bontenbal M, Planting AS, et al. Phase II study of carboplatin and etoposide as a first line regimen in patients with metastatic breast cancer. *Ann Oncol* 1994;5:858–860.

728. Cocconi G, Bisagni G, Bacchi M, et al. Cisplatin and etoposide as first-line chemotherapy for metastatic breast carcinoma: a prospective randomized trial of the Italian Oncology Group for Clinical Research. *J Clin Oncol* 1991;9:664–669.

729. Perez EA, Hillman DW, Mailliard JA, et al. Randomized phase II study of two irinotecan schedules for patients with metastatic breast cancer refractory to an anthracycline, a taxane, or both. *J Clin Oncol* 2004;22:2849–2855.

730. Wolff AC, O'Neill A, Kennedy MJ, et al. Single-agent topotecan as first-line chemotherapy in women with metastatic breast cancer: final results of eastern cooperative oncology group trial E8193. *Clin Breast Cancer* 2005;6:334–339.

731. Munoz R, Shaked Y, Bertolini F, et al. Anti-angiogenic treatment of breast cancer using metronomic low-dose chemotherapy. *Breast* 2005;14:466–479.

732. Colleoni M, Orlando L, Sanna G, et al. Metronomic low-dose oral cyclophosphamide and methotrexate plus or minus thalidomide in metastatic breast cancer: antitumor activity and biological effects. *Ann Oncol* 2006;17:232–238.

733. Orlando L, Cardillo A, Rocca A, et al. Prolonged clinical benefit with metronomic chemotherapy in patients with metastatic breast cancer. *Anticancer Drugs* 2006;17:961–967.

734. Munoz R, Man S, Shaked Y, et al. Highly efficacious nontoxic preclinical treatment for advanced metastatic breast cancer using combination oral UFT-cyclophosphamide metronomic chemotherapy. *Cancer Res* 2006;66:3386–3391.

735. Bocci G, Tuccori M, Emmenegger U, et al. Cyclophosphamide-methotrexate "metronomic" chemotherapy for the palliative treatment of metastatic breast cancer. A comparative pharmacoeconomic evaluation. *Ann Oncol* 2005;16:1243–1252.

736. Emens LA. Chemotherapy and tumor immunity: an unexpected collaboration. *Front Biosci* 2008;13:249–257.

737. Curigliano G, Spitaleri G, Pietri E, et al. Breast cancer vaccines: a clinical reality or fairy tale? *Ann Oncol* 2006;17:750–762.

738. Avigan D, Vasir B, Gong J, et al. Fusion cell vaccination of patients with metastatic breast and renal cancer induces immunological and clinical responses. *Clin Cancer Res* 2004;10:4699–4708.

739. Narayanan K, Jaramillo A, Benshoff ND, et al. Response of established human breast tumors to vaccination with mammaglobin-A cDNA. *J Natl Cancer Inst* 2004;96:1388–1396.

740. Chopra A, Kim TS, O'Sullivan I, et al. Combined therapy of an established, highly aggressive breast cancer in mice with paclitaxel and a unique DNA-based cell vaccine. *Int J Cancer* 2006;118:2888–2898.

741. Mittendorf EA, Peoples GE, Singletary SE. Breast cancer vaccines: promise for the future or pipe dream? *Cancer* 2007;110:1677–1686.

742. Sugamura K, Ishii N, Weinberg AD. Therapeutic targeting of the effector T-cell co-stimulatory molecule OX40. *Nat Rev Immunol* 2004;4:420–431.

743. Knutson KL, Dang Y, Lu H, et al. IL-2 immunotoxin therapy modulates tumor-associated regulatory T cells and leads to lasting immune-mediated rejection of breast cancers in neu-transgenic mice. *J Immunol* 2006;177:84–91.

744. Zou W. Regulatory T cells, tumour immunity and immunotherapy. *Nat Rev Immunol* 2006;6:295–307.

745. Emens LA, Armstrong D, Biedrzycki B, et al. A phase I vaccine safety and chemotherapy dose-finding trial of an allogeneic GM-CSF-secreting breast cancer vaccine given in a specifically timed sequence with immunomodulatory doses of cyclophosphamide and doxorubicin. *Hum Gene Ther* 2004;15:313–337.

746. Manning EA, Ullman JG, Leatherman JM, et al. A vascular endothelial growth factor receptor-2 inhibitor enhances antitumor immunity through an immune-based mechanism. *Clin Cancer Res* 2007;13:3951–3959.

747. Peoples GE, Gurney JM, Hueman MT, et al. Clinical trial results of a HER2/neu (E75) vaccine to prevent recurrence in high-risk breast cancer patients. *J Clin Oncol* 2005;23:7536–7545.

748. Peoples GE, Khoo S, Dehqanzada ZA, et al. Combined clinical trial results of a HER2/neu (E75) vaccine for prevention of recurrence in high-risk breast cancer patients. *Breast Cancer Res Treat* 2006;100[Suppl 1]:S6(abst 4).

749. Cardoso F, Di LA, Lohrisch C, et al. Second and subsequent lines of chemotherapy for metastatic breast cancer: what did we learn in the last two decades? *Ann Oncol* 2002;13:197–207.

750. McLachlan SA, Pintilie M, Tannock IF. Third line chemotherapy in patients with metastatic breast cancer: an evaluation of quality of life and cost. *Breast Cancer Res Treat* 1999;54:213–223.

751. McQuellon RP, Muss HB, Hoffman SL, et al. Patient preferences for treatment of metastatic breast cancer: a study of women with early-stage breast cancer. *J Clin Oncol* 1995;13:858–868.

752. Slevin ML, Stubbs L, Plant HJ, et al. Attitudes to chemotherapy: comparing views of patients with cancer with those of doctors, nurses, and general public. *BMJ* 1990;300:1458–1460.

753. Moinpour CM, Feigl P, Metch B, et al. Quality of life end points in cancer clinical trials: review and recommendations. *J Natl Cancer Inst* 1989;81:485–495.

754. Donovan K, Sanson-Fisher RW, Redman S. Measuring quality of life in cancer patients. *J Clin Oncol* 1989;7:959–968.

755. Nayfield SG, Hailey BJ, eds. *Report of the workshop on quality of life research in cancer clinical trials*. Bethesda, MD: National Institutes of Health, 1990.

756. Coates A, Gebski V, Signorini D, et al. Prognostic value of quality-of-life scores during chemotherapy for advanced breast cancer. Australian New Zealand Breast Cancer Trials group. *J Clin Oncol* 1992;10:1833–1838.

757. Coates AS, Hurny C, Peterson HF, et al. Quality-of-life scores predict outcome in metastatic but not early breast cancer. International Breast Cancer Study Group. *J Clin Oncol* 2000;18:3768–3774.

758. Ganz PA, Lee JJ, Siau J. Quality of life assessment. An independent prognostic variable for survival in lung cancer. *Cancer* 1991;67:3131–3135.

759. Smith TJ, Hillner BE, Desch CE. Efficacy and cost-effectiveness of cancer treatment: rational allocation of resources based on decision analysis. *J Natl Cancer Inst* 1993;85:1460–1474.

760. Outcomes of cancer treatment for technology assessment and cancer treatment guidelines. American Society of Clinical Oncology. *J Clin Oncol* 1996;14:671–679.

761. Carlson RW. Quality of life issues in the treatment of metastatic breast cancer. *Oncology (Williston Park)* 1998;12:27–31.

762. Cella DF, Tulsky DS, Gray G, et al. The functional assessment of cancer therapy scale: development and validation of the general measure. *J Clin Oncol* 1993;11:570–579.

763. Aaronson NK, Ahmedzai S, Bergman B, et al. The European Organization for Research and Treatment of Cancer QLQ-C30: a quality-of-life instrument for use in international clinical trials in oncology. *J Natl Cancer Inst* 1993;85:365–376.

764. Radice D, Redaelli A. Breast cancer management. quality-of-life and cost considerations. *Pharmacoeconomics* 2003;21:383–396.

765. Anderson BO, Yip CH, Ramsey SD, et al. Breast cancer in limited-resource countries: health care systems and public policy. *Breast J* 2006;12[Suppl 1]:S54–S69.

766. Nole F, Munzone E, Zorzino L, et al. Variation of circulating tumor cell levels during treatment of metastatic breast cancer: prognostic and therapeutic implications. *Ann Oncol* 2008;19(5):891–897.

767. Bidard FC, Vincent-Salomon A, Sigal-Zafrani B, et al. Prognosis of women with stage IV breast cancer depends on detection of circulating tumor cells rather than disseminated tumor cells. *Ann Oncol* 2008;19(3):496–500.

768. Budd GT, Cristofanilli M, Ellis MJ, et al. Circulating tumor cells versus imaging—predicting overall survival in metastatic breast cancer. *Clin Cancer Res* 2006;12:6403–6409.

769. Kuukasjarvi T, Kononen J, Helin H, et al. Loss of estrogen receptor in recurrent breast cancer is associated with poor response to endocrine therapy. *J Clin Oncol* 1996;14:2584–2589.

770. Wu JM, Fackler MJ, Halushka MK, et al. Heterogeneity of breast cancer metastases: comparison of therapeutic target expression and promoter methylation between primary tumors and their multifocal metastases. *Clin Cancer Res* 2008;14:1938–1946.

Chapter 75
Treatment of HER2-Overexpressing Metastatic Breast Cancer

Sumanta Kumar Pal and Mark D. Pegram

In 2008 it is estimated that 184,450 cases of breast cancer will be diagnosed (1). Of these cases, approximately 6% will have metastatic disease at the time of initial presentation (2). Additionally, a substantial proportion of those patients with early stage disease will go on to develop metastatic breast cancer (MBC) despite appropriate locoregional therapy (3). Whereas traditional cytotoxic chemotherapy was originally the mainstay of treatment for these patients, targeted therapeutics emerging over the past decade have significantly improved prognosis for subsets of MBC patients (4).

A therapeutic target in MBC that has received intense research focus is the HER2 (ERBB) receptor, a member of the ERBB family of transmembrane receptors, including HER1 (ERBB1, or EGFR [epidermal growth factor receptor]), HER3 (ERBB3), and HER4 (ERBB4) (5). The ERBB family of receptors possesses a wide range of functions related to cell growth and proliferation. With the exception of HER2, ERBB family receptors undergo a conformational change in the ectodomain as a consequence of binding any of the 12 known ligands. This conformational change exposes a β-hairpin loop dimerization domain that facilitates EGFR, HER3, and HER4 to undergo homo- or heterodimerization (6) (Fig. 75.1). Dimerization leads to structural activation of the intracellular kinase domain, with subsequent activation of one of any number of signal transduction cascades including Ras-mitogen–activated protein kinase (Ras-MAPK), phosphatidyl 3′ kinase-protein kinase B (PI3K-PKB/Akt), and phospholipase C-protein kinase C (PLC-PKC) pathways (7). By contrast, HER2 does not bind to any of the ERBB-family ligands, and analysis of the crystal structure of the HER2 ectodomain demonstrates that the dimerization domain is natively exposed in an open conformation, suggesting that this transmembrane receptor species remains constitutively poised for dimerization (8). This property provides rationale for enhanced mitogenesis with increased HER2 expression, as observed in experiments utilizing HER2-transfected breast and ovarian xenograft models (9).

These laboratory observations have been bolstered by translational research involving clinical outcome data from breast cancer patients harboring amplification of the HER2 gene. Multivariate analyses of clinical data from 345 patients with lymph node–positive breast cancer demonstrated statistically significant decrements in disease-free survival (DFS) and overall survival (OS) in patients with HER2 gene amplification (10). These clinical data defining the role of HER2 in association with an aggressive tumor phenotype served as the impetus for development of HER2-targeted therapies. Given that approximately 20% of breast cancer patients globally demonstrate HER2 gene amplification, the clinical implications of such therapies are profound (11).

TRASTUZUMAB

Development of Trastuzumab

Initially, several murine monoclonal antibodies with antiproliferative activity specifically against HER2-overexpressing human cancer cell lines were identified (12,13). The complementarity determining regions from one of the most potent of these murine monoclonal antibodies were subsequently fused into a human immunoglobin G₁ (IgG₁) framework, resulting in a humanized HER2-directed monoclonal antibody, trastuzumab (14). Preclinical studies of trastuzumab demonstrated that following the humanization procedure, the activity of the antibody against HER2-overexpressing cancer cell lines and xenografts was retained, particularly when used in combination with other cytotoxic therapeutics (15). Numerous studies have been conducted that focused on the mechanisms of trastuzumab-related antitumor activity. Although no consensus exists at present, several plausible hypotheses have been suggested. Resolution of the crystal structure of trastuzumab complexed with HER2 has led to identification of a trastuzumab-binding site in the juxtamembrane region. It is possible that this juxtamembrane binding generates steric alteration of HER2 dimers to the extent that intracellular tyrosine kinase domains cannot efficiently interact and activate (8). Alternatively, preclinical data exist to support stimulation of antibody-dependent cellular cytotoxicity (ADCC) and modification of key cell cycle regulators (i.e., increased levels of p27, a Cdk2 inhibitor) subsequent to trastuzumab binding (16). Recent studies additionally suggest that inhibition of HER2 ectodomain cleavage may serve as a mechanism of trastuzumab activity, as the p95 fragment generated from cleavage retains intracellular activity (17).

Single-Agent Trastuzumab for Metastatic Breast Cancer

Pilot clinical trials suggested only modest activity of single-agent trastuzumab in the setting of heavily pretreated MBC with HER2 overexpression (Table 75.1). In this HER2-overexpressing population (defined in this study as those patients with immunohistochemical [IHC] staining for HER2 in >25% of cells), patients were treated with a loading dose of 250 mg, followed by 10 weekly doses of 100 mg. Patients with no evidence of disease progression were subsequently offered a maintenance dose of 100 mg weekly. Following single agent trastuzumab, objective responses were seen in 5 of 43 assessable patients (overall response rate [ORR] 11.5%), including one complete response (CR) and four partial responses (PRs) (18).

Subsequently, a much larger study in a pretreated MBC population explored a dosing regimen including a loading dose of 4 mg/kg followed by 2 mg/kg weekly maintenance therapy. Notably, the definition of HER2 overexpression differed in this study, including those patients with IHC scores of 2+ or 3+ (corresponding to moderate to strong membrane staining for HER2 protein). In a total of 213 treated patients, eight CRs and 22 PRs were observed (ORR 15%). The median duration of response was approximately 9.1 months, and median OS was 13 months (19). Common adverse events attributed to therapy included infusion-related fevers or chills, occurring in approximately 40% of patients, and these were treated successfully with pharmacologic intervention. Clinically significant cardiac dysfunction was noted in 4.7%

920

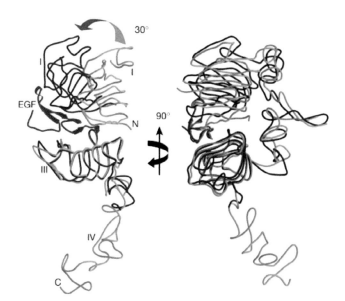

FIGURE 75.1. Orthogonal views of a ribbon diagram with the structure of HER2 (*green*) superimposed on the structured of EGFR (*blue*) bound to the ligand EGF (*red*). Note similarities in the structure of HER2 with activated EGFR, suggesting that HER2 (which lacks a ligand binding domain) retains a conformation in which it is constitutively active and poised for dimerization.

of patients, comprised of congestive heart failure (CHF), cardiomyopathy, or a decrease in ejection fraction (>10%). These observed cardiac events, along with events reported in a concurrent trial of trastuzumab in combination with chemotherapy, prompted further examination of potential risk factors for trastuzumab-associated cardiac toxicity (20). In a preliminary review of trastuzumab-related cardiac adverse events, 9 of 10 patients with cardiac events had prior anthracycline therapy and additionally had at least one risk factor for anthracycline-induced cardiomyopathy (including cumulative doxorubicin dose >400 mg/m^2, radiotherapy to the left chest, age >70 years, and history of hypertension) (19).

Whereas the previous two studies assessed a heavily pretreated population of patients, a separate trial assessed the use of trastuzumab as first-line monotherapy for HER2-overexpressing MBC. A total of 114 women were randomized to receive one of two trastuzumab dosing regimens: (a) a loading dose of 4 mg/kg followed by 2 mg/kg weekly, or (b) a loading dose of 8 mg/kg followed by 4 mg/kg weekly. Among 111 assessable patients, 7 CRs and 23 PRs were observed (ORR 26%). Accompanying this clinical trial was a retrospective analysis of HER2 gene amplification by fluorescence *in situ* hybridization (FISH). Differential benefit was noted among those patients with and without FISH amplification, with a response rate of 34% and 7%, respectively. Interestingly, a marked variation was seen among those patients with 3+ and 2+ IHC scores, with response rates of 35% and 0%, respectively. Again, the most frequently reported treatment-related adverse events were fevers and chills. Reports of cardiac dysfunction in the previously noted trials (19,20) led to an evaluation of cardiac events in this trial. Only two patients (2%) were noted to have clinically significant cardiac dysfunction, requiring no intervention other than discontinuation of trastuzumab. Of note, variations in trastuzumab dosing did not lead to significant differences in clinical endpoints. Median OS was 25.8 and 22.9 months in those who received 4 and 2 mg/kg, respectively (21).

Preclinical Rationale for Trastuzumab in Combination with Cytotoxic Therapy

As previously noted, initial studies of trastuzumab in cell lines suggested optimum efficacy of the antibody when combined with cytotoxic therapy (12). Initially, these experiments specifically assessed the combination of trastuzumab and cisplatin. Further preclinical studies have assessed several distinct chemotherapeutics in combination with trastuzumab against a panel of four HER2-overexpressing breast cancer cell lines (SKBR3, BT-474, MDA-MB 361, and MDA-MB 453) and confirmed *in vivo* in HER2 overexpressing xenograft models. Multiple drug effect/combination index isobologram analysis was used to quantify pharmacologic drug–drug interactions between trastuzumab and cytotoxic agents from multiple drug classes. Synergistic interactions were noted in all four cell lines when trastuzumab was combined with carboplatin, 4-hydroxycyclophosphamide, docetaxel, and vinorelbine. Additive interactions were noted with the combination of trastuzumab and doxorubicin, epirubicin and paclitaxel. Evaluation of the three-drug regimen of carboplatin, docetaxel, and trastuzumab also showed significant synergy (22). Variable interaction was noted for trastuzumab in combination with gemcitabine, with antagonism at high concentrations but synergy at low concentrations (23).

Separate but related methodologies have been used to assess the efficacy of trastuzumab-based combinations using *in vivo* models (24). In HER2-overexpressing xenografts, synergy has been observed using the combinations of trastuzumab with alkylating agents, platinum analogs, topoisomerase II inhibitors, and ionizing radiation. Additive interactions were observed with the combination of trastuzumab with taxanes and anthracyclines (25). Results of these experiments played a critical role in the design and conduct of subsequent clinical trials of trastuzumab in combination with cytotoxic chemotherapy.

Pivotal Trial of Trastuzumab with Chemotherapy

A pivotal phase III registration trial of trastuzumab and cytotoxic chemotherapy randomized patients to receive either standard chemotherapy alone or standard chemotherapy plus trastuzumab as first-line therapy for HER2-positive metastatic disease. HER2 overexpressors were defined as those possessing IHC scores of 2+ or 3+ using the same murine monoclonal antibody upon which trastuzumab was based as the primary detection antibody. In this trial, patients were stratified according to their prior adjuvant treatment. Patients who had not previously received adjuvant therapy with an anthracycline received doxorubicin or epirubicin and cyclophosphamide with or without trastuzumab, whereas in those patients who had previously received adjuvant anthracycline, a regimen of paclitaxel alone or paclitaxel in combination with trastuzumab was utilized. Trastuzumab was administered at a loading dose of 4 mg/kg, followed by a maintenance dose of 2 mg/kg weekly, until the observation of disease progression. Compared to nonrecipients of trastuzumab (N = 234), patients who received trastuzumab (N = 235) had a longer time to disease progression (7.4 vs. 4.6 months; *p* <.001), a higher rate of objective response (50% vs. 32%; *p* <.001), a longer mean duration of response (9.1 vs. 6.1 months; *p* <.001), and prolonged median OS (25.1 vs. 20.3 months; *p* = .046) (4) (Fig. 75.2). Along with the trastuzumab monotherapy noted above, these data supported the approval of trastuzumab for the treatment of HER2-positive MBC by the U.S. Food and Drug Administration (FDA) in 1998.

| Table 75.1 | KEY TRIALS OF TRASTUZUMAB THERAPY AND ASSOCIATED RESPONSE RATES |

Author (Reference)	Year	Study Type	N	1st Line?	Regimen	RR (%)
Phase II Studies						
Single-Agent Therapy						
Baselga et al. (18)	1999	Phase II	43	No	Trastuzumab 250 mg loading followed by 100 mg/wk $\times$ 10 wks	12
Cobleigh et al. (19)	1999	Phase II	213	No	Trastuzumab 4 mg/kg loading followed by 2 mg/kg/wk	15
Vogel et al. (21)	2002	Randomized phase II	111	Yes	Trastuzumab 4 mg/kg loading followed by 2 mg/kg/wk, or trastuzumab 8 mg/kg loading followed by 4 mg/kg/wk	26
Paclitaxel and Trastuzumab						
Leyland-Jones et al. (26)	2003	Phase II	32	No	Paclitaxel 175 mg/m^2 q3wks with trastuzumab 8 mg/kg loading followed by 6 mg/kg q3wks	59
Gasparini et al. (27)	2007	Randomized phase II	118	Yes	Paclitaxel 80 mg/m^2/wk alone or with trastuzumab 4 mg/kg loading followed by 2 mg/kg qwk	75[a]
Gori et al. (28)	2004	Phase II	25	No	Paclitaxel 60–90 mg/m^2/wk with trastuzumab 4 mg/kg loading followed by 2 mg/kg qwk	56
Seidman et al. (29)	2001	Phase II	88	No	Paclitaxel 90 mg/m^2/wk with trastuzumab 4 mg/kg loading followed by 2 mg/kg qwk	61
Docetaxel and Trastuzumab						
Esteva et al. (33)	2002	Phase II	30	Yes[b]	Docetaxel 35 mg/m^2/wk with trastuzumab 2 mg/kg/wk for 3 out of 4 wks/cycle	63
Tedesco et al. (34)	2004	Phase II	26	Yes[b]	Docetaxel 35 mg/m^2/wk for 6 wks followed by 2 wks rest with trastuzumab 4 mg/kg loading followed by 2 mg/kg qwk	50
Raff et al. (35)	2004	Randomized phase II	17	No	Docetaxel 35 or 40 mg/m^2/wk for 3 wks, then 1 wk off, with trastuzumab 4 mg/kg loading (day 1) followed by 2 mg/kg qwk (days 8 and 15) of a 28-d cycle	59
Montemurro et al. (36)	2004	Phase II	42	No	Docetaxel 75 mg/m^2 q3wks x 6 with trastuzumab 4 mg/kg loading followed by 2 mg/kg qwk	67
Marty et al. (37)	2005	Randomized phase II	186	Yes	Docetaxel 75 mg/m^2 q3wks alone or with trastuzumab 4 mg/kgloading followed by 2 mg/kg qwk	61[a]
Vinorelbine/trastuzumab						
Burstein et al. (38)	2001	Phase II	40	No	Vinorelbine 25 mg/m^2/wk with trastuzumab 4 mg/kg loading followed by 2 mg/kg qwk	75
Jahanzeb et al. (39)	2002	Phase II	40	Yes	Vinorelbine 30 mg/m^2/wk with trastuzumab 4 mg/kg loading followed by 2 mg/kg qwk	78
Burstein et al. (40)	2003	Phase II	54	Yes	Vinorelbine 25 mg/m^2/wk with trastuzumab 4 mg/kg loading followed by 2 mg/kg qwk	68
Chan et al. (41)	2006	Phase II	62	Yes	Vinorelbine 30 mg/m^2/wk with trastuzumab 4 mg/kg loading followed by 2 mg/kg qwk	63
De Maio et al. (42)	2007	Phase II	40	No	Vinorelbine 30 mg/m^2/wk on days 1 and 8 of a 3-wk cycle with trastuzumab 8 mg/kg loading followed by 6 mg/kg qwk	50
Papaldo et al. (43)	2006	Phase II (two-arm)	68	Yes	Vinorelbine 25 mg/m^2/wk alone or with trastuzumab 4 mg/kg loading followed by 2 mg/kg qwk	51
Capecitabine and Trastuzumab						
Schaller et al. (49)	2007	Phase II	27	No	Capecitabine 1,250 mg/m^2 bid for 14 d in a 21-d cycle given with trastuzumab 4 mg/kg loading followed by 2 mg/kg qwk	45
Bartsch et al. (50)	2007	Phase II	40	No	Capecitabine 1,250 mg/m^2 bid for 14 d in a 21-d cycle given trastuzumab 8 mg/kg loading followed by 6 mg/kg q3wks	20
Yamamoto et al. (51)	2008	Phase II	56	No	Capecitabine 1,657 mg/m^2 bid for 14 d in a 21 d cycle given with trastuzumab 4 mg/kg loading followed by 2 mg/kg qwk	50
Cisplatin and Trastuzumab						
Pegram et al. (52)	1998	Phase II	39	No	Cisplatin 75 mg/m^2 on days 1, 29, and 57 with trastuzumab 250 mg loading followed by 100 mg/wk for 9 wks	24
Gemcitabine and Trastuzumab						
Bartsch et al. (57)	2008	Phase II	26	No	Gemcitabine 1,250 mg/m^2 on days 1 and 8 of a 3-wk cycle with trastuzumab 8 mg/kg loading followed by 6 mg/kg q3wks	19
Three-Drug Regimens						
Perez et al. (54)	2005	Phase II	43	Yes	Paclitaxel 200 mg/m^2 q3wks and carboplatin (AUC 6 mg/mL) q3wks with trastuzumab 8 mg/kg loading followed by 6 mg/kg q3wks	65
			48	Yes	Paclitaxel 80 mg/m2/wk given with carboplatin (AUC w 2 mg/mL) every 3 out of 4 wks with trastuzumab 4 mg/kg loading followed by 2 mg/kg qwk	81

| Table 75.1 | KEY TRIALS OF TRASTUZUMAB THERAPY AND ASSOCIATED RESPONSE RATES (*Continued*) |

Author (Reference)	Year	Study Type	N	1st Line?	Regimen	RR (%)
Pegram et al. (56)	2004	Phase II	59	Yes[b]	Docetaxel 75 mg/m^2 q3wks with carboplatin (AUC 6 mg/mL) q3wks with trastuzumab 4 mg/kg loading followed by 2 mg/kg qwk	58
			62	Yes	Paclitaxel 75 mg/m2 q3wks with carboplatin (AUC 6 mg/mL) q3wks with trastuzumab 4 mg/kg loading followed by 2 mg/kg qwk	79
Miller et al. (58)	2001	Phase II	42	Yes	Gemcitabine 1,250 mg/m^2 on days 1 and 8 and paclitaxel 175 mg/m2 on day 1 of a 3-wk cycle with trastuzumab 4 mg/kg loading followed by 2 mg/kg qwk	67
Stemmler et al. (59)	2005	Phase II	20	No	Gemcitabine 750 mg/m2 with cisplatin 30 mg/m2 on days 1 and 8 of a 3-wk cycle with trastuzumab 4 mg/kg loading followed by 2 mg/kg qwk	40
Phase III Studies						
Slamon et al. (4)	2001	Phase III	469	No	Trastuzumab 4 mg/kg loading followed by 2 mg/kg/wk	32
					Taxane or anthracycline with cyclophosphamide given with trastuzumab 4 mg/kg loading followed by 2 mg/kg/wk	50
Robert et al. (55)	2006	Phase III	196	Yes	Paclitaxel 200 mg/m2 q3wks alone with trastuzumab 4 mg/kg loading followed by 2 mg/kg qwk	36
					Paclitaxel 200 mg/m2 q3wks with carboplatin (AUC 6 mg/mL) q3wks with trastuzumab 4 mg/kg loading followed by 2 mg/kg qwk	57
Burstein et al. (45)	2007	Phase III	81	Yes	Vinorelbine 25 mg/m2/wk with trastuzumab 4 mg/kg loading followed by 2 mg/kg qwk, or	51
					Docetaxel/paclitaxel, investigator preference, with trastuzumab 4 mg/kg loading followed by 2 mg/kg qwk	40
Pegram et al. (22)	2007	Phase III	263	Yes	Docetaxel 100 mg/m2 q3wks with trastuzumab 4 mg/kg loading followed by 2 mg/kg qwk	73
					Docetaxel 75 mg/m2 q3wks with carboplatin (AUC 6 mg/mL) q3wks with trastuzumab 4 mg/kg loading followed by 2 mg/kg qwk	73

AUC, area under the curve.
[a]Indicates RR for trastuzumab containing arm.
[b]Indicates first- and second-line treatment included.

In addition to providing strong support for the combination of trastuzumab with cytotoxic chemotherapy, the study also provided important insights related to cardiac toxicity. Of 63 patients who experienced symptomatic or asymptomatic cardiac dysfunction in this study, 39 had received the combination of anthracycline, cyclophosphamide, and trastuzumab (comprising roughly 27% of this subgroup). A much lower rate of cardiac dysfunction was observed in the remaining groups, with an incidence of 8%, 13%, and 1% in groups that had received anthracycline and cyclophosphamide alone, paclitaxel and trastuzumab, and paclitaxel alone, respectively. Grade III or IV New York Heart Association (NYHA) cardiac dysfunction was similarly observed at a much higher frequency in the group that received combined anthracycline and trastuzumab therapy. Increasing age was noted to be the only risk factor associated with cardiac dysfunction within this subgroup. Notably, cumulative anthracycline dose did not correlate with cardiac toxicity; however, the vast majority of patients in this treatment arm received the prescribed six doses of anthracycline treatment (4). Results from this trial led to caution in formulating further trials of trastuzumab therapy with concomitant anthracycline.

Trastuzumab and Paclitaxel

The aforementioned pivotal trial data suggests significant benefit with the combination of trastuzumab and conventional chemotherapy and further identifies a subgroup of trastuzumab recipients (those receiving the antibody in combination with paclitaxel) with more limited cardiac toxicity (4). Several follow-up trials expanded the data in support of the combination of paclitaxel and trastuzumab. A phase II study assessed a nearly identical paclitaxel regimen (at a dose of 175 mg/m^2) with an escalated 3-weekly dose of trastuzumab (8 mg/kg loading dose, followed by 6 mg/kg every 3 weeks) distinct from the pivotal trial. In 32 assessable patients, an ORR of 59% was observed, with a median response duration of 10.5 months and median TTP of 12.2 months (26). Several phase II studies have explored a regimen of trastuzumab and weekly paclitaxel. A randomized phase II trial assessed the efficacy of a weekly paclitaxel regimen in combination with trastuzumab as first-line therapy for MBC. HER2-overexpressing patients (characterized as 2+ or 3+ by IHC) received paclitaxel at a dose of 80 mg/m^2, either alone or in combination with a loading dose of trastuzumab of 4 mg/kg followed by a weekly dose of 2 mg/kg. ORR was noted to be significantly higher with combined therapy relative to single-agent paclitaxel (75% vs. 56.9%; $p = .037$), and this effect was noted to be more pronounced in the subset of patients with IHC scores of 3+ relative to 2+ (84.5% vs. 47.5%; $p = .0005$). Interestingly, no significant difference in TTP was observed in a combined analysis; however, when the subgroup with IHC score of 3+ was independently considered, the trastuzumab-receiving arm demonstrated prolonged TTP (13.2 vs. 9.7 months;

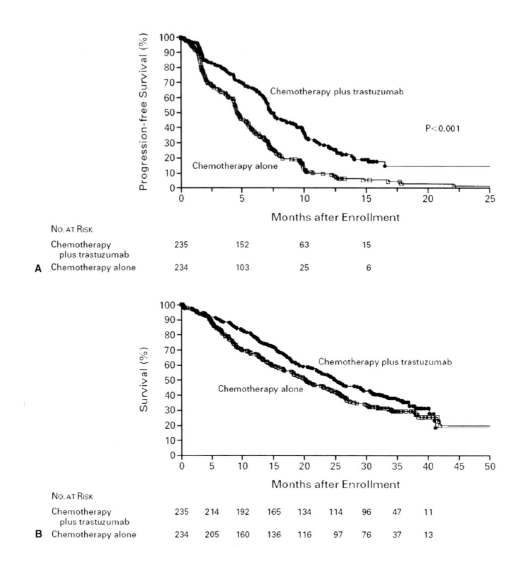

FIGURE 75.2. Kaplan-Meier estimates of progression-free survival **(A)** and overall survival **(B)** according to whether patients were assigned to receive chemotherapy plus trastuzumab or chemotherapy alone in a pivotal trial of trastuzumab.

$p = .03$). Median OS had not been reached at the time of original publication. In analysis of adverse events, no significant decreases in ejection fraction were noted on either arm of therapy. Notably, however, baseline ejection fractions in both treatments arms were relatively high (65% among trastuzumab recipients and 63% in trastuzumab nonrecipients) (27).

In the setting of heavily pretreated MBC patients, two separate phase II studies assess the efficacy of paclitaxel with trastuzumab. In the first, 25 HER2-overexpressing patients who previously received anthracycline- and taxane-based regimens were treated with trastuzumab (using a loading dose of 4 mg/kg and a subsequent weekly dose of 2 mg/kg) and paclitaxel (using a weekly regimen with doses between 60 to 90 mg/m²). An ORR of 56% was achieved, with a median duration of response of 10.4 months. In contrast to the limited cardiotoxicity seen with first-line therapy, two patients (8%) were removed from the study in light of grade III cardiotoxicity (28). A second phase II study utilized a similar patient population (i.e., anthracycline- and taxane-pretreated patients) with the exception of allowing non-HER2 overexpressors. Patients received a schedule of trastuzumab and paclitaxel (at 90 mg/m²) and an ORR of 61% was observed, comparable to the previous trial. However, when

stratified by HER2 status as determined by FISH and IHC, response rates appeared superior among HER2 overexpressors (67% to 81% vs. 41% to 16%; the wide intervals relate to different methodologies for HER2 characterization) (29).

Given comparable response data in phase II trials of weekly and 3-weekly paclitaxel in combination with trastuzumab, Cancer and Leukemia Group B (CALGB) protocol 9840 sought to determine which of the two regiments was more efficacious. In this complex phase III trial, patients were originally randomized to receive paclitaxel at 175 mg/m² every 3 weeks or 80 mg/m² weekly. Of note, the trial incorporates a "historical control" comprised of patients (N = 158) treated with paclitaxel at 175 mg/m² every 3 weeks who were previously enrolled on CALGB 9342 (a trial randomizing to three different doses of paclitaxel alone). Although the trial did not originally stipulate the necessity of HER2 testing, a protocol amendment was made after the enrollment of 171 patients requiring HER2 characterization by FISH or IHC. Patients determined to overexpress HER2 were treated uniformly with trastuzumab; non-HER2 overexpressors were randomized to receive paclitaxel and trastuzumab or paclitaxel alone. A total of 577 patients were treated on CALGB 9840, and with inclusion of 158 patients from CALGB 9342, a total of 735 patients were included in the final analysis. In the combined sample, weekly paclitaxel appeared to be superior to 3-weekly paclitaxel by ORR (42% vs. 29%; $p = .0004$), TTP (9 vs. 5 months; $p < .0001$), and median OS (24 vs. 12 months; $p = .0092$). Supporting results from the previously noted phase II study of weekly paclitaxel, trastuzumab therapy did not provide benefit in non-HER2-overexpressing patients (30). Although the trial design evoked a great deal of controversy, given inclusion of a large subset of patients from a previous study and treatment of non-HER2-overexpressing patients with trastuzumab (31), the trial did establish proof of concept that HER2 overexpression is *required* for response to paclitaxel and trastuzumab.

Trastuzumab and Docetaxel

Although preclinical data suggest that paclitaxel and trastuzumab have an additive effect *in vitro*, further drug interaction experiments with other taxanes documented synergism with the combination of trastuzumab and docetaxel (23). Accompanying the growing body of clinical data pertaining to paclitaxel and trastuzumab for HER2-expressing MBC, a large series of phase II studies assessing docetaxel and trastuzumab were conducted. The first published report utilized a docetaxel dosing regimen of 35 mg/m^2 per week with trastuzumab at 2 mg/kg per week delivered in 4-week cycles (3 weeks of treatment followed by a 1 week rest period) until the time of progression or unacceptable toxicity. An ORR of 63% was observed in 30 assessable HER2-overexpressing patients, comprised entirely of PRs. A slightly higher ORR (67%) was determined in a subset of patients (N = 24) who had HER2-amplified tumors determined retrospectively by FISH assay. The study included assays of serum levels of HER2 ectodomain, given previous data suggesting a predictive role of this moiety in the setting of antiestrogen therapy (32). Responses did, in fact, appear to be significantly higher in the group with higher levels of serum HER2 ectodomain (76% vs. 33%; $p = .04$) (33).

A second phase II study assessed a slightly different weekly schedule of docetaxel (35 mg/m^2 per week for 6 weeks, followed by 2 weeks of rest) in combination with trastuzumab administered as a loading dose (4 mg/kg loading) followed by 2 mg/kg weekly. Mirroring results from the previous study, an ORR of 50% was observed in 26 evaluable patients (with HER2 overexpression determined by both IHC and FISH), whereas a higher ORR (67%) was observed in those patients with HER2 amplified tumors determined by FISH (34). In both phase II trials, little cardiac toxicity was observed. A third phase II trial of weekly docetaxel for MBC includes an arm containing 17 HER2-overexpressing patients; the reported ORR was similar to the two previously noted trials (59%, comprised entirely of PRs) (35).

Alternative dosing of docetaxel using a 3-weekly regimen was assessed in a separate phase II trial. In this study, 42 women received docetaxel at 75 mg/m^2 every three 3 weeks for six cycles concomitant with a loading dose of trastuzumab at 4 mg/kg followed by a weekly dose at 2 mg/kg. In the intent to treat this population, ORR appeared to be comparable to weekly docetaxel with trastuzumab (67%), with a median progression-free survival (PFS) and duration of response of 9 months and 12 months, respectively (36). Supplementing these data, the largest published assessment of docetaxel and trastuzumab to date is a randomized phase II trial of 186 HER2-overexpressing patients receiving docetaxel at 100 mg/m^2 every 3 weeks, with or without weekly trastuzumab. The combination of trastuzumab and docetaxel was superior to docetaxel alone with respect to ORR (61% vs. 34%; $p = .0002$), median OS (31.2 vs. 22.7 months), and TTP (11.7 vs. 6.1 months) (Figure 75.3). In regard to toxicity, grade III to IV neutropenia and febrile neutropenia were seen more frequently with combination therapy (32% vs. 22%, and 23% vs. 17%, respectively). One patient on the combination arm incurred

symptomatic heart failure; a second patient developed symptomatic heart failure in association with disease progression 5 months after discontinuation of trastuzumab. However, this patient was receiving concurrent therapy with an investigational anthracycline (37). Thus, it appears that 3-weekly dosing of docetaxel with weekly trastuzumab is safe and efficacious. Although cardiac events related to therapy appear to be infrequent, consideration should be given to associated risks of myelosuppression when using docetaxel combinations.

Trastuzumab and Vinorelbine

Similar to docetaxel, synergy was noted with the combination of trastuzumab and vinorelbine in preclinical models (23). Several phase II trials support this experimental observation. The first published trial assessed 40 HER2-overexpressing women (classified as 2+ or 3+ by IHC), most with multiple prior therapies, who received a regimen of trastuzumab (4 mg/kg loading, followed by 2 mg/kg) in combination with weekly vinorelbine (25 mg/m^2, with dose adjustments for neutrophil counts). An impressive ORR of 75% was noted in the total population, with an even more substantial ORR in the subset of patients receiving trastuzumab and vinorelbine as first-line therapy (84%) and in the subset with HER2-overexpression characterized as 3+ by IHC (80%). As with docetaxel, hematologic toxicity was frequent, with grade III or IV adverse hematologic events recorded in 43% of patients. Notably, cardiac toxicity was only observed in a small fraction of patients who either had a lower baseline ejection fraction (between 50% and 59%) or a cumulative previous anthracycline dose greater than 240 mg/m^2 (38). A second phase II study utilized an identical regimen, with the exception of a slightly higher weekly dose of vinorelbine (30 mg/m^2). The trial included a similar number of patients (N = 40) and demonstrated comparable ORR (78%), again with a more pronounced ORR in the subset of patients with HER2-overexpression characterized as 3+ by IHC (82%). Adverse events were similar, with a preponderance of hematologic toxicities and limited cardiac toxicity (39).

Given encouraging results in heavily pretreated patients, subsequent efforts focused the combination of trastuzumab and vinorelbine for first-line therapy of MBC. In the first of several phase II reports, 54 women with HER2-overexpressing MBC received vinorelbine at a dose of 25 mg/m^2 weekly in combination with weekly trastuzumab. Of note, the study included more stringent criteria for characterization of HER2 overexpression, namely, IHC scores of 3+ or amplification demonstrated by FISH. No distinction in ORR was observed based on method of HER2 characterization and ORR was comparable to that observed in previous studies (68%). Only two patients incurred cardiac toxicity; declines in ejection fraction on echocardiogram performed at week 16 on protocol therapy were noted to predict these individuals (40). A second multinational phase II study used a nearly identical schema, with the exception of a slightly higher weekly dose of vinorelbine (30 mg/m^2) and inclusion of patients with HER2 overexpression characterized as 2+ (provided there was demonstration of HER2 amplification by FISH). Again, ORR was comparable to previous trials (62.9%), and hematologic toxicity was frequent (grade III or IV toxicity in 83% of patients) (41).

To ease patient burden associated with weekly therapy, a separate phase II trial assessed a regimen of vinorelbine (30 mg/m^2) administered on days 1 and 8 of a 3-week cycle combined with trastuzumab on day 1 (8 mg/kg loading, followed by 6 mg/kg). The ORR observed in this study was slightly lower than that observed in previous phase II studies (50%). Surprisingly, the decreased intensity of the vinorelbine regimen did not lead to substantial decreases in hematologic toxicity (grade III or IV toxicity was observed in 72% of patients) (42). Thus, it appears that the 3-weekly regimen of vinorelbine offers little advantage.

Although no phase III trials exist to specifically identify a benefit from the addition of trastuzumab to vinorelbine therapy in HER2-positive MBC, a two-arm phase II trial stratified according to HER2 status has been published. In this study of 68 women with no prior therapy for MBC, non-HER2 overexpressors received vinorelbine alone at 25 mg/m^2 weekly, whereas HER2 overexpressors received an identical dose of vinorelbine in combination with weekly trastuzumab. The ORR in patients receiving combination therapy was substantially higher than in those receiving vinorelbine alone (51.4% vs. 27.3%) (43). Although a potential explanation for these findings is an intrinsic difference in sensitivity to vinorelbine conferred by HER2 overexpression, an alternative explanation for these data is a change in the natural history of HER2-overexpressing disease (44) attributable to synergism of trastuzumab plus vinorelbine therapy.

The aforementioned phase II studies of vinorelbine in combination with trastuzumab show response data similar to previously noted combination trials with taxanes. The Trastuzumab and Vinorelbine or Taxane (TRAVIOTA) study sought to address this issue, although the effort was hampered by poor accrual. Originally planned for 250 patients, just 81 evaluable patients were ultimately enrolled who were randomized 1:1 to receive either weekly vinorelbine or weekly taxane therapy (either paclitaxel or docetaxel based on the investigator's preference) in combination with weekly trastuzumab. No significant differences were noted in response rates with vinorelbine- or taxane-based combination therapy (51% and 40%, respectively; $p = .37$). In general, toxicities incurred with vinorelbine and taxane therapy were similar to that noted in previous studies. Of note, two patients were removed from the study for cardiac toxicity, both from the vinorelbine arm. However, the small sample size makes it impossible to draw significant conclusions regarding the relative efficacy or the relative toxicity of the agents tested (45).

Trastuzumab and Capecitabine

In recent years, capecitabine (an orally administered prodrug of fluorouracil) (46) has emerged as an effective agent for the treatment of MBC (47,48). The ease of administration of this drug prompted interest in combination trials utilizing a regimen of capecitabine and trastuzumab. Three phase II clinical trials of this combination have been recently published. The first assessed a heavily pretreated population of patients with HER2-overexpressing MBC. A total of 27 patients received capecitabine dosed at 1,250 mg/m^2 twice daily for 14 days followed by a 7-day rest period. Trastuzumab was administered with a 4 mg/kg loading dose, followed by 2 mg/kg weekly. The ORR observed in this trial (45%) was relatively low as compared to combination trials including vinorelbine or taxane therapy, although rates of grade III and IV toxicity were substantially lower (49). A second phase II study used a similar capecitabine regimen in combination with 3-weekly trastuzumab The ORR in this heavily pretreated population was low (20%) (50). It is interesting to speculate whether or not these data set mirror expectations derived from preclinical studies, in which the combination of vinorelbine or taxane with trastuzumab showed synergy, whereas the combination of fluorouracil with trastuzumab showed antagonism.

A third data set from a phase II trial in Japan shows more encouraging results, particularly when capecitabine and trastuzumab are used in the first-line setting for MBC. In this study, patients received capecitabine at a dose of 1,657 mg/m^2 on days 1 through 21 of a 28-day cycle, in combination with weekly trastuzumab. The ORR observed in this trial was 50%, however, the subset of patients treated with capecitabine and trastuzumab as first-line therapy for MBC had a higher (65%) ORR (51). These results are notable inasmuch as the dosing regimen employed for capecitabine is substantially lower than the FDA-approved dose.

Trastuzumab and Cisplatin

The first experiments exploring synergy of HER2-receptor antibodies with conventional chemotherapy used an *in vitro* model of HER2-overexpressing cancer cells treated with cisplatin. Preincubation with anti-HER2 antibody specifically in HER2-overexpressing cells led to impairment of DNA repair mechanisms, and a resulting accumulation of platinum/DNA adducts that triggered an apoptotic response. This phenomena was termed *receptor-enhanced chemosensitivity* (12), and subsequent experiments using the combination of trastuzumab and cisplatin in HER2-positive human breast tumor xenograft models demonstrated a similar effect (15). Moreover, evaluation by multiple drug effect/combination index isobologram analysis revealed synergy in HER2-overexpressing cell line models (25).

Consequently, a multicenter phase II clinical trial was conducted to evaluate the efficacy of the combination of cisplatin and trastuzumab. In a heavily pretreated population of patients with HER2-overexpressing MBC, 39 patients were treated with a 250 mg loading dose of trastuzumab followed by 100 mg of trastuzumab weekly for 9 weeks, accompanied by cisplatin at 75 mg/m^2 on days 1, 29, and 57. An ORR of 24% was observed in 37 evaluable patients. Approximately 56% of patients enrolled experienced grade III or IV toxicity (comprised primarily of nausea, asthenia, and hematologic toxicity), and only one patient incurred cardiotoxicity (of note, this patient had received a cumulative anthracycline dose of 420 mg/m^2 prior to enrollment) (52). Beyond this initial data set, further exploration of platinum-based therapy for HER2-overexpressing MBC has focused on three-drug regimens incorporating carboplatin and trastuzumab (based on the previously observed preclinical synergy) (23).

Three-Drug Regimens Incorporating Trastuzumab

The design of clinical trials utilizing three-drug regimens including trastuzumab were based on multiple synergistic interactions noted with two distinct regimens: (a) paclitaxel, cisplatin, and trastuzumab, and (b) docetaxel, carboplatin, and trastuzumab (23,53). The combination of platinum, taxane, and trastuzumab was subsequently assessed in a series of clinical trials. With respect to paclitaxel, a multicenter phase II trial was conducted evaluating two distinct schedules of paclitaxel and carboplatin with trastuzumab in HER2-overexpressing patients. In the first regimen, paclitaxel at (200 mg/m^2) and carboplatin (with an area under the curve [AUC] of 6 mg/mL) was administered with trastuzumab (8 mg/kg loading followed by 6 mg/kg maintenance) every 3 weeks for eight cycles. The second regimen was comprised of paclitaxel (at 80 mg/m^2) and carboplatin (with an AUC of 2 mg/mL) administered with trastuzumab (4 mg/kg loading followed by 2 mg/kg maintenance) weekly for 3 weeks in a 4-week cycle, for a total of six cycles. The ORR was superior with weekly treatment (81% vs. 65%), as was median OS (3.2 vs. 2.3 years). Interestingly, this result was coupled with decreased overall toxicity in the arm receiving weekly therapy (54).

These encouraging results prompted assessment of a similar regimen in a phase III trial. In this study, 196 women with HER2-overexpressing MBC were randomized to receive paclitaxel (at 175 mg/m^2 every 3 weeks) and weekly trastuzumab (4 mg/kg loading followed by 2 mg/kg weekly maintenance) alone, or in combination with carboplatin (with an AUC of 6 mg/mL·min, administered every 3 weeks). Notably, the trial incorporated a 3-weekly regimen of carboplatin, paclitaxel, and trastuzumab that appeared to be inferior to a weekly regimen based on the aforementioned phase II data. Nonetheless, the three-drug regimen was found to be superior to paclitaxel plus trastuzumab in comparison of ORR (57% vs. 36%; $p = .03$) and median PFS (13.8 vs. 7.6 months; $p = .005$). Although both regimens were well tolerated, a significant increase in the incidence of febrile neutropenia was observed with the addition of carboplatin ($p < .01$). Cardiomyopathy developed in only two patients; both were enrolled on the paclitaxel and trastuzumab alone arm and were alive at most recent follow-up (55). Thus, the addition of carboplatin to paclitaxel and trastuzumab appears well tolerated and is associated with superior efficacy.

A phase II study utilizing a regimen of docetaxel, carboplatin, and trastuzumab was conducted by the University of California, Los Angeles Oncology Research Network (UCLA-ORN). In this study, 62 patients with HER2-overexpressing MBC were treated with a median of six cycles of docetaxel at 75 mg/m^2 and carboplatin at an AUC of 6 mg/mL every 3 weeks, concurrently with trastuzumab (with a 4 mg/kg loading dose, followed by 2 mg/kg weekly until the time of disease progression). The ORR in the UCLA-ORN study was 58%, with a median TTP of 12.7 months. Subset analysis showed a more pronounced response in patients with HER2 amplification documented by FISH. Of note, a companion study, Breast Cancer International Research Group (BCIRG) 101, assessed a similar docetaxel-based regimen, substituting cisplatin at 75 mg/m^2 for carboplatin. Comparable results were observed in this trial, with an ORR of 79% and median TTP of 9.9 months (56).

Data from these parallel phase II trials led to the design and completion of a phase III trial utilizing a docetaxel-carboplatin–based regimen in the experimental arm. This trial (BCIRG 007) included 263 patients with HER2 amplification by FISH assay who were randomized to receive either docetaxel and trastuzumab alone or in combination with carboplatin. In the docetaxel and trastuzumab alone arm, docetaxel was administered at a dose of 100 mg/m^2 every 3 weeks in combination with trastuzumab (given weekly at 2 mg/kg following an initial loading dose of 4 mg/kg). In the arm receiving carboplatin, a lower dose of docetaxel (75 mg/m^2) was administered with carboplatin at an AUC of 6 mg/mL every 3 weeks, along with trastuzumab on an identical weekly schedule. A first efficacy analysis after 204 events suggested no significant difference with the addition of carboplatin in ORR (73% in both arms) or median TTP (10.4 months with carboplatin vs. 11.1 months without; $p = .57$). Significant cardiac toxicity was not encountered with either regimen, and the most frequent grade III and IV toxicities encountered on both therapeutic arms included neutropenic infection, asthenia, thrombocytopenia, anemia, and diarrhea. At a median follow-up duration of 39 months, median OS was not significantly different (36 months) with either therapy (22) (Fig. 75.3). Thus, either docetaxel (100 mg/m^2) and trastuzumab or docetaxel (75 mg/m^2) with carboplatin represents highly efficacious regimens, both of which support preclinical hypotheses of synergism with trastuzumab (23).

Additional three-drug regimens incorporating trastuzumab have been devised, in particular regimens based on gemcitabine and trastuzumab combinations (23). In a heavily pretreated population of HER2-overexpressing patients, an ORR of 19.2% was observed in 26 patients treated with gemcitabine at a dose of 1,250 mg/m^2 on days 1 and 8 of a 3-week cycle along with trastuzumab on day 1 (57). Interestingly, phase II trials that assessed the addition of paclitaxel to this regimen produced much more encouraging data. One such trial including HER2-overexpressing MBC patients previously untreated for metastatic disease utilized a regimen of gemcitabine at 1,200 mg/m^2 on days 1 and 8 with paclitaxel at 175 mg/m^2 on day 1, combined with weekly trastuzumab. In 42 evaluable patients,

an ORR of 67% was achieved, with median OS estimated at approximately 27 months (58). Building on the synergy data for trastuzumab with cisplatin, a separate study assessed a regimen of gemcitabine at 750 mg/m^2 and cisplatin at 30 mg/m^2 on days 1 and 8 of a 21-day cycle in combination with weekly trastuzumab. The study enrolled 20 anthracycline- and taxane-pretreated patients with HER2-overexpressing MBC, and with a median of six cycles of therapy, an ORR of 40% was observed (59). In the setting of an anthracycline and taxane pretreated population, these data are encouraging (28,29,52).

Trastuzumab and Pegylated Liposomal Doxorubicin

In addition to traditional cytotoxic chemotherapy, numerous efforts have been made to combine novel therapeutics with trastuzumab to enhance efficacy. Studies of pegylated liposomal doxorubicin (PLD) represents one such effort. PLD was developed in an effort to curtail cardiac toxicities incurred with standard doxorubicin therapy. In a phase III trial of MBC patients randomized to receive either PLD or doxorubicin, similar OS was observed in both treatment arms, but the risk of cardiotoxicity was significantly higher with doxorubicin as compared to PLD (60). Thus theoretically, the combination of PLD and trastuzumab could yield efficacy comparable to that observed with trastuzumab and doxorubicin, while avoiding the associated risk of cardiac adverse events (4). A published phase II trial examined precisely this regimen, evaluating HER2-overexpressing women with MBC receiving PLD at a dose of 50 mg/m^2 every 4 weeks for six cycles in combination with weekly trastuzumab. The ORR was 52%, with a median PFS of 12.0 months (median OS had not been reached at the time of publication). In this trial, only three patients developed protocol-specified cardiotoxicity based on an absolute decline in ejection fraction greater than or equal to 15%. Of note, each of the three patients had received prior anthracycline therapy. Thus, the regimen of PLD and trastuzumab may warrant further exploration (61). Preclinical experiments do suggest an additive interaction between trastuzumab and anthracyclines (23).

Combinations of HER2-Targeting Agents with Endocrine Therapy

Preclinical studies suggest substantial crosstalk between pathways related to HER2 and hormone receptors. Overexpression of HER2 was demonstrated to cause ligand-independent down-regulation of estrogen receptor (ER) and, further, suppression of ER transcripts (62). Given this association, it is plausible that inhibition of HER2 activity may augment endocrine therapy by enhancing ER expression. As clinical validation of this hypothesis, the recently reported phase III TAnDEM study randomized HER2-overexpressing, hormone receptor–positive postmenopausal MBC patients to anastrazole alone or the combination of anastrazole and trastuzumab. At the time of progression, patients were given the option to continue on trastuzumab therapy if they were previously randomized to the monotherapy arm. Despite this crossover allowance, a moderate (although statistically insignificant) benefit in OS was yielded from combination therapy (28.5 vs. 23.9 months; $p = .325$). Interestingly, in a *post hoc* exploratory analysis assessing the effects of crossover, median OS was significantly less in the group that received no trastuzumab therapy (i.e., anastrazole alone with no crossover; median OS, 17.2 months) versus survival in groups receiving anastrazole and trastuzumab initially (median OS, 28.5 months) or at the time of crossover (median OS, 25.1 months) (63). Direct HER2-tyrosine kinase inhibition in combination with endocrine therapy is also currently being investigated; a phase I trial using the combination

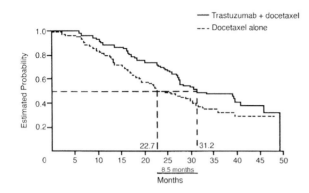

FIGURE 75.3. Kaplan-Meier estimates of overall survival according to whether patients were assigned to docetaxel and trastuzumab or docetaxel alone in M77001.

of lapatinib and letrozole suggested that the combination was safe and tolerable. In 34 patients assessed, PRs were observed in 6 individuals, 4 of whom had MBC (62).

Trastuzumab and EGFR Tyrosine Kinase Inhibitors

Whereas trastuzumab binds the extracellular domain of the HER2 moiety (8), a unique class of agents interacts with the intracellular domain of ERBB family proteins. Lapatinib, a dual inhibitor of EGFR and HER2 tyrosine kinase domains, is discussed later in this chapter (64). Gefitinib and erlotinib, two inhibitors with affinity for the EGFR tyrosine kinase domain, have demonstrable efficacy in non–small cell lung cancer (65,66). Response data for these agents in MBC, however, have been poor. In a pilot study of 22 patients with refractory MBC treated with erlotinib, no clinical responses were observed (67). Limited single-agent data exist for gefitinib in the setting of MBC; two trials report activity of the drug in combination with docetaxel, but it is challenging to determine response attributable to the EGFR antagonist (68,69). In the setting of HER2-overexpressing MBC, Eastern Cooperative Oncology Group (ECOG) study 1100 assessed a regimen of daily oral gefitinib combined with weekly trastuzumab, utilizing a phase I or II design. During a planned interim analysis, TTP parameters did not meet prespecified statistical end points for study continuation (70). More encouraging data were obtained from a phase I trial of erlotinib in combination with trastuzumab, spurned by preclinical data suggesting synergy between the agents in breast cancer cell lines (71). Among 14 evaluable patients with heavily pretreated HER2-overexpressing MBC, two partial responses were elicited, prompting initiation of an ongoing phase II study (72).

Trastuzumab and Bevacizumab

Recent studies have suggested the utility of antiangiogenic therapy in breast cancer. Specifically, a phase III trial randomizing patients to paclitaxel alone or in combination with bevacizumab (a monoclonal antibody directed at vascular endothelial growth factor [VEGF]) was recently reported. A total of 722 patients were enrolled in this study, and although no significant difference was observed in OS, a significantly prolonged PFS was observed with bevacizumab and paclitaxel as compared to paclitaxel alone (11.8 vs. 5.9 months; $p < .001$). An increased

frequency of objective responses were also seen with combination therapy (36.9% vs. 21.2%; $p < .001$) (73).

Although this study was performed in an unselected population, significant interest has been generated by translational research linking expression of the pro-angiogenic VEGF to HER2 expression. In an analysis of primary breast tumor lysates from 611 unselected patients, six VEGF isoforms were quantitated by enzyme-linked immunosorbent assay (ELISA) as was HER2 protein quantified by the same methodology. Overexpression of HER2 was shown to correlate with up-regulation of VEGF in human breast cancer specimens. In reviewing clinical data associated with these specimens, it became apparent that increasing VEGF was also associated with an aggressive clinical phenotype, especially among patients with increased HER2 expression (74).

These clinical and translational experiments served as the rational for the design of subsequent experiments combining antagonists to both VEGF and the HER2 receptor. An optimal dosing regimen for the combination of bevacizumab and trastuzumab was established in a phase I dose-escalation clinical trial. Based on the phase I pharmacokinetic and safety data, a phase II trial was subsequently conducted, representing the first phase II trial of two humanized monoclonal antibodies in combination given to human subjects. At an interim analysis with 37 patients enrolled, 1 CR and 19 PRs were noted, reflecting an ORR of 54.1%. However, in a stringent cardiac safety analysis, 13 cardiac adverse events were noted in this cohort, one of which was symptomatic (75).

The success encountered thus far with the combination of trastuzumab and bevacizumab has led to the design of further phase III trials in the metastatic and adjuvant settings. The BETH trial is a joint effort of the Cancer International Research Group (CIRG) and the National Surgical Adjuvant Breast and Bowel Project (NSABP) and will randomize HER2-overexpressing patients to receive six cycles of adjuvant docetaxel, carboplatin, and trastuzumab, with or without bevacizumab, with trastuzumab and bevacizumab continuing for a total of 1 year. Enrollment of approximately 3,000 patients is planned. The ECOG is currently conducting a randomized phase III trial of paclitaxel, carboplatin, and trastuzumab with or without bevacizumab as first-line treatment for HER2-positive MBC. Both of these phase III trastuzumab combined with bevacizumab study designs include early stopping rules for cardiac toxicity in the event that there are excess cardiac adverse events associated with this novel combination.

Sunitinib

The tyrosine kinase inhibitor sunitinib has been demonstrated in *in vitro* studies to antagonize the VEGF receptor, platelet-derived growth factor receptor (PDGFR), stem cell factor receptor (KIT), and colony-stimulating factor-1 receptor (76–78). The clinical efficacy of sunitinib has been established in several tumor types, most notably renal cell carcinoma (79). The use of sunitinib in breast cancer represents an intensive area of investigation, particularly with respect to HER2-overexpressing tumors. As previously described, HER2-overexpressing tumors appear to have increases in VEGF expression that are significantly associated with HER2 expression, and levels of HER2 and VEGF correlate with clinical outcome (74).

A multicenter, phase II study assessed the activity of sunitinib in MBC patients who had previously received anthracycline and taxane therapy. Using a dose scheme established from phase I studies in advanced solid tumors (specifically, 50 mg orally daily for 4 weeks followed by 2 weeks rest in repeated 6-week cycles), a total of 64 patients were treated with at least one dose of sunitinib. Most toxicities incurred were mild to moderate, and an ORR of 11% was observed, with seven PRs. With respect to the HER2-overexpressing subset of patients, the observed RR was higher (25%). Response data from this subset has prompted formulation of two trials specific to the HER2-overexpressing population. A phase II trial of daily sunitinib with weekly or 3-weekly trastuzumab in HER2-over-expressing MBC patients who have received one or fewer prior therapies for MBC is currently accruing. In parallel, a phase I trial is currently being conducted to explore the combination of trastuzumab, docetaxel, and sunitinib as first-line therapy for HER2-positive MBC (80).

Continuation of Trastuzumab Beyond Initial Progression

A majority of the aforementioned trials utilizing trastuzumab-based regimens mandate the continuation of trastuzumab therapy until the time of disease progression. Beyond the time of progression, the role of further trastuzumab-based regimens is unclear. Before the availability of salvage HER2-targeted therapy with lapatinib (discussed later), a frequently employed strategy was the continuation of trastuzumab beyond the initial time of disease progression. Use of this approach was addressed in an extension of the pivotal phase III trial of trastuzumab in combination with chemotherapy. A total of 247 patients with documented disease progression were enrolled in the extension study. Of these, 154 patients had originally received chemotherapy (group 1) and 93 had received chemotherapy and trastuzumab (group 2). The majority of patients enrolled in the extension trial received a combination of chemotherapy and trastuzumab, with the remainder receiving either trastuzumab alone or a combination of trastuzumab and palliative radiotherapy or hormonal therapy. The most commonly used chemotherapeutic agents used in the extension trial in combination with trastuzumab were paclitaxel, vinorelbine, docetaxel, and flu-orouracil, although 8% of patients received concomitant doxorubicin. Although efficacy information from the trial was limited (safety was the primary objective), 14% of patients in group 1 and 11% of patients in group 2 experienced an objective response. These responses were observed both when trastuzumab was combined with chemotherapy and when single-agent trastuzumab therapy was employed. The incidence of cardiac toxicity was relatively low, occurring in 9% of patients in group 1 and only 2% of patients in group 2 (81). A relatively small retrospective review of the Hellenic Cooperative Oncology Group (HCOG) experience offers a similar suggestion, implying a significant number of responses with second- and third-line therapy with trastuzumab leading to substantial improvements in median survival (82).

Despite these encouraging results, a separate retrospective review offers contrasting results. In a series of 184 HER2-over-expressing MBC patients who had received trastuzumab therapy over a 5-year period, relevant clinical end points such as time to second progression (TT-SP) and postprogression survival (PPS) were assessed. Among 132 patients who had progressed on trastuzumab-based therapy at the time of analysis, 21 patients experienced rapid progression and did not receive additional therapy, 40 patients received further trastuzumab-based regimens, and 71 patients received further non-trastuzumab-based regimens. In the latter two groups, there did not appear to be significant difference in TT-SP, PPS, ORR, or OS (83). Although these data are complicated by issues related to retrospective methodology, further trials may be necessary to clarify the role of trastuzumab therapy beyond the time of initial progression.

Further evidence in support of continuation of trastuzumab beyond the time of disease progression comes from a recently presented trial conducted in a population of patients with advanced, HER2-overexpressing breast cancer that had progressed during or after treatment with trastuzumab. Patients were randomized to receive either capecitabine (at 2,500 mg/m^2 on days 1 through 14 every 3 weeks) alone or in combination with trastuzumab (at 6 mg/kg every 3 weeks). Although the trial was closed prematurely secondary to slow accrual, a preplanned interim analysis of 112 patients suggested a moderate benefit in TTP with combination therapy (33 vs. 24 weeks; $p = .178$). No significant differences in serious adverse events were observed between the two arms, with the majority of the events surprisingly occurring in the capecitabine monotherapy arm (84).

Mechanisms of Trastuzumab Resistance

In the pivotal phase III trial comparing the combination of cytotoxic chemotherapy to trastuzumab alone, an impressive ORR of 50% was achieved with combined therapy, substantially improved relative to previous trials of monotherapy with trastuzumab. However, the median duration of response on this therapeutic arm was only 9.1 months (4). In response to these data, a significant body of evidence has focused on mechanisms of trastuzumab resistance. Several studies have implicated the role of loss of phosphatase and tensin homolog (PTEN) in trastuzumab resistance. Reduction of PTEN, a dual phosphatase negatively regulating PI3K and Akt activities, through antisense oligonucleotides led to trastuzumab resistance in *in vitro* and *in vivo* models. Additionally, IHC analyses of clinical specimens demonstrated that PTEN-deficient breast tumors had poorer responses to trastuzumab-based therapy relative to tumors with normal PTEN expression (85). As a potential therapeutic approach in patients with PTEN loss, it appears that inhibition of the PI3K-Akt pathway (e.g., through use of mammalian target of rapamycin [mTOR] inhibitors) may lead to restoration of trastuzumab sensitivity in preclinical assays (86).

Alternatively, aberrant signaling through the insulin-like growth factor-I receptor (IGF-IR) pathway, leading to PI3K-Akt pathway activation, may mediate trastuzumab resistance. An assay of MCF-7 and SKBR-3 breast cancer cell lines revealed that treatment with IGF-I (and subsequent activation of IGF-IR) led to a diminution in trastuzumab-induced cell growth inhibition (87). This is supported a separate preclinical study of IGF-IR inhibition in combination with trastuzumab therapy in MCF-7 cells, showing a synergistic interaction using dual receptor inhibition (88). Similar to IGF-IR overexpression, overexpression of the Met receptor may serve to decrease trastuzumab sensitivity by offering a "bypass mechanism" for cell growth and proliferation. A recently published report suggested that Met knockdown in breast cancer cell lines using RNA interference significantly enhanced trastuzumab sensitivity. Conversely, coactivation of Met and HER2 through use of the ligands hepatocyte growth factor (HGF) and neuregulin, respectively, led to substantial increases in cell growth (89).

Other purported mechanisms of trastuzumab resistance include limitations in drug distribution secondary to the size of the antibody. Fluorescently tagged trastuzumab injected in mice bearing MDA-MB 435 breast cancer xenografts displayed antibody accumulation in the periphery of tumors. Notably, this was not correlated with increased HER2 expression in peripheral regions. Additionally, vascular distribution of trastuzumab was highly irregular, and distribution of trastuzumab did not correlate with vascular density, as one would expect with unhindered trastuzumab transport (90). Approaches to HER2-overexpressing patients using small molecule inhibitors may circumvent such issues with drug delivery. In the next section, lapatinib therapy is addressed. Interestingly, preclinical studies

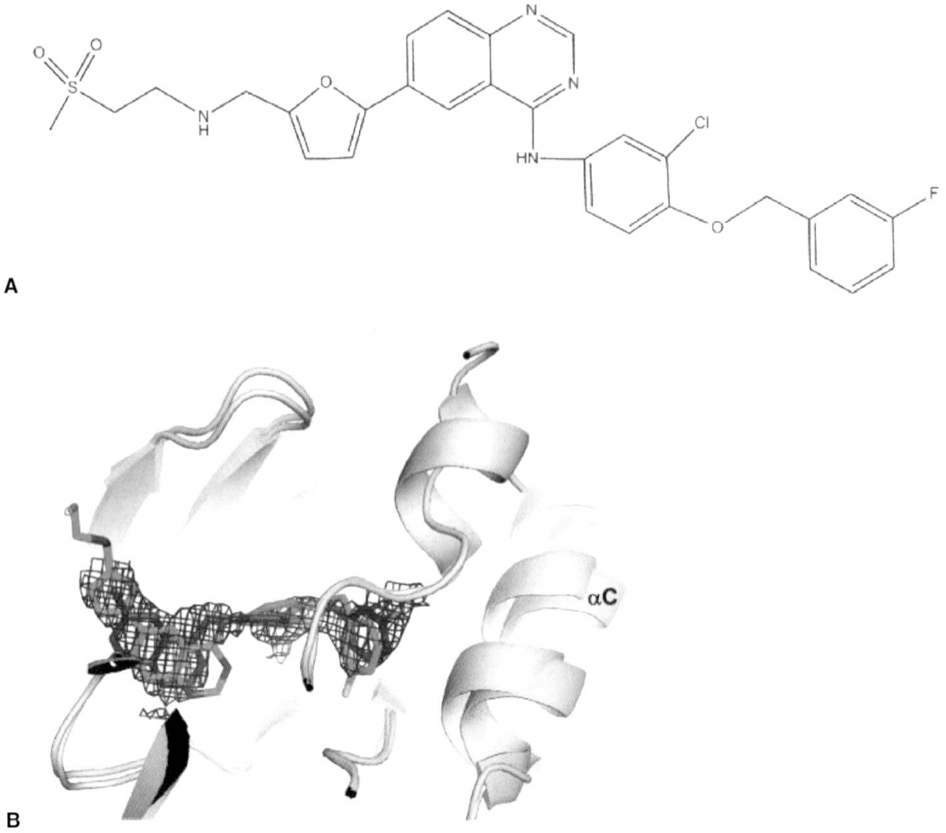

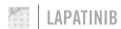

A

B

FIGURE 75.4. A: Chemical structure of lapatinib. **B:** Stick model of lapatinib (*red*). The structure of the EGFR kinase-lapatinib complex is superimposed with the EGFR kinase colored pale cyan and lapatinib green.

seem to indicate lapatinib has significant activity in trastuzumab refractory cell lines (91), supporting clinical observations in subsequent randomized trials (92).

LAPATINIB

Lapatinib Monotherapy

In contrast to trastuzumab, which binds an epitope located in the extracellular domain of the HER2 moiety (8), the orally active dual tyrosine kinase inhibitor lapatinib binds reversibly to the intracellular kinase domain of both HER2 and EGFR (93) (Fig. 75.4). Growth inhibition was observed with lapatinib therapy in HER2-overexpressing BT-474 breast cancer cell lines. Xenografts derived from BT-474 cell lines were similarly inhibited by lapatinib treatment (94). A separate analysis of HER2-overexpressing cell lines suggested marked reductions in tyrosine phosphorylation of EGFR and HER2 following exposure to lapatinib. Additionally, lapatinib led to inhibition of Erk1/2 and AKT, downstream effectors of cell proliferation and survival, respectively (95). In a phase I study, 67 patients with EGFR- or HER2-overexpressing tumors were randomly assigned to one of five dose cohorts of daily lapatinib therapy. A total of four PRs occurred among 57 evaluable patients; all were in patients with trastuzumab-refractory MBC. Stable disease occurred in a total of 24 patients, 10 of whom were patients with MBC. The most commonly observed adverse events were diarrhea and rash, the former in a dose-dependent fashion (64).

A correlative study accompanying the aforementioned phase I clinical trial of lapatinib monotherapy in solid tumor malignancies focused attention on the four patients attaining PR in the clinical trial. Analysis of serial biopsies performed in each of these patients suggested that each had elevated baseline levels of active, phosphorylated HER2 (determined by IHC). With lapatinib therapy, a decrease in the extent of HER2 phosphorylation was observed. In three of the four responders, inhibition of activated phospho-Akt and phosphor-Erk1/2 was noted, concordant with preclinical studies, suggesting these moieties were inhibited by lapatinib. In contrast to assessment of phosphorylated HER2, level of EGFR phosphorylation at baseline did not seem to distinguish responders from nonresponders. Notably, however, decrements in EGFR phosphorylation were seen in responding patients (96).

Encouraging data from this phase I trial within the subset of patients with MBC led to the implementation of a phase II clinical trial including both HER2-overexpressing and non-HER2-overexpressing MBC. In 140 patients with HER2-overexpressing disease, an ORR of 4.3% was determined by investigator assessment. All responders were noted to have overexpression of HER2 characterized as 3+ by IHC; five of six responders additionally had FISH amplification. No tumor responses occurred among 89 non-HER2-overexpressing MBC patients. As in the phase I monotherapy study, diarrhea and rash were the most commonly observed toxicities (97).

Lapatinib and Capecitabine

Given the limited data to support the clinical utility of lapatinib monotherapy, further efforts have focused on combinations of lapatinib with standard chemotherapeutics. In a series of preclinical experiments, four cancer cell lines with a range of HER2 and EGFR expression (MCF7/wt, BT-474, SKBR-3, and A-431) were exposed to varying concentrations and combinations of lapatinib, trastuzumab, epirubicin, gemcitabine, and 5-fluorouracil. Independent of HER2 and EGFR expression, lapatinib was noted to have synergy with 5-fluorouracil (98). This observation served as the rationale for a phase I trial of lapatinib and capecitabine in advanced solid tumors. Although only 7 of 45 patients enrolled (16%) carried a diagnosis of MBC, one CR and three confirmed PRs occurred; the CR occurred in a patient with MBC treated with lapatinib at 1,250 mg per day and capecitabine at 2,000 mg/m^2 per day, representing the optimally tolerated regimen. The most common toxicities incurred with this regimen were diarrhea, rash, nausea, palmar-plantar erythrodysesthesia, mucositis, vomiting, and stomatitis (99).

The observed activity of the combination of lapatinib and capecitabine in MBC led to the initiation of a randomized phase III trial. In this study, HER2-overexpressing patients with MBC who had progressed after regimens, including an anthracycline, a taxane, and trastuzumab, received either capecitabine alone (2,500 mg/m^2 per day on days 1 through 14 of a 21-day cycle) or in combination with lapatinib (with the optimal treatment regimen defined from the previous phase I trial). An interim analysis met prespecified criteria for early reporting given superiority of the group receiving combination therapy. At the time of this analysis, 49 events had occurred in the combination group as opposed to 72 events in the monotherapy group (hazard ratio [HR] 0.49; p <.001). Median TTP was prolonged from 4.4 months with monotherapy to 8.4 months with combination therapy (Fig. 75.5). The ORR was higher with combination therapy (22%) as compared to monotherapy (14%), although this was marginally significant (p = .09). In contrast to trastuzumab-containing regimens, no symptomatic cardiac events were observed with lapatinib therapy (92). In a recently published update of the trial, including attempts to correlate a response with various biomarkers, lapatinib response failed to correlate with baseline levels of soluble HER2 extracellular domain or EGFR amplification (100). Nonetheless, given its favorable safety profile in combination with the observed efficacy in combination with capecitabine, further trials of lapatinib therapy in HER2-overexpressing breast cancer are under way.

Lapatinib and Taxanes

Lapatinib exhibits a chemosensitizing effect when used in combination with paclitaxel in a model of resistant EGFR-overexpressing ovarian cancer cell lines (101). Similar preclinical observations led to the initiation of multiple clinical trials investigating the combination of lapatinib and paclitaxel. Although data from most of these trials are immature, an early safety analysis combining data from several of these clinical studies was recently reported. In 192 patients receiving either docetaxel or paclitaxel in combination with lapatinib, the rates of neutropenia and rash were similar to each agent alone, although the frequency of diarrhea was more pronounced. Although the analysis was centered on safety, a preliminary report from one trial that was assessed suggested a response rate of greater than 70% with the combination of lapatinib and paclitaxel (102).

Data from one placebo-controlled randomized trial combining lapatinib and paclitaxel have been reported thus far. Interestingly, this trial evaluates a population of patients with stage IIIb, IIIc, or IV at first diagnosis or relapse with either negative HER2 testing (0/1+ by IHC analysis, or no FISH amplification) or no prior testing. Central analysis of HER2 expression was performed in all available cases (representing 78% of test population). A total of 579 patients were randomized 1:1 to receive either lapatinib at a dose of 1,500 mg daily with paclitaxel at 175 mg/m^2 every 3 weeks, or placebo and paclitaxel on the same schedule. From the study population, HER2 overexpression was elicited in 17% of patients enrolled in the study. Within this small subset of patients, a trend toward benefit from lapatinib therapy was observed with respect to median OS (24 months with lapatinib vs. 19 months with placebo; p = .16). As anticipated, no such difference was observed in the larger subset of patients with normal HER2 expression (103). Although only a relatively small cohort of patients with HER2 overexpression was considered, these data are encouraging and support the implementation of further clinical trials in a selected population.

Novel Therapies for Breast Cancer in Combination with Lapatinib

As noted previously, PLD offers substantial advantages to therapy with doxorubicin, with similar clinical efficacy in the setting of MBC but significantly reduced cardiac toxicity (60). Although phase II data suggest the potential efficacy of trastuzumab in combination with PLD (61), trials are currently being undertaken to assess the safety and tolerability of combination therapy with lapatinib. In a phase I dose-escalation trial, patients were treated with one of four doses of PLD (20, 30, 45, or 60 mg/m^2) in combination with daily lapatinib. Among four evaluable patients, one PR has been observed thus far. The combination appears to be well tolerated; one patient had a significant decline in cardiac ejection fraction, but this was thought to be secondary to progressive disease (104). Although the data at present are immature, the regimen appears to hold promise, especially given preclinical studies supporting the combination of anthracycline and lapatinib (98).

Dual Targeting of the HER2 Receptor: Lapatinib and Trastuzumab

The rationale for dual inhibition of the HER2 receptor with monoclonal antibody and tyrosine kinase inhibitor treatment emerges from preclinical experiments assessing this combination in HER2-overexpressing BT-474 breast cancer cell lines. Treatment of BT-474 cell lines with lapatinib led to only a minimal increase in tumor cell apoptosis, with an associated minimal decrease in phosphorylated HER2, Akt, Erk1/2, and, most notably, survivin (a member of the inhibitor of apoptosis family of proteins). Similarly, treatment with trastuzumab had little effect on apoptosis or survivin concentration. However, the combination of lapatinib and trastuzumab led to markedly enhanced tumor cell apoptosis and down-regulation of survivin (105). In a separate series of experiments examining a broad panel of breast cancer cell lines (including cells maintained in trastuzumab-conditioned media), synergy with concomitant trastuzumab and lapatinib treatment was observed in four cell lines (106).

Although clinical data assessing the combination are limited, preliminary data from a phase I trial are available. This open label trial uses a two-stage design, with the initial stage comprised of lapatinib dose escalation to establish the

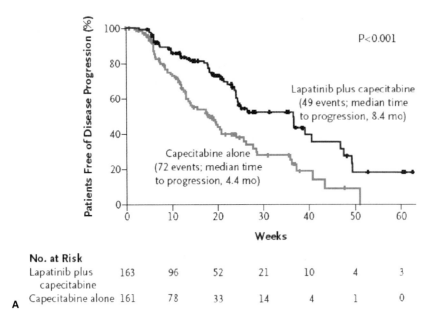

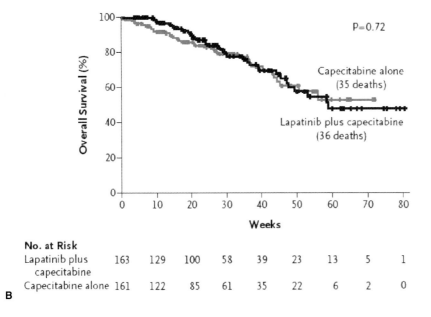

FIGURE 75.5. Kaplan-Meier estimates of disease-free progression **(A)** and overall survival **(B)** according to whether patients were assigned to capecitabine alone or in combination with lapatinib.

optimally tolerated dose. The second stage includes patients in an expansion cohort in which pharmacokinetic parameters are assessed. A total of 48 patients with HER2-overexpressing MBC were treated; among 27 evaluable patients, one CR and seven PRs were observed, all in trastuzumab-pretreated subjects. A lapatinib dose of 1,000 mg daily was identified as the optimally tolerated regimen for further trials in combination with trastuzumab (107). A subsequent report focused on cardiac safety suggested that the combination of trastuzumab and lapatinib results in no symptomatic cardiac events in a total of 238 patients registered in four separate trials (108).

Encouraging safety and efficacy data from the aforementioned trials in MBC prompted formulation of the Adjuvant Lapatinib and/or Trastuzumab Treatment Optimization (ALTTO)

trial. In this trial, patients are randomized to one of four arms after completion of standard adjuvant therapy:

1. Trastuzumab alone every 3 weeks for 52 weeks,
2. Lapatinib daily for 52 weeks,
3. Trastuzumab weekly for 12 weeks followed by a 6-week rest period, and then lapatinib daily for 34 weeks, or
4. Lapatinib daily and trastuzumab every 3 weeks for a total of 52 weeks.

Representing a collaboration of the Breast International Group (BIG) and the North Central Cancer Treatment Group (NCCTG), the ALTTO trial will be conducted at an estimated 1,300 sites in approximately 50 countries. Target accrual for the trial is approximately 8,000 patients (80).

CENTRAL NERVOUS SYSTEM METASTASES: THE ROLE OF HER2 AND TARGETED THERAPY

In data obtained from a large institutional review, it appears that the incidence of central nervous system (CNS) metastases in breast cancer varies with stage at diagnosis. Only 2.5% of patients with localized disease at initial presentation ultimately developed CNS metastases, in contrast to 13.4% of patients who had metastatic disease at the time of presentation (109). A separate review of an autopsy series including 144 patients carrying a diagnosis of breast cancer suggested an incidence of CNS metastases of 26%, contrasting with the previous estimate and suggesting a high frequency of clinically occult disease (110). Subsequent to the introduction of trastuzumab therapy, several retrospective reviews of patients receiving trastuzumab suggested an incidence of CNS disease in the range of 25% to 48%, substantially higher than the historically reported incidence (111–113). This increase in CNS metastases in HER2-overexpressing populations is supported by preclinical rationale. A subclone of the MDA-MB 231 breast cancer cell line, 231-BR, was generated with a property of selective metastasis to the brain. When this subclone was transfected with varying levels of HER2, the level of HER2 incorporated seemed to correlate with the size and extent of brain metastases after implantation in a mouse model (114).

Given discordance in the incidence CNS metastases in trastuzumab recipients and nonrecipients, concern may arise for the possibility of trastuzumab possibly enhancing the rate of CNS events. This was addressed by a retrospective review of NSABP-31, a large, randomized trial in which HER2-overexpressing patients received adjuvant chemotherapy alone or chemotherapy followed by 1 year of trastuzumab. In reviewing data among patients with distant recurrence, 28 CNS recurrences occurred in the arm receiving trastuzumab, whereas 35 occurred in the control arm ($p = .35$) (115). Thus, it does not appear that trastuzumab increases the risk of CNS relapse. Rather, although trastuzumab serves to reduce the overall clinical outcome of recipients (including those with CNS metastases) (116), the CNS may serve as a sanctuary site for trastuzumab therapy. Supporting this hypothesis, a recent study assessed six HER2-overexpressing MBC patients with CNS metastases who received whole brain radiation therapy (WBRT) after trastuzumab. The ratio of trastuzumab concentration in serum as compared to CSF was 420:1 prior to WBRT. Of note, this ratio declined substantially after WBRT to 76:1, suggesting that disruption of the blood–brain barrier with radiation may serve as a mechanism to more effectively deliver trastuzumab (117).

Outside of trastuzumab, lapatinib has been investigated as a potential approach to the patient with HER2-overexpressing MBC with CNS involvement. In the randomized trial of capecitabine alone or in combination with lapatinib, it was noted that 11 patients in the monotherapy group had CNS progression, as compared to only 4 patients with combination therapy. Although this was statistically nonsignificant ($p = .10$), these data encouraged further exploration of lapatinib and capecitabine for CNS disease (92). The National Cancer Institute Cancer Therapy Evaluation Program (NCI/CTEP) 6969 trial included patients with HER2-overexpressing MBC with new or progressive brain metastases and at least one measurable lesion greater than 1.0 cm. Patients received lapatinib at a dose of 750 mg oral twice daily, with tumor measurements by magnetic resonance imaging (MRI) on 8-week intervals (118). Of 39 patients enrolled, one PR in CNS disease by Response Evaluation Criteria in Solid Tumors (RECIST) criteria was recorded (ORR 2.6%). An additional 30% of patients were noted to have a decrease in the size of their initially noted CNS lesions that did not meet RECIST criteria. A radiographic volumetric analysis of CNS metastases suggested a greater than 30% decrement in tumor volume in three patients, and an additional seven patients had a decrease between 15% to 30% (119).

These encouraging data for lapatinib were supplemented by trial EGF105084, in which eligible patients had HER2-overexpressing MBC, prior treatment with trastuzumab and cranial irradiation, and radiographic evidence of progressive brain metastases with at least one measurable lesion greater than 1.0 cm. Again, serial imaging was obtained with MRI, and patients were treated with lapatinib at an identical dose as in NCI/CTEP 6969 (120). A recently updated analysis of 242 patients enrolled suggested a greater than 50% volumetric reduction in CNS tumor load in 15 patients (6%) and a greater than 20% reduction in 41 patients (17%). Given encouraging phase III trial data for the combination of lapatinib and capecitabine, the EGF105084 parent trial was modified to include an extension arm comprised of patients who were offered this combination therapy in the face of CNS progression on lapatinib monotherapy. In 51 patients assessed in the extension arm, 10 PRs were recorded (20%), and stable disease was observed in 20 patients (39%). Greater than 50% volumetric reduction in tumor load was seen in 10 patients (20%) (121). Although further prospective assessments are warranted, it appears that the combination of lapatinib with chemotherapy may be a viable option for patients with brain metastases.

OTHER NOVEL AGENTS TARGETING THE HER2 RECEPTOR

Pertuzumab

Pertuzumab in a humanized, monoclonal antibody that represents the first agent in a new class of targeted therapeutics termed HER dimerization inhibitors (HDIs) (122). The crystal structure of pertuzumab complexed to HER2 suggests a binding site that is distinct from that of trastuzumab. Whereas trastuzumab binds in the juxtamembrane region and may sterically inhibit intracellular contacts, pertuzumab binds to a more peripheral region in the extracellular domain and widely separates HER2 from potential dimerization partners. Structurally, pertuzumab differs in a region between the variable and constant regions of the Fab (~20% larger than in trastuzumab) (123). A phase I trial of pertuzumab suggested that the agent was well tolerated. In 21 patients, two PRs were observed (none among the three breast cancer patients treated) (124). Further phase II trials have reported mild activity in prostate cancer, ovarian cancer, and non–small cell lung cancer (125–127).

Of note, the original phase I trial of pertuzumab included a partial response in a patient with refractory ovarian carcinoma lacking HER2 overexpression. Thus, a second trial assessed the utility of pertuzumab in non-HER2 overexpressors. In this phase II study, patients were randomized to receive pertuzumab at one of two distinct loading doses. In 41 evaluable patients, 2 PRs were observed along with 18 cases of stable disease. There appeared to be no relationship between the dose of pertuzumab and response, nor was there a relationship between dose and toxicity (128). Given the seemingly limited efficacy of this regimen, further efforts to characterize the activity of pertuzumab should be undertaken in concert with chemotherapy or in selected populations.

Finally, a recently presented trial assessed the strategy of dual HER2 blockade with the combination of pertuzumab and trastuzumab. In this phase II multicenter trial, patients who had HER2-overexpressing MBC that had progressed on prior trastuzumab therapy received pertuzumab (840 mg loading dose followed by 420 mg weekly) and trastuzumab (either 2 mg/kg weekly or 6 mg/kg every 3 weeks). Most adverse events reported were mild to moderate. In 24 assessable patients, five PRs were achieved (21%) with a significant number of individuals achieving stable disease (50%) (129).

HKI-272

HKI-272 represents a novel tyrosine kinase inhibitor with affinity for EGFR, HER2, and HER4. In distinction from lapatinib, which reversibly binds to the intracellular domain of EGFR and HER2, binding of HKI-272 to these moieties is irreversible. Preclinical assessment suggests that treatment of HER2-overexpressing BT-474 cells with this agent results in inhibition of HER2 phosphorylation and subsequent downregulation of MAPK and Akt activity. Interestingly, inhibition of HER2 with HKI-272 appears to be highly dependent on the level of HER2 expression. Preclinical assessment of HKI-272 in MDA-MB 361 cell lines, which possesses roughly 40% of the HER2-receptors detected in BT-474 cells, suggests an 80-fold decrease in affinity. Experimental observations also suggest that affinity of the agent for EGFR is markedly lower than the affinity for HER2 (130).

A phase I study of HKI-272 in advanced solid tumors has recently been reported. Interestingly, the study selected for patients with expression of EGFR or HER2. The study reported a maximal tolerated dose of 320 mg daily; most toxicities incurred were mild to moderate. A total of 41 patients were enrolled, including 23 patients with MBC. Among these patients, two confirmed PRs and two unconfirmed PRs were observed (131). Given responses observed in the subset of patients with MBC, further trials are under way to assess the activity of HKI-272 in this setting. In addition to studies of monotherapy, HKI-272 is being studied in combination with paclitaxel and with trastuzumab (80).

Trastuzumab-DM1

Trastuzumab-DM1 represents a novel agent in the class of anticancer therapeutics termed antibody-drug conjugates (ADCs). Trastuzumab-DM1 is comprised of the monoclonal antibody trastuzumab chemically linked to the highly potent antimicrotubule drug DM1, derived from maytansine (132). Maytansine has independently been assessed in patients with breast cancer in a phase II study with minimal activity when used as a single agent in a heavily pretreated population (133). In this construct, however, maytansine is held to the trastuzumab through an MCC linker, which theoretically provides a stable bond between the two moieties, allowing for prolonged exposure and reduced toxicity. In a preliminary report from a phase I trial, trastuzumab-DM1 was administered to seven patients with a dose-limiting toxicity of grade IV thrombocytopenia (although this was rapidly reversible). One partial response has been observed thus far, with a duration of over 6 months. Further results from this trial are eagerly anticipated (132).

CONCLUSIONS

A number of therapeutic advances have been made in the treatment of HER2-overexpressing MBC in recent years. The efficacy of single-agent trastuzumab was enhanced through the addition of standard cytotoxic chemotherapy in rational combinations derived from preclinical assays. Combination of trastuzumab with other novel therapeutics, including endocrine

therapy and bevacizumab, holds potential promise; and the continuation of trastuzumab beyond the time of disease progression, although unproven, warrants further exploration. In the setting of trastuzumab-refractory disease, lapatinib in combination with chemotherapy represents a viable option. Current studies are exploring combinations of lapatinib with several standard therapeutics (including both cytotoxic and endocrine agents), and of great interest are studies utilizing the combination of trastuzumab and lapatinib. With respect to specific subpopulations of patients with HER2-overexpressing disease, lapatinib appears to have significant activity in those patients with CNS metastases. The future of HER2-targeted therapy of MBC includes a host of novel agents, including (but not limited to) trastuzumab-DM1, HKI-272, and pertuzumab, as well as other indirect approaches targeting HER2 such as hsp 90 inhibitors. The therapy of HER2-overexpressing breast cancer thus represents an exciting frontier in which numerous paradigms for anticancer therapy continue to be established.

MANAGEMENT SUMMARY

- HER2-overexpressing MBC should be treated with a combination of trastuzumab and cytotoxic chemotherapy, although caution must be exercised with concomitant use of anthracyclines given the potential for cardiac toxicity.
- Phase III trial data support the use of two three-drug regimens including trastuzumab: (a) paclitaxel, platinum, and trastuzumab, or (b) docetaxel, carboplatin, and trastuzumab.
- Concordant with preclinical observations, clinical trials of trastuzumab in combination with cisplatin, docetaxel, and vinorelbine show considerable efficacy, and these represent reasonable regimens for HER2-overexpressing MBC as well.
- A combination of HER2 and VEGF-directed therapies with trastuzumab and bevacizumab shows potential promise.
- There is preliminary evidence to suggest a benefit from trastuzumab beyond the time of disease progression.
- Lapatinib, an orally administered, small molecule tyrosine kinase inhibitor, has affinity for EGFR and HER2 and can be used in combination with capecitabine for trastuzumab-refractory HER2-overexpressing MBC.
- Preliminary data from trials combining lapatinib and trastuzumab have yielded promising results.
- HER2-overexpressing MBC patients with CNS metastases may benefit uniquely from lapatinib alone or in combination with capecitabine, whereas trastuzumab seems to provide little benefit in preventing CNS progression.
- A number of novel therapeutic agents including antibody-drug conjugates (trastuzumab-DM1), VEGFR inhibitors (sunitinib), irreversible small molecule HER2-tyrosine kinase inhibitors (HKI-272), and HER2 dimerization inhibitors (pertuzumab) show promise in the treatment of HER2-overexpressing MBC.

References

1. Jemal A, Siegel R, Ward E, et al. Cancer statistics, 2008. *CA Cancer J Clin* 2008;58:71–96.
2. Surveillance, Epidemiology, and End Results (SEER) Program. SEER*Stat Database: Incidence—SEER 17 Regs Limited-Use, Nov 2006 Sub (1973–2004 varying), National Cancer Institute, DCCPS, Surveillance Research Program, Cancer Statistics Branch, released April 2007, based on the November 2006 submission. Available at www.seer.cancer.gov.
3. Early Breast Cancer Trialists' Collaborative Group. Effects of chemotherapy and hormonal therapy for early breast cancer on recurrence and 15-year survival: an overview of the randomised trials. *Lancet* 2005;365:1687–1717.

4. Slamon DJ, Leyland-Jones B, Shak S, et al. Use of chemotherapy plus a monoclonal antibody against HER2 for metastatic breast cancer that overexpresses HER2. *N Engl J Med* 2001;344:783–792.
5. Mass RD. The HER receptor family: a rich target for therapeutic development. *Int J Radiat Oncol Biol Physics* 2004;58:932–940.
6. Pal SK, Pegram M. Targeting HER2 epitopes. *Semin Oncol* 2006;33:386–391.
7. Marmor MD, Skaria KB, Yarden Y. Signal transduction and oncogenesis by ERBB/HER receptors. *Int J Radiat Oncol Biol Physics* 2004;58:903–913.
8. Cho H-S, Mason K, Ramyar KX, et al. Structure of the extracellular region of HER2 alone and in complex with the Herceptin Fab. *Nature* 2003;421:756–760.
9. Pegram MD, finn RS, Arzoo K, et al. The effect of HER-2/neu overexpression on chemotherapeutic drug sensitivity in human breast and ovarian cancer cells. *Oncogene* 1997;15:537–547.
10. Slamon DJ, Godolphin W, Jones LA, et al. Studies of the HER-2/neu proto-oncogene in human breast and ovarian cancer. *Science* 1989;244:707–712.
11. Slamon DJ, Clark GM, Wong SG, et al. Human breast cancer: correlation of relapse and survival with amplification of the HER-2/neu oncogene. *Science* 1987;235:177–182.
12. Pietras RJ, Fendly BM, Chazin VR, et al. Antibody to HER-2/neu receptor blocks DNA repair after cisplatin in human breast and ovarian cancer cells. *Oncogene* 1994;9:1829–1838.
13. Hudziak RM, Lewis GD, Winget M, et al. p185 HER2 monoclonal antibody has antiproliferative effects *in vitro* and sensitizes human breast tumor cells to tumor necrosis factor. *Mol Cell Biol* 1989;9:1165–1172.
14. Carter P, Presta L, Gorman CM, et al. Humanization of an anti-p185 HER2 antibody for human cancer therapy. *Proc Natl Acad Sci* 1992;89:4285–4289.
15. Pietras RJ, Pegram MD, finn RS, et al. Remission of human breast cancer xenografts on therapy with humanized monoclonal antibody to HER-2 receptor and DNA-reactive drugs. *Oncogene* 1998;17:2235–2249.
16. Harari D, Yarden Y. Molecular mechanisms underlying ERBB2/HER2 action in breast cancer. *Oncogene* 2000;19:6102–6114.
17. Molina MA, Codony-Servat J, Albanell J, et al. Trastuzumab (Herceptin), a humanized anti-HER2 receptor monoclonal antibody, inhibits basal and activated HER2 ectodomain cleavage in breast cancer cells. *Cancer Res* 2001;61:4744–4749.
18. Baselga J, Tripathy D, Mendelsohn J, et al. Phase II study of weekly intravenous trastuzumab (Herceptin) in patients with HER2/neu-overexpressing metastatic breast cancer. *Semin Oncol* 1999;26:78–83.
19. Cobleigh MA, Vogel CL, Tripathy D, et al. Multinational study of the efficacy and safety of humanized anti-HER2 monoclonal antibody in women who have HER2-overexpressing metastatic breast cancer that has progressed after chemotherapy for metastatic disease. *J Clin Oncol* 1999;17:2639.
20. Slamon D, Leyland-Jones B, Shak S. Addition of Herceptin (humanized anti-HER2 antibody) to first line chemotherapy for HER2 overexpressing metastatic breast cancer (HER21/MBC) markedly increases anticancer activity: a randomized multinational controlled phase III trial. *Proc Am Soc Clin Oncol* 1998;17:(abst 377).
21. Vogel CL, Cobleigh MA, Tripathy D, et al. Efficacy and safety of trastuzumab as a single agent in first-line treatment of HER2-overexpressing motastatic breast cancer. *J Clin Oncol* 2002;20:719–726.
22. Pegram M, Forbes J, Pienkowski T, et al. BCIRG 007: first overall survival analysis of randomized phase III trial of trastuzumab plus docetaxel with or without carboplatin as first line therapy in HER2 amplified metastatic breast cancer (MBC). ASCO annual meeting proceedings. Part I. *J Clin Oncol* 2007;25(18S)[Suppl]:LBA1008.
23. Pegram MD, Konecny GE, O'Callaghan C, et al. Rational combinations of trastuzumab with chemotherapeutic drugs used in the treatment of breast cancer. *J Natl Cancer Inst* 2004;96:739–749.
24. Lopez AM, Pegram MD, Slamon DJ, et al. A model-based approach for assessing in vivo combination therapy interactions. *Proc Natl Acad Sci* 1999;96:13023–13028.
25. Pegram M, Hsu S, Lewis G, et al. Inhibitory effects of combinations of HER-2/neu antibody and chemotherapeutic agents used for treatment of human breast cancers. *Oncogene* 1999;18:2241–2251.
26. Leyland-Jones B, Gelmon K, Ayoub J-P, et al. Pharmacokinetics, safety, and efficacy of trastuzumab administered every three weeks in combination with paclitaxel. *J Clin Oncol* 2003;21:3965–3971.
27. Gasparini G, Gion M, Mariani L, et al. Randomized phase II trial of weekly paclitaxel alone versus trastuzumab plus weekly paclitaxel as first-line therapy of patients with HER-2 positive advanced breast cancer. *Breast Cancer Res Treat* 2007;101:355–365.
28. Gori S, Colozza M, Mosconi A, et al. Phase II study of weekly paclitaxel and trastuzumab in anthracycline- and taxane-pretreated patients with HER2-overexpressing metastatic breast cancer. *Br J Cancer* 2004;90:36–40.
29. Seidman AD, Fornier MN, Esteva FJ, et al. Weekly trastuzumab and paclitaxel therapy for metastatic breast cancer with analysis of efficacy by HER2 immunophenotype and gene amplification. *J Clin Oncol* 2001;19:2587–2595.
30. Seidman AD, Berry D, Cirrincione C, et al. Randomized phase III trial of weekly compared with every-3-weeks paclitaxel for metastatic breast cancer, with trastuzumab for all HER-2 overexpressors and random assignment to trastuzumab or not in HER-2 nonoverexpressors: final results of Cancer and Leukemia Group B protocol 9840. *J Clin Oncol* 2008;26:1642–1649.
31. Gonzalez-Angulo AM, Hortobagyi GN. Optimal schedule of paclitaxel: weekly is better. *J Clin Oncol* 2008;26:1585–1587.
32. Yamauchi H, O'Neill A, Gelman R, et al. Prediction of response to antiestrogen therapy in advanced breast cancer patients by pretreatment circulating levels of extracellular domain of the HER-2/c-neu protein. *J Clin Oncol* 1997;15:2518–2525.
33. Esteva FJ, Valero V, Booser D, et al. Phase II study of weekly docetaxel and trastuzumab for patients with HER-2-overexpressing metastatic breast cancer. *J Clin Oncol* 2002;20:1800–1808.
34. Tedesco KL, Thor AD, Johnson DH, et al. Docetaxel combined with trastuzumab is an active regimen in HER-2 3+ overexpressing and fluorescent *in situ* hybridization-positive metastatic breast cancer: a multi-institutional phase II trial. *J Clin Oncol* 2004;22:1071–1077.
35. Raff J, Rajdev L, Malik U, et al. Phase II study of weekly docetaxel alone or in combination with trastuzumab in patients with metastatic breast cancer. *Clin Breast Cancer* 2004;4:420–427.
36. Montemurro F, Choa G, Faggiuolo R, et al. A phase II study of three-weekly docetaxel and weekly trastuzumab in HER2-overexpressing advanced breast cancer. *Oncology* 2004;66:38–45.
37. Marty M, Cognetti F, Maraninchi D, et al. Randomized phase II trial of the efficacy and safety of trastuzumab combined with docetaxel in patients with human epidermal growth factor receptor 2-positive metastatic breast cancer administered as first-line treatment: the M77001 study group. *J Clin Oncol* 2005;23:4265–4274.
38. Burstein HJ, Kuter I, Campos SM, et al. Clinical activity of trastuzumab and vinorelbine in women with HER2-overexpressing metastatic breast cancer. *J Clin Oncol* 2001;19:2722–2730.
39. Jahanzeb M, Mortimer JE, Yunus F, et al. Phase II trial of weekly vinorelbine and trastuzumab as first-line therapy in patients with HER2+ metastatic breast cancer. *Oncologist* 2002;7:410–417.
40. Burstein HJ, Harris LN, Marcom PK, et al. Trastuzumab and vinorelbine as first-line therapy for HER2-overexpressing metastatic breast cancer: multicenter phase II trial with clinical outcomes, analysis of serum tumor markers as predictive factors, and cardiac surveillance algorithm. *J Clin Oncol* 2003;21:2889–2895.
41. Chan A, Martin M, Untch M, et al. Vinorelbine plus trastuzumab combination as first-line therapy for HER 2-positive metastatic breast cancer patients: an international phase II trial. *Br J Cancer* 2006;95:788–793.
42. De Maio E, Pacilio C, Gravina A, et al. Vinorelbine plus 3-weekly trastuzumab in metastatic breast cancer: a single-centre phase 2 trial. *BMC Cancer* 2007;7:50.
43. Papaldo P, Fabi A, Ferretti G, et al. A phase II study on metastatic breast cancer patients treated with weekly vinorelbine with or without trastuzumab according to HER2 expression: changing the natural history of HER2-positive disease. *Ann Oncol* 2006;17:630–636.
44. Slamon DJ, Clark GM. Amplification of c-ERBB-2 and aggressive human breast tumors? *Science* 1988;240:1795–1798.
45. Burstein HJ, Keshaviah A, Baron AD, et al. Trastuzumab plus vinorelbine or taxane chemotherapy for HER2-overexpressing metastatic breast cancer: the trastuzumab and vinorelbine or taxane study. *Cancer* 2007;110:965–972.
46. Blum JL. The role of capecitabine, an oral, enzymatically activated fluoropyrimidine, in the treatment of metastatic breast cancer. *Oncologist* 2001;6:56–64.
47. Blum JL, Dieras V, Mucci P, et al. Multicenter, phase II study of capecitabine in taxane-pretreated metastatic breast carcinoma patients. *Cancer* 2001;92:1759–1768.
48. Blum JL, Jones SE, Buzdar AU, et al. Multicenter phase II study of capecitabine in paclitaxel-refractory metastatic breast cancer. *J Clin Oncol* 1999;17:485.
49. Schaller G, Fuchs I, Gonsch T, et al. Phase II study of capecitabine plus trastuzumab in human epidermal growth factor receptor 2 overexpressing metastatic breast cancer pretreated with anthracyclines or taxanes. *J Clin Oncol* 2007;25:3246–3250.
50. Bartsch R, Wenzel C, Altorjai G, et al. Capecitabine and trastuzumab in heavily pretreated metastatic breast cancer. *J Clin Oncol* 2007;25:3853–3858.
51. Yamamoto D, Iwase S, Kitamura K, et al. A phase II study of trastuzumab and capecitabine for patients with HER2-overexpressing metastatic breast cancer: Japan Breast Cancer Research Network (JBCRN) 00 trial. *Cancer Chemother Pharmacol* 2008;61:509–514.
52. Pegram MD, Lipton A, Hayes DF, et al. Phase II study of receptor-enhanced chemosensitivity using recombinant humanized anti p185 HER2/neu monoclonal antibody plus cisplatin in patients with HER2/neu-overexpressing metastatic breast cancer refractory to chemotherapy treatment. *J Clin Oncol* 1998;16:2659–2671.
53. Konecny G, Pegram M, Beryt M. Therapeutic advantage of chemotherapy drugs in combination with Herceptin against human breast cancer cell with HER-2/neu overexpression. *Breast Cancer Res Treat* 1999;57:114(abst 467).
54. Perez E, Suman V, Rowland K, et al. Two concurrent phase II trials of paclitaxel/carboplatin/trastuzumab (weekly or every-3-week schedule) as first-line therapy in women with HER2-overexpressing metastatic breast cancer: NCCTG study 983252. *Clin Breast Cancer* 2005;6:425–432.
55. Robert N, Leyland-Jones B, Asmar L, et al. Randomized phase III study of trastuzumab, paclitaxel, and carboplatin compared with trastuzumab and paclitaxel in women with HER-2-overexpressing metastatic breast cancer. *J Clin Oncol* 2006;24:2786–2792.
56. Pegram MD, Pienkowski T, Northfelt DW, et al. Results of two open-label, multicenter phase II studies of docetaxel, platinum salts, and trastuzumab in HER2-positive advanced breast cancer. *J Natl Cancer Inst* 2004;96:759–769.
57. Bartsch R, Wenzel C, Gampenrieder S, et al. Trastuzumab and gemcitabine as salvage therapy in heavily pre-treated patients with metastatic breast cancer. *Cancer Chemother Pharmacol* 2008;62(5):903–910.
58. Miller KD, Sisk J, Ansari R, et al. Gemcitabine, paclitaxel, and trastuzumab in metastatic breast cancer. *Oncology (Williston Park)* 2001;15:38–40.
59. Stemmler H, Kahlert S, Brudler O, et al. High efficacy of gemcitabine and cisplatin plus trastuzumab in patients with HER2-overexpressing metastatic breast cancer: a phase II study. *Clin Oncol (R Coll Radiol)* 2005;17:630–635.
60. O'Brien MER, Wigler N, Inbar M, et al. Reduced cardiotoxicity and comparable efficacy in a phase III trial of pegylated liposomal doxorubicin HCl (CAELYXTM/Doxil(R)) versus conventional doxorubicin for first-line treatment of metastatic breast cancer. *Ann Oncol* 2004;15:440–449.
61. Chia S, Clemons M, Martin L-A, et al. Pegylated liposomal doxorubicin and trastuzumab in HER-2 overexpressing metastatic breast cancer: a multicenter phase II trial. *J Clin Oncol* 2006;24:2773–2778.
62. Chu Q, Goldstein L, Murray N, et al. A phase I, open-label study of the safety, tolerability and pharmacokinetics of lapatinib (GW572016) in combination with letrozole in cancer patients. 2005 ASCO annual meeting proceedings. Part I of II. *J Clin Oncol* 2005;23[16S Suppl]:3001.
63. Mackey JR, Kaufman B, Clemen M, et al. Trastuzumab prolongs preogression-free survival in hormone-dependent and HER2-positive metastatic breast cancer. Breast *Cancer Res Treat* 2006;100(sppl 1):abstract 3.
64. Burris HA 3rd, Hurwitz HI, Dees EC, et al. Phase I safety, pharmacokinetics, and clinical activity study of lapatinib (GW572016), a reversible dual inhibitor of epidermal growth factor receptor tyrosine kinases, in heavily pretreated patients with metastatic carcinomas. *J Clin Oncol* 2005;23:5305–5313.
65. Shepherd FA, Rodrigues Pereira J, Ciuleanu T, et al. Erlotinib in previously treated non–small cell lung cancer. *N Engl J Med* 2005;353:123–132.
66. Cappuzzo F, Ligorio C, Janne PA, et al. Prospective study of gefitinib in epidermal growth factor receptor fluorescence in situ hybridization-positive/phospho-Akt-positive or never smoker patients with advanced non-small-cell lung cancer: the ONCO BELL trial. *J Clin Oncol* 2007;25:2248–2255.
67. Tan AR, Yang X, Hewitt SM, et al. Evaluation of biologic end points and pharmacokinetics in patients with metastatic breast cancer after treatment with erlotinib, an epidermal growth factor receptor tyrosine kinase inhibitor. *J Clin Oncol* 2004;22:3080–3090.

68. Ciardiello FTT, Caputo F, De Laurentiis M, et al. Phase II study of gefitinib in combination with docetaxel as first-line therapy in metastatic breast cancer. *Br J Cancer* 2006;94:1604–1609.
69. Dennison S, Jacobs S, Wilson J, et al. A phase II clinical trial of ZD1839 (Iressa) in combination with docetaxel as first-line treatment in patients with advanced breast cancer. *Invest N Drugs* 2007;25:545–551.
70. Moulder SL, O'Neill A, Arteaga C, et al. final results of ECOG1100: a phase I/II study of combined blockade of the ERBB receptor network in patients with HER2-overexpressing metastatic breast cancer (MBC). ASCO annual meeting proceedings. Part I. *J Clin Oncol* 2007;25[18S Suppl]:1033.
71. Finn RS, Wilson CA, Sanders J, et al. Targeting the epidermal growth factor receptor (EGFR) and HER-2 with OSI-774 and trastuzumab, respectively, in HER-2 overexpressing human breast cancer cell lines results in a therapeutic advantage *in vitro*. *Proc Am Soc Clin Oncol* 2003;22:(abst 940).
72. Britten CD, Pegram M, Rosen P, et al. Targeting ERBB receptor interactions: a phase I trial of trastuzumab and erlotinib in metastatic HER2+ breast cancer. 2004 ASCO Annual Meeting Proceedings (Post-Meeting Edition). *J Clin Oncol* 2004;22[14S Suppl]:3045.
73. Miller K, Wang M, Gralow J, et al. Paclitaxel plus bevacizumab versus paclitaxel alone for metastatic breast cancer. *N Engl J Med* 2007;357:2666–2676.
74. Konecny GE, Meng YG, Untch M, et al. Association between HER-2/neu and vascular endothelial growth factor expression predicts clinical outcome in primary breast cancer patients. *Clin Cancer Res* 2004;10:1706–1716.
75. Pegram M, Chan D, Dichmann R, et al. Phase II combined biological therapy targeting the HER2 proto-oncogene and the vascular endothelial growth factor using trastuzumab (T) and bevacizumab (B) as first line treatment of HER2-amplified breast cancer. *Breast Cancer Res Treat* 2006;100[Suppl 1]:(abst 201).
76. Murray L, Abrams T, Long K, et al. SU11248 inhibits tumor growth and CSF-1R-dependent osteolysis in an experimental breast cancer bone metastasis model. *Clin Experiment Metastasis* 2003;20:757–766.
77. Mendel DB, Laird AD, Xin X, et al. In vivo antitumor activity of SU11248, a novel tyrosine kinase inhibitor targeting vascular endothelial growth factor and platelet-derived growth factor receptors: determination of a pharmacokinetic/pharmacodynamic relationship. *Clin Cancer Res* 2003;9:327–337.
78. Abrams TJ, Murray LJ, Pesenti E, et al. Preclinical evaluation of the tyrosine kinase inhibitor SU11248 as a single agent and in combination with "standard of care" therapeutic agents for the treatment of breast cancer. *Mol Cancer Ther* 2003;2:1011–1021.
79. Motzer RJ, Hutson TE, Tomczak P, et al. Sunitinib versus interferon alfa in metastatic renal-cell carcinoma. *N Engl J Med* 2007;356:115–124.
80. National Institutes of Health. Available at http://www.clinicaltrials.gov.
81. Tripathy D, Slamon DJ, Cobleigh M, et al. Safety of treatment of metastatic breast cancer with trastuzumab beyond disease progression. *J Clin Oncol* 2004;22: 1063–1070.
82. Fountzilas G, Razis E, Tsavdaridis D, et al. Continuation of trastuzumab beyond disease progression is feasible and safe in patients with metastatic breast cancer: a retrospective analysis of 80 cases by the hellenic cooperative oncology group. *Clin Breast Cancer* 2003;4:120–125.
83. Montemurro F, Donadio M, Clavarezza M, et al. Outcome of patients with HER2-positive advanced breast cancer progressing during trastuzumab-based therapy. *Oncologist* 2006;11:318–324.
84. von Minckwitz G, Vogel P, Schmidt M, et al. Trastuzumab treatment beyond progression in patients with HER-2 positive metastatic breast cancer the TBP study (GBG 26/BIG 3-05). *Breast Cancer Res Treat* 2007;106(abst 4056).
85. Nagata Y, Lan K-H, Zhou X, et al. PTEN activation contributes to tumor inhibition by trastuzumab, and loss of PTEN predicts trastuzumab resistance in patients. *Cancer Cell* 2004;6:117–127.
86. Lu C-H, Wyszomierski SL, Tseng L-M, et al. Preclinical testing of clinically applicable strategies for overcoming trastuzumab resistance caused by PTEN deficiency. *Clin Cancer Res* 2007;13:5883–5888.
87. Lu Y, Zi X, Zhao Y, et al. Insulin-like growth factor-i receptor signaling and resistance to trastuzumab (Herceptin). *J Natl Cancer Inst* 2001;93:1852–1857.
88. Camirand A, Lu Y, Pollak M. Co-targeting HER2/ERBB2 and insulin-like growth factor-1 receptors causes synergistic inhibition of growth in HER2-overexpressing breast cancer cells. *Med Sci Monit* 2002;8:BR521–526.
89. Shattuck DL, Miller JK, Carraway KL 3rd, et al. Met receptor contributes to trastuzumab resistance of HER2-overexpressing breast cancer cells. *Cancer Res* 2008;68:1471–1477.
90. Baker JHE, Lindquist KE, Huxham LA, et al. Direct visualization of heterogeneous extravascular distribution of trastuzumab in human epidermal growth factor receptor type 2 overexpressing xenografts. *Clin Cancer Res* 2008;14:2171–2179.
91. Nahta R, Yuan LXH, Du Y, et al. Lapatinib induces apoptosis in trastuzumab-resistant breast cancer cells: effects on insulin-like growth factor I signaling. *Mol Cancer Ther* 2007;6:667–674.
92. Geyer CE, Forster J, Lindquist D, et al. Lapatinib plus capecitabine for HER2-positive advanced breast cancer. *N Engl J Med* 2006;355:2733–2743.
93. Cockerill S, Stubberfield C, Stables J, et al. Indazolylamino quinazolines and pyridopyrimidines as inhibitors of the EGFr and c-ERBB-2. *Bioorg Med Chem Lett* 2001;11:1401–1405.
94. Rusnak DW, Lackey K, Affleck K, et al. The effects of the novel, reversible epidermal growth factor receptor/ERBB-2 tyrosine kinase inhibitor, GW2016, on the growth of human normal and tumor-derived cell lines *in vitro* and *in vivo*. *Mol Cancer Ther* 2001;1:85–94.
95. Xia W, Mullin R, Keith B, et al. Anti-tumor activity of GW572016: a dual tyrosine kinase inhibitor blocks EGF activation of EGFR/ERBB2 and downstream Erk1/2 and AKT pathways. *Oncogene* 2002;21:6255–6263.
96. Spector NL, Xia W, Burris H 3rd, et al. Study of the biologic effects of lapatinib, a reversible inhibitor of ERBB1 and ERBB2 tyrosine kinases, on tumor growth and survival pathways in patients with advanced malignancies. *J Clin Oncol* 2005; 23:2502–2512.
97. Burstein HJ, Storniolo AM, Franco S, et al. A phase II study of lapatinib monotherapy in chemotherapy-refractory HER2-positive and HER2-negative advanced or metastatic breast cancer. *Ann Oncol* 2008;19(6):1068–1074.
98. Budman DR, Soong R, Calabro A, et al. Identification of potentially useful combinations of epidermal growth factor receptor tyrosine kinase antagonists with conventional cytotoxic agents using median effect analysis. *Anticancer Drugs* 2006;17:921–928.
99. Chu QSC, Schwartz G, de Bono J, et al. Phase I and pharmacokinetic study of lapatinib in combination with capecitabine in patients with advanced solid malignancies. *J Clin Oncol* 2007;25:3753–3758.
100. Cameron D, Casey M, Press M, et al. A phase III randomized comparison of lapatinib plus capecitabine versus capecitabine alone in women with advanced breast cancer that has progressed on trastuzumab: updated efficacy and biomarker analyses. *Breast Cancer Res Treat* 2008;112(3):533–543.
101. Coley HM, Shotton CF, Ajose-Adeogun A, et al. Receptor tyrosine kinase (RTK) inhibition is effective in chemosensitising EGFR-expressing drug resistant human ovarian cancer cell lines when used in combination with cytotoxic agents. *Biochem Pharmacol* 2006;72:941–948.
102. Crown JP, Burris HA, Jones S, et al. Safety and tolerability of lapatinib in combination with taxanes (T) in patients with breast cancer (BC). ASCO annual meeting proceedings. Part I. *J Clin Oncol* 2007;25[18S Suppl]:1027.
103. Leo AD, Gomez H, Aziz Z, et al. Lapatinib (L) with paclitaxel compared to paclitaxel as first-line treatment for patients with metastatic breast cancer: a phase III randomized, double-blind study of 580 patients. 2007 ASCO annual meeting proceedings. Part I. *J Clin Oncol* 2007;25[18S Suppl]:1011.
104. Cianfrocca ME, Rosen ST, Roenn JH, et al. A phase I trial of pegylated liposomal anthracycline and lapatinib (L) combination in the treatment of metastatic breast cancer (MBC): first evaluation of an anthracycline and lapatinib combination in the treatment of MBC. 2007 ASCO annual meeting proceedings. Part I. *J Clin Oncol* 2007;25[18S Suppl]:1079.
105. Xia W, Gerard CM, Liu L, et al. Combining lapatinib (GW572016), a small molecule inhibitor of ERBB1 and ERBB2 tyrosine kinases, with therapeutic anti-ERBB2 antibodies enhances apoptosis of ERBB2-overexpressing breast cancer cells. *Oncogene* 2005;24:6213–6221.
106. Konecny GE, Pegram MD, Venkatesan N, et al. Activity of the dual kinase inhibitor lapatinib (GW572016) against HER-2-overexpressing and trastuzumab-treated breast cancer cells. *Cancer Res* 2006;66:1630–1639.
107. Storniolo A, Burris H, Pegram M, et al. A phase I, open-label study of lapatinib (GW572016) plus trastuzumab; a clinically active regimen. 2005 ASCO annual meeting proceedings. Part I of II. *J Clin Oncol* 2005;23[16S Suppl]:559.
108. Storniolo AM, Koehler M, Preston A, et al. Cardiac safety in patients (pts) with metastatic breast cancer (MBC) treated with lapatinib (L) and trastuzumab (TRA). 2007 ASCO annual meeting proceedings. Part I. *J Clin Oncol* 2007;25[18S Suppl]:514.
109. Barnholtz-Sloan JS, Sloan AE, Davis FG, et al. Incidence proportions of brain metastases in patients diagnosed (1973 to 2001) in the metropolitan Detroit cancer surveillance system. *J Clin Oncol* 2004;22:2865–2872.
110. Cho SY, Choi HY. Causes of death and metastatic patterns in patients with mammary cancer. Ten-year autopsy study. *Am J Clin Pathol* 1980;73:232–234.
111. Yau T, Swanton C, Chua S, et al. Incidence, pattern and timing of brain metastases among patients with advanced breast cancer treated with trastuzumab. *Acta Oncol* 2006;45:196–201.
112. Stemmler HJ, Kahlert S, Siekiera W, et al. Characteristics of patients with brain metastases receiving trastuzumab for HER2 overexpressing metastatic breast cancer. *Breast* 2006;15:219–225.
113. Clayton AJ, Danson S, Jolly S, et al. Incidence of cerebral metastases in patients treated with trastuzumab for metastatic breast cancer. *Br J Cancer* 2004;91: 639–643.
114. Palmieri D, Bronder JL, Herring JM, et al. Her-2 overexpression increases the metastatic outgrowth of breast cancer cells in the brain. *Cancer Res* 2007;67: 4190–4198.
115. Romond EH, Perez EA, Bryant J, et al. Trastuzumab plus adjuvant chemotherapy for operable HER2-positive breast cancer. *N Engl J Med* 2005;353:1673–1684.
116. Gori S, Rimondini S, De Angelis V, et al. Central nervous system metastases in HER-2 positive metastatic breast cancer patients treated with trastuzumab: incidence, survival, and risk factors. *Oncologist* 2007;12:766–773.
117. Stemmler J, Schmitt M, Willems A, et al. Brain metastases in HER2-overexpressing metastatic breast cancer: comparative analysis of trastuzumab levels in serum and cerebrospinal fluid. 2006 ASCO annual meeting proceedings. Part I. *J Clin Oncol* 2006;24[18S Suppl]:1525.
118. Lin NU, Carey LA, Liu MC, et al. Phase II trial of lapatinib for brain metastases in patients with HER2+ breast cancer. 2006 ASCO annual meeting proceedings. Part I. *J Clin Oncol* 2006;24[18S Suppl]:503.
119. Lin NU, Carey LA, Liu MC, et al. Phase II trial of lapatinib for brain metastases in patients with human epidermal growth factor receptor 2-positive breast cancer. *J Clin Oncol* 2008;26:1993–1999.
120. Lin NU, Dieras V, Paul D, et al. EGF105084, a phase II study of lapatinib for brain metastases in patients (pts) with HER2+ breast cancer following trastuzumab (H) based systemic therapy and cranial radiotherapy (RT). 2007 ASCO annual meeting proceedings. Part I. *J Clin Oncol* 2007;25[18S Suppl]:1012.
121. Lin N, Paul D, Dieras V, et al. Lapatinib and capecitabine for the treatment of brain metastases in patients with HER2+ breast cancer an updated analysis from EGF105084. *Breast Cancer Res Treat* 2008 (abst 6076).
122. Adams C, Allison D, flagella K, et al. Humanization of a recombinant monoclonal antibody to produce a therapeutic HER dimerization inhibitor, pertuzumab. *Cancer Immunol Immunother* 2006;55:717–727.
123. Franklin MC, Carey KD, Vajdos FF, et al. Insights into ERBB signaling from the structure of the ERBB2-pertuzumab complex. *Cancer Cell* 2004;5:317–328.
124. Agus DB, Gordon MS, Taylor C, et al. Phase I clinical study of pertuzumab, a novel HER dimerization inhibitor, in patients with advanced cancer. *J Clin Oncol* 2005; 23:2534–2543.
125. Agus DB, Sweeney CJ, Morris MJ, et al. Efficacy and safety of single-agent pertuzumab (rhuMAb 2C4), a human epidermal growth factor receptor dimerization inhibitor, in castration-resistant prostate cancer after progression from taxane-based therapy. *J Clin Oncol* 2007;25:675–681.
126. de Bono JS, Bellmunt J, Attard G, et al. Open-label phase II study evaluating the efficacy and safety of two doses of pertuzumab in castrate chemotherapy-naive patients with hormone-refractory prostate cancer. *J Clin Oncol* 2007;25:257–262.
127. Gordon MS, Matei D, Aghajanian C, et al. Clinical activity of pertuzumab (rhuMAb 2C4), a HER dimerization inhibitor, in advanced ovarian cancer: potential predictive relationship with tumor HER2 activation status. *J Clin Oncol* 2006;24: 4324–4332.
128. Cortes J, Baselga J, Kellokumpu-Lehtinen P, et al. Open label, randomized, phase II study of pertuzumab (P) in patients (pts) with metastatic breast cancer (MBC)

with low expression of HER2. 2005 ASCO annual meeting proceedings. Part I of II. *J Clin Oncol* 2005;23[16S Suppl]:3068.

129. Baselga J, Cameron D, Miles D, et al. Objective response rate in a phase II multicenter trial of pertuzumab (P), a HER2 dimerization inhibiting monoclonal antibody, in combination with trastuzumab (T) in patients (pts) with HER2-positive metastatic breast cancer (MBC) which has progressed during treatment with T. 2007 ASCO annual meeting proceedings. Part I. *J Clin Oncol* 2007;25[18S Suppl]:1004.

130. Rabindran SK, Discafani CM, Rosfjord EC, et al. Antitumor Activity of HKI-272, an orally active, irreversible inhibitor of the HER-2 tyrosine kinase. *Cancer Res* 2004;64:3958–3965.

131. Wong KK, Fracasso PM, Bukowski RM, et al. HKI-272, an irreversible pan ERBB receptor tyrosine kinase inhibitor: Preliminary phase 1 results in patients with solid tumors. 2006 ASCO annual meeting proceedings. Part I. *J Clin Oncol* 2006;24[18S Suppl]:3018.

132. Beeram M, Krop I, Modi S, et al. A phase I study of trastuzumab-MCC-DM1 (T-DM1), a first-in-class HER2 antibody-drug conjugate (ADC), in patients (pts) with HER2+ metastatic breast cancer (BC). 2007 ASCO annual meeting proceedings. Part I. *J Clin Oncol* 2007;25[18S Suppl]:1042.

133. Neidhart JA, Laufman LR, Vaughn C, et al. Minimal single-agent activity of maytansine in refractory breast cancer: a Southwest Oncology Group study. *Cancer Treat Rep* 1980;64:675–677.

Chapter 76
End-of-Life Considerations in Patients with Breast Cancer

Susan Urba

To cure sometimes, to heal often, to comfort always.
—Dame Cicely Saunders

Breast cancer is the most common cause of cancer in women in the United States, and it is the second most common cause of death after lung cancer. In 2006 it is estimated that 214,640 patients were diagnosed with breast cancer and 41,430 patients died of that disease (1). Breast cancer is a disease that may have several different outcomes, depending on the stage at which it is diagnosed, the molecular aggressiveness of the disease, and the patient's wishes for and tolerance of treatment modalities. Even in the face of incurable metastatic disease, most patients pursue some sort of palliative chemotherapy if their performance status allows it. However, for these patients the cancer will eventually spread and cause death. Clinicians have an obligation to support patients through all of their treatments, whether it is surgery, chemotherapy, radiation, symptom management, or therapy for psychosocial distress, from the time of their diagnosis to their death.

The traditional way of looking at the overview of a patient's care is illustrated in Figure 76.1. Most patients were considered to be in "active" treatment for their disease at first, and then when treatments failed or the cancer progressed, they were switched over to hospice care. Patients had crossed over some invisible threshold to the "end of life." Physicians often turned the care of their patients over to the hospice medical director, so it is no wonder that patients came to believe that as they neared the end of their lives their physicians abandoned them to hospice because there was "nothing left to do."

The more modern way of approaching patient care is to consider the patient's treatment (both "active" and "palliative") as a continuum, as depicted in Figure 76.2. At the time of diagnosis, if the patient is well enough to tolerate aggressive anticancer treatment, the surgery, radiation, or chemotherapy predominates, and most of the discussion in the doctor's office usually revolves around response rates and cure rates. However, usually there are other issues to be addressed that are more of a supportive or palliative nature. The patient may have pain or other symptoms that first brought her to her physician and led to the diagnosis of her breast cancer. She almost certainly will have distress and possibly depression regarding the diagnosis. Depending on her age and family status, she may have children who need to be told about their mother's health, which can add to her stress. Therefore, palliative care does indeed start early for patients who have a new diagnosis of breast cancer. Pain and symptom management and psychosocial counseling are needed early in the course of the disease and its treatment. Over the course of time, the chemotherapy options may dwindle and the need for symptom management will come to predominate, but the patient should never feel that all initial efforts are "active" and "hopeful," while all later efforts near the end of life are "passive" and "hopeless." Hospice care and family bereavement care continues to be the final part of the diagram.

Actually, hospice can even be concurrent with disease-modifying care and palliative care. Hospices are beginning to allow interventions such as palliative chemotherapy and radiation, intravenous hydration, and blood transfusions. Some hospices are starting to participate in symptom-management research or in trials done to determine the cost-effectiveness of enrolling patients early in hospice and allowing more "active" and expensive interventions. This allows earlier enrollment of patients who otherwise would have waited until much later.

Physicians, nurses, and social workers can continue to foster hope throughout their entire relationship with the patient. However, the nature of hope will change over the course of treatment. At first there is usually hope for cure or a good response to treatment, with resultant prolongation of life. Later, that hope may evolve to include good relief of pain and nonpain symptoms such as fatigue, dyspnea, or nausea. As the length of projected survival becomes shorter, patients may hope for strengthening of their relationships with family and friends. This can include the resolution of unfinished business in their lives, such as the repair of a damaged relationship or the achievement of a simple goal. And finally, the hope for a peaceful death, free of pain and fear, predominates.

END OF LIFE: CAN WE DEFINE IT? CAN WE PREDICT IT?

God, grant me the serenity to accept the things I cannot change, the courage to change the things I can, and the wisdom to know the difference.
—The Serenity Prayer

Occasionally, it is relatively easy to determine when the end of a patient's life is near. However, most data demonstrate that physicians are not good at predicting when a patient is going to die. Although there is no exact definition of the period of time called "end of life," some aspects are described in the National Institutes of Health State-of-the-Science Conference Statement on Improving End-of-Life Care (2). They point out that the patient has a chronic disease or persistent symptoms or functional impairment, and that these impairments result from underlying irreversible disease and require formal or informal care and can lead to death. Another simpler definition describes the end of life as a phase of life when a person is living with an illness that will worsen and eventually cause death and is not limited to the short period of time when the person is moribund (3).

Physicians are poor prognosticators and tend to be more optimistic than may be warranted (4). Christakis and Lamont (5) conducted a Robert Woods Johnson clinical scholar study to determine the accuracy of physicians' predictions for their patients. They reported data on 343 physicians who were asked to provide survival estimates for 468 terminally ill patients at the time of hospice referral into five different home hospices. Accuracy was defined as being within 33% of the patient's actual survival. The median survival for those patients was 24 days. Only 20% of the physicians' predictions were accurate. Sixty-three percent of the survival estimates were overly optimistic and 17% were overly pessimistic. The physicians tended to overestimate survival even up to a factor of 5. More experienced physicians tended to be more accurate. Predictions were inaccurate both for patients with cancer or nonmalignant disease. An interesting fact was that the longer a physician knew his or her patient, the less likely he or she was to correctly predict prognosis. On the one hand, it might be expected that the better a physician knew his or her patients, the better sense the physician should have of how sick that patient really is and how

938

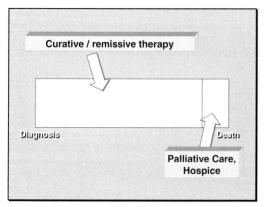

FIGURE 76.1. Traditional model of patient care. (Modified from Plenary 3: elements and models of end-of-life care: the Education in Palliative and End-of-Life Care (EPEC) Curriculum: EPEC Project, 1999, 2003.)

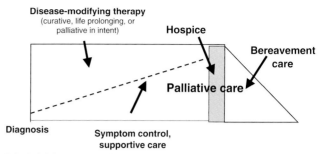

FIGURE 76.2. Current model of patient care. (From Plenary 3: elements and models of end-of-life care: the Education in Palliative and End-of-Life Care (EPEC) Curriculum: EPEC Project, 1999, 2003.)

much time she may have to live. However, what seems to be actually true is that the better a physician knows a patient, the more optimistic he or she will try to be, even subconsciously, about the patient's likely outcome.

There are some guidelines to help physicians determine a patient's prognosis to enable physicians to impart appropriate information to the patient and family regarding the need for making decisions that are necessary at the end of life. These decisions include resuscitation status, resolution of financial issues and finalization of wills, and attention to relationships that may need tending to in the patient's life. Much information exists in the literature regarding survival data for patients with metastatic cancer. The average survival duration for women treated for metastatic breast cancer is approximately 24 months, but it can range from a few months to many years (6).

Brain metastases occur in 25% to 35% of patients with cancer, and more commonly in those with breast or lung cancer. This confers a very poor prognosis. Without radiation, median survival is 1 to 2 months. With radiation, survival may be prolonged to 3 to 6 months (7). Historically, the 1-year survival has been only 20%. For patients with poor Karnofsky performance status, median survival is only 2.3 months. Radiation therapy can confer relief of symptoms such as headache, weakness, seizures, and mental status changes. However, patients also have to endure the side effects of the treatment, such as profound fatigue and anorexia or nausea.

Meningeal carcinomatosis also portends a poor prognosis. Breast cancer is the solid tumor most commonly associated with leptomeningeal metastases (8). Untreated, median survival is 4 to 6 weeks. Intrathecal chemotherapy or radiation of the neuraxis can slightly improve median survival to 12 weeks and palliate symptoms, but the treatment itself can cause neurologic complications, fatigue, and nausea.

Hypercalcemia occurs in 25% of breast cancer patients. Hypocalcemic agents seem to have little effect in decreasing mortality in these patients. However, the physician should be aware that hypercalcemia usually develops as a late complication of cancer, and it has grave prognostic significance (9). Fifty percent of patients with hypercalcemia die within 1 month, and 75% die within 3 months after starting hypocalcemic treatment. Many patients near the end of life do not choose to have their hypercalcemia treated and may opt for supportive care only.

Malignant pleural effusions are associated with a life expectancy of 4 to 12 months (10). Mortality is 54% at 1 month and 84% at 6 months. Survival is approximately 10 months if the pleural effusion is the first sign of the malignancy. However, the tumor type causing the malignant pleural effusion makes a difference in the outcome: breast cancer patients tend to do a

little better, compared to patients with lung cancer or gastric cancer. The American Society of Clinical Oncology Curriculum on Symptom Management states: "Nearly all patients with a malignant pleural effusion are eligible and suitable candidates for hospice referral."

Over the years, several studies have described ways in which symptoms can help us determine how close a patient may be to death. Reuben et al. (11) reported a case series of 1,592 consecutive patients who were assisted in hospice programs. Fourteen symptoms were assessed in those patients, and performance status, the global measure of a patient's functional capacity, was the most important prognostic factor predicting survival. Although symptoms may be interrelated to each other, 5 of these 14 symptoms maintained independent prognostic value in multivariate analysis. They were shortness of breath, dry mouth, anorexia, dysphagia, and weight loss.

Similarly, Vigano et al. (12) reviewed 22 studies that were concerned with prognostic factors in terminal cancer patients. These studies included 7,089 patients whose median survival was 1.8 to 11 weeks. One hundred and thirty-six variables were examined in these reports, and performance status was the predominant predictor. In particular, they found that low performance status is a reliable predictor of short-term survival. In patients enrolled in palliative care programs, Karnofsky performance status score of less than 50 suggested that life expectancy was less than 8 weeks. High Karnofsky performance status scores did not necessarily predict long survival; deterioration could occur unexpectedly and indicated serious worsening of prognosis. The other symptoms that were prognostic for short survival were dyspnea, dysphagia, xerostomia, anorexia, and delirium or cognitive failure, which is very similar to the findings of the previously described study.

Why is prediction of survival difficult? Patients who are becoming debilitated from their illness are frail and their immune systems are compromised, and they can be prone to sudden death from unexpected events such as infection or bleeding. Also, the connection between the mind and body is intangible and difficult for practitioners to fully understand. Many clinicians who work with terminally ill patients consider it possible that to some extent patients can "wait" to die until they have one last visit with a particular loved one. Or, they may "give up" the will to live and die shortly thereafter.

Why is it so important for a physician to try to predict probable length of survival? They owe it to their patients to provide as accurate information as possible so that informed decisions can be made. Patients with optimistic misperceptions of their prognosis request medical therapies most physicians consider futile because they have not been given the sense that these treatments *are* futile. These patients are 8.5 times as likely to request life-extending medical care than patients with more accurate survival estimates (13), and they are also more likely to die in the hospital on mechanical ventilation than those who have a more realistic survival estimate. When patients understand prognostic information, this influences their preferences with respect to cardiopulmonary resuscitation (14).

Physicians also need to be able to estimate when a patient may be eligible for hospice care in order to make a referral at the appropriate time. According to Medicare guidelines, hospice eligibility occurs when a patient is suffering from a chronic disease and estimated survival is 6 months or less if the disease follows its predicted course. Therefore, the treating physician must occasionally step back and reassess a patient's performance status, length of time since diagnosis, response to treatment, and subsequent progression of disease to determine more accurately when it is time to cease chemotherapy and increase supportive care efforts.

 ## HOW AND WHERE PEOPLE DIE

> The relief of suffering and the cure of disease must be seen as twin obligations of a medical profession that is truly dedicated to the care of the sick. Physicians' failure to understand the nature of suffering can result in medical intervention that (though technically adequate) not only fails to relieve suffering but becomes a source of suffering itself.
> —Eric J. Cassel, *The Nature of Suffering and the Goals of Medicine*

More than 90% of patients in the United States say that they want to die at home. However, in 2001, 50% of deaths occurred in the hospital, 23% in nursing homes, and another 23% at home (15).

The SUPPORT (Study to Understand Prognoses and Preferences for Outcomes and Risks of Treatments) trial was a large study that attempted to improve end-of-life decision making and reduce the frequency of a mechanically supported, painful, and prolonged process of dying (16). In this report, 4,301 patients were prospectively observed for 2 years. During this period of observation, documentation was recorded regarding shortcomings in communication, the frequency of aggressive treatment, and the characteristics of hospital deaths. Lack of communication was widespread. For example, only 47% of physicians knew when their patients preferred to avoid cardiopulmonary resuscitation (CPR). Forty-six percent of the do-not-resuscitate (DNR) orders were written within 2 days of death. Aggressive interventions were conducted on many patients: 38% of patients who died spent at least 10 days in an intensive care unit. And disappointingly, for 50% of conscious patients who died in the hospital, family members reported moderate to severe pain at least half the time.

After these observations were made, a 2-year phase II clinical trial was conducted in which 4,804 patients and their physicians were randomized to an intervention group or the control group. These patients were at the end of life, with an overall 6-month mortality rate of 47%. Physicians in the intervention group received estimates of the likelihood of 6-month survival, information on outcomes of cardiopulmonary resuscitation, and functional disability. A specifically trained nurse had multiple contacts with the patient, family, physician, and hospital staff to elicit preferences, improve understanding of outcomes, encourage attention to pain control and facilitate advance care planning and patient–physician communication. Disappointingly, these interventions did not result in improvement in patient–physician communication. Discussion of CPR preferences occurred with 37% of control patients and 40% of intervention patients. There was no difference between groups for the incidence or timing of written DNR orders, physicians'

knowledge of their patients' preferences not to be resuscitated, number of days spent in an intensive care unit receiving mechanical ventilation, or level of reported pain. Therefore, although enhancement of patient–physician communication was advocated as the major method for improving patient outcomes near the end of life, changes in communication were inadequate to change established practices.

As a result of this study, researchers have sought to understand what patients and families really want, need, and expect at the end of life (17). Some areas of concern identified by dying patients are avoiding prolongation of dying, strengthening relationships with loved ones, achieving a sense of control, minimizing burden, and managing pain (18). Other investigators reported that factors considered important by the patient–family unit at the end of life are pain and symptom management, good patient–physician communication, being prepared for what to expect, achieving a sense of completion in life, clear decision making, and being treated as a "whole" person (19).

THE EVOLUTION OF PALLIATIVE CARE

The World Health Organization give the following definition of palliative care: "Palliative care is an approach that improves the quality of life of patients and their families facing the problems associated with life-threatening illness, through the prevention and relief of suffering by means of early identification and impeccable assessment and treatment of pain and other problems, physical, psychosocial, and spiritual" (20). In 1959 Dame Cicely Saunders (21), who is generally considered the founder of the modern hospice movement, wrote her first major manuscript titled "The Management of Patients in the Terminal Stage." At that time, it was the only chapter on this topic in a six-volume series on cancer. However, it was just the beginning of many articles Saunders would write on terminal illness, human suffering, and hospice care. Fortunately, in the years since then, the palliative care movement has gained formal recognition as a specialty within internal medicine and provides guidelines for health practitioners involved in the care of dying patients.

PAIN MANAGEMENT

> Pain is a more terrible lord of mankind than even death itself.
> —Albert Schweitzer

The American College of Physicians published a new set of guidelines in 2008 describing evidence-based interventions to improve palliative care at the end of life (22). The first in the set of five recommendations from the guideline paper is: "In patients with serious illness at the end of life, clinicians should regularly assess patients for pain, dyspnea, and depression." The assessment and treatment approaches for these symptoms are described below.

Pain is experienced to some degree by the majority of cancer patients at the end of life. The concept of "total pain" was first introduced by Saunders, the founder of St. Christopher's Hospice in England (23). She pointed out that physical pain is often entwined with other dimensions of suffering: psychological (depression); social (family estrangement); and spiritual (loss of meaning in life). For example, pain from a metastatic tumor in the abdomen can become more intense and require more pain medication when the patient is experiencing distress over her child who has been arrested for drug abuse. Or, spiritual despair because of regrets over previous actions in the patient's life can worsen the patient's physical and psychological suffering. Although this can be true of all cancer patients at any time, it is particularly common in patients who are nearing death and who may become more introspective while trying to make sense of the meaning of their lives.

In 1982 the World Health Organization developed a global "Program for Cancer Pain Relief" and designated a three-step analgesic ladder for cancer pain: nonopioids for mild pain, mild opioids for intermediate pain, and strong opioids for severe pain (24). A simple visual analog scale can be used to determine the intensity of the pain, in which the patient ranks her pain on a scale of 0 to 10.

Since opioids are the mainstay of therapy for moderate to severe pain at end of life, it is necessary to be familiar with equianalgesic dosing and the possible adverse effects that can occur. The purpose of an equianalgesic table is to provide relative dose information for the health practitioner when it is necessary to change the route of administration of the opioid or when it is necessary to rotate to another opioid altogether. This type of table lists the relative equivalents for various opioids when administered orally or intravenously and the duration of the effect. There are numerous equianalgesic tables available, and while they are generally quite similar to one another, there may be an occasional minor variation in the numbers, depending on the source. Table 76.1 is an example. As shown on this table, if a patient were taking 30 mg of morphine orally every 4 hours and develops nausea and vomiting, it may be necessary to switch the morphine to intravenous administration. The equianalgesic table shows that 30 mg of oral morphine is equivalent to 10 mg of intravenous morphine, or a 3:1 ratio. Therefore, the patient would be given 10 mg of intravenous morphine every 4 hours, and equivalent pain control would be expected.

If a patient were taking morphine 30 mg orally every 4 hours and she develops nightmares that are likely to be related to the morphine, it is reasonable to switch her to another opioid, such as oxycodone. The equianalgesic table shows that the comparable dose of oxycodone would be 20 mg every 4 hours.

The only dose conversion that is somewhat more difficult to list in an equianalgesic table is the relation between the fentanyl transdermal patch and oral opioids. The confusion stems from the fact that the patch is applied every 3 days, yet the fentanyl is actually released into the patient on a microgram-per-hour basis. A simple approach is to consider the ratio between oral morphine and the fentanyl patch to be either 2:1 or 3:1. Therefore, a patient who is taking a total of 100 mg of oral morphine per day may need to be switched to a fentanyl patch because of increasing debility and difficulty swallowing. Using a 2:1 ratio, the correct conversion would be to use a fentanyl patch 50 μg/per hour, applied every 3 days. Using a 3:1 ratio, the proper dosage for the transdermal patch would be 37 μg (this dose could be achieved by applying a 25 μg patch and a 12 μg patch).

Opioid analgesics should be administered on a scheduled basis around the clock, rather than on an as needed basis, for moderate to severe pain. This is typically best achieved with an extended-release opioid preparation. It is also necessary to supply a short-acting, immediate-release opioid to be taken in case pain occurs despite the long-acting medication. In order to calculate dose of the breakthrough medicine, 5% to 15% of the total 24-hour extended-release dose should be prescribed in an immediate release form, typically every 3 to 4 hours as needed. The time to reach maximal serum concentration (C_{max}) of the opioid varies according to the route of administration. Oral morphine can be redosed hourly during a pain crisis; subcutaneous or intramuscular medication can be redosed in 30 minutes, and intravenous opioid should have its maximal effect in 10 minutes. It is no use waiting longer than the time it takes to achieve the C_{max} before repeating the dose of the opioid if the patient's pain is relentless and unrelieved by the previous dose of medication.

If a dose increase is warranted because of increasing pain, this can be done safely in one of two ways. For the patient who has been taking extended-release medication as well as breakthrough medication, the total extra milligrams of opioid taken as breakthrough dosing in a 24-hour period should be added up. That amount should then be added into the extended-release regimen. For example, consider a patient who has been taking extended-release morphine 100 mg twice a day; fluctuating periods of pain throughout the day have required her to take an average of an extra 80 mg of immediate-release morphine over a 24-hour period. This pattern has recurred for several days. The extra 80 mg should be added to the extended-release dosing, by adding an extra 40 mg to each of the twice a day doses. The patient's new dose would be extended-release morphine 140 mg orally twice a day.

If the physician does not have any idea how much extra pain medication the patient has been requiring in the form of breakthrough medication because she has not been keeping track of it, then a 25% to 50% increase is generally a safe increment that may relieve the pain without causing respiratory depression or excessive sedation. "Start low, and go slow" is a general guideline for opioid administration, particularly in elderly or debilitated patients at the end of life.

The possibility of adverse effects resulting from opioid administration must be considered at the time the opioid is being prescribed. The most common adverse effect is constipation, occurring in more than 90% of patients if no prophylaxis is given. Laxatives are the mainstay of prevention of opioid-related constipation. They should be prescribed to be taken automatically, without waiting for constipation to first occur. Senna-containing products are very effective; if they do not work at first, they should be titrated up to the maximum dose before adding another type of agent to relieve constipation. A new agent, methylnaltrexone bromide, has just been approved by the U.S. Food and Drug Administration (FDA) in April 2008. It can help restore bowel function in patients with late-stage, advanced illness who are receiving opioids on a continuous basis to help alleviate their pain. Opioids interfere with normal bowel elimination function by relaxing the intestinal smooth muscles and preventing them from contracting and pushing out waste products. Methylnaltrexone bromide acts by blocking opioid entrance into the cells, thus allowing the bowels to continue to function normally. It is an injectable medication that can be administered as needed, but not to exceed one dose in a 24-hour period. The recommended starting schedule is one dose every other day as needed for patients with late-stage advanced illness.

Another common side effect is opioid-induced nausea, which occurs in approximately one third of patients treated with opioids. The nausea may gradually subside on its own within a week after starting the pain medication and may not require further treatment. However, most patients who experience this side effect prefer to be treated with antinausea medication, such as prochlorperazine, metoclopramide, or dexamethasone.

	Dose (Parenteral)	Dose (Oral)	Duration of Effect (hrs)
Table 76.1 **EXAMPLE OF AN EQUIANALGESIC TABLE**			
Morphine	10	30	4–6
Hydromorphone	1.5	7.5	4–6
Oxycodone	—	20	4–6
Hydrocodone	—	30	4–6

Although patients and physicians are concerned about respiratory depression and "overdose" of opioids, this is in fact a very rare problem. Undertreatment of pain occurs more commonly than overtreatment. If recommended starting dosages are used when initiating therapy in an opioid-naive patient, there is little chance of causing respiratory depression.

The liver conjugates morphine to an active metabolite, morphine-6-glucoronide, which is cleared via the kidneys. At the end of life, it is not uncommon for dehydration to occur, which leads to progressive renal insufficiency. Therefore, it may be necessary to decrease the dose of an opioid in an elderly patient whose liquid intake decreases as she gets sicker to avoid accumulation of active morphine metabolites. If the family notices that the patient is becoming more lethargic, it may be due to the dying process or it may be due to increased effect from a previously tolerated dose of morphine. If this is suspected, it would be reasonable to try to decrease the morphine dose to see if the sensorium improves without compromise of the pain control. If the pain worsens with this maneuver, then it should be increased back to its original dose.

In the last days or weeks of life, many patients cannot swallow very well and stop taking many of their medications orally. Thus, pain medicine that was previously given by mouth must now be delivered via another route. Morphine elixir delivered sublingually can be very effective because the sublingual cavity is rich in blood vessels and is nonkeratinized, thus eliminating an important barrier to drug absorption (25). Even if the patient does not swallow the medication, the morphine can cross the mucosa and enter the systemic circulation directly. This route of administration also avoids hepatic first-pass metabolism and, therefore, potentially increases bioavailability relative to the oral route.

Other methods of drug delivery are also possible. Some oral pain medications can be given as a rectal suppository when the patient stops swallowing. Or severe pain that requires continuous opioid delivery may be treated by intermittent subcutaneous injections or a continuous infusion subcutaneously. There is usually no reason to give pain medication intramuscularly because this is the most painful method, and there is no kinetic advantage over subcutaneous administration. The transdermal method of delivery is useful at the end of life, although patients who are very cachectic have little fatty tissue through which to absorb the medication, and the absorption of the opiate may be erratic with less effective pain control.

Neuropathic Pain

Like pain assessment in any other patient, the type of physical pain syndrome should be established for a terminally ill patient by determining the location, quality, and exacerbating factors of the pain. Nociceptive pain is typically treated with acetaminophen, nonsteroidal anti-inflammatory medications and opioids. Neuropathic pain is characterized by a burning, stinging, or shooting quality and may be experienced by patients who have been treated with chemotherapy regimens containing cisplatin or paclitaxel or whose tumor involves the brachial plexus or has impinged directly on a nerve. This pain is usually treated with opioids, in conjunction with adjuvant medications such as anticonvulsants, antidepressants, or corticosteroids.

Some of the initial work in the pharmacologic management of neuropathic pain utilized tricyclic antidepressants. Amitriptyline was identified as being an effective agent for patients with diabetic neuropathy, but the anticholinergic side-effect profile limited its use in some patients, particularly the elderly. Nortriptyline (100 to 150 mg at bedtime) or desipramine (100 to 300 mg at bedtime) is somewhat better tolerated and also affords some relief of burning neuropathic pain. However, more recently anticonvulsants have been used for these patients with good relief and with a generally better side-effect profile. Gabapentin is currently indicated for the treatment of postherpetic neuralgia, but it also has been used in palliative care settings for the relief of neuropathic pain related to cancer or chemotherapy. Pregabalin is a newer medication currently approved for neuropathic pain associated with diabetic neuropathy or postherpetic neuralgia and is also effective for cancer-related neuropathy.

Bone Pain

Bone metastases occur in many women with advanced breast cancer and can lead to deterioration of quality of life. Bisphosphonates have been recommended for the management of bone pain as well as the prevention of skeletal complications in patients with metastatic bone disease (26,27). The use of bisphosphonates in a study of breast cancer patients resulted in improved quality of life compared with that of patients not using bisphosphonates (28). In that study, changes in quality of life and bone pain due were assessed in 466 women who were randomized to receive placebo or two different doses of ibandronate, a third-generation bisphosphonate. Bone pain, functional status (physical, emotional, and social), fatigue, and overall global status were improved for patients receiving the higher dose of the bisphosphonate. The medication was a well-tolerated palliative treatment.

The bisphosphonates most frequently used in general clinical practice are clodronate, pamidronate, and zoledronic acid. The second recommendation in the American College of Physicians' palliative care guidelines is: "In patients with serious illness at the end of life, clinicians should use therapies of proven effectiveness to manage pain. For patients with cancer, this includes nonsteroidal anti-inflammatory drugs, opioids, and bisphosphonates." A summary of pain management is given in Table 76.2.

PALLIATIVE SEDATION

> I will tell him, the doctor, that he must think of something else. It's impossible, impossible, to go on like this.
> —Leo Tolstoy, *The Death of Ivan Ilyich*

In general, pain and many symptoms can be adequately managed in most dying patients. However, occasionally a patient may experience physical pain or suffering in all its domains that is refractory to standard palliative measures. Rarely, a patient's pain near the end of life may escalate out of control, despite the liberal and judicious use of pain medications, aggressive treatment of the opioid side effects, consultation with interventional pain specialists, psychosocial therapy, and nonpharmacologic measures. No matter how well controlled pain and symptoms may have been for most of the patient's illness, if she dies in severe pain and distress, that is what the family will remember, and it will be a "bad" death. In a situation like this, relief of symptoms may prevail over all other considerations, including maintenance of consciousness. Palliative sedation may afford a more comfortable and dignified death.

What is palliative sedation? Palliative sedation is an option of last resort when all efforts to control symptoms have failed (29). According to the American Academy of Hospice and Palliative Medicine, it is the use of sedating medications intended to decrease a patient's level of consciousness to mitigate the experience of suffering, but not to hasten the end of life. The Hospice and Palliative Nurses Association defines palliative sedation as the monitored use of medications intended to induce varying degrees of unconsciousness, but not death, for relief of refractory and unendurable symptoms in imminently dying patients.

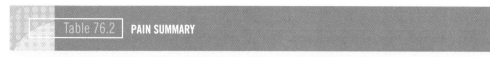

Table 76.2	**PAIN SUMMARY**

Assess total pain: physical, spiritual, psychological.

Physical pain intensity assessment: Visual analog scale (rank pain on a scale of 0 to 10)

Mild: 1–3	**Moderate: 4–6** Codeine,	**Severe: 7–10** Morphine,
Non-opioids: NSAID's, acetaminophen	hydrocodone	hydromorphone, oxycodone, fentanyl

Principles of opioid therapy:
- Extended-release opioid around the clock.
- Immediate-release opioid for breakthrough pain as needed (dose is 5%–15% of the 24-hour extended-release dose)

Use equianalgesic table for:
- conversion between oral and parenteral administration of opioids
- conversion between two different opioid preparations

Opioid side effects
- Constipation: prevention with stimulant laxatives
- Nausea: treat with antinausea medications

Routes of administration: other routes are possible if patient stops swallowing
- Transdermal
- Transmucosal
- Rectal

Physical pain quality assessment: nociceptive vs. neuropathic (described as burning, stinging, electrical, hot, cold). If neuro pathic, consider anticonvulsants, antidepressant

Bone metastases: treat with bisphosphonate

Typically, a medication such as a benzodiazepine or a barbiturate is used as the sedating agent. Examples include midazolam, lorazepam, or phenobarbital. A bolus is administered intravenously or subcutaneously, followed by a continuous infusion or scheduled intermittent maintenance dosing. The purpose of the medication schedule is to have the patient sleep and have relief of her suffering. If she is very close to death, it is possible to continue the sedation until death comes. After the patient's death, some may raise the question whether the sedating medications contributed to and perhaps even caused the death. The answer is that the sedating medication was administered only to achieve the level of sedation that would relieve the suffering. The patient was dying already, and that natural course of dying continued to take place. The intent of the action of administering sedation is explained in the concept of *double effect*.

The doctrine of double effect was developed by the Roman Catholic Church, dating back to the 16th century. It is acknowledged that it may be impossible to avoid all potentially harmful actions, and one may be preferable to another. For example, the more harmful action may be letting a patient die in unbearable suffering, and the less harmful action may be administering medication to allow her to sleep until death, without intent of hastening her death. Double effect is intrinsic to the distinction between assisted suicide and terminal sedation. Four conditions should be present (30,31):

1. The nature of the act must be good or morally neutral (administration of medication to relieve pain).
2. The secondary untoward effect (possible death) must not be the means to accomplish the primary goal, which is relief of suffering.
3. There must be proportionality between the intended primary effect and the unintended but foreseen secondary effect. With palliative sedation, proportionality is established by the terminal condition of the patient, the urgent need to relieve suffering, and the consent of the patient or proxy.
4. There must be no less harmful option for achieving the goal of relieving suffering. Of course, informed consent is considered essential, and palliative sedation is only initiated after a frank discussion with the patient and/or surrogate decisionmaker.

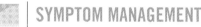

SYMPTOM MANAGEMENT

Dyspnea

Dyspnea is a frequent symptom in patients with advanced illness, and it has documented prognostic value. Patients describe this very distressing symptom as air hunger, suffocating, or choking and is of course very distressing (32). There are many reasons why women with breast cancer may experience dyspnea near the end of life. The cancer itself can cause this symptom due to extensive lung metastases, pleural effusions, pericardial effusion, lymphangitic spread, or pulmonary embolism. Treatment for the cancer may result in inflammation or fibrosis of the lung: this can be a long-term side effect of radiation, particularly if the field includes a moderate to large portion of the lungs. However, there are also a certain number of patients who simply experience a sensation of breathlessness in the last few weeks of life without an obvious identifiable cause. A component of anxiety can certainly exacerbate the sensation of shortness of breath. Treatments directed to the specific cause of the dyspnea should be given if they are available. Corticosteroids can be tried for radiation pneumonitis or carcinomatous lymphangitic spread in the lungs. Bronchodilators can be used if there is a component of bronchospasm. However, no matter what the cause, there are general principles of assessment and treatment that should also be applied.

The only reliable measure of shortness of breath is patient self-report. Patients may complain of dyspnea, with normal objective measures of respiratory function. When oxygenation is measured with pulse oximetry, the results may show an oxygen saturation of 90% or higher, yet the patient is clearly uncomfortable and in need of palliation. Arterial blood gas results also do not always correlate with the patient's level of distress, and so the symptom must simply be believed because the patient reports it (33).

There are three components to dyspnea:

1. A central mechanism, based in the respiratory center in the medulla, which coordinates the diaphragm and intercostal muscles;

2. A peripheral mechanism involving the muscles and blood vessels; and
3. An emotional overlay in which fear, worry, and panic can magnify the discomfort of the symptom.

Of course the first obligation is to treat the underlying cause of the dyspnea if possible. However, if the cancer itself has caused the dyspnea, and chemotherapy or radiation has been ineffective, then the primary palliative intervention for the patient is symptomatic management to improve the oxygenation or relieve the sensation of shortness of breath. The cornerstones of treatment are oxygen and opioids. Although there are minimal data to support the effectiveness of anxiolytics in the treatment of dyspnea, these agents have some success in patients who have a high component of anxiety. Opioids themselves are not anxiolytic, particularly when used on a chronic basis. Nonpharmacologic interventions are also useful to restore a sense of adequacy of air intake and calmness.

Oxygen

A therapeutic trial of oxygen is necessary, regardless of whether or not hypoxemia has been documented by pulse oximetry. Unfortunately, many insurance companies will not pay for the oxygen supply unless there is verification that the patient's oxygen saturation is less than a predetermined level: for example, in the low to mid-80s. Oxygen is expensive. Concentrators can cost $240 to $450 per month, a regulator can cost $15 to $80 per month, with an additional charge of $15 per oxygen tank. One of the benefits of hospice insurance coverage is that the oxygen can be provided to the patient for the palliation of dyspnea without numerical proof of hypoxemia. After the oxygen is initiated, pulse oximetry may or may not be helpful in assessing response. The best assessment of response is the patient's self-report regarding whether she perceives relief.

Opioids

Opioids are another cornerstone of palliation of dyspnea (2). This class of drugs can relieve dyspnea without a measurable effect on the respiratory rate or blood gas. It is possible that oxygen consumption may be decreased, or that the perception of dyspnea is altered and improved. Many health practitioners think of morphine as the primary opioid for the treatment of dyspnea, and while it is an excellent choice, other medications in the same class can be used. Table 76.3 lists some typical starting doses for opiate therapy, which is actually very similar to the starting doses for pain therapy. If the patient is elderly, a 10% to 30% lower dose should be used for initiation of treatment. If adjustments are required to give better relief, titrations should be made more slowly for patients with severe pulmonary disease to ensure that they tolerate the medication. If the patient is already on a fixed schedule of an opioid for pain, add a short-acting opioid equivalent to 30% to 50% of the baseline opioid taken over 4 hours and give it every hour as needed. For instance, if the patient is already taking morphine 20 mg every 4 hours as needed for pain, it would be reasonable to use 5 to 10 mg every hour as needed for severe shortness of breath. Of course, the patient would have to be monitored for sedation and other side effects after these medication changes were being made.

Nebulized morphine is of interest because there are many opioid receptors in the lungs, and so theoretically direct delivery of morphine to the lung might be able to induce relief of dyspnea without the side effects typical of systemic morphine. It could be used relatively easily in hospice and does not require the patient to swallow or have an intravenous catheter. Several trials have been reported, although most of them have been quite small. In a relatively recent trial 11 patients were initially treated with either subcutaneous morphine or nebulized morphine, and then crossed over to the other treatment so that they served as their own control. No difference was found between the two interventions. Within 30 minutes, both modalities provided relief as measured on a scale of 0 to 10, but neither was superior (34). Currently, there is no evidence to support the use of nebulized morphine for the relief of dyspnea (35). If the patient does experience relief from a nebulized treatment, it may be the result of the nebulized humidity itself, with or without the morphine.

The clinical practice guideline published by the American College of Physicians for improvement in palliative care specifically addressed dyspnea. In its assessment of dyspnea, the college noted that 13 studies show a valuable effect of morphine for dyspnea, but nebulized opioids compared with oral opioids showed no additional benefit.

Nonpharmacologic Interventions

Nonpharmacologic approaches can also help terminally ill patients gain the sense that they are breathing more easily (36). A fan should be at the patient's bedside so that she can experience the flow of cool air, which can eliminate the sensation of stuffiness or smothering. The air movement stimulates the V2 branch of the fifth cranial nerve, inhibiting the sensation of breathlessness. The head of the bed should be raised or numerous pillows placed behind her to prop her up. The temperature in the room should be reduced slightly, without chilling the patient, because heat and stuffiness can exacerbate the sensation of shortness of breath. Light and an aura of space can also improve how the patient feels. If possible, the patient's bed should be located near a window or at least have a clear line of vision to a window. If weather permits the window could be open.

As the patient nears death, it is common for many friends and relatives to congregate, but the number of people in the room should be limited for the dyspneic patient to minimize the sensation of being closed in. On the other hand, the presence of a few people can be helpful to alleviate the fright and distress a patient may feel if she is laboring to breathe while she is alone. These interventions may seem obvious, but it is not uncommon for a hospice nurse to receive an urgent call from a dyspneic patient, only to arrive at her house can find her laying flat in bed in a warm, darkened room without a window, crowded with anxious relatives. A few quick changes to the environment can improve the patient's well-being even before oxygen is started or a dose of opioid is given.

The American College of Physicians makes the following recommendation about dyspnea in terminally ill patients: In patients with serious illness at the end of life, clinicians should use therapies of proven effectiveness to manage dyspnea, which include opioids and oxygen for short-term relief of hypoxemia.

Depression

Physicians are not very good at suspecting, identifying, and diagnosing depression (37). Many oncologists think that most

Table 76.3	OPIOIDS FOR PALLIATION OF DYSPNEA

Opiate	Possible Starting Dose
Hydrocodone	5 mg po q 4 hrs
Codeine	30 mg po q 4 hrs
Morphine	5–10 mg po q 4 hrs
Oxycodone	5 mg po q 4 hrs
Hydromorphone	0.5–1 mg po q 4 hrs

patients with a diagnosis of cancer near the end of their lives are bound to be depressed, and so they do not aggressively treat this condition. However, although depression may be a natural reaction to a very difficult situation, this does not mean that treatment would not be helpful. Fifteen percent to 25% of terminally ill cancer patients experience full depression. More than 60% of cancer patients report experiencing distress, and this is highly correlated with a poor quality of life (38).

Treatment of depression is both pharmacological and non-pharmacological. Pharmacologic interventions include psychostimulants, selective serotonin reuptake inhibitors, and tricyclic antidepressants. For depressed patients who have a very short projected life span, psychostimulants such as methylphenidate or pemoline are used more often than usual because they can have a more immediate effect. Sometimes the improvement in mood can occur even within 24 hours of starting treatment.

Clinicians should consider several things when addressing the patient's depression. Pain control is of utmost importance because uncontrolled pain is a major risk for depression and suicide in terminally ill patients. The physician or nurse should ask their patients about their possible fears of death and dying and find out what concerns they may have regarding what they envision happening to their family after their death. Psychological support can be provided by a member of the health team, whether it is a psychiatrist, psychologist, social worker, hospice personnel, or the oncologist or family practitioner (39).

The American College of Physicians' Clinical Practice Guideline makes this recommendation for patients with depression: In patients with serious illness at the end of life, clinicians should use therapies of proven effectiveness to manage depression. For patients with cancer, this includes tricyclic antidepressants, selective serotonin reuptake inhibitors, or psychosocial intervention (22).

Fatigue

Fatigue is one of the most common and debilitating symptoms experienced by patients with cancer (40). In a study of 763 women who survived breast cancer, 35% reported fatigue 1 to 5 years after treatment, and 34% reported it 5 to 10 years after treatment completion (41). Generally, until the last few days of the patient's life when she may be totally bedridden, patients and families find it very distressing to deal with fatigue so pronounced that even mild social interaction such as quiet conversation may be difficult. Rather than accept this as the inevitable result of terminal disease, it is possible for the health practitioner to recommend some minor interventions that may improve the quality of the patient's life by maximizing what energy she may have. Structured aerobic exercise can lead to better quality of life and less fatigue (42). Patients and their families tend to think that fatigue must be treated with rest. However, a minimal amount of structured exercise, if tolerated, is actually preferable and yields better results. The prescription should be simple, such as walk 20 minutes a day, which would be 10 minutes going out and 10 minutes coming back. By setting realistic goals, the patient may be able to find more energy.

Other coexisting conditions that may cause fatigue should be considered: depression, pain, sleep disorder, severe anemia, medications that may depress the central nervous system, and distressing psychosocial issues. Depending on how close to death the patient appears to be, the physician and patient may or may not decide to add a new medication or intervention. A patient with insomnia or a reversed sleep pattern may want to be treated with a sleeping pill at night in order to be more rested in the morning. An anemic patient who may have several months to live may desire a blood transfusion to maximize her ability to stay as active as possible as long as possible. A patient with many psychosocial concerns who has trouble sleeping and ends up being exhausted most of the time could benefit from counseling with a social worker or psychiatrist.

Medications such as methylphenidate may be administered in small doses to try to combat disease-related fatigue. In summary, the physician must assess for fatigue, evaluate its cause, and offer possible interventions when appropriate in order to maximize the patient's quality of life during the last period of her life.

Anorexia

Near the end of life, anorexia is a very common problem that may reduce a patient's quality of life. Cachexia may occur in up to 80% of patients with advanced cancer (43). An aspect of suffering associated with anorexia that may not be readily obvious is the diminishment of social interactions, especially at mealtime. Interpersonal communication often occurs around the table during a meal, and patients who cannot partake in this can develop a sense of isolation. The anorexia can also lead to fatigue, which just compounds the problem. Instead of being able to join her family at the table during mealtime, even if she does not eat, the patient may prefer to rest on the couch or in bed. Anorexia itself is not really physically uncomfortable. Ninety-seven percent of dying patients who stopped eating experienced either no hunger or hunger only initially (44).

What can the physician do to help the patient deal with anorexia? If the patient is very concerned and wishes to increase her intake, counseling the patient and family about appropriate foods and setting small goals may be helpful. Patients should be advised to eat lightly and avoid protein-rich foods. Many women will find that they have a particular taste aversion or a category of food they cannot tolerate, so the family should be counseled to respect that. Even if a particular food used to be her favorite, physiologic changes near the end of life may mean that she simply cannot eat that food anymore. The family can be educated that the patient is not starving to death. The patient should eat what she can and not be pressured to do more if she cannot.

Some young breast cancer patients who have small children may want very aggressive intervention and request parenteral hyperalimentation. This approach to nutrition does not have a role in advanced cancer care at the end of life. Proinflammatory cytokines are part of a wasting syndrome and lead to failure of artificial feeding interventions. The only rare patient who may benefit is a woman with a hepatic or abdominal metastasis compressing her stomach, causing severe early satiety due to the partial obstruction. If the patient has a short-term goal that she adamantly wants to achieve before dying, such as being present at a special event for her child that will occur in the very near future, a short period of intravenous hydration or hyperalimentation may be considered. But in general, prospective randomized trials failed to show benefit for parenteral alimentation for most cancer patients. A meta-analysis reached the same conclusion for both parenteral and enteral nutrition; neither intervention affected morbidity or mortality (45). The complications of intravenous catheter placement and maintenance must be considered, such as pneumothorax, blood clot, bacteremia, and sepsis. A patient receiving hyperalimentation must have blood tests checked frequently to assess for electrolyte and fluid imbalance, and as the patient gets weaker near the end of life those blood draws can become more distressing.

Few prospective trials have been done to evaluate the benefits of enteral feeding tubes in patients with advanced cancer. However, for the patient who insists on trying to maintain some nutrition, particularly if her prognosis seems to be measured in months rather than weeks or days, a feeding tube has fewer complications, is less expensive, and delivers nutrients in a more physiologic manner. However, the problems it can cause include aspiration, particularly in patients with delayed gastric emptying, diarrhea or constipation, nausea, abdominal cramps, and bloating. Some patients require metoclopramide before each feeding to help with gastric emptying.

Some pharmacologic interventions may help stimulate the appetite. Megestrol acetate has been tested in at least 12 controlled clinical trials for cancer patients and was administered anywhere from 1 to 12 weeks, depending on the study. It can improve appetite and increase caloric intake, which leads to increased body weight (mostly fat). Many patients describe an improved sense of well-being, and sometimes this occurs even without weight gain. In studies of terminally ill patients, lower doses than are typically prescribed (160 to 480 mg per day) can improved appetite, fatigue, and general well-being without causing weight gain (46). For some patients, the benefits of increased appetite may be dose related, with the optimal dose being 800 mg orally each day. However, there are good reasons to try to limit the dose. Side effects of megestrol acetate, although infrequent, are probably dose related, and include deep venous thrombosis (particularly if the patient has a history of thromboembolic disease), peripheral edema, increased glucose in a diabetic, and breakthrough bleeding. The medication can also be expensive, particularly for a hospice. Thus, a reasonable approach would be to start with a lower dose and titrate to response.

Corticosteroids such as dexamethasone, prednisolone, and methylprednisolone have been tested for their effect on appetite in five randomized trials. It has been demonstrated that they can cause increased appetite and food intake, improved sense of well-being, and even improved performance status, although sometimes the effect disappears within 4 weeks (47). Weight gain has typically not been observed. And short-term use of steroids has other benefits that may affect terminally ill patients: suppressing nausea, improving asthenia, and suppressing pain. So, for patients in whom weight gain is not the objective but rather improved sense of well-being, there is a rationale for starting a steroid (typically prednisone or dexamethasone) with a 1-week trial and then tapering off if there is no response. The total daily dose can be given with breakfast or in divided doses after breakfast and lunch, in order to avoid the insomnia that can be associated with evening doses.

Lastly, dronabinol is synthetic THC (tetrahydrocannabinol), which is the active ingredient in cannabis. Its FDA indications are for AIDS-related weight loss and refractory nausea and vomiting secondary to cancer chemotherapy, but can have some benefit for cancer-related anorexia as well (48). Again, these interventions for anorexia at the end of life are typically more appropriate for a patient who is not in her last weeks or days, but rather has the probability of a longer survival and wishes to maximize every aspect of her nutrition.

SPIRITUAL ISSUES

> Do not go gentle into that good night
> Old age should burn and rave at close of day.
> Rage, rage against the dying of the light.
> —Dylan Thomas, *Do Not Go Gentle Into that Good Night*

Spiritual pain or suffering is common, particularly at the end of life. There are several components to this suffering: loss of being, loss of relationships, loss of self, loss of purpose, and awareness of death. However, there is also the possibility of the discovery and realization of a life-affirming and transcending purpose (49). Although medical staff may not feel equipped or knowledgeable to address deep issues of spirituality, it is important to recognize that these issues may rise very strongly to the forefront of a patient's concerns as she comes closer to the end of her life. The topic should at least be brought up and referrals made as appropriate. Chaplain support is one of the key pieces of total patient care offered by a hospice team.

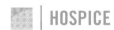

HOSPICE

> What tormented Ivan Ilych most was the deception, the lie, which for some reason they all accepted, that he was not dying but was simply ill, and he only need keep quiet and undergo a treatment and then something very good would result. He however knew that do what they would nothing would come of it, only still more agonizing suffering and death. This deception tortured him—their not wishing to admit what they all knew and what he knew, but wanting to lie to him concerning his terrible condition, and wishing and forcing him to participate in that lie. Those lies—lies enacted over him on the eve of his death and destined to degrade this awful, solemn act to the level of their visitings, their curtains, their sturgeon for dinner—were a terrible agony for Ivan Ilych. And strangely enough, many times when they were going through their antics over him he had been within a hairbreadth of calling out to them: "Stop lying! You know and I know that I am dying. Then at least stop lying about it!" But he had never had the spirit to do it.
> —Leo Tolstoy, *The Death of Ivan Ilych*

Hospice care is a continuation of medical care, consisting of a set of comprehensive services designed to address physical, emotional, and spiritual needs of individuals and their families who face a life-threatening illness. A fundamental point is that hospice care focuses on the patient and family as a unit, and priority is placed on managing pain, symptoms, psychosocial issues, and grief.

The word *hospice* has the same linguistic root as the word hospitality (50). It was originally used to describe a place of shelter for weary and sick travelers returning from religious pilgrimages. In the 19th century, hospices were places where the dying were cared for, often run by religious orders. The modern hospice movement began in the 1970s when Saunders started St. Christopher's Hospice in London. Florence Wald, a former dean of Yale University School of Nursing, started the first U.S. hospice in New Haven, Connecticut, in 1974. In 1982 the federal government began reimbursing for hospice care for Medicare beneficiaries. By 1994 the Health Care Financing Administration (HCFA) reported 1682 Medicare-certified hospices were operating in the United States, serving 20% of dying patients. Of all patients dying of cancer in the United States, only 40% are referred to hospice.

Christakis and Escarce (51) examined the length of hospice enrollment for 6,451 hospice patients. The median survival after enrollment in hospice for these patients was 36 days. Fifteen percent died within 7 days, and 15% lived longer than 6 months. This demonstrates that most patients enter hospice late during the course of their terminal illnesses. This deprives the hospice team of the chance to get to know the patient and family well enough to maximize the quality of the care they are capable of delivering.

Early enrollment in hospice is resisted by some patients and families who may not fully understand its infrastructure. The spouse of a terminally ill breast cancer patient may decline hospice because he feels he is capable of providing the medical care she needs, such as administering medications, helping with her personal care, and assisting her in getting around the house. That is why the interdisciplinary nature of the staff should be emphasized, because the care goes far beyond giving medication or checking blood pressure. A typical hospice staff includes a registered nurse on call 24 hours a day, a social worker, medical director, nurse's aide (who can provide personal care up to 20 hours per week), spiritual counselor, physical therapist, occupational therapist, grief support counselors (who provide ongoing support for at least 13 months after a loss), and volunteers who can sit with the patient so the caregiver can get out of the house. Earlier enrollment may enhance the quality of life for the patient and the cost-effectiveness.

For most patients, hospice care is a benefit covered by their insurance, including Medicare (Part A), Medicaid, Blue Cross/Blue Shield, most health maintenance organizations (HMOs), and most private insurance companies. If a person lacks insurance, many hospices have a "compassionate" fund to provide care, usually as a result of community fund raising.

There are two criteria for admission to hospice care: life expectancy of 6 months or less if the disease continues its normal course, and the patient's choice to change the focus of care from treating the disease to supportive care. Many patients seem to think that enrolling in hospice somehow ensures that they will die in 6 months. It is important to explain to the patient and family that the 6-month criterion is an artificial guideline established by Medicare, and many patients who are hospice appropriate live longer than 6 months. It is impossible for physicians to be accurate for each patient's true prognosis, particularly for breast cancer, which has a wide range of biological behavior, from aggressive to indolent. Consequently, initial hospital enrollment is for one 90-day certification period, and then ongoing assessment of prognosis continues. Recertification is required at the end of each period. The first two enrollment periods are effective for 90 days, and then an unlimited number of 60-day renewals are possible. The patient may withdraw from hospice at any time. Some patients change their mind and revoke hospice in order to pursue "curative" treatment.

When enrolling in hospice, the patient signs a statement choosing hospice care instead of routine Medicare-covered benefits. The hospice benefit then pays for the patient's care, equipment, and medications related to the "terminal" diagnosis. Her "nonhospice" health insurance covers treatment for any other health problems that are current or may develop. Patients often express the concern that hospice means "no care" and that simple ailments such as a urinary tract infection will not be treated. However, hospices do treat the patient according to the patient's wishes and within reasonable guidelines and give antibiotics for infections if warranted. Patients who take anticoagulants for thromboembolism or pulmonary embolus are of course continued on that medication, and blood tests are done regularly to check coagulation values.

Besides hospice care in the home, the hospice benefit allows the patient the opportunity to receive 5 days of respite care in a hospital, inpatient hospice, or nursing home. This allows the caregiver to get a break or go out of town if needed and know that the patient is well cared for. A third type of care option for patients whose symptoms are difficult to control in the home setting is general in-patient care. This allows short-term inpatient treatment of recalcitrant symptoms.

There appear to be some possible racial or cultural differences in preferences for care at the end of life (52). In a data analysis of African American and white patients discharged from VITAS Innovative Hospice Care programs over a 4-year period of time, the association between race and discharge disposition defined as hospice revocation to pursue aggressive care (such as emergency medical care, chemotherapy, or invasive medical intervention) versus all other discharges was examined. African American patients had 70% higher odds of leaving hospice to pursue life-prolonging therapies (odds ratio 1.70; 95% confidence interval, 1.57–1.84). In a subgroup analysis of survival 1 year after hospice revocation, 48.4% of the enrollees who revoked hospice to pursue life-prolonging therapies were still alive.

It is possible that differences in care choices at the end of life may also be socioeconomic: higher income people who have had easier access to treatment may be more likely to feel comfortable ending care. Lower income people who may have developed a distrust of the medical system because of financial difficulties getting care paid for may be more reluctant to give up any future options.

Fiscal responsibility is an important factor in all of health care, including hospice care. Medicare pays the hospice a daily rate for each hospice patient, which at the time of this writing is approximately $149 per day for routine care. When a patient is admitted for general inpatient care to take care of acute symptoms, the rate is increased to $660 per day. For the 5 days of respite care, the hospice is reimbursed $151 per day. Therefore, when a hospice patient requests an aggressive or expensive intervention, the hospice administrator and team must consider the request from two vantage points. Philosophically, they must consider whether the treatment is likely to improve the patient's comfort. And second, they simply must consider whether they will be able to bear the extreme expense. Generally, if the intervention is the right thing to do for the patient, the hospice will bear the cost. However, if there are alternate, less-expensive possibilities, the hospice will consider these. For example, a patient who is already on total parenteral nutrition (TPN) may want to enroll in hospice but not give up her intravenous feedings. The TPN costs more than $1,000 per day, which must be balanced against the $149 per day that the hospice will be paid from Medicare. In view of the lack of data for benefit for parenteral nutrition in dying patients and the extraordinary cost, it is fairly rare for a patient to be in hospice with parenteral alimentation. Of course, there may be some exceptions to this general rule.

Another example of an expensive palliative intervention is radiation therapy. Generally, patients have completed this sort of treatment before entering hospice. However, if a new unexpected problem such as spinal cord compression should occur after hospice enrollment, the patient will be referred emergently for radiation therapy to prevent paralysis, if she wishes. The patient's fears should be allayed that hospice does not do nothing if there are palliative interventions available that will improve her quality of life.

It is physicians' responsibility to evaluate patients as they near the end of life to determine hospice appropriateness. Not everyone will wish to enroll in hospice, but it should not be because the subject was never brought up. It is explained to the patient that in this day and age earlier hospice enrollments are encouraged to maximize excellent symptom management and psychosocial interventions. When survival is limited, the patient needs to assess what goals she would like to achieve, if any, before death. For many women, this may include leaving a legacy for their children or families. Members of the hospice staff are attuned to this and can assist the patient in life review. Then she can record those memories in a journal, letter, or scrapbook to leave for her family. Some child life specialists work with the children to help them complete a scrapbook with their mother, which accomplishes two things: the children get the extra time with their mother reviewing memories while they select the photos or art work for the scrapbook, and then the book or letter provides a tangible memory of their life with their mother. Many patients and families state that in retrospect, they wish they had requested hospice sooner.

CHILDREN

A substantial number of patients dying from breast cancer are relatively young, compared to other cancers that tend to affect older patients. Therefore, a good percentage of terminally ill breast cancer patients may have children young enough to still be living at home. Issues related to their care and worry about their psychological reaction to her illness can consume a large part of the mother's time and energy. First, it is wise for the health practitioner to have a discussion with the patient early on regarding whether she has talked to her child at all about her illness. What does she think her child understands about her illness, and does she need help communicating information about her disease? Not uncommonly, the word "cancer" may not have been used yet around the child for fear of frightening him or her. Or, the seriousness of the illness may have been minimized, although the patient is terminally ill and death may come soon.

What do children and teenagers need when a family member is dying? Long before most people realize it, children become aware of death. Many people do not like to talk about things that upset them, and so they hide their feelings and say nothing (53). But they are still communicating, because children are great observers, and when they notice that their parents are avoiding talking about something that is obviously upsetting, they hesitate to bring up the subject themselves or ask questions. They need at least some accurate information about the illness, and the extent to which this is delivered depends on the child's age and maturity. Child life specialists or social workers can often provide the exact language that can be used to talk to children to explain serious illness.

The information might typically include the name of the disease, its location, and the effect that it is having on the patient's body. Reassurance should be given that breast cancer is not contagious. Some children may have magical thinking that they were somehow responsible for their mother or relative getting the cancer because of some bad behavior, thoughts, feelings, or wishes. They need to be reassured that they had nothing to do with the cause of the cancer. Information about treatments such as pain medication is helpful, so that the child can understand why her mother may be more tired or sedated than usual. Most children should be kept updated about the course of events in a simple and straightforward way. Children will imagine things usually even worse than reality if they are not given some information.

If appropriate, children should be encouraged to spend time with the patient if she is strong enough for it. They could even be involved in some minor aspects of her care, such as getting her something to drink or bringing her medications to her. Children derive some benefit and comfort in maintaining their daily routine; they need organization and structure that will preserve the activities that matter most to them (54). They need permission to do some things that they might otherwise be hesitant to do: socialize or play with their friends, ask questions, express their feelings, and talk about death.

Most importantly, children need reassurance that they will continue to be cared for after their mother dies. It can be helpful to answer their questions ahead of time regarding who they will live with or drive them to their events. In the Academy Award winning movie *Terms of Endearment*, a young mother played by Debra Winger has breast cancer and is told by her doctor at one point that there are "no more treatment options" and that she should make appropriate plans for the future. The first thing she says through her tears is that she needs to try to find someone to take care of her children. This concern can override all others, and if a mother is without an obvious caregiver such as a husband, she may need help from the health care team identifying appropriate care for her children.

WHAT IS A GOOD DEATH?

The concept of a "good death" has been contemplated throughout history. The Ars Moriendi, translated from Latin as "art of dying," is a body of Christian literature that provided practical guidance for the dying and those attending them in the early 15th century. These manuals informed the dying about what to expect and prescribed prayers, actions, and attitudes that would lead to a "good death" and salvation. In modern times, the topic continues to carry great interest for patients and health practitioners alike. There can be no single definition of a good death that could include everyone's personal preferences. For instance, for some patients talking

about death is very important because it brings satisfaction and rest. Others do not wish to ever talk about death, or at least not too long; they would rather discuss other things (55). The challenge for the clinician is to come to some understanding of the patient and her wishes so that the right amount of discussion can take place.

End-of-life research has identified some commonalities and themes that seem to hold true for many patients and families. The Institute of Medicine gave its definition in its report on end-of-life care: "A decent or good death is one that is: free from avoidable distress and suffering for patient, families, and caregivers; in general accord with patients' and families' wishes; and reasonably consistent with clinical, cultural, and ethical standards" (56). The principal aim of Saunders and those who worked with her in England was to make the experience of dying better, which meant free of pain and unpleasant symptoms, and relief from the "total pain" caused by physical, spiritual, and psychosocial suffering (57).

The doctor who attends to terminally ill patients must be aware of the patient's loneliness, which becomes one of the most important components of the pain these patients can experience (58). Patients have the knowledge that they are in the last days of their lives, and this can be terrifying because it is a process, it continues for a time. Therefore, some patients wish death to be quick so that they will not have to prolong the experience of being aware that they are dying. And, after all, even a good death is *death*.

An analysis of the concept of a good death was done by a method called concept analysis, in which 42 articles were reviewed (59). There was strong agreement that a good death was highly individual, changeable over time, and based on perspective and experience. They reported that the attributes of a good death, listed in order of frequency of appearance in the literature, were:

1. being in control,
2. being comfortable,
3. sense of closure,
4. affirmation/value of the dying person recognized,
5. trust in care providers,
6. recognition of impending death,
7. beliefs and values honored,
8. burden minimized,
9. relationships optimized,
10. appropriateness of death,
11. leaving a legacy, and
12. family care.

THE LAST DAYS AND HOURS

The care of patients in their last weeks of life is a fundamental palliative care skill (60). One of the most important goals for health care professionals involved in the care of the dying is to ensure that the patient and family are informed and knowledgeable about what may occur during the last weeks, days, and hours of life.

The patient often begins to withdraw from the things and people around her. She may first lose interest in worldly things, such as reading or watching television. Gradually, she may begin to separate herself from people and state that she is too tired for visits from friends and neighbors. Eventually, she may want limited contact even with some family members. If the family has not been educated about this common phenomenon ahead of time, they may feel rejected and left out. But this separation process is commonly seen, as the dying patient sleeps more and spends more time internally.

Communication will decrease, and her eyes will be closed more and more. Some of the time is spent sleeping, but some of the time she may simply be uninterested in talking. She will use fewer words when she does speak. If the patient is on high-dose opioids, this may contribute to some impairment of communication. Of course each patient is different and may not display this behavior, but it would not be unexpected for this type of withdrawal to occur.

Decreased eating is one of the hardest things for families and friends to watch. They often equate poor nutritional intake with starvation, not realizing that the patient stops eating *because* she is dying, not the other way around. Nothing may taste good anymore, and intermittent cravings for certain foods may occur. Liquids may be preferred to solids, which can also be hard for the family to accept because most people consider solid food to be the main source of nutrition. Over time it makes the last days of life easier if the family is not constantly fighting with the patient to eat.

Physical changes occur as the body nears death (61). The blood pressure becomes lower, and the pulse may become either very high or very low. The patient's temperature may become cool. Her skin may be flushed or pale. Her hands and feet may become mottled and bluish. Breathing may increase to a rapid rate or become slow and agonal, often scaring those who are keeping vigil with her. It is difficult for a dying patient to clear her secretions, and so with each breath she may emit a rattling or gurgling sound, called the *death rattle*. This can be treated with anticholinergic medications such as scopolamine or atropine to dry the secretions. Although there is no evidence that patients find this condition disturbing, the noises may be disturbing to the patient's visitors and caregivers who may fear that the patient is choking to death. The death rattle is a good predictor that death is near; one study suggested that the median time from onset of death rattle to death was 16 hours.

Confusion and disorientation occur frequently in the last days of life. The patient may sleep a lot and yet wake easily. She may start talking about someone or something she dreamt about, confusing the dream for reality. She may talk to people who have already died ahead of her. If her confusion increases, she may even become agitated, pick at the blankets, and try to get out of bed. Some patients require sedation to keep them safe from falling or injuring themselves. She may appear to be actively dying, and then she may have a temporary clearing of her sensorium, sitting up and talking with people for the first time in quite a while. She may eat something, and her friends and relatives may hope that she is going to live after all. However, most typically this is a temporary situation and she soon reverts back to her former level of decreased consciousness. Her eyes may be closed, or they may remain open and become glassy.

Terminal delirium can be divided into hyperactive type, with restlessness and agitation, or hypoactive type, with somnolence. If there is a concern that the patient's pain control is poor, then her pain medication should be optimized as the first intervention. Family members are typically advised to stay near the patient's bedside to continually reorient her if she intermittently wakes and is confused. The agitation may need to be treated pharmacologically with a medication such as lorazepam (62). If she cannot tolerate or has a paradoxical reaction to a benzodiazepine, then a neuroleptic medication such as haloperidol can be used (63).

GUIDANCE FOR CAREGIVERS

The National Cancer Institute provides some guidance to caregivers regarding ways that they can provide emotional comfort to the dying patient they are taking care of (64). The guideline points out that patients have fear of abandonment and fear of being a burden. They are concerned about loss of dignity and loss of control. Therefore, caregivers can provide comfort in the following ways:

- Keep the person company; talk, watch movies, read, or just be with the person.
- Allow the person to express fears and concerns about dying. Be prepared to listen.
- Be willing to reminisce about the person's life.
- Avoid withholding difficult information. Most patients prefer to be included in discussions about issues that concern them.
- Reassure the patient that you will honor advance directives.
- Ask if there is anything you can do.
- Respect the person's need for privacy.

The dying individual's final moments can be profound, special, and memorable for the survivors who spend that time with her (65). In some cases this does not occur simply because the family is not present at the time of death or because other medical factors, such as discussion about whether to resuscitate the patient, took place at the time of death. This reinforces the reasons for not hesitating to speak with the patient and family about prognosis and resuscitation issues well ahead of time if possible so that the opportunity for sacred, shared moments between the dying patient and her loved ones at the time of death may occur.

SUMMARY

The role of a health care clinician taking care of a breast cancer patient changes over time. The role does not decrease as the patient's disease progresses and she comes close to the end of her life. The responsibilities of the clinician become more multifaceted and take on a different focus. Communication takes on a new importance as the issues being discussed become more emotionally complicated in nature. The physician owes it to the patient to make a reasonable judgment about prognosis and convey that to her so she has the opportunity to take care of unfinished business in her life, which may involves such areas a relationships, finances, and advance planning. The patient's wishes for resuscitation efforts must be discussed and documented, the earlier the better. Pain is a common problem, and so good pain management skills are essential. The extreme frequency of other nonpain symptoms at the end of life ensure that the review of systems will almost certainly identify a substantial number of issues that require pharmacologic or psychosocial intervention. When appropriate, hospice should be introduced to the patient as early as possible. This allows the multidisciplinary hospice team to have the chance to get to know the patient and family in order to provide the best possible care for the physical, psychosocial, and spiritual needs of the patient and family unit. The doctor–patient relationship should never be abandoned because the patient has come close to her time of death. For the physician, this is a time rich with the possibility of improving the quality of the patient's life and the quality of her death.

MANAGEMENT SUMMARY

- Treatment of a breast cancer patient nearing the end of life is a continuum of active and palliative care. Anticancer options may start declining while the need for symptom management and psychological support begins to increase.
- Typically doctors are poor prognosticators of life expectancy, but hospice regulations require a survival estimate of 6 months of life or less. Poor prognostic

features in breast cancer patients include brain metastases, meningeal carcinomatosis, hypercalcemia, and malignant pleural effusion.

- Pain management is extremely important for end-of-life care. Total pain should be assessed, which includes physical, psychological, and spiritual suffering. This is best achieved through a multidisciplinary team if available.

- Physical pain should be assessed and diagnosed as nociceptive or neuropathic. For both types, opioids are the mainstay of treatment. However, if the pain is neuropathic, adjuvant medications should also be considered. These include anticonvulsants (gabapentin or pregabalin), antidepressants (nortriptyline, desipramine), and corticosteroids.

- Extended-release opioids should be administered around the clock, and an immediate release opioid (5% to 15% of the total 24-hour scheduled dose) should be prescribed for use on an as needed basis for breakthrough pain.

- The health practitioner should be familiar with the use of an equianalgesic table to facilitate changing routes of opioid administration or to calculate dosage when it is necessary to change from one opioid to another.

- Common opioid side effects include constipation and nausea, and both should be treated preventively. Respiratory depression is rare and can be avoided by avoiding sudden, large increases in the opioid dose.

- Bone metastases are frequent, and treatment should include a bisphosphonate such as clodronate, pamidronate, or zoledronic acid.

- Breast cancer patients near the end of life must be frequently assessed for symptoms. Some of the most common symptoms are dyspnea, depression, fatigue, and anorexia.

- Dyspnea is best evaluated by the patient's report or breathlessness, rather than depending on measurement of her oxygen level. Treatment includes oxygen, opioids, and nonpharmacologic interventions.

- Depression is extremely common and should be asked about during clinic visits. Antidepressants, psychostimulants, and psychological support should be offered.

- Fatigue should be treated with moderate structured exercise if possible, insomnia medication, and a mild psychostimulant may be helpful.

- Anorexia is very common and perhaps the most difficult symptom for family members to deal with. The family will require psychological and educational support if they are concerned that the patient is starving to death. Pharmacologic interventions are available for those who want them: megestrol acetate, corticosteroids, or dronabinol.

- Hospice care is a set of comprehensive services for the patient–family unit who face a life-threatening illness. Two requirements are an estimated prognosis of 6 months or less and the patient's desire for supportive care only. Early hospice referral allows the multidisciplinary team to provide optimal care.

- The children of breast cancer patients need to be given information about the medical situation. Depending on their age, children should be encouraged to spend time with the patient, and they should be reassured about what will happen to them after the patient dies. Because dying mothers often find it difficult to bring up this topic to their children, the health practitioner should try to help facilitate this communication.

- The last days and hours of life often need intense symptom management. The family can benefit from education regarding what to expect: the dying patient may withdraw from talking and eating, and confusion and disorientation are possible. Physical changes include low blood pressure, slow or rapid pulse, and cool extremities.

- Caregivers for dying patients should be given guidance regarding how best to care for the patient. They often need psychological support themselves because of the difficulties and intensity of the caregiver role.

References

1. SEER cancer statistics review, 1975–2003. Available at http://seer.cancer.gov/csr/1975_2003/.
2. National Institutes of Health State-of-the-Science Conference Statement on Improving End-of-Life Care. December 6–8, 2004. Available at http://consensus.nih.gov/2004/2004EndOfLifeCareSOS024html.htm.
3. Lorenz KA, Lynn J, Dy SM, et al. Evidence for improving palliative care at the end of life: a systematic review. *Ann Intern Med* 2008;148:147–159.
4. Vigano A, Dorgan, M, Bruera E, et al. The relative accuracy of the clinical estimation of the duration of life for patients with end of life cancer. *Cancer* 1999;86:170–176.
5. Christakis NA, Lamont EB. Extent and determinants of error in doctor's prognoses in terminally ill patients: prospective cohort study. *BMJ* 2000;320:469–472.
6. Gennari A, Conte P, Rosso R, et al. Survival of metastatic breast carcinoma patients over a 20-year period. *Cancer* 2005;104:1742.
7. Weissman DE. Determining prognosis in advanced cancer. Fast fact and concept 13. 2nd ed. July 2005. End-of-Life Palliative Education Resource Center. Available at www.eperc.mcw.edu.
8. Lin NU, Bellon JR, Winer EP. CNS metastases in breast cancer. *J Clin Oncol* 2004;22:3608–3617.
9. National Cancer Institute. Hypercalcemia. Available at http://www.cancer.gov/cancertopics/pdq/supportivecare/hypercalcemia/healthprofessional.
10. Burrows C, Mathews WC, Colt HG. Predicting survival in patients with recurrent symptomatic malignant pleural effusions: an assessment of the prognostic values of physiologic, morphologic, and quality of life measures of extent of disease. *Chest* 2000;117:73–78.
11. Reuben DB, Mor V, Hiris J. Clinical symptoms and length of survival in patients with terminal cancer. *Arch Intern Med* 1988;148:1586–1591.
12. Vigano A, Dorgan M, Buckingham J, et al. Survival prediction in terminal cancer patients: a systematic review of the medical literature. *Palliat Med* 2000;14:363–374.
13. Weeks JC, Cook EF, O'Day SJ. Relationship between cancer patients' predictions of prognosis and their treatment preferences. *JAMA* 1998;279:1709–1714.
14. Murphy DJ, Burrows D, Santilli S, et al. The influence of the probability of survival on patient's preferences regarding CPR. *N Engl J Med* 1994;330:545–549.
15. Brown Atlas of Dying. Available at http://www.chcr.brown.edu/dying/brownatlas.htm.
16. The SUPPORT principal investigators. A controlled trial to improve care for seriously ill hospitalized patients: the study to understand prognoses and preferences for outcomes and risks of treatments (SUPPORT). *JAMA* 1995;274:1591–1598.
17. Collins LG, Parks SM, Winter L. The state of advance care planning: one decade after SUPPORT. *Am J Hospice Palliat Med* 2006;23:378–384.
18. Singer PA, Martin DK, Lavery JV, et al. Reconceptualizing advance care planning from the patient's perspective. *Arch Intern Med* 1998;158:879–884.
19. Steinhauser KE, Clipp EC, McNeilly M, et al. In search of a good death: observations of patients, families, and providers. *Ann Intern Med* 2000;132:825–832.
20. Sepulveda C, Marlin A, Yoshida T, et al. Palliative care: the World Health Organization's global perspective. *J Pain Symptom Manage* 2002;24:91–96.
21. Saunders C. The management of patients in the terminal stage. In: Raven R, ed. *Cancer*. vol. 6. London: Butterworth and Company, 1960:403–417.
22. Qaseem A, Snow V, Shekelle P, et al. Evidence-based interventions to improve palliative care of pain, dyspnea, and depression at the end of life: a clinical practice guideline from the American College of Physicians. *Ann Intern Med* 2008;148:141–146.
23. Clark D. "Total pain," disciplinary power and the body in the work of Cicely Saunders 1958–1967. *Soc Sci Med* 1999;49:727–736.
24. Clark D. From margins to centre: a review of the history of palliative care in cancer. *Lancet Oncol* 2007;8:430–438.
25. Reisfield GM, Wilson GR. Rational use of sublingual opioids in palliative medicine. *J Palliat Med* 2007;10:465–475.
26. National Cancer Institute. Pain: pharmacologic management. 2008. Available at http://www.cancer.gov/cancertopics/pdq/supportivecare/pain/HealthProfessional/page4.
27. Ripamonti C, Fulfaro F. Malignant bone pain: pathophysiology and treatments. *Curr Rev Pain* 2000;4:187–196.
28. Diel IJ, Body JJ, Lichinitser MR, et al. Improved quality of life after long-term treatment with the bisphosphonate ibandronate in patients with metastatic bone disease due to breast cancer. *Eur J Cancer* 2004;40:1704–1712.
29. Fabbro ED, Reddy SG, Walker P, et al. Palliative sedation: when the family and consulting service see no alternative. *J Palliat Med* 2007;10:488–492.
30. Lo B, Rubenfield G. Palliative sedation in dying patients. *JAMA* 2005;294:1810–1816.
31. Boyle J. Medical ethics and double effect: the case of terminal sedation. *Theor Med Bioethics* 2004;25:51–60.
32. Fabbro ED, Dalal S, Bruera E. Symptom control in palliative care. Part III: dyspnea and delirium. *J Palliat Med* 2006;9:422–437.
33. Coyne PJ, Viswanathan R, Smith TJ. Nebulized fentanyl citrate improves patients' perception of breathing, respiratory rate, and oxygen saturation in dyspnea. *J Pain Symptom Manage* 2002;23:157–160.
34. Bruera E, Sala R, Spruyt O, et al. Nebulized versus subcutaneous morphine for patients with cancer dyspnea: a preliminary study. *J Pain Symptom Manage* 2005;29:613–618.
35. National Cancer Institute. Supportive care in cancer, dyspnea. Available at http://www.cancer.gov/cancertopics/pdq/supportivecare/cardiopulmonary/HealthProfessional.
36. LeGrand SB, Walsh D. Palliative management of dyspnea in advanced cancer. *Curr Opin Oncol* 1999;11:250.
37. Emanuel, EJ. Depression, euthanasia, and improving end-of-life care. *J Clin Oncol* 2005;23:6456–6458.

38. Portenoy RK, Thaler, HT, Kornblith AB, et al. Symptom prevalence, characteristics and distress in a cancer population. *Qual Life Res* 1994;3:183–189.

39. Block SD. Assessing and managing depression in the terminally ill patient. *Ann Intern Med* 2000;132:209–218.

40. Hofman M, Ryan JL, Figueroa-Moseley CD, et al. Cancer-related fatigue: the scale of the problem. *Oncologist* 2007;12[Suppl]:4–10.

41. Bower JE, Ganz PA, Desmon KA, et al. Fatigue in long-term breast carcinoma survivors: a longitudinal investigation. *Cancer* 2006;106:751–758.

42. Mustian KM, Morrow GR, Carroll JK, et al. Integrative nonpharmacologic behavioral interventions for the management of cancer-related fatigue. *Oncologist* 2007; 12[Suppl]:52–67.

43. Fabbro ED, Dalal S, Bruera E. Symptom control in palliative care. Part II: cachexia/anorexia and fatigue. *J Palliat Med* 2006;9:409–421.

44. McCann RM, Hall WJ, Groth-Junker A. Comfort care for terminally ill patients: the appropriate use of nutrition and hydration. *JAMA* 1994;272:1263–1266.

45. Lipman TO. Clinical trials of nutritional support in cancer. Parenteral and enteral therapy. *Hematol Oncol Clin North Am* 1991;5:91–102.

46. Loprinzi CL, Micholok JC, Schaid DJ, et al. Phase III evaluation of four doses of megestrol acetate as therapy for patients with cancer anorexia and/or cachexia. *J Clin Oncol* 1993;11:762–767.

47. Popiela T, Lucchi R, Giongo F. Methylprednisolone as an appetite stimulant in patients with cancer. *Eur J Cancer Clin Oncol* 1989;25:1823–1829.

48. Walsh D, Nelson K, Mahmoud FA. Established and potential therapeutic applications of cannabinoids in oncology. *Support Care Cancer* 2003;11:137–143.

49. Millspaugh D. Assessment and response to spiritual pain, parts I and II. *J Palliat Med* 2005;8:919–923, 1110–1117.

50. National Hospice and Palliative Care Organization. History of hospice. Available at www.nhpco.org.

51. Christakis NA, Escarce JJ. Survival of Medicare patients after enrollment in hospice programs. *N Engl J Med* 1996;335:172–178.

52. Johnson KS, Kuchibhatla M, Tanis D, et al. Racial differences in hospice revocation to pursue aggressive care. *Arch Intern Med* 2008;168:218–224.

53. Talking to children about death. Patient information publications. Bethesda, MD: Clinical Center National Institutes of Health, 2006.

54. The critical need to communicate effectively with the children of cancer patients. *J Support Oncol* 2006;4:75–76.

55. Goldsteen M, Houtepen R, Proot IM, et al. What is a good death? Terminally ill patients dealing with normative expectations around death and dying. *Patient Educ Counsel* 2006;64:378–386.

56. Field MJ, Cassel CK. *Approaching death: improving care at the end of life*. Washington, DC: National Academy Press, 1997.

57. Walters G. Is there such a thing as a good death? *Palliat Med* 2004;18: 404–408.

58. Aitini E, Cetto GL. Editorial: a good death for cancer patients: still a dream? *Ann Oncol* 2006;17:733–734.

59. Kehl KA. Moving toward peace: an analysis of the concept of a good death. *Am J Hospice Palliat Care* 2006;23:277–286.

60. Plonk WM, Arnold RM. Terminal care: the last weeks of life. *J Palliat Med* 2005;8: 1042–1054.

61. Moneymaker KA. Understanding the dying process: transitions during final days to hours. *J Palliat Med* 2005;8:1079.

62. Ferris FD, von Gunten CF, Emanuel LL. Competency in end-of-life care: last hours of life. *J Palliat Med* 2003;6:605–613.

63. Emanuel L, Ferris FD, von Gunten C, et al. The last hours of living: practical advice for clinicians. Available at http://www.medscape.com/viewprogram/5808. Adapted from EPEC-O: education in palliative and end-of-life care for oncology, Module 6: last hours of living. The EPEC Project, Chicago, IL, 2005.

64. National Cancer Institute. End-of-life care: questions and answers, Question 3. Available at http://www.cancer.gov/cancertopics/factsheet/Support/end-of-life-care.

65. Valentine C. The "moment of death." *Omega* 2007;55:219–236.

Chapter 77
Management Summary for Metastatic Disease for the Care of Patients with Metastatic Disease

Marc E. Lippman

Almost without exception, metastatic breast cancer is incurable, and, therefore, the primary goals of therapy are the alleviation of symptoms, the avoidance of complications of disease progression, and the prolongation of quality of life as long as possible. The consequences of a diagnosis of metastatic disease are so life-altering for a patient and her family that formal histologic documentation by biopsy is required in virtually every case. Furthermore, the determination of specific biological markers, which may guide therapy such as estrogen receptor, progesterone receptor, and *ERBB2* (formerly *HER2/neu*) status, provide an additional indication for biopsy. Additional biological data are very likely to result in further refinement of treatment with the increased usage of targeted therapies that will inevitably occur over the next several years.

Local symptoms are often best treated by specific local therapy, which commonly is associated with less toxicity than systemic therapies. Whenever possible, multidisciplinary discussion and review with appropriate team members, including surgeons, radiation oncologists, medical oncologists, and other supportive caregivers, such as skilled oncology nurses, social workers, psychologists, and physical therapists, should be used. As systemic therapy has improved, the role for ablative approaches (such as surgery, stereotactic radiosurgery, stereotactic body radiation therapy, and radiofrequency ablation) to limited metastases in the central nervous system, liver, lung, and spine is expanding. In patients who present with metastatic disease at diagnosis, the role for surgery of the primary tumor is unproven; although retrospective evidence suggests a benefit.

The choice of optimal systemic therapy is rarely limited to a specific option, and a careful balancing of patient expectations, urgency of the need for response, prior therapies and responses previously seen, and values for appropriate biological markers are all important in arriving at reasonable recommendations. In general, endocrine therapies are less toxic than chemotherapies and should be chosen first for patients with a reasonable likelihood of obtaining benefit. In general, sequential single agents have not been shown to be inferior to combinations in most settings and are often better tolerated by patients. The field is rapidly changing and potential combinations of biological agents (e.g., lapatinib and trastuzumab) and chemotherapeutics with either biologic agents such as trastuzumab or bevacizumab are rapidly evolving. Given this, the treating oncologist needs to monitor the literature closely for the latest findings.

Adroit and effective management of symptoms with antiemetics, neuroleptics, antidepressants, and optimal nutritional support is essential and frequently incompletely attended to. Careful review of patient symptomatology is of paramount importance in order to elicit symptoms, including those that patients may be reluctant to discuss. Bisphosphonates are generally warranted in patients with documented metastases to bone.

Chapter 78
Angiogenesis Inhibition in Breast Cancer

Sofyan M. Radaideh, Kathy D. Miller, Bryan P. Schneider, and George W. Sledge, Jr.

Angiogenesis, the process of new vessel formation, is an intricate and multiply redundant process that plays a major role in fetal development, as well as wound healing, endometrial proliferation, and pregnancy in adults. It has also become apparent that this process is vital to both local tumor growth and metastasis (1). Without new vessel formation, tumors cannot grow to more than 2 to 3 mm (2). The angiogenic cascade is divided in two phases: activation and resolution. *Activation* requires degradation of the basement membrane, endothelial cell migration, and invasion of the extracellular matrix, with endothelial cell proliferation and capillary lumen formation. *Resolution* involves maturation and stabilization of the new vasculature by pericytes, with inhibition of further endothelial proliferation, reconstitution of the basement membrane, and junctional complex formation (3). These processes are tightly regulated, and many of the factors involved have been identified.

Tumor angiogenesis differs from physiologic angiogenesis, because it tends to be a disorganized process. The tumoral microvessels frequently lack complete endothelial linings and basement membranes. They are irregular and tortuous, with arteriovenous shunts and blind ends. Blood flow is sluggish, and the tumor-associated capillaries are more permeable than those in normal tissues (4). Tumor angiogenesis offers a new target for cancer therapy, with widespread activity, low potential toxicity, and possibly a synergistic effect when combined with classic cytotoxic therapy and radiotherapy.

TARGETS FOR ANTIANGIOGENIC THERAPY

Many agents have been identified in preclinical studies that may interfere with tumor angiogenesis, and a growing number of these agents have entered clinical trials. Several of these agents have entered phase III trials in breast cancer and other human malignancies, and antiangiogenic therapy now plays an established role in the treatment of human cancer. The agents that specifically target angiogenesis may be grouped into several mechanistic categories: growth factor or receptor pathway antagonists, protease inhibitors, endothelial toxins, and natural inhibitors of angiogenesis.

Vascular Endothelial Growth Factor Antagonists

Vascular endothelial growth factor (VEGF), the best-studied angiogenic factor, has a proven significance in breast cancer. The VEGF/VEGF receptor axis plays a crucial role in vascular endothelial growth, migration, and survival, as well as in lymphangiogenesis (Fig. 78.1). There are many possible ways to target VEGF, and numerous agents have entered into the clinic, for patients with breast cancer. Several potential points of attack

on the interaction of VEGF with its receptor (VEGF-R) are under examination; including blockade of the ligand, the external membrane of VEGF-R, the internal (tyrosine kinase) portion of VEGF-R, VEGF receptor message, downstream intermediates, and indirect inhibition of upstream regulators of VEGF.

Of these approaches, ligand sequestration has been the most thoroughly studied. *Bevacizumab* (Avastin, rhuMAb VEGF) is a recombinant humanized monoclonal antibody that recognizes all known isoforms of VEGF-A. Phase I trials have been conducted with bevacizumab, both as a single agent and in combination with chemotherapeutic agents (5,6). Toxicities reported with bevacizumab (in phase I and subsequent trials) have included rare infusion reactions, hypertension (generally mild, but on occasion requiring therapeutic intervention), proteinuria, arterial and venous thromboembolic phenomena, bowel perforation (predominantly in trials of colon and ovarian cancer), and significant bleeding episodes (when combined with chemotherapy in non–small-cell lung cancer). After initial trials demonstrated safety, a phase II trial of bevacizumab monotherapy was performed in patients with heavily pretreated (anthracycline- and taxane-refractory) metastatic breast cancer (7). This trial demonstrated the ability of bevacizumab to induce both complete and partial remissions in patients with advanced disease, with an additional population of patients undergoing prolonged stabilization of metastatic disease.

Subsequently, a phase III trial was initiated in the refractory metastatic setting. This trial randomized patients with anthracycline- and taxane-refractory metastatic breast cancer to receive either the fluoropyrimidine capecitabine alone or in combination with bevacizumab (8). This trial failed to meet its primary end point of improvement in time to progression. A secondary end point, objective response rate, was significantly increased, confirming the biologic effect seen in the phase II setting.

Heavily pretreated breast cancer may have been the wrong place to test antiangiogenic agents, or indeed any new agent. Tumor progression, with an associated increase in proangiogenic factors produced by breast cancers (9), may render VEGF redundant or irrelevant as a driver of angiogenesis. If timing were an essential element of the angiogenesis cascade, then perhaps blocking this pathway in first-line metastatic disease might show true clinical benefits compared with heavily pretreated disease. This realization led to a second phase III trial, the (E2100) trial, which investigated the role of bevacizumab as a front-line treatment in metastatic breast cancer (10). E2100 trial was a North American Breast Cancer Intergroup led by the Eastern Cooperative Oncology Group, which randomized 722 women with locally recurrent or metastatic breast cancer to receive either paclitaxel alone or paclitaxel plus bevacizumab. In this trial, paclitaxel plus bevacizumab significantly prolonged progression-free survival (the primary end point) as compared with paclitaxel alone (median, 11.8 vs. 5.9 months; $p < .001$) (Fig. 78.2), and increased the objective response rate (36.9% vs.

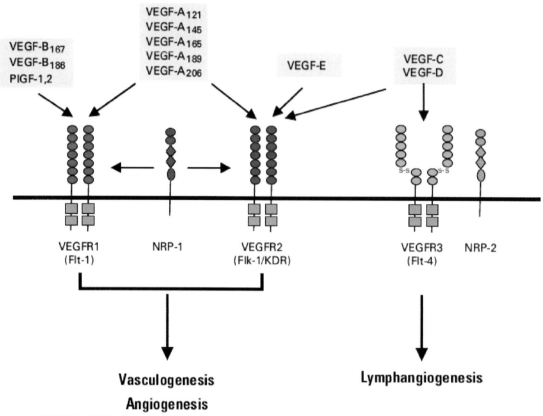

FIGURE 78.1. VEGF family members and their receptors. (From Hicklin DJ, Ellis L. Role of vascular endothelial growth factor pathway in tumor growth and angiogenesis. *J Clin Oncol* 2005;23:1011–1027, with permission.)

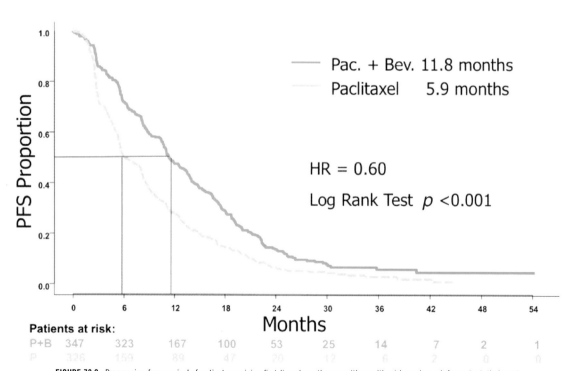

FIGURE 78.2. Progression-free survival of patients receiving first-line chemotherapy with or without bevacizumab for metastatic breast cancer, the primary endpoint of the E2100 trial. Bev, bevacizumab; PFS, progression free survival; HR, hazard ration; Pac, paclitaxel.

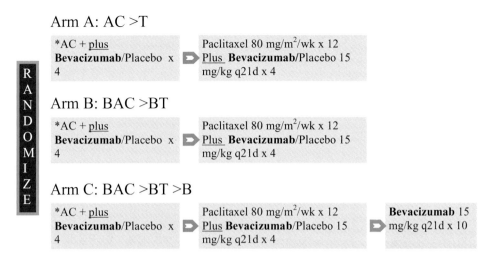

FIGURE 78.3. E1503; Bevacizumab treatment in the adjuvant setting. A, Doxorubicin; C, Cyclophosphamide; T, Paclitaxel; AC, Adriamycin and Cyclophosphamide; BAC, Bevacizumab, Adriamycin, and Cyclophosphamide; BT, Bevacizumab and Paclitaxel.

21.2%, $p < .001$). The overall survival rate, however, was similar in the two groups (median, 26.7 vs. 25.2 months; $p = .16$). The safety profile of the combination was similar to that reported in previous randomized trials. Most side effects were minimal, rarely limited therapy, and did not have a detrimental effect on overall quality of life, with hypertension representing the most common grade 3/4 toxicity. Rare life-threatening or fatal events included arterial thromboembolic phenomena and bowel perforation. Toxic effects of anti VEGF therapy for breast cancer are discussed at greater length below.

Based on the positive results of E2100, confirmatory trials were launched to examine other aspects of front-line therapy with bevacizumab. The AVADO ("AVAstin and DOcetaxel") trial randomized women with front-line metastatic breast cancer to receive docetaxel alone or docetaxel plus either a lower or a higher dose of bevacizumab (10a). This trial demonstrated a statistically significant improvement in progression-free survival for both bevacizumab-containing arms of the trial compared to the parent (docetaxel) arm, providing confirmation of the results obtained in E2100. Nevertheless, the improvement in progression-free survival was less than that seen in E2100, perhaps due to the difference in drug (docetaxel vs. paclitaxel), schedule (every 3 week vs. weekly administration), or to duration of therapy (longer in E2100 than AVADO).

Although the E2100 patients were receiving their first chemotherapy for metastatic breast cancer, only a third had never received any chemotherapy. As a result, first-line therapy for metastatic breast cancer is not truly "early" in the natural history of breast cancer. Recent laboratory studies suggest that the initial events in the development of metastasis are VEGF-dependent (11,12). If this is also true in the clinic, then the most successful application of angiogenesis inhibitors is likely to be in patients with micrometastatic disease in the adjuvant setting.

Exploration of the role of bevacizumab in the adjuvant setting is already under way. An Eastern Cooperative Oncology Group (ECOG) pilot trial (E2104) has been performed in patients with lymph node-positive, resected primary breast cancers. The study examined the incidence of clinical congestive heart failure, changes in left ventricular ejection fraction (LVEF) and noncardiac toxicity when bevacizumab was combined with doxorubicin-containing adjuvant chemother-apy. Preliminary results suggested that incorporation of bevacizumab into anthracycline-containing adjuvant therapy was feasible (13). However, continued cardiac monitoring is required in the future's large trials to define the true impact of bevacizumab on cardiac function in the adjuvant setting.

Based on the positive results of E2100 and the safety seen in E2104; the North American Breast Cancer Intergroup has recently initiated a phase III randomized controlled trial (E5103) for women with lymph node-positive or high-risk, lymph node-negative breast cancer. This trial randomizes women with estrogen-receptor positive or negative and ERBB2 (formerly HER2)-negative breast cancer, to one of three groups. The first group receives doxorubicin and cyclophosphamide followed by paclitaxel. A second group receives the same backbone chemotherapy regimen combined with bevacizumab during the course of chemotherapy only. The third group receives the same backbone chemotherapy regimen, in addition to a total of 1 year treatment of adjuvant bevacizumab (Figure 78.3).

Other phase III adjuvant bevacizumab trials are currently in development in both the adjuvant and neoadjuvant settings in breast cancer. Once data are available, it is hoped it will determine the right combinations and schedules of agents that work best in conjunction with bevacizumab in breast cancer patients.

Toxic Effects of Anti-Vascular Endothelial Growth Factor Therapy and Their Management

Vascular endothelial growth factor blockade, although generally well tolerated, is associated with specific side effects that are mechanistic in nature. The E2100 trial offers a window into VEGF-related toxicity, as demonstrated in (Table 78.1), below. In this trial, patients receiving bevacizumab in addition to paclitaxel-based chemotherapy had statistically significant increases in grade 3 and 4 toxicities for infection, fatigue, sensory neuropathy, hypertension, cerebrovascular ischemia, headache, and proteinuria. It seems likely that the increased rates of infection, fatigue, and sensory neuropathy seen in E2100 were a function of prolonged exposure to chemotherapy, because patients receiving bevacizumab not only had prolonged progression-free survival, but also received increased duration of taxane-based chemotherapy.

Table 78.1	**GRADE 3 AND 4 TOXICITY OF BEVACIZUMAB IN E2100**		
Effect	Paclitaxel + Bevacizumab (%)	Paclitaxel (%)	*p*-value
Infection	9.3%	2.9%	<.001
Fatigue	9.1%	4.9%	.04
Sensory neuropathy	23.8%	17.7%	.05
Hypertension	14.8	0	<.001
Cerebrovascular ischemia	1.9	0	.02
Headache	2.2	0	.008
Proteinuria	3.5	0	<.001

In contrast to toxic side-effects related to increased chemotherapy duration, it seems likely that the remaining toxicities were VEGF-related and mechanistic in nature (i.e., were a function of a ligand-receptor interaction in a normal tissue organ). These side effects included hypertension, cerebrovascular ischemia, headache, and proteinuria.

Of these side effects, hypertension is certainly the one most commonly faced by patients receiving anti-VEGF therapies such as bevacizumab (although the side effect has also been reported with other VEGF-targeting agents). Hypertension is generally mild-to-moderate in nature, although very rarely severe hypertension (malignant hypertension) has been reported. Hypertension is thought to be related to alterations in endothelial function related to blockade of the nitric oxide pathway downstream from the VEGF receptor (14). In contrast to anti-VEGF therapy, VEGF infusions are associated with decreases in blood pressure. Management of anti-VEGF–related hypertension has not been carefully studied in the clinic, although it appears responsive to standard antihypertensive agents, and is reversible on discontinuation of anti-VEGF therapy. For patients experiencing mild-to-moderate degrees of hypertension, anti-VEGF therapy may be continued in the presence of appropriate antihypertensive therapy.

Central nervous system effects of anti-VEGF therapy, although relatively uncommon, may be serious and life-threatening. Cerebrovascular ischemia reported with bevacizumab may involve either transient ischemic attacks or stroke. These toxicities, unsurprisingly, are more common in the elderly and in patients with underlying risk factors. Management of these complications is similar to that in patients not receiving anti-VEGF therapy. In contrast to hypertension, which is generally readily manageable, we recommend discontinuation of VEGF-targeted therapy in the presence of cerebrovascular ischemia.

Women receiving VEGF-targeted therapy frequently experience headaches, and occasionally these headaches may prove severe. These headaches are traditionally migraine-like in nature, and anecdotally respond to antimigraine agents, such as serotonin receptor-active agents. Headaches may recur, and patients experiencing headaches may require chronic antimigraine medications, such as beta blocker therapy, if the patient's cancer continues to respond to anti-VEGF therapy.

Reversible posterior leukoencephalopathy syndrome (RPLS) is a rare central nervous system complication of anti-VEGF therapy. RPLS is a subacute neurologic syndrome typically consisting of headache, cortical blindness, and seizures, and it has been reported anecdotally in patients receiving VEGF-targeting therapy. The etiology of RPLS is not well understood at present, nor is its relationship to VEGF inhibition, although it has been suggested that vasospasm of the posterior cerebral arteries may be important. Immediate cessation of anti-VEGF therapy,

and appropriate antihypertensive management (a potential predisposing factor) are indicated (15,16).

Nephrotoxicity, in the form of proteinuria, is common in patients receiving prolonged anti-VEGF therapy, with as many as 40% of patients having at least some degree of proteinuria. More severe protein loss (e.g., nephrotic syndrome) is rare, occurring in approximately 1% to 2% of patients. Although not well studied, proteinuria is reversible when anti-VEGF therapy is held, and patients may be re-challenged. A standard approach has been to discontinue bevacizumab temporarily if urine protein excretion is 2 g/24 hours or greater and then resumed when protein excretion is less than 2 g/24 hour. Bevacizumab treatment should be discontinued if nephrotic-range proteinuria develops. From a mechanistic standpoint, VEGF is important in renal glomerular homeostasis, so the renal effects of anti-VEGF therapy are expected (17).

Additional toxicities that have been reported for anti-VEGF therapies include pulmonary hemorrhage and bowel perforations. These toxicities are commonly related to disease type (lung carcinoma for pulmonary hemorrhage and colorectal cancer and ovarian cancer for bowel perforation), and have been reported only rarely in women receiving bevacizumab for treatment of breast carcinoma. When these toxicities occur, they may prove fatal and therefore represent a standard part of the informed consent for anti-VEGF therapies.

Vascular Endothelial Growth Factor Receptor Antagonists

In addition to VEGF ligand-binding agents, numerous other drugs have targeted the VEGF pathway. Monoclonal antibodies have also been developed against both VEGF-R types 1 and 2 (VEGF-R1, R2) (18,19), and many clinical trials have been initiated with these agents. In addition, many receptor tyrosine kinase inhibitors have been developed, targeting the internal membrane tyrosine kinase portion of VEGF-R1 and VEGF-R2 (20–24). Some target more than one receptor, such as ZD6474, which targets VEGF-R2 (flk-1/kdr) and the epidermal growth factor receptor (EGFR). However, ZD6474 showed limited monotherapy activity in patients with refractory metastatic breast cancer (25).

Sunitinib (SU11248, Sutent), a multitargeted tyrosine-kinase inhibitor that blocks VEGF-receptors, platelet-derived growth factor receptor (PDGFR), *c-kit* and *Flt*-3, has recently been approved for the treatment of gastrointestinal stromal tumors and renal cell carcinoma. Based on early data suggesting activity of antiangiogenesis in breast cancer, a phase II trial of single-agent sunitinib was performed, which demonstrated activity in 64 heavily pretreated patients with refractory metastatic breast cancer (26). In this trial, patients received sunitinib at a dose of 50 mg/day in 6-week cycles (4 weeks on, then 2 weeks off treatment). Overall, seven patients (11%) achieved a partial response and three additional patients (5%) maintained stable disease for 6 months or more. Based on these results, a phase III trial has been initiated comparing the new standard of paclitaxel plus bevacizumab with paclitaxel and sunitinib. Sorafenib, another multitargeted tyrosine-kinase inhibitor (for VEGF receptors and RAF kinase), has been approved by the U.S. Food and Drug Administration for renal cell carcinoma and hepatoma. This agent is undergoing development in metastatic breast cancer. A recently reported phase II trial demonstrated a low response rate in patients with heavily pretreated metastatic breast cancer (27). Axitinib, a small molecule receptor tyrosine kinase inhibitor, has been examined in a randomized phase II trial comparing docetaxel with docetaxel plus axitinib in a front-line metastatic breast cancer setting (28). In this trial, patients receiving combined therapy had superior response rates and progression-free survival, although the size of this study prevents any definitive conclusions with regard to efficacy.

Other Inhibitors of Vascular Endothelial Growth Factor/Vascular Endothelial Growth Factor Receptor Pathway

Inhibition of the VEGF receptor message has been attempted with ribozyme (catalytic RNA). Angiozyme is a synthetic ribosome that cleaves the messenger RNA for the VEGF *Flt*-1 receptor. Preclinical studies confirmed inhibition of both primary tumor growth and metastasis (29,30). A phase II trial in breast cancer has been reported with this agent and, however, showed no evidence of clinical activity (31).

Production of VEGF is regulated by other transmembrane receptor tyrosine kinases, through which it might be possible to produce indirect inhibition of VEGF. Stimulation or overexpression of the EGFR (ERBB1) and ERBB2 (*c-erb*-b2, *neu*) increases production of VEGF and induces angiogenesis in human cancers in preclinical models (32–35). Inhibition of these receptors reduces VEGF production and angiogenesis in preclinical models, which suggests that targeting these receptors might lead to indirect inhibition of angiogenesis and potentially a synergistic effect with direct inhibitors (36–39). A phase I trial combining the anti-ERBB2 agent trastuzumab with bevacizumab, as well as a subsequent phase II extension (40,41), explored this theory in patients with ERBB2-positive metastatic breast cancer. The results of these trials, as recently reported, suggest that this combination is both feasible and active. More recently, the ECOG has initiated a phase III trial (E1105) exploring the combination of bevacizumab and trastuzumab in the context of front-line chemotherapy for ERBB2-positive metastatic breast cancer.

Protease Inhibitors

The inhibitors of the matrix metalloproteins (MMP) can be grouped into three categories:

1. Collagen peptidomimetics and nonpeptidomimetics
2. Tetracycline derivatives
3. Bisphosphonates

Marimastat is a peptidomimetic that chelates the zinc atom of the active site of the MMP; it has been the most studied MMP inhibitor. It inhibits a broad spectrum of the MMP and has activity in multiple human xenograft models (42). Phase I trials identified dose-limiting musculoskeletal toxicities (MST) including arthralgias or arthritis, tendonitis, and bursitis (43).

Two completed trials have evaluated the MMP inhibitor marimastat in breast cancer. The phase III trial (E2196) randomized patients with metastatic breast cancer who were responding or stable after initial chemotherapy to treatment with either marimastat or placebo. This trial failed to show any clinical benefit. Indeed, patients with higher marimastat levels exhibited MST, and MST was associated with inferior survival (44). In a limited institution pilot study, 63 patients with stage II breast cancer received marimastat at one of two dose levels, either following doxorubicin-based chemotherapy or concomitantly with tamoxifen. MST resulted in significant dose reductions and limited chronic administration yielding plasma levels below the target range (45).

BMS-275291 is another MMP inhibitor that was also examined for treatment of breast cancer. A pilot phase II trial similar to that performed with marimastat was conducted with BMS-275291 in the adjuvant setting for patients with stage I-IIIA, but it was terminated owing to MST (46).

The available clinical data with MMP inhibitors do not support a role for their use in patients with breast cancer (or in other human malignancies) and, in fact, these agents have largely been abandoned in active clinical investigation. Whether the failure of these agents is a function of inadequate drug levels, unexpected toxicity, or a more basic failure of the underlying hypothesis is uncertain.

Endothelial Toxins

TNP-470 (AGM-1470), a synthetic derivation of fungillin, was shown to inhibit tumor growth and metastasis in a preclinical model (47). It was one of the first antiangiogenic agents to enter phase I studies, however, it showed limited clinical benefit evident with only one objective response reported, although several patients showed stabilization of disease (48,49). Vitaxin, a humanized monoclonal antibody against α-V β-3 integrin, was well tolerated and showed limited activity in a phase I trial (50). EMD 121974 (cilengitide) is a cyclic Arg-Gly-Asp peptide with antiangiogenic activity, and it has been shown to synergize with radioimmunotherapy in breast cancer xenografts (51).

Natural Inhibitors

The administration of natural inhibitors of angiogenesis as therapeutics is also an area of intense research. A phase I trial of recombinant human angiostatin in patients with refractory solid tumors found no dose-limiting toxicities or changes in coagulation factors. No objective responses were reported, although some patients had measurable decreases in urine fibroblast growth factor-β (FGF-b) and VEGF levels (52).

2-Methoxyestradiol (2-ME$_2$) is a nonestrogenic metabolite of estradiol with antitumor and antiendothelial cell activity (53,54). Phase I study in patients with previously treated metastatic breast cancer showed no dose-limiting toxicity with doses ranging from 200 to 1,000 mg once daily, and metabolism was variable, with a half-life of approximately 10 to 12 hours. No objective responses were produced, although prolonged disease stabilization was achieved in several of the patients. A phase I study of 2-ME$_2$ in combination with docetaxel in patients with newly diagnosed metastatic breast cancer showed 2-ME$_2$, alone or in combination with docetaxel, is well tolerated in these patients, but systemic exposure remained below the expected therapeutic range (55).

ANTIANGIOGENIC ACTIVITY OF CHEMOTHERAPEUTIC AGENTS

Recent studies have suggested that several classes of chemotherapeutic drugs have antiangiogenic activity *in vitro* or *in vivo*, including several agents that are routinely used in breast cancer (56). It is, therefore, reasonably likely that antiangiogenic therapy represents an old rather than a new approach to the treatment of breast cancer.

The antiangiogenic effect of chemotherapeutics may require a different dose and schedule than typically used for cytotoxic effect. Preclinical studies suggest that prolonged exposure to low drug concentrations—exactly the opposite to the maximal tolerated doses administered to target the tumor compartment—may be necessary (57). This approach has been termed *metronomic therapy* (58). Three reports (59–61) confirm the importance of schedule for chemotherapy's antiangiogenic effects. In all three of these, the combination of low, frequent dose chemotherapy plus an agent targeting the endothelial compartment controlled tumor growth better than the cytotoxic agent alone.

An "antiangiogenic schedule" (170 mg/kg every 6 days) of cyclophosphamide was more effective than the conventional maximal tolerated dose (150 mg/kg every other day for three doses every 21 days) in Lewis lung carcinoma and L1210 leukemia models; the antiangiogenic dosing was three times more effective in controlling growth of chemotherapy-resistant

Lewis lung carcinoma and EMT-6 breast cancer cell lines (59). The addition of TNP-470 to the antiangiogenic schedule of cyclophosphamide induced endothelial cell apoptosis within tumors, an effect that preceded apoptosis of drug-resistant Lewis lung carcinoma. Low-dose vinblastine (0.75 mg/m^2 intraperitoneal with 1-mg/m^2 continuous infusion for 3 weeks followed by 1.5 mg/m^2 intraperitoneal twice per week) plus an antibody against VEGF-R2 controlled growth of neuroblastoma xenografts during 210 days of therapy (60). Similar findings have been reported with carboplatin plus a VEGF-neutralizing antibody (61).

Only a few clinical trials have formally tested the metronomic schedules (58). Hanahan et al. (58) and Fennelly et al. (62) reported that 4 of 13 patients with ovarian cancer who had received and subsequently relapsed from prior paclitaxel therapy responded when treated with increasing doses of paclitaxel administered weekly. Moreover, two of these patients had disease progression while receiving paclitaxel. Prolonged infusion of paclitaxel (140 mg/m^2 over 96 hours) induced responses in 7 of 26 patients who had relapsed within a median of 1 month short of taxane infusions (63).

The European Organization for Research and Treatment of Cancer studied two cyclophosphamide, methotrexate, and fluorouracil regimens: a classic 28-day regimen of daily cyclophosphamide for 14 days and a modified intravenous schedule with bolus cyclophosphamide every 3 weeks. The overall response rate and survival clearly favored the classic regimen (64). Although generally viewed as a test of dose intensity (the classic regimen delivered higher total doses of both cyclophosphamide and 5-fluorouracil), this study may also be considered a test of an antiangiogenic versus bolus schedule. A phase II study of low-dose methotrexate (2.5 mg twice a day for 2 days each week) and cyclophosphamide (50 mg daily) in patients with heavily pretreated metastatic breast cancer found an overall response rate of 19% (and additional 13% of patients were stable for 6 months). Serum VEGF levels decreased in all patients remaining on therapy for at least 2 months but did not correlate with response (65).

More recently, the Dana Farber group reported results from a phase II, randomized study comparing metronomic-scheduled, oral cyclophosphamide and methotrexate with and without the addition of bevacizumab in patients with advanced breast cancer (66). Results demonstrated clear improvements in response rates for the combination arm compared with metronomic therapy alone. The group reported two partial responses (PR) for the chemotherapy alone group (10%), compared with 10 PR for the chemotherapy plus bevacizumab arm (29%). Median time-to-progression was also increased in the combined arm (5.5 vs. 2.0 months), and toxicities appeared minimal for both arms. Another adjuvant pilot trial comparing metronomic therapy with and without bevacizumab, in patients with residual disease after completion of neoadjuvant chemotherapy, has been proposed as a follow-up to this study. Trials such as this may lead the way for a new approach for patients for whom traditional cytotoxic agents cannot be used because of limiting comorbid conditions or when tumors are resistant to the *old* approach.

PREDICTION OF THERAPEUTIC BENEFIT

In an era of progressive therapeutic individualization driven by advances in genomic, proteomic, and pharmacogenomic technology, it seems reasonable to attempt such an approach for antiangiogenic therapy. Although antiangiogenic therapy was once touted as being "resistant to resistance" because it targeted endothelial cells rather than cancer cells, numerous mechanisms of resistance have been identified in the laboratory, and

clinical resistance is an unfortunate reality (67). Therefore, identification of women more or less likely to benefit from therapy would be immensely beneficial.

Both for breast cancer and for other human cancers, we currently lack reliable or reproducible means of identifying patients most likely to benefit from antiangiogenic therapy. Examinations of tumor VEGF and VEGF-R content have so far proved to be of little value in a variety of human cancers. Recent work by Schneider et al. (68), examining the E2100 proof-of-concept phase III metastatic trial, has suggested that host factors may play an important role in determining both toxicity and therapeutic outcome. In this analysis, the presence of specific VEGF single nucleotide polymorphisms (SNP) was associated both with the most common grade 3/4 toxicity (hypertension) and with overall survival. These data require independent confirmation, but suggest an interesting new approach to therapeutic individualization for anti-VEGF targeted therapies (68).

CONCLUSION

Antiangiogenic therapy for breast cancer—indeed, for all cancers—is still in its youth. Nevertheless, it is already apparent that this approach will play an important role in the treatment of patients with metastatic breast cancer, and is under active evaluation in the adjuvant setting. Progress in this field will require the completion of ongoing trials and continued improvement in our understanding of the biology of angiogenesis. Little question exists that angiogenesis is a crucial component of the progression of the disease. It seems likely that continued efforts to modulate angiogenesis will bring us closer to our goal of improving the survival of patients with breast cancer.

References

1. Folkman J. What is the evidence that tumors are angiogenesis dependent? *J Natl Cancer Inst* 1990;82(1):4–6.
2. Folkman J. Seminars in Medicine of the Beth Israel Hospital, Boston. Clinical applications of research on angiogenesis. *N Engl J Med* 1995;333(26):1757–1763.
3. Pepper MS, Mandriota SJ, Vassalli JD, et al. Angiogenesis-regulating cytokines: activities and interactions. *Curr Top Microbiol Immunol* 1996;213(Pt 2):31–67.
4. Brown JM, Giaccia AJ. The unique physiology of solid tumors: opportunities (and problems) for cancer therapy. *Cancer Res* 1998;58(7):1408–1416.
5. Margolin K, Gordon MS, Holmgren E, et al. Phase Ib trial of intravenous recombinant humanized monoclonal antibody to vascular endothelial growth factor in combination with chemotherapy in patients with advanced cancer: pharmacologic and long-term safety data. *J Clin Oncol* 2001;19(3):851–856.
6. Gordon MS, Margolin K, Talpaz M, Set al Phase I safety and pharmacokinetic study of recombinant human anti-vascular endothelial growth factor in patients with advanced cancer. *J Clin Oncol* 2001;19(3):843–850.
7. Sledge G, Miller K, Novotny W, et al. A phase II trial of single-agent rhuMAb VEGF (recombinant humanized monoclonal antibody to vascular endothelial cell growth factor) in patients with relapsed metastatic breast cancer. *Proc Am Soc Clin Oncol* 2000;19:3a.
8. Miller KD, Chap LI, Holmes FA, et al. Randomized phase III trial of capecitabine compared with bevacizumab plus capecitabine in patients with previously treated metastatic breast cancer. *J Clin Oncol* 2005;23(4):792–799.
9. Relf M, LeJeune S, Scott PA, et al. Expression of the angiogenic factors vascular endothelial cell growth factor, acidic and basic fibroblast growth factor, tumor growth factor beta-1, platelet-derived endothelial cell growth factor, placenta growth factor, and pleiotrophin in human primary breast cancer and its relation to angiogenesis. *Cancer Res* 1997;57(5):963–969.
10. Kathy Miller MD, Molin Wang, et al. Paclitaxel plus bevacizumab versus paclitaxel alone for metastatic breast cancer. *N Engl J Med* 2007;357(26):2666–2676.
10a. Miles D, Chan A, Romieu G, et al. Randomized, double-blind, placebo-controlled, phase III study of bevacizumab with docetaxel or docetaxel with placebo as first-line therapy for patients with locally recurrent or metastatic breast cancer (mBC): AVADO. *J Clin Oncol* 26:2008 (May 20 suppl; abstr LBA1011^).
11. Kaplan RN, Riba RD, Zacharoulis S, et al. VEGFR1-positive haematopoietic bone marrow progenitors initiate the pre-metastatic niche. *Nature* 2005;438(7069):820–827.
12. Steeg PS. Tumor metastasis: mechanistic insights and clinical challenges. *Nat Med* 2006;12(8):895–904.
13. Miller KD ONA, Perez EA, Seidman AD, et al. Phase II feasibility trial incorporating bevacizumab into dose dense doxorubicin and cyclophosphamide followed by paclitaxel in patients with lymph node positive breast cancer: a trial of the Eastern Cooperative Oncology Group (E2104) [Abstract 3036]. *Breast Cancer Res Treat* 2007;106(Suppl 1). Available at *www.sabcs.org*.
14. Mourad JJ, des Guetz G, Debbabi H, et al. Blood pressure rise following angiogenesis inhibition by bevacizumab. A crucial role for microcirculation. *Ann Oncol* 2008;19(5):927–934.

15. Glusker P, Recht L, Lane B. Reversible posterior leukoencephalopathy syndrome and bevacizumab. *N Engl J Med* 2006;354(9):980–982; discussion 980–982.
16. Allen JA, Adlakha A, Bergethon PR. Reversible posterior leukoencephalopathy syndrome after bevacizumab/FOLFIRI regimen for metastatic colon cancer. *Arch Neurol* 2006;63(10):1475–1478.
17. Zhu X, Wu S, Dahut WL, et al. Risks of proteinuria and hypertension with bevacizumab, an antibody against vascular endothelial growth factor: systematic review and meta-analysis. *Am J Kidney Dis* 2007;49(2):186–193.
18. Zhu Z, Witte L. Inhibition of tumor growth and metastasis by targeting tumor-associated angiogenesis with antagonists to the receptors of vascular endothelial growth factor. *Invest New Drugs* 1999;17(3):195–212.
19. Kozin SV, Boucher Y, Hicklin DJ, et al. Vascular endothelial growth factor receptor-2-blocking antibody potentiates radiation-induced long-term control of human tumor xenografts. *Cancer Res* 2001;61(1):39–44.
20. Smolich BD, Yuen HA, West KA, et al. The antiangiogenic protein kinase inhibitors SU5416 and SU6668 inhibit the SCF receptor (c-kit) in a human myeloid leukemia cell line and in acute myeloid leukemia blasts. *Blood* 2001;97(5):1413–1421.
21. Mendel DB, Laird AD, Smolich BD, et al. Development of SU5416, a selective small molecule inhibitor of VEGF receptor tyrosine kinase activity, as an anti-angiogenesis agent. *Anticancer Drug Res* 2000;15(1):29–41.
22. Shaheen RM, Davis DW, Liu W, et al. Antiangiogenic therapy targeting the tyrosine kinase receptor for vascular endothelial growth factor receptor inhibits the growth of colon cancer liver metastasis and induces tumor and endothelial cell apoptosis. *Cancer Res* 1999;59(21):5412–5416.
23. Drevs J, Hofmann I, Hugenschmidt H, et al Effects of PTK787/ZK 222584, a specific inhibitor of vascular endothelial growth factor receptor tyrosine kinases, on primary tumor, metastasis, vessel density, and blood flow in a murine renal cell carcinoma model. *Cancer Res* 2000;60(17):4819–4824.
24. Wood JM, Bold G, Buchdunger E, et al. PTK787/ZK 222584, a novel and potent inhibitor of vascular endothelial growth factor receptor tyrosine kinases, impairs vascular endothelial growth factor-induced responses and tumor growth after oral administration. *Cancer Res* 2000;60(8):2178–2189.
25. Miller KD, Trigo JM, Wheeler C, et al. A multicenter phase II trial of ZD6474, a vascular endothelial growth factor receptor-2 and epidermal growth factor receptor tyrosine kinase inhibitor, in patients with previously treated metastatic breast cancer. *Clin Cancer Res* 2005;11(9):3369–3376.
26. Burstein HJ, Elias AD, Rugo HS, et al. Phase II study of sunitinib malate, an oral multitargeted tyrosine kinase inhibitor, in patients with metastatic breast cancer previously treated with an anthracycline and a taxane. *J Clin Oncol* 2008;26(11): 1810–1816.
27. Bianchi GVL, S; Zamagni, C, et al. Phase II multicenter trial of sorafenib in the treatment of patients with metastatic breast cancer [Abstract 162]. *2007 Breast Cancer Symposium ASCO*, Sept. 8, 2007, San Francisco, CA.
28. Rugo HS, Stopeck A, Joy AA, et al. A randomized, double-blind phase II study of the oral tyrosine kinase inhibitor (TKI) axitinib (AG-013736) in combination with docetaxel (DOC) compared to DOC plus placebo (PL) in metastatic breast cancer (MBC). *J Clin Oncol* 2007;25(18S):003.
29. Sandberg JA, Sproul CD, Blanchard KS, et al. Acute toxicology and pharmacokinetic assessment of a ribozyme (ANGIOZYME) targeting vascular endothelial growth factor receptor mRNA in the cynomolgus monkey. *Antisense Nucleic Acid Drug Dev* 2000;10(3):153–162.
30. Sandberg JA, Bouhana KS, Gallegos AM, et al. Pharmacokinetics of an antiangiogenic ribozyme (ANGIOZYME) in the mouse. *Antisense Nucleic Acid Drug Dev* 1999;9(3):271–277.
31. Hortobagyi GN WD, Elias A, et al. Angiozyme treatment of stage IV metastatic breast cancer patients: assessment of serum markers of angiogenesis. *Breast Cancer Res Treat* 2002;76:S97.
32. Goldman CK, Kim J, Wong WL, et al. Epidermal growth factor stimulates vascular endothelial growth factor production by human malignant glioma cells: a model of glioblastoma multiforme pathophysiology. *Mol Biol Cell* 1993;4(1):121–133.
33. Maity A, Pore N, Lee J, et al. Epidermal growth factor receptor transcriptionally up-regulates vascular endothelial growth factor expression in human glioblastoma cells via a pathway involving phosphatidylinositol 3'-kinase and distinct from that induced by hypoxia. *Cancer Res* 2000;60(20):5879–5886.
34. Yen L, You XL, Al Moustafa AE, et al. Heregulin selectively upregulates vascular endothelial growth factor secretion in cancer cells and stimulates angiogenesis. *Oncogene* 2000;19(31):3460–3469.
35. Clarke K, Smith K, Gullick WJ, et al Mutant epidermal growth factor receptor enhances induction of vascular endothelial growth factor by hypoxia and insulin-like growth factor-1 via a PI3 kinase dependent pathway. *Br J Cancer* 2001;84(10):1322–1329.
36. Ciardiello F, Caputo R, Bianco R, et al Inhibition of growth factor production and angiogenesis in human cancer cells by ZD1839 (Iressa), a selective epidermal growth factor receptor tyrosine kinase inhibitor. *Clin Cancer Res* 2001;7(5):1459–1465.
37. Ciardiello F, Caputo R, Bianco R, et al. Antitumor effect and potentiation of cytotoxic drugs activity in human cancer cells by ZD-1839 (Iressa), an epidermal growth factor receptor-selective tyrosine kinase inhibitor. *Clin Cancer Res* 2000;6(5):2053–2063.
38. Bruns CJ, Solorzano CC, Harbison MT, et al. Blockade of the epidermal growth factor receptor signaling by a novel tyrosine kinase inhibitor leads to apoptosis of endothelial cells and therapy of human pancreatic carcinoma. *Cancer Res* 2000; 60(11):2926–2935.
39. Perrotte P, Matsumoto T, Inoue K, et al. Anti-epidermal growth factor receptor antibody C225 inhibits angiogenesis in human transitional cell carcinoma growing orthotopically in nude mice. *Clin Cancer Res* 1999;5(2):257–265.
40. Pegram M, Chan D, Dichmann RA, et al. Phase II combined biological therapy targeting the HER2 proto-oncogene and the vascular endothelial growth factor using trastuzumab (T) and bevacizumab (B) as first line treatment of HER2-amplified breast cancer [Abstract 3039]. *Breast Cancer Res Treat* 2006;100(Suppl 1). Available at www.sabcs.org.
41. Pegram MD, Yeon C, Ku NC, et al. Phase I combined biological therapy of breast cancer using two humanized monoclonal antibodies directed against HER2 proto-oncogene and vascular endothelial growth factor (VEGF) [Abstract 3039]. *Breast Cancer Res Treat* 2004;88(Suppl 1). Available at www.sabcs.org.
42. Ferrante K, Winograd B, Canetta R. Promising new developments in cancer chemotherapy. *Cancer Chemother Pharmacol* 1999;43(Suppl):S61–S68.
43. Naglich JG, Jure-Kunkel M, et al Inhibition of angiogenesis and metastasis in two murine models by the matrix metalloproteinase inhibitor, BMS-275291. *Cancer Res* 2001;61(23):8480–8485.
44. Sparano JA, Bernardo P, Stephenson P, et al. Randomized phase III trial of marimastat versus placebo in patients with metastatic breast cancer who have responding or stable disease after first-line chemotherapy: Eastern Cooperative Oncology Group trial E2196. *J Clin Oncol* 2004;22(23):4683–4690.
45. Miller KD, Gradishar W, Schuchter L, et al A randomized phase II pilot trial of adjuvant marimastat in patients with early-stage breast cancer. *Ann Oncol* 2002;13(8):1220–1224.
46. Miller KD, Saphner TJ, Waterhouse DM, et al. A randomized phase II feasibility trial of BMS-275291 in patients with early stage breast cancer. *Clin Cancer Res* 2004;10(6):1971–1975.
47. Singh Y, Shikata N, Kiyozuka Y, et al. Inhibition of tumor growth and metastasis by angiogenesis inhibitor TNP-470 on breast cancer cell lines *in vitro* and *in vivo*. *Breast Cancer Res Treat* 1997;45(1):15–27.
48. Bhargava P, Marshall JL, Rizvi N, et al A Phase I and pharmacokinetic study of TNP-470 administered weekly to patients with advanced cancer. *Clin Cancer Res* 1999;5(8):1989–1995.
49. Stadler WM, Kuzel T, Shapiro C, et al. Multi-institutional study of the angiogenesis inhibitor TNP-470 in metastatic renal carcinoma. *J Clin Oncol* 1999;17(8): 2541–2545.
50. Gutheil JC, Campbell TN, Pierce PR, et al. Targeted antiangiogenic therapy for cancer using Vitaxin: a humanized monoclonal antibody to the integrin alphavbeta3. *Clin Cancer Res* 2000 Aug;6(8):3056–3061.
51. Burke PA, DeNardo SJ, Miers LA, et al. Cilengitide targeting of alpha(v)beta(3) integrin receptor synergizes with radioimmunotherapy to increase efficacy and apoptosis in breast cancer xenografts. *Cancer Res* 2002;62(15):4263–4272.
52. DeMoraes ED, Fogler WE, Grant D, et al. Recombinant human angiostatin: a phase I clinical trial assessing safety, pharmacokinetics and pharmacodynamics. *Proc Am Soc Clin Oncol* 2001;20:3a.
53. Yue TL, Wang X, Louden CS, et al. 2-Methoxyestradiol, an endogenous estrogen metabolite, induces apoptosis in endothelial cells and inhibits angiogenesis: possible role for stress-activated protein kinase signaling pathway and Fas expression. *Mol Pharmacol* 1997;51(6):951–962.
54. Klauber N, Parangi S, Flynn E, et al. Inhibition of angiogenesis and breast cancer in mice by the microtubule inhibitors 2-methoxyestradiol and taxol. *Cancer Res* 1997;57(1):81–86.
55. James J, Murry DJ, Treston AM, et al. Phase I safety, pharmacokinetic and pharmacodynamic studies of 2-methoxyestradiol alone or in combination with docetaxel in patients with locally recurrent or metastatic breast cancer. *Invest New Drugs* 2007;25:41–48.
56. Miller KD, Sweeney CJ, Sledge GW Jr. Redefining the target: chemotherapeutics as antiangiogenics. *J Clin Oncol* 2001;19(4):1195–1206.
57. Slaton JW, Perrotte P, Inoue K, et al. Interferon-alpha-mediated down-regulation of angiogenesis-related genes and therapy of bladder cancer are dependent on optimization of biological dose and schedule. *Clin Cancer Res* 1999;5(10):2726–2734.
58. Hanahan D, Bergers G, Bergsland E. Less is more, regularly: metronomic dosing of cytotoxic drugs can target tumor angiogenesis in mice. *J Clin Invest* 2000;105(8):1045–1047.
59. Browder T, Butterfield CE, Kraling BM, et al. Antiangiogenic scheduling of chemotherapy improves efficacy against experimental drug-resistant cancer. *Cancer Res* 2000;60(7):1878–1886.
60. Klement G, Baruchel S, Rak J, et al. Continuous low-dose therapy with vinblastine and VEGF receptor-2 antibody induces sustained tumor regression without overt toxicity. *J Clin Invest* 2000;105(8):R15–R24.
61. Wild R, Dings RP, Subramanian I, Ramakrishnan S. Carboplatin selectively induces the VEGF stress response in endothelial cells: potentiation of antitumor activity by combination treatment with antibody to VEGF. *Int J Cancer* 2004;110:343–351.
62. Fennelly D, Aghajanian C, Shapiro F, et al. Phase I and pharmacologic study of paclitaxel administered weekly in patients with relapsed ovarian cancer. *J Clin Oncol* 1997;15(1):187–192.
63. Seidman AD, Hochhauser D, Gollub M, et al. Ninety-six-hour paclitaxel infusion after progression during short taxane exposure: a phase II pharmacokinetic and pharmacodynamic study in metastatic breast cancer. *J Clin Oncol* 1996;14(6): 1877–1884.
64. Engelsman E, Klijn JC, Rubens RD, et al. "Classical" CMF versus a 3-weekly intravenous CMF schedule in postmenopausal patients with advanced breast cancer. An EORTC Breast Cancer Co-operative Group Phase III Trial (10808). *Eur J Cancer* 1991;27(8):966–970.
65. Colleoni M, Rocca A, Sandri MT, et al. Low-dose oral methotrexate and cyclophosphamide in metastatic breast cancer: antitumor activity and correlation with vascular endothelial growth factor levels. *Ann Oncol* 2002;13:73–80.
66. Burstein HJ, Spigel D, Kindsvogel K, et al. Metronomic chemotherapy with and without bevacizumab for advanced breast cancer: a randomized phase II study [Abstract 4]. *Breast Cancer Res Treat* 2005;94(Suppl 1). Available at www.sabcs.org.
67. Schneider BP, Sledge GW Jr. Drug insight: VEGF as a therapeutic target for breast cancer. *Nat Clin Pract Oncol* 2007;4(3):181–189.
68. Schneider BP, Radovich M, Sledge GW, et al. Association of polymorphisms of angiogenesis genes with breast cancer. *Breast Cancer Res Treat* 2008;111: 157–163.

Carlos L. Arteaga

Protein tyrosine kinases catalyze the transfer of the γ-phosphate of adenosine triphosphate (ATP) to hydroxyl groups of tyrosines on cellular substrates. They are important regulators of intracellular signal transduction pathways mediating cell proliferation, differentiation, migration, metabolism, survival, and multicellular communication. Indeed, tyrosine phosphorylation of proteins is rare and is tightly regulated in quiescent cells, but abundant in rapidly proliferating or transformed cells. Intramolecular control of the kinases involved in the phosphorylation of tyrosyl proteins involves multiple autoinhibitory mechanisms to safeguard against inappropriate or unwanted kinase activation (1). A search of the human genome for tyrosine kinase coding elements has identified 90 unique kinase genes, encoding transmembrane receptor or cytoplasmic nonreceptor tyrosine kinases (2). The receptor tyrosine kinases contain an extracellular ligand-binding domain, which is usually glycosylated. The ligand-binding region is connected to the cytoplasmic domain by a single transmembrane helix. The cytoplasmic domain contains a conserved protein tyrosine kinase core and additional regulatory motifs that are the target of autophosphorylation or phosphorylation by heterologous protein kinases (3). Signaling by receptor tyrosine kinases requires ligand-induced receptor oligomerization, resulting in autophosphorylation of tyrosine residues in the cytoplasmic domain (4). This results in activation of the receptor's catalytic activity, whereas these phosphorylated tyrosine residues become the *docking sites* for the specific binding of cytoplasmic signaling proteins containing Src homology-2 (SH2) and protein tyrosine-binding (PTB) domains.

Signaling pathways regulated by protein tyrosine kinases are the frequent target of somatic mutations, leading to many human cancers. Of the more than 100 dominant oncogenes known to date, many encode protein tyrosine kinases (3). Several mechanisms lead to aberrant function by protein tyrosine kinases and subsequent oncogenic transformation. These include

- Genomic rearrangements resulting in oncogenic fusion proteins that include the kinase catalytic domain and an unrelated protein that provides an activation function
- Gain-of-function mutations in the juxtamembrane or kinase domains or small deletions of regulatory regions
- Overexpression with or without gene amplification
- Loss of the normal autoinhibitory and regulatory constraints of kinase activation

At this time, several tyrosine kinase inhibitors (TKI) of variable target specificity have been approved by the U.S. Food and Drug Administration (FDA) for treatment of patients with a variety of cancers.

Several receptor protein and cytoplasmic tyrosine kinases are known to be mutated or overexpressed in human breast cancer. These include the epidermal growth factor receptor (EGFR; *ERBB1*), ERBB2 (formerly HER2/neu), insulin and insulin-like growth factor (IGF) receptors, fibroblast growth factor receptor-2 (FGFR-2), FGFR-4, Src, Brk, and Syk, among others. In many examples reviewed below, inactivation of several of these tyrosine kinases with exogenous inhibitors has resulted in an antitumor effect in preclinical models of breast cancer and in patients with breast cancer. Several conditions are generally considered before the selection of a tyrosine kinase as a therapeutic target against which drugs are developed. First, the kinase should be a *gain-of-function* oncogene,

causal to tumor development and tumor maintenance, or both. It should be differentially expressed in tumor versus nontumor tissue and identifiable in cancer tissue. Importantly, it should not have a critical role in postnatal or adult physiology, thus providing an exploitable therapeutic window. Structure-function knowledge of the molecular target should be in hand to develop mechanism-based inhibitors. In general, TKI have consisted of neutralizing antibodies and low molecular weight ATP-mimetics, which will be reviewed below.

ERBB2 INHIBITORS: TRASTUZUMAB (HERCEPTIN)

The ERBB2 is a member of the ErbB family of transmembrane receptor tyrosine kinases, which also includes the epidermal growth factor receptor (EGFR, ErbB1), ERBB3, and ERBB4. Binding of ligands to the extracellular domain of EGFR, ERBB3, and ERBB4 induces the formation of kinase active homo- and heterodimers to which activated ERBB2 is recruited as a preferred partner (5). Although ERBB2 does not bind any of the ErbB ligands directly, its potent catalytic activity amplifies signaling by ErbB-containing heterodimers via increasing ligand binding affinity or receptor recycling and stability (5). These functions make ERBB2 a critical therapeutic target within the ErbB receptor network. Amplification of the *ERBB2* gene occurs in approximately 25% of invasive breast cancers and is associated with poor patient outcome (6).

Trastuzumab (Herceptin), a humanized monoclonal antibody that binds the ectodomain of the ERBB2 receptor, has been approved by the FDA for the treatment of ERBB2-overexpressing breast cancer in both the adjuvant and metastatic settings. Trastuzumab binds to an epitope in the juxtamembrane region of the ERBB2 receptor. Treatment with this antibody alone has been shown to induce clinical responses in patients with ERBB2-overexpressing breast cancers. The joint efficacy analysis of the pivotal North Central Cancer Treatment Group (NCCTG) N9831 and the National Surgical Adjuvant Breast and Bowel Project (NSABP) B-31 trials demonstrated that the addition of trastuzumab to standard adjuvant chemotherapy (doxorubicin, cyclophosphamide, paclitaxel) reduced disease recurrence by 52% and the risk of death by 33% compared with chemotherapy alone in patients with ERBB2-overexpressing breast cancer (7). On this basis, trastuzumab in combination of standard adjuvant chemotherapy was approved by the FDA for treatment of patients of surgically-resected ERBB2-positive early breast cancer (extensively discussed in Chapters 51 and 75).

Proposed mechanisms of action of the antibody include downregulation of ERBB2 receptors from the cell surface, blockade of metalloprotease-mediated cleavage at the juxtamembrane region of ERBB2 (8), interference of ErbB receptor heterodimerization, and inhibition of the phosphatidylinositol-3 kinase (PI3K)/Akt survival pathway (9), recruitment of FcR-III-expressing immune effector cells that mediate antibody-dependent cell mediated cytotoxicity (ADCC) (10), and inhibition of the production of angiogenic factors (11). Little published data exist to support any of these mechanisms as operative *in situ* in patients treated with trastuzumab. Further, the antibody-induced downregulation of ERBB2 has been challenged by a recent paper suggesting that neither the internalization nor the cell surface expression of ERBB2 is altered when bound by trastuzumab (12).

In a neoadjuvant trial, 40 patients with locally advanced ERBB2-positive breast cancer were treated with weekly single-agent trastuzumab for 3 weeks, at which time docetaxel was added for a total of 12 weeks before surgery (13). In this study, sequential core biopsies at weeks 1 and 3 after initiation of trastuzumab were taken. Clinical responses at 12 weeks correlated with an increase in tumor cell apoptosis at week 1 as measured by cleaved caspase-3 immunohistochemistry (IHC). Interestingly, P-Erk and P-Akt, as measured by IHC with phospho-specific antibodies, were reduced by treatment, thus supporting an antisignaling effect of the antibody *in vivo*. In a recent study, 54 patients with *EERBB2* gene-amplified breast cancer receiving trastuzumab plus a taxane for metastatic disease were evaluated for genotype of the Fcγ receptor, which is necessary for the engagement of cells that mediate ADCC. The FcγRIIIa-158 V/V genotype correlated with objective response and progression-free survival. The ADCC analysis of patients' peripheral blood mononuclear cells (PBMC) also showed that PBMC from patients with this polyphormism exhibited significantly higher ADCC than PBMC harboring different genotypes (14).

The clinical efficacy of trastuzumab appears limited to breast cancers that overexpress ERBB2 as measured by intense membrane staining in most tumor cells with ERBB2 antibodies (3+ by IHC) or two or more copies of the *ERBB2* gene determined by fluorescent *in situ* hybridization (FISH). Therefore, ERBB2 overexpression determined by IHC or FISH is the biomarker predictive of good odds of response to treatment with the antibody. However, a recent reanalysis of patients enrolled in a large adjuvant trial comparing chemotherapy versus chemotherapy plus trastuzumab (7) showed that 9.7% of patients enrolled had tumors that did not meet criteria for *ERBB2* amplification by FISH (two or more gene copies) nor scored 3+ for the ERBB2 protein by IHC (15). Interestingly, these patients also benefited from treatment with trastuzumab. This somewhat surprising result suggests a possible discordance in the levels of ERBB2 expression (and thus, ERBB2 dependence) between the primary tumor and its micrometastases. This possibility is further suggested by a study by Meng et al. (16) where 9 of 24 patients with breast cancer whose primary tumor was ERBB2-negative acquired *ERBB2* gene amplification in their circulating tumor cells during cancer progression. Of nine patients, four were treated with trastuzumab-*containing* regimens. One had a complete and two had a partial response (16). Based on data such as these, a randomized trial has been proposed by the NSABP in which patients with 1+ or 2+ ERBB2 by IHC (HercepTest) and no gene amplification (FISH-negative) will be randomized to adjuvant chemotherapy followed by 1 year of trastuzumab or placebo (Soon Paik, NSABP, personal communication, May 2008).

Cardiac toxicity has been the main side effect of trastuzumab. Cardiac safety and risk factors in the NCCTG N9831 adjuvant trial were recently reported (17). Cardiac events were defined as symptomatic congestive heart failure (CHF), definite or probable cardiac death, and/or a reduction in the left ventricular ejection fraction (LVEF) of 15 percentage points below the pretreatment values, irrespective of whether it fell above or below the institutional lower limits of normal. Among 1,944 patients, the 3-year cumulative incidence of cardiac events was 0.3%, 2.8%, and 3.3%, respectively. Cardiac function improved in most cases of CHF following discontinuation of the antibody and administration of cardiac medication. Factors associated with an increased risk of trastuzumab-associated cardiotoxicity were older age, prior or current antihypertensive medications, and a lower LVEF at registration into the trial. Incidence of asymptomatic reductions in LVEF that merited temporary discontinuation of trastuzumab was 8% to 10%. LVEF recovered and the drug was restarted in approximately 50% of these subjects (17). This is also discussed in Chapter 55.

The reversible nature of this toxicity implies that this type of dysfunction differs from the more permanent doxorubicin-induced cardiomyopathy. Indeed, one study showed that trastuzumab can often be continued or restarted in patients who had developed cardiac dysfunction with no subsequent cardiac events (18). In the HERceptin Adjuvant (HERA) trial, a similar low incidence of cardiac events of 2.6% was reported in the arm of the study receiving 1 year of adjuvant trastuzumab (19). The Breast Cancer International Research Group (BCIRG) 006 three-arm trial compared standard adriamycin/cyclophosphamide (AC) followed by docetaxel plus trastuzumab and carboplatin plus docetaxel plus trastuzumab (TCH). The incidence of grade 3/4 CHF was 1.9%, 0.4%, and 0.4%, respectively (20). This difference was significant between the AC/docetaxel plus trastuzumab versus the TCH arm of the trial.

Lapatinib

Another approach to block ERBB2 is the use of ATP-competitive, small molecule TKI. Lapatinib is a recently approved dual TKI against both EGFR and ERBB2 (21); it has shown antitumor activity both *in vitro* and *in vivo* against cancer cells and tumors that overexpress ERBB2 (22,23). It is also active as a single agent in patients with ERBB2-positive cancers, either as first-line therapy or after escape from trastuzumab (24,25). O'Shaughnessy et al. (26) reported a randomized trial of lapatinib plus trastuzumab versus lapatinib monotherapy in patients with heavily pretreated ERBB2-positive metastatic breast cancer that had progressed while patients were on trastuzumab. A 12.4% clinical benefit rate (CBR) was found in the single-agent lapatinib arm. Treatment with the combination improved the progression free survival (PFS) from 8.1 to 12 months, doubled the CBR to 25%, and marginally improved survival (26), overall suggesting that a complete inhibition of the ERBB2 pathway improves outcome of patients with ERBB2-positive tumors.

Some mechanistic studies have shed light on trastuzumab-resistant ERBB2 signaling mechanisms blocked by lapatinib that can explain action of the TKI against trastuzumab-refractory cancers. For example, in some ERBB2-positive tumors, the oncogene product expresses as a kinase-active, 95-kDa cytosolic fragment that lacks the trastuzumab binding epitope and, therefore, can potentially allow the cancer cell to escape antibody action. These fragments of an approximate molecular weight of 95 kDa are kinase-active, but lack the trastuzumab binding epitope and, therefore, can potentially allow the cancer cell to escape antibody action. Lapatinib potently inhibits the catalytic activity of p95^{ERBB2} (27). Notably, a retrospective analysis of a cohort of patients with metastatic ERBB2-positive breast cancer treated with trastuzumab and chemotherapy showed an 11% (1/9) versus 51% (19/37) response rate in tumors with and without evidence of cytosolic p95^{ERBB2}, respectively (27). Further, in breast cancer cells that develop resistance to trastuzumab as a result of overexpression of ErbB ligands and EGFR, lapatinib still inhibited ERBB2 activity and growth of the resistant cells (28). This result also underscores the potent effect of lapatinib on the catalytic activity of the ERBB2 tyrosine kinase. Mechanistic differences between trastuzumab, lapatinib, and other ERBB2 inhibitors are summarized in Table 79.1.

In the study that led to its registration by the FDA, women with ERBB2-positive, locally advanced or metastatic breast cancer that had progressed after treatment with regimens containing anthracyclines, taxanes, and trastuzumab were randomized to capecitabine plus lapatinib (25). Progression-free survival and time to progression were almost doubled by the addition of the ERBB2 antagonist without an increase in severe

Table 79.1	MOLECULAR AND CLINICAL CHARACTERISTICS OF ERBB2 INHIBITORS[a]		
	Trastuzumab	Lapatinib	Pertuzumab
Receptor downregulation	In some cells	May increase cell surface ERBB2	Unknown
ERBB2 heterodimerization	Does not block	Inhibits signaling output from ERBB2-containing heterodimers	Inhibits
Antibody-mediated cell-mediated cytotoxicity (ADCC)	Yes	No	Unknown
Ectodomain cleavage	Inhibits	No effect	No effect
Postreceptor signaling (in vivo)	Partial inhibitor	Strong inhibitor	Not reported
Inhibit p95[ERBB2]	No	Yes	No
Cardiotoxicity	Rare	Rare	Rare
Diarrhea	Uncommon	Dose-limiting toxicity	Dose-limiting toxicity

[a]ERBB2, formerly HER2.

toxicity or symptomatic cardiac events. Patients enrolled in this study had their eligibility (3+ ERBB2 by IHC or gene amplification by FISH) confirmed centrally. In 241/315 (77%) of patients, ERBB2 overexpression was confirmed; in these, lapatinib plus capecitabine was better than capecitabine alone. However, benefit from lapatinib was not detected in 74/315 (23%) patients with cancers where ERBB2 overexpression as defined by the protocol was not confirmed centrally. Similar results were observed in a randomized trial of paclitaxel plus lapatinib in patients treated with first-line therapy for metastatic breast cancer. Outcome was similar between both arms of the study in 401 patients with ERBB2-negative tumors. In 91 patients with ERBB2-overexpressing cancers, the addition of lapatinib, however, improved the median time to progression to 8.1 months compared with 5.8 months in the paclitaxel arm (29). Thus, as for trastuzumab-treated patients, the benefit of lapatinib appears to be limited to patients with ERBB2-overexpressing breast cancer.

Although central nervous system (CNS) metastases developed in a few patients in the registration trial, they occurred in fewer women in the combination arm than in the monotherapy arm (25), suggesting a potential difference between lapatinib and trastuzumab as it applies to recurrences in the CNS. Lin et al. (30) reported a phase II trial of lapatinib in 39 patients with ERBB2-positive breast cancer and brain metastases (30). One patient achieved a partial response in the brain and seven patients (18%) were progression-free at 16 weeks. This clinical outcome plus volumetric changes observed by magnetic resonance imaging (MRI), suggested antitumor activity not previously seen in this site of metastases. At the time of this writing, additional prospective studies of lapatinib plus trastuzumab in patients with ERBB2-positive brain metastases are in progress.

Single-agent lapatinib has also shown activity in patients with recurrent inflammatory ERBB2-positive tumors (31). In this trial, patients coexpressing P-ERBB2 and P-ERBB3 were more likely to respond to lapatinib. Prior trastuzumab therapy, baseline serum levels of the ERBB2 ectodomain, and loss of phosphatase and tensin homolog (PTEN), as measured by IHC, did not preclude response to the ERBB2 TKI (31,32). Finally, a neoadjuvant trial of lapatinib plus chemotherapy in 36 newly diagnosed ERBB2-positive breast cancers was recently completed (Jenny Chang, Baylor College of Medicine; personal communication, June 2008). In this trial, lapatinib was given alone for the first 6 weeks. Of patients, 60% exhibited a partial response at the end of 6 weeks. Median tumor size was 9.5 cm and most of the clinical responses were significant. Currently, two large world-wide randomized studies, ALTTO and Neo-ALTTO (**A**djuvant **L**apatinib and/or **T**rastuzumab **T**reatment **O**ptimization), are testing lapatinib alone or in combination with trastuzumab in the neoadjuvant and adjuvant settings in patients with early ERBB2-positive breast cancer.

Main side effects of lapatinib are diarrhea and fatigue. Interestingly, rash, an almost universal side effect of EGFR inhibitors, is less common with lapatinib. This feature plus the lack of reported activity in non-small cell lung cancer (NSCLC), a tumor type where EGFR inhibitors are approved, and the structural data indicating that lapatinib binds to the inactive conformation of the EGFR (33) raise questions about the potency of lapatinib to block the EGFR in vivo. The cardiac safety data of lapatinib was reported recently by Perez et al. (34). LVEF was monitored by echocardiogram or multi-gated acquisition (MUGA) scan in 3,558 patients treated with the TKI for an average of 13.7 weeks (range 0.6–56.8). A total of 58/3,558 (1.6%) patients exhibited a decrease in LVEF (mean 18.7%; range 11% to 32%); this was symptomatic in only 7/3,558 (0.2%). In all cases, both symptoms and the reduction in LVEF were reversible, either spontaneously or with standard therapy for heart failure. In this cohort, 598 patients had received prior anthracyclines and 759 prior trastuzumab; a reduction in LVEF was observed in only 1.5% and 1.8% of these groups, respectively. No risk factors were associated with a reduction in LVEF.

Other ERBB2 Inhibitors

One mechanism of ERBB2 activation is via heterodimerization with ligand-activated EGFR or ERBB3. Structural data using ErbB receptor extracellular domain crystals and data with cancer cell lines have shown that trastuzumab is unable to block ligand-induced EGFR/ERBB2 and ERBB2/ERBB3 heterodimers (35). Pertuzumab is a humanized IgG$_1$ that specifically binds an epitope in the dimerization domain of ERBB2 and, therefore, can block transactivation of ERBB2 by its ErbB coreceptors in cells with low and high ERBB2 levels (36,37). The main toxicity associated with pertuzumab has been diarrhea. In a recent trial, the addition of pertuzumab to trastuzumab in patients with ERBB2-overexpressing breast cancers whose disease had progressed on trastuzumab therapy resulted in a 40% clinical benefit rate (38). Whether pertuzumab has any activity in breast cancers with low ERBB2 levels remains to be determined.

Trastuzumab-DM1 (T-DM1) is a novel ERBB2 antibody-conjugate designed to combine trastuzumab action with targeted delivery of a highly potent antimicrotubule maytansine derivative DM1 (39) to ERBB2 overexpressing cells. It is proposed that after binding to ERBB2, T-DM1 undergoes receptor-mediated internalization followed by intracellular release of DM1. T-DM1 has activity in trastuzumab-sensitive and -resistant breast cancer cell lines (CL Arteaga, unpublished data). In a recent phase I study of T-DM1, 6 of 24 patients previously treated with trastuzumab exhibited a partial response (40). Grade 2 or greater nausea, alopecia, neuropathy, or cardiotoxicity were not observed. Reversible grade 4 thrombocytopenia was dose limiting. Currently, phase II trials of T-DM1 in patients with ERBB2-positive metastatic breast cancer are underway.

CI-1033, CL-387,785, and HKI-272 are irreversible dual inhibitors of the EGFR and ERBB2 tyrosine kinases. Their mechanism of action involves the covalent association with a cysteine residue in the kinase domain that is specific to ErbB receptors (41). This modification interferes with ATP binding and, in some cells, leads to ubiquitylation, accelerated endocytosis, and intracellular degradation of the ERBB2 receptor (42). HKI-272 and CI-1033 are active against cells expressing a mutant form of ERBB2 with an insertion in exon 20 (43, 44). Of these, HKI-272, from Wyeth, is in clinical development. In a phase I trial with this TKI, diarrhea, nausea, and fatigue were the main side effects. Partial responses were observed in heavily pretreated patients with trastuzumab-resistant ERBB2-overexpressing breast cancer (45), suggesting that these advanced tumors remained dependent on the ERBB2 oncogene.

Epidermal Growth Factor Receptor Inhibitors

Compared with ERBB2, there is less experimental evidence that the EGFR is a critical molecule in the pathogenesis or maintenance of breast cancer. Nonetheless, EGFR antagonists have been widely tested in patients with breast cancer. The EGFR TKI gefitinib and erlotinib have shown, at best, very modest clinical activity in patients with heavily pretreated metastatic disease (46–50). In one of these trials using gefitinib (500 mg/day) monotherapy, sequential IHC studies in skin and tumor biopsies demonstrated complete inhibition of EGFR activity as measured with receptor phospho-specific antibodies. However, tumor cell proliferation measured by Ki67 IHC was reduced in skin but not in tumor cells after 28 days of therapy (50). Because of its relative overexpression in breast cancers with a basal type gene expression signature (51), the EGFR has been proposed as a therapeutic target in tumors that lack detectable hormone receptors and ERBB2. In two recent trials in patients with this triple negative, basal-type metastatic breast cancer, the addition of the EGFR antibody cetuximab did not, however, appreciably add to the effect of chemotherapy (52,53).

Recent pharmacodynamic studies with EGFR inhibitors have provided some clues that might be of clinical use of these compounds in combinatorial therapies. Guix et al. (54) administered erlotinib for 6 to 14 days to women with operable untreated breast cancer to determine a biomarker associated with evidence of drug-mediated cellular activity in the surgical specimen. Erlotinib inhibited cell proliferation (Ki67), P-EGFR, P-MAPK, P-Akt, and P-S6 only in estrogen receptor (ER)-positive but not in ERBB2-positive or triple-negative tumors. These data are consistent with at least three reports showing clinical activity of gefitinib limited against ER-positive breast cancers (48,49,55). Interestingly, erlotinib inhibited phosphorylation of ERα in Ser[118]. Similar results had been reported by Polychronis et al. (55) in ER-positive/EGFR-positive newly diagnosed breast cancers treated for 6 weeks with neoadjuvant gefitinib. Because phosphorylation of this site is mainly regulated by MAPK (56), these results are evidence of operative cross-talk between ER and ErbB receptor signaling early in the natural history of hormone-dependent breast cancer. In addition, they imply that clinical trials of EGFR antagonists in combination with antiestrogens should be explored further. Along those lines, the Eastern Cooperative Oncology Group (ECOG) is conducting a trial in which fulvestrant plus gefitinib is compared with anastrozole plus gefitinib as first-line therapy for metastatic ER-positive postmenopausal breast cancer. End points of the trial are time to progression and biomarker analysis. Combination of EGFR inhibitors and endocrine therapies are further discussed below in this chapter.

THERAPEUTIC RESISTANCE

The therapeutic inactivation of oncogenic kinases essential for tumor cell survival creates selective pressures for the development of mechanisms of acquired resistance. Further, as it applies to type I receptor tyrosine kinases (i.e., ErbB receptors), they do not act as autonomous units but as an interconnected regulatory systems endowed with compensatory feedback loops that counteract or negate the action of therapies that target a single molecule within these networks. As it applies to TKI, these mechanisms of escape include gene amplification, production of a secondary mutation in the targeted kinase, substitution of the signaling function of the targeted kinase(s) by upregulation of compensatory signaling pathways, and overexpression of transporters involved in drug efflux, among others. There are several examples where the molecular profiling of either cancer cell lines selected in the presence of a TKI or after treatment recurrent tumors has led to the discovery of clinically relevant, targetable mechanisms of drug resistance. These include the T315I mutation in the Bcr/Abl kinase in chronic myelogenous leukemia (CML), a T790M secondary mutation and *MET* gene amplification, both in NSCLC with a gefitinib-sensitive activating mutation in EGFR (57), and insulin-like growth factor I receptor (IGF-IR) in cancer cells with wild-type *EGFR* gene amplification (58). Efforts to discover acquired mutations in the *ERBB2* gene are on their way by focusing on biopsies of metastatic recurrences in patients treated with adjuvant trastuzumab or after disease progression on lapatinib. A graphic representation of the mechanisms described below is shown in Figure 79.1.

Many patients with *ERBB2* gene-amplified metastatic breast cancers do not respond or eventually escape trastuzumab, suggesting both *de novo* and acquired mechanisms of therapeutic resistance. Several studies have already reported or speculated on potential mechanisms of resistance to trastuzumab (28). For example, overexpression of the IGF-I receptor or increased levels of IGF-IR/ERBB2 heterodimers, which potently activate PI3K and its downstream effector Akt, abrogate trastuzumab action when transfected into antibody-sensitive breast cancer cells. Amplification of PI3K signaling as a result of loss or low levels of the lipid phosphatase PTEN and *PIK3CA* activating mutations in primary tumors is also associated with lower odds of response to trastuzumab (59,60). Exogenous ligands of the EGFR, HRBB3, and ERBB4 coreceptors have been shown to rescue from the antiproliferative effect of the antibody. This is consistent with structural and cellular data using ErbB receptor ectodomains and different ERBB2 monoclonal antibodies which show that trastuzumab is unable to block ligand-induced EGFR/ERBB2 and ERBB2/ERBB3 heterodimers. Consistent with this notion, we recently reported trastuzumab-resistant ERBB2-overexpressing BT-474 human breast cancer cells generated *in vivo*. The resistant cells retained *ERBB2* gene amplification and trastuzumab binding. They exhibited higher levels of P-EGFR and EGFR/ERBB2 heterodimers as well as overexpression of EGFR, tumor growth factor alpha (TGFα), heparin binding EGF (HB-EGF), and heregulin RNA compared with the parental trastuzumab-sensitive cells (28), suggesting enhanced EGFR- and ERBB3-mediated activation of ERBB2.

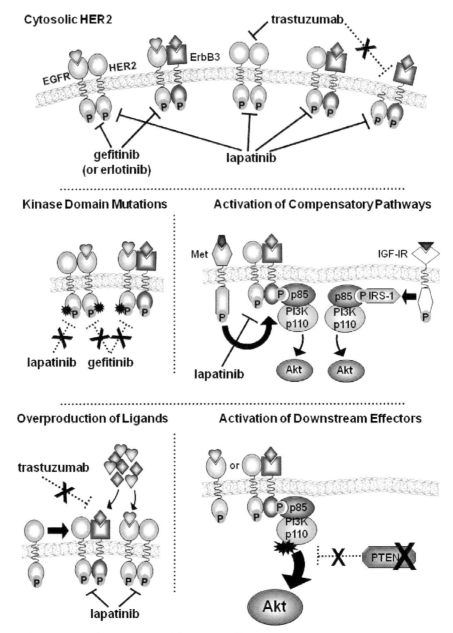

FIGURE 79.1. Mechanisms of resistance to ERBB2 (previously HER2) inhibitors. Cytosolic ERBB2: Lapatinib inhibits the catalytic activity of full-length ERBB2 and p95^{ERBB2} regardless of its dimeric partner. Trastuzumab binds an epitope in the juxtamembrane domain IV of ERBB2 not present in p95^{ERBB2}. **Kinase Domain Mutations**: Kinase domain mutations can potentially interfere with lapatinib binding. Insertions in exon 20 of ERBB2 have been reported to be resistant to lapatinib. **Activation of Compensatory Pathways**: Receptor tyrosine kinasases such as amplified Met can engage ERBB3 (97) and bypass lapatinib-mediated inhibition of the ERBB2 tyrosine kinase. Further, overexpressed insulin-like growth factor I receptor (IGF-IR) can engage the PI3K/Akt pathway directly and mediate resistance to lapatinib and trastuzumab. **Overproduction of Ligands**: Because of the location of its binding epitope, trastuzumab is unable to block ERBB2 that is engaged by heterodimerization with hyperactivated EGFR and/or ERBB3. Lapatinib should be able to block the signaling output of ERBB2-containing heterodimers where ERBB2 is the more potent kinase. **Activation of Downstream Effectors**: Loss of PTEN (or activating mutations in the *PIK3CA* gene) should derepress PI3K/Akt signaling output and generate resistance to both lapatinib and trastuzumab.

The ERBB2 TKI lapatinib and the ERBB2 antibody pertuzumab, which blocks ERBB2 heterodimerization with ErbB coreceptors (36,37), inhibited growth of the antibody-resistant cells, suggesting that, although resistant to trastuzumab, the cells were still dependent on ERBB2-dependent interactions with the ErbB receptor network (28).

To abrogate an EGFR-mediated mechanism of escape and enhance the response to trastuzumab or its duration, EGOG conducted a phase I/II trial of the EGFR TKI gefitinib in combination trastuzumab in patients with metastatic ERBB2-positive metastatic breast cancer (61). Gefitinib (250 mg/day) was the maximal dose that can be safely administered with full-dose weekly trastuzumab. Interim analysis of the efficacy suggested that the combination was unlikely to result in clinical benefit over that reported from trastuzumab alone. These results did not support the use of this combination in patients with ERBB2-positive metastatic breast cancer. There are molecular mechanisms that might explain the lack of benefit of this combination. In a recent report, Sergina et al. (62) showed that, in ERBB2-overexpressing breast cancer cells, the inhibition of ERBB2 phosphorylation induced by gefitinib is followed by feedback upregulation of activated ERBB3 (ErbB3) and Akt, thus limiting the inhibitory effect of the EGFR TKI (62). Consistent with this, in mice bearing breast cancer xenografts with high levels of ERBB2, Arpino et al. (64) added pertuzumab, an antibody that blocks ERBB2-ERBB3 heterodimerization (37,63), to gefitinib and trastuzumab. Only the triple therapy completely eradicated the established xenografts (64). In a recent trial, the addition of pertuzumab to trastuzumab in patients with ERBB2-overexpressing breast cancers whose disease had progressed in trastuzumab resulted in a 40% clinical response rate (38), further implying that ERBB3 signaling, as a result of ERBB2-ERBB3 crosstalk, is a possible mechanism of escape from trastuzumab therapy. Inhibition of ERBB2-mediated transactivation of ERBB3 would also explain the antitumor effect of lapatinib observed against ERBB2-positive tumors that had escaped trastuzumab (25). These results suggest that additional therapies to trastuzumab, such as those targeting the ERBB2 tyrosine kinase directly or the interaction between ERBB2 and ERBB3, will be more synergistic than gefitinib or erlotinib when combined with trastuzumab.

A more recent paper showed overexpression of the Met receptor in ERBB2-overexpressing breast cancer. Met overexpression induced resistance to trastuzumab, as inhibition of Met sensitized cells to ERBB2 antibody, whereas Met activation protected cells against trastuzumab action. Interestingly, ERBB2-overexpressing breast cancer cells rapidly upregulated Met expression on treatment with trastuzumab, thus promoting their own resistance (65). Finally, Anido et al. (66) reported the presence of ERBB2 C-terminal fragments, which result from alternative translation initiation from methionines near the transmembrane domain of the full-length receptor molecule. These fragments of an approximate molecular weight of 95 kDa are kinase-active but lack the trastuzumab binding epitope and, therefore, can potentially allow the cancer cell to escape antibody action. A retrospective analysis of a cohort of patients with metastatic ERBB2-positive breast cancer treated with trastuzumab and chemotherapy showed an 11% (1/9) versus 51% (19/37) response rate in tumors with and without evidence of cytosolic p95^{ERBB2}, respectively (27). Despite these important leads, however, no biomarker(s) yet exist that can reliably predict lack of benefit from trastuzumab which, in turn, can be used for subsequent clinical trial development or individual therapeutic decisions.

Less is known about mechanisms of *de novo* or acquired resistance to lapatinib or whether these will overlap with mechanisms of escape to other ERBB2 TKI. Because of its recent approval, at this time no lapatinib-treated tumor cohorts with adequate follow-up exist where one can ask this question retrospectively in unbiased fashion. Unlike trastuzumab, low levels of PTEN were not associated with lack of response to lapatinib in a recent clinical trial in patients with ERBB2-overexpressing inflammatory breast cancer (31).

Other data suggest that on acquisition of resistance to anti-ERBB2 drugs, ERBB2-positive cancer cells rely on ER signaling for growth and survival. For example, treatment with trastuzumab has been shown to restore detectable ER levels to some ER-negative tumors that went on to respond to aromatase inhibitors (67). Treatment with lapatinib upregulates ER transcription and PgR levels in BT-474 breast cancer cells (68). In this last study, growth of some of the lapatinib-resistant populations was inhibited by RNA interference (RNAi) of ERα and treatment with the pure antiestrogen fulvestrant delayed the emergence of resistance to the TKI.

INSULIN AND INSULIN-LIKE GROWTH FACTOR RECEPTORS

The insulin-like growth factor (IGF) network is composed of the ligands insulin, IGF-I, and IGF-II; the insulin, IGF-I, and IGF-I transmembrane receptor tyrosine kinases; and the IGF binding proteins (IGFBP). The ligands IGF-I and IGF-II bind the IGF-IR. The IGF-I receptor is closely related to the insulin receptor (IR), which is activated by insulin and IGF-II. In normal physiology, ligand-induced activation of the IGF-IR plays a role in fetal growth and linear growth of the skeleton and other organs, whereas insulin acts via the IR to regulate glucose homeostasis. The local bioavailability of IGF ligands is abnormally high in some cancers; IGFBP and IGFBP proteases are important for regulating ligand bioavailability. Abundant evidence suggests that IGF-IR signaling is important in maintaining tumor cells *in vivo* and that inhibition of IGF-IR signaling affects growth and motility of cancer cells both *in vitro* and in mouse models (69). Although IGF-IR activating mutations have not been reported in human tumors, there are reports of genetic polymorphisms in genes encoding IGF-I and IGFBP3 proteins associated with a higher risk of breast cancer.

Several approaches have been proposed and developed to block IGF-IR signaling. The stimulation of the IR by insulin or IGF-II also enhances mitogenesis and survival of cancer cells, suggesting that dual targeting of both IGF-IR and IR might be required for complete blockade of the IGF network in cancer cells (70,71). Therapeutic approaches targeted to this network include ATP mimetics that inhibit the IGF-IR tyrosine kinase, IGF-IR neutralizing antibodies, dominant-negative mutants, recombinant IGFBP, antisense oligonucleotides, growth hormone-releasing hormone (GHRH) antagonists, antibodies against IGF-I and IGF-II, and soluble receptor fusion proteins. The two types of inhibitors that hold the most promise in translating to clinical use are the receptor TKI and the IGF-IR neutralizing antibodies. The small molecule TKI block IGF-IR's catalytic activity by blocking ATP binding to the ATP site in the kinase domain or by blocking substrate binding to the activated receptor. It is highly likely that because of receptor homology, they will cross-react with the IR resulting in glucose intolerance. Several of the antibodies in preclinical and clinical development have been shown to induce downregulation of IGF-IR via the endocytic pathway, thus diminishing cell surface receptors available for stimulation by exogenous ligands (70).

Experimental evidence suggests that IGF-IR antagonists will be effective in combination with other targeted therapies. For example, IGF-IR overexpression can confer resistance to trastuzumab (discussed above). Cell lines and primary tumors that either acquire resistant or do not respond to trastuzumab, overexpress IGF-IR (72,73). Inhibition of the serine or threonine kinase TOR induces IRS-1 expression and P-Akt in cancer cell lines and in primary tumors in patients treated with rapamycin, CCI-779, or RAD001 (74,75). This feedback upregulation of P-Akt can enhance IGF-IR signaling output and negate the antitumor effect of target of rapamycin (TOR) inhibitors. Higher levels of IGF-IR, IRS-1, and IGF-II have been detected in ER-positive human breast cancer cells that adapted to hormonal deprivation or that became resistant to tamoxifen (76,77). Thus, IGF-IR antagonists may prevent or delay resistance to ERBB2 and TOR inhibitors and to endocrine therapy. At the time of this writing, many IGF-IR antagonists are in variable phases of clinical development as both single agents and in combination with standard anticancer therapies in patients with breast and other carcinomas. They are summarized in Table 79.2 below.

Table 79.2	IGF-IR INHIBITORS IN CLINICAL DEVELOPMENT		
Type of Drug	Drug	Phase of Development	Source
MAb	CP-751,871	Phase III	Pfizer
MAb	IMC-A12	Phase II (colorectal)	ImClone Systems
MAb	R1507	Phase II	Roche
MAb	AMG479	Phase II (Ewing's)	Amgen
MAb	H7C10 (MK-0646)	Phase II	Merck/Pierre Fabre
MAb	SCH 717454 (19D12)	Phase II (sarcoma)	Schering-Plough
MAb	AVE1642	Pre-clinical	Sanofi-Aventis
MAb	BIIB022	Phase I	Biogen IDEC
TKI	OSI-906	Phase I	OSI Pharmaceuticals
TKI	NVP-AEW541	Clinical development stopped	Novartis
TKI	BMS-554417; BMS-536924	Both pre-clinical	Bristol Myers Squibb
TKI	XL-228	Phase I	Exelixis
Recombinant IGFBP-3	INSM-rhIGFBP-3	Phase I	INSMED

IGF-IR, insulin-like growth factor I receptor; IGFBP, IGF binding proteins; MAb, monoclonal antibody; TKI, tyrosine kinase inhibitor.

COMBINATORIAL THERAPIES

One area in which TKI have added or are expected to add to current standards of care is in combination with antiestrogen therapy in hormone-dependent breast cancer. Preclinical models or acquired resistance to tamoxifen and aromatase inhibitors have shown upregulation of polypeptide growth factor receptor signaling, including the ErbB receptor network. The addition of EGFR inhibitors to antiestrogen therapy has been mentioned above. As it applies to other members of the ErbB receptor family, about 10% of tumors that relapse early while on adjuvant tamoxifen exhibit high levels of ERBB2 in the biopsy of the recurrent cancer (78). Patients with ER-positive metastatic breast cancer treated with letrozole or tamoxifen who convert to ERBB2-positive in their serum at the time of disease progression exhibit a shorter survival compared with those who do not convert (79). Preliminary analysis of patients enrolled in the Breast International Group (BIG) I-98 and Arimidex, Tamoxifen Alone or in Combination (ATAC), two large randomized trials of adjuvant endocrine therapy in ER-positive breast cancers where aromatase inhibitors and tamoxifen were used, has shown a superior disease-free survival in patients with ER-positive/ERBB2-negative than those with ER-positive/ERBB2-positive tumors (80,81). Ellis et al. (82) reported the effect of neoadjuvant endocrine therapy in postmenopausal patients with stage II-III breast cancer who were not candidates for breast conservation. The clinical response after 4 months of neoadjuvant therapy with letrozole or tamoxifen was no different between ER-positive/ERBB2-negative and ER-positive/ERBB2-positive tumors. However, the ER-positive/ERBB2-positive cancers did not show suppression of tumor cell proliferation as measured by Ki67 IHC in the surgical specimen, suggesting continuous growth despite endocrine therapy.

A randomized phase III study (TAnDEM) was performed to evaluate the efficacy of trastuzumab plus anastrozole compared with anastrozole alone in postmenopausal women with ERBB2-positive and ER-positive and/or PgR-positive metastatic breast cancer (82a). Patients in the combination arm had significant improvement in progression-free survival, objective response rate, and clinical benefit rate compared with patients in the anastrozole arm. Median survival was not statistically different between both arms of the study, although this comparison was questionable because 70% of patients in the anastrozole arm were treated with trastuzumab at the time of progression.

In a phase I study in heavily pretreated patients, the combination of lapatinib and letrozole was well tolerated. Main toxicities were grade 1 skin rash and grade 1/2 diarrhea (83). Three of 18 patients with ER-positive/ERBB2-positive tumors exhibited stable disease lasting more than 6 months and negative pharmacokinetic interactions occurred between both drugs. A large randomized, double-blind, placebo-controlled, multicenter study of letrozole plus lapatinib versus letrozole plus placebo in postmenopausal hormone receptor-positive (ER-positive or PgR-positive)/ERBB2-positive metastatic breast cancer (EGF30008) recently completed accrual. This study started in 2003 and enrolled 1,286 patients of which approximately 18% (>200) had ERBB2-overexpressing cancers. It is powered to detect a 30% improvement in time to disease progression in patients treated with the combination. At the time of this writing, there are not sufficient tumor progressions to determine if there is a difference between the treatment arms (J.D. Meltzman, GlaxoSmithKline, personal communication, April 2008). In this trial, many patients are still on active treatment, some of them in excess of 2 years.

Cristofanilli et al. (84) recently reported the results of a randomized phase II study of anastrozole plus gefitinib versus anastrozole plus placebo in postmenopausal women with hormone receptor-positive metastatic breast cancer. Fifty patients received anastrozole plus placebo and 43 the aromatase and the EGFR inhibitor combined. Patients treated with this combination showed a median PFS of 14.5 versus 8.1 months in the anastrozole plus placebo control arm of the trial. Follow-up was too short to report overall survival (84). A similar randomized phase II trial of was reported by Osborne et al. (85). Patients with new metastatic disease or those who had recurrence after adjuvant tamoxifen or had recurred during or after adjuvant therapy with an aromatase inhibitor were randomized to tamoxifen plus or minus gefitinib. The PFS was 10.9 versus 8.8 months in the combination versus the tamoxifen arm with a PFS hazard ratio of 0.84 (85). The results of these two studies in patients with ER-positive metastatic disease should be contrasted with those of a 16-week neoadjuvant trial of anastrozole plus or minus gefitinib in patients with stage I-IIIB ER-positive breast cancer. In this study, objective response showed a nonsignificant trend against the combination versus the anastrozole arm (48% vs. 61%). This difference was statistically significant in the PgR-positive group (86). Lack of patient selection, prior adjuvant therapy, the different stage of disease (i.e., localized vs. metastatic) and study end points (i.e., response vs. PFS) are potential reasons to explain these discrepant results.

Inhibition of vascular endothelial growth factor (VEGF) has also been tested as a means of enhancing the effect of endocrine therapy and abrogating the emergence of resistance to it. A phase II study of letrozole and bevacizumab reported evidence of modest antitumor activity (87). Efficacy in this trial was limited because previous use of an aromatase inhibitor without evidence of progression was allowed and most patients enrolled had had prior treatment with letrozole or anastrozole. Currently, the Cancer and Leukemia Group B (CALGB) is conducting a randomized comparison of letrozole or tamoxifen plus or minus bevacizumab as first-line therapy in women with ER-positive metastatic breast cancer. Other phase II trials are combining letrozole with vatalanib, a pan-inhibitor of VEGF receptor (VEGFR) kinases, or with imatinib, a small molecule that inhibits the Abl, c-Kit, and PDGFR tyrosine kinases. Finally, a trial of anastrozole and sorafenib is ongoing. All these studies have been summarized recently (88,89). Sorafenib is a multikinase inhibitor that inhibits VEGFR, PDGFR, and the Raf kinase. One limitation of these studies is that other than ER, no other biomarker potentially predictive of benefit from the addition of the TKI is being used for patient selection or stratification.

Signaling downstream the ErbB receptor network regulated VEGF transcription (90). As a result of this, tumors with *ERBB2* gene amplification overexpress VEGF and exhibit enhanced angiogenesis. Further, VEGF overexpression adds to the predictive value of poor patient outcome conferred by high ERBB2 levels (91). Therefore, bevacizumab has been combined with trastuzumab in a phase I/II trial as first-line therapy for metastatic ERBB2-positive breast cancer. An interim analysis of the first 37 patients enrolled in this trial showed an overall response rate of 54%. There were 13 of 37 cardiac adverse events reported; all were grade 1 or 2 and asymptomatic except one, which was a case of florid congestive heart failure. Accrual of 50 patients has been completed, but a final efficacy analysis is not available at the time of this writing (Mark Pegram, University of Miami, personal communication, April 2008). In addition, ECOG is leading a large intergroup phase III study where patients with metastatic ERBB2-positive breast cancer are randomized to chemotherapy (carboplatin and taxol or physician's choice) with trastuzumab plus or minus bevacizumab, using survival as an end point. This recently initiated trial has early stopping rules and frequent cardiac surveillance as part of its design.

STRATEGIES FOR THE CLINICAL DEVELOPMENT OF TYROSINE KINASE INHIBITORS

A number of considerations differentiate the clinical development of TKI from that of conventional anticancer chemotherapy. The potential dependence of cancers on the function of the target tyrosine kinase compared with normal host tumor tissues suggest that the TKI will be less toxic and better tolerated than chemotherapy and are, therefore, deliverable over a longer period. Second, the optimal biological dose at which the TKI modulate their molecular target should not match their maximal tolerated dose, a concentration at which off-target toxicities are likely to occur. Third, knowledge of the drug target implies that drug action can be monitored with appropriate pharmacodynamic biomarkers that, in turn, may guide drug development and therapeutic intervention. In the cases where TKI have been most successful, they have been developed in tumors known to be highly dependent on the drug target, such as the Bcr/Abl inhibitor imatinib in CML, trastuzumab, lapatinib in ERBB2-positive breast cancer, and erlotinib in non–small-cell lung cancer harboring activating *EGFR* gene mutations. We should recognize, however, that for most TKI currently in clinical development, a profile of kinase dependence that will identify tumors likely to

derive clinical benefit is not clearly recognizable or has not been established *a priori*.

All these considerations suggest that the current process of drug development used for conventional chemotherapy does not fully apply to that of mechanism-based TKI. They also suggest that a biomarker profile should be developed before or during early phases of drug development to select patients into phase II efficacy trials of TKI alone or in combinatorial therapies that include them. Several data suggest that short-term, tissue-based pharmacodynamic trials provide information that can be used later for patient selection or exclusion into early trials with novel TKI. For example, administration of antiestrogens for a period of 1 to 3 weeks has been shown to induce a significant antiproliferative effect, as measured by Ki67 IHC, in ER-positive but not ER-negative breast cancers (92–94). Treatment-induced tumor cell apoptosis, as measured by cleaved caspase-3 IHC 1 week after administration of trastuzumab correlated with clinical response of ERBB2-overexpressing breast cancers (13). The neoadjuvant IMPACT (immediate preoperative Arimidex compared with tamoxifen) trial compared anastrozole, tamoxifen, and the combination of both drugs. Drug-induced inhibition of Ki67 IHC *in situ* after 2 weeks of therapy was better in anastrozole-treated patients compared with the patients in the other two arms (95). Interestingly, this result after only 2 weeks of therapy mirrors the results of the large adjuvant ATAC trial in which relapse-free survival was also better in the anastrozole arm of the study (96).

All these considerations and the clinical examples mentioned above point to some creative approaches in the design of exploratory trials with novel TKI to ensure that critical end points in their clinical development are measured. For example, after a safe dose of a TKI has been defined in a conventional phase I study, patients with operable breast cancer who are not candidates for neoadjuvant therapy can be treated with the investigational TKI for a period of time adequate for the drug to achieve steady-state levels in plasma. Effects on cell proliferation (Ki67), apoptosis (TUNEL, cleaved caspase-3 IHC), and inhibition of the drug target *in situ* (with phospho-specific antibodies) can be easily assessed in formalin-fixed cores from the surgical specimen. A gene expression signature indicative to kinase inactivation can be generated from fixed or frozen tumor material not further required for clinical purposes. Evidence of inhibition of the molecular target of the TKI will validate the phase II dose selected by the phase I process. Lack of inhibition of the target *in situ* would suggest that the drug is not reaching its target despite adequate drug levels (also testable) or other pharmacologic limitation. Addressing this hurdle would be critically important before engaging in larger and (potentially) uninformative efficacy trials. Evidence of inhibition of cell proliferation (Ki67), induction of apoptosis (e.g., TUNEL), or both can be correlated with routine clinical markers, such as ER, PgR, and ERBB2 levels to determine if the drug has or has not activity against an obvious subtype of breast cancer. In turn, this can potentially inform of subtypes in which the clinical development should be focused or subtypes that can be enriched for in early phase II studies. A flow diagram of this presurgical approach for the testing of novel TKI during the preapproval process of clinical development is shown in Figure 79.2 below.

Although not of a *therapeutic* intent, the short duration of therapy and the previously assessed safety of these TKI (during their conventional phase I development) make this presurgical trial design highly feasible. Clearly, this approach requires additional examples and experience. Speculatively, however, this strategy may expedite the development of TKI by confirming target inactivation in tumors and informing of conventional and novel biomarkers that can be used for the selection of patients likely to respond in subsequent phase II trials. Finally and also importantly, this approach may also inform of tumor types that

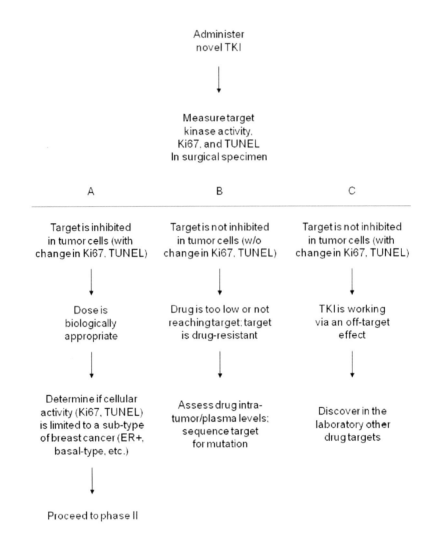

FIGURE 79.2. Presurgical (after phase I) clinical trial design for molecular target validation, discovery of predictive biomarkers of response, and identification of subgroups of breast cancer with and without cellular sensitivity to novel tyrosine kinase inhibitors (TKI). This design allows the assessment of tyrosine kinase inhibition in tumors. This can be done by measuring the kinase itself with site-specific phospho-antibodies (i.e., P-EGFR, P-ERBB2) or a surrogate marker of its activity (i.e., P-FAK for the Src tyrosine kinase). **A**, **B**, and **C** represent three possible outcomes of this clinical study design. (Modified from Sawyers CL. Opportunities and challenges in the development of kinase inhibitor therapy for cancer. *Genes Dev* 2003;17:2998, with permission.)

are unlikely to respond. The profile of those tumors can, in turn, be used to exclude patients from early efficacy trials because they are likely to dilute the net signal of clinical activity of the investigational TKI or a combination that includes it. Such scenario, the equivalent of developing trastuzumab in tumors without ERBB2 gene amplification, would threaten the clinical development of therapeutic TKI in breast cancer.

Supported by NIH R01 grants CA62212 and CA80195, an ACS Clinical Research Professorship Grant CRP-07-234, Breast Cancer Specialized Program of Research Excellence (SPORE) grant P50 CA98131, and Vanderbilt-Ingram Comprehensive Cancer Center Support grant P30 CA68485.

References

1. Hunter T. The Croonian Lecture 1997. The phosphorylation of proteins on tyrosine: its role in cell growth and disease. *Philos Trans R Soc Lond B Biol Sci* 1998;353(1368):583–605.
2. Robinson DR, Wu YM, Lin SF. The protein tyrosine kinase family of the human genome. *Oncogene* 2000;19(49):5548–5557.
3. Blume-Jensen P, Hunter T. Oncogenic kinase signalling. *Nature* 2001;411(6835):355–365.
4. Schlessinger J. Cell signaling by receptor tyrosine kinases. *Cell* 2000;103(2):211–225.
5. Yarden Y, Sliwkowski MX. Untangling the ErbB signalling network. *Nat Rev Mol Cell Biol* 2001;2(2):127–137.
6. Ross JS, Fletcher JA. The HER-2/neu oncogene in breast cancer: prognostic factor, predictive factor, and target for therapy. *Stem Cells* 1998;16(6):413–428.
7. Romond EH, Perez EA, Bryant J, et al. Trastuzumab plus adjuvant chemotherapy for operable HER2-positive breast cancer. *N Engl J Med* 2005;353(16):1673–1684.
8. Molina MA, Codony-Servat J, Albanell J, et al. Trastuzumab (Herceptin), a humanized anti-Her2 receptor monoclonal antibody, inhibits basal and activated Her2 ectodomain cleavage in breast cancer cells. *Cancer Res* 2001;61(12):4744–4749.
9. Yakes FM, Chinratanalab W, Ritter CA, et al. Herceptin-induced inhibition of phosphatidylinositol-3 kinase and Akt Is required for antibody-mediated effects on p27, cyclin D1, and antitumor action. *Cancer Res* 2002;62(14):4132–4141.
10. Clynes RA, Towers TL, Presta LG, et al. Inhibitory Fc receptors modulate *in vivo* cytoxicity against tumor targets. *Nat Med* 2000;6(4):443–446.
11. Izumi Y, Xu L, di Tomaso E, et al. Tumour biology: herceptin acts as an anti-angiogenic cocktail. *Nature* 2002;416(6878):279–280.
12. Austin CD, De Maziere AM, Pisacane PI, et al. Endocytosis and sorting of ErbB2 and the site of action of cancer therapeutics trastuzumab and geldanamycin. *Mol Biol Cell* 2004;15(12):5268–5282.
13. Mohsin SK, Weiss HL, Gutierrez MC, et al. Neoadjuvant trastuzumab induces apoptosis in primary breast cancers. *J Clin Oncol* 2005;23(11):2460–2468.
14. Musolino A, Naldi N, Bortesi B, et al. Immunoglobulin G fragment C receptor polymorphisms and clinical efficacy of trastuzumab-based therapy in patients with HER-2/neu-positive metastatic breast cancer. *J Clin Oncol* 2008;26(11):1789–1796.
15. Paik S, Kim C, Wolmark N. HER2 status and benefit from adjuvant trastuzumab in breast cancer. *N Engl J Med* 2008;358(13):1409–1411.
16. Meng S, Tripathy D, Shete S, et al. HER-2 gene amplification can be acquired as breast cancer progresses. *Proc Natl Acad Sci U S A* 2004;101(25):9393–9398.

17. Perez EA, Suman VJ, Davidson NE, et al. Cardiac safety analysis of doxorubicin and cyclophosphamide followed by paclitaxel with or without trastuzumab in the North Central Cancer Treatment Group N9831 adjuvant breast cancer trial. *J Clin Oncol* 2008;26(8):1231–1238.

18. Ewer MS, Vooletich MT, Durand JB, et al. Reversibility of trastuzumab-related cardiotoxicity: new insights based on clinical course and response to medical treatment. *J Clin Oncol* 2005;23(31):7820–7826.

19. Smith I, Procter M, Gelber RD, et al. 2-year follow-up of trastuzumab after adjuvant chemotherapy in HER2-positive breast cancer: a randomised controlled trial. *Lancet* 2007;369(9555):29–36.

20. Robert N, Leyland-Jones B, Asmar L, et al. Randomized phase III study of trastuzumab, paclitaxel, and carboplatin compared with trastuzumab and paclitaxel in women with HER-2-overexpressing metastatic breast cancer. *J Clin Oncol* 2006;24(18):2786–2792.

21. Rusnak DW, Lackey K, Affleck K, et al. The effects of the novel, reversible epidermal growth factor receptor/ErbB-2 tyrosine kinase inhibitor, GW2016, on the growth of human normal and tumor-derived cell lines *in vitro* and *in vivo*. *Mol Cancer Ther* 2001;1(2):85–94.

22. Spector NL, Xia W, Burris H, 3rd, et al. Study of the biologic effects of lapatinib, a reversible inhibitor of ErbB1 and ErbB2 tyrosine kinases, on tumor growth and survival pathways in patients with advanced malignancies. *J Clin Oncol* 2005;23(11):2502–2512.

23. Konecny GE, Pegram MD, Venkatesan N, et al. Activity of the dual kinase inhibitor lapatinib (GW572016) against HER2-overexpressing and trastuzumab-treated breast cancer cells. *Cancer Res* 2006;66(3):1630–1639.

24. Gomez HL, Doval DC, Chavez MA, et al. Efficacy and safety of lapatinib as first-line therapy for ErbB2-amplified locally advanced or metastatic breast cancer. *J Clin Oncol* 2008;26(18):2999–3005.

25. Geyer CE, Forster J, Lindquist D, et al. Lapatinib plus capecitabine for HER2-positive advanced breast cancer. *N Engl J Med* 2006;355(26):2733–2743.

26. O'Shaughnessy J, Blackwell KL, Burstein H, et al. A randomized study of lapatinib alone or in combination with trastuzumab in heavily pretreated HER2+ breast cancer progressing on trastuzumab therapy. *Proceeding of the American Society of Clinical Oncology* 2008;26(15S):44s.

27. Scaltriti M, Rojo F, Ocana A, et al. Expression of p95HER2, a truncated form of the HER2 receptor, and response to anti-HER2 therapies in breast cancer. *J Natl Cancer Inst* 2007;99(8):628–638.

28. Ritter CA, Perez-Torres M, Rinehart C, et al. Human breast cancer cells selected for resistance to trastuzumab in vivo overexpress epidermal growth factor receptor and ErbB ligands and remain dependent on the ErbB receptor network. *Clin Cancer Res* 2007;13(16):4909–4919.

29. Di Leo A, Gomez H, Aziz Z, et al. Lapatinib (L) with paclitaxel compared to paclitaxel as first-line treatment for patients with metastatic breast cancer: a phase III randomized, double-blind study of 580 patients. *Proceeding of the American Society of Clinical Oncology* 2007;25(18S):34s.

30. Lin NU, Carey LA, Liu MC, et al. Phase II trial of lapatinib for brain metastases in patients with human epidermal growth factor receptor 2-positive breast cancer. *J Clin Oncol* 2008;26(12):1993–1999.

31. Johnston S, Trudeau M, Kaufman B, et al. Phase II study of predictive biomarker profiles for response targeting human epidermal growth factor receptor 2 (HER-2) in advanced inflammatory breast cancer with lapatinib monotherapy. *J Clin Oncol* 2008;26(7):1066–1072.

32. Cameron D, Casey M, Press M, et al. A phase III randomized comparison of lapatinib plus capecitabine versus capecitabine alone in women with advanced breast cancer that has progressed on trastuzumab: updated efficacy and biomarker analyses. *Breast Cancer Res Treat* 2007;106(Suppl 1):S22.

33. Wood ER, Truesdale AT, McDonald OB, et al. A unique structure for epidermal growth factor receptor bound to GW572016 (Lapatinib): relationships among protein conformation, inhibitor off-rate, and receptor activity in tumor cells. *Cancer Res* 2004;64(18):6652–6659.

34. Perez EA, Koehler M, Byrne J, et al. Cardiac safety of lapatinib: pooled analysis of 3,689 patients enrolled in clinical trials. *Mayo Clin Proc* 2008;83(6):679–686.

35. Cho HS, Mason K, Ramyar KX, et al. Structure of the extracellular region of HER2 alone and in complex with the Herceptin Fab. *Nature* 2003;421(6924):756–760.

36. Adams CW, Allison DE, Flagella K, et al. Humanization of a recombinant monoclonal antibody to produce a therapeutic HER dimerization inhibitor, pertuzumab. *Cancer Immunol Immunother* 2006;55(6):717–727.

37. Franklin MC, Carey KD, Vajdos FF, et al. Insights into ErbB signaling from the structure of the ErbB2-pertuzumab complex. *Cancer Cell* 2004;5(4):317–328.

38. Baselga J, Cameron D, Miles D, et al. Objective response rate in a phase II multicenter trial of pertuzumab, a HER2 dimerization inhibiting monoclonal antibody, in combination with trastuzumab in patients with HER2-positive metastatic breast cancer which has progressed during treatment with trastuzumab. *Proceeding of the American Society of Clinical Oncology* 2007;25 (18S):33s.

39. Widdison WC, Wilhelm SD, Cavanagh EE, et al. Semisynthetic maytansine analogues for the targeted treatment of cancer. *J Med Chem* 2006;49(14):4392–4408.

40. Krop IE, Beermam M, Modi S, et al. A phase I study of trastuzumab-DM1, a first-in-class HER2 antibody-drug conjugate, in patients with advances HER2+ breast cancer. *Breast Cancer Res Treat* 2007;106 (Suppl. 1):S33.

41. Smaill JB, Rewcastle GW, Loo JA, et al. Tyrosine kinase inhibitors. 17. Irreversible inhibitors of the epidermal growth factor receptor: 4-(phenylamino) quinazoline- and 4-(phenylamino) pyrido. *J Med Chem* 2000;43(7):1380–1397.

42. Citri A, Alroy I, Lavi S, et al. Drug-induced ubiquitylation and degradation of ErbB receptor tyrosine kinases: implications for cancer therapy. *EMBO J* 2002;21(10):2407–2417.

43. Wang SE, Narasanna A, Perez-Torres M, et al. HER2 kinase domain mutation results in constitutive phosphorylation and activation of HER2 and EGFR and resistance to EGFR tyrosine kinase inhibitors. *Cancer Cell* 2006;10(1):25–38.

44. Shimamura T, Ji H, Minami Y, et al. Non-small-cell lung cancer and Ba/F3 transformed cells harboring the ERBB2 G776insV_G/C mutation are sensitive to the dual-specific epidermal growth factor receptor and ERBB2 inhibitor HKI-272. *Cancer Res* 2006;66(13):6487–6491.

45. Wong KK, Fracasso PM, Bukowski RM, et al. HKI-272, an irreversible pan erbB receptor tyrosine kinase inhibitor: preliminary phase I results in patients with solid tumors. *Proceeding of the American Society of Clinical Oncology* 2006;24:125s.

46. Albain K, Elledge R, Gradishar WJ, et al. Open label, phase II multicenter trial of ZD1839 ('Iressa') in patients with advanced breast cancer. *Br Cancer Res Treat* 2002;76 (Suppl. 1):S33.

47. Winer EP, Cobleigh M, Dickler M, et al. Phase II multicenter study to evaluate the efficacy and safety of Tarceva (erlotinib, OSI-774) in women with previously treated locally advanced or metastatic breast cancer. *Breast Cancer Res Treat* 2002;76:445A.

48. Agrawal A, Gutteridge E, Cheung KL, et al. Efficacy and tolerability of gefitinib in oestrogen receptor negative and tamoxifen resistant oestrogen receptor positive locally advanced or metastatic breast cancer. *Breast Cancer Res Treat* 2005;24:S61.

49. Ciardiello F, Troiani T, Caputo F, et al. Phase II study of gefitinib in combination with docetaxel as first-line therapy in metastatic breast cancer. *Br J Cancer* 2006; 94(11):1604–1609.

50. Baselga J, Albanell J, Ruiz A, et al. Phase II and tumor pharmacodynamic study of gefitinib in patients with advanced breast cancer. *J Clin Oncol* 2005;23(23): 5323–5333.

51. Livasy CA, Perou CM, Karaca G, et al. Identification of a basal-like subtype of breast ductal carcinoma *in situ*. *Hum Pathol* 2007;38(2):197–204.

52. Carey LA, Mayer E, Marcom PK, et al. TBCRC 001: EGFR inhibition with cetuximab in metastatic triple negative (basal-like) breast cancer. *Breast Cancer Res Treat* 2007;106(Suppl 1):S32.

53. O'Shaughnessy J, Weckstein DJ, Vukelja SJ, et al. Preliminary results of a randomized phase II study of weekly irinotecan/carboplatin with or without cetuximab in patients with metastatic breast cancer. *Breast Cancer Res Treat* 2007;106 (Suppl 1):S32.

54. Guix M, Granja Nde M, Meszoely I, et al. Short preoperative treatment with erlotinib inhibits tumor cell proliferation in hormone receptor-positive breast cancers. *J Clin Oncol* 2008;26(6):897–906.

55. Polychronis A, Sinnett HD, Hadjiminas D, et al. Preoperative gefitinib versus gefitinib and anastrozole in postmenopausal patients with oestrogen-receptor positive and epidermal-growth-factor-receptor-positive primary breast cancer: a double-blind placebo-controlled phase II randomised trial. *Lancet Oncol* 2005;6(6): 383–391.

56. Sarwar N, Kim JS, Jiang J, et al. Phosphorylation of ERalpha at serine 118 in primary breast cancer and in tamoxifen-resistant tumours is indicative of a complex role for ERalpha phosphorylation in breast cancer progression. *Endocr Relat Cancer* 2006;13(3):851–861.

57. Arteaga CL. HER3 and mutant EGFR meet MET. *Nat Med* 2007;13(6):675–677.

58. Guix M, Faber AC, Wang SE, et al. Acquired resistance to EGFR tyrosine kinase inhibitors in cancer cells is mediated by loss of IGF-binding proteins. *J Clin Invest* 2008;118(7):2609–2619.

59. Nagata Y, Lan KH, Zhou X, et al. PTEN activation contributes to tumor inhibition by trastuzumab, and loss of PTEN predicts trastuzumab resistance in patients. *Cancer Cell* 2004;6(2):117–127.

60. Berns K, Horlings HM, Hennessy BT, et al. A functional genetic approach identifies the PI3K pathway as a major determinant of trastuzumab resistance in breast cancer. *Cancer Cell* 2007;12(4):395–402.

61. Arteaga CL, O'Neill A, Moulder SL, et al. A phase I-II study of combined blockade of the ErbB receptor network with trastuzumab and gefitinib in patients with HER2 (ErbB2)-overexpressing metastatic breast cancer. *Clin Cancer Res* 2007;13: 4909–4919.

62. Sergina NV, Rausch M, Wang D, et al. Escape from HER-family tyrosine kinase inhibitor therapy by the kinase-inactive HER3. *Nature* 2007;445(7126): 437–441.

63. Agus DB, Akita RW, Fox WD, et al. Targeting ligand-activated ErbB2 signaling inhibits breast and prostate tumor growth. *Cancer Cell* 2002;2(2):127–137.

64. Arpino G, Gutierrez C, Weiss H, et al. Treatment of human epidermal growth factor receptor 2-overexpressing breast cancer xenografts with multiagent HER-targeted therapy. *J Natl Cancer Inst* 2007;99(9):694–705.

65. Shattuck DL, Miller JK, Carraway KL, 3rd, et al. Met receptor contributes to trastuzumab resistance of Her2-overexpressing breast cancer cells. *Cancer Res* 2008;68(5):1471–1477.

66. Anido J, Scaltriti M, Bech Serra JJ, et al. Biosynthesis of tumorigenic HER2 C-terminal fragments by alternative initiation of translation. *EMBO J* 2006;25(13):3234–3244.

67. Munzone E, Curigliano G, Rocca A, et al. Reverting estrogen-receptor-negative phenotype in HER-2-overexpressing advanced breast cancer patients exposed to trastuzumab plus chemotherapy. *Breast Cancer Res* 2006;8(1):R4.

68. Xia W, Bacus S, Hegde P, et al. A model of acquired autoresistance to a potent ErbB2 tyrosine kinase inhibitor and a therapeutic strategy to prevent its onset in breast cancer. *Proc Natl Acad Sci U S A* 2006;103(20):7795–8000.

69. Pollak MN, Schernhammer ES, Hankinson SE. Insulin-like growth factors and neoplasia. *Nat Rev Cancer* 2004;4(7):505–518.

70. Sachdev D, Yee D. Disrupting insulin-like growth factor signaling as a potential cancer therapy. *Mol Cancer Ther* 2007;6(1):1–12.

71. Tao Y, Pinzi V, Bourhis J, Deutsch E. Mechanisms of disease: signaling of the insulin-like growth factor 1 receptor pathway—therapeutic perspectives in cancer. *Nat Clin Pract Oncol* 2007;4(10):591–602.

72. Jerome L, Alami N, Belanger S, et al. Recombinant human insulin-like growth factor binding protein 3 inhibits growth of human epidermal growth factor receptor-2-overexpressing breast tumors and potentiates Herceptin activity *in vivo*. *Cancer Res* 2006;66(14):7245–7252.

73. Harrris LN, You F, Schnitt SJ, et al. Preoperative therapy for HER2-overexpressing early-stage breast cancer: Multigene profiling may identify predictors of resistance to trastuzumab and vinorelbine therapy. *Clin Cancer Res* 2006;12.

74. O'Reilly KE, Rojo F, She QB, et al. mTOR inhibition induces upstream receptor tyrosine kinase signaling and activates Akt. *Cancer Res* 2006;66(3):1500–1508.

75. Shi Y, Yan H, Frost P, et al. Mammalian target of rapamycin inhibitors activate the AKT kinase in multiple myeloma cells by up-regulating the insulin-like growth factor receptor/insulin receptor substrate-1/phosphatidylinositol 3-kinase cascade. *Mol Cancer Ther* 2005;4(10):1533–1540.

76. Martin LA, Pancholi S, Chan CM, et al. The anti-oestrogen ICI 182,780, but not tamoxifen, inhibits the growth of MCF-7 breast cancer cells refractory to long-term oestrogen deprivation through down-regulation of oestrogen receptor and IGF signalling. *Endocr Relat Cancer* 2005;12(4):1017–1036.

77. Knowlden JM, Hutcheson IR, Barrow D, et al. Insulin-like growth factor-I receptor signaling in tamoxifen-resistant breast cancer: a supporting role to the epidermal growth factor receptor. *Endocrinology* 2005;146(11):4609–4618.

78. Gutierrez MC, Detre S, Johnston S, et al. Molecular changes in tamoxifen-resistant breast cancer: relationship between estrogen receptor, HER-2, and p38 mitogen-activated protein kinase. *J Clin Oncol* 2005;23(11):2469–2476.

79. Lipton A, Leitzel K, Ali SM, et al. Serum HER-2/neu conversion to positive at the time of disease progression in patients with breast carcinoma on hormone therapy. *Cancer* 2005;104(2):257–263.

80. Rasmussen BB, Regan MM, Lykkesfeldt AE, et al. Central assessment of ER, PgR and HER2 in BIG I-98 evaluating letrozole (L) compared to tamoxifen (T) as initial adjuvant endocrine therapy for postmenopausal women with hormone receptor-positive breast cancer. *Proceeding of the American Society of Clinical Oncology* 2007;25 (18S).

81. Dowsett M, Allred, C. Relationship between quantitative ER and PgR expression and HER2 status and recurrence in the ATAC trial. *Breast Cancer Res Treat* 2006;100:S21.

82. Ellis MJ, Tao Y, Young O, et al. Estrogen-independent proliferation is present in estrogen-receptor HER2-positive primary breast cancer after neoadjuvant letrozole. *J Clin Oncol* 2006;24(19):3019–3025.

82a. Kaufman et al. 2008 meeting of the European Society of Medical Oncology (ESMO).

83. Chu QS, Cianfrocca ME, Goldstein LJ, et al. A phase I and pharmacokinetic study of lapatinib in combination with letrozole in patients with advanced cancer. *Clin Cancer Res* 2008;14(14):4484–4490.

84. Cristofanilli M, Valero V, Mangalik A, et al. A phase II multi-center, double-blind, randomized trial to compare anastrozole plus gefitinib with anastrozole plus placebo in postmenopausal women with hormone receptor-positive (HR+) breast cancer (MBC) *Proceeding of the American Society of Clinical Oncology* 2008; 26(15S):44s.

85. Osborne K, Neven P, Dirix L, et al. Randomized phase II study of gefitinib (IRESSA) or placebo in combination with tamoxifen in patients with hormone receptor positive metastatic breast cancer. *Breast Cancer Res Treat* 2007; 106(Suppl 1):S107.

86. Smith IE, Walsh G, Skene A, et al. A phase II placebo-controlled trial of neoadjuvant anastrozole alone or with gefitinib in early breast cancer. *J Clin Oncol* 2007;25(25):3816–3822.

87. Traina TA, Dickler MN, Caravelli JF, et al. A phase II trial of letrozole in combination with bevacizumab, an anti-VEGF antibody, in patients with hormone receptor positive metastatic breast cancer. *Breast Cancer Res Treat* 2005;94 (Suppl 1):47.

88. Leary AF, Sirohi B, Johnston SR. Clinical trials update: endocrine and biological therapy combinations in the treatment of breast cancer. *Breast Cancer Res* 2007;9(5):112.

89. Johnston SR, Martin LA, Leary A, et al. Clinical strategies for rationale combinations of aromatase inhibitors with novel therapies for breast cancer. *J Steroid Biochem Mol Biol* 2007;106(1–5):180–186.

90. Petit AM, Rak J, Hung MC, et al. Neutralizing antibodies against epidermal growth factor and ErbB-2/neu receptor tyrosine kinases down-regulate vascular endothelial growth factor production by tumor cells *in vitro* and *in vivo*: angiogenic implications for signal transduction therapy of solid tumors. *Am J Pathol* 1997;151(6):1523–1530.

91. Konecny GE, Meng YG, Untch M, et al. Association between HER-2/neu and vascular endothelial growth factor expression predicts clinical outcome in primary breast cancer patients. *Clin Cancer Res* 2004;10(5):1706–1716.

92. Dowsett M, Dixon JM, Horgan K, et al. Antiproliferative effects of idoxifene in a placebo-controlled trial in primary human breast cancer. *Clin Cancer Res* 2000;6(6):2260–2267.

93. Dowsett M, Bundred NJ, Decensi A, et al. Effect of raloxifene on breast cancer cell Ki67 and apoptosis: a double-blind, placebo-controlled, randomized clinical trial in postmenopausal patients. *Cancer Epidemiol Biomarkers Prev* 2001;10(9):961–966.

94. DeFriend DJ, Howell A, Nicholson RI, et al. Investigation of a new pure antiestrogen (ICI 182780) in women with primary breast cancer. *Cancer Res* 1994;54(2):408–414.

95. Dowsett M, Ebbs SR, Dixon JM, et al. Biomarker changes during neoadjuvant anastrozole, tamoxifen, or the combination: influence of hormonal status and HER-2 in breast cancer—a study from the IMPACT trialists. *J Clin Oncol* 2005;23(11):2477–2492.

96. Howell A, Cuzick J, Baum M, et al. Results of the ATAC (Arimidex, Tamoxifen, Alone or in Combination) trial after completion of 5 years' adjuvant treatment for breast cancer. *Lancet* 2005;365(9453):60–62.

97. Engelman JA, Zejnullahu K, Mitsudomi T, et al. MET amplification leads to gefitinib resistance in lung cancer by activating ERBB3 signaling. *Science* 2007;316(5827):1039–1043.

José Baselga

Advances in the understanding of the molecular alterations that lead to malignant transformation and the development of cancer have resulted in the development of targeted therapies directed against these alterations. In breast cancer, initial validation of this approach has been achieved with the anti-ERBB2 (formerly HER2) monoclonal antibody (MAb) trastuzumab in patients with ERBB2 overexpressing tumors and, to a lesser degree, with the anti-angiogenic MAb bevacizumab (1,2).

The cellular and molecular processes that lead to cancer, the already classic "hallmarks of malignancy" proposed by Hanahan and Weinberg (3), include self-sufficiency in growth signals, insensitivity to antigrowth factor signals, evasion of apoptosis, lack of senescence, invasion and metastasis, and sustained angiogenesis. All these processes can be potentially targeted with a variety of therapeutic strategies and novel agents. Moreover, many of these agents are being developed in breast cancer, mainly owing to its improved molecular classification, which greatly facilitates the rational development of targeted therapeutics.

This chapter highlights novel targeted agents against breast cancer that are furthest along in their early clinical development. Some of these agents, including monoclonal antibodies against growth factor receptors (ERBB2 and insulin-like growth factor receptor) and anti-angiogenesis approaches are not discussed here because they are being presented elsewhere in this book. In this chapter, we will review novel agents that target nonreceptor tyrosine kinases, signaling pathways downstream from growth factor receptors, DNA-repair mechanisms, apoptosis, and agents that induce enhanced degradation and processing of oncogenic proteins (Fig. 80.1 and Table 80.1). These compounds are all in early stages of clinical development, but some of them are beginning to demonstrate evidence of clinical activity suggesting that they will play a role in the therapy for patient with breast cancer (Table 80.2). It is highly likely that some of these agents will move forward in their clinical development and be incorporated into our current approved armamentarium of anticancer agents.

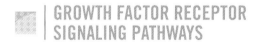

GROWTH FACTOR RECEPTOR SIGNALING PATHWAYS

Inhibitors of the Phosphatidyl Inositol 3-kinase (PI3K)/Akt Pathway

Phosphatidyl inositol 3-kinase (PI3K) is a major signaling component downstream of growth factor receptor tyrosine kinases (4). The PI3K-Akt signaling pathway regulates many normal cellular processes, including cell proliferation, survival, growth, and motility—processes that are critical for tumorigenesis. Indeed, the role of this pathway in oncogenesis has been extensively investigated and altered expression or mutation of many components of this pathway have been implicated in human cancer (5–9). PI3K is composed of a 110-kDa catalytic subunit and an 85-kDa adaptor subunit. When growth factors (e.g. epidermal growth factor [EGF] or insulin growth factor [IGF] bind to their cognate receptor, the p85 adaptor subunit is recruited to the intracellular part of the growth factor receptor. Subsequent dimerization with the p110 subunit then leads to full enzymatic activity of PI3K.

Once recruited to the membrane, the p110 catalytic subunit of PI3K phosphorylates phosphatidylinositol-4,5-bisphosphate (PIP2) at the 3′ position of the inositol ring, thus generating PIP3. The resulting PIP3 serves to recruit phospholipid-binding domain containing proteins to the plasma membrane. In particular, serine/threonine kinase Akt (also known as protein kinase B) is recruited to the membrane and successively fully activated by PDK1 before moving to the cytoplasm and to the nucleus where it promotes protein synthesis and cell growth by alleviating TSC1/2 suppression of the mammalian target of rapamycin (mTOR), allowing the latter to act as part of the mTOR–raptor complex on 4EBP1 and ribosomal protein S6 kinases (S6K) (10). In addition, Akt reduces cell cycle inhibitors p27 and p21, and promotes cell cycle proteins c-Myc and cyclin D1, resulting in enhanced cellular proliferation (11). Its influence extends to a host of pro- and antiapoptotic proteins, such as the Bcl-2 family member Bad, limiting programmed cell death and boosting cellular survival (11).

PI3K is negatively regulated at the level of PIP3 by phospholipid phosphatases, such as phosphatase and tensin homologe (PTEN) (12). The underlying mechanism is the dephosphorylation of PIP3 into its inactive form PIP2. In addition, signaling through the PI3K pathway is modulated by the cross-talk with other signals and pathways, including hormones, integrins, and ras-dependent mitogen activated protein kinase (MAPK/ERK) pathway (13).

As mentioned above, growing evidence indicates that uncontrolled activation of the PI3K/Akt/mTOR pathway, achieved via numerous genetic and epigenetic alterations, contributes to the development and progression of human cancers, including breast cancer (14). These genetic alterations include PTEN deletions (15,16) and *hot-spots* mutations of the PI3K gene (5), which have been shown to have transforming capacity *in vitro* and *in vivo* (17,18). Further, these alterations may result in resistance to upstream antireceptor agents. For example, trastuzumab depends on intact PTEN for its action in ERBB2-overexpressing breast cancer and PTEN loss predicts for trastuzumab resistance in preclinical models as well as in patients (19,20).

The frequent dysregulation of the PI3K/Akt/mTOR pathway in human breast cancer has made components of this pathway attractive for therapeutic targeting (21). Clinical trials are currently underway with mTOR, PI3K, and Akt inhibitors. Among them, mTOR inhibitors are further ahead in development. Rapamycin derivatives, such as everolimus, temsirolimus, and deforolimus, are potent inhibitors of mTOR (22–24). In an unselected and heavily pretreated patient population with breast cancer, these agents have shown modest antitumor activity in the range of approximately 10% (25,26). Although these early results are an indication that mTOR inhibitors are active in breast cancer, a need exists either to identify the subset of patients that may benefit from these agents or to design appropriate combinatorial approaches.

Based on the cross-talk between the estrogen receptor and the PI3K/Akt/mTOR pathways, clinical trials with mTOR inhibitors have explored the combination of rapamycin analogues and aromatase inhibitors. A randomized phase II study compared oral temsirolimus combined with letrozole with letrozole alone in 104 patients with hormonal receptor positive metastatic breast cancer (27). Because of the toxicity of the high-dose schedule that resulted in dose delays or reductions

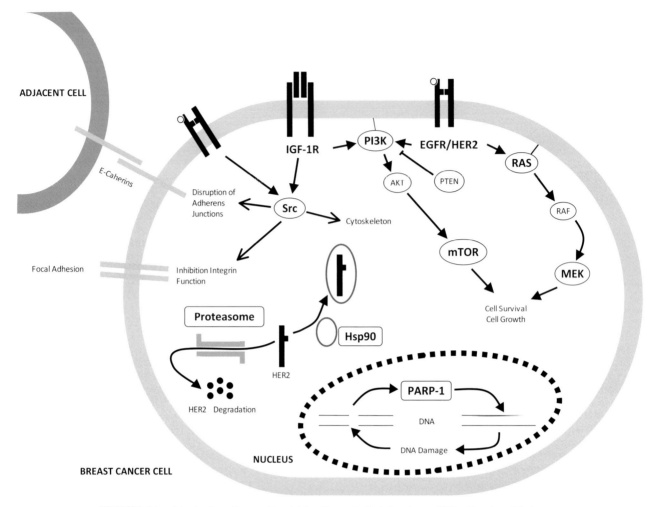

FIGURE 80.1. Intracellular signaling pathways and targeted drugable opportunities in breast cancer EGFR, epidermal growth factor receptor; HERBB2, epidermal growth factor receptor type 2; Hsp90, heat shock protein-90; IGF-1R, insulin-like growth factor 1 receptor; MEK, MAPK/extracellular signal regulated kinase kinase; mTOR, mammalian target of rapamycin; PARP-1, poly(ADP-ribose) polymerase-1; PI3K, phosphoinositide-3 kinase.

Table 80.1 | **SUMMARY OF NOVEL AGENTS BEING DEVELOPED IN BREAST CANCER**

Growth Factor Receptor Signaling Inhibitors

—PI3K/Akt Pathway Inhibitors
- **Rationale**: Critical survival pathway downstream of growth factor receptors; PI3K activating mutations/PTEN deletions frequent in breast cancer
- **Agents**: mTOR, PI3K, dual mTOR/PI3K, and Akt inhibitors
- **Clinical activity**: mTOR inhibitors active in breast cancer (modest). Activity of other agents not reported
- **Future directions**: Pilot studies with patients with PI3K mutations. Combination studies with anti-ERBB2 (previously HER2) and anti-IGFR-1 agents

—Src Inhibitors
- **Rationale**: src mediates processes important for tumor progression, such as cellular adhesion, motility, survival and proliferation.
- **Agents**: Src tyrosine kinase inhibitors
- **Clinical activity**: Not yet reported
- **Future directions**: Novel study designs to detect prevention of metastasis

—RAF/MEK/MAPK (ERK) Pathway Inhibitors
- **Rationale**: Critical signaling pathway downstream of growth factor receptors
- **Agents**: RAF and MEK kinase inhibitors
- **Clinical activity**: Sorafenib has modest activity as single agent. Other compounds not yet reported.

- **Future directions**: Sorafenib in combination with chemotherapy and hormones. Combinations with PI3K inhibitors

—Hsp90 Inhibitors
- **Rationale**: Oncoproteins, such as Akt and ERBB2, are repaired by Hsp90
- **Agents**: Geldanamycin derivates
- **Clinical activity**: Activity reported in combination with trastuzumab in patients with ERBB2 amplified breast cancer and trastuzumab resistance
- **Future directions**: Registration studies likely to be initiated in ERBB2 breast cancer

DNA-Repair Interfering Agents. PARP Inhibitors
- **Rationale**: PARP inhibition leads to cell death in *BRCA* deficient tumors
- **Agents**: PARP-1 inhibitors
- **Clinical activity**: Activity reported in *BRCA* mutant ovarian cancer
- **Future directions**: Studies in BRCA mutant breast cancer. Studies in basal type breast cancer in combination with platinum agents

Inducers of Apoptosis
- **Rationale**: Evasion of apoptosis is one of the hallmarks of cancer
- **Agents**: Activating TRAIL receptor monoclonal antibodies
- **Clinical activity**: Not yet reported in breast cancer
- **Future directions**: Early in development. Combination studies with chemotherapy and growth factor receptor inhibitors being planned

Hsp90, heat shock protein 90; IGFR, IGF-1R, insulin-like growth factor 1 receptor; MEK, mitogen activated protein kinase [MAPK]/extracellular signal regulated kinase kinase; mTOR, mammalian target of rapamycin; PARP-1, poly(ADP-ribose) polymerase-1; PI3K, phosphoinositide-3 kinase; PTEN, phosphatase and tensin homolog; RAF, receptor activation factor (RAF) kinase; TRAIL, tumor necrosis factor-related apoptosis-inducing ligand.

Table 80.2	**TARGETED THERAPIES IN DEVELOPMENT**			
Target	**Agents Under Study**	**Company**	**Route**	**Study Phase**
PI3K	BEZ235*	Novartis	Oral	Phase I
	PX866	ProlX Pharmaceuticals	Oral	Phase I
	BGT226	Novartis	Oral	Phase I
	XL765*	Exelixis	Oral	Phase I
	XL147	Exelixis	Oral	Phase I
mTOR	CCI-779 (Temsirolimus)	Wyeth Pharmaceuticals	IV	Phase III
	RAD001 (Everolimus)	Novartis	Oral	Phase III
	BEZ-235*	Novartis	Oral	Phase I
	XL765*	Exelixis	Oral	Phase I
	AP23573	ARIAD Pharmaceuticals	IV	Phase I
	OSI-027	OSI Pharmaceuticals	Oral	Phase I
Akt	Perifosine	Keryx Biopharmaceuticals	Oral	Phase I
	GSK-690693	GlaxoSmithKline	IV	Phase I
	VQD-002	VioQuest Pharmaceuticals	IV	Phase I
Src	BMS-354825 (Dasatinib)	Bristol-Myers Squibb	Oral	Phase II
	XL228	Exelixis	Oral	Phase I
	AZD0530	AstraZeneca	Oral	Phase I
	KX2-391	Kinex Pharmaceuticals	Oral	Phase I
	SKI-606 (Bosutinib)	Wyeth Pharmaceuticals	Oral	Phase I
Raf	BAY 43-9006 (Sorafenib)	Bayer Pharmaceuticals	Oral	Phase III
	XL281	Exelixis	Oral	Phase I
	RAF265	Novartis	Oral	Phase I
MEK	CI-1040	Pfizer	Oral	Phase II
	XL518	Exelixis/Genentech	Oral	Phase I
	AZD6244	AstraZeneca	Oral	Phase I
	PD-325901	Pfizer	Oral	Phase I
Hsp90	KOS-953 (Tanespimycin)	Kosan Biosciences	IV	Phase II
	KOS-1022 (Alvespimycin)	Kosan Biosciences	Oral	Phase I
	IPI-504	AstraZeneca	IV	Phase I
	STA-9090	Synta Pharmaceuticals	IV	Phase I
	AUY922	Novartis	IV	Phase I
PARP	AZD2281 (KU-0059436)	AstraZeneca	Oral	Phase I
	ABT-888	Abbott	Oral	Phase I
	AG014699	Pfizer	IV	Phase I
	BSI-201	BiPar Sciences	IV	Phase I
TRAIL	TRM-1 (Mapatuzumab)	Human Genome Sciences	IV	Phase I
	LBY135	Novartis	IV	Phase I
	AMG-655	Amgen	IV	Phase I
	AMG-655	Amgen	IV	Phase I

*Dual PI3K and mTOR inhibitors.

or discontinuations, the protocol was amended to low-dose schedules. After the amendment, early data from 92 patients suggested that progression-free survival (PFS) could be longer for the combination arms than for the letrozole alone, and, therefore, a large phase III trial was initiated. However, this study was terminated before accrual was completed owing to lack of efficacy for the combination. The lack of benefit of an mTOR inhibitor in combination with an aromatase inhibitor observed in this trial could be an indication of a lack of efficacy of this strategy but it could also be potentially explained by a suboptimal exposure to the mTOR inhibitors owing to the dose reduction of temsirolimus that was implemented. In the case of everolimus, another mTOR inhibitor, a series of well-conducted pharmacokinetic and pharmacodynamic studies that analyzed mTOR inhibition in tumors as well as in surrogate tissues led to the identification of a dose of 10 mg/day as optimal for further clinical development (28). In a subsequent phase II, double

blind randomized study of everolimus in combination with letrozole versus placebo and letrozole in the neoadjuvant setting, the combination arm proved to be superior over letrozole and placebo with a higher statistically significant response rate (68% vs. 59%) (29). This study incorporated carefully conducted pre- and on-study tumor biopsies and pharmacodynamic studies demonstrated a near doubling of response rate by decreases in the cell cycle indicator Ki67 in the everolimus treated group. This is potentially important because Ki67 drops in the neoadjuvant setting have been recently demonstrated to correlate with long-term outcome (30). The safety profile of the combination was acceptable and in line with the known side effects of rapamycin analogues (stomatitis, rash, thrombocytopenia, asthenia, and medically manageable hypercholesterolemia). Other potentially active combinations with mTOR inhibitors include a combination with trastuzumab in patients with trastuzumab-refractory disease. In a phase I study in patients with trastuzumab and taxane-refractory disease, the addition of everolimus has resulted in a high response rate and this combination is now being explored in the phase II setting (31).

A potential explanation for the limited activity of mTOR inhibitors in breast cancer and other tumor types may be related to a *collateral effect* of mTOR blockade. mTOR inhibition blocks the natural negative feedback on IGF-1R signaling impinging on PI3K (32,33). The result is an increase in PI3K and Akt activation, which could potentially counteract the inhibition of mTOR. In preclinical models, dual inhibition of both IGF-1 signaling, with either MAb or tyrosine kinase inhibitors, and mTOR results in a superior antiproliferative effect over each single strategy (32). This combination is now being explored in phase I trials.

In terms of PI3K inhibitors, the use of high throughput screening of chemical libraries and structural information, combined with extensive medicinal chemistry efforts, have led to the discovery of new pan-PI3K and isoform-selective inhibitors with improved specificity, potency, and pharmaceutical properties (33). Some of these compounds have already been studied in early clinical trials. Among them, NVP-BEZ235 is a potent dual PI3K/mTOR inhibitor that exhibits potent antiproliferative activity against a broad panel of tumor cell lines both *in vitro* and *in vivo* (34) and is also highly active in breast cancer cells harboring activating PI3K mutations (35). Other agents under study include XL765, also a dual PI3K/mTOR inhibitor (36), and XL147, a more pure PI3K inhibitor (37). Initial data from early developmental phase I studies seem to suggest that these agents are safe and that PI3K signaling inhibition is achieved in patients (38). To date, no clinical data have been released with a variety of Akt inhibitors although they are currently in clinical development.

Src-family Tyrosine Kinases Inhibitors

The v-Src (Rous sarcoma virus) tyrosine kinase was the first oncogenic gene discovered (39). The corresponding cellular gene, c-Src, is a non-receptor signaling kinase that functions at the hub of a vast array of signal transduction pathways that influence cellular proliferation, differentiation, motility, and survival (40). Other biological functions mediated by Src activity in tumor cells include epithelial-to-mesenchymal transition, which is implicated in the development of metastasis (41).

Several mechanisms lead to increased Src activity in tumors. Src is downstream from growth factor receptors, including platelet-derived growth factor (PDGF) receptor (PDGFR), epidermal growth factor receptor (EGFR), insulin-like growth factor-1 receptor (IGF-1R), and hepatocyte growth factor/scatter factor receptor (HGFR) (42). In many tumor types, including breast cancer, overexpression of these receptors, their ligands, or both is frequent (43). Additional mechanisms of Src activation include, overexpression of Src binding partners, such as focal adhesion kinase (44).

Several indications suggest that Src may play a role in breast cancer. High levels of Src activity and expression are present in breast cancer (45,46) and Src activity is increased in human breast cancer tissues compared with benign breast tumors or adjacent normal breast tissues (45,47). In experimental models, transgenic mice with polyoma middle T antigen under the control of mouse mammary tumor virus promoter were found to develop highly metastatic mammary tumors with increased Src activity (48). Moreover, when these mice were cross-bred with Src-deficient mice, the resulting chimeric mice no longer developed mammary tumors (48). In addition, mice overexpressing the ERBB2 oncogene develop highly metastatic mammary tumors that have elevated Src activity (49). Finally, in tamoxifen resistant cells, Src promotes cellular invasion and motility, which is reversed by Src inhibitors (50).

Src inhibitors are in clinical development, either given alone or in combination with other therapies. As with other kinase inhibitors, src inhibitors differ among themselves by their specificity. Dasatinib (BMS-354825) is a synthetic small-molecule inhibitor of Src and abl, as well as other kinases, with a broad antiproliferative activity against hematologic and solid tumor cell lines (51). Dasatinib induces hematologic and cytogenetic responses in patients with imatinib-refractory chronic myelogenous leukemia and Philadelphia chromosome-positive acute lymphoid leukemia (52). Preclinical evidence suggests that dasatinib could be effective in breast cancer cell lines of a basal-like subtype, a tumor subtype that is categorized as being aggressive and with a lack of effective targeted treatments (53). Because basal-like tumors frequently lack expression of estrogen and progesterone receptor as well as ERBB2 (also known in the clinic as *triple-negative* breast cancer), there is a scientific rationale for the clinical development of dasatinib in the treatment of patients with triple negative breast cancer.

More selective src inhibitors are also being developed. AZD-0530 is a highly selective, dual-specific, orally available small molecule inhibitor of Src kinase and Bcr-Abl (54). A phase I clinical study has shown that the agent is safe. Pharmacodynamic end points, such as activation of the Src downstream targets, paxillin and focal adhesion kinase, which are mediators of cell motility and invasion, have allowed the identification of a dose that is biologically relevant (55). Interestingly, one of the important roles of src is to promote bone resorption. In patients, AZD-0530 has been shown to decrease the levels of bone resorption markers in serum and urine, suggesting a potential effect on osteoclasts (55,56). This may be a desirable effect of src inhibitors in cancer patients because it could potentially interfere with bone disease progression and delay the occurrence of pathologic fractures. Nevertheless, the challenges with developing src inhibitors in breast cancer are considerable, namely the expected lack of classic antitumor activity and the technical difficulties and lack of expertise in developing agents that may prevent metastasis as their main mechanism of action.

RAF/MEK/MAPK (ERK) Pathway Inhibitors

The RAS proteins are members of a large superfamily of GTP-binding proteins that play a complex role in the normal transduction of growth factor receptor-induced signals (57–59). Stimulation of several growth factor receptors, such as ERBB2 and the closely related EGFR, causes activation of RAS by stimulating its binding to GTP. RAS, in its active, GTP-bound state, binds several key target proteins, which results in the subsequent activation of several downstream pathways, including those mediated by RAF/MAPK, PI3kinase, and RAL-GDS pathways (57–60). Engagement of these pathways leads to stimulation of cell cycle progression, desensitization of the cell to proapoptotic stimuli, changes in cytoskeletal organization and invasion, and other processes required for cell proliferation. Different agents have been developed to target the Ras/Raf/MAPK (ERK) pathway owing to the aberrant activation of this pathway in a large number of human tumors. These agents include farnesyltransferase inhibitors, Raf inhibitors, and MEK/MAPK inhibitors.

It has been a fruitless task so far to develop sufficiently clinically active RAS inhibitors. After the synthesis of the pro-RAS protein, a series of post-translational biochemical processes convert this protein to a more hydrophobic one that permits its localization to the cytoplasmic membrane where it becomes activated. The first modification of this process is catalyzed by the farnesyltransferase (FT) enzyme (61) and, as a consequence, FT inhibitors were developed as a therapeutic strategy to inhibit RAS activation. Several RAS FT inhibitors have been developed with modest results (62–64).

In advanced breast cancer, a phase II trial with the oral farnesyltransferase inhibitor tipifarnib (R115777) showed a modest activity with a low toxicity profile, consisting mainly in neuropathy and myelosuppression. The objective response rates ranged from 10% to 14%, with an additional 9% to 15% of patients with stable disease for at least 6 months (64). In a different setting, a phase II clinical trial evaluated the efficacy of tipifarnib in combination with doxorubicin and cyclophosphamide in patients with advanced and locally advanced breast cancer (65). The regimen was safe and clinically active. Pathologic complete response in the breast was observed in 7 of 21 (33%) patients. None of these results were felt to be sufficiently conclusive to continue the development of this class of agents in breast cancer. The lack of activity may because RAS is alternatively prenylated by the FT-related enzyme geranylgeranyltransferase I, which may render cells resistant to FT inhibition.

An alternate strategy is to target downstream members of the RAS signaling pathway, such as RAF and MEK/MAPK. Sorafenib (Bay 43-9006) is a small kinase inhibitor that blocks signaling proteins and receptors, including B-RAF, vascular endothelial growth factor (VEGF) receptor 2 (VEGFR2), VEGFR3, PDGFR-b, KIT, FLT-3, and RET (66). Sorafenib is in clinical development in a wide range of solid tumors. For example, in advanced renal cell carcinoma, sorafenib increases progression-free survival compared with placebo (67). In breast cancer, a phase II trial was conducted to assess the efficacy and safety of sorafenib monotherapy in 54 patients with metastatic breast cancer previously treated (68). One patient had a partial response and 20 (37%) patients had a stable disease as their best response, with prolonged stabilization observed in 22% and 11% of patients at 4 and 6 months, respectively. Sorafenib was safe and well tolerated, with a manageable toxicity profile in heavily pretreated patients with metastatic breast cancer (MBC). Studies investigating this agent in combination with chemotherapeutic agents in the treatment of metastatic breast cancer are ongoing in a series of randomized phase II studies. Agents being studied in combination with sorafenib in breast cancer include capecitabine, taxanes, aromatase inhibitors, and bevacizumab. Additional potent RAF inhibitors are in clinical development (69).

CI-1040 (PD184352) is an oral, selective MEK inhibitor of both isoforms. Preclinical activity was demonstrated in breast cancer cell lines (70), and mild gastrointestinal, skin, and constitutional side effects were observed in a phase I trial (71). A phase II study was conducted in patients with advanced colorectal, non–small-cell lung, and pancreatic cancer, including a cohort of 14 patients with metastatic breast cancer treated with two prior chemotherapy regimens. However, no clinical responses were observed (72). Other agents that inhibit MEK and that are in clinical development include XL518 (73) and AZD6244 (74). In the initial phase I study with XL518, MEK signaling in tumor and hair samples was inhibited by XL518, suggesting that pERK may have utility as a clinical biomarker (73).

Heat Shock Protein (Hsp) 90 Inhibitors

Hsp90 is a molecular chaperone that is required for the refolding of proteins under conditions of environmental stress and for the conformational maturation of a subset of key signaling proteins (75). Many of these client proteins, such as AKT, HER2, c-KIT, EGFR, and PDGFR-α, are oncoproteins and important cell-signaling proteins deregulated in cancer (76,77). As signal transducers and molecular switches, these client proteins are inherently unstable. Hsp90 keeps unstable signaling proteins poised for activation until they are stabilized by conformational changes associated with the formation of signal transduction complexes. Conversely, inhibition of adenosine triphosphate (ATP) binding to Hsp90 prevents the formation of

the mature complex and results in the proteasome-dependent degradation of associated client proteins. Consequently, Hsp90 is a single molecular target that is a central integrator of multiple pathways important to cancer.

Ansamycin antibiotics, such as 17-allylaminogeldanamycin (17-AAG), bind to Hsp90 and regulate its function, resulting in the proteasomal degradation of a subset of signaling proteins that require Hsp90 for conformational maturation (78,79). Ansamycins induce rapid degradation of ERBB2 and a concomitant loss in ERBB3 associated PI3 kinase activity (79). In murine xenograft models, 17-AAG also reduces the expression of ERBB2 and phosphorylation of Akt and inhibits tumor growth (79). Thus, pharmacologic inhibition of Akt activation is achievable with ansamycins and may be useful for the treatment of ERBB2 driven tumors. In addition to their capacity to induce degradation of full length ERBB2, Hsp90 inhibitors also degrade a truncated version of ERBB2, known as p95ERBB2, that lacks the extracellular domain of the receptor and that is present in up to one-third of ERBB2 overexpressing tumors (80). The degradation by Hsp90 inhibitors of truncated versions of ERBB2 has potential clinical applications because these forms have been shown in patients to result in trastuzumab resistance (81).

In the clinic, initial studies with the Hsp90 inhibitor tanespimycin (KOS-953) (82) and the second-generation Hsp90 inhibitor, alvespimycin (KOS-1022), (83) have demonstrated antitumor activity and tolerability in combination with trastuzumab in patients with trastuzumab-refractory ERBB2-positive metastatic breast cancer. Other Hsp90 inhibitors are also entering the clinic. The major challenge with these agents in ERBB2-positive disease is how to develop them strategically because a plethora of new agents against ERBB2 have shown activity in patients with ERBB2-amplified tumors that have progressed with trastuzumab.

DNA-REPAIR INTERFERING AGENTS

Polyadenosine 5′-diphosphoribose (Poly[ADP-ribose])Polymerase 1 (PARP-1) Inhibitors

Poly-(ADP–ribose) or PAR polymerization is a unique post-translational modification of histones and other nuclear proteins that contributes to the survival of proliferating and nonproliferating cells following DNA damage. This event represents an immediate cellular response to DNA damage and involves the modification of glutamate, aspartate, and lysine residues, with the addition of long chains of adenosine diphosphate (ADP)-ribose units, derived from nicotine adenine dinucleotide (NAD)$^+$, onto the DNA-binding proteins. The enzymes that catalyze this process, poly(ADP-ribose) polymerases (PARP), are regulatory components in DNA damage repair and other cellular processes (84). Of the various members of the PARP enzyme family, only PARP-1 and PARP-2 work as DNA damage sensor and signaling molecules.

PARP-1 is a nuclear enzyme consisting of three domains, the N-terminal DNA-binding domain containing two zinc fingers, the automodification domain, and the C-terminal catalytic domain. It binds to both single and double-stranded DNA breaks through the zinc-finger domain. PARP-1 catalyzes the cleavage of NAD+ into nicotinamide and ADP-ribose, the latter is then synthesized to form branched nucleic acid-like polymers covalently attached to nuclear acceptor proteins. This branched ADP-ribose polymer is highly negatively charged, which in turn leads to the unwinding and repair of the damaged DNA through the base excision repair pathway (84). Cells deficient in PARP-1 have been shown to have delayed DNA repair function. In addition, PARP-1 is also known to bind double-stranded DNA breaks, preventing accidental recombination of homologous DNA (85). On binding DNA breaks, the catalytic activity of PARP-1 is stimulated more than 500-fold (86). Enhanced PARP-1 expression or activity has been observed in a number of different tumor cell lines and could provide a greater level of resistance to both endogenous genotoxic stress as well as to DNA damage-inducing therapeutic agents.

The PARP inhibitors have been developed to investigate the role of PARP-1 in cell biology and to overcome DNA repair-mediated resistance of cancer cells to genotoxic agents (87). PARP inhibitors have been shown to enhance, in human cancer cell models, the antitumor activity of DNA-methylating agents, such as temozolomide, platinums, topoisomerase poisons, and ionizing radiation (88), and to restore sensitivity of tumors resistant to methylating agents or topoisomerase I inhibitors, two classes of agents being used for the treatment of breast cancer. Studies of PARP expression in various tumor types have identified that breast cancers with negative estrogen receptor, progesterone receptor, and ERBB2 expression were much more likely to overexpress PARP (89). Recent studies indicate that PARP inhibition in *BRCA1* and *BRCA2* homozygous null cells, but not the isogenic *BRCA* heterozygous cells, leads to selective cell death. The *BRCA1* and *BRCA2* genes encode proteins that are implicated in homologous DNA strand break repair, known as homologous recombination. *BRCA1* or *BRCA2* dysfunction profoundly sensitizes cells to PARP inhibition, leading to chromosomal instability, cell cycle arrest, and apoptosis (89). This seems to be because the inhibition of PARP leads to the persistence of DNA lesions normally repaired by homologous recombination.

Initial phase I studies with the PARP inhibitor AZD2281 (KU-0059436) have shown that this agent is safe in patients with advanced breast cancer or ovarian cancer associated with an inherited mutation in one of the cancer genes, *BRCA1* or *BRCA2* (90). Preliminary data from 11 evaluable patients with hereditary *BRCA*-associated ovarian cancer demonstrated a response rate of 55%. First responses were observed at 100 mg twice daily on an intermittent schedule (14 days dosing in 21-day cycles) and subsequently at twice daily 200 mg and 400 mg continuous dosing. Other phase II studies are now underway to define further the activity of PARP inhibitors in patients with hereditary breast and ovarian cancer. In addition, based on the strong rationale to combine cisplatin with PARP inhibitors and the emerging data in triple-negative breast cancer showing high level of activity of cisplatinum therapy, a neoadjuvant study with cisplatin in combination with AZD2281 in patients with this subtype of breast cancer is currently underway.

Targeting Programmed Cell Death (Apoptosis)

Apoptosis or programmed cell death is an evolutionarily conserved process for removing unwanted cells from the body and the mechanisms responsible for the control of cell number (91). Apoptosis is necessary in processes such as embryonic development and tissue turnover (92). Apoptosis may also be triggered by external stimuli, such as cytotoxic agents or radiation. Evasion of apoptosis is associated with many human cancers; it is one of the hallmarks of the malignant phenotype and may play a role in the observed chemoradioresistance that occurs in many tumors (93). Therefore, (re)induction of apoptosis is a promising anticancer strategy.

Apoptosis occurs via two separate yet interlinked signaling mechanisms: the extrinsic pathway, activated by death receptors (DR) at the cellular surface, and the intrinsic pathway, activated by mitochondrial signals from within the cell in response to severe cell stress (e.g., DNA damage). The intrinsic pathway is controlled by interactions between pro- and antiapoptotic members of the Bcl-2 protein family. Extrinsic and intrinsic pathways converge through effector caspases, which are modulated by several cell-endogenous factors, including inhibitor of apoptosis (IAP) proteins, such as XIAP and ML-IAP, and cellular FLIP (c-FLIP), which inhibit caspases and procaspases, respectively (94).

Tumor necrosis factor (TNF)-related apoptosis-inducing ligand (TRAIL) receptor 2 (TR-2/DR5) is a member of the TNF super family of receptors. TRAIL is the natural ligand for the death receptor DR5; TRAIL binding to DR5 initiates an intracellular caspase cascade and induces apoptosis in many human transformed cell lines but not most normal cells (95). Activating DR5 may be an effective anticancer therapy in humans (96). Recombinant human Apo2/TRAIL has been studied in different preclinical models and has shown its ability to induce apoptosis in cell lines from a broad spectrum of human cancers, including breast cancer, without affecting normal cells (97). At present, mapatumumab (HGS-ETR1, TRM-1), a fully human immunoglobulin G1 lambda agonist MAb, has been developed to bind with high affinity to the extracellular domain of TRAIL receptor-1, activating the extrinsic apoptotic pathway. A phase I clinical trial has shown the safety of this drug in patients with solid tumors (98). Similarly, AMG655 AMG 655, a fully human monoclonal agonist antibody that binds human TRAIL receptor-2 (TR-2/DR5), has shown to be safe in a phase I study and has some early evidence of clinical activity (99). As with other classes of agents presented in this chapter, the optimal way to administer these agents, either alone or in combination with chemotherapy, it is not known. In addition, some theoretical considerations support combining proapoptotic agents with growth factor receptor inhibitors.

CONCLUSIONS

Over the past several years, significant advances have been made in our understanding of a growing number of critical pathways involved in breast cancer. These advances have led to the development of novel therapies that are being collectively known as *molecularly targeted therapies*. This nomenclature highlights their target specificity and their capacity to interfere with key molecular oncogenic events responsible for the malignant phenotype.

These novel therapies hold substantial promise as efficacious and nontoxic agents against breast cancer. They also bring new challenges when compared with conventional cytotoxic therapies that require a different clinical development strategy.

First, the optimal dose and schedule of these agents may be difficult to determine and pharmacodynamic markers of target engagement are being incorporated in most of the initial studies in patients. This need will be even more apparent with agents such as src inhibitors that are not expected to have antitumor activity because their main mechanism of action is via prevention of invasion and metastasis. Second, these agents, unlike chemotherapy, will only be effective in a subset of tumors that show dependency on the target to which the therapy is being directed. This is well exemplified by the anti-ERBB2 agent trastuzumab, only active in tumors with high levels of expression and amplification of the ERBB2 gene. Because ERBB2 is overexpressed in only 25% of breast tumors, if trastuzumab would have been developed in an unselected patient population, its antitumor activity would have been missed owing to a dilutional effect brought in by the non-ERBB2 overexpressing population. This implies that patient selection strategies will be of paramount importance. Each class of agents may require a different strategy, ranging from restricting entry criteria to only a subset of tumors with a given molecular alteration (i.e., PI3K mutations) or, at the very minimum, to collecting tumor blocks in all patients. Third, therapy end points with these novel therapies need to be revisited. Some of these agents are not expected to result in tumor shrinkage (or response) and, therefore, clinical response may not be an optimal end point. To further complicate things, some of these agents will have limited activity by themselves and yet have the capacity to markedly enhance the antitumor activity of conventional agents such as chemotherapy or even other biological agents. This later point is well exemplified by the antiangiogenic MAb bevacizumab, which has no activity as a single agent and yet is clinically active when combined with chemotherapy.

Finally, we should consider to study these new agents in less heavily pretreated patients. In the past, we had studied new agents in breast cancer in patients whose disease had progressed to all approved lines of therapies. However, with the increased availability of multiple lines of therapy in breast cancer, novel agents are being tested in increasingly more heavily pretreated patients. This patient population with advanced disease that has been extensively pretreated may not be the ideal population to detect the clinical efficacy of novel agents because their tumors may have already evolved to a state of high resistance to any type of therapy. It is also difficult to conduct repeat tumor sampling in this setting with the goal to identify new biomarkers of target engagement and sensitivity to these novel agents. Although a solution to this problem is unresolved at this time, pilot studies of novel agents in the neoadjuvant setting in breast cancer are increasingly being conducted, either as a window study, where the study agent is given for a short period of time, or in combination with either endocrine or chemotherapy agents.

References

1. Slamon DJ, Leyland-Jones B, Shak S, et al. Use of chemotherapy plus a monoclonal antibody against her2 for metastatic breast cancer that overexpresses HER2. *N Engl J Med* 2001;344:783–792.
2. Miller K, Wang M, Gralow J, et al. Paclitaxel plus bevacizumab versus paclitaxel alone for metastatic breast cancer. *N Engl J Med* 2007;357:2666–2676.
3. Hanahan D, Weinberg R. The hallmarks of cancer. *Cell* 2000;100:57–70.
4. Cantley LC. The phosphoinositide 3-kinase pathway. *Science* 2002;296:1655–1657.
5. Samuels Y, Wang Z, Bardelli A, et al. High frequency of mutations of the PIK3CA gene in human cancers. *Science* 2004;304:554.
6. Bachman K, Argani P, Samuels Y, et al. The PIK3CA gene is mutated with high frequency in human breast cancers. *Cancer Biol Ther* 2004;3:772–775.
7. Lee JW, Soung YH, Kim SY, et al. PIK3CA gene is frequently mutated in breast carcinomas and hepatocellular carcinomas. *Oncogene* 2004;24:1477–1480.
8. Campbell IG, Russell SE, Choong DYH, et al. Mutation of the PIK3CA gene in ovarian and breast cancer. *Cancer Res* 2004;64:7678–7681.
9. Philp AJ, Campbell IG, Leet C, et al. The phosphatidylinositol 3′-kinase p85 α gene is an oncogene in human ovarian and colon tumors. *Cancer Res* 2001;61:7426–7429.
10. Inoki K, Li Y, Zhu T, et al. TSC2 is phosphorylated and inhibited by Akt and suppresses mTOR signalling. *Nat Cell Biol* 2002;4:648–657.
11. Vivanco I, Sawyers CL. The phosphatidylinositol 3-kinase-Akt pathway in human cancer. *Nat Rev Cancer* 2002;2:489.
12. Cantley LC, Neel BG. New insights into tumor suppression: PTEN suppresses tumor formation by restraining the phosphoinositide 3-kinase/AKT pathway. *Proc Natl Acad Sci U S A* 1999;96:4240–4245.
13. Vivanco I, Sawyers CL. The phosphatidylinositol 3-Kinase-AKT pathway in human cancer. *Nat Rev Cancer* 2002;2:489–501.
14. Hennessy BT, Smith DL, Ram PT, et al. Exploiting the PI3K/AKT pathway for cancer drug discovery. *Nat Rev Drug Discov* 2005;4:988–1004.
15. Engelman JA, Luo J, Cantley LC. The evolution of phosphatidylinositol 3-kinases as regulators of growth and metabolism. *Nat Rev Genet* 2006;7:606–719.
16. Liaw D, Marsh D, Li J, et al. Germline mutations of the PTEN gene in Cowden disease, an inherited breast and thyroid cancer syndrome. *Nat Genet* 1997;16:64–67.
17. Samuels Y, Diaz JLA, Schmidt-Kittler O, et al. Mutant PIK3CA promotes cell growth and invasion of human cancer cells. *Cancer Cell* 2005;7:561–573.
18. Bader AG, Kang S, Vogt PK. Cancer-specific mutations in PIK3CA are oncogenic in vivo. *Proc Natl Acad Sci U S A* 2006;103:1475–1479.
19. Nagata Y, Lan K-H, Zhou X, et al. PTEN activation contributes to tumor inhibition by trastuzumab, and loss of PTEN predicts trastuzumab resistance in patients. *Cancer Cell* 2004;6:117–127.
20. Berns K, Horlings HM, Hennessy BT, et al. A functional genetic approach identifies the PI3K pathway as a major determinant of trastuzumab resistance in breast cancer. *Cancer Cell* 2007;12:395–402.
21. Dillon RL, White DE, Muller WJ. The phosphatidyl inositol 3-kinase signaling network: implications for human breast cancer. *Oncogene* 2007;26:1338–1345.
22. Tabernero J, Rojo F, Calvo E, et al. Dose- and schedule-dependent inhibition of the mammalian target of rapamycin pathway with everolimus: a phase I tumor pharmacodynamic study in patients with advanced solid tumors. *J Clin Oncol* 2008; 26:1603–1610.
23. Temsirolimus: CCI 779, CCI-779, cell cycle inhibitor-779. *Drugs R D* 2004;5: 363–367.
24. Mita MM, Mita AC, Chu QS, et al. Phase I trial of the novel mammalian target of rapamycin inhibitor deforolimus (AP23573; MK-8669) administered intravenously daily for 5 days every 2 weeks to patients with advanced malignancies. *J Clin Oncol* 2008;26:361–367.
25. Chan S, Scheulen ME, Johnston S, et al. Phase II study of temsirolimus (CCI-779), a novel inhibitor of mTOR, in heavily pretreated patients with locally advanced or metastatic breast cancer. *J Clin Oncol* 2005;23:5314–5322.
26. Raymond E, Alexandre J, Faivre S, et al. Safety and pharmacokinetics of escalated doses of weekly intravenous infusion of cci-779, a novel mTOR inhibitor, in patients with cancer. *J Clin Oncol* 2004;22:2336–2347.
27. Carpenter JT, Roche H, Campone M, et al. Randomized 3-arm, phase 2 study of temsirolimus (CCI-779) in combination with letrozole in postmenopausal women with locally advanced or metastatic breast cancer. *Proceeding of the American Society of Clinical Oncology* 2005;23:A564.
28. Tabernero J, Rojo F, Calvo E, et al. dose- and schedule-dependent inhibition of the mammalian target of rapamycin pathway with everolimus: a phase I tumor pharmacodynamic study in patients with advanced solid tumors. *J Clin Oncol* 2008; 26:1603–1610.
29. Baselga J, Semiglazov V, van Dam P, et al. Phase II double-blind randomized trial of daily oral RAD001 (everolimus) plus letrozole (LET) or placebo (P) plus LET as neoadjuvant therapy for ER+ breast cancer [Abstract 2066]. San Antonio Breast Cancer Symposium 2007.
30. Dowsett M, Smith IE, Ebbs SR, et al. prognostic value of Ki67 expression after short-term presurgical endocrine therapy for primary breast cancer. *J Natl Cancer Inst* 2007;99:167–170.
31. André F, Campone M, Hurvitz SA, et al. Multicenter phase I clinical trial of daily and weekly RAD001 in combination with weekly paclitaxel and trastuzumab in patients with HER2-overexpressing metastatic breast cancer with prior resistance to trastuzumab [Abstract 1003]. *J Clin Oncol* 2008;26:1003.
32. Di Cosimo S, Scaltriti M, Val D, et al. The PI3-K/AKT/mTOR pathway as a target for breast cancer therapy. In: American Society of Clinical Oncology Meeting Abstracts 2007;25:3511.
33. Sauveur-Michel Maira S-M, Voliva C, et al. Class IA phosphatidylinositol 3-kinase: from their biologic implication in human cancers to drug discovery. *Expert Opin Ther Targets* 2008;12(2):223–238.
34. Maira S-M, Stauffer F, Brueggen J, et al. Identification and characterization of NVP-BEZ235, a new orally available dual PI3K/mTor inhibitor with potent *in vivo* antitumor activity. *Mol Cancer Ther* 2008;7(7):1851–1863.
35. Serra V, Markman B, Scaltriti M, et al. NVP-BEZ-235, a dual PI3K/mTOR inhibitor, prevents PI3K signaling and inhibits growth of cancer cells with activating PI3K mutations. *Cancer Res* 2008;68(19):8022–8030.
36. Laird AD. XL765 targets tumor growth, survival, and angiogenesis in preclinical models by dual inhibition of PI3K and mTOR. *Cancer Res* 2008;68(19):8022–8030.
37. Shapiro G, Edelman G, Calvo E, et al. Targeting aberrant PI3K pathway signaling with XL147, a potent, selective and orally bioavailable PI3K inhibitor. *Cancer Res* 2008;68(19):8022–8030.
38. Papadopoulos KP, Markman B, Tabernero J, et al. A phase I dose-escalation study of the safety, pharmacokinetics (PK), and pharmacodynamics (PD) of a novel PI3K inhibitor, XL765, administered orally to patients (pts) with advanced solid tumors [Abstract 3510]. *J Clin Oncol* 2008;26.
39. Martin GS. The hunting of the Src. *Nat Rev Mol Cell Biol* 2001;2:467–475.
40. Thomas SM, Brugge JS. Cellular functions regulated by Src family kinases. *Annu Rev Cell Dev Biol* 1997;13:513–609.
41. Yeatman TJ. A renaissance for SRC. *Nat Rev Cancer* 2004;4:470–480.
42. Bromann PA, Korkaya H, Courtneidge SA. The interplay between Src family kinases and receptor tyrosine kinases. *Oncogene* 2004;23:7957.
43. Blume-Jensen P, Hunter T. Oncogenic kinase signalling. *Nature* 2001;411:355–365.
44. Avizienyte E, Frame MC. Src and FAK signalling controls adhesion fate and the epithelial-to-mesenchymal transition. *Curr Opin Cell Biol* 2005;17:542–547.
45. Verbeek B, Vroom T, Adriaansen-Slot S, et al. c-Src protein expression increased in human breast cancer. An immunohistochemical and biochemical analysis. *J Pathol* 1996;180:383–388.
46. Ottenhoff-Kalff AE, Rijksen G, van Beurden EACM, et al. Characterization of protein tyrosine kinases from human breast cancer: involvement of the c-src oncogene product. *Cancer Res* 1992;52:4773–4778.
47. Rosen N, Bolen JB, Schwartz AM, et al. Analysis of pp60c-src protein kinase activity in human tumor cell lines and tissues. *J Biol Chem* 1986;261:13754–13759.
48. Guy CT, Muthuswamy SK, Cardiff RD, et al. Activation of the c-Src tyrosine kinase is required for the induction of mammary tumors in transgenic mice. *Genes Dev* 1994;8:23–32.
49. Muthuswamy SK, Siegel PM, Dankort DL, et al. Mammary tumors expressing the neu proto-oncogene possess elevated c-Src tyrosine kinase activity. *Mol Cell Biol* 1994;14:735–743.
50. Hiscox S, Morgan L, Green T, et al. Elevated Src activity promotes cellular invasion and motility in tamoxifen resistant breast cancer cells. *Breast Cancer Res Treat* 2006;97:263–274.
51. Lombardo LJ, Lee FY, Chen P, et al. Discovery of N-(2-chloro-6-methyl- phenyl)-2-(6-(4-(2-hydroxyethyl)-piperazin-1-yl)-2-methylpyrimidin-4-ylamino)thiazole-5-carboxamide (BMS-354825), a dual Src/Abl kinase inhibitor with potent antitumor activity in preclinical assays. *J Med Chem* 2004;47:6658–6661.
52. Talpaz M, Shah NP, Kantarjian H, et al. dasatinib in imatinib-resistant Philadelphia chromosome-positive leukemias. *N Engl J Med* 2006;354:2531–2541.
53. Huang F, Reeves K, Han X, et al. Identification of candidate molecular markers predicting sensitivity in solid tumors to dasatinib: rationale for patient selection. *Cancer Res* 2007;67:2226–2238.
54. Hennequin LF, Allen J, Breed J, et al. N-(5-chloro-1,3-benzodioxol-4-yl)-7-[2-(4-methylpiperazin-1-yl)ethoxy]-5-(tetrahydro-2H-pyran-4-yloxy)quinazolin-4-amine, a novel, highly selective, orally available, dual-specific c-Src/Abl kinase inhibitor. *J Med Chem* 2006;49:6465–6488.
55. Tabernero J, Cervantes A, Hoekman K, et al. Phase I study of AZD0530, an oral potent inhibitor of Src kinase: first demonstration of inhibition of Src activity in human cancers. *Proceeding of the American Society of Clinical Oncology* 2007:a3520.
56. Eastell R, Hannon RA, Gallagher N, et al. The effect of AZD0530, a highly selective, orally available Src/Abl kinase inhibitor, on biomarkers of bone resorption in healthy males. *Proceeding of the American Society of Clinical Oncology* 2007;a3041:2005.
57. Downward J. Targeting RAS signalling pathways in cancer therapy. *Nat Rev Cancer* 2003;3:11–22.

58. Schubbert S, Shannon K, Bollag G. Hyperactive Ras in developmental disorders and cancer. *Nat Rev Cancer* 2007;7:295–308.
59. Malumbres M, Barbacid M. RAS oncogenes: the first 30 years. *Nat Rev Cancer* 2003;3:459–465.
60. Izumi Y, Hirata M, Hasuwa H, et al. A metalloprotease-disintegrin, MDC9/meltrin-gamma/ADAM 9 and PKC delta are involved in TPA-induced ectodomain shedding of membrane-anchored heparin-binding EGF-like growth factor. *EMBO J* 1998; 17:7260–7272.
61. Barbacid M. Ras genes. *Annu Rev Biochem* 1987;56:779–827.
62. Rowinsky EK, Windle JJ, D. Von Hoff D. Ras protein farnesyltransferase: a strategic target for anticancer therapeutic development. *J Clin Oncol* 1999;17:3631–3652.
63. Tabernero J, Rojo F, Marimon I, et al. Phase I pharmacokinetic and pharmacodynamic study of weekly 1-hour and 24-hour infusion BMS-214662, a farnesyltransferase inhibitor, in patients with advanced solid tumors. *J Clin Oncol* 2005;23: 2521–2533.
64. Johnston SRD, Hickish T, Ellis P, et al. Phase II study of the efficacy and tolerability of two dosing regimens of the farnesyl transferase inhibitor, R115777, in advanced breast cancer. *J Clin Oncol* 2003;21:2492–2499.
65. Sparano JA, Moulder S, Kazi A, et al. Targeted inhibition of farnesyltransferase in locally advanced breast cancer: a phase I and II trial of tipifarnib plus dose-dense doxorubicin and cyclophosphamide. *J Clin Oncol* 2006;24:3013–3018.
66. Wilhelm SM, Carter C, Tang L, et al. BAY 43-9006 exhibits broad spectrum oral antitumor activity and targets the RAF/MEK/ERK pathway and receptor tyrosine kinases involved in tumor progression and angiogenesis. *Cancer Res* 2004;64: 7099–7109.
67. Escudier B, Eisen T, Stadler WM, et al. Sorafenib in advanced clear-cell renal-cell carcinoma. *N Engl J Med* 2007;356:125–134.
68. Bianchi G, Loibl S, Zamagni C, et al. Phase II multicenter trial of sorafenib in the treatment of patients with metastatic breast cancer [Abstract 164]. American Society of Clinical Oncology Breast Cancer Symposium 2007.
69. Stuart DD, Aardalen K, Venetsanakos E, et al. RAF265 is a potent Raf kinase inhibitor with selective anti-proliferative activity *in vitro* and *in vivo* [Abstract 4876]. American Association for Cancer Research Annual Meeting Abstracts; Washington, D.C., April 1, 2006.
70. Lee FA, Judith S-L, Mark BM. CI-1040 (PD184352), a targeted signal transduction inhibitor of MEK (MAPKK). *Semin Oncol* 2003;30:105–116.
71. LoRusso PM, Adjei AA, et al. Phase I and pharmacodynamic study of the oral MEK inhibitor CI-1040 in patients with advanced malignancies. *J Clin Oncol* 2005;23:5281–5293.
72. Rinehart J, Adjei AA, LoRusso PM, et al. Multicenter phase II study of the oral MEK inhibitor, CI-1040, in patients with advanced non-small-cell lung, breast, colon, and pancreatic cancer. *J Clin Oncol* 2004;22:4456–4462.
73. Rosen LS, Galatin P, Fehling JM, et al. A phase I dose-escalation study of XL518, a potent MEK inhibitor administered orally daily to subjects with solid tumors [Abstract 14585]. *J Clin Oncol* 2008;26(Suppl):14585.
74. Schad K, Baumann Conzett K, Enderlin V, et al. Continuous MEK inhibition by AZD6244 (ARRY-142886) results in exhaustion of the cutaneous keratinocytic stem cell pool and resembles senescence driven skin aging [Abstract 9075]. *J Clin Oncol* 2008;26:9075.
75. Neckers L, Kern A, Tsutsumi S. Hsp90 inhibitors disrupt mitochondrial homeostasis in cancer cells. *Chem Biol* 2007;14:1204–1206.
76. Zhang H, Burrows F. Targeting multiple signal transduction pathways through inhibition of Hsp90. *J Mol Med* 2004;82:488–499.
77. Maloney A, Workman P. HSP90 as a new therapeutic target for cancer therapy: the story unfolds. *Expert Opin Biol Ther* 2002;2:3–24.
78. Neckers L. Effects of geldanamycin and other naturally occurring small molecule antagonists of heat shock protein 90 on HER2 protein expression. *Breast Dis* 2000;11:49–59.

79. Basso AD, Solit DB, Munster PN, et al. Ansamycin antibiotics inhibit Akt activation and cyclin D expression in breast cancer cells that overexpress HER2. *Oncogene* 2002;21:1159–1166.
80. Chandarlapaty S, Scaltriti M, Baselga J, et al. Extracellular cleaved HER2 (p95) confers partial resistance to trastuzumab but not HSP90 inhibitors in models of HER2 amplified breast cancer. *J Clin Oncol* 2007;25(Suppl):10515.
81. Scaltriti M, Rojo F, Ocana A, et al. Expression of p95HER2, a truncated form of the HER2 receptor, and response to anti-HER2 therapies in breast cancer. *J Natl Cancer Inst* 2007;99:628–638.
82. Modi S, Stopeck AT, Gordon MS, et al. Combination of trastuzumab and tanespimycin (17-AAG, KOS-953) is safe and active in trastuzumab-refractory HER-2 overexpressing breast cancer: a phase I dose-escalation study. *J Clin Oncol* 2007;25:5410–5417.
83. Miller K, Rosen LS, Modi S, et al. Phase I trial of alvespimycin (KOS-1022; 17-DMAG) and trastuzumab (T). *Proceeding of the American Society of Clinical Oncology* 2007:a1115.
84. Virag L, Szabo C. The therapeutic potential of poly(ADP-ribose) polymerase inhibitors. *Pharmacol Rev* 2002;54:375–429.
85. Yang Y-G, Cortes U, Patnaik S, et al. Ablation of PARP-1 does not interfere with the repair of DNA double-strand breaks, but compromises the reactivation of stalled replication forks. *Oncogene* 2004;23:3872–3882.
86. Schreiber V, Dantzer Fo, Ame J-C, de Murcia G. Poly(ADP-ribose): novel functions for an old molecule. *Nat Rev Mol Cell Biol* 2006;7:517–528.
87. Ratnam K, Low JA. Current development of clinical inhibitors of poly(ADP-ribose) polymerase in oncology. *Clin Cancer Res* 2007;13:1383–1388.
88. Graziani G, Szabo C. Clinical perspectives of PARP inhibitors. *Pharmacol Res* 2005;52:109.
89. Farmer H, McCabe N, Lord CJ, et al. Targeting the DNA repair defect in BRCA mutant cells as a therapeutic strategy. *Nature* 2005;434:917–921.
90. Yap TA, Boss DS, Fong PC, et al. First in human phase I pharmacokinetic (PK) and pharmacodynamic (PD) study of KU-0059436 (Ku), a small molecule inhibitor of poly ADP-ribose polymerase (PARP) in cancer patients (p), including BRCA1/2 mutation carriers. *Proceeding of the American Society of Clinical Oncology* 2007:a3529.
91. Okada H, Mak TW. Pathways of apoptotic and non-apoptotic death in tumour cells. *Nat Rev Cancer* 2004;4:592–603.
92. Vaux DL, Strasser A. The molecular biology of apoptosis. *Proc Natl Acad Sci U S A* 1996;93:2239–2244.
93. Pommier Y, Sordet O, Antony S, et al. Apoptosis defects and chemotherapy resistance: molecular interaction maps and networks. *Oncogene* 2004;23: 2934–2949.
94. Ashkenazi A, Herbst RS. To kill a tumor cell: the potential of proapoptotic receptor agonists. *J Clin Invest* 2008;118:1979–1990.
95. Kelley SK, Ashkenazi A. Targeting death receptors in cancer with Apo2L/TRAIL. *Curr Opin Pharmacol* 2004;4:333–339.
96. Fesik SW. Promoting apoptosis as a strategy for cancer drug discovery. *Nat Rev Cancer* 2005;5:876–885.
97. Nicholson DW. From bench to clinic with apoptosis-based therapeutic agents. *Nature* 2000;407:810–816.
98. Tolcher AW, Mita M, Meropol NJ, et al. Phase I pharmacokinetic and biologic correlative study of mapatumumab, a fully human monoclonal antibody with agonist activity to tumor necrosis factor related apoptosis-inducing ligand receptor-1. *J Clin Oncol* 2007;25:1390–1396.
99. LoRusso P, Hong D, Heath E, et al. First-in-human study of AMG 655, a pro-APOptotic TRAIL receptor-2 agonist, in adult patients with advanced solid tumors [Abstract 3534]. *J Clin Oncol* 2007;25(Suppl):3534.

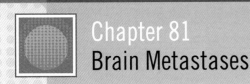
Chapter 81
Brain Metastases

Nancy U. Lin and Naren R. Ramakrishna

Despite major improvements in the therapeutic options available for patients with advanced breast cancer, brain metastases remain a challenging clinical problem. Because of their unique location, even relatively small tumors in the central nervous system (CNS) may result in neurological symptoms that negatively impact quality of life (QOL). The goals of treatment are to improve or stabilize patient symptoms while minimizing treatment-related toxicities. Intracranial involvement with breast cancer can also occur as leptomeningeal involvement and this is covered in Chapter 83.

Historically, brain metastases most commonly occurred late in the natural history of breast cancer and in the presence of progressive extracranial disease. In this setting, the principal therapeutic modality was whole brain radiotherapy (WBRT). As systemic therapies for breast cancer have improved and overall survival lengthens, it appears that:

1. the incidence of brain metastases is increasing,
2. a greater proportion of patients have controlled extracranial disease at the time of their CNS diagnosis, and
3. CNS recurrence after initial treatment is becoming more frequent (1–3).

These factors have led to debates on how best to sequence existing strategies, including surgery, stereotactic radiosurgery (SRS), and WBRT, as well as renewed interest in the development of systemic therapies, including cytotoxic chemotherapy and targeted approaches.

INCIDENCE AND EPIDEMIOLOGY

Because of incomplete reporting, the true incidence of brain metastases is difficult to estimate with certainty (4). Registry data from The Netherlands and the United States indicate that among patients with primary lung, breast, melanoma, renal, and colorectal cancers presenting at any stage, the combined incidence of brain metastases is between 8.5% and 9.6% (4,5). Thus, metastatic disease to the brain is a far more common cause of intracranial neoplasms than are primary brain tumors.

Of patients diagnosed with brain metastases, between 13% and 20% will carry a primary diagnosis of breast cancer, making breast cancer the second most common cause of CNS involvement, after lung cancer (4,6,7). As expected, the risk of developing brain metastases varies according to stage at initial diagnosis. In patients presenting with localized, early stage breast cancer, less than 3% will ultimately be diagnosed with brain metastases; this risk increases to 7% to 8% in women with locally advanced or high-risk disease (4,8–10). Of patients with advanced breast cancer, 10% to 16% will eventually be diagnosed with brain metastases (4,11,12). Prospective studies evaluating the frequency of screen-detected, asymptomatic brain metastases over time have not been reported. However, among heavily pretreated patients with advanced breast cancer who

underwent brain imaging at a single time point as part of eligibility screening for clinical trials, 14.8% were found to have occult CNS involvement (13). In contrast to the clinical estimates, autopsy series from the 1970s and 1980s indicate that up to 30% of patients have CNS involvement at the time of death (11,14). Many of these patients died of progressive systemic disease, and the CNS diagnosis was made only at the time of death. However, improvements in systemic therapy have already resulted in better and more sustained control of extracranial disease and prolonged overall survival, raising concerns that there will be additional time for formerly occult CNS lesions to become clinically symptomatic. Indeed, for a subset of women with advanced breast cancer, control of CNS disease has become a vital component of overall disease control and quality of life.

RISK FACTORS FOR CENTRAL NERVOUS SYSTEM INVOLVEMENT

Clinical factors such as young age and African American ethnicity are associated with an increased risk of developing brain metastases (4,11,15). Among patients aged 20 to 39 at initial breast cancer diagnosis (of any stage) within the Metropolitan Detroit Cancer Surveillance System, the incidence proportion percentage of brain metastases was 10%, compared to less than 3% of patients over the age of 70 (4). In one small study of patients with metastatic breast cancer, 43% of women under age 40 were ultimately diagnosed with brain metastases (15). It is conceivable that the observed increased risk in these populations relates to the higher proportion of aggressive tumor subtypes, including HER2-positive, estrogen receptor (ER)–negative, and triple-negative (i.e., ER-, PR [progesterone receptor]-, and HER2-negative) tumors, compared to the breast cancer population at large (16–18).

Biological risk factors include ER-negativity, HER2-positivity, and high grade (3,10,19–24). Of these factors, the association between HER2 status and brain metastasis has been most studied, but there are accumulating data regarding ER-negative and triple-negative breast cancers as well.

Since the introduction of trastuzumab for the treatment of metastatic, HER2-positive breast cancer, multiple groups have reported a 25% to 40% incidence of CNS relapse, which is significantly higher than expected compared to historical controls of unselected patients with advanced breast cancer (2,25–29). Of note, in the majority of cases, the appearance of brain metastases occurred in the setting of controlled extracranial disease, implicating the CNS as a sanctuary site (2,26,28). Indeed, although trastuzumab is highly active against HER2-positive breast cancer, it does not appear to penetrate the blood–brain barrier due to its large molecular weight (30,31). Further support for this sanctuary hypothesis comes from the early stage setting (8,9,22). In the National Surgical Adjuvant

979

Breast and Bowel Project (NSABP) B-31, N9831, and HERceptin adjuvant (HERA) trials, a trend toward an increase in the frequency of brain metastases as first event was observed in the trastuzumab treated arms, although the absolute incidence was still quite low overall (8,9). Beyond treatment-related factors, HER2 overexpression itself appears to confer a higher likelihood of CNS spread. In preclinical models, the expression of HER2 leads to increased outgrowth of breast cancer metastases in the brain (32). And in studies of early breast cancer patients treated in the pretrastuzumab era, HER2 was still a risk factor for CNS relapse (23,33). It is the combination of a biological subtype that is predisposed to spread to the CNS and effective systemic therapies that do not cross the blood–brain barrier that likely explain the higher incidence of brain metastases observed in HER2-positive patients treated in the current era, compared to historical controls.

There is also emerging evidence that basal-like tumors are associated with an increased risk of CNS relapse. Tsuda et al. (34) compared the clinical features of 20 high-grade carcinomas with large, central acellular zones to 40 matched high-grade carcinomas without these zones. The presence of acellular zones appeared to be highly correlated to a myoepithelial (i.e., basal) immunophenotype, and these tumors were more likely to metastasize to the brain. A higher incidence of CNS metastases has also been observed in African Americans and in *BRCA1* mutation carriers; of note, basal-like tumors are more common in these groups than in the general population (4,18,35,36). More direct evidence comes from two recent reports comparing patients presenting with primary, basal-like tumors, as assessed by CK5/6 and CK14, to patients with non-basal tumors (37,38). In both studies, basal phenotype was associated with an increased risk of brain metastases.

METHOD OF SPREAD AND DISTRIBUTION

Parenchymal brain metastases are thought to arise from hematogenous dissemination of tumor cells. Consistent with this hypothesis, the distribution of lesions mirrors overall blood flow in the brain, such that supratentorial lesions are the most common site of involvement (80%), followed by the cerebellum (15%), and brainstem (5%) (11,39,40). In addition, the vascular border zones and the gray and white matter junction are common areas of metastatic involvement, which is thought to be due to changes in vessel diameter and flow (41).

Older studies indicated that approximately half of patients with brain metastases presented with a single lesion (39). However, with the introduction of magnetic resonance imaging (MRI), a significantly more sensitive technique, current series indicate that only about one third to one fourth of patients with brain metastases have a confirmed single lesion (42–44). The term solitary brain metastasis indicates a single brain lesion in the absence of systemic metastases.

CLINICAL MANIFESTATIONS

Because brain imaging is not part of routine clinical care for asymptomatic patients with breast cancer, brain metastases are most commonly diagnosed in the setting of new neurological symptoms. The range of symptoms is wide and includes headache, focal neurologic dysfunction, cognitive dysfunction, and seizures. As a result of higher inpatient and outpatient costs, the economic burden of brain metastases from breast cancer is estimated at more than double that of patients with metastatic breast cancer without CNS involvement (45).

Headaches are present in up to half of patients with brain metastases and are commonly bifrontal (46). In patients with a single metastasis or a dominant lesion, there may be a predominance of the pain on the side of the metastasis (47). Coexisting nausea or emesis occurs in about half of patients with headaches and is a predictive factor for the presence of brain metastases (47,48). Although a tension-type headache has been frequently described, this finding has not been consistently replicated (48).

Focal neurologic dysfunction is the presenting symptom in 20% to 40% of patients (49). Hemiparesis is the most common complaint. The distribution of symptoms depends on the location of the metastases and the presence or absence of surrounding edema.

Cognitive dysfunction, including mental status changes, memory problems, or mood or personality changes, is the presenting symptoms in one third of patients (49). Frequently, neurological examination will elicit additional deficits of which the patient is unaware (50). However, medications, metabolic abnormalities, and infections are more common causes of encephalopathy in cancer patients than brain metastases and should be included in the differential diagnosis of altered mental status (51).

Seizures are the presenting symptom in 10% to 20% of patients with brain metastases, and an additional 10% to 26% will develop seizures at some time during the course of their illness (52–55). Supratentorial involvement increases the risk of seizure, whereas seizures are quite uncommon in patients with posterior fossa lesions (52).

In contrast to melanoma or choriocarcinoma, brain metastases from breast cancer tend not to bleed; therefore, acute cerebral hemorrhage is rarely a presenting symptom (56).

DIAGNOSTIC EVALUATION

In patients presenting with suspicious neurological signs or symptoms, evaluation with computed tomography (CT) or contrast-enhanced MRI is indicated. Of these approaches, MRI is the more sensitive noninvasive, diagnostic test (42,57,58).

MRI detects more lesions in the posterior fossa, where beam-hardening artifact can make CT difficult to interpret (58). MRI is also superior in defining the number of CNS lesions, a distinction that may dramatically affect clinical recommendations. For example, in a study of 23 patients who underwent both double-dose delayed CT and contrast-enhanced MRI, MRI detected more than 67 definite lesions, compared to only 37 lesions on CT, and three of the patients with five or fewer lesions on CT had "too numerous to count" lesions on MRI (57).

The differential diagnosis of enhancing mass lesions in a patient with breast cancer includes metastasis, primary brain tumor, abscess, demyelinating disorders, cerebral infarction, hemorrhage, progressive multifocal leukoencephalopathy, and posttreatment change (i.e., radiation necrosis, postsurgical change). Radiographic features that may differentiate brain metastases from other CNS lesions include the presence of multiple lesions (which helps to distinguish metastases from primary brain tumors), localization at the junction of the gray and white matter, circumscribed margins, and relatively large amounts of vasogenic edema compared to the size of the lesion (49). The clinical history can also be helpful in guiding appropriate diagnostic testing. For patients with advanced breast cancer who present with multiple brain lesions, further testing may not be necessary. For patients without evidence of extracranial involvement by breast cancer, consideration should be given to tissue sampling to distinguish between metastatic breast cancer versus metastasis from a nonbreast primary, primary brain tumor, or nonmalignant cause. A tissue diagnosis should also be strongly considered for patients presenting with a single brain lesion. In a randomized trial evaluating the role of surgical resection for single brain metastasis, 11% of patients were found to have an alternate diagnosis on pathologic review (59). Finally, the differential diagnosis of dural-based lesions includes meningiomas. Because the incidence of meningioma has been reported to be somewhat higher in breast cancer patients than the general population, and because imaging studies may be inconclusive, tissue diagnosis may be required (60). Thus, in any patient in whom the diagnosis of brain metastases is in doubt, based on the radiographic appearance of the lesion(s), the presence of a single lesion, or the clinical history, obtaining tissue is important to establish the diagnosis conclusively.

Another clinical dilemma exists in patients who have previously received radiotherapy or SRS for brain metastases and now present with an equivocal MRI scan. One approach is to consider supplemental imaging with either positron emission tomography (PET), single photon emission CT (SPECT), functional MRI, or MR spectroscopy (61). With a detection rate of only 61% to 68% compared to contrast-enhanced MRI, ^{18}F-flurorodeoxyglucose (FDG)-PET does not appear sufficiently sensitive for use as a screening tool for brain metastases (62,63). However, FDG-PET may be helpful in distinguishing radiation necrosis from tumor progression. In a study of 32 patients with brain metastases from any solid tumor, FDG-PET with MRI coregistration had a sensitivity of 86% and specificity of 80%, although not all groups have been able to replicate these findings (64,65). Another potentially useful tool is Tl-201 SPECT. In one study of 72 patients, the sensitivity was reported at 91% for differentiating between radiation necrosis and tumor progression (66). Finally, a variety of newer techniques are under evaluation, including the use of alternative PET tracers (i.e., ^{18}F-fluorocholine, ^{18}F-flurorothymidine, or L-[methyl-^{11}C] methionine) and quantification of blood vessel tortuosity (61,67). In cases in which the imaging studies remain equivocal, management options include following the patient carefully over time versus proceeding to a biopsy for tissue diagnosis. Choosing between these options depends on several factors, including the accessibility of the lesion and the presence or absence of associated symptoms.

PROGNOSIS

Historically, CNS involvement tended to occur late in the course of metastatic breast cancer, and median survival was poor, on the order of 4 to 6 months (21,68–70). Predictive factors for prolonged survival include Karnofsky performance status greater than 70, solitary brain metastasis, systemic tumor control, longer disease-free interval, and ER positivity. As will be discussed below, treatment of brain metastases with radiotherapy or surgery is also associated with prolonged survival, compared to supportive care only.

In recent years, some, although not all, studies have suggested that the prognosis for patients with CNS metastases from breast cancer may be improving. In a series of 74 patients treated at the University of California San Francisco between 1997 to 2005, the median survival after brain metastasis diagnosis was 14.4 months (71). Several groups have explored the impact of HER2 status on prognosis after CNS relapse. Kirsch et al. (72) examined the outcomes of 95 women at Massachusetts General Hospital diagnosed with brain metastases between 1998 and 2003. Median survival after CNS diagnosis was 22.4 months in patients with HER2-positive disease, compared to 9.4 months in patients with HER2-negative disease ($p = .0002$). Of interest, the survival advantage in the HER2-positive subset could not be explained by superior CNS control and was felt to be due primarily to improved systemic control with trastuzumab. Gori et al. (26) report similar findings: median time to death from CNS diagnosis was 23 months in patients with HER2-positive breast cancer. These findings contrast with those of Tham et al. (21), who reported a median survival of

only 5.5 months after CNS diagnosis in unselected patients and shorter survival in HER2-positive patients. One potential explanation for the difference between studies is that the Tham study predated the widespread use of trastuzumab. Together, these data, although retrospective in nature, suggest that (a) improvements in systemic therapy are allowing some patients to live longer than previously seen, and (b) pursuing more aggressive approaches in the CNS among breast cancer patients with well-controlled systemic disease may be reasonable.

 # MANAGEMENT

The management of patients with brain metastases can be divided into symptomatic and definitive therapy. Symptomatic therapy includes the use of corticosteroids for the treatment of peritumoral edema and anticonvulsants for control of seizures, whereas definitive therapy includes treatments such as surgery, radiotherapy, SRS, chemotherapy, targeted therapy, and radiosensitizers directed at eradicating the tumor itself.

Symptomatic Therapy

Corticosteroids

Corticosteroids are indicated in patients with symptomatic edema and are thought to exert their effect by reducing capillary permeability, restoring arteriolar tone, and facilitating transport of fluid into the ventricular system, where it can be cleared by cerebrospinal fluid bulk flow (73–75). Most patients will improve symptomatically within 24 to 72 hours, although improvement of edema on imaging studies may not be immediately apparent (76).

Of the corticosteroids, dexamethasone is the most widely used because of its relatively weak mineralocorticoid activity, which reduces the potential for fluid retention. The usual starting dose is 4 mg every 6 hours and may be preceded by a 10 mg load, depending on clinical circumstances. Because of potential adverse effects, such as myopathy, hyperglycemia, insomnia, fluid retention, gastritis, acne, and immunosuppression, the dose of corticosteroids should be kept to the minimum effective dose and tapered during or after definitive therapy. Corticosteroid use also increases the risk of *Pneumocystis jiroveci* pneumonia. In two case series, the median duration of dexamethasone therapy was only 10 weeks before onset of symptoms from *P. jiroveci*, and symptoms commonly appeared during tapering of steroid therapy (77,78). Therefore, *P. jiroveci* prophylaxis should be considered for patients for whom the anticipated duration of steroid use exceeds 4 to 5 weeks.

Anticonvulsants

Approximately 10% to 20% of patients with brain metastases present with seizures, and an additional 10% to 26% will develop seizures at some time during the course of their illness (52–55). For most patients, confirmation of the diagnosis with electroencephalography is not necessary, and the use of standard anticonvulsants is generally indicated.

However, about one third of patients experience at least one adverse effect from anticonvulsant therapy, including rash, hepatoxicity, myelosuppression, nausea, headache, somnolence, or cognitive dysfunction. Stevens-Johnson's syndrome has been reported in association with both phenytoin and carbamazepine use (79). Overall, 24% of patients given anticonvulsants will ultimately either switch therapy or discontinue anticonvulsants altogether as a result of drug-related toxicity (80).

In addition, via their effect upon the cytochrome P450 system, the enzyme-inducing antiepileptic drugs (EIAEDs) (e.g., phenobarbital, phenytoin, carbamazepine) accelerate the metabolism of many commonly used chemotherapy drugs, including doxorubicin, paclitaxel, cyclophosphamide, methotrexate, topotecan, and irinotecan, potentially reducing their efficacy (80). EIAEDs also increase the metabolism of many of the newer targeted agents, such as gefitinib, lapatinib, tipifarnib, and others in the pipeline. Interactions may also occur with a wide range of commonly prescribed medications, including corticosteroids, macrolide antibiotics, antifungal agents, oral contraceptives, antidepressants, anxiolytics, and anticoagulants, potentially leading to reduced efficacy, significant toxicity, or breakthrough seizures (81).

To determine whether the routine use of anticonvulsants is indicated in patients without a prior history of seizure, the Quality Standards Subcommittee of the American Academy of Neurology reviewed the results of 12 studies that addressed this question (80). None of the individual studies indicated a significant reduction in seizure incidence between the prophylaxis and nonprophylaxis groups. A meta-analysis of the four randomized trials indicated no difference in seizure incidence (odds ratio [OR] 1.09; 95% confidence interval [CI], 0.63–1.89; p = .8), seizure-free survival (OR 1.03; 95% CI, 0.74–1.44; p = .9), or overall survival (0.93; 95% CI, 0.65–1.32; p = .7). Because of the known potential for adverse effects and drug interactions and the lack of clear benefit, the routine use of anticonvulsants is not recommended in patients without a history of seizures. A possible exception includes patients with lesions in areas of high epileptogenicity (e.g., motor cortex), although a benefit in this subset has not been clearly demonstrated in clinical studies.

Venous Thromboembolic Disease

Venous thromboembolic (VTE) disease occurs in approximately 20% of patients with brain metastases (82). Because of the concern for intracranial hemorrhage (ICH), many clinicians are reluctant to fully anticoagulate patients. However, mechanical approaches, such as the placement of an inferior vena cava (IVC) filter, are reported to be associated with complications in two thirds of patients (83). In addition, VTE recurs in up to 40% of patients with brain metastases treated with an IVC filter alone (84).

Compared to IVC filter placement, anticoagulation is associated with a lower rate of recurrent VTE, and for most patients with breast cancer, the risk of hemorrhage appears acceptable. In a series of 42 patients with brain metastases from a variety of solid tumors treated at Memorial Sloan-Kettering Cancer Center in New York who were anticoagulated for VTE, only three patients (7%) experienced ICH, including two patients in the setting of supratherapeutic anticoagulation (84). Consequently, the data, although limited, suggest that anticoagulation is generally preferable to IVC filter placement in breast cancer patients who develop clinically significant VTE.

DEFINITIVE TREATMENT

The goals of definitive treatment of brain metastases are to relieve or stabilize neurological symptoms and to achieve long-term tumor control while minimizing toxicity. The choice of therapy is influenced by:

1. the size, number, and location of lesions,
2. the presence or absence of symptoms,
3. the patient's life expectancy, including the patient's performance status and the status of the patient's extracranial disease,
4. prior treatment, and
5. expected toxicities of treatment.

Given these complex considerations, the optimal care of patients with brain metastases involves close multidisciplinary collaboration in order to avoid overtreatment of patients with a limited life expectancy, as well as potential undertreatment of patients with well-controlled systemic disease and significant CNS-related morbidity.

Whole Brain Radiotherapy

For over five decades, WBRT has played a central role in the management of brain metastases. Early case series supported a survival benefit for brain metastases in patients treated with WBRT compared to supportive care only (85). Breast cancer brain metastases in particular appear to be relatively responsive to WBRT. A study of volumetric response rates of brain metastases to WBRT by Nieder et al. (86) revealed breast cancer to have favorable response rates in relation to other histologies, such as non–small cell lung and melanoma, with an overall complete or partial remission rate of 93%. For patients with brain metastases from breast cancer, estimates of the median expected survival following treatment with WBRT alone is between 4 to 6.5 months versus 1 to 2 months with supportive care only (87). In addition to a survival benefit, WBRT provides effective palliation of neurological symptoms, with durable improvement, or stability of neurological symptoms observed in approximately 70% to 90% of patients (55,88,89). For patients presenting with cranial nerve deficits, approximately 40% may have an improvement with WBRT (89). For breast cancer patients who develop cranial neuropathies, prompt MRI should be performed to evaluate for meningeal or skull base involvement. Should these be present, corticosteroids and radiotherapy should be initiated promptly to increase the likelihood of symptom palliation (55).

A wide range of WBRT dose-fractionation schedules, ranging from 2,000 cGy in five fractions to 4,000 cGy in 20 fractions, have been compared for efficacy and toxicity in two Radiation Therapy Oncology Group (RTOG) randomized trials (Table 81.1) (87,90). Although the various schedules showed no significant difference in median survival or duration of symptom palliation, symptomatic relief occurred sooner in patients treated with larger fractions. Even when breast cancer patients were analyzed in a subgroup analysis, time to progression of neurologic function or death did not differ by schedule (90). Further shortened WBRT courses such as 1,000 cGy in a single fraction or 1,200 cGy in two fractions achieve similar survival and palliative benefit as more extended fractionation schemes, but appear to be associated with inferior duration of symptom improvement and time to neurological progression (91). In addition, large fraction size may increase the risk of neurocognitive dysfunction (92). A randomized trial comparing accelerated hyperfractionated WBRT to 3,000 cGy in 10 fractions showed no benefit to survival or palliation, even among favorable prognostic groups (93). The current standard therapy of 3,000 cGy in 10 300-cGy fractions over 2 weeks provides a balance between prompt palliation and acceptably low acute side effects (94). Although 3,000 cGy in 10 fractions may be appropriate for patients with expected survivals of less than 6 months, the dose fractionation schedule should be individualized, and for patients who may be long-term survivors, a more extended dose fractionation, such as 3,750 cGy in 250-cGy fractions or 4,000 cGy in 200-cGy fractions may decrease neurocognitive sequelae (95).

The toxicity of WBRT is generally divided into acute, early delayed, and late effects (96). The most debilitating acute and early delayed effects are fatigue and somnolence, which can be profound. They may arise within the first week of therapy and persist for weeks or months (97). Other prominent acute and early delayed effects of WBRT that impact adversely on quality of life include hair loss, skin erythema, loss of taste, and

Table 81.1 SUMMARY OF SELECTED PROSPECTIVE RANDOMIZED CLINICAL TRIALS EVALUATING MANAGEMENT STRATEGIES FOR BRAIN METASTASES

Trial (Reference)	Study Design	Patients	Total No. of Patients	No. of Patients with Breast Cancer	Results
Trials evaluating whole brain radiotherapy dose-fractionation schedules[a]					
Borgelt et al., 1980 (87)					
First study	30 Gy/10 fractions vs. 30 Gy/15 fractions vs. 40 Gy/15 fractions vs. 40 Gy/20 fractions	Solid tumors	910	166	More rapid symptom improvement with larger fractions (55% of patients achieved improved symptoms at 2 weeks with 30 Gy/10 fractions compared to 43% for other regimens, $p = .06$). No difference in OS among treatment schedules.
Second study	20 Gy/5 fractions vs. 30 Gy/10 fractions vs. 40 Gy/15 fractions	Solid tumors	902	146	More rapid symptom improvement with larger fractions (64% of patients achieved improved symptoms at 2 weeks with 20 Gy/5 fractions compared to 54% for the other regimens, $p = .01$). No difference in OS among treatment schedules.
Borgelt et al., 1981 (91)					
First study	10 Gy/1 fraction vs. protracted course (20, 30, or 40 Gy/10–20 fractions)	Solid tumors	26[b]	2	No difference in rate of symptom improvement or OS. Shorter duration of improvement (4 vs. 10 wks, $p = .02$) and TTP (median 8 vs. 11.5 wks, $p = .07$) with high dose radiation.
Second study	12 Gy/2 fractions vs. protracted course (20, 30, or 40 Gy/10–20 fractions)	Solid tumors	33[a]	1	No statistically significant difference in rate of symptom improvement, duration of improvement, or OS with high-dose radiation.
Murray et al., 1997 (93)	32 Gy/20 fractions over 10 days followed by boost (24.4 Gy/14 fractions over 7 days) vs. 30 Gy/10 fractions	Solid tumors	429	43	No difference in OS with accelerated hyperfractionation ($p = .52$).
Trials evaluating the role of surgery in addition to WBRT					
Patchell et al., 1990 (59)	Surgery followed by WBRT (36 Gy/12 fractions) vs. WBRT alone	Solid tumors, single brain metastasis	48	3	Improved local control 52% vs. 20% ($p < .02$), OS (median 40 vs. 15 wks, $p < .01$), and functionally independent survival (median 38 vs. 8 wks, $p < .005$).
Noordijk et al., 1994 (103)	Surgery followed by WBRT (40 Gy/20 fractions over 10 days) vs. WBRT alone	Solid tumors, single brain metastasis	63	12	Improved OS (median 10 vs. 6 mos, $p = .04$) and functionally independent survival (7.5 vs. 3.5 mos, $p = .06$).
Mintz et al., 1996 (104)	Surgery followed by WBRT (30 Gy/10 fractions) vs. WBRT alone	Solid tumors, single brain metastasis	84	10	No difference in OS (median 5.6 vs. 6.3 mos, $p = .24$) or proportion of functionally independent days (mean 0.32 for both arms, $p = .98$).
Trials evaluating the role of WBRT in addition to local therapy					
Patchell et al., 1998 (100)	Surgery + WBRT (50.4 Gy/28 fractions) vs. surgery alone	Solid tumors, single brain metastasis status post complete surgical resection	95	9	Improved local control (recurrence in tumor bed 10% vs. 46%, $p < .001$) and distant control (recurrence in other sites in the brain 14% vs. 37%, $p < .01$). Decreased death due to neurologic causes (14% vs. 44%, $p = .003$). No difference in OS (median 48 vs. 43 wks, $p = .39$) or functionally independent survival (median 37 vs. 35 wks, $p = .61$).
Aoyama et al., 2006 (122)	WBRT (30 Gy/10 fractions) + SRS (with 30% dose reduction) vs. SRS alone	Solid tumors, 1–4 lesions, all ≤3 cm	132	9	Improved local control (89% vs. 73%, $p = .002$) at 1 year. Decreased likelihood of recurrence of tumor anywhere in the brain at 1 year (47% vs. 76%, $p < .001$), and decreased requirement for salvage therapy (15% vs. 43%, $p < .001$). No difference in preservation of neurologic function. No difference in primary endpoint of OS (7.5 vs. 8.0 mos, $p = .42$). No difference in death due to neurologic causes (22.8% vs. 19.3%, $p = .64$).
Trials evaluating dose intensification of radiotherapy					
Kondziolka et al., 1999 (120)	WBRT (30 Gy/12 fractions) + SRS vs. WBRT alone	Solid tumors, 2–4 lesions, all ≤2.5 cm	27	4	Improved local control (local recurrence rate at 1 year 8% vs. 100%; median time to local recurrence 36 vs. 6 mos, $p = .0005$). Longer time to recurrence of tumor anywhere in the brain (34 vs. 5 mos, $p = .002$). No difference in OS (11 vs. 7.5 mos, $p = .22$).
Andrews et al., 2004 (121)	WBRT (37.5 Gy/15 fractions) + SRS vs. WBRT alone	Solid tumors, 1–3 lesions, largest ≤4 cm	333	34	Improved local control at 1 year (82% vs. 71%, $p = .01$). Higher likelihood of stable or improved performance status at 6 months (43% vs. 27%, $p = .03$). No difference in primary end point of OS (6.5 vs. 5.7 mos, $p = .14$). Survival advantage observed in subgroup of patients with a single brain metastasis (median 6.5 vs. 4.9 mos, $p = .04$).
Trials evaluating radiosensitizers					
Mehta et al., 2003 (155)	WBRT (30 Gy/10 fractions) + motexafin gadolinium vs. WBRT alone	Solid tumors	401	75	No difference in OS (median 5.2 vs. 4.9 mos, $p = .48$), time to neurologic progression (median 9.5 vs. 8.3 mos, $p = .95$), or death due to neurologic causes (49% vs. 52%, $p = .60$).
Suh et al., 2006 (156)	WBRT (30 Gy/10 fractions) + efaproxiral vs. WBRT alone	Solid tumors, RPA class I or II	515	107	No difference in OS (median 5.4 vs. 4.4 mos, $p = .16$), time to neurological progression, or death due to neurologic causes. In an exploratory subgroup analysis, improved OS (HR for death 0.51, $p = .003$) and response rate (54% vs. 41%, $p = .01$) in breast cancer patients.
Knisely et al., 2008 (154)	WBRT (37.5 Gy/15 fractions) + thalidomide vs. WBRT alone	Solid tumors, multiple (>3), large (>4 cm), or midbrain metastases	175	31	No difference in OS (median 3.9 mos for both arms), or in deaths due to neurologic causes.

OS, overall survival; TTP, time to progression; WBRT, whole brain radiotherapy; SRS, stereotactic radiosurgery; HR, hazard ratio
[a]All fractions given once daily unless otherwise specified.
[b]Represents number of patients assigned to the high-dose arm. These patients were compared to 143 control patients who received a more protracted course of radiation.

decreased appetite. Although the acute and early delayed effects are generally reversible, the late effects are generally permanent and may be progressive. Of particular concern are the risks of radiation-related leukoencephalopathy and necrosis that may manifest clinically as significant neurologic or neurocognitive dysfunction (97).

The potential for neurocognitive dysfunction following WBRT is of substantial concern, particularly for patients who may have long survival. The actual risk of WBRT-induced neurocognitive dysfunction is difficult to estimate as most brain metastases patients do not survive sufficiently long to realize such risks. DeAngelis et al. (92) described 12 cases of progressive dementia that developed at a median of 14 months following treatment with WBRT alone or surgery plus WBRT. All patients displayed cortical atrophy and also developed urinary incontinence and ataxia, and seven patients died of these complications with no evidence of tumor recurrence. Their treatment was done with relatively large fraction sizes ranging from 300 to 600 cGy and total doses of 2,500 to 3,900 cGy. Other factors that may increase the risk of late radiation toxicity from whole brain radiotherapy include age, extent of disease, diabetes mellitus, concomitant chemotherapy, and multiple sclerosis (97–99).

Following surgical resection of a solitary brain metastasis, postoperative WBRT has frequently been employed with the goal of decreasing the risk of both local and distant recurrence in the brain. (Local refers to a recurrence at the original site of metastasis and distant to a recurrence elsewhere in the brain.) A randomized trial by Patchell et al. (100) further clarified the effects of postoperative WBRT for patients with a surgically resected solitary brain metastasis (Table 81.1). In this study, 95 patients were randomized to either WBRT or no further treatment following complete resection of a solitary brain metastasis. The addition of WBRT decreased the risk of local recurrence (10% vs. 46%; p <.01), distant brain recurrence, that is, the appearance of a new CNS lesions outside the resection site (14% vs. 37%; p <.01), and the risk of neurological death (14% vs. 44%; p = .003). Although no significant difference in overall survival was found, the higher risk of neurological death observed with surgery alone has been suggested as a justification for combined therapy in this group of patients. The impact, however, of the elevated risk of local or distant brain recurrence on QOL compared to the toxicity from the addition of WBRT, particularly in patients with long expected survival, remains unclear, especially when other low morbidity salvage therapies such as SRS may be effective. Also, localized boost therapy to the surgical resection cavity using SRS or fractionated stereotactic radiotherapy without WBRT may decrease the risk of local recurrence to levels comparable or less than that achieved with WBRT (101). The possibility that WBRT may be omitted in select patients, particularly those undergoing SRS for limited brain metastatic disease, is an area of active clinical investigation and is discussed further below. Another approach under investigation is the use of hippocampal-sparing techniques, given the very low likelihood of hippocampal involvement in patients with brain metastases and the prospect for decreased neurocognitive toxicity with WBRT (102).

Surgery

The role of surgery in patients with brain metastases is to provide relief of symptoms resulting from mass effect of the tumor, to establish a histologic diagnosis, to improve local control, and to provide a potential benefit to survival.

Three prospective, randomized trials have been conducted to evaluate the role of surgery in patients with brain metastases (Table 81.1). The first trial, reported by Patchell et al. (59), randomly assigned 48 patients with a single brain metastasis (6% with a breast primary) to either surgery followed by WBRT versus WBRT alone. Patients in the combined-modality arm

achieved better local control (20% vs. 52%; p <.02), improved median duration of functional independence (38 vs. 8 weeks; p <.005), and longer overall survival (40 vs. 15 weeks, p <.01), compared to the patients who received WBRT alone. These findings were replicated in a study of 63 patients (19% with breast primaries) led by Noordijk et al. (103), in which patients treated with surgery and WBRT achieved prolonged survival (median 10 vs. 6 months; p = .04) and functionally independent survival (7.5 vs. 3.5 months; p = .06) compared to patients treated with WBRT alone. Of note, only patients with stable or absent extracranial disease appeared to derive a survival benefit from surgery; patients with progressive extracranial disease experienced a median survival of only 5 months irrespective of the allocated treatment. A third study reported no difference in either survival or functionally independent survival with the addition of surgery to WBRT (104). In contrast to the first two trials, nearly half of the patients in this study were enrolled with coexisting extracranial metastases, and approximately 40% of patients had a Karnofsky performance status of 70% or less at study entry. In addition, the presence of a single brain lesion was categorized based on CT rather than MRI (which could have missed multiple lesions), and 10 of 43 patients randomly assigned to radiotherapy underwent surgical resection at some point in their disease course, which may have further confounded the results.

In addition to the randomized trial data, the positive impact of surgical resection on survival has also been observed in large, retrospective studies and retains its significance even after adjusting for other prognostic factors (105). Although there have been no trials of surgical resection limited to breast cancer patients, the totality of the data strongly indicates that surgical resection should be considered in patients with a single metastasis and stable extracranial disease.

In patients with multiple brain metastases, the role of surgery remains controversial, and the data are limited to retrospective series. In a series of 56 patients who underwent resection of multiple lesions, patients who had had all of their brain metastases resected experienced improved survival compared to patients who had one or more lesions left unresected. These patients also experienced comparable survival to a series of 26 patients who had undergone resection for a single metastases and who were matched for type of primary tumor and systemic disease status (106). Iwadate et al. (107) reported similar results: patients with multiple metastases who underwent total or subtotal resection and had remaining tumors less than 2 cm achieved a median survival of 12.4 months, compared to 9.6 months in patients with a single metastasis treated with surgical resection, and 4.5 months in patients with multiple metastases and who had more than 2 cm of residual cancer after surgery. Wronski et al. (108) reported the largest retrospective series limited to patients with brain metastases from breast cancer (n = 70) and found no statistical difference in survival between patients treated with surgical resection with single lesions and those with multiple lesions. In contrast, Hazuka et al. (109) noted that the median survival of 18 patients undergoing resection of multiple metastases was only 5 months, far shorter than that observed in 28 patients undergoing resection of a single lesion. In summary, although some of the retrospective data are encouraging, in the absence of randomized data, it is difficult to distinguish between a true effect from surgery versus selection bias; that is, patients with technically resectable lesions and who are candidates for resection may have a better prognosis irrespective of the surgical intervention received.

The potential benefits of surgical resection must be weighed against the risks. Fortunately, advances in surgical techniques, including preoperative functional MRI, intraoperative neuronavigational devices, intraoperative cortical mapping, and intravenous sedation anesthesia, have improved the safety of surgical resection of brain metastases and in some cases can allow resection of lesions located in eloquent areas (110). In a retrospective cohort study of 13,685 admissions for the resection of metastatic brain tumors from the Nationwide Inpatient Sample, the overall in-hospital mortality rate fell from 4.6% in 1988 to 1990 to 2.3% in 2000 (111). Consistent with other studies of surgical intervention, mortality and morbidity were also lower in higher-volume centers and with higher-volume surgeons.

Stereotactic Radiosurgery

SRS has come to play an increasingly important role in the management of brain metastases, in many cases offering an alternative to surgery, WBRT, or both. SRS involves the delivery of a single large dose of focused radiation to one or more tumor masses with rapid dose fall-off beyond the tumor margin (Fig. 81.1). Tumors are targeted for treatment with the aid of a minimally invasive stereotactic frame (112,113) or using x-ray image guidance together with mask immobilization (114,115). The precise dose localization and shaping afforded by this technique minimize the treatment-related morbidity that may result from normal tissue irradiation. Overall, SRS is thought to have a local control rate of approximately 85%; local control is optimal with doses greater than or equal to 1,800 cGy (116). SRS has the potential for noninvasive local tumor control, while allowing targeting of multiple lesions, and has been evaluated for its potential to supplement, replace, or defer both WBRT and surgery.

Treatment-related morbidity using SRS depends on tumor size and location, radiosurgery dose, and prior treatment. The RTOG performed an SRS dose escalation study to determine the maximum tolerated dose (MTD) in patients previously irradiated for either a primary brain tumor or a solitary metastasis (117). Dose was escalated in 3 Gy increments such that grades 3, 4, and 5 toxicity 3 months following SRS remained less than 20%. For tumors 3 to 4 cm in diameter, the MTD was 15 Gy, for those 2 to 3 cm in diameter the MTD was 18 Gy, and for those less than 2 cm the MTD was 24 Gy. On multivariate analysis, increased dose, worsening Karnofsky performance status, and increasing tumor diameter were associated with higher risk of grade 3 to 5 neurotoxicity. The actuarial incidence of radionecrosis at 12 months post-SRS was 8%, and at 24 months it was 11%.

Although surgical resection would be expected to be superior palliation for tumors with symptomatic mass effect, it is unclear if SRS is equivalent to surgery for patients with single small to medium-sized lesions without symptomatic mass effect. A 2003 retrospective series from Mayo Clinic evaluated outcomes for patients with solitary brain metastases less than 35 mm treated with either surgery or radiosurgery (118). The use of WBRT following surgery or SRS (82% in surgery arm vs. 96% in SRS arm; $p = .17$) was not significantly different between the groups. Although patients treated with either modality had similar survival, a significant improvement in local control was observed in the SRS group with no local recurrences (0/26) versus 15% (11/74) in the surgery arm. However, the overall recurrence rates including distant brain recurrence were not significantly different: 29% in the SRS arm and 30% in the surgery arm.

Although no randomized trials have been performed to directly compare surgery to SRS, several studies have evaluated whether SRS combined with WBRT results in a similar outcome to surgery and WBRT for patients with a solitary brain metastasis. To adjust for the bias of treating smaller or unresectable lesions with SRS as opposed to surgery, Auchter et al. (119) reviewed 122 patients with a surgically resectable solitary brain metastasis treated with SRS followed by WBRT. The median survival following SRS plus WBRT treatment was 1.1 years, comparing favorably to the expected survival for similar patients treated with surgery and WBRT. Of note, the overall local control rate within the SRS volume was 86% and the rate of intracranial recurrence outside the SRS volume was 22%, comparable to that observed in the first Patchell et al. (59) study.

Patients with multiple brain metastases who were treated with WBRT alone in the past, with SRS reserved for intracranial recurrence, are now more likely to receive WBRT and initial SRS based on the rationale that SRS should improve local tumor control and potentially survival. Early data to support this view came from a single institution randomized trial reported by Kondziolka et al. (120) that evaluated WBRT alone versus WBRT plus SRS for patients with two to four lesions less than 2.5 cm in size. Study accrual was terminated at 60% (27 patients) following interim evaluation that revealed a significant improvement in local control with combined treatment. Patients receiving both SRS and WBRT had a local recurrence rate at 1 year of only 8% versus 100% for those receiving WBRT alone. The median time to local recurrence was 6 months for WBRT alone and 36 months following WBRT plus SRS ($p = .005$). Despite the substantial difference in local control, no significant difference in survival between the treatment groups was found in this small study population.

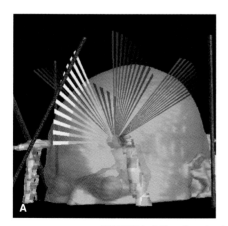 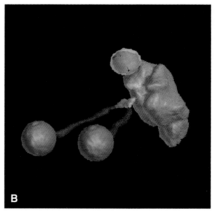 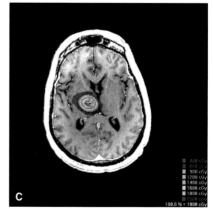

FIGURE 81.1. A: Three-dimensional rendering of patient anatomy contoured on computed tomography and magnetic resonance imaging (MRI) studies for a linear accelerator (LINAC) radiosurgery treatment. The target is shown in magenta. The convergent blue and yellow fans represent the arc sweeps used to deliver the radiation. **B:** Three-dimensional rendering of target and critical structures (optic tract and brainstem) for a LINAC radiosurgery treatment. Shown in translucent green is the three-dimensional dose envelope that tightly conforms to the target (in magenta). **C:** MRI with dose wash: Axial MRI showing contoured target volume (thick magenta line) and overlayed with the dose distribution for the radiosurgery treatment. The prescription dose of 1,800 cGy is shown in orange. (Images courtesy of Fred Hacker, PhD.)

To determine if WBRT plus SRS could also result in a survival benefit, the RTOG 95-08 trial randomized a total of 333 patients with one to three brain metastases to WBRT plus SRS or WBRT alone with the primary end point of overall survival (Table 81.1) (121). The 1-year local control was increased for the combined treatment group (82% vs. 71%; *p* = .01), a smaller improvement than that observed in the prior study reported by Kondziolka et al. (120). Although no significant difference in overall survival or cause of death was observed, several subgroups were identified that showed benefit from combined treatment. Patients with a solitary metastasis derived a survival benefit from the addition of SRS to WBRT, with a median survival of 6.9 versus 4.5 months (*p* = .04), analogous to the results observed in the first Patchell et al. (59) randomized trial comparing surgery plus WBRT with WBRT alone. In addition, patients in recursive partitioning analysis (RPA) class I (defined as Karnofsky performance status 70 or higher, age <65, controlled primary cancer, and no extracranial metastases), age less than 50, or those with squamous or non–small cell histology showed significant survival benefit from combined treatment. Patients undergoing combined treatment were more likely to have stable or improved performance status at 3 months (50% vs. 33%; *p* = .02) and 6 months (43% vs. 27%; *p* = .03). These results suggest that a survival benefit of combining WBRT plus SRS may be limited to select patients, while the probability of maintaining a stable or increased performance status may be a more general benefit of combined treatment.

The capacity of SRS to achieve local control of multiple intracranial tumors has prompted re-examination of the role of WBRT in palliative CNS radiotherapy. Does treatment with SRS allow WBRT to be deferred or eliminated in select patients? A randomized trial evaluating SRS alone versus SRS plus WBRT in patients with one to four brain metastases was reported by Aoyama et al. (122) (Table 81.1). A total of 132 patients were randomized, although it should be noted that breast cancer patients comprised only 7% of the study population. The primary end point was survival, and patients were stratified by number of metastases, extracranial disease status, and primary site. The radiosurgery dose was reduced by 30% in the combined treatment group relative to the recommendations from the RTOG 90-05 dose escalation study in order to decrease the risk of toxicity (117). There was no difference in overall survival, neurologic survival, or functional preservation between the groups. As expected, the risk of developing a new brain metastasis was higher in the SRS-alone arm versus the combined treatment arm (63.7% vs. 41.5%; *p* = .03). In addition, 12-month local control was greater for combined treatment than SRS alone (88.7% vs. 72.5%; *p* = .002). The neurocognitive function of patients in both arms were followed by Mini-Mental Status Examination (MMSE) (123). Although there was no significant difference in rate of improvement of MMSE posttreatment, among patients whose MMSE deteriorated by three points or more, the SRS-alone arm experienced a shorter time to deterioration (7.6 vs. 16.5 months; *p* = .05), likely reflecting the increased likelihood of symptomatic recurrence in the brain. Of the patients who were enrolled in the SRS-alone arm, 44% underwent salvage therapy versus 17% for the combined arm. WBRT was used for salvage in 16% of patients randomized to the SRS-alone arm. These study findings show that the use of SRS alone for patients with one to four brain metastases may not compromise survival, but it does result in increased risk of distant and local recurrence in the brain. Should SRS alone be used, clinical and radiographic follow-up every 2 to 4 months to detect brain recurrence is warranted.

The choice of deferring WBRT and treating with SRS alone must take into consideration the risk of increasing distant brain recurrence (DBR). The impact of early DBR versus the morbidity of WBRT on QOL is not well understood and must be considered

a crucial consideration in determining appropriate treatment. In a study aimed at determining the effects of DBR occurring after SRS alone, Regine et al. (124) assessed the recurrence pattern and symptomatic effects of recurrence in 36 patients treated with SRS alone. They found that 71% of patients displayed a symptomatic recurrence, of which 59% had an associated neurological deficit. Further supporting the importance of extracranial disease status, they report that the rate of symptomatic recurrence was 80% in patients with active disease in the brain only versus 35% for patients with active extracranial disease (*p* = .03). A comprehensive neurocognitive assessment of patients treated with WBRT in the phase III trial PCI-P120-9801 evaluating the radiosensitizer motexafin gadolinium revealed that patients with better than median local and distant tumor control displayed significantly improved preservation of executive and fine motor function relative to patients with less than median response to treatment (125). These results support the notion that optimizing local and distant brain tumor control is an important facet of preserving neurocognitive function.

Another clinical setting well suited for SRS is the treatment of post-WBRT intracranial recurrences. The use of WBRT retreatment, typically with total doses of 2,000 to 2,500 cGy in 200 cGy fractions, is associated with significant morbidity and a posttreatment median survival of only 3.5 to 5 months (55,126). Reirradiation of less than five brain metastases is best accomplished with SRS, which has far less toxicity than WBRT retreatment (127,128). Bhatnagar et al. (129) reported a retrospective review of 205 patients who underwent radiosurgery for treatment of four or more metastases in the initial or reirradiation setting. The median overall survival was 8 months and median time to disease progression in the brain was 9 months. Interestingly, the total volume of metastases rather than total number was predictive for survival. Recursive partitioning analysis identified a favorable subgroup consisting of 43% of patients with median survival of 13 months who had less than seven tumors and less than 7 cc of cumulative tumor volume versus 6 months median survival for the remaining patients (130). The increased use of SRS for treatment of patients with recurrent brain metastases and more than four lesions should provide further evidence to guide treatment in this challenging subgroup.

Hormonal Therapy

Many hormonal agents cross the blood–brain barrier. No prospective trials have been conducted in patients with brain metastases from breast cancer; however, several case reports describe responses in the CNS to tamoxifen and megestrol acetate (131–133). Aromatase inhibitors, which act via inhibition of peripheral conversion of androgens to estrogen, also have been reported to have anecdotal activity in the CNS (134). In animal models, fulvestrant does not appear to cross the blood–brain barrier, and no reports of CNS activity have been published to date (135).

Chemotherapy

The delivery of chemotherapeutic agents through the blood–brain barrier is limited by intrinsic drug characteristics, including molecular weight, lipid solubility, and plasma protein binding, as well as host and tumor characteristics, such as active efflux transport and interstitial fluid pressure (136). For these reasons, it has been widely postulated that the generally disappointing results of chemotherapy for brain metastases are related to inadequate penetration through the blood–brain barrier. However, in comparison to normal brain, tumor-associated vasculature is frequently disrupted with disordered, highly tortuous, and more permeable vessels (67). The leakage of water-soluble contrast agents through the blood–tumor barrier and the reported responses in the literature to a variety of chemotherapeutic agents too large or hydrophilic to cross the intact blood–brain barrier support the concept that a key principle in choosing systemic therapy is to prioritize agents with activity against breast cancer. In practice, this principle can be challenging to fulfill, as patients in the modern era are often already heavily pretreated by the time systemic therapy is being considered for the treatment of progressive CNS disease.

To date, no chemotherapeutic agents have gained FDA approval for the treatment of brain metastases from breast cancer. Data are available from case reports, case series, and small prospective trials. Rosner et al. (137) treated 100 consecutive patients with brain metastases from breast cancer with several regimens, which included cyclophosphamide, 5-fluorouracil, and prednisone. The objective response was 50%, with a median duration of response of 7 months. Of note, because of the time period during which patients were treated, just over half of the patients were evaluated by CT and the remainder were evaluated with a radionuclide brain scan only. Additionally, patients were relatively untreated compared to the current era: only 7% of patients had received adjuvant chemotherapy and just under half had received any prior chemotherapy for metastatic disease.

Boogerd et al. (138) treated 22 patients with either CMF (cyclophosphamide, methotrexate, and 5-fluorouracil) or CAF (cyclophosphamide, doxorubicin, and 5-fluorouracil). Seven patients had progressive disease after WBRT. The objective response rate by imaging criteria was 54%. When compared to a matched group of historical controls treated with WBRT, median survival was longer (25 vs. 10 weeks). However, the radiotherapy group was treated between 1980 to 1987, whereas the chemotherapy group was treated between 1987 to 1990. In addition, the radiotherapy group did worse than would have been expected based on other series from that time period. Therefore, no definitive conclusions can be drawn with respect to the comparison of WBRT and chemotherapy.

The efficacy of temozolomide for brain metastases has been evaluated in multiple phase II studies including a broad range of solid tumors. The published studies have indicated only minimal activity against breast cancer (139–142). Several reports presented in abstract form indicate a potentially higher level of activity (143). However, unless these reports are confirmed, temozolomide at the current dosing schedule is not likely to have a major role as a single agent in the treatment of brain metastases from breast cancer.

In contrast, several case reports and a single prospective study support a potential role for capecitabine in this setting (144–146). Rivera et al. (146) evaluated the maximally tolerated dose of capecitabine in combination with temozolomide in a phase I study of patients with brain metastases from breast cancer. Of 22 patients evaluable for response, 4 achieved a complete or partial response in the CNS.

Other chemotherapeutic agents that have been examined in prospective trials include cisplatin and topotecan. A detailed discussion of investigational methods to enhance delivery of agents to the CNS is outside the scope of this chapter, but approaches being studied include convection-enhanced delivery, targeted ultrasound blood–brain barrier disruption, and global osmotic blood–brain barrier disruption (136).

Overall, the paucity of prospective studies evaluating systemic therapy for CNS disease makes any definitive recommendations difficult. It would seem reasonable to base the choice of chemotherapy on a patient's prior therapy for breast cancer, with priority given to drugs that have had some reported activity in the CNS.

Targeted Therapy

A growing number of targeted agents have entered clinical development in breast cancer, including those inhibiting the HER2, Ras/Raf, PI3 kinase, and angiogenesis pathways. However, with few exceptions, the initial clinical trials have excluded patients with active brain metastases.

Two prospective, phase II studies have evaluated the safety and efficacy of lapatinib, a dual inhibitor of epidermal growth factor receptor (EGFR) and HER2, in patients with HER2-positive breast cancer and progressive brain metastases. In the first study (n = 39), one patient achieved an objective response in the CNS by predefined modified Response Evaluation Criteria in Solid Tumors (RECIST) criteria (147). In the second study (n = 242), 6% of patients achieved an objective response by composite criteria, including 50% or more reduction of CNS tumor volume (148). Patients who had progressed on this study were given the option of participating in an extension phase in which capecitabine was added to lapatinib. Of 50 evaluable patients, 10 (20%) achieved an objective response in the CNS (149). Of interest, in a phase III trial comparing capecitabine alone versus capecitabine plus lapatinib in patients with progressive extracranial disease, a trend toward fewer CNS relapses was observed in the combination arm (6% vs. 2%; $p = .045$) (150). Together, these results indicate a potential role for lapatinib or other small molecule HER2 inhibitors in the treatment or prevention of brain metastases from HER2-positive breast cancer. Further studies are ongoing.

Angiogenesis inhibitors represent another potentially promising avenue for investigation. In preclinical models, breast cancer cell lines selected for brain metastasis potential were found to release significantly more vascular endothelial growth factor A (VEGF-A) and were associated with increased vessel density (151). Furthermore, administration of a VEGF receptor TKI led to a decrease in brain tumor burden. Vredenburgh et al. (152) conducted a phase II trial of bevacizumab plus irinotecan in 35 patients with recurrent glioblastoma. In this study, the 6-month progression-free survival was 46%, higher than would have been expected based on historical controls, and 57% of patients achieved an objective response. CNS hemorrhage was observed in only one patient. Other angiogenesis inhibitors are under investigation in glioblastoma, including AZD2171, a pan-VEGF receptor TKI that appears to normalize tumor vasculature and reduce peritumoral edema (153). Because of the concern for intracranial hemorrhage, patients with brain metastases have been excluded from nearly all trials of angiogenesis inhibitors. However, data from the glioblastoma studies support the exploration of angiogenesis inhibitors in patients with brain metastases in the context of clinical trials.

Radiosensitizers

Another approach to maximize the efficacy of radiation is the use of systemic agents such as radiosensitizers (Table 81.1). In order to investigate the combination of antiangiogenic therapies with radiotherapy, the RTOG conducted a phase III study of WBRT with or without thalidomide for patients with brain metastases from solid tumors. The study was closed early after an interim analysis indicated a very low likelihood of demonstrating a survival advantage in the experimental arm (154). Mehta et al. (155) randomly assigned 401 patients (75 with breast cancer) to WBRT (3000 cGy) with or without motexafin gadolinium, a redox active drug that is thought to generate reactive oxygen species via futile redox cycling. No difference in overall survival or time to neurologic progression was noted in the overall study population. Finally, Suh et al. (156) conducted a similar phase III trial utilizing efaproxiral (RSR13), an allosteric modifier of hemoglobin. Efaproxiral shifts the hemoglobin–oxygen dissociation curve, thereby leading to release of oxygen into the bloodstream and improved tissue oxygenation. In the overall study population (n = 515), there was no difference in survival, the primary end point. Exploratory subset analysis of 115 patients with breast cancer suggested a possible benefit in this subgroup (median survival 8.7 vs. 4.6 months) (157). A confirmatory phase III study has completed accrual and results are pending.

Other agents under investigation include temozolomide and lapatinib. In a randomized, phase II trial (n = 48; five with breast cancer), the addition of temozolomide was associated with a higher objective response rate than WBRT alone (158). Studies limited to breast cancer patients have not been reported. A phase I study of WBRT with lapatinib in patients with HER2-positive breast cancer is ongoing, but neither safety nor efficacy data are yet available.

CONCLUSIONS AND FUTURE DIRECTIONS

Brain metastases may lead to significant morbidity in patients with advanced cancer, and it is a particularly feared site of recurrence by patients. HER2-positive and ER-negative tumors appear to be especially likely to spread to the CNS. Advances in surgery and radiotherapy have reduced treatment-related morbidity and allow for treatment of lesions that may have previously been considered unamenable to treatment. However, as patients live longer with metastatic breast cancer, it is likely that an increasing number of patients will develop CNS progression after standard first-line therapies. Thus, the optimal management of patients will increasingly require close, multidisciplinary collaborations. Furthermore, there is a greater need than ever to evaluate novel approaches to CNS metastases in the context of well-designed clinical trials.

MANAGEMENT SUMMARY

- In a breast cancer patient with signs or symptoms of brain metastases, a prompt contrast-enhanced MRI is indicated.
- Twenty percent of patients with brain metastases develop VTE disease. In patients with clinically significant VTE disease, anticoagulation is indicated.
- Initial treatment of brain metastases is influenced by lesion number, location, size, and upon the status of a patient's systemic disease.
- Supportive therapy includes corticosteroids for patients with symptomatic edema and anticonvulsants for patients with a history of seizures. In patients without a seizure history, the routine use of prophylactic anticonvulsants is not recommended. Prophylaxis for *Pneumocystis jiroveci* pneumonia should be considered for patients for whom the anticipated duration of steroid use exceeds 4 to 5 weeks.
- In patients with single or solitary brain lesions, good performance status, and stable extracranial disease, surgical resection or SRS is recommended. Surgery is preferred for lesions with symptomatic mass effect, larger lesions, and when the risk of operative morbidity is acceptably low. WBRT after local therapy reduces the risk of intracranial recurrence but does not appear to affect overall survival.
- For patients with a limited number of lesions, good performance status, and favorable extracranial disease status, consideration should be given to aggressive intracranial therapy, with either WBRT followed by SRS, or SRS alone. Initial WBRT reduces the risk of subsequent intracranial recurrence and improves local tumor control in the brain but does not appear to prolong survival. The potential long-term neurotoxicities associated with WBRT must be weighed against the cognitive impairment associated with progressive disease in the CNS. Consideration

should also be given to participation in a clinical trial evaluating the use of radiosensitizers given in conjunction with WBRT

- For patients with suboptimal control of extracranial disease, poor performance status, and short expected survival, therapy should be directed toward optimal palliation, such as a course of WBRT alone and consideration of hospice referral.
- For patients with recurrent or new CNS lesions after WBRT, the standard of care is not well defined. Because of the complexity of potential options, including SRS, surgical resection, systemic therapy, or WBRT retreatment, multidisciplinary management is appropriate, particularly in patients with favorable extracranial disease status. Consideration should also be given to participation in the increasing number of clinical trials targeted to this patient population.

References

1. Giordano SH, Buzdar AU, Smith TL, et al.. Is breast cancer survival improving? *Cancer* 2004;100(1):44–52.
2. Bendell JC, Domchek SM, Burstein HJ, et al. Central nervous system metastases in women who receive trastuzumab-based therapy for metastatic breast carcinoma. *Cancer* 2003;97(12):2972–2977.
3. Lin NU, Winer EP. Brain metastases: the HER2 paradigm. *Clin Cancer Res* 2007;13(6):1648–1655.
4. Barnholtz-Sloan JS, Sloan AE, Davis FG, et al. Incidence proportions of brain metastases in patients diagnosed (1973 to 2001) in the Metropolitan Detroit Cancer Surveillance System. *J Clin Oncol* 2004;22(14):2865–2672.
5. Schouten LJ, Rutten J, Huveneers HA, et al. Incidence of brain metastases in a cohort of patients with carcinoma of the breast, colon, kidney, and lung and melanoma. *Cancer* 2002;94(10):2698–2705.
6. Zimm S, Wampler GL, Stablein D, et al. Intracerebral metastases in solid-tumor patients: natural history and results of treatment. *Cancer* 1981;48(2):384–394.
7. Nussbaum ES, Djalilian HR, Cho KH, et al. Brain metastases. Histology, multiplicity, surgery, and survival. *Cancer* 1996;78(8):1781–1788.
8. Romond EH, Perez EA, Bryant J, et al. Trastuzumab plus adjuvant chemotherapy for operable HER2-positive breast cancer. *N Engl J Med* 2005;353(16):1673–1684.
9. Smith I, Procter M, Gelber RD, et al. 2-year follow-up of trastuzumab after adjuvant chemotherapy in HER2-positive breast cancer: a randomised controlled trial. *Lancet* 2007;369(9555):29–36.
10. Gonzalez-Angulo AM, Cristofanilli M, Strom EA, et al. Central nervous system metastases in patients with high-risk breast carcinoma after multimodality treatment. *Cancer* 2004;101(8):1760–1766.
11. Tsukada Y, Fouad A, Pickren JW, et al. Central nervous system metastasis from breast carcinoma. Autopsy study. *Cancer* 1983;52(12):2349–2354.
12. Patanaphan V, Salazar OM, Risco R. Breast cancer: metastatic patterns and their prognosis. *South Med J* 1988;81(9):1109–1112.
13. Miller KD, Weathers T, Haney LG, et al. Occult central nervous system involvement in patients with metastatic breast cancer: prevalence, predictive factors and impact on overall survival. *Ann Oncol* 2003;14(7):1072–1077.
14. Posner JB, Chernik NL. Intracranial metastases from systemic cancer. *Adv Neurol* 1978;19:579–592.
15. Evans AJ, James JJ, Cornford EJ, et al. Brain metastases from breast cancer: identification of a high-risk group. *Clin Oncol (R Coll Radiol)* 2004;16(5):345–349.
16. Love RR, Duc NB, Dinh NV, et al. Young age as an adverse prognostic factor in premenopausal women with operable breast cancer. *Clin Breast Cancer* 2002;2(4):294–298.
17. Clark GM, Osborne CK, McGuire WL. Correlations between estrogen receptor, progesterone receptor, and patient characteristics in human breast cancer. *J Clin Oncol* 1984;2(10):1102–1109.
18. Carey LA, Perou CM, Livasy CA, et al. Race, breast cancer subtypes, and survival in the Carolina Breast Cancer Study. *JAMA* 2006;295(21):2492–2502.
19. Slimane K, Andre F, Delaloge S, et al. Risk factors for brain relapse in patients with metastatic breast cancer. *Ann Oncol* 2004;15(11):1640–1644.
20. Sanna G, Franceschelli L, Rotmensz N, et al. Brain metastases in patients with advanced breast cancer. *Anticancer Res* 2007;27(4C):2865–2869.
21. Tham YL, Sexton K, Kramer R, et al. Primary breast cancer phenotypes associated with propensity for central nervous system metastases. *Cancer* 2006;107(4):696–704.
22. Gabos Z, Sinha R, Hanson J, et al. Prognostic significance of human epidermal growth factor receptor positivity for the development of brain metastasis after newly diagnosed breast cancer. *J Clin Oncol* 2006;24(36):5658–5663.
23. Pestalozzi BC, Zahrieh D, Price KN, et al. Identifying breast cancer patients at risk for central nervous system (CNS) metastases in trials of the International Breast Cancer Study Group (IBCSG). *Ann Oncol* 2006;17(6):935–944.
24. Lin NU, Bellon JR, Winer EP. CNS metastases in breast cancer. *J Clin Oncol* 2004;22(17):3608–3617.
25. Stemmler HJ, Kahlert S, Siekiera W, et al. Characteristics of patients with brain metastases receiving trastuzumab for HER2 overexpressing metastatic breast cancer. *Breast* 2006;15(2):219–225.
26. Gori S, Rimondini S, De Angelis V, et al. Central nervous system metastases in HER-2 positive metastatic breast cancer patients treated with trastuzumab: incidence, survival, and risk factors. *Oncologist* 2007;12(7):766–773.
27. Altaha R, Crowell E, Ducatman B, et al. Risk of brain metastases in HER2/neu-positive breast cancer. *J Clin Oncol* 2004;22(14S):47s.

28. Clayton AJ, Danson S, Jolly S, et al. Incidence of cerebral metastases in patients treated with trastuzumab for metastatic breast cancer. *Br J Cancer* 2004; 91(4):639–643.

29. Yau T, Swanton C, Chua S, et al. Incidence, pattern and timing of brain metastases among patients with advanced breast cancer treated with trastuzumab. *Acta Oncol* 2006;45(2):196–201.

30. Pestalozzi BC, Brignoli S. Trastuzumab in CSF. *J Clin Oncol* 2000;18(11): 2349–2351.

31. Stemmler J, Schmitt M, Willems A, et al. Brain metastases in HER2-overexpressing metastatic breast cancer: comparative analysis of trastuzumab levels in serum and cerebrospinal fluid. *J Clin Oncol* 2006;24(18S):(abst 1525).

32. Palmieri D, Bronder JL, Herring JM, et al. Her-2 overexpression increases the metastatic outgrowth of breast cancer cells in the brain. *Cancer Res* 2007; 67(9):4190–4198.

33. Kallioniemi OP, Holli K, Visakorpi T, et al. Association of c-erbB-2 protein overexpression with high rate of cell proliferation, increased risk of visceral metastasis and poor long-term survival in breast cancer. *Int J Cancer* 1991;49(5):650–655.

34. Tsuda H, Takarabe T, Hasegawa F, et al. Large, central acellular zones indicating myoepithelial tumor differentiation in high-grade invasive ductal carcinomas as markers of predisposition to lung and brain metastases. *Am J Surg Pathol* 2000;24(2):197–202.

35. Albiges L, Andre F, Balleyguier C, et al. Spectrum of breast cancer metastasis in BRCA1 mutation carriers: highly increased incidence of brain metastases. *Ann Oncol* 2005;16(11):1846–1847.

36. Foulkes WD, Stefansson IM, Chappuis PO, et al. Germline BRCA1 mutations and a basal epithelial phenotype in breast cancer. *J Natl Cancer Inst* 2003;95(19): 1482–1485.

37. Luck AA, Evans AJ, Green AR, et al. The influence of basal phenotype on the metastatic pattern of breast cancer. *Clin Oncol (R Coll Radiol)* 2008;20(1):40–45.

38. Fulford LG, Reis-Filho JS, Ryder K, et al. Basal-like grade III invasive ductal carcinoma of the breast: patterns of metastasis and long-term survival. *Breast Cancer Res* 2007;9(1):R4.

39. Delattre JY, Krol G, Thaler HT, et al. Distribution of brain metastases. *Arch Neurol* 1988;45(7):741–744.

40. Cairncross J, Posner J. The management of brain metastases. In: Walker M, ed. *Oncology of the nervous system.* Boston: Nijhoff, 1983:341.

41. Hwang TL, Close TP, Grego JM, et al. Predilection of brain metastasis in gray and white matter junction and vascular border zones. *Cancer* 1996;77(8):1551–1555.

42. Sze G, Milano E, Johnson C, et al. Detection of brain metastases: comparison of contrast-enhanced MR with unenhanced MR and enhanced CT. *AJNR Am J Neuroradiol* 1990;11(4):785–791.

43. Akeson P, Larsson EM, Kristoffersen DT, et al. Brain metastases—comparison of gadodiamide injection-enhanced MR imaging at standard and high dose, contrast-enhanced CT and non-contrast-enhanced MR imaging. *Acta Radiol* 1995;36 (3):300–306.

44. Schellinger PD, Meinck HM, Thron A. Diagnostic accuracy of MRI compared to CCT in patients with brain metastases. *J Neurooncol* 1999;44(3):275–281.

45. Pelletier EM, Shim B, Goodman S, et al. Epidemiology and economic burden of brain metastases among patients with primary breast cancer: results from a US claims data analysis. *Breast Cancer Res Treat* 2007;108(2)297–305.

46. Forsyth PA, Posner JB. Headaches in patients with brain tumors: a study of 111 patients. *Neurology* 1993;43(9):1678–1683.

47. Argyriou AA, Chroni E, Polychronopoulos P, et al. Headache characteristics and brain metastases prediction in cancer patients. *Eur J Cancer Care (Engl)* 2006;15(1):90–95.

48. Christiaans MH, Kelder JC, Arnoldus EP, et al. Prediction of intracranial metastases in cancer patients with headache. *Cancer* 2002;94(7):2063–2068.

49. Wen PY, Black PM, Loeffler JS. Treatment of metastatic breast cancer: metastatic brain cancer. In: DeVita VT, Hellman S, Rosenberg SA, eds. *Cancer: principles and practice of oncology.* 6th ed. Philadelphia: Lippincott William & Wilkins, 2001:2655–2670.

50. Jeyapalan SA, Batchelor TT. Diagnostic evaluation of neurologic metastases. *Cancer Invest* 2000;18(4):381–394.

51. Tuma R, DeAngelis LM. Altered mental status in patients with cancer. *Arch Neurol* 2000;57(12):1727–1731.

52. Cohen N, Strauss G, Lew R, et al. Should prophylactic anticonvulsants be administered to patients with newly-diagnosed cerebral metastases? A retrospective analysis. *J Clin Oncol* 1988;6(10):1621–1624.

53. Glantz MJ, Cole BF, Friedberg MH, et al. A randomized, blinded, placebo-controlled trial of divalproex sodium prophylaxis in adults with newly diagnosed brain tumors. *Neurology* 1996;46(4):985–991.

54. Forsyth PA, Weaver S, Fulton D, et al. Prophylactic anticonvulsants in patients with brain tumour. *Can J Neurol Sci* 2003;30(2):106–112.

55. Coia LR. The role of radiation therapy in the treatment of brain metastases. *Int J Radiat Oncol Biol Phys* 1992;23(1):229–238.

56. Mandybur TI. Intracranial hemorrhage caused by metastatic tumors. *Neurology* 1977;27(7):650–655.

57. Davis PC, Hudgins PA, Peterman SB, et al. Diagnosis of cerebral metastases: double-dose delayed CT vs contrast-enhanced MR imaging. *AJNR Am J Neuroradiol* 1991;12(2):293–300.

58. Sze G, Shin J, Krol G, et al. Intraparenchymal brain metastases: MR imaging versus contrast-enhanced CT. *Radiology* 1988;168(1):187–194.

59. Patchell RA, Tibbs PA, Walsh JW, et al. A randomized trial of surgery in the treatment of single metastases to the brain. *N Engl J Med* 1990;322(8):494–500.

60. Custer BS, Koepsell TD, Mueller BA. The association between breast carcinoma and meningioma in women. *Cancer* 2002;94(6):1626–1635.

61. Herholz K, Coope D, Jackson A. Metabolic and molecular imaging in neurooncology. *Lancet Neurol* 2007;6(8):711–724.

62. Rohren EM, Provenzale JM, Barboriak DP, et al. Screening for cerebral metastases with FDG PET in patients undergoing whole-body staging of non-central nervous system malignancy. *Radiology* 2003;226(1):181–187.

63. Griffeth LK, Rich KM, Dehdashti F, et al. Brain metastases from non-central nervous system tumors: evaluation with PET. *Radiology* 1993;186(1):37–44.

64. Chao ST, Barnett GH, Liu SW, et al. Five-year survivors of brain metastases: a single-institution report of 32 patients. *Int J Radiat Oncol Biol Phys* 2006;66(3):801–809.

65. Ross DA, Sandler HM, Balter JM, et al. Imaging changes after stereotactic radiosurgery of primary and secondary malignant brain tumors. *J Neurooncol* 2002;56 (2):175–181.

66. Serizawa T, Saeki N, Higuchi Y, et al. Diagnostic value of thallium-201 chloride single-photon emission computerized tomography in differentiating tumor recurrence from radiation injury after gamma knife surgery for metastatic brain tumors. *J Neurosurg* 2005;102[Suppl]:266–271.

67. Bullitt E, Lin NU, Smith JK, et al. Blood vessel morphologic changes depicted with MR angiography during treatment of brain metastases: a feasibility study. *Radiology* 2007;245(3):824–830.

68. DiStefano A, Yong Yap Y, Hortobagyi GN, et al. The natural history of breast cancer patients with brain metastases. *Cancer* 1979;44(5):1913–1918.

69. Mahmoud-Ahmed AS, Suh JH, Lee SY, et al. Results of whole brain radiotherapy in patients with brain metastases from breast cancer: a retrospective study. *Int J Radiat Oncol Biol Phys* 2002;54(3):810–817.

70. Altundag K, Bondy ML, Kau SW, et al. Clinicopathologic characteristics and prognostic factors in 420 metastatic breast cancer patients with central nervous system metastases. *Breast Cancer Res Treat* 2005;94[Suppl 1]:(abst 3056).

71. Melisko ME, Chew K, Baehner F, et al. Clinical characteristics and molecular markers predicting the development and outcome of breast cancer brain metastases. *Breast Cancer Res Treat* 2005;94[Suppl 1]:S55.

72. Kirsch DG, Ledezma CJ, Mathews CS, et al. Survival after brain metastases from breast cancer in the trastuzumab era. *J Clin Oncol* 2005;23(9):2114–2146.

73. Galicich J, French L, Melby J. Use of dexamethasone in the treatment of cerebral edema associated with brain tumors. *Lancet* 1961;81:46–53.

74. Hedley-Whyte ET, Hsu DW. Effect of dexamethasone on blood-brain barrier in the normal mouse. *Ann Neurol* 1986;19(4):373–377.

75. Ostergaard L, Hochberg FH, Rabinov JD, et al. Early changes measured by magnetic resonance imaging in cerebral blood flow, blood volume, and blood–brain barrier permeability following dexamethasone treatment in patients with brain tumors. *J Neurosurg* 1999;90(2):300–305.

76. Vecht CJ, Verbiest HB. Use of glucocorticoids in neuro-oncology. In: Wiley R, ed. *Neurological complications of cancer.* New York: Marcel Dekker, 1995:199.

77. Henson JW, Jalaj JK, Walker RW, et al. Pneumocystis carinii pneumonia in patients with primary brain tumors. *Arch Neurol* 1991;48(4):406–409.

78. Schiff D. Pneumocystis pneumonia in brain tumor patients: risk factors and clinical features. *J Neurooncol* 1996;27(3):235–240.

79. Micali G, Linthicum K, Han N, et al. Increased risk of erythema multiforme major with combination anticonvulsant and radiation therapies. *Pharmacotherapy* 1999;19(2):223–227.

80. Glantz MJ, Cole BF, Forsyth PA, et al. Practice parameter: anticonvulsant prophylaxis in patients with newly diagnosed brain tumors. Report of the Quality Standards Subcommittee of the American Academy of Neurology. *Neurology* 2000;54(10):1886–1893.

81. Anderson GD. Pharmacogenetics and enzyme induction/inhibition properties of antiepileptic drugs. *Neurology* 2004;63[10 Suppl 4]:S3–S8.

82. Sawaya R, Zuccarello M, Elkalliny M, et al. Postoperative venous thromboembolism and brain tumors: part I. Clinical profile. *J Neurooncol* 1992;14(2):119–125.

83. Levin JM, Schiff D, Loeffler JS, et al. Complications of therapy for venous thromboembolic disease in patients with brain tumors. *Neurology* 1993;43(6): 1111–1114.

84. Schiff D, DeAngelis LM. Therapy of venous thromboembolism in patients with brain metastases. *Cancer* 1994;73(2):493–498.

85. Chao J, Phillips R, Nickson J. Roentgen ray therapy of cerebral metastases. *Cancer* 1954;7:682–689.

86. Nieder C, Berberich W, Schnabel K. Tumor-related prognostic factors for remission of brain metastases after radiotherapy. *Int J Radiat Oncol Biol Phys* 1997;39(1):25–30.

87. Borgelt B, Gelber R, Kramer S, et al. The palliation of brain metastases: final results of the first two studies by the Radiation Therapy Oncology Group. *Int J Radiat Oncol Biol Phys* 1980;6(1):1–9.

88. Coia LR, Aaronson N, Linggood R, et al. A report of the consensus workshop panel on the treatment of brain metastases. *Int J Radiat Oncol Biol Phys* 1992;23 (1):223–227.

89. Cairncross JG, Kim JH, Posner JB. Radiation therapy for brain metastases. *Ann Neurol* 1980;7(6):529–541.

90. Gelber RD, Larson M, Borgelt BB, et al. Equivalence of radiation schedules for the palliative treatment of brain metastases in patients with favorable prognosis. *Cancer* 1981;48(8):1749–1753.

91. Borgelt B, Gelber R, Larson M, et al. Ultra-rapid high dose irradiation schedules for the palliation of brain metastases: final results of the first two studies by the Radiation Therapy Oncology Group. *Int J Radiat Oncol Biol Phys* 1981;7(12): 1633–1638.

92. DeAngelis LM, Delattre JY, Posner JB. Radiation-induced dementia in patients cured of brain metastases. *Neurology* 1989;39(6):789–796.

93. Murray KJ, Scott C, Greenberg HM, et al. A randomized phase III study of accelerated hyperfractionation versus standard in patients with unresected brain metastases: a report of the Radiation Therapy Oncology Group (RTOG) 9104. *Int J Radiat Oncol Biol Phys* 1997;39(3):571–574.

94. Tsao MN, Lloyd N, Wong R, et al. Whole brain radiotherapy for the treatment of multiple brain metastases. *Cochrane Database Syst Rev* 2006;3:CD003869.

95. Schultheiss TE, Kun LE, Ang KK, et al. Radiation response of the central nervous system. *Int J Radiat Oncol Biol Phys* 1995;31(5):1093–1112.

96. Sheline GE, Wara WM, Smith V. Therapeutic irradiation and brain injury. *Int J Radiat Oncol Biol Phys* 1980;6(9):1215–1228.

97. Cross NE, Glantz MJ. Neurologic complications of radiation therapy. *Neurol Clin* 2003;21(1):249–277.

98. Crossen JR, Garwood D, Glatstein E, et al. Neurobehavioral sequelae of cranial irradiation in adults: a review of radiation-induced encephalopathy. *J Clin Oncol* 1994;12(3):627–642.

99. Murphy CB, Hashimoto SA, Graeb D, et al. Clinical exacerbation of multiple sclerosis following radiotherapy. *Arch Neurol* 2003;60(2):273–275.

100. Patchell RA, Tibbs PA, Regine WF, et al. Postoperative radiotherapy in the treatment of single metastases to the brain: a randomized trial. *JAMA* 1998;280(17):1485–1489.

101. Soltys SG, Adler JR, Lipani JD, et al. Stereotactic radiosurgery of the postoperative resection cavity for brain metastases. *Int J Radiat Oncol Biol Phys* 2008; 70(1):187–193.

102. Ghia A, Tome WA, Thomas S, et al. Distribution of brain metastases in relation to the hippocampus: implications for neurocognitive functional preservation. *Int J Radiat Oncol Biol Phys* 2007;68(4):971–977.

103. Noordijk EM, Vecht CJ, Haaxma-Reiche H, et al. The choice of treatment of single brain metastasis should be based on extracranial tumor activity and age. *Int J Radiat Oncol Biol Phys* 1994;29(4):711–717.

104. Mintz AH, Kestle J, Rathbone MP, et al. A randomized trial to assess the efficacy of surgery in addition to radiotherapy in patients with a single cerebral metastasis. *Cancer* 1996;78(7):1470–1476.

105. Lagerwaard FJ, Levendag PC, Nowak PJ, et al. Identification of prognostic factors in patients with brain metastases: a review of 1,292 patients. *Int J Radiat Oncol Biol Phys* 1999;43(4):795–803.

106. Bindal RK, Sawaya R, Leavens ME, et al. Surgical treatment of multiple brain metastasis. *J Neurosurg* 1993;79(2):210–216.

107. Iwadate Y, Namba H, Yamaura A. Significance of surgical resection for the treatment of multiple brain metastases. *Anticancer Res* 2000;20(1B):573–577.

108. Wronski M, Arbit E, McCormick B. Surgical treatment of 70 patients with brain metastases from breast carcinoma. *Cancer* 1997;80(9):1746–1754.

109. Hazuka MB, Burleson WD, Stroud DN, et al. Multiple brain metastases are associated with poor survival in patients treated with surgery and radiotherapy. *J Clin Oncol* 1993;11(2):369–373.

110. Black PM, Johnson MD. Surgical resection for patients with solid brain metastases: current status. *J Neurooncol* 2004;69(1–3):119–124.

111. Barker FG 2nd. Craniotomy for the resection of metastatic brain tumors in the U.S., 1988–2000: decreasing mortality and the effect of provider caseload. *Cancer* 2004;100(5):999–1007.

112. Tsai JS, Buck BA, Svensson GK, et al. Quality assurance in stereotactic radiosurgery using a standard linear accelerator. *Int J Radiat Oncol Biol Phys* 1991;21(3):737–748.

113. Leksell L. The stereotaxic method and radiosurgery of the brain. *Acta Chir Scand* 1951;102(4):316–319.

114. Verellen D, Soete G, Linthout N, et al. Quality assurance of a system for improved target localization and patient set-up that combines real-time infrared tracking and stereoscopic x-ray imaging. *Radiother Oncol* 2003;67(1):129–141.

115. Adler JR Jr, Chang SD, Murphy MJ, et al. The CyberKnife: a frameless robotic system for radiosurgery. *Stereotact Funct Neurosurg* 1997;69(1–4, Pt 2):124–128.

116. Boyd TS, Mehta MP. Radiosurgery for brain metastases. *Neurosurg Clin North Am* 1999;10(2):337–350.

117. Shaw E, Scott C, Souhami L, et al. Single dose radiosurgical treatment of recurrent previously irradiated primary brain tumors and brain metastases: final report of RTOG protocol 90-05. *Int J Radiat Oncol Biol Phys* 2000;47(2):291–298.

118. O'Neill BP, Iturria NJ, Link MJ, et al. A comparison of surgical resection and stereotactic radiosurgery in the treatment of solitary brain metastases. *Int J Radiat Oncol Biol Phys* 2003;55(5):1169–1176.

119. Auchter RM, Lamond JP, Alexander E, et al. A multi-institutional outcome and prognostic factor analysis of radiosurgery for resectable single brain metastasis. *Int J Radiat Oncol Biol Phys* 1996;35(1):27–35.

120. Kondziolka D, Patel A, Lunsford LD, et al. Stereotactic radiosurgery plus whole brain radiotherapy versus radiotherapy alone for patients with multiple brain metastases. *Int J Radiat Oncol Biol Phys* 1999;45(2):427–434.

121. Andrews DW, Scott CB, Sperduto PW, et al. Whole brain radiation therapy with or without stereotactic radiosurgery boost for patients with one to three brain metastases: phase III results of the RTOG 9508 randomised trial. *Lancet* 2004;363(9422):1665–1672.

122. Aoyama H, Shirato H, Tago M, et al. Stereotactic radiosurgery plus whole-brain radiation therapy vs stereotactic radiosurgery alone for treatment of brain metastases: a randomized controlled trial. *JAMA* 2006;295(21):2483–2491.

123. Aoyama H, Tago M, Kato N, et al. Neurocognitive function of patients with brain metastasis who received either whole brain radiotherapy plus stereotactic radiosurgery or radiosurgery alone. *Int J Radiat Oncol Biol Phys* 2007;68(5):1388–1395.

124. Regine WF, Huhn JL, Patchell RA, et al. Risk of symptomatic brain tumor recurrence and neurologic deficit after radiosurgery alone in patients with newly diagnosed brain metastases: results and implications. *Int J Radiat Oncol Biol Phys* 2002;52(2):333–338.

125. Li J, Bentzen SM, Renschler M, et al. Regression after whole-brain radiation therapy for brain metastases correlates with survival and improved neurocognitive function. *J Clin Oncol* 2007;25(10):1260–1266.

126. Cooper JS, Steinfeld AD, Lerch IA. Cerebral metastases: value of reirradiation in selected patients. *Radiology* 1990;174(3, Pt 1):883–885.

127. Noel G, Proudhom MA, Valery CA, et al. Radiosurgery for re-irradiation of brain metastasis: results in 54 patients. *Radiother Oncol* 2001;60(1):61–67.

128. Alexander E 3rd, Moriarty TM, Davis RB, et al. Stereotactic radiosurgery for the definitive, noninvasive treatment of brain metastases. *J Natl Cancer Inst* 1995;87(1):34–40.

129. Bhatnagar AK, Flickinger JC, Kondziolka D, et al. Stereotactic radiosurgery for four or more intracranial metastases. *Int J Radiat Oncol Biol Phys* 2006;64(3):898–903.

130. Bhatnagar AK, Kondziolka D, Lunsford LD, et al. Recursive partitioning analysis of prognostic factors for patients with four or more intracranial metastases treated with radiosurgery. *Technol Cancer Res Treat* 2007;6(3):153–160.

131. Lien EA, Wester K, Lonning PE, et al. Distribution of tamoxifen and metabolites into brain tissue and brain metastases in breast cancer patients. *Br J Cancer* 1991;63(4):641–645.

132. Salvati M, Cervoni L, Innocenzi G, et al. Prolonged stabilization of multiple and single brain metastases from breast cancer with tamoxifen. Report of three cases. *Tumori* 1993;79(5):359–362.

133. Stewart DJ, Dahrouge S. Response of brain metastases from breast cancer to megestrol acetate: a case report. *J Neurooncol* 1995;24(3):299–301.

134. Madhup R, Kirti S, Bhatt ML, et al. Letrozole for brain and scalp metastases from breast cancer—a case report. *Breast* 2006;15(3):440–442.

135. Howell A, Osborne CK, Morris C, et al. ICI 182,780 (Faslodex): development of a novel, "pure" antiestrogen. *Cancer* 2000;89(4):817–825.

136. Muldoon LL, Soussain C, Jahnke K, et al. Chemotherapy delivery issues in central nervous system malignancy: a reality check. *J Clin Oncol* 2007;25(16):2295–2305.

137. Rosner D, Nemoto T, Lane WW. Chemotherapy induces regression of brain metastases in breast carcinoma. *Cancer* 1986;58(4):832–839.

138. Boogerd W, Dalesio O, Bais EM, et al. Response of brain metastases from breast cancer to systemic chemotherapy. *Cancer* 1992;69(4):972–980.

139. Christodoulou C, Bafaloukos D, Kosmidis P, et al. Phase II study of temozolomide in heavily pretreated cancer patients with brain metastases. *Ann Oncol* 2001;12(2):249–254.

140. Abrey LE, Olson JD, Raizer JJ, et al. A phase II trial of temozolomide for patients with recurrent or progressive brain metastases. *J Neurooncol* 2001;53(3):259–265.

141. Trudeau ME, Crump M, Charpentier D, et al. Temozolomide in metastatic breast cancer (MBC): a phase II trial of the National Cancer Institute of Canada–Clinical Trials Group (NCIC-CTG). *Ann Oncol* 2006;17(6):952–956.

142. Friedman HS, Evans B, Reardon D, et al. Phase II trial of temozolomide for patients with progressive brain metastases. *Proc Am Soc Clin Oncol* 2003;22:102(abst 408).

143. Siena S, Landonio G, Beaietta E, et al. Multicenter Phase II study of temozolomide therapy for brain metastasis in patients with malignant melanoma, breast cancer, and non-small cell lung cancer. *Proc Am Soc Clin Oncol* 2003;22:(abst 407).

144. Wang ML, Yung WK, Royce ME, et al. Capecitabine for 5-fluorouracil-resistant brain metastases from breast cancer. *Am J Clin Oncol* 2001;24(4):421–424.

145. Ekenel M, Hormigo AM, Peak S, et al. Capecitabine therapy of central nervous system metastases from breast cancer. *J Neurooncol* 2007;85(2):223–227.

146. Rivera E, Meyers C, Groves M, et al. Phase I study of capecitabine in combination with temozolomide in the treatment of patients with brain metastases from breast carcinoma. *Cancer* 2006;107(6):1348–1354.

147. Lin NU, Carey LA, Liu MC, et al. Phase II trial of lapatinib for brain metastases in patients with human epidermal growth factor receptor 2-positive breast cancer. *J Clin Oncol* 2008;26(12):1993–1999.

148. Lin NU, Dieras V, Paul D, et al. EGF105084, a phase II study of lapatinib for brain metastases in patients (pts) with HER2+ breast cancer following trastuzumab (H) based systemic therapy and cranial radiotherapy (RT). *J Clin Oncol* 2007;25(18S):35s(abst 1012).

149. Lin NU, Paul D, Dieras V, et al. Lapatinib and capecitabine for the treatment of brain metastases in patients with HER2+ breast cancer: an updated analysis from EGF105084. *Breast Cancer Res Treat* 2007;106[Suppl 1]:(abst 6076).

150. Cameron D, Martin A-M, Newstat B, et al. Lapatinib (L) plus capecitabine (C) in HER2+ advanced breast cancer (ABC): updated efficacy and biomarker analyses. Presented at American Society of Clinical Oncology annual meeting. June 1–5, 2007. Chicago. Abst 1035.

151. Kim LS, Huang S, Lu W, et al. Vascular endothelial growth factor expression promotes the growth of breast cancer brain metastases in nude mice. *Clin Exp Metastasis* 2004;21(2):107–118.

152. Vredenburgh JJ, Desjardins A, Herndon JE 2nd, et al. Phase II trial of bevacizumab and irinotecan in recurrent malignant glioma. *Clin Cancer Res* 2007;13(4):1253–1259.

153. Batchelor TT, Sorensen AG, di Tomaso E, et al. AZD2171, a pan-VEGF receptor tyrosine kinase inhibitor, normalizes tumor vasculature and alleviates edema in glioblastoma patients. *Cancer Cell* 2007;11(1):83–95.

154. Knisely JP, Berkey B, Chakravarti A, et al. A phase III study of conventional radiation therapy plus thalidomide versus conventional radiation therapy for multiple brain metastases (RTOG 0118). *Int J Radiat Oncol Biol Phys* 2008;71(1):79–86.

155. Mehta MP, Rodrigus P, Terhaard CH, et al. Survival and neurologic outcomes in a randomized trial of motexafin gadolinium and whole-brain radiation therapy in brain metastases. *J Clin Oncol* 2003;21(13):2529–2536.

156. Suh JH, Stea B, Nabid A, et al. Phase III study of efaproxiral as an adjunct to whole-brain radiation therapy for brain metastases. *J Clin Oncol* 2006;24(1):106–114.

157. Scott C, Suh J, Stea B, et al. Improved survival, quality of life, and quality-adjusted survival in breast cancer patients treated with efaproxiral (Efaproxyn) plus whole-brain radiation therapy for brain metastases. *Am J Clin Oncol* 2007;30(6):580–587.

158. Antonadou D, Paraskevaidis M, Sarris G, et al. Phase II randomized trial of temozolomide and concurrent radiotherapy in patients with brain metastases. *J Clin Oncol* 2002;20(17):3644–3650.

Chapter 82
Epidural Metastases

Patrick Y. Wen, Brian J. Scott, Craig D. McColl, and Ronnie John Freilich

Epidural spinal cord compression (ESCC), resulting from tumor growth in the spinal epidural space, is one of the true neurologic emergencies that can arise in patients with breast cancer. Because the prognosis for good functional outcome is primarily dependent on the degree of impairment at the commencement of treatment, clinicians who care for patients with breast cancer must remain vigilant about the possible presence of ESCC. More than 91% of patients with ESCC have symptoms for longer than 1 week before a diagnosis is made (1), with pain lasting for a mean duration of 6 weeks (2). Compromise of the conus medullaris and cauda equina by epidural metastasis is generally included in a discussion of ESCC because the natural history and management of these problems are similar to those of compression of the spinal cord itself. ESCC is discussed in more detail in several recent reviews (3–6).

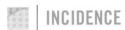

INCIDENCE

The incidence of ESCC in patients with cancer is approximately 5% (7,8). A similar incidence (4%) has been reported in patients with breast cancer (1). Breast cancer accounts for 7% to 32% of all cases of ESCC in patients with cancer (4,9–16). The median time from the diagnosis of breast cancer to the onset of ESCC is 42 months, with a range of 0 to 28 years (1). ESCC usually occurs in the setting of widely metastatic disease (17), although rarely ESCC may be the initial presentation of cancer; this occurs more frequently in a general hospital than in a specialized cancer center (9,10). In some instances, biopsy of an epidural metastasis is required to establish the diagnosis of cancer.

PATHOLOGY

Epidural metastases most commonly arise from metastases to the vertebral column (85%). They arise less commonly from metastases to the paravertebral space (5% to 10%) that either secondarily invade bone and then grow into the epidural space or invade the epidural space directly through the intervertebral foramen. In rare instances, direct hematogenous spread to the epidural space or parenchyma of the spinal cord occurs (18,19), but this presentation is more likely with lymphoma than with breast cancer. If ESCC develops as the first manifestation of cancer, the absence of bony or skeletal metastases makes breast cancer an unlikely diagnosis. The vertebral column is the most common site of metastases to bone (20). Vertebral metastases occur in up to 41% of all patients with cancer (21) and in 60% of patients with breast cancer (13). The incidence in patients with advanced breast cancer may be as high as 84% (18). This high incidence relates to the fact that cancers of the breast (and cancers of the pelvis) are in communication with Batson's vertebral plexus (22), a low-pressure valveless venous system that fills when thoracoabdominal pressure is raised (e.g., by maneuvers such as coughing, straining, and lifting). The presence of growth factors in bone marrow may also be a contributing factor (23). Of patients with breast cancer and ESCC, 93% have known bone metastases at the onset of their neurologic deficit, with a median time from the first bone metastasis to ESCC of 11 months (range, 0 to 7.5

years). Breast cancer is commonly associated with multilevel vertebral metastases, as compared with lung cancer, in which a single level is usually involved (9). Stark et al. (9) demonstrated noncontiguous vertebral involvement in 50% of patients with breast cancer who had abnormal plain spine radiography, and epidural tumor was multifocal in 29%. As would be anticipated from their origin in the vertebral bodies, most epidural metastases are situated anterior or anterolateral to the spinal cord (10), which has important implications for their surgical management. Sixty percent of epidural metastases arise in the thoracic spine and another 30% in the lumbosacral region. These figures are proportionate to the volume of bone in each of these spinal regions (4).

Spinal cord damage in ESCC is due primarily to direct compression of the spinal cord by tumor and rarely to compression of radicular arteries that pass through the intervertebral foramen (18). Axonal swelling and white matter edema occur early in animal models of ESCC, whereas gray matter damage occurs later (24). Prolonged cord compression results in necrosis of both gray and white matter. Early spinal cord damage is likely caused by venous stasis, whereas arteriolar compression by tumor is probably responsible for the late stage of tissue necrosis (24).

CLINICAL SYMPTOMS AND SIGNS

As noted earlier, ESCC due to breast cancer occurs most commonly in the thoracic spine (9,10,25), in part because this is the longest section of the vertebral column but also because of the pattern of drainage from Batson's plexus and the proximity of the primary tumor to the thoracic vertebrae. The principal symptom of ESCC is pain (Table 82.1). It is the initial symptom in 96% of patients and precedes other symptoms by a mean of 6 weeks (2). Pain is of three types: local, radicular, and referred. Local back pain is usually a constant ache and occurs in almost all patients. Radicular pain is caused by involvement of nerve roots by the tumor mass and is typically described as a shooting pain. It is more common with cervical and lumbosacral lesions than with thoracic lesions (10). With cervical or lumbosacral epidural metastases, radicular pain is typically unilateral. With thoracic disease, however, radicular pain is commonly bilateral, producing a band-like pain or tightness that may be felt more at the lateral or anterior chest wall than in the back itself. Referred pain occurs at a distant site from the lesion and does not radiate. For example, T12-L1 vertebral lesions may be referred to both iliac crests or both sacroiliac joints, whereas C7-T1 lesions may be referred to the interscapular region or to both shoulders (26). The pain of epidural metastasis is often worsened by lying supine, possibly because of filling of vertebral veins in this position. Patients typically report that they are unable to sleep lying down and need to sleep sitting up; this information is often not volunteered by patients but must be sought by direct questioning. The pain tends to be most prominent at night and into the morning, with resolution or improvement over the course of the day (27). The Valsalva maneuver (coughing, sneezing, or straining at stool) exacerbates the pain of epidural metastases, as it fills vertebral veins and raises intracranial pressure, which is then transmitted to the already compromised spinal canal. Pain is also worsened by stretching maneuvers, such as neck flexion in the case

		SYMPTOMS AND SIGNS OF EPIDURAL SPINAL CORD COMPRESSION IN 130 PATIENTS WHO PRESENTED TO A LARGE CANCER HOSPITAL		
Symptom/Sign	First Symptom (%)	Symptoms at Diagnosis (%)	Signs at Diagnosis (%)	
Pain	96	96	—	
Weakness	2	76	87	
Autonomic dysfunction	0	57	—	
Sensory loss	0	51	78	
Ataxia	2	3	7	
Herpes zoster	0	2	2	
Flexor spasms	0	1	1	

Table 82.1

From Barron KD, Hirano A, Araki S, et al. Experiences with metastatic neoplasms involving the spinal cord. *Neurology* 1959;9:91, with permission.

of cervical or upper thoracic tumors and straight-leg raising with lumbosacral or thoracic lesions. Escalating back pain in patients with cancer is a particularly ominous indicator of the possibility of ESCC. Tenderness may be present over the vertebral column at the site of the lesion, and there may be referred tenderness at the site of referred or radicular pain. Pain that worsens substantially with movement of the neck or back may be a sign of mechanical instability of the spinal column, which can occur in the setting of vertebral or epidural metastases (27).

The spinal cord usually ends at the level of L1. Therefore, ESCC above L1 will produce a myelopathy, whereas lesions below this level result in a cauda equina syndrome. Myelopathic symptoms include limb weakness in a pyramidal distribution, numbness and paresthesias, and sphincter disturbance (urinary retention, urinary urgency, constipation, or fecal urgency). At the time of diagnosis, 76% of patients complain of weakness, 87% are weak on examination, 57% have autonomic dysfunction, 51% have sensory symptoms, and 78% have sensory deficits on examination (10). In many series, fewer than 50% of patients are ambulatory at diagnosis, and up to 25% are paraplegic (1,2,10); these figures are significant because prognosis is related to clinical deficit at presentation. Outcomes might be improved if patients were encouraged to seek treatment earlier.

Signs of a myelopathy include paraparesis or quadriparesis, increased tone, clonus, hyperreflexia, extensor-plantar responses, a distended bladder, or a sensory level. A patch of hyperesthesia may be present at the upper aspect of the sensory level. The sensory, motor, and reflex levels are only an approximate indication of the site of pathology; because sensory fibers retain their somatotopic organization as they ascend in the cord, the actual site of cord compression may be several segments above the apparent sensory level. Furthermore, there may be multiple sites of epidural disease. The entire spinal cord should, therefore, be imaged in all patients with myelopathy.

The myelopathy may be incomplete, and it is a serious error to dismiss the possibility of ESCC on the basis that any particular sign is absent. Neither a sensory level nor an extensor plantar response is necessary to make the clinical diagnosis of ESCC. Dorsal column sensation (vibration and proprioception) and spinothalamic sensation (pain and temperature) must be assessed independently in all patients with cancer and back pain. Because the subjective appreciation of light touch involves both sensory pathways, light-touch sensation may be reasonably well preserved, even in the presence of a clear cut sensory level for pain or vibration sense when these are tested separately. A hemicord or Brown-Séquard's syndrome (characterized by ipsilateral weakness and proprioception loss, and contralateral loss of pain and temperature) may occur, although this is rare in ESCC (9,10). In an oncologic population,

Brown-Séquard's syndrome is more typical of intramedullary cord metastasis or radiation myelopathy (28). Involvement of spinocerebellar tracts in the spinal cord can lead to lower extremity ataxia out of proportion to the degree of weakness. Dorsal column involvement can lead to a sensory ataxia with positive rombergism while sparing power and reflexes. Both of these clinical presentations may focus the attention of the unwary examiner on the cerebellum, thereby delaying diagnosis (29). Patients may also present with herpes zoster, presumably as a result of reactivation of latent virus by compression of the dorsal root ganglion by tumor (10).

ESCC at the conus medullaris and cauda equina produces different neurologic symptoms and signs, although pain is still a prominent feature, particularly with cauda equina lesions. Conus lesions typically present with early and marked sphincter disturbance and perineal sensory loss. Anal sphincter tone may be lax, and there may be an absent anal wink. Cauda equina lesions produce patchy lower motor neuron signs related to the lumbar and sacral nerve roots—hyporeflexia or areflexia, myotomal leg weakness, and dermatomal sensory loss; sphincter disturbance tends to occur late and to be less marked than in conus lesions. When the signs include a mixture of upper and lower motor neuron features or dermatomal sensory loss as well as a sensory level, the possibility of coexistent nerve root involvement and cord compression should be considered.

INVESTIGATIONS

The serious consequences of untreated ESCC, paraplegia or quadriplegia, necessitate an orderly and expeditious investigation of all patients in whom this diagnosis is suspected. The imaging modalities that can be used in the investigation of ESCC include plain spinal radiographs, radionuclide bone scans, and computed tomography (CT) of the spine, as well as techniques that definitively image the epidural space: myelography (with or without CT) and magnetic resonance imaging (MRI). Because most patients with ESCC present with back pain, the investigation of ESCC can be regarded as the investigation of patients with cancer and back pain. It is not practical or appropriate to perform definitive imaging of the epidural space in every patient with cancer who has back pain, and this has led to the development of algorithms for the investigation and treatment of these patients (18,30–33), as shown in Figure 82.1. However, as the availability of MRI has increased, most patients are evaluated with MRI as the only imaging modality. When discussing the available investigational tools, the clinician should consider the following clinical presentations: isolated back pain with a normal neurologic examination, radiculopathy, plexopathy, and myelopathy.

Isolated Back Pain

Plain Spine Radiographs

Several studies have demonstrated the clinical usefulness of plain radiographs in the assessment of possible epidural disease. Of patients with epidural metastases, 85% have a vertebral body metastasis seen on plain radiography at the appropriate level (9,10). This figure varies depending on the type of tumor: Epidural disease caused by breast cancer has been associated with visible vertebral metastases in 94% to 98% of patients (9,34), whereas only 32% of patients with lymphoma and ESCC have bony abnormalities on plain radiographs (35). Plain radiographs may be less sensitive in detecting bony disease at certain sites, particularly the C7-T1 vertebrae (which are commonly involved in breast cancer), because overlying bone and mediastinal shadows may obscure the image of these

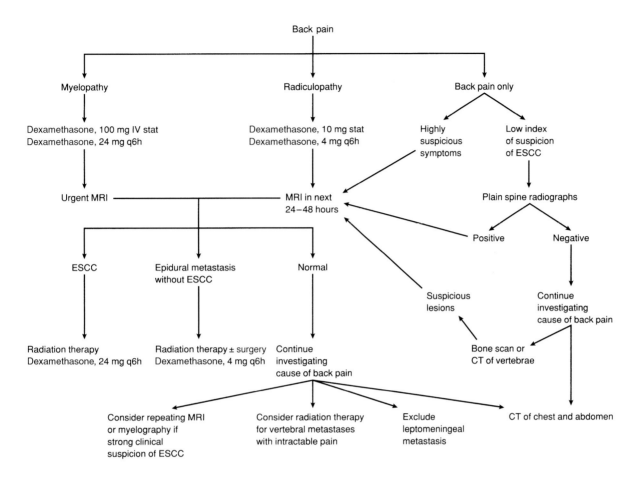

FIGURE 82.1. Algorithm for the investigation and treatment of patients with breast cancer and back pain. CT, computed tomography; ESCC, epidural spinal cord compression; IV, intravenously; MRI, magnetic resonance imaging; stat, immediately.

vertebrae. Rodichok et al. (36) found epidural metastases in 25 of 34 (74%) patients with isolated back pain, no neurologic abnormalities, and an abnormal plain radiograph. In contrast, Graus et al. (37) found ESCC in only 12 of 35 (34%) patients in this setting. When Graus et al. (37) classified the x-ray abnormalities by the types of changes seen, however, they found that epidural metastases were present in 7 of 8 (87%) patients with more than 50% vertebral collapse and 4 of 13 (31%) patients with isolated pedicle destruction, but only 1 of 14 (7%) patients with metastasis restricted to the vertebral body without severe collapse. Both studies demonstrated an incidence of epidural metastasis of 3% or less in patients with normal plain radiographs. If plain radiographs of the spine are abnormal, more definitive imaging must be arranged on an urgent basis (Fig. 82.1).

Radionuclide Bone Scans

Bone scintigraphy is more sensitive than plain radiography in the detection of epidural metastasis (38). On occasion, however, scintigraphy fails to detect metastatic breast cancer if the metastases produce purely lytic bone lesions (39). Scintigraphy may also be insensitive after radiotherapy (33). Furthermore, scintigraphy is less specific than radiography (38). In patients with an abnormal bone scan but a normal plain radiograph, Portenoy et al. (38) found epidural metastases in only 1 of 9 (12%) symptomatic segments (defined as vertebral segments that produce pain or neurologic signs) and 0 of 22 asymptomatic

segments. It was concluded that bone scans may, however, play a role in the assessment of back pain. For example, normal findings on bone scan may confirm that an epidural metastasis is unlikely in patients with normal findings on radiography. In the study of Rodichok et al. (36), epidural metastases were demonstrated in 15 of 26 (58%) patients with back pain, no neurologic signs, and abnormal findings on bone scan, compared to 2 of 10 (20%) patients with normal findings on bone scan. Bone scans were not performed in many cases because the clinical picture and plain radiographs led immediately to myelography. The authors determined that bone scans do not contribute significantly to the information obtained from plain radiographs. Portenoy et al. (38) recommend that asymptomatic spinal metastases discovered on staging bone scans should be characterized further with plain radiography.

Computed Tomographic Scanning

CT scanning without the instillation of myelographic dye is more sensitive than plain radiographs in detecting vertebral and paravertebral metastases, and it has been demonstrated that cortical disruption adjacent to the epidural space is a useful marker of epidural metastasis (31,40). CT does not visualize the epidural space adequately, however. Furthermore, CT produces axial images, and thus, only a limited area of the spine can be imaged by this technique. CT scans may be useful in differentiating vertebral collapse due to tumor from that due to osteoporosis.

Magnetic Resonance Imaging

In patients with widely metastatic disease and whose pain is suggestive of ESCC, MRI is the imaging modality of choice.

SUMMARY

In patients with breast cancer and isolated back pain without neurologic abnormalities, plain spine radiographs are occasionally the appropriate first line of investigation. Definitive imaging of the epidural space should be performed if plain films are abnormal. In patients with a clinical picture that is strongly suggestive of epidural metastasis (e.g., back pain that is significantly exacerbated by lying flat and worsened by the Valsalva maneuver), definitive imaging of the epidural space should still be performed even if a plain radiograph is normal; in fact, it is reasonable to proceed straight to MRI in this situation. The potential difficulties in interpreting changes at the C7-T1 vertebrae should be considered if this is the site of clinical suspicion. In patients with local back pain with characteristics that are not strongly suggestive of epidural metastasis, definitive imaging of the epidural space is not indicated if a plain radiograph is normal. Investigations must proceed, however, to determine the cause of the back pain. Bone scan, CT scan of the vertebrae, or MRI of the spine may be performed. Other investigations that may be useful include CT scan of the chest or abdomen to exclude lesions such as paravertebral or visceral metastases. The differential diagnosis of back pain also includes leptomeningeal metastases, but there are usually other clinical clues to suggest this diagnosis.

Radiculopathy

Radiculopathy is associated with a high incidence of epidural metastases. In the Rodichok et al. (36) series of patients with cancer and back pain, 27 of 43 (63%) patients with radiculopathy and without signs of spinal cord involvement were found to have epidural metastases, compared with 27 of 61 (44%) patients with local back pain alone. When plain radiographs were abnormal, epidural metastases were found in 20 of 22 (91%) patients with radiculopathy. Similarly, in patients with abnormal findings on plain radiographs, Graus et al. (37) found epidural metastases in 47 of 67 (70%) patients with radiculopathy, compared with 12 of 35 (34%) patients with local back pain alone. Importantly, in the series by Graus et al. (37) and Rodichok et al. (36), epidural metastases were found in 9% to 33% of patients with radiculopathy and normal findings on plain radiographs (36,37).

Given the high incidence of epidural metastases in patients with radiculopathy, even in those with normal findings on plain radiographs, it is reasonable to proceed straight to definitive imaging of the epidural space with MRI in all patients with breast cancer and radiculopathy. It is important to remember that in the thoracic spine, which is the most common site of ESCC in breast cancer, radiculopathy commonly presents as bilateral, band-like dermatomal pain and that, in some situations, lateral or even anterior chest pain may be more prominent than back pain.

Plexopathy

The possibility of epidural metastasis must be considered in patients with breast cancer and a malignant brachial plexopathy because tumor may infiltrate directly along the plexus to the epidural space. Brachial plexus lesions present with pain (usually in the shoulder girdle and radiating to the elbow, medial side of the forearm, and medial two digits) as well as weakness and sensory symptoms in a segmental distribution.

Clinical clues to the presence of epidural metastases in the setting of brachial plexopathy include a panplexopathy (as compared to the more usual lower plexopathy with involvement of C7, C8, and T1 nerve roots) and the presence of Horner's syndrome (indicating more proximal involvement) (41). The presence of back pain also suggests that the tumor has grown proximally, but back pain may be absent with epidural extension. Patients with brachial plexopathy require imaging of the brachial plexus with CT or MRI and, if vertebral body collapse or erosion is present, at the C7-T1 levels, or if a paraspinal mass is seen, then definitive imaging of the epidural space should be performed. Epidural tumor is present in approximately one third of patients with paraspinal lesions and a normal plain radiograph (37). If MRI is used to image the brachial plexus, the cervical and upper thoracic spine can be imaged at the same time.

Myelopathy

Definitive Imaging of the Epidural Space: Magnetic Resonance Imaging and Myelography

Definitive imaging of the epidural space is required in patients with myelopathy and in other patients in whom the clinical presentation or investigations strongly suggest the presence of epidural metastases. Myelography was the traditional mainstay of investigation of ESCC, but MRI is now the investigation of choice. Myelography is performed by the instillation of a contrast agent into the subarachnoid space through a lumbar spinal puncture (Fig. 82.2). Water-soluble contrast agents, such as iohexol (Omnipaque [GE Healthcare Ltd, Buckinghamshire, UK]), are used rather than the older lipid-soluble agents, which produced complications such as arachnoiditis. CT can be performed after myelography to provide axial images through

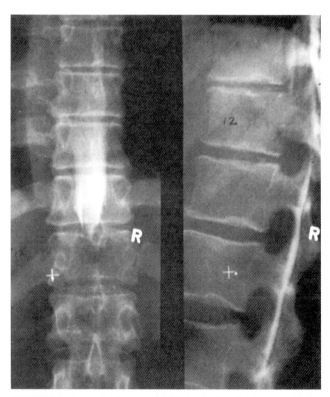

FIGURE 82.2. Myelogram showing a complete block to the flow of contrast material. The upper level of the block at T11-12 is delineated by a C1-2 injection (*left*), whereas the lower level of the block at T12-L1 is demonstrated by a lumbar injection (*right*). Note the right T12 pedicle erosion seen on the left side of the diagram.

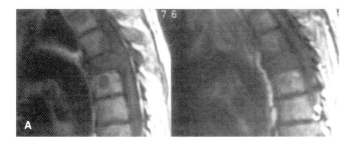

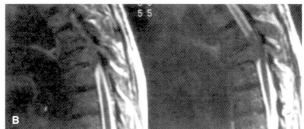

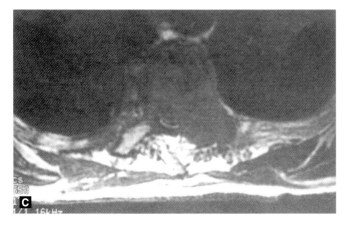

FIGURE 82.3. **A:** Sagittal T1-weighted magnetic resonance imaging (MRI) scans demonstrating epidural spinal cord compression. The vertebral body is completely replaced by tumor and appears hypodense. Tumor extends posteriorly from the vertebral body to compress the spinal cord from its anterior aspect; this is the most common pathology encountered with epidural metastases. The two scans shown are 4 mm apart; the degree of spinal cord compression appears less severe on the scan on the right, emphasizing the inadequacy of a single midline sagittal image as a "screening test" for epidural metastasis. Note the hypodense signal in multiple vertebral bodies indicative of diffuse bony metastases in this patient. **B:** In this sagittal T2-weighted MRI sequence, cerebrospinal fluid is white and the spinal cord is gray; pathology is better demonstrated on T2-weighted than on T1-weighted images. **C:** This axial T1-weighted image shows the vertebral canal to be almost completely obliterated by tumor extending posteriorly from the vertebral body.

abnormal regions. If a complete spinal block is present on myelography, a cisternal C1-2 puncture must be performed to identify the upper border of the block to allow for adequate treatment planning. CT scanning after myelography may assist in the delineation of this upper border, as enough contrast material may get past the block to be seen on CT; however, this occurs in fewer than 50% of patients with complete block (42). Cerebrospinal fluid should be collected when myelography is performed to exclude leptomeningeal metastasis. Myelography may be contraindicated in patients with a coagulopathy and in individuals with raised intracranial pressure from intracerebral metastases. A spinal tap performed in patients with a complete block may worsen the neurologic deficit as a result of the creation of a pressure differential between the spinal canal above and below the block (43).

MRI has a number of advantages over myelography: It is noninvasive, it produces excellent delineation of soft tissue planes, it is very sensitive in the detection of vertebral and paravertebral metastases, and it provides imaging in three planes (sagittal, coronal, and axial) (Fig. 82.3). Furthermore, MRI is useful in discriminating between benign and malignant vertebral collapse (44). Several early studies that compared MRI with myelography in the evaluation of patients with suspected ESCC suggested that MRI was not as sensitive as myelography (45,46). The scanning protocols for these studies did not, however, routinely include axial images; sagittal images (with or without coronal images) may easily miss a small or laterally placed metastasis. Other investigators, on the other hand, have shown MRI to be as sensitive as myelography in the detection of epidural metastases, including the detection of small lesions and metastases that produce nerve root compression (47,48). In some instances, MRI has been shown to be superior to myelography in the detection of epidural metastases, in accurately determining the upper border of a complete block, in imaging multiple sites of spinal block, and in the detection of paravertebral and vertebral metastases (46–48). Furthermore, the quality of MRI technology has continued to improve since its introduction (44), casting doubt on original estimates of its utility. A retrospective cost-effectiveness study concluded that when the results of incorrect or delayed

diagnoses were taken into account, the cost of diagnosing ESCC in a U.S. institution was 65% higher in the pre-MRI era than since MRI became available in 1985 (49). The use of MRI was calculated to produce a similar saving (40%) in a British context (50). Although MRI is recommended as the investigation of choice in ESCC, it is important to remember that, in some situations, MRI scanning may give a false-negative result, and repeated MRI or myelography may be indicated if a strong clinical suspicion of epidural metastases remains, particularly if the MRI scan was degraded by artifact. Furthermore, if MRI is not readily available or cannot be performed (e.g., in patients with pacemakers or the occasional patient with severe claustrophobia), myelography should be performed.

An unenhanced MRI scan can establish the diagnosis of ESCC. However, a contrast-enhanced scan using gadolinium-DTPA (diethylenetriamine penta-acetic acid) should also be obtained to look for leptomeningeal metastasis, which may mimic the presentation of ESCC. The entire spine should be imaged, as epidural disease may be present at multiple levels, and the spinal level indicated by clinical examination may be several segments below the level of the lesion (51). It is important to obtain axial scans in addition to sagittal images. A "screening" midline sagittal scan is inadequate; multiple sagittal scans using thin slices should be performed. Coronal images of the spine are not required routinely. Adequate analgesia (including corticosteroids) should be administered before the MRI is performed because the patient must lie motionless for the scan, and lying flat may worsen the back pain. If the patient cannot tolerate the full procedure, or if there is not enough time to perform an MRI of the entire spine, the area of interest should be imaged first, followed at a later time by imaging of the remainder of the spine. When ordering radiologic investigations, a clear distinction should be made between the suspected neurologic level of involvement and the suspected vertebral level; the discrepancy between these is greatest at the inferior end of the spinal cord. Because the spinal cord terminates at the first lumbar vertebra, all of the lumbar segments and some of the sacral segments of the cord are usually situated within the thoracic spine.

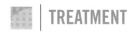 **TREATMENT**

Corticosteroids

Corticosteroids, usually in the form of dexamethasone, are used routinely in the management of ESCC because they reduce pain and sometimes stabilize or improve neurologic deficits (3,14,18). Although one animal model of ESCC showed no effect of high-dose glucocorticoids on spinal cord water content (52), other models have shown that these drugs do reduce the vasogenic edema associated with ESCC, primarily by decreasing capillary permeability (53–55). The effect on vasogenic edema was found to be dose dependent when intramuscular dexamethasone was given to animals in doses equivalent to human doses of 1.5, 15, and 150 mg twice a day (55). The clinical signs of ESCC in the animals were stabilized or improved by the high-dose dexamethasone regimen (53,54), and this effect has been shown to be dose dependent (55).

Extrapolating the experimental data to humans suggests a role for the use of high-dose dexamethasone in acute ESCC. One 1980 study demonstrated that a bolus dose of 100 mg dexamethasone intravenously, followed by a tapering schedule starting with 96 mg a day in four divided doses for 3 days, has a significant and rapid effect on the pain associated with ESCC (14). In a 1989 study, no difference in pain, ambulation, or bladder function was seen in 37 patients with ESCC who received either a 10- or a 100-mg bolus of dexamethasone intravenously (56). A randomized controlled trial in 1994, however, showed that in 57 patients with ESCC who proceeded to radiotherapy, high-dose dexamethasone significantly increased the proportion of patients who remained ambulant after treatment (57). Although it has been suggested that it might be feasible to withhold steroids in patients with good motor function who are proceeding directly to radiotherapy, this approach has been assessed in only one small uncontrolled study (58).

In general, a bolus dose of 100 mg of dexamethasone is recommended for patients with suspected ESCC who present with significant deficits, followed by a maintenance dose of 24 mg every 6 hours. Steroids may then be tapered over 2 to 3 weeks while the patient receives definitive therapy. In general, the dose may be halved approximately every 3 days. In patients who have persistent or worsening pain, steroids may need to be increased or tapered more slowly. Patients with minimal deficits can probably be safely treated with a 10-mg bolus of dexamethasone, followed by an initial maintenance dose of 8 to 16 mg daily. The bolus dose of steroids is given once the clinical diagnosis is made and before an MRI is performed. Patients with radicular pain receive a 10-mg bolus of dexamethasone, followed by a dose of 4 mg four times a day that is subsequently tapered, pending the results of neuroimaging. If MRI demonstrates cord compression (or if myelography shows a block of more than 80%), the high-dose regimen may be used, whereas the low-dose regimen is used for patients with epidural disease without cord compression (or a block on myelography of more than 80%).

The only difference between oral and intravenous administration of dexamethasone is that systemic availability is slowed by approximately 30 minutes when it is given orally. Intravenous dexamethasone is recommended for the initial bolus to provide analgesia quickly, but unless the patient has a nonfunctioning gut, oral dexamethasone is generally used at other times. Prolonged use of high-dose dexamethasone is associated with more side effects than low-dose dexamethasone, but for short-term use, the toxicity of the doses is similar (18). In areas in which *Pneumocystis jiroveci* (formerly *Pneumocystis carinii*) infection is common, patients who are receiving steroids should receive prophylaxis against this opportunistic pathogen (59). The recommended regimen is trimethoprim-sulfamethoxazole, one double-strength tablet once or twice a day, 3 days a week. Some authors recommend H_2 blockers, such as ranitidine, to reduce the risk of peptic ulceration during steroid therapy (60).

Surgery and Radiation Therapy

Decompressive laminectomy (with or without radiation therapy) was the mainstay of treatment for ESCC until the mid-1980s, with clinical improvement noted in 30% to 40% of patients (61). However, several studies demonstrated that the outcome achieved by radiation alone is as good as that of laminectomy and radiation combined; this applied not only to radiosensitive tumors, such as breast cancer, but also to more radioresistant tumors (1,10,62,63). The outcome for radiosensitive tumors, however, is better than that for radioresistant tumors, regardless of the treatment modality used (10). The poor response to laminectomy is due, at least in part, to the anterior or anterolateral location of most epidural metastases; epidural metastases are difficult to remove using the posterior approach of a laminectomy, and a posterior decompression does not relieve the anterior spinal cord compression. Laminectomy may further weaken a spine that is already compromised by vertebral destruction. Overall, surgery is associated with a higher complication rate than radiation therapy, particularly in the setting of steroid use (10,63). Considering all tumor types, one review concluded that surgery for ESCC was associated with a mortality of 6% to 24% and a nonneurologic complication rate of approximately 10% (64). These observations have led to the use of radiation therapy as the initial treatment of choice for most patients with ESCC.

To circumvent the problems associated with laminectomy, an anterolateral surgical approach to ESCC has been developed using vertebral body resection and stabilization of the spine with methylmethacrylate (65–68). Bone grafts have been used for stabilization and are recommended in patients in whom survival beyond 6 months is anticipated, but the grafts may not tolerate subsequent radiation therapy, particularly in the first 3 to 6 weeks after grafting (69,70). Several nonrandomized studies indicated that vertebral body resection (with or without radiation therapy) is superior to radiation alone in terms of ambulation and sphincter control, with some studies showing significant recovery of ambulation in paraplegic patients (26,66–68,71–73). It has also been claimed that in patients with a variety of tumor types, aggressive surgery can improve long-term survival (73). These studies have used surgery in highly selected patients, however, and have often used historical controls for comparison. Furthermore, surgical morbidity with this approach may be considerable, with postoperative complication rates of 10% to 48% reported for vertebral body resection (68,73).

A posterolateral approach has also been proposed as a less aggressive alternative to vertebral body resection, with removal of the lamina, facet joint, and pedicle on the involved side, followed by instrumentation to achieve stability (74). Only small series of patients treated in this manner have been reported, with limited follow-up, but the technique may find a role in the palliation of patients with advanced disease (73).

In 2005 Patchell et al. (75) reported a phase III prospective, randomized controlled trial comparing surgical decompression followed by radiation therapy (RT) to RT alone in patients with solid tumor ESCC. Patients with at least one neurological symptom of ESCC (including pain) and evidence of a solitary epidural metastasis following whole spine MRI were given high-dose steroids and then randomized to receive surgery followed by RT (n = 50) versus RT alone (n = 51). Patients with multiple lesions, nerve root compression, radiosensitive tumors (lymphoma, leukemia, multiple myeloma, and germ cell tumors), and paraplegia more than 48 hours prior to entry were excluded.

In contrast to previous studies, many of which had only used a posterior approach, the surgical approach was chosen by the surgeon based on the location of the tumor (anterior, lateral, or posterior). The study population included 13 breast cancer patients, equally distributed between groups (seven had surgery plus RT, six had RT alone). The primary end point was the ability to walk immediately following radiation, with duration of ambulation and survival time among the secondary end points. In the group who received surgery, 84% were able to ambulate at the end of RT, compared to 57% of those who received RT alone ($p = .001$). The median duration of ambulation was 122 days with surgery plus RT, compared to 13 days with RT alone ($p = .003$). Stability of Frankel functional scale and American Spinal Injury Association (ASIA) motor scores as well as decreased need for opiates and corticosteroids were seen more often in those who received surgery. Overall survival was better in the surgery plus RT group (126 days vs. 100 days with RT alone; $p = .033$). Importantly, surgery did not result in prolonged hospitalization; the median hospital stay was 10 days in both the surgery group (interquartile range 2 to 51 days) and the radiation group (0 to 41 days; $p = .86$). Based on superior posttreatment ambulatory rate in the surgically treated group, the study was stopped at the midpoint analysis and concluded that surgery plus RT is superior to RT alone in the treatment of malignant ESCC (78).

This study suggests that patients with ESCC treated with radical direct decompressive surgery plus postoperative radiotherapy retained the ability to walk longer than patients treated with radiation alone. Surgery permitted most patients to remain ambulatory and continent for the remainder of their lives, whereas patients treated with radiation alone spent approximately two thirds of their remaining time unable to walk and incontinent. In patients who have multiple metastases, or in institutions without the surgical resources to perform emergency anterior decompression in patients with ESCC routinely, the benefit of surgery is less clear. Also, whether the benefit of surgery applies to radiosensitive tumors such as breast cancer remains to be seen, since breast cancer patients comprised only 13% of the study group. Nonetheless, this is an important study that provides evidence to support surgical decompression in certain patients with ESCC.

In general, patients with breast cancer undergoing focal radiation therapy receive a dose of up to 3,000 cGy (30 Gy) administered over 2 weeks. Short-course radiotherapy involving two doses of 800 cGy has also been proposed, producing results comparable to those obtained with higher doses in uncontrolled studies (76,77). Three- and 4-week regimens administering up to 40 Gy have also been described, without benefit in motor function, local control of disease, or survival over the standard 2-week regimen (78). No dose fractionation schedule has proven to be significantly more efficacious than others (28). One approach is to recommend the course of radiation based on the patient's expected survival and ability to tolerate treatments. Short-course RT may be most appropriate for those with an estimated survival of less than 6 months, since the main benefit of long-course RT is reduced local recurrence (77).

Rades et al. (77) performed a retrospective review of 335 breast cancer patients who had received radiation to determine significant prognostic factors. They found that slower development of motor deficit (>14 days) and ability to ambulate prior to initiating RT were associated with a better functional outcome. A short course of radiation (8 Gy in one dose vs. 30 to 40 Gy over 3 to 4 weeks) did not significantly impact functional status after treatment, but was associated with a higher in-field rate of recurrence (20% at 2 years vs. 10% with standard course RT). Median overall survival was 20 months, but was lessened in patients with visceral metastases, deterioration of motor function after RT, rapid development of motor deficits (1 to 7 days), and poor performance status (77).

Radiation therapy should begin on an urgent basis. In situations in which patients present in the middle of the night, when it is logistically difficult to obtain neuroimaging or commence radiation therapy, the high-dose steroid regimen may be commenced; the radiation oncologists can be notified about the patient and an MRI performed first thing the following morning.

The use of radiation therapy for recurrent ESCC, when this involves reirradiating a previously treated segment of spinal cord, poses a significant risk of producing radiation myelopathy (79) and is generally not recommended. Reirradiation has been used with some success by Schiff et al. (80), however, who suggest that myelopathy is unlikely to occur within the limited life expectancy of this population. Radiotherapy is also recommended for asymptomatic patients with radiologic evidence of cord compression (81).

Surgery is recommended for patients whose disease progresses or relapses despite radiation therapy, for those with unstable spines due to fracture dislocation of the vertebrae, and for patients in whom the spinal cord compression is largely caused by bony fragments in the epidural space rather than tumor. Surgery for patients who are nonambulatory at presentation is probably beneficial, although the data are inconclusive (81). In patients who were treated soon after the onset of paraplegia (<48 hours), the Patchell et al. (75) study showed improved outcomes in those who underwent surgery with RT. Of those who entered the study unable to walk (32 patients), 10 of 16 (32%) regained the ability to walk in the surgery group compared to 3 of 16 (19%) who received RT alone ($p = .012$). Additionally, the surgical group maintained ambulation for a median 59 days, compared to 0 days in those receiving only RT ($p = .04$). Treatment decisions therefore must be individualized, taking into account the risk of surgery and the patient's overall condition and ability to tolerate therapy. Surgery may be indicated in patients with an unknown primary malignancy, as it provides diagnostic and therapeutic benefit, although a percutaneous needle biopsy under radiologic guidance will be informative in most cases and will have fewer complications than an open procedure (84,85). One retrospective study in 1996 showed significantly better functional outcomes with emergency surgery than with surgery postponed to the next elective operating list within 24 hours (86). This finding may have reflected selection bias, but, nevertheless, it is generally recommended that surgery be performed as soon as possible.

Chemotherapy and Hormonal Therapy

Chemotherapy does not play a significant role in the treatment of ESCC cause by metastatic breast cancer, although Boogerd et al. (87) describe protracted remission of epidural metastases in four patients with breast cancer who received chemotherapy. Chemotherapy may be a more important treatment modality in highly chemosensitive tumors, such as germ cell tumors, lymphoma, and neuroblastoma (3,4,88,89). There are also anecdotal reports of patients with ESCC from breast cancer benefiting from hormonal therapy (90).

Supportive Therapy

Patients with myelopathy resulting from ESCC require close attention to analgesia, bowel and bladder care, and the prevention of pressure sores. Prophylaxis against venous thromboembolism should always be considered in bed-bound patients.

PROGNOSIS

The outcome of ESCC is directly related to the patient's clinical condition at the commencement of treatment (Table 82.2).

| Table 82.2 | TREATMENT OUTCOME AS INFLUENCED BY PRETREATMENT AMBULATORY STATUS |

| | | | | Patients Ambulant After Treatment | | | |
| | | | | Nonambulant Before Treatment | | | |
Author (Ref)	No. of Patients	Tumor Type	Ambulant before Treatment	Overall	Paretic	Plegic	Treatment Modality
Hill et al. (1)	70	Breast	96% 22/23	45% 13/29	—	—	RT = Laminectomy
Kim et al. (2)	59	All	100% 13/13	26% 12/46	35% 11/31	7% 1/15	RT ± Laminectomy
Gilbert et al. (10)	235	All	75% 60/80	35% 54/155	45% 52/116	5% 2/39	RT = Laminectomy + RT
Maranzano et al. (58)	158	All	79% 33/42	14% 16/116	18% 16/89	0% 0/27	Radiotherapy
Young et al. (62)	72	All	81% 34/42	62% 21/32	62% 21/32	—	Vertebral body resection
Sundaresan et al. (68)	110	All	≥94% ≥ 58/62	84% 32/48	—	—	Vertebral body resection
Gokaslan (70)	49	All	91% 21/23	38% 10/26	50% 10/20	0% 0/6	RT ± Surgery
Janjan (79)	345	All	79% 103/131	18% 38/214	21% 35/165	6% 3/49	RT = Laminectomy ± RT
Schiff et al. (80)	105	All	96% 48/50	47% 26/55	56% 25/45	10% 1/10	RT
Loblaw and Laperriere (81)	56	Breast	97% 29/30	69% 18/26	74% 17/23	33% 1/3	RT
Yaada etal. (82)	153	All	91% 72/79	28% 21/74	—	—	RT ± Laminectomy

RT, radiotherapy; =, treatments are equally effective; ±, with or without.

Patients who are ambulant are far more likely to remain ambulant after treatment. 79% to 100% of patients who are ambulant before treatment remain so, whereas only 18% to 69% of nonambulant patients regain the ability to walk (1–4,10, 91–95). In most series, fewer than 10% of patients who are paraplegic or quadriplegic before treatment regain the ability to walk (1–4,10,89–92), although vertebral body resection has been associated with ambulation rates of 24% to 56% in initially paraplegic patients (75,81). In addition, in one study, 6 of 13 paraplegic patients became ambulant after receiving vertebral body resection and radiation therapy (66).

The prognosis for patients with breast cancer treated with radiation therapy alone has been characterized by Maranzano et al. (93). The likelihood of responding to radiation therapy is dependent on the pretreatment ambulatory status, whereas duration of response is dependent on the post-treatment ambulatory status (93). In the study by Maranzano et al. (93), 18 of 26 (69%) patients who were nonambulant before treatment became at least partially ambulant with treatment (walking alone or with support). Only 1 ambulant patient of 30 (3%) became nonambulant despite treatment, underscoring the value of early diagnosis. The median duration of response was 12 months for all patients, 15 months for patients who were ambulant after treatment, and only 2 months for those who were nonambulant after treatment (93). Bladder control was regained in 67% of patients with sphincter dysfunction.

The mean survival of patients with breast cancer in whom ESCC develops is 5 to 14 months (1,16,91,92). The time from diagnosis of breast cancer to the development of ESCC has been found to be a predictor of survival, with patients who develop ESCC after 3 or more years having a better survival (1). One study suggests a longer survival in patients treated with both laminectomy and radiation therapy compared with patients treated by either laminectomy or radiation alone, but these differences may be explained by selection bias (91). One study has demonstrated no survival difference in patients treated with surgery or radiation (1). Proponents of vertebral body resection have claimed that this technique may prolong

survival (73). The absolute survival benefit seen in the Patchell et al. (75) study with surgery (126 days vs. 100 days) was statistically significant ($p = .033$). Although this is important, perhaps the more clinically relevant benefit seen with surgical decompression was the improved duration of ambulation after therapy for those who had surgery (122 days vs. 13 days), and that patients who had surgery generally required lower doses of corticosteroids and opiates.

Posttreatment ambulatory status is the most important factor influencing survival in patients with breast cancer (1,93). In the study by Maranzano et al. (93), the median survival was 13 months for all patients, 17 months for patients who were ambulant after treatment, and only 2 months for those who were nonambulant after treatment. The 1-year survival of posttreatment ambulant patients in this study was 66% versus 10% for nonambulant patients. However, local control of the breast cancer at the site of spinal metastasis did not appear to be responsible for the improved survival in ambulant patients because most deaths were due to progression of systemic disease rather than relapse in the irradiated spine (93). In another series reported by Maranzano et al. (92), which included patients with ESCC due to other cancer types, median survival was better in patients with breast cancer (12 months) than in patients with other tumor types (3 to 7 months). This relatively long survival, in association with the fact that early diagnosis may preserve ambulatory status, underscores the potential value of prompt investigation and treatment of ESCC in patients with breast cancer.

MANAGEMENT SUMMARY

- Early diagnosis and treatment of epidural spinal cord compression is very important in preventing serious neurologic disability. Functional outcome is primarily dependent on the degree of neurologic impairment at the commencement of treatment. Optimal outcomes occur when no neurologic findings are present at the time of diagnosis.

- Epidural spinal cord compression should be suspected in any breast cancer patient with back or neck pain, particularly if there is myelopathy or radiculopathy.
- In patients with pain and myelopathy, dexamethasone 100 mg intravenously should be administered immediately, followed by 24 mg orally every 6 hours, with a spine MRI obtained urgently.
- In patients with pain and radiculopathy or with highly suspicious symptoms, dexamethasone 10 mg intravenously should be administered immediately followed by 4 mg orally every 6 hours and a spine MRI obtained within 24 hours.
- In patients with pain and a low index of suspicion for epidural spinal cord compression, plain spine radiographs or a bone scan should be obtained.
- If epidural spinal cord compression is confirmed on MRI, treatment is generally radiation therapy to a dose equivalent to 3,000 cGy in 10 treatments.
- Surgical decompression should be considered in patients with a single lesion, unstable spine, and paraplegia for less than 48 hours.
- Chemotherapy has a limited role in epidural spinal cord compression due to metastatic breast cancer.
- For patients with neurologic compromise, ensure patients receive adequate analgesia, bowel and bladder care, and prevention of pressure sores. Prophylaxis against venous thromboembolism should be considered in bed-bound patients.

References

1. Hill ME, Richards MA, Gregory WM, et al. Spinal cord compression in breast cancer: a review of 70 cases. *Br J Cancer* 1993;68:969.
2. Kim RY, Spencer SA, Meredith RF, et al. Extradural spinal cord compression: analysis of factors determining functional prognosis—prospective study. *Radiology* 1990;176:279.
3. Mut M, Schiff D, Shaffrey ME. Metastasis to nervous system: spinal epidural and intramedullary metastases. *J Neurooncol* 2005;75(1):43–56.
4. Sherman J, Aregawi DG, Shaffrey ME, et al. Spinal metastases. In: Schiff D, Kesari S, Wen PY, eds. *Cancer neurology in clinical practice.* 2nd ed. Totowa, NJ: Humana Press, 2008:163–180.
5. Kwok E, Tibbs PA, Patchell RA. Clinical approach to metastatic epidural spinal cord compression. *Hematol Oncol Clin North Am* 2006;20:1297.
6. Byrne TN, Borges LF, Loeffler JS. Metastatic epidural spinal cord compression: update on management. *Semin Oncol* 2006;33:307.
7. Barron KD, Hirano A, Araki S, et al. Experiences with metastatic neoplasms involving the spinal cord. *Neurology* 1959;9:91.
8. Bach F, Larsen BH, Rohde K, et al. Metastatic spinal cord compression: occurrence, symptoms, clinical presentations and prognosis in 398 patients with spinal cord compression. *Acta Neurochir (Wien)* 1990;107:37.
9. Stark RJ, Henson RA, Evans SWJ. Spinal metastases: a retrospective survey from a general hospital. *Brain* 1982;105:189.
10. Gilbert RW, Kim J-H, Posner JB. Epidural spinal cord compression from metastatic tumor: diagnosis and treatment. *Ann Neurol* 1978;3:40.
11. Torma T. Malignant tumors of the spine and spinal extradural space. *Acta Chir Scand Suppl* 1957;225:1.
12. White WA, Patterson RH, Bergland RM. Role of surgery in the treatment of spinal cord compression by metastatic neoplasm. *Cancer* 1971;27:558.
13. Fornasier VL, Horne JG. Metastases to the vertebral column. *Cancer* 1975;36:590.
14. Greenberg HS, Kim JH, Posner JB. Epidural spinal cord compression from metastatic tumor: results with a new treatment protocol. *Ann Neurol* 1980;8:361.
15. Dunn RC, Kelly WA, Wohns RNW, et al. Spinal epidural neoplasia: a 15-year review of the results of surgical therapy. *J Neurosurg* 1980;52:47.
16. Constans JP, de Divitiis E, Donzelli R, et al. Spinal metastases with neurological manifestations: review of 600 cases. *J Neurosurg* 1983;59:111.
17. Lu C, Stomper PC, Drislane FW, et al. Suspected spinal cord compression in breast cancer patients: a multidisciplinary risk assessment. *Breast Cancer Res Treat* 1992; 51:121–131.
18. Posner JB. Spinal metastases. In: *Neurologic complications of cancer.* Philadelphia: FA Davis, 1995:111.
19. Byrne TN. Spinal cord compression from epidural metastases. *N Engl J Med* 1992; 327:614.
20. Dethy S, Piccart MJ, Paesmans M, et al. History of brain and epidural metastases from breast cancer in relation with the disease evolution outside the central nervous system. *Eur Neurol* 1995;35:38.
21. Byrne TN, Waxman SG. Spinal cord compression: diagnosis and principles of management. In: Byrne TN, Waxman SG. *Contemporary neurology series.* Vol. 33. Philadelphia: FA Davis, 1990.
22. Batson OV. The vertebral venous system: Caldwell lecture, 1956. In: Weiss L, Gilbert HA, eds. *Bone metastasis.* Boston: GK Hall, 1981:21.
23. Arguello F, Baggs RB, Duerst RE, et al. Pathogenesis of vertebral metastasis and epidural spinal cord compression. *Cancer* 1990;65:98.
24. Kato A, Ushio Y, Hayakawa T, et al. Circulatory disturbance of the spinal cord with epidural neoplasm in rats. *J Neurosurg* 1985;63:260.
25. Sundaresan N, Digiacinto GV, Hughes JE, et al. Treatment of neoplastic spinal cord compression: results of a prospective study. *Neurosurgery* 1991;29:645.
26. Foley KM. Pain syndromes in patients with cancer. In: Bonica JJ, Ventafridda V, eds. *Advances in pain research and therapy.* Vol. 2. New York: Raven Press, 1979:59.
27. Bilsky M, Smith M. Surgical approach to epidural spinal cord compression. *Hematol Oncol Clin North Am* 2006;20:1307.
28. Schiff D, Batchelor T, Wen P. Neurologic emergencies in cancer patients. *Neurol Clin North Am* 1998;16:449.
29. Hainline B, Tuszynski MH, Posner JB. Ataxia in epidural spinal cord compression. *Neurology* 1992;42:2193.
30. Lewis DW, Packer RJ, Raney B, et al. Incidence, presentation, and outcome of spinal cord disease in children with systemic cancer. *Pediatrics* 1986;78:438.
31. O'Rourke T, George CB, Redmond J, et al. Spinal computed tomography and computed tomographic metrizamide myelography in the early diagnosis of metastatic disease. *J Clin Oncol* 1986;4:576.
32. Portenoy RK, Lipton RB, Foley KM. Back pain in the cancer patient: an algorithm for evaluation and management. *Neurology* 1987;37:134.
33. Redmond JR, Friedl KE, Cornett P, et al. Clinical usefulness of an algorithm for the early diagnosis of spinal metastatic disease. *J Clin Oncol* 1988;6:154.
34. Harrison KM, Muss HB, Ball MR, et al. Spinal cord compression in breast cancer. *Cancer* 1985;55:2839.
35. Haddad P, Thaell JF, Kiely JM, et al. Lymphoma of the spinal extradural space. *Cancer* 1976;38:1862.
36. Rodichok LD, Ruckdeschel JC, Harper GR, et al. Early detection and treatment of spinal epidural metastases: the role of myelography. *Ann Neurol* 1986;20:696.
37. Graus F, Krol G, Foley KM. Early diagnosis of spinal epidural metastasis (SEM): correlation with clinical and radiological findings. *Proc Am Soc Clin Oncol* 1985;4:269(abst).
38. Portenoy RK, Galer BS, Salamon O, et al. Identification of epidural neoplasm: radiography and bone scintigraphy in the symptomatic and asymptomatic spine. *Cancer* 1989;64:2207.
39. Tryciecky EW, Gottschalk A, Ludema K. Oncologic imaging: interactions of nuclear medicine with CT and MRI using the bone scan as a model. *Semin Nucl Med* 1997; 2:142.
40. Weissman DE, Gilbert M, Wang H, et al. The use of computed tomography of the spine to identify patients at high risk for epidural metastases. *J Clin Oncol* 1985; 3:1541.
41. Kori SH, Foley KM, Posner JB. Brachial plexus lesions in patients with cancer: 100 cases. *Neurology* 1981;31:45.
42. Kori SH, Shah CP. Efficacy of metrizamide CT in delineating upper level of epidural metastatic disease. *Neurology* 1987;37[Suppl 1]:337(abst).
43. Hollis PH, Malis LI, Zappulla RA. Neurological deterioration after lumbar puncture below complete spinal subarachnoid block. *J Neurosurg* 1986;64:253.
44. Traill Z, Richards MA, Moore NR. Magnetic resonance imaging of metastatic bone disease. *Clin Orthop* 1995;312:76.
45. Krol G, Heier L, Becker R, et al. MRI and myelography in the evaluation of epidural extension of primary and metastatic tumors. In: Valk J, ed. *Neuroradiology 1985/1986.* Amsterdam: Elsevier Science, 1986:91.
46. Heier LA, Krol G, Sundaresan N, et al. MR imaging in evaluation of epidural lesions: comparison with myelography. *Radiology* 1985;157:150(abst).
47. Carmody RF, Yang PJ, Seeley GW, et al. Spinal cord compression due to metastatic disease: diagnosis with MR imaging versus myelography. *Radiology* 1989;173:225.
48. Williams MP, Cherryman GR, Husband JE. Magnetic resonance imaging in suspected metastatic spinal cord compression. *Clin Radiol* 1989;40:286.
49. Jordan JE, Donaldson SS, Enzmann DR. Cost effectiveness and outcome assessment of magnetic resonance imaging in diagnosing cord compression. *Cancer* 1995; 75:2579.
50. Podd TJ, Walkden SE. The use of MRI in the investigation of spinal cord compression [Letter]. *Br J Radiol* 1992;65:187.
51. Cook AM, Lau TN, Tomlinson MJ, et al. Magnetic resonance imaging of the whole spine in suspected malignant spinal cord compression: impact on management. *Clin Oncol* 1998;10:39.
52. Siegal T, Shohami E, Shapira Y, et al. Indomethacin and dexamethasone treatment in experimental neoplastic spinal cord compression: part 2. Effect on edema and prostaglandin synthesis. *Neurosurgery* 1988;22:334.
53. Ushio Y, Posner R, Posner JB, et al. Experimental spinal cord compression by epidural neoplasm. *Neurology* 1977;27:422.
54. Ushio Y, Posner R, Kim JH, et al. Treatment of experimental spinal cord compression caused by extradural neoplasms. *J Neurosurg* 1977;47:380.
55. Delattre JY, Arbit E, Thaler HT, et al. A dose–response study of dexamethasone in a model of spinal cord compression caused by epidural tumor. *J Neurosurg* 1989; 70:920.
56. Vecht CJ, Haaxma-Reiche H, van Putten WLJ, et al. Initial bolus of conventional versus high-dose dexamethasone in metastatic spinal cord compression. *Neurology* 1989;39:1255.
57. Sorensen S, Helweg-Larsen S, Mouridsen H, et al. Effect of high-dose dexamethasone in carcinomatous metastatic spinal cord compression treated with radiotherapy: a randomised trial. *Eur J Cancer* 1994;1:22.
58. Maranzano E, Latini P, Beneventi S, et al. Radiotherapy without steroids in selected metastatic spinal cord compression patients. *Am J Clin Oncol* 1996;19:179.
59. Sepkowitz KA, Brown AE, Telzak EE, et al. *Pneumocystis carinii* pneumonia among patients without AIDS at a cancer hospital. *JAMA* 1992;267:832.
60. Ciezki J, Macklis RM. The palliative role of radiotherapy in the management of the cancer patient. *Semin Oncol* 1995;2[Suppl 3]:82.
61. Gorter K. Results of laminectomy in spinal cord compression due to tumours. *Acta Neurochir (Wien)* 1978;42:177.
62. Young RF, Post EM, King GA. Treatment of spinal epidural metastases: randomized prospective comparison of laminectomy and radiotherapy. *J Neurosurg* 1980;53:741.
63. Findlay GF. Adverse effects of the management of malignant spinal cord compression. *J Neurol Neurosurg Psychiatry* 1984;47:761.
64. Podd TJ, Carpenter DS, Baughan CA, et al. Spinal cord compression: prognosis and implications for treatment fractionation. *Clin Oncol* 1992;6:341.
65. Siegal T, Siegal T, Robin G, et al. Anterior decompression of the spine for metastatic epidural cord compression: a promising avenue of therapy? *Ann Neurol* 1982;11:28.
66. Harrington KD. Anterior cord decompression and spinal stabilization for patients with metastatic lesions of the spine. *J Neurosurg* 1984;61:107.

67. Siegal T, Siegal T. Surgical decompression of anterior and posterior malignant epidural tumors compressing the spinal cord: a prospective study. *Neurosurgery* 1985;17:424.

68. Sundaresan N, Galicich JH, Lane JM, et al. Treatment of spinal metastases by vertebral body resection. *J Neurosurg* 1985;63:676.

69. Bell GR. Surgical treatment of spinal tumours. *Clin Orthop* 1997;335:54.

70. Gokaslan ZL. Spine surgery for cancer. *Curr Opin Oncol* 1996;8:178.

71. Sundaresan N, Scher H, DiGiacinto GV, et al. Surgical treatment of spinal cord compression in kidney cancer. *J Clin Oncol* 1986;4:1851.

72. Saengnipanthkul S, Jirarattanaphochai K, Rojviroj S, et al. Metastatic adenocarcinoma of the spine. *Spine* 1992;17:427.

73. Sundaresan N, Sachdev VP, Holland JF, et al. Surgical treatment of spinal cord compression from epidural metastasis. *J Clin Oncol* 1995;13:2330.

74. Shaw B, Mansfield FL, Borges L. One-stage posterolateral decompression and stabilization for primary and metastatic vertebral tumors in the thoracic and lumbar spine. *J Neurosurg* 1989;70:405.

75. Patchell R, Tibbs PA, Regine WF, et al. Direct decompressive surgical resection in the treatment of spinal cord compression caused by metastatic cancer: a randomized trial. *Lancet* 2005;366:643.

76. Maranzano E, Latini P, Perucci E, et al. Short-course radiotherapy (8 Gy × 2) in metastatic spinal cord compression: an effective and feasible treatment. *Int J Radiat Oncol Biol Phys* 1997;38:1037.

77. Rades D, Veninga T, Stalpers LJA, et al. Prognostic factors predicting functional outcomes, recurrence-free survival, and overall survival after radiotherapy for metastatic spinal cord compression in breast cancer patients. *Int J Radiat Oncol Biol Phys* 2006;64(1):182.

78. Rades D, Karstens JH, Hoskin PJ, et al. Escalation of radiation dose beyond 30 Gy in 10 fractions for metastatic spinal cord compression. *Int J Rad Oncol Biol Phys* 2007;67(2)525.

79. Janjan NA. Radiotherapeutic management of spinal metastases. *J Pain Symptom Manage* 1996;1:47.

80. Schiff D, Shaw EG, Cascino TL. Outcome after spinal reirradiation for malignant epidural spinal cord compression. *Ann Neurol* 1995;37:583.

81. Loblaw DA, Laperriere NJ. Emergency treatment of malignant extradural spinal cord compression: an evidence-based guideline. *J Clin Oncol* 1998;16:1613.

82. Yaada Y, Lovelock DM, Bilsky MH. A review of image-guided intensity-modulated radiotherapy for spinal tumors. *Neurosurgery* 2007;61(2):226.

83. Gerszten PC, Burton SA, Ozhasoglu C, et al. Radiosurgery for spinal metastases: clinical experience in 500 cases from a single institution. *Spine* 2007;32:193.

84. Fyfe I, Henry A, Mulholland R. Closed vertebral biopsy. *J Bone Joint Surg* 1983;65:140.

85. Findlay GF, Sandeman DR, Buxton P. The role of needle biopsy in the management of malignant spinal compression. *Br J Neurosurg* 1988;2:479.

86. Harris JK, Sutcliffe JC, Robinson NE. The role of emergency surgery in malignant spinal extradural compression: assessment of functional outcome. *Br J Neurosurg* 1996;10:27.

87. Boogerd W, van der Sande JJ, Kröger R, et al. Effective systemic therapy for spinal epidural metastases from breast carcinoma. *Eur J Cancer Clin Oncol* 1989;25:149.

88. Sanderson IR, Pritchard J, Marsh HT. Chemotherapy as the initial treatment of spinal cord compression due to disseminated neuroblastoma. *J Neurosurg* 1989;70:688.

89. Cooper K, Bajorin D, Shapiro W, et al. Decompression of epidural metastases from germ cell tumors with chemotherapy. *J Neurooncol* 1990;8:275.

90. Boogerd W, van der Sande JJ, Kröger R. Early diagnosis and treatment of spinal epidural metastasis in breast cancer: a prospective study. *J Neurol Neurosurg Psychiatry* 1992;55:1188.

91. Srensen PS, Brgesen SE, Rohde K, et al. Metastatic epidural spinal cord compression: results of treatment and survival. *Cancer* 1990;65:1502.

92. Maranzano E, Latini P, Checcaglini F, et al. Radiation therapy in metastatic spinal cord compression: a prospective analysis of 105 consecutive patients. *Cancer* 1991;67:1311.

93. Maranzano E, Latini P, Checcaglini F, et al. Radiation therapy of spinal cord compression caused by breast cancer: report of a prospective trial. *Int J Radiat Oncol Biol Phys* 1992;24:301.

94. Helweg-Larsen S. Clinical outcome in metastatic spinal cord compression: a prospective study in 153 patients. *Acta Neurol Scand* 1996;94:26.

95. Rades D, Veninga T, Stalpers LJA, et al. Outcome after radiotherapy alone for metastatic spinal cord compression in patients with oligometastases. *J Clin Oncol* 2007;25(1):50.

Chapter 83
Leptomeningeal Metastasis

Rebecca Fisher and Lisa M. DeAngelis

Leptomeningeal metastasis (LM) occurs when tumor spreads to the subarachnoid space and cerebrospinal fluid (CSF) that surround the brain and spinal cord. It may be the sole site of central nervous system (CNS) metastasis or may coexist with brain, dural, or parenchymal spinal cord metastases. LM is an increasingly important neurologic complication of solid tumors in addition to its well-recognized association with hematopoietic malignancies. Enhanced clinical detection with improved neuroimaging and prolonged patient survival with better control of systemic cancer contribute to the increased frequency of LM in patients with solid tumors, particularly breast cancer.

The frequency of LM in clinical series of patients with breast cancer is estimated at 8%; but autopsy series of these patients reveal an incidence of 3% to 40% (1). LM usually coexists with disseminated systemic disease, but it can also occur as an isolated site of relapse. The CNS is being recognized as a sanctuary site for metastatic disease in patients with breast cancer whose systemic tumor has been controlled with effective systemic therapies (2,3). The growing repertoire of active agents to treat breast cancer typically consists of water-soluble drugs that do not penetrate the blood–brain barrier. In addition, P-glycoprotein is highly expressed by brain capillary endothelium and acts as an enzymatic pump, mediating efflux of some active breast cancer chemotherapeutic agents such as anthracyclines, taxanes, and vinca alkaloids (4). These agents can eradicate disease in systemic sites, but if microscopic tumor resides in the CNS, they do not cross the intact blood–brain barrier; thus, these agents allow the CNS tumor to grow, leading to subsequent brain or leptomeningeal metastases. Once CNS tumor reaches a macroscopic size, the blood–brain barrier is typically disrupted, and occasionally systemically administered drugs can be effective against CNS metastases. However, sequestration of microscopic tumor behind an intact blood–brain barrier is likely a major explanation for the rising frequency of brain and leptomeningeal metastases in patients with otherwise well-controlled breast cancer.

Determining the diagnosis of LM is often difficult because the presenting neurologic signs can be confused with other CNS complications of breast cancer. Neuroimaging and laboratory tests aid in establishing the diagnosis but are limited by a lack of sensitivity, specificity, or both. Optimal therapy has not been defined; difficulties of drug distribution in the CSF, intrinsic drug resistance of the metastases, and neurotoxicity are important factors that limit the success of standard therapies. Nevertheless, in some patients, an aggressive approach is rewarding, and prolonged survival is possible. This chapter reviews the clinical presentation of this disorder, the methods of diagnosis, and the recommended therapeutic approaches.

CLINICAL SETTING

CNS metastases in breast cancer have been associated with younger age, premenopausal status, infiltrating ductal histology, estrogen- and progesterone-receptor negativity, aneuploidy, altered p53, and epidermal growth factor receptor (EGFR) overexpression (5). Lobular type breast cancer has a predilection for LM compared to other histologic types of breast cancer. In a study done by Altundag et al. (6), 3.8% of 420 breast cancer patients with CNS metastases had a tumor of lob-ular histologic type, but 31.6% of these patients presented with isolated LM, compared to 7% of all patients in the series.

Recent studies have shown an apparent increase in CNS metastases in women with *ERBB2* (formerly HER2/*neu*) positive breast cancer (6,7). Using magnetic resonance imaging (MRI) or computed tomography (CT), breast cancer patients without known CNS involvement were screened, and *ERBB2* overexpression and an increased number of systemic metastatic sites were predictive of CNS involvement (8). The increased incidence may be multifactorial and includes biologic factors, as well as treatment-related factors: trastuzumab is a monoclonal antibody directed against the *ERBB2* receptor. Due to its high molecular weight, it does not cross the blood–brain barrier. There are conflicting reports of a higher incidence of CNS involvement in patients who received trastuzumab; some studies have documented a 25% to 40% incidence of CNS metastases; however, a study done by Lai et al. (9) found no association between trastuzumab therapy and subsequent CNS metastases. Review of the most current data suggests that trastuzumab does not increase the risk of CNS relapse directly, but rather improves systemic control and overall survival, leading to an unmasking of occult brain metastases that would otherwise remain clinically silent (6,10).

A wide time interval between the diagnosis of breast cancer and the occurrence of LM has been reported; in large series, it ranges from a few weeks to more than 15 years (1). In rare instances, LM is the initial manifestation of breast cancer. Many patients with a solid tumor have widespread metastatic disease when LM is diagnosed, but in patients with breast cancer, the systemic tumor may be inactive or responding to chemotherapy. Of 40 patients with breast cancer with leptomeningeal metastasis reported by Yap et al. (11), the systemic disease was responding or stable in 14 (35%), and there was no evidence of active systemic tumor in 12 (30%); the remainder had concurrent systemic relapse.

PATHOPHYSIOLOGY

The cerebral and spinal meninges are composed of the dura mater, arachnoid, and pia mater. The leptomeninges include the arachnoid and pia mater. The pia mater is a thin lining, closely adherent to the surface of the brain and spinal cord, separated from the arachnoid by fine trabeculae. It follows the sulci of the cerebral cortex and penetrates the parenchyma of the CNS in association with arterioles. The associated parenchymal perivascular space is termed the Virchow-Robin space (Fig. 83.1). Pathologic evidence suggests several methods by which tumor cells reach the leptomeninges:

1. Hematogenous spread to the vessels of the arachnoid or to the choroid plexus of the ventricles (the latter produces dissemination of malignant cells to the leptomeninges by normal CSF flow);
2. Direct extension from adjacent metastasis in the cerebral parenchyma or dura or the lymphatic paraspinal region;
3. Retrograde access to the subarachnoid space by tumor cells infiltrating the venous system from adjacent calvarial or spinal metastases; or
4. Iatrogenic spread after resection of a brain metastasis.

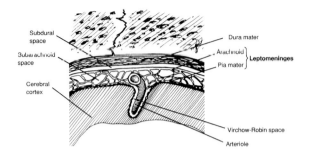

FIGURE 83.1. Relation of the cerebral meninges to the brain.

Tumor dissemination into the CSF after surgical procedures is primarily associated with removal of cerebellar lesions, in which the subsequent development of leptomeningeal disease may be as high as 67% (12).

Autopsy studies demonstrate that leptomeningeal tumor grows in a sheet-like fashion along the surface of the brain, spinal cord, and nerve roots (13). It usually disseminates widely, but it may be limited to portions of the cerebral or spinal leptomeninges. When tumor cells are closely adherent to one another, multifocal nodules may form, particularly on the cauda equina or ventricular surface of the brain. LM is usually accompanied by a fibroblastic proliferation of the meninges. An inflammatory response may be seen pathologically in the leptomeninges, and occasionally reactive lymphocytes accompany malignant cells in a CSF specimen. Tumor may ensheath meningeal arteries and veins within the subarachnoid space and may extend into the Virchow-Robin spaces, with resulting perivascular tumor cuffing and parenchymal invasion. Tumor also may encase or invade the spinal and cranial nerves.

CLINICAL MANIFESTATIONS

The clinical hallmark of LM is the simultaneous occurrence of multifocal abnormalities at more than one level of the neuraxis (cerebral, cranial nerve, and spinal). A careful neurologic examination often reveals more signs than suggested by the clinical symptoms. Spinal symptoms are the most common presentation of LM (Table 83.1), typically limb weakness, usually involving the legs, and may be accompanied by paresthesias and pain in the affected limb. Neurologic examination may

reveal asymmetric depression of deep-tendon reflexes, radicular limb weakness, and sensory loss. Signs of meningeal irritation, such as nuchal rigidity, are rare. The most common finding of cerebral dysfunction is a change in mentation. Seizures occur in fewer than 10% of patients. Cerebral symptoms of LM often result from the obstruction of CSF flow and include headache, changes in mentation (lethargy, confusion, and memory loss), nausea and vomiting, and ataxia. These symptoms often indicate elevated intracranial pressure, which may occur with or without hydrocephalus. The most common cranial nerve symptom is diplopia. Hearing loss, vision loss, and facial numbness also occur. Paresis of the extraocular muscles is the most common cranial nerve abnormality, followed by facial weakness and diminished hearing (1).

METHODS OF DIAGNOSIS

The diagnosis of LM often requires a high index of suspicion. Initial testing may not reveal the diagnosis, and the physician must often resort to a variety of tests combined with clinical findings to establish the diagnosis. Occasionally, a presumptive diagnosis is made and treatment is initiated if the clinical picture is typical, other diagnoses are excluded, and the CSF is abnormal despite a negative CSF cytologic examination (Table 83.2).

Neuroimaging with gadolinium-enhanced MRI should be the first test obtained in a patient with cancer who has new neurologic symptoms. Specific findings on MRI may be sufficient to establish the diagnosis of LM and may eliminate the need for CSF analysis. Neuroimaging is also essential to exclude parenchymal brain (Chapter 81) or spinal epidural lesions (Chapter 82), which may produce a similar clinical picture and may occasionally coexist with LM. Gadolinium-enhanced MRI is the best technique for either cranial or spinal imaging (14). CT may occasionally reveal leptomeningeal tumor, but it is less sensitive and is not useful for spinal imaging unless contrast material has been instilled in the subarachnoid space (15,16).

Definitive imaging findings that establish the diagnosis of LM include:

1. Enhancement of the leptomeninges over the convexities or within the cerebral or cerebellar sulci;
2. Tumor nodules or diffuse enhancement of the brainstem, spinal cord, or cauda equina (Figs. 83.2 and 83.3);
3. Enhancement of the cranial nerves; and
4. Enhancement of the basal cisterns or subependymal area.

Despite the sensitivity of MRI, it is negative in 25% to 30% of patients with positive CSF cytology, but it is negative in only 10% of patients with solid tumors compared with 55% of

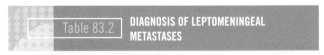 **PRESENTING SYMPTOMS AND SIGNS OF LEPTOMENINGEAL METASTASES** (Table 83.1)	
Symptom or Sign	Percentage
Spinal radiculopathy	48
Cranial nerves	45
III, IV, VI	22
VII	23
Headache	40
Cerebral symptoms or signs	38
Limb weakness	38
Mental change	29
Difficulty walking	26
Cerebellar signs	24
Sensory abnormalities	23
Seizures	6

Modified from Jayson GC, Howell A. Carcinomatous meningitis in solid tumors. *Ann Oncol* 1996;7:773, with permission.

Table 83.2   DIAGNOSIS OF LEPTOMENINGEAL METASTASES

Neuroimaging: magnetic resonance imaging or computed tomography
 Enhancement of cerebrospinal fluid in sulci
 Tumor nodules on cauda equina
 Enhancement of spinal cord surface
 Enhancement of basal cisterns
 Enhancement of ependymal surface
Cerebrospinal fluid
 Positive cytology
 Tumor markers
  CA-15-3
  Carcinoembryonic antigen
Aneusomy by fluorescence *in situ* hybridization

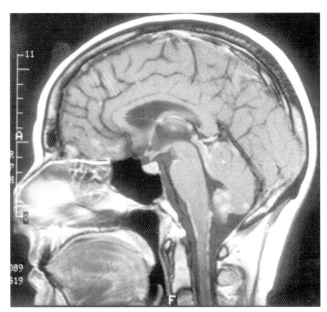

FIGURE 83.2. Leptomeningeal metastases from breast cancer. Sagittal gadolinium-enhanced brain magnetic resonance imaging reveals diffuse linear enhancement of the tectum, ventral and dorsal medulla, and upper cervical cord. Patchy enhancement can also be seen coating the cerebellum and inferior frontal lobe. This image is diagnostic.

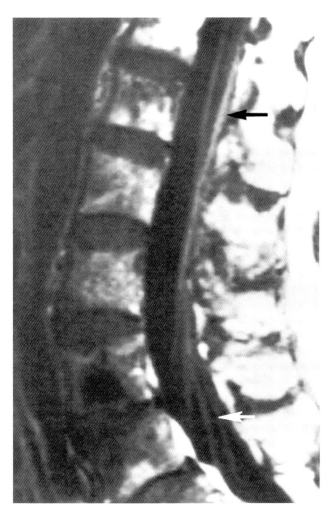

FIGURE 83.3. Sagittal gadolinium-enhanced spine magnetic resonance imaging reveals thickening and linear enhancement of the leptomeninges adjacent to the distal spinal cord (*dark arrow*) and on the lumbosacral nerve roots (*white arrow*).

patients with hematologic malignancies (14–16). Rarely, ^{18}F-florodeoxyglucose (FDG) positron emission tomography (PET) CT may establish a diagnosis of LM (17).

In the absence of diagnostic radiographic abnormalities, other imaging findings that suggest LM include hydrocephalus or small superficial metastases deep in sulci. Patients clinically suspected of having LM need to undergo CSF analysis to establish the diagnosis when neuroimaging is negative or inconclusive. Even definitive radiographic findings in patients not known to have systemic cancer cannot automatically be attributed to metastasis because primary leptomeningeal tumors, infection, postoperative conditions, or even changes after lumbar puncture can mimic subarachnoid metastases. These patients require CSF documentation of malignancy to establish the diagnosis.

The established gold standard to diagnose LM is the demonstration of malignant cells in the CSF, typically obtained by lumbar puncture. Malignant cells are not identified in the CSF of patients with parenchymal, dural, or epidural metastasis, and they indicate metastasis to the subarachnoid space (18). The initial lumbar CSF cytologic examination gives positive results in up to 50% of patients with LM, but the yield increases to 90% if three lumbar punctures are performed (1). The detection of malignant cells can increase when larger volumes (>10 cc) of CSF are available for analysis and occasionally when a CSF sample is taken from an alternate site; examination of cisternal CSF can be more sensitive, particularly in those patients with cerebral or cranial nerve symptoms (1). The failure to detect malignant cells in the CSF may be a sampling error because tumor cells are not equally distributed throughout the CSF due to adherence of the cells to CNS structures, or it may indicate that the tumor is localized. In an autopsy study of 30 patients with LM, Glass et al. (18) found a positive CSF cytologic evaluation in 76% of patients with multifocal or disseminated LM, but in only 58% of those with focal disease.

Newer technologies have been used to improve detection of malignant cells in the CSF, including monoclonal antibodies for immunohistochemical analysis, flow cytometry, which measures the chromosomal content of cells, fluorescence *in situ* hybridization (FISH), which detects aneusomy of chromosome 1, and polymerase chain reaction (PCR) in which genetic alterations of the tumor cells are used for amplification (19). FISH of chromosome 1 is most likely to be helpful in patients with solid tumors, whereas the other techniques are usually more effective in patients with hematopoietic malignancies.

Despite these modern techniques, approximately 5% to 10% of patients with LM do not have detectable malignant cells in their CSF. If CSF results are repeatedly negative and pathologic confirmation is required, leptomeningeal biopsy may be performed for definitive diagnosis, but it can also give a false-negative because the disease is not evenly distributed.

The CSF of most patients with LM has abnormalities of the routine chemistries and white blood cell count (1). An elevated protein concentration is the most common abnormality but is usually less than 100 mg/dL; there is a normal gradient of protein along the CSF axis, and a normal ventricular CSF protein concentration is less than 20 mg/dL. Up to one-half of patients have pleocytosis, usually mononuclear. About one-third of patients have a low CSF glucose concentration, defined as less than 70% of a simultaneous serum glucose concentration. Elevation of β-glucuronidase, total lactic acid dehydrogenase (LDH) or the percentage of the LDH-5 isoenzyme, and β_2-microglobulin can be indirect indicators of LM. However, these biomarkers are nonspecific and may be elevated in infections and other disorders of the CNS (20,21). Carcinoembryonic antigen (CEA) and the breast cancer antigen (CA15-3) are elevated in the CSF of some patients with breast cancer (22), but the CSF levels must be compared with serum concentrations because extremely elevated serum levels can cross the blood–brain barrier and be detected in the CSF. Like CSF protein levels, tumor marker values are lower in the ventricular than lumbar CSF, thus making interpretation from this region difficult.

Other CSF markers reported to aid in the diagnosis of LM include telomerase (23), glucosephosphate isomerase (24), creatine kinase BB isoenzyme (25), and tissue polypeptide antigen (26); none are specific for breast cancer.

Occasionally a combination of markers can be useful. One study found vascular endothelial growth factor (VEGF) concentrations increased, and tissue plasminogen activator (tPA) concentrations decreased; combining these two markers predicted leptomeningeal disease with 100% sensitivity. There was, however, a false-positive rate up to 27% (27).

CSF protein profiles of soluble adhesion molecules, cytokines, and chemokines have been used to discriminate between LM and other processes (28). Mass spectrometry–based methods have looked at protein expression patterns in CSF from breast cancer patients with and without LM and have found reproducible peptide profiles that might assist in diagnosing LM (29).

CSF is usually sampled in patients suspected of LM to establish the diagnosis with the demonstration of malignant cells. However, lumbar puncture may be necessary to measure the intracranial pressure. Headache, nausea, vomiting, and lethargy may be clinical indicators of increased intracranial pressure in patients with LM. Plateau waves, which are marked increases in intracranial pressure often triggered by a change in body position, may be manifest as transient decreased consciousness, visual disturbances, or gait difficulties; they are often confused with seizures because of their brief duration. Elevated intracranial pressure may be a consequence of hydrocephalus resulting from impairment of CSF flow. Hydrocephalus is almost always communicating in this situation and is easily diagnosed on cranial imaging. However, marked elevation of intracranial pressure can occur in patients with LM in the *absence* of hydrocephalus. These patients may have normal or small-appearing ventricles on MRI or CT scans. In these patients, lumbar puncture is needed to measure the elevated intracranial pressure. Elevated intracranial pressure requires specific therapeutic intervention and is an absolute contraindication to intrathecal chemotherapy until the condition is corrected (discussed below). Failure to diagnose increased intracranial pressure is a common mistake in the management of patients with LM and can be the cause of persistent neurologic symptoms, failure to respond to treatment, and treatment-related neurotoxicity.

TREATMENT

Vigorous treatment of LM can improve neurologic function and prevent further deterioration; however, sustained remissions are rare, and patients usually succumb to their neurologic disease. Two categories of treatment can be considered: symptomatic and definitive. Symptomatic treatment may include anticonvulsants for those who have had a seizure, and pain medication to relieve painful radiculopathies. Corticosteroids are usually ineffective in treating LM because there is little edema in the underlying CNS parenchyma. Consequently, glucocorticoids rarely improve neurologic function in patients with LM the way they do in patients with brain metastasis. However, steroids can rapidly ameliorate symptoms associated with raised intracranial pressure. Definitive treatment is directed against the cancer and often involves radiotherapy plus chemotherapy, intrathecal or systemic.

All patients with LM should undergo enhanced MRI of the entire neuraxis to search for bulky disease. Radiation should be administered to symptomatic areas (i.e., cranial irradiation for

cranial neuropathies), whether or not structural disease is identified on imaging, and to bulky disease because radiotherapy is usually the most effective modality for treating focal LM nodules. It is also the most reliable modality for the relief of symptoms, especially pain.

Bulky tumor deposits impair CSF flow and cause an accumulation of drug proximal to the flow obstruction; focal radiotherapy can occasionally restore normal CSF dynamics (30). The use of complete neuraxis radiotherapy is discouraged because it does not control the disease and is associated with acute morbidities such as esophagitis and severe myelosuppression, particularly in patients who are heavily pretreated or who are receiving systemic chemotherapy. Whole brain radiotherapy can enhance the neurotoxicity of chemotherapy administered into the CSF and should be used only when the patient has symptoms from the brain or cranial nerves or when cranial CSF flow is obstructed. Intrathecal chemotherapy should not be administered concurrently with whole brain radiotherapy to reduce the risk of neurotoxicity. Radiotherapy is effective at treating a region of LM, but the process involves the entire neuraxis, and therefore treatment must encompass the whole subarachnoid space. Chemotherapy is often used to accomplish this.

Bulky leptomeningeal tumor develops its own vascular supply which has a disrupted blood–brain barrier. Therefore, intravenous chemotherapy may reach an enhancing subarachnoid nodule, but most systemic drugs do not achieve sufficiently high levels in the CSF and cannot eradicate tumor cells floating in the CSF or clusters less than 1 mm thick that do not generate their own blood vessels. For this reason, chemotherapy has been administered directly into the CSF. Direct CSF instillation achieves a higher concentration of drug in the subarachnoid space because the initial volume of distribution is smaller than the vascular compartment and the clearance half-life is longer in the spinal fluid for some agents (31). In addition, intra-CSF instillation often reduces or spares systemic toxicity, although the CSF can act as a reservoir for some drugs, such as methotrexate, that can slowly leak into the peripheral circulation and cause mucositis and myelosuppression. A disadvantage of chemotherapy administration into the CSF is the frequent occurrence of CSF flow abnormalities, which may result in nonuniform distribution of the drug throughout the CSF pathways, thereby reducing efficacy and increasing local toxicity, particularly at the skull base; flow obstruction can cause drug instilled in the ventricle to penetrate slowly into the periventricular tissue and cause leukoencephalopathy (30, 32–34). Moreover, intra-CSF chemotherapy does not penetrate into bulky tumor deposits of infiltrated roots or cranial nerves and therefore cannot treat nodular disease effectively.

Despite these limitations, there is still a role for intrathecal chemotherapy, particularly in patients with minimal bulky disease. However, there must be normal CSF flow before the drug is instilled. Radionuclide CSF flow studies using indium should be performed prior to intrathecal chemotherapy administration because they often demonstrate abnormalities of CSF dynamics that result in compartmentalization of CSF pathways (30, 32,33). CSF flow abnormalities usually correlate with bulky disease identified by neuroimaging, and flow disruption should be presumed in these patients. However, impaired CSF flow can be present despite normal neuroimaging. Areas of bulky tumor that cause CSF flow impairment may respond to involved-field radiotherapy that can restore normal CSF flow and can thus permit normal distribution of intra-CSF chemotherapy throughout the subarachnoid space.

Intra-CSF chemotherapy can be instilled directly into the lumbar subarachnoid space or the ventricular system through an Ommaya reservoir. Intraventricular administration is recommended because this approach ensures delivery of drug into the CSF and allows for simple repetitive administration. Lumbar punctures result in inadvertent epidural or subdural injection in 10% of procedures. Most important, delivery of drug into the ventricular system ensures more reliable and uniform drug distribution (35). Three agents are routinely instilled into the CSF: methotrexate, thiotepa, and cytarabine (including liposomal cytarabine, or DepoCyt). Only methotrexate and thiotepa have intrinsic activity against breast cancer. Intra-CSF administration of methotrexate usually is performed twice a week initially, and the frequency is gradually tapered. The dose is fixed at 12 to 15 mg because the volume of CSF is identical for all patients regardless of size.

Continuous intrathecal administration of methotrexate via a subcutaneous port delivering 10 mg over 5 consecutive days achieved a more stable CSF drug concentration, avoided peak concentrations, and reduced complications (36).

Intra-CSF thiotepa has been studied in patients with LM from solid tumors, including breast carcinoma. The dosage is usually 10 mg and is administered twice weekly initially. The frequency is decreased over 1 to 3 months. In a comparative randomized study of intraventricular methotrexate versus thiotepa in 52 patients with solid tumors, 25 of whom had breast carcinoma, Grossman et al. (37) found a slight survival advantage with methotrexate. Thiotepa has a rapid half-life in the CSF that may limit its effectiveness. No evidence shows that combination intra-CSF chemotherapy is better than single-agent therapy, and toxicity is additive (38,39).

DepoCyt is a sustained-release form of cytarabine that maintains cytotoxic levels in the CSF for 10 days or more. The dose is administered at 50 mg twice monthly, and then is decreased to monthly treatments. Adverse side effects include arachnoiditis and headaches, which can be severe (19). All patients must be treated with dexamethasone 4 mg twice a day beginning 2 days prior and continuing at least 2 days following each dose of DepoCyt. In an open label trial of DepoCyt, 110 patients, 34% with breast cancer, had a response rate comparable to twice weekly methotrexate. An increased time to neurological progression was seen, favoring DepoCyt; this may be due to prolonged tumor exposure to cytotoxic concentrations of cytarabine (40).

Areas of investigation include tumor selective radioimmunotherapy, including intrathecal iodine-labeled monoclonal antibodies; these targeted therapies may inhibit leptomeningeal tumor growth, but none have been developed specifically for breast cancer (41). Yang et al. (42) examined the potential role of reovirus in breast cancer treatment. Breast cancer cell lines are susceptible to reovirus, a naturally occurring virus that usurps the activated RAS-signaling pathway of tumor cells; cell lysis occurs following infection. In experimental animals, intrathecal administration caused mild local inflammation and communicating hydrocephalus. Intratumoral administration reduced tumor size and prolonged survival.

Other agents being explored for intrathecal administration include mafosfamide, diaziquone, topotecan, and immunotherapy using interleukin-2 and interferon alfa (19). A single patient with HER2 overexpressing breast cancer and LM was treated with 5 mg of intrathecal trastuzumab, followed by gradual dose escalation to 20 mg. She did well for 11 months until disease progression (43), and the treatment was well tolerated.

An increasingly important approach to the treatment of LM is the use of systemic drugs, which are either lipophilic and can penetrate the subarachnoid space or are administered in high doses to reach the leptomeninges (44–46). This approach has the benefits of reaching the entire CSF, regardless of CSF flow dynamics, and treating both bulky and microscopic disease. However, it can subject patients to the systemic toxicities of chemotherapy. High-dose methotrexate is the best-studied agent and was reported to give a median survival of 13.8 months, far superior to standard intrathecal chemotherapy with a median survival of only 2.3 months (44). This study included only one patient with breast cancer.

Lassman et al. (47) studied high-dose methotrexate at 3.5 g/m^2 in 32 patients with or without radiotherapy and intrathecal chemotherapy, 29 of whom had breast cancer. Patients had recurrent parenchymal or leptomeningeal metastases. An objective response or stable disease was seen in nine patients (28%), and median overall survival was 19.9 weeks with one patient alive more than 135 weeks; most of these patients had breast cancer and LM with or without brain metastases and had stable or improved disease, with reasonable toxicity. Treatment with higher doses of methotrexate (8g/m^2) has been associated with 84% cytologic clearing of CSF and survival of 23.7 weeks (44).

Capecitabine, an oral analog of 5-flurorouracil (5-FU), has been effective despite limited penetration of 5-FU into the CNS. In one study, patients with parenchymal or LM received 1,000 mg/m^2 twice daily for 14 days in a 21-day treatment cycle; 43% of patients had a complete response and 43% had stable disease. Treatment was well tolerated, with no observed neurological toxicity. Median overall survival was 13 months, with a median of 8-month progression-free survival (48).

Hormonal manipulation can be effective occasionally; letrozole is a nonsteroidal aromatase inhibitor that reduces estrogen synthesis. In one case report, a woman with lobular carcinoma and LM was treated with letrozole 2.5 mg per day. Within the first 2 months of treatment, she had resolution of her neurological symptoms including dizziness, headaches, and diplopia. Treatment was stopped after 16 months due to non-CNS disease recurrence (49).

Elevated intracranial pressure can occasionally be corrected with whole brain radiotherapy, but usually antitumor treatment cannot restore adequate CSF dynamics to normalize intracranial pressure. Many of these patients must be treated with a ventriculoperitoneal (VP) shunt to correct the elevated pressure. Omuro et al. (50) looked at 640 patients with LM and 6% had VP shunt placement; 62% of these patients had breast cancer. After VP shunt placement, 77% had improvement of their symptoms with decreased headache, nausea and vomiting, and improved level of alertness. Three patients had shunt malfunction, and one developed a subdural hematoma. No deaths were attributed to complications of the procedure.

Placement of a VP shunt can be lifesaving, however, it can complicate subsequent treatment for LM, particularly involving the administration of intrathecal chemotherapy. A subcutaneous reservoir with an on-off device may be placed in series with the shunt valve, but these devices often function poorly. The newer programmable shunts can be opened and closed easily, but they are programmed with an external magnet, and each time the patient has an MRI scan, the shunt must be reprogrammed to ensure flow through the shunt. Alternatively, when a shunt is in place, intra-CSF chemotherapy can be administered by lumbar puncture, but it will not reach the entire CSF compartment. In patients with a shunt, systemic chemotherapy may be a better option because it does not require normal CSF flow to distribute the agent throughout the subarachnoid space.

PROGNOSIS

Response criteria in LM are not standardized. Most reported studies define complete response as the normalization of CSF and improvement of clinical symptoms. Sixty percent to 80% of patients show response after intra-CSF methotrexate, with or without radiation (11,51). Response may be durable, even if only a partial response is obtained (52).

The median survival in patients with untreated LM is 6 weeks to 2 months (1). There are conflicting data regarding the efficacy of intrathecal or systemic chemotherapy or radiotherapy in the treatment of LM. Of solid tumors, breast cancer responds best to treatment with a median survival of 6 months, and 15% of patients survive more than 1 year. Other reports also suggest that a patient's clinical condition is a greater determinant of outcome than the use of intrathecal chemotherapy (53). Early diagnosis and treatment may improve outcome (19).

Systemic and intrathecal chemotherapy are the only treatment modalities shown to improve survival in LM when compared to spinal and whole brain radiotherapy (54). However, RT relieves symptoms more effectively. Methotrexate seems to provide an improved survival compared with no therapy in most studies, with a median survival ranging from 3 months to 6 months (11,35,55) and a median survival of 15 months in those who respond (11,51). Boogerd et al. (56) randomized 35 patients to receive appropriate systemic therapy and radiotherapy to clinically relevant sites, with or without intrathecal methotrexate. Patients who received intrathecal chemotherapy did not have additional survival benefit or improved neurological response, but did have an increased risk of neurotoxicity.

 ## TOXICITY

Toxicity from treatment of LM is primarily neurologic, and systemic toxicities arise primarily from systemic chemotherapy, typically myelosuppression. Systemic complications of intrathecal methotrexate include stomatitis and myelosuppression. Low-dose oral leucovorin protects against these toxicities in patients receiving intrathecal methotrexate, and the authors typically administer 10 mg of leucovorin twice daily for eight doses to all patients receiving intrathecal methotrexate. Intra-CSF thiotepa can cause myelosuppression, particularly when concurrent systemic chemotherapy is administered.

Spinal radiotherapy can contribute to depressed bone marrow function, particularly if the patient is heavily pretreated or receiving concurrent systemic therapy. Mucositis can also occur with radiotherapy to the cervical or upper thoracic region. Fatigue is almost universal and can be exacerbated by any of the treatment modalities used against LM.

Neurotoxicity after irradiation of the nervous system, or after intra-CSF or systemic chemotherapy, is a significant obstacle to treating patients with LM aggressively. The most common neurologic complication of intra-CSF chemotherapy is transient aseptic meningitis, which develops within hours of injection and produces headache, fever, stiff neck, and confusion. It does not necessarily recur on subsequent injections, and corticosteroids can prevent or ameliorate the reaction (1). Intra-CSF methotrexate causes leukoencephalopathy, but any drug instilled into the subarachnoid space can cause neurotoxicity. The risk of leukoencephalopathy rises with increasing total methotrexate dose, prolonged CSF methotrexate levels, and concurrent cranial radiotherapy (57,58). Leukoencephalopathy can often be identified first on cranial MRI in which increased signal, predominantly in the periventricular white matter, can be seen on T2-weighted or fluid-attenuated inversion recovery (FLAIR) images (Fig. 83.4). Patients develop apathy, memory loss, gait disturbance, and, later, urinary incontinence. Clinical abnormalities correlate loosely with the severity of changes seen radiographically. Focal leukoencephalopathy can result from high local cerebral concentrations of methotrexate around an Ommaya reservoir catheter, particularly if inadvertent separation of the catheter occurs or if intraventricular pressure is elevated (53,59). Clinically significant complications related to the Ommaya reservoir are uncommon but include infection of the reservoir, bacterial meningitis, and intracerebral hemorrhage (60). Any drug can also cause myelopathy after lumbar injection (61).

If neurologic decline occurs, treatment-related toxicity must be distinguished from progressive leptomeningeal tumor. If the

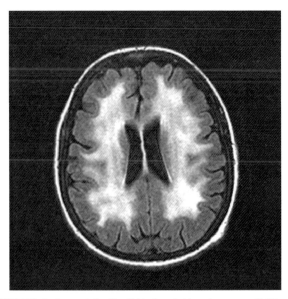

FUGURE 83.4. Leukoencephalopathy. Fluid-attenuated inversion recovery (FLAIR) magnetic resonance image of a patient with breast cancer treated with intrathecal methotrexate only for leptomeningeal metastasis. There is extensive white matter hyperintensity that is bilateral and symmetric. She had no cognitive impairment.

latter occurs, the chemotherapy agent should be changed, radiation administered to bulky areas, or both. Patients must also be monitored for progression of their systemic disease, although in large series (1), most patients with breast cancer died of progressive leptomeningeal disease.

 ## MANAGEMENT SUMMARY

- Leptomeningeal metastasis is an increasingly common complication of breast cancer.
- Early diagnosis is important before the patient develops severe neurologic deficits that cannot be reversed with treatment.
- Diagnosis can be established by the demonstration of tumor nodules or enhancing disease in the subarachnoid space on MRI or the finding of tumor cells in the CSF.
- Treatment usually requires focal radiotherapy to symptomatic sites or areas with bulky disease followed by chemotherapy.
- The optimal choice of chemotherapy depends on a thorough assessment of the neurologic extent of disease. Patients with multiple nodules may be treated best with systemic chemotherapy, whereas those with positive CSF cytology, but negative imaging, can be treated well with intra-CSF chemotherapy alone and thus spared the toxicity of systemic intravenous drug administration. Intrathecal methotrexate, thiotepa, and cytarabine have all been reported to have some efficacy.
- Despite treatment, most patients do poorly, and the median survival is about to 4 to 6 months although some survive for years with vigorous treatment.

References

1. Posner JB. *Neurologic Complications of Cancer.* New York: Oxford University Press, 1995.
2. Freilich RJ, Seidman AD, DeAngelis LM. Central nervous system progression of metastatic breast cancer in patients treated with paclitaxel. *Cancer* 1995;76:232.

3. Kosmas C, Malamos NA, Tsavaris N, et al. Chemotherapy-induced complete regression of choroidal metastases and subsequent isolated leptomeningeal carcinomatosis in advanced breast cancer: a case report and literature review. *J Neurooncol* 2000;47:161.

4. Lin N, Bellon JR, Winer EP. CNS metastases in breast cancer. *J Clin Oncol* 2004;22:3608–3617.

5. Tham YL, Sexton K, Kramer R, et al. Primary breast cancer phenotypes associated with propensity for central nervous system metastases. *Cancer* 2006;107:696–704.

6. Altundag K, Bondy M, Mirza N, et al. Clinicopathologic characteristics and prognostic factors in 420 metastatic breast cancer patients with central nervous system metastasis. *Cancer* 2007;110:2640–2647.

7. Duchnowska R, Szczylik C. Central nervous system metastases in breast cancer patients administered trastuzumab. *Cancer Treat Rev* 2005;31:312–318.

8. Miller KD, Weather T, Haney LG, et al. Occult central nervous system involvement in patients with metastatic breast cancer: prevalence, predictive factors and impact on overall survival. *Ann Oncol* 2003;14:1072–1077.

9. Lai R, Dang CT, Malkin MG, et al. The risk of central nervous system metastases after trastuzumab therapy in patients with breast carcinoma. *Cancer* 2004;101:810–816.

10. Lin NU, Winer EP. Brain metastases: the HER2 paradigm. *Clin Cancer Res* 2007;13:1648–1655.

11. Yap HY, Yap BS, Rasmussen S, et al. Treatment for meningeal carcinomatosis in breast cancer. *Cancer* 1982;49:219.

12. van der Ree TC, Dippel DW, Avezaat CJ, et al. Leptomeningeal metastasis after surgical resection of brain metastases. *J Neurol Neurosurg Psychiatry* 1999;66:225.

13. Olson ME, Chernik NL, Posner JB. Infiltration of the leptomeninges by systemic cancer. *Arch Neurol* 1974;30:122.

14. Freilich RJ, Krol G, DeAngelis LM. Neuroimaging and cerebrospinal fluid cytology in the diagnosis of leptomeningeal metastasis. *Ann Neurol* 1995;38:51.

15. Chamberlain MC, Sandy AD, Press GA. Leptomeningeal metastasis: a comparison of gadolinium-enhanced MR and contrast-enhanced CT of the brain. *Neurology* 1990;40:435.

16. Sze G, Soletsky S, Bronen R, et al. MR imaging of the cranial meninges with emphasis on contrast enhancement and meningeal carcinomatosis. *AJNR* 1989;10:965.

17. Shah S, Rangarajan V, Purandare N, et al. ^{18}F-FDG uptakes in leptomeningeal metastases from carcinoma of the breast on a positron emission tomography/computerized tomography study. *Indian J Cancer* 2007;44:115–118.

18. Glass JP, Melamed M, Chernik NL, et al. Malignant cells in cerebrospinal fluid (CSF): the meaning of a positive CSF cytology. *Neurology* 1979;29:1369.

19. Chamberlain M. Neoplastic meningitis. *Neurologist* 2006;12:179–187.

20. Twijnstra A, van Zanten AP, Hart AAM, et al. Serial lumbar and ventricle cerebrospinal fluid lactate dehydrogenase activities in patients with leptomeningeal metastases from solid and haematological tumors. *J Neurol Neurosurg Psychiatry* 1987;50:313.

21. Twijnstra A, van Zanten AP, Nooyen WJ, et al. Cerebrospinal fluid beta-2-microglobulin: a study in controls and patients with metastatic and non-metastatic neurological diseases. *Eur J Cancer Clin Oncol* 1986;22:387.

22. Twijnstra A, Nooyen WJ, van Zanten AP, et al. Cerebrospinal fluid carcinoembryonic antigen in patients with metastatic and nonmetastatic neurological diseases. *Arch Neurol* 1986;43:269.

23. DeAngelis LM, Posner JB. Telomerase activity in brain and leptomeningeal metastases. *J Neurol Sci* 1998;161:114.

24. Newton HB, Fleisher M, Schwartz MK, et al. Glucosephosphate isomerase as a CSF marker for leptomeningeal metastasis. *Neurology* 1991;41:395.

25. Bach F, Bjerregaard B, Soletormos G, et al. Diagnostic value of cerebrospinal fluid cytology in comparison with tumor marker activity in central nervous system metastases secondary to breast cancer. *Cancer* 1993;72:2376.

26. Bach F, Soletormos G, Dombernowsky P. Tissue polypeptide antigen activity in cerebrospinal fluid: a marker of central nervous system metastases of breast cancer. *J Natl Cancer Inst* 1991;83:779.

27. Van de Langerijt B, Gijtenbeek JM, de Reus HPM, et al. CSF levels of growth factors and plasminogen activators in leptomeningeal metastases. *Neurology* 2006;67:114–119.

28. Brandsma D, Voest EE, de Jager W, et al. CSF protein profiling using multiplex immuno-assay: a potential new diagnostic tool for leptomeningeal metastases. *J Neurol* 2006;253:1177–1184.

29. Dekker LJ, Boogerd W, Tockhammer G, et al. MALDI-TOF mass spectrometry analysis of cerebrospinal fluid tryptic peptide profiles to diagnose leptomeningeal metastases in patients with breast cancer. *Mol Cell Proteomics* 2005;4:1341–1349.

30. Mason WP, Yeh SDJ, DeAngelis LM. Indium-diethylenetriamine pentaacetic acid cerebrospinal fluid flow studies predict distribution of intrathecally administered chemotherapy and outcome in patients with leptomeningeal metastases. *Neurology* 1998;50:438.

31. Poplack DG, Bleyer WA, Horowitz ME. Pharmacology of antineoplastic agents in cerebrospinal fluid. In: Wood JH, ed. *Neurobiology of Cerebrospinal Fluid.* New York: Plenum, 1980:561.

32. Chamberlain MC, Corey-Bloom J. Leptomeningeal metastasis: 111 indium-DTPA CSF flow studies. *Neurology* 1991;41:1765.

33. Grossman SA, Trump DL, Chen DCP, et al. Cerebrospinal fluid flow abnormalities in patients with neoplastic meningitis. *Am J Med* 1982;73:641.

34. Glantz MJ, Hall Wa, Cole BF, et al. Diagnosis, management, and survival of patients with leptomeningeal cancer based on cerebrospinal fluid-flow status. *Cancer* 1995;75:2919.

35. Shapiro WR, Young DF, Mehta BM. Methotrexate: distribution in cerebrospinal fluid after intravenous, ventricular and lumbar injections. *N Engl J Med* 1975;293:161.

36. Shinoura N, Tabei Y, Yamada R, et al. Continuous intrathecal treatment with methotrexate via subcutaneous port: implication for leptomeningeal dissemination of malignant tumors. *J Neurooncol* 2008;87(3):309–316.

37. Grossman SA, Finkelstein DM, Ruckdeschel JC, et al. Randomized prospective comparison of intraventricular methotrexate and thiotepa in patients with previously untreated neoplastic meningitis. *J Clin Oncol* 1993;11:561.

38. Giannone L, Greco FA, Hainsworth JD. Combination intraventricular chemotherapy for meningeal neoplasia. *J Clin Oncol* 1986;4:68.

39. Trump DL, Grossman SA, Thompson G, et al. Treatment of neoplastic meningitis with intraventricular thiotepa and methotrexate. *Cancer Treat Rep* 1982;66:1599.

40. Jaeckle KA, Batchelor T, O'Day SJ, et al. An open label trial of sustained-release cytarabine (DepoCyt) for the intrathecal treatment of solid tumor neoplastic meningitis. *J Neurooncol* 2002;57:231.

41. Kramer K, Humm JL, Souweidane MM, et al. Phase I study of targeted radioimmunotherapy for leptomeningeal cancers using intra-Ommaya 131-I-3F8. *J Clin Oncol* 2007;25:5465–5470.

42. Yang WQ, Senger DL, Lun XQ, et al. Reovirus as an experimental therapeutic for brain and leptomeningeal metastases from breast cancer. *Gene Ther* 2004;11:1579–1589.

43. Stemmler HJ, Schmitt M, Harbeck N, et al. Application of intrathecal trastuzumab for treatment of meningeal carcinomatosis in HER2 overexpressing metastatic breast cancer. *Oncol Rep* 2006;15:1373–1377.

44. Glantz MJ, Cole BF, Recht L, et al. High-dose intravenous methotrexate for patients with nonleukemic leptomeningeal cancer: is intrathecal chemotherapy necessary? *J Clin Oncol* 1998;16:1561.

45. Grant R, Naylor B, Greenberg HS, et al. Clinical outcome in aggressively treated meningeal carcinomatosis. *Arch Neurol* 1994;51:457.

46. Tetef ML, Margolin KA, Doroshow JH, et al. Pharmacokinetics and toxicity of high-dose intravenous methotrexate in the treatment of leptomeningeal carcinomatosis. *Cancer Chemother Pharmacol* 2000;46:19.

47. Lassman A, Abrey LE, Shah GG, et al. Systemic high-dose intravenous methotrexate for central nervous system metastases. *J Neurooncol* 2006;78:255–260.

48. Ekenel M, Hormigo AM, Peak S, et al. Capecitabine therapy of central nervous system metastases from breast cancer. *J Neurooncol* 2007;85:223–227.

49. Ozdogan M, Samur M, Bozcuk H, et al. Durable remission of leptomeningeal metastasis of breast cancer with letrozole: a case report and implications of biomarkers on treatment selection. *Jpn J Clin Oncol* 2003;33:229–231.

50. Omuro AMP, Lallana EC, Bilsky MH, et al. Ventriculoperitoneal shunt in patients with leptomeningeal metastasis. *Neurology* 2005;64:1625–1627.

51. Ongerboer de Visser BW, Somers R, Nooyen WH, et al. Intraventricular methotrexate therapy of leptomeningeal metastasis from breast carcinoma. *Neurology* 1983;33:1565.

52. Siegal T, Lossos A, Pfeffer MR. Leptomeningeal metastasis: analysis of 31 patients with sustained off-therapy response following combined-modality therapy. *Neurology* 1994;44:1463.

53. de Waal R, Algra PR, Heimans JJ, et al. Methotrexate induced brain necrosis and severe leukoencephalopathy due to disconnection of an Ommaya device. *J Neurooncol* 1993;15:269.

54. Rudnicka H, Niwinska A, Murawska M. Breast cancer leptomeningeal metastasis—the role of multimodality treatment. *J Neurooncol* 2007;84:57–62.

55. Fizazi K, Asselain B, Vincent-Salomon A, et al. Meningeal carcinomatosis in patients with breast carcinoma. *Cancer* 1996;77:1315.

56. Boogerd W, van den Bent MJ, Koehler PJ, et al. The relevance of intraventricular chemotherapy for leptomeningeal metastasis in breast cancer: a randomized study. *Eur J Cancer* 2004;40:2726–2733.

57. Bleyer WA. Neurological sequelae of methotrexate and ionizing radiation: a new classification. *Cancer Treat Rep* 1981;65:89.

58. Shapiro WR, Chernik NL, Posner JB. Necrotizing encephalopathy following intraventricular instillation of methotrexate. *Arch Neurol* 1973;28:96.

59. Lemann W, Wiley RG, Posner JB. Leukoencephalopathy complicating intraventricular catheters: clinical, radiographic and pathologic study of 10 cases. *J Neurooncol* 1988;6:77.

60. Sandberg DI, Bilsky MH, Souweidane MM, et al. Ommaya reservoirs for the treatment of leptomeningeal metastases. *Neurosurgery* 2000;47:49.

61. Hahn AF, Feasby TE, Gilbert JJ. Paraparesis following intrathecal chemotherapy. *Neurology* 1983;33:1032.

Nathan I. Cherny and Oded Olsha

In patients with cancer, symptoms and signs of brachial plexus injury may be attributable to acute brachial neuritis, trauma to the plexus during surgery or anesthesia, metastatic spread of tumor, transient or permanent radiation injury, or radiation-induced tumors. In patients with breast cancer, metastatic spread of tumor, radiation injury to the plexus, and second primaries are the most common causes of such signs. Careful evaluation of the clinical history, symptoms and signs, as well as electrodiagnostic and imaging studies are helpful in diagnosing the cause of a brachial plexopathy.

TUMOR INFILTRATION OF THE BRACHIAL PLEXUS (METASTATIC BRACHIAL PLEXOPATHY)

Despite the proximity to the draining axillary lymph nodes, tumor infiltration of the plexus remains relatively uncommon (1). Even among specialist consultation services in a major cancer center this diagnosis represented only 5% of the neurologic consultations evaluated by the neurology consultation service (2) and 4% of patients referred to a cancer pain service (3). Early and accurate diagnosis is critical in preventing irreversible nerve damage and chronic neuropathic pain and in determining the prognosis and treatment of the tumor.

Clinical Symptoms and Signs

Pain

Eighty-five percent of patients with tumor infiltration present with pain that is moderate to severe, often preceding neurologic signs or symptoms for up to 9 months (4–8). The pain distribution depends on the site of plexus involvement. Typically the pain radiates in the sensory distribution of the lower plexus, usually involving the shoulder girdle and radiating to the elbow, medial side to the forearm, and the fourth and fifth fingers (consistent with involvement of the lower plexus C7,C8,T1) (4–6).

Other less common clinical presentations are occasionally observed including pain localized to the posterior aspect of the arm or to the elbow, a burning or freezing sensation and hypersensitivity of the skin along the ulnar aspect of the arm, or pain referred to either the shoulder girdle or the tip of either the index finger or thumb (consistent with infiltration of the upper plexus C5-6 by tumor rising in the supraclavicular nodes).

By the time of diagnosis of a brachial plexus lesion, 98% of patients have pain that is most often reported as severe. In the series by Kori et al. (4) 2 of 78 patients with malignant brachial plexopathy had pain as the only symptom or sign of tumor recurrence and required exploration and biopsy of the plexus to establish the diagnosis.

Parasthsesias

Paresthesias occur as a presenting symptom in 15% of patients with tumor, in an ulnar distribution from infiltration of the lower plexus, or with a median nerve distribution in lesions of the upper plexus.

Lymphedema

Lymphedema is rarely a presenting symptom of tumor infiltration of the brachial plexus (4,5), but it does occur in about 10% of patients, most often in patients who have had previous radiation therapy to the plexus and who subsequently develop recurrent tumor.

Weakness

Focal weakness, atrophy, and sensory changes in the distribution of the C7, C8, and T1 roots occur in more than 75% of patients. In one series of patients with brachial plexopathy arising from any tumor type, 25% of patients presented with whole-plexus motor weakness (panplexopathy) (4).

Horner's Syndrome

Patients with a panplexopathy or Horner's syndrome have a higher likelihood of epidural extension and should undergo imaging of the epidural space as part of their evaluation.

Palpable Masses

Careful physical examination commonly reveals palpable supraclavicular or axillary lymphadenopathy. Occasionally, tumor infiltration in the distal plexus is associated with a palpable mass or fullness in the clavipectoral triangle. In all cases, these areas need careful evaluation.

Relation to Natural History

In 12 of 78 patients with tumor infiltration of the brachial plexus included in the Kori et al. (4) series, the plexus lesion was the only evidence of tumor, and other metastases appeared only after several months. In two patients, the plexus lesion was the only sign of recurrence for 4 years. In one patient, surgical exploration after 2 years of plexopathy signs proved to be normal, but because of progressive worsening of neurologic signs, a second exploration was carried out, confirming tumor recurrence.

RADIATION INJURY TO THE BRACHIAL PLEXUS

Pathophysiology of Radiation Injury

Sensitivity to a given dose of radiation is dependent on several factors, including age, the radiation dose, the size of the port, and especially, the premorbid state of the irradiated nerve (9). Although very little of the plexus is usually exposed in a chest wall port, radiation to the supraclavicular, infraclavicular, or axillary nodes do expose substantial portions of the plexus to the potential for radiation damage (10).

In cases of radiation injury to the brachial plexus, the predominant findings are in the upper plexus. This is because the divisions of the lower trunk run a shorter course through standard ports and are partially protected by the clavicle.

There are three possible types of peripheral nerve damage after radiation therapy (11):

1. A very high dose of radiation may cause severe vascular damage to the blood vessels that supply a segment of a nerve. This type of peripheral nerve damage occurs within months to years after irradiation.
2. Extensive fibrosis of the adjacent and overlying connective tissues may damage a peripheral nerve trunk situated within intact tissue. This tends to be a very late phenomenon, occurring many years after radiation.
3. Extensive fibrosis of the adjacent and overlying connective tissues may damage a peripheral nerve trunk situated within tissues previously subjected to surgical dissection. The microvascular disruption caused by the previous dissection makes these tissues more vulnerable and consequently fibrosis may develop more rapidly, after a few months to years.

Fibrosis and decreased vascularity may destroy peripheral nerves and prevent the regeneration of their proximal normal portions. The degree of connective tissue injury at the time of or preceding radiation therapy may be important in influencing the subsequent development of connective tissue fibrosis.

Three distinct clinical syndromes of brachial plexopathy related to radiation therapy have been reported in patients with breast cancer: (a) reversible or transient brachial plexopathy, (b) radiation fibrosis or radiation injury to the brachial plexus, and (c) acute ischemic brachial plexopathy (4,7,12,13). All three are uncommon clinical entities, each with a characteristic clinical presentation and course.

Transient Radiation Injury

A transient brachial plexopathy has been described in breast cancer patients immediately following radiotherapy to the chest wall and adjacent nodal areas. In retrospective studies, the incidence of this phenomenon has been variably estimated as 1% to 20% (6,12,14); clinical experience suggests that lower estimates are more accurate. In a review of 565 patients who were treated with moderate doses (5,000 cGy in 5 weeks) of supervoltage radiation therapy, Salner et al. (12) identified eight (1.4%) cases of transient brachial plexopathy, with the onset of symptoms occurring 3 to 14 months following irradiation (median, 4.5 months). The clinical symptoms included paresthesias in the arm and hand and, less commonly, weakness and pain. Seven of eight patients received adjuvant chemotherapy; in six patients, symptoms began following drug treatment. There was a temporal clustering of these cases, possibly suggesting a neurotropic viral component. The symptoms and signs of paresthesias and weakness did not conform to any anatomical pattern but most commonly affected the distribution of the lower plexus. Weakness occurred in five of eight patients and was profound in two patients. All patients regained full strength. In three patients, residual paresthesias persisted. In a long-term follow-up of 1,624 patients, Pierce et al. (15) found that radiation-induced plexopathy was transient in 16 cases. Mild symptoms, with minimal pain and weakness, were predictive of resolution. Similarly, in a series of 419 patients who received radiation to the axillary nodal bed, Galper et al. (14) reported that five (1.2%) patients developed a transient brachial plexopathy.

In contrast to these experiences in which the prevalence was very low, Fulton (6), in a retrospective study of 63 patients, reported radiation-induced plexopathies in 19, 14 of whom had transient plexopathy and 5 of whom had a permanent plexopathy. He suggested that transient plexopathy did not appear to predispose patients to the development of a radiation-induced permanent plexopathy.

Radiation Fibrosis

Radiation fibrosis of the brachial plexus results in progressive and irreversible neurologic dysfunction of the brachial plexus. This entity has been well described in the literature (4,6,7,9, 16–23). The risk of development of chronic brachial plexopathy has been variably estimated as 0.6% to 14% (4,7,12,16,18, 23–28). Among 140 patients receiving supraclavicular radiation therapy Bajrovic et al. (29) reported an annual incidence of 2.9% per year for mild plexopathy and 0.8% per year for moderate to severe symptoms that did not abate over time.

Time Course and Natural History

Symptoms usually develop months to years after radiotherapy (7,16,18,22,28,30), although in many cases no latency is apparent (20,31). In the series by Kori et al. (4), the interval from the last dose of radiation to the first symptoms of plexus disorder in patients with radiation fibrosis ranged from 3 months to 26 years, with a median of 4 years. They observed that 5 of the 7 patients who received radiation therapy because of local disease developed radiation damage within 1 year, whereas 13 of 15 patients who received radiation therapy to the plexus as prophylaxis developed symptoms after 1 year. There is no good explanation for this finding.

Dose and Schedule Relationship

Scheduling factors associated with an increased relative risk of subsequent plexopathy include high total dose (19,28,32) and larger fraction size (>1,900 cGy per day) (20,26,28,33–35). Powell et al. (30) compared the incidence of radiation-induced brachial plexopathy in 449 patients who had been randomized to either 4,600 cGy in 15 fractions or 5,400 cGy in 27 to 30 fractions. The incidence of radiation plexopathy was only 1% in the high-dose, small fraction group, as compared to 5.9% in the low-dose, large fraction cohort; thus concluding that fractional dose is the major scheduling risk factor. The literature regarding the risk of radiation fibrosis with hypofractionated schedules was recently reviewed by Galecki et al. (36). Overall they found that the use of fractional doses of 2.2 to 4.58 Gy, with the total doses between 43.5 and 60 Gy, was associated with a significantly elevated risk of brachial plexus injury (1.7% to 73%)

Other factors associated with an increased relative risk include younger age of treatment (20,31) and concurrent cytotoxic therapy (6,15,20).

Symptoms and Signs

Weakness

Arm weakness is the dominant symptom of radiation fibrosis. Motor weakness typically involves the muscles innervated by the upper plexus alone or both the upper and lower plexus (4–7,18,20,22,25,31). Weakness in a distribution of the lower plexus alone is uncommon (20,31).

Pain

Although pain is a presenting symptom in less than 20% of patients with radiation injury to the brachial plexus, its prevalence increases with time (4,20,21,31). The pain is commonly described as mild discomfort associated with aching pain in the shoulder or hand. At the time of diagnosis, 65% of patients will report discomfort or pain in the arm; in 35% it is severe (4).

Parasthesias

In over 50% of affected patients a prominent symptom is paresthesias (4). They are commonly reported to occur in the thumb and forefinger, but often involve the entire hand. These symptoms are often confused with carpal tunnel syndrome, but may be differentiated clinically and by electrodiagnostic studies.

Lymphedema

Lymphedema of the ipsilateral arm was observed in 16 of 22 of patients with radiation fibrosis in the series by Kori et al. (4) and in a substantial proportion of those reported by others (5). Olsen et al. (31) found that lymphedema is a common late consequence of radiation therapy that occurs in approximately 25% of patients, and that it was not predictive of brachial plexus fibrosis.

Radiation Skin Changes

Radiation skin changes were noted in approximately one third of the patients with radiation injury, but these changes were not predictive of an underlying plexopathy (4).

Uncommon

Osteoradionecrosis of the ribs and rarely of the humeral head can be noted on plain radiographs (17). Horner's syndrome is rarely observed (5,20,25,31).

Natural History

The natural history of brachial plexus fibrosis is variable. Motor dysfunction may be incomplete, or may progress to a severe paresis (20,21,31). In a long-term follow-up study of 71 patients radiated to 57 Gy, 11 of the 12 surviving patients had severe arm paralysis (28). Even with advanced radiation fibrosis, severe pain is relatively uncommon, and its presence should prompt evaluation of the patient for recurrent tumor (4).

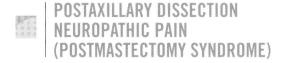

POSTAXILLARY DISSECTION NEUROPATHIC PAIN (POSTMASTECTOMY SYNDROME)

Prevalence

Chronic pain of variable severity is a common sequel of surgery for breast cancer. Although chronic pain has been reported to occur after almost any surgical procedure on the breast (from lumpectomy to radical mastectomy), it is most common after procedures involving axillary dissection (5,37–39). This is a common pain syndrome after axillary lymph node dissection, occurring in 30% to 70% of patients (37,40–48).

The risk for, and severity of, pain is correlated positively with the number of lymph nodes removed (28,49) and is inversely correlated with age (43,46,49). There are conflicting data as to whether preservation of the intercostobrachial nerve during axillary lymph node dissection can reduce the incidence of this phenomenon (48,50–54). The incidence is reduced, but not avoided, when axillary dissection is avoided either by sentinel node excision without full dissection (55–58) or when nodes are irradiated without dissection (59).

Clinical Features

The pain is usually characterized as a constricting and burning discomfort that is localized to the medial arm, axilla, and anterior chest wall (39,60–63). Pain may begin immediately or as late as many months following surgery. The natural history of this condition appears to be variable, and both subacute and chronic courses are possible (64,65). The onset of pain later than 18 months following surgery is unusual, and a careful evaluation to exclude recurrent chest wall disease is recommended in this setting. On examination, there is often an area of numbness within the region of the pain (52,56,62,66). Chronicity of

pain is related to the intensity of the immediate postoperative pain (44,67), postoperative complications, and subsequent treatment with chemotherapy and radiotherapy (45).

Etiology

Postaxillary node dissection pain is most commonly associated with neuropraxia of the intercostobrachial nerve during the process of axillary lymph node dissection (39,62,68). There is marked anatomic variation in the size and distribution of the intercostobrachial nerve, and this may account for some of the variability in the distribution of pain observed in patients with this condition (69).

Differential Diagnosis

This syndrome must be differentiated from postmastectomy frozen shoulder (70,71), axillary web syndrome (72), and breast cellulitis (73). In some cases of pain after breast surgery a trigger point can be palpated in the axilla or chest wall.

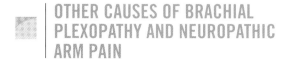

OTHER CAUSES OF BRACHIAL PLEXOPATHY AND NEUROPATHIC ARM PAIN

Second Primaries

Uncommonly a malignant peripheral nerve tumor or a second primary tumor in a previously irradiated site can account for pain recurring late in the patient's course (74–76). Primary tumors of the brachial plexus are uncommon (77–80), and nerve sheath tumors that occur years after radiation therapy are generally thought to be a late effect of the therapy (74). This condition must be differentiated from recurrence of breast cancer, which may also occur in a plexus previously damaged by radiation fibrosis (81).

Carpal Tunnel Syndrome

Among patients with a past medical history of breast cancer who were referred for evaluation of arm pain, 4 of 30 were found to have carpal tunnel syndrome (5). Although electrophysiological abnormalities that are consistent with carpal tunnel syndrome occur twice as frequently ipsilateral to the resection among women who have undergone mastectomy (82), it is an infrequent cause of arm pain in this population and the diagnosis requires demonstration of a prolonged sensory latency that is greater than that recorded for the radial and ulnar nerves (83,84).

Lymphedematous Brachial Plexus Compression

Some authors have suggested that lymphedema alone can produce a compression injury of the brachial plexus (5,82). Ganel et al. (82) performed a series of electromyographic studies on women who had undergone mastectomies with or without subsequent radiation therapy. On the basis of an increased prevalence of F-wave latency abnormalities ipsilateral to previous mastectomy in women with lymphedema, they proposed that the lymphedema may indeed cause an entrapment brachial plexopathy. Vecht (5) inferred this diagnosis in 1 of 28 patients evaluated for arm pain on the basis of negative imaging studies and a nonprogressive neurological deficit in a patient with lymphedema. In the absence of demonstrable reversibility of the neurologic deficit with effective management of the lymphedema or surgical evaluation of the plexus to exclude recurrent tumor or radiation fibrosis, this diagnosis should be approached with clinical skepticism.

Radiation Induced Ischemic Brachial Plexopathy

Gerard et al. (13) have reported a case of subclavian artery occlusion occurring 19 years after a patient with breast cancer was treated with 4,000 cGy irradiation to the breast and axillary area, following a radical mastectomy. The patient's symptoms occurred acutely after carrying a heavy object and holding her left arm outstretched above the shoulder. The lesion appeared to be acute in onset and nonprogressive and was painless, in contrast to the typical progressive nature of radiation fibrosis and the associated pain in up to 35% of patients in that group. Rubin et al. (85) recently described an episode of radiation-induced arteritis of large vessels and brachial plexopathy occurring 21 years after local radiation for breast cancer. Arteriography revealed arteritis, with ulcerated plaque formation at the subclavian–axillary artery junction, consistent with radiation-induced disease and diffuse irregularity of the axillary artery.

Pathologic Fracture of the Humerus

Pathological fractures or fracture dislocations of the humerus may traumatize adjacent nerves of the infraclavicular plexus (86). Fractures or dislocations of the neck of the humerus may cause axillary nerve compression, whereas midshaft fractures, which are less common, may damage radial or ulnar terminal nerves.

DIAGNOSTIC INVESTIGATIONS

There are many potential causes of plexopathy in cancer patients, the most common of which are tumor infiltration and radiation fibrosis. Often patients with symptoms suggestive of plexopathy have received prior radiotherapy and in these patients it is important to distinguish between tumor infiltration and radiation induced fibrosis. When radiological findings are nondiagnostic, electrophysiological studies may assist in making the distinction.

Cross-sectional imaging is essential in all patients with symptoms or signs compatible with plexopathy. Both magnetic resonance imaging (MRI) and computed tomography (CT) scanning are commonly used in these settings, and there are few comparative data addressing the sensitivity and specificity in this setting (87,88). MRI has the theoretical advantage of reliably assessing the integrity of the adjacent epidural space. This is particularly important when there are clinical or radiological features suggestive of epidural encroachment through the intervertebral foramina.

Magnetic Resonance Imaging

Although comparative data on the sensitivity and specificity of MRI to CT in evaluating lesions of the brachial plexus are not available, MRI is widely thought to be the best choice for evaluating the anatomy and pathology of the brachial plexus (89–91). MRI is a noninvasive procedure that can assess the integrity of the vertebral bodies and may differentiate tumor from radiation fibrosis as well as fully visualize the adjacent epidural space (89). Additional advantages include its superior soft tissue resolution and the ability to readily reconstruct images in multiple planes.

T1-weighted images best define the relationship of tumor to the surrounding structures (92). Both tumor and radiation fibrosis generate intense images. Contrary to initial reports, increased T2 signal in or near the plexus is commonly seen in both radiation plexopathy and tumor infiltration and is not useful in this distinction (93,94).

There are some data to suggest that dynamic gadolinium-enhanced T1-weighted imaging can help differentiate tumor from radiation fibrosis: recurrent tumors demonstrate early increased signal intensity of the lesion within 3 minutes after bolus injection, whereas fibrosis generates no substantial enhancement on postcontrast T1-weighted images (95).

Even with contemporary techniques and equipment, there are divergent experiences in the sensitivity and specificity of MRI in the detection of malignant brachial plexopathy (96,97): a prospective study of MRI used for detection of malignant brachial plexopathy yielded a sensitivity of 96%, specificity of 95%, positive predictive value of 96%, and negative predictive value of 95% (96). The most common findings observed with radiation fibrosis are thickening and diffuse enhancement of the brachial plexus without a focal mass or soft tissue changes with low signal intensity on both T1- and T2-weighted images (90,98).

Since patients with brachial plexus lesions are at high risk for developing epidural cord compression from direct tumor infiltration along the plexus into the epidural space or from hematogenous spread of tumor to the vertebral body (4,99,100), imaging should include the adjacent epidural space. Imaging of the epidural space is essential if spinal cord compression is suspected and in the evaluation of patients who have any of the clinical findings that are commonly associated with this complication, including panplexopathy, Horner's syndrome, vertebral body erosion or collapse at the C7-T1 levels, or a paraspinal mass detected on CT scanning. Accurate imaging with MRI determines the extent of epidural encroachment (which influences prognosis and may alter the therapeutic approach) and defines the appropriate radiation portals.

Computed Tomography Scan

Recent years have witnessed tremendous improvements in the techniques of CT imaging that have enhanced the value of this modality in the imaging of the brachial plexus. Modern spiral CT enables simultaneous x-ray source rotation and patient table translation as well as retrospective multiplanar and three-dimensional reconstruction. In many cases, these approaches are very helpful particularly in the identification of mass lesions in the plexus and adjacent infiltration of the neural foramina. Modern CT imaging is often a good initial option, particularly in situations when MRI is not readily available.

CT scanning techniques to image the brachial plexus should include both bone and soft tissue windows and should be contrast enhanced to give a clear definition of vascular structures. Adequate imaging requires scanning from C4 to T6 vertebral bodies using a large gantry aperture to include both axillary fossae (101) so that the symptomatic plexus may be compared with the asymptomatic one. Vascular enhancement allows for identification of vascular structures that relate to the plexus. Since a high concentration of contrast can produce a streaking artifact, some experts recommend that intravenous contrast should be administered contralateral to the suspected lesion (101). The elements of the brachial plexus are depicted as nodular or linear areas of soft tissue density that can be difficult to identify.

The typical appearance of radiation fibrosis of the plexus on CT studies is a diffuse infiltration and loss of tissue planes without a mass lesion (24). There is often associated lymphedema in the arm, evident on CT, and occasionally, radiation necrosis of the clavicle or rib or humeral head occurs at the adjacent level (17). Tumor infiltration of the plexus cannot be differentiated from radiation fibrosis by CT studies when diffuse infiltration is noted. In such cases CT-guided biopsy of brachial plexus mass may be helpful (102).

Ultrasound

In skilled hands ultrasound also can be a useful modality for evaluation of the brachial plexus. The nerves are localized at the level of the vertebral foramina can then be followed longitudinally and axially down to the axillary region. In a study of 28 patients with clinical findings of brachial plexopathy who subsequently underwent surgery, abnormal findings were detected in 20 of 28 patients (103). Focal masses within a nerve or adjacent to it and diffuse thickening of the nerve were the findings in primary and secondary tumors. Postirradiation changes presented as nerve thickening. Color Doppler was useful in detecting internal vascularization within masses and relation of a mass to adjacent vessels.

Ultrasound examination of the axilla is a useful technique for the identification of metastatic axillary nodes (104,105). In the evaluation of the axilla for nodal disease ultrasound has been observed to be more sensitive than mammography (106) and digital subtraction angiography, but less sensitive than CT scanning (107). Hypoechoic masses frequently indicate tumor. Hyperechoic lesions are much less specific and may be either malignant or benign (107). Color Doppler ultrasonography can detect alterations in blood flow around axillary nodes infiltrated with tumor. In a prospective study involving 75 patients who subsequently underwent axillary dissection (105), this technique demonstrated a sensitivity of 70%, a specificity of 98%, and a positive predictive value of 96%. These impressive results are substantially better than those observed using other imaging modalities and suggest a potential utility of this technique in the assessment of patients with brachial plexopathy that is worthy of further evaluation.

Positron Emission Tomography Scanning

Compared to conventional imaging techniques, positron emission tomography (PET) and PET/CT scanning has both greater sensitivity and specificity in detecting metastases from breast cancer (108–110). The fused ^{18}F-fluorodeoxyglucose (FDG)-PET and CT images give two pieces of critical information within a single study: the extent of viable tumor and its exact location. Because it provides biological and functional information, FDG-PET often is complementary to CT or MRI. This is particularly true when trying to differentiate between post-treatment scar and recurrent tumor.

Despite these generalizations, published information specific to the detection of brachial plexopathy is limited (111). In a study of 19 patients with symptoms suggestive of brachial plexopathy, 14 had abnormal uptake of FDG in the region of the symptomatic plexus. Of those with abnormal findings in the plexus, only 33% had a lesion identifiable on CT imaging (112).

Electrophysiologic Studies

Electrophysiological studies may be useful in distinguishing tumor infiltration from radiation fibrosis (113). Electrodiagnostic studies in patients with radiation fibrosis have been demonstrated to show signs of fibrillation and positive waves associated with denervation. Widespread myokymia is strongly suggestive of radiation-induced plexopathy (25,114–117). Roth et al. (117) assessed electrodiagnostically a patient with radiation fibrosis following radiation therapy for breast cancer who had clinical myokymia, cramps, and pain. They related the myokymia to the existence of a persistent conduction block of several years duration. Streib et al. (118) also reported conduction blocks in two patients treated for breast cancer. Plexus exploration in one of the patients did not reveal constrictive connective tissue or other sources of nerve entrapment. The exact cause of conduction block is not fully understood. A study comparing H reflexes of the flexor carpi radialis muscle among 52 controls and 25 patients with radiation-induced brachial plexopathy found decreased conduction velocity in 13 of the effected patients (119).

In malignant plexopathy electromyography typically reveals fibrillation potentials and positive waves characteristic of denervation in the distribution of the brachial plexus that is consistent with plexus signs and symptoms (24,25,114,120). A normal electromyogram in the cervical paraspinal muscles is usually adequate to exclude the presence of root disease. In the rare instances that myokymia is observed in patients with tumor infiltration of the brachial plexus, it is localized and may be isolated to one muscle group alone (114), whereas widespread myokymic discharges are strongly suggestive of radiation-induced plexopathy (25,114–116).

Median somatosensory-evoked potentials may be helpful in differentiating between radiculopathy and brachial plexus injury. In a series of studies in 49 patients with suspected unilateral brachial plexus problems, median somatosensory-evoked potentials were always normal in injuries of upper trunk and root avulsions confined to one or two root levels and were abnormal in generalized plexopathies, multiple trunk lesions, and multiple root avulsions (121). This test may be useful in patients with pain but without evidence of neurologic abnormalities who are at risk for tumor infiltration of the brachial plexus. Indeed, exploration of the plexus should be considered for select patients who have suggestive clinical findings and abnormal median somatosensory-evoked potentials.

Surgical Exploration

The differential diagnosis of tumor infiltration from radiation injury to the plexus may be made in the majority of cases using the clinical criteria, imaging, and electrophysiological studies. However, if these diagnostic approaches fail to define the nature of the neurologic disorder, exploration of the plexus may occasionally be diagnostic (75,122). In additional to traditional open exploration, minimally invasive laparoscopic methods have been developed and described (123). Such exploration should be undertaken only under the following circumstances:

1. The CT, MRI, and PET scans are normal or show no evidence of change from before the onset of symptoms.
2. A work-up including tumor markers establishing the full extent of disease has been completed and shows no evidence of diffuse metastatic disease.
3. The site of neurologic involvement is certain (for example, a lesion that can be localized to either the upper or lower plexus). This factor is important in determining the appropriate surgical approach. Upper plexus dysfunction may best be assessed through a supraclavicular approach, whereas involvement of the lower plexus is best assessed through a posterior scapular approach or a high posterior thoracotomy, commonly used to explore apical tumors of the lung (124).

TREATMENT OF BRACHIAL PLEXOPATHY IN BREAST CANCER

The care of patients with brachial plexopathy requires an integrated approach involving primary therapy appropriate to the specific diagnosis along with symptomatic treatment of pain.

Primary Therapies

Treatment of Radiation Fibrosis

The management of patients with radiation fibrosis begins with the establishment of an accurate diagnosis to rule out metastatic disease. There are no proven methods to reverse neurologic damage. Splinting the arm at the chest wall, preventing subluxation of the shoulder joint, and using intensive physical therapy to manage lymphedema are common approaches to managing the musculoskeletal pain syndromes associated with this disorder (125,126).

Some authors have suggested the use of neurolysis with pedicle omentoplasty to treat radiation fibrosis (127–130). Cumulative anecdotal data suggest that this procedure frequently results in reduced pain, and that progression of neurologic deficit can be arrested in some cases (21,127–130). In the largest series, Le-Quang (127) reported 60 patients followed 2 to 9 years and advocated early surgery as soon as possible after the onset of paresthesias. Surgical exploration of the brachial plexus is difficult, and further injury to the nerve may be associated with a worsening pain syndrome following surgically induced nerve injury (131). Further studies are necessary to assess the usefulness of this technique to preserve neurologic function and to treat pain.

Hyperbaric oxygen therapy has been shown to be beneficial to areas of radiation damage. It improves tissue oxygen gradients and oxygen tension, enabling fibroblast proliferation, collagen formation, and angiogenesis at the wound edges, further improving oxygenation and re-epithelialization. Despite positive experience in other regions (132,133), a double-blinded randomized trial of hyperbaric therapy did not yield substantial relief in patients with radiation-induced brachial plexopathy (134).

There are some data that show that antioxidant therapy with a combination of pentoxifylline and vitamin E may partially reverse radiation fibrosis, particularly when treatment is started soon after the initial radiation insult (135,136). No specific experience has been reported using this approach in radiation-induced plexopathy.

Treatment of Tumor Infiltration

The treatment of tumor infiltration of the brachial plexus depends on the status of the patient's disease, the extent of neurologic involvement, and any prior history of radiation therapy to the brachial plexus. In patients with tumor infiltration of the brachial plexus with evidence of metastatic disease in other sites, systemic chemotherapy is a reasonable approach. In those who have undergone previous radiation therapy to the region, systemic therapies involving either cytotoxic or hormonal therapies may offer the only reasonable antitumor treatment. However, in a patient who has not previously been irradiated if the neurologic signs are rapidly progressive or if there is evidence of epidural spinal cord compression, radiation therapy is the procedure of choice. As stated, MRI or myelography should be used to define the exact radiation ports in these cases.

The dose of radiation therapy employed varies. In the reported series, a dose of 3,000 cGy, delivered over a 3-week period, or 5,000 cGy delivered over a 5-week period represent the most commonly used dose ranges (4,12,120,137). There is clinical evidence to suggest that steroids provide pain relief in patients with tumor infiltration of the brachial plexus, and they are often used to provide analgesia during therapy (138). If the diagnosis of brachial plexus tumor infiltration is made early and effective therapy is instituted, the patient's neurologic symptoms should resolve, and a marked reduction in pain should be noted.

There are conflicting data on the likelihood of benefit from palliative radiotherapy for malignant brachial plexopathy in breast cancer. In a review of the published experience to date and his own experience, Ampil (137) reported that the total delivered dose, rather than the width of the therapy port, was the most important factor in achieving optimal symptomatic palliation. In his series of 23 patients, significant pain relief was achieved in 77.2% of patients for a median of 3 months; the observed objective response rate was 46%. In the series by Nisce and Chu (139), 12 of 47 patients (25.5%) with metastatic brachial plexopathy and breast cancer had complete pain relief for a mean duration of 15 months, and 23 (49%) had partial

pain relief for a mean duration of 6 months. These researchers suggested that higher doses of irradiation (5,000 cGy) were more effective than lower doses. In retrospective review of Kori et al. (4), radiation treatment in doses of 2,000 to 5,000 cGy delivered to the plexus relieved pain in 46% of cases. Neurologic improvement was minimal, and persistent, chronic pain was the most significant problem. In Fulton's (6) experience with 44 breast cancer patients with definite (n = 31) or probable (n = 13) brachial plexopathy, 9 of the 17 patients treated with radiation therapy improved. Among patients in whom radiation therapy was no longer a therapeutic option because of prior radiation therapy, the yield from systemic therapies was low: two of seven patients responded to hormonal therapy and only one of six patients responded to chemotherapy. In a small series of five patients in Israel, all had substantial pain relief (122).

There are no published reports on the specific effects of chemotherapy or hormonal therapy on malignant brachial plexopathy. Anecdotally, clinical experience indicates that patients with malignant infiltration of the plexus who respond to systemic therapy generally have substantial relief of plexopathy-related pain. Since most responses are partial and subsequently followed by relapse, pain often returns when disease recurs. Indeed, worsening pain is often the earliest indicator of recurrence or progression.

MANAGEMENT OF PAIN ASSOCIATED WITH BRACHIAL PLEXOPATHY

Analgesic Pharmacotherapy

Primary antitumor therapies should be considered for patients with tumor invasion of the brachial plexus. All patients with pain should initially be treated with analgesic pharmacotherapy in accordance with the World Health Organization's three-step analgesic ladder (140).

Opioids in the Management of Brachial Plexus Pain

A trial of opioid therapy should be administered to all patients with pain of moderate or greater severity, irrespective of the pathophysiological mechanism underlying the pain (141). Patients who present with severe pain are usually treated with an opioid customarily used in step 3 of the analgesic ladder. Until recently, patients with moderate pain have been conventionally treated with a combination product containing acetaminophen or aspirin plus codeine, dihydrocodeine, hydrocodone, oxycodone, or propoxyphene. The doses of these combination products can be increased until the maximum dose of the nonopioid coanalgesic is attained (e.g., 4,000 mg acetaminophen); beyond this dose, the opioid contained in the combination product could be increased as a single agent, or the patient could be switched to an opioid conventionally used for strong pain. Recent years have witnessed the proliferation of new opioid formulations that may improve the convenience of drug administration for patients with moderate pain. These include controlled-release formulations of codeine, dihydrocodeine, oxycodone, morphine, and tramadol in dosages appropriate for moderate pain.

Opioids should be administered by the least invasive and most convenient route capable of providing adequate analgesia for the patient. In routine practice, the oral route is usually the most appropriate. Parenteral routes of administration should be considered for patients who have impaired swallowing or gastrointestinal obstruction, those who require the rapid onset of analgesia, and highly tolerant patients who require doses that cannot otherwise be conveniently administered.

Patients with continuous or frequently recurring pain generally benefit from scheduled around-the-clock dosing. All patients who receive an around-the-clock opioid regimen should also be offered a *rescue dose*, a supplemental dose given on an as-needed basis to treat pain that breaks through the regular schedule. The rescue drug is typically identical to that administered on a continuous basis, with the exception of transdermal fentanyl and methadone; the use of an alternative short half-life opioid is recommended for the rescue dose when these drugs are used. Patient-controlled analgesia is a technique of parenteral drug administration in which the patient controls a pump that delivers bolus doses of an analgesic according to parameters set by the physician.

Patients in severe pain who are opioid naive should generally begin one of the opioids conventionally used for severe pain at a dose equivalent to 5 to 10 mg intramuscular morphine every 3 to 4 hours. If a switch from one opioid drug to another is required, the equianalgesic dose table (Table 84.1) is used as a guide to the starting dose. The persistence of inadequate pain relief should be addressed through a stepwise escalation of the opioid dose until adequate analgesia is reported or unmanageable side effects supervene. The severity of the pain should determine the rate of dose titration. An understanding of the strategies used to prevent or manage common opioid toxicities is needed to optimize the balance between analgesia and side effects.

Adjuvant Analgesics

Even with optimal management of adverse effects, some patients do not attain an acceptable balance between pain relief and side effects. Several types of noninvasive interventions including adjuvant analgesics, a switch to another opioid, and the use of psychological, physiatric, or noninvasive neurostimu-latory techniques should be considered for their potential to improve this balance by reducing the opioid requirement. Adjuvant analgesics are drugs that have a primary indication other than pain but have analgesic effects in some painful conditions. The use of adjuvant analgesics can contribute substantially to the successful management of pain caused by brachial plexopathy.

Corticosteroids

Corticosteroids are frequently used in the management of neuropathic pain due to infiltration or compression of neural structures by tumor (142). Patients with advanced cancer who experience pain and other symptoms that may respond to steroids are usually given relatively small doses (e.g., dexamethasone 1 to 2 mg twice daily). A very short course of relatively high doses (e.g., dexamethasone 100 mg intravenously followed initially by 96 mg per day in divided doses) can be used to manage a severe exacerbation of pain associated with malignant brachial plexopathy (138). The dose should be gradually lowered following pain reduction to the minimum needed to sustain relief.

Centrally Acting Adjuvant Analgesics Used for Neuropathic Pain

Neuropathic pain is generally less responsive to opioid therapy than nociceptive pain, and in many cases the outcome of pharmacotherapy may be improved by the addition of a centrally acting adjuvant analgesic. This subject has been recently reviewed by the neuropathic pain working group of the International Association for the Study of Pain (143). Several antidepressants and calcium channel $\alpha_2\delta$ ligands are included in their list of first-line medications.

Table 84.1 **OPIOIDS CONVENTIONALLY USED IN THE MANAGEMENT OF SEVERE PAIN (STEP 3 OF THE ANALGESIC LADDER)**

| Drug | Dose (mg) Equianalgesic to 10 mg i.m. Morphine | | Half-life (hr) | Duration of Action (hr) | Comments |
	i.m.	p.o.			
Morphine sulfate	10	30 (repeated dose) 60 (single dose)	2–3	3–4	M6G accumulation in renal failure may predispose to additional toxcity; wide range of formulations; on WHO essential drug list
Oxycodone hydrochloride	15	30	2–3	2–4	Formulated as single agent; can be used for severe pain
Hydromorphone hydrochloride	1.5	7.5	2–3	2–4	Wide range of formulations; useful in the elderly
Methadone hydrochloride	10	20	15–190	4–8	Plasma accumulation may lead to delayed toxicity; dosing should be initiated on a PRN basis
Meperidine hydrochloride	75	300	2–3	2–4	*Not recommended for cancer pain;* normeperidine toxicity limits use; contraindicated in patients with renal failure and those receiving MAO inhibitors
Oxymorphone hydrochloride	1	10 (p.r.)	2–3	3–4	No oral formulation available; less histamine release than other opioids
Levorphanol tartrate	2	4	12–15	4–8	Plasma accumulation may lead to delayed toxicity
Fentanyl transdermal system	a	—	—	48–72	Patches available to deliver 25, 50, 75, and 100 μg/hr

MAO, monoamine oxidase; PRN, as needed; WHO, World Health Organization.
[a] Transdermal fentanyl, 100 μg/hr.
Modified from Cherny NI, Portenoy RK. Cancer pain management: current strategy. *Cancer* 1993;72[Suppl]:3393, with permission.

Antidepressant drugs are commonly used to manage neuropathic pains, and the evidence for analgesic efficacy is greatest for the tertiary amine tricyclic drugs, such as amitriptyline, doxepin, and imipramine. The secondary amine tricyclic antidepressants (such as desipramine, clomipramine, and nortriptyline) have fewer side effects and are preferred when concern about sedation, anticholinergic effects, or cardiovascular toxicity is high. Duloxetine, a selective serotonin and norepinephrine reuptake inhibitor (SSNRI), has demonstrated potential efficacy in neuropathic pain. It is generally well tolerated and dosing is simple; starting at 30 mg per day and titrated after 1 week to 60 mg per day. The potential efficacy of venlafaxine, another SSNRI, has also been demonstrated at dosages of 150 to 225 mg per day.

Gabapentin and pregabalin both bind to the $\alpha_2\delta$ subunit of voltage-gated calcium channels, decreasing the release of glutamate, norepinephrine, and substance P (48). Gabapentin is generally well tolerated, and the main adverse effects are somnolence and dizziness. Several weeks can be required to reach an effective dosage, which is usually between 1,800 and 3,600 mg per day (administered in three divided doses). When it is effective, pain relief may be seen as early as the second week of therapy, but peak effect usually occurs approximately 2 weeks after a therapeutic dosage is achieved.

Pregabalin produces similar dose-dependent side effects similar to those of gabapentin. Treatment can be initiated at 75 mg twice daily and can be titrated up to 300 mg twice daily. The onset of pain relief with pregabalin can be more rapid than with gabapentin.

The so-called second-line adjuvant analgesics all have less evidence of potential efficacy. Second-line anticonvulsants include carbamazepine, lamotrigine, oxcarbazepine, topiramate, and valproic acid. Second-line antidepressant medications include bupropion, citalopram, and paroxetine. Other agents that may be considered in this setting include mexiletine and baclofen.

Experience with other drugs in the treatment of cancer-related neuropathic pain is very limited. Clonidine, an α_2 adrenergic agonist available in oral or transdermal formulations, has antinociceptive effects in the management of diverse pains, but like the tricyclic antidepressants, it is conventionally used for continuous neuropathic pain in the cancer population (144). Calcitonin (200 IU per day) has been shown to be an active analgesic in the management of some neuropathic pains, and pimozide, a phenothiazine neuroleptic, has activity against lancinating neuropathic pain. The latter drug is not preferred due to a high incidence of adverse effects, including physical and mental slowing, tremor, and parkinsonian symptoms.

Anesthetic and Neurosurgical Techniques

Invasive anesthetic and neurosurgical techniques should only be considered for patients who are unable to achieve a satisfactory balance between analgesia and side effects from systemic analgesic therapies. Techniques such as intraspinal opioid and local anesthetic administration, locoregional infusion of local anesthetic (145–148), intrapleural local anesthetic (149,150), or intraventricular opioid administration (151) can potentially achieve this end without compromising neurological integrity. The use of neurodestructive procedures such as brachial plexus blockade (152,153), chemical, surgical or radiofrequency rhizotomy (154), or a dorsal root entry zone lesion (155,156) should be based on an evaluation of the likelihood and duration of analgesic benefit, the immediate and long-term risks, the likely duration of survival, and the anticipated length of hospitalization.

Rarely, patients have been treated with a forequarter amputation of the limb for relief of the discomfort of a lymphedematous, functionless arm, but this approach is not successful in providing significant pain relief but does improve patient complaints of a heavy lymphedematous useless extremity (157–160).

MANAGEMENT SUMMARY

- Early diagnosis of tumor infiltration of the brachial plexus is important to prevent the development of chronic neuropathic pain and neurological dysfunction.
- Evaluation consists of a careful history, a detailed neurological examination, and MRI or CT. Electrodiagnostic studies should be performed if the radiographic studies are negative for both soft tissue and bony disease. An evaluation to assess for evidence of metastatic disease should follow and, if negative, surgical exploration should be considered to allow for biopsy of adjacent lymph nodes and soft tissue.
- In patients presenting with brachial plexopathy after previous radiation therapy, the history and physical findings and follow-up on CT and MRI may be helpful to distinguish tumor recurrence from radiation fibrosis, but none of these may be definitive. Surgical exploration should be considered if the diagnosis will effect the treatment decision (e.g., in a patient with progressive symptoms of brachial plexopathy but without other evidence of distant metastases in whom documentation recurrent disease will result in a decision to initiate anticancer treatment).

References

1. Chua B, Ung O, Boyages J. Competing considerations in regional nodal treatment for early breast cancer. *Breast J* 2002;8(1):15–22.
2. Clouston PD, DeAngelis LM, Posner JB. The spectrum of neurological disease in patients with systemic cancer. *Ann Neurol* 1992;31(3):268–273.
3. Gonzales GR, Elliott KJ, Portenoy RK, et al. The impact of a comprehensive evaluation in the management of cancer pain. *Pain* 1991;47(2):141–144.
4. Kori SH, Foley KM, Posner JB. Brachial plexus lesions in patients with cancer: 100 cases. *Neurology* 1981;31(1):45–50.
5. Vecht CJ. Arm pain in the patient with breast cancer. *J Pain Symptom Manage* 1990;5(2):109–117.
6. Fulton DS. Brachial plexopathy in patients with breast cancer. *Develop Oncol* 1987;51:249–257.
7. Bagley FH, Walsh JW, Cady B, et al. Carcinomatous versus radiation-induced brachial plexus neuropathy in breast cancer. *Cancer* 1978;41(6):2154–2157.
8. Tsairis P, Dyck PJ, Mulder DW. Natural history of brachial plexus neuropathy. Report on 99 patients. *Arch Neurol* 1972;27(2):109–117.
9. Maruyama Y, Mylrea MM, Logothetis J. Neuropathy following irradiation. An unusual late complication of radiotherapy. *Am J Roentgenol Radium Ther Nucl Med* 1967;101(1):216–219.
10. Erven K, Van Limbergen E. Regional lymph node irradiation in breast cancer. *Future Oncol* 2007;3(3):343–352.
11. Cavanagh JB. Effects of x-irradiation on the proliferation of cells in peripheral nerve during Wallerian degeneration in the rat. *Br J Radiol* 1968;41(484):275–281.
12. Salner AL, Botnick LE, Herzog AG, et al. Reversible brachial plexopathy following primary radiation therapy for breast cancer. *Cancer Treat Rep* 1981;65(9–10):797–802.
13. Gerard JM, Franck N, Moussa Z, et al. Acute ischemic brachial plexus neuropathy following radiation therapy. *Neurology* 1989;39(3):450–451.
14. Galper S, Recht A, Silver B, et al. Is radiation alone adequate treatment to the axilla for patients with limited axillary surgery? Implications for treatment after a positive sentinel node biopsy. *Int J Radiat Oncol Biol Phys* 2000;48(1):125–132.
15. Pierce SM, Recht A, Lingos TI, et al. Long-term radiation complications following conservative surgery (CS) and radiation therapy (RT) in patients with early stage breast cancer. *Int J Radiat Oncol Biol Phys* 1992;23(5):915–923.
16. Bates T, Evans RG. Audit of brachial plexus neuropathy following radiotherapy. *Clin Oncol (R Coll Radiol)* 1995;7(4):236.
17. Schulte RW, Adamietz IA, Renner K, et al. [Humeral head necrosis following irradiation of breast carcinoma. A case report]. *Radiologe* 1989;29(5):252–255.
18. Thomas JE, Colby MY Jr. Radiation-induced or metastatic brachial plexopathy? A diagnostic dilemma. *JAMA* 1972;222(11):1392–1395.
19. Basso-Ricci S, della Costa C, Viganotti G, et al. Report on 42 cases of postirradiation lesions of the brachial plexus and their treatment. *Tumori* 1980;66(1):117–122.
20. Olsen NK, Pfeiffer P, Johannsen L, et al. Radiation-induced brachial plexopathy: neurological follow-up in 161 recurrence-free breast cancer patients. *Int J Radiat Oncol Biol Phys* 1993;26(1):43–49.
21. Killer HE, Hess K. Natural history of radiation-induced brachial plexopathy compared with surgically treated patients. *J Neurol* 1990;237(4):247–250.
22. Fathers E, Thrush D, Huson SM, et al. Radiation-induced brachial plexopathy in women treated for carcinoma of the breast. *Clin Rehabil* 2002;16(2):160–165.
23. Senkus-Konefka E, Jassem J. Complications of breast-cancer radiotherapy. *Clin Oncol (R Coll Radiol)* 2006;18(3):229–235.
24. Cascino TL, Kori S, Krol G, et al. CT of the brachial plexus in patients with cancer. *Neurology* 1983;33(12):1553–1537.
25. Lederman RJ, Wilbourn AJ. Brachial plexopathy: recurrent cancer or radiation? *Neurology* 1984;34(10):1331–1335.
26. McDermot RS. Cobalt 60 bean therapy: post-radiation effects in breast cancer patients. *J Can Assoc Radiol* 1971;22(3):195–198.
27. Uematsu M, Bornstein BA, Recht A, et al. Long-term results of post-operative radiation therapy following mastectomy with or without chemotherapy in stage I-III breast cancer. *Int J Radiat Oncol Biol Phys* 1993;25(5):765–770.

28. Johansson S, Svensson H, Larsson LG, et al. Brachial plexopathy after postoperative radiotherapy of breast cancer patients—a long-term follow up. *Acta Oncol* 2000;39(3):373–382.
29. Bajrovic A, Rades D, Fehlauer F, et al. Is there a life-long risk of brachial plexopathy after radiotherapy of supraclavicular lymph nodes in breast cancer patients? *Radiother Oncol* 2004;71(3):297–301.
30. Powell S, Cooke J, Parsons C. Radiation-induced brachial plexus injury: follow-up of two different fractionation schedules. *Radiother Oncol* 1990;18(3):213–220.
31. Olsen NK, Pfeiffer P, Mondrup K, et al. Radiation-induced brachial plexus neuropathy in breast cancer patients. *Acta Oncol* 1990;29(7):885–890.
32. Bentzen SM, Dische S. Morbidity related to axillary irradiation in the treatment of breast cancer. *Acta Oncol* 2000;39(3):337–347.
33. Svensson H, Westling P, Larsson LG. Radiation-induced lesions of the brachial plexus correlated to the dose-time-fraction schedule. *Acta Radiol Ther Phys Biol* 1975;14(3):228–238.
34. Cohen L, Svensson H. Cell population kinetics and dose-time relationships for post-irradiation injury of the brachial plexus in man. *Acta Radiol Oncol Radiat Phys Biol* 1978;17(2):161–166.
35. Gillette EL, Mahler PA, Powers BE, et al. Late radiation injury to muscle and peripheral nerves. *Int J Radiat Oncol Biol Phys* 1995;31(5):1309–1318.
36. Galecki J, Hicer-Grzenkowicz J, Grudzien-Kowalska M, et al. Radiation-induced brachial plexopathy and hypofractionated regimens in adjuvant irradiation of patients with breast cancer—a review. *Acta Oncol* 2006;45(3):280–284.
37. Maunsell E, Brisson J, Deschenes L. Arm problems and psychological distress after surgery for breast cancer. *Can J Surg* 1993;36(4):315–320.
38. Hladiuk M, Huchcroft S, Temple W, et al. Arm function after axillary dissection for breast cancer: a pilot study to provide parameter estimates. *J Surg Oncol* 1992; 50(1):47–52.
39. Vecht CJ, Van de Brand HJ, Wajer OJ. Post-axillary dissection pain in breast cancer due to a lesion of the intercostobrachial nerve. *Pain* 1989;38(2):171–176.
40. Kakuda JT, Stuntz M, Trivedi V, et al. Objective assessment of axillary morbidity in breast cancer treatment. *Am Surg* 1999;65(10):995–998.
41. Keramopoulos A, Tsionou C, Minaretzis D, et al. Arm morbidity following treatment of breast cancer with total axillary dissection: a multivariated approach. *Oncology* 1993;50(6):445–449.
42. Kuehn T, Klauss W, Darsow M, et al. Long-term morbidity following axillary dissection in breast cancer patients—clinical assessment, significance for life quality and the impact of demographic, oncologic and therapeutic factors. *Breast Cancer Res Treat* 2000;64(3):275–286.
43. Warmuth MA, Bowen G, Prosnitz LR, et al. Complications of axillary lymph node dissection for carcinoma of the breast: a report based on a patient survey. *Cancer* 1998;83(7):1362–1368.
44. Tasmuth T, von Smitten K, Kalso E. Pain and other symptoms during the first year after radical and conservative surgery for breast cancer. *Br J Cancer* 1996; 74(12):2024–2031.
45. Tasmuth T, von Smitten K, Hietanen P, et al. Pain and other symptoms after different treatment modalities of breast cancer. *Ann Oncol* 1995;6(5):453–459.
46. Smith WC, Bourne D, Squair J, et al. A retrospective cohort study of post mastectomy pain syndrome. *Pain* 1999;83(1):91–95.
47. Carpenter JS, Andrykowski MA, Sloan P, et al. Postmastectomy/postlumpectomy pain in breast cancer survivors. *J Clin Epidemiol* 1998;51(12):1285–1292.
48. Taylor KO. Morbidity associated with axillary surgery for breast cancer. *ANZ J Surg* 2004;74(5):314–317.
49. Hack TF, Cohen L, Katz J, et al. Physical and psychological morbidity after axillary lymph node dissection for breast cancer. *J Clin Oncol* 1999;17(1):143–149.
50. Temple WJ, Ketcham AS. Preservation of the intercostobrachial nerve during axillary dissection for breast cancer. *Am J Surg* 1985;150(5):585–588.
51. Salmon RJ, Ansquer Y, Asselain B. Preservation versus section of intercostal-brachial nerve (IBN) in axillary dissection for breast cancer—a prospective randomized trial. *Eur J Surg Oncol* 1998;24(3):158–161.
52. Ivanovic N, Granic M, Randelovic T, et al. [Functional effects of preserving the intercostobrachial nerve and the lateral thoracic vein during axillary dissection in breast cancer conservative surgery]. *Vojnosanit Pregl* 2007;64(3):195–198.
53. Freeman SR, Washington SJ, Pritchard T, et al. Long term results of a randomised prospective study of preservation of the intercostobrachial nerve. *Eur J Surg Oncol* 2003;29(3):213–215.
54. Torresan RZ, Cabello C, Conde DM, et al. Impact of the preservation of the intercostobrachial nerve in axillary lymphadenectomy due to breast cancer. *Breast J* 2003;9(5):389–392.
55. Langer I, Guller U, Berclaz G, et al. Morbidity of sentinel lymph node biopsy (SLN) alone versus SLN and completion axillary lymph node dissection after breast cancer surgery: a prospective Swiss multicenter study on 659 patients. *Ann Surg* 2007;245(3):452–461.
56. Baron RH, Fey JV, Borgen PI, et al. Eighteen sensations after breast cancer surgery: a 5-year comparison of sentinel lymph node biopsy and axillary lymph node dissection. *Ann Surg Oncol* 2007;14(5):1653–1661.
57. Schulze T, Mucke J, Markwardt J, et al. Long-term morbidity of patients with early breast cancer after sentinel lymph node biopsy compared to axillary lymph node dissection. *J Surg Oncol* 2006;93(2):109–119.
58. Lucci A, McCall LM, Beitsch PD, et al. Surgical complications associated with sentinel lymph node dissection (SLND) plus axillary lymph node dissection compared with SLND alone in the American College of Surgeons Oncology Group Trial Z0011. *J Clin Oncol* 2007;25(24):3657–3663.
59. Albrecht MR, Zink K, Busch W, et al. [Dissection or irradiation of the axilla in postmenopausal patients with breast cancer? Long-term results and long-term effects in 655 patients]. *Strahlenther Onkol* 2002;178(9):510–516.
60. Wood KM. Intercostobrachial nerve entrapment syndrome. *South Med J* 1978;71(6): 662–663.
61. Paredes JP, Puente JL, Potel J. Variations in sensitivity after sectioning the intercostobrachial nerve. *Am J Surg* 1990;160(5):525–528.
62. van Dam MS, Hennipman A, de Kruif JT, et al. [Complications following axillary dissection for breast carcinoma (see comments)]. *Ned Tijdschr Geneeskd* 1993;137(46): 2395–2398.
63. Granek I, Ashikari R, Foley KM. Postmastectomy pain syndrome: clinical and anatomic correlates. *Proc Am Soc Clin Oncol* 1983;3:(abst 122).
64. International Association for the Study of Pain. Subcommittee on taxonomy. Classification of chronic pain. *Pain* 1986;3[Suppl]:135–138.
65. Ernst MF, Voogd AC, Balder W, et al. Early and late morbidity associated with axillary levels I-III dissection in breast cancer. *J Surg Oncol* 2002;79(3):151–156.
66. Schell SR. Patient outcomes after axillary lymph node dissection for breast cancer: use of postoperative continuous local anesthesia infusion. *J Surg Res* 2006; 134(1):124–132.
67. Stevens PE, Dibble SL, Miaskowski C. Prevalence, characteristics, and impact of postmastectomy pain syndrome: an investigation of women's experiences. *Pain* 1995;61(1):61–68.
68. Bratschi HU, Haller U. [Significance of the intercostobrachial nerve in axillary lymph node excision]. *Geburtshilfe Frauenheilkd* 1990;50(9):689–693.
69. Assa J. The intercostobrachial nerve in radical mastectomy. *J Surg Oncol* 1974; 6(2):123–126.
70. Deutsch M, Flickinger JC. Shoulder and arm problems after radiotherapy for primary breast cancer. *Am J Clin Oncol* 2001;24(2):172–176.
71. Johansen J, Overgaard J, Blichert-Toft M, et al. Treatment of morbidity associated with the management of the axilla in breast-conserving therapy. *Acta Oncol* 2000;39(3):349–354.
72. Moskovitz AH, Anderson BO, Yeung RS, et al. Axillary web syndrome after axillary dissection. *Am J Surg* 2001;181(5):434–439.
73. Hughes LL, Styblo TM, Thoms WW, et al. Cellulitis of the breast as a complication of breast-conserving surgery and irradiation. *Am J Clin Oncol* 1997;20(4):338–341.
74. Gorson KC, Musaphir S, Lathi ES, et al. Radiation-induced malignant fibrous histiocytoma of the brachial plexus. *J Neurooncol* 1995;26(1):73–77.
75. Payne R, Foley KM. Exploration of the brachial plexus in patients with cancer. *Neurology* 1986;36[Suppl 1]:329.
76. Hussussian CJ, Mackinnon SE. Postradiation neural sheath sarcoma of the brachial plexus: a case report. *Ann Plast Surg* 1999;43(3):313–317.
77. Zbaren P, Becker M. Schwannoma of the brachial plexus. *Ann Otol Rhinol Laryngol* 1996;105(9):748–750.
78. Sell PJ, Semple JC. Primary nerve tumours of the brachial plexus. *Br J Surg* 1987; 74(1):73–74.
79. Sharma BS, Banerjee AK, Kak VK. Malignant schwannoma of brachial plexus presenting as spinal cord compression. *Neurochirurgia (Stuttg)* 1989;32(6):189–191.
80. Horowitz J, Kline DG, Keller SM. Schwannoma of the brachial plexus mimicking an apical lung tumor. *Ann Thorac Surg* 1991;52(3):555–556.
81. Brennan MJ. Breast cancer recurrence in a patient with a previous history of radiation injury of the brachial plexus: a case report. *Arch Phys Med Rehabil* 1995;76(10):974–976.
82. Ganel A, Engel J, Sela M, et al. Nerve entrapments associated with postmastectomy lymphedema. *Cancer* 1979;44(6):2254–2259.
83. Dawson DM. Entrapment neuropathies of the upper extremities [see comments]. *N Engl J Med* 1993;329(27):2013–2018.
84. de Araujo MP. Electrodiagnosis in compression neuropathies of the upper extremities. *Orthop Clin North Am* 1996;27(2):237–244.
85. Rubin DI, Schomberg PJ, Shepherd RF, et al. Arteritis and brachial plexus neuropathy as delayed complications of radiation therapy. *Mayo Clin Proc* 2001;76(8): 849–852.
86. Chen CH, Lai PL, Niu CC, et al. Simultaneous anterior dislocation of the shoulder and fracture of the ipsilateral humeral shaft. Two case reports. *Int Orthop* 1998;22(1):65–67.
87. Amrami KK, Port JD. Imaging the brachial plexus. *Hand Clin* 2005;21(1):25–37.
88. Ajar A, Hoeft M, Alsofrom GF, et al. Review of brachial plexus anatomy as seen on diagnostic imaging: clinical correlation with computed tomography-guided brachial plexus block. *Reg Anesth Pain Med* 2007;32(1):79–83.
89. van Es HW. MRI of the brachial plexus. *Eur Radiol* 2001;11(2):325–336.
90. Wittenberg KH, Adkins MC. MR imaging of nontraumatic brachial plexopathies: frequency and spectrum of findings. *Radiographics* 2000;20(4):1023–1032.
91. Todd M, Shah GV, Mukherji SK. MR imaging of brachial plexus. *Top Magn Reson Imaging* 2004;15(2):113–125.
92. Posniak HV, Olson MC, Dudiak CM, et al. MR imaging of the brachial plexus. *AJR Am J Roentgenol* 1993;161(2):373–379.
93. Thyagarajan D, Cascino T, Harms G. Magnetic resonance imaging in brachial plexopathy of cancer. *Neurology* 1995;45(3, Pt 1):421–427.
94. Wouter van Es H, Engelen AM, Witkamp TD, et al. Radiation-induced brachial plexopathy: MR imaging. *Skeletal Radiol* 1997;26(5):284–288.
95. Dao TH, Rahmouni A, Campana F, et al. Tumor recurrence versus fibrosis in the irradiated breast: differentiation with dynamic gadolinium-enhanced MR imaging. *Radiology* 1993;187(3):751–755.
96. Qayyum A, MacVicar AD, Padhani AR, et al. Symptomatic brachial plexopathy following treatment for breast cancer: utility of MR imaging with surface-coil techniques. *Radiology* 2000;214(3):837–842.
97. Lingawi SS, Bilbey JH, Munk PL, et al. MR imaging of brachial plexopathy in breast cancer patients without palpable recurrence. *Skeletal Radiol* 1999;28(6):318–323.
98. Hoeller U, Bonacker M, Bajrovic A, et al. Radiation-induced plexopathy and fibrosis. Is magnetic resonance imaging the adequate diagnostic tool? *Strahlenther Onkol* 2004;180(10):650–654.
99. Hagen N, Stulman J, Krol G, et al. The role of myelography and magnetic resonance imaging in cancer patients with symptomatic and asymptomatic epidural disease. *Neurology* 1989;39:309.
100. Kanner R, Martini N, Foley KM. Nature and incidence of postthoracotomy pain. *Proc Am Soc Clin Oncol* 1982;1:(abst 590).
101. Krol G. Evaluation of neoplastic involvement of brachial and lumbar plexus: Imaging aspects. *J Back Musculoskel Rehab* 1993;3(3):25–32.
102. Cole JW, Quint DJ, McGillicuddy JE, et al. CT-guided brachial plexus biopsy. *AJNR Am J Neuroradiol* 1997;18(8):1420–1422.
103. Graif M, Martinoli C, Rochkind S, et al. Sonographic evaluation of brachial plexus pathology. *Eur Radiol* 2004;14(2):193–200.
104. Yang WT, Ahuja A, Tang A, et al. High resolution sonographic detection of axillary lymph node metastases in breast cancer [published erratum appears in *J Ultrasound Med* 1996;15(9):644]. *J Ultrasound Med* 1996;15(3):241–246.
105. Walsh JS, Dixon JM, Chetty U, et al. Colour Doppler studies of axillary node metastases in breast carcinoma. *Clin Radiol* 1994;49(3):189–191.
106. Rissanen TJ, Makarainen HP, Mattila SI, et al. Breast cancer recurrence after mastectomy: diagnosis with mammography and US. *Radiology* 1993;188(2):463–467.
107. Tohnosu N, Okuyama K, Koide Y, et al. A comparison between ultrasonography and mammography, computed tomography and digital subtraction angiography for the detection of breast cancers. *Surg Today* 1993;23(8):704–710.
108. Gallowitsch HJ, Kresnik E, Gasser J, et al. F-18 fluorodeoxyglucose positron-emission tomography in the diagnosis of tumor recurrence and metastases in the follow-up of patients with breast carcinoma: a comparison to conventional imaging. *Invest Radiol* 2003;38(5):250–256.

109. Siggelkow W, Zimny M, Faridi A, et al. The value of positron emission tomography in the follow-up for breast cancer. *Anticancer Res* 2003;23(2C):1859–1867.

110. Dose J, Bleckmann C, Bachmann S, et al. Comparison of fluorodeoxyglucose positron emission tomography and "conventional diagnostic procedures" for the detection of distant metastases in breast cancer patients. *Nucl Med Commun* 2002;23(9):857–864.

111. Luthra K, Shah S, Purandare N, et al. F-18 FDG PET-CT appearance of metastatic brachial plexopathy in a case of carcinoma of the breast. *Clin Nucl Med* 2006;31(7):432–434.

112. Ahmad A, Barrington S, Maisey M, et al. Use of positron emission tomography in evaluation of brachial plexopathy in breast cancer patients. *Br J Cancer* 1999; 79(3–4):478–482.

113. Krarup C, Crone C. Neurophysiological studies in malignant disease with particular reference to involvement of peripheral nerves. *J Neurol* 2002;249(6):651–661.

114. Harper CM Jr, Thomas JE, Cascino TL, et al. Distinction between neoplastic and radiation-induced brachial plexopathy, with emphasis on the role of EMG. *Neurology* 1989;39(4):502–506.

115. Albers JW, Allen AA, et al. Limb myokymia. *Muscle Nerve* 1981;4(6):494–504.

116. Flaggman PD, Kelly JJ Jr. Brachial plexus neuropathy. An electrophysiologic evaluation. *Arch Neurol* 1980;37(3):160–164.

117. Roth G, Magistris MR, Le Fort D, et al. [Post-radiation branchial plexopathy. Persistent conduction block. Myokymic discharges and cramps.] *Rev Neurol (Paris)* 1988;144(3):173–180.

118. Streib EW, Sun SF, Leibrock L. Brachial plexopathy in patients with breast cancer: unusual electromyographic findings in two patients. *Eur Neurol* 1982;21(4): 256–263.

119. Ongerboer de Visser BW, Schimsheimer RJ, Hart AA. The H-reflex of the flexor carpi radialis muscle; a study in controls and radiation-induced brachial plexus lesions. *J Neurol Neurosurg Psychiatry* 1984;47(10):1098–1101.

120. Son YH. Effectiveness of irradiation therapy in peripheral neuropathy caused by malignant disease. *Cancer* 1967;20(9):1447–1451.

121. Synek VM. Validity of median nerve somatosensory evoked potentials in the diagnosis of supraclavicular brachial plexus lesions. *Electroencephalogr Clin Neurophysiol* 1986;65(1):27–35.

122. Meller I, Alkalay D, Mozes M, et al. Isolated metastases to peripheral nerves. Report of five cases involving the brachial plexus. *Cancer* 1995;76(10):1829–1832.

123. Krishnan KG, Pinzer T, Reber F, et al. Endoscopic exploration of the brachial plexus: technique and topographic anatomy—a study in fresh human cadavers. *Neurosurgery* 2004;54(2):401–409.

124. Dubuisson AS, Kline DG, Weinshel SS. Posterior subscapular approach to the brachial plexus. Report of 102 patients. *J Neurosurg* 1993;79(3):319–330.

125. Brennan MJ. Lymphedema following the surgical treatment of breast cancer: a review of pathophysiology and treatment. *J Pain Symptom Manage* 1992;7(2): 110–116.

126. Daane S, Poltoratszy P, Rockwell WB. Postmastectomy lymphedema management: evolution of the complex decongestive therapy technique. *Ann Plast Surg* 1998;40(2):128–134.

127. Le-Quang C. [Post-radiotherapy lesions of the brachial plexus. Classification and results of surgical treatment]. *Chirurgie* 1993;119(5):243–251.

128. Narakas AO. Operative treatment for radiation-induced and metastatic brachial plexopathy in 45 cases, 15 having an omentoplasty. *Bull Hosp Jt Dis Orthop Inst* 1984;44(2):354–375.

129. Terzis JK, Maragh H. Strategies in the microsurgical management of brachial plexus injuries. *Clin Plast Surg* 1989;16(3):605–616.

130. Brunelli G, Brunelli F. Surgical treatment of actinic brachial plexus lesions: free microvascular transfer of the greater omentum. *J Reconstr Microsurg* 1985;1(3): 197–200.

131. Match RM. Radiation-induced brachial plexus paralysis. *Arch Surg* 1975;110(4): 384–386.

132. Videtic GM, Venkatesan VM. Hyperbaric oxygen corrects sacral plexopathy due to osteoradionecrosis appearing 15 years after pelvic irradiation. *Clin Oncol (R Coll Radiol)* 1999;11(3):198–199.

133. Suzuki K, Kurokawa K, Suzuki T, et al. Successful treatment of radiation cystitis with hyperbaric oxygen therapy: resolution of bleeding event and changes of histopathological findings of the bladder mucosa. *Int Urol Nephrol* 1998;30(3): 267–271.

134. Pritchard J, Anand P, Broome J, et al. Double-blind randomized phase II study of hyperbaric oxygen in patients with radiation-induced brachial plexopathy. *Radiother Oncol* 2001;58(3):279–286.

135. Delanian S, Porcher R, Rudant J, et al. Kinetics of response to long-term treatment combining pentoxifylline and tocopherol in patients with superficial radiation-induced fibrosis. *J Clin Oncol* 2005;23(34):8570–8579.

136. Delanian S, Balla-Mekias S, Lefaix JL. Striking regression of chronic radiotherapy damage in a clinical trial of combined pentoxifylline and tocopherol. *J Clin Oncol* 1999;17(10):3283–3290.

137. Ampil FL. Radiotherapy for carcinomatous brachial plexopathy. A clinical study of 23 cases. *Cancer* 1985;56(9):2185–2188.

138. Rousseau P. The palliative use of high-dose corticosteroids in three terminally ill patients with pain. *Am J Hosp Palliat Care* 2001;18(5):343–346.

139. Nisce LZ, Chu FC. Radiation therapy of brachial plexus syndrome from breast cancer. *Radiology* 1968;91(5):1022–1025.

140. World Health Organization. *Cancer pain relief.* 2nd ed. Geneva: World Health Organization, 1996.

141. Cherny NI. The management of cancer pain [see comments]. *CA Cancer J Clin* 2000;50(2):70–120.

142. Watanabe S, Bruera E. Corticosteroids as adjuvant analgesics. *J Pain Symptom Manage* 1994;9(7):442–445.

143. Dworkin RH, O'Connor AB, Backonja M, et al. Pharmacologic management of neuropathic pain: evidence-based recommendations. *Pain* 2007;132(3):237–251.

144. Owen MD, Fibuch EE, McQuillan R, et al. Postoperative analgesia using a low-dose, oral-transdermal clonidine combination: lack of clinical efficacy. *J Clin Anesth* 1997;9(1):8–14.

145. Fischer HB, Peters TM, Fleming IM, et al. Peripheral nerve catheterization in the management of terminal cancer pain. *Reg Anesth* 1996;21(5):482–485.

146. Vranken JH, van der Vegt MH, Zuurmond WW, et al. Continuous brachial plexus block at the cervical level using a posterior approach in the management of neuropathic cancer pain. *Reg Anesth Pain Med* 2001;26(6):572–575.

147. Nadig M, Ekatodramis G, Borgeat A. Continuous brachial plexus block at the cervical level using a posterior approach in the management of neuropathic cancer pain. *Reg Anesth Pain Med* 2002;27(4):446.

148. Wang MY, Teitelbaum GP, Loskota WJ, et al. Brachial plexus catheter reservoir for the treatment of upper-extremity cancer pain: technical case report. *Neurosurgery* 2000;46(4):1009–1012.

149. Myers DP, Lema MJ, de Leon-Casasola OA, et al. Interpleural analgesia for the treatment of severe cancer pain in terminally ill patients. *J Pain Symptom Manage* 1993;8(7):505–510.

150. Dionne C. Tumour invasion of the brachial plexus: management of pain with intrapleural analgesia [letter]. *Can J Anaesth* 1992;39(5, Pt 1):520–521.

151. Cramond T, Stuart G. Intraventricular morphine for intractable pain of advanced cancer. *J Pain Symptom Manage* 1993;8(7):465–473.

152. Mullin V. Brachial plexus block with phenol for painful arm associated with Pancoast's syndrome. *Anesthesiology* 1980;53(5):431–433.

153. Cooper MG, Keneally JP, Kinchington D. Continuous brachial plexus neural blockade in a child with intractable cancer pain. *J Pain Symptom Manage* 1994;9(4): 277–281.

154. Sindou M, Fobe JL. Rhizotomies and dorsal route entry zone lesions in the management of cancer related pain. In: Arbit E, ed. *Management of cancer-related pain.* Mount Kisko: Futura, 1993:341.

155. Zeidman SM, Rossitch EJ, Nashold BS Jr. Dorsal root entry zone lesions in the treatment of pain related to radiation-induced brachial plexopathy. *J Spinal Disord* 1993;6(1):44–47.

156. Teixeira MJ, Fonoff ET, Montenegro MC. Dorsal root entry zone lesions for treatment of pain-related to radiation-induced plexopathy. *Spine* 2007;32(10):E316–319.

157. Fanous N, Didolkar MS, Holyoke ED, et al. Evaluation of forequarter amputation in malignant diseases. *Surg Gynecol Obstet* 1976;142(3):381–384.

158. Merimsky O, Kollender Y, Inbar M, et al. Palliative major amputation and quality of life in cancer patients. *Acta Oncol* 1997;36(2):151–157.

159. Soucacos PN, Dailiana ZH, Beris AE, et al. Major ablative procedures in orthopaedic surgery. *Bull Hosp Jt Dis* 1996;55(1):46–52.

160. Wittig JC, Bickels J, Kollender Y, et al. Palliative forequarter amputation for metastatic carcinoma to the shoulder girdle region: indications, preoperative evaluation, surgical technique, and results. *J Surg Oncol* 2001;77(2):105–114.

Beryl A. McCormick and David H. Abramson

The most common malignant lesion of the human eye is metastatic cancer, and the primary cancer with the highest incidence of ocular involvement is breast cancer. A recent study reviewing all published articles in the English language from 1975 to 2006 found breast cancer associated with 47% to 81% of all uveal tract metastases. Although the true prevalence is unknown, in part because most of these studies are based on referrals to an ophthalmology group, the same review reported 5% to 9% (1).

INCIDENCE

Most metastases to the eye occur in the vascular layer of the eye because the source of most metastases is hematogenous dissemination. This layer, the uveal tract, includes the middle choroidal layer of the globe, the ciliary body, and the iris of the eye. In a study from Demirci et al. (2), based on referrals to the Ocular Oncology Service at Wills Eye Hospital, 264 patients with 361 eyes exhibiting metastases to the uveal tract from breast cancer were identified over a 27-year period. The mean time from primary diagnosis to development of ocular disease was 65 months, and 38% of cases involved both eyes.

Frequently, the choroid is diffusely filled with many metastatic deposits. Simultaneous metastatic involvement of the central nervous system (CNS) and the eye is common. Because of the therapeutic implications once ocular disease has been diagnosed, computed tomography (CT) or magnetic resonance imaging (MRI) should be performed to rule out concomitant CNS involvement. Ten of 32 patients with breast cancer with ocular metastases had CNS involvement in one series (3). The Demirci et al. (2) series found 6% of ocular metastases cases associated with brain metastases prior to ocular diagnosis and 28% with brain involvement post ocular diagnosis. Almost 90% of the uveal tract metastases involve the choroid; in the Demirci et al. (2) series, only 3%, had iris metastases and less than 1% had ciliary body metastases. Multiple sites in the uvea were involved in 11% of cases.

Rarely, breast cancer can metastasize to other parts of the eye and orbit, including the optic disc, the conjunctiva (4,5), the lacrimal gland, and the orbital structures including fat, muscle, bone, and optic nerve (6). Breast cancer also is the most likely primary tumor to involve the eyelids. In a series by Riley (7), 38% of metastatic lesions in the eye lids were found to be from breast cancer.

In cases of metastases to the CNS, cells may travel with the cerebral spinal fluid around the optic nerve and present in the optic head, simulating papilledema (Fig. 85.1). Occasionally, these cells will fill the vitreus without ever involving the choroid or retina.

DIAGNOSIS

Virtually all ocular tumors are diagnosed without a biopsy. Accuracy rates using clinical examination and ultrasound are reported to be higher than 99% (8). The indirect ophthalmoscope with photography is the gold standard. Ocular ultrasound (performed by the ophthalmologist) is often helpful.

Ocular metastases are usually diffuse, multifocal, and often bilateral (Fig. 85.2). They are rarely pigmented, in contrast to the most common primary tumor of the eye, ocular melanoma,

which is always solitary, unilateral, and usually pigmented. The metastatic tumor in the eye appears creamy and may involve hundreds of metastatic foci in a single eye that may coalesce and form a solitary larger tumor. Characteristic mottling of the retinal pigment epithelium, called *peau d'orange*, is diagnostic. Retinal detachments caused by the tumor mass in the underlying choroid layer are commonly seen.

Ultrasound can be helpful in the work-up but is not diagnostic. The diffuse nature of metastases associated with retinal detachment can be detected with ultrasound, although this is also evident ophthalmoscopically. Reflectivity on the A-scan ultrasound biometry may be higher than that seen in melanomas but is also not diagnostic.

Because most intraocular metastases are only a few millimeters high, CT scans, MRI, and even positron emission tomography (PET) scans may completely miss these tumors, although any associated retinal detachment may be detected. Such studies are helpful with extrabulbar intraorbital disease.

Fluorescein angiography is often performed by ophthalmologists. It is useful in clarifying the sites of metastases and occasionally can identify sites not appreciated with the ophthalmoscope, but this study is rarely diagnostic and thus not required for the diagnosis.

Table 85.1 presents the most common symptoms that bring the patient to the ophthalmologist for breast cancer metastatic to various sites in the eye. These include decreased visual acuity, metamorphopsia (image distortion), a notable blind spot, diplopia, and less often pain, headache, and photophobia (9–11). For patients with metastatic disease in the orbital soft tissues, the most common presenting symptoms are proptosis, ptosis, pain, diplopia, and clinical evidence of a mass (9,10). Rarely, a scirrhous carcinoma may cause retraction of the soft tissues and enophthalmos (12). Imaging of the orbits by contrast-enhanced CT or MRI (13) is essential in the work-up of orbital masses.

TREATMENT AND PROGNOSIS

Appropriate treatment for most ocular metastases has been a course of external beam radiation therapy. However, as the systemic therapy options for women with stage IV breast cancer increase, more case reports are appearing that document treatment response in the eye from both hormone and chemotherapy agents.

Radiation Options

External beam radiation is the most widely reported treatment option. In the Demirci et al. (2) series, this was the treatment used in 59% of all patients. Sixty-four percent of eyes demonstrated regression after radiation and an additional 18% stable disease. In the Kanthan et al. (1) review, visual acuity stabilized or improved in 57% to 100% of all cases treated (breast and other histologies).

Treatment planning for the common choroidal metastases should begin with a review of the ophthalmologist's findings on examination, especially in the situation where the disease is not demonstrated on CT or MRI scans. Because of the multifocal nature of breast metastases, the goal of treatment planning is to design a field that encompasses all of the involved choroid while avoiding multiple entry and exit-beam pathways that

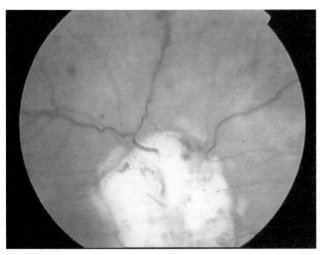

FIGURE 85.1. Optic nerve metastasis stimulating papilledema.

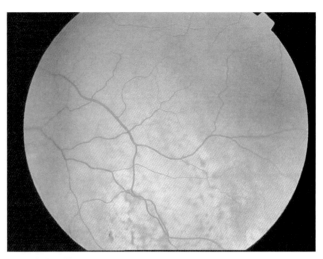

FIGURE 85.2. Diffuse intraocular breast metastases.

may compromise a course of palliative radiation at a later time to adjacent anatomic sites. Lateral fields suffice in most cases. For patients with concurrent CNS disease, shaped opposed fields that encompass the eyes and the brain are used.

Several centers have published reports of more focused radiation techniques, such as stereotactic radiosurgery, proton beam treatment, and the use of episcleral brachytherapy plaques, for uveal tract metastasis. Cases selected for such treatments should be well circumscribed and solitary. Shields et al. (14) treated 36 patients of whom breast cancer repre-

sented the most common primary tumor, using radioactive plaque therapy that delivered a mean dose of 68.8 Gy to the tumor apex and a mean dose of 235 Gy to the base in a mean time of 86 hours. Tumor regression occurred in all patients, but visual acuity improved in only 19%, stabilized in 39%, and decreased in 42%. Within a mean of 8 months, 8% developed a cataract and 8% radiation retinopathy, papillopathy, or both.

A group from Heidelberg reported using stereotactic radiation therapy in 10 patients with solitary metastatic disease to the choroid. Both a single dose (12 to 20 Gy) and a fractionated

Table 85.1	SYMPTOMS AND SIGNS OF OCULAR METASTASES	
Site	**Symptoms**	**Signs**
Iris	Asymptomatic Blurred vision	Iris mass (usually superior) Uveitis Glaucoma Pseudo-hypopyon
Ciliary body	Asymptomatic Blurred vision, pain	Dome-shaped or sessile mass (usually inferiorly) Uveitis Glaucoma Sectorial cataract Lens subluxation Shallow anterior chamber
Vitreous	Floaters Blurred vision	Vitritis
Choroid	Asymptomatic Blurred vision Metamorphopsia Pain, diplopia (rare)	Yellow placoid lesions (usually superior and temporal) Serous retinal detachment Alteration of retinal pigment epithelium Choroidal detachment Glaucoma
Retinal	Blurred vision Floaters	Vitritis Black infiltrative retinal mass with retinitis-like appearance
Optic disc	Asymptomatic Blurred vision	Diffuse or localized disc swelling Disc haemorrhages Disc oedema
Extraocular	Diplopia	Proptosis or enophthalmos Heterotropia
Cerebral	Field defects Hemineglect Abnormal color vision Blurred vision Diplopia	Strabismus Field loss

dose (30 Gy in 10 fractions) was studied. Tumor regression as assessed by ultrasound or MRI was noted in eight patients, and no late side effects were seen (15). Gragoudas (16) reported using a proton beam to treat selected choroidal lesions, with a dose of 28 Gy total delivered in two fractions. With limited follow-up, results appear similar to those of conventional external beam therapy. As with plaque therapy, surgical localization is sometimes required with proton beam treatment; in patients with a relatively short life span, use of external beam therapy would seem the better choice in most clinical situations.

Side effects were seen in only a small number of patients and included transient keratoconjunctivitis, subconjunctival hemorrhage, radiation retinopathy, optic neuropathy, exposure keratopathy, neovascularization of the iris, and cataracts. The series by Rudoler et al. (17) had two cases of narrow angle glaucoma, one requiring an enucleation. They concluded that Caucasian race, increased intraocular pressure at diagnosis, and diagnosis by biopsy predisposed for radiation complications on univariate analysis, but the small number of events did not support a multivariate analysis.

Shields et al. (18) also reported results of external beam radiation to the metastatic disease in the iris of 40 patients, with breast again the most common primary tumor. Similar to the results in the choroid, local control was 100%, and the median survival from the time of eye metastases was 13 months.

For patients with orbital soft tissue metastases, a wedged-pair arrangement of photon beams will provide good coverage of the orbit. Depending on the location of the metastasis on imaging, conformal treatment planning to avoid normal structures is also useful. Doses are similar to those used in the treatment of choroidal disease. The anticipated side effects of orbital radiation include periorbital edema, excessive tearing, and radiation-related inflammation of the conjunctiva. Corneal irritation and permanent dry eye are rare in this dose range; radiation-induced cataracts can also be observed in longer-term survivors.

Systemic Therapy Results

Most of the reports of systemic therapy for ocular metastases are case reports. However, the Wills Eye Group has a series of 17 women treated with an aromatase inhibitor 13 of whom had prior treatment with tamoxifen. They reported response in 10 of the patients, after an average treatment time of 2 months. The authors described the ocular response as "concordant" with the systemic response in most of the responders (19).

Of interest is a case report of intravitreal bevacizumab use for a solitary choroidal metastasis; this is based on the success of this treatment for macular degeneration. The patient had a dramatic reduction in the measured size of her lesion and improved visual acuity (20).

Figure 85.3 demonstrates the survival from diagnosis of ocular metastasis in the Wills Eye series of 264 women, regardless of local treatment.

MANAGEMENT SUMMARY

Patients with breast cancer metastatic to the eye are almost always symptomatic. The most common site of ocular metastasis is the choroid layer, and the diagnosis is best made by ophthalmoscopic examination, with supporting photography and ultrasound. Biopsy is not appropriate within the globe. Work-up should also include an imaging study to rule out brain metastasis.

Although external beam radiation therapy is the treatment of choice for this group of patients, with the growing number of effective systemic therapies available to patients, an alternative

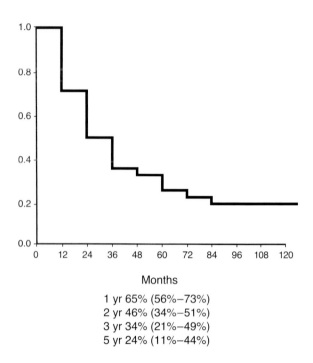

FIGURE 85.3. Survival following diagnosis of uveal metastasis from breast cancer, using Kaplan Meier estimates.

management strategy would be careful monitoring of the ocular disease while on appropriate systemic chemo- or hormone therapy for systemic stage IV disease.

References

1. Kanthan G, Jayamohan J, Yip D, et al. Management of metastatic carcinoma of the uveal tract: an evidence-based analysis. *Clin Exper Ophthalmol* 2007;35:553–565.
2. Demirci H, Shields C, Chao A, et al. Uveal metastasis from breast cancer in 264 patients. *Am J Ophthalmol* 2003;136:264–271.
3. Ratanatharathorn V, Powers W, Grimm J, et al. Eye metastasis from carcinoma of the breast: diagnosis, radiation treatment and results. *Cancer Treat Rev* 1991;18:261.
4. Kiratli H, Shields C, Shields J, et al. Metastatic tumours to the conjunctiva: report of 10 cases. *Br J Ophthalmol* 1996;80:5–8.
5. Shields J, Shields C, Singh. Metastatic neoplasms in the optic disc: the 1999 Bjerrum lecture: part 2. *Arch Ophthalmol* 2000;118:217–224.
6. Backhouse O, Simmons I, Frank A, et al. Optic nerve breast metastasis mimicking meningioma. *Aust N Z Ophthalmol* 1998;26:247–249.
7. Riley FG. Metastatic tumors of the eye lids. *Am J Ophthalmol* 1970;69:140.
8. The Collaborative Ocular Melanoma Study Group. Accuracy of diagnosis of choroidal melanomas in the COMS study. *Arch Ophthalmol* 1990;108:1268–1273.
9. Freedman M, Folk J. Metastatic tumors to the eye and orbit. *Arch Ophthalmol* 1987;105:1215.
10. Glasburn J, Klionsky M, Brady L. Radiation therapy for metastatic disease involving the orbit. *Am J Clin Oncol* 1984;7:145.
11. Shields C, Shields J, Gross N, et al. Survey of 520 eyes with uveal metastases. *Ophthalmology* 1997;104:1265–1276.
12. Chang B, Cunniffe G, Hutchinson C. Enophthalmos associated with primary breast carcinoma. *Orbit* 2002;21:307–310.
13. Char D, Miller T, Kroll S. Orbital metastases: diagnosis and course. *Br J Ophthalmol* 1997;81:386–390.
14. Shields C, Shields J, De Potter P, et al. Plaque radiotherapy for the management of uveal metastasis. *Arch Ophthalmol* 1997;115:203–209.
15. Bellmann C, Fuss M, Holz F, et al. Stereotactic radiation therapy for malignant choroidal tumors: preliminary, short-term results. *Ophthalmology* 2000;107:358–365.
16. Gragoudas E. Current treatment of metastatic choroidal tumors. *Oncology* 1989;3:103–108.
17. Rudoler S, Shields C, Corn B, et al. Functional vision is improved in the majority of patients treated with external beam radiotherapy for choroid metastases: a multivariate analysis of 188 patients. *J Clin Oncol* 1997;15:1244–1251.
18. Shields J, Shields C, Kiratli H, et al. Metastatic tumors to the iris in 40 patients. *Am J Ophthalmol* 1995;119:422–430.
19. Manquez M, Brown M, Shields C and Shields J. Management of choroidal metastases from breast carcinomas using aromatase inhibitors. *Curr Opin Ophthal* 2006;17:251–256.
20. Amselem L, Cervera E, Diaz-Llopis M, et al. Intravitreal bevacizumab for choroidal metastasis secondary to breast carcinoma: short-term follow up [Letter]. *Eye* 2007;21:566–567.

Steven J. Mentzer and Lawrence N. Shulman

The pathologic accumulation of fluid in the pleura, pericardium, or peritoneum is a common management problem in patients with metastatic breast cancer. The reported incidence of malignant pleural effusions in breast cancer patients has been estimated at 2% to 12% (1). Although the incidence of clinically significant malignant pericardial effusions (2) and malignant ascites (3) appears to be less, the number of patients with new malignant effusions will likely exceed 20,000 to 30,000 in the United States in 2008. The annual incidence of malignant effusions of all causes is estimated to be greater than 150,000 (4).

The clinical consequences of malignant effusions range from mild dyspnea to life-threatening compromise of lung and heart function. The most common complaint of patients with malignant pleural or pericardial effusions is dyspnea. Defined as the uncomfortable awareness of breathing, dyspnea is common in patients with metastatic breast cancer (5). Dyspnea is particularly common in advanced disease where the incidence of dyspnea correlates with disease progression (6).

A practical clinical problem is distinguishing the symptoms caused by advanced disease from the reversible symptoms related to excess fluid accumulation. This chapter will review a practical approach to the diagnosis and treatment of malignant effusions of the pleura, pericardium, and peritoneum.

MALIGNANT PLEURAL EFFUSIONS

In normal circumstances, the volume of lung parenchyma fills the chest cavity leaving little room for pleural fluid. The fluid between the visceral and parietal pleural surfaces is extremely thin and may vary between 5 and 35 μm (7). The fluid in the pleural cavity, totaling only 10 to 20 mL, functions as a lubricant during ventilation. The normal pleural fluid enters the pleural space as a filtrate generated by the capillaries in the parietal pleura lining of the chest wall. Some of the fluid may be reabsorbed by visceral pleural capillaries; however, most fluid is drained by lymphatic stomata in the parietal and mediastinal pleura. The recirculation of this lubricant is driven by gravity as well as ventilatory and cardiogenic motions.

Three pathophysiological processes are known to contribute to the development of pleural effusions. A common mechanism is the perturbation of passive Starling forces (8). Effusions that develop from Starling forces reflect an unfavorable balance between hydrostatic fluid filtration and oncotic reabsorption. This process typically results in bilateral pleural effusions. Other pathophysiological processes commonly result in unilateral effusions. One of these processes is functional impairment in lymphatic drainage. A mechanical obstruction of regional lymphatics or a relative rise in lymph resistance (e.g., elevated central venous pressures) can decrease lymphatic clearance. Another cause of unilateral pleural effusions is an increase in tumor-related capillary permeability (9). In most tumors, intratumoral capillaries demonstrate enhanced blood flow and permeability (10).

BILATERAL PLEURAL EFFUSIONS

Bilateral pleural effusions are generally the result of an imbalance in transpleural fluid filtration. The clinical problems associated with an increase in fluid filtration include conditions that increase hydrostatic pressure such as heart failure and hypervolemic states. Bilateral effusions can also result from a pathologic decrease in oncotic pressure. Low oncotic pressure can occur in renal failure, hepatic failure, or nutritional deficiencies. In all of these clinical problems, the accumulation of pleural effusion is the result of fluid filtration in excess of reabsorption.

Bilateral pleural effusions can also occur in breast cancer patients, but are commonly the result of advanced disease including bilateral parenchymal involvement, lymphangitic disease, or mediastinal lymphatic obstruction. Only approximately 10% of patients with breast cancer related malignant effusions present with bilateral pleural effusions, and over 80% of these patients have known metastatic disease (11).

Patients who have unexplained bilateral pleural effusions should have a systemic evaluation with particular attention to cardiac, renal, and hepatic function. Following a chest computed tomography (CT) scan to confirm the presence of the pleural effusion, thoracentesis may provide symptomatic benefit and an opportunity to assess the protein content in the fluid. Because the filtration occurs across an endothelial barrier, the fluid has a decreased protein content. A typical patient may have a protein content of 2 g/dL in the effusion and a serum protein content of 6 g/dL. If the protein concentration of the effusion is less than half the serum concentration, a diagnosis of a transudative effusion is established.

The significance of identifying a transudative effusion is that surgical intervention is rarely beneficial beyond therapeutic thoracentesis. A tube thoracostomy, or chest tube, offers little benefit over thoracentesis in a patient who has a transudative effusion. In the setting of edematous and poorly compliant lungs, a chest tube will further compromise ventilatory mechanics. In contrast, a therapeutic thoracentesis will provide symptomatic relief while the appropriate end organ therapy is instituted. Appropriate medical therapy should target the organ dysfunction that is causing the imbalance in fluid filtration.

UNILATERAL PLEURAL EFFUSIONS

Unilateral pleural effusions are commonly the result of an impairment in lymphatic drainage or an increase in capillary permeability. Although unilateral malignant pleural effusions can occur in the hemithorax ipsilateral or contralateral to the original breast cancer, there appears to be a slightly increased incidence of malignant pleural effusions ipsilateral to the primary breast cancer (11–13).

Breast cancer–related malignant pleural effusions may occur as a result of obstruction of lymphatic stoma. Pleural lymphatic stoma are most prevalent along the mediastinal pleura, diaphragmatic pleural surface, and the anterior chest wall (7). Another mechanism of pleural effusion is an increase in capillary permeability. Increased capillary permeability has been demonstrated in intratumoral capillaries (14). Both mechanisms are associated with a relatively increased protein concentration in the pleural fluid. Pleural fluid with a protein content at least half of the serum concentration (>3 g/dL) is commonly referred to as an exudative pleural effusion.

Diagnosis

The presence of a unilateral pleural effusion is typically detected by chest radiograph. In most patients who have a continuous pleural space, 150 to 200 mL of pleural fluid will cause a blunting of the costophrenic angle in an upright chest radiograph. The chest radiograph should be interpreted cautiously as the unilateral opacity may be the result of a pleural effusion or parenchymal lung collapse. Collapsed or atelectatic lung can be distinguished from pleural effusions by an assessment of the volume of the ipsilateral hemithorax. Collapsed lung is associated with tracheal deviation (mediastinal shift), an elevated hemidiaphragm, and narrowed intercostal spaces. If there is evidence of decreased lung volumes (i.e., a small hemithorax), chest CT scanning with contrast is useful to assess the relative contribution of the pleural effusion and underlying atelectatic lung to the opacity. Chest CT scans can also provide a relative assessment of any potential pericardial effusion or pulmonary emboli.

In the setting of a unilateral pleural effusion, a diagnostic thoracentesis is often indicated. A diagnostic thoracentesis provides insight into the etiology of the effusion, the contribution of the effusion to the patient's symptoms, and the function of the underlying lung. To achieve these goals, the initial diagnostic thoracentesis should remove as much of the fluid as possible. Radiographic heterogeneity or variable echogenicity often is mistakenly interpreted as loculated fluid. Despite the presence of fibrinous septa, most pleural effusions are contiguous fluid collections and can be drained completely by thoracentesis alone.

To help establish the etiology of the effusion, chemical analysis of the fluid can distinguish exudative and transudative pleural effusions. The protein content of an exudative effusion is typically greater than 75% of the serum protein concentration. In chronic inflammation, such as a *Mycobacterium tuberculosis* infection, the pleural fluid protein concentration may exceed serum concentrations. Additional chemical tests such as pH, glucose, and lactate dehydrogenase (LDH) add little information. Low pH and glucose may simply reflect the chronicity of the effusion. Similarly, the LDH level may be useful in lymphomas (15), but is unlikely to be elevated in breast cancer patients.

In the setting of an unexplained exudative effusion, the most effective diagnostic approach involves the examination of the cells in the pleural fluid. The diagnostic yield of cytologic examination of pleural fluid cells exceeds 50% in most types of malignant pleural effusion (16). The yield increases modestly with repeated thoracentesis. Alternatively, the detection of numerous polymorphonuclear leukocytes in the pleural fluid suggests the presence of an acute inflammatory process. The presence of abundant mononuclear cells can be the most problematic finding. Mononuclear cells may represent normal lymphoid cells in a chronic effusion, reactive cells in a tuberculous infection, or even small cell carcinoma.

Treatment

The complete evacuation of the pleural fluid provides an opportunity to assess the contribution of the effusion to the patient's dyspnea. With the rapid removal of effusions greater than 800 mL, the patient may reflexively cough. The forewarned patient is likely to perceive the coughing as a positive sign. On occasion, however, the withdrawal of the fluid results in angina-like chest discomfort. Although the etiology of the pain is unclear, the thoracentesis should be stopped. In most cases, the pain rapidly abates.

The symptomatic benefit of thoracentesis may be delayed because re-expansion of the lung can be associated with regional or "negative pressure" pulmonary edema. Negative pressure pulmonary edema is most commonly observed when thoracentesis is performed ill-advisedly in the setting of a malignant proximal airway obstruction; however, it also may be observed in patients who have functional small airway obstruction. The simplest physiologic explanation for this observation is that the negative pressure that is applied to the pleural catheter creates a pressure gradient from the alveolar space to the pleural space. Because the transalveolar pressure cannot be equilibrated by air flow, continued expansion of the

lung occurs at the expense of fluid accumulation in the lung interstitium. The fluid may not be apparent immediately, but accumulate over hours, suggesting the advisability of ongoing monitoring. Negative pressure pulmonary edema responds to diuretic therapy and typically resolves within 24 to 48 hours. Parenchymal edema that persists for longer than 48 hours may represent infection or lymphangitic tumor.

Lung parenchyma that has been compressed by pleural fluid for weeks to months may not have sufficient compliance to fill the pleural space despite the removal of the fluid. Post-thoracentesis radiographs may show a pneumothorax that is mistakenly ascribed to lung injury as a result of the thoracentesis. The pneumothorax does not reflect acute lung injury but rather chronic entrapment of the lung. The underlying lung is entrapped, not by a fibrinous peel, as seen in pleural empyema, but by the remodeling of the underlying lung parenchyma from chronic volume loss. Although the mechanisms that are involved in lung remodeling are unclear, the process seems to be dependent on the degree of parenchymal inflammation (17). Tumor-related entrapment of the lung can also occur and is a reflection of advanced disease (11). This is more likely to occur with longstanding malignant effusions.

A useful assessment of the pleural space is performed using video thoracoscopy. In most cases, a 5-mm thoracoscope can inserted through a 1-cm access port. The thoracoscope permits visualization of the visceral and parietal pleural surfaces. Directed biopsies of the pleura can be performed if there is any diagnostic uncertainty. The thoracoscope also can provide a visual assessment of lung recruitment maneuvers, typically prolonged end-inspiratory pauses, to increase lung volumes. Lungs that fail to fill a resting (anesthetized) hemithorax, despite maximal positive pressure insufflation, are entrapped. An assessment of pleural apposition is important because it is a prerequisite to any subsequent attempts at mechanical or chemical pleurodesis.

PLEURODESIS

In patients who demonstrate visceral-parietal pleural apposition, a pleurodesis procedure is a common therapeutic option. The goal of the procedure is the prevention of fluid reaccumulation by fusing the visceral and parietal pleural surfaces. Pleurodesis procedures may be either mechanical or chemical. Mechanical approaches use abrasives, such as coarse gauze sponges, to denude the pleural mesothelium and facilitate scarring. In most cases, the utility of mechanical pleurodesis tends to be restricted to clinical situations in which localized or focal pleural symphysis is desired.

Chemical pleurodesis has been performed with numerous compounds, including antibiotics, chemotherapeutic agents, and fine-grained minerals. In the past, the antibiotics included tetracycline and doxycycline; however, tetracycline is no longer available in the United States in a liquid form. Both of these antibiotics can be associated with intense pleuritic pain. The chemotherapeutic agents include bleomycin and cisplatin. The use of bleomycin, the only agent that is approved by the U.S. Food and Drug Administration for the prevention of recurrent effusions, is limited by its expense. Numerous studies suggest that all categories of sclerosing agents, including immunotherapy, seem to be similarly effective (18–28). A meta-analysis of pleurodesis studies reported in 1994 suggested that approximately two thirds of patients benefit from pleurodesis, and that talc, tetracycline, and bleomycin are comparably effective (29).

Because of cost considerations, availability, and ease of use, talc is the most commonly used agent in the setting of malignancy. Talc is a fine-grained mineral that is composed of hydrated magnesium silicate. Sterilized talc can be introduced into the pleural space as a dry powder by insufflation or in a liquid slurry; both routes of administration appear to be comparably effective (28). Completely evacuating the effusion and insufflating dry talc at the time of thoracoscopy eliminates the uncertain dose effects of bedside talc slurry therapy. Ideally, the talc can be introduced into the pleural space while the patient is spontaneously ventilating under general anesthesia. This results in an even distribution of the talc that can be confirmed by video thoracoscopy. Pleural drainage tubes are placed in the apex and across the diaphragm and are maintained on –20 cm H_2O suction for 48 hours.

Talc and the other sclerosing agents stimulate pleural inflammation that often is associated with pleuritic pain, fever, and hypoxia. The relative hypoxia, which may persist for several days, appears to reflect an inflammation-associated intrapulmonary shunt. In most cases, the morbidity is mild if the contralateral lung is normal. In contrast, a pleurodesis-induced intrapulmonary shunt may result in several days of life-threatening hypoxemia in the setting of contralateral lung disease. A pleural catheter without active pleurodesis may be a preferable strategy in this group of patients.

The efficacy of talc and the other chemical sclerosing agents seems to be dependent on pleural apposition, the effective delivery of the sclerosing agent, and the adequacy of the inflammatory reaction. Although two thirds of patients seem to have a symptomatic benefit (28,30), the degree of effective pleural symphysis is variable. The most reliable pleurodesis occurs laterally and apically, whereas residual fluid is observed commonly across the diaphragm. These observations suggest that pleural movement, particularly the motion of a functioning diaphragm, inhibits pleural symphysis.

Indwelling Catheter

An alternative to chemical or mechanical pleurodesis is the placement of an indwelling pleural catheter. The pleural catheters, similar in design to indwelling Hickman central venous catheters, have a subcutaneous cuff that seals the external portion of the catheter (31). Typically, the catheter is placed in the operating room to ensure sterility. In most patients, general anesthesia and selective lung ventilation are used for placement of the catheter. A light general anesthetic is used to control patient ventilation and to facilitate bronchoscopy. Bronchoscopy is performed to assess the airway for possible tumor obstruction and to aspirate re-expansion secretions. Also, bronchoscopy provides an opportunity to evaluate parenchymal abnormalities with bronchoalveolar lavage cytology and culture.

The catheter can be drained intermittently with the use of a properly configured syringe or a proprietary suction bottle. In either case, pleural catheters that are drained several times per week over 6 to 9 weeks can show significant increases in the volume of the underlying lung. This gradual recruitment of lung volume is potentially useful in facilitating pleural apposition and recruiting lung function. The surface tension that is produced by the simple apposition of visceral and parietal pleura may contribute to limiting the reaccumulation of pleural fluid. After the pleural catheter has stopped draining, it can be removed. Although no active pleurodesis has been performed, recurrence of the pleural effusion is rare.

▨ | MALIGNANT PERICARDIAL EFFUSIONS

Breast cancer is the second leading cause of malignant pericardial disease, accounting for 25% of malignant effusions, with lung cancer being the most common cause (33%) (2,32). Patients with breast cancer can develop pericardial effusions because of lymphatic obstruction, direct tumor involvement of the pericardium, or radiation pericarditis. The impairment of heart function as a result of fluid or blood in the pericardial sac is referred to as tamponade.

Pericardial involvement by breast cancer is present in approximately 25% of patients with metastatic disease at the time of death, but it is responsible for death in fewer than 5% of patients with breast cancer (33). In a large series from the Mayo Clinic, patients with breast cancer and an incidental pericardial effusion rarely developed life-threatening pericardial tamponade (5%) (2). In contrast, patients with symptomatic pericardial effusion frequently required surgical management as pericardiocentesis is associated with a high relapse rate. The median survival of patients with known malignant pericardial involvement was 17 months; median survival was 20 months for patients who had surgical management of their effusions.

Similar pathophysiologic processes are responsible for the accumulation of fluid in the pleura and pericardium. The most significant difference is that transudative effusions in the pericardium are generally asymptomatic (34). Probably because of the compliance of the pericardium, pericardial fluid volumes can increase more than 20-fold without overt cardiac signs or symptoms (34). In contrast, an impairment of lymphatic drainage or an increase in mesothelial and capillary endothelial permeability often results in more rapid fluid accumulation and a greater likelihood of effusion-related signs and symptoms.

Diagnosis

Dyspnea is the most common initial complaint of patients who have malignant pericardial effusions (35). The clinical manifestations of pericardial tamponade are dyspnea, tachycardia, and peripheral edema. Dyspnea and tachycardia are greatly exacerbated with even minimal activity because the heart is unable to adequately increase cardiac output when tamponade is present. The components of Beck's triad (hypotension, active jugular veins, diminished heart sounds) also are present in most patients with advanced disease. In addition, the cardiac impulse is almost never felt in patients with tamponade. Presence of a palpable cardiac impulse makes tamponade very unlikely. Regardless of the findings on clinical examination, however, the potential diagnosis of pericardial effusion and cardiac tamponade should be considered in patients who have cancer and progressive dyspnea that is out of proportion to the change in their chest radiograph.

The diagnosis of a pericardial effusion can be suggested by chest radiograph and established by chest CT scanning or echocardiography. The diagnosis of cardiac tamponade, however, must be established by correlating clinical signs with echocardiographic findings. Two-dimensional echocardiography may show a pericardial effusion, but the diagnosis of cardiac compression may be unclear. Echocardiographic findings of early diastolic collapse of the right ventricular free wall has a specificity of 84% to 100%, but a sensitivity of 38% to 48% (32). In contrast, late diastolic compression of the right atrium has a sensitivity of 55% to 60% and a specificity of 50% to 68% (32). Also, a substantial augmentation of right-sided flow with inspiration (Kussmaul sign) may be noted on echocardiography. Any of these signs is suggestive of clinically significant tamponade (36).

Treatment

The hemodynamic consequences of the pericardial effusion can be established by percutaneous drainage. Image-guided pericardiocentesis should be performed in all patients who demonstrate evidence of tamponade. Pericardiocentesis confirms the presence of the effusion, provides fluid for diagnostic studies, and decreases the risks of any subsequent general anesthesia. In some cases, pericardiocentesis provides definitive diagnosis and treatment. For example, radiation therapy or chemotherapy can cause pericarditis without malignant involvement of the pericardium. Radiation therapy is usually associated with radiation doses to the pericardium in excess of 30 Gy. This is a dose of radiation that can be seen in the treatment of lung, esophageal, or breast cancer. In many of these cases, the pericardiocentesis decompresses the pericardium and the inflammation-associated effusion resolves without the need for further intervention.

Because cardiac tamponade restricts normal compensatory mechanisms, general anesthesia can be associated with life-threatening hypotension. As a result, all patients who have cardiac dysfunction secondary to a pericardial effusion should have a percutaneous pericardiocentesis performed before general anesthesia and definitive surgical intervention.

Pericardiocentesis is associated with recurrent pericardial effusions in 20% to 50% of patients (37–40). Patients who have recurrent pericardial effusions should be considered for surgical pericardiotomy. The goal of definitive surgical drainage of a pericardial effusion is to re-establish the lymphatic drainage of the pericardial sac. This can be achieved by creating communication (or window) between the pericardium and the pleural space or the pericardium and adjacent subcutaneous tissues.

The pericardial–pleural window can be performed by video thoracoscopy or anterior thoracotomy (Fig. 86.1) (13). A portion of the pericardium is excised anterior to the phrenic nerve. In situations in which the pericardium is loculated, a second window posterior to the phrenic nerve may be indicated. The relative value of drains that are placed in the pericardium at the time of surgery is uncertain. Drains that are placed in the properly decompressed pericardium typically have little output and are removed within 24 to 48 hours.

Because of the common pathophysiology of pleural and pericardial effusions, 50% of patients who have pericardial effusions present with a coexistent pleural effusions (41). Video thoracoscopy of the left hemithorax provides an opportunity to treat both effusions. The theoretical disadvantage of this approach is that the effusions usually are the consequence of common lymphatic obstruction. Because of the diffuse lymphatic disease, the creation of a pericardial–pleural window on the same side as a pleural effusion may not result in reabsorption of the fluid; however, the pericardium is decompressed and the secondary effects that are related to cardiac tamponade are improved.

In patients who have limited thoracoscopic access to the pericardium, a subxiphoid pericardial window is an alternative approach (42,43). The subxiphoid approach involves a midline

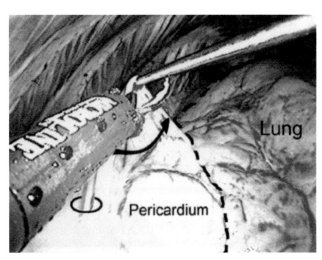

FIGURE 86.1. Thoracoscopic pericardial window. View from the left hemithorax with pericardium, anterolateral to the left lung, tented upward with a retraction forceps. The thoracoscopic scissors approaching the pericardium are shown. The planned pericardiotomy, posterior to the phrenic nerve (*circle*), is illustrated with the arrow.

incision that extends 4 cm below the xiphoid process. The pericardial window is created by excising 10 to 15 cm² of anterior pericardium. This approach is believed to have a recurrence rate of approximately 30% in 3 months. The recurrence rates decrease with larger pericardial windows. The smallest recurrence rates are achieved when anterior pericardium is excised from one phrenic nerve to the other phrenic nerve. In addition to removing a larger portion of pericardium, the phrenic nerve to phrenic nerve approach also may have the advantage of exposing the pericardial fluid to the lymphatic drainage of both pleural spaces.

In selected patients, the pericardial effusion can be controlled by draining the pericardial space and sclerosing the pericardium. The rationale for this approach is similar to that applied in the pleural space. Tetracycline has been the most commonly used sclerosing agent for malignant pericardial effusions; however, the sclerosing agents are generally the same as those used in pleural disease. Although this approach may be the only option in some patients who have end-stage disease, there is a concern that sclerosing the pericardial space may produce a loculated pericardium. In the setting of an incompletely fused pericardium, a recurrent effusion may not be safely accessible by thoracoscopy. This concern is unlikely to be a practical problem if the patient's life expectancy is limited to a few weeks. Pericardial sclerotherapy has been reported to control fluid reaccumulation in 70% to 80% of patients for 30 days (40).

MALIGNANT ASCITES

Ascites in patients with breast cancer can occur either from peritoneal serosal implants or from extensive hepatic metastases and resultant portal hypertension. Extensive hepatic metastases with portal hypertension usually occur as a terminal event. Unless systemic chemotherapy is rapidly effective in reducing the tumor burden, fatal hepatic failure ensues. In this circumstance, ascites is of secondary concern.

The peritoneum is a continuous mesothelial membrane lining the potential space between the intra-abdominal viscera and the abdominal wall. In men, this is a completely closed cavity, whereas in women, it is interrupted by the lumina of the fallopian tubes. The parietal layer covers the abdominal wall, whereas the visceral peritoneum coats the intestine and intra-abdominal organs. The peritoneum is a dialyzing membrane and constantly secretes and reabsorbs serous fluid (3). Accumulation of this fluid, known as ascites, can be found in metastatic breast cancer.

Diagnosis

Ascites from peritoneal tumor implants is uncommon in patients with breast cancer (44). The abdominal bloating associated with ascites is uncomfortable and often causes early satiety, resulting in decreased oral intake. Upward pressure on the diaphragm, which prevents full expansion of the lungs, can cause dyspnea. The ascites itself is usually not life-threatening, because the peritoneal implants are generally only one manifestation of disseminated metastatic disease. Other sites of involvement are often more concerning. Ascites may be confirmed on clinical examination, abdominal ultrasound, or abdominopelvic CT.

Treatment

In patients with metastatic breast cancer and ascites, the most effective therapy is systemic chemotherapy or hormonal therapy directed at reducing tumor mass, which results in a reduced amount of ascites. In the absence of effective systemic therapy, symptomatic ascites can be palliated with paracentesis. Paracentesis is performed using local anesthesia and sterile technique. The patient is usually placed in a left semidecubitus position with the head of the bed elevated. A needle or needle-catheter system similar to that used for thoracentesis is used. The ascitic fluid may be drained manually or using a vacuum bottle system. Occasionally, paracentesis is performed with ultrasound guidance for more precise localization of the ascites. Without control of the underlying tumor, however, ascitic fluid reaccumulates. The rate of reaccumulation and the duration of symptomatic benefit is variable. Some patients experience relief of their symptoms for several days and benefit from repeated paracenteses.

Because of the systemic distribution of disease, intra-abdominal chemotherapy has not been considered an option for most patients with breast cancer.

Peritoneovenous shunts have been described as therapy for patients with malignant ascites and have been shown to reduce abdominal girth and number of paracenteses in selected patients (45). Complications can be serious, however, with significant numbers of patients developing disseminated intravascular coagulation, sepsis, and congestive heart failure. Shunts frequently occlude, and the theoretical concern exists that shunts will disseminate peritoneal tumor cells (46). In practice, peritoneovenous shunts are rarely used to relieve ascites in patients with metastatic breast cancer.

MANAGEMENT SUMMARY

- Malignant pleural effusions are a common complication of metastatic breast cancer and frequently cause dyspnea and chest pain.
- If systemic therapy is not successful at controlling malignant pleural effusions, drainage and sclerosis can be undertaken by a variety of approaches. Video-assisted thoracoscopic surgery together with talc sclerosis is a favored approach.
- Malignant pericardial effusions are common complications of metastatic breast cancer and can be life-threatening, leading to sudden and rapid cardiac decompensation when intrapericardial pressures rise above critical values.
- Malignant pericardial effusions that cause cardiac compromise are medical emergencies. Percutaneous catheter drainage can provide transient relief and cardiovascular stabilization. Placement of a pericardial window using a variety of possible surgical approaches, including video-assisted thoracoscopic surgery and the subxyphoid approach, is usually successful at relieving symptoms for a prolonged period of time.
- Ascites is an uncommon manifestation of metastatic breast cancer and usually results either from peritoneal spread of carcinoma cells or portal hypertension from liver involvement with cancer. This is best managed by controlling the metastatic breast cancer with systemic therapy.

References

1. Antony VB, Loddenkemper R, Astoul P, et al. Management of malignant pleural effusions. *Eur Respir J* 2001;18:402–419.
2. Buck M, Ingle JN, Giuliani ER, et al. Pericardial effusion in women with breast cancer. *Cancer* 1987;60:263–269.
3. Aslam N, Marino CR. Malignant ascites: new concepts in pathophysiology, diagnosis, and management. *Arch Intern Med* 2001;161:2733–2737.
4. American Thoracic Society. Management of malignant pleural effusions. *Am J Respir Crit Care Med* 2000;162:1987–2001.
5. Escalante CP, Martin CG, Elting LS, et al. Dyspnea in cancer patients. Etiology, resource utilization, and survival-implications in a managed care world. *Cancer* 1996;78:1314–1319.
6. Heyes Moore L. Respiratory symptoms. In: Saudners C, ed. *The management of terminal malignant disease*. London: Edward Arnold, 1984:113–118.
7. Lai-Fook SJ. Pleural mechanics and fluid exchange. *Physiol Rev* 2004;84:385–410.
8. Starling EH. On the absorption of fluids from the convective tissue spaces. *J Physiol (Lond)* 1896;19:312–326.
9. Zocchi L. Physiology and pathophysiology of pleural fluid turnover. *Eur Respir J* 2002;20:1545–1558.
10. Dvorak HF, Nagy JA, Berse B, et al. Vascular permeability factor, fibrin, and the pathogenesis of tumor stroma formation. *Ann N Y Acad Sci* 1992;667:101–111.
11. Fentiman IS, Rubens RD, Hayward JL. The pattern of metastatic disease in patients with pleural effusions secondary to breast cancer. *Br J Surg* 1982;69:193–194.
12. Cantö-Armengod A. Macroscopic characteristics of pleural metastases arising from the breast and observed by diagnostic thoracoscopy. *Am Rev Respir Dis* 1990;142:616–618.
13. DeCamp MM Jr, Mentzer SJ, Swanson SJ, et al. Malignant effusive disease of the pleura and pericardium. *Chest* 1997;112:291S–295S.
14. Furman-Haran E, Margalit R, Grobgeld D, et al. Dynamic contrast-enhanced magnetic resonance imaging reveals stress-induced angiogenesis in MCF7 human breast tumors. *Proc Natl Acad Sci U S A* 1996;93:6247–6251.
15. Mentzer SJ, Reilly JJ, Skarin AT, et al. Patterns of lung involvement by malignant lymphoma. *Surgery* 1993;113:507–514.
16. Dines DE, Pierre RV, Franzen SJ. The value of cells in the pleural fluid in the differential diagnosis. *Mayo Clin Proc* 1975;50:571–572.
17. Polunovsky VA, Chen B, Henke C, et al. Role of mesenchymal cell death in lung remodeling after injury. *J Clin Invest* 1993;92:388–397.
18. Aelony Y, King R, Boutin C. Thoracoscopic talc poudrage pleurodesis for chronic recurrent pleural effusions. *Ann Intern Med* 1991;115:778–782.
19. Figlin R, Mendoza E, Piantadosi S, et al. Intrapleural chemotherapy without pleurodesis for malignant pleural effusions: LCSG trial 861. *Chest* 1994;106[Suppl]:363S–366S.
20. Gravelyn TR, Michelson MK, Gross BH, et al. Tetracycline pleurodesis for malignant pleural effusions. A 10-year retrospective study. *Cancer* 1987;59:1973–1977.
21. Heffner JE, Standerfer RJ, Torstveit J, et al. Clinical efficacy of doxycycline for pleurodesis. *Chest* 1994;105:1743–1747.
22. Koldsland S, Svennevig JL, Lehne G, et al. Chemical pleurodesis in malignant pleural effusions: a randomised prospective study of mepacrine versus bleomycin. *Thorax* 1993;48:790–793.
23. Martinez-Moragon E, Aparicio J, Rogado MC, et al. Pleurodesis in malignant pleural effusions: a randomized study of tetracycline versus bleomycin. *Eur Respir J* 1997;10:2380–2383.
24. Ohri SK, Oswal SK, Townsend ER, et al. Early and late outcome after diagnostic thoracoscopy and talc pleurodesis. *Ann Thorac Surg* 1992;53:1038–1041.
25. Torre M, Belloni P. Nd:YAG laser pleurodesis through thoracoscopy: new curative therapy in spontaneous pneumothorax. *Ann Thorac Surg* 1989;47:887–889.
26. van de Brekel JA, Duurkens VA, Vanderschueren RG. Pneumothorax. Results of thoracoscopy and pleurodesis with talc poudrage and thoracotomy. *Chest* 1993;103:345–347.
27. Webb WR, Ozmen V, Moulder PV, et al. Iodized talc pleurodesis for the treatment of pleural effusions. *J Thorac Cardiovasc Surg* 1992;103:881–886.
28. Zimmer PW, Hill M, Casey K, et al. Prospective randomized trial of talc slurry vs. bleomycin in pleurodesis for symptomatic malignant pleural effusions. *Chest* 1997;112:430–434.
29. Walker-Renard PB, Vaughan LM, Sahn SA. Chemical pleurodesis for malignant pleural effusions. *Ann Intern Med* 1994;120:56–64.
30. Hartman DL, Gaither JM, Kesler KA, et al. Comparison of insufflated talc under thoracoscopic guidance with standard tetracycline and bleomycin pleurodesis for control of malignant pleural effusions. *J Thorac Cardiovasc Surg* 1993;105:743–748.
31. Putnam JB Jr, Walsh GL, Swisher SG, et al. Outpatient management of malignant pleural effusion by a chronic indwelling pleural catheter. *Ann Thorac Surg* 2000;69:369–375.
32. Chiles C, Woodard PK, Gutierrez FR, et al. Metastatic involvement of the heart and pericardium: CT and MR imaging. *Radiographics* 2001;21:439–449.
33. Hagemeister FB Jr, Buzdar AU, Luna MA, et al. Causes of death in breast cancer: a clinicopathologic study. *Cancer* 1980;46:162–167.
34. Bisel HF, Wroblewski F, Ladue JS. Incidence and clinical manifestations of cardiac metastases. *J Am Med Assoc* 1953;153:712–715.
35. Warren WH. Malignancies involving the pericardium. *Semin Thorac Cardiovasc Surg* 2000;12:119–129.
36. Sagrista-Sauleda J, Merce J, Permanyer-Miralda G, et al. Clinical clues to the causes of large pericardial effusions. *Am J Med* 2000;109:95–101.
37. Anderson TM, Ray CW, Nwogu CE, et al. Pericardial catheter sclerosis versus surgical procedures for pericardial effusions in cancer patients. *J Cardiovasc Surg (Torino)* 2001;42:415–419.
38. Celermajer DS, Boyer MJ, Bailey BP, et al. Pericardiocentesis for symptomatic malignant pericardial effusion: a study of 36 patients. *Med J Aust* 1991;154:19–22.
39. Girardi LN, Ginsberg RJ, Burt ME. Pericardiocentesis and intrapericardial sclerosis: effective therapy for malignant pericardial effusions. *Ann Thorac Surg* 1997;64:1422–1428.
40. Martinoni A, Cipolla CM, Civelli M, et al. Intrapericardial treatment of neoplastic pericardial effusions. *Herz* 2000;25:787–793.
41. Mentzer SJ, Swanson SJ, Sugarbaker DJ. Malignant effusive disease of the pleura and pericardium. *Chest* 1997;112:291S–295S.
42. Campbell PT, Van Trigt P, Wall TC, et al. Subxiphoid pericardiotomy in the diagnosis and management of large pericardial effusions associated with malignancy. *Chest* 1992;101:938–943.
43. Wall TC, Campbell PT, O'Connor CM, et al. Diagnosis and management (by subxiphoid pericardiotomy) of large pericardial effusions causing cardiac tamponade. *Am J Cardiol* 1992;69:1075–1078.
44. Parsons SL, Watson SA, Steele RJ. Malignant ascites. *Br J Surg* 1996;83:6–14.
45. Souter RG, Wells C, Tarin D, et al. Surgical and pathologic complications associated with peritoneovenous shunts in management of malignant ascites. *Cancer* 1985;55:1973–1978.
46. Tarin D, Price JE, Kettlewell MG, et al. 1984. Mechanisms of human tumor metastasis studied in patients with peritoneovenous shunts. *Cancer Res* 1984;44:3584–3592.

Steven J. Mentzer and Lawrence N. Shulman

Discrete tumors of 3 cm or less in the peripheral lung are commonly referred to as solitary pulmonary nodules. The nodules are typically asymptomatic and are identified by routine radiographic examinations. Solitary pulmonary nodules are not associated with atelectasis or hilar adenopathy. If the nodule is new, based on comparisons with previous chest radiographs, the solitary pulmonary nodule most likely represents either a cancer or a benign granuloma (1–3).

In patients with a history of breast cancer, solitary pulmonary nodules may represent recurrent breast cancer. The lung is a common site for breast cancer metastases (4–6). The lung is the first site of recurrence in 15% to 25% of patients with metastatic breast cancer (7–9). Clinical series have demonstrated that pulmonary metastases are second only to bone is a first site of recurrent breast cancer. In more than half of the patients with lung recurrence, a solitary pulmonary nodule is the presenting sign. Other common intrathoracic sites of metastatic disease include the pleura, mediastinal, pericardium, and internal mammary lymph nodes (7–9).

The pulmonary nodule may also represent a primary lung cancer. Lung cancer in women is both common and frequently fatal. Lung cancer represents 15% of all cancers in women and 26% of all cancer deaths in women (10). The radiographic appearance of the tumor and the patient's clinical risk factors are generally not useful in excluding the possible diagnosis of lung cancer. Approximately 10% to 15% of patients with lung cancer present with a solitary pulmonary nodule; 20% of these patients are nonsmokers. The current data suggest that a solitary pulmonary nodule represents a primary lung cancer in more than 50% patients with a history of breast cancer (1,11–14).

The most common benign pathologic diagnosis of a solitary pulmonary nodule is a granuloma. Granulomas can occur in response to inhaled particulate matter or a variety of infectious pathogens. The histopathologic evaluation of granulomatous lesions typically involve special histochemical studies to exclude acid-fast bacilli, fungal forms, or foreign material. Although granulomas lesions can be routinely cultured, most granulomas are sterile and do not require further therapy.

DIAGNOSIS

Although the patient's risk factors cannot exclude the possibility of lung cancer, the patient's antecedent cancer history increases the likelihood that a solitary pulmonary nodule represents cancer (15,16). In a series from the authors' institution, the probability that a solitary pulmonary nodules was benign was cut in half with a prior history of cancer (17). The malignant diagnosis was linked to the prior cancer in 82% of patients with a history of lung cancer and 79% of patients with a history of extrapulmonary malignancy (17).

Pulmonary nodules are commonly evaluated by chest computed tomography (CT). The CT scan is particularly useful in identifying benign characteristics. Granulomas can be totally calcified or have central or laminar calcification. These observations virtually exclude the diagnosis of malignant diseases (3).

Chest CT scans are more sensitive than chest radiography in detecting pulmonary metastases (18,19). Chest CT scans can detect peripheral nodules as small as 2 to 3 mm. In patients with a discrete nodule on chest radiography and a history of extrathoracic malignancy, CT may detect additional nodular lesions (20,21). A limitation of chest CT scans is that many of these nodules are benign (19–21). Further, the chest CT scan cannot distinguish between primary and metastatic nodules. Despite these limitations, the specificity of CT can be enhanced with attention to other clinical factors. Chest CT scans are also essential for surgical planning.

When malignant disease is a possibility, CT scans of the chest, abdomen, and pelvis can provide important staging information not only for sites of intrathoracic involvement, but also other common metastatic sites for breast cancer, specifically, the liver, peritoneum, and bones (7–9,21). Common metastatic sites for lung cancer include intrathoracic lymph nodes, pleura, liver, bones, and adrenal glands.

Magnetic resonance imaging (MRI) has been used to evaluate lung nodules. This preliminary work suggests that conventional MRI does not have sufficient resolution to provide any additional spatial information to that provided by CT. More recent use of functional scans suggest the utility of MRI scans in assessing pulmonary ventilation and perfusion (22). In addition, dynamic MRI scans provide "washout" information that may help discriminate benign and malignant nodules (23). Despite these potential applications, the additional time and expense of chest MRI has precluded its routine use.

Positron emission tomography (PET) scans are useful in detecting malignancy. Major clinical trials have established a sensitivity greater than 92% for detecting malignancy (24,25). The specificity of PET scans in the lung, however, drops to 76% to 92% because PET scans can be falsely positive in a variety of inflammatory lung diseases such as sarcoidosis and tuberculosis. Conversely, PET scans can be falsely negative in bronchoalveolar carcinoma and may also be negative in malignant lesions of less than 1 cm in diameter (26). PET scans are clinically useful for identifying a lesion as potentially malignant as well as providing extracranial staging information. An integrated PET and CT scan provides additional benefit because the physiological information obtained with ^{18}F-fluorodeoxyglucose (FDG) avidity can be combined with precise topographic localization.

DIAGNOSTIC PROCEDURES

Cytologic studies to confirm a malignant diagnosis have limited value in evaluating the solitary pulmonary nodule. Cytologic specimens are typically obtained from sputum, bronchoscopic washing, and transthoracic needle biopsy. Specimens for sputum cytologic study should be obtained from early morning sputum on 3 consecutive days. Specimens should be appropriately collected to prevent oral contamination and carefully preserved to facilitate interpretation (27). Sputum cytology can yield a malignant diagnosis in 80% of patients with a large central tumor (28). The yield of sputum cytology decreases to less than 25% with more peripheral lesions and diminishing size of the malignancy (28). In patients undergoing bronchoscopic examination, endoscopic brushings and airway lavage can improve the cytologic yield from a peripheral lesion to more than 70% (29). The accuracy of both sputum and bronchial cytology is limited by small sample size. In addition, inflammatory exudates, excessive blood, or poor preservation decrease the tumor detection rate. Cytologically atypical cells in the lung often are associated with inflammatory disorders, further complicating the cytologic diagnosis of malignancy.

Transthoracic needle biopsy performed by fluoroscopic or CT guidance provides the cytologic specimen directly from the peripheral lung nodule. Needle aspiration cytology provides the positive diagnosis of malignancy in 80% to 90% of patients with a malignant nodule (30–32). The procedure is performed on an outpatient basis with a small risk of pneumothorax (about 10%) (33). The major problem with transthoracic needle biopsy is the appreciable false-negative rate (34). For example, Charig et al. (30) have shown that in 38 patients with no malignant cells identified by the technique, 25 were subsequently confirmed to have a lung malignancy. Further, the needle aspiration cytology can differ from the resected specimens in as many as 35% of cases (35). Another problem is that cytologic studies rarely positively establish a benign diagnosis. Even when bacterial or fungal forms are identified in a cytologic specimen, it is difficult to exclude the possibility of a coexistent malignant disease.

Bronchoscopy also has a limited role in evaluating the solitary pulmonary nodule. Bronchoscopy can facilitate cytologic diagnosis by airway washing, cytologic brushings, or bronchoalveolar lavage. These diagnostic approaches may be useful in establishing a diagnosis of infection caused by pulmonary pathogens such as *Mycobacterium tuberculosis*. Although infections with *M. tuberculosis* commonly result in nodular lesions, the patient must be carefully monitored to exclude coexistent carcinoma. An additional bronchoscopic approach is fluoroscopically directed transbronchial biopsy. Transbronchial biopsies are useful in documenting diffuse parenchymal disease, such as lymphangitic carcinoma in the lung. The diagnostic yield of transbronchial biopsy in peripheral lung nodules falls to about 20% to 50%, depending on the size and location of the lesion (3,36). Other limitations of transbronchial biopsy in solitary pulmonary nodules are the small sample size (about 300 alveoli), the small risk of pneumothorax, and the potential delay in establishing a definitive diagnosis.

The most reliable approach to establishing a definitive diagnosis in a patient with a solitary pulmonary nodule is surgical resection. Surgery provides an adequate tissue for cytomorphologic, immunohistochemical, and protein receptor studies. In contrast to other diagnostic approaches, surgery avoids the sampling and interpretative errors that might delay definitive therapy. In the past, the major limitation with surgery was the morbidity associated with a standard thoracotomy. This limitation has resolved with the development of video-assisted thoracoscopic surgery.

THORACOSCOPY

The thoracoscope provides an opportunity to diagnose and treat diseases of the chest with minimal morbidity. Thoracoscopic surgery involves a video thoracoscope and generally two working ports to facilitate manipulation of the lung and other intrathoracic structures (37–40) (Fig. 87.1). Minimally invasive procedures performed through two or three access ports are generally referred to as thoracoscopic operations. The advantages of thoracoscopic video optics and miniaturized instrumentation have led to their incorporation in a variety of thoracic surgical procedures. Because these procedures are performed with variable incision lengths, this spectrum of surgical procedures has led to the more inclusive term of video-assisted thoracic surgery (VATS) (41).

Video thoracoscopy is a surgical approach that requires general anesthesia and a fully equipped operating room. Bronchoscopy is routinely performed at the beginning of the procedure to confirm placement of the double-lumen endotracheal tube or the bronchial blocker. Bronchoscopy also provides an opportunity to identify any potential occult endobronchial

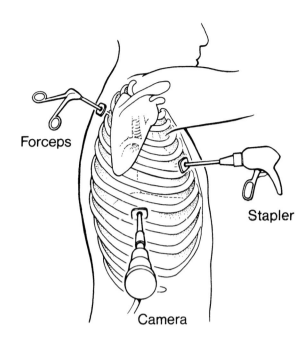

FIGURE 87.1. Video thoracoscopy is performed in the lateral thoracotomy position. Thoracoscopy access ports are positioned to triangulate the area of interest and to facilitate the manipulation of intrathoracic structures. With single-lung ventilation, deflation of the ipsilateral lung provides an opportunity to examine the contents of the hemithorax. The solitary pulmonary nodule can be identified and resected to facilitate the histopathologic diagnosis. If the preliminary frozen section diagnosis is consistent with a primary lung metastasis, the thoracoscope can be used to surgically stage the ipsilateral hemithorax.

lesions (42). Because bronchoscopy is routinely performed at the time of surgery, outpatient bronchoscopy is rarely necessary.

The morbidity of thoracoscopy is minimized by the small incisions used in this procedure. When pulmonary resections are performed, a variable-sized chest drain is used to evacuate residual air and facilitate lung expansion. Depending on the extent of the resection and the condition of the remaining lung, the drain may be indwelling for less than an hour or for more than a few days.

The primary benefit of thoracoscopy is the enhanced flexibility it provides in illuminating difficult diagnostic problems. Video thoracoscopy provides a panoramic view of the ipsilateral hemithorax. This view includes the visceral and parietal pleural surfaces, the internal chest wall, and the internal mammary, hilar, and paratracheal lymph nodes. In the patient with a history of breast cancer, video thoracoscopy provides an opportunity to examine the pleural surfaces for any evidence of malignancy. Small amounts of pleural fluid can be sent for cytologic examination, and biopsy can be performed directly on pleural nodules. Internal mammary, hilar, and paratracheal lymph nodes can be inspected and biopsied. In most cases, the solitary pulmonary nodule can be identified and removed. Histologic margins can be assessed histologically to ensure complete resection.

In the patient with a definitive diagnosis of lung cancer, a VATS anatomic resection can be performed during the same anesthetic. The anatomic resection of a segment or lobe of the lung can be performed with significantly less morbidity than is associated with a standard thoracotomy. The development of improved thoracoscopic instruments have made VATS anatomic resections commonplace. If an accurate histopathologic diagnosis cannot be established at the time of the thoracoscopic procedure, any further resection should be delayed. An advantage of video thoracoscopy is that the procedure presents few limitations for subsequent thoracotomy or VATS lobectomy.

The aggressive natural history of primary lung cancer underscores the importance of establishing a definitive histopathologic diagnosis of lung carcinoma. A definitive diagnosis, however, may be difficult to establish with peripheral adenocarcinomas. Peripheral adenocarcinomas can be ambiguous lesions, presenting a challenge to the pathologist and clinician in discriminating breast metastases from primary lung cancer.

PATHOLOGY EVALUATION

Primary tumors of the lung with squamous cell or small cell cytomorphologic features are easy to distinguish from breast cancer; however, a pathologic diagnosis of adenocarcinoma occurs in 60% to 70% of primary lung cancers (43). Similarly, 80% of the metastatic lesions in the lung are adenocarcinomas (4). Because of their histologic similarity, the distinction between primary lung adenocarcinoma and metastatic breast cancer can be difficult. The association of a peripheral location, pleural retraction, anthracotic pigment, and central scarring were previously thought to be characteristic of lung primaries. These features, however, can be mimicked by metastatic adenocarcinoma of the breast (44).

Special studies occasionally can be helpful in distinguishing primary lung carcinoma from metastatic breast cancer. A problem with immunohistochemical (IHC) stains for estrogen- and progesterone-receptor protein studies is that breast cancer metastases can lose the expression of these distinguishing features. In addition, recurrent breast cancers in the lung are estrogen-receptor positive in only 25% of cases (45). Confounding this observation is the finding that primary lung cancers can express a variety of unexpected proteins. For example, estrogen receptors are expressed in 18% to 30% of primary lung adenocarcinomas (46), although these tumors generally have weak expression of the estrogen receptor, and strong staining suggests a primary breast cancer (47). Similarly, progesterone receptors have been described in about 15% of primary lung cancers (47).

In addition to diagnostic cytomorphologic features, the most discriminating pathologic feature of breast metastases to the lung is immunohistochemical staining for gross cystic disease fluid protein (GCDFP) (48–50). GCDFP is a small molecular weight protein that is associated with apocrine differentiation. It has not been reported in primary lung carcinomas and can effectively exclude the diagnosis of a lung primary (49–51). The limitation of staining for GCDFP is that the antigen is present in only 30% to 50% of breast cancer patients (51–53). Furthermore, primary breast cancers that express this protein may lose antigen expression when they recur systemically.

A more practical test for discriminating lung and breast origin is immunohistochemistry for thyroid transcription factor-1 (TTF-1). TTF-1 is a transcription factor expressed in epithelial cells of the thyroid and lung. Expression of TTF-1 helps distinguish primary lung cancers from metastatic adenocarcinoma from other primary sites (54). The TTF-1 antibodies stain approximately 75% to 85% of pulmonary adenocarcinomas with little or no reactivity with metastatic breast adenocarcinomas (46,55,56). The present data suggest that TTF-1 staining, when positive, is a reliable indicator of a primary lung adenocarcinoma.

RESECTION OF A SOLITARY PULMONARY NODULE

In patients with a solitary breast metastasis, resecting the nodule may have some therapeutic value. Staren et al. (57) report a mean survival of 58 months after resection of a solitary pulmonary nodule. Lanza et al. (58) reviewed 37 cases of surgical resection of a solitary nodule and found a 49.5% actuarial 5-year survival rate. These authors (58) as well as others (59,60) have found a correlation between a longer disease-free interval and improved survival after metastasectomy. This relationship is consistent with studies of metastases of other histologic types (39,58,61). Although these retrospective studies are preliminary, the results suggest that the surgical resection of solitary pulmonary nodules may result in long-term survival benefit for selected patients.

The potential benefit of multiple metastasectomies has been proposed for sarcoma, germ cell tumors, and other selected tumors (39,59,61). These tumors, however, are unique in their tropism for the lung. In contrast to these diseases, breast cancer does not demonstrate a selective pattern of pulmonary metastasis. A potential therapeutic value of the resection of multiple metastases in breast cancer is unlikely (59).

MANAGEMENT SUMMARY

- In a patient with a history of breast cancer, a solitary pulmonary nodule could represent a benign lesion, an isolated metastasis from a known breast cancer or an occult cancer from elsewhere in the body, or a primary lung cancer.
- The focus of the diagnostic evaluation is distinguishing these possibilities. A CT is indicated for this purpose. A PET-CT scan can sometimes be helpful in this situation.
- If, on staging, there is no indication of metastatic disease elsewhere and the nodule appears malignant, then histologic confirmation and potential resection are options that should be explored.
- Minimally invasive surgical approaches (VATS) can be useful to provide a definitive histologic diagnosis, anatomic staging information, and the potential for therapeutic resection.

References

1. Swensen SJ, Jett JR, Payne WS, et al. An integrated approach to evaluation of the solitary pulmonary nodule. *Mayo Clin Proc* 1990;65:173–186.
2. Anderson RW, Arentzen CE. Carcinoma of the lung. *Surg Clin North Am* 1980; 60:793–814.
3. Swensen SJ, Silverstein MD, Ilstrup DM, et al. The probability of malignancy in solitary pulmonary nodules. Application to small radiologically indeterminate nodules. *Arch Intern Med* 1997;157:849–855.
4. Abrams HL, Spiro R, Goldstein N. Metastases in carcinoma. Analysis of 1,000 autopsied cases. *Cancer* 1950;3:74–85.
5. Warren S, Witham EM. Studies on tumor metastasis. 2. The distribution of metastases in cancer of the breast. *Surg Gynecol Obstet* 1933;57:81–85.
6. Saphir O, Parker ML. Metastasis of primary carcinoma of the breast with special reference to spleen, adrenal glands and ovaries. *Arch Surg* 1941;42:1003–1018.
7. Kamby C, Vejborg I, Kristensen B, et al. Metastatic pattern in recurrent breast cancer. Special reference to intrathoracic recurrences. *Cancer* 1988;62:2226–2233.
8. Kamby C, Rose C, Ejlertsen B, et al. Stage and pattern of metastases in patients with breast cancer. *Eur J Cancer Clin Oncol* 1987;23:1925–1934.
9. Nikkanen TA. Recurrence of breast cancer. A retrospective study of 569 cases in clinical stages I–III. *Acta Chir Scand* 1981;147:239–245.
10. Jemal A, Siegel R, Ward E, et al. Cancer statistics, 2008. *CA Cancer J Clin* 2008; 58:71–96.
11. Cahan WG, Castro EB, Huvos AG. Primary breast and lung carcinoma in the same patient. *J Thorac Cardiovasc Surg* 1974;68:546–555.
12. Cahan WG, Castro EB. Significance of a solitary lung shadow in patients with breast cancer. *Ann Surg* 1975;181:137–143.
13. Casey JJ, Stempel BG, Scanlon EF, et al. The solitary pulmonary nodule in the patient with breast cancer. *Surgery* 1984;96:801–805.
14. Chang EY, Johnson W, Karamlou K, et al. The evaluation and treatment implications of isolated pulmonary nodules in patients with a recent history of breast cancer. *Am J Surg* 2006;191:641–645.
15. Gould MK, Fletcher J, Iannettoni MD, et al. Evaluation of patients with pulmonary nodules: when is it lung cancer?: ACCP evidence-based clinical practice guidelines (2nd ed.). *Chest* 2007;132:108S–130S.
16. Khokhar S, Vickers A, Moore MS, et al. Significance of non-calcified pulmonary nodules in patients with extrapulmonary cancers. *Thorax* 2006;61:331–336.
17. Mery CM, Pappas AN, Bueno R, et al. Relationship between a history of antecedent cancer and the probability of malignancy for a solitary pulmonary nodule. *Chest* 2004;125:2175–2181.
18. Chalmers N, Best JJ. The significance of pulmonary nodules detected by CT but not by chest radiography in tumour staging. *Clin Radiol* 1991;44:410–412.
19. Davis SD. CT evaluation for pulmonary metastases in patients with extrathoracic malignancy. *Radiology* 1991;180:1–12.
20. Fernandez EB, Colon E, McLeod DG, et al. Efficacy of radiographic chest imaging in patients with testicular cancer. *Urology* 1994;44:243–249.
21. Scott WW Jr, Fishman EK. Detection of internal mammary lymph node enlargement: comparison of CT scans and conventional roentgenograms. *Clin Imaging* 1991;15:268–272.

22. Fain SB, Korosec FR, Holmes JH, et al. Functional lung imaging using hyperpolarized gas MRI. *J Magn Reson Imaging* 2007;25:910–923.
23. Schaefer JF, Schneider V, Vollmar J, et al. Solitary pulmonary nodules: association between signal characteristics in dynamic contrast enhanced MRI and tumor angiogenesis. *Lung Cancer* 2006;53:39–49.
24. Czernin J, Phelps ME. Positron emission tomography scanning: current and future applications. *Annu Rev Med* 2002;53:89–112.
25. Fletcher JW, Kymes SM, Gould M, et al. A comparison of the diagnostic accuracy of ^{18}F-FDG PET and CT in the characterization of solitary pulmonary nodules. *J Nucl Med* 2008;49:179–185.
26. Fischer BM, Mortensen J, Dirksen A, et al. Positron emission tomography of incidentally detected small pulmonary nodules. *Nucl Med Commun* 2004;25:3–9.
27. Walts AE. Cytologic techniques for the diagnosis of pulmonary neoplasms. In: Marchevsky AM, ed. *Lung biology in health and disease. Surgical pathology of lung neoplasms.* New York: Marcel Dekker, 1990:29–61.
28. Ng AB, Horak GC. Factors significant in the diagnostic accuracy of lung cytology in bronchial washing and sputum samples. II. Sputum samples. *Acta Cytol* 1983;27:397–402.
29. Ng AB, Horak GC. Factors significant in the diagnostic accuracy of lung cytology in bronchial washing and sputum samples. I. Bronchial washings. *Acta Cytol* 1983;27:391–396.
30. Charig MJ, Stutley JE, Padley SP, et al. The value of negative needle biopsy in suspected operable lung cancer. *Clin Radiol* 1991;44:147–149.
31. Cristallini EG, Ascani S, Farabi R, et al. Fine needle aspiration biopsy in the diagnosis of intrathoracic masses. *Acta Cytol* 1992;36:416–422.
32. Zakowski MF, Gatscha RM, Zaman MB. Negative predictive value of pulmonary fine needle aspiration cytology. *Acta Cytol* 1992;36:283–286.
33. Collins CD, Breatnach E, Nath PH. Percutaneous needle biopsy of lung nodules following failed bronchoscopic biopsy. *Eur J Radiol* 1992;15:49–53.
34. Veale D, Gilmartin JJ, Sumerling MD, et al. Prospective evaluation of fine needle aspiration in the diagnosis of lung cancer. *Thorax* 1988;43:540–544.
35. Horrigan TP, Bergin KT, Snow N. Correlation between needle biopsy of lung tumors and histopathologic analysis of resected specimens. *Chest* 1986;90:638–640.
36. Wang KP, Haponik EF, Britt EJ, et al. Transbronchial needle aspiration of peripheral pulmonary nodules. *Chest* 1984;86:819–823.
37. DeCamp MM Jr, Jaklitsch MT, Mentzer SJ, et al. The safety and versatility of video-thoracoscopy: a prospective analysis of 895 consecutive cases. *J Am Coll Surg* 1995;181:113–120.
38. Landreneau RJ, Mack MJ, Hazelrigg SR, et al. Video-assisted thoracic surgery: basic technical concepts and intercostal approach strategies. *Ann Thorac Surg* 1992;54:800–807.
39. Mentzer SJ, Antman KH, Attinger C, et al. Selected benefits of thoracotomy and chemotherapy for sarcoma metastatic to the lung. *J Surg Oncol* 1993;53:54–59.
40. Rena O, Papalia E, Ruffini E, et al. The role of surgery in the management of solitary pulmonary nodule in breast cancer patients. *Eur J Surg Oncol* 2007;33:546–550.
41. McKneally MF, Lewis RJ, Anderson RJ, et al. Statement of the AATS/STS Joint Committee on Thoracoscopy and Video Assisted Thoracic Surgery. *J Thorac Cardiovasc Surg* 1992;104:1.
42. King DS, Castleman B. Bronchial involvement in metastatic pulmonary malignancy. *J Thorac Surg* 1943;12:305–315.
43. Edwards BK, Howe HL, Ries LA, et al. Annual report to the nation on the status of cancer, 1973–1999, featuring implications of age and aging on U.S. cancer burden. *Cancer* 2002;94:2766–2792.
44. Marchevsky AM. Metastatic tumors of the lung. In: Marchevsky AM, ed. *Lung biology in health and disease. Surgical pathology of lung neoplasms.* New York: Marcel Dekker, 1990:231–245.
45. Johnson FE, Rosen PP, Menendez-Botet C, et al. Estrogen receptor protein in visceral metastases from breast carcinoma. *Am J Surg* 1981;142:252–254.
46. Lau SK, Chu PG, Weiss LM. Immunohistochemical expression of estrogen receptor in pulmonary adenocarcinoma. *Appl Immunohistochem Mol Morphol* 2006;14:83–87.
47. Beattie CW, Hansen NW, Thomas PA. Steroid receptors in human lung cancer. *Cancer Res* 1985;45:4206–4214.
48. Wick MR, Lillemoe TJ, Copland GT, et al. Gross cystic disease fluid protein-15 as a marker for breast cancer: immunohistochemical analysis of 690 human neoplasms and comparison with alpha-lactalbumin. *Hum Pathol* 1989;20:281–287.
49. Brown RW, Campagna LB, Dunn JK, et al. Immunohistochemical identification of tumor markers in metastatic adenocarcinoma. A diagnostic adjunct in the determination of primary site. *Am J Clin Pathol* 1997;107:12–19.
50. Pagani A, Sapino A, Eusebi V, et al. PIP/GCDFP-15 gene expression and apocrine differentiation in carcinomas of the breast. *Virchows Arch* 1994;425:459–465.
51. Chaubert P, Hurlimann J. Mammary origin of metastases. Immunohistochemical determination. *Arch Pathol Lab Med* 1992;116:1181–1188.
52. Monteagudo C, Merino MJ, LaPorte N, et al. Value of gross cystic disease fluid protein-15 in distinguishing metastatic breast carcinomas among poorly differentiated neoplasms involving the ovary. *Hum Pathol* 1991;22:368–372.
53. Fiel MI, Cernaianu G, Burstein DE, et al. Value of GCDFP-15 (BRST-2) as a specific immunocytochemical marker for breast carcinoma in cytologic specimens. *Acta Cytol* 1996;40:637–641.
54. Holzinger A, Dingle S, Bejarano PA, et al. Monoclonal antibody to thyroid transcription factor-1: production, characterization, and usefulness in tumor diagnosis. *Hybridoma* 1996;15:49–53.
55. Harlamert HA, Mira J, Bejarano PA, et al. Thyroid transcription factor-1 and cytokeratins 7 and 20 in pulmonary and breast carcinoma. *Acta Cytol* 1998;42:1382–1388.
56. Bejarano PA, Baughman RP, Biddinger PW, et al. Surfactant proteins and thyroid transcription factor-1 in pulmonary and breast carcinomas. *Mod Pathol* 1996;9:445–452.
57. Staren ED, Salerno C, Rongione A, et al. Pulmonary resection for metastatic breast cancer. *Arch Surg* 1992;127:1282–1284.
58. Lanza LA, Natarajan G, Roth JA, et al. Long-term survival after resection of pulmonary metastases from carcinoma of the breast. *Ann Thorac Surg* 1992;54:244–248.
59. Friedel G, Linder A, Toomes H. The significance of prognostic factors for the resection of pulmonary metastases of breast cancer. *Thorac Cardiovasc Surg* 1994;42:71–75.
60. Schlappack OK, Baur M, Steger G, et al. The clinical course of lung metastases from breast cancer. *Klin Wochenschr* 1988;66:790–795.
61. Brandt B, Ehrenhaft JL. Surgical management of pulmonary metastasis. *Curr Probl Cancer* 1980;4:1–25.

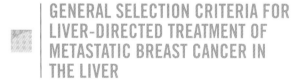

Chapter 88
Management of Isolated Liver Metastases

Rebecca Miksad, Douglas Hanto, Robert D. Timmerman, and Steven Come

About half of all patients with metastatic breast cancer develop liver metastases (1–3), and this development generally portends a poor prognosis. Median overall survival (OS) after the diagnosis of liver metastases ranges from 4 to 17 months (4,5). In comparison, median survival after the diagnosis of extrahepatic metastases may be as long as 29 to 48 months for bone-only disease (6,7). Since liver metastases commonly occur in the setting of concurrent extrahepatic metastases, liver involvement is generally considered to be a manifestation of disseminated disease, and patients are usually treated with systemic therapy (4,5,8,9) (see Chapters 73–80). However, a minority of patients present with metastatic breast cancer limited to the liver (5% to 12%) (3–5,10). In an effort to improve disease control in these patients, localized, liver-directed therapy for breast cancer has been explored. Published studies have evaluated the safety and benefit of hepatic resection, radiofrequency ablation (RFA), transarterial chemoembolization (TACE) or intra-arterial chemotherapy, stereotactic body radiation therapy (SBRT), and interstitial laser therapy (ILT) to treat liver metastases from breast cancer. However, the comparative efficacies of these approaches remain controversial because there have been no randomized controlled trials. Furthermore, identifying appropriate patients for treatment remains a challenge (3,9,11) and the carefully selected patients in published series may represent good prognosis subgroups independent of the therapeutic approach.

Nevertheless, studies suggest that treatment of metastatic breast cancer limited to the liver may benefit some patients. In addition, as improvements in systemic therapies offer better control of metastatic disease and longer survival, more patients may need localized management of liver metastases. This chapter reviews localized, liver-directed treatment of metastatic breast cancer limited to the liver, details specific clinical considerations for each treatment option, and describes the available data for common and emerging approaches.

GENERAL SELECTION CRITERIA FOR LIVER-DIRECTED TREATMENT OF METASTATIC BREAST CANCER IN THE LIVER

Careful patient selection is essential to optimize the risk–benefit ratio of liver-directed approaches. The patients most likely to benefit from these approaches have a good overall prognosis (see Chapters 31 and 32). Specifically, candidates should have controlled primary disease, limited metastatic disease in the liver (both number and size of lesions), longer disease-free intervals, a younger age, and a higher performance status (3,5,12–15). The presence of extrahepatic metastatic or residual primary breast cancer is commonly (16,17), although not always (18,19), considered a contraindication to liver-directed therapy, an approach supported by the more extensive experience in colorectal cancer (20,21).

Preprocedure work-up should define the extent of disease as well as its (known or potential) responsiveness to systemic therapy to aid risk assessment and decision making. Commonly used imaging studies are computed tomography (CT) imaging of the chest to rule out pulmonary and mediastinal disease; triphasic CT scan of the abdomen and pelvis to evaluate the number and location of liver metastases in order to facilitate procedure planning and to rule out other intra-abdominal disease; and a bone scan to rule out bone metastases. A positron emission tomography (PET) scan may also be useful to identify extrahepatic disease (see Chapters 34 and 35). The need for thorough staging was highlighted in a series of 90 breast cancer patients evaluated for resection of liver metastases: 60% were deemed ineligible preoperatively due to extrahepatic metastases, 22% had unresectable extrahepatic disease at exploratory laparotomy, and only 10% ultimately underwent resection (15).

Palliative liver-directed treatment may be beneficial if the hepatic disease impairs the patient's quality of life. However, recent improvements in outcomes for endocrine-responsive and for *ERBB2* (formerly *HER2/neu*) amplified cancers, as well as a trend toward palliative single-agent chemotherapy, render systemic therapy more effective and better tolerated than previously (22–24). Thus, the risks and benefits of liver-directed therapies should be compared to systemic treatment options (5) (see Chapters 73 through 80).

SURGICAL TREATMENT OPTION: HEPATIC RESECTION

Hepatic resection (metastectomy) is the most commonly available liver-directed treatment option for patients with isolated liver lesions. The morbidity and mortality of hepatic resection has declined significantly over the past two decades due to improvements in (a) understanding of intrahepatic segmental anatomy; (b) imaging techniques (three-dimensional CT and intraoperative ultrasound) to characterize the tumor; (c) anesthetic management; (d) surgical techniques (preoperative portal vein embolization, segmental and anatomic resections, vascular inflow occlusion, maintenance of low central venous pressure, devices for safer division of the liver parenchyma and for maintenance of hemostasis); (e) laparoscopic hepatic resection approaches; (f) understanding of negative risk factors (steatosis, remnant liver volume, and preoperative chemotherapy); and (g) postoperative care (25). As a result, surgical resection is a technically safe option for patients with metastatic breast cancer limited to the liver.

Patients deemed to be surgical candidates after preoperative screening undergo additional evaluation in the operating room. Prior to hepatic resection, patients are often explored to rule out extrahepatic, intra-abdominal disease. Intraoperative ultrasound may identify additional liver lesions not imaged preoperatively, can characterize the exact location of the lesion(s), and is able to define the proximity of lesions to venous structures. The value of this additional exploration was demonstrated by a series of 108 breast cancer patients considered for hepatic resection after extensive preoperative evaluation with imaging (26). Over a 20-year period, 23% were found to have unresectable extrahepatic or hepatic disease during abdominal exploration and an additional 13% had unexpected, but resectable, intra-abdominal disease (26). Of the 85 patients who ultimately underwent hepatic resection, an R0 (microscopically negative margin) resection was only attained in 65%, while an R1 (microscopically positive margin) resection was achieved in 18% and an R2 resection (macroscopically positive margin) was accomplished in 17% (26).

Selection Criteria for Hepatic Resection

In addition to the general selection criteria outlined above, hepatic resection candidates must have lesions that can be completely resected while leaving an adequately sized liver remnant. Because the function and architecture of the liver are integrated, adequate liver function can be maintained if there is a critical volume of intact liver and a contiguous bile duct system (20% of a normal liver, 40% of the liver if steatosis is present). If a small liver remnant is anticipated, a patient may benefit from preoperative portal vein embolization (right or left) of the lobe to be resected. This causes hypertrophy of the opposite lobe (the lobe that will become the liver remnant), thereby decreasing the risk of postoperative hepatic insufficiency (27).

Although there are limited data, the combination of hepatic resection and RFA has been explored for metastatic disease in both lobes or in those who have one or more lesions that are technically unresectable (16). In addition, while patients with extrahepatic metastases are traditionally excluded from resection, some series include patients with controlled extrahepatic disease (26).

Outcome of Hepatic Resection for Metastatic Breast Cancer

Most published series of outcomes after hepatic resection for metastatic breast cancer involve small, non-uniform patient populations (Table 88.1). The survival data reflect this heterogeneity: median overall survival in 19 published series (total of 495 patients) ranges from 15 to 63 months and the 5-year survival rate ranges from 18% to 61% (12–16,26,28–40). The postoperative mortality is commonly 0% (13,14,16,26), although rates of 3% (n = 34) (32) to 6% (n = 17) (12) in small series have been reported. Morbidity rates range from 0% (12) to 29% (32).

Despite the limits of case series data, several favorable prognostic factors have emerged for hepatic resection of metastatic breast cancer. Consistent with the colorectal and primary liver tumor literature, smaller metastatic breast cancer liver lesions and a lower number of liver lesions are associated with a better prognosis with hepatic resection (12,13). In addition, a longer length of time between initial diagnosis and the development of liver metastases (more than 1 year [12], 3 years [14], or 4 years [13,15]) is associated with improved survival in some series, but not all (16,26,35). The type of resection attained may also be important: an R0 resection (22% to 43% 5-year survival) conferred improved survival compared to an R2 resection (0% to 16% 5-year survival) (26,32). However, an earlier series of 54 patients did not demonstrate the same benefit: median survival was 40 months for R0 resections and 31 months for R1 and R2 resections (p = .56) (37). In this series, the only significant prognostic predictor of median survival was hormone-receptor status: 44 months if positive and 19 months if negative. This result was substantiated in two series published subsequently for 5-year survival (49% for estrogen receptor [ER]-positive primary tumors compared to 23% for ER negative [p = 0.10]) (26) and median survival (3.52 years for ER positive compared to 1.5 years for ER negative [p = 0.02]) (40).

In the largest (n = 85) and most recent series of liver resection for metastatic breast cancer, the median survival was 32 months and the 5-year survival was 37% (26). Multivariate analysis identified three factors correlated with poor outcome: (a) the absence of response to preresection chemotherapy (p = .008); (b) an R2 resection (p = .0001); and (c) lack of repeat resection for recurrent liver disease (p = .01). The most important predictor of survival in this series was the completeness of the resection, with only 10% of R2 resection patients surviving 5 years, compared with 42% of R1 and 43% of R0 patients. Patients who developed recurrent liver metastases and then underwent reresection had a 5-year survival of 81%, while those who did not had a 5-year survival of 29%. Although the presence of extrahepatic disease did not affect prognosis in this multivariate analysis, the subset of patients with extrahepatic disease at the time of hepatectomy had a

| Table 88.1 | SUMMARY OF HEPATIC RESECTION FOR METASTATIC BREAST CANCER TO THE LIVER |

Author (Reference)	Year	Type of Study	No. of Patients (N)	Median Survival (mos)	5-Year Survival (%)
Schneebaum et al. (29)	1994	CR	6	42	—
Lorenz et al. (30)	1995	CR	8	15	12
Elias et al. (31)	1995	CS	21	26	22
Raab et al. (32)	1998	CS	34	27	18
Seifert et al. (33)	1999	CR	15	57	54 (3 yrs)
Kondo et al. (34)	2000	CR	6	36	40
Maksan et al. (15)	2000	CS	9	—	51
Selzner et al. (12)	2000	CS	17	25	22
Yoshimoto et al. (35)	2000	CS	25	34	27
Pocard et al. (13)	2000	CR	65	47	46 (4 yrs)
Carlini et al. (36)	2002	CS	17	53	46
Elias et al. (37)	2003	CS	54	34	50 (3 yrs)
Vlastos et al. (16)	2004	CR	31	63	61
d'Annibale et al. (14)	2005	CS	18	32	30
Ercolani et al. (38)	2005	CR	21	42	25
Okaro et al. (84)	2005	CS	6	31	—
Sakamoto et al. (39)	2005	CR	34	36	21
Adam et al. (26)	2006	CR	85	32	37
Martinez et al. (40)	2006	CR	20	32	33

CR, chart review; CS, case series.
Note: Table 88.1 has been expanded and updated from Table 80.1, *Diseases of the Breast*, 3rd Edition.

lower 5-year survival (16%) compared to patients with resected or controlled extrahepatic disease (25%) and those without extrahepatic disease (43%).

Although the data are limited to case series, hepatic resection for metastatic breast cancer can be performed safely and may result in favorable median and 5-year survival rates for appropriately selected patients. However, hepatic resection has not been compared in a randomized trial with systemic chemotherapy or with nonsurgical, liver-directed options.

 # NONSURGICAL, LIVER-DIRECTED, LOCALIZED TREATMENT OPTIONS

The data for nonsurgical, liver-directed, localized therapy are most thoroughly developed for primary hepatocellular cancer (HCC) (41) and for metastatic colon cancer (42,43). However, there are emerging data for metastatic breast cancer. The lack of randomized, controlled clinical trials limits interpretation of survival benefit and comparative efficacy. In general, nonsurgical, liver-directed therapies can be done percutaneously, allowing for a shorter recovery time and facilitating the administration of systemic treatment when planned.

Transarterial Chemoembolization and Intraarterial Chemotherapy

In contrast to the normal liver parenchyma, which is primarily fed by the portal vein, tumors in the liver are supplied by the hepatic artery. TACE takes advantage of this blood supply pattern by instilling cytotoxic agents mixed with iodized oil into the hepatic artery feeding the tumor and then embolizing this vessel (often with gelatin sponge particles) to cut off the tumor blood supply (44). Because of the differential blood supply, the normal liver parenchyma suffers relatively little harm. Intraarterial chemotherapy follows the same principles as TACE, but embolization is not performed. Chemotherapy may be distilled once during a single procedure, or a pump may be placed for longer-term, continuous infusion.

The technical success of TACE is demonstrated by the presence of hyperattenuating iodized oil within the tumor on unenhanced CT (45). Because the size of the liver tumor may not change after liver-directed therapy (46), the European Association for the Study of the Liver (EASL) has been proposed as an alternative to the Response Evaluation Criteria in Solid Tumors (RECIST). Originally developed for HCC, the EASL recommends that the standard for determining treatment response after liver-directed therapy be lesion enhancement (47). A surrogate end point for response is the apparent diffusion coefficient (ADC), which measures the mobility of water in tissues: viable tumor cells restrict the mobility of water while necrotic tumor cells allow increased diffusion (45). In one study of TACE for patients with metastatic breast cancer (n = 14, prospective chart review), no tumors met the RECIST criteria for complete response, but the ADC increased by a mean of 27% after treatment (45).

Overall treatment efficacy may be improved by combining TACE with other localized treatments such as radiofrequency ablation (48) and SBRT. However, the best sequencing of and the optimal interval between each therapy are unknown.

Selection Criteria for Transarterial Chemoembolization

Although TACE and intra-arterial chemotherapy techniques were developed to spare the normal liver, common complications stem from liver damage, especially if there is inadequate functional reserve or poor blood flow to the liver. In addition to the general selection criteria for localized treatment of liver metastases, commonly accepted contraindications to TACE for metastatic breast cancer are derived from the literature for other malignancies: absence of hepatopetal blood flow (portal vein thrombosis); encephalopathy; and biliary obstruction (44). Relative contraindications are serum bilirubin greater than 2 mg/dL; lactate dehydrogenase greater than 425 U/L; aspartate aminotransferase greater than 100 U/L; tumor burden involving more than 50% of the liver or both lobes of the liver; cardiac or renal insufficiency; ascites; recent variceal bleed; and significant thrombocytopenia (49). Although there are limited prognostic data for metastatic breast cancer treated with TACE, these contraindications are primarily related to technical issues and the patient's ability to tolerate liver injury incurred from the procedure.

Potentially serious complications from TACE are liver failure, tumor rupture, encephalopathy, acute cholecystitis, acute pancreatitis, and arterial damage (44). More commonly, patients experience fever, nausea, and abdominal pain. Because of these potential complications, patients are often observed overnight in the hospital after the procedure (44). However, the complication rate for TACE tends to be lower than for long-term arterial infusion (46). In a series from 2000 of 484 patients who underwent TACE for recurrent HCC, complication and death rates were 23% and 4%, respectively (44).

Outcome of Transarterial Chemoembolization for Metastatic Breast Cancer

The largest study of TACE in metastatic breast cancer is a retrospective chart review of 48 patients with primary breast carcinoma who underwent either TACE (n = 28) or systemic chemotherapy (n = 20) (criteria for treatment choice not described) (50). With no grade 3 or 4 adverse events, TACE had a 35.7% response rate (30% 2-year survival) while systemic chemotherapy had a 7.1% response rate (11% 2-year survival). Response rates were calculated according to World Health Organization (WHO) criteria for patients who experienced disappearance of the tumor, termed complete remission (CR), or a decrease in tumor size of more than 50%, termed partial remission (PR) (50). A chart review of eight patients treated with TACE demonstrated a median OS of 6 months, with no patient surviving longer than 14 months (46). Recently, a study of 14 patients with 27 lesions using magnetic resonance imaging (MRI) showed a median survival of 25 months and a 35% OS at 3 years (45). Once again, it is difficult to establish a survival benefit for TACE in the absence of randomized, controlled trials. A summary of nonsurgical locoregional treatments for metastatic breast cancer to the liver is given in Table 88.2.

Radiofrequency Ablation

RFA is a minimally invasive technique that uses extreme heat to destroy cancer cells. An electrode is inserted into the tumor and high-frequency alternating current is transmitted from the tip of the probe into the surrounding tissue (51). As the tissue molecules become excited, heat (>60°C) is generated and coagulative necrosis occurs. The amount of tissue

| Table 88.2 | SUMMARY NONSURGICAL LOCOREGIONAL TREATMENTS FOR METASTATIC BREAST CANCER TO THE LIVER |

Author (Reference)	Year	Type of Study	No. of Patients (N)	Median Survival (mos)	Survival (Time Point)
Radiofrequency Ablation (RFA)					
Livraghi et al. (65)	2001	NRT	24	—	96% (4 to 44 mos)
Lawes et al. (66)	2006	NRT	19	—	41% (2.5 yrs)
Gunabushanam et al. (85)	2007	NRT	14	—	64% (1 yrs)
Sofocleous et al. (19)	2007	CR	12	60	30% (5 yrs)
Transarterial Chemoembolization (TACE)					
Giroux et al. (46)	2004	CR	8	6	0% (13 mos)
Li et al. (50)	2005	CR	48	28	30% (2 yrs)
Buijs et al. (45)	2007	CR	14	25	35% (3 yrs)
Stereotactic Body Radiation Therapy (SBRT)					
Wulf et al. (81)	2001	NRT	23	—	61% tumor control at 24 mos
Herfurth et al. (80)	2004	NRT	37	—	67% tumor control at 18 mos
Katz et al. (82)	2007	CR	69	14.5	57% tumor control at 20 mos
Interstitial Laser Therapy (ILT)					
Mack et al. (49)	2004	NRT	232	4.3 yrs	41% (5 yrs)
Hepatic Arterial Infusion (HAI)					
Fraschini et al. (86)	1987	NRT	31	11	—
Ikeda et al. (87)	1999	NRT	28	25.3	—
Camacho et al. (88)	2007	NRT	10	—	All developed tumor progression

NRT, nonrandomized trial; CS, case series; CR, chart review; PS, pilot study.
Note: Table 88.2 has been expanded and updated from Table 80.1, *Diseases of the Breast*, 3rd Edition.

destroyed is related to the impedance properties of the tissue and the distance of the tissue from the electrode. Tissue destruction may be modulated by the cooling effect of a heat sink, such as blood vessels located adjacent to the tumor: heat is carried away and the necessary temperature for coagulative necrosis may not be reached (52,53).

Sites treated with RFA frequently cavitate after the procedure, forming a distinctive scar band. The risk of complications increases with proximity to the porta hepatis. Rarely, hepatitis, infection, and injury to larger bile ducts and nearby bowels may occur. Patients with pre-existing liver damage such as cirrhosis and those with larger tumors are more likely to experience complications (54). Although not typical, needle track seeding has been reported (54). Given the generally limited risks, RFA can be done as an outpatient.

Selection Criteria for Radiofrequency Ablation

In addition to the general selection criteria for localized treatment of liver metastases, tumor size and the number of liver metastases are important selection criteria for other tumor types treated with RFA, both for achieving local control and for predicting a survival benefit. However, there are few prognostic data for metastatic breast cancer. In colorectal cancer, fewer lesions and smaller tumors were associated with improved survival: the 5-year survival rate was 56% for solitary colorectal liver metastases less than 2.5 cm in size, 13% for larger lesions, and 11% for multiple lesions (55). Similar size limitations were observed for HCC: RFA induced a CR in 80% of HCC tumors 3 cm or less (56) but was substantially less effective in HCC tumors larger than 3 cm (50% response) (57). It is unclear if these experiences can be extrapolated to the metastatic breast cancer setting.

Outcome of Radiofrequency Ablation for Metastatic Breast Cancer

Although RFA has been extensively studied for colorectal liver metastases (20,58–63), there is growing case series evidence for metastatic breast cancer (Table 88.2). After a median follow-up of 16 months, 64% of patients were alive in a group of 14 patients with 16 tumors treated with RFA (64). In a larger case series of 24 breast cancer patients with 64 liver metastases treated with RFA and followed for a median of 19 months, 58% developed new metastases, the majority of which occurred in the liver (71%) (65). However, most patients with disease limited to the liver were disease free at last follow-up.

In contrast, a separate series demonstrated good survival for both those with and without extrahepatic metastases at the time of RFA: six of eleven patients with extrahepatic disease were disease free after a median follow-up of 15 months (66).

In most reported cases for metastatic breast cancer, RFA was used in combination with systemic chemotherapy, and very few side effects (mild right upper quadrant discomfort and asymptomatic pleural effusion) were noted but none required specific treatment (19,64). RFA has also been combined with surgical resection (16). Based on these data and the experience in other malignancies, RFA for metastatic breast cancer limited to the liver may be beneficial for select patients. The data for patients with concurrent extrahepatic disease are mixed.

Stereotactic Body Radiation Therapy

SBRT approaches evolved from intracranial stereotactic radiosurgery (SRS) and stereotactic radiotherapy (SRT) to treat tumors outside of the cranium and therefore, subject to physiologic movement (67–69). The term *stereotactic* describes the correlation of the tumor target position to fiducials with a reliable and readily known position (70). Unlike conventionally fractionated radiotherapy (CFRT), stereotactic radiation is completed with a limited number of high-dose fractions with a steep dose gradient (71).

Although a large safety margin can be added to CFRT to compensate for tumor motion, the potent radiation dose in each fraction (10 to 20 Gy) of SBRT means that the tumor must be tracked to accommodate its motion while minimizing damage to normal tissue (70). Fiducials, often gold seeds, are placed in a way that they maintain the same relationship to the tumor, despite physiologic movement, in order to accurately define the tumor target. Fiducials define a coordinate system used in SBRT treatment and planning to achieve a conformal and compact dose distribution that treats effectively, controls for motion (four-dimensional therapy), and minimizes normal tissue damage (72,73).

Patient Selection for Stereotactic Body Radiation Therapy

Because SBRT relies on imaging to precisely define the target lesion(s) to accommodate physiologic motion, candidates for this approach should have tumors with well-delineated borders and must also be willing and able to have fiducials placed. Theoretically, the primary size limitation for SBRT is the size of the remaining liver after treatment. Based on the surgical literature, this critical liver volume is considered to be about one third of the liver (around 500 to 700 cm^3) (74,75) and damaging more than this amount may cause liver failure (76). Other potential SBRT complications are radiation damage, bile duct injury (rare), and damage to organs adjacent to the tumor such as the stomach, kidney, or lung (rare).

Early CT follow-up to assess response after SBRT can be hindered by a zone of *hypo*density corresponding to the normal tissue volume that received approximately 30 Gy (74,77). This phenomenon is of uncertain etiology, and there is no known clinical consequence (77). After a few months, the adjacent normal tissue may appear to have increasing *hyper*density (77).

Outcome of Stereotactic Body Radiation Therapy for Metastatic Breast Cancer

Data for SBRT of breast cancer metastatic to the liver are limited. However, there are several prospective trials of SBRT that include a mix of primary tumor types, including metastatic breast cancer (Table 88.2). After retrospective results showed promise for SBRT (76,78), 37 patients with 60 lesions (4 primary liver tumors and 56 metastatic tumors, 14 of which were breast cancer) were prospectively treated with a single fraction of SBRT (dose escalated from 14 to 25 Gy) (79). No major complications were reported, and the actuarial freedom from local failure rate at 18 months was 67%, with failures mainly occurring in patients treated with lower doses. An updated report with long-term follow-up, however, showed higher rates of recurrence (80).

A higher dose (about 30 Gy in three fractions) was used in a series of 23 patients who received SBRT for liver metastases, 6 (26%) of which were metastatic breast cancer, and achieved actuarial local control rates at 1 and 2 years of 76% and 61%, respectively (81). Although there was one case of self-limited grade 2 hepatitis at 6 weeks, no patient experienced a grade 3 or higher toxicity. However, in a phase II study of colorectal metastases treated with SBRT (69% with metastases to the liver) one patient died of hepatic failure, one patient required surgery for a colonic perforation, and two patients were conservatively treated for duodenal ulcerations (18). A prospective SBRT study of 69 patients (16 [23%] with metastatic breast cancer) with a total of 174 metastases in the liver, achieved a local control rate of 57% at 20 months and a median survival of 14.5 months (82). Subsequent subset analysis suggested that breast cancer lesions had better survival and control compared to metastases from other primary sites: 2- and 4-year survival rates were 72% and 64% in patients with breast cancer compared to 38% and 18%, respectively, for other primary sites (82). With the higher radiation doses, SBRT may offer a benefit to select patients.

Interstitial Laser Therapy

Localized tumor destruction can also be achieved through hyperthermic coagulative necrosis caused by laser light delivered through quartz diffusing laser fibers placed directly in the tumor (49). ILT has been used to treat tumors up to 5 cm and can be performed through a variety of modalities: percutaneously with local anesthesia in the outpatient setting, laparoscopically, or intraoperatively (49). The reported ILT serious complication rate (1.5%) is low, with four symptomatic pleural effusions, two liver abscesses, one bile duct injury, and no deaths occurring in a series of 452 patients (49). However, there were 41 (9%) asymptomatic pleural effusions and 20 (4%) asymptomatic subcapsular hematomas incidentally detected on follow-up imaging (49).

Accurate positioning of the laser can be ensured using real-time imaging; MRI is preferred over CT and ultrasonography due to the heat sensitivity of the MRI sequence and its ability to demonstrate the degree of necrosis by rapidly depicting temperature changes. Monitoring with MRI also minimizes radiation exposure thereby increasing safety (49).

Patient Selection for Interstitial Laser Therapy

Patient selection for ILT follows general guidelines for liver-directed therapy; and some suggest less than five lesions, with none measuring more than 40 mm in diameter (83).

Results of Interstitial Laser Therapy for Metastatic Breast Cancer

The largest published experience with ILT for metastatic breast cancer included 232 patients with 578 liver metastases treated with ILT and systemic chemotherapy (1993 to 2002) (Table 88.2). Although 31% of patients had concurrent bone metastases, all patients had five or fewer hepatic metastases with no lesion larger than 5 cm in diameter (49). The rate of local liver recurrence at 6 months after ILT was less than 5%, the median survival was 4.3 years, and the 5-year survival rate was 41% (calculated from the date of diagnosis of the target liver metastasis rather than the date of ILT treatment) (49). Although ILT may be promising, data are limited for metastatic breast cancer to the liver.

MANAGEMENT SUMMARY

Localized, liver-directed therapy of metastases from breast cancer has been used successfully in carefully selected patients, with low morbidity and encouraging survival rates. Although there is substantial experience with liver-directed treatment of colorectal cancer metastases in the liver and for primary liver tumors, the metastatic breast cancer literature is limited to a relatively small number of case series. Hepatic resection remains the most commonly available localized, liver-directed treatment for metastatic breast cancer limited to the liver, and it has been available the longest and has the largest amount of supporting data. However, techniques such as RFA, SBRT, and ILT may offer an advantage because they are less invasive. The relative paucity of data and the lack of randomized, controlled trials for all liver-directed treatments of metastatic breast cancer limit interpretation of survival data and analysis of prognostic factors.

Given the natural history of breast cancer, few patients have metastatic disease limited to the liver. Although the case series evidence suggests a benefit for metastatic disease limited to the liver, there are conflicting data about the benefit of liver-directed therapy in the setting of extrahepatic metastases. Therefore, a thorough staging evaluation with chest CT, triphasic CT of the abdomen and pelvis, bone scan, and, possibly, Positron Emission Tomography is important for risk assessment. Extrapolating from the surgical resection literature, patients most likely to benefit from liver-directed, localized therapy are those who are responsive to preprocedure

systemic treatment; those whose tumor is completely eradicated by the procedure; and those who have recurrent liver lesions eradicated. Survival data appear promising, but in the absence of randomized controlled trials it is difficult to estimate a survival benefit for localized, liver-directed therapy.

Despite the paucity of clinical trial data, techniques for liver-directed therapy are increasingly available and are improving with respect to morbidity and local disease control. In parallel, systemic therapy options are also improving, with enhanced efficacy and patient tolerance. Thus, the decision to proceed with a liver-directed approach, particularly as an alternative to systemic therapy, must be made after carefully balancing the risks and benefits of all options and should take advantage of local expertise. Given the biology of metastatic breast cancer, the authors believe that a bias toward systemic therapy is an appropriate starting point and have developed a proposed treatment algorithm (Fig. 88.1) based on the available data and our clinical experience. The authors advocate the development of and enrollment in prospective clinical trials to address the unanswered question of comparative efficacy between the various liver-directed treatment options and systemic treatment, as outlined in Table 88.3.

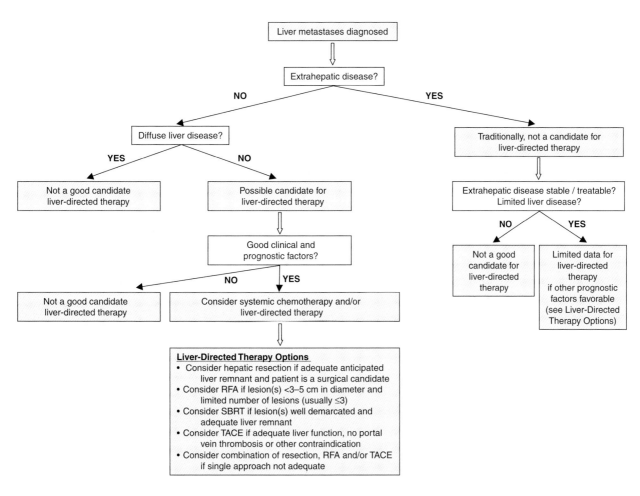

FIGURE 88.1. Liver-directed treatment options for breast cancer metastatic to the liver. The decision to proceed with a liver-directed approach for the treatment of breast cancer metastatic to the liver must be made after carefully balancing the risks and benefits all options. Given the biology of metastatic breast cancer and the paucity of clinical trial data about liver-directed treatment options, the authors believe that a bias toward systemic therapy is an appropriate starting point and this proposed algorithm should be individualized for each patient and take advantage of local expertise. RFA, radiofrequency ablation; SBRT, stereotactic body radiation therapy; TACE, transarterial chemoembolization.

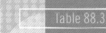

Table 88.3   COMPARATIVE EFFICACY OF TREATMENT OPTIONS

Liver-Directed Treatment Therapies:

1. **Surgical Resection**
   A. **Pros:**
      I. Data available from a large number of case series over 20+ years
      II. Compared to other liver-directed treatment options, more extensive data suggesting a 5-year survival benefit in appropriately selected patients
      III. Relatively available
   B. **Cons:**
      I. Invasive procedure requiring hospitalization
      II. Risk of postoperative complications and decreased liver function
      III. Many patients not eligible due to comorbidities and extent of liver disease
      IV. Best results obtained for patients with small and/or few lesions

2. **Nonsurgical Liver-Directed Therapies (General)**
   A. **Pros:**
      I. Less invasive than surgical resection
      II. More patients may be eligible
      III. Compared to surgical resection, decreased risk of postprocedure complications and of decreased liver function
      IV. Procedure may be accomplished in outpatient setting or with short hospital stay
      V. Efficacy may be improved by combining modalities
      VI. Approaches supported by data for colorectal and hepatocellular cancer
   B. **Cons:**
      I. Data in breast cancer limited to relatively few, heterogeneous case series
      II. Data for survival and tumor control are mixed
      III. Treatment modalities and operator expertise may not be readily available
      IV. Despite generally good safety results, serious complications have been reported

3. **Patient Selection Guidelines for Liver-Directed Therapies (General)**
   A. **General selection guidelines associated with best outcomes:**
      I. Good overall prognosis
      II. Good performance status and few comorbidities
      III. Documented response to preprocedure systemic therapy
      IV. Smaller lesions and fewer number of lesions in the liver
      V. Metastatic disease isolated to the liver only
      VI. Longer disease free interval between treatment of primary cancer and development of hepatic metastasis
      VII. Liver lesions that can be completely eradicated by the procedure
   B. **Additional, procedure-specific guidelines**
      I. **Resection**
         1. Adequate anticipated liver remnant (may be able to enhance with preoperative embolization)
         2. Good operative risk
      II. **Radiofrequency ablation**
         1. Lesion size less than 3 to 5 cm in diameter
         2. Limited number of lesions (usually three or less)
      III. **Transarterial chemoembolization**
         1. Adequate liver function
         2. No portal vein thrombosis or other contraindication
      IV. **Stereotactic body radiation therapy**
         1. Well demarcated
         2. Adequate anticipated liver remnant

References

1. Viadana E, Cotter R, Pickren JW, et al. An autopsy study of metastatic sites of breast cancer. *Cancer Res* 1973;33:179–181.
2. Winston CB, Hadar O, Teitcher JB, et al. Metastatic lobular carcinoma of the breast: patterns of spread in the chest, abdomen, and pelvis on CT. *AJR Am J Roentgenol* 2000;175:795–800.
3. Atalay G, Biganzoli L, Renard F, et al. Clinical outcome of breast cancer patients with liver metastases alone in the anthracycline-taxane era: a retrospective analysis of two prospective, randomised metastatic breast cancer trials. *Eur J Cancer* 2003;39:2439–2449.
4. Pentheroudakis G, Fountzilas G, Bafaloukos D, et al. Metastatic breast cancer with liver metastases: a registry analysis of clinicopathologic, management and outcome characteristics of 500 women. *Breast Cancer Res Treat* 2006;97:237–244.
5. Wyld L, Gutteridge E, Pinder SE, et al. Prognostic factors for patients with hepatic metastases from breast cancer. *Br J Cancer* 2003;89:284–290.
6. Sherry MM, Greco FA, Johnson DH, et al. Breast cancer with skeletal metastases at initial diagnosis. Distinctive clinical characteristics and favorable prognosis. *Cancer* 1986;58:178–182.
7. Elder EE, Kennedy CW, Gluch L, et al. Patterns of breast cancer relapse. *Eur J Surg Oncol* 2006;32:922–927.
8. Hoe AL, Royle GT, Taylor I. Breast liver metastases—incidence, diagnosis and outcome. *J R Soc Med* 1991;84:714–716.
9. Eichbaum MH, Kaltwasser M, Bruckner T, et al. Prognostic factors for patients with liver metastases from breast cancer. *Breast Cancer Res Treat* 2006;96:53–62.
10. Zinser JW, Hortobagyi GN, Buzdar AU, et al. Clinical course of breast cancer patients with liver metastases. *J Clin Oncol* 1987;5:773–782.
11. Hortobagyi GN. Progress in systemic chemotherapy of primary breast cancer: an overview. *J Natl Cancer Inst* 2001;30:72–79.
12. Selzner M, Morse MA, Vredenburgh JJ, et al. Liver metastases from breast cancer: long-term survival after curative resection. *Surgery* 2000;127:383–389.
13. Pocard M, Pouillart P, Asselain B, et al. Hepatic resection in metastatic breast cancer: results and prognostic factors. *Eur J Surg Oncol* 2000;26:155–159.
14. d'Annibale M, Piovanello P, Cerasoli V, et al. Liver metastases from breast cancer: the role of surgical treatment. *Hepatogastroenterology* 2005;52:1858–1862.
15. Maksan SM, Lehnert T, Bastert G, et al. Curative liver resection for metastatic breast cancer. *Eur J Surg Oncol* 2000;26:209–212.
16. Vlastos G, Smith DL, Singletary SE, et al. Long-term survival after an aggressive surgical approach in patients with breast cancer hepatic metastases. *Ann Surg Oncol* 2004;11:869–874.
17. Elias D, Baton O, Sideris L, et al. Local recurrences after intraoperative radiofrequency ablation of liver metastases: a comparative study with anatomic and wedge resections. *Ann Surg Oncol* 2004;11:500–505.
18. Hoyer M, Roed H, Traberg Hansen A, et al. Phase II study on stereotactic body radiotherapy of colorectal metastases. *Acta Oncol* 2006;45:823–830.
19. Sofocleous CT, Nascimento RG, Gonen M, et al. Radiofrequency ablation in the management of liver metastases from breast cancer. *AJR Am J Roentgenol* 2007;189:883–889.
20. Gillams AR, Lees WR. Radio-frequency ablation of colorectal liver metastases in 167 patients. *Eur Radiol* 2004;14:2261–2267.
21. Siperstein AE, Berber E, Ballem N, et al. Survival after radiofrequency ablation of colorectal liver metastases: 10-year experience. *Ann Surg* 2007;246:559–567.
22. Berry DA, Cronin KA, Plevritis SK, et al. Effect of screening and adjuvant therapy on mortality from breast cancer. *N Engl J Med* 2005;353:1784–1792.
23. Chia SK, Speers CH, D'Yachkova Y, et al. The impact of new chemotherapeutic and hormone agents on survival in a population-based cohort of women with metastatic breast cancer. *Cancer* 2007;110:973–979.
24. Cassier PA, Chabaud S, Trillet-Lenoir V, et al. A phase-III trial of doxorubicin and docetaxel versus doxorubicin and paclitaxel in metastatic breast cancer. results of the ERASME 3 study. *Breast Cancer Res Treat* 2008;109(2):343–350.
25. Kuvshinoff B, Fong Y. Surgical therapy of liver metastases. *Semin Oncol* 2007;34:177–185.
26. Adam R, Aloia T, Krissat J, et al. Is liver resection justified for patients with hepatic metastases from breast cancer? *Ann Surg* 2006;244:897–907.
27. Hemming AW, Reed AI, Howard RJ, et al. Preoperative portal vein embolization for extended hepatectomy. *Ann Surg* 2003;237:686–691.
28. Stehlin JS Jr, de Ipolyi PD, Greeff PJ, et al. Treatment of cancer of the liver. Twenty years' experience with infusion and resection in 414 patients. *Ann Surg* 1988;208:23–35.
29. Schneebaum S, Walker MJ, Young D, et al. The regional treatment of liver metastases from breast cancer. *J Surg Oncol* 1994;55:26–32.
30. Lorenz M, Wiesner J, Staib-Sebler E, et al. [Regional therapy breast cancer liver metastases.] *Zentralblatt Chirurgie* 1995;120:786–790.
31. Elias D, Lasser PH, Montrucolli D, et al. Hepatectomy for liver metastases from breast cancer. *Eur J Surg Oncol* 1995;21:510–513.
32. Raab R, Nussbaum KT, Behrend M, et al. Liver metastases of breast cancer: results of liver resection. *Anticancer Res* 1998;18:2231–2233.
33. Seifert JK, Weigel TF, Gonner U, et al. Liver resection for breast cancer metastases. *Hepatogastroenterology* 1999;46:2935–2940.
34. Kondo S, Katoh H, Omi M, et al. Hepatectomy for metastases from breast cancer offers the survival benefit similar to that in hepatic metastases from colorectal cancer. *Hepatogastroenterology* 2000;47:1501–1503.
35. Yoshimoto M, Tada T, Saito M, et al. Surgical treatment of hepatic metastases from breast cancer. *Breast Cancer Res Treat* 2000;59:177–184.
36. Carlini M, Lonardo MT, Carboni F, et al. Liver metastases from breast cancer. Results of surgical resection. *Hepatogastroenterology* 2002;49:1597–1601.
37. Elias D, Maisonnette F, Druet-Cabanac M, et al. An attempt to clarify indications for hepatectomy for liver metastases from breast cancer. *Am J Surg* 2003;185:158–164.
38. Ercolani G, Grazi GL, Ravaioli M, et al. The role of liver resections for noncolorectal, nonneuroendocrine metastases: experience with 142 observed cases. *Ann Surg Oncol* 2005;12:459–466.
39. Sakamoto Y, Yamamoto J, Yoshimoto M, et al. Hepatic resection for metastatic breast cancer: prognostic analysis of 34 patients. *World J Surg* 2005;29:524–527.
40. Martinez SR, Young SE, Giuliano AE, et al. The utility of estrogen receptor, progesterone receptor, and HER-2/neu status to predict survival in patients undergoing hepatic resection for breast cancer metastases. *Am J Surg* 2006;191:281–283.
41. Curley SA, Izzo F, Delrio P, et al. Radiofrequency ablation of unresectable primary and metastatic hepatic malignancies: results in 123 patients. *Ann Surg* 1999;230:1–8.
42. de Baere T, Elias D, Dromain C, et al. Radiofrequency ablation of 100 hepatic metastases with a mean follow-up of more than 1 year. *AJR Am J Roentgenol* 2000;175:1619–1625.
43. Decadt B, Siriwardena AK. Radiofrequency ablation of liver tumours: systematic review. *Lancet Oncol* 2004;5:550–560.
44. Poon RT, Fan ST, Tsang FH, et al. Locoregional therapies for hepatocellular carcinoma: a critical review from the surgeon's perspective. *Ann Surg* 2002;235:466–486.
45. Buijs M, Kamel IR, Vossen JA, et al. Assessment of metastatic breast cancer response to chemoembolization with contrast agent enhanced and diffusion-weighted MR imaging. *J Vasc Interv Radiol* 2007;18:957–963.
46. Giroux MF, Baum RA, Soulen MC. Chemoembolization of liver metastasis from breast carcinoma. *J Vasc Interv Radiol* 2004;15:289–291.

47. Bruix J, Sherman M, Llovet JM, et al. Clinical management of hepatocellular carcinoma. Conclusions of the Barcelona-2000 EASL conference. European Association for the Study of the Liver. *J Hepatol* 2001;35:421–430.
48. Vogl TJ, Mack MG, Balzer JO, et al. Liver metastases: neoadjuvant downsizing with transarterial chemoembolization before laser-induced thermotherapy. *Radiology* 2003;229:457–464.
49. Mack MG, Straub R, Eichler K, et al. Breast cancer metastases in liver: laser-induced interstitial thermotherapy—local tumor control rate and survival data. *Radiology* 2004;233:400–409.
50. Li XP, Meng ZQ, Guo WJ, et al. Treatment for liver metastases from breast cancer: results and prognostic factors. *World J Gastroenterol* 2005;11:3782–3787.
51. Gillams AR. The use of radiofrequency in cancer. *Br J Cancer* 2005;92:1825–1829.
52. Goldberg SN, Hahn PF, Tanabe KK, et al. Percutaneous radiofrequency tissue ablation: does perfusion-mediated tissue cooling limit coagulation necrosis? *J Vasc Interv Radiol* 1998;9:101–111.
53. Dupuy DE, Goldberg SN. Image-guided radiofrequency tumor ablation: challenges and opportunities—part II. *J Vasc Interv Radiol* 2001;12:1135–1148.
54. Poon RT, Ng KK, Lam CM, et al. Radiofrequency ablation for subcapsular hepatocellular carcinoma. *Ann Surg Oncol* 2004;11:281–289.
55. Lencioni RA. Tumor Radiofrequency Ablation Italian Network (TRAIN): long-term results in hepatic colorectal cancer metastases. Paper presented at Radiological Society of North America, 90th Scientific Assembly and Annual Meeting. Chicago, IL. November 28–December 3, 2004.
56. Lu DS, Yu NC, Raman SS, et al. Radiofrequency ablation of hepatocellular carcinoma: treatment success as defined by histologic examination of the explanted liver. *Radiology* 2005;234:954–960.
57. Sala M, Llovet JM, Vilana R, et al. Initial response to percutaneous ablation predicts survival in patients with hepatocellular carcinoma. *Hepatology (Baltimore)* 2004;40:1352–1360.
58. Abdalla EK, Vauthey JN, Ellis LM, et al. Recurrence and outcomes following hepatic resection, radiofrequency ablation, and combined resection/ablation for colorectal liver metastases. *Ann Surg* 2004;239:818–827.
59. Berber E, Pelley R, Siperstein AE. Predictors of survival after radiofrequency thermal ablation of colorectal cancer metastases to the liver: a prospective study. *J Clin Oncol* 2005;23:1358–1364.
60. Elias D, Sideris L, Pocard M, et al. Results of R0 resection for colorectal liver metastases associated with extrahepatic disease. *Ann Surg Oncol* 2004;11:274–280.
61. Machi J, Oishi AJ, Sumida K, et al. Long-term outcome of radiofrequency ablation for unresectable liver metastases from colorectal cancer: evaluation of prognostic factors and effectiveness in first- and second-line management. *Cancer J* 2006;12:318–326.
62. Oshowo A, Gillams A, Harrison E, et al. Comparison of resection and radiofrequency ablation for treatment of solitary colorectal liver metastases. *Br J Surg* 2003;90:1240–1243.
63. Yu NC, Kim YJ, Raman SS, et al. Intraoperative radiofrequency ablation of unresectable liver metastases from colorectal carcinoma: long-term results in 50 patients. Paper presented at Radiological Society of North America, 92nd Scientific Assembly and Annual Meeting. Chicago, IL. November 26–December 1, 2006.
64. Gunabushanam G, Sharma S, Thulkar S, et al. Radiofrequency ablation of liver metastases from breast cancer: results in 14 patients. *J Vasc Interv Radiol* 2007;18:67–72.
65. Livraghi T, Goldberg SN, Solbiati L, et al. Percutaneous radio-frequency ablation of liver metastases from breast cancer: initial experience in 24 patients. *Radiology* 2001;220:145–149.
66. Lawes D, Chopada A, Gillams A, et al. Radiofrequency ablation (RFA) as a cytoreductive strategy for hepatic metastasis from breast cancer. *Ann R Coll Surg Engl* 2006;88:639–642.
67. Nagata Y, Takayama K, Matsuo Y, et al. [Stereotactic body radiotherapy (SBRT).] *Gan To Kagaku Ryoho* 2006;33:455–461.
68. Potters L, Timmerman R, Larson D. Stereotactic body radiation therapy. *J Am Coll Radiol* 2005;2:676–680.
69. Song DY, Kavanagh BD, Benedict SH, et al. Stereotactic body radiation therapy. Rationale, techniques, applications, and optimization. *Oncology (Williston Park)* 2004;18:1419–1430.
70. Papiez L, Timmerman R, DesRosiers C, et al. Extracranial stereotactic radioablation: physical principles. *Acta Oncol* 2003;42:882–894.
71. Schefter TE, Kavanagh BD, Timmerman RD, et al. A phase I trial of stereotactic body radiation therapy (SBRT) for liver metastases. *Int J Radiat Oncol Biol Phys* 2005;62:1371–1378.
72. Timmerman R, Galvin J, Michalski J, et al. Accreditation and quality assurance for Radiation Therapy Oncology Group: multicenter clinical trials using stereotactic body radiation therapy in lung cancer. *Acta Oncol* 2006;45:779–786.
73. Potters L, Steinberg M, Rose C, et al. American Society for Therapeutic Radiology and Oncology and American College of Radiology practice guideline for the performance of stereotactic body radiation therapy. *Int J Radiat Oncol Biol Phys* 2004;60:1026–1032.
74. Kavanagh BD, McGarry RC, Timmerman RD. Stereotactic radiosurgery (stereotactic body radiation therapy) for oligometastases. *Semin Radiat Oncol* 2006;16:77–84.
75. Kavanagh BD, Bradley J, Timmerman RD. Stereotactic irradiation of tumors outside the central nervous system. In: Halperin E, Perez C, Brady L, et al., eds. *Perez and Brady's principles and practice of radiation oncology.* Baltimore: Lippincott Williams & Wilkins, 2007:389–396.
76. Blomgren H, Lax I, Goranson H, et al. Radiosurgery for tumors in the body: clinical experience using a new method. *J Radiosurg* 1998;1:63–74.
77. Herfarth KK, Hof H, Bahner ML, et al. Assessment of focal liver reaction by multiphasic CT after stereotactic single-dose radiotherapy of liver tumors. *Int J Radiat Oncol Biol Phys* 2003;57:444–451.
78. Blomgren H, Lax I, Naslund I, et al. Stereotactic high dose fraction radiation therapy of extracranial tumors using an accelerator. Clinical experience of the first thirty-one patients. *Acta Oncol* 1995;34:861–870.
79. Herfarth KK, Debus J, Lohr F, et al. Stereotactic single-dose radiation therapy of liver tumors: results of a phase I/II trial. *J Clin Oncol* 2001;19:164–170.
80. Herfarth KK, Debus J, Wannenmacher M. Stereotactic radiation therapy of liver metastases: update of the initial phase-I/II trial. *Front Radiat Ther Oncol* 2004;38:100–105.
81. Wulf J, Hadinger U, Oppitz U, et al. Stereotactic radiotherapy of targets in the lung and liver. *Strahlenther Onkol* 2001;177:645–655.
82. Katz AW, Carey-Sampson M, Muhs AG, et al. Hypofractionated stereotactic body radiation therapy (SBRT) for limited hepatic metastases. *Int J Radiat Oncol Biol Phys* 2007;67:793–798.
83. Vogl TJ, Mack MG, Straub R, et al. Magnetic resonance imaging–guided abdominal interventional radiology: laser-induced thermotherapy of liver metastases. *Endoscopy* 1997;29:577–583.
84. Okaro AC, Durkin DJ, Layer GT, et al. Hepatic resection for breast cancer metastases. *Ann R Coll Surg Engl* 2005;87:167–170.
85. Gunabushanam G, Sharma S, Thulkar S, et al. Radio frequency ablation of liver metastases from breast cancer: results in 14 patients. *J Vasc Interv Radiol* 2007;18:67–72.
86. Fraschini G, Fleishman G, Yap HY, et al. Percutaneous hepatic arterial infusion of cisplatin for metastatic breast cancer. *Cancer Treat Rep* 1987;71:313–315.
87. Ikeda T, Adachi I, Takashima S, et al. A phase I/II study of continuous intra-arterial chemotherapy using an implantable reservoir for the treatment of liver metastases from breast cancer: a Japan Clinical Oncology Group (JCOG) study 9113. JCOG Breast Cancer Study Group. *Jpn J Clin Oncol* 1999;29:23–27.
88. Camacho L, Kurzrock R, Cheung A, et al. Pilot study of regional, hepatic intra-arterial paclitaxel in patients with breast carcinoma metastatic to the liver. *Cancer* 2007;109:2190–2196.

Chapter 89
Bone-Directed Therapy and Breast Cancer: Bisphosphonates, Monoclonal Antibody, and Radionuclides

Richard L. Theriault

Bone health has become a prominent issue for patients with breast cancer and clinicians who care for them. For those diagnosed with primary breast cancer who subsequently develop metastases, bone is the most common site of disease. Complications of bone metastases include hypercalcemia of malignancy and skeletal-related events such as pathologic fractures, spinal cord compression, and nerve root compression (1). In addition to bone metastases, bone loss as a consequence of primary treatment for breast cancer has been recognized as a significant clinical problem with the potential to lead to osteopenia, osteoporosis, and increased fracture risk.

 ## BREAST CANCER AND BONE METASTASES

Bone metastases are the most common site of metastatic disease in women with a primary diagnosis of breast cancer. Approximately 47% to 85% of patients with metastases will have bone disease. Bone is also the most frequent first site of metastatic disease, and there is a strong predilection for metastases to develop in the bone marrow–rich microenvironment of the pelvis, ribs, thoracic lumbar cervical spines, skull, and long bones.

Patients who develop bone metastases have a prolonged period of survival, a median of 24 to 30 months, placing them at substantial risk of skeletal morbidity (2). Skeletal morbidity may include pathologic fractures in the spine, long bones, pelvis, and ribs, and multiple fractures are common. In addition, spinal cord and nerve root compression may develop as a consequence of vertebral instability and pathologic fracture.

Hypercalcemia of malignancy is associated with altered mental status, renal failure, and death.

Domchek et al. (3) reported on an unselected population of patients with metastatic breast cancer focusing on the development of skeletal complications. A group of 718 women were followed for a median of 107 months. Reported skeletal complications included pathologic fracture, hypercalcemia of malignancy, spinal cord compression, and surgery or radiation therapy to bone. Half of the patients in this series had skeletal complications. More than 50% of those with skeletal complications had multiple complications.

Radiation therapy to bone was a frequent occurrence (40.8% incidence), while pathologic fracture reportedly occurred in 7.8% of the patients. The median time to first skeletal complications was reported to be 27 months overall and 11 months for those with bone only disease. Median survival of patients with bone only metastases was 26 months.

Bone metastases, characteristically, have an osteolytic or osteoblastic appearance on radiographics, with osteolytic lesions predominating (4). Even with lesions that appear purely osteolytic, generally an osteoblastic component is present. The osteoblastic activity results in increased uptake of radionuclide and visualization of abnormalities on bone scan, allowing detection of bone metastases.

Perturbations in bone remodeling occur as a consequence of bone metastases development. These include activation of osteo-clastogenesis, excessive numbers of osteoclasts and, excessive osteoclastic activity resulting in destruction of bone (5,6).

The factors responsible for the proclivity of breast cancer to metastasize to bone are not completely elucidated, but this is an area of active research (7). It is clear that high blood flow in areas of red marrow, the adhesive molecules noted on breast cancer cells, and a number of cytokines help to promote bone metastases development within the marrow spaces. In addition a variety of growth factors are involved in metastasis development (6,8). Moieties of the integrin cell adhesion receptors have been shown experimentally to promote metastases development, presumably due to extracellular matrix binding (9). Parathyroid hormone–related protein (PTHrP), vascular endothelial growth factor; transforming growth factor β (TGF-β), and interleukins 8 and 11 have all been implicated in the bone metastases cascade (5,10,11).

Guise et al. (12) have reported that tumor-secreted endothelin-1 may result in the development of osteoblastic metastases. PTHrP has been shown to be up-regulated by TGF-β released from bone as a consequence of increased osteolysis. TGF-β receptors on the surface of breast cancer cells within the microenvironment facilitate up-regulation of PTHrP expression with resulting amplification of osteolytic activity (13).

Interleukin 11, interleukin 8, and transforming growth factor α have been shown to be osteoclast activators (13). Receptor activator of nuclear factor κB ligand (RANKL) induces osteoclasogenesis. RANKL is a member of the tumor necrosis factor family of cytokines and is produced by bone marrow stromal cells and osteoblasts (5,14).

Osteoclast activity occurs in relation to osteoblast production of RANKL. Osteoclast and osteoclast precursors have receptors for RANKL. Upon binding to receptors, osteoclastogenesis and osteoclastic activity are increased (15). RANKL binds to osteoclast precursors at the RANK receptor site and under the influence of granulocyte-macrophage colony-stimulating factor (GM-CF) osteoclast precursors increase in number and differentiate into active multinucleate osteoclasts. Osteoclast differentiation, activation, and functional activity are reduced when the natural inhibitor of RANKL, osteoprotegerin, binds ligand, preventing binding to the RANK receptor. Osteoprotegerin (OPG) is also a member of the tumor necrosis factor cytokine family and a direct inhibitor of RANKL. Tumor cells can activate osteoblast production of RANKL. Osteolysis releases bone-derived growth factors, which then potentiate tumor cell growth, leading to further activation of osteoblast RANKL production.

OPG provides a soluble inhibitor receptor for RANKL in circulation and is produced by a number of cell types. The relative osteoclastigenic activity of RANKL is controlled by OPG. Bone metastases results in continuous activation of osteoclasts by tumor cells and bone marrow microenvironmental factors (8). As a consequence, breast cancer bone metastases are associated with an increase in the number and functional activity of osteoclasts in the region of metastatic disease. The final common pathway for bone destruction in metastatic disease is continuous osteolysis.

Dysregulation of bone formation and bone destruction lead to the clinical presentations of hypercalcemia of malignancy, skeletal events, including pathologic fractures, spinal cord compression, and nerve root compression and the need for surgery and radiation to bone.

CANCER TREATMENT–INDUCED BONE LOSS

Treatment for primary breast cancer may result in accelerated bone loss as a consequence of estrogen deprivation. In premenopausal women, this may occur as a result of premature ovarian failure associated with the use of gonadotoxic chemotherapy, luteinizing hormone-releasing hormone agonists to suppress ovarian function or oophorectomy (16–20). In postmenopausal women the use of aromatase inhibitors results in a profound hypoestrogenic state and bone loss (21–24).

Cancer treatment–induced bone loss (CTIBL) occurs as a consequence of premature menopause in women treated with multiagent chemotherapy in the adjuvant or neoadjuvant setting. Shapiro et al. (25) reported a 4% reduction in bone mineral density within 6 months of breast cancer treatment with cytotoxic chemotherapy. Breast cancer diagnosis itself tends to place patients at increased risk of osteopenia and osteoporosis and fracture. Kanis et al. (26) reported the incidence of vertebral fractures in breast cancer patients receiving standard adjuvant therapy in the United Kingdom and Canada. Three hundred fifty patients who did not develop metastases were shown to have an odds ratio for experiencing a vertebral fracture nearly five times greater than an age-matched control group. Patients who had extraskeletal recurrence without overt evidence of bone metastases had a 20 times greater risk of vertebral fracture than the matched control group.

Permanent ovarian failure occurs most often with use of alkylating agents such as cyclophosphamide. The incidence of ovarian failure is related to the total cumulative dose of the drug and the age of the patient when exposed to treatment.

For women who have received classic CMF (cyclophosphamide, methotrexate, and 5-fluorouracil) chemotherapy, the cumulative cyclophosphamide dose will reach greater than 8 g/m^2. Therefore, they are at substantial risk for developing ovarian failure.

Premature ovarian failure has been reported with the use of TAC (docetaxel, doxorubicin, and cyclophosphamide), FAC (fluorouracil, doxorubicin, and cyclophosphamide), and FEC (fluorouracil, epirubicin, and cyclophosphamide) chemotherapy administered in the adjuvant or neoadjuvant setting (17). Although many premenopausal women receiving chemotherapy will experience amenorrhea, this is more likely to be transient in younger women (16).

Age is a predominant factor in development of permanent ovarian failure, with a 0% to 40% incidence for women under the age of 40 and a 70% to 90% incidence for women over the age of 40 (17).

The use of tamoxifen in premenopausal women has been shown to have a negative impact on bone integrity (27,28). The negative effects of tamoxifen on bone may be due to a greater antagonist effect from tamoxifen in the presence of higher estrogen levels in premenopausal woman, while bone agonistic properties may predominate in the low estrogen environment of postmenopausal women.

For postmenopausal women, the use of aromatase inhibitors has become a standard adjuvant endocrine therapy (29,30). The use of aromatase inhibitors as first adjuvant endocrine therapy or in sequence with tamoxifen has been shown to result in increased bone loss, development of osteopenia or osteoporosis, and increase in fracture risk for postmenopausal women (22,31).

Unlike bone metastasis studies for which skeletal events serve as end points, the end point evaluation for CTIBL has been bone mineral density (BMD) (32,33). BMD as measured by dual energy x-ray absorptiometry (DEXA) reflects an individual's risk of osteopenia or osteoporosis. The U.S. Prevention Services Task Force recommends measurement of BMD for all

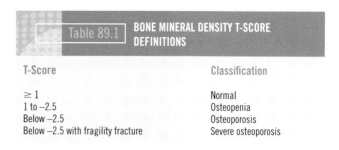

Table 89.1	BONE MINERAL DENSITY T-SCORE DEFINITIONS

T-Score	Classification
≥ 1	Normal
1 to −2.5	Osteopenia
Below −2.5	Osteoporosis
Below −2.5 with fragility fracture	Severe osteoporosis

women 65 years of age or older and women 60 to 64 years of age who are at increased risk of osteoporosis.

The American Society of Clinical Oncology bone health guidelines indicate that most women with primary breast cancer are at risk for osteoporosis due to age or cancer treatment (34). Screening with DEXA is recommended for these women. BMD is interpreted according to T-score and Z-score. T-score compares bone density of the patient with that of an average healthy adult. Z-score compares patient bone density with an age-matched control. T-score is used in the World Health Organization definitions of osteopenia and osteoporosis (Table 89.1). A T-score of less than −2.5 with a fragility fracture is considered severe osteoporosis.

INTERVENTIONS FOR BONE LOSS: BISPHOSPHONATES

Bisphosphonates are a modification of pyrophosphate (Fig. 89.1). The substitution of carbon for phosphorus makes these compounds resistant to breakdown by endogenous phosphatases in circulation (35). Bisphosphonates are not well absorbed with oral administration, hence their bioavailability is limited when taken by mouth. Bisphosphonates bind to hydroxyapatite at sites of active bone remodeling and metabolic activity. Bisphosphonate hydroxyapatite is resistant to the effects of osteoclast lysozymes produced at the ruffled border of osteoclast adhesion sites. Bisphosphonates inhibit osteoclast activity, including differentiation, adhesion to bone, and osteoclast activation as well as the production and secretion of lysozyme at the bone binding site (36–38). They reduce the number and functional activity of osteoclasts as well as the depth of osteoclastic resorption cavities and hence inhibit bone degradation.

The degree of inhibition of osteoclast function has been shown to vary in relation to bisphosphonate structure (Fig. 89.1). The amino-containing agents are more potent with zoledronic acid, the most potent inhibitor of osteoclast function (39,40). Bisphosphonate function is assessed in an *in vivo* rat model system (41). Of the proposed mechanisms of action, inhibition of the mevalonic pathway, essential for cholesterol synthesis and protein prenylation, may be significant (42). The lipid modification of G-proteins is essential for cell growth and differentiation. Inhibition of prenylation alters osteoclast morphology and function and induces apoptosis. Dunford et al. (43) have demonstrated a correlation between inhibition of farnesyl diphosphate synthase and inhibition of bone resorption by bisphosphonates. Zoledronic acid is a potent inhibitor of prenylation. Bisphosphonates also have been shown to activate caspases, which are functionally involved in apoptosis. Up-regulation of osteoprotegerin production by osteoblasts occurs with bisphosphonate exposure.

Bisphosphonates are the most widely used agents in the palliative treatment of bone metastases. Bisphosphonate effects on skeletal morbidity due to bone metastases have been assessed

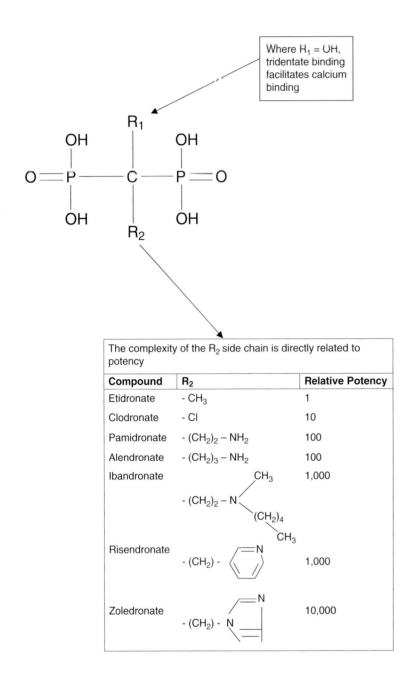

Where $R_1 = OH$, tridentate binding facilitates calcium binding

The complexity of the R_2 side chain is directly related to potency

Compound	R_2	Relative Potency
Etidronate	- CH_3	1
Clodronate	- Cl	10
Pamidronate	- $(CH_2)_2$ – NH_2	100
Alendronate	- $(CH_2)_3$ – NH_2	100
Ibandronate	- $(CH_2)_2$ – N, CH_3, $(CH_2)_4$, CH_3	1,000
Risendronate	- (CH_2) -	1,000
Zoledronate	- (CH_2) - N	10,000

FIGURE 89.1. Bisphosphonate structure and relative potencies.

in randomized and nonrandomized trials and have been a subject of systematic reviews including Cochrane reviews (44–54).

Evaluation of bone pain, fracture risk, hypercalcemia, the need for radiation therapy to bone, and need for surgery to bone have been the end points of clinical relevance in assessing bisphosphonate benefits for patients with breast cancer metastases.

Bisphosphonates in Breast Cancer Bone Metastases

Clodronate

Clodronate has been used for bone metastases in studies that have included oral or intravenous administration of the drug. Elomaa et al. (44) reported a prospective controlled trial in which

clodronate was found to have a substantial benefit for patients with bone disease. Improvements in bone pain, reduction in new lytic disease, and decreased frequency of hypercalcemia and pathologic fracture were noted.

Iveson et al (55) reported a randomized study of oral clodronate versus placebo. The frequency of all skeletal events was less in the clodronate group. The events monitored included radiotherapy for bone pain, number of nonvertebral and vertebral fractures, and number of episodes of hypercalcemia.

Similar results were reported by Paterson et al. (45) in a randomized, double-blind, controlled trial of clodronate. Studies examining bone pain relief have reported substantial analgesic effects of clodronate in patients with refractory bone pain treated with intravenous or oral preparations.

In a review of bisphosphonate use, oral administration is reported to appear less effective than intravenously administered drug due to poor oral bioavailability of bisphosphonates (56).

Although clodronate has been shown to be effective in reducing skeletal morbidity, it is not available for use in the United States.

Pamidronate

The use of pamidronate and its impact on skeletal morbidity has been assessed with oral and intravenous administration in randomized studies of patients with breast cancer bone metastases. Reduction in bone pain, pathologic fracture, and need for radiation to bone as well as reduction in frequency of episodes of hypercalcemia have been reported.

Two large double-blind, randomized, placebo-controlled trials have been reported for breast cancer patients with bone metastases (46,47). These evaluated the use of intravenous pamidronate versus placebo in two patient populations; one receiving chemotherapy for metastatic disease and one receiving endocrine therapy for metastatic disease. Both groups had demonstrable osteolytic bone disease by plain radiography. Pamidronate was administered at a dose of 90 mg intravenously over 2-hour infusion time.

In the chemotherapy plus pamidronate or placebo trial reported by Hortobagyi et al. (46), the efficacy end points included skeletal related events (i.e., pain and analgesic scores), fractures, need for radiation to bone, need for surgery to bone, spinal cord compression, and hypercalcemia malignancy. The chemotherapy trial compared the proportion of total events at 12 months for patients in each treatment group (i.e., pamidronate vs. placebo). The time to first skeletal-related event was longer for those in the pamidronate group: 13.1 months versus 7 months for those in the placebo group ($p = .005$). The proportion of patients with any skeletal event was less in the pamidronate than placebo group (43% vs. 56%; $p = .008$), and improvements in bone pain and analgesic scores were associated with the use of pamidronate.

In the parallel trial for patients receiving endocrine therapy for osteolytic metastatic disease, 372 patients were randomly allocated to pamidronate or placebo in a double-blind fashion with pamidronate 90 mg or placebo administered intravenously over 2 hours. Twenty-four–month efficacy and safety data reported reductions in skeletal morbidity rate at 12, 18, and 24 months. Patients receiving pamidronate had a decrease in the proportion of skeletal events at 24 months (56% vs. 67%; $p = .027$).

Lipton et al. (48) reported an analysis of the combination of these studies and noted substantial reduction in the proportion of skeletal events in patients treated with pamidronate (51% vs. 64% for placebo). Time to pathologic fracture was 25.2 months for the pamidronate group versus 12.8 in the placebo group, and the median time to need for radiation therapy was "not reached" for pamidronate versus 16 months with placebo.

Pamidronate is approved by the U.S. Food and Drug Administration (FDA) for use in breast cancer bone metastases. The dose and schedule of administration are 90 mg intravenously, over at least 2 hours, once every 4 weeks, with appropriate monitoring of renal function and electrolytes.

Zoledronic Acid

Zoledronic acid is more potent than pamidronate in inhibiting osteoclastic activity. This is presumed to be related to its heterocyclic imidazole ring side change on the pyrophosphate backbone (Fig. 89.1).

In addition to its antiosteoclast activity, zoledronic acid has been shown to decrease the viability of human MDA-MB231 breast cancer cells and induce apoptosis in human HS578T breast cancer cells (57).

Zoledronic acid has been compared to pamidronate in a randomized trial for treatment of hypercalcemia malignancy. It was shown to have a more rapid onset of hypocalcemic effect and a longer duration of effect than pamidronate (58).

Dose ranging studies with zoledronic acid compared 0.4, 2, and 4 mg doses administered on a 4 weekly schedule with 90 mg of pamidronate on the same schedule. Zoledronic acid administered in 2 and 4 mg doses decreased the need for radiation therapy to bone. Increases in bone mineral density and decrease in the bone resorption marker N-telopeptide were shown to be similar for the 2 and 4 mg zoledronic acid dose (59,60).

A subsequent randomized clinical trial comparing zoledronic acid and pamidronate enrolled patients with metastatic breast cancer to bone and multiple myeloma. Patients were randomly allocated to receive pamidronate 90 mg intravenously over 2 hours or zoledronic acid 4 or 8 mg intravenously over 5 minutes in a double-blind, double dummy fashion (61). Because of unexpected renal toxicity at the 8 mg zoledronic acid dose, the intravenous infusion time was lengthened from 5 to 15 minutes and the infusion volume increased to 100 mL. Subsequently, the 8-mg dose was replaced with the 4-mg dose because of continued renal toxicity. This study was designed as a noninferiority trial. Results demonstrated that 44% of patients treated with zoledronic acid compared to 46% of patients treated with pamidronate had skeletal-related events. The proportion of patients who developed fracture, required radiation therapy to bone, surgery for bone, or spinal cord compression was statistically the same in each group.

In a subsequent analysis, patients with osteolytic disease included in the zoledronic acid group were compared with those patients with osteolytic disease who had previously been enrolled in the pamidronate studies. The pamidronate studies required at least one radiographically demonstrable osteolytic lesion for eligibility. A comparison of 190 patients in the zoledronic acid studies who had a radiographically confirmed osteolytic lesion to the 162 patients in the pamidronate studies previously reported showed the proportion of skeletal events was 48% for zoledronic acid and 58% for pamidronate ($p = .058$). The time to first skeletal event for the pamidronate group was 174 days and for zoledronic acid 310 days ($p = 0.013$) (62).

Long-term data, up to 25 months, on zoledronic acid use has demonstrated superior efficacy compared to pamidronate in regard to skeletal events and no significant difference in toxicity (63).

Zoledronic acid is approved by the FDA for use in bone metastases for breast cancer. The dose and schedule of administration are 4 mg intravenously over 15 minute every 4 weeks.

Ibandronate

The use of oral and intravenous ibandronate for bone metastases from breast cancer has been assessed in randomized controlled trials. An early report by Coleman et al. (64) assessed the efficacy of oral ibandronate in patients with metastatic bone disease (64). In this study 110 patients, 77 of whom had breast cancer, were treated with doses of oral ibandronate or placebo. Ibandronate was administered at 5, 10, 20, and 50 mg doses. The primary end points of the study were urinary calcium excretion, and in addition, bone breakdown products including pyridinoline, deoxypyridinoline, and N-telopeptide were measured. The authors concluded that the oral ibandronate reduced bone resorption markers and that further evaluation of this oral agent was warranted in metastatic bone disease.

Two randomized phase III trials of oral ibandronate have been combined and reported by Body et al. (65). In these studies, more than 500 patients were randomized to receive oral ibandronate 50 mg daily or a placebo. Skeletal morbidity rate was used as the primary end point. Oral ibandronate was shown to significantly reduce skeletal morbidity rate with a significant reduction in number of events of radiotherapy and surgery for bone.

Intravenous ibandronate has been evaluated in placebo-controlled phase III trials. A review of these data by Tripathy et al. (66) included studies randomized with ibandronate or placebo in patients with bone metastases from breast cancer. Intravenous ibandronate at 6 mg was infused over 1 to 2 hours every 3 to 4 weeks. Significant reductions in skeletal complications were reported as measured by skeletal morbidity rate.

The long-term use of intravenous ibandronate for metastatic breast cancer has been reported by Pecherstorfer et al. (67). They reported an extension study following the use of ibandronate in a randomized, double-blind fashion comparing placebo to ibandronate 6 mg intravenously over 1 to 2 hours every 3 to 4 weeks. All patients who completed the initial randomized controlled trial were then offered open-label treatment with ibandronate in the extension phase. The 96-week open-label, safety study following the phase III program demonstrated that long-term use of intravenous ibandronate was well tolerated. Importantly, no substantial renal toxicity was reported with up to 4 years of ibandronate administration.

Ibandronate is not approved by the FDA for use in breast cancer bone metastases.

A recent Cochrane review of bisphosphonate use for breast cancer included randomized studies comparing bisphosphonates and placebo or different bisphosphonates in women with metastatic disease. In addition to efficacy data, toxicity data were recorded. Twenty-one randomized studies were included. Skeletal events were reduced by the use of bisphosphonates 17% (relative risk [RR] 0.83; 95% confidence interval [CI], 0.78–0.89; $p < .00001$). Studies including intravenous pamidronate, intravenous zoledronic acid, and oral clodronate were shown to have clinically beneficial effects on skeletal events. For women with metastatic breast cancer and clinically evident bone metastases, bisphosphonates reduced the risk of skeletal events and the skeletal event rate and delayed the time to first skeletal event.

A Cochrane review assessing the relief of pain with the use of bisphosphonates included 30 randomized, controlled trials with more than 3,600 patients. Analysis indicated that the proportion of patients with pain relief was increased with bisphosphonate use, with the number needed to treat at 4 weeks of 11 patients and at 12 weeks of 7 patients. The number needed to harm was reported to be 16. The authors concluded that there is evidence to support the effectiveness of bisphosphonates in providing some pain relief in patients with metastatic disease to bone. They did not recommend the use of bisphosphonates for immediate effect or as first-line therapy (53).

The American Society of Clinical Oncology has reviewed the role of bisphosphonates and bone health issues in women with breast cancer and noted that bisphosphonates provide a supportive benefit to patients with bone metastases. However, a review of Surveillance, Epidemiology, and End Results (SEER) data suggests not all women who may be candidates for bisphosphonate administration are receiving these agents. Giordano et al. (73) report that older women were less likely to receive bisphosphonates, and that these agents may be underused in this population of patients.

Bisphosphonates for Cancer Treatment–Induced Bone Loss

Clodronate

Oral and intravenous clodronate have been shown to have a beneficial effect on bone loss in patients with breast cancer. In an early study, 149 premenopausal women treated with CMF were randomized to receive either oral clodronate at the standard dose of 1,600 mg per day or no bone-targeted treatment. BMD was assessed in the lumbar spine and femoral neck and measured before therapy at 1 and 2 years posttherapy (53,69). At 2 years the women who had chemotherapy-induced amenorrhea

or oligomenorrhea and were in the control arm had a loss of 9.5% in bone mineral density at the lumbar spine and 4.6% at the femoral neck. In the clodronate group a loss of 5.9% and 0.4% at lumbar and femoral regions, respectively, was noted. These observations on preserving bone density were confirmed at the 3- and 5-year analyses of patient data. At 5 years patients in the clodronate group had significantly less bone loss in the lumbar spine (19).

Powles et al. (70) also reported on clodronate use to prevent bone loss. In a randomized, double-blind trial women were treated with oral clodronate, 1,600 mg per day, or placebo. Preservation of bone mineral density was confirmed at 1 and 2 years' follow-up. Clodronate increased bone mineral density at the lumbar spine, total hip, and the trochanter.

Short-term intravenous clodronate, 1,500 mg for seven cycles, did not seem to ameliorate CTIBL in chemotherapy-treated patients (71).

Risedronate

Risedronate is a more potent oral bisphosphonate and is widely used in the treatment of postmenopausal osteoporosis. Delmas et al. (72) conducted a placebo-controlled, randomized study in 53 breast cancer patients who had chemotherapy-induced ovarian failure. Patients were randomized to receive either risedronate or placebo on 2-week cycles of therapy. Bone mineral density was the end point of the study, which also included measurement of bone turnover markers. Stratification for use of tamoxifen was included. There was no change in bone mineral density at the lumbar spine in the risedronate-treated patients. The mean annual rate of change in the placebo-treated group was −1.4 compared to the risedronate group +0.3. In a randomized phase II trial of risedronate to assess its effectiveness in preventing bone loss, significant decreases in bone mineral density occurred in the lumbar spine and hip in the placebo-treated group, while an increase in bone mineral density was noted in the risedronate group.

Oral risedronate has been assessed in the prevention of bone loss as reported by Greenspan et al. (73) in a randomized controlled trial involving 87 postmenopausal women postchemotherapy who were treated with weekly risedronate 35 mg or placebo. In this study the primary outcome measure was change in bone mineral density in the lumbar spine and hip at 12 months. For women treated with risedronate there was an increase in spine and hip bone density of 1.2% and 1.3%, respectively. Significant decreases in bone density were observed in women in the placebo group. The authors concluded that risedronate once weekly was effective in preventing bone loss in women who have been treated with chemotherapy for breast cancer.

Two recently reported studies with risedronate reached different conclusions. Hines et al. (74) examined the use of risedronate or placebo in premenopausal women receiving adjuvant chemotherapy for stage I to III breast cancer. Risedronate 35 mg weekly had no effect on bone density when assessed at 1 year. Greenspan et al. (75) noted that weekly risedronate reduced bone loss in postmenopausal women treated with risedronate 35 mg weekly whether or not they received an aromatase inhibitor.

Ibandronate

Ibandronate for prevention of bone loss in postmenopausal women has been reported by Lester et al. (76). In this randomized, placebo-controlled trial 131 women were given either monthly ibandronate 150 mg or placebo. Baseline bone density results included 68 women with normal BMD T-scores. In those with osteopenia or osteoporosis (50 and 13 patients, respectively) there were significant increases in BMD (p <.01) at the lumbar spine and hip at 1 and 2 years of the study.

Pamidronate and Zoledronic Acid

The effectiveness of pamidronate and zoledronic acid in preventing CTIBL has been assessed in randomized, controlled trials. Intravenous pamidronate 60 mg every 3 months maintained bone mineral density and prevented bone loss at the lumbar spine and hip (77).

Inhibition of bone loss has been assessed with zoledronic acid in pre- and postmenopausal women. In a randomized, controlled, open-label phase III trial reported by Gnant et al. (78), premenopausal women were randomized to receive tamoxifen 20 mg daily plus goserelin 3.6 mg subcutaneously every 28 days with or without zoledronic acid 4 mg intravenously every 6 months versus anastrozole 1 mg daily and goserelin with or without zoledronic acid for 3 years. Four hundred one patients were included in the bone mineral density subprotocol. Endocrine treatment without zoledronic acid resulted in significant bone loss with a reduction in bone mineral density of 14.4% at 36 months and a mean bone mineral density T-score reduction of −1.4. Women receiving anastrozole plus goserelin had a greater reduction in bone mineral density than those receiving tamoxifen plus goserelin. In the women treated with zoledronic acid, bone mineral density was reported to remain stable compared to endocrine therapy alone (p = .0001). The authors concluded that zoledronic acid 4 mg intravenously every 6 months effectively inhibited bone loss in women who were premenopausal with endocrine responsive breast cancers treated with tamoxifen plus goserelin or an aromatase inhibitor plus goserelin.

A late-breaking abstract from the Austrian Breast and Colorectal Cancer Study Group reported on 1,801 premenopausal women treated with adjuvant ovarian suppression and randomized to goserelin plus tamoxifen or goserelin plus anastrozole. The women were randomized to receive zoledronic acid 4 mg intravenously every 6 months for 3 years. At a median follow-up of 60 months those randomized to zoledronic acid had improved disease-free survival (137 events vs. 42 events; p = .01) In addition a nonsignificant trend in overall survival favored the zoledronic acid–treated patients (p = .10) (79).

Brufsky et al. (80) reported on the use of zoledronic acid in postmenopausal women with endocrine responsive breast cancers treated with letrozole. In this randomized, controlled, trial, women receiving letrozole were assigned to receive zoledronic acid 4 mg intravenously every 6 months either at the start of letrozole treatment (the upfront group), or begin zoledronic acid when lumbar spine or total hip T-scores decreased to less than −2 (the delayed group). The end point of the study was change in lumbar spine bone mineral density at month 12. Three hundred one patients were included in the upfront and delayed groups. Results demonstrated preservation of bone mineral density in the upfront group. It was 4.4% higher in the group treated with zoledronic acid at the beginning of letrozole administration compared to the delayed group. Similarly, total hip bone mineral density was 3.3% higher in the upfront group. The authors concluded that administration of zoledronic acid at the start of letrozole therapy prevented bone loss in the lumbosacral spine.

A study of similar design has been reported by Bundred et al. (81) and included 1,065 patients who received adjuvant letrozole and were randomized to immediate start or delayed start of zoledronic acid (81). They noted that at 12 months the lumbar spine bone mineral density increased in those patients who received immediate administration of zoledronic acid and concluded that immediate zoledronic acid prevented bone loss in women receiving letrozole as adjuvant therapy for endocrine sensitive primary breast cancers.

A combined analysis of these studies confirmed the benefit of upfront zoledronic acid for preservation of BMD in postmenopausal women treated with letrozole (82). In this report 1,667 women were included, demonstrating improved BMD in the lumbar spine and hip at the 12 month time point. Interestingly, the authors also report fewer recurrences in the zoledronic acid upfront-treated patients compared to the delayed-treated group (7 vs. 17; p = .0401).

In a review of cancer treatment–induced bone loss, Michaud and Goodin (83,84) noted that early identification and intervention for cancer treatment–induced bone loss may be essential to decrease fracture risk. The use of calcium, vitamin D, regular exercise, and oral or intravenous bisphosphonates should be considered for this population. None of the bisphosphonates have been approved by the FDA for the treatment of cancer treatment–induced bone loss.

Bisphosphonates for the Prevention of Metastases

The adjuvant use of bisphosphonates has been assessed in a number of randomized controlled trials. A study by Diel et al. (85) randomized 302 patients who had cytokeratin positive cells in bone marrow at the time of primary surgery for breast cancer. Randomization was to oral clodronate 1,600 mg per day for 2 years or no bisphosphonate therapy. Standard therapy for primary breast cancer, including surgery, clinically indicated endocrine therapy or chemotherapy was provided. In their initial report, there was a reduction in distant metastases, bone metastases, visceral metastases, and an improvement in survival for patients treated with oral clodronate. An update of these data, at a median follow-up of 53 months, indicated a continued significant reduction in bone metastases development and a reduction of mortality for the clodronate treated patients (86). No effect on visceral metastases was noted. Diel et al. (87) have presented the rationale for the use bisphosphonates as preventive agents.

Powles et al. (88,89) reported a randomized, placebo-controlled trial of oral clodronate in primary breast cancer patients. In this study 1,069 patients with primary breast cancer were randomly assigned to oral clodronate 1,600 mg per day or placebo for a period of 2 years. During administration of clodronate there was a substantial reduction in development of bone metastases. At 5 years a significant reduction of bone metastases was reported. In addition the clodronate-treated patients had a more favorable survival. They concluded that there was no effect of clodronate on visceral metastases development or a statistically significant survival advantage, but there was an effect on development of bone metastases during administration of clodronate.

Saarto et al. (90) have reported a randomized controlled trail for node-positive breast cancer patients treated with oral clodronate 1,600 mg daily for 3 years. The control group did not receive placebo. After primary and local therapy for breast cancer treatment, premenopausal women were treated with adjuvant CMF and postmenopausal women received either adjuvant tamoxifen or toremifene for 3 years. They reported no reduction in bone metastases or nonbone metastases and a decrease in overall survival in the clodronate-treated group. The authors concluded that adjuvant clodronate had no effect on the development of bone metastases but appeared to have a negative effect on disease-free survival and an increase in nonskeletal metastases. The 10-year results of this trial also demonstrated no benefit for clodronate-treated patients in preventing bone metastasis and no significant difference in survival (91). This study has been criticized for the treatment assignment of endocrine therapy in postmenopausal women regardless of estrogen-receptor value.

Zoledronic acid has been used in the adjuvant setting in a feasibility study of patients with disseminated tumor cells in the bone marrow. Tumor cells were detected in a single bone marrow aspiration. Patients were given zoledronic acid 4 mg intravenously monthly for 2 years. Twenty-five of 32 patients had decreased tumor cells at 1-year follow-up and 12 of 17 had a significant decrease at 2-year follow-up. The authors concluded that zoledronic acid decreased the number of disseminated tumor cells in this patient group. This study included 45 patients. Clearly further study is needed before changing practice.

The recent reports of Gnant et al. (79) and Brufsky et al. (82) will add to the intrigue of prevention of metastases with the use of bisphosphonates.

A recent meta analysis of clodronate and breast cancer survival was reported by Ha and Li (92). They examined clinical trials that compared 2 to 3 years of oral clodronate therapy at 1,600 mg per day for patients with primary or metastatic breast cancer. Those who did not receive bisphosphonate therapy, with or without placebo, were the control group. A meta-analysis was carried out separately for patients with advanced and metastatic breast cancer and those with primary disease. They concluded that oral clodronate resulted in no statistically significant difference in overall survival, bone metastases–free survival, or nonskeletal metastases–free survival in patients with advanced breast cancer who received adjuvant oral clodronate therapy. Clodronate in the setting of primary breast cancer had no substantial benefit.

The National Surgical Adjuvant Breast and Bowel Project (NSABP) has completed accrual (>3,000 patients) on a randomized clinical trial (NSABP B-34) of clodronate versus placebo for patients with primary breast cancer treated with systemic chemotherapy and/or tamoxifen or no therapy. Analyses will stratify for participant age, hormone receptor status, and number of positive lymph nodes. Results of this trial are eagerly awaited.

Similarly the Southwest Oncology Group (SWOG) has initiated a randomized trial of adjuvant bisphosphonate therapy for patients with primary breast cancer. Participants are randomized to receive clodronate 1,600 mg orally per day, zoledronic acid 4 mg intravenously every 4 weeks for 6 months, then every 3 months for 2.5 years or ibandronate 50 mg orally daily. This is an ongoing phase III study. Total accrual is expected to include 6,000 participants.

The AZURE (Adjuvant Zoledronic acid reduce Recurrence) trial will assess the role of zoledronic acid as adjuvant therapy in addition to adjuvant or neoadjuvant chemotherapy and/or endocrine therapy. In this study 360 patients have been accrued, and the first report indicated that zoledronic acid could be given safely with chemotherapy without increased myelotoxicity or negative effects on chemotherapy dose. It is hoped that the results of these large randomized trials will determine the relative benefit of adjuvant bisphosphonate therapy for patients with primary breast cancer (93).

Bisphosphonates Adverse Events: Long-Term Safety and Efficacy

Bisphosphonate toxicities include systemic and organ specific effects. Toxicities include transient increases in bone pain, myalgias, and acute febrile reactions. These occur in more than 5% of patients. Fatigue and nausea occur more frequently with bisphosphonate administration than with placebo. In addition, anemia and neutropenia have been reported. Reported electrolyte imbalances include hypocalcaemia and hypophosphatemia.

Renal dysfunction has resulted in increases in both serum urea nitrogen and creatinine values. Azotemia developing as a consequence of bisphosphonate administration has lead the FDA to include a black box warning indicating that creatinine needs to be monitored for all patients receiving intravenous bisphosphonates. Renal dysfunction appears to be more prominent with intravenous administration and amino bisphosphonates.

Dose adjustment for the use of zoledronic acid in patients with multiple myeloma or metastatic bone disease from solid tumors include reducing the dose to 3.5 mg in patients with a creatinine clearance of 50 to 60 mL per minute; 3.3 mg dose for creatinine clearance of 40 to 49 mL per minute, and 3 mg dose for those with a creatinine clearance of 30 to 39 mL per minute.

Zoledronic acid and pamidronate are not recommended for use in patients with a creatinine of greater than 3 mg/dL. The FDA recommends that serum creatinine be measured prior to each administration of zoledronic acid.

Recent reports of severe toxicity associated with use of bisphosphonates have included the documentation of osteonecrosis of the jaw. In a systematic review Woo et al. (94) assessed the reported cases of osteonecrosis of the jaw in association with bisphosphonate use. They noted that although oral and intravenous bisphosphonate had been linked to osteonecrosis of the jaw amino-bisphosphonate and intravenous administration had the most frequent reports of this complication. They reported that 38.8% of the patients with osteonecrosis of the jaw had metastatic breast cancer, and that 66% of the patients had received zoledronic acid or pamidronate while an additional 28% had receive pamidronate and zoledronic acid. They estimated a prevalence of osteonecrosis in patients with cancer at 6% to 10%. More than half of the cases occur after some type of dental alveolar surgery. They suggested preventive strategies, including careful attention to dental infection, before beginning bisphosphonate therapy but noted that there are no data to support discontinuation of bisphosphonate therapy if this complication occurs.

Wilkenson et al. (95) identified 16,000 cancer patients diagnosed between 1986 and 2002 treated with intravenous bisphosphonates, pamidronate, or zoledronic acid. They matched these to 28,698 bisphosphonate nonusers in a 2 to 1 ratio. Results of their study, which were based on SEER data, indicated a hazard ratio of 3.15 for an increased risk of diagnosis of an inflammatory condition of the jaw or osteomyelitis.

Weitzman et al. (96) recommended that patients have a dental examination prior to initiating bisphosphonate therapy, complete any necessary dental procedures prior to the therapy beginning, and receive regular dental visits during bisphosphonate therapy. An additional recommendation was made for good oral hygiene, minimization of any jaw trauma, and avoidance of dental surgery during treatment.

There are limited long-term safety and efficacy data for the use of bisphosphonates in breast cancer patients. Ali et al. (97) reported on 22 patients who received a bisphosphonate at a median duration of 3.6 years who had been evaluated for toxicity and safety. No significant perturbations in calcium and phosphorous or other electrolytes were reported. White blood cell counts were reported to be normal. Decrease in hemoglobin and platelet counts and increase in creatinine were reported but were considered clinically insignificant. There were no stress fractures of long bones encountered with the long duration of administration.

As noted previously, the use of ibandronate for up to 4 years has not been associated with any substantial long-term delayed complications or morbidity (67).

Bisphosphonate Cost and Resource Utilization Considerations

Data on the cost and benefits of bisphosphonates are limited. Hillner et al. (98) reported the cost-effective analysis of pamidronate in breast cancer bone metastases, concluding that pamidronate costs exceeded the cost savings for prevention of skeletal events. They noted, however, that the analysis was "most sensitive" to the cost of pamidronate and treatment of pathologic fractures.

In an analysis of resource utilization associated with zoledronic acid administration, shorter infusion time with zoledronic acid compared to pamidronate was associated with time savings for patients. "Opportunity benefits" were reported to favor the zoledronic acid group (99). A retrospective analysis of the impact of pamidronate on inpatient and outpatient services was reported by Beusterien et al. (100). In this study, a review of medical records of 295 patients with bone metastases from primary breast cancer compared nonpamidronate treated patients to patients who received pamidronate in an early group (i.e., within 3 months of diagnosis of bone metastases) and a late group (i.e., more than 3 months after diagnosis of metastases). Utilization of resources among the groups was assessed using multivariate regression analysis. The early pamidronate group was reported to be much less likely to have unplanned office visits as compared to the late pamidronate and the nonpamidronate group. For the nonpamidronate group compared to the late pamidronate group, hospitalization with bone disease was reduced by approximately 50%. For those who received pamidronate, length of hospitalization was reported to be shorter in both pamidronate groups than in the nonpamidronate group.

Wardley et al. (101) reported significant improvement in pain score and quality of life with community administration versus hospital administration of bisphosphonate. No safety concerns were noted and no increase in frequency of renal or other toxicity was noted in the community setting compared to the hospital setting. The authors conclude that safety and quality of life benefits in breast cancer patients were confirmed, especially when the agent was administered in the community setting.

A recent "Guidance" on bisphosphonate use in solid tumors provides a framework for their application based on expert opinion (102).

MONOCLONAL ANTIBODY TREATMENT OF BONE DISEASE

Denosumab, a human monoclonal antibody to the RANKL, has been shown to suppress bone resorption. Hamdy (103) reported a dose-dependent, rapid, and sustained inhibition of bone resorption with subcutaneous administration of denosumab. Lewiecki et al. (104) reported that denosumab is a potential treatment for osteoporosis. Body et al. (105) assessed the effects of a single subcutaneous dose of denosumab (0.1, 0.3, 1.0, or 3.0 mg/kg) on bone resorption as measured by N-telopeptide levels. They demonstrated a rapid onset of action and prolonged effect, 84 days, for a single administration. Lipton et al. (106) evaluated denosumab in a phase II randomized trial evaluating five dosing regimens of denosumab in patients with breast cancer–related bone metastases. Two hundred fifty-five women were assessed in the five denosumab cohorts and one intravenous bisphosphonate cohort. The end point was change in the bone turnover marker N-telopeptide. At week 13 of the study, the median percentage reduction in N-telopeptide was greater than 70% in denosumab groups and 79% for the intravenous bisphosphonate group. The authors concluded that subcutaneous denosumab administration has similar effectiveness to intravenous bisphosphonate and no substantially greater toxicity was reported.

Ellis et al. (107) reported the results of a randomized, phase III trial of denosumab in women receiving adjuvant aromatase inhibitor therapy. In addition to the aromatase inhibitor patients received either placebo or denosumab 60 mg subcutaneously every 6 months for four doses. Patients receiving denosumab showed increases in BMD at 12 months compared to placebo, irrespective of patient age, duration of menopause, or initial BMD T-score.

Ongoing phase III trials of denosumab compared to bisphosphonates will assess efficacy in regard to skeletal-related events as well as further clarify toxicity associated with the administration of the monoclonal antibody.

RADIONUCLIDE THERAPY FOR PAIN RELIEF IN PATIENTS WITH BONE METASTASES

Bone-seeking radiopharmaceuticals have been assessed for efficacy in relieving bone pain in multiple clinical trials for patients with metastatic carcinoma of the breast and prostate cancer. These agents bind with high affinity to active metastatic disease sites. The agents tested include samarium-153, strontium-89, rhenium-188, and rhenium-186. In the past phosphorous 32 labeled phosphates have been given for bone metastases with substantial benefit in relief of pain, but there is an increased risk of hematologic toxicities (108).

In a recent comparative study reported by Liepe and Kotzerke (109) four radionuclides were compared in a total of 79 patients, 18 of whom were noted to have breast cancer. Seventy-three percent of the patients were reported to experience bone pain relief and 15% were reported to be able to discontinue analgesics and remain pain free. Thrombocytopenia and neutropenia were seen between the second and fifth weeks after radionuclide administration. Among the agents, no significant differences in palliation of pain or Karnofsky performance status were reported.

In a systematic review of radiopharmaceuticals for bone pain, Bauman et al. (110) reviewed the published English literature to assess the efficacy of radiopharmaceuticals in the palliation of metastatic bone pain. They included six randomized, phase III trials and two randomized, phase II trials. Strontium-89 and samarium-153 were used in the randomized controlled trials. Five percent to 10% of the patients were noted to have metastatic breast cancer, but the majority of patients had metastatic prostate cancer and a minority had metastatic lung cancer. The authors concluded that single-agent radiopharmaceutical strontium-89 or samarium-153 is an option for palliation of multiple sites of bone pain when pain control with conventional analgesic medications is unsatisfactory.

A systematic review by Finlay et al. (111) evaluated the use of strontium-89 and samarium-153 for palliation of pain for metastatic bone disease. They reported that pain relief responses varied between 40% to 95%, that pain relief onset began within 1 to 4 weeks of administration of the radiopharmaceutical, and that relief may last for as long as 18 months.

Samarium-153 and strontium-89 are commercially available. Strontium is reported to mimic calcium uptake into bone and its renal excretion. A presumed antitumor effect would be exerted because it is a β-emitter with a half-life of about 50 days and has a tissue penetration of approximately 8 mm. The amount of strontium retained in the body has been correlated with the extent of metastatic involvement. In patients with extensive metastatic disease only 10% to 20% of strontium is eliminated over 100 days.

Samarium-153 is commercially available, has a high affinity for skeletal tissue, and concentrates in areas of enhanced bone metabolic activity by associating with hydroxyapatite crystals.

Retreatment with samarium for painful boney metastasis may be undertaken in 2 to 3 months if an initial beneficial response had been noted and recovery for hematologic toxicity has been confirmed.

As with systemic endocrine therapy, a flare response (i.e., transient increase in bone pain after administration of systemic radionuclide) has been reported in approximately 10% of patients.

Samarium-153 and strontium-89 have received FDA approval for adult and pediatric use for relief of metastatic bone pain. Rhenium-186 and rhenium-188 are investigational agents and are not available commercially in the United States.

A Cochrane database review noted that most studies of radiopharmaceuticals have been with small numbers of patients and have limited duration of follow-up. Nevertheless, single-agent radiopharmaceuticals should be considered an option for bone pain palliation when conventional pain medications are inadequate and bone scan activity confirms metastatic disease sites (110).

SUMMARY

Bone health has become a prominent clinical consideration for women with breast cancer. For primary breast cancer, premenopausal women treated with gonadotoxic chemotherapy, luteinizing hormone-releasing hormone agonists with tamoxifen or aromatase inhibitor should be monitored for bone loss. Assessment of bone mineral density by DEXA is recommended. In postmenopausal women in whom an aromatase inhibitor is to be used as adjuvant therapy, monitoring of bone health with bone mineral density is also recommended.

Bisphosphonates are the most widely used bone-directed therapeutic agents and have wide application in clinical use (Table 89.2). Randomized, controlled trials show a benefit of administration of zoledronic acid in women treated with letrozole in the adjuvant setting. Oral bisphosphonate may be considered in this setting. Randomized, controlled trials of clodronate and risedronate have been shown to be of clinical value. Women who develop osteopenia or osteoporosis should be considered for treatment with bisphosphonates (risedronate, alendronate ibandronate, pamidronate, or zoledronic acid).

For patients who develop bone metastases, the use of intravenous bisphosphonate is recommended. Pamidronate 90 mg intravenously over 2 hours every 4 weeks or zoledronic acid 4 mg intravenously over 15 minutes every 4 weeks is recommended. The optimal duration and schedule of the administration remains unknown and subject to further clinical research.

All patients receiving bisphosphonates require dental examinations prior to treatment. Frequent monitoring of renal function with serum creatinine is recommended.

Bone pain can be managed with adjunctive bisphosphonate therapy or, for those with intractable bone pain, radiopharmaceuticals.

Adjuvant bisphosphonate use is being assessed in phase III clinical trials.

FUTURE DIRECTIONS

The biology of bone metastases and the microenvironmental factors that provide a predilection for the development of bone metastases from breast cancer are subject to intense research. The relationships among osteoclast, osteoblast, tumor cells, the role of growth factors, including PTHrP, TGF-β, vascular endothelial growth factor, granulocyte colony-stimulating factor, granulocyte-macrophange colony-stimulating factor, and cytokines, will continue to be investigated and may lead to new insights for treatment and prevention of bone disease.

Further well-planned research is required to determine the optimal duration of administration of bisphosphonates in the metastatic setting as well as the optimal frequency and the duration of administration of bisphosphonates in the setting of cancer treatment–induced bone loss. Cost-effectiveness analyses or cost-benefit ratios need to be examined in a prospective fashion. Biotechnology may lead to further enhancement of bone-directed therapy as evidenced by the development of denosumab and the early clinical trials that include this agent.

References

1. Coleman RE. Clinical features of metastatic bone disease and risk of skeletal morbidity. *Clin Cancer Res* 2006;12:6243s–6249s.
2. Coleman RE. Metastatic bone disease: clinical features, pathophysiology and treatment strategies. *Cancer Treat Rev* 2001;27:165–176.
3. Domchek SM, Younger J, Finkelstein DM, et al. Predictors of skeletal complications in patients with metastatic breast carcinoma. *Cancer* 2000;89:363–368.
4. Scheid V, Buzdar AU, Smith TL, et al. Clinical course of breast cancer patients with osseous metastasis treated with combination chemotherapy. *Cancer* 1986;58:2589–2593.
5. Roodman GD. Mechanisms of bone metastasis. *N Engl J Med* 2004;350:1655–1664.
6. David RG. Role of stromal-derived cytokines and growth factors in bone metastasis. *Cancer* 2003;97:733–738.
7. Moreau J, Anderson KM, Mauney JR, et al. Studies of osteotropism on both sides of the breast cancer-bone interaction. *Ann N Y Acad Sci* 2007;1117:328–344.
8. Siclari VA, Guise TA, Chirgwin JM. Molecular interactions between breast cancer cells and the bone microenvironment drive skeletal metastases. *Cancer Metastasis Rev* 2006;25:621–633.
9. White DE, Muller WJ. Multifaceted roles of integrins in breast cancer metastasis. *J Mammary Gland Biol Neoplasia* 2007;12:135–142.
10. Rose AA, Siegel PM. Breast cancer-derived factors facilitate osteolytic bone metastasis. *Bull Cancer* 2006;93:931–943.
11. Kingsley LA, Fournier PG, Chirgwin JM, et al. Molecular biology of bone metastasis. *Mol Cancer Ther* 2007;6:2609–2617.
12. Guise TA, Kozlow WM, Heras-Herzig A, et al. Molecular mechanisms of breast cancer metastases to bone. *Clin Breast Cancer* 2005;5[Suppl]:S46–S53.
13. Kozlow W, Guise TA. Breast cancer metastasis to bone: mechanisms of osteolysis and implications for therapy. *J Mammary Gland Biol Neoplasia* 2005;10:169–180.
14. Dougall WC, Chaisson M. The RANK/RANKL/OPG triad in cancer-induced bone diseases. *Cancer Metastasis Rev* 2006;25:541–549.
15. Roodman GD. Biology of osteoclast activation in cancer. *J Clin Oncol* 2001;19:3562–3571.
16. Hortobagyi GN, Buzdar AU, Marcus CE, et al. Immediate and long-term toxicity of adjuvant chemotherapy regimens containing doxorubicin in trials at M.D. Anderson Hospital and Tumor Institute. *NCI Monogr* 1986;(1):105–109.
17. Stearns V, Schneider B, Henry NL, et al. Breast cancer treatment and ovarian failure: risk factors and emerging genetic determinants. *Nat Rev Cancer* 2006;6:886–893.
18. Sverrisdottir A, Fornander T, Jacobsson H, et al. Bone mineral density among premenopausal women with early breast cancer in a randomized trial of adjuvant endocrine therapy. *J Clin Oncol* 2004;22:3694–3699.
19. Vehmanen L, Saarto T, Elomaa I, et al. Long-term impact of chemotherapy-induced ovarian failure on bone mineral density (BMD) in premenopausal breast cancer patients. The effect of adjuvant clodronate treatment. *Eur J Cancer* 2001;37:2373–2378.
20. Howell S, Shalet S. Gonadal damage from chemotherapy and radiotherapy. *Endocrinol Metab Clin North Am* 1998;27:927–943.
21. Perez EA, Weilbaecher K. Aromatase inhibitors and bone loss. *Oncology (Williston Park)* 2006;20:1029–1039.
22. Coleman RE, Banks LM, Girgis SI, et al. Skeletal effects of exemestane on bone-mineral density, bone biomarkers, and fracture incidence in postmenopausal women with early breast cancer participating in the Intergroup Exemestane Study (IES): a randomised controlled study. *Lancet Oncol* 2007;8:119–127.

Table 89.2	BISPHOSPHONATES, APPROVED INDICATIONS, DOSES, AND SCHEDULES	
Agent	**Indication**	**Dose, Route, and Schedule**
Zoledronic	Metastases	4 mg IV, over 15 min, every 4 wks
Pamidronate	Metastases	90 mg IV over 2 hours every 4 wks
Zoledronic acid	Osteoporosis	5 mg IV once yearly
Alendronate	Osteopenia/osteoporosis	5 mg PO daily 70 mg PO weekly
Risedronate	Osteopenia/osteoporosis	5 mg PO daily 35 mg PO daily
Ibandronate	Osteopenia/osteoporosis	2.5 mg PO daily 150 mg PO once monthly

IV, intravenous; PO, by mouth.

23. Shapiro CL. Aromatase inhibitors and bone loss: risks in perspective. *J Clin Oncol* 2005;23:4847–4849.
24. Eastell R, Adams JE, Coleman RE, et al. Effect of anastrozole on bone mineral density: 5-year results from the anastrozole, tamoxifen, alone or in combination trial 18233230. *J Clin Oncol* 2008;26:1051–1057.
25. Shapiro CL, Manola J, Leboff M. Ovarian failure after adjuvant chemotherapy is associated with rapid bone loss in women with early-stage breast cancer. *J Clin Oncol* 2001;19:3306–3311.
26. Kanis JA, McCloskey EV, Powles T, et al. A high incidence of vertebral fracture in women with breast cancer. *Br J Cancer* 1999;79:1179–1181.
27. Love RR, Mazess RB, Tormey DC, et al. Bone mineral density in women with breast cancer treated with adjuvant tamoxifen for at least two years. *Breast Cancer Res Treat* 1988;12:297–302.
28. Powles TJ, Hickish T, Kanis JA, et al. Effect of tamoxifen on bone mineral density measured by dual-energy x-ray absorptiometry in healthy premenopausal and postmenopausal women. *J Clin Oncol* 1996;14:78–84.
29. Winer EP, Hudis C, Burstein HJ, et al. American Society of Clinical Oncology technology assessment on the use of aromatase inhibitors as adjuvant therapy for postmenopausal women with hormone receptor-positive breast cancer: status report 2004. *J Clin Oncol* 2005;23:619–629.
30. Rieber AG, Theriault RL. Aromatase inhibitors in postmenopausal breast cancer patients. *J Natl Compr Cancer Netw* 2005;3:309–314.
31. Coleman RE, Body JJ, Gralow JR, et al. Bone loss in patients with breast cancer receiving aromatase inhibitors and associated treatment strategies. *Cancer Treat Rev* 2008;34:S31–S42.
32. Theriault RL, Biermann JS, Brown E, et al. NCCN task force report: bone health and cancer care. *J Natl Compr Cancer Netw* 2006;4[Suppl 2]:S1–S20.
33. Carlson RW, Hudis CA, Pritchard KI. Adjuvant endocrine therapy in hormone receptor-positive postmenopausal breast cancer: evolution of NCCN, ASCO, and St. Gallen recommendations. *J Nat .Compr Cancer Netw* 2006;4:971–979.
34. Hillner BE, Ingle JN, Chelbowski RT, et al. American Society of Clinical Oncology 2003 update on the role of bisphosphonates and bone health issues in women with breast cancer. *J Clin Oncol* 2003;21:4042–4057.
35. Fleisch H. Bisphosphonates: pharmacology and use in the treatment of tumour-induced hypercalcaemic and metastatic bone disease [review]. *Drugs* 1991;42: 919–944.
36. Rogers MJ, Gordon S, Benford HL, et al. Cellular and molecular mechanisms of action of bisphosphonates. *Cancer* 2000;88:2961–2978.
37. Selander K, Lehenkari P, Vaananen HK. The effects of bisphosphonates on the resorption cycle of isolated osteoclasts. *Calcif Tissue Int* 1994;55:368–375.
38. Murakami H, Takahashi N, Sasaki T, et al. A possible mechanism of the specific action of bisphosphonates on osteoclasts: tiludronate preferentially affects polarized osteoclasts having ruffled borders. *Bone* 1995;17:137–144.
39. Schenk R, Eggli P, Fleisch H, Rosini S. Quantitative morphometric evaluation of the inhibitory activity of new aminobisphosphonates on bone resorption in the rat. *Calcif Tissue Int* 1986;38:342–349.
40. Russell RG, Xia Z, Dunford JE, et al. Bisphosphonates: an update on mechanisms of action and how these relate to clinical efficacy. *Ann N Y Acad Sci* 2007;1117: 209–257.
41. Green JR. Chemical and biological prerequisites for novel bisphosphonate molecules: results of comparative preclinical studies [review]. *Sem Oncol* 2001;48:4–10.
42. Russell RG, Watts NB, Ebetino FH, et al. Mechanisms of action of bisphosphonates: similarities and differences and their potential influence on clinical efficacy. *Osteoporos Int* 2008;19(6):733–759.
43. Dunford JE, Thompson K, Coxon FP, et al. Structure-activity relationships for inhibition of farnesyl diphosphate synthase in vitro and inhibition of bone resorption in vivo by nitrogen-containing bisphosphonates. *J Pharmacol Exp Ther* 2001; 296:235–242.
44. Elomaa I, Blomqvist C, Porkka L, et al. Treatment of skeletal disease in breast cancer: a controlled clodronate trial. *Bone* 1987;8:S53–S56.
45. Paterson AHG, Popwles TJ, Kanis JA, et al. Double-blind controlled trial of oral clodronate in patients with bone metastases from breast cancer. *J Clin Oncol* 1993;11:59.
46. Hortobagyi GN, Theriault RL, Porter L, et al. Efficacy of pamidronate in reducing skeletal complications in patients with breast cancer and lytic bone metastases. Protocol 19 Aredia Breast Cancer Study Group. *N Engl J Med* 1996;335:1785–1791.
47. Theriault RL, Lipton A, Hortobagyi GN, et al. Pamidronate reduces skeletal morbidity in women with advanced breast cancer and lytic bone lesions: a randomized, placebo-controlled trial. Protocol 18 Aredia Breast Cancer Study Group. *J Clin Oncol* 1999;17:846–854.
48. Lipton A, Theriault RL, Hortobagyi GN, et al. Pamidronate prevents skeletal complications and is effective palliative treatment in women with breast carcinoma and osteolytic bone metastases: long term follow-up of two randomized, placebo-controlled trials. *Cancer* 2000;88:1082–1090.
49. Hortobagyi GN, Theriault RL, Lipton A, et al. Long-term prevention of skeletal complications of metastatic breast cancer with pamidronate. Protocol 19 Aredia Breast Cancer Study Group. *J Clin Oncol* 1998;16:2038–2044.
50. Hultborn R, Gundersen S, Ryden S, et al. Efficacy of pamidronate in breast cancer with bone metastases: a randomized, double-blind placebo-controlled multicenter study. *Anticancer Res* 1999;19:3383–3392.
51. Murad AM, Andfade-Filho ACC, Santos MO, et al. Phase II multicentric trial of the use of intravenous clodronate by single fifteen-day interval infusions in patients with bone osteolysis. *J Clin Oncol* 1997;16.
52. Rizzoli R, Forni M, Schaad MA, et al. Effects of oral clodronate on bone mineral density in patients with relapsing breast cancer. *Bone* 1996;18:531–537.
53. Wong R, Wiffen PJ. Bisphosphonates for the relief of pain secondary to bone metastases. *Cochrane Database Syst Rev* 2002;CD002068.
54. Pavlakis N, Stockler M. Bisphosphonates for breast cancer. *Cochrane Database Syst Rev* 2002;CD003474.
55. Iveson TJ, Powle TJ, Tidy A, et al. Clodronate decreases the incidence of bone metastases in patients with advanced or metastatic breast cancer but no clinical evidence of bone metastases. *Br J Cancer* 1994;71[Suppl 24]:15(abst).
56. Major PP, Lipton A, Berenson J, et al. Oral bisphosphonates: a review of clinical use in patients with bone metastases. *Cancer* 2000;88:6–14.
57. Senaratne SG, Pirianov G, Mansi JL, et al. Bisphosphonates induce apoptosis in human breast cancer cell lines. *Br J Cancer* 2000;82:1459–1468.
58. Major P, Lortholary A, Hon J, et al. Zoledronic acid is superior to pamidronate in the treatment of hypercalcemia of malignancy: a pooled analysis of two randomized, controlled clinical trials. *J Clin Oncol* 2001;19:558–567.
59. Berenson JR, Bescio RA, Rosen LS, et al. A phase I dose-ranging trial of monthly infusions of zoledronic acid for the treatment of osteolytic bone metastases. *Clin Cancer Res* 2001;7:478–485.
60. Berenson JR, Rosen LS, Howell A, et al. Zoledronic acid reduces skeletal-related events in patients with osteolytic metastases. *Cancer* 2001;91:1191–1200.
61. Rosen LS, Gordon D, Antonio BS, et al. Zoledronic acid versus pamidronate in the treatment of skeletal metastases in patients with breast cancer or osteolytic lesions of multiple myeloma: a phase III, double-blind, comparative trial. *Cancer J* 2001;7:377–387.
62. Rosen LS, Gordon DH, Dugan W Jr, et al. Zoledronic acid is superior to pamidronate for the treatment of bone metastases in breast carcinoma patients with at least one osteolytic lesion. *Cancer* 2004;100:36–43.
63. Rosen LS, Gordon D, Kaminski M, et al. Long-term efficacy and safety of zoledronic acid compared with pamidronate disodium in the treatment of skeletal complications in patients with advanced multiple myeloma or breast carcinoma: a randomized, double-blind, multicenter, comparative trial. *Cancer* 2003;98:1735–1744.
64. Coleman RE, Purohit OP, Black C, et al. Double-blind, randomised, placebo-controlled, dose-finding study of oral ibandronate in patients with metastatic bone disease. *Ann Oncol* 1999;10:311–316.
65. Body JJ, Diel IJ, Lichinitzer M, et al. Oral ibandronate reduces the risk of skeletal complications in breast cancer patients with metastatic bone disease: results from two randomised, placebo-controlled phase III studies. *Br J Cancer* 2004;90: 1133–1137.
66. Tripathy D, Body JJ, Bergstrom B. Review of ibandronate in the treatment of metastatic bone disease: experience from phase III trials. *Clin Ther* 2004;26: 1947–1959.
67. Pecherstorfer M, Rivkin S, Body JJ, et al. Long-term safety of intravenous ibandronate acid for up to 4 years in metastatic breast cancer: an open-label trial. *Clin Drug Investig* 2006;26:315–322.
68. Giordano SH, Fang S, Duan Z, et al. Use of intravenous bisphosphonates in older women with breast cancer. *Oncologist* 2008;13:494–502.
69. Saarto T, Blomqvist C, Valimaki M, et al. Chemical castration induced by adjuvant cyclophosphamide, methotrexate, and fluorouracil chemotherapy causes rapid bone loss that is reduced by clodronate: a randomized study in premenopausal breast cancer patients. *J Clin Oncol* 1997;15:1341–1347.
70. Powles TJ, McCloskey E, Paterson AH, et al. Oral clodronate and reduction in loss of bone mineral density in women with operable primary breast cancer. *J Natl Cancer Inst* 1998;90:704–708.
71. Vehmanen L, Saarto T, Risteli J, et al. Short-term intermittent intravenous clodronate in the prevention of bone loss related to chemotherapy-induced ovarian failure. *Breast Cancer Res Treat* 2004;87:181–188.
72. Delmas Pd, Balena R, Confravreux E, et al. Bisphosphonate risedronate prevents bone loss in women with artificial menopause due to chemotherapy of breast cancer: a double-blind, placebo-controlled study. *J Clin Oncol* 1997;15:955–962.
73. Greenspan SL, Bhattacharya RK, Sereika SM, et al. Prevention of bone loss in survivors of breast cancer: a randomized, double-blind, placebo-controlled clinical trial. *J Clin Endocrinol Metab* 2007;92:131–136.
74. Hines SL, Mincey BA, Sloan JA, Thomas SP, Chottiner CL, et al. A phase III randomized, placebo-controlled, double-blind trial of risedronate for prevention of bone loss in premenopausal women undergoing adjuvant chemotherapy for breast cancer (BC). *J Clin Oncol* 2008;26[15 Suppl]:525.
75. Greenspan SL, Brufsky A, Lembersky BC, et al. Risedronate prevents bone loss in breast cancer survivors: a 2 year, randomized, double-blind, placebo-controlled clinical trial. *J Clin Oncol* 2008 Jun 1;26(16):2644–2652.
76. Lester D, Dodwell D, Purohit OP, et al. Use of monthly oral ibandronate to prevent anastrozole-induced bone loss during adjuvant treatment for breast cancer: two-year results from ABIRON study. *J Clin Oncol* 2008;26[15 Suppl]:554.
77. Fuleihan G, Salamoun M, Mourad YA, et al. Pamidronate in the prevention of chemotherapy-induced bone loss in premenopausal women with breast cancer: a randomized controlled trial. *J Clin Endocrinol Metab* 2005;90:3209–3214.
78. Gnant MF, Mlineritsch B, Luschin-Ebengreuth G, et al. Zoledronic acid prevents cancer treatment-induced bone loss in premenopausal women receiving adjuvant endocrine therapy for hormone-responsive breast cancer: a report from the Austrian Breast and Colorectal Cancer Study Group. *J Clin Oncol* 2007;25:820–828.
79. Gnant M, Mlineritsch B, Schippinger W, et al. Adjuvant ovarian suppression combined with tamoxifen or anastrozole, alone or in combination with zoledronic acid, in premenopausal women with endocrine-responsive, stage I and II breast cancer: first efficacy results from ABCSG-12. *J Clin Oncol* 2008;26(15 Suppl):LBA4.
80. Brufsky A, Harker WG, Beck JT, et al. Zoledronic acid inhibits adjuvant letrozole-induced bone loss in postmenopausal women with early breast cancer. *J Clin Oncol* 2007;25:829–836.
81. Bundred NJ, Campbell ID, Davidson N, et al. Effective inhibition of aromatase inhibitor-associated bone loss by zoledronic acid in postmenopausal women with early breast cancer receiving adjuvant letrozole: ZO-FAST study results. *Cancer* 2008;112:1001–1010.
82. Brufsky A, Bundred N, Coleman R, et al. Integrated analysis of zoledronic acid for prevention of aromatase inhibitor-associated bone loss in postmenopausal women with early breast cancer receiving adjuvant letrozole. *Oncologist* 2008;13:503–514.
83. Michaud LB, Goodin S. Cancer-treatment-induced bone loss, part 1. *Am J Health Syst Pharm* 2006;63:419–430.
84. Michaud LB, Goodin S. Cancer-treatment-induced bone loss, part 2. *Am J Health Syst Pharm* 2006;63:534–546.
85. Diel IJ, Solomayer EF, Costa SD, et al. Reduction in new metastases in breast cancer with adjuvant clodronate treatment. *N Engl J Med* 1998;6:357–363.
86. Diel IJ, Solomayer E, Gollan C, et al. Bisphosphonates in the reduction of metastases in breast cancer—results of the extended follow-up of the first study population. *Proc Am Soc Clin Oncol* 2000;19:82a.
87. Diel IJ, Solomayer EF, Bastert G. Bisphosphonates and the prevention of metastasis: first evidences from preclinical and clinical studies. *Cancer* 2000;88: 3080–3088.
88. Powles T, Paterson S, Kanis JA, et al. Randomized, placebo-controlled trial of clodronate in patients with primary operable breast cancer. *J Clin Oncol* 2002;20: 3219–3224.
89. Powles T, Paterson A, McCloskey E, et al. Reduction in bone relapse and improved survival with oral clodronate for adjuvant treatment of operable breast cancer (ISRCTN 83688026). *Breast Cancer Res* 2006;8:R13.
90. Saarto T, Blomqvist C, Virkkunen P, et al. Adjuvant clodronate treatment does not reduce the frequency of skeletal metastases in node-positive breast cancer patients: 5-year results of a randomized controlled trial. *J Clin Oncol* 2001;19:10–17.

91. Saarto T, Vehmanen L, Virkkunen P, et al. Ten-year follow-up of a randomized controlled trial of adjuvant clodronate treatment in node-positive breast cancer patients. *Acta Oncol* 2004;43:650–656.

92. Ha TC, Li H. Meta-analysis of clodronate and breast cancer survival. *Br J Cancer* 2007;96:1796–1801.

93. Coleman R, Thorpe H, Cameron D, et al. Zoledronic acid is well tolerated and can be safely administered with adjuvant chemotherapy—first safety data from AZURE trial (BIG01/04). *Breast Cancer Res Treat* 2006;100(1):S107 (abst).

94. Woo SB, Hellstein JW, Kalmar JR. Narrative [corrected] review: bisphosphonates and osteonecrosis of the jaws. *Ann Intern Med* 2006;144:753–761.

95. Wilkinson GS, Kuo YF, Freeman JL, et al. Intravenous bisphosphonate therapy and inflammatory conditions or surgery of the jaw: a population-based analysis. *J Natl Cancer Inst* 2007;99:1016–1024.

96. Weitzman R, Sauter N, Eriksen EF, et al. Critical review: updated recommendations for the prevention, diagnosis, and treatment of osteonecrosis of the jaw in cancer patients—May 2006. *Crit Rev Oncol Hematol* 2007;62:148–152.

97. Ali SM, Esteva FJ, Hortobagyi G, et al. Safety and efficacy of bisphosphonates beyond 24 months in cancer patients. *J Clin Oncol* 2001;19:3434–3437.

98. Hillner BE, Weeks JC, Desch CE, et al. Pamidronate in prevention of bone complications in metastatic breast cancer: A cost-effectiveness analysis. *J Clin Oncol* 2000;18:72–79.

99. Des Harnais CL, Bajwa K, Markle JP, et al. A microcosting analysis of zoledronic acid and pamidronate therapy in patients with metastatic bone disease. *Support Care Cancer* 2001;9:545–551.

100. Beusterien KM, Hill MC, Ackerman SJ, et al. The impact of pamidronate on inpatient and outpatient services among metastatic breast cancer patients. *Support Care Cancer* 2001;9:169–176.

101. Wardley A, Davidson N, Barrett-Lee P, et al. Zoledronic acid significantly improves pain scores and quality of life in breast cancer patients with bone metastases: a randomised, crossover study of community vs. hospital bisphosphonate administration. *Br J Cancer* 2005;92:1869–1876.

102. Aapro M, Abrahamsson PA, Body JJ, et al. Guidance on the use of bisphosphonates in solid tumours: recommendations of an international expert panel. *Ann Oncol* 2008;19:420–432.

103. Hamdy NA. Denosumab: RANKL inhibition in the management of bone loss. *Drugs Today (Barc.)* 2008;44:7–21.

104. Lewiecki EM, Miller PD, McClung MR, et al. Two-year treatment with denosumab (AMG 162) in a randomized phase 2 study of postmenopausal women with low BMD. *J Bone Miner Res* 2007;22:1832–1841.

105. Body JJ, Facon T, Coleman RE, et al. A study of the biological receptor activator of nuclear factor-kappa B ligand inhibitor, denosumab, in patients with multiple myeloma or bone metastases from breast cancer. *Clin Cancer Res* 2006;12:1221–1228.

106. Lipton A, Steger GG, Figueroa J, et al. Randomized active-controlled phase II study of denosumab efficacy and safety in patients with breast cancer-related bone metastases. *J Clin Oncol* 2007;25:4431–4437.

107. Ellis GK, Bone HG, Chlebowski RT, et al. Subgroup analysis of a randomized, phase III study of the effect of denosumab in women with nonmetastatic breast cancer receiving aromatase inhibitor (AI) therapy. *J Clin Oncol* 2008;26(15S):17s.

108. Silberstein EB. The treatment of painful osseous metastases with phosphorus-32-labeled phosphates. *Semin Oncol* 1993;20:10.

109. Liepe K, Kotzerke J. A comparative study of 188Re-HEDP, 186Re-HEDP, 153Sm-EDTMP, and 89Sr in the treatment of painful skeletal metastases. *Nucl Med Commun* 2007;28:623–630.

110. Bauman G, Charette M, Reid R, et al. Radiopharmaceuticals for the palliation of painful bone metastasis—a systemic review. *Radiother Oncol* 2005;75:258–270.

111. Finlay IG, Mason MD, Shelley M. Radioisotopes for the palliation of metastatic bone cancer: a systematic review. *Lancet Oncol* 2005;6:392–400.

Chapter 90
Local Management of Bone Metastases

Janet Sybil Biermann, Albert J. Aboulafia, and James A. Hayman

Since the last publication of this textbook only a few short years ago there has been an explosion in the understanding of the evaluation and treatment of patients with skeletal metastases resulting from breast cancer. Historically, published information and clinical trials relating to the skeletal complications of malignancy combined data that included a variety of different primary sites. Many of the diagnostic and treatment strategies that were recommended for patients with metastatic bone disease as a whole are not applicable today for the unique group of patients with metastases secondary to breast cancer. It is only recently, and not widely, appreciated that skeletal metastases that result from breast primary differ dramatically from the other primary sites with respect to clinical presentation, prognosis, and treatment. Additionally, the introduction of bisphosphonates has dramatically changed the treatment strategy for patients with metastatic breast cancer to the skeleton, rendering much of the prior literature less useful. Only recently have published articles relating to the treatment of skeletal metastases focused on the cohort of patients with primary breast cancer rather than combining data with patients with skeletal metastases from any primary site. Table 90.1 presents Web site resources for patients.

Although there has been an increasing appreciation for the differences in treatment among patients with metastatic bone disease from breast and other primary sites, the goals of treatment remain the same. They include relief of pain, restoration or maintenance of function, and avoiding hypercalcemia, metabolic derangements, bone marrow invasion, spinal cord compression, and pathological fracture.

More widespread use of sensitive imaging techniques such as magnetic resonance imaging (MRI) and positron emission tomography (PET) has created the ability to detect bone metastases at an earlier stage, often identifying asymptomatic disease. Although in general the number of patients coming to surgery for skeletal stabilization has decreased, carefully selected patients will reap major benefits from surgical intervention in terms of pain control and function.

INCIDENCE

It is estimated that there will be 1.2 million new cases of cancer diagnosed in the United States in 2008. Half of those cancers will include breast, kidney, lung, thyroid, and prostate, which have a proclivity for skeletal metastases. This number far exceeds the estimated number of primary sarcomas of bone (2,700 per year), with many occurring in patients under the age of 40 years. Breast cancer is the most common cancer and the second leading cause of cancer-related morbidity among women in North America and Western Europe. In those patients who develop metastases, the skeleton is the most frequently involved site. Radiographic studies have demonstrated skeletal metastases in 70% to 80%, and autopsy studies as high as 85%, of patients who die of their disease. The most common sites of skeletal involvement include the spine and long bones (i.e., femur and humerus) (1). In part, due to the long survival of patients with breast cancer, bone metastases are common, and their potential impact on quality of life, morbidity, and mortality is significant. Certainly not all skeletal metastases will require treatment. Although the spine is the most common site of metastases from breast to bone, it is estimated that only one third of spinal metastases will become symptomatic during the

course of the patients life. The treatment of a given skeletal lesion depends on a variety of factors including the clinical presentation.

CLINICAL PRESENTATION

The clinical presentation of a patient with skeletal metastases will depend on a variety of factors. For the majority of patients with metastatic breast cancer, the primary is known before skeletal metastases become symptomatic. The clinical presentation of a patient with skeletal metastases from breast cancer may be initiated due to the onset of a symptomatic bone lesion (i.e., pain, radiculopathy or pathological fracture) or the result of an imaging study that was performed as part of a staging evaluation (at the time of initial diagnosis or routine follow-up), or less commonly for unrelated reasons. The diagnostic work-up and treatment for these conditions will depend greatly on whether the scenario takes place in the setting of a known history of breast cancer or not and whether the bone lesion is solitary or not. It is fundamentally important that in evaluating a patient with a destructive lesion of bone, a logical, thorough, and meticulous algorithm be followed in order to avoid major errors in diagnosis and treatment and minimize potential complications (2).

The majority of patients presenting with bone metastases report pain as an initial symptom, although there may be asymptomatic identification if the patient has a subsequent bone scan. In evaluating the treatment choices for patients with long bone (humerus, femur, tibia) metastasis, it is particularly important to identify whether the pain is associated with weight bearing and relived by rest, as this is one prognostic indicator of the likelihood of pathologic fracture (3). Careful assessment of the patient's analgesic use relative to pain reporting is important, as large doses of narcotics may obfuscate the severity of the symptoms and lead to undertreatment locally.

The various clinical presentations that a patient with suspected metastatic breast cancer to bone may present include the following:

1. New onset of skeletal pain *with* a known history of breast cancer (symptomatic);
2. New onset of skeletal pain *without* a known history of breast cancer (symptomatic);
3. Discovery of an asymptomatic lesion in a patient *with* a known history of breast cancer (as part of routine staging or follow-up or less likely an incidental finding);
4. Discovery of an asymptomatic lesion in a patient *without* a known history of breast (cancer as part of routine staging or follow-up or less likely an incidental finding).

DIAGNOSIS AND IMAGING OF BONE METASTASIS

Diagnostic Evaluation

Although it is true that for any patient over age 40 with a destructive bone lesion the most likely diagnosis is metastatic tumor or myeloma, the presumptive diagnosis of metastatic disease is strengthened if the patient has a history of breast cancer. However, all too often the assumption is made that a

| Table 90.1 | **RELEVANT PATIENT INFORMATION WEB SITES** |

Entity	Description	Website
American Cancer Society	General overview of bone metastasis for patients, including symptoms, diagnosis, treatments from the American Cancer Society	http://www.cancer.org/docroot/CRI/content/CRI_2_4_1X_What_Is_bone_metastasis_66.asp
Novartis	Commercial site with general information on symptoms, diagnosis, imaging studies	http://www.us.novartisoncology.com/info/coping/bone_metastasis.jsp?usertrack.filter_applied=true&NovaId=3350119511325999391
American Academy of Orthopaedic Surgeons	Physician authored site with general information on bone metastases for patients	http://www.orthoinfo.org/topic.cfm?topic=A00093
National Cancer Institute	Overview of metastatic cancer, including to bone	http://www.cancer.gov/cancertopics/factsheet/Sites-Types/metastatic
University of Michigan	General information on bone metastasis including symptoms, diagnosis, treatments, glossary of terms	http://www.cancer.med.umich.edu/cancertreat/tissue_bone/bonegeneral.shtml

bone lesion is metastatic in a patient with a history of breast cancer and the assumption proves to be wrong. Conversely, a patient with a very remote history of breast cancer (20 years or more) and bone pain is not suspected of having potential metastases due to the lack of appreciation of the potential delayed presentation of skeletal metastases in breast cancer. As with any patient with a potentially malignant bone lesion, the patient with breast cancer requires a logical and systematic approach to evaluation in order to optimize outcomes, avoid unnecessary procedures and expenses, and expedite medical and emotional support.

The first step in evaluating a patient with a skeletal lesion requires a careful history and physical examination. The history should include the presence or absence of prior cancer diagnosis, the stage of disease, the histology, and accounting of any prior imaging studies and treatment to date. Although generally nonspecific, the presence or absence of pain, the character of pain, the onset, duration, aggravating, and alleviating factors, and response to analgesics should be noted. Pain related to skeletal metastases is usually described as a dull aching pain that may be exacerbated with activity or weight-bearing when the lower extremities are involved. Night pain is more common in metastatic disease than in conditions such as arthritis, mechanical low back pain, or tendonitis. A general history regarding risk factors for other cancers should also be elicited such as smoking, alcohol abuse, sun or toxin exposure, obesity, and family history.

Plain Radiographs

Plain films are the initial study to be obtained in the patient with suspected bone metastasis. Bone metastases from breast cancer may be lytic, blastic, or mixed. Use of bisphosphonates may result in a shift of the spectrum to a higher incidence of sclerotic metastases (4).

Typically lesions are poorly marginated, originate within the medullary space but cause some adjacent cortical destruction, with a characteristic "moth-eaten" appearance. Especially in the setting of pathologic fracture or insufficiency of bone, there may be adjacent periosteal reaction. Soft tissue masses extending outside the bone may be present, particularly in deposits of long-standing.

Approximately 30% to 50% of the bone must be destroyed prior to the lesion being evident on the plain film. Generally surgical intervention is not considered in cases with less bone destruction. Although plain films are arguably the best modality for determining necessity of surgical intervention, they are not as sensitive as other modalities, particularly MRI, for determining the presence or absence of metastases.

Bone Scan

Bone scans remain relatively nonspecific as indicators of metastatic disease, with positive findings present on bone scans with unrelated causation, including arthritis, occult insufficiency fractures, and prior bone trauma. Additionally, bone scan, being a test of metabolic function, does not indicate the degree of structural damage, information important in determining which treatment modality might be most appropriate. Most skeletal metastases from breast cancer show increase radiotracer uptake at the site of involvement. Exceptions to this generalization include extremely aggressive lytic metastases (that would like be apparent on plain radiographs) and some estrogen receptor–negative metastases, particularly those involving the cervical spine (5).

Computed Tomography Scanning

In patients with known metastatic breast cancer being followed with chest, abdomen, and pelvis computed tomography (CT) scanning, CT detected metastatic bone lesions in 43 of 44 (98%) patients with bone metastases. The remaining patient had a solitary, asymptomatic bony metastasis in shaft of femur. Bone scan was positive in all patients with bone metastases. There were 11 cases of false-positive findings on bone scan. These findings suggest that in patients with known metastases, CT scanning alone is likely sufficient to evaluate bone metastases and, in fact, bone scanning is more likely to lead to findings of false positivity (6).

Magnetic Resonance Imaging

MRI is the single best imaging modality to assess bone marrow. However, changes within the bone marrow due to skeletal metastases may be difficult to distinguish from marrow changes from nonneoplastic conditions. Benign conditions that may alter the appearance of the bone marrow on MRI include trauma, infection, radiation, the administration of growth factors (i.e., pegfilgrastim [Neulasta], filgrastim [Neupogen], granulocyte colony-stimulating factor), and osteoporosis.

With regard to decision making for intervention for symptomatic metastases, however, MRI is less useful. MRI signals are determined by paramagnetic qualities and on vascularity, depending on the sequences used, rather than structural factors. Cortical bone is relatively poorly imaged by MRI. In fact, MRI may artifactually indicate or overstate cortical erosions or bone destruction. Although MRI plays an important role in the assessment of etiology of local bone pain, it is of minimal utility in determining which patients may benefit from surgery.

Positron Emission Tomography, with or without Computed Tomography

PET scan and PET-CT are indicated for evaluating the response to treatment for patients with metastatic breast cancer. As a result, PET scans and PET-CT scans that have been performed for patients being followed with visceral metastases are discovering asymptomatic skeletal lesions. Both the PET scan and the CT scan portion of the PET are capable of discovering bone metastases prior to their becoming symptomatic. The sensitivity of PET and PET-CT compared with other imaging modalities such as the bone scan have not been well studied. Siggelkow et al. (7), in a study involving 57 patients with breast cancer found that PET scan had a relatively low positive predictive value of 74.5% and a relatively high predictive value of 98.3%. It is likely that the combination of the PET and CT will prove to be sensitive and specific when read by an experienced clinician.

EXTERNAL BEAM RADIATION THERAPY

Because bone metastases are so prevalent among women with metastatic breast cancer, treatment with external beam radiation in such patients is not uncommon. Although a number of systemic options are now available for treating diffuse bony metastatic disease, such as bisphosphonates and radionuclides, external beam radiation remains the least invasive and most effective established local therapy for the treatment of localized bony metastases. The most common reason for its use in this setting is pain control, but it can also be used to prevent progression of lesions that if left untreated could lead to fracture or spinal cord or cauda equina compression. Accordingly, the primary objective of such treatment should be to improve or maintain patients' quality of life and physical function for the duration of their lives with the least toxicity and inconvenience.

There are a surprising number of issues to consider when assessing whether such treatment has been successful. Not only is there the degree of pain relief but also the rapidity of its onset as well as its durability. One must also take into account potential acute (e.g., nausea and vomiting) and late toxicities (e.g., fracture or spinal cord damage), the possible need for retreatment, the potential to reduce dependence on narcotics thereby reducing any associated side-effects, how well such treatment results in the ability of patients to maintain or improve their physical function, and the convenience of treatment. When surveyed, patients with bone metastases ranked from most to least important the duration of pain relief, likelihood of complications, degree of pain relief, mobility, dependence on narcotics, and lastly the length of treatment (8).

When making decisions about who to treat and how best to treat them, there are a number of issues to consider. One important factor is the natural history of the patient's disease. In the case of metastatic breast cancer, survival is typically longer than for the average patient with bone metastases, with median survival on the order of 2 to 3 years. Although physicians are not very good at estimating patients' life expectancies (9), it still needs to be taken into account when deciding how best to manage these patients. The number of bony lesions and the presence of visceral metastases are also relevant, as are the extent of bone destruction and the presence of an associated soft tissue mass. The site of the lesion can also influence the likelihood of toxicity (e.g., spine versus extremity). Other issues to consider include the patients' performance status, any comorbidities, prior treatment with adjuvant or palliative radiation, and their ability and willingness to come for daily treatment. At the societal level, there are also the direct medical costs of treatment, the burden on family and friends, and the ability to access a nearby treatment facility in a timely fashion to consider.

When making decisions about where to treat, it is necessary to pay particular attention to patients' symptoms and any recent imaging studies, including plain x-ray images, CT scans, MRI scans, bone scans, or fluorodeoxyglucose (FDG)-PET scans. CT and MRI are especially helpful in defining the extent of any associated soft tissue mass. Typically, the field arrangements used to treat patients with bone metastases are relatively straightforward and often consist of two opposed treatment fields or sometimes even a single rectangular field.

Conventional External Beam Radiation

Although there is general consensus regarding its efficacy, there is controversy about how best to deliver external beam radiation for the treatment of painful bone metastases. Numerous studies have reported overall response rates in the range of 60% to 70%, with complete response rates between 20% to 30% (10). The onset of pain relief usually occurs within 3 weeks of the completion of treatment, and the duration of pain relief is typically on the order of 3 to 5 months (11). The likelihood and severity of acute toxicity depends on the site and size of the field being treated but is generally tolerable. The likelihood of patients developing significant late complications is also very low, with pathologic fracture and spinal cord compression rates in the range of only 2% to 3%.

When it comes to treatment with radiation, higher doses typically result in improved outcomes. However, this does not necessarily appear to be the case for palliative radiation for bony metastases. In a study completed over 20 years ago, the Radiation Therapy Oncology Group (RTOG) randomized 266 patients with solitary bone metastases to 40.5 Gy in 15 fractions or 20 Gy in 5 fraction and 750 patients with multiple bone metastases to 30 Gy in 10 fraction, 15 Gy in 5 fractions, 20 Gy in 5 fractions, or 25 Gy in 5 fractions and initially reported no differences in outcomes (12). Of note, in this trial pain was assessed by the treating physician, not the patient. Interestingly, these results did not lead to the use of short-course radiation. Instead, practice patterns in the United States over the past several decades have been heavily influenced by an unplanned reanalysis of these data in which patients with both solitary and multiple bone metastases were combined into a single group and the primary end point was redefined; it reported longer-course radiation (e.g., 30 Gy in 10 fractions) to be more effective (13).

Over the past decade, evidence has been mounting in patients with uncomplicated bony metastases, typically defined as lesions that have not been previously irradiated and have or will not soon result in fracture or spinal cord compression or require surgical intervention, that single-dose radiation treatment is just as effective as fractionated radiation therapy. In the Bone Pain Working Group trial 765 patients with painful bone metastases, 36% of whom had breast cancer, were randomized to 8 Gy in 1 fraction or either 20 Gy in 5 or 30 Gy in 10 fractions (14). They found no differences in terms of patient-reported time to improvement in pain, maximal pain relief, time to progression of pain, analgesics used, acute toxicity, pathologic fracture, or spinal cord compression. Patients treated with single fractions were retreated at a rate of 23% versus 10% for those receiving multiple fractions, although it was unclear whether this represented lower efficacy of single fractions or just a lower threshold to retreat patients after a single fraction.

The Dutch Bone Metastasis Study randomized 1,171 patients, 39% of whom had breast cancer, to either a single 8 Gy fraction or 24 Gy in six fractions and reported nearly identical results (15). Again, differences in patient-reported response rates, duration of response, use of pain medication, side effects, and quality of life were nonexistent between the two arms, while the retreatment rate was higher in the single fraction group (25% vs. 7%). One difference in this study was that the rate of pathologic fractures was twice as high as in the single fraction group; however, the absolute rates were still extremely low (4% vs. 2%). In a follow-up study, these investigators found that single fraction patients who did not respond or who had progressive pain were much more likely to be retreated than multiple fraction patients (35% vs. 8% and 22% vs. 10%, respectively), supporting the assertion that physicians are more willing to retreat patients with single fractions (16). They also reported that retreatment with radiation is highly effective in both patients without either an initial response (66% response rate after single fractions and 33% after multiple fractions) or progressive pain after an initial response (70% for single fractions and 57% after multiple fractions). Another issue especially relevant to patients with breast cancer, who, as noted above, often have prolonged survival, is whether single fractions provide pain relief that is as durable as fractionated radiation. To address this issue, the Dutch investigators looked specifically at 320 patients enrolled in their study who survived for greater than 52 weeks, 63% of whom had breast cancer (17). The mean duration of response and progression rates in this subgroup were similar between single and multiple fraction patients, 29 versus 30 weeks and 55% and 53%, respectively, again with high response rates following retreatment. Therefore, while the rates of progression among patients with prolonged survival are relatively high, these data suggest that it may be preferable to retreat those patients who progress rather than initially treating all patients with longer treatment courses. These investigators also examined cost and quality of life issues associated with single versus multiple fraction radiation using data from their trial and concluded that single fractions are less costly, associated with comparable quality-adjusted survival, and therefore are more cost-effective (18).

More recently the RTOG conducted another bone metastases trial limited to patients with either breast (50%) or prostate cancer and randomized 898 such patients to either a single 8 Gy fraction or 30 Gy in 10 fractions (19). Again the response rates were similar, while the retreatment rate was higher in the patients treated with single fractions (18% vs. 9%). Interestingly, the rate of acute toxicity was greater in the multiple fraction arm than in the single fraction arm (17% vs. 10%). Data from a Canadian trial confirmed this result and also found that the prophylactic use of antiemetics reduced the likelihood of nausea and vomiting when treating the lumbar or pelvic region (20).

In addition to the studies mentioned above, at least 12 other randomized trials have been performed examining this issue. The results of these trials have been summarized in several systematic reviews (10,21), and meta-analyses (11,22), all of which fail to demonstrate a difference between single and multiple fractions. These data led Cancer Care Ontario to develop evidence-based guidelines on fractionation for palliation of bone metastases that recommended the use of single fractions for symptomatic uncomplicated bone metastases (23). It is therefore interesting to note that when radiation oncologists are surveyed regarding the use of single fractions in this setting many are reluctant to use them (24), and these results have been confirmed by several population-based studies of actual treatment records (25,26). When patients are surveyed, some have expressed a preference for single fractions, while others favor multiple fractions (24).

To date, treatment of so-called complicated bone metastases has been less well studied. As noted above, significant experience now exists regarding the efficacy of retreating bone metastases with radiation. However, the optimal retreatment regimen has not yet been identified but is currently the subject of a large international randomized trial comparing retreatment with single versus multiple fractions. As discussed elsewhere in this chapter, patients with bone metastases that have or are about to cause a pathologic fracture often undergo surgical stabilization.

Although the data supporting its use in this setting are limited, multiple fraction radiation is typically employed postoperatively (27).

Another related issue that is also not well studied concerns bone remineralization. In the only randomized study to investigate remineralization, Koswig and Budach (28) reported significantly more remineralization 6 months following 30 Gy in 10 fractions than 8 Gy in a single fraction (173% vs. 120% mean increase in bone density, respectively) and suggested that multiple fractions be considered when this is felt to be an important issue. Radiotherapy is also frequently used to treat bone metastases that are causing actual or impending spinal cord or cauda equina compression. In all these settings, it is still generally accepted that patients be treated with conventional fractionated radiation (e.g., 30 Gy in 10 fractions).

Stereotactic Body Radiation Therapy

Advances in the delivery of external beam radiation have recently led to interest in treating spine metastases more aggressively with radiation using an approach known as stereotactic body radiation therapy. Based on the same principles as stereotactic radiosurgery, stereotactic body radiation therapy generally refers to the use of very precise, highly conformal radiation therapy delivered to an extracranial site in one to five treatments. To achieve these goals patients typically need to be reproducibly immobilized, imaged at least immediately prior to, and sometimes during, treatment to confirm proper patient positioning, and treated with multiple, often noncoplanar and unopposed, static beams or dynamic arcs to achieve highly conformal treatment plans that spare adjacent critical normal tissues. Although initially developed for treating lung lesions, this approach is also starting to be used to treat spine metastases in patients who have previously received dose-limiting treatment to the spinal cord or in those who are felt to have such a good prognosis that more aggressive treatment may be considered.

Preliminary results from several centers in breast cancer patients have been encouraging with response rates upward of 90%, response duration of 13 months, little to no long-term toxicity, and retreatment rates between 0% to 15% (29,30).

Hemibody Radiation Therapy

At the other end of the spectrum, hemibody irradiation has been used in the past to treat diffuse bony disease and is effective in that setting with response rates of 70% to 90% (31,32). However, because of newer systemic options (e.g., bisphosphonates, radionuclides) as well as concerns regarding acute toxicity, mostly gastrointestinal, and the ability to deliver subsequent myelosuppressive chemotherapy, its use has generally declined.

SURGICAL MANAGEMENT

A large proportion of patients with metastatic breast cancer will require some type of intervention for symptomatic disease to bone. Wedin et al. (33) looked at a population of patients in Sweden with metastatic breast cancer to bone, and of 641 patients with breast carcinoma presenting with symptomatic skeletal metastasis during 1989 to 1994, 107 (17%) subsequently underwent surgery. Metastases were located in long bones (77 patients), spine (14 patients), and pelvis (6 patients). The median survival postoperatively was 6 months. It is likely that the rate of operation in this population is diminishing. In another study of patients presenting with bone metastases, Cazzaniga et al. (34) reported on a series of 459 patients presenting with metastatic breast cancer, and in their 28-month follow-up, new skeletal-related events were observed in 122 patients (26.6%).

Patients can be expected to have a relatively lengthy survival on average after surgical intervention, and surgical efforts should be directed at reasonably durable reconstructions. Durr et al. (35), looking at a group of patients undergoing orthopaedic surgery for fractures or impending fractures secondary to metastatic breast cancer, noted survival rates of 59% after 1 year, 36% after 2 years, 13% after 5 years, and 7% after 10 years.

The evaluation of the outcomes of surgical intervention in patients with bone metastases has been markedly hampered by the variability in presentation of patients with regard to site and disease status and the variability in treatment approaches. No prospective randomized data are available to compare outcomes of surgical interventions with different techniques, or even comparing surgical intervention to nonsurgical care. The participation of a multidisciplinary team can help address issues of integration of imaging findings, prognosis, coordination with other forms of care, and examination of potential surgical benefit versus morbidity (36).

The health care costs of skeletal-related events in the metastatic breast cancer population are significant. Delea et al. (37) evaluated a group of 617 patients with breast cancer and metastatic disease to bone, about half of whom had had one or more skeletal-related events. After matching cases based on propensity scores, there were 201 patients each in the skeletal-related events and no skeletal-related events groups, with mean follow-up of 13.8 and 11.0 months, respectively. In the skeletal-related events group, costs of treatment of skeletal-related events were $13,940 (95% confidence interval [CI], $11,240–$16,856) per patient. Total medical care costs were $48,173 (95% CI, $19,068–$77,684) greater in skeletal-related events versus no skeletal-related events patients ($p = .001$). Along the same lines, Zhou et al. (38) evaluated a group of women with breast cancer who presented with fractures, and for older women with early-stage breast carcinoma, the direct costs for bone fracture were estimated at $45,579, and 57% of those costs came from treating the bone fracture (32% came from inpatient hospital costs, and 25% came from noninpatient hospital costs), 25% came from other excess treatment costs, and 18% came from excess long-term care costs.

There are special considerations in the management of pathologic fractures secondary to malignancy compared to conventional fracture management in normal, traumatized bone. Typically fixation is more difficult in the involved bone, not only at the site of the metastatic deposit but also in adjacent bone, which is often osteoporotic in the metastatic breast cancer population. In contrast to traumatic fractures, fracture healing in the metastatic setting is relatively poor due to multiple factors, including local tumor regrowth, effects of chemotherapy and radiation therapy, and overall catabolic state of the patient. Additionally, the prolonged time for immobilization and protected limb function is unacceptable in the palliative setting of a patient with limited lifespan in whom prompt restoration of function is paramount. Because of this, excision of bone and prosthetic reconstruction is more frequently utilized, as well as load-sharing intramedullary devices (rather than load-bearing plate and screw constructs, which also require screw fixation in bone). Prosthetic replacement may be preferable in some situations where long bones are fractured adjacent to a joint in such a way that fixation in the small, periarticular segment cannot be achieved. Definitive fixation with prosthetic implants allows for immediate weightbearing and may be associated with a lower reoperation rate than with use of intramedullary fixation (39). In general, functional outcomes are better in the lower extremities than in the humerus with this approach (40).

Preoperative Assessment And Counseling

In considering patients for possible surgical intervention, multiple levels of assessment must take place in order to ensure an intervention that provides effective palliation, has an acceptable complication risk, and is consonant with the patient's wishes.

It is difficult to document when or if surgical intervention for bone metastasis may be associated with prolonged survival. For the most part, goals of surgical intervention in long bones is with the goal of providing pain relief and improving function. However, this is not always apparent to the patient and family, and in order to ensure that expectations of all parties are aligned, detailed preoperative counseling regarding the palliative nature of the intervention is necessary. In most cases of intervention, a nonsurgical alternative can be provided for consideration, which typically includes altered or protected weightbearing (sometimes wheelchair status) and an increase in narcotic use.

The identification of the bone metastasis and its contribution to the pain and disability the patient is experiencing is critical and typically can be achieved only by a careful history and musculoskeletal examination. It is important not to assume that the metastasis is *de facto* the source the pain, but rather to exclude other potential causes of pain including arthrosis of adjacent joints, tendinopathies, bursitis, and other bone, joint, and soft tissue maladies.

The risks of surgery should be carefully itemized, including the possibility of life-threatening complications or a possible clinical deterioration, leading to failure to leave the hospital, as high as 10% in some series. Infection, particularly in arthroplasty, can be catastrophic, requiring long-term suppressive antibiotics at best, and necessitating multiple reoperations and even amputation, at worst.

Anticipated prognosis must be carefully weighed against surgical recovery and surgical risks. Typically, patients should have a minimum expected 6-week longevity in order to benefit from long bone stabilization with intramedullary devices, and about 3 months in order to benefit from arthroplasty.

The patient must be sufficiently robust to withstand surgery. If a patient is nonambulatory, the reasons for this and the duration should be carefully assessed preoperatively before considering surgery to restore lower limb long bone function. If general fatigue and disability are limiting factors rather than the skeletal issues, or if the patient has been nonambulatory for a considerable period of time, the prognosis for restoration of ambulation may be quite poor.

Chemotherapy effects must be considered. Platelets normally should be above 50,000 in order to withstand surgical blood loss and may need to be higher (100 K) for pelvic or open spine cases. Neutrophils must be over 1 K in order to adequately guard against infection. If the patient is on myelosuppressive therapy, this should be discontinued in such a time frame that a nadir below this level will not be anticipated.

Site-Specific Surgical Considerations

Pelvis

Reconstruction of the fractured or severely involved pelvis secondary to bone metastases remains one of the more challenging aspects of orthopaedic oncology. Successful surgical restoration involves effective transfer of loads normally three times body weight from the femur to the sacrum, bypassing or reconstructing damaged or missing bone.

A number of reconstructive options have been described, including the use of Steinmann pins threaded through remaining intact pelvis combined with cement and protrusion rings to create sufficient integrity for hip replacement (41). Another option is to excise the affected area of the pelvis entirely and replace it with a saddle prosthesis that spans the gap between femoral shaft and upper ileum. A minimum of 2.5 cm of intact ileum is necessary to stabilize the pelvis, and complications of this procedure include dislocation of the saddle element off the pelvis. All reconstructions for the pelvis entail relatively lengthy operative times and the potential for significant blood loss. In selected highly symptomatic patients with limited ambulatory goals, girdlestone resection can be contemplated for palliation and improved sitting.

In selected patients with lytic lesions of the acetabulum refractory to radiation who may be poor surgical candidates, percutaneous cementoplasty can be considered. In this procedure, liquid polymethylmethacrylate (PMMA) is injected percutaneously into the lytic defect with the intent of providing some structural support without an extensive surgical procedure to completely reconstruct the acetabulum. This can provide pain relief and immediate improvement in structural support (42,43). This technique is primarily suited to periacetabular lesions.

Radiofrequency ablation has been reported in combination with cementoplasty in a small series of bone metastatic patients with 100% initial pain relief (44), but more research is needed to evaluate this combined modality approach (45).

Femur

Proximal Femur (Neck and Peritrochanteric)

In contrast to pathologic fractures arising from osteoporosis of the femoral neck in the elderly, pathologic fractures of the femoral neck, even nondisplaced fractures, should be considered for hemiarthroplasty. Fixation with screws along the femoral neck, while effective in nondisplaced osteoporotic fractures, is fraught with the complications of persistent pain, non-

healing, and need for additional surgery. In contrast, replacement of the proximal femur (femoral neck) with hemiarthroplasty results in predictable pain relief and early functional recovery (Figs. 90.1 and 90.2) (46). Use of a long stemmed prosthesis can guard against subsequent fractures distal to the implant. Resurfacing of the acetabulum is usually unnecessary unless there is coexistent, symptomatic arthritis.

With regard to femoral shaft fractures, or impending shaft fractures, treatment has been described with a number of intramedullary implants (47). Although in past decades, surgical treatment algorithms for long bone metastases focused on open procedures and cement augmentation, newer fixation options allow for excellent fixation proximally and distally, with implants inserted proximally or distally to the fracture site with smaller incisions and less necessity for augmentation locally with bone cement. With the opportunity to bypass the fractured site there is in general a lower blood loss and speedier recovery. In a series of 182 surgical interventions for metastatic disease of the femur, treatment of 97 impending pathologic fractures yielded better results than treatment of 85 completed pathologic fractures with less average blood loss (438 cc vs. 636 cc), shorter hospital stay (7 vs. 11 days), greater likelihood of discharge to home as opposed to an extended care facility (79% vs. 56%), and greater likelihood of resuming support-free ambulation (35% vs. 12%). Prophylactic intramedullary nailing of the femur, rather than intramedullary nailing of completed fractures, results in shorter hospital stays, lower perioperative complication rates, and better functional outcomes (48).

Femoral nailing of pathologic fractures or impending fractures can be associated with hypoxia and pulmonary complications thought to be related to tumor and fat embolism. Acute oxygen desaturation and hypotension occurred in 11 of 45 patients in a small series of patients in whom this was rigorously

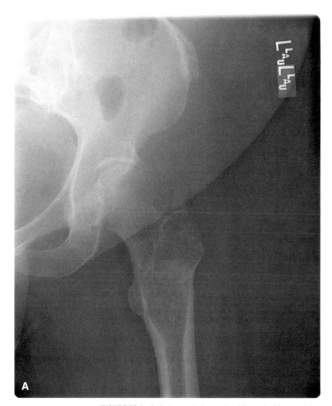
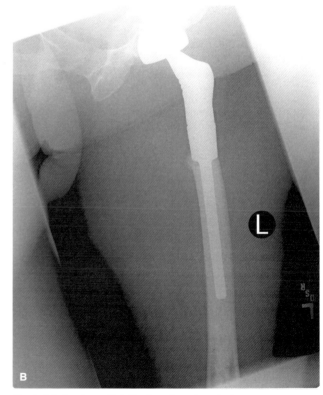

FIGURE 90.1. A: Anteroposterior proximal femur in 60-year-old woman with metastatic breast caner. Plain film shows disease in proximal femur extending into femoral neck and head. Patient had prior external beam therapy and presentation with 3-week history of debilitating groin pain and inability to walk. **B:** Postoperative plain film shows long stemmed hemiarthroplasty. Patient was able to return to ambulatory status prior to succumbing to disease 1 year later.

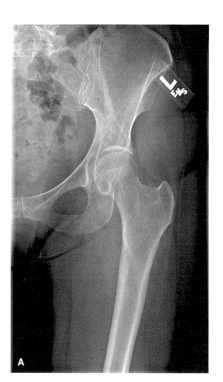

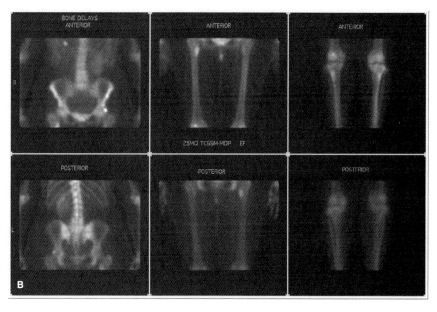

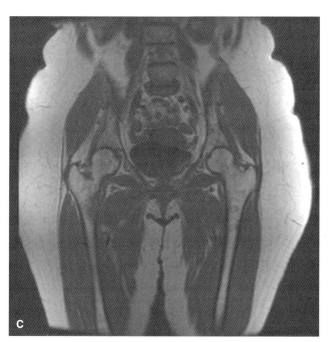

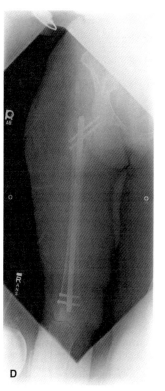

FIGURE 90.2. A: Anteroposterior proximal femur in 56-year-old woman with 2-month history of increasing weightbearing pain in the femur and a history of breast cancer treated 1 year previously. Lytic destructive disease present extending from trochanter to proximal shaft. **B:** Tc 94m methylene-diphosphonate (MDP) scan shows uptake in proximal right femur subtrochanteric region. **C:** Coronal T1-weighted magnetic resonance image shows marrow replacement of proximal shaft of femur as well as other lesions in ilium. **D:** Anteroposterior femur plain radiograph following intermedullary nailing of the femur. Percutaneous biopsy prior to nail placement confirmed metastatic breast cancer. Patient resumed ambulation without pain.

studied (49). In prophylactic intramedullary nailing of the femur, venting (creation of small distal "vent" in the bone) may decrease intramedullary pressures and the risk of fat and tumor embolization (50).

Lesions of the distal femur, including the condyles and of the proximal, periarticular tibia, are relatively less common. Lesions refractory to external beam therapy or those that have fractured can be treated with segmental replacement or resurfacing arthroplasty. Due to the high rate of wound healing complications following radiation and the disastrous results of infection, liberal use of soft tissue flaps, generally the gastrocnemius, should be considered for reconstructions in this location.

Humerus

The humerus is more typically involved later in the disease process in bone metastasis. Considerations include the potential for considerable disability, particularly if the dominant extremity is involved, in activities of daily living, and the potential to lose the ability to live independently.

Disease in the proximal humerus typically is extensive and requires excision of the involved bone rather than stabilization. Involvement of the attachments of the rotator cuff to the humerus leads to difficulty in reconstructing this defect with a conventional shoulder replacement, and segmental replacing systems should be considered. Regaining of full functional range of motion of the shoulder is rarely a possibility due to muscle insertion loss; however, regaining a stable, painless shoulder will allow the patient to use the elbow, wrist, and hand more successfully and free the opposite limb from a "tending" function.

From the proximal one sixth of the humerus to the distal fourth of the humerus, stabilization of destructive lesions can be carried out using an intramedullary nail. These devices are inserted through small incisions in the shoulder area typically with relatively short operative times and minimal blood loss. The limb can be used for light activities within days.

In the distal fourth of the humerus, due to the unique anatomical considerations compounded with the adjacent elbow joint, interlocked nails are not an option. Approaches to the distal humerus include open curettage and plating and segmental replacement of the distal humerus with elbow joint replacement. Although generally done under tourniquet to reduce blood loss, these interventions have longer operative times and higher complication rates than locked nailing.

Spine

The vertebral column is the most common of all sites of bone metastases to the spine, with the spine metastases present in the majority of patient succumbing to metastatic disease from breast cancer. Manifestations of spinal involvement include pain, vertebral collapse, and neurological compromise from either tumor or extruded fracture fragments.

Pain is the most common presenting symptom from spinal metastases. While bony involvement may be treated with radiation therapy, the symptoms arising from vertebral collapse are likely to be refractory to radiation treatment and more responsive to measures to reintroduce more normal height to the vertebrae. Often patients are able to localize the offending levels, which is very helpful in targeting treatment in the patient with diffuse spine involvement. Vertebral compressions fractures can cause pain, spinal deformity (kyphosis, due to forward collapse, or scoliosis due to rotatory or sagittal plane bending), loss of height, or pulmonary or visceral compromise due to volume restrictions. Nerves exiting the spinal column may experience compression due to loss of height. Spinal cord compression can occur from either direct epidural extension of tumor, from collapsed fracture fragments forced into the spinal canal, or from tenting of the spinal cord due to deformity, most commonly kyphosis. Careful examination of the patient to ascertain the cause of pain and presence or absence of myelopathy is essential in the initial evaluation and management of the patient with spinal metastasis.

Surgical intervention potential for spinal metastatic disease has changed greatly in the past decade. Newer surgical approaches allow for improved access to all spinal levels. Improved instrumentation systems that allow for better fixation in compromised bone and more intraoperative flexibility are now available. Vertebral body replacing systems have allowed for greater opportunity to remove diseased segments with safe, structural supports (51).

Surgical intervention can be considered even in patients with multiple levels of disease or with relatively advance stage cancers. Sciubba et al. (52) reported on a series of 87 patients undergoing 125 spinal surgeries to evaluate prognostic variables. Presence of visceral metastases, multiplicity of bony lesions, presence of estrogen receptors (ER), and segment of spine (cervical, thoracic, lumbar, sacral) in which metastases arose were compared with patient survival. Those with ER positivity had a longer median survival after surgery compared to those with ER negativity. Patients with cervical location of metastasis had a shorter median survival compared with those having metastases in other areas of the spine. The presence of visceral metastases or a multiplicity of bony lesions did not have prognostic value.

Preoperative functional status likely has an impact on the effectiveness of spinal decompression procedures, and early surgical intervention should be considered in patients with spinal metastases and neurological findings. North et al. (53) evaluated results in 61 open spinal procedures for spine metastases. Preoperatively, 53 of 61 (87%) patients in the study population suffered neurological symptoms (e.g., weakness) and 52 (85%) were ambulatory. Postoperatively, 59 (97%) were ambulatory. Most patients who survived 6 months (81%) remained ambulatory, as did 66% of those alive at 1.6 years. The median postoperative survival was 10 months. The risk factors for loss of ambulation were preoperative loss of ambulatory ability, recurrent or persistent disease after primary radiotherapy of the operative site, a procedure other than corpectomy, and tumor type other than breast cancer. Prognostic factors for reduced survival were surgical intervention extending over two or more spinal segments, recurrent or persistent disease after primary radiotherapy involving the operative site, diagnosis other than breast cancer, and a cervical spinal procedure.

Percutaneous structural options for the symptomatic treatment of painful collapse of spinal vertebrae without neurological abnormalities include vertebroplasty and kyphoplasty. Percutaneous vertebroplasty is a radiographically image-guided procedure in which the surgeon or radiologist injects liquid PMMA into the collapsed vertebrae under image intensification with the intention of improving pain by increasing the structural integrity of the affected bone. Vertebroplasty was initially used for benign vascular tumors, but its use has spread to osteoporotic fractures as well as vertebral collapse secondary to metastatic or myelomatous bone tumors. Complications from vertebroplasty largely result from inadvertent extrusion of the PMMA into undesirable and unplanned areas outside the vertebral body, inducing posterior leakage with the potential disastrous consequence of cord trauma.

Kyphoplasty was introduced to essentially perform vertebroplasty in a more controlled fashion. In kyphoplasty, a small balloon or "bone tamp" is introduced under fluoroscopic guidance into the vertebral body through a percutaneous transpedicular approach and then inflated to create a "space" into which the PMMA can then be injected. It offers the advantage of significantly greater height restoration (54) and a lower rate of cement extrusion and leakage outside the vertebral body (55). The inflatable tamp compresses adjacent compromised bone and potentially occludes alternative pathways for the cement to extrude while creating a space for the cement to occupy. Due to the increased procedural time and instrumentation, kyphoplasty is associated with higher expense and increased exposure to radiographic contrast agents. Randomized trials comparing vertebroplasty and kyphoplasty, or, indeed, either of these procedures compared to nonoperative management, have yet to be performed. However, reports of kyphoplasty have indicated that it is associated with safe, reliable pain relief, restoration of vertebral height, and even when cement is extruded it is generally without neurologic complication (56–58).

MANAGEMENT SUMMARY

- Asymptomatic breast cancer metastases may occur, particularly in the setting of widespread metastases to bone, and can be managed medically.

- Pain that is controlled by analgesics and not weightbearing in nature or associated with spinal compression may be improved with the initiation of bisphosphonates or the beginning of new systemic therapy; bone metastases in these situations may be observed and followed radiographically to assess whether systemic treatment may be sufficient. Progression in pain or radiographic findings would indicate the potential indication for radiation or surgery or both.
- External beam radiotherapy usually improves pain due to bone metastases.
- Strong consideration should be given to treating patients with uncomplicated painful bone metastases with a single 8 Gy fraction.
- Multiple fraction radiation should still be used for patients at significant risk for pathologic fracture, following surgical stabilization and for patients with spinal cord or cauda equina compression.
- Prophylactic surgery for stabilization should be considered in medically appropriate candidates with weight-bearing pain in the long bones, particularly the femur.
- Spinal decompression surgery should be strongly considered for patients with spinal involvement and neurologic compromise.
- Patients with frank long bone or pelvic fractures should be considered for stabilization of fractures or joint-replacing surgery.
- Percutaneous kyphoplasty can be considered for patients with symptomatic vertebral collapse secondary to bone metastatic involvement without neurologic involvement.
- Radiofrequency ablation is a relatively new technique available at selected centers and may be considered in selected patients with failed radiation therapy who do not have lesions requiring surgical stabilization.

References

1. Namer M. Clinical consequences of osteolytic bone metastases. *Bone* 1991;12 [Suppl 1]:S7.
2. Rougraff BT, Kneisl JS, Simon MA. Skeletal metastases of unknown origin. A prospective study of a diagnostic strategy. *J Bone Joint Surg Am* 1993;75(9):1276–1281.
3. Damron TA, Morgan H, Prakash D, et al. Critical evaluation of Mirels' rating system for impending pathologic fractures. *Clin Orthop Relat Res* 2003;415[Suppl]:S201–S207.
4. Quattrocchi CC, Piciucchi S, Sammarra M, et al. Bone metastases in breast cancer: higher prevalence of osteosclerotic lesions. *Radiol Med (Torino)* 2007;112(7):1049–1059.
5. Petren-Mallmin M, Andreasson I, Nyman R, et al. Detection of breast cancer metastases in the cervical spine. *Acta Radiol* 1993;34(6):543–548.
6. Bristow AR, Agrawal A, Evans AJ, et al. Can computerised tomography replace bone scintigraphy in detecting bone metastases from breast cancer? A prospective study. *Breast* 2008;17(1):98–103.
7. Siggelkow W, Zimny M, Faridi A, et al. The value of positron emission tomography in the follow-up for breast cancer. *Anticancer Res* 2003;23(2C):1859–1867.
8. Barton MB, Dawson R, Jacob S, et al. Palliative radiotherapy of bone metastases: an evaluation of outcome measures. *J Eval Clin Pract* 2001;7(1):47–64.
9. Chow E, Davis L, Panzarella T, et al. Accuracy of survival prediction by palliative radiation oncologists. *Int J Radiat Oncol Biol Phys* 2005;61(3):870–873.
10. Chow E, Harris K, Fan G, et al. Palliative radiotherapy trials for bone metastases: a systematic review. *J Clin Oncol* 2007;25(11):1423–1436.
11. Wu JS, Wong R, Johnston M, et al. Meta-analysis of dose-fractionation radiotherapy trials for the palliation of painful bone metastases. *Int J Radiat Oncol Biol Phys* 2003;55(3):594–605.
12. Tong D, Gillick L, Hendrickson FR. The palliation of symptomatic osseous metastases: final results of the study by the Radiation Therapy Oncology Group. *Cancer* 1982;50(5):893–899.
13. Blitzer PH. Reanalysis of the RTOG study of the palliation of symptomatic osseous metastasis. *Cancer* 1985;55(7):1468–1472.
14. Bone Pain Trial Working Party. Eight Gy single fraction radiotherapy for the treatment of metastatic skeletal pain: randomised comparison with a multifraction schedule over 12 months of patient follow-up. *Radiother Oncol* 1999;52(2):111–121.
15. Steenland E, Leer JW, van Houwelingen H, et al. The effect of a single fraction compared to multiple fractions on painful bone metastases: a global analysis of the Dutch Bone Metastasis Study. *Radiother Oncol* 1999;52(2):101–109.
16. van der Linden YM, Lok JJ, Steenland E, et al. Single fraction radiotherapy is efficacious: a further analysis of the Dutch Bone Metastasis Study controlling for the influence of retreatment. *Int J Radiat Oncol Biol Phys* 2004;59(2):528–537.
17. van der Linden YM, Steenland E, van Houwelingen HC, et al. Patients with a favourable prognosis are equally palliated with single and multiple fraction
18. van den Hout WB, van der Linden YM, Steenland E, et al. Single- versus multiple-fraction radiotherapy in patients with painful bone metastases: cost-utility analysis based on a randomized trial. *J Natl Cancer Inst* 2003;95(3):222–229.
19. Hartsell WF, Scott CB, Bruner DW, et al. Randomized trial of short- versus long-course radiotherapy for palliation of painful bone metastases. *J Natl Cancer Inst* 2005;97(11):798–804.
20. Kirkbride P, Warde P, Panzarella A, et al. A randomised trial comparing the efficacy of single fraction radiation therapy plus ondansetron with fractionated radiation therapy in the palliation of skeletal metastases. *Int J Radiat Oncol Biol Phys* 2000;48[Suppl 3]:185(abst).
21. Wai MS, Shelley M, Held I, et al. Palliation of metastatic bone pain: single fraction versus multifraction radiotherapy—a systematic review of the randomised trials. *Cochrane Database Syst Rev* 2004;2:CD004721.
22. Sze WM, Shelley M, Held I, et al. Palliation of metastatic bone pain: single fraction versus multifraction radiotherapy—a systematic review of randomised trials. *Clin Oncol (R Coll Radiol)* 2003;15(6):345–352.
23. Wu JS, Wong RKS, Lloyd NS,et al. Radiotherapy fractionation for the palliation of uncomplicated painful bone metastases—an evidence-based practice guideline. *BMC Cancer* 2004;4:71.
24. Bradley NM, Husted J, Sey MS, et al. Review of patterns of practice and patients' preferences in the treatment of bone metastases with palliative radiotherapy. *Support Care Cancer* 2007;15(4):373–385.
25. Kong W, Zhang-Salomons J, Hanna T, et al. A population-based study of the fractionation of palliative radiotherapy for bone metastasis in Ontario. *Int J Radiat Oncol Biol Phys* 2007;69(4):1209–1217.
26. Williams MV, James ND, Summers E, et al. National survey of radiotherapy fractionation practice in 2003. *Clin Oncol (R Coll Radiol)* 2006;18(1):3–14.
27. Townsend PW, Smalley SR, Cozard SC, et al. Role of postoperative radiation therapy after stabilization of fractures caused by metastatic disease. *Int J Radiat Oncol Biol Phys* 1995;31(1):43–49.
28. Koswig S, Budach V. [Remineralization and pain relief in bone metastases after after different radiotherapy fractions (10 times 3 Gy vs. 1 time 8 Gy). A prospective study.] *Strahlenther Onkol* 1999;175(10):500–508.
29. Gerszten PC, Burton SA, Welch WC, et al. Single-fraction radiosurgery for the treatment of spinal breast metastases. *Cancer* 2005;104(10):2244–2254.
30. Ryu S, Jin R, Jin JY, et al. Pain control by image-guided radiosurgery for solitary spinal metastasis. *J Pain Sympt Man* 2008;35(3):292–298.
31. Poulter CA, Cosmatos D, Rubin P, et al. A report of RTOG 8206: a phase III study of whether the addition of single dose hemibody irradiation to standard fractionated local field irradiation is more effective than local field irradiation alone in the treatment of symptomatic osseous metastases. *Int J Radiat Oncol Biol Phys* 1992;23(1):207–214.
32. Salazar OM, Rubin P, Hendrickson FR, et al. Single-dose half-body irradiation for palliation of multiple bone metastases from solid tumors. Final Radiation Therapy Oncology Group report. *Cancer* 1986;58(1):29–36.
33. Wedin R, Bauer HC, Rutqvist LE. Surgical treatment for skeletal breast cancer metastases: a population-based study of 641 patients. *Cancer* 2001;92(2):257–262.
34. Cazzaniga ME, Dogliotti L, Cascinu S, et al. Diagnosis, management and clinical outcome of bone metastases in breast cancer patients: results from a prospective, multicenter study. *Oncology* 2006;71(5–6):374–381.
35. Dürr HR, Müller PE, Lenz T, et al. Surgical treatment of bone metastases in patients with breast cancer. *Clin Orthop Relat Res* 2002;396:191–196.
36. Papageloupoulos PJ, Mavrogenis AF, Galanis EC, et al. Advances and challenges in diagnosis and management of skeletal metastases. *Orthopedics* 2006;29(7):609–622.
37. Delea T, McKiernan J, Brandman J, et al. Retrospective study of the effect of skeletal complications on total medical care costs in patients with bone metastases of breast cancer seen in typical clinical practice. *J Support Oncol* 2006;4(7):341–347.
38. Zhou Z, Redaelli A, Johnell O, et al. A retrospective analysis of health care costs for bone fractures in women with early-stage breast carcinoma. *Cancer* 2004;100(3):507–517.
39. Wedin R. Surgical treatment for pathologic fracture. *Acta Orthop Scand Suppl* 2001;72(302):1–29.
40. Camnasio F, Scotti C, Peretti GM, et al. Prosthetic joint replacement for long bone metastases: analysis of 154 cases. *Arch Orthop Trauma Surg* 2008;128(8):787–793.
41. Harrington KD. Orthopaedic management of extremity and pelvic lesions. *Clin Orthop Relat Res* 1995;312:136–147.
42. Harris K, Pugash R, David E, et al. Percutaneous cementoplasty of lytic metastasis in left acetabulum. *Curr Oncol* 2007;14(1):4–8.
43. Harty JA, Brennan D, Eustace S, et al. Percutaneous cementoplasty of acetabular bony metastasis. *Surgeon* 2003;1(1):48–50.
44. Toyota N, Naito A, Kakizawa H, et al. Radiofrequency ablation therapy combined with cementoplasty for painful bone metastases: initial experience. *Cardiovasc Intervent Radiol* 2005;28(5):578–583.
45. Callstrom MR, Charboneau JW, Goetz MP, et al. Painful metastases involving bone: feasibility of percutaneous CT- and US-guided radio-frequency ablation. *Radiology* 2002;224(1):87–97.
46. Chrobok A, Spindel J, Mrozek T, et al. Partial long-stem resection Austin-Moore hip endoprosthesis in the treatment of metastases to the proximal femur. *Ortop Traumatol Rehabil* 2005;7(6):600–603.
47. Samsani SR, Panikkar V, Venu KM, et al. Breast cancer bone metastasis in femur: surgical considerations and reconstruction with long gamma nail. *Eur J Surg Oncol* 2004;30(9):993–997.
48. Ward WG, Holsenbeck S, Dorey FJ, et al. Metastatic disease of the femur: surgical treatment. *Clin Orthop Relat Res* 2003;415[Suppl]:S230–S244.
49. Barwood SA, Wilson JL, Molnar RR, et al. The incidence of acute cardiorespiratory and vascular dysfunction following intramedullary nail fixation of femoral metastasis. *Acta Orthop Scand* 2000;71(2):147–152.
50. Roth SE, Rebello MM, Kreder H, et al. Pressurization of the metastatic femur during prophylactic intramedullary nail fixation. *J Trauma* 2004;57(2):333–339.
51. Khan SN, Donthineni R. Surgical management of metastatic spine tumors. *Orthop Clin North Am* 2006;37(1):99–104.
52. Sciubba DM, Gokaslan ZL, Suk I, et al. Positive and negative prognostic variables for patients undergoing spine surgery for metastatic breast disease. *Eur Spine J* 2007;16(10):1659–1667.
53. North RB, LaRocca VR, Schwartz J, et al. Surgical management of spinal metastases: analysis of prognostic factors during a 10-year experience. *J Neurosurg Spine* 2005;2(5):564–573.

54. Belkoff SM, Mathis JM, Jasper LE, et al. An ex vivo biomechanical evaluation of a hydroxyapatite cement for use with vertebroplasty. *Spine* 2001;26(14):1542–1546.

55. Phillips FM, Todd Wetzel F, Lieberman I, et al. An in vivo comparison of the potential for extravertebral cement leak after vertebroplasty and kyphoplasty. *Spine* 2002;27(19):2173–2179.

56. Fourney DR, Schomer DF, Nader R, et al. Percutaneous vertebroplasty and kyphoplasty for painful vertebral body fractures in cancer patients. *J Neurosurg* 2003;98 [1 Suppl]:21–30.

57. Pflugmacher R, Beth P, Schroeder RJ, et al. Balloon kyphoplasty for the treatment of pathological fractures in the thoracic and lumbar spine caused by metastasis: one-year follow-up. *Acta Radiol* 2007;48(1):89–95.

58. De Negri P, Tirri T, Paternoster G, et al. Treatment of painful osteoporotic or traumatic vertebral compression fractures by percutaneous vertebral augmentation procedures: a nonrandomized comparison between vertebroplasty and kyphoplasty. *Clin J Pain* 2007;23(5):425–430.

Chapter 91
Breast Cancer in Older Women

Gretchen G. Kimmick, Kevin S. Hughes, and Hyman B. Muss

BACKGROUND

Increasing age is a major risk factor for breast disease and for breast cancer incidence and mortality. One-third to one-half of breast cancer diagnoses occur in women age 65 years and older, the geriatric population (1,2). According to United States (U.S.) cancer statistics from 2001 to 2003, 1 in 15 women aged 70 years and older will develop breast cancer, compared with 1 in 27 women aged 60 to 69 years, 1 in 25 women aged 40 to 49, and 1 in 210 women younger than 39 years (1). Furthermore, the U.S. Census Bureau predicts that the number of women in the age groups of 65 to 84 years will nearly double and in the 85 and older age group will nearly quadruple by 2050 (Fig. 91.1)—leading to a substantial increase in the number of breast cancer diagnoses. The good news is that breast cancer-specific mortality rates declined in the early 21st century. The puzzle, however, is that breast cancer-specific survival is inversely proportional to age and, although breast cancer-specific mortality rates improved overall, the change for the better occurred preferentially in women diagnosed at ages younger than 70 years (3). Breast cancer is, therefore, a noteworthy health concern in the geriatric population.

Explaining the overall poorer breast cancer-specific survival in the geriatric population is complicated and may be related to diagnosis at more advanced stage, lower screening mammography rates, less aggressive management, and poorer overall health status of older women, which limits treatment options (4,5). Although reports are not entirely consistent, stage for stage, it appears that both older and younger women fare well with early-stage disease, but that as stage increases, mortality rates may diverge and older women fare worse (6–8). In the Finnish Cancer Registry, for instance, relative 10-year survival was approximately 80% and constant across age groups in women with node-negative breast cancer, but in women with node-positive breast cancer, older women fared worse; with node-positive breast cancer, 10-year survival was 49% for women aged 46 to 50 years versus 35% for women older than age 75 years (p <.001) (8). A large population-based series from British Columbia Cancer Agency, on the other hand, reported that 5-year breast-cancer specific survival was similar across age groups for stage III and IV breast cancer, but worse for older age groups for stages I and II: 5-year breast cancer-specific survival for stages I and II breast cancer were 94.8% and 82.5% for age 50 to 64 years, 95.1% and 80.8% for age 65 to 74 years, 93.6% and 79.1% for age 75 to 84 years, and 82.0% and 68.5% for age 85 years and older (p <.0001 and p = .0032) (9). Evidence from the Surveillance, Epidemiology, and End Results (SEER) program, between 1990 and 2003, suggests that risk of breast cancer mortality varies by age and estrogen receptor (ER) status (3); in women with ER-positive breast cancer, there was a decline in breast cancer mortality in younger and older women, but, in women with ER-negative breast cancer, decrease in mortality was seen among women younger than age 70 years, and not among women age 70 and older. Taken together, this evidence suggests that older women with more advanced disease or ER-negative disease are at risk for higher breast cancer-specific mortality, which leads to examination of treatment patterns.

In multiple reports, older age is a risk factor for *less than standard* management, even after controlling for factors such as comorbidity, cognitive status, social support, and functional status (5,10–16). Older women are less likely to undergo breast-conserving surgery, as compared with mastectomy, more likely not to have adjuvant radiation after breast-conserving surgery, and less likely to receive systemic therapy, particularly chemotherapy. These deviations from standard therapy are likely multifactorial (17,18). One explanation is that older women, in general, are perceived as having less aggressive breast cancers, which do not require as aggressive therapy. A second explanation is that it is difficult to weigh benefits and risks of therapy in older women who may have other illnesses or frailty. A third predicament is the lack of data from randomized clinical trials (19). Thus, high-level evidence to guide practice patterns for breast cancer is sparse for women older than age 70 years, leaving us unable to draw firm conclusions about treatment. In older women, therefore, treatment is sometimes tailored to what appears to be appropriate, but is actually inadequate. This is demonstrated by a study of 407 breast cancer patients age 80 and older in the Geneva Cancer Registry, in which undertreatment was directly proportional to disease-specific survival (11). In this study, 12% of women received no treatment for breast cancer, 32% received tamoxifen only, 7% had breast-conserving surgery alone, 33% had mastectomy, and 14% had breast-conserving surgery and adjuvant therapy; corresponding 5-year breast cancer-specific survival rates were 46%, 51%, 82%, and 90%, respectively. Hence, controversy exists about what constitutes appropriate care for breast cancer in older women, but data from prospective randomized trials are needed, because disease-specific outcome may be compromised by delivering less than what is standard care.

Tumor biology is important to choice of treatment and affects response to treatment. As a group, older women with breast cancer have tumors with less aggressive biologic characteristics. Indices of cell proliferation indicate slower growth: thymidine-^{3}H labeling indices are lower, and tumors are more frequently diploid and of lower histologic grade (5,20–22). Genetic alterations in tumor cells generally reflect less aggressive histology, including normal p53 expression and absence of expression of epidermal growth factor receptor-1 (EGF-1) and EGF-2 (HER-2, c-erb-b2, formerly HER-2/*neu*) (21). Breast cancers in postmenopausal women are more likely to express hormone receptors (21,22). Despite the apparent biologic pattern of a less aggressive phenotype, in a large report, spanning 60 years and including 2,136 elderly women treated with surgery and without adjuvant systemic therapy at the University of Chicago, the rate of distant metastases and the likelihood of

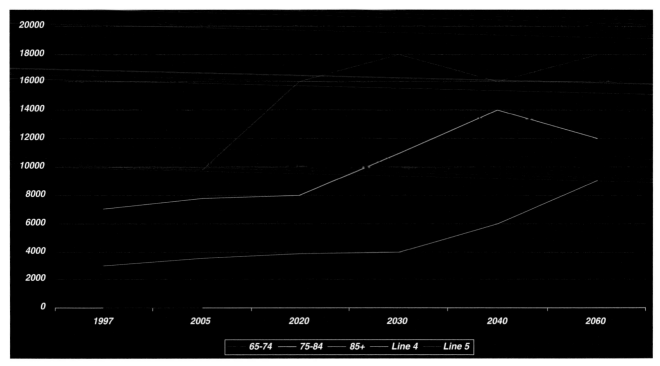

FIGURE 91.1. Population projections for women in the United States (in thousands). (Data from United States Bureau of the Census. *Statistical abstracts of the United States,* 117th ed. Washington, DC: U.S. Government Printing Office, 1997;and *The national data book.* Washington, DC: Hoover's Business Press, 1997.)

developing distant metastases were similar in women over age 70 years as compared with women age 40 to 70 years (23). One potential biologic explanation for this finding is proposed by Honma et al. (24), who reported that breast cancers in women older than 85 years are less frequently progesterone receptor-(PR) positive and are more frequently androgen receptor positive (24). The estrogen receptor-α (ER-α) and PR status of tumors in older women distinctly differed from those of premenopausal women. These authors postulated that this pattern of hormone receptor expression is related to the extremely low endogenous estrogen levels in very old women and that androgen and androgen receptor may play significant roles in the pathogenesis of breast carcinomas in this age group. This is an area of research that may eventually help us better explain the etiology and natural history of breast cancer in older women.

Infiltrating ductal cancer is the most common histologic type of breast cancer in older women. The more indolent histologic types, such as mucinous and papillary carcinomas, are also encountered more frequently (20,24). Mucinous carcinomas represent only 1% of breast cancers in premenopausal women, but 4% to 5 % in women aged 75 to 85 years and approximately 6% in women more than 85 years of age (20,25). Papillary cancers are very rare in all age groups: 0.3% of cancers in premenopausal women and less than 1% in older women (25).

Few data are available regarding preinvasive breast cancer in older women. Those available suggest that recurrence after diagnosis of ductal carcinoma *in situ* (DCIS) is less likely (26–29). In one study, local recurrence rates after excision of DCIS were lower, although pathologic features did not appear more indolent in older women (26). Some authors attributed the lower local recurrence rate to immunohistochemical and genetic differences; ERBB2 is less often overexpressed in DCIS in older patients, whereas ER, PR, *bcl*-2, cyclin D1, Ki-67, and p53 expression is similar (27).

Of note, although, in general, histologic characteristics and behavior of breast cancers in older women are more indolent, aggressive tumors do occur and require treatment. For instance, overexpression of ERBB2 in breast cancers is less common in older women; when it does occur, it portends higher recurrence risk and lower cancer-specific survival compared with tumors that are negative for ERBB2, just as in younger women (30).

 LIFE EXPECTANCY AND COMORBIDITY

In Western societies, average life expectancy is approximately 15.1 years at age 70 years and 9.1 years at age 80 years (31) (Table 91.1). Increasing age is generally considered a major determinant of health status on its own, although functional status, disability, and other existing illnesses are also important determinants of mortality. As age increases, there is a consistent decline in functional status, and disability rates increase (32,33). Poor functional status is a strong and significant indicator of an increased mortality rate (34–36). Pijls et al. (34) reported that self-rated health was an independent risk factor for cancer mortality and mortality from other causes. Compared with those rating themselves as "healthy," the relative risk of cancer-related mortality for patients rating themselves as "moderately healthy" or "not healthy" was 4.2 (95% confidence interval [CI], 1.9–9.4), and the relative risk of mortality from other causes was 3.0 (95% CI, 1.2–7.8), even after adjusting for the presence of major chronic diseases, age, medication use, smoking, alcohol consumption, physical activity, body mass index, systolic blood pressure, serum cholesterol concentration, education, marital status, and family history of chronic diseases. Life expectancy is also limited in women who have moderate and severe dementia and among women experiencing progressive functional decline (37–39). Functional status in older persons, therefore, constitutes an important indicator of the overall health condition and reflects the degree of a person's independence and his or her ability to use health care services.

Table 91.1	AVERAGE REMAINING LIFETIME AT VARIOUS AGES[a]	
Age (yr)	Life Expectancy, Men and Women (yr)	Life Expectancy, Women (yr)
60	22.5	24.0
65	18.7	20.0
70	15.7	16.2
75	11.9	12.8
80	9.1	9.8
85	6.8	7.2
90	5.0	5.2
95	3.6	3.7
100	2.6	2.6

[a]Table shows average number of years of life remaining at the beginning of the age interval. Modified from United States National Center for Health Statistics. *Vital Statistics of the United States.* Washington, DC: United States Census Bureau, 2004, with permission.

The number of coexisting illnesses (comorbidity) a patient may have increases with advancing age; the result is that deaths unrelated to breast cancer are more likely in patients older than 65 years than in those younger than 65 years (20% vs. 3%, p <.001) (40). Moreover, comorbid conditions that impose functional limitations and that may be expected to progress, such as diabetes with end-organ damage, steroid- or oxygen-dependent chronic obstructive pulmonary disease, or a known terminal illness, definitely limit survival (41). With age, heart and cerebrovascular diseases become increasingly important as causes of death (42) (Fig. 91.2).

In a series of studies, Satariano et al. (41,43,44) explored the association of comorbid illness and mortality in women with breast cancer. Two years after an assessment of comorbidity of 463 patients with breast cancer aged 55 to 84 years, women who died were more likely to have previously reported one or

more comorbid conditions than were survivors (62% vs. 38%) (43). The greater the number of comorbid conditions, the higher was the risk of death from all causes, including breast cancer, independent of age and breast cancer stage. Compared with women with no comorbid conditions, women reporting one comorbid condition were 2.5 times more likely to die, and those reporting two or more comorbid conditions were 3.4 times more likely to die. After 4 years of follow-up, women with two or more concurrent conditions were 2.2 times more likely to die of breast cancer (95% CI, 1.13–4.18) after adjustment for other factors. Heart disease was a major risk factor; women with symptomatic heart disease that limited daily activity were 2.4 times more likely to die of breast cancer (95% CI, 1.07–5.52). In addition, an interaction was found between comorbidity and stage of disease at diagnosis, such that the effect of comorbidity on survival varied depending on the stage of breast cancer at diagnosis (41). Among patients with three or more comorbid conditions, stage of disease had little additional effect on survival; an early breast cancer diagnosis in women with a high level of comorbidity conferred no survival disadvantage.

Increased prevalence of comorbidity and functional impairment in older cancer patients increases the risk of treatment-related complications and mortality (45,46). Poor social support, limited access to transportation, and impaired cognition are associated with delays in diagnosis and they increase the likelihood of inadequate treatment of cancer in patients aged 65 and older (47). Yet, with improvements in health care and current excellent life expectancies, more persons reach old age without measurable loss of functional capacity and free of severe medical conditions (48). Several instruments have been proposed to monitor comorbid conditions, but none has been widely accepted by the oncology community. The Italian Group for Geriatric Oncology evaluated the use of a Comprehensive Geriatric Assessment scale among elderly cancer patients (49). These investigators found a statistically significant association between comorbidity as measured by the modified Satariano index and functional status as measured by activities of daily living and instrumental activities of daily living. No association was found between performance

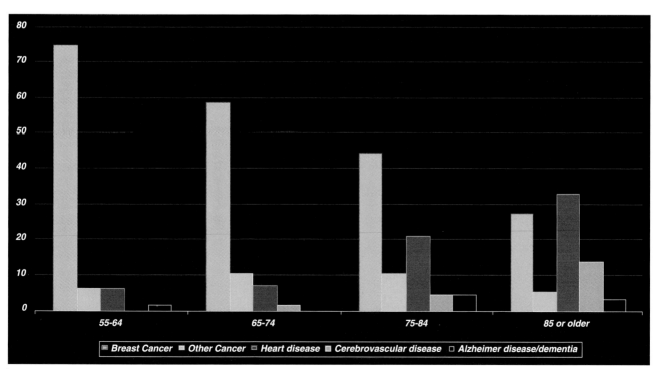

FIGURE 91.2. Cause of death within age-groups. (From Yancik R, Wesley MN, Ries LAG, et al. Effect of age and comorbidity in postmenopausal breast cancer patients aged 55 years and older. *JAMA* 2001;285:885–892, with permission.)

status and comorbidity, however. This finding is concerning because oncologists use performance status to estimate whether a patient is likely to tolerate treatment, such as chemotherapy. Several groups of experts, including the International Society of Geriatric Oncology (SIOG) and the National Comprehensive Cancer Network, recommend some form of comprehensive geriatric assessment be performed in older patients with cancer (50,51).

Recognizing the intertwining factors, including communication, that affect management of an older patient with breast cancer is extremely important. An essential component of the patient physician interaction mandates that the physician provides accurate, understandable information; such open interactions have been associated with many desirable outcomes of medical care, including reduced postoperative pain and hospital stays (52), improved functional status (53), and better quality of life (54). Reports have noted that older patients receive less interactive informational support from their physicians compared with younger patients (55). Future work should focus on methods of effective information exchange tailored to older patients.

 ## PREVENTION

Chemoprevention of breast cancer is reviewed in Chapter 22. The selective estrogen receptor modulators (SERM), tamoxifen and raloxifene, decrease the incidence of breast cancer, with differential benefit in decreasing hormone receptor-positive breast cancers and not hormone receptor-negative breast cancers, but the effect on mortality is probably small and has not yet been proved by any trial. Four breast cancer prevention trials have been reported, comparing tamoxifen and placebo (56–59). The largest of these trials, the National Surgical Adjuvant Breast and Bowel Project Prevention trial (NSABP P-1), showed dramatic reductions in the incidence of invasive and noninvasive breast cancer in women taking tamoxifen; at 7 years of follow-up, relative risks were 0.57 (95% CI, 0.46–0.70) and 0.63 (95% CI, 0.45–0.89), respectively (56). All women aged 60 years and older were eligible to participate, regardless of other risk factors, and the benefit was seen across age groups. Yet, only 30% of trial participants were older than 60 years, and only 6% were older than 70 years. Women who received tamoxifen also had a 32% reduction in risk of osteoporotic fractures, but a two times higher risk of pulmonary embolism and three times higher risk of endometrial cancer than women who received placebo. Similarly, at 96-month median follow-up, the International Breast Cancer Intervention Study (IBIS-I) showed a 28% reduction in the incidence of breast cancers for women taking tamoxifen (95% CI, 9%–42%), but noted a significant increase in deep-vein thrombosis and pulmonary embolism (relative risk [RR] 2.26, 95% CI, 1.36–3.87) (58). Interestingly, subgroup analysis by age 50 years or less and more than 50 years showed more benefit for the younger group than the older (RR 0.65, 95% CI, 0.45–0.94 vs. 0.79; 95% CI, 0.59–1.06). The Royal Marsden and Italian Trials also found some benefit of tamoxifen, although effects were noted only after extended follow-up (57,59). Only after follow-up of 20

years did the Royal Marsden prevention trial report positive results (HR = 0.77, 95% CI, 0.48–1.23, during the 8-year treatment period versus HR = 0.48, 95% CI, 0.29–0.79, in the post-treatment period, for ER-positive breast cancer), describing benefits that occurred predominantly during the post-treatment follow-up (59). The Italian Prevention Trial reported decreased risk of breast cancer only among women they defined as high risk for hormone receptor-positive breast cancer (RR 0.24, 95% CI, 0.10–0.59); these were women who were taller than 160 cm, had at least one intact ovary, were younger than age 14 years at menarche, and had no full-term pregnancy before age 24 years (57). Overall, the risk-to-benefit ratio for the use of preventive tamoxifen in older women is still unclear.

Another SERM, raloxifene, may have less of an estrogenic effect on the uterus and offer a more favorable risk-to-benefit ratio than tamoxifen in the preventive setting. The STAR (Study of Tamoxifen and Raloxifene) trial, compared 5 years of preventive treatment with tamoxifen or raloxifene in postmenopausal women. With a median follow-up of 3.9 years, the annual event rate was low and no significant difference was seen between the drugs with respect to benefits or risks (60). Raloxifene was more commonly associated with musculoskeletal complaints, dyspareunia, and weight gain. Women on tamoxifen claimed more gynecologic problems, vasomotor symptoms, leg cramps, and bladder control problems. In general, however, vasomotor symptoms and sexual complaints were less of an issue in women over age 60 years, compared with younger women.

A model developed by Gail et al. (61) can help the physician to estimate the risk of breast cancer and then determine if the benefits of tamoxifen outweigh the risks in women of different age-groups. Table 91.2 shows the minimal 5-year risk of invasive breast cancer for the benefit of preventive tamoxifen to exceed the risks in the general population. These risks were calculated for women with similar thromboembolic risk as in the NSABP P1 trial. For example, the Gail model 5-year risk of invasive breast cancer for a 72-year-old woman with an intact uterus must be 7% or more for the benefits of tamoxifen to outweigh its risks.

Current trials are exploring the use of aromatase inhibitors (AI) in breast cancer prevention, with careful attention to their effect on bone mass and osteoporosis risk (62).

SCREENING

Breast cancer screening, also discussed in Chapter 11, involves serial mammography, clinical breast examination, and breast self-examination. For older postmenopausal women, the higher probability of developing breast cancer, as compared with younger postmenopausal women, translates to a greater likelihood that a new lump is cancer and that an abnormal mammogram indicates the presence of cancer. Comparing mammographic results of women aged 50 to 64 years (n = 21,226) and of women aged of 65 years and older (n = 10,914), for instance, Faulk et al. (63) found that mammography had a higher positive predictive value, a higher yield of positive biopsies, and a greater cancer detection rate per 1,000 studies in older women. Finding

Table 91.2	MINIMAL 5-YEAR RISK OF INVASIVE BREAST CANCER FOR TAMOXIFEN'S BENEFIT TO EXCEED RISK IN THE GENERAL POPULATION, BY AGE				
Age (yr)	35–39	40–49	50–59	60–69	70–79
Uterus intact	1.5	1.5	4.0	>7.0	>7.0
No uterus	1.5	1.5	1.5	3.5	6.0

From Gail MH, Costantino JP, Bryant J, et al. Weighing the risks and benefits of tamoxifen treatment for preventing breast cancer. *J Natl Cancer Inst* 1999;91:1829–1846, with permission.

an early cancer in an older woman, however, may not lengthen or improve her life. The current questions about screening older women are as follows:

1. Do older women who are screened live longer than those who are not screened (because of finding cancers at a more curable stage)?
2. Do older women who are screened have a higher quality of life than women who are not screened (owing to finding cancers earlier when they require less aggressive treatment)?
3. Do older women require screening less frequently than yearly (because of slower growing cancers)?
4. Is there an age at which screening mammography should cease?

Large randomized trials show that routine annual or biannual mammography in women aged 50 to 75 years is associated with a reduction in breast cancer-related mortality of 25% to 30% within 5 to 6 years of initiation (64). Because only two of these trials included women older than 75 years, the optimal upper age limit for mammographic screening is still a matter of debate. Recommendations, therefore, are based on retrospective data and the results of small studies with surrogate end points. Several retrospective reviews suggest that, in older women, tumors detected by mammography are smaller and earlier in stage than tumors detected by other means (65–67). Wilson et al. (66), in a retrospective study of 62 women older than 75 years, for example, showed that mammographically detected breast cancers were of earlier stage. Because earlier stage cancers generally have a better prognosis and require less extensive local and systemic therapy, the use of screening mammography is supported in healthy older women.

The frequency of screening mammography in women older than age 75 is an area of debate. A retrospective study of Field et al. (68) supported the use of annual mammography in this age group; smaller, earlier-stage tumors were found by annual mammography than by biennial screening. Prospective data to support screening mammography in older women do not exist.

In 1991, Medicare made screening mammography every 2 years a covered benefit and, in 1999, annual screening was a covered benefit. During the first years of Medicare coverage, most older women were unaware that screening was a Medicare benefit (69), which led to the Health Care Financing Administration publicizing mammography coverage (70). Self-reported, 2-year mammography screening rates for women more than 65 years of age increased from 43% in 1990 to 64% in 1998 (71). Even with screening mammography as a covered benefit and after several national informational campaigns, 60% of a sample of 1,000 older female Medicare beneficiaries in Michigan between 1993 and 1997 either had not had a mammogram or had had only one (72). Although Medicare endorses screening mammography, screening rates are low.

Mammography rates decrease with increasing age, continuing to decline into the ninth decade of life (73,74). Rates as low as 26.7% in a 2-year period for women 75 and older have been reported (74). Poor level of function; limitations in activities of daily living; poor general health; a history of stroke, hip fracture, or dementia; older age; low income; low education level; underestimation of risk; fewer primary care visits; lack of a place to go for health care; and failure of physicians to recommend or discuss mammography are directly associated with lower screening rates (73–80). A history of hypertension, diabetes mellitus, or myocardial infarction was not associated with mammography use (74). Attention to factors associated with lower mammography use improves screening rates. The physician's recommendation, however, is probably the most important stimulus for obtaining screening mammography in older women. On-site mobile mammography and personalized mailings have also proved useful (81,82). Emphasizing the reassurance that mammography brings recipients may also be helpful in improving screening rates (83).

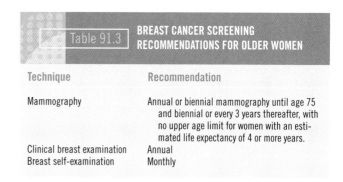

Table 91.3	BREAST CANCER SCREENING RECOMMENDATIONS FOR OLDER WOMEN
Technique	**Recommendation**
Mammography	Annual or biennial mammography until age 75 and biennial or every 3 years thereafter, with no upper age limit for women with an estimated life expectancy of 4 or more years.
Clinical breast examination	Annual
Breast self-examination	Monthly

Modified from American geriatrics society clinical practice committee. AGS position statement: breast cancer screening in older women. *J Am Geriatr Soc* 2000;48:842–844, with permission.

Low screening rates are probably related to physician and patient perception that the benefits of screening mammogram decrease with increasing age. Some experts recommend mammography for healthy women up to age 85 years, and not after that (84). Because the average 85-year-old woman in the United States is expected to live 9.2 more years and because survival benefits for mammographic screening are evident after 5 to 6 years of follow-up, an age cut-off based on life expectancy should be used (44). A decision analysis, constructed to compare the utility of breast cancer screening using mammography with that of physical breast examination in older women, also addressed this questions. The benefits of screening mammography outweighed the financial costs for older women, irrespective of age, but the magnitude of benefit decreased with increasing age and comorbidity (85).

Based on these reports, the American Geriatrics Society Clinical Practice Committee published guidelines for breast cancer screening in older women that are presented in Table 91.3 (87). The Committee recommended annual or biennial mammography until age 75 years and then biennially or every 3 years thereafter in women with a life expectancy of 4 or more years. Overall, whereas it is less clear that mammography saves lives in women over age 75, it definitely finds cancers at an earlier stage, thus allowing less aggressive treatment and perhaps a better quality of life. Longer intervals between mammograms are likely adequate. Mammography for women with a life expectancy of at least 5 years, intact mental function, and mobility makes good medical sense.

TREATMENT OF THE PRIMARY LESION IN THE OLDER PATIENT

After the publication of the NSABP Protocol B-06 in 1985 (87), it became accepted that women with invasive breast cancer should be offered the choice between modified radical mastectomy and breast conservation (lumpectomy, axillary sampling, and breast radiation). Since that time, breast conservation has become the more common surgical approach, and axillary dissection has been replaced by sentinel node biopsy (with delayed axillary dissection, if sentinel node is positive) (88). Women aged 70 and older are also more likely to choose breast conservation than mastectomy (89). Older women should be offered the option of breast preservation, because body image and the loss of a breast are important issues regardless of age. In addition, breast preservation is a much less morbid procedure, mostly done as an out-patient procedure, and is thus preferable in the older individual with comorbidities. Individualization of treatment is appropriate, and decisions should be made based on patient preference, overall health, tumor stage, and biology.

Today, most older patients can receive effective surgical treatment with minimal mortality risk and morbidity. Operative mortality rates for breast surgery are very low, at 1% to 2% (90,91). The main factor influencing surgical morbidity is not age but the presence of comorbidity (25,92) and frailty. There may be at least a short-term decrease in cognitive function after general anesthesia in elderly patients (93), and even a slight decrease in cognition in an older frail patient may mean the difference between independence and consignment to assisted or total care. Attention should be paid to functional status and comorbid illnesses in making decisions about surgical management.

MANAGEMENT OF THE AXILLA IN OLDER PATIENTS

In the management of invasive breast cancer in general, it is agreed that sentinel node biopsy is preferred in the patient with clinically node-negative disease, and that axillary dissection should be reserved for those with known positive axillary nodes (see Chapters 41 and 42). In the elderly, however, axillary evaluation may not always be necessary. The nuances of axillary management in the elderly will be discussed.

Axillary lymph node dissection may lead to arm morbidity and other complications, especially in the elderly. In a longitudinal cohort study of 571 patients with stage I and II breast carcinoma who were 67 years of age and older, for instance, the risk of arm dysfunction during the 2 years after initial treatment was more than four times higher (83% vs. 17%, $p = .0001$) for women who underwent axillary dissection compared with women without axillary dissection (94). In a study that randomized women age 60 and older to axillary clearance or not, however, after the first postoperative visit (at which point the physician and patient assessment of quality of life related to arm symptoms was worse for women who had the axillary dissection), disruptions in quality of life disappeared within 6 to 12 months and there was no long-term difference in arm movement or pain (95). Thus, despite the potential morbidity, for elderly women with clinically positive axillary lymph nodes who can tolerate surgery, axillary dissection represents the best treatment. Alternative treatments, such as radiation and tamoxifen (if the tumor is ER- or PR-positive) may play a role in controlling disease for a short time in patients too ill to have surgical treatment.

For older women with clinically negative nodes and a hormone receptor-positive tumor, in whom chemotherapy is unlikely to be used, axillary evaluation may be superfluous, and add morbidity without benefit. A retrospective study of patients treated with lumpectomy plus tamoxifen, but without radiation or axillary dissection, for instance, found low rates of recurrence in the ipsilateral axilla at 5 and 10 years; axillary relapse rates were 4.3% and 5.9%, respectively (96). Axillary recurrence was also low among older women who did not have axillary surgery in the Cancer and Leukemia Group B (CALGB 9343) trial (97). This trial included women age 70 and older with small (≤2 cm), clinically node-negative, ER-positive or PR-positive primary breast cancers treated by lumpectomy plus tamoxifen who were then randomized to receive breast radiation or not. Axillary surgery was not a requirement for study entry. In the radiation arm of the trial, 200 women did not undergo axillary dissection, and none had axillary recurrence, whereas 4 of 204 women who did not undergo axillary clearance and did not receive breast radiation had axillary recurrence. Finally, the International Breast Cancer Study Group (IBCSG) trial 10-93 actually randomized women age 60 and older with clinically node-negative, operable breast cancer, in whom adjuvant tamoxifen was indicated, to axillary clearance

or not (95). Of participants in this trial, 80% had hormone receptor-positive breast cancer. At a median follow-up of 6.6 years, axillary recurrence (~2% overall), disease-free (67% vs. 66%; HR 1.06, $p = .69$) survival, and overall (75% vs. 73%; HR 1.05, $p = .77$) survival were not significantly affected by axillary surgery. Even in the absence of axillary evaluation or treatment, therefore, axillary recurrence is rare in older women with small, ER-positive tumors treated with tamoxifen, radiation, or both.

In summary, for older women with ER-positive or PR-positive cancers that are 2 cm or less, for whom chemotherapy is unlikely regardless of node status (patients >75 chronologically, or physiologically impaired), axillary evaluation, even with sentinel node biopsy, has little utility. For tumors more than 2 cm, or ER-negative and PR-negative tumors, sentinel node biopsy has utility for determining who might benefit from adjuvant chemotherapy. For the node-positive patient, axillary dissection remains the standard for those who can tolerate the procedure.

BREAST RADIATION AFTER LUMPECTOMY

Older women tolerate breast irradiation as well as younger women (98,99), but consigning an older person to 4 to 6 weeks of radiation therapy may be exhausting and detrimentally affect her quality of life. The schedule and duration of adjuvant breast radiation may be obstacles for older patients. The question remains whether older women need radiation after breast preservation. Standard local treatment for breast cancer has similar disease-free and overall survival benefits in older and younger women, but older women have more deaths from illness other than breast cancer (11% vs. 2%; $p = .0006$) (100,101). Of note is the lower risk of ipsilateral in breast tumor recurrence (IBTR) in older women, with or without radiation. A regimen of breast-conserving surgery and breast irradiation was found to yield a 10-year rate of local treatment failure of 4% in older women compared with 13% in women younger than 65 years (100). Similar findings were seen in the Milan trial 3: In women treated with quadrantectomy without breast irradiation, those younger than 45 years had an IBTR rate of 17.5% versus 3.8% for women older than 55 years (102).

One approach to this problem has been the development of radiation therapy schedules that are more tolerable for older patients. Two retrospective analyses examined the use of once-weekly radiation schedules (103,104). Rostom et al. (104) reported the use of once-weekly irradiation for 84 older patients with breast cancer (stages I to IV) (104). Treatment was well tolerated. Reactive fibrosis, skin thickening, or both occurred in 25 patients; symptomatic pneumonitis was reported in 4 patients; and brachial plexopathy occurred in 1 patient. Among patients with stage I and II tumors, local tumor control and cosmetic results were encouraging. Maher et al. (103) evaluated a regimen that included once-weekly radiation therapy for a total of seven fractions and concurrent tamoxifen in a group of older women with a mean age of 81 years (range, 64 to 91 years). At a median follow-up of 36 months, the overall survival rate was 87%, the disease-specific survival rate was 88%, and the local recurrence rate was 14%. With the high dose per fraction, 39% of patients experienced moderate fibrosis at the primary site. No rib fractures, radiation pneumonitis, or brachial plexopathy were seen.

Another approach to decreasing the inconvenience and possibly the morbidity of radiation therapy is accelerated partial breast irradiation (PBI), which treats only the affected area of the breast and completes therapy in about 1 week (105). In the elderly, where local recurrence is less of an issue, this may be an ideal approach, if radiation is needed at all. Further studies are in progress to determine the efficacy and morbidity of this approach.

An alternative approach has been to use tamoxifen alone after lumpectomy as a means of obviating the need for radiation therapy in women with hormone receptor-positive tumors. A retrospective study of patients treated with lumpectomy plus tamoxifen, but without radiation, demonstrated ipsilateral breast cancer recurrence rates of 5.4% and 8.7%, and incidences of distant metastases of 6.2% and 13.4%, 5 and 10 years after initial surgery, respectively (96). In a controlled clinical trial comparing quadrantectomy versus quadrantectomy plus radiotherapy in postmenopausal women older than 55 years with breast cancers smaller than 2.5 cm, a low local relapse rate (3.8%) was found for patients who had quadrantectomy alone at a median follow-up of 39 months (102). Two other small studies addressing the same issue, however, showed higher locoregional recurrence rates (~10%) in women older than 70 years who were treated with local excision and tamoxifen alone, without adjuvant radiation (106,107).

This question has been more completely studied by CALGB 9343 (97), which randomly assigned 636 women 70 years of age or older with clinical stage I (T1N0M0), ER-positive breast carcinoma treated by lumpectomy plus tamoxifen and radiation (317 women) or tamoxifen alone (319 women). The only significant difference between the two groups was in the incidence of locoregional recurrence, 4 (1%) in the group randomized to tamoxifen plus radiation and 23 (7%) in the group randomized to tamoxifen alone, (p <.001). The difference in the incidence of mastectomy after local recurrence (4 [1%] vs. 9 [3%], p = .07) did not reach statistical significance. No significant differences were seen between the two groups with regard to distant metastases (9 [3%] vs. 11 [3%], p = .59), all-cause mortality (86 [27%] vs. 82 [26%], p = .84), or breast cancer-specific mortality (5 [2%] vs. 5 [2%], p = .92). Although decreasing IBTR by a little over 5% (p <.001), radiation did not have an impact on ultimate breast conservation, distant metastases, or death from other causes, and, of the 180 women who have died, 94% died of causes other than breast cancer. It should be noted that this trial accepted minimal margins (no ink on tumor) and that margins of 1 to 2 mm might yield even lower IBTR. Today, we would recommend wider margins (1 to 2 mm) and would use either tamoxifen or an AI. We would anticipate even less IBTR.

Wide excision of the primary tumor alone in older women has resulted in local control rates ranging from 71% to 97% (102,108–110). In general, these results are inferior to those of other treatments, such as lumpectomy and breast radiation or lumpectomy plus hormonal therapy, but wide excision alone may be considered for patients with progressive localized breast cancer that is ER- and PR-negative who have significant comorbidity, to minimize and potentially prevent complications of locally advanced breast cancer.

ENDOCRINE THERAPY ALONE AS PRIMARY TREATMENT

The use of tamoxifen alone as initial treatment for localized breast cancer was first studied in women who were not candidates for surgery or who refused surgical treatment and this approach is still appropriate in these settings today. In women with hormone receptor-positive breast cancer, response rates are high and responses are usually evident within a couple of months of starting therapy (111–116). Response is also a good indicator of survival; in one study, actuarial 5-year survival rate was 49.4% and was highest for those showing an initial complete response (92%) (117). Response duration of 10 to 50 months, however, is usually the limiting factor to this approach

in most patients (111,118,119), although regression can persist up to 5 years in one-third of patients (117). Because most patients develop progressive local disease necessitating salvage therapy with radiotherapy or surgery, removal of the primary tumor is preferable, if possible.

Better local control with surgery is also the conclusion of randomized trials comparing primary hormonal therapy with surgery. Two randomized trials from the European Organization for Research and Treatment of Cancer (EORTC) confirmed that surgery yields better local control than hormonal therapy, but no benefit with respect to survival. The first compared modified radical mastectomy with tamoxifen as sole initial therapy for operable breast cancer in women age 70 and older (114). At 10 years median follow-up, progression (29% vs. 68%, logrank p <.0001) and local progression (11% vs. 92%, logrank p <.0001) were more common with tamoxifen alone; overall survival was similar in the two groups (73% vs. 61%). The other was a randomized trial of standard surgery, defined as modified radical mastectomy (MRM) versus less extensive surgery, wide local excision (WLE) and tamoxifen (T) (115). At a median follow-up of approximately 10 years, there were significantly more locoregional relapses in the WLE-T group (16% vs. 26%), but more distant metastases in the MRM group (28% vs. 13%). Survival rates were similar (72% vs. 69%). The Italian Group for Research on Endocrine Therapy in the Elderly (GRETA) trial reported inferior results with tamoxifen alone, at median follow-up of 80 months, compared with adjuvant tamoxifen after surgery (112). Local progression was more common in the tamoxifen arm (11% vs. 45%). At a median follow-up of 12.7 years, the Cancer Research Campaign also reported more relapses (56.1% vs. 24.9%) and more deaths (30% vs. 19%) in women randomized to tamoxifen alone versus optimal surgery plus tamoxifen (120). A Cochrane meta-analysis on this topic, including seven eligible randomized trials comparing primary endocrine therapy with surgery, with or without adjuvant endocrine therapy, in women aged 70 years and older with early breast cancer who were fit for surgery, confirmed the superiority of surgery to tamoxifen with respect to local control, but not overall survival (121). The hazard ratios for overall survival did not reach statistical significance: HR for surgery alone versus primary endocrine therapy was 0.98 (95% CI, 0.74–1.30) and for surgery plus endocrine therapy versus primary endocrine therapy was 0.86 (95% CI, 0.73–1.00). The HR for progression-free survival showed the benefit of surgery over endocrine therapy alone: HR for surgery alone versus primary endocrine therapy was 0.55 (95% CI, 0.39–0.77) and for surgery plus endocrine therapy versus primary endocrine therapy was 0.65 (95% CI, 0.53–0.81). In summary, primary tamoxifen alone is inadequate treatment for patients able to tolerate surgery; both local control and survival are adversely affected when surgery is omitted from primary therapy. Primary use of hormonal agents is indicated only when life expectancy is severely limited.

Data suggest that aromatase inhibitors may be superior to tamoxifen in treating primary breast cancer. In a prospective, randomized trial of 327 postmenopausal women with ER- or PR-positive tumors reported by Eiermann et al (122), complete and partial responses assessed by breast examination were 55% with letrozole compared with 36% with tamoxifen. Aromatase inhibitors also appear to be superior to tamoxifen in postmenopausal patients with hormone receptor-positive metastatic breast cancer (123,124) and in the adjuvant setting (125). It is logical, therefore, to consider AI as an alternative to tamoxifen as preoperative or definitive therapy for older women with hormone receptor-positive lesions. Thus, the use of tamoxifen or an AI, instead of surgery, for older women with receptor-positive breast cancer may obviate the need for surgical intervention in women with severe comorbidities and limited life expectancies, especially frail patients.

The trials reported by Eiermann et al. (122) and Ellis et al. (126) support the use of preoperative endocrine therapy to improve a women's chance for breast conservation. In the study by Eiermann et al. (122), all patients were considered to have inoperable disease at the time of entry into the study, 45% had breast-conserving therapy after preoperative letrozole, compared with only 35% after preoperative tamoxifen. Ellis et al. (127) studied 250 postmenopausal women with hormone receptor-positive primary breast cancer who were ineligible for breast-conserving surgery and reported tumor regression in 60% and 41% and breast-conserving surgery in 48% and 36% of women randomized to letrozole or tamoxifen, respectively. Differences in response between letrozole and tamoxifen were most marked for tumors that were ErbB-1 and/or ErbB-2 positive and ER positive (88% vs. 21%, $p = .0004$).

In summary, primary hormonal therapy is not an ideal management approach for older women who are fit for surgery, but it offers the chance of disease control to women who have hormone receptor-positive breast cancer and are not able to undergo surgery.

ADJUVANT THERAPY

Recommendations for adjuvant therapy in women older than 70 years are outlined in Table 91.4 and are discussed below. The 2000 updated meta-analysis of adjuvant therapy trials by the Early Breast Cancer Trialists' Collaborative Group (EBCTCG), clearly shows the benefit of adjuvant tamoxifen therapy and adjuvant chemotherapy in improving relapse-free and overall survival in postmenopausal women with early-stage, hormone receptor-positive breast cancer (127). For older women with hormone receptor-positive breast cancer, endocrine therapy represents the major consideration for adjuvant treatment. Tamoxifen therapy significantly decreases both local and distant relapse and improves survival in women aged

70 years and older. The EBCTCG overview of randomized trials of tamoxifen reported that 5 years of adjuvant tamoxifen in women 70 years of age and older decreased the annual risk of recurrence by 54% (standard deviation [SD], 13) and the annual risk of death by 34% (SD, 13) (127). The proportional reductions in breast cancer relapse and mortality were similar for women with node-negative and node-positive tumors. Only patients with ER-positive tumors or ER-unknown status benefited from tamoxifen; women with tumors devoid of ER derived no benefit from tamoxifen therapy regardless of age.

The third-generation AIs (anastrozole, letrozole, and exemestane) have improved outcomes as adjuvant endocrine therapy for postmenopausal women. Several trials comparing AI with tamoxifen, as either initial adjuvant endocrine therapy or after 2 to 3 years of tamoxifen, have shown significant improvements in relapse-free survival averaging about 3% to 5% for AI therapy. As initial therapy, AIs have not been associated with improved overall survival (128), but one trial showed a survival improvement for patients changed to exemestane after 2 to 3 years of tamoxifen when compared with 5 years of tamoxifen alone (129). Another trial comparing letrozole with placebo in women who had completed 5 years of adjuvant tamoxifen therapy showed a significant improvement in relapse rate for letrozole for all patients and for overall survival in node-positive patients (130). Unlike tamoxifen, AIs are not associated with endometrial cancer or thromboembolism, but they do increase the risk of fracture. In one study, specifically looking at outcomes by age, women older than 70 years treated with letrozole did not have an increase in side effects when compared to placebo (131). The most common toxicity of AIs is arthralgia and myalgia, which can be severe in some patients but which are less common in elderly patients. The American Society of Clinical Oncology (ASCO) guidelines suggest that AI be used as adjuvant therapy in postmenopausal women, although no recommendations concerning the use of specific agents or schedules were made (132).

The excellent therapeutic index of endocrine therapy makes it a treatment consideration for most women with hormone receptor-positive breast cancer. Under-use of adjuvant endocrine therapy may put older patients with breast cancer at higher risk of disease recurrence and death (133). Older women with hormone-receptor positive breast cancer with estimated survivals of 5 years or less, who are frail, or who have well differentiated tumors 1 cm or smaller are unlikely to benefit, however. A careful discussion of the risks and benefits on endocrine therapy is mandatory; in one study women older than 80 years were half as likely as younger women to report a discussion about tamoxifen with their doctor (134). Compliance is also an issue in older patients. Of postmenopausal women, 15% discontinue tamoxifen; patients reporting side effects and those with poor physical function are more likely to discontinue treatment (135). In another study, approximately 20% of patients taking AI were not compliant (136). With the increasing longevity of the oldest old, adjuvant hormonal therapy should be discussed and offered to suitable candidates and compliance should be encouraged and monitored.

The decision to use adjuvant chemotherapy in older patients is more complicated because of the potential for increased toxicity with chemotherapy as compared with endocrine therapy. The latest EBCTCG meta-analysis of adjuvant therapy included only about 1,000 women age 70 years or older in trials comparing polychemotherapy with no chemotherapy (129). This sample size was insufficient to clearly define the benefits of chemotherapy in this age group. The proportional benefits of chemotherapy for patients aged 70 years and older are unlikely, however, to be different than those for postmenopausal women 50 to 69 years of age. For patients aged 50 to 69 years, the proportional risk reductions were 20% (SD, 3%) for recurrence and 11% (SD, 3%) for overall mortality. This mortality reduction

	RECOMMENDATIONS FOR ADJUVANT THERAPY IN WOMEN OLDER THAN 70 YEARS		
Table 91.4			

Risk Category	Definition	Treatment
Node negative and ERBB2 negative		
Minimal or low	<1 cm, ER or PR positive, grade I	No treatment or hormonal therapy
Moderate	>1 cm and <2 cm, ER or PR positive, grade I or II	Hormonal therapy ± chemotherapy Consider GEP, if ER or PR positive
High	>2 cm or grade II or III (any ER or PR)	Hormonal therapy ± chemotherapy if ER or PR positive; chemotherapy if ER or PR negative Consider GEP, if ER or PR positive
Node positive and ERBB2 negative		
ER positive	Any	Hormonal therapy ± chemotherapy
ER negative	Any	Chemotherapy
ERBB2 positive	≥1 cm, any ER or PR	Consider chemotherapy and trastuzumab Hormonal therapy, if ER or PR positive

ER, estrogen receptor; GEP, genetic expresión profiling; PR, progesterone receptor.

translates into a 2% and 3% net gain in 10-year survival for women with node-negative and node-positive breast cancer, respectively.

The overview analyses also clearly showed that in women with hormone receptor-positive tumors, the combination of tamoxifen and chemotherapy was significantly better than the use of either modality alone (127). The proportional reductions in recurrence and death were 22% (SD, 4%) versus 12% (SD, 4%) for chemotherapy versus no adjuvant chemotherapy; 19% (SD, 3%) versus 11% (SD, 4%) for chemotherapy and tamoxifen versus tamoxifen alone; and 52% versus 47% for chemotherapy and tamoxifen versus chemotherapy alone (127). Anthracycline-containing chemotherapy was associated with a small but significant further reduction in the risk of recurrence (12%; SD, 4%) and a marginal reduction in mortality (11%; SD, 5%; p = .02) compared with chemotherapy using cyclophosphamide, methotrexate, and 5-fluorouracil (CMF). Although these differences are significant, they are small; non–anthracycline-containing regimens may be preferable in many older patients, in whom the risk of anthracycline cardiac toxicity is higher than in younger patients (137). The CALGB analyzed data from four randomized trials of adjuvant chemotherapy in 6,489 patients with node-positive disease, including three trials that included anthracyclines. These four trials compared different doses, schedules, and chemotherapeutic agents; patients receiving more treatment (higher doses of therapy or anthracyclines in addition to CMF regimens, or taxanes in addition to doxorubicin and cyclophosphamide) had superior relapse-free and overall survival compared with patients receiving less treatment. Patients 65 years and older fared significantly better with more chemotherapy compared with less chemotherapy (31% risk reduction in relapse for those receiving more treatment; 95% CI for risk reduction, 9%–47%) as did those 51 to 64 years of age (14% reduction; 95% CI, 1%–25%) and those 50 years of age and younger (11% risk reduction; 95% CI, 0%–20%). However, about 1% of older patients died of treatment-related toxicities (138). A recent meta-analysis of the EBCTCG in women with ER-poor breast cancer showed a significant benefit for polychemotherapy in both women less than 50 years and those 50 to 69 years. The 10-year risks of recurrence and death from breast cancer for those treated with polychemotherapy versus no chemotherapy (about six cycles of CMF or cyclophosphamide, doxorubicin, plus fluorouracil [CAF]) were 33% vs. 45%, and 24% vs. 32% for those less than 50 years, and 42% vs. 52%, and 36% vs. 42% for those 50 to 69 years, respectively (140). Tamoxifen was of no benefit in these patients and there was no information on ERBB2 status.

SELECTING ADJUVANT CHEMOTHERAPY

As in younger women, adjuvant therapy decisions should be based on risk of recurrence, estimated survival, and the potential benefits and toxicities of treatment. For patients with hormone receptor-positive, HER-2-negative disease, the major consideration for adjuvant treatment is endocrine therapy. Few patients with node-negative, hormone receptor-positive disease will benefit from chemotherapy; however, older women with estimated survivals exceeding 10 years should be considered for a gene-based assay (Oncotype DX, Genomic Health) as some may have high 10-year risks of metastases and breast cancer death with endocrine therapy alone and may derive great benefit from chemotherapy (140,141). The decision is more difficult in patients with node-positive disease. Use of the web-based program adjuvantonline.com can be of great help in this decision, because life span based on age and comorbidity can be calculated and used to define more precisely the benefits of chemotherapy in these older, higher risk patients. For women with hormone receptor-negative breast cancer, chemotherapy is

of greater value and is likely to be of value both in node-positive and high-risk node-negative disease (139,142,143). Desch et al. (144) reported that the cost-to-benefit ratio of adjuvant chemotherapy in women with ER-negative, node-negative breast cancer who were between 60 and 80 years of age was high, but within the range of other commonly reimbursed procedures (144). For ERBB2-positive disease, the major consideration for therapy, in addition to endocrine therapy, is the use of chemotherapy and trastuzumab. Older patients with ERBB2-positive tumors are more likely to derive benefits from chemotherapy and trastuzumab because such tumors are generally less responsive to endocrine therapy. Older patients have greater risk of cardiac toxicity with trastuzumab and require careful monitoring (145). Older patients with small ERBB2-positive, node-negative, hormone receptor-positive tumors (T1a and T1b) are not likely to derive major benefit from trastuzumab. Older women with hormone receptor-negative, ERBB2-positive tumors are likely to derive the greatest benefit from chemotherapy and trastuzumab. The use of trastuzumab alone in lower risk, ERBB2-positive older patients has not been studied and trials are underway exploring the role of trastuzumab alone in this setting.

Other estimates of the value of adjuvant chemotherapy may be helpful. Using a Markov model, Extermann et al. (146) studied the threshold risk of relapse at which adjuvant tamoxifen and chemotherapy offered benefit to women up to age 85 years, including those with and without comorbidity (Fig. 91.3). Using data from the 1992 overview analysis (147), these investigators examined the threshold risk for a 1% benefit in 5-year or 10-year relapse-free survival; the model assumed was that the tumor was ER positive and that 5 years of tamoxifen therapy, standard chemotherapy, or both were used. For tamoxifen, the threshold risks of relapse were 11% and 20% for a 1% benefit in 10-year survival for healthy and sick women at age 65 years, respectively. At age 85 years, the threshold risks of relapse were 28% and 35% for a 1% benefit in 5-year survival for healthy and sick women, respectively (no 10-year survival benefit was seen in this age group). For chemotherapy, the threshold risk of relapse was 19% for a healthy 65-year-old patient and 62% for a sick 85-year-old patient. Overall, comorbidity increased the threshold risk of relapse by approximately 10% for tamoxifen therapy and by 20% for chemotherapy. This analysis supports the view that chemotherapy benefits are likely to be very small in patients 75 years and older whose tumors are ER- or PR-positive.

Newer trials of adjuvant therapy focused on older patients are needed. The French Adjuvant Study Group compared tamoxifen alone with tamoxifen and a low-dose weekly epirubicin regimen in women older than 65 years with operable breast cancer (148). Toxicity was minimal with the epirubicin regimen, and, at a median follow-up of 64 months, disease-free (26.5% vs. 22.1%, p = .02), but not overall survival (80.9% and 82.8%, p = .67), was significantly improved. This trial was underpowered to detect

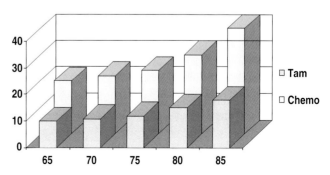

Extermann et al, JCO 2000 12:1709

FIGURE 91.3. Ten-year risk of breast cancer relapse needed to improve mortality by 1% in patients with estrogen receptor–positive tumors.

Table 91.5	TRIALS OF ADJUVANT CHEMOTHERAPY FOR BREAST CANCER IN OLDER WOMEN		
Trial	**Treatment**	**Target accrual**	**Status**
CALGB 49907	AC or CMF vs. capecitabine	600	Closed
ICE (BIG)	Ibandronate ± capecitabine	1,400	Any node status
			Any ER status
ELDA (NCI-Naples)	Docetaxel vs. CMF	300	Moderate to high-risk patients
ACTION (UK)	AC or EC vs. none	1,000	ER negative

ACTION, Adjuvant Cytotoxic Chemotherapy in Older Women; ELDA, Elderly Breast Cancer-Docetaxel in Adjuvant Treatment; ICE, Study in Elderly Patients with Early Breast Cancer; NCI, National Cancer Institute.

small but meaningful differences in overall survival, but it is important in suggesting that a low-dose, weekly, minimally toxic anthracycline schedule was associated with a significant decrease in relapse. A randomized trial (Clinical Trials Support Unit/CALGB 49907) comparing standard chemotherapy with the oral fluoropyrimidine, capecitabine, has completed accrual. Patients randomized to standard therapy were treated with a standard CMF regimen (using oral cyclophosphamide) or with doxorubicin and cyclophosphamide, according to patient and physician preference CALGB 49907 results are available and were added to the first paragraph in the left-hand column of page 1068: Initial results showed that standard chemotherapy resulted in significantly superior relapse free and overall survival. The three year absolute differences in relapse free survival was 85% vs. 68% and overall survival was 91% vs. 86%, favoring standard chemotherapy (148a). As part of this trial, quality of life, comorbidity, and compliance with oral chemotherapy (cyclophosphamide and capecitabine) are also being measured. Other trials of chemotherapy are underway in Europe in the elderly population and will add to our knowledge in this area (Table 91.5). Consensus recommendations for adjuvant therapy in elderly patients have recently been published (149) and the topic recently reviewed (150).

TREATMENT OF METASTATIC DISEASE

Metastatic breast cancer is incurable. All women, regardless of age, should be managed using the principles outlined in Chapter 77. Treatment should focus on maintaining the highest quality of life while controlling symptoms. Endocrine therapy is the mainstay of treatment for hormone receptor-positive metastatic breast cancer in older women, but older patients should be offered chemotherapy when metastases become refractory to endocrine treatment. The response rates and toxicity profiles of the standard chemotherapy regimens for metastatic breast cancer are similar in younger and older women who are in reasonably good health (151–153). A detailed review of the pharmacology of chemotherapeutic agents in older patients has been published (154). Most cytotoxic agents are metabolized in the liver. Caution should be exercised and dose modification considered for patients with liver dysfunction (as evidenced by bilirubin or transaminases greater than twice the upper limits of normal) who are treated with anthracyclines or taxanes. Methotrexate excretion is dependent on renal function; before methotrexate is administered to older women, creatinine clearance should be measured. Gelman and Taylor (155) modified methotrexate dosage on the basis of renal function in older women with advanced breast cancer without compromise of its therapeutic effect. In the metastatic setting, the risk of anthracycline-related cardiotoxicity is not convincingly higher in otherwise healthy older women than in younger women. However, weekly anthracycline regimens or liposomal preparations are safer than higher dose every-3-week regimens and are worthy of consideration. Older women with ERBB2-positive metastatic breast cancer should be considered for trastuzumab in addition to chemotherapy with a taxanes or vinorelbine, or as a single agent; patients with disease progression on such treatment should be considered for chemotherapy plus lapatinib.

The severity and duration of myelosuppression are increased in older patients treated with chemotherapy, but these effects have not resulted in major differences in mortality related to neutropenia, sepsis, or bleeding (151,152). Nausea and vomiting may be less frequent in older patients (156), and psychosocial adjustment to chemotherapy appears better for older than for younger women (157).

After the first chemotherapy regimen for metastases, response rates to subsequent *salvage* chemotherapy regimens are generally poor. Taxanes have shown substantial activity, however, even in heavily pretreated patients and weekly schedules are more effective and better tolerated (158,159). In women older than 65 years, vinorelbine had similar pharmacokinetics and a favorable toxicity profile in older women when compared with younger women (160). Liposome-encapsulated doxorubicin is being tested in older patients because it is less cardiotoxic than other anthracyclines and easy to administer (161). Capecitabine, an oral fluorouracil prodrug, also represents an excellent treatment choice for older patients; it is well tolerated, although hand-foot syndrome and diarrhea occur frequently and can be dose limiting (162).

MANAGEMENT SUMMARY

Screening

- Yearly clinical breast examination and monthly breast self-examination are recommended for all women.
- Yearly mammography is recommended up to age 75 years.
- Mammography every 2 or 3 years is recommended for women over age 75 years who have minimal limiting comorbid conditions.
- Compliance with mammography is best if it is recommended by the primary physician.
- In women with multiple comorbidities, the benefit of screening mammography should be weighed against estimated life expectancy.

Local Definitive Therapy

- No single approach for managing the primary lesion fits all older women with breast cancer. Recommendations to help define treatment options for some of the more common subgroups of older patients are presented in Table 91.6.

Table 91.6	TREATMENT RECOMMENDATIONS FOR MANAGEMENT OF THE PRIMARY LESION

Breast Conservation Possible	ER/PR	Clinical Node Status	Health Status[a]	Suggested Treatment
No	Positive	Any	Poor	Hormonal therapy[b]
No	Positive	Likely negative	Good	Simple mastectomy with sentinel node biopsy or Preoperative hormonal therapy to try to convert to BCS[c] or Preoperative chemotherapy to try to convert to BCS, if tumor characteristics would otherwise warrant chemotherapy be given[c]
No	Negative	Likely negative	Good	Simple mastectomy with sentinel node biopsy or Preoperative chemotherapy to try to convert to BCS, if tumor characteristics would otherwise warrant chemotherapy be given[c]
No	Positive	Positive or likely positive[d]	Good	Mastectomy and axillary dissection or Preoperative hormonal therapy if ER/PR positive, or chemotherapy to try to convert to BCS[c]
Yes	Positive	Any	Poor	Hormonal therapy[b]
Yes	Any	Likely negative	Good	Lumpectomy with or without sentinel node biopsy
Yes	Any	Positive or likely positive[d]	Good	Lumpectomy and axillary dissection

BCS, breast-conserving surgery; ER/PR, estrogen receptor or progesterone receptor.
[a]Poor health means limited life expectancy.
[b]Hormonal therapy usually consisting of an aromatase inhibitor or tamoxifen.
[c]In cases where preoperative systemic therapy is delivered, node assessment with direct biopsy, image-guided biopsy, or sentinel lymph node (SLN) mapping and sampling should be considered up front, to guide need for axillary dissection at the time of definitive surgery.
[d]Positive confirmed by biopsy.

- Patients with large tumors that cannot be treated with breast conservation, who have positive lymph nodes clinically, or who are likely to have positive nodes, are best treated by modified radical mastectomy if they are sufficiently healthy to undergo surgery or with hormonal agents (tamoxifen or aromatase inhibitors) if they are too sick to have surgery or if their life expectancy is short. Preoperative tamoxifen or aromatase inhibitors may be tried in an effort to make breast-conserving therapy possible.
- Patients with large tumors that cannot be treated with breast conservation, who have clinically negative lymph nodes, and who are likely to have pathologically negative nodes and whose tumors are ER positive are best treated by simple mastectomy, with sentinel node biopsy, if they are sufficiently healthy to undergo surgery or with hormonal agents (tamoxifen or aromatase inhibitors) if they are too sick to have surgery or if their life expectancy is short. Preoperative tamoxifen or aromatase inhibitors may be tried in an effort to make breast-conserving therapy possible.
- Candidates for breast conservation include most patients with smaller tumors. Those who have clinically positive lymph nodes should have a node biopsy to confirm

involvement, and then are best treated by lumpectomy and axillary node dissection (if patients are sufficiently healthy to undergo surgery), followed by breast radiation.
- For ER-negative and PR-negative cancers, clinically N0 cancers, lumpectomy and sentinel node biopsy (axillary dissection if node positive) followed by breast irradiation is recommended.
- For the patient with a T1, clinically node-negative, ER-positive or PR-positive cancers, we recommend lumpectomy and sentinel node biopsy (axillary dissection if node positive), if the patient is a candidate for chemotherapy. The use of hormonal therapy, or radiation (full course or abbreviated) is likely equivalent, and should be discussed with the patient. The use of both hormonal therapy and radiation is likely more than is needed.
- For the patient with a T1, clinically node-negative, ER-positive or PR-positive cancer where chemotherapy is not being seriously considered, lumpectomy is adequate surgical therapy, and sentinel node biopsy should be avoided. The use of hormonal therapy, or radiation (full course or abbreviated) is likely equivalent, and should be discussed with the patient. The use of both hormonal therapy and radiation is likely more than is needed.

- Primary hormonal therapy (tamoxifen or an aromatase inhibitor) may be offered to patients with hormone receptor-positive tumors who are too frail to have surgery or who have a limited life expectancy. Some patients are too frail for surgery when they present for treatment, and their tumors are ER negative. Individualized treatment and frank discussions with the patient and family are essential.

Systemic Adjuvant Therapy

- Adjuvant hormonal therapy should be considered in all older women with hormone receptor-positive tumors. Only older women with a very low risk of distant metastases (<10%) or severe comorbid illness should not be offered tamoxifen or an aromatase inhibitor.
- Adjuvant chemotherapy should be considered for older women whose risk of systemic breast cancer recurrence is sufficiently high and who are in good general health (estimated survival of at least 5 years). Chemotherapy is most beneficial in older women who have ER- or PR-negative tumors. For older women with hormone receptor-positive tumors, however, only a small added value to chemotherapy is seen, even in patients with positive lymph nodes; the added value of chemotherapy in these patients should be estimated from available models (i.e., www.adjuvantonline.com).
- Trastuzumab and chemotherapy should be considered for older women with ERBB2 positive tumors.

Treatment of Metastatic Disease

- Endocrine therapy is the standard front-line treatment for almost all women with hormone receptor-positive metastatic breast cancer.
  - Patients with hormone receptor-negative metastatic breast cancer whose metastases are not rapidly progressive or life-threatening should also be considered for at least one trial of endocrine therapy, because no survival disadvantage to this approach exists and false–negative ER and PR assays still occur.
  - The sequence of endocrine therapy should be an aromatase inhibitor → tamoxifen or fulvestrant → megestrol acetate → estrogens or corticosteroids (in selected patients).
  - Patients who have responded to endocrine therapy can be rechallenged with the same agent or a similar agent (i.e., a steroidal aromatase inhibitor in a patient whose disease has progressed during treatment with a nonsteroidal inhibitor).
- Systemic chemotherapy for metastatic breast cancer should be reserved for women with symptomatic disease who have progression of metastases during endocrine therapy.
  - The sequential use of single agents is the preferred strategy for these patients.
- Adjunct therapies for metastatic breast cancer involving bone include bisphosphonates, strontium chloride-89, and radiation therapy.

References

1. Jemal A, Siegel R, Ward E, et al. Cancer statistics, 2007. *CA Cancer J Clin* 2007;57(1):43–66.
2. Ferlay J, Autier P, Boniol M, et al. Estimates of the cancer incidence and mortality in Europe in 2006. *Ann Oncol* 2007;18(3):581–592.
3. Jatoi I, Chen BE, Anderson WF, et al. Breast cancer mortality trends in the United States according to estrogen receptor status and age at diagnosis. *J Clin Oncol* 2007;25(13):1683–1690.
4. Freyer G, Braud AC, Chaibi P, et al. Dealing with metastatic breast cancer in elderly women: results from a French study on a large cohort carried out by the 'Observatory on Elderly Patients'. *Ann Oncol* 2006;17(2):211–216.
5. Gennari R, Curigliano G, Rotmensz N, et al. Breast carcinoma in elderly women. Features of disease presentation, choice of local and systemic treatments compared with younger postmenopausal patients. *Cancer* 2004;101(6):1302.
6. Herbsman H, Feldman J, Seldera J, et al. Survival following breast cancer surgery in the elderly. *Cancer* 1981;47:2358.
7. Masetti R, Antinori A, Terribile D, et al. Breast cancer in women 70 years of age or older. *J Clin Oncol* 1996;13:2722.
8. Holli K, Isola J. Effect of age on the survival of breast cancer patients. *Eur J Cancer* 1997;33(3):425.
9. Bernstein V, Truong P, Speers C, et al., BC Cancer Agency V, BC, Canada. Breast cancer biology, treatment, and survival in elderly women [Abstract 985]. *Proceeding American Society of Clinical Oncology* 2001;20.
10. Giordano SH, Hortobagyi GN, Kau SW, et al. Breast cancer treatment guidelines in older women. *J Clin Oncol* 2005;23(4):783–791.
11. Bouchardy C, Rapiti E, Fioretta G, et al. Undertreatment strongly decreases prognosis of breast cancer in elderly women. *J Clin Oncol* 2003;21(19):3580.
12. Mandelblatt JS, Hadley J, Kerner JF, et al. Patterns of breast carcinoma treatment in older women. *Cancer* 2000;89(3):561.
13. Du XL, Key CR, Osborne C, et al. Discrepancy between consensus recommendations and actual community use of adjuvant chemotherapy in women with breast cancer. *Ann Intern Med* 2003;138(2):90–97.
14. Enger SM, Thwin SS, Buist DS, et al. Breast cancer treatment of older women in integrated health care settings. *J Clin Oncol* 2006;24(27):4377–4383.
15. Wyld L, Garg DK, Kumar ID, et al. Stage and treatment variation with age in postmenopausal women with breast cancer: compliance with guidelines. *Br J Cancer* 2004;90(8):1486–1491.
16. Lavelle K, Todd C, Moran A, et al. Non-standard management of breast cancer increases with age in the UK: a population based cohort of women > or =65 years. *Br J Cancer* 2007;96(8):1197–1203.
17. Bickell NA, McEvoy MD. Physicians' reasons for failing to deliver effective breast cancer care. A framework for underuse. *Med Care* 2003;41:442.
18. Velanovich V, Gabel M, Walker EM, et al. Causes for the undertreatment of elderly breast cancer patients: tailoring treatments to individual patients. *J Am Coll Surg* 2002;194(1):8.
19. Kimmick G, Kornblith A, Mandelblatt J, et al. A randomized controlled trial of an educational program to improve accrual of older persons to cancer treatment protocols: CALGB 360001. *J Clin Oncol* 2004;22(14):739S.
20. Diab SG, Elledge RM, Clark GM. Tumor characteristics and clinical outcome of elderly women with breast cancer. *J Natl Cancer Inst* 2000;92(7):550.
21. Lyman GH, Lyman S, Balducci L, et al. Age and the risk of breast cancer recurrence. *Cancer Control* 1996;3(5):421.
22. Pierga JY, Girre V, Laurence V, et al. Characteristics and outcome of 1755 operable breast cancers in women over 70 years of age. *Breast* 2004;13(5):369–375.
23. Singh R, Hellman S, Heimann R. The natural history of breast carcinoma in the elderly—implications for screening and treatment. *Cancer* 2004;100(9):1807.
24. Honma N, Sakamoto G, Akiyama F, et al. Breast carcinoma in women over the age of 85: distinct histological pattern and androgen, oestrogen, and progesterone receptor status. *Histopathology* 2003;42:120.
25. Yancik R, Ries LG, Yates JW. Breast cancer in aging women. A population-based study of contrasts in stage, surgery, and survival. *Cancer* 1989;63:976.
26. Vicini FA, Recht A. Age at diagnosis and outcome for women with ductal carcinoma-in-situ: a critical review of the literature. *J Clin Oncol* 2002;20:2736.
27. Rodrigues NA, Dillon D, Carter D, et al. Differences in the pathologic and molecular features of intraductal breast carcinoma between younger and older women. *Cancer* 2003;97:1393.
28. Solin LJ, Fourquet A, Vicini FA, et al. Mammographically detected ductal carcinoma in situ of the breast treated with breast-conserving surgery and definitive breast irradiation: long-term outcome and prognostic significance of patient age and margin status. *Int J Radiat Oncol Biol Phys* 2001;50(4):991–1002.
29. Smith BD, Gross CP, Smith GL, et al. Effectiveness of radiation therapy for older women with early breast cancer. *J Natl Cancer Inst* 2006;98(10):681–690.
30. Poltinnikov IM, Rudoler SB, Tymofyeyev Y, et al. Impact of Her-2 Neu overexpression on outcome of elderly women treated with wide local excision and breast irradiation for early stage breast cancer: an exploratory analysis. *Am J Clin Oncol* 2006;29(1):71–79.
31. Arias E. *United States Life Tables, 2004.* Hyattsville, MD: National Center for Health Statistics, 2007.
32. Bild DE, Fitzpatrick A, Fried LP, et al. Age-related trends in cardiovascular morbidity and physical functioning in the elderly—the Cardiovascular Health Study. *J Am Geriatr Soc* 1993;41(10):1047.
33. Strawbridge WJ, Kaplan GA, Camacho T, et al. The dynamics of disability and functional change in an elderly cohort—results from the Alameda County Study. *J Am Geriatr Soc* 1992;40(8):799.
34. Pijls LTJ, Feskens EJM, Kromhout D. Self-rated health, mortality, and chronic diseases in elderly men—the Zutphen Study, 1985–1990. *Am J Epidemiol* 1993;138(10):840.
35. Reuben DB, Rubenstein LV, Hirsch SH, et al. Value of functional status as a predictor of mortality—results of a prospective study. *Am J Med* 1992;93(6):663.
36. Inouye SK, Peduzzi PN, Robison JT, et al. Importance of functional measures in predicting mortality among older hospitalized patients. *JAMA* 1998;279(15):1187.
37. Ferrucci L, Guralnik JM, Cecchi F, et al. Constant hierarchic patterns of physical functioning across seven populations in five countries. *Gerontologist* 1998;38(3):286.
38. Bernard SL, Kincade JE, Konrad TR, et al. Predicting mortality from community surveys of older adults: the importance of self-rated functional ability. *J Gerontol B Psychol Sci Soc Sci* 1997;52(3):S155.
39. Dunlop DD, Hughes SL, Mannheim LM. Disability patterns in activities of daily living: patterns of change and a hierarchy of disability. *Am J Public Health* 1997;87:378.
40. Fish EB, Chapman JA, Link MA. Competing causes of death for primary breast cancer. *Ann Surg Oncol* 1998;5(4):368.
41. Satariano WA, Ragland DR. The effect of comorbidity on 3-year survival of women with primary breast cancer. *Ann Intern Med* 1994;120:104.
42. Yancik R, Wesley MN, Ries LAG, et al. Effect of age and comorbidity in postmenopausal breast cancer patients aged 55 years and older. *JAMA* 2001;285(7):885.
43. Satariano WA, Ragheb NE, Dupuis MA, et al. Comorbidity in older women with breast cancer: an epidemiologic approach. In: Yancik R, Yates JW (eds.) *Cancer in the elderly: approaches to early detection and treatment.* New York: Springer, 1989:71.

44. Satariano WA. Aging, comorbidity, and breast cancer survival: an epidemiologic view. *Adv Exp Med Biol* 1993;330:1.
45. Bergman L, Dekker G, van Leeuwen FE, et al. The effect of age on treatment choice and survival in elderly breast cancer patients. *Cancer* 1991;67:2227.
46. Guralnik JM. Assessing the impact of comorbidity in the older population. *Ann Epidemiol* 1996;6(5):376.
47. Goodwin JS, Hunt WC, Samet JM. Determinants of cancer therapy in elderly patients. *Cancer* 1993;72:594.
48. Yancik R, Ganz PA, Varicchio CG, et al. Perspectives on comorbidity and cancer in older patients: Approaches to expand the knowledge base. *J Clin Oncol* 2001;19(4):1147.
49. Repetto L, Fratino L, Audisio RA, et al. Comprehensive geriatric assessment adds information to Eastern Cooperative Oncology Group performance status in elderly cancer patients: An Italian group for geriatric oncology study. *J Clin Oncol* 2002;20(2):494.
50. Extermann M, Aapro M, Bernabei R, et al. Use of comprehensive geriatric assessment in older cancer patients: recommendations from the task force on CGA of the International Society of Geriatric Oncology (SIOG). *Crit Rev Oncol Hematol* 2005; 55(3):241–252.
51. Carreca I, Balducci L, Extermann M. Cancer in the older person. *Cancer Treat Rev* 2005;31(5):380–402.
52. Egbert LD, Battit GE, Welch CE, et al. Reducation of postoperative pain by encouragement and instrucion of patients. *N Engl J Med* 1964;270:825.
53. Greenfield S, Kaplan S, Ware JE. Expanding patient involvement in care—effects on patient outcomes. *Ann Intern Med* 1985;102(4):520.
54. Kerr J, Engel J, Schlesinger-Raab A, et al. Communication, quality of life and age: results of a 5-year prospective study in breast cancer pateints. *Ann Oncol* 2003;14:421.
55. Maly RC, Leake B, Silliman RA. Health care disparities in older patients with breast carcinoma - Informational support from physicians. *Cancer* 2003;97(6):1517.
56. Fisher B, Costantino JP, Wickerham DL, et al. Tamoxifen for the prevention of breast cancer: current status of the National Surgical Adjuvant Breast and Bowel Project P-1 study. *J Natl Cancer Inst* 2005;97(22):1652–1662.
57. Veronesi U, Maisonneuve P, Rotmensz N, et al. Tamoxifen for the prevention of breast cancer: late results of the Italian Randomized Tamoxifen Prevention Trial among women with hysterectomy. *J Natl Cancer Inst* 2007;99(9):727–737.
58. Cuzick J, Forbes JF, Sestak I, et al. Long-term results of tamoxifen prophylaxis for breast cancer—96-month follow up of the randomized IBIS-I trial. *J Natl Cancer Inst* 2007;99(4):272–282.
59. Powles TJ, Ashley S, Tidy A, et al. Twenty-year follow-up of the Royal Marsden randomized, double-blinded tamoxifen breast cancer prevention trial. *J Natl Cancer Inst* 2007;99(4):283–290.
60. Vogel VG, Costantino JP, Wickerham DL, et al. Effects of tamoxifen vs. raloxifene on the risk of developing invasive breast cancer and other disease outcomes: the NSABP Study of Tamoxifen and Raloxifene (STAR) P-2 trial. *JAMA* 2006;295(23): 2727–2741.
61. Gail MH, Costantino JP, Bryant J, et al. Weighing the risks and benefits of tamoxifen treatment for preventing breast cancer. *J Natl Cancer Inst* 1999;91(21):1829.
62. Cuzick J. Aromatase inhibitors for breast cancer prevention. *J Clin Oncol* 2005; 23(8):1636–1643.
63. Faulk RM, Sickles EA, Sollitto RA, et al. Clinical efficacy of mammographic screening in the elderly. *Radiology* 1995;194:193.
64. Kerlikowske K, Grady D, Rubin SM, et al. Efficacy of screening mammography. A meta-analysis. *JAMA* 1995;273:149.
65. Hwang ES, Cody HS, 3rd. Does the proven benefit of mammography extend to breast cancer patients over age 70? *South Med J* 1998;91(6):522.
66. Wilson TE, Helvie MA, August DA. Breast cancer in the elderly patient: early detection with mammography. *Radiology* 1994;190(1):203.
67. Peer PG, Holland R, Hendriks JH, et al. Age-specific effectiveness of the Nijmegen population-based breast cancer-screening program: assessment of early indicators of screening effectiveness. *J Natl Cancer Inst* 1994;86:436.
68. Field LR, Wilson TE, Strawderman M, et al. Mammographic screening in women more than 64 years old: a comparison of 1- and 2-year intervals. *AJR Am J Roentgenol* 1998;4:961.
69. American Association of Retired P. *Older women and Medicare mammography benefit: 1992 awareness and usage levels.* Washington, DC: American Association of Retired Persons, 1993.
70. Trontell AE, Franey EW. Use of mammography services by women aged greater-than-or-equal-to-65 years enrolled in Medicare—United States, 1991–1993 (Reprinted from *MMWR* 1995;44:777–781). *JAMA* 1995;274(18):1420.
71. National Center for Health S. *Health, United States, 2000 with adolescent health chartbook.* Hyattsville, MD: National Center for Health Statistics, 2000.
72. Van Harrison R, Janz NK, Wolfe RA, et al. 5-year mammography rates and associated factors for older women. *Cancer* 2003;97(5):1147.
73. Burns RB, McCarthy EP, Freund KM, et al. Variability in mammography use among older women. *J Am Geriatr Soc* 1996;44:922.
74. Blustein J, Weiss LJ. The use of mammography by women aged 75 and older: factors related to health, functioning, and age. *J Am Geriatr Soc* 1998;46:941.
75. Burg MA, Lane DS, Polednak AP. Age group differences in the use of breast cancer screening tests. *J Aging Health* 1990;2(4):514.
76. Mor V, Pacala JT, Rakowski W. Mammography for older women: who uses, who benefits? *J Gerontol* 1992;47(Spec No):43.
77. Coleman EA, Feuer EJ. Breast cancer screening among women from 65 to 74 years of age in 1987–88 and 1991. NCI Breast Cancer Screening Consortium. *Ann Intern Med* 1992;117:961.
78. Fox SA, Roetzheim RG. Screening mammography and older Hispanic women. Current status and issues. *Cancer* 1994;74:2028.
79. Friedman LC, Neff NE, Webb JA, et al. Age-related differences in mammography use and in breast cancer knowledge, attitudes, and behaviors. *J Cancer Educ* 1998;13(1):26.
80. Satariano WA. Comorbidity and functional status in older women with breast cancer: implications for screening, treatment, and prognosis. *J Gerontol* 1992; 47(Spec No):24.
81. Reuben DB, Bassett LW, Hirsch SH, et al. A randomized clinical trial to assess the benefit of offering on-site mobile mammography in addition to health education for older women. *AJR Am J Roentgenol* 2002;179(6):1509.
82. Van Harrison R, Janz NK, Wolfe RA, et al. Personalized targeted mailing increases mammography among long-term noncompliant medicare beneficiaries—a randomized trial. *Med Care* 2003;41(3):375.
83. Thomas LR, Fox SA, Leake BG, et al. The effects of health beliefs on screening mammography utilization among a diverse sample of older women. *Women Health* 1996;24(3):77.
84. van Dijck JA, Broeders MJ, Verbeek AL. Mammographic screening in older women. Is it worthwhile? *Drugs Aging* 1997;10(2):69.
85. Mandelblatt JS, Wheat ME, Monane M, et al. Breast cancer screening for elderly women with and without comorbid conditions. A decision analysis model. *Ann Intern Med* 1992;116:722.
86. American Geriatrics Society Clinical Practice C. AGS Position Statement: Breast cancer screening in older women. *J Am Geriatr Soc* 2000;48:842.
87. Fisher B, Bauer M, Margolese R, et al. Five-year results of a randomized clinical trial comparing total mastectomy and segmental mastectomy with or without radiation in the treatment of breast cancer. *N Engl J Med* 1985;312:665.
88. Bourez RL, Rutgers EJ, van de Velde CJ. Will we need lymph node dissection at all in the future? *Clin Breast Cancer* 2002;3(5):315.
89. Sandison AJ, Gold DM, Wright P, et al. Breast conservation or mastectomy: treatment choice of women aged 70 years and older. *Br J Surg* 1996;83(7):994.
90. Amsterdam E, Birkenfeld S, Gilad A, et al. Surgery for carcinoma of the breast in women over 70 years of age. *J Surg Oncol* 1987;35:180.
91. Svastics E, Sulyok Z, Besznyak I. Treatment of breast cancer in women older than 70 years. *J Surg Oncol* 1989;41:19.
92. Bergman L, Kluck HM, van Leeuwen FE, et al. The influence of age on treatment choice and survival of elderly breast cancer patients in south-eastern Netherlands: a population- based study. *Eur J Cancer* 1992;28A:1475.
93. Dijkstra JB, Houx PJ, Jolles J. Cognition after major surgery in the elderly: test performance and complaints. *Br J Anaesthesia* 1999;82(6):867.
94. Mandelblatt JS, Edge SB, Meropol NJ, et al. Sequelae of axillary lymph node dissection in older women with stage 1 and 2 breast cancer. *Cancer* 2002;95: 2445.
95. Rudenstam CM, Zahrieh D, Forbes JF, et al. Randomized trial comparing axillary clearance versus no axillary clearance in older patients with breast cancer: first results of International Breast Cancer Study Group Trial 10-93. *J Clin Oncol* 2006;24(3):337–344.
96. Martelli G, DePalo G, Rossi N, et al. Long-term follow-up of elderly patients with operable breast cancer treated with surgery without axillary dissection plus adjuvant tamoxifen. *Br J Cancer* 1995;72(5):1251.
97. Hughes KS, Schnaper LA, Berry D, et al. Lumpectoy plus tamoxifen with or without irradiation in women 70 years of age or older with early breast cancer [Abstract 11]. *Breast Cancer Res Treat* 2006;100S.
98. Lindsey AM, Larson PJ, Dodd MJ, et al. Comorbidity, nutritional intake, social support, weight, and functional status over time in older cancer patients receiving radiotherapy. *Cancer Nurs* 1994;17(2):113.
99. Wyckoff J, Greenberg H, Sanderson R, et al. Breast irradiation in the older woman: a toxicity study. *J Am Geriatr Soc* 1994;42:150.
100. Merchant TE, McCormick B, Yahalom J, et al. The influence of older age on breast cancer treatment decisions and outcome. *Int J Radiat Oncol Biol Phys* 1996; 34(3):565.
101. Solin LJ, Schultz DJ, Fowble BL. Ten-year results of the treatment of early-stage breast carcinoma in elderly women using breast-conserving surgery and definitive breast irradiation. *Int J Radiat Oncol Biol Phys* 1995;33(1):45.
102. Veronesi U, Luini A, Del Vecchio M, et al. Radiotherapy after breast-preserving surgery in women with localized cancer of the breast. *N Engl J Med* 1993; 328:1587.
103. Maher M, Campana F, Mosseri V, et al. Breast cancer in elderly women: a retrospective analysis of combined treatment with tamoxifen and once-weekly irradiation. *Int J Radiat Oncol Biol Phys* 1995;31:783.
104. Rostom AY, Pradhan DG, White WF. Once weekly irradiation in breast cancer. *Int J Radiat Oncol Biol Phys* 1987;13:551.
105. Kozak KR, Smith BL, Adams J, et al. Accelerated partial-breast irradiation using proton beams: initial clinical experience. *Int J Radiat Oncol Biol Phys* 2006;66(3): 691–698.
106. Dunser M, Haussler B, Fuchs H, et al. Tumorectomy plus tamoxifen for the treatment of breast cancer in the elderly. *Eur J Surg Oncol* 1993;19:529.
107. Sader C, Ingram D, Hastrich D. Management of breast cancer in the elderly by complete local excision and tamoxifen alone. *Aust N Z J Surg* 1999;69(11):790.
108. Kantorowitz DA, Poulter CA, Sischy B, et al. Treatment of breast cancer among elderly women with segmental mastectomy or segmental mastectomy plus postoperative radiotherapy. *Int J Radiat Oncol Biol Phys* 1988;15:263.
109. Clark RM, McCulloch PB, Levine MN, et al. Randomized clinical trial to assess the effectiveness of breast irradiation following lumpectomy and axillary dissection for node-negative breast cancer. *J Natl Cancer Inst* 1992;84:683.
110. Reed MW, Morrison JM. Wide local excision as the sole primary treatment in elderly patients with carcinoma of the breast. *Br J Surg* 1989;76:898.
111. Ciatto S, Cirillo A, Confortini M, et al. Tamoxifen as primary treatment of breast cancer in elderly patients. *Neoplasma* 1996;43(1):43.
112. Mustacchi G, Ceccherini R, Milani S, et al. Tamoxifen alone versus adjuvant tamoxifen or operable breast cancer of the elderly: long-term results of the phase III randomized controlled multicenter GRETA trial. *Ann Oncol* 2003;14(3):414.
113. Preece PE, Wood RA, Mackie CR, et al. Tamoxifen as initial sole treatment of localized breast cancer in elderly women: a pilot study. *BMJ Clinical Research ed* 1982;284:869.
114. Fentiman IS, Christiaens MR, Paridaens R, et al. Treatment of operable breast cancer in the elderly: a randomised clinical trial EORTC 10851 comparing tamoxifen alone with modified radical mastectomy. *Eur J Cancer* 2003;39(3):309.
115. Fentiman IS, van Zijl J, Karydas I, et al. Treatment of operable breast cancer in the elderly: a randomised clinical trial EORTC 10850 comparing modified radical mastectomy with tumorectomy plus tamoxifen. *Eur J Cancer* 2003; 39(3):300.
116. Salmon RJ, Remvikos Y, Campana F, et al. Neo adjuvant Tamoxifen in post menopausal patients with operable breast cancer. *Eur J Surg Oncol* 2003;29(10): 831.
117. Horobin JM, Preece PE, Dewar JA, et al. Long-term follow-up of elderly patients with locoregional breast cancer treated with tamoxifen only. *Br J Surg* 1991;78:213.
118. Akhtar SS, Allan SG, Rodger A, et al. A 10-year experience of tamoxifen as primary treatment of breast cancer in 100 elderly and frail patients. *Eur J Surg Oncol* 1991;17:30.
119. Bergman L, van Dongen JA, van Ooijen B, et al. Should tamoxifen be a primary treatment choice for elderly breast cancer patients with locoregional disease? *Breast Cancer Res Treat* 1995;34(1):77.

120. Fennessy M, Bates T, MacRae K, et al. Late follow-up of a randomized trial of surgery plus tamoxifen versus tamoxifen alone in women aged over 70 years with operable breast cancer. *Br J Surg* 2004;91(6):699.

121. Hind D, Wyld L, Beverley CB, et al. Surgery versus primary endocrine therapy for operable primary breast cancer in elderly women (70 years plus). *Cochrane Database Syst Rev* 2006(1):CD004272.

122. Eiermann W, Paepke S, Appfelstaedt J, et al. Preoperative treatment of postmenopausal breast cancer patients with letrozole: a randomized double blind multicenter study. *Ann Oncol* 2001;12(11):1527.

123. Nabholtz JM, Buzdar A, Pollak M, et al. Anastrozole is superior to tamoxifen as first-line therapy for advanced breast cancer in postmenopausal women: results of a North American multicenter randomized trial. Arimidex Study Group. *J Clin Oncol* 2000;18(22):3758–3767.

124. Mouridsen H, Gershanovich M, Sun Y, et al. Phase III study of letrozole versus tamoxifen as first-line therapy of advanced breast cancer in postmenopausal women: analysis of survival and update of efficacy from the International Letrozole Breast Cancer Group. *J Clin Oncol* 2003;21(11):2101–2109.

125. Baum M, Buzdar AU, Cuzick J, et al. Anastrozole alone or in combination with tamoxifen versus tamoxifen alone for adjuvant treatment of postmenopausal women with early breast cancer: first results of the ATAC randomised trial. *Lancet* 2002;359(9324):2131.

126. Ellis MJ, Coop A, Singh B, et al. Letrozole is more effective neoadjuvant endocrine therapy than tamoxifen for ErbB-1- and/or ErbB-2-positive, estrogen receptor-positive primary breast cancer: evidence from a phase III randomized trial. *J Clin Oncol* 2001;19(18):3808.

127. Abe O, Abe R, Enomoto K, et al. Effects of chemotherapy and hormonal therapy for early breast cancer on recurrence and 15-year survival: an overview of the randomised trials. *Lancet* 2005;365(9472):1687.

128. Howell A, Cuzick J, Baum M, et al. Results of the ATAC (Arimidex, Tamoxifen, Alone or in Combination) trial after completion of 5 years' adjuvant treatment for breast cancer. *Lancet* 2005;365(9453):60.

129. Coombes RC, Paridaens R, Jassem J, et al. First mature analysis of the Intergroup Exemestane Study. *Proceeding American Society of Clincal Oncology* 2006;24:933S.

130. Goss PE, Ingle JN, Martino S, et al. Randomized trial of letrozole following tamoxifen as extended adjuvant therapy in receptor-positive breast cancer: updated findings from NCIC CTG MA.17. *J Natl Cancer Inst* 2005;97(17):1262–1271.

131. Muss HB, Tu D, Ingle JN, et al. The benefits of letrozole in postmenopausal women with early stage breast cancer who have had five years of tamoxifen are independent of age. *Breast Cancer Res Treat* 2006; S23.

132. Winer EP, Hudis C, Burstein HJ, et al. American Society of Clinical Oncology technology assessment on the use of aromatase inhibitors as adjuvant therapy for postmenopausal women with hormone receptor-positive breast cancer: status report 2004. *J Clin Oncol* 2005;23(3):619–629.

133. Hebert-Croteau N, Brisson J, Latreille J, et al. Compliance with consensus recommendations for systemic therapy is associated with improved survival of women with node-negative breast cancer. *J Clin Oncol* 2004;22(18):3685–3693.

134. Silliman RA, Guadagnoli E, Rakowski W, et al. Adjuvant tamoxifen prescription in women 65 years and older with primary breast cancer. *J Clin Oncol* 2002;20(11):2680.

135. Demissie S, Silliman RA, Lash TL. Adjuvant tamoxifen: predictors of use, side effects, and discontinuation in older women. *J Clin Oncol* 2001;19(2):322.

136. Partridge AH, Lafountain A, Mayer E, et al. Adherence to initial adjuvant anastrozole therapy among women with early-stage breast cancer. *J Clin Oncol* 2008; 24(4):556.

137. Von Hoff DD, Layard MW, Basa P, et al. Risk factors for doxorubicin-induced congestive heart failure. *Ann Intern Med* 1979;91:710.

138. Muss HB, Woolf SH, Berry DA, et al. Older women with node positive breast cancer get similar benefits from adjuant chemotherapy as younger patients: The Cancer and Leukemia Group B experience. *Proceedings American Society of Clinical Oncology* 2003;22:1.

139. Early Breast Cancer Trialists' Collaborative G, Clarke M, Coates AS, Darby SC, et al. Adjuvant chemotherapy in oestrogen-receptor-poor breast cancer: patient-level meta-analysis of randomised trials. *Lancet* 2008;371(9606):29–40.

140. Paik S, Shak S, Tang G, et al. A multigene assay to predict recurrence of tamoxifen-treated, node-negative breast cancer. *N Engl J Med* 2004;351(27):2817–2826.

141. Paik S, Tang G, Shak S, et al. Gene expression and benefit of chemotherapy in women with node-negative, estrogen receptor-positive breast cancer. *J Clin Oncol* 2006;24(23):3726–3734.

142. Elkin EB, Hurria A, Mitra N, et al. Adjuvant chemotherapy and survival in older women with hormone receptor-negative breast cancer: assessing outcome in a population-based, observational cohort. *J Clin Oncol* 2006;24(18):2757–2764.

143. Giordano SH, Duan Z, Kuo YF, et al. Use and outcomes of adjuvant chemotherapy in older women with breast cancer. *J Clin Oncol* 2006;24(18):2750–2756.

144. Desch CE, Hillner BE, Smith TJ, et al. Should the elderly receive chemotherapy for node-negative breast cancer? A cost-effectiveness analysis examining total and active life-expectancy outcomes. *J Clin Oncol* 1993;11:777.

145. Telli ML, Hunt SA, Carlson RW, et al. Trastuzumab-related cardiotoxicity: calling into question the concept of reversibility. *J Clin Oncol* 2007;25(23):3525–3533.

146. Extermann M, Balducci L, Lyman GH. What threshold for adjuvant therapy in older breast cancer patients? *J Clin Oncol* 2000;18(8):1709.

147. Systemic treatment of early breast cancer by hormonal, cytotoxic, or immune therapy. 133 randomized trials involving 31,000 recurrences and 24,000 deaths among 75,000 women. Early Breast Cancer Trialists' Collaborative Group. *Lancet* 1992;339:1–15,71–85.

148. Fargeot P, Bonneterre J, Roche H, et al. Disease-free survival advantage of weekly epirubicin plus tamoxifen versus tamoxifen alone as adjuvant treatment of operable, node-positive, elderly breast cancer patients: 6-year follow-up results of the French adjuvant study group 08 trial. *J Clin Oncol* 2004; 22(23):4622–4630.

148a. Muss HB, Berry DL, Cirrincione C, et al: Standard chemotherapy (CMF or AC) versus capecitabine in early-stage breast cancer (BC) patients aged 65 and older: Results of CALGB 49907. *J Clin Oncol* 26:Abstract 507, 2008.

149. Wildiers H, Kunkler I, Biganzoli L, et al. Management of breast cancer in elderly individuals: recommendations of the International Society of Geriatric Oncology. *Lancet Oncol* 2007;8(12):1101–1115.

150. Crivellari D, Aapro M, Leonard R, et al. Breast cancer in the elderly. *J Clin Oncol* 2007;25(14):1882–1890.

151. Christman K, Muss HB, Case LD, et al. Chemotherapy of metastatic breast cancer in the elderly. The Piedmont Oncology Association experience. *JAMA* 1992; 268:57.

152. Ibrahim NK, Frye DK, Buzdar AU, et al. Doxorubicin-based chemotherapy in elderly patients with metastatic breast cancer. Tolerance and outcome. *Arch Intern Med* 1996;156(8):882.

153. Giovanazzi-Bannon S, Rademaker A, et al. Treatment tolerance of elderly cancer patients entered onto phase II clinical trials: an Illinois Cancer Center study. *J Clin Oncol* 1994;12:2447.

154. Kimmick GG, Fleming R, Muss HB, et al. Cancer chemotherapy in older adults—a tolerability perspective. *Drugs Aging* 1997;10(1):34.

155. Gelman RS, Taylor SG. Cyclophosphamide, methotrexate, and 5-fluorouracil chemotherapy in women more than 65 years old with advanced breast cancer: the elimination of age trends in toxicity by using doses based on creatinine clearance. *J Clin Oncol* 1984;2:1404.

156. Begg CB, Cohen JL, Ellerton J. Are the elderly predisposed to toxicity from cancer chemotherapy? An investigation using data from the Eastern Cooperative Oncology Group. *Cancer Clinical Trials* 1980;3:369.

157. Nerenz DR, Love MR, Leventhal H, et al. Psychosocial consequences of cancer chemotherapy for elderly patients. *Health Serv Res* 1986;20:961.

158. Ravdin PM, Valero V. Review of docetaxel (Taxotere), a highly active new agent for the treatment of metastatic breast cancer. *Semin Oncol* 1995;22(Suppl 4):17.

159. Hortobagyi GN, Holmes FA. Single-agent paclitaxel for the treatment of breast cancer: an overview. *Semin Oncol* 1996;23(1 Suppl 1):4.

160. Sorio R, Robieux I, Galligioni E, et al. Pharmacokinetics and tolerance of vinorelbine in elderly patients with metastatic breast cancer. *Eur J Cancer* 1997;33 (2):301.

161. Ranson MR, Carmichael J, O'Byrne K, et al. Treatment of advanced breast cancer with sterically stabilized liposomal doxorubicin: results of a multicenter phase II trial. *J Clin Oncol* 1997;15(10):3185.

162. Blum JL, Buzdar AU, LoRusso PM, et al. A multicenter phase II trial of XelodaTM (capecitabine) in paclitaxel-refractory metastatic breast cancer. *Proceedings American Society of Clinical Oncology* 1998;17:125a.

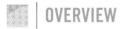

Chapter 92
Breast Cancer in Younger Women

Ann H. Partridge, Aron Goldhirsch, Shari Gelber, and Richard D. Gelber

OVERVIEW

Breast cancer rarely occurs in young women. Of the hundreds of thousands of breast cancers diagnosed worldwide, fewer than 0.1% occur in women under age 20 years; 1.9% between 20 and 34; and 10.6% between 35 and 44 (1,2). Although fewer than 7% of women diagnosed with breast cancer are younger than 40 years, more than 14,000 young women are diagnosed annually with invasive or noninvasive breast cancer in the United States alone, with thousands more diagnosed worldwide (3–5). Incidence rates appear to be stable over the past several decades in young women in the Western world, despite increases in mammography and reproductive and lifestyle trends (2,6) (Fig. 92.1) (3). A suggestion is that rates are increasing among young women, particularly in less-developed countries, but this may be owing to improvements in awareness, diagnosis, and reporting (7,8).

Despite the relative rarity of breast cancer in young women, it is the leading cause of cancer-related deaths in women under 40, and survival rates for young women with breast cancer are lower than for their older counterparts (4,9). The 5-year relative survival rate for women with breast cancer diagnosed before age 40 years is 82% compared with 89% for women diagnosed at age 40 or older (4). Although controversial, accumulating evidence suggests that young age is an independent risk factor for disease recurrence and death, despite that young women have conventionally received more intensive treatment than older women (10–12). Delays in diagnosis and the lack of effective screening in younger women may contribute to the poorer prognosis because they are more likely to present with larger tumors and more involved lymph nodes (13). However, survival differences more likely reflect biological differences in the type of breast cancer developed in young women. Young women are more likely to develop more aggressive subtypes of breast cancer with unfavorable prognostic features, and are less responsive to conventional therapy compared with disease arising in older premenopausal or postmenopausal women (14–16). Specifically, tumors in young women are more likely to be high-grade, hormone receptor(HR)-negative, and have high proliferation fraction and more lymphovascular invasion. Evidence is mixed about the proportion of ERBB2 (formerly HER-2/*neu*) overexpressing tumors, with more modern studies suggesting similar rates across age cohorts (14–19) A population-based registry study in Korea of young women diagnosed with breast cancer, consisting of 1,444 women age less than 35 years, and 8,441 women age 35 to 50 years, revealed significant differences in clinicopathologic characteristics by age at diagnosis. Women younger than 35 were more likely to have greater T stage (*p* <.001) and N stage (*p* <.001) tumors. Furthermore, in the younger age group, 32.4% were estrogen receptor (ER)-positive, 30.6% ER-negative, and 37.0% unknown compared with 36.6% ER-positive, 27.8% ER-negative, and 35.5% ER-unknown in the older group (*p* = .002). In addition the younger age group was 29.9% PR-positive, 31.9 PR-negative, and 38.2 unknown, compared with 36.6% PR-positive, 27.6 PR-negative, and 35.8 unknown in the older group (*p* <.001). ERBB2 status, as determined by immunohistochemistry score, did not differ between the 263 women in those younger than 35 years compared with the 1,947 women in the older age group for whom ERBB2 status was available (*p* = .238) (15). A recent preliminary investigation

suggests that breast cancer arising in young women may represent a distinct biologic entity with unique patterns of deregulated signaling pathways, such as through the Src and E2F oncogenic pathways, which may affect prognosis (20).

Also, increasing evidence suggests that biologic subtypes of breast cancer vary by race as a function of age. In a large, population-based study of breast cancer subtypes within age and racial subsets, the basal-like breast cancer subtype (ER-, PR-, ERBB2-, cytokeratin 5/6 positive, and/or ERBB1+), was more prevalent among premenopausal black women (39%) compared with postmenopausal black women (14%) and non-black women (16%) of any age (*p* <.001), whereas the better prognosis luminal A subtype (ER+ and/or PR+, ERBB2-) was less prevalent (36% vs. 59% and 54%, respectively). This higher prevalence of basal-like breast tumors and lower prevalence of luminal A tumors likely contributes to the poorer prognoses of young black women with breast cancer (21) (see Chapter 32, Prognostic and Predictive Factors: Molecular).

In addition to being at higher risk of dying from breast cancer, despite conventionally receiving more aggressive therapy, young women face a variety of problems unique to, or accentuated by, their young age. They are more likely to be diagnosed at a life stage when role functioning in the home and work can be threatened or disrupted by the diagnosis and treatment of breast cancer. Issues such as attractiveness and fertility may be of substantial importance. Young women are more likely to have young children for whom they are responsible, or desire to have biologic children following treatment. They also have an increased risk of harboring a genetic risk factor for breast cancer, and often suffer from a relative lack of information regarding treatment and survivorship issues compared with older patients. These concerns may contribute to the greater psychosocial distress seen in younger women at both diagnosis and in follow-up (22–25).

Research to date on breast cancer in young women is limited by generally small sample sizes and heterogeneous cut-offs used to differentiate between young and old. Although, age is a continuum and any cut-off is somewhat arbitrary. Many investigators have chosen up to age 35 or 40 to define breast cancer in younger women, recognizing that previous work focusing on premenopausal women is composed primarily of women in their 40s owing to the higher incidence of the disease in older premenopausal women.

 ## RISK FACTORS FOR EARLY ONSET BREAST CANCER AND GENETICS ISSUES

Aside from female gender, increasing age is the strongest risk factor for developing breast cancer. Consequently, younger women are at much lower risk even when compared with older premenopausal women. An average woman has a 1 in approximately 1,800 risk of developing breast cancer in her 20s, 1 in 230 in her 30s, and 1 in 70 in her 40s (4). Family history is the primary risk factor for developing breast cancer at young age, particularly when breast cancer has occurred in a first-degree relative at a young age. Although 5% to 10% of breast cancers are attributable to germ-line mutations such as *BRCA1* and *BRCA2* on chromosomes 17 and 13, respectively, another 15% to 20% of breast cancers are associated with the presence of

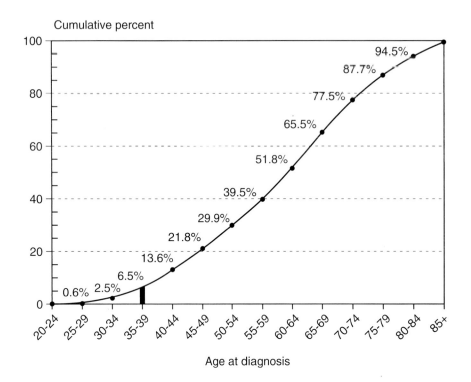

Cumulative percent

0.6% 2.5% 6.5% 13.6% 21.8% 29.9% 39.5% 51.8% 65.5% 77.5% 87.7% 94.5%

Age at diagnosis

FIGURE 92.1. Cumulative distribution of breast cancer diagnoses by age. (From Hankey BF, Miller B, Curtis R, et al. Trends in breast cancer in younger women in contrast to older women. *J Natl Cancer Inst Monogr* 1994;16:7–14, with permission.)

gene polymorphisms and environmental factors (e.g., radiation; see later). By virtue of her age alone, a young woman diagnosed with breast cancer has a greater probability of carrying a *BRCA* mutation. In an unselected group of women under 40 having surgery for early breast cancer, 9% harbored a deleterious *BRCA1* or *BRCA2* mutation (26). Other factors, including a personal or family history of ovarian cancer, bilateral breast cancer, or Ashkenazi Jewish ancestry, may increase that risk. The meaning of an unknown variant of the *BRCA1* or *BRCA2* genes may also vary by race (27). Young women with breast cancer should consider genetic counseling and testing for *BRCA1* and *BRCA2*, particularly if they have a family history of breast or ovarian cancer. Please see Chapters 18 and 19 for more details.

Some rare genetic disorders may predispose younger women to develop breast cancer. These include Cowden disease (*PTEN* gene mutation on chromosome 10 and associated with hamartomas, as well as with breast or thyroid cancer at a young age), and Li-Fraumeni syndrome (mutation of *TP53* gene on chromosome 17, with increased incidence of soft tissue and bone sarcomas, brain tumors, adrenocortical tumors, and breast cancers) (28) (see Chapter 18 for more detail). Young women exposed to ionizing radiation during childhood and teenage years, such as survivors of pediatric Hodgkin disease treated with mantle field irradiation, are also at high risk of developing breast cancer (29). Despite preconceptions, most cases of breast cancer occurring in young women appear to be spontaneous and not clearly related to either carcinogens in the environment or family cancer syndromes (30). However, environmental and hormonal risk factors for breast cancer are not well characterized for younger women, but appear to be somewhat different than for older women. Although breastfeeding appears to be protective against breast cancer at any age, pregnancy appears to have a dual effect on the risk of breast cancer. Large epidemiologic studies indicate that earlier age at first live birth has a long-term protective effect on the lifetime risk of breast cancer, yet it transiently increases the risk immediately following childbirth for 3 to 15 years postpartum, but reduces

the risk in later years (24,31–34). The excess transient early risk of breast cancer is most pronounced among women who are older at the time of their first delivery. Thus, pregnancy has a protective effect for postmenopausal breast cancer and is a risk factor for premenopausal breast cancer, particularly for older premenopausal women. The biologic mechanism for this is not well elucidated. Also contrary to what has been demonstrated in older women, weight gain and higher body mass index appear to be protective against the development of breast cancer at younger age (35–37).

 ## BREAST DIAGNOSTIC ISSUES FOR YOUNG WOMEN

Most lesions arising in the breasts of young premenopausal women will be benign (see Chapter 10 on Benign Breast Disease). Mammography is often of limited value in this population because of high breast tissue density, and targeted ultrasound or magnetic resonance imaging can provide additional discriminatory information in the workup of a breast abnormality (38–40). Breast cancers may be more extensive in younger patients, although it is not clear whether they are at higher risk of multicentricity or bilateral disease, in the absence of a hereditary predisposition, and no evidence indicates that multifocality affects survival in this population (41–46).

 ## TREATMENT ISSUES

Many clinical trials have divided patient populations based on menopausal status, or age greater or less than 50. Virtually no published clinical trials have focused on treatment issues for the youngest women. Trials reporting results of treatments for premenopausal women largely reflect outcomes for patients in their 40s. Thus, findings from studies that consider average results for premenopausal women may not be directly applicable to very young patients.

Local Therapy Issues

Partly owing to inadequate screening options for young women, breast cancer tends to be larger and more often locally advanced. Consequently, young women may more likely need or benefit from preoperative systemic therapy than older women, although available data in this area are limited. Despite the large benefit that young women obtain from an irradiation boost to the tumor bed, most studies continue to indicate that young age is a risk factor for local recurrence, for both invasive and noninvasive disease (47–53) (Fig. 92.2). No evidence suggests, however, that mastectomy in young women improves survival compared with breast conservation, likely because these women are also at increased risk of systemic recurrence. In a population-based Danish cohort of 9,285 premenopausal women with breast cancer, the incidence of local recurrence was 15.4% after breast-conserving therapy among the 719 women under age 35 compared with 3.0% in women ages 45 to 49, although no difference was found in the risk of death between the two age groups (54). Thus, young age alone is not a contraindication to breast conservation. Nonetheless, an increasing number of young women are opting not only for mastectomy, but for contralateral prophylactic mastectomy (55). Reasons for this trend are not completely clear, nor is there evidence that such aggressive surgical measures will improve outcomes. For some young women, local therapy

decisions may be influenced by the presence or absence of a known genetic risk for new primary breast cancer (i.e., a *BRCA1* or *BRCA2* mutation). Thus, prompt genetic counseling and testing for young women at risk for harboring a deleterious genetic mutation should be considered, especially for women for whom the results would have an impact on local therapy decisions. Bilateral prophylactic mastectomy and oophorectomy are increasingly considered for young women with known *BRCA1* or *BRCA2* mutations, despite the current lack of clear benefits of such risk-reducing strategies in breast cancer survivors (56,57).

At present, no relevant data are available on the late effects of radiation therapy plus modern systemic therapy (including anthracyclines, taxanes, and trastuzumab) on cardiac functioning in young women. Moreover, other effects of radiation therapy in patients with very long life expectancy must be taken into account (58).

Attention to margin status may be particularly important for young women undergoing breast conservation treatment. In one evaluation including 37 women younger than 35 with lymph node-negative breast cancer having breast-conserving therapy, local recurrence rates were 50.0% for women with positive margins compared with 20.8% for those with negative margins (51). In a more recent publication, women age 40 or younger with invasive disease had 10-year local recurrence-free survival of 84.4% with negative margins versus 34.6% with positive margins, whereas women over 40 years had local recurrence-free survival of 94.7% if margins were negative compared with 92.6% if margins were positive (52). These findings translated to a 10-year distant disease-free survival (DFS) of 72.0% for younger women with negative margins

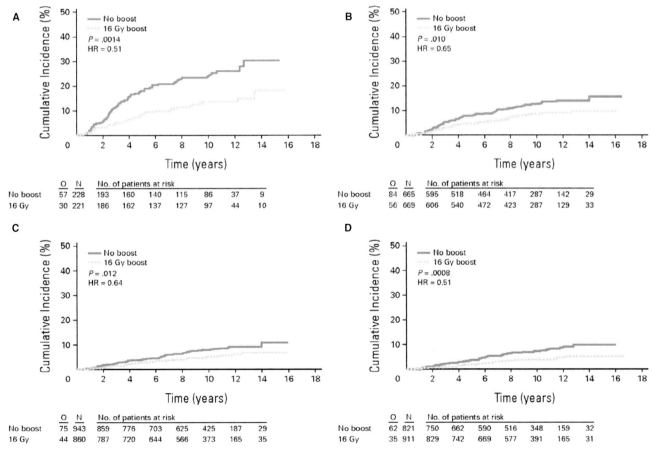

FIGURE 92.2. Cumulative incidence of ipsilateral breast cancer recurrence according to age. Age (**A**) ≤40, (**B**) 41 to 50, (**C**) 51 to 60, and (**D**) > 60 years. (From Bartelink, H. et al. *J Clin Oncol* 2007;25:3259–3265, with permission.)

compared with 39.7% (relative risk [RR] = 3.4) for the younger age group with positive margins, whereas for older women, no significant difference was seen in DFS among those with negative compared to positive margins.

Systemic Therapy Issues

Adjuvant treatment recommendations are based on tumor and patient characteristics predicting the risk of systemic recurrence and potential responsiveness to therapy, as well as the patient's preferences and values. Increasingly, treatments are tailored, regardless of age, to the phenotypic subtype of the tumor as assessed by conventional factors, such as grade, proliferation rate, estrogen and progesterone receptors, and ERBB2 expression. More recent application of genetic signature technology has provided additional predictive information regarding the degree of risk and responsiveness to therapy (see Chapter 32). However, most of the data on adjuvant treatment response was obtained during an era when details related to endocrine responsiveness were either incomplete or imprecise. Even today, endocrine responsiveness evaluation requires improved reporting of steroid hormone receptors and a better understanding of the role of ERBB2 overexpression and amplification (59,60). Currently it is recommended that the estimation of endocrine responsiveness should be the first consideration in tailoring adjuvant therapies for patients with breast cancer, regardless of age (61). Adjuvant chemotherapy has historically been used extensively in premenopausal patients because of its overwhelming beneficial effects on outcome (62,63). The incremental benefits of newer cytotoxic drugs and regimens, including the addition of the taxanes, dose density, and trastuzumab, appear to be present across age groups, although data for very young women are limited (64–68).

Adjuvant Systemic Therapy in Patients with Hormone Receptor-Negative Disease

For premenopausal women with hormone receptor (HR)-negative disease, adjuvant chemotherapy is a very important component of successful treatment. Only one trial, however, has prospectively tested the use of chemotherapy in women with HR-negative, node-negative disease (National Surgical Adjuvant Breast and Bowel Project [NSABP] B13) (69,70). Table 92.1 displays the relative risk of relapse for the chemotherapy-treated group compared with the surgery alone group. No difference was found between the risk for very young compared with the older premenopausal patients, with a 38% reduction in the risk of recurrence from the use of chemotherapy. Novel biologic and chemotherapeutic regimens (e.g., platinum agents) that have shown early promise in women with early (e.g., trastuzumab) and advanced disease (e.g., bevacizumab, platinum agents) may also be particularly relevant in the treatment of young women

with breast cancer, because this population is more likely to develop HR-negative disease (71).

Adjuvant Systemic Therapy in Patients with Hormone Receptor-Positive Disease: Chemotherapy and Endocrine Therapy

Controversy exists about the optimal management of young women with HR-positive breast cancer (72). Since the 1990s, adjuvant tamoxifen has been the mainstay of endocrine therapy for premenopausal women when the Early Breast Cancer Trialists' Collaborative Group (EBCTCG) overview, a large meta-analysis consisting of dozens of randomized trials, revealed a beneficial effect in women under 50 similar to the benefit seen for older women (62,73). The first adjuvant systemic therapy for premenopausal women with breast cancer was ovarian ablation, but its use was almost abandoned in the mid-1970s when the benefits of adjuvant cytotoxic chemotherapy became clear. When the results of all trials of ovarian ablation were summarized by the EBCTCG meta-analysis, the beneficial effect of ovarian ablation appeared to be large in the absence of chemotherapy, whereas no apparent advantage was seen when ovarian ablation was added to cytotoxic chemotherapy (74). More than 80% of the women in this chemotherapy alone group experienced ovarian function suppression with the cytotoxic treatment, however, and the cohort was also a mixture of women with ER-positive and ER-negative disease (75). The International Breast Cancer Study Group (IBCSG) evaluated treatment outcome for very young women compared with older premenopausal women who received adjuvant chemotherapy alone. Very young premenopausal women (<35 years of age) with HR-positive tumors had a worse outcome compared with older premenopausal women, and compared with both older and younger women with HR-negative disease (76). This led to the hypothesis that the effects of cytotoxic chemotherapy on ovarian function, and the timing and duration of treatment related-amenorrhea differ between older and younger premenopausal women. Very young women are much less likely to experience ovarian dysfunction with chemotherapy resulting in a poorer prognosis in the absence of additional endocrine therapy (77–79) (see Chapter 96: Reproductive Issues in Breast Cancer Survivors). To confirm the interaction between age and ER status in premenopausal women treated with chemotherapy alone, the IBCSG, NSABP, Eastern Cooperative Oncology Group (ECOG), and Southwestern Oncology Group (SWOG) conducted a pooled analysis of 9,864 patients. Table 92.2 summarizes the results from all four cooperative groups. In each analysis, the relative risk of an event, estimated from a Cox proportional hazards regression model stratified by study and treatment group, was substantially higher for young patients with ER-positive tumors compared with the reference population of older patients with ER-positive tumors. This phenomenon was not observed for

---

| Table 92.1 | RELATIVE RISK OF RELAPSE COMPARING PATIENTS IN THE CHEMOTHERAPY GROUP (METHOTREXATE → FLUOROURICIL) VERSUS THE NO ADJUVANT THERAPY GROUP: RESULTS FROM THE NATIONAL SURGICAL ADJUVANT BREAST AND BOWEL PROJECT TRIAL B-13 FOR ESTROGEN RECEPTOR–NEGATIVE, NODE-NEGATIVE CASES | | | | |

Age-Group	Patients (N)	Events (N)	Relative Risk	95% Confidence Interval	p-Value
<35	69	28	0.62	(0.29, 1.30)	.21
35–49	371	107	0.62	(0.42, 0.91)	.01

From Goldhirsch A, Gelber RD, Yothers G, et al. Adjuvant therapy for very young women with breast cancer: need for tailored treatments. *J Natl Cancer Inst Monogr* 2001;30:44–51, with permission.

Table 92.2	RELATIVE RISK OF RELAPSE[a] AND CORRESPONDING 5-YEAR DISEASE-FREE SURVIVAL[b] FOR PREMENOPAUSAL WOMEN IN CHEMOTHERAPY ALONE GROUPS IN TRIALS CONDUCTED BY THE INTERNATIONAL BREAST CANCER STUDY GROUP (IBCSG), THE NATIONAL SURGICAL ADJUVANT BREAST AND BOWEL PROJECT (NSABP), THE EASTERN COOPERATIVE ONCOLOGY GROUP (ECOG), AND THE SOUTHWEST ONCOLOGY GROUP (SWOG)[c]

		ER-positive		ER-negative		
Group	Total Patients (N)	<35	≥35[b]	<35	≥35[b]	Interaction p-Value
		Relative Risk of Relapse (Number of Events/Number of Patients)				
IBCSG	2,233	1.84 (72/96)	1.00 (737/1353)	1.13 (50/88)	1.02 (370/696)	.009
NSABP	5,849	1.72 (254/402)	1.00 (1210/2716)	1.27 (214/441)	1.12 (1045/2290)	.0001
ECOG	1,112	1.54 (42/71)	1.00 (274/602)	1.40 (40/73)	1.26 (195/366)	.17
SWOG	670	2.67 (11/29)	1.00 (48/293)	0.81 (7/55)	1.13 (52/293)	.012

ECOG, Eastern Cooperative Oncology Group; ER, estrogen receptor; IBCSG, International Breast Cancer Study Group; NSABP, National Surgical Adjuvant Breast and Bowel Project; SWOG, Southwest Oncology Group.

[a] Includes breast cancer relapses, second primary breast tumors, and deaths without relapse for IBCSG (also includes nonbreast second primaries), ECOG, and SWOG; includes only breast cancer relapses (other events are censored) for NSABP.

[b] Premenopausal ≥35 years of age for IBCSG, ECOG, and SWOG; 35 to 49 years for NSABP. Chemotherapy regimens of the various trials included in the collaboration: IBCSG: classic CMF (cyclophosphamide, methotrexate, fluorouracil) for 12, 9, 6, or 3 courses; NSABP: melphalan + fluorouracil ± methotrexate × 12; melphalan + fluorouracil + doxorubicin × 12; AC (doxorubicin + cyclophosphamide) × 4 ± CMF (given intravenously on day 1, 8 q 28 days) × 6; classic CMF × 6; AC "intensified dose" × 4; AC "intensified dose" with growth factors × 4; ECOG: classic CMF × 12 or 6 courses; CAF × 6 courses; intensive "16-week regimen"; SWOG: classic CMF × 6 courses; CAF × 6 courses.

[c] Cohorts defined by age and estrogen receptor status are compared with the reference population of older women with estrogen receptor-positive tumors (number of events/number of patients are shown in parentheses).

From Goldhirsch A, Gelber RD, Yothers G, et al. Adjuvant therapy for very young women with breast cancer: need for tailored treatments. *J Natl Cancer Inst Monogr* 2001;30:44–51, with permission.

patients with ER-negative tumors. In recent years, it has become clear that in patients with HR-positive disease, the beneficial effects of cytotoxic agents are probably a result of a complex mixture of cytotoxic and endocrine effects of chemotherapy. IBCSG Trial VIII compared sequential chemotherapy followed by the gonadotropin-releasing hormone agonist goserelin with each modality alone in 1,063 pre- and perimenopausal women with lymph node-negative breast cancer (80). Women were randomized to goserelin for 24 months (n = 346), six courses of "classic" CMF (cyclophosphamide, methotrexate, 5-fluorouracil) chemotherapy (n = 360), or six courses of classic CMF followed by 18 months of goserelin. (CMF → goserelin; n = 357). (A fourth no adjuvant treatment arm with 46 patients was discontinued early). Of patients, 20% were aged 39 years or younger and median follow-up was 7 years. Patients with ER-negative tumors had better DFS if they received CMF (5-year DFS for CMF = 84%, 95% confidence interval [CI], 77%–91%; 5-year DFS for CMF → goserelin = 88%, 95% CI, 82%–94%) than if they received goserelin alone (5-year DFS = 73%, 95% CI, 64%–81%). By contrast, for patients with ER-positive disease, chemotherapy alone and goserelin alone provided similar outcomes (5-year DFS for both treatment groups = 81%, 95% CI, 76%–87%), whereas sequential therapy (5-year DFS = 86%, 95% CI, 82%–91%) provided a statistically nonsignificant improvement compared with either modality alone, primarily because of the results among younger women (Fig. 92.3). The DFS results shown in Figure 92.3 according to treatment group illustrate that outcomes for older premenopausal women with ER-positive disease cannot be used to define appropriate treatment choices for younger women (in this example, ≤39 years). For some young patients, endocrine therapy alone may suffice, or a combined endocrine therapy approach may be optimal (61,80–83).

Tamoxifen

Tamoxifen, the most thoroughly studied selective ER modulator (SERM), has not been specifically investigated in very young patients. This drug typically increases the estradiol

secretion from premenopausal ovaries. The updated EBCTCG meta-analysis of all randomized trials of adjuvant tamoxifen has revealed that 2 to 5 years of treatment has similar efficacy in all age groups, including patients less than 40 years of age (62). However, several analyses have suggested that the youngest women in various treatment groups seem to get less benefit from tamoxifen alone (15,16,70). These findings suggest an opportunity to improve on treatment results for this patient population. It is also important to note that, although risks associated with tamoxifen (e.g., blood clot, stroke, and uterine cancer) tend to be much lower in younger patients than older patients, younger women are more likely to develop ovarian cysts because of high estradiol levels resulting in ovarian hyperstimulation while on tamoxifen (84,85).

Adjuvant Ovarian Ablation (Suppression) with or without Tamoxifen

The combination of ovarian suppression or ablation and tamoxifen has been tested in advanced disease and proved superior to either treatment alone (86). In a trial conducted in Asia, the combination of oophorectomy and tamoxifen compared with no adjuvant therapy resulted in an 11% absolute benefit in DFS and an 18% benefit in overall survival (OS) at 10 years (87). In the subset of patients with ER-positive tumors, 10-year DFS probabilities were 66% in the treated group compared with 47% in the control group, corresponding to 10-year OS rates of 82% and 49%, respectively. In a subset analysis from this same study, ERBB2 overexpression appeared to have a favorable influence on response to adjuvant oophorectomy and tamoxifen in women with ER-positive disease (88).

Acceptance of ovarian function suppression, tamoxifen, or the combination may be a significant problem for premenopausal women in general and for younger patients in particular (89). Issues include objective and subjective symptoms of menopause, psychological distress, and adjustment to changes in personal and family plans. Chemotherapy seems

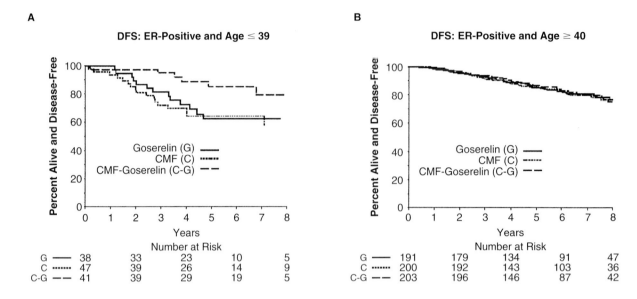

FIGURE 92.3. Kaplan-Meier plots of disease-free survival (DFS) for the ER-positive cohort enrolled in International Breast Cancer Study Group (IBCSG) Trial VIII comparing six courses of cyclophosphamide, methotrexate, and 5-fluorouracil (C), 24 months of goserelin (G), and six courses of C followed by 18 months of goserelin (C-G) at 7 years of median follow-up. Results for subgroups according to age less than 39 years **(A)** and age 40 years or more **(B)** are shown. (From International Breast Cancer Study Group (IBCSG). Adjuvant chemotherapy followed by goserelin versus either modality alone for premenopausal lymph node-negative breast cancer: a randomized trial. *J Natl Cancer Inst* 2003;95:1833–1846, with permission.)

easier to offer to younger patients because of its shorter duration and lesser degree of long-term effects on endocrine function than ovarian suppression, although recent evidence suggests most premenopausal healthy women would choose ovarian suppression over CMF chemotherapy, hypothetically (90). Long-term symptoms of acute ovarian suppression may be a particular problem for some patients. However, in an evaluation of 874 pre- and perimenopausal women in IBCSG Trial VIII (see previous section in this chapter), patients receiving goserelin alone showed a marked improvement or less deterioration in quality of life (QOL) measures over the first 6 months than those patients treated with CMF, yet no differences were seen at 3 years except for hot flashes (91). As reflected in the hot flashes scores, patients in all three treatment groups experienced induced amenorrhea, but the onset of ovarian function suppression was slightly delayed for patients receiving chemotherapy. Of note, in this study, younger patients (<40 years) who received goserelin alone returned to their premenopausal status at 6 months after the cessation of therapy, whereas those who received CMF showed only marginal changes from their baseline hot flashes scores, likely indicative of minimal ovarian dysfunction.

The ongoing study Suppression of Ovarian Function Trial (SOFT) randomizing premenopausal women with HR-positive disease to tamoxifen, tamoxifen and ovarian suppression, or exemestane and ovarian suppression should further elucidate the role of ovarian suppression, and optimal endocrine therapy in young women with breast cancer. (www.ibscg.org) The lack of acceptability resulting in premature closure of the Premenopausal Endocrine Responsive Chemotherapy Trial (PERCHE), a randomized trial evaluating the role of chemotherapy in the setting of combined endocrine therapy, will hamper the availability of more definitive evidence regarding the benefits and risks of chemotherapy in addition to endocrine therapy in very young patients. The optimal duration and the timing of adjuvant endocrine therapy options in very young patients with HR-positive disease, also remain open questions.

 ## BREAST CANCER DIAGNOSED DURING PREGNANCY

It is more likely that younger rather than older premenopausal women will be faced with concurrent pregnancy and the diagnosis of breast cancer, although the issues are similar, irrespective of age. Cytotoxic treatments have been safely administered, beginning in the second trimester, after the completion of organogenesis, although there are risks (92–94). Tamoxifen is contraindicated during pregnancy, because it has been associated with teratogenicity. Reportedly, however, many babies have been born without obvious abnormality after *in utero* exposure (95). Issues regarding whether to maintain the pregnancy and the timing of breast cancer treatment are complex both from a medical and psychosocial standpoint (for additional details, see Chapter 68).

 ## BREAST DISEASE IN ADOLESCENTS

Breast disease in adolescent females is fortunately uncommon, with most presenting lesions being benign, most commonly fibroadenomas (96,97). For most breast lesions in children and adolescents, open biopsy can be avoided (98). Breast cancer is very rare in this population. Because of this, neither the prognosis nor optimal management of the disease in this age group is clear. Available case series suggest that adolescents with breast tumors comprise a mix of histologic subtypes including cystosarcoma phyllodes, and more commonly, adenocarcinomas including invasive intraductal, invasive lobular, signet ring, and secretory adenocarcinomas (99,100). Treatment recommendations should be tailored to the specific histology, and attention to psychosocial issues, including adherence with therapy, is prudent in the care of teenagers with breast cancer.

BREAST CANCER IN CHILDHOOD CANCER SURVIVORS

Young women with a history of treatment for childhood cancer, in particular those treated with chest ("mantle") irradiation for Hodgkin's Disease, are at dramatically increased risk of early onset breast cancer (101,102) (See Chapter 20 in this text). Treatment considerations in this unique subgroup may be complicated by previous systemic therapy, recommendations against further radiation therapy, and psychosocial issues.

TREATMENT OF YOUNG WOMEN WITH ADVANCED DISEASE

Very young women who present with metastatic disease are generally treated using an algorithm reflecting the general incurability of the disease, and employing ovarian function suppression together with other treatment options if the disease is endocrine responsive (see Chapter 73 and 74 in this text). The sequential use of endocrine therapy followed at the time of disease progression by chemotherapy, similar to the conventional approach in older premenopausal and post-menopausal women, is reasonable, although this has not been specifically tested in younger patients. Young patients with metastatic disease may be particularly vulnerable to psychosocial distress, particularly if they have young dependents (103).

QUALITY OF LIFE AND PSYCHOSOCIAL ISSUES

A growing body of evidence suggests that younger women with breast cancer are at increased risk of psychosocial distress compared with older women, both at diagnosis and follow-up (104–110). In a large prospective cohort study, women age 40 and younger who developed breast cancer

experienced significant declines in their QOL compared with age-matched women without breast cancer (111). Adjusting for disease severity and treatment factors, young women who developed breast cancer had the largest relative declines in QOL following diagnosis compared with middle-aged and elderly women who developed breast cancer. In a survey of women who were 50 years or younger at diagnosis and disease-free at 6 years follow-up, women generally reported high levels of physical functioning, but the youngest women (ages 25–34 at diagnosis) exhibited the greatest degree of psychosocial distress, particularly with social and emotional functioning as well as vitality (22). Many young women also feel isolated and lacking information (112). When they attend breast cancer support groups, their issues are often substantially different from those of the older women. Others in their age cohort are planning for the future, whereas young women with breast cancer are facing a life-threatening and physically mutilating disease. Little information is available regarding work and life decisions made by these women. And although access to psychosocial support is associated with a better QOL in breast cancer survivors, these results have not been presented separately for the youngest patients (113–116).

FERTILITY AND PREGNANCY AFTER BREAST CANCER

Young women with breast cancer may face the risk of becoming amenorrheic with treatment, either temporarily or permanently, resulting in potential infertility, onset of menopausal symptoms, problems with sexual functioning, and exposure to long-term risks of early menopause. The risk of amenorrhea is related to increasing patient age and treatment received (117,118) (Fig. 92.4). For some young women, cessation of menses may be welcome and may improve outcomes for women with HR-positive disease. For many young women, however, the threat or experience of infertility may be devastating. Discussion of this important survivorship issue should

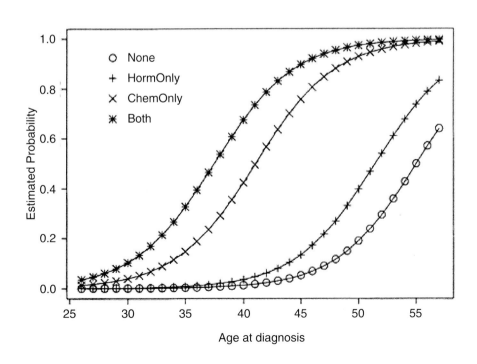

FIGURE 92.4. Probability of menopause during the first year after diagnosis (according to a model). (From Goodwin PJ, Ennis M, Pritchard KI, et al. Risk of menopause during the first year after breast cancer diagnosis. *J Clin Oncol* 1999;17: 2365–2370, with permission.)

commence early in the treatment decision process because some women may elect to try to preserve fertility through intervention or forgo some therapy (119,120). However, available fertility preservation strategies including gonadotropin-releasing hormone (GnRH) agonist treatment during chemotherapy, as well as cryopreservation of embryos, oocytes, or ovarian tissue are hampered by either limited efficacy, safety concerns, or both (121). Young breast cancer survivors can be reassured that at the present time no clear risk in having a biologic child exists. However, studies are limited by substantial biases, including the *healthy mother* bias, and concerns remain for some (122,123). Pregnancy after breast cancer is a very complex and personal decision for a woman who remains at risk for recurrent disease (for additional details, see Chapter 96 Reproductive Issues in Breast Cancer Survivors).

 ## MENOPAUSAL SYMPTOMS AND SEXUAL FUNCTIONING

Menopausal symptoms and sexual dysfunction are common in breast cancer survivors. To date, most breast cancer survivors included in evaluations of sexual dysfunction have been over age 40, reflecting the demographics of breast cancer. Little information is available focusing on sexual dysfunction in very young breast cancer survivors, and no intervention studies have been conducted. Research has, however, identified risk factors for sexual dysfunction in breast cancer survivors including younger age, premature menopause, and the use of chemotherapy (124). The use of tamoxifen and type of breast surgery may also have an impact on sexual functioning, especially in young breast cancer survivors. In a survey of 371 women diagnosed with breast cancer age 40 and younger (mean age at diagnosis 33 years and mean age at follow-up 36 years) where 77% of these women were premenopausal at follow-up, many reported bothersome sexual functioning or menopausal-type symptoms (125). In particular, 46% of women reported hot flashes and 39% reported dyspareunia. Current ovarian suppression, menopausal status, baseline anxiety before the diagnosis, pregnancy after the diagnosis, prior chemotherapy, and lower perceived financial status were associated with more bothersome symptoms. Evidence indicates that intervention to improve menopausal symptoms and sexual functioning is effective, although limited research to date focuses on very young women (126).

CONCLUSIONS

When a very young woman is diagnosed with breast cancer, she may face several threats to her future health and well-being. Most concerning, a young woman with breast cancer is more likely than an older woman to have an adverse prognosis. The differential in prognosis by age may reflect, in part, biological differences between breast cancer that develops in a younger compared with an older woman. Prognosis may, however, also be affected by suboptimal therapy, particularly endocrine therapy, in the youngest patients who are least likely to lose ovarian functioning as a result of systemic therapy. Because of the relative rarity of breast cancer in young women, large pooled analyses and multinational clinical trials are necessary to address the many controversies and improve therapy for younger patients. Late health and psychosocial effects of breast cancer in young women should also be considered in this vulnerable population.

 ## MANAGEMENT SUMMARY

Local Therapy

- Consider preoperative systemic therapy for women with locally advanced disease or those with large tumors who desire breast preservation.
- Careful attention to margin status and boost irradiation after lumpectomy is warranted to minimize the higher risk of local recurrence associated with young age.

Systemic Therapy

- Consider the endocrine as well as the direct cytotoxic effects of chemotherapy.
- Optimize endocrine therapy given evidence for benefits in young women with hormone receptor-positive disease.

Psychosocial and Survivorship Issues

- Evaluate concerns about future fertility early on and refer for consideration of fertility preservation strategies as needed before systemic therapy.
- Consider genetic testing (e.g., *BRCA1* or *BRCA2* testing), early on if it would have an impact on a woman's treatment decisions.
- Provide psychosocial support and referrals given the increased distress often seen in young women with breast cancer.

References

1. Ries LAG, Melbert D, Krapcho M, et al. SEER Cancer Statistics Review, 1975–2004. Bethesda, Maryland: National Cancer Institute. Based on November 2006 SEER data submission, posted to the SEER web site, 2007; 2007. Available at http://seer.cancer.gov/csr/1975_2004/.
2. Stat bite: Breast cancer in young U.S. women. *J Natl Cancer Inst* 2006;98(24): 1762.
3. Hankey BF, Miller B, Curtis R, et al. Trends in breast cancer in younger women in contrast to older women. *J Natl Cancer Inst Monogr* 1994(16):7–14.
4. American Cancer Society. Breast cancer facts and figures 2007–2008. Atlanta: American Cancer Society, Inc.
5. American Cancer Society. Breast cancer facts and figures 2004–2005. Atlanta: American Cancer Society, Inc.
6. Tarone RE. Breast cancer trends among young women in the United States. *Epidemiology* 2006;17(5):588–590.
7. Colonna M, Delafosse P, Uhry Z, et al. Is breast cancer incidence increasing among young women? An analysis of the trend in France for the period 1983–2002. *Breast* 2008;17(3):289–292.
8. Porter P. "Westernizing" women's risks? Breast cancer in lower-income countries. *N Engl J Med* 2008;358(3):213–216.
9. Jemal A, Siegel R, Ward E, et al. Cancer statistics, 2007. *CA Cancer J Clin* 2007; 57(1):43–66.
10. Adami HO, Malker B, Holmberg L, et al. The relation between survival and age at diagnosis in breast cancer. *N Engl J Med* 1986;315(9):559–563.
11. Jayasinghe UW, Taylor R, Boyages J. Is age at diagnosis an independent prognostic factor for survival following breast cancer? *Aust N Z J Surg* 2005;75(9): 762–7.
12. Han W, Kim SW, Park IA, et al. Young age: an independent risk factor for disease-free survival in women with operable breast cancer. *BMC Cancer* 2004;4(1):82.
13. Zabicki K, Colbert JA, Dominguez FJ, et al. Breast cancer diagnosis in women < or = 40 versus 50 to 60 years: increasing size and stage disparity compared with older women over time. *Ann Surg Oncol* 2006;13(8):1072–1077.
14. Sidoni A, Cavaliere A, Bellezza G, et al. Breast cancer in young women: clinico-pathological features and biological specificity. *Breast* 2003;12(4):247–250.
15. Ahn SH, Son BH, Kim SW, et al. Poor outcome of hormone receptor-positive breast cancer at very young age is due to tamoxifen resistance: nationwide survival data in Korea—a report from the Korean Breast Cancer Society. *J Clin Oncol* 2007;25(17):2360–2368.
16. Colleoni M, Rotmensz N, Peruzzotti G, et al. Role of endocrine responsiveness and adjuvant therapy in very young women (below 35 years) with operable breast cancer and node negative disease. *Ann Oncol* 2006;17(10):1497–1503.
17. Agrup M, Stal O, Olsen K, et al. C-erbB-2 overexpression and survival in early onset breast cancer. *Breast Cancer Res Treat* 2000;63(1):23–29.
18. Klauber-DeMore N. Tumor biology of breast cancer in young women. *Breast Dis* 2005;23:9–15.
19. Hartley MC, McKinley BP, Rogers EA, et al. Differential expression of prognostic factors and effect on survival in young (< or =40) breast cancer patients: a case-control study. *Am Surg* 2006;72(12):1189–1194; discussion 94–95.
20. Anders CK, Acharya CR, Hsu DS, et al. Age-specific differences in oncogenic pathway deregulation seen in human breast tumors. *PLoS ONE* 2008;3(1):e1373.

21. Carey LA, Perou CM, Livasy CA, et al. Race, breast cancer subtypes, and survival in the Carolina Breast Cancer Study. *JAMA* 2006;295(21):2492–2502.
22. Ganz PA, Greendale GA, Petersen L, et al. Breast cancer in younger women: reproductive and late health effects of treatment. *J Clin Oncol* 2003;21(22):4184–4193.
23. Connell S, Patterson C, Newman B. Issues and concerns of young Australian women with breast cancer. *Support Care Cancer* 2006;14(5):419–426.
24. Woo JC, Yu T, Hurd TC. Breast cancer in pregnancy: a literature review. *Arch Surg* 2003;138(1):91–98; discussion 99.
25. Avis NE, Crawford S, Manuel J. Psychosocial problems among younger women with breast cancer. *Psychooncology* 2004;13(5):295–308.
26. Golshan M, Miron A, Nixon AJ, et al. The prevalence of germline BRCA1 and BRCA2 mutations in young women with breast cancer undergoing breast-conservation therapy. *Am J Surg* 2006;192(1):58–62.
27. Haffty BG, Silber A, Matloff E, et al. Racial differences in the incidence of BRCA1 and BRCA2 mutations in a cohort of early onset breast cancer patients: African American compared to white women. *J Med Genet* 2006;43(2):133–137.
28. Nusbaum R, Vogel KJ, Ready K. Susceptibility to breast cancer: hereditary syndromes and low penetrance genes. *Breast Dis* 2006;27:21–50.
29. Travis LB, Hill D, Dores GM, et al. Cumulative absolute breast cancer risk for young women treated for Hodgkin lymphoma. *J Natl Cancer Inst* 2005;97(19):1428–1437.
30. Bleyer A, Viny A, Barr R. Cancer in 15- to 29-year-olds by primary site. *Oncologist* 2006;11(6):590–601.
31. Newcomb PA, Storer BE, Longnecker MP, et al. Lactation and a reduced risk of premenopausal breast cancer. *N Engl J Med* 1994;330(2):81–87.
32. Leon DA, Carpenter LM, Broeders MJ, et al. Breast cancer in Swedish women before age 50: evidence of a dual effect of completed pregnancy. *Cancer Causes Control* 1995;6(4):283–291.
33. Albrektsen G, Heuch I, Kvale G. The short-term and long-term effect of a pregnancy on breast cancer risk: a prospective study of 802,457 parous Norwegian women. *Br J Cancer* 1995;72(2):480–484.
34. Lambe M, Hsieh C, Trichopoulos D, et al. Transient increase in the risk of breast cancer after giving birth. *N Engl J Med* 1994;331(1):5–9.
35. Swerdlow AJ, De Stavola BL, Floderus B, et al. Risk factors for breast cancer at young ages in twins: an international population-based study. *J Natl Cancer Inst* 2002;94(16):1238–1246.
36. Coates RJ, Uhler RJ, Hall HI, et al. Risk of breast cancer in young women in relation to body size and weight gain in adolescence and early adulthood. *Br J Cancer* 1999;81(1):167–174.
37. Brinton LA, Swanson CA. Height and weight at various ages and risk of breast cancer. *Ann Epidemiol* 1992;2(5):597–609.
38. Johnstone PA, Moore EM, Carrillo R, et al. Yield of mammography in selected patients age < or = 30 years. *Cancer* 2001;91(6):1075–1078.
39. Morrow M, Wong S, Venta L. The evaluation of breast masses in women younger than forty years of age. *Surgery* 1998;124(4):634–640; discussion 640–641.
40. Wright H, Listinsky J, Rim A, et al. Magnetic resonance imaging as a diagnostic tool for breast cancer in premenopausal women. *Am J Surg* 2005;190(4):572–575.
41. Nielsen M, Thomsen JL, Primdahl S, et al. Breast cancer and atypia among young and middle-aged women: a study of 110 medicolegal autopsies. *Br J Cancer* 1987;56(6):814–819.
42. Fukutomi T, Akashi-Tanaka S, Nanasawa T, et al. Multicentricity and histopathological background features of familial breast cancers stratified by menopausal status. *Int J Clin Oncol* 2001;6(2):80–83.
43. Guenther JM, Kirgan DM, Giuliano AE. Feasibility of breast-conserving therapy for younger women with breast cancer. *Arch Surg* 1996;131(6):632–636.
44. Lesser ML, Rosen PP, Kinne DW. Multicentricity and bilaterality in invasive breast carcinoma. *Surgery* 1982;91(2):234–240.
45. Litton JK, Eralp Y, Gonzalez-Angulo AM, et al. Multifocal breast cancer in women < or =35 years old. *Cancer* 2007;110(7):1445–1450.
46. Lehman CD, Gatsonis C, Kuhl CK, et al. MRI evaluation of the contralateral breast in women with recently diagnosed breast cancer. *N Engl J Med* 2007;356(13):1295–1303.
47. Bartelink H, Horiot JC, Poortmans P, et al. Recurrence rates after treatment of breast cancer with standard radiotherapy with or without additional radiation. *N Engl J Med* 2001;345(19):1378–1387.
48. Huston TL, Simmons RM. Locally recurrent breast cancer after conservation therapy. *Am J Surg* 2005;189(2):229–235.
49. Bollet MA, Sigal-Zafrani B, Mazeau V, et al. Age remains the first prognostic factor for loco-regional breast cancer recurrence in young (<40 years) women treated with breast conserving surgery first. *Radiother Oncol* 2007;82(3):272–280.
50. Bartelink H, Horiot JC, Poortmans PM, et al. Impact of a higher radiation dose on local control and survival in breast-conserving therapy of early breast cancer: 10-year results of the randomized boost versus no boost EORTC 22881-10882 trial. *J Clin Oncol* 2007;25(22):3259–3265.
51. Leong C, Boyages J, Jayasinghe UW, et al. Effect of margins on ipsilateral breast tumor recurrence after breast conservation therapy for lymph node-negative breast carcinoma. *Cancer* 2004;100(9):1823–1832.
52. Jobsen JJ, Van Der Palen J, Ong F, et al. Differences in outcome for positive margins in a large cohort of breast cancer patients treated with breast-conserving therapy. *Acta Oncol* 2007;46(2):172–180.
53. Omlin A, Amichetti M, Azria D, et al. Boost radiotherapy in young women with ductal carcinoma in situ: a multicentre, retrospective study of the Rare Cancer Network. *Lancet Oncol* 2006;7(8):652–656.
54. Kroman N, Holtveg H, Wohlfahrt J, et al. Effect of breast-conserving therapy versus radical mastectomy on prognosis for young women with breast carcinoma. *Cancer* 2004;100(4):688–693.
55. Tuttle TM, Habermann EB, Grund EH, et al. Increasing use of contralateral prophylactic mastectomy for breast cancer patients: a trend toward more aggressive surgical treatment. *J Clin Oncol* 2007;25(33):5203–5209.
56. Robson M, Svahn T, McCormick B, et al. Appropriateness of breast-conserving treatment of breast carcinoma in women with germline mutations in BRCA1 or BRCA2: a clinic-based series. *Cancer* 2005;103(1):44–51.
57. Pierce LJ, Levin AM, Rebbeck TR, et al. Ten-year multi-institutional results of breast-conserving surgery and radiotherapy in BRCA1/2-associated stage I/II breast cancer. *J Clin Oncol* 2006;24(16):2437–2443.
58. Darby SC, McGale P, Taylor CW, et al. Long-term mortality from heart disease and lung cancer after radiotherapy for early breast cancer: prospective cohort study of about 300,000 women in US SEER cancer registries. *Lancet Oncol* 2005;6(8):557–565.
59. Wolff AC, Hammond ME, Schwartz JN, et al. American Society of Clinical Oncology/College of American Pathologists guideline recommendations for human epidermal growth factor receptor 2 testing in breast cancer. *J Clin Oncol* 2007;25(1):118–145.
60. Ross JS, Symmans WF, Pusztai L, et al. Standardizing slide-based assays in breast cancer: hormone receptors, HER2, and sentinel lymph nodes. *Clin Cancer Res* 2007;13(10):2831–2835.
61. Goldhirsch A, Wood WC, Gelber RD, et al. Progress and promise: highlights of the international expert consensus on the primary therapy of early breast cancer 2007. *Ann Oncol* 2007;18(7):1133–1144.
62. Early Breast Cancer Trialists' Collaborative Group (EBCTCG). Effects of chemotherapy and hormonal therapy for early breast cancer on recurrence and 15-year survival: an overview of the randomised trials. *Lancet* 2005;365(9472):1687–1717.
63. Kroman N, Jensen MB, Wohlfahrt J, et al. Factors influencing the effect of age on prognosis in breast cancer: population based study. *BMJ* 2000;320(7233):474–478.
64. Martin M, Pienkowski T, Mackey J, et al. Adjuvant docetaxel for node-positive breast cancer. *N Engl J Med* 2005;352(22):2302–2313.
65. Henderson IC, Berry DA, Demetri GD, et al. Improved outcomes from adding sequential Paclitaxel but not from escalating Doxorubicin dose in an adjuvant chemotherapy regimen for patients with node-positive primary breast cancer. *J Clin Oncol* 2003;21(6):976–983.
66. Citron ML, Berry DA, Cirrincione C, et al. Randomized trial of dose-dense versus conventionally scheduled and sequential versus concurrent combination chemotherapy as postoperative adjuvant treatment of node-positive primary breast cancer: first report of Intergroup Trial C9741/Cancer and Leukemia Group B Trial 9741. *J Clin Oncol* 2003;21(8):1431–1439.
67. Piccart-Gebhart MJ, Procter M, Leyland-Jones B, et al. Trastuzumab after adjuvant chemotherapy in HER2-positive breast cancer. *N Engl J Med* 2005;353(16):1659–1672.
68. Romond EH, Perez EA, Bryant J, et al. Trastuzumab plus adjuvant chemotherapy for operable HER2-positive breast cancer. *N Engl J Med* 2005;353(16):1673–1684.
69. Fisher B, Dignam J, Mamounas EP, et al. Sequential methotrexate and fluorouracil for the treatment of node-negative breast cancer patients with estrogen receptor-negative tumors: eight-year results from National Surgical Adjuvant Breast and Bowel Project (NSABP) B-13 and first report of findings from NSABP B-19 comparing methotrexate and fluorouracil with conventional cyclophosphamide, methotrexate, and fluorouracil. *J Clin Oncol* 1996;14(7):1982–1992.
70. Goldhirsch A, Gelber RD, Yothers G, et al. Adjuvant therapy for very young women with breast cancer: need for tailored treatments. *J Natl Cancer Inst Monogr* 2001;(30):44–51.
71. Colleoni M, Rotmensz N, Robertson C, et al. Very young women (<35 years) with operable breast cancer: features of disease at presentation. *Ann Oncol* 2002;13(2):273–279.
72. Parton M, Smith IE. Controversies in the management of patients with breast cancer: adjuvant endocrine therapy in premenopausal women. *J Clin Oncol* 2008;26(5):745–752.
73. Tamoxifen for early breast cancer: an overview of the randomised trials. Early Breast Cancer Trialists' Collaborative Group. *Lancet* 1998;351(9114):1451–1467.
74. Ovarian ablation in early breast cancer: overview of the randomised trials. Early Breast Cancer Trialists' Collaborative Group. *Lancet* 1996;348(9036):1189–1196.
75. Chemotherapy with or without oophorectomy in high-risk premenopausal patients with operable breast cancer. Ludwig Breast Cancer Study Group. *J Clin Oncol* 1985;3(8):1059–1067.
76. Aebi S, Gelber S, Castiglione-Gertsch M, et al. Is chemotherapy alone adequate for young women with oestrogen-receptor-positive breast cancer? *Lancet* 2000;355(9218):1869–1874.
77. Goldhirsch A, Gelber RD, Castiglione M. The magnitude of endocrine effects of adjuvant chemotherapy for premenopausal breast cancer patients. The International Breast Cancer Study Group. *Ann Oncol* 1990;1(3):183–188.
78. Pagani O, O'Neill A, Castiglione M, et al. Prognostic impact of amenorrhoea after adjuvant chemotherapy in premenopausal breast cancer patients with axillary node involvement: results of the International Breast Cancer Study Group (IBCSG) Trial VI. *Eur J Cancer* 1998;34(5):632–640.
79. Walshe JM, Denduluri N, Swain SM. Amenorrhea in premenopausal women after adjuvant chemotherapy for breast cancer. *J Clin Oncol* 2006;24(36):5769–5779.
80. Castiglione-Gertsch M, O'Neill A, Price KN, et al. Adjuvant chemotherapy followed by goserelin versus either modality alone for premenopausal lymph node-negative breast cancer: a randomized trial. *J Natl Cancer Inst* 2003;95(24):1833–1846.
81. Bao T, Davidson NE. Adjuvant endocrine therapy for premenopausal women with early breast cancer. *Breast Cancer Res* 2007;9(6):115.
82. Cuzick J, Ambroisine L, Davidson N, et al. Use of luteinising-hormone-releasing hormone agonists as adjuvant treatment in premenopausal patients with hormone-receptor-positive breast cancer: a meta-analysis of individual patient data from randomised adjuvant trials. *Lancet* 2007;369(9574):1711–1723.
83. Thürlimann B, Price KN, Gelber RD, et al. Is chemotherapy necessary for premenopausal women with lower-risk node-positive, endocrine responsive breast cancer? 10-year update of International Breast Cancer Study Group Trial 11-93. *Breast Cancer Res Treat* 2008;113(1):137–144.
84. Mourits MJ, de Vries EG, Willemse PH, et al. Ovarian cysts in women receiving tamoxifen for breast cancer. *Br J Cancer* 1999;79(11–12):1761–1764.
85. Gail MH, Costantino JP, Bryant J, et al. Weighing the risks and benefits of tamoxifen treatment for preventing breast cancer. *J Natl Cancer Inst* 1999;91(21):1829–1846.
86. Klijn JG, Blamey RW, Boccardo F, et al. Combined tamoxifen and luteinizing hormone-releasing hormone (LHRH) agonist versus LHRH agonist alone in premenopausal advanced breast cancer: a meta-analysis of four randomized trials. *J Clin Oncol* 2001;19(2):343–353.
87. Love RR, Van Dinh N, Quy TT, et al. Survival after adjuvant oophorectomy and tamoxifen in operable breast cancer in premenopausal women. *J Clin Oncol* 2008;26(2):253–257.
88. Love RR, Duc NB, Dinh NV, et al. Young age as an adverse prognostic factor in premenopausal women with operable breast cancer. *Clin Breast Cancer* 2002;2(4):294–298.
89. Fellowes D, Fallowfield LJ, Saunders CM, et al. Tolerability of hormone therapies for breast cancer: how informative are documented symptom profiles in medical notes for 'well-tolerated' treatments? *Breast Cancer Res Treat* 2001;66(1):73–81.
90. Fallowfield L, McGurk R, Dixon M. Same gain, less pain: potential patient preferences for adjuvant treatment in premenopausal women with early breast cancer. *Eur J Cancer* 2004;40(16):2403–2410.

91. Bernhard J, Maibach R, Thurlimann B, et al. Patients' estimation of overall treatment burden: why not ask the obvious? *J Clin Oncol* 2002;20(1):65–72.
92. Theriault R, Hahn K. Management of breast cancer in pregnancy. *Curr Oncol Rep* 2007;9(1):17–21.
93. Hahn KM, Johnson PH, Gordon N, et al. Treatment of pregnant breast cancer patients and outcomes of children exposed to chemotherapy in utero. *Cancer* 2006;107(6):1219–1226.
94. Ring A. Breast cancer and pregnancy. *Breast* 2007;16(Suppl 2):S155–S158.
95. Partridge AH, Garber JE. Long-term outcomes of children exposed to antineoplastic agents in utero. *Semin Oncol* 2000;27(6):712–726.
96. Foxcroft LM, Evans EB, Hirst C, et al. Presentation and diagnosis of adolescent breast disease. *Breast* 2001;10(5):399–404.
97. Elsheikh A, Keramopoulos A, Lazaris D, et al. Breast tumors during adolescence. *Eur J Gynaecol Oncol* 2000;21(4):408–410.
98. Ravichandran D, Naz S. A study of children and adolescents referred to a rapid diagnosis breast clinic. *Eur J Pediatr Surg* 2006;16(5):303–306.
99. Corpron CA, Black CT, Singletary SE, et al. Breast cancer in adolescent females. *J Pediatr Surg* 1995;30(2):322–324.
100. Rivera-Hueto F, Hevia-Vazquez A, Utrilla-Alcolea JC, et al. Long-term prognosis of teenagers with breast cancer. *Int J Surg Pathol* 2002;10(4):273–279.
101. Kenney LB, Yasui Y, Inskip PD, et al. Breast cancer after childhood cancer: a report from the Childhood Cancer Survivor Study. *Ann Intern Med* 2004;141(8):590–597.
102. Maule M, Scelo G, Pastore G, et al. Risk of second malignant neoplasms after childhood leukemia and lymphoma: an international study. *J Natl Cancer Inst* 2007;99(10):790–800.
103. Turner J. Children's and family needs of young women with advanced breast cancer: a review. *Palliat Support Care* 2004;2(1):55–64.
104. Wenzel LB, Fairclough DL, Brady MJ, et al. Age-related differences in the quality of life of breast carcinoma patients after treatment. *Cancer* 1999;86(9):1768–1774.
105. Bloom JR, Stewart SL, Chang S, et al. Then and now: quality of life of young breast cancer survivors. *Psychooncology* 2004;13(3):147–160.
106. Mor V, Malin M, Allen S. Age differences in the psychosocial problems encountered by breast cancer patients. *J Natl Cancer Inst Monogr* 1994(16):191–197.
107. Schag CA, Ganz PA, Polinsky ML, et al. Characteristics of women at risk for psychosocial distress in the year after breast cancer. *J Clin Oncol* 1993;11(4):783–793.
108. Ganz PA, Desmond KA, Leedham B, et al. Quality of life in long-term, disease-free survivors of breast cancer: a follow-up study. *J Natl Cancer Inst* 2002;94(1):39–49.
109. Vinokur AD, Threatt BA, Caplan RD, et al. Physical and psychosocial functioning and adjustment to breast cancer. Long-term follow-up of a screening population. *Cancer* 1989;63(2):394–405.
110. Avis NE, Crawford S, Manuel J. Quality of life among younger women with breast cancer. *J Clin Oncol* 2005;23(15):3322–3330.
111. Kroenke CH, Rosner B, Chen WY, et al. Functional impact of breast cancer by age at diagnosis. *J Clin Oncol* 2004;22(10):1849–1856.
112. Gould J, Grassau P, Manthorne J, et al. 'Nothing fit me': nationwide consultations with young women with breast cancer. *Health Expect* 2006;9(2):158–173.
113. Wong-Kim EC, Bloom JR. Depression experienced by young women newly diagnosed with breast cancer. *Psychooncology* 2005;14(7):564–573.
114. Baucom DH, Porter LS, Kirby JS, et al. Psychosocial issues confronting young women with breast cancer. *Breast Dis* 2005;23:103–113.
115. Bloom JR, Stewart SL, Johnston M, et al. Sources of support and the physical and mental well-being of young women with breast cancer. *Soc Sci Med* 2001;53(11):1513–1524.
116. Allen SM, Shah AC, Nezu AM, et al. A problem-solving approach to stress reduction among younger women with breast carcinoma: a randomized controlled trial. *Cancer* 2002;94(12):3089–3100.
117. Goodwin PJ, Ennis M, Pritchard KI, et al. Risk of menopause during the first year after breast cancer diagnosis. *J Clin Oncol* 1999;17(8):2365–2370.
118. Petrek JA, Naughton MJ, Case LD, et al. Incidence, time course, and determinants of menstrual bleeding after breast cancer treatment: a prospective study. *J Clin Oncol* 2006;24(7):1045–1051.
119. Partridge AH, Gelber S, Peppercorn J, et al. Web-based survey of fertility issues in young women with breast cancer. *J Clin Oncol* 2004;22(20):4174–4183.
120. Thewes B, Meiser B, Taylor A, et al. Fertility- and menopause-related information needs of younger women with a diagnosis of early breast cancer. *J Clin Oncol* 2005;23(22):5155–5165.
121. Blumenfeld Z. How to preserve fertility in young women exposed to chemotherapy? The role of GnRH agonist cotreatment in addition to cryopreservation of embryo, oocytes, or ovaries. *Oncologist* 2007;12(9):1044–1054.
122. Sankila R, Heinavaara S, Hakulinen T. Survival of breast cancer patients after subsequent term pregnancy: "healthy mother effect". *Am J Obstet Gynecol* 1994;170(3):818–823.
123. Partridge AH, Ruddy KJ. Fertility and adjuvant treatment in young women with breast cancer. *Breast* 2007;16(Suppl 2):S175–S181.
124. Schover LR. Premature ovarian failure and its consequences: vasomotor symptoms, sexuality, and fertility. *J Clin Oncol* 2008;26(5):753–758.
125. Leining MG, Gelber S, Rosenberg R, et al. Menopausal-type symptoms in young breast cancer survivors. *Ann Oncol* 2006;17(12):1777–1782.
126. Ganz PA, Greendale GA, Petersen L, et al. Managing menopausal symptoms in breast cancer survivors: results of a randomized controlled trial. *J Natl Cancer Inst* 2000;92(13):1054–1064.

Jeanne Mandelblatt, Wenchi Liang, Vanessa B. Sheppard, Judy Wang, and Claudine Isaacs

It has been more than three decades since the war on cancer was first declared by President Nixon with the passage of the National Cancer Act in 1975 (1). Twenty years later, President Clinton announced a bold initiative to end ethnic and racial disparities in health (2). For breast cancer, this goal was to be achieved through a combination of prevention, increased use of screening, and improved access to treatment for all Americans. However, despite important progress, these goals have not been met and the elimination of racial and ethnic disparities in breast cancer remains elusive.

As the fight against cancer and elimination of disparities continues in the 21st century, new tools in our armamentarium have begun to influence research and our understanding of observed racial and ethnic variation in patterns of breast cancer incidence, morbidity, and mortality. Only a 0.1% genetic difference could account for some of the within-species race or ethnic group differences in cancer risk and response to treatment (3–6). Thus, current breast cancer disparities research focuses more on how differences of phenotype and gene–environment interactions contribute to the disparity in mortality and survival rates between race and ethnic groups. Disentangling these factors from the simultaneous contextual and behavioral determinants of breast cancer outcomes remains a research challenge (5).

Given these complexities, we have adapted Glass and McAtee's multidimensional hierarchical model of human behavior to guide our review of breast cancer in race and ethnic minority women (Fig. 93.1) (7). In this context, race and ethnicity encompass several social constructs that may affect breast cancer risk and expression, including the *collective culture* of a minority group within a larger society, the *ethnic origin*, or place of ancestry, *racial* or *ethnic identity* and skin color, and shared physical environments (6,8). In this model, expression of breast cancer in racial and ethnic minority women is a composite of interactive feedback between levels of social, built, and natural environments; factors that modulate risk via the opportunities and constraints they impose on minority women's behavior; and the impact of behavior and exposures on the expression of biologic systems (7,9).

Relationships between and across levels are illustrated by one population study that found that late-stage breast cancer diagnoses increased in periods of high unemployment and that African American women were three times more likely to be diagnosed with late-stage breast cancer than whites in these periods (10). As other examples of multilevel interactions, immigration debates in the U.S. Congress will have an influence on disparities in breast cancer because Latinos are now the largest minority group in the United States. Likewise, chronic under-funding of national and state agencies charged with collecting surveillance data and developing strategies to implement cancer control activities could further widen disparities (11). Budget constraints, including cuts to research grants, could also lead scientists to reduce needed sample sizes for meaningful racial or ethnic-specific analysis. Fiscal constraints also affect material conditions, such as reduced educational opportunities, and contribute to continued chronic shortages of minority scientists. Such conditions, in turn, perpetuate suboptimal participation in research by minorities who may be at high risk (12), and hamper progress in the war on cancer.

In this updated overview, we assess what is known about minority women at risk of developing or with breast cancer in light of this broad framework, highlighting new research developments. For this review, we include women of African, Hispanic, Asian, and Pacific Island descent as "racial and ethnic minority women" and compare their experiences to that of white, non-Hispanic women (hereinafter referred to as *white*). We acknowledge, however, the enormous variability within each of these broad groupings of minority women and highlight within minority group differences *where data are available*.

In the following sections, we examine the epidemiology, tumor biology, and social context of breast cancer in relation to race and ethnicity and state-of-the-art breast cancer prevention, early detection, diagnosis, and treatment services. This synthesis is intended to highlight key issues along the spectrum of cancer control for minority women and to inform future directions in research and dissemination.

EPIDEMIOLOGY AND RISK FACTORS

Breast cancer disparities are especially evident among young African American women, who have the highest breast cancer incidence and mortality rates. It is possible that these disparities are associated with race and ethnic differences in biological, lifestyle, and environmental risk factors. The following section summarizes recent breast cancer trends and risk factor variations among racial and ethnic groups in the United States.

Disease Trends

Important differences in disease incidence and mortality trends exist between minority women and whites. For example, although overall breast cancer incidence is highest in white women, African American women younger than age 40 experience a higher incidence than their white counterparts. In the years 2000 to 2004, the incidence rate ratio for African American compared with white women ranged from 1.5 before age 25 to 1.1 by ages 35 to 39; after age 40 rates were similar to or lower than those for whites. Thus, African American women are younger at diagnosis than white women, with median ages of 56 and 63 years, respectively (13). For other ethnic minority groups, incidence is generally lower than whites at all ages, although the small numbers of cases at younger ages make estimates somewhat unstable (14).

Overall breast cancer mortality is higher in African American women (33.8/100,000) than in white women (25/100,000). Gaps in mortality rates between African American and white women have been widening since 1980 (15) and age-specific mortality is also higher at every age except those 85 years and older (16). Mortality rate ratios for African Americans versus whites are most pronounced for younger women, but remain well above 1 for all ages, indicating widening disparities in outcomes after diagnosis for this minority group (17). The mortality rate for Hispanic women is intermediate (16.1), followed by American Indians and Alaska Natives (13.8) and Asian and Pacific Islander women (12.6) (16,18,19).

Risk Factors

Traditionally, family history, reproductive history, and lifestyle factors have been considered the primary risk factors for breast cancer. More recently, mammography density and ductal hyperplasia have been recognized as potential risk factors;

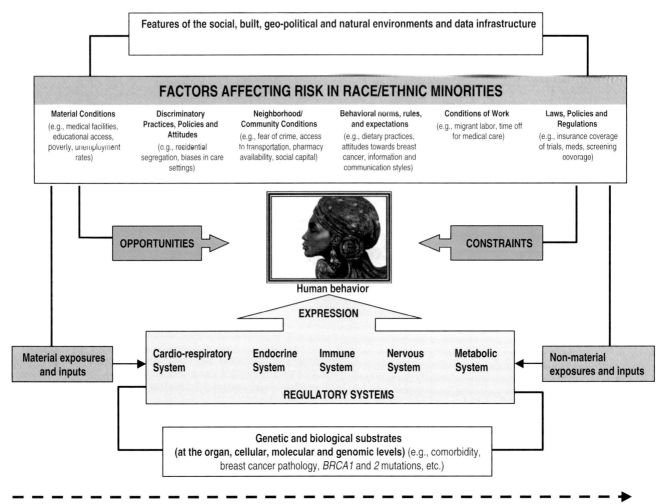

FIGURE 93.1. Multi-dimensional hierarchical model of human behavior. (Adapted from Glass TA, McAtee MJ. Behavorial science at the cross-roads in public health: extending horizons, envisioning the future. *Soc Sci MED* 2006;62(7):1650–1671.)

evidence about environmental risk factors is less clear. Studies that have examined risks for breast cancer in minorities suggest that the effects of established breast cancer risk factors (e.g., early menarche, late age at first full-term pregnancy, and nulliparity) do not vary by race or ethnicity (20–24).

Reflective of the temporal dimension depicted in Figure 93.1, the timing of reproductive events appears to affect risk of disease development. High parity reduces postmenopausal breast cancer risk for all ethnicities except Hispanic women (21,22,24,25). In contrast, studies have suggested a transient increase in premenopausal risk with each pregnancy owing to hormonal stimulation, especially if cells have already experienced a neoplastic transformation or *hit*. Because African American women generally give birth to more children and at an earlier age than white women, this premenopausal parity effect is thought to influence the higher incidence of breast cancer in young African American women, with a crossover to lower rates after age 40 relative to whites (24,26). However, a recent case-control study demonstrated a significant reduction of breast cancer risk per full-term pregnancy for younger and older white and African American women, so this issue is not absolute (25).

The impact of breast-feeding on breast cancer risk also may have temporal trends. Earlier studies examining lactation in African American women showed a strong protective effect

among African American women aged 20 to 39, but no effect in those ages 40 to 54 (20). Among Hispanic women, protective effects have only been observed for premenopausal women (23), whereas in Asian American women, lactation seems to be protective at all ages (21). However, a recent large case-control study shows a similar effect of lactation in both premenopausal and postmenopausal white and African American women (25). Lactation duration appears to be protective for both white and African American women aged 35 to 49 years but had no effect at age 50 and older (25), suggesting that timing of exposures is important in cancer risk, but results are inconsistent across race and ethnic groups.

Mammographic density has been found to be highest in Asian women and similar in white and Hispanic women (27,28). However, some found African American women to have the lowest density (27,29), whereas one study found their density similar to whites (28). The inconsistent results for African Americans are probably owing to lack of or incomplete control for body mass index (BMI), because African Americans have high rates of obesity and obese women generally have lower breast density (see below for discussion of impact of BMI on risk) (27,30). Asian American women generally have smaller regions of breast density than whites, but because of their smaller average breast size, their mean percent breast density is larger (31).

In terms of how these patterns of breast density affect cancer risk, one study found that mammography density had similar effects in African American and white women, but larger effects in Asian American women, with risk increasing from 11% and 15% to 30%, respectively, for each 10% increase in percent density, especially for women over age 50 (32). However, these race and ethnic differences virtually disappear when women with the highest BMI are excluded. Understanding breast density will become more important as new diagnostic technologies evolve (e.g., digital mammography is more sensitive than mammography for women 50 and younger with dense breasts) (33).

Although most studies among white women find that high BMI increases postmenopausal breast cancer risk (34), no effect has been seen in most studies of African American women and it is not clear if this is a true absence of effect or lack of power to detect small, but meaningful increases in risk (20,35,36). In contrast, among Hispanic women risk increases with BMI regardless of age (37). For Asians, risk also increases with BMI (38), but recent data show the link only applies to postmenopausal Asians (39). Height, one component of the BMI, has consistently been shown to be a risk factor for postmenopausal white (40–42) and Asian American women (43), whereas effects in premenopausal women have been inconsistent (44). The converse has been true among African American women (35,45). Resolution of these somewhat contradictory data on the effects of height and weight (BMI) on breast cancer risk will be important in understanding how best to reduce disparities in incidence (and mortality) by race and ethnicity, for obesity (defined as a BMI of 30 or more) is increasing at alarming rates for all U.S. women and there are striking differences in the rates of obesity both before and after menopause among the different race and ethnic groups (46).

High physical activity, a correlate of lower BMI, is associated with decreased premenopausal and postmenopausal breast cancer in African American (47), Hispanic (48), and Asian women (39,48), an effect similar to that observed in white women (48,49). Not all studies in white women have observed protective effects (50,51), however, and effects have varied according to the definition of activity, age at which the activity occurred, and BMI or adiposity (48).

Evaluation of risk factors related to energy balance (age at menarche, BMI, physical activity, height, energy intake) is complicated because they are all closely inter-related and reflect diverse exposures and behaviors at different stages of life (Fig. 93.1) (52). Risk attributable to these exposures may also be modified by the age at which the risk factor is assessed. For instance, virtually all studies find that being overweight (BMI >25 and <30) or obese (BMI of 30+) is strongly linked to early age at menarche among all race and ethnic groups. However, race and ethnic differences remain even after controlling for obesity, with African Americans are still twice as likely to have reached early menarche compared with whites (53).

The use of hormone replacement therapy (HRT) is another risk factor for breast cancer for whites, Asian Americans, and Hispanics (39,54,55), but this association is inconsistent for African Americans (56). The sharp decrease of breast cancer incidence observed in 2003 is largely felt to be owing to a significant decrease in HRT use (57,58) following the release of a 2002 report indicating the adverse effect of HRT on breast cancer that resulted in early termination of the large prospective Women's Health Initiative study (54).

In addition to biological and lifestyle factors, certain environmental factors may contribute to breast cancer, but results have not been consistent. For instance, shift work or light at night has been found to be associated with increased breast cancer risk (59), but the Long Island breast cancer case-control study recently reported mixed results (60). On the other hand, exposure to traffic emissions at menarche or at first live birth increases a women's risk for developing pre- or postmenopausal breast cancer (61).

These factors may help explain disparities in breast cancer incidence, because minorities, especially younger African Americans, are more likely to live in more polluted areas, such as inner cities or industrial areas (62).

Summary: Epidemiology and Risk Factors

Despite some race and ethnic differences in the epidemiology of breast cancer, the current thinking is that this primarily represents a differential prevalence of risk factors, rather than differential effects in producing the observed ethnic differences in breast cancer incidence. For instance, late age at first live birth is most frequent for Asian Americans, followed by whites, African Americans, and Hispanics, and the order reversed for the prevalence of high parity. Asian American women have the lowest alcohol intake and BMI, and high levels of physical activity (22,34,63). This is exemplified by a recent finding that a revised breast cancer risk assessment tool created by using African American breast cancer data better predicts breast cancer risk for African American women than the original Gail model, although the risk factors included in both models remain the same (64). Thus, understanding breast cancer disparities requires more race and ethnicity-specific research on complex interactions among biological, social, and environmental aspects of breast cancer risk.

TUMOR BIOLOGY

Breast cancer is a heterogeneous disease, with a growing number of subtypes identified using DNA microarrays (65). These different subtypes are associated with various immunohistochemical biomarkers (66). A growing body of evidence suggests that minority women are at a higher risk of having poor prognosis disease subtypes and biomarkers than white women. Alternatively, there may be yet undiscovered gene–environment interactions (e.g., exposures, reproductive patterns, and lifestyle risks) that produce the observed patterns of disease and tumor markers by race and ethnicity. In this section, we review what is currently known about breast cancer tumor biology among minority women.

Prognostic Markers

Estrogen (ER) and progesterone receptors (PR) and human epidermal growth factor receptor-2 (ERBB2, previously HER2) are the most clinically used markers and they vary by race or ethnicity. Tumor and nuclear grade also show race and ethnic variations. There are also other emerging markers, but these are not included here because of the preliminary nature of race and ethnic comparisons (67).

Studies have consistently shown that, regardless of age and menopausal status, white and Asian American women have the highest incidence of favorable prognosis ER- and PR-positive tumors, whereas African American women have the lowest incidence, and Hispanic women have intermediate levels (Table 93.1) (55,66,68–70). One recent study observed that breast tumors in African American women had decreased ER-β and increased ER-α, relative to normal tissue, and that these differences were more pronounced than among whites. Because ER-β is associated with response to tamoxifen and ER-α is associated with an adverse prognostic profile, these differences could influence the lower survival rates with ER-positive tumors observed for African American women compared with whites (69).

The population-based Carolina Breast Cancer Study (CBCS) recently reported associations between race, tumor subtypes, and survival (66). The study found that African American women were significantly more likely to have basal type breast

Table 93.1	ESTIMATED PREVALENCE RATES (%) OF DIFFERENT BREAST CANCER MORPHOLOGIC TYPES AND TUMOR MARKERS BY RACE AND ETHNICITY				
		White	African American	Hispanic	Asian American
Morphologic Type[a]	Tumor Marker		Range of Prevalence Rates (%)		
	ER+	76.4 ~ 79.5[a,b,c]	58.9 ~ 63.4[a,b]	68.0 ~ 70.9[b,c]	73.0[b]
Luminal A	ERBB2−[d]	58.1[a]	50.0[a]	—	—
Luminal B	ERBB2+	18.6[a]	13.4[a]	—	—
	ER−	20.5 ~ 23.6[a,b,c]	36.6 ~ 41.1[a,b]	29.1 ~ 32.0[b,c']	27.0[b]
Basal type	ERBB2−	17.2[a]	28.0[a]		
ERBB2+/ER−	ERBB2+	6.1[a]	8.6[a]	—	—

[a]Data source: Carolina Breast Cancer Study, 1993–1996. From Carey LA, Perou CM, Livasy CA, et al. Race, breast cancer subtypes, and survival in the Carolina Breast Cancer Study. *JAMA* 2006;295(21):2497–2502, with permission.
[b]Data source: 11 SEER cancer registries, 1992–1996. From Miller BA, Hankey BF, Thomas TL. Impact of sociodemographic factors, hormone receptor status, and tumor grade on ethnic differences in tumor stage and size for breast cancer in U.S. women. *Am J Epidemiol* 2002;155(6):534–545, with permission.
[c]Data source: Arizona Cancer Registry, 1995–2003. From Martinez ME, Nielson CM, Nagle R, et al. Breast cancer among Hispanic and non-Hispanic White women in Arizona. *J Health Care Poor Underserved* 2007;18[4 Suppl]:130–145, with permission.
[d]Formerly HER2.

cancer (*triple negative*) than non-African Americans (adjusted odds ratio [OR] 2.1, 95% confidence interval [CI] 1.3–3.4). This finding was owing to the high prevalence of basal tumors in premenopausal African American women (39%); rates were comparable in postmenopausal African Americans (14%) and pre- and postmenopausal non-African American women (16%) (*p* <.001), indicating a significant race by menopausal status interaction. Even when diagnosed with stage I disease, premenopausal African American women were more likely than other groups of women diagnosed at stage I to have triple negative disease (66). Interestingly, there were no race differences in ER- and PR-negative disease that was ERBB2 positive (52% vs. 75% for triple negative) (66). ERBB2 overexpression appears to occur with similar frequency among white, Hispanic, African American (68,71–73), and Asian American women (74) and has been linked to survival in Asians (75). Further large-scale research is needed to confirm that no race or ethnic variations exist in ERBB2 expression or its impact on outcomes (76).

Of note, after considering tumor biology and stage, African American women still had significantly lower survival in the CBCS than non-African Americans (64% and 81% vs. 81% and 91% for pre- and postmenopausal cases, respectively, *p* <.001). Similarly, African-American women have been noted to have higher histologic and nuclear grade tumors than whites, even within the same stage of disease. Even after considering stage and grade, they still have lower within-stage survival (77). These types of findings suggest that currently understood tumor biological differences cannot fully account for observed survival disparities (78).

Genetic Susceptibility Markers

Breast cancers that occur at younger ages, as are seen in African American women, may be caused more by genetic mutations than environmental, lifestyle, or behavior factors. Genetic mutations may also account for some of the within-stage survival differences seen for racial and ethnic minority women, especially when disparities persist after controlling for the quality of and access to treatment (79). We review the few studies that have explored ethnic differences in genetic susceptibility markers, such as p53, *BRCA1* and *BRCA2*, and *CYP1A1*.

TP53 is a tumor suppressor gene. Mutations of its protein, p53, lead to cell immortalization and carcinogenesis and are the most common somatic mutations associated with breast cancer (found in 50% of tumors) (80). Older studies have consistently shown p53 *somatic* mutation prevalence to be similar in tumors from African American, Hispanic, and white women (68,74). Studies of the prognostic value of p53 (74) or its mutation spectra (81) have been too small to discern reliably the ethnic differences, although some data suggest the specific genetic alterations in p53 somatic mutations vary by race (74,82). Recent studies have found that p53 mutations are most likely to be seen in ER-negative tumors, including triple negative tumors that are more common in younger African American women than other groups (66).

Germline mutations in the *BRCA1* or *BRCA2* genes also confer a markedly high risk of breast cancer, especially at young ages (83), but each hereditary breast cancer gene seems to be associated with a different tumor profile. *BRCA1* carriers appear to have higher rates of poor prognosis basal cell cancers (triple negative), whereas those with *BRCA2* have tumors with a less distinct profile and, similar to sporadic breast cancers, are more often ER positive (84). Among women with breast cancer, it appears that African Americans have rates of *BRCA1* mutations that are lower than or similar to those in whites, depending on family history (85). In a population-based, case-control study of sporadic breast cancer, *BRCA1* was detected in 2.5% of 120 white women and 0% of 88 African American women (86). A recent review found that, of the 26 *BRCA1* and 18 *BRCA2* known pathogenic mutations observed in African Americans, 58% and 56%, respectively, appear not to occur in other racial or ethnic groups (87). The 185delAG mutation that is common in Ashkenazi Jews has been detected in a high percentage (60%) of *BRCA1* mutations in women of Spanish or Latin American ancestry (88). Studies of women in Asian countries suggest that Asian women have similar or somewhat lower mutation frequencies than Western women, with a number of unique mutations identified (89,90).

A study estimating population prevalence of *BRCA1* mutations found an average rate of 8.3% among Ashkenazi Jewish women of all ages. Among minority women, Latinos had the highest rates (3.5%) and Asians the lowest (0.5%), suggesting the Latinos (of diverse ancestry) may have some unrecognized Ashkenazi Jewish ancestry (Table 93.2). The study also noted that, in minority patients diagnosed before age 35, the highest *BRCA1* prevalence was seen among African Americans (16.7% vs. 7.2% in non-Ashkenazi Jewish whites) (91).

Despite these surprisingly high rates of mutations among Latinos and young African Americans, only 10% of current *BRCA1* testing is done in minorities (92) and little is known

Table 93.2	ESTIMATED PREVALENCE RATES OF BRCA1 MUTATIONS BY RACE AND ETHNICITY IN A POPULATION-BASED SAMPLE OF PATIENTS UNDER AGE 65 WITH INVASIVE BREAST CANCER[a]				
	White Ashkenazi	non-Ashkenazi	Latino[b]	African American[c]	Asian American[d]
	n = 41	n = 508	n = 393	n = 341	n = 444
Prevalence Rate (95% CI)					
All ages	8.3% (3.1–20.1)	2.2% (0.7–6.9)	3.5% (2.1–5.8)	1.3% (0.6–2.6)	0.5% (0.1–2.0)
Under 35 years	66.7 (15.4–95.7)	7.2 (0.7–6.9)	8.9 (3.8–19.7)	16.7 (7.1–34.3)	2.4 (0.3–15.4)
50–64 years	4.8 (1.2–18.0)	0.3 (0.1–0.9)	3.0 (1.2–7.2)	0.0	0.0

[a]Weighted average of women with high and low pretest probability of having a mutation and getting tested.
[b]Latino includes third-generation U.S. born (n = 95), Mexican (n = 200), Central American (n = 49), South American (n = 28), Spain, Caribbean, and other (n = 21).
[c]Predominately U.S. born to U.S. parents (n = 331).
[d]Asian includes Chinese (n = 200), Filipino (n = 151), Japanese (n = 66), Vietnamese (n = 10), Korean (n = 3) and other (n = 14).
From John EM, Miron A, Gong G, et al. Prevalence of pathogenic BRCA1 mutation carriers in 5 US racial/ethnic groups. *JAMA* 2007;298[24]:2869–2876, with permission.

about how to recruit minorities to hereditary breast cancer research (93). Disparities in testing and use by race or ethnicity, in turn, can distort our understanding of true population prevalence and perpetuate inequities in breast cancer survival in the subgroups of women with mutations by limiting access to needed prevention, surveillance, and surgical treatment options for women unaware of their risk (94). Moreover, as noted above, prediction models that serve as the basis for counseling minority women for genetic testing have, until very recently, only been based on data from nonminority populations, leading to validity questions (94).

Making prediction even more complex for minority woman are observations that there appear to be a different spectrum of *BRCA1* mutations by race or ethnicity along with variability in mutation penetrance by group (83,95,96). It appears that the rates of *BRCA1* mutations in African Americans are not as high as would be expected based on their higher representation of tumors at early ages with aggressive features (similar to those seen in common with *BRCA1* mutations and triple negative disease). Environmental interactions or other pathways may explain the observed patterns. It will also be important to determine whether the etiologic significance of the genes is similar in women with different African or Hispanic ancestry, and create screening criteria accordingly, just as has been done in recognition of the increased risk of *BRCA1* mutations in Ashkenazi Jewish women. Thus, more data, especially population-based data, are needed to understand fully how much *BRCA* mutations (and other genetic factors) contribute to racial and ethnic disparities in biology and outcomes (79).

A number of *CYP1A1* gene polymorphisms (involved with estrogen metabolism pathways) have also been related to breast cancer risk, but results of comparisons between African Americans and whites have been inconsistent (97,98). Overall, race-related variations in gene polymorphisms might account for some differences in breast cancer risk and biology, but data are currently insufficient to be conclusive and there is a paucity of data on minority groups other than African Americans.

Gene Expression Profiling

Gene expression profiling has further highlighted the biologic heterogeneity of breast cancer and has begun to usher in the possibility for individualized therapy (99). Although several gene expression profiles have been developed, only a few are presently being evaluated in phase III clinical trials, and the predictive validity of these tests is an evolving science (e.g., Mammaprint, Oncotype DX) (100). Initial findings suggest that gene expression profiles are a better predictor of clinical out-

come than any currently used criteria or guidelines (e.g., St. Gallens, National Cancer Comprehensive Network [NCCN]) (100). However, to date we have little data regarding patterns of use of gene expression profiling in general or minority populations. A recent retrospective study by O'Neill et al. (101) suggests that minorities are equally as interested as nonminorities in genomic profiling when making treatment decisions, although this study included only 19 minority patients. The ability to provide targeted therapy could potentially contribute to reducing racial and ethnic disparities in survival.

Summary: Tumor Biology

Overall, advances in tumor profiling and genomic technology have led to a recent explosion of our understanding of breast cancer tumor biology. Data are emerging for African American women, but less information is available for other race and ethnic minority women; this will be an important research priority into the future. It will also be important to ensure that missing data on tumor biology are not differentially missing by race and ethnicity, so that conclusions about cross-group differences in tumor characteristics are not biased. Likewise, increasing accrual of minority women to correlative science studies will maximize the probability that results seen are generalizable to broader populations.

Data on tumor biology are important for ensuring that the most appropriate treatment regimens are applied for women of all race and ethnic groups, especially as more molecular targeted therapies, such as trastuzumab, are developed. These advances in knowledge of tumor biology have also generated new research on the risk factors for specific tumor profiles. As these data mature, they should generate new and exciting avenues for targeted primary prevention for minority (and other) women that consider interactions between lifestyle and other risks, environment and genes.

EARLY DETECTION OF BREAST CANCER, CLINICAL FOLLOW-UP OF ABNORMAL SCREENING, AND DIAGNOSIS

Historically, African American and Hispanic women have been observed to present with larger tumors and a more advanced stage at diagnosis than white and Asian American women (102–104). Some of these differences may be attributable to the tumor biologic factors described in the preceding section, but some are associated with psychosocial factors that affect minority women in obtaining regular screening (18,105,106) and prompt diagnostic follow-up after an abnormal result (103,107). In this section, we review the current state of the science in the early detection and clinical follow-up of minority women, with an emphasis on the contextual factors depicted on Figure 93.1.

Early Detection—Rates and Determinants

Recent mammography screening rates are close to the Healthy People 2010 goal of 70% of the population having had a mammogram within the past 1 to 2 years. By the year 2005, recent screening rates for African Americans (65%) were similar to those of whites (68%), but rates were lower for Latino (60%) and Asian women (54%) (15), perhaps because of a higher proportion of non-English speakers in these latter two minority groups (108).

According to the cross-sectional data from the Centers for Disease Control and Prevention (CDC) Behavioral Risk Factor and Surveillance Survey (BRFSS) (109) and the National Health Interview Survey (NHIS) (110), breast cancer screening rates have steadily increased over time. The current national surveillance mechanisms, however, do not assess minority women's regular screening behaviors. These population surveys are also plagued by under-representation of the most vulnerable (e.g., low education, recent immigrants, and non-English speaking minorities), and so may not accurately reflect the extent of screening problems. Thus, the data infrastructure for tracking progress in national goals for cancer screening and for eliminating disparities in early detection is inherently limited and cannot help evaluate progress for certain segments of the population.

For all race and ethnic groups, having a regular source of primary care provides key opportunities for having recent (and regular) screening, but minority women are less likely to have a regular source of care than others (104,111). Within primary care, the settings of care and provider behavior have been shown to affect screening in minority women. For example, Gemson et al. (112) reported that physician practices with 50% or higher African American patient populations were less likely to follow mammography guidelines than practices where 50% or more of the patients were white and, within the same practice, physicians were more likely to order mammograms for their white than for their African American patients. Similar results have been reported in managed care practices, where minority women are screened less often than whites (113,114), but are more likely to have regular screening than their counterparts in non-managed care settings (115,116). Among the Medicare population, physicians also order fewer mammograms for minority and low income older women than they do for white and high income older women (117).

Psychosocial, cognitive, and knowledge-related factors also affect minority women's screening behaviors (118,119). Additional barriers to mammography in minority women include lack of health insurance, the price of mammography, inconvenience, absence of symptoms, perceived low risk for breast cancer, and life conditions related to recent immigration (120–122). For instance, because 67.4% of Asian Americans and 40.2% of Hispanics are immigrants, their English proficiency and acculturation levels will all affect mammography use (108,123,124). Cultural context can also provide opportunities or impose constraints on minority women's screening behaviors (125,126). For example, cultural beliefs held more by African American women than whites (e.g., folk beliefs, religious beliefs, relationships with men, fatalism, beliefs about treatment, and knowledge) accounted for much of observed race difference in screening and stage at presentation (127,128). Other culturally related beliefs, such as reliance on self-care and modesty, also affect minority women's screening

behaviors (123,124,126). For example, Asian women report that compression of the breasts during mammography is embarrassing and harmful to their body, leading them to prefer Eastern self-care; such views are associated with low use of regular screening (124).

Socioeconomic context also explains race difference in early detection. As seen on Figure 93.1, neighborhood conditions can also constrain screening opportunities. For instance, African, Latin, and Asian Americans often live segregated or in areas of poverty and urban blight. Living in socioeconomically deprived areas, with high unemployment and crime, can lead to a life view focused on day-to-day survival and an erosion of social cohesion, community participation, and trust (i.e., *social capital*) (129). Such perspectives can represent a barrier to seeking cancer screening services, follow-up of any abnormal test results, or when symptoms develop, to a delay in obtaining needed care (130). In addition, these areas often have fewer screening facilities than other areas (131). Even after adjusting for such neighborhood socioeconomic differences, some disparities persist and within-race or -ethnic group variability in screening practices (132,133). Such results strongly suggest that there are additional levels of institutional or medical or nonmedical contextual forces, including discrimination, that affect screening in minority groups. Thus, multiple levels of factors affect screening patterns and must be considered in interventions to optimize screening use.

Early Detection in Minority Women with or at Risk for *BRCA1* and *BRCA2* Mutations

Most of the research on surveillance screening among women at high risk of breast cancer owing to *BRCA1* and *BRCA2* mutations has been done in nonminority populations. As with other groups of women, women at risk for (or with) *BRCA1* or *BRCA2* mutations are most likely to adhere to screening surveillance if they have a recommendation from a primary physician (134). Psychological stress has been noted to be negatively associated with adherence to mammography in this high risk group (135–137). However, a normal mammogram can also reassure women at high risk and reduce stress, enhancing return for the next screening (138). Similar factors may affect counseling and testing for breast cancer susceptibility mutations and subsequent mammography use among high-risk minority women (139–141). This will be an important area for further research as more minority women are tested for genetic susceptibility mutations.

Evidence-based Interventions to Increase Screening in Minority Populations

Numerous innovative interventions have been developed to increase use of screening (123,142,143). These interventions have been targeted to women, their providers, or both, and have included in-reach approaches within medical settings and outreach to at-risk communities. A full review of this literature is beyond the scope of this chapter, but the reader is referred to the National Cancer Institute (NCI)-American Cancer Society(ACS)-CDC sponsored web site called Cancer Control "PLANET" for a summary of effective approaches (144). In general, combining several approaches seems to yield the greatest effectiveness in minority groups, but the range of effect sizes is only modest (10% to 20%), indicating the complexity of health behaviors (145–147).

Follow-up After Abnormal Screening

There are several steps from the discovery of an abnormal breast screening finding to diagnostic resolution (and treatment for cancer). On average, two procedures are performed to evaluate each abnormal breast screening examination finding (148), but the appropriate time span from notification of abnormal results to diagnostic resolution has not been established. Thus, the end point of this period is variously defined in the literature as time to first diagnostic test, time to biopsy, time to completion of workup, or time to diagnostic resolution (149).

Using different time intervals, numerous studies indicate that minority women are much more likely to experience delays in diagnosis and treatment than are white women (103,107). These results have been attributed to a variety of interactions of structural, material, and behavioral factors (150). For example, research found that women who believed that treatment was unnecessary because "only God could cure cancer" were more likely to indicate that they would delay presentation for evaluation of a breast mass (128). In a study of Medicare claims, Gorin et al. (103) found that older African American women had a median of 29 day delay in biopsy confirmation of diagnosis compared with 21 days among whites and Asian Americans and Pacific Islanders (AAPI) and differences persisted after controlling for age, comorbidities, stage, city, and area poverty. Inadequate patient-provider communication, low levels of trust in the medical system, and fears of testing may also affect women's decisions to seek follow-up care (151,152). Other factors that affect delay in seeking care include lack of social support, type of medical services, health care access, and perceptions of racism (153,154).

Interventions to Improve Clinical Follow-up of Abnormal Screening Results

In the past decade, navigating women with abnormal screening to diagnostic services has gained increasing attention and has been the focus of new legislation and interventions (155,156). Recent interventions have included intensive individual counseling (157) and navigation (158), and each of these increases timely follow-up among women with breast abnormalities. For example, in one randomized, controlled trial, a patient navigation intervention with low-income and minority women with abnormal mammograms significantly increased adherence to diagnostic resolution (159). The NCI Center for Reducing Cancer Health Disparities has also funded a 5-year, national initiative to evaluate a variety of patient navigation models; results should be available around 2011 (156). Ultimately, for navigation interventions to be effective in reducing race and ethnic mortality disparities, it will be necessary to reach women who would not otherwise receive any diagnostic follow-up or to decrease clinically meaningful delays.

Summary: Early Detection of Breast Cancer, Clinical Follow-up of Abnormal Screening, and Diagnosis

Significant strides have been made in screening for minority women, although there are gaps for certain subgroups based on language, immigration status, or other factors. As screening rates have increased, attention has shifted to ensuring that all women have prompt and appropriate clinical follow-up and are able to navigate the health care system to obtain diagnostic resolution of any abnormal screening results.

TREATMENT

Once minority women are diagnosed with breast cancer, beyond disease biology and stage, survival outcomes depend on the timeliness, completeness and quality of treatment, and receipt of treatment that is appropriately targeted to tumor

markers. However, recent data demonstrate that African American and other minority patients with breast cancer often experience greater delays in treatment initiation, have more under use of appropriate adjuvant therapy, and have worse survival rates than white women, even, as noted previously, after considering tumor biology and stage (77,103,104,160–164). In this section, we review the literature on breast cancer local and systemic treatment among race and ethnic minority patients, highlighting systemic neoadjuvant and adjuvant therapy, because these modalities are largely credited with improving breast cancer survival in this phase of care and can make the most difference for minority women with poor prognosis markers (165). Most data on treatment differences by race focus on African American women; we note any relevant literature for other race or ethnic groups where data are available.

Limited data exist that describe patterns of use of neoadjuvant therapy in minority women, although most studies have shown it as an effective tool in down-staging breast cancers and decreasing the number of mastectomies performed for all race and ethnic groups (166). There may be survival differences, however, as suggested by a study comparing survival outcomes from neoadjuvant and adjuvant doxorubicin-based chemotherapy among a group of white, Hispanic, and African American women. In that trial, African Americans in the neoadjuvant group had lower rates of response to neoadjuvant chemotherapy, a lower 10-year distant metastasis-free survival rate, and a worse 10-year overall survival rate than Hispanics and whites, even after considering stage and biomarkers. Hispanic women had equivalent outcomes to white women in both the neoadjuvant and adjuvant arms (118).

If neoadjuvant therapy is not indicated, then local therapy with surgery is the next step in treatment. Some differences have been noted by race and ethnicity for primary local therapy (167,168). Several studies have noted lower use of breast conserving surgery (BCS) among Asian subgroups (e.g., Vietnamese, Filipino, Chinese, and Japanese) when compared with whites (169), but breast size differences are likely to have affected these surgical patterns. However, because lumpectomy and mastectomy have equivalent survival, these variations are not likely to explain any disparities. Local control for women who receive lumpectomy also includes radiotherapy. For example, we found that older African American Medicare beneficiaries were less likely to receive radiation after lumpectomy than older whites (170), increasing the risk of local recurrences. Of note, these older African American women also reported higher perceptions of ageist and racist attitudes during their local breast cancer treatment than older white women (170). Although this difference in the process of care is important, this finding should be considered with a note of caution, however, because a recent clinical trial for older women demonstrated that radiation and hormone therapy were equivalent to hormone therapy in women aged 65 years and older in terms of recurrence risk (171). Hispanic, Asian, and African American women have also been noted in several studies to have lower rates of breast reconstruction after mastectomy than do whites (172). Thus, the major differences in local treatment by race or ethnicity are most likely to affect quality and not quantity of life.

After local therapy, systemic hormonal and nonhormonal therapy is recommended for virtually all women with invasive breast cancer and, as with other phases of care, race and ethnic variations exist in patterns of care. For example in a 2007 study, Bickell et al. (173) found more African American and Hispanics experienced under-use of all adjuvant therapies. Prehn et al. (169) found that Chinese women were more likely than other AAPI groups and whites to have systemic therapy omitted.

For minority women with ER-negative tumors, failure to receive nonhormonal adjuvant treatment could have a significant adverse impact on survival (174). African American and other minority women have also been noted to have lower use of consultations with medical oncologists (174), receive less aggressive chemotherapy regimens (175), and be more likely than white women to discontinue chemotherapy early, resulting in lower survival (55,175,176). No evidence suggests, however, that chemotherapy pharmacokinetics differ by race or influence treatment effectiveness (177,178). For instance, Dignam et al. (178,179) demonstrated equal efficacy of adjuvant tamoxifen and chemotherapy in African American and white patients with breast cancer treated in cooperative group trials. Thus, failure of many minority women to receive standard adjuvant care may account for a portion of the mortality differential by race or ethnicity.

When African American women receive similar adjuvant chemotherapy treatments as whites (based on tumor, node, and markers), their outcomes are more comparable (179,180), although some studies in equal access health care systems still show disparities. Such results suggest that factors from other levels of influence, such as institutional discrimination, are also important (55,104,161,177,181–183).

African American women, especially those with low incomes, are also less likely to receive hormonal therapy than are white women (184), but this pattern can be changed through positive interactions with providers. For example, women whose physicians are more positive about therapy benefits, and women who are seen by an oncologist are more likely receive endocrine therapy (185). It is important to note that adherence to adjuvant endocrine therapy may differ from chemotherapy in several ways. For example, tamoxifen is an oral medication that is taken daily for a 5-year period (186). As an oral medication, a pharmacy must be accessible and its costs (up to $1,200 annually) may not be fully covered by insurance (187). Additionally, self-efficacy may have an impact on adherence to daily use. In a study of Medicaid patients, only 50% of women were adherent to their prescribed hormonal therapy after 4 years and African American women were significantly less likely to be adherent than were white women (185).

Overall, there is a paucity of data to explain these suboptimal patterns of care. From what we do know, it appears that characteristics of the social context, material constraints, and other factors that affect behavior combine to influence use of services. For instance, compared with whites, African American patients with breast cancer are more likely to list a publicly funded facility as a usual source of care. African Americans also have more comorbid illnesses, are more likely to be overweight, and are more likely to be current smokers. All of these factors affect treatment options and patterns (167,175,188). The expression of biological systems also influences treatment patterns. As one example, Griggs et al. (175) noted that African American women received lower doses of chemotherapy compared with white women, even after considering other factors. They felt that the low baseline white blood cell counts (25% to 40% lower than whites), may have limited the administration of full dose chemotherapy and the risk of infectious or hematologic toxicities (160). Alternative explanations include bias or lower acceptance of toxicity by minority patients.

A few studies have noted findings that support the idea that minority women experience bias in obtaining breast cancer treatment. One study interviewed surgeons and found that they were less likely to recommend adjuvant therapy for their minority patients (163). Physicians' perceptions that minority (and poor) patients are less likely to be compliant than whites could also lead to lower rates of adjuvant therapy referrals and fewer prescriptions for hormonal therapy (189). Interestingly, in some settings, physicians have been observed to be more contentious in their communication with their African American patients; such communicative difficulties, if also seen in oncology consultations, could decrease adherence to treatment recommendations (190). For non-English speaking Latinos and AAPI, language barriers only add to communica-

tion difficulties during the treatment process. Material constraints that lead to having few minority cancer providers could also affect recommendations for treatment and patient adherence to recommendations.

Minority patients, in turn, sometimes view the health care system as cold, unfriendly, and insensitive to their particular cultural needs (191,192). Distrust of the health care system is linked with noncompliance (193). Differences in preferences for information and expectations about care may also influence patient treatment behaviors. For example, compared with whites and African Americans, Latinos tend to rely more on family members than doctors in decisions about breast cancer treatment (194). Additionally, less acculturated Latinas are even more likely to rely on their family for treatment decision-making than more acculturated Latinas (194).

Summary: Treatment

Advances in breast cancer treatments (particularly systemic therapy) have led to greater survival from this disease. Evidence of racial disparities in receipt of treatment exists, however, especially adjuvant therapies, although we know little about treatment patterns among Asians and Latinas. In most studies, disparities in treatment are not completely explained by racial and ethnic variation in the prevalence of clinical risk factors and prognostic markers. Thus, inequities in access to state-of-the art treatment may partly explain disparities in survival among racial and ethnic minorities. Improving access and adherence to treatment may be amenable to patient- or provider-focused interventions. This will be an important area of future research. Scientific advances in genomics have led to critical information regarding gene expression, which in turn, is informing chemotherapy regimens. Further data in this area may lead to more individualized and targeted therapies. As treatment for breast cancer continues to improve and become individualized, it will be important to reduce current disparities and ensure wide-spread access to emerging therapies.

 DISCUSSION

Despite significant advances in the war against breast cancer, an understanding of the complex environmental, biologic, psychological, behavioral, and sociocultural processes and interactive pathways whereby race and ethnicity exert their influence on breast cancer outcomes remains elusive and disparities persist (104,195,196). Evidence in support of differences in tumor biology between minorities and whites is mounting and recent studies have documented distinct tumor characteristics among African American women (66). Additional population-based studies are urgently needed for other racial and ethnic subpopulations.

When resources are limited, triaging and tailoring research and service resources to those patients and communities with the greatest breast cancer burden would appear to be a logical first step. However, in the absence of any serious progress toward health care reform, and in the absence of a sustainable infrastructure for community-based participatory research and collection of surveillance data, those who need the most will undoubtedly continue to receive the least. Only efforts to involve these high-risk populations as partners in cutting-edge cancer research can ensure that the research findings will be accepted by the community and that the interventions tested have a reasonable chance of proving themselves cost-effective and sustainable after the research funding has ended.

Whether focused on service delivery or inclusion in research, comprehensive cancer centers are in a position to take the lead in forging partnerships with the medically underserved communities in their regional service areas to address disparities in cancer outcomes and to ensure delivery of laboratory and clinical innovations to populations at risk for poor cancer outcomes (197–200). Several cancer centers are developing disparities programs and community partnerships (201). The model evolving for such programs includes bringing together researchers from basic sciences to population sciences together with community stakeholders to address disparities issues using frameworks such as that depicted in Figure 93.1 (202). As we move forward, it will be important to evaluate the success of these models in improving outcomes for minority women at risk for, or with, breast cancer and for training a new generation on minority scientists to continue the war on this disease.

References

1. Greenwald P, Sondik E. Cancer control objectives for the nation: 1985–2000. *NCI Monographs* 1986;1986(2).
2. United States Department of Health and Human Services. Call to action: eliminating racial and ethnic disparities in health. Washington, DC, 1998.
3. Olopade OI, Schwartsmann G, Saijo N, et al. Disparities in cancer care: a worldwide perspective and roadmap for change. *J Clin Oncol* 2006;24(14):2135–2136.
4. Human Genome. Human Genome Project, www.genome.gov/10001722. Accessed January 1997.
5. Mountain JL, Risch N. Assessing genetic contributions to phenotypic differences among 'racial' and 'ethnic' groups. *Nat Genet* 2004;36(11 Suppl):S48–S53.
6. Tate SK, Goldstein DB. Will tomorrow's medicines work for everyone? *Nat Genet* 2004;36(11 Suppl):S34–S42.
7. Glass TA, McAtee MJ. Behavioral science at the crossroads in public health: extending horizons, envisioning the future. *Soc Sci Med* 2006;62(7):1650–1671.
8. Rebbeck TR, Halbert CH, Sankar P. Genetics, epidemiology, and cancer disparities: is it black and white? *J Clin Oncol* 2006;24(14):2164–2169.
9. Freeman HP. Poverty, race, racism, and survival. *Ann Epidemiol* 1993;3(2):145–149.
10. Catalano RA, Satariano WA. Unemployment and the likelihood of detecting early-stage breast cancer. *Am J Public Health* 1998;88(4):586–589.
11. Institute of Medicine. Ensuring quality cancer care. In: Hewitt M, Simone J, eds. Washington, DC: National Academy Press, 1999.
12. Moorman PG, Newman B, Millikan RC, et al. Participation rates in a case-control study: the impact of age, race, and race of interviewer. *Ann Epidemiol* 1999;9(3):188–195.
13. Ries LAG, Eisner M, Kosary CL, et al. SEER Cancer Statistics Review, 1975–2000. Bethesda, MD: National Cancer Institute, 2003.
14. National Cancer Institute. SEER *stat database: incidence—SEER 7 regs limited-use, November 20006 sub (2000–2004), National Cancer Institute, DCCPS, Surveillance Research Program, Cancer Statistics Branch, released April 2007, based on the November 2006 submission. Accessed December 2007.
15. American Cancer Society. ACS 2007–2008 breast cancer fact sheets based on National Health Interview Survey public data files. 2005.
16. Ries L, Melbert D, Krapcho M, et al. SEER Cancer Statistics Review, 1975–2004—based on November 2006 SEER data submission, posted to the SEER web site, 2007. Accessed January 2008.
17. National Cancer Institute, DCCPS SRP, Cancer Statistics Branch. SEER stat database: mortality—all COD, public use with state, total U.S. (1990–2004). Cancer Statistics Branch, released April 2007. Underlying mortality data provided by NCHS. Accessed December 2007.
18. Howe HL, Wu X, Ries LA, et al. Annual report to the nation on the status of cancer, 1975–2003, featuring cancer among U.S. Hispanic/Latino populations. *Cancer* 2006;107(8):1711–1742.
19. Smigal C, Jemal A, Ward E, et al. Trends in breast cancer by race and ethnicity: update 2006. *CA Cancer J Clin* 2006;56(3):168–183.
20. Trock BJ. Breast cancer in African American women: epidemiology and tumor biology. *Breast Cancer Res Treat* 1996;40(1):11–24.
21. Wu AH, Ziegler RG, Pike MC, et al. Menstrual and reproductive factors and risk of breast cancer in Asian-Americans. *Br J Cancer* 1996;73(5):680–686.
22. Pike MC, Kolonel LN, Henderson BE, et al. Breast cancer in a multiethnic cohort in Hawaii and Los Angeles: risk factor-adjusted incidence in Japanese equals and in Hawaiians exceeds that in whites. *Cancer Epidemiol Biomarkers Prev* 2002;11(9):795–800.
23. Gilliland FD, Hunt WC, Baumgartner KB, et al. Reproductive risk factors for breast cancer in Hispanic and non-Hispanic white women: the New Mexico Women's Health Study. *Am J Epidemiol* 1998;148(7):683–692.
24. Palmer JR, Wise LA, Horton NJ, et al. Dual effect of parity on breast cancer risk in African American women. *J Natl Cancer Inst* 2003;95(6):478–483.
25. Ursin G, Bernstein L, Wang Y, et al. Reproductive factors and risk of breast carcinoma in a study of white and African American women. *Cancer* 2004;101(2):353–362.
26. Pathak DR, Osuch JR, He J. Breast carcinoma etiology: current knowledge and new insights into the effects of reproductive and hormonal risk factors in black and white populations. *Cancer* 2000;88(5 Suppl):1230–1238.
27. del Carmen MG, Hughes KS, Halpern E, et al. Racial differences in mammographic breast density. *Cancer* 2003;98(3):590–596.
28. El Bastawissi AY, White E, Mandelson MT, et al. Variation in mammographic breast density by race. *Ann Epidemiol* 2001;11(4):257–263.
29. Habel LA, Capra AM, Oestreicher N, et al. Mammographic density in a multiethnic cohort. *Menopause* 2007;14(5):891–899.
30. Titus-Ernstoff L, Tosteson AN, Kasales C, et al. Breast cancer risk factors in relation to breast density (United States). *Cancer Causes Control* 2006;17(10):1281–1290.
31. Maskarinec G, Meng L, Ursin G. Ethnic differences in mammographic densities. *Int J Epidemiol* 2001;30(5):959–965.
32. Ursin G, Ma H, Wu AH, et al. Mammographic density and breast cancer in three ethnic groups. *Cancer Epidemiol Biomarkers Prev* 2003;12(4):332–338.
33. Pisano ED, Hendrick RE, Yaffe MJ, et al. Diagnostic accuracy of digital versus film mammography: exploratory analysis of selected population subgroups in DMIST. *Radiology* 2008;246(2):376–383.
34. Bernstein L, Teal C, Joslyn S, et al. Ethnicity-related variation in breast cancer risk factors. *Cancer* 2003;97(1 Suppl):222–229.
35. Hall IJ, Newman B, Millikan RC, et al. Body size and breast cancer risk in black women and white women: the Carolina breast cancer study. *Am J Epidemiol* 2000;151:754–764.
36. Palmer JR, Adams-Campbell LL, Boggs DA, et al. A prospective study of body size and breast cancer in black women. *Cancer Epidemiol Biomarkers Prev* 2007;16(9):1795–1802.
37. Wenten M, Gilliland FD, Baumgartner K, et al. Associations of weight, weight change, and body mass with breast cancer risk in Hispanic and non-Hispanic white women. *Ann Epidemiol* 2002;12(6):435–444.
38. Ziegler RG, Hoover RN, Nomura AM, et al. Relative weight, weight change, height, and breast cancer risk in Asian-American women. *J Natl Cancer Inst* 1996;88(10):650–660.
39. Wu AH, Yu MC, Tseng CC, et al. Body size, hormone therapy and risk of breast cancer in Asian American women. *Int J Cancer* 2007;120(4):844–852.
40. van den Brandt PA, Spiegelman D, Yaun SS, et al. Pooled analysis of prospective cohort studies on height, weight, and breast cancer risk. *Am J Epidemiol* 2000;152(6):514–527.
41. Friedenreich CM. Review of anthropometric factors and breast cancer risk. *Eur J Cancer Prev* 2001;10(1):15–32.
42. Swerdlow AJ, De Stavola BL, Floderus B, et al. Risk factors for breast cancer at young ages in twins: an international population-based study. *J Natl Cancer Inst* 2002;94(16):1238–1246.
43. Galanis DJ, Kolonel LN, Lee J, et al. Anthropometric predictors of breast cancer incidence and survival in a multi-ethnic cohort of female residents of Hawaii, United States. *Cancer Causes Control* 1998;9(2):217–224.
44. Baer HJ, Rich-Edwards JW, Colditz GA, et al. Adult height, age at attained height, and incidence of breast cancer in premenopausal women. *Int J Cancer* 2006;119(9):2231–2235.
45. Palmer JR, Rao RS, Adams-Campbell LL, et al. Height and breast cancer risk: results from the Black Women's Health Study (United States). *Cancer Causes Control* 2001;12(4):343–348.
46. Ogden CL, Carroll MD, Curtin LR, et al. Prevalence of overweight and obesity in the United States, 1999–2004. *JAMA* 2006;295(13):1549–1555.
47. Adams-Campbell LL, Rosenberg L, Rao RS, et al. Strenuous physical activity and breast cancer risk in African American women. *J Natl Med Assoc* 2001;93(7–8):267–275.
48. Slattery ML, Edwards S, Murtaugh MA, et al. Physical activity and breast cancer risk among women in the southwestern United States. *Ann Epidemiol* 2007;17(5):342–353.
49. McTiernan A. Associations between energy balance and body mass index and risk of breast carcinoma in women from diverse racial and ethnic backgrounds in the U.S. *Cancer* 2000;88(5 Suppl):1248–1255.
50. Colditz GA, Feskanich D, Chen WY, et al. Physical activity and risk of breast cancer in premenopausal women. *Br J Cancer* 2003;89(5):847–851.
51. Mertens AJ, Sweeney C, Shahar E, et al. Physical activity and breast cancer incidence in middle-aged women: a prospective cohort study. *Breast Cancer Res Treat* 2006;97(2):209–214.
52. Chang SC, Ziegler RG, Dunn B, et al. Association of energy intake and energy balance with postmenopausal breast cancer in the prostate, lung, colorectal, and ovarian cancer screening trial. *Cancer Epidemiol Biomarkers Prev* 2006;15(2):334–341.
53. Anderson SE, Dallal GE, Must A. Relative weight and race influence average age at menarche: results from two nationally representative surveys of U.S. girls studied 25 years apart. *Pediatrics* 2003;111(4 Pt 1):844–850.
54. Rossouw JE, Anderson GL, Prentice RL, et al. Risks and benefits of estrogen plus progestin in healthy postmenopausal women: principal results From the Women's Health Initiative randomized controlled trial. *JAMA* 2002;288(3):321–333.
55. Li CI, Malone KE, Daling JR. Differences in breast cancer stage, treatment, and survival by race and ethnicity. *Arch Intern Med* 2003;163(1):49–56.
56. Moorman PG, Kuwabara H, Millikan RC, et al. Menopausal hormones and breast cancer in a biracial population. *Am J Public Health* 2000;90(6):966–971.
57. Ravdin PM, Cronin KA, Howlader N, et al. The decrease in breast-cancer incidence in 2003 in the United States. *N Engl J Med* 2007;356(16):1670–1674.
58. Glass AG, Lacey JV Jr, Carreon JD, et al. Breast cancer incidence, 1980–2006: combined roles of menopausal hormone therapy, screening mammography, and estrogen receptor status. *J Natl Cancer Inst* 2007;99(15):1152–1161.
59. Davis S, Mirick DK. Circadian disruption, shift work and the risk of cancer: a summary of the evidence and studies in Seattle. *Cancer Causes Control* 2006;17(4):539–545.
60. O'Leary ES, Schoenfeld ER, Stevens RG, et al. Shift work, light at night, and breast cancer on Long Island, New York. *Am J Epidemiol* 2006;164(4):358–366.
61. Nie J, Beyea J, Bonner MR, et al. Exposure to traffic emissions throughout life and risk of breast cancer: the Western New York Exposures and Breast Cancer (WEB) study. *Cancer Causes Control* 2007;18(9):947–955.
62. Woodruff TJ, Parker JD, Kyle AD, et al. Disparities in exposure to air pollution during pregnancy. *Environ Health Perspect* 2003;111(7):942–946.
63. Hall IJ, Moorman PG, Millikan RC, et al. Comparative analysis of breast cancer risk factors among African American women and white women. *Am J Epidemiol* 2005;161(1):40–51.
64. Gail MH, Anderson WF, Garcia-Closas M, et al. Absolute risk models for subtypes of breast cancer. *J Natl Cancer Inst* 2007;99(22):1657–1659.
65. Perou CM, Sorlie T, Eisen MB, et al. Molecular portraits of human breast tumours. *Nature* 2000;406(6797):747–752.
66. Carey LA, Perou CM, Livasy CA, et al. Race, breast cancer subtypes, and survival in the Carolina Breast Cancer Study. *JAMA* 2006;295(21):2492–2502.
67. Furberg H, Millikan RC, Geradts J, et al. Environmental factors in relation to breast cancer characterized by p53 protein expression. *Cancer Epidemiol Biomarkers Prev* 2002;11(9):829–835.
68. Elledge RM, Clark GM, Chamness GC, et al. Tumor biologic factors and breast cancer prognosis among white, Hispanic, and black women in the United States. *J Natl Cancer Inst* 1994;86:705–712.
69. Miller BA, Hankey BF, Thomas TL. Impact of sociodemographic factors, hormone receptor status, and tumor grade on ethnic differences in tumor stage and size for breast cancer in U.S. women. *Am J Epidemiol* 2002;155(6):534–545.

70. Martinez ME, Nielson CM, Nagle R, et al. Breast cancer among Hispanic and non-Hispanic White women in Arizona. *J Health Care Poor Underserved* 2007;18(4 Suppl):130–145.
71. Lai H, Lai S, Ma F, et al. Prevalence and spectrum of p53 mutations in white Hispanic and non-Hispanic women with breast cancer. *Breast Cancer Res Treat* 2003;81(1):53–60.
72. Weiss SE, Tartter PI, Ahmed S, et al. Ethnic differences in risk and prognostic factors for breast cancer. *Cancer* 1995;76:268–274.
73. Peredo R, Sastre G, Serrano J, et al. Her-2/neu oncogene expression in Puerto Rican females with breast cancer. *Cell Mol Biol (Noisy-le-grand)* 2001;47(6):1025–1032.
74. Shiao YH, Chen VW, Scheer WD, et al. Racial disparity in the association of p53 gene alterations with breast cancer survival. *Cancer Res* 1995;55(7):1485–1490.
75. Selvarajan S, Wong KY, Khoo KS, et al. Over-expression of c-erbB-2 correlates with nuclear morphometry and prognosis in breast carcinoma in Asian women. *Pathology* 2006;38(6):528–533.
76. Millikan R, Eaton A, Worley K, et al. HER2 codon 655 polymorphism and risk of breast cancer in African Americans and whites. *Breast Cancer Res Treat* 2003; 79(3):355–364.
77. McBride R, Hershman D, Tsai WY. Within-stage racial differences in tumor size and number of positive lymph nodes in women with breast cancer. *Cancer* 2007; 110(6):1201–1208.
78. Ihemelandu CU, Leffall LD Jr, DeWitty RL, et al. Molecular breast cancer subtypes in premenopausal African American women, tumor biologic factors and clinical outcome. *Ann Surg Oncol* 2007;14(10):2994–3003.
79. Ademuyiwa FO, Olopade OI. Racial differences in genetic factors associated with breast cancer. *Cancer Metastasis Rev* 2003;22(1):47–53.
80. Thor AD, Yandell DW. Prognostic significance of p53 overexpression in node-negative breast carcinoma: preliminary studies support cautious optimism. *J Natl Cancer Inst* 1993;85(3):176–177.
81. Hussain SP, Harris CC. Molecular epidemiology of human cancer: contribution of mutation spectra studies of tumor suppressor genes. *Cancer Res* 1998;58(18): 4023–4037.
82. Jones BA, Kasl SV, Howe CL, et al. African American/white differences in breast carcinoma: p53 alterations and other tumor characteristics. *Cancer* 2004;101(6): 1293–1301.
83. Chen S, Parmigiani G. Meta-analysis of BRCA1 and BRCA2 penetrance. *J Clin Oncol* 2007;25(11):1329–1333.
84. Hedenfalk I, Duggan D, Chen Y, et al. Gene-expression profiles in hereditary breast cancer. *N Engl J Med* 2001;344(8):539–548.
85. Panguluri RC, Brody LC, Modali R, et al. BRCA1 mutations in African Americans. *Hum Genet* 1999;105(1–2):28–31.
86. Newman B, Mu H, Butler LM, et al. Frequency of breast cancer attributable to BRCA1 in a population-based series of American women. *JAMA* 1998;279(12):915–921.
87. Olopade OI, Fackenthal JD, Dunston G, et al. Breast cancer genetics in African Americans. *Cancer* 2003;97(1 Suppl):236–245.
88. Mullineaux LG, Castellano TM, Shaw J, et al. Identification of germline 185delAG BRCA1 mutations in non-Jewish Americans of Spanish ancestry from the San Luis Valley, Colorado. *Cancer* 2003;98(3):597–602.
89. Ikeda N, Miyoshi Y, Yoneda K, et al. Frequency of BRCA1 and BRCA2 germline mutations in Japanese breast cancer families. *Int J Cancer* 2001;91(1):83–88.
90. Zhi X, Szabo C, Chopin S, et al. BRCA1 and BRCA2 sequence variants in Chinese breast cancer families. *Hum Mutat* 2002;20(6):474.
91. John EM, Miron A, Gong G, et al. Prevalence of pathogenic BRCA1 mutation carriers in 5 U.S. racial/ethnic groups. *JAMA* 2007;298(24):2869–2876.
92. Huo D, Olopade OI. Genetic testing in diverse populations: are researchers doing enough to get out the correct message? *JAMA* 2007;298(24):2910–2911.
93. Hughes C, Peterson SK, Ramirez A, et al. Minority recruitment in hereditary breast cancer research. *Cancer Epidemiol Biomarkers Prev* 2004;13(7):1146–1155.
94. Hall MJ, Olopade OI. Disparities in genetic testing: thinking outside the BRCA box. *J Clin Oncol* 2006;24(14):2197–2203.
95. Fackenthal JD, Olopade OI. Breast cancer risk associated with BRCA1 and BRCA2 in diverse populations. *Nat Rev Cancer* 2007;7(12):937–948.
96. Nanda R, Schumm LP, Cummings S, et al. Genetic testing in an ethnically diverse cohort of high-risk women: a comparative analysis of BRCA1 and BRCA2 mutations in American families of European and African ancestry. *JAMA* 2005;294(15): 1925–1933.
97. Taioli E, Bradlow HL, Garbers SV, et al. Role of estradiol metabolism and CYP1A1 polymorphisms in breast cancer risk. *Cancer Detect Prev* 1999;23(3):232–237.
98. Bailey LR, Roodi N, Verrier CS, et al. Breast cancer and CYPIA1, GSTM1, and GSTT1 polymorphisms: evidence of a lack of association in Caucasians and African Americans. *Cancer Res* 1998;58(1):65–70.
99. Piccart-Gebhart MJ, Sotiriou C. Adjuvant chemotherapy—yes or no? Prognostic markers in early breast cancer. *Ann Oncol* 2007;18(Suppl 12):xii2–xii7.
100. Morris SR, Carey LA. Gene expression profiling in breast cancer. *Curr Opin Oncol* 2007;19(6):547–551.
101. O'Neill SC, Brewer NT, Lillie SE, et al. Women's interest in gene expression analysis for breast cancer recurrence risk. *J Clin Oncol* 2007;25(29):4628–4634.
102. Lantz PM, Mujahid M, Schwartz K, et al. The influence of race, ethnicity, and individual socioeconomic factors on breast cancer stage at diagnosis. *Am J Public Health* 2006;96(12):2173–2178.
103. Gorin SS, Heck JE, Cheng B, et al. Delays in breast cancer diagnosis and treatment by racial/ethnic group. *Arch Intern Med* 2006;166(20):2244–2252.
104. Hahn KM, Bondy ML, Selvan M, et al. Factors associated with advanced disease stage at diagnosis in a population-based study of patients with newly diagnosed breast cancer. *Am J Epidemiol* 2007;166(9):1035–1044.
105. Smith-Bindman R, Miglioretti DL, Lurie N, et al. Does utilization of screening mammography explain racial and ethnic differences in breast cancer? *Ann Intern Med* 2006;144(8):541–553.
106. Sarker M, Jatoi I, Becher H. Racial differences in breast cancer survival in women under age 60. *Breast Cancer Res Treat* 2007;106(1):135–141.
107. Jacobson JS, Grann VR, Hershman D, et al. Breast biopsy and race/ethnicity among women without breast cancer. *Cancer Detect Prev* 2006;30(2):129–133.
108. Jacobs EA, Karavolos K, Rathouz PJ, et al. Limited English proficiency and breast and cervical cancer screening in a multiethnic population. *Am J Public Health* 2005;95(8):1410–1416.
109. Center for Disease Control and Prevention, Available at http://apps.nccd.cdc.gov/brfss/race.asp?cat=WH&yr=2006&qkey=4421&state=UB. Accessed January 2008.
110. Breen N, Yabroff KR, Meissner HI. What proportion of breast cancers are detected by mammography in the United States? *Cancer Detect Prev* 2007;31(3):220–224.
111. Ward E, Halpern M, Schrag N, et al. Association of insurance with cancer care utilization and outcomes. *CA Cancer J Clin* 2008;58(1):9–31.
112. Gemson DH, Elinson J, Messeri P. Differences in physician prevention practice patterns for white and minority patients. *J Community Health* 1988;13:53–64.
113. Fox SA, Stein JA. The effect of physician-patient communication on mammography utilization by different ethnic groups. *Med Care* 1991;29(11):1065–1082.
114. Schneider EC, Zaslavsky AM, Epstein AM. Racial disparities in the quality of care for enrollees in Medicare managed care. *JAMA* 2002;287(10):1288–1294.
115. O'Malley AS, Forrest CB, Mandelblatt J. Adherence of low-income women to cancer screening recommendations. *J Gen Intern Med* 2002;17(2):144–154.
116. Haas JS, Phillips KA, Sonneborn D, et al. Effect of managed care insurance on the use of preventive care for specific ethnic groups in the United States. *Med Care* 2002;40(9):743–751.
117. Coleman EA, O'Sullivan P. Racial differences in breast cancer screening among women from 65 to 74 years of age: trends from 1987–1993 and barriers to screening. *J Women Aging* 2001;13(3):23–39.
118. Consedine NS, Magai C, Spiller R. Breast cancer knowledge and beliefs in subpopulations of African American and Caribbean women. *Am J Health Behav* 2004;28(3):260–271.
119. Farmer D, Reddick B, D'Agostino R, et al. Psychosocial correlates of mammography screening in older African American women. *Oncol Nurs Forum* 2007;34(1): 117–123.
120. Ogedegbe G, Cassells AN, Robinson CM, et al. Perceptions of barriers and facilitators of cancer early detection among low-income minority women in community health centers. *J Natl Med Assoc* 2005;97(2):162–170.
121. Lee-Lin F, Menon U, Pett M, et al. Breast cancer beliefs and mammography screening practices among Chinese American immigrants. *J Obstet Gynecol Neonatal Nurs* 2007;36(3):212–221.
122. Cui Y, Peterson NB, Hargreaves M, et al. Mammography use in the Southern Community Cohort Study (United States). *J Health Care Poor Underserved* 2007;18(4 Suppl):102–117.
123. Wang JH, Liang W, Schwartz MD, et al. Development and evaluation of a culturally tailored educational video: changing breast cancer-related behaviors in Chinese women. *Health Educ Behav* 2008;35(6):806–820.
124. Liang W, Wang JH, Chen MY, et al. Developing and validating a measure of Chinese cultural views of health and cancer. *Health Educ Behav* 2008;35(3): 361–375.
125. Guidry JJ, Greisinger A, Aday L, et al. Barriers to cancer treatment: a review of published research. *Oncol Nur Forum* 1996;23(9):1393–1398.
126. Simon CE. Breast cancer screening: cultural beliefs and diverse populations. *Health Soc Work* 2006;31(1):36–43.
127. Lannin DR, Mathews HF, Mitchell J, et al. Influence of socioeconomic and cultural factors on racial differences in late-stage presentation of breast cancer. *JAMA* 1998;279(22):1801–1807.
128. Mitchell J, Lannin DR, Mathews HF, et al. Religious beliefs and breast cancer screening. *J Womens Health (Larchmt)* 2002;11(10):907–915.
129. Kawachi I, Kennedy BP, Lochner K, et al. Social capital, income inequality, and mortality. *Am J Public Health* 1997;87(9):1491–1498.
130. Womeodu RJ, Bailey JE. Barriers to cancer screening. *Med Clin North Am* 1996;80(1):115–133.
131. Mandelblatt J, Andrews H, Wallace R, et al. Impact of access and social context on breast cancer stage at diagnosis. *J Health Care Poor Underserved* 1995;6(3): 342–351.
132. Wells KJ, Roetzheim RG. Health disparities in receipt of screening mammography in Latinas: a critical review of recent literature. *Cancer Control* 2007;14(4):369–379.
133. Gomez S, Tan S, Keegan TH. Disparities in mammographic screening for Asian women in California: a cross-sectional analysis to identify meaningful groups for targeted intervention. BMC *Cancer* 2007;7(1):201.
134. Tinley ST, Houfek J, Watson P, et al. Screening adherence in BRCA1/2 families is associated with primary physicians' behavior. *Am J Med Genet A* 2004;125(1): 5–11.
135. Thorpe JM, Kalinowski CT, Patterson ME, et al. Psychological distress as a barrier to preventive care in community-dwelling elderly in the United States. *Med Care* 2006;44(2):187–191.
136. Schwartz MD, Taylor KL, Willard KS. Prospective association between distress and mammography utilization among women with a family history of breast cancer. *J Behav Med* 2003;26(2):105–117.
137. Gil F, Mendez I, Sirgo A, et al. Perception of breast cancer risk and surveillance behaviours of women with family history of breast cancer: a brief report on a Spanish cohort. *Psychooncology* 2003;12(8):821–827.
138. Tyndel S, Austoker J, Henderson BJ, et al. What is the psychological impact of mammographic screening on younger women with a family history of breast cancer? Findings from a prospective cohort study by the PIMMS Management Group. *J Clin Oncol* 2007;25(25):3823–3830.
139. Kendall J, Kendall C, Catts ZA, et al. Using adult learning theory concepts to address barriers to cancer genetic risk assessment in the African American community. *J Genet Couns* 2007;16(3):279–288.
140. Halbert C, Kessler L, Collier A, et al. Psychological functioning in African American women at an increased risk of hereditary breast and ovarian cancer. *Clin Genet* 2005;68(3):222–227.
141. Kinney AY, Bloor LE, Mandal D, et al. The impact of receiving genetic test results on general and cancer-specific psychologic distress among members of an African American kindred with a BRCA1 mutation. *Cancer* 2005;104(11):2508–2516.
142. Wilkin HA, Valente TW, Murphy S, et al. Does entertainment-education work with Latinos in the United States? Identification and the effects of a telenovela breast cancer storyline. *J Health Commun* 2007;12(5):455–469.
143. Darnell JS, Chang CH, Calhoun EA. Knowledge about breast cancer and participation in a faith-based breast cancer program and other predictors of mammography screening among African American women and Latinas. *Health Promot Pract* 2006;7(3 Suppl):201S–212S.
144. National Cancer Institute, Centers for Disease Control and Prevention, American Cancer Society. Cancer Control "PLANET." Accessed data January 2008.
145. Mandelblatt JS, Yabroff KR. Effectiveness of interventions designed to increase mammography use: a meta-analysis of provider-targeted strategies. *Cancer Epidemiol Biomarkers Prev* 1999;8(9):759–767.
146. Yabroff KR, O'Malley A, Mangan PA, et al. Inreach and and outreach interventions to improve mammography use. *J Am Med Womens Assoc* 2001;56(4):166–173.
147. Yabroff KR, Mandelblatt JS. Interventions targeted toward patients to increase mammography use. *Cancer Epidemiol Biomarkers Prev* 1999;8(9):749–757.

148. Kerlikowske K, Grady D, Barclay J, et al. Positive predictive value of screening mammography by age and family history of breast cancer. *JAMA* 1993;270(20):2444–2450.

149. Kerlikowske K. Timeliness of follow-up after abnormal screening mammography. *Breast Cancer Res Treat* 1996;40(1):53–64.

150. Strzelczyk JJ, Dignan MB. Disparities in adherence to recommended follow-up on screening mammography: interaction of sociodemographic factors. *Ethn Dis* 2002;12(1):77–86.

151. Padgett DK, Yedidia MJ, Kerner J, et al. The emotional consequences of false positive mammography: African American women's reactions in their own words. *Women Health* 2001;33(3–4):1–14.

152. Kerner JF, Yedidia M, Padgett D, et al. Realizing the promise of breast cancer screening: clinical follow-up after abnormal screening among black women. *Prev Med* 2003;37(2):92–101.

153. Bastani R, Yabroff KR, Myers RE, et al. Interventions to improve follow-up of abnormal findings in cancer screening. *Cancer* 2004;101(5 Suppl):1188–1200.

154. Kaplan CP, Eisenberg M, Erickson PI, et al. Barriers to breast abnormality follow-up: minority, low-income patients' and their providers' view. *Ethn Dis* 2005;15(4):720–726.

155. Kaiser Daily Health Policy Report. Available: from http://www.kaisernetwork.org/Daily_reports/rep_index.cfm?DR_ID=30975. Accessed January 2008.

156. National Cancer Institute, National Institutes of Health. Center to Reduce Cancer Health Disparities. Patient Navigator Research Program. http://crchd.cancer.gov/pnp/pnrp-index.html. Accessed January 2007.

157. Ell K, Padgett D, Vourlekis B, et al. Abnormal mammogram follow-up: a pilot study in women with low income. *Cancer Pract* 2002;10(3):130–138.

158. Battaglia TA, Roloff K, Posner MA, et al. Improving follow-up to abnormal breast cancer screening in an urban population. A patient navigation intervention. *Cancer* 2007;109(2 Suppl):359–367.

159. Ell K, Vourlekis B, Lee PJ, et al. Patient navigation and case management following an abnormal mammogram: a randomized clinical trial. *Prev Med* 2007;44(1):26–33.

160. Hershman D, Weinberg M, Rosner Z, et al. Ethnic neutropenia and treatment delay in African American women undergoing chemotherapy for early-stage breast cancer. *J Natl Cancer Inst* 2003;95(20):1545–1548.

161. Griggs JJ, Culakova E, Sorbero ME, et al. Effect of patient socioeconomic status and body mass index on the quality of breast cancer adjuvant chemotherapy. *J Clin Oncol* 2007;25(3):277–284.

162. Griggs JJ, Culakova E, Sorbero ME, et al. Social and racial differences in selection of breast cancer adjuvant chemotherapy regimens. *J Clin Oncol* 2007;25(18):2522–2527.

163. Bickell NA, LePar F, Wang JJ, et al. Lost opportunities: physicians' reasons and disparities in breast cancer treatment. *J Clin Oncol* 2007;25(18):2516–2521.

164. Lyman GH, Dale DC, Crawford J. Incidence and predictors of low dose-intensity in adjuvant breast cancer chemotherapy: a nationwide study of community practices. *J Clin Oncol* 2003;21(24):4524–4531.

165. Barrett RE, Cho YI, Weaver KE, et al. Neighborhood change and distant metastasis at diagnosis of breast cancer. *Ann Epidemiol* 2008;18(1):43–47.

166. Cance WG, Carey LA, Calvo BF, et al. Long-term outcome of neoadjuvant therapy for locally advanced breast carcinoma: effective clinical downstaging allows breast preservation and predicts outstanding local control and survival. *Ann Surg* 2002;236(3):295–302.

167. Bradley CJ, Given CW, Roberts C. Race, socioeconomic status, and breast cancer treatment and survival. *J Natl Cancer Inst* 2002;94(7):490–496.

168. Shavers VL, Harlan LC, Stevens JL. Racial/ethnic variation in clinical presentation, treatment, and survival among breast cancer patients under age 35. *Cancer* 2003;97(1):134–147.

169. Prehn AW, Topol B, Stewart S, et al. Differences in treatment patterns for localized breast carcinoma among Asian/Pacific islander women. *Cancer* 2002;95(11):2268–2275.

170. Mandelblatt JS, Kerner JF, Hadley J, et al. Variations in breast carcinoma treatment in older Medicare beneficiaries: is it black or white. *Cancer* 2002;95(7):1401–1414.

171. Hughes KS, Schnaper LA, Berry D, et al. Lumpectomy plus tamoxifen with or without irradiation in women 70 years of age or older with early breast cancer. *N Engl J Med* 2004;351(10):971–977.

172. Joslyn SA. Patterns of care for immediate and early delayed breast reconstruction following mastectomy. *Plast Reconstr Surg* 2005;115(5):1289–1296.

173. Bickell NA, Wang JJ, Oluwole S, et al. Missed opportunities: racial disparities in adjuvant breast cancer treatment. *J Clin Oncol* 2006;24(9):1357–1362.

174. Pierce L, Fowble B, Solin LJ, et al. Conservative surgery and radiation therapy in black women with early stage breast cancer. Patterns of failure and analysis of outcome. *Cancer* 1992;69(11):2831–2841.

175. Griggs JJ, Sorbero ME, Stark AT, et al. Racial disparity in the dose and dose intensity of breast cancer adjuvant chemotherapy. *Breast Cancer Res Treat* 2003;81(1):21–31.

176. Mandelblatt J, Hadley J, Kerner J, et al. Patterns of breast carcinoma treatment in older women: patient preferences and clinical and physician influences. *Cancer* 2000;89(3):561–573.

177. Dignam JJ. Efficacy of systemic adjuvant therapy for breast cancer in African American and Caucasian women. *J Natl Cancer Inst Monogr* 2001;(30):36–43.

178. Dignam JJ, Redmond CK, Fisher B, et al. Prognosis among African American women and white women with lymph node negative breast carcinoma: findings from two randomized clinical trials of the National Surgical Adjuvant Breast and Bowel Project (NSABP). *Cancer* 1997;80(1):80–90.

179. Dignam JJ. Differences in breast cancer prognosis among African American and Caucasian women. *CA Cancer J Clin* 2000;50(1):50–64.

180. Banerjee M, George J, Yee C, et al. Disentangling the effects of race on breast cancer treatment. *Cancer* 2007;110(10):2169–2177.

181. Newman LA, Singletary SE. Overview of adjuvant systemic therapy in early stage breast cancer. *Surg Clin North Am* 2007;87(2):499–509, xi.

182. Du W, Simon MS. Racial disparities in treatment and survival of women with stage I-III breast cancer at a large academic medical center in metropolitan Detroit. *Breast Cancer Res Treat* 2005;91(3):243–248.

183. Curtis E, Quale C, Haggstrom D, et al. Racial and ethnic differences in breast cancer survival: how much is explained by screening, tumor severity, biology, treatment, comorbidities, and demographics? *Cancer* 2008;112(1):171–180.

184. Silliman RA, Guadagnoli E, Rakowski W, et al. Adjuvant tamoxifen prescription in women 65 years and older with primary breast cancer. *J Clin Oncol* 2002;20(11):2680–2688.

185. Partridge AH, Wang PS, Winer EP, et al. Nonadherence to adjuvant tamoxifen therapy in women with primary breast cancer. *J Clin Oncol* 2003;21(4):602–606.

186. Early Breast Cancer Trialists' Collaborative Group. Tamoxifen for early breast cancer: an overview of the randomised trials. *Lancet* 1998;351:1451–1467.

187. Cardinale B. Drug topics red book-pharmacy fundamental reference. Montvale NJ: Medical Economics Company, 1998.

188. Ghafoor A, Jemal A, Cokkinides V, et al. Cancer statistics for African Americans. *CA Cancer J Clin* 2002;52(6):326–341.

189. Price JH, Desmond SM, Snyder FF, et al. Perceptions of family practice residents regarding health care and poor patients. *J Fam Pract* 1988;27(6):615–621.

190. Street RL Jr, Gordon H, Haidet P. Physicians' communication and perceptions of patients: is it how they look, how they talk, or is it just the doctor? *Soc Sci Med* 2007;65(3):586–598.

191. Blendon RJ, Buhr T, Cassidy EF, et al. Disparities in health: perspectives of a multi-ethnic, multi-racial America. *Health Aff (Millwood)* 2007;26(5):1437–1447.

192. Johnson RL, Saha S, Arbelaez JJ, et al. Racial and ethnic differences in patient perceptions of bias and cultural competence in health care. *J Gen Intern Med* 2004;19(2):101–110.

193. Armstrong K, Ravenell KL, McMurphy S, et al. Racial/ethnic differences in physician distrust in the United States. *Am J Public Health* 2007;97(7):1283–1289.

194. Maly RC, Umezawa Y, Ratliff CT, et al. Racial/ethnic group differences in treatment decision-making and treatment received among older breast carcinoma patients. *Cancer* 2006;106(4):957–965.

195. Chlebowski RT, Chen Z, Anderson GL, et al. Ethnicity and breast cancer: factors influencing differences in incidence and outcome. *J Natl Cancer Inst* 2005;97(6):439–448.

196. Tammemagi CM. Racial/ethnic disparities in breast and gynecologic cancer treatment and outcomes. *Curr Opin Obstet Gynecol* 2007;19(1):31–36.

197. The DC Cancer Coalition. DC Cancer Control Plan 2005–2010. Accessed January 2008.

198. Sheppard VB, Cox LS, Kanamori MJ, et al. Brief report: if you build it, they will come: methods for recruiting Latinos into cancer research. *J Gen Intern Med* 2005;20(5):444–447.

199. Kreling BA, Canar J, Catipon E, et al. Latin American Cancer Research Coalition. Community primary care/academic partnership model for cancer control. *Cancer* 2006;107(8 Suppl):2015–2022.

200. Betancourt JR, Maina AW. The Institute of Medicine report "Unequal treatment": implications for academic health centers. *Mt Sinai J Med* 2004;71(5):314–321.

201. Emmons KM, Burns WK, Benz EJ. Development of an integrated approach to cancer disparities: one cancer center's experience. *Cancer Epidemiol Biomarkers Prev* 2007;16(11):2186–2192.

202. Plowfield LA, Wheeler EC, Raymond JE. Time, tact, talent, and trust: essential ingredients of effective academic-community partnerships. *Nurs Educ Perspect* 2005;26(4):217–220.

Chapter 94
Nursing Care in Patient Management and Quality of Life

Karen M. Meneses

Nurses have an integral role in the interdisciplinary management of patients from prevention, screening, and early detection through diagnosis, treatment, recurrence, and survivorship. This chapter is divided into patient care management during early-stage disease, with focuses on patient care during surgery, radiation therapy, chemotherapy, targeted therapy, and hormonal therapy; and patient care management during advanced disease. Each section emphasizes patient management issues related to education, symptom management, and psychosocial support.

 PATIENT CARE MANAGEMENT IM EARLY-STAGE BREAST CANCER

Education

Practice guidelines for the treatment of early-stage breast cancer are well publicized and are available to patients and their families (1). Patients who are best able to make decisions about treatment are those who can express and communicate their beliefs, feelings, and preferences, who actively listen to information shared by their oncology team, and who search out additional information or second opinions from trusted and respected sources (1,2). Likewise, clinicians who are best able to assist patients in making reasonable decisions about treatment are those who recognize that decision-making is a process that occurs over time and who acknowledge patients' vulnerability in making decisions (3–5).

Numerous patient teaching materials are available in print (e.g., books, pamphlets, and brochures) and in audiovisual (tapes and audiocassettes), computer-assisted, and web-based formats to help patients in making decisions about treatment (4–6). In addition, electronic support groups, face-to-face support groups, counselors, and individual networking efforts contribute to helping patients find information. The sheer volume of information available can be overwhelming and can sometimes hinder decision-making (7). Clinicians can foster patient decision-making by on-going assessment of their patients' developmental stage, educational level, degree of anxiety, energy level, personal coping styles, past experiences, and family history (5,6). Nurses can help patients and their families discern what is useful during this stressful time and what can be used at a later date by knowing what resources are available in their institution, in the community, and regionally and nationally.

Preoperative Teaching

Specific preoperative teaching focuses on information about the procedure, incision and drain care, pain management, lymphedema prevention and management, and prosthetic devices (8–10). In the United States, length of stay for mastectomy is about a day. Thus, preoperative teaching ideally begins in the surgeon's office. Patients generally find that a simple pamphlet, brochure, or video that illustrates the surgical experience beginning with admission, surgery, and recovery helps to orient them to the surgical facility and procedures.

Patient teaching before surgery may include instructions about stopping use of any aspirin-containing products, vitamin E, and herbal preparations for at least 7 days preoperatively. Because postoperative pain medications that contain opioids, such as acetaminophen (Tylenol) with codeine, morphine, and hydrocodone (Vicodin), can cause constipation, it is helpful for patients to drink several glasses of water before midnight the night before surgery. Similar to other surgical procedures, no solid food or drink may be ingested at least 6 hours preoperatively.

On the day of surgery, patients may feel comfortable wearing a loose-fitting blouse with front tab buttons for ease of comfort, particularly when axillary node dissection is planned. The National Lymphedema Network (NLN) (11) suggests that patients measure both arms in specific areas preoperatively. The measurement can serve as a baseline to monitor for changes in arm measurement during treatment and follow-up.

Symptom Management after Mastectomy

Incisional Wound and Drain Care

Nurses can provide specific information about dressing changes, measurement and recording of drainage, monitoring for signs and symptoms of infection, and personal hygiene (9,10). Patients generally prefer a description of what their surgical incision will look like, and an appropriate visual diagram or photograph helps to illustrate the anticipated results. Postoperatively, patients need instruction on how to care for the Jackson-Pratt drain, how to empty the drain, and how to record the amount of fluid. Patients are very sore after surgery, however, and may find the drains difficult to manage or empty. Patients need to prevent or minimize unnecessary pressure, to prevent accidental dislodgement.

Patients find it helpful to have a family member or friend close by to help them with physical care, personal hygiene, and monitoring for potential postoperative complications (i.e., seroma, hematoma, increased pain or discomfort, or fever). Eating light foods such as clear broth or soup, fruit juices, and soft foods may help ease postanesthesia effects such as nausea. For general comfort, patients find it helpful to use lots of pillows to support the affected arm and back. In case of an emergency, patients should be provided with after-hours telephone numbers to contact the surgeon and team.

Pain Management and Comfort Measures

Postoperative pain varies widely, depending on individual and cultural characteristics, the surgical procedure, and pain medication relief (12,13). Some patients have relatively little discomfort with lumpectomy and require mild analgesics, whereas others may have pain after mastectomy and reconstruction that requires stronger analgesia. A plan for postsurgical pain management is best individualized between the clinician and patient with regular monitoring of pain relief.

Postoperative sensations and pain, such as muscle tightness, difficulty in lifting of the arm, and soreness around the shoulder, are to be expected (13). Support for the arm and shoulder during the first 24 postoperative hours and avoidance of active stretching or pulling until after the drains are removed are helpful. Gentle stretching exercises can usually begin soon after surgery (usually 48 hours) and should be individualized to reflect the extent of the operation, the presence of drains, and the preoperative capabilities of the patient. For patients who will receive radiation therapy as part of their treatment, regaining adequate range of motion is extremely important because the radiation treatment position requires the arm to be abducted at a 160-degree angle. The reader is referred to Chapter 45 for information related to Lymphedema.

Prosthetic Fitting

Prosthetic fitting for women who have had mastectomy and reconstruction is generally done around the first postoperative follow-up appointment or when the incision has healed. However, women benefit from receiving specific information about how, when, and where to purchase a prosthesis and from having a temporary prosthesis in hand before hospital discharge. Many different prosthetics are available, such as soft forms and self-adhering forms, in a variety of colors and textures. There are also stylish and specially designed lingerie and bathing suits that can accommodate the prosthesis. Having a sample of a breast prosthesis and mastectomy bra to use during preoperative teaching is useful.

Care after Breast Reconstruction

Although breast reconstruction approximates the look of the natural breast, it cannot duplicate the same look and feel (13). After reconstruction, patients may start home exercises such as brisk walking, stationary bike riding, and gentle stretching exercises. Avoiding high-impact aerobics, jogging, and lifting weights above 5 to 10 pounds is recommended for several weeks after reconstruction (14). Baron and Vaziri (14) suggest that patients avoid the use of health spas and public swimming pools until after the incision lines and drain sites are healed.

Psychosocial Recovery

Detailed discussions of patients' psychological reaction and support programs are found elsewhere in the text. Specific preoperative discussions in which clinicians can engage with their patients include attending to the emotional impact of the initial diagnosis and treatment of breast cancer and acknowledging that the surgical experience marks the beginning of a long recovery period. Other psychosocial strategies include the following: helping patients to reframe their time sequence; reordering priorities about work, family, and social activities; and encouraging short-term thinking (e.g., practice 1 day at a time, practice thought-stopping that provokes anxiety, and think through the process of the events of the week and the time it takes to accomplish tasks).

 # PATIENT CARE MANAGEMENT DURING RADIATION THERAPY

Education

Teaching patients about radiation therapy ideally begins during the consultation visit, when the role of radiation therapy in the overall treatment plan, additional diagnostic studies needed, and treatment planning are discussed. Patients may be apprehensive about starting radiation but generally are relieved to learn that side effects are well tolerated (15). Information about radiation treatment planning includes the rationale for simulation, the need to minimize radiation dose to vital organs such as the lung and heart, and the construction of immobilization devices to keep the limbs in consistent position during treatment. Patients must plan to spend sufficient time for the simulation procedure, must be prepared to feel some discomfort while lying on a hard simulation table, must understand that the radiation therapist will place a permanent tattoo or skin markings (e.g., the size of a freckle) directly on their skin surface to help reproduce the treatments on a daily basis, and must realize that simulation is *not* a radiation treatment (16,17).

Jahraus et al. (15) evaluated the impact of an education program on knowledge of patients with breast cancer who were receiving radiation therapy. Subjects (n = 79) completed questionnaires before and after an education program. The education consisted of a 20-minute interactive video (first session); individualized education, including technical procedures and self-care (second session); and a 1-hour class (third session). Individual teaching as required was provided afterward during radiation therapy. These investigators found an increase in knowledge scores, a finding indicating that the program was effective.

After simulation is completed, patients receive an appointment to start treatment that will be given daily, 5 days a week. Patients find it helpful when the radiation oncology nurse gives information about a typical day or week's treatment so that they can obtain a mental picture of the experience. Patients also find it helpful to keep a diary of daily activities and appointments. Some patients also prefer to bring a tape player to listen to their relaxation tapes or music during treatment. The first treatment generally takes about 30 to 45 minutes; subsequent treatments take about 15 minutes. Patients often feel uncomfortable while lying on a hard treatment table. They may be disconcerted by the sounds emanating from the radiation treatment machine. Patients need reassurance that although they are alone during treatment, the radiation therapists remain in contact with them by screen monitor and intercom. Today, radiation oncology departments are often located on the ground floor, with natural light, serene wall colors, and artwork. Soothing background music helps to allay patients' anxiety.

Symptom Management During Radiation Therapy

Symptom management includes teaching about the potential side effects of radiation therapy, self-care measures to manage the side effects, and managing the overall radiation therapy experience. The acute physical side effects of radiation therapy are skin reactions and fatigue.

Skin Reactions

Radiation-induced skin effects range from slight peeling, dryness, tanning and itchiness, and breast tenderness and fullness to moist desquamation (17–23). The severity of skin reactions is related to radiation factors (i.e., total dose, fractionation, energy beam, bolus treatment, and volume of tissue treated), patient factors (e.g., breast size, age, nutritional state, presence of comorbid disease), and treatment factors, such as previous or concurrent chemotherapy. Particularly susceptible areas of skin breakdown include the inframammary fold and supraclavicular areas.

Teaching patients self-care skin management during radiation ideally begins before or at the start of treatment. The radiation oncology team examines patients for acute side effects on a weekly basis and as needed as therapy progresses. Whereas patients often believe that natural products or creams are more beneficial, Heggie et al. (24) found no differences with respect to the efficacy of topical aloe vera gel compared with aqueous cream on radiated skin. Although there are variations in practice, some general teaching guidelines for skin care during radiation therapy are listed on Table 94.1.

Fatigue

Fatigue is recognized as one of the most prevalent symptom of cancer and its treatment (25–29). Fatigue can be a chronic problem that results from several causes (i.e., treatment and pathophysiologic, behavioral, and emotional factors). It occurs during treatment and persists even after treatment ends. Patients with cancer report that fatigue has a negative influence on quality of life: It can impair the ability to function or maintain daily routines (e.g., weakness, no energy), influence emotional reaction (e.g., sadness, irritability), and interrupt work schedules (e.g., poor attention or concentration). Although rest can restore a normal level of functioning in the healthy person, this restorative capacity is diminished in patients with cancer. Patients receiving radiation therapy report a usual pattern of fatigue that gradually rises by the third week of treatment and gradually declines after therapy ends. Some patients experience less fatigue on weekends, when radiation is not delivered.

The National Comprehensive Cancer Network (NCCN) practice guidelines for cancer-related fatigue (25) use a treatment algorithm of regular patient evaluation and a brief screening instrument. These guidelines for cancer-related fatigue can be

---

| Table 94.1 | **SKIN CARE INTERVENTIONS DURING RADIATION THERAPY** |

Side Effect	Onset after Start of Radiation Therapy	Appearance/Presentation	Intervention
Erythema	2 wk	Mild redness progressing to bright redness; mild to moderate discomfort	Cleanse skin with unscented soap (e.g., Basis, Pears, Neutrogena) Use lukewarm water in shower and bath Lubricate skin with water-based moisturizer containing no perfumes Do not use deodorant in underarm of treated breast Wear loose-fitting cotton garments and avoid wool and other scratchy fabrics against skin Protect radiated skin from sun, wind, and temperature extremes
Hyperpigmentation	2 wk	Mild to deep tanning; more pronounced in dark-skinned patients; dark brown dots on skin surface	Same as above
Folliculitis	2 wk	Itchy skin; red dots appear in sternal, infraclavicular, and supraclavicular areas	Apply cool wet packs to skin Oatmeal colloidal-based soap (e.g., Aveeno)
Antihistamine for generalized itching may be taken at bedtime			0.5% corticosteroid cream to affected area; apply thin layer *after* radiation treatment Unscented moisturizer Aloe vera gel
Dryness or dry desquamation	2–3 wk	Dry, flaking, peeling skin; accompanies folliculitis; most often occurs in supraclavicular areas	Unscented moisturizer Aloe vera gel
Moist desquamation	4–5 wk; may occur after radiation therapy during chemotherapy	Moist peeling of skin; denuded areas exposed; associated with moderate discomfort particularly in inframammary fold	Cleanse area with quarter-strength hydrogen peroxide solution Keep area dry with a soft dressing Moisture vapor permeable dressing may be applied Do not use tape directly on area of skin breakdown Nonsteroidal anti-inflammatory drug for moderate to severe discomfort
Breast fullness or heaviness			Use firm, athletic support bra

Modified from O'Rourke N, Robinson L. Breast cancer and the role of radiation therapy. In: Dow KH, ed. *Contemporary issues in breast cancer.* Sudbury, MA.: Jones & Bartlett, 1996, with permission.

accessed at www.nccn.org. Basic cancer-related information is given after initial screening. A more focused evaluation is done when the patient has moderate or higher levels of fatigue. Patients are evaluated based on five factors known to be associated with fatigue: pain, emotional distress, sleep disturbance, anemia, and hypothyroidism. The presence of any of these factors requires treatment with patient reevaluation. If none of the factors is present or if the fatigue is unresolved, a more comprehensive assessment is recommended, including a thorough review of systems, review of medications, assessment of comorbidity, nutritional and metabolic evaluation, and assessment of activity level.

Specific causes of fatigue such as infection, fluid and electrolyte imbalances, or cardiac dysfunction are treated accordingly. Nonpharmacologic and pharmacologic treatment of the fatigue is considered when specific causes are not identified. Nonpharmacologic interventions may include a moderate exercise program to improve functional capacity and activity tolerance, restorative therapies to decrease cognitive alterations and improve mood state, and nutritional and sleep interventions for patients with disturbances in eating or sleeping. Pharmacologic therapy may include drugs such as antidepressants for depression or erythropoietin for anemia.

Patients may also experience problems with physical functioning, sleep, and attention, for which exercise and sleep hygiene programs are being evaluated (30–34). Effective management of cancer-related fatigue involves an informed and supportive oncology care team that assesses patients' fatigue levels regularly and systematically and incorporates education and counseling regarding strategies for coping with fatigue (25).

Psychosocial and Family Support

Radiation treatments require daily visits over a 4- to 5-week period that may require adjustment in work, family, and social patterns. Patients welcome assistance in helping them reorganize their work schedules to accommodate daily treatment (35,36). Strategies include scheduling radiation treatment at either the beginning or end of the workday, shortening the workday schedule when possible, or even taking a temporary leave of absence from work during radiation. Because of the daily imposition of the radiation treatment schedule, other patients may need assistance with home management and child care. Older patients or those with mobility problems may additionally require assistance in traveling to and from daily treatment.

PATIENT CARE MANAGEMENT DURING CHEMOTHERAPY

Symptom Management during Chemotherapy

The most common physical symptoms experienced are nausea and vomiting, bone marrow depression, hair loss, fatigue, weight gain, mucositis, neurotoxicity, menopausal symptoms, and, rarely, hemorrhagic cystitis. Managing vascular access devices (VAD) and decreasing risk of extravasation are also important aspects of clinical care.

Bone Marrow Depression

Neutropenia is a dose-limiting toxicity of chemotherapy. The nadir is predictable and occurs about 10 to 14 days after treatment, with recovery occurring about 3 to 4 weeks later. Signs and symptoms of infection include fever, pain and tenderness,

change in elimination of urine and stool, lethargy, myalgia, and malaise. Observed signs of infection are generally absent in moderate to severe neutropenia because of the lack of circulating neutrophils.

Ongoing and early assessment, identification, and patient education about the signs and symptoms of infection, handwashing, and meticulous personal hygiene are essential components in preventing and reducing neutropenia-related infections (37,38). The NCCN Myeloid Growth Factors Guidelines examined therapeutic efficacy and clinical benefit (37). The practice guidelines include risk assessment, prophylaxis of high risk patients, and judicious use of myeloid growth factors.

Nausea and Vomiting

With the widespread use of serotonin antagonists, nausea and vomiting are manageable side effects of chemotherapy (39–47). Chemotherapy-induced nausea and vomiting are categorized as acute (during treatment), delayed (>24 hours after therapy), and anticipatory (a classic conditioned response as a result of inadequate antiemetic therapy). The risks of nausea and vomiting are related to the type and dose of chemotherapy used and individual patient factors, such as female gender, younger age, previous chemotherapy, and history of motion sickness (43–45). The emetogenic potential of chemotherapeutic agents is classified from high to low. Typical chemotherapeutic agents used to treat breast cancer, such as cisplatin, cyclophosphamide, doxorubicin, and methotrexate, have either moderate to high emetogenic potential. Although several antiemetic regimens are available, they must be individualized for each patient (46). Inadequate control of nausea and vomiting during treatment can lead to anticipatory nausea and vomiting, which is more difficult to manage (46).

The serotonin antagonists, used either alone or in combination with corticosteroids, have led to a substantial improvement in the control of nausea and vomiting. These agents are highly selective for 5-HT$_3$ receptors and are best used with highly emetogenic chemotherapeutic regimens. The serotonin antagonists do not have the extrapyramidal reactions more commonly associated with dopamine antagonists.

Other classes of antiemetics include dopamine antagonists (i.e., metoclopramide, phenothiazines, and butyrophenones), corticosteroids, benzodiazepines, and cannabinoids. Centrally acting agents, such as phenothiazine and metoclopramide, have untoward side effects, such as sedation, dizziness, extrapyramidal reactions, and anticholinergic effects such as dry mouth and constipation (46). Dopamine antagonists alone or in combination help to relieve moderate and delayed nausea and vomiting.

Nonpharmacologic interventions for nausea and vomiting are used as an adjunct to pharmacologic measures and include behavioral interventions (e.g., hypnosis, passive relaxation), acupressure, and dietary modifications (46,47). Dibble et al. (47) found acupressure to be an adjunct to pharmacologic management of nausea and vomiting, particularly delayed nausea and vomiting.

Metoclopramide and dexamethasone have improved efficacy compared with the serotonin antagonists with delayed nausea and vomiting. Benzodiazepines have some efficacy in anticipatory nausea and vomiting. Although anticipatory nausea and vomiting (ANV) is less likely to occur in patients receiving short-term adjuvant chemotherapy (45), ANV may occur in patients with metastatic disease who are receiving ongoing therapy.

Mucositis

Mucositis is a general term that refers to an inflammation of the mucosa. The incidence of chemotherapy-induced mucositis increases with high-dose chemotherapy (48–50). Agents that are considered highly stomatotoxic are the antimetabolites, anthracyclines, plant alkaloids, and taxanes. Patient factors that are considered to confer a higher risk of developing mucositis include older age, alcohol and tobacco use, poor oral hygiene, poor nutritional status, use of ill-fitting dentures, and compromised renal function (48–49).

Consistent use of an oral care regimen offers the best protection against mucositis. Pretreatment strategies to prevent and decrease the incidence of oral complications include a baseline oral assessment, treatment of preexisting dental disease, and patient education (48). Effective oral care protocols include a combination of a cleansing method, use of lubricants, measures to relieve pain and inflammation, and measures to prevent or treat infection (48).

In an extensive Cochrane Database systematic review of the literature on the use of Chinese medicinal herbs to treat side effects of chemotherapy, including mucositis, in breast cancer patients, Zhang et al. (50) found highly limited evidence about the effectiveness of medicinal herbs in alleviating chemotherapy side effects.

Neurotoxicity

Patients receiving 5-fluorouracil and paclitaxel are at risk of neurotoxic complications (51). Peripheral neuropathies present with loss of sensation that begins at the fingertips and spreads to the wrist and starts from the toes and spreads to the ankles. With additional therapy, progressive muscle pain, weakness, motor changes, and hypersensitivity to heat and intolerance to cold can occur (51).

Neurotoxicity associated with paclitaxel includes numbness and paresthesias in the hands and feet that can worsen over time with treatment. Treatment of neurotoxicity has included changes in dose and timing (51). One study evaluated vitamin-E prophylaxis against chemotherapy-induced neuropathy demonstrating a neuroprotective effect (52).

Alopecia

Alopecia includes body hair loss (e.g., eyelashes and eyebrows, axillary, and pubic hair). The literature continues to demonstrate that hair loss remains one of the most distressing side effects of chemotherapy (53). Although a mastectomy scar is devastating, hair loss can be publicly stigmatizing. Hair loss is often viewed as an assault to one's physical appearance, body image, self-esteem, and sexuality. Although patients may cognitively prepare for hair loss, the actual occurrence is most often a difficult emotional experience.

Chemotherapeutic agents can cause either partial or complete atrophy of the hair root bulb constricting the hair shaft, which can break easily. Different chemotherapy agents have the differential ability to induce hair loss based on their route of administration, dosing schedules, and peak blood levels. For example, doxorubicin is most commonly linked to alopecia. Patterns of doxorubicin-associated hair loss generally occur 2 to 3 weeks after initial treatment, with continued hair loss occurring over time. Conversely, paclitaxel-associated hair loss often occurs dramatically and suddenly. Methotrexate and fluorouracil are associated with minimal hair loss. Oral cyclophosphamide is related to hair thinning, particularly at the crown.

Patient teaching should stress and reassure that hair loss is temporary. Useful interventions for hair loss include the following:

Before Hair Loss Occurs
- Cut hair in a manageable and easy to maintain style before chemotherapy.
- Use a mild, protein-based shampoo and conditioner.
- Use an electric hair dryer on the lowest setting.
- Avoid electric curlers and curling irons, hair spray, and hair dye that may increase the fragility of hair.

- Avoid excessive brushing and hair combing.
- Purchase a wig to fit one's normal hair color and style.
- Consider accessing the American Cancer Society's program, "Look Good . . . Feel Better" for additional tips on managing hair loss.

After Hair Loss Occurs
- Protect exposed scalp from excessive temperature changes.
- Use emollient or lotion to moisturize the scalp.
- Reduce scalp itching by using an oatmeal-based colloidal soap.
- Use scarves and turbans as an alternative to wigs.

Arthralgia and Myalgia

Myalgias and arthralgias can occur in patients receiving paclitaxel (54). Symptoms are dose related. Paclitaxel, at doses less than 170 mg/m^2, is associated with mild discomfort, whereas doses greater than 200 mg/m^2 are associated with more severe discomfort and pain. Effects occur 48 to 72 hours after infusion and can persist for up to 7 days. Effects occur primarily in large joints, but they can involve the whole body. Pharmacologic interventions, such as nonsteroidal analgesics or narcotics, are usually required. Nonpharmacologic interventions include warm baths, relaxation techniques, and massage therapy.

Hemorrhagic Cystitis

Hemorrhagic cystitis is an uncommon complication of chemotherapy that can occur more often in patients receiving high-dose chemotherapy. Symptoms range from microscopic hematuria to frank bleeding. Maintaining adequate hydration of at least 80 ounces of fluid daily and patient education are key factors in preventing this side effect. High-risk patients require hyperhydration, frequent voiding, dipstick testing, and diuresis. Patients should also be instructed to report dysuria, bladder irritation, or suprapubic pain promptly.

Behavioral Symptoms

Behavioral symptoms during adjuvant chemotherapy and after treatment include changes in energy, sleep, mood, depressive symptoms, and cognition (55–58). Behavioral symptoms are related to a serious disruption in quality of life and can persist for many years after treatment. Treatment and cancer survivorship plans include information about the range of anticipated time that behavioral sequelae occur. Behavioral symptom management relies on cognitive-behavioral strategies.

Management Issues in Chemotherapy Administration

Central venous catheters and vascular access devices are commonly used, which increases comfort and ease during chemotherapy and blood product administration (59). Several VAD are readily available, and the choice depends on the specific need for chemotherapy and blood products and length of time required for VAD. The various types of VAD available include tunneled central venous catheters (e.g., Hickman, Groshong), peripherally inserted central catheters, implantable ports (e.g., Port-A-Cath), and peripheral ports (PAS Port), which are used for long-term continuous or intermittent therapy. Peripheral needle and peripheral catheters are generally selected for short-term access. Management of VAD requires knowledge of their selection, placement, port-insertion care, accessing, flushing, site care, troubleshooting, and repairing (59). Patient factors must also be taken into account. For example, external devices must be flushed, cleaned, and cared for, and thus, the patient's ability to understand instructions, properly care for the catheter, and purchase supplies are important.

Occlusion and infection are the complications that occur with VAD. Intraluminal catheter occlusion or the inability to withdraw blood or to infuse fluid is the general result of a blood clot, precipitant, or an unknown factor (59). When this occurs with a port, the general cause is improper placement of the needle in the septum rather than the portal. Although the risk of infection is less with a VAD, nevertheless these devices can become locally infected at the catheter exit site. Symptoms include redness, warmth, swelling, and discomfort. Management may require appropriate blood culture and antibiotics.

Minimizing Extravasation

Extravasation is defined as "the accidental injection or leakage of drugs into the perivascular or subcutaneous spaces during an intravenous administration" (60,61). It is a serious complication, causing pain, swelling, erythema, paresthesias, and ulceration of tissue. The reported incidence of extravasation ranges from 0.01% to 6% (60). Factors influencing the degree of extravasation include the type of vesicant, the dose, and the concentration.

Chemotherapeutic agents are classified as either vesicants (drugs causing tissue damage if extravasated) or irritants (drugs that cause redness and inflammatory reaction at the injection site without necrosis or ulceration). The anthracyclines are the chemotherapeutic agents used in breast cancer that are classified as vesicants (60,61). Because vesicants cause extensive tissue damage, major efforts are made to prevent that complication. When extravasation occurs, antidotes differ depending on the chemotherapeutic agent.

Irritants include fluorouracil, mitoxantrone, and etoposide. Irritants are more readily metabolized, removed from the injection site, and excreted compared with vesicants. Assessment parameters to differentiate extravasation from irritation or flare reaction include pain, redness, ulceration, swelling, and blood return. An extravasation kit should be readily available and generally includes 10% or 25% sodium thiosulfate, hyaluronidase (stored in refrigerator), 5- and 10-mL syringes, sterile water, sterile saline, and 19- and 25-gauge needles (61).

Hypersensitivity Reactions

Hypersensitivity reactions can occur within a few seconds after the start of paclitaxel infusion, usually within the first 10 minutes. Vital signs monitoring is recommended every 15 minutes for the first hour of infusion, followed by every 30 minutes in the second hour of infusion. Paclitaxel is formulated in Cremophor EL, which causes the polyvinylchloride intravenous tubing and bag to leach into the infusion fluid. Thus, this agent is administered in either glass or polyolefin containers using a 0.22-μ filter and polyethylene-lined intravenous administration sets. Premedication regimens of oral steroids, diphenhydramaine, and cimetidine have decreased the incidence of hypersensitivity reactions (62).

Psychosocial Support

Psychosocial response during chemotherapy is considered the most difficult to manage. The associated acute physical side effects combined with the longer duration of chemotherapy contribute to a deeper psychological burden compared with the effects from radiation therapy or surgery alone. Patients need encouragement to pace their activities, to incorporate their treatment into their daily family and work routines, and, most of all, to be encouraged to ask for and receive assistance. Many patients appreciate the support they receive from others who have *been there* or who are going through similar experiences.

Others take comfort in their family and interpersonal relationships. Breast cancer patients are increasingly using electronic means of support through chat rooms and blogs (63). Most patients prefer to maintain a normal lifestyle during chemotherapy. They may continue to work as long as they desire, but may request a treatment schedule that permits recovery from side effects on days off from work. Other patients may request that their chemotherapy treatment be given on weekends or evenings. Clinicians support patients by accommodating their reasonable requests as much as possible.

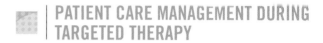

PATIENT CARE MANAGEMENT DURING TARGETED THERAPY

Symptom Management

Targeted therapies have differential side effects. Trastuzumab can cause heart damage and must be used cautiously in patients receiving anthracyclines (64,65). Bevacizumab can cause delay in wound healing, high blood pressure, or kidney damage (66). Lapatinib can cause side effects, such as diarrhea and acneiform skin reactions, and red and painful hands and feet (67). Lapatinib is an oral agent that can have several drug–drug interactions. Patients on herbal products such as St. John's wort should discontinue use while on lapatinib. Diarrhea can become severe. Patients must contact their oncologist immediately with symptoms of dehydration. They are also restricted from eating grapefruit or grapefruit juice while on lapatinib.

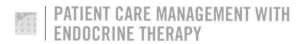

PATIENT CARE MANAGEMENT WITH ENDOCRINE THERAPY

Symptom Management

Tamoxifen and aromatase inhibitors (AI) have similar side effect profiles with both classes of endocrine therapy showing similar effects on quality of life (68,69). Hot flashes are common to both tamoxifen and AI. Nonhormonal treatments have included antidepressants and gabapentin (70). Sexual dysfunction, such as vaginal dryness and dyspareunia, have been reported (71). Increased bone turnover, reduced bone density, and increase in fractures have been reported with AI (72). In addition, adherence to endocrine therapy over time has been a challenge to clinicians (73).

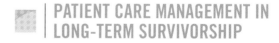

PATIENT CARE MANAGEMENT IN LONG-TERM SURVIVORSHIP

Education

The end of treatment is associated with a decline in physical side effects, such as nausea and vomiting, hair loss, and bone marrow depression. It is also associated with a return to some semblance of order and routine. However, breast cancer survivors often experience many physical and psychosocial adjustments after treatment ends (72–76). Physiologic effects that can persist include sexuality issues, menopausal symptoms, weight gain, and fertility issues in younger women (77–84). Psychosocial adjustments may be marked by feelings of sadness, grief, loss, emotional letdown, and uncertainty over the future. Furthermore, social adjustments and concerns about managing relationships with spouse or significant others,

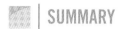

children, family members and friends, sexuality issues, dealing with work and insurance concerns, and the existential focus of finding meaning in the experience of breast cancer are very real and expected tasks of managing illness demands in the after-treatment period.

Psychosocial Support

Responses of Spouse or Significant Other

Breast cancer exerts its effect on the spouse or significant other, particularly during active treatment (73–76,85–87). Family research indicates that spouses assume many of the daily home responsibilities during active treatment. When treatment ends, however, the responsibilities shift back to patients. Rarely does a diagnosis of breast cancer lead to major disruption of a marital or intimate relationship. Relationships that were stable before the diagnosis tend to remain stable after treatment. Conversely, relationships that were marked by discord continue to experience strain after treatment ends. Although women may take advantage of the social support groups available for breast cancer survivors, spouses and significant others do so less often. One promising avenue for spouses to find information and exchange concerns is through web-based discussions and chat rooms dedicated to breast cancer survivors.

Children's Concerns

Mothers with breast cancer report various concerns about their children that range from daily disruptions (becoming sick during chemotherapy) to existential questions about dying and leaving the children behind (85,88,89). The day-to-day concerns center on how to talk to their children about breast cancer without unnecessarily frightening them. A child's strengths and vulnerabilities, cognitive capacities, developmental level age, and gender are the major influences of children's response to mother's breast cancer.

Adjustment to Work

Work issues can be major hurdles in adjustment after breast cancer (90–92). Breast cancer survivors may desire to continue working or may seek new work or professional employment after treatment ends. Worry about health insurance and benefits poses a high priority concern. Several cancer advocacy organizations, particularly the National Coalition for Cancer Survivorship, have excellent pamphlets and books that discuss the insurance, employment, legal, and financial matters of high concern to cancer survivors that are well worth the cost of having copies in one's organization patient lending library.

Meaning in Illness

Patients have used many resources and avenues in helping them manage the breast cancer survivorship experience. Some become active in breast cancer advocacy; others volunteer at a local cancer organization to give talks, to meet other breast cancer survivors, and to coach others through the experience; whereas others choose to spend time with close family and friends. The means are as varied and as individual as the women themselves. The main point to convey to other breast cancer survivors is that there *is* life after cancer (93). Although life may be different from before the breast cancer experience, it can be an inherently fulfilling and satisfying experience. Women can choose to dwell on the negative aspects if they desire, but in many breast cancer survivors' published experiences, many rewards were unforeseen or unknown at the time of their diagnosis. Only in reflecting back on their experiences were they able to identify the many strengths and rewards.

SUMMARY

In summary, the human dimension of living through and beyond the breast cancer experience is more than management of acute physical side effects. It is the careful attention to *persons* with breast cancer, their unique personality, preference, choices, decisions, experiences, and insight that give meaning, shape, and form to the illness and disease. On a day-to-day basis, oncology nurses are a vital component to the oncology team by helping to coordinate patient care, manage symptoms and psychosocial distress, manage the daily patient ebb and flow, evaluate quality-of-life outcomes, and add the critical dimension of caring to oncology care.

References

1. National Comprehensive Cancer Network Practice Guidelines. Accessed at http://www.nccn.org February 1, 20207.
2. Mellink WA, Dulmen AM, Wiggers T, et al. Cancer patients seeking a second surgical opinion: results of a study on motives, needs, and expectations. *J Clin Oncol* 2003; 21(8):1492–1497.
3. Whelan T, Sawka C, Levine M, et al. Helping patients make informed choices: a randomized trial of a decision aid for adjuvant chemotherapy in lymph node-negative breast cancer. *J Natl Cancer Inst* 2003;95:581.
4. Sepucha KR, Belkora JK, Aviv C, et al. Improving the quality of decision making in breast cancer: consultation planning template and consultation recording template. *Oncol Nurs Forum* 2003;30:99.
5. Davison BJ, Degner LF. Feasibility of using a computer-assisted intervention to enhance the way women with breast cancer communicate with their physicians. *Cancer Nurs* 2002;25:417.
6. Charles CA, Whelan T, Gafni A, et al. Shared treatment decision making: what does it mean to physicians? *J Clin Oncol* 2003;21:932.
7. Rees CE, Bath PA. Information-seeking behaviors of women with breast cancer. *Oncol Nurs Forum* 2001;28:899.
8. Murphy A, Holcombe C. Effects of early discharge following breast surgery. *Prof Nurse* 2001;16:1087–1090.
9. Chapman D, Purushotham AD. Acceptability of early discharge with drain in situ after breast surgery. *Br J Nurs* 2001–2002;10:1447.
10. Lynn J. Surgery techniques. In: Dow KH, ed. *Contemporary issues in breast cancer*, 2nd ed. Sudbury, MA: Jones & Bartlett, 2004.
11. National Lymphedema Network. Accessed at: http://www.lymphnet.org/ February 1, 2007.
12. Kwekkeboom K. Postmastectomy pain syndromes. *Cancer Nurs* 1996;19:37.
13. Baron RH, Fey JV, Raboy S, et al. Eighteen sensations after breast cancer surgery: a comparison of sentinel lymph node biopsy and axillary lymph node dissection. *Oncol Nurs Forum* 2002;29:65.
14. Baron R, Vaziri N, Reconstructive surgery. In: Dow KH ed. *Contemporary issues in breast cancer*, 2nd ed. Sudbury, MA, Jones & Bartlett, 2004:90–108.
15. Jahraus D, Sokolosky S, Thurston N, et al. Evaluation of an education program for patients with breast cancer receiving radiation therapy. *Cancer Nurs* 2002;25:266.
16. McQuestion M. Evidence-based skin care management in radiation therapy. *Semin Oncol Nurs* 2006;22:163–173.
17. Lopez E, Guerrero R, Nunez M, et al. Early and late skin reactions to radiotherapy for breast cancer and their correlation with radiation-induced DNA damage in lymphocytes. *Breast Cancer Res* 2005;7:R690–R698.
18. Bentzen S, Overgaard J. Patient-to-patient variability in the expression of radiation-induced normal tissue injury. *Semin Radiat Oncol* 1994;4:69.
19. Sitton E. Early and late radiation-induced skin alterations: I. Mechanisms of skin changes. *Oncol Nurs Forum* 1992;19:801.
20. Sitton E. Early and late radiation-induced skin alterations: II. Nursing care of irradiated skin. *Oncol Nurs Forum* 1992;19:907.
21. Archambeau J, Pezner R, Wasserman T. Pathophysiology of irradiated skin and breast. *Int J Radiat Oncol Biol Phys* 1995;31:1171.
22. Aistars J. The validity of skin care protocols followed by women with breast cancer receiving external radiation. *Clin J Oncol Nurs* 2006;10:487–492.
23. Porock D, Kristjanson L. Skin reactions during radiotherapy for breast cancer: the use and impact of topical agents and dressings. *Eur J Cancer Care (Engl)* 1999;8:143.
24. Heggie S, Bryant GP, Tripcony L, et al. A phase III study on the efficacy of topical aloe vera gel on irradiated breast tissue. *Cancer Nurs* 2002;25:442.
25. Cancer-related fatigue. NCCN clinical practice guidelines in oncology. Accessed at nccn.org/professionals/physicians_gls/PDF/fatigue.pdf. February 1, 2008.
26. Minton O, Stone P. How common is fatigue in disease-free breast cancer survivors? A systematic review of the literature. *Breast Cancer Res Treat* 2008;112:5–13.
27. Woo B, Dibble SL, Piper BF, et al. Differences in fatigue by treatment methods in women with breast cancer. *Oncol Nurs Forum* 1998;25:915.
28. Vogelzang, NJ, Breitbart, W, Cella, D, et al. Patient, caregiver, and oncologist perceptions of cancer-related fatigue: results of a tri-part assessment survey. *Semin Hematol* 1997;34(Suppl 2):4.
29. Jacobsen PB, Donovan KA, Small BJ, et al. Fatigue after treatment for early stage breast cancer: a controlled comparison. *Cancer* 2007;110:1851–1859.
30. Mock V, Hassey Dow K, Meares C, et al. Effects of exercises on fatigue, physical functioning, and emotional distress during radiation therapy for breast cancer. *Oncol Nurs Forum* 1997;24:991.
31. Quesnel C, Savard J, Simard S, et al. Efficacy of cognitive-behavioral therapy for insomnia in women treated for nonmetastatic breast cancer. *J Consult Clin Psychol* 2003;71:189.
32. Berger AM, VonEssen S, Kuhn BR, et al. Adherence, sleep, and fatigue outcomes after adjuvant breast cancer chemotherapy: results of a feasibility intervention study. *Oncol Nurs Forum* 2003;30:513.

33. Courneya K, Segal R, Mackey J, et al. Effects of aerobic and resistance exercise in breast cancer patients receiving adjuvant chemotherapy: a multicenter randomized controlled trial. *J Clin Oncol* 2007;25:4396–4404.

34. Donovan K, Small B, Andrykowski M, et al. Utility of a cognitive-behavioral model to predict fatigue following breast cancer treatment. *Health Psych* 2007;26:464–472.

35. Wengstrom Y, Haggmark C, Forsberg C. Coping with radiation therapy: effects of a nursing intervention on coping ability for women with breast cancer. *Int J Nurs Pract* 2001;7:8.

36. Kolcaba K, Fox C. The effects of guided imagery on comfort of women with early stage breast cancer undergoing radiation therapy. *Oncol Nurs Forum* 1999;26:67.

37. NCCN Practice Guidelines in Oncology–v.1.2008. Meyloid growth factors. Available at http://nccn.org/professionals/physicians_gls/PDF/myeloid_growth.pdf. Accessed February 1, 2008.

38. Burstein H. Myeloid growth factor support for dose-dense adjuvant chemotherapy for breast cancer. *Oncology (Williston Park)* 2006;14(Suppl 9):13–15.

39. Pisters KM, Kris MG. Management of nausea and vomiting caused by anticancer drugs: state of the art. *Oncology* 1992;6:99.

40. Gregory RE, Ettinger DS. 5-HT3 receptor antagonists for the prevention of chemotherapy-induced nausea and vomiting: a comparison of their pharmacology and clinical efficacy. *Drugs* 1998;55:173.

41. Levitt M, Warr D, Yelle L, et al. Ondansetron compared with dexamethasone and metoclopramide as antiemetics in the chemotherapy of breast cancer with cyclophosphamide, methotrexate, and fluorouracil. *N Engl J Med* 1993;328:1081.

42. Harvey RD 3rd, Lindley CL. Serotonin antagonists: an update. *Cancer Pract* 1998; 6:133.

43. Cubeddu LX, Hoffman IS, Fuenmayor NT, et al. Antagonism of serotonin S3 receptors with ondansetron prevents nausea and emesis induced by cyclophosphamide-containing chemotherapy regimens. *J Clin Oncol* 1990;8:1721.

44. Booth C, Clemons M, Dranitsaris G et al. Chemotherapy-induced nausea and vomiting in breast cancer patients: a prospective observational study *J Support Oncol* 2007;5:374–380.

45. Bloechl-Daum B, Deuson RR, Mavros P et al. Delayed nausea and vomiting continue to reduce patients' quality of life after highly and moderately emetogenic chemotherapy despite antiemetic treatment. *J Clin Oncol* 2006;24:4472.

46. Wickham R. Nausea and vomiting. In: Groenwald S, Frogge M, Goodman M, et al, eds. *Cancer symptom management*. Sudbury, MA: Jones & Bartlett, 1996:218.

47. Dibble S, Luce J, Cooper B, et al. Acupressure for chemotherapy-induced nausea and vomiting: a randomized clinical trial. *Oncol Nurs Forum* 2007;34:813.

48. Smith S, Teresi M. Acute leukemias. In: Dipiro J, Talbert R, Yee G, et al, eds. *Pharmacotherapy: a pathophysiologic approach*. Stamford, CT: Appleton & Lange, 1997:2603.

49. Larson PJ, Miaskowski C, MacPhail L, et al. The PRO-SELF Mouth Aware program: an effective approach for reducing chemotherapy-induced mucositis. *Cancer Nurs* 1998;21:263.

50. Zhang M, Liu X, Li J, et al. Chinese medicinal herbs to treat the side-effects of chemotherapy in breast cancer patients. *Cochrane Database Syst Review* 2007;2:CD004921.

51. Argyriou A, Chroni E, Koutras A. Vitamin E for prophylaxis against chemotherapy-induced neuropathy: A randomized controlled trial. *Neurology* 2005;64:26.

52. Pace A, Nistico C, Cuppone F et al. Peripheral neurotoxicity of weekly paclitaxel chemotherapy: A schedule or a dose issue? *Clin Breast Cancer* 2007;7:550.

53. Lemieux J, Maunsell E, Provencher L. Chemotherapy-induced alopecia and effects on quality of life among women with breast cancer: a literature review. *Psychooncology*; 2007:August 22. Epub.

54. Leyland-Jones B, Glemon K, Ayoub JP, et al. Pharmacokinetics, safety, and efficacy of trastuzumab administered every three weeks in combination with paclitaxel. *J Clin Oncol* 2003; 21:3965.

55. Bower JE. Behavioral symptoms in patients with breast cancer and survivors. *J Clin Oncol* 2008;26:768.

56. Janz N, Mujahid M, Chung L, et al. Symptom experience and quality of life following breast cancer treatment. *J Womens Health (Larchmt)* 2007;16:1348.

57. Avis N, Crawford S, Manuel J. Quality of life among younger women with breast cancer. *J Clin Oncol* 2005;23:3322.

58. Savard J, Simard S, Ivers H, Morin C. Randomized study of the efficacy of cognitive-behavioral therapy for insomnia secondary to breast cancer. Part I: Sleep and psychological effects. *J Clin Oncol* 2005;23:6083.

59. Reymann P. Chemotherapy: principles of administration. In: Groenwald S, Frogge M, Goodman M, et al, eds. *Cancer Nursing: principles and practice*, 3rd ed. Sudbury, MA: Jones & Bartlett, 1996:293.

60. McDonald A. Skin ulceration. In: Groenwald S, Frogge M, Goodman M, et al, eds. *Cancer nursing: principles and practice*, 3rd ed. Sudbury, MA: Jones & Bartlett, 1996:364.

61. Powel L. *Cancer chemotherapy guidelines and recommendations for practice*. Pittsburgh, PA: Oncology Nursing Press, 1996.

62. Bookman M, Kloth D, Kover P, et al. Intravenous prophylaxis for paclitaxel-related hypersensitivity reactions. *Ann Oncol* 1997:8:611.

63. Wise M, Han Y, Shaw B. et al. Effects of using online narrative and didactic information on health care participation for breast cancer patients. *Patient Educ Couns* 2008;70:348.

64. Senqupta P, Northfelt D, Gentile F, et al. Trastuzumab-induced cardiotoxicity: heart failure at the crossroads. *Mayo Clin Proc* 2008;83:197.

65. Kelly H, Kimmick G, Dees E, et al. Response and cardiac toxicity of trastuzumab given in conjunction with weekly paclitaxel and doxorubicin/cyclophosphamide. *Clin Breast Cancer* 2006;7:237.

66. Miller K, Wang, M, Gralow J, et al. Paclitaxel plus bevacizumab versus paclitaxel alone for metastatic breast cancer. *J Engl J Med* 2007;357:2666.

67. Burstein H, Storniolo A, Franco S. A phase II study of lapatinib monotherapy in chemotherapy-refractory HER-2 positive and HER2-negative advanced or metastatic breast cancer. *Ann Oncol* 2008;19:1068–1074.

68. Whelan TJ, Goss PE, Ingle JN, et al. Assessment of quality of life in MA.17: A randomized placebo-controlled trial of letrozole after five years of tamoxifen in postmenopausal women. *J Clin Oncol* 1999;23:6931.

69. Fallowfield L, Cella D, Cuzick J, et al. Quality of life of postmenopausal women in the Arimidex, Tamoxifen, Alone or in Combination (ATAC) adjuvant breast cancer trial. *J Clin Oncol* 2004;22:4261.

70. Coates AS, Keshaviah A, Thurliman B, et al. Five years of letrozole compared with tamoxifen as initial adjuvant therapy for postmenopausal women with endocrine-responsive early breast cancer: Update of study BIG 1-98. *J Clin Oncol* 2007; 25:486.

71. Bordeleau L, Pritchard K, Goodwin P, et al. Therapeutic options for the management of hot flashes in breast cancer survivors: an evidence-based review. *Clin Ther* 2007;29:230.

72. Perez E, Josse R, Pritchard K, et al. Effect of letrozole versus placebo on bone mineral density in women with primary breast cancer completing 5 or more years of adjuvant tamoxifen: a companion study to NCIC CTG MA.17. *J Clin Oncol* 2006;24:3629.

73. Partridge A, Wang P, Winer E, et al. Nonadherence to adjuvant tamoxifen therapy in women with primary breast cancer. *J Clin Oncol* 2003;21:602.

74. Ganz PA, Hahn EE. Implementing a survivorship care plan for patients with breast cancer. *J Clin Oncol* 2008;26:759.

75. Meneses K, McNees P, Loerzel V, et al. Transition from treatment to survivorship: Effects of a psychoeducational intervention on quality of life in breast cancer survivors *Oncol Nurs Forum* 2007;34:1007.

76. Dow KH, Ferrell BR, Leigh S, et al. Quality of life in long-term survivors of breast cancer. *Breast Cancer Res Treat* 1996;261.

77. Schover LR. Premature ovarian failure and its consequences: vasomotor symptoms, sexuality, and fertility. *J Clin Oncol* 2008;26:753.

78. Dow KH, Kuhn D. Fertility options in young breast cancer survivors: a review of the literature. *Oncol Nurs Forum* 2004;31:E46.

79. Carpenter JS, Storniolo AM, Johns S, et al. Randomized, double-blind, placebo-controlled crossover trials of venlafaxine for hot flashes after breast cancer. *Oncologist* 2007;12:124.

80. Carpenter JS, Neal JG, Payne J, et al. Cognitive-behavioral interventions for hot flashes. *Oncol Nurs Forum* 2007;34:37.

81. Dow KH, Lafferty P. Quality of life, survivorship, and psychosocial adjustment of young women with breast cancer after breast-conserving surgery and radiation therapy. *Oncol Nurs Forum* 2000;27:1555.

82. Gadducci A, Cosio S, Genazzani AR. Ovarian function and childbearing issues in breast cancer survivors. *Gynecol Endocrinol* 2007;23:625.

83. Makari-Judson G, Judson C, Mertens W. Longitudinal patterns of weight gain after breast cancer diagnosis: observations beyond the first year *Breast J* 2007;13:258.

84. Trentham-Dietz A, Newcomb P, Nichols H, et al. Breast cancer risk factors and secondary primary malignancies among women with breast cancer. *Breast Cancer Res Treat* 2007;105:195.

85. Hilton B, Gustavson K. Shielding and being shielded: children's perspectives on coping with their mother's cancer and chemotherapy. *Can Oncol Nurs J* 2002;12:198.

86. Mellon S. Comparisons between cancer survivors and family members on meaning of the illness and family quality of life. *Oncol Nurs Forum* 2002;29:1117.

87. Mellon S, Northouse LL, Weiss LK. A population-based study of the quality of life of cancer survivors and their family caregivers. *Cancer Nurs* 2006;29:120.

88. Cimprich B, Janz N, Northouse L et al. Taking CHARGE: a self-management program for women following breast cancer treatment. *Psychooncology* 2005;14:704.

89. Zahlis EH. The child's worries about mother's breast cancer: sources of distress in school-age children. *Oncol Nurs Forum* 2001;208:1019.

90. Johnsson A, Fornander T, Olsson M, et al. Factors associated with return-to-work after treatment for breast cancer. *Acta Oncol* 2007;46:90.

91. Bouknight R, Bradley C, Luo Z. Correlates of return to work for breast cancer survivors *J Clin Oncol* 2006;24:345.

92. Maunsell E, Drolet M, Brisson C, et al. Work situation after breast cancer. Results from a population-based study. *J Natl Cancer Inst* 2004;96:1813.

93. Jim HS, Andersen B. Meaning in life mediates the relationship between social and physical functioning and distress in cancer survivors. *Br J Health Psychol* 2007; 12:363.

Julia H. Rowland and Mary Jane Massie

Breast cancer, the most common form of cancer among American women, will be diagnosed in a projected 184,450 women in the year 2008. Incidence rates, flat for a number of years, appear to be rising again. Despite this, fewer than 41,000 women will die of the disease, and mortality rates continue to decline (1). Women with a history of breast cancer represent the largest constituency (24%) of the estimated 11.1 million cancer survivors in the United States and represent 43% of the 6.1 million women living with a history of cancer (2). Although an exact understanding of the causes and control of breast cancer continues to elude researchers, advances in detection and treatment have led to increases in disease-free survival (DFS). Most women diagnosed can expect to be cured of, or live for long periods with, their disease. Unlike treatment for other chronic diseases, however, many treatments for cancer are toxic and intensive. Practice trends have moved toward use of multidrug regimens delivered over shorter periods (dose intensity), sometimes in combination with higher doses of drug (dose density), resulting in increasing demands on patients' physical, psychological, and social resources, both short and long term. (See chapters on adjuvant therapy in Section VII.)

Several developments in breast cancer care have drawn attention to the key role of psychosocial factors in prevention, detection, treatment, and outcome. Improvements in, and broader use of, screening mammography have led not only to an increase in the number of women whose cancers are diagnosed at earlier stages, but also to questions of who gets screened, who does not, and who pays for it. Because of the earlier stage of diagnosis consequent to more mammographic detection; new developments in surgical, radiotherapeutic, and medical approaches; and the greater use of preoperative systemic therapy, more women are confronted with a variety of treatment choices. This includes choices such as sentinel node biopsy versus full axillary dissection; lumpectomy plus irradiation versus mastectomy; mastectomy with or without breast reconstruction with implants or autologous tissue or both; tamoxifen versus an aromatase inhibitor (AI) and for how long. All of this serves to increase the importance of the woman's role in the decision-making process and the critical role of patient–doctor and family communication as well as patient adherence in breast cancer care. Finally, the identification of genetic markers of breast cancer risk and the evaluation of chemopreventive agents have raised awareness of the psychological toll on unaffected women who are at increased risk for this disease (3). All of these changes have occurred in the context of greater cost-containment efforts and heightened attention to privacy, ethical, and informed consent issues in the delivery of care. There is now greater awareness of the psychosocial aspects of care, as evidenced by the more routine use of quality-of-life assessment in treatment trials and the more frequent articles in the medical literature on this topic. With the publication in 2008 of the Institute of Medicine's report, *Cancer Care for the Whole Patient: Meeting Psychosocial Health Needs*, a new standard has been set for oncology practice, one that acknowledges that the patient herself—her needs, hopes and desires—is as important as, and at times more important than, the tumor in planning and delivering optimal care (4).

Although breast cancer is a major stress for any woman, there is great variability in women's psychological responses. This chapter outlines the normal and abnormal responses to breast cancer and factors that may increase a woman's risk for poor adaptation. In addition, the role of social support in adaptation, in particular that from family members, and concerns related to sexual functioning and post-treatment survivorship are addressed.

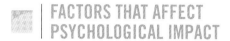

FACTORS THAT AFFECT PSYCHOLOGICAL IMPACT

Three sets of factors contribute to psychological response: the sociocultural context in which treatment options are offered, the psychological and psychosocial factors that the woman and her environment bring to the situation, and the medical factors or physical facts the woman must confront in terms of disease stage, treatment, response, and clinical course (Table 95.1). To provide comprehensive care, each of these areas must be assessed and problems encountered must be evaluated and addressed over the course of the patient's illness.

Sociocultural Context and Psychosocial Issues in Decision-Making

To understand and interpret the data on women's responses to breast cancer, an appreciation of the medical and social context within which diagnosis and treatment occur is critical. The broader changes in public attitudes toward cancer that occurred over the last century have resulted in major changes:

- Greater emphasis on the patient's role in decision-making.
- Demand for, and public involvement in, the assessment of research into the prevention and treatment of breast cancer.
- Substantial federal support for research on the psychosocial and behavioral aspects of cancer.

Many of these changes were championed by breast cancer advocates whose activism, starting in the early 1990s, helped to ensure that women today have more information about, understanding of, and resources to manage their breast cancer illness and recovery than ever before.

Over the course of care, women face three major decision points, each of which precipitates its own set of related choices to be considered (Table 95.2). The first is encountered at the time of initial discovery of a lump or symptom suggestive of breast cancer. The woman needs to determine whether or not this is worrisome and when to seek further evaluation. Most women consult their gynecologist or primary care provider (PCP) when this occurs. However, how quickly a woman decides to seek evaluation of her symptom or to follow up on a recommended course of action depends on a number of variables, including sociodemographic status (perhaps the most important factor related to this is access to care); knowledge, attitudes, and beliefs about cancer; personality and coping style; and the nature of the existing doctor–patient relationship (5). A number of factors have been identified that predict for delay in seeking care. Women who are older (>65 years), have a symptom other than a breast lump, do not disclose the symptom to someone else, have negative attitudes toward, or a poor relationship with, their PCP, and are fearful of cancer treatments are at risk for delay in seeking care (5). Further, language barriers, inadequate resources, and inaccurate beliefs may disproportionally affect Latina and black women

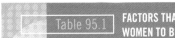

Table 95.1	FACTORS THAT CONTRIBUTE TO THE PSYCHOLOGICAL RESPONSES OF WOMEN TO BREAST CANCER

Current Sociocultural Context, Treatment Options, and Decision Making
- Changes in surgical and medical management from a uniform approach (e.g., breast-conserving management; introduction of sentinel node biopsies and neoadjuvant therapy; more therapeutic options and acknowledged uncertainty)
- Social attitudes
- Public figures openly sharing their breast cancer experience
- Autobiographic accounts of and "how to" guides for dealing with and surviving breast cancer in the popular press
- Ethical imperative for patient participation in treatment issues; legal imperative for knowledge of treatment options
- Variations in care by ethnicity, location, age
- Public awareness of treatment and research controversies; advocacy for more funding and lay oversight

Psychological and Psychosocial Factors
- Type and degree of disruption in life-cycle tasks caused by breast cancer (e.g., marital, childbearing, work)
- Psychological stability and ability to cope with stress
- Prior psychiatric history
- Availability of psychological and social support (partner, family, friends)

Medical Factors
- Stage of cancer at diagnosis
- Treatment(s) received: mastectomy or lumpectomy and radiation, adjuvant chemotherapy, hormonal therapy
- Availability of rehabilitation
  - Psychological (partner, support groups)
  - Physical (reconstruction; arm mobility and lymphedema prevention)
- Psychological support provided by physicians and staff

(6,7). Other factors that may contribute to delay in seeking consultation include less education, absence of a lump, lower perceived risk, less spirituality, cost, and not wanting to think about breast symptoms (8). If a delay in early detection has occurred, a woman's guilt over her role or anger at her physician's role can interfere with adaptation to treatment. Helping her focus on the fact that she is receiving care now is important in enabling a woman to engage in the recovery process.

At the time of consultation with a surgeon, a woman typically faces her second set of decisions: what treatment(s) to undergo (Table 95.2). The first of these is how to treat the breast and axilla. Most women today report being given a choice in primary treatment (mastectomy vs. limited resection and irradiation). Differences, however, still persist in the types of breast cancer treatment received by a woman, based on geography, age, and race. Women who live distant from major treatment centers or reside in specific parts of the country may receive care that is different from that recommended by national guidelines or that received by women in other regions (9). Black women are less likely to receive breast conservation and, when they do, radiation therapy may more often be omitted as part of their care (10). Black women with less education are at risk for receipt of non–guideline-concordant adjuvant chemotherapy regimens, potentially contributing to worse outcomes (11). Older women are less likely to receive treatment consistent with guidelines (12). Those older than 65 to 70 years may not undergo lymph node dissection and be less likely to receive adjuvant tamoxifen (13). Further, although comorbidity and age appear to be significant predictors of treatment in older women, these are not necessarily correlated (14).

At this juncture, some women must also decide whether to seek a second opinion or care elsewhere. Access to support networks, now widely available across the country, helps women locate reputable breast specialists in their area. Also, women's access to online information about current standard therapies and clinical trials helps patients and families organize their thinking and questions to more effectively use first and second opinions. A number of insurance carriers mandate a second opinion before the performance of any elective procedure. Motivation to seek second opinions at times may be driven by anxiety, as well as by less satisfactory experience with other providers, need for a more active role in the process, or desire to hear a different recommendation (15). Surgeons often help set limits on excessive information gathering by setting a stop date to the search.

A number of cancer centers across the United States offer multidisciplinary breast clinics that address the need for women

Table 95.2	MAJOR DECISION POINTS ACROSS THE COURSE OF BREAST CANCER CARE

Detection and Diagnosis of a Suspicious Symptom
- What constitutes a worrisome symptom
- Whether to seek attention for a symptom (or delay)
- Whom to consult
- What type of procedure(s) to use to confirm cancer (e.g., MRI, type of biopsy, biomarkers, etc.)

Selection of Treatment Options
- Local therapy
  1. How to treat the breast
     a. Mastectomy with or without reconstruction, and if reconstruction: type and timing
     b. Breast conservation, with or without irradiation
  2. How to treat the axilla
     a. Sentinel node biopsy
     b. Full axillary dissection
     c. No assessment
- Systemic therapy
  1. Chemotherapy: type and duration
  2. Hormonal therapy: type and duration
- Other considerations
  1. Clinical trial participation
  2. Second opinions
  3. Genetic testing and/or prophylactic surgery

Post-treatment Follow-up Care
- Whether to seek follow-up care or follow recommendations
- Who should perform follow-up:
  1. Oncologist (medical, radiation, surgical)
  2. Primary care physician
  3. Both
  4. Other (nurse practitioner)
- How often follow-up should occur?
- What tests should be performed or services provided and with what periodicity?

to seek opinions from diverse specialists. Women are usually seen after their initial biopsy and meet with a surgeon, medical oncologist, radiation oncologist, and in some centers, other specialists, including a pathologist, plastic surgeon, mental health professional, genetic counselor, or clinical research nurse. This one-stop visit provides the woman with information about all of her treatment options and outlines for her treatment that is tailored to her specific cancer and personal needs. Clinical experience suggests that such programs are helpful in reducing stress and facilitating information gathering. However, studies have yet to be conducted that demonstrate the benefits of this approach. Decision aids provide another format for communicating information about treatment options. These tools define the risks and benefits of surgical treatment options and provide standardized information that can be used to supplement the patient–physician dialogue. Research suggests that use of these adjuncts to counseling women increases the likelihood that women with early-stage disease will consider breast-conserving surgery and enhances knowledge of treatment options (16). Use of decision aids is also associated with less decisional conflict and greater satisfaction with the decision made (17). Finally, work is ongoing at various centers to develop instructional kits, videotapes, and online educational tools designed to walk a woman through the various treatment options of specific interest to her using easy-to-understand and even interactive communication formats (18,19). Surveys suggest that patients, their caregivers, and providers embrace these supplemental technologies (20), although discussing Internet information adds time to physician visits (21). Research also underscores the importance of providing treatment information in various formats (e.g., printed, audiotape, videotape, and compact disc) and using different language (e.g., positive and negative framing, percentiles and proportions, and simple terms and survival figures) (22,23).

The emphasis on informed decision-making places a responsibility on the physician to be cognizant of the individual woman's physical and psychological needs and to tailor accordingly the discussion and recommendations made. At times, it may mean tempering a woman's demands for unrealistic treatment, acquiescing to another woman's desire to defer a final decision to her physician or significant other, or in some cases, reassuring a woman that she need not reach a decision immediately, but has a few days to research her options and come to an appropriate choice. As desire for information and preference about decision-making roles can change over time, asking about them periodically is important (24). For example, although uncomfortable with extensive details at the outset, a woman may find she wants more information and the opportunity to provide greater input into decisions as time goes on. (A broader review of patients' response styles and physician–patient communication issues is provided elsewhere ([25]).

The increasing complexity of care and vast array of information resources available to physicians and patients alike make good patient–doctor communication more important than ever. The documented benefits of effective communication include improved patient comprehension of, and adherence to, treatment recommendations, enhanced physical and emotional well-being, and increased patient and physician satisfaction. Poor communication is a key factor in litigation and medical complaints (26). Fortunately, the medical community is beginning to provide formal communication skills training to oncologists (27,28).

The time between diagnosis and initiation of treatment is one of the most stressful periods in the breast cancer experience, exceeded in degree of stress only by the period of waiting for surgical or other test results (29). For a woman paralyzed by the decision-making process and overwhelmed by the knowledge that she has a potentially life-threatening illness, referral for psychiatric consultation can be useful. It is sometimes helpful for these women to have the pressure temporarily removed by postponing surgery and then to review the events and possi-

ble treatments in a setting in which they can express concerns and fears and identify the reasons for their response.

Although the decision-making process may be stressful, research indicates that women who are given a choice about treatment do the same as or better psychologically than those who are not (30–33). Studies show that the quality of physician communication during this phase is a critical determinant of subsequent psychological well-being in patients with breast cancer (34,35). It is important to note, however, that although most women confronted with breast cancer want to have information, clinicians must be aware that not all women want to make the final decision about treatment (36–38). A woman's need for information must be assessed separately from her desire to participate in or delegate treatment choice. Whatever the process, physician recommendation continues to play a critical role in women's choice of treatment.

Psychological Variables in Adaptation

In 1980, Meyerowitz (39) delineated three broad areas of psychosocial impact of breast cancer:

- Psychological discomfort (anxiety, depression, and anger).
- Changes in life patterns (consequent to physical discomfort, marital or sexual disruption, and altered activity level).
- Fears and concerns (mastectomy or loss of breast, recurrence, and death)

Although women diagnosed today have many more treatment options and resources for support, the psychological concerns remain the same. In addition to these variables, the life stage at which the cancer occurs, previous emotional stability (personality and coping style), and presence of interpersonal support also affect adaptation (Table 95.3).

Age, or the point in the life cycle at which breast cancer occurs, is of prime importance (40–42). Unlike most cancers, breast cancer affects women across a broad age range, from

---

Table 95.3 **RISK FACTORS FOR POOR ADAPTATION**

Medical
- More advanced disease
- More intense or aggressive treatment
- Other or multiple comorbid medical conditions
- Fewer rehabilitative options
- Poor doctor–patient relationship

Personal
- Prior psychiatric history
- Past trauma history (especially physical or sexual abuse)
- Rigid or limited coping capacity
- Helpless or hopeless outlook
- Low income or education
- Multiple competing demands (e.g., work, child or other family care, economic)
- Poor marital or interpersonal relationship
- Younger age (<40) or older age (>80)

Social
- Lack of social support (and/or religious affiliation)
- Limited access to service resources
- Cultural biases
- Social stigma or illness taboo

Breast Cancer Specific
- Prior breast cancer experience
  - Recurrence or second breast cancer
  - Loss of family or friends to breast cancer
- High investment in body image, in particular breasts

Adapted from Weisman D. Early diagnosis of vulnerability in cancer patients. *Am J Med Sci* 1976;271:187, with permission.

teenagers to centenarians. Concerns about the threat to life and future health, as well as fears of potential disfigurement, disability, and distress associated with treatment, are common to all women diagnosed with breast cancer. These concerns, however, are often more pronounced in younger women for whom a cancer diagnosis is seen as "off-timed" in the normal life course (43). In younger patients, there is a sense of disruption in their primary role as caregiver and partner and, increasingly, as breadwinner; they often perceive having more to lose (including career and the chance to have and see offspring grow up) than older patients do (44). Feeling different or isolated is a theme also voiced by younger women. (See Chapter 92 on Breast Cancer in Younger Women.) Although almost half of breast cancer survivors are age 65 years or older, scant psychosocial research focuses on this cohort (45). Historically, researchers have suggested that older patients may experience less distress because of greater life experience, including familiarity with medical settings (46), but this has not been clearly established. Breast cancer diagnosed in a woman older than 80 years may be experienced in the presence of other major losses, particularly of a spouse, and concurrent chronic medical conditions. Older women with breast cancer experience greater decrements in their health-related quality of life and lower psychosocial well-being than unaffected peers (47), and they are at risk for significantly higher rates of decline in upper body function (48). This pattern, coupled with the observation that older women are significantly less likely to receive appropriate surgical care or rehabilitation (49,50), suggests that patients at both ends of the age continuum are at increased risk for problems in adaptation. Finally, although threats to body image, sense of femininity, and self-esteem may be great in younger women, particularly those who are single or without a partner, these threats are concerns of many older women as well (51). (See Chapter 91 on Breast Cancer in Older Women.)

The second variable contributing to adaptation relates to the patient herself, that is, her personality and unique coping patterns. Women who are flexible and use active problem-solving approaches to the stresses of breast cancer exhibit less distressed mood and better adaptation (52–54). Balancing coping styles over time may also be important (55,56). For example, although distraction is a helpful coping technique while waiting for test results and in managing the stress of a chemotherapy infusion, this would not work well when attention to changes in treatment details is needed. Finally, women who are able to draw on and use available social resources and support adapt better and may even live longer than women who do not (57,58). By contrast, women at risk for poor coping include those who

- Exhibit a passive, helpless, hopeless, or pessimistic stance in the face of illness
- Are rigid in their use of coping strategies
- Tend to be socially isolated or to reject help when it is offered

Prior trauma and current stressful life events also may adversely affect a woman's adaptation to breast cancer (59). Women who manifest persistent depressive symptoms in the face of cancer may be at risk not only of poor quality of life but also premature death (60,61). Such patients should be considered promptly for professional psychological assessment and support.

The relationship between attitude, cancer risk, and survival remains an area of public interest and active research. Because breast cancer is a prevalent neoplasm with significant psychological impact and inadequately defined causative factors, the possible role of psychological variables in vulnerability to breast cancer and its progression has been explored in medical studies and has received much attention from patients and in the press. Many women express concern that they "brought it on themselves" or that their bad attitude or lifestyle may be making the cancer worse. Stewart et al. (62) found that 42.2% of the 378 breast cancer survivors surveyed believed that stress caused cancer and 27.9% felt that stress reduction could prevent a recurrence, confirming work done 20 years earlier. Epidemiologic studies, however, have failed to find an association between stress and breast cancer development (63) or survival (64). These data notwithstanding, concerns about the adverse general health effects of chronic stress suggest that addressing this when it occurs is important. Stress management for breast cancer survivors is discussed later in this chapter.

The belief that she may be responsible for her own illness and its outcome can become an added psychological burden for many women with breast cancer. Some, based on these beliefs, seek questionable and unproved therapies as primary treatment, either never starting or discontinuing conventional treatments. Conflicting reports in the media about the relationship between emotions and breast cancer are a growing concern. For these reasons, oncologists should be alert to these possible concerns in their patients and provide both clarification and reassurance to patients that currently no medical evidence indicates that stress causes cancer. Other important factors in adaptation are a patient's prior experiences with breast cancer and body image. The memory of a mother, sister, or grandmother's death from breast cancer or that of a close friend or colleague can make the diagnosis seem more ominous and may result in greater levels of psychological distress during and after treatment. Some women with a high investment in their bodies cannot tolerate even the idea of loss or damage to a breast. They may delay seeking consultation for a symptom and may be at risk for problems after treatment if attempts to preserve cosmetic appearance are less successful than expected.

A woman's sociocultural background can further influence her breast cancer experience. How cancer is viewed in her community of affiliation (for example, if cancer is seen as stigmatizing or is never discussed) will affect her adaptation response. Although a needed and growing area of research, the interpretation of between-group differences in studies conducted among ethnoculturally diverse samples is complicated because ethnicity is often confounded with variables, such as income, education, and treatment, known to be predictors of or associated with quality of life (65,66). (For a full discussion of this topic, see also Chapter 93, Breast Cancer in Minority Women.)

Two understudied minority groups are lesbian breast cancer survivors and survivors living in rural communities. Some data suggest that lesbian breast cancer survivors may be more comfortable with body image and perceive greater social support than their heterosexual peers. They, however, also tend to experience more difficulty interacting with physicians (67). Survivors in rural areas are at greater risk for relationship problems, lack of support, and feelings of isolation (68). In addition to the demands felt by all women dealing with breast cancer, they are vulnerable to concerns about how partners and family will cope during absences for treatment, the burden of running farms or property alone, and the financial strain of transportation and health care costs (69–71).

Finally, adjustment depends on the response from other significant people, from spouse or partner, family and friends. Because of the importance of social support to women's adaptation, this is addressed at greater length in the section Role and Care of the Family, later in this chapter.

Prolonged anxiety or depression is not an expected reaction to a cancer diagnosis (72). The common stress reactions around the time of diagnosis and onset of treatment usually can be evaluated and managed by the patient's physicians, nurses, or social worker. Some women, however, have greater problems and can benefit from psychological management by psychiatrists and psychologists, who often are collaborating members of the treatment team (Table 95.4).

If a patient's anxiety or insomnia interferes with functioning, low-dose anxiolytic medication (e.g., lorazepam [0.25 to 1.0 mg

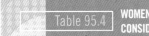

Table 95.4	WOMEN WITH BREAST CANCER WHO SHOULD BE CONSIDERED FOR PSYCHIATRIC EVALUATION

1. Those who present with current symptoms or a history of the following:
   - Depression or anxiety
   - Suicidal thinking (attempt)
   - Substance or alcohol abuse
   - Confusional state (delirium or encephalopathy)
   - Mood swings, insomnia, or irritability from steroids
2. Those who
   - Have a family history of breast cancer
   - Are very young, old, pregnant, nursing, single, or alone
   - Are adjusting to multiple losses and managing multiple life stresses
   - Seem paralyzed with cancer treatment decisions
   - Fear death during surgery or are terrified by loss of control under anesthesia
   - Request euthanasia
   - Seem unable to provide informed consent

orally three to four times a day] or clonazepam [0.25 to 1.0 mg orally twice daily]) or a hypnotic (e.g., zolpidem [5 to 10 mg]) usually reduces symptoms to a manageable level. When anxiety and insomnia cannot be controlled with these medications, or when surgical or medical staff observe symptoms of depression, such as frequent crying episodes, irritability, inability to concentrate, or remarks indicating hopelessness or helplessness or suicidal thoughts, psychiatric consultation is indicated. Psychiatric consultants combine support of the patient and evaluation and support of her significant others with medication to restore a woman to her prior level of function. The selective serotonin reuptake inhibitors (SSRI) (e.g., fluoxetine, paroxetine, sertraline, fluvoxamine, citalopram, escitalopram) and novel or mixed action antidepressants (venlafaxine, duloxetine, bupropion) are considered first-line treatment because they are better tolerated in patients with comorbid depression and medical conditions. Venlafaxine is currently believed to be the antidepressant that should be prescribed to the depressed woman (or the woman with hot flashes) who is taking tamoxifen because venlafaxine appears to affect tamoxifen metabolism less than other antidepressants do. (See Chapter 54 Management of Menopause Symptoms in Breast Cancer Survivors for management of hot flashes.)

Medical Variables in Adaptation

The stage of breast cancer at diagnosis, the treatment required, the prognosis, and the available rehabilitative opportunities constitute important medical variables that influence psychological adjustment. However, central to successful adaptation is a woman's relationship with her treating physicians (surgeon, radiation oncologist, medical oncologist), and the degree to which they are sensitive to her individual concerns, communicate clearly, and monitor emotional and physical well-being. The length and intensity of current treatments and the recognition that women treated for breast cancer must be followed for extended periods of time have placed an added burden on health care providers. In some settings, nurse clinicians provide continuity of care and serve as patient advocates. In others, patients are screened for psychosocial needs and triaged to psychological care as indicated. Preliminary guidelines for psychosocial care across the cancer continuum have been developed (73). However, these guidelines were created with highly resourced comprehensive cancer centers in mind. Adherence to such guidelines even in these specialized settings is reported as being low, with only 20% of National Comprehensive Cancer Network sites surveyed reporting routine use of screening of all patients for distress (74). The extent to which such guidelines

are being adopted or even adapted and applied more broadly remains unknown but appears to be low (75). Further, concerns about the cost of providing the recommended psychosocial and supportive care and who should pay for this continue to be significant barriers to optimal service delivery.

Surgery

Mastectomy

Mastectomy is now performed in fewer than half of women diagnosed with early-stage breast cancer. Of late, however, the number of women selecting ipsilateral mastectomy with contralateral prophylactic mastectomy has increased (76). Part of this increase is related to greater use of preoperative magnetic resonance imaging (MRI) (77). Further, for women who do have a mastectomy, more will undergo breast reconstruction than previously, although some data suggest that many mastectomy patients are not made aware of their reconstruction options. Considerable research exists on the impact of loss of one or both breasts on women's physical, social, and emotional functioning. Among the effects documented are feelings of mutilation and altered body image, diminished self-worth, loss of a sense of femininity, decreases in sexual attractiveness and function, anxiety, depression, hopelessness, guilt, shame, and fear of recurrence, abandonment, and death (39,78). Although mourning for the loss of a cherished body part and the threat to life are universal, the extent to which other sequelae are experienced is variable. Current data reveal that women who are well adjusted before they have a mastectomy and whose disease is in an early stage can expect at 1 year to have a quality of life equal to that of unaffected peers (79,80). Today, a woman's persistent issues generally have less to do with the type of surgery received and more to do with her personal and social characteristics and the adjuvant therapy given. Issues related to the latter are discussed in the treatment-specific chapters and in the section Breast Cancer Survivors, later in this chapter.

Research suggests that in addition to a number of medical factors (e.g., tumor size, location, and aggressiveness), several other characteristics may distinguish women who have mastectomy from those who receive breast-sparing surgery. These include older age, fear of irradiation, preferring to have no therapy beyond surgery, being black or Hispanic (or possibly low income), and among older women, living with extended or nonfamily members or in an assisted-living setting (10).

Breast-conserving Therapy (Lumpectomy and Irradiation)

Until recently, the number of women undergoing breast-conserving therapy (BCT) steadily increased; however, in many areas of the country, the use of mastectomy has recently begun to increase. A significant factor in what type of surgery is performed is the nature of the care that is available. For women diagnosed in communities that are removed from major medical centers, mastectomy may simply be a more practical and safe treatment choice. Another deciding factor may be the availability of high-quality irradiation therapy. Further, restricted access to plastic surgeons can limit the availability of reconstructive options. Another factor determining choice is the knowledge and availability of genetic testing for mutations in *BRCA1* and *BRCA2*, where patients with mutations now generally undergo bilateral mastectomy. Cultural and ethnic values may also direct or even dictate choice, although the role of these is poorly understood (81). Physician recommendation continues to exert the most significant influence on treatment choice for most women.

Despite the variability in methods used or cohorts studied, women who receive BCT are less self-conscious about their appearance, have a better body image, and report greater satisfaction with sexual activity. In particular, women in the conservation group tend to feel they are less sexually inhibited, have sex more often, and report that their husbands are more interested in them sexually and more affectionate than women who have had mastectomy. Early reports suggested that women in BCT groups manifest a somewhat better overall adjustment than those in mastectomy groups (82). Longer term follow-up of more current cohorts of breast cancer survivors has, however, failed to show differences in overall quality of life based on type of surgery alone (83–85). A consistent finding is that psychosocial variables are for the most part much stronger predictors of psychosocial outcomes than are medical factors (86). These latter studies further suggest that benefits to sexual function associated with BCT may be less than previously believed (87–89). Among survivors undergoing BCT, satisfaction with surgical results can have a marked bearing on psychosexual morbidity (90). This is expected, given that BCT is often selected because it is perceived as less disfiguring than mastectomy. A significant confound to examining the impact of surgery on women's quality-of-life outcomes is that younger women, known to be at increased risk for psychosocial problems in adaptation to breast cancer, tend to elect to undergo BCT. These young patients are also more likely to receive adjuvant chemotherapy, which has a significant negative impact on sexual functioning. What we have learned is that BCT is not a psychosocial panacea; rather, it is a surgical and cosmetic option that may facilitate adaptation for many women.

Two critical factors that continue to influence the surgical decision-making process are attitudes about cancer and irradiation. The thought of leaving tumor cells in the breast is intolerable for some women, who feel more secure with mastectomy. Other women fear irradiation or are unable to devote 6 weeks to daily irradiation treatments because of family, work demands, or distance from a treatment center. Personality characteristics also influence a woman's decision. Women who select BCT over mastectomy have been found to be more concerned about insult to body image and more dependent on their breasts for self-esteem and believe they would have had difficulty adjusting to loss of the breast to mastectomy. In contrast, patients who choose mastectomy perceive the breast containing cancer as an offending part that should be removed, and they are more fearful of the side effects of irradiation.

Women undergoing irradiation are at risk for psychological disturbance, in particular depressive symptoms. These symptoms may be, in part, side effects of the irradiation, or more likely secondary to persistent fears about their disease and the risk of recurrence. Providing a reassuring environment, orientation to care, and strong support promotes optimal adaptation. Most women undergoing radiation therapy experience initial anxiety related to the treatment, which diminishes after a few treatments only to return toward the conclusion of therapy because of fear of regrowth of tumor without treatment, as well as in anticipation of the loss of close observation by the doctor and treatment staff. To ease this transition, patients should be made aware of the paradoxical increase in feelings of distress. Staff should remain available by telephone and through follow-up appointments. Fears of disease recurrence remain high in many women and reach distressing levels before follow-up visits, before follow-up mammograms and scans, and while waiting for test results.

When discussing women's reactions to irradiation, one additional factor that is important to consider is the risk for upper extremity lymphedema. Women who develop lymphedema are at high risk for problems in both psychological and social functioning (91). Fortunately, the proportion of women affected by this problem has decreased with the use of sentinel node biopsy. However, patients with a positive sentinel node biopsy typically undergo a complete axillary dissection. Women having both axillary irradiation and surgical resection

of axillary lymph nodes are at highest risk of developing lymphedema and should be educated about measures they can take to reduce this risk. On the other hand, patients who are receiving irradiation just to the breast can be reassured that such treatment will not increase their risk of lymphedema. Data from two small pilot studies suggest that participation in an upper-body exercise program does not increase arm circumference or volume in women who already have lymphedema and may improve their quality of life. Additional larger-scale studies are needed to confirm this effect and, importantly, to develop evidence-based guidelines for care that might benefit hundreds of women (92,93). (See Chapters 43 and 45 for more details regarding management of axillary irradiation and lymphedema, respectively.)

Reconstruction

Postmastectomy breast reconstruction is an important rehabilitative option pursued by a significant subset of women undergoing mastectomy. In the study by Ganz et al. (80) of women treated for early-stage breast cancer in Los Angeles or the greater Washington, DC area, 41.7% who received a mastectomy went on to have breast reconstruction. Some evidence suggests, however, that reconstruction is not being routinely addressed in the surgical decision-making process. In their Surveillance, Epidemiology and End Results (SEER)-based sample, Alderman et al. (94) found that only a third of patients reported that their general surgeon discussed this option with them during the decision-making process. Younger, more educated women with larger tumors were more likely to report that this discussion took place. Further, patients whose surgeon did cover this option were four times more likely to have a mastectomy.

Relatively few studies have systematically examined the psychosocial impact of mastectomy alone compared with mastectomy plus reconstruction. Contemporary studies seek to evaluate psychosocial and sexual outcomes for women selecting one of the three different surgical options (lumpectomy vs. mastectomy alone vs. mastectomy with reconstruction) (85,95–100). In one study, which looked only at body image and self-esteem, patients who underwent BCT reported more positive body image than women in either the mastectomy or the immediate reconstruction groups (97). Interestingly, this difference was not significant for the delayed reconstruction group, suggesting that these women may use a different standard for comparison. No differences were seen between groups on self-esteem, which was uniformly high. Parker et al. (85), using a prospective longitudinal research design, describe similar subtle differences in early adaptation among women undergoing each of the three different procedures, but note that few differences could be seen among groups 2 years after treatment (85). In general, aspects of quality of life other than body image are not better in women who have undergone BCT or mastectomy with reconstruction. In what remains the largest three-way comparison study, investigators found no differences in women's emotional, social, or role functions by type of surgery (87). Women in both mastectomy groups (with or without reconstruction) complained of more physical symptoms related to their surgeries than women undergoing lumpectomy. Consistent with others' findings, women in the mastectomy with reconstruction group were most likely to report that breast cancer had a negative impact on their sex lives (45.4% vs. 41.3% for mastectomy alone and 29.8% for lumpectomy). An important factor in women's sexual outcomes is that mastectomy with or without reconstruction results in permanent loss of sensation in the breast area. Further, as discussed in Chapters 39 and 47, the use of postmastectomy radiation therapy generally decreases the cosmetic results with reconstruction, particularly with implants. At the same time, the use of immediate breast reconstruction can compromise effective and safe delivery of postmastectomy radiation therapy for patients with left-sided breast cancer.

Research suggests there are sociodemographic differences between women who do and do not undergo postmastectomy reconstruction. Women undergoing mastectomy with reconstruction are generally younger, are better educated, have higher incomes, are more likely to be partnered, and have earlier stage of disease (87,101,102). Women who are older, Hispanic, or born outside the United States appear less likely to have reconstruction (103). Fewer black women undergo reconstruction; this may often be owing to economic and access barriers (including lower rates of referral for these procedures), but is also potentially related to lower interest in having reconstruction (104,105). Asian women are also less likely than white women to undergo reconstruction. Some data suggest that among sexual minority women (self-identified as lesbian or bisexual), there may be more decisional regrets among those who choose reconstruction versus mastectomy alone, leading to more adjustment problems (106). We already know that where you live will determine rates of reconstruction as well. Fewer women living in the Midwest and South are offered or receive reconstruction, whereas more women living proximate to National Cancer Institute (NCI)-designated cancer centers will be offered and undergo this option (107). Regrettably, few efforts have been made to understand the psychological variables associated with who does and does not seek reconstruction, in particular in the present era in which autologous tissue procedures and immediate reconstruction represent standard options for care. Further, additional research is needed on the impact on women's satisfaction and functioning related to the extent of surgery performed (e.g., unilateral versus bilateral transverse rectus abdominis myocutaneous [TRAM] flap surgery, TRAM with or without implant) and procedures used to achieve good symmetry (e.g., nipple–aureolar complex reconstruction, contralateral breast reduction, or mastopexy).

In addition to local treatment choice (e.g., BCT vs. mastectomy with or without reconstruction), the impact on psychosocial function of timing and type of reconstruction performed has been examined.

Timing of Reconstruction: Immediate versus Delayed. Research with women undergoing immediate reconstruction has shown high levels of patient satisfaction with surgical results and less psychosocial morbidity than in those who undergo mastectomy alone, although as noted in discussions above, these differences diminish over time (108). Patients undergoing immediate reconstruction report being less depressed and anxious and experience less impairment of their sense of femininity, self-esteem, and sexual attractiveness than their peers who delay or do not seek reconstruction. Al-Ghazal et al. (98) reported that 76% of women who delayed surgery would have preferred immediate reconstruction, whereas only 5% of the immediate group wished they had delayed surgery. Researchers have noted that initial differences in adjustment may be minimal and disappear over time. At least one study has suggested that satisfaction with technical aspects of the reconstructive outcome may be slightly lower among women undergoing immediate versus delayed reconstruction (109). This may reflect the fact that women with immediate reconstruction compare the result with their original breast, whereas those undergoing delayed surgery use the mastectomy site as their basis for comparison.

Type of Reconstruction: Implant versus Transverse Rectus Abdominis Myocutaneous Flap. The research evaluating psychosocial outcomes for women undergoing reconstruction using TRAM flap surgery has also been an area of interest. In our own research, we looked at 146 women on average 3 years after undergoing reconstruction; 95 (64%) had an implant and 51 (35%) under-

went TRAM surgery (110). No differences were seen between groups in satisfaction with the appearance or feel of their breasts or the overall impact of breast cancer on their sex lives, although a consistent tendency was noted for the women with TRAM reconstructions to report greater comfort and satisfaction. This pattern is consistent with others' findings and the observation that timing of reconstruction may be more important than procedure on women's long-term adaptation (108). However, women who had an implant were significantly more worried about having a problem with their reconstruction; 25% of women with implants indicated they worried a fair amount to very much about the future versus only 8% of the TRAM group. Longer-term follow-up of cosmetic outcomes for implant recipients would appear to confirm these fears. Clough et al. (111) report that overall cosmetic outcome was rated as acceptable in 86% at 2 years but had declined to 54% by 5 years in their study sample. Further, 23% of the 334 women in their study underwent implant exchange (excluding those with expanders). A similar pattern was not observed among TRAM reconstructions, in which assessment of cosmetic outcome remained stable over time (111). Ongoing research is needed not only to document women's long-term psychosocial outcomes after reconstruction, including response to newer surgical flap techniques (e.g., deep inferior epigastric perforator), but also to help elucidate trends in, and the interplay between, type and timing of surgery (108).

Regardless of the type of reconstructive surgery proposed or selected, women need to be well informed about what to expect. Key concerns of women about reconstruction include the cost of the surgery, the length of time under anesthesia, the number of procedures required, the cosmetic results achievable, and the safety of the techniques used, both in terms of potential for complications and, in the case of implants, risk of masking recurrent cancer or promoting recurrent autoimmune disease. Surgeons differ in their approach to informing women about cosmetic results. Some prefer to use written materials only, and others show pictures of reconstructed breasts. Many use some combination of these approaches and, at times, may refer a woman to a patient who has previously had reconstruction for more details. Wider availability of video and online tools for decision-making are beginning to provide a unique way to educate women about choices that allow them to tailor the information they receive (e.g., access pictures and obtain details about specific aspects of a given surgery, recovery, and outcomes) to suit their information needs. Many of these formats include personal vignettes by women who have undergone different procedures and share their rationale for their particular decision. In our experience and that of others, several additional issues appeared important in counseling women who were considering or undergoing these procedures. These include the need for discussion of all facets of the surgical steps (including number and length of hospitalizations and follow-up office visits or procedures) and a thorough review of the nature and timing of any planned symmetry and nipple-reconstruction procedures.

Adjuvant Chemotherapy

When a patient receives a recommendation for adjuvant chemotherapy, it requires adjustment to an additional and toxic therapeutic modality, a lengthened treatment period, and greater awareness of the threat to life. Some women in this group describe their early weeks of treatment as having been characterized by "one piece of bad news after another." Deciding whether to undergo adjuvant or systemic therapy, and if so, which drugs or protocol to use, constitutes one of the major decision points related to treatment decision-making (Table 95.2).

Psychological preparation for chemotherapy is essential and should incorporate patient educational materials, nursing input, and an outline by the physician of the disease and treatment-related expectations. Anticipation of chemotherapy can be difficult. Women's fears of the side effects arise from knowledge of the acute sequelae of chemotherapy (e.g., nausea, hair loss, anemia) which, although transient, are nonetheless distressing. With greater awareness and discussion of these, fear of chemotherapy's persistent effects (e.g., fatigue, pain, memory problems, sexual dysfunction, sleep disturbance, depression) also can cause major concern (112). Reactive anxiety and depression should be treated to assist in the woman's adjustment. Because many women with node-negative, early-stage breast cancer now receive some form of adjuvant therapy, the past association of these treatments with "more serious disease" has diminished.

Clinical experience suggests that most women cope with the short-term adverse psychological effects by focusing on delayed benefits (e.g., reassurance that they have done everything possible to eradicate their disease). Clinicians need to be aware, however, that for some women declines in health-related quality of life during treatment increase risk for discontinuation of chemotherapy (113). Monitoring for problems and addressing these promptly are important in ensuring adherence to the planned course of care.

Nausea and vomiting, once common side effects of adjuvant chemotherapy, feared and dreaded by patients, are now well controlled with pharmacologic and behavioral interventions (114,115). Five additional troublesome side effects of adjuvant therapy that have psychological consequences, however, warrant special attention. These include hair loss, weight gain, problems with concentration, premature menopause, and fatigue. Although anticipated, the impact of alopecia is often devastating. Some women report this as more distressing than their breast surgery because it is a visible, overtly disfiguring indicator of disease. Some women even rate hair loss as being as distressing as learning of their diagnosis. Early discussion of the expected changes, information about wigs, including that these are often covered as prosthetic devices by most insurers if prescribed, and referral to the American Cancer Society's *Look Good . . . Feel Better* program can help reduce distress caused by hair loss.

The cause of weight gain with chemotherapy remains unclear. A study by Huntington (116) revealed that 50% of patients gained more than 10 pounds. Because of the added insult to self-esteem posed by significant weight gain, and more importantly data suggesting that overweight leads to worse prognosis (117), greater attention is being paid to this problem. Physical activity and exercise programs during chemotherapy are increasingly being recommended, along with nutritional guidance. The introduction of exercise programs during chemotherapy is feasible and well tolerated (118). Remaining physically active provides significant benefit to women in controlling weight gain, improving functional and cardiac status, and potentially enhancing quality of life. The demonstrated benefit of exercise in alleviating moderate symptoms of depression in noncancer populations can increase the appeal of this intervention in the cancer setting, in which at times the breast cancer patient may be reluctant to take more medications. Additional benefits of exercise include greater exposure to healthful vitamin D from the sun if done outdoors and social support if done with a companion. (See Chapter 53 for broader discussion of lifestyle interventions.)

Difficulty with attention, concentration, memory, and processing speed is also reported by many women undergoing chemotherapy. These troubling neurocognitive effects, which may also be chemotherapy dose related, are the focus of active research (119–123) (see also Chapter 55 on Side Effects of Systemic Therapy). The symptoms may be associated with the stress of illness, antiemetic drugs, hormonal changes secondary to chemotherapy-induced menopause, and, principally, treatment-induced alterations in neurochemical and brain function (124). In some women, this effect may be mediated by

a genetic predisposition (125). Important in this literature is the finding that women's complaints about cognitive compromise are not consistently associated with neuropsychological test performance (126). To date, the incidence of complaints is higher than the documented rate of cognitive deficits (127). Nevertheless, if cognitive dysfunction is found to persist over time or, as some studies suggest, worsen (128), this troubling side effect may become a dose-limiting factor in treatment decisions and care (129).

A further troublesome effect of chemotherapy in premenopausal women is premature menopause (130). (See Chapter 54 on Management of Menopause Related to Systemic Therapy.) The threatened or actual loss of fertility and acute onset of menopause anticipated with adjuvant chemotherapy often cause distress in the woman who is premenopausal at diagnosis. Iatrogenic acute estrogen deficiency may, in a few patients, be associated with psychiatric syndromes, depression in particular (131). The hot flashes, night sweats, and vaginal dryness and atrophy caused by chemotherapy-induced menopause can produce severe physical discomfort. The latter symptoms can lead to dyspareunia. Although instruction on the use of vaginal lubricants can be helpful, thinning of the vaginal mucosa may still result in irritation on intercourse. Although controversial, use of topical vaginal estrogen (e.g., Estring, Pfizer, New York, NY, Vagifem, Novo Nordisk Pharmaceuticals Inc., Princeton, NJ) may be recommended for women experiencing severe dyspareunia. Studies indicate that the levels of circulating estrogens observed with this intervention are not expected to alter breast cancer recurrence patterns (132).

Hot flashes are among the most common acute and long-term side effects of breast cancer treatment. This symptom is seen secondary to chemotherapy-induced premature menopause, secondary to exposure to tamoxifen or raloxifene, or consequent to cessation of hormone replacement therapy (HRT) following diagnosis (133). Hot flashes can be profoundly debilitating for some women. Clonidine, venlafaxine, paroxetine, fluoxetine, mirtazapine, and gabapentin are nonhormonal agents that have demonstrated efficacy in small controlled and uncontrolled trials in reducing hot flashes and should be considered in patients unwilling or unable to take hormonal therapies (134–139). An accumulating body of evidence suggests, however, that several SSRI antidepressant drugs, especially fluoxetine and paroxetine, might interfere with tamoxifen metabolism by inhibiting the CYP2D6 enzyme. Venlafaxine and mirtazapine are antidepressants that minimally affect CYP2D6 activity and are a reasonable consideration for women taking tamoxifen (136). Soy-based phytoestrogens, on the other hand, appear to provide little relief of hot flashes compared with placebo (140). A further effect of chemotherapy is loss of libido, which is likely associated with a reduction in circulating androgens (141). For many women, loss of desire is the most difficult sequel to treat.

A final troubling side effect of systemic therapy is fatigue. Increased use of multidrug adjuvant therapies that are both more dose dense and more intense is leading to more women complaining of prolonged fatigue (142). Fatigue was once expected to resolve within months of completion of treatment, but reports of persistent fatigue among breast cancer survivors are growing. Longer follow-up studies of chemotherapy-exposed groups have shown that fatigue may be a chronic effect of treatment, lasting many months and even years after treatment ends (143). Noted clinically, the prevalence, etiology, and treatment of post-treatment fatigue continue to be needed areas of research (144). This symptom often occurs in the absence of evidence of anemia, although this should always be ruled out as a cause, and does not usually respond to increased rest. In one of the largest prospective studies to date, follow-up of women on average 7 years post-treatment found that 20% experienced persistent fatigue over the follow-up period, and that this persistent effect was associated with depression, cardiovascular problems, and prior treatment with both radiation and chemotherapy (143).

A final note in this area is that continued follow-up of cohorts of breast cancer survivors is necessary to provide us with needed information on both the chronic and potential late effects of newer therapies. This would include, for example, documentation of the course of pain syndromes, such as neuropathies seen in association with use of taxanes, as well as in women exposed to growth products (e.g., granulocyte colony-stimulating factor, Neupogen, and Epogen) during chemotherapy. Introduction of molecularly targeted agents, alone or in combination with chemotherapy (e.g., trastuzumab), will also increase our need for longitudinal outcome data among women treated, especially given early reports of troubling side effects even with these supposedly less toxic therapies (145,146). Although overall level of functioning and quality of life among long-term, disease-free breast cancer survivors remains high many years after primary therapy, past systemic adjuvant treatment was associated with persistent poorer performance in several domains, including physical activity and function, pain, and general health (83,147). These findings need to be taken into account when counseling women about treatment choice, particularly when disease is limited.

As critical as it is to prepare women well for the commencement of treatment, it is equally important to anticipate and plan for emotional reactions to ending treatment, when fears of recurrence peak. Our clinical experience suggests that women experience more severe reactive anxiety and depression during this part of the treatment than at an earlier period, perhaps because of their greater awareness of prognosis. In this regard, women who go on to adjuvant hormonal therapies may gain a sense of relief, knowing that they are still doing something active to prevent recurrence. A number of other factors also contribute to anxiety (Table 95.5). In recognition of the many persistent effects of modern breast cancer treatment, some clinicians routinely advise women anticipating the end of treatment to allot as many months for their recovery as were spent being treated for their cancer. This may be particularly important advice to help women negotiate the *re-entry* phase of their recovery, as they struggle to regain a sense of what will be their *new normal* and constructively interact with family members, friends, and colleagues, who may expect everything to return to usual shortly after the termination of treatment. Developing and discussing a treatment summary and follow-up care plan (issues discussed in greater detail under the survivorship section below) can also help ease the distress of women as they make the transition to recovery. Two booklets that form part of the NCI's *Facing Forward* series, *Life After Cancer Treatment*, and *When Someone You Love Has Completed Cancer Treatment*, provide useful information for the woman and her family about what to expect after initial therapy ends.

Adjuvant Hormonal Therapy

Increasing and even longer-term use (beyond 5 years) of tamoxifen, AIs, or both in the adjuvant setting has drawn attention to the psychological and sexual impact of these therapies. Once used mostly with postmenopausal patients, tamoxifen is now routinely given to premenopausal women with hormone receptor-positive breast cancer as part of their adjuvant therapy. Tamoxifen, an antiestrogen, has weak estrogenic effects on the vaginal mucosa. Some older women find that the associated increase in hot flashes with tamoxifen (or an AI) is a limiting factor in its use. By contrast, some younger patients report that tamoxifen provides relief from the vaginal dryness and decreased libido that accompany chemotherapy-induced premature menopause. Problems with tamoxifen-related hot flashes are more common among women who have a history of moderate to severe hot flashes with menopause and a history of estrogen therapy use. It is important to note that a small subset of women become depressed with use of tamoxifen, which can require temporary or even permanent discontinuation of its use (148). The impact of tamoxifen exposure on brain function is also beginning to come under examination (149–151). Reports of a small number of deaths from tamoxifen-related uterine cancer, as well as concern over other toxicities, have made many patients and physicians anxious about continued or long-term use of this drug. Rates of discontinuation or nonpersistence of use of tamoxifen, whether owing to problems with drug side effects or some other reason, may be higher than believed (152,153). (See Chapter 48 for a discussion of appropriate monitoring for these potential complications.)

Less is known about the psychological and sexual impact of the newer class of hormonal agents, the AIs (154,155). These agents have been associated with troubling joint and muscle pain symptoms (156,157). One report found that as many as 10% of women had discontinued AI use because of these side effects (158). The impact of these newer therapies on women's sense of well-being as well as adherence patterns among breast cancer survivors with respect to long-term adjuvant hormonal use are areas warranting future research.

RECURRENT AND ADVANCED DISEASE

With more women living longer after treatment for breast cancer, the numbers of those treated subsequently for recurrent local and distant disease have grown. Although previously neglected, the research examining women's reactions to these events has grown as well (159). When breast cancer patients learn of a recurrence, they are usually "devastated." Overall quality-of-life recovery is slower following a recurrence compared with recovery following initial diagnosis and treatment. Despite the physical burden of recurrence, during the year after diagnosis women show steady improvement in psychological functioning, reflecting the adaptive capacity of survivors (159). The associated distress with recurrence can come in many forms and affect multiple quality-of-life domains (160). Compared with disease-free survivors, women with recurrent breast cancer report poorer physical functioning and perceived health, more impairment in emotional well-being, more problems in relationships with family and health care providers, and less hope. Even when disease is localized, significant levels of psychiatric morbidity may occur (159,161,162). Family members of these women also report high levels of emotional distress (161). Whereas much research has been done on the role of social support and women's response to breast cancer, research among women suffering a recurrence suggests that their emotional distress can also affect the support received. When psychological distress persists in the context of a recurrence, it may serve to drive away rather than elicit support

---

Table 95.5	**CHALLENGES RELATED TO ENDING TREATMENT**

1. Fear that the cancer will return
2. Concern about ongoing monitoring (e.g., whom to call if a problem or symptom arises)
3. Loss of a supportive environment (including relationships with staff and fellow patients)
4. Diminished sense of well-being because of treatment effects (often feeling less well than when treatment was initiated)
5. Social demands: "re-entry" problems (dealing with expectations of family and friends that the breast cancer patient will quickly be back to "normal" and resume full function equivalent to pre-illness levels)

from a social network (163). Women with recurrent disease, whether local or distant, are a particularly vulnerable group for whom active psychosocial intervention is warranted. Any planned assistance should include attention to the strain on family members.

Supportive care for patients with advanced breast cancer is aimed at comfort and control of symptoms. Different metastatic sites, especially bone, lungs, and brain, present special supportive problems. As discussed in the section Interventions, participation in support groups may improve quality of survival significantly in this group of women, although the effect of such groups on length of survival appears limited (164).

Advanced care is often provided at home with support from the family or in a hospice setting (see Chapter 76). Central to the success of a home care program is continuity of care with physicians and staff and continued support of family and friends. Psychiatric consultation should be considered when distress (anxiety and depression) is not responsive to the usual supportive measures. Depression in particular may reach significant proportions in these settings (165). Although suicide is unusual, suicidal ideation is common. A management approach that combines psychological support with use of antidepressants and anxiolytics (particularly clonazepam and lorazepam) is often helpful. Agitated behavior associated with metabolic encephalopathy, resulting often from hypercalcemia, brain metastases, or narcotic or steroid side effects, may require use of a neuroleptic.

Because pain is such a common companion of people living with advanced stages of disease, attention to its management is critical to patient care (166). Cancer pain is perceived by the American public to be the worst type of pain (167) and the most feared symptom. Patients with cancer who experience pain are more likely to exhibit higher levels of mood disturbance and functional disability than those who have little or no pain. Spiegel and Bloom (168) found that for women with metastatic breast cancer, beliefs about the meaning of the pain in relation to the illness predicted level of pain better than site of metastasis. Glajchen et al. (169) found that 64% of patients surveyed cited communication barriers as an impediment to pain relief. This may be exacerbated if the physician does more talking than listening (170). Attitudinal barriers to compliance with medical treatment were cited by more than half of the respondents, including stoicism and fear of narcotic addiction. Thus, addressing the meaning and response to pain from the perspective of the patient is as important as providing an explanation of proposed control techniques.

INTERVENTIONS

The use and variety of psychosocial and behavioral interventions applied in the cancer setting in general and in breast cancer care in particular continue to grow (171). Population-based data demonstrate cancer to be one of several chronic illnesses that precipitate the need for, and use of, mental health services (172,173). Young age at diagnosis, being a younger survivor (<65 years), being formerly married, and having a chronic comorbid illness all are associated with increased use of mental health services in the context of cancer. Despite documented need, as many as one in six survivors may fail to receive mental health services because of cost (172).

Although varying greatly by type (e.g., individual vs. group), orientation (e.g., behavioral vs. cognitive vs. supportive), mode of delivery (in person vs. remote, e.g., by phone, Internet, or teleconference), duration (time limited vs. open ended), and timing (e.g., before, during, or after treatment), as well as target populations served (early vs. advanced, <40 years vs. older, partnered vs. single, or mixed), the fundamental purpose of interventions developed has been the same—to provide each

woman with the skills or resources necessary to cope with her illness and improve the quality of her life and health. The various types of psychosocial and behavioral interventions used in the cancer setting and their efficacy in improving targeted outcomes are well reviewed elsewhere (174–176). Most of these interventions have been developed specifically for patients with breast cancer or have included patients with breast cancer. Detailed review of the use of different interventions in the care of patients with breast cancer is beyond the scope of this chapter. However, three points must be made regarding the use of such programs in the overall care of patients with breast cancer and their families.

First, researchers have found that patients who received an intervention designed to improve knowledge or coping or to reduce distress do better than those who did not. Specifically, patients provided or randomized to some form of individual or group intervention experienced less anxiety and depression, had an increased sense of control, had improved body image and better sexual function, reported greater satisfaction with care, and exhibited improved medication adherence (176,177). Importantly, in no studies to date have women who received additional help fared worse than their peers who received *standard care*. If anything, these studies have demonstrated that *usual* care is often inadequate for many women and that additional education and support have the potential to significantly enhance women's function and well-being. Significant attention needs to be brought to bear on the development and delivery of psychosocial care models if we are to understand who needs what, delivered by whom, and when in the course of care (178,179). Further, understanding the economic impact of these programs or services in terms of delivery, changes in health care utilization, and out-of-pocket expenses may be critical if we are to expect broader uptake of these into routine practice (180,181).

Second, use of psychosocial interventions continues to grow, especially in the setting of breast cancer. Use of these services reflects not only patient demand for supportive care, but also growing recognition that addressing psychosocial issues may improve outcomes for patients (4). At one point, it was hoped that such interventions would result in life extension. In their seminal study, Spiegel et al. (182) found that women with metastatic breast cancer who participated in 1 year of weekly supportive-expressive group therapy that included instruction in self-hypnosis for pain (N (patient/group numbers)=50) survived an average of 18 months longer from time of randomization compared with a control group (N=36). Two replication studies, however, one conducted by Goodwin et al. (164) in Toronto and the second by Spiegel et al. (183), have failed to demonstrate a survival benefit of supportive-expressive group therapy. Both teams did, nevertheless, find significant benefit to women in overall quality of life and pain management (184). The current consensus is that psychosocial interventions do not prolong survival (185). In breast cancer, because so many women do well or live for longer periods even with more advanced disease, the incremental benefit to survival conferred by receipt of these interventions may be harder to detect.

The newest wave of research seeks to understand the psychoneuroimmunologic interface between behavioral or supportive interventions and survivors' health, to enable better understanding of exactly how these interventions work (186–188). Provocative, but admittedly preliminary, research in the area of psychoneuroimmunology and cancer suggested that psychological variables (e.g., perceived stress, mood) might modify disease outcomes (189,190). However, efforts to design interventions to address this interface have produced mixed results. Despite the growing number of trials reported, meta-analyses provide only modest evidence that psychosocial or behavioral interventions reliably alter immune parameters.

The most consistent evidence has come from hypnosis and conditioning trials (191). Because of their key role in breast cancer, a better understanding of the impact of psychosocial interventions on endocrine functioning and disease outcomes warrants further pursuit. Finding and recruiting appropriate participants, selecting the most promising biologic system measures, and designing and delivering methodologically rigorous studies will be key challenges to advancing this science (191).

Third, although it might be argued that an individually tailored intervention should result in the best outcome for any given patient, this may not be feasible, suitable, or even desirable in all cases. Some patients with cancer resist being singled out for individual therapy and feel burdened by any label that might suggest that they are mentally ill and not simply medically ill. Furthermore, increasing evidence shows that participation in group activity offers a uniquely supportive and normalizing experience for many patients with cancer struggling to deal with the realities of their new or continued status as cancer survivors. In studies that have specifically compared use of individual interventions with group interventions, groups were as effective as individual counseling or support in reducing patient distress (192). Use of new communication technologies, in particular the Internet, but also established ones, such as teleconferencing and telephone (193,194), to provide group support represents the new frontier in intervention research. These technologies not only extend the capacity to reach women isolated by geography or physical limitations, but also (in the case of phone and Internet) permit some degree of anonymity and content control for those women more hesitant to engage in face-to-face programs. In addition to providing medical information, the Internet may offer a unique vehicle to improve access to information and social support and reduce isolation (195–197).

Research suggests that four key elements are vital to achieving optimal outcomes for all cancer survivors:

- Access to state-of-the-art cancer care
- Active coping, in particular active participation or engagement in one's care, even if this means delegating decision-making
- Use of social support (although it is recognized that the perception that this is available may be sufficient) (198)
- Having a sense of meaning or purpose in life (this can include someone to live for, spiritual belief or connectedness, or a way to make sense of illness and health and one's place in the world)

Many of the psychosocial and behavioral interventions developed in cancer are designed to foster or reinforce some or all of these core needs. However, access to these remains a problem. Clinician awareness about, and referral of patients to, even such well-established programs as the American Cancer Society's Reach to Recovery is variable (199). Providers in one health maintenance organization report referring 70% of their patients to system-provided services and estimated that 40% of patients used these, when in fact fewer than 10% of patients reported this was the case. Further, patient barriers to service use cited in this study were lack of awareness of the service and lack of provider referral. Individuals who already felt they had adequate support also made less use of services when they were provided (200).

Key to the development of an effective intervention is the recognition that for many women, cancer represents a transitional event. As defined by Andrykowski et al. (201), cancer is "a traumatic event that alters an individual's assumptive world with the potential to produce long-lasting changes of both a positive as well as negative nature." As such, the primary goal in any intervention is to use this teachable moment to help minimize the negative and enhance the positive impact of illness on recovery and well-being.

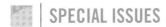

SPECIAL ISSUES

Three changes in how breast cancer is diagnosed and treated have important ramifications for clinicians in their treatment of patients. These include increased awareness of the familial nature of breast cancer, greater involvement of family in patient care, and growing attention to the impact of breast cancer treatment on women's sexual functioning. (Psychological issues related to being at genetic risk for breast cancer are covered in Chapter 19.) In the remaining sections, the special issues related to the care of other family members and the role of sexual quality of life in rehabilitation are reviewed. In addition, a final section touches on the burgeoning interest in, and information on, the well-being of our growing population of long-term breast cancer survivors.

Role and Care of the Family

Social support has been found to be integral not only to positive adjustment, but also to length of survival (202) in women with breast cancer. When people are ill, they tend to feel less in control and less confident, especially when they must rely on others. At the same time, serious illness of any kind increases the ill person's need for closeness to others to counteract feelings of insecurity and vulnerability. The need for love and support often heightens in patients over time, as a reaction to the effects of disease and treatment and the fear that they will no longer be loved or cared for. Fears of abandonment and rejection are often keenly felt by the patient with cancer. Absence of social support or loss of a significant person who withdraws during the patient's illness becomes an additional stressor that may be more emotionally painful than the illness itself.

Active involvement of the family clearly serves a range of patient needs, from the most basic—namely, provision of emotional support (the "psychic fuel" that keeps a patient going) to the practical (e.g., financial resources and transportation to treatment) to the more abstract (e.g., providing meaningful roles and hence functional goals toward which the patient can strive). Despite the recognized importance of the role of partners and family in caring for women with breast cancer, this subject remains the focus of only a modest number of studies (203–205). Further, even less is known about family adaptation long-term because most studies conducted have examined the acute or early post-treatment period. Once treatment ends, family members must adapt to the changes brought on by cancer (e.g., role shifts, economic shifts, ongoing care needs), deal with their loved one's lingering effects of illness (altered appearance, function, or behavior), and learn to live with potential uncertainty about the future (206). Family caregivers may experience lower quality of life, more fear of cancer recurrence, and less support than their loved one with cancer does (207). The strongest predictors for survivors' quality of life were family stressors, social support, meaning of the illness, and employment status, whereas the strongest predictors for family caregivers' quality of life were fear of recurrence and social support. Of note, survivors' and caregivers' quality of life contributed independently to the others' (207).

Partners' adaptation, similar to patients,' varies over time. In a comparison study between couples' adaptation to benign versus malignant disease, those facing breast cancer reported greater decreases in marital and family functioning, more uncertain appraisals, and more illness-related adjustment problems. The strongest predictors of adjustment for women were severity of the illness and hopelessness, and for husbands, their own baseline level of adjustment (208). In a separate study, Mellon and Northouse (209) reported that risk for spousal distress was increased in cases in which the wife's illness was more severe, she experienced more distress, there were more limited resources available (e.g., for economic and social support), and greater stresses on the family. Work by Lewis et al. (210) indicates that spouses who are older, less well educated, more recently married, or in less well-adjusted marriages; who expressed heightened fears over their wife's well being; who worried about their job performance; or were more uncertain about their future were more likely to be depressed (210).

The impact of cancer on the couple may be observed long after treatment ends. In their work, Northouse et al. (211) found that couples who reported high levels of distress or a greater number of role problems at diagnosis were at risk for high distress as much as 1 year later. Further, they found that patients' and husbands' levels of adjustment were significantly related. Other factors influence couples' adaptation as well. Ben-Zur et al. (212) report that husbands' perception of their wives' coping as emotion focused was associated with low psychosocial function, whereas perception of her coping as problem focused was linked to husbands' higher psychosocial functioning. Husbands' over- or underestimation of wives' adjustment also may have a negative impact on wives' mood (213). Northouse (214) reported that when asked what helped them cope with illness during hospitalization and 1 month later, both patients and husbands identified emotional support, information, attitude, and religion as being important factors. Satisfaction with the partner's helping relationship is also associated with patients' psychological well-being (215). However, younger couples may be at particular risk of having problems (216).

Open dialogue, characterized by high empathy and low withdrawal, appears to be critical to optimal outcomes. Sabo et al. (217) found that the tendency for some men to assume a "protective guardian" stance was sometimes a deterrent to effective and open communication. On the reverse side, avoidant coping in husbands was associated with worse adaptation in these men (218). Kagawa-Singer and Wellisch (219) stress the importance of appreciating cultural differences when interpreting couples' adaptation. They found that Asian American women (specifically those of Chinese and Japanese descent) were expected to be self-sacrificing and nurturing of husband and family regardless of illness, whereas European American women were allowed to be more dependent. Further, Asian American women emphasized a goal of harmony over intimacy, whereas European American women embraced the reverse, and in communication preferred nonverbal versus the verbal communication style valued by European American women. These studies indicate that families may require assistance both with role adjustment and in addressing maladaptive communication styles in the face of life-threatening illness. Early work on interventions to promote coping conducted with family caregivers alone (220–222) or in combination with the survivor (223,224) document modest benefits. In a few of these studies, patients or family members also appeared to benefit from the caregiver's participation in the intervention, even though they were not part of the intervention, suggesting a ripple effect of these programs (220,221). Interventions to reduce distress among caregivers of older women with cancer have the potential to reduce patients' hospital readmissions and interruptions in cancer therapy and to improve both patients' and caregivers' emotional health (225). More research in this promising adjunct to quality care is needed (226,227).

Although many couples describe being on an "emotional roller coaster" across the course of care, most spouses rise to the myriad challenges of breast cancer in their mate. One study found that a significant number (42%) of couples felt that breast cancer brought them closer (228). Although research into marital breakdown or divorce after cancer is sparse, partners generally do not abandon the marriage (229). Rather, the data thus far indicate that most marital relationships remain stable and, in some cases, may be strengthened by the cancer experience. The evidence does suggest, however, that a preexisting history of marital discord is a risk factor for breakdown following a cancer diagnosis (229,230). Taylor-Brown et al. (231) surmise that two additional factors may lead the woman to dissolve a partnership. The first of these is life review. Cancer is very "permission giving" to many survivors. The woman who uses this event to examine her satisfaction with a preexisting partnership may, if she finds it lacking or emotionally dissatisfying, decide to make a major life change and exit the relationship. In a similar vein, desire to reduce the stress in her life, felt by many women to be a causal factor in risk for cancer, may precipitate a drive to make major life changes. If a woman feels that her marriage is adding to and not serving to reduce the stress of illness, she may feel compelled to get out of this situation to safeguard her health.

It is critical to remember that support is a two-way street; the source of the problem may arise in the provider of support (family member) or in the recipient and commonly involves both (232,233). The impact of cancer can be as devastating to a family member as to the patient herself, and sometimes worse. Although the woman can obtain support from multiple sources and control her anxiety through focus on just getting through treatment, partners often receive less attention and report feeling uncertain what to do and helpless in their role as observers. Spouses may feel angry, ashamed, and vulnerable to illness themselves. Clinicians who work with families of patients with cancer suggest that they may at times need to be viewed as second-order patients. Furthermore, their needs may vary across the course of illness and recovery. It is helpful for staff to acknowledge the difficult task faced by family members, to provide opportunities for them to talk about questions and reactions both with the patient and alone, and to ensure that backup supports are available and that provision is made to give family members relief, especially if care is going to be complex or long term. It is also important to permit family members to limit care to those areas in which they are most comfortable and effective.

The traumatic effect on children, both sons and daughters, is considerable when the mother develops breast cancer. Behavioral problems (including regressive and acting-out behavior), conflicts with parents, and other symptoms of emotional distress (anxiety, depression, and diminished self-esteem) have been seen to increase during illness in a parent (234–238). A number of factors may affect a child's response to maternal breast cancer, including disease severity, family and child coping reactions, the child's age, and parent and family characteristics, in particular their communication or expressiveness (239,240).

Lichtman et al. (241) noted deterioration of the mother–child relationship in 12% of women with breast cancer they studied. Problems were more likely to arise in those situations in which the mother had a poor prognosis, extensive surgery, poor psychological adjustment, or to a smaller extent, difficulty in adjusting to chemotherapy or radiotherapy. A history of parent–child conflicts also placed the relationship at risk during the mother's illness. Mothers' relationships with their daughters were significantly more stressed than those with their sons. Daughters were more likely to show signs of fearfulness, withdrawal, and hostility, emanating perhaps from their greater fears of developing the disease and the greater demands placed on the daughters. These findings parallel those reported by Litman (235) and Wellisch (242), who noted that mothers rely more often on daughters than on sons during illness and that adolescent daughters may be particularly vulnerable to disruption in their lives. In a series of longitudinal studies, Armsden and Lewis (243) found that, although rated as better behaved by their mothers and nurse observers than children of healthy parents or those with noncancer illness, young and preadolescent children (ages 6–12 years) were especially susceptible to feelings of low self-esteem when dealing with their mother's early-stage breast cancer. Children's reports of distress and poor self-concept persisted over an 8-month period (243). The relationship between the mother's illness and her child's coping is often complex. In one study, women who were more depressed, were single heads of household, and reported greater illness-related demands on their family were more likely to have a child with lower self-worth and social acceptance; these mothers were also more likely to report lower quality in parenting their children (244). In this study, many single women, when interviewed, said they were besieged by feelings of self-deprecation because of the breast cancer and felt alone with their disease.

The monitoring of all children, especially when the mother's breast cancer is advanced, is important. The opportunity for parents to discuss how and what to tell their children about the mother's illness early in the course of care is also important and should include advice on tailoring these conversations to meet appropriate developmental needs of their offspring. Specific interventions to help a mother and her children cope with illness may be helpful (245). A number of books addressing this topic and a publication of the NCI, *When Someone in Your Family Has Cancer,* may be useful in this process. Many mental health professionals recommend that key staff at the child's school be informed when a parent has cancer. Teachers and school counselors can assist in monitoring the child's behavior and response to this family stressor. This task may be more difficult when the offspring is an adolescent. Some work suggests that this age group may have many unmet needs when the parent is ill (239).

Finally, concern about what impact breast cancer may have on a mother's survival may be complicated by worry about its meaning for an offspring's future well-being. Many women diagnosed with breast cancer are the first in their family to have the disease and report feeling guilty about having "brought the disease into the family." At the same time, adult offspring, in particular daughters, may feel angry about, or frightened by, the potential implications of their mother's illness on their risk of the disease. With the growth of high-risk genetic clinics, attention has focused on the overall psychological adjustment and quality of life of female first-degree relatives of patients. These patterns of response in female family members warrant special attention, because excessive psychological distress potentially can interfere both with family function and with adherence to subsequent breast cancer screening, an issue addressed in greater detail in Chapter 19. Whereas the information needs of women treated for breast cancer are well documented, those of their family members bear further study.

Quality of Life and Sexual Functioning

The impact of disease and treatment on women's sexual functioning, once rarely discussed or addressed, has garnered growing research attention. Interest in this previously neglected topic is both a function of past advocacy by women for greater attention to these issues and consequent to the increasing numbers of women for whom treatment is causing significant problems in this valued area of function.

Several large studies inform our knowledge of this area of breast cancer survivors' health and functioning. Data gathered by Ganz et al. (79,246) among 227 patients with early-stage breast cancer suggest that a subset of women may be at risk for psychosexual distress after treatment. At-risk women, evaluated shortly after diagnosis, were identified as having more physical, psychosocial, medical interaction, sexual, and marital problems. One year later, problems and frequencies for the at-risk group included not feeling sexually attractive (54%), not being interested in having sex (44%), decreased frequency of sexual intercourse (58%), difficulty in becoming sexually aroused (42%), difficulty with lubrication (50%), and difficulty in achieving orgasm (41% low risk and 56% at risk). Important in their research was the finding that, whereas survivors

appear to attain maximal recovery from the physical and emotional trauma by 1 year after surgery, a number of specific problems persist beyond 1 year, in particular those amenable to sexual rehabilitation (e.g., body image, lubrication, orgasm).

In a subsequent large-scale follow-up study, conducted among 864 breast cancer survivors on average 3 years after diagnosis, Ganz et al. (84) found survivors' sexual functioning to be similar to that of age-matched healthy women. However, younger women who experienced chemotherapy-induced menopause and women of any age who received chemotherapy reported poorer sexual functioning (84). Problems in sexual comfort (lubrication and pain with intercourse) persisted in these latter groups of women even years after completion of chemotherapy (83). In addition to treatment received, predictors of sexual health after breast cancer include a number that are mutable to change, including vaginal dryness, emotional health, body image, the quality of the partnered relationship, and sexual problems in the partner (247).

In their review of sexuality and cancer in women, Weijmar Schultz et al. (248) describe the range of psychological reactions to cancer that threaten sexual function, including threats to

- Sexual identity and self-esteem, such as disturbances of mood, gender, and sexual identity and body image
- Personal control over body functions, such as disease-related symptoms (e.g., pain, fatigue, and nausea) that interfere with or inhibit sexual functioning
- Intimacy, such as loss of social contacts that have potential for intimate physical expression, the disintegration of established patterns of achieving physical pleasure and intimacy, or myths related to contagion
- Reproductive function, such as the direct impairment of fertility or the fear of recurrence with pregnancy

In addition to these psychological reactions, some women experience less joy and vigor, as well as an underlying uncertainty about their health and the vulnerability of their bodies to further assault (249). The emotional distress, pain, fatigue, and insult to the patient's body image and self-esteem caused by the diagnosis and treatment of breast cancer can damage sexual functioning, even among individuals who had a strong and satisfying sexual relationship before illness. When illness occurs in the context of preexisting problems or before relationships are fully established, the outcome may be devastating. Despite heightened sensitivity to sexual issues, in practice, provision of effective sexual interventions remains highly variable. Further, research to guide the delivery and evaluate the impact of care in this area is limited.

A central challenge to addressing sexual dysfunction when it occurs is avoidance of this sensitive topic by both provider and patient. In addition to the discomfort most people feel when discussing sex, practitioners must contend with limited time and at times privacy to raise these issues, lack of awareness that sexual problems are being encountered, or when present, knowledge about local resources to address these. It is hoped that this last barrier is dissipating as education about effective therapies for problems such as vaginal dryness, hot flashes, painful intercourse, and lack of desire becomes more broadly acknowledged and available. Finally, belief that the patient is principally (or solely) concerned with her cancer, despite well-documented evidence in the President's Cancer Panel as well as Institute of Medicine survivorship reports (250,251) refuting this, prevents other staff from raising sexual issues.

Special training in sex therapy techniques is not a prerequisite for discussing sexual dysfunction; only information about and willingness to refer women for help with these issues is needed. For women still in their childbearing years, American Society of Clinical Oncology (ASCO) guidelines are now available about asking and referring these individuals for fertility preservation options and counseling (252). (See Chapter 96 on Reproductive Issues in Breast Cancer Survivors for discussion of management of fertility and breast cancer.) Health care professionals should be reassured that their patients often feel an enormous sense of relief to have a problem acknowledged and to know that it is not uncommon and that help is available through suitable referral. Because sexual problems tend to worsen, not improve, over time, sexual rehabilitation needs to start early. Ideally, this should occur before treatment starts for those patients for whom specific impairment of sexual function can be anticipated (e.g., premature menopause in the premenopausal or perimenopausal woman). Raising the topic of sexual function early, by letting the patient know it is an appropriate focus of concern and that the health care provider is willing to discuss it, opens the door for future dialogue in this area. It also helps ensure that problems with sexual function will be addressed. Auchincloss (253) cautions, however, against initiating sexual discussions during periods of acute stress (e.g., treatment setbacks, recurrences, and family or work crises) and places a high premium on finding a private space for conducting such dialogues. Some teams may find it practical to designate one staff member to initiate conversations or to follow up on those introduced by the primary physician. The primary nurse often is best suited for this position. Establishing this role is important because it is as undesirable to have everyone asking about sexual function as to have no one inquire about this area of concern. When specific questions arise, the nurse needs to know what the patient has been told and by whom, to focus questions for patients, direct their inquiries to the appropriate staff member, clarify or reinforce information provided, and serve as an advocate for the patient. Above all, this designated member should know about resources for help in this area and, as needed, coordinate input with that of others (254).

BREAST CANCER SURVIVORS

Growing attention is being focused on cancer survivors and the experience of living through and beyond their illness and its treatment (250,251,255,256). A number of reasons exist for this. One is the large and increasing number of survivors, a figure that already includes more than 2.5 million women with a history of breast cancer in the United States alone (2). A second reason is that more of these individuals are surviving longer after treatment. Among current breast cancer survivors, almost 343,000 were diagnosed 20 or more years ago (2). A third reason is that as more women live longer after breast cancer, they are surviving sufficiently long to experience the persistent and late consequences of their cancer treatments. As this population has grown, so too has our understanding of cancer's long-term and late effects on patients' health and well-being (257).

Although women vary widely in their response to diagnosis and treatment, it is remarkable that most return to lives that are as full as and often richer personally than before their illness; in many cases, survivors' social and emotional functioning was found to be better than that of control or comparison samples of unaffected peers. Although some women leave jobs following a cancer diagnosis, either by choice or because of disability (258), employment patterns show that breast cancer survivors who continue to work may work longer hours even than their unaffected peers (259). Besides being a vital source of income and often of needed health care coverage, work can also be an important source of social support and self-esteem as well as distraction from illness during treatment. Those in manual labor jobs (which often includes women with lower education and income) may experience more limitations, but most find that employers are accommodating to their needs

(260), suggesting that many of the myths about cancer's adverse impact on survivors' functional capacity are beginning to be dispelled (261). However, counseling around work-related issues and referral for help in negotiating workplace issues are important in aiding women's continued employment as desired (262).

In general, the current generation of studies has led clinicians to realize that concern about high rates of subsequent marked impairment in treated women may have been exaggerated (263–265). Our own work and that of others has shown that breast cancer does not appear to lead to the development of a post-traumatic stress disorder in significant numbers of women (29,266,267). Striking to many clinical researchers involved in the conduct of long-term follow-up studies is the enormous resilience evidenced by women. In the words of one survivor, "It sure has a way of putting your life's priorities in order! Shame it had to happen, but in many ways my life is better. I'm no longer a workaholic, more loving, kinder to others, much more spiritual. I spend much more time with family. I'm more comfortable and 'centered' in my life. I fell in love with my husband all over again" (84). Indeed, responses such as these have generated an entire genre of studies examining what is referred to as post-traumatic growth or benefit-finding (268,269). Some data suggest that black women in particular may be able to find meaning in their cancer experience (65,270). Also impressive has been the willingness of women to share important details about their cancer experience and recovery. Whereas some of the willingness to share is driven by altruistic motives and the hope of many survivors to improve the lives of women who will be diagnosed and treated after them, it also stems from a desire to bring to the attention of the medical community the need to document and, when needed, address the potential late effects of breast cancer on women's lives into the future. The growing interest in cancer survivorship, as reflected in the number of programs offered by the NCI-designated cancer centers designed specifically to address survivors' needs after treatment, is testament that survivors' call to action is being heard (http://cancercenters. cancer.gov/documents/Survivorship%20Appendix%20D.pdf). Services provided focus on two main areas: (*a*) surveillance and (*b*) health and well-being after treatment.

Follow-up Care and Surveillance After Treatment

Although concern about disease recurrence may diminish over time, for most breast cancer survivors, this never fully goes away. In our research among women on average 3 years after diagnosis, 42% said they worried a fair amount to very much that the cancer would come back. Younger women and those exposed to chemotherapy were more likely to worry about a future recurrence (84). Degree of worry may fluctuate and be triggered by a variety of sources, including continuing physical problems after treatment (271) (Table 95.6). At the same time, family members' fear of recurrence in the survivor can have a direct and adverse affect on family quality of life, whereas the survivor's fear of recurrence affected family meaning of cancer illness that in turn adversely affected quality of life (207). When activated, fear can lead to disruptive behavior, such as heightened body monitoring (frequent self-examination for signs and symptoms of a recurrence), anxiety well in advance of a doctor visit, and worry about the future, or, in some instances, severely disabling reactions, including hypochondriac-like preoccupation with health at one extreme, or avoidance and denial at the other, inability to plan for the future, and despair. Surprisingly, despite its prevalence, relatively few interventions have been developed that specifically target this aspect of women's recovery. The one exception to this general pattern is work by Mishel (272) who, along with her colleagues, has been developing interventions to help women successfully cope with uncertainty. Although other

Table 95.6	TRIGGERS FOR FEAR OF RECURRENCE

1. Routine follow-up visits and tests
2. Anniversary dates (e.g, date of diagnosis, end of cancer treatment, birthday)
3. Worrisome or "suspicious" symptoms
4. Persistent treatment-related side effects (especially fatigue or pain)
5. Change in health (e.g., weight loss, fatigue)
6. Illness in a family member
7. Death of a fellow survivor/prominent cancer survivor
8. Times of stress
9. Idiosyncratic triggers (e.g., "learned responses" such as the smell of alcohol due to association with receipt of chemotherapy; sight of the treatment center)

interventions that effectively reduce distress and improve a sense of well-being might be expected to result in decreased worry about disease recurrence, this remains to be tested.

Part of this persistent anxiety may be attributable to the fact that breast cancer survivors understand that their cancer could recur at any time after treatment and that medical follow-up must continue for life. Data support the appropriateness of this concern. As women live longer after their initial breast cancer diagnosis, they are at higher risk than women with no cancer history of developing a second cancer, most often a second breast cancer (273). In this context, it is important to note that not all women post-treatment for breast cancer consider or think of themselves as "survivors." Although some women embrace this language and are proud of their status, others reject being so labeled. Still others fear that calling themselves survivors before 5 years might invite a recurrence. More important is that each woman treated recognizes the need for follow-up for life. Involvement in the decision-making around follow-up care itself, the third major decision point in the breast cancer patient's illness pathway (Table 95.2), has been shown to be associated with improved quality of life (274). Failing to plan for follow-up care sets clinicians up to fail to meet survivors' needs (275). Observational data show that receipt of post-treatment surveillance mammograms reduces breast cancer-related mortality in older survivors treated for early-stage disease (276).

In response to the recommendation in both the President's Cancer Panel Report (250) and the Institute of Medicine (IOM) adult cancer survivorship report (251) that survivors receive a treatment summary and plan for future care at the end of treatment, ASCO released templates for the generation of this information (277) and plans to make their use one of their quality oncology practice indicators (QOPI). However, what type of follow-up care should be provided to which survivors and at what periodicity is a major topic of debate (278) (see Chapter 70 on Evaluation of Patients After Primary Therapy). The primary purpose of follow-up care historically was to provide surveillance for recurrent disease. With the growth of survivorship research, this approach has undergone a major transition. Increasingly, it is recognized that women also need to be followed and treated for adverse long-term or persistent (e.g., fatigue, premature menopause, sexual dysfunction) and late occurring (second nonbreast cancer malignancies, lymphedema, cardiac toxicity, premature aging effects) sequelae of treatment. The status and challenge of this new area of care are well described in the thoughtful review of Kattlove and Winn (279). They note that optimal follow-up care must address women's needs in the following domains: surveillance, genetic counseling and testing, detection and treatment of second primaries, treatment complications, physiologic alterations, and psychosocial problems. Ganz and Hahn (280) provide guidance on how to implement these more comprehensive

care plans for breast cancer survivors transitioning to recovery. Among the questions for the future will be to determine where this care is best delivered and by whom: in primary care, specialty clinics, or some combination of these (281–283). Research will also be needed on the cost, both economic and with respect to women's sense of well-being, of the models developed for follow-up care.

Greater attention in the general medical community to the potential physical late effects of treatment will likely generate new information for women into the future. Persistent problem areas reported by women include fatigue, dealing with menopausal symptoms, coming to terms with body image changes, and negotiating strategies to reduce risk for work and health insurance discrimination. In addition to providing valuable data on the health-related quality-of-life outcomes for women treated, the growing population of survivors has created a resource both for other survivors and for those who are newly diagnosed with breast cancer. Use of experienced veteran-to-rookie counselors and role models can provide a vital complement to the comprehensive care of patients.

An important take-home message in all of the research discussed in this last section is that a cancer diagnosis represents for many a "teachable moment" for health care providers along with breast cancer survivors themselves (284), a moment currently being missed by many oncology practitioners (285,286). The crisis of cancer often creates a window of receptivity during which health care professionals can provide patients with educational messages about and support for pursuing healthy lifestyle choices. Although these activities, if adopted, may not alter length of breast cancer survival, they do carry the potential to reduce individual risk significantly for treatment-related or other chronic illness-related morbidities and potentially other cancers. To take full advantage of this opportunity to intervene, it will be vital to understand what women identify as important for them to address (e.g., weight, diet, stress, exercise, and tobacco and alcohol use), the types of information and resources needed to promote and maintain change in these identified areas, and how to most effectively deliver these interventions. Encouraging breast cancer survivors to take control of what they can in their lives may enable them to live with better health in, and less fear of, the future.

Health Behavior after Cancer

One of the newest topics in breast cancer follow-up care is the role of health promotion (see also Chapter 53). This has been spurred largely by survivors' interest in, and growing requests for, informed guidance about what they can do to reduce their risk of cancer-related morbidity and mortality. Many breast cancer survivors already report taking better care of themselves in the wake of cancer, with particular focus on adopting healthier lifestyles, reducing stress, eating better, and exercising regularly. As Maunsell et al. (287) point out, these changes are often adopted independent of physician advice. In our research with long-term ($\geq$5 years after diagnosis) breast cancer survivors, the areas in which the experience of cancer had the most positive impact were in diet, exercise activities, and religious beliefs. The greatest negative impact was felt in the domains of love life and, for younger survivors, on work life or career and financial situation (83).

Two areas receiving significant research attention with respect to their impact on women's health outcomes are stress management and physical activity interventions. As noted earlier, many women believe the stress in their lives can precipitate or exacerbate breast disease. For these survivors, reducing stress is seen as potentially life-saving. Researchers at the University of Miami's Mind Body Center have developed a standardized 10-week training program that equips women with the cognitive and behavioral skills necessary to identify, analyze, and manage stress (288,289). In a slightly different model, Jacobsen et al. (290) found that a self-administered form of stress management may be as effective as or more effective than, as well as less costly than, a professionally delivered program in improving role functioning, mental health, and physical well-being.

A second avenue to stress reduction is staying active during or becoming physically active after cancer treatment. One of the fastest growing areas of behavioral research in general (291) and with respect to cancer in particular (292,293), physical activity interventions have taken on even greater importance as the nation struggles with rising rates of obesity (294). Research shows that physical activity, often begun now during treatment, can improve mood (reduce anxiety and depression), enhance cardiovascular function, control weight, improve body image and self-esteem, reduce nausea and fatigue, and potentially alter immune function (295–297). Weight, diet, and to a more variable extent, exercise have been linked to breast cancer risk and mortality (298–300). To date, two observational studies (301,302) and one randomized clinical trial (303) have found a survival benefit for women who became or remained moderately physically active after breast cancer treatment.

As the evidence of its benefits for survivors mounts, lifestyle changes (in particular physical activity, smoking cessation, weight control, and to some extent, lower fat and more fruit and vegetable consumption) are being recommended after treatment (304,305). As mentioned earlier, many have begun to argue that cancer may well represent a "teachable moment" for those diagnosed, a time when those affected may be open and willing to make significant lifestyle and behavioral changes with the potential to improve their current and future health (306–308). Although population-based data both in the United States and Canada suggest that survivors may be more active than their peers without a cancer history, both groups remain well below the recommended levels of daily activity; smoking and dietary practices also lag behind recommended patterns (292,309,310). American Cancer Society guidelines for nutrition and physical activity were updated in 2005 (311), although it is expected that learning to tailor these to vulnerable subpopulations will be needed (312).

Use of complementary and alternative medicine (CAM), estimated as applied by one-third to as many as 83% of patients during active cancer treatment (313–316), is also seen in the post-treatment setting (317). In our longer-term follow-up sample (83), most women reported using some form of vitamins (86.6%) and followed diets or took dietary supplements (60.7%). The most commonly used dietary practices were following a low-fat (48.4%), low-calorie (20.4%), or low-salt (18.6%) diet. Many also took herbal preparations (49.3%), often using more than one remedy (62%). Of note, women who reported using St. Johns Wort (9.8%) also reported significantly more symptoms of emotional distress than nonusers. This finding, similar to others' reports of poorer psychological functioning among patients with cancer using CAM remedies (318,319), suggests that some women may be self-medicating depressive symptoms. Asking about what CAM practices or products a woman may be pursuing is important to guiding her care. Many women state they value their oncologist's opinion about use of these therapies and practices (320).

As noted earlier, many breast cancer survivors seek ways to reduce the stress in their lives after diagnosis. Reducing alcohol exposure is also common in this population. Surprisingly, because few survivorship studies inquire about smoking, we have very little information on women's practices in this regard. Data from the National Health Interview Survey (NHIS) indicate that, although overall smoking rates are lower in survivors than adults without a cancer history (19.7% vs. 23.8%), many cancer survivors continue to smoke after treatment. Such behavior appears to be of particular concern among younger survivors (19 to 40 years of age), in whom the rate of smoking

after treatment (40.5%) was significantly higher than estimates for their cancer-free peers (27.1%) (321). The NHIS data and those of others suggest that survivors who smoke want to stop (322). Provocative data among survivors of lung cancer suggest that smoking cessation after diagnosis can dramatically improve survival (and may even be as effective as chemotherapy in altering disease progression) (323), reminding us that it is never too late to realize a health benefit by quitting. Those caring for breast cancer survivors need to ask about this behavior and intervene as appropriate (324,325).

CONCLUSION

Breast cancer, the most common cancer in women, has a unique and at times complex psychological impact, but one to which psychologically healthy women respond well without the development of serious psychological symptoms. Increased use of local treatment of breast-conserving and reconstructive procedures is reducing the negative effect on self-image and body image. Broader dissemination of information from psychological studies of adaptation to the available treatment options can help in efforts to determine the best treatment to meet patients' physical and emotional needs. Addressing the psychosocial and psychosexual needs of patients with breast cancer improves quality of survival and may even enhance length of survival from other comorbid conditions and events, even if not from cancer. As newer therapies, such as the molecularly targeted treatments of the future, are introduced, research on their immediate and delayed psychosocial impact is needed. Finally, with the increasing demand for their involvement in care, special attention must be directed to the psychological well-being of the immediate relatives of women with breast cancer, especially their partners and offspring.

In closing, clinicians should be reminded that their relationship with a given patient remains paramount above all the considerations outlined previously. A physician's style, behavior, attitudes, and beliefs can dramatically affect a woman's experience. Toward this end, it is important for the health care professional to view himself or herself as part of the treatment. By acquiring and honing the communication skills necessary to engage a patient in her own care, while being respectful and observant of her needs (and those with whom she presents), clinicians can increase the opportunity to minimize psychological trauma, enhance treatment adherence, and obtain the best possible outcome for each woman treated.

MANAGEMENT PRINCIPLES

- Although most women diagnosed and treated for breast cancer do well psychologically and socially, one-fourth of women with breast cancer have psychological symptoms that warrant psychiatric intervention.
- Clues to identifying women with psychological distress include previous treatment for depression or anxiety, symptoms of depression and anxiety that seem out of the *normal* range, and psychological symptoms that are worsening over time.
- The diagnosis and treatment of breast cancer cause psychological distress for all women; recovery from physical and emotional symptoms usually occurs gradually during the 12 months after the completion of cancer treatment. Patients should be told that asking for psychological help is a sign of strength, not weakness.
- Offer psychological and social support services to all women (availability of support services varies depending on your location and type of practice).

- Consider using brief, easily scored distress screening tools periodically across the course of care to help you identify women who are most in need of psychological treatment.
- Psychological support comes in many forms and is delivered by many professionals. Encourage your available psychosocial support members to become active participants in your multidisciplinary team.
- Symptoms of anxiety and insomnia during the diagnostic, pretreatment, and treatment phases often can be rapidly and effectively treated with low-dose anxiolytics and hypnotics.
- Symptoms of depression should be evaluated by a psychiatrist or a psychologist; safe and effective antidepressants are available for women who are being treated or have been treated for breast cancer.
- Inform women who are receiving dexamethasone that it can cause psychological symptoms (anxiety, depression, mood swings); ask women to report these symptoms if they occur because they can be rapidly and effectively treated.
- Family members' responses to a woman's illness are important to her adaptation. These need to be monitored and support provided if there are signs of distress.
- The oncologist can play an important role in encouraging the patient's early resumption of sexual activity after breast surgery or chemotherapy. Encourage the patient's partner to attend diagnostic planning and follow-up visits. Sometimes partners need referral for psychological support so they can better support your patient.
- Menopausal symptoms are highly distressing for many women. Mood swings, irritability, insomnia, and hot flashes can be effectively treated with a variety of medications. Some of these patients benefit from referral to a psychiatrist for evaluation.
- Women value communication with their physicians. The most satisfied patients are those who feel they were compassionately warned about potential side effects of treatment.
- Be aware that some women emotionally "sail" through treatment and then develop symptoms of distress; symptoms develop in some of these women at the anniversary of their diagnosis or during the following year. Ask women during their 3-month post-treatment and 1-year follow-up visits how they are doing emotionally and refer as appropriate.
- Psychological symptoms, such as anxiety, are common at the conclusion of cancer treatment. Women feel vulnerable and less protected when not being seen regularly by their radiation or medical oncologist. Provide women with information on what to expect when treatment ends.
- It is useful to provide each woman with a survivorship care plan that includes a written summary of the treatments received and recommendations for follow-up care. This can help breast cancer survivors negotiate the transition to recovery and plan appropriately for future health care needs.

References

1. American Cancer Society. *Cancer facts and figures—2008*. Atlanta: American Cancer Society, Inc., 2008.
2. Ries LAG, Melbert D, Krapcho M, et al., eds. SEER cancer statistics review, 1975–2005. 2008. Available at: http://seer.cancer.gov/csr/1975_2005/.
3. Vadaparampil ST, Miree CA, Wilson C, et al. Psychosocial and behavioral impact of genetic counseling and testing. *Breast Dis* 2006;27:97–108.
4. Adler NE, Page AEK, eds. *Cancer care for the whole patient: meeting psychosocial health needs*. Washington, DC: National Academies Press, 2008.
5. Bish A, Ramirez A, Burgess C, et al. Understanding why women delay in seeking help for breast cancer symptoms. *J Psychosom Res* 2005;58:321–326.
6. Ashing-Giwa KT, Padilla GV, Bohorquez DE, et al. Understanding the breast cancer experience of Latina women. *J Psychosoc Oncol* 2006;24:19–52.
7. Reifenstein K. Care-seeking behaviors of African American women with breast cancer symptoms. *Res Nurs Health* 2007;30:542–557.
8. Friedman LC, Kalidas M, Elledge R, et al. Medical and psychosocial predictors of delay in seeking medical consultation for breast symptoms in women in a public sector setting. *J Behav Med* 2006;29:327–334.
9. Goodwin JS, Freeman JL, Mahnken JD, et al. Geographic variations in breast cancer survival among older women: implications for quality of breast cancer care. *J Gerontol A Biol Sci Med Sci* 2002;57:M401–406.
10. Mandelblatt JS, Hadley J, Kerner JF, et al. Patterns of breast carcinoma treatment in older women: patient preference and clinical and physical influences. *Cancer* 2000;89:561–573.
11. Griggs JJ, Culakova E, Sorbero ME, et al. Social and racial differences in selection of breast cancer adjuvant chemotherapy regimens. *J Clin Oncol* 2007;25:2522–2527.
12. Yancik R, Wesley MN, Ries LA, et al. Effect of age and comorbidity in postmenopausal breast cancer patients aged 55 years and older. *JAMA* 2001;285:885–892.
13. Silliman RA, Guadagnoli E, Rakowski W, et al. Adjuvant tamoxifen prescription in women 65 years and older with primary breast cancer. *J Clin Oncol* 2002;20:2680–2688.
14. Hurria A, Leung D, Trainor K, et al. Factors influencing treatment patterns of breast cancer patients age 75 and older. *Crit Rev Oncol Hematol* 2003;46:121–126.
15. Mellink WA, Dulmen AM, Wiggers T, et al. Cancer patients seeking a second surgical opinion: results of a study on motives, needs, and expectations. *J Clin Oncol* 2003;21:1492 1497.
16. Waljee JF, Rogers MA, Alderman AK. Decision aids and breast cancer: do they influence choice for surgery and knowledge of treatment options? *J Clin Oncol* 2007;25:1067–1073.
17. O'Leary KA, Estabrooks CA, Olson K, et al. Information acquisition for women facing surgical treatment for breast cancer: influencing factors and selected outcomes. *Patient Educ Couns* 2007;69:5–19.
18. Samarel N, Fawcett J, Tulman L, et al. A resource kit for women with breast cancer: development and evaluation. *Oncol Nurs Forum* 1999;26:611–618.
19. Wise M, Han JY, Shaw B, et al. Effects of using online narrative and didactic information on health care participation for breast cancer patients. *Patient Educ Couns* 2008;70:348–356.
20. Monnier J, Laken M, Carter CL. Patient and caregiver interest in Internet-based cancer services. *Cancer Pract* 2002;10:305–310.
21. Helft PR, Hlubocky F, Daugherty CK. American oncologists' views of Internet use by cancer patients: a mail survey of American Society of Clinical Oncology members. *J Clin Oncol* 2003;21:942–947.
22. Lobb EA, Butow PN, Kenny DT, et al. Communicating prognosis in early breast cancer: do women understand the language used? *Med J Aust* 1999;171:290–294.
23. Hack TF, Whelan T, Olivotto IA, et al. Standardized audiotape versus recorded consultation to enhance informed consent to a clinical trial in breast oncology. *Psychooncology* 2007;16:371–376.
24. Vogel BA, Bengel J, Helmes AW. Information and decision making: patients' needs and experiences in the course of breast cancer treatment. *Patient Educ Couns* 2008;71:79–85.
25. Epstein RM, Street RL, Jr. *Patient-centered communication in cancer care: promoting healing and reducing suffering*. Bethesda, MD: National Cancer Institute. NIH Publication No. 07-6225, 2007.
26. Levinson W. Doctor–patient communication and medical malpractice: implications for pediatricians. *Pediatr Ann* 1997;26:186–193.
27. Fallowfield L, Jenkins V. Current concepts of communication skills training in oncology. *Recent Results Cancer Res* 2006;168:105–112.
28. Back AL, Arnold RM, Baile WF, et al. Efficacy of communication skills training for giving bad news and discussing transitions to palliative care. *Arch Intern Med* 2007;167:453–460.
29. Green BL, Rowland JH, Krupnick JL, et al. Prevalence of posttraumatic stress disorder in women with breast cancer. *Psychosomatics* 1998;39:102–111.
30. Ashcroft JJ, Leinster SJ, Slade PD. Breast cancer—patient choice of treatment: preliminary communication. *J R Soc Med* 1985;78:43–46.
31. Morris J, Royle GT. Offering patients a choice of surgery for early breast cancer: a reduction in anxiety and depression in patients and their husbands. *Soc Sci Med* 1988;26:583–585.
32. Owens RG, Ashcroft JJ, Leinster SJ, et al. Informal decision analysis with breast cancer patients: an aid to psychological preparation for surgery. *J Psychosoc Oncol* 1987;5:23–33.
33. Fallowfield LJ, Hall A, Maguire GP, et al. Psychological outcomes of different treatment policies in women with early breast cancer outside a clinical trial. *BMJ* 1990;301:575–580.
34. Liang W, Burnett CB, Rowland JH, et al. Communication between physicians and older women with localized breast cancer: implications for treatment and patient satisfaction. *J Clin Oncol* 2002;20:1008–1016.
35. Lerman C, Daly M, Walsh WP, et al. Communication between patients with breast cancer and health care providers. Determinants and implications. *Cancer* 1993;72:2612–2620.
36. Petrisek AC, Laliberte LL, Allen SM, et al. The treatment decision-making process: age differences in a sample of women recently diagnosed with nonrecurrent, early-stage breast cancer. *Gerontologist* 1997;37:598–608.
37. Bilodeau BA, Degner LF. Information needs, sources of information, and decisional roles in women with breast cancer. *Oncol Nurs Forum* 1996;23:691–696.
38. Deber RB, Kraetschmer N, Irvine J. What role do patients wish to play in treatment decision making? *Arch Intern Med* 1996;156:1414–1420.
39. Meyerowitz BE. Psychosocial correlates of breast cancer and its treatments. *Psychol Bull* 1980;87:108–131.
40. Rowland JH. Developmental stage and adaptation: adult model. In: Holland JC, Rowland JH, eds. *Handbook of psychooncology: psychological care of the patient with cancer*. New York: Oxford University Press, 1989:25–43.
41. Mosher CE, Danoff-Burg S. A review of age differences in psychological adjustment to breast cancer. *J Psychosoc Oncol* 2005;23:101–114.
42. Kornblith AB, Powell M, Regan MM, et al. Long-term psychosocial adjustment of older vs younger survivors of breast and endometrial cancer. *Psychooncology* 2007;16:895–903.
43. Avis NE, Crawford S, Manuel J. Quality of life among younger women with breast cancer. *J Clin Oncol* 2005;23:3322–3330.
44. Mor V, Malin M, Allen S. Age differences in the psychosocial problems encountered by breast cancer patients. *J Natl Cancer Inst Monogr* 1994:191–197.

45. Bellizzi KM, Rowland JH. Role of comorbidity, symptoms and age in the health of older survivors following treatment for cancer. *Aging Health* 2007;3:625–635.
46. Ganz PA, Schag CC, Heinrich RL. The psychosocial impact of cancer on the elderly: a comparison with younger patients. *J Am Geriatr Soc* 1985;33:429–435.
47. Robb C, Haley WE, Balducci L, et al. Impact of breast cancer survivorship on quality of life in older women. *Crit Rev Oncol Hematol* 2007;62:84–91.
48. Westrup JL, Lash TL, Thwin SS, et al. Risk of decline in upper-body function and symptoms among older breast cancer patients. *J Gen Intern Med* 2006;21:327–333.
49. Bradley CJ, Clement JP, Lin C. Absence of cancer diagnosis and treatment in elderly Medicaid-insured nursing home residents. *J Natl Cancer Inst* 2008;100:21–31.
50. Schmitz KH, Cappola AR, Stricker CT, et al. The intersection of cancer and aging: establishing the need for breast cancer rehabilitation. *Cancer Epidemiol Biomarkers Prev* 2007;16:866–872.
51 Figueiredo MI, Cullen J, Hwang YT, et al. Breast cancer treatment in older women: does getting what you want improve your long-term body image and mental health? *J Clin Oncol* 2004;22:4002–4009.
52. Schnoll RA, Knowles JC, Harlow L. Correlates of adjustment among cancer survivors. *J Psychosoc Oncol* 2002;20:37–59.
53. Stanton AL, Danoff-Burg S, Huggins ME. The first year after breast cancer diagnosis: hope and coping strategies as predictors of adjustment. *Psychooncology* 2002;11:93–102.
54. Ransom S, Jacobsen PB, Schmidt JE, et al. Relationship of problem-focused coping strategies to changes in quality of life following treatment for early stage breast cancer. *J Pain Symptom Manage* 2005;30:243–253.
55. Astin JA, Anton-Culver H, Schwartz CE, et al. Sense of control and adjustment to breast cancer: the importance of balancing control coping styles. *Behav Med* 1999;25:101–109.
56. Manuel JC, Burwell SR, Crawford SL, et al. Younger women's perceptions of coping with breast cancer. *Cancer Nurs* 2007;30:85–94.
57. Falagas ME, Zarkadoulia EA, Ioannidou EN, et al. The effect of psychosocial factors on breast cancer outcome: a systematic review. *Breast Cancer Res* 2007; 9:R44.
58. Kroenke CH, Kubzansky LD, Schernhammer ES, et al. Social networks, social support, and survival after breast cancer diagnosis. *J Clin Oncol* 2006;24:1105–1111.
59. Green BL, Krupnick JL, Rowland JH, et al. Trauma history as a predictor of psychologic symptoms in women with breast cancer. *J Clin Oncol* 2000;18:1084–1093.
60. Brown KW, Levy AR, Rosberger Z, et al. Psychological distress and cancer survival: a follow-up 10 years after diagnosis. *Psychosom Med* 2003;65:636–643.
61. Groenvold M, Petersen MA, Idler E, et al. Psychological distress and fatigue predicted recurrence and survival in primary breast cancer patients. *Breast Cancer Res Treat* 2007;105:209–219.
62. Stewart DE, Cheung AM, Duff S, et al. Attributions of cause and recurrence in long-term breast cancer survivors. *Psychooncology* 2001;10:179–183.
63. Garssen B. Psychological factors and cancer development: evidence after 30 years of research. *Clin Psychol Rev* 2004;24:315–338.
64. Lillberg K, Verkasalo PK, Kaprio J, Tet al. Stressful life events and risk of breast cancer in 10,808 women: a cohort study. *Am J Epidemiol* 2003;157:415–423.
65. Giedzinska AS, Meyerowitz BE, Ganz PA, et al. Health-related quality of life in a multiethnic sample of breast cancer survivors. *Ann Behav Med* 2004;28:39–51.
66. Meyerowitz BE, Richardson J, Hudson S, et al. Ethnicity and cancer outcomes: behavioral and psychosocial considerations. *Psychol Bull* 1998;123:47–70.
67. Fobair P, O'Hanlan K, Koopman C, et al. Comparison of lesbian and heterosexual women's response to newly diagnosed breast cancer. *Psychooncology* 2001;10: 40–51.
68. Bettencourt BA, Schlegel RJ, Talley AE, et al. The breast cancer experience of rural women: a literature review. *Psychooncology* 2007;16:875–887.
69. Burman ME, Weinert C. Concerns of rural men and women experiencing cancer. *Oncol Nurs Forum* 1997;24:1593–1600.
70. McGrath P, Patterson C, Yates P, et al. A study of postdiagnosis breast cancer concerns for women living in rural and remote Queensland. Part I: personal concerns. *Aust J Rural Health* 1999;7:34–42.
71. McGrath P, Patterson C, Yates P, et al. A study of postdiagnosis breast cancer concerns for women living in rural and remote Queensland. Part II: support issues. *Aust J Rural Health* 1999;7:43–52.
72. Jacobsen PB, Jim HS. Psychosocial interventions for anxiety and depression in adult cancer patients: achievements and challenges. *CA Cancer J Clin* 2008;58:214–230.
73. Holland JC, Andersen B, Breitbart WS, et al. Distress management. *J Natl Compr Canc Netw* 2007;5:66–98.
74. Jacobsen PB, Ransom S. Implementation of NCCN distress management guidelines by member institutions. *J Natl Compr Canc Netw* 2007;5:99–103.
75. Pirl WF, Muriel A, Hwang V, et al. Screening for psychosocial distress: a national survey of oncologists. *J Support Oncol* 2007;5:499–504.
76. Tuttle TM, Habermann EB, Grund EH, et al. Increasing use of contralateral prophylactic mastectomy for breast cancer patients: a trend toward more aggressive surgical treatment. *J Clin Oncol* 2007;25:5203–5209.
77. Kuhl C, Kuhn W, Braun M, Schild H. Pre-operative staging of breast cancer with breast MRI: one step forward, two steps back? *Breast* 2007;16(Suppl 2):S34–S44.
78. Moyer A, Salovey P. Psychosocial sequelae of breast cancer and its treatment. *Ann Behav Med* 1996;18:110–125.
79. Ganz PA, Coscarelli A, Fred C, et al. Breast cancer survivors: psychosocial concerns and quality of life. *Breast Cancer Res Treat* 1996;38:183–199.
80. Ganz PA, Rowland JH, Meyerowitz BE, et al. Impact of different adjuvant therapy strategies on quality of life in breast cancer survivors. *Recent Results Cancer Res* 1998;152:396–411.
81. Long E. Breast cancer in African American women. Review of the literature. *Cancer Nurs* 1993;16:1–24.
82. Moyer A. Psychosocial outcomes of breast-conserving surgery versus mastectomy: a meta-analytic review. *Health Psychol* 1997;16:284–298.
83. Ganz PA, Desmond KA, Leedham B, et al. Quality of life in long-term, disease-free survivors of breast cancer: a follow-up study. *J Natl Cancer Inst* 2002;94:39–49.
84. Ganz PA, Rowland JH, Desmond K, et al. Life after breast cancer: understanding women's health-related quality of life and sexual functioning. *J Clin Oncol* 1998; 16:501–514.
85. Parker PA, Youssef A, Walker S, et al. Short-term and long-term psychosocial adjustment and quality of life in women undergoing different surgical procedures for breast cancer. *Ann Surg Oncol* 2007;14:3078–3089.
86. Carver CS, Smith RG, Petronis VM, et al. Quality of life among long-term survivors of breast cancer: different types of antecedents predict different classes of outcomes. *Psychooncology* 2006;15:749–758.
87. Rowland JH, Desmond KA, Meyerowitz BE, et al. Role of breast reconstructive surgery in physical and emotional outcomes among breast cancer survivors. *J Natl Cancer Inst* 2000;92:1422–1429.
88. Arora NK, Gustafson DH, Hawkins RP, et al. Impact of surgery and chemotherapy on the quality of life of younger women with breast carcinoma: a prospective study. *Cancer* 2001;92:1288–1298.
89. Thors CL, Broeckel JA, Jacobsen PB. Sexual functioning in breast cancer survivors. *Cancer Control* 2001;8:442–448.
90. Al-Ghazal SK, Fallowfield L, Blamey RW. Does cosmetic outcome from treatment of primary breast cancer influence psychosocial morbidity? *Eur J Surg Oncol* 1999;25:571–573.
91. McWayne J, Heiney SP. Psychologic and social sequelae of secondary lymphedema: a review. *Cancer* 2005;104:457–466.
92. McKenzie DC, Kalda AL. Effect of upper extremity exercise on secondary lymphedema in breast cancer patients: a pilot study. *J Clin Oncol* 2003;21:463–466.
93. Ahmed RL, Thomas W, Yee D, et al. Randomized controlled trial of weight training and lymphedema in breast cancer survivors. *J Clin Oncol* 2006;24:2765–2772.
94. Alderman AK, Hawley ST, Waljee J, et al. Understanding the impact of breast reconstruction on the surgical decision-making process for breast cancer. *Cancer* 2008;112:489–494.
95. Fallowfield LJ. Psychosocial adjustment after treatment for early breast cancer. *Oncology (Williston Park)* 1990;4:89–97.
96. Margolis G, Goodman RL, Rubin A. Psychological effects of breast-conserving cancer treatment and mastectomy. *Psychosomatics* 1990;31:33–39.
97. Mock V. Body image in women treated for breast cancer. *Nurs Res* 1993;42:153–157.
98. Al-Ghazal SK, Fallowfield L, Blamey RW. Comparison of psychological aspects and patient satisfaction following breast conserving surgery, simple mastectomy and breast reconstruction. *Eur J Cancer* 2000;36:1938–1943.
99. Nissen MJ, Swenson KK, Ritz LJ, et al. Quality of life after breast carcinoma surgery: a comparison of three surgical procedures. *Cancer* 2001;91:1238–1246.
100. Yurek D, Farrar W, Andersen BL. Breast cancer surgery: comparing surgical groups and determining individual differences in postoperative sexuality and body change stress. *J Consult Clin Psychol* 2000;68:697–709.
101. Morrow M, Scott SK, Menck HR, et al. Factors influencing the use of breast reconstruction postmastectomy: a National Cancer Database study. *J Am Coll Surg* 2001; 192:1–8.
102. Morrow M, Mujahid M, Lantz PM, et al. Correlates of breast reconstruction: results from a population-based study. *Cancer* 2005;104:2340–2346.
103. Greenberg CC, Schneider EC, Lipsitz SR, et al. Do variations in provider discussions explain socioeconomic disparities in postmastectomy breast reconstruction? *J Am Coll Surg* 2008;206:605–615.
104. Desch CE, Penberthy LT, Hillner BE, et al. A sociodemographic and economic comparison of breast reconstruction, mastectomy, and conservative surgery. *Surgery* 1999;125:441–447.
105. Tseng JF, Kronowitz SJ, Sun CC, et al. The effect of ethnicity on immediate reconstruction rates after mastectomy for breast cancer. *Cancer* 2004;101:1514–1523.
106. Boehmer U, Linde R, Freund KM. Breast reconstruction following mastectomy for breast cancer: the decisions of sexual minority women. *Plast Reconstr Surg* 2007;119:464–472.
107. Polednak AP. Geographic variation in postmastectomy breast reconstruction rates. *Plast Reconstr Surg* 2000;106:298–301.
108. Atisha D, Alderman AK, Lowery JC, et al. Prospective analysis of long-term psychosocial outcomes in breast reconstruction: two-year postoperative results from the Michigan Breast Reconstruction Outcomes Study. *Ann Surg* 2008;247:1019–1028.
109. Rowland JH, Holland JC, Chaglassian T, et al. Psychological response to breast reconstruction. Expectations for and impact on postmastectomy functioning. *Psychosomatics* 1993;34:241–250.
110. Rowland JH, Meyerowitz BE, Ganz PA, et al. Body image and sexual functioning following reconstructive surgery in breast cancer survivors (BCS) [Abstract 163]. *Proc Am Soc Clin Oncol* 1996;15:124.
111. Clough KB, O'Donoghue JM, Fitoussi AD, et al. Prospective evaluation of late cosmetic results following breast reconstruction: II. TRAM flap reconstruction. *Plast Reconstr Surg* 2001;107:1710–1716.
112. Bower JE. Behavioral symptoms in patients with breast cancer and survivors. *J Clin Oncol* 2008;26:768–777.
113. Richardson LC, Wang W, Hartzema AG, et al. The role of health-related quality of life in early discontinuation of chemotherapy for breast cancer. *Breast J* 2007;13: 581–587.
114. Wiser W, Berger A. Practical management of chemotherapy-induced nausea and vomiting. *Oncology (Williston Park)* 2005;19:637–645.
115. Figueroa-Moseley C, Jean-Pierre P, Roscoe JA, et al. Behavioral interventions in treating anticipatory nausea and vomiting. *J Natl Compr Canc Netw* 2007;5: 44–50.
116. Huntington MO. Weight gain in patients receiving adjuvant chemotherapy for carcinoma of the breast. *Cancer* 1985;56:472–474.
117. Majed B, Moreau T, Senouci K, et al. Is obesity an independent prognosis factor in woman breast cancer? *Breast Cancer Res Treat* 2007 October 16. Epub ahead of print.
118. Schmitz KH, Ahmed RL, Hannan PJ, et al. Safety and efficacy of weight training in recent breast cancer survivors to alter body composition, insulin, and insulin-like growth factor axis proteins. *Cancer Epidemiol Biomarkers Prev* 2005;14:1672–1680.
119. Castellon SA, Silverman DH, Ganz PA. Breast cancer treatment and cognitive functioning: current status and future challenges in assessment. *Breast Cancer Res Treat* 2005;92:199–206.
120. Tannock IF, Ahles TA, Ganz PA, et al. Cognitive impairment associated with chemotherapy for cancer: report of a workshop. *J Clin Oncol* 2004;22:2233–2239.
121. Jansen C, Miaskowski C, Dodd M, et al. Potential mechanisms for chemotherapy-induced impairments in cognitive function. *Oncol Nurs Forum* 2005;32:1151–1163.
122. Stewart A, Bielajew C, Collins B, et al. A meta-analysis of the neuropsychological effects of adjuvant chemotherapy treatment in women treated for breast cancer. *Clin Neuropsychol* 2006;20:76–89.
123. Vardy J, Rourke S, Tannock IF. Evaluation of cognitive function associated with chemotherapy: a review of published studies and recommendations for future research. *J Clin Oncol* 2007;25:2455–2463.
124. Wieneke MH, Dienst ER. Neuropsychological assessment of cognitive functioning following chemotherapy for breast cancer. *Psychooncology* 1995;4:61–66.
125. Ahles TA, Saykin AJ, Noll WW, et al. The relationship of APOE genotype to neuropsychological performance in long-term cancer survivors treated with standard dose chemotherapy. *Psychooncology* 2003;12:612–619.

126. Castellon SA, Ganz PA, Bower JE, et al. Neurocognitive performance in breast cancer survivors exposed to adjuvant chemotherapy and tamoxifen. *J Clin Exp Neuropsychol* 2004;26:955–969.
127. Van Dam FSAM, Schagen SB, Muller MJ, et al. Impairment of cognitive function in women receiving adjuvant treatment for high-risk breast cancer: high-dose versus standard-dose chemotherapy. *J Natl Cancer Inst* 1998;90: 210–218.
128. Hermelink K, Untch M, Lux MP, et al. Cognitive function during neoadjuvant chemotherapy for breast cancer: results of a prospective, multicenter, longitudinal study. *Cancer* 2007;109:1905–1913.
129. Ganz PA. Cognitive dysfunction following adjuvant treatment of breast cancer: a new dose-limiting toxic effect? *J Natl Cancer Inst* 1998;90:182–183.
130. Schover LR. Sexuality and body image in younger women with breast cancer. *J Natl Cancer Inst Monogr* 1994:177–182.
131. Duffy LS, Greenberg DB, Younger J, et al. Iatrogenic acute estrogen deficiency and psychiatric syndromes in breast cancer patients. *Psychosomatics* 1999;40: 304–308.
132. Pritchard KI. The role of hormone replacement therapy in women with a previous diagnosis of breast cancer and a review of possible alternatives. *Ann Oncol* 2001;12:301–310.
133. Carpenter JS, Andrykowski MA, Cordova M, et al. Hot flashes in postmenopausal women treated for breast carcinoma: prevalence, severity, correlates, management, and relation to quality of life. *Cancer* 1998;82:1682–1691.
134. Loprinzi CL, Barton DL, Rhodes D. Management of hot flashes in breast-cancer survivors. *Lancet Oncol* 2001;2:199–204
135. Loprinzi CL, Sloan JA, Perez EA, et al. Phase III evaluation of fluoxetine for treatment of hot flashes. *J Clin Oncol* 2002;20:1578–1583.
136. Stearns V, Johnson MD, Rae JM, et al. Active tamoxifen metabolite plasma concentrations after coadministration of tamoxifen and the selective serotonin reuptake inhibitor paroxetine. *J Natl Cancer Inst* 2003;95:1758–1764.
137. Biglia N, Kubatzki F, Sgandurra P, et al. Mirtazapine for the treatment of hot flushes in breast cancer survivors: a prospective pilot trial. *Breast J* 2007;13: 490–495.
138. Butt DA, Lock M, Lewis JE, et al. Gabapentin for the treatment of menopausal hot flashes: a randomized controlled trial. *Menopause* 2008;15:310–318.
139. Bordeleau L, Pritchard K, Goodwin P, et al. Therapeutic options for the management of hot flashes in breast cancer survivors: an evidence-based review. *Clin Ther* 2007;29:230–241.
140. Van Patten CL, Olivotto IA, Chambers GK, et al. Effect of soy phytoestrogens on hot flashes in postmenopausal women with breast cancer: a randomized, controlled clinical trial. *J Clin Oncol* 2002;20:1449–1455.
141. Kaplan HS. A neglected issue: the sexual side effects of current treatments for breast cancer. *J Sex Marital Ther* 1992;18:3–19.
142. Minton O, Stone P. How common is fatigue in disease-free breast cancer survivors? A systematic review of the literature. *Breast Cancer Res Treat* 2007 December 7. Epub ahead of print.
143. Bower JE, Ganz PA, Desmond KA, et al. Fatigue in long-term breast carcinoma survivors: a longitudinal investigation. *Cancer* 2006;106:751–758.
144. Bower JE. Prevalence and causes of fatigue after cancer treatment: the next generation of research. *J Clin Oncol* 2005;23:8280–8282.
145. Perik PJ, de Korte MA, van Veldhuisen DJ, et al. Cardiotoxicity associated with the use of trastuzumab in breast cancer patients. *Expert Rev Anticancer Ther* 2007;7:1763–1771.
146. Bird BR, Swain SM. Cardiac toxicity in breast cancer survivors: review of potential cardiac problems. *Clin Cancer Res* 2008;14:14–24.
147. Michael YL, Kawachi I, Berkman LF, et al. The persistent impact of breast carcinoma on functional health status: prospective evidence from the Nurses' Health Study. *Cancer* 2000;89:2176–2186.
148. Cathcart CK, Jones SE, Pumroy CS, et al. Clinical recognition and management of depression in node negative breast cancer patients treated with tamoxifen. *Breast Cancer Res Treat* 1993;27:277–281.
149. Ernst T, Chang L, Cooray D, et al. The effects of tamoxifen and estrogen on brain metabolism in elderly women. *J Natl Cancer Inst* 2002;94:592–597.
150. Paganini-Hill A, Clark LJ. Preliminary assessment of cognitive function in breast cancer patients treated with tamoxifen. *Breast Cancer Res Treat* 2000;64:165–176.
151. Jenkins V, Shilling V, Fallowfield L, et al. Does hormone therapy for the treatment of breast cancer have a detrimental effect on memory and cognition? A pilot study. *Psychooncology* 2004;13:61–66.
152. Owusu C, Buist DS, Field TS, et al. Predictors of tamoxifen discontinuation among older women with estrogen receptor-positive breast cancer. *J Clin Oncol* 2008;26: 549–555.
153. Barron TI, Connolly R, Bennett K, et al. Early discontinuation of tamoxifen: a lesson for oncologists. *Cancer* 2007;109:832–839.
154. Buijs C, de Vries EG, Mourits MJ, et al. The influence of endocrine treatments for breast cancer on health-related quality of life. *Cancer Treat Rev* 2008 May 29. Epub ahead of print.
155. Mok K, Juraskova I, Friedlander M. The impact of aromatase inhibitors on sexual functioning: current knowledge and future research directions. *Breast* 2008 May 14. Epub ahead of print.
156. Winters L, Habin K, Gallagher J. Aromatase inhibitors and musculoskeletal pain in patients with breast cancer. *Clin J Oncol Nurs* 2007;11:433–439.
157. Crew KD, Greenlee H, Capodice J, et al. Prevalence of joint symptoms in postmenopausal women taking aromatase inhibitors for early-stage breast cancer. *J Clin Oncol* 2007;25:3877–3883.
158. Henry NL, Giles JT, Ang D, et al. Prospective characterization of musculoskeletal symptoms in early stage breast cancer patients treated with aromatase inhibitors. *Breast Cancer Res Treat* 2007 October 6. Epub ahead of print.
159. Yang HC, Thornton LM, Shapiro CL, et al. Surviving recurrence: psychological and quality-of-life recovery. *Cancer* 2008;112:1178–1187.
160. Mahon SM, Cella DF, Donovan MI. Psychosocial adjustment to recurrent cancer. *Oncol Nurs Forum* 1990;17:47–52.
161. Northouse LL, Mood D, Kershaw T, et al. Quality of life of women with recurrent breast cancer and their family members. *J Clin Oncol* 2002;20:4050–4064.
162. Bull AA, Meyerowitz BE, Hart S, et al. Quality of life in women with recurrent breast cancer. *Breast Cancer Res Treat* 1999;54:47–57.
163. Brady SS, Helgeson VS. Social support and adjustment to recurrence of breast cancer. *J Psychosoc Oncol* 1999;17:37–55.
164. Goodwin PJ, Leszcz M, Ennis M, et al. The effect of group psychosocial support on survival in metastatic breast cancer. *N Engl J Med* 2001;345:1719–1726.
165. Wilson KG, Chochinov HM, Skirko MG, et al. Depression and anxiety disorders in palliative cancer care. *J Pain Symptom Manage* 2007;33:118–129.
166. Breitbart W, Payne DK. Pain. In: Holland JC, Breitbart W, Jacobsen PB, et al., eds. *Psycho-oncology*. New York: Oxford University Press, 1998:450–467.
167. Levin DN, Cleeland CS, Dar R. Public attitudes toward cancer pain. *Cancer* 1985;56:2337–2339.
168. Spiegel D, Bloom JR. Group therapy and hypnosis reduce metastatic breast carcinoma pain. *Psychosom Med* 1983;45:333–339.
169. Glajchen M, Peyser S, Calder K. Multidimensional management of cancer pain. In: Holland JC, Lesko LM, Massie MJ, eds. *Current concepts in psycho-oncology IV Syllabus of the postgraduate course* [Abstract 263]. New York: Memorial Sloan-Kettering Cancer Center, 1991.
170. Berry DL, Wilkie DJ, Thomas CR Jr, et al. Clinicians communicating with patients experiencing cancer pain. *Cancer Invest* 2003;21:374–381.
171. Stanton AL. Psychosocial concerns and interventions for cancer survivors. *J Clin Oncol* 2006;24:5132–5137.
172. Hewitt M, Rowland JH. Mental health service use among adult cancer survivors: analyses of the National Health Interview Survey. *J Clin Oncol* 2002;20:4581–4590.
173. Owen JE, Goldstein MS, Lee JH, et al. Use of health-related and cancer-specific support groups among adult cancer survivors. *Cancer* 2007;109:2580–2589.
174. Tapper VJ. Psychotherapeutic trials specific to women with breast cancer: the state of the science. *J Psychosoc Oncol* 1999;17:85–99.
175. Barsevick AM, Sweeney C, Haney E, et al. A systematic qualitative analysis of psychoeducational interventions for depression in patients with cancer. *Oncol Nurs Forum* 2002;29:73–84.
176. Osborn RL, Demoncada AC, Feuerstein M. Psychosocial interventions for depression, anxiety, and quality of life in cancer survivors: meta-analyses. *Int J Psychiatry Med* 2006;36:13–34.
177. Rehse B, Pukrop R. Effects of psychosocial interventions on quality of life in adult cancer patients: meta analysis of 37 published controlled outcome studies. *Patient Educ Couns* 2003;50:179–186.
178. Scholten C, Weinlander G, Krainer M, et al. Difference in patient's acceptance of early versus late initiation of psychosocial support in breast cancer. *Support Care Cancer* 2001;9:459–464.
179. Zimmermann T, Heinrichs N, Baucom DH. "Does one size fit all?" moderators in psychosocial interventions for breast cancer patients: a meta-analysis. *Ann Behav Med* 2007;34:225–239.
180. Carlson LE, Bultz BD. Benefits of psychosocial oncology care: improved quality of life and medical cost offset. *Health Qual Life Outcomes* 2003;1:8.
181. Mandelblatt JS, Cullen J, Lawrence WF, et al. Economic evaluation alongside a clinical trial of psycho-educational interventions to improve adjustment to survivorship among patients with breast cancer. *J Clin Oncol* 2008;26:1684–1690.
182. Spiegel D, Bloom JR, Kraemer HC, et al. Effect of psychosocial treatment on survival of patients with metastatic breast cancer. *Lancet* 1989;2:888–891.
183. Spiegel D, Butler LD, Giese-Davis J, et al. Effects of supportive-expressive group therapy on survival of patients with metastatic breast cancer: a randomized prospective trial. *Cancer* 2007;110:1130–1138.
184. Bordeleau L, Szalai JP, Ennis M, et al. Quality of life in a randomized trial of group psychosocial support in metastatic breast cancer: overall effects of the intervention and an exploration of missing data. *J Clin Oncol* 2003;21:1944–1951.
185. Smedslund G, Ringdal GI. Meta-analysis of the effects of psychosocial interventions on survival time in cancer patients. *J Psychosom Res* 2004;57:123–135.
186. Varker KA, Terrell CE, Welt M, et al. Impaired natural killer cell lysis in breast cancer patients with high levels of psychological stress is associated with altered expression of killer immunoglobin-like receptors. *J Surg Res* 2007;139:36–44.
187. Carlson LE, Speca M, Faris P, et al. One year pre-post intervention follow-up of psychological, immune, endocrine and blood pressure outcomes of mindfulness-based stress reduction (MBSR) in breast and prostate cancer outpatients. *Brain Behav Immun* 2007;21:1038–1049.
188. Giese-Davis J, Wilhelm FH, Conrad A, et al. Depression and stress reactivity in metastatic breast cancer. *Psychosom Med* 2006;68:675–683.
189. Levy SM, Herberman RB, Lippman M, et al. Immunological and psychosocial predictors of disease recurrence in patients with early-stage breast cancer. *Behav Med* 1991;17:67–75.
190. Miller AH, ed. Biological mechanisms of psychosocial effects on disease: implications for cancer control. *Brain Behav Immun* 2003;17:1–134.
191. Miller GE, Cohen S. Psychological interventions and the immune system: a meta-analytic review and critique. *Health Psychol* 2001;20:47–63.
192. Trijsburg RW, van Knippenberg FC, Rijpma SE. Effects of psychological treatment on cancer patients: a critical review. *Psychosom Med* 1992;54:489–517.
193. Sandgren AK, McCaul KD, King B, et al. Telephone therapy for patients with breast cancer. *Oncol Nurs Forum* 2000;27:683–688.
194. Donnelly JM, Kornblith AB, Fleishman S, et al. A pilot study of interpersonal psychotherapy by telephone with cancer patients and their partners. *Psychooncology* 2000;9:44–56.
195. Gustafson DH, McTavish FM, Stengle W, et al. Reducing the digital divide for low-income women with breast cancer: a feasibility study of a population-based intervention. *J Health Commun* 2005;10(Suppl 1):173–193.
196. Owen JE, Klapow JC, Roth DL, et al. Randomized pilot of a self-guided internet coping group for women with early-stage breast cancer. *Ann Behav Med* 2005;30:54–64.
197. Meier A, Lyons EJ, Frydman G, et al. How cancer survivors provide support on cancer-related Internet mailing lists. *J Med Internet Res* 2007;9:e12.
198. Sammarco A. Perceived social support, uncertainty, and quality of life of younger breast cancer survivors. *Cancer Nurs* 2001;24:212–219.
199. Fernandez BM, Crane LA, Baxter J, et al. Physician referral patterns to a breast cancer support program. *Cancer Pract* 2001;9:169–175.
200. Eakin EG, Strycker LA. Awareness and barriers to use of cancer support and information resources by HMO patients with breast, prostate, or colon cancer: patient and provider perspectives. *Psychooncology* 2001;10:103–113.
201. Andrykowski MA, Curran SL, Studts JL, et al. Psychosocial adjustment and quality of life in women with breast cancer and benign breast problems: a controlled comparison. *J Clin Epidemiol* 1996;49:827–834.
202. Weihs KL, Enright TM, Simmens SJ. Close relationships and emotional processing predict decreased mortality in women with breast cancer: preliminary evidence. *Psychosom Med* 2008;70:117–124.
203. Northouse L, Mellon S, Harden J, et al. Effects of cancer on families of adult cancer survivors. In: Miller SM, Bowen DJ, Croyle RT, et al., eds. *Handbook of cancer control and behavioral science: a resource for researchers, practitioners, and policy makers*. Washington, DC: American Psychological Association, 2008.

204. Given B, Sherwood P, Given C. Family care during cancer care. In: Miller SM, Bowen DJ, Croyle RT, et al., eds. *Handbook of cancer control and behavioral science: a resource for researchers, practitioners, and policy makers*. Washington, DC: American Psychological Association, 2008.

205. Lewis FM. The effects of cancer survivorship on families and caregivers. *Cancer Nurs* 2006;29:20–21, 23–25.

206. Walker BL. Adjustment of husbands and wives to breast cancer. *Cancer Pract* 1997;5:92–98.

207. Mellon S, Northouse LL, Weiss LK. A population-based study of the quality of life of cancer survivors and their family caregivers. *Cancer Nurs* 2006;29:120–131.

208. Northouse L, Templin T, Mood D. Couples' adjustment to breast disease during the first year following diagnosis. *J Behav Med* 2001;24:115–136.

209. Mellon S, Northouse LL. Family survivorship and quality of life following a cancer diagnosis. *Res Nurs Health* 2001;24:446–459.

210. Lewis FM, Fletcher KA, Cochrane BB, et al. Predictors of depressed mood in spouses of women with breast cancer. *J Clin Oncol* 2008;26:1289–1295.

211. Northouse LL, Templin T, Mood D, et al. Couples' adjustment to breast cancer and benign breast disease: a longitudinal analysis. *Psychooncology* 1998;7:37–48.

212. Ben-Zur H, Gilbar O, Lev S. Coping with breast cancer: patient, spouse, and dyad models. *Psychosom Med* 2001;63:32–39.

213. Romero C, Lindsay JE, Dalton WT, et al. Husbands' perceptions of wives' adjustment to breast cancer: the impact on wives' mood. *Psychooncology* 2008;17:237–243.

214. Northouse LL. The impact of breast cancer on patients and husbands. *Cancer Nurs* 1989;12:276–284.

215. Pistrang N, Barker C. The partner relationship in psychological response to breast cancer. *Soc Sci Med* 1995;40:789–797.

216. Northouse LL. Breast cancer in younger women: effects on interpersonal and family relations. *J Natl Cancer Inst Monogr* 1994:183–190.

217. Sabo D, Brown J, Smith C. The male role and mastectomy: support groups and men's adjustment. *J Psychosoc Oncol* 1986;4:19–32.

218. Dalton WT, 3rd, Nelson DV, Brobst JB, et al. Psychosocial variables associated with husbands' adjustment three months following wives' diagnosis of breast cancer. *J Cancer Educ* 2007;22:245–249.

219. Kagawa-Singer M, Wellisch DK. Breast cancer patients' perceptions of their husband's support in a cross-cultural context. *Psychooncology* 2003;12:24–37.

220. Bultz BD, Speca M, Brasher PM, et al. A randomized controlled trial of a brief psychoeducational support group for partners of early stage breast cancer patients. *Psychooncology* 2000;9:303–313.

221. Blanchard CG, Toseland RW, McCallion P. The effects of a problem-solving intervention with spouses of cancer patients. *J Psychosoc Oncol* 1996;14:1–21.

222. Lewis FM, Cochrane BB, Fletcher KA, et al. Helping her heal: a pilot study of an educational counseling intervention for spouses of women with breast cancer. *Psychooncology* 2008;17:131–137.

223. Hoskins CN, Haber J, Budin WC, et al. Breast cancer: education, counseling, and adjustment—a pilot study. *Psychol Rep* 2001;89:677–704.

224. Bucher JA, Loscalzo M, Zabora J, et al. Problem-solving cancer care education for patients and caregivers. *Cancer Pract* 2001;9:66–70.

225. Given B, Sherwood PR. Family care for the older person with cancer. *Semin Oncol Nurs* 2006;22:43–50.

226. Northouse L. Helping families of patients with cancer. *Oncol Nurs Forum* 2005; 32:743–750.

227. Cochrane BB, Lewis FM. Partner's adjustment to breast cancer: a critical analysis of intervention studies. *Health Psychol* 2005;24:327–332.

228. Dorval M, Guay S, Mondor M, et al. Couples who get closer after breast cancer: frequency and predictors in a prospective investigation. *J Clin Oncol* 2005;23: 3588–3596.

229. Dorval M, Maunsell E, Taylor-Brown J, Kilpatrick M. Marital stability after breast cancer. *J Natl Cancer Inst* 1999;91:54–59.

230. Manne S. Cancer in the marital context: a review of the literature. *Cancer Invest* 1998;16:188–202.

231. Taylor-Brown J, Kilpatrick M, Maunsell E, et al. Partner abandonment of women with breast cancer. Myth or reality? *Cancer Pract* 2000;8:160–164.

232. Fisher JD, Nader A, Whitcher-Alagna S. Recipient reactions to aid. *Psychol Bull* 1982;91:27–54.

233. Coyne JC, Wortman CB, Lerman DR. The other side of support: emotional overinvolvement and miscarried helping. In: Gottlieb BH, ed. *Marshaling social support: formats, processes, and effects*. Newbury Park: Sage Publications, 1988;305–330.

234. Wellisch DK. Family relationships of the mastectomy patient: interactions with the spouse and children. *Isr J Med Sci* 1981;17:993–996.

235. Litman TJ. The family as a basic unit in health and medical care: a social-behavioral overview. *Soc Sci Med* 1974;8:495–519.

236. Lewis FM. The impact of cancer on the family: a critical analysis of the research literature. *Patient Educ Couns* 1986;8:269–289.

237. Howes MJ, Hoke L, Winterbottom M, et al. Psychosocial effects of breast cancer on the patient's children. *J Psychosoc Oncol* 1994;12:1–21.

238. Lewis FM, Hammond MA, Woods NF. The family's functioning with newly diagnosed breast cancer in the mother: the development of an explanatory model. *J Behav Med* 1993;16:351–370.

239. Osborn T. The psychosocial impact of parental cancer on children and adolescents: a systematic review. *Psychooncology* 2007;16:101–126.

240. Grabiak BR, Bender CM, Puskar KR. The impact of parental cancer on the adolescent: an analysis of the literature. *Psychooncology* 2007;16:127–137.

241. Lichtman RR, Taylor SE, Wood JV, et al. Relations with children after breast cancer: the mother-daughter relationship at risk. *J Psychosoc Oncol* 1984;2:1–19.

242. Wellisch DK. Adolescent acting out when a parent has cancer. *Int J Fam Therapy* 1979;1:230–241.

243. Armsden GC, Lewis FM. Behavioral adjustment and self-esteem of school-age children of women with breast cancer. *Oncol Nurs Forum* 1994;21:39–45.

244. Lewis FM, Zahlis EH, Shands ME, et al. The functioning of single women with breast cancer and their school-aged children. *Cancer Pract* 1996;4:15–24.

245. Lewis FM, Casey SM, Brandt PA, et al. The enhancing connections program: pilot study of a cognitive-behavioral intervention for mothers and children affected by breast cancer. *Psychooncology* 2006;15:486–497.

246. Ganz PA, Hirji K, Sim MS, et al. Predicting psychosocial risk in patients with breast cancer. *Med Care* 1993;31:419–431.

247. Ganz PA, Desmond KA, Belin TR, et al. Predictors of sexual health in women after a breast cancer diagnosis. *J Clin Oncol* 1999;17:2371–2380.

248. Weijmar Schultz WCM, Van de Wiel HBM, Hahn DEE, et al. Sexuality and cancer in women. *Annu Rev Sex Res* 1992;3:151–200.

249. Quigley KM. The adult cancer survivor: psychosocial consequences of cure. *Semin Oncol Nurs* 1989;5:63–69.

250. Reuben SH. *Living beyond cancer: finding a new balance—President's Cancer Panel 2003–2004 annual report*. 2004.

251. Hewitt M, Greenfield S, Stovall E, eds. *From cancer patient to cancer survivor—lost in transition*. Washington, DC: Institute of Medicine, National Research Council, 2006.

252. Lee SJ, Schover LR, Partridge AH, et al. American Society of Clinical Oncology recommendations on fertility preservation in cancer patients. *J Clin Oncol* 2006;24:2917–2931.

253. Auchincloss SS. Sexual dysfunction in cancer patients: issues in evaluation and treatment. In: Holland J, Rowland JH, eds. *Handbook of psychooncology: psychological care of the patient with cancer*. New York: Oxford University Press, 1989;383–413.

254. Jenkins VA, Fallowfield LJ, Poole K. Are members of multidisciplinary teams in breast cancer aware of each other's informational roles? *Qual Health Care* 2001; 10:70–75.

255. Rowland JH, Bellizzi KM. Cancer survivors and survivorship research: a reflection on today's successes and tomorrow's challenges. *Hematol Oncol Clin North Am* 2008;22:181–200.

256. Rowland JH, Hewitt M, Ganz PA. Cancer survivorship: a new challenge in delivering quality cancer care. *J Clin Oncol* 2006;24:5101–5104.

257. Ganz PA, ed. *Cancer survivorship: today and tomorrow*. New York: Springer, 2007.

258. Short PF, Vasey JJ, Belue R. Work disability associated with cancer survivorship and other chronic conditions. *Psychooncology* 2008;17:91–97.

259. Bradley CJ, Bednarek HL, Neumark D. Breast cancer and women's labor supply. *Health Serv Res* 2002;37:1309–1328.

260. Bouknight RR, Bradley CJ, Luo Z. Correlates of return to work for breast cancer survivors. *J Clin Oncol* 2006;24:345–353.

261. Bradley CJ, Bednarek HL. Employment patterns of long-term cancer survivors. *Psychooncology* 2002;11:188–198.

262. Main DS, Nowels CT, Cavender TA, et al. A qualitative study of work and work return in cancer survivors. *Psychooncology* 2005;14:992–1004.

263. Schover LR. Myth-busters: telling the true story of breast cancer survivorship. *J Natl Cancer Inst* 2004;96:1800–1801.

264. Knobf MT. Psychosocial responses in breast cancer survivors. *Semin Oncol Nurs* 2007;23:71–83.

265. Lemieux J, Bordeleau LJ, Goodwin PJ. Medical, psychosocial, and health-related quality of life issues in breast cancer survivors. In: Ganz PA, ed. *Cancer survivorship: today and tomorrow*. New York, NY: Springer, 2007;122–144.

266. Tjemsland L, Soreide JA, Malt UF. Posttraumatic distress symptoms in operable breast cancer III: status one year after surgery. *Breast Cancer Res Treat* 1998;47: 141–151.

267. Kornblith AB, Herndon JE, 2nd, Weiss RB, et al. Long-term adjustment of survivors of early-stage breast carcinoma, 20 years after adjuvant chemotherapy. *Cancer* 2003;98:679–689.

268. Aspinwall LG, MacNamara A. Taking positive changes seriously. *Cancer* 2005; 104:2549–2556.

269. Bellizzi KM, Blank TO. Predicting posttraumatic growth in breast cancer survivors. *Health Psychol* 2006;25:47–56.

270. Ashing-Giwa K, Ganz PA, Petersen L. Quality of life of African American and white long term breast carcinoma survivors. *Cancer* 1999;85:418–426.

271. Gill KM, Mishel M, Belyea M, et al. Triggers of uncertainty about recurrence and long-term treatment side effects in older African American and Caucasian breast cancer survivors. *Oncol Nurs Forum* 2004;31:633–639.

272. Mishel MH, Germino BB, Gil KM, et al. Benefits from an uncertainty management intervention for African-American and Caucasian older long-term breast cancer survivors. *Psychooncology* 2005;14:962–978.

273. Mariotto AB, Rowland JH, Ries LA, et al. Multiple cancer prevalence: a growing challenge in long-term survivorship. *Cancer Epidemiol Biomarkers Prev* 2007;16: 566–571.

274. Andersen MR, Urban N. Involvement in decision-making and breast cancer survivor quality of life. *Ann Behav Med* 1999;21:201–209.

275. Earle CC. Failing to plan is planning to fail: improving the quality of care with survivorship care plans. *J Clin Oncol* 2006;24:5112–5116.

276. Lash TL, Fox MP, Buist DS, et al. Mammography surveillance and mortality in older breast cancer survivors. *J Clin Oncol* 2007;25:3001–3006.

277. American Society of Clinical Oncology. Chemotherapy treatment plan and summary. 2008. Available at: http://www.asco.org/ASCO/About+ASCO/ASCO +Information/Annual+Reports/2006–2007+Annual+Report/Section+1.+Quality +Care/Treatment+Plan+and+Summary and http://www.asco.org/ASCO/Quality +Care+%26+Guidelines/Quality+Measurement+%26+Improvement/Chemotherapy +Treatment+Plan+and+Summary/Breast+Cancer+Treatment+Plan+and+ Summary+Resources?cpsextcurrchannel=1.

278. Hewitt M, Ganz PA, eds. *Implementing cancer survivorship care planning: workshop summary: A National Coalition for Cancer Survivorship and Institute of Medicine National Cancer Policy Forum Workshop in partnership with the Lance Armstrong Foundation and the National Cancer Institute*. Washington, DC: National Academies Press, 2007.

279. Kattlove H, Winn RJ. Ongoing care of patients after primary treatment for their cancer. *CA Cancer J Clin* 2003;53:172–196.

280. Ganz PA, Hahn EE. Implementing a survivorship care plan for patients with breast cancer. *J Clin Oncol* 2008;26:759–767.

281. Grunfeld E, Mant D, Yudkin P, et al. Routine follow up of breast cancer in primary care: randomised trial. *BMJ* 1996;313:665–669.

282. Earle CC, Burstein HJ, Winer EP, et al. Quality of non-breast cancer health maintenance among elderly breast cancer survivors. *J Clin Oncol* 2003;21:1447–1451.

283. Oeffinger KC, McCabe MS. Models for delivering survivorship care. *J Clin Oncol* 2006;24:5117–5124.

284. Ganz PA. A teachable moment for oncologists: cancer survivors, 10 million strong and growing! *J Clin Oncol* 2005;23:5458–5460.

285. Ganz PA, Kwan L, Somerfield MR, et al. The role of prevention in oncology practice: results from a 2004 survey of American Society of Clinical Oncology members. *J Clin Oncol* 2006;24:2948–2957.

286. Sabatino SA, Coates RJ, Uhler RJ, et al. Provider counseling about health behaviors among cancer survivors in the United States. *J Clin Oncol* 2007;25:2100–2106.

287. Maunsell E, Drolet M, Brisson J, et al. Dietary change after breast cancer: extent, predictors, and relation with psychological distress. *J Clin Oncol* 2002;20:1017–1025.

288. Antoni MH, Lehman JM, Kilbourn KM, et al. Cognitive-behavioral stress management intervention decreases the prevalence of depression and enhances benefit finding among women under treatment for early-stage breast cancer. *Health Psychol* 2001;20:20–32.
289. Antoni MH, Lechner SC, Kazi A, et al. How stress management improves quality of life after treatment for breast cancer. *J Consult Clin Psychol* 2006;74:1143–1152.
290. Jacobsen PB, Meade CD, Stein KD, et al. Efficacy and costs of two forms of stress management training for cancer patients undergoing chemotherapy. *J Clin Oncol* 2002;20:2851–2862.
291. King AC. The coming of age of behavioral research in physical activity. *Ann Behav Med* 2001;23:227–228.
292. Courneya KS, Katzmarzyk PT, Bacon E. Physical activity and obesity in Canadian cancer survivors: population-based estimates from the 2005 Canadian Community Health Survey. *Cancer* 2008;112:2475–2482.
293. Galvao DA, Newton RU. Review of exercise intervention studies in cancer patients. *J Clin Oncol* 2005;23:899–909.
294. Rock CL, Demark-Wahnefried W. Nutrition and survival after the diagnosis of breast cancer: a review of the evidence. *J Clin Oncol* 2002;20:3302–3316.
295. Courneya KS, Friedenreich CM. Physical exercise and quality of life following cancer diagnosis: a literature review. *Ann Behav Med* 1999;21:171–179.
296. Schwartz AL. Physical activity after a cancer diagnosis: psychosocial outcomes. *Cancer Invest* 2004;22:82–92.
297. McTiernan A. Physical activity after cancer: physiologic outcomes. *Cancer Invest* 2004;22:68–81.
298. Pischon T, Nothlings U, Boeing H. Obesity and cancer. *Proc Nutr Soc* 2008;67:128–145.
299. Murtaugh MA, Sweeney C, Giuliano AR, et al. Diet patterns and breast cancer risk in Hispanic and non-Hispanic white women: the Four-Corners Breast Cancer Study. *Am J Clin Nutr* 2008;87:978–984.
300. Breslow RA, Ballard-Barbash R, Munoz K, et al. Long-term recreational physical activity and breast cancer in the National Health and Nutrition Examination Survey I epidemiologic follow-up study. *Cancer Epidemiol Biomarkers Prev* 2001;10:805–808.
301. Holmes MD, Chen WY, Feskanich D, et al. Physical activity and survival after breast cancer diagnosis. *JAMA* 2005;293:2479–2486.
302. Holick CN, Newcomb PA, Trentham-Dietz A, et al. Physical activity and survival after diagnosis of invasive breast cancer. *Cancer Epidemiol Biomarkers Prev* 2008;17:379–386.
303. Pierce JP, Stefanick ML, Flatt SW, et al. Greater survival after breast cancer in physically active women with high vegetable-fruit intake regardless of obesity. *J Clin Oncol* 2007;25:2345–2351.
304. Mahon SM. Tertiary prevention: implications for improving the quality of life of long-term survivors of cancer. *Semin Oncol Nurs* 2005;21:260–270.
305. Kellen E, Vansant G, Christiaens MR, et al. Lifestyle changes and breast cancer prognosis: a review. *Breast Cancer Res Treat* 2008 April 4. Epub ahead of print.
306. Demark-Wahnefried W, Aziz NM, et al. Riding the crest of the teachable moment: promoting long-term health after the diagnosis of cancer. *J Clin Oncol* 2005;23:5814–5830.
307. Demark-Wahnefried W, Pinto BM, et al. Promoting health and physical function among cancer survivors: potential for prevention and questions that remain. *J Clin Oncol* 2006;24:5125–5131.
308. Demark-Wahnefried W, Jones LW. Promoting a healthy lifestyle among cancer survivors. *Hematol Oncol Clin North Am* 2008;22:319–342.
309. Bellizzi KM, Rowland JH, Jeffery DD, et al. Health behaviors of cancer survivors: examining opportunities for cancer control intervention. *J Clin Oncol* 2005;23:8884–8893.
310. Mayer DK, Terrin NC, Menon U, et al. Health behaviors in cancer survivors. *Oncol Nurs Forum* 2007;34:643–651.
311. Doyle C, Kushi LH, Byers T, et al. Nutrition and physical activity during and after cancer treatment: an American Cancer Society guide for informed choices. *CA Cancer J Clin* 2006;56:323–353.
312. Stull VB, Snyder DC, Demark-Wahnefried W. Lifestyle interventions in cancer survivors: designing programs that meet the needs of this vulnerable and growing population. *J Nutr* 2007;137:243S–248S.
313. Lee MM, Lin SS, Wrensch MR, et al. Alternative therapies used by women with breast cancer in four ethnic populations. *J Natl Cancer Inst* 2000;92:42–47.
314. Goldstein MS, Lee JH, Ballard-Barbash R, et al. The use and perceived benefit of complementary and alternative medicine among Californians with cancer. *Psychooncology* 2008;17:19–25.
315. Velicer CM, Ulrich CM. Vitamin and mineral supplement use among U.S. adults after cancer diagnosis: a systematic review. *J Clin Oncol* 2008;26:665–673.
316. Boon HS, Olatunde F, Zick SM. Trends in complementary/alternative medicine use by breast cancer survivors: comparing survey data from 1998 and 2005. *BMC Womens Health* 2007;7:4.
317. Matthews AK, Sellergren SA, Huo D, et al. Complementary and alternative medicine use among breast cancer survivors. *J Altern Complement Med* 2007;13:555–562.
318. Burstein HJ, Gelber S, Guadagnoli E, et al. Use of alternative medicine by women with early-stage breast cancer. *N Engl J Med* 1999;340:1733–1739.
319. Montazeri A, Sajadian A, Ebrahimi M, et al. Depression and the use of complementary medicine among breast cancer patients. *Support Care Cancer* 2005;13:339–342.
320. Edgar L, Remmer J, Rosberger Z, et al. Resource use in women completing treatment for breast cancer. *Psychooncology* 2000;9:428–438.
321. Hewitt M, Rowland JH, Yancik R. Cancer survivors in the United States: age, health, and disability. *J Gerontol A Biol Sci Med Sci* 2003;58:82–91.
322. Cox LS, Africano NL, Tercyak KP, et al. Nicotine dependence treatment for patients with cancer. *Cancer* 2003;98:632–644.
323. Dresler CM. Is it more important to quit smoking than which chemotherapy is used? *Lung Cancer* 2003;39:119–124.
324. Schnoll RA, Zhang B, Rue M, et al. Brief physician-initiated quit-smoking strategies for clinical oncology settings: a trial coordinated by the Eastern Cooperative Oncology Group. *J Clin Oncol* 2003;21:355–365.
325. Carter CL, Key J, Marsh L, et al. Contemporary perspectives in tobacco cessation: what oncologists need to know. *Oncologist* 2001;6:496–505.

Ann H. Partridge and Elizabeth S. Ginsburg

Breast cancer is one of the most commonly diagnosed malignancies in women of childbearing age. Approximately 10% of women diagnosed with breast cancer are younger than age 45, translating to more than 23,000 women in the United States yearly and tens of thousands more worldwide (1,2). In light of improvements in the diagnosis and treatment of breast cancer and an increasing focus on survivorship issues, combined with the sociodemographic trend of delaying childbearing, an increasing number of young breast cancer survivors are interested in future fertility. Breast cancer treatment can diminish or destroy a woman's reproductive potential owing to direct gonadal toxicity or the natural waning of fertility during the time needed to receive optimal therapy. Many young women remain premenopausal and fertile for at least some period of time after breast cancer treatment, and some are interested in interventions to preserve fertility (3). Because of the intricate relationship between breast cancer and hormones, consideration of fertility and reproductive issues in this population is complex. Reproductive factors are associated with the risk of developing breast cancer, and hormonal manipulations and medications are a mainstay of breast cancer treatment. Amenorrhea is associated with improved prognosis compared with women who continue to menstruate through chemotherapy, in the absence of tamoxifen (4–6). (See Chapter 92 on breast cancer in young women and Chapter 50 on chemoendocrine issues.) Nevertheless, for some young women with breast cancer, the threat or experience of infertility may be particularly distressing (3,7). The founder of Fertile Hope, an advocacy organization that supports fertility preservation for cancer patients, proclaimed about her cancer diagnosis, "The thought of being sterile was almost as devastating as my cancer diagnosis itself" (www.fertilehope.org). Some women are also interested in avoiding potential ill-health effects of premature menopause, including menopausal symptoms, bone thinning, cardiovascular problems, and mental health issues (3,8–10).

EFFECT OF BREAST CANCER TREATMENT ON OVARIAN FUNCTION

Fertility in young women with breast cancer may be affected by several factors. First, the time required to receive systemic breast cancer treatment can last months (e.g., conventional cytoxic chemotherapy) to years (e.g., biologic therapy, including trastuzumab or adjuvant tamoxifen). During treatment, while pregnancy is contraindicated because of the risks of teratogenicity, ovarian function and fertility are declining owing to the natural decrease in ovarian reserve with aging (Fig. 96.1). The average age of menopause in Western societies is 51 years. Adjuvant chemotherapy results in direct toxicity to the ovary, and potentially premature menopause. The degree of damage to the ovaries will determine whether amenorrhea is temporary or permanent. Chemotherapy interferes with dividing cells in the ovary, generally maturing follicles (11). Because alkylating agents, such as cyclophosphamide, are not cell-cycle specific, they may also directly kill oocytes and pregranulosa cells of primordial follicles.

Evidence is mixed about whether chemotherapy given during the follicular phase of the menstrual cycle is more injurious to ovarian function (12–14). Reports of the risk of menopause, meaning a permanent loss of menses associated with an absence of residual functional follicles, range between 10% and 90%, depending on the regimen given, the age of the patients, and the definition used for menopause. Most studies are limited by having used chemotherapy-related amenorrhea (CRA) as a surrogate for menopause and infertility. Treatment regimens vary substantially, and follow-up is heterogeneous, and usually relatively short. CRA may be temporary, especially in very young women, and older women are more likely to have permanent amenorrhea. Chronically, anovulatory women may remain fertile even if they are not having menstrual cycles, and ongoing menses are a poor surrogate for fertility, especially as women age, because of waning egg quality. Available data confirm that risk of CRA is related to increasing age and increasing cumulative dose of cytotoxic chemotherapy, in particular, alkylating agents (15). A prospective longitudinal survey of 595 women in the United States with breast cancer diagnosed at age 25 to 40 undergoing adjuvant chemotherapy confirmed that menstrual cycles were less likely to persist at 1 year among women treated with regimens containing higher cumulative doses of cyclophosphamide (i.e., cyclophosphamide, methotrexate and 5-fluorouracil [CMF] or 5-fluorouracil, doxorubicin; and cyclophosphamide [FAC] rather than doxorubicin and cyclophosphamide [AC], doxorubicin, cyclophosphamide, and paclitaxel [ACT]; or doxorubicin, cyclophosphamide, and docetaxel [ACD]) (odds ratio [OR] .37, 95% confidence interval [CI], .37–.67), although women who received CMF were more likely than those on AC, ACT, or ACD to bleed during the 1 month following chemotherapy (~50% vs. 20%, OR, 2.9, 95% CI, 1.7–5) (16) (Fig. 96.2). Rates of menstrual bleeding 6 months after completion of chemotherapy were also strongly related to patient age, with approximately 85% having ongoing menses among women age younger than 35 years, 61% in women ages 35 to 40, and less than 25% in those older than 40 (Fig. 96.3). Recent evidence suggests that the addition of the taxanes, including paclitaxel in particular, to anthracycline-based adjuvant chemotherapy confers little or no increased risk of CRA, although data are mixed (17–20). Table 96.1 details risk of CRA with common adjuvant therapy regimens by age (15).

Even among women who remain premenopausal after cytotoxic therapy, menopause may ensue sooner than would have been expected. An analysis of International Breast Cancer Study Group (IBCSG) Trials V and VI revealed that 227 women who were menstruating and disease free at 2 years after diagnosis and treatment with six to seven cycles of CMF had earlier menopause compared with controls (21). For a woman who was age 30 at the time of diagnosis, and menstruating 24 months after six cycles of CMF, there was a 37% risk of menopause only 3 years later (at age 35), and an 84% risk at age 40. Accumulating data indicate that ovarian reserve is diminished even in young women who remain premenopausal after chemotherapy for breast cancer (22–25). Hormonal treatments appear to primarily impact fertility owing to delaying childbearing, allowing natural waning of ovarian function (26).

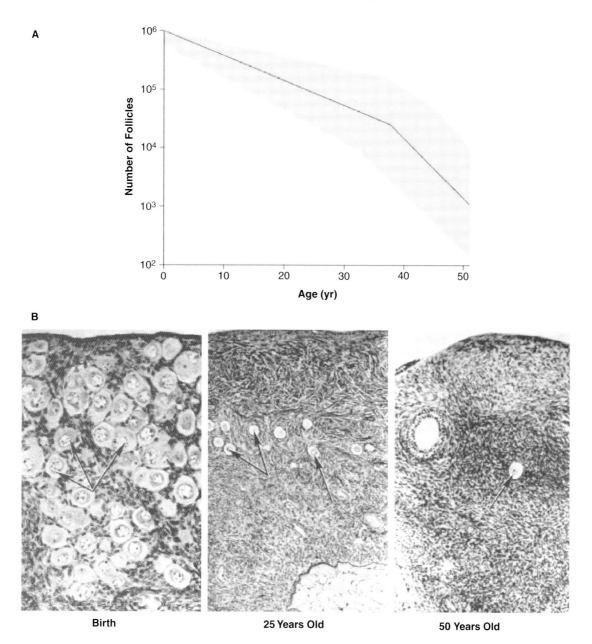

FIGURE 96.1. Natural decline in oocytes over time from birth to menopause. (Adapted from Lobo RA. Potential options for preservation of fertility in women. *N Engl J Med* 2005;353(1):64–73, with permission.) **Panel A** depicts the decline in human ovarian oocytes by age (Data from Faddy MJ, Gosden RG, Gougeon A, et al. Accelerated disappearance of ovarian follicles in mid-life: implications for forecasting menopause. *Hum Reprod* 1992;7(10):1342–1346, with permission.) **Panel B** shows histologic specimens of oocytes (*arrows*) from birth, age 25 years, and age 50 years. (Adapted from Erickson GF. Ovarian anatomy and physiology. In: Lobo RA, Kelsey J, Marcus R, eds. *Menopause: biology and pathobiology.* San Diego: Academic Press, 2000:13–32, with permission.)

CONSIDERATIONS FOR WOMEN WHO DESIRE TO HAVE A FUTURE BIOLOGICAL CHILD

The American Society of Clinical Oncology (ASCO) has published recommendations regarding fertility preservation considerations for cancer patients (27). For women with breast cancer, strategies for fertility preservation have scarce efficacy or safety information. These limitations may hamper discussion of these issues, referrals to reproductive specialists, and the enthusiasm for patients and providers to utilize them (28–30). The first step in counseling breast cancer patients regarding their fertility is to determine the patient's desire for a future biological child (Fig. 96.4). The risk of premature menopause and infertility associated with various treatment options must be understood so that a patient can weigh the pros and cons of fertility-sparing strategies, in the risk-to-benefit analysis of her cancer treatment options. Some women may elect to forego some therapy if the incremental benefits are modest and the risk of subsequent infertility is high (3). For those who desire a future biological child and need systemic therapy which will put them at risk for premature menopause, fertility preservation strategies are available. Although studied in other cancer populations, limited enthusiasm exists in utilizing oral contraceptives through chemotherapy in young

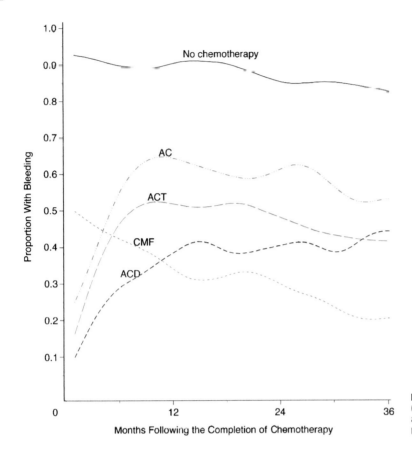

FIGURE 96.2. Menstrual bleeding by chemotherapy regimen received. (Adapted from Petrek JA, Naughton MJ, Case LD, et al. Incidence, time course, and determinants of menstrual bleeding after breast cancer treatment: a prospective study. *J Clin Oncol* 2006;24(7):1045–1051, with permission.)

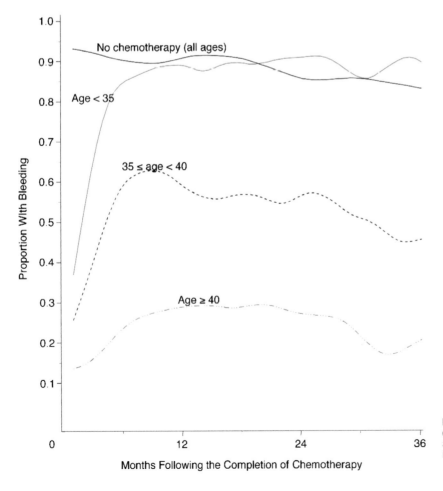

FIGURE 96.3. Menstrual bleeding by patient age at receipt of chemotherapy. (Adapted from Petrek JA, Naughton MJ, Case LD, et al. Incidence, time course, and determinants of menstrual bleeding after breast cancer treatment: a prospective study. *J Clin Oncol* 2006;24(7):1045–1051, with permission.)

	ESTIMATED RATES OF CHEMOTHERAPY-
Table 96.1	RELATED AMENORRHEA (CRA) WITH MODERN
	CHEMOTHERAPY REGIMENS BY AGE

Chemotherapy Regimen	CRA (%), Age ≤30[a]	CRA (%), Age 30–40[a]	CRA (%), Age ≥40[a]
None	~0	<5	20–25
AC × 4	~0	13	57–63
AC × 4 followed by T × 4	15		>38
AC × 4 followed by D × 4	6	12	35–50
CMF × 6	19	31–38	76–96
CAF/CEF × 6	23–47		75–89
FEC × 6	38		73
TAC × 6	51		

AC × 4, four cycles of adriamycin and cyclophosphamide (intravenously [IV]); T × 4, four cycles of paclitaxel; D × 4, four cycles of docetaxel; CMF × 6, six cycles of cyclophosphamide (oral), methotrexate, 5-fluorouracil; CAF/CEF × 6, six cycles of cyclophosphamide (oral), adriamycin or epirubicin, 5-fluorouracil; FEC × 6, six cycles of 5-fluorouracil, epirubicin, cyclophosphamide (IV); TAC × 6, six cycles of docetaxel, adriamycin, cyclophosphamide.
[a]Studies varied by inclusion of persons aged 30, 40, or 50 years in the younger or older age categories (5,15–17,26,74,75).
Adapted from Partridge AH, Ruddy KJ. Fertility and adjuvant treatment in young women with breast cancer. *Breast* 2007;16[Suppl 2]:S175–S181, with permission.

women with newly diagnosed breast cancer, given the concerns that excess hormones may worsen prognosis (31). Ovarian suppression with gonadotropin releasing-hormone (GnRH-) agonists (e.g., leuprolide acetate) is widely available and can be administered during cytotoxic chemotherapy. Several small studies have shown mixed results with regard to the efficacy of this strategy (32). For example, Fox et al. (33) reported that 23 of 24 premenopausal young patients with early-stage breast cancer given leuprolide through treatment remained premenopausal by 12 months after chemotherapy (33). However, of the 21 patient not lost to follow-up or death, at a mean of 34 months, 5 women had been pregnant (1 twice),

with three of these six pregnancies requiring assisted reproduction techniques. There are ongoing clinical trials to evaluate the efficacy of this strategy (www.cancer.gov/clinicaltrials/SWOG-S0230; www.isdscotland.org/isd/1663.html).

Cryopreservation of either ovarian tissue or oocytes, the latter of which requires ovarian stimulation before treatment, is also an option where available. For both of these strategies, there has been only limited success to date and these procedures should be considered experimental. Cryopreservation of oocytes may be particularly appealing for patients who do not have a male partner and do not wish to use donor sperm. To date, efficacy has been only approximately 1.6% live births per frozen oocyte, three to four times lower than embryo cryopreservation (27,34). Ovarian tissue cryopreservation, in theory, could allow preservation of hundreds of primordial follicles (containing immature eggs) before chemotherapy without ovarian stimulation and the associated concerns about high hormone levels, and treatment delay, other than to remove the ovarian tissue. However, thus far only two live births have occurred following this technique, which suffers from substantial technical limitations (35,36). This technique is also associated with theoretical concerns of reintroduction of cancer cells in the reimplanted ovarian tissue removed. Cryopreservation of embryos following *in vitro* fertilization (IVF) is a standard procedure with a relatively high success rate in infertile women, at 15% to 30% pregnancy rate per transfer of two to three thawed embryos, depending on maternal age (www.sart.org). In women with breast cancer, there has been concern that ovarian stimulation for cryopreservation of oocytes or embryos, with the associated supraphysiologic estradiol and other hormone levels, might increase the risk of cancer recurrence, particularly in the setting of hormone receptor-positive disease. Estradiol levels during traditional stimulated IVF cycles can be greater than 2000 pg/mL, whereas levels average less than 200 pg/mL in the normal menstrual cycle.

Because natural cycle IVF (not utilizing ovarian stimulation) has much lower embryo yield compared with stimulated cycles,

Communicate with patient and elicit preferences regarding fertility, premature menopause
Assess of risk with treatment
Discuss avoidance of conception during breast cancer treatment and counsel regarding family planning

↓

Patient at risk for infertility, ovarian dysfunction
Patient interested in fertility, ovarian function preservation

↓

Refer to specialist with expertise in fertility preservation
Consider pros and cons of available fertility preservation strategies

Options	Considerations
Embryo cryopreservation	-Requires sperm source, ovarian stimulation with associated concern of prognostic effect
Oocyte cryopreservation	-Requires ovarian stimulation; limited efficacy, experimental
Ovarian tissue cryopreservation	-Invasive, potential for reintroduction of cancerous cells; limited efficacy, experimental
Ovarian suppression	-Menopausal symptoms and bone thinning; efficacy unknown, studies ongoing

↓

Provide ongoing counseling and support regarding fertility, menopausal and family planning concerns and decisions in follow-up

FIGURE 96.4. Management summary for premenopausal women with breast cancer regarding issues. (Adapted from Lee SJ, Schover LR, Partridge AH, et al. American Society of Clinical Oncology recommendations on fertility preservation in cancer patients. *J Clin Oncol* 2006;24(18):2917–2931, with permission.)

research evaluating alternative stimulation strategies has been conducted. Tamoxifen and letrozole have been utilized for ovarian stimulation in women with recently diagnosed early breast cancer before IVF and preliminary results are reassuring because there is a lack of clear early risks or effect on overall survival and recurrence (37–40). The 2- to 6-week period required for this procedure before beginning systemic breast cancer treatment may not be prudent in some disease settings (e.g., inflammatory breast cancer), although is reasonable without undue delays in other settings, such as in the interval between surgery and the start of chemotherapy (41).

Infertility can be devastating for some individuals and relationships, and limited research in cancer survivors suggests infertility in this population is also quite distressing (42,43). Many young women with breast cancer struggle with the competing interests of optimizing personal survival, and the powerful desire to have a future biological child (44). For some women, modifications of treatment, or intervention aimed at fertility preservation, or a combination, may be appropriate. Many other women and their loved ones choose to avoid any potential personal risk, and modify expectations regarding future biologic children, often considering alternatives such as adoption.

 ## ASSESSMENT OF OVARIAN FUNCTION AND FERTILITY AFTER BREAST CANCER

Many survivors are interested in understanding their reproductive potential, but assessment of fertility and even menopausal status after treatment for breast cancer can be complicated and imprecise. Interruptions in menstrual cycles are not sensitive or specific for infertility. Temporary amenorrhea is common after chemotherapy, even in women who resume menstrual functioning, and hormonal treatments make the presence or absence of menses a less accurate reflection of reproductive potential. In a prospective cohort of 595 premenopausal women age 20 to 40 at diagnosis of early breast cancer, women experiencing monthly bleeding decreased from 90% to 40% following the first dose of chemotherapy (16). The rates of monthly bleeding rose to 55% over the next 15 months, but then 5 years after diagnosis slowly declined to 35%. Women who were taking tamoxifen were 15% less likely to be menstruating at 1 year, presumably because of temporary ovarian dysfunction during treatment. Follicle-stimulating hormone (FSH) level less than 20 mIU/mL, luteinizing-hormone (LH) less than 20 mIU, and estradiol (E2) more than 20 pg suggest that ovulation is still possible (45). However, even within the normal ranges of these hormones, there may be a correlation between higher levels and poorer chance of conception (46). Women with decreased ovarian reserve often have shorter menstrual cycles because of accelerated follicle development. FSH levels on the third day of menses greater than 10 mIU/mL, resulting in E2 levels greater than 75 pg/mL, cause early ovulation, which is associated with limited fertility. Inhibin levels and anti-mullerian hormone (AMH) levels may also clarify fertility status. Inhibin A is primarily secreted during the luteal phase, whereas inhibin B is primarily secreted during the follicular phase. Levels of both decrease during chemotherapy, but increase to normal range in those who eventually resume menses (47,48). AMH is produced by early-stage ovarian follicles and, therefore, reflects ovarian reserve present as reflected by the pool of remaining primordial follicles (49). Vaginal ultrasound can be used to measure antral follicle counts (AFC) on the third day of the menstrual cycle. The number of follicles measuring 3 to 10 mm or greater correlates with potential fertility (50). Hormonal manipulation can

have a major impact on these values. Estradiol can be four to five times higher and FSH can be markedly suppressed on tamoxifen. Consequently, AFC while on tamoxifen may not accurately reflect ovarian reserve. AMH is produced by very early follicles and is not influenced by menstrual cycle phase, so it may be the best indicator of ovarian reserve in a woman who has been on tamoxifen, although only limited research exists to date in this area (51).

 ## FAMILY PLANNING AND BIRTH CONTROL AFTER BREAST CANCER

Hormonal methods of contraception generally are not recommended for breast cancer survivors because of concerns about a potential effect on breast cancer outcomes, including new primary disease. Barrier methods of contraception or insertion of a nonhormonal intrauterine device (IUD) can be considered to prevent unwanted pregnancy, which can be particularly onerous for young survivors (52). Although no clear evidence indicate that ovulation induction or IVF increases the risk of breast cancer, there has been concern that IVF may increase risk of breast cancer in a person with a personal or family history of the disease (53). IVF has been conducted in cancer survivors, although response to stimulation, and subsequent embryo yield have been suboptimal (54).

 ## SAFETY OF PREGNANCY AFTER BREAST CANCER

Concern exists that pregnancy after breast cancer may worsen prognosis, especially among women with hormone receptor-positive disease. To date, the effect of pregnancy after a diagnosis of breast cancer on relapse and survival has not been reported prospectively. Evidence from several retrospective studies on pregnancy following breast cancer has not shown a decrease in survival or an increase in recurrence; however, these studies are all limited by significant biases (55–67). Table 96.2 presents recent studies evaluating survival among breast cancer survivors who have a subsequent pregnancy compared with survivors who do not have a pregnancy after breast cancer. Although not all studies reach statistical significance, they all suggest that women who have a pregnancy after breast cancer may have lower risk of recurrence and death. In a large population-based study in western Australia, 2,539 women under 45 years of age diagnosed with breast cancer between 1982 and 2000 were evaluated for subsequent pregnancy and disease outcomes (67). In this study, 123 of the 2,539 women (5%) became pregnant after breast cancer and, of these, only 50 (41%) of these women had received chemotherapy. Consistent with previous studies, women who had a pregnancy after breast cancer were more likely to be alive in follow-up, and this effect was stronger if a woman waited at least 2 years after diagnosis to have a pregnancy (hazard ratio [HR] for death 0.48, 95% CI, 0.27–0.83), but was also present at trend level if the delay was between 6 and 24 months (HR = 0.45, 95% CI, 0.16–1.28). Although these data are reassuring, all studies are confounded by the "healthy mother" effect, that women who become pregnant after breast cancer are healthier and less likely to develop a recurrence at baseline compared with women who do not become pregnant (56). It is possible that there is a beneficial biologic effect from the high hormonal levels of pregnancy. High-dose estrogen and progestins are effective treatment for breast cancer, and an antitumor effect has been seen in *in vitro* and animal models, possibly owing to signaling via the insulin growth factor pathway (68). Ongoing prospective studies

Table 96.2	RECENT STUDIES EVALUATING SAFETY OF PREGNANCY AFTER BREAST CANCER		
Study (Reference)	Breast Cancer Survivors with Subsequent Pregnancy (N)	Controls (N)	Relative Risk (95% CI) of Recurrence or Death
Sankila, 1994 (56)	91	471	0.20 (0.10–0.50)
Von Schoultz, 1995 (57)	50	2,119	0.48 (0.18–1.29)
Kroman, 1997 (55)	173	5,514	0.55 (0.28–1.06)
Valentgas, 1999 (60)	53	265	0.80 (0.30–2.30)
Gelber, 2001 (63)	94	188	0.44 (0.21–0.46)
Mueller, 2003 (65)	438	2,775	0.54 (0.41–0.71)
Blakely, 2004 (66)	47	323	0.70 (0.25–1.95)
Ives, 2007 (67)	123	2,416	0.59 (0.37–0.95)

CI, confidence interval.
Adapted from Partridge AH, Ruddy KJ. Fertility and adjuvant treatment in young women with breast cancer. *Breast* 2007;16[Suppl 2]:S175–S181, with permission.

may help to elucidate further the potential risks and benefits of pregnancy after breast cancer.

A common recommendation is for breast cancer survivors to wait at least 2 years after treatment before attempting a pregnancy, in an effort to get them beyond the period of highest risk of recurrence. However, the available data have not revealed any detriment in disease outcomes from pregnancy sooner. Given that many women with breast cancer are at risk of recurrence long beyond the first few years after diagnosis, and that fertility wanes with age, some women elect not to wait a substantial period of time to become pregnant after diagnosis. For women with hormone receptor-positive disease, 5 years of tamoxifen therapy is often recommended, during which time pregnancy is contraindicated. This approach is problematic for many women, given the decline in fertility over time and some may elect to forgo completion of a 5-year course of tamoxifen to try to become pregnant sooner rather than later.

PREGNANCY AND LACTATION AFTER BREAST CANCER

Whether a breast cancer survivor who is interested in future fertility ultimately becomes pregnant is complicated by a range of medical and psychosocial issues. Sparse data exist on fertility and pregnancy outcomes among women with a history of breast cancer. Findings from select populations of young women with breast cancer suggest that approximately 5% to 15% of young breast cancer survivors will become pregnant at least once after their diagnosis (33,67,69). No increased rate of birth defects among offspring conceived has been found. Three large studies including nearly 4,000 total offspring of childhood cancer survivors, excluding clearly hereditary cancers, revealed no statistically significant increase in cancers or malformations (70). Some *BRCA1* or *BRCA2* mutation carriers will consider preimplantation or prenatal genetic testing (71). Women who have been treated with cytotoxic agents in the past may be at increased risk of peripartum complications (e.g., cardiomyopathy owing to prior anthracycline and trastuzumab) although no data are available. Future research in this area is warranted, and women with a history of breast cancer treatment should consider receiving *high-risk* obstetric care during a pregnancy.

Breast cancer survivors who have a baby may be interested in breast-feeding (52). The degree to which local therapy has affected the normal breast anatomy will dictate the ability of that breast to produce milk. Women who have had a mastectomy can lactate from the opposite breast. Milk production may be limited by the lack of the second breast, and substantial asymmetry may result between the engorged, lactating breast and the contralateral chest wall, or reconstructed breast during the period of lactation. For women who have undergone breast-conserving therapy (BCT), resection of centrally located tumors, particularly if affecting the nipple–areolar complex, is more likely to impair lactation. Radiation therapy can cause lobular sclerosis and atrophy within breast tissue, which may also limit milk production (72). Asymmetry may be a problem in this situation as well with the treated breast less engorged. In a multicenter, retrospective review of 53 women who became pregnant after BCT, one-third had some lactation from the affected breast. Many of these women reported low milk output or the baby preferring the untreated breast, and only 25% of women were able to successfully breast-feed from the treated breast (62,73). Although it is evident that lactation is protective against breast cancer risk in both pre- and postmenopausal women, because the numbers are so small, no efforts have been made to evaluate the benefits of lactation in breast cancer survivors.

CONCLUSION

Young women with breast cancer have a strong desire to not only decrease their risk of recurrence, but to go on and live satisfying lives. This goal may entail the ability to have a biological child in the future, or to avoid premature menopause. Discussions about these issues should be tailored to each patient's preferences, taking into account the baseline risk of her disease, risk reduction from recommended therapy, as well as risk of infertility from treatment. Because of the time-sensitive nature of beginning treatment and some fertility preservation strategies, early referral to a fertility specialist is prudent for those interested (27). For some patients, a combination of fertility preservation strategies may be optimal, whereas many patients will elect to forgo any such intervention. Regardless, shared informed decision-making not only about conventional risks of treatment, but including these important issues is likely to lead to more realistic expectations, and better psychosocial outcomes for young breast cancer survivors.

References

1. Ries LAG, Melbert D, Krapcho M, et al. SEER Cancer Statistics Review, 1975–2004. In: National Cancer Institute. Bethesda, MD. http://seer.cancer.gov/csr/1975_2004/.

2. American Cancer Society. Breast Cancer Facts and Figures 2007–2008. Atlanta: American Cancer Society, Inc.

3. Partridge AH, Gelber S, Peppercorn J, et al. Web-based survey of fertility issues in young women with breast cancer. *J Clin Oncol* 2004;22(20):4174–4183.

4. Pagani O, O'Neill A, Castiglione M, et al. Prognostic impact of amenorrhoea after adjuvant chemotherapy in premenopausal breast cancer patients with axillary node involvement: results of the International Breast Cancer Study Group (IBCSG) Trial VI. *Eur J Cancer* 1998;34(5):632–640.

5. Parulekar WR, Day AG, Ottaway JA, et al. Incidence and prognostic impact of amenorrhea during adjuvant therapy in high-risk premenopausal breast cancer: analysis of a National Cancer Institute of Canada Clinical Trials' Group Study—NCIC CTG MA.5. *J Clin Oncol* 2005;23(25):6002–6008.

6. Parton M, Smith IE. Controversies in the management of patients with breast cancer: adjuvant endocrine therapy in premenopausal women. *J Clin Oncol* 2008; 26(5):745–752.

7. Avis NE, Crawford S, Manuel J. Psychosocial problems among younger women with breast cancer. *Psychooncology* 2004;13(5):295–308.

8. Chen WY, Manson JE. Premature ovarian failure in cancer survivors: new insights, looming concerns. *J Natl Cancer Inst* 2006;98(13):880–881.

9. Rocca WA, Bower JH, Maraganore DM, et al. Increased risk of cognitive impairment or dementia in women who underwent oophorectomy before menopause. *Neurology* 2007;69(11):1074–1083.

10. Schover LR. Premature ovarian failure and its consequences: vasomotor symptoms, sexuality, and fertility. *J Clin Oncol* 2008;26(5):753–758.

11. Himelstein-Braw R, Peters H, Faber M. Morphological study of the ovaries of leukaemic children. *Br J Cancer* 1978;38(1):82–87.

12. Di Cosimo S, Alimonti A, Ferretti G, et al. Incidence of chemotherapy-induced amenorrhea depending on the timing of treatment by menstrual cycle phase in women with early breast cancer. *Ann Oncol* 2004;15(7):1065–1071.

13. Hrushesky WJ, Vyzula R, Wood PA. Fertility maintenance and 5-fluorouracil timing within the mammalian fertility cycle. *Reprod Toxicol* 1999;13(5):413–420.

14. Mehta RR, Beattie CW, Das Gupta TK. Endocrine profile in breast cancer patients receiving chemotherapy. *Breast Cancer Res Treat* 1992;20(2):125–132.

15. Walshe JM, Denduluri N, Swain SM. Amenorrhea in premenopausal women after adjuvant chemotherapy for breast cancer. *J Clin Oncol* 2006;24(36): 5769–5779.

16. Petrek JA, Naughton MJ, Case LD, et al. Incidence, time course, and determinants of menstrual bleeding after breast cancer treatment: a prospective study. *J Clin Oncol* 2006;24(7):1045–1051.

17. Fornier MN, Modi S, Panageas KS, et al. Incidence of chemotherapy-induced, long-term amenorrhea in patients with breast carcinoma age 40 years and younger after adjuvant anthracycline and taxane. *Cancer* 2005;104(8):1575–1579.

18. Abusief ME, Missmer SA, Ginsburg ES, et al. Chemotherapy-related amenorrhea in women with early breast cancer: the effect of paclitaxel or dose density. *J Clin Oncol* 2006 ASCO Annual Meeting Proceedings (Post-Meeting Edition) 2006; 24(18S):10506.

19. Reh A, Oktem O, Oktay K. Impact of breast cancer chemotherapy on ovarian reserve: a prospective observational analysis by menstrual history and ovarian reserve markers. *Fertil Steril* 2007;90(5):1635–1639.

20. Tham YL, Sexton K, Weiss H, et al. The rates of chemotherapy-induced amenorrhea in patients treated with adjuvant doxorubicin and cyclophosphamide followed by a taxane. Am *J Clin Oncol* 2007;30(2):126–132.

21. Partridge A, Gelber S, Gelber RD, et al. Age of menopause among women who remain premenopausal following treatment for early breast cancer: long-term results from International Breast Cancer Study Group Trials' V and VI. *Eur J Cancer* 2007;43(11):1646–1653.

22. Oktay K, Oktem O, Reh A, et al. Measuring the impact of chemotherapy on fertility in women with breast cancer. *J Clin Oncol* 2006;24(24):4044–4046.

23. Anderson RA, Themmen AP, Al-Qahtani A, et al. The effects of chemotherapy and long-term gonadotrophin suppression on the ovarian reserve in premenopausal women with breast cancer. *Hum Reprod* 2006;21(10):2583–2592.

24. Lutchman Singh K, Muttukrishna S, Stein RC, et al. Predictors of ovarian reserve in young women with breast cancer. *Br J Cancer* 2007;96(12):1808–1816.

25. Ruddy KJ, Partridge AH, Gelber G, et al. Ovarian reserve in women who remain premenopausal after chemotherapy for early stage breast cancer [Abstract 9571]. *J Clin Oncol* 2008;26:(May 20 Suppl) p. 519s.

26. Goodwin PJ, Ennis M, Pritchard KI, et al. Risk of menopause during the first year after breast cancer diagnosis. *J Clin Oncol* 1999;17(8):2365–2370.

27. Lee SJ, Schover LR, Partridge AH, et al. American Society of Clinical Oncology recommendations on fertility preservation in cancer patients. *J Clin Oncol* 2006; 24(18):2917–2931.

28. Partridge AH, Winer EP. Fertility after breast cancer: questions abound. *J Clin Oncol* 2005;23(19):4259–4261.

29. Thewes B, Meiser B, Taylor A, et al. Fertility- and menopause-related information needs of younger women with a diagnosis of early breast cancer. *J Clin Oncol* 2005; 23(22):5155–5165.

30. Duffy CM, Allen SM, Clark MA. Discussions regarding reproductive health for young women with breast cancer undergoing chemotherapy. *J Clin Oncol* 2005; 23(4):766–773.

31. Behringer K, Breuer K, Reineke T, et al. Secondary amenorrhea after Hodgkin's lymphoma is influenced by age at treatment, stage of disease, chemotherapy regimen, and the use of oral contraceptives during therapy: a report from the German Hodgkin's Lymphoma Study Group. *J Clin Oncol* 2005;23(30): 7555–7564.

32. Partridge AH, Ruddy KJ. Fertility and adjuvant treatment in young women with breast cancer. *Breast* 2007;16(Suppl 2):S175–S181.

33. Fox KR, Scialla J, Moore H. Preventing chemotherapy-related amenorrhea using leuprolide during adjuvant chemotherapy for early-stage breast cancer [Abstract 50]. *Proceeding of the American Society of Clinical Oncology* 2003;22:13.

34. Ozmen B, Schopper B, Schultz-Mosgau A, et al. A live birth after transfer of a day 2 embryo derived from frozen-thawed zygotes that had undergone polar body biopsy: a case report. *Fertil Steril* 2008;90(4):1201.e 9–11.

35. Donnez J, Dolmans MM, Demylle D, et al. Live birth after orthotopic transplantation of cryopreserved ovarian tissue. *Lancet* 2004;364(9443):1405–1410.

36. Meirow D, Levron J, Eldar-Geva T, et al. Pregnancy after transplantation of cryopreserved ovarian tissue in a patient with ovarian failure after chemotherapy. *N Engl J Med* 2005;353(3):318–321.

37. Oktay K, Buyuk E, Davis O, et al. Fertility preservation in breast cancer patients: IVF and embryo cryopreservation after ovarian stimulation with tamoxifen. *Hum Reprod* 2003;18(1):90–95.

38. Oktay K, Buyuk E, Libertella N, et al. Fertility preservation in breast cancer patients: a prospective controlled comparison of ovarian stimulation with tamoxifen and letrozole for embryo cryopreservation. *J Clin Oncol* 2005;23(19):4347–4353.

39. Oktay K, Hourvitz A, Sahin G, et al. Letrozole reduces estrogen and gonadotropin exposure in women with breast cancer undergoing ovarian stimulation before chemotherapy. *J Clin Endocrinol Metab* 2006;91(10):3885–3890.

40. Azim AA, Costantini-Ferrando M, Oktay K. Safety of fertility preservation by ovarian stimulation with letrozole and gonadotropins in patients with breast cancer: a prospective controlled study. *J Clin Oncol* 2008;26(16):2630–2635.

41. Madrigrano A, Westphal L, Wapnir I. Egg retrieval with cryopreservation does not delay breast cancer treatment. *Am J Surg* 2007;194(4):477–481.

42. Schover LR. Psychosocial aspects of infertility and decisions about reproduction in young cancer survivors: a review. *Med Pediatr Oncol* 1999;33(1):53–59.

43. Canada AL, Schover LR. Research promoting better patient education on reproductive health after cancer. *J Natl Cancer Inst Monogr* 2005(34):98–100.

44. Partridge AH. Fertility preservation: a vital survivorship issue for young women with breast cancer. *J Clin Oncol* 2008;26(16):2612–2613.

45. Speroff L, Fritz MA, eds. *Clinical gynecology endocrinology and fertility*. Philadelphia: Lippincott Williams & Wilkins, 2004.

46. Weghofer A, Margreiter M, Fauster Y, et al. Age-specific FSH levels as a tool for appropriate patient counselling in assisted reproduction. *Hum Reprod* 2005;20(9): 2448–2452.

47. Blumenfeld Z, Ritter M, Shen-Orr Z, et al. Inhibin A concentrations in the sera of young women during and after chemotherapy for lymphoma: correlation with ovarian toxicity. *Am J Reprod Immunol* 1998;39(1):33–40.

48. Blumenfeld Z, Dann E, Avivi I, et al. Fertility after treatment for Hodgkin's disease. *Ann Oncol* 2002;13(Suppl 1):138–147.

49. van Rooij IA, Broekmans FJ, te Velde ER, et al. Serum anti-Mullerian hormone levels: a novel measure of ovarian reserve. *Hum Reprod* 2002;17(12):3065–3071.

50. Scheffer GJ, Broekmans FJ, Looman CW, et al. The number of antral follicles in normal women with proven fertility is the best reflection of reproductive age. *Hum Reprod* 2003;18(4):700–706.

51. Cook CL, Siow Y, Taylor S, et al. Serum mullerian-inhibiting substance levels during normal menstrual cycles. *Fertil Steril* 2000;73(4):859–861.

52. Connell S, Patterson C, Newman B. A qualitative analysis of reproductive issues raised by young Australian women with breast cancer. *Health Care Women Int* 2006; 27(1):94–110.

53. Salhab M, Al Sarakbi W, Mokbel K. In vitro fertilization and breast cancer risk: a review. *Int J Fertil Womens Med* 2005;50(6):259–266.

54. Ginsburg ES, Yanushpolsky EH, Jackson KV. In vitro fertilization for cancer patients and survivors. *Fertil Steril* 2001;75(4):705–710.

55. Kroman N, Jensen MB, Melbye M, et al. Should women be advised against pregnancy after breast-cancer treatment? *Lancet* 1997;350(9074):319–322.

56. Sankila R, Heinavaara S, Hakulinen T. Survival of breast cancer patients after subsequent term pregnancy: "healthy mother effect." *Am J Obstet Gynecol* 1994;170(3): 818–823.

57. von Schoultz E, Johansson H, Wilking N, et al. Influence of prior and subsequent pregnancy on breast cancer prognosis. *J Clin Oncol* 1995;13(2):430–434.

58. Petrek JA. Pregnancy safety after breast cancer. *Cancer* 1994;74(1 Suppl):528–531.

59. Gemignani ML, Petrek JA. Pregnancy after breast cancer. *Cancer Control* 1999; 6(3):272–276.

60. Velentgas P, Daling JR, Malone KE, et al. Pregnancy after breast carcinoma: outcomes and influence on mortality. *Cancer* 1999;85(11):2424–2432.

61. Dow KH, Harris JR, Roy C. Pregnancy after breast-conserving surgery and radiation therapy for breast cancer. *J Natl Cancer Inst Monogr* 1994;16:131–137.

62. Higgins S, Haffty BG. Pregnancy and lactation after breast-conserving therapy for early stage breast cancer. *Cancer* 1994;73(8):2175–2180.

63. Gelber S, Coates AS, Goldhirsch A, et al. Effect of pregnancy on overall survival after the diagnosis of early-stage breast cancer. *J Clin Oncol* 2001;19(6):1671–1675.

64. Upponi SS, Ahmad F, Whitaker IS, et al. Pregnancy after breast cancer. *Eur J Cancer* 2003;39(6):736–741.

65. Mueller BA, Simon MS, Deapen D, et al. Childbearing and survival after breast carcinoma in young women. *Cancer* 2003;98(6):1131–1140.

66. Blakely LJ, Buzdar AU, Lozada JA, et al. Effects of pregnancy after treatment for breast carcinoma on survival and risk of recurrence. *Cancer* 2004;100(3):465–469.

67. Ives A, Saunders C, Bulsara M, et al. Pregnancy after breast cancer: population based study. *BMJ* 2007;334(7586):194.

68. Yuri T, Tsukamoto R, Miki K, et al. Biphasic effects of zeranol on the growth of estrogen receptor-positive human breast carcinoma cells. *Oncol Rep* 2006;16(6): 1307–1312.

69. Partridge A, Gelber S, Peppercorn J, et al. Fertility outcomes in young women with breast cancer: a web-based survey [Abstract 6085]. *Proceeding of the American Society of Clinical Oncology* 2004;23:538.

70. Arora NK, Gustafson DH, Hawkins RP, et al. Impact of surgery and chemotherapy on the quality of life of younger women with breast carcinoma: a prospective study. *Cancer* 2001;92(5):1288–1298.

71. Offit K, Sagi M, Hurley K. Preimplantation genetic diagnosis for cancer syndromes: a new challenge for preventive medicine. *JAMA* 2006;296(22):2727–2730.

72. Schnitt SJ, Connolly JL, Harris JR, et al. Radiation-induced changes in the breast. *Hum Pathol* 1984;15(6):545–550.

73. Tralins AH. Lactation after conservative breast surgery combined with radiation therapy. *Am J Clin Oncol* 1995;18(1):40–43.

74. Burstein HJ, Winer EP. Primary care for survivors of breast cancer. *N Engl J Med* 2000;343(15):1086–1094.

75. Martin M, Pienkowski T, Mackey J, et al. Adjuvant docetaxel for node-positive breast cancer. *N Engl J Med* 2005;352(22):2302–2313.

76. Lobo RA. Potential options for preservation of fertility in women. *N Engl J Med* 2005;353(1):64–73.

77. Faddy MJ, Gosden RG, Gougeon A, et al. Accelerated disappearance of ovarian follicles in mid-life: implications for forecasting menopause. *Hum Reprod* 1992;7(10): 1342–1346.

78. Erickson GF. Ovarian anatomy and physiology. In: Lobo RA, Kelsey J, Marcus R, eds. *Menopause: biology and pathobiology*. San Diego: Academic Press, 2000:13–32.

Chapter 97
Medical Legal Aspects of Breast Cancer Evaluation

R. James Brenner

Delay in diagnosis of breast cancer remains the most common reason that physicians in the United States are sued for malpractice (1), and this is a rising legal issue in different countries. Although the relatively high prevalence of breast cancer combined with rising expectations for early detection and cure promoted in good faith by many organizations may contribute to this situation, more often than not liability is found because physicians either ignore or are not deliberate about management of potential signs and symptoms of breast cancer or radiologists do not detect cancer, misinterpret imaging findings, or fail to communicate information properly (2–4). Both clinicians and imagers involved in interventional procedures may also incur liability for failing to reconcile tissue diagnoses with clinical or imaging findings (2,5).

The law of negligence governs most medical malpractice cases. Although pejorative in connotation, the "tort" or civil law of negligence reflects four elements; namely, duty, breach of duty, causation, and damages. Although an adverse outcome often triggers a lawsuit, it is the conduct of the physician, not the outcome, that determines liability. The benchmark for this analysis, whether employed by a judge or jury, is forseeability; in other words, were clinical conditions or imaging findings sufficiently foreseeable that certain conduct was required as a standard of care? The law is predicated on the notion that the standard of care is an objective one, defined as what a reasonable and prudent physician would do under similar circumstances. Because those circumstances vary, so too does the reasonable duty (6). The dispositive concept in this analysis is not accuracy, but reasonableness.

The duty of the primary care physician is to obtain a proper history, perform a reasonable clinical examination of the breast and regional lymph nodes, and develop a deliberate management plan. Patient history is becoming more important as genetic profiles and predispositions are better studied (7) and its relationship to a management plan is illustrated by the duty, for example, to order screening mammography, especially in postmenopausal women. The ordering of screening mammography for younger women may be more controversial from an outcomes analysis with different guidelines developed by different specialty societies. From a risk management perspective, however, the ordering of such an examination obviates the allegation that a screening mammogram that was not ordered might have detected cancer at an earlier stage. For women with a lifetime cancer risk of 20% to 25%, the American Cancer Society has suggested a role for magnetic resonance imaging (MRI) screening (8). Payer plans may not reimburse for such an expensive procedure, but the duty to discuss the relative merits of MRI and facilitate a referral is not necessarily obviated by financial considerations (9). Likewise, screening ultrasound has been reported as having potential value (10), a perspective that will be modified with the anticipated final results of a National Cancer Institute (NCI)-sponsored trial (American College of Radiology Imaging Network [ACRIN] 6666) with results expected in 2009. A rising

interest in breast density as an independent risk factor that may prompt medical interventions has emerged and, with the development of digital mammography techniques which offer the feasibility of a quantitative density assessment, may need to be considered in the near future (11). Where reimbursement may not be immediately forthcoming, careful and documented discussions with the patient, inviting alternative approaches (e.g., self-pay) may evidence reasonable care. In addition, such new information which has already become incorporated into quantitative risk models (12), may prompt additional screening needs, such as MRI, as discussed above.

Most legal redress against clinicians relate to either the omission of a proper clinical breast examination or physical findings that do not prompt reasonable action. Because screening for breast cancer is not synonymous with mammography (13)—some cancers are only detectable by physical examination and may be confirmed by targeted ultrasound only after the lump is identified—regular examinations are considered standard of care. Women with multiple lumps and bumps (fibrocystic change) may require serial examinations to identify a dominant mass. A deliberate dynamic plan may not intercept such a lesion at a first visit, but it is an indication of reasonable care (6). Asking a patient to return "prn" may not support such a conclusion. Thus, proper instructions, medical record documentation, and efforts at follow-up of questionable findings provide a basis for reasonable care, even when a cancer diagnosis may be delayed.

Imaging errors occur in detection, diagnostic interpretation, and communication. Considerable variability exists in screening detection, and methods such as double reading or computer-aided detection have invited variable results (14,15). Thus, although such efforts may reduce legal risk, they are not currently considered standard of care; however, discriminate use of such approaches may introduce complicating factors that modify this conclusion (16). In like manner, certain thresholds of diagnosis, such as a spiculated mass (in the absence of trauma) or clustered pleomorphic calcifications are customary indications to recommend biopsy, the failure of which often results in liability. Other circumstances might involve nonspecific imaging findings on mammography. The integration of clinical examination findings may have an important impact and failure to triage patients appropriately based on such information is a common basis for legal redress (17).

Evolving technology often presents both the clinician and imager with issues regarding reasonable care. Although full field digital mammography (FFDM) has shown relative equivalency to traditional film-screen analogue mammography, results have also indicated a potential superiority for evaluation of dense breasts, with sensitivity possibly less than film screen studies for breasts consisting primarily of fat, given the processing algorithms available at the time (18). Given the higher costs of FFDM, which has been more readily absorbed in the United States than other countries, the lack of uniform adoption mitigates its role as the standard of care. In women with dense breasts, it may be preferable (including advance platforms such as tomosynthesis), but as with many evolving technologies, it likely does not necessarily reflect what a reasonable and prudent physician would do under current circumstances. Similar arguments apply to MRI. This discussion should neither discourage implementation of either technology nor indicate that such developments will not rise to a standard of care (e.g., use of MRI for detecting breast cancer metastatic to axillary lymph nodes with a negative mammogram and physical examination) in the future.

Treatment issues follow a similar analysis. Sentinel node biopsy, which may decrease the complication of arm edema associated with full axillary node dissection, may be seen as *a* standard of care, but not necessarily *the* standard of care at the present time (19); as in the ultrasound evaluation of axillary lymph nodes, this paradigm too may evolve (20). Use of new adjuvant techniques, such as accelerated partial breast irradiation or new adjuvant or neoadjuvant therapies, are usually introduced and appropriately applied under regulated protocols (21); the use outside of protocols may incur liability. With common acceptance, evidenced by prevailing expert opinion and published data, such approaches may rise to a threshold standard of care, but do not represent such a bar presently (22). In like manner, therapy based on minimal positive immunohistochemical staining of sentinel axillary lymph nodes represents a works in progress with future outcomes better defining the conditions under which treatment for regional involvement may require certain therapy regimens (23).

As can be deduced from this discussion, essential elements of diagnosis and treatment constitute reasonable and prudent care. Variations should be well documented and may provide a basis for different types of care based on the legally accepted concept of "alternative school of thought." The rapid evolution of technology—including imaging, personalize treatment regimens, and genomics—will influence where the bar is placed regarding standard of care issues and analysis of actual harm consequent to deviations from such care, but only after persuasive if not convincing demonstration of efficacy.

References

1. Physicians Insurance Association of America. *Breast cancer study.* Rockville, MD: Physicians Insurers Association of America, 2002.
2. Brenner RJ. Breast cancer and malpractice: a guide to the clinician. *Seminars in Breast Disease* 1998;1:3–14.
3. Brenner RJ. Mammography and malpractice litigation: current status, lessons, and admonitions *Am J Roentgenol AJR* 1993;161:931–935.
4. Brenner RJ, Bartholomew L. Communication errors in radiology: liability and cost assessment. *J Am Coll Radiol* 2005;2:428–431.
5. Brenner RJ. Interventional procedures of the breast: medical legal considerations. *Radiology* 1995;195:611–615.
6. Brenner RJ. Medical legal aspects of breast imaging. *Surg Oncol Clin N Am* 1994;3:67–85.
7. Plevritis SK, Kurian AW, Sigal BM, et al. Cost-effectiveness of screening BRCA1/2 mutation carriers with breast magnetic resonance imaging. *JAMA* 2006;295:2374–2384.
8. Saslow D, Boetes C, Burke W, et al. American Cancer Society guidelines for breast cancer screening with MRI as an adjunct to mammography. *CA Cancer J Clin* 2007;57:75–89.
9. Wickline v State of California, 183 Cal App 1064, 118 Cal Rptr 661 (1986).
10. Gordon PB. Ultrasound for breast cancer screening and staging. *Radiol Clin North Am* 2002;40:431–441.
11. Boyd N, Guo H, Martin LJ, et al. Mammographic density and the risk and detection of breast cancer. *N Engl J Med* 2007;356:227–236.
12. Palomares MR, Pratt KD, Lehman CD, et al. Mammographic density correlates with Gail model: implications for a new marker of breast cancer [Abstract 1689]. *Proceeding of the American Society of Clinical Oncology* 2001.
13. Morrison AS, Brisson J, Khalid N. Breast cancer incidence and mortality in the breast cancer detection demonstration project. *J Natl Cancer Inst* 1988;80:1540–1547.
14. Fenton JJ, Taplin SH, Careny PA, et al. Influence of computer-aided detection on performance of screening mammography. *N Engl J Med* 2007;356:1399–1409.
15. Warren Burhenne LJ, Wood SA, D'Orsi CJ, et al. Potential contribution of computer-aided detection to the sensitivity of screening mammography. *Radiology* 2000;215:554–562.
16. Brenner RJ. Computer-assisted detection in clinical practice: medical legal considerations. *Semin Roentgenol* 2007;42:280–286.
17. Brenner RJ. False-negative mammograms: medical, legal, and risk management implications. *Radiol Clin N Am* 2000;38:741–758.
18. Pisano ED, Gatsonis C, Hendrick E, et al. Diagnostic performance of digital versus film mammography for breast cancer screening. *N Engl J Med* 2005;353:1772–1783.
19. Newman EL, Kahn A, Diehl KM, et al. Does the method of biopsy affect the incidence of sentinel lymph node metastases. *Breast J* 2006;12:53–57.
20. Alvarez S, Anorbe E, Alcorta P, et al. Role of sonography in the diagnosis of axillary lymph node metastases: a systematic review. *AJR Am J Roentgenol* 2006;186:1342–1348.
21. Kuerer HM, Julian TB, Strom EA, et al. Accelerated partial breast irradiation after conservative surgery for breast cancer. *Ann Surg* 2004;239:338–351.
22. Brenner RJ. The Expert Witness, Understanding the Rationale, *J Am Col Radiol* 2007;4:612–616.
23. Calhoun KE, Hansen NM, Turner RR, et al. Nonsentinel node metastases in breast cancer patients with isolated tumor cells in the sentinel node: implications for complete axillary dissection. *Am J Surg* 2005;190:588–591.

Chapter 98
Cost and Cost-Effectiveness Considerations

Bruce E. Hillner

Escalating health care costs have been a persistent and openly discussed worry in American health care since the 1980s. During the 1990s, managed care in its various forms was able temporarily to slow the growth rate in health care costs. Since 2000, health care costs have again begun to grow substantially faster than overall inflation. In 2004, health expenditures were about 16% of the United States gross domestic product, and it is projected to reach 20% within the next 7 years.

Current expenditures for cancer are estimated in the United States to be about $100 billion. Three areas in particular have been the primary sources of the rapid growth in cancer care costs: new cytotoxic and biological therapies; supportive drugs, such as erythroid growth factors; and the increased use of assorted imaging techniques. Each of these will be discussed in this chapter.

Since 2000, for breast cancer patients innovative approaches to adjuvant therapy have emerged using a new class of hormonal therapies (aromatase inhibitors), new schedules of delivering chemotherapy (dose-dense therapy), and targeted treatments at specific newly identified features of the breast cancer cells (trastuzumab). The financial price of these new interventions has been an increase in costs of five- to tenfold compared with the preceding standard approach. Marked increases in adjuvant therapy costs are a microcosm of broader trends pushing up health care costs in the United States—patients continue to want the newest (and most expensive) drugs and medical devices; patients are relatively protected from the prices of new agents (excluding potential copayments); the U.S. Food and Drug Administration (FDA) does not regulate or negotiate prices as part of its approval process for new agent; and Medicare does not consider costs in any of its reimbursement decisions. Outside the United States, cost-effectiveness projections are increasingly used in the decision to include new interventions in a national formulary. Either explicitly or implicitly, all societies have to address the issue of allocation of limited resources.

This chapter contains a review and commentary on reports addressing cost issues in breast cancer care published in the period 2003 to 2007. The review will discuss in a stepwise manner reports by the clinical question (e.g., the cost of radiation therapy). The goal is introduce the reader to the extent that research on economic issues have or have not tracked the evolution of breast cancer treatment. A 2007 special issue of the *Journal of Clinical Oncology* presents an excellent overview of the current debate of costs of all types of cancer care delivery. Readers interested in the technical issues of performing and reporting cost-effectiveness analyses should seek out the introductory and advanced sources listed in the bibliography (1–3).

TYPES OF ECONOMIC ANALYSIS

Table 98.1 summarizes the five common categories of cost studies in health care. The first category of *cost of illness* studies describes the financial burden or consequences of illness, but do not make any comparison with other conditions. A *cost comparison* report does not explicitly address the relative benefit of the two approaches or populations subject to comparison. A *cost minimization* reports either explicitly or implicitly, but assumes no difference in the benefit (or harm) incurred between two different approaches. By comparing the costs

incurred, the lowest cost strategy will, by definition, be preferred because it has the lowest cost.

Cost-effectiveness analysis (CEA) and *cost-utility analysis* (CUA) estimate the additional cost per unit benefit associated with the use of a given intervention as compared with the alternative. The intervention of interest can be of any type: prevention, screening, diagnosis, treatment, or symptom control. CEA consider either a specific health effect (e.g., disease-free survival) without assigning a specific value to it or using years of life. CUA is a specific type of cost-effectiveness analysis that combines mortality and morbidity into a single multidimensional measure called a quality adjusted life-year (QALY).

The result of a CEA is usually expressed as a ratio of the difference in cost between the two competing strategies divided by the difference in benefit. A CEA is of most interest when the new intervention is more effective and more costly than the reasonable alternative strategy. The lower the ratio of the additional cost of the new intervention to gain the additional benefit, the more appealing to society as a whole is it to add the intervention to current medical approaches.

A common criticism of the entire area of medical cost-effectiveness analysis has been the lack of standards in the performing them and the quality of reporting the results. Although standards have been promulgated, they have not always been followed. In this chapter, we will attempt to highlight where selected reports illustrate good and occasional bad examples of the field. Three recurring themes will be stressed. First, in cost minimization studies was it appropriate to assume the two strategies are equally effective? Second, was the data used to guide the efficacy estimates accurate, representative, and credible? Third, was the default strategy representative? It should be the strategy most likely to have been used had the new intervention not be available. Additional detailed elements to look for are summarized in the 16-point checklist summarized in Table 98.2.

INTERVENTIONS AND TESTING IN HIGH-RISK WOMEN

In the 1990s, the identification of germ-line mutations revolutionized the care for women with strong family histories of breast cancer. Women with germ-line mutations are estimated to account for 5% to 10% of patients diagnosed with breast cancer in the United States. Because women who develop cancer associated with these mutations do so at a relatively young age, these mutations account for a disproportionate share of life-years lost from cancer. Cohort studies continue to define better the relative penetrance of risk for women with *BRCA1*, *BRCA2*, and newer mutations.

Anderson and colleagues (4) reported a cost-effectiveness analysis comparing combinations of prophylactic surgery or chemoprevention to a hypothetical cohort of carriers of *BRCA1* or *BRCA2* mutations who were age 35 to 50 years. They compared tamoxifen, oral contraceptives, bilateral salpingo-oophorectomy, mastectomy, both surgeries, and standard surveillance.

They found that oophorectomy alone or with mastectomy resulted in the best balance between costs and benefits for 35-year old women. When patient utilities for quality of life were included in the model, bilateral oophorectomy was the dominant strategy. When survival alone was considered, oophorectomy

Table 98.1	CATEGORIES OF COST STUDIES IN HEALTH CARE		
Type of Analysis	**Units of Costs**	**Units of Benefit**	**Results**
Cost of illness	$	Not addressed	$
Cost comparison	$	Not addressed	$
Cost minimization	$	Assumed to be identical	$
Cost effectiveness	$	Effect of interest (e.g., years of life)	$/Unit of effect
Cost-utility	$	Quality adjusted life years (QALY)	$/QALY

plus mastectomy was dominant with a cost-effective (CE) ratio of $2,300 per LY. When older women who have not yet developed cancer were modeled, the incremental CE ratio rapidly increased to $73,700 per LY in those 50 years of age.

Other reports addressed the costs of clinical genetic services in a variety of European settings. Sevilla et al. (5) from France highlighted the direct sequencing method for *BRCA1* and *BRCA2* testing is currently limited to a single U.S. company. They assessed alternative testing approaches available at three French centers. They found that they could reduce the cost per mutation detected by four- to sevenfold, but would miss an estimated 2% to 13% of cases.

Gronwald (6) from Poland reported on a novel approach to get women to increase their awareness about hereditary breast cancer. Genetic testing was offered to 5,024 women thorough an announcement in a popular women's magazine. They found 3.9% of the cohort to be *BRCA* mutation carriers. The overall cost of the program was only $125,000, leading to a cost per mutation detected of $630, which is about 50 to 100 times lower than programs in the United States.

In the United Kingdom, a randomized comparison of genetic counseling given by a nurse counselor compared with that given by a clinical geneticist led to equivalent patient satisfaction and reduction in anxiety at a lower cost (7). A second report addressed the costs of adding genetic risk counseling into women in Wales (8). They found that additional personal cost where patients were seen in the clinic was low—less than 20 pounds per patient. However, the major new incurred costs were the counseling or testing of other family members that increased costs an additional threefold.

Magnetic Resonance Screening

More recently, the use of dedicated magnetic resonance imaging (MRI) has been shown to be more sensitive than mammography in detecting breast cancer in high-risk women. The cancers detected by MRI are more often at a less advanced stage (stage I, node negative). MRI is also expensive, with charges typically exceeding $1,500 per test. In addition to cost, MRI has relatively poor specificity or high false–positive rates. To date, no evidence indicates that MRI screening improves overall survival owing to the short-term follow-up.

Given these concerns, investigators have estimated the cost per cancer detected and anticipated cost effectiveness based on the anticipated survival advantage of cancer detection at an earlier stage. Griebsch et al. (9) used data collected from a multicenter evaluation of MRI and mammography in 649 women aged 35 to 49 years at high risk of breast cancer who had annual testing for between 2 and 7 years. For all women, the incremental cost per cancer detected was 28,400 pounds and less than 15,300 if a *BRCA* mutation carrier. The cost per MRI study was 405 pounds (9).

Table 98.2	QUALITY CHECKLIST OF REPORTS ADDRESSING COST AND COST-EFFECTIVENESS ANALYSIS	
Transparency Criteria	**Description**	
Objective	Was this presented in clear, specific, and measurable manner?	
Perspective	Was the perspective stated and reasons for its selection?	
Data sources	Were the best available sources used (i.e., RCT)?	
Subgroup data	Were the subgroups prespecified at the beginning of the study?	
Uncertainty	1. Statistical analysis to address random events	
	2. Sensitivity analysis to cover a range of assumptions	
Incremental analysis	Were the alternatives for resources and costs assessed incrementally?	
Data abstraction	Were the methods used for data abstraction and values of health states stated?	
Time horizon	Did horizon allow for all relevant outcomes? Were benefits and costs beyond 1 year discounted?	
Costing	Were the measures used appropriate and described for quantities and unit costs	
Primary outcome	Was this clearly stated? Were the major short-term, long-term, and negative outcomes included?	
Outcome scales	Were the outcome measures valid and reliable? If not, was a justification given?	
Structure	Were the model's structure, methods, analysis, and the components of the numerator and denominator displayed in a transparent manner?	
Assumptions and limitations	Were the choice of the model, main assumptions, and limitations stated and justified?	
Potential biases	Were the direction and magnitude of potential biases explicitly discussed?	
Conclusions	Were these justified and based on the study results?	
Funding source	Was there a statement disclosing the source of funding?	

RCT, randomized clinical trial.
Modified from Chiou CF, Hay JW, Wallace JF, et al. Development and validation of a grading system for the quality of cost-effectiveness studies. *Med Care* 2003;41(1):32-44, with permission.

Plevritis SK et al. (10) reported a decision model cost-effectiveness projection from the United States perspective of a hypothetical cohort of *BRCA1* or *BRCA2* mutation carriers, age ranging from 25 to 69 years who decline prophylactic surgery. The key assumptions were that MRI increased the sensitivity of annual testing from 35% to 85%, the proportion of cancers detected with negative axillary node involvement increased from 57% to 81%, and a false–positive rate of 5% to 25% depending on patient age when tested. This modeling approach was more complex than those later described in addressing the cost-effectiveness of adjuvant aromatase inhibitors. The primary result was that incorporating annual MRI has an incremental cost-effectiveness that widely varies based on patient age and specific *BRCA* mutation. The strategy with the lowest ratio was annual MRI for 10 years from ages 40 to 49 years at a cost of $43,500 for *BRCA1* carriers and $111,600 for *BRCA2* carriers.

The role of tamoxifen for primary prevention of cancer in high-risk women without germ-line mutations was revisited in two papers. Each used a base case scenario of 50-year-old women. Melnikow et al. (11) used the minimum 5-year projected risk of breast cancer of 1.66% necessary to enter the National Surgical Adjuvant Breast and Bowel Project (NSABP) P-1 trial, whereas Cykert et al. (12) used a risk that was twice as high. As with prior projections, the incremental CE ratios markedly changed based on the costs of tamoxifen assigned, if the duration of benefit was limited to the 5 years of treatment or beyond, and baseline breast cancer risk. Melnikow concluded that tamoxifen was less costly and more effective only for women with 5-year breast cancer risks of greater than 4%. Cykert projected a CE ratio of $43,000 per QALY at a 5-year cancer risk of 3.4%.

Mammography

A mixture of methods addressed distinct mammography questions. These are summarized in Table 98.3. No new efficacy data were reported about screening mammography. Woo et al. (13) embraced the framework of a fixed budget to address the relative benefits and costs of cancer screening in general (breast, colorectal, and cervical) and how to optimize the resources spent in Hong Kong. They found that for the same amount of money currently being spent in Hong Kong on cancer screening, reallocating the same dollars could increase double cancer-associated life years saved. They also found that mammography should take a secondary role after first providing pap coverage every 4 years and 30% coverage for colonoscopy every 10 years after age 50. Wong et al. (14) in a independent report used mammography efficacy estimates done in Western countries (relative risk reduction of 30%) and applied these to Chinese women and local financial data. Their CE ratios for the rest of China were about double those of Woo in Hong Kong.

Relevant to the United States, Stout et al. (15) developed a complex discrete event simulation model that attempted to estimate the impact of gradual temporal increases in the number of women participating in routine screening and changes in survival associated with greater use of adjuvant therapy. Their model addressed numerous combinations of age at first screen, age at last screen, and screening interval. Between 1990 and 2000, about 50% of U.S. women participated in screening for which they estimated an incremental CE ratio of $58,000 per QALY for women age 40 to 80 with an intend to offer annual screening and no adverse effect on quality of life for an abnormal screen. How much, if any, quality of life penalty for short-term pain and anxiety associated with evaluation for a false–positive finding on a mammogram is one of the key factors in their analysis, which can greatly attenuate the QALY benefits of mammography.

Mandelblatt et al. (16–18) issued several reports related to mammography for older women. They reported a meta-analysis of 15 years of CE projections of biennial screening for women age 65 to 75 or 80 years. The assumed efficacy of mammography was consistently about 30%. Given this inferred efficacy, the

Author (Reference)	Question	Country	Conclusion
Wong (14)	Biannual screening in China	China	Screening women aged 40–60 had a CE ratio of $61,600 per QALY
Woo (13)	Cancer screening policy comparing different tests and frequency	China	Mammography every 2 years is lower priority than pap coverage or colonoscopy every 10 years
Groenewoud (21)	Double reading strategies	Dutch	For discordant readings, immediate referral projected CE 4,200 Euro per LY
Jacobi (58)	Screening in younger women	Dutch	In younger women with *BRCA1/2* mutations, annual screening is only CE in women with two affective relatives
Ciatto (21)	Discordant double readings	Italy	Arbitration by a third mammographer, for every cancer missed owing to false–negative arbitration, 151 unnecessary recalls and 21,248 euro saved
Neeser (59)	Structured screening vs. *ad hoc*	Switzerland	Formal screening vs. opportunistic screening CE ratio of $73,000 to $118,000 per LY
Lindfor (19)	Computer-aided diagnosis of mammograms	United States	If the relative efficacy of CAD is 29%, its CE ratio was $19,000 per LY
Mandelblatt (17)	Improving breast cancer outcomes	United States	If 76% of women getting biannual mammograms, reminder interventions have CE ratio >100,000 per LY
Mandelblatt	Extending age of screening	United States	>$100,000 per LY after age 79
Mandelblatt (16)	Meta-analysis of cost-effectiveness projections in older women	United States	Biennial screening from age 65 to 75 or 80 years, $ per LY $34,000 to $88,000
Saywell (60)	Mammography adherence	United States	In-person counseling most effective
Saywell (61)	Improve mammography attendance	United States	A tailored mail letter was the most cost-effective $.39 per 1% increase in screening
Stout (15)	CE projections from actual screening behavior	United States	If all ages are aggregated, CE ratio of $36,700 per LY
Wu (62)	Improve mammography attendance	United States	Tailored telephone counseling lowest cost yet effective strategy

CAD, computer aided diagnosis; CE, cost-effectiveness; LY, life-years; QALY, quality adjusted life-year.

estimated CE ratios were between $34,000 and $88,000 per LY, which increased with age. In other reports, they noted that extending screening beyond age 79 will have CE ratios greater than $100,000 per LY and that reminders to these women are relatively high costs as well.

Whether computer aided diagnosis (CAD) of digital mammograms is an effective technique remains controversial. Lindfors et al. (19) suggested that if the relative efficacy of cancer detection is increased 29%, then CAD will have an attractive CE ratio (19).

Double reading of mammograms is an increasing worldwide trend. However, the preferred strategy whether there is disagreement is debated. This debate was illustrated by a Dutch approach suggesting immediate referral for biopsy has had projected CE ratio of 4,200 euros per LY, whereas an Italian study (20) concluded that arbitration by a third reader would lead to 151 fewer biopsies per missed cancers and save over 21,000 euros (21).

Axillary Node Staging

The adoption of sentinel lymph node biopsy (SLNB) into routine breast cancer management has been rapidly embraced. The optimal approach to SLNB continues to be debated. One approach is for an intraoperative pathologic analysis thorough frozen section or touch imprint cytology, which if found positive, the surgeon proceeds to an immediate complete axillary dissection. Alternatively, the surgeon may decide that the likelihood of node-positive disease is low using patient risk factors and await pathologic analysis of paraffin permanent sections. These options were compared in a decision analysis model from M.D. Anderson Cancer Center that used their experience from 342 consecutive patients for the relevant probabilities; the cytology had a 0.43 sensitivity and 0.99 specificity (22). They found that, given the low false–positive rate of cytology, that intraoperative touch cytology had a CE ratio of $13,800 for women with preoperative T1 size cancer and $7,100 for T2 cancers. If the sensitivity approached 60%, the cytology strategy would become dominant (more effective and less costly).

Radiation Therapies

Because of the increasing use of screening mammography, the number of women with ductal carcinoma *in situ* (DCIS) being identified is also growing. Large randomized trials have shown that adjuvant radiation therapy reduces the relative risk of invasive and noninvasive ipsilateral recurrences after breast-conserving surgery (BCS), but does not have an impact on overall survival. Therefore, the CE of radiation therapy (RT) is dependent on the relative value of improving local control and reducing the need for costly salvage therapy, which needs to be weighed against the added costs of RT. This clinical situation is a classic scenario for a CUA.

Hayman et al. (23) have provided the needed preferences or utility scores for the risks and benefits of RT. They prospectively collected utilities from 120 patients and 210 nonpatients for eight relevant health states. The differences in the utilities between patients and nonpatients were minimal. Their key finding was that the principal benefit associated with adding RT to BCS is the ability of RT to reduce actual invasive recurrences. That is, actual invasive recurrences have a substantial negative effect (Table 98.4).

These utilities were used by Suh et al. (24) in developing a cost-utility model using the increasing common Markov or state-transition approach. The base case scenario was a cohort of 55-year-old women with DCIS and projected a lifetime horizon. The relative efficacy of RT was based on the NSABP B-17 trial and direct medical costs of the 2002 Medicare fee schedule plus non-medical time and transportation costs. The base case result

Table 98.4	**UTILITY SCORES RELEVANT TO MANAGING DUCTAL CARCINOMA *IN SITU***

	Mean Score
Breast-conserving Surgery and Radiation	
Without recurrence	
Patients	0.93
Nonpatients	0.90
Invasive Breast Cancer recurrences	
Patients	0.75
Nonpatients	0.84

Modified from Hayman JA, Kabeto MU, Schipper MJ, et al. Assessing the benefit of radiation therapy after breast-conserving surgery for ductal carcinoma-in-situ. *J Clin Oncol* 2005;23(22):5171-5177, with permission.

found that adding RT to BCS had an incremental cost-utility ratio of $36,700 per QALY. When patient-derived utilities were used instead of nonpatient utilities, the CE ratio declined to $5,200 per QALY. The key sensitivity analysis was the uncertainty in the relative efficacy of RT in reducing invasive local recurrences. When the 95% confidence intervals around this point estimate were used, the CE ratios ranged from $20,300 (upper limit efficacy) to $128,500 (lower limit efficacy). Not surprisingly, the CE ratios also changed dramatically based on the relative cost of RT. These two papers (23,24) are unusually transparent in their exploration of the economic and clinical tradeoffs.

New Forms of Radiation Therapy

Compared with traditional RT, proton beam therapy offers distinct clinical advantages at substantial higher financial costs. Proton therapy offers more precise dose distribution and should reduce treatment-associated heart and lung toxicity. The risk of radiation-induced cardiac diseases, especially for left-sided breast cancer, is well established (25). In addition to reduced toxicity, several of the new approaches of partial breast irradiation can be given over a shorter period, which reduces patient time and costs. The relative efficacy in these techniques in reducing long-term breast cancer and toxicity-associated outcomes has not been established. The NSABP and Radiation Therapy Oncology Group (RTOG) have agreed to jointly sponsor a randomized trial of partial breast irradiation, which provides equivalent local tumor control and survival compared with conventional whole breast irradiation in the local management of early-stage breast cancer (NSABP B-39). Two reports addressing costs associated with proton beam therapy were found. Lundkvist et al. (26) developed a Markov model of the potential benefits of proton therapy from a Swedish perspective. This model's value is limited because the relative efficacy for the various breast cancer outcomes was assumed equivalent. The authors' projected 76% benefit in reducing the treatment-associated risk of coronary artery disease was based on a small, single center series solely on dose comparisons. Despite this large relative effect, the model found that the projected CE ratios were high at 67,000 euros per LY (26).

In the United States, several partial breast RT techniques can be given outside the research setting, therefore a cost comparison of alternative approaches is relevant to payer's and patients. Suh et al. (27) performed a cost comparison of four whole breast and four partial breast techniques. Their projections included a detail tracking of the technical and professional codes with 2003 Medicare reimbursement rates as well as projections for a patient's typical travel and lost employment time. Table 98.5 shows that the costs estimates vary almost threefold. The technical component for the brachytherapy approaches accounted for the marked differences. If the

Table 98.5	**2003 TOTAL DIRECT COSTS OF DIFFERENT BREAST RADIATION REGIMENS**	
	Payer's Costs ($)	Patient's Costs ($)
Whole breast without boost	7,400	1,100
Whole breast with boost	9,500	1,400
Whole breast with accelerated schedule	5,400	700
Whole breast with intensity modulated	17,900	1,400
Accelerated partial breast irradiation (APBI) using Mammosite system	17,800	500
APBI with interstitial brachytherapy	16,800	500
APBI with high dose rate intensity-modulation	9,200	500
APBI with three-dimensional conformal	7,200	500

Modified from Suh WW, Pierce LJ, Vicini FA, et al. A cost comparison analysis of partial versus whole-breast irradiation after breast-conserving surgery for early-stage breast cancer. *Int J Radiat Oncol Biol Phys* 2005;62(3):790-796, with permission.

randomized comparisons demonstrate equivalent efficacy, the financial winners and losers are easy to identify from this report.

Adjuvant Therapies

Hormonal Therapy

Three biologically similar, but distinct, aromatase inhibitors (AI) were assessed in several large randomized trials. These trials compared AI therapy with tamoxifen therapy or following tamoxifen therapy in women with estrogen receptor (ER)-positive breast cancers. These trials have had three distinct designs: the upfront use of an AI instead of tamoxifen for 5 years (28,29), switching to an AI after 2 or 3 years of tamoxifen (30), or the late addition or extended therapy with an AI after 5 years of tamoxifen (31,32). In all settings, an AI was found to be beneficial in reducing breast cancer disease-free survival; however, only in the extended therapy patients has an overall survival benefit yet been shown. These trials are reviewed in detail in Chapter 48.

Soon after publication of the initial trial results, a series of economic analyses began appearing that addressed the anticipated long-term benefits of individual AI and the timing of their use. These trials are summarized in Table 98.6.

Table 98.6	**AROMATASE INHIBITOR ECONOMIC ANALYSES**							
Author (Reference)	AIS	Time Frame	Model Type	Country	AI Efficacy	Utility	CE Ratio (Currency per QALY)	
First-line Metastatic								
Dranitsaris (63)	Letrozole	Lifetime	Markov	Canada	Meta-analysis		12,500 C	
Karnon (64)	Letrozole	Lifetime	Markov	United Kingdom.	Trial	Yes	8,500 P	
Simons (65,66)	Anastrozole	Lifetime		United States	Trial	No	$9,000 to $14,000/LY	
Marchietti (4)	Anastrozole or letrozole	Lifetime	Markov	Italy	Trials	Yes	10,800 E Anastrozole 16,900 E Letrozole	
Okubo (67)	Letrozole	Lifetime	Markov	Japan	Trials	Yes	$5,000/LY	
Adjuvant	**Crossover**							
Gill (68)	AI	Lifetime	Markov	Spain	Trial	Yes	EXE lowest CE 30,000	
Lonning (69)	AI	Lifetime	Markov	Norway	Trials	Yes	Crossover at 2–3 years lower CE Ratio than extended AI therapy	
Lundkvist (70)	Exemestane	Lifetime	Markov	Sweden	Trial	Yes	20,000 E/QALY	
Risebrough (71)	Exemestane	Lifetime	Markov	Canada	Trial	Yes	28,100 C	
Skedgel (72)	Exemestane	Lifetime	Markov	Canada	Indirect	Yes	EXE following Tam has lower CE ratio than upfront anastrozole	
Skedgel (73)	Exemestane	Lifetime	Markov	Belgium	Indirect	Yes	Tam followed by EXE has lowest CE ratio	
Thompson (74)	Exemestane	Lifetime	Markov	United States	Trial	Yes	20,100	
Younis (75)	AI	Lifetime	Markov	United Kingdom	Indirect	Yes	Tam-AI for low risk, upfront AI high risk	
Adjuvant	**First-line**							
Hillner (76)	Anastrozole	Lifetime	Markov	United States	Trial	Yes	$40,600/LY $74,000/QALY	
Piskur (77)	Anastrozole		Decision tree	Slovenia	Trial	No	Costs of AI 1.75: 1 of Tam	
Rochi (78)	Anastrozole	Lifetime	Markov	Canada	Trial	Yes	28,000 C/QALY	
Delea (79)	Letrozole	Lifetime	Markov	United States	Trial	Yes	$23,700/QALY	
Hind (80)	Anastrozole	Lifetime	Markov	United Kingdom	Trial	Yes	19,200 to 23,200 P	
Mansel (81)	Anastrozole	Lifetime	Markov	United Kingdom	Trial	Yes	17,600 P	
Extended Adjuvant								
Delea (79)	Letrozole	Lifetime	Markov	United States	Trial	Yes	$28,700	
El Ouagari (82)	Letrozole	Lifetime	Markov	Canada	Trial	Yes	34,000 C	
Hind (80)	Letrozole	Lifetime	Markov	United Kingdom	Trial	Yes	9,800 P	

AI, aromatase inhibitor; C, Canadian dollars; CE, cost-effectiveness; E, Euros; EXE, exemestane; P, English pounds; QALY, quality adjusted life-year; Tam, tamoxifen.

Table 98.7	ADJUVANT TRASTUZUMAB COST-EFFECTIVENESS REPORTS

Author (Reference)	Strategy	Funding	Model Type	Country	Relative Efficacy	Time Frame	CE Ratio (Currency per QALY)
Dedes (83)	ERBB2[a]	None	Markov	Switzerland	ERBBA, Finnish	15 yr	20,000 E[b] Cost savings using 9-week schedule
Garrison (84)	ERBB2+	Industry	Markov	United States.	NSABP	20 yr or lifetime	34,200 at 20 yr
Kurian (85)	ERBB2+	None	Markov	United States	NSABP	40 yr	40,000
Liberato (86)	ERBB2+	None	Markov	Italy	NSABP	15 yr	19,000
Miller (87)	ERBB2+	None	Markov	Australia	NSABP	Lifetime	22,800 A 1,700 A for 9 week schedule
Norum (88)	ERBB2+	None	Spreadsheet	Norway	NSABP	Lifetime	8,200 E to 30,300 E

CE, cost-effective; NSABP, National Surgical Adjuvant Breast and Bowel Project.
[a]Formerly HER2.
[b]A, Australian dollars; E, Euros; if not stated U.S. dollars.

The commonality of the general evaluative approach is notable (33). Almost all evaluations used a Markov decision model framework to extrapolate the observed rates of relapse and adverse events from the relevant clinical trials to extended time horizon to estimate lifetime costs and benefits. Almost all models considered separate contralateral breast cancers, local recurrences, and systemic recurrences, including occasionally different sites of metastases. Although most models considered the known toxicities of tamoxifen, notable differences were found in the frequency of AI toxicities on bone loss and osteoporotic fractures. Most importantly, the models differed in how long the benefit of the AI persisted in reducing breast cancer recurrences—ranging from 5 years to indefinitely. All the models assumed that a reduction in breast cancer recurrence will eventually lead to a long-term reduction in breast cancer deaths.

For front-line therapy with anastrozole or letrozole, the different investigators projected costs per LY gained ranging from $28,000 Canadian, about 20,000 pounds, or $40,600. The assessments of cross-over strategies found that these lead to lower CE ratios than front-line therapy, but overall CE ratios were consistently less than $30,000 per LY. Extended adjuvant letrozole's CE ratios varied between the U.S., Canadian, and British assessment owing almost completely to the higher drug pricing in the United States and Canadian.

In summary, the cost-effectiveness of adjuvant AI have been extensively and carefully evaluated in a variety of countries, which generally suggests that for patients with the risk of systemic recurrences similar to those participating in the clinical trials, AI are cost-effective. Of note, the percent of women in these randomized clinical trials with node-positive disease ranged from 34% to 46%. The optimal CE strategy for low risk (node negative, <10 mm tumors) ER-positive women and those with pre-existing osteoporosis remains uncertain.

Trastuzumab

At the 2005 annual American Society of Clinical Oncology (ASCO) meeting and its subsequent publication 6 months later, the initial results of the two large randomized trials of adjuvant trastuzumab were ground breaking (34,35). These trials showed that trastuzumab was associated with an unprecedented reduction of about one-half in the risk of breast cancer recurrences. This is discussed in detail in Chapter 51.

Given that the drug costs alone for 1 year of trastuzumab use exceed the average lifetime costs of the typical breast cancer patient of 10 to 15 years ago, these results were obvious candidates for CE projections to assist policy makers in their decision-making to adopt wide-spread use of trastuzumab.

Subsequently, a third trial from Finland found a similar relative risk reduction with adjuvant trastuzumab when given for only 9 weekly infusions (36). This led to additional CE projections involving indirect comparisons of the duration and costs of therapy.

The different CE models are summarized in Table 98.7. These models predominantly used Markov transition models to project lifetime costs and benefits. Patient age was generally assumed identical to trial participants or an age of about 50 years. All but one of the reports assumed the benefit of trastuzumab would persist only for 5 years because this is well supported by the Early Breast Cancer Trialists' Meta-analysis (37). Although different approaches to the relative risk of recurrence, patterns of treatment, and associated survival beyond year 5, the overall conclusions were striking similar—CE ratios between $20,000 and $40,000 per LY for the 1-year schedule and less than $5,000 per LY for the 9-week schedule.

We noted in an editorial commentary that the primary conclusion that adjuvant trastuzumab is 'cost effective' likely represents 'icing on the cake' to American oncologists who have rapidly embraced trastuzumab (38). From early 2005 to mid-2006, United States sales of trastuzumab have increased by 250% or an additional approximate $750 million per year—the absolute increase in annual sales approximates our estimate of treating all U.S. women with new node positive, ERBB2 (formerly HER2)-positive breast cancer independent of age or comorbidity.

Despite the relatively favorable CE ratios, expanded use of trastuzumab will have a major impact on budgets of countries or payers of cancer care. A shorter duration of trastuzumab using the Finnish 9-week approach dramatically lowers overall costs and CE ratios. The duration of trastuzumab therapy is not being addressed in current U.S. trials, but is being addressed in a French trial comparing 6- with 12-month therapy.

Chemotherapy

Benefits

Only three reports were found addressing issues in adjuvant chemotherapy. Two of these reports addressed the advantage of using a FEC-1000 (fluorouracil, epirubicin, cyclophosphamide) compared with either FEC-50 or traditional cyclophosphamide, methotrexate and 5-fluorouracil (CMF) in women axillary node-positive disease. The industry-sponsored comparison of FEC-100 versus FEC-50 is notable for only using the primary efficacy point estimate (hazard rate [HR] = 0.80) without exploring the confidence interval around it (39). The Norwegian analysis used indirect evidence of the superiority of FEC leading to 3% to 7% increase in 5-year survival. If this magnitude of benefit is accurate, the CE ratios projected were 3,600 to 15,100 euros per LY (40).

The third paper took a national health policy perspective in addressing the impact of changes in the national guidelines for adjuvant therapy in The Netherlands from 1994 to 2001 (41). The revised guidelines were associated with an 80% relative increase in the total number of breast cancer patients eligible for adjuvant therapy. The guidelines were projected to increase 10-year overall survival by 10% and would have a CE ratio of about 5,000 euros per LY. Their projection, however, is an under-estimate of current treatment patterns because the drug costs for current chemotherapy, such as FEC-100 or taxanes, regimens are much higher than CMF.

Venous Access and Toxicities

Venous port device technology revolutionized the convenience and safety of giving infusional chemotherapy. Installation of external tunneled catheter usually into the subclavian vein became a standard approach in the 1990s. In recent years, peripherally inserted central catheters usually inserted by interventional radiology have been increasingly used. Although direct comparisons in a randomized trial are needed to compare the long-term patency, thrombosis, and infectious complications, an indirect comparison of 200 consecutive breast cancer patients having these procedures is an important contribution (42). The overall major complication rates with the central or peripheral approaches were 7% to 12%, including sepsis, deep vein thrombosis, and skin dehiscence. The overall cost for insertion without future complications was about 230 euros, which is less than U.S. professional fees. The average costs of complications approximately equal the costs of insertion.

The benefits of adjuvant hormonal and chemotherapy observed in clinical trials have been successfully translated in routine care, with evidence in multiple countries of a 25% decline in breast cancer mortalities in middle-aged women since the 1990s. The other half of the benefit-to-risk discussion that must occur between patient and provider is about the short- and long-term toxicities, including death with adjuvant chemotherapy. The relative frequencies of grade 3 or 4 toxicities in clinical trials are commonly used source when the toxicities are quantitatively discussed with patients or modeled. In an important and novel paper, Hassett et al. (43) addressed whether the toxicity in routine practice (effectiveness) is similar to or different than the clinical trial estimates (efficacy). This report used a unique database—an aggregation of medical claims from America's largest corporations that self-insure their employees and their dependents. This large cohort, although not a fully representative cross-section, has unique strengths—a diverse profile of individuals in the work force (age <65 years), broad geographic locations, and a range of health care plans contracted to oversee the delivered care.

This study using more than 12,000 women from 1998 to 2002 evaluated hospitalizations and emergency room visits associated with the period that women would be eligible for adjuvant therapy after primary surgical therapy. The authors carefully match the patients getting chemotherapy (based on their drug and procedure claims) with other women not getting chemotherapy using propensity scores. The results were striking: hospitalizations in the year after breast cancer diagnosis were 8.4% for fever, 5.5% for neutropenia or thrombocytopenia, 2.5% for dehydration, and 2.4% for other gastrointestinal toxicities. About 40% of the hospitalizations were attributed to chemotherapy toxicity, and the remainder were owing to surgery-related toxicities. The financial costs of these adverse effects averaged an additional $1,271 per patient undergoing chemotherapy, and the average amount spent by patients experiencing complications because of chemotherapy was about $14,000.

Gene Assays

Since the first reporting in 2002, the use of microarray analyses of genetic patterns of individual breast cancers to stratify women into good or bad prognosis groups has exploded. These assays have been used for two distinct goals that are complementary, but not necessarily identical: prognosis and prediction. Although many individual prognostic factors exist for breast cancer patients, currently only estrogen-receptor and ERBB2 are clinically useful predictors of treatment response. This important distinction is emphasized when the three CE analyses summarized in Table 98.8 are compared.

Each of these reports describes a decision analyses mode for different cohorts of breast cancer patients considering adjuvant therapy. The Oestreicher et al. (44) model compared hypothetical cohorts—one whose treatment was guided by National Institutes of Health (NIH) guidelines or the Dutch 70-gene microarray profile (44). If given, the costs for chemotherapy reflected higher U.S. prices and the shift to using taxanes in most patients. They found that, although the gene profiling patients received more targeted treatment, the 10-year recurrence-free survival was improved by 5% (29% vs. 34%) and saved $2,900 per patient using the NIH guidelines. This leads to a *reverse* CE ratio: the new strategy leads to a lower benefit but is less costly—$13,800 per LY.

The two industry-sponsored assessments of the 21-gene profiling utilizing reverse transcription-polymerase chain reaction (RT-PCR) address the question of benefits from chemotherapy in addition to tamoxifen in the largest subgroup of new breast cancer cases—axillary node-negative, ER positive disease (45,46). Two reports compared using the gene assay either following the NCCN guidelines, universal tamoxifen only, or chemotherapy. The Oncotype DX assay predictive power was assessed in 651 patients from a NSABP trial and discussed in more detail in Chapter 32. Patients were stratified patients by prognosis and benefit from chemotherapy. The low-risk group representing about one-half of patients did not benefit at all from chemotherapy, whereas the high-risk group representing about one-quarter of patients had a huge benefit (relative risk reduction of 74%) from chemotherapy. Given the remarkable differences in benefits, it is no surprise that the CE ratios were low. At the end of 2007, the ASCO recommendations for the use of tumor markers in breast cancer endorsed the use of the assay for the subgroup modeled (47).

Metastatic Disease

For women with recurrent breast cancer that was originally hormone responsive, the same decision point between tamoxifen and an AI occurs similar to the adjuvant setting. Economic analyses using either patient level primary data or decision modeling all found that the incremental CE ratios were relatively favorable less than $20,000 per LY (Table 98.6).

Bisphosphonates

The costs associated with bisphosphonates for women with metastatic bone disease were addressed in several studies. Depending on the country and drug pricing, oral bisphosphonate may or may not have a major cost advantage. In the United States, de Lemos et al. (48), in a retrospective series of 169 patients, found that pamidronate given in a 1-hour infusion compared with the FDA approved standard of 2 hours was safe and a net lower cost to an infusion center than zoledronate given over 15 minutes. Finally, a retrospective analysis of a larger U.S. health insurer (see discussion by Hassett et al. [43] of chemotherapy toxicity) addressed the burden of illness and costs for women having skeletal related complications. These were estimated at about $14,000 per patient (49).

Table 98.8	GENE-PROFILING COST-EFFECTIVENESS ANALYSES						
Author	Target Group	Intervention	Standard	Testing ($)	Chemotherapy ($)	Benefit (QALY)	CE Ratio ($ per LY)
Hornberger (45)	ER+, node (−)	Recurrence Score Guided	NCCN Guideline	3,450	15,700	0.86	Cost Saving
Lyman (46)	ER+, node (−)	Recurrence Score Guided	Tamoxifen only	3,450	NA	2.2	$2,000 per LY
		Recurrence Score Guided	Tamoxifen and Chemotherapy	3,450	10,000	Similar	Cost Savings
Oestreicher (44)	Premenopausal Stage I, II	Gene Expression Profiling	NIH Guidelines	3,460	22,000	−0.21	−13,800

SUMMARY

Studies of cost and cost-effectiveness are done to influence clinical practice. A recurring challenge to the reader of these studies is the difficulty in integrating individual reports into defining a comprehensive breast cancer benefits package. Such a benefits package has been previously proposed for screening, local primary therapy, radiotherapy, and adjuvant systemic therapy (50,51). No United States insurer, however, has yet adopted a similar concept. Relative effectiveness has been shown repeatedly to be the dominant driver of the CE or cost-utility ratios. Therefore, effectiveness, predominantly a change in overall survival, remains the gold standard. Consistent prolonged improvements in patient quality of life or utility as discussed herein are often harder to establish. Prioritizing allocation of health care dollars to and away from specific elements or type of breast cancer care compared with other major diseases of adults will require discussions that American's have yet been willing to discuss openly.

Such a discussion will likely occur after the recent FDA approval of bevacizumab for use with paclitaxel in first treatment of metastatic disease (52). Chapter 78 discusses in detail the randomized trial showing patients treated with bevacizumab and paclitaxel compared with paclitaxel had an improved progressive-free survival, which was its primary end point (53). The trial was too small, however, to detect modest increases in overall survival, although 1-year survival was increased (81.2% vs. 73.4%, $p = .01$) (54). The cost for bevacizumab treatment is approximately $7,700 per month.

The spectrum of breast cancer issues that have been the focus of economic analyses has generally paralleled the growth in randomized trial evidence supporting a new intervention. The overall report quality has steadily improved with greater transparency and detail. This is particularly true for work published in the higher impact peer-reviewed journals. At the same time, the volume of work being published is increasing, the consistency of identifying funding sources relatively weak, and many analyses fall short of the standards discussed in the beginning of this chapter.

The goals of economic analyses in cancer care continue to be utilitarian—seeking to provide the most value for the dollar spent. Evaluations of the costs and quality of life during clinical trials and in routine practice continue to be infrequently prospectively collected. The United Kingdom's National Institute for Clinical Excellence provides an attractive model should the United States ever politically decide to address health care prioritizing explicitly. The mismatch between what the United States spends on cancer care and technology assessment of it appears to be both unwise and unsustainable (55,56).

ACKNOWLEDGMENT

Dr. Hillner's preparation of this work was supported in part by a Research Scholar Grant for Health Services, Health Policy, and Outcomes Research (RSGHP-04-003-01-CPHPS) from the American Cancer Society.

References

1. Drummond MF. *Methods for the economic evaluation of health care programmes*, 2nd ed. Oxford; New York: Oxford University Press, 1997.
2. Gold MR, Siegel JE, Russell LB, et al. *Cost-effectiveness in health and medicine*. New York: Oxford University Press, 1996.
3. Petitti DB. *Meta-analysis, decision analysis, and cost-effectiveness analysis*, 2nd ed. New York: Oxford University Press, 2000.
4. Anderson K, Jacobson JS, Heitjan DF, et al. Cost-effectiveness of preventive strategies for women with a BRCA1 or a BRCA2 mutation. *Ann Intern Med* 2006;144(6):397–406.
5. Sevilla C, Julian-Reynier C, Eisinger F, et al. Impact of gene patents on the cost-effective delivery of care: the case of BRCA1 genetic testing. *Int J Technol Assess Health Care* 2003;19(2):287–300.
6. Gronwald J, Huzarski T, Byrski T, et al. Direct-to-patient BRCA1 testing: the Twoj Styl experience. *Breast Cancer Res Treat* 2006;100(3):239–245.
7. Balmana J, Sanz J, Bonfill X, et al. Genetic counseling program in familial breast cancer: analysis of its effectiveness, cost and cost-effectiveness ratio. *Int J Cancer* 2004;112(4):647–652.
8. Cohen D, Barton G, Gray J, Brain K. Health economics and genetic service development: a familial cancer genetic example. *Fam Cancer* 2004;3(1):61–67.
9. Griebsch I, Brown J, Boggis C, et al. Cost-effectiveness of screening with contrast enhanced magnetic resonance imaging vs. x-ray mammography of women at a high familial risk of breast cancer. *Br J Cancer* 2006;95(7):801–810.
10. Plevritis SK, Kurian AW, Sigal BM, et al. Cost-effectiveness of screening BRCA1/2 mutation carriers with breast magnetic resonance imaging. *JAMA* 2006;295(20):2374–2384.
11. Melnikow J, Kuenneth C, Helms LJ, et al. Chemoprevention: drug pricing and mortality: the case of tamoxifen. *Cancer* 2006;107:950–958.
12. Cykert S, Phifer N, Hansen C. Tamoxifen for breast cancer prevention: a framework for clinical decisions. *Obstet Gynecol* 2004;104(3):433–442.
13. Woo PPS, Kim JJ, Leung GM. What is the most cost-effective population-based cancer screening program for Chinese women? *J Clin Oncol* 2007;25(6):617–624.
14. Wong IO, Kuntz KM, Cowling BJ, et al. Cost effectiveness of mammography screening for Chinese women. *Cancer* 2007;110(4):885–895.
15. Stout NK, Rosenberg MA, Trentham-Dietz A, et al. Retrospective cost-effectiveness analysis of screening mammography. *J Natl Cancer Inst* 2006;98(11):774–782.
16. Mandelblatt J, Saha S, Teutsch S, et al. The cost-effectiveness of screening mammography beyond age 65 years: a systematic review for the U.S. Preventive Services Task Force. *Ann Intern Med* 2003;139(10):835–842.
17. Mandelblatt JS, Schechter CB, Yabroff KR, et al. Toward optimal screening strategies for older women. Costs, benefits, and harms of breast cancer screening by age, biology, and health status. *J Gen Intern Med* 2005;20(6):487–496.
18. Mandelblatt JS, Schechter CB, Yabroff KR, et al. Benefits and costs of interventions to improve breast cancer outcomes in African American women. *J Clin Oncol* 2004;22(13):2554–2566.

19. Lindfors KK, McGahan MC, Rosenquist CJ, et al. Computer-aided detection of breast cancer: a cost-effectiveness study. *Radiology* 2006;239(3):710–717.
20. Ciatto S, Ambrogetti D, Risso G, et al. The role of arbitration of discordant reports at double reading of screening mammograms. *J Med Screen* 2005;12(3):125–127.
21. Groenewoud JH, Otten JD, Fracheboud J, et al. Cost-effectiveness of different reading and referral strategies in mammography screening in The Netherlands. *Breast Cancer Res Treat* 2007;102(2):211–218.
22. Jeruss JS, Hunt KK, Xing Y, et al. Is intraoperative touch imprint cytology of sentinel lymph nodes in patients with breast cancer cost effective? *Cancer* 2006;107(10):2328–2336.
23. Hayman JA, Kabeto MU, Schipper MJ, et al. Assessing the benefit of radiation therapy after breast-conserving surgery for ductal carcinoma-in-situ. *J Clin Oncol* 2005;23(22):5171–5177.
24. Suh WW, Hillner BE, Pierce LJ, et al. Cost-effectiveness of radiation therapy following conservative surgery for ductal carcinoma in situ of the breast. *Int J Radiat Oncol Biol Phys* 2005;61(4):1054–1061.
25. Early Breast Cancer Trialists' Collaborative G. Effects of radiotherapy and surgery in early breast cancer—an overview of the randomized trials. *N Engl J Med* 1995;333(22):1444–1456.
26. Lundkvist J, Ekman M, Ericsson SR, et al. Economic evaluation of proton radiation therapy in the treatment of breast cancer. *Radiother Oncol* 2005;75(2):179–185.
27. Suh WW, Pierce LJ, Vicini FA, et al. A cost comparison analysis of partial versus whole-breast irradiation after breast-conserving surgery for early-stage breast cancer. *Int J Radiat Oncol Biol Phys* 2005;62(3):790–796.
28. Howell A, Cuzick J, Baum M, et al. Results of the ATAC (Arimidex, Tamoxifen, Alone or in Combination) trial after completion of 5 years' adjuvant treatment for breast cancer. *Lancet* 2005;365(9453):60–62.
29. Coates AS, Keshaviah A, Thurlimann B, et al. Five years of letrozole compared with tamoxifen as initial adjuvant therapy for postmenopausal women with endocrine-responsive early breast cancer: update of study BIG 1-98. *J Clin Oncol* 2007;25(5):486–492.
30. Coombes R, Hall E, Gibson L, et al. A randomized trial of exemestane after two to three years of tamoxifen therapy in postmenopausal women with primary breast cancer. *N Engl J Med* 2004;350(11):1081–1092.
31. Goss P, Ingle J, Martino S, et al. A randomized trial of letrozole in postmenopausal women after five years of tamoxifen therapy for early-stage breast cancer. *N Engl J Med* 2003;349(19):1793–1802.
32. Goss PE, Ingle JN, Martino S, et al. Efficacy of letrozole extended adjuvant therapy according to estrogen receptor and progesterone receptor status of the primary tumor: National Cancer Institute of Canada Clinical Trials Group MA.17. *J Clin Oncol* 2007;25(15):2006–2011.
33. Karnon J. Aromatase inhibitors in breast cancer: a review of cost considerations and cost effectiveness. *Pharmacoeconomics* 2006;24(3):215–232.
34. Piccart-Gebhart MJ, Procter M, Leyland-Jones B, et al. Trastuzumab after adjuvant chemotherapy in HER2-positive breast cancer. *N Engl J Med* 2005;353(16):1659–1672.
35. Romond EH, Perez EA, Bryant J, et al. Trastuzumab plus adjuvant chemotherapy for operable HER2-positive breast cancer. *N Engl J Med* 2005;353(16):1673–1684.
36. Joensuu H, Kellokumpu-Lehtinen P-L, Bono P, et al. Adjuvant docetaxel or vinorelbine with or without trastuzumab for breast cancer. *N Engl J Med* 2006;354(8):809–820.
37. Early Breast Cancer Trialists' Collaborative Group (EBCTCG) Effects of chemotherapy and hormonal therapy for early breast cancer on recurrence and 15-year survival: an overview of the randomised trials. *Lancet* 2005;365(9472):1687–1717.
38. Hillner BE, Smith TJ. Do the large benefits justify the large costs of adjuvant breast cancer trastuzumab? *J Clin Oncol* 2007;25(6):611–613.
39. Bonneterre J, Bercez C, Bonneterre ME, et al. Cost-effectiveness analysis of breast cancer adjuvant treatment: FEC 50 versus FEC 100 (FASG05 study). *Ann Oncol* 2005;16(6):915–922.
40. Norum J, Holtmon M. Adjuvant fluorouracil, epirubicin and cyclophosphamide in early breast cancer: is it cost-effective? *Acta Oncol* 2005;44(7):735–741.
41. Kievit W, Bolster MJ, van der Wilt GJ, et al. Cost-effectiveness of new guidelines for adjuvant systemic therapy for patients with primary breast cancer. *Ann Oncol* 2005;16(12):1874–1881.
42. Marcy PY, Magne N, Castadot P, et al. Radiological and surgical placement of port devices: a 4-year institutional analysis of procedure performance, quality of life and cost in breast cancer patients. *Breast Cancer Res Treat* 2005;92(1):61–67.
43. Hassett MJ, O'Malley AJ, Pakes JR, et al. Frequency and cost of chemotherapy-related serious adverse effects in a population sample of women with breast cancer. *J Natl Cancer Inst* 2006;98(16):1108–1117.
44. Oestreicher N, Ramsey SD, Linden HM, et al. Gene expression profiling and breast cancer care: what are the potential benefits and policy implications? *Genet Med* 2005;7(6):380–389.
45. Hornberger J, Cosler LE, Lyman GH. Economic analysis of targeting chemotherapy using a 21-gene RT-PCR assay in lymph-node-negative, estrogen-receptor-positive, early-stage breast cancer. *Am J Manag Care* 2005;11(5):313–324.
46. Lyman GH, Cosler LE, Kuderer NM, et al. Impact of a 21-gene RT-PCR assay on treatment decisions in early-stage breast cancer: an economic analysis based on prognostic and predictive validation studies. *Cancer* 2007;109(6):1011–1018.
47. Harris L, Fritsche H, Mennel R, et al. American Society of Clinical Oncology 2007 Update of Recommendations for the Use of Tumor Markers in Breast Cancer. *J Clin Oncol* 2007;25(33):5287–5312.
48. de Lemos ML, Taylor SC, Barnett JB, et al. Renal safety of 1-hour pamidronate infusion for breast cancer and multiple myeloma patients: comparison between clinical trials and population-based database. *J Oncol Pharm Pract* 2006;12(4):193–199.
49. Delea T, McKiernan J, Brandman J, et al. Retrospective study of the effect of skeletal complications on total medical care costs in patients with bone metastases of breast cancer seen in typical clinical practice. *J Support Oncol* 2006;4(7):341–347.
50. Kattlove H, Liberati A, Keeler E, et al. Benefits and costs of screening and treatment for early breast cancer. Development of a basic benefit package. *JAMA* 1995;273:142–148.

51. Malin JL, Keeler E, Wang C, et al. Using cost-effectiveness analysis to define a breast cancer benefits package for the uninsured. *Breast Cancer Res Treat* 2002;74(2):143–153.
52. http://www.accessdata.fda.gov/scripts/cder/drugsatfda/index.cfm?fuseaction=Search. Label_ApprovalHistory#apphist. Accessed July 26, 2007.
53. Miller K, Wang M, Gralow J, et al. Paclitaxel plus bevacizumab versus paclitaxel alone for metastatic breast cancer. *N Engl J Med* 2007;357(26):2666–2676.
54. Haines IE, Miklos GLG, Rossi A, et al. Paclitaxel plus bevacizumab for metastatic breast cancer. *N Engl J Med* 2008;358(15):1637–1638.
55. Emanuel EJ, Fuchs VR, Garber AM. Essential elements of a technology and outcomes assessment initiative. *JAMA* 2007;298(11):1323–1325.
56. Garber A, Goldman DP, Jena AB. The promise of health care cost containment. *Health Aff (Millwood)* 2007;26(6):1545–1547.
57. Chiou CF, Hay JW, Wallace JF, et al. Development and validation of a grading system for the quality of cost-effectiveness studies. *Med Care* 2003;41(1):32–44.
58. Jacobi CE, Nagelkerke NJ, van Houwelingen JH, et al. Breast cancer screening, outside the population-screening program, of women from breast cancer families without proven BRCA1/BRCA2 mutations: a simulation study. *Cancer Epidemiol Biomarkers Prev* 2006;15(3):429–436.
59. Neeser K, Szucs T, Bulliard JL, et al. Cost-effectiveness analysis of a quality-controlled mammography screening program from the Swiss statutory health care perspective: quantitative assessment of the most influential factors. *Value Health* 2007;10(1):42–53.
60. Saywell RM Jr, Champion VL, Zollinger TW, et al. The cost effectiveness of 5 interventions to increase mammography adherence in a managed care population. *Am J Manag Care* 2003;9(1):33–44.
61. Saywell RM Jr, Champion VL, Skinner CS, et al. A cost-effectiveness comparison of three tailored interventions to increase mammography screening. *J Womens Health (Larchmt)* 2004;13(8):909–918.
62. Wu JH, Fung MC, Chan W, et al. Cost-effectiveness analysis of interventions to enhance mammography compliance using computer modeling (CAN*TROL). *Value Health* 2004;7(2):175–185.
63. Dranitsaris G, Verma S, Trudeau M. Cost utility analysis of first-line hormonal therapy in advanced breast cancer: comparison of two aromatase inhibitors to tamoxifen. *Am J Clin Oncol* 2003;26(3):289–296.
64. Karnon J, Jones T. A stochastic economic evaluation of letrozole versus tamoxifen as a first-line hormonal therapy: for advanced breast cancer in postmenopausal patients. *Pharmacoeconomics* 2003;21(7):513–525.
65. Simons WR, Jones D, Buzdar A. Cost-effectiveness of anastrozole versus tamoxifen as first-line therapy for postmenopausal women with advanced breast cancer. *Clin Ther* 2003;25(11):2972–2987.
66. Marchetti M, Caruggi M, Colombo G. Cost utility and budget impact of third-generation aromatase inhibitors for advanced breast cancer: a literature-based model analysis of costs in the Italian National Health Service. *Clin Ther* 2004;26(9):1546–1561.
67. Okubo I, Kondo M, Toi M, et al. Cost-effectiveness of letrozole versus tamoxifen as first-line hormonal therapy in treating postmenopausal women with advanced breast cancer in Japan. *Gan To Kagaku Ryoho* 2005;32(3):351–363.
68. Gil JM, Rubio-Terres C, Del Castillo A, et al. Pharmacoeconomic analysis of adjuvant therapy with exemestane, anastrozole, letrozole or tamoxifen in postmenopausal women with operable and estrogen receptor-positive breast cancer. *Clin Transl Oncol* 2006;8(5):339–348.
69. Lonning PE. Comparing cost/utility of giving an aromatase inhibitor as monotherapy for 5 years versus sequential administration following 2–3 or 5 years of tamoxifen as adjuvant treatment for postmenopausal breast cancer. *Ann Oncol* 2006;17(2):217–225.
70. Lundkvist J, Wilking N, Holmberg S, et al. Cost-effectiveness of exemestane versus tamoxifen as adjuvant therapy for early-stage breast cancer after 2–3 years treatment with tamoxifen in Sweden. *Breast Cancer Res Treat* 2007;102(3):289–299.
71. Risebrough NA, Verma S, Trudeau M, et al. Cost-effectiveness of switching to exemestane versus continued tamoxifen as adjuvant therapy for postmenopausal women with primary breast cancer. *Cancer* 2007;110(3):499–508.
72. Skedgel C, Rayson D, Dewar R, et al. Cost-utility of adjuvant hormone therapies for breast cancer in post-menopausal women: sequential tamoxifen-exemestane and upfront anastrozole. *Breast Cancer Res Treat* 2007;101(3):325–333.
73. Skedgel C, Rayson D, Dewar R, et al. Cost-utility of adjuvant hormone therapies with aromatase inhibitors in post-menopausal women with breast cancer: upfront anastrozole, sequential tamoxifen-exemestane and extended tamoxifen-letrozole. *Breast* 2007;16(3):252–261.
74. Thompson D, Taylor DC, Montoya EL, et al. Cost-effectiveness of switching to exemestane after 2 to 3 years of therapy with tamoxifen in postmenopausal women with early-stage breast cancer. *Value Health* 2007;10(5):367–376.
75. Younis T, Rayson D, Dewar R, et al. Modeling for cost-effective-adjuvant aromatase inhibitor strategies for postmenopausal women with breast cancer. *Ann Oncol* 2007;18(2):293–298.
76. Hillner BE. Benefit and projected cost-effectiveness of anastrozole versus tamoxifen as initial adjuvant therapy for patients with early-stage estrogen receptor-positive breast cancer. *Cancer* 2004;101(6):1311–1322.
77. Piskur P, Sonc M, Cufer T, et al. Pharmacoeconomic aspects of adjuvant anastrozole or tamoxifen in breast cancer: a Slovenian perspective. *Anticancer Drugs* 2006;17(6):719–724.
78. Rocchi A, Verma S. Anastrozole is cost-effective vs. tamoxifen as initial adjuvant therapy in early breast cancer: Canadian perspectives on the ATAC completed-treatment analysis. *Support Care Cancer* 2006;14(9):917–927.
79. Delea TE, Karnon J, Smith RE, et al. Cost-effectiveness of extended adjuvant letrozole therapy after 5 years of adjuvant tamoxifen therapy in postmenopausal women with early-stage breast cancer. *Am J Manag Care* 2006;12(7):374–386.
80. Hind D, Ward S, De Nigris E, et al. Hormonal therapies for early breast cancer: systematic review and economic evaluation. *Health Technol Assess* 2007;11(26):iii–iv, ix–xi, 1–134.
81. Mansel R, Locker G, Fallowfield L, et al. Cost-effectiveness analysis of anastrozole vs. tamoxifen in adjuvant therapy for early stage breast cancer in the United Kingdom: the 5-year completed treatment analysis of the ATAC

('Arimidex,' Tamoxifen alone or in combination) trial. *Br J Cancer* 2007;97(2):152–161.

82. El Ouagari K, Karnon J, Delea T, et al. Cost-effectiveness of letrozole in the extended adjuvant treatment of women with early breast cancer. *Breast Cancer Res Treat* 2007;101(1):37–49.

83. Dedes KJ, Szucs TD, Imesch P, et al. Cost-effectiveness of trastuzumab in the adjuvant treatment of early breast cancer: a model-based analysis of the HERA and FinHer trial. *Ann Oncol* 2007;18(9):1493–1499.

84. Garrison LP Jr, Lubeck D, Lalla D, et al. Cost-effectiveness analysis of trastuzumab in the adjuvant setting for treatment of HER2-positive breast cancer. *Cancer* 2007;110(3):489–498.

85. Kurian AW, Thompson RN, Gaw AF, et al. A cost-effectiveness analysis of adjuvant trastuzumab regimens in early HER2/neu-positive breast cancer. *J Clin Oncol* 2007;25(6):634–641.

86. Liberato NL, Marchetti M, Barosi G. Cost effectiveness of adjuvant trastuzumab in human epidermal growth factor receptor 2-positive breast cancer. *J Clin Oncol* 2007;25(6):625–633.

87. Millar JA, Millward MJ. Cost effectiveness of trastuzumab in the adjuvant treatment of early breast cancer: a lifetime model. *Pharmacoeconomics* 2007;25(5):429–442.

88. Norum J, Olsen JA, Wist EA, et al. Trastuzumab in adjuvant breast cancer therapy. A model based cost-effectiveness analysis. *Acta Oncol* 2007;46(2):153–164.

Index